REBECCA BIRKAN

W9-CTX-174

Collaborative Health Care

Gerontologic Considerations

Applying Research to Nursing Practice

Applying Rehabilitation Principles to Medical/ Surgical Nursing

Special Illustrations

Pathophysiology Illustrated

Multisystem Effects of Disease

Medical-Surgical Nursing

Critical Thinking in Client Care

Priscilla LeMone, RN, DSN
Sinclair School of Nursing
University of Missouri – Columbia
Columbia, Missouri

Karen M. Burke, RN, MS
Clatsop Community College
Astoria, Oregon

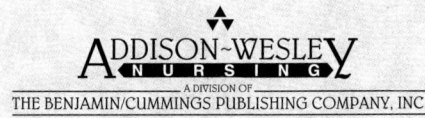
ADDISON-WESLEY
NURSING
A DIVISION OF
THE BENJAMIN/CUMMINGS PUBLISHING COMPANY, INC.

Menlo Park, California • Reading, Massachusetts • New York
Don Mills, Ontario • Wokingham, UK • Amsterdam • Bonn
Paris • Milan • Madrid • Sydney • Singapore • Tokyo
Seoul • Taipei • Mexico City • San Juan, Puerto Rico

Executive editor: *Patricia L. Cleary*
Senior developmental editor: *Mark F. Wales*
Associate developmental editors: *Laura Bonazzoli,*
  Mary Helen Bond
Associate editor: *Virginia Simione Jutson*
Editorial assistant: *Marla Nowick*
Managing editor: *Wendy Earl*
Production supervisor: *Sharon Montooth*
Text and page designers: *Juan Vargas and Edie Williams*
Cover designer: *Yvo Riezebos Design*
Art coordinator: *Michele Mangelli*
Photo coordinator: *Kelli d'Angona*
Copy editors: *Sally Peyrefitte and Antonio Padial*
Proofreader: *Martha Ghent*
Indexer: *Katherine Pitcoff*
Senior manufacturing supervisor: *Merry Free Osborn*
Compositor and prepress supplier: *GTS Graphics*
Production coordinator/GTS Graphics: *Sandie Sigrist*
Printer and binder: *Rand McNally, Inc.*
Cover printer: *Color Dot Litho*
Cover quilt: *Wings of Mystery* by Setsuko Segawa. Image
  supplied by Mitsumura Suiko Shoin Co., Kyoto, Japan.

Photographic and art credits follow the index.

Care has been taken to confirm the accuracy of information presented in this book. The authors, editors, and the publisher, however, cannot accept any responsibility for errors or omissions or for the consequences from application of the information in this book and make no warranty, express or implied, with respect to its contents.

The authors and publisher have exerted every effort to ensure that drug selections and dosages set forth in this text are in accord with current recommendation and practice at time of publication. However, in view of ongoing research, changes in government regulations, and the constant flow of information relating to drug therapy and drug reactions, the reader is urged to check the package inserts of all drugs for any change in indications of dosage and for added warnings and precautions. This is particularly important when the recommended agent is a new and/or infrequently employed drug.

Copyright © 1996 by Addison-Wesley Nursing, A Division of The Benjamin/Cummings Publishing Company, Inc.

All rights reserved. No part of this publication may be reproduced, stored in a retrieval system, or transmitted, in any form or by any means, electronic, mechanical, photocopying, recording, or any other media or embodiments now known or hereafter to become known, without the prior written permission of the publisher. Manufactured in the United States of America. Published simultaneously in Canada.

Library of Congress Cataloging-in-Publication Data

Medical-surgical nursing : critical thinking in client care / [edited
  by] Priscilla LeMone, Karen M. Burke.
      p.   cm.
    Includes bibliographical references and index.
      ISBN 0-8053-4150-1. -- ISBN (invalid) 0-8053-0349-0
      1. Nursing.   2. Surgical nursing.   3. Critical thinking.
  I. LeMone, Priscilla. II. Burke, Karen M.
      [DNLM: 1. Surgical Nursing--handbooks. 2. Nursing Care-
  -handbooks.   WY 49 M4889 1996]
    RT41.M493   1996
    610.73'677--dc20
    DNLM/DLC
    for Library of Congress   95-26501
                                                        CIP

ISBN 0-8053-4150-1
1 2 3 4 5 6 7 8 9 10–RNV–99 98 97 96 95

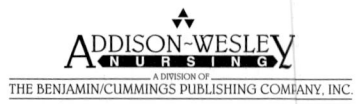

2725 Sand Hill Road, Menlo Park, California 94025

Contributors

■ ■

Phyllis C. Adams, RN, BSN, MSN, EdD, CNS
University of Texas, Houston
  Health Science Center
Houston, Texas

Suzanne C. Beyea, RN, CS, PhD
Saint Anselm College
Manchester, New Hampshire

Fay L. Bower, DNSc, FAAN
Clarkson College
Omaha, Nebraska

Eileen Breslin, RNC, PhD
Northern Arizona University
Flagstaff, Arizona

Tonya Buttry, RNC, MSN
Southeast Missouri Hospital
College of Nursing
Cape Girardeau, Missouri

Nancy Collins, RN, BLA, BSN, MSN
Aurora University
Aurora, Illinois

Anne Walendy Davis, RN, PhD, C
East Central University
Ada, Oklahoma

Claire Dyer, RN
St. Francis Memorial Hospital
Bothin Burn Center
San Francisco, California

Nancy Evans, BS
Medical Writer/Editor
San Francisco, California

Joyce Heise, RN, MSN, CCRN
Kent State University, East
  Liverpool Center
East Liverpool, Ohio

Reneé Semonin Holleran, RN, PhD, CEN, CCRN, CFRN
University Air Care
University of Cincinnati
  Medical Center
Cincinnati, Ohio

Elaine Jackson, RN, PhD
Southeast Missouri State University
Cape Girardeau, Missouri

Joanne M. Johnson, RNC, BSN, MSN
Cincinnati State Technical
  and Community College
Cincinnati, Ohio

Karen C. Johnson-Brennan, RN, Ed
San Francisco State University
San Francisco, California

Karen Van Dyke Lamb, ND, RN, CS
Rush University College of Nursing
Chicago, Illinois

Frances Jean Kelley, RN, PhD
University of Texas, Houston
Houston Health Science Center
Houston, Texas

Valerie Matthiesen, RN, DNSc
Rush College of Nursing
Chicago, Illinois

Gloria J. McNeal, BSN, MSN, CS, PhD(c)
Thomas Jefferson University
Philadelphia, Pennsylvania

Ann Mabe Newman, RN, DSN
University of North Carolina,
  Charlotte
Charlotte, North Carolina

Diana Roberts, RN, CNS
St. Francis Memorial Hospital
Wound Center
San Francisco, California

Julia G. Robinson, RN, MS, FNPC, PhD(c)
California State University,
  Bakersfield
Bakersfield, California

Jane Rose, RNC, MSN
Southeast Missouri State
  University
Cape Girardeau, Missouri

Mary Ellen Santucci, RN, MSN, CRRN
Thomas Jefferson University
Philadelphia, Pennsylvania

Dawn M. Specht, RN, MSN, CEN, CCRN
Episcopal Hospital
Thomas Jefferson University
Philadelphia, Pennsylvania

Ann D. Sprengel, RN, EdD
Southeast Missouri State University
Cape Girardeau, Missouri

Maryfran McKenzie Stulginsky, RN, MS
Bon Secours Home Health/Hospice
Baltimore, Maryland

Virginia Sullivan, RN, MSN, CS
University of North Carolina,
  Charlotte
Charlotte, North Carolina

Cathy J. Thompson, RN, MSN, CCRN
University of Texas, Houston
Houston, Texas

Mae E. Timmons, RN, EdD
Clarkson College
Omaha, Nebraska

Steve R. Toussiant, RN, MSN, OCN
Linfield College
Portland, Oregon

Suzanne M. K. Tracy, RN, MN, MA
Rivier College-St. Joseph School
  of Nursing
Nashua, New Hampshire

Sharon Wahl, RN, EdD
San Jose State University
San Jose, California

Janet R. Weber, RN, BSN, MSN, EdD
Southeast Missouri State University
Cape Girardeau, Missouri

Linda Wessel, RN, CETN, BSN
Southeast Missouri Hospital
Cape Girardeau, Missouri

Susan Karm Wieczorek, RN, AAN, BSN, MSN
Health Education Consulting
  Institute
Fortson, Georgia

Terri J. Woods, RN, MSN, EdD
Southeast Missouri State University
Cape Girardeau, Missouri

Consultants

Joanne M. Johnson, RNC, BSN, MSN
Cincinnati State Technical and
  Community College
Cincinnati, Ohio

Johanna K. Stiesmeyer, RN, MS, CCRN
Camino Healthcare System
Mountain View, California

Reviewers

Sheila Acheson, RN, BSN, MA
Phillips Beth Israel School of
    Nursing
New York, New York

Phyllis C. Adams, RN, BSN, MSN,
    EdD, CNS
University of Texas, Houston
    Health Science Center
Houston, Texas

Kathleen E. Andrews, RN, MN,
    CCRN
Missouri Western State College
St. Joseph, Missouri

Roberta H. Anding, MS, RD/LD, CDE
University of Texas, Houston
Houston, Texas

Janet Azar, RN, BSN, MNEd
Tidewater Community College
Portsmouth, Virginia

Catherine F. Bennett, RNC, MSN
Lansing Community College
Lansing, Michigan

Nancy Berger, RNC, MSN
Charles E. Gregory School of
    Nursing
Perth Amboy, New Jersey

Kathie M. Bitker, RN, MSN,
    ARNP/CNS
Wichita State University
Wichita, Kansas

Dorothy S. Bonner, RN, MN
LSUMC School of Nursing
New Orleans, Lousiana

Mildred Wernet Boyd, RN, MSN, MSA
Essex Community College
Baltimore, Maryland

Louise K. Brentin, RN, BSN, MSN
Delta College
University Center, Michigan

Gracia Buffleben, RN
Veterans Administration Medical
    Center
Livermore, California

Susan M. Burchiel, MSN, RN, C
Cuesta College
San Luis Obispo, California

Patricia E. Camp, RN, DSN
Samford University
Birmingham, Alabama

Susan Kasal Chrisman, RN, MSN,
    BSN, PhD(c)
Research College of Nursing
Kansas City, Missouri

Sandra Marshall Cifelli, RN,
    BSN, MSN
Louise Harkey School of
    Nursing
Concord, North Carolina

Norma L. Cole, RN, MA
Johnson County Community
    College
Overland Park, Kansas

Pat Colledge, RN, MSN
Idaho State University
Pocatello, Idaho

Joan W. Conklin, RNC, EdD
Bloomfield College
Bloomfield, New Jersey

Dianne G. Copenhaver, RN, PhD
Coppin State College
Baltimore, Maryland

Sandra Kay Croyle, RN, PhD
Butler County Community
    College
Butler, Pennsylvania

Patricia Cryer, RN, BSN, MS
Tyler Junior College
Tyler, Texas

Rick Daniels, RN, PhD
Oregon Health Sciences University,
    Ashland
Ashland, Oregon

Nancy Darland, RNC, MSN, CNS
Louisiana Tech University
Ruston, Louisiana

Margaret Davey, RN, MAppsc
Curtin University of Technology
Bentley, Western Australia

Jamie T. Davis, rn, msn
Columbia State Community
    College
Columbia, Tennessee

Kathleen A. DeLorenzo, RN, PhD, CS
Abilene Intercollegiate
    School of Nursing
Abilene, Texas

Janet Duffy Dionne, RN, MS, CCRN
Community College of Denver
Denver, Colorado

Colleen Duggan, RN, MSN
Johnson County Community College
Overland Park, Kansas

Lorna Eppert, RN, BSN, MSN
Good Samaritan Hospital
    School of Nursing
Cincinnati, Ohio

Martha L. Goodnetter, RN, MS, OCN
Cardinal Stritch College
Milwaukee, Wisconsin

Divina Gracia S. Grossman, PhD,
    RN, CS
Florida International University
Miami, Florida

Carol A. Harvell, ARNP, BSN, MSN
Hillsborough Community College
Tampa, Florida

Frank D. Hicks, RN, PhD(c), CCRN
Niehoff School of Nursing,
    Loyola University
Chicago, Illinois

Melissa Homan, RN, MSN, CCRN
Jamestown Community College
Jamestown, New York

Betty L. Hopping, EdD
Retired, Beth-El College of Nursing
Colorado Springs, Colorado

Tana W. Hunter, RN, MS, CS
Brigham Young University
Provo, Utah

Elizabeth Miller Jenkins, RN, MS
University of Delaware
Newark, Delaware

Peggy Jenkins, CCRN, MS
Harwick College
Oneonta, New York

M. Regina Jennette, RN, MA, MSN
West Virginia Northern
    Community College
Wheeling, West Virginia

Karen C. Johnson-Brennan, RN, Ed
San Francisco State University
San Francisco, California

Cynthia Jones, RN, MN
Arkansas Tech University
Russellville, Arkansas

Frances Jean Kelley, RN, PhD
Georgetown University
Washington, DC

Mary Lee S. Kirkland, RN, EdD
Medical University of South
 Carolina
Charleston, South Carolina

Mary Kuhl, RN, PhD
Kaskaskia College
Centralia, Illinois

RuthAnne Kuiper, RN, MN, CCRN
Presbyterian Hospital School of
 Nursing
Charlotte, North Carolina

Elisa A. Mancuso, RNC, MSN, FNS
Suffolk Community College
Brentwood, New York

Elizabeth (Penny) Marcum, RN,
 BSN, MSN
Louise Obici School of Nursing
Suffolk, Virginia

Cedaliah Melton-Freeman, RN, BSN,
 MSN
Eastern Kentucky University
Richmond, Kentucky

Sue Ellen Miller, RN, MSN
Catawba Valley Community College
Hickory, North Carolina

Aletta Linger Moffett, RN, BSN, MSN,
 CS
Fairmont State College
Fairmont, West Virginia

Ruthanne Oglesby, RN, ASN, BSN,
 MSN, EdD
University of Florida, Gainesville
Gainesville, Florida

Patricia O'Leary, RN, DSN
Middle Tennessee State University
Murfreesboro, Tennessee

Nancy Otterness, RN, MS
Boise State University
Boise, Idaho

Alice Palmer, RN, OCN, MS
Cincinnati State Technical and
 Community College
Cincinnati, Ohio

Kathleen S. Pangle, RN, MSEd, MSN
West Shore Community College
Scottville, Michigan

Carolyn S. Powell, RN, BSN, MSN
Abraham Baldwin College
Tifton, Georgia

M. Patricia B. Quigley, RN, BSN, MN,
 Ed
Salve Regina University
Newport, Rhode Island

Jane E. Ransom, BSN, MSN
Medical College of Ohio School
 of Nursing
Toledo, Ohio

Julia Ann Raithel, RN, MSN
Deaconess College of Nursing
St. Louis, Missouri

Betty L. Redding, RN, MSN
Mississippi Gulf Coast Community
 College
Gautier, Mississippi

Katherine Dentoni Ricossa, RN, C,
 BSN, PHN
Mission College, Santa Clara,
 California
Good Samaritan Hospital, San Jose,
 California

Roberta Ronayne, RN, Msc(A)
University of Ottawa
Ontario, Canada

Norma Russell, RN, MSN, ANP
University of Wisconsin, Oshkosh
Oshkosh, Wisconsin

Patricia L. Ryan, RN, MA, MSN, C
Gwynedd-Mercy College
Gwynedd Valley, Pennsylvania

Muriel P. Shaul, RN, PhD
University of Texas
Austin, Texas

Denice C. Sheehan, RN, MSN,
 CRNH
Ursuline College
Pepper Pike, Ohio

Kathy J. Shutler, RN, BSN, MSN
Belmont Technical College
St. Clairsville, Ohio

April Sieh, RN, MSN
Delta College
University Center, Michigan

Lynn A. Templeton, RN, BSN, MSN,
 CFNP
Arizona State University
Tempe, Arizona

Yvonne Tolson-Myers, RN, MSN,
 CCRN
Ohio Valley Hospital School of
 Nursing
Steubenville, Ohio

Suzanne M. K. Tracy, RN, MN, MA
Rivier College-St. Joseph School of
 Nursing
Nashua, New Hampshire

Sharon Vincent, RN, ASN, BSN,
 MSN
Augusta College
Augusta, Georgia

Jill J. Webb, RN, BSN, MSN, CS
Union University
Jackson, Tennessee

Mildred Wicks, RN, BSN, MN, Ed
Community College of Allegheny
 County
Pittsburgh, Pennsylvania

Jeanne Widener, RN, MSN,
 CCRN
Eastern Kentucky University
Richmond, Kentucky

Alvin F. Wong, Pharm.D
University of California, San
 Francisco
San Francisco, California

Ruth C. Yanos, RN, BSN, MSN, CS
Delaware Technical and
 Community College
Dover, Delaware

Mali Ziglari, RN, MSN, ARNP/CNS
Neosho County Community
 College
Chanute, Kansas

Preface

Introduction

In a society characterized by change, perhaps nothing is changing more rapidly than health care. Changes in the health care environment encompass an emphasis on healthy living, a focus on wellness, a move toward providing care for clients in a variety of settings, and increased attention to collaboration among health care providers. To meet people's needs for health promotion and health restoration, the nursing profession is reshaping not only its current practice but also its education of future nurses.

Medical-surgical nursing is the broadest and most complex area of learning in nursing education. Students are expected to apply prerequisite or concurrently acquired knowledge of anatomy and physiology, chemistry, pharmacology, sociology, and psychology to the care of adults who are ill or injured. At the same time, students must learn to synthesize new knowledge to provide individualized care that addresses a myriad of human responses to potential or actual alterations in health. Faculty teaching medical-surgical nursing must find the most effective means of presenting an enormous amount of content within the time constraints of the course, while helping students to become effective problem solvers and skilled practitioners of nursing.

This text is carefully crafted to meet the learning needs of students and the challenges that educators face in a rapidly changing health care environment. The book is also designed to be used as a reference by practicing nurses in any care setting.

Our Vision

Our purpose in writing this book is to provide nursing knowledge that can be applied in the clinical setting when caring for real people. We envisioned a text that would

- Reflect current knowledge of the science and art of nursing in today's world.

- Provide clear explanations of the pathophysiologic processes of various disorders.

- Emphasize the nurse's role in collaborative care.

- Prioritize nursing interventions specific to altered human responses to illness.

- Foster critical-thinking skills.

- Offer visual tools for learners.

Medical-Surgical Nursing: Critical Thinking in Client Care is that text. To achieve our goals, we have provided focused discussions of nursing interventions along with highlighted rationales, a case-study approach to the nursing process, and an emphasis on client and family teaching. Critical-thinking challenges also are integrated throughout the book. Newly developed, full-color art and photographs are strategically placed in each chapter to reinforce the student's understanding of key concepts and processes.

Organized to Facilitate Student Learning

This text is organized within a broad framework of **functional health patterns.** Unit One introduces the roles of the medical-surgical nurse, the factors influencing human responses to health and illness, and nursing care of the adult client in the home setting. Unit Two focuses on common alterations in health patterns; these chapters provide the knowledge that serves as the foundation for the nursing care chapters.

The remaining units address alterations in the function of body systems. Each unit begins with an assessment chapter designed to support the clinical chapters that follow. In the clinical chapters, the discussion of each major disorder follows a consistent pattern, beginning with pathophysiology and moving to collaborative care and then to nursing care. We believe that this framework facilitates learning by enabling students to integrate assessment skills with knowledge of pathophysiology, diagnostic tests, pharmacology, and medical treatment when planning and implementing nursing care.

Key Components of Our Teaching and Learning Framework

- **Physical assessment.** The assessment chapters that open each clinical unit provide an overview of basic anatomy and physiology, focused interview questions for the nursing history based on functional health patterns, guidelines for conducting the physical assessment, potential abnormal findings, and an overview of variations in assessment findings for the older adult. Each assessment chapter is supported by **full-color illustrations** and photos of anatomy and assessment procedures.

- **Pathophysiology.** Each nursing care chapter includes a section on the pathophysiology of each major disorder discussed. This section covers definitions, pathologic changes in human structure and function, incidence, etiology, manifestations, and possible complications. *Clinical Manifestations* boxes are provided to reinforce the student's understanding of the disorder's manifestations and complications. In addition, our eye-catching *Pathophysiology Illustrated* feature and *Multisystem Effects* diagrams provide visual pathways to help the student learn about the causes and consequences of major disease processes.

- **Collaborative care.** The nursing care chapters also include discussions of collaborative care for each disorder. The Collaborative Care sections present information about laboratory and diagnostic tests, pharmacology, and such treatment options as surgery, radiation, dietary management, and conservative care. Although medical interventions are fully considered, the focus of this section is the role of the nurse in providing collaborative care. This section also includes *Nursing Implications* boxes and *Nursing Care* boxes for major laboratory and diagnostic tests, pharmacology, and surgery. The Nursing Implications boxes for diagnostic tests and surgery highlight client preparation, client and family teaching, and nursing care.

- **Rationale-based nursing care.** Our nursing care discussions are primarily organized around *prioritized nursing diagnoses*. This approach is consistent with practices mandated by the present health care system in which nurses must focus on the client's critical responses to illness rather than on all potential problems. Each priority nursing diagnosis includes both *interventions and rationales* to help the student understand which nursing actions to perform and why to perform them. A list of other possible nursing diagnoses follows the discussions of priority nursing diagnoses. Client and family teaching, an essential component of nursing care, rounds out each nursing care discussion. When alternative approaches to care are required to meet the needs of older adults, these considerations are discussed in the text and in accompanying *Gerontologic Considerations* boxes.

- **Case study approach to the nursing process.** Discussions of many major disorders conclude with a *case study* and a narrative nursing care plan illustrating how to apply the nursing process to the care of a particular client. Each step of the nursing process is related to the client represented in the case study, which concludes with *critical-thinking questions* that draw the student into the decision-making process. This innovative presentation of nursing care encourages the student to view the client as a person, not just as a medical or nursing diagnosis. The case studies also portray nurses acting in the real world — assessing and monitoring the status of their clients, planning and providing direct care in a variety of settings, and teaching clients and their family members how to provide self-care.

- **Critical pathways.** To address the trend toward providing collaborative, outcome-driven client care, we include *critical pathways* for certain major disorders in selected clinical chapters. Each critical pathway establishes a time-sequenced approach to organizing multidisciplinary interventions that includes diagnostic testing, medication administration, treatments, consultations, client education, and discharge planning.

Special Features That Promote Learning

We include a variety of features throughout our book to facilitate student learning.

- **Pharmacology.** Specialized pharmacology boxes in the clinical chapters provide disorder-specific discussions of drugs. Each box summarizes the pharmacologic effects of a category of drugs and outlines related nursing responsibilities and considerations for client and family teaching. Because dosages are highly individualized and subject to change, they are not discussed in these boxes.

- **Collaborative Care.** Included selectively as part of the collaborative care discussions for major disorders, these boxes introduce the roles of key members of the health care team and illustrate the coordination of multidisciplinary interventions. This feature is also designed to encourage communication and interaction between the nurse and other members of the health care team.

- **Gerontologic Considerations.** Nurses are providing care to an expanding population of older clients. We acknowledge this trend by including in selected chapters Gerontologic Considerations boxes that are designed to sensitize nurses to the older client's special needs. This feature complements our focus on enabling the nurse to provide age-sensitive care.

- **Clinical Manifestations.** These boxes summarize the primary manifestations and potential complications of major disorders.

- **Nursing Research.** Nursing research provides the knowledge base for nursing actions and is an integral component of client care. We feature nursing research boxes in nearly every clinical chapter to help students understand how research findings can improve everyday nursing practice. The critical-thinking questions that conclude each research box encourage students, at this formative stage in their careers, to apply the findings of nursing research to the care of their clients.

- **Rehabilitation Principles.** With the trend toward shorter inpatient stays and longer recovery periods in the home, nurses are placing more emphasis on rehabilitation principles in planning care. Boxes in selected clinical chapters show students how to adapt basic principles of rehabilitation in order to provide better care.

Teaching/Learning Package

To supplement the text and facilitate active involvement in the learning process, we include a variety of student learning aids in our comprehensive supplements package.

For the Nurse Educator

- **Instructor's Manual** by Margie H. Ng, RN, MS

    The instructor's manual includes creative teaching strategies to assist nursing faculty in using the text. Each chapter contains an overview, learning objectives, chapter outline, small group and classroom discussions for clinical activities, teaching aids, and a list of additional readings.

- **Test Bank** by Johanna K. Stiesmeyer, RN, MS, CCRN

    The test bank contains 1500 questions. Each question is freestanding and coded to indicate cognitive level, nursing process step, and client need. The questions are presented in the current NCLEX format. In addition, the test bank is available on IBM 3.5-inch and 5.25-inch disk formats.

- **Transparency Package**

    The transparency package contains 56 full-color acetate transparencies of selected art from the text.

For the Student and Practicing Nurse

- **Clinical Handbook for Medical-Surgical Nursing** by Susan Gauthier, RN, MSN, PhD

    This pocket-sized handbook provides a succinct review of 163 diseases and disorders. Each discussion considers pathophysiology, nursing diagnoses and interventions, and client teaching and discharge planning. Entries are arranged alphabetically for easy reference.

- **Student Study Guide** by Suzanne C. Beyea, RN, CS, PhD; Elizabeth Ayello, RN, PhD; Carl A. Kirton, RN, MA, CCRN; and Susanne M. K. Tracy, RN, MN, MA

    This study guide reinforces the clinical applications of key concepts presented in the text. It also offers additional case studies, study tips, and multiple-choice, matching, and fill-in exercises.

- **Fluid and Electrolyte and Acid-Base Case Study Module** by Audrey Jean Berman, RN, PhD, OCN; and Karen Van Leuven, RN, PhDc

    This learning module uses community-based case studies and application questions to help students solve problems related to fluid and electrolyte and acid-base disorders.

Acknowledgments

As each of us grows into adulthood, the efforts and influence of all those who love, guide, and teach us help shape us into who we become. So too does a textbook develop. Although the process of creating a book — like the process of growing up — is often long and painful, this end product is one of which we are immensely proud.

We want to thank the editorial staff at Addison-Wesley Nursing, including Patti Cleary, Peggy Adams, Mark Wales, Laura Bonazzoli, Mary Helen Bond, Ginnie Simione Jutson, and Marla Nowick. The beautiful book you are holding is the result of the production teamwork of Wendy Earl, Sharon Montooth, Michele Mangelli, Edie Williams, Kelli d'Angona, Sally Peyrefitte, and Antonio Padial. Special thanks to our designer, Juan Vargas, and to our artists, especially Wendy Hiller Gee, who created the dazzling Pathophysiology Illustrated feature. Without the steady guidance, support, and invaluable knowledge of all these people, our dream would not have come true.

A special thank-you to all the contributors, consultants and reviewers for your expert knowledge and faith in the book. Lastly, our thanks to students past, present, and future — you inspired this book, and it is primarily for each of you that it is written.

Priscilla LeMone
Karen Burke

For Steve and the kids.
Without your love, support,
patience, and understanding,
this could not have happened.
— Karen Burke

With all my love, for Jacque
— Priscilla LeMone

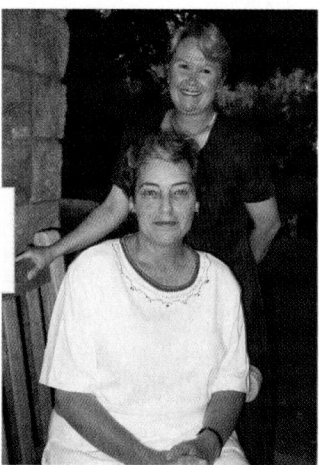

Brief Contents

■ ■

To the Student

This book will help you acquire the knowledge and skills needed for success in medical-surgical nursing practice. The content and features introduce and spotlight two closely related kinds of information: the science and art of nursing and the nurse's role in collaborative care.

The Science and Art of Nursing

Physical Assessment

The assessment chapters that begin each clinical unit survey normal anatomy and physiology and offer you carefully structured approaches to interviewing and assessing your clients.

ASSESSMENT TECHNIQUE	POSSIBLE ABNORMAL FINDINGS
Thyroid Gland ■ **Palpate the thyroid gland for size and consistency.** Stand behind the client, and place your fingers on either side of the trachea below the thyroid cartilage (Figure 19–4). Ask the client to tilt the head to the right. Now ask the client to swallow. As the client swallows, displace the left lobe while palpating the right lobe. Repeat to palpate the left lobe. 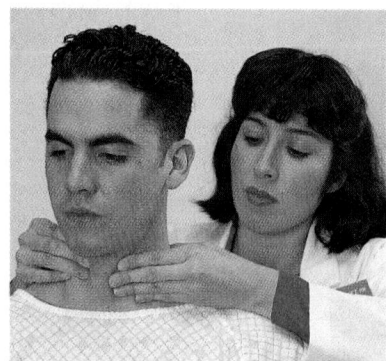 **Figure 19–4** Palpating the thyroid gland from behind the client.	**Exophthalmos** (protruding eyes) may be seen in hyperthyroidism. The thyroid may be enlarged in clients with Graves' disease or a goiter. Multiple nodules may be seen in metabolic disorders, whereas the presence of only one nodule may indicate a cyst or a benign or malignant tumor. One enlarged nodule suggests malignancy.

Pathophysiology

Discussions: The clearly written coverage of diseases and disorders is easy to locate. Important clinical manifestations are highlighted in boxes.

Pathophysiology

Approximately 85% of all primary renal tumors are renal cell carcinomas. These tumors arise in the epithelium of the proximal convoluted tubules. Males are affected more than females by a 2:1 ratio. The highest incidence is seen in people over the age of 55 years. Smoking has been identified as an environmental risk factor; the chronic irritation associated with renal calculi may also contribute.

Renal tumors are often silent, with few clinical manifestations. The classic triad of symptoms, gross hematuria, flank pain, and a palpable abdominal mass, is seen in only about 10% of people with renal cell carcinoma. Hematuria, often microscopic, is the most consistent manifestation. Systemic manifestations include fever without evidence of infection, fatigue, and weight loss. Laboratory findings may include either anemia or polycythemia along with an elevated sedimentation rate. See the accompanying clinical manifestations box.

> **Clinical Manifestations of Renal Tumors**
>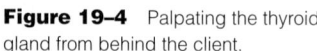
> - Microscopic or gross hematuria
> - Flank pain
> - Palpable abdominal mass
> - Fever
> - Fatigue
> - Weight loss
> - Anemia or polycythemia

Pathophysiology Art: You'll find powerful visual reinforcement of selected disorder discussions in the *Multisystem Effects* art and the *Pathophysiology Illustrated* art.

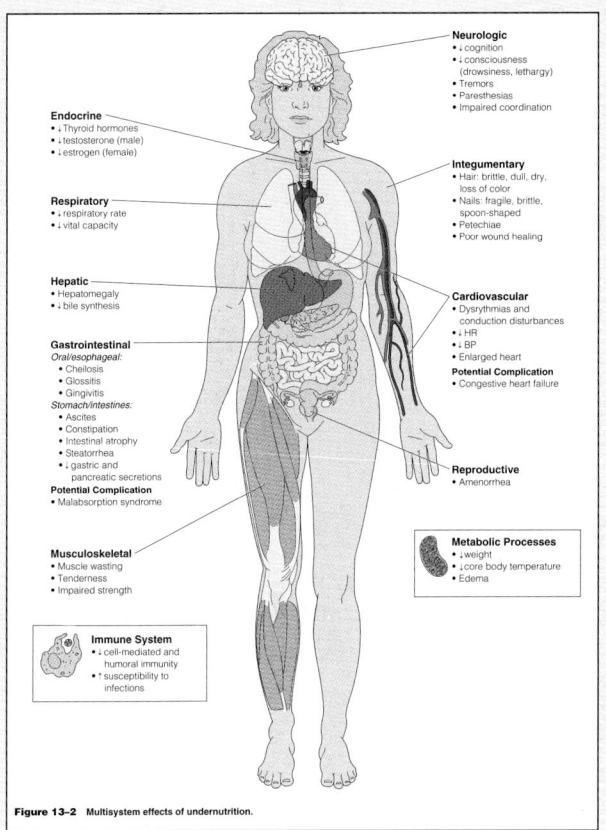

Figure 13–2 Multisystem effects of undernutrition.

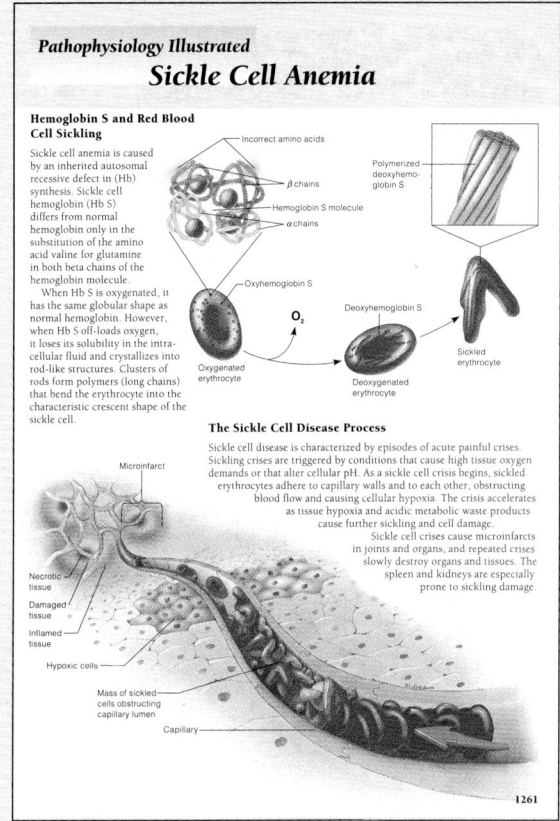

Rationale-Based Nursing Care

The nursing care discussions for most disorders are organized around prioritized nursing diagnoses. This approach will help you focus on the client's critical responses to illness. The interventions following each priority diagnosis include rationales, which are highlighted in italic type.

Nursing Care

As noted earlier, peritonitis is a serious illness. Clients require intensive nursing and medical interventions to recover fully. Without aggressive management, the infectious or septic process of peritonitis may lead to multiple organ systems failure. Nursing interventions for these clients address pain; disruptions in fluid balance; altered protection due to the presence of an infection, drains, and possibly repeated surgeries; and anxiety.

Pain

Abdominal distention and the acute inflammatory process contribute to the pain experienced by a client with peritonitis. If surgery has been performed, the client also experiences pain related to disruption of abdominal muscles and other tissues. As with any acutely ill or surgical client, managing the client's pain is necessary to promote healing as well as comfort and to prevent complications from immobility.

Nursing interventions with rationales follow:

- Assess the client's pain, including its location, severity, and type. *A change in the location or type of pain or an in-*crease *in its severity may indicate further infection, abscess formation, or other complications of peritonitis. Report these to the primary care provider.*

- Place the client in a Fowler's or semi-Fowler's position with the knees and feet elevated. *This position helps minimize stress on abdominal structures and facilitate respirations, promoting comfort.*

- Once the diagnosis has been established, administer analgesics as ordered on a routine basis or using patient-controlled analgesia (PCA). *Analgesics typically are withheld or minimized to avoid masking symptoms until the diagnosis has been made. Thereafter, routine administration of analgesics helps maintain pain control, facilitating healing and movement.*

- Teach and assist the client to use alternative pain management techniques along with pharmacologic interventions. *Techniques such as meditation, visualization, massage, and progressive relaxation augment analgesics and increase the client's level of comfort.*

Applying the Nursing Process: Case Studies

Case studies are an integral part of the nursing care discussions for major disorders. Each case shows how the nursing process is used to care for actual clients in a variety of settings. Critical thinking questions located at the end of each case will draw you into the care planning process.

Applying the Nursing Process

Case Study of a Client with Hypothyroidism: Jane Lee

Jane Lee is a 60-year-old retired nurse living with her husband and daughter on a farm that has been in the family for four generations. Jane has gained 10 lb (4.5 kg) in the past few months, even though she is rarely hungry and eats much less than normal. She is always cold, tired, and weak—so tired that she has not even been able to help with the chores on the farm or do housework. She is concerned about her appearance and the way she sounds when she talks.

Assessment

Brian Henning, RN, completes the admission assessment for Mrs. Lee at the health center. He finds that she now weighs 150 lb (68 kg), an increase of 10 lb (4.5 kg) over her weight at her last visit 6 months earlier. Mrs. Lee states that she always feels cold, tired, and weak. She also states that she is constipated, has difficulty remembering things, and looks different. Physical assessment findings included a palpable and bilaterally enlarged thyroid; dry, yellowish skin; nonpitting edema of the face and lower legs; and slow, slurred speech. Diagnostic tests revealed the following abnormal findings: T_3, 56 ng/dL (normal range: 80 to 200 ng/dL); T_4, 3.1 (normal range: 5 to 12 μg/dL); TSH, 6.2 μU/mL (normal range: 2.0 to 5.4 μU/mL). The medical diagnosis of hypothyroidism is made, and Mrs. Lee is started on levothyroxine 100 mg daily.

Diagnosis

The nursing diagnoses for Mrs. Lee include the following:

- *Constipation* related to decreased peristalsis, as evidenced by hard, formed stools every 4 days
- *Impaired Verbal Communication* related to changes in speech patterns and enlarged tongue
- *Self-Esteem Disturbance* related to changes in physical appearance and activity intolerance

Expected Outcomes

The expected outcomes established in the plan of care specify that Mrs. Lee will:

- Regain normal bowel elimination patterns, having a soft, formed stool at least every other day.
- Experience improvement in verbal communication.
- Regain positive self-esteem as medications reduce physical changes and increase activity levels.

Planning and Implementation

In teaching Mrs. Lee to care for herself at home, Mr. Henning plans and implements the following interventions:

- Teach Mrs. Lee how to increase fluids, bulk, and fiber in her diet to help her regain a normal bowel elimination pattern of a soft, formed stool every other day.
- Teach her to take medications as prescribed and not to expect immediate reversal of symptoms affecting speech.

Evaluation

On her return visit to the health center 2 months later, Mrs. Lee tells Mr. Henning that she is no longer constipated but that she is continuing to drink six glasses of water and eating oatmeal every day. She no longer feels cold, is regaining her normal energy, and even feels well enough to plant her garden. Her speech is clear and easy to understand. As she leaves the examining room, Mrs. Lee says, "It's hard to believe that I have changed so much—now I look and feel like the 'old' me!"

Critical Thinking in the Nursing Process

1. What physical changes that normally occur with aging are similar to the manifestations of hypothyroidism?
2. Describe the factors that put Mrs. Lee's safety at risk. What alterations in her home environment would you suggest to promote safety until the prescribed medication takes effect?
3. The client taking oral thyroid medications may become hyperthyroid. List the signs and symptoms you

---

The Nurse's Role in Collaborative Care

Nursing Implications for Pharmacology

Unlike the information found in a drug guide, the nursing responsibilities and the client teaching recommendations found in this feature are tailored to the needs of clients receiving medications for specific disorders.

Nursing Implications for Pharmacology: Nonsteroidal Anti-Inflammatory Drugs

NSAIDs

aspirin (acetylsalicylic acid)
fenoprofen calcium (Nalfon)
ibuprofen (Motrin)
naproxen sodium (Anaprox)
piroxicam (Feldene)
ketorolac tromethamine (Toradol)
naproxen (Naprosyn)

The NSAIDs have anti-inflammatory, analgesic, and antipyretic effects. It is believed that they inhibit the enzyme cyclooxygenase, thereby decreasing synthesis of prostaglandins. These drugs provide analgesic effects by reducing inflammation and by perhaps blocking the generation of noxious impulses.

Nursing Responsibilities

- Do not administer aspirin with other NSAIDs.
- Assess and document if the client is taking a hypoglycemic agent or insulin; the NSAIDs may increase the hypoglycemic effect.
- Administer with meals, milk, or a full glass of water to decrease gastric irritation.
- Assess clients who are also taking anticoagulants for bleeding; the NSAIDs increase this risk.

Client and Family Teaching

- Drugs may cause gastrointestinal bleeding (report nausea, vomiting of blood, dark stools), visual disturbances (report blurred or diminished vision), hearing problems, dizziness, skin rash, and renal problems (report weight gain or edema).
- Take medications with meals to decrease gastric irritation.
- Avoid drinking alcohol or taking any over-the-counter drug unless approved by the health care provider.
- The desired effects may not appear for 3–5 days, and the full effects may not appear for 2–4 weeks.
- Maintain regular health care appointments.

Nursing Care Boxes

Your clients will often require nursing care related to the effects of diagnostic tests or medical procedures such as surgery. This feature outlines selected nursing care and client teaching considerations before, during, and after major medical procedures.

Nursing Care of the Client Having an Adrenalectomy

PREOPERATIVE CARE

- Request a dietary consultation to discuss with the client about a diet high in vitamins and proteins. If hypokalemia exists, include foods high in potassium. *Glucocorticoid excess increases catabolism. Vitamins and proteins are necessary for tissue repair and wound healing following surgery.*

- Use careful medical and surgical asepsis when providing care and treatments. *Cortisol excess increases the risk of infection.*

- Monitor the results of laboratory tests of electrolytes and glucose levels. *Electrolyte and glucose imbalances are corrected before the client has surgery.*

- Teach the client to turn, cough, and perform deep-breathing exercises. *Although they are important for all surgical clients, these activities are even more important for the client who is at risk for infection. Having the client practice and demonstrate the activities increases postoperative compliance.*

POSTOPERATIVE CARE

- Take and record vital signs, measure intake and output, and monitor electrolytes on a frequent schedule, especially during the first 48 hours after surgery. *Removal of an adrenal gland, especially a bilateral adrenalectomy, results in adrenal insufficiency. Addisonian crisis and hypovolemic shock may occur. Cortisol is often given on the day of surgery and in the postoperative period to replace inadequate hormone levels. Intravenous fluids are also administered.*

- Assess body temperature, WBC levels, and wound drainage. Change dressings using sterile technique. *Impaired wound healing increases the risk of infection in clients with adrenal disorders. Use aseptic technique to decrease this risk.*

Collaborative Care Boxes

This feature introduces the members of the health care team who may be involved in caring for a client with a specific disorder. You will also find information designed to facilitate communication with other care providers.

Collaborative Health Care: The Client with Thyroid Disorders

Health Care Team	Client-Centered Goals
Endocrinologist	Responsible for evaluation, treatment, and management of thyroid disorders. Orders diagnostic tests and evaluates results. Prescribes appropriate medication.
General surgeon	For clients requiring surgery, conducts preoperative assessment, performs surgery removing or resecting tumor, manages postoperative course, monitors surgical outcomes following discharge.
RN and health care team communications	Reports any adverse effects from medications. Reports any difficulty breathing or speaking, and/or signs and symptoms of hemorrhage following surgery. Advises dietitian regarding client's intake and food preferences. Alerts social worker to any home care needs.
Dietitian	Provides client with diet that promotes achieving or maintaining ideal body weight. Teaches client and family strategies to maintain a well-balanced diet inclusive of all food groups. Provides snacks appropriate to calorie recommendations.

Critical Pathways

Health care is an increasingly collaborative, outcome-driven process. The critical pathways introduce you to a time-sequenced method of organizing multidisciplinary interventions for clients.

Critical Pathway for Client Following Thyroidectomy

	Date _____ 1st Day Postoperative	Date _____ 2nd Day Postoperative	Date _____ 3rd Day Postoperative
Expected length of stay: 3 days			
Daily outcomes	Client will • Be afebrile. • Have clean, dry wound with well-approximated edges healing by first intention. • Recover from anesthesia, as evidenced by return of vital	Client will • Be afebrile. • Have clean, dry wound with well-approximated edges healing by first intention. • Demonstrate cooperation with turning, coughing,	Client will • Be afebrile. • Have a dry, clean wound with well-approximated edges healing by first intention. • Manage pain with nonpharmacologic measures.

Detailed Contents

Part Two
Nutrition and Metabolic Patterns   411

Part Three
Elimination Patterns   755

Part Four
Activity and Exercise Patterns   1001

Part Five
Cognitive and Perceptual Patterns   1657

continued

PART
ONE

Medical-Surgical Nursing Practice

Dimensions of Medical-Surgical Nursing

The Medical-Surgical Nurse

LEARNING OBJECTIVES

After completing this chapter, you will be able to

- Describe the activities and characteristics of the nurse's roles as caregiver, educator, advocate, leader and manager, and researcher.
- Explain the importance of quality assurance in medical-surgical nursing.
- Discuss the steps of the nursing process—assessment, diagnosis, planning, implementation, and evaluation—when used in client care, and provide a rationale for the use of the nursing process in clinical practice.

- Describe the importance of codes for nursing and nursing standards in medical-surgical nursing care.
- Discuss some of the legal and ethical dilemmas in client care.
- Discuss current issues and trends in medical-surgical nursing practice, including changes in populations requiring care, trends and issues in health care delivery, the use of computers in nursing, and nursing's role in health care reform.

Medical-surgical nursing is the health care and the illness care of adults, based on knowledge derived from the arts and sciences and shaped by knowledge from nursing. The focus of medical-surgical nursing is the adult client's response to actual or potential alterations in health. In this textbook, those human responses are structured within the framework of functional health patterns, and nursing care is presented within the context of nursing diagnoses.

Medical-surgical nursing encompasses many different interrelated components. The adult client—the person with whom and for whom nursing care is designed and implemented—ranges in age from the late teens to the early 100s. The human responses that nurses must consider when planning and implementing care result from changes in the structure and/or function of all body systems, as well as the interrelated effects of those changes on the social, cultural, economic, and personal life of the client. The wide range of ages and the variety of health care needs specific to individual clients make medical-

surgical nursing an ever-changing and challenging area of nursing practice.

The information in this chapter serves as a broad overview of medical-surgical nursing practice. The topics addressed include the roles of the nurse, the nursing process, and legal and ethical guidelines in providing care. As preparation for the constant changes in health care and nursing that all nurses will face, a discussion of issues and trends in medical-surgical nursing concludes the chapter.

Roles of the Nurse in Medical-Surgical Practice

■ ■ ■

Health care today is a vast and complex system. It reflects changes in society, changes in the populations requiring nursing care, and a philosophical shift toward health promotion rather than illness care. The roles of the medical-

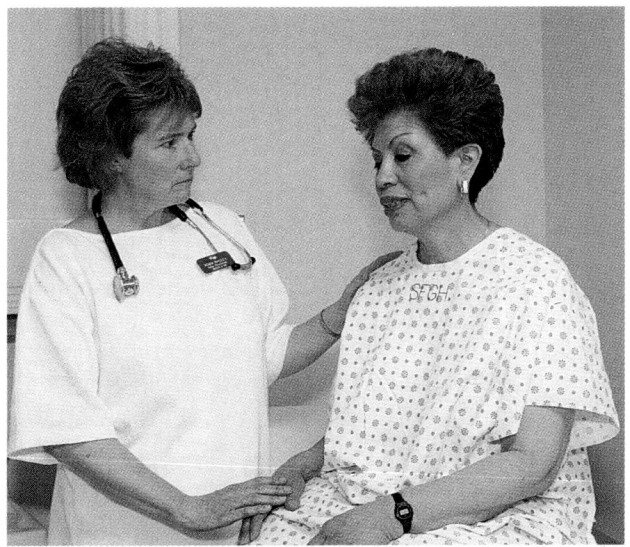

Figure 1–1 In the role of caregiver, the nurse provides comprehensive, individualized care to the adult client.

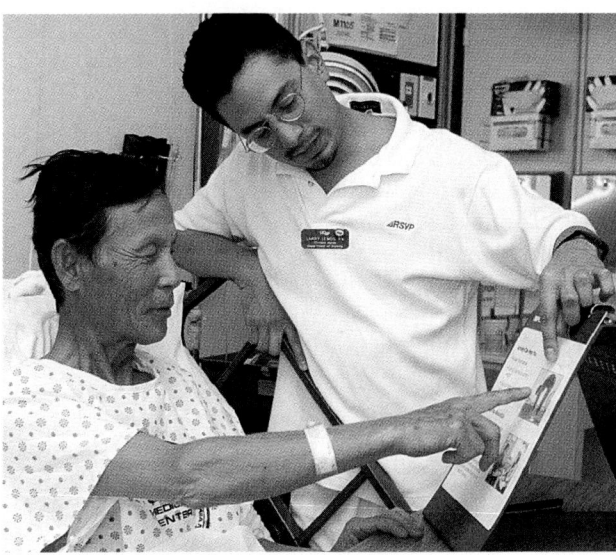

Figure 1–2 The nurse's role as educator is an essential component of care. As part of the discharge planning process, this nurse is providing teaching for self-care at home.

surgical nurse have broadened and expanded in response to these changes. Medical-surgical nurses are not only caregivers but also educators, advocates, leaders and managers, and researchers. The nurse assumes these various roles to promote and maintain health, to prevent illness, and to facilitate coping with disability or death for adults in any setting.

The Nurse as Caregiver

Nurses have always been *caregivers*. However, the activities carried out within the caregiver role have changed tremendously in this century. From 1900 to the 1960s, the nurse was almost always female and was regarded primarily as the person who gave personal care and carried out physicians' orders. This dependent role has changed over the past 40 years as a result of the increased education of nurses, research in and the development of nursing knowledge, and the recognition that nurses are autonomous and informed professionals.

The caregiver role for the nurse today is both independent and collaborative. Nurses independently make assessments and plan and implement client care based on nursing knowledge and skills (Figure 1-1). Nurses also collaborate with other members of the health care team to implement and evaluate care.

As a caregiver, the nurse is a practitioner of nursing both as a science and as an art. Using the nursing process as the framework for care, the nurse provides interventions to meet not only the physical needs but also the psychosocial, cultural, spiritual, and environmental needs of clients and families. (See the box on page 6.) This consideration of all aspects of the client ensures a holistic

approach to nursing. Holistic nursing care is based on **holism,** the philosophical view that interacting wholes are greater than the sum of their parts. A holistic approach also emphasizes the uniqueness of the individual.

In providing comprehensive, individualized care, the nurse uses critical-thinking skills to analyze and synthesize knowledge from the arts, the sciences, and nursing research and theory. The science of nursing (that is, the knowledge base of nursing) is translated into the art of nursing through caring. Caring is the means by which the nurse is connected with and concerned for the client (Benner & Wrubel, 1989). Thus, the nurse as caregiver is knowledgeable, skilled, empathic, and caring.

The Nurse as Educator

The nurse's role as *educator* is becoming increasingly important for several reasons. Individuals as well as local, state, and federal governments are placing greater emphasis on health promotion and illness prevention; hospital stays are becoming shorter; and the number of chronically ill in our society is increasing. All these factors make the educator role essential to maintaining the health and well-being of clients.

The framework for the role of educator is the teaching-learning process. Within this framework, the nurse assesses learning needs, plans and implements teaching methodologies to meet those needs, and evaluates the effectiveness of the teaching. To be an effective educator, the nurse must have effective interpersonal skills and be familiar with adult learning principles (Figure 1–2).

A major component of the educator role today is discharge planning. **Discharge planning** is a systematic

Culturally Sensitive Nursing

■ ■ ■

The primary focus of nursing care is the client as the client relates to the environment and experiences events or situations related to health or illness. These experiences are given shape and personal meaning by culture, the socially inherited characteristics of a human group. These characteristics include the beliefs, practices, habits, likes, dislikes, customs, and rituals people learn from their families and pass on to their children. Cultural background is an essential component of a person's ethnic identity. A person's ethnic identity includes belonging to a social group within a culture and a social system and sharing a common religion, language, ancestry, and physical characteristics.

The health care system encompasses clients who are culturally diverse. This diversity includes differences in country of origin, health beliefs, sexual orientation, race, socioeconomic level, and age. Despite increasing diversity, nursing has been slow to address the need for culturally sensitive care. Many different factors account for this inattention, including ethnocentrism (people's belief that their own cultural group's beliefs and values are the only acceptable ones) and prejudice. The health care system is itself a culture, primarily made up of white middle-class people, and it often serves as a barrier to culturally sensitive care.

The 1992 American Academy of Nursing Expert Panel on Culturally Competent Nursing Care identified several reasons why it has become increasingly important that nurses plan culturally sensitive care:

- The demographic and ethnic composition of the population of the world in general, and the United States in particular, has changed markedly, and there is a lack of ethnic representation in health care professionals in the health care system. Information on and knowledge about values, beliefs, experiences, and health care needs of various populations is limited.
- There is a growing awareness and acceptance of diversity and an increased willingness to maintain and support ethnic and cultural heritage.
- People of color and immigrants are facing increasing unemployment, decreasing opportunity, and

limited access to health care. These conditions may contribute to the establishment of new minorities, such as the homeless.

- The international focus on providing health care for all people by the year 2000 (within the context of inequity, barriers, and lack of access) may have raised the consciousness of health care professionals to some of the inequities inherent in health care systems in both developing countries and developed countries.
- Nurses make up the largest force in the delivery of health care and therefore have the potential to contribute to the changing inequities in and inaccessibility to health care.
- Consumers are becoming increasingly aware of what is competent and sensitive health care.

This same panel of experts proposed general principles for nurses in becoming sensitive to cultural diversity and to providing culturally sensitive care. For example:

- Nurses must learn to appreciate intergroup and intragroup cultural diversity and commonalties in racial/ethnic minority populations.
- Nurses must understand how social structure factors shape health behaviors and practices among members of racial/ethnic minorities.
- Nurses must confront their own ethnocentrism and racism.
- Nurses must begin rehearsing, practicing, and evaluating service provided to cross-cultural populations.

People of every culture have the right to have their cultural values known, respected, and addressed appropriately in nursing and other health care services (Leininger, 1991). To provide nursing care that is culturally sensitive, nurses must develop a sensitivity to personal fundamental values about health and illness; must accept the existence of differing values; and must be respectful of, interested in, and understanding of other cultures without being judgmental.

---

method of preparing the client and family for exit from the health care agency and for maintaining continuity of care after they leave the setting (Zarle, 1989). Although teaching is a major part of discharge planning, discharge planning also involves making referrals, identifying com-

munity and personal resources, and arranging for necessary equipment and supplies for home care. Because education is such an important aspect of medical-surgical nursing, sections on client and family teaching are included throughout this textbook.

The Nurse as Advocate

The **client** (a person requiring health care services) entering the health care system is often unprepared to make independent decisions. The nurse as *client advocate* actively promotes the client's rights to autonomy and free choice. The nurse as advocate "speaks for the patient, mediates between the patient and other persons, and/or protects the patient's right to self-determination" (Ellis & Hartley, 1991, p. 270). The goals of the nurse as advocate are to

- Assess the need for advocacy.
- Communicate with other health care team members.
- Provide client and family teaching.
- Assist and support client decision making.
- Serve as a change agent in the health care system.
- Participate in health policy formulation.

The nurse must practice advocacy based on the belief that clients have the right to choose treatment options without coercion. The nurse must also accept and respect the decision of the client, even though it may differ from the decision the nurse would make.

The Nurse as Leader and Manager

All nurses are *leaders* and *managers*. They practice leadership, and they manage time, people, resources, and the environment in which they provide care. Nurses carry out these roles by directing, delegating, and coordinating activities. Nurses also evaluate the quality of care provided.

Models of Nursing Practice

Nurses are leaders and managers of client care within a variety of models of nursing practice. Two models often used are primary nursing and case management.

Primary Nursing   **Primary nursing** is a model of care that allows the nurse to provide individualized direct care to a small number of clients during their entire inpatient stay. This model was developed to reduce the fragmentation of care experienced by the client and to facilitate family-centered continuity of care. In primary nursing, the nurse provides care; communicates with clients, families, and other health care providers; and carries out discharge planning.

Case Management   In contrast to primary nursing, **case management** focuses on management of a caseload (group) of clients as well as the members of the health care team caring for those clients. The nurse who is case manager is usually a clinical specialist, and the caseload consists of clients with similar health care needs. As case manager, the nurse manages the quality of care provided, including accuracy, timeliness, and cost. The case manager also is in contact with clients after discharge, ensuring continuity of care and health maintenance.

Quality Assurance

In the role of leader and manager, the nurse is responsible for the quality of client care through a process called quality assurance. **Quality assurance** consists of the quality-control activities that evaluate, monitor, or regulate the standard of services provided to the consumer. Clients are assured of quality care through professional and technical licensure of individual care providers; accreditation of hospitals (for example, by the Joint Commission on Accreditation of Healthcare Organizations [JCAHO]; licensure of hospitals, pharmacies, and nursing homes; and certification in specialty areas.

Quality-assurance methods also are used to evaluate the care of clients. These methods commonly evaluate actual care against an established set of standards of care. This evaluation is made by reviewing documentation, by conducting client surveys and nurse interviews, and/or by direct observation of nurse or client performance. The data are then used to identify differences between actual practice and established standards and to develop a plan of action to resolve the differences. The actions are then assessed to determine whether they were effective in improving practice.

The Nurse as Researcher

Nurses have always identified problems in client care. Although they have developed interventions to meet specific needs, the activities often have not been conducted within a scientific framework or communicated to other nurses through nursing literature. To develop the science of nursing, nursing knowledge must be established through clinical research and then published, so that the findings can be used by all nurses to improve client care.

To be relevant, nursing research must have a goal to improve the care that nurses provide clients. This means that all nurses must consider the *researcher* role to be integral to nursing practice. Summaries of relevant nursing research are therefore included in almost all the nursing care chapters of this textbook. After the summary and discussion of each study, a critical-thinking section specifically related to the findings of the study encourages the student to apply the findings to the clinical setting.

Framework for Practice: The Nursing Process

■ ■ ■

The **nursing process** is the series of activities nurses perform as they provide care to clients. This section discusses the nursing process as a framework for the nursing care of adult medical-surgical clients. The discussion focuses on a nursing model of care, differentiating nursing from other helping professions.

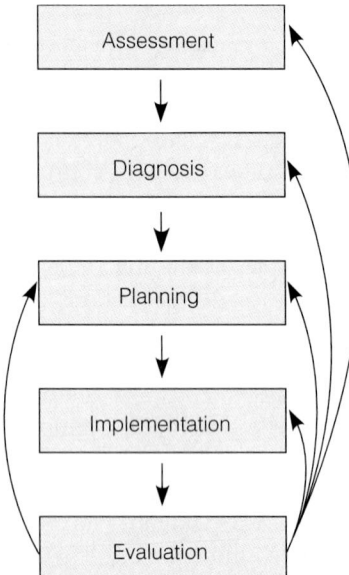

Figure 1-3 Steps of the nursing process. Notice that the steps are interrelated and interdependent. For example, evaluation of the client might reveal the need for further assessment, additional nursing diagnoses, and/or a revision of the plan of care.

The nursing process can be used in any setting in which the nurse provides care. The purpose of that care may be to promote wellness, maintain health, restore health, or facilitate coping with disability or death. Regardless of the purpose of care, the planned process of nursing allows for the inclusion of activities that are specific, individualized, and holistic in nature.

Steps of the Nursing Process

There are five steps, or phases, in the nursing process: assessment, diagnosis, planning, implementation, and evaluation. These steps are not discrete; they are interrelated and interdependent. The steps are most often used in a cyclic manner, as illustrated in Figure 1-3. Each step is discussed in detail below.

The five-step nursing process used today has evolved over the past 40 years. The nursing process was named by Hall in the 1950s (Hall, 1955), and in the 1960s it was divided into four steps—assessment, planning, implementation, and evaluation (Yura & Walsh, 1967). Continued work by nursing theorists and authors led to the addition of the diagnosis step during the 1970s. Assessment, diagnosis, planning, implementation, and evaluation are now accepted as the five steps of the process. The steps have been legitimized by the *Standards of Practice* (American Nurses Association, 1991), state nursing practice acts, and licensing examinations that are structured on a nursing model of care based on the nursing process.

This textbook assumes that the student already has a basic understanding of the nursing process and is now ready to expand and apply that knowledge to adult clients with medical-surgical health problems. The following discussion is intended to serve only as a review; for more information, consult books specifically focused on the use of the nursing process, and read the case studies in the nursing care chapters throughout this textbook.

Assessment

Assessment is the first step of the nursing process. It is a nursing activity that begins with the client's first encounter with the health care system and continues as long as the client requires care. During assessment, data (pieces of information) about health status are collected, validated, organized, clustered into patterns, and communicated either verbally or in written form. Assessment serves as the basis for deriving accurate nursing diagnoses, for planning and implementing both initial and ongoing individualized care, and for evaluating the care that is given. An example of a nursing admission data form is shown in Figure 1-4. An example of a client assessment flowsheet is provided in Figure 1-5.

The data that the nurse collects must be holistic in nature; that is, all dimensions of an individual must be considered carefully. The data collected are both objective and subjective. Information that the nurse perceives by the senses is objective data; it is seen, heard, touched, or smelled, and can be verified by another person—for example, blood pressure, temperature, pulse, or the presence of infected drainage. Information that is perceived only by the person experiencing it—for example, pain, dizziness, or anxiety—is subjective data.

Nurses assess clients in two ways: through an initial assessment and through focused assessments. The *initial assessment* of the client, conducted through a nursing history and physical assessment, is necessary for

- Accumulation of comprehensive data about health responses.

- Identification of specific factors that contribute to these responses in a specific individual.

- Facilitation of mutually established goals and outcomes of care. (Iyer et al., 1994)

Focused assessments are ongoing and continuous, occurring whenever the nurse interacts with the client. They enable the nurse to evaluate nursing actions and make decisions about whether to continue or change interventions to meet outcomes. They also provide structure for the documentation of nursing care. In addition, focused assessments enable the nurse to identify responses to a disease process or a treatment modality that was not present during the initial assessment or to monitor the status of an actual or potential problem previously identified (Alfaro, 1994).

NURSING ADMISSION DATA

Personal Belongings	With Patient	Sent Home	In Safe	N/A
Dentures				
Glasses/Contacts				
Hearing Aid				
Billfold/Purse				
Jewelry				
Clothing				
Other				
Description:				

DATE_____ TIME_____
☐ ADMISSION   ☐ OBSERVATION
☐ AMBULATORY   ☐ WHEELCHAIR   ☐ STRETCHER

ADMITTED FROM: ☐ HOME   ☐ NURSING FACILITY
                        ☐ EMERGENCY ROOM   ☐ OTHER_____
INFORMATION GIVEN BY: ☐ FAMILY MEMBER   ☐ FRIEND   ☐ PATIENT
☐ UNABLE TO TAKE HISTORY – PATIENT UNRESPONSIVE/CONFUSED/
        NOT ACCOMPANIED BY FAMILY OR FRIEND
        ☐ PREVIOUS MEDICAL RECORD

ORIENTATION TO ROOM
☐ VISITING HOURS   ☐ CALL LIGHT IN REACH/EXPLAINED
☐ OPERATION OF BED AND SIDE RAILS   ☐ USE OF PHONE
☐ PATIENT HANDBOOK   ☐ INTRODUCED TO ROOMMATE

CLINICAL DATA
HEIGHT _____
WEIGHT _____ ☐ BEDSCALE ☐ STANDING ☐ APPROXIMATE
TEMP: _____   PULSE: _____ RESPIRATIONS _____
BLOOD PRESSURE (RIGHT ARM) _____ (LEFT ARM) _____
            ☐ SITTING   ☐ LYING
NURSE ASSIST. SIGNATURE: _____

ALLERGEN: (DRUGS, FOOD, TAPES, DYES, OTHERS)

ALLERGEN	SYMPTOMS

CURRENT MEDICATIONS, SUPPLEMENTS, NON-PRESCRIPTION DRUGS:

Name	Dose/Route/Frequency	Last Dose	Started

FAMILY PRACTICE PHYSICIAN_____
MEDICAL HISTORY
ADMITTED MEDICAL DIAGNOSIS_____
_____
PREVIOUS SURGERIES:_____
_____
_____
_____

☐ Medication to Pharmacy   ☐ Medication sent home   ☐ Not Here
Medication info from: ☐ Bottles   ☐ Verbally
                        ☐ Written list   ☐ Transfer sheet   ☐ Other

PAST MEDICAL HISTORY: EXPLAIN.
☐ Cardiovascular_____
☐ Respiratory_____
☐ Neurological_____
☐ Musculoskeletal_____
☐ Gastrointestinal_____
☐ Genitourinary_____
☐ Hematological_____
☐ Cancer_____
☐ Diabetes_____

☐ Hypertension_____
☐ Skin_____
☐ Ear, Eyes, Nose, Throat_____
☐ Reproductive _____
☐ Other_____
_____
_____
MOST RECENT HOSPITALIZATION_____
NURSE'S SIGNATURE: _____ RN/LPN

Figure 1–4 An example of a nursing admission data form, completed on the client's admission to the hospital. A complete database also requires the physician's history and physical examination, a comprehensive nursing history, laboratory and radiologic data, and any additional information from other members of the health care team.

PATIENT ASSESSMENT FLOWSHEET

INITIALS/SIGNATURE _____

_____

_____

_____

Date _____

INITIAL ASSESSMENT	2300–0700 TIME/INITIALS _____	0700–1500 TIME/INITIALS _____	1500–2300 TIME/INITIALS _____
NUTRITION/ METABOLIC PATTERN	SKIN: ☐ Dry ☐ Intact ☐ Warm ☐ Cold ☐ Other _____ Turgor: _____ ☐ N/V _____ TUBES: (feeding) _____ IV SITE: _____ IV FLUIDS: _____ WOUNDS/DRSGS: _____	SKIN: ☐ Dry ☐ Intact ☐ Warm ☐ Cold ☐ Other _____ Turgor: _____ ☐ N/V _____ TUBES: (feeding) _____ IV SITE: _____ IV FLUIDS: _____ WOUNDS/DRSGS: _____	SKIN: ☐ Dry ☐ Intact ☐ Warm ☐ Cold ☐ Other _____ Turgor: _____ ☐ N/V _____ TUBES: (feeding) _____ IV SITE: _____ IV FLUIDS: _____ WOUNDS/DRSGS: _____
RESPIRATORY/ CIRCULATORY PATTERN	BREATH SOUNDS: _____ RESPIRATIONS: _____ OXYGEN: _____ PULSE OX: _____ ☐ Cough ☐ Sputum APICAL PULSE: _____% ☐ Regular ☐ Irregular TELEMETRY: _____ NAILBED COLOR: ☐ Pink ☐ Pale ☐ Blue PEDAL PULSES: R ☐ – ☐ + _____ L ☐ – ☐ + EDEMA: R ☐ – ☐ + _____ L ☐ – ☐ + CALF R ☐ – ☐ + TENDERNESS: L ☐ – ☐ +	BREATH SOUNDS: _____ RESPIRATIONS: _____ OXYGEN: _____ PULSE OX: _____ ☐ Cough ☐ Sputum APICAL PULSE: _____% ☐ Regular ☐ Irregular TELEMETRY: _____ NAILBED COLOR: ☐ Pink ☐ Pale ☐ Blue PEDAL PULSES: R ☐ – ☐ + _____ L ☐ – ☐ + EDEMA: R ☐ – ☐ + _____ L ☐ – ☐ + CALF R ☐ – ☐ + TENDERNESS: L ☐ – ☐ +	BREATH SOUNDS: _____ RESPIRATIONS: _____ OXYGEN: _____ PULSE OX: _____ ☐ Cough ☐ Sputum APICAL PULSE: _____% ☐ Regular ☐ Irregular TELEMETRY: _____ NAILBED COLOR: ☐ Pink ☐ Pale ☐ Blue PEDAL PULSES: R ☐ – ☐ + _____ L ☐ – ☐ + EDEMA: R ☐ – ☐ + _____ L ☐ – ☐ + CALF R ☐ – ☐ + TENDERNESS: L ☐ – ☐ +

SEE NURSES' NOTES FOR
FURTHER ASSESSMENT,
ABNORMALS, OR CHANGES IN
HEALTH STATUS

CODE: LOC – LEVEL OF CONSCIOUSNESS
MAE – MOVES ALL EXTREMITIES
NA – NOT APPLICABLE
BILAT – BILATERAL
INSP: INSPIRATORY EXP: EXPIRATORY

\+ POSITIVE
– NEGATIVE
× TIMES

Figure 1–5 A flowsheet for assessment of the hospitalized client. On each shift, the nurse checks feeding tubes, IV sites, dressings, respirations, pulses, and other factors as appropriate for each client.

To make accurate and holistic assessments, nurses must have and use a wide variety of knowledge and skills. The ability to assess the physical status of the client is essential, as is the ability to use effective communication techniques. Nurses must be knowledgeable in pathophysiology and pharmacology and be able to identify abnormal laboratory and diagnostic test data. Finally, nurses must have a solid foundation of nursing knowledge and skill that will enable them to interpret assessment data and to use that interpretation as the basis for individualized care.

Diagnosis

The American Nurses Association (ANA) has defined nursing as "the diagnosis and treatment of human responses to actual or potential health problems" (1980, p. 9). These human responses have four perspectives: normal physiologic regulatory responses, pathophysiologic responses, experiential responses, and behavioral responses (Mitchell et al., 1991). The nurse identifies the responses by applying one or more **nursing diagnoses,** defined by the North American Nursing Diagnosis Association (NANDA) as "a clinical judgment about individual, family, or community responses to actual or potential health problems/life processes. Nursing diagnoses provide the basis for selection of nursing interventions to achieve outcomes for which the nurse is accountable" (NANDA, 1990, p. 5).

The nurse analyzes data collected during the assessment step to support appropriate nursing diagnoses. During analysis, the nurse organizes, or clusters, data into categories of information that can be used to identify actual or potential alterations in health. Data can be organized within a variety of frameworks and methods for identifying patterns of human behavior (Wilkinson, 1992). Methods commonly used are basic human needs (Maslow, 1970), body systems, human response patterns, and functional health patterns (Gordon, 1982). The broad organizational structure used to categorize information in this book is based on Gordon's functional health patterns, described in the accompanying box.

Making a diagnosis is a complex process and always involves uncertainty. Therefore, the nurse uses diagnostic reasoning to choose nursing diagnoses that best define the individual client's health problems. Diagnostic reasoning is a form of clinical judgment (Radwin, 1990) used to make decisions about which label (or diagnosis) best describes the patterns of data. Radwin's review of research about diagnostic reasoning in nursing found that elements of the clinical judgment process include data gathering and validation, data categorization, intuition, and prior clinical experience.

There is no single universally accepted list of diagnoses used in nursing. However, the work of NANDA is widely used. This group has been working since 1973 to identify, develop, and classify nursing diagnoses. The diagnoses

Functional Health Patterns
■ ■ ■

1. *Health-perception–health-management pattern.* Describes client's perceived pattern of health and well-being and how health is managed.

2. *Nutritional-metabolic pattern.* Describes pattern of food and fluid consumption relative to metabolic need and pattern indicators of local nutrient supply.

3. *Elimination pattern.* Describes pattern of excretory function (bowel, bladder, and skin).

4. *Activity-exercise pattern.* Describes pattern of exercise, activity, leisure, and recreation.

5. *Cognitive-perceptual pattern.* Describes sensory-perceptual and cognitive patterns.

6. *Sleep-rest pattern.* Describes patterns of sleep, rest, and relaxation.

7. *Self-perception–self-concept pattern.* Describes self-concept pattern and perceptions of self (e.g., body comfort, body image, feeling state).

8. *Role-relationship pattern.* Describes patterns of role-engagements and relationships.

9. *Sexuality-reproductive pattern.* Describes client's patterns of satisfaction and dissatisfaction with sexuality; describes reproductive patterns.

10. *Coping–stress-tolerance pattern.* Describes general coping pattern and effectiveness of the pattern in terms of stress tolerance.

11. *Value-belief pattern.* Describes patterns of values, beliefs (including spiritual), or goals that guide choices or decisions.

Note. Adapted from *Nursing Diagnosis: Process and Application* by M. Gordon, 1982, New York: McGraw-Hill.

are classified by a taxonomy; that is, they are grouped into classes and subclasses based on patterns and relationships. Work on both the nursing diagnoses and the taxonomy is ongoing. The NANDA system was accepted in 1988 by the ANA as the official system of diagnosis for the United States. Nursing diagnoses within the NANDA taxonomy are used in this book and are listed in Table 1–1 Appendix B.

A nursing diagnosis is "a clinical diagnosis made by a professional nurse that describes actual or potential health problems which the nurse, by virtue of her [or his] education and experience, is capable and licensed to treat" (Gordon, 1987, p. 8). A diagnosis is written in two parts joined by the phrase "related to." The first part of

Table 1–1   NANDA Taxonomy of Nursing Diagnoses

Pattern 1:	**Exchanging**
1.1.2.1	Altered Nutrition: More than Body Requirements
1.1.2.2	Altered Nutrition: Less than Body Requirements
1.1.2.3	Altered Nutrition: Potential for More Than Body Requirements
1.2.1.1	Risk for Infection
1.2.2.1	Risk for Altered Body Temperature
1.2.2.2	Hypothermia
1.2.2.3	Hyperthermia
1.2.2.4	Ineffective Thermoregulation
1.2.3.1	Dysreflexia
1.3.1.1	Constipation
1.3.1.1.1	Perceived Constipation
1.3.1.1.2	Colonic Constipation
1.3.1.2	Diarrhea
1.3.1.3	Bowel Incontinence
1.3.2	Altered Urinary Elimination
1.3.2.1.1	Stress Incontinence
1.3.2.1.2	Reflex Incontinence
1.3.2.1.3	Urge Incontinence
1.3.2.1.4	Functional Incontinence
1.3.2.1.5	Total Incontinence
1.3.2.2	Urinary Retention
1.4.1.1	Altered (Specify Type) Tissue Perfusion (Renal, Cerebral, Cardiopulmonary, Gastrointestinal, Peripheral)
1.4.1.2.1	Fluid Volume Excess
1.4.1.2.2.1	Fluid Volume Deficit
1.4.1.2.2.2	Risk for Fluid Volume Deficit
1.4.2.1	Decreased Cardiac Output
1.5.1.1	Impaired Gas Exchange
1.5.1.2	Ineffective Airway Clearance
1.5.1.3	Ineffective Breathing Pattern
1.5.1.3.1	Inability to Sustain Spontaneous Ventilation
1.5.1.3.2	Dysfunctional Ventilatory Weaning Response (DVWR)
1.6.1	Risk for Injury
1.6.1.1	Risk for Suffocation
1.6.1.2	Risk for Poisoning
1.6.1.3	Risk for Trauma
1.6.1.4	Risk for Aspiration
1.6.1.5	Risk for Disuse Syndrome
1.6.2	Altered Protection
1.6.2.1	Impaired Tissue Integrity
1.6.2.1.1	Altered Oral Mucous Membrane
1.6.2.1.2.1	Impaired Skin Integrity
1.6.2.1.2.2	Risk for Impaired Skin Integrity
1.7.1	Decreased Adaptive Capacity: Intracranial
1.8	Energy Field Disturbance
Pattern 2:	**Communicating**
2.1.1.1	Impaired Verbal Communication
Pattern 3:	**Relating**
3.1.1	Impaired Social Interaction
3.1.2	Social Isolation
3.1.3	Risk for Loneliness
3.2.1	Altered Role Performance
3.2.1.1.1	Altered Parenting
3.2.1.1.2	Potential Altered Parenting
3.2.1.1.2.1	Risk for Altered Parent/Infant/Child Attachment
3.2.1.2.1	Sexual Dysfunction
3.2.2	Altered Family Processes
3.2.2.1	Caregiver Role Strain
3.2.2.2	Risk for Caregiver Role Strain
3.2.2.3.1	Altered Family Process: Alcoholism
3.2.3.1	Parental Role Conflict
3.3	Altered Sexuality Patterns
Pattern 4:	**Valuing**
4.1.1	Spiritual Distress (Distress of the Human Spirit)
4.2	Potential for Enhanced Spiritual Well-Being
Pattern 5:	**Choosing**
5.1.1.1	Ineffective Individual Coping
5.1.1.1.1	Impaired Adjustment

the statement is the particular human response that has been identified from the analysis of data. It identifies what needs to change in a specific client as a result of nursing interventions, and it also identifies the client outcomes that measure the change. The part of the statement that follows the "related to" phrase identifies the physical, psychosocial, cultural, spiritual, and/or environmental factors (etiologies) that cause or contribute to the occurrence of the response.

Two types of nursing diagnoses are used: those that identify actual human responses, and those that identify potential human responses. Nurses develop and implement a plan of care for actual responses; they also plan interventions to support health concerns and prevent illness concerns for potential human responses (Popkess-Vawter, 1989). Examples of nursing diagnoses are found throughout this textbook.

The *PES method* of writing a nursing diagnosis is frequently used in nursing practice (Gordon, 1987). Diagnoses written according to this method consist of three components:

1. The problem (P), which is the NANDA label.
2. The etiology (E) of the problem, which names the related factors and is indicated by the phrase "related to."
3. The signs and symptoms (S), which are the defining characteristics and are indicated by the phrase "as manifested by."

The following are examples of nursing diagnoses that are written using the PES method:

- *Anxiety* related to hospitalization as manifested by statements of nervousness and by crying

Table 1-1 (continued)

5.1.1.1.2	Defensive Coping
5.1.1.1.3	Ineffective Denial
5.1.2.1.1	Ineffective Family Coping: Disabling
5.1.2.1.2	Ineffective Family Coping: Compromised
5.1.2.2	Family Coping: Potential for Growth
5.1.3.1	Potential for Enhanced Community Coping
5.1.3.2	Ineffective Community Coping
5.2.1	Ineffective Management of Therapeutic Regimen (Individuals)
5.2.1.1	Noncompliance (Specify)
5.2.2	Ineffective Management of Therapeutic Regimen: Families
5.2.3	Ineffective Management of Therapeutic Regimen: Community
5.2.4	Ineffective Management of Therapeutic Regimen: Individual
5.3.1.1	Decisional Conflict (Specify)
5.4	Health Seeking Behaviors (Specify)

Pattern 6: Moving

6.1.1.1	Impaired Physical Mobility
6.1.1.1.1	Risk for Peripheral Neurovascular Dysfunction
6.1.1.1.2	Risk for Perioperative Positioning Injury
6.1.1.2	Activity Intolerance
6.1.1.2.1	Fatigue
6.1.1.3	Risk for Activity Intolerance
6.2.1	Sleep Pattern Disturbance
6.3.1.1	Diversional Activity Deficit
6.4.1.1	Impaired Home Maintenance Management
6.4.2	Altered Health Maintenance
6.5.1	Feeding Self-Care Deficit
6.5.1.1	Impaired Swallowing
6.5.1.2	Ineffective Breastfeeding
6.5.1.2.1	Interrupted Breastfeeding
6.5.1.3	Effective Breastfeeding
6.5.1.4	Ineffective Infant Feeding Pattern
6.5.2	Bathing/Hygiene Self-Care Deficit
6.5.3	Dressing/Grooming Self-Care Deficit
6.5.4	Toileting Self-Care Deficit
6.6	Altered Growth and Development

6.7	Relocation Stress Syndrome
6.8.1	Risk for Disorganized Infant Behavior
6.8.2	Disorganized Infant Behavior
6.8.3	Potential for Enhanced Organized Infant Behavior

Pattern 7: Perceiving

7.1.1	Body Image Disturbance
7.1.2	Self-Esteem Disturbance
7.1.2.1	Chronic Low Self-Esteem
7.1.2.2	Situational Low Self-Esteem
7.1.3	Personal Identity Disturbance
7.2	Sensory/Perceptual Alterations (Specify) (Visual, Auditory, Kinesthetic, Gustatory, Tactile, Olfactory)
7.2.1.1	Unilateral Neglect
7.3.1	Hopelessness
7.3.2	Powerlessness

Pattern 8: Knowing

8.1.1	Knowledge Deficit (Specify)
8.2.1	Impaired Environmental Interpretation Syndrome
8.2.2	Acute Confusion
8.2.3	Chronic Confusion
8.3	Altered Thought Processes
8.3.1	Impaired Memory

Pattern 9: Feeling

9.1.1	Pain
9.1.1.1	Chronic Pain
9.2.1.1	Dysfunctional Grieving
9.2.1.2	Anticipatory Grieving
9.2.2	Risk for Violence: Self-directed or directed at others
9.2.2.1	Risk for Self-Mutilation
9.2.3	Post-Trauma Response
9.2.3.1	Rape-Trauma Syndrome
9.2.3.1.1	Rape-Trauma Syndrome: Compound Reaction
9.2.3.1.2	Rape-Trauma Syndrome: Silent Reaction
9.3.1	Anxiety
9.3.2	Fear

- *Bowel Incontinence* related to loss of sphincter control as manifested by involuntary passage of stool
- *Fatigue* related to the side effects of chemotherapy as manifested by the inability to carry out normal daily routines and statements of overwhelming exhaustion

Planning

During the **planning** step, the nurse develops a list of nursing interventions and client outcomes to promote healthy responses and prevent, reverse, or decrease unhealthy responses. *Outcomes,* which are mutually established by the client and nurse, identify what the client will be able to do as a result of the nursing interventions. Both outcomes and nursing interventions are documented in a written plan of care that directs nursing activities, directs nursing documentation, and provides a tool for evaluation (Alfaro, 1994).

Nurses plan interventions for two types of client problems: those that require nursing management, stated as nursing diagnoses; and those that require collaborative management, which may be referred to as collaborative or clinical problems. Nursing diagnoses provide the basis for selecting nurse-initiated interventions to achieve outcomes for which the nurse is accountable (NANDA, 1990). **Collaborative problems** are pathophysiologic, treatment-related, personal, environmental, and maturational situations that nurses monitor for detection of onset or changes in status. Both physician-initiated and nurse-initiated interventions minimize the complications of collaborative problems (Carpenito, 1991).

Outcome criteria for nursing diagnoses are client centered, time specific, and measurable. They are classified into three domains: cognitive ("knowing"), affective ("feeling"), and psychomotor ("doing"). The nurse considers all three domains to ensure holistic care.

Outcome criteria for collaborative problems are nursing goals, usually written as statements that begin with "to detect and report early signs and symptoms of potential complications of . . ." and "to implement preventive and corrective nursing interventions ordered by . . ." (Alfaro, 1994). In many instances, these goals are not written down as part of the plan of care. Preventive and corrective nursing interventions for collaborative problems may be ordered by the physician or by institutional policy, procedures, protocols, or standards.

The nursing interventions that are planned must be specific and individualized. If, for example, the nurse identifies that a client is at risk for fluid volume deficit, it is not enough that the nurse simply encourage the client to drink increased amounts of fluid. The nurse and the client together must identify those liquids the client prefers, the times that will be best for drinking them, and the amount of fluid (in ounces or milliliters); this information must be documented as a nursing order on the written care plan. Only then does care truly become a part of the plan of care.

Implementation

The **implementation** step is the action or "doing" phase of the nursing process, during which the nurse carries out planned interventions. Ongoing assessment of the client before, during, and after the intervention is an essential component of implementation. Although the plan may be appropriate, there are many variables that may modify or negate any planned intervention, making a change in the plan necessary. For example, the nurse would not be able to force fluids if the client were nauseated or vomiting.

When implementing the planned interventions, the nurse follows several important principles:

- Set daily priorities, based on initial assessments and on the client's condition as reported during the change of shift report and/or documented in the client's chart. Ensure that critical assessments (such as status of invasive lines, fluids infusing, or changes in health status during the preceding shift) take first priority.

- Be aware of the interrelated nature of nursing interventions. For example, while giving a bath the nurse can also assess physical and psychologic status, use therapeutic communication, teach the client, do range-of-motion exercises, and provide skin care.

- Determine the most appropriate interventions for each individual client, based on health status and illness treatment. Examples of appropriate interventions include the following:
  a. Directly performing the activity for the client
  b. Assisting the client to perform the activity
  c. Supervising the client/family while they are performing the activity
  d. Teaching the client/family about health care
  e. Monitoring the client at risk for potential complications or problems

- Use available resources to provide interventions that are realistic for the situation and practical in terms of equipment available, financial status of the client, and resources available (including staff, agency, family, and community resources).

- Provide interventions that are appropriate to the needs of each client and are based on sound rationale.

Documenting interventions is the final component of implementation, and it is a legal requirement. There are many different ways of documenting care. The traditional narrative source-oriented and problem-oriented charting methods are used, as are such newer methods as focused charting, charting by exception, and computer-assisted documentation.

Evaluation

The **evaluation** step of the nursing process allows the nurse to determine whether the plan was effective and either to continue the plan, to revise the plan, or to terminate the plan. The outcome criteria that were established during the planning step provide the basis for evaluation. Although evaluation is listed as the last part of the nursing process, in actuality it takes place continuously throughout client care.

To evaluate a plan, the nurse collects data from the client, reviews the chart, and observes the client. The nurse then compares the status of the client with the written outcomes. If the outcomes have been accomplished, the nurse may either continue or terminate the plan. If the outcomes have not been accomplished, the nurse must modify the nursing diagnoses, outcomes, or plan.

Benefits of the Nursing Process

The nursing process benefits nurses providing care, clients receiving care, and settings in which care is provided. As nurses gain increasing autonomy in their practice, the use of the nursing process helps them identify their independent practice domain. The nursing process also provides a common reference system and a common terminology to serve as a base for improving clinical practice through research. In addition, the nursing process can serve as a framework for the evaluation of quality care.

The nursing process also benefits the client receiving care and the agency or institution providing that care. The client is the recipient of planned, individualized interventions, is involved in all steps of the process, and is assured continuity of care through the written care plan. The nursing process benefits the health care institution through better resource utilization, increased client satisfaction, and improved documentation of care.

As the 21st century approaches, increased research and theory development will continue to refine the nursing process, providing a consistent framework for identifying client responses to actual or potential health problems and delineating the unique role of the nurse in providing care.

The Nursing Process in Clinical Practice

With experience, the nursing process becomes an integral part of providing care; the nurse does not consciously stop and consider each step. Rather, using the process as a framework, the nurse provides care based on the client's specific, individualized needs. For example, when caring for a client who is hemorrhaging, the nurse uses all five steps simultaneously to meet critical, life-threatening needs. In contrast, when considering long-term needs for a client with a chronic illness or disability, the nurse makes in-depth assessments, mutually determines goals with the client, and provides documentation through a written plan of care that can be developed and revised as necessary by all nurses providing care. As a nurse becomes an expert practitioner, the nursing process becomes so much a part of the nurse that the nurse may not even consciously consider it while providing care; the practice *is* the process (Benner, 1984).

Guidelines for Nursing Practice

■ ■ ■

Nursing practice is structured by standards and codes of ethics that guide nursing practice and protect the public. This section presents some of those guidelines, specifically, codes for nurses and standards of nursing practice. These guidelines are especially important because nurses encounter legal and ethical problems almost daily. A discussion of representative issues also is included.

Codes for Nurses

An established code of ethics is one criterion that defines a profession. *Ethics* are principles of conduct. Ethical behavior is concerned with moral duty, values, obligations, and the distinction between right and wrong. *Codes of ethics* for nurses provide a frame of reference for "professionally valued and ideal nursing behaviors that are congruent with the principles expressed in the Code for Nurses" (Ketefian, 1987, p. 13).

The large number of ethical issues facing nurses in clinical practice makes the established codes for nurses critical to moral and ethical decision making. The codes also help define the roles of nurses. The codes of ethics presented here were developed by and for members of the International Council of Nurses, the American Nurses Association, and the Canadian Nurses' Association.

The International Council of Nurses Code

The *International Council of Nurses (ICN) Code for Nurses* was developed in 1953 and most recently revised in 1973 (see the box on page 16). This code helps guide nurses in setting priorities, making judgments, and taking action when they face ethical dilemmas in clinical practice.

The American Nurses Association Code

The *American Nurses Association (ANA) Code for Nurses* states principles of ethical concern (see the box on page 17). First published in 1950, the code was most recently revised in 1985. It guides the behavior of nurses and also defines nursing for the general public.

The Canadian Nurses' Association Code

The *Canadian Nurses' Association (CNA) Code of Ethics for Nursing* (Values: Standards section) was developed in 1980 and revised in 1991 (see the box on page 18). Its purposes are the same as those of the ICN and ANA codes.

Standards of Nursing Practice

A *standard* is a statement or criterion that can be used by a profession and by the general public to measure quality of practice. Established *standards of nursing practice* make each individual nurse accountable for practice. This means that each nurse providing care has the responsibility or obligation to account for his or her own behaviors within that role. Professional nursing organizations develop and implement standards of practice to identify clearly the nurse's responsibilities to society.

The ANA standards of clinical nursing practice (1991b) are outlined in the box on page 19. The CNA standards for nursing practice also are shown on page 19. These standards allow objective evaluation of nursing licensure and certification, institutional accreditation, quality assurance, and public policy.

Legal and Ethical Dilemmas in Nursing

A *dilemma* is a choice between two unpleasant alternatives. Nurses providing adult medical-surgical nursing care face dilemmas almost daily—so many that a complete discussion of them is impossible here; however, many of those commonly experienced involve caring for the client with acquired immune deficiency syndrome

The International Council of Nurses Code for Nurses

■ ■ ■

The fundamental responsibility of the nurse is four-fold: to promote health, to prevent illness, to restore health, and to alleviate suffering. The need for nursing is universal. Inherent in nursing is respect for life, dignity, and the rights of man. It is unrestricted by considerations of nationality, race, creed, color, age, sex, politics, or social status. Nurses render health services to the individual, the family, and the community and coordinate their services with those of related groups.

Nurses and People

The nurse's primary responsibility is to those people who require nursing care. The nurse, in providing care, promotes an environment in which the values, customs, and spiritual beliefs of the individual are respected. The nurse holds in confidence personal information and uses judgment in sharing this information.

Nurses and Practice

The nurse carries responsibility for nursing practice and for maintaining competence by continual learning. The nurse maintains the highest standards of nursing care possible within the reality of a specific situation. The nurse uses judgment in relation to individual competence when accepting and delegating

responsibilities. The nurse when acting in a professional capacity should at all times maintain standards of personal conduct that reflect credit upon the profession.

Nurses and Society

The nurse shares with other citizens the responsibility for initiating and supporting action to meet the health and social needs of the public.

Nurses and Coworkers

The nurse sustains a cooperative relationship with coworkers in nursing and other fields. The nurse takes appropriate action to safeguard the individual when his care is endangered by a coworker or any other person.

Nurses and the Profession

The nurse plays the major role in determining and implementing desirable standards of nursing practice and nursing education. The nurse is active in developing a core of professional knowledge. The nurse, acting through the professional organization, participates in establishing and maintaining equitable social and economic working conditions in nursing.

Note. From *ICN Code for Nurses: Ethical Concepts Applied to Nursing* by International Council of Nurses, 1973, Geneva: Imprimeries Populaires.

(AIDS), client rights, and issues of dying and death. The nurse must use ethical and legal guidelines to make decisions about moral actions when providing care in these and in many other situations.

Caring for the Client with AIDS

The number of people with AIDS continues to increase and is rapidly reaching epidemic proportions. No longer is AIDS thought to occur only in male homosexuals or drug addicts; AIDS occurs in both heterosexual and homosexual men and women of all ages and at all socioeconomic levels. Because there is no cure for AIDS, and because it inflicts such great physical, emotional, financial, and social havoc, the disease inspires great fear.

For nurses, AIDS poses a moral and ethical dilemma: Caring for the person with AIDS is a nursing responsibility, yet possible infection with the virus is a real and ever-

present danger. According to the ANA, the nurse has a moral obligation to provide care for the client with AIDS unless the risk exceeds the responsibility. The ANA (1986) lists four criteria for deciding when the nurse must provide care:

1. The patient is at significant risk of harm, loss, or damage if the nurse does not assist.
2. The nurse's intervention or care is directly relevant to preventing harm.
3. The nurse's care will probably prevent harm, loss, or damage to the patient.
4. The benefit the patient will gain outweighs any harm the nurse might incur and does not present more than minimal risk to the health care provider.

The nurse is morally obligated to provide care to the client with AIDS when all four of these criteria are met. In

---

The American Nurses Association Code for Nurses

■ ■ ■

1. The nurse provides services with respect for human dignity and the uniqueness of the client, unrestricted by considerations of social or economic status, personal attributes, or the nature of health problems.

2. The nurse safeguards the client's right to privacy by judiciously protecting information of a confidential nature.

3. The nurse acts to safeguard the client and the public when health care and safety are affected by the incompetent, unethical, or illegal practice of any person.

4. The nurse assumes responsibility and accountability for individual nursing judgments and actions.

5. The nurse maintains competence in nursing.

6. The nurse exercises informed judgment and uses individual competence and qualifications as criteria in seeking consultation, accepting responsibilities, and delegating nursing activities to others.

7. The nurse participates in activities that contribute to the ongoing development of the profession's body of knowledge.

8. The nurse participates in the profession's efforts to implement and improve standards of nursing.

9. The nurse participates in the profession's efforts to establish and maintain conditions of employment conducive to high-quality nursing care.

10. The nurse participates in the profession's effort to protect the public from misrepresentation and to maintain the integrity of nursing.

11. The nurse collaborates with members of the health professions and other citizens in promoting community and national efforts to meet the health needs of the public.

Note. From *Code for Nurses with Interpretive Statements* by American Nurses Association, 1985, Kansas City, MO: ANA.

---

almost all instances, care must be provided. In addition, most health care agencies have a written policy requiring nurses to provide care to clients with AIDS, except in certain circumstances, such as the nurse's pregnancy.

Ensuring Client Rights

Nurses respect the right to confidentiality of client information found in the client's record or secured during interviews. (In most instances, state nursing practice acts legally require nurses to uphold this right.) However, the rights of the client as an individual can result in dilemmas for the nurse in the clinical setting. For example, the right to privacy and confidentiality becomes a dilemma when the nurse does not have access to information concerning the presence of AIDS or HIV in clients being cared for. The current law in most states mandates that HIV test results can be given to another person only if the client provides written consent for the release of that information. Many health care providers believe that this law violates their own right to personal safety and are actively working to change the law.

The right to refuse treatment (including surgery, medication, medical therapy, and food/fluids) is another client right that raises nursing dilemmas. The nurse, as client advocate, must first establish that the client is competent. If the client is competent, the situation, the alternatives, and the potential harm from refusal must be carefully explained. By law, the client must establish an advance directive on admission to a health care agency stating the client's choice about preserving or prolonging life. An advance directive, or living will, is a document in which a client formally states preferences for health care in the event that he or she later becomes mentally incapacitated. The client also names a person who has durable power of attorney to serve as a substitute decision-maker to implement the client's stated preferences (McCrary & Botkin, 1989). This document becomes a part of the client's hospital record and is honored even if the client becomes incompetent during the period of treatment. However, several states assert that artificial feeding is not a procedure that may be rejected under living will statutes. The nurse must take responsiblity for remaining currently informed about laws in this area of practice.

Coping with Issues Involving Dying and Death

Questions about who lives, who dies, and who decides often arise in the health care setting. The issues surrounding death and dying have become increasingly pressing as advances in technology extend the lives of people with chronic debilitating illness and major trauma. These changes have altered concepts of living and dying, resulting in ethical conflicts regarding quality of life and death with dignity versus technologic methods of preserving life in any form.

Canadian Nurses' Association Code of Ethics for Nursing (Values: Standards)

■   ■   ■

Clients

1. A nurse is obliged to treat clients with respect for their individual needs and values.

2. Based upon respect for clients and regard for their right to control their own care, nursing care should reflect respect for the right of choice held by clients.

3. The nurse is obliged to hold confidential all information regarding a client learned in the health care setting.

4. The nurse has an obligation to be guided by consideration for the dignity of clients.

5. The nurse is obligated to provide competent care to clients.

6. The nurse is obliged to represent the ethics of nursing before colleagues and others.

7. The nurse is obligated to advocate the client's interest.

8. In all professional settings, including education, research, and administration, the nurse retains a commitment to the welfare of clients. The nurse bears an obligation to act in such a fashion as will maintain trust in nurses and nursing.

Health Team

9. Client care should represent a cooperative effort, drawing upon the expertise of nursing and other health professions. Acknowledging personal or professional limitations, the nurse recognizes the perspective and expertise of colleagues from other disciplines.

10. The nurse, as a member of the health care team, is obliged to take steps to ensure that the client receives competent and ethical care.

The Social Context of Nursing

11. Conditions of employment should contribute to client care and to the professional satisfaction of nurses. Nurses are obliged to work toward securing and maintaining conditions of employment that satisfy these connected goals.

Responsibilities of the Profession

12. Professional nurses' organizations recognize a responsibility to clarify, secure, and sustain ethical nursing conduct. The fulfillment of these tasks requires that professional organizations remain responsive to the rights, needs and legitimate interests of clients and nurses.

Note. From *Code of Ethics for Nursing* by Canadian Nurses' Association, 1985, Ottawa, Ontario: CNA.

Even if the client is competent and requests that no heroic measures be used to maintain life, many questions arise in nursing care. What constitutes a heroic measure? Should nursing interventions to provide comfort include administering narcotics at a level known to depress respirations? Should a feeding tube be placed in the client who is terminally ill? These and other questions are being debated not only within the health care system but also in the courts.

Issues and Trends in Medical-Surgical Nursing

■   ■   ■

Health care is a vast and complicated system, affected by, and reflecting changes in, society. The trends and issues facing medical-surgical nurses are ones that will shape both the philosophy and the providing of care as the world enters the 21st century. Of the many different trends and issues affecting nursing care today, only a selected few are discussed here: changes in the population requiring care, trends and issues in health care delivery, the use of computers in nursing, and nursing's role in health care reform.

Changes in the Population Requiring Care

In the last 10 years, the characteristics of the population requiring nursing care have changed dramatically. Fifty percent of all people admitted to acute care facilities are over the age of 75, and 45% of people admitted to critical care units are over the age of 65 (Callahan, 1987). The US Bureau of the Census (1992) projects that the demand for hospital services for the elderly will increase by 40% from 1987 to 2000. The number of Americans infected with

---

American Nurses Association
Standards of Clinical Nursing Practice
■ ■ ■

Standards of Care

Assessment: The nurse collects client health data.

Diagnosis: The nurse analyzes the assessment data in determining diagnoses.

Outcome Identification: The nurse identifies expected outcomes individualized to the client.

Planning: The nurse develops a plan of care that prescribes interventions to attain expected outcomes.

Implementation: The nurse implements the interventions identified in the plan of care.

Evaluation: The nurse evaluates the client's progress toward attainment of outcomes.

Standards of Professional Performance

Quality of Care: The nurse systematically evaluates the quality and effectiveness of nursing practice.

Performance Appraisal: The nurse evaluates his/her own nursing practice in relation to professional practice standards and relevant statues and regulations.

Education: The nurse acquires and maintains current knowledge in nursing practice.

Collegiality: The nurse contributes to the professional development of peers, colleagues, and others.

Ethics: The nurse's decisions and actions on behalf of clients are determined in an ethical manner.

Collaboration: The nurse collaborates with the client, significant others, and health care providers in providing care.

Research: The nurse uses research findings in practice.

Resource Utilization: The nurse considers factors related to safety, effectiveness, and cost in planning and delivering client care.

Note. From *Standards of Clinical Practice* by American Nurses Association, 1991, Kansas City, MO: ANA.

HIV is rising rapidly, with current statistics suggesting that there are more than 1.5 million people infected with HIV. The US Centers for Disease Control (CDC) expects the number to increase by 100,000 new cases per year by the mid-1990s (CDC, 1993). In addition, the number of medically indigent—those without any type of public or private insurance and who cannot pay for health care out of pocket—has doubled from an estimated 25 million to over 50 million in the past 10 years. Finally, the number of homeless is estimated to range from 250,000 to 3 million (Rafferty, 1989). All of these changes have had profound effects on the practice of nursing.

The Older Adult

The number of older adults (age 65 and over) in the total population has increased significantly since the early 1900s. Older adults now make up over 12% of the total population, and it is projected that by the year 2030, people over the age of 65 will outnumber those under the age of 18 (23% and 18% of the population, respectively). Of those 65 and older, the greatest increase will be in those over 75 (Spencer, 1989).

Canadian Nurses' Association
Standards for Nursing Practice
■ ■ ■

1. Nursing practice requires that a conceptual model(s) for nursing be the basis of practice.

2. Nursing practice requires the effective use of the nursing process.

3. Nursing practice requires that the helping relationship be the nature of the nurse-client interaction.

4. Nursing practice requires nurses to fulfill professional responsibilities.

Note. From *A Definition of Nursing Practice: Standards for Nursing Practice* by Canadian Nurses' Association, 1987, Ottawa, Ontario: CNA.

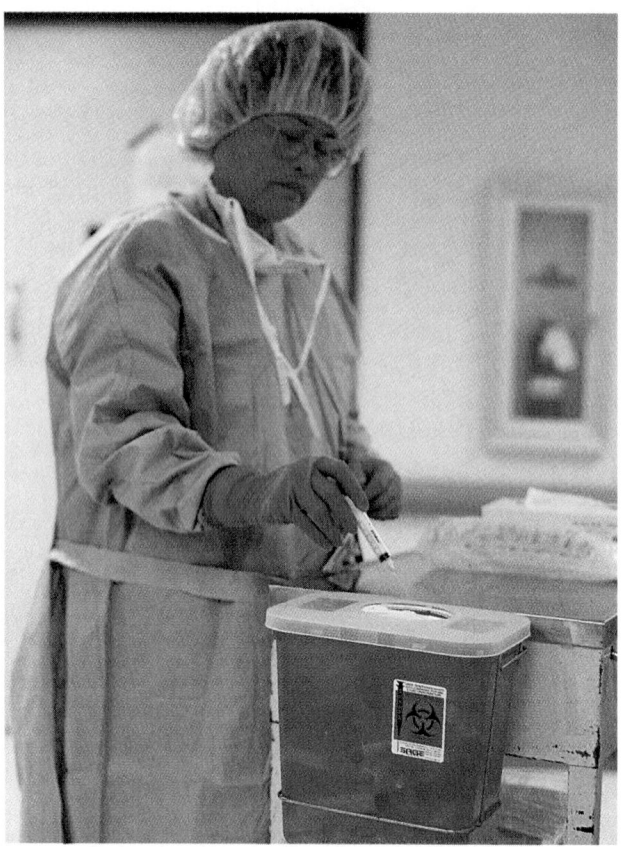

Figure 1-6 This nurse is disposing of a needle and syringe in a special container, a necessary practice to avoid the transmission of HIV through needle sticks with contaminated needles.

Older adults have more chronic illnesses and recover less rapidly from acute illnesses than young and middle adults. Treatment of illness requires a large number of hospital beds; the possibility exists that hospitals will become intensive care settings for older adults. Older adults also require more long-term care, community services, and home care. As a result, nursing care will be increasingly geared toward meeting the needs of the older adult in health and illness. The older adult is discussed at length in Chapter 2, and in special boxes that occur throughout the book to emphasize nursing care for this population.

The Client with AIDS

The emergence of AIDS, a disease caused by the human immunodeficiency virus (HIV), has resulted in a crisis in health care and has required permanent changes in the way nurses give care to others. Initially reported in the United States in 1981, the disease now affects more than 100,000 adolescents and adults in the US and 8–10 mil-

lion people worldwide (CDC, 1994). Initially, AIDS was believed to affect only homosexual men and intravenous drug users (especially in urban areas). Now the disease is found in heterosexual men and women, and the incidence in suburban and rural areas is increasing.

The epidemic has changed the practice of every nurse today. For example, nurses must now wear gloves whenever they come into contact with blood or other body fluids; they must exercise caution when handling contaminated clothing, bed linens, or dressings; and they must remember never to recap needles (Figure 1–6). Universal precautions to prevent transmission of HIV are published by the US Department of Health and Human Services; the most current recommendations are found on the inside of the back cover of this book. A full discussion of the client with AIDS is included in Chapter 8.

The Indigent Client

A major factor in accessing and using health care services is the ability to pay. The indigent client most often has neither personal resources nor insurance for health care. As a result, the indigent client either does not seek preventive and restorative health care interventions or receives them too late to avoid serious illness.

The medically indigent are composed of three groups: the nonworking uninsured, the medically uninsurable, and the employed uninsured. These three groups also are more likely to be living below the poverty line. Characteristic of those classified as poor are ever-increasing numbers of families headed by single-parent mothers, children, members of minority groups, and the elderly. Inner-city welfare recipients represent only a small part of the nation's poor; the working poor tend to be minimum-wage, semieducated people working in agriculture or the private sector. The number of poor who work has increased by 52% in the last decade, accounting for 7 million Americans (Malloy, 1990).

The numbers of medically indigent are increasing as a result of the high rate of unemployment in the United States. The loss of a job usually means not only the loss of income but also the loss of health insurance. Losing a job often causes a crisis; unemployment has been associated with physical illness; increased drug and alcohol use; increased incidence of child, spouse, or elder abuse and/or neglect; and increased mortality rates. However, because of insufficient income and lack of health insurance, these physical and psychosocial health care needs are neglected. In addition, the loss of income often precipitates homelessness.

The poor and the homeless are at increased risk for illness for many reasons, including the following:

■ The failure to seek preventive health care, such as immunizations, prenatal care, well-baby check ups, and health screenings.

- The failure to seek treatment for illness, resulting in an increased incidence of chronic illness and disability.

- Overcrowding, substandard housing, or lack of shelter, which increases the risk of illness from environmental hazards (rats, insects, sewage, extremes of temperature, polluted water).

- Poor living conditions, which contribute to an increased incidence of violence, resulting in abuse (child, spouse, elder) and death.

- A lack of transportation to secure food, coupled with inadequate food storage, which increases the risk of malnutrition. A diet that is high in calories and high in fat (protein is more expensive to buy) increases the risk of obesity and elevated cholesterol levels; both of these conditions are risk factors for hypertension and cardiovascular disease.

One of the social and political topics of debate in the United States is whether health care is a right or a privilege. The current system has, in effect, rationed health care by making it accessible primarily to those with adequate health insurance. It is obvious that a large segment of the population does not have the means to provide for adequate health care and that a solution must be found. Health care reform legislation is moving toward solving this problem.

Nurses can play a major role in finding solutions to health care problems by participating in policy formation and by designing innovative health care models. These models would focus on health promotion and disease prevention for the poor, the homeless, and the elderly in nurse-managed clinics (Malloy, 1990).

The Homeless Client

The problem of homelessness escalated throughout the 1980s and continues to be a significant factor in the changing health care system today. Homelessness affects men, women, and families; it cuts across racial and cultural boundaries and affects people of all ages and previous income levels. In the United States, homelessness affects an estimated 3 million people, one-third of whom are members of homeless families. And 85% of homeless families are headed by single women (Institute of Medicine, 1988).

What Is Homelessness?   *Homelessness,* defined by the National Academy of Sciences (NAS), is the condition experienced by an individual who:

1. Lacks a fixed, regular, and adequate nighttime residence, or

2. Has a primary nighttime residence that is designed to provide temporary living accommodations (including welfare hotels, congregate shelters, and transitional housing for the mentally ill).

3. Has as a primary nighttime residence in an institution that provides a temporary residence for individuals intended to be institutionalized.

4. Has as a primary nighttime residence in a public or private place not designed for or ordinarily used as regular sleeping accommodations for human beings. (Institute of Medicine, 1988)

Homeless people may be temporarily homeless, episodically homeless, or chronically homeless. Temporary homelessness may be the result of a natural disaster, such as fire or flood. Migrant workers and teenage runaways are examples of episodically homeless groups. The chronically homeless are those without permanent residences for a year or more (Institute of Medicine, 1988).

Factors Contributing to Homelessness   The factors that contribute to homelessness are complex and interrelated. Stanhope and Lancaster (1992) identified the following factors: individual health status (alcoholism and mental illness); immediate social environment (unemployment, poverty, family dysfunction, lack of low-income housing); and health and social policies (deinstitutionalization, reduced health and welfare benefits).

Health Problems of the Homeless   Homelessness has a negative effect on health. A study of the homeless by the Institute of Medicine (1988) found that homelessness and health interact as follows: (1) Some health problems, such as severe alterations in mental health, may lead to homelessness; (2) homelessness may lead to illness or to exacerbation of a chronic illness; and (3) homelessness makes treatment and care of any illness almost impossible.

Health problems in the homeless population include both physical and mental alterations. Homeless people are more prone to injuries and to acute illnesses, such as respiratory infections, food poisoning, and skin infestations. Chronic problems affecting the homeless include high blood pressure, chronic respiratory problems (including tuberculosis), heart and peripheral vascular disorders, and malnutrition. Mental health problems that contribute significantly to physical alterations are schizophrenia, depression, and substance abuse. Health problems of the homeless elderly are discussed in the box on page 22.

Nursing Care for the Homeless   Nursing care for the homeless is provided by city and county hospitals, hospital emergency rooms, ambulatory clinics, on-site health care teams, mobile outreach services, and community agencies (Berne, et al., 1990). Most care is provided by community health nurses (Figure 1–7). Although nurses who provide care for the homeless face many problems (including poor working conditions and professional isolation), there are also many personal rewards.

Applying Research to Nursing Practice
Homeless Elderly Men

■ ■ ■

To identify the universal self-care requisites of homeless elderly men, researchers interviewed ten homeless men, 65 or older, and analyzed the information collected (Harris & Williams, 1991). The themes identified by the subjects were finding clean water, finding enough nutritious food, resting enough, getting some exercise, finding ways to use time better, finding people to trust and have as a friend, being aware of health needs and finding help, getting medicines and being treated, protecting themselves, meeting needs in the winter, having a safe place to stay at night, getting money, keeping clean, and having clean clothes.

Implications for Nursing

As the number of both elderly and homeless people rises, the population of homeless elderly will continue to escalate. Findings of this study support that universal self-care requisites are common to all individuals, regardless of age or living conditions. Only limited research has been conducted on the needs of the homeless elderly. More information is needed from which nursing interventions specific to this population can be developed. An important nursing intervention in caring for the homeless elderly is linking them with appropriate community agencies and resources. Therefore, nurses must be informed about such resources in the community.

Critical Thinking in Client Care
1. What factors in the elderly population might precipitate homelessness?
2. In general, would you expect to find more elderly men or elderly women homeless, and why? (Do men or women tend to live longer?)
3. What community agencies and resources are available in your area or city to help the homeless?

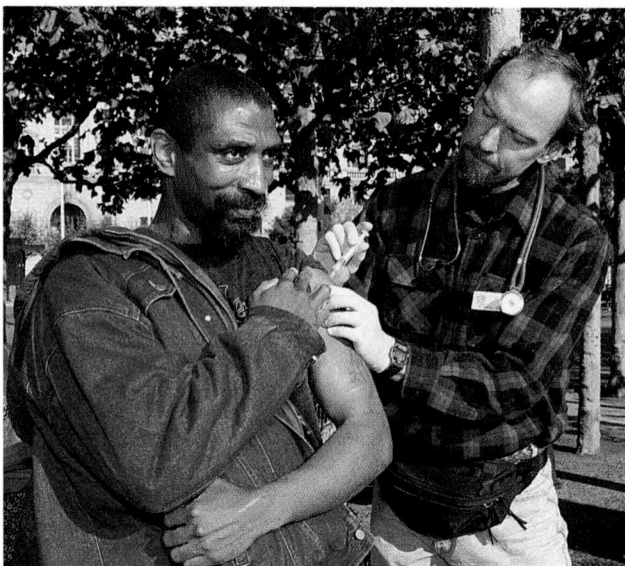

Figure 1-7 Care for the homeless is often provided by nurses working in the community setting.

- Reforms in cost and reimbursement of physician services. For example, third-party payers will reimburse physician services only to the amount that has been established as equitable. The American Medical Association (AMA) suggests that physicians post the costs of services in waiting rooms so that consumers may compare costs prior to requesting care.

- Changes in health care financing through expanded Medicaid coverage, universal health insurance plans, mandated employer's insurance, or a national comprehensive health plan to try to answer the problem of uncompensated care.

- Increased support for ambulatory services, with hospitals becoming centers that focus on two major areas: ambulatory care and intensive care with rehabilitation.

- A shortage of nurses prepared at the master's or doctoral levels for advanced practice roles.

- Increased government intervention in quality assurance in hospitals and in community-based settings. Quality-assurance programs in health care agencies are required for accreditation and refer to the quality, quantity, appropriateness, and cost of services provided.

- A decrease in the health of the population, resulting in part from illiteracy, violence, drug use, poverty, and unemployment. (Anderson, 1994; Kelly, 1991; Moccia, 1989, 1992; Perkins & Perkins, 1992)

Critical Pathways

A recent trend in health care is to provide care from multidisciplinary, managed action plans. Critical pathways,

Trends and Issues in Health Care Delivery

There are so many trends and issues in health care delivery that it is impossible to include all of them here. The list below includes only the most significant trends and issues discussed in current nursing literature:

also called critical paths, multidisciplinary plans, anticipated recovery plans, multidisciplinary action plans, and action plans, are one model for this approach to health care. Such pathways are generally developed for specific diagnoses—usually high volume, high risk, and high cost case types—with the collaboration of members of the health care team. This client care management tool describes how resources will be used to achieve predetermined outcomes. It also establishes the sequence of multidisciplinary interventions, including education, discharge planning, consultations, medication administration, diagnostics, therapeutics, and treatments.

Critical pathways have several goals:

- Achieve realistic, expected client and family outcomes.
- Promote professional and collaborative practice and care.
- Ensure continuity of care.
- Guarantee appropriate use of resources.
- Reduce costs and length of stay.
- Provide the framework for continuous improvement.

Critical pathways are often used in conjunction with case management models and/or quality improvement efforts. The overall goal is to design pathways that facilitate a reproducible standard of care for specific client populations and improve the quality and proficiency of that care.

When clients do not achieve expected outcomes, variances from the critical pathways are recorded and studied by the multidisciplinary team. Variances are often grouped as either system, provider, or client variances. A typical system variance would be the unavailability of diagnostic testing. A provider variance might relate to a practitioner's level of experience. A client variance may result from an unexpected change in condition. In many agencies, critical pathways are designed so that interventions and variances can be easily documented. Most documentation systems require a check off when interventions are performed or variances occur.

The agency determines the process for developing a critical pathway. Information imperative to the development of any critical pathway includes literature reviews, chart reviews, expert opinion, and insurance reimbursements for the designated case type. A typical approach is to first identify high cost, high volume, and high risk case types for the agency. Next, a multidisciplinary team, including physicians, develops a consensus around the management of the case type and a critical pathway. The pathway is then piloted with a designated group of clients, and revisions are based on the number and types of variances. The goal is to develop a pathway that best meets the needs of clients, in the particular practice setting.

In many agencies, critical pathways or similar models are replacing the traditional nursing care plan. The advantages of critical pathways are that they are outcome-driven and provide a time line to achieve specified goals. Additionally, critical pathways provide opportunities for health care workers to collaborate and establish dynamic plans of care that consider all of the clients' needs. Although initially developed for acute hospitalizations, critical pathways are now developed to manage clients in home health, outpatient, and long-term settings. Because of their growing importance in all areas of nursing, examples of critical pathways for major health problems are provided throughout this book.

The Use of Computers in Nursing

Nurses not only provide nursing care, but also must document the assessments that they make and the care that they give. The statement "If you didn't chart it, you didn't do it" has meant that nurses must spend a substantial amount of their time documenting. For many nurses, one of the less desirable aspects of nursing is the amount of time that they must take to document ongoing assessments and care—time that most nurses believe would be better spent with the client. Computerization of hospital management systems and records may be the answer to this problem.

Computers in health care institutions are used to

- Program the administration rate of fluids.
- Order supplies and services (for example, diets and diagnostic tests) for clients.
- Store and provide immediate access to the results of diagnostic tests.
- Develop and implement client acuity-classification systems, which are used to predict staffing needs of nursing personnel.
- Generate staffing schedules.
- Provide continuing education programs.
- Provide medication documentation records.
- Document ongoing nursing assessments and care, including vital signs.
- Develop individualized nursing care plans.

By having the computer at the bedside, nurses can document assessments and care immediately and efficiently. Bedside computers cut down on both the time required to document and the potential for documentation errors. The nurse can review the entire client record at the bedside, as well as at terminals in central locations. Computers can also save nurses time by automatically calculating intake and output and titration of drugs by factors such as body surface area, weight, and/or blood pressure; further information is provided through graphic printouts of trends across time.

Computerized documentation is also used for discharge planning, discharge summary, and client teaching protocols. Records of previous admissions can be easily accessed, facilitating continuity of care. Finally, computerized nursing-process programs enable the nurse to develop individualized care plans from a database of defining characteristics, related factors, diagnostic labels (nursing diagnoses), outcomes of care, and nursing interventions to meet the outcomes.

Despite the advantages, the use of computer technology has raised some concerns. Computerized decision making for nursing care plans is based solely on scientific facts and thus negates the humanistic, caring aspect of nursing. The potential exists for nurses to interact more with machines than they do with clients, coming to regard the client as the extension of a machine. Lastly, confidentiality of client health care information is threatened by access to records from multiple sources, including insurance companies, employers, and the government (Murphy, 1990).

The Role of Nursing in Health Care Reform

America's health care system has many strengths. It also has many weaknesses. As the largest number of care providers in the health care system, nurses have long recognized that more needs to be done to improve the health of the people of the United States. In 1991, the ANA published *Nursing's Agenda for Health Care Reform*. This document presents a plan for focusing on health (rather than illness) care, increases collaborative efforts toward health between consumers and providers, describes new health care delivery arrangements, and ensures services that focus on consumer needs.

The basic components of nursing's "core of care" include the following:

- A restructured health care system.
- A federally defined standard package of essential health care services available to all citizens and residents of the United States, provided and financed through an integration of public and private plans and sources.
- A phase-in of essential services.
- Planned change to anticipate health service needs that correlate with changing national demographics.
- Steps to reduce health care costs.
- Case management required for those with continuing health care needs. Case management will reduce the fragmentation of the present system, promote consumers' active participation in decisions about their health, and create an advocate on their behalf.

- Provisions for long-term care.
- Insurance reforms to improve access to coverage.
- Establishment of public/private sector review to determine resource allocation, cost-reduction approaches, allowable insurance premiums, and fair and consistent reimbursement levels for providers.

Nurses can make a difference in the health of individuals, families, communities, and the nation. To do so, nursing must focus on health-oriented care as an integral component of the health care system.

Bibliography

■ ■ ■

Alfaro, R. (1994). *Applying nursing diagnoses and nursing process: A step-by-step guide.* (2nd ed.). Philadelphia: Lippincott.

American Academy of Nursing Expert Panel on Culturally Competent Nursing Care. (1992). Culturally competent health care. *Nursing Outlook, 40*(6), 277–283.

American Nurses Association. (1980). *A social policy statement.* Kansas City, MO: ANA.

———. (1985). *Code for nurses.* Kansas City, MO: ANA.

———. (1986). *Committee on ethics: Statement regarding risk versus responsibility in providing nursing care.* Kansas City, MO: ANA.

———. (1988). *Ethics in nursing: Position statements and guidelines.* Kansas City, MO: ANA.

———. (1991a). *Nursing's agenda for health care reform.* Kansas City, MO: ANA.

———. (1991b). *Standards of clinical nursing practice.* Kansas City, MO: ANA.

———. (1994). Health care reform shapes HOD debate. *American Nurse,* (July/August), 1, 21.

Anderson, C. (1994). Advanced practice: Quality control. *Nursing Outlook, 42*(2), 54–55.

Bagis-Smith, J., & McKeehan, K. M. (1990). Continuity of care across hospital-community boundaries. In J. C. McCloskey & H. K. Grace (Eds.), *Current issues in nursing* (pp. 181–186). St Louis: Mosby.

Barrick, B. (1990). Light at the end of a decade. *American Journal of Nursing, 90*(11), 37–40.

Benner, P. (1984). *From novice to expert: Excellence and power in clinical nursing practice.* Redwood City, CA: Addison-Wesley Nursing.

Benner, P., & Wrubel, J. (1989). *The primacy of caring: Stress and coping in health and illness.* Redwood City, CA: Addison-Wesley Nursing.

Berne, A. S., Dato, C., Mason, D. J., & Rafferty, M. (1990). A nursing model for addressing the health needs of homeless families. *Image: Journal of Nursing Scholarship, 22*(1), 8–13.

Callahan, D. (1987). *Setting limits: Medical goals in an aging society.* New York: Simon & Schuster.

Canadian Nurses' Association. (1991). *Code of ethics for nurses.* Ottawa, Ontario: CNA.

———. (1987). *A definition of nursing practice: Standards for nursing practice.* Ottawa, Ontario: CNA.

Care, S. (1991). Death by choice. *American Journal of Nursing, 91*(7), 33–34.

Carpenito, L. J. (1991). *Nursing care plans and documentation: Nursing diagnoses and collaborative problems.* Philadelphia:. Lippincott.

———. (1992). *Nursing diagnosis: Application to clinical practice.* (4th ed.). Philadelphia: Lippincott.

Cassanego, M., & Zlotnick, C. (1992). Unemployment and health. *Nursing & Health Care, 13*(2), 78–82.

Crummer, M. B., & Carter, V. (1993). Critical pathways—the pivotal tool. *Journal of Cardiovascular Nursing, 7*(4), 30–37.

Donovan, N. M. (1991). Confidentiality vs. duty to warn: Whose life is it anyway? *Nursing & Health Care, 12*(8), 432–436.

Ellis, J. R., & Hartley, C. L. (1991). *Managing and coordinating nursing care.* Philadelphia: Lippincott.

Esper, P. S. (1988). Discharge planning—a quality assurance program. *Nursing Management, 19*(10), 66–68.

Farley, S. (1993). The community as partner in primary health care. *Nursing & Health Care, 14*(5), 244–249.

Friedman, E. (1990a). Nursing: New power, old problems. *Journal of the American Medical Association, 264,* 2977–2978, 2981–2982.

———. (1990b). Troubled past of "invisible" profession. *Journal of the American Medical Association, 264,* 2851–2858.

Gordon, M. (1982). *Nursing diagnosis: Process and application.* New York: McGraw–Hill.

———. (1987). *Nursing diagnosis: Process and application.* (2nd ed.). New York: McGraw–Hill.

Grindel, C. G., & McGuffin, B. (1992). Standards of clinical nursing practice. *MEDSURG Nursing, 1*(1), 23–28.

Hall, L. E. (1955, June). Quality of nursing care. *Public Health News.* Newark, NJ: State Department of Health.

Halloran, E. J. (1988). Computerized nursing assessments. *Nursing & Health Care, 9*(9), 497–499.

Harris, J. L., & Williams, L. K. (1991). Universal self-care requisites as identified by homeless elderly men. *Journal of Gerontological Nursing, 17*(6), 39–43.

Hoffman, P. A. (1993). Critical path method: An important tool for coordinating clinical care. *Journal on Quality Improvement 19*(7), 235–246.

Institute of Medicine. (1988). *Homelessness, health, and human needs.* Washington, DC: National Academy Press.

International Council of Nurses. (1973). *ICN code for nurses: Ethical concepts applied to nursing.* Geneva: Imprimeries Populaires.

Iyer, P. W., Taptich, B. J., & Bernocchi-Losey, D. (1994). *Nursing process and care planning.* (2nd ed.). Philadelphia: Saunders.

Kazanowski, M. K. (1992). A nursing department's response to risks associated with human immunodeficiency virus. *Nursing Outlook, 40*(1), 42–44.

Kelly, L. S. (1991). Another look at the future of health care. *Nursing Outlook, 39*(4), 150–151.

Ketefian, S. (1987). Moral behavior in nursing. *Advances in Nursing Science, 9,* 10–19.

Lamb, G., & Stempel, J. (1994). Nurse case management from the client's view: Growing as insider-expert. *Nursing Outlook, 42*(1), 7–13.

Leininger, M. (1991). Transcultural care principles, human rights, and ethical considerations. *Journal of Transcultural Nursing, 3,* 21–23.

Lindberg, J. B., Hunter, M. L., & Kruszewski, A. Z. (1990). *Introduction to nursing: Concepts, issues, and opportunities.* Philadelphia: Lippincott.

Malloy, C. (1990). Indigent care. In J. C. McCloskey & H. K. Grace (Eds.), *Current issues in nursing* (pp. 607–611). St. Louis: Mosby.

Maslow, A. (1970). *Motivation and personality.* New York: Harper & Row.

Mayhew, P. A. (1993). The importance of the practicing nurse in nursing research. *MEDSURG Nursing, 2*(3), 210–211, 246.

McCrary, S. V., & Botkin, J. R. (1989). Hospital policy on advance directives: Do institutions ask patients about living wills? *Journal of the American Medical Association, 262*(17), 2411–2414.

Meyer, C. (1991). Nursing and AIDS: A decade of caring. *American Journal of Nursing, 91*(12), 26–31.

Mezey, M., Evans, L., Golub, Z., Murphy, E., & White, G. (1994). The patient self-determination act: Sources of concern for nurses. *Nursing Outlook, 42*(1), 30–38.

Mitchell, P. H., Gallucci, B., & Fought, S. G. (1991). Perspectives on human response to health and illness. *Nursing Outlook, 39*(4), 154–157.

Moccia, P. (1989). 1989: Shaping a human agenda for the nineties. Trends that demand our attention as managed care prevails. *Nursing & Health Care, 10*(1), 15–17.

———. (1992). In 1992 a nurse in every school. *Nursing & Health Care, 13*(1), 14–18.

Murphy, C. P. (1990). Technological advances and ethical dilemmas. In J. C. McCloskey & H. K. Grace (Eds.), *Current issues in nursing* (pp. 587–591). St Louis: Mosby.

Nightingale, F. (1859/1969). *Notes on nursing: What it is, what it is not.* New York: Dover Publications.

North American Nursing Diagnosis Association. (1987). *Taxonomy I.* St Louis: NANDA.

———. (1990). *Taxonomy I—Revised, 1990.* St Louis: NANDA.

Pender, N. J. (1993). Health care reform: One view of the future. *Nursing Outlook, 41*(2), 56–57.

Perkins, C. B., & Perkins, K. C. (1992). Uncompensated care: The millstone around the neck of U.S. health care. *Nursing & Health Care, 13*(1), 20–23.

Popkess-Vawter, S. (1989). Nursing diagnosis: Its development and future. In C. E. Lambert, Jr. & V. A. Lambert (Eds.), *Perspectives in nursing: The impacts on the nurse, the consumer, and society* (pp. 93–118). Norwalk, CT: Appleton & Lange.

Radwin, L. E. (1990). Research on diagnostic reasoning in nursing. *Nursing Diagnosis, 1*(2), 70–77.

Rafferty, M. (1989). Standing up for America's homeless. *American Journal of Nursing, 89*(12), 1614–1617.

Schwarz, J. K. (1992). Living wills and health care proxies: Nurse practice implication. *Nursing & Health Care, 13*(2), 92–96.

Smith, P., Pass, C. M., Pounovich-Stream, C., & Jones, B. (1992). Implementing nurse case management in a community hospital. *MEDSURG Nursing, 1*(1), 47–52.

Spector, R. E. (1991). *Cultural diversity in health and illness.* (3rd ed.). Norwalk, CT: Appleton & Lange.

Spencer, G. (1989). Projections of the population of the United States by age, sex, and race: 1988 to 2080. *Current Population Reports Series P-25. No. 1018.* Washington, DC: US Bureau of the Census.

Sprayberry, L. D. (1993). Nursing's dual role in health care policy. *Nursing & Health Care, 14*(5), 250–254.

Stanhope, M., & Lancaster, J. (1992). *Community health nursing: Process and practice for promoting health.* (3rd ed.). St Louis: Mosby.

Sullivan, E. J., & Decker, P. J. (1988). *Effective management in nursing.* (3rd ed.). Redwood City, CA: Addison-Wesley Nursing.

Ugarriza, D., & Fallon T. (1994). Nurses' attitudes toward homeless women: A barrier to change. *Nursing Outlook, 42*(1), 26–29.

US Bureau of the Census. (1992). *Statistical Abstract of the United States.* (112th ed.). Washington, DC: US Government Printing Office.

US Centers for Disease Control. (1990). HIV prevalence estimates and AIDS case projections for the United States. *Morbidity and Mortality Weekly Report, 39,* (RR-16), 1.

———. (June 7, 1991). The HIV/AIDS epidemic: The first ten years. *Morbidity and Mortality Weekly Report, 40,* 357.

———. (1993). Update: Acquired immunodeficiency syndrome—United States, 1992. *Morbidity and Mortality Weekly Report 42,* 547–551, 557.

———. (1994). Update: Impact of the expanded AIDS surveillance case definition for adolescents and adults on case reporting—United States, 1993. *Morbidity and Mortality Weekly Report 43,* 160–170.

Wilkinson, J. M. (1992). *Nursing process in action: A critical thinking approach.* Redwood City, CA: Addison–Wesley Nursing.

Wilson, H. S. (1991). Identifying problems for clinical research to create a nursing tapestry. *Nursing Outlook, 39*(6), 280–282.

Yura, H., & Walsh, M. (1967). *The nursing process: Assessing, planning, implementing, evaluation.* New York: Appleton–Century–Crofts.

Zarle, E. T. (1989). Continuity of care: Balancing care of elders between health care settings. *Nursing Clinics of North America, 24,* 697–705.

Zlotnick, C., & Cassanego, M. (1992). Unemployment and health. *Nursing & Health Care, 13*(2), 78–82.

The Adult Client in Health and Illness

LEARNING OBJECTIVES

After completing this chapter, you will be able to

- Describe the physical status, risks for alterations in health, assessment guidelines, and healthy behaviors of the young adult, middle adult, and older adult.
- Discuss the definitions, functions, and developmental stages and tasks of the family.
- Define health, incorporating the health-illness continuum and the concept of high-level wellness.
- Identify factors affecting health status.
- Describe the nurse's role in health promotion.
- Describe the primary, secondary, and tertiary levels of illness prevention.
- Compare and contrast illness and disease.
- Describe illness behaviors in acute illness.
- Discuss chronic illness, including characteristics, needs and tasks of the chronically ill, and the effects on the family.
- Discuss the role of the nurse in planning and implementing care as a part of rehabilitation.

Gordon Hight, a 21-year-old college student, is admitted to the emergency room with multiple injuries and head trauma following a motorcycle accident. Mary Green, a 38-year-old homemaker, arrives at same-day surgery for biopsy of a tumor in her left breast. Sam Rosengarten, a 55-year-old attorney, is in the intensive care unit for treatment of a myocardial infarction. Margarite Schlefer, age 82, is in a long-term care facility following a fall that fractured her right hip. These examples demonstrate the striking variety among adult clients—the focus of care in medical-surgical nursing.

This chapter discusses the adult client at different developmental stages, providing an overview of physical status, risks for alterations in health, broad assessment guidelines, and health promotion activities. Information on the family of the client includes definitions and functions of the family, as well as developmental tasks and related health risk factors. A discussion of the client in health and illness summarizes health, illness, factors af-

fecting health, acute illness, chronic illness, and rehabilitation.

The Adult Client

■ ■ ■

Although growth and development are continuous processes throughout life, the adult years commonly are divided into three stages: the young adult (age 18 to 40), the middle adult (age 40 to 65), and the older adult (over age 65). Although the developmental markers are not as clearly delineated in the adult as in the infant or child, specific changes do occur in intellectual, psychosocial, and spiritual development, as well as in physical structures and functions, with aging.

The developmental theories specific to the adult, with related stages and tasks, are listed in Table 2–1. The

Table 2–1   Theories of Adult Development

	Theorist	Age	Task
Psychosocial Development	Erikson	18–25	Identity versus role confusion ■ Establishing an intimate relationship with another person ■ Committing oneself to work and to relationships
		25–65	Generativity versus stagnation ■ Accepting one's own life as creative and productive ■ Having concern for others
		65–death	Integrity versus despair ■ Accepting worth of one's own life ■ Accepting inevitability of death
Spiritual Development	Fowler	After 18	■ Having a high degree of self-consciousness ■ Constructing one's own spiritual system
		After 30	■ Being aware of truth from a variety of viewpoints
	Westerhoff	Young adult	Searching Faith ■ Acquiring a cognitive and an affective faith through questioning one's own faith
		Middle–Older Adult	Owned Faith ■ Putting faith into action and standing up for beliefs
Moral Development	Kohlberg	Adult	Post-Conventional Level Social contract/legalistic orientation ■ Defining morality in terms of personal principles ■ Adhering to laws that protect the welfare and rights of others
			Universal-Ethical Principles ■ Internalizing universal moral principles ■ Respecting others; believing that relationships are based on mutual trust
Developmental Tasks	Havighurst	18–35	■ Selecting and learning to live with a mate ■ Starting a family and rearing children ■ Managing a home ■ Starting an occupation ■ Taking on civic responsibility ■ Finding a congenial social group
		35–60	■ Achieving civic and social responsibility ■ Establishing and maintaining an economic standard of living ■ Assisting teenage children in becoming responsible and happy adults ■ Developing leisure-time activities ■ Relating to one's spouse as a person ■ Accepting and adjusting to the physiologic changes of middle age ■ Adjusting to aging parents
		60 and over	■ Meeting civic and social obligations ■ Establishing an affiliation with one's own age group ■ Establishing satisfactory physical living arrangements ■ Adjusting to decreasing physical strength, health, retirement, reduced income, death of spouse

Note. Adapted from *Childhood and Society* (2nd ed.) by E. Erickson, 1963, New York: Norton; *Stages of Faith: The Psychology of Human Development and the Quest for Meaning* by J. W. Fowler, 1981, New York: Harper & Row; *Human Development and Education* (3rd ed.) by R. J. Havighurst, 1972, New York: Longman; *The Meaning of Measurement of Moral Development* by L. Kohlberg, 1979, New York: Clark University; and *Will Our Children Have Faith?* by J. Westerhoff, 1976, New York: Seabury Press.

Table 2–2	Physical Status and Changes in the Young Adult Years	
Assessment	**Status During the 20s**	**Status During the 30s**
Skin	Smooth, even temperature	Wrinkles begin to appear
Hair	Slightly oily, shiny Balding may begin	Graying may begin Balding may begin
Vision	Snellen 20/20	Some loss of visual acuity and accommodation
Musculoskeletal	Strong, coordinated	Some loss of strength and muscle mass
Cardiovascular	Maximum cardiac output 60–90 beats/min Mean BP: 120/80	Slight decline in cardiac output 60–90 beats/min Mean BP: 120/80
Respiratory	Rate: 12–20 Full vital capacity	Rate: 12–20 Decline in vital capacity

application of a variety of developmental theories is important to the holistic care of the adult client when nurses perform assessments, implement care, and provide teaching for clients and families.

The Young Adult as Client

Physical Status
From age 18 to 25, the healthy *young adult* is at the peak of physical development. All body systems are functioning at maximum efficiency. Then, during the 30s, some normal physiologic changes begin to occur. A comparison of physical status for young adults during their 20s and 30s is shown in Table 2–2.

Risks for Alterations in Health
The young adult is at risk for alterations in health from accidents, sexually transmitted diseases, substance abuse, and physical or psychosocial stressors. These risk factors may be interrelated.

Accidents   Accidents are the leading cause of injury and death in people between ages 15 and 24 (Hales, 1994). Most injuries and fatalities occur as the result of motor vehicle accidents, but injuries and death also result from drowning, fire, use of firearms, occupational accidents, and exposure to environmental hazards. Accidental injury or death is often associated with the use of alcohol or other chemical substances, or with psychologic stress. Figure 2–1 is a self-assessment for risk factors for motor vehicle accidents.

Sexually Transmitted Diseases   Sexually transmitted diseases include genital herpes, chlamydia, gonorrhea, syphilis, and AIDS. The young adult who is sexually active with a variety of partners and who does not use condoms is at greatest risk for development of these diseases.

Substance Abuse   Substance abuse is a major cause for concern in the young adult population. Although alcohol abuse occurs at all ages, it is greater in the 20s than during any other decade of the life span (Freiberg, 1987). Alcohol contributes to motor vehicle accidents and physical violence, and it is damaging to the developing fetus in pregnant women. It can also cause liver disease and nutritional deficits.

Other substances that are commonly abused include nicotine, marijuana, amphetamines, cocaine, and crack. Smoking increases the risk of respiratory and cardiovascular diseases. Cocaine and crack can cause death from cardiovascular effects (increased heart rate and ventricular dysrhythmias), and can lead to addiction and health problems in the baby born to an addicted mother.

Physical and Psychosocial Stressors   The young adult is subjected to a wide variety of physical and psychosocial stressors. Physical stressors that increase the risk of illness include environmental pollutants and work-related risks (for example, electrical hazards, mechanical injuries, or exposure to toxins or infectious agents). Other physical stressors include exposure to the sun, ingestion of chemical substances (e.g., caffeine, alcohol, nicotine), and pregnancy.

Many different and individualized psychosocial stressors may affect the young adult. Choices must be made about education, occupation, relationships, independence, and life-style. The young adult without adequate education or job skills may face unemployment, poverty, homelessness, and limited access to health care. Divorces in the United States are increasing. Three out of every five marriages end in divorce, and this number is even higher among young adults (Edelman & Mandle, 1990). Divorce often results in loneliness, feelings of failure, financial difficulties, domestic violence, and child abuse. The inability of the young adult to cope with these stressors may re-

RISK FACTOR	⟶		INCREASING RISK	⟶	
Alcohol consumption*	Nondrinker	Occasionally small to moderate consumption	Frequently small to moderate consumption	Occasionally heavy consumption	Frequently heavy consumption
Mileage driven/yr*	Under 5000 miles/yr	5001–10,000 miles/yr		10,001–20,000 miles/yr	Over 20,000 miles/yr
Use of seat belt*	Always	Usually		Occasionally	Never
Use of shoulder harness*	Always	Usually		Occasionally	Never
Use of drugs or medication that decrease alertness*	No use	Occasional use		Moderate use	Frequent use

*Indicates risk factors that can be fully or partially controlled.

Figure 2–1 This component of a health appraisal estimates the risk for automobile accidents. A check mark is placed in the box that best describes current behavior.

sult in suicide, which ranks next to accidents as a major cause of death in this age group. Although difficult to prove, it is believed that some accidental deaths, especially when associated with substance abuse, are actually suicides.

Assessment Guidelines

The guidelines below are useful in assessing the achievement of significant developmental tasks in the young adult. Does the young adult:

- Feel independent from parents?
- Have a realistic self-concept?
- Like himself or herself and the direction in which life is going?
- Interact well with family?
- Cope with the stresses of constant change and growth?
- Have well-established bonds with significant others, such as marriage partners or close friends?
- Have a meaningful social life?
- Have a well-established career or occupation?
- Demonstrate emotional, social, and economic responsibility for own life?
- Have a set of values that guide behavior?
- Have a healthy life-style? (Kozier et al., 1995, p. 626)

Physical assessment of the young adult includes height and weight with related food-intake patterns, blood pressure, and vision. During the health history, specific questions should be asked about substance use, sexual concerns, exercise, menstrual history and patterns, coping mechanisms, and any familial chronic illnesses.

Promoting Healthy Behaviors in the Young Adult

The nurse promotes health in the young adult by teaching the behaviors listed in the box on page 30. Information about health for the young adult is primarily provided in community settings. Examples are

- Health-related courses and seminars at colleges and universities that include information on the use of sports and exercise facilities, alcohol and drug abuse, smoking cessation, mental health, and sexual health.
- Workplace programs that include blood pressure monitoring, exercise, smoking cessation, cafeteria nutrition guidelines, and stress-reduction activities.
- Community programs that include media information, health fairs, support groups, and information about risk factors for disease and injury.

The Middle Adult as Client

Physical Status

The *middle adult,* age 40 to 65, has physical status and function similar to that of adults in their 20s and 30s. However, many changes take place between ages 40 and 65. Table 2–3 lists the physical changes that normally occur in the middle years.

Risks for Alterations in Health

The middle adult is at risk for alterations in health from obesity, cardiovascular disease, cancer, substance abuse, and psychosocial stressors. These factors may be interrelated.

Obesity   The middle adult often has a problem maintaining a healthy weight. Weight gain in middle adult-

Healthy Behaviors in the Young Adult

■ ■ ■

- Choose foods from all food groups, and eat a variety of foods.
- Choose a diet low in fat (30% or less of total calories), saturated fat (less than 10% of calories), and cholesterol (less than 300 mg daily).
- Choose a diet that each day includes at least three servings of vegetables, two servings of fruits, and six servings of grains.
- Use sugar, salt, and sodium in moderation.
- For females, increase to or maintain 18 mg of iron daily in the diet.
- Make exercise a regular part of life, carrying out activities that increase the heart rate to a set target, and maintain that rate for 30–60 minutes three or four times a week.
- Include exercise as part of any weight-reduction program.

- Have regular physical examinations, including assessment for cancer of the thyroid, ovaries, lymph nodes, and skin (every 3 years).
- Have a vision examination every 2–4 years.
- Have an annual dental checkup.
- For females, have a baseline mammogram between age 35 and 39 and a breast examination every 3 years.
- For females, have Pap tests as recommended by a physician: annually until three or more consecutive normal results, and then at physician's discretion.
- For males, have testicular and prostate examinations every 5 years.
- Conduct breast or testicular self-examination monthly.

hood is usually the result of continuing to consume the same number of calories while decreasing physical activity and experiencing a decrease in basal metabolic rate. Obesity affects all the major organ systems of the body, increasing the risk of atherosclerosis, hypertension, elevated cholesterol and triglyceride levels, and diabetes. Obesity is also associated with heart disease, osteoarthritis, and gallbladder disease.

Cardiovascular Disease   The major cardiovascular risk factors, especially for coronary artery disease, include age, male gender, cigarette smoking, hypertension, elevated blood cholesterol levels, and diabetes. Other contributing factors include obesity, stress, and lack of exercise. The middle adult is at risk for disorders of peripheral vascular, cerebrovascular, and cardiovascular disease. A self-assessment of risk factors for cardiovascular disease is shown in Figure 2–2.

Cancer   Cancer is the third leading cause of death in adults between ages 25 and 64 in the United States, with one-third of cases occurring between ages 35 and 64. Cancers of the breast, colon, lung, and reproductive system are common in the middle years. The middle adult is at risk for cancer from environmental toxins as a result of increased length of exposure and is also at risk from alcohol and nicotine use.

Substance Abuse   Although the middle adult may abuse a variety of substances, the most commonly abused

are alcohol, nicotine, and prescription drugs. Excess alcohol use in the middle adult contributes to an increased risk of liver cancer, cirrhosis, pancreatitis, hyperlipidemia, and anemia. Alcoholism also increases the risk of accidental injury or death and disrupts careers and relationships. Cigarette smoking increases the risk of cancer of the larynx, lung, mouth, pharynx, bladder, pancreas, esophagus, and kidney; of chronic obstructive pulmonary disorders; and of cardiovascular disorders. The most commonly abused class of prescription drugs is tranquilizers.

Physical and Psychosocial Stressors   The middle adult years are ones of change and transition, frequently resulting in stress. Both men and women must adapt to changes in physical appearance and function and accept their own mortality. Children may leave home or, as is becoming more common, choose to remain at home. Parents are aging, with illness and death probable. The middle adult thus becomes what has been called "the sandwich generation," caught between the need to care for both children and aging parents. Both men and women may make career changes, and approaching retirement becomes a reality. Divorce in the middle years is a major emotional, social, and financial stressor.

Assessment Guidelines
The following guidelines are useful in assessing the achievement of significant developmental tasks in the middle adult. Does the middle adult:

Table 2–3	Physical Changes in the Middle Adult Years
Assessment	**Changes**
Skin	■ Decreased turgor, moisture, and subcutaneous fat result in wrinkles. ■ Fat is deposited in the abdominal and hip areas.
Hair	■ Loss of melanin in hair shaft causes graying. ■ Hairline recedes in males.
Sensory	■ Visual acuity for near vision decreases (presbyopia) during the 40s. ■ Auditory acuity for high-frequency sounds decreases (presbycusis); more common in men. ■ Sense of taste diminishes.
Musculoskeletal	■ Skeletal muscle mass decreases by about age 60. ■ Thinning of intervertebral discs results in loss of height (about 1 inch [2.5 cm]). ■ Postmenopausal women may have loss of calcium and develop osteoporosis.
Cardiovascular	■ Blood vessels lose elasticity. ■ Systolic blood pressure may increase.
Respiratory	■ Loss of vital capacity (about 1 L from age 20 to 60) occurs.
Gastrointestinal	■ Large intestine gradually loses muscle tone; constipation may result. ■ Gastric secretions are decreased.
Genitourinary	■ Hormonal changes occur: menopause, women (↓ estrogen); andropause, men (↓ testosterone).
Endocrine	■ Gradual decrease in glucose tolerance occurs.

■ Accept the aging body?

■ Feel comfortable with and respect himself or herself?

■ Enjoy some new freedom to be independent?

■ Accept changes in family roles?

■ Enjoy success and satisfaction from work and/or family roles?

■ Interact well and share companionable activities with a partner?

■ Expand or renew previous interests?

■ Pursue charitable and altruistic activities?

■ Consider plans for retirement?

■ Have a meaningful philosophy of life?

■ Follow preventive health care practices? (Kozier et al., 1995, p. 633)

Physical assessment of the middle adult includes all body systems, with careful measurement of blood pressure patterns, vision, and hearing. Monitoring for cancer symptoms is essential. During the health history, specific questions should be asked about food intake and exercise habits, substance abuse, sexual concerns, changes in the reproductive system, and coping mechanisms.

Promoting Healthy Behaviors in the Middle Adult

The nurse promotes health in the middle adult by teaching the behaviors listed in the box on page 33. Informa-tion about health for the middle adult may be provided in a variety of community settings, including outpatient clinics, occupational health clinics, and private practice. Examples are

■ Programs that emphasize accepting responsibility for one's own health. This type of teaching can be in a seminar or on a one-to-one basis, and includes information specific to a group of individuals with an identified need, such as smokers, women who have just entered the work force, or men nearing retirement.

■ Community and industry information about safety hazards in the home and workplace, as well as during leisure activities.

■ Literature about community resources available for health promotion, including programs offered at alcohol/drug abuse treatment centers, clinics and health centers, counseling services, crisis intervention centers, spouse abuse programs, and health education and promotion agencies (such as American Red Cross, American Cancer Society, American Heart Association, YWCA, YMCA).

The Older Adult as Client

Physical Status

The *older adult* period begins at age 65, but it can be further divided into three periods: the "young-old" (age 65 to 74), the "middle-old" (age 75 to 84), and the "old-old"

RISK FACTOR		⟶ INCREASING RISK ⟶					
Sex and age		Female under 40	Female 40–50	Male 25–40	Female after menopause	Male 40–60	Male 61 or over
Family history (mother, father, brothers, sisters)	High blood pressure	No relatives with condition		One relative		Two relatives	Three relatives
	Heart attack	No relatives with condition	One relative with condition after 60	Two relatives with condition after 60	One relative with condition before 60	Two relatives with condition before 60	
	Diabetes	No relatives with condition	One or more relatives with maturity onset diabetes		One or more relatives with preadolescent or adolescent onset		
Blood pressure*	Systolic	≤ 120	121–140	141–160	161–180	181–200	> 200
	Diastolic	≤ 70	71–80	81–90	91–100	101–110	> 110
Diabetes*		No diagnosis	Maturity onset, controlled	Maturity onset, uncontrolled	Adolescent onset, controlled	Adolescent onset, uncontrolled	
Weight*		At or slightly below recommended weight	10% overweight	20% overweight	30% overweight	40% overweight	50% overweight
Cholesterol*† level (mg/100 mL)		< 180	181–200	201–220	221–240	241–260	261–280	> 280
Serum triglycerides* (mg/100 mL) fasting		≤ 150		151–400		401–1000	> 1000
Percent of fat in diet*		20–30%		31–40%		41–50%	> 50%
Frequency of exercise*	Recreational	Intensive recreational exertion (35–45 min at least 4 times/wk)		Moderate recreational exertion		Minimal recreational exertion	No recreational exertion
	Occupational	Intensive occupational exertion		Moderate occupational exertion		Minimal occupational exertion	Sedentary occupation
Sleep patterns*		7 or 8 hr sleep/night		> 8 hr sleep/night		4–6 hr sleep/night	
Cigarette smoking*	No./day	Nonsmoker	1–10/day	11–20/day	21–30/day	31–40/day	Over 40/day
	No. of yr smoked	Nonsmoker	< 10 yr	11–15 yr	16–20 yr	21–30 yr	≥ 31 yr
Stress*	Domestic	Minimal		Moderate		High	Very high
	Occupational	Minimal		Moderate		High	Very high
Behavior pattern* (particularly males)		**Type B:** Relaxed, appropriately assertive, not time-dependent, moderate to slow speech			**Type A:** Excessively competitive, aggressive, striving, hyperalert, time-dependent, loud, explosive speech		
Air pollution*		Low		Moderate		High	
Use of oral contraceptives* (females)		Do not use oral contraceptives		Under 40 and use oral contraceptives		Over 40 and use oral contraceptives	

* Indicates risk factors that can be fully or partially controlled.
† Serum lipid analysis is also recommended to determine low-density (beta) and high-density (alpha) lipoprotein levels. Evidence suggests that high-density lipoprotein (HDL) carries cholesterol from tissues for metabolism and excretion. An inverse correlation appears to exist between HDL and coronary artery disease.

Figure 2–2   This component of a health appraisal estimates the risk for cardiovascular disease. A check mark is placed in the box that best describes current behavior or situations.

Healthy Behaviors in the Middle Adult

■ ■ ■

- Choose foods from all food groups, and eat a variety of foods.

- Choose a diet low in fat (30% or less of total calories), saturated fat (less than 10% of calories), and cholesterol (less than 300 mg daily). Adjust daily calorie intake to maintain healthy weight.

- Choose a diet that each day includes at least three servings of vegetables, two servings of fruits, and six servings of grains.

- Use sugar, salt, and sodium in moderation.

- Increase calcium intake (in perimenopausal women) to 800 mg daily.

- Consume high-fiber foods.

- Make exercise a part of life, carrying out regular exercise that is moderately strenuous, is consistent, and avoids overexertion; exercise for 30 minutes at least three times a week.

- Include exercise as part of any weight-reduction program.

- Have an annual vision examination.

- Have an annual dental checkup.

- Have a physical examination annually, including assessment for cancer of the thyroid, testes, prostate, mouth, ovaries, skin, colon, and lymph nodes.

- For females, have a mammogram every 1–2 years from age 40 to 49, and annually from age 50 on. Have a breast examination annually.

- For females, have a Pap test as recommended for the young adult (see box on page 30).

- Have a digital rectal examination and stool blood test annually. After age 50, have a proctoscopic examination every 3–5 years after normal results are obtained from two consecutive annual examinations.

- For males, have testicular and prostate examinations annually.

- Conduct breast or testicular self-examination every month. (The perimenopausal woman should set a specific date each month for the exam, as menstrual periods may be irregular or absent.)

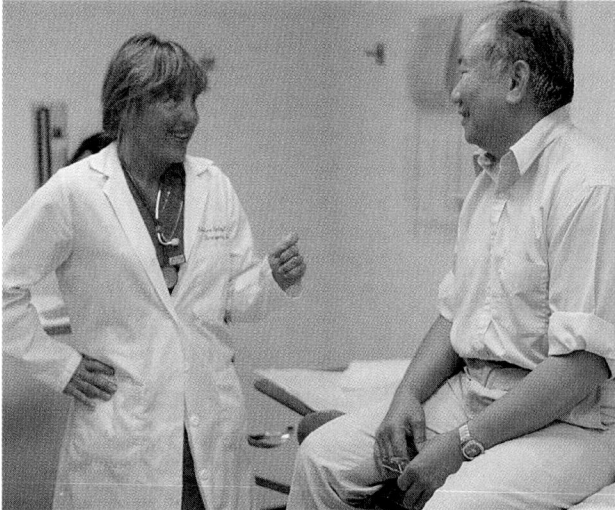

Figure 2–3   The older adult population is increasing more rapidly than any other age group, making gerontologic nursing an integral component of medical-surgical nursing practice.

(age 85 and over). With increasing age, a number of normal physiologic changes occur, as listed in Table 2–4.

The older adult population is increasing more rapidly than any other age group. Within this century, the number of adults in the United States living to age 65 or older has increased from 4% in 1900 to 12% (28 million) in 1984. That percentage is projected to be slightly more than 18% (66 million) by the year 2030, with the largest increase occurring in adults over the age of 75. Currently, the life expectancy in North America is 71.5 years for males and 78.3 years for females (AARP, 1990; US Bureau of the Census, 1987, 1989).

The increase in numbers of older adults has important implications for nursing. Clients needing health care in all settings will be older, requiring nursing interventions and teaching specifically designed to meet needs that differ from those of young and middle adults. Although *gerontologic nursing* (care of the older adult) is a nursing specialty area, it is also an integral component of medical-surgical nursing (Figure 2–3).

Risks for Alterations in Health

The older adult is at risk for alterations in health from a variety of causes. Approximately 90% of all older adults have at least one chronic illness (Eliopoulos, 1987). The most frequently occurring conditions in the older adult are arthritis, hypertension, hearing impairments, heart disease, cataracts, sinusitis, orthopedic disorders, visual impairments, and diabetes (AARP, 1990). The leading causes of death in this population are heart disease, cancer, and stroke.

Like the middle adult, the older adult is at risk for alterations in health from obesity, cardiovascular disease,

Table 2–4	Physical Changes in the Older Adult Years

Assessment	Changes
Skin	▪ Decreased turgor and sebaceous gland activity result in dry, wrinkled skin. Melanocytes cluster, causing "age spots" or "liver spots."
Hair and Nails	▪ Scalp, axillary, and pubic hair thins; nose and ear hair thickens. Women may develop facial hair. ▪ Nails grow more slowly; may become thick and brittle.
Sensory	▪ Visual field narrows, and depth perception is distorted. ▪ Pupils are smaller, reducing night vision. ▪ Lenses yellow and become opaque, resulting in distortion of green, blue, and violet tones and increased sensitivity to glare. ▪ Production of tears decreases. ▪ Sense of smell decreases. ▪ Age-related hearing loss progresses, involving middle- and low-frequency sounds. ▪ Threshold for pain and touch increases. ▪ Alterations in proprioception (sense of physical position) may occur.
Musculoskeletal	▪ Loss of overall mass, strength, and movement of muscles occurs; tremors may occur. ▪ Loss of bone structure and deterioration of cartilage in joints result in increased risk of fractures and in limitation of range of motion.
Cardiovascular	▪ Systolic blood pressure rises. ▪ Cardiac output decreases. ▪ Peripheral resistance increases, and capillary walls thicken.
Respiratory	▪ Continued loss of vital capacity occurs as the lungs become less elastic and more rigid. ▪ Anteroposterior chest diameter increases; kyphosis. ▪ Although blood carbon dioxide levels remain relatively constant, blood oxygen levels decrease by 10% to 15%.
Gastrointestinal	▪ Production of saliva decreases, and decreased number of taste buds decrease accurate receptors for salt and sweet. ▪ Gag reflex is decreased, and stomach motility and emptying are reduced. ▪ Both large and small intestines have some atrophy, with decreased peristalsis. ▪ The liver decreases in weight and storage capacity; gallstones increase; pancreatic enzymes decrease.
Genitourinary	▪ Kidneys lose mass, and the glomerular filtration rate is reduced (by nearly 50% from young adulthood to old age). ▪ Bladder capacity decreases, and the micturition reflex is delayed. Urinary retention is more common. ▪ Women may have stress incontinence; men may have an enlarged prostate gland. ▪ Reproductive changes in men occur: — Testosterone decreases. — Sperm count decreases. — Testes become smaller. — Length of time to achieve an erection increases; erection is less full. ▪ Reproductive changes in women occur: — Estrogen levels decrease. — Breast tissue decreases. — Vagina, uterus, ovaries, and urethra atrophy. — Vaginal lubrication decreases. — Vaginal secretions become alkaline.
Endocrine	▪ Pituitary gland loses weight and vascularity. ▪ Thyroid gland becomes more fibrous, and plasma T_3 decreases. ▪ Pancreas releases insulin more slowly; increased blood glucose levels are common. ▪ Adrenal glands produce less cortisol.

and cancer. Other risk factors specific to this age group include injuries and pharmacologic therapy.

Injuries Injuries in the older adult cause many different problems: illness, financial burden, hospitalization, self-care deficits, loss of independence, and even death. The risk of injury is increased by normal physiologic changes that accompany aging, pathophysiologic alterations in health, environmental hazards, and lack of support systems. The three major causes of injury in the older adult are falls, fires, and motor vehicle accidents. Of these causes, falls with resultant hip fractures are the most significant in terms of long-term disability and death.

Pharmacologic Therapy The average older adult in the community has 11 prescriptions filled each year; although older adults constitute 12% of the total population, they consume 32% of all prescriptions (Eliopoulos, 1990). While these medications do make life more comfortable for the older adult, they are a risk factor because of adverse drug reactions and interactions. Other factors contributing to drug therapy problems in this age group include decreased metabolism, nutritional problems, visual deficits, memory changes, cost, and noncompliance.

Physical and Psychosocial Stressors The older adult is at risk for alterations in health from many physical and psychosocial stressors. The older adult is exposed to the same environmental hazards as the young and middle adult, but the accumulation of years of exposure may now appear. For example, exposure to the sun in earlier years may be manifested by skin cancer, and the long-term effects of exposure to noise pollution can result in impaired hearing. The older adult (especially the older male) is at increased risk for respiratory disorders as a result of years of smoking, or from air pollution from such pollutants as coal or asbestos dust. Living conditions and economic constraints may prevent the older adult from having necessary heating and cooling, contributing to thermal-related illness and even death. Elder abuse and neglect further increase the risk of injury or illness (Edelman & Mandle, 1990).

Psychosocial stressors for the older adult include the illness or death of a spouse, decreased or limited income, retirement, isolation from friends and family because of lack of transportation or distance, return to the home of a child, or relocation to a long-term health care facility. A further stressor may be role loss or reversal—for example, when the wife becomes the caretaker of her chronically ill husband. Figure 2–4 is a self-assessment tool for signs of stress.

Assessment Guidelines

The following guidelines are useful in assessing the achievement of significant developmental tasks in the older adult. Does the older adult:

Mood and Disposition Signs

_____ I become overexcited.

_____ I worry.

_____ I feel insecure.

_____ I have difficulty sleeping at night.

_____ I become easily confused and forgetful.

_____ I become very uncomfortable and ill-at-ease.

_____ I become nervous.

Musculoskeletal Signs

_____ My fingers and hands shake.

_____ I can't sit or stand still.

_____ I develop twitches.

_____ My head begins to ache.

_____ I feel my muscles become tense or stiff.

_____ I stutter or stammer when I speak.

_____ My neck becomes stiff.

Visceral Signs

_____ My stomach becomes upset.

_____ I feel my heart pounding.

_____ I sweat profusely.

_____ My hands become moist.

_____ I feel light-headed or faint.

_____ I experience cold chills.

_____ My face becomes "hot."

_____ My mouth becomes dry.

_____ I experience ringing in my ears.

_____ I get a sinking feeling in my stomach.

Figure 2–4 A checklist such as this one identifies responses to stress. The client is able to assess his or her stress level by tallying the number of checkmarks.

- Adjust to the physiologic changes related to aging?
- Manage retirement years in a satisfying manner?
- Have satisfactory living arrangements and income to meet changing needs?
- Participate in social and leisure activities?
- Have a social network of friends and support persons?
- View life as worthwhile?
- Have high self-esteem?

Healthy Behaviors in the Older Adult

■ ■ ■

- Choose foods from all food groups, and eat a variety of foods. Include some high-quality protein at each meal, such as low-fat milk and cheese, peanut butter, meat, fish, or poultry.

- Choose a diet low in fat (30% or less of total calories), saturated fat (less than 10% of calories), and cholesterol (less than 300 mg daily). Adjust daily caloric intake to balance energy expenditure, and maintain healthy weight. A daily caloric intake of 1200 kcal is recommended, but it may vary according to body build and activity level.

- Choose a diet that each day includes at least three servings of vegetables, two servings of fruits, and six servings of grains. Increased amounts of high-fiber foods may be necessary; if so, fluid intake should also be increased.

- Use sugar, salt, and sodium in moderation.

- Increase calcium intake to at least 800 mg per day (1000–1500 mg per day may be recommended).

- Make exercise a part of life, following a regular program of moderate exercise, such as walking or swimming. Avoid overexertion.

- Have an annual vision examination.

- Have an annual dental checkup.

- Have an annual physical examination that includes urinalysis and assessment for cancer of the thyroid, testes, prostate, mouth, ovaries, skin, colon, and lymph nodes.

- For females, have a breast examination and a mammogram annually.

- For females, have Pap tests as recommended by physician.

- For males, have an annual testicular and prostate examination.

- Have a digital rectal examination and stool blood test annually. Have a proctoscopic examination as recommended for the middle adult (see box on page 33).

- Conduct breast or testicular self-examination every month.

- Maintain immunizations for diphtheria and tetanus by having boosters every 10 years.

- Obtain annual immunizations against pneumococcal pneumonia and influenza, especially with a history of chronic cardiovascular or respiratory illness.

- Practice the following to avoid injury:
  a. Have adequate lighting in all rooms of the house including stairs, basements, and bedrooms.
  b. Avoid sitting or standing rapidly; if dizziness occurs, remain in one position until dizziness is gone.
  c. Have handrails installed by the toilet and in the shower or bathtub.
  d. Do not use throw rugs.
  e. Install smoke alarms.
  f. Never step into a tub or shower without checking the temperature of the water.
  g. Always wear corrective lenses and/or hearing aids when driving.
  h. Do not drive a car after taking medications that cause drowsiness or dizziness.

- Have the abilities to care for self or to secure appropriate help?
- Gain support from a value system or spiritual philosophy?
- Adapt life-style to diminishing energy and ability?
- Accept and adjust to the death of significant others? (Kozier et al., 1995, p. 651)

Physical assessment of the older adult includes a careful examination of all body systems. During the health history, specific questions should be asked about usual dietary patterns; elimination; exercise and rest; use of alcohol, nicotine, over-the-counter medications, and prescription drugs; sexual concerns; financial concerns; and support systems.

Promoting Healthy Behaviors in the Older Adult

The nurse promotes health in the older adult by teaching the behaviors listed in the accompanying box. Older adults get the same benefits from health teaching that young adults and middle adults do; they should never be viewed as being "too old" for healthy living practices. Nurses should, however, structure teaching activities to meet age-related physiologic changes, such as using charts and literature with large print. Health education for the older adult is provided in hospitals, long-term care facilities, retirement centers, outpatient clinics, senior citizen centers, and other community settings. Examples are

- Educational seminars about accident prevention in the home, in automobiles, and when taking public transportation.

- Health screenings and information in health fairs specifically for the older adult.

- Community programs that provide immunization for influenza.

- Literature about financial assistance for health care, crisis hot lines, community services and resources (as described earlier for the middle adult) transportation, and nutrition (such as Meals-on-Wheels).

The Family of the Adult Client

■ ■ ■

Although some clients are totally alone in the world, most have one or more people who are significant in their lives. These significant others may be related or bonded to the client by birth, by adoption, by marriage, or by friendship. Although not always meeting traditional definitions, people (or even pets) significant to the client are the client's family. The nurse includes the family as an integral component of care in all health care settings. This section discusses definitions and functions of the family, family developmental tasks, and family-specific risk factors with related health problems.

Definitions and Functions of the Family

What is a **family**? The definitions of a family are changing as society changes. According to one definition, a family is a unit of people related by marriage, birth, or adoption (Duvall, 1977). An expanded definition states that "a family is composed of two or more people who are emotionally involved with each other and live in close geographical proximity" (Friedman, 1981, p. 8). In a global society, it may not be possible for family members to live in close proximity, but they do remain emotionally involved.

Although every family is unique, all families have certain structural and functional features in common. **Family structure** (family roles and relationships) and **family function** (interactions among family members and with the community) provide the following:

- *Interdependence.* The behaviors and level of development of individual family members constantly influence and are influenced by the behaviors and level of development of all other members of the family.

- *Maintenance of boundaries.* The family creates boundaries that guide its members, providing a distinct and unique family culture. This culture, in turn, provides values.

- *Adaptation to change.* The family changes as new members are added, current members leave, and the development of each member progresses.

- *Performance of family tasks.* Essential tasks maintain the stability and continuity of the family. These tasks include physical maintenance of the home and the people in the home, the production and socialization of family members, and the maintenance of the psychologic well-being of members.

The family carries out the tasks that are necessary for its survival and continuity (Duvall, 1977):

- Providing shelter, food, clothing, and health care

- Allocating money, time, and space according to each member's needs

- Determining the roles and responsibilities of each member for the support, management, and care of the home and other family members

- Ensuring the socialization of members through the internalization of increasingly mature roles in the family and in society

- Establishing socially acceptable ways to interact with others through communication and the expression of feelings in areas such as love, anger, and sexuality

- Rearing and releasing children appropriately

- Relating to the community (neighborhood, school, church, work) and establishing rules for relatives, guests, and friends

- Maintaining morale and motivation, rewarding achievement, dealing with personal and family crises, setting attainable goals, and developing family loyalties and values

Family Developmental Stages and Tasks

The family, just like the individual, has developmental stages and tasks. Each stage brings change, requiring adaptation; each new stage also brings family-related risk factors for alterations in health. The nurse must consider both the needs of the client at a specific developmental stage and the needs of the client within a family with specific developmental tasks. Family developmental stages and developmental tasks are described below; related risk factors and health problems for each stage are listed in Table 2–5.

Couple
Two people, living together with or without being married, are in a period of establishing themselves as a couple. The developmental tasks of the couple include adjusting to living together as a couple, establishing a mutually satisfying relationship, relating to kin, and deciding whether or not to have children.

Family with Infants and Preschoolers
The family with infants or preschoolers must adjust to having and supporting the needs of more than two members. Other developmental tasks of the family at this stage

Table 2–5   Family-Related Risk Factors for Alterations in Health

Stage	Risk Factors	Health Problems
Couple, or Family with Infants and Preschoolers	■ Lack of knowledge about family planning, contraception, sexual and marital roles ■ Inadequate prenatal care ■ Altered nutrition: inadequate nutrition, overweight, underweight ■ Smoking, alcohol/drug abuse ■ First pregnancy before age 16 or after age 35 ■ Low socioeconomic status ■ Lack of knowledge about child health and safety ■ Rubella, syphilis, gonorrhea, AIDS	Premature pregnancy Low-birth-weight infant Birth defects Injury to infant or child Accidents
Family with School-Age Children	■ Unsafe home environment ■ Working parents with inappropriate or inadequate resources for child care ■ Low socioeconomic status ■ Child abuse or neglect ■ Multiple, closely spaced children ■ Repeated infections, accidents, and hospitalizations ■ Unrecognized and unattended health problems ■ Poor or inappropriate nutrition ■ Toxic substances in the home ■ Immature, dependent parents ■ Generational pattern of using social agencies as a way of life	Behavior problems Speech and vision problems Learning disabilities Communicable diseases Physical abuse Cancer Developmental delay Obesity, underweight
Family with Adolescents and Young Adults	■ Family values of aggressiveness and competition ■ Racial and ethnic family origin ■ Socioeconomic factors contributing to peer relationships ■ Life-style and behavior leading to chronic illness (substance abuse, inadequate diet) ■ Lack of problem-solving skills ■ Conflicts between parent and children	Violent death and injury Alcohol/drug abuse Unwanted pregnancy Suicide Sexually transmitted diseases
Family with Middle Adults	■ High-cholesterol diet ■ Overweight ■ Hypertension ■ Smoking, alcohol abuse ■ Physical inactivity ■ Genetic predisposition, heredity ■ Personality patterns related to stress ■ Habits: low-fiber and high-cholesterol diet; charcoal grilling ■ Exposure to environment: sunlight, radiation, asbestos, water or air pollution ■ Depression ■ Gingivitis	Cardiovascular disease (coronary artery disease and cerebral vascular disease) Cancer Accidents Suicide Mental illness Periodontal disease, loss of teeth
Family with Older Adults	■ Age ■ Depression ■ Drug interactions ■ Metabolic and endocrine disorders ■ Chronic illness ■ Death of spouse ■ Reduced income ■ Poor nutrition ■ Lack of exercise ■ Past environment and life-style	Impaired vision and hearing Hypertension Acute illness Chronic illness Infectious diseases (influenza, pneumonia) Injuries from burns and falls Depression

Note. Adapted from *Healthy People: The Surgeon General's Report on Health Promotion and Disease Prevention,* Health and Human Services Pub. No. 79-55071, 1992, Washington, DC: US Government Printing Office, and *Healthy People 2000: National Health Promotion and Disease Prevention Objectives (Summary),* American Public Health Association, 1990, Washington, DC: US Government Printing Office.

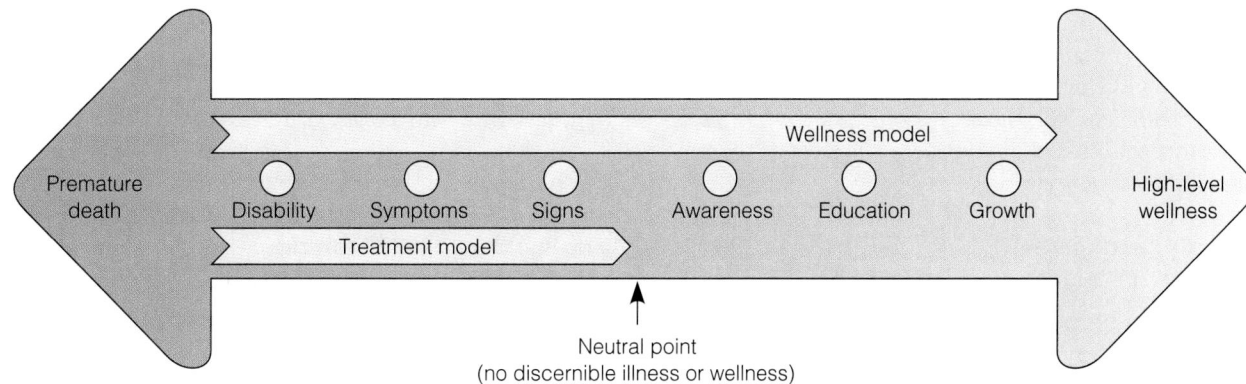

Figure 2–5 The health-illness continuum.

are developing an attachment between parents and children, adjusting to the economic costs of having more members, coping with energy depletion and lack of privacy, and carrying out activities that enhance growth and development of the children.

Family with School-Age Children
The family with school-age children has the developmental tasks of adjusting to the expanded world of children in school and encouraging educational achievement. A further task is promoting joint decision making between children and parents.

Family with Adolescents and Young Adults
The developmental tasks of the family with adolescents and young adults focus on transition. While providing a supportive home base and maintaining open communications, parents must balance freedom with responsibility and release adult children as they seek independence.

Family with Middle Adults
The family with middle adults (in which the parents are middle-aged and children are no longer at home) has the developmental tasks of maintaining ties with older and younger generations and planning for retirement. If the family consists of just the middle-aged couple, they have the developmental task of reestablishing the relationship and (if necessary) acquiring the role of grandparents.

Family with Older Adults
The older adult family has the developmental tasks of adjusting to retirement, adjusting to aging, and coping with the loss of a spouse. If a spouse dies, further tasks include adjusting to living alone or closing the family home.

Health and Illness in the Adult Client

■ ■ ■

This section provides an overview of health and illness. Definitions of health and factors affecting health in the adult are given. The discussion of illness includes causes of disease, acute and chronic alterations in health, and rehabilitation from illness in the adult client.

Health

The World Health Organization (WHO) defines **health** as "a state of complete physical, mental, and social well-being, and not merely the absence of disease or infirmity" (WHO, 1974, p. 1). This definition, formulated more than 20 years ago, is still used as the classic descriptor of a state of health. Even so, it does not take into account the many different levels of health a person may experience, or that a person may be clinically described as ill and still define himself or herself as well. These additional factors, which greatly influence nursing care, include the health-illness continuum and high-level wellness.

The Health-Illness Continuum and High-Level Wellness
The **health-illness continuum** represents health as a dynamic process, with high-level wellness at one extreme of the continuum and death at the opposite extreme (Figure 2–5). Individuals place themselves at different locations on the continuum at specific points in time.

The concept of a continuum of health and illness was expanded by Dunn (1959) in his description of *high-level wellness*. Dunn conceptualized **wellness** as an active process influenced by the environment. He differentiated good health from wellness:

> Good health can exist as a relatively passive state of freedom from illness in which the individual is at peace with his environment. . . . Wellness is an integrated method of functioning which is oriented toward maximizing the potential of which the individual is capable, within the environment where he is functioning. (1959, p. 4)

A variety of factors influence wellness, including self-concept, environment, culture, and spiritual values. Providing care based on a framework of wellness facilitates active involvement by both the nurse and the client in promoting, maintaining, or restoring health. It also supports the philosophy of holistic health care, in which all aspects of a person (physical, psychosocial, cultural, spiritual, and intellectual) are considered as essential components of individualized care.

Factors Affecting Health

Many different factors affect a person's health or level of wellness. These factors often interact to promote health or to become risk factors for alterations in health. The factors affecting health are described below.

Genetic Makeup   Each person has a genetic makeup that influences health status throughout life. Genetic makeup affects personality, temperament, body structure, intellectual potential, and susceptibility to the development of hereditary alterations in health. Examples of chronic illnesses that are associated with genetic makeup include sickle-cell disease, hemophilia, diabetes mellitus, and cancer.

Cognitive Abilities and Educational Level   Although cognitive abilities are determined prior to adulthood, the level of cognitive development affects whether people view themselves as healthy or ill; cognitive levels also may affect health practices. Cognitive abilities may be altered by injuries to and illnesses affecting the brain. Educational level affects the ability to understand and follow guidelines for health. For example, if an individual is functionally illiterate, written information about healthy behaviors and health resources is worthless.

Race, Ethnicity, and Cultural Background   Certain diseases occur at a higher rate of incidence in some races and ethnic groups than in others. For example, in the United States, hypertension is more common in African Americans, tuberculosis and diabetes mellitus are among the leading causes of illness in Native Americans, and eye disorders are more prevalent in Chinese Americans.

The ethnic and cultural background of an individual also influences health values and behaviors, life-style, and illness behaviors. Every culture defines health and illness in a way that is unique; in addition, each culture has its own health beliefs and illness treatment practices.

Age, Gender, and Developmental Level   Age, gender, and developmental level are factors in health and illness. Cardiovascular disorders are uncommon in young adults, but the incidence increases after the age of 40. Myocardial infarctions are more common in men than women until women are past menopause. Some diseases occur only in one gender or the other, for example, prostate cancer in men and cervical cancer in women. The older adult has increased incidence of chronic illness and increased potential for serious illness or death from infectious illnesses (such as influenza and pneumonia).

Life-Style and Environment   The components of a person's life-style that affect health status include patterns of eating, use of chemical substances (alcohol, nicotine, caffeine, legal and illegal drugs), exercise and rest patterns, and coping methods. Examples of altered responses are the relationship of obesity to hypertension, cigarette smoking to chronic obstructive pulmonary disease, a sedentary life-style to heart disease, and a high-stress career to alcoholism.

The environment has a major influence on health. Occupational exposure to toxic substances (such as asbestos and coal dust) increases the risk of pulmonary disorders. Air, water, and food pollution increases the risk of respiratory disorders, infectious diseases, and cancer. Environmental temperature variations can result in hypothermia or hyperthermia, especially in the older adult.

Socioeconomic Background   Both life-style and environmental influences are affected by one's income level. The culture of poverty, which crosses all racial and ethnic boundaries, negatively influences health status. Living at or below the poverty level often results in crowded, unsanitary living conditions or homelessness. Housing is often overcrowded, lacks adequate heating or cooling, and is infested with insects and rats. Crowded living conditions increase the risk of transferring communicable diseases. Other problems include lack of infant and child care, lack of medical care for injuries or illness, inadequate nutrition, use of addictive substances, and violence.

Geographic Area   The geographic area in which one lives influences health status. Such illnesses as malaria are more common in tropical areas of North America, whereas multiple sclerosis occurs with greater frequency in the northern United States and Canada. Other geographic influences are seen in the number of skin cancers in people living in sunny, hot areas and sinus infections in people living in areas of high humidity.

Health Promotion and Maintenance

For many years, the emphasis in nursing was on care of the acutely ill client in the hospital setting. With changes in society and in health care, this emphasis is shifting toward preventive, community-based care. Although the focus of this book is not community health nursing, the importance of teaching health maintenance and providing continuity of care as a client moves among health care settings is an essential component of medical-surgical nursing. This section lists healthy living practices, summarizes a national agenda to promote health, and introduces the concept of illness prevention.

Healthy Living   Certain practices are known to promote health and wellness:

- Eating three balanced meals a day and including foods according to the Food Guide Pyramid (Figure 2–6)

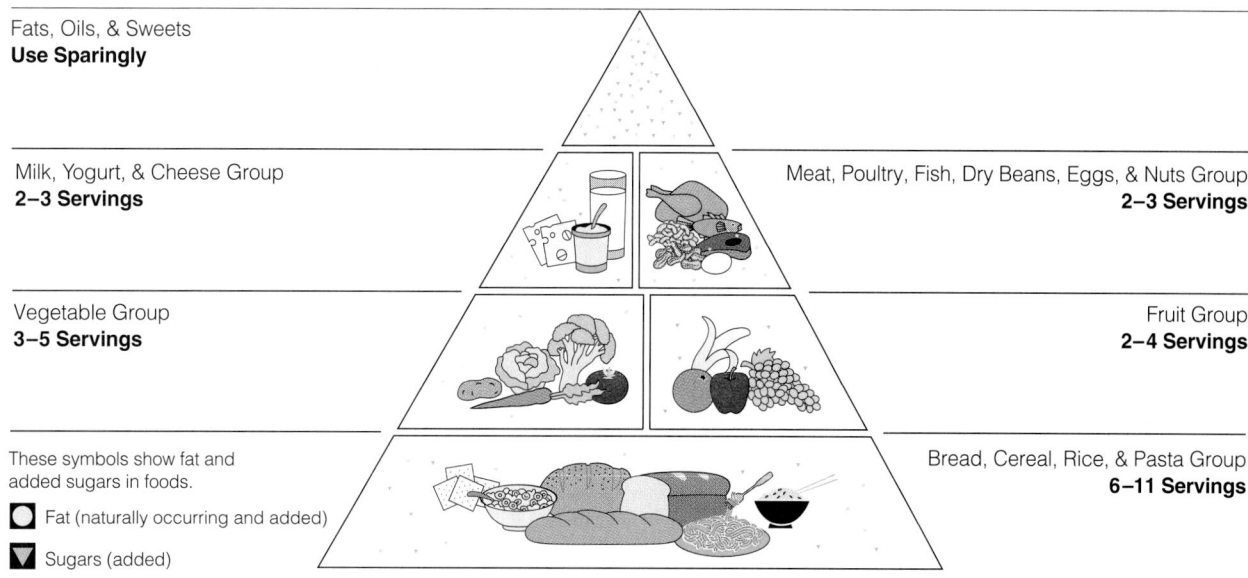

Fats, Oils, & Sweets
Use Sparingly

Milk, Yogurt, & Cheese Group
2–3 Servings

Meat, Poultry, Fish, Dry Beans, Eggs, & Nuts Group
2–3 Servings

Vegetable Group
3–5 Servings

Fruit Group
2–4 Servings

These symbols show fat and
added sugars in foods.

○ Fat (naturally occurring and added)

▽ Sugars (added)

Bread, Cereal, Rice, & Pasta Group
6–11 Servings

Figure 2–6   The food guide pyramid is designed to be used as a guide when buying foods and preparing meals. The recommended servings provide 1600–1800 kcal/day.

- Eating moderately to maintain a healthy weight
- Exercising moderately, following a regular routine
- Sleeping 7–8 hours each day
- Limiting alcohol consumption to a moderate amount
- Eliminating smoking
- Keeping sun exposure to a minimum

The nurse promotes health by teaching the activities that maintain wellness, by providing information about the characteristics and consequences of diseases when risk factors have been identified, and by supplying specific information about decreasing risk factors (Pender, 1987). (Examples of health-promotion behaviors for adults at various developmental levels were discussed earlier in the chapter.) The nurse also promotes health by following healthy practices and serving as a role model.

National Health Promotion   The US Department of Health and Human Services (1990) published national health objectives for the year 2000. A selected list of recommendations is included in the box on page 42.

Illness Prevention

Activities to prevent illness include any measures that limit the progression of an illness at any point of its course. (Illness is discussed in detail later in the chapter.) Three levels of illness prevention have been defined (Leavell & Clark, 1965). Each level of prevention occurs at a distinct point in the development of a disease process and requires specific nursing interventions (Edelman & Mandle, 1990). The levels are as follows:

1. *Primary level of prevention.* The primary level includes generalized health-promotion activities as well as specific actions that prevent or delay the occurrence of a disease. Below are examples of primary prevention activities:
   a. Protecting oneself against environmental risks, such as air and water pollution
   b. Eating nutritious foods
   c. Protecting oneself against industrial hazards
   d. Obeying seat-belt laws
   e. Obtaining sex counseling
   f. Obtaining immunizations
   g. Undergoing genetic screenings
   h. Eliminating the use of alcohol and cigarettes

2. *Secondary level of prevention.* Activities at this level emphasize early diagnosis and treatment of an illness that is already present to stop the pathologic process and enable the person to return to his or her former state of health as soon as possible. Below are examples of secondary prevention activities:
   a. Undergoing screenings for diseases such as hypertension, diabetes mellitus, and glaucoma
   b. Obtaining physical examinations and diagnostic tests for cancer
   c. Performing self-examination for breast and/or testicular cancer
   d. Obtaining tuberculosis skin tests
   e. Obtaining specific treatment of illness (for example, the treatment of streptococcal infections of the throat will prevent secondary infections involving the heart and/or kidneys)

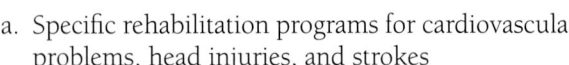

Examples of National Health Promotion and Disease Prevention Objectives

■ ■ ■

- Increase to at least 20% the proportion of people age 18 and older who engage in physical activity that promotes the development and maintenance of cardiopulmonary fitness three or more days per week for 20 minutes or more per occasion.

- Reduce overweight to no more than 20% among people age 20 and older.

- Reduce dietary fat intake to an average of 30% or less of calories and average saturated fat intake to less than 10% of calories.

- Increase to at least 85% the proportion of people age 18 and older who use food labels to make nutritious food selections.

- Reduce deaths caused by alcohol-related motor vehicle crashes to no more than 8.5 per 100,000 people.

- Reduce cigarette smoking to a prevalence of no more than 15% among people age 20 and older.

- Increase years of healthy life to at least 65 years.

- Increase to at least 90% the proportion of people age 65 and older who had the opportunity to participate the preceding year in at least one organized health promotion program through a senior center, life-care facility, or other community-based setting that serves older adults.

- Reduce physical abuse directed at women by male partners to no more than 27 per 1000 couples.

- Increase to at least 90% the proportion of adults who have had their blood pressure measured within the preceding 2 years and can state whether their blood pressure is normal or high.

Note: From *Healthy People 2000* by US Department of Health and Human Services, 1990, Washington, DC: US Department of Health and Human Services.

---

a. Specific rehabilitation programs for cardiovascular problems, head injuries, and strokes
b. Work training programs following illness or injury
c. Educating the public to employ rehabilitated people to the fullest possible extent

Disease and Illness

Disease and *illness* are terms that are often used interchangeably, but in fact they have different meanings. In general, nursing is concerned with illness, while medicine is concerned with disease.

Disease

Disease (literally meaning "without ease") is a medical term describing alterations in structure and function of the body or mind. Diseases may have mechanical causes, biologic causes, or normative causes. Mechanical causes of disease result in damage to the structure of the body and are the result of trauma or extremes of temperature. Biologic causes of disease affect body function and are the result of genetic defects, the effects of aging, infestation and infection, alterations in the immune system, and alterations in normal organ secretions. Normative causes are psychologic but involve a mind-body interaction, so that physical manifestations occur in response to the psychologic disturbance.

The cause of many diseases is still unknown. The following are generally accepted as common causes of disease:

- Genetic defects
- Developmental defects resulting from exposure to viruses, chemicals, or drugs that affect the developing fetus
- Biologic agents or toxins (including viruses, bacteria, rickettsia, fungi, protozoa, and helminths)
- Physical agents, such as temperature extremes, radiation, and electricity
- Chemical agents, such as alcohol, drugs, strong acids or bases, and heavy metals
- Generalized response of tissues to injury or irritation
- Alterations in the production of antibodies, resulting in allergies or hypersensitivities
- Faulty metabolic processes (for example, a production of hormones or enzymes above or below normal)
- Continued, unabated stress

Diseases may be classified as acute or chronic, communicable, congenital, degenerative, functional, malignant, psychosomatic, idiopathic, or iatrogenic. These classifications are defined in Table 2–6. In all types of disease, alterations in structure or function cause signs and symptoms that prompt a person to seek treatment from a

3. *Tertiary level of prevention.* The tertiary level focuses on stopping the disease process and returning the affected individual to a useful place in society within the constraints of any disability. The activities primarily revolve around rehabilitation. Below are examples of tertiary prevention measures:

Table 2–6   Disease Classification Definitions

Classification	Definition
Acute	A disease that has a rapid onset, lasts a relatively short period of time, and is self-limiting
Chronic	A disease that has one or more of these characteristics: (1) is permanent, (2) leaves permanent disability, (3) causes nonreversible pathophysiology, (4) requires special training of the client for rehabilitation, (5) requires a long period of care
Communicable	A disease that can spread from one person to another
Congenital	A disease or disorder that exists at or before birth
Degenerative	A disease that results from deterioration or impairment of organs or tissues
Functional	A disease that affects function or performance but does not have manifestations of organic illness
Malignant	A disease that tends to become worse and cause death
Psychosomatic	A psychologic disease that is manifested by physiologic symptoms
Idiopathic	A disease that has an unknown cause
Iatrogenic	A disease that is caused by medical therapy

physician or traditional healer. Although both subjective symptoms and objective signs commonly appear with disease, objective signs often predominate. Examples include bleeding, vomiting, diarrhea, limitation of movement, swelling, visual disturbances, changes in elimination. However, pain (a subjective symptom) is often the primary reason that prompts a person to seek health care.

Illness

Illness is the response a person has to a disease. This response is highly individualized, as the person responds not only to his or her own perceptions of the disease but also to the perceptions of others. Illness integrates pathophysiologic alterations; psychologic effects of those alterations; effects on roles, relationships, and values; and cultural and spiritual beliefs. A person may have a disease and not categorize himself or herself as ill, or may validate feelings of illness through the comments of others ("You don't look as though you feel well today").

Acute Illness

An **acute illness** occurs rapidly, lasts for a relatively short period of time, and is self-limiting. The condition responds to self-treatment or to medical-surgical intervention. Clients with uncomplicated acute illnesses usually have full recovery and return to normal preillness functioning.

The experience of being acutely ill is described as a sequential pattern of illness behaviors. **Illness behaviors** are the way people cope with the alterations in health and function caused by the disease. Included in the behaviors are the perception of the illness, an evaluation of the seriousness of the symptoms, acceptance of the need for assistance in regaining health, and resumption of normal activities upon recovery. Illness behaviors are highly individualized and are influenced by age, gender, family values, economic status, culture, educational level, and mental status. The sequence of illness behaviors is given below (Suchman, 1972).

Experiencing Symptoms   In the first stage of an acute illness, a person experiences one or more signs or symptoms (also called manifestations) that serve as cues for an awareness that a change in normal health is occurring. The most significant of these is pain. Examples of other manifestations that signal an illness are bleeding, difficulty with breathing, swelling, or fever. If the manifestations are mild or are familiar (such as symptoms of the common cold or influenza), the person usually uses over-the-counter medications or a folk remedy for self-treatment. If the symptoms are relieved, no further action is taken. However, if the symptoms are severe or become worse, the person moves to the next stage.

Assuming the Sick Role   In the second stage of the sequence, the person assumes the sick role. This role assumption signals acceptance of the symptoms as proof that an illness is present. The person usually validates this belief with others and seeks support for the need to have professional treatment or to stay at home from school or work.

Self-preoccupation is characteristic of this stage, and the person focuses on alterations in function resulting from the illness. If the illness is resolved, the person validates a return to health with others and resumes normal activities. However, if manifestations remain or increase in severity and others agree that no improvement has occurred, the person moves to the next stage by seeking medical care.

Seeking Medical Care   In our society, validation of illness is most often provided by a physician. People who believe themselves to be ill (and who are encouraged by others to contact a health care provider) make the medical contact for diagnosis, prognosis, and treatment of the illness. If the medical diagnosis is of an illness, the person moves to the next stage. If the medical diagnosis does not support illness, the client may return to normal functioning or may seek validation from a different health care provider.

Assuming a Dependent Role   The stage of assuming a dependent role begins when a person accepts the diagnosis and planned treatment of the illness. As the severity of the illness increases, so does the dependent role. Dependence falls into the following categories (Wu, 1973):

- Complying with the demands of others
- Needing physical assistance with activities of daily living and care
- Needing emotional support through approval, reassurance, physical closeness, and protection

It is during this stage that the person may enter the hospital for treatment and care. The responses of the person to care depend on many different variables: the severity of the illness, the degree of anxiety or fear about the outcome, the loss of roles, the support systems available, individualized reactions to stress, and previous experiences with illness care.

Achieving Recovery and Rehabilitation   The final stage of an acute illness is recovery and rehabilitation. Institutional health care focuses on the acute care needs of the ill client, with recovery beginning in the hospital and completed at home. This focus makes client education and continuity of care a major goal for nursing. It has also contributed to the shift in settings for nursing care, with increasing numbers of nurses providing care in community settings and the home.

The person now gives up the dependent role and resumes normal roles and responsibilities. As a result of education during treatment and care, the person may be at a higher level of wellness after recovery is complete. There is no set timetable for recovery from an illness; each person responds differently. The degree of severity of the illness and the method of treatment both affect the length of time required, as does the person's compliance with treatment plans and motivation to return to normal health.

Chronic Illness

Chronic illness is an umbrella term that encompasses many different lifelong pathologic and psychologic alterations in health. It is the leading health problem in the world today, and the number of persons with chronic illnesses is estimated to triple by the year 2040 (Jennings et al., 1988). Current trends affecting an increased incidence of chronic illnesses include diseases of aging, diseases of life-style and behavior, the AIDS epidemic, and environmental factors (Shugars et al., 1991).

Definition   Most descriptions of chronic illness are based on the definition by the National Commission on Chronic Illness (1956), which states that a chronic illness is any impairment or deviation from normal functioning that has one or more of the following characteristics:

- It is permanent.
- It leaves permanent disability.
- It is caused by nonreversible pathologic alterations.
- It requires special training of the client for rehabilitation.
- It may require a long period of care.

Chronic illness is also characterized by impaired function in more than one body system; responses to this impaired function may occur in sensory perception, self-care abilities, mobility, cognition, and social skills. The demands on the individual and family as a result of these responses are often lifelong (Miller, 1983).

The intensity of a chronic illness and its related symptoms ranges from mild to severe, and the illness is usually characterized by periods of remission and exacerbation. During periods of remission, the person does not experience symptoms, even though the disease is still clinically present. With periods of exacerbation, the symptoms reappear. These periods of change in symptoms do not appear in all chronic diseases.

Needs of the Chronically Ill Person   Each person with a chronic illness has a unique set of responses and needs. The response of the person to the illness is influenced by many different factors. These factors are presented below (Melvin & Nagi, 1970):

- The point in the life cycle at which the onset of the illness occurs
- The type of limitations imposed by the illness
- The degree of limitation imposed by the illness
- The visibility of impairment or disfigurement
- The stigma attached to the impairment or disfigurement
- The pathophysiology causing the illness
- The relationship between the impairment and functioning in social roles
- Pain and fear

These factors are highly complex. They are interrelated within each person, resulting in individualized illness behaviors and needs. Because there are so many different chronic diseases and because the experience of each person with the illness is a composite of individualized responses, it is difficult to generalize about needs. However, almost all people with a chronic illness will need to

- Live as normally as possible, despite the symptoms and treatment that make the person with a chronic illness feel alienated, lonely, and different from others without the illness.

■ Learn to adapt activities of daily living and self-care activities.

■ Grieve over the loss of physical function and structure, income, status, roles, and dignity.

■ Learn to live with chronic pain.

■ Comply with a medical treatment plan.

■ Maintain a positive self-concept.

■ Maintain a sense of hope.

■ Maintain a feeling of being in control.

■ Confront the inevitability of death. (Miller, 1983; Pollock, 1986)

Tasks of the Chronically Ill Person   The person with a chronic illness must accomplish certain tasks (Strauss et al., 1984). These tasks are listed below; the box on page 46 lists guidelines for the assessment of task achievement.

■ Preventing and managing a medical crisis

■ Carrying out prescribed regimens

■ Controlling symptoms

■ Reordering time

■ Adjusting to changes in the course of the disease

■ Preventing social isolation

■ Attempting to normalize interactions with others

Some people with chronic illness successfully meet health-related needs and perform tasks, whereas others do not. Research indicates that adaptation is influenced by variables such as anger, depression, denial, self-concept, locus of control, hardiness, and disability. Nursing interventions for the person with a chronic illness focus on education to promote independent functioning, reduce health care costs, and improve well-being and quality of life (Braden, 1990; Pollock et al., 1990).

The Family of the Client with a Chronic Illness   The client with a chronic illness is hospitalized for diagnosis and treatment of acute exacerbations, but the care of the client is primarily provided at home. "Although it is the individual who is diagnosed with the chronic disease, the entire family experiences life with the illness" (Woods et al., 1989, p. 46). Chronic illness in a family member is a major stressor that may cause changes in family structure and function, as well as changes in performing family developmental tasks.

Many different factors affect family responses to chronic illness; family responses in turn affect the client's response to and perception of the illness. Factors influencing response to chronic illness include personal, social, and economic resources; the nature and course of the disease; and demands of the illness as perceived by family members.

Support for the family is essential. The following information should be considered when performing any family assessment and developing a client's plan of care:

■ Cohesiveness of the family

■ Open communication patterns within the family

■ Family interactions that support self-care

■ Number of friends and relatives available

■ Participation in community and leisure activities

■ Family values and beliefs about health and illness

■ Cultural and spiritual beliefs

■ Developmental level of the client and family

Client and family teaching is integrated throughout this book, specific to responses to alterations in health. It is important to remember that standardized teaching plans may not be effective. Rather, chronically ill clients and families should be given the freedom to choose appropriate literature, self-help or support groups, and interactions with others with the same illness. Information provided by the nurse must be individualized to specific, current needs (Burckhardt, 1987; Forsyth et al., 1984).

Rehabilitation

Rehabilitation is the process of learning to live to one's maximum potential with a chronic impairment and its resultant functional disability. Rehabilitation nursing is based on a philosophy that each person has a unique set of strengths and abilities that can enable that person to live with dignity, self-worth, and independence. This philosophy provides a framework for recovery and rehabilitation of clients with both acute and chronic illnesses. However, nursing care to promote rehabilitation primarily focuses on clients with chronic illnesses or impairments.

Definition of Terms

The terms *impairment, disability,* and *handicap* are often used as synonyms, but they have different meanings. An **impairment** is a disturbance in structure or function resulting from physiologic or psychologic abnormalities. A **disability** is the degree of observable and measurable impairment. A **handicap** is the total adjustment to disability that limits functioning at a normal level (Stanhope & Lancaster, 1992, p. 537). For example, following a motorcycle accident, Kim Rushin had damage to her left leg that resulted in an impairment in the ability to flex her knee. This resulted in a 50% disability of that leg and caused a handicap, because Kim was a school bus driver and could no longer operate the bus safely.

Guidelines for Assessing Task Achievement in the Chronically Ill Person

■ ■ ■

Preventing and Managing a Medical Crisis

Does the chronically ill person

- Comply with prescribed medical therapy?
- Know the symptoms of the onset of a crisis?
- Have a plan for resolving the crisis?
- Have one or more support people to assist with crisis management?
- Accept dependence on others for care during a crisis?

Carrying Out Prescribed Regimens

Does the chronically ill person

- Verbalize accurate information about medication administration (time, route, side effects)?
- Demonstrate an ability to use required equipment?
- Allot time for care realistically?
- Understand the energy needed to carry out prescribed care?
- Accept the discomfort or untoward side effects of medical care (such as giving self-injections or having sexual dysfunction from medications for hypertension)?
- Accept the need to continue treatment even when symptoms are controlled?

Controlling Symptoms

Does the chronically ill person

- Plan activities of daily living, work schedules, and participation in social activities to facilitate symptom control?
- Design a schedule for self-care that reduces visibility of treatment modalities (e.g., insulin injections, dialysis treatments, colostomy irrigations)?
- Know about and use assistive devices to make symptom control manageable?
- Have access to community resources?

- Have necessary financial resources?
- Verbalize acceptance of own limitations?

Reordering Time

Does the chronically ill person

- Participate in family and community activities if the illness results in loss of work?
- Verbalize the time necessary for care?
- Develop a flexible plan to meet treatment demands and also meet personal needs?

Adjusting to Changes in the Course of the Disease

Does the chronically ill person

- Label self as a person with a chronic illness?
- Accept life-style changes resulting from the effects of the chronic illness?
- Accept the unpredictability of the disease?

Preventing Social Isolation

Does the chronically ill person

- Participate in family and community activities?
- Communicate with others about the disease?
- Verbalize feelings about the reaction of others?

Attempting to Normalize Interactions with Others

Does the chronically ill person

- Maintain normal behavior and an optimal level of functioning within limits imposed by the disease?
- Carry out roles and responsibilities within the family and the community?
- Verbalize acceptance of role changes?
- Have access to counseling, if necessary?

Rehabilitation: A Team Approach to Care

Rehabilitation promotes reintegration into the client's family and community through a team approach. Many different aspects of the client's life are included in the plan of care, including physical function, mental health, interpersonal relationships, social interactions, and vocational status. This comprehensive consideration of the client requires the expertise of a team of health care providers.

The rehabilitation team usually meets weekly to discuss the achievement of client goals (Figure 2–7). As a part of this comprehensive plan of care, the following are included:

- Assessing the level of function
- Developing an individualized and holistic plan of care, with ongoing evaluation of outcomes
- Including the family in the plan of care
- Implementing discharge planning to ensure a smooth transition to home

The Nursing Process in Rehabilitation

The nurse provides care for the chronically ill client of all ages and with many types of disability. The 20-year-old men with quadriplegia from a spinal cord injury has needs that are different from the 75-year-old woman who has had a stroke and is unable to move her left arm or speak. However, the plan of care developed for each of these clients considers common factors in assessing and planning individualized interventions.

Assessment   Assessment of the client's needs begins with the initial contact and is ongoing throughout care. Assessment of the client and family includes functional level and self-care abilities, educational needs, psychosocial needs, and the home environment. It is critical to determine the priorities of needs from the client and family perspective before establishing any plan of care. Questions for assessment include the following:

- What is the client's present level of physical function (mobility, self-care, communication, skin integrity, bowel and bladder function)?
- What are the client and family goals (short-term and long-term)?
- Are goals realistic and attainable?
- What concerns are verbalized by the client and family (financial, work, housing, school, transportation, sexual activities, social activities, relationships)?
- What stage of grief and loss is present (denial, anger, bargaining, acceptance)?
- What educational levels have the client and family members achieved? What is the learning style of the client and family?
- What home environment will the client be going to?
- What resources are available to facilitate reintegration (personal, support, community, federal)?

Interventions   Nursing interventions to facilitate rehabilitation are revised to meet client and family needs as the client progresses toward reintegration. In the acute care stage, the nurse focuses on interventions to prevent complications. As recovery progresses, the nurse develops and implements individualized teaching plans for the client and family. General areas of interventions include the following:

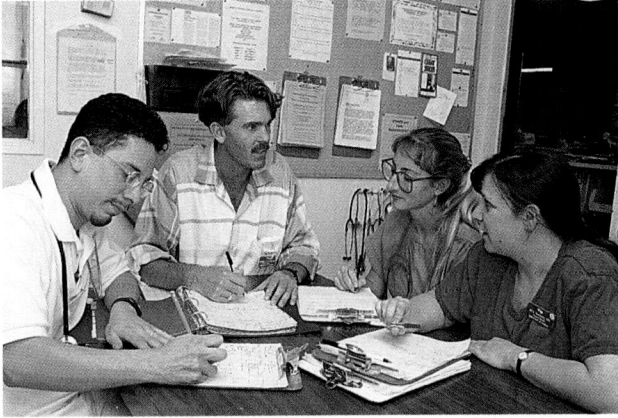

Figure 2-7   The rehabilitation team discusses the individualized plan of care and achievement of goals.

- Preventing complications
   a. Recognizing symptoms of complications
   b. Preventing infection
   c. Maintaining correct body alignment and position and range of motion
   d. Preventing skin breakdown
   e. Providing adequate nutrition and fluids
- Providing care as necessary and appropriate, with the goal of achieving a level of independence realistic for the client
   a. Bathing, brushing teeth, grooming
   b. Toileting
   c. Eating
   d. Position change and mobility
- Implementing individualized teaching plans, with emphasis on care at home
   a. Physical exercises
   b. Use of assistant devices (including crutches, walkers, wheelchairs, prostheses)
   c. Use of equipment (safety rails, raised toilet seats, special beds) and home modifications
   d. Referrals to community agencies (nursing care, special equipment or supplies, support groups, counseling, physical therapy, occupational therapy, respiratory therapy, vocational guidance, house cleaning, meals)
- Providing information about the disease process or disability, and about health promotion and health maintenance activities

To ensure continuity of care during rehabilitation, the community health nurse is involved in the plan of care during the acute care stage. Continued education and support of the client and family are essential; the achievement of self-care and mobility does not guarantee independence in all areas of human functioning.

Bibliography

■ ■ ■

Alford, D., & Futressl, M. (1992). Wellness and health promotion in the elderly. *Nursing Outlook, 40*(5), 221–226.

American Association of Retired Persons. (1990). *A profile of older Americans.* Washington, DC: American Association of Retired Persons.

American Cancer Society. (1990). *Summary of current guidelines for the cancer-related checkup: Recommendations.* Atlanta, GA: American Cancer Society.

American College Health Association. (1990). *Eating 101: The basics of good nutrition.* Rockville, MD: American College Health Association.

Artinian, N. (1994). Selecting a model to guide family assessment. *Dimensions in Critical Care Nursing, 14*(1), 4–12.

Bennett, E. G., & Woolf, D. (Eds.). (1991). *Substance abuse: Pharmacologic, developmental and clinical perspectives.* (2nd ed.). Albany, NY: Delmar.

Braden, C. J. (1990). A test of the self-help model: Learned response to chronic illness experience. *Nursing Research, 39*(1), 42–47.

Bronstein, K. S., Popovich, J. M., & Stewart-Amidei, C. (1991). *Promoting stroke recovery: A research-based approach for nurses.* St. Louis: Mosby.

Burckhardt, C. S. (1987). Coping strategies of the chronically ill. *Nursing Clinics of North America, 22,* 543–550.

Dietary Guidelines Advisory Committee. (1990). Report of the dietary guidelines advisory committee on the *Dietary guidelines for Americans, 1990.* Hyattsville, MD: US Department of Agriculture Human Nutrition Information Service.

Dunn, H. (1959). High-level wellness for man and society. *American Journal of Public Health, 49,* 786–972.

Duvall, E. M. (1977). *Marriage and family development.* Philadelphia: J. B. Lippincott.

Edelman, C. L., & Mandle, C. L. (1990). *Health promotion throughout the lifespan.* (2nd ed.). St. Louis: Mosby.

Eliopoulos, C. (1987). *A guide to the nursing of the aging.* Baltimore: Williams & Wilkins.

———. (1990). *Caring for the elderly in diverse care settings.* Philadelphia: Lippincott.

Erikson, E. (1963). *Childhood and society.* (2nd ed.). New York: Norton.

Forsyth, G. L., Delaney, K. D., & Gresham, M. L. (1984). Vying for a winning position: Management style of the chronically ill. *Research in Nursing and Health, 7,* 181–188.

Fowler, J. W. (1981). *Stages of faith: The psychology of human development and the quest for meaning.* New York: Harper & Row.

Freiberg, K. L. (1987). *Human development: A life-span approach.* (3rd ed.). Boston: Jones and Bartlett.

Friedman, M. (1981). *Family nursing: Theory and assessment.* New York: Appleton-Century-Crofts.

Fryback, P., & Reinert, B. (1993). Facilitating health in people with terminal diagnoses by encouraging a sense of control. *MEDSURG Nursing, 2*(3), 197–201.

Girduno, D. A., & Everly, G. S. (1979). *Controlling stress and tension: A holistic approach.* Bowie, MD: Robert T. Brady.

Hales, D. (1994). *An invitation to health.* (5th ed.) Redwood City, CA: Benjamin/Cummings.

Hartweg, D. (1993). Self-care actions of healthy middle-aged women to promote well-being. *Nursing Research, 42*(4), 221–227.

Havighurst, R. J. (1972). *Human development and education.* (3rd ed.). New York: Longman.

Healthy people: The Surgeon General's report on health promotion and disease prevention. (1982). Health and Human Services Pub. No. 79-55071. Washington, DC: US Government Printing Office.

Healthy people 2000: National health promotion and disease prevention objectives (summary). (1990). American Public Health Association. Washington, DC: US Government Printing Office.

Holloway, C., & Pokorny, M. (1994). Early hospital discharge and independence: What happens to to the elderly? *Geriatric Nursing, 15*(1), 24–27.

Hughes, F. P., & Noppe L. D. (1991). *Human development across the life span.* New York: Merrill.

Jennings, B., Callahan, D., & Caplan, A. L. (1988). Ethical issues in chronic illness. *Hastings Center Report, 18*(1), 1–16.

Jensen, L., & Allen, M. (1993). Wellness: The dialectic of illness. *Image: Journal of Nursing Scholarship, 25*(3), 220–224.

Kohlberg, L. (1979). *The meaning and measurement of moral development.* New York: Clark University.

Kozier, B., Erb, G., & Olivieri, R. (1995). *Fundamentals of nursing: Concepts, process and practice.* (5th ed.). Redwood City, CA: Addison-Wesley Nursing.

Leavell, H., & Clark, A. E. (1965). *Preventive medicine for doctors in the community.* New York: McGraw-Hill.

Loomis, M. E., & Conco, D. (1991). Patients' perceptions of health, chronic illness, and nursing diagnoses. *Nursing Diagnosis, 2*(4), 162–170.

Melvin, J., & Nagi, S. (1970). Factors in behavioral responses to impairments. *Archives of Physical Medicine and Rehabilitation, 51,* 552–557.

Meyer, C. (1993). The changing face of rehabilitation nursing. *American Journal of Nursing, 93*(2), 76–78, 80, 82.

Miller, J. F. (1983). *Coping with chronic illness: Overcoming powerlessness.* Philadelphia: F. A. Davis.

Pender, N. J. (1987). *Health promotion in nursing practice.* (2nd ed.). Norwalk, CT: Appleton & Lange.

Pender, N. J., Barkauskas, V. H., Hayman, L., Rice, V. H., & Anderson, E. T. (1992). Health promotion and disease prevention: Toward excellence in nursing practice and education. *Nursing Outlook, 40*(3), 106–112, 120.

Pollock, S. E. (1986). Human responses to chronic illness: Physiologic and psychosocial adaptation. *Nursing Research, 35*(2), 90–95.

Pollock, S. E., Christian, B. J., & Sands, D. (1990). Responses to chronic illness: Analysis of psychological and physiological adaptation. *Nursing Research, 39*(5), 300–304.

Redeker, N. S. (1988). Health beliefs and adherence to chronic illness. *Image: Journal of Nursing Scholarship, 20*(1), 31–35.

Robertson, J. F. (1991). Promoting health among the institutionalized elderly. *Journal of Gerontological Nursing, 17*(6), 15–19.

Ryan, R. S., & Travis, J. W. (1981). *Wellness workbook for health professionals.* Berkeley, CA: Ten Speed Press.

Salsberry, P. (1993). Assuming responsibility for one's health: An analysis of a key assumption in Nursing's Agenda for Health Care Reform. *Nursing Outlook, 41*(5), 212–216.

Schraeder, B. D., Heverly, M. A., & Rappaport, J. (1990). Patterns of functioning in families with a chronically ill parent: An exploratory study. *Research in Nursing and Health, 13*(1), 35–44.

Shugars, D. A., O'Neil, E. H., & Bader, J. D. (Eds.). (1991). *Healthy America: Practitioners for 2005, an agenda for action for US health professional schools.* Durham, NC: The Pew Health Professions Commission.

Stanhope, M., & Lancaster, J. (1992). *Community health nursing: Process and practice for promoting health.* St Louis: Mosby.

Strauss, A. L., et al. (1984). *Chronic illness and the quality of life.* St Louis: Mosby.

Stuifbergen, A. K. (1990). Patterns of functioning in families with a chronically ill parent: An exploratory study. *Research in Nursing and Health, 13*(1), 35–44.

Suchman, E. A. (1972). Stages of illness and medical care. In E. G. Jaco (Ed.). *Patients, physicians, and illness.* New York: Free Press.

Swanson, K. (1993). Nursing as informed caring for the well-being of others. *Image: Journal of Nursing Scholarship, 25*(4), 353–357.

US Bureau of the Census. (July 1987). Money, income, and poverty status of families and persons in the United States: 1986. *Current Population Reports Series P-60.* No. 152. Washington, DC: US Bureau of the Census.

———. (1989). *Statistical abstract of the United States.* (109th ed.). Washington, DC: US Government Printing Office.

US Department of Health and Human Services. (1990). *Healthy people 2000.* Washington, DC: US Department of Health and Human Services.

Westerhoff, J. (1976). *Will our children have faith?* New York: Seabury Press.

Woods, N. F., Yates, B. C., & Primomo, J. (1989). Supporting families during chronic illness. *Image: Journal of Nursing Scholarship, 21*(1), 46–50.

World Health Organization. (1974). *Constitution of the World Health Organization: Chronicle of the World Health Organization.* Geneva: World Health Organization.

Wu, R. (1973). *Behavior and illness.* Englewood Cliffs, NJ: Prentice Hall.

CHAPTER 3

Nursing the Adult Client in the Home

LEARNING OBJECTIVES

After completing this chapter, you will be able to

- Discuss the health care trends that have led to an increase in the number of medical-surgical clients receiving nursing care in the home.
- Describe the nature of home health nursing.
- Describe the components of the home health care system, including referral and reimbursement sources.
- Discuss the roles of the home health nurse and the impact of reimbursement on these roles.
- Discuss some of the standards and laws that guide nursing practice in the home.

- Discuss the impact of the home setting on nursing practice.
- Apply the practical wisdom offered by home health nursing experts to care of the client in the home.
- Apply the nursing process to care of the client in the home.
- Describe and explain the rationale for high-technology home care, hospice care, and home care for clients with AIDS.

In recent years, nursing care of the adult client has steadily moved from the hospital into the home setting, responding to demographic, technologic, and socioeconomic developments. Clients once considered too sick to leave the hospital or who required high-technology care that mandated institutional care are now living at home and receiving that care from nurses and other health care providers. Consider the following example that illustrates the complex needs of clients receiving care at home.

Margaret Ford, a 77-year-old retired salesperson, lives alone in her own apartment. Her medical history includes advanced pancreatic cancer with uncontrolled pain, a complicated cardiac history, and a dermatologic condition called prurigo. Her son and daughter, who live nearby, honor their mother's desire for independence but worry about her safety. Mrs. Ford currently has profound lower extremity edema due to the pancreatic tumor mass impeding venous return. As a result, stasis ulcers have de-veloped on her lower legs, and fluid is constantly draining through the prurigo lesions located there. Several weeks ago, contact dermatitis appeared. It is suspected that the dermatitis is the result of either the irritating draining edema or the paper towels Mrs. Ford decided to use as bandages. Mrs. Ford's current nursing needs include frequent assessment, pain and symptom management, health teaching, and treatment of her lower legs.

Mrs. Ford has a variety of medical-surgical problems, but she is not being cared for in an inpatient setting. Mrs. Ford is a client of a home health agency that provides a variety of skilled medical services for people at home.

This chapter provides information about the home health care system, roles of the home health nurse, and nursing practice for the adult client in the home. Specialized home care nursing for clients who require high-technology interventions, are terminally ill, or have acquired immune deficiency syndrome (AIDS) is also discussed.

The Home Health Care System

■ ■ ■

Current Trends

The health care system is changing, and so are settings for medical-surgical nursing practice. Not long ago, clients with acute health problems were hospitalized until their conditions no longer required physician or nursing care. Shortly before discharge, nurses taught clients how to care for themselves at home. If their condition deteriorated at home, they were once again admitted to the hospital. At that time, nursing students, whose learning experiences often exposed them to a variety of clinical settings, looked principally to hospitals for employment opportunities on graduation. This is no longer realistic.

An aging population, the use of diagnosis-related groups (DRGs) as a basis for reimbursement, and "quicker and sicker" discharges from hospitals have had a profound effect on the health care system. Cost-effectiveness and the ability to deliver high-technology interventions at home are changing the face of health care (Humphrey, 1988; Lindeman, 1992). Insurers now accept the home as a legitimate place to enter the health care system (Knollmueller, 1993; National Association for Home Care, 1993). This position change, coupled with the overwhelming consumer preference for home over institutionalized care, makes home care one of the fastest growing industries in the health care market (Morgan & McClain, 1993; Weinstein, 1993). In addition, much health care reform legislation focuses on alternatives to institutional care and promises to provide home health services to an increasing number of Americans (Brent, 1994). The US Department of Health and Human Services (1991) predicts that 8000 more home health nurses will be needed by the year 2000. Given these developments, it is debatable whether 8000 will be nearly enough.

In the recent past, two-thirds of all registered nurses worked in hospitals. Today, one-third of all hospital beds are empty on any given night (Zusy, 1994). With the downsizing of acute care facilities, fewer hospital positions are available for new graduates. Nurses must now think beyond acute care for employment, and those in acute care must keep the home and community continuously in sight.

Professional organizations are encouraging nurses to hone their clinical skills, advance their education, and look to alternative clinical settings (public health, home care, school nursing, health maintenance organizations, and the private sector) in order to stay employed within the "scrambled health care system of the nineties" (Zusy, 1994). Nurse educators are being urged to expand their home and community health content (Brent, 1994), put greater emphasis on client education, help nurses find and explore alternative practice settings, and foster the development of refined critical-thinking skills that can be applied across multiple practice settings (Zusy, 1994).

For some nurses, these dramatic changes are a source of anxiety. However, nursing in the 21st century holds great promise for growth. The home and community focus of tomorrow's health care may better ground acute care providers. Career opportunities both in hospitals and the community may expand, increasing the demand for case managers, health promotion consultants, directors of community care facilities, and other specialists and creating new employment opportunities never before envisioned by nurses. Although the possibilities are many, one thing is certain: The 21st century promises to be a history-making era for nurses.

Definitions

Home care in today's society is not easily defined. It is not simply illness care at home, nor is it the act of setting up a hospital room in someone's house. Contemporary definitions tend to reflect the opinions of the leading professional and trade organizations in the industry.

The National Association for Home Care (1987) defines home care as services for recovering, disabled, or chronically ill people in need of treatment or support to function effectively in the home environment. Home care is appropriate for adults and children in danger of abuse or neglect or for any person who needs either short-term or long-term assistance that cannot be provided by family members or friends.

The American Medical Association (1986) definition of home care points out that home health care services are requested and are under the medical direction of a physician. The personnel who provide the services operate as a team in assessing and implementing the plan of care.

The US Department of Health and Human Services (1980) places home care along a continuum of health care. Home care is provided in the client's place of residence for the purpose of promoting, maintaining, or restoring health or of maximizing the level of independence while minimizing the effects of disability and illness, including terminal illness.

Home care is both professional and technical. Professional home care is provided by people who are practice-driven and guided by professional standards based on scientific theory and ethics. Professional home care providers are licensed, are certified, and/or have special qualifications. Nurses, therapists, social workers, and home health aides are considered professional providers.

Technical home care providers are business- and product-driven. Customer satisfaction, field service, reimbursement, and profits are their primary concerns. Durable medical equipment companies (businesses that deliver medical equipment to homes) are technical providers.

Because home care was initially the focus of community health nursing, there is debate over whether **home health nursing** is part of, synonymous with, or completely different from community health nursing (Clark, 1991; Green & Diggers, 1989; Burbach & Brown, 1988; Humphrey, 1988; Stanhope & Lancaster, 1988). One definition of home health nursing reflects its origins in community health nursing: Home health nursing is the providing of nursing care to acute and chronically ill clients of all ages in their home while integrating community health nursing principles that focus on environmental, psychosocial, economic, cultural, and personal health factors affecting an individual's and family's health status (Humphrey & Milone-Nuzzo, 1991).

According to a simpler definition, the primary concern of home health nursing is the health of people (Clark, 1991). Home health nurses enter the home for the purpose of providing care for a specific illness. A broader definition of home health nursing has been derived from recent research involving practicing home health nurses: Home health nursing is the branch of nursing that meets both the acute and chronic health care needs of clients and families in their home environment (Stulginsky, 1993a). Inherent in this definition is an appreciation for the family's psychosocial resources, the neighborhood in which the family lives, and the availability of community services.

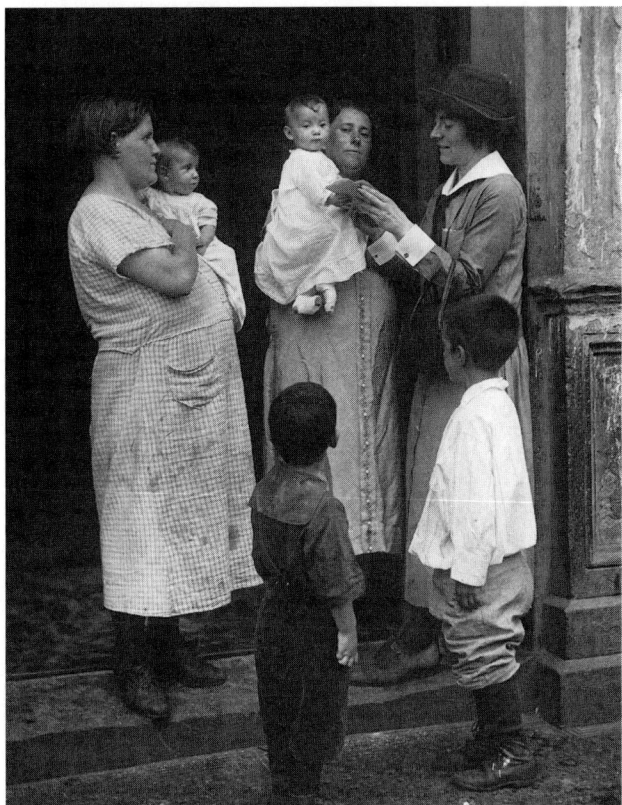

Figure 3–1 In the 19th century, philanthropic individuals and organizations sponsored nurses to visit the sick poor in their own homes.

History of Home Care

The concept of nurses meeting health care needs in the home and community is not new. Rather, it is a legacy left us by our predecessors in public health nursing (Zerwekh, 1992). Although many sources date the birth of home care in the United States with the opening of the Boston Dispensary's first home care program in 1796, it wasn't until the establishment of visiting nursing associations in the late 1800s that care of the sick in their own homes took hold (Humphrey & Milone-Nuzzo, 1991).

At that time, few hospitals were available to handle the health and illness problems of a nation experiencing both rapid growth in its cities and a large influx of immigrants. Illness and hygiene problems seemed to abound as a result of substandard living and working conditions. In response, several philanthropic individuals and organizations sponsored nurses to visit the sick poor in their homes (Figure 3–1). The role of the nurse then, as it is today, was to be an advocate for the client, a provider of direct care, and an educator. Both illness care and health promotion were the nurse's principal focus (Zerwekh, 1992).

Home care services continued to develop and grow in the 20th century with the provision of home care benefits to policyholders by the Metropolitan Life Insurance Company, the introduction of visiting nursing services by the American Red Cross, the establishment of the Frontier Nursing Service, and the decline of physician home visits during World War II. In 1946, the concept of a "hospital without walls" was introduced with the establishment of a posthospitalization home care program developed by Montefiore Hospital in New York City.

These and many other milestones mark the historical growth and development of home health care in the United States. In recent years, the passage of Medicare in 1965, Medicaid in 1970, the addition of hospice benefits in 1973, and the introduction of diagnosis-related groups (DRGs) in 1983 have dramatically affected home care. In 1965, Medicare legislation entitled the nation's elderly to home care services, primarily skilled nursing and other therapies of a curative or restorative nature. This same benefit was extended to certain disabled younger Americans in 1973. As a result, between 1967 and 1980, the number of Medicare-certified home health agencies nearly doubled.

This number doubled again when DRGs were introduced (National Association for Home Care, 1993). DRGs are categories for reimbursement of inpatient services. The DRG system pays the same predetermined amount of money for the care of different persons with the same medical diagnosis. DRGs were introduced in an effort to control the spiraling cost of health care. Prior to their introduction, Medicare reimbursed hospitals on a cost-plus basis, paying for the actual cost of caring for an individual plus other allowable expenses, such as depreciation of facilities and administrative costs. Many changes in the health care system have been attributed to the introduction of DRGs, including earlier discharge from hospitals and the increased need for home care services. In 1992, nearly 14,000 home health providers delivered services to some 6 million clients at a cost of $21 billion (National Association for Home Care, 1993).

Nurses who practice home care do so within a system that includes clients, referral sources, physicians, home health agencies, and reimbursement sources. The system is interactive and, like any other, functions best when its members communicate, cooperate, and collaborate with one another.

Clients

Home health clients represent a diverse population including psychiatric clients, infants, children, perinatal clients, the disabled, and acutely and chronically ill adults.

Health Problems

Although home care clients represent a wide variety of health care needs, statistics on typical diagnoses on admission to home care demonstrate a dramatic incidence of medical-surgical problems. Table 3–1 lists the percentage of clients receiving home or hospice care for various medical-surgical diagnoses. Today, almost any medical-surgical issue dealt with in a formal clinical setting can be addressed in the home. The box on page 53 lists the core health problems that nurses working in home care encounter.

Age

Currently, home care is provided to clients of all ages. Nevertheless, age and functional disability are the primary predictors of need for home care services. Information from a national survey conducted by the Agency for Health Care Policy and Research found that about half of all home care clients are over the age of 65 and that the number of home care services clients need seems to increase with age (National Association for Home Care, 1993).

Family

The client in home health is the person receiving care and the person's family. Some sources identify the person and the family as primary and secondary clients, respectively

Table 3–1	Percentage of Clients Receiving Home or Hospice Care by Diagnosis (1992)

Diagnosis	% Clients Receiving Home or Hospice Care
Neoplasms	72.3
Circulatory disorders	38.1
Endocrine, nutritional, metabolic, and immune disorders	9.8
Musculoskeletal and connective tissue disorders	9.3
Neurologic and sensory disorders	9.0
Injury and poisoning	7.3
Respiratory disorders	6.5
Infection and parasitic diseases	5.9
Skin and subcutaneous disorders	4.6
Digestive disorders	3.5
Diseases of the blood and blood-forming organs	2.9
Genitourinary disorders	2.2

Note. Survey conducted by the National Center for Health Statistics. Printed in *Basic Statistics About Home Care* by National Association for Home Care, 1993, Washington, DC: National Association for Home Care.

(Clark, 1991). The recognition that the family is also a client acknowledges the powerful influence that families exert on the wellness situation. Despite this dual focus, client advocacy grounds care. Clients are the "controlling center around which a circle of providers take direction" (Stulginsky, 1993a).

A client's family is not limited to persons related by birth, adoption, or marriage. In the home, family members may include lovers, friends, colleagues, other significant people, and even animals who hold the potential of greatly affecting the health care environment.

Referral Sources

A *referral source* is a person recommending home health services and supplying the agency with details about the client's needs. A referral source can be a physician, nurse, social worker, therapist, or discharge planner. Families sometimes generate their own referrals, either by approaching one of the sources already mentioned or by calling a home health agency directly to make an inquiry. When the family seeks a referral and the agency feels that the client qualifies for services, usually the agency contacts the client's physician and requests a referral on the client's behalf.

Core Home Health Problems (Identified for Nurses Preparing for the ANA Home Health Nurses Certification Examination)

■ ■ ■

Coronary artery disease/angina pectoris

Myocardial infarction

Congestive heart failure

Hypertension

Cardiomyopathy

Valvular heart disease

Pacemakers

Invasive interventions

Cardiac rehabilitation

Asthma/bronchitis

Chronic obstructive pulmonary disease

Pneumonia

Pulmonary edema

Pulmonary embolus

Pleural effusion

Mechanical ventilation at home

Cerebrovascular accident

Seizure disorders

Alzheimer's disease

Mental illnesses

Diabetes mellitus

Ostomies

Cancer

Acquired immune deficiency syndrome

Terminal illness

Perinatal care

Nutritional disorders

Enteral/parenteral needs

Medicare's Required Data for the Plan of Care

■ ■ ■

1. All pertinent diagnoses
2. A notation of the beneficiary's mental status
3. Types of services, supplies, and equipment ordered
4. Frequency of visits to be made
5. Client's prognosis
6. Client's rehabilitation potential
7. Client's functional limitations
8. Activities permitted
9. Client's nutritional requirements
10. Client's medications and treatments
11. Safety measures to protect against injuries
12. Discharge plans
13. Any other items the home health agency or physician wishes to include

---

Note. Medicare Health Insurance Manual-11, Section 204.2

At the nursing assessment visit, the nurse begins to formulate the plan of care. The box above lists Medicare's required data for the nursing plan of care. Once formulated, the plan of care is sent back to the physician for review and approval. The physician's signature on the plan of care authorizes the home health agency's providers to continue with services and also serves as a contract indicating agreement to participate in the care of the client on an ongoing basis.

Home Health Agencies

Home health agencies are either public or private organizations engaged in providing skilled nursing and other therapeutic services in the client's home (Harris, 1988). There are several different types of home health agencies; however, they differ only in the way their programs are organized and administered. All home health agencies are similar in that they must meet uniform standards for licensing, certification, and accreditation (Stanhope & Lancaster, 1988). Home health agencies include the following:

- *Official or public agencies.* These are agencies operated by state or local governments, financed primarily by tax funds. Most official agencies offer home care,

Physicians

Home care cannot begin without a physician's order, nor can it proceed without a physician-approved treatment plan. This is a legal and reimbursement requirement.

Once a referral is made and an initial set of physician orders is obtained, a nursing assessment visit is scheduled to identify the client's needs. If the input of another provider, such as a physical therapist, is necessary to complete the initial assessment, the nurse arranges for this visit.

health education, and disease-prevention programs in the community.

- *Voluntary or private not-for-profit agencies.* These agencies are supported by donations, endowments, charities such as the United Way, and third-party reimbursement. They are governed by a volunteer board of directors, which usually represents the community they serve. Because these agencies are not-for-profit, they are exempt from federal income tax.

- *Private, proprietary agencies.* Most of these agencies are for-profit organizations and are governed by either individual owners or national corporations. Although some of these agencies participate in third-party reimbursement, others rely on "private-pay" sources.

- *Institution-based agencies.* These agencies operate under a parent organization, such as a hospital. The home health agency is governed by the sponsoring organization and the mission of both is similar. Often, the majority of home health referrals comes from the parent organization.

Home health agency personnel typically include administrators, managers, professional providers, paraprofessionals, and business office staff. While the professional providers coordinate and deliver the client's health care services, the office staff handle the daily business operations of the agency (which includes billing for reimbursement).

Depending on the agency and geographic location, professional providers may include registered nurses, practical nurses, nurse practitioners, enterostomal therapists, physical therapists, occupational therapists, speech therapists, respiratory therapists, social workers, a chaplain or pastoral minister, dietitians, and home health aides. It is not unusual for clients to require the services of several professionals simultaneously; however, no matter how many providers are in the home, the responsibility for case coordination (also called *case management*) remains with the registered nurse.

Reimbursement Sources

A *reimbursement source* is a party that pays for home health services. Medicare is home care's largest single reimbursement source. Although there are other sources as well (Medicaid, other public funding, private insurance, and public donation), it is interesting to note that the second largest source of payment after Medicare is out-of-pocket funds (National Association for Home Care, 1993).

The treatment plan (formulated by the home health agency providers and authorized by the physician) is used by the reimbursement source. Only interventions identified on the treatment plan are paid for. The reimbursement source evaluates each treatment plan to determine whether the goals and plans set forth by the professional providers match the needs assessed. Periodically the reimbursement source may ask for the home health provider's notes to substantiate what is being done in the home. This is one reason why accurate documentation is critical.

Roles of the Home Health Nurse

■ ■ ■

The role expectations of the home health nurse are similar to those of the professional nurse in any setting. On behalf of clients in the home, the nurse serves as an advocate, a provider of direct care, an educator, and a coordinator of services (Morgan & McClain, 1993; Humphrey & Milone-Nuzzo, 1991).

Advocate

As client advocate, the nurse explores, informs, supports, and affirms the choices of clients. Advocacy begins on the first visit, when clients are introduced to the philosophy and process of home care, that is, to empower, enable, and enhance self-care (Wasik et al., 1990). As a protector of client rights, the nurse discusses advance medical directives, living wills, and durable power of attorney for health care. The home health agency's bill of rights also needs to be discussed. The box on page 58 provides an example of a home health agency's bill of rights.

During the course of care, clients may need help negotiating the complex medical system (especially in regard to medical insurance), accessing community resources, recognizing and coping with required changes in lifestyle, and making informed decisions. Because advocacy can be approached from many nursing models, it is beneficial for practicing nurses to identify which individual or combination of models best fits their own personal philosophy and to incorporate those concepts into their nursing practice (Morgan & McClain, 1993).

When the family's desires differ from those of the client, advocacy can be a challenge. It is impossible for the nurse to please everyone. If a conflict arises, the nurse must remain the primary client's advocate, regardless of any negative response from the family (Stulginsky, 1993a).

Provider of Direct Care

Home health nurses usually are not involved in providing personal care for clients (bathing, changing linens, and so on). Routine personal care usually is provided by the family or a home health aide arranged for by the nurse. If a personal care need arises during the course of the skilled visit (for example, if a client experiences an incontinent episode), the nurse typically either bathes and changes the client or assists the caregiver to do so before moving on to the skilled activities planned for the visit.

As a provider of direct care, the professional nurse uses the nursing process to assess, diagnose, plan care, intervene, and evaluate client needs. During the course of this process, home health nurses frequently are involved in performing specific procedures and treatments, such as physical assessments, care of intravenous lines, ostomy care, wound care, pain management, and so on. However, most of the home health nurse's time is spent teaching.

Educator

Illness care, as well as disease prevention, is the educational focus of the home health nurse. Many nurse experts profess that their role as teacher is the crux of their nursing practice (Hellwig, 1990) and that "nurses in the home are always teaching" (Carr, 1990) (Figure 3–2). For this reason, it is important that home health nurses develop expertise in the theory and principles of client education.

For the home health nurse, the greatest educational challenge frequently is motivating the client. Discovering what it takes to make the client want to learn and focusing the client on what is most important can tax the ingenuity of even the most dedicated nurse. Despite the work involved, nurses are rewarded by the knowledge that through their efforts, clients have learned to manage independently. Because the nurse's role as educator is becoming increasingly important, guidelines for client and family teaching are included in the discussion of each major disorder addressed in this text. Much of this content is applicable in the home care setting.

Coordinator of Services

As a coordinator of services, the home health nurse is the main contact with the client's physician and all other providers involved in the treatment plan. It is the responsibility of the registered nurse case coordinator (or clinical case manager) to report client changes, to discuss responses, and to develop and secure treatment plan revisions on an ongoing basis. This is accomplished both formally, through scheduled case and team conferences, and informally (often over the phone) with concerned providers. Documentation of all coordination activities is legally required.

Impact of Reimbursement on Nursing Roles

Medicare's regulations for reimbursement are the model for many other third-party payors. Medicare has specifi-

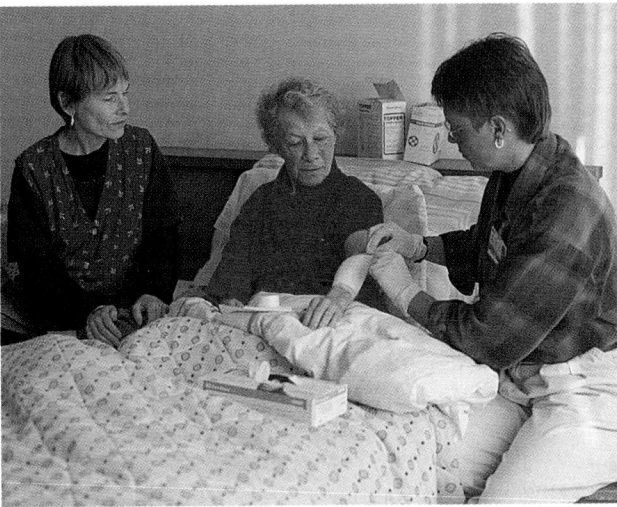

Figure 3–2 The home health nurse often provides client education. This nurse is teaching the client and family member how to apply dressings.

cally defined what skilled services will be reimbursed in home health. Medicare does not reimburse visits made to support general health maintenance, health promotion, or clients' emotional or socioeconomic needs. There are very specific criteria that both client and nurse must meet in order to secure Medicare reimbursement. The client must meet all of the following criteria:

- The client must be in need of "reasonable and necessary" home care with a "skilled need."
- The client must be essentially homebound.
- The client must have a plan of care that meets the necessary Medicare criteria.
- The client must require intervention on an intermittent basis only.

Medicare will reimburse only when the skilled provider performs at least one of the following tasks:

- Teaching about a new or acute situation
- Assessing an acute process or a change in the client's condition
- Performing a skilled procedure or a hands-on service requiring the professional skill, knowledge, ability, and judgment of a registered nurse (Morgan & McClain, 1993)

The reimbursement guidelines present problems because they are not sensitive to the full scope of nursing practice. Today, many of the client and family needs nurses encounter during home visits are complex and time consuming, reflecting both intense psychosocial and economic concerns. No longer the exception, these situations seem to be the norm (Smith, 1987; Stulginsky,

1993a and 1993b) and cannot be ignored by the conscientious nurse. This situation presents a profound dilemma. Shouldn't it be nursing, not reimbursement, that drives practice in the home? But if so, how are nurses to reconcile spending time on issues for which their agency will receive no payment? How are they to meet agency home visit productivity standards when each home they enter requires more and more from them? How are they to document activities and interventions that are not considered "skilled"? This issue places nurses in a moral and ethical vise (Anderson, 1992; Collopy et al., 1990). Despite the costs and difficulties, it is imperative that home health nursing not succumb to the industry's tendency to become reimbursement driven. Although this requires nurses to live with a great deal of mixed feelings, in the interest of remaining true to home health nursing's professional practice standards, nurses must learn to accept them. The accompanying box describes one nurse's attempt to balance her professional standards with Medicare's definition of a "skilled need."

Nursing Practice in the Home

■ ■ ■

Guidelines

Home health nurses are responsible for adhering to the same codes and standards that guide all other nurses. These codes and standards, which were provided in Chapter 1, have a twofold purpose: to guide nursing practice and to protect the public. In addition to these guidelines, other codes and statements give specific guidance on issues that impact care in the home.

American Nurses Association Standards of Practice

The American Nurses Association (ANA) Standards for Home Health Nursing Practice (see the box on page 57) are used in conjunction with the ANA Standards of Community Health Nursing as a basis for the practice of nursing in the home. The standards address the nursing process, interdisciplinary collaboration, quality assurance, professional development, and research. These standards reflect the current state of knowledge in the field of home and community health nursing and should be the criteria for characterizing, measuring, and guiding the achievement of quality care. The standards speak to two levels of practice (generalist, prepared on the baccalaureate level, and specialist, prepared on the graduate level) and outline what achievements are expected of the professional nurse in the home (Humphrey & Milone-Nuzzo, 1991).

National Association for Home Care Bill of Rights

Another source of guidance regarding home care is the National Association for Home Care (NAHC) Bill of

---

Balancing Professional Practice Beliefs and Medicare Requirements: An Interview with a Home Health Nurse

■ ■ ■

"Home health nurses don't get paid for what they really do. Neither do agencies. They get reimbursed for something that goes along the medical model. But that's the least of what we do.

"The most wonderful visit I ever had was with a diabetic in a row home in Baltimore. The client was new to insulin, and I went into the home to teach. There was no heat, hot water, or electricity, and he didn't know what to do. He had paid his rent.

"He gave me the business card of the landlord. I recognized his name in connection with scandals. He was considered a slum lord. There was no phone number on his card, just a post office box. So I made a few phone calls to some public agencies. It took about fifteen minutes.

"The next day, I came back and the client had heat, hot water, and electricity."

Obviously, Medicare would not have reimbursed your agency for what you did on that visit. It wasn't skilled nursing. How did you handle that?

"To get reimbursement? I documented that I gave him a list of his medications and instructed him regarding frequency and dosage."

Does that bother you in any way?

"No, it doesn't bother me at all. What I did was much more valuable than teaching him about diabetes. Although I probably gave him the list, no teaching occurred. He was just too distracted."

What you're saying is that you couldn't have walked out of the home without addressing that issue.

"No, and we have many situations like this."

You mean the way the regulations are written we're forced into certain situations out of ethical need?

"Exactly right."

Note. From "Nurses' home health experience—part II: The unique demands of home visits" by M. Stulginsky, 1993, *Nursing and Healthcare, 14*(9), pp. 484–485.

Rights. In 1982, the NAHC adopted a comprehensive code of ethics to which all members subscribed. The Home Care Bill of Rights grew out of that code, and in 1987 Congress made its use a requirement for all home health agencies. Although home health agencies are permitted to make additions to the NAHC's original Bill of Rights, they are required by law to address the concepts

ANA Standards for Home Health Nursing Practice

■ ■ ■

Standard I. Organization of Home Health Services

All home health services are planned, organized, and directed by a master's-prepared professional nurse with experience in community health and administration.

Standard II. Theory

The nurse applies theoretical concepts as a basis for decision in practice.

Standard III. Data Collection

The nurse continuously collects and records data that are comprehensive, accurate, and systematic.

Standard IV. Diagnosis

The nurse uses health assessment data to determine nursing diagnoses.

Standard V. Planning

The nurse develops care plans that establish goals. The care plan is based on nursing diagnoses and incorporates therapeutic, preventive, and rehabilitative nursing actions.

Standard VI. Intervention

The nurse, guided by the care plan, intervenes to provide comfort, to restore, improve, and promote health, to prevent complications and sequelae of illness, and to effect rehabilitation.

Standard VII. Evaluation

The nurse continually evaluates the client's and family's responses to interventions in order to determine progress toward goal attainment and to revise the database, nursing diagnoses, and plan of care.

Standard VIII. Continuity of Care

The nurse is responsible for the client's appropriate and uninterrupted care along the health care continuum, and therefore uses discharge planning, case management, and coordination of community resources.

Standard IX. Interdisciplinary Collaboration

The nurse initiates and maintains a liaison relationship with all appropriate health care providers to assure that all efforts effectively complement one another.

Standard X. Professional Development

The nurse assumes responsibility for professional development and contributes to the professional growth of others.

Standard XI. Research

The nurse participates in research activities that contribute to the profession's continuing development of knowledge of home care.

Standard XII. Ethics

The nurse uses the code for nurses established by the American Nurses Association as a guide for ethical decision making in practice.

Note. From *Standards for Home Health Nursing Practice* by American Nurses Association, 1986, Kansas City, MO: ANA.

---

in the NAHC Bill of Rights with all home health clients on the initial visit.

The box on page 58 provides an example of a home health agency's bill of rights.

American Nurses Association Position Statements

The ANA has published position statements addressing moral, ethical, and legal issues faced by home and community health nurses. These include the following:

- *A Statement on the Scope of Home Health Nursing Practice* (1992)
- *Nursing Care and Do Not Resuscitate Decisions* (1992)
- *Foregoing Artificial Nutrition and Hydration* (1992)

Legal Considerations

The legal considerations within home health center around issues of privacy and confidentiality, the client's

A Home Health Agency's Bill of Rights

▪ ▪ ▪

The agency acknowledges the client's rights and encourages the client and family to participate in their plan of care through informed decision making. In accordance with this belief, each client/family member will receive, prior to admission, the following bill of rights and responsibilities.

1. The client and the client's property will be treated with respect by the program's staff.

2. The client will receive care without regard to race, color, creed, age, sex, religion, national origin, or mental or physical handicap.

3. The client has the right to be free from mental and physical abuse.

4. The client's medical record and related information is maintained in a confidential manner by the program.

5. The client will receive a written statement of the program's objectives, scope of services, and grievance process prior to admission.

6. The client, family, or guardian has the right to file a complaint regarding the services provided by the program without fear of disruption of service, coercion, or discrimination.

7. The client will be advised of the following in advance of service:
   a. Description of services and proposed visit frequency
   b. Overview of the anticipated plan of care and its likely outcome
   c. Options that may be available

8. The client/family is encouraged to participate in the plan of care. The client will receive the necessary information concerning the client's condition and will be encouraged to participate in changes that may arise in care.

9. The program shall provide for the right of the client to refuse any portion of planned treatment to the extent permitted by law without relinquishing other portions of the treatment plan, except where medical contraindications exist. The client will be informed of the expected consequences of such action.

10. The client has a right to continuity of care:
    a. Services provided within a reasonable time frame
    b. A program that is capable of providing the level of care required by the client
    c. Timely referral to alternative services, as needed
    d. Information regarding impending discharge, continuing care requirements, and other services, as needed

11. The client will be informed of the extent to which payment will be expected for items or services to be furnished to clients by Medicare, Medicaid, and any other program that is funded partially or fully with federal funds. Upon admission, the client will be informed orally and in writing of any charges for items and services that the program expects will not be covered upon admission. The client will be informed of any change in this amount as soon as possible, but no later than within 25 days after the program is made aware of the change.

12. Upon request, the client may obtain
    a. An itemized bill.
    b. The program's policy for uncompensated care.
    c. The program's policy for disclosure of the medical record.
    d. Identity of health care providers with which the program has contractual agreements, insofar as the client's care is concerned.
    e. The name of the responsible person supervising the client's care and how to contact this person during regular business hours.

13. The client has the right to obtain medical equipment and other health-related items from the company of the client's choice and assumes financial responsibility for such. The program's staff will assist in obtaining supplies and physician approvals as needed.

14. The client/family is responsible for
    a. Giving the progam accurate, necessary information.
    b. Being available and cooperative during scheduled visits.
    c. Assisting, as much as possible, in the plan of care.
    d. Alerting the staff to any problems as soon as possible.

Note. Adapted from the Patient Bill of Rights and Responsibilities, Bon Secours Home Health and Hospice, Baltimore, MD.

access to health information, the client's freedom from unreasonable restraint, witnessing of documents, informed consent, and matters of negligence and/or malpractice. Although many nurses find the solitary nature of home health practice unsettling, numerous sources suggest that nurses can best avoid lawsuits by familiarizing themselves with the standards of practice, providing care that is consistent with both the standards and their agency's policies, and documenting all care fully and accurately according to agency guidelines (Morgan & McClain, 1993).

Preparing Clients to Go Home

The old adage that discharge plans begin at admission makes more sense today than ever before. With shortened lengths of hospital stay, it is imperative that all clients be evaluated for their ability to manage at home. Nurses preparing to send clients home need to consider many of the following questions:

- Does the client have any overt need for follow-up therapy, treatments, or client education?

- What equipment, supplies, or information about community resources seems necessary?

- Are there any teaching tools that can be sent home? Are they written at an acceptable reading level? Do they come in other languages?

- What cognitive abilities do the client and the caregiver seem to possess? Are there any sensory deprivations that impede learning?

- Was the caregiver present during and included in instruction? How have the client and caregiver responded to health teaching thus far? Have they comprehended what has been taught? Was their stress level such that they could not listen?

- Was health education cut short because of early discharge? Was it rushed?

- Who will be the principal caregiver in the home? Is there one? Are all caregivers comfortable in doing what needs to be done? If not, what support do they need to become comfortable?

- Is a preexisting caregiving situation already in the home?

- What is the stage of the family life cycle now?

- Has a devastating diagnosis and/or prognosis just been determined?

- Is high-technology intervention necessary?

The answers to these questions suggest two equally important nursing interventions: initiating a client referral and teaching the client and family.

Initiating Referrals

The nurse considers making a referral to either a home health agency, a hospice, or a community resource if the client seems to have a need for formal follow-up beyond the present clinical setting. Hospital discharge planners, social workers, organizations for the aged, and local nonprofit agencies usually have a good command of the services and support groups available in their communities.

The nurse must talk to clients and their caregivers about their concerns related to home management. It is not unusual for one member of the family to think that no additional help is necessary and for another to feel differently. Among the steps the nurse can take are to facilitate an informal family meeting in which everyone shares concerns and to make inquiries about the family's insurance coverage for home health care. Suggesting services families have no funds to pay for only adds to the problem. For clients with limited means, the nurse can identify staff in the institution who are most knowledgeable about funding and consult with them. In every instance, it is important that the nurse avoid making assumptions: Intelligent, well-educated, and financially secure clients can be just as overwhelmed by illness as the less learned and poor. Everyone is a referral candidate.

If the family feels that no help is necessary and the nurse feels otherwise, the nurse may ask them to consider an evaluation visit, explaining that they may look at the situation differently once the client is home. If family members continue to refuse, the nurse can let them know that the door is never closed and give them contacts in the community that they can access independently should their needs change.

Teaching the Client and Family

Clients need assistance with understanding their situations, making health care decisions, and changing health behaviors (Redman, 1988). However, it is unrealistic to believe that clients can be taught everything they need to know during today's shortened hospital stays. The nurse should therefore recommend a home health referral for anyone in need of follow-up teaching. Prioritized teaching is essential: Even under the best of circumstances, clients generally forget about one-third of what is said to them, and their recall of specific instructions and advice is less than 50% (Morra, 1985). Comprehensive information related to client and family teaching is included in most of the following chapters in this text. This can be used as a guide in planning teaching.

When preparing clients for discharge, the nurse focuses on safety and survival first. Even if health education is to continue with home care, a day or two may elapse before the nurse arrives, and clients must be able to manage by themselves until then. The nurse must not discharge clients without giving them the right information and supplies to get them through the first few days at home.

Differences in Home Health Nursing

■ ■ ■

- Nurses are invited into the setting where care takes place.
- Control belongs to the client.
- Practice is solitary.
- Intimacy and shared humanity are nurtured.
- Family issues are more visible.
- Nurses must play a greater variety of roles.
- Families of one require more support than in the institutional setting.
- Caregiver burden becomes obvious.
- Substandard conditions affect care.

Additionally, clients should not be discharged without complete information related to their medications and the manifestations of complications they should report to their doctor. Finally, all clients should be able to manage at least minimally any necessary treatments. Management includes not only performing procedures safely but also knowing how to obtain necessary supplies in the community.

The Impact of Setting

Nursing practice in the home is a unique experience that differs in many ways from nursing practice in a hospital setting. These differences are summarized in the accompanying box.

Nurses are invited into homes. They are guests and cannot assume entry, as they do in formal clinical settings. The environment belongs to the client, who retains control. Every nursing action must communicate respect for these boundaries. To negotiate both repeated entry and a share of power in the client's domain, the nurse must establish trust and rapport quickly. This is often difficult, because most home health nurses are with each client for only 1 hour a few times a week.

Home health nursing is solitary. In the home, there are no colleagues present to consult, to assist, or to rely on for support. The home is a practice setting where nurses learn to trust their theoretical and intuitive knowledge and to be totally accountable.

The home is one of the richest symbols in Western culture. The very word generates strong feelings of ownership, control, security, family history, independence, comfort, protection, and conflict (Rubenstein, 1990). The family perceives a sharing of self when they consistently allow entry to a stranger. Because clients and nurses most often meet during periods of vulnerability and crisis, and because socializing is such an integral part of the home visit process (Leahy et al., 1982), nurse providers are often perceived as friends or extended family members, blurring the boundaries of practice.

Intimacy and shared humanity are nurtured in the home. During the course of establishing rapport and getting to know each other as people, the nurse-client relationship often becomes something more. Nurses and clients end up giving to each other and learning from each other through the simple sharing of "ordinary things" (Taylor, 1992). By connecting as human beings, they touch each other's spirits in profound ways (Carson, 1989). In home health, it is not unusual for nurses to realize suddenly not only that they do things to create a healing environment but also that their very presence has become the healing environment (Quinn, 1992).

Family issues and relationships are more visible in the home. Over time, as the nurse becomes a familiar presence and the family's behavior relaxes, the nurse can gain a clearer and more complete picture of family relationships, dynamics, life-style choices, and coping patterns. Multigenerational behavior patterns are more obvious, and working around them can become quite a feat.

In the home, nurses play a variety of roles. Although they focus on providing health care, home health nurses also understand that promoting the client's optimal wellness often necessitates interventions that are not treatment oriented. Nurses report that they find themselves functioning as social workers, friends, spiritual comforters, psychologists, financial counselors, and interpreters of medical information (Green & Diggers, 1989).

"Families of one" are a worrisome reality for home health nurses. Today more older adults are living alone. Some may have current or potential caregivers nearby, whereas others, for any of various reasons, have no one. These people often require considerable nursing support to remain strong, independent, and resourceful (Caserta, 1989). Caring for "families of one" can take a toll on even the strongest home health nurse. Some nurses have reported calling between visits, keeping in touch after discharge, and driving by on days off because they have such difficulty "letting go" their concerns about these clients.

Caregiver burden is not easily hidden in the home. In more than 7 million American households, people are taking care of disabled relatives and friends (Matthis, 1991). Many of these caregivers are themselves older adults. Health care planners visualize the home as a place where all kinds of medical services can occur but may give little thought to how people manage. Few ever ask whether families can cope with the level of care they are expected to assume (Gubrium & Sankar, 1990). Caregiving has only recently been acknowledged as a complex activity, requiring adjustment in family living patterns, relationships, and finances. For some families, the crisis of caregiving is short lived, but for others it lasts for years. As a result, caregivers are at great risk for both physical and emotional illness (Eisdorfer, 1991; Ferrell et al., 1991). Because the success of home care heavily depends on the supports in place (Hewner, 1986), addressing the needs of the support network is imperative.

Care in the home sometimes is inadequate. Personal health habits, living conditions, resources, and support systems may leave much to be desired. It is not unusual for home health nurses to face unchanged dressings, undertreated infections, off-and-on self medication, poor nutrition, filthy conditions, and unreliable caregivers. No matter how vigilant nurses may be, practice settings like these work against their best efforts. If the conditions cannot be changed, the nurse usually has just two choices: to withdraw from the situation or to continue to practice within the environment. Because home health nurses rarely withdraw, they typically are forced to cope with these substandard conditions visit after visit and often experience increasing levels of stress and frustration.

Practical Wisdom

In 1993, a research study of practicing home health nurses was conducted to solicit knowledge about the art and science of home health nursing from their lived experience. This research (Stulginsky, 1993a and 1993b) was initiated in response to the discovery that the nursing literature contained very little current information about home visits.

The results, culled from rich and poignant stories, have added a practical dimension to many of the interventions home health nurses typically implement during the course of client care. The practical suggestions gleaned from this research and from other home health experts follow.

Establish Trust and Rapport

To establish trust and rapport in the client's home, nurses must try to find common ground (Price & Braden, 1978) and to let go of ethnocentric ("My culture's way is the best way") views (Carey, 1989). They must make sure everything they say and do communicates an understanding that the nurse is a guest: offering suggestions in a way that acknowledges the client's right to say no; sensing "where people are" and honoring that; maintaining a respectful distance; and noticing and honoring family customs ("Gee, no one wears shoes in your house; I'll take mine off, too."). Nurses should try to negotiate their schedules around the family's needs; nursing should enhance family coping, not complicate it. Above all, nurses should validate clients' illness experiences, remembering that everyone needs someone who is willing to listen and say, "I hear what you are saying, and I think I have a sense of how you feel."

Proceed Slowly

The nurse must enter the home with an awareness that the first contact is important (Berg & Helgeson, 1984). On the first nursing visit, the nurse can suggest to clients that they have someone else present "to help them listen." To avoid overwhelming clients with too much information, the nurse stresses the essential information and repeats it on subsequent visits. When making suggestions, the nurse offers clients the pluses and minuses of each alternative. Informed decisions are difficult to make if people are too overwhelmed to think of their options. The nurse speaks slowly, directly, and within the client's range of vision (they may have to lip-read) and refrains from shouting at hearing-impaired clients. The nurse must allow time for families to process the information they receive.

Set Goals and Boundaries

The nurse explores clients' expectations of home care. In particular, the nurse explains the primary goal (to achieve self-care), defines nurse and client roles within this framework, and discusses limitations: "No, a home health nurse is not the same as private duty nurse." And "Home health nurses don't routinely do that, but today I'll make an exception." It is important that the nurse stress mutual accountability, choice, and negotiation as part of the process.

Assess the Home Environment

The nurse surveys the overall home environment, using common sense, intuition, and imagination (Keeling, 1978). Among the variables to note are sights, sounds, smells, dress, tone of voice, body language, and the use of touch; visiting patterns among family members; significant relationships; what is sacred and what is not; the appearance of the house, yard, sidewalk, and neighborhood; and the effect of illness on the family (Bayer, 1973; Lentz & Meyer, 1979; Clark, 1991). The nurse asks questions and listens carefully to stories and offhand remarks.

Prioritize

It is important that nurses be flexible and realize they cannot tackle everything. Although it is necessary to enter the home with a plan in mind, nurses must be prepared to modify the plan according to conditions they encounter once inside. Safety, issues that are of concern to clients, and those problems that can most easily be solved should be addressed first (Clark, 1991). Alternatively, the nurse can focus on safety first, then short-term and long-term goals (Carr, 1989). If the priorities that are set are primarily the nurse's and not the client's, they may not be met.

Promote Learning

Instead of just teaching the client, the nurse tries actively to promote the client's ability to learn by, for example, identifying what is most important to the client and teaching that. Survival takes first priority; the nurse teaches the information people need to ensure their safety until the next visit. The nurse prioritizes material on a needs-to-know, wants-to-know, ought-to-know basis, assessing and responding to learner readiness.

Timing is important; people who are not ready to listen cannot be taught. In addition, the nurse must allow a sufficient amount of time to teach, ask clients how and when they learn best, use appropriate methods and materials when possible, and capitalize on the client's frustration and desire to regain control of self-care (Hellwig, 1990). Whenever possible, the nurse teaches while providing care.

The nurse can empower clients to learn by talking them through learning tasks, encouraging them to listen to their own bodies and to ask questions, and urging them to write down things they want to know and to bring them up at the next visit or doctor's appointment.

Limit Distractions

Homes are full of events or circumstances that divert a person's attention from the job at hand (Pruitt et al., 1987). Such distractions as children, animals, noise, clutter, and controlling, manipulative, or aggressive mannerisms can try even the most experienced nurse. However, environmental and behavioral distractions can yield useful information about people, their relationships, and their values. For example, a dirty house could indicate a lack of interest in housekeeping, outright neglect and abuse, depression, or increased disability (Lentz & Meyer, 1979).

Distractions should be limited as much as possible. For example, the nurse might ask a client, "May I please turn off your television while we visit?" or, "I'd like to schedule my next visit for a time when the children are in school. Is that all right with you?" The nurse must be truthful about allergies, fear of a client's pet, or difficulty hearing in a particular room but should not debate the priority of the visit over the distraction (such as a favorite television show); the nurse not only may not change the client's views but also risks losing the client's trust and rapport. If all efforts at limiting distractions fail, the nurse should leave the home and return on another day: "I can see this isn't going to work for us today. I'll need to leave."

If any distraction originates with the nurse, such as fear of harm, reaction to the client's life-style, preoccupation with role or a feeling of being overwhelmed by the situation in the home, the nurse should seek out a colleague to discuss the problem. Often, another perspective is all that is needed to deal with the issue.

Put Safety First

Nurses must focus on safety and survival first, for themselves as well as their clients, in all that they do. When traveling in the community, the nurse takes such precautions as keeping car doors locked, keeping supplies out of sight, and staying inside the car in potentially dangerous situations. Colleagues, families, and community members can offer useful guidelines for maintaining safety and self-protection.

It is important to avoid overwhelming families with numerous health care providers in the home. Most people don't want a lot of strangers in their home, no matter how helpful they may seem to be. The nurse can help families manage moments of crisis by staying as close as possible. If abuse is suspected, the nurse must notify authorities and/or remove clients from potentially dangerous situations.

Make Do

Nurses must learn to be resourceful and cost conscious with equipment, supplies, and services in the home. When needing to "make do" or improvise, they should do so in a low-key manner to avoid causing the family any additional anxiety. The nurse must make every effort to convey the message that the situation is under control; after leaving the home, the nurse can react as necessary.

Special Issues in the Home

Safety

Safety assessment in the home is a nursing responsibility and a legal requirement. Nurses cannot close their eyes to an unsafe environment. Upon entering the home and on a continuing basis, it is imperative that the nurse alert the family to unsafe and hazardous conditions, suggest remedies, and document in the clinical record the family's response to the nurse's suggestions.

In particular, nurses must remain alert to the following conditions:

- How clients handle stairs
- How they manage their own care if they are alone
- The presence of a smoke detector in the home (the fire department will often install one free if notified)
- The presence of bathroom safety equipment
- Electrical hazards
- Slippery throw rugs, clutter, or a furniture arrangement that may cause a fall
- A supply of expired medications
- Inappropriate clothing or shoes
- Cooking habits that may precipitate a fire
- An inadequate food supply
- Poorly functioning utilities
- Chipping paint
- Signs of abusive behavior

Obviously, nurses cannot go into homes and change the family's living space and life-style, but they can register their concern and react appropriately if the situation suggests that an injury is about to occur or if they suspect abuse or neglect. Within the home and community setting, ignoring an unsafe environment is considered nursing negligence.

The disposal of toxic medications and sharp objects (such as needles used for injections) is also a safety issue in the home, especially if young children are present. Once again, it is imperative that the nurse address this with the client, demonstrate safe disposal, and provide the necessary equipment to accomplish that end.

Documentation should address what information the nurse has covered, the family's response to the teaching, and assessment of their ongoing practice of safety precautions.

Infection Control

Infection control in the home centers around protecting clients, caregivers, and the community from the spread of disease. Within the home, nurses may encounter clients with infectious or communicable diseases, clients who are immunocompromised, and/or clients having multiple access devices, drainage tubes, or draining wounds. The home presents a challenging environment in which to practice infection control for several reasons: Families typically are set in their own ways of doing things; caregivers often lack any formal education on the subject; the setting itself may not be conducive; and the facilities for even the most basic of aseptic practices (hand washing) may be lacking. Without doubt, the single most important nursing intervention in controlling infection is health teaching. Clients and caregivers need to know the importance of effective hand washing, the use of gloves, the disposal of wastes and soiled dressings, the handling of linens, and the practice of universal precautions (see Appendix A). Unfortunately, the imparting of important information does not always bring about a change in behavior. Trying to change a family's values frequently demands a great deal of ingenuity from the nurse.

Applying the Nursing Process in the Home

The nursing process used in home care is no different from that practiced in any other setting. The unique challenges of home care present themselves chiefly in the implementation step. Generally, the differences lie in assessing how the home's unique environment impacts the need or problem and using outcome criteria and mutual participation to plan goals and delineate interventions.

Assessment

In home health care, nursing assessment and data collection center chiefly around the first home visit. This is not to say that nurses do not collect information on an ongoing basis, but because most agencies require the submission of a plan of care within 48 hours of the initial evaluation, the first visit carries tremendous weight. Under ideal circumstances, a preliminary review of background information initiates the assessment process; the reality in home health, however, is that few clients are referred with copies of either their medical records or their discharge summaries. If the client has received home health services in the past, records may be available, but often all the nurse has prior to initiating care is the referral form describing the present problem, some notations about past medical history, and a projection of the skilled interventions needed. Therefore, it falls to the nurse to try to obtain as complete a clinical picture as possible when meeting the client.

Assessment begins when the nurse calls the client to arrange a visit. That telephone call can yield much information to the nurse who pays close attention. How alert, oriented, and stressed does the client (and/or family) seem to be? Does the client know the reason for the home health referral? How open to intervention do the client and family seem to be? Have they encountered any difficulties since discharge from the prior setting? Are there any supplies they need on the first visit?

During the visit, much of the assessment process centers around collecting the information requested on the tools and forms contained in the agency's admission packet. Many such packets include a physical and psychosocial database; a medication sheet; forms for pain assessment, spiritual assessment, and financial assessment; and a family roster. It is extremely important that the data collected be as complete and accurate as possible and reflect subjective, objective, current, and historical information. Through interviewing, direct observation, and physical assessment, the nurse can achieve the goal of the initial visit, namely, to gain as clear and accurate a clinical picture of the client as possible.

Diagnosis

Once the initial assessment is completed, the nurse must then identify the real and/or potential client problems that emerge from the data. Within some agencies problems are identified by using the approved listing of nursing diagnoses published by the North American Nursing Diagnosis Association (NANDA); in other agencies, problems are identified from the gathered information using the PES system. No matter which method is used, meaningful statements describing the client's issues, based on data collection, must be part of the home health record both to organize care and to justify reimbursement.

In almost all home care situations, Knowledge Deficit is an appropriate nursing diagnosis. The box on page 64 lists some nursing interventions for *Knowledge Deficit* specific to a client with Alzheimer's disease and the client's family.

Interventions for the Nursing Diagnosis Knowledge Deficit

▪ ▪ ▪

Nursing Diagnosis

Knowledge Deficit related to lack of information about Alzheimer's disease process and care

Outcome Criteria

- Short term: Adequate knowledge, as evidenced by family's stating disease progression and treatment (expected within 1 week)
- Long term: Adequate knowledge, as evidenced by family following the recommended interventions throughout illness course (within 1 month) or by discharge from home health

Nursing Interventions

1. Alert the family to both environmental hazards and client habits that could threaten safety. (first visit)
2. Provide the family with specific recommendations for keeping the client safe, for example, serving foods warm, not hot; allowing client to eat with fingers; cutting food in small pieces; wearing an ID bracelet; discouraging daytime sleep. (first visit)
3. Discuss the disease course (degenerative), the prognosis (incurable), typical issues of concern (promoting adequate nutrition, activity, rest, safety, and independence; supporting cognitive function; communication, socialization, and family caregiving; the supportive care available; and the ultimate need for long-term placement with disease progression. (first visit)
4. Discuss local resources, including adult day care, support groups, and Alzheimer's Disease Association. Give family a list of these resources. (first visit)

5. Include all family members or significant persons in teaching and planning care. (each visit)
6. Prepare the family for typical types of Alzheimer's disease behaviors: forgetfulness, disorientation, agitation, screaming, crying, physical or verbal abuse, accusations of infidelity. (subsequent visits)
7. Teach the family specific interventions for dealing with these behaviors: calm, unhurried manner, music, stroking, rocking, structuring the environment, distracting the client. (subsequent visits)
8. Stress the importance of both exercise and recreation in terms of quality of life and decreasing nighttime restlessness. (subsequent visits)
9. Reinforce the client's continued needs for socialization and intimacy. (subsequent visits)
10. Suggest specific interventions for meeting socialization needs: limiting visitors to one or two at a time, pet therapy, use of the phone. (subsequent visits)
11. Research and suggest useful interventions that are described in the literature and/or that are utilized in more formal Alzheimer's disease settings and may also be helpful in the home. (subsequent visits)
    a. Keep the environment safe for the client.
    b. Use reality orientation with client several times a day, and post clocks, calendars, and telephone numbers within easy sight of the client.
    c. Give client simple directions, using simple sentences and a quiet, monotonal voice so as not to excite the client.
    d. Allow the use of the telephone, because calls will help orient the client.
    e. Permit hoarding. Permit behaviors linked to past life.

Note. Some material in this care plan is adapted from *Home Health Nursing Care Plans* by Marie S. Jaffe and Linda Skidmore-Roth, 1988, St Louis: Mosby.

Planning

Planning in home health includes setting priorities, establishing goals, and deciding on intervention strategies designed to meet the needs of the client. Advice from experts indicates that the greatest level of success is achieved when clients feel an ownership of the suggested plan (Pesznecker et al., 1989). For this reason, planned

interventions and outcome criteria should be client centered, realistic, achievable, and mutually agreed on (Carey, 1989). The nurse works with the client to

1. Identify significant issues and needs.
2. Set mutually agreed-upon goals.
3. Make and initiate acceptable plans to meet them.

How to Set Mutually Acceptable Goals with Clients

■ ■ ■

- Do not assume that by virtue of your expertise and knowledge you know what is best for clients.

- Recognize that clients have the ultimate responsibility for managing their own lives.

- Own your values, but realize that they are not necessarily shared by others, nor are they superior to the values of others.

- Send a message of respect. If you respect the client, then you should trust that the client has the ability to determine what is best and to make good decisions based on what the client believes.

- Accept people as they are. Work *with* families rather than working *on* them.

- Remember that people generally resist being told what to do.

- Recall that people who make their own decisions tend to be accountable for them.

- Prepare yourself to feel angry when clients make choices that diverge from your value system and expertise, or when clients expend less energy and exhibit less ability than you expect.

- Learn both to understand your feelings and to avoid expressing them inappropriately.

- Use a process to set mutually acceptable goals. Ask families what they feel they want or need to work on; alternatively, share your assessment data, suggest possible goals, and use these as a starting point to which the family can react.

Note. Ideas extracted from "How Values Affect the Mutual Goal-setting Process with Multiproblem Families" by R. Carey, 1989, *Journal of Community Health Nursing, 6*(1), pp. 7–14.

The accompanying box provides guidelines for setting goals with clients.

Goals and outcome criteria also should be stated to clients and documented clearly and concisely, in timed, measurable, and observable terms. These measures help clients and care providers better focus their work together and appraise the effectiveness of care. In addition, outcome criteria provide the reimbursement source a measurable standard from which to judge the appropriateness of the plan of care.

Implementation

The home health nurse implements most of the intervention strategies arrived at in the planning stage. However, some of the interventions may be carried out by another agency provider, by a paraprofessional introduced into the setting by the nurse case manager, or by the client.

Nurses and clients reach an agreement about the implementation of care through a process called **contracting**, the negotiation of a cooperative working agreement between the nurse and client that is continuously renegotiated (Sloan & Schummer, 1975). Contracting is a concept used often in, but not exclusive to, many home and community health settings. Contracting can occur both formally and informally. It involves an exploration of a need, establishment of goals, evaluation of resources, development of a plan, division of responsibilities, agreement of a time frame, and, finally, evaluation or termination. Contracting requires the nurse to relinquish control as the expert and consider the client as an equal partner in the process.

Obviously, contracting is not appropriate with all clients. It is certainly inadvisable if the nurse-client relationship is to be short lived (no more than two visits) or if the client has limited cognitive abilities. However, contracting is useful for clients who demonstrate a willingness to be active participants in their health care. It is certainly empowering, can save time, and keeps the nursing goals directed and focused.

The box on page 66 provides an example of verbal contracting.

Evaluation

Evaluation in home health is both formative and summative. *Formative evaluation* is the systematic ongoing comparison of the plan of care with the goals actually being achieved from visit to visit. In *summative evaluation*, the nurse reviews the total plan of care and the client's progress toward goals in order to determine the client's eligibility for discharge.

Reimbursement guidelines may be helpful in driving the evaluation process. Because reimbursement sources require that all skilled services be justified, many home health agencies have designed their clinical notes to include areas for evaluation of the client's response to the visit's interventions and documentation of a plan of care for the next scheduled visit.

Specialized Home Care Nursing

■ ■ ■

High-Technology Home Care

The changes responsible for the growth of the home care industry itself have also brought about a new subspe-

Contracting

■ ■ ■

Nurse: Mr. Ford, your mother is no longer safe alone in her home and requires help performing many of her activities of daily living. I can initiate home health aide services three times a week for 2 hours a day under Medicare, but she will need more assistance than that. Services beyond what Medicare provides must be contracted for by you on a private-pay basis.

Mr. Ford: Can you arrange that for us?

Nurse: I can give you a list of agencies here in the community that provide home health aide services, and I can recommend the ones that our clients have used successfully in the past, but the responsibility for choosing a service and negotiating hours and fees belongs to the family.

Mr. Ford: I really don't know much about this. I'd really feel better if you did this for us.

Nurse: Mr. Ford, why don't the two of us discuss your mother's needs so that you'll have a clearer understanding of what type of help you want to try to arrange. I can tell you about the local agencies we frequently refer our clients to, and I can give you suggestions about what questions to ask. We can also discuss the typical costs involved. This way, when you call to make inquiries, you'll be equipped with the right information.

Mr. Ford: I still would rather you do this.

Nurse: Mr. Ford, this is something the family must do. What I will do is teach whomever you hire what they will need to know about caring for your mother. Can we agree that by my next visit, you will have made some inquiries and will be ready to discuss what agency will best meet your family's situation?

Mr. Ford: All right. I'll start making some calls. Give me 2 or 3 days.

Nurse: Fine, then I'll plan for a longer visit Thursday so we can discuss what you find out.

cialty, high-technology home care. Therapies that in the past could be performed only in acute care settings and required prolonged hospital stays now are being performed consistently at home. This trend is expected to increase because of the cost-effectiveness of high-technology home care and the development of advanced equipment technology that has simplified such cumbersome equipment as ventilators, monitors, suction machines, intravenous pumps, nebulizers, and dialysis machines (Lindeman, 1992). Some of the treatments involved in high-technology home care include enteral feedings, intravenous therapy (chemotherapy, antibiotic therapy, pain management, hyperalimentation, and hydration therapy), oxygen therapy, phototherapy, tracheostomy care, home ventilation, and renal dialysis.

The benefits of high-technology care in the home are easily identifiable and include increased client comfort and lower financial costs. There are liabilities, however, and the decision to recommend high-technology home care should not be made without careful consideration. Commitment is necessary for everyone involved—client, nurse, and physician. Safety factors in the environment and the physical, mental, and emotional resources of the family are critical considerations. The availability of the proper equipment is important; not every family lives in an area where the technology is both available and can be routinely serviced. Teaching is also critical. Because the family's ability to use the equipment is related to the knowledge and the skill of the person doing the teaching, a technically skilled resource person must be available.

Specialized high-technology home care agencies have developed in response to these new needs. In some cases, clients are managed exclusively by these groups. In others, the high-technology agency works in coordination with a home health agency or hospice. In the latter situation, the primary nurse case manager assumes responsibility for the client's care, and the high-technology nurse acts as a consultant. Although the responsibility for teaching is often shared, it is the primary nurse who usually maintains the therapy once initiated, monitors the client's response to treatment, assesses the family's management in the home, maintains the bulk of documentation, and acts as a liaison between client, family, physician, agency personnel, and the equipment suppliers.

High-technology machinery, with its numerous strange sounds and alarms, can produce anxiety in many clients (especially older adults). Often, the greatest nursing challenge is to demystify the technology and bring a sense of calm management to the setting (Figure 3–3).

Hospice Care

Hospice care is another subspecialty of home care. The hospice originated in medieval times as a place for weary travelers to seek refuge on their journeys. Hospice care in the United States began with a home care program in New Haven, Connecticut, in 1974 modeled after the world-renowned Saint Christopher's Hospice in London.

Hospice care generally refers to "a way of caring for people near the end of their journey through life, faced with dying and in need of refuge" (Vines & Hartzell, 1981). Hospice care blends expertise in pain and symptom management with traditional principles of compassion, individualized care, and concern for dignity (Humphrey & Milone-Nuzzo, 1991). Although hospice care can and is provided in inpatient facilities and acute care settings, the model for hospice care in the United States has become hospice home care.

Hospice nursing requires a firm foundation in home health principles, the ability to function as a member of an interdisciplinary team, and a special sensitivity for and aptitude in dealing with the emotional issues that center around the dying. The interdisciplinary team includes physicians, nurses, social workers, home health aides, pastoral ministers, and volunteers focusing on the physical, psychologic, social, economic, and spiritual needs of the client and family. Promoting quality of life is the principal concern. Twenty-four-hour, 7-day-a-week availability is considered critical to hospice care. So too is bereavement follow-up that usually lasts up to 1 year following the death of the client (or until services are no longer needed).

In 1973, a special reimbursement plan for hospice care was developed by Medicare because it was recognized that the regulations and restrictions mandated by the traditional Medicare benefit did not adequately address the needs of the terminally ill. Through informed consent, the Medicare Hospice Benefit is now available to any person with a terminal diagnosis, a prognosis of 6 months or less, and a physician's referral. The Medicare Hospice Benefit covers nursing and other support services, therapies considered necessary by the hospice team, prescription drugs related to the terminal illness, and medical equipment. Although the Medicare Hospice Benefit can be utilized in an inpatient setting, it is most often utilized to reimburse hospice services delivered in the home.

It is the mission of hospice home care and the nurse to assist the family in their efforts to care for their dying loved one at home. For this reason, the goal of every hospice nurse is twofold: to help clients and their families achieve the experience they desire during this final journey and to be present in such a way as to make their journey less lonely.

AIDS Home Care

The first acquired immune deficiency syndrome (AIDS) home care and hospice program in the United States was established by the Visiting Nurses and Hospice of San Francisco in 1984. At that time, the average daily census was 18. In 1992, the average daily census exceeded 240. Today there are many programs specializing in the home and hospice care of AIDS clients. In addition, most of the same programs that care for clients for a variety of other illnesses also care for clients with AIDS.

Nursing management of the AIDS client in the home includes acute care, chronic care, and hospice care. Although many of the goals and interventions vary accord-

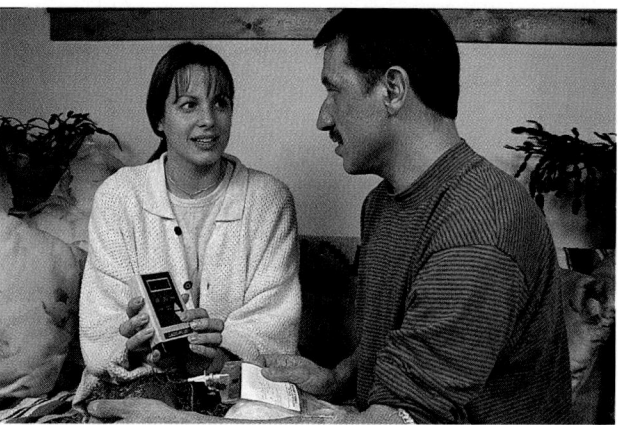

Figure 3–3 Demystifying high-technology home care equipment is a nursing challenge. Here, a nurse demonstrates the use of a patient-controlled analgesia (PCA) pump used in management of chronic pain.

ing to the stage of illness, care always centers around support and education of the client and family. See Chapter 8 for a discussion of specific nursing interventions for the client with AIDS.

Bibliography

■ ■ ■

American College of Physician Health and Public Policy Committee (1986). Home health care position paper. *Annals of Internal Medicine, 105,* 454–460.

American Nurses Association. (1986). *Standards for Home Health Nursing Practice.* Kansas City, MO: ANA.

———. (1986). *Standards for Community Health Nursing.* Kansas City, MO: ANA.

Anderson, K. (1992). Deceptive documentation in home healthcare nursing. *Home Healthcare Nurse, 10*(6), 31–35.

Bayer, M. (1973). Community diagnosis through sight, sense and sound. *Nursing Outlook, 21*(11), 712–713.

Berg, C. & Helgeson, D. (1984). That first home visit. *Journal of Community Health Nursing, 1*(3), 207–215.

Brent, N. (1994). Healthcare reform: Implications for home health care nursing and agencies. *Home Healthcare Nurse, 12*(1), 10–11.

Burbach, C. & Brown, B. (1988). Community health and home health nursing: Keeping the concepts clear. *Nursing and Health Care, 9*(2), 97–100.

Carey, R. (1989). How values affect the mutual goal setting process with multiproblem families. *Journal of Community Health Nursing, 6*(1), 7–14.

Carr, P. (1989). Priorities. *Home Healthcare Nurse, 6*(6), 42–44.

———. (1990). Needs to know, wants to know, ought to know. *Home Healthcare Nurse, 8*(4), 34.

Carson, V. B. (1989). *Spiritual Dimensions of Nursing Practice.* Philadelphia: WB Saunders.

Caserta, J. E. (1989). Families. *Home Healthcare Nurse, 9*(3),5.

Clark, M.J. (1991). The home visit process. In *Nursing in the Community* (pp. 143–159). Norwalk, CT: Appleton & Lange.

Collopy, B., Dubler, N., & Zuckerman, C. (1990). The ethics of home care: Autonomy and accommodation. *Hastings Center Report, 20*(2), 1–14.

Eisdorfer, C. (1991). Caregiving: An emerging risk factor for emotional and physical pathology. *Bulletin of the Menninger Clinic, 55,* 238–247.

Ferrell, B., Rhiner, M., Cohen, M. Z., & Grant, M. (1991). Pain as a metaphor for illness. Part I: Impact of cancer pain on family caregivers. *Oncology Nursing Forum, 18*(8), 1303–1308.

Garvey, E., & Logue, J. (1988). The community health nurse in home health and hospice care. In Stanhope, M. & Lancaster, J. (eds.), *Community Health Nursing: Process and practice for promoting health.* St Louis, Mosby.

Green, J., & Diggers, B. (1989). All visiting nurses are not alike: Home health and community health nursing. *Journal of Community Health Nursing, 6*(2), 83–93.

Gubrium, J., & Sankar, A. (1990). *The Home Care Experience: Ethnography and Policy.* Newberry Park, CA: Sage Publications.

Harris, M. D. (1988). *Home Health Administration.* Owings Mills, MD: National Health Publishing.

Hellwig, K. (1990). Health teaching: The crux of home care nursing. *Home Healthcare Nurse, 8*(4), 35–37.

Hewner, S. (1986). Bringing home the health care. *Journal of Gerontological Nursing, 12*(2), 29–34.

Humphrey, C. (1988). The home as the setting for practice: Clarifying the boundaries of practice. *Nursing Clinics of North America, 23*(2), 305–314.

Humphrey, C., & Milone-Nuzzo, P. (1991). *Home Care Nursing: An orientation to practice.* Norwalk, CT: Appleton & Lange.

Jaffe, M. S., & Skidmore-Roth, L. (1988). *Home Health Nursing Care Plans.* St Louis, Mosby.

Keeling, B. (March 1978). Making the most of the first home visit. *Nursing 78,* 24–28.

Knollmueller, R. (1993). The role of prevention in home health care nursing practice. *Home Healthcare Nurse, 11*(1), 21–23.

Leahy, K. M., Cobb, M. M., & Jones, M. C. (1982). *Community Health Nursing.* St Louis, Mosby.

Lentz, J. R., & Meyer, E. A. (1979). The dirty house. *Nursing Outlook, 27*(9), 590–593.

Lindeman, C. (1992). Nursing and technology, moving into the 21st century. *Caring Magazine, 11*(9), 5–10.

Matthis, E. (1991). Family caregivers want education for their caregiving roles. *Home Health Care 10*(4), 19–22.

Medicare Home Health Agency Manual. Pub. 11. (April, 1989). Washington, DC: Home Care Financing Adminstration.

Morgan, K., & McClain, S. (1993). *Core Curriculum for Home Health Care Nursing.* Gaithersburg, MD: Aspen Publishers.

Morra, M. E. (1985). Making choices: The consumer's perspective. *Cancer Nursing, 8*(Suppl. 1), 54–59.

National Association for Home Care. (1987). *National Association for Home Care Definition.* Washington, DC: National Association for Home Care.

——— . (1993). *Basic Statistics About Home Care, 1993.* Washington, DC: National Association for Home Care.

Pesznecker, B., Zerwekh, J., & Horn, B. (1989). The mutual participation relationship: Key to facilitating self-care practices in client and families. *Public Health Nursing, 6*(4), 197–203.

Price, J., & Braden, C. (1978). The reality of home visits. *American Journal of Nursing, 78*(9), 1536–1538.

Pruitt, R., Keller, L., & Hale, S. (1987). Mastering distractions that mar home visits. *Nursing and Health Care, 8*(6), 345–347.

Quinn, J. (1992). Holding sacred space: The nurse as healing environment. *Holistic Nursing Practice, 4*(6), 26–36.

Redman, B. D. (1988). The place of patient education in healthcare. In *The Process of Patient Education* p. 1. St. Louis, Mosby.

Rubenstein, R. (1990). Culture and disorder in the home care experience: The home as sickroom. In Gubrium, J. & Sankar, A. (eds.) *The home care experience: ethnography and policy.* (pp. 37–57). Newberry Park, CA: Sage Publications.

Sloan, M. R., & Schummer, B. T. (1975). The process of contracting in community nursing. In Spradley, V., (ed.), *Contemporary Community Nursing.* Boston: Little, Brown.

Smith, J. B. (1987). Home care is more than Medicare regs. *American Journal of Nursing, 87*(3), 305–306.

Stanhope, M. & Lancaster, J. (1988). *Community health nursing: process and practice for promoting health.* St Louis, Mosby.

Stulginsky, M. M. (1993a). Nurses' home health experience—Part I: The practice setting. *Nursing and Healthcare, 14*(8), 402–407.

——— . (1993b). Nurses' home health experience—Part II: The unique demands of home visits. *Nursing and Healthcare, 14*(9), 476–485.

Taylor, B. (1992). Relieving pain through ordinariness in nursing: A phenomenologic account of a comforting nurse-patient encounter. *Advanced Nursing Science, 15*(1), 33–43.

US Department of Health and Human Services. (1991). *Health personnel in the U. S.: eighth report to congress.* DHHS No. HRS-P-00-92-1. Rockville, MD: US Government Printing Office.

Vines, E., & Hartzell, D. H. (March 1981). The hospice movement in the United States. *National Health Standards and Quality Information Clearinghouse Information Bulletin.*

Wasik, B., Bryant, D., & Lyons, C. (1990). Philosophy of home visiting. In *Home visiting: procedures for helping families* pp. 45–68. Newberry Park, CA: Sage Publications.

Weinstein, S. (1993). A coordinated approach to home infusion care. *Home Healthcare Nurse 11*(1), 15–20.

Zerwekh, J. (1992). Public health nursing legacy: Historical practical wisdom. *Nursing & Healthcare, 13*(2), 84–91.

Zusy, M. J. April 18, 1994. Staying employed in nursing in the nineties. *The Nursing Spectrum,* 5.

Alterations in Patterns of Health

Nursing Care of Clients in Pain

LEARNING OBJECTIVES

After completing this chapter, you will be able to

- Give a variety of definitions of pain and terminology related to pain.
- Discuss the pain experience, including the anatomic and physiologic bases of pain.
- Discuss the theories of pain transmission and perception.
- Compare and contrast five types of pain.
- Discuss a variety of factors that may affect a client's response to pain.

- Explore several myths and misconceptions about pain.
- Discuss collaborative measures to reduce or relieve pain, including pharmacology, surgery, and others.
- Describe pain rating scales and their use in assessing pain.
- Explain how relaxation, distraction, and cutaneous stimulation may be helpful in reducing or relieving pain.
- Use the nursing process as a framework for providing individualized nursing care for clients experiencing pain.

Pain is a subjective response to both physical and psychologic stressors. All people feel pain at some point during their lives. Although pain typically is experienced as uncomfortable and unwelcome, it also serves a powerful protective role, warning of potentially health-threatening conditions. Each individual pain event is a distinct and personal experience that is influenced by physiologic, psychologic, cognitive, sociocultural, and spiritual factors. Pain is the symptom most associated with describing oneself as ill, and it is the most common reason for seeking health care.

Pain presents a difficult challenge to caregivers because it is a subjective phenomenon that has no reliable objective indicators. As health care providers, nurses commonly assess objective manifestations, such as blood pressure, laboratory values, or skin color. In contrast, to assess pain, nurses must rely on the verbal report and

nonverbal cues of the client as the most critical indicators of the type, location, duration, and intensity of pain.

Nurses have the responsibility to minimize or eliminate pain, based on standards established by the US Department of Health and Human Services (1992). The guidelines serve as the basis for nursing care of all clients with pain. The goals of the pain management standards are to

- Reduce the incidence and severity of clients' postoperative, posttraumatic, or illness-related pain.
- Educate clients about the need to communicate unrelieved pain so that they can receive prompt evaluation and effective treatment.
- Enhance client comfort and satisfaction.
- Reduce postoperative complications and, in some cases, shorten stays after surgical procedures.

Definitions of Pain

■ ■ ■

There are many accepted definitions of pain. The International Association for Study of Pain (1979) described pain as an unpleasant sensory and emotional experience associated with actual or potential tissue damage. This widely accepted medical definition of pain is limited by its focus on pain as an indicator of actual or potential tissue damage. However, pain is not always an indicator of tissue damage; psychogenic pain, for example, and some forms of headache pain are not associated with tissue damage. Sternbach (1968) stated that pain is a personal, private sensation of hurt that signals current or impending tissue damage and serves to protect one from harm. Although this definition properly focuses on the personal, private nature of pain, it too is limited in its focus on pain as an indicator of current or impending tissue damage. McCaffery (1979, p. 11) defined pain as "whatever the person experiencing it says it is, and existing whenever the person says it does." This definition acknowledges the client as the only person who can accurately define and describe his or her own pain and serves as the basis for nursing assessment and care of clients in pain. It also supports the values and beliefs about pain necessary for holistic nursing care, including the following:

■ Pain can be experienced only by the person affected; that is, pain has a personal meaning.

■ If the client says he or she has pain, the client is in pain. All pain is real.

■ Pain has physical, emotional, cognitive, sociocultural, and spiritual dimensions.

■ Pain affects the whole body, usually negatively.

■ Pain may serve as both a response to and a warning of actual or potential trauma.

Neurophysiology of Pain

■ ■ ■

Nerve receptors for pain are called *nociceptors*. They are located at the ends of small afferent neurons and are woven throughout all the tissues of the body except the brain. Nociceptors are especially numerous in the skin and muscles.

Stimuli

Pain occurs when nociceptors are stimulated by biologic, mechanical, thermal, electrical, or chemical factors (Table 4–1). The intensity and duration of the stimuli determine the sensation; long-lasting, intense stimulation produces

Table 4–1	Pain Stimuli
Causative Factor	**Example**
Microorganisms (e.g., bacteria, viruses)	Meningitis
Inflammation	Sore throat
Impaired blood flow	Angina
Invasive tumor	Colon cancer
Radiation	Radiation for cancer
Heat	Sunburn
Obstruction	Kidney stone
Spasm	Colon cramping
Compression	Carpal tunnel syndrome
Decreased movement	Pain after cast removal
Stretching or straining	Sprained ankle
Fractures	Fractured hip
Swelling	Arthritis
Deposits of foreign tissue	Endometriosis
Chemicals	Skin rash
Electricity	Electrical burn
Conflict, difficulty in life	Psychogenic pain

greater pain than does brief, mild stimulation. Nociceptors are stimulated either by direct damage to the cell or by the local release of biochemicals secondary to cell injury. *Bradykinin*, an amino acid, appears to be the most abundant and potent pain-producing chemical; other biochemical sources of pain include prostaglandins, histamine, hydrogen ions, and potassium ions. It is believed that in response to noxious stimuli, these biochemicals bind to nociceptors, causing them to initiate pain impulses.

Pain Pathway

The neural pathway of pain is illustrated in Figure 4–1 and is summarized as follows:

1. Pain is perceived by the nociceptors in the periphery of the body, for example, in the skin or viscera. Cutaneous pain is transmitted through small afferent A-delta and even smaller C nerve fibers to the spinal cord. *A-delta fibers* are myelinated and transmit impulses rapidly. They produce sharp, well-defined pain sensations, such as those that result from cuts, electric shocks, or the impact of a blow. A-delta fibers are associated with acute pain. *C fibers* are not myelinated and thus transmit pain impulses more slowly. The pain from deep body structures (such as

Figure 4–1 *A*, Cutaneous nociceptors generate pain impulses that pass via A-delta and C fibers to spinal cord's dorsal horn. *B*, Secondary neurons in dorsal horn pass impulses across spinal cord to anterior spinothalamic tract. *C*, Slow pain impulses ascend to the thalamus, while fast pain impulses ascend to the cerebral cortex. The reticular formation in the brainstem integrates the emotional, cognitive, and autonomic responses to pain.

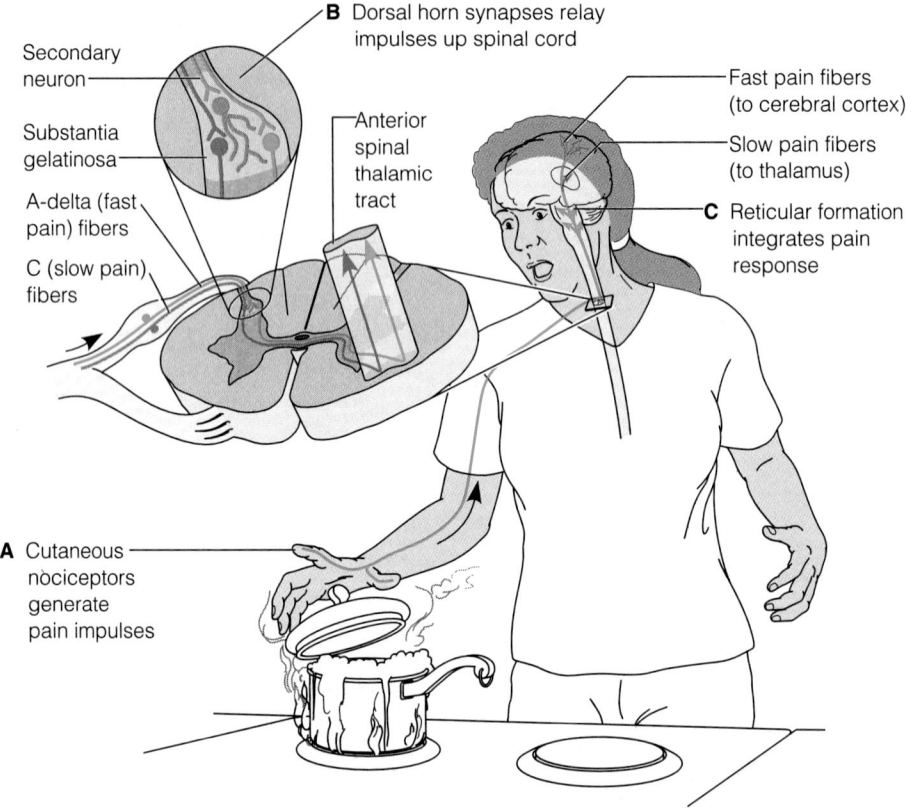

muscles and viscera) is primarily transmitted by C fibers, producing diffuse burning or aching sensations. C fibers are associated with chronic pain. Both A-delta and C fibers are involved in most injuries. For example, if a person bangs the elbow, A-delta fibers transmit this pain stimulus within 0.1 second. The person feels this pain as a sharp, localized, smarting sensation. One or more seconds after the blow, the person experiences a duller, aching, diffuse sensation of pain impulses carried by the C fibers.

2. Secondary neurons transmit the impulses from the afferent neurons through the dorsal horn of the spinal cord, where they synapse in the *substantia gelatinosa*. The impulses then cross over to the anterior and lateral spinothalamic tracts.

3. The impulses ascend the anterior and lateral spinothalamic tracts and pass through the medulla and midbrain to the thalamus.

4. In the thalamus and cerebral cortex, the pain impulses are perceived, described, localized, and interpreted, and a response is formulated. A noxious impulse becomes pain when the sensation reaches conscious levels and is perceived and evaluated by the person experiencing the sensation.

Some pain impulses ascend along the paleospinothalamic tract in the medial section of the spinal cord. These impulses enter the reticular formation and the limbic systems, which integrate emotional and cognitive responses to pain. Interconnections in the autonomic nervous system may also cause an autonomic response to the pain. In addition, deep nociceptors often converge on the same spinal neuron, resulting in pain that is experienced in a part of the body other than its origin.

Inhibitory Mechanisms

Efferent fibers run from the reticular formation and midbrain to the substantia gelatinosa in the dorsal horns of the spinal cord. Along these fibers, pain may be inhibited or modulated. The *analgesia system* is a group of midbrain neurons that transmits impulses to the pons and medulla, which in turn stimulate a pain inhibitory center in the dorsal horns of the spinal cord. The exact nature of this inhibitory mechanism is unknown.

The most clearly defined chemical inhibitory mechanism is fueled by *endorphins* (endogenous morphines), naturally occurring opioid peptides present in neurons in the brain, spinal cord, and gastrointestinal tract. Endorphins in the brain are released in response to afferent noxious stimuli, whereas endorphins in the spinal cord are released in response to efferent impulses. Endorphins work by binding with opiate receptors on the neurons to inhibit pain impulse transmission (Figure 4–2).

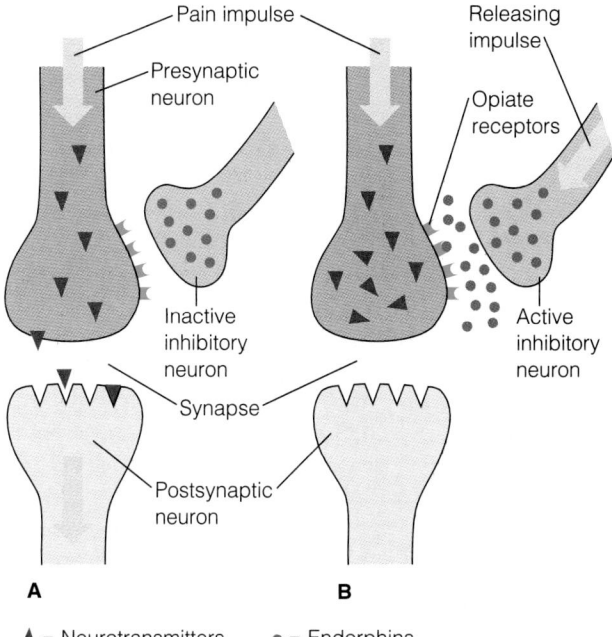

A = Neurotransmitters   **●** = Endorphins

Figure 4–2   *A*, Pain impulse causes presynaptic neuron to release burst of neuro-transmitters across synapse. These bind to postsynaptic neuron and propagate impulse. *B*, Inhibitory neuron releases endorphins, which bind to presynaptic opiate receptors. Neurotransmitter release is inhibited, and pain impulse interrupted.

Theories of Pain

■ ■ ■

Several theories related to pain transmission and modulation have been proposed. The theories discussed in this chapter are the specificity theory, the pattern theory, and the gate-control theory.

Specificity Theory

The most widely accepted theory of pain transmission through the end of the 19th century, the **specificity theory,** advances the idea that the body's neurons and pathways for pain transmission are as specific and unique as those for other body senses, such as taste or touch. The specificity theory proposes that free nerve endings in the skin act as pain receptors, accept sensory input, and transmit this input along highly specific nerve fibers. These fibers synapse in the dorsal horns of the spinal column, and cross over to the anterior and lateral spinothalamic tracts. The pain impulses then ascend to the thalamus and cerebral cortex, where painful sensations are perceived. This is a simplification of the pathway discussed earlier and shown in Figure 4–1. It is important to note that the specificity theory does not explain the differences in pain perception among individuals, nor does it satisfactorily account for the effect of psychologic variables, the effect of previous experience with pain, phantom limb pain, or peripheral neuralgias.

Pattern Theory

The **pattern theory,** proposed in the early 1900s, identifies two major types of pain fibers: rapidly conducting fibers and slowly conducting fibers. (Recall the A-delta and C fibers discussed earlier.) The stimulation of these fibers forms a "pattern." This theory also introduces the concept of *central summation:* Peripheral impulses from many fibers of both types are combined at the level of the spinal cord, and from there a summation of these impulses ascends to the brain for interpretation. This theory, like the specificity theory, does not account for individual perceptual differences or psychologic factors.

Gate-Control Theory

The **gate-control theory** suggests that pain and its perception are determined by the interaction of two systems (Melzack & Wall, 1965, 1968). The first of these interrelated systems is the substantia gelatinosa in the dorsal horns of the spinal cord. The substantia gelatinosa regulates impulses entering or leaving the spinal cord. The second system is an inhibitory system within the brain stem.

As discussed earlier, small-diameter A-delta and C fibers carry fast and slow pain impulses. In addition, large-diameter A-beta fibers carry impulses for tactile stimulation from the skin. In the substantia gelatinosa, these impulses encounter a "gate" thought to be opened and closed by the domination of either the large-diameter touch fibers or the small-diameter pain fibers. If impulses along the small-diameter pain fibers outnumber impulses along the large-diameter touch fibers, the gate is open, and pain impulses travel unimpeded to the brain. If impulses from the touch fibers predominate, they will close the gate, and the pain impulses will be "turned away" at the gate (Figure 4–3). This explains why massaging a stubbed toe can reduce the intensity and duration of the pain.

The second system described by the gate-control theory is thought to be located in the brain stem. It is believed that cells in the midbrain, activated by a variety of factors, such as opiates, psychologic factors, or even simply the presence of pain itself, signal receptors in the medulla. These receptors in turn stimulate nerve fibers in the spinal cord to block the transmission of pain fibers. It is hypothesized that this brain stem regulatory system may help explain why even severe pain may not be perceived under certain circumstances, such as when an athlete fails to notice an injury until the competition is over.

Recent research has shown that the control and modulation of pain is much more complex than the description

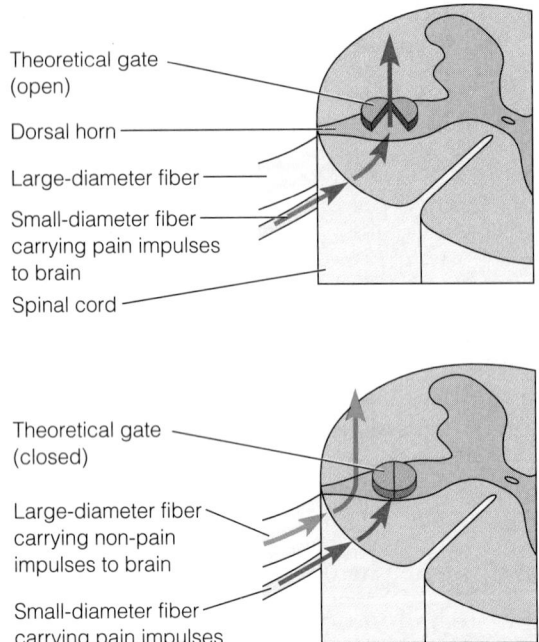

Figure 4–3 The spinal cord component of the gate-control theory. Pain transmission by small-diameter fibers is blocked when large-diameter fibers carrying touch impulses dominate, closing the gate in the substantia gelatinosa.

set forth in the gate-control theory. Tactile information is now known to be transmitted by both large- and small-diameter fibers, and significant interactions between sensory neurons of various sources is known to occur at multiple levels of the central nervous system (Porth, 1994).

Types of Pain

■ ■ ■

The two major classifications of pain are acute pain and chronic pain. Each of these types of pain has different causes and effects and yields different physical and psychologic responses.

Acute Pain

Acute pain is usually temporary, has a sudden onset, and is localized. Pain that lasts for less than 6 months and has an identified cause is classified as acute pain. It most often results from tissue injury from trauma, surgery, or inflammation. The three major types of acute pain are somatic pain, visceral pain, and referred pain.

Somatic pain arises from nerve receptors originating in the skin or close to the surface of the body. Somatic pain may be either sharp and well localized, or dull and diffuse. It is often accompanied by nausea and vomiting.

Visceral pain arises from body organs. Visceral pain is dull and poorly localized because of the low number of nociceptors. The viscera are sensitive to stretching, inflammation, and ischemia but relatively insensitive to cutting and temperature extremes. Visceral pain is associated with nausea and vomiting, hypotension, and restlessness. It often radiates or is referred.

Referred pain is pain that is perceived in an area distant from the site of the stimuli. It commonly occurs with visceral pain as visceral fibers synapse at the level of the spinal cord, close to fibers innervating other subcutaneous tissue areas of the body (Figure 4–4). Pain in a spinal nerve may be felt cutaneously in any body area innervated by sensory neurons that share that same spinal nerve route. Body areas defined by spinal nerve route are called *dermatomes* (see Chapter 39).

Acute pain serves as a warning of actual or potential injury to tissues. As a stressor, it initiates the fight-or-flight autonomic stress response. Characteristic physical responses occur, including tachycardia, rapid and shallow respirations, increased blood pressure, dilated pupils, sweating, and pallor. In addition, the person experiencing the acute pain responds to this threat with anxiety and fear. This psychologic response may further increase the physical responses to acute pain.

Chronic Pain

Chronic pain is prolonged pain, usually lasting longer than 6 months. It is not always associated with an identifiable cause and is often unresponsive to conventional medical treatment. Unlike acute pain, chronic pain has a much more complex and poorly understood purpose.

Chronic pain can be subdivided into four categories:

- *Recurrent acute pain* is characterized by relatively well defined episodes of pain interspersed with pain-free episodes. Examples of recurrent acute pain include migraine headaches and sickle-cell crises.

- *Ongoing time-limited pain* is identified by a defined time period. Some examples are cancer pain, which ends with control of the disease or death, and burn pain, which ends with rehabilitation or death.

- *Chronic nonmalignant pain*, also known as *chronic benign pain*, is non-life-threatening pain that nevertheless persists beyond the expected time for healing. Chronic lower back pain falls into this category.

- *Chronic intractable nonmalignant pain syndrome* is similar to simple chronic nonmalignant pain but is characterized by the person's inability to cope well with the pain and sometimes by physical, social, and/or psychologic disability resulting from the pain.

The client with chronic pain often is depressed, withdrawn, immobile, irritable, and/or controlling. Although

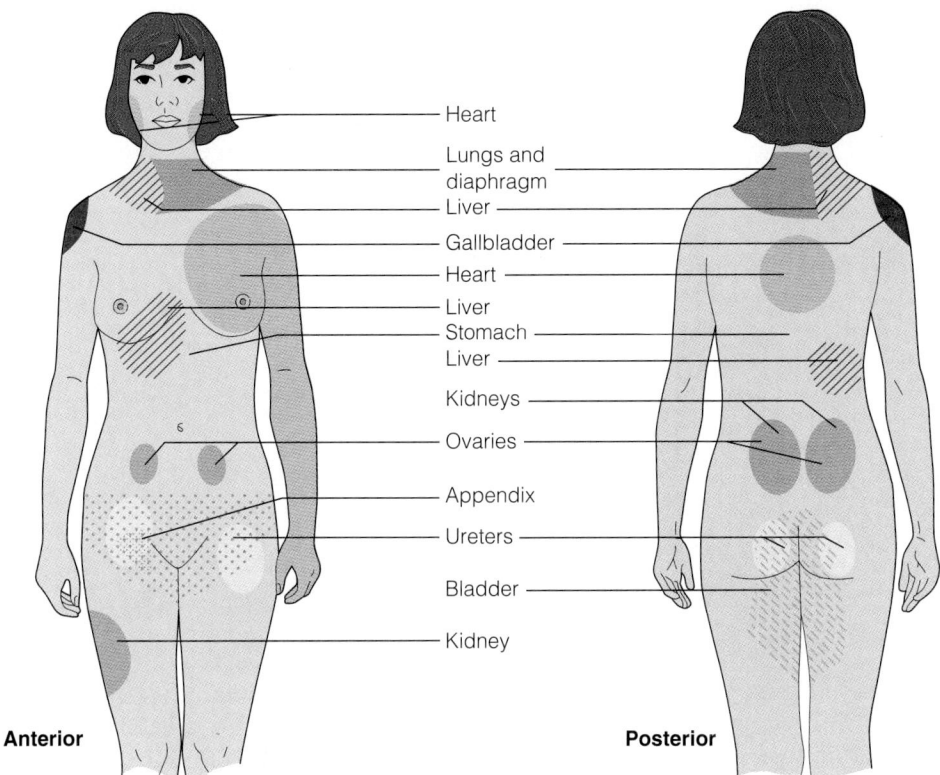

Heart
Lungs and diaphragm
Liver
Gallbladder
Heart
Liver
Stomach
Liver
Kidneys
Ovaries
Appendix
Ureters
Bladder
Kidney

Anterior

Posterior

Figure 4–4   Referred pain is the result of the convergence of sensory nerves from certain areas of the body before they enter the brain for interpretation. For example, a toothache may be felt in the ear, pain from inflammation of the diaphragm may be felt in the shoulder, and pain from ischemia of the heart muscle (angina) may be felt in the left arm.

chronic pain may range from mild to severe and may be continuous or intermittent, the unrelenting presence of the pain often results in the pain itself becoming the pathologic process requiring intervention.

The most common chronic pain condition is lower back pain. Other common chronic pain conditions include the following (McCance & Huether, 1994):

- *Neuralgias* are painful conditions that result from damage to a peripheral nerve caused by infection or disease. Postherpetic neuralgia (following shingles) is an example.

- *Reflex sympathetic dystrophies* are characterized by continuous severe, burning pain. These conditions follow peripheral nerve damage and present the symptoms of pain, vasospasm, muscle wasting, and vasomotor changes (vasodilation followed by vasoconstriction).

- *Hyperesthesias* are conditions of oversensitivity to tactile and painful stimuli. Hyperesthesias result in diffuse pain that is usually increased by fatigue and emotional lability.

- *Myofascial pain syndrome* is a common condition marked by injury to or disease of muscle and fascial tissue. Pain results from muscle spasm, stiffness, and collection of lactic acid in the muscle. Fibromyalgia is an example.

- *Cancer* often produces chronic pain usually due to factors associated with the advancing disease. These fac-

tors include a growing tumor's pressing on nerves or other structures, stretching of viscera, obstruction of ducts, or metastasis to bones. The malignant tumor also may mechanically stimulate pain or the production of biochemicals that cause pain. Pain also may be associated with chemotherapy and radiation therapy.

- *Chronic postoperative pain* is rare but may occur following incisions in the chest wall, radical mastectomy, radical neck dissection, and surgical amputation.

A comparison of the functions of, treatment of, and responses to acute and chronic pain is found in Table 4–2.

Central Pain

Central pain is related to a lesion in the brain that may spontaneously produce high-frequency bursts of impulses that are perceived as pain. Thalamic pain is one of the most common types. Central pain may be caused by a vascular lesion, tumor, trauma, or inflammation. Thalamic pain is severe, spontaneous, and often continuous. Hyperesthesia may occur on the side of the body contralateral to the lesion in the thalamus. Kinesthetic proprioception can also be lost.

Phantom Pain

Phantom pain is a confusing pain syndrome that occurs following surgical or traumatic amputation of a limb. The

Table 4–2   Comparison of Acute and Chronic Pain

Acute Pain	Chronic Pain
May serve to warn client.	May prompt client to seek information about self-care.
May prompt client to seek medical help for condition.	May prompt client to seek medical help for pain relief.
Easily diagnosed with current methods.	May be difficult and confusing to diagnose with current methods.
Treatment available through traditional MD, RN, PT team.	May require a nontraditional multidisciplinary team for management.
Health team is in charge of client.	Self-management is key to recovery.
Pain lasts less than 6 months.	Pain lasts more than 6 months.
Endorphins are stimulated.	Endorphins are depressed.
Blood pressure, pulse, and respiration are increased.	Vital signs are normal.
Pupils are dilated.	Pupils are normal.
Skin is diaphoretic, pale, cool.	Skin is dry, warm, normal color.
Mood is restless, anxious, distressed.	Mood is depressed, despairing.

client experiences pain in the missing body part even though there is complete mental awareness that the limb is gone. This pain may include itching, tingling, or pressure sensations, or it may be more severe, including burning or stabbing sensations. In some cases, the client may describe a sensation that the amputated limb is twisted or cramped. It is thought that this phenomenon may be due to stimulation of the severed nerves at the site of the amputation. Treatment is complex and often unsuccessful.

Psychogenic Pain

Psychogenic pain is pain that is experienced in the absence of any diagnosed physiologic cause or event. Typically psychogenic pain involves a long history of complaints of severe pain. It is thought that the client's emotional needs prompt the pain sensations. Psychogenic pain is real, not pretended, and may in turn lead to physiologic changes, such as muscle tension, which may produce further pain. This condition may result from interpersonal conflicts, a need for support from others, or a desire to avoid a stressful or traumatic situation. Depression is often present, and psychogenic pain may also be present in other family members.

Factors Affecting Client Response to Pain

■ ■ ■

The client's physical response to pain involves specific and often predictable neurologic changes. In fact, everyone has the same *pain threshold;* in other words, everyone perceives pain stimuli at the same stimulus intensity. For example, heat is perceived as painful at 44–46 C, the range at which it begins to damage tissue (Marieb, 1995). What varies, then, is the client's perception of and reaction to pain. The client's response to pain is shaped by multiple and interacting factors, including age, sociocultural influences, emotional state, past experiences with pain, the source and meaning of the pain, and the client's knowledge base. When one describes a person as highly sensitive to pain, one is referring to the person's *pain tolerance,* which is the amount of pain a person can endure before outwardly responding to it. The ability to tolerate pain may be decreased by repeated episodes of pain, fatigue, anger, anxiety, and sleep deprivation. Pain tolerance may be increased by medications, alcohol, hypnosis, warmth, distraction, and spiritual practices.

Age

The age of the person experiencing pain influences that person's perception and expression of pain. The older adult with normal age-related changes in neurophysiology may have decreased perception of sensory stimuli and a higher pain threshold. In addition, chronic disease processes more common in the older adult, such as peripheral vascular disease or diabetes, may interfere with normal nerve impulse transmission. Individuals in this age group may have atypical responses to pain: decreased perception of acute pain, heightened perceptions of chronic pain, and/or increased incidence of referred pain.

Often believing that pain is a part of growing older, the client may ignore pain or self-medicate with over-the-counter medications. As a result of these responses, the older adult is at increased risk of injury or serious illness. Table 4–3 lists some age-related changes and their effects on pain.

Table 4–3   Age-Related Changes and Their Effects on Pain

Factors Related to Aging	Effects	Outcomes
Decreased blood flow	Ischemia, decreases in brain function	Client forgets to take medication
Changes in neurotransmitters related to sleep and mood	Decreased sleep resulting in vulnerability to pain	Greater risk of chronic pain, fatigue, increased withdrawal
Reduced levels of norepinephrine	Lowered transmission of pain	Less likely to notice an injury
Changes in sensory interpretation	Lowered pain sensation	Client may not take appropriate protective action
Decreased peripheral nerve conduction	Lowered response to pain	Not seeking appropriate care
Slowed reaction time	Slower avoidance response	Client receives more serious injury
Reduced movement	Increased risk for muscle wasting	May cause immobility

Sociocultural Influences

Each person's response to pain is strongly influenced by the family, community, and culture. Sociocultural influences affect the way in which a client tolerates pain, interprets the meaning of pain, and reacts verbally and nonverbally to the pain.

For example, if the family of origin believes that males should not cry and must tolerate pain stoically, the male client often will appear withdrawn and will refuse pain medication. If a family encourages open and intense emotional expression, the client may cry freely and appear comfortable requesting pain medication. Cultural standards also teach an individual how much pain to tolerate, what types of pain to report, to whom to report the pain, and what kind of treatment to seek. For example, clients of northern European ancestry may value "being a good patient," which may cause them to avoid "complaining" about their pain, whereas clients of Jewish ancestry may value seeking information about their pain, which may cause them to discuss their pain often and in detail. Note, however, that behaviors vary greatly within a culture and from generation to generation. The nurse should approach each client as an individual, observing the client carefully, taking the time to ask questions, and avoiding assumptions.

The nurse also has a set of sociocultural values and beliefs about pain. If these values and beliefs differ from those of the client, the assessment and management of pain may be based on the values of the nurse rather than on the needs of the client. The nurse must be familiar with ethnic and cultural diversity in pain expression and management and respect cultural differences. It is particularly important to remember that pain behaviors are not an objective indicator of the amount of pain present for any individual client. Finally, most experts agree that cultural differences in the expression of, response to, and interpretation of the meaning of pain need further research.

Emotional Status

The client's emotional status influences the perception of pain. The sensation of pain may be blocked by intense concentration (during sports activities, for example) or may be increased by anxiety or fear. Pain often is increased when it occurs in conjunction with other illnesses or physical discomforts such as nausea or vomiting. Emotional status and the perception of pain also may be altered by the presence or absence of support people or caregivers who genuinely care about pain management.

The association between anxiety and pain is well documented. Anxiety may increase the client's perception of pain, and pain in turn may cause anxiety. In addition, the muscle tension common with anxiety can create its own source of pain. This association explains why nonpharmacologic interventions such as relaxation or guided imagery are helpful in relieving or decreasing pain.

Fatigue and sleeplessness also are related to pain experiences. On the one hand, pain interferes with the person's ability to fall asleep and stay asleep and thus induces fatigue. On the other hand, fatigue can lower the client's pain tolerance.

Depression is clearly linked to pain: Serotonin, a neurotransmitter, is involved in the modulation of pain in the central nervous system. In clinically depressed clients, serotonin is decreased, leading to an increase pain sensations. The reverse is also true: In the presence of pain, depression is quite common.

Finally, a client who perceives advantages from the sick role may be motivated to maintain pain. These advantages, called *secondary gain,* may include support from others or avoidance of disagreeable work.

Past Experiences with Pain

Previous experiences with pain are likely to influence the person's response to a current pain episode. If the person's childhood experiences with pain were responded to appropriately by supportive adults, the adult usually will have a healthy attitude to pain. If, however, the person's developmental experiences with pain have been responded to with exaggerated emotions or neglectful indifference, that person's future responses to pain may be exaggerated or denied. Note that a precise response based on developmental factors is impossible to predict.

The responses of professional caregivers to the person in pain can influence the person's response during the next pain episode. If caregivers respond to the pain with effective strategies and a caring attitude, the client will remain more comfortable during any subsequent pain episode, and the complicating anxiety will be avoided. If, however, the pain is not adequately relieved, or if the client feels that empathetic care was not given, anxiety about the next pain episode sets up the client for a more complex and therefore more painful event.

Source and Meaning

The meaning associated with the pain influences the experience of pain. For example, the pain of labor to deliver a baby is experienced differently from the pain following removal of a major organ for cancer. Because pain is the major signal for health problems, it is strongly linked to all of the associated meanings of health problems, such as disability, loss of role, and death. For this reason, it is important to explain to clients the etiology and prognosis for the pain assessed.

If the client perceives the pain as deserved (e.g., "just punishment for sins"), the client may actually feel relief that the "punishment" has commenced. If the client believes that the pain will relieve him or her from an unrewarding job, dangerous military service, or even stressful social obligations, there may similarly be a feeling of relief. In contrast, pain that is perceived as meaningless—for example, chronic low back pain or the unrelieved pain of arthritis—can cause anxiety and depression.

Knowledge Deficit

A lack of understanding of the source, outcome, and meaning of the pain can contribute negatively to the pain experience. If the client has a clear and accurate perception of the pain, it is far easier for professionals to increase the client's knowledge of both the significance of the pain and the strategies the client can use to diminish discomfort in a timely way. It is important for the staff caring for the client to assess the client's readiness to learn, use methods of teaching the client that are effective for the individual client and family, and evaluate carefully the adequacy of the learning. This teaching must include the process of the pain, its predictable course (if possible), and the proposed plan of care for the client. In addition,

clients are encouraged to communicate preferences for pain relief. Learning how to let significant others know of the presence of pain and how to use their help can also promote the effective management of pain.

Myths and Misconceptions About Pain

■ ■ ■

Among both clients and professionals, myths and misconceptions about pain and its management abound. They present significant problems in addressing the pain. The most common of these myths are included here.

- "Pain is a result, not a cause." According to the traditional view of pain, pain is only a symptom of a condition. However, it is now recognized that unrelieved or poorly relieved pain itself sets up further responses, such as immobility, anger, and anxiety; pain may also delay healing and rehabilitation.

- "Chronic pain is really a masked form of depression." As explained earlier, serotonin plays a chemical role in pain transmission. Serotonin is also the major modulator of depression. Therefore, pain and depression are chemically related, not mutually exclusive. It is quite common to find them coexisting.

- "Narcotic medication is too risky to be used in chronic pain." This common misconception often deprives clients of the most effective source of pain relief. It is true that other methods should be tried first; if, however, they prove ineffective, narcotics should be considered as an appropriate alternative.

- "People who take a lot of drugs at home will need more pain medication in the clinical setting." Sanford and Schlicher (1986) report that clients who take either legal or illegal drugs are no more likely to need additional pain relief than the general population.

- "It is best to wait until a client has pain before giving medication." It is now widely accepted that anticipating pain has a noticeable effect on the amount of pain a client experiences. Offering pain relief before a pain event is well on its way can lessen the pain.

- "Many clients lie about the existence or severity of their pain." Very few clients lie about their pain.

- "The same physical stimulus will produce the same quality, intensity, and duration of pain in different people." As mentioned previously, the threshold for pain is the same for everyone; however, the quality, intensity, and duration of pain vary greatly in different individuals.

- "Postoperative pain is best treated with intramuscular injections." The most commonly used postoperative pain relief for many years was meperidine (Demerol)

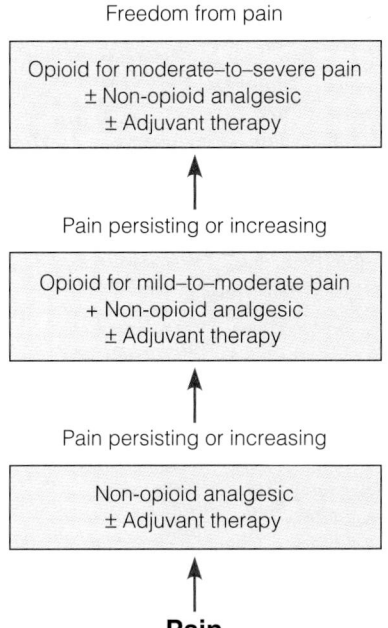

Freedom from pain

Opioid for moderate–to–severe pain
± Non-opioid analgesic
± Adjuvant therapy

Pain persisting or increasing

Opioid for mild–to–moderate pain
+ Non-opioid analgesic
± Adjuvant therapy

Pain persisting or increasing

Non-opioid analgesic
± Adjuvant therapy

Pain

Figure 4–5 The WHO analgesic ladder illustrates the process for selection of analgesic medications for pain management.

given intramuscularly. McCaffery (1987) explains that this was a poor choice because it has many adverse effects, such as irritating tissues and producing the central nervous system (CNS) stimulant normeperidine. In addition, meperidine is short acting. Most contemporary experts do not recommend its use.

These and many other myths and misconceptions continue to place barriers in the way of effective pain relief. It is the nurse's responsibility to explore any data with appropriate research and clinical experience.

Collaborative Care

■ ■ ■

Effective pain relief is a result of collaboration among a variety of health professionals as well as specialized professional groups. *Pain clinics* are discrete centers staffed by a team of health care professionals who use a multidisciplinary approach to managing chronic pain. Therapies may include traditional pharmacologic agents as well as herbs, vitamins, and other dietary supplements; nutritional counseling; psychotherapy; biofeedback; hypnosis; acupuncture; massage; and other treatments. *Hospices* for dying clients also provide a multifaceted approach to pain management.

Pharmacology

Medication is the most common approach to pain management. A variety of drugs with many kinds of delivery

Terms Associated with Pain Medication

■ ■ ■

- *Addiction:* The compulsive use of a substance despite negative consequences, such as health threats or legal problems.
- *Drug abuse:* The use of any chemical substance for other than a medical purpose.
- *Physical drug dependence:* A biologic need for a substance. If the substance is not supplied, physical withdrawal symptoms occur.
- *Psychologic drug dependence:* A psychologic need for a substance. If the substance is not supplied, psychologic withdrawal symptoms occur.
- *Drug tolerance:* The process by which the body requires a progressively greater amount of a drug to achieve the same results.
- *Equianalgesic:* Having the same pain-killing effect when administered to the same individual. Drug dosages are equianalgesic if they have the same effect as morphine sulfate 10 mg administered intramuscularly.
- *Pseudoaddiction:* Behavior involving drug-seeking; a result of receiving inadequate pain relief.

systems are available to the professional pain relief team. These drugs include nonsteroidal anti-inflammatory drugs (NSAIDs), narcotics, synthetic narcotics, antidepressants, and local anesthetic agents. In addition to administering the prescribed medications, the nurse may act independently in choosing the dosage and timing. The nurse is also responsible for assessing the side effects of the medications, evaluating the medication's effectiveness, and providing client teaching. The nurse's role in pain relief is client advocate as well as direct caregiver.

The use of medications is effectively guided by the World Health Organization (WHO) "ladder of analgesia" (WHO, 1986/1990) (Figure 4–5). NSAIDs and narcotic pain medications are used progressively until pain is relieved, a fact that reflects the interactive nature of these two types of analgesics. The box above describes terms associated with pain medication.

Types of Medications
The pharmacologic agents most commonly used in pain relief are the nonsteroidal anti-inflammatory drugs (NSAIDs), narcotics, antidepressants, and local anesthetics.

Table 4–4   Factors to Consider When Selecting an NSAID

Chemical Class	Half Life (Hours)	Time-To-Peak Level (Hours)	Usual Dosing Interval (Times per Day)	Recommended Maximum Daily Dose (Mg)
Salicylates				
Acetylated				
Aspirin	0.25±0.03	1–2	4–6	3600–5400
Aspirin, buffered				
Aspirin, enteric coated				
Aspirin, sustained release				
Nonacetylated				
Choline salicylate (Arthropan)		1–2	4–6	4800–7200
Choline magnesium trisalicylate				
(Trilisate)	2–19	2	1–3	4500
Diflunisal (Dolobid)	13±2	2–3	2	1500
Salsalate (Disalcid)	2–19		2–3	4000
Magnesium salicylate			3–4	various
Sodium salicylate			4–6	various
Propionic Acids				
Fenoprofen (Nalfon)	2.5±0.5	1–2	3–4	3200
Flurbiprofen (Ansaid)	3.8±1.2	1.5	2–4	300
Ibuprofen (Motrin, others)	2±0.5	1–2	3–4	3200
Ketoprofen (Orudis)	1.8±0.3	0.5–2	3–4	300
Ketoprofen SR (Oruvail)	—		1	200
Naproxen (Naprosyn)	14±1	2–4	2	1500
Naproxen sodium (Anaprox)	14±1	1–2	2	1650
Oxaprozin (Daypro)	50–60	NA	1	1800
Acetic Acids				
Diclofenac sodium (Voltaren)	1.1±0.2	2–3	2–4	200
Etodalac (Lodine)	7	2–4	2–4	1200
Indomethacin (Indocin)	2.4±0.4	1–2		200
Indomethacin SR (Indocin SR)	—	2–4		150
Ketoralac (Toradol)	4.5	0.5–1	4–6	40
Sulindac (Clinoril, others)	15±4	2–4	1–2	400
Tolmetin (Tolectin)	4.9±4	0.5–1	3–4	2000
Fenamates (Anthranilic Acids)				
Meclofenamate (Meclomen)	3	0.5–1	4–6	400
Mefenamic acid (Ponstel)	3	2–4	4	1000
Oxicams				
Piroxican (Feldene)	48±8	3–5	1–2	30–40
Nonacidic (Naphthylkanone)				
Nabumetone (Relafon)	26±5	2.5–4	1–2	2000
Pyrazolones				
Phenylbutazone (Butazolidin)	68±25	0.5–1	3–4	400

Note. From "Selecting and Monitoring Nonsteroidal Anti-Inflammatory Drugs" by R. Fischer, 1994, *ADVANCE for Nurse Practitioners, 26.*

Nonsteroidal Anti-Inflammatory Drugs (NSAIDs)
NSAIDs act on peripheral nerve endings and minimize pain by interfering with prostaglandin synthesis. Examples are aspirin, ibuprofen, and indomethacin. NSAIDs are the treatment of choice for mild pain and continue to be effective when combined with narcotics for moderate to severe pain. Factors to consider when selecting an NSAID are provided in Table 4–4. Nursing implications for NSAIDs are found in the accompanying pharmacology box.

Nursing Implications for Pharmacology: Nonsteroidal Anti-Inflammatory Drugs

NSAIDs

aspirin (acetylsalicylic acid)

fenoprofen calcium (Nalfon)

ibuprofen (Motrin)

naproxen sodium (Anaprox)

piroxicam (Feldene)

ketorolac tromethamine (Toradol)

naproxen (Naprosyn)

indomethacin (Indocin)

ketoprofen (Orudis)

sulindac (Clinoril)

The NSAIDs have anti-inflammatory, analgesic, and antipyretic effects. It is believed that they inhibit the enzyme cyclooxygenase, thereby decreasing synthesis of prostaglandins. These drugs provide analgesic effects by reducing inflammation and by perhaps blocking the generation of noxious impulses.

Nursing Responsibilities

- Do not administer aspirin with other NSAIDs.

- Assess and document if the client is taking a hypoglycemic agent or insulin; the NSAIDs may increase the hypoglycemic effect.
- Administer with meals, milk, or a full glass of water to decrease gastric irritation.
- Assess clients who are also taking anticoagulants for bleeding; the NSAIDs increase this risk.

Client and Family Teaching

- Drugs may cause gastrointestinal bleeding (report nausea, vomiting of blood, dark stools), visual disturbances (report blurred or diminished vision), hearing problems, dizziness, skin rash, and renal problems (report weight gain or edema).
- Take medications with meals to decrease gastric irritation.
- Avoid drinking alcohol or taking any over-the-counter drug unless approved by the health care provider.
- The desired effects may not appear for 3–5 days, and the full effects may not appear for 2–4 weeks.
- Maintain regular health care appointments.

Narcotics (Opioids) Narcotics, or opioids, are derivatives of the opium plant. These drugs (and their synthetic forms) are the pharmacologic treatment of choice for moderate to severe pain. Examples are morphine, codeine, and fentanyl. Narcotic analgesics produce analgesia by binding to opioid receptors both within and outside the CNS. A summary of narcotic drugs, their usual dosages, peak effect, and nursing considerations is provided in Table 4–5.

A common myth among health care professionals is that the use of narcotics for pain treatment poses a real threat of addiction. Actually, when the medications are used as recommended, there is little to no risk of addiction. Rather, if pain is not adequately treated, the client may seek more and more narcotic relief, thus increasing the risk of addiction. Nursing implications for narcotics are found in the box on page 83.

Antidepressants Antidepressants within the tricyclic and related chemical groups act on the production and retention of serotonin in the CNS, thus inhibiting pain sensation. They also promote normal sleeping patterns, further alleviating the suffering of the client in pain.

Local Anesthetics Drugs such as benzocaine and zylocaine are part of a large group of substances that block the initiation and transmission of nerve impulses in a local area, thus blocking pain as well. Local anesthetics can be delivered by a variety of methods. They are sometimes used to enable a client to begin moving and using a painful area in order to diminish long-term pain.

Duration of Action

Each of the pharmacologic agents has a unique absorption and duration of action. The nurse caring for the client in pain must understand that no drug will have a wholly predictable course of action, because different clients absorb, metabolize, and excrete medications at different dosage levels. The only way to obtain reliable data about the effectiveness of the medication for the individual client is to assess how that client responds. Therefore, the best choice is to *individualize the dosing schedule.*

The two major descriptors of dosing schedules are around-the-clock (ATC) or as-necessary (PRN). (PRN stands for *pro re nata,* Latin for "as circumstances may require.") ATC administration is appropriate if the client experiences pain constantly and predictably during a 24-hour period. PRN administration is appropriate for pain that is not predictable or constant. PRN medication should be administered as soon as the pain begins.

Table 4–5   Equianalgesic Drug Chart

Analgesic	Dosage (mg)	Peak (min)	Duration (h)	Nursing Considerations
Morphine sulfate	10 IM 30–60 PO	30–60 IM 60–120 PO	4–5 IM 4–5 PO	PO dose is 3–6 times the IM dose. A lower dose may be appropriate for older clients with chronic pain. Contraindicated in clients with acute bronchial asthma or upper-airway obstruction.
Butorphanol tartrate (Stadol)	2 IM N/A PO	30–60 IM	3–4 IM	May cause withdrawal in clients physically dependent on narcotics. May cause hallucinations. Increases cardiac workload. Contraindicated in clients with myocardial infarction.
Codeine	130 IM 200 PO	30–60 IM 60–120 PO	4 IM 4 PO	PO dose is about 1.5 times the IM dose. Often given synergistically with aspirin or acetaminophen for best effect. More toxic in high doses than morphine. Causes more nausea and vomiting than morphine and is constipating.
Hydromorphone HCl (Dilaudid)	1.5 IM 7.5 PO	15–30 IM 30 PO	4 IM 4 PO	PO dose is 5 times IM dose. Shorter acting than morphine. May cause loss of appetite. Contraindicated in clients with increased intracranial pressure or status asthmaticus.
Levorphanol tartrate (Levo-Dromoran)	2 IM 4 PO	60 IM 90–120 PO	4–5 IM 4–5 PO	Longer acting than morphine when given in repeated, regular doses. Accumulates, so analgesic effect may increase. SC recommended over IM route. Warn client drug has bitter taste. Contraindicated in clients with respiratory depression, asthma, alcoholism, or increased intracranial pressure.
Meperidine HCl (Demerol)	75 IM 300 PO	30–50 IM 60–90 PO	2–4 IM 2–4 PO	Metabolized to normeperidine, a toxic CNS stimulant which may cause CNS hyperexcitability. Normeperidine's effects increased, not reversed, by naloxone. Use with caution in clients with renal disease. PO dose of 300 not recommended.
Methadone HCl (Dolophine)	10 IM 20 PO	60–120 IM 90–120 PO	4–6 IM 4–6 PO	Initial PO dose is twice IM dose. Accumulates, so analgesic effect may increase. Warn client drug has bitter taste. Also used for heroin detoxification and temporary maintenance. Oral liquid form is legally required in maintenance programs.
Nalbuphine HCl (Nubain)	10 IM N/A PO	30–60 IM	3–6 IM	Longer acting and less likely to cause hypotension than morphine. Respiratory depression does not increase with increased dosages as compared to morphine. Similar to butorphanol, but does not increase cardiac workload.
Oxycodone HCl	N/A IM 30 PO	60 PO	3–6 PO	Now available as a single-entity product in tablet or liquid form. Also available in 5-mg dose in drugs such as Percodan and Percocet. Has faster onset and higher peak effect than most PO narcotics.
Oxymorphone HCl (Numorphan)	1–1.5 IM N/A PO	30–60 IM	3–6 IM	Also available as rectal suppository (10 mg equianalgesic), but more effective if given IM.
Pentazocine HCl	60 IM 180 PO	30–60 IM 30–90 PO	3–4 IM 3–4 PO	PO dose is 3 times IM dose. May produce withdrawal in clients physically dependent on narcotics. May cause confusion, hallucinations, anxiety. Contraindicated in clients with head injury or increased intracranial pressure. Use with caution in clients with cardiac problems.
Propoxyphene HCl (Darvon)	N/A IM 500 PO	120 PO	4–6 PO	Available only in oral form in United States. Never give as much as 500 mg PO. PO dose of 65–130 mg recommended. Used for mild to moderate pain. May cause false decreases in urinary steroid excretion tests. Report suspected propoxyphene abuse; propoxyphene in excessive doses ranks second to barbiturates as a cause of drug-related deaths.

Note. Morphine sulfate 10 mg IM is the analgesic dose to which all other IM and PO doses in this table are considered equianalgesic.

Note. Table compiled with data from Analgesic Study Section, Sloan-Kettering Institute for Cancer Research, New York; M. McCaffery, & A. Beebe, *Pain: Clinical Manual for Nursing Practice* (St Louis: Mosby, 1989); and R. Alfaro-LeFevre et al., *Drug Handbook: A Nursing Process Approach* (Redwood City, CA: Addison-Wesley Nursing, 1992).

Nursing Implications for Pharmacology: Narcotic Analgesics

NARCOTIC ANALGESICS

buprenorphine HCl (Buprenex)

codeine

hydromorphone HCl (Dilaudid)

meperidine HCl (Demerol)

propoxyphene HCl (Darvon)

morphine sulfate

nalbuphine HCl (Nubain)

oxymorphone HCl (Numorphan)

pentazocine (Talwin)

propoxyphene napsylate (Darvocet-N)

Narcotic analgesics are used to treat severe pain. The drugs in this category include opium, morphine, codeine, opium derivatives, and synthetic substances. Morphine and codeine are pure chemical substances isolated from opium. These drugs decrease the awareness of the sensation of pain by binding to opiate receptors in the brain and spinal cord. It is also believed that they diminish the transmission of pain impulses by altering cell membrane permeability to sodium and by affecting the release of neurotransmitters for efferent nerves sensitive to noxious stimuli. Narcotic analgesics affect the central nervous system, causing analgesia, euphoria, drowsiness, mental clouding, and lethargy. They also have various other effects: depending on the drug used, the narcotics depress respirations, stimulate the vomiting center, depress the cough reflex, induce peripheral vasodilatation (resulting in hypotension), constrict the pupil, and decrease intestinal peristalsis. The narcotics are addictive, causing psychologic and physical dependence.

Nursing Responsibilities

- Narcotics are regulated by federal law; the nurse must record the date, time, client name, type and amount of the drug used, and sign the entry in a narcotic inventory sheet. If the drug must be wasted after it is signed out, the act must be witnessed and the narcotic sheet signed by the nurse and the witness. Computerized narcotic documentation methods are also available.

- Keep a narcotic antagonist, such as naloxone, immediately available to treat respiratory depression.

- Assess allergies or adverse effects from narcotics previously experienced by the client.

- Assess for any respiratory disease, such as asthma, that might increase the risk of respiratory depression.

- Assess the characteristics of the pain and the effectiveness of drugs that have been previously used to treat the pain.

- Take and record baseline vital signs before administering the drug.

- Administer the drugs, following established guidelines.

- Monitor vital signs, level of consciousness, pupillary response, nausea, bowel function, urinary function, and effectiveness of pain management.

- Teach noninvasive methods of pain management for use in conjunction with narcotic analgesics.

- Provide for client safety.

Client and Family Teaching

- The use of narcotics to treat severe pain is unlikely to cause addiction.

- Do not drink alcohol.

- Do not take over-the-counter medications unless approved by the health care provider.

- Increase intake of fluids and fiber in the diet to prevent constipation.

- The drugs often cause dizziness, drowsiness, and impaired thinking; use caution when driving or making decisions.

- Report decreasing effectiveness or the appearance of side effects to the physician.

Giving analgesics before the pain occurs or increases allows the client to experience a confidence in the certainty of pain relief and thereby avoid some of the untoward effects of pain. The benefits of a preventive approach can be summarized as follows:

- The client may spend less time in pain.

- Frequent analgesic administration may allow for smaller doses and less analgesic administration.

- Smaller doses will in turn mean fewer side effects.

- The client's fear and anxiety about the return of pain will decrease.

- The client will probably be more physically active and avoid the difficulties caused by immobility.

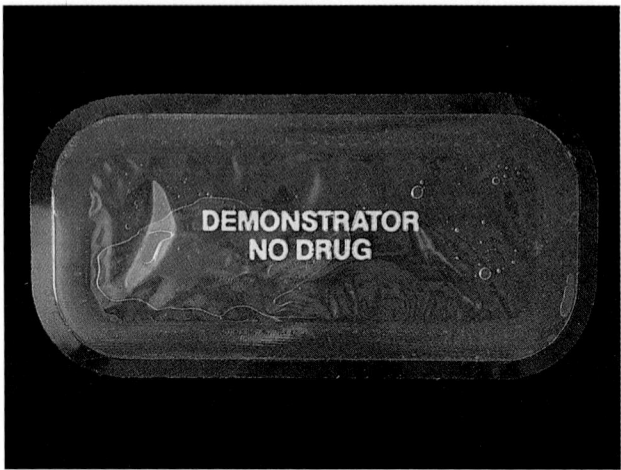

Figure 4–6 The transdermal patch administers medication in predictable doses.

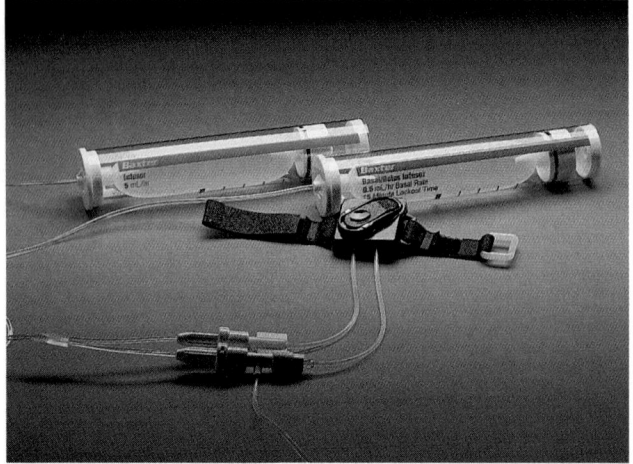

Figure 4–7 PCA units allow the client to self-manage severe pain. These units may be portable or mounted on intravenous poles.

The side effects of a drug can become difficult to manage if the dosage is too high. The best formula for adequate dosage is a balance between effective pain relief and minimal side effects. Within prescribed limits, the nurse can choose the correct dose according to the client's response. It is also the role of the nurse to inform the physician if the prescribed dosage does not meet the client's needs.

Routes of Administration

The route of administration significantly affects how much of the medication is needed to relieve pain. For example, oral doses of some narcotics must be up to five times greater than parenteral doses to achieve the same degree of pain relief. Of course, different narcotics have different recommended dosages. Consulting an *equianalgesic dosage chart* helps ensure that dosages of different narcotics administered by different routes will have the same analgesic effect when administered to the same client. Table 4–5 is an example of an equianalgesic chart.

Oral The simplest route for both client and nurse is the oral (PO) route. Special nursing care is still required, because some medications must be given with food, some are irritating to the gastrointestinal system, and some clients have trouble swallowing pills. Liquid and timed-release forms are available for special applications. The nurse must always be sure that the medication given is actually swallowed.

Rectal The rectal route is helpful for clients who are unable to swallow. Several of the opioid narcotics are available in this form. The rectal route is effective and simple, but the client and family may not accept it. To be effective, any rectal medication must be placed above the rectal sphincter.

Transdermal The transdermal, or "patch," form of medication is increasingly being used because it is simple, painless, and delivers a continuous level of medication (Figure 4–6). Although expensive, transdermal medications are easy to store and apply. Additional short-acting medication is often needed for breakthrough pain.

To apply a medication transdermally, the nurse or client must clip any hair from the area, clean the site (which should be on the upper torso) with clear water, dry the cleansed area, apply the patch immediately upon opening the package, and ensure that the contact is complete, especially around the edges. A patch lasts for 72 hours, and the next patch should be applied on a different site.

Sublingual Placement of the drug between the gum and the cheek, or beneath the tongue, is a potentially viable means of administration; however, in the United States no analgesic drugs currently are available in this form.

Nasal As a route for administering pain medications, the nasal route is currently under investigation.

Intramuscular Once the most popular route for pain medication administration, the intramuscular (IM) route is being reconsidered. Its disadvantages include uneven absorption from the muscle, discomfort on administration, and time consumed to prepare and administer the medication.

Intravenous The intravenous (IV) route provides the most rapid onset, usually ranging from 1 to 15 minutes. Medication can be given by drip, bolus, or **patient-controlled analgesia (PCA)**, a pump with a control mechanism that affords the client self-management of pain (Figure 4–7). Studies of PCA use for postoperative

Nursing Care of the Client Receiving Intraspinal Analgesia

Intraspinal analgesia is used to manage chronic and intractable cancer and severe postoperative pain. The intraspinal route may be either intrathecal (into the subarachnoid space) or epidural (into the epidural space). With the infusion of a narcotic into these spaces, there is a direct effect on the opiate receptors in the dorsal horn of the spinal cord; the narcotics are also absorbed systemically and affect the brain. This method provides complete pain relief but has some potentially dangerous side effects.

PROCEDURE

The physician places a catheter into the epidural space. Tubing is attached to an infusion pump, and the prescribed medication is administered. A portable or implantable pump may be used for narcotic administration that lasts more than a few days.

NURSING CARE

- Monitor vital signs every 15 minutes for the first 2–3 hours and every hour for the first 24 hours; the client is at risk for respiratory depression, which may not manifest itself for several hours.
- Ensure that naloxone, a narcotic antagonist, is immediately available to reverse respiratory depression.
- Monitor the effectiveness of the pain management.
- Monitor intake and output. Intraspinal narcotics may block the micturition reflex, causing urinary retention and necessitating the insertion of a Foley catheter.
- Use sterile technique to care for the catheter.

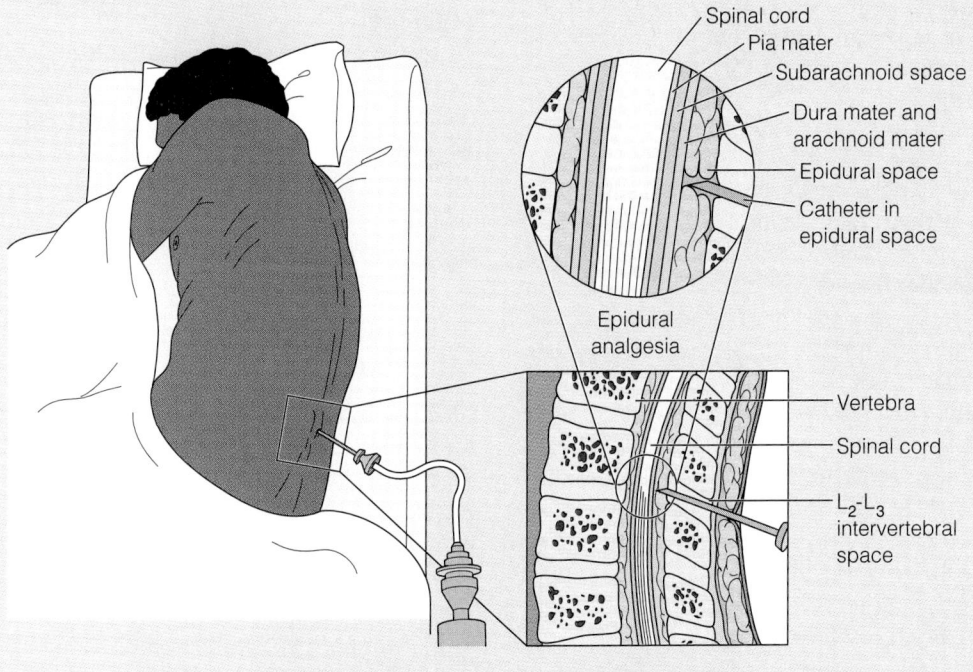

Spinal cord
Pia mater
Subarachnoid space
Dura mater and arachnoid mater
Epidural space
Catheter in epidural space

Epidural analgesia

Vertebra
Spinal cord
L₂-L₃ intervertebral space

Placement of the catheter in the epidural space.

pain have shown that clients require less overall medication because of the even blood level of medication maintained, the feeling of control maintained by the client, and the absence of anxiety. Several drugs are available for this route. The disadvantages are the nursing care needed for any intravenous line, the potential for infection, and the cost of disposable supplies. The PCA method of administration requires careful client teaching.

Subcutaneous   The subcutaneous (SC) route is accepted, but it is less commonly used than other methods. Its advantages and disadvantages are similar to those of the intravenous route.

Intraspinal   The intraspinal route is invasive and requires more extensive nursing care. The accompanying box provides nursing implications for clients receiving intraspinal analgesia.

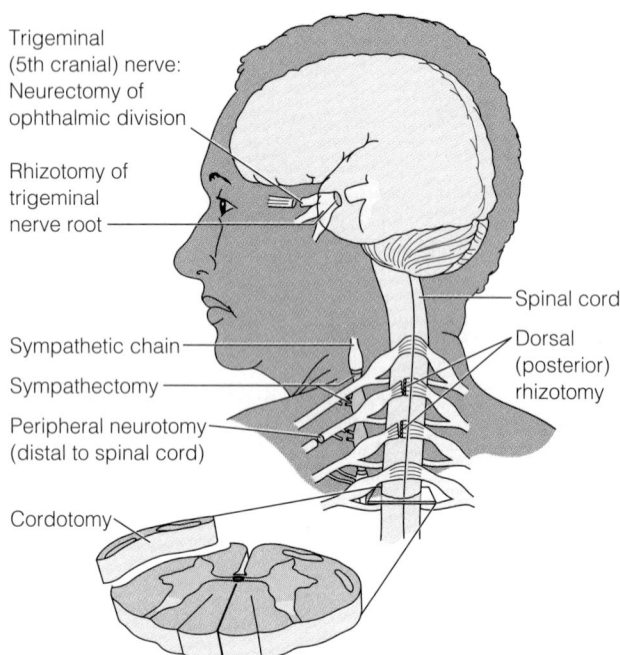

Trigeminal
(5th cranial) nerve:
Neurectomy of
ophthalmic division

Rhizotomy of
trigeminal
nerve root

Spinal cord

Sympathetic chain

Dorsal
(posterior)
rhizotomy

Sympathectomy

Peripheral neurotomy
(distal to spinal cord)

Cordotomy

Figure 4–8   Surgical procedures are used to treat severe pain that does not respond to other types of management. They include cordotomy, neurectomy, sympathectomy, and rhizotomy.

Nerve Blocks   In a nerve block, anesthetics, sometimes in combination with steroidal anti-inflammatory drugs, are injected by a physician or nurse anesthetist into or near a nerve, usually in an area between the nociceptor and the dorsal root. The procedure sometimes is performed to determine the precise location of the source of the pain: Pain relief indicates that the injection site is the site of the source of the pain. Temporary (local) nerve blocks may give the client enough relief to (1) develop a more hopeful attitude that pain relief is possible, (2) allow local procedures to be performed without causing discomfort, or (3) exercise and move the affected part. Nerve blocks may also be performed to predict the results of neurosurgery. For long-term pain relief, a permanent neurolytic agent is used. Neurolytic blocks usually are reserved for terminally ill clients because of the risks of weakness, paralysis, and bowel and bladder dysfunction.

Surgery

As a pain-relief measure, surgery usually is performed only after all other methods have failed. Clients need thorough knowledge of the implications of the use of surgery for pain relief. For example, motor function loss is an unwelcome side effect of some surgeries.

Some common surgical procedures used to relieve pain are shown in Figure 4–8 and include the following:

Cordotomy

A *cordotomy* is an incision into the anterolateral tracts of the spinal cord to interrupt the transmission of pain. Because it is difficult to isolate the nerves responsible for upper body pain, this surgery is most often performed for pain in the abdominal region and legs, including severe pain from terminal cancer. A *percutaneous cordotomy* produces lesions of the anterolateral surface of the spinal cord by means of a radio frequency current.

Neurectomy

A *neurectomy* is the removal of a nerve. It is sometimes used for pain relief. A peripheral neurectomy is the severing of a nerve at any point distal to the spinal cord.

Sympathectomy

The sympathetic nerves play an important role in producing and transmitting the sensation of pain. A *sympathectomy* involves destruction by injection or incision of the ganglia of sympathetic nerves, usually in the lumbar region or the cervicodorsal region at the base of the neck.

Rhizotomy

Rhizotomy is surgical severing of the dorsal spinal roots. It is most often performed to relieve the pain of cancer of the head, neck, or lungs. A rhizotomy may be performed not only by surgically cutting the nerve fibers but also by injecting a chemical such as alcohol or phenol into the subarachnoid space or by using a radio frequency current to selectively destroy pain fibers.

Transcutaneous Electrical Nerve Stimulation (TENS)

A **transcutaneous electrical nerve stimulation (TENS)** unit consists of a low-voltage transmitter connected by wires to electrodes that are placed by the client as directed by the physical therapist (Figure 4–9). The client experiences a gentle tapping or vibrating sensation over the electrodes. The client can adjust the voltage to achieve maximum pain relief.

The gate-control theory described earlier can clarify how TENS works. It is believed that TENS electrodes stimulate the large-diameter A-beta touch fibers to close the gate in the substantia gelatinosa. It is also theorized that TENS stimulates endorphin release by inhibitory neurons.

A TENS unit is most commonly used to relieve chronic benign pain and acute postoperative pain. In either case, thorough client teaching is essential, including an explanation of manufacturer's directions, instructions on where to place the electrodes, and the importance of placing the electrodes on clean, unbroken skin. The client should assess the skin daily for signs of irritation.

TENS offers several advantages: avoidance of drug side effects, client control, and good interaction with other therapies. Disadvantages are its cost and the need for expert training for initiation.

Acupuncture

Acupuncture is an ancient Chinese system involving the stimulation of certain specific points on the body to enhance the flow of vital energy (*chi*) along pathways called meridians. Acupuncture points can be stimulated by the insertion and withdrawing of needles, the application of heat, massage, laser, electrical stimulation, or a combination of these methods (Murray & Pizzorno, 1991). Only care providers with special training can use this method. Until recently, there were few practitioners in the United States; however, acupuncture is now becoming a more widely accepted therapy, especially for the treatment of pain.

Biofeedback

Biofeedback is an electronic method of measuring physiologic responses, such as brain waves, muscle contraction, and skin temperature, and then "feeding" this information back to the client. Most biofeedback units consist of electrodes placed on the client's skin and an amplification unit that transforms data into visual cues, such as colored lights. The client thus learns to recognize stress-related responses and to replace them with relaxation responses. Eventually, the client learns to repeat independently those actions that produce the desired brain wave effect.

Relaxation helps the client avoid the anxiety that often accompanies and complicates pain. Additionally, biofeedback provides the client with a measure of control over the response to pain.

Hypnotism

Hypnosis is a trance state in which the mind becomes extremely suggestible. To achieve hypnosis, the client sits or lies down in a dimly lighted, quiet room. The therapist suggests that the client relax and fix attention on an object. The therapist then repeats in a calm, soothing voice simple phrases, such as instructions to relax and listen to the therapist's voice. The client gradually becomes more and more relaxed and falls into a trance in which the client is no longer aware of the physical environment and hears only the therapist's voice. During this state, the therapist may make suggestions to encourage pain relief. It is possible to achieve complete anesthesia or to modify pain in a variety of ways through hypnotism. For the technique to work, however, the client must be fully relaxed and must want to be hypnotized.

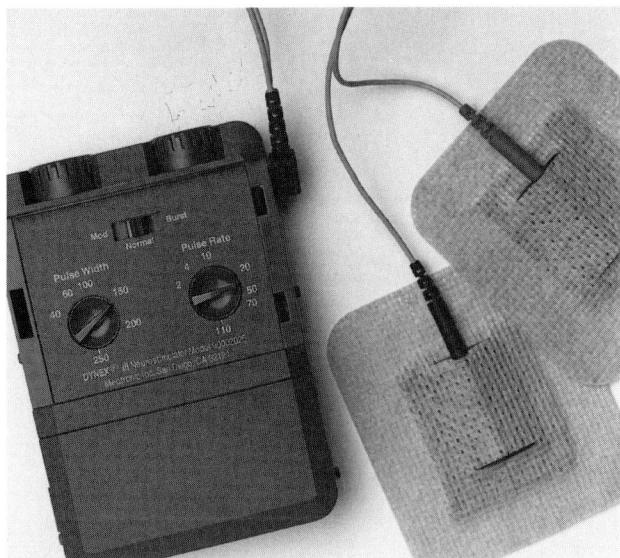

Figure 4–9 The TENS unit is believed to assist in pain management through the gate-control theory. Electrodes that deliver low-voltage electrical stimuli are placed directly on the client over painful areas.

Advantages include client control and lack of side effects. Disadvantages include the need for a skilled practitioner. However, some clients can learn to hypnotize themselves to achieve pain relief.

Nursing Care

Nursing care of the client with pain presents perhaps more of a challenge than almost any other type of illness or injury. Regardless of the type of pain, the goal of nursing care is to assist the client to achieve optimal control of the pain. The nursing process is used to organize the pain-relief strategies, and the nurse-client relationship is used to deliver effective care to help the client attain optimal comfort levels.

Assessment

First in the process of relieving pain for any client is the accurate, unbiased, and thorough assessment of the client's pain. A comprehensive approach to pain assessment is essential to ensure adequate and appropriate interventions. The four assessment areas are client perceptions, physiologic responses, behavioral responses, and the client's attempts to manage the pain and the effectiveness of these pain-management strategies.

Client Perceptions
The most reliable indicator of the presence and degree of pain is the client's own statement about the pain. The

Figure 4–10 The McGill Pain Questionnaire.

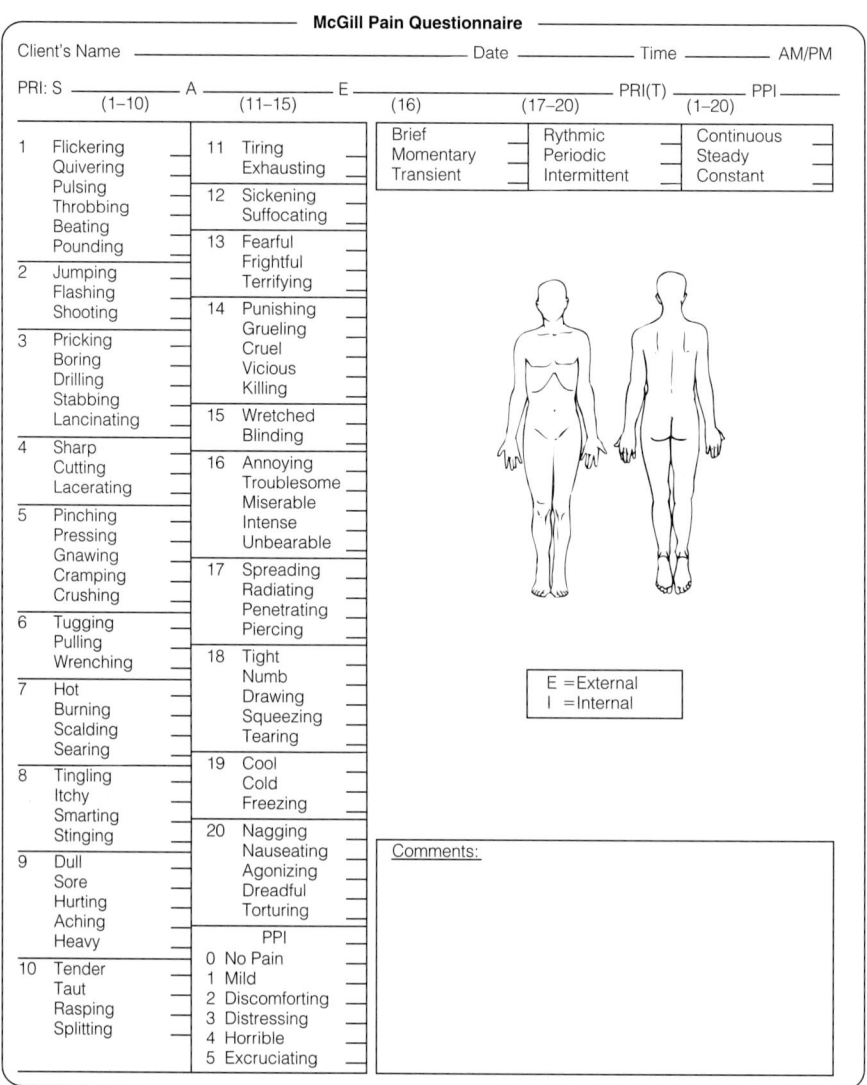

McGill Pain Questionnaire is a useful tool in assessing the client's subjective experience of the pain. It asks the client to locate the pain, to describe the quality of the pain, to indicate how the pain changes with time, and to rate the intensity of the pain (Figure 4–10).

The client's perception of the pain can also be assessed by using the PQRST technique (Murray, 1983):

P   What *precipitated* (triggered, stimulated) the pain? Has anything *palliated* (relieved) the pain? What is the *pattern* of the pain?

Q   What are the *quality* and *quantity* of the pain? Is it sharp, stabbing, aching, burning, stinging, deep, crushing, viselike, gnawing?

R   What is the *region* (location) of the pain? Does the pain *radiate* to other areas of the body?

S   What is the *severity* of the pain?

T   What is the *timing* of the pain? When does it begin, how long does it last, and how is it related to other events in the client's life?

The most common method to assess the severity of pain is a *pain rating scale*. Several scales are illustrated in Figure 4–11. For clients who do not understand English or numerals, a scale using colors (e.g., light blue for no pain through bright red for worst possible pain) may be helpful. The following nursing interventions will help the nurse use a pain rating scale to achieve optimal results:

- Explain the primary purpose of a pain rating scale, which is to provide consistent, prompt communication between the client and the care provider. Encourage the client to make a factual report of pain so as to avoid stoicism and exaggeration.

- To ensure consistent communication, explain the specific pain rating scale being used. If a word descriptor

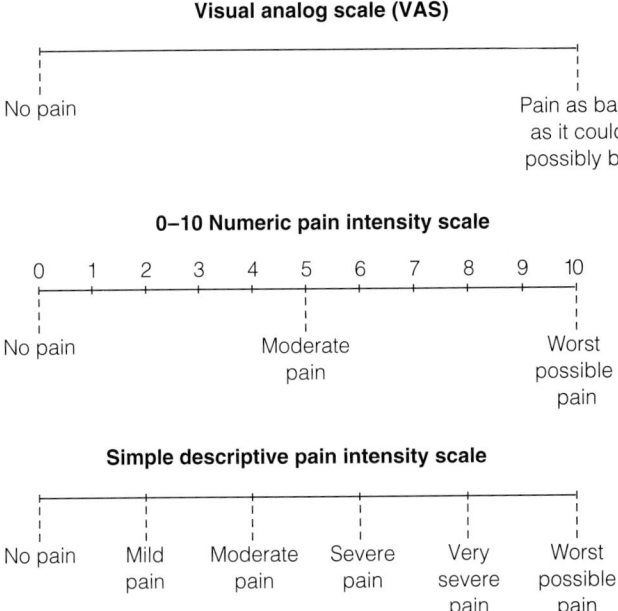

Figure 4–11   Examples of commonly used pain scales.

scale is used, verify that the client can read the language being used. If a numerical scale is used, be sure the client can count to 10.

- Discuss the definition of the word *pain* to ensure that the client and the provider are communicating on the same level. It is often helpful to use the client's own words when describing the pain.

- Explain to the client that the report of pain is important for promoting recovery, not just for achieving temporary comfort.

A thorough pain assessment will ensure a complete database for pain management.

Physiologic Responses

Predictable physiologic changes do occur in the presence of acute pain. These may include muscle tension; tachycardia; rapid, shallow respirations; increased blood pressure; dilated pupils; sweating; and pallor. Over time, however, the body will adapt to the pain stimulus. Thus, these physiologic changes may be extinguished in clients with chronic pain.

Behavioral Responses

There is a group of behaviors so typical of persons in pain that the behaviors are referred to as *pain behaviors*. They include bracing or guarding the painful part, taking medication, crying, moaning, grimacing, withdrawing from activity and socialization, becoming immobile, talking about pain, holding the painful area, breathing with increased effort, exhibiting a sad facial expression, and being restless.

Behavioral responses to pain may or may not coincide with the client's report of pain and are not very reliable cues to the pain experience. For example, one client may rate pain at an 8 on a 1–10 scale while laughing or walking down the hall; another may deny pain completely while tachycardic, hypertensive, and grimacing. Discrepancies between the client's report of pain and behavioral responses may be the result of cultural factors, coping skills, fear, denial, or the utilization of relaxation or distraction techniques.

Clients may deny pain for a variety of reasons, including fear of injections, fear of drug/narcotic addiction, misinterpretation of terms (the client may not think that aching, soreness, or discomfort qualify as pain), or the misconception that health care providers know when clients experience pain. Some clients may deny pain as part of an attempt to deny that there is something wrong with them. Other clients, by contrast, may think that "as needed" medications will be given only if their pain rating is high. Clients may also use pain as a mechanism to gain attention from family and health care providers.

Client Attempts at Pain Management

The client's attempts to manage pain are useful additions to the assessment database. This information is individualized and client specific, including many factors such as culture, age, and client knowledge. The nurse should obtain detailed descriptions of actions the client or significant others took, when and how these measures were applied, and how well they worked.

Diagnosis

Nursing diagnoses that may apply to the client with pain include the following:

- *Pain* related to inflammation and swelling of abdominal incision

- *Pain* related to muscle spasms following fracture of the femur

- *Chronic pain* related to recurring migraine headaches

- *Anxiety* related to lack of knowledge about pain management in the postoperative period

- *Powerlessness* related to inability to control chronic pain

- *Fatigue* related to inability to rest or have uninterrupted sleep secondary to severe pain

- *Ineffective Individual Coping* related to failure of medications to control chronic pain

- *Constipation* related to side effects of narcotic analgesics

- *Self-Care Deficit: Bathing/Hygiene* related to inability to use upper extremities secondary to the pain from rheumatoid arthritis

- *Hopelessness* related to lack of relief of cancer pain
- *Impaired Physical Mobility* related to pain from cancer metastasis to spine
- *Risk for Self-Directed Violence* related to long-term chronic pain

Planning and Implementation

The nurse, the client, and the family members must all be actively involved in any plan designed for pain management and must mutually establish goals. The outcomes of the plan should be based on the specific needs of the client (for example, partial or complete pain relief, ability to rest or sleep, or avoidance of narcotics), and criteria should be established to determine whether the goals have been attained.

Noninvasive Interventions
Various noninvasive nursing interventions are available for the management of pain. These interventions include relaxation, distraction, and cutaneous stimulation.

Relaxation   Relaxation involves the learning of activities that deeply relax the body and mind. Relaxation distracts the client, lessens the effects of stress from pain, increases pain tolerance, increases the effectiveness of other pain relief measures, and increases perception of pain control. In addition, by teaching the client relaxation techniques, the nurse acknowledges the client's pain and provides reassurance that the client will receive help in managing the pain (McCaffery & Beebe, 1989). Some examples of relaxation activities are as follows:

- *Diaphragmatic breathing* can relax muscles, improve oxygen levels, and provide a feeling of release from tension. The use of diaphragmatic breathing is more effective when the client either lies down or sits comfortably, remains in a quiet environment, and keeps the eyelids closed. Inhaling and exhaling slowly and regularly is also helpful. The technique for diaphragmatic breathing is described and illustrated in Chapter 7.
- *Progressive muscle relaxation* may be used alone or in conjunction with deep breathing to help manage pain. The client should be taught to tighten one group of muscles (such as those of the face), hold the tension for a few seconds, then relax the muscle group completely. The client should repeat these actions for all parts of the body. This method is also more effective when the client lies or sits comfortably, is in a quiet environment, and keeps the eyelids closed. There are some tapes that are available that will help the client with this relaxation process.
- *Guided imagery*, also called *creative visualization,* is the use of the imaginative power of the mind to create a scene or sensory experience that relaxes the muscles

and moves the attention of the mind away from the pain experience. To use guided imagery, the client must be able to concentrate, use the imagination, and follow directions. The nurse can facilitate this technique by asking the client for some descriptions of what the client finds most relaxing. The nurse then speaks to the client in a calm, soothing voice about those places or situations. The client usually must close the eyes to reduce visual stimulation so that the mind can picture the situation in as much detail as possible. There are tapes that are available that will assist the client with guided imagery.

- *Meditation* is a process whereby the client empties the mind of all sensory data and, typically, concentrates on a single object, word, or idea. This activity produces a deeply relaxed state in which oxygen consumption decreases, muscles relax, and endorphins are produced. At its deepest level, the meditative state may resemble a trance. A variety of exercises can induce the meditative state, and all are relatively easy to learn. Many books and tapes that the client can use to learn meditation are available commercially.

Distraction   Distraction involves the redirection of the client's attention away from the pain and onto something that the client finds more pleasant. Examples of distracting activities are practicing focused breathing, listening to music, or doing some form of rhythmic activity to music. For example, the client using recorded music for distraction may sing along with the song, tap out the rhythm with the fingers or foot, clap to the music, conduct the music, or add harmony. Full participation in the music is key to pain relief.

Participating in an activity that promotes laughter, such as reading a joke book or viewing a comedy, has been found to be highly effective in pain relief. Laughing for 20 minutes or more is known to produce an increase in endorphins that may continue pain relief even after the client stops laughing.

Cutaneous Stimulation   It is believed that stimulation of the skin is effective in relieving pain because it prompts closure of the gate in the substantia gelatinosa. Cutaneous stimulation may be accomplished by massage, vibration, application of heat and cold, and therapeutic touch. See Table 4–6 for descriptions, advantages, and disadvantages of these techniques.

Nursing Interventions with Rationales
The following is a list of nursing interventions with rationales that are appropriate for the client in pain.

- Assess the characteristics of the pain:
  a. Ask the client to point to the pain location or to mark the pain location on a figure drawing. *Pain*

Table 4–6	Methods of Cutaneous Stimulation		
Method	**Technique**	**Advantages**	**Disadvantages**
Touch	Nurse places hands on client's body or less than 1 inch (about 2.5 cm) above client's body to realign energy.	May initiate gate closure. Communicates caring.	None.
Pressure	Nurse places hand firmly on or around the area where the client feels the pain.	May relieve pain, decrease bleeding, and prevent swelling.	Benefits are temporary: when pressure is lifted, pain returns.
Massage	Nurse gently or briskly stimulates client's subcutaneous tissues by kneading, pulling, or pressing with fingers, palms, or knuckles.	May initiate gate closure. Promotes relaxation and sedation. Minimal side effects.	Time consuming.
Vibration	Nurse uses an electrical or battery-operated vibrator to stimulate the client's subcutaneous tissues.	May initiate gate closure. Low risk of tissue damage. Less costly than TENS.	Expense of equipment.
Heat	Nurse applies a hot-water bottle, heating pad, or hot towels to client's body. A hot shower or hot bath may also be effective. A heat lamp or other heat-generating device may also be used.	May reduce muscle spasm and pain. Works best for localized pain.	Contraindicated if bleeding or swelling are present.
Cold	Nurse applies dry or moist cold packs, gel packs, towels, or bags of ice chips to the client's body.	May reduce muscle spasm and pain. Cold may slow the transmission of pain impulses, and is more effective than heat for pain relief.	Cannot be used on ischemic tissues.

location provides information about the etiology of the pain and the type of pain being experienced.

b. Ask the client to rate the intensity of the pain by using a pain scale (1 to 10, with 10 being the worst pain ever experienced), a visual analog scale (a scale on which pain is marked on a continuum from no pain to severe pain), or with word descriptors (such as the McGill Pain Questionnaire). Use the same scale with each assessment. *The intensity of pain is a subjective experience. The perception of the intensity of pain is affected by the client's degree of concentration or distraction, state of consciousness, and expectations. Some body tissues are more sensitive than others. The research box on page 94 describes the effects of nurses' own pain experiences on their assessment of their clients' pain.*

c. Ask the client to describe the quality of the pain, saying, for example, "Describe what your pain feels like." If necessary, provide word descriptors for the client to select. *Descriptive terms provide insight into the nature and perception of the pain. In addition, the location and type of pain (for example, acute versus chronic) affect the quality.*

d. Ask the client to describe the pattern of the pain, including time of onset, duration, persistence, and times without pain. It is also important to ask whether the pain is worse at regular times of the day and whether it has any relationship to activity. *The pattern of pain also provides clues about cause and location.*

e. Ask the client to describe any precipitating or relieving factors. *Precipitating factors include sleep deficits, anxiety, temperature extremes, excessive noise, anxiety, fear, depression, and activity.*

f. Ask the client to describe the meaning of the pain, including its effects on life-style, self-concept, roles, and relationships. Other questions should explore how the client believes the pain will affect the future, how stressful it is, and what usual coping mechanism and support systems the client has. *Clients with acute pain may believe the pain is a normal response to injury or that it signals serious illness and death. Pain is a stressor that may affect the ability of the client to cope effectively. The client with chronic pain often has concerns about addiction to pain medication, costs, social interactions, sexual activities, and relationships with significant others.*

■ Monitor manifestations of pain by taking vital signs; assessing skin temperature and moisture; observing pupils; observing facial expressions, position in bed, guarding of body parts; and noting restlessness. *Autonomic responses to pain may result in an increased blood pressure, tachycardia, rapid respirations, perspiration, and*

PAIN FLOWSHEET

DATE 5/31/96

PURPOSES: 1) Record the patient's pain levels.
2) Provide data to titrate the analgesic's dosage.
3) Evaluate adverse reactions to the analgesic.

Patient's pain rating goal: __2 or less__

JOHN D. ELLIOT   Name
1000 ELM STREET   Address
ALBERT, MICHIGAN

RM. 301/DR. DIRK

DATE TIME INITIALS	ANALGESIC DOSE ROUTE	PAIN RATING 0 – 10 0 = No Pain 10 = Unbearable Pain	VITAL SIGNS			LEVEL OF AROUSAL/ ACTIVITY	MISCELLANEOUS: Adverse reactions, bowel function, other pain relief measures, care plan, and comments
			R	P	BP		
5/31/96 TJ. 2p	MS 10 mg IM	8	14	90	130/80	Restless	Describes severe pain
TJ. 245p		6	14				
TJ. 4p		4					Describes moderate pain
RS 5p	M.S. 15 mg. IM	8		84	126/80		Describes increased pain
RS 6¹⁵p		4	12		124/76		
RS 7 p		1	12			Relaxed, dozing	
RS 8¹⁰p	M.S. 15 mg. IM	5			130/80		
RS 9 p		2					
RS 9⁴⁵p		1	12	84	120/80	Sitting up, reading	
RS 11 p	M.S. 15 mg. IM	2					
							pt. states pain
	continued on M.S.						just about gone

Figure 4–12   A flowsheet for nursing documentation of pain management.

dilated pupils. *Other responses to pain include grimacing, clenching the hands, muscle rigidity, guarding, restlessness, and nausea. The client with chronic pain may have an unexpressive, tired facial appearance.*

■ Communicate belief in the client's pain by verbally acknowledging the presence of the pain, listening care-fully to the description of pain, and acting to help the client manage the pain. *Because pain is a personal, subjective experience, the nurse must convey belief in the client's pain. All pain is real, no matter what its cause. By conveying belief in the client's pain, the nurse reduces anxiety and thereby lessens pain.*

- Provide optimal pain relief with prescribed analgesics, determining the preferred route of administration. Provide pain-relieving measures for severe pain on a regular around-the-clock basis or by self-administration (such as with a PCA pump). A flowsheet for pain management is provided in Figure 4–12. *The client is a part of the decision-making process and can exert some control over the situation by choosing the administration route. The oral route is usually preferred. If frequent injections are necessary, the intravenous route is preferred because it is less painful and yields the maximum effect of the drug. Analgesics are usually most effective when they are administered before pain occurs or becomes severe. Around-the-clock administration has been proven to provide better pain management for both acute and chronic pain.*

- Teach the client and family noninvasive methods of pain management, such as relaxation, distraction, and cutaneous stimulation. *These techniques are especially useful when used in conjunction with pain medications and may also be useful in managing chronic pain.*

- Provide comfort measures, such as changing positions, back massage, oral care, skin care, and changing bed linens. *Basic comfort measures for personal cleanliness, skin care and mobility promote physical and psychosocial well-being, lessening the perception of pain.*

- Provide client and family teaching, and make referrals if necessary to assist with coping, financial resources, and care. *The client (and family) with pain requires information about medications, noninvasive techniques for pain management, and sources of assistance with home-based care. The client with acute pain requires information about the expected course of pain resolution.*

Client and Family Teaching

■   ■   ■

Provide information about impending pain and pain management to the client and family to lessen anxiety about the unknown and to provide the client with a means of controlling the pain. Explain what will happen, when it will happen, what it feels like, and what to do to help oneself during the event. Studies have demonstrated that providing this information has increased pain tolerance and reduced the amount of medication needed.

Teaching the client and family includes

- Specific drugs to be taken, including the frequency, potential side effects, possible drug interactions, and any special precautions to be taken (such as taking with food or avoiding alcohol).

- How to administer the drugs (if they are administered by any route other than by mouth).

- The importance of taking pain medications before the pain becomes severe.

- An explanation that the risk of addiction to pain medications is very small when they are used for pain relief and management.

- The importance of scheduling periods of rest and sleep.

- The name of a person to contact if pain is not controlled.

The client and family may obtain additional information about pain from the community resources listed in their local phonebook.

Applying the Nursing Process

Case Study of a Client with Pain: Susan Akers

Susan Akers is currently being seen at an outpatient clinic for chronic nonmalignant pain. She is 37 years old and is employed by a local paper factory. She has a 3-year history of neck and shoulder pain that usually is accompanied by headaches. She believes the pain is related to lifting objects at work, but it is now precipitated by activities of daily living. Ms. Akers is absent from work approximately three times a month and states that the absences are due to her pain and headaches. She has been seeking care in the local emergency department on the average of twice monthly for Demerol injections. She does not regularly use medications but does take Darvocet-N 100 and Valium as needed (usually two to three times a day.) Ms. Akers is divorced and has two children. She states that she has several friends in the area, but her parents and siblings live in another part of the United States.

Assessment

During the nursing history, Ms. Akers rates her pain during an acute episode as a 7 on a 1–10 scale. She states that lifting objects and moving her hands and arms above shoulder level precipitates sharp pain. The pain never really goes away, but it does decrease with upper extremity rest. She says that when she has to do a lot of lifting at work, she has difficulty sleeping at night. She takes 2 Darvocet-N 100 tablets every 4 hours when the pain is severe but does not get complete relief.

Diagnosis

The primary diagnosis identified for Ms. Akers is: *Chronic pain* related to muscle inflammation as manifested by pain scores, increase in pain on exertion, and client description of pain.

Expected Outcomes

The expected outcomes established in the plan of care specify that Ms. Akers will

- Return for follow-up visits with a journal of activities and pain experiences.

- After 3 to 5 days on regularly scheduled doses of narcotics, report a decrease in the level of pain from 7 to 3–4 on a 1–10 scale.

- Decrease number of absences from work.

- Modify activities at work and at home, especially when pain is intense.

Planning and Implementation

The following interventions are planned and implemented for Ms. Akers:

- Allow Ms. Akers to verbalize pain, and acknowledge belief in her report of pain.

- Consult with a physician for a nonnarcotic analgesic that Ms. Akers can take with a minimum of side effects, and instruct her in maintaining regular dosing schedules. Ask the physician also for a narcotic for use with acute episodes.

- For episodes of acute pain, instruct Ms. Akers to take narcotic analgesics as soon as the pain begins and every 4 hours, while continuing her dosage of nonnarcotic analgesic.

- List the therapeutic effects and possible side effects of prescribed medications.

- Teach one relaxation technique that is useful for Ms. Akers.

- Explore with Ms. Akers distraction techniques, such as listening to music, watching comedies, or reading.

- Introduce pacing by encouraging Ms. Akers to give priority to maintaining safe care of her children and going to work, spending less energy on housekeeping and delegating some chores to her children.

- Instruct Ms. Akers to contact the clinic by phone if her pain is unrelieved with narcotic and nonnarcotic analgesics.

Evaluation

Ms. Akers returns for scheduled follow-up visits with a completed journal of her activities and associated pain. She reports that taking oral narcotic analgesics has relieved her pain and that within 3 weeks nonnarcotic analgesics brought her pain under control. She also reports that her supervisor has reassigned her to a position that requires no lifting. She now rates her pain at 2–3 on a 1–10 scale. She has missed only 1 day of work in the last 3 months and reports that her children and friends have helped with her household tasks when she has requested they do so.

Applying Research to Nursing Practice Effect of Personal Pain Experience on Pain Assessment

■ ■ ■

A study was conducted to determine the effect of nurses' personal pain experiences on the assessment of their clients' pain (Holm et al., 1989). Demographic data and information from questionnaires were collected from 134 nurses who were employed in three Midwestern hospitals. The nurses were asked to state whether they had experienced painful situations such as surgery, fractures, and menstrual distress and, if so, to describe the intensity and frequency of pain as well as the degree of relief. The nurses were also asked about family members who had experienced pain, their own pain tolerance, and self-management of pain. Data were further collected through a questionnaire that asked the nurses to rate their perception of physical pain and psychologic distress as described in vignettes of people in pain.

The major finding of the study was that nurses who had experienced intense pain were generally more sympathetic to clients in pain.

Implications for Nursing

Nurses tend to underestimate and undermedicate pain. Findings from this study support the contention that nurses who have experienced pain are more understanding of and likely to assess physical and psychologic pain more accurately. As the health care providers most likely to assess pain, nurses must become more aware of factors affecting their own perceptions of the pain of others, as well as biases about pain that might interfere with effective pain management.

Critical Thinking in Client Care

1. What personal experiences with pain do you think will most affect your assessment and interventions for pain?

2. Considering the differences in acute and chronic pain described in this chapter, why do nurses tend to underestimate the characteristics of chronic pain?

3. How would you respond to the client in severe pain who refuses to take medication because "this is what I deserve"?

4. You are caring for a client who is diagnosed with terminal cancer. Another nurse says that he gives only half of the ordered dose of narcotics for pain relief because of the danger of respiratory depression. What would you do?

Critical Thinking in the Nursing Process

1. Describe three factors that support the statement "Pain is a personal experience." It may help to read the research box on page 94 on nurses' personal pain experiences.

2. Support or reject the common belief that each person has a different pain threshold.

3. Ms. Akers asks you how often she should take her pain medications. You tell her to (a) take them on a regular basis or (b) wait until she experiences pain. Which action would you choose, and why?

4. It has been suggested that Ms. Akers might manage pain better by using a TENS unit. Describe the physiologic basis for the effectiveness of this method.

5. Develop a care plan for Ms. Akers for the nursing diagnosis of *Constipation*.

Bibliography

■ ■ ■

Albert, L. (1988). Restraining pain. *Diabetes Forecast, 1*(88) 39–41.

Alfaro-LeFevre, R., Blicharz, M., Flynn, N., & Boyer, M. (1992). *Drug handbook: A nursing process approach.* Redwood City, CA: Addison-Wesley Nursing.

American Psychiatric Association. (1987). *Diagnostic and statistical manual of mental disorders IV.* Washington, DC: American Psychiatric Association.

Clements, S. & Cummings, S. (1991). Helplessness and powerlessness: Caring for clients in pain. *Holistic Nursing Practice, 6*(1), 76–85.

Corfman, J. (1990). Acute pain: A nursing challenge. *South Carolina Nurse, 5*(2), 32–33.

East, E. (1992). How much does it hurt? *Nursing Times, 88*(40), 48–49.

Faucett, J. (1991). Care of the critically ill patient in pain: The importance of nursing. In K. S. Puntillo (Ed.), *Pain in the Critically Ill: Assessment and Management* (pp. 115–136). Gaithersburg, MD: Aspen Publishers.

Fischer, R. (March 1994). Selecting and monitoring nonsteroidal anti-inflammatory drugs. *Advance for Nurse Practitioners, 26.*

Fishman, S. M. & Carr, D. B. (1992). Basic mechanisms of pain. *Hospital Practice, 27*(10), 63–66, 69–70, 75–76.

Greipp, M. E. (1992). Undermedication for pain: An ethical model. *Advances in Nursing Science, 15*(1), 44–53.

Gropper, E. I. (1992). Promoting health by promoting comfort. *Nursing Forum, 27*(2), 5–8.

Hofland, S. L. (1992). Elder beliefs: Blocks to pain management. *Journal of Gerontological Nursing, 18*(6), 19–24, 39–40.

Holm, K., Cohen, F., Dudas, S., Medema, P., & Allen, B. (1989). Effect of personal pain experience on pain assessment. *Image: Journal of Nursing Scholarship, 21*(2), 72–75.

International Association for Study of Pain. (1979). Pain terms: A list with definitions and notes on usage. *Pain, 6,* 249–252.

Jacques, A. (1992). Do you believe I'm in pain? Nurses' assessment of patients in pain. *Professional Nurse, 7*(4), 249–251.

Jaros, J. A. (1991). The concept of pain, *Critical Nursing Clinical of North America, 3*(1), 1–10.

Kaiko, R. F. (1980). Age and morphine analgesia in cancer patients with postoperative pain. *Clinical Pharmacology and Therapeutics, 28,* 823–826.

Kaiser, K. S. (1992). Assessment and management of pain in the critically ill trauma patient. *Critical Care Nursing Quarterly, 15*(2), 14–34.

Lenehan, G. P. (1992). On making pain a nursing priority. *Journal of Emergency Nursing, 18*(2), 91–92.

Lunse, C. P. & Price, P. (1992). Pain and the critically ill. *Canadian Nurse, 88*(7), 22–25.

Mahon, S. (1994). Concept analysis of pain: Implications related to nursing diagnoses. *Nursing Diagnosis, 5*(1), 14–23.

Marieb, E. N. (1995). *Human anatomy and physiology.* (3rd ed.). Redwood City, CA: Benjamin/Cummings.

McCaffery, M. (1979). *Nursing management of the patient with pain.* Philadelphia: Lippincott.

———. (September 1980). Understanding your patient's pain. *Nursing 80,* 26–31.

———. (June 1987). Giving meperidine for pain: Should it be so mechanical? *Nursing 87,* 51–61.

———. (1992a). *Pain: Assessment and intervention in clinical practice.* Unpublished manuscript.

———. (1992b). RN's assessment is critical in pain control. *American Nurse, 24*(2), 4, 12.

McCaffery, M. & Beebe, A. (1989). *Pain: Clinical manual for nursing practice.* St Louis: Mosby.

McCaffery, M. & Ferrell, B. R. (1991). Patient age: Does it affect your pain-control decisions? *Nursing, 21*(9), 44–48.

McCance, K. L. & Huether, S. E. (1994). *Pathophysiology: The biologic basis for disease in adults and children* (2nd ed.). St Louis: Mosby.

McGuire, L. (1994). The nurse's role in pain relief. *Medsurg Nursing, 3*(2), 94–98.

Melzack, R. (1975). The McGill Pain Questionnaire: Major properties and scoring methods. *Pain, 1,* 272–281.

Melzack, R. & Wall, P. D. (1965). Pain mechanisms: A new theory, *Science, 150,* 971–979.

———. (1968). Gate control theory of pain. In A. Soulairac, J. Cahn, & J. Carpentier (eds). *Pain: Proceedings of the international association on pain.* Baltimore: Williams & Wilkins.

Miaskowski, C. (1993). Current concepts in the assessment and management of acute pain. *Medsurg Nursing, 2*(1), 28–32.

Morrison, S. B. & Knop, J. C. (1992). Concern about pain management underscored: On making pain a nursing priority. *Journal of Emergency Nursing, 18*(5), 372–374.

Murray, M. (1983). Chest pain, dyspnea, confusion: When should you sound the alarm? *RN 1,* 67–74.

Murray, M. & Pizzorno, J. (1991). *Encyclopedia of Natural Medicine.* Rocklin, CA: Prima.

Olsson, G., et al. (1989). Nursing management of patients receiving epidural narcotics. *Heart and Lung, 18*(2), 130–138.

Paice, J. A. (1991) Unraveling the mystery of pain. *Oncology Nursing Forum, 18*(5), 843–849.

Porth, C. M. (1990). *Pathophysiology: Concepts of altered health states.* (3rd ed.) Philadelphia: Lippincott.

Romyn, D. (1992). Pain management: Know the facts. *Canadian Nurse, 88*(6), 26–27.

Sanford, K., & Schlicher, C. (1986). Pain management: Are your biases showing? *Nursing Life, 86*(6), 47–50.

Slack, J. & Faut-Callahan, M. (1991). Pain management: Update on drug interventions. *Nursing Clinics of North America, 26*(2), 463–476.

Sternbach, R. A. (1968). *Pain: A psychophysiological analysis.* New York: Academic.

US Department of Health and Human Services. (1992). *Acute pain management: Operative or medical procedures and trauma.* Rockville, MD: US Department of Health and Human Services.

Walding, M. (1991). Pain, anxiety, and powerlessness. *Journal of Advanced Nursing, 16,* 388–397.

Wallace, K. G. (1992). The pathophysiology of pain. *Critical Care Nursing Quarterly, 15*(2), 1–13.

Whipple, B. (1990). Neurophysiology of pain. *Orthopedic Nursing, 9*(4), 21–25.

Wilkie, D., Savedra, M., Holzemer, W., Tesler, M., & Paul, S. (1990). Use of the McGill Questionnaire to measure pain: A meta-analysis. *Nursing Research, 39*(1), 36–41.

World Health Organization. (1986/1990). *Cancer pain relief.* Geneva: WHO.

Nursing Care of Clients with Alterations in Fluid, Electrolyte, or Acid-Base Balance

LEARNING OBJECTIVES

After completing this chapter, you will be able to

- Discuss the functions, compartments, and regulatory mechanisms that maintain water balance in the body.
- Compare and contrast the causes, effects, and care of the client with fluid volume deficit and fluid volume excess.
- Describe the pathophysiology of imbalances of sodium, potassium, calcium, magnesium, and phosphorus.
- Compare and contrast the manifestations of electrolyte imbalances.
- Identify the causes and effects of acid-base imbalances.

- Identify laboratory and diagnostic tests used to diagnose and monitor treatment of fluid, electrolyte, and acid-base disorders.
- Recognize normal values, as well as values representing a deficit or excess, of electrolytes in the blood.
- Use arterial blood gas findings to identify the type of acid-base imbalance present in a client.
- Provide teaching about diet and medications used to treat or prevent electrolyte disorders.
- Use the nursing process as a framework to provide individualized nursing care to clients with fluid, electrolyte, or acid-base disorders.

Disorders of the normal composition of the body frequently occur as responses to illness and trauma and are encountered often in clinical practice. These disorders involve changes in the fluid balance of the intracellular and extracellular compartments of the body; changes in different elements or compounds, called electrolytes; and changes in the body's hydrogen ion concentration (pH), called acid-base imbalances. Normal physiologic processes are dependent on a relatively stable state within the

internal environment of the body, maintained in part through constancy of fluid volume, electrolyte, and acid-base balance. The fluid volumes, the electrolyte compositions, and the pH of both intracellular and extracellular spaces must remain constant within a relatively narrow range to maintain health and life.

Understanding fluid, electrolyte, and acid-base imbalances is based on a knowledge of the concept of homeostasis. **Homeostasis** is a term describing the stability of the internal processes of the body. Homeostasis is the body's tendency to maintain a state of physiologic balance in the presence of constantly changing conditions. Homeostasis is necessary for the body to function optimally at a cellular level and as a total organism. The maintenance of homeostasis is dependent on multiple factors in both the external environment and internal environment. For example, the relative concentration of oxygen, carbon dioxide, and available nutrients and wastes, as well as normal body temperature, must be maintained if the body is to continue to function. Homeostasis is reflected in the normal volume, composition, distribution, and pH of body fluids.

The goal in managing fluid, electrolyte, and acid-base imbalances is to reestablish and maintain a normal balance. Nursing care is directed toward assessing clients who are likely to develop imbalances, monitoring clients for early manifestations, and implementing collaborative and nursing interventions to prevent or correct imbalances. Effective nursing interventions are based on an understanding of the multiple interactive regulatory processes that maintain fluid, electrolyte, and acid-base balance and an understanding of the causes and treatment of imbalances that occur.

This chapter is divided into three principal sections addressing fluid volume disorders, electrolyte disorders, and acid-base disorders. Each section begins with a discussion of normal anatomy and physiology, which serves as the foundation for understanding the altered responses that are discussed in the rest of the section. Basic concepts are described and common terminology defined. The homeostasis of fluids, electrolytes, and acid-base balance is not easily separated into discrete parts, however; for this reason, discussions of these processes are interwoven throughout the chapter. For each disorder, potential complications as well as pertinent nursing diagnoses are presented. In addition, a box at the end of this chapter discusses normal age-related changes that contribute to the older adult's increased risk for disorders of fluid, electrolyte, and acid-base balance.

Fluid Volume Disorders

This section of the chapter provides an overview of body fluid balance and then discusses alterations in the body's fluid status: fluid volume deficit and fluid volume excess. A case study of a client with fluid volume excess is included to illustrate the application of the nursing process in client care.

An Overview of Fluid Balance in the Body

Fluid balance in the body involves the interrelationship of body water and fluids, fluid compartments and fluid spacing, membranes and transport systems, osmolarity and osmolality, tonicity, and the role of regulatory mechanisms.

Body Water and Fluids

The major fluid constituent of the body is water. Body fluid, which is composed of water and various dissolved substances (solutes), constitutes the intracellular and extracellular environments. Water functions in a number of ways to maintain normal cellular function. Body fluid

- Provides a medium for the transport and exchange of nutrients and other substances, such as oxygen, carbon dioxide, and metabolic wastes to and from cells.

- Provides a medium in which metabolic reactions may occur.

- Assists in regulating body temperature through the evaporation of perspiration.

- Provides form for body structure and acts as a shock absorber.

- Provides insulation.

- Acts as a lubricant.

Total body water constitutes about 60% of the total body weight, but this amount varies with age, gender, and amount of body fat present. Aging and tissue loss bring about a decrease in total body water; in people over the age of 65, body water may decrease to 45% to 50% of total body weight (Welty, 1992). Fat cells contain comparatively little water; in the slender person, therefore, the proportion of water to total body weight is greater than in the person of average weight. Conversely, in the obese person, the proportion of water to total body weight is smaller. Adult females have a lower percentage of body water content than males because they have a greater ratio of fat to lean tissue mass.

To maintain normal fluid balance, body water intake and output should be approximately equal. Although researchers do not all agree on the recommended amounts, the average fluid intake and output usually is about 2500 mL over a 24-hour period. Table 5–1 shows the sources of fluid gain and loss.

Table 5-1	Balanced Fluid Gain and Loss for an Adult	
	Source	**Amount (mL)**
Gain	Fluids taken orally	1200
	Water in food	1000
	Water as by-product of food metabolism	300
		↓
		2500
		↑
Loss	Urine	1500
	Feces	200
	Perspiration	300
	Respiration	500

Fluid Compartments and Fluid Spacing

Fluid Compartments

Body fluid is classified by its location inside or outside of cells. The *intracellular fluid compartment* designates all the fluid contained within cells and accounts for approximately 40% of total body weight. The *extracellular fluid compartment* designates all the fluid located outside of cells and accounts for approximately 20% of the total body weight (Figure 5–1). Extracellular fluid is in turn classified according to its location in the body.

- *Interstitial fluid* is the fluid in the spaces between most of the cells of the body. It accounts for approximately 15% of total body weight.
- *Intravascular fluid,* called plasma, is the fluid contained within the arteries, veins, and capillaries. It accounts for approximately 5% of total body weight.

Total body fluids = 60% of body weight

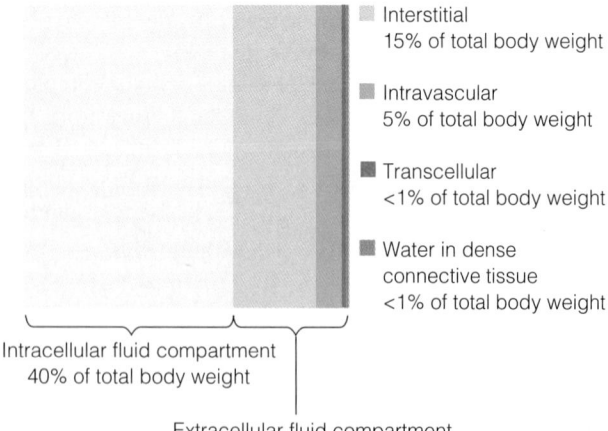

- Interstitial
  15% of total body weight
- Intravascular
  5% of total body weight
- Transcellular
  <1% of total body weight
- Water in dense
  connective tissue
  <1% of total body weight

Intracellular fluid compartment
40% of total body weight

Extracellular fluid compartment
20% of total body weight

Figure 5–1 A comparison of the major fluid compartments of the body.

- *Transcellular fluid* includes urine; digestive secretions; perspiration; and cerebrospinal, pleural, synovial, intraocular, gonadal, and pericardial fluids.
- Water contained in bone, cartilage, and other dense connective tissues; this water is not exchangeable with other body fluid compartments.

The cell wall membrane separates the intracellular from the extracellular fluid in the interstitial space. Interstitial fluid is separated from the plasma by capillary membranes. Transcellular fluid is distinctive in that it is separated from blood by both capillary endothelium and epithelium (Kokko & Tannen, 1990).

Third-Spacing

Third-spacing is the accumulation and sequestration of trapped extracellular fluid in an actual or potential body space as a result of disease or injury. The trapped fluid represents a volume loss and is unavailable for normal physiologic processes. Fluid may become trapped in such body spaces as the pericardial, pleural, peritoneal, or joint cavities; the bowel; and the abdomen. Fluid may also become trapped within soft tissues following trauma or burns. Assessing the magnitude of intravascular fluid loss that results from third-spacing is difficult. It may not be reflected in either changes in weight or by intake-and-output records, and it may not become apparent until after organ malfunction occurs (Metheney, 1992).

Edema

An excess accumulation of fluid in the interstitial space is called **edema.** Edema is classified as localized or generalized. Localized edema occurs secondary to traumatic injury from accidents or surgery, local inflammatory processes, and burns. *Anasarca* (generalized edema) is an excessive accumulation of fluid in the interstitial space throughout the body secondary to such conditions as cardiac failure and renal failure.

Membranes and Transport Processes

Membranes

Several types of membranes separate the body fluid compartments, and a number of processes play a role in maintaining the balance of water and solutes between these compartments. The membranes separating the body fluid compartments are classified as follows:

- *Cell membranes* separate interstitial fluid from intracellular fluid.
- *Capillary membranes* separate plasma from interstitial fluid.
- *Epithelial membranes* separate transcellular fluid from interstitial fluid and plasma. Epithelial membranes include the mucosal epithelium of the stomach, in-

testines, and gallbladder; the pleural, peritoneal, and synovial membranes; and the tubules of the kidney (Keyes, 1985).

A cell membrane consists of layers of lipid and protein molecules. The layering of these molecules controls the passage of fluid and solutes between the cell and interstitial fluid. The cell membrane is *selectively permeable;* that is, it allows the passage of water, oxygen, carbon dioxide, and small water-soluble molecules but bars the passage of proteins and other intracellular colloids.

The capillary membrane separating the plasma from the interstitial space is made of squamous epithelial cells. Pores in the membrane allow the passage of solute molecules (such as glucose and sodium), dissolved gases, and water. Minute amounts of albumin and other proteins can also pass through the pores of a capillary membrane, but normally the plasma proteins stay in the intravascular compartment.

Membrane Transport Processes

Four chemical and physiologic processes transport fluid, electrolytes, and other molecules across membranes between the intracellular and interstitial space and the interstitial space and plasma. These processes are osmosis, diffusion, filtration, and active transport.

Osmosis is a transport process by which water moves across a membrane that is permeable to water but impermeable to dissolved substances (solutes). The net shift of water is from an area of lower solute concentration to an area of higher solute concentration. The process continues as long as the solute concentration on both sides of the membrane is unequal. For example, if a solution of pure water and a solution of sodium chloride are separated by a selectively permeable membrane, water molecules will move across the membrane to the sodium chloride solution. Osmosis is the force most responsible for the movement of body fluid between the intracellular and the extracellular fluid compartments.

In the body, intravascular proteins exert an osmotic attraction on surrounding interstitial fluid. This *osmotic activity* is an important factor in maintaining the fluid balance between the interstitial and intravascular spaces. The composition of interstitial spaces and the intravascular spaces is essentially the same except for a higher concentration of proteins in the plasma. Because of the presence of plasma proteins (and especially albumin), the intravascular compartment has a slightly higher number of particles than does interstitial fluid. Plasma proteins, along with the osmotic activity generated by the presence of sodium, help to hold water within the vascular system.

Diffusion is the process in which molecules move down a concentration gradient from an area of high concentration to an area of low concentration to become evenly distributed (Figure 5–2). There are two types of diffusion: simple diffusion and facilitated diffusion. *Simple diffusion*

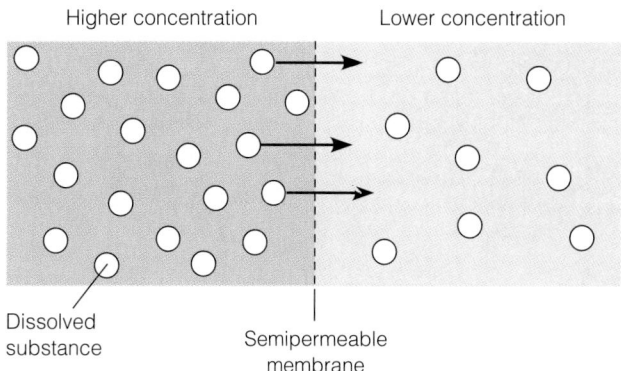

Higher concentration   Lower concentration

Dissolved substance   Semipermeable membrane

Figure 5–2   Molecules tend to move away from areas of higher concentration and toward areas of lesser concentration. They become evenly distributed through the process of diffusion.

is the random (kinetic) movement of particles in all directions through a solution or gas. In simple diffusion, water and solutes move through the cell membrane by passing through protein channels or by dissolving in the lipid membrane. Lipid-soluble materials, such as oxygen, nitrogen, carbon dioxide, and alcohol—as well as water—enter and leave the cell in this way. Water, permeable gases (carbon dioxide and oxygen), and solutes diffuse between the plasma and interstitial space through the capillary membrane.

Facilitated diffusion, also called carrier-mediated diffusion, is the process whereby large water-soluble molecules, such as glucose and amino acids, diffuse across cell membranes. A carrier is a substance that facilitates the diffusion of these substances across the cell membrane (Guyton, 1991). Proteins embedded in the cell membrane function as carriers in aiding molecules to cross the membrane. The rate of diffusion is influenced by a number of factors, including the availability of the carrier substance in the cell membrane. The effect of both simple and facilitated diffusion is the tendency to establish equal concentrations of the molecules on both sides of the membrane.

Filtration is the process by which water and dissolved substances (solutes) move out of a solution with higher hydrostatic pressure into a solution of comparatively lower hydrostatic pressure. Generally, filtration occurs across capillary membranes. Hydrostatic pressure, the pressure created by the pumping action of the heart and gravity against the capillary wall, is the force that moves fluid and electrolytes from the arterial end of the capillary to interstitial fluid and enables the kidneys to carry out glomerular filtration of the plasma.

The forces responsible for the movement of water between the intravascular and interstitial spaces in the capillary beds of the body are hydrostatic (filtration) pressure, the interstitial fluid pressure, and osmotic pressure (the pressure created by differences in the concentration

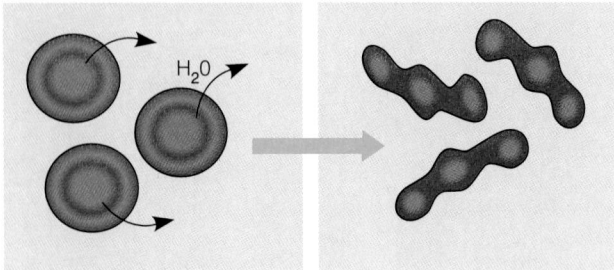

A Hypertonic solution

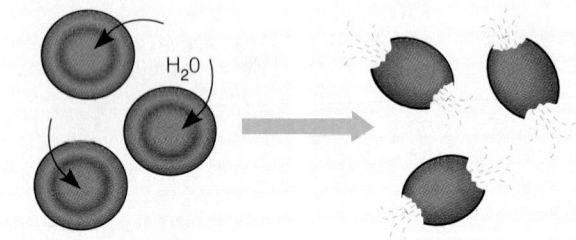

B Hypotonic solution

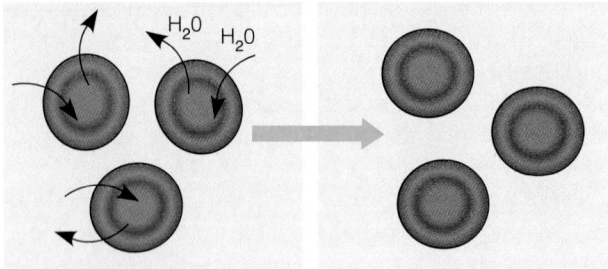

C Isotonic solution

Figure 5–3   Solutions of varying concentrations affect living cells in different ways. This example depicts the effects on red blood cells: *A,* Cells lose water and shrink in size (crenate) in hypertonic solutions. *B,* Cells absorb water, swell, and burst (hemolyze) in hypotonic solutions. *C,* Cells neither gain nor lose water, size, or shape in isotonic solutions.

of solutes on the two sides of a membrane). Hydrostatic pressure is higher at the arterial end of the capillary than at the venous end of the capillary, a fact that favors movement of water into the interstitial space. The interstitial hydrostatic pressure opposes this movement to some degree. At the venous end of the capillary, the osmotic force of the plasma proteins (in this case, called oncotic pressure) favors movement of fluid into the capillary.

Active transport is the process by which molecules are moved against a concentration gradient across cell membranes and absorptive epithelial membranes (Keyes, 1985). Like facilitated diffusion, substances cross the membrane by means of a carrier. Active transport differs from facilitated diffusion in that the movement of solutes

is not favored by a concentration gradient and requires the use of energy. A high concentration of a substance is maintained on one side of the membrane by the use of energy in the form of adenosine triphosphate (ATP).

Osmolarity and Osmolality

The concentration of a solution may be expressed as the osmolarity or osmolality of a solution. *Osmolarity* refers to the number of osmoles of solute per liter of solution; the total volume of solution is equal to the amount of water plus the amount of solute. Osmolarity is reported in milliosmoles per liter (mOsm/L) in a solution (Horne et al., 1991).

Osmolality refers to the number of osmoles of solute per kilogram of water; it is equal to the volume of the solution plus the relatively small amount of solute present. Osmolality is reported in milliosmoles per kilogram (mOsm/kg). The normal osmolality of both intracellular and extracellular fluids ranges between 275 and 295 mOsm/kg. The osmolality of the extracellular fluid depends chiefly on sodium concentration. The sodium concentration is approximately 142 mEq/L and rarely fluctuates more than 3% per day. Serum osmolality may be estimated by doubling the serum sodium concentration. The term *osmolality* will be used throughout this text.

Tonicity

Tonicity is the term used to refer to the tension or effect that the osmotic pressure of a solution exerts on cell size as a result of water movement across the cell membrane. *Isotonic* (or isoosmolar) solutions have the same concentration of solutes as the blood. With isotonic solutions, there is no net transfer of water across two compartments separated by a semipermeable membrane. *Hypertonic* (or hyperosmolar) solutions have a greater concentration of solutes than does the blood. With hypertonic solutions, a net transfer of water will occur from the area of lesser solute concentration to that of greater solute concentration. *Hypotonic* (or hypoosmolar) solutions have a lesser concentration of solutes than does the blood. With hypotonic solutions, the net transfer of water will be in the direction of greater solute concentration.

The effect of solute concentration is illustrated by what happens to red blood cells when they are placed in solutions of different tonicities (Figure 5–3). If red blood cells are placed in an isotonic solution, there is no net gain or loss of water, and no cell volume change occurs (cells neither swell nor shrink). Red blood cells placed in a hypertonic solution lose water because of the higher solute concentration outside the cell membrane, and as a result they become crenated (wrinkled and shrunken). When red blood cells are placed in a hypotonic solution, water moves into the cells, causing them to swell and rupture.

An understanding of tonicity is important in understanding the pathophysiologic changes that occur with fluid and electrolyte imbalances. For example, a change in the tonicity of extracellular fluid secondary to changes in sodium concentration causes a shift of water from the intracellular to the extracellular fluid compartment. Treatment of fluid and electrolyte problems often involves the use of intravenous solutions varying in tonicity. Intravenous solutions that are equal in osmolality to body fluids, for example, 0.9% sodium chloride (NaCl), are referred to as isotonic. Those with an osmolality less than that of body fluids, for example, 0.45% NaCl, are referred to as hypotonic. Hypertonic solutions, for example, 3% NaCl, are those that have an osmolality greater than that of body fluids.

Regulatory Mechanisms

Constancy of body water volume and osmolality depends on a number of regulatory mechanisms that preserve the balance between water intake and excretion. These mechanisms include thirst, the kidneys, the renin-angiotensin-aldosterone mechanism, antidiuretic hormone, and the atrial natriureteic factor. These complex mechanisms affect the volume, distribution, and composition of body fluid compartments and are only briefly summarized in this discussion.

Thirst

Thirst, the primary regulator of water intake, plays an important role in preventing dehydration and hyperosmolality of body fluids. Thirst is normally experienced when the plasma osmolality reaches 295 mOsm/kg (Kokko & Tannen, 1990).

The mechanisms largely responsible for stimulating the sensation of thirst are volume depletion (decreased extracellular fluid volume or hypovolemia) and stimulation of osmoreceptors located in the hypothalamus by hyperosmolality (Figure 5–4). Basically, the sensation of thirst is due to the processes of the renin-angiotensin-aldosterone mechanism.

The Kidneys and the Renin-Angiotensin-Aldosterone Mechanism

The kidneys are primarily responsible for the regulation of fluid volume and electrolyte balance in the body. Large amounts of plasma are filtered through the glomeruli (at a rate of 170 liters per 24 hours). However, because of selective reabsorption of water and solutes in the renal tubules, about 99% of this glomerular filtrate is reabsorbed, the osmolality and volume of body fluids are maintained, and only a comparatively small amount of urine is produced (1500 mL per 24 hours).

The *renin-angiotensin-aldosterone mechanism* works to maintain intravascular fluid balance and blood pressure.

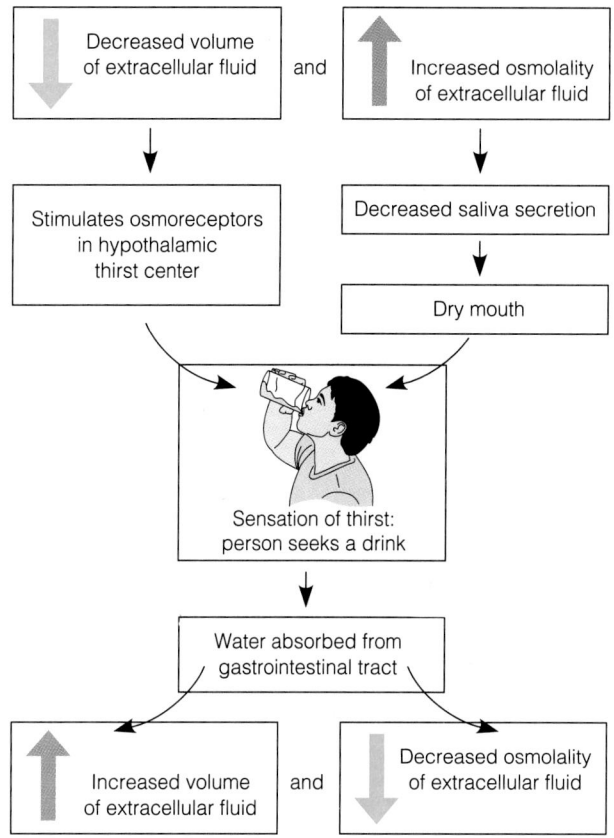

Figure 5–4   Factors stimulating water intake through the thirst mechanism.

Basically, this mechanism is initiated by a decrease in blood volume, resulting in decreased renal perfusion, which stimulates the renin-angiotensin system. Renin, an enzyme synthesized and released from the kidneys, combines with angiotensinogen (a plasma protein) in the circulating blood to form angiotensin I. Angiotensin I travels through the blood stream to the lung, where it is converted to angiotensin II. Angiotensin II stimulates the hypothalamus to release substances that arouse the sensation of thirst and activates the sympathetic nervous system to initiate vasoconstriction and raise blood pressure. Angiotensin II also directly affects the kidneys to retain sodium and water and stimulates the adrenal cortex to release aldosterone. Aldosterone is responsible for long-term regulation of sodium and water retention (Figure 5–5).

The Antidiuretic Hormone Mechanism

Antidiuretic hormone (ADH) is secreted by the posterior pituitary in response to increased osmolality. Solute concentration of the extracellular fluid increases secondary to water loss, resulting in decreased extracellular fluid volume. Osmoreceptors located in the hypothalamus sense

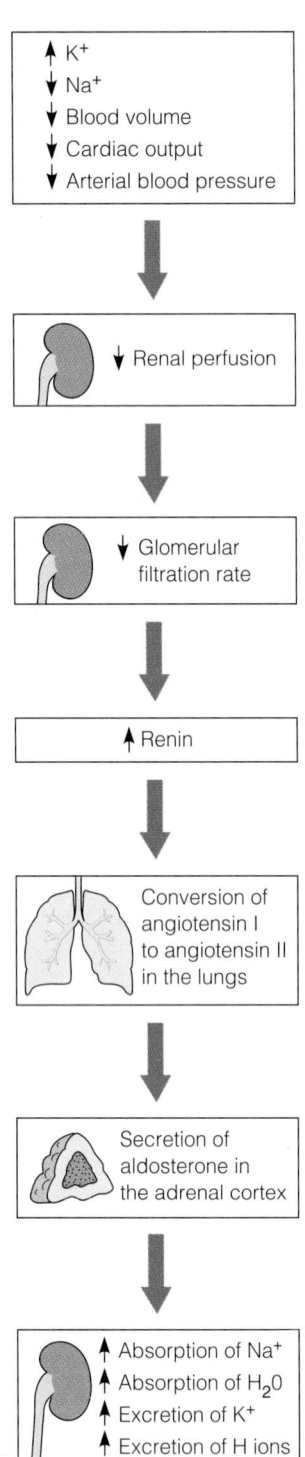

Figure 5–5 The renin-angiotensin-aldosterone mechanism. Decreased blood volume and renal perfusion, accompanied by increased serum potassium (K$^+$) and decreased serum sodium (Na$^+$), set off a chain of reactions leading to release of aldosterone from the adrenal cortex. Increased levels of aldosterone regulate serum K$^+$ and Na$^+$, blood pressure, and water balance through effects on the kidney tubules. See page 116 for a discussion of glomerular filtration rate and sodium balance.

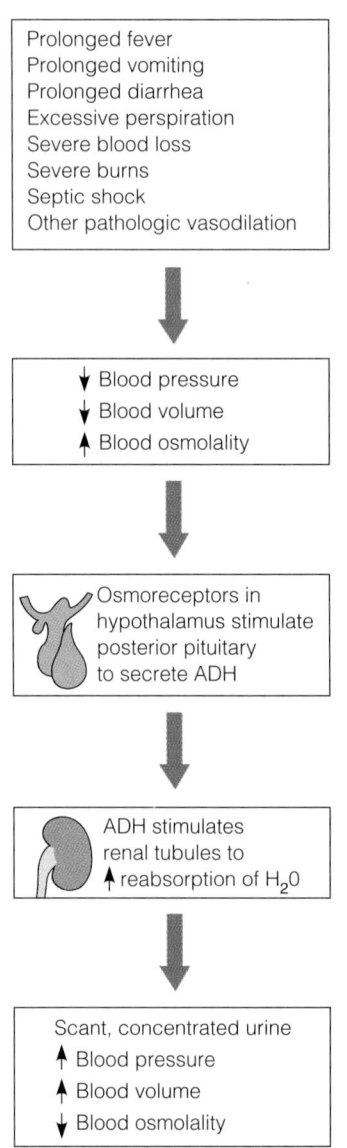

Figure 5–6 Antidiuretic hormone (ADH) release. Many different pathophysiologic conditions trigger the mechanisms that control ADH release. ADH stimulates the kidney tubules to increase reabsorption of water, increasing the blood volume.

increases in blood osmolality and decreases in blood volume, causing the release of ADH by the posterior pituitary. Antidiuretic hormone acts on the distal tubules of the kidney to increase water reabsorption. Increased reabsorption of water restores blood volume and corrects the osmolality (Figure 5–6).

Two disorders of water balance in which abnormal production of ADH is known to occur illustrate this effect. Diabetes insipidus is a condition characterized by a deficiency in ADH production. The deficiency in ADH causes a failure of the distal tubules and collecting ducts of the kidney to reabsorb water, resulting in the output of dilute urine of low osmolality. The hyperosmolality of the extracellular fluid that occurs does not trigger ADH release. However, it does stimulate the thirst mechanism. Thus, the client drinks additional fluids, and the cycle of high urine output and hyperosmolality continues. In the syndrome of inappropriate ADH secretion (SIADH), the release of ADH is unrelated to plasma osmolality or volume deficit. ADH release is inappropriate because it does not occur secondary to normal osmotic or volume stimuli, such as increased plasma osmolality and decreased extracellular fluid volume; rather, ADH release results from ADH production by disease. The increased reabsorption of water that occurs results in increased fluid volume and increased urine concentration. These diseases of the pituitary gland are discussed in Chapter 20.

Atrial Natriuretic Factor

The *atrial natriuretic factor* also affects water balance in the body. This substance is a hormone released by cardiac muscle cells in response to atrial distension from fluid overload. The atrial natriuretic factor affects several body systems, including the cardiovascular, renal, neural, gastrointestinal, and endocrine systems, but it primarily affects the renin-angiotensin-aldosterone system. Atrial natriuretic factor opposes this system by blocking the secretion and sodium-retaining effects of aldosterone, inhibiting renin secretion and causing vasodilatation (Birney & Penney, 1990).

The Client with Fluid Volume Deficit

■ ■ ■

Fluid volume deficit may result from the loss of fluids from the body or from fluid shifts within or outside the intravascular space as a result of regulatory mechanisms or from active fluid loss. These situations cause actual or potential vascular, intracellular, or extracellular dehydration (excessive loss of water from the body tissues). Fluid volume deficit in the extracellular fluid often causes hypovolemia (decreased circulatory volume). It is a relatively common problem that may exist alone or in combination with other electrolyte or acid-base imbalances.

Pathophysiology

Fluid volume deficits may be due to excessive fluid losses, insufficient fluid intake, or a combination of both. Excessive fluid loss may result from gastrointestinal tract disorders, renal or endocrine disorders, failure of regulatory mechanisms, hemorrhage, burns, medications (e.g., diuretics), infections and fevers, wound drainage, or third-spacing. Insufficient fluid intake may be the result of personal or environmental factors.

The most common cause of fluid volume deficit is excessive loss of gastrointestinal fluids from vomiting, diarrhea, gastrointestinal suctioning, intestinal fistulas, and intestinal drainage. These losses may be accompanied by hypokalemia (a decrease in serum potassium concentration), hyponatremia (a decrease in serum sodium concentration), and alkalosis (a decreased hydrogen ion serum concentration and increased pH) or acidosis (an increased hydrogen ion serum concentration and decreased pH), depending on which type of fluids are being lost. Imbalances of potassium, sodium, and acid-base balance are discussed in later sections of this chapter.

Other causes of fluid volume deficit include

- Excessive renal losses of sodium and water from diuretic therapy, certain polyuric renal disorders, uncontrolled diabetic ketoacidosis, hypoaldosteronism, and diabetes insipidus.
- Water loss during sweating from excessive exercise or increased environmental temperature.
- Hemorrhage.
- Third-space shifts secondary to burns, trauma, and inflammation.
- Chronic abuse of laxatives and/or enemas.

Inadequate fluid intake may result from lack of access to fluids, an inability to request fluids, an inability to swallow liquids, oral trauma, or altered thirst mechanisms.

The systemic effects of fluid volume deficit are essentially those of hypovolemia and of the related electrolyte and/or acid-base disorder that may occur secondary to the fluid loss (Figure 5–7). The development of manifestations of volume depletion depends on the severity and the rapidity of onset, as well as the age and general condition of the client.

Failure of regulatory mechanisms leads to initial manifestations of dilute urine, increased urinary output (followed by concentrated urine and decreased urine output as fluid volume deficit occurs), and sudden weight loss. Other possible manifestations include the following:

- Hypotension
- Decreased venous filling
- Tachycardia
- Decreased skin turgor
- Decreased pulse volume
- Increased body temperature
- Dry skin
- Dry mucous membranes
- Weakness
- Thirst
- Edema

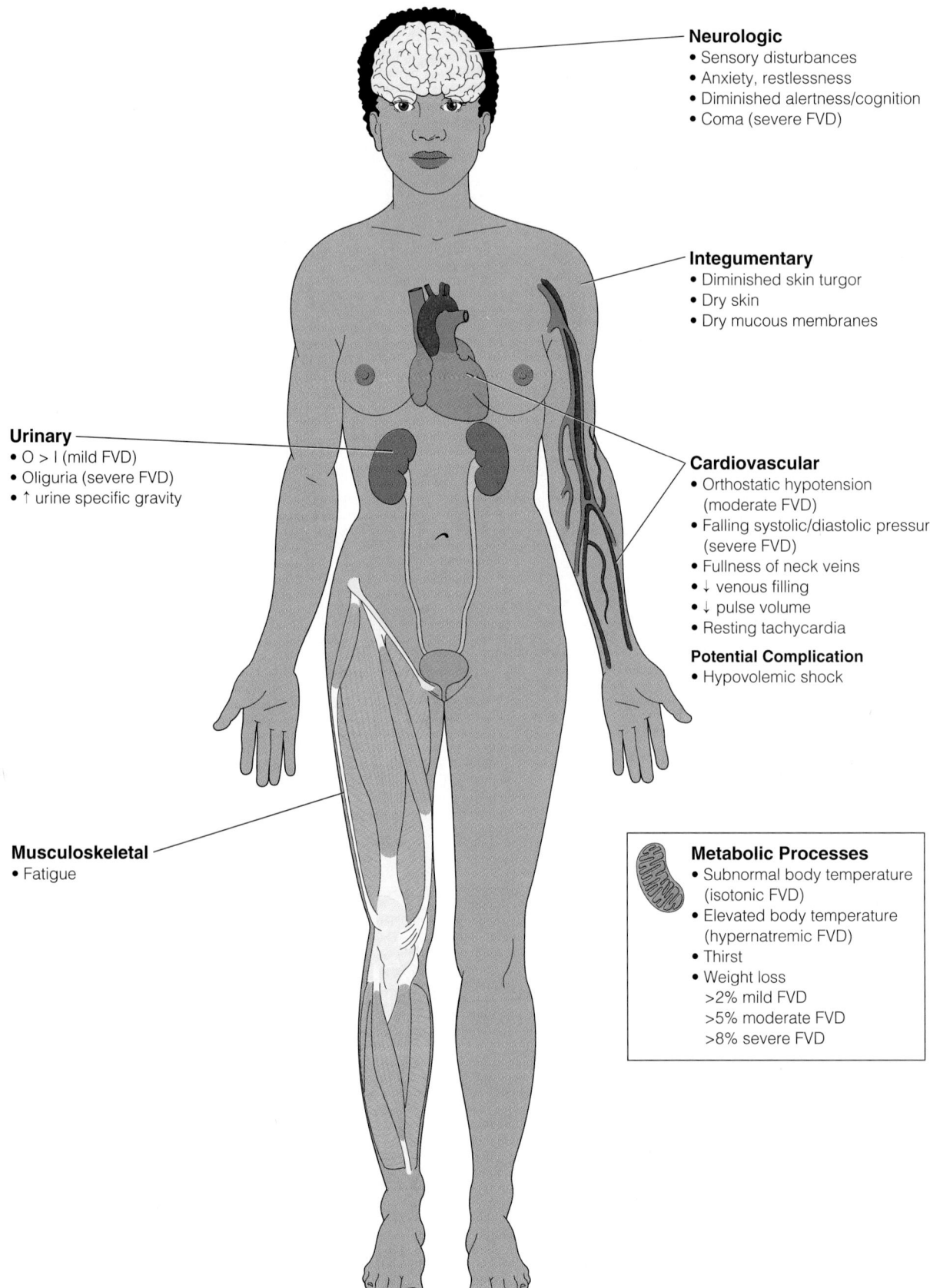

Neurologic
- Sensory disturbances
- Anxiety, restlessness
- Diminished alertness/cognition
- Coma (severe FVD)

Integumentary
- Diminished skin turgor
- Dry skin
- Dry mucous membranes

Urinary
- O > I (mild FVD)
- Oliguria (severe FVD)
- ↑ urine specific gravity

Cardiovascular
- Orthostatic hypotension (moderate FVD)
- Falling systolic/diastolic pressure (severe FVD)
- Fullness of neck veins
- ↓ venous filling
- ↓ pulse volume
- Resting tachycardia

Potential Complication
- Hypovolemic shock

Musculoskeletal
- Fatigue

Metabolic Processes
- Subnormal body temperature (isotonic FVD)
- Elevated body temperature (hypernatremic FVD)
- Thirst
- Weight loss
  >2% mild FVD
  >5% moderate FVD
  >8% severe FVD

Figure 5–7   Multisystem effects of fluid volume deficit.

Fluid deficit from active fluid loss also results in the following:

- Concentrated urine
- Decreased urine output
- Decreased venous filling
- Increased serum sodium
- Output greater than intake
- Sudden weight loss
- Altered mental status

A comparison of assessment findings for fluid deficit and fluid excess is found in Table 5–2.

Collaborative Care

The primary goals in managing fluid volume deficit are to identify clients at risk and prevent the deficit, to correct the underlying cause, and to correct existing deficits. Depending on the acuity of the imbalance, treatment may include replacement of fluids and electrolytes by the intravenous, oral, or enteral route. In nonacute circumstances, appropriate interventions may include the administration of fluids through a nasogastric tube (for clients who are unable to swallow) or oral replacement (for clients who are able to swallow). In acute situations, intravenous fluid administration is necessary.

Laboratory and Diagnostic Tests
The following laboratory tests may be ordered:

- *Serum electrolytes* are measured, with a focus on sodium and potassium levels. Deviations depend on the type of fluid lost and the causative factor. Decreases in sodium and potassium are common.

- *Serum hemoglobin and hematocrit* may be measured; in clients with fluid volume deficit from both regulatory mechanism failure and active fluid loss, the levels are elevated as a result of hemoconcentration.

- *Arterial blood gases (ABGs)* may be measured to detect changes in pH, carbon dioxide, and bicarbonate that occur in alterations in acid-base balance accompanying a fluid volume deficit. Alterations reflect the type of fluid lost and the severity of the deficit.

- *Urine specific gravity and osmolality* are measured and increase if the renal output of urine decreases and the urine becomes concentrated, or decrease if the urine is dilute.

The following diagnostic studies may be conducted to determine fluid volume deficit:

- *A fluid challenge test* may be conducted to establish fluid volume adequacy in clients who have questionable cardiac or renal function, manifested by severe

Table 5–2   Comparison of Assessment Findings in Clients with Fluid Imbalance

Assessment	Fluid Deficit	Fluid Excess
Blood pressure	Decreased systolic Decreased pulse pressure Postural hypotension	Increased
Blood pressure	Decreased systolic Decreased pulse	Increased
Respirations	Normal	Moist Crackles Wheezes
Jugular vein	Flat	Distended
Edema	Rare	Dependent
Skin turgor	Loose, poor turgor	Taut
Intake and output (I & O)	O > I	O < I
Urine specific gravity	High	Low
Weight	Loss	Gain

fluid deficit and decreased urinary output. Fluid volume must be established prior to initiating therapy in order to prevent serious imbalances; for example, fluid volume overload may occur if renal function is compromised. Various protocols for this test exist, but generally the test includes

  a. Obtaining baseline vital signs, breath sounds, urine output, and mental status.
  b. Administering (by intravenous infusion) an initial fluid volume of 200 to 300 mL over a 5- to 10-minute period.
  c. Reevaluating baseline data at the end of the 10-minute infusion periods.
  d. Administering additional fluid until a specified volume is infused or the desired hemodynamic parameters are achieved.

- *Central venous pressure (CVP)* is measured to determine the fluid status of the body. Central venous pressure is a direct measurement of the mean pressure in the right atrium.

The technique for measuring CVP is outlined in the box on page 106.

Pharmacology
Intravenous fluids are often prescribed to correct fluid volume deficit. Table 5–3 describes the types, tonicity, and uses of commonly administered intravenous fluids.

Measuring Central Venous Pressure (CVP) with a Manometer

■ ■ ■

Normal Values

When CVP is measured by a manometer, normal values range from 2 to 8 cm water. A low CVP indicates inadequate venous return from either actual fluid deficit and hypovolemia or from relative hypovolemia due to excessive peripheral vasodilatation. A high CVP indicates fluid overload, cardiac problems that decrease cardiac contractility, or pulmonary disorders that increase pulmonary vascular resistance.

General Information

CVP is a hemodynamic monitoring method for evaluating fluid volume status. It measures mean right atrial pressure and right ventricular end-diastolic pressure by means of a catheter. The CVP catheter is inserted by a physician, most often at the client's bedside, into the antecubital, internal jugular, or subclavian vein. Although institutional policies and procedures differ, nursing responsibilities include explaining the procedure to the client and family and monitoring the pressure at regular intervals. The steps in measuring CVP are as follows:

1. Explain to the client and family what is being done.

2. Prior to the first measurement, take baseline vital signs, and measure the level of the right atrium on the client's thorax. This is usually at the fourth intercostal space on the lateral chest wall, midway between the anterior and posterior chest. This site is marked and must be used for each measurement to ensure accuracy; it is the reference point for all measurements.

3. Place the bed in the same position for each reading, usually with the client supine and the head of the bed flat. The base of the manometer must be level with the marked site on the thorax (see accompanying figure).

4. Use a carpenter's level to check the level of the measuring device to make sure the 0 on the manometer is level with the reference point on the client's chest.

5. Remove any air bubbles in the line.

6. Turn the stopcock on the manometer so that fluid flows from the fluid source (intravenous fluids) into the manometer, filling it a few centimeters above the expected reading. Then turn the stopcock to open the line between the manometer and the client. The fluid level will fall and then reach a point at which it fluctuates with the client's respirations. This point is recorded as the CVP.

7. After the measurement is taken, turn the stopcock so that the fluid can again flow from the fluid source to the client.

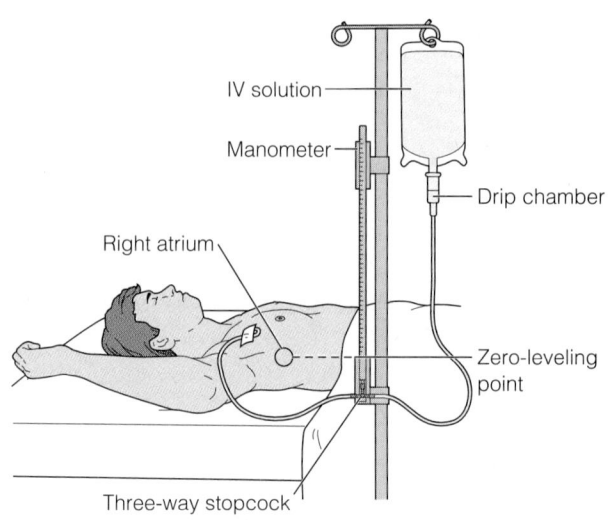

Measuring central venous pressure (CVP) with a manometer.

Isotonic electrolyte solutions (0.9% NaCl or Ringer's solution) are used to expand plasma volume in hypotensive clients or to replace abnormal losses, which are usually isotonic in nature. Five percent dextrose in water (D5W) is given to provide water to treat total body water deficits. D5W is isotonic (similar in tonicity to the plasma) and thus does not provoke hemolysis of red blood cells. The dextrose is metabolized to carbon dioxide and water, leaving free water available for tissue needs.

Hypotonic saline solution (0.45% NaCl with or without added electrolytes) or hypotonic mixed electrolyte solutions are used as maintenance solutions. These solutions provide additional electrolytes, such as potassium, a buffer (lactate or acetate) as needed, and water.

Table 5–3	Commonly Administered Intravenous Fluids	
	Fluid and Tonicity	**Uses**
Dextrose in Water Solutions	5% dextrose in water (D5W) Isotonic	Replaces water losses Reestablishes plasma volume Provides free water necessary for renal excretion of solutes Lowers sodium in hypernatremia
	10% dextrose in water (D10W) Hypertonic	Provides free water Provides nutrition (supplies 340 kcal/L)
	20% dextrose in water (D20W) Hypertonic	Supplies 680 kcal/L May cause diuresis
	50% dextrose in water (D50W) Hypertonic	Supplies 1700 kcal/L; often used if client very hypoglycemic
Saline Solutions	0.45% sodium chloride Hypotonic	Provides free water to replace hypotonic fluid losses Maintains levels of plasma sodium and chloride
	0.9% sodium chloride Isotonic	Expands intravascular volume Replaces water lost from extracellular fluid Used with blood transfusions Replaces large sodium losses (as from burns)
	3% sodium chloride Hypertonic	Corrects serious sodium depletion
Combined Dextrose and Saline Solution	5% dextrose & 0.45% sodium chloride Hypotonic	Provides free water Provides sodium chloride Maintenance fluid of choice if there are no electrolyte imbalances
Multiple Electrolyte Solutions	Ringer's solution Isotonic (electrolyte concentrations of sodium, potassium, chloride, and calcium are similar to plasma levels)	Expands the intracellular fluid Replaces extracellular fluid losses
	Lactated Ringer's solution Isotonic (similar in composition of electrolytes to plasma but does not contain magnesium)	Replaces fluid losses from burns and the lower gastrointestinal tract Fluid of choice for acute blood loss

Nursing Care

Nursing care of the client with a fluid volume deficit centers on the client's responses to the systemic effects of the disorder. Although individual client needs may differ, the problems and related nursing interventions most commonly encountered are *Fluid Volume Deficit, Risk for Altered Tissue Perfusion,* and *Risk for Injury.*

Fluid Volume Deficit

In general, fluid volume deficits are categorized into those that result from a decreased intake and those that result from abnormal losses. Identification of clients at risk and early intervention are necessary to prevent this disorder. Clients with abnormal losses require immediate and ongoing fluid replacement.

Nursing interventions and rationales are as follows:

- Assess for factors contributing to abnormal fluid losses, such as excessive losses from the gastrointestinal tract, kidneys, skin surface, and wounds and from decreased intake in clients with decreased level of consciousness, disorientation, nausea and anorexia, and physical limitations. *Identifying clients at risk enables the nurse to prevent fluid deficits or provide early intervention should they occur.*

- Assess intake and output accurately at scheduled intervals, and evaluate closely for reduced urine output and for a positive or negative fluid balance on 24-hour calculations. Hourly assessment of intake and output may be indicated. A urine output of less than 30 mL per hour should be reported to the primary health care provider. Measure urine specific gravity. *In the absence of renal failure, urine output should be in the range of 30 to*

60 mL per hour. Inadequate renal perfusion, cardiac failure, and fluid shifts contribute to a decreased urine output. Urine output of less than 400 mL in 24 hours is oliguria; urine output of less than 100 mL in 24 hours is anuria. Urine specific gravity varies with concentration of solutes and thus is a valuable index of the hydration status. A urine specific gravity of 1.010 to 1.025 is indicative of adequate hydration.

- Assess vital signs, CVP, and volume of peripheral arteries every 4 hours. *Hypotension, tachycardia, and low-volume, easily obliterated peripheral pulses are indicative of hypovolemia. CVP is a guide to fluid replacement.*

- Assess for indicators of dehydration: thirst, poor skin turgor, coated tongue. *These manifestations are indicators of decreased extracellular fluid.*

- Weigh client daily under standard conditions (same time of day, approximately the same clothing, balanced scale), and compare with 24-hour fluid balance. *Changes in weight may or may not accurately reflect changes in intravascular fluid volume. Third-space fluids represent a loss of intravascular fluid volume, but the loss may not be reflected by a change in weight.*

- Administer and monitor the intake of oral fluids as prescribed. Determine the client's beverage preferences, and provide these on a set schedule. *Oral fluids relieve thirst and dry mucous membranes and augment intravenous fluid replacement.*

- Administer intravenous fluids as prescribed using an electronic infusion pump (a machine for administering a specified volume of intravenous fluid at a controlled rate of flow). Assess for indicators of fluid overload from excessively rapid replacement: dyspnea, tachypnea, tachycardia, increased CVP, jugular vein distension, and edema. *Excessively rapid fluid replacement may lead to hypervolemia, resulting in pulmonary edema and cardiac failure, particularly in clients with compromised cardiac and renal function.*

- Assess laboratory values: electrolytes, serum osmolality, pH, partial pressure of carbon dioxide ($PaCO_2$), bicarbonate levels, and hematocrit. *Changes in electrolytes, serum osmolality, pH, and $PaCO_2$ occur with rehydration. Decreases in the hematocrit accompanied by decreases in serum sodium, osmolality, and blood urea nitrogen (BUN) occur with rehydration.*

Risk for Altered Tissue Perfusion

Decreased perfusion to the renal, cerebral, and peripheral tissues may occur with dehydration and resultant hypovolemia. Changes in mental status and cognitive function result from decreased cerebral perfusion and may include restlessness, anxiety, agitation, excitability, confusion, vertigo, fainting, and weakness.

Nursing interventions and rationales are as follows:

- Assess for restlessness, anxiety, and agitation, as well as changes in muscle strength. *Changes indicative of inadequate tissue perfusion may reflect imminent circulatory collapse and shock and necessitate immediate interventions.*

- Assess for hypotension and tachycardia when the client is in the supine position. Assess for orthostatic hypotension (a decrease in blood pressure when the client moves from a supine to a sitting position). With hypovolemia, a marked change in blood pressure (a drop of more than 15 mm Hg) and a change in pulse rate (an increase of more than 15 beats per minute) may occur when the client moves from a supine to a sitting position. *Postural hypotension accompanied by tachycardia is an indicator of hypovolemia. With severe hypovolemia, hypotension and tachycardia are present even in the supine position.*

Risk for Injury

The client with fluid volume deficit is at risk for injury because of dizziness and loss of balance resulting from decreased cerebral perfusion secondary to hypovolemia.

Nursing interventions and rationales are as follows:

- Institute safety precautions, including keeping the bed in low position, using side rails, and slowly raising the client from supine to sitting or sitting to standing position. *Using safety devices, such as side rails, and taking measures to allow for adjustment in blood pressure, such as changing the client's position slowly, lessens the risk of injury.*

- Teach the client and family members to avoid dehydration by replacing fluids lost as a result of, for example, exercise or hot weather, avoiding alcohol and caffeinated fluids (coffee, tea, cola); and avoiding prolonged exposure to intense heat (baths, showers, electric blankets). *These preventive measures are especially useful for the client at risk for fluid volume deficit.*

- Teach client and family members how to reduce orthostatic hypotension:
  a. Move from one position to another in stages; for example, raise the head of the bed before sitting up, and sit for a few minutes before standing.
  b. Use a walker or other assistive walking device.
  c. Avoid prolonged standing.
  d. Rest in a recliner rather than in bed during the day.
  e. Use assistive devices to pick up objects from the floor rather than stooping.

By teaching measures to reduce orthostatic hypotension, the nurse can reduce variables that increase risk for injury. Prolonged bed rest increases skeletal muscle weakness and decreases venous tone, contributing to postural hypotension. Prolonged standing allows blood to pool in the legs, reducing venous return and cardiac output.

Other Nursing Diagnoses

Examples of other nursing diagnoses that are appropriate for the client with fluid volume deficit include the following:

- *Fatigue* related to decreased cardiac output secondary to severe dehydration
- *Anxiety* related to lack of knowledge about the need to increase fluid intake when taking diuretics
- *Risk for Fluid Volume Deficit* related to loss of fluids secondary to large draining abdominal wound
- *Risk for Constipation* related to decreased oral intake of fluids
- *Activity Intolerance* related to dizziness and hypotension
- *Altered Mucous Membranes* related to loss of fluids from vomiting secondary to gastroenteritis
- *Potential Complication: Fluid and Electrolyte Imbalance* related to long-term vomiting and diarrhea (Carpenito, 1992).

Client and Family Teaching

Teaching the client and family about fluid volume deficit focuses on prevention. Emphasize the importance of maintaining adequate fluid intake, and teach them the signs and symptoms of fluid imbalance, the steps to take to prevent fluid deficit, and the importance of following the prescribed medication therapy. Prior to initiating a teaching plan, assess the client's understanding of the type of fluid loss that has been experienced and the fluids that provide replacement.

Provide both verbal and written instruction, including the following information:

- The amount and type of fluids to take each day.
- Avoid overexposure to heat and exercise.
- Increase fluid intake in hot weather.
- Decrease activity level during extremely hot weather.
- If vomiting, take small frequent amounts of ice chips or clear liquids, such as weak tea, flat cola, or ginger ale.
- Coffee, tea, alcohol, and large amounts of sugar increase urine output and can cause fluid loss.
- If the risk for fluid volume deficit is present, measure and record intake and output, ensuring an intake of at least 2000 mL of oral fluids and an output of at least 1000 to 1500 mL of urine each 24 hours.
- Replace fluids lost through diarrhea with fruit juices or bouillon rather than large amounts of tap water.

The older adult is at risk for fluid volume deficit from a variety of factors and requires teaching to prevent it from occurring. The factors include

- A general decrease in the perception of thirst.
- Age-related decrease in body fluids, resulting in decreased reserve.
- Age-related changes in body structure and function: decreased renal blood flow and glomerular filtration, decreased ability to concentrate urine, and impaired ability to regulate body temperature.
- Self-limiting of fluids due to fear of incontinence, with the majority of fluids taken in between 6:00 a.m. and 6:00 p.m.
- An increase in physical disabilities from age-related illnesses, such as arthritis, that limit access to fluids.
- Cognitive impairments that can interfere with recognition of thirst sensations.

Older adults and their caregivers must be taught who is most at risk and what specific interventions can be taken to meet the needs of this population. Those who are most at risk are older adults who are confused, are depressed, are tube fed, have self-care deficits, are on bed rest, or are taking medications (especially sedatives, tranquilizers, diuretics, and laxatives). The older adult who has no means of cooling the environmental temperature is also at risk for fluid volume deficit during extremely hot weather. Teaching for fluid replacement specific to the older adult includes offering preferred fluids on a regular basis over a 24-hour period; using alternative sources of liquid (such as gelatin, broth, or ice cream); and monitoring intake, output, and weight (Eliopoulos, 1987).

The Client with Fluid Volume Excess

■ ■ ■

Fluid volume excess (overhydration) is related to excessive fluid intake, excessive sodium intake, or disease states that compromise the regulatory mechanisms. The increased fluid volume may be reflected in fluid excess in the interstitial tissue spaces (for example, in edema or pulmonary congestion) and/or in the intravascular fluid space (hypervolemia). In most cases of water excess, the osmolality of blood has decreased, and water moves from the intravascular and interstitial spaces into the cells.

Pathophysiology

Fluid volume excess may be isotonic, hypotonic, or hypertonic. In isotonic volume excess (also called hypervolemia), isotonic fluids are ingested or retained, causing expansion of the extracellular compartment only. The primary manifestations are circulatory overload and interstitial edema. In *hypotonic volume excess* (also called water intoxication), both the extracellular and the intracellular compartments experience expansion. The manifestations of hypotonic volume excess are the result of circulatory overload, interstitial and cellular edema, and changes in electrolytes. In *hypertonic volume excess,* with ingestion of hypertonic solutions, the extracellular compartment expands, and the intracellular compartment contracts.

Fluid volume excess results from a wide variety of conditions that cause the retention of both sodium and water. These conditions include administration of steroids, cardiac failure, cirrhosis of the liver, renal failure, adrenal gland disorders, and stress conditions causing the release of ADH and aldosterone. Other causes include an excessive intake of sodium-containing foods, an intake of proprietary drugs high in sodium, and the administration of large amounts of intravenous fluids high in sodium (0.9% NaCl; isotonic Ringer's solution) in clients with compromised adaptive mechanisms.

Manifestations of extracellular fluid volume excess vary according to cause but, in general, include the following:

- Anasarca, the result of generalized interstitial fluid accumulation; pitting edema resulting from displacement of water in the interstitial spaces from finger pressure; or nonpitting edema

- A constant, irritating cough; dyspnea (labored or difficult breathing); orthopnea (shortness of breath when in the recumbent position); and crackles and wheezes (abnormal sounds heard on auscultation of the lungs) due to an accumulation of fluid in the lungs

- Weight gain in excess of 5% of usual body weight due to retention of fluid

- Elevated blood pressure, full and bounding pulse, jugular venous distention, and increased CVP due to increased intravascular volume

- Ascites due to an accumulation of fluid in the peritoneal cavity

- Pleural effusion due to an accumulation of fluid in the pleural space

- Changes in mental status with lethargy and confusion progressing to disorientation and coma as a result of the effect of fluid overload on the brain

Fluid volume excess is rarely a problem in healthy adults, but those at risk include the older adult, adults with chronic or debilitating illnesses, individuals with excessive ADH secretion in response to severe physical or emotional stress, and any client receiving intravenous therapy.

Collaborative Care

Managing fluid volume excess focuses on identifying clients at risk in order to prevent its occurrence; treating manifestations; and correcting the underlying cause. Management includes limiting sodium and water intake and administering diuretics.

Laboratory and Diagnostic Tests

The following laboratory tests may be ordered:

- *Serum electrolyte levels,* especially sodium, are measured, as is serum osmolality. Serum sodium and serum osmolality remain normal with hypertonic expansion or may decrease as a result of water dilution (hypotonic expansion).

- *Serum hematocrit and hemoglobin* are measured. In most cases of fluid volume excess, they are decreased as a result of plasma dilution from hypotonic expansion of extracellular fluid volume.

- *ABGs* may be measured. Changes in the ABGS include decreased pH and increased $PaCO_2$ secondary to respiratory dysfunction.

Pharmacology

In addition to the restriction of sodium and water intake, treatment for fluid volume excess may include the administration of diuretic drugs. The administration of diuretics in treating edema and fluid overload in specific disease conditions is discussed in Chapter 28 (cardiac disorders), Chapter 15 (hepatic disorders), and Chapter 26 (renal disorders). General information and client and family teaching for the client taking diuretics are outlined in the accompanying pharmacology box.

Nursing Care

Nursing care of clients with fluid volume excess focuses on identifying clients at risk and interventions to prevent its occurrence and on managing problems resulting from systemic effects. Nursing diagnoses and collaborative problems discussed in this section center around actual or potential complications related to the effects of an excess of body fluid: fluid volume excess, increased risk for impaired skin integrity, and respiratory insufficiency.

Fluid Volume Excess

Clients with actual or potential fluid volume excess include those receiving large amounts of intravenous isotonic saline or isotonic Ringer's solution over a short period of time and those with hepatic disease, cardiac failure, or renal failure. Monitoring the client for the presence or worsening of an existing fluid volume excess is important. This is particularly critical in older clients because of the age-related decline in cardiac and renal compensatory responses.

In addition to providing collaborative interventions, nursing interventions may include client education relative to (1) limiting the dietary intake of sodium, (2) the

Nursing Implications for Pharmacology: The Client Taking Diuretics

DIURETICS

Diuretics are drugs that increase urinary excretion of water and sodium. They are categorized into five groups: carbonic anhydrase inhibitors, loop diuretics, osmotic diuretics, potassium-sparing diuretics, and thiazide and thiazide-like diuretics. Diuretics are used to enhance renal function (although they may enhance the function of a healthy kidney, they do not restore function to a failing kidney) and to treat vascular fluid overload and edema. General side effects include rash, urticaria, orthostatic hypotension, dehydration, electrolyte imbalance, and hyperglycemia. Diuretics should be used with caution in the older adult.

Carbonic Anhydrase Inhibitors

Acetazolamide (Diamox)

Dichlorphenamide (Daranide)

Carbonic anhydrase inhibitors are mild diuretics that have a short activity time. They are used to reduce intraocular pressure in the eye; to promote kidney excretion of bicarbonate, sodium, potassium, and water; and as a mild anticonvulsant.

Loop Diuretics

Furosemide (Lasix)

Bumetanide (Bumex)

Loop diuretics inhibit sodium and chloride reabsorption in the ascending loop of Henle and increase potassium loss in the distal tubule (see Chapter 24 for the anatomy of the kidneys). As a result, loop diuretics promote the excretion of sodium, chloride, potassium, and water.

Osmotic Diuretics

Mannitol (Osmitrol)

Urea (Ureaphil)

Osmotic diuretics increase the osmotic pressure of glomerular filtrate to promote the excretion of sodium,

chloride, potassium, and water. This osmotic effect also occurs in the bloodstream, so that fluid is drawn from tissues into the vascular system, reducing intraocular and intracranial pressure.

Potassium-Sparing Diuretics

Spironolactone (Aldactone)

Amiloride HCl (Midamor)

Potassium-sparing diuretics promote excretion of sodium and water by inhibiting sodium-potassium exchange in the distal tubule.

Thiazide and Thiazide-like Diuretics

Thiazide	*Thiazide-like*
Chlorothiazide (Diuril)	Chlorthalidone (Hygroton)
Hydrochlorothiazide (HydroDIURIL)	Metolazone (Diulo)

Thiazide and thiazide-like diuretics promote the excretion of sodium, chloride, potassium, and water by decreasing absorption in the distal tubule.

Client and Family Teaching

- The drug will increase the amount and frequency of urination.
- The drugs must be taken even when you feel well.
- Take the drugs in the morning and afternoon to avoid having to get up at night to urinate.
- Change position slowly to avoid dizziness.
- Report the following to your primary health care provider: dizziness; trouble breathing; or swelling of face, hands, or feet.
- Weigh yourself every day, and report sudden gains or losses.
- Try to avoid using the salt shaker when eating.
- If the drug increases potassium loss, eat foods high in potassium, such as orange juice and bananas.

use of diuretics, and (3) self-monitoring and reporting of signs and symptoms of a deteriorating physical status.

Nursing interventions with rationales are as follows:

- Assess intake and output hourly. Note decreased urine output under 30 mL per hour or a positive fluid bal-

ance on 24-hour total intake and output calculations. *Cardiac failure and inadequate renal perfusion may result in decreased urine output and fluid retention.*

- Assess for edema, particularly in the pretibial, sacral, and periorbital areas. *Localized edema tends to occur in the dependent portions of the body—in the lower extremities of ambulatory clients and over the sacrum in bedridden clients. Periorbital edema is indicative of anasarca.*

- Assess vital signs, heart sounds, CVP, and volume of peripheral arteries. *Hypertension and bounding, high-volume peripheral pulses that are difficult to obliterate are indicative of hypervolemia. An S_3 gallop rhythm (third heart sound) on cardiac assessment indicates an inability of the heart to pump effectively. CVP is a guide to fluid replacement.*

- Assess weight daily under standard conditions (same time of day, approximately the same clothing, balanced scale). *Daily weights are one of the most important gauges of fluid balance. Acute weight gain or loss represents fluid gain or loss. Two kilograms of weight gain is equivalent to 2 liters of fluid gain.*

- Administer oral fluids cautiously. If fluid restriction is prescribed, institute and adhere to a 24-hour schedule for fluid intake. Instruct the client and significant others in the total volume that may be taken, the rationale for the fluid restriction, and methods for accurately measuring fluid volumes. *All sources of fluid intake, including ice chips, should be strictly monitored to avoid excess fluid intake and limit fluid intake to that which is prescribed.*

- Provide oral hygiene as needed. *Dry mucous membranes may contribute to client's desire to increase intake. Oral hygiene contributes to client comfort and keeps mucous membranes intact; it also helps relieve thirst if fluids are restricted.*

- Assess the client's needs for learning, and provide the client and significant others with appropriate instructions about
  a. Sodium restriction (discussed in the following section of the chapter)
  b. Fluid restriction
  c. Use of salt substitutes
  d. Use of prescribed medications and the reporting of side effects of medications
  e. Signs and symptoms of fluid retention, such as peripheral edema and acute weight gain
  f. Symptoms to report to the primary health care provider that indicate respiratory dysfunction, such as easy fatigability, shortness of breath, or a persistent, nonproductive cough

  When regulatory mechanisms are compromised, symptomatic control of fluid retention is essential. Sodium restriction decreases fluid retention, and diuretics increase fluid output. Knowledge of the purposes for therapy and of the correct use of prescribed drugs promotes client compliance.

Risk for Impaired Skin Integrity

Edema of the skin, which results from the accumulation of fluid in the interstitial spaces, decreases delivery of nutrients to tissues and increases susceptibility to injury.

Nursing interventions with rationales are as follows:

- Reposition the client at least every 2 hours. *Frequent change of position minimizes tissue pressure.*

- Assess vulnerable pressure areas—particularly tissues over bony prominences—with each position change, and provide skin care. *Edematous tissue over bony prominences is more prone to tissue breakdown.*

- Institute measures to minimize tissue pressure, such as providing eggcrate mattresses, foot cradles, and other devices. *An egg crate mattress distributes pressure over a wider area of the body surface and reduces pressure over bony prominences. A foot cradle minimizes the pressure that bedding can exert on the feet and lower extremities.*

Potential Complication: Respiratory Insufficiency

With fluid volume excess, impaired gas exchange may occur as a result of alveolar-capillary membrane changes secondary to pulmonary vascular congestion. Acute pulmonary edema is a serious and potentially life-threatening complication of pulmonary congestion.

Nursing interventions and rationales are as follows:

- Auscultate lungs for presence or worsening of crackles and wheezes; auscultate heart for extra heart sounds. *Crackles and wheezes are indicative of pulmonary congestion and edema. A gallop rhythm (S_3) is indicative of diastolic overloading of the ventricles secondary to fluid volume excess.*

- Maintain client in a semi-Fowler's position if dyspnea or orthopnea is present. *The semi-Fowler's position improves lung expansion by decreasing the pressure of abdominal contents on the diaphragm, facilitating lung expansion.*

- Evaluate ABGS for a decrease in the partial pressure of oxygen (PaO_2), an increase in pH, and a decrease in $PaCO_2$. Administer and monitor oxygen therapy. *Hypoxemia (decreased PaO_2) and respiratory alkalosis (increased pH and decreased $PaCO_2$) are indicative of a need for supplemental oxygen. Impairment of oxygen exchange at the alveolar-capillary membrane leads to hypoxemia; a compensatory increase in respiratory rate secondary to hypoxemia contributes to respiratory alkalosis.*

Other Nursing Diagnoses

Examples of other nursing diagnoses appropriate for the client with fluid volume excess include the following:

- *Anxiety* related to dyspnea secondary to pulmonary edema
- *Ineffective breathing pattern* related to pulmonary edema secondary to fluid overload
- *Activity Intolerance* related to fatigue secondary to impaired gas exchange
- *Risk for Impaired Physical Mobility* related to pitting edema of lower extremities
- *Risk for Altered Tissue Perfusion: Cerebral,* related to fluid retention
- *Body Image Disturbance* related to generalized edema
- *Potential Complication: Hypernatremia*

Client and Family Teaching

Teaching the client and family about fluid volume excess focuses on prevention. Any teaching plan must be based on the underlying cause of the fluid volume excess. Among the topics to address are the signs and symptoms of fluid imbalance and the steps to take to prevent excess. Emphasize the importance of taking medications as prescribed and avoiding foods that are high in sodium. In addition, teach the client and family methods of preventing or decreasing edema and preventing injury to edematous tissues.

Provide both verbal and written instructions that include the following information:

- Amount and type of fluids to take each day, with a specific plan for amounts and times if fluids are restricted.
- Methods of changing food purchases and food preparation to decrease overall sodium intake (see the box on page 119 for foods high in sodium).
- Methods of decreasing dependent edema:
  a. Frequently change positions.
  b. Avoid clothing that constricts circulation.
  c. Avoid crossing the legs when sitting.
  d. Wear support stockings or hose.
  e. Elevate the feet and legs above heart level when sitting.
- Measures to protect edematous skin from injury:
  a. Do not walk barefoot.
  b. Buy shoes that do not require "breaking in," and buy them in the afternoon rather than in the morning.
- If orthopnea is a problem, use more than one pillow when sleeping.
- If the risk of fluid excess is present, measure and keep a record of intake and output.
- Weigh daily, and report sudden increases in weight of more than 2 lb (0.9 kg) to the primary care provider.

Applying the Nursing Process

Case Study of a Client with Fluid Volume Excess: Dorothy Rainwater

Dorothy Rainwater is a 45-year-old woman who was the principal of a large high school before she developed a serious renal infection that resulted in acute renal failure. Ms. Rainwater has been hospitalized and is expected to recover from this acute illness, but she has very little urine output. Ms. Rainwater is a widow and the mother of two teenage sons. Until her illness, she was active in the care of her family as well as in school-related and community activities.

The application of the nursing process in this case study focuses on the alteration in fluid volume resulting from the client's renal failure, not on the disease itself.

Assessment

Mike Penning, the nurse assigned to care for Ms. Rainwater from 3:00 p.m. to 11:00 p.m., reviews her chart before beginning his assessment at the start of his shift. He notes that Ms. Rainwater is being treated for an acute infection of the kidneys (glomerulonephritis) and is in the oliguric phase of the illness, meaning that she has a greatly reduced urinary output. Her output for the previous 24 hours is 250 mL; this low output has been constant for the past 8 days. She has gained 1 lb (0.45 kg) in the past 24 hours. The laboratory findings from that morning are as follows: sodium, 155 mEq/L (normal limits are 136 to 148 mEq/L); potassium, 5.3 mEq/L (normal limits are 3.5 to 5.0 mEq/L); calcium, 7.6 mg/dL (normal limits are 8.0 to 10.5 mg/dL) and urine specific gravity 1.008 (normal limits are 1.010 to 1.030). Ms. Rainwater also has increased levels of blood urea nitrogen (BUN) and creatinine, whereas ABGs are within normal limits. The treatment for Ms. Rainwater's fluid excess is a restriction of fluids to less than 500 mL in 24 hours and the administration of furosemide (Lasix) intravenously.

Mr. Penning enters the room, introduces himself, and begins the assessment. He records the following findings in the bedside computer:

T 98.6 F.

P 102, with obvious neck vein distention.

R 28, with crackles and wheezes; head of bed elevated 30 degrees to facilitate respirations.

BP 160/92.

Skin: Edema present in both periorbital areas and in the sacrum; 3+ pitting edema present in feet bilaterally; skin pale and shiny.

Mental status: Alert, oriented; responds appropriately to questions.

Other: Client states she is thirsty, slightly nauseated, and extremely tired.

Mr. Penning reviews and continues the established plan of care for Ms. Rainwater.

Diagnosis

The current nursing diagnoses for Ms. Rainwater are as follows:

- *Fluid Volume Excess* related to acute renal failure
- *Risk for Impaired Skin Integrity* related to fluid retention and edema
- *Risk for Impaired Gas Exchange* related to pulmonary congestion
- *Activity Intolerance* related to fluid volume excess, fatigue, and weakness

Expected Outcomes

The expected outcomes for the plan of care specify that Ms. Rainwater will

- Regain fluid balance, as evidenced by weight loss, decreasing edema, a urine specific gravity between 1.010 and 1.030, and normal vital signs.
- Experience decreased dyspnea.
- Maintain intact skin and mucous membranes.
- Increase activity levels as prescribed.

Planning and Implementation

The following nursing interventions are planned and implemented for Ms. Rainwater:

- Take and record Dorothy's weight each morning at 6:00 a.m. and each evening at 6:00 p.m. Use bed scales until energy level increases.
- Take and record vital signs and breath sounds every 4 hours.
- Measure and record intake and output every 4 hours.
- Measure and record urine specific gravity every 8 hours.
- Restrict fluids as follows: 200 mL from 7:00 a.m. to 3:00 p.m.; 200 mL from 3:00 p.m. to 11:00 p.m.; 100 mL from 11:00 p.m. to 7:00 a.m. Ms. Rainwater prefers water or apple juice.

- Turn Ms. Rainwater from side to back to side every 2 hours, following schedule posted at the head of her bed. Inspect edematous areas, and provide skin care as needed; do not vigorously massage edematous areas.
- Provide oral care every 2 to 4 hours; allow Ms. Rainwater to brush her own teeth (caution not to swallow water) and use moistened applicators as desired.
- Maintain head of bed at 30 to 40 degrees; Ms. Rainwater prefers to use two small soft pillows under her head.
- Consult with Ms. Rainwater's physician about activity allowed; if prescribed, get Ms. Rainwater up in a reclining chair for 20 minutes twice a day. Monitor carefully for fatigue and weakness when increasing her activity level.

Evaluation

At the end of the shift, Mr. Penning evaluates the effectiveness of the plan of care and continues all diagnoses and interventions. Ms. Rainwater gained no weight, and her urinary output during his shift is 300 mL. Her urine specific gravity ranges from 1.031 to 1.033. Her vital signs remain unchanged, but her crackles and wheezes have decreased, and she states that she can breathe more easily. Her skin and mucous membranes are intact. Mr. Penning has discussed activity with Ms. Rainwater's physician, who wrote an order specifying that she be up for 15 minutes twice a day, beginning the following morning, and increase activity as tolerated.

Critical Thinking in the Nursing Process

1. What is the pathophysiologic basis for Ms. Rainwater's increased respiratory rate, blood pressure, and pulse?
2. Explain how elevating the head of the bed 30 degrees facilitates respirations.
3. Outline a plan for teaching Ms. Rainwater about diuretics.
4. Suppose Ms. Rainwater says, "I would really like to have all my fluids at once instead of spreading them out." What would be your reply, and why?
5. Develop a care plan for Ms. Rainwater for the nursing diagnosis *Powerlessness*.

▚▚▚ Electrolyte Disorders ▚▚▚

This section of the chapter provides an overview of electrolyte balance and then discusses alterations in sodium, potassium, calcium, phosphate, and magnesium balance. Normal values for electrolytes and serum osmolality are outlined in Table 5–4.

Body fluids contain both water molecules and chemical compounds. These chemical compounds can either remain intact in solution or separate (dissociate) into discrete particles. **Electrolytes** are substances that dissociate in solution to form charged particles, also called *ions*.

Cations are positively charged electrolytes; *anions* are negatively charged electrolytes. For example, sodium chloride (NaCl) in solution dissociates into a sodium ion, a cation carrying a positive charge (Na^+); and a chloride ion, an anion carrying a negative charge (Cl^-). Electrolytes may be *univalent* and carry only one electrical charge, such as sodium (Na^+) and chloride (Cl^-); or they may be *divalent,* carrying two electrical charges, such as magnesium (Mg^{2+}) and phosphate (HPO_4^{2+}).

Electrolytes have many functions:

- They assist in regulating water balance.
- They assist in regulating acid-base balance.
- They contribute to enzyme reactions.
- They are essential to neuromuscular activity.

Electrolytes are found in the intracellular and extracellular fluid compartments, but the electrolyte composition of intracellular and extracellular fluid differs significantly, as shown in Figure 5–8.

Sodium and chloride are the principal extracellular electrolytes. Sodium is the predominant extracellular cation, and chloride and bicarbonate (HCO_3^-) are the major extracellular anions. The high sodium concentration in the extracellular space is essential to the regulation of body fluid volume, contributing approximately 90% to the osmolality of the extracellular fluid (Metheney, 1992). Potassium (K^+) is maintained at a low concentration in the extracellular space. Although the composition of intracellular fluid differs somewhat from tissue to tissue, the principal intracellular electrolytes are potassium and magnesium.

High concentrations of intracellular potassium and extracellular sodium are maintained against an electrochemical gradient by an active transport mechanism located in the cell membranes. The sodium-potassium pump is an important example of active transport (Figure 5–9 on page 116). By this mechanism, cells actively transport potassium from interstitial fluid (an area of low concentration of potassium [5 mEq/L]) to the intracellular fluid compartment (an area of high concentration of potassium [150 mEq/L]). Sodium-potassium ATPase, an enzyme that is located in the cell membrane and that activates ATP, is the carrier mechanism for the transport of sodium and potassium across the cell membrane.

Disorders of sodium, potassium, calcium, magnesium, and phosphorus are summarized in Table 5–5.

Sodium Disorders

▪ ▪ ▪

Sodium, the principal regulator of extracellular fluid volume in the body, is primarily responsible for regulating the osmolality of extracellular fluids and is an important

Table 5–4	Normal Values for Electrolytes and Serum Osmolality	
Serum Component		**Values**
Electrolytes		
Sodium (Na^+)		136–148 mEq/L
Chloride (Cl^-)		98–106 mEq/L
Bicarbonate (HCO_3)		22–26 mEq/L
Calcium (Ca^{2+}) (total)		4.3–5.3 mEq/L
Potassium (K^+)		3.5–5.0 mEq/L
Phosphate/inorganic phosphorous (PO_4^{3-})		1.7–2.6 mEq/L
Magnesium (Mg^{2+})		1.3–2.1 mEq/L
Serum osmolality		275–295 mOsm/kg

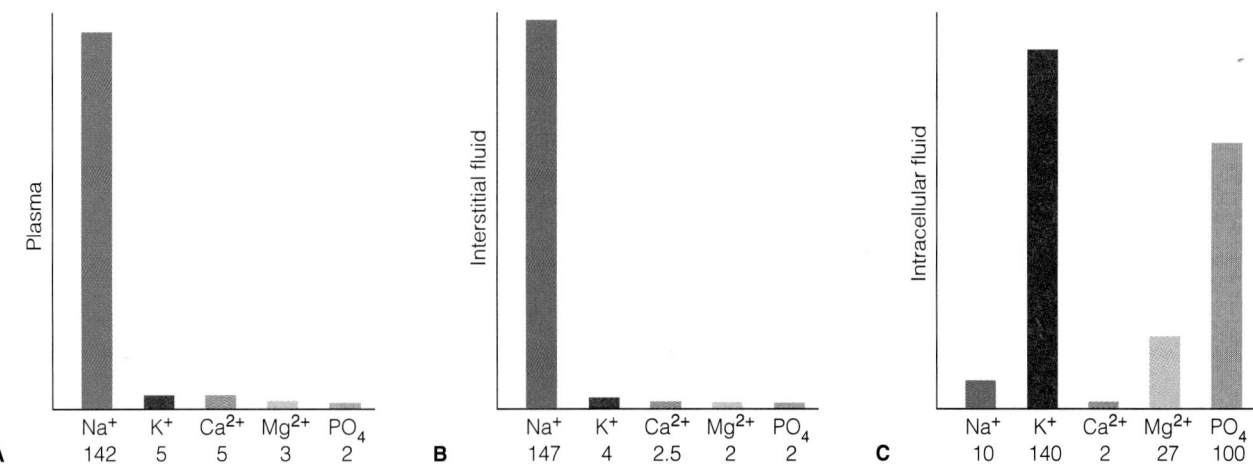

Figure 5–8   Electrolyte composition of *A*, plasma; *B*, interstitial fluid; and *C*, intracellular fluid in milliequivalents.

A	Na+	K+	Ca2+	Mg2+	PO4
	142	5	5	3	2

B	Na+	K+	Ca2+	Mg2+	PO4
	147	4	2.5	2	2

C	Na+	K+	Ca2+	Mg2+	PO4
	10	140	2	27	100

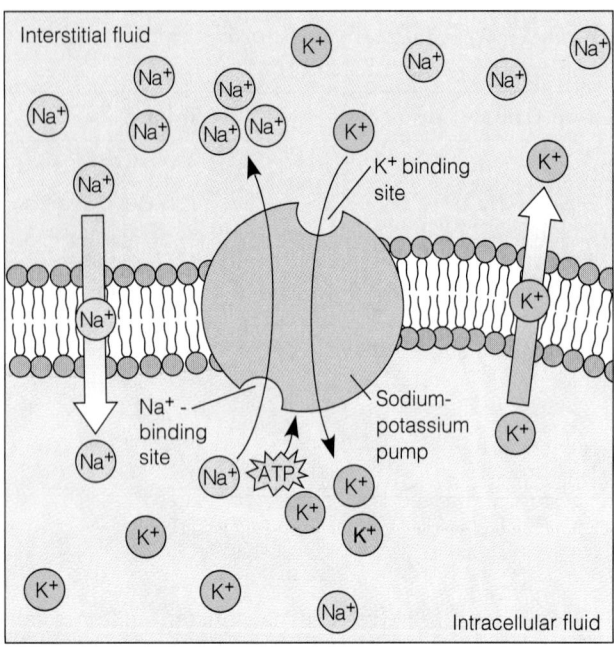

Figure 5–9   The sodium-potassium pump. Sodium and potassium ions are moved across the cell membranes against their concentration gradients. This active transport process is fueled by energy from adenosine triphosphate (ATP).

factor in maintaining neuromuscular activity and acid-base balance. Because of the close interrelationship between sodium and water balance, disorders of fluid volume and sodium often occur together.

This section of the chapter discusses sodium balance in the body, sodium deficit (hyponatremia), and sodium excess (hypernatremia). A case study and nursing care plan is not included; refer to the case study of the client with fluid volume excess in the preceding section.

Sodium Balance in the Body

The normal range of serum sodium concentration is approximately 136 to 148 mEq/L. Serum sodium levels are maintained by the mechanisms that regulate water intake and excretion, including renal excretion of water in response to hyponatremia and release of antidiuretic hormone (ADH), and stimulation of the thirst mechanism secondary to hypernatremia.

Serum sodium values reflect the concentration of sodium in the extracellular fluid; thus, fluid deficit causes an increase in the concentration of sodium even if the total body sodium is unchanged, and fluid excess causes a decrease in sodium concentration even though sodium has not been lost from the body. Sodium imbalances alter the osmolality of the extracellular fluid and affect water distribution between the fluid compartments. Body water moves from areas of lower osmolality, to areas of higher

osmolality, and water concentration in the intracellular fluid space changes.

Regulation of Sodium Balance

Extracellular fluid volume is maintained by mechanisms that regulate sodium balance and, therefore, the osmolality of body fluids. The two major mechanisms for the regulation of sodium balance are the glomerular filtration rate and the secretion of the hormone aldosterone.

The *glomerular filtration rate (GFR)* is the rate at which plasma is filtered through the renal glomeruli. Glomerular filtration rate is dependent on renal perfusion; renal perfusion is dependent on blood volume, cardiac output, and arterial blood pressure. GFR is also dependent on sodium and potassium levels. Increases and decreases in water intake change blood volume, cardiac output, and blood pressure, thus affecting the glomerular filtration rate. Hypovolemia (low blood volume) reduces renal perfusion and triggers the renin-angiotensin-aldosterone mechanism discussed earlier (see Figure 5–5).

Aldosterone, a hormone produced by the adrenal cortex, stimulates the cells of the distal tubules and collecting ducts of the kidney to increase both the rate of sodium and water absorption and the rate of potassium and hydrogen excretion. A decreased secretion of aldosterone causes an increase in the excretion of sodium and water and an increase in the absorption of potassium and hydrogen ions.

A number of factors stimulate aldosterone secretion; however, angiotensin II, produced by the renin-angiotensin-aldosterone system, is the most immediate regulator of aldosterone secretion.

Adrenocorticotropic hormone (ACTH), a hormone secreted by the anterior pituitary in response to stress, plays a minor role in regulating aldosterone secretion. Its main effect is to stimulate the release of cortisol (a glucocorticoid) by the adrenal gland. However, when ACTH is secreted in large amounts—for example, following significant accidental trauma or the trauma of major surgery—it causes the secretion of a small amount of aldosterone (Keyes, 1985).

Factors in Sodium Imbalances

Most of the sodium in the body comes from dietary intake. Although a sodium intake of 500 mg per day is usually sufficient to meet the body's needs, the average intake of sodium by adults in the United States is 12 to 30 times the daily requirement (Porth, 1994). Other sources of excess sodium are prescription medications, intravenous saline solutions, or self-prescribed remedies that contain sodium. Fortunately, the healthy kidney is able to maintain homeostasis even with excess sodium intake.

Sodium loss occurs through the kidneys, the skin, and the gastrointestinal tract. Changes in renal function may result in either an increase or a decrease in sodium excretion. Excessive sweating or loss of skin surface (as in

Table 5-5   Electrolyte Imbalances with Abnormal Values, Causes, and Results

Ion/ Normal Value	Abnormality/ Serum Value	Possible Causes	Results
Sodium 136–14 mEq/L	Hypernatremia ($Na^+ > 148$ mEq/L) Hyponatremia ($Na^+ < 136$ mEq/L)	Uncommon in healthy individuals; most often a result of excessive NaCl administration by intravenous route Excessive Na^+ loss through burned skin, excessive sweating, vomiting, diarrhea, tubal drainage of stomach, and as a result of excessive use of diuretics; deficiency of aldosterone (Addison's disease); renal disease	Increased blood pressure; water leaves cells to enter ECF; edema; congestive heart failure in cardiac patients Dehydration; decreased blood volume and blood pressure (shock); if sodium is lost and water is not, symptoms are the same as with water excess (mental confusion, giddiness, muscular twitching, convulsions, coma)
Potassium 3.5–5.0 mEq/L	Hyperkalemia ($K^+ > 5.0$ mEq/L) Hypokalemia ($K^+ < 3.5$ mEq/L)	Renal failure; deficit of aldosterone; rapid intravenous infusion of KCl; burns or severe tissue injuries, which cause K^+ to leave cells Gastrointestinal tract disturbances (vomiting, diarrhea), gastrointestinal suction; chronic stress; Cushing's disease; inadequate dietary intake (starvation); hyperaldosteronism; diuretic therapy	Bradycardia; cardiac arrhythmias, depression, and arrest; skeletal muscle weakness, flaccid paralysis Cardiac arrhythmias, possible cardiac arrest; muscular weakness; alkalosis; hypoventilation
Magnesium 1.3–2.1 mEq/L	Hypermagnesemia ($Mg^{2+} > 2.1$ mEq/L) Hypomagnesemia ($Mg^{2+} < 1.3$ mEq/L)	Rare (occurs when Mg is not excreted normally); deficiency of aldosterone; excessive ingestion of Mg^{2+}-containing antacids Alcoholism; loss of intestinal contents, severe malnutrition; diuretic therapy	Lethargy; impaired CNS functioning, coma, respiratory depression Tremors, increased neuromuscular excitability, convulsions
Chloride 98–106 mEq/L	Hyperchloremia (Cl^- excess in ECF: >106 mEq/L) Hyperchloremia (Cl^- deficit in ECF: <98 mEq/L)	Increased retention or intake; hypekalemia Vomiting; hypokalemia; excessive ingestion of alkaline substances	Metabolic acidosis due to enhanced loss of bicarbonate; stupor; rapid, deep breathing; unconsciousness Metabolic alkalosis due to bicarbonate retention
Calcium 4.3–5.3 mEq/L	Hypercalcemia ($Ca^{2+} > 5.3$ mEq/L) Hypocalcemia ($Ca^{2+} < 4.3$ mEq/L)	Hyperparathyroidism; excessive vitamin D; prolonged immobilization; renal disease (decreased excretion); malignancy; Paget's disease; Cushing's disease accompanied by osteoporosis Burns (calcium trapped in damaged tissues); increased renal excretion in response to stress and increased protein intake; diarrhea; vitamin D deficiency; alkalosis	Tetany, bone wasting, pathological fractures; flank and deep thigh pain; kidney stones, nausea and vomiting, cardiac arrhythmias and arrest; depressed respiration, coma Tingling of fingers, tremors, tetany, convulsions; depressed excitability of the heart, bleeder's disease
Phosphate 1.7–2.6 mEq/L	Hyperphosphatemia ($PO_4 > 2.6$ mEq/L) Hypophosphatemia ($PO_4 < 1.7$ mEq/L)	Acute or chronic renal insufficiency; hypoparathyroidism (decrease in calcium and increase in phosphorus); increased phosphorus intake and absorption; hyperthyroidism; respiratory or lactic acidosis; cellular release of phosphorus (cytotoxic drugs, catabolism from diabetic ketoacidosis, etc.) Transfer of phosphate into cells secondary to cellular anabolism, increased GI loss from antacid use, decreased intestinal absorption, respiratory or metabolic alkalosis, increased renal excretion (diuretic therapy, etc.), alcoholism	Muscle cramps and pain, paresthesias, tingling around the mouth (symptoms occur as a result of low serum calcium due to phosphate binding with ionized calcium) Calcification of soft tissues Apprehension; slurred speech; confusion; seizures; coma; paresthesias; muscle weakness; chest pain; dysrhythmias; heart failure; shock; metabolic alkalosis; hemolytic anemia; granulocytopenia; platelet destruction; anorexia, dysphagia; nausea and vomiting; gastric atony; and ileus

Note. Adapted from *Human Anatomy and Physiology* (2nd ed.) (p. 924) by E. N. Marieb, 1992, Redwood City, CA: Benjamin/Cummings.

Clinical Manifestations of Hyponatremia

■ ■ ■

General Manifestations, Depending on Serum Sodium Levels

- Anorexia
- Nausea and vomiting
- Abdominal cramping
- Diarrhea
- Headache
- Altered mental status
- Hyperreflexia
- Muscle twitching
- Tremors
- Convulsions
- Decreasing levels of consciousness

Hyponatremia with Decreased Extracellular Fluid

- Thirst
- Postural hypotension
- Tachycardia
- Dizziness
- Weakness

Hyponatremia with Increased Extracellular Fluid

- Hypertension
- Bounding pulse
- Edema
- Weight gain

---

burns) can cause excessive sodium loss. Because sodium is absorbed as gastrointestinal contents move down the intestines, conditions such as vomiting, diarrhea, and gastrointestinal suction increase sodium loss. Sodium may also be lost from the gastrointestinal tract when gastrointestinal tubes are irrigated with water instead of saline or when repeated tap water enemas are given (Porth, 1994). In addition, sodium loss or gain may occur in adrenal diseases (see Chapter 20).

The Client with Hyponatremia

■ ■ ■

Hyponatremia is a serum sodium level of less than 136 mEq/L. Hyponatremia most commonly results from a loss of sodium from the body, but it may also be caused by fluid volume excess, resulting in sodium dilution.

Pathophysiology

Causes of hyponatremia associated with a decreased extracellular fluid volume include those that result from renal losses of sodium (due to diuretics, adrenal insufficiency, or salt-losing renal diseases) and extrarenal losses of sodium (sweating, vomiting, diarrhea, and third-space sequestration of fluids).

The causes of low serum sodium levels with normal or increased extracellular volume (and resultant hemodilution) include the following:

- Edematous conditions, such as those accompanying congestive heart failure, renal failure, and cirrhosis of the liver, which result in hyponatremia from increased extracellular fluid volume
- Syndrome of inappropriate secretion of antidiuretic hormone (SIADH), with normal or increased fluid volume
- Excessive administration of hypotonic intravenous fluids, causing increased fluid volume

The manifestations of hyponatremia are primarily the result of serum hypoosmolality, which causes a movement of water into the cell. The manifestations that result depend on the rapidity of onset, the severity, and the cause of the hyponatremia. If the condition develops slowly, manifestations are usually not experienced until the serum sodium levels reach 125 mEq/L. Early signs and symptoms of hyponatremia are the result of an alteration in gastrointestinal function and include anorexia, nausea and vomiting, abdominal cramping, and diarrhea.

As sodium levels continue to decrease, the brain and nervous system are affected by increases in intercellular water. Neurologic manifestations progress rapidly when the serum sodium level falls below 120 mEq/L. Neurologic manifestations occur as a result of the osmotic gradient that develops across the blood–brain barrier and increases the water content of the brain cells. Manifestations of altered neurologic function include headache, depression, dulled sensorium, personality changes, irritability, lethargy, hyperreflexia, muscle twitching, and tremors. If serum sodium falls to very low levels, convulsions and coma are likely to occur.

In hyponatremia associated with decreased extracellular fluid volume, the manifestations are those associated with hypovolemia. The client may experience dry mucous membranes, thirst, postural hypotension and dizziness, weakness, and tachycardia.

In hyponatremia associated with expansion of extracellular fluid volume, manifestations include those of hypervolemia: bounding pulse, elevated blood pressure, peripheral or generalized edema, weight gain, and increased CVP. The accompanying box summarizes the clinical manifestations of hyponatremia.

Collaborative Care

Collaborative management of hyponatremia is aimed at returning the client to a normovolemic (normal blood volume) state. Treatment measures include the administration of fluids and diuretics (depending on the cause) and increasing the intake of high-sodium foods.

Laboratory and Diagnostic Tests

The following laboratory tests may be ordered:

- *Serum sodium and osmolality* are decreased in hyponatremia (serum sodium <136 mEq/L; serum osmolality <275 mOsm/kg). However, normal or increased serum osmolality is associated with hyponatremia due to renal failure because of the accumulation of waste products in the serum.

- *A 24-hour urine specimen* shows decreased sodium (<40 mEq/L over 24 hours) or increased sodium (>220 mEq/L over 24 hours), depending on the cause of the hyponatremia. For example, in conditions associated with normal or increased extracellular volume (such as SIADH), urinary sodium is increased; in conditions resulting from losses of isotonic fluids (sweating, diarrhea, vomiting, and third-space fluid accumulation), by contrast, urinary sodium is decreased.

Pharmacology

Hypovolemic hyponatremia is treated by fluid volume replacement with sodium-containing fluids. These fluids are administered by mouth, nasogastric tube, or by the intravenous route. Therapy may include replacement of other electrolyte losses that may have occurred.

When plasma volume is decreased, isotonic Ringer's solution or isotonic saline (0.9% NaCl) solution may be administered. Cautious administration of intravenous 3% or 5% NaCl solution may be necessary in clients who have very low plasma sodium levels (110 to 115 mEq/L).

The management of hypervolemic hyponatremia, or hyponatremia associated with normal plasma volume, includes the use of loop diuretics, which induce isotonic diuresis and fluid volume loss without hyponatremia (see the pharmacology box on page 111). Thiazide diuretics are avoided because they cause a relatively greater sodium loss in relation to water loss.

Treatment of hyponatremia due to inappropriate ADH secretion (see Chapter 20) is directed at correcting the underlying cause. If this is not possible or if the condition is severe, hypervolemia is treated with fluid restriction and loop diuretics or the administration of small amounts of 3% or 5% NaCl and loop diuretics.

Dietary Management

If hyponatremia is mild, increased intake of foods high in sodium may restore normal sodium balance (see the accompanying box). An increased intake of dietary sodium is usually accompanied by the restriction of oral fluids. Dietary increases in sodium are not effective in reversing severe hyponatremia or hyponatremia resulting from nonrenal pathophysiologic disorders.

Foods High in Sodium
■ ■ ■

High in Added Sodium

Processed Meat and Fish
- Bacon
- Luncheon meat and other cold cuts
- Sausage
- Smoked fish

Selected Dairy Products
- Buttermilk
- Cheeses
- Cottage cheese
- Ice cream

Processed Grains
- Graham crackers
- Most dry cereals

Most Canned Goods
- Meats
- Soups
- Vegetables

Snack Foods
- Salted popcorn
- Potato chips/pretzels
- Nuts
- Gelatin desserts

Condiments and Food Additives
- Barbecue sauce
- Catsup
- Chili sauce
- Meat tenderizers
- Worcestershire sauce
- Saccharin
- Pickles
- Soy sauce
- Salted margarine
- Salad dressings

Naturally High in Sodium

- Brains
- Kidney
- Clams
- Crab
- Lobster
- Oysters
- Shrimp
- Dried fruit
- Spinach
- Carrots

Nursing Care

Nursing care of the client with hyponatremia focuses on identifying clients at risk and managing problems resulting from the systemic effects of the disorder.

Risk for Fluid Volume Deficit or Excess

It is important to remember that hyponatremia may occur in clients with a variety of diseases or injuries and is often associated with excessive intravenous intake of hypotonic fluids, abnormal water retention, or excessive fluid loss. Clients at risk for mild hyponatremia include older clients, those who are having surgery and are allowed nothing by mouth (NPO) for several days, and those taking potent diuretics.

Nursing interventions and rationales are as follows:

- For clients who are receiving normal saline or those with cardiovascular disease who are receiving sodium-containing intravenous solutions for treatment of hyponatremia, monitor for signs of circulatory overload (increased blood pressure and CVP, tachypnea, tachycardia, gallop rhythm, shortness of breath, crackles). *Hypertonic saline solutions may cause a lethal hypervolemia. In clients with cardiovascular and renal disease, mechanisms for excretion of sodium and water are compromised.*

- For clients requiring fluid restriction, explain why fluid intake must be limited, how much fluid is allowed over 24 hours; and how to measure fluid volumes. *Client education increases compliance to prescribed interventions.*

- Monitor intake and output, weigh daily, and calculate 24-hour fluid balance. *Fluid excess or deficit may occur with hyponatremia.*

For additional nursing interventions that may apply to the client with hyponatremia, review the discussions of fluid volume deficit and fluid volume excess.

Risk for Sensory/Perceptual Alterations

Secondary to changes in the osmotic gradient across the blood–brain barrier, brain cells swell, and the client may exhibit symptoms of altered neurologic function.

- Assess the client for neurologic changes, such as lethargy, altered or decreased level of consciousness, confusion, and convulsions. Monitor behavior, mental status, and orientation. *Baseline data, as well as ongoing assessments, are critical in determining the neurologic effects of hyponatremia. Neurologic manifestations often occur with rapidly falling sodium levels and may be manifested by either increased or decreased activity.*

- Assess neuromuscular status for changes in muscle strength, muscle tone, and deep tendon reflexes. Assess muscle strength and tone by asking client to squeeze your hands, to hold the arms flexed while you pull downward, and to push both feet against your hands. Reflexes are assessed by using a reflex hammer (see Chapter 39). *Generalized muscular weakness and decreased deep tendon reflexes occur in response to hyponatremia. Muscle weakness is usually bilateral and more pronounced in peripheral muscle groups.*

- Maintain a quiet environment, and institute safety precautions in clients at risk for injury from seizure. *A quiet environment reduces neurologic stimulation. Safety precautions, such as ensuring that side rails are up and having an airway readily available, reduce risk of injury from seizure.*

Other Nursing Diagnoses

Examples of other nursing diagnoses that are appropriate for the client with hyponatremia include the following:

- *Fatigue* related to muscle weakness
- *Decreased Cardiac Output* related to alterations in plasma volume
- *Altered Thought Processes* related to the effect of hyponatremia on the central nervous system
- *Risk for Injury* related to muscle weakness and mental confusion
- *Self-Care Deficit: Bathing/Hygiene,* related to muscle weakness and confusion
- *Risk for Altered Mucous Membranes* related to fluid restriction

Client and Family Teaching

Client and family education focuses on the underlying cause of the sodium deficit and, often, on prevention. Clients at risk for hyponatremia as well as those who are experiencing hyponatremia require teaching.

People who are at risk for mild hyponatremia may be healthy but sometimes participate in activities that increase fluid loss through excessive perspiration (diaphoresis) and then replace those losses by drinking large amounts of water. This includes athletes, people who do heavy labor in high environmental temperatures, and the older adult who does not have access to environmental cooling during hot weather. Teaching to prevent mild hyponatremia includes

- The manifestations of mild hyponatremia, including nausea, cramps in the abdomen, and muscle weakness.

- The importance of drinking liquids containing sodium and other electrolytes at frequent intervals when the client is perspiring heavily, when environmental temperatures are high, and/or when the client has experienced several days of watery diarrhea.

- The importance of having regular laboratory tests to monitor electrolytes if the client is taking a potent diuretic or on a low-sodium diet.

- Types of foods and fluids to take orally if dietary sodium is not restricted.

The Client with Hypernatremia

■ ■ ■

Hypernatremia is a serum sodium concentration in excess of 148 mEq/L. It is sometimes classified as a hyperosmolar imbalance because it is associated with a hypertonicity of body fluids. Hypernatremia may occur from water loss or sodium gain. This condition causes cellular dehydration.

Pathophysiology

Hypernatremia results from either a gain in serum sodium in excess of water or a loss of water in excess of serum sodium. Because disorders that can cause acute changes in the serum sodium can also cause changes in the extracellular fluid volume, hypernatremia may occur with a fluid volume excess, a fluid volume deficit, or with a near-normal extracellular fluid volume. In all instances, hyperosmolality of the plasma occurs. With the increase in plasma osmolality, water moves out of the cell, leading to cellular dehydration.

Hypertonicity from pure water loss is relatively uncommon because of body processes that preserve water. Therefore, hypertonicity from pure water loss usually occurs in people who have a decrease in water intake, such as those with an altered thirst mechanism (e.g., the older adult), those who are unable to verbalize thirst (e.g., the unconscious person), and those who are unable to obtain water (e.g., individuals who are too sick to seek water or have no access to water). In these people, water loss may be increased by losses from extrarenal sources, such as the skin (fever with insensible loss, burns, diaphoresis), the gastrointestinal tract (watery diarrhea), and the lungs (hyperventilation, improperly humidified ventilators). Renal sources, too, may exacerbate pure water loss; examples include diabetes insipidus, osmotic diuresis secondary to hyperglycemia or increased urea level from high protein tube feedings, the use of intravenous contrast media for radiographic studies, and the use of intravenous mannitol and dextran.

Hypernatremia may result from the excessive oral intake of sodium from, for example, oral electrolyte solutions and hyperosmolar enteric formulas. Hypernatremia may also result from excessive intravenous infusion of sodium-containing fluids, such as sodium bicarbonate used in cardiac arrest or as treatment of lactic acidosis, and the administration of 3%, 5%, 0.9% intravenous saline solutions, or from medications high in sodium, such as sodium polystyrene sulfonate (Kayexalate). Excessive sodium retention may occur secondary to adrenal hyperfunction,which results in an increase in aldosterone production.

The primary manifestations of hypernatremia are those related to alterations in neurologic function secondary to dehydration of brain cells (thirst, restlessness, weakness, disorientation, lethargy, stupor, convulsions, coma) and those resulting from increased excitability and conduction of nerve cells (muscle irritability and twitching). Other findings include peripheral and pulmonary edema (hypernatremia associated with fluid volume excess),

---

Clinical Manifestations of Hypernatremia

■ ■ ■

- Thirst
- Restlessness
- Weakness
- Altered mental status
- Decreasing level of consciousness
- Muscle twitching
- Convulsions
- Postural hypotension
- Dyspnea
- Weight gain
- Elevated CVP

---

postural hypotension (hypernatremia associated with fluid volume deficit), weight gain, dyspnea, and elevated CVP. Neurologic manifestations are more likely to occur with a sudden increase in plasma sodium. Acute elevations of plasma sodium occurring over a period of less than 24 hours are often fatal. The accompanying box summarizes the chief clinical manifestations of hypernatremia.

Collaborative Care

The treatment of hypernatremia depends on its cause and includes oral administration of water and intravenous administration of hypotonic fluids (5% D5W or 0.45% NaCl solution) to correct the water deficit. Diuretics may also be administered to increase sodium excretion, and a low-sodium diet may be prescribed for long-term maintenance.

Correction of hypernatremia is done slowly (over a 48-hour period) to avoid deterioration of brain function from cerebral edema secondary to a shift of water into the brain cells.

Laboratory and Diagnostic Tests
The following laboratory and diagnostic tests may be ordered:

- *Serum sodium levels* are measured. In hypernatremia, serum sodium levels are greater than 148 mEq/L. The elevated serum sodium is indicative of the hypertonicity of the plasma.

- *Serum osmolality* is measured. In hypernatremia, serum osmolality is greater than 295 mOsm/kg.

- *The dehydration test* is conducted. In this test, water is withheld for 16 to 18 hours, and ADH is then administered. One hour after the ADH has been given, serum and urine osmolality are measured. This test is used to identify the cause of diseases that increase urine output, such as diabetes insipidus (a pituitary disorder).

Teaching Clients to Follow a Low-Sodium Diet

■ ■ ■

- Reducing sodium intake will help the body excrete excess sodium.

- The body needs less than one-tenth of a teaspoon of salt per day.

- Approximately one-third of sodium intake comes from salt added to foods during cooking and at the table; one-fourth to one-third comes from processed foods; and the rest comes from food and water naturally high in sodium.

- Sodium compounds are used in foods as preservatives, leavening agents, and flavor enhancers.

- Many nonprescription drugs (such as aspirin, cough medicine, laxatives, and antacids) as well as toothpastes and mouthwashes contain high amounts of sodium.

- Low-sodium salt substitutes are not really sodium free and may contain half as much sodium as regular salt.

- Use salt substitutes sparingly; larger amounts often taste bitter instead of salty.

- The preference for salt will eventually diminish.

- Salt, monosodium glutamate, baking soda, and baking powder contain substantial amounts of sodium.

- Read labels.

- In place of salt or salt substitutes, use herbs, spices, lemon juice, vinegar, and wine as flavoring when cooking.

Pharmacology

The principal treatment of hypernatremia is oral or intravenous water replacement. Occasionally, diuretics are used in combination with water replacement.

Nursing Care

Nursing care of the client with hypernatremia focuses on identifying clients at risk and on applying diagnoses relevant to the client with hypernatremia. Some nursing diagnoses and associated interventions applicable to the client with hypernatremia are similar to those clients with fluid volume deficit or fluid volume excess. Consult the earlier discussions of these disorders for more information.

Altered central nervous system function may result from hypernatremia itself or from the cerebral edema that occurs when the condition is corrected too rapidly. In both instances, it is extremely important that the client be closely monitored and that precautions to reduce risk of injury be instituted.

Risk for Injury Related to Altered Cerebral Function

- Monitor and maintain oral and intravenous fluid replacement to within the prescribed limits. Monitor serum sodium levels and osmolality; report rapid declines in serum sodium and osmolality. *Body water should be replaced gradually. Incremental replacement of body water to restore sodium and water balance prevents rapid decrease in serum sodium and serum osmolality and prevents cerebral edema.*

- Monitor neurologic function, assessing for altered mental status, lethargy, headache, nausea, vomiting, elevated blood pressure, and decreased pulse rate. *Swelling of the cells of the central nervous system alters neurologic function. Early intervention is based on timely identification of cerebral edema.*

- Institute safety precautions as necessary—keep the bed in its lowest position, side rails up and padded, and airway at the bedside. *Preventing trauma to clients is based on anticipating possible problems and preparing to prevent or treat injury.*

- Keep clocks, calendars, and familiar objects at the bedside. Provide orientation, and tell the client and family members that the disorientation is usually temporary. *A disruption in the quality and quantity of incoming stimuli can affect thought processes. Measures to increase normal perceptions of time and place facilitate reorientation.*

Other Nursing Diagnoses

Other applicable nursing diagnoses include the following:

- *Self-Care Deficit* related to altered neurologic function
- *Fluid Volume Excess* related to increased intake of sodium and water
- *Fluid Volume Deficit* related to decreased fluid intake
- *Anxiety* related to increased cerebral irritability
- *Impaired Physical Mobility* related to muscle weakness
- *Risk for Injury* related to increased neuromuscular irritability secondary to hypernatremia

Client and Family Teaching

Client and family teaching for the prevention of hypernatremia is conducted primarily for people who have some underlying pathophysiologic condition that interferes with normal sodium balance and who must be on a low-sodium diet. Teach the client and family members to read labels for sodium content, to avoid foods and proprietary medications high in sodium, to cook without salt, and to use spices to flavor foods. Instruct clients to discuss the use of salt substitutes with their primary health care provider. When developing a teaching plan to assist the client with a low-sodium diet, consider cultural dietary sources and identify nondietary sources of sodium, such as softened water or over-the-counter medications. The box on page 122 summarizes teaching for clients on a low-sodium diet.

Potassium Disorders

■ ■ ■

Potassium, the primary intercellular cation, plays a vital role in cell metabolism and helps determine the membrane potential of nerve and muscle cells. The ratio of intracellular potassium to extracellular potassium helps determine the resting membrane potential of nerve and muscle cells; either a deficit or an excess of potassium can adversely affect neuromuscular and cardiac function (Figure 5–10). Potassium is unique in that it can be either life-supporting or toxic and life-threatening, depending on its level in the body. The normal serum potassium level is 3.5 to 5.0 mEq/L.

The largest reservoir of body potassium is within the intracellular space (approximately 3500 mEq, or 90%). The intracellular potassium concentration is 140 to 150 mEq/L; the plasma concentration of the extracellular fluid fluctuates from 3.5 to 5 mEq/L. The concentrations of potassium in each of these body fluid compartments is maintained by the sodium-potassium pump.

To maintain the homeostatic balance of potassium in the body, there has to be a source of intake and a means of elimination. Normally, potassium is supplied in the foods ingested. Virtually all foods contain potassium, although some foods and fluids are richer sources of potassium than others. The kidneys are the principal regulators of potassium and eliminate potassium very efficiently; even when potassium intake is stopped, the kidneys continue to excrete potassium. Because the kidneys do not conserve potassium well, significant amounts may be lost through this route. This is most likely to happen when a person stops eating and drinking as, for example, on a crash diet. Potassium loss may also occur secondary to the effects of drugs, especially potassium-losing diuretics. Because the kidneys are the principal organs involved in the elimination of potassium, both renal failure and potassium-sparing diuretics (such as spironolactone) can lead to potentially serious elevations of serum potassium.

Normally only small amounts of potassium are lost in the feces, but substantial amounts may be lost from the gastrointestinal tract under abnormal circumstances. For example, large amounts of potassium-rich gastrointestinal fluid may be lost with diarrhea or through drainage from an ileostomy (a permanent opening into the small bowel).

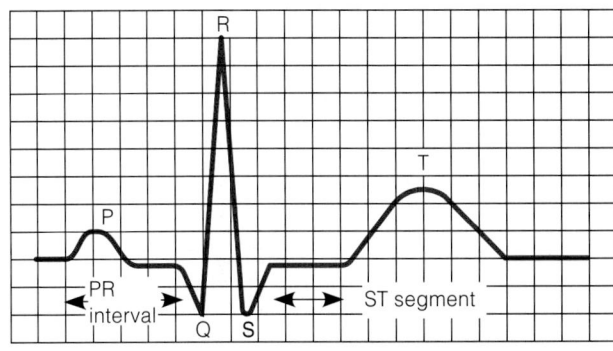

Figure 5–10   The effects of changes in potassium on electrocardiogram (ECG) tracings: *A*, normal ECG, *B*, ECG in hyperkalemia, *C*, ECG in hypokalemia.

Although dietary intake and renal output affect serum potassium levels, it is crucial to remember that movement of potassium into and out of the cells is potentially a greater source of serum potassium changes. For example, when acidosis (decreased pH from increased hydrogen ion concentration) is present, the body responds by moving potassium out of the cell into the serum (in exchange for hydrogen ions), leading to an increased serum potassium level (hyperkalemia). When alkalosis (increased pH from decreased hydrogen ion concentration) is present, the body responds by moving potassium from the serum into the cells in exchange for hydrogen ions, leading to a decreased serum potassium level (hypokalemia).

Aldosterone assists the kidneys in controlling the level of potassium concentration in the body through a feedback mechanism (see Figure 5–5). An increase in extracellular potassium levels stimulates the adrenal gland to increase production of aldosterone. In turn, aldosterone stimulates the kidneys to increase their excretion of potassium. Accordingly, hypersecretion or hyposecretion of aldosterone profoundly affects the serum potassium level. Clients with primary aldosteronism (from an aldosterone-secreting tumor of the adrenal gland) produce excessive amounts of aldosterone, which leads to excessive depletion of serum potassium levels. Conversely, clients with adrenal insufficiency (Addison's disease) have decreased aldosterone production and elevated serum potassium levels. See Chapter 20 for further information about these conditions.

The Client with Hypokalemia

■ ■ ■

Hypokalemia is an abnormally low level of serum potassium (less than 3.5 mEq/L). Hypokalemia is most often due to potassium loss from the body; in healthy people, inadequate intake rarely leads to hypokalemia.

Pathophysiology

Hypokalemia may result from many different factors, including

- Urinary loss of potassium secondary to drug therapy (such as potassium-losing diuretics, large doses of intravenous penicillins, aminoglycosides, cisplatin, and glucocorticoids), conditions that produce osmotic diuresis (such as diabetes mellitus), and conditions associated with hyperaldosteronism.

- Abnormal loss of gastrointestinal secretions from severe vomiting and diarrhea and from excessive ileostomy drainage.

In addition, potassium intake may be inadequate when the client undergoes extended parenteral fluid therapy with potassium-free solutions, for example, intravenous administration of D5W or 5% dextrose with 0.45% NaCl without added potassium. A temporary shift of potassium into the intracellular space resulting in a decreased serum potassium concentration may be caused by

- Alkalosis (the potassium ion is exchanged for the hydrogen ion).

- Situations of rapid tissue repair following burns, trauma, and starvation (potassium moves into the cells).

- Situations in which there is a persistently high level of insulin in the blood; for example, in clients receiving high-carbohydrate hyperalimentation solutions with added insulin.

All clients with serum potassium values of 3.5 mEq/L or less should be closely monitored. A serum potassium concentration of less than 2.5 mEq/L is potentially serious because of the disruption of cardiac rhythm and myocardial contraction.

The manifestations of hypokalemia are the result of alteration in the transmission of nerve impulses, which interferes with the normal contractility of smooth, skeletal, and cardiac muscle. Signs and symptoms of hypokalemia include generalized muscle weakness progressing to paralysis and ileus, leg cramps, nausea and vomiting, paresthesias, decreased bowel sounds, and decreased reflexes (Figure 5–11).

Cardiovascular effects include dysrhythmias; irregular, rapid, weak pulse; and decreased blood pressure. Characteristic cardiac effects seen in the electrocardiogram (ECG) pattern are flattened and inverted T waves, prominent U waves, depressed ST segment, peaked P waves, and a prolonged QT interval. However, the ECG pattern is not as reliable an indicator of the severity of hypokalemia as it is for hyperkalemia.

Because hypokalemia enhances the effect of digitalis, a medication used to treat congestive heart failure, hypokalemia in the client receiving digitalis can lead to digitalis toxicity. If these clients are also receiving potassium-losing diuretics, the risk for digitalis toxicity is increased, and close monitoring for both hypokalemia and the toxic effects of digitalis is crucial.

Collaborative Care

The management of hypokalemia focuses on prevention and/or definitive potassium replacement therapy.

Laboratory and Diagnostic Tests
The following laboratory and diagnostic tests may be ordered:

- *Serum potassium* is measured and is used to monitor potassium levels in clients who are at risk for developing potassium imbalances and in those who are being treated for correction of hypokalemia. Serum potassium values that are less than 2.5 mEq/L are associated with serious pathophysiologic disorders.

- *ABGs* are measured to determine the acid-base status of the client, because hydrogen ion imbalances frequently coexist with potassium imbalances. Laboratory test results should be monitored for the presence of increased pH, increased bicarbonate, and decreased chloride.

- *ECG recordings* are conducted and will reveal signs of hypokalemia and digitalis toxicity.

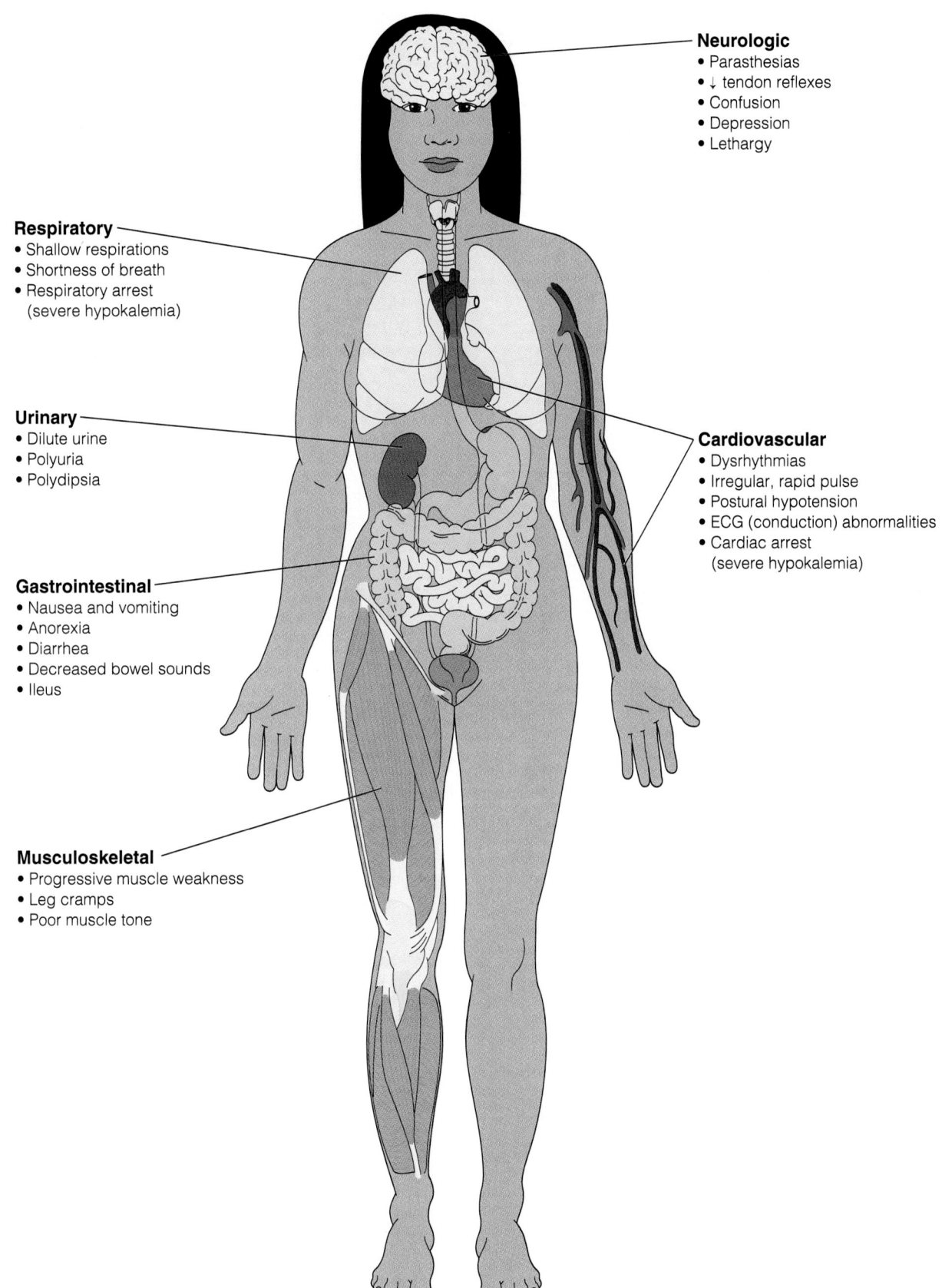

Neurologic
• Parasthesias
• ↓ tendon reflexes
• Confusion
• Depression
• Lethargy

Respiratory
• Shallow respirations
• Shortness of breath
• Respiratory arrest
  (severe hypokalemia)

Urinary
• Dilute urine
• Polyuria
• Polydipsia

Cardiovascular
• Dysrhythmias
• Irregular, rapid pulse
• Postural hypotension
• ECG (conduction) abnormalities
• Cardiac arrest
  (severe hypokalemia)

Gastrointestinal
• Nausea and vomiting
• Anorexia
• Diarrhea
• Decreased bowel sounds
• Ileus

Musculoskeletal
• Progressive muscle weakness
• Leg cramps
• Poor muscle tone

Figure 5–11 Multisystem effects of hypokalemia.

Nursing Implications for Pharmacology: The Client with Hypokalemia

POTASSIUM SOURCES

Potassium acetate (Tri-K)

Potassium bicarbonate (K+ Care, Klor-Con/EF)

Potassium citrate (K-Lyte)

Potassium chloride (Micro-K, K+ 10, Kaochlor, Kaon)

Potassium gluconate (Kaon Elixir, Royonate)

Potassium is rapidly absorbed from the gastrointestinal tract; potassium chloride is the agent of choice, because low chloride often accompanies low potassium. Potassium is used to treat hypokalemia, in replacement therapy with parenteral nutrition and potassium-losing diuretics, and prophylactically after major surgery.

Nursing Responsibilities

- When giving oral forms of potassium:
  a. Dilute or dissolve liquid potassium in fruit or vegetable juice.
  b. Chill to increase palatability.
- When giving parenteral forms of potassium:
  a. Administer slowly.
  b. Do not administer undiluted.
  c. Assess injection site frequently for signs of pain and inflammation.
  d. Use an infusion control device.
  e. Have sodium polystyrene sulfonate (Kayexalate) on hand if needed for treatment of hyperkalemia.
- Assess for abdominal pain, distention, gastrointestinal bleeding; if present, do not administer medication. Notify health care provider.
- Monitor fluid intake and output.
- Assess for manifestations of hyperkalemia: weakness, feeling of heaviness in legs, mental confusion, hypotension, cardiac arrhythmias, changes in ECG, increased serum potassium levels.

Client and Family Teaching

- Do not take potassium supplements if you are also taking a potassium-sparing diuretic.
- When parenteral potassium is discontinued, eat potassium-rich foods.
- Do not chew enteric-coated tablets or allow them to dissolve in the mouth; this may affect the potency and action of the medications.
- Do not use salt substitutes when taking potassium (most salt substitutes are potassium based).

Pharmacology

Administration of parenteral and/or oral potassium both prevents hypokalemia and treats established hypokalemia. Commonly prescribed potassium supplements, their actions, and nursing implications are described in the accompanying pharmacology box. When hypokalemia is present, treatment includes daily maintenance replacement and replacement of the current losses and existing deficit. Several days of therapy may be required to correct established hypokalemia.

In the surgical client who is receiving intravenous therapy, hypokalemia can be prevented through the addition of 40 mEq of potassium chloride to the 24-hour intravenous fluid allowance. Clients who are receiving total parenteral nutrition or enteric nutrition or who have fluid losses from the gastrointestinal tract (through nasogastric suction or ileostomy drainage) may require additional potassium supplements, depending on individual needs.

Dietary Management

Although increasing the dietary intake of potassium is not a treatment for actual hypokalemia, foods high in potassium may be used to prevent its occurrence or to supplement pharmacologic therapy. Foods and fluids high in potassium are listed in the box on page 127.

Nursing Care

Nursing care of clients at risk for developing hypokalemia is directed toward prevention. Nursing care differs somewhat for clients who have developed hypokalemia and, therefore, require potassium replacement therapy. The focus is on identifying clients at risk for hypokalemia and on preventng hypokalemia and the problems resulting from the systemic effects it exerts.

Decreased Cardiac Output

The client with hypokalemia is at risk for alteration in cardiac output. The cardiac effects of hypokalemia (prolonged cardiac repolarization and decreased strength of myocardial contraction) result in reduced cardiac output and hypotension. Hypokalemia also alters the response to cardiac drugs, such as digitalis and the antidysrhythmics.

Nursing interventions with rationale are as follows:

- Monitor vital signs at regular intervals, including peripheral pulses. *The pulse is thready and weak in clients with hypokalemia; hypotension on sitting or standing is noted first and then becomes generalized.*

- Monitor clients taking digitalis for digitalis toxicity. Monitor clients taking antidysrhythmics, such as lidocaine, procainamide, and quinidine, for resistance to the effects of these drugs. *Hypokalemia potentiates digitalis effects and increases resistance to certain antidysrhythmics.*

- In clients on ECG rate and rhythm monitors, observe for the characteristic pattern indicating hypokalemia. *Decreased conduction through the myocardium is exhibited by ST segment depression, broadened, flatter T waves, and U waves, giving the appearance of a prolonged QT interval. Life-threatening dysrhythmias may develop.*

- Monitor the rate of intravenous potassium administration closely. Intravenous potassium should be diluted and administered via an electronic infusion device. *Do not administer undiluted potassium directly into the vein. Concentrations of 20 to 40 mEq/L of infusion solution is the usual concentration and should not exceed 60 mEq/L. (For rapid replacement, the concentration of potassium in the solution may be higher.) The rate of infusion should not exceed 20 to 40 mEq per hour. The client's serum potassium level and clinical symptoms should be evaluated frequently during replacement therapy. In clients requiring rapid potassium replacement, the ECG is monitored for evidence of deadly cardiac effects. Inadvertent hyperkalemia secondary to replacement therapy may result in severe cardiac dysrhythmias and death.*

- Control discomfort over the infusion site. In the event that the infusion cannot be administered through a central vein, local irritation may occur over the infusion site. If the infusion cannot be slowed, discomfort may be controlled by applying an ice pack. *Potassium may cause local irritation to the vein wall.*

Potential Complication: Electrolyte Imbalance: Hypokalemia

Nursing interventions with rationales are as follows:

- Assess clients taking oral medications, potassium-losing diuretics, and other oral drugs associated with potassium loss (for example, cisplatin and glucocorticoids) for manifestations of hypokalemia. Additionally, question the client regarding compliance to prescribed potassium supplements and for dietary intake of foods and fluids. *Ingestion of potassium-losing diuretics without oral potassium replacement is frequently a cause of hypokalemia. Noncompliance to prescribed potassium supplements and lack of dietary intake of potassium-rich foods*

Foods High in Potassium

■ ■ ■

Fruits and Fruit Juices

■ Apple juice	■ Grapefruit	■ Pears
■ Apricots	■ Honeydew melon	■ Plums
■ Apricot nectar	■ Nectarines	■ Prunes
■ Avocados	■ Oranges	■ Prune juice
■ Bananas	■ Orange juice	■ Raisins
■ Cantaloupe		■ Strawberries
■ Dates	■ Papayas	■ Tangerines
■ Figs	■ Peaches	■ Watermelon

Vegetables and Vegetables Juices

■ Artichokes	■ Greens	■ Rhubarb
■ Asparagus	■ Mushrooms	■ Tomatoes
■ Broccoli	■ Okra	■ Turnips
■ Dry beans	■ Peas	■ V-8 Juice
■ Cauliflower	■ Potatoes	■ Yams
■ Eggplant	■ Pumpkin	■ Zucchini

Meats

■ Beef	■ Liver	■ Tuna
■ Chicken	■ Lobster	■ Turkey
■ Kidney	■ Pork loin	■ Salmon

Milk Products

■ Buttermilk	■ Low-fat yogurt
■ Chocolate milk	■ Milk
■ Evaporated milk	

---

may be contributing factors. Preventive nursing intervention for hypokalemia is predicated on the identification and assessment of individuals known to be at risk.

- Monitor clients receiving intravenous potassium-losing diuretics and/or intravenous drugs, such as amphotericin B and the penicillin derivatives, that induce potassium loss. *The diuretics frequently used for intravenous therapy have powerful potassium-losing properties. The side effects of certain drugs include potassium loss.*

- Identify clients at risk for hypokalemia to anticipate losses and need for potassium replacement. Monitor laboratory values, including serum potassium levels, and acid-base status, particularly alkalosis, indicated by an increased pH and bicarbonate. Assess client for potassium intake, urine output, excessive fluid losses from the gastrointestinal system (gastrointestinal suction, vomiting, excessive ileostomy drainage, and diarrhea), intravenous drugs causing potassium depletion, and fluid replacement without supplemental potassium. *Gastrointestinal fluids are rich in potassium, and excessive losses may lead to hypokalemia. Excessive loss of hydrogen ions from the upper gastrointestinal tract through suctioning or excessive vomiting is a cause of metabolic alkalosis; alkalosis results in the movement of potassium into the cell in exchange for hydrogen and results in potassium loss as the kidneys attempt to save hydrogen ions in exchange for potassium ions. The kidneys do not conserve potassium. Therefore, clients who are on fluid replacement and who are not ingesting adequate food or fluids require intravenous potassium supplements.*

- Monitor respiratory rate, depth, and effort; heart rate and rhythm; blood pressure; intestinal function (presence of bowel sounds); and skeletal muscle strength, movement, and sensation. *Hypokalemia results in an alteration in skeletal and smooth muscle function. Alteration in skeletal muscle function in turn results in muscle weakness, leading to marked generalized weakness. An abrupt onset of hypokalemia may lead to total muscle paralysis and include respiratory arrest. Paralytic ileus with changes in peristalsis may occur as a result of altered smooth muscle functioning.*

- Maintain accurate intake and output records. *Gastrointestinal fluid losses, particularly if combined with stress, can lead to significant potassium losses. Accurate intake and output records serve as a guide to the calculation of needs for replacement.*

- Encourage intake of foods and fluids with high potassium content, including salt substitutes containing potassium and prescribed oral potassium supplements for clients on long-term diuretic therapy. Educate clients regarding the need for the replacement and appropriate administration. Dilute liquid potassium supplements with water or juices. Educate clients in the need to follow through on laboratory tests as ordered by the physician. *In nonacute situations, potassium may be replaced and serum levels maintained through the diet and/or the use of potassium supplements. Liquid potassium supplements must be diluted because undiluted liquid potassium replacements can lead to gastric irritation.*

Other Nursing Diagnoses

Nursing diagnoses that are appropriate for the client with hypokalemia include the following:

- *Anxiety* related to knowledge deficit of manifestations of hypokalemia
- *Risk for Altered Health Maintenance* related to insufficient knowledge of supplemental sources of potassium
- *Activity Intolerance* related to muscle weakness.

- *Altered Nutrition: Less than Body Requirements* related to anorexia and paralytic ileus
- *Fluid Volume Deficit* related to excessive gastrointestinal fluid loss

Client and Family Teaching

Home care management of clients at risk for developing hypokalemia is based on preventive interventions. Discharge planning focuses on teaching the client to assume self-care practices, including compliance with prescribed medications and diet and the need for regular follow-up assessments.

Include the following information when teaching the client and family:

- If the client is taking digitalis, the pulse must be counted before taking the medication, and a rate of less than 60 must be reported to the primary health care provider. If the client is also taking a potassium-losing diuretic, high-potassium food or fluids must be included in the daily diet.

- Diarrhea increases potassium loss.

- If the oral potassium supplements are unpalatable, a powdered potassium salt can be mixed with orange sherbet or gelatin.

- If approved by the health care provider, potassium intake can be supplemented with potassium-containing salt substitutes; it is essential to read the label to be sure potassium is included in the preparation.

- Potassium levels must be measured at regular intervals.

<hr>

Applying the Nursing Process

Case Study of a Client with Hypokalemia: Rose Ortiz

Rose Ortiz is a 72-year-old widowed grandmother who lives in a modest dwelling by herself but in close proximity to her daughter's home. Her daughter demonstrates her concern for Ms. Ortiz's welfare by making daily telephone calls to check on her mother and visiting frequently. Ms. Ortiz has been diagnosed with mild congestive heart failure and is being treated with digoxin (Lanoxin) 0.125 mg, hydrochlorothiazide (Oretic) 75 mg orally (PO) daily, and a mildly restricted sodium diet (2 g daily). For the last several weeks, Ms. Ortiz has complained to her daughter that she feels weak and sometimes faint, light-headed, and dizzy. A serum electrolyte test ordered by her clinic physician reveals a potassium level of 2.4 mEq/L. Potassium chloride solution (Kaochlor 10%, 20 mEq/15 mL) PO twice daily is prescribed, and Ms. Ortiz is referred to Nancy Walters, a clinic nurse, for follow-up care.

Assessment

The health history obtained by Miss Walters reveals that Ms. Ortiz has rigidly adhered to her sodium-restricted diet and has been compliant in taking her prescribed medications, with the exception of occasionally taking an additional "water pill" when her ankles swell. She takes a laxative every evening to insure a daily bowel movement. She states that she is reluctant to take the potassium chloride the doctor has ordered because her neighbor complains of gastric distress when taking a potassium supplement his doctor prescribed. Physical assessment findings included T 98.4, P 70, R 20, and BP 138/84.

Diagnosis

Miss Walters makes the following nursing diagnoses for Ms Ortiz:

- *Risk for Injury* related to muscle weakness
- *Risk for Altered Health Maintenance* related to lack of knowledge of side effects of diuretic therapy and laxative use
- *Risk for Altered Health Maintenance* related to lack of knowledge of foods high in potassium

Expected Outcomes

The expected outcomes for the plan of care specify that Ms. Ortiz will

- Have a potassium level within normal limits (3.5 to 5.0 mEq/L).
- Regain normal muscle strength.
- Avoid traumatic physical injury.
- Verbalize understanding of the side effects of diuretic therapy and of the need for supplemental potassium.
- Verbalize understanding of the measures to avoid gastrointestinal irritation when taking oral potassium.
- Identify potassium-rich foods.

Planning and Implementation

The following nursing interventions are planned and implemented for Ms. Ortiz:

- Explain to Ms. Ortiz the need to use caution when ambulating, particularly when climbing or descending stairs. Clarify with her the probable cause of the muscle weakness, and explain that it will resolve with potassium supplement therapy.
- Discuss with Ms. Ortiz the side effects of diuretic therapy, and explain how taking additional diuretics may have contributed to her hypokalemia. Describe how laxatives may contribute to hypokalemia, and caution her about daily use. Caution her against changing prescribed drug therapy for purposes of self-treatment and taking laxatives. Discuss with her the effect of ad-

equate intake of high-fiber foods and fluids on bowel function, and explain that these will eliminate the need for a laxative.

- Explain to Ms. Ortiz the need for the prescribed potassium and its role in reversing her muscle weakness.
- Teach Ms. Ortiz to take the prescribed potassium supplement after breakfast and supper, to dilute it in 4 oz of juice or water, and to sip it slowly over a 5- to 10-minute period. Instruct her that if gastric irritation occurs, she is to call for other suggestions.
- Discuss dietary sources of potassium with Ms. Ortiz, and supply her with a list of potassium-rich foods (see the box on page 127).

Evaluation

On a follow-up clinic visit 1 week later, Ms. Ortiz discusses her progress with the nurse. The muscle weakness, dizziness, and other symptoms she has been experiencing are resolved. She is taking all of the prescribed drugs as directed and is taking laxatives only two or three times a week. Ms. Ortiz reports that she has increased her intake of potassium-rich foods and fluids and of high-fiber foods. Her potassium level is within normal limits.

Critical Thinking in the Nursing Process

1. What is the pathophysiologic basis for Ms. Ortiz's feelings of weakness and dizziness?
2. How may the chronic overuse of laxatives contribute to hypokalemia?
3. Describe the interaction of digitalis, diuretics, and potassium.
4. Develop a plan of care for Ms. Ortiz for the nursing diagnosis *Constipation*.

The Client with Hyperkalemia

■ ■ ■

Hyperkalemia is an abnormally high level of serum potassium (greater than 5 mEq/L). The effects of hyperkalemia on body functions are similar to those of hypokalemia and are the result of altered neuromuscular and cardiac function.

Pathophysiology

Hyperkalemia can result from inadequate excretion of potassium, excessively high intake of potassium, or a shift of potassium from the intracellular to the extracellular space. Causes of inadequate excretion include decreased renal excretion secondary to renal disease or renal failure, hypovolemia, the use of potassium-sparing diuretics, and

---

Clinical Manifestations of Hyperkalemia

∎ ∎ ∎

- Dysrhythmias
- Possible heart block
- Abdominal cramping
- Diarrhea
- Anxiety

- Paresthesias
- Muscle twitching and tremors
- Flaccid paralysis
- Dyspnea

---

adrenal insufficiency. Intake-related hyperkalemia may occur following the rapid transfusion of blood, the plasma portion of which is high in potassium because of the intracellular potassium that has escaped from hemolyzed red blood cells.

In metabolic acidosis, the excess hydrogen ions move into the cell to be buffered in exchange for the potassium ion, causing potassium to shift from the intracellular to the extracellular space. This occurs, for example, in diabetic ketoacidosis. Potassium also is released from cells following crush injuries, surgical trauma, burns, severe infections, chemotherapy with cytotoxic drugs, and conditions causing increased tissue catabolism. Hyperkalemia may also arise secondary to hyperglycemia from insulin deficit.

The most harmful consequence of hyperkalemia is its effect on cardiac function. The ECG changes seen early in hyperkalemia include the development of peaked, narrow T waves, particularly in the precordial leads; later changes include prolongation of the PR interval (atrioventricular block), widened QRS interval (interventricular block) progressing to complete heart block, and atrial asystole. Acidosis, low serum calcium and sodium, and high serum magnesium levels exaggerate the effects of hyperkalemia on cardiac function. Hyperkalemia also interferes with the action of digitalis on the heart.

The clinical manifestations of hyperkalemia are the result of altered nerve transmission. The effects of hyperkalemia on skeletal muscle function are primarily the result of heightened neuromuscular activity. Early manifestations include diarrhea, colic (abdominal cramping), anxiety, paresthesias, irritability, and muscle tremors and twitching. With increasing serum potassium levels, muscle weakness occurs, which then progresses to flaccid paralysis and respiratory paralysis. Pathophysiology related to specific collaborative problems is discussed further in the nursing care section. The accompanying box summarizes the clinical manifestations of hyperkalemia.

Collaborative Care

The management of hyperkalemia focuses on returning the serum potassium level to normal by treating the un-

derlying cause and avoiding additional potassium intake. The choice of therapy for existing hyperkalemia is based on the severity of the excess potassium.

The seriousness of the condition is determined by the level of serum potassium and the ECG findings. Mild hyperkalemia exists when the serum level is between 5 and 6.5 mEq/L and the ECG changes are limited to peaking of the T wave. Hyperkalemia is considered moderate when the serum level is between 6.5 and 8 mEq/L and the ECG changes are restricted to peaking of the T wave. Severe hyperkalemia is defined as a serum potassium level of greater than 8 mEq/L and an ECG pattern with absent P waves and widened QRS pattern (Petersdorf et al., 1991).

Mild hyperkalemia may be reversed by treating the cause (e.g., existing metabolic acidosis) or discontinuing the intake of potassium-sparing diuretics. Diuretics such as furosemide (Lasix) may be employed to enhance renal excretion of potassium.

Laboratory and Diagnostic Tests

The following laboratory and diagnostic tests may be ordered:

- *Serum electrolytes* are measured. With hyperkalemia, the serum potassium level is greater than 5.0 mEq/L. Low calcium and sodium levels may augment the effects of hyperkalemia; therefore, these electrolytes are usually measured as well.

- *ABGs* are measured. Because acidosis and hyperkalemia may coexist, ABGs are measured to determine whether acidosis is present.

- *ECG monitoring* is conducted. Cardiac rate and rhythm are monitored to determine the severity of the effects of hyperkalemia on cardiac function and to guide therapy. Correction of the hyperkalemia will reverse the cardiac effects.

Pharmacology

The objective of pharmacologic intervention for hyperkalemia is to reduce the serum potassium level and to reverse the effects of potassium on neuromuscular membranes. Commonly prescribed drugs, their actions, and nursing implications are summarized in the accompanying pharmacology box.

For moderate to severe hyperkalemia, short-term aggressive emergency measures are taken to lower the serum potassium temporarily by pushing potassium into the cells and counteracting the effects of hyperkalemia on the heart. Measures that favor the intracellular shift of potassium include the intravenous administration of hypertonic dextrose, the administration of regular insulin, and the intravenous administration of sodium bicarbonate. Glucose and insulin facilitate movement of potassium into the cell. Sodium bicarbonate may be used to treat acidosis; it favors the shift of potassium into the cell as

Nursing Implications for Pharmacology: The Client with Hyperkalemia

DIURETICS

Potassium-losing diuretics, such as furosemide (Lasix), may be used to enhance renal excretion of potassium.

Nursing Responsibilities

- Monitor serum electrolytes for diuretic effects on serum potassium level.
- Monitor and record body weight at regular intervals under standard conditions (same time of day, balanced scale, same clothing).
- Monitor intake and output.

INSULIN, HYPERTONIC DEXTROSE, AND SODIUM BICARBONATE

Insulin, hypertonic dextrose (10% to 50%), and sodium bicarbonate are used in the emergency treatment of moderately severe hyperkalemia. Both the intravenous administration of insulin and hypertonic glucose and the use of intravenous sodium bicarbonate cause a temporary shift of potassium into the cell in exchange for sodium, thus lowering the serum potassium level. Insulin promotes the transfer of potassium into the cell, and glucose prevents hypoglycemia. The onset of action of insulin and hypertonic dextrose occurs within 30 minutes and is effective for approximately 6 hours.

Sodium bicarbonate elevates the serum pH; potassium is moved into the cell in exchange for hydrogen. Sodium bicarbonate is particularly useful in the client with metabolic acidosis. The sodium provided helps reverse the cardiac effects of hyperkalemia. Onset of effects occurs within 15 to 30 minutes and is effective for approximately 2 hours.

Nursing Responsibilities

- Administer intravenous insulin and dextrose over prescribed interval of time using a rate volume infusion pump.
- Administer sodium bicarbonate as prescribed. It may be administered as an intravenous bolus or added to a dextrose-in-water solution and given by infusion.
- In clients receiving sodium bicarbonate, monitor for sodium overload, particularly in clients with hypernatremia, congestive heart failure, and renal failure.

- Monitor the ECG pattern closely for indications of the effectiveness of interventions.
- Monitor serum electrolytes (K^+, Na^+, Ca^{2+}, Mg^{2+}, and particularly serum K^+) frequently during therapy.

CALCIUM GLUCONATE AND CALCIUM CHLORIDE

Intravenous calcium gluconate or calcium chloride is used as a temporary emergency measure in treating severe hyperkalemia to counteract the toxic effects of potassium on myocardial contractility and on nerves and muscles.

Nursing Responsibilities

- Closely monitor the ECG of the client with severe hyperkalemia receiving intravenous calcium, particularly for bradycardia.
- Calcium should be used cautiously in clients receiving digitalis, because calcium increases the cardiotonic effects of digitalis and may precipitate digitalis toxicity, leading to dysrhythmias.

SODIUM POLYSTYRENE SULFONATE (KAYEXALATE) AND SORBITOL

Sodium polystyrene sulfonate (Kayexalate) is used in the treatment of moderate or severe hyperkalemia. Categorized as a cation exchange resin, Kayexalate exchanges sodium or calcium for potassium in the gastrointestinal tract. Sorbitol is given in conjunction with Kayexalate to promote bowel elimination, thus removing the potassium-containing resin. Kayexalate and sorbitol may be administered orally, through a nasogastric tube, or rectally as a retention enema. The usual dosage is 20 g three or four times a day with 20 mL of 70% sorbitol solution.

Nursing Responsibilities

- Because Kayexalate contains sodium, monitor clients with congestive heart failure and edema closely for water retention.
- Monitor serum electrolytes (K^+, Na^+, Ca^{2+}, Mg^{2+}) frequently during therapy.
- Restrict sodium intake in clients who are unable to tolerate increased sodium load (e.g., those with CHF or hypertension).

potassium ions are exchanged for hydrogen ions. Slow intravenous administration of calcium gluconate is used to suppress temporarily the toxic effects of potassium on the heart. Calcium gluconate should be administered cautiously and discontinued if bradycardia occurs.

To remove potassium from the body, drugs such as sodium polystyrene sulfonate (Kayexalate) may be administered orally or rectally. In the client with renal failure, hemodialysis and peritoneal dialysis are used to manage hyperkalemia.

Nursing Care

Nursing care for the client with hyperkalemia is oriented primarily around collaborative problems and the client's responses to the systemic effects of the elevated serum potassium. Nursing diagnoses and collaborative problems discussed in this section focus on identifying clients at risk for hyperkalemia, preventing hyperkalemia, and on addressing problems resulting from the systemic effects of hyperkalemia. (Individual needs may vary from client to client.)

Decreased Cardiac Output

The effects of hyperkalemia on myocardial function are the result of altered atrial and ventricular depolarization. The most critical effect of toxic levels of hyperkalemia are cardiac dysrhythmias with ventricular fibrillation and cardiac arrest. Harmful myocardial effects are more pronounced with rapid elevation of the serum potassium level.

Significant cardiac effects of hyperkalemia begin to occur at a serum potassium level of 7 mEq/L and are usually present at a level of 8 mEq/L. Low serum sodium and calcium levels, high serum magnesium levels, and acidosis contribute to the adverse effects of hyperkalemia on the heart muscle.

Nursing interventions with rationales are as follows:

- Monitor the ECG rate and rhythm for indications of hyperkalemia, such as development of peaked, narrow T waves, prolongation of the PR interval, depression of the ST segment, widened QRS interval, and loss of the P wave. Notify the physician of changes. *The most serious systemic effect of hyperkalemia is altered cardiac function resulting in dysrhythmias. The ECG and serum potassium levels are used as a guide to therapy.*

- Monitor clients receiving sodium bicarbonate closely for fluid volume excess. *Increased sodium from injection of a hypertonic sodium bicarbonate solution can cause a shift of water into the extracellular space.*

- Monitor the administration of calcium gluconate closely, particularly in patients who may be receiving digitalis. *Calcium augments the cardiotonic effects of digitalis; in patients receiving digitalis, this may lead to digitalis toxicity.*

Potential Complication: Electrolyte Imbalance: Hyperkalemia Secondary to Potassium Retention

Clients whose renal elimination of potassium is compromised are particularly at risk for hyperkalemia. Nursing care that focuses on early detection of hyperkalemia is essential.

- Closely monitor serum potassium levels, blood urea nitrogen, creatinine, and fluid intake and urine output of clients at risk for decreased urine output (those with hypovolemia and/or renal failure). Notify the physician of a serum potassium level of greater than 5 mEq/L or of urine output of less than 30 mL/h. Avoid giving potassium if oliguria (scant urine output) or anuria (no urine output) is present. For hypovolemic clients who are able to take fluids, increase fluid intake. *The kidneys are the major organs of excretion of potassium from the body. Oliguria or anuria resulting from hypovolemia or from renal failure may result in hyperkalemia.*

- Instruct clients taking supplemental forms of potassium and potassium-sparing diuretics to use with caution salt substitutes containing potassium. *Additional intake of potassium in clients taking these drugs may result in hyperkalemia.*

- Instruct clients with hyperkalemia from any cause to avoid salt substitutes and foods high in potassium content. *Elimination of dietary sources of potassium helps control hyperkalemia.*

- Instruct clients with chronic renal failure on potassium-restricted diets to avoid foods high in potassium. Provide the client with a list of these foods and of salt substitutes that contain potassium. *Avoiding external sources of potassium facilitates a decrease in the serum potassium level and helps prevent recurrence of hyperkalemia.*

- Monitor clients receiving cation exchange resins and sorbitol for fluid volume excess. *The resin exchanges potassium for sodium or calcium in the bowel. Excessive sodium and water retention may occur.*

Potential Complication: Electrolyte Imbalance: Hyperkalemia Secondary to Extracellular Shift of Potassium

As previously discussed, a number of conditions can cause an extracellular shift of potassium. Because serious complications secondary to hyperkalemia can develop, early identification and treatment of this condition is critical. Nursing care includes monitoring the client at risk closely and reporting significant signs and symptoms to the physician.

- Monitor serum electrolyte levels of clients at risk for hyperkalemia and acidosis. *Early detection and treatment of hyperkalemia can prevent serious alterations in neuromuscular function.*

- Monitor respiratory rate and depth. Elevate the head of the bed, and encourage deep breathing. *Hypoventilation and retained secretions may occur as a consequence of muscular weakness and shallow respirations. Carbon dioxide retention secondary to hypoventilation results in respiratory acidosis.*

Other Nursing Diagnoses

Other nursing diagnoses appropriate for the client with hyperkalemia include the following:

- *Activity Intolerance* related to muscle weakness and fatigue
- *Anxiety* related to altered sensation (paresthesias) in face, tongue, hands, and feet
- *Pain* related to intestinal cramping
- *Risk for Fluid Volume Deficit* related to diarrhea
- *Diarrhea* related to increased peristalsis

Client and Family Teaching

An important dimension of discharge planning for the client at risk for hyperkalemia is teaching directed toward preventing recurrence. Depending on the needs of the client, it may be necessary to include the family, a significant other, or a caregiver. Provide both written and verbal instructions on dietary restrictions and medications to be avoided, including a list of salt substitutes and foods high in potassium with instructions to avoid these.

Applying the Nursing Process

Case Study of a Client with Hyperkalemia: Montigue Longacre

Montigue Longacre, a 51-year-old male of African ancestry, is experiencing the effects of severe hypertension and end-stage renal disease. He arrives at the emergency clinic with complaints of shortness of breath on exertion and extreme weakness.

Assessment

During the admission history, Mr. Longacre reveals to the nurse, Janet Allen, that he normally receives dialysis three times a week. He skipped his last treatment, however, to attend the funeral of his father in a nearby city. During the last several days, he has eaten a large number of fresh oranges he received as a gift. Physical assessment findings revealed the following: T 99.2, P 100, R 28, BP 168/96, 2+ pretibial edema, and a 6 lb (3.6 kg) weight gain since his last hemodialysis treatment 3 days ago. The emergency clinic physician requests serum electrolytes, ABGs, BUN and creatinine level, and an ECG to be done immediately. The results of these diagnostic tests are as follows:

K^+, 6.5 mEq/L (normal range: 3.5 to 5 mEq/L)

BUN, 118 mg/dL (normal range: 7 to 18 mg/dL)

creatinine, 14 mg/dL (normal range: 0.7 to 1.3 mg/dL)

HCO_3^-, 17 mEq/L (normal range: 22 to 26 mEq/L)

ECG showing peaked T wave.

Mr. Longacre is placed on continuous ECG monitoring, and the physician prescribes hemodialysis. As an interim measure to lower the serum potassium, the physician prescribes D50W (25 g of dextrose), one ampule, to be administered with 20 units of regular insulin slowly by the intravenous route; sodium bicarbonate (Na_2HCO_3) 44 mEq, one ampule, intravenously over 3 to 5 minutes; and sodium polystyrene sulfonate (Kayexalate) and sorbitol as a retention enema.

Diagnosis

Mrs. Allen identifies the following nursing diagnoses for Mr. Longacre:

- *Activity Intolerance* related to skeletal muscle weakness
- *Potential for Injury* related to skeletal muscle weakness
- *Risk for Decreased Cardiac Output* related to existing hyperkalemia or to hypokalemia secondary to rapid correction of hyperkalemia
- *Risk for Altered Health Maintenance* related to knowledge deficit of causes and treatment of hyperkalemia
- *Fluid Volume Excess* related to oliguria/anuria

Expected Outcomes

The expected outcomes for the plan of care specify that Mr. Longacre will

- Gradually resume usual physical activities.
- Remain free of physical injury.
- Have a return of serum potassium levels to within normal range.
- Verbalize causes of hyperkalemia, the importance of compliance to hemodialysis regimen, and the role of diet in prevention of hyperkalemia.

Planning and Implementation

The following nursing interventions are planned and implemented for Mr. Longacre:

- Monitor intake and output every 2 hours.
- Monitor serum potassium and ECG closely during treatment to correct hyperkalemia.
- Monitor breath sounds for indications of worsening of pulmonary edema following injection of sodium bicarbonate and use of sodium polystyrene sulfonate, (Kayexalate).

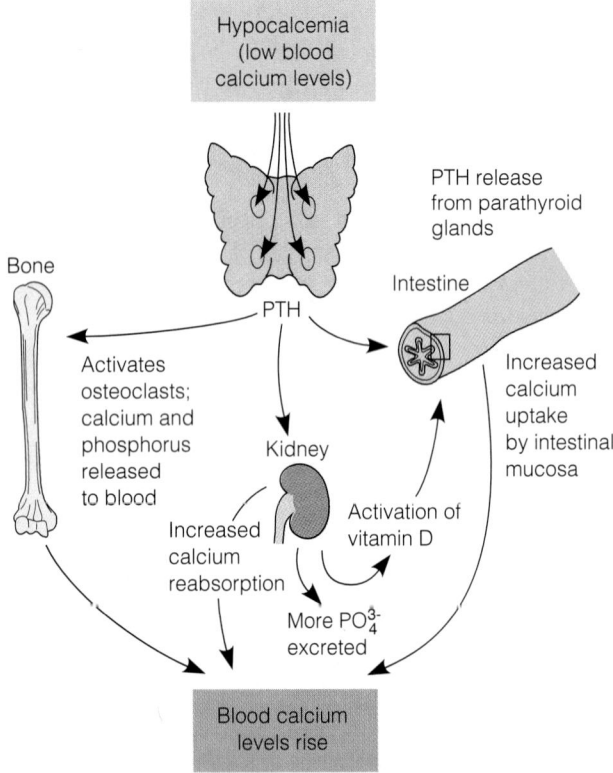

Figure 5–12 Low calcium levels (hypocalcemia) trigger the release of parathyroid hormone (PTH), increasing calcium ion levels through stimulation of bones, kidneys, and intestines.

- Administer sodium polystyrene sulfonate (Kayexalate) and sorbitol as a retention enema using a urinary retention catheter with balloon inflated to facilitate retention.

- Teach Mr. Longacre about the causes of hyperkalemia and the importance of continued medical management.

- Discuss foods high in potassium and the necessity of avoiding these to prevent or control hyperkalemia.

Evaluation

Following the emergency treatment measures and hemodialysis, Mr. Longacre's ECG and serum potassium level have returned to normal. His muscle strength has returned to near normal, and he verbalizes an understanding of the necessity of adhering to the prescribed hemodialysis regimen. Mrs. Allen provides him with verbal and written information on the causes of hyperkalemia, the importance of complying with the hemodialysis regimen, and the importance of limiting intake of dietary sources of potassium in renal failure. She also furnishes him with a list of foods high in potassium and cautions him against using potassium-containing salt substitutes and nonprescription drugs.

Critical Thinking in the Nursing Process

1. What information given by Mr. Longacre to Mrs. Allen might have led her to suspect hyperkalemia?

2. What temporary treatments were instituted to prevent fatal toxic effects of hyperkalemia on the heart?

3. Why was continuous ECG monitoring instituted as an emergency measure?

4. Why is the risk of pulmonary edema increased with the use of sodium bicarbonate and sodium polystyrene sulfonate (Kayexalate)?

5. Develop a care plan for Mr. Longacre for the nursing diagnosis *Anxiety*.

Calcium Disorders

■ ■ ■

Calcium is one of the most abundant ions in the body, with approximately 98% of calcium bound to phosphorus to form the minerals of the bones and teeth. The remaining 1% to 2% of calcium is in the extracellular fluid and is in three forms: protein-bound calcium (approximately 50%), ionized calcium (50%), and a trace of calcium bound to phosphate and other anions. Clinical laboratories usually report the *total* serum calcium (all three forms as one value). The normal adult total serum calcium concentration is 8.8 to 10.0 mg/dL.

Ionized calcium is responsible for almost all of the physiologic effects of calcium; it is essential to a number of body processes. Calcium in this form influences the level of neuromuscular irritability, the transmission of nerve impulses, skeletal and muscle contraction, and blood coagulation.

Serum calcium levels are governed by levels of parathyroid hormone (PTH) and calcitonin. Under normal conditions, an inverse relationship is maintained between calcium and phosphorus. When serum calcium levels increase, serum phosphorus levels decrease; the reverse occurs when serum calcium levels decrease. In response to a decrease in serum ionized calcium, the parathyroid gland increases PTH secretion, causing mobilization of skeletal calcium stores, increased intestinal absorption of calcium, and calcium conservation and phosphorus excretion by the kidneys (Figure 5–12). Vitamin D facilitates this process by stimulating calcium absorption by the intestines, and promoting PTH-induced mobilization of skeletal calcium.

Calcitonin is secreted in response to high serum calcium levels and is antagonistic to the effects of PTH. It lowers serum calcium levels by slowing bone resorption, increasing the urinary secretion of calcium, and reducing intestinal absorption of calcium.

The Client with Hypocalcemia

■ ■ ■

Hypocalcemia is a total serum calcium level of less than 8.8 mg/dL. This decrease in the serum calcium level can result from a decrease in the level of total body calcium or a reduction in the level of serum ionized calcium. The systemic effects of hypocalcemia, however, are a result of a decrease in ionized calcium.

Certain populations of people are at greater risk for hypocalcemia: older adults, older women, and people with lactose intolerance. Older adults are more likely to take over-the-counter medications, prescription medications, and laxatives and thereby experience a resulting change in electrolyte balance. Older adults are also at increased risk because of reduced dietary intake of calcium. Older women tend to lose calcium from bones, probably the result of the decrease in estrogen levels after menopause as well as the decrease in carrying out weight-bearing activities. People with lactose intolerance are more prone to have a genetic deficiency of the enzyme lactase. Intolerance to lactose (found in milk and milk products) causes diarrhea; if lactose intolerance is severe and the person is unable to consume any milk products, calcium deficiency may result.

Pathophysiology

Causes of hypocalcemia include the following:

- Changes in the level of ionized calcium occurring secondary to
  a. Massive transfusion with citrated blood. (Citrate, a compound added to stored whole blood to prevent clotting, binds with calcium.)
  b. Decreased production of parathyroid hormone (from surgical removal of the parathyroid glands).
  c. Alkalosis. (Calcium ionization decreases with increased serum carbonate and high pH levels; each 0.1 rise in pH lowers ionized calcium levels approximately 3% to 8%.)
  d. Rapid administration of intravenous phosphate to treat hypophosphatemia. (The level of ionized calcium decreases as a result of calcium-phosphate binding.)
- Drug therapy, including cimetidine, phenytoin, heparin, loop diuretics, magnesium sulfate, gentamicin, and cisplatin.
- Hemodilution following volume replacement with normal saline as a treatment for hemorrhage.
- Decreased absorption of calcium from the intestines secondary to gastric and intestinal resection, fatty stools, small bowel disease, deficient intake of vitamin D, altered metabolism of vitamin D secondary to liver disease, and chronic renal failure.

- Increased calcium loss from the kidney (e.g., due to the use of loop diuretics or to acute renal disease).
- Phosphate retention associated with renal failure. (Elevated serum phosphorus levels cause a reciprocal drop in the serum calcium level.)
- Acute pancreatitis. (Pancreatic lipase breaks down fat into fatty acids and glycerol; the fatty acids combine with calcium to form insoluble calcium soaps.)
- Hypoalbuminemia secondary to cirrhosis and nephrotic syndrome. (Total serum calcium is decreased, but the level of ionized calcium is unaffected.)
- Altered liver metabolism of vitamin D from the hepatic side effects of drugs or chronic alcoholism. (Serum calcium level decreases secondary to decreased concentration of vitamin D.)

Common causes of hypocalcemia are hypoparathyroidism (see Chapter 20) resulting from surgery (parathyroidectomy, thyroidectomy, radical neck dissection) and acute pancreatitis. In the client who has undergone surgery, symptoms of hypocalcemia usually occur within the first 24 to 48 hours but may be delayed.

Clinical manifestations begin when a decrease in the level of ionized calcium alters neuromuscular irritability, stimulating nerve and muscle cells. Decreased calcium also lowers the threshold of excitation of peripheral sensory nerve fibers. The most serious consequences of these changes in neuromuscular function are tetany (tonic muscular spasms) and convulsions. Indications of tetany are tingling and numbness of the circumoral area and extremities, muscle spasms of the face and extremities, and hyperactive reflexes. Contraction of the facial muscles from irritation of the facial nerve (positive Chvostek's sign) may be produced by tapping the facial nerve in front of the ear. Ischemia-induced corpopedal spasm (positive Trousseau's sign) may be elicited by inflating a blood pressure cuff on the upper arm to 20 mm Hg above systolic blood pressure for 2 to 5 minutes. These diagnostic assessments are discussed and illustrated in Chapter 19.

The client with tetany may develop bronchial muscle spasms simulating an asthma attack and visceral muscle spasms producing acute abdominal pain. A serious complication is airway obstruction from laryngospasm leading to respiratory arrest. Hyperventilation and respiratory alkalosis due to emotional stress and exercise may precipitate tetany because of the binding of ionized calcium that occurs with an increase in pH. The box on page 136 summarizes the clinical manifestations of hypocalcemia.

Collaborative Care

Management of hypocalcemia is directed toward correcting the underlying cause. Treatment of hypocalcemia involves administering oral or intravenous calcium. The route of administration and specific calcium salt used

---

Clinical Manifestations of Hypocalcemia

■ ■ ■

- Tetany
- Convulsions
- Dyspnea
- Laryngospasm
- Abdominal pain
- Respiratory arrest

---

depends on the severity of the hypocalcemia. In the asymptomatic client with chronic hypocalcemia, selected foods high in calcium, vitamin D, and oral calcium salts with or without vitamin D supplementation are prescribed. The symptomatic client with severe hypocalcemia is treated with intravenous calcium to prevent life-threatening problems, such as airway obstruction.

Laboratory and Diagnostic Tests

The laboratory and diagnostic tests that may be ordered and the resultant findings for hypocalcemia are as follows:

- *Serum calcium* will be less than 8.5 mg/dL (normal range: 8.5 to 10.0 mg/dL). Because 50% of serum calcium is combined with albumin, albumin and calcium levels are measured together. With lower levels of albumin, the serum calcium decreases. Ionized calcium is not measured independently of the total serum calcium; rather, it is estimated. Therefore, even if the total serum calcium does not change, the client may experience symptoms of hypocalcemia because less ionized calcium is available—as, for example, in the client with alkalosis. Conversely, even if the total serum calcium decreases—as, for example, in the client with hypoalbuminemia—the client may remain asymptomatic if the concentration of ionized calcium is unchanged.
- The *ECG* shows manifestations of hypocalcemia as a prolonged QT interval secondary to prolongation of the ST segment.
- *Serum magnesium* is measured because hypocalcemia is often associated with hypomagnesemia. A magnesium level of less than 1 mEq/L (normal range: 1.3 to 2.1 mEq/L) can induce hypocalcemia (Metheney, 1992).
- *Serum phosphate* is measured. Normal serum phosphate levels range from 2.7 to 4.5 mg/dL. Because of the reciprocal relationship between phosphorus and calcium levels, hyperphosphatemia (phosphorus levels greater than 4.5 mg/dL) is an associated finding in hypocalcemia.
- *Parathyroid hormone (PTH)* is measured primarily to establish a diagnoses of hyperparathyroidism, but a decrease in PTH occurs with some forms of hypocal-

cemia. Reports of PTH levels vary from laboratory to laboratory, and findings also vary with the method of analysis and the form of PTH that is being measured.

Pharmacology

In acute hypocalcemia, intravenous calcium is given to prevent or treat tetany and convulsions. Available intravenous calcium agents include calcium chloride, available in 10-mL ampules containing 13.6 mEq (272 mg) of calcium; calcium gluconate, available in 10-mL ampules containing 4.5 mEq (90 mg) of calcium; and calcium gluceptate, available in 5-mL ampules containing 4.5 mEq (90 mg) of calcium.

Serious complications that can occur with use of these drugs are severe necrosis and sloughing of tissues with extravascular injection, and bradycardia and cardiac arrest resulting from an excessively rapid infusion of the drug (overcorrection resulting in hypercalcemia). In clients taking digitalis preparations, intravenous calcium can precipitate digitalis toxicity because of the additive cardiotonic effects of calcium on the myocardium. When treating clients with hypocalcemia due to a magnesium deficit, replacement of magnesium in addition to calcium may be necessary.

In the client with chronic hypocalcemia, supplemental oral calcium preparations (calcium lactate, calcium gluconate, calcium carbonate, and others), an increase in the dietary intake of calcium, and oral vitamin D are used to restore normal serum calcium levels. Calcium supplements may be combined with vitamin D, or vitamin D may be given alone to increase gastrointestinal absorption of calcium.

Nursing implications, as well as a discussion of calcium salts, are found in the accompanying pharmacology box.

Nursing Care

Nursing management of the client with hypocalcemia focuses on client and family education, monitoring of individuals at risk, and monitoring the client's response to therapy. The following nursing diagnoses and collaborative problems apply to the client with hypocalcemia:

- *Potential Complication: Electrolyte imbalance: Hypocalcemia*
- *Decreased Cardiac Output* related to decreased myocardial contractility secondary to hypocalcemia, bradycardia, and atrioventricular block from overcorrection, or toxicity secondary to the augmented effect of digitalis from correction of hypocalcemia (Carpenito, 1992)
- *Risk for Injury* related to tetany and seizures
- *Risk for Impaired Gas Exchange* related to deficient oxygen supply secondary to laryngospasm

Nursing Implications for Pharmacology: The Client with Hypocalcemia

CALCIUM SALTS

Calcium carbonate (BioCal, Calsam, Caltrate, OsCal)

Calcium chloride

Calcium citrate

Calcium glubionate

Calcium gluceptate

Calcium gluconate

Calcium lactate

Calcium salts are used to increase calcium levels when there is a deficit in the body. Appropriate calcium levels are necessary to maintain many different body processes, including cell membrane permeability, enzyme activation, renal function, blood coagulation, cardiac rhythm, and skeletal muscle contraction. Calcium is absorbed well from the gastrointestinal tract; however, in cases of tetany, intravenous administration of calcium gluconate is necessary. Calcium is contraindicated in clients receiving digitalis.

Nursing Responsibilities

- Give oral calcium 1 to 1.5 hours after meals.
- Administer intravenous calcium slowly.
- Assess for use of other medications; document and report concomitant use of digitalis.

Client and Family Teaching

- Calcium requirements are best met by dietary intake of milk; however, if you are taking calcium salts, do not drink large amounts of milk.
- Older adults require decreased amounts of calcium.
- Calcium absorption is decreased if calcium is taken with meals high in fat or with certain drugs, such as corticosteroids and the tetracyclines.
- Adequate Vitamin D intake increases calcium absorption.

- *Knowledge Deficit* related to lack of understanding of how the disease process causes hypocalcemia
- *Risk for Noncompliance* related to lack of understanding of treatment regimen for hypocalcemia
- *Risk for Alterated Nutrition: Less than Body Requirements* related to inadequate dietary intake of calcium, vitamin D, and protein

Clients at risk for hypocalcemia are assessed for the following:

- Cardiac rate and rhythm.
- Respiratory rate, rhythm, and effort.
- Manifestations of neuromuscular irritability (tingling around mouth and fingers, muscle twitching or cramps, hyperreflexes).
- Serum calcium, magnesium, and albumin levels.
- ABGs.
- Response to therapeutic interventions, such as intravenous calcium.

Safety precautions include providing a quiet environment to reduce central nervous system stimuli, promoting relaxation to decrease stress and the potential for hyperventilation (and resultant respiratory alkalosis), and keeping tracheostomy equipment and intravenous calcium readily available.

Client and Family Teaching

To promote the client's highest level of wellness, the nurse provides information on dietary sources of calcium and vitamin D; reviews dietary intake of vitamins and fat, explains the relationship between fat, vitamin D, and calcium absorption; and encourages the client to take prescribed oral calcium and vitamin D replacements as directed.

The Client with Hypercalcemia

Hypercalcemia is a serum calcium value greater than 10.0 mg/dL. The condition occurs from an excess amount of ionized calcium in the serum and can have widespread systemic effects.

Pathophysiology

Hypercalcemia can result from a number of causes, including increased reabsorption of calcium from the bones, increased calcium intake, or decreased renal excretion of calcium.

Increased reabsorption of calcium from the bones most often is due to hyperparathyroidism secondary to a parathyroid adenoma or hyperplasia, or to malignant neoplastic disease that results in mobilization of calcium

---

Clinical Manifestations of Hypercalcemia

- Muscle weakness
- Fatigue
- Altered mental status
- Ataxia
- Personality changes
- Decreasing levels of consciousness
- Abdominal pain
- Nausea and vomiting
- Constipation
- Weight loss
- Dysrhythmias

---

from the skeletal reservoir. Other causes of increased reabsorption are lack of stress on the bone, which can result from prolonged immobilization or from Paget's disease, a disorder characterized by bone reabsorption followed by rapid rebuilding of bone.

An increase in calcium intake may result from overuse of calcium-containing antacids, excessive ingestion of milk, and excessive intravenous calcium administration in treatment of cardiopulmonary arrest. Both high doses of vitamin D and hyperparathyroidism cause increased gastrointestinal calcium uptake.

Decreased urinary excretion of calcium occurs in renal failure, in hyperparathyroidism, in milk-alkali syndrome, and with the use of drugs, such as the thiazide diuretics. Acidosis increases the ratio of ionized calcium to the total serum calcium.

The major consequences of chronic hypercalcemia are bone demineralization (called osteitis fibrosa cystica), renal nephropathy resulting from deposition of calcium in the renal parenchyma, and recurrent renal stones. Additionally, hypercalcemia has a depressive effect on the central and peripheral nervous systems and causes gastrointestinal symptoms, behavior changes, and myocardial conduction changes.

The systemic effects of hypercalcemia include neuromuscular changes secondary to decreased excitability at the myoneural junction. This results in muscle weakness and fatigue. Confusion, decreased memory, ataxia (the inability to coordinate movements), mild personality disturbances (apathy, depression, irritability), severe psychosis, stupor, or coma may occur as a result of central nervous system depression. Gastrointestinal effects of hypercalcemia include abdominal pain, anorexia, nausea, vomiting, constipation, pancreatitis, peptic ulcer disease, and weight loss. Cardiac effects of hypercalcemia include shortened ST segments and QT intervals and the enhancement of the effects of digitalis. Sinus bradycardia and various degrees of atrioventricular block may occur. The accompanying box summarizes the clinical manifestations of hypercalcemia.

Collaborative Care

The management of hypercalcemia focuses on correcting the underlying cause and reducing the serum calcium level. Treatment is particularly important in clients who have one or more of the following: serum calcium levels greater than 12 mg/dL, overt symptoms of hypercalcemia, compromised renal function, and an inability to maintain an adequate fluid intake (Wilson, 1992). Definitive treatment for hypercalcemia caused by parathyroid adenoma or hyperplasia is surgical removal of the affected gland(s).

Laboratory and Diagnostic Tests

The laboratory and diagnostic tests that may be ordered and the resultant findings are as follows:

- *Serum electrolytes* are measured. In hypercalcemia total serum calcium is greater than 10.0 mg/dL (normal range: 8.5 to 10.0 mg/dL). In clients with renal failure, the BUN and creatinine levels may be increased.

- *PTH* may be measured. Serum levels of PTH are measured to distinguish nonparathyroid from parathyroid causes of hypercalcemia (Fischbach, 1992).

- An *ECG* is conducted. ECG findings in hypercalcemia include a shortened QT interval secondary to shortening of the ST segment, depressed ST segment, and widened T wave. Bradydysrhythmias (heart rate slower than normal) and complete heart block may occur. Levels of calcium greater than 20 mg/dL may cause cardiac arrest.

Pharmacology

In acute hypercalcemia, increased urinary excretion of calcium is accomplished by administering intravenous saline solution (0.45% or 0.9%) to dilute the serum and administering diuretics (furosemide, ethacrynic acid) to increase urinary excretion of calcium and saline.

Rapid reversal of hypercalcemia in emergency situations may be accomplished by intravenous administration of sodium phosphate or potassium phosphate. Calcium binds to phosphate, and serum calcium levels thereby decrease. Paradoxically, complications of this therapy can include fatal hypocalcemia resulting from binding of the ionized calcium and soft tissue calcifications.

Other drug therapies include the use of intravenous plicamycin (Mithracin) to inhibit bone resorption. Glucocorticoids (cortisone), which compete with vitamin D, and a low-calcium diet may be prescribed to decrease gastrointestinal absorption of calcium and to increase urinary calcium excretion. Also, calcitonin may be prescribed to decrease skeletal mobilization of calcium and phosphorus and to increase renal output of calcium and phosphorus.

Nursing Care

As with hypocalcemia, nursing management of the client with hypercalcemia concentrates on client instruction, monitoring individuals at risk, preserving client safety, and continuous assessment of client's response to therapy. Both nursing diagnoses and collaborative problems are applicable to the client with hypercalcemia and include the following:

- *Potential Complication: Electrolyte Imbalance: Hypercalcemia*
- *Potential Complication: Renal Insufficiency* secondary to renal nephropathy from hypercalcemia
- *Decreased Cardiac Output* secondary to changes in myocardial contractility
- *Risk for Constipation* related to decreased peristalsis secondary to hypercalcemia
- *Risk for Altered Nutrition: Less than Body Requirements* related to anorexia secondary to hypercalcemia
- *Risk for Injury* related to altered sensorium and muscle weakness secondary to hypercalcemia
- *Risk for Fluid Volume Excess* related to rapid administration of intravenous saline
- *Risk for Fluid Volume Deficit* related to use of diuretics
- *Risk for Noncompliance* related to lack of understanding of treatment regimen for hypercalcemia

Clients at risk for hypercalcemia are assessed for the following:

- Cardiac rate and rhythm to identify sinus dysrhythmias and atrioventricular (AV) block
- Level of consciousness (confusion, coma) and neuromuscular responses
- Manifestations of personality changes (depression, apathy, irritability)
- Serum electrolytes: calcium, magnesium, and phosphate levels
- Intake and output to calculate fluid balance
- Indications of fluid volume excess, such as acute weight gain and edema, in clients receiving intravenous saline solutions
- Indications of fluid volume deficit, such as decreased blood pressure and increased heart rate, in clients receiving diuretics (e.g., furosemide)
- Renal function (i.e., BUN and creatinine level, urinary output, and severe flank pain indicative of renal stones) to identify signs of nephropathy
- Bowel function to identify constipation
- Prescribed treatment regimens, such as correct administration of intravenous saline

---

Foods High in Calcium

▪ ▪ ▪

- Cottage cheese
- Cheese
- Milk
- Cream
- Yogurt
- Ice Cream
- Molasses
- Canned sardines and salmon
- Rhubarb
- Broccoli
- Collard greens
- Soy flour
- Spinach
- Tofu

Safety precautions include providing safety measures for clients who are at risk for convulsions, who experience weakness, or who are at increased risk for fracture because of bone reabsorption.

Client and Family Teaching

To promote the client's highest level of wellness, teach the client and family which foods and over-the-counter antacids are rich in calcium, and instruct them to avoid these. Caution the client not to take massive doses of vitamin D supplements and to increase fluid intake to 2000 to 3000 mL over 24 hours. Instruct clients who are at high risk for renal stone formation to increase the intake of acid-ash foods (meats, fish, poultry, eggs, cranberries, plums, prunes). Finally, instruct the client to increase dietary fiber and fluid to maintain normal bowel function and avoid constipation. Foods high in calcium are listed in the accompanying box.

Phosphorus Disorders

▪ ▪ ▪

Phosphorus is found in all body tissues, but 85% of the total amount of phosphorus in the body is combined with calcium in bones and teeth. Another 14% is found in intracellular fluid; phosphorus is the primary anion of the intracellular fluid. The remainder (1%) is in the extracellular fluid space. Normal serum phosphorus levels in adults range from 2.5 to 4.5 mg/dL.

Phosphorus is essential to a wide range of body processes: the formation of bone and teeth, the production of adenosine triphosphate (ATP), and the formation of the red blood cell enzyme 2,3-diphosphoglycerate (2,3-DPG), which expedites oxygen delivery to tissues. Phosphorus is a constituent of enzymes that function in fat, carbohydrate, and protein metabolism, assists in the

> ### Clinical Manifestations of Hypophosphatemia
>
> - Increased bruising and bleeding
> - Slurred speech
> - Decreasing levels of consciousness
> - Seizures
> - Chest pain
> - Dysrhythmias
> - Increased rate and depth of respirations
> - Anorexia
> - Nausea and vomiting
> - Dysphagia
> - Decreased or absent bowel sounds

maintenance of acid-base balance, and is essential to normal nerve and muscle activity.

An inverse relationship exists between phosphorus and calcium levels: When one increases, the other decreases. Thus, regulatory mechanisms for the maintenance of calcium levels in the body also influence phosphorus levels. Serum phosphorous levels are influenced by intestinal absorption (under the influence of vitamin D) and parathyroid hormone (PTH) control of bone reabsorption. The kidneys exert major control over the regulation of serum phosphorus levels by excreting excess phosphorus or reabsorbing phosphorus when a phosphorus deficit exists. Phosphorus levels vary with age, gender, and diet.

The Client with Hypophosphatemia

Hypophosphatemia is a serum phosphorus level of less than 2.5 mg/dL. The condition results from a number of medical disorders but can also occur as a consequence of therapeutic interventions. The net movement of phosphorus into the cells is the most common cause of hypophosphatemia. Hypophosphatemia occurs with the use of total parenteral nutrition that contains insufficient phosphorus. (Cellular anabolism accelerates, causing an intracellular shift of phosphorus.) The administration of highly concentrated glucose solutions can also lead to hypophosphatemia. Other causes include

- Increased intestinal losses from use of antacids (protracted use of aluminum- and magnesium-containing antacids causes binding of phosphorus in the intestine) and severe vomiting and diarrhea
- Decreased intestinal absorption (deficiency of vitamin D, malabsorption disorders, starvation)

- Respiratory/metabolic alkalosis (intracellular phosphorus shift)
- Increased renal excretion (hyperparathyroidism, hypomagnesemia, hypokalemia, diuretic therapy, renal disorders, polyuria, and glycosuria from uncontrolled diabetic ketoacidosis)
- Alcoholism, especially during withdrawal
- Poor dietary intake (malnutrition)

Pathophysiology

Hypophosphatemia is defined as a serum phosphorus level of less than 2.5 mg/dL. The manifestations of acute hypophosphatemia are related to a combination of a depletion of ATP, which impairs cellular energy supplies, and a decrease in the level of 2,3-DPG in the red blood cell, which influences the release of oxygen from the hemoglobin. Severe hypophosphatemia alters virtually every major organ system. Signs and symptoms begin to appear when the serum phosphorus is less than 2.0 mg/dL. Hypophosphatemia can exert the following effects:

- Hematologic effects: hemolytic anemia secondary to increased fragility of red blood cells; altered functioning of granulocytes, which increases the risk of infection; and platelet dysfunction and destruction, which results in increased bruising and bleeding
- Central nervous system effects: apprehension, slurred speech, confusion, seizures, and coma
- Neuromuscular changes: muscle weakness, tremors, and numbness and tingling around the mouth and in the extremities
- Cardiovascular system effects: chest pain and dysrhythmias secondary to decreased oxygenation; heart failure and shock secondary to decreased myocardial contractility
- Respiratory effects: respiratory alkalosis due to increased rate or depth of respirations in response to hypoxia; respiratory muscle fatigue leading to respiratory failure
- Gastrointestinal effects: anorexia; dysphagia (difficulty swallowing); nausea and vomiting; gastric atony and ileus due to reduced gastrointestinal motility

The accompanying box summarizes the clinical manifestations of hypophosphatemia.

Collaborative Care

The management of hypophosphatemia focuses on prevention or definitive interventions to correct it. Measures to prevent its occurrence include adding appropriate amounts of phosphorus to total parenteral nutrition solutions and avoiding the use of phosphorus-binding antacids in clients at risk for developing hypophosphatemia. Depending on the degree, hypophosphatemia is treated with either intravenous replacement of phosphorus or the administration of oral supplements of phosphorus.

Nursing Care

Nursing care of the client with hypophosphatemia includes assessing for manifestations of phosphorus deficit and monitoring laboratory measurements of serum phosphorus. Nursing diagnoses that are appropriate for the client with hypophosphatemia are as follows:

- *Impaired Physical Mobility* related to bone pain and fractures secondary to movement of phosphorus out of bones
- *Impaired Gas Exchange* related to weakened muscles of respiration
- *Decreased Cardiac Output* related to the effect of hypophosphatemia on myocardial functioning
- *Risk for Injury* related to sensory or neuromuscular dysfunction

Client and Family Teaching

To promote the client's highest level of wellness, teach the client and family to recognize manifestations of hypophosphatemia. Discuss the importance of avoiding phosphorus-binding antacids, unless prescribed. If a high-phosphorus diet is encouraged, provide a list of foods high in phosphorus. See the accompanying box.

The Client with Hyperphosphatemia

■ ■ ■

Hyperphosphatemia is a serum phosphate level greater than 4.5 mg/dL. The most common cause of hyperphosphatemia is acute or chronic renal insufficiency. Other causes include

- Hypoparathyroidism, causing a decrease in calcium levels and an increase in phosphorus levels
- Increased phosphorus intake and absorption resulting from an excessive intake of vitamin D, the use of phosphate-containing enemas or laxatives (particularly in clients with compromised renal function), or excessive intake of phosphorus supplements
- Hyperthyroidism
- Increased movement of phosphorus out of the cells, as occurs in respiratory or lactic acidosis

---

> **Foods High in Phosphorus**
>
> ■ ■ ■
>
> - Organ meats (brain, liver, kidney)
> - Fish
> - Poultry
> - Milk and milk products
> - Whole grains
> - Nuts
> - Eggs
> - Dried beans

> **Clinical Manifestations of Hyperphosphatemia**
>
> ■ ■ ■
>
> - Muscle cramping and pain
> - Paresthesias
> - Tetany
> - Calcifications in soft tissues

- Cellular release of phosphorus following cellular destruction, which occurs with neoplastic diseases, such as leukemia treated with cytotoxic agents; conditions causing catabolism, such as starvation and diabetic ketoacidosis; and hemolytic anemia

Pathophysiology

Excessive serum phosphate levels cause few specific symptoms. The effects of high serum phosphate levels on nerves and muscles (muscle cramps and pain, paresthesias, tingling around the mouth, muscle spasms, tetany) are more the result of hypocalcemia that develops secondary to an elevated serum phosphorus level. The phosphate in the serum combines with ionized calcium, and the ionized serum calcium level falls.

A complication of hyperphosphatemia is calcification of soft tissues. In the presence of an increased calcium level, an increased phosphate level can cause calcium to bind with phosphate and precipitate in soft tissue. Calcifications in the brain, kidneys, joints, skin, cornea, arteries, heart, and skin may occur. The accompanying box summarizes the clinical manifestations of hyperphosphatemia.

Collaborative Care

The management of hyperphosphatemia is directed toward reducing the serum phosphate level. The best approach to management is to treat the underlying cause. In situations where this is not possible, alternative approaches to treatment include reducing phosphorus intake, increasing gastrointestinal and renal elimination of phosphorus, and removing it from the blood through hemodialysis.

In the client with renal failure, measures to reduce serum phosphate levels include hemodialysis, restriction and/or elimination of the dietary sources of phosphate, and the use of antacids (aluminum-containing antacids, calcium gels) to bind phosphate in the gastrointestinal tract. Hyperphosphatemia secondary to use of cytotoxic drugs for treating neoplastic disease is counteracted by maintaining the client's fluid volume to preserve adequate urine output, along with the use of allopurinol (Zyloprim), a drug that decreases the production of uric acid, preventing the formation of uric acid calculi in the kidney and uric acid nephropathy.

Nursing Care

When providing nursing care for the client with hyperphosphatemia, the nurse monitors the client for laboratory data revealing an excess of phosphorus and a deficit of calcium, as well as the signs of hypocalcemia.

Client and Family Teaching

Teach the client and family about the purpose of phosphate-binding drugs, the necessity of avoiding phosphate enemas and over-the-counter medications containing phosphate or phosphorus, and the importance of eliminating foods high in phosphorus from the diet.

Magnesium Disorders

■ ■ ■

In a healthy person, 50% of the magnesium in the body is contained in bones, 45% is in the intracellular space, and 5% is in the extracellular space. Magnesium is the second most abundant intracellular cation (next to potassium) and is active in a number of vital intracellular enzyme systems. It also decreases or blocks the release of the neurotransmitter acetylcholine at nerve endings, thus acting as a sedative on nerves and muscles. The normal serum concentration of magnesium ranges from 1.3 to 2.1 mEq/L. Approximately two-thirds of serum magnesium is ionized, and the remainder is bound to protein. Like calcium, the ionized fraction of magnesium affects neuromuscular irritability and contractility. An excess in serum magnesium depresses skeletal muscle contraction and central nervous system activity. A deficit results in increased irritability of the nervous system, cardiac dysrhythmias, and peripheral vasodilatation.

In addition to its effects on neuromuscular and central nervous system function, magnesium participates in a number of other significant physiologic processes. It is a cofactor in the activation of a number of enzyme systems, particularly those involving carbohydrate metabolism and protein synthesis, and it affects sodium and potassium transport across the cellular membrane by activating the sodium-potassium pump. Magnesium deficits frequently parallel potassium and/or calcium imbalances. Therefore, along with the potassium and calcium levels, magnesium levels in clients with these disorders should be monitored.

The Client with Hypomagnesemia

■ ■ ■

Hypomagnesemia is a magnesium level of less than 1.3 mEq/l. The causes of hypomagnesemia may be categorized into those that occur secondary to deficient magnesium intake and/or absorption, excessive renal excretion, excessive losses of body fluids other than urine, and miscellaneous causes.

Chronic alcoholism is one of the most common causes of hypomagnesemia. A combination of factors are thought to contribute to hypomagnesemia that accompanies alcoholism, including malabsorption, limited intake of magnesium, diarrhea and/or emesis, and the use of diuretics. Other causes of hypomagnesemia include those that occur secondary to

- Impaired intestinal absorption of magnesium from conditions such as gastrointestinal cancer, inflammatory bowel disease, small bowel resection, or chronic pancreatitis; or from drugs such as cisplatin and gentamicin
- Increased intestinal losses of magnesium from chronic diarrhea, ileostomy, and intestinal fistulas
- Increased renal excretion of magnesium from drugs such as ethacrynic acid and furosemide, the tubular necrosis phase of acute renal failure, volume expansion from hyperaldosteronism, or osmotic diuresis from hyperglycemia associated with diabetes mellitus
- Decreased intake of magnesium due to a lack of magnesium supplement in continuous intravenous therapy and with parenteral nutrition, which causes movement of extracellular magnesium into the cells

Pathophysiology

The manifestations of hypomagnesemia usually do not occur until the serum level drops below 1 mEq/L. However, bodily magnesium depletion may exist even in the presence of normal serum magnesium levels. Magnesium deficiency may contribute to the development of low serum levels of calcium, potassium, and phosphate. Therefore, a deficiency in these ions may be responsible for the cluster of signs and symptoms accompanying hypomagnesemia.

The pathophysiologic effects of hypomagnesemia are due mainly to increased neuromuscular responsiveness, and they parallel those of hypocalcemia. An increase in neuromuscular irritability leads to tremors, hyperreactive reflexes, positive Chvostek's sign, tetany, and convulsions. A positive Trousseau's sign is a rare finding in hypomagnesemia (Rice, 1983).

The cardiovascular effects of hypomagnesemia include ventricular dysrhythmias (supraventricular tachycardia, premature ventricular contractions, and ventricular fibrillation). In clients receiving digitalis preparations, hypomagnesemia increases susceptibility to digitalis toxicity and dysrhythmias; the potential for digitalis toxicity may be increased; as a result of increased renal losses of both magnesium and potassium secondary to the concomitant treatment with diuretics. Central nervous system changes accompanying hypomagnesemia include mood changes (apathy, depression, apprehension, agitation), confusion, hallucinations, psychoses, and paresthesias.

Hypomagnesemia also affects gastrointestinal function, but these changes are most likely due to concomitant hypokalemia. The gastrointestinal manifestations include nausea, vomiting, anorexia, diarrhea, and abdominal distention. The hypokalemia is in part due to failure of the sodium-potassium pump at the cell membrane. The accompanying box summarizes the clinical manifestations of hypomagnesemia.

Collaborative Care

The management of hypomagnesemia is directed toward prevention or the identification of an existing deficiency and its treatment through magnesium replacement therapy. Hypomagnesemia in clients receiving total parenteral nutrition is prevented by the addition of magnesium to the solution.

In clients who are able to eat, a mild deficiency may be corrected by increasing the intake of foods rich in magnesium (see the accompanying box), or the use of oral magnesium supplements (for example, magnesium-containing antacids, such as magnesium trisilicate). However, oral magnesium supplements may cause diarrhea and their use in therapy is therefore limited.

Clients with overt signs and symptoms of hypomagnesemia are treated with either an intravenous infusion or an intramuscular injection of magnesium sulfate. The concentration of solutions for parenteral use vary between 10% and 50%. Fifty percent solutions are suitable for intramuscular injection but should not be given undiluted intravenously. Clients with mild signs and symptoms are treated with intramuscular magnesium sulfate.

Clinical Manifestations of Hypomagnesemia

- Muscle tremors
- Tetany
- Convulsions
- Dysrhythmias
- Mood and personality changes
- Paresthesias
- Anorexia
- Nausea and vomiting
- Diarrhea

Foods High in Magnesium

- Green, leafy vegetables
- Seafood
- Meat
- Wheat bran
- Milk
- Legumes
- Bananas
- Oranges
- Grapefruit
- Chocolate
- Molasses
- Coconut
- Refined sugar

In clients with severe magnesium deficiency who are exhibiting neurologic changes or cardiac dysrhythmias, intravenous therapy is initiated as an emergency measure and may be continued over several days.

Nursing Care

The nursing care of clients experiencing problems resulting from hypomagnesemia centers on the client's responses to the systemic effects of a magnesium deficit. The following nursing diagnoses are applicable to the client with hypomagnesemia:

- *Altered Nutrition: Less than Body Requirements* for magnesium related to inadequate intake
- *Knowledge Deficit* of the need for magnesium in the diet and of foods high in magnesium
- *Risk for Injury* related to neuromuscular irritability and sensory changes secondary to hypomagnesemia
- *Decreased Cardiac Output* related to altered myocardial contractility secondary to hypomagnesemia

Nursing interventions for hypomagnesemia focus on carefully monitoring individuals at risk, assessing significant signs and symptoms, implementing safety measures

---

Clinical Manifestations of Hypermagnesemia

■ ■ ■

- Hypotension
- Flushing and sweating
- Dysrhythmias
- Nausea and vomiting

- Decreasing levels of consciousness
- Areflexia
- Respiratory depression
- Cardiac arrest

---

for the client exhibiting signs of neuromuscular irritability, client and family teaching, and administering prescribed medications.

For clients at risk for hypomagnesemia, carry out the following assessments:

- Monitor serum magnesium levels.

- Assess the client for manifestations of neuromuscular excitability, such as muscle twitching, tremors, grimaces, paresthesias (numbness and tingling sensation about the lips and in the extremities), leg cramps, and hyperactive reflexes.

- Monitor the client for changes in gastrointestinal function, such as nausea, vomiting, anorexia, diarrhea, and abdominal distention.

- Monitor the client for changes in cardiovascular function, such as premature atrial and ventricular beats and tachycardias; changes in the ECG, such as broad, flat, or inverted T waves, depressed ST segments, and prolonged QT intervals. In clients receiving digitalis, monitor for digitalis toxicity (Rice, 1983).

- Monitor laboratory results for electrolyte imbalances, particularly hypokalemia.

Clients receiving intravenous solutions of magnesium should be closely monitored for serum magnesium levels and deep-tendon reflexes. Depressed tendon reflexes indicate a high serum magnesium level. Intravenous administration of magnesium sulfate can potentiate an existing hypocalcemia; therefore, it is important to monitor serum calcium levels and to watch for signs of neuromuscular irritability. Nursing measures to decrease stimuli that augment neuromuscular irritability and to maintain client safety have been discussed in previous sections of the chapter.

Client and Family Teaching

To promote the client's maximum level of wellness, teach the client experiencing mild hypomagnesemia to increase dietary intake of foods high in magnesium, and provide information about magnesium supplements. In addition, if alcohol abuse has precipitated a magnesium deficit, a discussion with the client and family members about Alcoholics Anonymous, Al-Anon, and/or Al-a-Teen may be appropriate.

The Client with Hypermagnesemia

■ ■ ■

Hypermagnesemia is a magnesium blood serum level in excess of 2.1 mEq/L. Decreased renal excretion of magnesium and increased magnesium intake may cause the condition. Elevated serum magnesium is commonly associated with some degree of renal failure, which decreases excretion of magnesium. Hypermagnesemia is also seen in clients taking magnesium-containing antacids; however, this is rare.

In the client with chronic renal failure, magnesium excess may be due to the use of magnesium-containing antacids (such as Maalox), cathartics (magnesium hydroxide), or enemas. Magnesium excess may also result from the use of parenteral solutions containing magnesium.

Untreated diabetic ketoacidosis may lead to transient hypermagnesemia. In diabetic ketoacidosis, both the catabolic release of intracellular magnesium and the volume deficit that occurs secondary to osmotic diuresis from the elevated blood sugar contribute to the elevated serum magnesium levels. Other causes of transient elevations of serum magnesium secondary to volume depletion include adrenal insufficiency (Addison's disease) and overuse of diuretics.

Pathophysiology

Elevated serum magnesium levels interfere with neuromuscular transmission and depress the central nervous system. Effects on the cardiovascular system, such as hypotension, flushing, sweating, and bradydysrhythmias, also occur.

A predictable pattern of signs and symptoms accompanies progressive elevations of serum magnesium. With lower levels, nausea and vomiting, hypotension, facial flushing, sweating, and a feeling of warmth occur. With increasing levels, signs of central nervous system depression appear (weakness, lethargy, drowsiness, weak or absent deep-tendon reflexes). With marked elevation in serum magnesium, respiratory depression and coma ensue, and cardiac function is compromised (as evidenced by prolonged PR, QRS, and QT intervals on the ECG, bradycardia, heart block, and cardiac arrest). The accompanying box summarizes the clinical manifestations of hypermagnesemia.

Collaborative Care

The management of hypermagnesemia focuses on identifying and treating the underlying cause. All medications or compounds containing magnesium (such as antacids, intravenous solutions, or enemas) should be withheld in clients with elevated serum magnesium levels to prevent toxicity. In the client with renal failure, hemodialysis or peritoneal dialysis is instituted to remove the excess magnesium.

Therapy for diabetic ketoacidosis, such as administration of insulin and intravenous fluids containing dextrose, halts the cellular catabolism that results from elevated serum magnesium levels. Rehydration increases urine output, which will correct the hypermagnesemia. Too rapid a correction, however, may lead to hypomagnesemia. Emergency intervention for clients with possible fatal effects from magnesium toxicity (respiratory depression, cardiac arrest) includes the use of intravenous calcium gluconate (10% solution) to counteract the cardiac effects of magnesium and ventilatory support for respiratory failure.

Nursing Care

In the client with hypermagnesemia, nursing care related to identified nursing diagnoses centers on the client's responses to the systemic effects of excess magnesium. The following nursing diagnoses are appropriate for clients with hypermagnesemia:

- *Decreased Cardiac Output* related to altered myocardial conduction
- *Risk for Impaired Gas Exchange* related to respiratory depression secondary to hypermagnesemia
- *Risk for Injury* related to muscular weakness and altered level of consciousness

---

Medications Containing Magnesium

Antacids	Laxatives
▪ Gelusil	▪ Milk of Magnesia
▪ Maalox No. 1	▪ Magnesium oxide
▪ Maalox Plus	▪ Haley's M-O
▪ Riopan	▪ Magnesium citrate
▪ Milk of Magnesia	▪ Epsom salts
▪ Mylanta	
▪ Di-Gel	
▪ Gaviscon	

- *Risk for Altered Health Maintenance* related to knowledge deficit of possible hypermagnesemia associated with use of magnesium-containing antacids, laxatives, and enemas

Nursing care includes monitoring for potential problems related to hypermagnesemia, providing interventions to reduce the risk of hypermagnesemia, and providing measures to ensure the client's safety.

Client and Family Teaching

Education of the client with hypermagnesemia focuses on instructions to avoid magnesium-containing medications, including antacids, mineral supplements, cathartics, and enemas. Provide the client with a list of common magnesium-containing medications (see the accompanying box).

Acid-Base Disorders

Normal dietary intake and metabolic activities continually contribute acids to the body fluids (Figure 5–13). In spite of the continuous addition of these acids, the hydrogen concentration (pH) of these fluids is held to within a narrow range of between 7.35 and 7.45. A number of mechanisms operate to maintain this delicate homeostatic balance, which is essential to optimal cellular function. Increasing or decreasing the pH beyond this normal range can change the structure of the cellular enzymes and thereby affect cellular metabolism and alter the function of hormone systems.

Because acid-base imbalances are usually not primary disorders but the result of one or more pathophysiologic processes, some parts of this section of the chapter differ from the usual sequence found in other chapters. The nursing care sections include general assessments and care and provide examples of appropriate nursing diagnoses. Client and family teaching is not included but is discussed with specific disorders throughout the book. A case study of a client with respiratory acidosis is included to illustrate application of the nursing process.

Regulation of Acid-Base Balance

An *acid* is a molecule that can contribute a hydrogen ion. A *base* is a molecule that can accept or remove a hydrogen

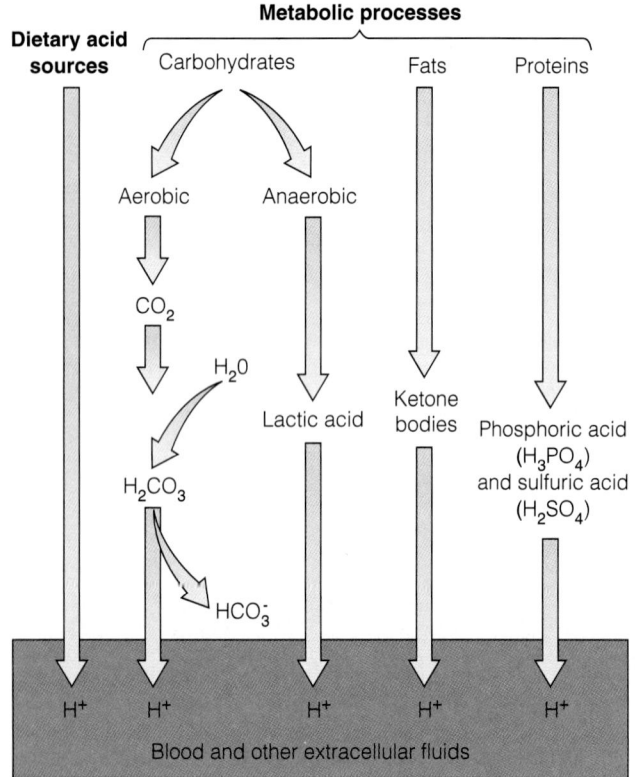

Figure 5-13 Hydrogen ion sources in the body include acids from dietary sources and from metabolism of carbohydrates, proteins, and fats.

ion (Porth, 1994). The degree to which an acid dissociates and donates a hydrogen ion, or a base dissociates and accepts a hydrogen ion, is determined by whether the acid is strong or weak. Two types of acids are produced during metabolic processes: volatile respiratory acids and nonvolatile metabolic acids.

Volatile respiratory acids are acids that can be excreted from the body as a gas. Carbonic acid, a volatile respiratory acid, dehydrates to carbon dioxide and water in the lungs, where carbon dioxide is excreted. Nonvolatile acids must be metabolized or excreted from the body in a water fluid; all acids found in the body fluids other than carbonic acid (such as lactic acid or acetoacetic acid) are classified as nonvolatile metabolic acids. Most of the body's acids and bases are weak; the most important of these are carbonic acid and bicarbonate.

A *buffer* is a substance or group of substances that controls the hydrogen ion concentration in a solution by absorbing hydrogen ions when a base is added or by releasing hydrogen ions when an acid is added. Special buffer systems of the body function constantly to maintain a stable pH, acting within 1 second after pH is altered. These systems comprise both the buffer systems in all body fluids that constantly adjust to changes in pH and the respiratory and renal systems that eliminate excess acids and bases. The kidneys also selectively conserve bicarbonate.

Body Buffer Systems

Buffers for regulating acid-base balance exist in all tissues and in the intracellular and extracellular fluids of the body. A buffer system is made of a weak acid and the alkali salt of that acid, or of a weak base and its acid salt. To prevent large pH changes, the system trades a strong acid for a weak acid or a strong base for a weak base (Porth, 1994, p. 631). The major buffer systems of the body are the bicarbonate buffer system, the phosphate buffer system, and the protein buffers.

The Bicarbonate Buffer System

The bicarbonate buffer system uses carbonic acid as its weak acid and bicarbonate as its weak base. This system operates in both the lungs and the kidneys. When volatile acids (such as carbonic acid produced by hydration of carbon dioxide in the body) and nonvolatile acids (such as those produced from the normal metabolism of dietary proteins, ketoacids, and lactic acid) are added to the extracellular fluid, this system is capable of readjusting the pH within seconds. The lungs eliminate or retain carbon dixoide, and the kidneys excrete or form bicarbonate.

The parts of the bicarbonate buffer system consist of 20 parts of base bicarbonate (HCO_3^-) to 1 part of carbonic acid (H_2CO_3). Normally, the serum concentration of bicarbonate is 24 mEq/L, and that of carbonic acid is 1.2 mEq/L. Thus, the ratio of bicarbonate to carbonic acid is 20:1. It is this ratio that maintains the pH at a normal level of 7.40 (Figure 5-14).

The respiratory system increases or decreases hydrogen ion concentration through changes in respiratory rate and depth. The effect of increasing or decreasing ventilation is that carbon dioxide is either retained or eliminated. More carbonic acid is formed with decreased ventilation and the retention of carbon dioxide. With increased ventilation, more carbon dioxide is eliminated (H_2CO_3 is converted to CO_2 and H_2O and eliminated). A change in the amount of carbonic acid formed is reflected in the Pa_{CO_2}. When carbon dioxide is retained, the Pa_{CO_2} increases (Pa_{CO_2} >45 mm Hg), indicating an increase in carbonic acid formation. When carbon dioxide is eliminated, the Pa_{CO_2} decreases (Pa_{CO_2} <35 mm Hg), indicating a decrease in carbonic acid formation.

The regulation of carbon dioxide excretion and, therefore, the control of the level of carbonic acid in the bicarbonate buffer system is performed by the respiratory center in the medulla oblongata. Hydrogen ions act directly on the respiratory center. A decrease in the pH to the acid side stimulates the respiratory center, causing an increase in the rate and depth of respirations, which removes carbon dioxide from the body. When the pH rises to the alkaline side, respirations decrease, and less carbon dioxide is removed via the lungs.

Respiratory compensation for eliminating carbonic acid is more effective than compensation for retaining it.

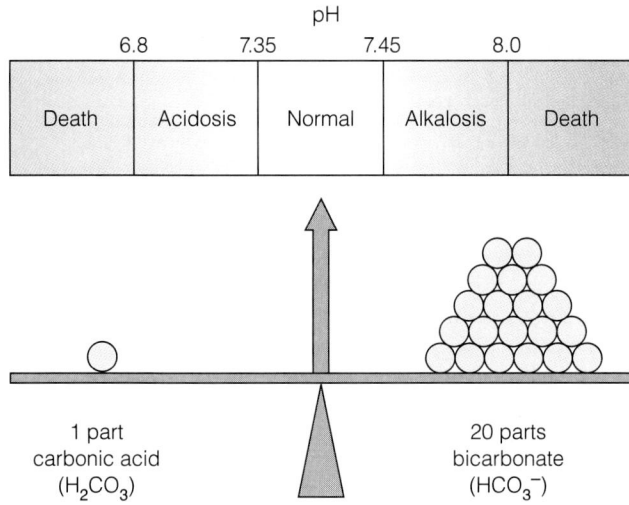

Figure 5–14 Normal acid-base balance ranges from 7.35 to 7.45. The normal ratio of bicarbonate to carbonic acid is 20:1.

Increasing the pH to the alkaline side has a minimal effect on the normal rate of respirations. Thus, compensatory mechanisms for metabolic acidosis (causing an increase in the rate and depth of respiration) are much more effective than for metabolic alkalosis (causing a decrease in the rate and depth of respiration).

The respiratory response to changes in hydrogen ion concentration occurs within a matter of minutes but is only about 50% to 75% effective. Although respiratory compensation will not reverse metabolic acidosis, it is effective in raising the pH toward normal. Conversely, in metabolic alkalosis, respiratory compensation is limited because decreasing the rate and depth of respiration will lead to hypoxemia (decreased oxygen content of the blood), and hypoxemia is itself a stimulus to respirations.

The kidneys also regulate acid-base balance by secreting hydrogen ions into the renal tubular fluid, where it combines with bicarbonate ions to form carbon dioxide and water. The water is eliminated in the urine; and the carbon dioxide diffuses into tubular cells, combines with water, and forms another bicarbonate and hydrogen ion.

Phosphate and Ammonia Buffer Systems

The phosphate and ammonia buffer systems are important in buffering fluids in the kidney tubules. Renal control of hydrogen ion concentration is based on mechanisms for increasing or decreasing the excretion of hydrogen ions. When the pH of the urine becomes acidic, hydrogen ions combine with buffers and are excreted in the urine. The major buffers are phosphate and ammonia.

Protein Buffers

Proteins are made up of amino acids, some of which have free acidic radicals that can dissociate into hydrogen ions and base ions. Protein buffers are found in hemoglobin, plasma proteins, and intracellular proteins. They buffer

hydrogen and carbon dioxide when they diffuse across the cell membrane into the cell.

Classification of Acid-Base Disorders

Acid-base disorders fall into two major categories: *acidosis* and *alkalosis*. **Acidosis** occurs when the hydrogen ion concentration increases above normal (reflected in a pH below 7.35). **Alkalosis** occurs when the hydrogen ion concentration decreases below normal (reflected in a pH above 7.45). The classification of acidosis and alkalosis into metabolic acidosis or alkalosis and respiratory acidosis or alkalosis is based on measurements of changes in the bicarbonate buffer system. Acid-base disorders with possible causes are described throughout this section of the chapter and are outlined in Table 5–6.

Metabolic acidosis and metabolic alkalosis are disorders in which the primary change is in the concentration of bicarbonate (Figure 5–15). *Metabolic alkalosis* is an abnormal increase in bicarbonate concentration (reflected in a serum bicarbonate level of more than 26 mEq/L) or a decrease in hydrogen ion concentration. *Metabolic acidosis* is an abnormal decrease in bicarbonate concentration (reflected in a serum bicarbonate level of less than 22 mEq/L) or an increase in hydrogen ion concentration.

Respiratory acidosis and respiratory alkalosis are disorders in which there is a primary change in the concentration of carbonic acid (Figure 5–16). With *respiratory alkalosis,* a loss of carbonic acid causes a fall in the carbon dioxide level (reflected in a $PaCO_2$ if less than 35 mm Hg), and increases the pH. Conversely, a retention of carbonic acid causes an increase in the carbon dioxide level (reflected in a $PaCO_2$ of more than 45 mm Hg), decreases the pH, and is called *respiratory acidosis.*

Acid-base disorders are further defined as primary (simple) and mixed. Primary (simple) disorders usually are due to one cause and affect only one part of the bicarbonate-carbonic acid buffer system. With primary disorders, compensatory changes in the other part of the system occur. *Mixed disorders* occur from a number of combinations of respiratory and metabolic disturbances. The result of mixed disorders may be that a disturbance in one part of the system is intensified by a superimposed disorder, but the net effect on the body is manifested as one disorder or the other.

Arterial Blood Gas (ABG) Measurement

Acid-base disorders are assessed and evaluated primarily through measuring arterial blood gases, using an arterial blood sample. The elements measured are pH, the $PaCO_2$, the PaO_2, bicarbonate levels, and oxygen saturation. These measurements reflect the functional status of alveolar ventilation, alveolar-capillary diffusion, pulmonary circulation, and pulmonary gas exchange. Oxygen and

Table 5-6   Acid-Base Disorders

Imbalance	Causes/Discussion
Metabolic acidosis ($HCO_3^- <22mEqL$; pH <7.35	*Severe diarrhea:* bicarbonate-rich intestinal (and pancreatic) secretions rushed through digestive tract before their solutes can be reabsorbed; bicarbonate ions are replaced by removal from blood *Renal disease:* failure of kidneys to rid body of acids formed by normal metabolic processes *Untreated diabetes mellitus:* lack of insulin or inability of tissue cells to respond to insulin, resulting in inability to use glucose; fats are used as primary energy fuel, and ketoacidosis occurs *Starvation:* lack of dietary nutrients for cellular fuels; body proteins and fat reserves are used for energy —both yield acidic metabolites as they are broken down for energy *Excess alcohol ingestion:* results in excess acids in blood *High ECF potassium concentrations:* potassium ions compete with H^+ for secretion in renal tubules; when ECF levels of K^+ are high, H^+ secretion is inhibited
Metabolic alkalosis ($HCO_3^- >26$ mEqL; pH <7.45	*Vomiting of chloride-containing gastric contents:* loss of stomach HCl requires that H^+ be withdrawn from blood to replace stomach acid; thus, H^+ decreases and HCO_3^- increases proportionately *Selected diuretics:* cause rapid reabsorption of Na^+ in distal tubule segments, leaving behind an excess of buffers in tubules that can combine with H^+ and thus remove excessive amounts *Ingestion of excessive amount of sodium bicarbonate:* bicarbonate moves easily into ECF, where it enhances natural alkaline reserve *Constipation:* prolonged retention of feces, resulting in increased amounts of HCO_3^- being reabsorbed *Excess aldosterone (e.g., adrenal tumors):* promotes excessive reabsorption of Na^+, which pulls increased amount of H^+ into urine
Respiratory acidosis ($Pco_2 >45$ mm Hg; pH<7.35	*Any condition that impairs gas exchange or lung ventilation (chronic bronchitis, cystic fibrosis, emphysema):* increased airway resistance and decreased expiratory air flow, leading to retention of carbon dioxide *Rapid, shallow breathing:* tidal volume markedly reduced *Narcotic or barbiturate overdose or injury to brain stem:* depression of respiratory centers, resulting in hypoventilation and respiratory arrest
Respiratory alkalosis ($Pco_2 <35$ mm Hg; pH>7.45)	*Direct cause is always hyperventilation:* hyperventilation in asthma, pneumonia, and at high altitude represents effort to raise Po_2 at the expense of excessive carbon dixoide excretion *Brain tumor or injury:* abnormality of respiratory controls

Note. From *Human Anatomy and Physiology* (2nd ed.) (p. 924) by E. N. Marieb, 1992, Redwood City, CA: Benjamin/Cummings.

carbon dioxide concentrations are also influenced by hemoglobin concentration, percent saturation, and the hemoglobin dissociation curve. Analysis of ABGs not only identifies acid-base disorders but also is useful in identifying the probable cause, determining the extent of the disturbance, and monitoring the effects of treatment.

The $Paco_2$ is a measure of the pressure exerted by dissolved carbon dioxide in the blood and is directly related to the carbon dioxide produced by the tissues. $Paco_2$ levels are regulated by the lungs and indicate the amount of carbonic acid available to the acid-base buffer system. Measurements of $Paco_2$ are used to determine whether the acidosis or alkalosis is metabolic or respiratory. The normal value for arterial $Paco_2$ is 35 to 45 mm Hg. Values less than 35 mm Hg indicate alkalosis; values greater than 45 mm Hg indicate acidosis.

The Pao_2 is a measure of the pressure exerted by oxygen in its free form that is dissolved in the plasma. Most oxygen in the blood is carried by hemoglobin; both the Pao_2 and the hemoglobin level are a measure of total oxygen content. The normal value for Pao_2 is 80 to 90 mm Hg. Measurements that are less than 60 mm Hg result from anaerobic metabolism resulting from hypoxemia.

The serum bicarbonate reflects the ability of the renal system to compensate for changes in the pH. A decrease in bicarbonate is indicative of acidosis, whereas an increase in bicarbonate is indicative of alkalosis. The normal value is 22 to 26 mEq/L. Measurements of less than 22 reflect acidosis; those greater than 26 reflect alkalosis.

Oxygen saturation is the ratio of oxygen present in the blood in comparison to the total amount of oxygen the blood is capable of holding. The ratio is related to the ability of hemoglobin to form oxyhemoglobin when exposed to oxygen in the alveolar air or when completely saturated with oxygen under test conditions. The normal values for oxygen saturation for arterial blood are 95% to 98%. Oxygen saturation decreases when the Pao_2 is less than 60%.

The base excess is a calculated value also known as buffer base capacity. The measurement of base excess reflects the degree of acid-base imbalance by indicating the status of the body's total buffering capacity. It represents the amount of acid or base that must be added to a blood sample to achieve a pH of 7.4. This is essentially a measure of increased or decreased bicarbonate. The normal value for base excess for arterial blood is −3.0 to +3.0.

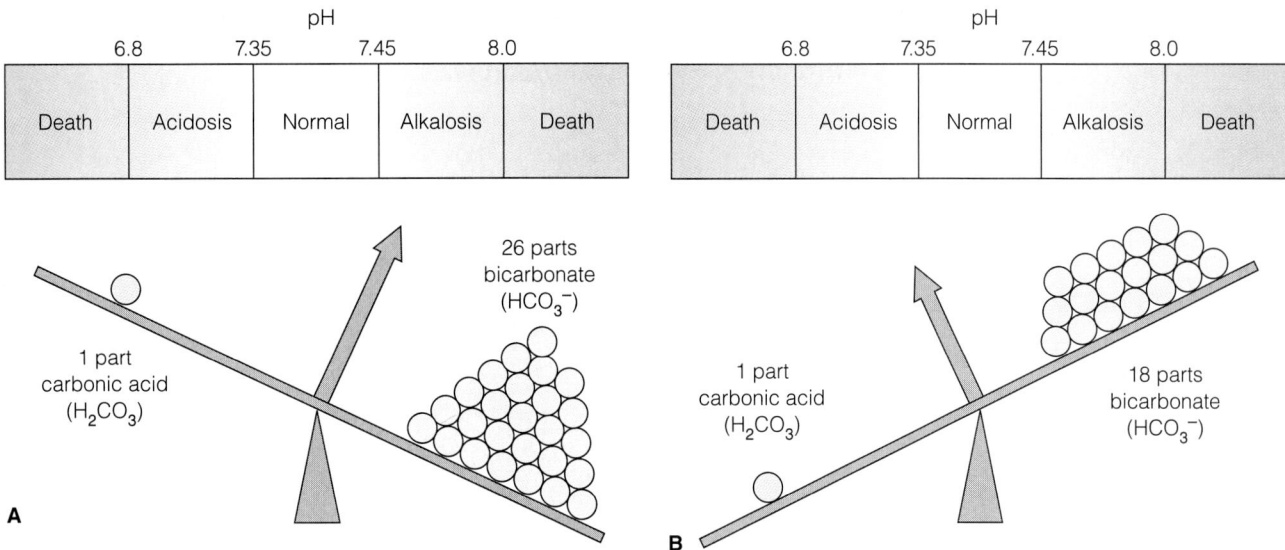

Figure 5–15   Metabolic acid-base imbalances: *A*, metabolic alkalosis. *B*, metabolic acidosis.

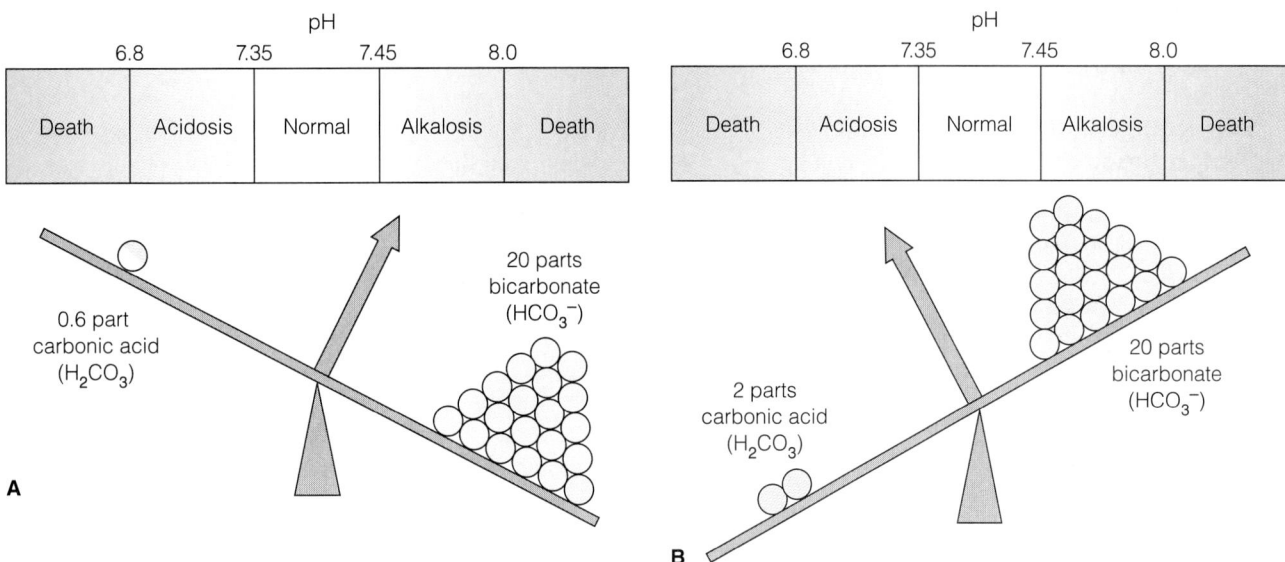

Figure 5–16   Respiratory acid-base imbalances: *A*, respiratory alkalosis. *B*, respiratory acidosis.

Measurements above +3.0 indicate metabolic alkalosis; values below −3.0 indicate metabolic acidosis.

A method of determining the acid-base status of a client, based on the ABG measurement, is outlined in the box on page 150.

The Client with Metabolic Alkalosis

■ ■ ■

Metabolic alkalosis is defined as a pathophysiologic process that occurs when there is a primary excess in the extracellular fluid of bicarbonate due to loss of acid (hydrogen ions) or the addition of excess bicarbonate. The

bicarbonate increases to above 26 mEq/L, and the pH is more than 7.45.

Pathophysiology

There are many causes for an increase in the bicarbonate ion in the extracellular fluid, including the following:

- Hydrogen ion losses from the gastrointestinal system (for example, through gastrointestinal suctioning or vomiting)

- Hydrogen ion losses from use of diuretics, mineralocorticoid excess, or hypercalcemia

- Hydrogen ion loss from a shift of hydrogen into the cells as a result of hypokalemia or carbohydrate refeeding after starvation

Interpretation of Arterial Blood Gases

■ ■ ■

Step 1: Evaluate the pH

pH <7.35 = acidosis

pH >7.45 = alkalosis

Step 2: Evaluate Respiratory Function (Ventilation)

Pa_{CO_2} >45 mm Hg = ventilatory failure and respiratory acidosis

Pa_{CO_2} <35 mm Hg = hyperventilation and respiratory alkalosis

Step 3: Evaluate Metabolic Processes

Serum bicarbonate <22 mEq/L and/or base excess < −3 mEq/L = metabolic acidosis

Serum bicarbonate >26 mEq/L and/or base excess > −3 mEq/L = metabolic alkalosis

Step 4: Determine the Primary and Compensating Disorder

To identify the primary disorder when both the Pa_{CO_2} and the bicarbonate deviate from normal, determine which ABG value (Pa_{CO_2} or bicarbonate) follows the deviation in pH and deviates the most from normal. The value that follows the deviation in pH and has the greatest deviation from normal identifies the primary

disturbance. For example, a client's ABGs are:

pH: 7.28 (acidosis)

Pa_{CO_2}: 28.9 mm Hg (respiratory alkalosis)

Bicarbonate: 11 mEq/L (metabolic acidosis)

Base excess: −13

Interpretation: The pH is less than 7.35, indicating acidosis. The Pa_{CO_2} is greater than 40 mm Hg, indicating a respiratory alkalosis; however, the bicarbonate is less than 26 mEq/L, indicating a metabolic acidosis. Because the bicarbonate value indicates acidosis, it follows the deviation in pH; it also shows the greatest deviation from normal. Therefore, the primary process is metabolic acidosis, and the compensatory process is respiratory alkalosis.

Step 5: Evaluate Oxygenation

The oxygenation status of the client is assessed by checking the Pa_{O_2} and Sa_{O_2} (oxygen saturation of hemoglobin) to determine whether they are within normal limits, decreased, or increased. Normally, the Pa_{O_2} remains between 80 and 100 mm Hg, with a normal Sa_{O_2} of 95% or greater indicating adequate oxygenation of tissue. Hypoxia at the cellular level can occur if the Pa_{O_2} decreases to less than 60 mm Hg, because it is accompanied by a marked decrease in the Sa_{O_2}.

■ Bicarbonate retention from administration of bicarbonate or massive blood transfusions

However, the most frequent causes of metabolic alkalosis are excessive losses of gastric secretions with a concomitant loss of hydrogen and chloride ions from vomiting and nasogastric suction, and excessive diuresis from diuretic therapy (with a concomitant loss of potassium, hydrogen, and chloride ions). Other causes include an excessive ingestion of alkaline drugs, such as antacids containing sodium bicarbonate, and excessive levels of aldosterone (adrenal hyperfunction), which promotes the reabsorption of bicarbonate and sodium and increases the excretion of potassium, hydrogen, and chloride ions. In metabolic alkalosis, the bicarbonate level increases to greater than 26 mEq/L, and the pH increases to more than 7.45. (The compensatory response to metabolic alkalosis is retention of carbon dioxide, reflected in a Pa_{CO_2} greater than 45 mm Hg.)

Metabolic alkalosis is often intensified by the presence of hypokalemia. Hypokalemia contributes to maintaining

metabolic alkalosis in two ways. In the first, potassium is exchanged for hydrogen ions at the cellular level to correct the hypokalemia. (Potassium ions leave the cell, and hydrogen ions enter the cell—an exchange of a cation for a cation.) The decrease in extracellular hydrogen ions intensifies the alkalosis. In the second, the kidneys excrete hydrogen ions in exchange for potassium ions (a cation for a cation) to conserve potassium. The loss of hydrogen ions augments the alkalosis.

Chloride depletion and volume depletion, such as that which occurs secondary to nasogastric suction, severe vomiting, diarrhea, and diuretic therapy, also contributes to the continuation of the metabolic alkalosis and hypokalemia. With the volume depletion, sodium ion reabsorption is stimulated to restore the fluid volume. Normally, reabsorption of sodium is accompanied by chloride, but because of the lack of the chloride ion in the renal tubule, hydrogen ions are exchanged for sodium ions (a cation for a cation) resulting in a loss of hydrogen ions. With excessive loss of potassium from the gastrointestinal tract and kidneys, hypokalemia occurs. In the presence of hypokalemia, potassium ions are exchanged for hydrogen ions, intensifying the metabolic alkalosis.

Manifestations of metabolic alkalosis may be absent, or if present, they may be related to volume depletion or hypokalemia. Severe metabolic alkalosis causes neurologic manifestations, including mental confusion, hyperactive reflexes, tetany, and spasm of the hands and feet. If the pH exceeds 7.55, respiratory failure, dysrhythmias, seizures, and coma may occur. The accompanying box summarizes the clinical manifestations of metabolic alkalosis.

Collaborative Care

The management of metabolic alkalosis focuses on diagnosing and correcting the underlying cause.

Laboratory and Diagnostic Tests

The following laboratory and diagnostic tests may be ordered:

- *ABGs* are measured to establish the diagnosis of metabolic alkalosis. In metabolic alkalosis, the bicarbonate level is greater than 26 mEq/L, and the pH is higher than 7.45. With severe metabolic alkalosis, the pH may be greater than 7.50, and the bicarbonate equal to or greater than 40 mEq/L. Compensatory hypoventilation in response to metabolic alkalosis varies greatly from individual to individual, depending on the presence of other conditions. With compensatory hypoventilation, carbon dioxide is retained, and the $Paco_2$ is greater than 45 mm Hg.

- *Serum electrolytes* are measured. Depending on the cause of the metabolic alkalosis, various changes are observed. A decreased serum potassium (<3.5 mEq/L) and decreased chloride (<95 mEq/L) are often present. A decrease in sodium (<135 mEq/L) may also be present.

- A *urinalysis* may be performed. Analysis of the urine chloride levels is used to distinguish metabolic alkalosis caused from hypovolemia from that which is the result of excessive aldosterone production or severe hypokalemia. In clients with excessive aldosterone production and severe hypokalemia, the urinary chloride is greater than 20 mmol/L (Petersdorf et al., 1991).

- An *ECG* is conducted. Changes in the ECG pattern are similar to those seen with hypokalemia. These changes may be due to hypokalemia or to the alkalosis (Petersdorf et al., 1991).

Pharmacology

In metabolic alkalosis caused by hypokalemia and volume depletion, therapy consists of the administration of saline solutions and potassium replacement. Clients with diuretic-induced metabolic alkalosis from long-term di-

---

Clinical Manifestations of Metabolic Alkalosis

■ ■ ■

- Hypotension
- Tachycardia
- Confusion
- Decreasing levels of consciousness
- Hyperreflexia
- Tetany
- Dysrhythmias
- Seizures
- Respiratory failure

---

uretic therapy are treated with oral potassium supplements.

In clients with hypokalemia and metabolic alkalosis from increased aldosterone production, treatment focuses on correcting the underlying adrenal disorder. Prolonged, severe metabolic alkalosis may require intravenous therapy with acidifying drugs, such as dilute hydrochloric acid, or acidifying salts, such as lysine hydrochloride, particularly in clients with significant hypoventilation (Wyngaarden et al., 1992).

Nursing Care

The nursing care of clients with metabolic alkalosis centers on the client's responses to its systemic effects, principally those related to volume depletion and hypokalemia. The nursing diagnoses that are applicable to the client with metabolic alkalosis include the following:

- *Fluid Volume Deficit* related to excessive loss of gastrointestinal fluid

- *Decreased Cardiac Output* related to volume depletion and altered myocardial conduction secondary to dysrhythmias induced by hypokalemia or alkalosis

- *Knowledge Deficit* related to appropriate use and potential side effects of potassium-losing diuretics

- *Risk for Impaired Gas Exchange* related to compensatory hypoventilation secondary to severe metabolic alkalosis

- *Risk for Injury* related to postural hypotension secondary to volume depletion

The Client with Metabolic Acidosis

■ ■ ■

Metabolic acidosis is defined as a pathophysiologic process that occurs when there is a primary loss of bicarbonate from the extracellular fluid due to increased acid

---

Clinical Manifestations of Metabolic Acidosis

∎ ∎ ∎

- Anorexia
- Nausea and vomiting
- Abdominal pain
- Weakness
- Altered mental status

- Decreasing levels of consciousness
- Dysrhythmias
- Bradycardia
- Warm, flushed skin
- Hyperventilation

---

production. It exists when the bicarbonate is less than 22 mEq/L and the pH is less than 7.35. Metabolic acidosis is rarely a primary disorder; rather, it usually develops during the course of another disease.

Pathophysiology

Metabolic acidosis occurs in conditions in which the following are present:

- An increased production of metabolic acids from
  a. Fasting and starvation states
  b. Diabetic ketoacidosis
  c. Salicylate poisoning
- Impaired excretion of metabolic acids from renal failure
- An increased bicarbonate loss from
  a. Loss of intestinal secretions in diarrhea, intestinal suction, intestinal fistula, and biliary or pancreatic drainage
  b. Increased renal losses
- An increased chloride level from
  a. Abnormal renal function
  b. Saline infusions
  c. Treatment with ammonium chloride
  d. Parenteral hyperalimentation

In acute conditions, the bicarbonate level decreases to less than 22 mEq/L, and the pH decreases to less than 7.35. The compensatory response to an acute metabolic acidosis is hyperventilation (a cardinal sign of acute metabolic acidosis) reflected in a $PaCO_2$ of less than 35 mm Hg, which adjusts the pH toward normal (recall that it is the ratio of carbonic acid to bicarbonate that affects the pH).

To identify the cause of metabolic acidosis in a client, it is helpful to classify the disorder into one of two groups: acidosis exhibiting an increased anion gap (*increased an-*

ion-gap acidosis) or acidosis exhibiting a normal anion gap (*normal anion-gap acidosis,* also called *hyperchloremic metabolic acidosis*). The *anion gap* (8 to 12 mEq/L) depicts the unmeasured anions of albumin, sulfates, phosphates, and organic acids. It represents the difference (gap) between the concentration of the cation sodium and the anions of chloride and bicarbonate and is calculated by the formula:

$$\text{anion gap} = Na^+ - (HCO_3^- + Cl^-).$$

Increased anion-gap acidosis is caused by an increased internal production of metabolic acids, as occurs with lactic acidosis and ketoacidosis; by the addition of acids from the ingestion of certain drugs and toxins; or by the decreased excretion of metabolic acids, as occurs in renal failure. Bicarbonate is displaced in increased anion-gap metabolic acidosis by the unmeasured anions of these acids. Again, these unmeasured anions are not measured with the serum electrolytes and are identified only by an increase in the anion gap or an increase in the difference between the measured cation sodium and the measured anions bicarbonate and chloride. For example, using the formula for calculating the anion gap and given a sodium level of 140 mEq/L, a bicarbonate level of 16 mEq/L, and a chloride level of 104 mEq/L, the anion gap will be

$$\text{anion gap} = 140 - (16 + 104) = 20.$$

Normal anion-gap (hyperchloremic) metabolic acidosis is usually caused by gastrointestinal losses of bicarbonate (diarrhea, fluid losses from the pancreas or biliary tract, other gastrointestinal losses); renal bicarbonate loss (early renal failure; adrenal insufficiency; renal tubular acidosis; therapy with drugs, such as amphotericin B, acetazolamide, spironolactone; and other renal losses); or the administration of exogenous acids (total parenteral nutrition solutions, ammonium chloride, and hydrochloric acid or its precursors). In normal anion-gap metabolic acidosis, the anion gap is unchanged.

Metabolic acidosis exerts effects on the gastrointestinal system, the neural system, the cardiovascular system, and the skin. Signs of compensation also appear. Gastrointestinal manifestations include anorexia, nausea, vomiting, and abdominal pain. Depression of neural function causes manifestations of weakness, lethargy, confusion, coma, and depression of vital signs. Cardiovascular manifestations include dysrhythmias, bradycardia, and decreased cardiac output. The skin is often warm and flushed. Signs of compensation are hyperventilation (a respiratory rate that is more rapid than normal, causing increased intake of oxygen and increased blowing off of carbon dioxide), decreased $PaCO_2$, and increased amounts of ammonia in the urine. The accompanying box summarizes the clinical manifestations of metabolic acidosis.

Collaborative Care

The management of metabolic acidosis is dependent on the underlying cause of the pathophysiologic process and whether it is acute or chronic in nature. The focus of treatment for acute metabolic acidosis is to treat the underlying cause.

Laboratory and Diagnostic Tests

The following laboratory and diagnostic tests may be ordered:

- *ABGs* are measured, with typical findings including a bicarbonate level of less than 22 mEq/L, pH of less than 7.35, and a compensatory decrease in $PaCO_2$ to less than 35 mm Hg. In lactic acidosis, the PaO_2 is decreased as a result of decreased blood oxygenation and inadequate tissue perfusion.

- *Serum electrolytes* are measured. The serum potassium is usually increased to more than 5 mEq/L as a result of a shift of potassium ions out of the cells in exchange for hydrogen ions. Calculation of the unmeasured ions (anion gap) is useful in determining the cause of the metabolic acidosis.

- *An ECG* is conducted. If the hyperkalemia that accompanies metabolic acidosis is severe, it may be reflected in changes in the ECG.

Pharmacology

Treatment for diabetic ketoacidosis includes insulin administration, fluid replacement, and correction of hypokalemia with a potassium replacement. Alcoholic ketoacidosis is treated with saline solutions and glucose. In clients with lactic acidosis from decreased tissue perfusion secondary to a severe respiratory or circulatory disorder—as, for example, respiratory or cardiac arrest—the focus of treatment is to correct the underlying disorder and improve tissue perfusion.

It is important to avoid overtreatment with intravenous bicarbonate. Overtreatment may lead to metabolic alkalosis, hypokalemia (because hydrogen ions move out of the cell and potassium enters the cell), and a resulting increase in the risk of dysrhythmias, hypocalcemia with increased risk of neuromuscular irritability, and fluid overload (hypervolemic hypernatremia) caused by hypertonicity of extracellular fluid. The hypertonic sodium bicarbonate causes a fluid shift from the intracellular to the intravascular space.

Clients with chronic renal failure and mild or moderate metabolic acidosis may or may not require treatment. Treatment may include oral alkali (for example, sodium bicarbonate) when the bicarbonate decreases to less than 16 to 18 mEq/L.

If the metabolic acidosis is due to diarrhea, treatment includes correcting the underlying cause and providing fluid and electrolyte replacement. Treatment for metabolic acidosis due to toxic ingestions depends on the drug or poison ingested.

Mechanical Ventilation

Although mechanical ventilation may be necessary, it is important to allow the client's compensatory hyperventilation to continue so that acidosis will not continue to increase. If the client is placed on a ventilator, the rate of respirations should be set lower than the client's spontaneous rate, and the tidal volume should be large enough to maintain the compensatory hyperventilation until the underlying cause is treated. (Mechanical ventilators are fully discussed in Chapter 34.)

Nursing Care

The nursing care of clients with metabolic acidosis centers on the client's responses to the underlying cause and its physiologic effects. Nursing diagnoses applicable to the client with metabolic acidosis include the following:

- *Decreased Cardiac Output* secondary to dysrhythmias from hyperkalemia and/or fluid volume deficit

- *Risk for Sensory/Perceptual Alterations* related to changes in central nervous system function secondary to acidosis

- *Risk for Injury* related to confusion, restlessness, seizures, and weakness

- *Risk for Altered Oral Mucous Membranes* related to hyperventilation

- *Risk for Fluid Volume Deficit* secondary to excessive gastrointestinal fluid loss

Nursing care includes closely monitoring the client and implementing interventions to prevent or correct problems. Assessment includes monitoring the client for particular signs and symptoms of complications and for response to therapy. The following are assessed and monitored:

- Vital signs, particularly changes in respiratory depth and rate (deep, rapid respirations are a compensatory response to acute metabolic acidosis)

- Bowel sounds and function to detect changes secondary to hypokalemia

- Neurologic function and mental status

- Fluid intake, output, and daily weight

- ECG rate and rhythm

- Serum electrolytes

Clinical Manifestations of Respiratory Alkalosis

▪ ▪ ▪

- Dizziness
- Diaphoresis
- Palpitations
- Dyspnea
- Anxiety/panic
- Tetany
- Convulsions

Nursing care also may include providing measures to protect the client from injury and administering intravenous fluids and electrolytes.

The Client with Respiratory Alkalosis

▪ ▪ ▪

Respiratory alkalosis is a condition existing when serum bicarbonate is less than 24 mEq/L, arterial $PaCO_2$ is below 35 mm Hg, and serum pH is greater than 7.45. Respiratory alkalosis can exist when bicarbonate levels are normal (Metheney, 1992). The condition occurs when there is an increase in the rate of alveolar ventilation in relation to the rate of carbon dioxide production. It is caused by a decrease in dissolved carbon dioxide, or a carbonic acid deficit.

Pathophysiology

Respiratory alkalosis often occurs during acute and chronic conditions associated with hyperventilation. It is most commonly related to hyperventilation associated with anxiety (called the "hyperventilation syndrome"). Other causes include the following:

- Respiratory center stimulation from fever, salicylate intoxication, or trauma of the central nervous system
- Infection
- Excessive mechanical ventilation in clients on ventilators

In acute conditions, the $PaCO_2$ decreases to less than 35 mm Hg, and the pH increases to greater than 7.45. In chronic conditions, the pH may remain normal as the kidneys adjust the serum bicarbonate level.

The manifestations of respiratory alkalosis are associated with a decreased cerebral blood flow and hyperexcitability of the nervous system. The client experiences dizziness, sweating, palpitations, panic, and dyspnea. If the alkalosis is severe, tetany, convulsions, and periods of

apnea may occur. The accompanying box summarizes the clinical manifestations of respiratory alkalosis.

Collaborative Care

The management of respiratory alkalosis focuses primarily on correcting the underlying cause. Definitive treatment is directed toward clients with severe hyperventilation who develop central nervous system manifestations or neuromuscular manifestations.

Laboratory and Diagnostic Tests

The following laboratory and diagnostic tests may be ordered:

- *ABGs* are measured. Typical findings in respiratory alkalosis from acute hyperventilation are a pH greater than 7.45 and a $PaCO_2$ less than 35 mm Hg. In chronic hyperventilation, there is a compensatory decrease in serum bicarbonate to less than 22 mEq/L and a return of the pH to normal.
- *Serum electrolytes* are measured. The major change is a decrease of bicarbonate as a compensatory response to chronic respiratory alkalosis.

Pharmacology

Sedatives or tranquilizers may be prescribed for clients who have anxiety-induced respiratory alkalosis.

Rebreathing Carbon Dioxide

The treatment for people who experience anxiety-producing respiratory alkalosis is to rebreathe carbon dioxide through an oxygen mask with an attached carbon dioxide reservoir. Self-care can be provided by having the client breathe into a paper bag to rebreathe his or her own expired carbon dioxide.

Oxygen Therapy

If hypoxia is the underlying cause of respiratory alkalosis, oxygen is administered by mask or cannula.

Nursing Care

In clients with respiratory alkalosis, applicable nursing diagnoses and interventions are those that relate to the underlying cause. In clients who experience hyperventilation caused by nervousness and anxiety or who are at risk for developing tetany, nursing diagnoses include the following:

- *Sensory/Perceptual Alterations* related to neurologic deficits
- *Altered Thought Processes* related to cerebral hyperexcitation
- *Ineffective Breathing Pattern* related to hyperventilation

- *Anxiety* related to effect of alkalosis on central nervous system
- *Risk for Injury* related to weakness or seizures
- *Risk for Injury* related to tetany

In the client with anxiety, the nursing care is directed toward providing support and reassurance and assisting with definitive therapy. Nursing care of clients at high risk for injury from tetany includes instituting safety precautions.

The Client with Respiratory Acidosis

■ ■ ■

Respiratory acidosis is serum $PaCO_2$ exceeding 45 mm Hg and serum pH less than 7.35. This condition occurs when there is a reduction in the rate of alveolar ventilation in relation to the rate of carbon dioxide production. Respiratory acidosis is caused by an accumulation of dissolved carbon dioxide, or carbonic acid.

Pathophysiology

Both acute and chronic respiratory acidosis are the result of carbon dioxide retention caused by alveolar hypoventilation. Hypoxemia (low oxygen in the arterial blood) frequently accompanies alveolar hypoventilation. A sudden failure of ventilation from any cause leads to acute respiratory acidosis. It is associated with a number of disorders, including the following:

- Depression of the respiratory center from general anesthesia, narcotic overdose, or head trauma
- Cardiac arrest
- Structural alterations in the thorax and lungs from thoracic injuries, obstruction of the airway (laryngospasm, aspiration of foreign objects), or pneumothorax
- Lung disorders, such as pulmonary edema, asthma, emphysema, chronic bronchitis, and pneumonia
- Neuromuscular impairment of the muscles of respiration from paralyzing drugs, Guillain-Barré syndrome, myasthenic crisis, amyotrophic lateral sclerosis, or severe hyperkalemia
- Improperly regulated mechanical ventilators

Chronic respiratory acidosis caused by pulmonary diseases such as chronic bronchitis and emphysema is the result of a decline in effective alveolar ventilation and a mismatched ventilation-perfusion ratio occurring over time. Other causes of chronic respiratory acidosis include diseases or conditions that restrict ventilation (scleroderma, prolonged pneumonia, and severe distortions of the thorax, such as kyphoscoliosis), neuromuscular con-

---

Clinical Manifestations of Respiratory Acidosis

■ ■ ■

- Warm, flushed skin
- Tachycardia
- Papilledema
- Headache
- Altered mental status
- Decreasing levels of consciousness
- Muscle twitching

---

ditions affecting respiratory movement (amyotrophic lateral sclerosis, multiple sclerosis, poliomyelitis), and conditions affecting the respiratory center (brain tumor, stroke). The majority of clients with chronic long-standing respiratory acidosis have chronic obstructive pulmonary disease secondary to chronic bronchitis and emphysema.

The level of elevation of the $PaCO_2$ that occurs with respiratory acidosis is indicative of the degree of ventilatory function. The extent to which the elevated $PaCO_2$ changes the pH is correlated with the rapidity of the onset of the ventilatory failure and the ability of the body to compensate for it.

In chronic respiratory acidosis (compensated) a decrease in effective alveolar ventilation or a ventilation-perfusion mismatch occurs over time, such as in chronic obstructive pulmonary disease. $PaCO_2$ levels increase over time and remain elevated. Renal compensatory mechanisms elevate the bicarbonate level, and eventually the pH approaches (but never quite reaches) normal.

Because acute respiratory acidosis occurs with the sudden onset of hypoventilation—as, for example, with cardiopulmonary or respiratory arrest—it results in a sudden rise in $PaCO_2$ and a marked change in pH. The serum bicarbonate is unchanged.

The manifestations of respiratory acidosis depend on whether the cause is acute or chronic and on how rapidly it occurs. The skin is warm and flushed, and the cardiac rate increases. Increased carbon dioxide crosses the blood–brain barrier to change the pH of cerebral fluids and increase blood flow; if this condition is long-standing, papilledema (swelling of the optic nerve) and increased cerebral spinal fluid pressure may result. Other neurologic manifestations include headache, irritability, muscle twitching, behavioral changes, confusion, lethargy, and coma. The accompanying box summarizes the clinical manifestations of respiratory acidosis.

Collaborative Care

Clients with acute respiratory failure usually require emergency interventions and are seen and treated either in intensive care units or the emergency department. The focus is on treating the underlying cause and restoring normal acid-base balance.

Laboratory and Diagnostic Tests

The following laboratory and diagnostic tests may be ordered:

- *ABGs* are measured. Typical findings in acute respiratory acidosis are a pH of less than 7.35 and a $PaCO_2$ of more than 45 mm Hg. Initially, the bicarbonate level in acute respiratory acidosis is within normal range but may increase over time if the condition persists. If the acute respiratory acidosis is superimposed on a chronic respiratory acidosis, the bicarbonate level is elevated in addition to the decreased pH and increased $PaCO_2$.

- *Serum electrolytes* are measured. The major change is an increase in bicarbonate levels to greater than 26 mEq/L as a compensatory response to persistent respiratory acidosis.

Pharmacology

Treatment of clients with chronic respiratory acidosis who develop acute respiratory acidosis is directed toward correcting the precipitating cause, such as pneumonia, and may include the use of antibiotics and bronchodilators.

Respiratory Support

Because severe respiratory acidosis is secondary to ventilatory failure, it is often accompanied by hypoxemia. Treatment is focused on restoring the alveolar ventilation and correcting the $PaCO_2$ and administering oxygen to reverse the hypoxemia. Pulmonary measures, such as providing breathing treatments and increasing fluid intake, may be instituted. If supplemental oxygen is used, it should be administered with extreme caution to the client with chronic respiratory acidosis. In these clients, the primary stimulus to breathe is hypoxemia, and elevating the PaO_2 eliminates the hypoxic drive. Overcorrection of the respiratory acidosis may result in metabolic alkalosis and should be avoided. Intubation and mechanical ventilation may be necessary in clients with acute ventilatory failure superimposed on chronic respiratory acidosis.

Nursing Care

In clients with respiratory acidosis, applicable nursing diagnoses and interventions are those that relate to the underlying cause.

Examples of nursing diagnoses and collaborative problems that apply to the client with acute respiratory acidosis include the following:

- *Anxiety* related to breathlessness
- *Potential Complication: Respiratory Insufficiency* secondary to acute hypoventilation (Carpenito, 1992)

- *Impaired Gas Exchange* related to alveolar hypoventilation
- *Sensory/Perceptual Alterations* related to acid-base imbalance
- *Altered Oral Mucous Membranes* related to abnormal breathing pattern
- *Ineffective Airway Clearance* related to thick pulmonary secretions and fatigue

Assessment includes monitoring the client for the manifestations of complications and for response to therapy; monitoring the client's respiratory rate, depth, and effort; breath sounds; level of consciousness; ECG rate and rhythm; serum electrolytes; and ABGs. Nursing care may include the administration of oxygen, intravenous fluids and electrolyte solutions, and medications.

Applying the Nursing Process

Case Study of a Client with Respiratory Acidosis: Marlene Hitz

Marlene Hitz, age 76, is eating lunch with her friends when she suddenly begins to choke and becomes unable to breathe. An attendant at the senior center successfully carries out the Heimlich maneuver to dislodge some meat caught in Ms. Hitz's throat. Ms. Hitz is transported to the emergency room of the local hospital by ambulance, because she had been unable to breathe for 4 minutes, is having shallow respirations, and is disoriented.

Assessment

On admission to the emergency department, Ms. Hitz is placed in an observation room. Oxygen is administered per nasal cannula at the rate of 4 L/min, blood is drawn for stat ABGs, a chest X-ray study is ordered, and intravenous fluids of 5% dextrose and 0.45% NaCl are administered at the rate of 50 mL per hour. David Love, the nurse admitting Ms. Hitz, makes the following assessments: T 98.2, P 102, R 36 and shallow, BP 146/92. Skin is warm and dry. Ms. Hitz is alert but not oriented to time or place and responds slowly to questions. She is restless.

The chest X-ray film shows no abnormality. ABG studies yield the following findings:

pH:	7.38 (normal: 7.35 to 7.45)
$PaCO_2$:	48 (normal: 35 to 45 mm Hg)
PaO_2:	92 (normal: 80 to 100 mm Hg)
Bicarbonate:	24 (normal: 22 to 26 mEq/L)

Although these findings indicate acute respiratory acidosis, Ms. Hitz is not cyanotic or lethargic, so Mr. Love continues to observe Ms. Hitz. Mr. Love also speaks with one of Ms. Hitz's friends from the senior center, who tells

Fluid, Electrolyte, and Acid-Base Disorders in the Older Adult

■ ■ ■

Because of normal age-related physiologic changes, particularly in sodium and water regulation, the older client is at increased risk for fluid and electrolyte imbalances. Several age-related changes also affect the older adult's ability to regulate acid-base balance. Under normal circumstances, homeostasis is maintained, but because of age-related decreases in functional reserves, the capacity of the older adult to respond to acute illness and other stressors is compromised.

Normal age-related changes that affect fluid, electrolyte, and acid-base balance include the following:

- A decrease in total body water related to an increase in body fat relative to a decline in lean body mass (intracellular water decreases)
- A decline in all parameters of renal function, including decreased renal concentrating capacity, impaired sodium conservation, decreased glomerular filtration rate, altered acid-base regulation (decreased ammonia production), and a reduced response to antidiuretic hormone
- A decrease in total potassium content related to a decline in lean body mass
- Decreased respiratory function related to altered lung volumes and reduced ventilation rate at rest and during physical exercise
- Decreased sensible and insensible water loss from the skin secondary to a decrease in the number and functional efficiency of sweat glands

- Decreased gastrointestinal motility and hydrochloric acid production.

The following fluid and electrolyte disorders are frequently encountered in the older adult:

- Fluid volume deficit (dehydration) and hypernatremia due to inadequate fluid intake or free-water losses accompanied by restricted water intake secondary to hyperglycemia, diarrhea, vomiting, or diuresis
- Hyponatremia due to inadequate sodium intake; increased sodium loss secondary to vomiting, diarrhea, or renal factors; overhydration from intravenous fluid therapy; impaired water excretion secondary to cardiac, renal, or hepatic disease; excessive diuretic therapy, or SIADH
- Hypokalemia due to excessive diuretic therapy or prolonged use of laxatives

Age-related functional changes in the lungs and kidneys diminish the older adult's ability to compensate for acid-base imbalances. There is a decrease in the compensatory respiratory response to acidosis and alkalosis. In the kidney, the decrease in ammonia production makes less available to combine with hydrogen ions to compensate for acidosis.

---

him that Ms. Hitz has always been very active, lives alone, and is "as sharp as a tack."

Diagnosis

Mr. Love makes the following nursing diagnoses:

- *Impaired Gas Exchange* related to hypoventilation secondary to respiratory arrest
- *Sensory/Perceptual Alteration* related to physiologic changes from acidosis
- *Anxiety* related to sudden change in health status and emergency hospital admission
- *Risk for Injury* related to confusion

Expected Outcomes

The expected outcomes established in the plan of care specify that Ms. Hitz will

- Have a normal or baseline gas exchange at rest and with exercise.
- Regain orientation to time, place, and person.
- Demonstrate a return to normal mental status.
- Rest more calmly in bed.
- Remain free of injury.

Planning and Implementation

Mr. Love plans and implements the following interventions in caring for Ms. Hitz:

- Monitor ABGs, which are to be redrawn in 2 hours.
- Monitor vital signs every hour. Note presence of bradycardia, hypotension, or respiratory distress.
- Assess color of skin, nail beds, and oral mucous membranes every hour.

- Assess mental status and degree of orientation every hour.

- Monitor anxiety level as evidenced by restlessness and agitation.

- Maintain a calm, quiet environment.

- Provide reorientation, and explain all activities when interacting with Ms. Hitz.

- Keep side rails in place, and place call bell so that Ms. Hitz can reach it.

Evaluation

Ms. Hitz remains in the emergency department for 6 hours. Her ABGs are still abnormal, and Mr. Love now notes the presence of respiratory crackles and wheezes. She is less anxious, and responds appropriately when asked who and where she is. Because she has not regained normal gas exchange, Ms. Hitz is admitted to the hospital for continued observation and treatment.

Critical Thinking in the Nursing Process

1. What age-related changes put Ms. Hitz at increased risk for acidosis (see the box on page 157)?

2. Describe the effect of acidosis on mental function.

3. Is the measurement of Ms. Hitz's oxygen status a true indicator of her respiratory function? Why, or why not?

4. Design a care plan for Ms. Hitz for the nursing diagnosis *Post-trauma Response*.

Bibliography

■ ■ ■

Abbott Laboratories (1970). *Fluids and electrolytes: Some practical guides to clinical use*. North Chicago: Abbott Laboratories.

Anderson, S. (1990). Six easy steps to interpreting blood gases. *American Journal of Nursing, 90*(8), 42–45.

Angelucci, D., & Todaro, A. (1993). Reversing acute dehydration. *Nursing, 23*(6), 33.

Birney, M. H., & Penney, D. G. (1990). Atrial natriuretic peptide: A hormone with implications for clinical practice. *Heart & Lung, 90*(2), 174–183.

Bullock, B. L. , & Rosendahl, P. P. (1992). *Pathophysiology: Adaptations and alterations in function* (3rd ed.). Philadelphia: Lippincott.

Carpenito, L. J. (1992). *Nursing diagnosis: Application to nursing practice* (4th ed.). Philadelphia: Lippincott.

Catchpole, A. (1982). Electrolytes, their physiological action and interaction: A review. *Journal of Intravenous Nursing, 50*(5), 476–481.

Cerrato, P. (1993). Vitamins and minerals. *RN, 56*(6), 28–33.

Clinical Insights. (1990). Respiratory acidosis. *Nursing, 20*(9), 52–53.

DeAngelis, R. (1991). Hypokalemia. *Critical Care Nurse, 11*(7), 71–75.

Dubose, T. D., Harrington, J. T., & Slovis, C. M. (1992). Acid-base emergencies. *Patient Care, 26*(3), 214–231.

Eliopoulos, C. (1987). *A guide to the nursing of the aging*. Baltimore, MD: Williams & Wilkins.

Fischbach, F. T. (1992). *Laboratory diagnostic tests* . (4th ed.). St. Louis: Lippincott.

Goldberger, E. (1986). *A primer of water, electrolyte and acid-base syndromes* (7th ed.). Philadelphia: Lea & Febiger.

Groer, M. W., & Shekleton, M. E. (1989). *Basic pathophysiology: A conceptual approach* (3rd ed.). St. Louis: Mosby.

Guyton, A. C. (1991). *Textbook of medical physiology* (8th ed.). Philadelphia: WB Saunders.

Horne, M. M., Heitz, U. E., & Swearingen, P. I. (1991). *Fluid, electrolyte, and acid-base balance: A case study approach*. St. Louis: Mosby.

Keyes, J. L. (1985). *Fluid, electrolyte, and acid-base regulation*. Monterey, CA: Wadsworth.

Kokko, J. P., & Tannen, R. L. (1990). *Fluids and electrolytes* (2nd ed.). Philadelphia: Saunders.

Marieb, E. N. (1992). *Human anatomy and physiology.* (2nd ed.). Redwood City, CA: Benjamin/Cummings.

Masiak, M. J., Naylor, M. D., & Hayman, L. L. (1985). *Fluids and electrolytes throughout the life cycle*. Norwalk, CT: Appleton–Century–Crofts.

Maxwell, M. H., Kleeman, C. R., & Narins, R. G. (1987). *Clinical disorders of fluid and electrolyte metabolism* (4th ed.). New York: McGraw-Hill.

Metheney, N. M. (1992). *Fluid and electrolyte balance: Nursing considerations*. Philadelphia: Lippincott.

Miller, M. (1987). Fluid and electrolyte balance in the elderly. *Geriatrics, 42*(11): 65–76.

Owens, M. W. (1993). Keeping an eye on magnesium. *American Journal of Nursing, 93*(2), 66–67.

Paul, A. A., & Southgate, D. A. (1978). *McCance and Widdowson's the composition of food* (4th ed.). New York: Elsevier/North-Holland Biomedical Press.

Pestana, C. (1989). *Fluids and electrolytes in the surgical patient* (4th ed.). Baltimore: Williams & Wilkins.

Petersdorf, R. G., Adams, R. D., Braunwald, E., Isselbacher, K. J., Martin, J. B. & Wilson, J. D. (Eds.). (1991). *Harrison's principles of internal medicine* (12th Ed.). St. Louis: McGraw-Hill.

Pfister, S. M. & Bullas, J. B. (1989). Arterial blood gas evaluation: Metabolic acidemia. *Critical Care Nurse, 9*(1), 70–72.

Porth, C. M. (1994). *Pathophysiology: Concepts of altered health states* (4th ed.). Philadelphia: Lippincott.

Rice, V. (1983). Magnesium, calcium, and phosphate imbalances; their clinical significance. *Critical Care Nurse, 3*(3), 90–112.

———. (1987). Acid-base derangements in the patient with cardiac arrest. *Focus on Critical Care, 14*(6), 53–61.

Rossman, I. (1986). *Clinical geriatrics* (3rd ed.). Philadelphia: Lippincott.

Russell, J. M. (1991). Successful methods of arterial blood gas interpretation. *Critical Care Nursing, 11*(4), 14–19.

Rutherford, C. (1989). Fluid and electrolyte therapy: Considerations for patient care. *Journal of Intravenous Nursing, 12*(3), 178–188.

Schwartz, M. (1987). Potassium imbalances. *American Journal of Nursing, 87*(10), 1292.

Shoemaker, W. C., Ayres, S., Grenvik, A., Holbrook, P. R., & Thompson, W. L. (Eds.). (1989). *Textbook of critical care*. (2nd ed.). Philadelphia: Saunders.

Spencer, R. T., Nichols, L. W., Gladys, B. L., Henderson, H. S. & West, F. M. (1993). *Clinical pharmacology and nursing management* (4th ed.). Philadelphia: Lippincott.

Stein, E. (1987). *Clinical electrocardiography*. Philadelphia: Lea & Febiger.

Stringfield, Y. N. (1993). Back to basics: Acidosis, alkalosis, and ABGs. *American Journal of Nursing, 93*(11), 43–44.

Tasota, F., & Wesmiller, S. (1994). Assessing ABGs: Maintaining the delicate balance. *Nursing 94, 24*(5), 34–45.

Terry, J. (1991). The other electrolytes: Magnesium, calcium, and phosphorus. *Journal of Intravenous Nursing, 14*(3), 167–175.

Timiras, P. S. (1988). *Physiological basis of geriatrics*. New York: Macmillan.

Todd, B. (1989). Diuretic dangers. *Geriatric Nursing, 10*(4), 212–214.

Watt, B. K., & Merrill, A. L.: (1975). *Composition of foods—raw, processed, prepared*. Agriculture Handbook No. 8. US Department of Agriculture. New York: Dover.

Weinstein, S. M. (1993). *Plumer's principles and practice of intravenous therapy.* (5th ed.). Philadelphia: Lippincott.

Welty, N. J. (1992). *Body fluids and electrolytes: A programmed presentation*. (6th ed.). St. Louis: Mosby.

Wilson, R. F. (1992). *Critical care manual: Applied physiology and principles of therapy* (2nd ed.). Philadelphia: Davis.

Wyngaarden, J. B., Smith, L. H., & Bennett, J. C. (Eds.). (1992). *Cecil's textbook of medicine* (19th ed.). Philadelphia: Saunders.

Nursing Care of Clients in Shock

● ●

LEARNING OBJECTIVES

After completing this chapter, you will be able to

- Describe the sequence of pathologic events and compensatory mechanisms that occurs in shock.
- Discuss the risk factors, etiologies, and pathophysiology of hypovolemic shock, cardiogenic shock, septic shock, neurogenic shock, and anaphylactic shock.
- Compare assessment findings for various types of shock.

- Outline the emergency nursing care of the client in shock.
- Discuss nursing implications for medications and for fluid replacement solutions used to treat the client in shock.
- Use the nursing process as a framework for providing individualized care to clients with various types of shock.

Shock is a response of the body to illness or injury. Shock begins as a compensatory response to changes in the delivery or use of oxygen by tissues. Unless the conditions precipitating the response are treated, however, shock rapidly becomes a critical condition. As shock progresses, multisystem organ failure follows, and death may result.

This chapter discusses the pathophysiology of shock, the different types of shock, the collaborative care provided to detect and treat shock, and the nursing care implemented to meet the needs of clients in shock. Nursing care for the client at risk for shock focuses on assessment and monitoring to prevent the onset of shock and on providing interventions to meet the physical and psychosocial needs of the client in shock.

The Client in Shock

■ ■ ■

Shock is a clinical syndrome characterized by a systemic imbalance between oxygen supply and demand. This im-

balance results in a state of inadequate blood flow to the peripheral tissues, causing life-threatening cellular dysfunction, hypotension, and oliguria.

To maintain cellular metabolism, cells of all body organs and tissues require a regular and consistent supply of oxygen and the removal of metabolic wastes. This homeostatic regulation is maintained primarily by the cardiovascular system and depends on four physiologic components:

1. A cardiac output that is sufficient to meet bodily requirements

2. An uncompromised vascular system, in which the vessels have a diameter that is sufficient to allow unimpeded blood flow and have good tone (the ability to constrict or dilate to maintain normal pressure).

3. A volume of blood that is sufficient to fill the circulatory system, and a blood pressure that is adequate to maintain blood flow

4. Tissues that are able to extract and use the oxygen delivered through the capillaries

In a healthy person, these components function as a system to maintain tissue perfusion. During shock, however, one or more of these components are disrupted. Before considering the pathophysiology of shock, let's review the basics of hemodynamics:

- *Stroke volume (SV)* is the amount of blood pumped into the aorta with each contraction of the left ventricle.
- *Cardiac output (CO)* is the amount of blood pumped per minute into the aorta by the left ventricle. CO is determined by multiplying the stroke volume (SV) by the heart rate (HR); (CO = SV × HR).
- *Mean arterial pressure (MAP)* is the product of cardiac output and *systemic vascular resistance (SVR)*; (MAP = CO × SVR). When CO, SVR, or total blood volume rises, MAP and tissue perfusion increase. Conversely, when CO, SVR, or total blood volume falls, MAP and tissue perfusion decrease.
- The sympathetic nervous system maintains the smooth muscle surrounding the arteries and arterioles in a state of partial contraction called *sympathetic tone*. Increased sympathetic stimulation increases vasoconstriction and SVR; decreased sympathetic stimulation allows vasodilation, which decreases SVR.

When one or more of the cardiovascular components do not function properly, the body's hemodynamic properties are altered. Consequently, tissue perfusion may be inadequate to sustain normal cellular metabolism. The result is the clinical syndrome known as shock. The manifestations of shock result from the body's attempts to maintain vital organs (heart and brain) and to preserve life following a drop in cellular perfusion. However, if the injury or condition triggering shock is severe enough or of long enough duration, cellular hypoxia and cellular death occur. If shock is not stopped, organ failure and death may result.

Pathophysiology

The Stages of Shock

Shock advances through four stages: initial, compensatory, progressive, and irreversible (see the accompanying box). Shock is triggered by a sustained drop in mean arterial pressure. This drop can occur after a decrease in cardiac output, a decrease in the circulating blood volume, or an increase in the size of the vascular bed due to peripheral vasodilation. If intervention is timely and effective, the sequence of physiologic events that characterizes shock may be stopped; if not, shock may lead to death.

The Initial Stage The *initial stage* of shock begins when baroreceptors in the aortic arch and the carotid sinus detect a sustained drop in MAP of less than 10 mm Hg from normal levels. The circulating blood volume may decrease (usually to less then 500 mL), but not enough to cause serious effects.

The body reacts to the decrease in arterial pressure as it would to any physical stressor. Mechanisms that respond to stressors are initiated by the cerebral integration center, causing the sympathetic nervous system to increase the heart rate and the force of cardiac contraction, thus increasing cardiac output. Sympathetic stimulation also causes peripheral vasoconstriction, resulting in increased systemic vascular resistance and a rise in arterial pressure. The net result is that the perfusion of cells, tissues, and organs is maintained.

Symptoms are almost imperceptible during the initial stage of shock. The pulse rate may be slightly elevated. If the injury is minor or of short duration, arterial pressure is usually maintained, and no further symptoms occur.

The Compensatory Stage The *compensatory stage* of shock begins after MAP falls 10 to 15 mm Hg below normal levels. The circulating blood volume is reduced by 25% to 35% (1000 mL or more), but compensatory mechanisms are able to maintain blood pressure and tissue perfusion to vital organs, thereby preventing cell damage.

Sympathetic Nervous System Stimulation Stimulation of the sympathetic nervous system results in the release of epinephrine from the adrenal medulla and the release of norepinephrine from the adrenal medulla and the sympathetic fibers. Both hormones rapidly stimulate the alpha- and beta-adrenergic fibers.

- Stimulated alpha-adrenergic fibers cause *vasoconstriction* in the blood vessels supplying the skin and most of the abdominal viscera. Perfusion of these areas decreases.
- Stimulated beta-adrenergic fibers cause *vasodilation* in vessels supplying the heart and skeletal muscles (beta one response), and increase the heart rate and force of cardiac contraction (beta two response). Further, blood vessels in the respiratory system dilate, and the respiratory rate increases (beta two response).

Thus, stimulation of the sympathetic nervous system results in increased cardiac output and oxygenation of these tissues.

Renin-Angiotensin Response The renin-angiotensin response occurs as the blood flow to the kidneys decreases.

- Renin released from the kidneys converts a plasma protein to angiotensin II (see Chapter 5).
- Angiotensin II causes vasoconstriction and stimulates the adrenal cortex to release aldosterone.
- Aldosterone causes the kidneys to reabsorb water and sodium and to lose potassium.

The absorption of water maintains circulating blood volume while increased vasoconstriction increases SVR, maintaining central vascular volume and raising blood pressure.

Four Stages of Shock

■ ■ ■

Pathophysiology

Manifestations

I. Initial Stage

1. Sustained decrease in MAP detected by baroreceptors
2. SNS stimulated and stress response initiated

- Slightly decreased pulse
- Normal to slightly decreased blood pressure
- Pale, cool, moist skin over face and extremities
- Thirst

II. Compensatory Stage

1. Continued decrease in MAP
2. SNS stimulation releases epinephrine and norepinephrine
3. Stimulated alpha-adrenergic fibers cause *vasoconstriction* of vessels in the skin and most abdominal organs
4. Stimulated beta-adrenergic fibers cause *vasodilation* of vessels in the heart, lungs, and skeletal muscles
5. Renal reabsorption of water and sodium, promoted by:
    - Renin-angiotensin response (kidneys)
    - ACTH release (hypothalamus), stimulating aldosterone release (adrenal glands)
    - ADH release (posterior pituitary)
6. Fluid shifts from interstitial space to capillaries

- Falling blood pressure
- Cool, pale skin over face, trunk, and extremities
- Poor skin turgor
- Diaphoresis
- Decreased bowel sounds
- Rapid, thready pulse
- Increased respirations
- Decreased urinary ouptut
- Thirst
- Anxiety, restlessness

III. Progressive Stage

1. Continued decrease in MAP
2. Vasoconstriction causes diffuse cellular hypoxia and anerobic metabolism
3. Cellular sodium-potassium pumps fail
4. Acididotic environment and diffusion of water into cells destroy cellular integrity
5. Fluid shifts out of capillaries back into interstitial space
6. Plasma proteins diffuse out of vascular space into interstitial space
7. Increasing SNS stimulation further reduces perfusion of skin, muscles, and visceral organs
8. Generalized cellular anoxia, ischemia, acidosis, and hyperkalemia

- Falling blood pressure
- Cool, pale skin
- Generalized edema
- Rapid, shallow respirations
- Rapid, thready pulse
- Diminished or absent peripheral pulse
- Dysrhythmias
- Oliguria
- Areflexia

IV. Irreversible Stage

1. Profound tissue anoxia and cellular death
2. Multisystem organ failure
3. Cardiac arrest and death

- Severe hypotension
- Rapid, weak, or irregular pulse
- Rapid, shallow respirations
- Crackles and wheezes
- Pallor and cyanosis
- Disorientation, lethargy, coma
- Areflexia
- Anuresis
- Cardiac arrest and death

Release of Hypothalamic and Pituitary Hormones

■ The hypothalamus releases adrenocorticotropic hormone (ACTH) which causes the adrenal glands to secrete aldosterone. Aldosterone promotes the reabsorption of water and sodium by the kidneys, preserving blood volume and pressure.

■ The posterior pituitary gland releases antidiuretic hormone (ADH), which increases renal reabsorption of water and causes peripheral vasoconstriction. The combined effects of hormones released by the hypothalamus and posterior pituitary glands work to conserve central vascular volume.

Volume Shift in Fluid Compartments   As MAP falls in the compensatory stage of shock, decreased capillary hydrostatic pressure causes a fluid shift from the interstitial space into the capillaries. The net gain of fluid raises the blood volume.

Working together, these compensatory mechanisms can maintain MAP for only a short period of time. During this period, the perfusion and oxygenation of the heart and brain are adequate. If effective treatment is provided, the process is arrested, and no permanent damage occurs. However, unless the underlying cause of shock is reversed, these compensatory mechanisms soon become harmful, and shock perpetuates shock.

The Progressive Stage   The *progressive stage* of shock occurs after a sustained decrease in MAP of 20 mm Hg or more below normal levels and a fluid loss of 35% to 50% (1800 to 2500 mL of fluid). Although the compensatory mechanisms in the previous state remain activated, they are no longer able to maintain MAP at a level sufficient to ensure perfusion of vital organs.

The vasoconstriction response that first helped sustain MAP eventually limits blood flow to the point that cells become oxygen deficient. To remain alive, the affected cells switch from aerobic to anaerobic metabolism. The lactic acid formed as a by-product of anaerobic metabolism contributes to an acidotic state at the cellular level. As a result, adenosine triphosphate (ATP), the source of cellular energy, is produced inefficiently. Lacking energy, the sodium-potassium pump fails. Potassium diffuses outward from the cell, whereas sodium and water diffuse inward. As this process continues, the cell swells, cell membrane integrity is lost, and cell organelles are damaged. Lysosomes within the cell spill out their digestive enzymes, which disintegrate any remaining organelles. Some enzymes spread to adjacent cells, where they erode and rupture cell membranes.

The acid by-products of anaerobic metabolism dilate the precapillary arterioles and constrict the postcapillary venules. This causes increased hydrostatic pressure within the capillary, and fluid shifts back into the interstitial space. The capillaries also become increasingly permeable, allowing serum proteins to shift from the vascular space into the interstitium. The buildup of plasma proteins increases the osmotic pressure in the interstitium, further accelerating the fluid shift out of the capillaries.

Throughout this period, the heart rate and vasoconstriction increase. However, perfusion of the skin, skeletal muscles, kidneys, and gastrointestinal organs is greatly diminished. Cells in the heart and brain become hypoxic while other body cells and tissues become ischemic and anoxic. A generalized state of acidosis and hyperkalemia ensues (see Chapter 5). Unless this stage of shock is treated rapidly, the client's chances of survival are poor.

The Irreversible Stage   If shock progresses to the *irreversible stage*, tissue anoxia becomes so generalized and cellular death so widespread that no treatment can reverse the damage. Even if MAP is temporarily restored, too much cellular damage has occurred to maintain life. Death of cells is followed by death of tissues, which results in death of organs. Death of vital organs contributes to subsequent death.

Effects of Shock on Body Systems

Whatever its causes, shock produces predictable effects on the body's organ systems (Figure 6–1).

Cardiovascular Effects   The perfusion and oxygenation of the heart, a vital organ, are adequate in the early stages of shock. As shock progresses, however, myocardial cells become hypoxic, and myocardial muscle function diminishes. Initially, the blood pressure may be normal or even slightly elevated (as a result of compensatory mechanisms) and the heart rate only slightly increased. Sympathetic stimulation increases the heart rate (a sinus tachycardia of 120 beats per minute is common) in an effort to increase cardiac output. As a result of vasoconstriction and decreased blood volume, the palpated pulse is rapid, weak, and thready; as shock progresses, peripheral pulses are usually nonpalpable.

Tachycardia reduces the time available for left ventricular filling and coronary artery perfusion, further reducing cardiac output. With progressive shock, the heart's electrical systems and contractility are adversely affected by altered acid-base balance, hypoxia, and hyperkalemia. Consequently, cardiac arrhythmias may develop. Decreased blood volume with decreased venous return also decreases cardiac output, and blood pressure falls.

The blood pressure changes produced by shock are characterized by a progressive decrease in both systolic and diastolic pressures and a narrowing pulse pressure. Auscultation of blood pressure is often difficult or impossible and is an inaccurate reflection of blood pressure status (see the nursing research box on page 164). For this reason, hemodynamic monitoring is usually instituted to follow the client's cardiovascular status accurately.

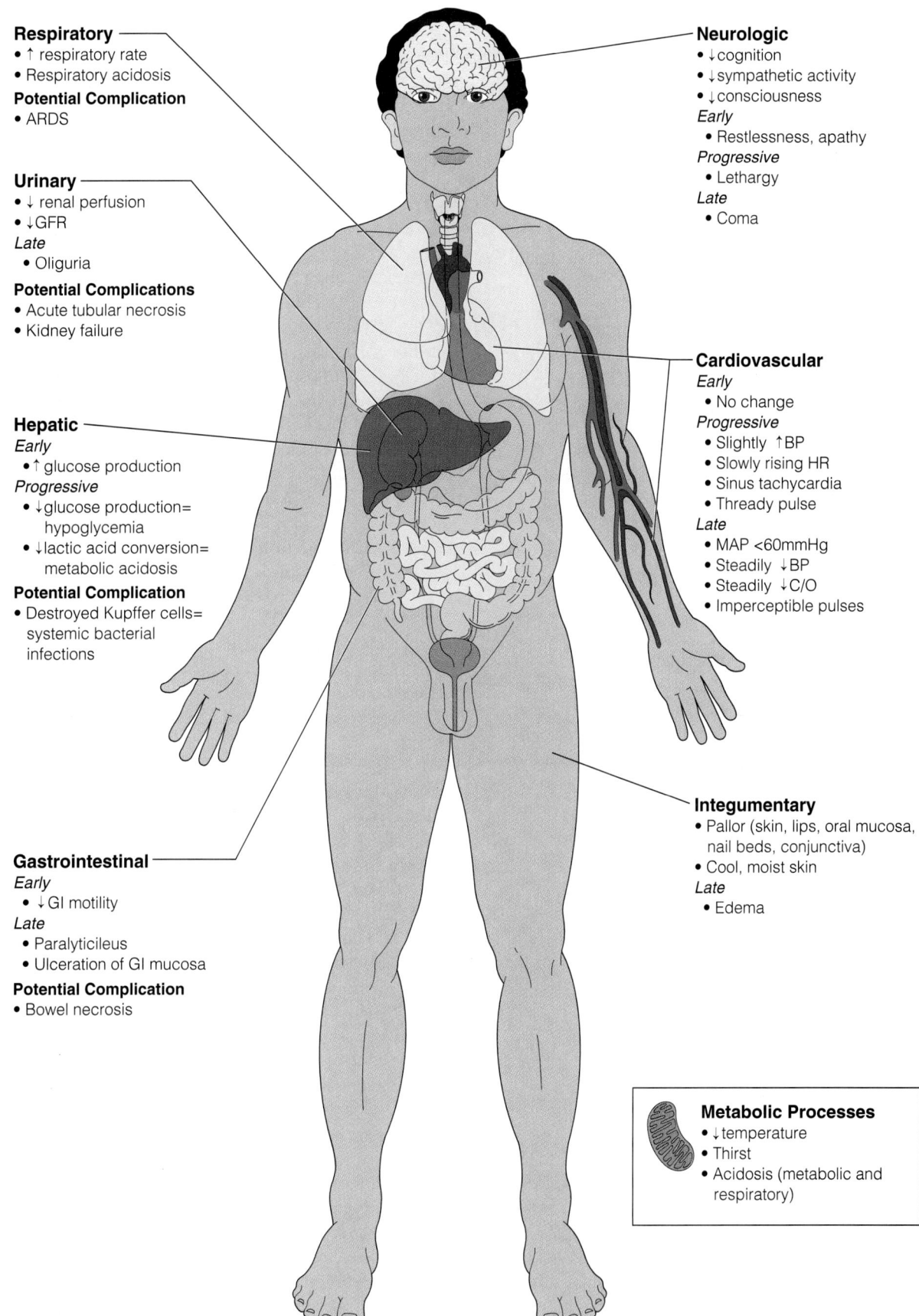

Respiratory
- ↑ respiratory rate
- Respiratory acidosis

Potential Complication
- ARDS

Urinary
- ↓ renal perfusion
- ↓GFR

Late
- Oliguria

Potential Complications
- Acute tubular necrosis
- Kidney failure

Hepatic
Early
- ↑ glucose production

Progressive
- ↓glucose production=
  hypoglycemia
- ↓lactic acid conversion=
  metabolic acidosis

Potential Complication
- Destroyed Kupffer cells=
  systemic bacterial
  infections

Gastrointestinal
Early
- ↓ GI motility

Late
- Paralyticileus
- Ulceration of GI mucosa

Potential Complication
- Bowel necrosis

Neurologic
- ↓cognition
- ↓sympathetic activity
- ↓consciousness

Early
- Restlessness, apathy

Progressive
- Lethargy

Late
- Coma

Cardiovascular
Early
- No change

Progressive
- Slightly ↑BP
- Slowly rising HR
- Sinus tachycardia
- Thready pulse

Late
- MAP <60mmHg
- Steadily ↓BP
- Steadily ↓C/O
- Imperceptible pulses

Integumentary
- Pallor (skin, lips, oral mucosa,
  nail beds, conjunctiva)
- Cool, moist skin

Late
- Edema

Metabolic Processes
- ↓temperature
- Thirst
- Acidosis (metabolic and
  respiratory)

Figure 6–1   Multisystem effects of shock.

Applying Research to Nursing Practice
Direct and Indirect Blood Pressure Measurement

■ ■ ■

Researchers conducted a study to determine the relationship between direct intra-arterial blood pressure readings and indirect auscultated blood pressure readings measured by using different listening pieces and auscultation sites (Byra-Cook et al., 1990). Fifty critical care clients, ages 18 to 70, who were undergoing hemodynamic monitoring had their blood pressure taken by auscultation using either the bell or the diaphragm of the stethoscope at the antecubital fossa and over the brachial artery. Auscultation of the blood pressure using the diaphragm of the stethoscope over the brachial artery in the upper arm (immediately superior to the internal medial condyle and medial to the biceps tendon) showed the highest overall correlation between direct and indirect blood pressure readings for both systolic and diastolic pressures.

Implications for Nursing

In all care settings, assessing blood pressure is an independent nursing action carried out to detect alterations in health. It is important that nurses use the most accurate technique and method of auscultation so that they can accurately determine changes in blood pressure. The findings in this study carry significant implications for the early detection of shock, as well as the ongoing monitoring of changes in blood pressure in clients in shock. This study is especially important for nurses practicing in general care and in critical care settings.

Critical Thinking in Client Care
1. What is the rationale for the use of the bell in auscultating blood pressure and heart sounds? For the use of the diaphragm?
2. Which would be expected to produce the highest blood pressure findings: direct or indirect measurement? Support your answer with appropriate rationale.
3. List potential sources of error in taking blood pressure.

Respiratory Effects During shock, oxygen delivery to cells may be impaired by a drop in circulating blood volume or, in the case of blood loss, by an insufficient number of red blood cells that carry oxygen. Although the respiratory rate increases as a result of compensatory mechanisms that promote oxygenation, the number of alveoli that are perfused decreases, and gas exchange is impaired. As a result, oxygen levels in the blood decrease, and carbon dioxide levels increase. As perfusion of the lungs diminishes, carbon dioxide is retained, and respiratory acidosis occurs.

A complication of decreased perfusion of the lungs is *adult respiratory distress syndrome (ARDS),* or *"shock lung."* The exact mechanism that produces ARDS is unknown, but some contributing factors have been identified. The pulmonary capillaries become increasingly permeable to proteins and water, resulting in noncardiac pulmonary edema. Production of surfactant (which controls surface tension within alveoli) is impaired, and the alveoli collapse or fill with fluid. This potentially lethal form of respiratory failure may result from any condition that causes hypoperfusion of the lungs, but it is more common in shock caused by hemorrhage, severe allergic responses, trauma, and infection (Perry, 1988). (ARDS is discussed further in Chapter 34.)

Gastrointestinal and Hepatic Effects Through the splanchnic circulation, the gastrointestinal organs normally receive 25% of the cardiac output. Shock, however, constricts the splanchnic arterioles and redirects arterial blood flow to the heart and brain. Consequently, gastrointestinal organs become ischemic and may be irreversibly damaged.

Gastric mucosa tends to ulcerate when it becomes ischemic. Lesions of the gastric and duodenal mucosa (called *stress ulcers*) can develop within hours of severe trauma, sepsis, or burns (Porth, 1994). Gastrointestinal ulcers may hemorrhage within 2 to 10 days following the original cause of shock. In addition, the permeability of damaged mucosa increases, allowing enteric bacteria or their toxins to enter the abdominal cavity and then progress to the circulation.

Gastric and intestinal motility is impaired during shock, and paralytic ileus may result. If the episode of shock is prolonged, necrosis of the bowel may occur. In many cases, alterations in the structure and function of the gastrointestinal tract impair absorption of nutrients, such as protein and glucose.

Shock also alters the metabolic functions of the liver. Initially, gluconeogenesis (the process of forming glucose from noncarbohydrate sources) and glycogenolysis (the breakdown of glycogen into glucose) increase. This process allows blood glucose levels to increase as the body attempts to respond to the stressor. However, as shock progresses, liver functions are impaired, and hypoglycemia develops. Metabolism of fats and protein is impaired, and the liver can no longer effectively remove lactic acid, contributing to the development of metabolic acidosis. A further problem results from the destruction of the liver's reticuloendothelial Kupffer cells. These cells (phagocytes that destroy bacteria) are unable to function, and bacteria may proliferate within the circulatory system. As a result, overwhelming bacterial infection and toxicity occur.

Neurologic Effects The primary effects of shock on the neurologic system involve changes in mental status and orientation. Cerebral hypoxia produces altered levels of consciousness, beginning with apathy and lethargy and progressing to coma. A common early symptom of cerebral hypoxia is restlessness. Continued ischemia of brain cells eventually causes swelling, resulting in cerebral edema, neurotransmitter failure, and irreversible brain cell damage.

As cerebral ischemia worsens, the sympathetic activity and vasomotor centers are depressed. This leads to a loss of sympathetic tone, causing systemic vasodilatation and pooling of blood in the periphery. As a result, venous return and cardiac output further decrease.

Renal Effects Blood that normally perfuses the kidneys is shunted to the heart and brain during the progressive stage of shock, resulting in renal hypoperfusion. The drop in renal perfusion is reflected in a corresponding decrease in the glomerular filtration rate. As a result, urine output is reduced, and the urine that is produced is highly concentrated. Oliguria of less than 20 mL per hour indicates progressive shock (Rice, 1991).

Healthy kidneys can tolerate a drop in perfusion for only about 20 minutes; thereafter, acute tubular necrosis develops (Porth, 1994). As tubular necrosis occurs, epithelial cells slough off and block the tubules, disrupting nephron function. The accumulating loss of functional nephrons eventually causes renal failure. Without normal renal function, metabolic waste products are retained in the plasma.

If treatment restores renal perfusion, the kidneys can regenerate the lost epithelial cells in the tubules, and renal function usually returns to normal. However, in the older or chronically ill client or in the client with sustained shock, loss of renal function may become permanent.

Effects on Skin, Temperature, and Thirst In most types of shock, blood vessels supplying the skin are vasoconstricted, and the sweat glands are activated. As a result, changes in skin color occur. The skin of Caucasian clients becomes pale. In persons with darker skin (such as those of African, Hispanic, or Mediterranean descent), shock-related skin color changes may be assessed as paleness of the lips, oral mucous membranes, nail beds, and conjunctiva. The skin is usually cool and moist and, in the later stages of shock, often edematous.

Two other physiologic alterations occur during shock. The body temperature decreases as shock progresses, the result of a decrease in overall body metabolism. Also, some persons in shock experience thirst. This symptom is probably a response to decreased blood volume and increased serum osmolality (Porth, 1994).

Types of Shock

Shock is identified according to its underlying cause. Types of shock include the following:

- Hypovolemic shock—caused by insufficient intravascular blood volume
- Cardiogenic shock—caused by failure of the heart's pumping action
- Septic shock—caused by infection-produced toxins
- Neurogenic shock—caused by alterations in vascular sympathetic tone
- Anaphylactic shock—caused by immunologic reactions

All types of shock progress through the same stages and exert similar effects on body systems. Any differences are noted in the following discussion.

Hypovolemic Shock **Hypovolemic shock** is caused by a decrease in intravascular volume of 15% or more (Porth, 1994). This form of shock is caused by the loss of whole blood, blood plasma, or extracellular fluid. During hypovolemic shock, the venous blood returning to the heart decreases, and ventricular filling drops. As a result, stroke volume, cardiac output, and blood pressure decrease. Hypovolemic shock is the most common type of shock, and it often occurs simultaneously with other types of shock.

The decrease in circulating blood volume that triggers hypovolemic shock may result from

- Loss of blood volume from hemorrhage (from surgery, traumatic injuries, gastrointestinal bleeding, blood coagulation disorders, ruptured esophageal varices).
- Loss of intravascular fluid from the skin due to injuries, such as burns (see Chapter 18).
- Loss of blood volume from severe dehydration.
- Loss of body fluid from the gastrointestinal system due to persistent and severe vomiting or diarrhea or continuous nasogastric suctioning.
- Renal losses of fluid due to the use of diuretics or to endocrine disorders such as diabetes insipidus (see Chapter 20).
- Conditions causing fluid shifts from the intravascular compartment to the interstitial space (see Chapter 5).
- *Third-spacing* due to such disorders as liver diseases with ascites, pleural effusion, or intestinal obstruction (see Chapter 5).

Hypovolemic shock affects all body systems. The effects of hypovolemic shock vary depending on the client's age, general state of health, extent of injury or severity of illness, length of time before treatment is provided, and the rate of volume loss.

The manifestations of hypovolemic shock are the direct result of the decrease in circulating blood volume and

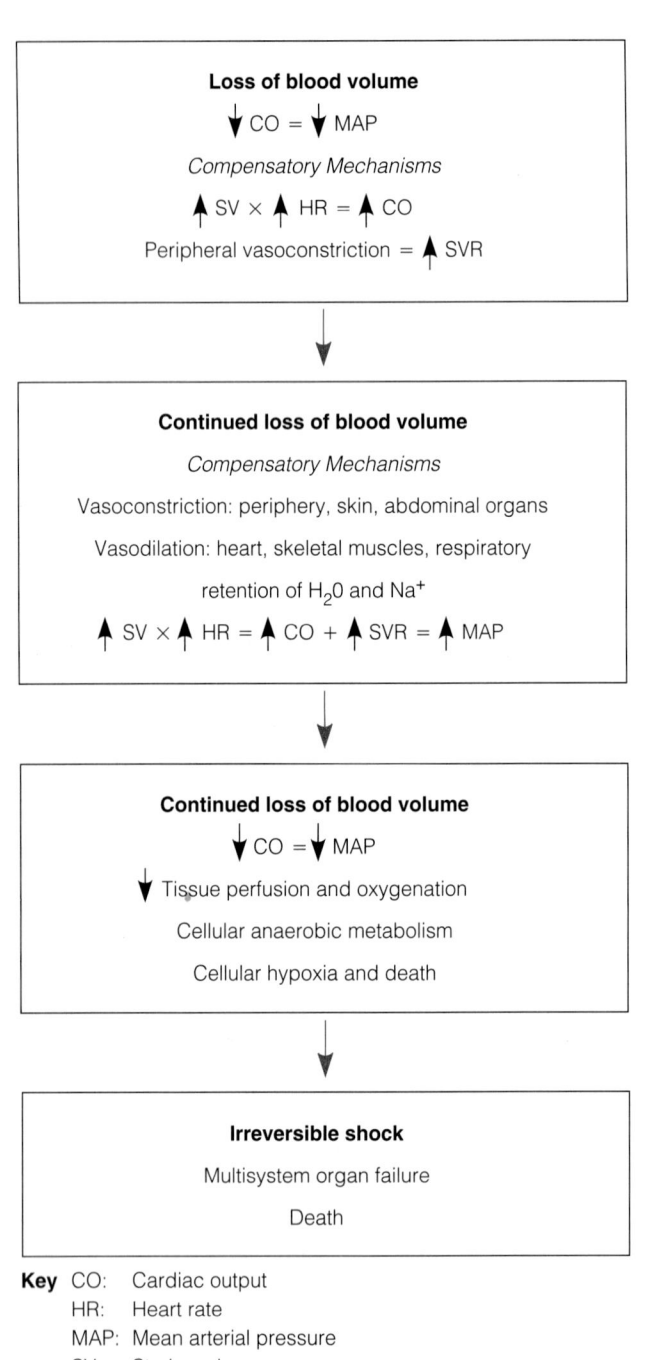

Loss of blood volume

$\downarrow$ CO = $\downarrow$ MAP

Compensatory Mechanisms

$\uparrow$ SV $\times$ $\uparrow$ HR = $\uparrow$ CO

Peripheral vasoconstriction = $\uparrow$ SVR

Continued loss of blood volume

Compensatory Mechanisms

Vasoconstriction: periphery, skin, abdominal organs

Vasodilation: heart, skeletal muscles, respiratory

retention of H_2O and Na^+

$\uparrow$ SV $\times$ $\uparrow$ HR = $\uparrow$ CO + $\uparrow$ SVR = $\uparrow$ MAP

Continued loss of blood volume

$\downarrow$ CO = $\downarrow$ MAP

$\downarrow$ Tissue perfusion and oxygenation

Cellular anaerobic metabolism

Cellular hypoxia and death

Irreversible shock

Multisystem organ failure

Death

Key CO: Cardiac output
HR: Heart rate
MAP: Mean arterial pressure
SV: Stroke volume
SVR: Systemic vascular resistance

Figure 6–2 The stages of hypovolemic shock.

the initiation of compensatory mechanisms (Figure 6–2). The loss of circulating blood volume reduces cardiac output by decreasing venous return to the heart. As a result, blood pressure drops. The decrease in blood pressure is sensed by the carotid and cardiac baroreceptors and is communicated to the vasomotor centers in the brain stem. The vasomotor centers then induce the sympathetic compensatory responses that characterize shock generally. If the fluid loss is less than 500 mL, activation of the

sympathetic response is generally adequate to restore cardiac output and blood pressure to near normal, although the heart rate may remain elevated (Price & Wilson, 1992).

With a sustained loss of blood volume (1000 mL or more), the shock stage progresses. Heart rate and vasoconstriction increase, and blood flow to the skin, skeletal muscles, kidneys, and abdominal organs decreases. Several renal mechanisms and a decline in capillary pressure help to conserve blood volume. Eventually, the amount of blood flowing to cells is too low to oxygenate them and sustain production of cellular energy. Anaerobic metabolism begins, producing an acidotic environment for cells. As a result, cells lose their physical integrity. If untreated, shock causes multiple organ failure, and death results. A summary of assessment findings in clients in various stages of hypovolemic shock is found in the accompanying box.

Cardiogenic Shock **Cardiogenic shock** occurs when the heart's pumping ability is compromised to the point that it cannot maintain cardiac output and adequate tissue perfusion. Cardiac disorders are discussed in Chapter 28; this section focuses only on the effects of shock caused by these disorders.

The loss of the pumping action of the heart may be caused by the following conditions:

- Myocardial infarction
- Cardiac tamponade
- Restrictive pericarditis
- Cardiac arrest
- Dysrhythmias, such as fibrillation or ventricular tachycardia
- Pathologic changes in the valves
- Cardiomyopathies from hypertension, alcohol, bacterial or viral infections, or ischemia
- Complications of cardiac surgery
- Chemical toxins
- Electrolyte imbalances (especially changes in normal potassium and calcium levels)
- Drugs affecting cardiac muscle contractility
- Head injuries causing damage to the cardioregulatory center

Of these causes, myocardial infarction is the most common cause of cardiogenic shock. Of clients admitted to the hospital for treatment of myocardial infarction, 15% to 20% develop cardiogenic shock. The severity and progression of shock are related to the amount of myocardial damage (Whitman, 1988).

Whatever the cardiogenic cause, the decrease in cardiac output causes a decrease in MAP. Heart rate may increase in response to compensatory mechanisms. How-

---

Assessment Findings in Clients in Hypovolemic Shock

■ ■ ■

Initial Stage   (Loss of 500 mL of Blood or Less)

- Blood pressure: normal to slightly decreased
- Pulse: slightly increased from baseline
- Respirations: normal (baseline)
- Skin: cool, pale (in periphery), moist
- Mental status: alert and oriented
- Urine output: slight decrease
- Other: thirst, decreased capillary refill time

Compensatory and Progressive Stages
(Loss of 25% to 35% of Circulating Blood Volume)

- Blood pressure: hypotension
- Pulse: rapid, thready
- Respirations: increased
- Skin: cool, pale (includes trunk); poor turgor with fluid loss, edematous with fluid shift
- Mental status: restless, anxious, confused, or agitated
- Urine output: oliguria (less than 30 mL/hour)
- Other: marked thirst, acidosis, hyperkalemia, decreased capillary refill time, decreased or absent peripheral pulses

Irreversible Stage   (Loss of 35% to 50% of Circulating Blood Volume)

- Blood pressure: severe hypotension (often, systolic pressure is below 80 mm Hg)
- Pulse: very rapid, weak
- Respirations: rapid, shallow; crackles and wheezes
- Skin: cool, pale, mottled with cyanosis
- Mental status: disoriented, lethargic, comatose
- Urine output: anuria
- Other: loss of reflexes, decreased or absent peripheral pulses

---

Assessment Findings in Clients in Cardiogenic Shock

■ ■ ■

- Blood pressure: hypotension
- Pulse: rapid, thready; distention of veins of hands and neck
- Respirations: increased, labored; crackles and wheezes; pulmonary edema
- Skin: pale, cyanotic, cold, moist
- Mental status: restless, anxious, lethargic progressing to comatose
- Urine output: oliguria to anuria
- Other: dependent edema; elevated CVP; elevated pulmonary capillary wedge pressure; arrhythmias

---

Cyanosis, however, is more common in cardiogenic shock, because stagnating blood increases extraction of oxygen from the hemoglobin at the capillary beds. As a result, the skin, lips, and nail beds may appear cyanotic. As cardiac failure (and cardiogenic shock) progresses, left ventricular end-diastolic pressure increases. The increase is transmitted to the pulmonary capillary bed, and pulmonary edema may occur. Retention of blood in the right side of the heart increases right atrial pressure, which leads to jugular venous distention as a result of backflow through the venae cavae. A summary of assessment findings in the client in cardiogenic shock is found in the box above.

Septic Shock   Septic shock is the result of the effect of toxins produced by an infectious agent. This condition more commonly results from infections with gram-negative bacteria such as *Pseudomonas aeruginosa, Escherichia coli,* and *Klebsiella pneumoniae.* However, a form of septic shock may also be caused by gram-positive cocci (such as *Clostridium, Staphylococcus aureus,* and *Streptococcus pneumoniae*). Less commonly, septic shock develops secondary to a systemic infection by the fungus *Candida albicans* (Barry, 1989; Evans, 1991). The pathophysiology of septic shock is complex and not completely understood.

Clients at risk for developing infections leading to septic shock include those who are hospitalized, have debilitating chronic illnesses, or have poor nutritional status. The risk is heightened after invasive procedures or surgery. Other clients at risk of septic shock include older adults and the immunocompromised. The following are portals of entry for infection that may lead to septic shock:

- The urinary system: catheterizations, suprapubic tubes, cystoscopy

---

ever, tachycardia increases myocardial oxygen consumption and decreases coronary perfusion. The myocardium becomes progressively depleted of oxygen, causing further myocardial ischemia and necrosis. The typical sequence of shock is essentially unchanged in cardiogenic shock.

Assessment Findings in Clients in Septic Shock

■ ■ ■

Early (Warm) Septic Shock

- Blood pressure: normal to hypotension
- Pulse: increased, thready
- Respirations: rapid and deep
- Skin: warm, flushed
- Mental status: alert, oriented, anxious
- Urine output: normal
- Other: increased body temperature; chills; weakness; nausea, vomiting, diarrhea; decreased CVP

Late (Cold) Septic Shock

- Blood pressure: hypotension
- Pulse: tachycardia, arrhythmias
- Respirations: rapid, shallow, dyspneic
- Skin: cool, pale, edematous
- Mental status: lethargic to comatose
- Urine output: oliguria to anuria
- Other: normal to decreased body temperature; decreased CVP

- The respiratory system: suctioning, aspiration, tracheostomy, endotracheal tubes, respiratory therapy, mechanical ventilators
- The gastrointestinal system: peptic ulcers, ruptured appendix, peritonitis
- The skin: surgical wounds, intravenous catheters, intra-arterial catheters, invasive monitoring, decubitus ulcers, burns, trauma
- The female reproductive system: elective surgical abortion, ascending infections from transmission of bacteria during the intrapartal and postpartal periods, tampon use, sexually transmitted diseases

Septic shock begins with *septicemia,* the presence of pathogens and their toxins in the blood. As pathogens are destroyed, their ruptured cell membranes allow endotoxins to leak into the plasma. The endotoxins disrupt the vascular system, coagulation mechanism, and immune system and trigger an immune and inflammatory response. For this reason, the initial effects of septic shock differ from those of hypovolemic and cardiogenic shock; cardiac output is high, and systemic vascular resistance is low.

Endotoxins directly damage the endothelial lining of small blood vessels first; the small blood vessels of the kidneys and lungs are most susceptible. Cellular damage stimulates the release of vasoactive proteins and activates coagulation factor XII. The vasoactive proteins stimulate peripheral vasodilation and increase capillary permeability; the activation of coagulation factors results in the production of multiple intravascular blood clots (Evans, 1991).

As a result of the increased capillary permeability and vasodilation, fluid shifts from the intravascular space to the interstitial space. Hypovolemia results as fluid volume is lost from the circulating blood. Hypovolemia and intravascular coagulation alter oxygenation and cellular metabolism, leading to anaerobic metabolism, lactic acidosis, and cellular death.

Septic shock has an early phase and a late phase. In *early septic shock* (sometimes called the *warm phase*), vasodilation results in weakness and warm, flushed skin, and the septicemia often causes high fever and chills. In *late septic shock* (sometimes called the *cold phase*), hypovolemia and activity of the compensatory mechanisms result in typical shock manifestations, including cold, moist skin; oliguria; and changes in mental status. Death may result from respiratory failure, cardiac failure, or renal failure. A summary of assessment findings in the client in septic shock is found in the accompanying box.

Toxic shock syndrome is an especially virulent form of septic shock, occurring most frequently in menstruating women who use tampons. It is thought that bacterial toxins diffuse from the site of infection in the vagina into the circulation. The toxins then trigger a widespread inflammatory response and septic shock. The manifestations of toxic shock syndrome include extreme hypotension, hyperpyrexia, headache, myalgia, confusion, skin rash, vomiting, and diarrhea (Porth, 1994).

Disseminated intravascular coagulation (DIC), a generalized response to injury, is a potential risk in septic shock. This condition is characterized by simultaneous bleeding and clotting throughout the vasculature. Sepsis injures blood cells, causing platelet aggregation and decreased blood flow. As a result, blood clots form throughout the microcirculation. The clotting slows circulation further while stimulating excess fibrinolysis. As the body's stores of clotting factors are depleted, generalized bleeding begins. DIC is further discussed in Chapter 31.

Neurogenic Shock Neurogenic shock (also called **vasogenic shock**) is the result of an imbalance between parasympathetic and sympathetic stimulation of vascular smooth muscle. If parasympathetic overstimulation or sympathetic understimulation persists, sustained vasodilation occurs, and blood pools in the venous and capillary beds.

Neurogenic shock causes dramatic reduction in systemic vascular resistance as the size of the vascular compartment increases. As systemic vascular resistance decreases, pressure in the blood vessels becomes too low to drive nutrients across capillary membranes, and impaired cellular metabolism occurs.

The following conditions can cause neurogenic shock by increasing parasympathetic stimulation or inhibiting sympathetic stimulation of the smooth muscle of blood vessels:

- Head injury
- Trauma to the spinal cord (spinal shock, a form of neurogenic shock, is described in Chapter 41)
- Insulin reactions (which cause hypoglycemia, decreasing glucose to the medulla)
- Central nervous system depressant drugs (such as sedatives, barbiturates, or narcotics)
- Spinal anesthesia
- General anesthesia
- Severe pain
- Prolonged exposure to heat

Bradycardia occurs early, but tachycardia ensues as compensatory mechanisms are initiated. Central venous pressure drops as veins dilate, venous return to the heart decreases, stroke volume decreases, and MAP falls. In early stages, the extremities are warm and pink (from the pooling of blood), but as shock progresses, the skin becomes pale and cool. A summary of assessment findings in the client in neurogenic shock is found in the accompanying box.

Anaphylactic Shock   **Anaphylactic shock** is the result of a widespread hypersensitivity reaction (called *anaphylaxis*). The pathophysiology in this type of shock includes vasodilation, pooling of blood in the periphery, and hypovolemia with altered cellular metabolism. These physiologic alterations occur when a sensitized person has contact with an *allergen* (a foreign substance to which an individual is hypersensitive). There are many different allergens that can cause anaphylactic shock. The most common include the following:

- Substances used to diagnose and treat disease:
  a. Antibiotics (e.g., penicillin, sulfa drugs)
  b. Vaccines, antitoxins
  c. Local anesthetics
  d. Iodine dyes used in diagnostic tests
  e. Blood and blood products
  f. Narcotics, such as morphine, meperidine hydrochloride (Demerol), and codeine
- Foods:
  a. Legumes (e.g., soybeans), nuts, seeds
  b. Shellfish (e.g., lobster, shrimp, clams, crabs)
  c. Egg white (albumen)

> ## Assessment Findings in Clients in Neurogenic Shock
> ■ ■ ■
>
> - Blood pressure: hypotension
> - Pulse: slow and bounding
> - Respirations: vary
> - Skin: warm, dry
> - Mental status: anxious, restless, lethargic progressing to comatose
> - Urine output: oliguria to anuria
> - Other: lowered body temperature

---

  d. Milk and milk products
  e. Chocolate
- Stings and bites of insects (e.g., bees, wasps, hornets, yellow jackets, fire ants, deerflies)
- Snake venom

Anaphylactic shock does not occur with the first exposure to an allergen. With the first exposure to a foreign substance (the antigen), the body produces specific immunoglobulin E (IgE) antibodies against this antigen. The person is thus sensitized to that specific antigen. With subsequent exposure, the antigen reacts with the already formed IgE antibodies, and cellular integrity is disrupted. In addition, large amounts of histamine and other vasoactive amines are released and distributed through the circulatory system. These substances cause increased capillary permeability and massive vasodilatation, resulting in profound hypotension and eventual vascular collapse.

Histamine also causes smooth muscles to constrict in the bladder, uterus, intestines, and bronchioles. Respiratory distress, bronchospasm, laryngospasm, and severe abdominal cramping result. Serotonin (a neurotransmitter with vasoconstrictive properties) is released, further affecting respiratory status by increasing capillary permeability in the lungs. As a result, plasma leaks into the alveoli, gas exchange is impaired, and pulmonary edema may ensue.

Anaphylactic shock begins and progresses rapidly. Manifestations may begin within 20 minutes of contact with an antigen. Unless appropriate intervention is provided, death can occur within a matter of minutes. Because anaphylaxis is rapid and potentially lethal, people with known allergies should carry some form of warning (such as a MedicAlert bracelet) informing others of their susceptibility. Health care providers should be extremely careful to assess and document allergies or previous drug reactions. A summary of assessment findings in the client in anaphylactic shock is found in the box on page 170.

Assessment Findings in Clients in Anaphylactic Shock

■ ■ ■

- Blood pressure: hypotension
- Pulse: increased, dysrhythmias
- Respirations: dyspnea, stridor, wheezes, laryngospasm, bronchospasm, pulmonary edema
- Skin: warm, edematous (lips, eyelids, tongue, hands, feet, genitals)
- Mental status: restless, anxious, lethargic to comatose
- Urine output: oliguria to anuria
- Other: paresthesias; pruritus; abdominal cramps, vomiting, diarrhea

---

Emergency Care of the Client in Hypovolemic Shock

■ ■ ■

1. Ensure adequate airway; provide assistance in breathing if necessary.
2. Assess for cause of hemorrhage, if present, and apply pressure at pressure points.
3. Assess for manifestations of shock, which may include
   a. Decreased systolic and diastolic blood pressure
   b. Rapid, thready pulse
   c. Rapid, shallow respirations
   d. Cold, pale, moist skin
   e. Thirst
   f. Restlessness
   g. Changes in level of consciousness
4. Maintain the client's position with trunk and head flat and legs slightly elevated (if no head injury is present).
5. Cover the client to maintain warmth.
6. Use touch and verbal communication to reduce apprehension and anxiety.
7. Seek immediate medical care.

Collaborative Care

Treatment of the client in shock focuses on treating the underlying cause, increasing arterial oxygenation, and improving tissue perfusion. Depending on the cause and type of shock, interventions include emergency care measures, use of an antishock device, oxygen therapy, fluid replacement, and pharmacologic therapy. Emergency care is often the first course of collaborative action taken to arrest shock.

Emergency Care

Emergency care of the client in shock focuses on maintaining a level of tissue perfusion adequate to sustain life. Hypovolemic shock is the most common type of shock and the type that most often requires emergency care as a result of trauma and hemorrhage. (Trauma and hemorrhage are discussed fully in Chapter 10.) An outline of the initial emergency care for the client in hypovolemic shock is found in the accompanying box.

The treatment of shock begins as soon as medical rescuers arrive on the scene and continues through transport for continued intensive care in an acute care facility. Because shock is sequential and progressive, the amount of time for reversing the pathophysiologic process is limited. To preserve life, treatment must be initiated and the client stabilized within the first hour of any injury that may cause death. This time limit is known as the "golden hour" of trauma care.

Laboratory and Diagnostic Tests

There are no specific laboratory and diagnostic tests that determine shock. However, laboratory data can assist the health care team in identifying the type of shock and assessing the client's physical status. The following laboratory tests may be ordered:

- *Blood hemoglobin and hematocrit.* Changes in hemoglobin and hematocrit concentrations usually occur in hypovolemic shock. These changes reflect the underlying etiology: In hypovolemic shock resulting from hemorrhage, the hemoglobin and hematocrit concentrations are lower than normal; in hypovolemic shock resulting from intravascular fluid loss, by contrast, the hemoglobin and hematocrit concentrations are higher than normal.

- *Arterial blood gases (ABGs)* are measured to determine oxygen and carbon dioxide levels and pH. The effects of shock and of the body's compensatory mechanisms cause a decrease in pH (indicating acidosis), a decrease in the partial pressure of oxygen (PaO_2) and in total oxygen saturation, and an increase in the partial pressure of carbon dioxide ($PaCO_2$).

- *Serum electrolytes* are measured to monitor the severity and progression of shock. As shock progresses, glucose levels decrease, sodium levels decrease, and potassium levels increase.

- *Blood urea nitrogen (BUN), serum creatinine levels, and urine specific gravity and osmolality.* These tests measure renal function. As perfusion of the kidneys is decreased and renal function is reduced, the BUN and creatinine levels increase as does urine specific gravity and osmolality.

- *Blood cultures* are performed to identify the causative organism in septic shock.

- *White blood cell count (WBC) and differential WBC* are measured in the client with septic or anaphylactic shock. The total WBC is increased in septic shock. Elevated neutrophils indicate acute infection, monocytes are increased in a bacterial infection, and eosinophils are increased in an allergic response.

- *Serum cardiac enzymes* are elevated in cardiogenic shock: lactate dehydrogenase (LDH), creatine phosphokinase (CPK), and serum glutamic-oxaloacetic transaminase (SGOT).

In addition to laboratory tests, diagnostic tests may be ordered to determine the extent of injury or damage or to locate the site of internal hemorrhage. These tests might include X-ray studies, computerized tomography (CT) scans, magnetic resonance imaging (MRI), endoscopic examinations, and echocardiograms.

Oxygen Therapy

Establishing and maintaining a patent airway and ensuring adequate oxygenation are critical interventions in reversing shock. All clients in shock (even those with adequate respirations) should receive oxygen therapy (usually by mask or nasal cannula) to maintain the PaO$_2$ at greater than 80 mm Hg during the first 4 to 6 hours of care (Dolan, 1991).

If the client's unassisted respiration cannot maintain PaO$_2$ at this level, ventilatory assistance may be necessary. Care of the client requiring ventilatory assistance is discussed in Chapter 34.

Military Antishock Trousers

Military antishock trousers (MAST) are a device used to treat hypovolemic shock resulting from trauma and hemorrhage (Figure 6–3). The device is an inflatable unit with an abdominal chamber and two leg chambers. Each of the chambers can be inflated separately. The device facilitates an increase in arterial pressure by

- Compressing vascular beds, which increases SVR.

- Redistributing blood flow from the peripheral circulation into the central circulation so that it is available for the heart and lungs.

It is recommended that this device be applied as soon as possible after the initial injury, preferably at the scene of the accident. However, the use of MAST is contraindicated in clients who are pregnant, have severe abdominal injuries, are seriously burned, or have obvious cardiovascular deficits. The device is applied only until fluid replacement has restored blood volume and arterial pres-

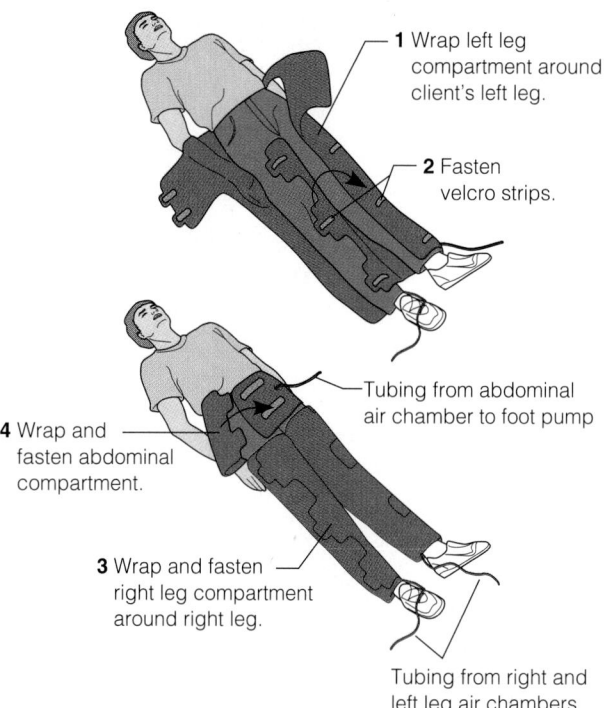

1 Wrap left leg compartment around client's left leg.

2 Fasten velcro strips.

Tubing from abdominal air chamber to foot pump

4 Wrap and fasten abdominal compartment.

3 Wrap and fasten right leg compartment around right leg.

Tubing from right and left leg air chambers

Figure 6–3   Military antishock trousers provide rapid, emergency treatment of shock.

sure. It is then slowly deflated, beginning with the abdominal section, and the client's blood pressure is carefully monitored for stability (Dolan, 1991).

Fluid Replacement

The most effective treatment for the client in hypovolemic shock is the administration of intravenous fluids or blood. Fluids are also given to the client with septic and neurogenic shock. However, the client with cardiogenic shock may require either fluid replacement or restriction, depending on the client's pulmonary artery pressure.

Various fluids may be administered alone or in combination as part of fluid replacement therapy in treating shock. Whole blood or blood products are administered to increase the oxygen-carrying capacity of the blood and thus increase oxygenation of cells. Fluid replacements, such as crystalloid and colloid solutions, are administered to increase circulating blood volume and tissue perfusion. Fluid replacements are administered in massive amounts through two large-bore peripheral lines or through a central line. (The administration of blood and blood products is discussed in Chapter 10. Intravenous solutions are discussed in Chapter 5.)

Crystalloid Solutions   *Crystalloid solutions* contain dextrose or electrolytes dissolved in water; they are either isotonic or hypotonic. Isotonic solutions include normal saline (0.9%), lactated Ringer's solution, and Ringer's solution. Hypotonic solutions include one-half normal saline (0.45%) and 5% dextrose in water (D5W).

Nursing Implications for Pharmacology: Colloid Solutions

COLLOID SOLUTIONS (PLASMA EXPANDERS)

Albumin 5% (Albuminar-5, Buminate 5%)

Albumin 25% (Albuminar-25, Buminate 25%)

Dextran 40 (Gentran 40)

Dextran 70 (Gentran 70, Macrodex)

Dextran 75 (Gentran 75)

Hetastarch (Hespan [HES])

Plasma protein fraction (Plasmanate, Plasma-Plex, Plasmatein, Protenate)

These solutions are blood volume expanders and are used to treat hypovolemic shock due to surgery, hemorrhage, burns, or other trauma. Albumin and plasma protein fraction are prepared from healthy blood donors. Dextran and hetastarch are synthetically prepared large molecules. The solutions promote circulatory volume and tissue perfusion by rapidly expanding plasma volume. They are often administered until whole blood is available.

Nursing Responsibilities

- Before infusion begins, establish baseline of vital signs, lung sounds, heart sounds, and (if possible) CVP and pulmonary artery wedge pressure.
- Start administration of ordered intravenous fluids, using a large-gauge (18- or 19-gauge) infusion needle.
- Take and record vital signs as required by institutional policy (usually every 15 to 60 minutes) and client status.
- Take and record intake and output every 1 to 2 hours.

- Monitor for manifestations of congestive heart failure or pulmonary edema (dyspnea, cyanosis, cough, crackles, wheezes). If these manifestations appear, stop the fluids and notify the physician immediately.
- Monitor for bleeding from new sites; an increase in blood pressure may cause bleeding in severed vessels that did not bleed with decreased blood pressure.
- Monitor for manifestations of dehydration (dry lips; scant, dark-colored urine; loss of skin turgor). Increased intravenous fluids are usually ordered if the client becomes dehydrated.
- Monitor for manifestations of circulatory overload (jugular vein distention, increase in CVP, increase in pulmonary artery wedge pressure). If these manifestations occur, slow rate of infusion and notify physician.
- Monitor prothrombin time, partial thromboplastin time, and platelet counts.
- If administering dextran or plasma protein fraction, have epinephrine and antihistamines readily available for any manifestations of a hypersensitivity reaction (fever, chills, rash, headache, wheezing, flushing).
- Maintain client on bed rest with side rails elevated.

Client and Family Teaching

- The solutions are given to replace lost serum protein, which helps maintain the volume of blood.
- The vital signs are taken frequently to ensure the safety of the client.

All crystalloid solutions increase fluid volume in both the intravascular and the interstitial space. Of the total amount infused, only about 25% remains in the intravascular system; the remaining 75% moves into the interstitial space. Consequently, fluid volume is only minimally expanded and the potential for peripheral edema is increased when crystalloid solutions are used. However, Ringer's lactate (an electrolyte solution) and 0.9% and 0.45% saline are often the fluids of choice in treating hypovolemic shock, especially in the emergency phase of care while blood is being typed and cross-matched. Large amounts of these solutions may be infused rapidly, increasing blood volume and tissue perfusion.

Colloid Solutions   *Colloid solutions* contain substances (colloids) that cannot diffuse through capillary walls. Hence, colloids remain in the vascular system and increase the osmotic pressure of the serum, causing fluid to move into the vascular compartment from the interstitial space. As a result, plasma volume expands. Colloid solutions used to treat shock include 5% albumin, 25% albumin, hetastarch, plasma protein fraction, and dextran.

Colloid products reduce platelet adhesiveness and have been associated with reductions in blood coagulation. Consequently, the client's prothrombin time (PT), platelet count, and partial thromboplastin time (PTT) should be monitored when these solutions are administered. The accompanying pharmacology box includes further information about colloid solutions and associated nursing responsibilities and client teaching.

Blood and Blood Products   If hypovolemic shock is due to hemorrhage, the infusion of blood and blood products may be indicated. The goal of blood administration is to keep the hematocrit at 30% to 35% and the hemoglobin level between 12.5 and 14.5 g/100 mL (Dolan, 1991, p. 994). Available blood and blood products include fresh whole blood, stored whole blood, packed red cells, platelet concentrate, fresh-frozen plasma, and cryoprecipitate. Often, packed red cells are given to provide hemoglobin concentration and are supplemented with crystalloids to maintain an adequate circulatory volume.

Blood administration has disadvantages. Blood is expensive and carries the risk of transfusion reactions, despite careful matching of the product with client blood. If large amounts of blood are transfused, the anticoagulant in the blood (to prevent clotting in storage) may cause coagulation defects and bleeding. Stored blood is also deficient in platelets and other clotting factors, further increasing the risk of clotting problems. If autotransfusions are used, there is increased risk of sepsis and emboli.

Pharmacology

When fluid replacement alone is not sufficient to reverse shock, *vasoactive* drugs (i.e., drugs causing vasoconstriction or vasodilation) and *inotropic* drugs (i.e., drugs improving cardiac contractility) may be administered. When used to treat shock, these drugs increase venous return through vasoconstriction of peripheral vessels; they also improve the pumping ability of the heart by facilitating myocardial contractility and by dilating coronary arteries to increase perfusion of the myocardium.

Drugs that are used to treat shock are discussed in the pharmacology box on page 174. Other drugs that may be administered to the client in shock include:

- Diuretics to increase urine output *after* fluid replacement has been initiated
- Sodium bicarbonate to treat acidosis
- Calcium to replace calcium lost as a result of blood transfusions
- Antiarrhythmic agents to stabilize heart rhythm
- Antibiotics to suppress organisms responsible for septic shock

The client with cardiogenic shock may also require a cardiotonic glycoside (such as digitalis) to treat cardiac failure. Steroids may be used to treat anaphylactic shock.

Nursing Care

Nursing interventions to prevent shock are an essential part of the nursing care of every client. Preventive interventions, as well as interventions for clients who are at greatest risk for developing shock include the following:

- *Hypovolemic shock*: Clients who have undergone surgery, have sustained multiple traumatic injuries, or have been seriously burned are most likely to develop hypovolemic shock. Assessing fluid status is essential in preventing shock and includes daily assessments of weight, fluid intake by all routes, measurable fluid loss (for example, urine, vomitus, wound drainage, gastric drainage, and chest tube drainage), and fluid loss that must be estimated, such as profuse perspiration and wound drainage.

- *Cardiogenic shock*: Clients with left anterior wall myocardial infarctions are at risk for developing cardiogenic shock. Nursing care to prevent the development of cardiogenic shock focuses on maintaining or improving myocardial oxygen supply. Interventions include providing immediate pain relief, maintaining rest, and administering supplemental oxygen.

- *Neurogenic shock*: The risk of neurogenic shock is increased in clients who have spinal cord injuries and those who have received spinal anesthesia. Preventive nursing care includes maintaining immobility of clients with spinal cord trauma and elevating the head of the bed 15 to 20 degrees following spinal anesthesia. (However, elevations of more than 20 degrees can potentiate spinal headaches and should be avoided.)

- *Septic shock*: Clients who are hospitalized, are debilitated, are chronically ill, and/or have undergone invasive procedures or tube insertions are at high risk for septic shock. Nursing care to prevent septic shock includes careful and consistent hand washing, the use of aseptic techniques for procedures (for example, catheterizations, suctioning, changing dressings, starting and maintaining intravenous fluids or medications), and monitoring for local and systemic manifestations of infection.

- *Anaphylactic shock*: Preventive nursing interventions for anaphylactic shock include collecting data during the initial interview to identify allergies, ensuring that this information is communicated to all other health care providers, and carefully monitoring the client receiving intravenous medications, blood, or blood products.

Nursing care for the client in shock focuses on assessing and monitoring overall tissue perfusion and on meeting psychosocial needs of the client and the family. This section discusses nursing diagnoses that are appropriate for the client with hypovolemic shock: *Decreased Cardiac Output, Altered Tissue Perfusion,* and *Anxiety.* The intervals between assessments differ according to the acuity of the client and institutional policy; therefore, some of the nursing interventions discussed in this chapter are not time framed.

Nursing Implications for Pharmacology: The Client in Shock

ADRENERGICS (SYMPATHOMIMETICS)

Adrenergic drugs (also called sympathomimetics) mimic the fight-or-flight response of the sympathetic nervous system, selectively stimulating alpha-adrenergic and beta-adrenergic receptors. Many of these drugs have both vasopressor (vasoconstricting) effects and positive inotropic effects (Table 6–1). Stimulation of alpha-adrenergic receptors results in vasoconstriction and increased systemic blood pressure. Stimulation of beta-adrenergic receptors increases the force and rate of myocardial contraction.

The physiologic effect of these drugs includes improved perfusion and oxygenation of the heart, with increased stroke volume and heart rate, and increased cardiac output. Increased cardiac output in turn increases tissue perfusion and oxygenation. The major disadvantage is that increases in stroke volume and heart rate also increase the oxygen requirements of the myocardium. These drugs may be used in the early stages of shock, especially in types of shock characterized by vasodilation.

Nursing Responsibilities

- Carefully monitor responses in the older adult, who may be especially sensitive to sympathomimetics and require lower doses.

- When administering these drugs by the subcutaneous route, carefully aspirate the injection site to avoid injecting the drug directly into a blood vessel.

Table 6–1   Adrenergic Drugs Used to Treat Shock

Action	Drug	Receptor
Vasoconstrictors	Norepinephrine (Levophed)	A
	Metaraminol (Aramine)	A
Inotropes	Dopamine (Inotropin)	A
	Dobutamine (Dobutrex)	B
	Isoprotenernol (Isuprel)	B

- Use the intravenous route only with continuous infusion pumps. Carefully adjust the dose to accommodate the client's cardiovascular status (as ordered by the physician or by written protocol).

- Document lung sounds, vital signs, and hemodynamic parameters before starting the medication, and then according to institutional policy (usually every 5 to 15 minutes).

- Record and monitor urine output; report output of less than 30 mL per hour.

- Be aware that the sympathomimetics are incompatible with sodium bicarbonate or alkaline solutions.

- When administering drugs that cause vasoconstriction, such as norepinephrine (Levophed) and metaraminol (Aramine), monitor the intravenous insertion site for infiltration. If infiltration does occur,

Decreased Cardiac Output

Decreased cardiac output is the primary problem for the client in shock. Although much of the care related to this diagnosis is collaborative, there are many independent nursing interventions that are critical to the care of the client in shock.

Nursing interventions with rationales are as follows:

- Assess and monitor cardiovascular function, including:
  a. Blood pressure
  b. Heart rate and rhythm
  c. Capillary refill time
  d. Peripheral pulses
  e. Hemodynamic monitoring of arterial pressures, pulmonary artery pressures, and central venous pressures (CVP).

A baseline assessment is necessary to establish the stage of shock. If palpable peripheral pulses and audible (to auscul-

tation) blood pressure are lost, inserting central arterial, venous, and pulmonary artery catheters is essential to establish progression of shock accurately and to evaluate the client's response to therapy.

- Measure and record intake and output (total output and urinary output) hourly. *A decrease in circulating blood volume with hypotension and the effect of the compensatory mechanisms associated with shock can cause renal failure. Urinary output of less than 30 mL per hour in an acutely ill adult indicates reduced renal blood flow.*

- Monitor bowel sounds, abdominal distention, and abdominal pain. *Decreased splanchnic blood flow reduces bowel motility and peristalsis; paralytic ileus may result.*

- Monitor for sudden sharp chest pain, dyspnea, cyanosis, anxiety, and restlessness. *Hemoconcentration and increased platelet aggregation may result in pulmonary emboli.*

Pharmacology: The Client in Shock (continued)

stop the infusion and notify the physician immediately. (Infiltration may cause ischemia and necrosis of tissue.)

Client Teaching

- Because these drugs mimic a physiologic reaction to stress, they may cause feelings of anxiety.
- Close monitoring to adjust the dose will be carried out by qualified nurses using written protocols.
- Report heart palpitations or chest pain immediately.

VASODILATORS

Nitroglycerin (Tridil)

Nitroprusside (Nipride)

Drugs that cause vasodilation act directly on smooth muscle, affecting both arterioles and veins. Peripheral resistance, cardiac output, and pulmonary wedge pressure are all reduced as a result of the vasodilation. These effects decrease the oxygen need of the heart and decrease pulmonary congestion. Vasodilators are used primarily in the treatment of cardiogenic shock and may be combined with a sympathomimetic (e g., dopamine).

Nursing Responsibilities

- Protect these drugs from light by wrapping the intravenous bag in the package that is provided.

- Mix with D5W only.
- Infuse with an infusion pump, and use within 4 hours of reconstitution.
- Do not add other medications to the solution.
- Assess mental status, blood pressure, and pulse prior to initiating medication. Thereafter, assess blood pressure and pulse according to institutional policy (usually every 5 minutes initially, then every 15 minutes until stable, and then every hour).
- Monitor for confusion, dizziness, tachycardia, arrhythmias, hypotension, and adventitious breath sounds. Report these immediately if they occur, and slow the rate of infusion to a keep-open rate.
- Monitor for signs of thiocyanate poisoning (nausea, disorientation, muscle spasms, decreased or absent reflexes) if infusion lasts longer than 72 hours.
- Keep client in bed with side rails up.

Client and Family Teaching

- It is important to stay in bed and change positions slowly to avoid dizziness.
- The blood pressure and pulse are taken frequently to adjust the dose of medication.
- Headache is a common side effect.

- Maintain client on bed rest, and provide (to the extent possible) a calm, quiet environment. Position the client in a supine position with the legs elevated to about 20 degrees, trunk flat, and head and shoulders elevated higher than the chest (Figure 6–4). *Limiting activity and ensuring rest decreases the workload of the heart. The supine position with legs elevated increases venous return. However, this position should not be used for clients in cardiogenic shock. The Trendelenburg position is no longer recommended, because it causes the abdominal organs to press against the diaphragm (limiting respirations), decreases filling of the coronary arteries, and initiates aortic and carotid sinus reflexes.*

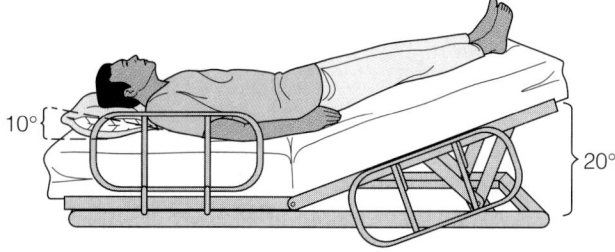

Figure 6–4   The client in shock should be positioned with the lower extremities elevated approximately 20 degrees (knees straight), trunk horizontal, and the head elevated about 10 degrees.

Altered Tissue Perfusion

As shock progresses, diminished tissue perfusion causes ischemia and hypoxia of major organ systems. Compensatory mechanisms initially decrease blood flow to the skin, abdominal organs, and kidneys. However, as shock worsens, blood flow and oxygenation of the lungs, heart, and brain are also impaired. Hypoxia and ischemia result from decreased tissue perfusion in the kidneys, brain, heart, lungs, gastrointestinal tract, and the periphery.

Nursing interventions with rationales are as follows:

- Monitor skin color, temperature, turgor, and moisture. *Decreased tissue perfusion is evidenced by the skin's becoming pale, cool, and moist; as hemoglobin concentrations decrease, cyanosis occurs.*

- Monitor cardiopulmonary function by assessing
  a. Blood pressure (by auscultation or by hemodynamic monitoring)
  b. Rate and depth of respirations
  c. Lung sounds
  d. Capillary refill
  e. Peripheral pulses (brachial, radial, dorsalis pedis, and posterior tibial); include presence, equality, rate, rhythm, and quality. If unable to palpate pulses, use a device such as a Doppler ultrasound flowmeter to assess peripheral arterial blood flow.
  f. Jugular vein distention
  g. CVP measurements
  Baseline vital signs are necessary to determine trends in subsequent findings. As shock progresses, the blood pressure decreases, and the pulse becomes rapid, weak, and thready. As perfusion of the lungs decreases, crackles, wheezes, and dyspnea are commonly assessed. Capillary refill is prolonged, and peripheral pulses are weak or nonpalpable. Neck veins that cannot be seen when the client is in the supine position indicate decreased intravascular volume. CVP is an accurate means of determining fluid status in the client in shock; the findings will be low (5 to 15 cm of water is normal) in hypovolemic shock because of the decreased blood volume. See Chapter 5 for a discussion of CVP.

- Monitor body temperature. *An elevated body temperature increases metabolic demands, depleting reserves of bodily energy. It also increases myocardial oxygen demand and may place the client with previous cardiac problems at even greater risk for hypoperfusion.*

- Monitor urinary output per Foley catheter hourly, using a urimeter. *Urine output is a reliable indicator of renal perfusion. A urine output of less than 30 mL per hour in an acutely ill adult client indicates a decrease in renal perfusion.*

- Assess mental status and level of consciousness. *The appropriateness of the client's behavior and responses reflects the adequacy of cerebral circulation. Restlessness and anxiety are common early in shock; in later stages, the client may become lethargic and progress to a comatose state. Altered levels of consciousness are the result of both cerebral hypoxia and the effects of acidosis on brain cells.*

Anxiety

Many clients in hypovolemic shock have experienced some form of major trauma and may have life-threatening, multiple injuries. Following on-the-scene treatment, the client is admitted to the health care setting usually through the emergency department. Surgery may be required to treat injuries, followed by care in a critical care unit. Throughout this sequence of crisis events, treatment is invasive, and contact with family is minimal.

Client and family responses to these situations of uncertainty, instability, and change include anxiety, fear, and powerlessness (Jillings, 1990). These responses are affected by age, developmental level, cultural and ethnic group, experience with illness and the health care system, and support systems.

Nursing interventions with rationales are as follows:

- Assess the cause(s) of the anxiety, and manipulate the environment to provide periods of rest. *Reducing stimuli that cause anxiety is calming and facilitates rest, which is necessary in the client at risk for bleeding.*

- Administer prescribed pain medications on a regular basis. *Pain precipitates and/or aggravates anxiety.*

- Provide interventions to increase comfort and reduce restlessness:
  a. Maintain cleanliness in the environment.
  b. Provide skin and oral care.
  c. Monitor the effectiveness of ventilation or oxygen therapy.
  d. Eliminate all nonessential activities.
  e. Remain with the client during procedures.
  f. Listen carefully to client.
  g. Speak slowly and calmly, using short sentences.
  h. Use touch to provide support.
  Unfamiliar sounds, sights, and odors can all increase anxiety. Damp skin or a dry mouth increases discomfort. Inadequate gas exchange with a decrease in oxygen or an increase in carbon dioxide in the blood may cause the client to experience a "feeling of doom." Activity increases the body's need for oxygen. Listening and touch provide support in an environment in which the client often feels alone and abandoned. Severe anxiety interferes with the ability to understand others and to respond appropriately.

- Support the client and the client's family:
  a. Provide time, space, and privacy for family members.
  b. Allow family members access to the client when feasible.
  c. Encourage the client and family to express their feelings and concerns. Provide anticipatory guidance to prepare for recovery or death and to support realistic hope.
  d. Acknowledge the beliefs, values, and expectations of the client and family.
  This broad category of nursing interventions is the cornerstone of psychosocial care. Allowing the family access to the client reduces anxiety and gives both the client and the family some feeling of control. If prognosis is poor, access and involvement allow the family to begin the grieving process. If recovery is expected, contact provides the client and family with a feeling of hope. Supporting the client and family

facilitates concrete problem solving, promotes acceptance of the illness and its implications, and helps them begin to establish ways of managing the illness experience (Jillings, 1990, p. 329).

- Provide information about the current setting to both the client and family; provide the family with information about resources that are available (such as pastoral care, social services, temporary housing, meals). *Knowing what to expect and how to control the environment to meet basic needs reduces anxiety.*

Other Nursing Diagnoses

Other nursing diagnoses that are appropriate for the client in shock, regardless of type, include the following:

- *Risk for Infection* related to multiple invasive procedures
- *Risk for Fluid Volume Excess* related to rapid infusion of massive amounts of intravenous fluids
- *Impaired Gas Exchange* related to fluid accumulation in lungs
- *Activity Intolerance* related to decreased oxygenation of tissues
- *Altered Thought Processes* related to decreased cerebral tissue perfusion secondary to hemorrhage
- *Altered Urinary Elimination* related to decrease in cardiac output
- *Fear* related to unknown future and possibility of death
- *Risk for Injury* related to altered level of consciousness

---

Applying the Nursing Process

Case Study of a Client with Septic Shock: Huang Mei Lan

Huang Mei Lan is a 43-year-old unmarried female who lives alone in a major West Coast city. Ms. Huang came to America 15 years ago from China and now speaks English well. Her family still lives in China. She worked in a neighborhood storefront sewing shop until 3 years ago, when she was diagnosed with breast cancer. Her treatment included mastectomy of the affected breast and follow-up chemotherapy.

Last month, Ms. Huang experienced a recurrence of cancer in the lymph glands of the affected side. Surgery to remove the glands was performed and chemotherapy started. Ms. Huang has a central line, a urinary catheter, and a surgical incision. She is underweight, weak, and depressed. Although she has multiple physical problems, she never complains or asks for any kind of medication.

Assessment

Ms. Huang's primary nurse, Tonda Canote, enters Ms. Huang's room early in the morning to make her initial assessment. Miss Canote finds Ms. Huang huddled in the middle of the bed, shivering violently. Her vital signs are: T 104 F, P 110, R 30, and BP 106/66. Her skin is hot, dry, and flushed with poor turgor. She is alert and oriented, but is restless and appears anxious. She states she is nauseated and suddenly begins vomiting and is incontinent with liquid stool. Laboratory data indicate leukocytosis, respiratory alkalosis, and reduced platelet count. Blood cultures, as well as cultures of Ms. Huang's sputum, urine, and wound drainage, are conducted. She is diagnosed as having septic shock.

Hetastarch is ordered per intravenous line, and intravenous broad-spectrum antibiotics are begun until the organism and its portal of entry can be determined. Despite treatment, Ms. Huang's condition worsens. Her blood pressure continues to drop, her skin becomes cool and cyanotic, and she begins to have periods of disorientation. She is transferred to the critical care unit. As she is being prepared for the transfer she begins to cry and asks, "Am I going to die?"

Diagnosis

As she provides care for Ms. Huang, Miss Canote makes the following nursing diagnoses:

- *Risk for Fluid Volume Deficit* related to vomiting, diarrhea, high fever, and shift of intravascular volume to interstitial spaces
- *Risk for Ineffective Breathing Pattern* related to rapid respirations and possibility of progression of septic shock
- *Risk for Altered Tissue Perfusion* related to progression of septic shock with decreased cardiac output, hypotension, and massive vasodilation
- *Anxiety* related to feelings that illness is worsening and is potentially life threatening and to transfer to critical care unit

Miss Canote communicates these diagnoses to the nurses in the critical care unit, where the at risk nursing diagnoses are restated as actual nursing diagnoses.

Expected Outcomes

The expected outcomes established in the plan of care specify that Ms. Huang will

- Maintain adequate circulating blood volume.
- Regain and maintain blood gas parameters within normal limits.
- Regain and maintain stable hemodynamic levels.
- Verbalize increased ability to cope with stressors.

Planning and Implementation

The following nursing interventions are planned and implemented for Ms. Huang by nurses in the critical care unit, with assessments made as often as necessary to monitor her condition:

- Monitor neurologic status, including mental status and level of consciousness.

- Monitor cardiovascular status, including arterial blood pressure; rate, rhythm, and quality of pulses; central venous pressure; pulmonary artery pressure; and cardiac output.

- Assess color and character of skin.

- Monitor results of arterial blood gases, blood counts, clotting times, and platelet counts.

- Monitor respiratory status, including respiratory rate, rhythm, and breath sounds.

- Monitor body temperature every 2 hours.

- Monitor urinary output hourly, reporting any output of less than 30 mL per hour.

- Remain with Ms. Huang during this period of acute stress, explaining procedures and providing comfort measures (oral care, skin care, turning, positioning).

Evaluation

Despite intensive nursing and medical care, Ms. Huang's condition remains critical. The interventions are continued.

Critical Thinking in the Nursing Process

1. What stage of shock was Ms. Huang experiencing when Tonda Canote first entered her room? Provide supporting evidence.

2. Vasopressors may be used in the treatment of septic shock. Explain the rationale for their use.

3. While monitoring Ms. Huang's arterial blood gases, the nurse notes that her PaO_2 is < 60 mm Hg, and her $PaCO_2$ was > 50. What do these findings indicate, and why have they occurred?

4. Ms. Huang has been given large amounts of colloids intravenously. Hemodynamic monitoring indicates a higher than normal CVP and pulmonary artery pressure. What do these findings indicate? What physical assessments would you make to confirm the changes?

5. Would the nursing diagnosis *Altered Skin Integrity* be appropriate for Ms. Huang? Why, or why not?

6. Sleep deprivation in the critical care unit may be a problem for some clients. Develop a care plan for Ms. Huang for the nursing diagnosis *Sleep Pattern Distur-*

bance. Consider the setting when developing interventions.

Bibliography

■ ■ ■

Anderson, S. (1990). ABGs: Six easy steps to interpreting blood gases. *American Journal of Nursing, 90*(8), 42–45.

Alfaro-LeFevre, R.; Blicharz, M. E.; Flynn, N. M.; & Boyer, M. J. (1992). *Drug handbook: A nursing process approach.* Redwood City, CA: Addison-Wesley Nursing.

Barry, S. (1989). Septic shock: Special needs of patients with cancer. *Oncology Nursing Forum, 16*(1), 31–35.

Byra-Cook, C. J., Dracup, K. A., & Lazik, A. J. (1990). Direct and indirect blood pressure in critical care patients. *Nursing Research, 39*(5), 285–288.

Carpenito, L. J. (1992). *Nursing diagnosis: Application to clinical practice.* (4th ed.). Philadelphia: Lippincott.

Dolan, J. T. (1991). *Critical care nursing: Clinical management through the nursing process.* Philadelphia: FA Davis.

Evans, C. F. (1991). Nursing management of the patient with septic shock. In J. T. Dolan, (Ed.), *Critical care nursing: Clinical management through the nursing process* (pp. 1360–1369). Philadelphia: FA Davis.

Fallon, L., & Waterman, J. (1991). Nursing management of the patient with anaphylactic shock. In J. T. Dolan, (Ed.), *Critical care nursing: Clinical management through the nursing process* (pp. 1370–1379). Philadelphia: FA Davis.

Jillings, C. R. (1990). Shock: Psychosocial needs of the patient and family. *Critical Care Nursing Clinics of North America, 2*(2), 325–330.

Kee, J. L. (1991). *Laboratory and diagnostic tests with nursing implications.* (3rd ed.). Norwalk, CT: Appleton & Lange.

Kidd, P. S., & Wagner, K. D. (1992). *High acuity nursing: Preparing for practice in today's health care settings.* Norwalk, CT: Appleton & Lange.

Lancaster, L. E., & Rice, V. (1990). Nursing care planning: Overview and application to the patient in shock. *Critical Care Nursing Clinics of North America, 2*(2), 279–286.

Littleton, M. (1988). Pathophysiology and assessment of sepsis and septic shock. *Critical Care Nursing Quarterly, 11*(1), 30–47.

McCormac, M. (1990). Managing hemorrhagic shock. *American Journal of Nursing, 90*(8), 22–27.

Metheny, N. M. (1990). Why worry about IV fluids? *American Journal of Nursing, 90*(6), 50–57.

Murphy, T. G., & Bennett, E. J. (1992). Low-tech, high-touch perfusion assessment. *American Journal of Nursing, 92*(5), 36–48.

O'Neal, P. (1994). How to spot early signs of cardiogenic shock. *American Journal of Nursing, 94*(5), 36–40.

Perry, A. G. (1988). Shock complications: Recognition and management. *Critical Care Nursing Quarterly, 11*(1), 1–8.

Porth, C. M. (1994). *Pathophysiology: Concepts of altered health states.* (4th ed.) Philadelphia: Lippincott.

Price, S. A., & Wilson, L. M. (1992). *Pathophysiology: Clinical concepts of disease processes.* St. Louis: Mosby.

Rice, V. (1991). Shock, a clinical syndrome: An update. Part 4. Nursing care of the shock patient. *Critical Care Nurse, 11*(7), 28–42.

Roberts, A. (1994). Systems of life: Blood: 1. *Nursing Times, 90*(19), 35–38.

Russell, S. (1994). Hypovolemic shock: Is your patient at risk? *Nursing94, 24*(4), 34–39.

———. (1994). Septic shock: Can you recognize the clues? *Nursing94, 24*(4), 40–48

Sarsany, S. L. (February 1988). Massive bleeding. *RN,* 36–38.

Summers, G. (1990). The clinical and hemodynamic presentation of the shock patient. *Critical Care Nursing Clinics of North America, 2*(2), 161–166.

Whitman, G. (1988). Tissue perfusion. In M. Kinney, D. Packa, & S. Dunbar (Eds.), *AACN clinical reference for critical care nursing* (2nd ed.). (p. 129). New York: McGraw-Hill.

Nursing Care of Clients Having Surgery

LEARNING OBJECTIVES

After completing this chapter, you will be able to

- Describe the various classifications of surgical procedures.
- Identify laboratory and diagnostic tests used in the perioperative period.
- Describe nursing implications for medications prescribed for the surgical client.
- Provide appropriate nursing care for the client in the

perioperative, intraoperative, and postoperative phases of surgery.

- Identify variations in perioperative care for the older adult.
- Describe principles of pain management specific to acute postoperative pain control.
- Discuss the differences and similarities between outpatient and inpatient surgery.
- Use the nursing process as a framework for providing individualized care for the client undergoing surgery.

Surgery is an invasive medical procedure performed to diagnose or treat illness, injury, or deformity. Although surgery is a medical treatment, the nurse assumes an active role in caring for the client before, during, and after surgery. Collaborative care and independent nursing care together prevent complications and promote optimal recovery of the surgical client.

Perioperative nursing is a specialized area of practice for providing nursing care to the surgical client. Perioperative nursing incorporates the three phases of the surgical experience: preoperative, intraoperative, and postoperative. The *preoperative phase* begins when the decision for surgery is made and ends when the client is transferred to the operating room. The *intraoperative phase* begins with the client's entry into the operating room and ends with admittance to the *postanesthesia care unit (PACU, or recovery room)*. The *postoperative phase* begins with the client's

admittance to the postanesthesia recovery area and ends with the client's complete recovery from the surgical intervention.

Surgical procedures can be classified according to *purpose, risk factor,* and *urgency* (Table 7–1). Based on this information, nursing care can be individualized to best meet client needs.

Although the perioperative nurse works in collaboration with other health care professionals to identify and meet the client's needs, the perioperative nurse has the primary responsibility and accountability for nursing care of the client undergoing surgery. An overview of perioperative nursing activities is provided in the box on page 181. This chapter addresses specific client needs and nursing care for each of the three distinct phases of the perioperative period, as well as for the client having outpatient surgery.

Table 7–1   Classification of Surgical Procedures

	Classification	Function	Examples
Purpose	Diagnostic	Determine or confirm a diagnosis	Breast biopsy, bronchoscopy
	Ablative	Remove diseased tissue, organ, or extremity	Appendectomy, amputation
	Constructive	Build tissue/organs that are absent (congenital anomalies)	Repair of cleft palate
	Reconstructive	Rebuild tissue/organ that has been damaged	Skin graft after a burn, total joint replacement
	Palliative	Alleviate symptoms of a disease (not curative)	Bowel resection in client with terminal cancer
	Transplant	Replace organs/tissue to restore function	Heart, lung, liver, kidney transplant
Risk Factor	Minor	Minimal physical assault with minimal risk	Removal of skin lesions, dilation and curettage (D&C), cataract extraction
	Major	Extensive physical assault and/or serious risk	Transplant, total joint replacement, cholecystectomy
Urgency	Elective	Suggested, though no foreseen ill effects if postponed	Cosmetic surgery, cataract surgery, bunionectomy
	Urgent	Necessary to be performed within 1 to 2 days	Heart bypass surgery, amputation resulting from gangrene, fractured hip
	Emergency	Performed immediately	Obstetric emergencies, bowel obstruction, ruptured aneurysm, life-threatening trauma

The Client Having Inpatient Surgery

■ ■ ■

Inpatient surgery requires admission to a hospital either one or more days before the scheduled procedure or, as is more common in recent years, early on the morning of the procedure. Generally a stay of one or more additional days is anticipated. Although the length of stay for surgical clients has declined during the past 2 decades, many procedures still require inpatient stays of 4 to 6 days or more following major surgery.

Throughout inpatient surgery, clients may experience any of a wide variety of responses to the initial health problem or the surgery itself. In addition, most clients have a strong emotional response to the prospect of inpatient surgery, which may in turn lead to physical and psychologic alterations. Thus, the complexity of the inpatient surgical experience requires exceptional collaborative and independent nursing care.

Collaborative Care

The client undergoing surgery receives care from a number of health care providers. The focus of this collaborative approach is to place the client in the best possible health status before, during, and after surgery.

Laboratory and Diagnostic Tests
Laboratory and diagnostic tests are performed prior to surgery to provide baseline data and/or detect problems that may place the client at additional risk during and af-

ter surgery. Because of the trend toward shortened hospital stays, many laboratory studies and diagnostic procedures are performed in a preadmission clinic within a week prior to elective surgery.

Complete blood counts, electrolyte studies, coagulation studies, and urinalysis are the most commonly performed perioperative laboratory tests. Table 7–2 discusses the significance and nursing implications of abnormal findings for these common tests. Additional laboratory tests may be performed as the history and physical findings dictate. For example, if the client has a low hemoglobin and hematocrit and significant blood loss during surgery is anticipated, the surgeon may order a type and cross-match of the client's blood for a possible transfusion.

In addition to laboratory tests, the client undergoing surgery typically has a chest X-ray examination performed. This radiologic procedure provides baseline information about the size, shape, and condition of the heart and lungs. The presence of pulmonary complications, such as lung disease, tuberculosis, calcification, infiltration, or pneumonia, may require that surgery be postponed to allow the client to undergo further evaluation or treatment. If findings are abnormal and the surgery cannot be postponed, information from the chest X-ray study can be used to determine the safest form of anesthesia.

Another commonly performed preoperative diagnostic procedure is the electrocardiogram (ECG). This test is ordered routinely on clients who are undergoing general anesthesia and who are over 40 years of age or have cardiovascular disease. The electrocardiogram provides an

Examples of Perioperative Nursing Activities

Preoperative Phase

Home/Clinic
- Initiate initial preoperative assessment.
- Plan teaching methods appropriate to client's needs.
- Involve family in interview.

Surgical Unit
- Perform complete preoperative assessment.
- Coordinate client teaching with other nursing staff.
- Explain phases in perioperative period and expectations.
- Develop a plan of care.

Surgical Suite
- Assess client's level of consciousness.
- Review chart.
- Identify client.
- Verify surgical site.
- Develop a plan of care.
- Provide psychologic support:
  a. Tell client what is happening.
  b. Determine psychologic status.
  c. Give prior warning of noxious stimuli.
  d. Communicate client's emotional status to other members of the health care team as appropriate.

Intraoperative Phase

Surgical Suite
Maintenance of safety:

- Ensure that sponge, needle, and instrument counts are correct.
- Position the client:
  a. Functional alignment
  b. Exposure of surgical site
  c. Maintenance of position throughout procedure
- Apply grounding device to client.
- Provide physical support.
- Maintain aseptic, controlled environment.

Physiologic monitoring:

- Calculate effects of excessive fluid loss.
- Distinguish normal from abnormal cardiopulmonary data.

- Report changes in client's pulse, respirations, temperature, and blood pressures.

Psychologic monitoring (prior to induction and if client is conscious):

- Provide emotional support to client.
- Stand near/touch client during procedures/induction.
- Continue to assess client's emotional status.
- Communicate client's emotional status to other members of the health care team as appropriate.

Postoperative Phase

PACU
Communication of intraoperative information:

- Give client's name.
- State type of surgery performed.
- Provide contributing intraoperative factors (i.e., drain, catheters).
- State physical limitations.
- State impairments resulting from surgery.
- Report client's preoperative level of consciousness.
- Communicate necessary equipment needs.

Evaluation:

- Determine client's immediate response to surgical intervention.

Surgical Unit
- Evaluate effectiveness of nursing care in the OR.
- Determine client's level of satisfaction with care given during perioperative period.
- Evaluate products used on client in the OR.
- Determine client's psychological status.
- Assist with discharge planning.

Home/Clinic
- Seek client's perception of surgery in terms of the effects of anesthetic agents, impact on body image, distortion, immobilization.
- Determine family's perception of surgery.

Note. From "A Model for Perioperative Nursing Practice," 1985, *AORN Journal, 41*(1): 189–94. Reprinted with permission of The Association of Operating Room Nurses, A Model for Perioperative Nursing Practice. Revised 3/88.

Table 7–2 Laboratory Tests for Perioperative Assessment

Test	Significance of Increased Values	Significance of Decreased Values	Nursing Implications
Hemoglobin (Hgb) and hematocrit (Hct)	Dehydration, excessive fluid plasma loss, polycythemia vera	Fluid overload, excessive blood loss, anemia	Monitor oxygenation, intake and output (I&O), and vital signs, and assess for bleeding.
White blood cell count (WBC)	Infectious/inflammatory processes, leukemia	Immune deficiencies	Monitor for signs of inflammation; monitor drainage, temperature, and pulse. Use strict universal precautions.
Platelet count	Malignancies, polycythemia vera	Clotting deficiency disorders, chemotherapy	If decreased, assess for bleeding at incision sites and drainage tubes, and assess for hematomas.
Carbon dioxide (CO_2)	Emphysema, chronic bronchitis, asthma, pneumonia, respiratory acidosis, vomiting, nasogastric suctioning	Metabolic acidosis, hyperventilation	Monitor respiratory status and arterial blood gases (ABGs).
Electrolytes Potassium (K^+)	Kidney dysfunction, dehydration, suctioning	Side effects of diuretics, vomiting, NG suctioning	Monitor K^+ level, cardiac and neurologic function, and preoperative diuretic therapy.
Sodium (Na^+)	Kidney dysfunction, normal saline-containing intravenous fluids	Side effects of diuretics, vomiting, NG suctioning	Monitor Na^+ level and I&O; assess for peripheral edema and effects of perioperative diuretic therapy.
Chloride (Cl^-)	Kidney dysfunction, dehydration, alkalosis	Side effects of diuretics, vomiting, NG suctioning	Monitor Cl^- level and I&O; assess for peripheral edema and perioperative diuretic therapy.
Prothrombin time (protime, or PT) and partial thromboplastin time (PTT)	Defect in mechanism for blood clotting, anticoagulant therapy (aspirin, heparin, warfarin), side effect of other drugs affecting clotting time	Hypercoagulability of the blood may lead to thrombus formation in the veins	If clotting time is elevated, monitor PT/PTT values. Assess for bleeding at incision site and drainage tubes and for hematomas. If clotting time is decreased, monitor for thrombus formation (pulmonary emboli, thrombophlebitis), and evaluate PT and PTT values.
Urinalysis	Varied	Varied	Used to detect abnormal substances (e.g., protein, glucose, red blood cells, or bacteria) in the urine. Notify surgeon if abnormalities are detected.

evaluation of the cardiac status of either new or preexisting cardiac conditions. The client's surgery may be cancelled or postponed if a life-threatening cardiac condition is discovered.

In addition to the chest X-ray study and ECG, other diagnostic tests may be performed perioperatively to gather further assessment data. For example, for clients who have chronic obstructive pulmonary disease, pulmonary function studies often are performed to determine the extent of respiratory dysfunction. This information guides the anesthesiologist before and during surgery in choosing the type of anesthetic to be used, and it will guide the surgeon and nursing staff in the recovery phase.

Pharmacology

The client having surgery receives medications before, during, and after surgery to achieve specific therapeutic outcomes.

Preoperative Pharmacology The surgical client usually is given preoperative medications 45 to 70 minutes before the scheduled surgery. Any delay in administration should be reported promptly to the surgical department. Preoperative medications may also be given in the surgical holding room to produce the desired effects.

A combination of preoperative drugs may be ordered to achieve the desired outcomes with minimal side effects. Such outcomes include sedating the client, reducing anxiety, inducing amnesia to minimize unpleasant surgical memories, increasing comfort during preoperative procedures, reducing gastric acidity and volume, increasing gastric emptying, decreasing nausea and vomiting, and reducing the incidence of aspiration by drying oral and respiratory secretions. Table 7–3 outlines commonly prescribed preoperative medications.

Intraoperative Pharmacology *Anesthesia* is used to produce unconsciousness, analgesia, reflex loss, and mus-

Table 7-3   Preoperative Medications

Generic	Trade	Dose and Route	Action by Category	Nursing Implications
Benzodiazepines				
Midazolam	Versed	3–5 mg IM	Decreases anxiety and produces sedation to some extent	Monitor for respiratory depression, hypotension, drowsiness, and lack of coordination.
Diazepam	Valium	5–20 mg PO	Induces amnesia	
Lorazepam	Ativan	1–4 mg IM or IV	May induce substantial amnesia	
Opioid Analgesics				
Morphine	Morphine	5–15 mg IM	Decreases discomfort of preoperative procedures	Monitor for respiratory depression, nausea, vomiting, orthostatic hypotension, and pruritus. Smaller doses may be given to frail or older clients.
Meperidine	Demerol	50–150 mg IM		
H$_2$-Receptor Antagonists				
Cimetidine	Tagamet	300 mg IV or PO	Increases gastric pH and decreases gastric volume	Monitor for confusion, particularly in the older client (uncommon side effect).
Famotidine	Pepcid	20 mg IV		
Ranitidine	Zantac	50 mg IV		
Nonparticulate Antacids				
Sodium citrate	Bicitra	15 mL PO	Increases gastric pH	Administer in 15 mL of water.
Antiemetics				
Metoclopramide	Reglan	10 mg IV	Enhances gastric emptying	Monitor for sedation and extrapyramidal reaction (involuntary movement, muscle tone changes, and abnormal posture).
Droperidol	Inapsine	10–15 mg PO 0.625– 2.5 mg IM	Tranquilizer	
Anticholinergics				
Atropine Sulfate	Atropine Sulfate	0.4–0.6 mg IM or IV	Reduces oral and respiratory secretions to decrease risk of aspiration	Monitor for confusion, restlessness, and tachycardia. Prepare client to expect a dry mouth.
Glycopyrrolate	Robinul	0.1–0.3 IM mg or IV		
Scopolamine	Scopolamine	0.4–0.6 mg IM or IV		

Note. Adapted from "What You Need to Know About Administering Preoperative Medications" by K. Litwick, 1991, *Nursing, 21,*(8): 44–47.

cle relaxation during a surgical procedure. General anesthesia produces all of the above effects, whereas regional anesthesia results in analgesia, reflex loss, and muscle relaxation but does not cause the client to lose consciousness. An anesthesiologist (physician) or certified registered nurse anesthetist (CRNA) administers the anesthetics during the intraoperative phase of surgery.

General Anesthesia   **General anesthesia** is most commonly administered by inhalation and, to a lesser extent, by the intravenous route. It produces central nervous system depression. As a result, the client loses consciousness and does not perceive pain, skeletal muscles relax, and reflexes diminish.

Advantages to general anesthesia include rapid excretion of the anesthetic agent and prompt reversal of its effects when desired. Additionally, general anesthesia can be used with all age groups and any type of surgical procedure. It produces amnesia.

Disadvantages of general anesthesia include risks associated with circulatory and respiratory depression. Clients with serious respiratory or circulatory diseases, such as emphysema or congestive heart failure, are at greater risk for complications.

The phases of general anesthesia are divided into three distinct categories: induction, maintenance, and emergence. During the *induction phase,* the client receives the anesthetic agent intravenously or by inhalation. During this phase, airway patency is achieved with endotracheal intubation. The next phase of general anesthesia is *maintenance.* During this period, the client is positioned, the skin is prepared, and surgery is performed. The anesthesiologist maintains the proper depth of anesthesia while constantly monitoring physiologic parameters such as heart rate, blood pressure, respiratory rate, temperature, and oxygen and carbon dioxide levels. The final phase of anesthesia is the client's *emergence* from this altered physiologic state. As the anesthetic agents are withdrawn or the effects reversed pharmacologically, the client begins to awaken. The endotracheal tube is removed (extubated) once the client is able to reestablish voluntary breathing. It is critical to ensure airway patency in this period, because extubation may cause bronchospasm or laryngospasm.

Regional Anesthesia **Regional anesthesia** is a type of local anesthesia in which medication is instilled around the nerves to block transmission of nerve impulses in a particular area. Regional anesthesia produces analgesia, relaxation, and reduced reflexes. The client is awake and conscious during the surgical procedure but does not perceive pain. Regional anesthesia may be classified further as follows:

- *Surface* or *topical anesthesia* is applied to the skin or mucous membranes to block nerve impulses at that site. Wounds of the skin or burns are anesthetized using a cocaine solution, lidocaine (Xylocaine), or benzocaine.

- *Local nerve infiltration* is achieved by injecting lidocaine or tetracaine around a local nerve to depress nerve sensation over a limited area of the body. This technique may be used when a skin or muscle biopsy is obtained or when a small wound is sutured.

- *Nerve blocks* are accomplished by injecting an anesthetic agent at the nerve trunk to produce a lack of sensation over a specific body area, such as an extremity.

- *Epidural blocks* are local anesthetic agents injected into the epidural space, which is located outside the dura mater of the spinal cord. This type of intraspinal anesthesia can be used for surgeries involving the abdomen and lower extremities. An advantage of the epidural block is a reduced risk of neurologic complications, such as headaches or hypotension. A disadvantage is the precise technical skill required to introduce the catheter into the epidural space.

- *Spinal anesthesia* is accomplished by injecting a local anesthetic agent into the subarachnoid space. Surgeries of the lower abdomen, perineum, and lower extremities are likely to use this type of regional anesthesia. Leakage of cerebrospinal fluid (CSF) from the needle insertion site may cause reduced CSF pressure and postoperative headaches. Bed rest, maintaining hydration, and applying pressure to the infusion site combat this common side effect.

Postoperative Pharmacology Pharmacologic management of acute postoperative pain follows the principles outlined below. For more information on pain management, see the nursing care section on managing acute

postoperative pain, pages 206–207. Also see Chapter 4.

Pain that is established and severe is more difficult to treat than pain that is at its onset. Therefore, postoperative analgesics should be administered initially at regular intervals to maintain a therapeutic blood level. Administering analgesics as needed (PRN) allows for a lowering of this therapeutic level; delays in the medication administration further increase pain intensity. Therefore, PRN administration of analgesics is not recommended in the first 36 to 48 hours postoperatively.

Nonsteroidal anti-inflammatory drugs (NSAIDs) should be administered to treat mild to moderate postoperative pain. This category of drugs should be given soon after surgery (orally, parenterally, or rectally) along with opioids unless contraindicated. Although NSAIDs, including acetaminophen, may not be sufficient to control pain completely, they allow for the use of lower doses of opioid analgesics and, therefore, fewer side effects. NSAIDs can be given safely to older clients, but the nurse should observe closely for side effects, particularly gastric and renal toxicity.

Opioid analgesics, such as morphine and meperidine (Demerol), are considered the foundation for managing moderate to severe postoperative pain. Opioid dosage requirements vary greatly from one client to another, so the dosage must be individually tailored. Later in the postoperative recovery period, opioid analgesics (oral or intramuscular) may be given PRN. In this way, pain relief can be maintained, while the potential for drug side effects is decreased.

Contrary to the belief of many health care providers (including nurses), physical dependence and tolerance to opioid analgesics is uncommon in short-term postoperative use. Additionally, opioid analgesics, when used to treat acute pain, rarely lead to psychologic dependence and addiction.

Older clients tend to be more sensitive to the analgesic effects of opioids, experiencing a higher peak effect with a longer duration of pain control. Nevertheless, in appropriate dosages, opioids can be given safely and effectively to older clients.

Informed Consent

Informed consent (often referred to as an *operative permit*) is a legal document required for certain diagnostic procedures or therapeutic measures, including surgery. This legal document serves to protect the client, nurse, physician, and health care facility. Informed consent includes the following information:

- The need for the procedure in relation to the diagnoses
- A description and purpose of the proposed procedure
- Possible benefits and potential risks
- Likelihood of a successful outcome
- Alternative treatments or procedures available

- Anticipated risks should the procedure not be performed
- Physician's advice as to what is needed
- Right to refuse treatment or withdraw consent

It is the responsibility of the surgeon who performs the procedure to obtain the client's informed consent. The surgeon should discuss the above information with the client and family in language they can understand.

Ideally, the nurse should be present when the information is presented. Later the nurse can discuss what was presented with the client and family, if necessary. If the client has questions or concerns that were not discussed or made clear, or if the nurse questions the client's understanding, the surgeon is responsible for supplying further information. If these situations arise, the nurse should contact the surgeon before having the client sign the informed consent form. Following a thorough discussion of the informed consent, the nurse witnesses the client's signature on the form (Figure 7–1). The nurse also signs the form, indicating that the correct person is signing the form and that the client was alert and aware of what was being signed. The accompanying box lists the elements necessary for a valid and legal informed consent.

The decision to have surgery is a major event in any person's life, especially the older client, who faces additional risks. Therefore, the nurse should allow adequate time for the client to process information, ask questions, and make decisions with the assistance of professionals and family members. Because the older client often receives a significant amount of advice from adult children and other family members, this input is almost always represented in the decision to proceed with surgery. The nurse works closely with both the client and family members to provide teaching and emotional support.

Nursing Care

Nursing care in each of the three phases of surgery will be discussed in the following section. A case study at the end of the section, in which one client is followed through the entire perioperative experience, brings this information together. Perioperative nursing diagnoses are provided in the box on page 187 to assist in identifying the needs of the surgical client. This is not an exhaustive list, but it can serve as a guide in identifying possible nursing diagnoses.

Preoperative Nursing Care

The client's response to planned surgery varies greatly. When planning and implementing nursing care, the nurse should consider individual psychologic and physical differences, the type of surgery, and the circumstances surrounding the need for surgery. Therefore, a thorough nursing assessment is needed to determine the most appropriate care for each client undergoing surgery.

Elements of Valid and Legal Informed Consent

■ ■ ■

- *Voluntary participation:* The client's participation in the decision-making process and the final decision itself must be voluntary. The client's giving or withholding permission is a free choice made without pressure, deceit, duress, or coercion.

- *Mental competence and legal age:* The client must be able to understand the information presented and to think rationally about the decision. Therefore, a minor* or a sedated, confused, unconscious, or mentally incompetent client cannot sign an informed consent. In such instances, a parent, spouse, next-of-kin, or legally appointed guardian can give consent. In emergency situations, telephone or court-ordered consents may be obtained.

---

*Guidelines for legal age vary by state in the United States and by province in Canada.

Physical and Psychologic Preparation   Prior to planning and implementing care for the surgical client, the nurse must first assess the needs of the client and the factors that may increase the risks associated with surgery. The nurse gathers assessment information by taking a nursing history and by performing a physical examination. From this information the nurse establishes baseline data, identifies physical needs, determines teaching needs and psychologic support for the client and family, and prioritizes nursing care. The type of surgical procedure directs the assessment and intervention planned by the nurse. However, a complete assessment is also necessary to identify risk factors and to determine the client's overall health status. Refer to Table 7–4 on page 188 for common risk factors for the client undergoing surgery, and the related nursing interventions and implications. For example, if a client is admitted for surgery on the right knee, it is of concern to the nurse that this client has diabetes, smokes one and a half packs of cigarettes per day, has numbness in the right foot, and takes insulin. This information should be incorporated into a care plan, using appropriate nursing diagnoses and interventions to meet all of the client's needs and assist the client toward full postoperative recovery.

Surgery is a significant and stressful event in the life of the client and family. Regardless of the nature of the surgery (whether major or minor), anxiety will be present. The degree of anxiety that the client and family will

---

M.R. # _____

Saint Francis Medical Center

Informed Consent to Operation, Administration of Anesthetics, and to the Rendering of Other Medical Services

1.   I do hereby authorize and direct _____ M.D./D.O./D.D.S., my physician, and/or such associates or assistants of his choice, to perform the following operation or procedure:
_____

_____

upon _____ (patient's name). I understand that the above named physician and his associates or assistants are employed by me and will be occupied solely with performing such operation or procedure.

2.   The nature of the operation or procedure has been explained to me and no warranty or guarantee has been made as to result or cure. I have been advised that additional surgical and/or medical procedures or treatment may be deemed necessary during the course of the operation or procedure consented hereto, and I fully consent to such additional procedures and treatment which, in the opinion of my physician, are deemed necessary or desirable for the well being of the patient. The possible risks and complications of the operation or procedure have been explained to me. The physician has explained to me the above medical terminology and I satisfactorily understand the type of operation/procedure.

3.   I hereby authorize and direct the above named physician and/or his associates or assistants or those working under his direction to provide for _____ (patient's name) such additional services as he or they may deem reasonable and necessary, including, but not limited to, the administration and maintenance of anesthesia, blood or blood derivatives, and the performance of services involving pathology and radiology and I hereby consent thereto. The possible risks and complications of blood transfusions and the administration of anesthetics have also been explained to me.

4.   I understand also that the persons in attendance at such operation or procedure for the purpose of administering anesthesia, and the radiologists in attendance at such operation or procedure for the purpose of performing radiological (x-ray) service are not the agents, servants or employees of St. Francis Medical Center nor of any physician, but are independent health care providers who are employed by me in the same way that my surgeon and physician are employed by me.

5.   I hereby authorize the Medical Center pathologist or personnel to use their discretion in the disposal of any severed tissue or member.

6.   I hereby grant permission for St. Francis Medical Center to obtain clinical photographs for educational purposes or for my patient record as deemed necessary by my physician.

7.   *The exception to this consent:* (If none, write "none".) _____

_____ and I assume full responsibility for these exceptions.

_____   _____
PATIENT'S SIGNATURE   DATE

If the patient is a minor or incompetent or is unable to sign, the following must be completed:

I hereby certify that I am the (relationship)_____ of the above named patient

who is unable to sign because _____ ,
and I am fully authorized to give the consent herein granted.

_____   _____
SIGNATURE   DATE

_____   _____
WITNESSED BY/date   WITNESSED BY/date

If signed in the physician's office, the following MUST be completed by the Medical Center.

_____   _____
REVIEWED BY (patient name)/date   WITNESSED BY /date

Figure 7–1 Informed consent form.

Examples of Perioperative Nursing Diagnoses

■ ■ ■

Preoperative

- Knowledge Deficit
- Anxielty
- Fear
- Anticipatory Grieving
- Decisional Conflict
- Ineffective Individual Coping
- Altered Sexuality Patterns
- Sleep Pattern Disturbance
- Altered Thought Processes
- Altered Family Processes

Intraoperative

- Knowledge Deficit
- Anxiety
- Fear
- Ineffective Airway Clearance
- Risk for Aspiration
- Decreased Cardiac Output
- Hypothermia
- Risk for Infection
- Altered Thought Processes
- Impaired Gas Exchange
- Altered Urinary Elimination
- Fluid Volume Deficit
- Fluid Volume Excess
- Impaired Verbal Communication

Postoperative

- Knowledge Deficit
- Pain
- Ineffective Breathing Pattern
- Ineffective Airway Clearance
- Impaired Skin Integrity
- Altered Nutrition: Less Than Body Requirements
- Altered Sexuality Patterns
- Sleep Pattern Disturbance
- Fatigue
- Urinary Retention
- Altered Urinary Elimination
- Impaired Adjustment
- Body Image Disturbance
- Impaired Physical Mobility
- Risk for Activity Intolerance
- Risk for Injury
- Self-Care Deficit
- Altered Health Maintenance
- Diversional Activity Deficit
- Social Isolation

---

experience is not necessarily proportional to the magnitude of the surgical procedure. For example, a client scheduled to have a biopsy to rule out cancer, which is considered minor surgery, may be more anxious than a client undergoing gallbladder removal, which is considered major surgery.

The nurse's ability to listen actively to both verbal and nonverbal messages is imperative to establishing a trusting relationship with the client and family. Therapeutic communication can help the client and family identify fears and concerns. The nurse can then plan nursing interventions and supportive care to reduce the client's anxiety level and assist the client to cope successfully with the stressors encountered during the perioperative period.

Preoperative Client and Family Teaching Client teaching is an essential nursing responsibility in the preoperative period. Client education along with emotional support have a positive effect on the client's physical and psychologic well-being, both before and after surgery. In an analysis of 102 studies, surgical clients receiving client education and/or supportive interventions had less pain and anxiety, experienced fewer complications, were discharged sooner, were more satisfied with their care, and returned to normal activities sooner than clients who did not receive this type of care (O'Connor et al., 1990). These positive outcomes may be attributed in part to the perceived sense of control the client gains through the nurse's teaching. Refer to the accompanying research box on page 190 for more information on the implications of this research for perioperative nursing practice.

Client teaching should be initiated as soon as the client is made aware of the upcoming surgery. Teaching may begin as early as in the physician's office or at the time of preadmission testing. Although the education process continues during postoperative care, most of the teaching is carried out prior to surgery, because pain and the effects of anesthesia can greatly diminish the client's ability to learn.

The amount of information desired varies from client to client. Therefore, it is the nurse's responsibility to assess the client's need for and readiness to accept informa-

Table 7–4 Nursing Implications for Surgical Risk Factors

Factor	Associated Risk	Nursing Implications
Advanced age	Older adults have age-related changes that affect physiologic, cognitive, and psychosocial responses to the stress of surgery; decrease tolerance of general anesthesia and postoperative medications; and delay wound healing.	Selected nursing interventions are summarized in Table 7–6 on page 208.
Obesity	The obese client is at increased risk for delayed wound healing, wound dehiscence, infection, pneumonia, atelectasis, thrombophlebitis, arrhythmias, and heart failure.	Promote weight reduction if time permits. Monitor closely for wound, pulmonary, and cardiovascular complications postoperatively. Encourage coughing, turning, and diaphragmatic breathing exercises and early ambulation.
Malnutrition	Reserves may not be sufficient to allow the body to respond satisfactorily to the physical assault of surgery; organ failure and shock may result. Increased metabolic demands may result in poor wound healing and infection.	With the physician and dietitian, promote weight gain by providing a well-balanced diet high in calories, protein, and vitamin C. Administer total parenteral nutrition intravenously, nutritional supplements, and tube feedings as prescribed. Daily weights and calorie counts also may be ordered.
Dehydration/ electrolyte imbalance	Depending on the degree of dehydration and/or type of electrolyte imbalance, cardiac dysrhythmia or heart failure may occur. Liver and renal failure may also result.	Administer intravenous fluids as ordered. Monitor I&O. Monitor client for evidence of electrolyte imbalance (see Chapter 5).
Cardiovascular disorders	Presence of cardiovascular disease increases the risk of hemorrhage and shock, hypotension, thrombophlebitis, pulmonary embolism, stroke (especially in the older client), and fluid volume overload.	Diligently monitor vital signs, especially pulse rate, regularity, and rhythm, and general condition of the client. Closely monitor fluid intake (oral and parenteral) to prevent circulatory overload. Assess skin color. Assess for chest pain, lung congestion, and peripheral edema. Observe for signs of hypoxia, and administer oxygen as ordered. Early postoperative ambulation and leg exercises reduce the risk of vascular problems, such as thrombophlebitis and pulmonary embolism.
Respiratory disorders	Respiratory complications such as bronchitis, atelectasis, and pneumonia are some of the most common and serious postoperative complications. Respiratory depression from general anesthesia and acid-base imbalance may also occur. Clients with pulmonary disease are more at risk for developing these complications.	Closely monitor respirations, pulse, and breath sounds. Also assess for hypoxia, dyspnea, lung congestion, and chest pain. Encourage coughing, turning, and diaphragmatic breathing exercises and early postoperative ambulation. Encourage the client to quit smoking or at least to reduce the number of cigarettes smoked.
Diabetes mellitus	Diabetics experience an increased risk for fluctuating blood glucose levels, which can lead to life-threatening hypoglycemia or ketoacidosis. Diabetics also tend to have more cardiovascular disease and are more susceptible to delayed wound healing and wound infection.	Monitor the client closely for signs and symptoms of hypoglycemia and hyperglycemia. Monitor blood glucose levels every 4 hours or as ordered. Administer insulin as prescribed. Encourage intake of food at the designated meal and snack times.

tion. The teaching will be directed in part by the particular surgical procedure that is being performed. However, the information in the accompanying box on page 191 is relevant to most clients undergoing major surgery.

In addition to teaching the client and family about measures that will decrease the risk of complications, the nurse provides other preoperative information to prepare the client and family for surgery. This information should include the following:

- Laboratory and diagnostic tests—reasons and preparations

- Time family should arrive if surgery is scheduled in early morning

Table 7-4   (continued)

Factor	Associated Risk	Nursing Implications
Renal and liver dysfunction	The client with renal or liver dysfunction may poorly tolerate general anesthesia, have fluid/electrolyte and acid-base imbalances, decreased metabolism and excretion of drugs, increased risk for hemorrhage, and delayed wound healing.	Monitor for fluid volume overload, I&O, and response to medication. Evaluate closely for drug side effects and evidence of acidosis or alkalosis.
Alcoholism	The alcoholic client may be malnourished and experience delirium tremens (acute withdrawal symptoms). The alcoholic may require more general anesthesia. Hemorrhage and delayed wound healing can result from liver damage and poor nutritional status.	Monitor closely for signs of delirium tremens. Encourage well-balanced diet. Monitor for wound complications. Administer supplemental nutrients parenterally as ordered.
Nicotine use	Cigarette smokers are at increased risk for respiratory complications such as pneumonia, atelectasis, and bronchitis because of increased mucus secretions and a decreased ability to expel them.	Ideally, the client should quit smoking. Be supportive of the client, and monitor closely for respiratory difficulties. Coughing, turning, and diaphragmatic breathing exercises with early ambulation are very important. Increase daily fluid intake to 2500–3000 mL (unless contraindicated) to help liquefy respiratory secretions to aid expectoration.
Medications	Anesthesia interaction with some medications can cause respiratory difficulties, hypotension, and circulatory collapse. Other medications can produce side effects that may increase surgical risk.	Inform the anesthesiologist of all prescribed or over-the-counter medications.
Anticoagulants (including aspirin)	May cause intraoperative and postoperative hemorrhage.	Monitor for bleeding. Assess PT/PTT values.
Diuretics (particularly thiazides)	May lead to fluid and electrolyte imbalances, producing altered cardiovascular response and respiratory depression.	Monitor I&O and electrolytes. Assess cardiovascular and respiratory status.
Antihypertensives (particularly phenothiazines)	Increase the hypotensive effects of anesthesia.	Closely monitor blood pressure.
Antidepressants (particularly monoamine oxidase inhibitors)	Increase the hypotensive effects of anesthesia.	Closely monitor blood pressure.
Antibiotics (particularly the "mycin" group)	May cause apnea and respiratory paralysis.	Monitor respirations.

- Preparations for the day of surgery: nothing by mouth (NPO) after midnight prior to a morning surgery, skin preparation, indwelling catheter or bladder elimination, start of intravenous infusion, preoperative medication, handling of valuables (rings, watch, money)
- Sedative/hypnotic medication to be taken the night before surgery to promote rest and sleep

- Informed consent
- Expected timetable for surgery and the recovery room
- Transfer to the surgery department
- Location of the surgical waiting room
- Transfer to recovery room

Applying Research to Nursing Practice
Effects of Client Education on Surgical Outcomes

▪ ▪ ▪

Increased perioperative teaching and psychologic support by staff nurses were found to shorten the hospital stay and reduce the use of sedatives, antiemetics, and hypnotics in postoperative clients (O'Connor et al., 1990). The study found that even though the nurses provided more education and support, there was no decrease in the time spent on other nursing activities. The effectiveness of increased education was demonstrated in the improved outcomes for surgical clients. The investigators urge further research on the effects of client education on these and other measurable outcomes.

Implications for Nursing

Numerous studies have shown that client education and supportive nursing interventions are cost-effective. Clients receiving supportive care and education experience less pain and anxiety, develop fewer complications, have shorter hospital stays, are more satisfied with their care, and return to their normal activities faster than those who do not receive this type of care. Nurses are the ideal providers of client education because of the close relationship they establish with clients. In an era when the need for justifying costs is increasing, the benefit the nurse provides as client educator further establishes the value of nursing in tangible ways.

Critical Thinking in Client Care

1. What types of supportive care and/or client education can reduce pain and nausea following surgery?

2. Which postoperative complications are most likely to be minimized or prevented by having clients participate in their own care?

3. How can the client's satisfaction with care affect the client's rate of recovery?

4. If you were to have surgery tomorrow, what would you want your nurse to tell you?

5. What effects can preadmission teaching have on the hospital experience?

- Anticipated postoperative routine and devices or equipment (drains, tubes, equipment for intravenous infusions, oxygen or humidifying mask, dressings, splints, casts)
- Plans for postoperative pain control

Preparation the Day of Surgery A *preoperative surgical checklist* serves as an outline for finalizing preparation of the client for surgery (Figure 7–2). The nurse completes the checklist before the client is transported to surgery. Nursing responsibilities the day of surgery include the following:

- Assist with bathing, grooming, and changing into operating room gown.
- Ensure that the client takes nothing by mouth (NPO).
- Provide additional teaching, and reinforce prior teaching.
- Remove nail polish, lipstick, and make-up to facilitate circulatory assessment during and after surgery.
- Ensure that identification, blood, and allergy bands are correct, legible, and secure.
- Remove hair pins and jewelry; a wedding ring may be worn if it is removed from the finger, covered with gauze, and then taped to the finger.

- Complete skin or bowel preparation as ordered.
- Insert an indwelling catheter, intravenous line, or nasogastric tube as ordered.
- Remove dentures, artificial eye, and contact lenses, and store them in a safe place.
- Leave a hearing aid in place if the client cannot hear without it, and notify the operating room nurse.
- Verify that the informed consent has been signed prior to administering preoperative medications.
- Verify that the client's height and weight are recorded in the chart (for dosage of anesthesia).
- Verify that all ordered laboratory and diagnostic test reports are in the chart.
- Have the client empty the bladder immediately before the preoperative medication is administered (unless an indwelling catheter is in place).
- Administer preoperative medication as scheduled. (Refer to the Preoperative Pharmacology section earlier in the chapter for commonly prescribed preoperative medications.)
- Ensure the safety of the client once the medication has been given by placing the client on bed rest with the side rails up and by placing the call light within reach.

Preoperative Client Teaching

Diaphragmatic Breathing Exercise

Diaphragmatic (abdominal) breathing exercises are taught to the client who is at risk for developing pulmonary complications, such as atelectasis or pneumonia. Risk factors for pulmonary complications include general anesthesia, abdominal or thoracic surgery, history of smoking, chronic lung disease, obesity, and advanced age.

In diaphragmatic breathing, the client inspires deeply while allowing the abdomen to expand outward. On expiration, the abdomen contracts inward as air from the lungs is expelled.

1. Explain to the client that the diaphragm is a muscle that makes up the floor of the abdominal cavity and assists in breathing. The purpose of diaphragmatic breathing is to promote lung expansion and ventilation and enhance blood oxygenation.
2. Position the client in a high or semi-Fowler's position (see figure below).
3. Ask the client to place the hands lightly on the abdomen.
4. Instruct the client to breathe in deeply through the nose, allowing the chest and abdomen to expand.
5. Have the client hold the breath for a count of 5.
6. Tell the client to exhale completely through pursed (puckered) lips, allowing the chest and abdomen to deflate.

7. Have the client repeat the exercise five times consecutively.

Encourage the client to perform diaphragmatic breathing exercises every 1 to 2 waking hours, depending on the client's needs and institutional protocol.

Coughing Exercise

Coughing exercises are also taught to the client who is at risk for developing pulmonary complications. The purpose of coughing is to loosen, mobilize, and remove pulmonary secretions. Splinting the incision decreases the physical and psychologic discomfort associated with coughing.

1. Assist the client in following steps 1 through 4 for diaphragmatic breathing.
2. Ask the client to splint the incision with interlocked hand or pillow (see figure below).
3. Tell the client to take three deep breaths and then cough forcefully.
4. Have the client repeat the exercise five times consecutively every 2 hours while awake, taking short rest periods between coughs, if necessary.

Leg, Ankle, and Foot Exercises

Leg exercises are taught to the client who is at risk for developing thrombophlebitis (inflammation of a vein,

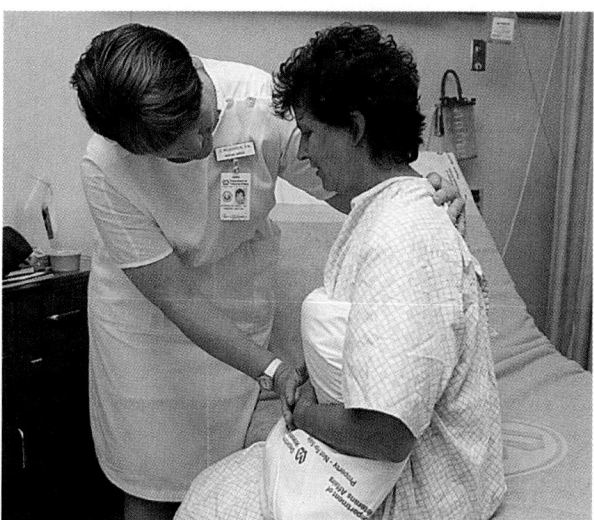

Diaphragmatic breathing exercise.

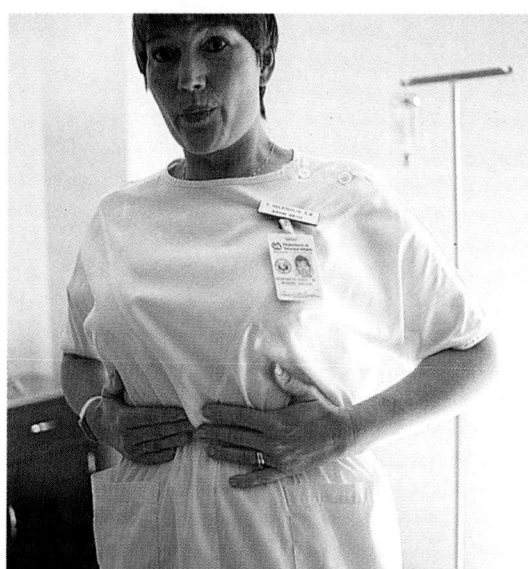

Splinting abdomen while coughing.

▶

Preoperative Client Teaching *Continued*

■ ■ ■

which is associated with the formation of blood clots). Risk factors for developing thrombophlebitis include decreased mobility preoperatively and/or postoperatively; a history of difficulties with peripheral circulation; and cardiovascular, pelvic, or lower extremity surgeries.

The purpose of leg exercises is to promote venous blood return from the extremities. As the leg muscles contract and relax, blood is pumped back to the heart, promoting circulation and reducing venous stasis. These exercises also maintain muscle tone and range of motion, which facilitate early ambulation.

Teach the client to perform the following exercises while lying in bed:

1. Muscle pumping exercise: Contract and relax calf and thigh muscles at least ten times consecutively.

2. Leg exercises:
   a. Bend the knee and raise it toward the chest (see figure below).
   b. Straighten out leg and hold for a few seconds before lowering the leg back to the bed.
   c. Repeat exercise five times consecutively prior to alternating to the other foot.

3. Ankle and foot exercises:
   a. Rotate both ankles by making complete circles, first to the right and then to the left (see figure below).
   b. Repeat five times and then relax.
   c. With feet together, point toes toward the head and then to the foot of the bed (see figure below).
   d. Repeat this pumping action ten times, and then relax.

Encourage the client to perform leg, ankle, and foot exercises every 1 to 2 hours while awake, depending on the client's needs and ambulatory status, the physician's preference, and institutional protocol.

Turning in Bed

The client who is at risk for circulatory, respiratory, or gastrointestinal dysfunction following surgery is taught to turn in bed. Although this may be a simple task prior to surgery, after surgery (particularly after abdominal surgery) the client may find it a difficult procedure. To make the procedure more comfortable, the client may need to splint the incision using the hand placed on a small pillow or blanket. Additionally, the client should be taught that analgesics can be given to ease postoperative discomfort involved with turning. Encourage the client to turn every 2 hours while awake.

1. Tell the client to grasp the side rail toward the direction to be turned, to rest the opposite foot on the mattress, and to bend the knee.

2. Instruct the client to roll over in one smooth motion by pulling on the side rail while pushing off with the bent knee.

3. Pillows may need to be positioned behind the client's back to help the client maintain a side-lying position. The older client may also need padding over pressure points between the knees and ankles to decrease the chance of decubitus ulcer formation from pressure.

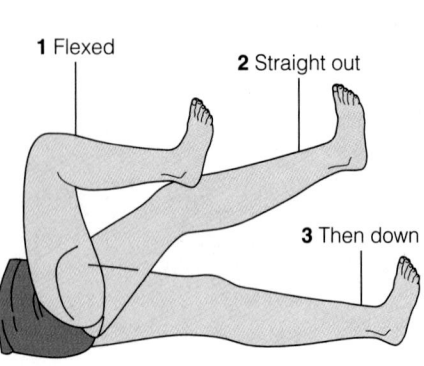

1 Flexed **2** Straight out **3** Then down

Leg exercises.

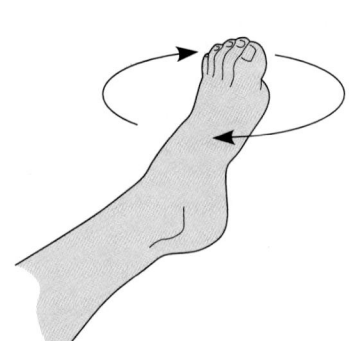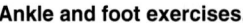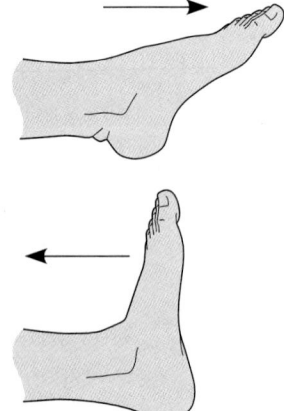

Ankle and foot exercises.

PRE-ADMISSION TESTING/ PRE-OP SURGICAL CHECKLIST

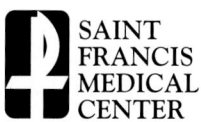

SAINT FRANCIS MEDICAL CENTER

PRE-OPERATIVE CHECKLIST

Arrival to Holding Room _____ To OR _____

OR Transport Tech _____ OR # _____

Nurse sending Patient to OR _____

OR	Date	ZONE/UNIT
	Review PATT Sheet with Patient _____	
	Alert & oriented _____	
	Pt. identifies self, surgery, surgeon	
	NPO since _____	
	ID bracelet, allergy bracelet, blood band	
	Operative consent signed, IOL permit	
	Shave Prep as appropriate	
	H & P: chart _____ dict _____ Med R. Call _____	
	Lab reports (as ordered):	
	CBC/Hgb ____ & Hct ____ on chart ____ pending ____	
	Urinalysis ____ ____	
	Culture & Sens. ____ ____	
	Profile/Lytes ____ ____	
	BUN/Creat./Kt + ____ ____ ____	
	Acid Phos. ____ ____	
	T3/T4 ____ ____	
	PT/PTT/Bleed Time ____ ____	
	Type Screen/Cross ____ ____	
	Autologous blood _____ # units _____	
	Blood release date _____ Other _____	
	Accucheck Blood Sugar Pre-op _____	
	Abnormal labs reported to: _____ when: _____	
	Pulmonary Functions as Ordered _____	
	Chest X-ray: report on chart ____ pending ____ on cart ____	
	report to: _____ x-rays called for _____	
	Other: _____	
	EKG report: on chart _____ pending _____ tracing _____	
	Anesthesia visit by: _____	
	Dentures: removed _____ family _____ locked _____	
	Glass/Con: removed _____ family _____ locked _____	
	Jewelry: taped _____ to family _____	
	Valuables to family _____ to Bus. Office _____	
	Makeup/Nailpolish, hairpins removed _____	
	Voided _____ Catheter _____	
	Pneumatic boots _____ TEDS _____ Leggins _____	
	Pre-Op Medication _____ Antibiotics _____	
	Old records to OR with patient _____	
	Family to WR _____ No family present _____	

ADDRESSOGRAPH

PRE-ADMISSION TESTING

PAT/Teaching completed per guidelines ____ Pre-op phone call completed ____

Patient/family indicates understanding _____

Pamphlets Provided:

SDS Patient Guide _____ Total Joint _____ T & A _____

Caring for You - Anesthesia _____ Surgery at SFMC _____

Neurosurgery _____ Hello Tubes _____ Ped. Hernia _____

Cysto _____ Fractures _____ Other: _____

Video:

You and Your Surgery _____ Cholecystectomy _____ Pediatric _____

ESWL ____ Understanding Total Hip/Knee ____ Other: _____

Nurse specialist visit: _____ Physical Therapy per order/policy _____

Previous P.T. instructions per Patient _____

Instructions Given:

NPO after: MN _____ Liquid Breakfast _____ Avoid Alcohol _____

Appropriate dress _____ Bra _____ No makeup/nailpolish/jewelry _____

Bring a driver _____ Shower _____ Shampoo _____ Scrub _____

Hibiclens _____ Phisohex _____ Phisoderm _____ Other _____

Laxative ____ Enema ____ Douche ____ Eye drops ____ Pre-op office visit ____

Adequate home care available? _____

Problems/concerns _____

Referrals _____

Notes: _____

_____

RN _____

Post-Op Phone Call: Date _____

No Problems Indicated _____ No Answer _____

Referral _____

Temp _____ Pulse _____ Resp _____ BP sup./sit _____

IV of _____ started/intact with # ____ Angio x # ____ Attempts ____

Site _____ RN _____

Pt. to OR per standards of care _____

Holding Room Nurse

Pulse Oximeter used _____ Strip on Chart _____

Notes: _____

_____

_____

_____

_____

_____

_____

Figure 7–2 Preoperative checklist.

PRE-OP NURSING NOTES

HC	LAB	B/P	TEMP
PULSE	RESP	HT	WT

ABN LAB REPORTED TO:	☐ N/A

LAST VOIDED TIME:

MENTAL STATUS ☐ Alert ☐ Responsive ☐ Not Responsive

☐ Confused ☐ Apprehensive

ID BAND CORRECT?	☐ YES	☐ NO
CONSENTS WRITTEN CORRECTLY?	☐ YES	☐ NO
PT CONFIRMS SURGERY/SITE AND SIDE?	☐ YES	☐ NO

NPO ☐ AFTER MIDNIGHT ☐ AFTER 0700 ☐ N/A

ALLERGIES ☐ NKA ☐ YES ☐ ALLERGY BAND

SMOKER ☐ YES ☐ NO

DENTURES ☐ CAPS ☐ GLASSES ☐ CONTACTS

RINGS ☐ PT WEARING

PRE-OPERATIVE CALL / DISCHARGE PLAN

Date _____

TIME 1st _____ 2nd _____ Spoke to _____

No anticipated needs after discharge ☐

Discussed discharge plans with pt. / S.O. ☐

Comments _____

Interviewed by _____ Reassessed by _____

Sponsor _____ Phone # _____

PRE-OPERATIVE NURSING ASSESSMENT   BY: DATE:

1 History of Diseases   Do you have any of the following?

a LUNG

_____ Bronchitis

_____ Emphysema

_____ Asthma

_____ TB

_____ Sinusitis

_____ Respiratory Infections

VASCULAR

_____ High Blood Pressure

_____ Heart Attack

_____ Heart Murmur

_____ Circulation Problems

_____ Heart Disease

_____ Sickle-Cell

SYSTEMIC

_____ Diabetes

_____ Endocrine

_____ Kidney/Bladder Problems

_____ Alcohol

_____ Stomach/Bowel Problems

_____ Hepatitis

_____ Convulsions

_____ Fainting

_____ Glaucoma

_____ Motion Sickness

b OTHER Last menstrual period _____

Other Medical Problems _____

_____

_____

Bleeding Tendencies _____

2 Drug History   Have you taken any of the following drugs in the last six months?

_____ Diuretics

_____ Hormones

_____ Steroids

_____ Anti-coagulants

_____ Tranquilizers

_____ Thyroid Medications

_____ Birth Control Pills

_____ Aspirin

_____ Narcotics

_____ Blood Pressure Medicines

_____ Antibiotics

_____ Arthritis Medications

_____ Diabetic Medicines

_____ Heart Medications

Other (specify) _____

_____

_____

ALLERGIES: _____

_____

_____

3 Personal History   (Include complications if indicated)

a Prior Surgery Date(s) _____

b Prior Anesthesia Date(s) _____

c Skin Integrity _____

d Physical Limitations/ROM _____

IV	SOLUTION	QUANTITY/cc ☐ 500ml ☐ 1000ml	WHEAL SALINE ☐ XYLOCAINE 5 ☐	GAUGE	LENGTH	SITE LT/RT ARM / HAND	NURSE

TIME	MEDICATION AMOUNT	ROUTE	GIVEN BY	ORDERED BY	SIGNATURE

NOTES

Figure 7–3 Preoperative nursing notes.

- Obtain and record vital signs.

- Provide ongoing supportive care to the client and the client's family.

- Document all preoperative care in the appropriate location, such as the preoperative surgical checklist, the medication record, or the narrative preoperative nursing notes (Figure 7–3).

- Verify with the surgical personnel the client's identity, and verify that all information is documented appropriately.

- Assist the surgical personnel in transferring the client from the bed to the gurney.

- Prepare the client's room for postoperative care, including making the surgical bed and ensuring that the anticipated supplies and equipment are in the room.

Intraoperative Nursing Care

The intraoperative phase of surgery begins when the client enters the operating room and ends when the client is transferred to the post-anesthesia recovery room (PACU). In the operating room, all of the surgical team members have a vital role in the overall success of the procedure. The surgeon and anesthesiologist maintain primary roles, but the nurses collaborating with the physicians are responsible for maintaining the safety of the client and the environment and providing physiologic monitoring and psychologic support (Figure 7–4).

Members of the Surgical Team   Because of the complexity of the intraoperative environment, members of the surgical team must function as a coordinated unit. The surgeon, surgical assistant(s), anesthesiologist or certified registered nurse anesthetist, circulating nurse, and scrub nurse or operating room technician constitute the surgical team. Each member provides specialized skills and is essential to the successful outcome of the surgery.

The *surgeon* is the physician performing the procedure. As head of the surgical team, all medical actions and judgments are the surgeon's responsibility.

The *surgical assistant* works closely with the surgeon in performing the operation. The number of assistants varies according to the complexity of the procedure. The assistant may be another physician, a nurse, a physician's assistant, or other trained personnel. The assistant performs such duties as exposing the operative site, retracting nearby tissue, sponging and/or suctioning the wound, ligating bleeding vessels, and suturing or assisting with suturing of the surgical wound.

The *anesthesiologist* or the *certified registered nurse anesthetist (CRNA)* relieves the surgeon of the responsibility for the client's general well-being, thus allowing the surgeon to focus on the technical aspects of the procedure. The anesthesiologist or CRNA evaluates the client preoperatively, administers the anesthesia and other required medications, transfuses blood or other blood products,

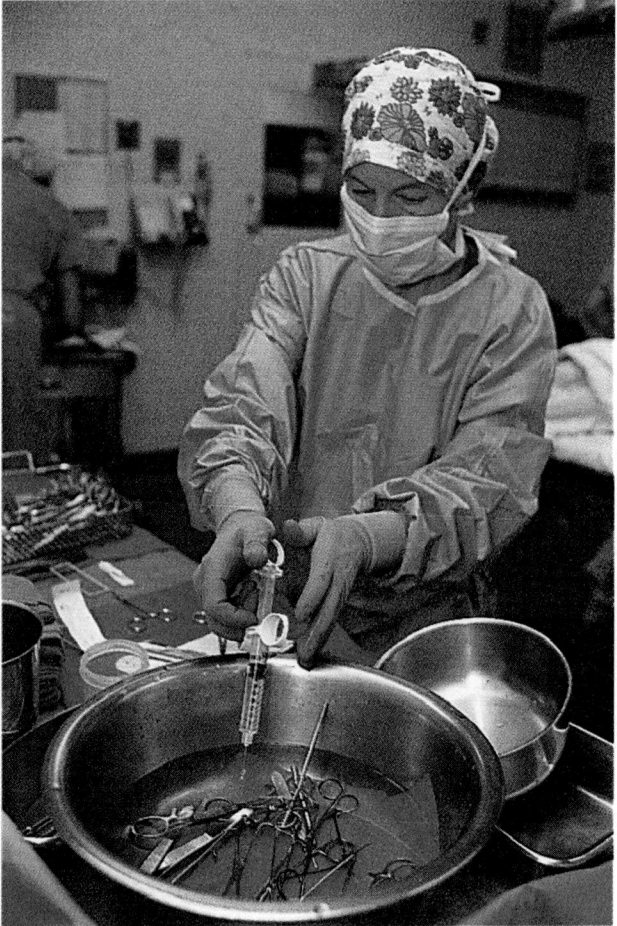

Figure 7–4   A scrub nurse in the operating room.

infuses intravenous fluids, continuously monitors the client's physiologic status, alerts the surgeon to developing problems and treats them as they may arise, and supervises the client's recovery in the PACU.

The *circulating nurse* is a highly experienced registered nurse who coordinates and manages a wide range of activities before, during, and after the surgical procedure. For example, the circulating nurse oversees the physical aspects of the operating room itself, including the equipment. The circulating nurse also assists with transferring and positioning the client, prepares the client's skin, ensures that no break in aseptic technique occurs, and counts all sponges and instruments. The circulating nurse assists all other team members, including the anesthesiologist or CRNA. Thorough documentation in the surgical area is essential, and the circulating nurse is responsible for documenting intraoperative nursing activities, medications, blood administration, placement of drains and catheters, and length of the procedure. (Figure 7–5 is a sample form for a circulating nurse's operating room notes.) The circulating nurse also formulates a care plan based on physiologic and psychosocial assessments of the

OPERATING ROOM NURSES NOTES

Pt. Name _____ Date _____

ALLERGIES
O.R. # _____
SURGEON(S): _____
ASSISTANT(S): _____
ANESTHESIOLOGIST: _____

	RELIEF	TIME
CIRCULATOR:		
1ST SCRUB:		
2ND SCRUB:		

ANES. TECH.: _____
OBSERVER(S): _____
PRE-OP DIAGNOSIS: _____

POST-OP DIAGNOSIS: _____

OPERATION: _____

ROOM TIME START: _____ END: _____

ANESTHESIA: ☐ General   ☐ Spinal   ☐ Epidural
            ☐ Local   ☐ MAC   ☐ Regional _____
            ☐ Endotracheal Tube ☐ Mask ☐ O₂ via nasal can
            ☐ Nasotracheal Tube

MONITORING DEVICES: ☐ S.A.R.A.   ☐ E.K.G.
                    ☐ Dynamap   ☐ Temp. _____
                    ☐ Pulse Oximeter ☐ Other _____

SURGICAL POSITION: ☐ Supine   ☐ Prone   Lateral:
                   ☐ Rt   ☐ Left _____
                   ☐ Lithotomy ☐ Jackknife   ☐ Other

TABLE: ☐ Amsco   ☐ Reliance

POSITIONAL AIDS: ☐ N/A   ☐ Head Pillow   ☐ Chest Rolls
                ☐ Bean Bag _____ ☐ Head Foam Pad
                ☐ Tape ☐ Ax. Roll ☐ Sandbag ☐ Foam Pads ☐ Gel
                Pads ___ ☐ Pillow Knees   ☐ Chan Rest
                ☐ Shoulder roll   ☐ Other

PRESSURE POINTS PADDED: ☐ N/A   ☐ Heels   ☐ Elbows
                        ☐ Popliteal   ☐ Other

SAFETY STRAP SECURED: ☐ N/A   ☐ Yes
        RT. ARM: ☐ Side ☐ Armboard ☐ Chest ☐ Support
        LT. ARM: ☐ Side ☐ Armboard ☐ Chest ☐ Support
        LEGS: ☐ Legs Uncrossed   ☐ Other

EQUIPMENT: ☐ N/A   ☐ Microscope   ☐ Video
    Laser ☐ Type _____ ☐ Other _____
    Hyperthermia Unit# _____ Temp. _____

ELECTROSURGICAL UNIT: ☐ N/A Unit # _____
        ☐ Monopolar   ☐ Bipolar   ☐ Ground
        ☐ COAG   ☐ CUT
        Skin Condition Post-op   ☐ WNL   ☐ See Comments

TOURNIQUET: ☐ N/A   ☐ Yes # _____
        LOCATION: ☐ Rt. Arm   ☐ Lt. Arm   ☐ Rt. Thigh
                  ☐ Left Thigh ☐ Rt. Calf ☐ Lt. Calf
        PRESSURE: (mm/Hg) _____ Skin Cond. Post-op ☐ WNL
        ☐ See Comments
        #1 Time Up _____ Time Down _____ Total _____ min.
        #2 Time Up _____ Time Down _____ Total _____ min.

PREP: ☐ N/A Solution: _____
        #1 _____ By: _____
        #2 _____ By: _____

MEDICATIONS GIVEN OTHER THAN BY ANESTHESIA:
☐ N/A _____

MED	ROUTE	ADMIN. BY

IRRIGATION SOLUTIONS: ☐ N/A   ☐ NaCl _____ cc
                      ☐ Ringer's   ☐ Other

URINARY DRAINAGE: ☐ N/A   ☐ Straight Cath
        Size _____ Fr. FOLEY: Size _____
        Inserted by: _____
        ☐ In place on arrival to O.R. _____
TOTAL OUTPUT IN O.R. _____ cc

PROSTHESIS/IMPLANTS: ☐ N/A _____
_____
_____
_____
_____
_____
_____

DRAINS: ☐ N/A   ☐ Jackson Pratt   ☐ Other _____
Site: _____

PACKING: ☐ N/A   ☐ Plain   ☐ Vaseline   ☐ Iodoform
            ☐ Adaptic ☐ Other _____
Site: _____

CASTING MATERIAL: ☐ N/A ☐ Plaster ☐ Fibercast ☐ OCL
SPLINT: ☐ Arm   ☐ Leg   CAST: ☐ Arm ☐ Long Leg ☐ Short Leg
                                ☐ Other _____
X-RAYS TAKEN IN O.R.   ☐ No   ☐ Yes ☐ Fluoroscan

BLOOD ADMINISTERED: ☐ N/A ☐ Autologous ☐ Other _____

COUNTS:	CIRCULATOR	SCRUB
SPONGES: ☐ N/A		
#1 ☐ Correct ☐ Not Correct _____		
#2 ☐ Correct ☐ Not Correct _____		
(If not correct, document) _____		
SHARPS: ☐ N/A _____		
#1 ☐ Correct ☐ Not Correct _____		
#2 ☐ Correct ☐ Not Correct _____		
INSTRUMENTS: ☐ N/A		
☐ Correct ☐ Not Correct _____		

WOUND CLASSIFICATION: ☐ I ☐ II ☐ III ☐ IV

ESTIMATED BLOOD LOSS: _____ cc

DRESSING: _____

CULTURE: ☐ Yes   ☐ No _____
SOURCE: _____
SPECIMEN: ☐ Yes   ☐ No   ☐ FS Source: _____
_____

REPORT GIVEN TO: _____
TRANSPORTED TO: ☐ PACU ☐ OBS _____
    VIA: ☐ PACU Bed ☐ Hospital Bed ☐ Reliance Stretcher
DENTURES: ☐ N/A ☐ Upper ☐ Lower ☐ Partial ☐ In ☐ Out
OTHER PROSTHESIS: ☐ N/A _____
RECEIVED BY: _____
PERIOPERATIVE NOTES/NURSE'S SIGNATURE: _____
_____

Figure 7–5 Operating room nurse's notes.

client. Finally, the circulating nurse is at all times an advocate for the safety and well-being of the client.

The role of the *scrub nurse* primarily involves technical skills, manual dexterity, and in-depth knowledge of the anatomic and mechanical aspects of a particular surgery. The scrub nurse handles sutures, instruments, and other equipment immediately adjacent to the sterile field. Although the title implies that the person who performs these duties is a nurse, the role of the scrub nurse may also be assumed by an *operating room technician (ORT),* depending on hospital policy and the complexity of the surgery.

The role of nurses in surgery continues to evolve to improve client care. In recent years, nurses have begun to specialize within the already specialized field of perioperative nursing. Specialty surgical teams have developed in response to the demands of increasingly complex technical surgeries. For example, a designated open heart surgical team may be responsible for all open heart cases and ordinarily not be involved with other procedures. The use of specialty surgical teams allows nurses to become highly skilled in a particular range of procedures.

Surgical Attire   Strict dress codes are necessary in the surgical department to provide infection control within the operating room suites, reduce cross-contamination between the surgery department and other hospital units or departments, and promote both personnel and client health and safety. All personnel in the surgical department must be in proper surgical attire. The design and composition of the surgical attire minimize bacterial shedding, thus reducing wound contamination.

The area in the surgical department is divided into unrestricted, semirestricted, and restricted zones. The *unrestricted zones* permit access by those in hospital uniforms or street clothes. These areas may also allow limited access for communicating with operating room personnel.

The *semirestricted zones* require scrub attire, including a scrub suit, shoe covers, and a cap or hood (Figure 7–6, *A*). Hallways, work areas, and storage areas are considered semirestricted.

Restricted zones are located within operating rooms. Personnel wear masks, sterile gowns, and gloves in addition to appropriate scrub attire (Figure 7–6, *B*). The entire surgical attire is changed between procedures or whenever it becomes soiled or wet.

The Surgical Scrub   The *surgical scrub* is performed to render hands and arms as clean as possible in preparation for a procedure. All personnel who participate directly in the procedure must perform a surgical scrub with a brush and antimicrobial soap. Skin cannot be rendered sterile, but it can be considered "surgically clean" following the scrub. The purposes of the surgical scrub are to

- Remove dirt, skin oils, and transient microorganisms from hands and forearms.

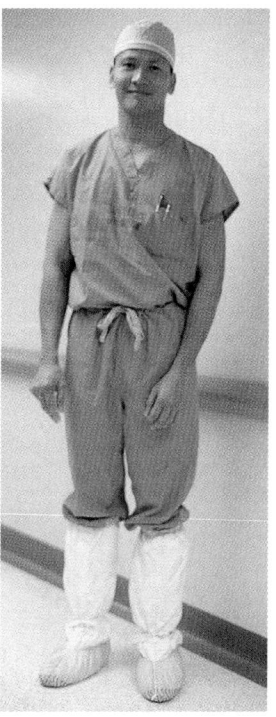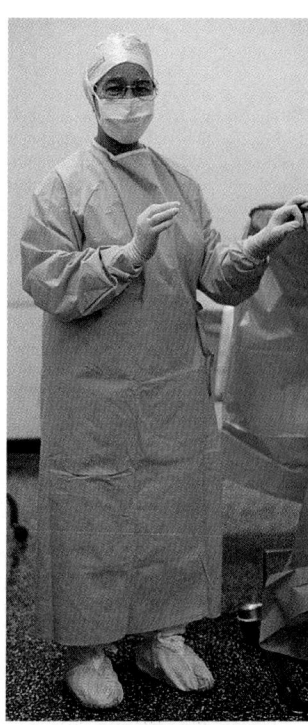

Figure 7–6   Surgical attire. *A,* Scrub attire includes scrub suit, shoe covers, and cap or hood to cover hair. *B,* Sterile attire includes scrub suit, shoe covers, and cap or hood, plus gown, gloves, and mask.

- Increase client safety by reducing microorganisms on surgical personnel.
- Leave an antimicrobial residue on the skin to inhibit growth of microbes for several hours.

Following the 5- to 10-minute surgical scrub, hands and arms are dried with sterile towels.

Preparing the Client   Although much preparation has taken place prior to the client's transfer to the surgical department, additional activities, such as shaving and positioning, may be performed. The skin preparation, which usually includes cleansing the area with a prescribed antimicrobial agent, already may have been performed, either by the client or by nursing personnel, prior to the transfer to the surgical department. Additional skin cleansing is performed in the surgical department to further decrease microorganisms on the skin and thereby reduce the possibility of wound infection.

The surgeon also may order the skin shaved in and around the proposed incision area (Figure 7–7). Shaving may be completed preoperatively, but more often it is performed in the surgical department. The extent to which the area is shaved varies. Generally, the area shaved is wider than the planned incision because of the possibility of unexpected extension of the incision. Disposable, sterile supplies are used, in accordance with aseptic techniques. However, the benefit of shaving the incisional site has become a controversial issue. Physical trauma to the

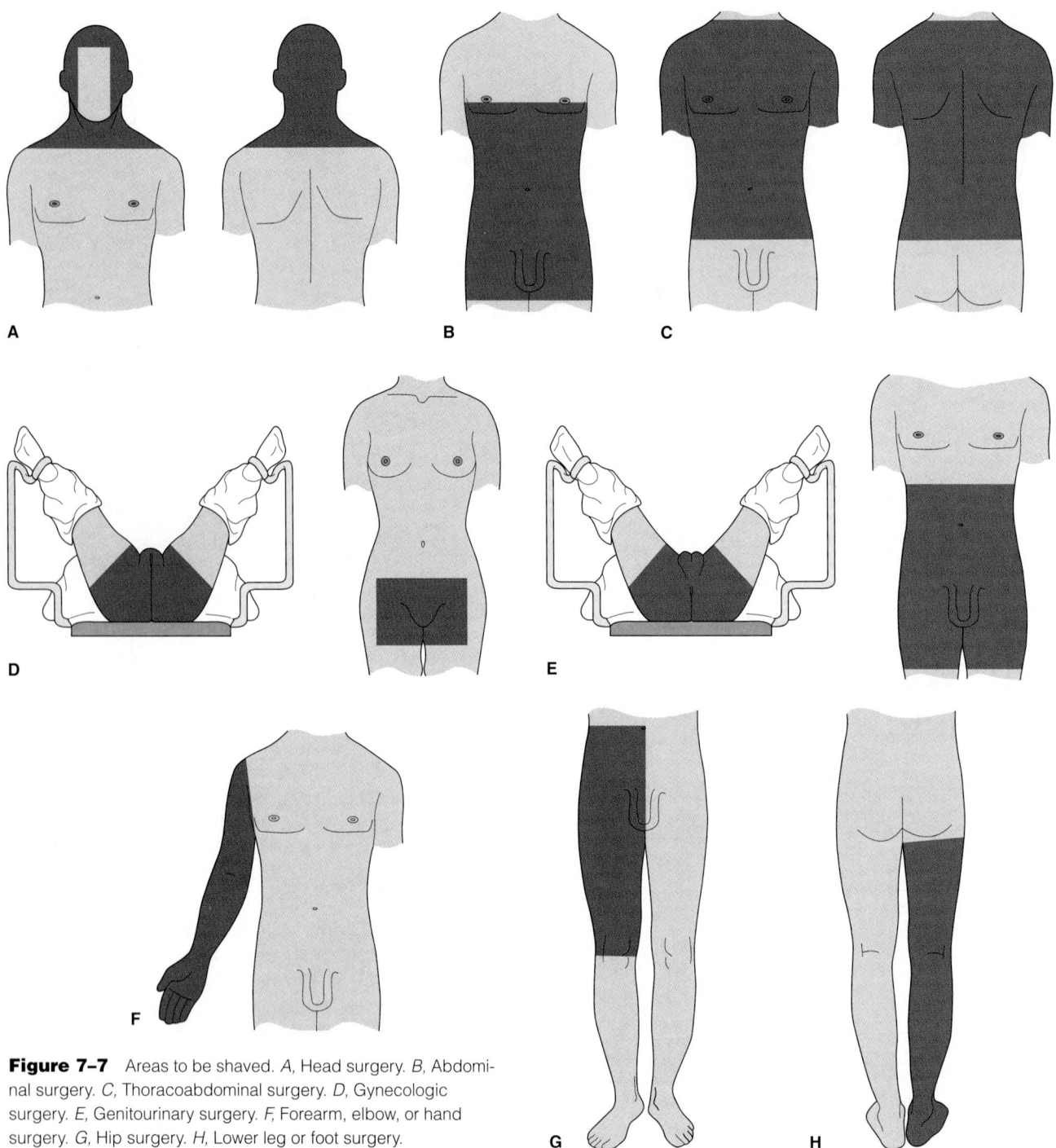

Figure 7–7 Areas to be shaved. *A*, Head surgery. *B*, Abdominal surgery. *C*, Thoracoabdominal surgery. *D*, Gynecologic surgery. *E*, Genitourinary surgery. *F*, Forearm, elbow, or hand surgery. *G*, Hip surgery. *H*, Lower leg or foot surgery.

shaved area can weaken the client's defense against organisms, thus increasing the chance of wound infection. An altered body image also may result from the physiologic trauma of a surgical shave, particularly if the shave involves the head or groin area. Hospital policy and surgeon preference should be followed.

Preparing the client for surgery also includes positioning the client on the operating table. Table 7–5 shows frequently used positions and describes corresponding surgical procedures and possible adverse effects. Positioning allows for exposure of the operative site and access for administration of anesthesia. Proper positioning is imperative to prevent injury to the client. Pressure, rubbing, and/or shearing forces can cause injury to the tissue over bony prominences. If positioning causes normal joint range of motion to be exceeded, injury to muscles and joints can occur. Improper positioning also can lead to sensory and motor dysfunction, resulting in nerve damage. Pressure on peripheral blood vessels can decrease venous return to the heart and negatively affect the client's

Table 7–5   Common Surgical Positions

Position and Use	Possible Adverse Effects and Nursing Interventions
(a) The *dorsal recumbent* (or *supine*) *position* is used for many abdominal surgeries (e.g., colostomy and herniorrhaphy) as well as for some thoracic surgeries (e.g., open heart surgery) and some surgeries on the extremities. 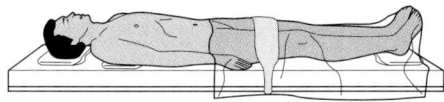	This position may cause excessive pressure on posterior bony prominences, such as the back of the head, scapulae, sacrum, and heels. Pad these areas with soft materials. To avoid compression of blood vessels and sluggish circulation, ensure that the knees are not flexed. Use trochanter rolls or other padding to avoid internal or external rotation of the hips and shoulders.
(b) The *semi-sitting position* is used for surgeries on the thyroid and neck areas. 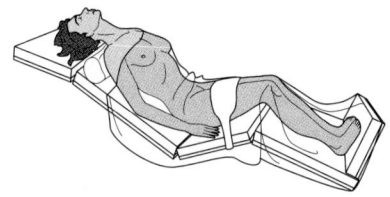	This position can lead to postural hypotension and venous pooling in the legs. It may promote skin breakdown on the buttocks. Sciatic nerve injury is possible. Assess for hypotension. Ensure that knees are not sharply flexed. Use soft padding to prevent nerve compression.
(c) The *prone position* is used for spinal fusions and removal of hemorrhoids. 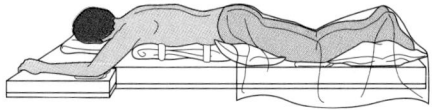	This position causes pressure on the face, knees, thighs, anterior ankles, and toes. Pad bony prominences, and support the feet under the ankles. To promote optimum respiratory function, raise the client's chest and abdomen, and support with padding. Corneal abrasion could occur if the eyes are not closed or are insufficiently padded.
(d) The *lateral chest position* is used for some thoracic surgeries, as well as hip replacements. 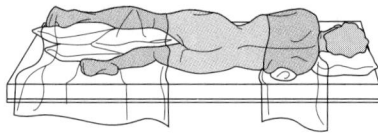	This may cause excessive pressure on the bony prominences on the side on which the client is positioned. Ensure adequate padding and support, especially of the downside arm. The weight of the upper leg may cause peroneal nerve injury on the downside leg. Both legs must therefore be padded.
(e) The *lithotomy position* is used for gynecologic, perineal, or rectal surgeries. 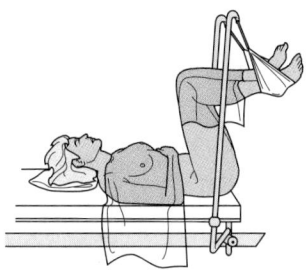	This position causes an 18% decrease (from a standing position) in vital capacity of the lungs. Monitor respirations, and assess for hypoxia and dyspnea. The lithotomy position can lead to joint damage, peroneal nerve damage, and damage to peripheral blood vessels. To avoid injury, ensure adequate padding, and manipulate both legs into the stirrups simultaneously.
(f) The *jackknife position* is used for proctologic surgeries, such as removal of hemorrhoids. 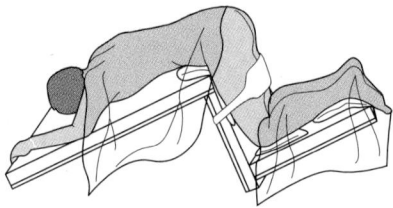	This position causes a 12% decrease (from a standing position) in vital capacity of the lungs. Monitor respirations, and assess for hypoxia and dyspnea. In this position, the greatest pressure is felt at the bends in the table. Therefore, the client is supported with pads at the groin and knees, as well as at the ankles. Padding of the chest and knees helps prevent skin breakdown. Padding and proper positioning help prevent pressure on the ear, the neck, and the nerves of the upper arm.

blood pressure. Additionally, oxygenation of the blood can be decreased if the client is not properly positioned to promote lung expansion.

Because the client is anesthetized and therefore cannot respond to discomfort, it is the surgical team's responsibility to position the client not only for the best surgical advantage but also for client safety and comfort. The circulating nurse refers to hospital policy, the surgeon's preference, and the client's history to ensure optimal positioning and continuously assesses the client.

Intraoperative Awareness Prior to induction of anesthesia, the circulating nurse establishes rapport with the client to assess the client's psychologic status. This assessment is continued throughout the surgical procedure. After anesthetic medications have been given, the client may appear oblivious to the surroundings; however, studies have shown that the client's awareness during the intraoperative period may be greater than once believed (Schultetus, 1987). *Intraoperative awareness* is the client's subconscious awareness of what is being said and done during surgery. Although most clients do not consciously remember what happened or what was said, psychologic trauma can result. Because there is no reliable method of preventing this phenomenon, conversations during surgery should be maintained on a professional level (Schultetus, 1987). Nothing should be said while the client is unconscious that would not be said if the client were awake.

Special Considerations for the Older Adult Because of cardiovascular and tissue changes that result from aging, surgeries lasting longer than 2 hours place the older adult at increased risk for complications. The older adult is more prone to hypotension, hypothermia, and hypoxemia resulting from anesthesia and the cool temperature in the operating room.

Other complications experienced by the older adult result from positioning. Intraoperative positioning of arthritic joints can account for postoperative joint pain that is unrelated to the operative site. Also, the longer the surgery, the greater the chance of decubitus ulcer (pressure sore) formation. The older client is at increased risk for developing pressure sores because of decreased subcutaneous fat tissue and reduced peripheral circulation.

Finally, the older adult often has some degree of hearing and/or visual impairment. These impairments coupled with a strange environment can make the operating room a frightening, disorienting place. By effectively communicating with the client, the nurse can provide support and reassurance to minimize these factors. To decrease confusion and assist in communication, hearing aids and glasses should be used when appropriate and possible.

Postoperative Nursing Care

Immediate Postoperative Care Immediate postoperative care begins when the client has been transferred from the operating room to the PACU. The nurse monitors the client's vital signs and surgical site to determine the response to the surgical procedure and to detect significant changes. Assessing mental status and level of consciousness is another ongoing nursing responsibility, and the client may require repeated orientation to time, place, and person. Emotional support also is essential, because the client is in a vulnerable and dependent position. Assessing and evaluating hydration status by monitoring intake and output is crucial to detecting cardiovascular or renal complications. In addition, the PACU nurse assesses the client's pain level. Careful administration of analgesics provides comfort yet does not compound the potential side effects from the anesthesia.

Continuing Postoperative Care After the client is stabilized and awakens, the client is transferred to his or her room. The PACU nurse communicates specific information regarding the client's condition and postoperative orders to the floor nurse prior to the client's arrival. This prepares the floor nurse for any additional problems or needed equipment.

Immediate and continuing assessment is essential to detect and/or prevent complications. In documenting assessment findings, the nurse completes a flow record specific to the individual client's situation. See Figure 7–8 for an example of a flow record used for clients undergoing common surgical procedures. Baseline data are obtained and compared to preoperative data. A postoperative head-to-toe assessment includes but may not be limited to the following:

- General appearance
- Vital signs
- Level of consciousness
- Emotional status
- Quantity of respirations
- Skin color and temperature
- Discomfort/pain
- Nausea/vomiting
- Type of intravenous fluids and flow rate
- Dressing site
- Drainage on the dressing and/or bed linen
- Urinary output (catheter or ability to urinate)
- Ability to move all extremities

The hospital policy or physician's orders dictate the frequency of follow-up assessments. However, after major

Name _____

M.R. # _____

SAINT FRANCIS MEDICAL CENTER

SPECIAL PROCEDURE FLOW RECORD

DATE AND TIME

PARAMETER											
Blood Pressure											
Pulse											
Respirations											
Temperature											

PROCEDURE KEY

ROUTINE POST-OP:
VS–As Ordered: Include c̄ VS IV–Fluids/Rate; Dressing Site; Drains: LOC; Pain*; Nausea/Vomiting; Output;Turn-Cough-Deep Breathe; Moves All Extremities

ANGIOGRAM:
VS q̄ 15 min x 4, q̄ 30 min x 4 q̄ 1H x 4; Include c̄ VS LOC: Peripheral Pulses; Dressing Site (Bleeding-Hematoma): IV; Output; Thigh Measurement q̄ 2H x 8; Chest Pain*; Neuro Checks c̄ Vital Signs for CEA's to include Speech, Grips, Motor Function of Unaffected Extremity

COLONOSCOPY:
VS–As Ordered: Include c̄ VS Abdominal Pain*; Bowel Sounds; Distention; Rectal Bleeding

PANENDOSCOPY/ERCP:
VS–As ordered: Include c̄ VS Abdominal Pain*; Bowel Sounds; Red or Coffee Ground Emesis

LIVER BIOPSY:
VS–As ordered: Include c̄ VS Biopsy Site (Swelling, Bleeding); Pain*; Referred Pain to RT Shoulder

BRONCH./THORACENTESIS:
VS–As Ordered: Include c̄ VS LOC; SOB; Chest Pain*; Hemoptysis

MYELOGRAM:
VS q̄ 30 min X 2 q̄ 4 hrs x 2; Include c̄ VS Neurological Checks (Excluding Babinskis); Sensation to Extremities; Numbness/Tingling; Nausea/Vomiting; headache; CBR 8/12 hrs HOB ↑30–45° as Ordered; Intake (F.F. 1000 cc/8 hrs); Output; Time of First Voiding

SEIZURE:
Body Part where Seizure began: Generalized/ Focal; Tonic/Clonic; Duration; LOC After: Confusion Drowsiness; Paralysis/Location; Incontinence; Tongue Biting

TONSILLECTOMY:
VS–As Ordered; Include c̄ VS HOB↑; Intake; Ice Collar; Active Bleeding; Pain*

TRACTION:
Type; AMT. of WT.; Length of Time: Proper Alignment, WTS Hanging Freely; Cond. of Pin Sites; Pin Site Care Done: Cond. of Pressure Points; Pts. Tolerance to Treatment

STOOL CHART:
AMT; Color; Consistency; Odor; Obvious Blood; Hemoccult +/-

CONTINUOUS BLADDER IRRIGATION:
Solution; Rate; Urine Color/Character; Pain*; Leakage

*PAIN: IF PRESENT DESCRIBE IN PT. CARE NOTES.

Figure 7–8   Special procedure flow record.

surgery, the nurse generally assesses the client every 15 minutes during the first hour and, if the client is stable, every 30 minutes for the next 2 hours, and then every hour during the subsequent 4 hours. Assessments are then carried out every 4 hours, subject to change according to the client's condition and protocol for the particular surgical procedure.

After carrying out the initial assessment and ensuring the client's safety by lowering the bed, raising the side rails, and placing the call light within reach, the nurse notes the physician's postoperative orders. These orders guide the nurse in the specific care of the postoperative client. For example, the orders specify activity level, diet, medications for pain and nausea, antibiotics, continuation of preoperative medications, frequency of vital sign assessments, administration of intravenous fluids, and laboratory tests, such as hemoglobin and potassium level. In most institutions, orders written prior to surgery must be reordered following surgery because the client's condition is presumed to have changed.

Common Postoperative Complications A number of factors place the client at risk for postoperative complications. Nursing care before, during, and after surgery is aimed at preventing and/or minimizing the effects of these complications. Preoperative care and teaching to decrease postoperative complications have been discussed. The following discussions address postoperative cardiovascular, respiratory, and wound complications, along with problems associated with elimination.

Cardiovascular Complications Common postoperative cardiovascular complications include shock, hemorrhage, deep venous thrombosis, and pulmonary embolism.

Shock is a life-threatening postoperative complication. It results from an insufficient blood flow to vital organs or an inability to use oxygen and nutrients or to rid tissues of waste material. Hypovolemic shock, the most common type of shock in the postoperative client, results from a decrease in circulating fluid volume. Decreased fluid volume develops with blood or plasma loss or, less commonly, from severe prolonged vomiting or diarrhea. Symptoms vary according to the severity of the shock; the greater the loss of fluid volume, the more severe the symptoms. Chapter 6 provides a detailed discussion of nursing care of the client with various types of shock.

Hemorrhage is an excessive loss of blood. A *concealed hemorrhage* occurs internally from a blood vessel that is no longer sutured or cauterized or from a drainage tube that has eroded a blood vessel. An *obvious hemorrhage* occurs externally from a dislodged or ill-formed clot at the wound. Hemorrhage also may result from abnormalities in the blood's ability to clot; these abnormalities may result from a pathologic condition, or they may be a side effect of medications.

Hemorrhage from a venous source oozes out quickly and is dark red, whereas an arterial hemorrhage is characterized by bright red spurts of blood pulsating with each heartbeat. Whether the hemorrhage is from a venous or an arterial source, hypovolemic shock will occur if sufficient blood is lost from the circulation.

Assessment findings commonly observed with hemorrhage depend on the amount and rate of blood loss. Restlessness and anxiety are observed in the early stage of hemorrhage. Frank bleeding will be present if the hemorrhage is external. Symptoms characteristic of shock also will be noted.

Care of the client who is hemorrhaging centers around stopping the bleeding and replenishing the circulating blood volume. Nursing care includes providing care associated with shock as well as one or more of the following:

- Applying one or more sterile gauze pads and a snug pressure dressing to the area

- Applying mechanical pressure with gloved hands (may be necessary for severe external bleeding)

- Preparing client and family for emergency surgery (in severe situations where bleeding cannot be stopped)

Deep venous thrombosis (DVT) is the formation of a thrombus (blood clot) that occurs in association with inflammation in deep veins. This complication most often occurs in the lower extremities of the postoperative client. It may result from the combination of several factors, including trauma during surgery, pressure applied under the knees, and sluggish blood flow during and after surgery. Those clients particularly at risk for developing DVT include those who are over age 40 and who

- Have undergone orthopedic surgery to lower extremities; urologic, gynecologic, or obstetric surgeries; or neurosurgery.

- Have varicose veins.

- Have a history of thrombophlebitis or pulmonary emboli.

- Are obese.

- Have an infection.

- Have a malignancy.

Common assessment findings reveal pain or cramping in the involved calf or thigh. Redness and edema of the entire extremity may occur along with a slightly elevated temperature. A positive *Homans' sign* (pain in the calf on dorsiflexion of the affected foot) may be noted.

Nursing care of the client with DVT focuses on preventing a portion of the clot from dislodging and becoming an embolus (traveling blood clot) circulating to the heart, brain, or lungs; preventing other clots from forming; and supporting the client's own physiologic mechanism for dissolving clots. Nursing care includes the following measures:

- Administer anticoagulants and analgesics as prescribed. (NSAIDs are not usually given along with anticoagulants, because doing so increases the anticoagulant effects.)

- Monitor laboratory values for clotting times.

- Maintain bed rest and keep affected extremity at or above heart level.

- Apply thigh-high antiemboli stockings or devices to stimulate venous return and continuing care based on protocol, if ordered.

- Ensure that the affected area is not rubbed or massaged.

- Apply moist heat as prescribed.

- Record bilateral calf or thigh circumferences every shift.

- Teach and support the client and family.

■ Assess color and temperature of involved extremity every shift.

A *pulmonary embolism* is a dislodged blood clot or other substance that lodges in a pulmonary artery. For the postoperative client with DVT, the threat that a portion of the thrombus may dislodge from the vein wall and travel to the lung, heart, or brain is a constant concern. Early detection of this potentially life-threatening complication depends on the nurse's astute, continuing assessment of the postoperative client.

Common assessment findings of the client experiencing a pulmonary embolism include mild to moderate dyspnea, chest pain, diaphoresis, anxiety, restlessness, rapid respirations and pulse, dysrhythmias, cough, and cyanosis. The severity of the symptoms is determined by the degree of pulmonary vascular blockage. Sudden death can occur if a major pulmonary artery becomes completely blocked.

Stabilizing respiratory and cardiovascular functioning while preventing the formation of additional emboli is of utmost importance in the care of the client with a pulmonary embolism. Nursing care includes the following measures:

■ Immediately notify the physician and nursing supervisor.

■ Frequently assess and record general condition and vital signs.

■ Maintain the client on bed rest, and keep the head of the bed elevated.

■ Provide oxygen as ordered.

■ Administer prescribed intravenous fluids to maintain fluid balance while preventing fluid overload.

■ Administer prescribed anticoagulants.

■ Maintain comfort by administering analgesics and sedatives (use caution to prevent respiratory depression).

■ Provide supportive measures for the client and family.

Refer to Chapter 34 for a detailed discussion of pulmonary embolism.

Respiratory Complications   Common postoperative respiratory complications include pneumonia and atelectasis.

Pneumonia is generally defined as the inflammation of lung tissue. Inflammation is caused either by an infection or by the presence of a foreign substance in the lung, which leads to an infection. A number of factors may be involved in the development of pneumonia, including aspiration infection, retained pulmonary secretions, failure to cough deeply, and impaired cough reflex and decreased mobility.

Common assessment findings of the client with pneumonia include

■ High fever

■ Rapid pulse and respirations

■ Chills (may be present initially)

■ Productive cough (may be present depending on the type of pneumonia)

■ Dyspnea

■ Chest pain

■ Crackles and wheezes

Treating the pulmonary infection, supporting the client's respiratory efforts, promoting lung expansion, and preventing the organisms' spread are the goals in the care of the client with pneumonia. Nursing care includes the following measures:

■ Obtain sputum specimens for culture and sensitivity testing.

■ Position client with the head of the bed elevated.

■ Encourage the client to turn, cough, and perform deep-breathing exercises at least every 2 hours.

■ Assist with incentive spirometry, intermittent positive pressure breathing (IPPB), and/or nebulizer treatments as ordered.

■ Ambulate client as condition permits and as prescribed.

■ Administer oxygen as ordered.

■ Assess vital signs, breath sounds, and general condition.

■ Maintain hydration to help liquefy pulmonary secretions.

■ Administer antibiotics, expectorants, antipyretics, and analgesics as ordered.

■ Provide or assist with frequent oral hygiene.

■ Prevent the spread of microorganisms by teaching proper disposal of tissues, covering mouth when coughing, and good hand-washing technique.

■ Provide supportive measures for the client and family.

Chapter 34 provides a detailed discussion of pneumonia.

Atelectasis is an incomplete expansion or collapse of lung tissue resulting in inadequate ventilation and retention of pulmonary secretions. Assessment findings commonly observed include dyspnea, diminished breath sounds over the affected area, anxiety, restlessness, crackles, and cyanosis.

Promoting lung expansion and systemic oxygenation of tissues is a goal in the care of the client with atelectasis. Nursing care includes the following measures:

■ Position the client with the head of bed elevated.

Primary intention

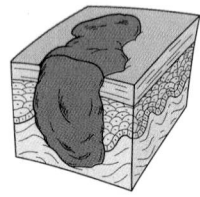 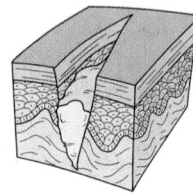 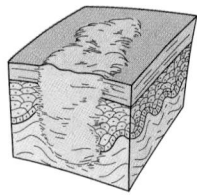

Clean incision   Early suture   "Hairline" scar

Secondary intention

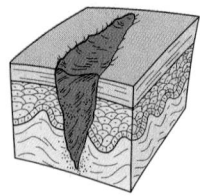 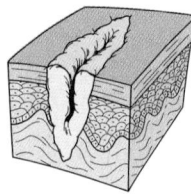 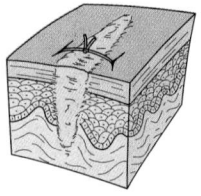

Gaping wound   Granulation tissue   Large scar
with blood clot   fills in wound

Tertiary intention

Contaminated wound   Granulation tissue   Closure with
                                                          wide scar

Figure 7–9   Wound healing by primary, secondary, and tertiary intention.

- Administer oxygen as prescribed.
- Encourage coughing, turning, and deep breathing every 2 hours.
- Ambulate the client as condition permits and as prescribed.
- Assist with incentive spirometry or other pulmonary exercises, such as inflating a balloon, as ordered.
- Administer analgesics as prescribed.
- Promote hydration.
- Provide supportive measures to the client and family.

Complications Associated with Elimination   Common postoperative complications associated with elimination include urinary retention and altered bowel elimination. The inability to urinate with *urinary retention* may occur postoperatively as a result of the recumbent position, effects of anesthesia and narcotics, inactivity, altered fluid balance, nervous tension, or surgical manipulation in the pelvic area. Nursing care centers around promoting nor-

mal urinary elimination and includes the following measures:

- Assess for bladder distention if the client has not voided within 7 to 8 hours after surgery or if the client is urinating small amounts frequently.
- Monitor intake and output.
- Maintain intravenous infusion if fluids are prescribed.
- Increase daily oral fluid intake to 2500 to 3000 mL if the client's condition permits.
- Insert a straight or indwelling catheter if ordered.
- Promote normal urinary elimination by
  a. Assisting and providing privacy when the client uses a bedpan.
  b. Assisting the client in using the bedside commode or ambulating to the bathroom.
  c. Assisting male clients to stand to void.
  d. Pouring a measured amount of warm water over the peritoneal area. (If urination occurs, subtract the amount of water from the total amount for an accurate output measurement.)

Bowel elimination frequently is altered after abdominal or pelvic surgery and sometimes after other surgeries, as well. Return to normal gastrointestinal function may be delayed by general anesthesia, narcotic analgesia, decreased mobility, or altered fluid and food intake during the perioperative period.

Nursing care centers around the return of normal bowel function and includes the following measures:

- Assess for the return of normal peristalsis:
  a. Auscultate bowel sounds every 4 hours while the client is awake.
  b. Assess the abdomen for distention. (A distended abdomen with absent or high-pitched bowel sounds may indicate paralytic ileus.)
  c. Determine whether the client is passing flatus.
  d. Monitor for passage of stool, including amount and consistency.
- Encourage early ambulation within prescribed limits.
- Facilitate a daily fluid intake of 2500 to 3000 mL (unless contraindicated).
- Provide privacy when the client is using the bedpan, bedside commode, or bathroom.

If no bowel movement has occurred by 3 to 4 days after surgery, a suppository or an enema may be ordered.

Wound Complications   Discussion of the complications associated with surgical wounds is preceded by an overview of wound healing, wound drainage, and nursing care of wounds.

Wounds heal by either primary, secondary, or tertiary intention (Figure 7–9). Healing by *primary intention* takes place when the wound is uncomplicated and clean and has sustained little tissue loss. The edges of the incision are well approximated (have come together well) with sutures or staples. This type of surgical incision heals quickly, and very little scarring is expected.

Secondary intention refers to the healing that occurs when the wound is large, gaping, and irregular. Tissue loss prevents wound edges from approximating; therefore, granulation takes place to fill in the wound. This type of wound takes longer to heal, is more prone to infection, and develops more scar tissue.

If enough time passes before a wound is sutured, healing by *tertiary intention* occurs. Infection is more likely to take place. Because the wound edges are not approximated, tissue is regenerated by the granulation process. Closure of the wound results in a wide scar.

From the time the surgical incision is made until the wound is completely healed, all wounds progress through four stages of healing. However, healing time varies according to many factors, such as age, nutritional status, general health, and the type and location of the wound. The accompanying box provides a summary of the stages of wound healing.

Wound drainage (exudate) results from the inflammatory process occurring in the first two stages of wound healing. The drainage is from the rich blood supply that surrounds the wound tissue and is composed of escaped fluid and cells. The drainage is described as serous, sanguineous, or purulent.

- *Serous* drainage contains mostly the clear serous portion of the blood. The drainage appears clear or slightly yellow and is thin in consistency.

- *Sanguineous* drainage contains a combination of serum and red blood cells and has a thick, reddish appearance. This is the most common type of drainage from a noncomplicated surgical wound.

- *Purulent* drainage is composed of white blood cells, tissue debris, and bacteria. Purulent drainage is the result of infection and tends to be of a thicker consistency, with various colors specific to the type of organism. It also may have an unpleasant odor.

The box on page 206 describes and illustrates various types of wound drainage devices. These devices decrease pressure in the wound area by removing excess fluid, which promotes healing and decreases complications.

Nursing care of the postoperative client with a surgical wound focuses on preventing and monitoring for wound complications. The nurse assumes a leading role in supporting the wound-healing process, providing emotional support to the client, and teaching wound care to the client.

Common assessment findings of an infected wound include purulent, odorous discharge and redness, warmth, and edema around the edges of the incision. Ad-

---

Stages of Wound Healing

■ ■ ■

- *Stage I: from surgery through day 2.* Inflammatory process occurs to prepare the surrounding tissue for healing. Blood vessels constrict, and clotting occurs. Vasodilation follows, bringing more blood, white blood cells, and fibroplastin to the wound site. Epithelial cells begin to form and reestablish blood flow in the wound tissue. A mild temperature elevation is normal.

- *Stage II: day 3 through day 14 following surgery.* Fewer white blood cells are present. Collagen tissue forms in the wound tissue. Granulation tissue, red with a rich blood supply, is established.

- *Stage III: day 15 to week 6 following surgery.* Collagen fibers continue to strengthen the wound. As the blood supply decreases, the scar tissue appears pink and somewhat raised.

- *Stage IV: several months to a year following surgery.* As the wound tissue constricts, the scar becomes flat, smaller, and white.

---

ditionally, the client may have a fever, chills, and increased respiratory and pulse rates. Nursing care includes the following measures:

- Maintain medical asepsis (for example, by using a good hand-washing technique).

- Follow Centers for Disease Control (CDC) guidelines for wound care.

- Observe aseptic technique during dressing changes and handling of tubes and drains.

- Assess vital signs, especially temperature.

- Evaluate the characteristics of wound discharge (color, odor, and amount).

- Assess the condition of the incision (approximation of the edges, sutures, staples, or drains).

- Clean, irrigate, and pack the wound in the prescribed manner. Sterile normal saline is often prescribed; povidone-iodine (Betadine) is no longer recommended for wound care.

- Maintain the client's hydration and nutritional status.

- Culture the wound prior to beginning antibiotic therapy.

- Administer antibiotics and antipyretics as prescribed.

- Provide supportive measures to client and family.

Wound Drainage Devices

■ ■ ■

A Penrose drain, used for passive wound drainage, promotes healing from the inside to the outside (see figure A below). The use of the drain decreases the chance of abscess formation. The safety pin in the Penrose drain prevents the exposed end from slipping down into the wound. Wound care focuses on cleaning around the drain with a prescribed solution, such as sterile normal saline, and replacing the precut gauze dressing as necessary to keep the surrounding skin dry and encourage further drainage. An absorbent dressing is placed over the drain and gauze (not shown).

Wound suction devices promote drainage of fluid from the incision site, decreasing pressure on healing tissues and reducing abscess formation. Shown are the Jackson-Pratt and Hemovac wound suction devices (see figures B and C below).

The frequency with which the nurse empties the device depends on the time elapsed since surgery, type of surgery, amount of drainage, and hospital policy. For example, immediately after surgery the nurse may empty the device every 15 to 60 minutes. With time, as drainage decreases, the device is emptied every 2 to 4 hours (per hospital policy). Amount, color, consistency, and odor of drainage are documented.

Usually, the nurse removes the drain on the second to fourth day after surgery (depending on hospital policy). Removal causes minor client discomfort. The drain site is cleaned, and a sterile dressing is applied.

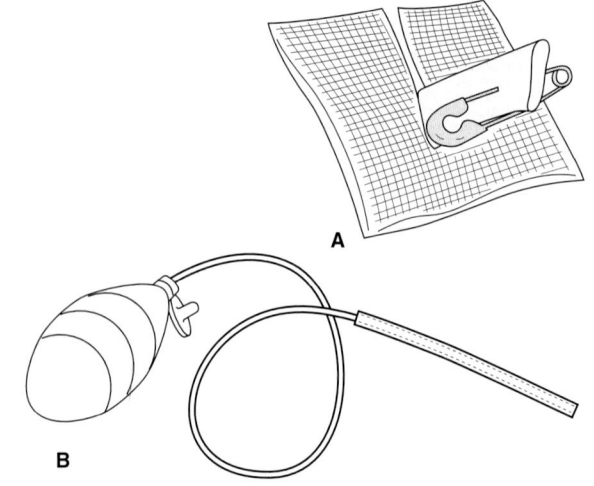

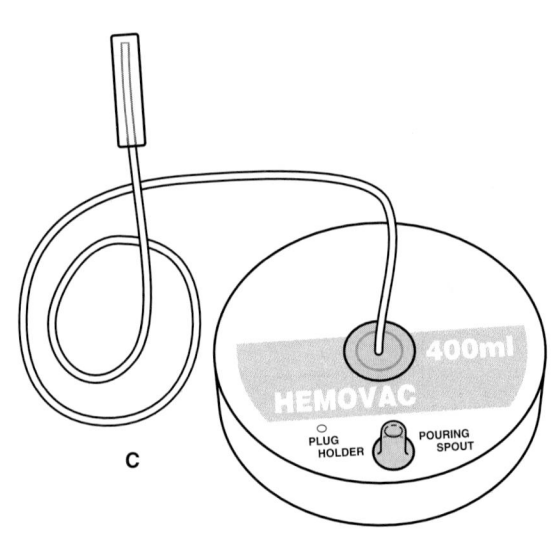

Wound drainage devices. *A*, Penrose passive wound drainage device. *B*, Jackson-Pratt wound suction device. *C*, Hemovac wound suction device.

Dehiscence is a separation in the layers of the incisional wound (Figure 7–10, A). Treatment depends on the extent of wound disruption. If the dehiscence is extensive, the incision must be resutured in surgery. **Evisceration** is the protrusion of body organs from a wound dehiscence (Figure 7–10, B). These serious complications may result from delayed wound healing or may occur immediately following surgery. They also may occur after forceful straining (coughing, sneezing, or vomiting). When dehiscence occurs, the wound should be covered immediately with a sterile dressing moistened with normal saline. Emergency surgery is performed to repair these conditions.

Either the nurse or physician removes sutures or staples after the wound has healed sufficiently (usually 5 to 10 days after surgery). Removal is performed using medical aseptic technique. Additional support may be provided to the incision by applying strips of tape (or Steri-Strips) as directed by institutional policy or by the physician.

Special Considerations for the Older Adult   Physiologic, cognitive, and psychosocial changes associated with the aging process place the older adult at increased risk for postoperative complications. These age-related changes with selected nursing interventions are summarized in Table 7–6. With an ever-increasing population of older adults, particularly the very old, the nurse must be aware of these normal changes and modify nursing care accordingly in an effort to provide safe, supportive care.

Managing Acute Postoperative Pain   Pain is expected after surgery. It is neither realistic nor practical to eliminate postoperative pain completely. Nevertheless, the client should receive substantial relief from and control of this discomfort. Controlling postoperative pain not only promotes comfort but also facilitates coughing, turning, deep-breathing exercises, earlier ambulation, and decreased length of hospitalization resulting in fewer postoperative complications, and therefore reducing health care costs. Despite the apparent benefits of effective pain control, recent studies indicate that about half of postoperative clients do not receive adequate pain relief or control (Acute Pain Management Guideline Panel, 1992).

Managing acute postoperative pain is an important nursing role before, during, and after surgery. Successful pain management involves the cooperative effort of the client, physician, and nurse. Preoperatively, the client should be made aware of how much pain to anticipate and what methods are available to control pain. After discussing options with the client, health care providers must respect the client's personal preferences. The information that follows is based on *Acute Pain Management in Adults: Operative Procedures* (Acute Pain Management Guideline Panel, 1992).

Postoperative pharmacologic agents were discussed earlier in this chapter. Various nonpharmacologic approaches to pain management are used alone or in combination to control acute postoperative pain. Relaxation, distraction, and imagery techniques can be successful in decreasing mild pain and anxiety. Massage and the application of heat or cold can also relieve postoperative pain. Transcutaneous electrical nerve stimulation (TENS) has been used successfully to decrease postoperative incisional pain. Other approaches include acupuncture, acupressure, and therapeutic touch. Additional information on pain management techniques is found in Chapter 4.

The client's input and participation in assessing pain and pain relief is essential to a successful pain control regime. For example, the client can rate the pain on a scale of 0 to 10 (where 0 signifies no pain and 10 signifies unbearable pain). Pain assessment should be completed and documented at scheduled intervals to determine the degree of pain control, to observe for drug side effects, and to assess the need for changes in the dosage and/or frequency of medication administration.

Postoperative Client and Family Teaching   Because the postoperative phase does not end until the client has recovered completely from the surgical intervention, the nurse plays a vital role as the client nears discharge. As the client prepares to recuperate outside the hospital, the nurse provides essential information and support to help the client successfully meet self-care demands. All aspects of teaching should be accompanied by written guidelines, directions, and information. This is particularly helpful

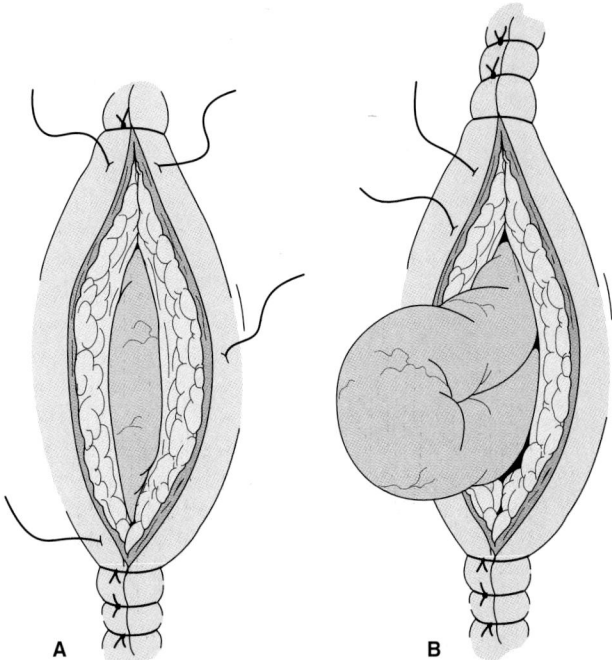

Figure 7–10   Wound complications. *A,* Dehiscence is a disruption in the incision resulting in a separation of the layers of the wound. *B,* Evisceration is a protrusion of a body organ through a surgical incision.

when a large amount of unfamiliar, detailed information is presented. Because the hospital stay is often brief, the nurse must make an organized, coordinated effort to educate the client and family. Teaching needs vary, but the most common needs include

- How to perform wound care. Teaching is more effective if the nurse first demonstrates and explains the procedure for the client and family or other caregiver. The client and family should then participate in the care. To evaluate the effectiveness of the teaching, the nurse should ask the client or caregiver to demonstrate the procedure in return. Ideally, teaching is carried out over several days, evaluated, and periodically reinforced.

- Signs and symptoms of a wound infection. The client should be able to determine what is normal and what should be reported to the physician.

- Method and the frequency of taking one's temperature.

- Limitations or restrictions that may be imposed on such activities as lifting, driving, bathing, sexual activity, and other physical activities.

- Control of pain. If analgesics are prescribed, the client should be instructed in the dosage, frequency, purpose, common side effects, and side effects to report to the physician. The nurse should reinforce the use of relaxation, distraction, imagery, or other pain-control techniques that the client has found useful in controlling postoperative pain.

Table 7–6 Nursing Interventions for Older Surgical Clients

System	Age-Related Changes	Nursing Intervention
General Appearance	Change in height, weight, and fat distribution	Assess physical parameters. Provide for warmth. Turn frequently.
Integument	Diminished integrity secondary to loss of subcutaneous fat and decreased oil production, elasticity, and hydration	Provide careful preoperative preparation to avoid trauma. Use other means to assess oxygenation and hydration, such as evaluation of mucous membranes, laboratory studies, and urine output.
Sensory-perceptual	Decline in vision and hearing ability; dryness of mouth	Compensate for sensory deficits: Speak low, not loud; minimize noise in environment; provide adequate room light; stay within client's field of vision when speaking; encourage client to wear hearing aid to the operating room. Provide comfort measures when NPO.
Respiratory	Decreased efficiency of cough reflex and decreased aeration of lung fields	Teach and encourage coughing and diaphragmatic breathing exercises. Assess baseline parameters. Constantly monitor lung sounds and respiratory status.
Cardiovascular	Less efficient, decreased adaptation to stress	Monitor for hypotension and shock. Assess for thrombus formation, cardiac dysrhythmias, peripheral pulses, and edema.
Gastrointestinal	Decline in gastric motility	Encourage intake of adequate fluids, nutritious meals, soft diet. Assist with feeding; monitor bowel function.
Genitourinary	Decreased efficiency of kidney; loss of bladder control	Monitor I&O and electrolyte levels. Assess for drug side effects. Assist with voiding as needed.
Musculoskeletal	Stiffness of joints; decrease in strength; brittleness of bones	Carefully position on OR table. Move carefully and gently. Prevent pressure sores.
Cognitive-psychosocial	Decreased reaction time; stable intellectual ability stable; proneness to delirium and altered mental status while in hospital	Provide ample time for making decisions. Implement safety measures. Talk to client as adult, not as child. Orient frequently.

Note. Adapted from "Perioperative Nursing Care for the Elderly Surgical Patient" by C. Dellasaga and C. Burgunder, 1991, *Today's O.R. Nurse, 13*(6): 12–17.

<table>
<tr><td>**Applying the Nursing Process**</td></tr>
</table>

Case Study of a Client Having Inpatient Surgery: Martha Overbeck

Martha Overbeck is a 74-year-old widow of German descent who lives alone in a senior citizens' housing complex. She is active in the housing complex's activities, as well as in the Lutheran Church. She is in good health and is independent; however, she has become progressively less active as a result of arthritic pain and stiffness. Mrs. Overbeck has degenerative joint changes that have particularly affected her right hip. On the recommendation of her physician and following a discussion with her friends, Mrs. Overbeck has been admitted to the hospital for an elective right total hip replacement. Her surgery has been scheduled for 8:00 a.m. the following day.

Mrs. Eva Jackson, a close friend and neighbor, accompanies Mrs. Overbeck to the hospital. Mrs. Overbeck explains that her friend will help in her home and assist her with the wound care and prescribed exercises.

Preoperative Phase

Assessment
Gloria Nobis, RN, completes the admission assessment for Mrs. Overbeck. Mrs. Overbeck appears to be an alert, oriented, healthy 74-year-old client. She is 30 pounds over her ideal weight. Mrs. Overbeck states she has pain and some stiffness in her weight-bearing joints, particularly the right hip. Enteric-coated aspirin 750 mg four times daily is the only medication she has been taking. Preadmission laboratory tests are normal, except for a slightly elevated clotting time (which suggests an increased risk of bleeding). The X-ray film of her right hip reveals degenerative joint changes indicative of osteoarthritis.

Mrs. Overbeck confides in Ms. Nobis that although she has faith that her surgery will be successful, she feels uneasy. She cannot identify exactly why she feels apprehensive. She states she has had a number of restless nights since her decision to have surgery. She has never had major surgery and is not familiar with the hospital routine.

Diagnosis

Ms. Nobis identifies the following nursing diagnoses for Mrs. Overbeck and includes them in her preoperative plan of care:

- *Anxiety* related to unfamiliar environment (hospital) and upcoming surgery
- *Knowledge Deficit* related to lack of information about the perioperative surgical experience
- *Sleep Pattern Disturbance* related to environmental changes (hospitalization) and anxiety response

Expected Outcomes

The expected outcomes established in the plan of care specify that Mrs. Overbeck will

- Describe an increase in psychologic and physiologic comfort.
- Verbalize an understanding of perioperative events to occur.
- Demonstrate turning, coughing, deep-breathing exercise, and leg exercises.
- Report sleeping soundly from 10:00 p.m. to 7:00 a.m.

Planning and Implementation

Ms. Nobis plans and implements the following interventions to assist Mrs. Overbeck in the preoperative surgical phase:

- Establish a therapeutic relationship with Mrs. Overbeck and her friend.
- Provide reassurance and comfort by acknowledging concerns and conveying understanding.
- Familiarize Mrs. Overbeck with hospital routines.
- Initiate perioperative teaching to include
  a. Preparation for surgery.
  b. A visit from the operating room nurse and anesthesiologist.
  c. Coughing, turning, and deep-breathing exercises.
  d. Leg exercises.
  e. Written materials describing total hip replacements.
- Help Mrs. Overbeck identify factors that interfere with her ability to sleep.
- Decrease noise, lighting, and disturbances between 10:00 p.m. and 7:00 a.m. as requested by Mrs. Overbeck.
- Encourage the use of the prescribed hypnotic/sedative medications to assist in sleep prior to surgery.

Evaluation

By the end of the shift, Ms. Nobis assesses that Mrs. Overbeck's anxiety has diminished. Mrs. Overbeck confirms that she feels more comfortable about the upcoming surgery. She is able to describe the preoperative prepara-

tions that will occur the following morning, events that are most likely to occur in surgery and the recovery room, and routine postoperative nursing care following her total hip replacement. She states that she will take the hypnotic/sedative prescribed to help her sleep. She asks Ms. Nobis to convey to the evening and night nurses that she would like to have her door closed and the lights off except for the one in the bathroom.

Critical Thinking in the Nursing Process

1. What teaching would you implement with Mrs. Overbeck and her friend to prepare them for the first 72 hours of postoperative recovery?
2. What consultations may be appropriate for you to make to other health care providers to assist Mrs. Overbeck before and after surgery?
3. Develop a care plan for Mrs. Overbeck for the nursing diagnosis *Knowledge Deficit* related to lack of information about preoperative care.

Intraoperative Phase

Assessment

The following morning Mrs. Overbeck has a right total hip replacement. In the operating room, Jim Arnold, RN, is the circulating nurse assigned to Mrs. Overbeck. Mr. Arnold completes the admission assessment, noting that her oral temperature is 98.3 F (36.8 C). Her extremities are cool with a rapid capillary refill time. Mr. Arnold determines that Mrs. Overbeck is at high risk for developing hypothermia because of her age and planned prolonged exposure to the cool surgical room. Mr. Arnold notes from her chart that she has osteoarthritis of both hips and knees.

Diagnosis

Mr. Arnold identifies the following nursing diagnoses:

- *Risk for hypothermia* related to cool operating room temperature and client's advanced age
- *Chronic pain* related to degenerative joint changes and inflammation of joints

Expected Outcomes

The expected outcomes established in the plan of care specify that Mrs. Overbeck will

- Maintain body temperature within normal limits.
- Communicate with the surgical team if position becomes uncomfortable (before induction of anesthesia).

Planning and Implementation

Mr. Arnold plans and implements the following interventions for the care of Mrs. Overbeck:

- Apply warm blankets on arrival to the operating room.
- Use a heating lamp to provide warmth to Mrs. Overbeck's extremities during surgery.
- Cover as much of Mrs. Overbeck's body surface as possible during her preparation and throughout the surgery.
- Administer warmed intravenous fluids and irrigants.
- Position Mrs. Overbeck in such a way as to decrease stress on the involved joints.

Evaluation

During the 2 hours in the operating room, Mrs. Overbeck's temperature is maintained at 98.0 F (36.7 C). No shivering is noted. Her skin is cool, but no pallor is noted. Capillary refill time is rapid in both feet. Mrs. Overbeck is positioned to decrease stress in her affected joints as much as possible. However, because of the location of the surgery and the length of time she must spend in one position, Mrs. Overbeck may experience joint pain in the unoperated joints.

Critical Thinking in the Nursing Process

1. What normal age-related physical changes place Mrs. Overbeck at risk for developing hypothermia or decubitus ulcers?

2. What nursing care during surgery can be implemented to protect Mrs. Overbeck from developing impaired skin integrity?

3. What assessments does Mrs. Overbeck's prolonged clotting time necessitate?

4. Develop a care plan for Mrs. Overbeck for the nursing diagnosis *Risk for Aspiration* related to decreased level of consciousness and diminished gag reflex.

Postoperative Phase

Assessment

Gloria Nobis, RN, is again assigned to Mrs. Overbeck's care on return to her room. Ms. Nobis performs a complete head-to-toe assessment and determines that Mrs. Overbeck is drowsy but oriented. Her skin is pale and slightly cool. Mrs. Overbeck states she is cold and requests additional covers. Ms. Nobis places a warmed cotton blanket next to Mrs. Overbeck's body, adds another blanket to her covers, and adjusts the room's thermostat to increase the room temperature. Mrs. Overbeck states that she is in no pain and would like to sleep. She has even, unlabored respirations and stable vital signs as compared to preoperative readings.

Mrs. Overbeck is NPO. An intravenous solution of dextrose and water is infusing at 100 mL/h per infusion pump. No redness or edema is noted at the infusion site. Ms. Nobis notes that the antibiotic ciprofloxacin hydrochloride (Cipro) is to be administered by mouth when the client is able to tolerate fluids. Mrs. Overbeck has a large gauze dressing over her right upper lateral thigh and hip with no indications of drainage from the wound. Tubing protrudes from the distal end of the dressing and is attached to a passive suctioning device (Hemovac). Ms. Nobis empties 50 mL of dark red drainage from the suctioning device and records the amount and characteristics on a flow record. Mrs. Overbeck has a Foley catheter in place with 250 mL of clear, light amber urine in the dependent gravity drainage bag.

When assessing Mrs. Overbeck's lower extremities, Ms. Nobis finds her feet slightly cool and pale with rapid capillary refill time bilaterally. Dorsalis pedis and posterior tibial pulses are strong and equal bilaterally. Ms. Nobis notes slight pitting edema in the right foot and ankle as compared to the left extremity. Sensation and ability to move both feet and toes also is noted, along with a lack of numbness and tingling (paresthesia).

Ms. Nobis records the above findings on a postoperative flowsheet. After ensuring that Mrs. Overbeck is safely positioned and can reach her call light, Ms. Nobis gives Mrs. Overbeck's friend, Mrs. Jackson, a progress report. They then go into Mrs. Overbeck's room.

Diagnosis

Ms. Nobis makes the following postoperative nursing diagnoses for Mrs. Overbeck:

- *Risk for Infection:* right hip wound related to disruption of normal skin integrity by the surgical incision
- *Risk for Injury* related to potential dislocation of right hip prosthesis secondary to total hip replacement
- *Pain* related to right hip incision and positioning of arthritic joints during surgery

Expected Outcomes

The expected outcomes established in the plan of care specify that Mrs. Overbeck will

- Regain skin integrity of the right hip incision without experiencing signs or symptoms of infection.
- Demonstrate (along with Mrs. Jackson) proper aseptic technique while performing the dressing change.
- Verbalize signs and symptoms of infection to be reported to her physician.
- Describe measures to be taken to prevent dislocation of right hip prosthesis.
- Report control of pain at incision and in arthritic joints.
- Remain afebrile.

Planning and Implementation

Ms. Nobis develops a care plan that includes the following interventions to assist Mrs. Overbeck during her postoperative recovery:

- Use aseptic technique while changing dressing.

- Monitor temperature and pulse every 4 hours to assess for elevation.

- Assess wound every 8 hours for purulent drainage and odor. Assess edges of wound for approximation, edema, redness, or inflammation in excess of expected inflammatory response.

- Teach Mrs. Overbeck and Mrs. Jackson how to use aseptic technique while assessing the wound and performing the dressing change.

- Teach Mrs. Overbeck and Mrs. Jackson the signs and symptoms of infection and when to report their findings to her physician.

- Review and discuss with Mrs. Overbeck the written materials on total hip replacement.

- Convey empathetic understanding of Mrs. Overbeck's incisional and arthritic joint pain.

- Medicate Mrs. Overbeck every 4 hours (or as ordered) to maintain a therapeutic analgesic blood level.

Evaluation

Throughout Mrs. Overbeck's hospitalization, Ms. Nobis works with Mrs. Overbeck and Mrs. Jackson to ensure that Mrs. Overbeck can care for herself after discharge from the hospital. Five days after her surgery, Mrs. Overbeck is discharged with a well-approximated incision with no indications of an infection. Prior to discharge, Ms. Nobis is confident that with Mrs. Jackson's help, Mrs. Overbeck can properly assess the incision. With minimal help, Mrs. Overbeck is able to replace the dressing using aspectic technique. She can cite the signs and symptoms of an infection, take her own oral temperature, and describe preventative measures to decrease the chances of dislocating her prosthetic hip. Because of her reduced mobility the past 5 days, Mrs. Overbeck states that she can tell the arthritis in her "old bones" is "acting up." She reports less pain in her right hip than before the surgery. Mrs. Overbeck tells Ms. Nobis she will be back the following winter to have her left hip replaced.

Critical Thinking in the Nursing Process

1. Describe risk factors for Mrs. Overbeck's safety; what changes in her home environment would you suggest to promote safety until she recovers more fully?

2. Why is Mrs. Overbeck placed on the antibiotic Cipro although she has no indications of an infection? What teaching would you do?

3. Mrs. Overbeck's clotting time is slightly elevated as a result of an ordered anticoagulant. Why would this medication be ordered? Consider the client's age and the area of surgery.

4. Mrs. Overbeck is 30 pounds above her ideal weight and has osteoarthritis. Develop a care plan for the

nursing diagnosis *Altered Health Maintenance* related to intake in excess of metabolic requirements.

The Client Having Outpatient Surgery

■ ■ ■

Outpatient, ambulatory, or *same-day surgery* is defined as a surgical procedure performed on a nonhospitalized client under local or general anesthesia. The surgical procedure is of short duration, usually 15 to 90 minutes. Following the surgical procedure, the client may be discharged immediately or remain for a short period of postoperative recovery and observation. Surgeries such as cataract removal with or without lens implants, hernia repairs, tubal ligations, vasectomies, dilation and curettage (D&C), and biopsies are routinely performed on an outpatient basis.

The number of outpatient surgeries has rapidly grown in the past decade, as part of the effort to contain the high costs of surgery. Moreover, increasingly complex surgeries on clients with complicated medical problems are now commonly performed on an outpatient basis. This increase in number of procedures and acuity level of the clients has presented a challenge to the perioperative nurse.

Outpatient surgery offers several advantages:

- Decreased cost to the client, hospital, and insuring agency

- Reduced risk of hospital-acquired infection

- Less interruption in the client's and family's routine

- Possible reduction in time lost from work and/or other responsibilities

- Less physiologic stress to the client and family

However, outpatient surgery does present some disadvantages:

- Less time for the nurse to establish rapport with client and family

- Less time for the nurse to assess, evaluate, and teach the client and family

- Lack of opportunity for the nurse to assess for the risk of postoperative complications that may occur after the client has been discharged

Many similarities exist between nursing care of the inpatient and outpatient surgical client. Physical care is provided in much the same manner in the preoperative, intraoperative, and postoperative phases of surgery. The major differences lie in the degree of teaching and emotional support that must be provided. In addition to the physiologic insult of surgery, the outpatient surgical client

OUTPATIENT CARE PLAN

Outpatient Surgery Center
Directions: Each unit, please check "Yes" or "No" and initial
appropriate space in column on right.

Patient's Name _____ Date _____

NURSING DIAGNOSES	PATIENT OUTCOME STANDARDS	Goal Met		OPTI	PRE-OP	OR	PACU	OBS
I. A. Anxiety related to knowledge deficit regarding surgical procedure. B. Fear related to risk of death, alteration of body image, or change in lifestyle. C. Impaired verbal communication related to anxiety. D. Impaired verbal communication related to preoperative medication/sedation. E. Impaired verbal communication related to language barrier. F. Ineffective individual or family coping related to perceived threat of surgery or surgical outcome. G. Noncompliance related to sensory alteration, fear, anxiety. H. Sensory-perceptual alteration related to inadequate tissue perfusion, or pre-existing deficits.	**I.** The patient demonstrates knowledge of the physiological and psychological responses to surgical intervention. Comments _____	Yes						
		No						
II. A. Potential for infection related to: Type of operative procedure Wound classification Tissues transected Length of procedure Pre-existing disease process Obesity Length of preoperative hospitalization Implants Presence/insertion of invasive/indwelling lines	**II.** The patient is free from infection. Comments _____	Yes						
		No						
III. A. Potential for impaired skin integrity related to: Positioning Pre-existing disease process Pooling of prep solutions under patient Improper placement of electrical dispersive pad Impaired circulation Poor tissue perfusion Allergic reactions to chemical agents	**III.** The patient's skin integrity is maintained. Comments _____	Yes						
		No						
IV. A. Potential for injury related to: Electrical hazards Positioning Retained foreign objects External constriction of peripheral circulation Chemical agents (ETO or Glutaraldehyde residuals, irritants, allergans) B. Impaired gas exchange related to: Positioning Inadequate airway Obesity C. Impaired physical mobility related to positioning.	**IV.** The patient is free from injury related to positioning, extraneous objects, or chemical, physical, and electrical hazards. Comments _____	Yes						
		No						
V. A. Potential for fluid and electrolyte imbalance related to: Type of surgical procedure Excessive blood loss Shock, trauma	**V.** The patient's fluid and electrolyte balance is maintained. Comments _____	Yes						
		No						
VI. A. Potential for altered or ineffective participation in rehabilitation related to: Ineffective coping mechanisms Anxiety due to surgical outcomes Lack of resources for self care after discharge	**VI.** The patient participates in the rehabilitation process. Comments _____	Yes						
		No						

Figure 7-11 An outpatient care plan form used in an outpatient surgery center.

must cope with the additional stress produced by the need to learn a great deal of information in a short span of time. The nurse teaches the client and family in both the preoperative and postoperative periods to enable the client to perform self-care following discharge. More extensive teaching and emotional support is mandated as clients requiring more complex surgical procedures and experiencing more complicated health problems undergo outpatient surgery. Figure 7–11 shows a standard outpatient care plan form.

Following outpatient surgery, the client is discharged after meeting the institution's criteria, which include:

- Vital signs are stable.
- Client is able to stand and begin to walk without dizziness or nausea.
- Pain is controlled or alleviated.
- Client is able to urinate.
- Client is oriented.
- Client demonstrates understanding of postoperative instructions.

Bibliography

■ ■ ■

A model for perioperative nursing practice. (1985). *AORN Journal 41,* (1), 189–194.

Acute Pain Management Guideline Panel. (1992). *Acute pain management in adults: Operative procedures. Quick reference guide for clinicians.* AHCPR Pub. No. 92-0019. Rockville, MD: Agency for Health Care Policy and Research, Public Health Service, US Department of Health and Human Services.

Badger, J. (1994). Calming the anxious patient. *American Journal of Nursing, 94*(5), 46–50.

Breemhaar, B. & Van den Borne, H. W. (1991). Effects of education and support for surgical patients: The role of perceived control. *Patient Education and Counseling, 18,* 199–210.

Caldwell, L. M. (1991). The influence of preference for information on preoperative stress and coping in surgical outpatients. *Applied Nursing Research, 4,* (4), 177–183.

———. (1991b.). Surgical outpatient concerns: What every perioperative nurse should know. *AORN Journal, 53*(3), 761–763, 766–767.

Carpenito, L. J. (1992). *Nursing diagnosis: Application to clinical practice.* (4th ed.). Philadelphia: Lippincott.

Cerrato, P. L. (1988). What diet does for wound healing. *RN, 51*(6), 73–76.

Cooper, D. M. (1990). Optimizing wound healing: A practice within nursing's domain. *Nursing Clinics of North America, 25*(1), 165–180.

Cuzzell, J. (1994). Back to basics: Test your wound assessment. *American Journal of Nursing, 94*(6), 34–35.

Cuzzell, J. Z., & Stotts, N. A. (1990). Wound care: Trial & error yields to knowledge. *American Journal of Nursing, 90*(10), 53–54.

Daake, D. R., & Gueldner, S. H. (1989). Imagery instruction and the control of postsurgical pain. *Applied Nursing Research, 2*(3), 114–120.

Davis, M. J., & Nomura, L. A. (1990). Vital signs of class I surgical patients. *Western Journal of Nursing Research, 12*(1), 28–41.

Dealey, C. (1991). Criteria for wound healing. *Nursing91, 4*(29), 20–22.

Dellasega, C. & Burgunder, C. (1991). Perioperative nursing care for the elderly surgical patient. *Today's O.R. Nurse, 13*(6), 12–17.

Farley, M. J. (1991). Teamwork in perioperative nursing: Understanding team development. *AORN Journal, 53*(3), 730–738.

Fincham, J. E. (1992). Perioperative implications of tobacco use. *AORN Journal, 56*(3), 531–538.

Fromm, C. G., & Metzler, D. J. (1993). Preparing your older patient for surgery. *RN, 56*(1), 38–42.

Gauthier, K. D., & LeMone, P. (1990). Trauma: The acute response. *AAOHN Journal, 38*(10), 475–481.

Groath, L., & Howery, D. (1992). 25 predictions for perioperative nursing. *Nursing92, 22*(1), 48–49.

Heidenreich, T., & Giuffre, M. (1990). Postoperative temperature measurement. *Nursing Research, 39*(3), 153–155.

Holmes, S. (1991). Nutrition and the surgical patient. *Nursing Standard, 5*(44), 30–32.

Jackson, M. F. (1988). High risk surgical patients. *Today's O.R. Nurse, 10*(2), 26–33.

———. (1989). Elderly care: Implications of surgery in very elderly patients. *AORN Journal, 50*(4), 859–869.

Jones, P. L., & Millman, A. (1990). Wound healing and the aged patient. *Nursing Clinics of North America, 25*(1), 263–277.

Kapp, M. B. (1990). Elder care: Informed, assisted delegated consent for elderly patients. *AORN Journal, 52*(4), 857–862.

Keene, A. (1991). Perioperative assessment and nursing implications for the elderly. *Plastic Surgical Nursing, 11*(4), 143–166.

Kenney, S. A. (1993). Nursing care of the postoperative patient receiving epidural analgesia. *Medsurg Nursing, 2*(3), 191–196.

Krasner, D. (1992). The 12 commandments of wound care. *Nursing92, 22*(12), 34–42.

Laufman, H. (1990). Environmental concerns in surgery in the 1990s. *Today's OR Nurse, 12*(10), 41–48, 50–51.

Litwack, K. (1991). What you need to know about administering preoperative medications. *Nursing, 21*(8), 44–47.

Marshall, M. (1993). Postoperative confusion: Helping your patient emerge from the shadows. *Nursing93, 23*(1), 44–47.

McCaffery, M., & Beebe, A. (1992). Do you know the value of a nonnarcotic? *Nursing92, 22*(10), 48–49.

Menyhert, L. R. (1988). Special considerations in geriatric care: An overview. *Journal of Post Anesthesia Nursing, 3*(3), 162–164.

Nyamathi, A., & Kashiwabara, A. (1988). Preoperative anxiety: Its affect on cognitive thinking. *AORN Journal, 47*(1), 164–170.

Oberle, K., Wry, J., Paul, P., & Grace, M. (1990). Environment, anxiety, and postoperative pain. *Western Journal of Nursing Research, 12*(6), 745–757.

O'Connor, F. W., Devine, E. C., Cook, T. D., Wenk, V. A., and Curtin, T. R. (1990). Enhancing surgical nurses' patient education: Development and evaluation of an intervention. *Patient Education and Counseling, 16,* 7–20.

Persaud, D. D., & Dawe, U. (1992). Effects of a surgical preoperative assessment clinic on patient care. *Hospital Topics, 70*(4), 37–40.

Polomano, R. C., Blumenthal, N. P., & Riegler, F. X. (1993). Interpleural analgesia for the management of postoperative pain. *Medsurg Nursing, 2*(3), 185–190.

Pope, K. E. (1990). Cost containment and the short-stay needs of surgical patients. *Nursing Management, 21*(3), 71–74.

Poss, C. (1991). Outpatient surgery documentation: Incorporating nursing diagnosis. *AORN Journal, 53*(1), 81, 83–86, 88–89.

Reeder, J. M. (1989). Ethical dilemmas in peri-operative nursing practice. *Nursing Clinics of North America, 24,* 999–1007.

Saltiel-Berzin, R. (1992). Managing a surgical patient who has diabetes. *Nursing92, 22*(4), 34–42.

Schultetus, R. R. (1987). Intraoperative awareness. *Today's O.R. Nurse, 9*(9), 22–27.

Shireff, A. (1990). Pre-operative nutritional assessment. *Nursing Times, 86*(8), 68, 70, 72.

Shireff, A. (1990). Pre-operative nutritional assessment. *Nursing Times, 86*(8), 78–82.

Smith, S. L. (1990). Postoperative perfusion deficits. *Critical Care Nursing Clinics of North America, 2*(4), 567–578.

Tanx, C. (1987). Quality patient care on surgery day. *Today's O.R. Nurse, 9*(12), 16–17.

Valenta, A. (1994). Using the vacuum dressing alternative for difficult wounds. *American Journal of Nursing, 94*(4), 44–45.

Walsh, J. (1993). Postop effects of OR positions. *RN, 56*(2), 50–58.

Willey, T. (1992). Use a decision tree to choose wound dressings. *American Journal of Nursing, 92*(2), 43–46.

Woundcare Update91, (1991). *Nursing91, 21*(4), 47–50.

Young, M. S., & Kindred, D. (1993). Malignant hyperthermia: Not just an operating room emergency. *Medsurg Nursing, 2*(1), 41–43, 46.

Nursing Care of Clients with Altered Immunity

The human body is continually challenged by a dizzying array of foreign substances, infectious agents, and abnormal cells. Fortunately, the body has defense mechanisms and alarm systems to protect it from invasion and takeover by these hostile forces. The immune system is the body's major defense mechanism against infectious organisms and abnormal or damaged cells.

Knowledge of the functions and responses of the immune system enables the nurse to provide preventive care, promote homeostasis, help the client maintain optimal wellness, and anticipate potential problems related to immune function. And for clients experiencing such problems, the nurse can prescribe appropriate rehabilitative measures, such as increased rest or attention to optimal nutrition. In addition, a thorough knowledge of the immune system can help the nurse teach clients and families to follow recommended treatment regimens, to promote and maintain health, and to prevent disease.

Recent years have seen the emergence of new diseases affecting the immune system. These diseases include human immunodeficiency virus (HIV) infection and altered strains of familiar diseases, such as multiple-drug-resistant tuberculosis. At the same time, understanding of the components of the immune system and specific immune responses is increasing. It is therefore all the more important that today's nurses understand the foundations of the immune system and the immune response.

Overview of the Immune System

The *immune system* is a complex and intricate network of specialized cells, tissues, and organs. Cells of the immune system seek out and destroy damaged cells and foreign

Table 8–1   Cells and Tissues of the Immune System

Component	Location	Function
Leukocytes		
Granulocytes		
Neutrophils	Circulation	Phagocytosis and chemotaxis
Eosinophils	Circulation, respiratory tract, and gastrointestinal tract	Phagocytosis
		Protection against parasites
		Involved in allergic response
Basophils	Circulation	Release of chemotactic substances
Monocytes and macrophages	Circulation (monocytes) and body tissue, such as skin (histocytes), liver (Kupffer's cells), alveoli, spleen, tonsils, lymph nodes, bone marrow, brain	Trapping and phagocytizing of foreign substances and cellular debris
		Secretion of interleukin-1 to stimulate lymphocyte growth
Lymphocytes		
T Cells (mature in thymus gland)	Circulation, lymph system, tissues	Activation of T and B cells
		Control of viral infections and destruction of cancer cells
		Involved in hypersensitivity reactions and graft tissue rejection
B Cells (mature in bone marrow)	Circulation, spleen	Production of antibodies (immunoglobulins) to specific antigens
NK (natural killer) Cells	Circulation	Cytotoxic; killing of tumor cells, fungi, viral-infected cells, and foreign tissue
Lymphoid Tissues		
Primary or central lymphoid structures	Bone marrow and thymus gland	Production of immune cells; sites for cell maturation
Secondary or peripheral lymphoid structures	Lymph nodes, spleen, tonsils, intestinal lymphoid tissue, lymphoid tissue in other organs	Sites for activation of immune cells by antigens

tissue yet recognize and preserve host cells (Porth, 1994). The immune system performs the following functions:

- Defending and protecting the body from infection by bacteria, viruses, fungi, and parasites
- Removing and destroying damaged or dead cells
- Identifying and destroying malignant cells, thereby preventing their further development into tumors

The immune system is activated by minor injuries, such as small lacerations or bruises, or by major injuries, such as burns, surgeries, and systemic diseases (e.g., pneumonia). The response of the immune system may be nonspecific or specific. Nonspecific responses prevent or limit the entry of invaders into the body, thereby limiting the extent of tissue damage and reducing the workload of the immune system. Inflammation is a nonspecific response activated by both minor and major injuries. When the inflammatory process is unable to destroy invading

organisms or toxins, a more specific response, called the immune response, is activated.

Immune System Components

The immune system consists of molecules, cells, and organs that function to produce the immune response (Table 8–1). These components may be involved in the nonspecific inflammatory response, the specific immunologic response, or both.

Leukocytes

Leukocytes, or white blood cells (WBCs), are the primary cells involved in both nonspecific and specific immune system responses. Like all blood cells, leukocytes derive from stem cells, the hemocytoblasts, in the bone marrow (Figure 8–1). Unlike red blood cells (RBCs), which are confined to the circulation, leukocytes use the circulation to transport themselves to the site of an inflammatory or immune response. As the mobile units of the immune

Figure 8–1 The development and differentiation of leukocytes from hemocytoblasts.

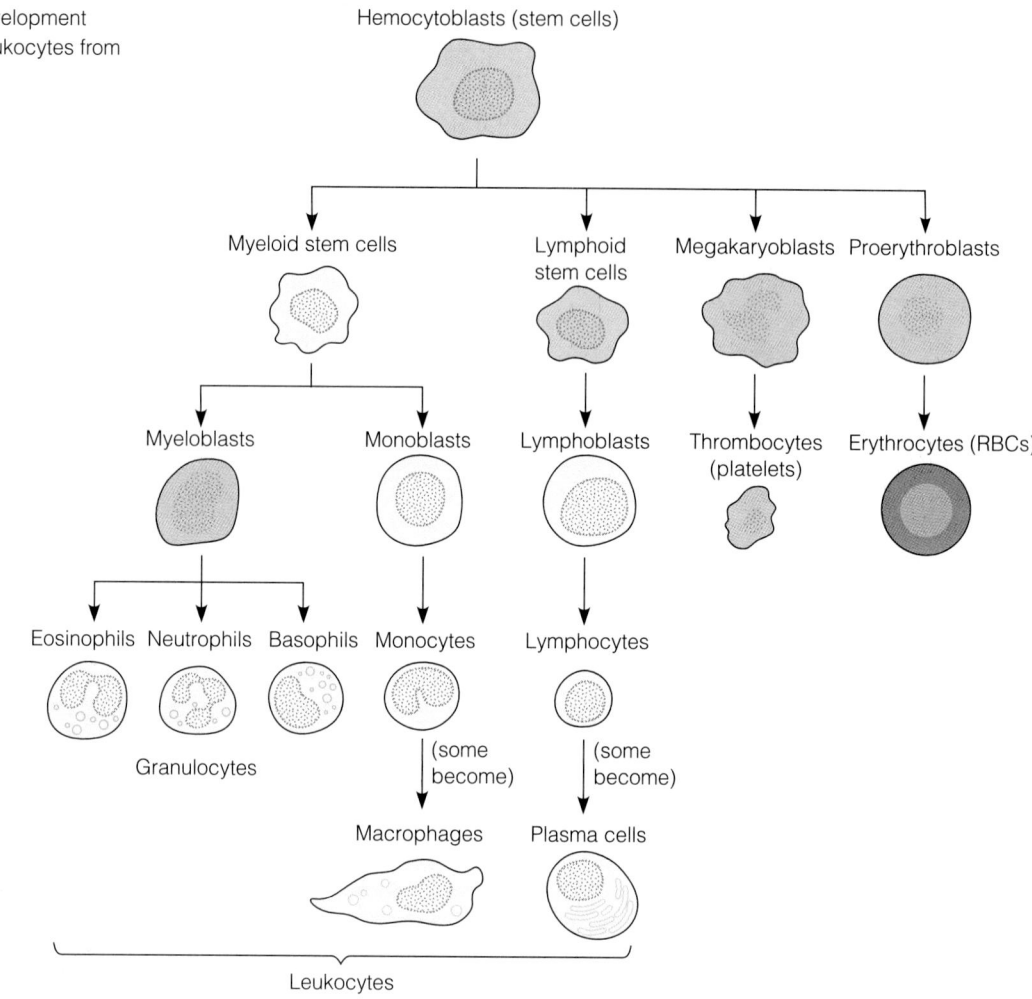

system, leukocytes detect, attack, and destroy anything that is recognized as "foreign." They are able to move through tissue spaces, locating damaged tissue and infection by responding to chemicals released by other leukocytes and damaged tissue.

The normal number of circulating leukocytes is 4000 to 10,000 cells per cubic millimeter (mm^3) of blood. Many more leukocytes are *marginated;* that is, they adhere to vascular epithelial cells along the vessel walls, in other tissue spaces, or in the lymph system. In the presence of an attack such as an infection, additional WBCs are released from the bone marrow, leading to **leukocytosis,** a WBC count of greater than $10,000/mm^3$. As WBCs move out of the bone marrow into the blood, the bone marrow increases its production of additional leukocytes. A decrease in the number of circulating leukocytes, known as **leukopenia,** occurs when bone marrow activity is suppressed or when leukocyte destruction increases.

Leukocytes are divided into three major groups: granulocytes, monocytes, and lymphocytes. The granulocytes and monocytes derive from the myeloid stem cells of the bone marrow and are instrumental in the inflammatory response. Lymphocytes derive from the lymphoid stem

cells of the bone marrow and are the primary cells involved in the specific immune response. In laboratory tests, the WBC count indicates the total number of circulating leukocytes. The WBC differential identifies the portion of the total represented by each type of leukocyte.

Granulocytes   *Granulocytes* constitute 60% to 80% of the total number of normal blood leukocytes. Their cytoplasm has a granular appearance, and their nuclei are distinctively multilobular (see Figure 8–1). Granulocytes have a short life span, measured in hours to days, compared to the life span of monocytes, which is measured in months to years. Granulocytes play a key role in protecting the body from harmful microorganisms during acute inflammation and infection. There are three types of granulocytes: neutrophils, eosinophils, and basophils.

Neutrophils, also called polymorphonuclear leukocytes (PMNs or polys), are the most plentiful of the granulocytes, constituting 55% to 70% of the total number of circulating leukocytes. Neutrophils are *phagocytic* cells, responsible for engulfing and destroying foreign agents, particularly bacteria and small particles. Neutrophils are the first phagocytic cells to arrive at the site of invasion, drawn by chemicals released by damaged tissue and invading organisms.

Neutrophils are produced in the bone marrow and released into the circulation when they mature. *Segmented neutrophils* (or "segs") are mature forms, and usually account for about 55% of total leukocytes. *Bands* are immature neutrophils and usually make up around 5% of leukocytes. It takes about 10 days for a neutrophil to mature and be released into the circulation. Once released, neutrophils have a circulating half-life of 6 to 10 hours. They cannot replicate and must be replaced constantly to maintain adequate numbers in the circulation. They do not return to the bone marrow.

Eosinophils account for 1% to 4% of the total number of circulating leukocytes. They mature in the bone marrow in 3 to 6 days before they are released into the circulation. Eosinophils have a circulating half-life of 30 minutes and a tissue half-life of 12 days. They too are phagocytic cells but are less efficient at this process than neutrophils. Eosinophils are found in large numbers in the respiratory and gastrointestinal tracts, where they are thought to be responsible for protecting the body from parasitic worms, including tapeworms, flukes, pinworms, and hookworms. Eosinophils surround the parasite and release toxic enzymes from their cytoplasmic granules. The parasite, although too large to be phagocytized, is destroyed. Eosinophils are also involved in a hypersensitivity response, inactivating some of the inflammatory chemicals released during the inflammatory response.

Basophils constitute about 0.5% to 1% of the circulating leukocytes. These cells are not phagocytic. Granules within basophils contain proteins and chemicals such as heparin, histamine, bradykinin, serotonin, and a slow-reacting substance of anaphylaxis (leukotrienes). These substances are released into the bloodstream during an acute hypersensitivity reaction or stress response.

Monocytes and Macrophages   *Monocytes* are the largest of the leukocytes and constitute 2% to 3% of circulating leukocytes. After their release from the bone marrow, monocytes are mobile for 1 to 2 days. They then migrate to various tissues throughout the body, attaching themselves to the tissues, where they remain for months or even years until they are activated. Monocytes mature into **macrophages** after settling into the tissues. Once they have migrated and matured, macrophages are differentiated by the tissues in which they reside. *Histiocytes* are tissue macrophages in the skin and subcutaneous tissues, *Kupffer cells* are found in the liver, *alveolar macrophages* in the lungs, and *microglia* in the brain. Tissue macrophages are also found in the spleen, tonsils, lymph nodes, and bone marrow.

Monocytes and macrophages are actively phagocytic, with the capacity to phagocytize large foreign particles and cell debris. Once they are in the tissue, macrophages can multiply to encapsulate and trap foreign matter that cannot be phagocytized. Like neutrophils, macrophages are drawn to an inflamed area by chemicals released from damaged tissue, a process known as *chemotaxis*. Monocytes and macrophages are particularly important in the body's defense against chronic infections, such as tuberculosis, viral infections, and certain intracellular parasitic infections.

Lymphocytes   Small and nondescript cells, the **lymphocytes** account for 20% to 40% of circulating leukocytes. Lymphocytes are the principal effector and regulator cells of specific immune responses. Along with monocytes and macrophages, lymphocytes protect the body from microorganisms, foreign tissue, and cell mutations or alterations. Lymphocytes monitor the body for cancerous cells, a process known as immune surveillance, and respond through a complex sequence of events initiated by contact with a foreign substance and resulting in its elimination or destruction.

Like other leukocytes, lymphocytes derive from the stem cells in the bone marrow (Figure 8–2). Lymphocytes have "homing" patterns. They constantly circulate then return to concentrate in lymphoid tissues: the lymph nodes, spleen, thymus, tonsils, Peyer's patches in the submucosa of the distal ileum, and the appendix. On contact with an **antigen,** a substance capable of evoking a specific immune response, lymphocytes are activated and mature into either *effector cells* (e.g., plasma cells or cytotoxic cells), which are instrumental in destruction of the antigen, or *memory cells*. Memory cells stay inactive, sometimes for years, but activate immediately with subsequent exposure to the same antigen. They then proliferate rapidly, producing an intense immune response. Memory cells are responsible for providing acquired immunity.

Although lymphocyte subtypes are difficult to distinguish by appearance, they have distinct differences in the following:

- How and where they mature
- Life cycle
- Surface characteristics
- Function

There are three types of lymphocytes: **T lymphocytes (T cells); B lymphocytes (B cells);** and **natural killer cells (NK cells** or null cells), which are also known as third-population cells.

T cells mature in the thymus gland, whereas B cells complete their maturation in the bone marrow. T cells and B cells are integral to the specific immune response and are discussed further in that section of this chapter.

NK cells are large, granular cells found in the spleen, lymph nodes, bone marrow, and blood. They constitute 5% to 10% of circulating lymphocytes. NK cells provide immune surveillance and resistance to infection, and they play an important role in the destruction of early

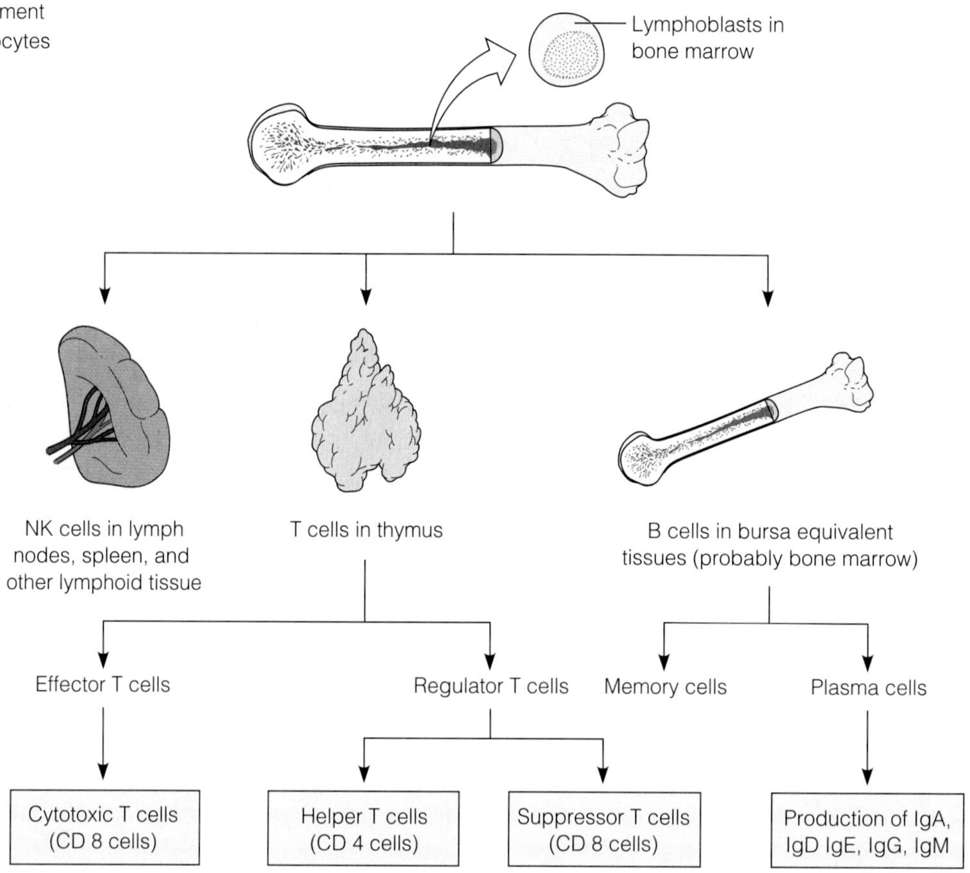

Figure 8–2 The development and differentiation of lymphocytes from the lymphoid stem cell (lymphoblasts).

Lymphoblasts in bone marrow

NK cells in lymph nodes, spleen, and other lymphoid tissue

T cells in thymus

B cells in bursa equivalent tissues (probably bone marrow)

Effector T cells

Regulator T cells

Memory cells

Plasma cells

Cytotoxic T cells (CD 8 cells)

Helper T cells (CD 4 cells)

Suppressor T cells (CD 8 cells)

Production of IgA, IgD IgE, IgG, IgM

malignant cells. Like B cells and T cells, NK cells are cytotoxic, but whereas T and B cells can attack only specific infected cells or malignant cells, NK cells can attack any target.

None of these cells acts independently. Their functions are closely interrelated.

The Lymphoid System

Lymphocytes tend to concentrate in lymphoid tissues. The lymph nodes, spleen, thymus, tonsils, lymphoid tissue scattered in connective tissues and mucosa, and the bone marrow constitute the *lymphoid system*. The thymus and bone marrow, in which T and B cells mature, are considered *primary* or *central lymphoid organs*. The spleen, lymph nodes, tonsils, and other peripheral lymphoid tissue are *secondary lymphoid organs* (Figure 8–3).

Lymph nodes, the most numerous elements of the lymphoid system, are small round or bean-shaped encapsulated bodies that vary in size from 1 mm up to 2 cm. Distributed throughout the body, lymph nodes generally occur in groups at the junction of the lymphatic vessels. They can be found in the neck, axillae, abdomen, and groin.

Lymph nodes have two functions: They filter foreign products or antigens from the lymph, and they house and support proliferation of lymphocytes and macrophages. *Lymph,* a clear, protein-containing fluid transported by

lymph vessels, enters the node through afferent lymphatic vessels. Inside the node, the lymph flows through sinuses in the cortex of the lymph node where T and B lymphocytes and macrophages are abundant, then through sinuses of the medulla of the lymph node, which contains macrophages and plasma cells. The presence of a foreign antigen stimulates lymphocytes and macrophages to proliferate in the lymph nodes. Macrophages destroy the antigen by phagocytosis. Immune cells, along with lymph, then leave the lymph node through efferent vessels. Lymphocyte movement is also facilitated by an abundant blood supply to the node.

The *spleen* is the largest lymphoid organ in the body and the only lymphoid organ that can filter blood. The spleen is located in the upper left quadrant of the abdomen. The spleen has two kinds of tissue, white pulp and red pulp. White pulp is lymphoid tissue that serves as a site for lymphocyte proliferation and immune surveillance. B cells predominate in the white pulp. Blood filtration occurs in the red pulp. In blood-filled venous sinuses, phagocytic cells dispose of damaged or aged RBCs and platelets. Other debris and foreign matter, such as bacteria, viruses, and toxins, are also removed from the blood. The spleen also stores blood and the breakdown products of RBCs for future use. The spleen is not essential for life; if it is removed because of disease or trauma, the liver and the bone marrow assume its functions.

The *thymus gland* is located in the superior anterior mediastinal cavity beneath the sternum. It reaches its maximum size at puberty, then begins to atrophy slowly. By adulthood, it is difficult to differentiate from surrounding adipose tissue even though it remains active. In the elderly, the vast majority of thymus tissue has been replaced by adipose and fibrous connective tissue. The main function of the thymus is to serve as a site for the maturation and differentiation of thymic lymphoid cells, the T cells, primarily during fetal life and childhood. *Thymosin*, an immunoregulatory hormone of the thymus, stimulates lymphopoiesis, the formation of lymphocytes or lymphoid tissue.

Bone marrow is soft organic tissue found in the hollow cavity of the long bones, particularly the femur and humerus, as well as the flat bones of the skull, sternum, ribs, and vertebrae. Bone marrow produces and stores hematopoietic stem cells, from which all cellular components of the blood are derived (see Figure 8–1).

Lymphoid tissues are also located at key sites of potential invasion by microorganisms: the submucosa of the genitourinary, respiratory, and gastrointestinal tracts and the skin. Plasma cells in these lymphoid tissues defend the body against bacterial invasion at areas exposed to the external environment. In general, these tissues are known as *mucosa-associated lymphoid tissue (MALT)*. Diffuse collections of lymphocytes, plasma cells, and phagocytes are scattered throughout the respiratory tract, concentrating at bifurcations of the bronchi and bronchioles. Gastrointestinal lymphoid tissue occurs as both diffusely scattered MALT and in more clearly defined tissues, such as the appendix and *Peyer's patches*, which are lymph nodules located on the distal ileum near its junction with the colon. Tonsils and adenoids protect the body from inhaled or ingested foreign agents. Skin-associated lymphoid tissue contains lymphocytes and *Langerhans cells* in the epidermis, which transport antigens to regional lymph nodes for phagocytosis.

The Nonspecific Inflammatory Response

Barrier protection is the body's first line of defense against infection. The skin is the primary barrier. When intact, it prevents invasion by external organisms. When the skin is damaged or lost (e.g., as a result of injury, surgery, or burns), infection is much more likely. The membranes lining inner surfaces of the body are protected by a barrier of mucus, which traps microorganisms and other foreign substances. These can then be removed by other protective mechanisms, such as ciliary movement or the washing action of tears or urine. In addition, many body fluids contain bactericidal substances that provide barrier protection. These include acid in gastric fluid, zinc in prostatic fluid, and lysozyme in tears, nasal secretions, and saliva (Roitt, 1994).

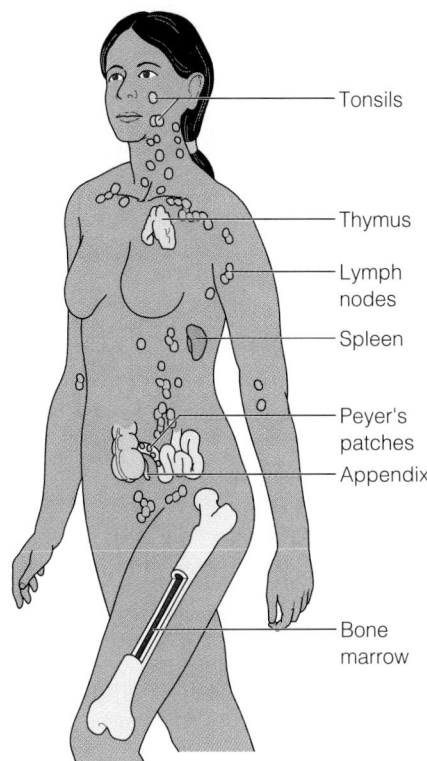

Figure 8–3   The lymphoid system: the central organs of the thymus and bone marrow, and the peripheral organs, including the spleen, tonsils, lymph nodes, and Peyer's patches.

When these first-line defenses are breached, resulting tissue damage or foreign material entering the body induces a nonspecific immune response. This is known as **inflammation.** Inflammation is an adaptive response to injury that brings fluid, dissolved substances, and blood cells into the interstitial tissues where the invasion or damage has occurred. The response is called nonspecific because the same events occur regardless of cause of the inflammatory process. Through the inflammatory reaction, the invader is neutralized and eliminated, destroyed tissue removed, and the process of healing and repair initiated.

There are three stages in the inflammatory response: (1) a vascular response characterized by vasodilation and increased permeability of blood vessels, (2) a cellular response and phagocytosis, and (3) tissue repair.

Vascular Response

After tissue cells become damaged, local blood vessels briefly constrict. Vasodilation follows almost immediately as inflammatory mediators such as histamine and kinins are released from damaged tissue (see the box on page 220). Increased blood flow causes vasocongestion at the injury site with resultant redness and heat. The congestion also increases local hydrostatic pressure. This, along

Inflammatory Mediators

■ ■ ■

Many of the manifestations of inflammation are produced by *inflammatory mediators,* which are chemicals released as a result of immunologic processes or tissue injury or damage. These inflammatory mediators are broadly classified as follows:

- Vasoactive substances produce smooth muscle constriction, postcapillary vasodilation, and increased capillary permeability.
- Chemotactic factors attract leukocytes to the damaged tissue.
- Plasma enzymes activate the clotting cascade, plasminogen system, and complement system.
- Miscellaneous cell products, for example, oxygen metabolites and lysosomal enzymes damage surrounding tissue.

Many of the outward manifestations of inflammation result from vasoactive substances such as *histamine, serotonin,* and *leukotrienes* (formerly known as slow-reacting substance of anaphylaxis, or SRS-A). Stored in mast cells, basophils, and platelets, histamine is released when an injury occurs or with stimulation by the immune system. An important component of the early inflammatory response, histamine causes vasodilation and vascular permeability in the affected area. Histamine is also a key factor in many hypersensitivity reactions. Serotonin is released from platelets and produces effects similar to those of histamine. The leukotrienes play a significant vasoactive role in the later stages of the inflammatory response.

Prostaglandins are chemotactic substances drawing leukocytes to the inflamed tissue. In addition, they play a vasoactive role and are pain and fever inducers. Aspirin and other nonsteroidal anti-inflammatory drugs (NSAIDs) as well as the glucocorticoids inhibit prostaglandin synthesis, thereby reducing fever, pain, and inflammation.

Plasma factors such as Hageman factor activate the clotting cascade, plasminogen system (involved in the lysis of clots), and complement system. With activation of the clotting cascade, bacteria and other foreign substances are trapped in the area of tissue damage. Fibrin, which has vasoactive by-products, is also released. (See Chapter 31 for a full description of the clotting process.) The complement system serves a chemotactic role and facilitates the phagocytic process.

Major chemical mediators of inflammation are summarized in Table 8–2.

Table 8–2   Major Chemical Mediators of Inflammation

Factor	Source	Effect
Histamine	Mast cells, basophils, and platelets	Vasodilation and increased capillary permeability, producing tissue redness, warmth, and edema
Kinins (bradykinin and others)	Plasma protein factors	Histaminelike effects; chemotaxis and pain inducers
Prostaglandins	Metabolism of anachidonic acid from cell membranes	Histaminelike effects; chemotaxis, pain, and fever inducers
Leukotrienes	Anachidonic acid metabolism	Smooth muscle constriction (especially bronchoconstriction), increased vascular permeability, chemotaxis

---

with the increased vessel permeability that results from chemical mediators, moves fluid out of the capillaries and into the interstitial spaces of the tissue. The escaping fluid, called *fluid exudate,* contains large amounts of protein and causes local edema. Fluid exudate has three functions: (1) It provides protection to the injured tissue by bringing certain nutrients needed for tissue healing; (2) it dilutes bacterial toxins, and (3) it transports cells needed for phagocytosis. With mild tissue damage, the fluid is *serous* in nature, made up primarily of plasma fluid and proteins. With moderate to severe tissue damage, fluid exudate is *sanguineous* or *hemorrhagic,* containing large amounts of RBCs. A mixture of RBCs and serum is referred to as *serosanguineous* exudate. *Fibrinous* exudates form a thick, sticky meshwork of fibrinogen, in effect "walling off" inflamed tissues and preventing the spread of infection (Porth, 1994). In more severe or acute inflammation, the fluid contains fibrin, RBCs, and dead

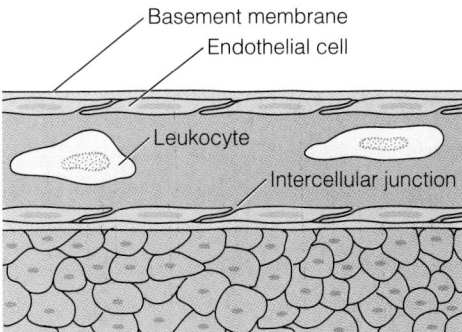

A Leukocytes in circulation

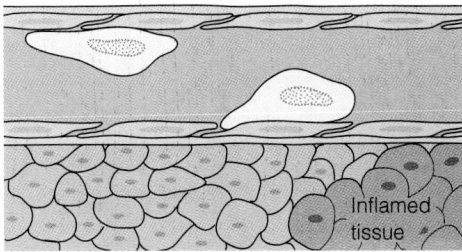

B Margination and pavementing

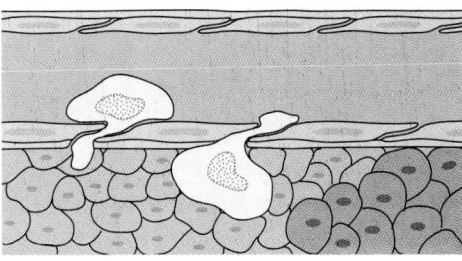

C Emigration

Figure 8–4   The process of leukocyte emigration at the site of inflammation. *A,* Normal blood flow with free movement of formed elements. *B,* As blood flow slows, leukocytes move toward the periphery of stream and begin to cling to capillary endothelium, a process known as margination and pavementing. *C,* Leukocytes emigrate from the vessel into inflamed tissues.

and live bacteria. This type of exudate, called *purulent* exudate, has an odor and color characteristic of the bacteria present.

The vascular response localizes invading bacteria and keeps them from spreading. Increased capillary permeability enhances the release of clotting factors such as fibrinogen, which converts to fibrin threads, entrapping the bacteria and walling them off from contact with the rest of the body.

Cellular Response

The cellular stage of the inflammatory process begins within less than an hour after the injury. This stage is marked by the margination and emigration of leukocytes into the damaged tissue, chemotaxis, and phagocytosis (Porth, 1994).

As serous fluid escapes the capillaries, the viscosity of blood in the area increases and its flow becomes more sluggish. Leukocytes marginate, moving to the edges of the blood vessels, and begin to adhere to the capillary endothelium. This process is known as *pavementing*. After margination and pavementing, leukocytes emigrate from the blood vessel into the tissue spaces (Figure 8–4). Within hours, millions of leukocytes emigrate into the area of inflammation (Price & Wilson, 1992).

Once leukocytes have emigrated, they are drawn to the damaged or inflamed tissues by chemotactic signals. Infectious agents, damaged tissues, and activated plasma substances such as complement fractions provide chemotaxic signals that attract an army of neutrophils, monocytes, and macrophages to the injury site.

The number of neutrophils around the site increases to about 15,000/mm³ to 25,000/mm³ (Guyton, 1990), and they begin their role in phagocytosis within a few hours. Monocytes become transient macrophages to augment the activity of the fixed macrophages; together they engulf dead cells, damaged tissue, nonfunctioning neutrophils, and invading bacteria.

Phagocytosis

Phagocytosis is a process by which a foreign agent or target cell is engulfed, destroyed, and digested. Neutrophils and macrophages, known as *phagocytes,* are the primary cells involved in phagocytosis. Once attracted to the inflammatory site, phagocytes select and engulf foreign material.

The following factors or processes help phagocytes differentiate foreign tissue from normal cells:

- *Smooth surface.* Normal tissue has a smooth surface that is resistant to phagocytosis, whereas the rough surface of a foreign agent or target cell promotes phagocytosis.

- *Surface charge.* Healthy body cells present an electronegative surface charge that repels phagocytes. Cellular debris and foreign agents, by contrast, have an electropositive charge that attracts them.

- *Opsonization.* This immune system process coats the surface of bacteria or target cells with a substance (an opsonin) such as complement (see the box on page 222). This surface coating enables the phagocyte to bind tightly with the foreign tissue, facilitating phagocytosis (Figure 8–5, *A*).

The Complement System

■ ■ ■

The *complement system* is composed of approximately 20 complex plasma proteins that are activated by a tissue injury or antigen-antibody reaction. The complement system is involved in both nonspecific and specific immune responses. Its activation results in the production of effector molecules that are involved in the processes of inflammation, phagocytosis, and cell lysis or destruction (Porth, 1994; Roitt, 1994). Specifically, complement activation leads to

- Mediation of the inflammatory response. When the complement system is activated, chemical mediators such as histamine are released from mast cells and basophils, leading to smooth muscle contraction, increased vascular permeability and edema, and the attraction of leukocytes.

- Opsonization (or coating) of antigen-antibody complexes to facilitate phagocytosis.

- Alteration of the cell membrane or viral capsule. When the cell surface is altered, lysis results. Bacteria and viruses are destroyed; certain normal cells, such as RBCs, platelets, and lymphocytes, that are damaged or old may also be destroyed through this process.

The complement system has two "arms," or pathways, of protein and enzyme reactions. The *classic pathway* is activated by antibody-containing immunoglobulins and other substances such as DNA and C-reactive protein. The *alternate pathway* is activated by tissue injury, polysaccharides, or enzymes. When either pathway is activated, the results are mediation of the inflammatory process, attraction of phagocytes, facilitation of phagocytosis, and lysis of microbes.

Phagocytes engulf the foreign agent or target cell by projecting pseudopodia ("false feet") in all directions around it (Figure 8–5, *B*). This produces a chamber called a *phagosome* containing the antigen, which is ingested into the cytoplasm (Figure 8–5, *C*). Once the phagosome has been engulfed, lysosomes fuse with the phagosome, killing any live organism and releasing digestive enzymes which destroy the antigen (Figure 8–5, *D*).

Phagocytes—in particular, neutrophils and macrophages—contain bactericidal agents that kill most of the bacteria they ingest before the bacteria can multiply and destroy the phagocyte itself. The phagocyte kills bacteria in a number of ways; for example, it alters the intracellular pH and produces bactericidal agents. Oxidizing

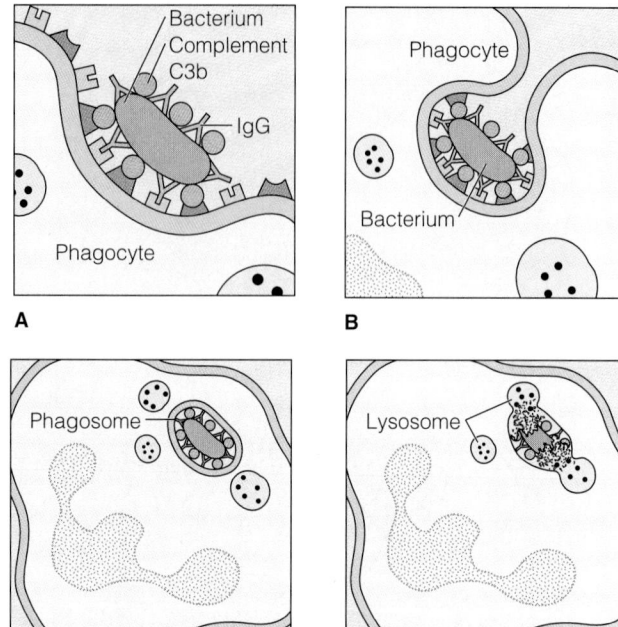

Figure 8–5 The process of phagocytosis. *A,* Opsonization coats the surface of the bacterium with IgG (an antibody) and complement. *B,* The bacterium is bound to and engulfed by the phagocyte. *C,* The phagosome is ingested into the cytoplasm of the phagocyte. *D,* Lysosomes fuse with the phagosome, releasing digestive enzymes and destroying the antigen.

agents, such as superoxide, hydrogen peroxide, and hydroxyl ions, are bactericidal. Two lysosomal substances that kill bacteria are lysozyme and phagocytin.

Some antigens, such as the tubercle bacterium, have coats or secrete substances that are resistant to lysosomal and bactericidal agents. To destroy such antigens, lysosomes release digestive enzymes into the phagosome. The lysosomes of neutrophils and macrophages contain an abundance of proteolytic (protein-destroying) enzymes that digest bacteria and other foreign protein components. The macrophage's lysosomes also contain lipases (fat-splitting enzymes) capable of digesting the thick lipid membranes of such bacteria as *Mycobacterium tuberculosis* and *Mycobacterium leprae.*

Once neutrophils have ingested toxic substances to their capacity, they in turn are killed. Neutrophils have the capacity to phagocytize 5 to 20 bacteria before they become inactive. Macrophages then digest the dead neutrophils. Monocytes or macrophages are capable of phagocytizing up to 100 bacteria. Because of their size, they can ingest larger particles than neutrophils can ingest, such as whole RBCs, necrotic tissue, cell fragments, malarial parasites, and dead neutrophils. Macrophages have the ability to extrude (release) the toxic substances and lysosomal enzymes within their phagosomes. As a result, they can continue to function for months and even years.

Healing

Inflammation is the first phase of the healing process. During the inflammatory process, particulate matter, bacteria, damaged cells, and inflammatory exudate are removed by phagocytosis. This process, called *debridement,* prepares the wound for healing.

The second phase of the healing process, known as *reconstruction,* may overlap the inflammatory phase. The ideal result of the healing process is *resolution,* the restoration of the original structure and function of the damaged tissue. Simple resolution occurs when there is no destruction of the normal tissue and the body is able to neutralize and remove the offending agent through the inflammatory process (Bullock & Rosendahl, 1992).

Resolution may also occur when the damaged tissue is capable of *regeneration.* The ability to regenerate, or replace lost parenchyma (functional tissue) with new, functional cells varies by tissue and cell type. *Labile cells* continue to regenerate throughout life. These cells are found in tissues where there is a daily turnover of cells—namely, bone marrow and the epithelial cells of the skin, mucous membranes, cervix, gastrointestinal tract, and genitourinary tract. *Stable cells* normally stop replicating when growth ceases but are capable of regeneration when stimulated by an injury. Osteocytes (which are found in bone) and parenchymal cells of the kidneys, liver, and pancreas are stable cells. *Permanent* or *fixed cells* are unable to regenerate. When these cells are destroyed, they are replaced by fibrous scar tissue. Nerve cells, skeletal muscle cells, and cardiac muscle cells are fixed cells (Porth, 1994).

When regeneration and complete resolution is not possible, healing occurs by replacement of the destroyed tissue with collagen scar tissue. This process is known as *repair.* Although tissue that has undergone repair does not have the physiologic function of the destroyed tissue, the scar fills the lesion and provides tensile tissue strength. The healing process is discussed further in Chapter 7.

Age-Related Changes in the Inflammatory Response

In the older adult, nonspecific immune defenses and the inflammatory response are reduced, and healing is therefore slower. The phagocytic activity of some granulocytes (neutrophils and eosinophils) may be diminished. A decreased fever response and altered cell growth and proliferation in older persons suggest age-associated defects in monocyte/macrophage function. Many inflammatory factors that have an immunosuppressive effect have been shown to be synthesized and released at higher levels in the older adult. This may account for some of the reduction in inflammatory response (Hazzard, Bierman, Blass, Ettinger, & Halter, 1994).

Most of the changes in the inflammatory response that are commonly attributed to aging are actually due to a loss of functional reserve and to chronic diseases. Neu-

trophil function is impaired by the hyperglycemia associated with diabetes mellitus; nearly 18% of the population over the age of 65 years has diabetes. Vascular disease (atherosclerosis in particular) is prevalent in aged populations. The reduced blood flow associated with vascular disease impairs local resistance to infection and wound healing (Abrams & Berkow, 1990; Hazzard et al., 1994). The older client is also more likely to take medications that interfere with inflammation and healing. The cardinal signs of inflammation—redness, heat, and swelling—tend to be diminished or absent in older adults.

The box on page 224 discusses other age related changes to the immune system.

The Specific Immune Response

The introduction of some foreign substances, namely antigens, into the body causes a more specific reaction than the nonspecific inflammatory response. On the first exposure to an antigen, a change occurs in the host, resulting in a specific and rapid response following subsequent exposures. This specific response is known as the *immune response.*

The immune response to an antigen has several distinctive properties:

- The immune response typically is directed against materials recognized as *foreign* (i.e., from outside the body) and is not usually directed against the *self* (i.e., cells or structures produced by the body). This property is known as *self-recognition.*

- The immune response is *specific.* It is initiated by and directed against particular antigens (such as a specific virus, bacterium, or transplanted tissue).

- Unlike a localized inflammatory response, the immune response is *systemic.* Immunity is generalized; it is not restricted to the initial site of infection or entry of foreign tissue.

- Finally, the immune response has *memory.* Repeated exposures to an antigen produce a more rapid response.

A client whose immune system is able to identify antigens and effectively destroy or remove them is said to be *immunocompetent.* Health problems may occur when the immune response is altered. Overreaction of the immune system leads to hypersensitivity disorders, such as allergies. When the immune system loses the ability to recognize self, autoimmune disorders may ensue. Immunodeficiency diseases or malignancies can develop when the immune system is incompetent or unable to respond effectively. All of these alterations in immunity are discussed later in this chapter.

Recognition of Self

The effectiveness of the immune system depends on its ability to differentiate normal host tissue from abnormal

Gerontologic Considerations: Clients with Infections

■ ■ ■

A decline in immune function is associated with aging. Consequently, older adults are more susceptible to infections. In fact, infections are among the top ten causes for hospitalization and one of the five leading causes of death among people over 65 years of age.

The presentation of infection in older adults may be obscured by age-related changes in structure and function, or by coexisting chronic conditions. Fever may be mild or absent altogether as a result of age-related alterations in metabolism, or from medications such as nonsteroidal anti-inflammatory agents and corticosteroids. The white blood count may be slightly elevated.

Confusion is one of the most frequent atypical signs of infection in older adults. Subtle changes in behavior, such as restlessness, may also be observed. The physician will initially order a chest X-ray, urinalysis and culture, and complete blood count to determine if infection is present and, if so, its source.

The nurse needs an accurate baseline assessment for comparison when changes related to infection occur. The nurse should be alert for subtle changes in the patient's mental status or behavior and perform a thorough mental status assessment. Other baseline assessments include the amount of fluids consumed, urinary output, activity levels, complaints of fatigue, and respiratory status.

Early diagnosis and prompt treatment of infection will result in improved outcomes for the older adult. Delay in treating infection may prolong the client's immobility and reduce the ability to perform activities of daily living.

Respiratory-Tract Infections

Older adults are particularly susceptible to pneumonia. Changes in the respiratory system associated with aging include rigidity of the chest wall with decreased expansion, decreased alveolar elasticity, and decreased ciliary movement. The cough reflex also decreases. As a result of these changes, the older adult who has pneumonia may not present with cough or sputum production.

Frail older adults, especially those with chronic respiratory conditions such as emphysema, are at risk for developing pneumonia as a complication of influenza. To prevent this complication, all persons over 65 should receive an annual immunization for influenza. In addition, pneumonia caused by pneumococcus bacteria can be deadly for older adults. To prevent pneumococcal pneumonia, it is recommended that individuals over the age of 65 receive immunization for this potentially fatal disease.

Urinary-Tract Infections

Older adults are also susceptible to urinary tract infection. Changes in the urinary system associated with aging include a reduced bladder capacity, increased residual urine, and decreased desire to void. In older men, benign prostatic hypertrophy is a common change which may cause urinary tract infection. In addition to these changes, chronic conditions and medications may contribute to retention, which can result in urinary tract infection.

Nosocomial Infections

Nosocomial (hospital acquired) infections are more common in older adults. Nursing interventions should focus on preventing nosocomial infection. The older adult should not be on prolonged bed rest unless the medical condition contraindicates mobilization. Promote respiratory clearance by encouraging clients to take deep breaths. Adequate fluids should be provided. Regular toileting schedules with good hygiene should be followed. The nurse must steadfastly adhere to principles of infection control.

Client and Family Teaching

To prevent infection, the older adult should be taught to:

- Eat a well-balanced diet.
- Drink adequate fluids.
- Get adequate rest.
- Obtain an annual influenza immunization.
- Use good hand-washing techniques.

Older adults and families should be taught to seek medical attention if they:

- Develop a fever or other signs and symptoms of infection.
- Exhibit changes in mental status and/or behavior.
- Experience fatigue or changes in activity levels.

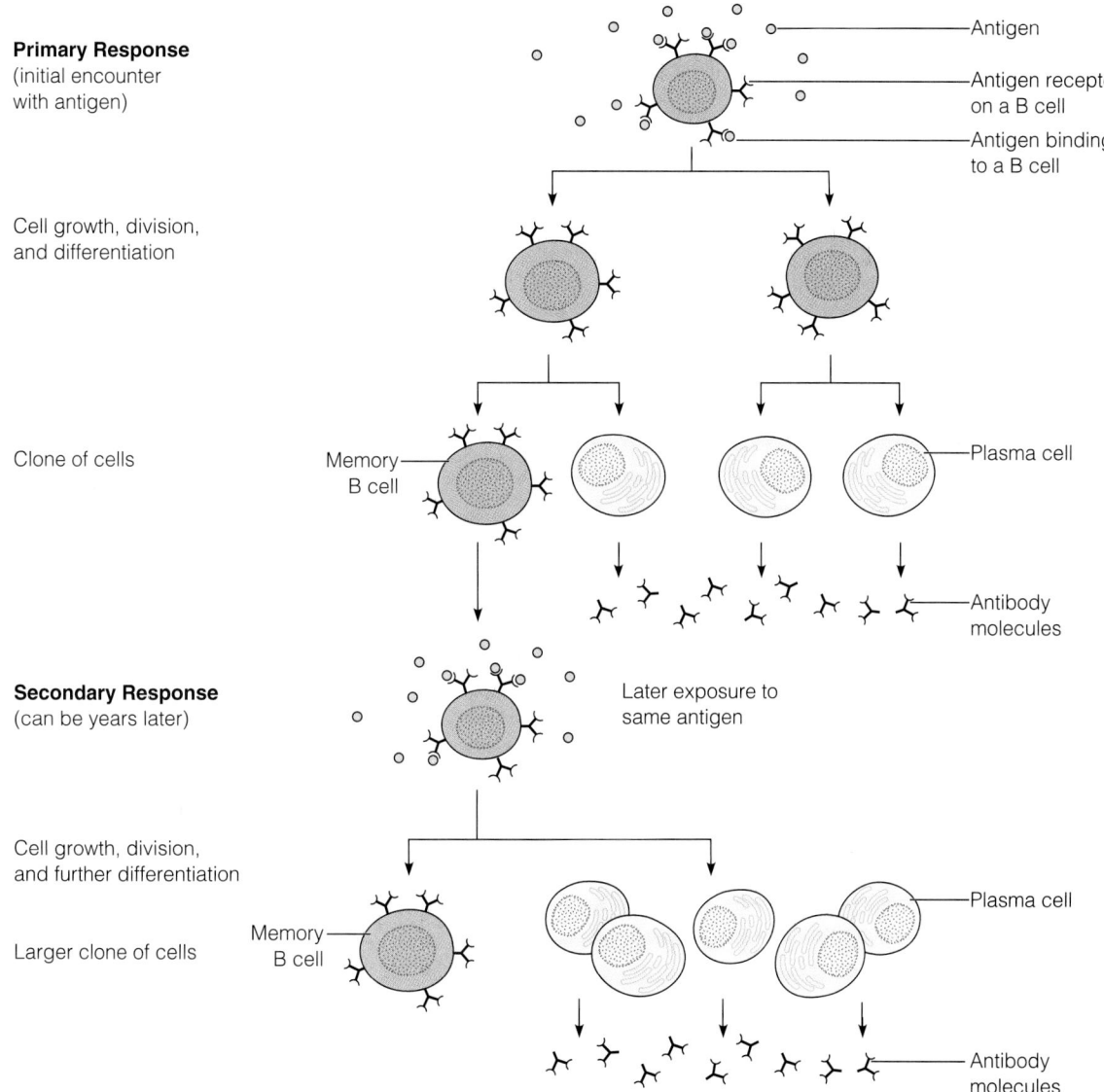

Primary Response
(initial encounter
with antigen)

————Antigen

————Antigen receptor
on a B cell

————Antigen binding
to a B cell

Cell growth, division,
and differentiation

Clone of cells

Memory
B cell

————Plasma cell

————Antibody
molecules

Secondary Response
(can be years later)

Later exposure to
same antigen

Cell growth, division,
and further differentiation

Larger clone of cells

Memory
B cell

————Plasma cell

————Antibody
molecules

Figure 8–6   Antibody-mediated (humoral) immunity. On initial exposure to the antigen, B cells with appropriate receptor sites are activated to become plasma cells and produce antibodies or memory cells. This is known as the primary response. With subsequent exposures, memory cells respond rapidly with antibody production. This is known as the secondary response.

or foreign tissue. Body cells, tissues, and fluids have antigenic properties that are unique and recognized by the immune system as "self." External agents, such as microorganisms, cells and tissues from other humans or animals, and some inorganic substances, have antigenic properties recognized by the immune system as "nonself."

Each body cell displays specific cell surface characteristics or markers that are unique to each person. These are known as *human leukocyte antigens (HLA)*. A person's HLA characteristics are coded within a large cluster of genes known as the *major histocompatibility complex (MHC)* located on chromosome 6. Recall that chromosomes are paired; each person inherits one member of the pair from

each parent. A chromosome pair contains multiple genes, each carrying instructions for production of one polypeptide chain. The number of genes in the MHC results in a multitude of HLA combinations. As a result, the possibility of two people having the same HLA type is extremely remote. Identical twins may be the exception, and some siblings have very similar HLA patterns. In tissue grafting and organ transplants, matching the HLA type as closely as possible tends to decrease rejection.

Antigens

As noted earlier, antigens are substances that are recognized as foreign or "nonself" and provoke a specific im-

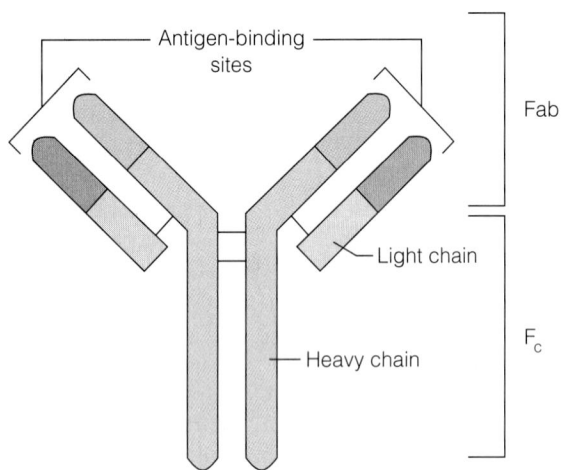

Figure 8–7 An antibody molecule. The Fab section is unique, providing an antigen-specific binding site. The Fc section is common to each class of immunoglobulin (IgG, IgA, IgM, IgD, IgE).

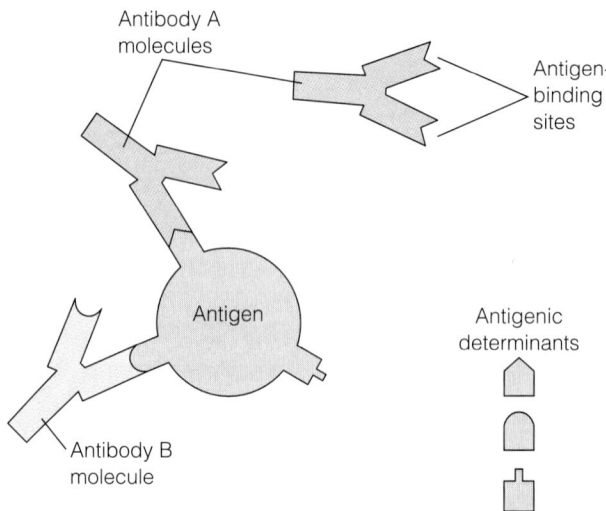

Figure 8–8 Antigen-antibody binding. The unique Fab site on the antibody binds with specific receptor sites on the antigen. As this illustration reveals, more than one kind of antibody may be produced to an antigen.

mune response when introduced into the body. Typically, antigens are large protein molecules, although polysaccharides, polypeptides, and nucleic acids may also be antigenic. Many antigens are proteins found on the cell membrane or cell wall of microorganisms or tissues. Other antigens include transplanted tissue or organs, incompatible blood cells, vaccines, pollen, egg white, and toxins such as bee or snake venom.

Complete antigens, known as *immunogens*, have two characteristics:

- *Immunogenicity*—the ability to stimulate a specific immune response
- *Specific reactivity*—stimulation of specific immune system components

The portion of an antigen that incites a specific immune response is called its antigenic determinant site (epitope): Complete antigens typically are large molecules with multiple antigenic sites; examples include proteins and certain polysaccharides. Small molecules, such as chemical toxins, drugs, and dust, that are unable to evoke an antigenic response alone may link to proteins to function as complete antigens. These substances are known as *haptans*.

When an antigen is encountered in the body, it is "recognized" by a specific receptor on a lymphocyte, and an immune response is generated. Two separate but overlapping immune responses may occur, depending on the antigen itself and the type of immune cell activated by contact with the antigen. Antigens such as bacteria, bacterial toxins, and free viruses usually activate B cells to produce **antibodies,** molecules that bind with the antigen and inactivate it. This is the **antibody-mediated (hu-**

moral) immune response. Other antigens, such as viral-infected cells, cancer cells, and foreign tissue, activate T cells, which are the primary agents of the **cell-mediated (cellular) immune response.** In this immune response, the lymphocytes themselves inactivate the antigen, either directly or indirectly.

The Antibody-Mediated Immune Response

The antibody-mediated immune response, also called the *humoral immune response,* is produced by B lymphocytes (B cells). B cells are constantly replaced through cell division and proliferation in the bone marrow. It is believed that B cells mature in the bone marrow and then migrate to the spleen to await activation. They normally constitute 10% to 15% of circulating lymphocytes.

B cells are activated by contact with an antigen and by T cells (discussed in the next section). Each B cell has receptor sites for a specific antigen or antigens. When the antigen is encountered, the activated B cell proliferates and differentiates into antibody-producing plasma cells and memory cells (Figure 8–6 on page 225). Plasma cells are short-lived, lasting only about 1 day. But while they are alive, they can produce thousands of antibody molecules per second. Memory cells retain antibody-producing information, allowing a rapid response if the antigen is again encountered.

The antibodies produced by B cells (see the box on page 227 and Figure 8–7) link with the antigen (Figure 8–8) and inactivate it through one of several processes:

- Promoting phagocytosis of the antigen by neutrophils
- Precipitation: combining with soluble antigens to form an insoluble complex or precipitate

Antibodies and Immunoglobulins

■ ■ ■

An *antibody* is an *immunoglobulin (Ig)* molecule with the ability to bind to and inactivate a specific antigen. Immunoglobulins make up the gamma globulin portion of the blood proteins. The immune system produces numerous antibodies, each active against a specific antigen. Antibodies fall into five classes of immunoglobulins: IgG, IgA, IgM, IgD, and IgE. Each has a slightly different structure and function.

Antibodies are Y-shaped molecules composed of two light and two heavy polypeptide chains (Figure 8–7). The top portion of the Y, called the *Fab* or *antigen-binding fragment,* is chemically variable and specific to the antigen. The lower portion, the *Fc* or *crystallizable fragment,* is constant for its class of immunoglobulin and directs the biologic activity of the immunoglobulin (the manner in which it functions). For example, the lower portion of immunoglobulin molecules produced against hepatitis A and hepatitis B are the same (IgG), but the upper portion is different and specific to the virus.

IgG, or *gamma globulin,* is the most abundant immunoglobulin, constituting about 75% of the total. IgG contains antibodies that are antiviral, antibacterial, and antitoxin in nature. It is the only immunoglobulin that can cross the placenta, and it provides a measure of immunologic protection for the neonate. Because of its abundance of antibodies, gamma globulin is often administered to provide *passive protection* when a client has been exposed to a disease.

IgA is often called *secretory immunoglobulin* because of its predominance in body fluids such as tears, saliva, and genital secretions. IgA provides localized protection against viral and bacterial infection, preventing organisms from binding with mucosal cells.

IgM is the first antibody formed during the initial encounter with an antigen and early infections. It is predominant for about 1 week, after which its levels decline. IgM forms antigen-antibody complexes and activates complement. This facilitates the phagocytic process by macrophages. IgM also forms natural antibodies (e.g., for ABO blood group antigens) and is an important component of the immune complexes seen in autoimmune disorders.

The exact function of *IgD* is unknown. It is speculated that IgD may be the receptor that binds antigens to the surfaces of B cells, thereby activating the cells.

Although the concentration of *IgE* is minute, about 0.004% of the total, it plays an important role in allergic and other hypersensitivity reactions. IgE binds with mast cells and basophils, causing them to release chemical mediators involved in immediate hypersensitivity reactions, such as anaphylaxis. Increased levels of IgE are also present in clients with parasitic infections, intestinal worms in particular.

The classes of immunoglobulins and their roles are summarized in Table 8–3.

- Neutralization: combining with a toxin to neutralize its effects; the antigen-antibody complex is then destroyed by the process of phagocytosis
- Lysis of the antigen cell membrane caused by combination with antibodies and complement
- Agglutination (clumping) of antigens to form a noninvasive aggregate
- Opsonization: coating of the antigen with antibodies and complement, making them more susceptible to phagocytosis

The complete antibody-mediated response occurs in two phases. With initial exposure to an antigen, the *primary response* develops. B cells are activated to proliferate and begin producing antibodies. There is a latency period of 3 to 6 days before antibodies become detectable in the blood. Levels then continue to rise, peaking at 10 to 14 days after the initial exposure. With many illnesses, such as chicken pox, this peak correlates with recovery.

Subsequent exposure to the same antigen elicits a *secondary response*. Memory cells (Figure 8–6) formed during the primary response stimulate the production of plasma cells, and an almost immediate rise in antibody levels occurs (Figure 8–9). This rapid secondary response is the basis of acquired immunity and is instrumental in preventing disease. It is also the mechanism through which vaccines provide protection from disease.

The Cell-Mediated Immune Response

Many antigens cannot stimulate the antibody-mediated response or are "hidden" from it because they live inside the body's cells (viruses and mycobacteria are examples of such antigens). The immune response providing protection against these antigens is the cell-mediated immune response, also called *cellular immunity*. T lymphocytes (T cells) are the initiators of this type of immune response.

Approximately 70% to 80% of circulating lymphocytes are T cells. T cells migrate to the thymus during fetal and

Table 8–3 Immunoglobulin Characteristics and Functions

Class	Percentage of Total	Characteristics and Function
IgG	75%	Most abundant Ig; also known as gamma globulin; found in blood, lymph, and intestines
		Active against bacteria, bacterial toxins, and viruses
		Activates complement
		The only Ig to cross the placenta, providing immune protection to neonate
IgA	10% to 15%	Found in saliva, tears, and bronchial, gastrointestinal, prostatic, and vaginal secretions, as well as blood and lymph
		Provides local protection on exposed mucous membrane surfaces and potent antiviral activity by preventing binding of the virus to cells of the respiratory and gastrointestinal tracts
		Levels decrease during stress
IgM	5% to 10%	Found in blood and lymph
		First antibody produced with primary immune response
		High concentrations early in infection, decreases within about a week
		Mediates cytotoxic response and activates complement
IgD	< 1%	Found in blood, lymph, and surfaces of B cells
		Exact function unknown; may be receptor binding antigens to B cell surface
IgE	< 0.1%	Found on mast cells and basophils
		Involved in release of chemical mediators responsible for immediate hypersensitivity (allergic and anaphylactic) response

early life, establishing the lifetime pool of cells. T cells have a life span measured in years, maintaining their numbers through proliferation, primarily in the lymph nodes.

T cells are much more complex than B cells. There are two major classes of T cells, *effector cells* and *regulator cells*. The main effector T cell is the *cytotoxic cell,* also called the *killer T cell*. Regulator T cells are further classified as *helper T cells* and *suppressor T cells.*

Proteins on the surface of the T cell help define its function and also provide a marker that can be used to identify the cell class. These proteins are known as the *cluster of differentiation antigen* or *CD antigen.* The two primary CD proteins are CD4 and CD8. Both cytotoxic and suppressor T cells carry the CD8 antigen. Helper T cells have the CD4 antigen and are often called CD4 cells.

T cells are antigen specific; that is, each subset is activated by a particular antigen. The antigens that activate T cells must be presented on another cell surface, such as pieces of virus presented on the surface of an infected cell, or the HLA antigen on a cell of transplanted tissue. When activated, T cells divide and proliferate, forming antigen-specific clones (Figure 8–10). (A *clone* is an exact copy of another cell.)

Killer T cells bind with cell surface antigens on virus-infected or foreign cells. Killer T cells destroy the antigen by combining with it and then either destroying its cell membrane or releasing cytotoxic substances into the cell. Killer T cells can destroy cancer cells, cells of transplanted

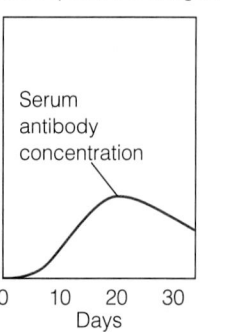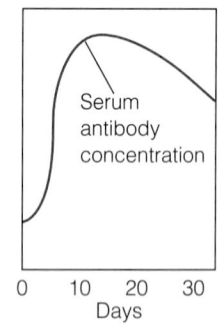

Initial exposure to antigen   Subsequent exposures to antigen

Serum antibody concentration

Serum antibody concentration

0 10 20 30
Days

0 10 20 30
Days

Figure 8–9 Antibody production in the primary and secondary responses of the antibody-mediated immune response. Note the more rapid and effective production following subsequent exposure.

organs, and grafted tissues. They are vital in the control of viral and bacterial infections.

Regulator T cells play a key role in controlling the immune response. The majority of regulator T cells are helper T (CD4) cells. CD4 cells are the most numerous of the T lymphocytes, making up 70% of the circulating population. They stimulate the proliferation of other T cells, amplify the cytotoxic activity of killer T cells, and activate B cells to proliferate and differentiate. They interact directly with B cells to promote their multiplication and conversion into plasma cells capable of producing antibodies.

Figure 8–10 Cellular immune response. *A,* An infected cell, abnormal cell, or phagocyte presents antigen on its surface that binds with a receptor site on a killer T or a helper T cell. The killer T cell is activated to proliferate into memory cells or mature cytotoxic cells. *B,* The helper T cell is activated to augment the cytotoxic response and stimulate the antibody-mediated immune response.

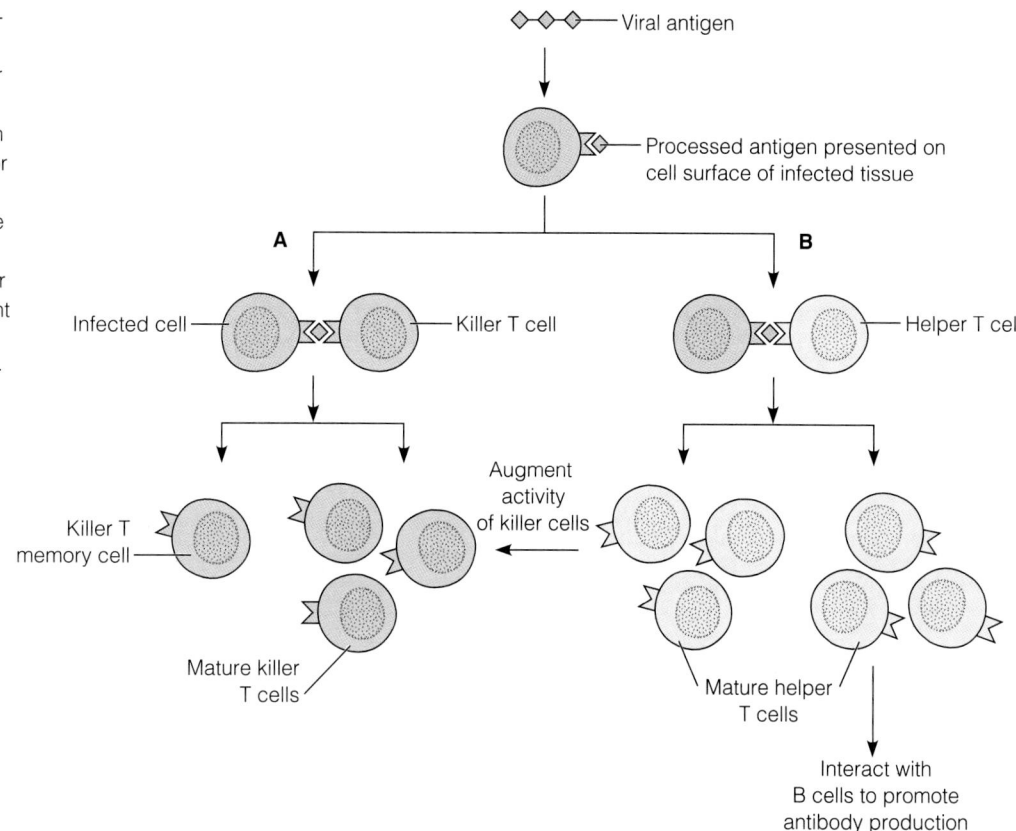

The other regulatory T cell group, suppressor T cells, provide negative feedback, making the immune response a self-limiting process. These cells are also important in preventing autoimmune disorders.

On activation, both effector and regulator T cells synthesize and release *lymphokines,* a type of soluble protein (see the box on page 230). Lymphokines secreted by cytotoxic and CD4 cells are important in amplifying the immune response and the nonspecific inflammatory response. They stimulate

- B cells to become plasma cells and produce antibodies.
- Macrophages to become activated macrophages (the most aggressive phagocyte).
- The proliferation of killer T cells.

Suppressor T cells release lymphokines which inhibit the activity of other T and B cells.

Although T cells can be activated only by specific antigens, much of the resulting effect is nonspecific—in other words, an enhanced inflammatory response. Like the antibody-mediated response, the cell-mediated response has memory. Subsequent exposures to an antigen result in a more rapid and effective inflammatory response as well as more effective phagocytosis by macrophages. This memory provides the basis for skin testing. A client previously exposed to tuberculosis, for example, develops a more pronounced inflammatory response when minute amounts are injected under the skin.

Age-Related Changes in Immune Function

A decline in immune function occurs with aging, although many of the mechanisms leading to this decline are not clear. External factors, such as nutritional status (see the nursing research box on page 231), and the effects of chemical exposure, ultraviolet radiation, and environmental pollution, affect the older adult's immune status. Internal factors affect it as well, including genetics, the function of the neurologic and endocrine systems, chronic and prior illnesses, and individual anatomic and physiologic variations. These myriad influences make it difficult to determine the effect of aging on the immune system. In some older individuals, the immune system is as effective as that of younger persons.

As noted previously, the thymus gland begins to involute or atrophy during adolescence. By age 50 to 60 years, thymic hormone levels are undetectable. Although the exact relationship of these events to T cell function is unclear, some T cell populations decrease or decline in function as the person ages. The ability of T cells to proliferate following activation also declines with advancing age; in addition, a portion of T cells cannot be activated in the elderly (Hazzard et al., 1994).

Cytokines

■ ■ ■

Cytokines are hormone-like polypeptides produced primarily by monocytes, macrophages, and T cells. Cytokines secreted by monocytes and macrophages may be called *monokines;* those secreted by T cells are known as *lymphokines.* Cytokines are also produced in small quantities in many different tissues throughout the body. Cytokines act as messengers of the immune system, facilitating communication between the cells to adjust or vary the inflammatory reaction or to initiate immune cell proliferation and differentiation. Cytokines are an essential component of an adequate immune response. The major cytokines and their functions are summarized in Table 8–4.

Interferons are a class of cytokine with broad antiviral effects. A number of different forms of interferon exist, broadly grouped as alpha, beta, and gamma interferons. Interferon is synthesized by cells infected with a virus and secreted into extracellular fluid. It then binds to specific receptors on uninfected neighboring cells, protecting them from infection. The spread of the virus is thus inhibited, and recovery from infection enhanced. It appears that interferons also moderate the activity of NK cells and may be involved in preventing the spread of abnormal malignant cells.

Table 8–4   Major Cytokines and Their Functions

Cytokine	Where Produced	Primary Functions
Interleukin-1 (IL-1)	Monocytes and macrophages; other cells	Activates T and B cells
		Induces fever and tissue catabolism
		Enhances NK activity
		Attracts neutrophils, macrophages, and lymphocytes
		Stimulates endothelial cell growth, collagen, and collagenases
Interleukin-2 (IL-2)	Helper T cells	Stimulates T and B cell proliferation
		Activates killer T and NK cells
Interleukin-3 (IL-3)	T cells	Stimulates growth and differentiation of bone marrow stem cells
Interleukin-4 (IL-4)	Activated helper T cells	Stimulates proliferation of T and B cells
		Increases IgE secretion by B cells
Interleukin-5 (IL-5)	T cells and activated mast cells	Promotes differentiation of B cells and eosinophils
		Stimulates production of IgA
Gamma interferon	T and NK cells	Stimulates phagocytosis by neutrophils and macrocytes
		Activates NK cells
		Augments B cell proliferation, enhancing both cellular and humoral immune responses
Alpha and beta interferons	Virus-infected cells; macrophages	Activate macrophages and endothelial cells
		Augment NK cell activity
		Act at gene level to protect neighboring cells from invasion by intracellular parasites, such as viruses, rickettsia, malaria
Tumor necrosis factor (TNF)	Activated macrophages, T cells, and NK cells	Major chemical mediator of inflammatory response
		Stimulates T cell activation, antibody production, and accumulation of leukocytes at inflammatory site
		Directly cytotoxic to some tumor cells
		Induces fever

Applying Research to Nursing Practice:
The Implications of Supplemental Nutrition for Immune Function

Optimal immune function is hampered in the client who is poorly nourished. Institutionalized and older clients are at risk for altered nutrition, which may contribute to an increased risk of infection.

A retrospective study of nursing home clients receiving oral nutritional supplements (such as Ensure) was conducted to determine why supplements were prescribed, how nutritional status was assessed, and whether supplements were effective (Johnson, Dooley, & Gleick, 1993). Weight loss and poor appetite were the primary reasons for initiating supplemental feedings. Other than serial weight, measurements, comparison of current weight to previous weight or "ideal body weight" standards, and subjective assessment of food consumption, little nutritional assessment was performed prior to the initiation of or during therapy.

Clients tended to gain weight while receiving oral supplements, achieving approximately their preadmission weight within 9 to 10 months. When compared with a control group of older clients, this more frail population showed no higher incidence of infections or hospitalizations. Although laboratory values were available on too few of the clients to provide statistically reliable data, several clients showed an improvement in albumin and total lymphocyte count.

Implications for Nursing

Nutritional assessment of older adults is vital in both acute and long-term care settings. Adequate nutrition plays an important role in healing and, it is believed, in maintaining immune function. Responsibility for monitoring and assessing nutritional status often falls to the nurse, primarily because of time spent with the client. Weights are not always an accurate measure of nutritional status, and anthropometric measurements may be difficult to obtain and interpret. Nurses need to be aware of laboratory studies and their relationship to the nutritional and immune status of the client. Clients with low total protein, albumin, cholesterol, hemoglobin, or WBC count are at risk for infection. Providing liquid oral nutritional supplements may help reduce this risk.

Critical Thinking in Client Care
1. Suggest cultural, ethnic, social, and psychological factors that might increase risk for altered nutrition in institutionalized and older clients.

2. Develop a nutritional assessment form for use in assessing nutritional status in nursing home clients.

3. If you are caring for a client who requires supplemental oral nutrition but has a limited income, what suggestions might you make that would be effective in increasing nutritional status and also be affordable for the client?

4. Describe sources of error in measuring body weight and develop a procedure that will more likely ensure reliable and consistent measurement.

With these changes, cell-mediated immune function declines. The client has reduced resistance to antigens such as *Mycobacterium tuberculosis*, influenza and varicella-zoster viruses, malignant cells, and tissue grafts.

Immunoglobulin levels remain relatively stable, but primary and secondary antibody responses decline with aging. This diminished antibody production has clinical implications in that immunizations (single-dose and booster) may not produce the expected protective immune response. Whereas the antibody response to foreign antigens is diminished, *autoantibodies* (antibodies that react to the client's own tissues) are more common in older persons. The presence of autoantibodies suggests impaired regulation of the immune system, but it is not associated with an increased incidence of autoimmune disorders (discussed later in this chapter) (Abrams & Berkow, 1990; Hazzard et al., 1994). Age-related changes in immune function are summarized in the box on page 232.

Assessing the Client's Immune System

Unlike body systems that are composed of a few closely related organs, the immune system is diverse and scattered. Optimal immune function depends on intact skin and mucous membrane barriers, adequate blood cell production and differentiation, a functional system of lymphatics and the spleen, and the ability to differentiate foreign tissue and pathogens from normal body tissue and flora. Because of this diversity of organs and function, as-

---

Age-Related Changes in Immune Function

■ ■ ■

- Involution of the thymus, with decreased hormone production

- Diminished production and response to lymphokines (IL-2 in particular)

- Decreased cell proliferation, with antigenic stimulation

- Decreased killer T cell cytotoxic activity

- Decreased levels of specific antibody response

- Increased levels of autoimmune antibodies

- Reduced or delayed hypersensitivity response

---

sessment of the immune system is often integrated throughout the history and physical examination.

Focused Interview

Prior to interviewing the client, review the biographic data, including age, sex, race, and ethnic background. This information can provide valuable clues about possible immunologic disorders. For example, many autoimmune disorders are more prevalent in women than in men. Family history is also important, because there is a genetic component in the etiology of many disorders affecting the immune system.

Many interview questions related to the immune system and disorders that affect it are of a sensitive nature. Be sure to provide for privacy of the client prior to the interview. If family members are present, request that they leave as well. Establish a trusting relationship with the client prior to asking the most sensitive questions (e.g., those related to the use of illicit drugs or sexual activity).

Health Perception–Health Management

Questions regarding the client's health perception–health management pattern which may be pertinent to the immune system include the following:

- *Perception of general health.* How has the client been feeling? How does the client perceive his or her health? Because the immune system plays a vital role in maintaining health and protection from disease, these questions can elicit important information.

- *Recent illnesses or changes in health status.* Have any changes in health status been noted? Has the client been sick recently?

- *Past illnesses/hospitalizations.* Has the client ever received a blood transfusion, organ transplant, or tissue transplant? Has the client ever had a transfusion reac-

tion? Has the client ever been turned away as a blood donor?

- *Allergies.* Is the client hypersensitive to anything, including medications, household dusts or danders, bee stings? If the client is hypersensitive, what type of reaction does the client experience? Does the client have a history of asthma, hay fever, or dermatitis?

- *Immunization status.* Has the client been fully immunized against measles, mumps, rubella, polio, tetanus, and hepatitis B? When did the client last receive any vaccines or immunizations?

- *Screening tests.* Have any screening tests, such as skin testing for tuberculosis or HIV serologic testing, been performed? When, and under what circumstances? What were the test results?

- *Occupation.* Is the client engaged in any occupation that may expose him or her to chemicals or other substances that may affect the immune system?

- *Current medications.* Is the client currently taking any medications; if so, what? Has the client ever experienced an adverse reaction, such as a rash or easy bruising, while taking a medication?

- *Recreational drug use.* Does the client currently use tobacco products, alcohol, or other recreational drugs? Does the client currently or has the client ever used drugs by injection or inhalation? Has the client ever shared needles or "works" with another person?

Nutritional-Metabolic

Related to the nutritional-metabolic health pattern, ask the client about

- Usual diet and recent weight changes.

- Any skin lesions, rashes, or impaired healing.

Activity-Exercise

In the activity-exercise health pattern, inquire about

- The client's exercise tolerance and any complaints of excessive or unusual fatigue or weakness.

- Frequent sore throats or upper respiratory illnesses.

- Swollen glands in the neck, axillae, or groin.

- Easy bruising or excessive bleeding from injuries or gums.

- Joint pain or swelling, morning stiffness, or backache.

Role-Relationship and Sexuality-Reproductive

Inquire about the client's living situation, including significant others and relationships. Ask the client in a tactful but straightforward manner about sexual relationships and practices. Question the client about the number of sexual partners and their gender. Ask about specific high-risk behaviors, such as anal intercourse, and any barrier protection used during sexual activity.

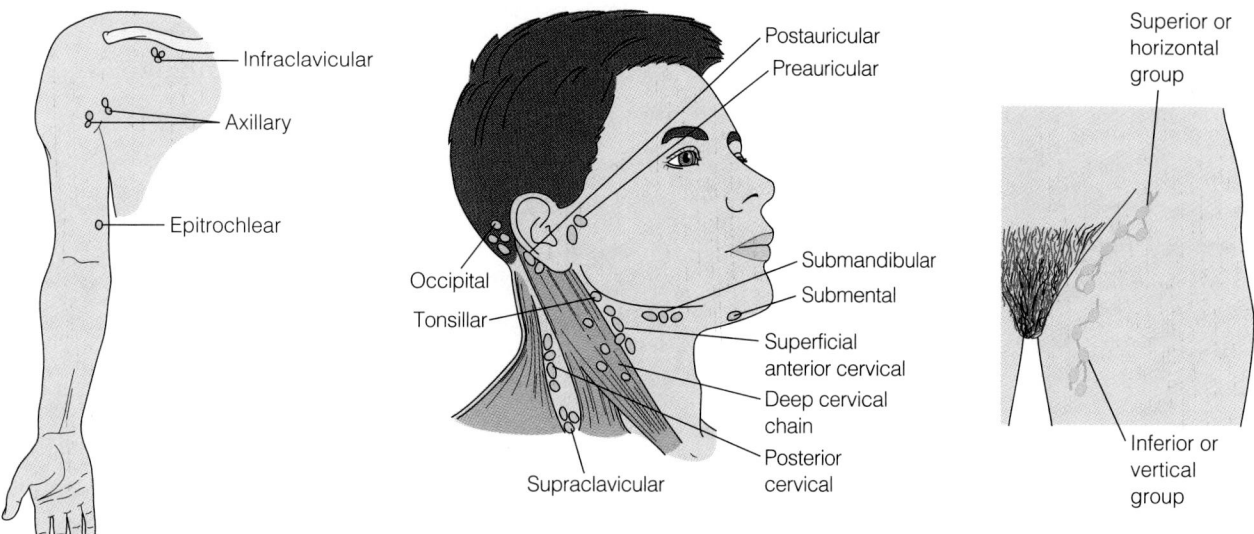

Figure 8–11   Lymph nodes that may be assessed by palpation.

Value-Belief

Ask the client about religious beliefs and practices. If the client specifies a religion with which you are unfamiliar, inquire about health-related issues, such as the belief in the use of medications and immunizations.

Physical Assessment

The techniques of inspection and palpation are especially important in assessing a client's immune system.

Assess the client's general appearance. Note whether the client's stated and apparent age coincide. Evident fatigue or weakness may indicate acute or chronic illness or immunodeficiency. Assess the client's height, weight, and body type for apparent weight loss or wasting. Observe the client's ease of movement, and note any evident stiffness or difficulty moving. Check the client's vital signs. An elevated temperature may indicate an infection or inflammatory response.

Assess skin color, temperature, and moisture. Pale or jaundiced skin may indicate a hemolytic reaction. Pallor may also indicate bone marrow suppression with accom-

panying immunodeficiency. Inspect the skin for evidence of rashes or lesions, such as petechiae, numerous bruises, purple or blue patches or lesions indicative of Kaposi's sarcoma, and wounds that are infected, inflamed, or unhealed. Note the location and distribution of any rashes or lesions noted.

Inspect the mucous membranes of the nose and mouth for color and condition. Pale, boggy (edematous) nasal mucosa is often associated with chronic allergies. Note petechiae, white patches, or lacy white plaques in the oral mucosa; they may indicate hemolysis or immunodeficiency.

Inspect and palpate the cervical lymph nodes for evidence of lymphadenopathy (swelling) or tenderness. Palpate the nodes of the axillae and groin as well (Figure 8–11).

Assess the musculoskeletal system by inspecting and palpating the joints for redness, swelling, tenderness, or deformity. Such changes may indicate an autoimmune disorder such as rheumatoid arthritis or systemic lupus erythematosus (SLE). Check joint range of motion as well, including that of the spine.

▪ ▪ ▪ Normal Immune Responses ▪ ▪ ▪

The Client with Tissue Inflammation and Healing

▪ ▪ ▪

As noted previously, inflammation is a nonspecific response to injury that serves to destroy, dilute, or contain the injurious agent or damaged tissue.

Inflammation may be either acute or chronic. Acute inflammation is a short-term reaction of the body to all types of tissue damage. It is immediate and aimed at protecting the body and preventing further invasion or injury. Acute inflammation usually lasts less than 1 to 2 weeks. Once the injurious agent is removed, the inflammation subsides. Healing with tissue repair or scar formation occurs, and the body functions in normal or near-normal capacity.

Chronic inflammation is slower in onset and may not have an acute phase. Its clinical manifestations occur over months or years. It involves cell proliferation and is debilitating, with long-term adverse effects. There is increased cellular exudate, necrosis, fibrosis, and sometimes tissue scarring, resulting in severe tissue damage.

Pathophysiology

The tissue damage that evokes an inflammatory response may be caused by specific or nonspecific agents. These agents may be *exogenous,* from outside the body, or *endogenous,* from within the body. Causes of inflammation include the following:

- Mechanical injuries, such as cuts or surgical incisions
- Physical damage, such as burns
- Chemical injury from toxins or poisons
- Microorganisms, such as bacteria, viruses, or fungi
- Extremes of heat or cold
- Immunologic responses, such as hypersensitivity reactions
- Ischemic damage or trauma, such as a stroke or myocardial infarction

Acute Inflammation

Regardless of the cause, location, or extent of the injury, the acute inflammatory response follows the previously outlined sequence of vascular response, cellular and phagocytic response, and healing.

Many of the manifestations of inflammation are produced by inflammatory mediators such as histamine and prostaglandins released when tissue is damaged (see Table 8–2 and the box on inflammatory mediators, page 220).

The *cardinal signs of inflammation* include:

- *Erythema* (redness)
- *Local heat* caused by the increased blood flow to the injured area (hyperemia)
- *Swelling* due to accumulated fluid at the site
- *Pain* from tissue swelling and chemical irritation of nerve endings
- *Loss of function* caused by the swelling and pain

The degree of functional loss depends on the location and extent of the injury. With increased tissue damage, more fluid exudate is formed, resulting in more swelling, pain, and functional impairment. Pain may be immediate or delayed. Prostaglandins intensify and prolong the pain. Kinins cause irritation to the nerve endings and contribute to the pain sensation.

Clinical Manifestations of Inflammation

Local Manifestations

- Erythema
- Warmth
- Pain
- Edema
- Functional impairment

Systemic Manifestations

- T >100.4 F (38 C) or <96.8 F (36 C)
- P >90/min
- R >20/min (tachypnea)
- WBC >12,000/mm³ or >10% bands

Dead neutrophils, necrotic tissue, and digested bacteria accumulate as a result of inflammation and phagocytosis, forming *pus.* It usually forms and remains until after the infection subsides. Pus may push itself to the surface of the body or become internalized. In the latter case, pus is gradually autolyzed (self-digested) by enzymes over a period of days. The end product is then absorbed by the body. On occasion, pus may remain after the infection is resolved. Pockets of pus, called abscesses, may need to be artificially drained with a procedure called *incision and drainage (I&D).* Ectopic calcifications are another possible result of residual collections of pus.

Systemic responses to inflammation include an increase in the size of lymph nodes due to the accumulation of bacteria, phagocytes, and destroyed lymph tissue. Enlarged lymph nodes are usually noted in the groin, axillae, and neck (Figure 8–11 on page 233). Fever, often precipitated by inflammatory mediators or bacterial toxins, inhibits the growth of many microorganisms and increases tissue repair functions. Loss of appetite and fatigue may occur in the effort to conserve energy during the inflammatory process. Leukocytosis occurs with increased WBC production to support inflammation and phagocytosis.

Local and systemic manifestations of inflammation are summarized in the accompanying box.

Chronic Inflammation

Whereas acute inflammation is a self-limiting process lasting less than 2 weeks, chronic inflammation tends to be self-perpetuating, lasting weeks to months or years. Chronic inflammation may develop when the acute inflammatory process has been ineffective in removing the offending agent. For example, mycobacteria have cell walls with high lipid and wax content, making them

Table 8–5   Factors That May Impair Healing

Factor	Effect
Malnutrition	
Protein deficit	Prolongs inflammation and impairs healing process
Carbohydrate and kilocalorie deficit	Impairs metabolic processes and promotes catabolism; proteins are used for energy rather than for healing
Fat deficit	Impairs cell membrane synthesis in tissue repair
Vitamin deficits	
Vitamin A	Limits epithelialization and capillary formation
B-Complex	Inhibits enzymatic reactions that contribute to wound healing
Vitamin C	Impairs collagen synthesis
Tissue hypoxia	Associated with an increased risk of infection and impaired healing, because oxygen is required to support cell function and collagen synthesis
Impaired blood supply	Inadequate delivery of oxygen and nutrients to healing tissues and removal of waste products
Impaired inflammatory and immune processes	Decreased phagocytosis and wound debridement; increased risk of infection; delayed healing

Note. Data are from *Pathophysiology: Concepts of Altered Health States* (4th ed.) by C. M. Porth, 1994, Philadelphia: Lippincott.

resistant to phagocytosis. Chronic inflammation and granuloma formation is common with *Mycobacterium tuberculosis* infection. Persistent irritation by chemicals, particulate matter, or physical irritants such as talc, asbestos, or silica may also result in chronic inflammation.

The chronic inflammatory process is characterized by a dense infiltration of the site by lymphocytes and macrophages. The macrophages mass or coalesce to form a multinucleated giant cell surrounded by lymphocytes, in a lesion called a *granuloma*. The granuloma is effective in walling off the offending agent, isolating it from the rest of the body. However, the infectious agent or offending irritant may not be destroyed and can survive within the granuloma for a long period of time. The granuloma formed in tuberculosis is called a tubercle. *Mycobacterium tuberculosis* may survive for many years within the tubercle, emerging when the client's immune system is no longer able to contain it.

Complications

Inflammation and wound healing are highly metabolic processes that may be affected by a number of factors.

Without adequate nutrition, blood supply, and oxygenation, tissues cannot effectively complete the process. Impaired inflammatory and immune processes can interfere with phagocytosis and preparation of the wound for healing. Infection prolongs the inflammatory process and delays healing.

Chronic diseases may also impair healing. Diabetes mellitus is a prominent example. With high blood glucose levels associated with poorly controlled diabetes, chemotaxic and phagocytic function is decreased. Collagen formation and tensile strength of the wound are also impaired. Small blood vessel disease is common in people with diabetes, a factor that further impairs the healing process.

Drug therapy, particularly corticosteroid medications, may suppress the immune and inflammatory responses, delaying healing (Porth, 1994). Other external factors, such as exposure to ionizing radiation and wound cleansing agents, can also affect healing. Table 8–5 summarizes major factors that affect the inflammatory process and wound healing.

Collaborative Care

Management of the client with inflamed tissue focuses on promoting healing. Care is generally supportive, allowing the client's own physiologic processes to remove foreign matter and damaged cells. Wound care may be minimal, involving only simple cleansing, or extensive, involving irrigations and debridement of necrotic tissue. The client is encouraged to rest to conserve energy and support healing, and to drink fluids to help dilute and remove waste products from the body. A well-balanced, nutritious diet with vitamin supplements also promotes healing. Anti-inflammatory medications are administered only when the inflammatory process has become problematic. Antibiotics may also be prescribed to help eliminate infectious causes of inflammation.

Laboratory and Diagnostic Tests

Laboratory and diagnostic tests may be needed to identify the source and extent of inflammation. The following laboratory tests may be ordered:

- *WBC count with differential* provides information about the type and extent of inflammatory response. With inflammation, the total WBC count typically increases, a condition known as leukocytosis. Leukopenia, a decreased WBC, occurs with bone marrow failure, overwhelming infections, malnutrition, and autoimmune disorders. Analysis of the differential count—that is, the percentage of the total WBC made up by each type of leukocyte—provides further clues about inflammatory processes (Table 8–6).

- *Erythrocyte sedimentation rate (ESR or sed rate)* is a nonspecific test used to detect inflammation. The rate at

Table 8-6   The White Blood Cell Count and Differential

Cell Type and Normal Value	Increased	Decreased
Total WBCs: 4000 to 10,000 per mm³	*Leukocytosis*: Infection or inflammation, leukemia, trauma or stress, tissue necrosis	*Leukopenia*: Bone marrow depression, overwhelming infection, viral infections, immunosuppression, autoimmune disease, dietary deficiency
Neutrophils (segs, PMNs, or polys): 55% to 70%	*Neutrophilia*: Acute infection or stress response, myelocytic leukemia, inflammatory or metabolic disorders	*Neutropenia*: Bone marrow depression, overwhelming bacterial infection, viral infection, Addison's disease
Eosinophils (eos): 1% to 4%	*Eosinophilia*: Parasitic infections, hypersensitivity reactions, autoimmune disorders	*Eosinopenia*: Cushing's syndrome, autoimmune disorders, stress, certain drugs
Basophils (basos): 0.5% to 1%	*Basophilia*: Hypersensitivity responses, chronic myelogenous leukemia, chickenpox or smallpox, splenectomy, hypothyroidism	*Basopenia*: Acute stress or hypersensitivity reactions, hyperthyroidism
Monocytes (monos): 2% to 8%	*Monocytosis*: Chronic inflammatory disorders, tuberculosis, viral infections, leukemia, Hodgkin's disease, multiple myeloma	*Monocytopenia*: Bone marrow depression, corticosteroid therapy
Lymphocytes (lymphs): 20% to 40%	*Lymphocytosis*: Chronic bacterial infection, viral infections, lymphocytic leukemia	*Lymphocytopenia*: Bone marrow depression, immunodeficiency, leukemia, Cushing's syndrome, Hodgkin's disease, renal failure

Note. Data are from *Laboratory Tests and Diagnostic Procedures* by C. C. Chernecky, R. L. Krech, and B. J. Berger, 1993, Philadelphia: W. B. Saunders; and *Mosby's Diagnostic and Laboratory Test Reference* by K. D. Pagana and T. J. Pagana, 1992, St Louis: Mosby-Year Book.

which RBCs fall to the bottom of a vertical tube is an indicator of inflammation. An increased plasma protein content occurs with acute inflammatory processes, causing RBCs to "stack," increasing their weight and speeding their descent. An increased ESR may indicate acute or chronic inflammation, tuberculosis, autoimmune disorders, some malignancies, and nephritis. Decreased ESR is associated with congestive heart failure, sickle-cell anemia, polycythemia vera, and low plasma protein. No specific client preparation is required for this blood test.

- *C-reactive protein (CRP) test* may be requested to detect this abnormal glycoprotein. CRP is produced by the liver and is excreted into the bloodstream during the acute phase of an inflammatory process from any cause. CRP can also be an indicator of the client's response to therapy, because it disappears rapidly when inflammation subsides (Chernecky, Krech, & Berger, 1993). The normal or expected result of this test is negative for CRP. A positive result indicates an acute or chronic inflammatory process. Factors that may cause false test results include pregnancy, oral contraceptive use, or the presence of an intrauterine device. Food and fluids are restricted for 4 to 8 hours before venipuncture to obtain the serum for this test.

In addition to the above laboratory tests, cultures of the blood and other body fluids may be ordered to determine whether infection is the cause of inflammation.

Pharmacology

Medications may be prescribed for the client with an inflammatory response to help alleviate distressing symptoms or destroy infectious agents.

Acetaminophen (Tylenol) may be administered to reduce the fever and pain associated with inflammation. Acetaminophen has no anti-inflammatory effect; it will not reduce the inflammatory process but rather only relieve associated symptoms. Acetaminophen decreases fever by acting directly on the hypothalamus heat-regulating center. It also works on the central nervous system to relieve pain sensations.

Antibiotics may be used either prophylactically to prevent infection from interfering with the healing process of damaged tissue, or therapeutically to treat the infection. If infection is present, the organism and its response or sensitivity to various antibiotics are used to guide therapy. Antibiotic therapy is discussed in greater depth in the section of this chapter that discusses infectious diseases.

Although inflammation is a beneficial process to prepare acutely injured tissue for healing, it can have damaging effects as well. When these effects are a concern or the manifestations of inflammation are deleterious to the client, anti-inflammatory medications may be prescribed. Anti-inflammatory medications fall into three broad groups: salicylates, such as aspirin; other nonsteroidal anti-inflammatory drugs (NSAIDs); and corticosteroids.

Aspirin (also called acetylsalicylic acid, or ASA) is an NSAID that also has antipyretic and analgesic effects. Its beneficial effects are largely dose related. Although 10 grains of aspirin may have little effect on inflammation, it is an effective analgesic and antipyretic dosage. To relieve pain, aspirin acts primarily on peripheral sensory nerves by inhibiting the synthesis of prostaglandins and kinins, which are chemical stimuli of sensory nerves. As an antipyretic, aspirin acts both centrally and peripherally. It inhibits the formation of pyrogenic substances that raise the hypothalamic thermostat. It also dilates peripheral blood vessels and promotes diaphoresis, increasing the dissipation of heat (Shlafer, 1993).

In therapeutic doses, aspirin mediates the inflammatory process by inhibiting the synthesis of prostaglandins and acting on the mobility and activation of leukocytes. Inflammation is reduced, along with the swelling, redness, and impaired function that accompanies it.

The other NSAIDs have activity similar to that of aspirin. They inhibit prostaglandin synthesis, reducing the inflammatory and pain response. NSAIDs fall into a number of different groups:

- Salicylates, which include aspirin and related compounds
- Acetic acids, including indomethacin (Indocin), ketorolac (Toradol), sulindac (Clinoril), and tolmetin (Tolectin)
- Propionic acids, including ibuprofen (Motrin and numerous nonprescription preparations), fenoprofen (Nalfon), and naproxen (Naprosyn)
- Fenamates, including meclofenamate (Meclomen)
- Pyrazoles, including phenylbutazone (Butazolidin)
- Oxicams, including piroxicam (Feldene)

Each group has a slightly different mode of action for prostaglandin inhibition. Clients may have varying degrees of relief with different NSAIDs; sometimes, several different agents must be tried before the most effective is identified. Side effects also differ to a certain extent; however, all have a potential cross-sensitivity with aspirin, all irritate the gastrointestinal tract, and all cause some degree of sodium and water retention. Indomethacin and phenylbutazone are the most toxic of the NSAIDs. Their use is limited to short-term therapy.

For acute hypersensitivity reactions, such as reactions to poison oak, or for inflammation that cannot be managed by aspirin or NSAID therapy, corticosteroid therapy may be prescribed. The glucocorticoids are hormones produced by the adrenal cortex that have widespread effects on body metabolism and the immune response. Glucocorticoids inhibit inflammation and may be lifesaving in acute fulminating or chronic progressive inflammation. They do not cure disease; they are palliative to manage the inflammatory process (Spencer, Nichols, Lipkin, Henderson, & West, 1993).

When glucocorticoids are prescribed to manage inflammation, the following principles are used to guide therapy:

- The smallest possible effective dose is used.
- If a local-acting preparation such as a topical agent or intra-articular injection will be effective, it is prescribed.
- To minimize suppression of adrenal gland activity, an alternate-day dose schedule is used whenever possible.
- High-dose corticosteroid therapy is never stopped abruptly but rather is tapered down, allowing the client's adrenal glands to resume normal function.
- The incidence of potentially harmful side effects increases with higher doses and prolonged therapy.

The nursing implications of caring for a client receiving aspirin, an NSAID, or corticosteroid medications are outlined in the box that begins on page 238.

Wound Care
Often an area of tissue inflammation requires little more care than gentle cleansing with soap and water. Some commonly used cleansing agents, such as povidone-iodine (Betadine) and hydrogen peroxide, have a drying effect on the tissue and may actually inhibit the process of healing. The granulation tissue present in a healing wound is fragile and bleeds easily. Normal or physiologic saline is the cleansing agent that is least damaging to healing tissues. Wound care is discussed in further detail in Chapter 7.

Nutrition
Healing depends on cell replication, protein synthesis, and the function of specific organs—the liver, heart, and lungs in particular. Weight loss and protein depletion are risk factors for poor healing and wound complications. Even a few days of severely impaired nutritional intake can noticeably affect healing (Way, 1994).

The client with an inflammatory process or healing wound requires a well-balanced diet of sufficient kilocalories to meet the metabolic needs of the body. See Table 8–5 on page 235. Inflammation often produces *catabolism,* a state in which body tissues are broken down. Healing, by contrast, is a process of *anabolism,* or building up. Without sufficient kilocalories and nutrients, catabolism may predominate, impairing healing.

Carbohydrates are important to meet energy demands, as well as to support leukocyte function. Adequate protein is necessary for tissue healing and the production of antibodies and WBCs. Lack of adequate protein increases the risk of infection. Complete protein sources, those which provide all the essential amino acids, are preferred. Dietary fats are used in the synthesis of cell membranes.

Vitamins A, B-complex, C, and K are also important to the healing process. Vitamin A is necessary for capillary

text continues on page 240

Nursing Implications for Pharmacology: Anti-Inflammatory Drugs

ASPIRIN

Aspirin (Ecotrin, Empirin, others) is a nonsteroidal anti-inflammatory drug (NSAID) with analgesic, antipyretic, and antiplatelet effects. Aspirin inhibits prostaglandin synthesis and activity, reducing inflammation. By reducing prostaglandin stimulation of peripheral sensory nerves and the hypothalamus, aspirin also provides an analgesic and antipyretic effect. In very low doses (as little as 80 mg per day), aspirin inhibits platelet aggregation and normal blood clotting.

Nursing Responsibilities

■ Prior to administering aspirin, assess the client for history of hypersensitivity to aspirin, bleeding disorders, peptic ulcer disease, gastritis, hepatic disease, or allergic asthma.

■ Assess for other drugs in the client's prescribed regimen that may interact with aspirin. Concurrent administration of any other anticoagulant (such as coumarin or heparin), or a thrombolytic (such as streptokinase) greatly increases the risk of bleeding. When administered with other NSAIDs, their antiarthritic effects may be antagonized (Shlafer, 1993).

■ Determine the use for which the aspirin is prescribed. For analgesic use, it is typically prescribed on a prn (as needed) basis. When prescribed as an antiplatelet medication (to prevent myocardial infarction or stroke), the recommended dosage is 80 mg per day or every other day. Anti-inflammatory effect requires much higher doses, as much as 650 to 1300 mg four or five times a day.

■ Administer aspirin crushed or whole with food or milk to prevent gastric irritation.

■ Evaluate for the desired response, for example, reduction of pain, fever, and inflammation.

■ Discontinue the drug and notify the physician for
  a. Signs of an allergic response including rash, urticaria, or anaphylaxis.
  b. Evidence of gastrointestinal bleeding: including coffee-ground emesis, black or overtly bloody stools, or anemia.
  c. Ototoxicity with tinnitus (ringing in the ears). A reduction in dose may relieve this manifestation.

■ Aspirin increases the risk of hypoglycemia. Teach clients who are also taking oral hypoglycemics to monitor blood glucose levels frequently.

Client and Family Teaching

■ Take the medication as prescribed. Even though it is available over-the-counter, aspirin is an effective medication with potentially serious side effects.

■ Always take aspirin with food or milk to avoid gastric irritation.

■ Do not substitute acetaminophen (Tylenol) for aspirin; acetaminophen does not have the anti-inflammatory or antiplatelet effects that aspirin does.

■ If gastric irritation and nausea is a problem, substituting enteric-coated aspirin may be helpful.

■ Report any dark stools, hematemesis, abnormal bleeding, blurred vision, ringing in the ears, rashes, or difficulty breathing to the physician.

■ Check the labels of other over-the-counter drugs carefully; many contain aspirin.

■ Do not use alcohol while taking aspirin: The combination greatly increases the risk of gastrointestinal bleeding.

NONSTEROIDAL ANTI-INFLAMMATORY DRUGS (NSAIDS)

Diclofenac sodium (Voltaren)

Diflunisal (Dolobid)

Fenoprofen calcium (Nalfon)

Flurbiprofen (Ansaid)

Ibuprofen (Motrin, others)

Indomethacin (Indocin)

Ketorolac tromethamine (Toradol)

Meclofenamate sodium (Meclomen)

Naproxen (Anaprox, Naprosyn)

Piroxicam (Feldene)

Sulindac (Clinoril)

Tolmetin sodium (Tolectin)

Although these drugs in the NSAID class are not salicylates, they share many of the same effects and side effects as aspirin. NSAIDs are widely used to manage arthritis and other causes of inflammation. They differ from one another by chemical composition, but all inhibit prostaglandin synthesis, thus effecting an anti-inflammatory response. All are more costly than aspirin, but they have a longer duration of action; therefore, fewer daily doses are required to achieve the desired

Pharmacology: Anti-Inflammatory Drugs (continued)

effect. Indomethacin (Indocin) is one of the most effective inhibitors of prostaglandin synthesis and therefore an extremely effective NSAID. Nevertheless, the short-term and long-term side effects of indomethacin limit its use to short-term therapy for an acute inflammatory response. Ketorolac tromethamine (Toradol) is the only NSAID used primarily for pain management. It has been shown to provide an analgesic effect equivalent to standard intramuscular doses of meperidine or morphine (Shlafer, 1993).

Nursing Responsibilities

- Assess the client for possible contraindications to NSAID therapy, including aspirin allergy (cross-sensitivity between these drugs and aspirin is common), asthma of allergic origin, peptic ulcer disease or gastritis, preexisting renal impairment, anticoagulant therapy, or antihypertensive therapy with beta blockers or angiotensin-converting enzyme (ACE) inhibitors.
- Obtain a baseline weight and vital signs prior to initiating therapy; all of these drugs can potentially cause sodium and water retention.
- Determine whether the client is taking other drugs with which the prescribed NSAID may interact. Although the specific effects vary among selected NSAIDs, monitor the following clients receiving NSAID therapy closely:
  a. Older clients, who are most likely to have chronic diseases or organ dysfunction, or take multiple medications.
  b. Clients who are on digoxin or an aminoglycoside antibiotic and have reduced renal function. The clearance of these drugs may be reduced, increasing the risk of toxicity.
  c. Clients on lithium or methotrexate; NSAID therapy may reduce the clearance of these drugs.
  d. Clients receiving diuretic therapy. The effects of the diuretic may be reduced, increasing the risk of edema and possible cardiac failure. With potassium-sparing diuretics, the risk of hyperkalemia is increased (Spencer et al., 1993).
- Administer these medications with food or milk to minimize their gastric irritant effects.
- Evaluate the client for the desired anti-inflammatory effect, including decreased pain, swelling, redness, and increased mobility.
- Assess for possible adverse effects of therapy, including evidence of gastrointestinal bleeding; im-

paired renal function; and central nervous system effects, such as drowsiness, dizziness, headache, nervousness, or sedation. Indomethacin may cause severe headache, confusion, or psychosis. Along with phenylbutazone, it is associated with possible bone marrow depression and leukopenia, anemia, and thrombocytopenia.

Client and Family Teaching

- Take these medications as prescribed; to achieve the most beneficial effect, therapeutic blood level needs to be maintained. Do not use them as pain relief agents.
- Several weeks of continuing therapy may be necessary before the full anti-inflammatory effect is recognized.
- Do not take these medications on an empty stomach; take with food or milk.
- Weigh at least weekly while taking these medications. Report to the physician any sudden weight gain of more than 3 to 5 lb.
- While taking NSAIDs, do not drive or operate machinery if drowsiness occurs.
- Promptly report to the physician any of the following: changes in vision, hearing, or mood; a change in urination or bloody urine; coffee-ground emesis or blood in the stool.
- Avoid the use of alcohol while taking NSAIDs; alcohol can increase the risk of central nervous system depression and gastric bleeding.
- Use acetaminophen as needed for pain relief; avoid aspirin.

CORTICOSTEROIDS

Methylprednisolone (Medrol, Solu-Medrol)

Prednisolone (Delta-Cortef)

Prenisone

Glucocorticoids are hormones normally produced by the cortex of the adrenal glands. These hormones affect the metabolism of carbohydrates, proteins, and fat in the body and are necessary for the stress response. Cortisol, the main glucocorticoid, has significant anti-inflammatory effects. As pharmacologic agents, the corticosteroids are used to treat many acute inflammatory and allergic conditions. Because of their multiple and significant side effects, their use as anti-inflammatory agents is limited to acute episodes and

➤

Pharmacology: Anti-Inflammatory Drugs *(continued)*

clients for whom other anti-inflammatory medications are ineffective.

Nursing Responsibilities

- Assess the client for conditions that may be adversely affected by corticosteroid administration: peptic ulcer disease, glaucoma or cataracts, diabetes mellitus, psychiatric disorders.

- Obtain baseline vital signs and weight; monitor both routinely while the client is on corticosteroid therapy. Hypertension and weight gain may result from salt and water retention.

- Monitor intake and output; assess for edema.

- Administer the medications as ordered. To reduce adrenal gland suppression, administer daily or alternate-day corticosteroids in the morning, when physiologic glucocorticoid levels are highest. Alternate-day schedules are preferred for long-term administration.

- Administer oral preparations with food to decrease gastrointestinal side effects. Antacids or histamine-receptor blocking agents such as cimetidine (Tagamet) may be prescribed while the client is on corticosteroid therapy.

- Monitor for desired effects of reduced inflammation and pain with increased mobility.

- Monitor for adverse effects, including
  a. Increased susceptibility to infection and masking of early signs of infection.
  b. Hyperglycemia.
  c. Hypokalemia. Muscle weakness, nausea, vomit-

ing, and cardiac rhythm disturbances are potential manifestations of hypokalemia.
  d. Edema, hypertension, and signs of cardiac failure due to fluid overload.
  e. Peptic ulcer formation and possible gastrointestinal hemorrhage. Monitor for abdominal pain, black or tarry stools, and signs of bleeding.
  f. Changes in mental status, including depression, euphoria, aggression, and behavioral changes.
  g. With long-term use, cushingoid effects, such as abnormal fat deposits in the face (moon face) and trunk (buffalo hump); muscle wasting and thinning of the extremities and skin; and osteoporosis.

Client and Family Teaching

- Take the drug as prescribed; do not change the dose or time of day. Do not stop the medication abruptly. The dose will be tapered down gradually when the drug is discontinued.

- Notify the physician if adverse or cushingoid effects occur.

- Take the medication with food or at mealtimes to decrease the gastrointestinal effects.

- Monitor body weight. If a gain of more than 5 lb is noted, notify the physician.

- Moderate salt intake and avoid foods high in sodium, such as processed meats and potato chips. Increase intake of foods high in potassium, such as fruits, vegetables, and lean meats.

- At all times, carry a card or wear a bracelet or tag identifying corticosteroid use.

formation and epithelialization. B-complex vitamins promote wound healing, and vitamin C is necessary for collagen synthesis. Vitamin K provides a vital component for the synthesis of clotting factors in the liver.

Although it has been established that minerals contribute to the inflammatory and healing processes, less is known about required amounts. Zinc appears to be important for tissue growth, skin integrity, cell-mediated immunity, and other general immune mechanisms (Lutz & Przytulski, 1994).

Nursing Care

The nursing care needs of the client with an inflammatory process are related to the manifestations of inflammation

(pain in particular) and altered tissue integrity. Priority nursing diagnoses include *Pain, Impaired Tissue Integrity,* and *Risk for Infection.*

Pain

Along with redness, warmth, swelling, and impaired function, pain is one of the cardinal manifestations of inflammation. Depending on the cause, affected area, and degree of inflammation, pain may be acute and immobilizing or chronic and demoralizing. It is important to remember that pain is a subjective experience and that client responses to pain vary. Refer to Chapter 4 for more information about pain and its management.

Nursing interventions with rationales follow:

- Assess the client's pain according to the client's reported rating of the pain (on a scale of 0 to 10, with 0 being no pain and 10 the worst pain). Note the character and location of the pain. *Because pain is subjective, the client provides the most accurate information regarding his or her pain experience.*

- Use physical and nonverbal cues to further assess the client's pain, especially if the client is nonverbal or tends to underreport pain.

- Administer anti-inflammatory medications as prescribed. *These medications help reduce the pain resulting from acute inflammation.*

- Administer analgesic medications as prescribed. *Although most analgesics do little to reduce inflammation, they provide additional pain relief by reducing the perception of pain.*

- Monitor the client for effectiveness of interventions. *Results may call for modifications in the regimen.*

- Provide comfort measures, such as back rubs, position changes, or relaxation techniques. *These measures reduce muscle tension, relieve areas of pressure, and provide distraction.*

- Encourage the client to engage in activities such as reading, watching television, and taking part in social interactions. *Such activities provide distraction from the pain experience.*

- Remind the client that rest is indicated for acutely inflamed tissue. *Strenuous activity or exercising an inflamed body part may increase discomfort and tissue damage.*

- If indicated, offer cold or heat as pain-relief measures. *For an acute injury, cold helps reduce swelling and relieve pain; after the initial stage, heat increases blood flow to the affected tissue and relieves pain and swelling by promoting absorption of edema fluid. Either heat or cold may be contraindicated with some inflammatory processes; for example, if the appendix is acutely inflamed, applying heat to the abdomen may prompt the appendix to rupture, increasing the risk of peritonitis. If unsure, check with the client's primary care provider.*

- Elevate the inflamed area if possible. *Elevation promotes venous return and reduces swelling.*

- Teach the client about the appropriate use and expected effects of anti-inflammatory medications. *If the client's pain continues after the initial doses of anti-inflammatory medication, the client may become discouraged and stop taking the medication before it becomes fully effective.*

Impaired Tissue Integrity

The inflammatory response can either precipitate or result from an impairment in the integrity of skin, support, or other tissues. Whatever the cause of the tissue alteration, it is vital that the nurse consider this alteration in delivering care.

Nursing interventions with rationales follow:

- Assess the skin and surrounding tissue, particularly in the area of inflammation, for integrity, edema, redness, and warmth. *Careful assessment is used to determine necessary care and protection measures.*

- Assess the client's general health and nutritional status. *Poor general health or chronic diseases such as diabetes mellitus or renal failure interfere with the healing processes and increase the risk of infection. A state of acute starvation lasting even only several days can impair healing as well.*

- Assess the client's respiratory and cardiovascular status, paying particular attention to the affected area. *Adequate tissue perfusion and oxygenation is necessary for healing.*

- Provide protection and support for inflamed tissue. *This reduces discomfort and decreases the risk of further tissue damage.*

- Clean inflamed tissue gently; if possible, use water or normal saline only. *Soap and harsh cleansing can cause further drying and tissue damage.*

- Keep the inflamed area dry, and expose it to air as much as possible. *This promotes healing and helps prevent infection.*

- Encourage the client to balance rest with the degree of mobility he or she can tolerate. *Rest decreases metabolic demands and allows for cell regeneration while mobility helps to promote oxygenation and perfusion of the tissues.*

- Provide supplemental oxygen as ordered. *Supplemental oxygen improves tissue oxygenation and reduces hypoxia.*

- Assist the client to eat a well-balanced diet with adequate kilocalories to meet the body's metabolic and healing needs. If the client is allowed nothing by mouth (NPO) or unable to consume an adequate diet, suggest parenteral nutrition, between-meal supplements, and/or multivitamin supplements. *Careful attention to diet and nutrient intake is important to provide the nutrients necessary for immune function and healing and to prevent catabolism.*

Risk for Infection

The inflammatory response often indicates that body defense mechanisms have been set in motion to protect against invading microorganisms. Wounds, whether traumatic or surgical in nature, are typically contaminated, as attested to by subsequent wound infections. The client with a healing wound is at particular risk for infection.

Nursing interventions with rationales follow:

- Assess the wound for the cardinal signs of inflammation and for specific signs of infection, including purulent drainage, odor, and poor healing. *The normal inflammatory response can indicate infection and, on occasion, mask its presence.*

- Assess the client's temperature every 4 hours. *In response to the inflammatory process the temperature rises, usually in the range of 99 F (37.2 C) degrees to 100.9 F (38.2 C). A temperature of 101.0 F (38.3 C) or above indicates infection.*

- Culture purulent or odorous wound drainage. *Wound culture is used to determine the infectious organism and to direct antibiotic therapy.*

- Apply dry or moist heat to the affected area for no longer than 20 minutes several times a day. *Heat increases the circulation of blood to and from the inflamed tissue. Time is limited to prevent burns.*

- Provide fluid intake of 2500 mL per day. *Adequate hydration helps maintain blood flow and nutrient supply to the tissues.*

- Assure adequate nutrition. *Adequate nutrition enhances the function and production of T cells and B cells, which are important in the immune response.*

- Use good hand-washing techniques. *Hand washing removes transient microorganisms and is the best mechanism to prevent the spread of infection to a susceptible person.*

- Wear sterile gloves when providing wound care. *Using sterile gloves helps prevent further contamination of the wound and the spread of infection to other clients.*

Other Nursing Diagnoses

The following are additional nursing diagnoses for the person with inflammation:

- *Activity Intolerance* related to loss of function of the inflamed area

- *Altered Nutrition: Less Than Body Requirements* related to malaise and general fatigue

- *Knowledge Deficit* about the cause of inflammation and treatment modalities

Client and Family Teaching

Client and family teaching enhances understanding of the inflammatory process, its cause, and its management. Teaching is also important to prevent further compromise that could result in infection.

Instructions, verbal and written, should include the following:

- Increase fluid intake to 2500 mL (approximately 2½ quarts) per day.

- Eat a well-balanced diet high in vitamins and minerals and with adequate protein and kilocalories for healing.

- Use good hand-washing techniques, particularly when caring for wounds or inflamed tissue and after using the bathroom.

- Elevate the inflamed area to reduce swelling and pain.

- Apply heat or cold for no longer than 20 minutes at a time to reduce the risk of tissue damage from burns or frostbite.

- Take all medications as prescribed, notifying the physician if adverse effects or hypersensitivity responses are noted.

- Rest acutely inflamed tissue; do not engage in strenuous activity until the inflammation has subsided.

The Client with Natural or Acquired Immunity

■ ■ ■

Immunity refers to the protection of the body from disease. Immunity to disease may be either natural or acquired, active or passive.

Immunity develops from the activation of the body's immune response. Depending on the antigen, antibody-mediated or cell-mediated responses are activated. The immune response typically involves components of both. In the immunocompetent client, these responses inactivate and remove the antigen, allowing recovery to occur or preventing the development of disease.

Pathophysiology

The processes of antibody-mediated and cell-mediated immunity result in the development of *acquired immunity* or **active immunity.** Active immunity occurs when the body produces antibodies or develops immune lymphocytes against specific antigens. Memory cells, which can produce an immediate immune response on reexposure to the antigen, provide long-term immunity.

Active immunity can be *naturally acquired*, resulting from contact with the disease-producing antigen and subsequent development of the disease. Naturally acquired immunity is common for diseases such as chickenpox and hepatitis A, in which the risk of developing the disease a second time is very small.

For many diseases, the potential consequences of a single disease episode on the individual and society make prevention desirable. This is especially true for highly contagious diseases capable of causing epidemics. In these instances, immunization or vaccination is used to provide *artificially acquired immunity.* The purpose of vaccination is to establish adequate levels of antibody and/or memory cells to provide effective immunity (Roitt, 1994). This is done by introducing the disease-producing antigen into the body in a manner that will stimulate the

Table 8–7   Types of Acquired Immunity

Type of Immunity		How Developed	Examples
Active Immunity	Natural	Acquired by infection with an antigen, resulting in the production of antibodies	Chickenpox, hepatitis A
	Artificial	Acquired by immunization with an antigen, such as attenuated live virus vaccine	MMR, polio, DPT, hepatitis B vaccines
Passive Immunity	Natural	Acquired by transfer of maternal antibodies to the fetus or neonate via the placenta or breast milk	Neonate initially protected against MMR if mother immune
	Artificial	Acquired by administration of antibodies or antitoxins in immune globulin	Gamma globulin injection following hepatitis A exposure

immune system to form antibodies and memory cells but will not produce disease. *Vaccines* may be made up of killed organisms or of live organisms that have been *attenuated* or modified to reduce their disease-producing capability. Typhoid is an example of a killed organism vaccine; measles-mumps-rubella (MMR) vaccine, by contrast, is made from attenuated organisms. Many newer vaccines use *subunits* of the antigen; these are portions of the organism that have antigenic properties but are unable to produce disease.

Passive immunity provides temporary protection against disease-producing antigens. Passive immunity is provided by antibodies produced by other people or animals. These acquired antibodies are used up; they either combine with the antigen or are naturally degraded by the body, and their protection is gradually lost. *Naturally acquired* passive immunity is provided by the transfer of maternal antibodies via the placenta and breast milk to the infant. Rabies human immune globulin and hepatitis B immune globulin (HBIG) are examples of immunizations used to provide *artificially acquired* passive immunity. The types of active and passive immunity are summarized in Table 8–7.

Collaborative Care

Collaborative care focuses primarily on assessing the client's immune status and ensuring acquired immunity to prevent disease.

Laboratory and Diagnostic Tests

A number of laboratory studies can be performed to assess the client's immune status. The most common studies include tests of serum proteins and immunoglobulins, antibody titers to evaluate antibody-mediated responses, and skin testing for cell-mediated responses:

- *Serum protein* is a measurement of the total protein in the blood. Normal levels for the adult and older adult

are 6 to 8 g/dL. *Albumin,* a protein formed in the liver, predominates, accounting for approximately 60% (3.2 to 4.5 g/dL) of the total serum protein. This protein is primarily responsible for the osmotic pressure of the blood. *Globulins* account for the majority of remaining serum protein, normally 2.3 to 3.4 g/dL. Globulins include all the immunoglobulins and the antibodies they contain. Total protein levels, albumin, and globulin are decreased in malnutrition. Liver disease also affects protein levels, decreasing the albumin to a greater extent than globulin. Decreased globulin levels are noted with immunologic deficiencies (Pagana & Pagana, 1992).

- *Protein electrophoresis* further breaks down globulin into its specific components, known as alpha$_1$, alpha$_2$, beta, and gamma globulin. Electrophoresis uses an electrical field to separate proteins by electrical charge, and molecular size and shape (Chernecky et al., 1993). Complement proteins, important in phagocytosis, are beta globulins. The immune globulins are gamma globulins. Gamma globulins subjected to further electrophoresis separate into immunoglobulins: IgA, IgD, IgE, IgG, and IgM. (See Table 8–3 on page 228.) Analysis of specific levels of each provides cues about the immune status of the client. IgG is the most prevalent, constituting approximately 75% of the total and containing the majority of circulating antibodies responsible for the humoral immune response.

- *Antibody testing* may be ordered to determine whether a client has developed antibodies in response to an infection or immunization. Some of the antibodies that may be identified include those for hepatitis, human immunodeficiency virus (HIV), rubella, toxoplasmosis, and *Treponema pallidum,* the organism responsible for syphilis. In the case of hepatitis and rubella, testing is often used to determine immunity. With the other disorders and hepatitis, it may also be used to determine if the client has the disease.

Table 8–8 Recommended Immunization for Adults

Vaccine	Type	Dose	Indications	Precautions and Nursing Implications
Measles-mumps-rubella (MMR)	Live virus	0.5 mL SC	All adults born after 1956, particularly those who are at risk for infection, such as college students and military recruits. Measles and mumps vaccination particularly recommended for males without history of previous infection; rubella vaccination recommended for all seronegative females.	As a live virus vaccine, should not be administered to pregnant women or immunocompromised clients. Do not administer to clients with a history of anaphylactic reaction to egg protein or neomycin.
Tetanus and diphtheria toxoids (Td)	Inactivated toxins	0.5 mL IM	Initial series of 3 injections (initial and at 1 and 6 months) if never immunized; booster every 10 years; following a major or contaminated wound if more than 5 years since last booster	Do not give in first trimester of pregnancy or to clients with a history of anaphylactic reaction to horse serum; administer deep IM in deltoid of dominant arm.
Hepatitis B (HB)	Inactive viral antigen	1.0 mL IM	Series of three doses: initial and at 1 and 6 months. Recommended for anyone at risk for exposure and for postexposure prophylaxis	Use with caution in pregnant or lactating females, older clients, and clients with active infection; have epinephrine 1:1000 available on unit in case of anaphylaxis and laryngospasm.
Influenza	Inactivated virus or viral components	0.5 mL IM	Yearly for all clients over age 65 and those at risk for complications, including debilitated clients and clients with chronic disease	Do not administer to acutely ill clients or clients with history of anaphylactic reaction to egg protein.
Pneumococcal	Bacterial polysaccharides	0.5 mL IM or SC	One dose for clients over age 65 and those at risk for pneumococcal pneumonia, including clients with chronic lung disease or other chronic diseases	Do not administer to pregnant women.

- *Skin testing* can be used to assess cell-mediated immunity. A known antigen such as streptokinase, tuberculin purified protein derivative (PPD) or candida is injected intradermally. The site is then observed for induration and erythema, which typically peaks at 24 to 48 hours. Typically, induration of at least 10 mm in diameter is a positive reaction indicating previous exposure and sensitization to the antigen. (For additional information on skin testing for hypersensitivity reactions, see pages 270 through 272; Figure 8–18 on page 271 illustrates induration and erythema.) *Anergy,* no reactivity to injected known antigens, indicates depressed cell-mediated immunity.

Immunizations

Vaccines are suspensions of whole or fractionated bacteria or viruses that have been treated to make them nonpathogenic. Vaccines are given to induce an immune response and subsequent immunity. Although vaccine development has been a major factor in improving public health, no vaccine is completely effective or entirely safe (Merck Research Laboratories, 1992). Table 8–8 outlines the vaccines recommended for the adult client to maintain optimal health and immune status.

Adults born before 1956 are generally considered to be immune to measles, mumps, and rubella by prior infection. For persons born after 1956 whose immunologic status is unclear or who are at significant risk of exposure to these diseases (e.g., persons entering health care careers), reimmunization is recommended (Merck Research Laboratories, 1992).

Tetanus and diphtheria toxoids are combined in a single immunization. The pediatric form of the vaccine is known as DT; the adult form, Td. The vaccine stimulates active immunity by inducing the production of antibodies and antitoxins. After an initial series of three immunizations, an intramuscular (IM) booster injection of 0.5 mL is recommended every 10 years to maintain protection.

Table 8–9   Preparations for Postexposure Prophylaxis

Disease	Preparation and Dose	Indications
Hepatitis A	Human immune globulin (IG), 0.02 mL/kg IM	Contacts in day care centers, households, custodial institutions; patrons of eating establishments known to have been exposed by infected food worker
Hepatitis B	Hepatitis B immune globulin (HBIG), 0.06 mL/kg IM	Possible percutaneous or sexual contact with blood or body fluids of an infected individual; usually given concurrently with hepatitis B vaccine
Varicella	Varicella-zoster immune globulin (VZIG), 12.5 units/kg; minimum dose 125 units, maximum 625 units	Susceptible adults exposed to varicella virus (e.g., chickenpox or shingles)
Tetanus	Tetanus immune globulin (TIG), 500 to 3000 units IM (part infiltrated around wound)	Clients with major or contaminated wounds who have no history of tetanus immunization or an unclear one that is not up-to-date; Td usually given as well
Rabies	Human rabies immune globulin (HRIG), 20 IU/kg, half IM, half infiltrated around wound	Persons with a significant exposure to a rabid or potentially rabid animal; followed with 5-dose course of rabies vaccine
Measles	Human immune globulin (IG), 0.25 mL/kg IM	Susceptible close contacts, especially people who are immunosuppressed; postpone immunization with measles vaccine until 3 months after IG
Rubella	Human immune globulin (IG), 0.55 mL/kg IM	Pregnant women exposed in first trimester when termination of pregnancy is not an option; does not ensure protection of fetus

Note. Table adapted from *Harrison's Principles of Internal Medicine* (12th ed.) by J. D. Wilson, E. Braunwald, K. J. Isselbacher, R. G. Petersdorf, J. B. Martin, A. S. Fauci, and R. K. Root (Eds.), 1991, New York: McGraw-Hill.

Older clients, particularly those who never entered the work force (e.g., older female adults), may have never received the initial series of DT vaccine.

Hepatitis B (HB) vaccine is given as a series of three or four immunizations to promote active immunity to hepatitis B. This vaccine is recommended for everyone at high risk for exposure through blood or other body fluids. It is mandated by the Occupational Health and Safety Administration (OSHA) for all health care workers at risk. Other high-risk populations include intravenous drug users, sexual partners of infected individuals, clients on hemodialysis, prison guards, and athletic coaches.

Influenza vaccine is recommended for persons at high risk for serious sequelae of influenza, including older adults, persons with lung disease or other chronic illness, and immunosuppressed individuals. The antigenic strain included in influenza vaccine varies each year according to the predicted predominant strains affecting the population. Yearly reimmunization is therefore required.

Pneumococcal vaccine is generally recommended for the same populations as influenza vaccine. A single dose of this vaccine confers lifetime immunity, although repeating immunization every 6 years may be considered for high-risk clients (Merck Research Laboratories, 1992).

In addition to routine immunizations, people traveling outside the United States and Canada should receive vaccines against diseases that are endemic in certain regions of the world.

Other immunologic substances may be administered as indicated. Immune globulins provide passive immunity as protection against a known or potential exposure to an antigen. Standard immune globulin is given to household contacts of clients with hepatitis A and persons traveling to areas in which it is endemic. Hepatitis B immune globulin (HBIG) contains higher titers of antibody to hepatitis B virus and is used for persons exposed by blood or sexual contact. Following confirmed or suspected contact with a pathogen, selected vaccines may be administered to stimulate an immediate immune response (Table 8–9).

For most vaccines, a sensitivity test should be performed prior to administration to detect sensitivity to substances such as horse serum or eggs. The substance is injected intradermally; if after 20 minutes there is no evidence of a reaction, the selected vaccine can be administered.

Moderate to severe local reactions may occur following administration of an immunization. Common reactions include redness, swelling, tenderness, and muscle ache. Administering the vaccine in the dominant arm of the client helps minimize local reactions, because use and movement of the arm facilitates absorption of the solution. Applying heat to the site is also beneficial. Occasionally local ulcerations occur; when they do, warm, wet pack, or sterile wet-to-dry dressings may be prescribed.

Nursing Care

Maintaining a population that is fully immunized against common, potentially epidemic, and devastating diseases is a major public health task for nursing. Nurses not only recommend and administer vaccines to individual clients and their families, but also plan and implement preventive care for whole communities.

Although this process may appear to be straightforward, multiple issues affect society's ability to immunize the entire population. For some people, for example, religious beliefs may preclude the use of immunizations to prevent disease. Also, people who are not citizens and the medically indigent population have difficulty accessing immunization services. Lack of immunization not only puts the individual at increased risk for infectious disease, but also increases the cost of medical services and the possibility of exposing immunocompromised people to disease.

Health-Seeking Behaviors: Immunization

For individual clients and their families, nurses promote immunocompetence by assessing immune status, recommending appropriate immunizations, and administering vaccines as ordered or indicated. Once a person reaches adulthood, routine immunizations often become a neglected part of health care.

Nursing interventions with rationales follow:

- Assess the client's immunization history and risk factors. *Assessment is necessary to determine what immunizations are appropriate.*

- Assess the client's and family's knowledge level, understanding, and attitudes about immunization. *This provides a basis for further education.*

- Determine whether the client has religious beliefs, a medical condition, or other factor that may contraindicate immunization.

- Discuss with the client and family the value and reasons for recommended immunizations. *Understanding promotes compliance.*

- Reinforce positive health-seeking behaviors of the client and family. *This will help promote future health-maintenance activities.*

- Using recommended immunization schedules, develop a plan for assisting the client to attain optimal immunization status. *Compliance with recommended schedules for immunization is important in preventing disease and disability.*

- Prior to administering prescribed vaccines:

  a. Assess for allergy to eggs, particularly if MMR or influenza vaccine is ordered. *Vaccines prepared from chicken or duck embryos will cause an allergic reaction in clients who are allergic to eggs.*

  b. Assess for hypersensitivity to horse serum. Clients sensitive to horse serum should not receive vaccines such as tetanus antitoxins. *This will cause a severe allergic reaction.*

- Withhold administration of active immunologic products when the client has an upper respiratory infection (URI) or other infection. *Active immunizations can cause a greater inflammatory reaction in the presence of infections.*

- Do not administer oral polio vaccines (OPV), MMR, or any live virus vaccine to immunosuppressed clients or to clients who are in close household contact with an immunosuppressed person. *Live virus vaccines can cause disease in the immunosuppressed client. The virus may be transmitted to close household contacts during the initial postvaccination period.*

- Do not administer live attenuated virus vaccines and passive immunizations such as gamma globulin simultaneously. *Passive antibodies interfere with the response of the live attenuated virus.*

- Observe the client for 20 to 30 minutes following inoculation. *This is the average time frame during which an adverse reaction may take place.*

- Keep epinephrine 1:1000 readily available when administering immunizations. *Epinephrine causes vasoconstriction and reduces laryngospasm; in acute anaphylaxis, it can be lifesaving.*

Other Nursing Diagnoses

Other nursing diagnoses that may be appropriate for the client with acquired immunity include the following:

- *Knowledge Deficit* related to advantages of immunizations

- *Pain* related to local inflammatory reaction to vaccine

- *Altered Health Maintenance* related to unknown immunization status

- *Risk for Infection* related to lack of current immunizations

Client and Family Teaching

Educating individual clients, families, and the public about the maintenance of immune status is a significant nursing responsibility. For individual clients and their families, instructions focus on the following areas:

- Appropriate immunizations and recommended schedules for initial vaccination and boosters.

- How and where to obtain immunizations. County or public health departments generally offer immunization clinics at a cost significantly lower than private physicians or urgent care clinics. Some allow a sliding scale fee based on the client's ability to pay.

- The need to observe the client for up to 30 minutes following a vaccine for possible adverse reactions.

- Possible side effects and adverse effects of the immunization administered.

- Self-care measures for side effects and postvaccination discomfort.

- Responses to immunization that should be reported immediately to the primary care provider.

- Maintenance of a permanent immunization record.

In the public health setting, the nurse looks at the immunization needs and illness risk for an entire community. Communities include not only cities and localities but also groups of people, such as college populations and employees in a workplace. Public education needs may be met through presentations to groups of people, feature articles in newspapers and other local publications, advertising, radio presentations and public service announcements, and one-to-one discussion and teaching.

Applying the Nursing Process

Case Study of a Client with Acquired Immunity: Terry Adams

Terry Adams is a 48-year-old executive who is planning a trip to central Africa. In preparation, he contacts his local health care provider to obtain the necessary immunizations. Jane Wong, the registered nurse in the clinic, obtains a nursing history on Mr. Adams.

Assessment

Mr. Adams's history reveals that he has always been very healthy and active, apart from a mild case of asthma. As an adult, he has had little problem with his asthma, "except for those rare occasions on which I am dumb enough to smoke more than one cigarette!" He is divorced and is not currently in a continuing relationship. He has two grown daughters with whom his relationship is good. Since contracting hepatitis A several years ago, he drinks alcohol only rarely, and never more than one or two drinks at any one time. He confesses to little organized exercise but plays golf two or three times a week and states that he is such a hyperactive workaholic that he rarely sits for any length of time. Mr. Adams has not seen a physician since recovering from the hepatitis and

doesn't know when he last received any immunizations. He does know that his parents saw to it that he had all recommended immunizations as a child, and recalls getting both Salk and Sabin polio vaccines when they came out. His physical examination reveals an alert and healthy individual with no abnormalities noted. His vital signs are as follows: BP, 142/82; P, 64; R, 14; and T, 97.4 F.

The physician orders the following immunizations for Mr. Adams:

- Measles-mumps-rubella (MMR)
- Combined tetanus and diphtheria toxoids (Td)
- Yellow fever vaccine
- Typhoid vaccine
- Meningococcal meningitis vaccine

Diagnosis

Ms. Wong develops the following nursing diagnoses for Mr. Adams:

- *Health-Seeking Behaviors:* immunization related to impending international travel
- *Altered Health Maintenance* related to apparent lapse in immunization status
- *Risk for Injury* related to adverse response to immunization

Expected Outcomes

The expected outcomes established in the plan of care specify that Mr. Adams will

- Obtain necessary immunizations.
- Verbalize a schedule for maintaining up-to-date immunization status.
- Experience no significant adverse effects from immunization.

Planning and Implementation

Ms. Wong plans and implements the following nursing interventions:

- Administer MMR, Td, and meningococcal meningitis vaccines prior to discharge from clinic.
- Observe closely for 30 minutes following immunization for potential adverse responses.
- Schedule return visit in 1 week for typhoid vaccine.
- Provide referral to a registered vaccination center for yellow fever vaccine and documentation of vaccination.
- Provide instructions for comfort measures to relieve local and systemic adverse effects of vaccines. Provide written instructions on manifestations that should be reported to the physician.

■ Document immunizations on a permanent record at the clinic and for the client.

Evaluation

Terry Adams completes his prescribed immunizations without major adverse effects, although he does complain of fever, malaise, and general achiness for several days following the typhoid vaccination. His trip to Africa is successful, and he returns to the United States without contracting any infectious diseases.

The Client with an Infection

■ ■ ■

In an effort to find a suitable environment in which to grow and reproduce, microorganisms—including bacteria, viruses, fungi, and parasites—often invade the human body. In most cases, contact between humans and microorganisms is incidental and may even be beneficial to both organisms. Resident bacteria of the skin, mucous membranes, and gastrointestinal tract are an important part of the body's defense system. However, many microorganisms are *virulent;* that is, they have the ability to cause disease. *Pathogens* are virulent organisms rarely found in the absence of disease. Some microorganisms known as *opportunistic pathogens* rarely, if ever, cause harm to persons with intact immune systems but are capable of producing infectious disease in the immunocompromised host (Porth, 1994).

Infectious disease has been pervasive throughout history. Modern medicine, antibiotic therapy, immunizations, and other public health measures to protect food and water supplies have significantly reduced the prevalence of infectious diseases in many parts of the world. Smallpox, once a frightening disease with long-term consequences, has been eradicated. Nevertheless, in spite of these advances, many infections, including malaria, typhoid, and tuberculosis, remain prevalent in developing nations. Sexually transmitted diseases (STDs) rage through modern cities and industrialized populations. New varieties and strains of pathogens, such as human immunodeficiency virus (HIV), evolve to cause disease. To a certain extent, modern medicine has contributed to the development of infectious diseases caused by antibiotic-resistant strains of microorganisms. Tuberculosis is again on the rise in the United States, partially because organisms have become resistant to standard therapies. Clients receive immunosuppressive therapy following organ or tissue transplant or in the treatment of neoplasms, making them more susceptible to infection. Metal and plastic prosthetic devices are implanted, providing potential sites for colonization by disease-producing organisms

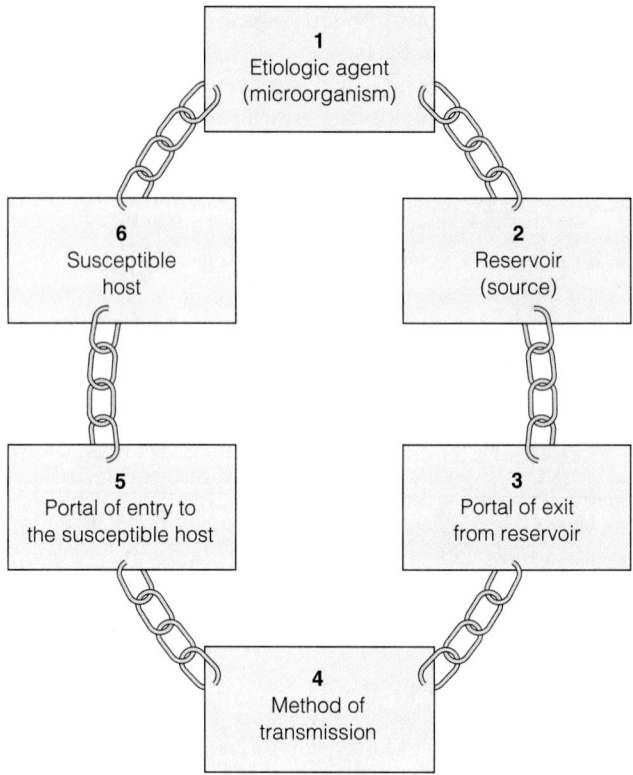

Figure 8–12   The chain of infection.

(Wilson et al., 1991). It has also become apparent that many diseases long considered unrelated to microorganisms may actually be infectious; for example, colonization of the gastric mucosa with *Helicobacter pylori* may be the predominant cause of peptic ulcer disease, and *oncogenic* viruses have the ability to transform normal cells into malignant cells.

Pathophysiology

Infection occurs when an organism is able to colonize and multiply within a host. The *host* can be any organism capable of supporting the nutritional and physical growth requirements of the microorganism—for example, humans. When the host experiences injury, pathologic changes, inflammation, or organ dysfunction in response to an infection or from intoxication by cellular poisons produced by a pathogen, it is called an *infectious disease.*

For a microorganism to cause infection, it must have disease-causing potential (virulence), be transmitted from its reservoir, and gain entry into a susceptible host. This is known as the *chain of infection* (Figure 8–12).

Pathogens

Pathogens capable of infecting and causing disease in a susceptible host include bacteria, viruses, mycoplasma,

Pathogenic Organisms

■ ■ ■

Bacteria

Bacteria are single-celled organisms capable of autonomous reproduction. Relatively small and simple organisms, they contain a single chromosome. A flexible cell membrane and rigid cell wall surrounds their cytoplasm, giving them a distinctive shape; some also have an extracellular capsule for additional protection. Bacteria have different characteristics and growth requirements: *aerobes* require oxygen for survival, whereas *anaerobes* cannot survive in the presence of oxygen; *gram-positive* bacteria stain purple when subjected to crystal violet stain, whereas *gram-negative* bacteria do not stain with crystal violet but turn red when subjected to safranin stain; the colonies formed by replicating bacteria differ from one another.

Viruses

Viruses are obligate intracellular parasites that are incapable of reproducing outside of a living cell. Viruses consist of a protein coat around a core of either DNA or RNA. Some viruses are shed continuously from infected cell surfaces; others, after inserting their genetic material into that of the infected cell, remain latent until they are stimulated to replicate. Viruses may or may not cause lysis and death of the host cell during replication. Oncogenic viruses are able to transform normal cells into malignant cells.

Mycoplasma

Although similar to bacteria, mycoplasma are smaller and have no cell wall, making them resistant to antibiotics that inhibit cell wall synthesis (e.g., penicillins).

Rickettsiae and Chlamydia

As obligate intracellular parasites with a rigid cell wall, rickettsiae and *Chlamydia* have some features of both bacteria and viruses. Rather than depending on the host cell for reproduction, they use vitamins, nutrients, or products of metabolism (e.g., ATP) from the host. *Chlamydia* are transmitted by direct contact, whereas many rickettsiae infect the cells of arthropods (e.g., fleas, ticks, and lice) and are transmitted from these vectors to humans.

Fungi

Fungi are prevalent throughout the world, but few are capable of causing disease in humans. Most fungal infections are self-limited, affecting the skin and subcutaneous tissue. Some fungi, such as *Pneumocystis carinii*, can cause life-threatening opportunistic infections in the immunocompromised host.

Parasites

The term *parasite* is typically applied to members of the animal kingdom that infect and cause disease in other animals. Protozoa, helminths, and arthropods are considered parasites. Protozoa are single-celled organisms transmitted via direct or indirect contact or an arthropod vector. Helminths are wormlike parasites: roundworms, tapeworms, and flukes are examples. They gain entry into humans primarily through ingestion of fertilized eggs or penetration of larvae through the skin or mucous membranes. Arthropod parasites, such as scabies (mites), lice, and fleas, typically infest external body surfaces, causing localized tissue damage and inflammation. Transmission is by direct contact with the arthropod or its eggs.

Note. Data summarized from *Pathophysiology: Concepts of Altered Health States* (4th ed.) by C. M. Porth, 1994, Philadelphia: Lippincott.

---

rickettsia, chlamydia, fungi, and parasites such as protozoa, helminths (worms), and arthropods (see the accompanying box). Each organism causes a different specific reaction in the host.

A number of different mechanisms have evolved in pathogens to facilitate their transmission and increase their ability to invade the host and cause disease. Factors influencing the transmission of an organism include its resistance to drying and to variations in environmental temperature. For example, spore-forming organisms are extremely resistant to drying.

Many microorganisms are capable of producing toxins or enzymes to facilitate their invasion of the host, increase their resistance to host defenses, and increase their ability to cause disease. Adhesion factors produced by or incorporated into the cell wall or membrane of the pathogen improve its ability to attach and colonize the host. Pathogens may also produce enzymes to enhance their spread to local tissues, chemicals to block specific immune processes or deplete neutrophils and macrophages, or extracellular capsules to discourage phagocytosis.

Pathogens are often capable of producing toxins that alter or destroy the normal function of host cells and promote colonization, proliferation, and invasion by the pathogen. Toxins often increase the disease-producing capability of the pathogen and, in some cases, are totally responsible for it; for example, cholera, tetanus, and botulism result from bacterial toxins, not from the direct effects of the infection. *Exotoxins* are soluble proteins secreted into surrounding tissue by the microorganism. Exotoxins are highly poisonous, causing cell death or dysfunction. *Endotoxins* are found in the cell wall of gram-negative bacteria which are released only when the cell is disrupted. Endotoxins have less specific effects than exotoxins, but they act as activators of many human regulatory systems, producing fever, inflammation, and potentially clotting, bleeding, or hypotension when released in large quantities.

Reservoir and Transmission

The reservoir or source, where the pathogen lives and multiplies, may be either endogenous or exogenous. Organisms that reside on skin or mucosal surfaces of the host are endogenous. Exogenous sources can include other humans, animals, soil, water, intravenous fluid, or equipment. Infectious diseases are usually transmitted from human sources, that is, persons who have clinical disease, subclinical infection, who are carriers. Carriers harbor the pathogen without showing evidence of clinical disease. Pathogens exit human hosts via respiratory secretions, body fluids from the gastrointestinal and genitourinary tracts, skin or mucous membrane lesions, the placenta, and blood.

Organisms may be transmitted from the source to the susceptible host by direct or indirect contact, droplet or airborne transmission, or a vector. Direct contact includes person-to-person spread or contact with infected body fluids, as well as transmission from contaminated food or water. Indirect contact occurs when the infectious agent is contracted by use of inanimate objects, such as dirty eating utensils. Sneezing, talking, and coughing allow transmission by droplet contact when the host is within 2 to 3 feet of the source. Smaller respiratory particles that stay suspended in air and are carried via air currents allow airborne transmission. Vectors are insects and animals such as flies, mosquitoes, or rodents that act as intermediate hosts between the source and host. Microorganisms usually first colonize the portal of entry, nonintact skin, wounds, mucous membranes, the respiratory, gastrointestinal, or genitourinary tracts.

Host Factors

The susceptible host is the final link in the chain of infection. Exposure to pathogens does not automatically cause infection or infectious disease. The outcome of contact with a pathogenic microorganism is determined by the balance of microbial virulence and host resistance. Factors that can enable the host to resist infection include the following:

- Physical barriers, such as the skin and mucous membranes
- The hostile environment created by acid stomach secretions, urine, and vaginal secretions
- Antimicrobial factors in saliva, tears, and prostatic fluid
- Respiratory defenses, including humidification, filtration, the mucociliary elevator, cough reflex, and alveolar macrophages
- Specific and nonspecific immune responses to pathogenic invasion

Stages of the Infectious Process

When infectious disease develops in the host, it typically follows a predictable course with stages based on the progression and intensity of manifestations.

The initial stage is the *incubation period,* during which the pathogen begins active replication but does not yet cause symptoms. Depending on the organism and host factors, the incubation period may last from hours, as with salmonella, to years, as with HIV infection.

The *prodromal stage* follows, during which symptoms first begin to appear. At this stage, symptoms are often nonspecific and include general malaise, fever, myalgias, headache, and fatigue.

Maximal impact of the infectious process is felt during the *acute phase* as the pathogen proliferates and disseminates rapidly. Toxic by-products of microorganism metabolism and cell lysis, along with the immune response, produce tissue damage and inflammation during this stage (Porth, 1994). Manifestations are more pronounced and specific to the infecting organism and site during the acute stage. Fever and chills may be significant during this phase. However, alcoholic clients and the very old may respond to severe infection by becoming hypothermic (Merck Research Laboratories, 1992). The client is often tachycardic and tachypneic because of increased metabolic demands. Localized manifestations are characteristic of the inflammatory response: redness, heat, swelling, pain, and impaired function. When the infectious disease affects an internal organ, manifestations are related to inflammatory changes in that organ and surrounding tissue. The client may experience tenderness to palpation over the site or show signs of impaired function, such as the hematuria and proteinuria characteristic of renal infections.

If the infectious process is prolonged, manifestations of the continuing immune response may become apparent. Catabolic and anorexic effects of the infection can lead to

---

Clinical Manifestations of Septic Shock

■ ■ ■

Early Manifestations

- Chills and fever
- Tachycardia and tachypnea
- Hypotension
- Skin warm and pink
- Urine output normal
- Altered mentation, with confusion, restlessness, and agitation

Later Manifestations

- Skin cool and pale or cyanotic
- Urine output <30 mL/h

---

loss of body fat and muscle wasting. Immune complexes may be deposited at sites other than the primary infection, resulting in an inflammatory process. Glomerulonephritis (e.g., following strep throat) and vasculitis are possible results. Another possible consequence of prolonged infection and immune response is the triggering of an autoimmune disease process (discussed later in this chapter), such as rheumatic cardiomyopathy or celiac disease. Juvenile-onset diabetes mellitus is thought to be the result of such a response (Wilson et al., 1991).

As the infection is contained and the pathogen eliminated, the *convalescent stage* of the disease occurs. During this stage, affected tissues are repaired and symptoms resolve. *Resolution* of the infection is total elimination of the pathogen from the body without residual manifestations. If a balance between organism and host factors occurs with neither predominating, chronic disease may develop or the organism be driven into a protected site, such as an abscess. A *carrier state* develops when host defenses eliminate the infectious disease but the organism continues to multiply on mucosal sites (Wilson et al., 1991).

Complications

Multiple and varied complications are associated with infectious diseases. They are typically specific to the infecting organism and the body system affected.

Acute invasion of the blood by certain microorganisms or their toxins can result in *septicemia* and *septic shock.* Whereas *bacteremia,* the presence of bacteria in the blood, may not have serious effects, septicemia refers to systemic disease associated with their presence or toxins. Septicemia is the 13th leading cause of death in the United States (Hazzard et al., 1994). Septic shock indicates a state of hypotension and impaired organ perfusion result-

ing from sepsis. Unless treated aggressively, septic shock leads to diffuse cell and tissue injury, and potentially to organ failure (Wilson et al., 1991).

The gram-negative organisms *Escherichia coli, Klebsiella, Proteus, Pseudomonas,* and *Serratia* are responsible for 60% to 70% of septic shock cases. Staphylococci, pneumococci, and streptococci are gram-positive microorganisms also frequently implicated (Tierney, McPhee, & Papadakis, 1994; Wilson et al., 1991). Endotoxins and exotoxins appear to be primarily responsible for the syndrome, by their multiple effects on tissues, cells, and plasma protein systems. Vasodilation reduces the peripheral vascular resistance and blood pressure; capillaries become more permeable, contributing to fluid loss and hypovolemia. Myocardial contractile function is depressed in about half of clients with septic shock (Wilson et al., 1991).

The usual signs of infection may not be evident before the client demonstrates the classic manifestations of septic shock: chills and fever, rapid pulse and respirations, hypotension, and altered mentation (see the accompanying box). Early in the course of the syndrome, the client's skin often is warm and pink, and the pulses full as a result of the vasodilation. As blood volume falls, classic signs of shock are seen: cool, clammy skin and reduced urine output. See Chapter 6 for further discussion of shock syndromes and their management.

Nosocomial Infections

Nosocomial infections are acquired in a health care setting, such as a hospital or nursing home. Currently, 3% to 7% of clients acquire a nosocomial infection while hospitalized (Tierney et al., 1994). Hospital-acquired infections add over 7.5 million hospital days, directly result in approximately 20,000 deaths, and contribute to 60,000 more deaths yearly in the United States (Wilson et al., 1991).

Clients entering hospitals are often the least able to mount immune defenses to infection. Immunologic responses may be compromised and normal defenses impaired in clients with, for example, cancer or chronic diseases, pressure ulcers, or organ transplants (Tierney et al., 1994). Nosocomial infections also occur when antibiotic therapy has altered natural defenses and impaired resistance to harmful microorganisms. Endogenous organisms outside normal habitat (such as in *Escherichia coli* in the urinary tract) become a threat to the client. Other pharmacologic and therapeutic procedures, such as chemotherapy, the use of corticosteroids, or radiation therapy, also contribute to nosocomial infections. Gram-negative enteric bacteria and gram-positive *Staphylococcus aureus* are the most common bacteria responsible.

Invasive procedures and altered immune defenses are the main factors contributing to infection. Urinary catheterization is the number-one cause; cardiac catheterization, peripheral and central intravenous lines, respiratory care procedures, and surgical procedures are also closely linked to nosocomial infection (see the accompanying box). Consequently, the urinary tract, surgical wounds, the respiratory tract, and invasive catheter sites on the skin are most often affected by hospital-acquired infection. Organisms causing the infection are often resistant to many drugs, not responding to antibiotics usually effective in treating infections acquired outside the hospital (Tierney et al., 1994).

Prevention is the most important control measure for nosocomial infections. The pathogens causing these infections are transmitted primarily by contact with hospital personnel (Wilson et al., 1991). *Effective hand washing is the single most important measure in infection control.* Although infections may also be transmitted by the airborne route, contaminated equipment, or from the environment, these are less significant causes. Invasive procedures and equipment should be used only when absolutely necessary; for example, it is not appropriate to insert an indwelling catheter when the only indication is incontinence. Peripheral intravenous equipment and sites are changed regularly. Intravenous bags and bottles are changed every 24 hours, tubing every 24 to 48 hours, and sites every 2 to 3 days.

Infectious Process in Older Adults

Older adults, particularly those over the age of 75 years, are at greater risk of acquiring an infection. Although the incidence of septicemia in the United States is increasing in all age groups, the greatest increase is among persons over the age of 65 years (Hazzard et al., 1994). Physiologic changes of aging that put the elderly at an increased risk for infection include the following:

- Cardiovascular changes, including loss of capillaries and decreased tissue perfusion
- Respiratory system changes, such as decreased mucociliary escalator, decreased elastic recoil, and a diminished cough reflex leading to decreased clearance of respiratory secretions
- Loss of muscle tone, reduced bladder contractility, altered bladder reflexes, and prostatic hypertrophy in men, leading to reduced bladder capacity and incomplete emptying
- Gastrointestinal system changes, including impaired swallow reflex, decreased gastric acidity, and delayed gastric emptying, which increase the risk of aspiration
- Skin and subcutaneous tissue changes with thinning of skin, decreased cushioning, and sensation, leading to increased risk of injury and ulceration
- Altered immune function
- Decreased phagocytosis by neutrophils and macrophages

Nosocomial Infections

■ ■ ■

- Nosocomial infections typically manifest after 48 hours of hospitalization.
- Urinary tract infection is the most common type, accounting for about 45% of all nosocomial infections.
- Pneumonia accounts for 15% of all nosocomial infections related to endotracheal or nasogastric intubation.
- Surgical wounds account for 30% of all nosocomial infections.
- Bacteremia accounts for 7% of all nosocomial infections related to invasive devices (e.g., intravenous catheters, arterial lines).
- Antibiotic-associated diarrhea accounts for less than 3% of all nosocomial infections related to prophylactic antibiotic doses.

- A reduced inflammatory response
- Slowed or impaired healing processes

In addition to these physiologic changes, other factors may contribute to the older adult's increased risk for infectious disease:

- Decreased activity level related to musculoskeletal, neurologic, or balance problems
- Poor nutrition and an increased risk of dehydration
- Chronic diseases, such as diabetes mellitus, cardiac disease, and renal disease
- Chronic medication use
- Lack of recent immunizations against preventable infectious diseases
- Altered mentation and dementias
- Hospitalization or residence in a long-term care facility
- Presence of invasive devices, such as indwelling urinary catheters and gastric tubes

The older adult not only is at increased risk for infection, but also may not exhibit classic manifestations of infection. Fever and chills occur less frequently because of age-related changes in the immune system, loss of central temperature control mechanisms, decreased muscle mass, and loss of shivering ability. The older adult may have only subtle signs of sepsis, including changes in mental status, disorientation, and tachypnea (Hazzard et al., 1994). Infectious diseases commonly seen in the elderly client are outlined in the box on page 253.

Common Infectious Diseases in Older Adults

■ ■ ■

- Pneumonia: The leading cause of infectious death in older adults; pneumococci, *Haemophilus influenzae,* and staphylococci are the leading causes of pneumonia in older adults.

- Urinary tract infection (UTI): The leading cause of bacteremia and sepsis in older adults; factors that contribute to UTI include immobility, poor hygiene, and incomplete bladder emptying.

- Intra-abdominal infections: Older adults have the highest incidence of gangrene of the appendix and gallbladder; diverticulitis also is common.

- Soft-tissue infection: Postoperative wound infections and decubitus ulcers are most prevalent in older adults.

- Tuberculosis: Relatively high incidence in older adults, especially those in long-term care settings; tuberculosis often occurs as reactivation or secondary tuberculosis when the immune system is no longer able to contain the bacteria.

Collaborative Care

The goals of care for the client with an infection are to identify the organ system affected by the infection and the causative agent and to achieve a cure by the least toxic, least expensive, and most effective means. Fortunately, most infectious diseases are self-limiting and will resolve with little or no medical care. However, medical treatment can be lifesaving in an overwhelming infection or immunocompromised host.

The body part or organ system affected by the infection is often obvious from the client's history and presenting signs and symptoms. Identifying the system allows the range of possible infecting organisms to be narrowed to those known to affect that system. The manner of presentation provides further cues as to the diagnosis. For example, pneumococcal pneumonia typically presents with an acute onset of chills, fever, and cough in a previously healthy adult, whereas the client with viral pneumonia relates a gradual onset of symptoms, with systemic manifestations such as muscle aches and headache often predominant. A history of recent activities also provides clues. Family members who all came down with vomiting and diarrhea within 12 hours after a picnic probably do not have the flu.

Once the infecting agent has been identified, either positively or by probability, therapy can be specifically tailored to the client's needs. Viral infections often resolve without treatment other than supportive care, such as providing rest and fluids. Skin infections may respond to a topical agent, avoiding the potential adverse effects of one administered systemically.

Laboratory and Diagnostic Tests

Laboratory studies are used to assess the client's response to infection, identify the infecting organism, and monitor the progress of therapy. The following laboratory tests may be ordered:

- *WBC count* provides clues about the infecting organism and the body's immune response to it (see Table 8–6). The normal WBC count ranges from 5,000 to 10,000 per mm^3. Leukocytosis, a WBC count of more than 10,000/mm^3, is common with acute bacterial infections. Leukopenia, a WBC count of less than 5000/mm^3, often accompanies viral infections. Leukopenia may also be seen in an overwhelming infection that impairs the ability of the bone marrow to respond adequately.

- *WBC differential* is also ordered (see Table 8–6). Neutrophilia, increased numbers of circulating neutrophils (or PMNs), is a common response with infection as the bone marrow responds to an increased need for phagocytes. Along with neutrophilia, a *shift to the left* is common in acute infection. This means that there are more immature neutrophils in circulation than normal (Figure 8–13), indicating an appropriate bone marrow response.

- *Cultures of the wound, blood, or other infected body fluids* may be obtained. After a swab or specimen for culture is obtained using sterile technique, it is placed in a culture medium to encourage growth of the organism outside the body. Once the organism has proliferated in the culture medium, it is inspected to determine its characteristics, such as shape, growth patterns, and Gram-staining qualities. The distinctive characteristics of each microorganism allow it to be identified. Once the organism has been cultured, it may be subjected to various antibiotics known to be effective against its particular strain to determine which antibiotic is likely to be most effective. This is known as *sensitivity* testing. Although culture and sensitivity testing is accurate, generally 24 to 48 hours are required to grow the organism, potentially delaying the institution of therapy. Any antibiotic (and possibly even oxygen therapy) may alter the ability to culture an organism, so specimens should be obtained before instituting treatment.

- *Serologic testing* provides an indirect means of identifying infecting agents by detecting antibodies to the suspected organism. When the antibody titer against a

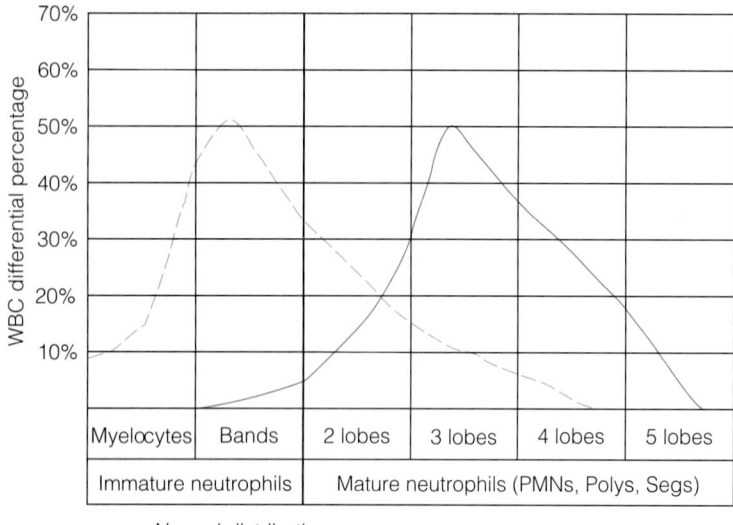

Type of WBC	Normal differential	Shift to left
Myelocytes	0%	Present
Band neutrophils (Bands)	3 to 5%	Increased
Segmented neutrophils (Segs, Polys, PMNs)	50 to 65%	May be stable, increased, or decreased

Figure 8-13 Neutrophils by stage of maturity and normal distribution in the blood.

specific organism rises during the acute phase of an infectious disease and begins to fall during convalescence, the diagnosis is supported. Although it is not as accurate as culture, serology is particularly useful for organisms that cannot easily be cultured, such as hepatitis B or HIV (Porth, 1994). The *enzyme-linked immunosorbent assay (ELISA),* a serologic test to detect antibodies to HIV, is the most widely used test for HIV infection.

- *Direct antigen detection methods* are in the process of being developed. These tests use monoclonal antibodies, which are purified antibody forms, to detect antigens in specimens from the diseased host (Porth, 1994). See the box on page 255. These tests offer rapid and accurate identification of the offending microorganism.

- *Antibiotic peak and trough levels* may be ordered to monitor for therapeutic blood levels of the prescribed medication(s). The *therapeutic range,* that is, the minimum and maximum blood levels at which the drug is effective, is known for a given drug. By measuring blood levels at the predicted peak (1 to 2 hours after oral administration, 1 hour after intramuscular administration, and 30 minutes after intravenous administration) and trough (lowest level, usually a few minutes before the next scheduled dose), health care personnel can determine that the client is maintaining a level within the therapeutic range at all times, ensuring maximal effect from the drug. It is also possible to determine whether the drug is reaching a toxic or harmful level during therapy, increasing the likelihood of adverse effects.

Diagnostic studies that may be ordered are generally specific to the organ system affected. These studies are discussed in further detail in other chapters of this book.

- *Radiologic examination of the chest, abdomen, or urinary system* may be ordered to detect organ abnormalities indicating an inflammatory response or tissue damage.

- *Lumbar puncture* may be performed to obtain cerebrospinal fluid (CSF) for examination and culture if a central nervous system (CNS) infection, such as meningitis or encephalitis, is suspected.

- *Ultrasonic examination* is a noninvasive diagnostic test for evaluation of organ function. An echocardiogram assesses cardiac function and may be ordered when pericarditis, myocarditis, or endocarditis is suspected. Renal ultrasonography may reveal distended kidneys or defects in the urinary tract predisposing the client to infection.

Pharmacology

Once the infecting organism and affected body system have been identified, specific therapy to cure the infectious disease can be instituted. The number of antimicrobial agents available makes choosing the appropriate one seem overwhelming. The perfect anti-infective agent would destroy pathogens while preserving host cells, would be effective against many different organisms while not promoting the development of resistance, would distribute to necessary tissues, and would remain in the body for relatively long periods (Spencer et al., 1993).

Because no currently available antimicrobial meets all the above criteria, physicians look for the agent that will be effective, have little toxicity, can be administered with

Monoclonal Antibodies

■ ■ ■

Antigens typically have numerous antigenic determinant sites, each capable of stimulating a different subset of B cells. Each clone secretes a slightly different antibody from the others. The immunoglobulin produced as a result is therefore *polyclonal,* with multiple different antibodies. In 1975, researchers devised a technique for making a single clone of "immortal" B cells that could be maintained indefinitely in a laboratory and would produce a single antibody to a specific antigen (see figure at right). This pure antibody, known as a *monoclonal* antibody, offers the following advantages:

■ It can target specific antigens.

■ It has a single, constant binding affinity for the antigen.

■ It can be diluted to a specific titer or concentration, because it is not mixed with other antibodies.

■ It can be purified to avoid adverse responses (McCance & Huether, 1994).

In addition to their use in providing passive protection from disease, multiple other uses are being identified for monoclonal antibodies, including the diagnosis and treatment of cancer, immunosuppression to prevent rejection of transplanted tissue or organs, immune response analysis, imaging techniques for diagnostic uses, and the early detection of viral infections (McCance & Huether, 1994; Roitt, 1994).

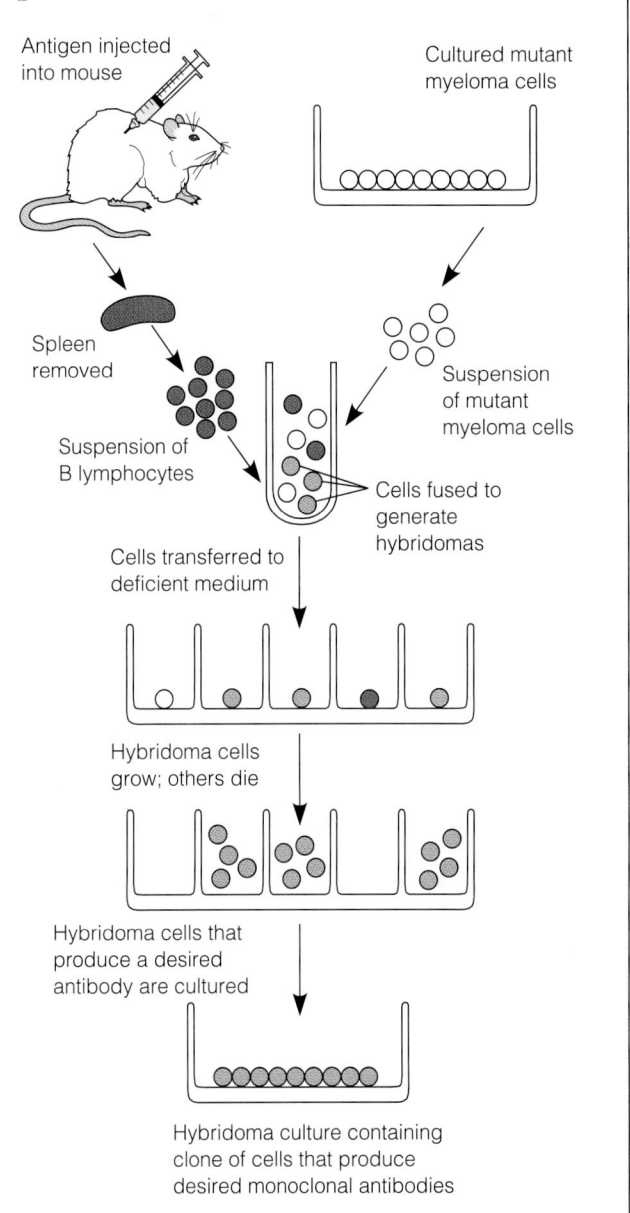

Antigen injected into mouse

Cultured mutant myeloma cells

Spleen removed

Suspension of B lymphocytes

Suspension of mutant myeloma cells

Cells fused to generate hybridomas

Cells transferred to deficient medium

Hybridoma cells grow; others die

Hybridoma cells that produce a desired antibody are cultured

Hybridoma culture containing clone of cells that produce desired monoclonal antibodies

---

relative convenience, and is cost-effective. Characteristics of both host and the infecting organism are considered in making the selection. The following host factors are considered in choosing an antimicrobial agent:

■ *History of hypersensitivity.* Previous hypersensitivity responses to an antimicrobial contraindicate the use of that agent or one of its class.

■ *The age and childbearing status of the client.* Sulfonamides and tetracyclines as well as some less common agents are contraindicated for pregnant women due to their possible effects on the fetus.

■ *Renal function.* Renal function is an important consideration because most antimicrobials are excreted through the kidneys. Impaired renal function may contraindicate a specific drug, such as an aminoglycoside antibiotic, because of its nephrotoxicity, or it may call for a reduced dosage.

■ *Hepatic function.* Hepatic function may alter the metabolism of a particular antimicrobial, increasing the risk of toxicity. Again, certain drugs are avoided with impaired hepatic function; others may dictate a reduced dosage.

- *Site of the infection.* The infection site is critical in choosing both the antimicrobial to be used and the route by which it is administered. Antimicrobials can be applied topically or administered by oral, intramuscular, intravenous, interperitoneal, or intrathecal routes. Oral and intravenous routes are most commonly used.

- *Other host factors.* For example, chronic diseases or other medications in the treatment regimen are also considered.

Antimicrobial preparations are broadly classified as bacteriostatic or bactericidal. *Bacteriostatic* agents inhibit the growth of the microorganism, leaving its destruction to the host's immune system. These agents are generally not indicated for the immunocompromised host. Tetracyclines, erythromycin, and chloramphenicol are bacteriostatic preparations. *Bactericidal* agents are capable of killing the organism without immune system intervention. These include the penicillins, cephalosporins, and aminoglycoside antibiotics (Shlafer, 1993).

The activity of antimicrobial agents on bacteria, fungi, and viruses falls under five basic mechanisms:

- Impairing cell wall synthesis, leading to lysis and cell destruction

- Protein synthesis inhibition, impairing microbial function

- Altering the permeability of the cell membrane, causing intracellular contents to leak

- Inhibiting the synthesis of nucleic acids

- Inhibiting other specific biochemical pathways of the organism, such as metabolic pathways (Shlafer, 1993)

Obviously, agents that work on the cell wall will not be effective against organisms that have no cell wall, such as mycoplasma and viruses. The antimicrobial's spectrum of activity is also considered in making a selection. Therapy is often initiated with a broad-spectrum antimicrobial until the specific organism is identified.

Finally, many microorganisms have the ability to develop resistance to an anti-infective agent; that is, the pathogen continues to live and grow in the presence of the anti-infective. Resistance develops as a result of a chance mutation by the pathogen, allowing a subpopulation of cells to survive. The chance of an organism's becoming resistant to an agent is partially related to the dose delivered. Resistance is less likely to occur when a lethal dose is administered; therefore, it is vital that clients understand the need to take all doses of the prescribed drug as ordered.

Antimicrobial medications are generally classified as antibacterial or antibiotic, antiviral, antifungal, and antiparasitic.

Antibiotic Medications used to treat bacterial infections are generally known as antibiotics. Their development and use began before World War II and has proliferated rapidly since. Most antibiotics are biologic substances, that is, substances produced by other microorganisms. Antibiotics fall into classes of drugs with related chemical structure and activity. Some are effective against only gram-positive bacteria, and others are effective against only gram-negative organisms. Newer broad-spectrum antibiotics have activity against a wide variety of bacteria, including both gram-positive and gram-negative forms. No antibiotic is totally safe. Hypersensitivity responses occur, and some drugs are toxic to organ systems, exhibiting hepatotoxicity, nephrotoxicity, ototoxicity, or bone marrow suppression.

The nursing implications for specific classes of antibiotics are outlined in the box beginning on page 257.

Antiviral Antiviral therapy is a relatively new phenomenon. Most antibiotics have little effect on viruses because the virus has no cell wall and no cytoplasm, produces no enzymes, and sequesters itself in a host cell to reproduce. Antiviral agents must be very selective in differentiating normal cellular activity from viral activity. In addition, the immune function of the host is a vital component in fighting viral infections; antiviral therapy may be relatively ineffective in the severely immunocompromised host. Making a timely diagnosis to allow institution of antiviral therapy can be an additional problem, because viruses are less easily identified using laboratory techniques. Antiviral agents in common use are summarized in the box on page 261.

Antifungal Antifungal agents are available in both topical and systemic forms. They act by interfering with the cytoplasmic membrane of the fungus. Topical agents include preparations for cutaneous use to treat candidiasis, tineas, and ringworm. Vaginal preparations to treat vulvovaginal candidiasis are also available, as are several nonprescription topical and vaginal antifungal agents.

Amphotericin B (Fungizone) is a systemic antifungal agent for parenteral administration. It is used to treat severe, life-threatening fungal infections including histoplasmosis, blastomycosis, candidiasis, and others. Another systemic antifungal in current use is flucytosine (Ancobon). Unlike amphotericin B, flucytosine can be administered orally. It is used to treat severe candidiasis infections such as candidae septicemia, endocarditis, pulmonary, or urinary tract infections, and *Cryptococcus* meningitis, pulmonary, or urinary tract infections.

Fluconazole (Diflucan) has the broadest use as an antifungal agent. It can be administered either orally or parenterally and is used to treat candidiasis infections as well as *Cryptococcus* meningitis. It is generally better tolerated than other systemic antifungal medications.

text continues on page 261

Nursing Implications for Pharmacology: Antibiotic Therapy

PENICILLINS

Penicillin G

Penicillin V

Amoxicillin (Amoxil)

Amoxicillin and potassium clavulanate (Augmentin)

Ampicillin (Polycillin)

Carbenicillin (Geopen, Geocillin)

Cloxacillin (Cloxapen, Tegopen)

Dicloxacillin (Dynapen)

Methicillin (Staphcillin)

Nafcillin (Unipen)

Piperacillin (Pipracil)

Ticarcillin (Ticar)

The penicillins were among the first antibiotics developed, ushering in the age of antibiotic therapy. Penicillins are bactericidal and work by interfering with cell wall synthesis and the enzymes involved in cell division and synthesis. Although many organisms have developed resistance to penicillins, these drugs remain important antibiotics and are considered to be safe, effective, and of low toxicity. Penicillins are particularly effective in treating gram-positive organisms.

Nursing Responsibilities

- Oral and parenteral forms of penicillin are available. Only aqueous solutions are appropriate for intravenous injection; intramuscular suspensions must not be used intravenously.

- Many strains of microorganisms are resistant to penicillins. Monitor for therapeutic response.

- Toxic reactions to penicillins are uncommon, especially with the naturally occurring penicillins, such as penicillin G or penicillin V. Hypersensitivity responses, however, are common. Assess the client for
  a. Local erythema and itching at the site of injection as an early indication of penicillin sensitivity.
  b. Skin rashes, urticaria (hives), and itching.
  c. Fever and chills.
  d. Anaphylactic shock with acute respiratory distress, hypotension, edema, tachycardia, cyanosis, or pallor.

- Observe all clients who receive parenteral penicillin for at least 30 minutes; have ventilatory support and epinephrine available.

- Discontinue the drug immediately if any hypersensitivity response occurs. Antihistamines or corticosteroids may be administered to relieve the symptoms of a mild reaction; epinephrine administered subcutaneously or intravenously and airway support is the treatment of choice for anaphylaxis.

- Do not administer penicillin, or administer the drug only with extreme caution, to anyone with a history of a hypersensitivity response to any form of the drug; a cross-reactivity may occur in clients allergic to cephalosporin antibiotics (Shlafer, 1993; Spencer et al., 1993).

- Although naturally occurring penicillins cross the placental barrier and may sensitize the fetus, their use in pregnancy is weighed against the benefit to the mother.

- The client receiving penicillin or other antibiotic therapy may develop a superinfection due to elimination of resident bacteria. Observe for signs of vaginitis, stomatitis, diarrhea and other gastrointestinal disturbances, especially in the older adult.

Client and Family Teaching

- Complete the entire prescribed course of therapy to increase the likelihood of eliminating the infection and to reduce the risk of developing penicillin-resistant organisms.

- If any signs of an allergic reaction develop, stop the drug and contact the physician.

- Penicillin may reduce the effectiveness of oral contraceptives. Alternative birth control measures should be used.

- Notify the physician if white patches are noted on the oral mucosa or if vaginitis develops. An antifungal drug may be prescribed and the antibiotic continued.

- Yogurt, buttermilk, or other lactobacilli-containing products may help maintain normal intestinal flora and prevent superinfection. To prevent inactivation of the bacterial culture, however, do not take these products within 1 hour of taking the drug (Spencer et al., 1993).

CEPHALOSPORINS

Cephalothin (Keflin)

Cefadroxil (Duricef)

Cefazolin (Ancef)

Cefaclor (Ceclor)

Cefoperazone (Cefobid)

Cefotaxime (Claforan)

Ceftazidime (Fortaz)

Ceftriaxone (Rocephin)

The cephalosporins are closely related to the penicillins structurally. Like penicillin, they inhibit cell wall synthesis. Some cross-sensitivity occurs with the two groups, and hypersensitivity responses to cephalosporins resemble those of penicillin. Cephalosporins are divided into three groups, or "generations," each having a somewhat different spectrum of activity. First-generation cephalosporins are effective primarily

Pharmacology: Antibiotic Therapy *(continued)*

against gram-positive organisms. Second- and third-generation drugs are more effective against gram-negative organisms, less so against gram-positive ones.

Nursing Responsibilities

- Check for previous hypersensitivity response to cephalosporins or penicillins. Monitor closely for cross-sensitivity. Hypersensitivity responses are similar to those seen with the penicillins.

- Gastrointestinal disturbances are the most common adverse effect of cephalosporins administered orally.

- Parenteral administration may cause phlebitis or local pain at intramuscular sites. Dilute and infuse intravenous preparations slowly to reduce the incidence of phlebitis. Rotate intramuscular sites and apply ice packs to reduce discomfort.

- Monitor laboratory results for evidence of adverse response, such as leukopenia and thrombocytopenia, nephrotoxicity (elevated BUN and serum creatinine), or hepatotoxicity (elevated bilirubin, LDH, ALT, AST, and alkaline phosphatase).

- Report adverse central nervous system effects such as headache, dizziness, malaise, and fatigue to the physician.

- Superinfections may develop, especially when therapy is prolonged. Monitor for evidence of gastrointestinal disturbances, stomatitis, and vaginitis.

Client and Family Teaching

- Complete the entire prescription unless signs of an adverse or allergic reaction occur. Report these promptly to the physician.

- Take the medication on an empty stomach, 1 hour before or 2 hours after meals.

- Space doses of the medication relatively evenly throughout the day and evening hours.

- Increase consumption of buttermilk or yogurt to prevent intestinal superinfection.

AMINOGLYCOSIDES

Amikacin (Amikin)   Neomycin (Neosporin)
Gentamicin (Garamycin)   Streptomycin (Stepolin)
Kanamycin (Kantrex)   Tobramycin (Nebcin)

The aminoglycoside antibiotics were the first important group of antibiotics found to be effective against gram-negative organisms. They remain an important class of antibiotics today. Aminoglycosides are bactericidal, interfering with protein synthesis in the pathogen. Aminoglycosides are not well absorbed from the gastrointestinal tract, so they are usually administered parenterally. They are often used in combination with other antibiotics to provide greater effect or a broader spectrum of activity. Hypersensitivity responses to the aminoglycosides are not as common as for penicillins and cephalosporin. However, they are ototoxic and nephrotoxic. The risk is highest for older adults, clients with preexisting renal disease, and persons receiving other ototoxic or nephrotoxic drugs (Shlafer, 1993; Spencer et al., 1993).

Nursing Responsibilities

- Assess the client for possible hypersensitivity to aminoglycoside antibiotics before and during therapy. Common hypersensitivity responses include rash, urticaria, generalized burning, fever, and eosinophilia. Stop the drug and notify the physician if the client develops signs of a hypersensitivity response.

- Assess the client's renal function before and during aminoglycoside therapy. Monitor intake and output, daily weight, BUN, and serum creatinine.

- Assess for evidence of adverse effects on the ear during therapy. Neural hearing loss with loss of perception of high tones, tinnitus, and vertigo are possible early indicators.

- Notify the physician if the client is receiving other nephrotoxic or ototoxic drugs such as furosemide (Lasix) and ethacrynic acid (Edecrin); aminoglycosides should not be administered concurrently.

- Administer intravenous preparations separately from other drugs; flush tubing before and after administration.

- Administer intramuscular injections deeply into a large muscle. Rotate sites to minimize tissue injury (Spencer et al., 1993).

Client and Family Teaching

- If signs and symptoms of an allergic response or manifestations of adverse or toxic effects occur, stop the drug and notify the physician.

- Monitor daily weights. A sudden weight gain may indicate adverse effects on the kidney and should be reported to the physician.

- Do not take any prescription or over-the-counter antiemetic medications while on aminoglycoside therapy; they may mask initial signs of ototoxicity (Shlafer, 1993).

Pharmacology: Antibiotic Therapy *(continued)*

TETRACYCLINES

Tetracycline HCl

Doxycycline
(Vibramycin)

Minocycline HCl
(Minocin)

Oxytetracycline
(Terramycin)

The tetracyclines, the first broad-spectrum antibiotics developed, are active against many gram-positive and gram-negative bacteria. They are also effective against organisms such as mycoplasma, rickettsiae, and *Chlamydia*. They are bacteriostatic, interfering with microbial protein synthesis (Wilson et al., 1991). Tetracycline is available only in oral forms; other preparations may be administered parenterally. They are not well absorbed when administered intramuscularly; the intravenous route is the preferred parenteral route. Tetracycline binds readily with metal and solid elements in the bowel, limiting its absorption when administered with food; the other preparations are highly soluble in lipids and can be administered with food.

Nursing Responsibilities

- When administering tetracycline, schedule doses 1 hour before or 2 hours after meals. Do not give with milk or milk products or antacids.

- Monitor for signs of superinfection: oral candidiasis (thrush), diarrhea, and skin or mucous membrane irritation. Report signs to the physician.

- Assess for skin rash due to hypersensitivity. Reassure the client that this does not indicate an allergy or a need to discontinue the medication.

- Tetracyclines potentiate the activity of anticoagulants. If the client is taking an anticoagulant medication, monitor prothrombin time, and monitor for signs of bleeding.

Client and Family Teaching

- While taking tetracycline, eat a few soda crackers with the medication to alleviate symptoms of gastrointestinal distress.

- Avoid excessive sun exposure while taking tetracyclines to reduce the risk of photosensitivity reactions.

ERYTHROMYCIN

Erythromycin
(E-Mycin, others)

Erythromycin salts (Ilosone,
E.E.S., Erythrocin, others)

Erythromycin is a very broad spectrum bacteriostatic antibiotic, effective against gram-positive and gram-negative organisms. Both oral and parenteral (intravenous) preparations are available. Erythromycin is used primarily to treat streptococcal pharyngitis in the client who is allergic to penicillin and, in combination with sulfonamides, to treat otitis media (Wilson et al., 1991). Toxicity is rare, as are serious adverse effects. Gastric upset is common, and may be relieved by substitution of a different form of the drug.

Nursing Responsibilities

- Administer erythromycin on an empty stomach or immediately before meals unless otherwise indicated.

- Give the drug with a full glass of water. Do not administer with acidic fruit juice.

- Administer intravenous preparations by slow infusion to minimize venous irritation (Shlafer, 1993).

Client and Family Teaching

- Gastric distress is a common side effect of erythromycin therapy and does not indicate an allergy to the drug.

- If gastric upset is significant, notify the physician; a different preparation may be substituted.

SULFONAMIDES AND TRIMETHOPRIM

Mafenide (Sulfamylon)

Silver sulfadiazine (Silvadene)

Sulfamethoxazole (Gantanol; in combination with trimethoprim, TMP-SMZ, Bactrim, Septra, others)

Sulfasalazine (Azulfidine, Sulfadyne)

Sulfisoxazole (Gantrisin, Pediazole)

Developed in the 1930s, sulfonamides were the first effective systemic antibacterial agents. They remain in widespread use despite many adverse effects and resistant pathogenic strains. Sulfonamides are bacteriostatic, inhibiting the growth of pathogens by interfering with their folic acid metabolism.

Trimethoprim is an antibiotic effective against most gram-positive and many gram-negative organisms. It is often combined with sulfamethoxazole. This combination is effective for urinary tract infections, *Pneumocystis carinii* pneumonia (PCP), otitis media, and other infections. It is also used prophylactically in the HIV-positive client with a CD4 cell count of less than 200 to prevent PCP. Hypersensitivity reactions are common in clients receiving sulfonamide preparations and tend to occur more frequently in persons with AIDS. Skin

➤

Pharmacology: Antibiotic Therapy (*continued*)

rashes and pruritus are the most common reactions. More severe responses include drug fever, exfoliative dermatitis, and Stevens-Johnson syndrome (a severe, potentially fatal form of erythema multiforme with skin and mucous membrane lesions that may lead to extensive denuding of the skin).

Nursing Responsibilities

- Assess for history of hypersensitivity to sulfonamides and related medications, such as thiazide diuretics and hypoglycemic preparations.

- Administer intravenous doses in dilute solution over at least 1 hour.

- Monitor intake and output. Maintain a fluid intake of at least 1500 mL per day.

- Check urine pH periodically, and administer alkalinizing agents as ordered to prevent crystalluria.

- Assess for evidence of bleeding, easy bruising, or systemic infection, and monitor blood count for possible bone marrow depression.

- Monitor for possible interactions when administered concurrently with anticoagulant (increased effect), phenytoin (increased risk of toxicity), and oral hypoglycemic agents (increased risk of hypoglycemia).

Client and Family Teaching

- Take the medication on an empty stomach, 1 hour before or 2 hours after meals. Take any missed dose as soon as the omission is discovered.

- Take each dose of medication with a full glass of water. Maintain a fluid intake of at least 2 quarts per day.

- Protect the skin from excessive sun exposure with clothing and sunscreens to reduce the risk of photosensitivity.

- Stop the drug and notify the physician if skin rash, itching, hives, easy bruising, bleeding gums, or other manifestations of adverse reaction develop.

METRONIDAZOLE (FLAGYL)

Metronidazole was originally introduced for the treatment of *Trichomonas* infection. It was later found to be effective against both amebiasis and giardiasis; still later, it was identified as an effective agent against most anaerobic gram-negative bacteria. Metronidazole is commonly used to prevent and treat infections following intestinal surgery. Metronidazole is bactericidal, as well as trichomonacidal and amebicidal.

Nursing Responsibilities

- Assess the client for a history of hypersensitivity response to this or related drugs and for preexisting neurologic problems. Metronidazole may cause central nervous system effects of dizziness, vertigo, syncope, and ataxia, as well as changes in mentation, such as confusion, depression, and irritability. Peripheral neuropathy is also common.

- Assess blood count and renal and liver function studies prior to initiating therapy. Bone marrow depression can occur with metronidazole, as can nephrotoxicity.

- Administer the drug as prescribed. When given orally, administer it after meals to minimize gastric distress and metallic taste. Infuse intravenous metronidazole over 60 minutes.

- Evaluate for therapeutic or adverse responses. Discontinue the medication and notify the physician if hypersensitivity or neurologic reactions occur. Hypersensitivity responses include chills and fever, rash, and itching.

- Ensure an adequate fluid intake of at least 2500 mL per day to minimize the risk of nephrotoxicity.

- Alert the primary care provider if this drug is ordered for clients taking warfarin (Coumadin); metronidazole may potentiate the anticoagulant effects.

- Monitor for toxic effects in the client who is also taking cimetidine, which inhibits metabolism of metronidazole.

Client and Family Teaching

- This medication may turn urine reddish brown; this is expected and not harmful.

- Discontinue the drug and notify the physician if hypersensitivity reaction or adverse effects occur, such as changes in mentation or coordination, painful or frequent urination, painful or difficult intercourse, impotence.

- Do not drink alcohol while taking this medication; an Antabuse-type reaction (flushing, sweating, headache, vomiting, and abdominal cramps) may occur.

- Maintain a fluid intake of 2.5 to 3 quarts per day.

- When the drug is prescribed for *Trichomonas* infections, treatment of both partners is necessary.

- While taking metronidazole, use condoms to prevent cross-contamination during intercourse.

Commonly Used Antiviral Agents

■ ■ ■

Amantadine (Symmetrel)

Amantadine is used to prevent and treat influenza A. It has been shown to be 55% to 80% or more effective in preventing the disease. When administered within 24 to 72 hours after the onset of symptoms, it reduces common manifestations of influenza. It is generally well tolerated; minimal central nervous system side effects, such as dizziness, anxiety, insomnia, and difficulty concentrating, may occur (Wilson et al., 1991).

Acyclovir (Zovirax) and Ganciclovir (Cytovene)

Acyclovir and ganciclovir are related compounds used primarily in the treatment of herpesviruses. Acyclovir is prescribed mainly in the treatment of genital herpes simplex infections. Although it does not kill the virus, acyclovir is effective in reducing the severity, duration, and frequency of recurrence of symptoms. Ganciclovir is indicated primarily in the treatment of cytomegalovirus infection. Although acyclovir is generally well tolerated with little toxicity, ganciclovir may profoundly suppress bone marrow function, and its use is therefore limited.

Zidovudine (AZT, Retrovir)

Zidovudine inhibits replication of HIV, although it does not kill it. Zidovudine's use is limited to clients with symptomatic HIV infection or CD4 cell counts of less than 200/mm^3. Zidovudine may be administered either orally or parenterally. Many clients are unable to tolerate recommended doses because of the drug's adverse effects, including nausea, vomiting, diarrhea, headache, fever, and skin rashes. Zidovudine is also potentially toxic to the kidneys and bone marrow. Zidovudine may be administered in combination with other HIV-replication inhibitors, including dideoxycytidine (ddC) and dideoxyinosine (ddI).

Vidarabine (Vira-A)

Vidarabine inhibits viral DNA synthesis and is effective against many herpesvirus infections. Its primary use is in treatment of herpes simplex encephalitis.

Interferons

Interferons are naturally produced cytokines whose use as antiviral agents is being explored. When administered intranasally, interferons have been shown to be effective in preventing rhinovirus upper respiratory infections. Other uses being explored include treatment of human papillomavirus (genital warts) and preventing or reducing Kaposi's sarcoma in clients with AIDS.

Antiparasitic   Drugs used to treat parasitic infections are as varied as the organisms that cause them. Generally, agents classified as antiparasitic are both expensive and likely to be toxic. Quinine was one of the first antiparasitic drugs developed in the treatment of malaria. Quinine is very toxic, but newer forms such as chloroquine (Aralen, Chlorocon) and hydroxychloroquine (Plaquenil) are widely used as antimalarial drugs. Metronidazole (Flagyl, others) is used to treat infections of protozoan parasites, including trichomoniasis, amebiasis, and giardiasis. This drug is also effective against most gram-negative bacteria and is widely used in the treatment of peritoneal and pelvic infections. Nursing responsibilities related to metronidazole are included in the pharmacology box on page 260.

Isolation Techniques

Controlling the spread of infectious diseases in the hospital or long-term care setting is particularly important to preventing nosocomial infection. *Hand washing is the single most important factor in preventing the transmission of infections.* Not all infectious diseases spread readily, necessitating special techniques or procedures. However, diseases such as chickenpox (varicella) and pulmonary tuberculosis are highly contagious and are spread by the airborne route, requiring special precautions to protect other hospitalized clients.

In determining the need for isolation precautions, health care personnel consider the usual reservoir or source of the microorganism, the mode of transmission, and susceptibility of hospital staff and other clients. For example, clients with *Pneumocystis carinii* pneumonia do not require isolation, because immunocompetent persons are not susceptible to this infection.

The Centers for Disease Control and Prevention (CDC) has published guidelines for isolation precautions to be used in health care facilities. These guidelines include both *universal precautions* and *category-specific isolation precautions.*

Universal Precautions *Universal Precautions for the Prevention of Transmission of Human Immunodeficiency Virus, Hepatitis B Virus, and Other Blood Borne Pathogens in Health Care Settings,* published by the CDC, provides guidelines for the handling of blood and other body fluids. These guidelines are employed with *all clients,* whether they are known to have an infectious disease or not. The guidelines were developed in light of the realization that many clients with an infectious disease such as HIV or hepatitis B have no apparent symptoms but can transmit the disease to others. Universal precautions are used by all health care workers who have direct contact with clients or with their body fluids or have indirect contact, such as by emptying trash, changing linens, or cleaning the room.

Universal precautions apply to the following:

- Blood
- Body fluids containing visible blood
- Semen and vaginal secretions, tissues, CSF, pleural fluid, synovial fluid, peritoneal fluid, pericardial fluid, and amniotic fluid

Unless visible blood is present, it is not necessary to use universal precautions with feces, nasal secretions, sputum, saliva, sweat, tears, urine, or vomitus.

Barrier protection is used to prevent exposing skin and mucous membrane surfaces to blood and body fluids. Barrier protection involves using gloves for touching or handling body fluids and adding other protection such as gowns, masks, or goggles if splashing or spraying is likely. Needles and other sharp objects are not recapped or bent but rather are disposed of in puncture-proof containers to prevent inadvertent percutaneous (needle-stick) exposure. Universal precautions are outlined in the accompanying box.

Category-Specific Isolation Precautions The nature and spread of some infectious diseases require that special techniques in addition to hand washing and universal precautions be employed to protect uninfected clients and workers. The CDC identifies seven categories of isolation precautions: strict isolation, contact isolation, respiratory isolation, acid-fast bacillus (tuberculosis) isolation, drainage and secretion precautions, blood and body fluid precautions, and enteric precautions. The last three of these categories now generally fall under universal precautions and are rarely used in the adult hospital populations of the United States. Indications for the use of category-specific isolation and specific precautions to be taken are outlined in Table 8–10.

Nursing Care

Nursing management related to infectious disease has two foci: (1) prevention and (2) health promotion and main-

---

Universal Precautions
■ ■ ■

Universal precautions, also known as body substance isolation, are to be used by all health care workers who have either direct contact with the client or body fluids or indirect contact through emptying trash, changing linens, or cleaning the room. These precautions apply to *all clients,* whether they are known to have an infectious disease or not.

Essential elements of universal precautions include the following:

- Use barrier protection to prevent exposure of skin and mucous membrane surfaces to blood and body fluids. Wear gloves when touching or handling body fluids; if splashing or spraying is likely, use additional protection, such as gowns, masks, or goggles.
- To prevent inadvertent percutaneous (needle-stick) exposure, dispose of needles and other sharp objects in puncture-proof containers without recapping or bending.
- Immediately and thoroughly wash hands and any other skin surfaces contaminated by blood, high risk body fluids, or fluids containing visible blood. Use an antibacterial soap or detergent. Mop up blood or body fluid spills using disposable towels; wash the surface with soap and water, and then disinfect with a bleach solution or other antiseptic preparation.

Universal precautions apply to the following:

- Blood
- Body fluids containing visible blood
- Semen and vaginal secretions, body tissues, cerebrospinal fluid, pleural fluid, synovial fluid, peritoneal fluid, pericardial fluid, and amniotic fluid

Unless visible blood is present, it is not necessary to use universal precautions with feces, nasal secretions, sputum, saliva, sweat, tears, urine, or vomitus.

---

tenance. Prevention focuses on assessing the client's risk for infection based on underlying condition, immune function, and prophylactic measures such as immunizations. Assessment for risks of nosocomial infection from invasive procedures and therapies is critical. Health promotion and maintenance activities include the following:

Table 8–10   Category-Specific Isolation

Category	Infectious Diseases	Purpose and Duration	Precautions
Strict isolation	Chickenpox, diphtheria, viral hemorrhagic fevers, such as Lassa fever; varicella zoster	Prevents spread of highly communicable diseases or pathogens readily transmitted by contact or airborne routes. Continued for duration of illness, until all lesions are crusted or two negative cultures are obtained (diphtheria).	Private room with closed door; gowns, masks, and gloves indicated for all persons entering room; hand washing; disposable supplies or decontamination of all articles leaving room.
Contact isolation	Herpes zoster, disseminated herpes simplex, wound or respiratory infection with highly virulent or multiple-drug-resistant pathogen, rabies	Prevents spread of easily transmissible organisms not requiring strict isolation. Generally continued for duration of illness.	As for strict isolation, depending on type of infection and degree of contact; gowns, masks, and gloves indicated for close contact or contact with infective material.
Respiratory isolation	Measles, meningitis, mumps, pneumonia, rubella, selected pneumonias	Prevents spread of microorganisms transmitted by direct contact or droplets. Duration varies from 24 hours after starting effective therapy to 4 to 9 days with viral infections such as measles, mumps, and rubella.	Private room; masks indicated for all persons entering room.
Tuberculosis isolation	Pulmonary tuberculosis	Prevent spread of *Mycobacterium tuberculosis* by airborne droplet nuclei. Continued for 2 weeks after initiation of therapy.	Room with special ventilation that does not allow air to circulate to general hospital ventilation; masks and gowns indicated only if client does not reliably cover mouth when coughing.

- Monitoring vital signs for alterations in temperature and other parameters
- Administering prescribed antibiotics and evaluating the client's response to therapy
- Implementing and maintaining aseptic technique and infection control measures, such as universal precautions
- Encouraging a balance of rest and activity, good nutritional intake, and other general health measures to support immunologic function and healing

The key nursing diagnoses are *Risk for Infection, Anxiety,* and *Pain.*

Risk for Infection
The spread of infection is a risk in any facility housing many people. It is a particular risk in hospitals, where many clients have at least some degree of immunosuppression and many drug-resistant strains of pathogens are prevalent. It is vital that nurses use good hand-washing techniques at all times, employ universal precautions with all clients, and use category-specific isolation techniques as indicated to prevent infectious spread to other clients, themselves, and their families.
Nursing interventions with rationales follow:

- Admit clients with known or suspected infections to a private room. *This is important to minimize the risk to other clients.*
- Wash hands thoroughly on entering and leaving the client's room, using a 10- to 15-second vigorous scrub with soap or antibacterial scrub solution. *A 10- to 15-second scrub removes transient microorganisms from the skin and helps prevent transmission of infection to or from the client.*
- Use universal precautions and personal protective devices to reduce the risk of transmission during client care. *Gloves, gowns, and masks are to be worn whenever there is a risk of skin or mucous membrane contamination by direct contact with infectious material, airborne spread of organisms, or droplet nuclei.*
- Inform the client and family about the reasons for and importance of isolation procedures during hospitalization. *Clients with isolation precautions may feel neglected, dirty, or shunned. Explanation of reasons and procedures can enhance the client's and family's understanding and acceptance.*
- Place a mask on the client and/or cover all infectious lesions or wounds completely when transporting the client to other parts of the facility for diagnostic or

treatment procedures. *These measures help minimize air contamination and the risk to visitors and personnel.*

- Collect a culture and sensitivity (C&S) specimen as ordered or indicated by purulent drainage, pyuria, or other manifestations of infection. *C&S is performed to determine the presence and type of infectious organisms as well as antibiotics most likely to be effective in eradicating it. Collect the specimen before the first dose of antibiotics is administered to ensure adequate organisms for culture.*

- Administer prescribed anti-infective agents. *Anti-infectives are used to destroy the invading microorganism.*

- Inform all personnel having contact with the client of the diagnosis. *This is particularly important for a client with a disease requiring category-specific isolation so that personnel can take appropriate precautions.*

- Ensure that visitors don appropriate protective wear before they enter the client's room. *Protective wear reduces their risk of infection.*

- Use appropriate measures for disposing of contaminated tissues, dressings, or other material and for removing soiled linens and equipment from the client's room. Check hospital policy or published guidelines for category-specific isolation.

- Teach the client the importance of complying with prescribed treatment for the entire course of the regimen. *Because anti-infective agents kill only a portion of the pathogen population with each dose, completion of the entire course of therapy is necessary to reduce the risk of relapse and creating drug-resistant organisms.*

Anxiety

The client with an infectious disease may experience anxiety related to his or her symptoms, treatment measures, the prognosis and expected outcome of the disease (Klein, Lee, Manton, & Parker, 1994). The diagnosis of an infection can be traumatic, causing the client to experience feelings of uneasiness, isolation, guilt (e.g., in regard to sexually transmitted diseases), apprehension, or depression.

Nursing interventions and rationales follow:

- Assess the client's level of anxiety. *The level of anxiety influences the client's response to and interpretation of the situation and degree of threat it poses.*

- Discuss the infection, treatments, prognosis, and outcomes. *Discussions help to allay fears and misconceptions.*

- Support and enhance the client's coping strategies. *A person uses intrapersonal and interpersonal mechanisms to reduce or relieve anxiety.*

- Include the client and significant others in the plan of care. *Inclusion of the client and family members provides assurance and confidence, and promotes understanding of the unknown.*

- Explain isolation procedures, and answer the client's and family's concerns. *Isolation may be necessary to prevent the spread of infection but can cause great anxiety for the client and family members.*

- Provide referrals as needed for continuing care, for example, to home health agencies, for dressing changes or periodic assessment.

Pain

The inflammatory process that generally accompanies infection can cause the client to experience general or localized discomfort or both.

Nursing interventions and rationales follow:

- Assess the client's pain. *Assessment is necessary to determine the location, severity, and client's response to pain.*

- Administer a mild analgesic as prescribed or indicated. *Analgesia is useful to relieve the discomfort of edematous tissue, myalgias, or headache.*

- Allow for rest periods. *Rest encourages healing and increases energy reserve.*

- Administer prescribed antipyretic as indicated for elevated temperature. *Although antipyretics lower the temperature and enhance comfort for the client, this benefit must be weighed against the possible beneficial effect of an elevated temperature in the immune response. Fever increases the motility and activity of WBCs, stimulates the production of interferon, and activates T cells. In addition, temperatures above the normal range inhibit the growth of many microorganisms (Porth, 1994).*

Other Nursing Diagnoses

Additional nursing diagnoses applicable to the person with an infection or infectious disease include:

- *Impaired Skin Integrity* related to injury and inflammation

- *Knowledge Deficit* of prescribed therapeutic regimen

- *Impaired Physical Mobility* related to swelling and edema

- *Risk for Altered Tissue Perfusion* related to septicemia

Client and Family Teaching

Client and family teaching is directed toward helping the client recover from the infection or disease, preventing its spread to others, and preventing life-threatening complications.

Verbal and/or written instructions should include the following:

- Use good hand-washing techniques, particularly after touching infected wounds or lesions, coughing, sneezing, blowing the nose, or using the bathroom. Wash hands thoroughly before eating or performing any procedures such as dressing changes.

- Take all prescribed antibiotics as ordered even after symptoms have subsided. Notify your health care provider if
  a. Symptoms do not improve within 24 to 48 hours after antibiotic therapy is instituted.
  b. Itching, rash, difficulty breathing, or other manifestations of antibiotic allergy occur.
  c. Adverse responses, such as gastrointestinal distress, interfere with completion of the prescription.
  d. Signs of superinfection, such as vaginitis, oral candidiasis, or diarrhea, occur.
  e. Manifestations of infection recur after the client completes the prescribed antibiotic.
  f. Any change in urination, skin color, easy bruising, or other manifestation of drug toxicity appears.
- Observe any skin lesions or wounds for further signs of infection such as drainage or swelling around the site. Report a persistent high fever.
- Increase fluid intake to at least 2500 mL (2.5 quarts) per day.

- Prevent the spread of infection to others by
  a. Avoiding crowds and contact with susceptible persons, especially those who are immunosuppressed (e.g., persons who have HIV infection, are undergoing therapy for cancer, or have had an organ transplant).
  b. Using disposable tissues to contain respiratory secretions when coughing or sneezing.
  c. Using appropriate food-handling precautions for diseases spread via the fecal-oral route, such as hepatitis A.
  d. Avoiding contact with or sharing of body fluids. For example, do not share needles or razors; use a condom during sexual activity, or abstain; each person should clean their own blood spills or wounds if possible.
- Check immunization records for all family members, and take measures to ensure up-to-date status for all. Contact local primary care provider or community health department to find resources for immunization.

Altered Immune Responses

Considering the complexity of the immune system, it is not surprising that abnormal or deleterious responses occur. Altered immune system responses include those characterized by hyperresponsiveness of the immune system and those characterized by an impaired immune response. Allergies, autoimmune disorders, and reactions to organ or tissue transplants are all examples of hyperresponsive immune function. AIDS and other immunodeficiency disorders result from impairment of the immune system.

The Client with a Hypersensitivity Reaction

Hypersensitivity is an altered immune response to an antigen that results in harm to the client. When the antigen is environmental or exogenous, it is called an **allergy**, and the antigen is referred to as an *allergen*. The tissue response to a hypersensitivity reaction may be simply irritating or bothersome, causing a runny nose or itchy eyes, or it may be life threatening, leading to blood cell hemolysis or laryngospasm.

Hypersensitivity reactions are primarily classified by the type of immune response that occurs on contact with the allergen. They may also be classified as immediate or delayed hypersensitivity responses. Anaphylaxis and transfusion reactions are examples of immediate hypersensitivity reactions; contact dermatitis is a typical delayed response. Allergies are sometimes referred to by the affected organ system (e.g., allergic rhinitis) or the allergen involved, as in hay fever. Classification by immunologic response is the most accurate and preferred means of studying allergies (Tierney et al., 1994).

Pathophysiology

In a hypersensitivity reaction, an antigen-antibody or antigen-lymphocyte interaction causes a response that is damaging to body tissues. Antigen-antibody responses characterize types I, II, and III, also known as immediate hypersensitivity responses. Type IV hypersensitivity is an antigen-lymphocyte reaction, resulting in a delayed hypersensitivity response.

Type I IgE-Mediated Hypersensitivity
Common hypersensitivity reactions, such as allergic asthma, allergic rhinitis (hay fever), allergic conjunctivitis, hives, and anaphylactic shock, are typical of type I or IgE-mediated hypersensitivity. This type of hypersensitivity response is triggered when an allergen interacts with IgE bound to mast cells and basophils. The antigen-antibody complex prompts release of histamine and other chemical

Sensitization stage

Antigen (allergen) invades body.

Plasma cells produce large amounts of class IgE antibodies against allergen.

IgE antibodies attach to mast cells in body tissues.

Subsequent (secondary) responses

More of same allergen invades body.

Allergen combines with IgE attached to mast cells, which triggers release of histamine (and other chemicals) from mast cell granules.

Histamine causes blood vessels to dilate and become leaky, which promotes edema; stimulates release of large amounts of mucus; and causes smooth muscles to contract (if respiratory system is site of allergen entry, asthma may ensue).

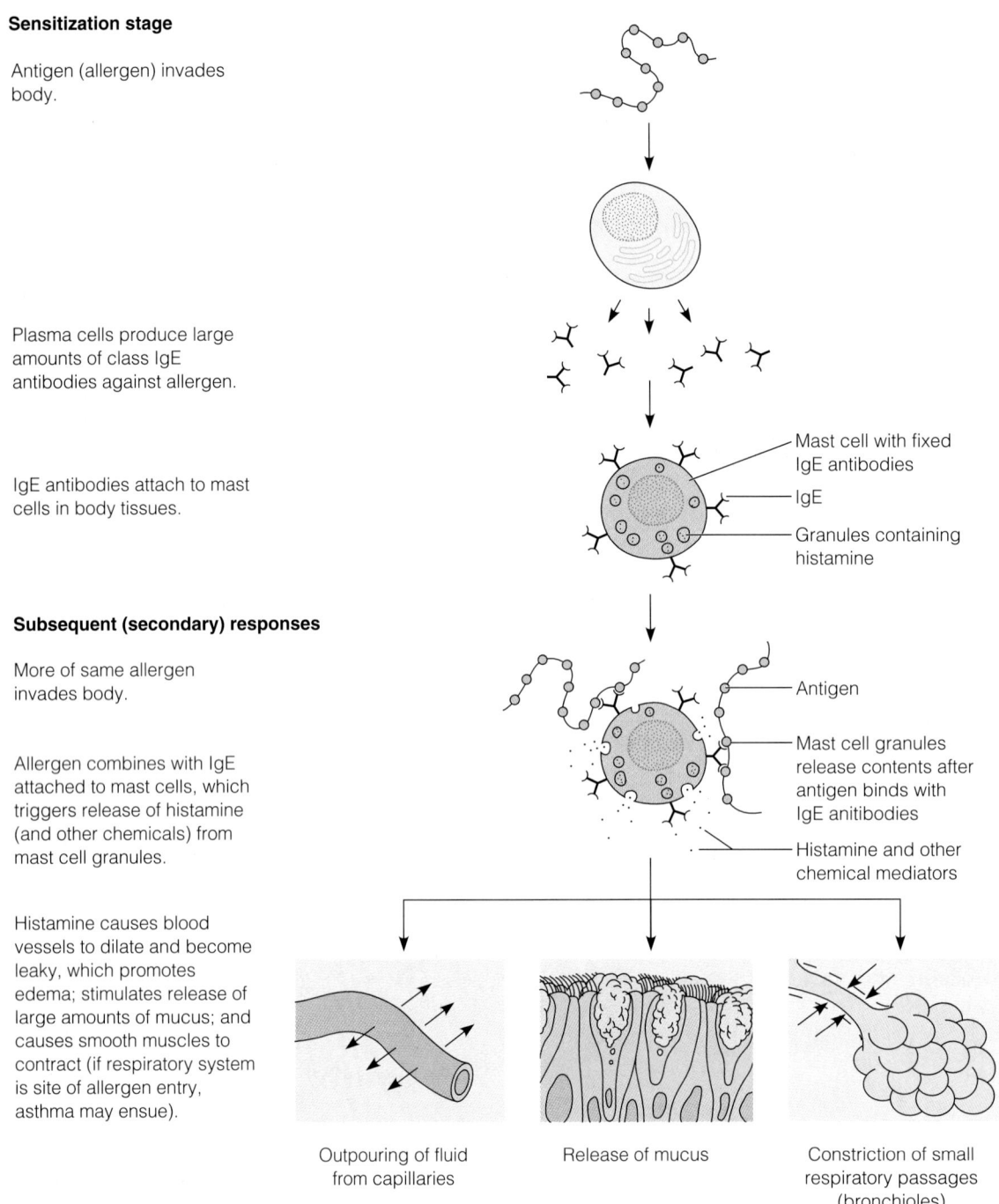

Mast cell with fixed IgE antibodies

IgE

Granules containing histamine

Antigen

Mast cell granules release contents after antigen binds with IgE anitbodies

Histamine and other chemical mediators

Outpouring of fluid from capillaries

Release of mucus

Constriction of small respiratory passages (bronchioles)

Figure 8–14 Type I IgE-mediated hypersensitivity response.

mediators, complement, acetylcholine, kinins, and chemotactic factors (Figure 8–14).

When a potent allergen such as bee or wasp venom or a drug is injected, resulting in widespread antibody-antigen reaction and response to these chemical mediators, a systemic response such as anaphylaxis, urticaria, or angioedema results.

Anaphylaxis is an acute systemic type I response that occurs in highly sensitive persons following injection of a specific antigen. Substances known to trigger anaphylaxis are summarized in the box on page 267. Anaphylaxis rarely follows oral ingestion, although this is possible. The reaction begins within minutes of exposure to the allergen and may be almost instantaneous. The release of

Substances Known to Trigger Anaphylaxis in Sensitized Persons

■ ■ ■

Hormones

- Insulin
- Vasopressin
- Parathormone

Enzymes

- Trypsin
- Chymotrypsin
- Penicillinase

Pollens

- Ragweed
- Grass
- Trees

Foods

- Eggs
- Seafoods
- Nuts
- Grains
- Beans
- Cottonseed oil
- Chocolate

Insect Venom

- Yellow jacket
- Hornet
- Paper wasp
- Honey bee

Vitamins

- Thiamine
- Folic acid

Occupational Agents

- Rubber products
- Industrial chemicals (ethylenes)

Antibiotics

- Penicillins
- Cephalosporins
- Amphotericin B
- Nitrofurantoin

Local Anesthetics

- Procaine
- Lidocaine

Medical Diagnostic Agents

- Sodium dehydrocholate
- Sulfobromophthalein

Antiserum

- Antilymphocyte gamma globulin

hibits air hunger, stridor and wheezing, and a barking cough. These respiratory effects can be lethal if the reaction is severe and intervention is not immediately available. Vasodilation and fluid loss from the vascular system can lead to impaired tissue perfusion and hypotension, a condition known as *anaphylactic shock.*

Fortunately, *localized responses* are more common manifestations of Type I hypersensitivity. These are typically *atopic* responses; that is, they have a strong genetic predisposition. Atopic reactions are the result of localized, rather than systemic, IgE-mediated responses to an allergen. They are prompted by contact of the allergen with cell-bound IgE in the bronchial tree, nasal mucosa, and conjunctival tissues. Chemical mediators are released locally, producing symptoms such as asthma, allergic rhinitis (hay fever), conjunctivitis, or atopic dermatitis. Allergens commonly associated with atopic reactions of this type include pollens, fungal spores, house dust mites, animal dander, and feathers (Porth, 1994). Food allergens can also cause localized responses, such as diarrhea or vomiting. If the gastrointestinal mucosa is altered by a local allergic response, the allergen may be absorbed, leading to a systemic reaction. Urticaria (hives) is the most common systemic response to food allergies.

Type II Cytotoxic Hypersensitivity

A hemolytic transfusion reaction to blood of an incompatible type is characteristic of a type II or cytotoxic hypersensitivity reaction. IgG or IgM type antibodies are formed to a cell-bound antigen such as the ABO or Rh antigen. When these antibodies bind with the antigen, the complement cascade is activated, resulting in destruction of the target cell (Figure 8–15).

Type II reactions may be stimulated by an exogenous antigen, such as foreign tissue or cells, or a drug reaction, in which the drug forms an antigenic complex on the surface of a blood cell, stimulating the production of antibodies. The affected cell is then destroyed in the resulting antigen-antibody reaction; for example, hemolytic anemia is sometimes associated with the administration of chlorpromazine (Thorazine). Withdrawal of the drug stops the reaction and cell destruction (Roitt, 1994).

Endogenous antigens can also stimulate a Type II reaction, resulting in an autoimmune disorder such as Goodpasture's syndrome, in which antigens are formed to specific tissues in the lungs and kidneys. Hashimoto's thyroiditis and autoimmune hemolytic anemia are additional examples of autoimmune type II reactions.

Type III Immune Complex–Mediated Hypersensitivity

Type III hypersensitivity reactions result from the formation of IgG or IgM antibody-antigen immune complexes in the circulation. When these complexes are deposited in vessel walls and extravascular tissues, complement is

histamine and other mediators causes vasodilation and increased capillary permeability, smooth muscle contraction, and bronchial constriction. These chemical mediators cause the client to experience the typical manifestations of anaphylaxis. Initially, a sense of foreboding or uneasiness, lightheadedness, and itching palms and scalp may be noted. Hives may develop, along with angioedema (localized tissue swelling) of the eyelids, lips, tongue, hands, feet, and genitals. Swelling can also affect the uvula and larynx, impairing breathing. This is further complicated by the bronchial constriction. The client ex-

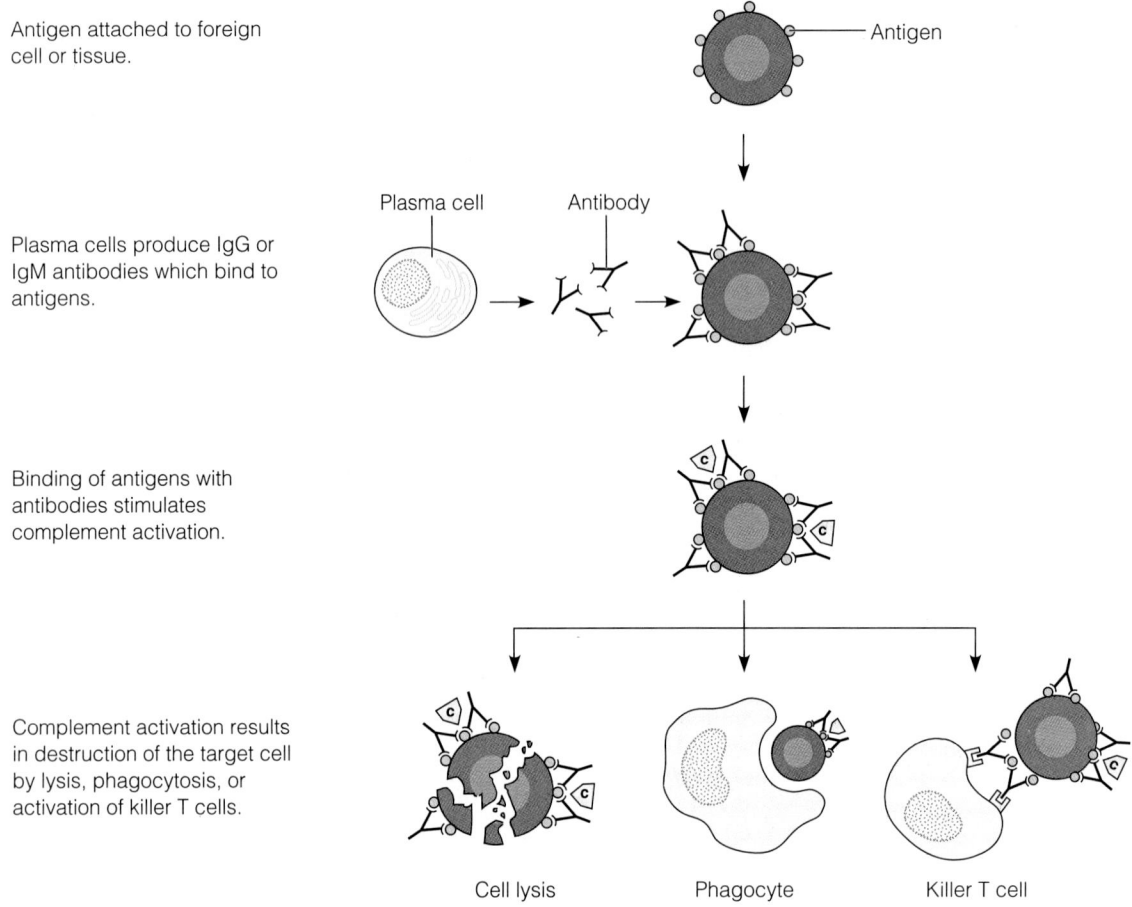

Antigen attached to foreign cell or tissue.

Antigen

Plasma cell

Antibody

Plasma cells produce IgG or IgM antibodies which bind to antigens.

Binding of antigens with antibodies stimulates complement activation.

Complement activation results in destruction of the target cell by lysis, phagocytosis, or activation of killer T cells.

Cell lysis

Phagocyte

Killer T cell

Figure 8–15   Type II cytotoxic hypersensitivity response.

activated and chemical mediators of inflammation such as histamine are released. Chemotactic factors attract neutrophils to the site of inflammation. When neutrophils attempt to phagocytize the immune complexes, lysosomal enzymes are released, increasing tissue damage (Figure 8–16).

Either systemic or local responses may be seen with type III reactions. Serum sickness is a systemic response, so named because it was first identified after administration of foreign serum, for example, horse antitetanus toxin. Although foreign serums are no longer administered, serum sickness occurs in response to some drugs, such as penicillin and sulfonamides. Immune complexes are deposited in walls of small blood vessels, the kidneys, and joints. Manifestations of serum sickness include fever, urticaria or rash, arthralgias, myalgias, and lymphadenopathy.

Localized responses may occur at a number of different sites. As immune complexes accumulate in the glomerular basement membrane of the kidneys—for example, following a streptococcal infection or with systemic lupus erythematosus—glomerulonephritis develops. When an antigen such as the dust from moldy hay or from pigeon feces is inhaled, an acute alveolar inflammatory response can occur, as in farmer's lung.

Type IV Delayed Hypersensitivity

Type IV reactions differ from other hypersensitivity responses in two ways. First, these reactions are cell mediated rather than antibody mediated, involving T cells of the immune system. Second, type IV reactions are delayed rather than immediate, with an onset 24 to 48 hours after exposure to the antigen. Type IV hypersensitivity responses result from an exaggerated interaction between an antigen and normal cell-mediated mechanisms. This exaggerated interaction results in the release of soluble inflammatory and immune mediators (from the lysozymes within the macrophages) and recruitment of killer T cells, causing local tissue destruction (Figure 8–17 on page 270).

Contact dermatitis is a classic example of a type IV reaction. Intense redness, itching, and thickening affect the skin in the area exposed to the antigen. Fragile vesicles are often present as well. Many antigens can provoke this response; poison ivy is a prime perpetrator. Other examples of cell-mediated responses include a positive tuberculin test and graft rejection episodes.

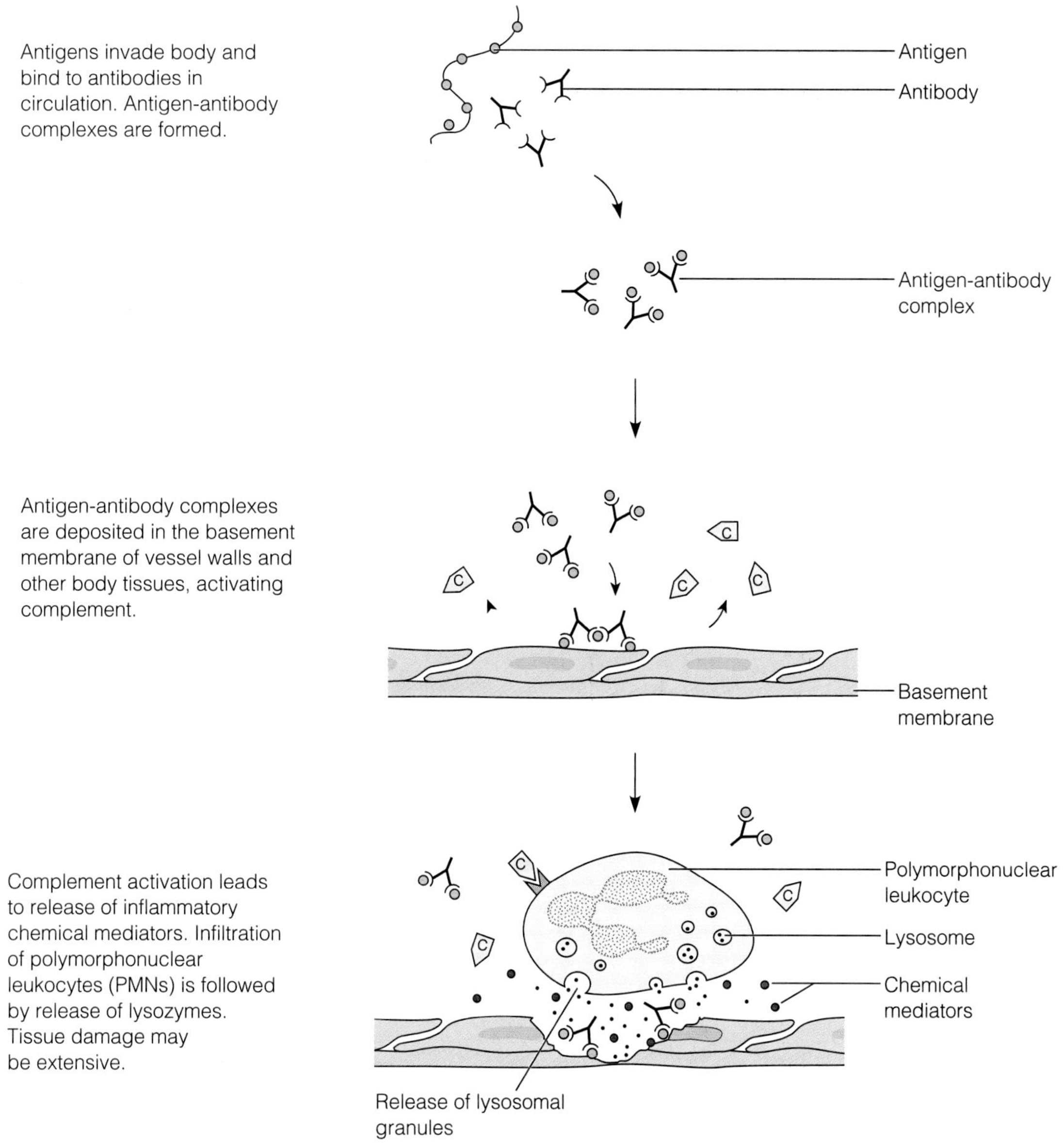

Antigens invade body and bind to antibodies in circulation. Antigen-antibody complexes are formed.

Antigen

Antibody

Antigen-antibody complex

Antigen-antibody complexes are deposited in the basement membrane of vessel walls and other body tissues, activating complement.

Basement membrane

Complement activation leads to release of inflammatory chemical mediators. Infiltration of polymorphonuclear leukocytes (PMNs) is followed by release of lysozymes. Tissue damage may be extensive.

Polymorphonuclear leukocyte

Lysosome

Chemical mediators

Release of lysosomal granules

Figure 8–16   Type III immune complex-mediated hypersensitivity response.

Collaborative Care

The focus of care for clients with allergic responses is to

- Minimize exposure to the allergen.
- Prevent a hypersensitivity response.
- Provide prompt, effective interventions for allergic responses when they occur.

Identifying allergens for the individual to reduce the likelihood of exposure is a key aspect of management. A complete history of all of the client's allergies is obtained, including medications, foods, animals, plants, and other materials. The type of hypersensitivity response is documented, as is onset, manifestations, and usual treatment.

In the presence of a documented or suspected hypersensitivity reaction, the allergen (e.g., intravenous medication or transfusion) is withdrawn immediately. With a type I hypersensitivity response, managing the client's airway takes highest priority, followed by maintaining cardiac output. Type II hypersensitivity responses may necessitate aggressive management of bleeding or renal failure. Type III (immune complex) reaction is treated by removing the offending antigen and interrupting the inflammatory response.

With a hypersensitivity response, supportive care is important to relieve the client's discomfort. This often involves the administration of selected antihistamine or anti-inflammatory medications. Other therapies, such as plasmapheresis, may be prescribed in selected instances.

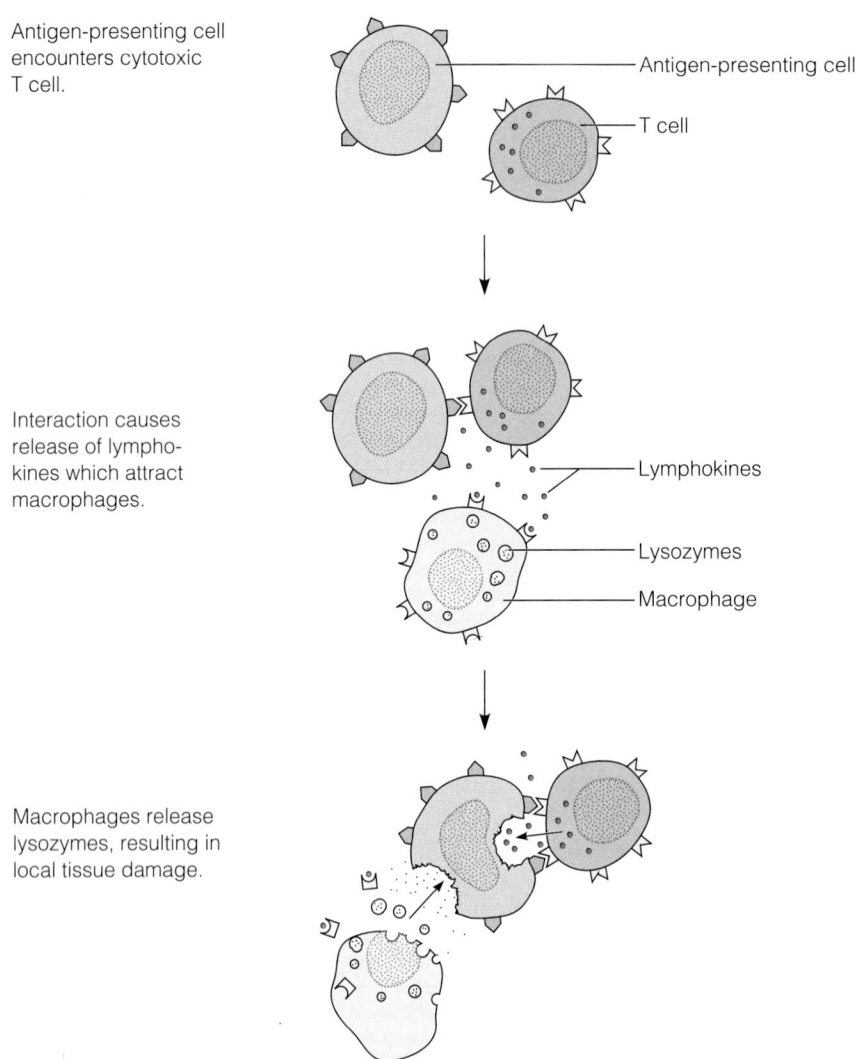

Antigen-presenting cell encounters cytotoxic T cell.

Antigen-presenting cell

T cell

Interaction causes release of lympho-kines which attract macrophages.

Lymphokines

Lysozymes

Macrophage

Macrophages release lysozymes, resulting in local tissue damage.

Figure 8–17   Type IV delayed hypersensitivity response.

Laboratory and Diagnostic Tests

To identify possible allergens or hypersensitivity reactions, the following laboratory tests may be ordered:

- *WBC count with differential* is performed to detect possible high levels of circulating eosinophils. Normally, eosinophils constitute a very small percentage (1% to 4%) of the total WBCs. Eosinophilia, however, is often present in clients with type I hypersensitivities.

- *Radioallergosorbent test (RAST)* may be performed to measure the amount of IgE directed toward specific allergens. The suspected allergen is added to a sample of the client's blood. The amount of IgE bound to the allergen is then measured to identify hypersensitivities. Although this test is considerably more expensive than skin testing and takes longer to complete, it poses no risk of an anaphylactic reaction, because testing is done outside the client's body. RAST is particularly useful in detecting allergies to some occupational chemicals and toxic allergens (Tierney et al., 1994).

- *Blood type and crossmatch* are ordered prior to any anticipated transfusions. The client's ABO blood group and Rh status are determined. Two major antigens, designated A and B, may be present on RBCs. Clients with the A antigen are designated as blood type A; those with blood type B have the B antigen. When neither antigen is found on the RBCs, the person is identified as type O. A third major RBC antigen is the Rh antigen. Persons with this antigen are called Rh-positive; those without are Rh-negative. Because a blood transfusion is actually a transplant of living tissue, antigen matching is vital to prevent significant hypersensitivity reactions. Once blood type is determined, a sample of the client's blood is mixed with a sample of matching donor blood and observed for antigen-antibody reactions in the crossmatch portion of this test. Although this procedure greatly reduces the risk of a hemolytic transfusion reaction (type II hypersensitivity), it does not totally eliminate it (Chernecky et al., 1993; Pagana & Pagana, 1992).

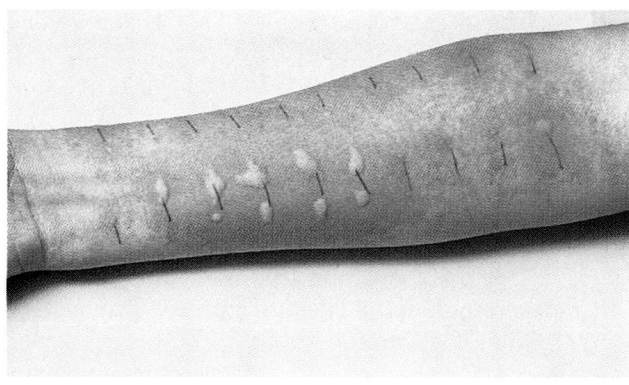

Figure 8–18 Skin testing on the forearm showing induration and erythema typical of a positive response to an antigen.

- *Indirect Coombs' test* detects the presence of circulating antibodies (other than ABO antibodies) against RBCs. The client's serum is mixed with the donor's RBCs. If antibodies to an RBC antigen are present in the client's serum, agglutination (clumping together) will occur. This is called a positive response. The normal value is negative, or no agglutination. This test is also part of the crossmatch portion of a blood type and crossmatch.

- *Direct Coombs' testing* is used to detect antibodies on the client's RBCs that can result in damage and destruction to the cells. This examination is used following a suspected transfusion reaction to detect antibodies coating the transfused RBCs. It is also used to identify possible reasons for hemolytic anemia when the cause is unknown. In the direct Coombs' test, the client's RBCs are mixed with Coombs' serum, which contains antibodies to IgG and several complement components. Agglutination will occur if the client's RBCs are coated with antibodies, resulting in a positive test. As with the indirect Coombs' test, the normal test result is negative (Chernecky et al., 1993; Pagana & Pagana, 1992).

- *Immune complex assays* may be performed to detect the presence of circulating immune complexes in suspected type III hypersensitivity responses. The assays are particularly useful in diagnosing suspected autoimmune disorders. Nonspecific assays of IgG-, IgM-, and IgA-containing immune complexes, which do not detect specific antibodies, as well as specific antibody assays may be done. The expected or normal result is a test negative for circulating immune complexes. A negative test does not, however, rule out an immune complex hypersensitivity response. In some cases, a negative result may indicate that the disease process has reached a later stage, in which complexes are no longer circulating but have initiated extensive tissue damage, such as glomerulonephritis (Wilson et al., 1991).

- *Complement assay* is also useful in detecting immune complex disorders. In these disorders, complement is, in effect, "used up" by the development of antigen-antibody complexes. Decreased levels are seen on examination. Both total complement level and amounts of individual components of the complement cascade can be determined.

Although laboratory tests are useful to confirm a hypersensitivity response, diagnostic tests, such as skin tests, are used to determine causes of hypersensitivity reactions. These tests are used to identify specific allergens to which a person may be sensitive. Allergens for testing are selected according to the client's history. Test solutions made from extracts of inhaled, ingested, or injected materials, such as pollens, mites, venoms, or some drugs, are used for the prick test and intradermal testing. Epicutaneous testing (prick testing) is generally done first to avoid a systemic reaction; it is followed by intradermal testing of allergens with a negative response to prick testing (Tierney et al., 1994).

- *Prick (epicutaneous or puncture) test:* A drop of diluted allergenic extract is placed on the skin, and the skin is then pricked or punctured through the drop. With a positive test, a localized pruritic wheal and erythema occurs. The response is maximal at 15 to 20 minutes.

- *Intradermal:* A small amount (just enough to create a wheal) of allergen extract at a 1:500 or 1:1000 dilution is injected on the forearm or intrascapular area. If several allergens are being tested, ½- or ¼-inch intervals are spaced between injections. As control measures, plain diluent (negative control) and histamine (positive control) are also injected. If there is no response to a particular allergen at 15 to 20 minutes, the test is negative. The appearance of a wheal and erythema, with a wheal diameter at least 5 mm greater than that produced by the control, indicates a positive response (Merck Research Laboratories, 1992) (Figure 8–18).

- *Patch:* A 1-inch patch impregnated with the allergen (e.g., perfume, cosmetics, detergents, or clothing fibers) is applied to the skin for 48 hours. Absence of a response indicates a negative test result. Positive responses are graded from mild (erythema in the exposed area), to severe (erythema, papules, vesicles, or ulceration).

- *Food allergy testing* is done when the client is suspected of having a food allergy but the source or implicated food item has not been clearly identified. Food allergy symptoms are typically demonstrated within hours of eating. Initially, the client is asked to keep a diary of foods consumed and allergic responses for a week. An elimination diet is then prescribed. The diet excludes most common food allergens and all suspected foods for one week. Any foods that may contain allergens in combination, such as breads, are also eliminated. If the client's symptoms do not improve, a different variation of the elimination diet is prescribed. If symptoms are relieved, foods are reintroduced to the diet one at a time until symptoms recur, indicating allergy to that food (Merck Research Laboratories, 1992).

Pharmacology

When it is impossible to avoid the offending allergen and allergic manifestations are severe or disrupt the client's activities of daily living (ADLs), pharmacologic intervention is prescribed.

Immunotherapy, also called hyposensitization or desensitization, consists of injecting an extract of the allergen(s) in gradually increasing doses. Immunotherapy is used primarily for allergic rhinitis or asthma related to inhaled allergens. It has also been shown to be effective in preventing anaphylactic responses to insect venom. With weekly or biweekly subcutaneous injections of the allergen, the client develops IgG antibodies to the allergen that appear to block effectively the allergic IgE-mediated response. Once a therapy plateau is reached, injections are continued indefinitely either monthly or bimonthly.

Antihistamines are the major class of drugs used in treating the symptoms of hypersensitivity responses, type I in particular. They are also useful to some extent in relieving manifestations (such as urticaria) of some type II and type III reactions.

Antihistamines block H_1-histamine receptors, acting as a competitive antagonist to histamine. They do not affect the production or release of histamine. Antihistamines are particularly useful in relieving allergic rhinitis and urticaria, although they are not effective in all clients. Their use is limited by their side effects, especially drowsiness and dry mouth. Several different groups of antihistamines are available; if one group is not effective for the client, another may be. Antihistamines are often combined with a sympathomimetic agent such as pseudoephedrine to improve their decongestant activity and counteract their sedative effect. Nursing care for the client receiving antihistamines is outlined in the pharmacology box on page 273.

The immediate treatment for anaphylaxis is parenteral epinephrine. Epinephrine is an adrenergic agonist (sympathomimetic) drug that has both vasoconstricting and bronchodilating effects. These qualities, combined with its rapid action, make epinephrine ideal for treating an anaphylactic reaction. For mild reactions with wheezing, pruritus, urticaria, and angioedema, a subcutaneous injection of 0.3 to 0.5 mL of 1:1000 epinephrine is generally sufficient. For clients with an injected toxin such as a bee sting, an additional amount equivalent to one-half the above may be injected directly into the site of the sting and a tourniquet applied above it to prevent further systemic absorption. Intravenous epinephrine using a

1:100,000 concentration may be used in the client with a more severe anaphylactic reaction.

Clients who have experienced an anaphylactic reaction to insect venom or other potentially unavoidable allergen should carry a kit (commonly called a "bee sting kit") for immediate treatment of future exposures. This kit typically includes a prefilled syringe of epinephrine and an epinephrine nebulizer, allowing prompt self-treatment (Merck Research Laboratories, 1992).

Cromolyn sodium (Intal, Nasalcrom) is a drug used to treat allergic rhinitis and asthma. Cromolyn sodium acts by stabilizing the mast cell membrane, preventing chemical mediator release (Skidmore-Roth, 1993). Because it is effective only when applied directly to involved tissue, it is delivered by inhaler or nasal spray. It has few side effects and a wide margin of safety, making it a good choice for clients in whom it is effective (Tierney et al., 1994).

Glucocorticoids are used in both systemic and topical forms for many types of hypersensitivity responses. It is their anti-inflammatory effects that are of most benefit, rather than immunosuppressive effects. A short course of corticosteroid therapy is often used for severe asthma, allergic contact dermatitis, and some immune-complex disorders (Tierney et al., 1994). Corticosteroids in topical forms or delivered by inhaler may be used for longer periods of time with few side effects; however, systemic absorption can occur.

Other Therapies

Other treatments used for hypersensitivity responses are generally dictated by the severity of the response and the organ system affected.

Airway management takes highest priority for the client with an acute anaphylactic reaction. Insertion of an endotracheal tube or emergency tracheostomy may be required to maintain airway patency with severe laryngospasm. Because anaphylaxis places the person at risk for vasomotor collapse and significant hypotension, it is necessary to insert an intravenous line and initiate fluid resuscitation with an isotonic solution, such as Ringer's lactate.

Plasmapheresis, the removal of harmful components in the plasma, may be used to treat immune complex responses such as glomerulonephritis and Goodpasture's syndrome. The glomerular-damaging antibody-antigen complexes are removed from the client's blood along with the plasma by passing the blood through a blood cell separator. An equal amount of albumin or human plasma is returned to the client along with the client's RBCs. This procedure is usually done in a series rather than as a one-time only treatment. It is not without risk, and informed consent is required. Potential complications of plasmapheresis include those associated with the placement of intravenous catheters, shifts in fluid balance, and alteration of blood clotting.

Nursing Implications for Pharmacology: Antihistamine Therapy

ANTIHISTAMINES

Ethanolamines: Diphenhydramine (Benadryl), clemastine (Tavist)

Ethylenediamine: Tripelennamine (PBZ-SR, Pelamine)

Alkylamines: Brompheniramine (Bromfed, Dimetane, others); chlorpheniramine (Chlor-Trimeton, others); triprolidine (Actidil, Bayidyl)

Phenothiazine: Promethazine (Phenergan, others)

Piperazine: Hydroxyzine (Vistaril)

Piperidines: Terfenadine (Seldane); astemizole (Hismanal); azatadine (Optimine); cyproheptadine (Periactin)

Diphenhydramine is considered the prototype antihistamine. It and other antihistamines are widely used in treatment of hypersensitivity responses and are available in both prescription and nonprescription preparations. The preferred route of administration is oral, although diphenhydramine and others can be given parenterally, particularly when immediate action is needed, as in anaphylaxis. Antihistamines are effective in alleviating the systemic effects of histamine, such as urticaria and angioedema. They also dry respiratory secretions through an anticholinergic effect. Antihistamines are *not* effective in relieving asthmatic responses to allergens and may actually worsen symptoms by their drying effect on respiratory secretions. Most antihistamines cause drowsiness, some more than others. Diphenhydramine and promethazine can cause significant drowsiness; terfenadine and astemizole are recently developed antihistamines which produce little sedative effect.

Nursing Responsibilities

- Assess for actual or potential contraindications to diphenhydramine prior to administering:
  a. Acute asthma or other lower respiratory disease, which may be aggravated by drying of respiratory secretions
  b. Hypersensitivity to antihistamines
  c. Glaucoma (increased intraocular pressure)
  d. Impaired gastrointestinal motility or obstruction, which may be worsened by the anticholinergic effects of diphenhydramine
  e. Prostatic hypertrophy or other urinary tract obstruction

  f. Cardiac disease or hyperthyroidism (diphenhydramine and other antihistamines may worsen tachycardia)
- Administer with caution to older clients, who are more likely to be taking other medications, have glaucoma or urinary tract obstruction, or have slowed gastrointestinal motility. Paradoxic central nervous system stimulation is common in older clients taking diphenhydramine (Shlafer, 1993).
- Administer with great caution to clients receiving other central nervous system depressants, such as barbiturates, narcotics, hypnotics, tricyclic antidepressants, or alcohol. Promethazine is very sedating, requiring reduction in doses of any other central nervous system depressant drugs.
- If giving intravenously, administer diphenhydramine at no more than 25 mg per minute undiluted.
- Monitor intake and output. Discontinue if the client develops urinary retention or frequency.
- Monitor for thrombocytopenia, agranulocytosis, or hemolytic anemia.
- Terfenadine and astemizole are the least sedating antihistamines and are most appropriate for clients who must remain alert while on antihistamine therapy.
- Promethazine has good antiemetic effects as well as antihistamine effects.
- Hydroxyzine is used primarily as an antianxiety agent, antiemetic, and potentiator of narcotic effects.

Client and Family Teaching

- Use hard candy, gum, ice chips, and frequent mouth rinses with cool water to relieve dryness.
- While taking this medication, do not drive or operate machinery if drowsiness occurs.
- Stop the drug and notify the physician if confusion, excessive sedation, chest tightness, wheezing, easy bruising, or excessive bleeding occurs.
- Do not take other over-the-counter antihistamines or use alcohol while taking prescribed antihistamines.

Nursing Care

Nursing care related to hypersensitivity reactions is first and foremost directed toward prevention, early identification, and providing prompt, effective treatment. Prior to administering any medication or treatment, ascertain the client's history of hypersensitivity reactions. If the client indicates a previous hypersensitivity response to a drug or to a closely related drug, investigate further. Ask the client to describe the response and its treatment. If it appears to have been a true hypersensitivity response, such as the development of a rash, hives, or difficulty breathing, check with the physician prior to administering the drug. Close observation is needed if the client is receiving a new medication for the first time. Remember that with IgE-mediated responses, the client may have received the drug in the past without developing noticeable hypersensitivity responses and nevertheless be at risk for anaphylaxis. The components of products used in the hospital (e.g., skin cleansers, radiopaque dyes) should be made known to the client in case of potential hypersensitivity responses.

Priority nursing diagnoses will vary according to the type of hypersensitivity reaction experienced by the client. Because nurses are most likely to become involved with a client experiencing a type I or type II response, this section focuses on diagnoses for these clients. Airway, breathing, and circulation (the ABCs) are of greatest importance for the client with an anaphylactic reaction. When a hemolytic reaction to an incompatible blood transfusion occurs, the client is at risk for injury.

Ineffective Airway Clearance

In anaphylactic reactions, the airway may be obstructed due to facial angioedema, bronchospasm, or laryngeal edema. Establishing and maintaining a patent airway is of highest priority.

Nursing interventions with rationales follow:

- Place the client in Fowler's to high-Fowler's position. *This position allows optimal lung expansion and ease of breathing.*
- Administer oxygen per nasal cannula at a rate of 2 to 4 L/min. *This increases the alveolar oxygen and its availability to cells of the body.*
- Assess the client's airway by observing for respiratory rate and pattern, level of consciousness and anxiety, nasal flaring, use of accessory muscles of respiration, chest wall movement, audible stridor; palpate for respiratory excursion; auscultate lung sounds and any adventitious sounds, such as wheezes. *Extreme anxiety or agitation, nasal flaring, stridor, and diminished lung sounds indicate air hunger and possible airway obstruction, necessitating immediate intervention.*

- Insert a nasopharyngeal or oropharyngeal airway, and arrange for immediate intubation as indicated by the client's status. *Assuring an adequate airway is vital to preserve the client's life.*
- Administer subcutaneous epinephrine 1:1000, 0.3 to 0.5 mL as prescribed. This may be repeated in 20 to 30 minutes if necessary. Administer parenteral diphenhydramine (deep intramuscular or intravenous) as prescribed. *Epinephrine is a potent vasoconstrictor and bronchodilator, counteracting the effects of histamine. Diphenhydramine is an antihistamine that blocks histamine receptors and its effect. These medications can be effective in rapidly reversing manifestations of anaphylaxis.*
- Provide calm reassurance to the client. *Hypoxemia and air hunger are terrifying for the client. Anxiety can impair the client's ability to cooperate with treatment and increase the respiratory rate, making breathing less effective.*

Decreased Cardiac Output

Peripheral vasodilation and increased capillary permeability from the release of histamine can significantly impair the client's cardiac output. When it falls to the degree that tissue perfusion becomes impaired and hypoxia results, a state of anaphylactic shock exists.

Nursing interventions with rationales follow:

- Monitor vital signs frequently, assessing for changes such as a fall in blood pressure, decreasing pulse pressure, tachycardia, and tachypnea. *These vital sign changes may indicate shock.*
- Assess skin color, temperature, capillary refill, edema, and other indicators of peripheral perfusion.
- Monitor the client's level of consciousness. *A change in level of consciousness (lethargy, apprehension, or agitation) is often the first indicator of decreased cardiac output.*
- Insert one or more large-bore (18-gauge or larger) intravenous catheters. *It is important to insert intravenous catheters as soon as possible to provide sites for rapid fluid replacement.*
- Administer warmed intravenous solutions, such as lactated Ringer's or normal saline, as prescribed. *These isotonic solutions help maintain intravascular volume. Warmed solutions are used to prevent hypothermia from the rapid administration of large amounts of fluid at room temperature (about 70 F, or 21.1 C).*
- Insert an indwelling catheter, and monitor urinary output frequently. *As the cardiac output drops, the glomerular filtration rate (GFR) falls. With an output of less than 30 mL per hour, the client is at risk for acute renal failure from ischemia.*
- Place a tourniquet above the site of an injected venom (such as a bee sting), and infiltrate the site with

epinephrine as prescribed. *Use of a tourniquet and the vasoconstriction resulting from epinephrine infiltration reduce further absorption of the allergen.*

- Once breathing is established, place the client flat with the legs elevated. *This position enhances perfusion of the central organs, such as the brain, heart, and kidneys.*

- As the client's status begins to improve, assess for shortness of breath and crackles in the lungs. *Aggressive fluid therapy may lead to hypervolemia and pulmonary edema.*

Risk for Injury

As noted before, the potential for hypersensitivity responses is high in clients subjected to medical treatments. Because a blood transfusion is a transplant of living tissue, the risk for adverse immunologic response and injury to the client is particularly significant.

Nursing interventions with rationales follow:

- Obtain and record a thorough history of previous blood transfusions and any reactions experienced, **no matter how mild.** *The client who has received prior blood transfusions is at increased risk for a hypersensitivity reaction, because antibody production may have been stimulated by prior exposure to antigens.* Alert the physician if previous transfusion reactions have occurred.

- Check for a signed informed consent to administer blood or blood products. *It is important to obtain informed consent for this invasive and risky procedure.*

- Using two licensed health care professionals, double-check the type, Rh factor, crossmatch, and expiration date for all blood and blood components received from the blood bank with the client's data. *This is an important safety measure to reduce the risk of a hemolytic transfusion reaction due to incompatible blood types.*

- Administer blood within 30 minutes of its delivery from the blood bank. *Bacteria can grow rapidly in living tissue, including blood. Administer blood promptly to reduce the chances of bacterial contamination.*

- Take and record vital signs within 15 minutes prior to initiating the blood infusion. *This provides a baseline for evaluating any changes related to the blood transfusion.*

- Infuse blood into a site separate from any other intravenous infusion. Use at least an 18-gauge catheter for the infusion. *This reduces the risk of damage to the blood cells due to incompatibility with other intravenous solutions or physical trauma. When blood is administered with dextrose solutions (e.g., D5W, D5NS), blood cell hemolysis and aggregation occurs; administration with lactated Ringer's can cause agglutination of cells.*

- Administer 50 mL of blood during the first 15 minutes of the transfusion. *Reactions generally occur within the first 15 minutes.*

- Assess the client during transfusion for complaints of back or chest pain, an increase in the temperature of more than 1.8 degrees F, chills, tachycardia, tachypnea, wheezing, hypotension, hives, rashes, or cyanosis. *These signs may indicate an adverse reaction to the blood transfusion.*

- Stop the blood transfusion immediately if a reaction occurs, no matter how mild, keeping the intravenous line open with normal saline. Notify the physician and the blood bank.

- If a reaction is suspected, send the blood and administration set to the laboratory along with a freshly drawn blood sample and urine specimen from the client. *These will be used to identify the cause of the reaction as well as its effect on the client.*

- If no adverse reaction occurs, administer the transfusion within a 4-hour period. *As noted previously, this is important to limit the risk of bacterial growth.*

Other Nursing Diagnoses

Other nursing diagnoses that may apply to the client experiencing a hypersensitivity response include:

- *Risk for Altered Thought Processes* related to reduced cerebral blood flow
- *Impaired Skin Integrity* related to hypersensitivity response
- *Anxiety* related to difficulty breathing
- *Health-Seeking Behaviors:* Testing and possible immunotherapy to prevent hypersensitivity responses
- *Altered Role Performance* related to hypersensitivity responses
- *Risk for Suffocation* related to potential anaphylactic reactions

Client and Family Teaching

The vast majority of hypersensitivity responses are appropriately treated by the client and/or family members with little or no medical intervention. Teaching, therefore, is a vital component of care. If the client is at risk for anaphylaxis, involving the family in teaching is essential because the response may occur with such rapidity that the client will be unable to provide self-care.

Assist the client to identify possible allergens that prompt a hypersensitivity response. Discuss possible strategies to avoid these allergens if at all possible. Clients with food allergies should meet with a dietitian to discuss necessary dietary changes and ways to continue meeting nutrient needs. Emphasize the need to notify health care personnel of all allergens. People who experience anaphylactic reactions should wear a bracelet or tag at all times identifying the substance or substances that provoke this response.

Instruct the client with anaphylactic reactions to insect venoms, food allergies, or other environmental allergens to carry an anaphylaxis kit containing epinephrine and antihistamines in injectable, inhaler, and oral forms to self-treat severe hypersensitivity reactions. Teach the client and family members how to inject the medication and use the inhaler. Emphasize the need for prompt treatment when initial symptoms occur. Instruct the client to seek medical attention after obtaining immediate treatment.

Teach the client about the use of prescription and nonprescription antihistamines and decongestants for symptom relief. Stress that these medications are not effective in relieving asthmatic symptoms and may actually worsen them. Emphasize the need to take precautions if drowsiness is a problem and to avoid other CNS depressants, such as alcohol. Discuss measures to relieve the anticholinergic side effects of these medications, such as dry mouth.

For clients anticipating surgery, discuss the advantages of autologous blood transfusion and "banking" their own blood prior to surgery. Instruct the client receiving a transfusion about symptoms to report immediately. To help allay the client's anxiety, explain the reason for close observation and taking frequent vital signs during the transfusion.

The client with an immune complex reaction needs information about the specific manifestations and body systems affected. Teach clients about the importance of treating disorders such as strep throat fully to reduce the risk of an immune complex response such as glomerulonephritis.

For the client with contact dermatitis, teaching focuses on providing appropriate skin care, preventing infection in affected skin, and promoting comfort. Include the following measures:

- Expose affected areas to air and sun as much as possible to promote healing.
- Avoid direct contact with people who have an infection.
- Wear cool, light, nonrestrictive clothing of natural fibers, such as cotton, to avoid irritating affected areas. Avoid wool, which can be irritating and may increase heat production, increasing the itching sensation.
- Avoid exposure to extremes of heat or cold.
- When bathing, use bath oils or plain water instead of soaps and detergents. Highly fatted soaps such as Dove are also less irritating.
- Use tub baths in cool to lukewarm water rather than showers to help provide an antipruritic effect.
- To decrease pruritus, maintain a cool environment and avoid exercising.
- Trim fingernails to reduce the risk of skin damage from scratching.

The Client with an Autoimmune Disorder

■ ■ ■

Maintaining optimal health and preventing disease depend not only on the immune system's ability to recognize and destroy foreign tissues and other antigens, but also on the immune system's ability to recognize self. When this self-recognition is impaired and immune defenses are directed against normal host tissue, the result is an **autoimmune disorder.**

Autoimmune disorders can affect any tissue in the body. Some are tissue- or organ-specific, affecting particular tissue or a particular organ. Hashimoto's thyroiditis is an example of an organ-specific autoimmune disorder. Circulating antibodies are formed to certain thyroid components, resulting ultimately in destruction of the gland. In other cases, autoantibodies are formed that are not tissue specific but tend to accumulate and cause an inflammatory response in certain tissue, for example, the renal glomerulus or the hepatic small bile ductules. Autoimmune disorders may also be systemic, with neither antibodies nor the resulting inflammatory lesions confined to any one organ. Rheumatologic disorders, such as rheumatoid arthritis and systemic lupus erythmatosus (SLE), are characteristic of systemic autoimmune disorders (Roitt, 1994). A list of selected autoimmune disorders is included in Table 8–11.

Pathophysiology

The mechanism that causes the immune system to recognize host tissue as a foreign antigen is not clear. The following factors are under study as possible contributors to the development of autoimmune disorders:

- The release of previously "hidden" antigens into the circulation, such as DNA or other components of the cell nucleus, which elicits an immune response
- Chemical, physical, or biologic changes in host tissue that cause self-antigens to stimulate the production of autoantibodies
- The introduction of an antigen, such as a bacteria or virus, whose antigenic properties closely resemble those of host tissue, resulting in the production of antibodies which target not only the foreign antigen but also normal tissue
- A defect in normal cellular immune function that allows B cells to produce autoantibodies unchecked
- Initiation of the autoimmune response by very slow-growing mycobacteria

Although the exact mechanism producing autoimmunity is unclear, several characteristics of autoimmune diseases are known. It is apparent that genetics plays a role,

Table 8–11	Selected Autoimmune Disorders	
More organ Specific	Hashimoto's thyroiditis	A chronic progressive inflammatory disease of the thyroid with lymphocyte infiltration and gradual destruction of the gland. See Chapter 20.
	Primary myxedema	Thyroid deficiency resulting from destruction of the thyroid gland due to an autoimmune process, often Hashimoto's thyroiditis. See Chapter 20.
	Thyrotoxicosis	Hyperthyroidism resulting from thyroid-stimulating immunoglobulins that stimulate activity of the gland. See Chapter 20.
	Pernicious anemia	Anemia resulting from absence of intrinsic factor associated with loss of parietal cells; most clients have antibodies to parietal cells. See Chapter 31.
	Addison's disease	Atrophy and hypofunction of the adrenal cortex, probably autoimmune in origin. See Chapter 20.
	Myasthenia gravis	A disease characterized by episodic muscle weakness caused by antibodies to the acetylcholine receptor of the neuromuscular junction. See Chapter 42.
	Insulin-dependent diabetes mellitus	Impaired insulin secretion, often the result of islet cell destruction by antibodies directed at the cell surface or cytoplasm. See Chapter 21.
	Goodpasture's syndrome	A type II hypersensitivity disorder with pulmonary hemorrhage and progressive glomerulonephritis characterized by circulating antiglomerular basement membrane antibodies. See Chapter 26.
	Multiple sclerosis	A probable autoimmune process resulting in disseminated patches of demyelination in the brain and spinal cord and varied neurologic manifestations. See Chapter 42.
	Idiopathic thrombocytopenic purpura	A chronic disorder characterized by petechiae, purpura, mucosal bleeding, and antibodies against platelets. See Chapter 31.
	Primary biliary cirrhosis	Inflammation and fibrosis of the bile ducts, probably of autoimmune origin. See Chapter 15.
	Active chronic hepatitis	A serious liver disease often resulting in hepatic failure and/or cirrhosis; may be autoimmune with infiltration by T cells and plasma cells. See Chapter 15.
Less organ specific	Ulcerative colitis	A chronic inflammatory disease of colon mucosa, possibly of autoimmune origin. See Chapter 23.
	Sjogren's syndrome	A systemic inflammatory disorder characterized by dryness of the mouth, eye, and other mucous membranes with lymphocyte infiltration of affected tissues. See Chapter 38.
	Rheumatoid arthritis	A chronic syndrome with inflammation of peripheral joints and generalized manifestations, characterized by infiltration of synovium by lymphocytes and plasma cells. See Chapter 38.
	Scleroderma	Diffuse fibrosis, degenerative changes, and vascular abnormalities of skin, joint structures, and internal organs; probably of autoimmune origin. See Chapter 38.
Non–organ specific	Systemic lupus erythematosus	An inflammatory connective tissue disorder characterized the presence of antinuclear antibodies. See Chapter 38.

because a higher incidence is seen in family members of people with autoimmune disorders. Autoimmune disorders are far more prevalent in females than in males. The disorders tend to overlap, so that the client with one autoimmune disorder may develop another or some manifestations of another. The onset of an autoimmune disorder is frequently associated with an abnormal stressor, either physical or psychologic. Autoimmune disorders are frequently progressive relapsing-remissing disorders characterized by periods of exacerbation and remission.

Specific autoimmune disorders are discussed in the sections of this text related to the affected organ systems or functional disruption (see Table 8–11).

Collaborative Care

For the most part, the diagnosis of an autoimmune disorder is based on the clinical manifestations demonstrated by the client. Serum assays are useful to identify autoantibodies. Other laboratory and diagnostic tests are generally specific to the suspected disorder and to identifying the degree of tissue damage and destruction. Although the manifestations of these disorders can often be managed, a cure typically is not possible unless the affected target tissue is removed (e.g., colectomy for the client with ulcerative colitis).

Laboratory and Diagnostic Tests

Serologic assays are used to identify and measure antibodies directed toward host tissue antigens or normal cellular components. Many autoantibodies that can be detected are not specific to a single autoimmune disorder and are used to establish the autoimmune process rather than the specific disorder. Although healthy persons often have low levels of autoantibodies, levels are much higher in clients affected by an autoimmune disorder. The following serologic assays may be ordered:

- *Antinuclear antibody (ANA)* is used to detect antibodies produced to DNA and other nuclear material. These antibodies can cause tissue damage characteristic of autoimmune disorders, such as SLE. The client's serum is combined with nuclear material and tagged antihuman antibody to detect ANA-antihuman antibody complexes. Although a few complexes may be detected in undiluted serum of normal clients, none should be seen with a dilution greater than 1:20 or 1:32. This is identified as a negative, or normal, result. When complexes are detected at higher levels of dilution, the test is positive for ANA. This test is not specific for SLE, because high levels of ANA may be present in other autoimmune disorders, such as rheumatoid arthritis and chronic active hepatitis nevertheless, 95% of clients with SLE have a positive ANA titer.

- *Lupus erythematosus (LE) cell prep* is also used to detect SLE and monitor its treatment. Neutrophils that contain large masses of phagocytized DNA from the nuclei of PMNs are called LE cells. Like the ANA, the LE cell prep is nonspecific for SLE. A positive result may also be seen in rheumatoid arthritis or with medications such as isoniazid, penicillamine, phenytoin, procainamide, streptomycin, or sulfonamide drugs.

- *Rheumatoid factor (RF)* is an immunoglobulin present in the serum of approximately 80% of clients with rheumatoid arthritis. It may be present in very low amounts in clients without an autoimmune disease and in the elderly, but when RF is detected at a dilution of 1:20 or higher, it indicates rheumatoid arthritis or another autoimmune process, such as SLE.

- *Complement assay* may also be useful in identifying autoimmune disorders. In these disorders, complement may be consumed in the development of antigen-antibody complexes. Decreased levels are seen on examination. Both total complement level and amounts of

individual components of the complement cascade can be determined.

Many other immunoglobulin and antibody assays can also be performed. These are specific to the suspected autoimmune process.

Pharmacology

A variety of approaches is used in the treatment of autoimmune disorders. Anti-inflammatory medications such as aspirin, NSAIDs, and corticosteroids may be prescribed to reduce the inflammatory response and minimize tissue damage. These drugs and nursing responsibilities related to their use are discussed in further detail in the pharmacology box on page 238. When these agents are not effective or well tolerated by the client, slow-acting anti-inflammatory medications may be prescribed. Slow-acting or antirheumatic drugs include such medications as gold salts, hydroxychloroquine (Plaquenil), and penicillamine. Their use is further detailed in Chapter 38. Cytotoxic drugs may be used in combination with plasmapheresis in treating many autoimmune disorders. Cytotoxic drugs are discussed in further detail in the next section of this chapter.

Nursing Care

Nursing care measures for the client with an autoimmune disorder are individualized and tailored to needs dictated by manifestations of the disorder. Nurses often will be involved with the client in an outpatient setting such as an office or home, evaluating the client's response to therapy and self-care management.

Consider the following nursing diagnoses in planning care for the client with an autoimmune disorder:

- *Activity Intolerance* related to inflammatory effects of autoimmune disorder
- *Ineffective Individual Coping* related to chronic disease process
- *Altered Family Processes* related to lack of understanding about autoimmune disorder and its effects
- *Altered Protection* related to disordered immune function
- *Risk for Ineffective Individual Management of Therapeutic Regimen* related to lack of understanding

Client and Family Teaching

Because many autoimmune disorders are chronic, teaching the client and family about the disorder and its management is a key nursing care component. The client may be taking drugs with multiple side effects or long-term effects, necessitating effective teaching. Clients with autoimmune disorders often do not appear to be ill, making

Table 8–12   Organ Transplants

Organ	Graft Type	Indications for Transplant	Success Rate
Kidney	Allograft; may be isograft	End-stage renal disease	80% to 90% at 1 year
Heart	Allograft	End-stage cardiac disease refractory to medical management	74% at 5 years
Lung	Allograft	Pulmonary hypertension, cystic fibrosis, pulmonary fibrosis, chronic obstructive pulmonary disease	70% at 1 year for combined heart-lung; 60% for single lung
Liver	Allograft	Severe liver dysfunction due to chronic active hepatitis, primary biliary cirrhosis, sclerosing cholangitis	70% to 90% 1-year survival
Bone marrow	Autograft or allograft	Leukemia, aplastic anemia, congenital immunologic defects	40% to 75% at 1 year
Skin	Autograft, allograft, or xenograft	Severe burns, plastic surgery	>95% at 5 years
Cornea	Allograft	Corneal ulceration and opacification	>95% at 5 years
Pancreas	Allograft	Pancreatic insufficiency, diabetes	65% at 1 year

Note. Summarized from *Current Medical Diagnosis and Treatment* (33rd ed.) by L. M. Tierney, S. J. McPhee, and M. A. Papadakis, 1994, Norwalk, CT: Appleton & Lange.

it difficult for friends and families to understand their care needs. The chronicity of these disorders also puts the client at high risk for unproven remedies and quackery. Nurses can provide psychologic support, listening, teaching, and referral to local support groups and state or national agencies.

The Client with a Tissue Transplant

■ ■ ■

Since the first kidney transplant performed from one identical twin to the other in 1954, organ and tissue transplantation has become an increasingly popular and viable treatment option. The transplantation of avascular tissues, such as skin, cornea, bone, and heart valves, is considered routine, with little need for tissue matching and immunosuppression. Transplants of organs—for example, the kidney, heart, heart and lung, liver, and bone marrow—are increasingly common and are no longer considered experimental or extraordinary procedures. Common organ transplants are outlined in Table 8–12.

Transplant success is closely tied to obtaining an organ with tissue antigens as close to those of the recipient as possible. As noted earlier in this chapter, every body cell has cell surface antigens known as HLA antigens that are unique to the individual. Although identical twins may have the same HLA type, the chance is reduced to 1 in 4 for siblings, and less than 1 in several thousand for unrelated individuals (Tierney et al., 1994). Matching the HLA

type of the donor and recipient as closely as possible decreases the potential for rejection of the transplanted organ or tissue but does not eliminate it.

Pathophysiology

An **autograft,** a transplant of the client's own tissue, is the most successful type of tissue transplant. Skin grafts are the most common examples of autografts. Increasingly, autologous bone marrow transplants and blood transfusions are being used to reduce immunologic responses. When the donor and recipient are identical twins, the term **isograft** is used. Because of the high likelihood of an HLA match, the success of these grafts is good and rejection episodes are mild. Few people, however, have an identical twin waiting in the wings to provide tissue for donation. And when the need is for an organ such as the heart, liver, or lungs, a living-donor transplantation is not possible. Most often, organ and tissue transplants are **allografts,** which are grafts between members of the same species but who have different genotypes and HLA antigens. Allografts may come from living donors; examples are bone marrow, blood, and a kidney. Most often, however, organs for transplantation are obtained from a cadaver. Donors are typically persons who meet the criteria for brain death; are less than 65 years old; and are free of systemic disease, malignancy, or infection, including HIV, hepatitis B, or hepatitis C. The organ is removed immediately before or after cardiac arrest and preserved until transplanted into the waiting recipient. Finally, **xenograft** is a transplant from an animal species to a human. These transplants are the least successful but may be used in

Table 8–13   Transplant Rejection Episodes

Type	Cause	Presentation	Treatment
Hyperacute	Preexisting antibodies to donor ABO or HLA antigens	Occurs within minutes to hours or days of the transplant Rapid deterioration of organ function	The transplant usually cannot be saved; prevent with crossmatch, and use antimetabolites or anti-inflammatory drugs before surgery.
Acute	Primarily a cell-mediated immune response to HLA antigens; antibody-mediated response may also contribute	Occurs within days to months after the transplant Signs of inflammation and impaired organ function	Increase immunosuppression using steroids, cyclosporine, monoclonal antibodies, or anti-lymphocyte globulins.
Chronic	Probably antibody-mediated response; may also involve inflammatory damage to vessel endothelium	Occurs 4 months to years after the transplant Gradual deterioration of organ function	None; loss of graft will occur, requiring retransplant.

selected instances, such as the use of pig skin as a temporary covering for a massive burn.

Tissue typing is used to determine the *histocompatibility,* which is the ability of cells and tissues to survive transplantation without immunologic interference by the recipient. Tissue typing is performed in an attempt to match the donor and recipient as closely as possible for HLA type, blood type (ABO, Rh) and to identify preformed antibodies to the donor's HLA antigens.

Both antibody-mediated and cell-mediated immune responses are involved in the complex process of transplant rejection. Host macrophages process donor antigen, presenting it to T and B lymphocytes. Activated lymphocytes lead to both antibody- and cell-mediated effects. Killer T cells bind with cells of the transplanted organ, resulting in cell lysis. Helper T cells stimulate the multiplication and differentiation of B cells, and antibodies are produced to graft endothelium. Complement activation or antibody-dependent cell-mediated cytotoxicity leads to transplant cell destruction (Shaefer & Williams, 1991). Rejection typically begins after the first 24 hours of the transplant, although it may present immediately. Rejection episodes are characterized as hyperacute, acute, or chronic, as summarized in Table 8–13.

Hyperacute tissue rejection occurs immediately to 2 to 3 days after the transplant of new tissue. Hyperacute rejection is due to preformed antibodies and sensitized T cells to antigens in the donor organ. Hyperacute rejection is most likely to occur in clients who have had a previous organ or tissue transplant, such as a blood transfusion. Hyperacute rejection may be evident even before the transplant procedure is completed. The grafted organ initially appears pink and healthy, but soon becomes soft and cyanotic as blood flow is impaired. Organ function deteriorates rapidly, and the client begins to experience symptoms of organ failure.

Acute tissue rejection is the most common and treatable type of rejection episode. It occurs between 4 days and 3 months after the transplant. Acute rejection is mediated primarily by the cellular immune response, resulting in transplant cell destruction. The client experiencing acute rejection demonstrates manifestations of the inflammatory process, with fever, redness, swelling, and tenderness over the graft site. Signs of impaired function of the transplanted organ may be noted (e.g., elevated blood urea nitrogen [BUN] and creatinine, liver enzyme and bilirubin elevations, or elevated cardiac enzymes and signs of cardiac failure).

Chronic tissue rejection occurs from 4 months to years after transplant of new tissue. Chronic rejection is most likely the result of antibody-mediated immune responses. Antibodies and complement are deposited in transplant vessel walls, causing narrowing and decreased function of the organ due to ischemia. The gradual deterioration of transplanted organ function is seen with chronic tissue rejection.

Graft-versus-host disease (GvHD) is a frequent and potentially fatal complication of bone marrow transplant. When there is no close match between donor and recipient HLA antigen, immunocompetent cells in the grafted tissue recognize host tissue as foreign and mount a cell-mediated immune response. If the host is immunocompromised, as is often the case when a bone marrow transplant is performed, host cells are unable to destroy the graft and instead become the targets of destruction. Of clients with very closely matched bone marrow, 30% to 60% nevertheless develop GvHD. Acute GvHD occurs within the first 100 days following a transplant and primarily affects the skin, liver, and gastrointestinal tract. The client develops a maculopapular pruritic rash beginning on the palms of the hands and soles of the feet. The rash may spread to involve the entire body and lead to desquamation. Gastrointestinal manifestations include abdominal pain, nausea, and bloody diarrhea. GvHD of longer than 100 days duration is said to be chronic. If it is limited to the skin and liver, the prognosis is good. If multiple organs are involved, the prognosis is poor (Porth, 1994; Roitt, 1994).

Collaborative Care

Pretransplant care and posttransplant care are directed toward reducing the risk that transplanted tissue will be rejected or result in GvHD. Laboratory and diagnostic studies are directed first at identifying a suitable donor, then at monitoring the immune response to the transplant. Immunosuppressive therapy with medications is a vital part of posttransplant care. Indeed, it is the development of effective immunosuppressive drugs that is responsible for the success of organ transplants using allografts.

Laboratory and Diagnostic Tests

The following laboratory studies may be ordered prior to organ or tissue transplantation:

- *Blood type and Rh factor* of both the donor and recipient are determined. Although there is some question about the benefit of histocompatibility testing prior to transplant of a cadaver organ, there is no question about the need for ABO blood group compatibility.

- *Crossmatching* of the client's serum against the donor's lymphocytes is performed to identify any preformed antibodies against antigens on donor tissues. If present, these antibodies would likely result in an immediate or hyperacute graft rejection with probable loss of the transplant.

- *HLA histocompatibility testing* (see the earlier section of this chapter on recognition of self, pages 223 through 224) is used to identify donors with an HLA type close to that of the recipient. Not particularly practical and of questionable value for cadaver transplants, HLA histocompatibility testing is used primarily to identify living donors for bone marrow and kidney transplant. Because of GvHD, histocompatibility tests to identify an identical or very close HLA match are particularly important in bone marrow transplant. HLA tests are performed using lymphocytes from a blood sample. The sample should not be obtained within 72 hours of a blood transfusion, because this will interfere with results.

- *Mixed lymphocyte culture (MLC) assay tests* also are used to determine histocompatibility between the donor and the recipient. This test is used to identify whether mononuclear cells of the recipient will react against the potential donor's leukocyte antigens. The disadvantage of this test is that results cannot be obtained until 7 to 10 days later (Chernecky et al., 1993). Factors that could interfere with the results of this test include use of oral contraceptives, a radioisotope scan within 1 week prior to the test, and chemotherapy.

Various diagnostic tests may be ordered to detect signs of transplant rejection. Ultrasonography or magnetic resonance imaging (MRI) of the transplanted organ may be performed to evaluate its size, perfusion, and function. Tissue biopsies of the transplanted organ are performed routinely to assess for evidence of tissue rejection.

Pharmacology

Prior to transplantation, several antibiotic and antiviral drugs may be prescribed, including the following:

- Trimethoprim-sulfamethoxazole (Septra, Bactrim), which decreases the incidence of gram-negative bacterial infections

- Acyclovir (Zovirax), which prevents the development of herpes simplex virus (HSV) pneumonia in bone marrow transplant recipients

- Ganciclovir (Cytovene), which prevents the development of cytomegalovirus (CMV) pneumonia with bone marrow transplant recipients

The mainstays of drug therapy for clients following a tissue or organ transplant are immunosuppressive agents. Varying regimens of these drugs are used, depending on the transplanted tissue and the medical center; however, a combination of corticosteroids and cyclosporine is common for maintenance therapy. Antilymphocyte therapy and the use of monoclonal antibodies are increasingly common in the immediate posttransplant period and for treating steroid-resistant rejection episodes.

Corticosteroids, primarily prednisone (Deltasone, others) and methylprednisolone (Solu-Medrol, others) were among the first medications employed to prevent transplant rejection, and they remain important agents today. Although the exact anti-inflammatory and immunosuppressive activity of corticosteroids is unknown, they are known to suppress production of interleukin 1 and 2, decrease monocyte migration, and suppress proliferative and cytotoxic T cell activity (Shaefer & Williams, 1991). Although they are very effective, the large doses of corticosteroids used posttransplant are associated with significant adverse effects. Wound healing is impaired, and the metabolism of fats, proteins, and carbohydrates is altered. Fat distribution changes, producing a cushingoid appearance with moon facies, increased truncal fat, and "buffalo hump." Fluid retention and hypertension are potential problems, as are osteoporosis, gastrointestinal bleeding, and emotional disturbances. Nursing responsibilities related to corticosteroid administration are outlined in the pharmacology box on page 239.

Azathioprine (Imuran) has been in use as an immunosuppressant for more than 25 years and continues to be a component of many regimens. Azathioprine inhibits both cell-mediated and antibody-mediated immunity, although its activity is more specific for T cells than B cells. As a drug that is rapidly metabolized by the liver, azathioprine can be given to clients with impaired renal function but may not be effective in clients with impaired hepatic function. Bone marrow suppression is the most common adverse effect of this drug, necessitating frequent evaluation of the CBC. Hepatotoxicity, pancreatitis, and increased risk of neoplasm are also associated with azathioprine administration. Nursing responsibilities related to azathioprine are included in the pharmacology box on page 283.

Cyclosporine has contributed significantly to the success of organ transplantation since its introduction in the 1970s. Cyclosporine inhibits T-cell function and the normal cell-mediated immune response. The incidence of cyclosporine toxicity and side effects is related to blood levels, so blood levels are monitored closely. Cyclosporine is both nephrotoxic and hepatotoxic, especially at high doses. Observable toxic effects include hypertension and CNS symptoms, such as flushing or tingling of the extremities, confusion, visual disturbances, and seizures or coma (Shaefer & Williams, 1991).

Muromonab-CD3, also known as OKT3 or Orthoclone, is the first monoclonal antibody produced for therapeutic use in humans (Shaefer & Williams, 1991). As a monoclonal antibody, OKT3 is specific to T cells, blocking their generation and function. It binds with a surface antigen on T cells, inactivating and removing them from circulation. It also blocks killer T cells attached to the graft. Because of significant side effects, the use of OKT3 is limited primarily to treatment of steroid-resistant rejection (Way, 1994).

Polyclonal antilymphocyte antibodies are also used as adjunctive immunosuppressant therapy. These are administered as antilymphocyte globulin (ALG) or antithymocyte globulin (ATG). These globulins contain antibodies against both T cells and B cells, as well as other mononuclear leukocytes. When administered, they deplete circulating lymphocytes, platelets, and granulocytes (Shaefer & Williams, 1991). Antilymphocyte globulins are used both to induce immunosuppression following a transplant and to treat steroid-resistant rejection episodes.

Nursing Care

The client who has an organ or tissue transplant has both immediate and long-term nursing care needs. Both the client and the family must be considered in providing nursing care. Because of the continuing risk of transplant rejection and the need for immunosuppression, *Altered Protection* and *Risk for Impaired Tissue Integrity* are priority nursing care foci.

The client's underlying disease process, the transplant, and the continuing need for immunosuppressive drug therapy also have emotional and psychologic consequences. Many nursing diagnoses, such as *Powerlessness* or *Ineffective Individual Coping* may be appropriate. The diagnosis *Anxiety* related to potential transplant rejection is considered in this section.

Altered Protection

Altered protection is a problem for the transplant client at all stages. Before the transplant occurs, failure of the affected organ may put the client at risk for infection and other multisystemic problems. Incisions and invasive perioperative procedures impair skin and mucous membrane protection from infectious organisms and other antigens. Immunosuppressive drugs given postoperatively to prevent graft rejection disarm the immune response to a certain extent, increasing the risk of infections and neoplastic growths.

Nursing interventions with rationales follow:

- Wash hands on entering the client's room and before providing direct care. *Hand washing removes transient organisms from the skin, reducing the risk of transmission to the client.*

- Use strict aseptic technique in changing dressings and caring for invasive catheters such as intravenous lines and indwelling urinary catheters. *Aseptic technique offers protection against external and resident host microorganisms.*

- Assess the client frequently for signs and symptoms of infection. Monitor the temperature and vital signs every 4 hours. Assess for evidence of inflammation, abnormal wound drainage, changes in urine or other body secretions, complaints of pain, or behavior changes that may indicate infection. Culture abnormal wound drainage. *The client on immunosuppressive therapy is more susceptible to infection, and usual signs and symptoms may not be evident. Both the temperature and inflammatory response can be suppressed by therapy. Prompt identification and intervention for infection is important in the immunosuppressed client.*

- Monitor laboratory values, including CBC and tests of organ function; report changes to the physician. *An elevation in the WBC count with a shift-to-the-left or a decline in function of the transplanted organ (e.g., a rising BUN and creatinine in the renal transplant client) may be early indications of infection or transplant failure.*

- Initiate reverse or protective isolation procedures as indicated by the client's immune status. *These procedures further protect the severely immunocompromised client from infection.*

- Instruct ill family members and visitors to avoid contact with the client. *A "minor" upper respiratory infection*

text continues on page 285

Nursing Implications for Pharmacology: Immunosuppressive Agents

CYTOTOXIC AGENTS

Azathioprine (Imuran)

Cyclophosphamide (Cytoxan)

Cyclosporine (Sandimmune)

Certain drugs that are identified as cytotoxic or antineoplastic agents are effective as immunosuppressive agents. They act by decreasing the proliferation of cells within the immune system and are widely used to prevent rejection following a tissue or organ transplant. They are usually administered concurrently with corticosteroid therapy, allowing lower doses of both preparations and resulting in fewer side effects.

Nursing Responsibilities

- Monitor the client's blood count, with particular attention to the WBC and platelet counts. Notify the physician if WBCs fall below 4000 or platelets below 75,000.
- Monitor renal and liver function studies, including creatinine, BUN, creatinine clearance, and liver enzymes. Report abnormal levels to the physician.
- Administer the drug as ordered. Administer oral preparations with food to minimize gastrointestinal effects. Antacids may be ordered.
- Increase fluids to maintain good hydration and urinary output.
- Monitor intake and output.
- Monitor for signs of abnormal bleeding: bleeding gums, bruising, petechiae, joint pain, hematuria, and black or tarry stools.
- Use meticulous hand washing and other appropriate measures to protect the client from infection. Assess for signs of infection.
- Pulmonary fibrosis is a potential adverse effect of cyclophosphamines. Therefore, monitor respiratory function using pulmonary function studies and clinical signs of dyspnea or cough.

Client and Family Teaching

- Avoid large crowds and situations where exposure to infection is probable.
- Report signs of infection, such as chills, fever, sore throat, fatigue, or malaise, to the physician.
- Use contraceptive measures to prevent pregnancy while on immunosuppressive therapy; these drugs are teratogenic.
- Avoid the use of aspirin or ibuprofen while taking these drugs. Report any signs of bleeding to the physician.

- With cyclophosphamide, amenorrhea may occur during therapy. The menses will resume after the drug is discontinued.
- If taking cyclophosphamide, report difficulty breathing or cough to the physician.

MONOCLONAL ANTIBODY

Muromonab-CD3 or OKT3 (Orthoclone)

This monoclonal antibody against T cells is formed by immunizing a mouse with an antigen to produce a specific antibody. Lymphocytes producing the antibody, OKT3, are cloned, and the antibody is harvested. When injected into humans, OKT3 binds with a surface antigen on T cells, removing them from circulation and inactivating those bound to allograft cells. Due to the high incidence of adverse effects, the first two doses of OKT3 are administered by a physician and the client closely observed for 2 hours following each dose.

Nursing Responsibilities

- Be sure a chest X-ray study has been performed within 24 hours preceding initiation of OKT3 therapy and that no congestion is present. The risk of anaphylaxis is greater in the client with fluid overload.
- Premedicate the client as ordered with hydrocortisone, acetaminophen, and diphenhydramine to reduce potential adverse effects.
- Position a crash cart or code cart with emergency medications in the client's room or in close proximity to it.
- After each of the first two doses, monitor vital signs every 15 minutes for 2 hours, then every 30 minutes for 2 hours.
- After the first two doses, administer a 2.5- to 10-mg dose by intravenous push over 1 to 2 minutes.
- Observe the client closely for potential adverse effects, including chills and fever; tachycardia; headache and tremor; hypertension or hypotension; nausea, vomiting, and diarrhea; chest pain, dyspnea, and wheezing.
- OKT3 can also cause anaphylaxis; observe for evidence of urticaria, angioedema, laryngeal edema, wheezing, or other signs of anaphylactic reaction.
- Monitor CBC for evidence of leukopenia or pancytopenia.
- Assess for infection. Remember that typical signs of infection such as fever and inflammation may be

Pharmacology: Immunosuppressive Agents (*continued*)

masked or reduced by immunosuppressive therapy (Shaefer & Williams, 1991).

Client and Family Teaching

- Teach about the drug and its purpose.
- Discuss potential adverse and side effects, and emphasize the need to report symptoms promptly.
- Inform the client that adverse effects are most likely to occur following the first two doses, necessitating close observation at that time. Reassure the client that this is standard protocol for this medication.

ANTILYMPHOCYTE GLOBULINS

- Antithymocyte globulin or ATG (ATGAM)
- Antilymphocyte globulin or ALG

These globulins containing antilymphocyte antibodies are produced by immunizing horses (the main source), rabbits, or sheep with human lymphocytes to stimulate production of antibodies (see figure at right). Serum from the animal is then recovered, and the active IgG fraction is isolated, purified, and administered parenterally to the client. It binds with peripheral lymphocytes and mononuclear cells, removing them from circulation (Shaefer & Williams, 1991; Way, 1994).

ATG or ALG is used both to induce immunosuppression immediately following a transplant and to treat steroid-resistant rejection episodes. As with monoclonal antibody, multiple side effects are associated with ATG or ALG.

Nursing Responsibilities

- Perform a skin test for sensitivity to horse serum prior to initial dose. Report any positive reaction to the physician, and hold administration until desensitization therapy has been completed.
- Premedicate the client as ordered with acetaminophen and diphenhydramine prior to each dose. Steroids may also be administered before the initial dose. Have epinephrine and hydrocortisone injections available at the client's bedside in case of anaphylactic reaction.
- Administer by intravenous infusion into a central line over 4 to 6 hours.
- Monitor vital signs hourly while medication is infusing.
- Assess for adverse effects, including chills and fever, erythema, and pruritus. Notify the physician; these may be treated symptomatically.
- Monitor the client's CBC daily; notify the physician

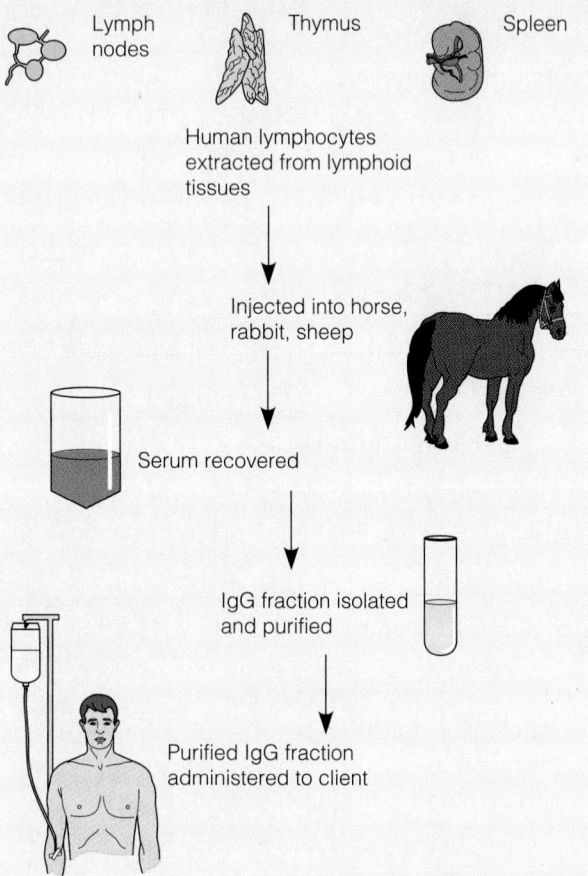

A horse is inoculated with washed human lymphocytes, stimulating the production of immunoglobulin with polyclonal antilymphocyte antibodies. These are then extracted from horse serum, purified, and administered intravenously to the client.

if WBC falls to less than 3000/mm³ or platelet count to less than 100,000/mm³. The medication may be stopped or reduced (Shaefer & Williams, 1991).

- Assess renal function studies to monitor for serum sickness. Report complaints of joint pain.
- Monitor the client for signs of infection, and report any signs promptly.

Client and Family Teaching

- Explain the need for special precautions and close monitoring while this drug is being administered.
- Instruct the client to report any adverse effects, including malaise or joint pain, promptly.
- Ask the client to report any evidence of easy bruising, bleeding gums, or black stools.
- Teach family members about the importance of not exposing the client to persons with infectious diseases.

can present a significant illness to the immunocompromised host.

■ Help ensure an adequate nutrient intake, offering supplementary feedings as indicated or maintaining parenteral nutrition if necessary. *Adequate nutrition is important for healing and immune system function.*

■ Change intravenous bags and tubing at least every 24 hours, and change peripheral intravenous sites every 48 to 72 hours, unless contraindicated. Remove invasive catheters and lines as soon as they are no longer necessary. *Changing lines and sites is important to reduce bacterial contamination. Fewer invasive lines provide fewer sites for bacterial invasion of the body.*

■ Emphasize the importance of washing hands thoroughly after using the bathroom and before eating. *This reduces the risk of infection with endogenous organisms.*

■ Provide good mouth care. *Good mouth care reduces the population of oral microorganisms and helps maintain an intact mucous membrane lining.*

■ Monitor for potential adverse effects of medications, including
   a. Thrombocytopenia and possible bleeding.
   b. Fluid retention with edema and possible hypertension.
   c. Loss of bone density, osteoporosis, and possible pathologic fractures.
   d. Renal or hepatic toxicity.
   e. Cardiac effects, particularly in the client with fluid retention and hypervolemia.

Medications used to maintain immunosuppression and preserve the allograft have many potential adverse effects that can alter normal protective and homeostatic mechanisms.

Risk for Impaired Tissue Integrity: Allograft

As noted earlier, the risk for transplant rejection is highest in the initial postoperative period, but it is never completely eliminated for the client who has had an allograft. The client who has had a bone marrow transplant has the additional risk of developing graft-versus-host disease. GvHD can affect the integrity of skin, mucous membranes, and other organs.

Nursing interventions with rationales follow:

■ Administer immunosuppressive therapy as prescribed. *Suppression of the immune response is necessary to reduce the risk of graft destruction by normal immune responses and to preserve its function.*

■ Assess the client for evidence of graft rejection, including tenderness, erythema, and swelling over the site; sudden weight gain, edema, and hypertension; chills and fever; malaise; and an increased WBC count and sedimentation rate. Report any changes immediately. *Early identification of rejection allows adjustment of medication regimens and, possibly, preservation of the graft.*

■ Monitor results of laboratory studies for function of the transplanted organ. *With a functional graft, results (e.g., renal or liver function studies) will improve; a functional decline may be an early indicator of rejection.*

■ Assess for and report signs of GvHD immediately, including maculopapular rash, erythema of the skin and possible desquamation, hair loss, abdominal cramping and diarrhea, jaundice with elevated bilirubin and liver enzymes (AST, ALT). *GvHD is a potentially lethal complication in the immunosuppressed client and necessitates immediate intervention.*

■ Stress the importance of maintaining immunosuppressive therapy and reporting signs of graft rejection promptly to the client.

Anxiety

The client who undergoes an organ or tissue transplantation often faces the unwelcome choices of death from organ failure or receiving an organ that his or her body will likely attempt to reject. In most cases, the client understands that in order to receive this transplant, someone else must die *and* be willing to give up an organ. When the transplant comes from a living donor (bone marrow or kidney), the client may worry not only about himself or herself, but also about the condition of the donor. Fear of rejection and guilt may be even greater in this instance.

Nursing interventions with rationales follow:

■ Assess the client's level of anxiety by noting such cues as expressions of apprehension, fear, or inadequacy; facial expression, tension, or shakiness; difficulty focusing; helplessness; poor eye contact; and restlessness. *Clients may have difficulty identifying or verbalizing feelings of fear and anxiety. Nonverbal cues are often useful in recognizing states of anxiety.*

■ Provide opportunities for the client to express feelings. Use opening statements such as, "Facing an organ transplant must be very stressful." Listen attentively. *Encouragement and active listening allows the client to express feelings of anxiety or fear.*

■ Arrange tasks to allow as much time with the client as possible. When leaving, tell the client when you will return. *Time spent with the client facilitates the development of trust.*

■ Provide clear, concise directions. *Highly anxious clients have difficulty focusing and retaining information.*

■ Do not ask the client to make unnecessary decisions, but involve the client in care. *The client needs to feel a sense of control but may become irritated if asked to make decisions unrelated to the situation.*

■ Encourage family members to remain with the client as much as possible. *This can help reduce the client's anxiety.*

■ Encourage the use of coping behaviors that have been effective for the client in the past. *Coping mechanisms and behaviors help lower anxiety to a more acceptable level.*

- Reduce or eliminate environmental stressors to the extent possible. *This gives the client a better sense of control.*

- Assist the client with stress-reduction and relaxation techniques, such as guided imagery, meditation, and muscle relaxation. *These techniques help the client gain control over physical responses to anxiety.*

- Arrange for a counselor or mental health specialist to work with the client. *Counseling can help the client identify and deal with his or her feelings.*

Other Nursing Diagnoses

Other nursing diagnoses that may be appropriate for the client with an organ or tissue transplant include:

- *Knowledge Deficit* related to the side effects of immunosuppressive medications

- *Ineffective Individual Coping* related to continuing threat of transplant rejection

- *Risk for Fluid Volume Excess* related to medication side effects

- *Body Image Disturbance* related to the presence of a transplanted organ

- *Ineffective Individual Management of Therapeutic Regimen* due to multiple medications required to prevent graft rejection

Client and Family Teaching

Teaching of the client and family regarding an organ or tissue transplant begins well before the transplant and continues throughout hospitalization and follow-up treatment.

Initial teaching focuses on the options, risks, and potential benefits of the transplant itself. Include the procedure by which the organ is selected and obtained, as well as the procedure by which it is transplanted into the client. If a living related donor is an option, discuss the risks and benefits for both the client and the donor. Outline the posttransplant treatment regimen, including any life-style changes that may be necessary for the client.

Following the transplant, provide verbal and written instructions, including the following:

- The signs and symptoms of transplant rejection and the importance of notifying the physician should these occur.

- The importance of following the prescribed medication regimen and maintaining a medication record.

- Side effects of immunosuppressive drug therapy. Include management techniques for minor side effects, and indicate which of these should be reported to the physician.

- The importance of avoiding exposure to infectious diseases, particularly respiratory infections, such as a URI, influenza, or pneumonia. Wearing a mask when going outside is helpful. Good hand-washing technique is particularly important in avoiding infections.

- Wearing a medical alert bracelet or tag identifying the client as a transplant patient and on immunosuppressive drug therapy.

- The importance of follow-up visits to the physician or clinic.

Impaired Immune Responses

Disorders of impaired immune system responses may be either congenital or acquired. Often it is the function of either T cells or B cells that is impaired, reducing the body's ability to defend against foreign antigens or abnormal host tissue.

No matter what the cause, clients with immunodeficiency disorders demonstrate an unusual susceptibility to infection. When the antibody-mediated response is primarily affected, the client is at particular risk for severe and chronic bacterial infections. These clients also do not develop long-lasting immunity to such diseases as chickenpox and are prone to recurrent cases. Clients with a defect of cell-mediated immunity tend to develop disseminated viral infections, such as herpes simplex and cytomegalovirus (CMV). Candidiasis and other fungal infections are also common. Because T cells are involved with activating antibody-mediated immune responses as well, overwhelming bacterial infections may occur. Immunodeficiency in its most severe form occurs when both antibody-mediated and cell-mediated responses are impaired. Clients with combined immunodeficiency are susceptible to all varieties of infectious organisms, including those not normally considered to be pathogens (Isselbacher et al., 1994).

Most immunodeficiency diseases are genetically determined and rare. They affect children more than adults. The noted exception to this is acquired immune deficiency syndrome, or AIDS, an infectious disease caused by a virus.

The Client with HIV Infection

In 1981, five cases of *Pneumocystis carinii* pneumonia (PCP) and 26 cases of a rare cancer, Kaposi's sarcoma, were diagnosed in young, previously healthy homosexual males in Los Angeles and New York City. The term **acquired immune deficiency syndrome (AIDS)** was ascribed to this new phenomenon to describe the immune system deficits associated with these opportunistic disorders. Prior to this time, both PCP and Kaposi's had been seen only in elderly, debilitated, or severely immunodeficient people. Other groups at risk for AIDS were soon identified: injection drug users, persons with hemophilia, recipients of blood transfusions, and immigrants from Haiti.

Research to identify the cause of this apparently new disease progressed feverishly, and in 1983 a common antibody was identified in clients with AIDS. The **human immunodeficiency virus (HIV)** was isolated in 1984. It then became apparent that AIDS was the final, fatal stage of HIV infection.

> It began, like so many epidemics, with a few isolated cases, a whisper that caught the ear of only a few in medical research. Today, that whisper has become a roar heard around the world. AIDS—acquired immunodeficiency syndrome—is now the epidemic of our generation, invading our lives in ways we never imagined—testing our scientific knowledge, probing our private values, and sapping our strength. AIDS no longer attracts our attention—it commands it. (Novello, 1993)

As of December 1993, there have been 361,164 cases of AIDS reported in the United States. Of those, 220,736 people have died (CDC, 1993). It is currently estimated that 1 million people in the United States are infected with HIV. Worldwide, an estimated 10 million people are infected. Virtually every country in the world reports cases of AIDS, with the highest incidence occurring in the United States, western Europe, central Africa, South America, and Canada. In some urban areas of central and east Africa, as many as one-third of sexually active adults have HIV (Isselbacher et al., 1994; Tierney et al., 1994).

HIV infection was the eighth leading cause of death in the United States in 1993 for persons of all ages. Among males between the ages of 35 and 44 years, it ranked as the leading cause of death. Although approximately 60% of deaths from HIV infection were among white males, the largest increase in age-adjusted death rates between 1991 and 1992 occurred among black females (CDC, 1993). It is estimated that by the year 2000, HIV will become the second leading cause of death for women in the childbearing years.

HIV is a retrovirus transmitted by direct contact with infected blood and body fluids. Significant concentrations of the virus are present in blood, semen, vaginal and cervical secretions, and CSF of infected individuals. It is also found in breast milk and saliva. Sexual contact is the primary mode of transmission. HIV is also transmitted through contact with infected blood via needle sharing during injection drug use or transfusion. Approximately 15% to 30% of infants born to HIV-positive mothers are infected perinatally.

The risk factors for HIV infection are behavioral. Among adults in the United States, 55% of reported cases are in men who have sex with other men, including homosexuals, bisexuals, and such groups as prison populations. Unprotected anal intercourse is the major route of transmission in this group. Injection drug use is the second leading risk factor, accounting for approximately 20% of cases. Sharing of needles and other drug paraphernalia is the primary route of transmission in this group. Heterosexual intercourse with an infected drug user and exchanging sex for drugs are major risk factors for women. Hemophiliacs who require large amounts of intravenous clotting factors and people infected through blood transfusion account for a small number of cases, approximately 2% to 3%.

Among the general population of the United States, the prevalence of HIV infection is very low. Less than 0.04% of people voluntarily donating blood (a process that generally excludes people with high-risk behavior) are found to be HIV positive (Wilson et al., 1991). HIV is *not* transmitted by casual contact, nor is there any evidence of its transmission by vectors such as mosquitoes. Blood *donation* also poses no risk of contracting HIV to the donor, because only new, sterile equipment is used.

A small but real occupational risk exists for health care workers. Percutaneous exposure to infected blood or body fluids through a needle-stick injury or nonintact skin is the primary route of transmission. Documented evidence indicates that parenteral exposure poses a 0.27% to 0.5% risk of becoming HIV positive. Mucosal exposures, such as splashing in the eyes or mouth, pose a much smaller risk.

Pathophysiology

HIV is a *retrovirus,* which carries its genetic information in RNA. On entry into the body, the virus infects cells which have the CD4 antigen. Once inside the cell, the virus sheds its protein coat and uses an enzyme called *reverse transcriptase* to convert the RNA to DNA (Figure 8–19). This viral DNA is then integrated into host cell DNA and duplicated during normal processes of cell division. Within the cell, the virus may remain latent or become activated to produce new RNA and to form virions. The virus then buds from the cell surface, disrupting its cell membrane and leading to destruction of the host cell.

Although the virus may remain inactive in infected cells for years, antibodies are produced to its proteins, a process known as *seroconversion*. These antibodies are usually detectable 6 weeks to 6 months after the initial infection. The antibodies seem to have little effect on the virus.

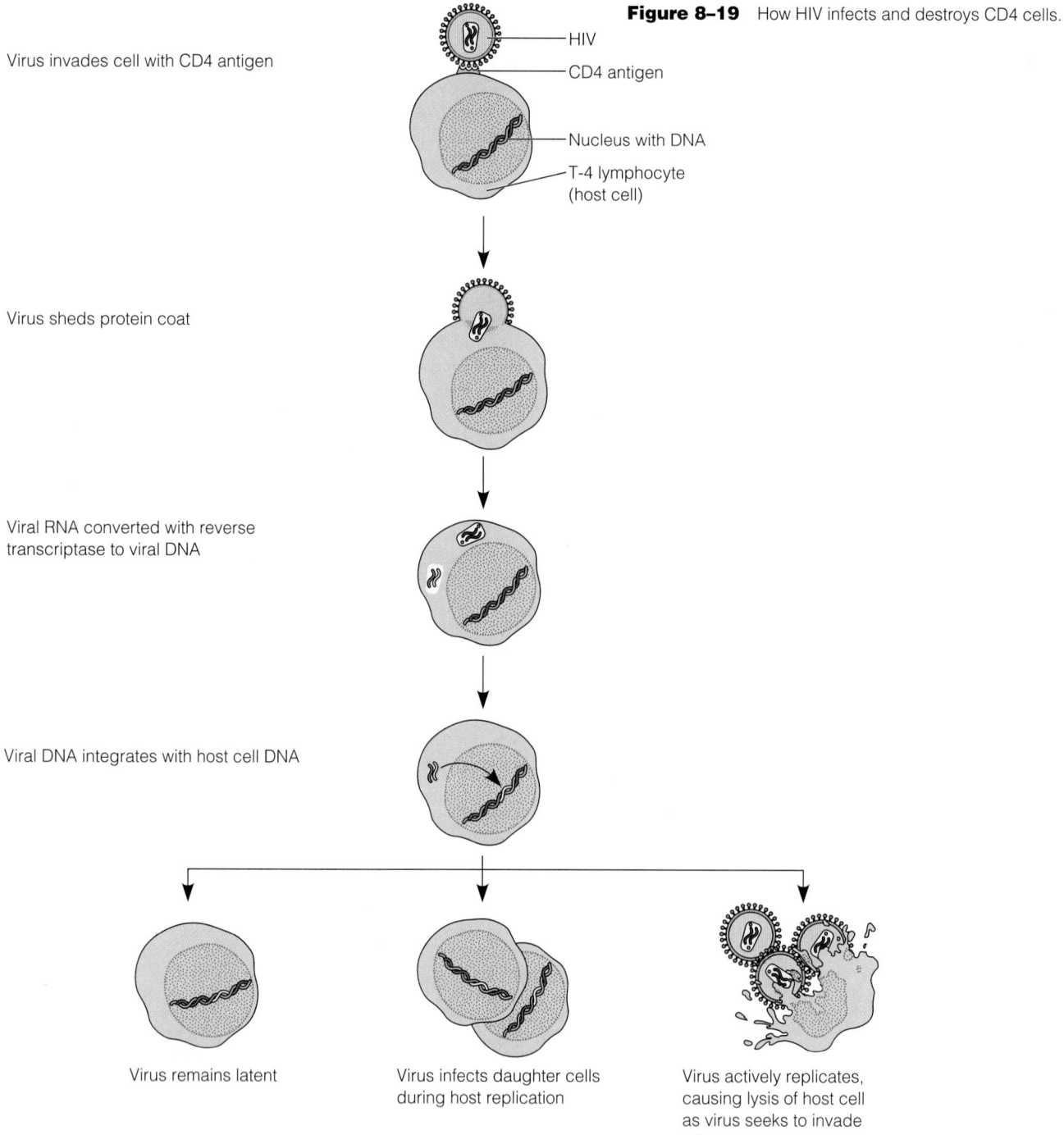

Figure 8–19 How HIV infects and destroys CD4 cells.

Virus invades cell with CD4 antigen

HIV

CD4 antigen

Nucleus with DNA

T-4 lymphocyte (host cell)

Virus sheds protein coat

Viral RNA converted with reverse transcriptase to viral DNA

Viral DNA integrates with host cell DNA

Virus remains latent

Virus infects daughter cells during host replication

Virus actively replicates, causing lysis of host cell as virus seeks to invade other cells

Helper T or CD4 cells are the primary cells infected by HIV. It also infects macrophages and certain cells of the CNS. Helper T cells play a vital role in normal immune system function, recognizing foreign antigens and infected cells, and activating antibody-producing B cells. They also direct cell-mediated immune activity and influence the phagocytic activity of monocytes and macro- phages. The loss of these helper T cells leads to the immunodeficiencies seen with HIV infection (Merck Research Laboratories, 1992; Porth, 1994). Figure 8–20 illustrates the typical course of HIV infection.

Pathologic changes are also noted in the CNS of many infected individuals. Although the mechanism of neurologic dysfunction is unclear, neurologic manifestations of

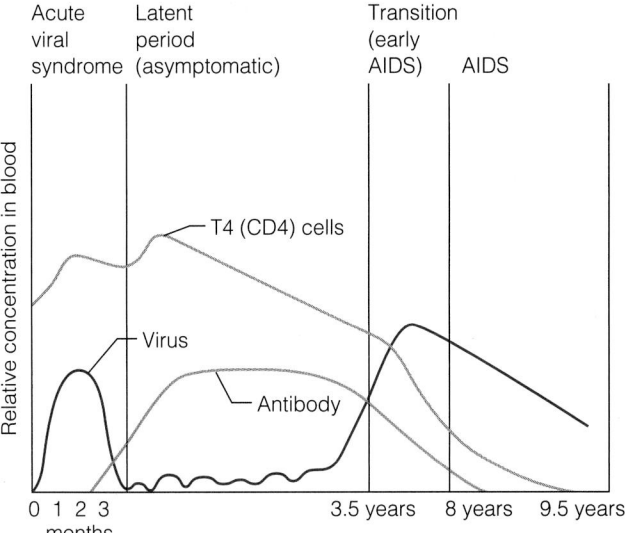

Figure 8–20   The progression of HIV infection. Acute illness develops shortly after the virus is contracted, corresponding with a rapid rise in viral levels. Antibodies are formed and remain present throughout the course of infection. Late in the disease, viral activation results in a marked increase in virus while CD4 (T4) cells diminish as they are destroyed with viral replication. Antibody levels gradually decrease as immune function is impaired.

HIV infection may be seen in clients who have no apparent immune deficiency (Porth, 1994; Tierney et al., 1994).

The clinical manifestations of HIV infection range from no symptoms to severe immunodeficiency with multiple opportunistic infections and cancers (see the clinical manifestations box on page 290). It appears that the majority of clients develop an acute mononucleosis-type illness within days to weeks after contracting the virus. Typical manifestations include fever, sore throat, arthralgias and myalgias, headache, rash, and lymphadenopathy. The client may also experience nausea, vomiting, and abdominal cramping. The client often attributes this initial manifestation of HIV infection to a common viral illness such as influenza, upper respiratory infection, or stomach virus.

Following this acute illness, clients enter a long-lasting asymptomatic period. Although the virus is present and can be transmitted to others, the infected host has few or no symptoms. Clearly, the majority of HIV infected persons are in this stage of the disease. The length of the asymptomatic period varies widely from individual to individual, but its mean length is estimated to be 8 to 10 years (Wilson et al., 1991).

Some clients with few other symptoms develop persistent generalized lymphadenopathy. This is defined as enlargement of two or more lymph nodes outside the inguinal chain with no other illness or condition to account for the lymphadenopathy.

The move from asymptomatic disease or persistent lymphadenopathy to AIDS is often not clearly defined. The client may complain of general malaise, fever, fatigue, night sweats, and involuntary weight loss. Persistent skin dryness and rash may be a problem. Diarrhea is common, as are oral lesions such as hairy leukoplakia, candidiasis, and gingival inflammation and ulceration.

With the development of significant constitutional disease, neurologic manifestations, or opportunistic infections or cancers, the client has manifestations that are characteristic of AIDS and a very poor prognosis (see the box on page 291). The average life span of the client upon diagnosis of AIDS is 20 months with an average cost of care during this period of approximately $85,000 in 1990 dollars (EMA Essay, 1991). Some estimates indicate that 99% of clients with HIV infection will develop AIDS. Of clients with AIDS, 95% die of opportunistic infections.

AIDS Dementia Complex and Neurologic Effects

Neurologic manifestations of HIV are common, affecting 40% to 60% of clients with AIDS. They result from both the direct effects of the virus on the nervous system and opportunistic infections.

AIDS dementia complex is the most common cause of mental status changes for clients with HIV infection. This dementia results from a direct effect of the virus on the brain and affects cognitive, motor, and behavioral functioning. Fluctuating memory loss, confusion, difficulty concentrating, lethargy, and diminished motor speed are typical manifestations of AIDS dementia complex. Clients become apathetic, losing interest in work and social and recreational activities. As the complex progresses, the client develops severe dementia with motor disturbances such as ataxia, tremor, spasticity, incontinence, and paraplegia (Porth, 1994; Price et al., 1988; Wilson et al., 1991).

Infections and lesions common with AIDS may also affect the CNS. Toxoplasmosis and non-Hodgkin's lymphoma are space-occupying lesions that may cause headache, altered mental status, and neurologic deficits. Cryptococcal meningitis and CMV infection also are common in people with AIDS.

Peripheral nervous system manifestations are also common in HIV-infected clients. Sensory neuropathies with manifestations of numbness, tingling, and pain in the lower extremities affect about 30% of clients with AIDS. A Guillain-Barré-type inflammatory demyelinating polyneuropathy can also occur, resulting in progressive weakness and paralysis.

Opportunistic Infections

Opportunistic infections are the most common manifestations of AIDS, often occurring simultaneously. The risk of opportunistic infections is predictable by the client's T4 or CD4 cell count. The normal CD4 cell count is greater

---

CDC Classification and Clinical Manifestations of HIV Infection

I. Acute Infection
- Fever
- Sore throat
- Arthralgias and myalgias
- Headache
- Rash
- Lymphadenopathy
- Nausea, vomiting, and abdominal cramping

II. Asymptomatic Infection
- None; converts to seropositive status

III. Persistent Generalized Lymphadenopathy
- Enlargement of two or more extrainguinal lymph nodes lasting 3 or more months

IV. Other Disease and AIDS

A. Constitutional Disease
- General malaise, fever, fatigue, and night sweats
- Involuntary weight loss
- Skin dryness and rashes
- Diarrhea
- Hairy leukoplakia, oral candidiasis, and gingival inflammation and ulceration

B. AIDS Dementia Complex
- Fluctuating memory loss, confusion, difficulty concentrating, apathy, and diminished motor speed
- Full dementia with impaired cognition, verbalization, and motor skills; headache, altered mental status, and focal neurologic deficits

C. Secondary Infectious Diseases
- *Pneumocystis carinii* pneumonia
- Cytomegalovirus (CMV)
- Candidiasis
- *Mycobacterium avium* complex (MAC)
- Tuberculosis
- Cryptococcus
- Toxoplasmosis
- Herpes simplex or herpes zoster

D. Secondary Cancers
- Kaposi's sarcoma
- Non-Hodgkin's lymphoma
- Cervical dysplasia and cervical cancer

E. Other Conditions
- Pelvic inflammatory disease
- Human papillomavirus

---

than 1000/mm³. When the CD4 count falls to less than 500/mm³, manifestations of immunodeficiency are seen. With a count of less than 200, opportunistic infections and cancers are likely.

***Pneumocystis carinii* Pneumonia** *Pneumocystis carinii* pneumonia (PCP) is the most common opportunistic infection affecting clients with AIDS. Approximately 75% to 80% of clients develop PCP at some point in their disease (Tierney et al., 1994; Wilson et al., 1991). It tends to be recurrent, and it is the cause of death in about 20% of clients with AIDS. PCP is caused by a common environmental fungus that is not pathogenic in clients with intact immune systems.

Unlike many pneumonias, the manifestations of PCP are nonspecific and may progress insidiously. Clients often present with fever, cough, shortness of breath, tachypnea, and tachycardia. Complaints of mild chest pain and sputum may also be present. Breath sounds may initially be normal. With severe disease, the client may present with cyanosis and significant respiratory distress.

Tuberculosis An estimated 4% of clients with AIDS develop tuberculosis, contributing significantly to the rise in incidence of this disease in the United States. In some clients, active tuberculosis results from reactivation of a prior infection. In other clients, it is a new, primary disease facilitated by impaired immune function. Rapid progression, diffuse pulmonary infiltrates, and disseminated disease occur more commonly in clients with AIDS. Multidrug-resistant strains of tuberculosis present a significant problem (Porth, 1994; Tierney et al., 1994).

Clients with pulmonary tuberculosis present with a cough productive of purulent sputum, fever, fatigue, weight loss, and lymphadenopathy. Disseminated disease affects the bone marrow, bone, joints, liver, spleen, CSF, skin, kidneys, gastrointestinal tract, lymph nodes, brain, and other sites.

Candidiasis *Candida albicans* infection is a very common opportunistic infection in clients with AIDS. It is usually manifested as oral thrush or esophagitis. In women, vaginal candidiasis is frequent and often recur-

CDC Case Definition of AIDS for Adults

■   ■   ■

1. Presence of any of the following disorders, with or without laboratory evidence of HIV infection:

   - *Pneumocystis carinii* pneumonia
   - Candidiasis of esophagus, trachea, bronchi, or lungs
   - Extrapulmonary cryptococcosis
   - Cryptosporidiosis with persistant diarrhea
   - Cytomegalovirus infection (other than of liver, spleen, or lymph nodes)
   - Herpes simplex virus infection with persistent skin lesion, bronchitis, pneumonitis, or esophagitis
   - *Mycobacterium avium* complex or disseminated *Mycobacterium kansasii* disease
   - Progressive multifocal leukoencephalopathy
   - Toxoplasmosis of the brain
   - Kaposi's sarcoma in client under 60 years old
   - Primary lymphoma of the brain in client under 60 years old

2. Presence of any of the following, with laboratory evidence of HIV infection:

   - HIV wasting syndrome
   - CD4 lymphocyte count of below 200 c/μL or below 14%
   - HIV encephalopathy
   - Pulmonary or extrapulmonary tuberculosis
   - Recurrent pneumonia
   - Disseminated coccidioidomycosis, disseminated histoplasmosis, or disseminated mycobacterial disease (other than *Mycobacterium tuberculosis*)
   - Recurrent *Salmonella* septicemia
   - Isosporiasis with persistent diarrhea
   - Kaposi's sarcoma or primary lymphoma of the brain, any age
   - Other non-Hodgkin's lymphoma
   - Invasive cervical cancer

rent. Oral thrush presents as white, friable plaques on the buccal mucosa or tongue and, in the HIV-infected client, is often the first indication of progression to AIDS. Clients with esophagitis have difficulty swallowing and substernal pain or burning which increases with swallowing.

***Mycobacterium avium* Complex**   *Mycobacterium avium* complex (MAC) affects up to 25% of clients with AIDS, typically occurring late in the course of the disease when CD4 cell counts are less than 50/μL to 100/μL. MAC is more common in women than men. MAC is caused by organisms commonly found in food, water, and soil. It is a major cause of "wasting syndrome" in persons with AIDS (Figure 8–21). Manifestations of MAC include chills and fever, weakness, night sweats, abdominal pain and diarrhea, and weight loss. Nearly every organ can be infected, and most people with MAC develop disseminated disease.

Other Infections   Herpes virus infections are common in clients with AIDS and may be severe. CMV can affect the retina, the gastrointestinal tract, or lungs. Disseminated herpes simplex or herpes zoster may occur, although severe mucocutaneous manifestations are more common.

Parasitic infections with *Toxoplasma gondii* and *Cryptococcus neoformans* commonly affect the CNS. Toxoplasmosis occurs as encephalitis or an intracerebral mass lesion. Changes in mental status, focal neurologic signs, and seizures may result. *Cryptococcus* infection may present as either meningitis or disseminated disease, primarily affecting the lungs. *Cryptosporidium,* a protozoon affecting the gastrointestinal tract, is an important cause of prolonged diarrhea in AIDS clients. Bacterial salmonella infections are also a relatively common cause of diarrhea (Wilson et al., 1991).

Women with AIDS have a high incidence of pelvic inflammatory disease (PID). Although the pathogens appear to be the same as those in PID affecting non-HIV-infected women, the disease is more severe. Inpatient treatment with intravenous antibiotics is often necessary.

Secondary Cancers

As cell-mediated immune function declines, the risk of malignancy increases. The CDC classification of AIDS currently includes four cancers: Kaposi's sarcoma, non-Hodgkin's lymphoma, primary lymphoma of the brain, and invasive cervical carcinoma.

Kaposi's Sarcoma   Kaposi's sarcoma (KS) is often the presenting symptom of AIDS. It remains the most common cancer associated with the disease. KS affects homosexual males with AIDS predominantly, occurring much less commonly in injection drug users and heterosexuals. At this time, the reason for the discrepancy is unknown.

A tumor of the endothelial cells lining small blood vessels, KS presents as vascular macules, papules, or violet lesions affecting the skin and viscera (Figure 8–22). The face is a common site for skin lesions, especially the tip of the nose and pinnae of the ears. Common sites for visceral disease include the gastrointestinal tract, lungs, and lymphatic system.

The lesions of KS are usually painless initially but may become painful as the disease progresses. Internally, the tumors may obstruct organ function or cause bleeding.

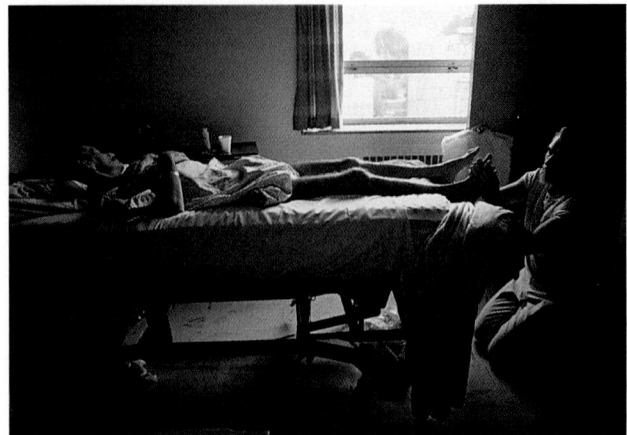

Figure 8–21   Wasting syndrome in a client with AIDS.

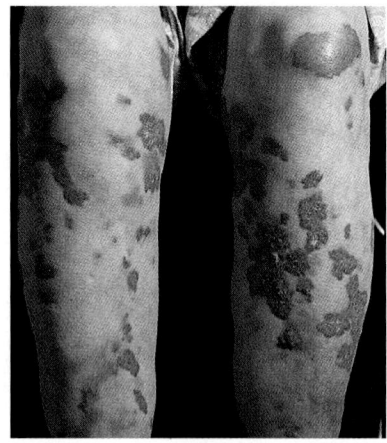

Figure 8–22   Kaposi's sarcoma lesions.

When the lungs are involved, gas exchange may be severely impaired, resulting in pulmonary hemorrhage. This disease may progress slowly or rapidly. KS is an indicator of late-stage HIV disease, with an average survival time of 18 months after diagnosis.

Lymphomas   *Lymphomas* are malignancies of the lymphoid tissue, including lymphocytes, lymph nodes, and the lymphoid organs such as the spleen and bone marrow. In AIDS, two lymphomas are common, non-Hodgkin's lymphoma and primary lymphoma of the brain. Hodgkin's disease also occurs five times more frequently in clients with HIV infection. The central nervous system is the usual site for these lymphomas, although they may be found in the bone marrow, gastrointestinal tract, liver, skin, and mucous membranes. They are aggressive tumors, growing and spreading rapidly. Headache and changes in mental status are common early symptoms of lymphomas affecting the CNS.

Cervical Cancer   Of women with HIV infection, 40% have cervical dysplasia. Cervical cancer develops frequently and tends to be aggressive. Women with concurrent HIV infection and cervical cancer usually die of the cervical cancer, not AIDS. Because of this, it is recommended that women with HIV infection have Papanicolaou (Pap) smears every 6 months and aggressive treatment of cervical dysplasia with colposcopic examination and cone biopsy.

Collaborative Care

Although multiple research studies to identify a cure for HIV infection and AIDS are under way, no cure is currently available. This fact, plus the apparent universally fatal nature of the disease, make prevention a vital strategy in HIV care.

The goals of care for the client with HIV disease are as follows:

- Early identification of the infection
- Promoting health-maintenance activities to prolong the asymptomatic period as long as possible
- Prevention of opportunistic infections
- Treatment of disease complications, such as cancers
- Providing emotional and psychosocial support

Prevention

To date, no safe immunization to protect against HIV infection has been developed. Education, counseling, and behavior modification are the primary tools for AIDS prevention.

The benefit of education and behavior modification is evident in the homosexual male population. The incidence of new HIV infections in this population has declined dramatically in high-prevalence cities such as San Francisco. Nurses play a vital role in providing education about this epidemic and infection prevention for individuals and communities.

All sexually active individuals need to know how HIV is spread. The following are the only totally safe sex practices:

- No sex
- Long-term mutually monogamous sexual relations between two uninfected people
- Mutual masturbation without direct contact

Clients who do engage in sexual activity need to know and practice safer sex (see the box on page 293). Reducing the number of sexual partners—for example, by entering into and remaining in a long-term mutually monogamous relationship with an uninfected partner—reduces the risk. Clients should not engage in unprotected sex, especially if the HIV status of the partner is unknown. Latex condoms have been shown to reduce the risk of transmitting HIV. Their effectiveness is improved when nonoxynol-9, a spermicide, is used for lubrication. However, nonoxynol-9 may cause genital ulcers that may

Gene Therapy for AIDS

■ ■ ■

HIV is a virus that is able to mutate quickly, eluding conventional therapies for infectious disease. HIV integrates itself into chromosomal DNA, a fact that suggests that molecular biology and gene therapy may prove to be more effective in combating this disease. Several studies are currently planned or in progress using gene therapy strategies (Kolata, 1994).

In one study, the infected WBCs are treated to interfere with the production of rev, a protein that transports copies of the virus's genetic messages from the cell nucleus to the surrounding cytoplasm. Without rev, the genetic messages necessary to make new viruses are unable to escape the cell nucleus and direct the virus production.

In a second study, a specially designed antibody that inactivates the rev protein is inserted into WBCs. The antibody stops infected cells from producing HIV.

A third gene therapy approach under study uses a gene that produces ribozymes, which are strands of DNA that can function as enzymes, attacking other DNA strands at specific sites. A ribozyme that attacks HIV RNA without harming normal cellular DNA is under development.

Although gene therapy holds the potential for the development of a successful treatment for HIV disease, it is likely to be years before such a treatment is proved effective and made readily available.

Guidelines for Safer Sex

■ ■ ■

- Practice mutual monogamy; if you are not in a mutually monogamous relationship, limit the number of sexual partners.
- Do not engage in unprotected sex, especially if HIV status of partner is unknown (remember that a person may be infected and infective for up to 6 months before converting to seropositive status).
- When entering into a new monogamous relationship, both partners should undergo HIV testing initially. If both are negative, practice abstinence or safer sex for 6 months, followed by retesting. If results still indicate that both partners are negative, sexual activity can probably be considered safe.
- Use latex condoms for oral, vaginal, or anal intercourse; avoid natural or animal skin condoms, which allow HIV to pass through.
- For vaginal or anal sex, lubricate the condom with the spermicidal agent nonoxynol-9 for additional protection.
- Do not use an oil-based lubricant such as petroleum jelly, which can result in condom damage; water-based lubricants are acceptable.
- Women should carry and use a female condom.
- Remember that use of other means of birth control, such as oral contraceptives, provide no protection against HIV; barrier protection with a condom is necessary.
- Engage in safer sexual practices that are less damaging to sensitive tissues (e.g., mutual masturbation, avoiding anal or oral sex).
- Do not use drugs or alcohol.
- Do not share needles, razors, toothbrushes, sexual toys, or other items that may be contaminated with blood or body fluids.
- If HIV positive:
  a. Do not engage in unprotected sexual activity.
  b. Inform all current and former sexual partners of HIV status.
  c. Inform all health care personnel—primary care providers, physicians, and dentists in particular—of HIV status.
  d. Do not donate blood, plasma, blood products, sperm, organs, or tissue.
  e. If female, do not become pregnant.

facilitate HIV transmission. To be effective, condoms must be used with every sexual encounter involving vaginal, oral, or anal intercourse. They also need to be applied and removed properly. A female condom is also available for use.

The most difficult group of high-risk people to reach and educate has been injection drug users. People in this group should never share needles, syringes, or other drug paraphernalia. Many cities have initiated needle-exchange programs, providing a sterile needle and syringe in exchange for a used one. A fresh solution of household bleach and water in a 1:10 ratio is effective to clean "works" when sterile supplies are not available. It is important to also teach people in this population about safer sex practices, because most heterosexual HIV transmission occurs between injection drug users and their partners.

Screening of voluntary blood donors and donated blood supplies has reduced the risk of transmission by transfusion to 1 in 100,000. Because current blood-screening methods use antibody testing, receiving donated blood continues to carry a small risk. Clients in the *window period* between contraction of the virus and the development of detectable antibodies are able to transmit the virus to others, even though they do not yet test positive for HIV. This window period usually lasts from 6 weeks to 6 months; rarely, it lasts up to 1 year. Whenever possible, clients should be encouraged to use autologous transfusion, donating their own blood prior to an anticipated surgery. Seeking donations from family members is not encouraged for several reasons. Family members may have engaged in high-risk behaviors but lie about their risk because of embarrassment or fear of discovery. Furthermore, the family member may have a different blood type or have other contraindications to donating.

Health care workers can prevent most exposures to HIV by using universal precautions (see the box on page 262). Testing to determine HIV status remains voluntary and relies on the use of antibody-screening methods. It is therefore impossible to identify every client who is HIV positive. With universal precautions, all clients are treated alike, eliminating the need to know the client's HIV status. All high-risk body fluids are treated as if they are infectious, and barrier precautions are used to prevent skin, mucous membrane, or percutaneous exposure to them. Counseling and testing are provided to health care workers with a documented needle-stick exposure. Some clinicians and facilities recommend prophylactic AZT therapy after needle-stick or splash exposure; however, it must be initiated immediately, and its effectiveness has yet to be established.

Laboratory and Diagnostic Tests

Laboratory and diagnostic testing is used to screen and identify the infection, as well as to monitor the client's disease and immune status.

The following laboratory studies may be ordered:

- *Enzyme-linked immunosorbent assay (ELISA)* is the most widely used screening test for HIV infection. The ELISA test was developed in 1985 to screen blood donors. ELISA is a test for HIV antibodies; it does not detect the virus. Therefore, a client may have a negative ELISA test early in the course of infection, before detectable antibodies have developed. The test has a 99.5% or higher sensitivity when performed at least 12 weeks after infection. This means that more than 99.5% of tests performed on blood containing HIV antibodies will show a positive result. False positives can occur; therefore, an initial positive result is always tested repeatedly and confirmed using a different method of antibody detection, usually the Western blot.

- *Western blot antibody testing* is more reliable but more time-consuming and more expensive than ELISA. When combined with ELISA however, a specificity of

greater than 99.9% is achieved. Specificity is a measure of the probability that a negative test result indicates that no antibodies are present. In this test, the client's serum is mixed with HIV proteins to detect reaction. If antibodies to HIV are present, a detectable antigen-antibody response will occur.

- *Polymerase chain reaction (PCR)* testing is a newer technique used to detect viral nucleic acids in people who are infected but fail to produce detectable antibody. This is a very small population, estimated to be between 0.001% and 0.01% of those infected.

- *CBC* is performed to detect anemia, leukopenia, and thrombocytopenia, which are often present in HIV infection. Lymphopenia (or low levels of lymphocytes) is especially common in this disease.

- *CD4 cell count* is the most widely used test to monitor the progress of the disease and guide therapy. The CD4 cell count has been shown to correlate so closely with the immunodeficiency disorders seen in AIDS that in 1993 the CDC added it to the surveillance case definition for AIDS (see the box on page 291). AIDS is now defined not only by the presence of opportunistic infections and other diseases indicative of immunodeficiency, but also by HIV-seropositive status and a CD4 count of less than 200/mm^3 or a percentage of CD4 lymphocytes of less than 14%. CD4 counts are recommended every 3 to 6 months for all people with HIV disease.

In addition to the widely used tests listed above, several other laboratory studies may be performed:

- *Blood culture for HIV* provides the most specific diagnosis but is an expensive and cumbersome test that is not widely available in the United States.

- *Immune-complex-dissociated p24 assay* is a test for p24 (HIV) antigen in the blood. This antigen indicates active reproduction of HIV and tends to be positive prior to seroconversion and with advanced disease. It is most useful in monitoring disease progress and the antiviral activity of medications (Tierney et al., 1994).

Diagnostic testing is used primarily to detect secondary cancers and opportunistic infections in the client with HIV. Tests ordered are both general and specific to the client's manifestations and may include the following:

- *Tuberculin skin testing* to detect possible tuberculosis infection

- *Magnetic resonance imaging (MRI)* of the brain to identify lymphomas

- *Specific cultures and serology examinations for opportunistic infections* such as PCP, toxoplasmosis, and others

- *Pap smears* every 6 months for early detection of cervical cancer in women

Pharmacology

Pharmacologic management of the client with HIV disease has two primary foci: (1) to suppress the infection itself, decreasing symptoms and prolonging the life of the client; and (2) to treat opportunistic infections and malignancies.

For the first goal, antiretroviral treatment is used. A number of agents have been developed since the onset of the epidemic, and many more are currently in development and research stages. The drugs in common usage today are outlined here. Their nursing implications are outlined in the pharmacology box on page 297.

- Zidovudine (Retrovir, AZT) was the first antiretroviral agent approved for use with HIV infection. It remains in widespread use and has been shown to decrease symptoms and prolong the lives of clients with AIDS. Zidovudine is often given to clients with a CD4 cell count of less than 500 because there is evidence that it slows the progression to severe disease (Tierney et al., 1994). Zidovudine may also be used prophylactically following a documented parenteral exposure to HIV. The use of zidovudine is limited by its adverse effects and the development of resistance to the drug by the virus. It is toxic to the bone marrow, frequently resulting in anemia and granulocytopenia. Some clients develop myopathy with muscle tenderness, weakness, and wasting. With long-term use, for example, longer than 18 months, the virus appears to become resistant to the drug's effects, and the therapeutic response is reduced.

- Didanosine (ddI, Dideoxyinosine) also inhibits reverse transcriptase and viral replication. It is used in combination therapy with zidovudine. Didanosine is also given to clients who have developed resistance to zidovudine or who are unable to tolerate its adverse effects.

- Zalcitabine (ddC, Dideoxycytidine) is also a retroviral inhibitor that interferes with the reproduction of HIV. Although it has been shown to be less effective than zidovudine as single-agent therapy, it provides a valuable alternative and combination agent.

- Stavudine (d4T, Deoxythymidine) is an investigational retroviral inhibitor that has been shown to increase CD4 cell counts and decrease serum p24 antigen levels. Current use is for clients who are intolerant of zidovudine and didanosine or those with disease progression. Like didanosine and zalcitabine, stavudine has an associated risk of peripheral neuropathy, hepatitis, and pancreatitis.

Treatment regimens using combination therapies with zidovudine and zalcitabine or other antiretroviral drugs are becoming increasingly popular. Alternating regimens (e.g., 1 month of zidovudine therapy followed by 1 month of zalcitabine therapy) are also in use. As drugs are developed that act on different parts of the viral replication cycle, combination therapies will increase (Tierney et al., 1994). Other agents may also be administered in combination with antiretroviral therapy. Interferons, which are naturally occurring lymphokines, have been used alone and in combination. Alpha-interferon may be used to treat KS and in combination with zidovudine to slow disease progression. Gamma-interferon is also used.

A number of pharmacologic agents is used to prevent and treat opportunistic infections and malignancies in the client with HIV. These agents are outlined in Table 8–14.

Many clients at some point require an implanted venous access device, such as a Hickman catheter, to facilitate blood sampling, intravenous medication administration, transfusions, and parenteral nutrition. See Chapter 26 for nursing care of the client with an intravenous access device implant.

It is recommended that all HIV-infected clients receive pneumococcal, influenza, hepatitis B, and *Haemophilus influenzae b* vaccines. Persons with a positive PPD and negative chest X-ray film are given prophylactic isoniazid (INH). When the client's CD4 cell count falls to less than 200, prophylactic treatment for PCP is initiated, usually with trimethoprim-sulfamethoxazole. Clients with a CD4 count of less than 100 are started on prophylactic treatment for MAC.

Nursing Care

The client with HIV and AIDS has many care needs, including both physical and psychosocial support (see the research box on page 299). Because there is as yet no cure or effective treatment for HIV disease, many of these needs fall within the realm of nursing to promote knowledge and understanding, self-care, comfort, and quality of life. As with many diseases that have an ultimately fatal outcome, the course of HIV infection may well be affected by the client's social support systems, control, perceived self-efficacy in management, and coping mechanisms (O'Brien & Pheifer, 1993).

As the epidemic spreads, nurses are providing care for increasing numbers of clients with HIV infection. These clients are not only in special care settings, but also on general units, maternal-child units, hospice, and home settings. As clients with HIV disease live longer, nurses will increasingly encounter clients in whom HIV disease is a secondary diagnosis, with another primary diagnosis, for example, heart disease, diabetes mellitus, or an operative procedure.

Nursing care needs for the client with HIV infection change over the course of the disease. Preventive health care measures, health-maintenance activities, education, and support of coping mechanisms are important in the early stages of the disease. Counseling the client with a new diagnosis of HIV infection is vital. HIV infection and AIDS continue to carry a social stigma that may interfere

Table 8–14 Pharmacologic Treatment of Common Opportunistic Infections and Malignancies in HIV Disease

Condition	Treatment	Potential Adverse Effects
Infections		
Pneumocystis carinii pneumonia	Trimethoprim-sulfamethoxazole	Rash, neutropenia, anemia, thrombocytopenia, Stevens-Johnson syndrome
	Pentamidine	Hypotension, altered blood glucose levels, hypocalcemia, anemia and leukopenia, liver and renal toxicity, pancreatitis
Tuberculosis	Combination drug therapy using isoniazid, rifampin, ethambutol, pyrazinamide, or streptomycin	Multiple; see Chapter 34
Candidiasis		
Oral thrush	Clotrimazole troches	Few toxic responses noted for either medication
	Nystatin suspension	
Esophagitis or recurrent vaginitis	Ketoconazole	Hepatitis, adrenal insufficiency
	Fluconazole	Hepatitis
	Amphotericin B	Bone marrow toxicity, acute renal or hepatic failure; nausea, vomiting; chills, fever, headache
Mycobacterium avium complex	Combination therapy using	
	■ Clarithromycin, plus	■ Hepatitis, nausea, diarrhea
	■ Clofazimine	■ Diarrhea, nausea, vomiting; skin discoloration, pruritus, rash
	■ Ethambutol	■ Thrombocytopenia, hepatitis, optic neuritis
	■ Rifampin	■ Bone marrow depression, renal failure, hepatitis
	■ Ciprofloxacin	■ Nausea, rash
	■ Amikacin	■ Bone marrow depression, renal failure, ototoxicity, hepatitis
Cytomegalovirus	Ganciclovir	Bone marrow depression, fever
	Foscarnet	Renal failure, electrolyte imbalances, seizures
Herpes simplex or herpes zoster	Acyclovir	Nausea, vomiting, diarrhea; CNS effects; renal failure
Toxoplasmosis	Pyrimethamine, plus	Bone marrow depression, rash; respiratory failure; nausea, vomiting, abdominal pain; hematuria
	Sulfadiazine or clindamycin and folinic acid	
Malignancies		
Kaposi's sarcoma	Intralesional vinblastine	Inflammation and pain at injection site
Lymphoma	Combination chemotherapy	Nausea, vomiting; bone marrow toxicity; alopecia

Note. Summarized from *Mosby's Nursing Drug Reference* by L. Skidmore-Roth, 1993, St Louis: Mosby-Year Book; *Current Medical Diagnosis and Treatment* (33rd ed.) by L. M. Tierney, S. J. McPhee, and M. A. Papadakis, 1994, Norwalk, CT: Appleton & Lange; and *Harrison's Principles of Internal Medicine* (12th ed.) by J. D. Wilson, E. Braunwald, K. J. Isselbacher, R. G. Petersdorf, J. B. Martin, A. S. Fauci, and R. K. Root (Eds.), 1991, New York: McGraw-Hill.

with the client's usual support systems and coping mechanisms. As the disease progresses and the client experiences more physical symptoms, direct care needs become more important while the need for psychosocial support continues.

Ineffective Individual Coping

On receiving the test results indicating HIV seropositive status, the person with HIV infection is faced with multiple issues rarely affecting other clients. First and foremost, HIV is a disease for which there is no known cure

Nursing Implications for Pharmacology: The Client with HIV

ZIDOVUDINE (AZT, RETROVIR)

Zidovudine is the first antiretroviral agent developed to treat HIV infection. It interferes with reverse transcriptase, thus inhibiting replication of the virus. Zidovudine is used for clients with CD4 cell counts of less than 500/µL. The usual dose is 500 to 600 mg per day in divided doses. It is administered orally.

Nursing Responsibilities

- Assess the client for possible contraindications to therapy including allergic response or a CD4 count of greater than 500/mm³.
- Administer by mouth, instructing the client to swallow capsules whole.
- Assess for adverse effects. Nausea and headache are common. They may be self-limiting, decreasing with time, or significant and continuing, necessitating a change of therapy. Other adverse effects include insomnia, malaise, and confusion.
- Assess the client's CBC and differential. Notify the physician of significant changes.

Client and Family Teaching

- Zidovudine will not cure HIV infection but slows its progress and reduces significant symptoms.
- Take the drug as prescribed every 4 to 6 hours to maintain an effective blood level.
- Take the drug at least ½ hour before or 1 hour after meals if tolerated.
- With this and all antiretroviral drugs, it is important to emphasize that the client is still infective and can pass the infection to others. Use safer sex practices and other measures to prevent transmission to partners. Do not donate blood.
- Notify the physician if signs of an infection or adverse response to zidovudine develop: sore throat, swollen lymph glands, fever; unusual fatigue or weakness; easy bruising, bleeding gums, or an injury that will not heal; persistent or intractable nausea; muscle pain or wasting.
- Continue all scheduled follow-up visits and laboratory studies to monitor for drug toxicity.
- Check with the physician before taking any prescription or over-the-counter drug containing aspirin or other NSAID.

DIDANOSINE (DDI, VIDEX, DIDEOXYINOSINE)

As with zidovudine, didanosine does not kill HIV but inhibits its replication within the cells. Its activity is similar to that of zidovudine. Didanosine has been shown to increase CD4 cell counts and lower p24 antigen levels (Tierney et al., 1994). Didanosine is used alone for clients who are intolerant or resistant to zidovudine. It is also being used with zidovudine in combination therapy regimens. Didanosine does not cause the anemia associated with zidovudine, but it may cause granulocytopenia. Didanosine is also associated with an increased risk of pancreatitis, peripheral neuritis, and dry mouth.

Nursing Responsibilities

- Assess for possible contraindications to didanosine therapy, including previous episodes of pancreatitis and impaired renal or liver function.
- Administer as directed. Tablets are to be chewed thoroughly or dissolved in 1 ounce of water at room temperature. The powder form is dissolved in water prior to administration.
- Administer with caution to clients taking vincristine, rifampin, pentamidine, ethambutol, or metronidazole; the action of both drugs may be affected by concurrent administration. Intravenous pentamidine and trimethoprim-sulfamethoxazole taken concurrently may increase the risk of acute and fatal pancreatitis.
- Didanosine interferes with the absorption of ketoconazole and dapsone. Doses of these drugs should be scheduled at least 2 hours apart from didanosine doses.
- Evaluate for therapeutic response and possible adverse effects. Notify the physician if the client develops manifestations of peripheral neuropathy, diarrhea, depression, or other adverse effects.
- Stop the drug and notify the physician immediately if the client develops manifestations of pancreatitis or hepatic failure, including nausea and vomiting, severe abdominal pain, elevated bilirubin, or elevated serum enzymes (e.g., amylase, AST, ALT).

Client and Family Teaching

- Take the drug as directed. The prescribed two-tablet dose must always be taken to get the required amount of antacid to prevent the drug from being destroyed by stomach acid.
- Take on an empty stomach, at least 1 hour before or 2 hours after meals.
- Do not use alcohol while taking didanosine; alcohol may increase the risk of pancreatitis.

- Stop the drug and call the doctor immediately if nausea, vomiting, abdominal pain, or diarrhea develops. These may indicate pancreatitis.
- Call the doctor if extremity pain, weakness, numbness, or tingling occurs. These side effects usually disappear when didanosine is discontinued.
- Other side effects to report to the physician include unusual bleeding or bruising, fatigue, weakness, fever, or persistent sore throat.

ZALCITABINE (DDC, DIDEOXYCYTIDINE)

Another inhibitor of retroviral replication, zalcitabine is generally used in combination therapy regimens with zidovudine. It may also be used alone in clients who have become resistant to zidovudine. Unlike zidovudine and didanosine, zalcitabine is not toxic to the bone marrow, is inexpensive, and easy to administer (Tierney et al., 1994). It is however, associated with severe peripheral neuropathy and an increased risk of pancreatitis. Other adverse effects include stomatitis, rash, fever, and arthritis (Cohen, 1991).

Nursing Responsibilities

- Assess for possible contraindications to zalcitabine: history of pancreatitis or evidence of impaired hepatic function.

- Check with the physician prior to administering the drug concurrently with vincristine, rifampin, intravenous pentamidine, ethambutol, pyrimethamine, dapsone, acyclovir, or metronidazole.
- Administer as prescribed, generally every 8 hours.
- Evaluate for desired effect of increased CD4 counts and lower blood levels of p24 antigen.
- Notify the physician if the client develops evidence of pancreatitis, impaired hepatic function, or painful peripheral neuropathy.

Client and Family Teaching

- Take the medication on an empty stomach, 1 hour before or 2 hours after meals.
- Check with the physician before taking any other prescription or over-the-counter medication.
- Do not consume alcohol while taking this medication; alcohol increases the risk of pancreatitis.
- Notify the physician immediately if symptoms of peripheral neuropathy (see above section on didanosine) or pancreatitis develops.
- Report to the physician signs of infection or changes in condition.

and which is, at this time, thought to be almost universally fatal. As mentioned earlier, HIV and AIDS carry a social stigma that may interfere with the client's social support systems and family relationships. The disease may also affect the ability to obtain and retain useful work and health insurance. The client may experience guilt about his or her life-style and the way the disease was contracted. As the disease progresses, social isolation, fatigue, body image changes, medication side effects, and multiple other issues affect the client's abilities to cope. Nursing interventions with rationales follow:

- Assess the client's social support network and usual methods of coping. *This will help both the nurse and the client identify people and mechanisms that can help the client cope more effectively with the disease.*
- If possible, assign a primary nurse for the client, whether the setting is home health, hospice, or acute care. *This helps promote the development of a therapeutic and trusting relationship and provides for continuity of care (Sparks & Taylor, 1993).*

- Allow for consistent, uninterrupted time spent with the client. *Time and a consistent presence encourage the client to express feelings and work through issues related to HIV infection.*
- Interact with the client at every opportunity outside of providing specific nursing care treatments. *This purposeful interaction communicates caring and acceptance without fear of HIV disease.*
- Support the client's social network. *Nontraditional families may offer more support than the traditional family. This in turn may necessitate a liberal interpretation of the term "family" if unit policy is "immediate family only."*
- Promote interaction between the client, significant others, and family. *Hospitalization and manifestations of HIV disease may bring about isolation from others and decrease the client's ability to cope.*
- Encourage the client to obtain necessary information and make care decisions. *This gives the client a greater sense of self-worth and control over the situation, increasing coping abilities.*

Applying Research to Nursing Practice: The Client with HIV Disease

■ ■ ■

Public health experts project that in less than a decade the global count of people with the human immunodeficiency virus (HIV) may have reached as many as 110 million, no fewer than 38 million adults. It is also expected that worldwide there will be more than 10 million children who will have contracted HIV by the year 2000. (O'Brien & Pheifer, 1993, p. 303)

Although the future prospect for HIV disease looks grim, the reality is that clients with HIV have nursing care needs now. In one study, researchers sought to identify the physical and psychosocial issues affecting clients with HIV disease that were appropriate for nursing intervention (O'Brien & Pheifer, 1993). Through interviews with a study group of 138 HIV-infected people, the majority of whom were gay males and met diagnostic criteria for AIDS, the researchers identified multiple needs. The key physical and psychosocial issues that were most frequently identified by the study participants and are appropriate for nursing interventions follow:

- Fatigue
- Weight loss
- Self-concept
- Loneliness
- Sexual integrity
- Home maintenance communication
- Impaired management
- Spiritual distress

Implications for Nursing

It is apparent from this study, that while nurses often focus primarily on the physical needs of the client, particularly in the acute care setting, the client with HIV is more concerned about psychosocial needs. The nurse who does not address these needs in planning care is not treating the client as a holistic being.

Critical Thinking in Client Care

Most of the participants in this study were gay males. How do you think the results might have differed had the study population been:

1. Heterosexual males;
2. Pregnant females;
3. Women caring for families; or
4. Injection drug users?

- Set and maintain limits on manipulative and other destructive behaviors. *The client who is unable to limit inappropriate behaviors needs the external control established by setting limits (Sparks & Taylor, 1993).*

- Assist the client to accept responsibility for his or her actions without blaming others. *Effective coping cannot occur without accepting responsibility for one's actions.*

- Support positive coping behaviors, client decisions, actions, and achievements. *As the client's self-esteem is enhanced, coping improves.*

- Provide referral to counselors, support groups, and agencies. *These external support systems can help the client develop effective coping strategies.*

- Encourage the client, family, and significant others to participate in support groups. *Support groups decrease the risk of social isolation and enhance implementation of coping mechanisms.*

- Provide addresses and phone numbers for local and national information resources and hot lines (see the back endsheets). *This gives the client resources of persons and groups who can provide information and support.*

Impaired Skin Integrity

Dryness, malnutrition, immobility from fatigue, and skin lesions on pressure sites all contribute to impaired integrity of the skin for the client with HIV disease. Maintaining skin integrity is important because of the progressive and debilitating nature of the disease. It is also a consideration both as the first line of defense against infection in an immunosuppressed client and as a site for secondary manifestations, such as KS and herpes.

Nursing interventions with rationales follow:

- Assess the skin frequently for lesions and areas of breakdown. *Early identification of impaired skin integrity allows prompt intervention.*

- Monitor lesions for signs of infection or impaired healing. *Infection or poor tissue perfusion not only impairs healing but may lead to further skin breakdown.*

- Turn the client at least every 2 hours, more frequently if necessary. *Turning decreases unrelieved pressure on bony prominences and improves circulation to the tissues.*

- Use pressure-relieving devices, such as pressure and egg crate mattresses, or sheep skin pads for elbows and heels. *These devices provide prophylactic relief of pressure.*

- Keep skin clean and dry using mild, nondrying soaps or oils for cleansing. *Night sweats and diarrhea, if present, can cause breakdown and damage to the skin. Frequent cleansing with nondrying products discourages bacterial growth, reducing the risk of infection.*

- Massage around but not over affected pressure sites. *This increases circulation to the surrounding tissue. Massaging over the affected area can cause skin breakdown.*

- If blisters are noted, leave intact, and dress with a hydrocolloid (Duoderm) dressing. *Blisters provide natural sterile coverings for damaged tissue, improving healing and preventing bacterial invasion.*

- Caution the client against scratching. Trim fingernails and use mitts or soft restraints if necessary in the confused client to prevent scratching. Check for circulation of hands and fingers frequently if mitts or restraints are used. *Scratching and skin damage allow bacteria to be introduced into lesions, increasing the risk of infection. Tight or restrictive restraints or mitts may compromise circulation.*

- Avoid the use of heat or occlusive dressings. *Heat can further dry and damage the skin; occlusive dressings may impair circulation and lead to ulceration.*

- Prevent skin shearing by using a turnsheet and adequate personnel in repositioning client. *Shearing causes tissue trauma that can lead to decubitus ulcers.*

- Encourage ambulation if possible; if the client is confined to bed, encourage active or passive range-of-motion exercises. *Activity increases circulation, decreases pressure and skin breakdown, and helps maintain muscle tone.*

- Monitor nutritional intake as well as albumin levels. *Maintenance of optimal nutrition decreases the risk of tissue breakdown and improves resistance to infection.*

Altered Nutrition: Less Than Body Requirements

Many factors associated with HIV disease, as well as manifestations of the disease itself, put the client at risk for altered nutrition and weight loss. Nausea and anorexia may be manifestations of the disease or the result of antiretroviral therapy. Chronic diarrhea is a common manifestation of constitutional HIV disease. Wasting syndrome is also common. It is manifested by involuntary weight loss of greater than 10% to 15% of baseline weight, severe diarrhea, fever, and chronic fatigue and weakness. The exact cause of wasting syndrome is unclear, but the diarrhea and fatigue contribute, as does the increased metabolic rate associated with fever. Oral and esophageal candidiasis and KS of the gastrointestinal tract may cause painful swallowing, making eating difficult and thereby contributing to anorexia. Poor nutritional status in the client with HIV can ultimately result in altered comfort, a change in body image, muscle wasting, increased risk of infection, and higher mortality and morbidity (O'Brien & Pheifer, 1993).

Nursing interventions with rationales follow:

- Assess the client's nutritional status, including weight; body mass; caloric intake; and laboratory studies, such as total protein and albumin levels, hemoglobin, and hematocrit. *Assessment is necessary to provide baseline data to monitor the effectiveness of interventions.*

- Assess the client for possible causes of altered nutrition, including oral or esophageal lesions, fever, nausea, or diarrhea. *This assessment provides direction for planned interventions.*

- Administer prescribed medications for candidiasis and other manifestations as ordered. *Eliminating this opportunistic infection improves comfort and facilitates food intake. Topical viscous anesthetic can help reduce pain and improve oral intake.*

- Administer antidiarrheal medications after stools as ordered; administer antiemetics prior to meals. Provide antipyretics as needed to control fever. *Reducing diarrhea will improve nutrient absorption; preprandial medication with an antiemetic reduces nausea and improves food intake. Reduction of fever lowers the body's metabolic demands.*

- Provide a diet high in protein and kilocalories. *A high-protein, high-kilocalorie diet provides the necessary nutrients to meet the client's metabolic and tissue healing needs.*

- Offer soft foods, and serve small portions. *Soft foods are easily digested. Small portions are more appealing to the anorectic or nauseated client.*

- Provide foods that the client likes, encouraging the client to plan his or her own meals. Encourage significant others to bring favorite foods from home. *The client is more likely to consume adequate amounts of preferred foods. Allowing the client to choose foods enhances the client's sense of control.*

- Assist the client with eating as needed. *Fatigue and weakness can prevent the client from eating an adequate amount of food.*

- Provide supplementary vitamins and enteral feedings, such as Ensure. *This improves the client's nutritional status and caloric intake.*

- Provide or assist the client with frequent oral hygiene. *Oral hygiene improves comfort and appetite, as well as reducing the risk of mucosal lesions.*

- Monitor weight, caloric intake, and other indicators of nutritional status on a continuing basis.

Altered Sexuality Patterns

The diagnosis of HIV infection can significantly alter the client's expressions of sexuality. Guilt over the diagnosis may interfere with libido. The client may be angry with a significant other or partner if that person was the probable source of infection. The client may fear spreading the disease to others via sexual relations. As the disease progresses, its manifestations can affect the client's body image and self-esteem, impairing sexuality. Other symptoms, such as nausea, fatigue, and weakness, may also interfere with libido and sexual satisfaction.

Nursing interventions with rationales follow:

- Examine your feelings about sexuality, your role in dealing with a client's sexuality, the client's life-style, and sexual preferences. *To deal effectively with the client's concerns, it is vital that the nurse be comfortable with his or her own feelings of sexuality and be able to accept the client's life-style. Referring the client to another nurse or counselor may be necessary.*

- Establish a trusting, therapeutic relationship with the client through the use of time, active listening, caring, and self-disclosure. Maintain a nonthreatening, nonjudgmental attitude toward the client. *Sexuality is a very private issue that will be uncomfortable or impossible for the nurse and client to discuss without a mutually trusting relationship.*

- Provide the client and significant other with factual information about HIV infection and its effects. *This helps the client separate fears and myths from reality.*

- Discuss safer sex practices, including hugging, cuddling, nonsexual contact, the use of latex condoms and spermicidal lubricant, and mutual masturbation. *Alternative forms of sexual activity and expressing affection can allow the client and significant other to remain close throughout the course of the disease.*

- Encourage the client and significant other to discuss their fears and concerns with each other. *Open communication helps them to deal with issues related to sexuality.*

- For the client without a significant other, stress the need to continue to meet people and develop social relationships while practicing safe sex. *The risk of isolation is high in the client with HIV infection, and relationships with others help the client to cope with the disease.*

- Refer the client and significant other to local support groups for people and partners of people with HIV. *Support groups provide a social and support network of people facing the same issues.*

Other Nursing Diagnoses

With a disease such as HIV infection, the list of possible nursing diagnoses is long. The following nursing diagnoses may be appropriate:

- *Impaired Adjustment* related to inadequate support systems

- *Activity Intolerance* related to fatigue

- *Powerlessness* related to terminal disease

- *Pain* related to KS and peripheral neuropathy

- *Altered Thought Processes* related to AIDS dementia complex

- *Body Image Disturbance* related to significant weight loss and muscle wasting

- *Risk for Caregiver Role Strain* related to care needs of the client with HIV

- *Altered Family Processes* related to alternative life-style

- *Impaired Home Maintenance Management* related to fatigue and weakness

- *Altered Oral Mucous Membrane* related to candidiasis

- *Altered Role Performance* related to manifestations of disease

- *Social Isolation* related to fear of AIDS

- *Spiritual Distress* related to testing of spiritual beliefs

Client and Family Teaching

Teaching needs for both the client and significant other are extensive. The primary need is information about the disease, its spread, and its expected course. The client and family need current factual information to plan realistically and to combat myths, misperceptions, and prejudices. At the same time, it is important to include information about current research and progress in treating the disease to maintain a sense of hopefulness.

Discuss guidelines for safer sex practices, and stress the need to follow these practices at all times and in all relationships. Emphasize the need to abstain from donating blood, organs, or sperm. Discuss tactics to avoid exchange of body fluids by not sharing needles or other drug paraphernalia, not sharing razors, not obtaining a tattoo. Stress the importance of informing all medical personnel providing direct care (especially anyone performing a dental, surgical, or obstetric procedure) about the diagnosis.

Talk to the client and family about measures to maintain optimal health. Include discussion about diet and nutritional intake, a balance of rest and exercise, stress reduction, life-style changes, and maintaining a positive outlook. To reduce the risk of opportunistic and other infections, teach the client about the importance of washing hands and avoiding people with infectious diseases. Discuss the need for regular medical follow-up and monitoring of immune status.

Encourage the client to stop smoking and to eliminate the use of alcohol and recreational or illicit drugs. Provide referral to clinics, agencies, or counselors to assist with withdrawal.

Teach care providers to use gloves when handling the client's secretions or excretions and to wash hands before and after providing direct care. Wash linens soiled with secretions or excretions separately using a 10% bleach solution. Emphasize that it is not important to separate dishes, glassware, and utensils, provided that they are washed in hot, soapy water. There is no reason that the client cannot assist with food preparation as long as he or she is feeling well.

Discuss the signs and symptoms of opportunistic infections and malignancies, as well as other symptoms that should be reported: persistent fever or night sweats, swollen glands, diarrhea, chest pain, dyspnea, headaches, and skin lesions.

For the client with advanced disease, provide information about resources such as hospice agencies and respite care. Demonstrate the use and care of implanted venous access devices, total parenteral nutrition, intravenous pumps and continuous medication delivery systems, and intravenous or aerosolized medications. Teach the client and significant other about the use of prescribed medications, including their anticipated and adverse effects.

Provide referrals to local care providers, home health services, support groups, and social agencies as indicated by client needs and wishes.

Applying the Nursing Process

Case Study of a Client with HIV Infection: Sara Lu

Sara Lu is a 26-year-old elementary school teacher who lives with her parents and two younger sisters. Ms. Lu is very close to her parents and sisters; they share everything with each other. During the required physical for admission to graduate school, Ms. Lu tells her physician that lately she has felt fatigued. She also states that she has had a persistent sore throat, intermittent bouts of diarrhea, and mild shortness of breath for about a month. She does not take any routine medications other than a daily multivitamin and an occasional acetaminophen tablet for a headache. She is active in a drama club in her community, and jogs 3 miles three to four times a week. She is engaged to be married; her wedding date is set for 6 months away. Her fiancé is the only person with whom she has had sexual relations. Her sexual activity has been unprotected. Ms. Lu has a history of open heart surgery 7 years ago to correct a congenital valve defect. She has been physically healthy since that time, until about a month or two ago. The physician orders a mononucleosis test, enzyme-linked immunosorbent assay (ELISA), Western blot analysis, CD4 T-cell count, a p24 antigen test, and an erythrocyte sedimentation rate (ESR). She has been asked to return in 1 week for follow-up.

Assessment

On Ms. Lu's return for a follow-up visit, her nursing history is obtained by Carole Kee, RN. Ms. Lu continues to have flulike symptoms but has improved somewhat. She states that she just has not been as active as usual and is worried about her health. Her appetite has decreased be-

cause of soreness in her mouth, and she has noted some whitish patches on her tongue and cheeks.

A chest X-ray film reveals no abnormality. The results of her laboratory tests are as follows:

- ELISA: positive for antibodies against HIV
- Western blot analysis: positive for antibodies against HIV
- p24 antigen test: positive for circulating HIV antigens
- ESR: increased to 25 mm/h (normal for women is 15 to 20 mm/h; normal for men is 10 to 15 mm/h).
- CD4 T-cell count: 599/mm^3 (normal range is 600 to 1200).

Ms. Lu's physical examination reveals that she has enlarged lymph nodes in her neck and white patches on her oral mucosa. Her skin is warm to the touch. Her vital signs are as follows: BP, 120/78; R, 20; P, 84; T 99.9 F (37.7 C).

Ms. Lu is told of the results of her laboratory tests and the medical diagnosis of HIV infection. Ms. Lu is distressed and wants to know how this happened, its meaning, whether she has infected her loved ones, and whether she will get better.

Diagnosis

Ms. Kee develops the following nursing diagnoses for Ms. Lu:

- *Altered Nutrition: Less Than Body Requirements* related to soreness in mouth
- *Risk for Fluid Volume Deficit* related to decreased fluid intake and diarrhea
- *Risk for Infection* related to altered immune protection
- *Anxiety* related to diagnosis and fear
- *Knowledge Deficit* about the HIV disease process

Expected Outcomes

The expected outcomes established in the plan of care specify that Ms. Lu will

- Maintain adequate nutrition for optimal body and cellular function.
- Consume at least 2500 mL of fluid per day.
- Remain free of infections and their complications.
- Verbalize anxiety and employ appropriate coping mechanisms.
- Verbalize and demonstrate knowledge of HIV disease.
- Verbalize measures to prevent HIV transmission to others, including safer sex practices.

Planning and Implementation

Ms. Kee plans the following interventions to be implemented:

- Monitor daily weight and intake and output.

- Monitor dietary habits.

- Teach Ms. Lu the importance of consuming a nutritionally balanced diet and maintaining adequate fluid intake.

- Suggest strategies for coping with anorexia and nausea.

- Provide dietary consultation referral.

- Monitor serum albumin to determine the protein needed to support the immune system.

- Encourage oral care before and after meals.

- Monitor elimination pattern.

- Assess bowel sounds.

- Administer antiemetic and antimotility medications as prescribed, and monitor reactions.

- Monitor for signs of dehydration, such as poor skin turgor, oliguria, and orthostatic hypotension.

- Increase fluid to 2500 mL daily.

- Use strict aseptic technique for all invasive procedures.

- Teach Ms. Lu to avoid exposure to infection and people with known illnesses.

- Administer antiretroviral medications and antibiotics as prescribed, and monitor response.

- Encourage maintenance of regular physical exercise.

- Monitor vital signs daily.

- Provide opportunities for Ms. Lu to verbalize her feelings.

- Avoid false reassurances.

- Provide appropriate and adequate information about HIV/AIDS.

- Teach safer sex practices and other measures to prevent HIV transmission.

- Teach anxiety-controlling techniques, such as imagery, deep breathing, and meditation.

Evaluation

Ms. Lu is eager to learn about her illness and wants her family to come with her for further explanation. She states that she is sure her fiancé will be available as well. Ms. Lu is taking home antifungal medication, diet plans, and a schedule for increased exercise. She will return in 1 week for counseling and in 1 month for a follow-up physical.

Critical Thinking in the Nursing Process

1. How does age effect the body's response to fighting HIV? What other factors affect the risk of HIV infection and its progression? Consider life-style factors and their effect on immune status.

2. Are the laboratory results for Ms. Lu a true indication that she is HIV positive? What additional tests might be ordered?

3. What is the most likely source of Ms. Lu's infection? What measures are used to reduce this risk, and how did Ms. Lu contract HIV? What is another possible source of Ms. Lu's HIV infection?

4. Ms. Lu says that her fiancé would like to have a child. How will you counsel her regarding pregnancy and childbearing?

Bibliography

■ ■ ■

Abrams, D. I. (1989). The persistent lymphadenopathy syndrome and immune thrombocytopenia purpura in HIV-infected individuals. In J. A. Levy (Ed.), *AIDS: Pathogenesis and treatment.* New York: Marcel Dekker.

Abrams, W. B., & Berkow, R., (Eds.). (1990). *The Merck manual of geriatrics.* Rahway, NJ: Merck, Sharp & Dohme Research Laboratories.

Aerwekh, J. (1994, February). The truth-tellers: How hospice nurses help patients confront death. *American Journal of Nursing, 94*(2), 30–34.

Anastasi, J., & Lee, V. (1994, June). HIV wasting: How to stop the cycle. *American Journal of Nursing, 94*(6), 18–24.

Anastasi, J., & Rivera, J. (1994, February). Understanding prophylactic therapy for HIV infections. *American Journal of Nursing, 94*(2), 36–41.

Andreoli, T. E., Carpenter, C. C. J., Plum, F., & Smith, L. H., Jr. (1990). *Cecil Essentials of medicine* (2nd ed.) Philadelphia: W. B. Saunders.

Bates, B. (1987). *A guide to physical examination and history taking,* (4th ed.). Philadelphia: Lippincott.

Bellack, J. P., & Edlund, B. J. (1992). *Nursing assessment and diagnosis,* (2nd ed.). Boston: Jones and Barlett.

Benjamin, E., & Leskowitz, S. (1991). *Immunology.* New York: Wiley-Liss.

Bondmass, M. (1994, January). The cardiac manifestations of acquired immune deficiency syndrome and nursing implications. *MEDSURG Nursing, 3*(1), 42–48.

Brown, Katherine K. (1994, September). Septic shock: Stopping the deadly cascade. *American Journal of Nursing, 94*(9), 20–27.

Bullock, B. L., & Rosendahl, P. P. (1992). *Pathophysiology: Adaptations and alterations in function* (3rd ed.). Philadelphia: Lippincott.

Burakoff, S. J., Deeg, H. J., Ferrara, J., & Atkinson, K. (Eds.). (1990). *Graft-vs-host disease: Immunology, pathophysiology, and treatment.* New York: Marcel Dekker.

Burggraf, V., & Stanley, M. (Eds.). (1989). *Nursing the elderly: A care plan approach.* Philadelphia: Lippincott.

Carpenito, L. J. (1992). *Nursing diagnosis: Application to clinical practice* (4th ed.). New York: Lippincott.

Centers for Disease Control. (1992, December 18). *1993 revised classification system for HIV infection and expanded surveillance case definition for AIDS among adolescents and adults. Morbidity and Mortality Weekly Report, 41* (RR-17).

Centers for Disease Control. (1993, September 28). *Annual summary of births, marriages, divorces, and deaths: United States, 1992. Monthly Vital Statistics Report, 41*(13), 1–36.

Chapel, H., & Haeney, H. C. (1993). *Essentials of clinical immunology.* Boston: Blackwell.

Chernecky, C. C., Krech, R. L., & Berger, B. J. (1993). *Laboratory tests and diagnostic procedures.* Philadelphia: W. B. Saunders.

Clinical Update. (1993, February). Understanding HIV. Why healthy cells self-destruct. *Nursing 93, 23*(2), 51.

Cohen, F. L. (1991, June). The pharmacologic treatment of HIV infection and AIDS in adults. *Nursing Clinics of North America, 26*(2), 315–329.

da Cunha, M. F. (1990). Immunopathologic and clinical correlates in immunocompromised patients. *Anesthesia Today, 1*(3), 1,3–6.

Davis, M. (1993, November). Dropping the barrier between Jim and Us. *Nursing 93, 23*(11), 63–64.

Dawson, M. M. (1991). *Lymphokines and interleukins*. Boca Raton, FL: CRC Press.

Doan-Johnson, S. (1993, June). Predicting the future of HIV/AIDS nursing. *Nursing 93, 23*(6), 48–49.

Drug Update: T.B., H.I.V., and hepatitis B. (1993, October). *Nursing 93, 23*(10), 71.

Edwards, B. (1994, January). When the family can't let go. *American Journal of Nursing, 94*(1), 52–56.

Eliopoulos, C. (1987). *Gerontological Nursing* (2nd ed.). Philadelphia: Lippincott.

EMA essay. (1991, May). HIV infection and health-care workers. *15*(5), 1–6.

Evaluation and management of early HIV infection. (1994, January). Clinical Practice Guidelines. No. 7. U. S. Department of Health and Human Services. Public Health. AHCPR Publication No. 94-0572. Rockville, MD: Agency for Health Care Policy and Research, Public Health Service.

Flaskerud, J. H., & Ungvarski, P. J. (1992). *HIV/AIDS: A guide to nursing care* (2nd. ed). Philadelphia: W. B. Saunders.

Gauthier, A. M. (1992, October). Would you divulge confidential information about a patient's HIV status? *Nursing 92, 22*(10), 59.

Grimes, D. (1991). *Infectious diseases*. St. Louis: Mosby Year Book.

Gulanick, M., Klopp, A., Galanes, S., Gradishar, D., & Pugas, M. K. (1990). *Nursing care plans: Nursing diagnosis and intervention*. St. Louis: Mosby.

Guyton, A. C. (1990). *Textbook of medical physiology* (8th ed.). Philadelphia: W. B. Saunders.

Hazzard, W. R., Bierman, E. L., Blass, J. P., Ettinger, W. H., Jr., & Halter, J. B. (Eds.). (1994). *Principles of geriatric medicine and gerontology*. (3rd ed.). New York: McGraw-Hill.

Holloway, N. M. (1993). *Nursing the critically ill adult* (4th ed.). Redwood, CA: Addison-Wesley Nursing.

Hudak, C. M., & Gallo, B. M. (1994). *A handbook of critical care nursing*. Philadelphia: Lippincott.

Isselbacher, K. J., Braunwald, E., Wilson, J. D., Martin, J. B., Fauci, A. S., & Kasper, D. L. (Eds.). (1994). *Harrison's Principles of internal medicine*. New York: McGraw-Hill.

Johnson, L. E., Dooley, P. A., & Gleick, J. B. (1993, September). Oral nutritional supplement use in elderly nursing home patients. *Journal of the American Geriatrics Society, 41*(9), 947–952.

Joneja, J. M. V., & Bielory, L. (1990). *Understanding allergy, sensitivity, and immunity: A comprehensive guide*. New Brunswick: Rutgers University Press.

Klein, A. R., Lee, G., Manton, A., & Parker, J. G. (1994). *Emergency nursing care curriculum*. Philadelphia: W. B. Saunders.

Kolata, G. (1994, May 31). Genetic attacks on AIDS readied. *New York Times*, p. C1, C3.

Kumar, V., Cotran, R. S., & Robbins, S. L. (1992). *Basic pathophysiology* (5th ed.). Philadelphia: W. B. Saunders.

Lancaster, L. E. (1992, March). Immunogenetic basis of tissue and organ transplantation and rejection. *Critical Care Nursing Clinics of North America, 4*(1), 1–24.

Lee, J. (Ed.). *The HLA system: A new approach*. (1990). New York: Springer-Verlag.

Lutz, C. A., & Przytulski, K. R. (1994). *Nutrition and diet therapy*. Philadelphia: F. A. Davis.

Madhok, R., Forbes, C. D., & Evatt, B. L. (Eds.). (1994). *Blood, blood products, and HIV*. New York: Chapman & Hall.

Marieb, E. N. (1995). *Human anatomy and physiology* (3rd ed.). Redwood City, CA: Benjamin/Cummings.

Mathewson-Kuhn, M. (1994). *Pharmacotherapeutics: A nursing approach*. Philadelphia: F. A. Davis.

McCance, K., & Huether, S. E. (1994). *Pathophysiology: The biologic basis for disease in adults and children*. St. Louis: Mosby.

Merck Research Laboratories. (1992). *The Merck manual of diagnosis and therapy* (16th ed.). R. Berkow, Ed. in Chief. Rahway, NJ: Author.

Miller-Keane encyclopedia & dictionary of medicine, nursing, & allied health (5th ed.). (1992). M. O'Toole, Ed. Philadelphia: W. B. Saunders.

Morrison, C. (1993, June). Delivery systems for the care of persons with HIV infection and AIDS. *Nursing Clinics of North America, 28*(2), 317–333.

Morton, P. G. (1993). *Health assessment in nursing* (2nd ed.). Springhouse, PA: Springhouse.

Mudge-Grout, C. L. (1992). *Immunologic disorders*. St. Louis: Mosby-Year Book.

Nokes, K. M., Wheeler, K., & Kendrew, J. (1994). *Image: Journal of Nursing Scholarship, 26*(2), 133–138.

Novello, A. C. (1993, June). *Surgeon General's report to the American public on HIV infection and AIDS—extracts*. Rockville, MD: CDC National AIDS Clearinghouse.

O'Brien, M. E., & Pheifer, W. G. (1993, June). Physical and psychosocial nursing care for patients with HIV infection. *Nursing Clinics of North America, 28*(2), 303–316.

Pagana, K. D., & Pagana, T. J. (1992). *Mosby's diagnostic and laboratory test reference*. St. Louis: Mosby-Year Book.

Paul, W. E. (1993). *Fundamental immunology*. New York: Raven Press.

Physicians' desk reference (48th ed.). (1994). Montvale, NJ: Medical Economics Data Production Company.

Porth, C. M. (1994). *Pathophysiology: Concepts of altered health states* (4th ed.). Philadelphia: Lippincott.

Powers, D. C. (1994). *Aging, immunity, and infection*. New York: Springer.

Price, R. W., Brew, B., Sidtis, J., Rosenblum, M., Scheck, A. C., & Cleary, P. (1988, February). The brain in AIDS: Central nervous system HIV-1 infection and AIDS dementia complex. *Science, 239*, 586–591.

Price, S. A., & Wilson, L. M. (1992). *Pathophysiology: Clinical concepts of disease processes* (4th ed.). St. Louis: Mosby-Year Book.

Riley, M. W., Ory, M. G., & Zablotsky, D. (Eds.). *AIDS in an aging society*. New York: Springer.

Rodgers-Seidl, F. F. (1991). *Geriatric Nursing Care Plans*. St. Louis: Mosby-Year Book.

Roitt, I. (1994). *Essential immunology* (8th ed.). London: Blackwell.

Shaefer, M., & Williams, L. (1991, June). Nursing implications of immunosuppression in transplantation. *Nursing Clinics of North America, 26*(2), 291–314.

Shlafer, M. (1993). *The nurse, pharmacology, and drug therapy: A prototype approach* (2nd ed.). Redwood City: Addison-Wesley Nursing.

Skidmore-Roth, L. (1993). *Mosby's Nursing drug reference*. St. Louis: Mosby-Year Book.

Sparks, S. M., & Taylor, C. M. (1993). *Nursing diagnosis reference manual* (2nd ed.). Springhouse, PA: Springhouse.

Spencer, R. T., Nichols, L. W., Lipkin, G. B., Henderson, H. S., & West, F. M. (1993). *Clinical pharmacology and nursing management* (4th ed.). Philadelphia: Lippincott.

Thompson, J. M., McFarland, G. K., Hirsch, J. E., & Tucker, S. M. (1993). *Mosby's Clinical nursing* (3rd ed.). St. Louis: Mosby-Year Book.

Tierney, L. M., Jr., McPhee, S. J., & Papadakis, M. A. (Eds.) (1994). *Current medical diagnosis and treatment* (33rd ed.). Norwalk, CT: Appleton & Lange.

Tortora, G. L., & Grabowski, S. R. (1993). *Principles of anatomy and physiology* (7th ed.). New York: HarperCollins.

Ulrich, S. P., Canale, S. W., & Wendell, S. A. (1994). *Medical-surgical nursing care planning guides* (3rd ed.). Philadelphia: W. B. Saunders.

Wallace, J. I., Paauw, D., & Spach, D. H. (1993, June). HIV infection in older patients: When to suspect the unexpected. *Geriatrics, 48*(6), 61–70.

Way, L. M., (Ed.) (1994). *Current surgical diagnosis and treatment* (10th ed.). Norwalk, CT: Appleton & Lange.

Weir, D. M., & Stewart, J. (1993). *Immunology*. New York: Churchill Livingstone.

Wilson, J. D., Braunwald, E., Isselbacher, K. J., Petersdorf, R. G., Martin, J. B., Fauci, A. S., & Root, R. K. (Eds.) (1991). *Harrison's Principles of internal medicine* (12th ed.) New York: McGraw-Hill.

Workman, M. L., Ellerhorst-Ryan, J., & Hargrove-Koertge, V. (1993). *Nursing care of the immunocompromised patient*. Philadelphia: W. B. Saunders.

Zurlinden, J., & Verheggen, R. (1994, January). HIV vaccines: A report from the front. *RN, 57*(1), 36–40.

Nursing Care of Clients with Cancer

LEARNING OBJECTIVES

After completing this chapter, you will be able to

- Define cancer and differentiate benign from malignant neoplasms.
- Discuss the theories of carcinogenesis, known carcinogens, and risk factors for cancer.
- Compare the mechanisms and characteristics of normal cells with those of malignant cells.
- Describe the effects of cancer on the body.
- Describe the laboratory and diagnostic tests used to diagnose cancer.

- Discuss the role of chemotherapy in cancer treatment.
- Discuss the use of surgery, radiation therapy, immunotherapy, and photodynamic therapy in the treatment of cancer.
- Describe the nursing interventions required for oncologic emergencies.
- Provide teaching to the client and family experiencing cancer.
- Use the nursing process as a framework for providing individualized care to the client with cancer.

Cancer is a family of complex diseases with manifestations that vary according to the body system affected and the type of tumor cells involved. People of any age, gender, ethnicity, or geographic region can be affected by this disease. Despite research shedding more light on this dreaded disease, cancer still kills its victims 50% of the time.

The fear engendered by even the suggestion of a cancer diagnosis is considerable. Often referred to as "the big C," cancer brings forth feelings of dread and helplessness similar to those experienced by people in the Middle Ages confronting the plague, a disease whose prevention, cause, and treatment were then unknown.

This chapter looks at the general pathogenesis, pathophysiology, and etiology of cancer; identifies current diagnostic and treatment modalities; and discusses nursing care that is appropriate for most clients with cancer. Discussions of cancers that affect specific body systems (e.g., leukemia, lung cancer) can be found in corresponding body system chapters in the text.

Cancer, the Nurse, and the Health Care Team

Cancer is a disease that results when normal cells mutate into abnormal, deviant cells that then perpetuate within the body. Cancer can affect any body tissue. Providing cancer care is a potentially complex process, reflecting cancer's many different types and manifestations.

Nursing focuses on cancer not as one disease, but as many diseases. The nurse recognizes that cancer is a disruptive process that affects the whole person and that person's significant others. Nursing interventions reflect the fact that cancer is chronic and has acute episodes, that the client is often treated in the home, and that the client is treated with a combination of therapeutic modalities. Equally important, the nurse recognizes that caring for the client with cancer involves prevention, detection, rehabilitation, and terminal care (Siegel, 1990).

The study of cancer is called **oncology,** a term that derives from the Greek word *oncoma* ("bulk"). *Oncologists* are physicians who specialize in caring for clients with cancer. Oncologists may be medical doctors, surgeons, radiologists, immunologists, or researchers. Often, the client with cancer has the benefit of a team of physicians who collaborate to provide the most effective treatment.

Another very significant member of the oncology team is the *oncology nurse*, who has received specialized training in such cancer treatment modalities as chemotherapy. Oncology nurses also have special skills in assisting the client and family with the psychosocial issues associated with cancer and terminal illness.

Cancer Incidence and Trends

■ ■ ■

Cancer mortality rates are exceeded only by those for heart disease. Despite continuing research, the rates of death from some forms of cancer are rising.

The 1994 statistics from the American Cancer Society (ACS) show that in the United States, approximately 20% of all deaths are attributable to cancer, with a death rate of 174 per 100,000 population in 1990. Furthermore, the National Cancer Institute (NCI) estimated that in 1994 alone over 1.2 million new cases of cancer would occur, with a projected death rate of 538,000 (American Cancer Society [ACS], 1994).

As of 1994, prostate cancer surpassed lung and colon cancer for the position of highest incidence. In 1994, an estimated 200,000 cases of prostate cancer were predicted, an increase of 50% since 1980. This increase was attributed to earlier detection resulting from the extensive use of a new diagnostic test (see Chapter 46). Breast cancer is now second highest in incidence (182,000 new cases in 1994), followed by lung cancer (172,000 new cases) and colorectal cancer (149,000 new cases). Among men, prostate cancer has the highest incidence, followed by lung cancer and colorectal cancer. Among women, breast cancer continues to have the highest incidence, followed by colorectal cancer and lung cancer.

Mortality rates for different cancers vary according to their incidence. In 1994, lung cancer was predicted to have the highest mortality rate, with 153,000 estimated deaths. Following in order were colorectal cancer (56,000 deaths), breast cancer (46,300 deaths), and prostate cancer (38,000 deaths). Table 9–1 lists estimated new cancer cases and mortality rates for 1994.

The 5-year survival rate for all cancers together is only 50%. Race and economic factors, however, affect survival rates. For example, the 5-year cancer survival rate of African Americans is only 38%; that of poor Americans, regardless of race, is 35% to 40% (ACS, 1994).

Statistics on the incidence of cancer from 1973 to 1990 are even more discouraging. Despite significant accomplishments in diagnosis and treatment, the NCI reports that the incidence of all cancers has increased by 18% and that cancer deaths have increased by 7% during these years (Beardsley, 1994; NCI, 1991). Although the incidence of stomach and uterine cancers and some leukemias has declined, the incidence of other cancers has exploded. For example, the incidence of lung cancer has increased more than 100% among women. Malignant melanoma and prostate cancer have both increased by 80%.

Cancer is still considered a disease of aging, with 66% of cancer deaths occurring after age 65 (Garfinkel, 1991). This fact has considerable significance for health care as our elderly population increases. Figure 9–1 illustrates the changes in U.S. cancer death rates from 1973 to 1990 by site and differentiated by incidence in people over and under age 65.

The Client with Cancer

■ ■ ■

Cancer is a complex disease. Hundreds of agents can contribute to its pathogenesis. There are approximately 12 major and 50 minor types of cancer, each producing its own effect on the body. Despite decades of research, cancer is still poorly understood. Before we discuss the various theories of the causes of cancer, it is useful to review how normal cells divide and adapt to changing conditions.

Normal Cell Growth

Mature normal cells are uniform in size and have nuclei characteristic of the tissue to which the cells belong. Within the nucleus of normal cells, chromosomes containing *deoxyribo11nucleic acid (DNA)* molecules carry the genetic information that control the synthesis of polypeptides (proteins). Genes are subunits of chromosomes and consist of portions of DNA that specify the production of particular sets of proteins. Thus, genes control the development of specific traits. The genetic information coded in a portion of DNA first is copied into *messenger ribonucleic acid (mRNA)*, which carries the DNA message to the

Table 9–1   Estimated New Cancer Cases and Deaths, United States—1994

	Estimated New Cases			Estimated Deaths		
	Both Sexes	**Male**	**Female**	**Both Sexes**	**Male**	**Female**
All sites	1,208,000	632,000	576,000	538,000	283,000	255,000
Buccal cavity and pharynx	29,600	19,800	9,800	7,925	5,150	2,775
Digestive organs	233,300	123,100	110,200	121,450	64,550	56,900
Respiratory system	189,000	112,800	76,200	158,200	97,900	60,300
Larynx	12,500	9,800	2,700	3,800	3,000	800
Lung	172,000	100,000	72,000	153,000	94,000	59,000
Bone	2,000	1,100	900	1,075	600	475
Connective tissue	6,000	3,300	2,700	3,300	1,600	1,700
Melanoma of skin	32,000	17,000	15,000	6,900	4,300	2,600
Breast	183,000	1,000	182,000	46,300	300	46,000
Genitals and reproductive organs	283,400	208,100	75,300	68,725	38,525	25,200
Urinary organs	78,800	55,000	23,800	21,900	13,800	8,100
Eye	1,750	950	800	250	125	125
Brain and central nervous system	17,500	9,600	7,900	12,600	6,800	5,800
Endocrine glands	14,450	4,150	10,300	1,725	750	975
Leukemia	28,600	16,200	12,400	19,100	10, 500	8,600
Other blood and lymph tissues	65,600	35,900	29,700	32,550	17,100	15,450
All other and unspecified sites	43,000	24,000	19,000	41,000	21,000	20,000

Note. From *Cancer Facts and Figures—1994,* by the American Cancer Society, 1994, Atlanta: Author.

ribosomes in the cytoplasm outside the nucleus. Next, *ribosomal RNA (rRNA)* and *transfer RNA (tRNA)* translate the genetic message and build the DNA-designated proteins. Through this process, the *genetic code* in the DNA of every gene is translated into the protein structures that determine the type, maturity, and function of a cell. Any change or disruption in a gene can result in an inaccurate "blueprint" that can produce an aberrant cell, which may then become cancerous. The box on page 309 lists some of the functions of DNA.

The Cell Cycle

The *cell cycle* consists of two distinct activity periods. During *interphase*, the cell grows, carries out its metabolic activities, and replicates all of its DNA in preparation for cell division. During *mitosis*, the cell reproduces itself.

Interphase is sometimes called the "resting phase" because the cell is not actually dividing during this stage; however, the cell is actively reproducing its interior components in preparation for cell division. Interphase consists of three subphases: G_1 *(growth 1)*, S *(synthesis)*, and

G_2 *(growth 2)*. Figure 9–2 illustrates the phases of the cell cycle and the proteins that control and promote each phase.

The length of G_1 varies according to whether the cells grow slowly or rapidly. In all cells, however, G_1 is the longest of all the phases in the cycle. This is the time of lively internal growth, heightened metabolic activity, and rapid synthesis of RNA and proteins. G_1 is considered the part of the cell cycle dedicated to achieving the specialized functions of a given cell type (Marieb, 1992). Researchers also believe that G_1 is where the cell cycle may pause when defective DNA is repaired (Research News, 1994a).

During S, the major activity is DNA synthesis, ensuring that during cell division identical copies of the DNA will go to each new cell. G_2 is the shortest part of interphase. During this interval, the cell also synthesizes proteins and enzymes needed for mitosis.

Finally, with all preparation complete, the cell begins mitosis (M). This phase culminates in the division of the parent cell into two exact copies called daughter cells, each having identical genetic material (Marieb, 1992).

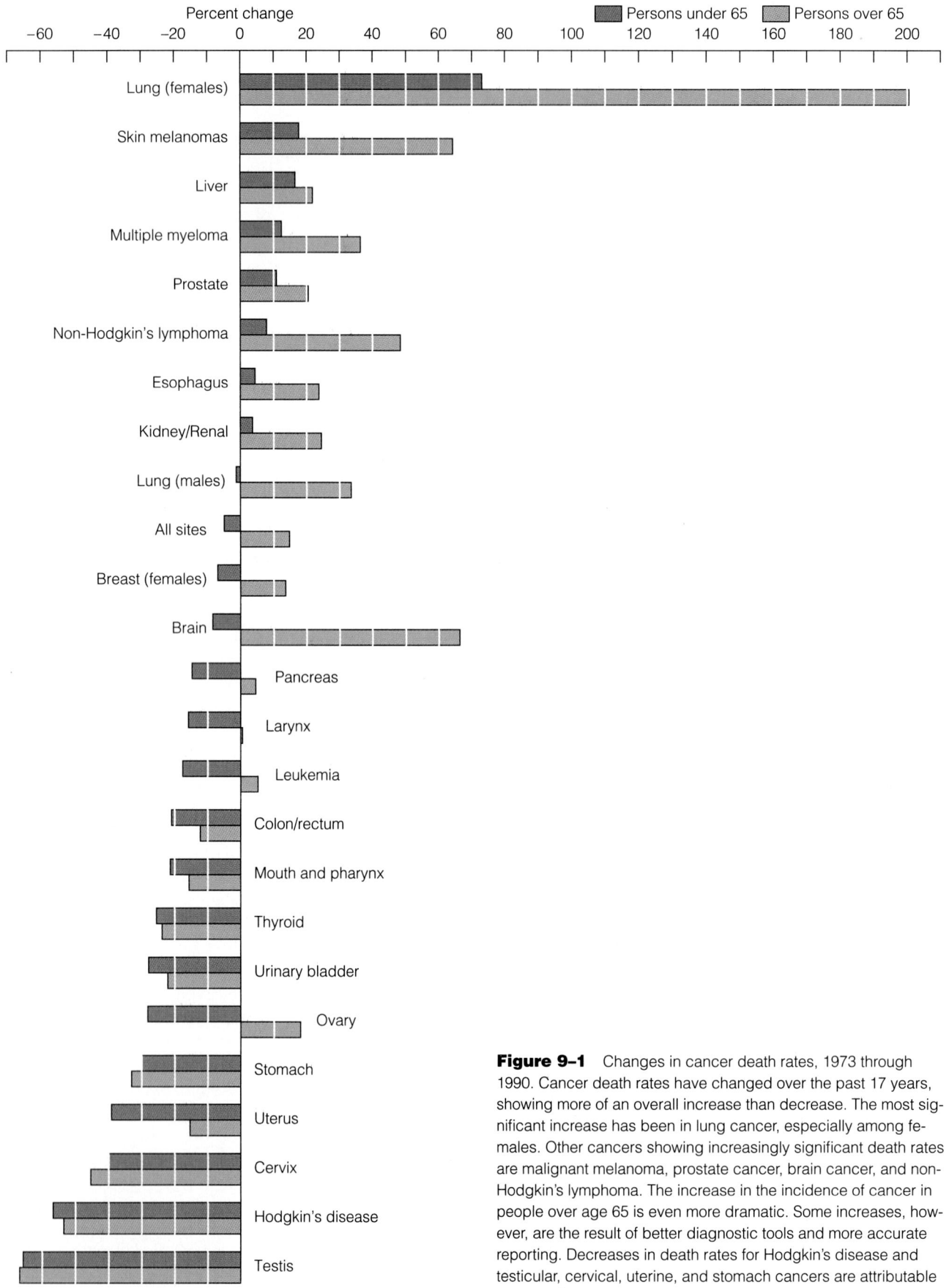

Figure 9-1 Changes in cancer death rates, 1973 through 1990. Cancer death rates have changed over the past 17 years, showing more of an overall increase than decrease. The most significant increase has been in lung cancer, especially among females. Other cancers showing increasingly significant death rates are malignant melanoma, prostate cancer, brain cancer, and non-Hodgkin's lymphoma. The increase in the incidence of cancer in people over age 65 is even more dramatic. Some increases, however, are the result of better diagnostic tools and more accurate reporting. Decreases in death rates for Hodgkin's disease and testicular, cervical, uterine, and stomach cancers are attributable to early diagnosis and more effective treatment.

Functions of DNA

■   ■   ■

- Orders production of enzymes.
- Instructs cells to produce specific chemicals.
- Instructs cells to develop specific structures.
- Determines individual traits and characteristics.
- Controls other DNA by telling a cell to "switch on" and use some portion of the genetic information stored in it.

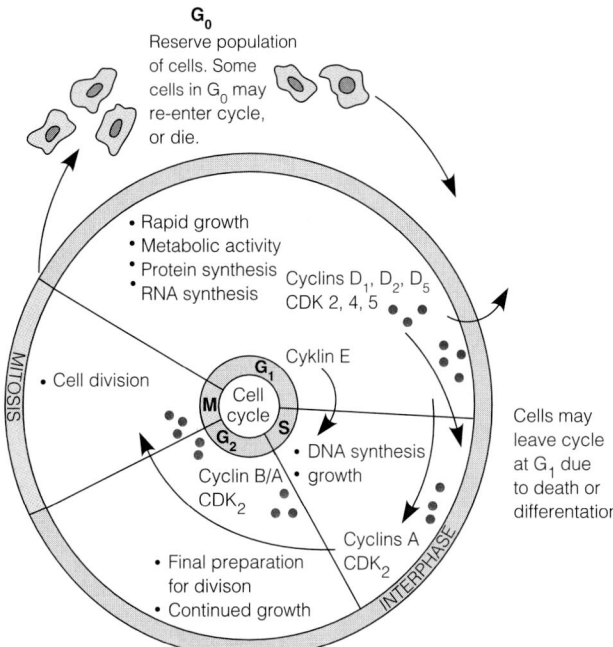

Figure 9–2   Phases of cell cycle. The cell cycle consists of two main phases: interphase and mitosis. Interphase consists of three subphases: G_1, S, and G_2. During each part of interphase, specific activities occur that contribute to cell growth and reproduction. Special proteins (CDK and cyclins) facilitate cell cycle activities and progression through each phase. During G_1, cells may leave the cycle because they have sustained irreparable damage or because they have completed differentiation. The cell cycle concludes with mitosis, the process by which two new identical cells are produced. Cells in G_0 are cells that are no longer reproducing. Although some of these cells are normal, others may be damaged and either undergoing repair or dying.

Biologists also speak of a G_0 phase. G_0 is used to denote nonproliferating cells that leave the cycle after dividing in mitosis. Their removal may be due to a mutation that needs to be repaired. Adverse conditions, such as the lack of a nutrient essential to the cells' proper development, may also cause cells to stall in the G_0 phase. Cells in G_0 do not respond to the signals that start the process of DNA synthesis. However, these cells continue to grow, make proteins, and carry out some of the differentiation functions of their particular cell type. These cells may die, or they may reenter the cycle as proliferating cells once the adverse condition is corrected. Unfortunately, some of the genetically damaged cells may not be repaired, thus giving rise to a pool of cancerous cells (Cooper & Cooper, 1991). These cells tend to hide in G_0, escaping the effects of most chemotherapy drugs. This could explain recurrence of cancers after extensive treatment.

Protein Regulators

Two groups of proteins, *cell division cycle (CDC) proteins* and *cyclins,* work together to initiate the chemical processes that produce the tasks of cell division. The cyclins received their name from the fact that their concentrations rise and fall along with the stages of the cell cycle, turning on enzymes called *cyclin-dependent kinases (CDKs)* at just the right moment. CDKs keep the cell moving through its cycle at a genetically determined rate. Thus, the cyclins, CDC proteins, and CDKs are considered the "engines" that drive growth and reproduction of the cell (Marieb, 1992; Research News, 1994a).

Several protein "brakes" have been identified that oppose the actions of the cyclins. For example, *p53* senses when DNA is damaged and stops cells from dividing until the DNA is repaired. It does this by stimulating the synthesis of another protein, *p21*, a CDK inhibitor. Another recently discovered protein, *p16*, binds to CDK-4, inhibiting cell growth. All of these proteins are encoded on and activated by the same gene (Cancer Research, 1992; Research News, 1994b).

A malfunction of any of these regulators of cell growth and division can result in the rapid proliferation of immature cells. In some cases, these cells are considered cancerous (malignant). Knowledge of cell cycle events is used in the development of chemotherapeutic drugs, which are designed to disrupt the cancer cells during different stages of their cell cycle. These drugs and their use are discussed later in the chapter. Discoveries of which genes control the promoting and inhibitory proteins of the cell cycle may spawn other new treatment modalities.

Differentiation

Differentiation is a normal process occurring over many cell cycles that allows cells to specialize in certain tasks. For example, some epithelial cells lining the lungs develop into tall columnar cells with cilia. These columnar cells sweep potentially dangerous debris out of the lungs. When adverse conditions occur in body tissues during differentiation, protective adaptations can produce alterations in cells. Some of these alterations are helpful, but in other cases the cells mutate beyond usefulness and become liabilities (Groer & Shekleton, 1989; Price & Wilson, 1992). Potentially unproductive cellular alterations occurring during cell differentiation are described below.

- **Hyperplasia** is an increase in the number or density of normal cells. Hyperplasia occurs in response to stress, increased metabolic demands, or elevated levels of hormones. Examples include the hyperplasia of myocardial cells in response to a prolonged increase in the body's demand for oxygen, and hyperplasia of uterine cells in response to rising levels of estrogen during pregnancy. Hyperplastic cells are under normal DNA control.

- **Metaplasia** is a change in the normal pattern of differentiation such that dividing cells differentiate into cell types not normally found in that location in the body. The metaplastic cell is normal for its particular type, but it is not in its normal location. Some metaplastic cells are less functional than the cells they replace. Metaplasia is a protective response to adverse conditions. Metaplastic cells are under normal DNA control and are reversible when the stressor or other disruptive condition ceases.

  One example of metaplasia occurs in the bronchial epithelium. Normal columnar ciliated cells are replaced by stratified squamous cells in response to inhaled pollutants, primarily cigarette smoke. The metaplastic squamous cells are more resistant to injury, but they lack cilia and the mucus-secreting function. These cells revert to normal when the irritant is removed but can eventually become cancerous if the person continues to smoke.

- **Dysplasia** represents a loss of DNA control over differentiation occurring in response to adverse conditions. Dysplastic cells show an abnormal degree of variation in size, shape, and appearance and a disturbance in the usual arrangement. Examples of dysplasia include changes in the cervix in response to continued irritation, such as from the human papillomavirus (HPV), or leukoplakia on oral mucous membranes in response to chronic irritation from smoking.

- **Anaplasia** is the regression of a cell to an immature or undifferentiated cell type. Anaplastic cell division is no longer under DNA control. Anaplasia usually occurs when a damaging or transforming event takes place inside the dividing, still undifferentiated cell. This results in a partial or complete interruption in the developmental pathway leading to full differentiation for future generations of the cell. Anaplasia may occur in response to overwhelmingly destructive conditions inside the cell or in surrounding tissue (Templeton & Weinberg, 1991).

Although hyperplasia, metaplasia, and dysplasia often reverse after the irritating factor is eliminated, they can lead to malignancy under certain conditions. This is especially true of dysplasia, which represents a loss of DNA control. Anaplasia is not reversible, but the degree of anaplasia determines the potential risk for cancer.

Etiology

The precise etiology of cancer is unknown. However, intensive research efforts during the past several decades has led to a cluster of increasingly credible and interrelated theories. In addition, research has identified numerous cancer-causing agents, or **carcinogens,** that may contribute to the development of the disease.

Although cancer research in the last two decades has brought new options for cancer treatment and improved clients' overall survival rate, it may have caused the perception that if a person gets cancer, it is somehow his or her "fault." Almost daily, people hear of research studies indicating that certain foods, habits, or environmental factors may cause cancer. Although much of this is true and is inspiring a welcome preventive focus to health care, it is not true that one can determine the specific factors that cause cancer in any individual. Seldom are people informed that genetic structure plays a prominent role in the strength of a person's immune system and his or her ability to destroy early cancerous cells. Nor are people told that the advances in medical treatment, which have eliminated many bacterial diseases (such as the plague), may be responsible for the unchecked proliferation of viruses implicated in the alteration of cellular DNA, which can be a precursor to cancer.

Although taking responsibility for one's own health is a positive step, it may have a negative result if clients feel so guilty and blameworthy that they fail to seek out early and appropriate health care. Also, clients who feel that their bodies have failed them may become depressed, and such feelings can impair the functioning of an already stressed immune system. People who feel responsible for having developed cancer can put their guilt in perspective by noting that most cancers result from a complex interaction between multiple environmental (exogenous) and host (endogenous) factors.

Theories of Carcinogenesis

Cellular Mutation   One theory suggests that carcinogens cause mutations in cellular DNA. It is believed that the carcinogenic process has two stages: *initiation* and *promotion.*

Initiation is a brief, but irreversible, interaction between a carcinogen and predisposed cells. A predisposed cell is one in which normal nucleic acids are altered, causing transformation of the cell into the first stage of a precancerous cell type. As the cell undergoes mitosis, this altered DNA is then incorporated into daughter cells. However, this event does not cause concern unless the cells or tissues are acted on by a promoter.

Promoters are agents that cause irreversibly initiated cells to grow and produce a tumor. However, promoters do not in themselves cause mutation and are therefore not considered carcinogenic. Promoters must be in continuous contact with the initiated cells to exert their cancer-generating effect. If the promoter is removed, its harmful effects often can be reversed. For example, when an individual quits smoking, the dozens of promoter substances in the smoke are slowly removed from the lungs, and the risk for lung cancer diminishes yearly.

A latent period occurs between the initiating event that damages the DNA and the manifestation of a tumor. The latent period may be as long as 10 to 20 years, a fact that may explain the tendency for many cancers to occur in older adults. Also, some researchers believe it takes at least five generations of mutant cells to result in enough damage to produce a cancer (Cohen, 1987; Rosenberg, 1992).

The Role of Oncogenes   Most cancer researchers believe that all cells in the body have **oncogenes**, which are genes capable of triggering cancerous characteristics. Normally, the actions of oncogenes are repressed. Adverse cellular conditions caused by invading viruses or other carcinogens may "switch on" a cell's oncogenes. Once activated, oncogenes produce proteins that accelerate the cell's rate of multiplication, heighten its responsiveness to growth hormones, and enable it to invade other tissues (Rosenberg, 1992).

Some normal genes are *proto-oncogenes*. These benign forms of oncogenes are necessary for some normal cellular functions, especially growth and development. However, proto-oncogenes are fragile; when exposed to carcinogens, they are easily damaged and mutate into oncogenes (Research News, 1994a).

Immune Response Failure   Some of the latest cancer research indicates that oncogenes may be remnants of embryonic cells that were not suppressed during fetal growth and development. In support of this theory, researchers point out that the human zygote displays many characteristics of a cancerous cell. It is aggressively invasive, sets up its own vascular network, takes nutrients from the host (mother) irrespective of the host's needs, and grows very rapidly. Thus, researchers have advanced the theory that oncogenes are normally active only during embryonic life. After birth, they are held in check by the body's T lymphocytes, a class of white blood cells of the immune system (Templeton & Weinberg, 1991).

The expression of oncogenes may be allowed by a decrease in the body's immune surveillance, which can oc-

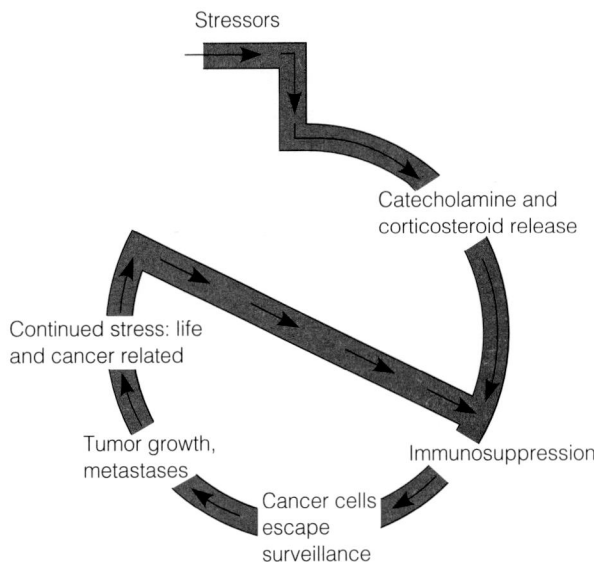

Figure 9–3   Relationship of stress to immunosuppression and continued cancer growth. After the cancer and emotional or other stressors have put increased pressure on the body's ability to respond physiologically to stress, the organism can no longer produce enough stress hormones to keep the body fighting the cancer. This causes a pattern of immunosuppression and increased cancer growth that continues unless it is interrupted by effective therapy or until the organism succumbs to the disease.

cur during times of stress or in response to certain carcinogens. For example, clients with acquired immune deficiency syndrome (AIDS), who have a decreased number of helper T lymphocytes, have a much higher than normal incidence of certain cancers, including non-Hodgkin's lymphoma and Kaposi's sarcoma (Groer & Shekleton, 1989). Figure 9–3 shows the relationship of stress to immunosuppression.

Furthermore, some researchers suspect that cancerous cells normally form continuously within the body. The healthy immune system recognizes these cells as "foreign" and develops tumor-specific immunoglobulins to destroy them. Only when a tumor is able to escape immune surveillance can it take hold and grow. It is thought that aberrant cells escape immune surveillance because their surfaces lack the proteins called human leukocyte antigens (HLA) that normally serve to help lymphocytes identify invaders to be destroyed. It is believed that certain oncogenic viruses reduce the expression of HLA markers in the altered cells (Herberman, 1991).

Finally, people who are immunocompromised, from whatever cause, experience a much greater incidence of cancer than the population as a whole. A competent immune response ensures that cancer cell destruction exceeds proliferation (Nossal, 1993).

Cancers Associated with Different Viruses

■ ■ ■

Herpes Simplex Virus Types I and II (HSV-1 and HSV-2)

- Carcinoma of the lip
- Cervical carcinoma
- Kaposi's sarcoma

Human Cytomegalovirus (HCMV)

- Kaposi's sarcoma
- Prostate cancer

Epstein-Barr Virus (EBV)

- Burkitt's lymphoma

Human Herpesvirus-6 (HHV-6)

- Lymphoma

Hepatitis B Virus (HBV)

- Primary hepatocellular cancer

Papillomavirus

- Malignant melanoma
- Cervical, penile, and laryngeal cancers

Human T-lymphotropic Viruses (HTLV)

- Adult T-cell leukemia and lymphoma
- T-cell variant of hairy-cell leukemia
- Kaposi's sarcoma

Derangements in Cell Cycle Machinery Investigators in cancer research are beginning to speculate that altered functioning of the cell cycle machinery may be the culprit in the development of many common cancers. Newly discovered mutations, defects, or absences of those genes that produce the proteins that inhibit cell growth—p53, p21, and p16—have been implicated in many common cancers. In addition, the genes for several of the cyclins are believed to be oncogenic. For example, excessive production of cyclin D1 commits the cell to DNA synthesis and division without further stimulus, resulting in the uncontrolled, rapid reproduction characteristic of malignant cells. Other cyclins are also capable of malfunction: D2 and D3, which block cell differentiation; E, which interferes with contact inhibition; and A, which promotes

the ability of cells to grow without being anchored to a surface. These discoveries have the potential for unlocking many of the mysteries of cancer biology. Researchers believe that derangement of the cell cycle machinery from the loss of inhibitor proteins such as p16 and p21, in combination with excessive production of the mutated, oncogenic cyclins, powerfully tips the balance in favor of developing a cancerous cell. These discoveries may lead to innovative ways to treat cancer as well as providing tumor "markers" that aid in diagnosis and prognosis (Cancer Research, 1992; Herberman, 1991; Research News, 1994a; Research News, 1994b).

Central to all these theories are two important concepts about the etiology of cancer. First, damaged DNA, whether inherited or from external sources, sets up the necessary initial step for cancer to occur. Second, impairment of the human immune system, from whatever cause, lessens its ability to destroy abnormal cells.

Known Carcinogens

A number of agents are known to cause cancer, or at least are strongly linked to certain kinds of cancers. These known carcinogens include viruses, drugs, hormones, and chemical and physical agents.

Carcinogens can be categorized in two groups: *Genotoxic* carcinogens directly alter DNA and cause mutations, and *promoter* substances cause other adverse biologic effects, such as cytotoxicity, hormonal imbalances, altered immunity, or chronic tissue damage. Promoter substances (which some researchers believe are not carcinogenic) do not cause cancer in the absence of previous cell damage (initiation) and often require high-level and long-term contact with the altered cells. Table 9–2 lists examples of genotoxic and promoter substances.

It should be noted that although everyone comes into contact with a vast number of substances that are considered carcinogenic, not everyone develops cancer. Other factors, such as genetic predisposition, impairment of the immune response, and repeated exposure to the carcinogen are all necessary for a cancer to develop.

Viruses Certain viruses can cause cancer by modifying the genes of the cells they invade. Retroviruses (viruses having genetic machinery composed of RNA, not DNA) make DNA copies of their own RNA by taking over a cell's DNA synthesis machinery. This viral DNA copy then enters a gene, making it a *virogene* (a normal gene containing a copy of a viral gene). The virogene may remain dormant for many years until activated. Several common viruses have been implicated as virogenes and have been associated with a variety of tumors. The human herpesvirus, varicella-zoster virus (VZV), has produced malignancies in laboratory studies but has not yet been associated with any human malignancy. The accompanying box identifies these viruses and the cancers they cause.

Table 9–2	Chemical Carcinogens and Relationship to Occupation	
Chemical Agent	**Action**	**Occupation Affected**
Polycyclic hydrocarbons (smoke, soot, tobacco, smoked foods) Benzopyrene	Genotoxic	Miners, coal gas workers, chimney sweeps, migrant workers, workers in offices where smoking is allowed in closed areas
Arsenic	Genotoxic	Pesticide manufacturers
Vinyl chloride polymers	Promotional	Plastics workers Artists
Methylaminobenzine	Genotoxic	Fabric workers Rubber and glue workers
Asbestos	Promotional	Construction workers, workers in old, run-down buildings with asbestos insulation, insulation makers
Wood and leather dust	Promotional	Woodworkers, carpenters, leather toolers
Chemotherapy drugs	Genotoxic	Drug manufacturers, pharmacists, nurses

In addition, viruses play a significant role in weakening immunologic defenses against neoplasms. For example, the human immunodeficiency virus (HIV), which infects helper T lymphocytes and monocytes, impairs the person's protection against certain cancers such as lymphoma and Kaposi's sarcoma.

Other viruses have also been associated with human malignancies. Hepatitis B virus (HBV) integrates its DNA with liver cell DNA and is believed to cause primary hepatocellular carcinoma. Papillomaviruses cause plantar, common, and flat warts, which are benign and usually regress spontaneously. However, they also cause genital warts and laryngeal papillomas, and they are associated with malignant melanoma and cervical, penile, and laryngeal cancers. The human T-lymphotropic viruses (HTLV) have been associated with adult T-cell leukemia and lymphoma as well as a T-cell variant of hairy-cell leukemia.

Although the role of viruses such as hepatitis B, Epstein-Barr virus, papillomaviruses, and human T-lymphotropic viruses (including HIV) is now firmly established, herpesviruses are still only suspected cancer causers. With the exception of hepatitis B, vaccines to prevent virus-induced cancers are still many years away. Because a long latency period may take place before tumors develop, it is difficult to evaluate the safety and effectiveness of potential vaccines (Rapp, 1991).

Drugs and Hormones Certain drugs can be either genotoxic or promotional. For example, chemotherapeutic drugs used to disrupt the cell cycle of malignant cells can be genotoxic for normal cells. They can also be promotional: By drastically reducing the number of leukocytes, they impair immune function. Examples of these chemotherapeutic drugs include busulfan, chlorambucil, and cycloposphamide. Some recreational drugs also are

implicated as carcinogens. These include the genotoxic betel nut chewed by many Pacific Islanders and the immunosuppressant promoters heroin and cocaine.

Hormones are also potential genotoxic carcinogens or promoters. Cancers of the reproductive organs are often mediated by gonadotropic hormones. Estrogen, both natural and synthetic, and diethylstilbestrol (DES) have been linked to cervical, endometrial, and breast cancers. Estrogen-containing contraceptive pills have been implicated in breast cancer, but they also have been shown to decrease the risk of ovarian cancer. Investigators have not reached a final conclusion as to the cancer risk posed by contraceptives. Newer research suggests that alterations in the molecular structure of testosterone in older men may be promotional in the development of prostate cancer. Also, glucocorticosteroids (cortisone) and anabolic steroids may act as promoters by altering the immune response or endocrine balance (Bostwick, 1990; Drago, 1990; Garnick, 1994; Gusberg & Runowicz, 1991; Zimny, 1991).

Chemical Agents Many chemicals have been demonstrated to be both genotoxic and promotional. Because many of these substances are encountered in the workplace, they constitute occupational hazards, which are discussed more thoroughly below. Examples of industrial and environmental carcinogens include polycyclic hydrocarbons, found in soot; benzopyrene, found in cigarette smoke; and arsenic, found in pesticides. These chemicals all have some genotoxic action; some alter DNA replication. Other industrial and environmental chemicals are considered promotional agents. These include wood and leather dust, polymer esters (used in plastics and paints), carbon tetrachloride, asbestos, and phenol.

Natural substances in the body may also be carcinogenic or promotional. For example, end products of metabolism that are produced in excess amounts and/or are ineffectively eliminated, such as bile acids from a high-fat diet, may promote cancer.

Some foods contain carcinogens that are added during preparation or preservation. Examples include the sugar substitute sodium saccharine and nitrosamines and nitrosindoles, which are found in pickled, salted foods. In some cases, food contaminants produce carcinogenic chemicals. Aflatoxin, a very potent carcinogen, is produced by the *Aspergillus* fungi. These organisms grow on improperly stored vegetable products, such as grains and peanuts.

Polycyclic aromatic hydrocarbons, nitrosamines, phenols, and other chemicals in tobacco act as either carcinogens or promoters of cancer. Table 9–2 lists the various genotoxic and promotional chemicals and gives examples of occupations affected by exposure to these chemicals.

Physical Agents   It has been well documented that excessive exposure to radiation causes increased rates of cancer by damaging the DNA in cells, by activating other oncogenetic factors, or by suppressing antitumor activity (protein inhibitors). Both solar radiation from ultraviolet rays and ionizing radiation from industrial or medical sources are carcinogenic. This fact has implications for workers exposed to these agents and for the population in general. Radon, a naturally formed radioactive gas found in the basements of many homes, is also a known carcinogen. People who have lived in areas where nuclear weapons testing has been carried out or whose ground water has been polluted by nuclear wastes are at risk for developing cancers. The worst known case of radiation poisoning and subsequent cancer development occurred at the end of World War II, when the atomic bomb was dropped on Nagasaki and Hiroshima. Many who survived the initial explosion later developed leukemia. There is also evidence that offspring of these survivors have suffered from significantly higher levels of cancer, suggesting that the radiation from these blasts also damaged survivors' reproductive cells.

Risk Factors

Risk factors make an individual or a population vulnerable to a specific disease or other unhealthy outcome. Risk factors can be divided into those that are controllable and those that are not controllable. Knowledge and assessment of risk factors are especially important in counseling clients and families about measures to prevent cancer.

Noncontrollable Risk Factors

Heredity   Inherited genetic defects are being identified as instrumental in the initiation of cancer (Blakeslee, 1994). It has been known for some time that breast and colon cancers tend to have a familial pattern, but for most

cancers, research has not yet distinguished true genetic transfer from environmental causes. One study did discover the absence of the gene for the tumor suppressor protein p21 in a woman with multiple episodes of malignant melanoma. To verify this finding, the investigators are now studying large families in Utah who have demonstrated familial melanoma (Cancer Research, 1992). So although much research is still needed to conclude that the inheritance of defective genes causes cancer, familial predisposition to certain diseases and malignancies should be counted among risk factors so that people at risk can reduce promotional behaviors. For example, a client who has a family history of lung cancer should be counseled to avoid smoking, to avoid areas where smoking is allowed, and to avoid working in an occupation that may expose the client to inhaled carcinogens.

Age   Approximately 66% of all cancers occur in people over age 65. A variety of factors is involved in this increased risk in older adults. One possible factor, as noted previously, is that at least five cycles of genetic mutations seem necessary to cause permanent damage to the afflicted cells. In addition, long-term exposure to high doses of promotional agents is usually necessary to allow the cancer to take hold. Also, evidence indicates that the immune response is altered with aging; the actions of the immune response become more generalized and less specific. Another problem is that *free radicals* (molecules resulting from the body's metabolic and oxidative processes) tend to accumulate in the cells over time, causing damage and mutation.

Hormonal changes that occur with aging can be associated with cancer. Postmenopausal women receiving exogenous estrogen have an increased risk for breast and uterine cancers. Older men are at risk for prostate cancer, possibly due to breakdown of testosterone into carcinogenic forms. See the accompanying box for a discussion about cancer and older adults.

Finally, severe and/or cumulative losses are implicated in promoting cancer. These losses, which are common to older adults, include the death of a spouse or friends, loss of position and status in society, and diminishment of physical abilities. (Rosenberg, 1992; Schuster & Ashburn, 1986; Selye, 1984).

Gender   Gender is a risk factor for certain types of cancer, rather than for acquiring cancer in general. For example, thyroid cancer occurs more commonly among females, whereas bladder cancer is seen more often among male clients. Chapters 46 and 47 provide more information on gender-specific cancers.

Poverty   Cancer statistics show that the poor are at higher risk for cancer than the population in general. Inadequate access to health care, especially preventive screening and counseling, may be a major factor. Although some of the other factors that may be involved,

Gerontologic Considerations: Clients with Cancer

■ ■ ■

Nurses need to be aware of how cancer and cancer treatments affect older adults. Cancer is the second leading cause of death in people over age 65. The incidence of cancer increases with advancing age, probably as a result of the accumulated exposure to carcinogens and to age-related declines in the action of the immune system. The most commonly seen cancers in older women are colorectal, breast, lung, pancreatic and ovarian. In older men, lung, colorectal, prostate, pancreatic and gastric cancers occur most frequently.

The importance of screening and early detection of cancer does not diminish with age. Unfortunately, many older adults do not receive adequate cancer screening. Because the older adult is closer to the end of life, some health care providers may believe that cancer screening is not as important as it is for the younger client. This attitude may result in delayed diagnosis and treatment.

Older adults may not participate in screening programs or seek treatment for cancer due to fear, depression, cognitive impairments, poor access to health care, or financial constraints. Some older adults (and healthcare providers) mistake cancer symptoms for normal age-related changes. Believing that little can be done, they do not seek healthcare for their symptoms. Fear of the cancer diagnosis also keeps older adults from seeking appropriate health care. When they do seek treatment, chronic conditions frequently seen in older adults may make the diagnosis of cancer more difficult by masking or confounding the usual symptoms associated with cancer.

Older adults are at greater risk for side-effects associated with cancer treatment because of age-related physiologic changes and chronic conditions associated with aging. This is particularly true for the side-effects of chemotherapeutic agents. Older adults have increased incidence of cardiotoxicity and toxicity of the central nervous system when undergoing chemotherapy than younger adults. The side-effects of chemotherapy can contribute to fatigue and cause problems related to immobility and functional decline. Alterations in the function of the immune system are also more frequent in older adults, which increases their risk for developing infection.

The problems associated with chemotherapy do not rule out its use, but the nurse must be aware of potential problems and monitor the client closely for the development of side-effects. The nurse needs to consider how the aging process will alter the response to the disease and treatment plan when planning care for older adults.

Client and Family Teaching

- Discuss the warning signs of cancer.
- Stress the importance of seeking health care, if any of the warning signs develop.
- Get an annual physical examination.
- For women, learn how to perform a breast self-exam and perform the exam every month.
- For men, undergo Prostate-specific antigen (PSA) screening for prostate cancer.

---

such as diet and stress, usually come under the category of controllable risks, these risks are frequently uncontrollable in this population.

Controllable Risk Factors

Stress Continuous unmanaged stress that keeps hormones, such as epinephrine and cortisol, at high levels can result in systematic "fatigue" and impaired immunologic surveillance. When the body attempts to adapt to physiologic and psychologic stressors, it goes through a series of stages called the general adaptation syndrome (GAS) (Seyle, 1984). First, the "alarm reaction" occurs, in which adrenal hormones increase, allowing the body to

cope with the stressor. Eventually, the body reaches the "stage of resistance," in which the stress hormones are significantly reduced, indicating that adaptation has occurred. If the physiologic adaptation is supported by appropriate coping strategies, the stressor is considered managed and body systems return to the prealarm functioning. However, if adaptation continues and the stress hormones remain elevated, the "stage of exhaustion" sets in. This stage will maintain life, but at great expense to body systems, resulting in general wear-and-tear as well as depression of the immune system (Seyle, 1984).

The literature mentions a type C, or "cancer personality," describing people who have unhealthy coping behaviors for life stressors. Type C people are identified as those who tend to others' needs to the exclusion of their own and who rarely ask for help or support, even in personal crises. These people tend to be emotionally, and sometimes even physically, isolated and have a great deal of buried, unexpressed anger. It is thought that this kind of behavior pattern has a harmful effect on the immune system over time, promoting vulnerability to cancer. Depression is also considered a major risk factor, especially depression that is chronic or related to multiple or major losses. Depression and hopelessness tend to shut down the energizing chemicals in the body and depress immune responses (Pasquali, Arnold, DeBasio, & Gorthey, 1985).

Diet   As previously mentioned, some foods are considered genotoxic, for example, the nitrosamines and nitrosindoles that are found in preserved meats and pickled, salted foods. Migrant workers have been found to have a high incidence of esophageal and gastric cancers related to their excessive consumption of these items. Other foods, such as high-fat, low-fiber foods—the mainstay of many Americans' diets—promote colon, breast, and sex hormone–dependent tumors. When fish and meat are excessively fried or broiled, potent carcinogenic compounds can form that may cause tumors in the mammary glands, colon, liver, pancreas, and bladder. Also, the repeated use of fat to fry foods at high temperatures produces high levels of polycyclic hydrocarbons, thereby increasing cancer risk considerably. Although many people profess to have changed their dietary habits, one only has to observe the large number of people who still lunch on cheeseburgers and french fries (and who teach their children to do the same) to realize that much more educational and motivational work is needed in this area. Other food-related substances that are believed to increase cancer risk include sodium saccharine, red food dyes, and both regular and decaffeinated coffee.

Occupation   Occupational risk can probably be considered either controllable or uncontrollable. For many people, their choice of occupation is limited by education and ability; during times of high unemployment, moreover, changing one's occupation because it poses risk factors may not be a viable option. Federal standards are designed to protect workers from hazardous substances, but many feel that these standards are not strict enough and inspections not frequent enough to prevent violations.

Specific risks vary according to the occupation. For example, outdoor workers, such as farmers and construction workers, are exposed to solar radiation; health care workers, such as X-ray technicians and biomedical researchers, are exposed to ionizing radiation and carcinogenic substances; and exposure to asbestos is a problem for people who work in old buildings with asbestos insulation in the walls. Table 9–2 correlates known carcinogens and occupations.

Infection   Because a number of viruses have been linked to some cancers, avoiding those specific infections will decrease risk. Although some infections may be unavoidable (Epstein-Barr, for example), others, such as genital herpes and papillomavirus-induced genital warts, can often be avoided by following safer-sex practices (e.g., the use of condoms).

Tobacco Use   Lung cancer is considered highly preventable because of the relationship of smoking and lung cancer. In addition, the carcinogenic substances in tobacco that are genotoxic are considered weak; therefore, stopping smoking can reverse the damage. However, many other substances in tobacco are highly promotional, so that the larger the dose and longer the use, the higher the risk for developing cancer. Longitudinal research has shown that the level of risk for a person who quits smoking will drop to that of a nonsmoker after 20 years of nonsmoking (Von Houtte, Salazar, Phillips, & Ashbury, 1983).

Tobacco is also related to other forms of cancer. Smokers face an increased risk for oropharyngeal, esophageal, laryngeal, gastric, pancreatic, and bladder cancers. Pipe and cigar smokers are especially susceptible to oropharyngeal and laryngeal cancers. Oral and esophageal cancers are increased among those who chew tobacco or use snuff. Smokers who have a genetic decrease in alpha-1 antitripsin (an enzyme that protects lung tissue) that results in emphysema face an even higher cancer risk than smokers without this defect.

More recent research has documented the deleterious effects of secondhand tobacco smoke. Tobacco-specific nitrosamines were recovered in the urine of children living with smokers. It is now accepted that nonsmokers who are exposed to tobacco smoke over long periods of time, whether in the workplace or the home, have an increased risk for lung or bladder cancers.

Alcohol Use   Alcohol acts as a promoter by modifying the metabolism of carcinogens in the liver and esophagus, thus increasing the effectiveness of the carcinogens in some tissues. People who both smoke and drink a considerable amount of alcohol daily have an increased risk for oral, esophageal, and laryngeal cancers.

Use of Recreational Drugs   Recreational drug use often promotes an unhealthy life-style that increases general cancer risk; for example, drug users often do not maintain adequate nutrition. Furthermore, recreational drugs are implicated as promoters because of their suppressive effect on the immune system. Although it has not been directly implicated in cancer development, marijuana has been demonstrated to cause chromosomal damage that may over time also result in cancer-causing DNA damage and genetic mutations. Marijuana smoke is also much more injurious to lung tissue than tobacco smoke.

Obesity Excessive body fat has been linked to an increased risk of hormone-dependent cancers. Because sex hormones are synthesized from fat, obese people often have excessive amounts of the hormones that feed hormone-dependent malignancies of the breast, bowel, ovary, endometrium, and prostate.

Sun Exposure As the protective ozone layer thins, more of the sun's damaging ultraviolet radiation reaches the earth. As a consequence, the rate of skin cancers has increased. Sun-related skin cancers are now considered to be a problem for all people, regardless of skin color, but people of Northern European extraction with very fair skin, blue or green eyes, and light-colored hair are most vulnerable. Elderly people with decreased pigment are also more at risk, even those with darker skin.

Figure 9–4 summarizes the interaction of factors that promote cancer.

Pathophysiology

Benign and Malignant Neoplasms

A **neoplasm** is a mass of new tissue (a collection of cells) that grows independently of its surrounding structures and has no physiologic purpose. The term *neoplasm* is often used interchangeably with *tumor*, from the Latin word meaning "swelling." Neoplasms are said to be autonomous because

- They grow at a rate uncoordinated with the needs of the body.
- They function independently of usual homeostatic controls.
- They share some of the properties of the parent cells but with altered size and shape.
- They do not benefit the host and in some cases are actively harmful.

Neoplasms are not completely autonomous, however, because they require a blood supply with nutrients and oxygen to sustain their growth. Neoplasms typically are classified as benign or malignant on the basis of their potential to damage the body and on their growth characteristics.

Benign Neoplasms *Benign neoplasms* are localized growths. They are cohesive (that is, they form a solid mass), have well-defined borders, and frequently are encapsulated. Benign neoplasms tend to respond to the body's homeostatic controls. Thus, they often stop growing when they reach the boundaries of another tissue (a process called *contact inhibition*). They grow slowly and often remain stable in size. Because they are usually encapsulated, benign neoplasms often are easily removed and tend not to recur.

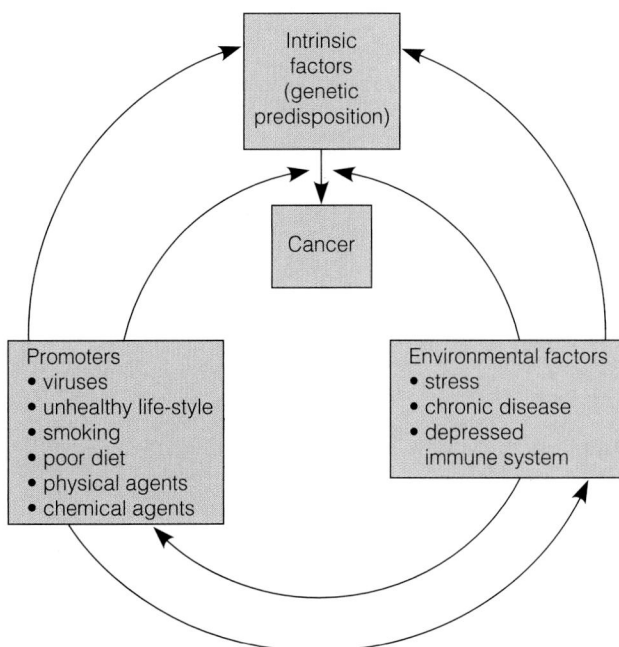

Figure 9–4 Interaction of factors that promote cancer. Most people have immune systems that are competent enough to resist the establishment of cancer from an initiated cell. Cancer takes hold when a number of promotional factors occur together and over enough time to weaken immune resistance. Like factors are grouped together for ease of presentation but may occur in any combination.

Although typically harmless, benign neoplasms nevertheless can be destructive if they crowd surrounding tissue and obstruct the function of organs. For example, a benign meningioma (from the meninges of the brain and spinal cord) can cause severely increased intracranial pressure (ICP), which progressively impairs the person's cerebral function. Unless the meningioma can be successfully removed, the steadily rising ICP will eventually lead to coma and death.

Malignant Neoplasms In contrast to benign neoplasms, *malignant neoplasms* grow aggressively and do not respond to the body's homeostatic controls. Malignant neoplasms are not cohesive, and they present with an irregular shape. Instead of slowly crowding other tissues aside, malignant neoplasms cut through surrounding tissues, causing bleeding, inflammation, and necrosis (tissue death) as they grow. This invasive quality of malignant neoplasms is reflected in the word origin of *cancer*, from the Greek *karkinos*, meaning "crab." When health care professionals use the term *cancer*, they are referring to a malignant neoplasm.

Malignant cells may break away from the primary tumor, traveling through the blood or lymph to invade other tissues and organs of the body and form a secondary tumor called a **metastasis**. This term also refers to

Table 9–3	Comparison of Benign and Malignant Neoplasms
Benign	**Malignant**
Local	Invasive
Cohesive	Noncohesive
Well-defined borders	Does not stop at tissue border
Pushes other tissues out of the way	Invades and destroys surrounding tissues
Slow growth	Rapid growth
Encapsulated	Metastasizes to distant sites
Easily removed	Not always easy to remove
Does not recur	Can recur

Characteristics of Malignant Cells
∎ ∎ ∎

- Loss of regulation of mitotic rate
- Loss of cell specialization
- Loss of contact inhibition
- Progressive acquisition of the cancerous phenotype and immortality
- Irreversibility of cancerous phenotype to greater aggressiveness
- Altered cell structure: differences in cell nucleus and cytoplasm
- Simplified metabolic activity
- Transplantability (metastasis)
- Ability to promote own survival

the process by which such spreading of malignant neoplasms—perhaps their most destructive trait—occurs. Malignant neoplasms can recur after surgical removal of the primary and secondary tumors and after other treatments. Table 9–3 compares benign and malignant neoplasms.

Malignant neoplasms vary in their degree of differentiation from the parent tissue. Highly differentiated cancer cells try to mimic the specialized function of the parent tissue, but undifferentiated cancers, consisting of immature cells, have almost no resemblance to the parent tissue and so perform no useful function. To make matters worse, undifferentiated cancers rob the body of its energy and nutrition as they grow. Undifferentiated anaplastic cells have little structural or functional relationship to the parent cells and are the basis of many malignant neoplasms. The degree of differentiation of anaplastic cells is a consideration in the classification and staging of neoplasms, discussed later in this chapter.

Characteristics of Malignant Cells

Malignant neoplasms may be identified by a number of predictable cellular characteristics:

- *Loss of regulation of the rate of mitosis.* This results in rapid cell division and growth of the neoplasm.
- *Loss of specialization and differentiation.* Malignant cells do not perform typical cellular functions. Many do produce hormones and enzymes similar to those of the parent tissue, but usually in excessive amounts, possibly revealing their presence.
- *Loss of contact inhibition.* Malignant cells do not respect other cellular boundaries. They easily invade and destroy other tissues.
- *Progressive acquisition of a cancerous phenotype.* Cellular mutation seems to be a sequential process involving

successive generations of cells, each generation becoming more deviant than the one before. Additionally, malignant cells seem to be "immortal"; that is, they do not stop growing and die as do normal cells, which have a genetically determined life span.

- *Irreversibility.* The transformation into a malignant cell is irreversible. Rarely does a malignant neoplasm revert to a benign state.
- *Altered cell structure.* Cytologic examination of malignant cells reveals distinct differences in the cell nucleus and cytoplasm as well as an overall cell shape that differs from that of normal cells of the particular tissue type.
- *Simplified metabolic activities.* The work of malignant cells is simpler than that of normal cells; they show an increased synthesis of substances needed for cell division, and they have no need to create proteins for the specialized functions of the tissues they invade.
- *Transplantability.* Malignant cells often break away from the primary tissue site and travel to other locations in the body, where they establish new growths.
- *Ability to promote their own survival.* Malignant cells may create ectopic sites to produce the hormones they need for their growth. By their very presence and their ability to initiate vascular permeability, malignant cells promote the development of nonneoplastic *stroma*, a connective tissue framework consisting of collagen and other components, which then supports the neoplasm. They may also create their own blood supply: tumor cells secrete a polypeptide *angiogenic growth factor* that stimulates blood vessels from surrounding normal tissue to grow into the tumor. Finally, malignant cells divert nutrition from the host to meet their own

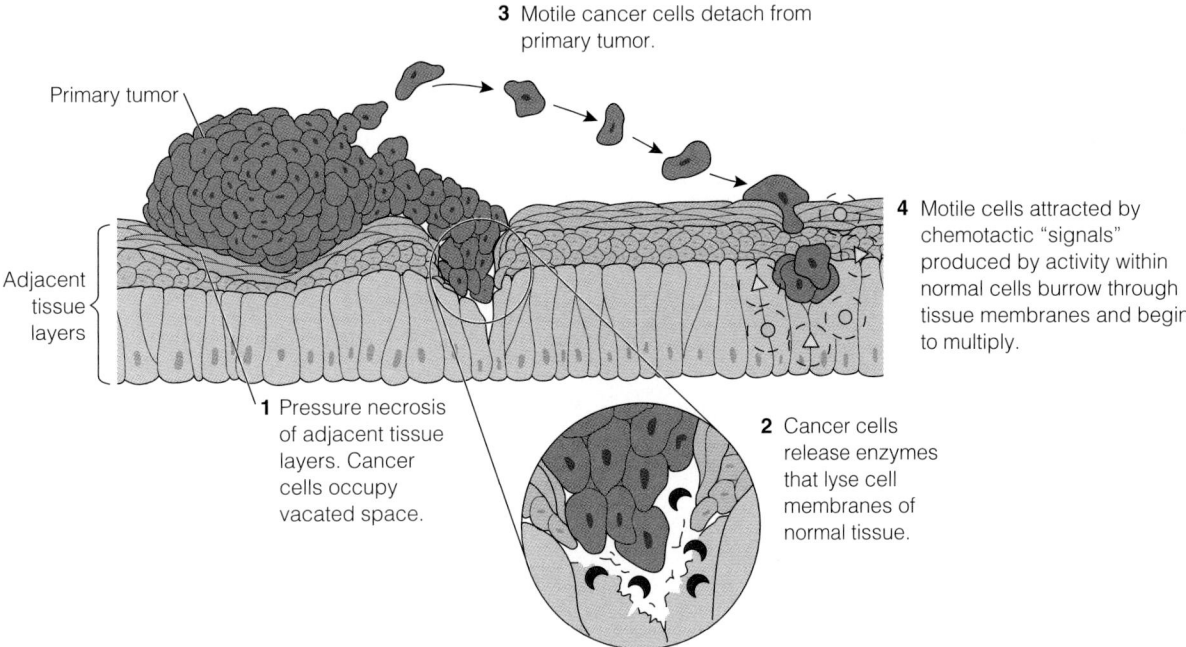

3 Motile cancer cells detach from primary tumor.

Primary tumor

Adjacent tissue layers

1 Pressure necrosis of adjacent tissue layers. Cancer cells occupy vacated space.

2 Cancer cells release enzymes that lyse cell membranes of normal tissue.

4 Motile cells attracted by chemotactic "signals" produced by activity within normal cells burrow through tissue membranes and begin to multiply.

Figure 9–5   How cancer cells invade normal tissue.

needs, by diffusion when the tumor is less than 1 mm and thereafter by means of the newly formed blood vessels. Malignant cells are parasitic and, if unchecked, eventually destroy their host.

The characteristics of malignant cells are summarized in the box on page 318.

Tumor Invasion and Metastasis

The ability of cancer cells to invade adjacent tissues and travel to distant organs is considered their most ominous characteristic. This quality makes treatment a considerable challenge.

Invasion   Aggressive tumors possess several qualities that facilitate invasion (Figure 9–5):

- *Ability to cause pressure atrophy.* From the pressure of its presence (decreased contact inhibition), a growing tumor can cause atrophy and necrosis of adjacent tissues. The malignancy then moves into the vacated space.

- *Ability to disrupt the basement membrane of normal cells.* Many cancer cells have the ability to bind to elements of the basement membrane and to secrete enzymes that degrade that physical barrier, thus facilitating their movement into normal tissues, lymph, and blood circulation.

- *Motility.* Because malignant cells are less tightly bound to each other than normal cells (reduced adhesive-

ness), they easily separate from the neoplasm and move into surrounding body fluids and tissues.

- *Response to chemical signals from adjacent tissues.* Chemotaxis (the movement of cells in response to a chemical stimulus) calls the tumor cells into the normal tissues, possibly as a result of the degrading of the basement membranes of the normal cells. This breakdown of normal cellular membranes releases the chemical stimulus that physiologically is designed to draw normal phagocytic cells to clean up the debris. (See Chapter 8 on the inflammatory response for more information on chemotaxis.) Malignant cells are also known to respond chemotactically to the end product of cellular metabolism. Some cancer cells even produce a substance called *autocrine motility factor*, which calls other malignant cells to a normal tissue. This substance is produced by the first invading cells and then actively draws other malignant cells from the primary tumor into the invaded normal tissue.

Metastasis   The factors that favor invasion also contribute to the process of metastasis. Metastasis can occur by means of one or more of three major mechanisms:

- Embolism in the blood or lymph
- Spread by way of body cavities
- Iatrogenesis

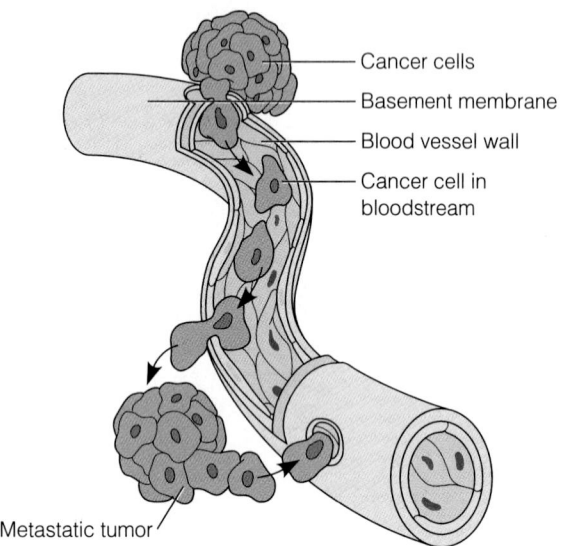

Cancer cells
Basement membrane
Blood vessel wall
Cancer cell in bloodstream

Metastatic tumor

Figure 9–6 Metastasis through the bloodstream. Cancer cells secrete enzymes and a motility factor that disrupt the basement membrane in the blood vessel. In this way, the cancer cells gain access into the circulation. Once in the blood, only about 1 cell in 1000 escapes immune detection, but that can be enough. Undetected cells move out of the blood, again secreting enzymes and cutting through the vessel wall into new tissue. The tissue selected for establishing a new tumor may be downstream from the original tumor, or a chemical attraction may cause the malignant cells to target a specific site. Once in the new site, the malignant cells multiply and establish a metastatic tumor.

A blood or lymph-borne metastasis allows a new tumor to be established in a distant organ. Figure 9–6 shows metastasis through the blood stream. A tumor's ability to metastasize in this manner requires the successful completion of the following steps:

1. Intravasation of malignant cells through blood or lymphatic vessel walls and into the circulation.

2. Survival of the malignant cells in the blood. To survive, the cells must escape the notice of the body's immune surveillance; only about 1 cell in 1000 does so.

3. Extravasation from the circulation and implantation in a new tissue.

The tumor cells tend to clump together, forming an embolus, and continue growing until they reach a point at which their size prevents further travel in the vessel or lymph channel. The growing neoplastic mass then uses its invasive abilities (secreting enzymes and motility factor) to move into the nearest organ.

About 60% of metastatic lesions tend to occur in a schema reflecting the pattern of blood or lymph circulation. However, it has been demonstrated that some malignant cells defy a blood-borne pattern and actually target specific organs to which they prefer to metastasize. For

Table 9–4 Various Cancers and Sites of Metastases

Primary Tumor	Common Metastatic Sites
Bronchogenic (lung)	Spinal cord, brain, liver, bone
Breast	Regional lymph nodes, vertebrae, brain, liver
Colon	Liver, lung, brain, ovary
Prostate	Bladder, bone (especially vertebrae), liver
Malignant melanoma	Lung, liver, spleen, regional lymph nodes

example, lung cancer frequently metastasizes to the adrenal glands. Such highly specific metastases may demonstrate a particular cancer's response to a specific organ's chemotatic signals. This response may be genetically programmed into the malignant cells. It is also theorized that a tumor's enzymes that promote invasion may work only with certain other tissues (Nowak & Handford, 1994).

Malignant cells that gain access to the lymph channels may travel to a preferred organ and then move into it the same way in which they emigrate through blood vessels. Alternatively, the malignant cells may become trapped in the lymph node and continue to grow. Eventually, the malignant cells replace the node's tissues. At this point, emboli from the cancerous node disseminate to other nodes, creating a cascade reaction. The malignant cascade causes widespread transfer of the tumor to uncharacteristic sites.

A malignant tumor may spread, breaking through the walls of the organ in which it is primarily housed and shedding cells into the nearby body cavity. The cells then are free to establish new growths in a distant area of that cavity. For example, malignant cells from a colon cancer may be seeded into the peritoneal cavity, establishing a new tumor in the mesenteric epithelium.

Iatrogenic metastases, which are not very common, can occur during surgical incision of a tumor or during a diagnostic biopsy. Awareness of this possibility has reduced the incidence of such occurrences.

Metastatic lesions are differentiated from primary neoplasms by cell morphology: Metastatic cells do not resemble the tissue in which they reside. The most common sites of metastasis are the lymph nodes, liver, lungs, bones, and brain. Table 9–4 lists different cancers and common sites of metastasis.

For metastasis to occur, the cancerous cells must avoid detection by the immune system. Thus, impairment or alteration of the immune system is a major factor in the establishment of metastatic lesions. Cells may escape detection in several different ways:

Factors That May Weaken or Alter the Immune Response
■ ■ ■

- Accumulated stress
- Depression
- Increased age
- Pregnancy
- Chronic disease
- Chemotherapy treatment for the primary cancer

- Aggressive cancer cells may compile a large mass (greater than 1 cm) so rapidly that the immune system is unable to overcome the tumor before it takes hold in a new tissue.

- For tumor cells to be recognized as foreign by the immune system, they must display on their surface a special antigen, called tumor-associated antigen (TAA). TAA marks tumor cells for destruction by the lymphocytes. Some oncogenic viruses depress the expression of TAA on infected cells. Also, some tumors in advanced stages of growth no longer display TAA. Thus, such tumor cells escape detection as they travel through the blood or lymph.

- If the person's immune response is weakened or altered, then a metastatic tumor may take hold with little opposition (Herberman, 1991; Janeway, 1993). Factors that may weaken or alter the immune response are listed in the accompanying box.

It is estimated that 50% of all cancers have already metastasized by the time the tumor is identified. This may account for the current 50% death rate and certainly supports the need for client education to facilitate early diagnosis. The time it takes for metatasis to occur is extremely variable and often difficult to predict. Some cancers, such as basal cell carcinomas, do not metastasize. The aggressiveness and location of the tumor, as well as the state of the person's immune system, determine whether and how rapidly metastasis takes place (Nowak & Handford, 1994).

Physiologic and Psychologic Effects of Cancer

Much of the nursing care for clients with cancer is related to the generalized effects of cancer on the body and the side effects of the treatments used to remove or destroy the cancer. Although pathophysiologic effects of the cancer vary with the type and location of the cancer, the following effects usually are observed.

Disruption of Function Physiologic functioning can be upset by obstruction or pressure. For example, a large tumor in the bowel can stop intestinal motility, resulting in a bowel obstruction. Prostatic tumors can obstruct the bladder neck or urethra, resulting in urine retention. Intracranial pressure can be dangerously increased by a glioma.

Obstruction or pressure can cause anoxia and necrosis of surrounding tissues, which in turn cause a loss of function of the involved organ or tissue. For example, a kidney tumor may progress to renal failure. Pressure against the superior vena cava from an adjacent lung tumor or tumor-infiltrated lymph nodes can interrupt the blood flow to the heart.

In the liver, either a primary hepatocellular cancer or metastatic lesion can have several significant effects:

- In liver parenchymal tissue, the multiple life-sustaining functions of the liver, such as carbohydrate metabolism, synthesis of plasma proteins, detoxification, and immunologic functions, are impaired. These functional impairments result in severe nutritional, hormonal, hematologic, and immunologic problems. (See Chapter 15 for a more complete discussion of liver functions and effects of disruption.)

- Because more than 1 liter of blood per minute passes through the liver via the portal vein, obstruction to this flow from a tumor can cause portal hypertension. This results in back-up of fluid and increased pressure in the splanchnic circulation. The end result is *ascites* (third-spaced fluid in the peritoneal cavity) and *varices* (friable, overdistended blood vessels) of the esophageal, gastric, mesenteric, and hemorrhoidal vessels.

Hematologic Alterations Hematologic alterations can impair the normal function of blood cells. For example, in *leukemia,* a malignant proliferative disease of the *hematopoietic* (blood cell-producing) system, the immature leukocytes are unable to perform the normal protective phagocytic functions. Thus, immunity is compromised. Additionally, the excessive numbers of immature leukocytes in the bone marrow diminish erythrocyte and thrombocyte (platelet) production, resulting in secondary anemia and clotting disorders (Mitus & Rosenthal, 1991; Pui & Rivera, 1991).

Other examples of hematologic alteration include the following:

- Gastrointestinal tumors disrupt the absorption of vitamin B_{12} and iron.

- Growing tumors need purines and folate and have a unique ability to accumulate and store these substances. Thus, the tumor deprives the bone marrow of these substances, which are needed for *erythropoiesis* (red blood cell production);

■ Renal cell carcinoma produces its own erythropoietin hormone, which causes an excessively large number of red blood cells to be produced and dumped into the bloodstream. The resulting polycythemia causes viscous blood, which impairs circulation, plugs up small capillaries, and promotes thrombus formation (Doweiko & Goldberg, 1991).

Infection If the tumor invades and connects two incompatible organs, such as the bowel and bladder, and thus creates a fistula, infection becomes a serious problem. As they destroy viable tissue and thus their source of nutrition, tumors may become necrotic, and septicemia may result. Also, some tumors are less efficient in creating capillaries; as a consequence, the center of the tumor may become necrotic and infected. When a tumor grows near the surface of the body, it may erode through to the surface, thus breaking down the natural defenses of intact skin and mucous membranes and providing a site for the entry of microorganisms. Any malignant involvement of the organs or tissues of immunity—such as the liver, bone marrow, Peyer's patches in the small intestine, spleen, or lymph nodes—can seriously impair the immune response, allowing infections to develop in vulnerable tissues.

Hemorrhage Tumor erosion through blood vessels can cause extensive bleeding, giving rise to severe anemia. Hemorrhage can be serious enough to cause life-threatening hypovolemic shock.

Anorexia-Cachexia Syndrome A characteristic feature of cancer is the wasted appearance of its victims, called **cachexia**. In many cases, unexplained rapid weight loss is the first symptom that brings the client to a health care provider. This can be due to a variety of problems associated with cancer, such as pain, infection, depression, or the side effects of chemotherapy and radiation. Usually, however, the emaciation, malnutrition, and loss of energy are attributed to the anorexia-cachexia syndrome.

The anorexia-cachexia syndrome is specific to cancer because of the effect of cancer cells on the metabolism of the host. The neoplastic cells inhibit food intake while they divert nutrition to their own use. Early in the disease, glucose metabolism is altered, causing an increase in serum glucose levels. Through the process of negative feedback, *anorexia* (loss of appetite) results. In addition, the tumor secretes substances that decreases appetite by altering taste and smell and producing early satiety. Pain, infection, and depression also contibute to anorexia. Some types of cancers cause specific food aversions, such as to red meat, coffee, or chocolate.

Avaricious cancer cells support their growth processes through widespread catabolism of the body's tissue and muscle proteins. This catabolism, coupled with inadequate nutrient intake, results in the typical cachexia. Normally, a starvation state reduces the body's basal metabolic rate. However, in many persons with cancer, the meta-

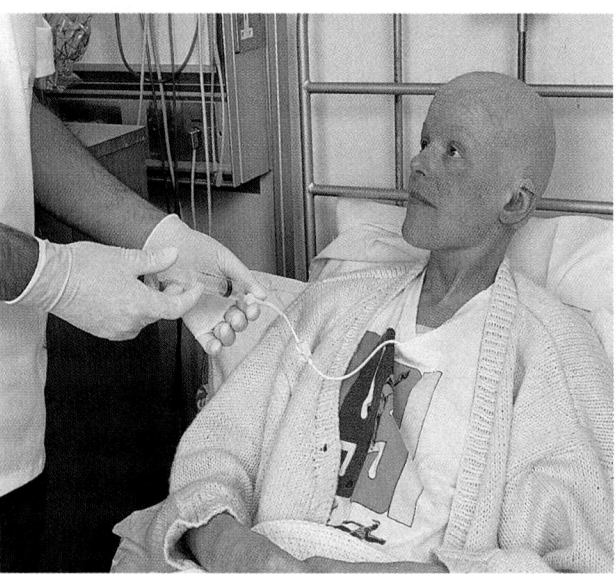

Figure 9–7 Cachexic person. Cancer robs its host of nutrients and increases body catabolism of fat and muscle to meet its metabolic needs.

bolic rate is increased, probably because of the hyperactive metabolic and reproductive activities of the malignant cells. One theory suggests that cytokinins produced by the body in response to the tumor presence are responsible for both early satiety and cachexia. One specific cytokine, called *tumor necrosis factor-alpha* or *cachectin*, is believed to enhance the increased metabolic consumption of nutrients. The anorexia-cachexia syndrome is further promoted by cancers of the gastrointestinal system, which decrease absorption and utilization of nutrients, and by the side effects of some treatment modalities (Daly & Shinkwin, 1991; Nowak & Handford, 1994). Figure 9–7 shows the characteristic appearance of a cachexic person.

Creation of Ectopic Sites Cancers can set up ectopic sites of hormone production that presumably are required for tumor growth but are not under the normal feedback control from the pituitary gland. These ectopic sites produce excessive amounts of the hormone, which prove harmful to the host. For example,

■ Breast, ovarian, and renal cancers may set up ectopic parathyroid hormone sites, causing severe hypercalcemia.

■ Oat cell and other lung cancers may produce ectopic secretions of insulin (causing hypoglycemia), parathyroid hormone (PTH), antidiuretic hormone (ADH, which causes excessive fluid retention, hypertension, and peripheral edema), and adrenocorticotropic hormone (ACTH). See Chapter 20 for the description of the multiple problems caused by excessive secretions of cortisone.

Table 9–5	Laboratory Indicators of Ectopic Functioning
Hormone	**Specific Laboratory Test**
Antidiuretic hormone (ADH)	Serum and urine osmolality
Adrenocorticotropic hormone (ACTH)	Plasma ACTH ACTH suppression test ACTH stimulation test Urine catecholamines
Calcitonin	Serum calcitonin
Insulin	Serum glucose Glucose tolerance test
Parathyroid hormone (PTH)	Serum PTH Serum calcium
Thyroxine	Serum thyroid-stimulating hormone (TSH), T_3, T_4

Types of Pain in Cancer Patients

Acute Pain

- Primary symptom associated with diagnosis
- Pain related to cancer treatment (surgery, radiation, chemotherapy)

Chronic Pain

- Pain related to cancer treatment
- A consequence of progression of the disease
- Preexisting pain related to other disorders
- Pain related to a history of drug abuse
- Cancer-related pain in the dying client

Note. Adapted from *The Treatment of Pain in the Patient with Cancer* by K. M. Foley, 1985, Atlanta: American Cancer Society.

Although the mechanisms by which cancers produce ectopic hormones is not clearly understood, some investigators believe that the cancer cells have embryonic genes that normally mask genetic information. Other investigators theorize that these ectopic hormones may be the result of abnormal differentiation (Templeton & Weinberg, 1991). See Table 9–5 for laboratory indicators of ectopic hormones.

Paraneoplastic Syndromes   Investigators have identified a number of tumor-related effects whose causative factors are not well understood:

- Lung and pancreatic tumors have been linked to leg vein thrombosis.
- Muscle and peripheral nerve problems have occurred in conjunction with breast and lung tumors.
- Some tumors distant from the brain produce increased intracranial pressure.

A possible explanation for these effects may rest with tumor toxins or antibody-antigen complexes in the affected tissues (Nowak & Handford, 1994).

Pain   Pain is ranked as one of the most serious concerns of clients, families, and oncology health care professionals. Because pain management for people with cancer has a reputation for being ineffective, the anticipation of pain engenders terror in even the most stoic of individuals (McCaffery, 1992). Many people fear pain and suffering even more than possible death; although pain management strategies have improved tremendously, a 1985 study noted that 60% to 90% of clients with advanced cancer reported substantial pain and approximately 25% of all cancer victims worldwide died without relief of severe pain (Foley, 1985). Research on pain with its devas-

tating statistics has led to great improvement in the pain management strategies currently practiced.

Types of Cancer Pain   Cancer pain can be divided into two main categories, acute and chronic pain, with subgroupings. These classifications serve to indicate appropriate therapeutic approaches. See the accompanying box. Acute pain has a well-defined pattern of onset, exhibits common signs and symptoms, and is often identified with hyperactivity of the autonomic system. Chronic pain, which lasts more than 6 months, frequently lacks the objective manifestations of acute pain, primarily because the autonomic nervous system adapts to this chronic stress. Unfortunately, chronic pain results in personality changes, alterations in functional abilities, and life-style disruptions that can seriously affect compliance with treatment and the quality of life.

Most cancer clients who cite acute pain as the primary symptom that led to the diagnosis tend to associate pain with the introduction to their disease (Foley, 1991). If these clients experience pain during the illness or after therapy, they often perceive the pain as introducing another cancer or as a recurrence of the original cancer. Other clients report experiencing pain as a component of cancer therapy. These clients often are able to endure the pain in anticipation of a successful outcome of treatment.

Clients with chronic pain may have pain related to treatment or indicating progression of the disease. Identifying the pain as treatment related rather than tumor related is extremely important because it has a definite effect on the client's psychologic outlook. For the client whose pain is due to the advancement of the disease, psychologic factors play an even more important role. Hopelessness and fear of impending death intensify physiologic pain and contribute to overall suffering (which goes well beyond just physical pain).

Three other categories used to classify clients with cancer pain are worth mentioning: clients with preexisting pain, those with a history of drug abuse, and dying clients with cancer-related pain. The first two groups may have altered perceptions of pain and may not have the anticipated response to pain medication. For the dying client, pain is strongly associated with both the client's and family's confronting of issues regarding hopelessness and death. This can intensify the perception of pain (see Chapter 11).

Causes of Cancer Pain   Direct tumor involvement accounts for approximately 70% of the pain experienced by persons with cancer. This includes metastatic bone disease, nerve compression, and involvement of visceral organs. The pain from tumor involvement is believed to be mechanical, resulting from stretching of tissues and compression. Chemicals from ischemia or tumor metabolites and toxins that activate and sensitize nociceptors and mechanoreceptors are also responsible for tumor pain. See Chapter 4 for a more complete discussion of the mechanics of pain.

Side effects or toxic effects of cancer therapies, such as surgery, radiation, and chemotherapy, are other causes of cancer pain. These are usually the result of traumatized tissue; one example is the oropharyngeal ulcerations that occur with some types of chemotherapy (Foley, 1991).

Physical Stress   When the immune system discovers the neoplasm, it tries to destroy it using the resources of the body. The body mounts an all-out assault on the foreign invader, calling on many resources:

- Multiple chemical mediators
- Hormones and enzymes
- Blood cells
- Antibodies
- Proteins of the general adaptation syndrome (stress response)
- Inflammatory and immune responses

These protective responses also mobilize fluid, electrolytes, and nutritional systems. This is a massive effort that requires tremendous energy. See Chapters 5 and 12 for specific information on these systems.

If the neoplasm is small enough, (i.e., microscopic) the immune system can destroy it, and a tumor will never manifest. However, a neoplasm of 1 cm is large enough to overwhelm most immune systems; the body will continue to try and fight it until it reaches the stage of exhaustion and is no longer able to (Selye, 1984). Thus, many clients

with cancer present with fatigue, weight loss, anemia, dehydration, and altered blood chemistries (e.g., decreases in electrolytes).

Psychologic Stress   People who are confronted with the diagnosis of cancer exhibit a variety of psychologic and emotional responses. Some people look on cancer as a death sentence and experience overwhelming grief, often giving up. Others feel guilt, considering the cancer a punishment for past behaviors, such as smoking or unhealthy eating habits, or for delaying diagnosis or treatment. Some feel guilty because they think that their immune system failure is somehow their fault. The person may experience anger, especially if the person believes that he or she had been practicing a healthful life-style; underneath that anger may reside feelings of powerlessness. Fear is common: fear of the outcome of the illness, fear of the effects of treatment, fear of pain, fear of death. Some people feel isolated because of the stigma of cancer and old beliefs of contagion. Body image concerns and sexual dysfunction may be present but often unexpressed, especially if the cancer is of the breast or sexual organs or causes visible body changes. The accompanying box summarizes the physiologic and psychosocial effects of cancer.

Collaborative Care

Collaborative care begins with a variety of specialized laboratory and diagnostic tests. Once cancer is diagnosed, medical treatment becomes a priority. The American Cancer Society identifies four major goals of medical treatment:

1. Eliminating the tumor or malignant cells
2. Preventing metastasis
3. Reducing cellular growth and the tumor burden
4. Promoting functional abilities and providing pain relief to those whose disease has not responded to treatment.

Laboratory and Diagnostic Tests

Diagnosis   Several procedures are used to diagnose cancer. X-ray imaging, computed tomography, ultrasonography, and magnetic resonance imaging can locate abnormal tissues or tumors. However, only microscopic histologic examination of the tissue reveals the type of cell and its structural difference from the parent tissue. Tissue samples are acquired through biopsy, shedded cells (e.g., Papanicolaou smear), or collections of secretions (e.g., sputum). Lymph nodes are also biopsied to determine whether metastasis has begun. Simple screening procedures can be used to pick up substances secreted by the tumor, such as the prostatic-specific antigen (PSA) blood test now being used to identify early prostatic cancers. Increases in enzymes or hormones released by normal tissues when they are damaged can also contribute to the diagnosis. Increased alkaline phosphatase noted in bone metastases and osteosarcoma is one example of an enzyme increase associated with cancer. Recent research has identified tumor markers that are being used both for early diagnosis and for devising immunologic treatments.

Some investigators studying chemical mediators of the immune system have noted that there seems to be communication between the chemical mediators and the emotional centers of the brain (Jaret, 1986; Rosenberg, 1992). A person who states, "I feel I have a cancer somewhere" should therefore be listened to, and the complaint investigated thoroughly.

To provide some standardization in diagnosis and treatment protocols, an elaborate identification system has been developed. This consists of naming the tumor (classification) and describing its aggressiveness (grading) and spread within or beyond the tissue of origin (staging).

Classification   Tumors are classified and named by the tissue or cell of origin. Tumor nomenclature often incorporates the Latin stem identifying the tissue from which the tumor arises. For example, a **carcinoma** arises from epithelial tissue; adjectives are added to further specify the location. A glandular malignancy arising from epithelial tissue is classified as an adenocarcinoma. A tumor arising from supportive tissues is called a **sarcoma**; the specific type of tissue is added as a prefix. For example, a cancer of fibrous connective tissue is called fibrosarcoma, and a smooth muscle cancer is a leiomyosarcoma. A tumor from seminal or germ tissue is called a **seminoma**. Table 9–6 compares the nomenclature of benign and malignant neoplasms.

Other names for tumors incorporate the name of the discoverer of that particular cancer, such as Burkitt's lymphoma or Hodgkin's disease. Hematopoietic malignancies (also known as "liquid tumors") are usually named by the type of immature blood cell that predominates. An example is myelocytic leukemia, named for the immature form of the granulocyte.

Grading and Staging   *Grading* evaluates the amount of differentiation (level of functional maturity) of the cell and estimates the rate of growth based on the mitotic rate. Cells which are the most differentiated—that is, most like the parent tissue and therefore the least malignant—earn a grade of 1. Grade 4 is reserved for the least differentiated and most aggressively malignant cells. Because of the differences inherent in tumor appearance and biologic behavior, grading criteria may vary with different locations and types of tumors.

Staging refers to the relative size of the tumor and extent of the disease. A tumor in situ is at stage 0, and stage IV indicates widespread metastases. The number system

Physiologic and Psychosocial Effects of Cancer

Note. Manifestations depend on the type and location of the cancer.

- Disruption of function (due to obstruction or pressure)
- Hematologic alterations
  a. Decreased leukocytes, erythrocytes, and thrombocytes
  b. Altered erythropoiesis
- Infections
  a. Fistula between noncompatible organs
  b. Necrosis of tumor center
  c. Malignant involvement of organs of immunity
- Hemorrhage (caused by erosion of neoplasm through blood vessels or surface of skin)
- Anorexia-cachexia syndrome
  a. Hyperglycemia
  b. Catabolism of tissue and muscle proteins
  c. Altered taste and smell
- Creation of ectopic sites of hormones
  a. PTH
  b. Insulin
  c. ADH
  d. ACTH
- Paraneoplastic syndromes
  a. Deep-vein thrombosis
  b. Peripheral nerve problems
  c. Increased intracranial pressure
- Pain
  a. Acute and chronic
  b. Caused by direct tumor involvement or side effects of therapy
- Physical stress
  a. Increased general adaptation syndrome activity
  b. Increased immunologic activity
  c. Increased inflammatory response activity
  d. Nutritional, fluid, and electrolyte alterations
- Psychologic stress
  a. Grief
  b. Hopelessness
  c. Guilt
  d. Anger
  e. Fear
  f. Isolation
  g. Body image concerns
  h. Sexual dysfunction

Table 9–6 Nomenclature for Benign and Malignant Neoplasms

	Tissue of Origin	Benign	Malignant
Ectoderm/Endoderm	Epithelium	Papilloma	Carcinoma
	Gland	Adenoma	Adenocarcinoma
	Liver cells	Hepatocellular adenoma	Hepatocellular carcinoma
	Neuroglia	Glioma	Glioma
	Melanocytes	Melanoma	Malignant melanoma
	Basal cells		Basal cell carcinoma
	Germ cells	Tetroma	Seminoma
Mesoderm	Connective tissue		
	Adipose tissue	Lipoma	Liposarcoma
	Fibrous tissue	Fibroma	Fibrosarcoma
	Bone tissue	Osteoma	Osteosarcoma
	Cartilage	Chondroma	Chondrosarcoma
	Muscle		
	Smooth muscle	Leiomyoma	Leiomyosarcoma
	Striated muscle	Rhabdomyoma	Rhabdomyosarcoma
	Neural tissue		
	Nerve cells	Ganglioneuroma	Neuroblastoma
	Endothelial tissues		
	Blood vessels	Hemangioma	Angiosarcoma
			Kaposi's sarcoma
	Meninges	Meningioma	Malignant meningioma
Hematopoietic Tissues	Granulocytes	Granulocytosis	Leukemia
	Plasma cells		Multiple myeloma
	Lymphocytes		Lymphomas

Table 9–7 TNM Staging Classification System

	Stage	Manifestations
Tumor	T_0	No evidence of primary tumor.
	T_{IS}	Tumor in situ.
	T_1, T_2, T_3, T_4	Ascending degrees of tumor size and involvement.
Nodes	N_0	No abnormal regional nodes.
	N_{1a}, N_{2a}	Regional nodes—no metastasis.
	N_{1b}, N_{2b}, N_{3b}	Regional lymph nodes—metastasis suspected.
	N_x	Regional nodes cannot be assessed clinically.
Metastasis	M_0	No evidence of distant metastasis.
	M_1, M_2, M_3	Ascending degrees of metastatic involvement of the host including distant nodes.

for staging is no longer in common use, having been replaced by the more useful TNM classification system. *T* stands for the relative tumor size, *N* indicates the presence and extent of lymph node involvement, and *M* denotes distant metastases. Table 9–7 shows the basic outline of the TNM system. Although the TNM system is generalized for all solid tumors, it is frequently adapted for specific types of cancers.

Other sophisticated systems have evolved, using specific coding to differentiate types and locations of tumors. These provide shorthand for the oncologist in staging and grading tumors and provide guidelines for treatment. For example, oncologists may use either an A-B-C-D staging system (which includes grading numbers) or a modified TNM system for evaluating prostate cancer (see Chapter 46). Duke's staging system for colorectal cancer also uses the A-B-C-D code, which focuses on the effectiveness of surgical treatment and the necessity of follow-up chemotherapy or radiation. See Chapter 23.

Cytologic Examination For the malignant tissues to be identified by name, grade, and stage, they must first be subjected to histologic and cytologic examination by light or electron microscope. Specimens are collected by three basic methods:

- Exfoliation from an epithelial surface. Examples include scraping cells from the cervix (Papanicolaou smear) or bronchial washings.

- Aspiration of fluid from body cavities or blood. Examples include white blood cells for evaluation of hema-

Table 9–8	Tumor-Derived Markers Associated with Specific Neoplasms	
	Tumor Marker	**Associated Neoplasm**
Oncofetal Antigens	Carcinoembryonic antigen (CEA)	Adenocarcinomas of colon, lung, breast, ovary, stomach pancreas
	Alpha-fetoprotein (AFP)	Hepatocellular carcinoma, gonadal germ cell tumors (seminoma)
Hormones	Human chorionic gonadotropin (HCG)	Gonadal germ cell tumors
	Calcitonin	Medullary cancer of thyroid
	Catecholamines/metabolites	Pheochromocytoma
Isoenzymes	Prostatic acid phosphatase (PAP)	Adenocarcinoma of prostate
	Neuron-specific enolase	Small-cell lung carcinoma, neuroblastoma
Specific Proteins	Prostate-specific antigen (PSA)	Adenocarcinoma of prostate
	Immunoglobin	Multiple myeloma
	CA 125	Epithelial ovarian cancer
	CA 19-9	Adenocarcinoma of pancreas, colon

Note. Adapted from "The Pathologic Evaluation of Neoplastic Disease" by J. D. Pfeifer and M. R. Wick, in *American Cancer Society Textbook of Clinical Oncology* by A. I. Holleb, D. J. Fink, and G. P. Murphy, Eds., 1991, pp. 7–24. Atlanta: American Cancer Society.

topoietic cancers, pleural fluid, and cerebral spinal fluid.

- Needle suction aspiration of solid tumors. This could include the breast, lung, or prostate.

Cytologic examination is also carried out on specimens from biopsied tissues or tumors and on collected body secretions, such as sputum or urine.

After collection, specimens are spread on a glass slide, fixed, and stained if necessary. The morphologic features of the cells are examined, with special attention to the nucleus and cytoplasm. Other special pathologic procedures can be carried out on the specimen, but they must be ordered ahead of time if special preparations of the specimen are necessary.

Several special diagnostic cytologic procedures are proving useful; chromosomal studies and DNA studies are examples. Research investigators are predicting the use of these studies for future treatment protocols (Pfeifer & Wick, 1991).

Tumor Markers   A *tumor marker* is a molecule detectable in serum or other body fluids. This protein marker is used as a biochemical indicator of the presence of a malignancy. Small amounts of tumor marker proteins are found in normal body tissues or benign tumors and are not specific for malignancy. However, high levels are suspicious and mandate follow-up diagnostic studies. Oncologists think that tumor markers are not specific enough to be used routinely for malignancy screening of the general population; rather, their primary use is to determine the client's response to therapy and to detect residual disease. However, one marker, *prostatic-specific antigen (PSA)* has received a great deal of media attention as a detector of prostate cancer. As a result, many health care practitioners are recommending it for screening of men over 40, much the same as Papanicolaou smears and mammograms are recommended for women.

Tumor markers fall into two general categories: those derived from the tumor itself, and those associated with host (immune) response to the tumor. Tumor-derived markers include the following:

- *Oncofetal antigens.* These are present in fetal tissue but normally are suppressed after birth. Thus, their presence in large amounts may reflect an anaplastic process in tumor cells. Alpha-fetoprotein (AFP) and carcinoembryonic antigen (CEA) are oncofetal antigens.

- *Hormones.* Hormones are, of course, present in considerable amounts in human blood and tissues, but very high levels not related to other conditions may signify the presence of a hormone-secreting malignancy. Some common hormones seen as tumor markers include human chorionic gonadotropin (HCG), antidiuretic hormone (ADH), parathyroid hormone (PTH), calcitonin, and catecholamines.

- *Tissue-specific proteins.* These narrow down the type of tissue that may be malignant, although they can also be increased in hyperplastic disorders. Examples of tissue-specific proteins include prostatic-specific antigen (PSA) and immunoglobin.

- *Isoenzymes.* Rapid, excessive growth of a tissue may cause some of the enzymes and isoenzymes normally present in that particular tissue to spill into the bloodstream. Elevated levels can point to either hyperplasia of the tissue or cancer. Prostatic acid phosphatase (PAP) and neuron-specific enolase (NSE) are examples. Table 9–8 compares selected tumor-derived markers with their presence in neoplasms and other conditions.

The second category of tumor markers (host-response) reflect the reaction of the body's defenses to the presence of the tumor. Host-response markers include substances such as serum ferritin, interleukin-2, tumor necrosis factor, C-reactive protein, and enzymes such as lactic dehydrogenase (Pfeifer & Wick, 1991).

Oncologic Imaging Because physical assessment procedures usually do not demonstrate the presence of a cancer until the tumor has reached a size that poses a major risk for metastasis, radiologic examination is extremely important in early diagnosis. This diagnostic process may involve routine X-ray imaging (usually for screening only), computed tomography, magnetic resonance imaging, ultrasonography, radioisotope scans, angiography, and tagged antibodies.

X-Ray Imaging Considered the least expensive and least invasive diagnostic procedure, film screen imaging (standard X-ray imaging) is the method of choice for screening such body areas as the breast (mammography), lung, and bone to identify changes in tissue density that may indicate malignancies. X-ray studies are limited in that they do not easily distinguish among calcifications, benign cystic growths, and true malignancies. However, as a screening tool, X-ray imaging can usually reassure the client if findings are negative or encourage follow-up studies if findings are suspicious. X-ray imaging is still the imaging method of choice for lung cancer. Unfortunately, it does not usually reveal tumors until they have reached about 1 cm in size, which is late in their development.

Computed Tomography Computed tomography (CT) has vastly advanced the effectiveness of traditional X-ray methods. By applying computers and mathematics to diagnostic imaging, CT allows the visualization of cross-sections of anatomy. Because CT scans reveal subtle differences in tissue densities, they provide much greater accuracy in tumor diagnosis. This procedure, although more expensive than X-ray imaging, is useful in the screening for some cancers such as renal cell and most gastrointestinal tumors. CT scans are especially useful to evaluate possible lymph node involvement.

Magnetic Resonance Imaging Like CT, magnetic resonance imaging (MRI) involves computerized mathematical technology; unlike CT, MRI produces images from radio frequency signals emitted by the body. Related diagnostic imaging procedures, positron emission tomography (PET), and single photon emission computed tomography (SPECT), create visible images by measuring electrical impulses from different body structures. Although MRI is relatively expensive, it is the diagnostic tool of choice for both screening and follow-up of cranial and head and neck tumors.

Some clients become claustrophobic during the MRI procedure because it requires that the client be placed inside the diagnostic imaging machine, an experience that has been likened to being encased in a small tube. In addition, some machines make loud thumping sounds that can be frightening if the client is not informed beforehand that this is normal.

Ultrasonography Ultrasonography is relatively safe and noninvasive. It measures the sound waves as they bounce off various body structures, giving an image of normal anatomy as well as revealing abnormalities that indicate tumors. Ultrasonography has been adapted for diagnosing some specific tumors. For example, transrectal ultrasonography has provided excellent imaging of early prostate cancers and is used to guide needle biopsy. Ultrasound imaging is also more useful for detecting masses in the denser breast tissue of young women.

Radioisotope Scans Radioisotope scans involve the use of a special scintillation scanner in conjunction with the ingestion or injection of specific radioactive isotopes. This is an invasive but usually safe diagnostic method for identifying tumors in various body tissues. For the client with a newly diagnosed cancer, the procedure is often used to check for possible bone or other organ metastases. This evaluation helps the health care provider determine appropriate treatment.

The principle underlying the technology is that certain isotopes have an affinity for specific tissues; for example, radioactive iodine (I 131) has an affinity for the thyroid gland. Malignancies in these tissues sequester an abnormally large amount of the isotope, which then can be traced and measured by the scintillation scanner. This procedure is considered safe because the amount of isotope used is small enough not to damage normal cells.

The procedure is usually minimally distressing for clients. Drinking the isotope solution is not pleasant but is tolerable, and some anxious clients may have difficulty lying still during the scan. Antianxiety medication may help. Some patients may experience nausea from drinking the isotope and require antiemetic drugs to complete the procedure. Client preparation may include allowing nothing by mouth or clear fluids only after midnight.

Angiography An expensive and invasive procedure, angiography is used infrequently for tumor diagnosis. Angiography is performed when the precise location of the tumor cannot be identified or there is a need to visualize the tumor's extent prior to surgery. The procedure involves injecting a radiopaque dye into a major blood vessel proximal to the organ or tissue to be examined. The movement of the dye through the vasculature of the organ or tissue is then traced by means of fluoroscopy or serial X-ray films. In some cases, small catheters are threaded through the vein under fluoroscopy to ensure the specific placement of the dye. Blockage to the flow of the dye indicates the tumor's location. Dye may also be used to identify blood vessels supplying a tumor, allowing the surgeon to know where to safely ligate vessels.

Angiography requires preparation similar to that for minor surgery: ensuring that the client takes in only fluids on the day of the examination, performing skin preparation at the insertion site, and administering sedative drugs prior to the procedure. Clients should be informed that injection of the dye used to enhance imaging may cause a hot, flushing sensation or nausea and vomiting. Although angiography is usually done on an outpatient basis, the client will be kept in a short-stay unit for several hours and monitored for such complications as bleeding at the catheter insertion site.

Tagged Antibodies An exciting new area of research in oncologic imaging is based on the concept of tumor markers. Investigators are working on developing monoclonal antibodies that will target a specific cancer and can be tagged with a radioactive isotope and administered to the client. After a designated period of time, the tagged antibodies find and react with the antigen. Then, nuclear scanning reveals a dense concentration of the radioisotopes and thus locates the cancer. This process is still under investigation, because targeting a cancer with a specific type of antibody is not easy. However, the process has been used with moderate success for imaging malignant melanoma (Hendee, Manaster, Harnsberger, Bragg, Thompson, & McClennan, 1991).

Direct Visualization Direct visualization procedures are invasive but do not require the use of radiography. Examples include the following:

- Sigmoidoscopy (viewing the sigmoid colon by use of a fiberoptic flexible sigmoidoscope)
- Cystoscopy (viewing the urethra and bladder)
- Endoscopy (viewing the upper gastrointestinal tract)
- Bronchoscopy (inspecting the tracheobronchial tree)

All of these methods allow the visual identification of the organs within the limits of the scope and usually permit biopsy of suspicious lesions or masses. Flexible fiberoptic scopes may be more useful, because they allow deeper penetration than do traditional scopes. These procedures all require some client preparation, cause moderate to considerable discomfort, and may require sedation or even anesthesia, as in the case of bronchoscopy. Some of the procedures, such as sigmoidoscopy and cystoscopy, may be performed in the physician's office and therefore cost less, making them more accessible screening procedures.

Client preparation includes a thorough bowel cleansing prior to the sigmoidoscopy and cystoscopy; the client may ingest only liquids the morning of the procedure. Because anesthesia may be required, clients undergoing bronchoscopy and endoscopy may be instructed to have nothing by mouth from midnight until the time of the procedure. These procedures are discussed in greater detail in later chapters of this text.

A more radical method of direct visualization for suspected malignancies is exploratory surgery with biopsy. The client undergoes the usual preoperative preparation (see Chapter 7) for the type of surgery anticipated. When the tumor is exposed, a sample of tissue (biopsy) is sent to the pathology laboratory for a "frozen-section" histologic examination. This can be done rapidly while the client remains on the operating table under anesthesia. If the initial report is negative, the benign mass is usually removed to prevent further symptoms. If the report is positive for cancer, the tumor and, often, adjacent lymph nodes are resected, along with any other suspicious tissue. The tumor, nodes, and any other specimens are sent to the pathology laboratory for more in-depth analysis. The client then receives the usual postoperative care.

Laboratory Tests Most laboratory tests of blood, urine, and other body fluids are used to rule out nutritional disorders and other noncancerous conditions that may be causing the client's symptoms. For example, a complete blood count (CBC) helps screen for such problems as anemia, infection, and impaired immunity. Blood chemistries can point out nutritional disturbances and electrolyte imbalances. However, when used in conjunction with other diagnostic studies, some laboratory tests can be quite useful in either screening for other pathologic conditions or for validating the cancer diagnosis. These tests include evaluating levels of enzymes such as alanine aminotransferase (ALT), aspartate aminotransferase (AST), and lactic dehydrogenase (LDH) for liver metastases; measuring special protein tumor markers, such as PSA for prostate cancer and CEA for colon cancer. Table 9–9 identifies some useful laboratory tests, their normal values, and their possible indications.

Psychologic Support During Diagnosis
Preparing for and awaiting the results of diagnostic tests can create extreme anxiety. Many clients compare the experience to that of a prisoner awaiting trial and sentencing: After they know what the "sentence" is, then they can prepare for the future. In addition to coping with the possibility of a life-threatening disease, or at least a life-altering one, clients often also face the prospect of uncomfortable, even painful, diagnostic procedures. They have important decisions to make that hang on the outcome of those tests. Many unspoken questions may exist:

- Do I have cancer?
- If so, what kind, and how serious?
- Has it spread?
- Will I survive?
- What kind of treatment is needed?
- How will this affect my life-style?

Table 9–9   Laboratory Tests Used for Cancer Diagnosis*

Test	Reference Value	Abnormality Indicated
Acid phosphatase (ACP)	0.0 to 0.8 U/L	Elevated in prostate, breast, and bone cancer and in multiple myeloma
Alanine aminotransferase (ALT)	5 to 35 U/mL (Frankel)	Moderate elevation in liver cancer
Albumin	3.5 to 5.0 g/dL	Decreased in malnutrition, metastatic liver cancer
Alkaline phosphatase (ALP)	20 to 90 U/L	Elevated in cancer of liver, bone, breast, and prostate, in leukemia, and in multiple myeloma
Alpha fetoprotein (AFP)	Male and nonpregnant female: <15 ng/mL	Elevated in germ cell tumors (e.g., seminoma), testicular cancer
Aspartate aminotransferase (AST)	5 to 40 U/mL (Frankel)	Elevated in liver cancer
Bilirubin	Total: 0.1 to1.2 mg/dL Direct: 0.0 to 0.3 mg/dL	Elevated in liver and gallbladder cancer
Bleeding time	Ivy method: 3 to 7 minutes	Prolonged in leukemia and metastatic liver cancer
Blood urea nitrogen (BUN)	5 to 25 mg/dL	Decreased in malnutrition; increased in renal cancer
Calcitonin	Male: <40 pg/mL Female: <20 pg/mL	Elevated to >500 pg/mL in thyroid medullary cancer, breast cancer, and lung cancer
Calcium (Ca)	4.5 to 5.5 mEq/L 9.0 to 11.0 mg/dL	Elevated in bone cancer and ectopic parathyroid hormone production (paraplastic syndrome)
Chloride (Cl)	95 to 105 mEq/L	Decreased in vomiting, diarrhea, syndrome of inappropriate antidiuretic hormone (SIADH)
C-reactive protein	>1:2 titer is positive	Elevated in metastatic cancer and Burkitt's lymphoma
Creatinine	0.5 to 1.5 mg/dL	Decreased in malnutrition; elevated in most cancers
Dexamethasone suppression test	>50% reduction in plasma cortisol	Nonsuppression in adrenal cancer and ACTH-producing tumors, severe stress
Estradiol-Serum	Female: 20 to 300 pg/mL Menopausal female: <20 pg/mL Male: 15 to 50 pg/mL	Elevated in estrogen-producing tumors and testicular tumors
Fibrinogen	200 to 400 mg/dL	Decreased in leukemia and as a side effect of chemotherapy
Gamma glutamyltransferase (GGT)	Male: 10 to 80 IU/L Female: 5 to 25 IU/L	Elevated in cancer of liver, pancreas, prostate, breast, kidney, lung, and brain
Fasting blood sugar	70 to 110 mg/dL	Decreased in malnutrition, cancer of stomach, liver, and lung
Haptoglobin	20 to 240 mg/dL	Elevated in Hodgkin's disease and cancer of lung, large intestine, stomach, breast, and liver
Hematocrit (Hct)	Male: 40% to 54% Female: 36% to 46%	Decreased in anemia, leukemia, Hodgkin's disease, lymphosarcoma, multiple myeloma, and malnutrition and as a side effect of chemotherapy

*All values refer to serum values unless otherwise indicated. Values are approximate; check the reference standards specified by your own agency's laboratory.

- How will this affect family members and friends?

Denial or intellectualization will serve some clients well, but others will display signs of anxiety and stress as they attempt to cope with this perceived menace.

The nurse can provide invaluable help during this very difficult stage by helping to keep clients actively involved in managing their life and disease. Sitting down with clients as soon as they enter the health care system, asking what they know already about what is going to happen, and soliciting questions is a good way to start. By initiating the interaction with objective questions and

Table 9–9   (continued)

Test	Reference Value	Abnormality Indicated
Hemoglobin (Hgb)	Male: 13.5 to 18 g/dL Female: 12 to 16 g/dL 1:3 ratio of Hgb:Hct	Decreased in anemia, many cancers, Hodgkin's disease, leukemia, and malnutrition and as a side effect of chemotherapy
Human chorionic gonadotropin (HCG)	Nonpregnant female <0.01 IU/L	Elevated in choriocarcinoma
Insulin	5 to 25 μU/mL	Elevated in insulinoma (islet cell tumor) and insulin-secreting cancers (e.g., lung cancer)
Lactic dehydrogenase (LDH)	100 to 190 IU/L	Elevated in liver, brain, kidney, muscle cancers, acute leukemia, anemia
Occult blood	Negative	Positive in gastric and colon cancers
Serum osmolality	280 to 300 mOsm/kg H_2O	Decreased in SIADH
Urine osmolality	50 to 1200 mOsm/kg H_2O	Increased in SIADH
Parathyroid hormone (PTH)	400 to 900 pg/mL	Increased in PTH-secreting tumors
Platelet (thrombocyte) count	150,000/mm^3 to 400,000/mm^3	Decreased in bone, gastric, and brain cancer, in leukemia, and as a side effect of chemotherapy
Potassium (K)	3.5 to 5.0 mEq/L	Decreased in vomiting and diarrhea and in malnutrition
Prostate-specific antigen (PSA)	0 to 4 ng/mL	Elevated from 10 to 120+ in prostate cancer
Total protein	6.0 to 8.0 g/dL	Decreased in malnutrition, gastrointestinal cancer, Hodgkin's disease; elevated in vomiting, diarrhea, multiple myeloma
Red blood cells (RBCs)	Male: 4.6 to 6.0 million/mm^3 Female: 4.0 to 5.0 million/mm^3	Decreased in anemia, leukemia, infection, multiple myeloma
Sodium (Na)	135 to 145 mEq/L	Decreased in SIADH, vomiting; elevated in dehydration
Uric acid	Male: 3.5 to 8.0 mg/dL Female: 2.8 to 6.8 mg/dL	Increased in leukemia, metastatic cancer, multiple myeloma, Burkitt's lymphoma, after vigorous chemotherapy

White Blood Cells (WBC)
    Total leukocytes
    Neutrophils
	4,500/mm^3 to 10,000/mm^3
	
	50% to 70%
		Elevated in acute infection, leukemias, tissue necrosis; decreased as a side effect of chemotherapy
		Elevated in bacterial infection Hodgkin's disease; decreased in leukemia and malnutrition and as a side effect of chemotherapy

Eosinophils
    Basophils
    Monocytes
	1% to 3%
	0.4% to 1.0%
	4% to 6%
		Elevated in cancer of bone, ovary, testes, and brain
		Elevated in leukemia and healing stage of infection
		Elevated in infection, monocytic leukemia and cancer; decreased in lymphocytic leukemia and as a side effect of chemotherapy

Lymphocytes	25% to 35%	Elevated in lymphocytic leukemia, Hodgkin's disease, multiple myeloma, viral infections, and chronic infections; decreased in malnutrition, cancer, and other leukemias and as a side effect of chemotherapy

encouraging clients to share what knowledge and experience they have, the nurse allows them to maintain control. From there, the nurse can obtain the information needed.

It is essential that clients thoroughly understand the preparation required for their tests, especially if they will be preparing at home. They also need to be informed of any unusual effects that may occur with the test, such as nausea from radioactive dye. If possible, a phone call the evening before to verify the client's understanding of the procedure and answer questions can be very supportive.

As clients begin to feel more comfortable with the

nurse, they may express concerns, fears, and other emotions. The nurse should avoid giving advice and false reassurance, but rather just listen and be supportive, sharing appropriate information when needed. For clients who are not ready to discuss concerns or for those who appear angry, being nonjudgmental and providing nonverbal support may facilitate more open communication. An atmosphere of calmness, warmth, caring, and respect can ease the tension and often unspoken terror of this initial period.

Support of and communication with the client's significant others is extremely important. Often they try to be strong for the client but have many fears and emotional concerns that they do not feel comfortable expressing. The nurse needs to be available to the family while the client is undergoing diagnostic procedures. Allowing them to talk without the need to edit for the client's benefit can help them manage their own difficulties in coping with their loved one's potential cancer diagnosis.

Chemotherapy

Chemotherapy involves the use of cytotoxic medications and chemicals to effect a cure in some cancers, such as leukemias, lymphomas, and some solid tumors; to decrease tumor size, adjunctive to surgery or radiation therapy; or to prevent or treat suspected metastases. Chemotherapy is also being used in conjunction with biologic response modifiers (BRMs) in some types of advanced cancers. BRMs are discussed shortly. All chemotherapy has side effects or toxic effects; the type and severity depend upon the drugs used.

Chemotherapy is used to disrupt the cell cycle in various phases by interrupting cell metabolism and replication. It also works by interfering with the ability of the malignant cell to synthesize needed enzymes and chemicals. Phase-specific drugs work during specific phases of the cell cycle; non-phase-specific drugs work through the entire cell cycle. Figure 9–8 lists the drugs that are useful in each phase of the cell cycle.

Most chemical treatment involves combinations of drugs in specific protocols that are given over varying periods of time. For example, one protocol for adult acute lymphocytic leukemia (ALL) uses the acronym DVPA: daunorubicin given on days 1 through 3; vincristine given on days 1, 8, 15, and 22; prednisone given on days 1 through 28, and asparaginase given on days 17 through 28. The treatment regimen is given in cycles with rest periods allowed, especially if toxic effects such as liver dysfunction or severe neutropenia occur. The treatment is continued until the disease goes into remission or this particular protocol is abandoned and a new one tried.

New research is exploring the possiblity of basing the administration of chemotherapy on the body's circadian rhythms. Some drugs work better if they follow the normal cyclic fluxations of body hormones during the night,

whereas others are more effective when given during daytime hours. Chemotherapy administration that follows circadian rhythms appears to be more potent in killing tumor cells and produces fewer side effects. In a study reported at the May 1994 annual meeting of the American Society of Clinical Oncology, people with advanced colon cancer who were treated in this cyclic fashion (called chronotherapy) demonstrated a 51% shrinkage in their tumors, compared with a shrinkage of only 28% in people who received chemotherapy in a steady dosage over 24 hours. These encouraging results are prompting continued research on the timing of chemotherapy with other types of cancers (Kolata, 1994b).

The *cell-kill hypothesis* explains why several courses of chemotherapy are necessary. A 1-cm tumor contains about 10^9 (ten billion) total cells, most of which are viable. During each cell cycle, the chemotherapy kills a fixed percentage of cells, always leaving some behind. With each reduction, the tumor burden of cells decreases until the number of viable, *clonogenic* cells (i.e., those that are able to clone daughter cells) becomes small enough to allow the body's immune system to finish the job. For this reason, oncologists usually give the maximum amount of chemotherapy that is tolerated by the client.

However, new research is challenging the accepted wisdom that increasing the amount of chemotherapy is more effective in promoting survival. In a random study of 2300 women with advanced breast cancer, a double dose of chemotherapy was no more effective than the standard dose. The investigators concluded that higher doses of chemotherapy, which significantly increase the adverse effects experienced by the client, are not justified. However, other researchers believe this issue is not closed and want more studies to compare increased dosages with survival outcomes (Kolata, 1994c).

Classes of Chemotherapeutic Drugs Chemotherapeutic agents fall basically into six major classes: alkylating agents, antimetabolites, cytotoxic antibiotics, plant alkaloids, hormones and hormone antagonists, and miscellaneous agents (Cooper & Cooper, 1991; Krakoff, 1992).

Alkylating Agents Alkylating agents are non-phase-specific and basically act on preformed nucleic acids by creating defects in tumor DNA. They cause cross-linking of DNA strands, which can permanently interfere with replication and transcription.

Alkylating agents work with both proliferating and nonproliferating cells (those in G_0 phase). Their toxicity relates to the ability to kill slowly cycling stem cells and manifests in delayed, prolonged, or permanent bone marrow failure. Toxicity can also cause a mutagenic effect on bone marrow stem cells, culminating in a treatment-resistant form of acute myelogenous leukemia. Because of the alkylating agents' effect on stem cells, they also cause irreversible infertility. Other common adverse effects include nephrotoxicity and hemorrhagic cystitis.

There are five subclasses of alkylating agents: nitrogen mustards (mechlorethamine), nitrosoureas (carmustine), alkyl sulfonates (busulfan), triazines (dacarbazine), and ethylenimines (thiotepa).

Antimetabolites Antimetabolites, a group of somewhat diverse drugs, are phase-specific, working best in the S phase and having little effect in G_0. They interfere with nucleic acid synthesis by either displacing normal metabolites at the regulatory site of a key enzyme or by substituting for a metabolite that is incorporated into DNA or RNA molecules.

Toxic effects usually do not occur until very high levels of the drug are administered. Toxicity is also more likely when the drugs accumulate in third-spaced fluid, such as pleural fluid (a characteristic that also makes them useful in treating malignant pleural effusions). Because the drug diffuses out slowly from the third-spaced fluid, exposure of the tissue to the drug is prolonged. Most toxic effects relate to rapidly proliferating cells, such as cells in the gastrointestinal tract, hair, and skin and white blood cells. Signs and symptoms include the following:

- Nausea and vomiting
- Stomatitis
- Diarrhea
- Alopecia
- Leukopenia

Some of the drugs can also cause liver and pulmonary toxicity.

The different classes of antimetabolites include folic acid analogues (methotrexate), pyrimidine analogues (5-fluorouracil), cytosine arabinoside (ARA-C), and purine analogues (6-mercaptopurine).

Cytotoxic Antibiotics Cytotoxic antibiotics all derive from various species of *Streptomyces* and are generally too toxic to be used as antibacterial agents. They are non-phase-specific and act in several ways: They disrupt DNA replication and RNA transcription; create free radicals, which generate breaks in DNA and other forms of damage; and interfere with DNA repair. In addition, these drugs bind to almost everything they contact and kill cells, probably through damaging the cell membrane. Their main toxic effect is damage to the cardiac muscle. This limits the amount and duration of treatment. Examples of these antibiotics include actinomycin D, doxorubicin, bleomycin, mitomycin-C, and mithramycin.

Plant Alkaloids Plant alkaloids consist of two main groups extracted from plant sources: *Vinca* alkaloids (e.g.,

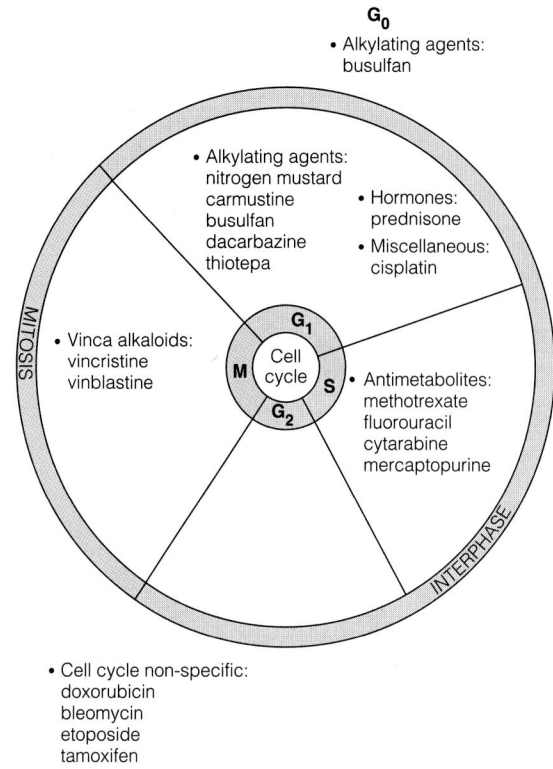

Figure 9–8 Chemotherapeutic drugs useful in each phase of the cell cycle. Based on their chemical makeup and biologic activity, different drugs used for cancer treatment act in specific phases and subphases of the cell cycle. Some drugs, called non-phase-specific drugs, are generalized and act throughout the cycle. Chemotherapy often involves combinations of drugs designed to attack the cancer cells at many different times in the cycle and thus to enhance effectiveness.

vincristine and vinblastine) and etoposide (also called VP-16). The *Vinca* alkaloids are phase-specific, acting during mitosis. They bind to a specific protein that promotes chromosome migration during mitosis and serves as a conduit for neurotransmitter transport along axons. The toxicity of these drugs is characterized by depression of deep-tendon reflexes, paresthesias (pain and altered sensation), motor weakness, cranial nerve disruptions, and paralytic ileus. Etoposide acts in all phases of the cell cycle, causing breaks in DNA and metaphase arrest. Although etoposide may cause bone marrow suppression and nausea and vomiting, the most common toxic effect is hypotension resulting from too rapid intravenous administration.

Hormones and Hormone Antagonists The main hormones used in cancer therapy are the corticosteroids (e.g., prednisone), which are phase-specific (G_1). These act by binding to specific intracellular receptors, repressing transcription of mRNA and thereby altering cellular function and growth. Corticosteroids have multiple side effects, such as impaired healing, hyperglycemia, hypertension, osteoporosis, and hirsutism.

Hormone antagonists work with hormone-binding tumors, usually those of the breast, prostate, and endometrium. They bind at the hormone's receptor site and thereby deprive the tumor of its hormones. These drugs do not cure but do cause regression of the tumor in about 40% of breast and endometrial tumors and 80% of prostate tumors. Tamoxifen competes with estradiol receptors in breast tumors. Diethylstilbestrol competes with hormone receptors in endometrial and prostate tumors. Antiandrogen (flutamide) and luteinizing hormone-releasing hormone (LHRH) block testosterone synthesis in prostate cancers. The main side effects of these drugs are alterations of the secondary sexual characteristics.

Miscellaneous Agents   The main miscellaneous drug is cisplatin, an inorganic drug containing platinum and chlorine atoms. It is most active in the G_1 subphase, but it is also non-phase-specific. Cisplatin binds to DNA and acts much like alkylating agents by forming intrastrand DNA crosslinks (gluing strands of DNA together so that they cannot separate). Its major toxic effect is reversible renal tubular necrosis. Cisplatin may be used alone or in combination with other chemotherapeutic drugs for testicular and ovarian cancers.

Effects of Chemotherapeutic Drugs   As described above, the side effects and toxic effects of chemotherapy vary with the drug used and the length of treatment. Because most of these drugs act on fast-growing cells, the side effects are manifestations of damage to normal rapidly dividing somatic cells. The side effects of hormones are expressions of the action of the hormone used or suppression of the normal hormone, such as the masculinizing effects of male hormones administered for ovarian cancers.

The tissues usually affected by cytotoxic drugs include the following:

- The mucous membranes of the mouth, tongue, esophagus, stomach, intestine, and rectum. This results in anorexia, loss of taste, aversion to food, erythema and painful ulcerations in any portion of the gastrointestinal tract, nausea, vomiting, and diarrhea.

- Hair cells, resulting in alopecia.

- Bone marrow depression affecting most blood cells (e.g., granulocytes, lymphocytes, thrombocytes, and erythrocytes). This results in an impaired ability to respond to infection, a diminished ability to clot blood, and severe anemia.

- Organs, such as heart, lungs, bladder, kidneys. This kind of damage is related to specific agents, such as cardiac toxicity with doxorubicin or pneumonitis with bleomycin.

- Reproductive organs, resulting in impaired reproductive ability or altered fetal development.

Table 9–10 gives the classifications of chemotherapeutic drugs, common examples, target malignancies, adverse effects and side effects, and nursing implications. Consult current pharmacology texts for additional drugs and for new combination therapies as they are developed.

Preparation and Administration   Many states or specific hospitals require that personnel be trained and certified to administer chemotherapy. Pharmacists in large hospitals and independent home care agencies usually prepare chemotherapeutic drugs for parenteral administration under specific safety guidelines established by the federal government or the Oncology Nursing Society. In some agencies, nurses are employed both to prepare and to administer these drugs. Because of the potential carcinogenic effects, it is usually recommended that the health care professional wear gloves, masks, and gowns while preparing and administering the drug and disposing of equipment. The nurse must use care when handling excretory products of clients undergoing chemotherapy and teach clients to dispose of their own body fluids safely. Oral medications pose a lesser risk of exposure, but a risk nonetheless, primarily through excretion in the urine.

Chemotherapeutic drugs can be administered orally, such as cyclophosphamide (Cytoxan) and chlorambucil (Leukeran). Some drugs, such as hormones or hormone-blocking agents, may also be given intramuscularly. However, many drugs require intravenous infusion or direct injection into intraperitoneal or intrapleural body cavities. Intravenous preparations can be given through large peripheral veins, but the risk of extravasation or irritation to the vein may preclude this method for long-term therapy. Many clients now receive vascular access devices (VADs), especially those undergoing treatment that requires several cycles over several weeks or months. VADs are also useful for adjunctive parenteral nutrition in the client who requires continuous intravenous infusions to manage pain or frequent blood drawing to monitor blood counts. Different types of VADs are available:

- Catheters that are inserted nonsurgically by threading them through a large peripheral vein into the vena cava. Called peripherally inserted central catheters (PICC), they have multiple lumens that facilitate blood drawing. Placement is usually monitored by fluoroscopy.

- Catheters tunneled under the skin on the chest into a major vein, such as the subclavian vein. Hickman or Groshong catheters may be used.

- Surgically implanted ports, such as Mediport, which are placed under the skin with a connected catheter inserted into a major vein. These are then accessed by

Table 9–10   Classifications of Chemotherapeutic Drugs

Drug Classification	Common Drugs	Target Malignancies	Adverse Effects or Side Effects	Nursing Implications
Alkylating agents	Mechlorethamine (Mustargen)	Hodgkin's disease Lymphosarcoma Lung cancer Chronic leukemia	Nausea and vomiting Leukopenia Thrombocytopenia Hyperuricemia	Maintain good hydration. Alkalinize urine. Administer antiemetics prior to chemotherapy. Monitor WBC, uric acid. Assess for infection.
	Busulfan (Myleran)	Chronic myelogenous leukemia	Leukopenia Thrombocytopenia Renal failure Pulmonary fibrosis	Monitor WBCs, BUN. Maintain adequate fluid intake. Assess for infection. Assess lungs for fibrotic (coarse, loud) rales.
	Cyclophosphamide (Cytoxan)	Lymphomas Multiple myeloma Leukemias Adenocarcinoma of lung and breast	Hemorrhagic cystitis Renal failure Alopecia Stomatitis Liver dysfunction	Encourage daily fluid intake of 2 to 3 liters during treatment. Monitor WBCs, BUN, liver enzymes. Teach ways to manage hair loss.
Antimetabolites	Methotrexate	Acute lymphoblastic leukemia Osteosarcoma Gestational trophoblastic carcinoma	Oral and gastrointestinal ulcerations Anorexia and nausea Leukopenia Thrombocytopenia Pancytopenia	Monitor CBC, WBC differential, BUN, uric acid, creatinine. Assess oral mucous membranes; treat ulcers prn. Assess for infection, bleeding.
	5-Fluorouracil (5-FU)	Colon carcinoma Rectal carcinoma Breast carcinoma Gastric carcinoma Pancreatic cancer	Stomatitis Alopecia Nausea and vomiting Gastritis Enteritis Diarrhea Anemia Leukopenia Thrombocytopenia	Monitor CBC with differential, BUN, uric acid. Administer antiemetics prn. Assess for bleeding; check stool occult blood. Evaluate hydration and nutrition status. Teach oral care for stomatitis. Assess for infection. Teach care for hair loss.
Antitumor antibiotics	Doxorubicin (Adriamycin)	Acute lymphoblastic leukemia (ALL) Acute myeloblastic leukemia Neuroblastoma Wilms' tumor Breast, ovarian, thyroid, lung cancer	Stomatitis Alopecia Nausea and vomiting Gastritis Enteritis Diarrhea Anemia Leukopenia Thrombocytopenia Cardiac toxicity	Monitor ECG; assess for arrythmias, gallops, and congestive heart failure (CHF). Monitor CBC with differential, BUN, uric acid. Administer antiemetics prn. Assess for bleeding; check stool for occult blood. Evaluate hydration and nutrition status. Teach oral care for stomatitis. Assess for infection. Teach care for hair loss.

➤

Table 9–10   (continued)

Drug Classification	Common Drugs	Target Malignancies	Adverse Effects or Side Effects	Nursing Implications
	Bleomycin (Blenoxane)	Squamous cell carcinoma Lymphosarcoma Reticulum cell sarcoma Testicular carcinoma Hodgkin's disease	Mucocutaneous ulcerations Alopecia Nausea and vomiting Chills and fever Pneumonitis and pulmonary fibrosis	Check for fever 3 to 6 hours after administration. Have chest X-ray films taken every 2 to 3 weeks. Assess respiratory status, and check for coarse rales. Evaluate hydration and nutrition status. Teach oral care for stomatitis. Assess for infection. Teach care for hair loss.
Plant alkaloids	Vincristine (Oncovin)	Combination therapy for acute leukemia, Hodgkin's and non-Hodgkin lymphomas, rhabdomyosarcoma, neuroblastoma, Wilm's tumor	Areflexia Muscle weakness Peripheral neuritis Constipation Paralytic ileus Mild bone marrow depression	Assess neuromuscular function. Monitor CBC with differential. Evaluate gastrointestinal function. Manage constipation.
	Vinblastin (Velban)	Combination therapy for Hodgkin's disease, lymphocytic and histocytic lymphoma, Kaposi's sarcoma, advanced testicular carcinoma, unresponsive breast cancer	Areflexia Alopecia Nausea and vomiting Bone marrow depression	Assess neuromuscular function. Monitor CBC with differential. Administer antiemetics prn. Teach ways to manage hair loss.
	Etoposide, also called VP-16 (VePesid)	Nonresponsive testicular tumors Small-cell lung cancer	Alopecia Hypotension with rapid infusion	Hydrate adequately before administration. Administer for 60 minutes. Monitor vital signs every 15 minutes during administration and every 2 to 4 hours thereafter. Teach ways to manage hair loss.

means of a special needle with a 90-degree bend inserted through the skin directly into the rubber dome of the port, which has a hard plastic back to prevent tissue damage.

Figure 9–9 shows examples of different catheters and vascular access ports.

Risk of infection, catheter obstruction, and extravasation are the main problems associated with VADs. Nurses therefore must teach clients and family members to observe for redness, swelling, pain, or exudate at the insertion site, which may indicate infection; to observe for swelling of neck or skin near the VAD for extravasation and infiltration; and to flush catheters and provide site care (cleaning and dressing changes) on a regular basis.

During each encounter with the client, the nurse always inspects the site; observes for infection, infiltration, and catheter occlusion; and provides site care whenever it is necessary.

Management of Clients Receiving Chemotherapy
In addition to providing the above nursing interventions, nurses assist in identifying and managing toxic effects or side effects of the drugs and provide psychosocial support. Careful assessment and monitoring of the client's signs and symptoms, including appropriate laboratory tests, alert the nurse to the onset of toxicity. Nausea and vomiting, diarrhea, inflammation and ulceration of oral mucous membranes, hair loss, skin changes, anorexia, and fatigue require specific medical and nursing actions.

| **Table 9–10** | (continued) | | | |

Drug Classification	Common Drugs	Target Malignancies	Adverse Effects or Side Effects	Nursing Implications
	Prednisone	Combination therapy for many tumors Leukemia Lymphoma	Fluid retention Hypertension Steroid diabetes Emotional lability Silent bleeding ulcers Increased risk for infection	Monitor vital signs. Administer diuretics prn. Check blood glucose regularly. Evaluate mental status. Administer oral medications with food. Administer hydrogen ion antagonist drugs (antacids) as ordered. Monitor WBC with differential. Check for signs of systemic infection.
	Diethylstilbestrol (DES)	Advanced breast and prostrate cancers	Fluid retention Feminization Uterine bleeding	Monitor vital signs. Administer diuretics prn as ordered. Explain reason for feminization to men, bleeding to women. Monitor for excessive bleeding.
	Tamoxifen (Nolvadex)	Breast cancer	Hot flashes Nausea and vomiting	Teach ways to manage hot flashes. Explain reason for hot flashes. Administer antiemetics as ordered.
Miscellaneous drugs	Cisplatin (CDDP) (Platinol)	Combination and single therapy for metastatic testicular and ovarian cancers, advanced bladder cancer, head and neck tumors, non-small-cell lung carcinoma, osteogenic sarcoma, neuroblastoma	Bone marrow depression: leukopenia and thrombocytopenia Renal tubular damage Deafness	Monitor WBC with differential and platelets, BUN, creatinine, uric acid. Watch for bleeding. Monitor for signs of infection. Evaluate hearing; check for tinnitus. Ensure that client is well hydrated before drug is administered. Encourage 2 to 3 liters of fluid intake daily.

These actions are discussed later in this chapter under the appropriate nursing diagnoses. Indicators of organ toxicities, such as nephrotoxicity, neurotoxicity, or cardiac toxicity, must be reported immediately to the physician.

Another aspect of managing clients undergoing chemotherapy is to teach them how to care for access sites and to dispose of used equipment and excretions safely. Nurses also teach clients to increase fluid intake to flush out the drugs; to get extra rest, which can both assist therapy and help the client avoid other illnesses; to identify major complications of their particular drug protocol; to know when to call the physician or emergency medical services; and, if their white blood cell count is low, to limit their exposure to other persons, especially those with infections or children.

During chemotherapy, a number of psychologic issues that can cause moderate to severe emotional distress may arise. The necessity to plan activities around chemotherapy treatments and the side effects can impair the client's ability to work, manage a household or care for family members, function sexually, or participate in social and recreational activities. Weight loss and alopecia may prompt feelings of powerlessness and depression. The nurse can assist by carefully evaluating symptoms, providing specific interventions as indicated, and allowing clients opportunities to express their fears, concerns, and feelings. Clients should be encouraged to participate in their care and maintain control over their life as much as possible (McCabe, 1991). Specific interventions will be discussed later in the chapter under the appropriate nursing diag-

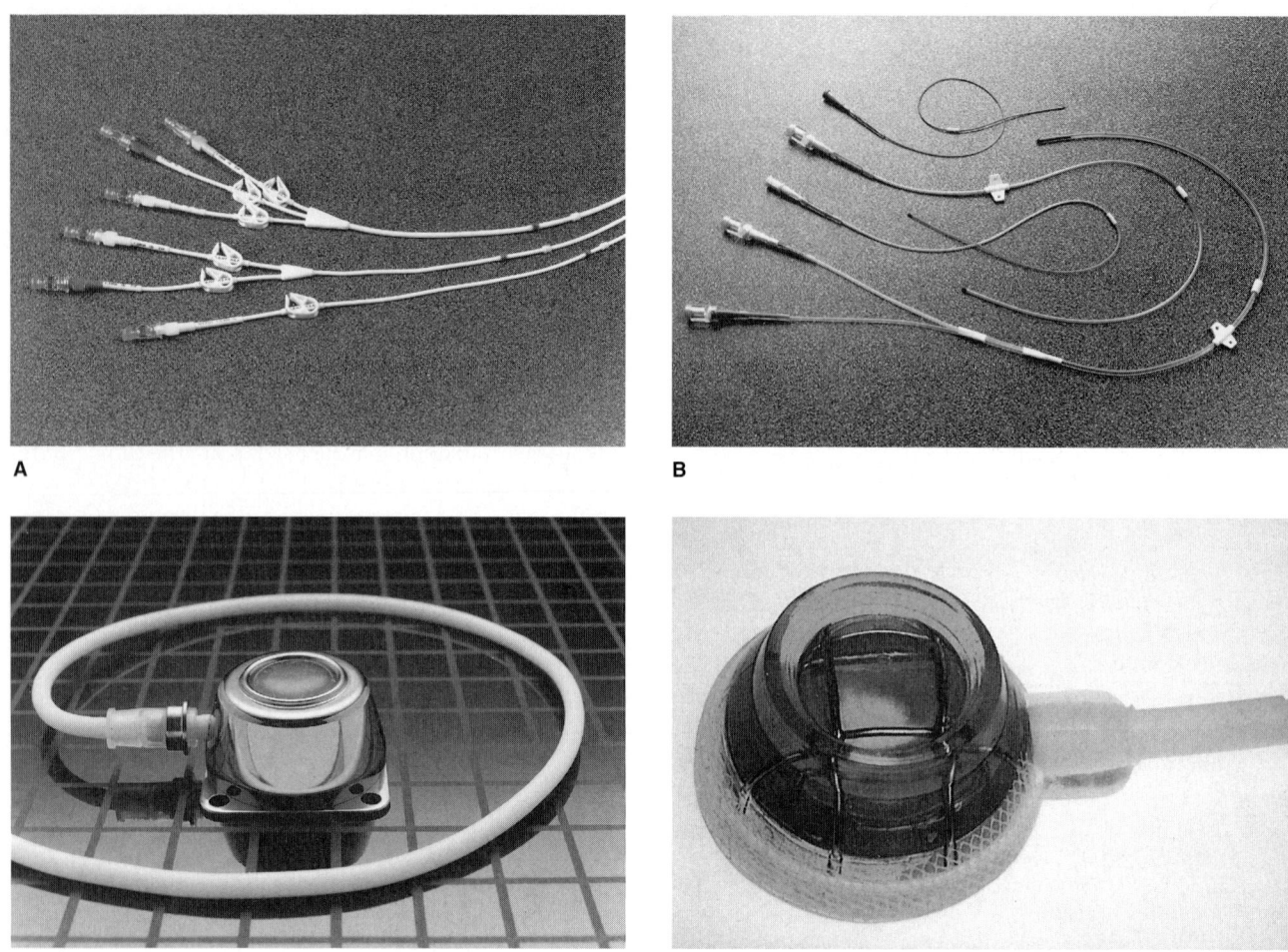

A

B

C

D

Figure 9–9 Vascular access devices. *A*, Single-, double-, and triple-lumen catheters;
B, single- and double-lumen Groshong catheters; *C*, Port-a-Cath Access System; *D*, Norport-SP, a
side-entrance port.

noses. Table 9–10 includes nursing implications for specific adverse effects of common chemotherapy drugs.

Surgery

Surgical resection is currently used for diagnosis and staging of more than 90% of all cancers and for primary treatment of more than 60%. Whenever possible, the tumor is
removed in its entirety. This sometimes necessitates mutilation of the body and the creation of new structures to
assume function of the lost structures. For example, removal of the distal sigmoid colon and rectum requires a
new means of bowel elimination, so the remaining
healthy segment of the bowel is brought out through a
created opening (stoma) in the abdominal wall, resulting
in a permanent colostomy (see Chapter 23). In like manner, when the bladder is removed, the ureters are transplanted into a created pouch just under the abdominal

wall. This serves as a continent ileostomy, a substitute
reservoir for urine (see Chapter 25). Surgery can also destroy sensitive nerve plexes, resulting in alteration or loss
of normal functioning; for example, prostate surgery may
result in incontinence and impotence.

Not all surgery results in such radical changes in functioning. There are several examples in which surgery can
eliminate cancer successfully with less distressing results:

- Removing a nonessential portion of the organ or tissue
  containing the tumor, such as in situ small bowel tumors
- Removing an organ whose function can be replaced
  chemically, such as the thyroid
- Resecting one of a pair of organs when the unaffected
  organ can take over the function of the missing one,
  such as a lung

Although the removal of any major body part has physiologic and psychologic consequences, the alternative—terminal disease—is usually less desirable.

If the tumor is in a nonresectable location or deeply invasive with metastases, surgery may be only a palliative measure to allow the involved organs to function as long as possible or to relieve pain. Surgery may also be done to reduce the bulk of the tumor in advanced disease, both at primary and metastatic sites. Decreasing the tumor size enhances the ability to control the remaining disease through other modalities. Surgery is often used in conjunction with other treatments to effect a more secure cure. When, for example, extensive removal of tissue is contraindicated (e.g., in surgical removal of a brain tumor), radiation may be used prior to surgery in an attempt to shrink the tumor first.

Other uses of surgical intervention include reconstruction and rehabilitation. One example is the construction of transabdominal mycocutaneous (TRAM) flaps in conjunction with or following modified radical mastectomy (see Chapter 48). For surgical interventions for cancers affecting specific body systems, refer to later chapters.

The future of surgery in cancer diagnosis and treatment is exciting. Surgical oncologists see much opportunity in working with researchers to identify premalignant disease earlier in high-risk populations and to acquire and process tissues to support studies on reversing oncogenic cell activity. Surgeons also work with molecular biologists using sophisticated techniques for obtaining tissues from obscure body locations to develop monoclonal antibodies from tissue antigenic material. Laser technology is being explored for use in different types of cancer surgery because it minimizes blood loss, reduces deformity, increases the accuracy of tissue resection, and speeds healing. This complex new tool is currently being investigated for radical prostatectomy in order to preserve urinary continence and sexual functioning. Another collaborative strategy under development is intraoperative radiation therapy, in which radiosensitive, nondiseased organs that may be damaged by radiation therapy are moved away from the radiation field and shielded. This technique allows more penetrating radiation to be directed to the malignant tumor with less trauma to normal vulnerable tissues or organs.

Nursing responsibilities focus on preparing the client physically and psychologically for the specific surgery, as well as teaching routine postoperative care in which the client is expected to participate. For example, the nurse teaches the client about respiratory care and the use of the incentive spirometer (e.g., a Triflow) to improve postoperative ventilation, early ambulation to prevent circulatory problems, and the manner in which the client will receive fluids and nutrition (intravenously or orally, depending on type of surgery). In addition, the nurse explains the specific surgical procedure and any anticipated alterations to the client's body, especially those that require major life-style adjustments, such as a colostomy. Before surgery, the nurse should give the client the opportunity to ask questions and to discuss concerns and fears. In some cases, the client may want to discuss alternative treatment options that are available. In the latter case, the nurse should avoid trying to persuade the client to accept any one option; rather, the nurse should contact the oncologist and the surgeon and set up a conference for the client prior to surgery.

Radiation Therapy

Still the treatment of choice for some tumors or by some oncologists, radiation may be used to kill the tumor, to reduce its size, to decrease pain, or to relieve obstruction. Lymph nodes and adjacent tissues are irradiated when beginning metastasis is suspected. Radiation therapy consists of delivering ionizing radiations of gamma and X-rays in one of two ways:

- *Teletherapy*. Also called external radiation, teletherapy involves placing the source of radiation at some distance from the client. A relatively uniform dosage is delivered.

- *Brachytherapy*. In brachytherapy, the radioactive material is placed directly into the tumor site, a technique that delivers a high dose to the tumor and a lower dose to the normal tissues. Brachytherapy is also referred to as internal, interstitial, or intracavitary radiation.

For many common neoplasms, a combination of these two therapies is used.

Lethal injury to DNA is believed to be the primary mechanism by which radiation kills cells, especially cells in faster growing tumors and tissues. As a result, when given over time, radiation can destroy not only rapidly multiplying cancer cells but also rapidly dividing normal cells, such as those of the skin and mucous membranes. A malignant tumor is considered cured when there are no surviving tumor stem cells. The goal of radiation therapy is to achieve maximum tumor control with a minimum of damage to normal tissue.

Implanted or ingested radiation can be dangerous for those living with, taking care of, or treating the client. Caregivers must protect themselves by, for example, shielding themselves from the source of radiation, limiting the time of exposure to the client, increasing the distance from the client, and using specific safety procedures for handling secretions. The box on page 340 identifies safety principles to be followed by those caring for clients undergoing internal radiation.

Tumors have differing sensitivities to radiation. Tumors that have the greatest number of rapidly proliferating cancer cells usually exhibit the best early response to radiation. The decision to use radiation as opposed to other

Safety Principles for Radiation

■ ■ ■

These recommendations apply to caregivers working with clients receiving internal radiation (brachytherapy).

- Maintain the greatest possible distance from the source of radiation.

- Spend the minimum amount of time close to the radiation source.

- Shield yourself from the radiation with lead gloves and aprons whenever possible.

- If you are pregnant, do not come into any contact with radiation sources.

- If you work routinely near radiation, wear a monitoring device to measure whole-body exposure.

- Avoid direct exposure with radioisotope containers; for example, do not touch the container.

- Keep clients with implanted radioisotopes in a private room with private bath and as far away from other hospitalized persons as possible.

- Dispose of body fluids of clients with unsealed implanted radioisotopes with special care and in specially marked containers.

- Handle bed linen and clothing with care and according to agency protocol.

- Use long-handled forceps to place any dislodged implants into a lead container.

- Consult with the radiation therapy department for any questions or problems in caring for clients with radioactive implants.

Degree of Radiosensitivity for Selected Cancers

■ ■ ■

Very Radiosensitive

- Neuroblastoma
- Lymphomas
- Chronic leukemia

Moderately Radiosensitive

- Bronchogenic carcinoma
- Esophageal carcinoma
- Squamous cell carcinoma
- Prostate carcinoma
- Cervical carcinoma
- Testicular carcinoma

Nonradiosensitive

- Many adenocarcinomas
- Fibrosarcoma
- Osteogenic carcinoma

exudate, a condition called radiation pneumonia. Occasionally, external radiation therapy may cause fistulas or necrosis of adjacent tissues. Implanted radioactive materials can lead to similar problems; moreover, the excretory products of these clients are usually considered dangerous and need special disposal. The accompanying box describes nursing implications for clients receiving radiation therapy.

modalities is based on balancing the probability of controlling the tumor against the probability of causing complications, such as tissue damage. The decision is usually reached by means of a risk-benefit analysis. Although this process may sound very scientific, it is often not exact. Radiation oncologists describe the prescription for radiation therapy as "giving the maximum dose that the normal tissues can tolerate and praying that it is sufficient to control the tumor" (Hendrickson & Withers, 1991). The accompanying box lists the degree of radiosensitivity for selected cancers.

The client receiving external radiation may experience skin changes such as blanching, erythema, desquamation, sloughing, or hemorrhage. Ulcerations of mucous membranes may cause severe pain; in addition, secretions can decrease, making the client more vulnerable to infection. Gastrointestinal effects include nausea and vomiting, diarrhea, or bleeding. Lungs may develop interstitial

Immunotherapy

Biologic response modifiers (BRMs) have been proposed as a fourth therapeutic modality for cancer (Brophy & Sharp, 1991; Jackson, Strauman, Frederickson, & Strauman, 1991). These agents are used to modify the biologic processes that result in malignant cells, primarily through enhancing the person's own immune responses. The development of these therapies was based on the immune surveillance hypothesis. Although it has been established that a competent immune system is the body's most important defense against any disease, the role that various immune cells play in combating different types of malignancies is not yet clear. Therefore, the use of BRMs is still experimental. Currently, they are used mainly to halt advanced and metastasizing disease.

It was originally believed that the body's resistance against tumors relied on lymphocytes, T cells in particular. Newer research, however, has shown that many

Nursing Implications for the Client Receiving Radiation Therapy

Nursing Responsibilities for Either External or Internal Radiation Therapy

- Carefully assess and manage any complications, usually in collaboration with the radiation oncologist.
- Assist in documenting the results of the therapy; for example, clients receiving radiation for metastases to the spine will show improved neurologic functioning as tumor size diminishes.
- Provide emotional support, relief of physical and psychologic discomfort, and opportunities to talk about fears and concerns. For some clients, radiation therapy is a last chance for cure or even just for relief of physical discomfort.

External Radiation

Prior to the start of treatments, the treatment area will be specifically located by the radiation oncologist and marked with colored semipermanent ink. Treatment is usually given 5 days per week for 15 to 30 minutes per day over 2 to 7 weeks.

Nursing Responsibilities

- Monitor for adverse effects: skin changes, such as blanching, erythema, desquamation, sloughing, or hemorrhage; ulcerations of mucous membranes; nausea and vomiting, diarrhea, or gastrointestinal bleeding.
- Assess lungs for rales, which may indicate interstitial exudate. Observe for any dyspnea or changes in respiratory pattern.
- Identify and record any medications that the client will be taking during the radiation treatment.
- Monitor white blood cell counts and platelet counts for significant decreases.

Client and Family Teaching

- Wash the skin that is marked as the radiation site only with plain water, no soap; do not apply deodorant, lotions, medications, perfume, or talcum powder to the site during the treatment period. Take care not to wash off the treatment marks.
- Do not rub, scratch, or scrub treated skin areas. If it is necessary to shave the treated area, use only an electric razor.
- Apply neither heat nor cold (e.g., heating pad or ice pack) to the treatment site.
- Inspect the skin for damage or serious changes, and report these to the radiologist or physician.

- Wear loose, soft clothing over the treated area.
- Protect skin from sun exposure during treatment and for at least 1 year after radiation therapy is discontinued. Cover skin with protective clothing during treatment; once radiation is discontinued, use sun-blocking agents with a sun protection factor (SPF) of at least 15.
- External radiation poses no risk to other people for radiation exposure, even with intimate physical contact.
- Be sure to get plenty of rest and eat a balanced diet.

Internal Radiation

The radiation source, called an implant, is placed into the affected tissue or body cavity and is sealed in tubes, containers, wires, seeds, capsules, or needles. An implant may be temporary or permanent. Internal radiation may also be ingested or injected as a solution into the bloodstream or a body cavity or be introduced into the tumor through a catheter. The radioactive substance may transmit rays outside the body or be excreted in body fluids.

Nursing Responsibilities

- Place the client in a private room.
- Limit visits to 10 to 30 minutes, and have visitors sit at least 6 feet from the client.
- Monitor for side effects such as burning sensations, excessive perspiration, chills and fever, nausea and vomiting, or diarrhea.
- Assess for fistulas or necrosis of adjacent tissues.

Client and Family Teaching

- While a temporary implant is in place, stay in bed and rest quietly to avoid dislodging the implant.
- For outpatient treatments, avoid close contact with others until treatment has been discontinued.
- If the radiologist indicates the need for such measures, dispose of excretory materials in special containers or in a toilet not used by others.
- Carry out daily activities as able; get extra rest if feeling fatigued.
- Eat a balanced diet; frequent, small meals often are better tolerated.
- Contact the nurse or physician for any concerns or questions after discharge.

different components of the immune system may be involved. A variety of immunotherapies is being tried, including combination therapies. For example, the *immunomodulator* chemical alpha interferon has been combined with the cytotoxic drug 5-fluorouracil (Brophy & Sharp, 1991).

Tumor immunology has several applications: detection screening in high-risk groups, differential diagnosis and classification of tumor cells, monitoring the course of the disease with early detection of recurrence, and active therapies to halt or limit the disease. The theory underlying tumor immunology is that most tumor cells have a structural appearance that is recognizable by the immune cells. Tumor-associated antigens (TAAs) exist on tumor cells but not on normal cells. TAAs elicit an immune response that, in a person with a competent immune system, will destroy or inhibit tumor growth. Thus, TAAs can be isolated from serum and used for both diagnosis and various treatment modalities. The prostate-specific antigen (PSA) is one such TAA currently in successful diagnostic use (Brawer & Lange, 1990).

Tumor cells are often in a stage of arrested development (i.e., in the differentiation stage) for the cell type they represent; thus, they express antigens characteristic of that particular stage of development. The immaturity of the cells provides the physician with information about the relative aggressiveness of the cancer.

Another aspect of immunotherapy is the development of monoclonal antibodies that enhance the immune system's ability to fight the cancer. Monoclonal antibodies are developed by inoculating an animal with the specific tumor antigen and recovering the specific antibodies produced. The antibodies are then given to the person with that cancer to assist in the destruction of the tumor. Monoclonal antibodies are also recreated, or cloned, in the genetic laboratory by recombining DNA to produce the specific antibody. Techniques involving recombinant DNA have been used to combine these antibodies with toxins and drugs that are then delivered selectively to the tumor sites.

A number of cytokines (normal growth-regulating molecules) with antitumor activity have been synthesized. Alpha interferon, bacillus Calmette-Guérin (BCG, which has been used for many years as an inoculation against tuberculosis), and interleukin-2 have shown some therapeutic benefit in eliciting increased immune responses. Combination strategies have also helped stimulate the function of the macrophages.

A most promising discovery has been the recently identified natural killer cells, called NK cells. These cells are like large granular lymphocytes but have a cell surface phenotype different from that of T lymphocytes or macrophages. They have demonstrated a spontaneous cytotoxic effect on some types of cancer cells. They also provide a strong resistance to metastasis and secrete cytokines.

When augmented by biologic response modifiers such as interleukin-2, they show increased tumor destructive activity (Herberman, 1991).

One other aspect of immunotherapy has been the use of hematopoietic growth factors, such as granulocyte colony-stimulating factor (G-CSF) and erythropoietin. These substances offset the suppression of granulocytes and erythrocytes that results from chemotherapy (Doweiko & Goldberg, 1991).

As promising as these new therapies are, they are accompanied by serious side effects and toxic effects. Interleukin-2 can cause acute alterations in renal, cardiac, liver, gastrointestinal, and mental functioning. Alpha interferon causes mental slowing, confusion, and lethargy and, when used in combination with 5-fluorouracil or interleukin-2, severe flulike symptoms—chills and fever of 103 F to 106 F (39.4 C to 41.1 C), nausea, vomiting, diarrhea, anorexia, severe fatigue, and stomatitis—may result. The toxic effects are probably exaggerations of the normal systemic effects that these substances cause when fighting infection. For example, interleukin-2 is known to raise body temperature substantially in an attempt to create a hostile environment for foreign invaders.

The accompanying box discusses nursing implications for clients receiving immunotherapy. For nursing care of specific problems, refer to the appropriate nursing diagnoses later in this chapter.

Photodynamic Therapy

Photodynamic therapy is a new method of treating certain kinds of superficial tumors. It goes by several different names: phototherapy, photoradiation, and photochemotherapy. Clients suffering from tumors growing on the surface of the bladder, peritoneal cavity, chest wall, pleura, bronchus, or head and neck are candidates for this treatment. The client is given an intravenous dose of a photosensitizing compound, Photofrin, which is selectively retained in higher concentrations in malignant tissue. This drug is activated by a laser treatment that is started 3 days after the drug injection and continued for 3 more days. The drug interacts with oxygen molecules in the tissue to produce a cytotoxic oxygen molecule called singlet oxygen.

At the time of the first intravenous injection, clients are observed for adverse hypersensitivity reactions, such as nausea, chills, and hives. Systemic or long-term toxicities are rare. The main side effects are local skin reactions and temporary photosensitivity, transiently elevated liver enzymes, and inflammatory responses of the tissues being treated, such as peritoneal or pleural tissues. This treatment is currently being used only on clients who have not responded to more traditional cancer treatments, but good results in decreasing the size of tumors have been reported (Dachowski & DeLaney, 1992).

Nursing Implications for Clients Receiving Immunotherapy

■ ■ ■

Immunotherapy

Immunotherapy can consist of various substances used alone, such as interleukin-2, or combination biotherapy, such as alpha interferon with 5-fluorouracil. The nurse's role is to enhance the client's quality of life.

Nursing Responsibilities

- Monitor for side effects: Alpha interferon may cause mental slowing, confusion, and lethargy; combination therapy of 5-fluorouracil or interleukin-2 and alpha interferon may cause severe flulike symptoms, with chills and fever of 103 F to 106 F (39.4 C to 41.1 C), nausea, vomiting, diarrhea, anorexia, severe fatigue, and stomatitis; erythropoietin may cause acute hypertension.

- Monitor enzymes and other appropriate biochemical indicators for acute alterations in renal, cardiac, liver, or gastrointestinal functioning, which can be side effects of interleukin-2.

- Evaluate response to therapy by conducting a thorough evaluation of clients' symptoms.

- Assess clients' coping behaviors and teach new strategies as needed.

- Manage fatigue and depression.

- Encourage self-care and participation in decision making.

- Provide close supervision for clients with altered mental functioning, either by caretakers or frequent nursing visits to the client's home.

- If client is unable to manage alone, teach medication administration and care of equipment to caregivers.

Client and Family Teaching

- Minimize symptoms by managing fever and flulike symptoms: increase fluid intake, take analgesic and antipyretic medications, and maintain bed rest until symptoms abate.

- Seek help for serious problems not managed by usual means, such as dehydration from diarrhea.

- Use correct techniques for providing subcutaneous injections.

- Identify how to work and care for ambulatory pumps when medication is administered through an intercatheter or vascular access device.

The major nursing responsibilities associated with photodynamic therapy are to address the client and family's anxiety about undergoing a relatively new treatment procedure and to educate them in managing side effects. The drug remains in the subcutaneous tissues for 4 to 6 weeks after injection. Any direct or indirect exposure to the sun activates the drug, resulting in a chemical sunburn. Clients are taught to protect themselves from sunlight (even on cloudy days) by covering themselves from head to toe in opaque clothing, including a wide-brimmed hat, gloves, shoes and stockings, and sunglasses with 100% ultraviolet block. Long-term care of treated skin includes the use of moisturizing lotions and protection from trauma or irritation.

Bone Marrow Transplantation

Bone marrow transplantation (BMT) is an accepted treatment to stimulate a nonfunctioning marrow or to replace marrow. BMT is given as an intravenous infusion of bone marrow cells from donor to patient. Most commonly used in leukemias, this therapy is being expanded to include treatment of solid tumors, such as breast tumors. Chapter 31 provides an in-depth discussion of this procedure.

Pain Management

Pain management is a very important component of medical oncology and is considered a crucial part of the collaborative treatment plan. There are three main categories of pain syndromes in clients with cancer, and the category influences the type of treatment (Foley, 1991):

- Pain associated with direct tumor involvement. The most common causes are metastatases to bone, nerve compression or infiltration, and involvement of hollow visceral organs.

- Pain associated with treatment. This may include postsurgical incisional or wound pain; peripheral neuropathy, ulceration of mucous membranes, and pain from herpes zoster outbreaks secondary to chemotherapy; and pain in nerve plexes, muscles, and peripheral nerves from radiation therapy.

- Pain from a cause not related to either the cancer or therapy, such as diabetic neuropathy.

The goal of pain therapy is to provide relief that is adequate to allow clients to function as they wish and, in the case of terminally ill clients, to die relatively free of pain. Drug therapy with opioid and nonopioid analgesics as

American Cancer Society CAUTION Model

■ ■ ■

Change in bowel or bladder habits

A sore that does not heal

Unusual bleeding or discharge

Thickening or lump in breast or elsewhere

Indigestion or difficulty in swallowing

Obvious change in wart or mole

Nagging cough or hoarseness

If you have a warning signal, see your doctor!

Note. From the American Cancer Society.

well as adjuvant medications (those that enhance the effect of the analgesic) is the basis of most physician-guided pain management. Other therapies include injection of anesthetic drugs into spinal cord or specific nerve plexes, surgical severing of nerves, radiation to reduce tumor size and pressure, and behavioral approaches. Pharmacologic pain management follows the following steps:

1. Conduct careful initial and ongoing assessment of the pain.
2. Evaluate the client's functional goals.
3. Set up a plan starting with combinations of nonnarcotic drugs (such as aspirin or ibuprofen) with adjuvants (such as corticosteroids or antidepressants).
4. Evaluate the degree of pain relief.
5. Progress to stronger drugs as needed, from mild narcotics such as oxycodone (Percodan) or propoxyphene (Darvon) to strong narcotics such as morphine or hydromorphone (Dilaudid).
6. Continue to try combinations and escalate dosages until maximal pain relief balanced with client's need to function is achieved.

Usually, medication is administered by the oral route as long as this route continues to be effective. Medication is given on a regular time schedule (e.g., every 4 hours) with additional medication prescribed to cover breakthrough pain. When the oral route alone becomes inadequate, the primary narcotic can be administered intramuscularly on an intermittent schedule or intravenously by means of a continuous drip, usually controlled by an infusion pump. Some of the newer pumps are portable, deliver medication continuously, and allow clients to control their breakthrough pain with a limited number of boluses.

When narcotic doses are increased gradually, there is no limit to the amount the client can receive, as long as adverse reactions can be managed. Clients have received up to 4800 mg (200 mg per hour) of morphine sulfate with up to six 200- to 400-mg breakthrough doses daily without major ill effects and with good pain control. The body develops tolerances to the sedative and respiratory depressive effects after a short period, and most clients are able to tolerate the level of medication needed to control the pain. Other side effects, such as constipation, nausea and vomiting, and itching, can be managed through the usual means and are discussed under the appropriate nursing diagnoses. If the client has persistent untoward side effects that do not respond to treatment, or if the client does not get adequate relief from the narcotic, different narcotics and combinations are tried. The drug of choice for long-term, high-dose therapy, both oral and parenteral, is morphine sulfate. It seems to provide the most effective pain management with the most manageable side effects (Fulton & Johnson, 1993).

Clients on high-dose narcotics should not have the medication abruptly stopped, because withdrawal symptoms will occur. If the drug needs to be stopped, it must be tapered gradually. For more information on pain management, and on alternative therapies in particular, see Chapter 4.

Nursing Care

Nurses face a major challenge in educating all clients about preventive measures and life-style changes to reduce the risk of cancer. At the same time, clients with cancer must be reassured that they are not responsible for having acquired cancer.

Once a cancer diagnosis is established, nurses have the responsibility to assist clients to recover and support them during the rehabilitation phase. In cases of terminal cancer, nurses provide comfort and facilitate positive growth for the client and significant others.

Early Detection

Early detection and treatment are considered the most important factors influencing the prognosis of those afflicted with cancer. However, many people do not seek early diagnosis and treatment because of denial, fear and anxiety, stigma, or the absence of specific early signs such as pain or weight loss (which usually are late signs). For this reason, screening procedures such as mammograms, the PSA blood test for prostatic cancer, occult blood stool tests, and sigmoidoscopy may be lifesaving.

The ACS promotes early detection through public education using the CAUTION model (see the accompanying box). This model encourages people to seek medical attention when they discover signs and symptoms that are characteristic of cancer. However, recently the ACS has published a stronger statement regarding screening:

"Each person should be aware of the cancer early detection guidelines that apply to them" (ACS, 1994). For people without symptoms, the ACS recommends a cancer checkup every 3 years for those ages 20 to 39 and yearly for those over 40. If a person is at special risk due to heredity, environment, occupation, or life-style, special tests or more frequent examinations may be necessary. A routine cancer checkup should include counseling to improve health behaviors and physical examination with related tests of the breast, uterus, cervix, colon, rectum, testes, prostate, skin, thyroid, and lymph nodes. The accompanying box lists the tests that are recommended for a cancer checkup. Nurses have a special role in public education and should encourage all with whom they come into contact not to forget their cancer checkup. Nurses must be familiar with the ACS guidelines so that they can advise clients, their families, and significant others.

Assessment

Focused Interview   During this initial phase of the nursing process, collect significant data about the client, including the following:

- History of the client's disease, including the signs and symptoms that led the client to seek health care
- Other current diseases, such as diabetes
- Current physical or psychologic problems resulting from the cancer, such as pain or depression
- Understanding of the treatment plan
- Expectations of the treatment plan
- Functional limitations due to illness or treatment
- Effect of the disease on current life-style
- Support systems or caretakers the client can rely on
- Coping strategies and how well they are working

Interview Questions   The following are appropriate questions to ask the client during the initial interview and at subsequent assessments:

- "What brought you in to see the doctor?" *Asking this question allows clients to tell their story in their own way, which may elicit more information than asking specific questions. The answer should elicit not only data about the signs and symptoms but also fears or concerns. If the cancer was discovered during a routine physical examination or checkup, the client may still have some difficulty accepting the disease, especially if there were no symptoms. For clients who offer insufficient information in response to this open-ended question, more specific questions may be necessary, such as "Did you have pain or any specific physical problems that caused you to seek health care?"*
- "Do you have any other medical conditions or problems that are troubling you at this time?" *It may be nec-*

American Cancer Society
Recommendations for Cancer Checkups
■ ■ ■

Breast

- Routine monthly breast self-examination starting at age 20
- Breast examination by a health care professional every 3 years from age 20 to 40 and yearly thereafter
- Screening mammography every 2 years from age 40 to 49 and yearly thereafter

Colon and Rectum

- Digital rectal exam yearly starting at age 40
- Stool occult blood test yearly after age 50
- Flexible sigmoidoscopy every 3 to 5 years after age 50

Uterus

- Yearly pelvic examination and Papanicolaou (Pap) test for sexually active girls and any women over 18; less often for women with three consecutive negative results
- An endometrial tissue sample at menopause for high-risk women with repeated samples at physician's discretion

Prostate

- Digital rectal exam yearly after age 50
- Prostate-specific antigen (PSA) test yearly after age 50

Note. From the American Cancer Society.

---

essary to ask about some specific diseases to help the client focus, for example, "Do you have high blood pressure?" or "Are you having any problems with your lungs?" Information gained from this question can help the nurse anticipate problems and potential nursing diagnoses related to other diseases that may interact with the cancer.

- "What kinds of physical problems are you having at this time? Do you have pain? Are you nauseated? Have you lost a great deal of weight? Are you so tired you have difficulty carrying on your daily activities? Are you feeling blue or discouraged because of your illness?" *For each positive response, ask follow-up questions to narrow down or define the exact nature of the problem.*

Two Scales of Functional Status for Cancer Clients

■ ■ ■

Karnofsky Scale: Criteria of Performance Status (PS)

100 Normal; no complaints; no evidence of disease.

90 Able to carry on normal activity; minor signs or symptoms of disease.

80 Able to carry on normal activity with effort; some signs or symptoms of disease.

70 Cares for self; unable to carry on normal activity or to do active work.

60 Requires occasional assistance but is able to care for most of own needs.

50 Requires considerable assistance and frequent medical care.

40 Disabled; requires special care and assistance.

30 Severely disabled; hospitalization indicated, although death not imminent.

20 Very sick; hospitalization necessary; active supportive treatment necessary.

10 Moribund; fatal processes progressing rapidly.

0 Dead.

Eastern Cooperative Oncology Group Scale (ECOG)

0 Fully active, able to carry on all predisease activities without restriction. (Karnofsky 90 to 100)

1 Restricted in physically strenuous activity, but ambulatory and able to carry out work of a light or sedentary nature, for example, light housework or office work. (Karnofsky 70 to 80)

2 Ambulatory and capable of all self-care, but unable to carry out work activities. Up and about more than 50% of waking hours. (Karnofsky 50 to 60)

3 Capable of only limited self-care, confined to bed or chair 50% or more of waking hours. (Karnofsky 30 to 40)

4 Completely disabled, cannot carry out any self-care, totally confined to bed or chair. (Karnofsky 10 to 20)

Note. Adapted from "The Use of Nitrogen Mustards in the Palliative Treatment of Carcinoma" by D. A. Karnofsky, L. Craver, & J. Burchenal, 1948, *Cancer, 1,* pp. 634–656.

Again, these data help identify what nursing diagnoses should be included in the care plan.

- "What options has your physician suggested for treating your cancer?" *The answer will indicate clients' knowledge about their treatment and, possibly, their communication with the physician or surgeon. Often, under the stress of a cancer diagnosis, clients do not hear or understand what the doctor is saying and are afraid to ask questions. Lack of knowledge indicates a need to collaborate with the physician to explain the information to the client in a manner that will enable the client to absorb and understand it. If the client does have a good understanding of the treatment plan, discussing how the client feels about it can be useful in exposing fears, concerns, and emotional responses.*

- "What do you expect to happen as a result of this treatment?" *The answer may reveal unrealistic expectations or lack of understanding of consequences of the treatment.*

- "What effect is the disease and/or treatment having on your ability to carry on with your usual daily activities?" *Additional questions may also be needed to pinpoint the types of limitations. The response to this question should indicate where the client belongs on a functional scale such as those shown in the accompanying box. This information can also be used to identify the need to collaborate with professionals from other disciplines. For example, if the client is the sole financial support of the family and is unable to work, a social worker may be able to help with resources; if the client is extremely weak, referral to a physical therapist may help with energy conservation strategies and strengthening exercises.*

- "Who is available to help you at home and run errands for you? Who can provide transportation for you to get to your appointments or treatments? Who can you rely on to be a good listener when you're sad or just to be a comfortable companion? Is there someone you would like to make health care decisions for you if there is a time that you are unable to make them for yourself?" *It often seems that the person who gets cancer is the one who takes care of everyone else; asking for help may be difficult for this person. This information can identify how much support and help the client has access to. The last question introduces the concept of advanced directives and durable power of attorney regarding health care (see Chapter 11).*

- "How do you manage your stress or your feelings of discomfort? What helps you feel better? Do you feel these measures work well for you?" *The responses to these questions provide information about the client's coping strategies and may identify maladaptive strategies such as alcohol or drug use. Lack of appropriate coping methods can interfere with the client's response to treatment and decrease overall quality of life.*

Other assessment questions may be useful at different stages of the client's illness. For example, if the client is

Table 9–11   Signs of Nutritional Status

System	Good Nutrition	Poor Nutrition
General	Alert, energetic, good endurance, psychologically stable	Withdrawn, apathetic, easily fatigued, irritable
	Weight within range for height, age, body size	Over- or underweight
Integumentary	Skin glowing, good turgor, smooth, free of lesions	Skin dull, pasty, scaly-dry, bruises, multiple lesions
	Hair shiny, lustrous, minimal loss	Hair brittle, dull, falls out easily
Head, eyes, ears, nose, and throat	Eyes bright, clear, no fatigue circles	Eyes dull, conjunctiva pale, discoloration under eyes
	Oral mucous membranes pink-red and moist	Oral mucous membranes pale
	Gums pink, firm	Gums red, spongy, and bleed easily
	Tongue pink, moderately smooth, no swelling	Tongue bright to dark red, swollen
Abdomen	Abdomen flat, firm	Abdomen flaccid or distended (ascites)
Musculoskeletal	Firm, well-developed muscles	Flaccid muscles, wasted appearance
	Good posture	Stooped posture
	No skeletal changes	Skeletal malformations
Neurologic	Good attention span, good concentration, astute thought processes	Inattentive, easily distracted, impaired thought processes
	Good reflexes	Paresthesias, reflexes diminished or hyperactive

not expected to survive the cancer, it is important to ask whether the client has made decisions about last wishes (e.g., for a funeral and burial), whether these have been discussed with significant others, and whether the client has made out a will.

Physical Assessment   As soon as the client is admitted to the health care service or agency, a complete physical assessment should be conducted to establish a baseline against which to evaluate later changes. It is especially important to document the nutritional status of the client using anthropomorphic measurements (i.e., frame size, height, weight, body fat, and muscle mass), and to evaluate laboratory results and note any specific signs and symptoms. Table 9–11 compares the signs and symptoms of good nutrition with those of malnutrition.

It is also important to assess the client's hydration status, especially if the client is not taking oral food and fluids well or is having bouts of vomiting. The box on page 348 lists specific assessments for hydration status.

Other recommended assessments are discussed under the specific nursing diagnoses that follow. They can also be found in other chapters that address specific body systems affected by the cancer. The box on page 348 identifies clinical manifestations of cancer, including some that are due to the side effects of treatment.

Nursing Diagnoses
Nursing goals focus on supporting the entire client system and managing specific problems such as pain, poor nutrition, dehydration, fatigue, adverse emotional responses, altered individual and family coping, and the side effects of medical treatment. Nursing also focuses on improving the quality of life by promoting rehabilitation for survivors of cancer and helping those who succumb to the disease maintain their dignity in the dying process. Because cancer affects the whole family, whether the client survives or not, nursing care includes everyone involved with the client from the onset of diagnosis through the entire disease and treatment process and the ultimate outcome. Many diagnoses are pertinent to clients with cancer; this section addresses only the most common diagnoses. Diagnoses specific to individual diseases can be found in their respective chapters.

Anxiety   Early in the disease continuum, for example, during diagnosis and treatment, threats to or changes in health status, physical comfort, role functioning, or even socioeconomic status can cause anxiety. Later on, anxiety may result from the anticipation of pain, disfigurement, and the ever-present threat of death. In particular, clients whose coping skills have been poor in the past (e.g., in managing anger) may now find themselves at a loss to manage this current crisis. The client may manifest overt signs of anxiety: trembling, restlessness, irritability, hyperactivity, stimulation of the sympathetic nervous system (increased blood pressure, pulse, respiration, excessive perspiration, pallor), withdrawal, worried facial expressions, and poor eye contact. The client may report insomnia and feelings of tension and apprehension, ex-

---

Factors to Consider in Assessing Hydration Status

■ ■ ■

- Intake and output
- Rapid weight changes
- Skin turgor and moisture
- Venous filling
- Vital sign changes
- Tongue furrows and moisture
- Eyeball softness
- Lung sounds
- Laboratory values

Clinical Manifestations of Cancer

■ ■ ■

- Hair loss
- Depression
- Fever
- Bleeding gums
- Oropharyngeal ulcerations
- Stomatitis
- Anorexia
- Nausea and vomiting
- Diarrhea
- Emaciation
- General weakness
- Flaccid muscles
- Stooped posture
- Pallor
- Excessive bruising
- Radiation burns
- Visible tumor (abdomen)
- Odor of decay
- Hypotension

---

pressing concerns regarding perceived changes brought about by the disease and fear of future events.

Nursing interventions with rationales follow:

- Carefully assess the client's level of anxiety (moderate anxiety, severe anxiety, or panic) and the reality of the threats represented in the client's current situation. *The level of anxiety and the reality of the perceived threat influence the type of intervention that is appropriate for the client. A client in panic may need medical intervention with appropriate medications, whereas those with moderate or even severe anxiety can probably be managed by the nurse through counseling and teaching new skills.*

- Establish a therapeutic relationship by conveying warmth and empathy and listening nonjudgmentally. *A client who feels safe in the relationship with the nurse more easily expresses feelings and thoughts. The client will be able to trust the nurse and perhaps be willing to try new behaviors as suggested. The amount of time this relationship may take to develop depends on the client's current emotional and mental state and the stage of the disease process.*

- Encourage the client to acknowledge and express feelings, no matter how inappropriate they may seem to the client. *Just by expressing their feelings, clients often can significantly diminish anxiety. Expressing feelings also allows the client to direct energy toward healing and thus has a positive therapeutic effect. Moreover, by acknowledging feelings, especially those the client considers unacceptable, the client can lay a groundwork for new coping behaviors.*

- Review the coping strategies the client has used in the past and build on past successful behaviors, introducing new strategies as appropriate. Explain why inap-

propriate strategies, such as repressing anger or turning to alcohol, are not helpful. *The client will be more willing to make changes that build on what has already worked in the past. The client will also be more willing to reject inappropriate strategies if he or she is given a persuasive reason why they have not had the desired effect in managing previous crises.*

- Identify resources in the community, such as crisis hotlines and support groups, that can help the client manage anxiety-producing situations. *The client may not have support systems available, or the client's significant others may be having their own difficulties in dealing with the cancer diagnosis. Programs such as "I Can Cope," sponsored by the American Cancer Society in most communities, provide education, counseling, and support in a group setting with other cancer patients.*

- Provide specific information for the client about the disease, its treatment, and what may be expected, especially for those clients with obvious misinformation. *Knowing what is to come gives the client a sense of control and enables the client to make decisions. Also, knowing that every effort will be made to keep the client as free of pain as possible can do a great deal to relieve anxiety.*

- Provide a safe, calm, and quiet environment for the client in panic. Stay with the client and administer antianxiety medications as ordered. *Staying with the client and displaying calmness and confidence can protect the client from injury and prevent further panic. If the panic does not subside with the nurse's presence and support, referral to the physician for medication management may be necessary.*

- Use crisis intervention theory to promote growth in the client and significant others, regardless of the outcome of the disease. *During a major crisis, people can, with assistance, transform the experience from one that causes defeat and despair to one that enhances personal and spiritual growth. If the nurse is not skilled in this area, a referral to an appropriate mental health professional is very helpful to the client and family.*

Body Image Disturbance   Cancer and cancer treatments frequently result in major physiologic and psychologic body image changes. Loss of a body part (e.g., amputation, prostatectomy, or mastectomy), skin changes and hair loss from chemotherapy or radiation therapy, or creation of unnatural openings on the body for elimination (e.g., colostomy or ileostomy) may have a major effect on the person's self-image. The gaunt, wasted appearance of the cachexic client and the draining, malodorous lesions that result when cancer breaks through the skin are other significant etiologies of body image disturbance. This may also give rise to fear of rejection, which plays a major role in sexual dysfunction. Thus, in addition to all of the other afflictions the cancer brings about, the client must endure major changes in appearance and function. The client may exhibit a visible physical alteration of some portion of the body, verbalize negative feelings about the body and/or fear of rejection by others, refuse to look at the affected site, and depersonalize the body change or lost part (e.g., by calling the colostomy "that thing").

Nursing interventions with rationales follow:

- Discuss with the client the meaning of the loss or change. *Doing so helps the nurse discover the best approach for this particular client and involves the client more actively in interventions. A small, seemingly trivial loss may have a big impact, especially when viewed in light of the other changes that are occurring in the client's life. Likewise, a major loss may not be as important as the nurse might imagine. It is a natural tendency for nurses to inject meanings of their own into client situations; to ensure more appropriate and individualized care, therefore, the nurse must evaluate each situation in terms of the reactions of the specific client.*

- Observe and evaluate the client's interaction with significant others. *On the one hand, people who are important to the client may reinforce negative feelings about body image; on the other hand, the client may be perceiving rejection where none exists.*

- If the client refuses to acknowledge the body change or loss, allow the client to engage in denial, but do not participate in the denial; for example, if a client does not want to look at the wound, the nurse may say, "I am going to change the dressing to your breast incision now." *During the initial stage of shock at the loss of a body part, denial is a protective mechanism and should not be challenged, but neither should it be promoted. A matter-of-*

fact approach and an empathetic attitude will go far to facilitate the client's eventual acceptance of the change.

- Assist the client and significant others to cope with the changes in appearance:
  a. Provide a supportive environment.
  b. Encourage the client and significant others to express feelings about the situation.
  c. Give matter-of-fact responses to questions and concerns.
  d. Identify new coping strategies to resolve feelings.
  e. Enlist family and friends in reaffirming the client's worth.

A supportive, safe environment in which feelings are respected and new coping strategies can be tried promotes acceptance, as does reaffirming that the client's worth is not diminished by any physical changes.

- Teach the client or significant others to participate in the care of the afflicted body area. Provide support and validation of their efforts. *Active involvement in providing care, such as changing a dressing or emptying a colostomy bag, empowers the client and/or significant others. This intimate involvement also desensitizes feelings about disfigurement and promotes acceptance. Involving significant others reduces the risk of their rejecting the client and can promote closeness. Positive reinforcement from the nurse encourages them to continue these behaviors.*

- Teach the client specific strategies for minimizing physical changes, such as providing skin care during radiation therapy and dressing to enhance appearance and minimize change in the body part. *Early intervention can limit the negative side effects of treatment and actually promote the client's recovery. Involving the client provides an additional way for the client to be in control of a difficult situation.*

- Teach clients ways to reduce the alopecia that results from chemotherapy and to enhance their appearance until the hair grows back (McCabe, 1991):
  a. Discuss the pattern and timing of hair loss. *This allows client to cope with changes and incorporate them into daily activities.*
  b. Use an ice cap or a tight headband during chemotherapy administration. *This decreases the amount of drug that reaches the hair follicles.*
  c. Encourage the client to wear cheerful, brightly colored head coverings; assist in color coordinating them with client's usual clothing. *Attractive head coverings protect the bald head while allowing the client to feel stylish and well-dressed.*
  d. Refer the client to a good wig shop before the client experiences hair loss. *Hair color and texture can be matched to minimize obvious changes in appearance.*
  e. Refer the client to support programs such as "Look Good . . . Feel Better," which is sponsored by the

American Cancer Society and the Cosmetic, Toilet, and Fragrance Association Foundation. *A support group can diminish feelings of isolation and provide practical tips for managing problems.* For a list of community resources available to clients with cancer, refer to a local phone book.

f. Reassure the client that hair will grow back after chemotherapy is discontinued, but also inform the client that the color and texture of the new hair may be different. *In one study, hair loss was identified as the most distressing symptom by 84% of 144 clients (Mc-Cabe, 1991). Interventions to reduce that loss can have a significant impact on body image concerns. Moreover, the client who knows what to expect may experience less anxiety and distress.*

Anticipatory Grieving   Anticipatory grieving is a response to loss that has not yet occurred. Overall, only 50% of people with cancer fully recover, and certain types of cancer have a much higher death rate; thus, the client with cancer is usually confronted by the necessity of facing death and making preparations. This can be a healthy response that allows the client and family to work through the dying process and achieve growth in the final stage of life. Perceived changes in body image and lifestyle also can prompt anticipatory grieving. The client or significant others may show sorrow, anger, depression, or withdrawal, expressing distress at the potential loss or verbalizing concern about unfinished life business.

Nursing interventions with rationales follow:

- Use the therapeutic communication skills of active listening, silence, and nonverbal support to provide an open environment for the client and significant others to discuss their feelings realistically and to express anger or other negative feelings appropriately. *This helps the client and family members get in touch with their feelings and confront the possibility of the loss or death.*

- Answer questions about illness and prognosis honestly, but always encourage hope. *This allows client and significant others to appraise their situation realistically and make plans, but it also helps combat feelings of hopelessness and depression.*

- Encourage the dying client to make funeral and burial plans ahead of time and to be sure the will is in order. Make sure the necessary phone numbers can be easily located. *This gives the client a sense of control and relieves family members of these concerns at a time when the client is most in need of their support and when they themselves are extremely stressed.*

- Encourage the client to continue taking part in activities he or she enjoys, including maintaining employment as long as possible. *This gives the client a sense of continuity of life even in the face of severe losses.*

Risk for Infection   Malnutrition, impaired skin and mucous membrane integrity, tumor necrosis, and suppression of the white blood cells from chemotherapy may all contribute to the risk for infection. Anorexia, as well as the disease itself, deprives the body of nutrients needed for healing, while impaired integrity of skin and mucous membranes (a result of chemotherapy and radiation therapy) compromise the first lines of defense against microbial invasion. Cells in the center of large or not very vascular tumors may die from malnutrition, eventually eroding through tissues to cause sepsis. Bone marrow depression resulting from the effects of certain types of cancers and from chemotherapy undermine the body's ability to respond to infection. The client may exhibit the classic signs of infection: lassitude, fever, anorexia, pain in the affected area, and physical evidence of infection, such as a purulent, draining lesion or wound.

Nursing interventions with rationales follow:

- Monitor the client's vital signs. *Fever and sympathetic nervous system responses, such as increased pulse and respiration, are usual early signs of impending infection. However, severely immunosuppressed clients may be unable to mount a fever; therefore, the absence of fever cannot rule out infection.*

- Monitor white blood cell counts frequently, especially for the client receiving chemotherapy that is known to cause bone marrow suppression. *This allows the nurse to notify the physician at the first sign of diminishing white blood cell counts so that corrective action can be taken.*

- Teach the client and significant others to avoid crowds, small children, and people with infections when the client's white blood cell count is at nadir (lowest point during chemotherapy) and to practice scrupulous personal hygiene. *During periods of leukopenia, the client may lose immunity to own home flora. Careful attention to hygiene reduces the risk. Crowds, which promote contact with a greater variety of infectious agents, and friends with minor infections can be very dangerous for the immunosuppressed client. Small children should be avoided because they often have microbes to which most people are usually immune but which the client cannot resist.*

- Protect skin and mucous membranes from injury. Teach the client and significant others appropriate skin care measures, such as good hygiene, use of a moisturizing lotion to prevent dryness and cracking, frequent changes of position for the bed-bound client, and immediate attention to skin breaks or lesions. *Ensuring intact skin strengthens the client's first line of defense against infection.*

- Encourage the client to consume a diet high in protein, minerals, and vitamins, especially vitamin C. *Improving nutrition decreases the risk of infection. Vitamin C has been shown to help prevent certain types of infection, such as colds.*

Risk for Injury In addition to infection, cancer can pose a risk for injury from, for example, obstruction by a large tumor or one that is located in a limited body space (e.g., in the brain, bowel, or bronchial airways). If the cancer is one that creates ectopic sites of hormones, elevated levels of hormones that are not under the control of the pituitary gland can injure the client in a variety of ways. Signs of obstruction depend on the organ involved: Bowel obstruction presents with pain, distention, and cessation of bowel activities; obstruction in the brain gives signs of increased intracranial pressure or personality/behavioral change; bronchial obstruction manifests as respiratory distress, cyanosis, and altered arterial blood gases. Ectopic production of parathyroid hormone manifests as high serum calcium levels as well as signs of hypercalcemia; ectopic production of antidiuretic hormone causes fluid retention and manifests as hypertension and peripheral and pulmonary edema.

Nursing interventions with rationales follow:

- Assess the client frequently for signs and symptoms indicating problems with organ obstruction. *Early detection of major problems allows the nurse to seek medical help for the client before the problem evolves into a physiologic crisis.*

- Teach the client and family to differentiate minor problems from those of a serious nature. Encourage them to consult with the nurse or physician if in doubt or to call 911 if the client becomes very ill. The accompanying box provides guidelines to help clients identify serious problems. *Having guidelines for when to call the doctor provides an anxiety-reducing safety net for the client and family and promotes early detection of complications.*

- Monitor laboratory values that may indicate the presence of ectopic functioning, and report abnormal findings to physicians immediately. (See Table 9–5 for laboratory indicators of ectopic functions.) *Early detection promotes early medical intervention and prevents serious consequences from the ectopic secretion.* Refer to Chapters 5, 19, and 20 for specific signs and symptoms of electrolyte imbalances and endocrine disorders.

Altered Nutrition: Less Than Body Requirements
The anorexia-cachexia syndrome (described earlier in this chapter) is a common cause of malnutrition in cancer clients. Metabolism increases in response to increased cancer cell reproduction while the cancer's parasitic activity reduces the nutrients available to the body. Loss of appetite, food aversion, nausea and vomiting, and painful oral lesions from chemotherapy contribute to impaired nutrition. Tumors of the gastrointestinal tract that affect absorption also contribute to the problem. Add to these

When to Call for Help
■ ■ ■

Instruct the client or family member to call the nurse or physician if any of the following signs or symptoms occur:

- Oral temperature greater than 101.5 F (38.6 C)
- Severe headache; significant increase in pain at usual site, especially if the pain is not relieved by the medication regimen; or severe pain at a new site
- Difficulty breathing
- New bleeding from any site, such as rectal or vaginal bleeding
- Confusion, irritability, or restlessness
- Withdrawal, greatly decreased activity level, or frequent crying
- Verbalizations of deep sadness or a desire to end life
- Changes in body functioning, such as the inability to void or severe diarrhea or constipation
- Changes in eating patterns, such as refusal to eat, extreme hunger, or a significant increase in nausea and vomiting
- Appearance of edema in the extremities or significant increase in edema already present

Instruct the client or family member to call 911 if the client

- Is having much difficulty breathing or if the lips or face has a bluish tinge.
- Becomes unconscious or has a convulsion.
- Exhibits unmanageable behavior, such as being physically abusive, hurting self, or engaging in uncontrollable activity.

the tremendous physical stress of fighting the cancer, and the result is a profound malnutrition. Signs and symptoms include wasted appearance, considerable weight loss over a relatively short period of time, anthropometric measurements below 85% of standard for fat and muscle tissue, decreases in serum proteins, and negative responses to antigen testing.

Nursing interventions with rationales follow:

- Assess the client's current eating patterns, including usual likes and dislikes, and identify factors that impair food intake. *This allows for a more individualized plan based on the client's needs and preferences.*

- Evaluate degree of malnutrition:
  a. Check laboratory values for total serum protein, serum albumin and globins, total lymphocyte count, serum transferrin, hemoglobin, and hematocrit. *These values represent the serum protein and blood cell counts that are most likely to decrease with malnutrition.*
  b. Evaluate immunologic response by antigen skin testing using common antigens such as *Candida,* PPD, mumps, and tetanus. A positive response— that is, more than 5 mm of induration and redness at the site of the intradermal injection—indicates immunocompetence. *Anergy,* no reaction to known antigens, indicates depressed immune function. *Suppression of the immune response can be related to malnutrition.*
  c. Calculate nitrogen balance and creatinine-height index. Calculate skeletal muscle mass, and compare findings to normal ranges. *Urinary creatinine is an index of lean body mass and decreases in malnutrition. Lean muscle mass is catabolized for energy in clients with cancer.*
  d. Take anthropometric measurements and compare them to standards: height, weight, elbow breadth, arm circumference, triceps skinfold thickness, and arm muscle mass. *This estimates the degree of wasting; findings below 85% of standard are considered malnutrition.* (See Chapter 12 for more information.)
- Teach the client the principles of maintaining good nutrition by using the Food Pyramid (see Chapter 2) and adapting the diet to the client's medical restrictions and current preferences. *This tailors the food plan to the client's needs and thereby promotes compliance.*
- Manage problems that interfere with eating:
  a. Encourage the client with food aversions to eat whatever appeals to him or her and to add nutritional supplements such as the Ensure or Isocal to diet. *It is better for the client to eat something even if it is not nutritionally balanced.*
  b. Eat small, frequent meals. *These are more easily digested and absorbed and usually better tolerated by the client with anorexia.*
  c. Encourage the client to try icy cold foods (such as ice cream) or those that are more highly seasoned if food has no taste. *Chemotherapy and radiation therapy may harm taste buds and render the client unable to distinguish the taste of foods. Strong seasonings and coldness make food more enjoyable to the client with diminished taste.*
  d. Encourage cold and bland semisoft and liquid foods for the client with painful oropharyngeal ulcers; have the client use an anesthetic mouthwash prior to eating. *These foods are less irritating to sensitive mucous membranes; deadening the pain can make chewing and swallowing easier.*
  e. Manage nausea and vomiting by administering antiemetic drugs (around-the-clock medication may be an effective preventive measure). Encourage the client to eat small, frequent, low-fat meals with dry foods such as crackers and toast, to avoid liquids with meals, and to sit upright for an hour after meals. Remove emesis basins, and encourage oral hygiene before eating. *Dry, low-fat foods are more readily tolerated by the nauseated client. Removing vomiting cues, such as odor and supplies associated with vomiting, can reduce nausea.*
- Teach client and family to supplement meals with nutritional supplements such as Ensure Plus or Isocal and to take multivitamin and mineral tablets with meals. Suggest increasing calories by adding ice cream or frozen yogurt to the liquid supplement or commercial protein-carbohydrate powders to milk or fruit juice. *Because the food intake of most cancer clients is usually less than that needed to maintain or gain weight, these supplements can add calories in a manner often tolerated by the client.*
- Teach client and family to keep a food diary to document client's daily intake. *If the client can see how little is being consumed, he or she may eat more. A food diary also helps the nurse keep a calorie count and alert the physician if more drastic nutritional measures, such as parenteral nutrition, need to be instituted.*
- Teach the client and family to administer parenteral nutrition via a central line or other VAD. Teach safety measures and care of the VAD, and explain how the pump delivering the solution works. Provide an emergency phone number for help with administration problems. (See Chapter 13 for safety guidelines for administering parenteral nutrition.) *The client with chronic or terminal cancer requiring parenteral nutrition is usually managed at home, so the client and family need information on how to manage the entire process.*

Impaired Tissue Integrity   The most common impairment of tissue integrity occurs in the oral-pharyngeal-esophageal mucous membranes. It is secondary to the effects of some chemotherapeutic drugs and radiation treatment to the head and neck. The oral-pharyngeal-esophageal tissues are lined with cells with a high mitotic turnover rate and are therefore very vulnerable to many cytotoxic chemotherapeutic drugs. Leukemias, bone marrow transplants, and herpes viral infections are other etiologic factors in the disruption of oral-pharyngeal-esophageal tissue. Manifestations of this problem may include the following:

- Small ulcers on the edges of the tongue and throughout the mucous membranes in the mouth and throat (due to chemotherapy)

- Herpes simplex type I lesions or vesicles that evolve to ulcerations
- Fungal infections, such as thrush (due to *Candida* infections), which is manifested by a white, yellow, or tan coating with dry, red, fissured tissue underneath
- Red, swollen, friable gums that bleed with minimal or no trauma (due to decreased platelets in leukemia);
- Xerostomia: excessive dryness of the mucous membranes (due to chemotherapy or radiation)

Nursing interventions with rationales follow:

- Carefully assess and evaluate the type of tissue impairment present. Identify possible sources, such as chemotherapy or radiation therapy to head and neck. *This allows the nurse to implement corrective measures appropriate to the type of problem.*
- Implement and teach measures for preventing oropharyngeal infection:
  a. Observe for systemic signs of infection. Be suspicious of any fever that has no apparent cause. *This facilitates early identification of an infection before it spreads.*
  b. Have client clean teeth gently and use a mouthwash several times a day: after waking up in the morning, after any oral intake, and before bedtime. The client should soak dentures nightly in hydrogen peroxide and floss gently with waxed floss after meals and bedtime; this measure is, however, contraindicated for people with leukemia or thrombocytopenia. *Disrupted mucous membranes allow the normal oral bacterial flora into the systemic circulation, which can result in sepsis in the immunocompromised person. Reducing the oral flora by frequent hygiene decreases the risk of infection.*
  c. Culture any oral lesions, and report the problem to physician. Herpes lesions may not follow a typical pattern in immunosuppressed clients. *Identifying the cause of the infection, whether viral, fungal, or bacterial, allows the physician to prescribe the appropriate treatment.*
- Implement and teach measures for reducing trauma to delicate tissues:
  a. Counteract dry mouth (xerostomia) with lubricating and moisturing agents, such as Gatoraid sugarless gum and Blistex. *This protects mucous membranes from infection and trauma.*
  b. Avoid putting sharp instruments in the mouth. Use smooth plastic spoons and forks for eating, especially for the client with a bleeding disorder. Dental work should be done by dental oncologists.
  c. Brush teeth with a very soft toothbrush, and obtain a new toothbrush monthly. If gums are friable and bleeding, clean teeth with a soft cloth and tooth-

---

Combination Mouthwashes for Oropharyngeal Pain Control

■ ■ ■

Kaiser Mouthwash
- Nystatin
- Hydrocortisone
- Tetracycline

Xyloxylin Suspension
- Benylin syrup
- Lidocaine
- Maalox suspension

Stanford Mouthwash
- Nystatin
- Tetracycline
- Lidocaine
- Hydrocortisone

Stomafate Suspension
- Sucralfate
- Sterile water
- Benylin syrup
- Maalox suspension

---

paste over finger. Chlorhexidine mouthwash (Peridex) may be used. *This protects gums from trauma and decreases risk of hemorrhage.*

- Administer specific medications as ordered to control infection and/or pain:
  a. Acyclovir is used for viral infections.
  b. Systemic antibiotics are used for bacterial infections.
  c. Nystatin or clotrimazole solution for "swish and swallow" or lozenges to be dissolved slowly in the mouth are used for fungal infections.
  d. Use viscous xylocaine or various combination mouthwashes before meals and as needed. *These agents reduce pain and inflammation. See the accompanying box for the ingredients of combination mouthwashes. Knowing the contents of each mouthwash can prevent hypersensitivity reactions (e.g., to lidocaine) and assist in patient teaching.*

Other Nursing Diagnoses   Other nursing diagnoses appropriate for clients with cancer include the following.

- *Caregiver Role Strain* related to severity or long-term nature of client's illness or to lack of support systems for caregiver.
- *Ineffective Individual Coping* related to lack of stress management strategies or to maladaptive stress management strategies.
- *Ineffective Denial* related to learned response pattern or to the presence of reality factors that are consciously intolerable.
- *Ineffective Family Coping: Compromised* related to prolonged disease of dominant family member or to dysfunctional family relationships.

Applying Research to Nursing Practice
Correlates of Fatigue in People with Breast or Lung Cancer

■ ■ ■

Fatigue in clients with cancer has been noted anecdotally for a long time, but little research has been done to identify the causative factors. In one study, researchers studied 77 clients with either breast or lung cancer to identify what factors correlated significantly with fatigue (Blesch, et al., 1991). Their findings showed that 99% of the study population experienced some level of fatigue, with 64% rating the fatigue as moderate to severe.

Previous research studies cited by the authors had identified a number of physiologic factors contributing to fatigue, such as anemia and malnutrition; these factors, however, did not have significance in this study. Although physiologic factors (as identified by laboratory studies and client reports) were present in the study population, the investigators found that the only statistically significant factors were pain, duration of illness, and mood alterations, such as anxiety, depression, and anger.

The authors believe that research regarding fatigue is in its infancy. They encourage others to develop more exact definitions of fatigue and more precise measurement tools. They also note that traditional nursing approaches to fatigue, such as scheduling tests to provide rest periods or not disturbing the client at night, may not be realistic. Rather, the authors suggest developing and testing innovative methods to manage fatigue.

Implications for Nursing

Adequate pain management can help control both the mood alterations that compound fatigue and the fatigue itself. Pain research has shown that regular, around-the-clock medications are more effective than sporadic dosing. Because the body adjusts to increasing amounts of pain medications within a day or two, teaching clients to take pain medications on a regular schedule, as opposed to waiting until severe pain is experienced, can improve their perception of fatigue.

Psychosocial interventions to improve mood and alleviate depression may also have a positive effect on relieving fatigue. Nurses can manage psychologic distress by the following interventions:

- Frequent supportive interactions with the client and family
- Listening to concerns, but not offering false reassurance
- Providing accurate information about the disease and treatment
- Correcting misconceived expectations
- Being realistic and straightforward, but encouraging hope
- Assessing client and family coping strategies and suggesting alternatives as needed
- Promoting independence in problem solving
- Encouraging the client and family to continue pleasurable activities as long as possible
- Being an advocate for the client in collaborations with the health care team in managing client problems related to the cancer or the treatment

Critical Thinking in Client Care

1. As a nursing diagnosis, fatigue is defined as an overwhelming sense of exhaustion and decreased capacity for physical and mental work. Discuss the effects and the treatment of the disease on this state.

2. Given the structured situation in acute care settings, suggest possible interventions to decrease fatigue in hospitalized clients.

3. Your home-care client is being treated for cancer of the breast with chemotherapy. Although she does not have pain, nausea is a problem. Describe the teaching you would do to help her understand how nausea and fatigue may be associated.

4. Fatigue, like pain, is a subjective experience. Develop an assessment guide to assess fatigue.

- *Fatigue* related to altered body chemistry (secondary to chemotherapy), increased energy requirements, overwhelming psychologic demands, or chronic pain. The accompanying research box provides information about documented causes of fatigue and implications for nursing practice.

- *Fluid Volume Deficit* related to excessive losses from vomiting or diarrhea or to diminished fluid intake.
- *Impaired Home Maintenance Management* related to fatigue or inadequate support systems.
- *Hopelessness* related to deteriorating physiologic condition or lost belief in transcendent values.

- *Knowledge Deficit* of treatment choices or of care at home.

- *Pain* and/or *Chronic Pain* related to disease process or treatment effects.

- *Impaired Physical Mobility* related to pain, fatigue, depression, or neuromuscular impairment.

- *Powerlessness* related to dependence on health care providers and significant others or to loss of control over life-style.

- *Self-Care Deficit: Feeding, Bathing/Hygiene, Dressing/ Grooming, and Toileting* related to decreased strength and endurance, neuromuscular impairment, or pain.

- *Sexual Dysfunction* related to altered body structure or function, effects of medication, or psychologic concerns.

- *Impaired Skin Integrity* related to malnutrition, impaired immunity, or effects of radiation.

- *Sleep Pattern Disturbance* related to pain, depression, or inactivity.

- *Impaired Social Interaction* related to self-concept disturbance or activity intolerance.

Nursing Interventions for Oncologic Emergencies

In caring for clients with cancer, nurses may encounter a number of emergency situations in which their role may be pivotal to the client's survival. Most of these emergencies require astute observations, accurate judgments, and rapid action once the problem has been identified. A brief description of some of the more common oncologic emergencies with nursing interventions follows. In all cases, immediate notification of the physician or emergency team is the first step.

Pericardial Effusions and Neoplastic Cardiac Tamponade

Malignant pericardial effusions that are secondary to lung or esophageal cancers or due to distant metastases can grow large enough to compress the heart, restrict heart movement, and result in a cardiac tamponade. The signs of cardiac tamponade are those of circulatory collapse or cardiogenic shock: hypotension, tachycardia, tachypnea, dyspnea, cyanosis, increased central venous pressure, anxiety, restlessness, and impaired consciousness. Interventions include the following:

- Start oxygen and alert respiratory therapy for other respiratory support as needed.

- Insert an intravenous catheter if one is not already in place.

- Monitor vital signs and initiate hemodynamic monitoring.

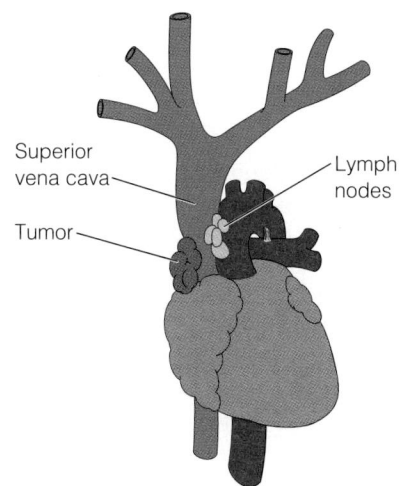

Figure 9–10 The superior vena cava syndrome. The enlargement of a tumor adjacent to the superior vena cava (usually in the lung or mediastinum) compresses that major blood vessel, which leads into the right atrium of the heart. As a result, blood backs up into the venous system behind the obstruction, diminishing blood flow into the heart.

- Prepare vasopressor drugs.

- Bring crash cart to bedside.

- Set up for and assist physician with a pericardial tap (pericardiocentesis). See Chapter 28.

- Reassure the client.

Superior Vena Cava Syndrome

The superior vena cava can be compressed by mediastinal tumors or adjacent thoracic tumors. The most common cause is small-cell or squamous-cell lung cancers. Occasionally the problem is caused by thrombus around a central venous catheter that then plugs up the vena cava, resulting in obstruction and back-up of the blood flowing into the superior vena cava.

Obstruction of the venous system produces pleural effusions; facial, arm, and tracheal edema; and, if untreated, cerebral edema and impaired cardiac filling. Signs and symptoms may develop slowly; facial and arm edema are early signs. As the problem progresses, pleural effusion and tracheal edema cause respiratory distress, dyspnea, cyanosis, and, eventually, altered consciousness and neurologic deficits. Figure 9–10 illustrates the superior venal cava syndrome.

Emergency measures include the following:

- Provide respiratory support with oxygen, and prepare for tracheostomy.

- Monitor vital signs.

- Administer corticosteroids (e.g., dexamethasone) to reduce edema.

- If the disorder is due to a clot, administer antifibrinolytic or anticoagulant drugs.
- Provide a safe environment, including seizure precautions.

After the emergency is managed, the client often receives radiation or chemotherapy to reduce the tumor size.

Sepsis and Septic Shock

Tumor necrosis coupled with an immunosuppressed and/or malnourished state can result in sepsis. Bacteria gain entrance to the blood, grow rapidly, and produce septicemia. Because malignant tumors are more likely to use anaerobic metabolic pathways, the bacteria of tumor sepsis are usually gram-negative and damage the body by a combination of bacterial endotoxins and an uncontrolled immune reaction. Gram-negative sepsis progresses to systemic shock and eventually results in multisystem failure. Signs and symptoms appear in two phases. The first phase, called hyperdynamic or warm shock, is characterized by vasodilation with vascular dehydration, high fever, peripheral edema, hypotension, tachycardia, tachypnea or Kussmaul's respirations, hot flushed skin with creeping mottling beginning in the lower extremities, and anxiety or restlessness. Without treatment, the shock progresses to the second phase, called hypodynamic or cold shock, which shows the more classic signs of shock: hypotension, rapid thready pulse, respiratory distress, cyanosis, subnormal temperature, cold clammy skin, decreased urinary output, and altered mentation. Identifying the problem while the client is still in the hyperdynamic state is crucial to the client's survival.

Interventions include the following:

- Fluid resuscitation with infusion of colloidal solutions (plasma volume expanders, such as albumin) and balanced salt solutions
- Hemodynamic monitoring to evaluate the effects of rehydration and to detect early signs of overload
- Oxygen and other respiratory support as needed
- Cultures of the source of infection and blood cultures
- Starting broad spectrum antibiotics until the specific organism is identified
- Vasopressor drugs, if blood pressure is not maintained by volume replacement
- Antiendotoxin serum to bind and inactivate the bacterial endotoxin
- Providing a safe environment for the client with altered mentation; providing support and reassurance for the anxious client (Wahl, 1989).

See Chapter 6 for further discussion of septic shock.

Spinal Cord Compression

Spinal cord compression is most commonly associated with pressure from expanding tumors of the breast, lung, or prostate; lymphoma; or metastatic disease. Spinal cord compression constitutes an emergency because of the potential for irreversible paraplegia. Early symptoms include progressive back and leg pain, numbness, paresthesias, and coldness. Later, bowel and bladder dysfunction occur and, finally, neurologic dysfunction progressing to weakness and paralysis. Treatment often consists of radiation or surgical decompression, but early detection is essential.

Nursing responsibilities include the following:

- Neurologic checks every shift for clients with advanced cancers of the breast, lung, prostate, or lymphoma
- Thorough assessment of all complaints of back pain or sensory changes
- Notification of physician if spinal cord compression is suspected and preparation for MRI
- Administration of cortisteroids (e.g., dexamethasone) to reduce cord edema and protect function

Obstructive Uropathy

Clients with intra-abdominal, retroperitoneal, or pelvic malignancies, such as prostate, cervical, or bladder cancers, may experience obstruction of the bladder neck or the ureters. Bladder neck obstruction usually manifests as urinary retention, flank pain, hematuria, or persistent urinary tract infections, but ureteral obstruction is not often evident until the client is in renal failure.

Interventions include the following:

- Investigate complaints of flank pain or urinary retention.
- Monitor serum blood urea nitrogen (BUN), creatinine, and potassium for elevated levels.
- Send a specimen of any foul-smelling urine for culture.
- Report hematuria to the physician immediately.
- Catheterize the client with acute retention as ordered.

Hypercalcemia

Hypercalcemia results from the excessive ectopic production of parathyroid hormone associated with cancers of the breast, lung, esophagus, thyroid, head, and neck and with multiple myeloma. Bone metastases may also cause hypercalcemia. When the rate of calcium mobilization from the bone exceeds the renal threshold for excretion, serum calcium levels can become dangerously elevated. Clients with hypercalcemia often present with nonspecific symptoms of fatigue, anorexia, nausea, polyuria, and constipation. Neurologic symptoms include muscle weakness, lethargy, apathy, and diminished reflexes. Without treatment, hypercalcemia progresses to alterations in mental status, psychotic behavior, cardiac arrythmias, seizures, coma, and death (see Chapter 5).

Nursing interventions include the following:

- Monitor serum calcium, phosphate, alkaline phosphatase, electrolytes, BUN, and creatinine levels.
- Monitor electrocardiogram for signs of hypercalcemia: decreased QT interval, widening of the T wave, prolonged PR interval, and bradycardia.
- Administer intravenous solutions of normal saline to increase urinary calcium excretion.
- Stop thiazide diuretics and vitamins A and D.
- Administer corticosteroids and calcitonin.
- Administer the chemotheraputic drug plicamycin (Mithracin) as ordered as a bolus through a freshly started intravenous line, and observe carefully for possible extravasation, which can ulcerate and sclerose underlying tissues.
- Maintain the client on bed rest until calcium levels decrease.

Hyperuricemia

Hyperuricemia usually is a complication of rapid necrosis of tumor cells after vigorous chemotherapy for lymphomas and leukemias. Hyperuricemia may be related to increased uric acid production or to the tumor lysis syndrome associated with Burkitt's lymphoma. Uric acid crystals are deposited in the urinary tract, causing renal failure and uremia. Clients with hyperuricemia manifest with nausea, vomiting, lethargy, and oliguria.

Nursing actions focus on prevention and include the following:

- Increase intravenous hydration to ensure urinary output of approximately 3 L a day for 48 hours prior to chemotherapy.
- Administer allopurinol (antigout drug) per recommended dosage and schedule for 48 hours prior to chemotherapy.
- Administer daily sodium bicarbonate to alkalinize the urine and thereby prevent uric acid crystallization.
- Monitor serum uric acid levels and urine pH.
- If signs of uremia occur, insert a Foley catheter and monitor urinary output as well as serum BUN, creatinine, and potassium levels.

Syndrome of Inappropriate Antidiuretic Hormone Secretion (SIADH)

Occurring in only about 2% of cancer patients, syndrome of inappropriate antidiuretic hormone secretion (SIADH) is related to an ectopic secretion of antidiuretic hormone (ADH) that is associated usually with small-cell lung carcinoma, but also occasionally with prostate and adrenal cancers. The kidney secretes an excessive amount of sodium and conserves a disproportionate amount of free water, causing profound hyponatremia. Signs and symptoms include anorexia, nausea, muscle aches, and subtle

---

American Cancer Society Dietary Guidelines to Prevent Cancer

■ ■ ■

- Avoid obesity.
- Cut down on total fat intake.
- Include a variety of vegetables and fruits in the daily diet.
- Eat more high-fiber foods, such as whole-grain cereals, vegetables, and fruits.
- Limit consumption of alcoholic beverages, if you drink at all.
- Limit consumption of salt-cured, smoked, and nitrate-cured foods.

Note. From the American Cancer Society.

---

neurologic symptoms that can progress to lethargy, confusion, seizures, and coma from cerebral edema (see Chapter 20).

Nursing interventions include the following:

- Monitor serum and urine sodium and osmolality as well as BUN, which will be low.
- Restrict water intake.

Client and Family Teaching

Prevention

The ACS makes specific recommendations for prevention in addition to the screening measures discussed earlier in this chapter. Based on these recommendations, nurses teach clients and families to decrease risk factors by

- Avoiding tobacco and excessive alcohol use.
- Avoiding situations where secondhand smoke is abundant.
- Eating a low-fat, high-fiber diet.
- Consuming ample amounts of antioxidant foods, such as those containing beta carotene (a vitamin A precursor), vitamins E and C, and omega-3 oils.
- Avoiding foods with carcinogenic additives, dyes, or chemicals used in processing. The accompanying box lists the ACS dietary guidelines.
- Taking certain medications and hormones, such as estrogen or tamoxifen, only under close medical supervision.
- Limiting exposure to radiation, including sun exposure.

- Using extreme caution if employed in an industry that uses carcinogenic chemicals or airborne particles (smoke). Seek new employment if at risk for related cancers.
- Protecting self from viral diseases known to cause cancer.
- Improving immunity by maintaining a healthy lifestyle and managing stress.

In addition, people should be encouraged to report to the public health department any known leaking of chemicals or radioactive materials into the water or air and any noted increase in the incidence of cancer, especially of one specific type, in their communities.

Rehabilitation and Survival

Rehabilitation from cancer not only involves regaining strength, recovering from surgery or chemotherapy, and learning to live with an altered body part or appliance, but also entails recovering from associated psychologic and emotional turmoil.

Rehabilitation centers provide physical therapy, occupational therapy, speech therapy, job retraining, and an opportunity to rest before resuming life responsibilities. In addition, many clients go home to convalesce and receive in-home support in the form of nursing supervision, direct care, and teaching. Hygiene and home maintenance can be provided by a certified home health aide. Physical and occupational therapists provide muscle strengthening and mobility training (especially with prostheses), and home safety teaching.

Psychologic rehabilitation of cancer survivors addresses quality of life issues. Three "seasons of cancer survival" have been described (Mullan, 1985). The first starts with diagnosis but is dominated by treatment. The second stage is one of extended survival, which occurs when treatment ends and the watchful waiting period begins. This period is characterized by fear of recurrence. Permanent survival is said to begin when the survival period has gone on long enough that the risk of recurrence is small. In this period, the client has to deal with secondary problems related to health and social issues resulting from the cancer experience. Employment may be a problem, health insurance may be cancelled, and life insurance may be difficult to get. Relationships may have suffered from the strain of the illness on significant others and the essential self-focusing required for recovery. However, both the client and significant others may have undergone a personal and spiritual growth that ushers in a new and enriching period of their lives.

New self-help groups are emerging in many communities to support others through their "seasons of survival." Many cancer survivors speak to groups about assisting other cancer survivors. Clients and families need to be informed about the many resources that are available through community agencies as well as the survivor support groups.

Discharge and Home Care Teaching

Before the client is discharged, teach both the client and significant others or caregivers to manage the client at home. Discuss problems that may result from the type of cancer and the treatment received, and provide information on how to manage these problems and when to call the physician. Teach wound care to the client with an open wound or draining lesion, and provide a referral to a home health nurse to monitor progress. Explain special diets clearly, or refer the client to a dietitian before discharge. Carefully review the physician's instructions with the client and family, making sure they understand medications to be taken, any other treatments, and when to see the doctor for follow-up care. Provide or order equipment and supplies needed for home care, especially any special bed or equipment for mobility and safety in the home. For the client who will need complex care, such as parenteral nutrition, provide a referral to a home health nurse before discharge. Because the hospital stay is often short, the client and family will benefit from follow-up phone calls for several days after the client arrives home; because people do not learn well under the stress of going home, provide the client and family with a number to call for concerns and questions.

Hospice Care

More and more cancer clients with terminal disease are electing to die at home. This decision has been made easier by the increased availability of hospice programs. When a client and family or significant others elect hospice care, they are usually precluding additional hospitalizations other than those required to manage reversible problems. Hospice clients also refuse resuscitation measures (CPR and other extraordinary measures).

Hospice care involves a multidisciplinary team and is designed to give the client comfort and to assist in a peaceful death with support to caretakers. The team usually consists of the following members:

- A nurse case manager, who manages the client's care, works directly with the client and family, and coordinates the activities of the other disciplines. The nurse is usually on call 24 hours a day by phone for the client or family and makes home visits frequently. The nurse is often with the family when the client dies.
- A physician, who makes periodic home visits and collaborates with the nurse manager regarding medications and treatments.
- An anesthesiologist or pharmacist, who manages pain control and watches for drug interactions.
- An infusion therapist, who provides equipment, supplies, solutions, and expertise for any parenteral nutri-

tion, intravenous medications, or blood products administered to the client. The infusion therapist, or designate, is usually on call 24 hours a day to troubleshoot equipment problems.

- A social worker, who helps with resources for the client and family, assists with financial concerns, helps with grief work, and provides general support and counseling as needed.
- A physical therapist, who teaches the family how to manage the immobilized client.
- A home health aide, who provides physical care to the client and assists the family with household chores.
- Volunteers, who provide companionship for the client and give respite to the family for short periods of time.

Many hospice services are connected with an inpatient respite care unit, where the client can receive 24-hour care for up to several weeks. This source provides the necessary care to the client if a family member becomes ill or needs to be relieved temporarily of the tremendous burden of caring for a dying loved one. Veterans Administration Medical Centers are very good models for these programs.

Studies of families that have participated in hospice services have found that family members were very positive about the experience. The aspects of hospice they most appreciated were the 24-hour accessibility and availability of the health team and the quality of communication from all team members. Family members emphasized that "the nurses listened, answered questions honestly, and prepared us for changes in the patient's condition." Team members were rated as very professional, but more relaxed and friendly than hospital staff; they sat down and talked with the family and displayed accepting, nonjudgmental attitudes. Team members were also seen as well informed, knowledgeable, and competent with excellent problem-solving skills (Hull, 1991).

Applying the Nursing Process

Case Study of a Client with Cancer: James Casey

James Casey is a 72-year-old man of Northern European heritage who has been under medical care for chronic obstructive pulmonary disease, chronic bronchitis, status post–myocardial infarction, and type I diabetes mellitus for over 15 years. He reports that he lost his wife from lung cancer 5 years ago and still "misses her terribly." He describes his bad habits as smoking two packs of cigarettes a day for 52 years (104 pack/years), one to two six-packs of beer a week, one "bourbon and water" a night, and "a lot of sugar-free junk food, like french fries." He as-

sures the nurse that he quit smoking 2 years ago, when he could no longer walk a block without considerable shortness of breath, and just quit drinking alcohol a few weeks ago at his physician's insistence. About a year ago, he had a basal-cell carcinoma removed from his right ear. Six months ago, cancerous tumors were discovered in his bladder, and he underwent two 6-week chemotherapy courses of bladder instillations of BCG. The latest report he received indicates that the tumors have grown back and no further chemotherapy would be useful. The urologist had considered surgery but believed that Mr. Casey's other medical problems would compromise his chances of survival. Mr. Casey decides to let the disease run its course and to be managed at home through hospice care. Because he lives alone in a modest home, he asks his daughter, Mary Walsh, and her family to move in with him to provide care and support during his final months. The daughter accepts, saying she is glad to be able to spend this time with her father; she has been informed of the physical and emotional stress this will entail.

Assessment

Glynis Jackson RN, the hospice nurse assigned as case manager for Mr. Casey, completes a health history and physical examination during her first two visits in his home, 1 day apart. She gathers this information over 2 days to conserve Mr. Casey's strength and allow more time for him and his daughter to talk about their concerns.

During the physical assessment, Ms. Jackson notes that Mr. Casey is pale with pink mucous membranes, thin with a wasted appearance and a strained, worried facial expression. He complains of severe back pain no longer adequately relieved by Percodan and Vicodin alternating every 2 to 4 hours. His blood pressure is 90/50, right arm in the reclining position with no significant orthostatic change; his apical pulse is 102, regular and strong; respiratory rate 24 and unlabored; breath sounds are clear but diminshed in the bases; oral temperature is 96.8 F.

A tunnelled Groshong catheter as a VAD is present in the right anterior chest. There is no drainage, redness, or swelling at the site. The catheter was placed last week when the client was at the anesthesiologist's office being evaluated for pain management, but no medication is running via the VAD.

His daughter, Ms. Walsh, reports that his urinary output is adequate. Approximately 200 mL of yellow, cloudy, nonmalodorous urine is present in the urinal at the bedside from his last voiding.

Mr. Casey states that he spends most of his time either in bed or sitting up in a chair in his room. He reports that he has no energy any more and is unable to walk to the bathroom unassisted, dress himself, or take care of his own personal hygiene. The nurse rates Mr. Casey's functional level at ECOG level 4: capable of only limited self-care, confined to bed or chair 50% or more of waking hours (Karnofsky 10 to 20). He tells the nurse that his daughter "is working day and night to help me and is looking awfully tired."

Ms. Walsh reports that Mr. Casey is eating very poorly: He has a small bowl of oatmeal with milk for breakfast and vegetable soup and crackers for lunch, but he tells her that he is too tired for dinner and wants only fruit juice. Mr. Casey tells the nurse that he has no appetite and eats just to please his daughter. He does drink at least three to four glasses of water a day plus juice. His finger-stick blood sugars remain within normal range.

His current weight is 120 pounds at 67 inches tall, down from 180 pounds a year ago. He has lost about 30 pounds over the last 2 months.

Available laboratory values from his visit with the doctor show the following:

Total protein: 4.1 (Normal range: 6.0 to 8.0 g/dL)

Albumin: 2.2 (Normal range: 3.5 to 5.0 g/dL)

Hemoglobin: 10.2 (Normal range: 13.5 to 18.0 g/dL)

Hematocrit: 30.5 (Normal range: 40.0 to 54.0%)

BUN: 30 (Normal range: 5 to 25 mg/dL slightly higher in older people)

Creatinine: 2.2 (Normal range: 0.5 to 1.5 mg/dL)

Diagnosis

The nursing diagnoses for Mr. Casey (and significant others) include the following:

- *Altered Nutrition: Less Than Body Requirements* related to anorexia and fatigue
- *Risk of Potential Caregiver Role Strain* related to severity of her father's illness and lack of help from other family members
- *Chronic Pain* related to progression of disease process
- *Impaired Physical Mobility* related to pain, fatigue, and beginning neuromuscular impairment
- *Risk for Impaired Skin Integrity* related to impaired physical mobility and malnourished state

Expected Outcomes

The expected outcomes established in the plan of care specify that

- Mr. Casey will increase his oral intake and show improvement in his serum protein values.
- His daughter will be able to maintain her supportive caretaking activities as long as Mr. Casey needs them.
- Mr. Casey will have minimal pain for the rest of his life.
- Mr. Casey will be able to continue his current activity level.
- Mr. Casey will have intact skin.

Planning and Implementation

The following interventions are planned and implemented during Mr. Casey's care:

- Ask Mr. Casey what his favorite foods are, and ask his daughter to offer him a small portion of one of these foods each day.
- Encourage Mr. Casey to drink up to four cans of Ensure Plus with Fiber a day, sipping them throughout the day.
- Talk with the physician about having Mr. Casey try a medication to stimulate the appetite.
- Have a home health aide come to the home, give him a shower or bed bath daily, and assist his daughter with some of the household chores.
- Talk with Ms. Walsh about having her adult son and daughter relieve her of the housework and stay with Mr. Casey so that she can get out of the house occasionally. Offer to talk with them if she is uncomfortable doing so.
- Request a volunteer to spend up to 4 hours a day, twice a week reading to Mr. Casey so that Ms. Walsh can attend to outside activities and chores.
- Talk with the anesthesiologist, and work out a pain-control program for Mr. Casey, using the VAD and a CADD-PCA infusion pump with a continuous morphine infusion.
- Call the infusion therapist to set up the equipment and supplies (including the medication) for the morphine infusion.
- Teach Mr. Casey and his daughter how to use the pump and about the side effects of the morphine infusion, including those that require a call to the nurse for assistance. Teach them which untoward effects should be reported.
- Leave detailed instructions regarding storage of the medication and care of the pump with Ms. Walsh, along with the telephone number of the infusion therapist.
- Request a physical therapy consultation to evaluate Mr. Casey's current level of functioning and determine how to maintain his current level.
- Instruct Ms. Walsh to allow ample rest periods between each activity Mr. Casey must carry out, such as taking a shower or using the commode.
- Order a hospital bed with electronic controls to be delivered to the house.
- Order a special foam pad for Mr. Casey's bed and chair and a bedside commode from the medical supply house.

- Instruct Ms. Walsh and the home health aide to inspect Mr. Casey's skin daily, give good skin care with emollient lotion after bathing, and report any beginning lesions immediately to the nurse.

Evaluation

Mr. Casey did increase his oral intake a little, sometimes eating the special treats his daughter prepared and drinking one or two cans of Ensure a day. However, his weight did not increase; it stayed at about 120 pounds until his death 2 weeks later. Ms. Walsh was very grateful for the extra help from the home health aide and the volunteer, though she could not bring herself to ask her son and daughter for help and did not want the nurse to do so. She did become more rested and reported that "Dad and I had some wonderful 3:00 a.m. talks when he couldn't sleep."

Mr. Casey was started on 20 mg of morphine per hour with boluses of 10 mg four times a day. This medication relieved his pain quite well; after 2 days he was alert enough most of the time to carry on a normal conversation and still walk to the bathroom with help up until 2 days before he died.

The hospital bed simplified Mr. Casey's care and made it much easier for him to rest comfortably and change position. His skin remained intact and in good condition.

Ms. Walsh reported that Mr. Casey died peacefully in his sleep, about 2 weeks after care was started. She said spending the last weeks of his life together was a healing experience for both of them.

Critical Thinking in the Nursing Process

1. What other tests could be done to evaluate Mr. Casey's nutritional status?

2. Mr. Casey had severe back pain. What were the possible pathophysiologic reasons for his pain?

3. One of the specified interventions was to consult the physician regarding medication to increase Mr. Casey's appetite. What medications might fulfill that function? What side effects might they have that would contraindicate these medications for Mr. Casey?

4. If Mr. Casey had developed signs and symptoms of sepsis, what manifestations would you expect to see? As the nurse making the home visits, what would be your nursing actions, and in what order of priority?

5. If Mr. Casey's daughter, Ms. Walsh, had a nursing diagnosis of *Ineffective Individual Coping,* what would you include in a teaching plan to help her learn new coping strategies?

Bibliography

■ ■ ■

American Cancer Society. (1994). *Cancer Facts and Figures—1994.* Atlanta: Author.

Beardsley, T. (1994, January). Trends in cancer epidemiology: A war not won. *Scientific American, 270*(1), 130–138.

Beart, R. W., Jr. (1991). Colorectal cancer. In A. I. Holleb, D. J. Fink, & G. P. Murphy (Eds.), *American Cancer Society textbook of clinical oncology* (pp. 213–218). Atlanta: American Cancer Society.

Beazley, R. M., & Cohn, I., Jr. (1991). Tumors of the liver. In A. I. Holleb, D. J. Fink, & G. P. Murphy (Eds.), *American Cancer Society textbook of clinical oncology* (pp. 237–244). Atlanta: American Cancer Society.

Begley, S. (1994, April 25). Beyond vitamins. *Newsweek*, pp. 45–49.

Blakeslee, S. (1994, May 17). Genes tell story of why some get cancer while others don't. *New York Times Medical Science*, pp. B6–7.

Blesch, K. S., Paice, J. A., Wickham, R., Harte, N., Schnoor, D. K., Purl, S., Rehwalt, M., Kopp, P. L., Manson, S., Coveny, S. B., McHale, M., & Cahill, M. (1991). Correlates of fatigue in people with breast or lung cancer. *Oncology Nursing Forum, 18*(1), 81–87.

Bostwick, D. G. (1990). The pathology of early prostate cancer. In G. P. Murphy (Ed.), *Prostate cancer: Pathology, detection, and diagnosis.* Atlanta: American Cancer Society Professional Education Publication.

Brawer, M. K., & Lange, P. H. (1990). Prostate-specific antigen and premalignant change: Implications for early detection. In G. P. Murphy (Ed.), *Prostate cancer: Pathology, detection, and diagnosis.* Atlanta: American Cancer Society Professional Education Publication.

Brophy, L. R., & Sharp, E. J. (1991). Physical symptoms of combination biotherapy: A quality-of-life issue. *Oncology Nursing Forum, 18*(1) (Suppl.), 25–30.

Cancer Research. (1992, November 13). Closing in on melanoma susceptibility gene(s). *Science, 258,* 1080–1081.

Champion, V. L. (1991). The relationship of selected variables to breast cancer detection behaviors in women 35 and older. *Oncology Nursing Forum, 18* (4), 733–739.

Cohen, L. A. (1987). Diet and cancer. *Scientific American, 257*(5), 42–48.

Consensus Conference. (1990). Oral complications of cancer therapies: Diagnosis, prevention, and treatment. *Oncology, 5* (7), 64–82.

Cooper, M. R., & Cooper, M. R. (1991). Principles of medical oncology. In A. I. Holleb, D. J. Fink, & G. P. Murphy (Eds.), *American Cancer Society textbook of clinical oncology* (pp. 47–68). Atlanta: American Cancer Society.

Dachowski, L. J., & DeLaney, T. F. (1992). Photodynamic therapy: The NCI experience and its nursing implications. *Oncology Nursing Forum, 19* (1), 63–66.

Daly, J. M., & Shinkwin, M. (1991). Nutrition and the cancer patient. In A. I. Holleb, D. J. Fink, & G. P. Murphy (Eds.), *American Cancer Society textbook of clinical oncology* (pp. 498–512). Atlanta: American Cancer Society.

Doenges, M. E., & Moorhouse, M. F. (1993). *Nurses pocket guide: Nursing diagnoses with interventions* (4th ed.). Philadelphia: F. A. Davis.

Dow, K. H. (1990). The enduring seasons in survival. *Oncology Nursing Forum, 17*(4), 511–516.

Doweiko, J. P., & Goldberg, M. A. (1991, August). Erythropoietin therapy in cancer patients. *Oncology, 5* (8), 31–37.

Drago, J. R. (1990). The role of new modalities in the early detection and diagnosis of prostate cancer. In G. P. Murphy (Ed.), *Prostate cancer: Pathology, detection, and diagnosis.* Atlanta: American Cancer Society Professional Education Publication.

Eberlein, T. J., & Wilson, R. E. (1991). Principles of surgical oncology. In A. I. Holleb, D. J. Fink, & G. P. Murphy (Eds.), *American Cancer Society textbook of clinical oncology* (pp. 25–34). Atlanta: American Cancer Society.

Ehmann, H. L., Sheehan, A., & Decker, G. M. (1991). Intervening with alopecia: Exploring an entrepreneurial role for oncology nurses. *Oncology Nursing Forum, 18* (4), 769–776.

Eyre, H. J., & Farver, M. L. (1991). Hodgkin's disease and non-Hodgkin's lymphomas. In A. I. Holleb, D. J. Fink, & G. P. Murphy

(Eds.), *American Cancer Society textbook of clinical oncology* (pp. 377–396). Atlanta: American Cancer Society.

Farber, L. P. (1991). Lung cancer. In A. I. Holleb, D. J. Fink, & G. P. Murphy (Eds.), *American Cancer Society textbook of clinical oncology*. Atlanta: American Cancer Society.

Foley, K. M. (1985). *The treatment of pain in the patient with cancer*. Atlanta: American Cancer Society Professional Education Publication.

Foley, K. M. (1991). Diagnosis and treatment of cancer pain. In A. I. Holleb, D. J. Fink, & G. P. Murphy (Eds.), *American Cancer Society textbook of clinical oncology*, (pp. 194–212). Atlanta: American Cancer Society.

Fulton, J. S., & Johnson, G. B. (1993). Using high-dose morphine to relieve cancer pain. *Nursing, 23* (8), 35–40.

Garfinkel, L. (1991). Cancer statistics and trends. In A. I. Holleb, D. J. Fink, & G. P. Murphy (Eds.), *American Cancer Society textbook of clinical oncology* (pp. 1–6). Atlanta: American Cancer Society.

Garnick, M. B. (1994, April). The dilemmas of prostate cancer. *Scientific American, 270*(4), 72–81.

Groenwald, S., Frogge, M., Goodman, M., & Yarbro, C. (1993). *Cancer nursing: Principles and practice,* (3rd ed.). Boston: Jones and Bartlett.

Groer, M. W., & Shekleton, M. E. (1989). *Basic pathophysiology: A holistic approach* (3rd ed.). St. Louis: Mosby.

Gusberg, S. B., & Runowicz, C. D. (1991). Gynecologic cancers. In A. I. Holleb, D. J. Fink, & G. P. Murphy (Eds.), *American Cancer Society textbook of clinical oncology* (pp. 481–497). Atlanta: American Cancer Society.

Held, J., & Volpe, H. (1991). Bladder preserving combined modality therapy for invasive bladder cancer. *Oncology Nursing Forum, 18*(1), 49–57.

Hendee, W. R., Manaster, B. J., Harnsberger, H. R., Bragg, D. G., Thompson, W. M., & McClennan, B. L. (1991). Oncologic imaging. In A. I. Holleb, D. J. Fink, & G. P. Murphy (Eds.), *American Cancer Society textbook of clinical oncology* (pp. 643–677). Atlanta: American Cancer Society.

Hendrickson, F. R., & Withers, H. R. (1991). Principles of radiation oncology. In A. I. Holleb, D. J. Fink, & G. P. Murphy (Eds.), *American Cancer Society textbook of clinical oncology* (pp. 35–46). Atlanta: American Cancer Society.

Herberman, R. B. (1991). Principles of tumor immunology. In A. I. Holleb, D. J. Fink, & G. P. Murphy (Eds.), *American Cancer Society textbook of clinical oncology* (pp. 69–79). Atlanta: American Cancer Society.

Hull, M. M. (1991). Hospice nurses: Caring support for caregiving families. *Cancer Nursing, 14*(2), 63–70.

Ignoffo, R. J., & Forni, P. J. (1989). *Cancer chemotherapy protocols: Drug administration regimens for physicians, nurses, and pharmacists*. San Francisco: Cetus Corporation.

Jackson, B. S., Strauman, J., Frederickson, K., & Strauman, T. J. (1991). Long-term biopsychosocial effects of interleukin-2 therapy. *Oncology Nursing Forum, 18* (4), 683–690.

Janeway, C. A., Jr. (1993). How the immune system recognizes invaders. *Scientific American, 269*(3), 72–79.

Jaret, P. (1986, June). Our immune system: The wars within. *National Geographic, 169*(6), 702–734.

Karnofsky, D., Abelmann, W., Craver, L., & Burchenal, J. (1948). The use of nitrogen mustard in the palliative treatment of carcinoma. *Cancer, 1,* 634–656.

Kee, J. L. (1994). *Handbook of laboratory and diagnostic tests with nursing implications* (2nd ed). Norwalk, CT: Appleton & Lange.

Kinne, D. W. (1991). *The surgical management of primary breast cancer*. Atlanta: American Cancer Society Professional Education Publication.

Kolata, G. (1994a, April 19). Big picture of cancer process is being seen for the first time. *New York Times Medical Science*.

Kolata, G. (1994b, May 17). Cancer therapy is hitched to rhythms. *New York Times Medical Science*.

Kolata, G. (1994c, May 17). Increasing chemotherapy may prove ineffective. *New York Times Medical Science*.

Krakoff, I. H. (1992). *Cancer chemotherapeutic and biologic agents*. Atlanta: American Cancer Society Professional Education Publication.

Loveys, B. J., & Klaich, K. (1991). Breast cancer: Demands of illness. *Oncology Nursing Forum, 18* (1), 75–80.

Mankin, H. J., Willett, C. G., & Harmon, D. C. (1991). Malignant tumors of the bone. In A. I. Holleb, D. J. Fink, & G. P. Murphy (Eds.), *American Cancer Society textbook of clinical oncology* (pp 355–358). Atlanta: American Cancer Society.

Marieb, E. N. (1992). *Human anatomy and physiology* (2nd ed.) Redwood City, CA: Benjamin/Cummings.

Mayer, D. K. (1992). The healthcare implications of cancer rehabilitation in the twenty-first century. *Oncology Nursing Forum, 19* (1), 23–27.

McCabe, M. S. (1991, July). Psychological support for the patient on chemotherapy. *Oncology, 5* (7), 91–107.

McCaffery, M. (1992, September). *Professional Oncology Conference: Managing Pain in the Cancer Patient*. Veterans Administration Hospital, Menlo Park, CA.

McCaffery, M., & Ferrell, B. (1994). How to use the new AHCPR guidelines. *American Journal of Nursing, 94*(7), 42–47.

Mitus, A. J., & Rosenthal, D. S. (1991). Adult leukemias. In A. I. Holleb, D. J. Fink, & G. P. Murphy (Eds.), *American Cancer Society textbook of clinical oncology* (pp. 410–432). Atlanta: American Cancer Society.

Mullan, F. (1985). Seasons of survival: Reflections of a physician with cancer. *New England Journal of Medicine, 313,* 270–273.

Musci, E. C., & Dodd, M. J. (1990). Predicting self-care with patients and family members' affective states and family functioning. *Oncology Nursing Forum, 17* (3), 394–400.

National Cancer Institute. (1991). *Cancer of the colon and rectum: Research report*. US Department of Health and Human Services: NCI Publication No. 92–95.

Nixon, D. W. (1990). *Nutrition and Cancer: American Cancer Society Guidelines, Programs, and Initiatives*. Atlanta: American Cancer Society Professional Education Publication.

Nossal, G. J. V. (1993). Life, death and the immune system. *Scientific American, 269* (3), 52–63.

Nowak, T. J., & Handford, A. G. (1994). *Essentials of pathophysiology: Concepts and applications for health care professionals*. Dubuque, IA: Wm. C. Brown.

Pasquali, E. A., Arnold, H. M., DeBasio, N., & Gorthey, E. (1985). *Mental health nursing: A holistic approach* (2nd ed.). St. Louis: Mosby.

Pfeifer, J. D. , & Wick, M. R. (1991). The pathologic evaluation of neoplastic diseases. In A. I. Holleb, D. J. Fink, & G. P. Murphy (Eds.), *American Cancer Society textbook of clinical oncology* (pp. 7–24). Atlanta: American Cancer Society.

Poland, J. (1991, July). Prevention and treatment of oral complications in the cancer patient. *Oncology, 5* (7), 45–62.

Price, S. A., & Wilson, L. M. (1992). *Pathophysiology: Clinical concepts of disease processes* (4th ed.). St. Louis: Mosby.

Pui, C-H, & Rivera, G. K. (1991). Childhood leukemias. In A. I. Holleb, D. J. Fink, & G. P. Murphy (Eds.), *American Cancer Society textbook of clinical oncology* (pp. 433 –452). Atlanta: American Cancer Society.

Ransohoff, J., Koslow, M., & Cooper, P. R. (1991). Cancer of the central nervous system and pituitary. In A. I. Holleb, D. J. Fink, & G. P. Murphy, Eds., *American Cancer Society textbook of clinical oncology* (pp. 329–337). Atlanta: American Cancer Society.

Rapp, F. (1991). Properties of viruses associated with human cancer. In A. I. Holleb, D. J. Fink, & G. P. Murphy (Eds.), *American Cancer Society textbook of clinical oncology* (pp. 133–152). Atlanta: American Cancer Society.

Research News. (1994, January 21). How cells cycle toward cancer. *Science, 263,* 319–321.

Research News. (1994b, April 15). New tumor-suppressor may rival p53. *Science, 264,* 344–345.

Rosenberg, S. A. (1992). *The transformed cell: Unlocking the mysteries of cancer*. New York: G. P. Putnam.

Roses, D. F., Gumport, S. L., Harris, M. N., & Kopf, A. W. (1989). *The diagnosis and management of common skin cancers*. Atlanta: American Cancer Society Professional Education Publication.

Scanlon, E. F. (1991). Breast cancer. In A. I. Holleb, D. J. Fink, & G. P. Murphy, Eds., *American Cancer Society textbook of clinical oncology* (pp. 177–193). Atlanta: American Cancer Society.

Schuster, C. S., & Ashburn, S. S. (1986). *The process of human development: A holistic life-span approach* (2nd ed.). Boston: Little, Brown.

Selye, H. (1984). *The stress of life* (rev. 2nd ed.). New York: McGraw-Hill.

Siegal, K. (1990). Psychosocial oncology research. *Social Work in Health Care, 15*(1), 21–43.

Singeltary, S. J., & Balch, C. M. (1991). Malignant melanoma. In A. I. Holleb, D. J. Fink, & G. P. Murphy (Eds.), *American Cancer Society textbook of clinical oncology* (pp. 263–270). Atlanta: American Cancer Society.

Sutton, J. D., Thalken, D. W., & Powell, M. C. (1993). *Nurses' IV drug manual.* Norwalk, CT: Appleton & Lange.

Templeton, D. J., & Weinberg, R. A. (1991). Principles of cancer biology. In A. I. Holleb, D. J. Fink, & G. P. Murphy (Eds.), *American Cancer Society textbook of clinical oncology* (pp. 678–689). Atlanta: American Cancer Society.

Terebelo, H. R. (1991). Alpha interferon: Perspectives in the biotherapy of chronic myelogenous leukemia. *Oncology Nursing Forum, 18* (1) (Suppl.), 5–8.

Torp-Pederson, S. T., & Siders, D. B. (1990). The role of transrectal ultrasound in the early detection of prostate cancer. In G. P. Murphy (Ed.), *Prostate cancer: Pathology, detection, and diagnosis.* Atlanta: American Cancer Society Professional Education Publication.

Von Houtte, P., Salazar, O. M., Phillips, C. E., & Asbury, R. F. (1983). Lung cancer. In P. Rubin, R. F. Bakemeier, & S. K. Krackov (Eds.), *Clinical oncology for medical students and physicians: A multidisciplinary approach* (6th ed.), (pp. 142–153). Atlanta: American Cancer Society.

Wahl, S. (1989). Septic shock: How to Detect it Early. *Nursing 89, 19* (1), 52–60.

Weinstein, I. B. (1981). *The scientific basis for carcinogen detection and primary cancer prevention.* Atlanta: American Cancer Society Professional Education Publication.

Wells, R. J. (1990). Rehabilitation: Making the most of time. *Oncology Nursing Forum, 17* (4), 503–507.

Wigzell, H. (1993, September). The immune system as a therapeutic agent. *Scientific American, 269* (3), 126–135.

Wilson, B. A., Shannon, M. T., & Stang, C. L. (1994). *Nurses' drug guide.* Norwalk, CT: Appleton & Lange.

Wilson, H. S., & Kneisl, C. R. (1992). *Psychiatric nursing.* Redwood City, CA: Addison-Wesley Nursing.

Winters, V., Peters, B., Coila, S., & Jones, L. (1990). A trial with a new peripheral implanted vascular access device. *Oncology Nursing Forum, 17* (6), 891–896.

Zimberg, M., & Berenson, S. (1990). Delirium in patients with cancer: Nursing assessment and intervention. *Oncology Nursing Forum, 17* (4), 529–538.

Zimny, M. E. (1991, August). Ovarian cancer: A nursing overview. *Oncology , 5* (8), 147–154.

CHAPTER 10

Nursing Care of Clients Experiencing Trauma

LEARNING OBJECTIVES

After completing this chapter, you will be able to

- Describe the three components of trauma and various types of trauma.
- Discuss some common effects of traumatic injury, their causes, and their initial management.
- Identify members of the trauma team.
- Describe assessments and interventions for prehospital care.
- Discuss laboratory and diagnostic tests used in assessing clients experiencing trauma.

- Describe collaborative interventions for clients experiencing trauma, including pharmacology, blood transfusion, and emergency surgery.
- Discuss the process of organ donation, including legal and ethical considerations.
- Discuss the teaching the nurse provides to the client and family experiencing trauma and outline teaching strategies to prevent traumatic injury.
- Use the nursing process as a framework for providing individualized care to clients with various types of traumatic injuries.

Trauma morbidity and mortality constitute a major health care challenge in the United States. Although significant strides have been made in combating heart disease and selected cancers, traumatic injury continues to be the number-one killer of the young. It is estimated that traumatic injury causes about 140,000 deaths per year. An additional 57 million people suffer nonfatal injuries each year (Trauma Nursing Coalition, 1992).

The cost of trauma has been estimated to be between $158 billion and $180 billion per year (Trauma Nursing Coalition, 1992). Trauma is costly in human lives, and productivity, as well (Cardona et al., 1994).

Traumatic injury usually occurs suddenly, leaving both the client and family with little time to prepare for its consequences. Nurses provide a vital link in both the physical and psychosocial care for the injured client and family. In caring for the client who has experienced trauma, nurses must consider not only the initial physical injury, but also

its long-term consequences, including rehabilitation and the client's return to his or her previous way of life.

The purpose of this chapter is to provide an introduction to the causes, effects, and management of trauma. The first three sections discuss the components of trauma, types of trauma, and common effects of traumatic injury. A discussion of trauma care follows, including prehospital and inpatient collaborative care of the client experiencing trauma; nursing care, which encompasses critical interventions, long-term care, and strategies to prevent trauma; and the teaching and discharge of the client and family experiencing trauma.

Components of Trauma

Traumatic injury results from an abnormal exchange of energy between a host and a mechanism within a predis-

Table 10–1	Common Mechanisms of Injury by Energy Source
Energy Source	**Common Mechanisms of Injury**
Mechanical	Motor vehicles Firearms Machines
Gravitational	Falls
Thermal	Heating appliances Fire Freezing temperatures
Electrical	Wires, sockets, and other electrical objects Lightning
Physical	Fists, feet, and other body parts (as in physical assault) Sharp objects, such as knives Ultraviolet radiation Ionizing radiation Water (drowning) Other submersion agents (e.g., grain) Explosions
Chemical	Drugs Poisons Industrial chemicals

Table 10–2	Common Mechanisms of Injury by Age of Adult Client
Age Group	**Mechanisms of Injury**
Young adult (15 to 24 years)	Motor vehicles Sports-related mechanisms (hockey pucks, baseball bats, fists and other body parts, e.g., in boxing, football) Penetrating objects (knives, guns)
Middle adult (25 to 64 years)	Motor vehicles Industrial equipment
Older adult (> 64 years)	Motor vehicles Falls

Note. Adapted from "Epidemiology of Trauma" by D. Stein in *A Comprehensive Curriculum for Trauma Nursing* (pp. 1–10) by E. Bayley and S. Turke (eds.), 1992, Boston: Jones and Bartlett; and from "Trauma in Childhood" by R. Semonin-Holleran in *Trauma Nursing: Art and Science* (pp. 527–553) by J. Neff and P. S. Kidd, (eds.), 1993, St Louis: Mosby-Year Book.

posing environment. These components—the host, the mechanism, and the environment—are discussed below.

Host

The *host* is the individual or group at risk of injury. Multiple factors influence the host's potential for injury: age, sex, race, economic status, preexisting illnesses, and use of substances such as alcohol. For example, a study of 263 trauma clients found that the majority were young and unemployed, were involved in substance abuse, were likely to be reinjured within 5 years of their first injury, and were at greater risk of dying young (Sims et al., 1989). The Major Trauma Outcome Study completed in 1990 found that trauma primarily afflicts males (Champion et al., 1990).

Mechanism

The *mechanism* is the source of the abnormal energy transmitted to the host. The energy exchanged can be mechanical, gravitational, thermal, electrical, physical, or chemical (Conroy, 1985). Table 10–1 lists the most common mechanisms for each type of energy. Table 10–2 lists the most common mechanisms by client age.

Mechanical energy is the most common type of energy transferred to a host in traumatic injury. The most common mechanical source of injury in all adult age groups is the motor vehicle. The box on page 366 lists the most predictable injuries resulting from motor vehicle accidents.

Guns are another common mechanical source of injury. Tragically, trauma from gunshot wounds has steadily increased over the past 20 years and has become a major reason for emergency department and trauma center admissions, especially in large cities.

Kinematics is the process of evaluating the amount of damage that may result from an abnormal exchange of mechanical energy with a host. Several principles of physics influence the amount of injury that a host may sustain (Rea, 1991):

- The greater the momentum of the moving object, the greater the amount of force that will be transferred to the object that is struck.

- The amount of damage that will result from the transfer of the energy varies at different parts of the body.

- As a force is applied to a body, there is a reciprocal force applied to another body.

A factor contributing to the description of any agent is *intention* (Stein, 1992). Examples of intentional injuries include most gunshot and stab wounds. It is important to remember, however, that some gunshot wounds are unintentional, such as those that occur when children play with their parents' guns. Even some stab wounds are unintentional, such as self-inflicted knife wounds that

Predictable Injuries from Motor Vehicle Accidents

■ ■ ■

Collision: Unrestrained Driver

- Head injuries
- Facial injuries
- Fractured larynx
- Fractured sternum
- Fractured clavicle
- Fractured patella and femur
- Cardiac contusion
- Lacerated liver or spleen
- Lacerated great vessels

Collision: Restrained Driver

- Pelvic injuries caused by lap restraints
- Spleen, liver, and pancreatic injuries caused by lap restraints
- Cervical fracture caused by shoulder restraints
- Rupture of mitral valve or diaphragm caused by shoulder restraints

Pedestrian Hit by Small Motor Vehicle

- Fractures of femur, tibia, and fibula on side of impact

Pedestrian Hit by Large Motor Vehicle or Dragged under Vehicle:

- Pelvic fractures

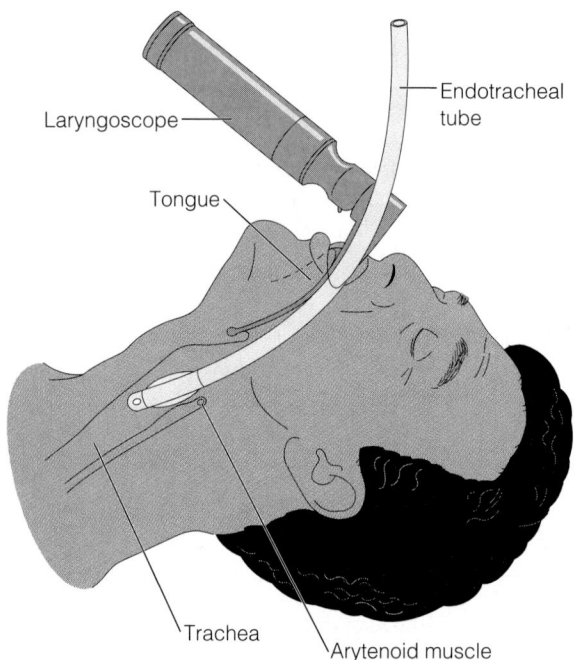

Figure 10–1 Placement of an oral endotracheal tube (ETT) for intubation. When the ETT is in place, air or oxygen can be blown into the external opening of the tube and enter the trachea.

occur during food preparation. Other common unintentional injuries result from motor vehicle crashes, falls, drowning, and fires.

Environment

The final component of trauma is the *environment*. The environment is composed of physical, cultural, and social realms. One example of a physical environment that may contribute to an injury is a road that has become slippery after a snowstorm. Occupation is an important environmental factor to consider when studying the epidemiology of trauma. Certain occupations face a high risk of traumatic injury; examples include police officers, professional athletes, and race car drivers. One's social and cultural environment also influences one's risk for injury. For example, one study found that there were no alcohol-related injuries among the Amish people because alcohol is forbidden to them and they therefore do not consume it. However, a significant number of Amish people suffered injuries from being kicked by a horse (Jones, 1990).

Types of Trauma

■ ■ ■

Whether intentional or accidental, trauma causes injury to one or more parts of the body. *Minor trauma* causes injury to a single part or system of the body and is usually treated in the hospital or emergency department. A fracture of the collarbone, a small second-degree burn, and a cut requiring stitches are all considered minor trauma. *Major* or *multiple trauma* involves serious single-system injury (such as the traumatic amputation of a leg) or multiple-system injuries. Multiple trauma (which is most often the result of a motor vehicle accident) requires immediate intervention that is specifically focused on ensuring the survival of the client. Clients who suffer multiple trauma receive immediate emergency care and often require long periods of intensive collaborative and nursing care.

Trauma also may be classified as either blunt or penetrating. *Blunt trauma* occurs when there is no communication from the damaged tissues to the outside environment. It is caused by a combination of forces including

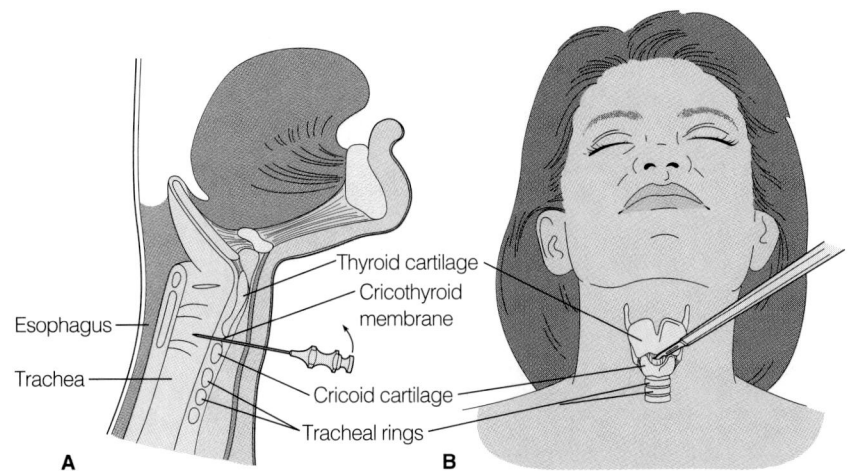

Figure 10–2 An emergency cricothyroidotomy may be performed if intubation is not successful in maintaining an open airway. This may be accomplished in two ways: *A,* inserting a 14-gauge needle into the trachea below the level of the obstruction; *B,* making an incision through the cricothyroid membrane and inserting a standard tracheostomy tube.

deceleration (a decrease in the speed of a moving object), *acceleration* (an increase in the speed of a moving object), *shearing* (forces occurring across a plane, with structures slipping across each other), *compression,* and *crushing.* Blunt forces often cause multiple injuries. Common blunt forces are motor vehicle accidents, falls, assaults, and sports activities. Blunt trauma often causes alterations in the anatomy and physiology of the head, spinal cord, bones, thorax, and abdomen.

Penetrating trauma occurs as the result of foreign objects set in motion. Penetration of tissues causes damage to body structures, most commonly the intestines, liver, spleen, and vascular system. Examples of penetrating trauma are gunshot wounds and low-velocity wounds, such as from stabbing or impalement.

Other types of trauma occur from inhalation, thermal changes, and blast forces. The respiratory system may be injured from inhalation of gases, smoke, and steam. Thermal injuries are manifested as burns or freezing. Injuries from blasts (explosions) are the result of the velocity of air movement and the force of projectiles from the explosion. Blast injuries are more severe in water than in air (the blast wave travels farther and faster in water) and enclosed spaces. The trauma from blast injuries includes pulmonary edema and hemorrhage, damage to abdominal organs, burns, penetrating injuries, and ruptured eardrums.

Effects of Traumatic Injury: Causes and Initial Management

■ ■ ■

As mentioned at the opening of this chapter, death is a common result of serious traumatic injury. Death from trauma may be immediate, early, or late. Immediate death is death at the scene from such injuries as a torn thoracic aorta or decapitation. Early death is death occurring within several hours of the injury from, for example, shock or lack of treatment for unrecognized injuries. Late death generally occurs 1 or more days after the injury and results from multiple organ failure.

Because of the serious consequences of a traumatic injury, it is important that the client's injuries be rapidly identified and appropriate interventions be instituted in a timely manner. Discussed below are some of the common effects of traumatic injury and some common interventions implemented by health care providers at the scene of the accident or in the emergency department.

Airway Obstruction

The trauma client's airway may become obstructed by the presence of blood, teeth, the tongue, and/or vomitus. After the client's cervical spine is immobilized (a procedure discussed later in this chapter), oxygen must be supplied. Airway interventions may include

- Clearing the airway by suctioning.

- Use of airway adjuncts, such as an oropharyngeal airway.

- Intubation with an oral endotracheal airway (Figure 10–1). This is the preferred method of airway management.

- Needle or surgical **cricothyroidotomy:** In needle cricothyroidotomy, a 14-gauge needle is inserted into the trachea below the level of the obstruction. Surgical cricothyroidotomy is the surgical incision of the cricothyroid membrane between the thyroid cartilage (visible externally as the Adam's apple) and the cricoid cartilage (Figure 10–2). This procedure is performed only after other methods are ineffective in opening and maintaining an open airway.

Figure 10–3 A needle thoracostomy may be used in the emergency treatment of a tension pneumothorax. *A,* A large-gauge needle is introduced, and air and fluid are aspirated. *B,* Alternatively a chest tube may be inserted and connected to a chest drainage system.

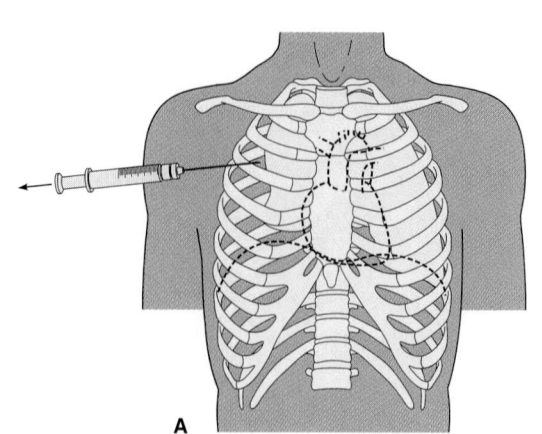
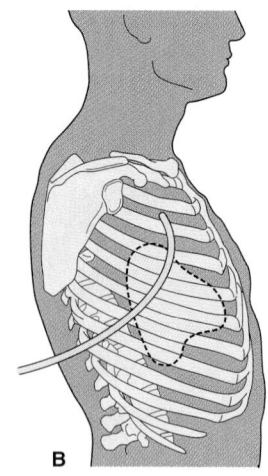

A   B

Tension Pneumothorax

A *pneumothorax* results from air in the pleural space from blunt and penetrating injuries to the chest. When a one-way valve is created so that air can enter the pleural space but not exit, a **tension pneumothorax** may develop. Many tension pneumothoraces result from blunt injury.

Immediate **needle thoracostomy** (insertion of a large-bore needle into the appropriate thoracic space) and chest tube insertion are performed. Most often, the needle is inserted into the second intercostal space at the midclavicular line or into the fifth intercostal space at the midaxillary line (Figure 10–3).

Hemorrhage

The American College of Surgeons Committee on Trauma (1993) has classified hemorrhage on a scale of I to IV: I is the mildest form of hemorrhage and IV is the most severe. Table 10–3 lists the signs and symptoms of each classification.

External Hemorrhage

When the client has suffered an injury that causes external hemorrhage, such as severing of an artery, the bleeding must be controlled immediately. Methods to achieve this include

- Applying direct pressure over the wound.
- Applying pressure over arterial pressure points (Figure 10–4).
- Elevating the injured limb.
- Clamping the bleeding vessel.
- Applying a tourniquet.

Internal Hemorrhage

Internal hemorrhage may result from either blunt or penetrating traumatic injury. Discovering the cause of, loca-

tion of, and extent of blood loss related to the injury are the most important concerns. Methods to discover the presence and location of internal hemorrhage include

- Diagnostic peritoneal lavage (discussed in the collaborative care section later in this chapter).
- Computerized tomography (CT) scans of the head, chest, and abdomen.

The body has several *potential spaces* that can accommodate large amounts of blood that may accumulate following injury. For example, bleeding into the pleural space may occur with chest trauma, and bleeding into the abdominal cavity may occur with abdominal trauma. A pelvic fracture may cause massive hemorrhage in the retroperitoneal region.

Once the source of internal hemorrhage has been recognized, interventions are initiated, including

- Operative control of bleeding.
- Continual assessment of the client, including physical assessment, vital signs, and serial laboratory work.

Hypovolemic Shock

A serious and potentially lethal complication of external and/or internal hemorrhage is hypovolemic shock. The most common cause of hypovolemic shock is traumatic injury. Factors that contribute to the development of hypovolemic shock include hemorrhage from blunt or penetrating injuries, long-bone or pelvic fractures, major vessel injuries, traumatic amputation, and plasma loss from tissue damage resulting from burns or crush injuries. The client who has suffered multiple injuries may develop shock from a combination of multiple sources of blood and fluid loss.

Care of the client who is experiencing hypovolemic shock may include rapid identification of the source of bleeding; fluid replacement; blood transfusion; and,

Table 10–3	Clinical Classification of Hemorrhage
Classification	**Signs and Symptoms**
I	Blood loss up to 750 mL Pulse rate less than 100 Blood pressure normal Capillary refill normal Respiratory rate 14 to 20 Normal urine output Slight anxiety
II	Blood loss 750 to 1500 mL Pulse rate greater than 100 Blood pressure normal Capillary refill decreased Respiratory rate 20 to 30 Urinary output decreased Anxiety
III	Blood loss 1500 to 2000 mL Pulse rate greater than 120 Blood pressure decreased Capillary refill decreased Respiratory rate 30 to 40 Urinary output decreased Confusion, lethargy
IV	Blood loss greater than 2000 mL Pulse rate greater than 140 Blood pressure decreased Capillary refill decreased Respiratory rate greater than 35 Urinary output decreased or absent Confusion, lethargy

Note. From "Perfusion: Cardiac and Vascular Injuries" by J. Neff in *Trauma Nursing: Art and Science* (pp. 195–262) by J. Neff and P. S. Kidd (eds.), 1993, St Louis: Mosby-Year Book.

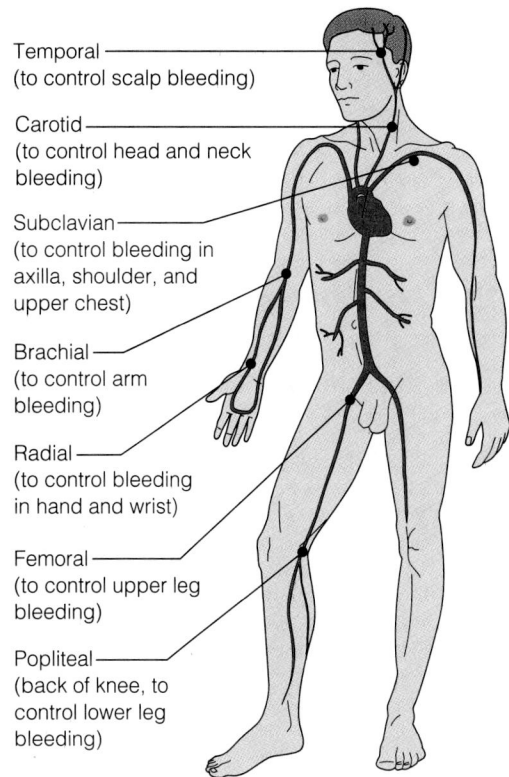

Temporal — (to control scalp bleeding)

Carotid — (to control head and neck bleeding)

Subclavian — (to control bleeding in axilla, shoulder, and upper chest)

Brachial — (to control arm bleeding)

Radial — (to control bleeding in hand and wrist)

Femoral — (to control upper leg bleeding)

Popliteal — (back of knee, to control lower leg bleeding)

Figure 10–4 The major pressure points used for the control of bleeding.

where indicated, operative intervention to control bleeding. Recent research has demonstrated that hypovolemic shock does not always necessitate aggressive fluid replacement. If the client is actively bleeding, rapid fluid volume replacement may actually worsen circulatory function and decrease a chance of survival, unless the bleeding can be controlled (Stern et al., 1993). It is imperative that the client be assessed before, during, and after fluid replacement to prevent further injury.

Hypovolemic shock is discussed in greater detail in Chapter 6.

Integumentary Effects

Injuries to the integument generally are not as serious as other injuries, with the exception of burns (see Chapter 18). The primary organ involved in integumentary trauma is the skin; however, underlying structures may also be injured. Injuries may result from either blunt or penetrating sources. It is important to evaluate all injuries to the integument because they may indicate a more serious injury, such as an open fracture. Additionally, large wounds may contribute to significant blood loss.

Four specific injuries to the integument include contusions, abrasions, puncture wounds, and lacerations (Figure 10–5). **Contusions** are superficial tissue injuries resulting from blunt trauma that causes the breakage of small blood vessels and bleeding into the surrounding tissue. **Abrasions** are partial-thickness denudations of an area of integument. They generally result from falls or scrapes. **Puncture wounds** occur when the integument is penetrated by a sharp or blunt object. **Lacerations** are open wounds that result from sharp cutting or tearing (Trott, 1991).

Injuries to the integument are at risk for contamination from dirt, debris, or foreign objects. The potential for infection may cause further stress to the client with multiple injuries. Interventions for injuries to the integument include

- Controlling any active bleeding.
- Immobilizing the affected area.
- Stabilizing any penetrating objects.
- Cleaning and irrigating the wound.

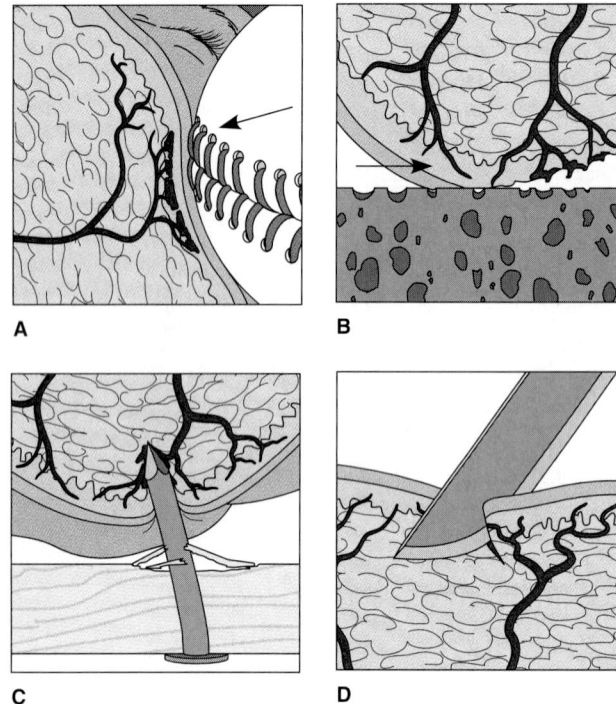

Figure 10–5 Traumatic injuries to the skin include: *A*, contusion; *B*, abrasion; *C*, puncture wound; and *D*, laceration.

- Applying the appropriate dressing.
- Administering tetanus immunization as indicated.
- Providing information about home wound care when the client is discharged.

Musculoskeletal Effects

Musculoskeletal injuries may occur alone or with multiple injuries as the result of blunt or penetrating mechanisms. Like injuries to the integument, musculoskeletal injuries usually are not considered a high priority in the care of the client with multiple injuries. Exceptions are the life- or limb-threatening musculoskeletal injury, such as a dislocated hip, or the musculoskeletal injury that may cause significant blood loss, such as a pelvic fracture (Rea, 1991).

Musculoskeletal injuries may provide clues to the presence of other serious injuries. For example, a fractured clavicle may indicate a thoracic injury.

Indications of musculoskeletal injuries include

- Swelling.
- Protrusion of bone.
- Obvious deformity.
- Abnormal motion.
- Pain.
- Pulseless extremity.
- Presence of crepitus.

Care of the client who has suffered a musculoskeletal injury is discussed fully in Chapter 37 and may include

- Assessing the neurovascular status of the injured extremity.
- Immobilizing the injured extremity.
- Applying ice to the injured extremity.
- Elevating the injured extremity.
- Providing medication for pain.

Neurologic Effects

Head injuries are one of the most common types of injury sustained as the result of trauma (Cardona et al., 1994). Injury to the spinal cord resulting in loss of neurologic function is one of the most devastating outcomes of trauma, but they are much less common than head injuries (Cardona et al., 1994).

The majority of head and spinal cord injuries result from blunt trauma and are sustained in motor vehicle crashes. Falls, sports injuries, and assault are some of the other sources of neurologic injury.

Loss of consciousness, altered mental status, and weakness or paralysis of the extremities are cardinal signs and symptoms of neurologic injury. Other indications of neurologic injury may include

- Changes in pupillary function.
- Scalp and/or facial wounds.
- Headache.
- Nausea and vomiting.
- Periorbital ecchymosis.
- Rhinorrhea and/or otorrhea (leakage of cerebrospinal fluid from the nose or ears).
- Mastoid ecchymosis (Battle's sign).
- Hemotympanum (blood behind the eardrum).
- Decreased sensation of pain and temperature.
- Weakness of the extremities and chest wall.
- Paralysis of the extremities and chest wall.
- Neck pain.
- Changes in vital signs (Cushing's triad: bradycardia, ataxic breathing, widening pulse pressure).

Care of the client who has sustained a neurologic injury is discussed in Chapters 40 and 41 and may include

- Assessing and managing the client's airway, breathing, and circulation.
- Immobilizing the client's cervical spine.
- Administering appropriate medications.

Effects on the Family

Traumatic injury usually occurs suddenly and with little warning. It may result in death or cause injury serious enough to alter dramatically both the client's and the family's lives. The suddenness and seriousness of the event are precipitating factors in the development of a psychologic crisis. Signs and symptoms of psychologic crisis include the following (Rea, 1991):

- Shock
- Numbness
- Guilt
- Anger

- Fear
- Anxiety
- Hostility

Immediate interventions include

- Establishing communication with the family as quickly as possible.
- Providing information about the client, the incident, and the care.
- Accompanying the family to see the client.

If the client has died, interventions include

- Allowing the family to view and touch the body if they desire.
- Explaining to the family local regulations that may require the death to be investigated (such as an autopsy).
- Helping the family to decide on the disposition of the body.

Over the past 10 years, some emergency departments have instituted care plans that allow families to participate as active members of the resuscitation team. This type of care is not without controversy, but it should be considered when appropriate. The accompanying nursing research box discusses the effectiveness of this practice.

Nursing interventions for clients suffering grief related to loss of a family member are discussed in detail in Chapter 11. Nursing interventions for clients suffering spiritual distress related to trauma are discussed later in this chapter.

Trauma Care

Care of the client experiencing trauma includes both collaborative and nursing interventions, which begin at the scene of the traumatic event. Victims of serious trauma may require care in an air or ground ambulance prior to their arrival at a hospital emergency department or trauma center. Surgery and postoperative care may be required, and some clients may also need long-term rehabilitative care.

Collaborative Care

Collaborative care of the trauma client depends on a team approach. Providing trauma care with a team focus helps

Applying Research to Nursing Practice
Family Presence During Resuscitation

■ ■ ■

Researchers conducted a study to evaluate the effect of the presence of the client's family during resuscitation in the emergency department (Hanson & Strawser, 1992). In the study, families of clients in cardiac arrest were allowed to remain with their loved ones during resuscitation if they so requested, if the resuscitation team permitted them to remain, and if a supportive individual such as a chaplain was also present. Family members were encouraged to talk to and touch their loved ones.

An evaluation completed by family members who participated found that 64% felt that their presence was beneficial to their loved one. In cases of client death, 76% of family members felt that their being present enabled them to accept their loved one's death more easily. Of the staff who were surveyed, 71% felt that the practice should continue, although they acknowledged that having the family present increased their stress levels and their emotional involvement in the resuscitation.

Implications for Nursing Practice

Providing emotional support during a crisis such as trauma resuscitation and possible death is one of the most difficult tasks that nurses face. Viewing the family as an important part of that process is a revolutionary idea in an age dominated by the technologic aspect of care. When family members are present during the client's resuscitation, they have the opportunity not only to participate in the client's care but also to observe the efforts of the emergency care team. Their presence affords family members some control in a situation that they feel may otherwise be totally out of their control.

Critical Thinking in Client Care

1. Describe the indications for allowing families to view a trauma resuscitation.
2. Describe some of the positive effects of allowing the family to view a trauma resuscitation.
3. What are your feelings about having family members present during trauma resuscitation?

each team member to be aware of his or her role. Prompt delegation of tasks and responsibilities improves the client's chances for survival and decreases the morbidity that may result from traumatic injuries.

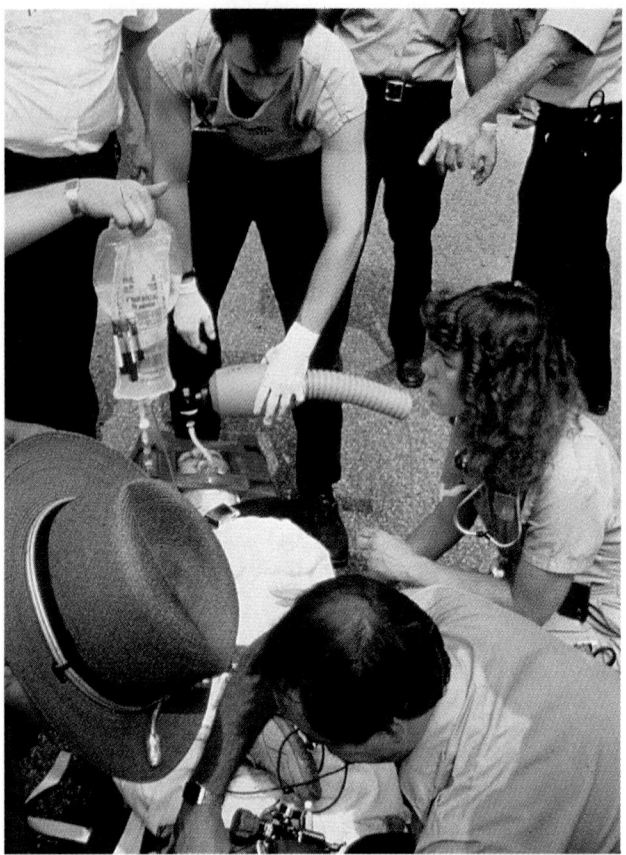

Figure 10–6 Flight nurses provide initial assessment, stabilization, and support for clients with trauma.

Table 10–4   Champion Revised Trauma Scoring System

Test	Score	Coded Value
Glasgow Coma Scale*	13 to 15	4
	9 to 12	3
	6 to 8	2
	4 to 5	1
	3	0
Systolic blood pressure	>89	4
	76 to 89	3
	50 to 75	2
	1 to 49	1
	0	0
Respiratory rate	10 to 29	4
	>29	3
	6 to 9	2
	1 to 5	1
	0	0
	Total score:	_____

The highest possible total score is 12. The lowest possible score is 0. The higher the total score, the greater the chance of survival.

* See Chapter 36 for instructions for using the Glasgow Coma Scale.

Note. From "A Revision of the Trauma Score" by H. Champion et al., 1989, *Journal of Trauma, 29*(5): 624.

Members of the Trauma Team

Nonnurse members of a **trauma team** may include the following emergency department staff: trauma surgeon, anesthesiologist, laboratory technicians, radiologist, and respiratory therapist. Nurses who are part of the trauma team include the prehospital care nurse, the flight nurse, the mobile intensive care nurse (MICN), the emergency nurse, the critical care nurse (including operating room and intensive care nurses), and the medical-surgical nurse.

The *prehospital care nurse* and *flight nurse* generally provide care for the trauma client before admission to the emergency department or the trauma unit. This care includes initial assessment, stabilization, and support (Figure 10–6). These nurses are skilled in advanced assessment techniques and such interventions as intubation, central line placement, and chest tube insertion.

The *mobile intensive care nurse (MICN)* is a specially educated nurse who not only provides client care in the field but also provides direction for other prehospital care providers via radio transmission. These nurses take reports from personnel in the field and provide advice and direction for client care based on protocols.

In a disaster setting with mass casualties, nurses may also carry out such tasks as *triage* (assessing and identifying those who need additional care) or serving as members of a *medical assistance team (MAT).* The MAT includes members of the American Red Cross who receive special training in caring for the injured in a disaster situation.

Prehospital Care

The survival of the client who has multiple injuries depends on an organized, comprehensive approach. Collaborative care of the injured client begins in the prehospital care environment.

The level of prehospital care varies throughout the United States as does the level of care that is provided in the field. Prehospital care providers include emergency medical technicians (EMTs), paramedics, nurses, and physicians. Prehospital care may provide rescue and either basic or advanced life support for the injured client, or a combination of both.

The major functions of prehospital care include

- Injury identification.
- Critical interventions.
- Rapid transport.

Injury Identification   Emergency care of the client experiencing trauma is based on rapid assessment to iden-

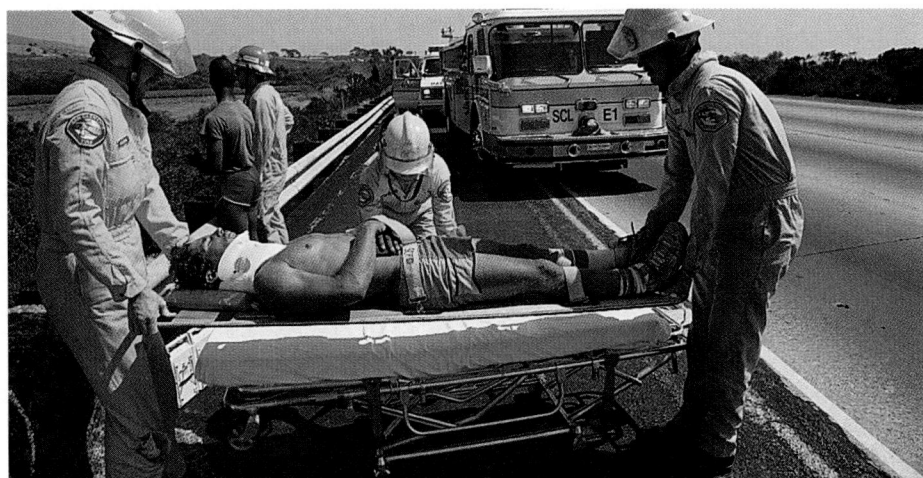

Figure 10–7 Immobilization of the cervical spine at the scene of the accident is essential to preventing further injury to the spinal cord. The combined use of a hard cervical collar, sandbags, and tape best restricts flexion, extension, rotation, and lateral bending of the neck.

tify injuries and initiate appropriate interventions. Injuries that indicate the need for trauma care include

- Penetrating injuries to the abdomen, pelvis, chest, neck, or head.
- Spinal cord injuries with deficit.
- Crushing injuries to the abdomen, chest, or head.
- Major burns (National Association of Air Medical Services Physicians, 1992).

Many methods are available to help health care providers determine the seriousness of the client's injuries and the potential for survival. These include the use of scoring systems, such as the Champion Revised Trauma Scoring System (Table 10–4).

In addition, the nurse performs a rapid but comprehensive trauma assessment organized into two steps, a primary and a secondary assessment. Both primary and secondary assessments may be used in the prehospital phase of client care, and both typically require advanced training in trauma nursing. Secondary assessment may continue into the emergency department and critical care phases.

Primary Assessment After ensuring that the cervical spine is immobilized, the nurse carries out a **primary assessment,** beginning with an assessment of the client's airway. The nurse assesses whether the client's airway is patent, maintainable, or nonmaintainable.

The next step in the primary assessment is evaluation of the client's breathing. The nurse assesses whether the client is breathing and what effort is required for ventilation. If the client is breathing, the nurse assesses whether the ventilations are impeded in any way, noting, for example, the presence of rib fractures or a collapsed lung.

Circulatory assessment follows; including palpating the client's peripheral and central pulses as well as assessing capillary refill. The nurse also examines the client's skin color and assesses the temperature of the client's skin.

A brief assessment of the client's neurologic status follows circulatory assessment. The nurse evaluates the client's level of consciousness and pupillary function.

In the next step of the primary assessment, the nurse exposes the client's integument to identify any obvious injuries and/or sites of uncontrolled bleeding.

Finally, the nurse obtains a brief history, including a description of what happened (that is, the agent of the injury), client allergies, and past medical history.

Secondary Assessment After the primary assessment has been completed and any life-threatening injuries have been stabilized, the caregiver performs the secondary assessment. The **secondary assessment** is a head-to-toe survey that includes a thorough evaluation of the client's anterior body and a brief assessment of the client's posterior body. During the secondary assessment, additional injuries are identified and appropriate interventions initiated. The steps of the complete secondary assessment are provided in the box on page 374.

Emergency Interventions As life-threatening problems are identified during the primary assessment, appropriate on-the-scene interventions must be performed immediately. These include providing basic life support and/or advanced cardiac life support, immobilizing the cervical spine, and managing the client's airway. *Basic life support (BLS)* consists of cardiopulmonary resuscitation (CPR). *Advanced cardiac life support (ACLS)* includes cardioversion; airway control, oxygenation, and ventilation; detection of arrhythmias; and drug therapy to treat hypotension, acid-base imbalance, fluid volume deficits, and arrhythmias.

Immobilization of the client's cervical spine is a primary intervention. The client is placed on a spine board, and a cervical collar and a head immobilizer are applied (Figure 10–7). The cervical spine may also be immobilized by logrolling the client onto a board, placing towel

Steps of the Secondary Assessment

■ ■ ■

The secondary assessment is a head-to-toe, anterior-to-posterior survey that may be conducted by a medical-surgical nurse. The nurse collects information primarily through inspection, palpation, and auscultation; subjective information (e.g., regarding pain) is also collected if the client is conscious. The assessment should proceed rapidly as follows.*

Head and Face

Soft-Tissue Injuries
■ Inspect for
   a. Lacerations
   b. Abrasions or contusions
   c. Avulsions
   d. Puncture wounds
   e. Impaled objects
   f. Ecchymosis
   g. Edema
   h. Pink or gray exposed tissue, which may indicate central nervous system disruption
■ Palpate for
   a. Crackling indicative of subcutaneous emphysema
   b. Tenderness

Bone Deformities
■ Inspect for
   a. Exposed bone
   b. Loose teeth or other material in the mouth that may compromise the airway
   c. Depressions
   d. Asymmetry of facial expressions and airway structures
■ Palpate for
   a. Depressions
   b. Angulation
   c. Tenderness

Eyes
■ Assess gross vision by holding up your fingers and asking the client how many you are holding up.
■ Inspect for
   a. Periorbital ecchymosis (raccoon's eyes)
   b. Subconjunctival hemorrhage
   c. Contact lenses
■ Check pupils for
   a. Size
   b. Shape
   c. Equality
   d. Reaction to light
■ Check extraocular movements (EOMs) by moving your finger into the client's visual field and having client follow your finger with the eyes.

Ears
■ Inspect for
   a. Ecchymosis behind the ears (Battle's sign)
   b. Skin avulsion and exposure of cartilage
   c. Blood or clear fluid in or draining from the external canal (if present, do *not* stop drainage, which may be cerebrospinal fluid)

Nose
■ Inspect for drainage of blood or clear fluid (if present, do *not* stop drainage, which may be cerebrospinal fluid)

Neck
■ Inspect for
   a. Surface or penetrating trauma
   b. Impaled objects
   c. Ecchymosis
   d. Edema
   e. Tracheal deviation
   f. Pulsating or distended neck veins
   g. Scars
■ Palpate for
   a. Tracheal deviation
   b. Tenderness
   c. Subcutaneous emphysema

Chest and Thorax

Soft-Tissue Injuries
■ Inspect the anterior and lateral thorax, including the axillae, for
   a. Lacerations
   b. Abrasions or contusions
   c. Avulsions
   d. Puncture wounds
   e. Impaled objects
   f. Ecchymosis
   g. Edema
   h. Scars
■ Palpate for
   a. Subcutaneous emphysema
   b. Tenderness
■ Inspect chest wall expansion and excursion during ventilation.
■ Inspect breathing for
   a. Rate
   b. Depth
   c. Degree of effort required
   d. Accessory or abdominal muscle use
   e. Paradoxical chest wall movement
■ Auscultate briefly for
   a. Breath and heart sounds
   b. Adventitious sounds, such as wheezing, rales, or rhonchi

*Note: A Glasgow Coma Scale score and trauma score should also be recorded in the medical record.

Steps of the Secondary Assessment (*continued*)

Bone Deformities

- Palpate the clavicles, sternum, and ribs.
- Palpate for tenderness, crepitus, and deformity.
- Inspect for expressions or reactions that indicate severe pain, which may indicate cardiac contusions, fractures, or damage to a great vessel.

Abdomen and Flank

- Inspect for
  a. Lacerations
  b. Abrasions or contusions
  c. Avulsions
  d. Puncture wounds
  e. Impaled objects
  f. Ecchymosis
  g. Exposed internal organs
  h. Distention
  i. Scars
- Auscultate briefly for bowel sounds. If none are present initially, reassess later during focused abdominal assessment.
- Palpate lightly for tenderness, rigidity, or masses.

Pelvis and Genitals

Soft Tissue Injuries

- Inspect for
  a. Lacerations
  b. Abrasions or contusions
  c. Avulsions
  d. Puncture wounds
  e. Impaled objects
  f. Ecchymosis
  g. Edema

Bone Deformities

- Inspect for exposed bone.
- Palpate for instability and tenderness over the iliac crests and pubic symphysis.

Bleeding

- Inspect
  a. Urethral meatus for blood (if present, do *not* insert indwelling urinary catheter)
  b. Vagina and rectum for evidence of bleeding

Altered Neurologic Function

- Inspect penis for priapism.
- Palpate rectal sphincter from anterior for loss of tone.

Altered Elimination

- Assess for
  a. Pain with bowel elimination
  b. Pain with urinary elimination
  c. Urge to void
  d. Inability to void

Extremities

Circulatory Status
(Do *not* remove properly applied splints that do not interfere with assessment.)

- Inspect for
  a. Color
  b. Skin temperature
  c. Symmetry
- Palpate for distal pulses.

Sensory Function

- Test gross sensory function by touching various parts of the injured extremity, especially fingertips and toes.
- Compare with the uninjured extremity.

Motor Function

- Inspect for spontaneous motor function of injured and uninjured extremities.
- Test presence and symmetry of motor strength and range of motion.

Soft-Tissue Injuries

- Inspect for
  a. Lacerations
  b. Abrasions or contusions
  c. Avulsions
  d. Puncture wounds
  e. Impaled objects
  f. Ecchymosis
  g. Edema
  h. Angulations
  i. Deformities
  j. Any open wound in proximity to a deformity
- Palpate for crepitus.

Posterior Assessment

- Observe cervical spine precautions, and splint suspected extremity fractures.
- Logroll client onto side or at least enough to assess
  a. Back
  b. Flanks
  c. Buttocks
  d. Thighs

  for

  a. Obvious bleeding
  b. Major wounds
  c. Impaled objects
- Palpate spine for tenderness and deformities.
- Palpate costovertebral angles for areas of tenderness.

Note. From *Trauma Nursing Core Course* by R. Rea, 1991, Chicago: Emergency Nurses Association.

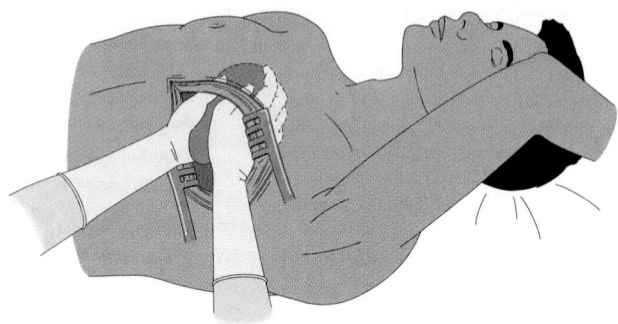

Figure 10–8 An emergency thoracotomy with internal cardiac massage may be necessary if the client in cardiac arrest does not respond to fluid replacement and external CPR.

rolls or a head immobilizer along the sides of the client's head, and securing the client to the board (Proehl, 1993).

If the client's airway is patent, high-flow oxygen is administered; high-flow oxygen systems provide all the inspired gas the client breathes. A nasogastric tube is inserted to prevent aspiration of stomach contents. Breathing interventions include assisting ventilations with a bag-valve mask until airway management is achieved. If a tension pneumothorax, hemothorax, or symptomatic pneumothorax is present, needle decompression or chest tube insertion is performed.

If the client does not respond to fluid and blood replacement and external CPR, **emergency thoracotomy** (surgical opening of the chest to perform internal CPR) may be considered. Emergency thoracotomy allows for the following (Ali, 1992, p. 697):

- Identification and treatment of pericardial tamponade (characterized by Beck's triad: distended neck veins, hypotension, and distant heart sounds)

- Internal cardiac massage (Figure 10–8)

- Identification and control of intrathoracic hemorrhage

- Cross clamping of the aorta to maintain cerebral cardiac perfusion

Circulation interventions include identifying and controlling active bleeding by direct pressure (for external bleeding) and surgery (for internal bleeding). Measures to reverse shock are initiated (see page 368 and Chapter 6). The client is placed on a cardiac monitor. A Foley catheter is inserted to measure urinary output. In some trauma centers, invasive catheters, such as central venous pressure (CVP) lines and/or pulmonary arterial catheters, are inserted for hemodynamic monitoring.

If the client was wearing a helmet at the time of injury, the helmet should remain in place until the client arrives at the hospital, unless the client's airway is at risk. If necessary, health care personnel remove the helmet by ma-

nipulating it over the client's nose and ears while holding the client's head and neck immobile; thus, safe removal requires at least two people. Improper removal puts the client at risk for injury or additional injury to the spinal cord.

If the client has positive neurologic findings, such as fixed and dilated pupils, pharmacologic interventions are initiated. Some neurosurgeons prefer that a burr hole procedure be performed (see Chapter 40). If the client is having any seizure activity, pharmacologic agents may control it.

Throughout the primary and secondary assessment, the emergency nurse closely monitors the client's body temperature and manages the environment around the client so that the client does not suffer any additional stress from cold. Warm blankets may be used to cover the client with multiple trauma to prevent hypothermia.

Rapid Transport   Clients who have multiple injuries must be transported as soon as possible to a regional trauma center. The most common modes of rapid transport are ground ambulances and air ambulances, which are helicopters specially staffed and equipped to care for trauma victims. Clients who are stable and within access of a ground ambulance are best transported by ground. Clients who are unstable and clients injured in wilderness areas or other areas in which ground access is difficult may best be transported by air. When these transport systems are unavailable, the client is transported by any available means.

The following other factors also influence the choice of the mode of transportation:

- The agent of injury

- The nature of the injury

- The number of accident victims

- The distance and time it will take to get the client to definitive care

- The time needed to extricate the client from the accident situation

- Traffic, road conditions, and weather

- Available modes of transportation in a given area

Laboratory and Diagnostic Tests
The laboratory and diagnostic tests that are ordered depend on the type of injury the client has sustained. The laboratory and diagnostic tests for specific types of trauma, such as burns or spinal cord injuries, are discussed in the appropriate chapters of this text. Additional tests that may be ordered for victims of trauma include the following:

- *Blood type and crossmatch,* which involves typing the client's blood for ABO antigens and Rh factor, screening the blood for antibodies, and crossmatching the client's serum and donor red blood cells (Neff, 1993, p. 235).

- **Blood alcohol level,** which measures the amount of alcohol in a client's blood. It has been found that between 20% and 50% of people who are injured may be intoxicated. Alcohol alters the client's level of consciousness and response to pain.

- *Drug screen* may also be ordered. Like alcohol, such drugs as cocaine alter the client's level of consciousness and overall response to the primary survey.

- *Pregnancy test* for any woman of childbearing age to rule out the potential for pregnancy and fetal injury.

The following diagnostic tests may be ordered to identify any injuries that the client may have sustained:

- *Diagnostic peritoneal lavage* is performed to determine the presence of blood in the peritoneal cavity, which may indicate abdominal injury. The test is generally done in the emergency department. To prepare the client for a peritoneal lavage, the nurse first inserts a nasogastric tube and connects it to suction. A Foley catheter is then inserted into the bladder and connected to a drainage system. The skin of the lower abdomen is shaved and scrubbed with a bactericidal solution. A local anesthetic (such as lidocaine) is injected subcutaneously, and a small incision is made. A catheter is placed into the peritoneal cavity, and any free blood is aspirated. If blood is found, the client is taken to the operating room for exploratory surgery. If no free blood is aspirated, 1 liter of an isotonic solution (Ringer's solution or normal saline) is rapidly infused into the peritoneal cavity and then allowed to drain by gravity. If the solution returns pink and is found to have a red blood cell count of from 20,000 to 100,000 mm^3, the test is considered positive, and the client is taken to the operating room for exploratory surgery.

- *Computerized tomography (CT) scans* are performed to discover injuries to the brain, skull, spinal cord, chest, and abdomen.

- *Magnetic resonance imaging (MRI) scans* are performed to discover injuries to the brain and spinal cord.

Pharmacology

The type of pharmacologic therapy used to treat the client who has experienced traumatic injury depends on the type and severity of the injuries, as well as the degree of traumatic shock that is present. The following general categories of medications may be used:

- Blood components and fluids are administered intravenously in the initial treatment of traumatic shock to replace intravascular volume. The administration of blood components is discussed in the following sec-

tion; the administration of intravenous fluids is discussed in Chapter 6.

- Inotropic drugs (drugs that increase myocardial contractility) are given to increase cardiac output and improve tissue perfusion. These drugs, often administered after fluid volume restoration, include dopamine, dobutamine, and isoproterenol (see Chapter 6).

- Vasopressors may be administered in conjunction with fluid replacement in the treatment of neurogenic, septic, or anaphylactic shock. Examples of vasopressors include dopamine, epinephrine, norepinephrine, and phenylephrine (see Chapter 6).

- Vasodilators are used if circulating blood volume is adequate. Vasodilators may improve blood flow to peripheral capillary beds, facilitate oxygen delivery, and decrease shock. However, they are not used in the treatment of the client with hemorrhage or hypovolemic shock and are not a part of initial trauma treatment. Vasodilators include nitroprusside and nitroglycerin (see Chapter 6).

In addition, medications are given to manage pain as soon as possible. However, the effects of the pain medications may alter client responses to injury and mask potential injuries. If pain medications are administered, they must be carefully regulated, and the client must be closely monitored. Pain medications are usually administered by a continuous infusion with opioid drugs (such as morphine, fentanyl, or meperidine), individually tailored to each client. An initial loading dose is administered and the infusion regulated to meet client needs. As soon as the client is alert and responsive, patient-controlled analgesia (PCA) should begin. Pain medications may also be administered by continuous epidural infusions; this route provides pain relief with less risk of effects on other body systems, such as respiratory depression or central nervous system sedation. Nursing care of the client in pain is discussed in Chapter 4.

Lastly, if the client has penetrating wounds, tetanus immunization status must be determined. If the client is unable to remember when the last tetanus immunization was given or is unable to answer, tetanus prophylaxis is prescribed and administered.

Blood Transfusions

Blood and blood components are substances that are initially produced in the body and then are donated for use by another person through a **transfusion** (an infusion of blood or blood components). A client may be given whole blood, red blood cells (RBCs), platelets, plasma, albumin, clotting factors, prothrombin, or cryoprecipitate (Table 10–5). Blood and blood components increase the amount of hemoglobin to carry oxygen to the cells, improve hemoglobin and hematocrit levels during active

Table 10–5 Types of Blood Components Used in Transfusion Therapy

Type	Use	Limitations
Whole blood	Replaces blood volume and oxygen-carrying capacity in hemorrhage and shock. Contains RBCs, plasma proteins, clotting factors, and plasma.	Contains few platelets or granulocytes; deficient in clotting factors V and VII. Greatest risks are for incompatibility or circulatory overload.
Red cells	Increase oxygen-carrying capacity in slow bleeding or in clients with anemia, with leukemia, or having surgery.	Has no viable platelets or granulocytes. Incompatibility may cause hemolytic reactions.
Platelets	Used to control or prevent bleeding in clients with platelet deficiencies.	If given for an extended period of time, antibodies may develop. Hypersensitivity reactions may occur.
Plasma	Expands blood volume; can be administered to any blood group or type. Contains all clotting factors and is used to restore those deficient in bleeding disorders.	May cause vascular overload, hypersensitivity reactions, or hemolytic reactions.
Albumin	Expands blood volume in shock and trauma. Used to treat clients in shock from trauma or infection and in surgery to replace blood volume and proteins.	Is not a substitute for whole blood. May cause hypersensitivity reactions.
Clotting factors	Factor VIII concentrate is used to treat clients with hemophilia A and von Willebrand's disease. Factor IX concentrate is used to treat clients with hemophilia B and other clotting factor deficiencies.	
Prothrombin complex	Contains prothrombin, clotting factors VII, IX, X, and part of XI. Used to treat clients with deficiencies of these factors.	
Cryoprecipitate	Contains factor VIII, factor XIII, von Willebrand's factor, and fibrinogen. Used to treat clients with clotting factor deficiencies.	May cause ABO incompatibilities.

bleeding, increase intravascular volume, and replace deficient substances, such as platelets and clotting factors.

The blood of each person is of one of four types: A, B, AB, and O. Blood group antigens A and B are present on RBC membranes and form the basis for the ABO blood categorization. The presence or absence of one or both of these inherited antigens determines one's blood type. Persons with blood type A have A antigens, those with blood type B have B antigens, those with type AB have both antigens, and those with neither antigen have blood type O.

ABO antibodies develop in the serum of persons whose RBCs lack the corresponding antigen; these antibodies are called anti-A and anti-B. The person with blood type B has A antibodies, the person with blood type A has B antibodies, the person with blood type O develops both types of antibodies, and the person with blood type AB has no antibodies.

A third antigen on the RBC membrane is D. People who are Rh positive have the D antigen, whereas people who are Rh negative do not. The presence of these antigens and antibodies may cause ABO and Rh incompatibilities when blood is administered. The incompatibilities cause hemolysis of the RBCs and agglutination of erythrocytes. (Agglutination is the clumping of cells that results from their interaction with specific antibodies.) The ABO blood group names and compatibilities are listed in Table 10–6.

Before RBCs or whole blood can be administered, a series of procedures are conducted to determine donor and recipient ABO types and Rh groups. These procedures, called a *type and crossmatch*, are performed by mixing the donor cells with the recipient's serum and watching for agglutination. If none occurs, the blood is considered compatible. The blood is also typed and tested for hepatitis A, hepatitis B, and human immunodeficiency virus (HIV).

Despite meticulous procedures for matching blood types and antigens, blood transfusion reactions may still occur. The most common of these is called a *febrile reaction*. Antibodies within the client receiving the blood are directed against the donor's white blood cells, causing fever and chills. Febrile reactions typically begin during the first 15 minutes of the transfusion. Future febrile reactions may be avoided by using leukocyte-poor blood. Hypersensitivity reactions result when antibodies in the client's blood react against proteins, such as immunoglobulin A, in the donor blood.

Hypersensitivity reactions may appear during or after the transfusion. The manifestations of hypersensitivity reaction include *urticaria* (the appearance of reddened wheals of various sizes on the skin) and itching.

Table 10–6	Blood Group Types and Compatibilities			
Blood Group	**RBC Agglutinogens**	**Serum Agglutinogens**	**Compatible Donor Blood Groups**	**Incompatible Donor Blood Groups**
A	A	Anti-B	A, O	B, AB
B	B	Anti-A	B, O	A, AB
AB	A, B	None	A, B, AB, O	None
O	None	Anti-A, Anti-B	O	A, B, AB

Note: Group O is often called the universal donor, and group AB is called the universal recipient.

Hemolytic reactions, the most dangerous transfusion reaction, usually result from an ABO incompatibility. The clumping of the RBCs blocks capillaries, decreasing blood flow to vital organs. In addition, macrophages engulf the clumped RBCs, releasing free hemoglobin into the circulating blood; the hemoglobin is then filtered by the kidneys and may block the renal tubules, causing renal failure. Hemolytic reactions usually begin after infusion of 100 to 200 mL of the incompatible blood. Manifestations of a hemolytic reaction include flushing of the face, a burning sensation along the vein, headache, urticaria, chills, fever, lumbar pain, abdominal pain, chest pain, nausea and vomiting, tachycardia, hypotension, and dyspnea. If any of these manifestations appear, the blood transfusion must be immediately discontinued.

Other risks to clients receiving blood include circulatory overload and electrolyte imbalances (see Chapter 5), and infectious diseases, such as hepatitis, cytomegalovirus, or HIV.

Clients who have experienced trauma of any degree of severity have had substantial blood loss and are usually in hypovolemic shock. Blood replacement is the treatment of choice to restore oxygen-carrying capacity. Clients in severe shock with active bleeding are given universal, type O red blood cells immediately. Clients with less severe injuries or bleeding may be stabilized with other types of fluids until type-specific or crossmatched blood is available.

Some emergency departments and trauma centers use autotransfusion equipment to provide blood for transfusions for the client with multiple injuries and/or severe shock. Autotransfusion is a method of blood administration in which special equipment returns the client's own blood to the client. The chest cavity is the typical source of blood to be autotransfused (Kitt & Proehl, 1993).

Nursing considerations for blood transfusion therapy are described in the pharmacology box on page 380.

Emergency Surgery

The need for immediate surgical intervention in the client with multiple injuries is indicated when the client remains in shock despite resuscitation and there is no obvious sign of blood loss (Moore et al., 1984). Abdominal and chest X-ray studies and a diagnostic peritoneal lavage or CT scan may be performed to help identify the potential source of the blood loss.

Nurses prepare the client for emergency surgery by

- Undressing the client and removing jewelry, dentures, or other loose objects.
- Placing an identification bracelet on the client.
- Providing the operating room nurse with any available information about the client, including mechanism of injury, allergies, past medical history, and interventions that have been performed.

It is important that the emergency or trauma nurse speak with the family as soon as possible and keep them informed about what is happening to their family member. Unfortunately, the need for emergency surgery may not allow time for family members or significant others to see their loved one before transfer to the operating room.

Organ Donation

In 1968, the **Uniform Anatomical Gift Act** was passed. This legislation ordained that people be informed about their options related to organ donation. In 1987, the act was revised to simplify the legal process surrounding organ donation. Under this act, consent for organ donation may be given not only by the donor but also by a spouse, adult children, parents, adult siblings, guardian, or any adult authorized to do so (Emergency Nurses Association, 1992). The act also encourages people to carry donor cards. Forty-five states have passed laws that require health care providers to ask family members about organ donation.

The increased success that has occurred over the past 30 years in organ transplant has made it a more common and valuable method of prolonging and improving life. However, many people are still waiting for organs, and many people who may be suitable organ donors die each year from traumatic injury.

Nursing Implications for Pharmacology: Blood Transfusion

The risk for and seriousness of blood transfusion reactions require that extreme caution be taken when blood is administered. Most fatal transfusion reactions are the result of human error. Although general guidelines are provided here, each institution has specific policies and procedures that must be followed. Prior to beginning the transfusion, the nurse must determine that typed and cross-matched blood is available and collect the needed equipment: a Y-tubing blood administration set with a filter (see the figure on page 381) a large-bore intravenous catheter, usually 18- or 19-gauge, and normal saline solution. Only normal saline is used with a blood transfusion: Dextrose causes clumping of RBCs, and distilled water causes hemolysis.

Nursing Responsibilities

- Assess for any previous reactions to blood.

- Explain the procedure to the client, and answer any questions.

- Prepare the intravenous equipment: Shut off one side of the Y-tubing, and attach the other side to the saline solution. Flush the tubing and filter with the saline.

- If venous access is not already in place, insert the intravenous needle (following body substance precautions), and begin administering the saline.

- Using institutional procedure, obtain the blood from the blood bank or laboratory. Administer the blood immediately; if this is not possible, return it to the blood bank or laboratory.

- Check and document that the donor and recipient blood have been tested and are compatible. This usually involves two nurses, each verifying that
  a. An order for blood has been written.
  b. Type and cross-match have been done.
  c. The name of the client and the name on the blood bag are identical.
  d. The number assigned to the unit of blood is identical to the one on the requisition for the blood.

  e. Blood type and Rh factor are compatible.
  f. The blood has not exceeded its expiration date.
  g The unit of blood is intact and has no bubbles or discoloration.

- Identify the client by reading the arm band and asking the client to tell you his or her name. Check the arm band against the unit of blood.

- Gently invert the blood bag several times to mix the plasma and RBCs.

- Take and record vital signs as a baseline.

- Attach the open side of the Y-tubing to the blood unit, and begin the transfusion at a slow rate of about 2 mL per minute. (Some trauma clients may have blood infused at a rapid rate. If blood is infused rapidly, it may need to be warmed prior to administration to prevent hypothermia.) Stay with the client for at least the first 15 minutes of the transfusion, monitoring for manifestations of a reaction and taking the client's vital signs.

- Continue to monitor the client during the transfusion, assessing for manifestations of hypersensitivity or hemolytic reactions and taking and recording vital signs as directed by institutional policy.

- After the first 15 minutes, the rate of infusion is increased. If there is no danger of fluid volume overload, most clients can tolerate an infusion of a unit of blood (ranging from 250 to 500 mL, depending on the blood component administered) in 2 hours. The unit of blood should be administered in 3 to 4 hours; after this time, it has warmed and begins to deteriorate.

- Take the following actions if manifestations of a reaction occur:
  a Stop the infusion of blood immediately, and notify the physician. Continue to infuse the saline.
  b. Take vital signs, and assess manifestations.
  c. Compare the blood slip with the unit of blood to ensure that an identification error was not made.

Organs and tissues that may be transplanted include the following (Hammond, 1992):

- Bones
- Eyes
- Skin
- Heart and heart valves
- Kidneys

- Liver
- Lungs
- Muscles and tendons
- Pancreas

The organ donation process begins with identification of the potential organ donor. Most people are potential organ donors. Exceptions include those who

- Currently abuse intravenous drugs.
- Have preexisting untreated infections, such as septicemia.
- Are HIV positive.

Pharmacology: Blood Transfusion (*continued*)

d. Save the blood bag and any remaining blood for return to the laboratory for further tests to determine the cause of the reaction.

e. Follow institutional policy for collecting urine and venous blood samples.

f. Continue to monitor the client and provide prescribed interventions to treat hypersensitivity or hemolytic manifestations.

■ Do not add medications to blood infusions or tubing.

■ When the blood is totally infused, use the saline to flush the tubing to ensure complete administration of the blood.

■ Return the empty blood bag to the blood bank or laboratory.

Client and Family

■ The possible risks of blood transfusions include infectious diseases and acquired immune deficiency syndrome (AIDS). However, because of careful handling and storage of blood, bacterial contamination is rare. Although hepatitis may be transmitted by contaminated blood, new tests for hepatitis antibodies in the donor blood are reducing this risk. Many people are afraid of contracting AIDS from blood; however, donor screening and HIV-antibody testing of donor blood has virtually eliminated the transmission of HIV by blood transfusion.

■ During the transfusion, immediately report any warm feelings, chills, itching, feelings of weakness or fainting, or difficulty breathing.

■ Report any signs of a delayed transfusion reaction: chills, fever, cough, difficulty breathing, hives, itching, or changes in circulation. Report difficulty with breathing, and seek medical care immediately.

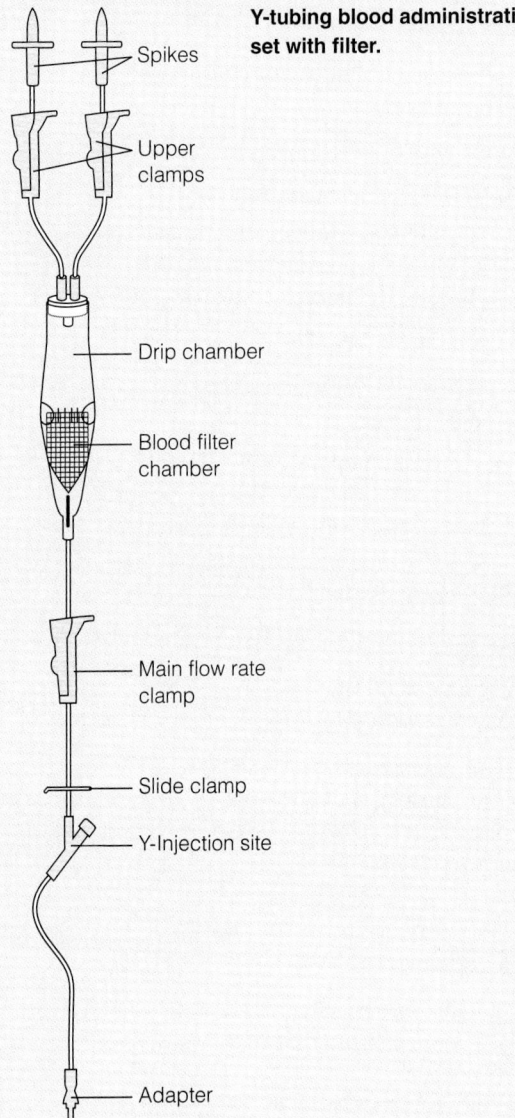

Y-tubing blood administration set with filter.

Spikes
Upper clamps
Drip chamber
Blood filter chamber
Main flow rate clamp
Slide clamp
Y-Injection site
Adapter

■ Have any malignancy other than a brain tumor.

■ Have active tuberculosis.

The Organ Procurement Organization should be notified as early as possible in the process. The national number is 1-800-24-DONOR. Nurses need to know which agency in their area of practice is responsible for organ procurement.

The family needs to be made aware of the client's prognosis and presented with the option of donating the client's organs. Both the family's and the client's feelings related to organ donation must be explored. Even if the client carries an organ donation card, many institutions will not remove any organs without a signature from a family member or other authorized person.

The nurse must always respect the family's concerns and feelings related to this process. Some members of

Brain Death Criteria

■ ■ ■

Clinical Signs

- Known cause of injury or condition
- Irreversible condition
- Apnea with a $PaCO_2$ greater than 60 mm Hg
- No response to deep stimuli
- No spontaneous movement (some spinal cord reflexes may be present)
- No gag or corneal reflex
- No oculocephalic or oculovestibular reflex
- Normothermic (body temperature greater than 32.2 C or 90 F)
- Acceptable levels of central nervous system depressants and neuromuscular blocking agents
- Absence of toxic or metabolic disorders

Confirmatory Tests

- Cerebral blood flow study
- Electroencephalogram
- Evoked response testing

Note. From *Trauma Resource Document* (p. 67) by Emergency Nurses Association, 1992, Park Ridge, IL: Emergency Nurses Association.

certain cultural groups may have religious constraints and/or issues of mistrust that may interfere with the donation process.

Before any organs can be removed, the client must be declared brain dead. **Brain death criteria** are clinical signs used to determine whether a comatose client is brain dead. The accompanying box lists brain death criteria. Once brain death has been confirmed, the family must also agree with the diagnosis and be allowed time to prepare for the client's death as well as they can.

When caring for an adult client who is an organ donor, the nurse carries out the following (Emergency Nurses Association, 1992):

- Maintain systolic blood pressure of 90 mm Hg to keep the client's organs perfused until removal.
- Maintain urine output at more than 30 mL per hour. This is usually accomplished by administering fluids and/or inotropic agents, such as dopamine.
- Maintain oxygen saturation at 90% or greater.

- Ensure that the client's body is not suffering from sepsis.

Because traumatic injuries and death are sudden and often occur to the young, approaching the family about potential organ donation is a very difficult process. Health care personnel can lessen the anxiety and stress that is a part of this process by being familiar with and following the hospital's established organ and tissue donation policy. By preplanning and providing appropriate guidance, nurses can help a family who is faced with sudden tragedy to make the life-affirming decision for organ transplant.

Forensic Considerations

Many injuries result from circumstances that require legal investigation to discover their source. In addition, many injuries, particularly penetrating trauma, may involve criminal activity. Therefore, it is important for the nurse to recognize the need to identify, store, and properly transfer potential evidence for medical-legal investigations.

Each item of clothing that is removed from the client must be placed in a breathable container, such as a paper bag, and documented appropriately. Bullets or knives should be labeled, with their source specified, and given to the proper authorities.

The client's hands may yield important evidence, such as powder burns on the skin or tissue or hair samples beneath the fingernails. It is recommended that paper bags be placed over the client's hands if the presence of evidence is suspected (Taylor & Jones, 1993).

The nurse observes for the presence of entrance and exit wounds and documents these findings. Some nurses find it easier to draw pictures than to provide written descriptions.

Finally, once the evidence has been collected, identified, and properly stored, the nurse needs to ensure that it is given to the appropriate authorities. A chain of custody needs to be maintained throughout the entire process. The chain of custody establishes documentation procedures that identify all those who come into contact with the evidence. The chain of custody also calls for the identification and labeling of the evidence, as well as a chronicle of where and in whose possession the evidence has been. For the chain of custody to remain intact, the evidence must remain in the continuous possession of identified people and be marked and sealed in tamper-proof containers (Taylor & Jones, 1993).

Nursing Care

Nursing care of the client who has been injured begins with a primary assessment and the initiation of collaborative interventions for any life-threatening injuries. Nursing care is directed toward the client's specific responses to trauma. Nursing diagnoses that are discussed in this section pertain to actual or potential problems with airway clearance, infection, mobility, spiritual distress, post-trauma response, and risk for trauma.

Ineffective Airway Clearance

The client who has suffered multiple injuries is at great risk for developing airway obstruction and apnea. Facial injuries, loose teeth, blood, and vomitus increase the risk for aspiration and obstruction. Neurologic injuries and cerebral edema alter the client's respiratory drive and ability to keep the airway clear.

Nursing interventions with rationales are as follows:

- Observe whether the client's airway is patent, maintainable, or nonmaintainable. Assess the client for signs and symptoms of airway obstruction:
  a. Facial trauma
  b. Debris in the airway, such as teeth, blood, or vomitus
  c. Stridor
  d. Tachypnea
  e. Bradypnea
  f. Cough
  g. Cyanosis
  h. Shortness of breath
  i. Decreased or absent breath sounds
  j. Altered mental status

  Assessing the airway and initiating interventions are the first steps in managing the client with multiple injuries. Because the airway is at risk for becoming obstructed by blood, teeth, or vomitus, suction and advanced airway equipment need to be available and used as indicated.

- Monitor oxygen saturation by placing the client on a pulse oximeter. *Changes in oxygen saturation as measured by the pulse oximeter indicate the effectiveness of the client's airway. Oxygen flow is adjusted to maintain the client's oxygen saturation from 94% to 100%.*

- Assess the client's level of consciousness. *An early sign of an ineffective airway is change in the client's behavior. If the client becomes anxious, combative, or unresponsive, the effectiveness of the airway needs to be immediately evaluated and appropriate interventions initiated.*

Risk for Infection

Traumatic injuries are considered dirty wounds. The trauma often occurs in a dirty environment. Projectiles enter the body through dirty surfaces and clothing, carrying dirt and debris into the wound. Open fractures provide a portal for the entry of bacteria and dirt. Even with surgical intervention, the wounds often remain contaminated (Holloway, 1993).

Nursing interventions with rationales are as follows:

- Use careful hand washing practices. *Hand washing remains the single most important factor in preventing the spread of infection.*
- Use strict universal precautions. *The use of universal precautions is essential in protecting the client and the nurse from infection.*
- When applying or changing dressings:
  a. Use strict aseptic technique.
  b. Monitor wounds for odor, redness, heat, swelling, and copious or purulent drainage.
  c. Monitor hidden wounds, such as those under casts, by asking the client whether the pain has increased and observing for increased drainage and heat over the area of the wound.
  d. Ensure that the dressing is appropriate for the size, shape, and location of the wound. Do not apply any dressing that might restrict circulation. Do not use tape; instead, use mesh or stretch gauze to hold dressings in place.
  e. Ensure that cross-contamination between wounds does not occur.
  f. Collect drainage in ostomy bags if it is copious. *The skin is the first line of defense against infection. Wounds from trauma provide a portal of entry for organisms. Risk factors for wound infection include contamination, inadequate wound care, and the condition of the wound at the time of closure (Carpenito, 1993). Aseptic techniques used in applying and changing dressings reduce the entry of organisms.*
- Take and record vital signs, including temperature, every 2 to 4 hours. *Vital signs, particularly an elevated body temperature, are indicators of the presence of an infection.*
- Provide adequate fluids and nutrition. *Adequate fluids, calories, and protein are essential to wound healing.*
- Assess for manifestations of gas gangrene: fever, pain, and swelling in traumatized tissues; drainage with a foul odor. *Gas gangrene is usually caused by the organism Clostridium perfringens. This bacterium is found in the soil and can be introduced into the body during a traumatic injury. The organism grows in the tissues, causing necrosis; hydrogen and carbon dioxide are released, with resultant swelling of tissues. If the infection continues, tissues are progressively destroyed, and death may result.*
- Assess status of tetanus immunization and administer tetanus toxoid or human toxin-antitoxin (TAT) as prescribed. *Tetanus is caused by an exotoxin produced by Clostridium tetani, usually introduced through an open wound. The organism is commonly found in the soil.*
- Use strict aseptic technique when inserting catheters, suctioning, administering parenteral medications, or performing any other invasive procedure. *Using aseptic technique during invasive procedures reduces the risk of entry of organisms.*

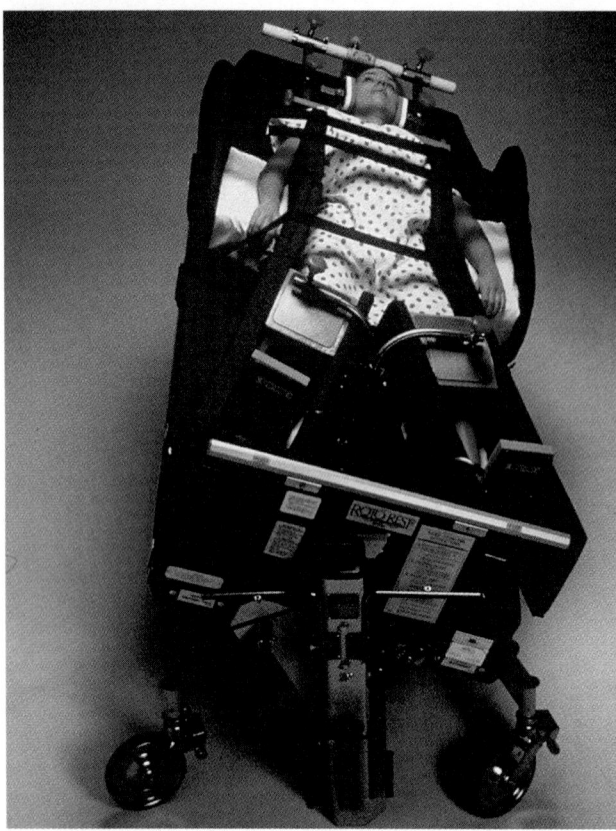

Figure 10–9 A kinetic continuous rotation bed provides a means of turning the client with multiple injuries to decrease the hazards of immobility.

Impaired Physical Mobility

The client with traumatic injuries is often unable to change positions independently and is at risk for complications of the integumentary, cardiovascular, gastrointestinal, respiratory, musculoskeletal, and renal systems. Clients at greatest risk are those who have had multiple injuries, spinal cord injuries, peripheral nerve injuries, and traumatic amputations. The nurse should collaborate with the physical therapist and occupational therapist (if available) to determine the most effective types and schedule of exercises and assistive devices.

Nursing interventions with rationales are as follows:

- Provide active or passive exercises to affected and unaffected extremities at least once every 8 hours. However, exercises should not be done if active bleeding or edema is present. *Exercise improves muscle tone, maintains joint mobility, improves circulation, and prevents contractures.*

- Turn, cough, and deep breathe at least every 2 hours. *Changing positions, coughing, and deep breathing reduce the risk of integumentary and respiratory complications.*

- If the client is unable to be moved and positioned, consider the use of a specialty bed, such as the kinetic continuous rotation bed (Figure 10–9). *The kinetic continuous rotation bed allows continuous turning of the client; the motion decreases pulmonary complications, venous stasis, postural hypotension, urinary stasis, muscle wasting, and bone demineralization (Holloway, 1993).*

- Monitor the lower extremities each day for manifestations of deep vein thrombosis: heat, swelling, and pain. Measure and record the circumference of the thigh and calf each day. If antiemboli stockings are used, they are removed for one hour during each shift and the skin assessed for changes. *Venous stasis in the client with impaired mobility results from an inability of surrounding muscles to contract and help move the blood through the veins. Thrombus (clot) formation in deep veins is a major risk for pulmonary embolism.*

Spiritual Distress

Trauma generally strikes with little or no warning and carries potentially devastating consequences ranging from severe alterations in the lives of the victim and family, to death. The traumatic death of a loved one may be the most difficult event a family may ever experience. The family's belief systems and psychologic stability are challenged when the family is faced with the decision to cease life support systems and/or to donate organs.

Nursing care of the family (or client) experiencing spiritual distress related to making the decision for organ donation includes the following:

- Provide the family with information about the option to donate the client's organs. *The decision to donate organs needs to be based on information about the client's condition, prognosis, and criteria by which brain death is determined. It is important to convey to family members that organ donation is only an option and that they should not feel they are obligated to consent or are doing something wrong if they do not consent (Emergency Nurses Association, 1992).*

- Encourage the family to ask questions and express their feelings related to making the decision. *Allowing families to express their feelings may help prevent long-term consequences, such as guilt.*

- Refer the family for follow-up care. *Long-term follow-up is important for the family facing the sudden death of a loved one. Grieving is not an overnight process, and providing the family with resources that may be used in the future may help prevent future crises and dysfunction. (For more information, see Chapter 11.)*

Post-Trauma Response

Post-Trauma response is an intense, sustained emotional response to a disastrous event. This response is characterized by emotions that range from anger to fear and by flashbacks or psychic numbing. In the initial stage, the client may be calm or may express feelings of anger, disbelief, terror, and shock. In the long-term phase, which begins anywhere from a few days to several months after the event, the client often experiences flashbacks and nightmares of the traumatic event. The client may call on ineffective coping mechanisms, such as the use of alcohol or drugs, and withdraw from relationships with others.

Nursing interventions with rationales are as follows:

- Assess the client's emotional responses while providing physical care. Observe for crying, suspiciousness, and fear during the initial phase of treatment. If the client is unconscious, encourage family members and friends to express their feelings. *These assessments provide valuable information about the client's ability to cope with the trauma.*

- Be available if the client wishes to talk about the trauma, and encourage the client to express his or her feelings when the client seems ready to do so. *The client may initially deny negative feelings; this denial is a coping mechanism in the initial phase of recovery.*

- Teach relaxation techniques, such as deep breathing, progressive muscle relaxation, or imagery. *These techniques are often useful in coping when thoughts of the trauma recur.*

- Refer the client and family members for counseling, psychotherapy, or support groups as appropriate. *Continued therapy may be necessary in allowing the client and family to resolve the acute and long-term effects of trauma.*

Risk for Trauma

Trauma is now viewed as a disease. As with other diseases, in addition to the research, time, and funding devoted to "cures," efforts are also being directed at the best method of nursing care: prevention. Nursing care directed at preventing injury includes:

- Observing for potential risk factors for traumatic injury (Kim et al., 1993). These include individual risk factors, such as
  a. Weakness.
  b. Poor vision.
  c. Lack of safety education.
  d. Lack of safety precautions.

  Potential risk factors also include environmental factors, such as
  a. Road conditions.
  b. Unsafe vehicles.
  c. Lack of restraining devices (e.g., car seats).
  d. Presence of guns or knives.
  e. Neighborhoods with high crime.

Identifying risk factors and developing interventions that decrease the potential for injury are initial steps in trauma prevention.

- Provide educational programs and information for clients (Kidd, 1993). Examples include distributing pamphlets on the correct use of a car seat or staging a prom drill for high school seniors. *Providing educational materials and programs offers an opportunity to disperse information about trauma prevention.*

- Monitor the pattern of injuries in the community:
  a. Participate in trauma registries.
  b. Perform chart reviews of injured clients.
  c. Collaborate with prehospital care providers for injury pattern identification.

A collaborative approach in identifying patterns of injury yields information about specific injuries or sources of trauma in the local environment. From these data, prevention strategies can be developed (Peclet et al., 1990).

Other Nursing Diagnoses

Other nursing diagnoses that are appropriate for the client who is experiencing trauma include the following:

- *Risk for Ineffective Breathing Pattern* related to mechanical obstruction from tension pneumothorax, hemothorax, or symptomatic pneumothorax

- *Risk for Fluid Volume Deficit* related to acute blood loss

- *Risk for Altered Family Processes* related to the crisis of trauma

- *Fear* related to unknown future and possibility of death

- *Risk for Injury* related to trauma resuscitation

- *Pain* related to multiple wounds and fractures

Client and Family Teaching

To prepare the client and family for discharge and promote maximum wellness

- Include the client and family in care during the hospitalization.

- Obtain information about the type of home environment to which the client will be returning. Determine whether any changes will be required to enable the client to function in that environment. For example, the client whose bedroom is on an upper floor may need to sleep in a room on the first floor until the healing process is complete.

- Provide information about the medications that the client will be taking at home. Be sure that the client and family members know when to take the medications and their potential side effects.

- If the client is to be on a special diet, provide information so that the family can adhere to the diet.

- Discuss the client's rehabilitation plan and its effect on the client's family. For example, if the client has to have physical therapy, discuss options for transportation.

- Have the client and/or family member demonstrate any dressing changes that must be done at home. Teach the client and family techniques for wound care and how to dispose of contaminated dressings properly.

- Ensure that the client and family know when they are to schedule follow-up appointments with the physician or at the trauma clinic.

- Discuss with the family some of the emotional changes that the client may undergo as a result of the trauma. For example, the client may experience changes in sleeping habits, nightmares, and reliving the incident. Refer the family to appropriate resources for management of these issues.

- Discuss the importance of allowing the client and family members to verbalize their feelings related to the incident, any fears or anxieties, and concerns about changes in body image.

- Provide the family who has lost a loved one with a referral for follow-up care.

Applying the Nursing Process

Case Study of a Client With Multiple Injuries: Jane Souza

Jane Souza is a 25-year-old married woman with two children who provides day care for preschool children in her home. As she is driving along an interstate road on which the speed limit is 65 miles per hour, a car comes across the median and strikes her vehicle head on. Ms. Souza, who is not wearing a seat belt, is thrown forward against the steering wheel. The front of her car is pushed up against her by the car that struck her, entrapping her lower extremities.

After extensive efforts to extricate her from the car, Ms. Souza is transported to the local trauma center. She is still conscious, is receiving high-flow oxygen by mask, and has one intravenous line in place. Her vital signs are a palpable systolic blood pressure of 80, a pulse rate of 120, and a respiratory rate of 36. On arrival, she states that she is having difficulty breathing.

Assessment

Ms. Souza's primary assessment yields the following information:

- *Airway:* Maintainable with high-flow oxygen in place.
- *Breathing:* Respiratory rate of 36, multiple bruising and abrasions on right side of her chest, decreased breath sounds on the right side.
- *Circulation:* No palpable radial pulses; +2 palpable brachial pulses. Monitor shows sinus tachycardia. No

active external bleeding noted. Skin color pale, cool to the touch, and diaphoretic.

- *Neurologic:* Moved her fingers when asked; complains of difficulty breathing; denies that she is hurt. Pupils 4 mm, equal, and react to light. Ms. Souza has a broken right arm and an open fracture of the left ankle; because of these injuries, extremity movement is limited.

Because of Ms. Souza's respiratory distress, she is intubated and ventilated with 100% oxygen. Another intravenous line is inserted and O-negative blood administered. Because her blood pressure continues to decrease, she is immediately transferred to the operating room.

Diagnosis

The emergency nursing staff make the following nursing diagnoses for Ms. Souza:

- *Ineffective Breathing Pattern* related to increased respiratory rate of 36, multiple bruises and abrasions on the right side of her chest, decreased breath sounds on the right, and respiratory difficulty
- *Fluid Volume Deficit* related to acute internal blood loss (presumed because no active bleeding can be found)
- *Risk for Injury* related to trauma resuscitation

Expected Outcomes

The expected outcomes established in the plan of care specify that Ms. Souza will

- Maintain adequate oxygenation.
- Maintain adequate circulating blood volume.

Planning and Implementation

The following nursing interventions are planned and implemented for Ms. Souza by the emergency nursing staff:

- Monitor Ms. Souza's airway, and assist the physician in any airway management she may need.
- Explain all procedures to Ms. Souza.
- Monitor the effects of fluid and blood administration, including any changes in Ms. Souza's blood pressure and pulse.
- Prepare Ms. Souza for transfer to the operating room for emergency surgery.
- Keep Ms. Souza's family informed about her condition.

Evaluation

Ms. Souza is transferred to the operating room, where it is determined that she has a ruptured spleen and a serious pelvic fracture. Ms. Souza's treatment continues in the operating room.

Critical Thinking in the Nursing Process

1. Both crystalloids and blood may be used to restore blood volume in the client with multiple injuries. Explain why O-negative blood was used in the emergency department.

2. During the primary assessment, it was found that Ms. Souza's blood pressure continued to decrease despite the administration of fluids. Why wasn't a secondary assessment completed before she went to the operating room?

3. Would the nursing diagnosis *Fluid Volume Deficit* be appropriate for Ms. Souza? Why, or why not?

4. The family of the client experiencing trauma has specific needs that need to be met by the nursing staff. Develop a care plan for Ms. Souza's family for the nursing diagnosis *Altered Family Processes*.

Bibliography

■ ■ ■

Ali, J. (1992). Priorities in multisystem trauma. In J. Hall, G. Schmidt, and L. Wood. *Principles of critical care* (pp. 693–703). New York: McGraw-Hill.

American College of Surgeons. (1993). *Advanced life support manual.* Chicago: American College of Surgeons.

American College of Surgeons, Committee on Trauma. (1989). *Advanced trauma life support manual.* Chicago: American College of Surgeons.

Cardona, V., Hurn, P., Mason, P., Scanlon, A., & Veise-Berry, S. (1994). *Trauma nursing: From resuscitation through rehabilitation.* Philadelphia: WB Saunders.

Carpenito, L. J. (1993). *Nursing Diagnosis: Applications to clinical practice.* (4th ed.). Philadelphia: Lippincott.

Champion, H., Copes, W., Gann, D., Gennarelli, T., & Flanagan, M. (1989). A revision of the trauma score. *Journal of Trauma, 29*(5), 624.

Champion, H., Copes, W., & Sacco, W. (1990). The major trauma outcome study: Establishing national norms for trauma care. *Journal of Trauma 11,*1356–1365.

Coffland, F., & Shelton, D. (1993). Blood component replacement therapy. *Critical Care Nursing Clinics of North America, 5*(3), 543–556.

Connell, K., Borg, M., Cavaliero, L., Ross, I., & Watchmaker, A. (1992). From coma to discharge: The story of a roller-coaster recovery. *Nursing92, 22*(6), 44–50.

Conroy, C. (1985). Trauma as a public health issue. *Emergency Care Quarterly, 1*(3), 69–75.

Emergency Nurses Association. (1992). *Trauma resource document.* Park Ridge, IL, Emergency Nurses Association.

Feliciano, D., Marx, J., & Sclarani, S. (1992). Abdominal trauma. *Patient Care, 26*(18), 44–48, 50, 56.

Gauthier, D., & LeMone, P. (1990). Trauma: The acute response. *AAOHN Journal, 38*(10), 475–482.

Hamilton, A. (1993). Trauma: Initial assessment skills. *Accident & Emergency Nursing, 1*(4), 183–192.

Hammond, L. (1992). Organ and tissue donation. In E. Bayley & S. Turcke (Eds). *A comprehensive curriculum for trauma nursing.* (pp. 238–252). Boston: Jones and Bartlett.

Hanson, C., & Strawser, D. (1992). Family presence during cardiopulmonary resuscitation: Foote Hospital Emergency Department's nine-year perspective. *Journal of Emergency Nursing, 18*(2), 104–106.

Holloway, N. M. (1993). *Nursing the critically ill adult.* (4th ed.). Redwood City, CA: Addison-Wesley Nursing.

Hurn, P. & Hartsock, R. (1993). Blunt thoracic injuries. *Critical Care Nursing Clinics of North America, 5*(4), 673–686.

Jones, M. (1990). A study of trauma in an Amish community. *Journal of Trauma, 7,* 899–902.

Judkins, D., & Iserson, K. (1991). Rapid admixture blood warming. *Journal of Emergency Nursing, 17*(3), 146–151.

Kaiser, K. (1992). Assessment and management of pain in the critically ill trauma patient. *Critical Care Nursing Quarterly, 15*(2), 14–34.

Kelly, D. (1993). Administration of blood products. In J. Proehl (Ed.). *Adult emergency nursing procedures.* (pp. 233–247). Boston: Jones and Bartlett.

Kidd, P. S. (1993). Prevention of traumatic injury. In J. Neff and P. S. Kidd (Eds.). *Trauma nursing: Art and science.* (pp.21–34). St Louis: Mosby-Year Book.

Kim, M., McFarland, G., & McLane, A. (1993). *Pocket guide to nursing diagnosis.* St Louis: Mosby-Year Book.

Kitt, S., & Proehl, J. (1993). General principles of autotransfusion. In J. Proehl (Ed.). *Adult emergency nursing procedures.* (pp. 255–256). Boston: Jones and Bartlett.

Misinski, M., Thompson, G., Talley, J., Lucich, S., & Johnson, R. (1993). Model for trauma outcomes management in patients with multiple trauma. *Critical Care Nursing Clinics of North America, 5*(4), 741–755.

Moore, E., Eiseman, B., & Van Way, C. (1984). *Critical decisions in trauma.* St Louis: Mosby-Year Book.

Moore, K., & Schwartz, K. (1993). Psychosocial support of trauma patients in the emergency department by nurses, as indicated by communication. *Journal of Emergency Nursing, 19*(4), 297–302.

Myers, M., & Norwood, S. (1994). Standing orders for trauma care. *Journal of Emergency Nursing, 20*(2), 111–117.

National Association of Air Medical Services Physicians. (1992). *Air Medical Dispatch: Prehospital and Disaster Medicine.* 7, 75–78.

Neff, J. (1993). Perfusion: Cardiac and vascular injuries. In J. Neff and P. Kidd (Eds.). *Trauma nursing: Art and science.* (pp. 195–262). St Louis: Mosby-Year Book.

Peclet, M., Newman, K., Eichelberger, M., Gotschall, S., Guzzetta, P., Anderson, V., Randolph, J., & Bowman, L. (1990). Patterns of injury in children. *Journal of Pediatric Surgery, 25*(3), 85–91.

Proehl, J. (1993). Mobility: Spinal and musculoskeletal injuries. In J. Neff & P. Kidd (Eds.). *Trauma nursing: Art and science.* (pp. 325–363). St Louis: Mosby-Year Book.

Rea, R. (1991). *Trauma nursing core course.* Chicago: Emergency Nurses Association.

Roberts, A. (1994). Systems of life: Blood: 1. *Nursing Times, 90*(19), 35–38.

Schrader, K. (1993). Penetrating chest trauma. *Critical Care Nursing Clinics of North America, 5*(4), 687–696.

Semonin-Holleran, R. (1993). Trauma in childhood. In J. Neff & P. Kidd (Eds.). *Trauma nursing: Art and science.* (pp. 527–553). St Louis: Mosby-Year Book.

Sims, D., Bivins, B., Obeid, F., Horst, H., Sorenson, V., & Fath, J., (1989). Urban trauma: A chronic recurrent disease. *Journal of Trauma, 29*(7), 946–947.

Stanik-Hutt, J. (1993). Strategies for pain management in traumatic thoracic injuries. *Critical Care Nursing Clinics of North America, 5*(4), 713–722.

Stein, D. (1992). Epidemiology of trauma. In E. Bayley & S. Turcke (Eds.). *A comprehensive curriculum for trauma nursing.* (pp. 1–10). Boston: Jones and Bartlett.

Stern, D., Dronen, S., Birrer, P., & Wang, X. (1993). Effect of blood pressure on hemorrhage volume and survival in a near-fatal hemorrhage model incorporating a vascular injury. *Annals of Emergency Medicine, 22*(2): 155–163.

Taylor, L., & Jones, A. (1993). Forensic aspects. In J. Neff & P. Kidd, (Eds.). *Trauma nursing: Art and science.* (pp. 61–78). St Louis: Mosby-Year Book.

Tippett, J. (1993). Spinal immobilization of the multiply injured patient. *Accident & Emergency Nursing, 1*(1), 25–33.

Toulson, S. (1993). A guide to advanced trauma life support. *Professional Nurse, 9*(2), 95–97.

Trauma Nursing Coalition. (1992). Nursing care of the trauma client.

Trott, A. (1991). *Wounds and lacerations.* St Louis: Mosby-Year Book.

Trunkey, D. (1983). Trauma. *Scientific American, 249,* 28–35.

CHAPTER 11

···

Nursing Care of Clients Experiencing Loss, Grief, and Death

LEARNING OBJECTIVES

After completing this chapter, you will be able to

- Define loss and grief.
- Describe theories of loss, grief, and dying.
- Discuss the relationship between age and loss.
- Discuss uncomplicated bereavement.
- Use the nursing process as a framework for providing

individualized care for clients and families experiencing loss, grief, or death.

- Describe some special interventions used in the care of dying clients.
- Describe the teaching the nurse provides to the client and family experiencing loss, grief, or death.
- Discuss legal and ethical issues related to loss, grief, and dying.

Grief as a response to loss is an inevitable dimension of the human experience. The loss of a job, a role (for example, the loss of the role of spouse, as occurs in divorce), a goal, body integrity, a loved one, or the impending loss of one's own life may trigger grief. Loss is also integral to death. Although death represents the ultimate loss, losses that occur in any phase of the life cycle may produce grief responses as intensely painful as those observed in the death experience.

Loss may be defined as an actual or potential situation in which a valued object, person, body part, or emotion that was formerly present is lost or changed and can no longer be seen, felt, heard, known, or experienced (Newman, 1993). A loss may be temporary or permanent, complete or partial, objectively verifiable or perceived, physical or symbolic. The meaning of the loss can be determined only by the person who experiences the loss.

Although the order of importance varies with the person, people most commonly fear the loss of the following:

- Health
- Social status
- Possessions
- Life-Style
- Sexual functioning
- Body part
- Death
- Marital relationship (i.e., through divorce)
- Reproductive functioning
- Stable relationships

Loss always results in change. The stress associated with the loss may be the precipitating factor leading to physiologic or psychologic change in the person or family. The effective or ineffective resolution of feelings surrounding the loss determines the person's ability to deal with the resulting changes.

Grief is the emotional response to loss and its accompanying changes. *Grieving* may be thought of as the internal process the person uses to work through the response to loss. In contrast, *mourning* describes the actions or expressions of the bereaved, including the symbols, clothing, and ceremonies that make up the outward manifestations of grief. Both grieving and mourning are healthy responses to loss (Newman, 1993) because they ultimately lead the person to invest energy in new relationships and to develop positive self-regard.

Theories of Loss, Grief, and Dying

■ ■ ■

Medical-surgical nurses practicing in acute care settings or in the community encounter clients exhibiting responses typical of various stages of the grieving process. Highly individual in quality and duration, the grief process may range from discomforting to debilitating, and it may last a day or a lifetime, depending on what the loss means to the person experiencing it. Although each person experiences loss in a different manner, knowledge of some of the major theories of loss, grief, and dying can provide the nurse with a framework for holistic care for the client and family experiencing or anticipating a loss.

Freud: Psychoanalytic Theory

In his classic paper *Mourning and Melancholia,* Freud (1917, 1957) wrote about grief and mourning as reactions to loss. His work provided valuable insights on the subject of grief. Freud described the process of mourning as one in which the person gradually withdraws attachment from the lost object or person. He observed that with normal grieving, this withdrawal of attachment is followed by a readiness to make new attachments. In comparing melancholia with the "normal emotions of grief, and its expression in mourning" (p. 124), Freud observed that the "work of mourning" is a nonpathologic condition that reaches a state of completion after a period of "inner labor" (p. 131). In addition to delineating the structure of grief, Freud characterized *melancholia* as a pathologic state, differentiating it from *grieving,* which he characterized as a nonpathologic state.

Bowlby: Protest, Despair, and Detachment

Bowlby (1973, 1980) studied the grief process in infants and children and its relationship to the grief process in adults. Bowlby believed that the grieving process initiated by a loss or separation from a loved object or person successfully ends when the grieving person experiences feelings of emancipation from the lost object or person.

Bowlby (1973) divided the grieving process into three phases and identified behaviors that are characteristic of each phase:

- *Protest.* The protest phase is marked by a lack of acceptance of the loss. All energy is directed toward protesting the loss. The client experiences feelings of anger toward self and others, and feelings of ambivalence toward the lost object or person. Crying and angry behaviors characterize this phase.
- *Despair.* The client's behavior becomes disorganized. Despair mounts as efforts to deny the loss compete with acceptance of permanent loss. Crying and sadness, coupled with a desire for the lost object or person to return, result in disorganized thoughts as the client recognizes the reality of the loss.
- *Detachment.* As the client realizes the permanence of the loss and gradually relinquishes attachment to the lost object, a reinvestment of energy occurs. Both the positive and negative aspects of the relationship are remembered. Expressions of hopefulness and readiness to move forward are characteristic of this phase.

Engel: Acute Grief, Restitution, and Long-Term Grief

The work of Engel (1964) was influenced by stress theories. Engel related the grief process to other methods of coping with stress: After the person perceives and evaluates the loss (the stressful event), the person adapts to it. Engel's recognition of the impact of cognitive factors on the grieving process was an important contribution to our understanding of grieving.

Engel also described three main stages in the grief process: an acute stage, a restitution stage, and a long-term stage. The *acute stage* occurs in two phases. The first phase, *shock and disbelief,* begins immediately after the person receives the news of the loss. The initial response may be denial, which may help the person to cope with the overwhelming pain. Alternatively, the grieving person in this phase may appear to accept the loss, making statements such as, "It was for the best," while repressing his or her feelings. This phase of shock and disbelief normally lasts only a few hours; however, it may continue for 1 or 2 days.

As the shock and disbelief begin to fade, the second phase, *developing awareness,* follows. The finality of the loss becomes a reality, and pain, anguish, anger, guilt, and blame surface. The person feels a need to make someone responsible for the loss. "If only" and "why" frequently punctuate the expressed or inner dialogue of the bereaved. Crying is common. "It is during this time that the greatest degree of anguish or despair, within the limits imposed by cultural patterns, is experienced or expressed" (p. 93). Culturally patterned behaviors, such as maintaining a stoic pose in public or weeping openly, characterize this phase.

The acute stage is followed by a stage of *restitution,* in which the mourning is institutionalized. Friends and family gather to support the grieving person through rituals dictated by the culture. As time passes, the mourner continues to feel a painful void and is preoccupied with thoughts of the loss. The mourner may join a support group or seek other social support for coping with the loss.

After the restitution stage, which lasts at least a year, the mourner begins to come to terms with the loss. In this *long-term stage,* interest in people and activities is renewed. The person puts the lost relationship in perspective as he or she begins to form new relationships. Engel observed that this period may last another 1 to 2 years.

Lindemann: Categories of Symptoms

Lindemann (1944) began his work on grieving by following the adjustment of people following a crisis. He interviewed people who had lost a loved one during the course of medical treatment; disaster victims, including those involved in a fire in a Boston nightclub in 1944; and relatives of members of the armed forces who had died. Lindemann's research led him to describe normal grief, anticipatory grieving, and morbid grief reactions.

Lindemann observed five categories of symptoms characteristic of *normal grief:*

1. Somatic distress
2. Preoccupation with the image of the deceased
3. Feelings of guilt
4. Hostile reactions
5. Loss of patterns of conduct

He defined the concept of *anticipatory grieving* as a cluster of predictable responses to an anticipated loss. These responses include the range of feelings experienced by the person or family preoccupied with an anticipated loss. For example, the client or family reviews the details of the anticipated loss and anticipates all of the adjustments that will be needed to cope with the loss.

Lindemann used the term *morbid grief reaction* to describe delayed and dysfunctional reactions to loss. He observed a variety of debilitating health problems in people who displayed excessive or delayed responses to loss.

Caplan: Stress and Loss

Caplan's (1990) theory of stress and its relationship to loss is useful in understanding the grief process. His work with Lindemann expanded the focus of the grief process to include not only bereavement but also other episodes of stress that people experience, such as may result from

surgery or childbirth. Caplan described these periods as "psychological crises precipitated by hazardous circumstances that lead to a temporary upset in the normal homeostatic balance of forces that characterizes transactions between an individual and his environment" (p. 28). He believed these "hazardous circumstances" lead to psychologic disequilibrium in some people because their coping skills are inadequate in helping them gain mastery over their predicament.

Caplan named three factors that influence the person's ability to deal with a loss. He believed these factors may cause distress for a year or more following the loss:

- The psychic pain of the broken bond and the agony of coming to terms with the loss
- Living without the assets and guidance of the lost person or resource
- The reduced cognitive and problem-solving effectiveness associated with the distressing emotional arousal

Caplan described the process of building new attachments to replace those that have been lost. This process involves two elements: a feeling of hope and the assumption of regular activity as a form of participating in ordinary living. Caplan further noted that "people who have an abiding commitment to supra-personal ideology such as religion or social and political affiliations usually have an easier time investing meaning in routine activities that act as bridges in linking them to the larger social framework within which they may eventually develop new individual attachments" (p. 37).

Bugen: Prediction Model

Bugen (1977) developed a model that can be used to predict the outcomes of the grieving process based on the significance of the relationships involved. The nurse can then use this information to plan appropriate interventions.

If the survivor views the relationship as *central,* the grieving process is extremely intense, and the survivor feels that life cannot be pursued in a meaningful way. When the relationship is *peripheral,* the grieving is less intense and progresses more rapidly to resolution. If the loss is viewed as *preventable,* the bereaved feel directly or indirectly responsible for it. The intensity and length of the grieving process are increased under these circumstances. If the loss is viewed as *unpreventable,* the lack of feelings of guilt or sense of responsibility for the loss produces a milder and briefer period of mourning.

Kübler-Ross: Research on Death and Dying

Kübler-Ross's (1969, 1978) research on death and dying has provided a framework for gaining insight about the stages of coping with an impending or actual loss. Her work has been widely used by health care providers. According to Kübler-Ross, not all people dealing with a loss go through these stages, and those who do may not experience the stages in the sequence described. In identifying the stages of death and dying, Kübler-Ross (1978) repeatedly stressed the danger of prematurely labeling a "stage" and emphasized that her goal was to describe her observations of how people come to terms with situations of loss.

She observed that some or all of the following reactions may occur during the grieving process and may reappear as the person experiences the loss:

- *Denial.* A person may react with shock and disbelief after receiving word of an actual or potential loss. After receiving a terminal diagnosis, notification of a death, or other serious loss, people may make such statements as "This can't be happening to me" or "This can't be true." This initial stage of denial serves as a buffer in helping the person or family mobilize defenses to cope with the situation.

- *Anger.* In the anger stage, the person resists the loss. The anger, behaviorally described as "acting out," is often directed toward family and health care providers.

- *Bargaining.* The bargaining stage serves as an attempt to postpone the reality of the loss. The person makes a secret bargain with God, expressing a willingness to do anything to postpone the loss or change the prognosis. This is the individual's plea for an extension of life or the chance to "make everything right" with a dying family member or friend.

- *Depression.* As the person realizes the full impact of the actual or perceived loss, the person enters a stage of depression. In this stage, the person prepares for the impending loss by working through the struggle of separation. While grieving over "what cannot be," the person may either talk freely about the loss or withdraw from others.

- *Acceptance.* Some people who are dying reach a stage of acceptance in which they may appear to be almost devoid of emotion. The struggle is past, and the emotional pain is gone. If the person has experienced the loss of a loved one or other valued object, he or she begins to come to terms with the loss and resumes activities with an air of hopefulness for the future.

Glaser and Strauss: Awareness Context

Glaser and Strauss (1965) identified the concept of *awareness* through their observations of the relationships between dying clients and their families. Glaser and Strauss distinguished four types of awareness in the relationships between the dying client and the family. The client and family may experience these types sequentially, or they may maintain one level of awareness throughout the dying process.

1. *Closed awareness.* Efforts are made to keep the terminally ill person from being aware of the impending death.

2. *Suspicious awareness.* The dying person becomes suspicious that information is being withheld.

3. *Mutual pretense.* The dying person and others know the condition is terminal but pretend otherwise.

4. *Open awareness.* The dying person and others know the condition is terminal and relate to each other openly.

Carter and Cody: Nurse Contributions

The work of Carter (1989), a nurse researcher, focused on identifying themes of bereavement expressed by grieving persons. She identified themes disclosed by people who had experienced the death of a loved one and compared them with the theoretical perspectives of Freud and Kübler-Ross and with existential theory based on the work of Frankl, Tillich, and others.

Carter's work identified features of bereavement that are different from or unaddressed by the other theoretical perspectives:

- Grief's changing character, including "waves" of intense pain that may be triggered years after the death by a photograph of the loved one, a favorite song, a fragrance, or anything that calls the loved one to mind.

- *Holding,* an individual process of preserving the fact and the meaning of the loved one's existence.

- Expectations, both social and personal, regarding how the bereaved should react to the experience.

- The critical importance of personal history in affecting the quality and meaning of individual bereavement.

Cody's (1991) research on grieving utilizes Parse's theory of nursing. Cody (1991, p. 62) suggests that grieving a personal loss is a process that involves the following:

- Finding meaning in what was lost in relation to what was, what is, and what is not yet to be

- Living daily life with others amid changing situations

- Moving forward in one's life through finding new ways to cope with loss

Cody found that the lived experience of grieving a personal loss involves "intense struggling in the flux of change," moving beyond the loss by accepting different possibilities for living without the loved one, and finally moving toward others (p. 67).

Table 11–1 summarizes the theories of loss, grief, and dying presented in this chapter.

Table 11–1   Summary of Theories of Loss

Theorist	Dynamics
Freud	Grief and mourning are reactions to loss. Grieving is the inner labor of mourning a loss. Inability to grieve a loss results in depression.
Bowlby	The successful grieving process initiated by a loss or separation during childhood ends with feelings of emancipation from the lost person or object.
Engel	After the person perceives and evaluates the loss, the person adapts to it. Shock and disbelief, developing awareness, and restitution occur during the first year following the loss; in the months following, the person puts the lost relationship into perspective.
Lindemann	A sequence of responses is experienced following a catastrophic event; defined concepts of anticipatory grieving and morbid grief reactions.
Caplan	Periods of psychologic crisis are precipitated by hazardous circumstances; successful resolution of grief involves feelings of hope and engaging in activities of ordinary living.
Bugen	The outcome of the grieving process can be predicted based on the significance of the relationship and whether the death was viewed as preventable.
Kübler-Ross	There are five stages defining the response to loss: denial, anger, bargaining, depression, and acceptance. Stages are not necessarily sequential.
Glaser and Strauss	Differing levels of awareness that influence communication patterns are observed in persons who are dying and their families: closed awareness, suspicious awareness, mutual pretense, open awareness.
Carter	Identified the quality of grief's changing character, the need to hold on to that which was good in the loved one's lost existence, expectations of how to react to the experience, and the ways in which personal history affects the quality and meaning of the loss.
Cody	Grieving a personal loss involves finding meaning with what was lost in relation to what was, what is, and what is yet to be; living daily life with others amid changing situations; and moving forward through finding new ways to live with the loss.

Table 11–2   Development of the Concept of Death

Age	Beliefs/Attitudes About Death
3	Fears separation; lacks comprehension of permanent separation.
3 to 5	Believes death is like sleeping and is reversible. Expresses curiosity about what happens to the body.
6 to 10	Understands finality of death. Views own death as avoidable. Associates death with violence. Believes wishes can be responsible for death.
11 to 12	Reflects views of death expressed by parents. Expresses interest in afterlife as an understanding of mortality develops. Recognizes death as irreversible and inevitable.
13 to 21	Usually has a religious and philosophic view of death but seldom thinks about it. Views own death as distant or a challenge, acting out defiance through reckless behavior. Previously held developmental awareness of death may still be present.
22 to 45	Does not think about death unless confronted with it. Emotionally distances self from death. Attitude toward death influenced by religious and cultural beliefs.
46 to 65	Experiences the death of parents or friends. Accepts own mortality. Experiences waves of death anxiety. Puts life in order to prepare for death and decrease anxiety.
66 and older	Fears lingering, incapacitating illness. Views death as inevitable but from a philosophical viewpoint: that is, as freedom from pain and illness or as a spiritual reunion with deceased friends and loved ones.

Relationship of Age to Loss

■ ■ ■

The age of the person experiencing the loss influences his or her understanding of and reaction to loss. Differences occur in each age group and are affected by the person's developmental stage. In general, as people experience life transitions, their ability to understand and accept the losses associated with the transitions increases. From the age of 3, the development of the concept of death as a loss proceeds rapidly. Table 11–2 outlines the development of the concept of death throughout the life span.

Collaborative Care

■ ■ ■

Grieving clients frequently enter the health care system with significant somatic symptoms. In some cases, the symptoms of grief and loss are overlooked until the client reaches a crisis state requiring psychiatric medical intervention. Collaborative care by the physician and the nurse early in the normal grieving process can help the client achieve an early and effective resolution of grief and avoid physical or psychiatric health problems.

Uncomplicated bereavement is the medical diagnosis physicians use when treating the client experiencing normal grieving after the death of a significant other. The physician uses the diagnostic criteria from the *Diagnostic and Statistical Manual of Mental Disorders (DSM-IV)* (American Psychiatric Association, 1994) to assess the client's symptoms. Before a differential diagnosis of uncomplicated bereavement is established as the focus of attention or treatment, other conditions not attributable to a mental disorder or to mood disorders must be ruled out. The etiology and the essential and diagnostic features of uncomplicated bereavement are provided in the accompanying box.

Nursing Care

■ ■ ■

Assessment

In planning and implementing nursing care for the client experiencing a loss, the nurse considers the individual responses, which may vary greatly. The approaches for obtaining assessment data as well as the nursing care depend on the age of the client and the circumstances under which the medical-surgical nurse encounters the client responding to a loss.

In an era of short acute care stays for clients, nurses may feel that an elaborate grief assessment is impossible or, at the least, impractical. But research and clinical experience suggest that clients who delay the grieving process after a loss are prone to have health problems that may last a lifetime. So whether caring for a client responding to a terminal diagnosis, the loss of a loved one, or a loss associated with an organ, limb, or body function, the nurse performs a thorough assessment of the client's physical and psychologic responses to the loss and uses that assessment as the basis for providing holistic care. The nurse in the acute care setting may have the opportunity only to begin the planning and intervention phase, but careful discharge planning for clients responding to a loss can make the difference in their successful resolution of grief.

DSM-IV: V62.82 Bereavement

■ ■ ■

This category can be used when the focus of clinical attention is a reaction to the death of a loved one. As part of their reactions to the loss, some grieving individuals present with symptoms characteristic of a Major Depressive Episode (e.g., feelings of sadness and associated symptoms such as insomnia, poor appetite, and weight loss). The bereaved individual typically regards the depressed mood as "normal," although the person may seek professional help for relief of associated symptoms such as insomnia or anorexia. The duration and expression of the "normal" bereavement vary considerably among different cultural groups. The diagnosis of Major Depressive Disorder is generally not given unless the symptoms are still present 2 months after the loss. However, the presence of certain symptoms that are not characteristic of a "normal" grief reaction may be helpful in differentiating bereavement from a Major Depressive Episode. These include

1. Guilt about things other than actions taken or not taken by the survivor at the time of death.

2. Thoughts of death other than the survivor feeling that he or she would be better off dead or should have died with the deceased person.

3. Morbid preoccupation with worthlessness.

4. Marked psychomotor retardation.

5. Prolonged and marked functional impairment.

6. Hallucinatory experiences other than thinking that he or she hears the voice of, or transiently sees the image of, the deceased person.

Note. From *Diagnostic and Statistical Manual of Mental Disorders DSM-IV*™ (4th ed.) (pp. 684–685) by American Psychiatric Association, 1994, Washington, DC: American Psychiatric Association.

Self-Assessment

The nurse may encounter the client at various stages of the grief process and may feel that crisis situations are not the time for self-reflection (Newman, 1993). However, because the nurse's conscious or unconscious reactions to the client's responses to the loss will influence the outcome of any interventions, nurses need to take time to analyze their own feelings and values related to loss and the expression of grief. When assessing the physical symptoms of grief, for example, the nurse may believe the client is exhibiting exaggerated behavior that is out of proportion to the loss suffered. As a consequence, the nurse may make a premature and inaccurate diagnosis of dysfunctional grieving (Newman, 1993). The nurse can promote self-awareness by asking the following questions:

- What are my personal feelings about how grief should be expressed?
- Am I making judgments about the meaning of this loss to the client?
- Are unresolved losses in my own life preventing me from relating therapeutically to the client?

The acute nature of the setting and the urgency required in caring for the client may not allow the nurse to resolve these questions completely; however, it is important to spend time in self-reflection to gain an awareness that the answers will affect interactions with the client. Even a brief moment of self-reflection will help the nurse approach the interaction in a less subjective manner.

Physical Assessment

Knowledge of the expected physical reactions to loss provides the nurse with a basis for identifying reactions requiring further assessment. To assess the extent of somatic distress, the nurse observes for changes in sensory processes and asks questions about the client's sleeping and eating patterns, activities of daily living, general health status, and pain.

Clients may experience one or more predictable somatic symptoms as they become aware of a loss. Gastrointestinal symptoms occur frequently. They may include indigestion, nausea or vomiting, anorexia, weight gain or loss, constipation, or diarrhea. The shock and disbelief that accompany a loss may cause shortness of breath, a choking sensation, hyperventilation, or loss of strength. Some clients also report insomnia, preoccupation with sleep, fatigue, and decreased or increased activity level (Carpenito, 1989).

Crying and sadness are observed during normal grief states. Crying may make the client feel exhausted and interfere with carrying out activities of daily living. However, a person who is unable to cry may have difficulty completing the mourning process. If the client does not express feelings of grief, somatic symptoms may increase. Also, overindulgence in alcohol or drugs may signal dysfunctional grief (Newman, 1993).

It is imperative that the client's concerns about pain be assessed, especially if the client has cancer or another painful illness. Knowledge of pain theories and pain assessment can help the nurse assess the need for pain medication (see Chapter 4). During the last stages of dying, the client usually becomes very weak, and sensations and reflexes decrease; these changes call for careful assessment of the client's physical needs.

Reactions to loss are not always obvious. For example, in a client admitted for a medical or surgical illness following a serious loss, assessment may reveal somatic complaints related to the grief state as well as the illness. When a person who has been healthy begins to develop patterns of increased illness, the nurse should be aware that this may signal dysfunctional grieving. This is especially common in the loss and grieving associated with a change in body image. In addition to making a physical assessment, the nurse needs to assess the client's perception of the alteration in body image. The loss of a body part, weight gain or loss, and scars from surgery or trauma can be difficult for the client to accept. Some clients may grieve the loss of hair that accompanies chemotherapy used in cancer treatment.

Changes in sensory processes may occur in response to the shock, denial, and disbelief created by the loss (Engel, 1964). When a client has been debilitated by illness, hearing and sight are sometimes diminished, especially in the client approaching death. Many clinicians, however, report an increased sensory perception in some dying clients. Because responses are highly individual, assessment of responses to sensory stimulation may produce varying data.

Spiritual Assessment

Because spiritual beliefs and practices greatly influence people's reaction to loss, it is important that the nurse explore them with the client when assessing a loss (Landrum et al., 1988). The spiritually healthy client has inner resources that help him or her work through the grief process. Faith, prayer, trust in God or a superior being, perception of a purpose in life, or belief in immortality are examples of the inner resources that may sustain the client during an actual or perceived loss (Newman, 1993).

Assessing the client's spiritual life and its significance to the client and family helps identify spiritual support systems. Some nurses are uncomfortable with assessing the client's spiritual needs; however, the following questions may be helpful (Newman, 1993):

- What are the spiritual aspects of the client's philosophy about life? Death?
- Are the values and beliefs about life and death congruent with those of people who are important to the client?
- Which spiritual resources and rituals have significance for the client?

Belief systems that are incompatible with those of family members can be an additional source of stress for clients who are dealing with a loss. The anger and resentment often observed among families who are faced with decisions concerning dying members may be avoided if the nurse assesses the potential impact of differing beliefs.

Clients coping with a loss often perceive that it is a punishment from God for their wrongdoing or for their failure to remain faithful to their religious practices.

Therefore, it is important to assess the level of guilt the client or family expresses. Assessing the client's comments regarding feelings of responsibility for the loss helps the nurse determine whether these feelings are an expected phase of grieving or indicate dysfunctional grieving.

Clients who had not considered themselves religious before the actual or perceived loss often turn to religion to seek comfort or to cope with feelings of despair, helplessness, hopelessness, or guilt. They may utter anguished statements such as "Why, God?" or "Please help me, God." The nurse continues to assess the client's verbalization of such feelings to determine the best interventions to help the client cope with the loss.

Psychosocial Assessment

When working through the grief process, clients can be overwhelmed by the fears associated with the loss and the changes it will produce. The client responding to an actual or perceived loss commonly expresses anxiety, that is, fear of the unknown. An extreme level of anxiety can threaten the client's well-being. Assessment includes helping client's openly acknowledge their fears. Some clients may fear the feelings they experience while proceeding through the grief process more than the loss iteslf. The most common fear expressed by clients facing a loss is that of losing self-control.

During the assessment phase, focusing on the meaning of the loss to the client is more important than attempting to place the client in a sequence or phase of grief. The degree of caring and sensitivity shown when asking questions about the meaning of the loss influences the amount of information the client will be willing to reveal. Asking such questions as "Why do you feel this way?" or "What does this loss mean to you?" is less helpful than making a statement such as "This must be difficult for you." The latter more effectively conveys the nurse's genuine interest in hearing how the client feels about the loss.

Awareness of the altered sensorium observed during the stage of shock and disbelief provides parameters for assessment. The nurse may note in the client feelings of numbness, unreality, emotional distance, intense preoccupation with the lost object, helplessness, loneliness, and disorganization. Also, as an awareness of the loss begins to develop, preoccupation with the lost person or object may increase, and self-accusation and ambivalence toward the lost person or object may follow. Bugen's (1977) model of grief, which describes the anger, ambivalence, and guilt felt toward the lost person or object, is helpful in assessing the level of these feelings.

Although the nurse may not be able to elicit much information during a brief initial contact with the client, as trust is built, the client will reveal the significance of the relationship and the circumstances surrounding the loss. By attempting to build trust during the first stages of the nurse-client relationship, the nurse will be better able to assess the impact of the loss. If the relationship was a sig- nificant one, the nurse will observe intense grief. The client may state, "I know I can't go on without him/her." The client may even feel anger at the person for having left, whether through death, divorce, or separation. The losses associated with changes in body image or loss of a work role may produce similar feelings.

Caregivers may have difficulty in assessing the grief of men, the elderly, or members of certain cultural groups who value stoicism and may be unable to express grief directly. The anger and sadness identified by Bowlby's (1973, 1980) theory of grief may be helpful in assessing these clients. Despair and detachment behaviors also provide guidance for planning care.

Anger As previously noted, anger is a part of the normal grieving process. The nurse can determine whether the anger is functional or dysfunctional by noting the extent, occurrence in the grieving process, and effect on the client. In Engel's (1964) framework of "developing awareness of the loss," the client's expression of anger can be viewed as a positive sign of working through the grief. Expressing anger (for example, asking "Why me?") may help the client gain a sense of control in managing the events surrounding the loss.

Guilt Guilt is frequently observed in the client responding to a loss. Whether justifiably or not, clients may blame themselves for what is happening. A statement such as "If only I had done more, this might not have happened" provides the nurse with subjective assessment data confirming the client's feelings of guilt. To assess the extent of the guilt, the nurse may need to ask a direct question such as "Are you saying you feel your loss is the result of something you did or didn't do?"

If guilt is not resolved, it may become dysfunctional, and the client will continue to lash out in anger at friends, family, and caregivers. Guilt can destroy a marriage, for example, if parents blame each other for the death of a child (Gifford & Cleary, 1990). In the normal grieving process, however, the guilt that was initially felt so intensely begins to subside as the grieving client begins to deal with the permanence of the loss.

Depression As the grieving process continues, preoccupation with thoughts surrounding the loss begins to replace the denial, anger, and guilt. This is the period of restitution in which the work of mourning continues (Engel, 1964). The client's unresponsiveness to visitors and decreased physical activity, which are normal reactions during this time, may be incorrectly assessed as symptoms of clinical depression. The nurse needs to be especially vigilant during this period and refrain from administering medications that interfere with the normal, painful work of grieving. This is a stage of depression in which the person grieves over "what cannot be" (Kübler-Ross, 1969). This stage is characterized either by the client's willingness to talk openly about the loss or by withdrawal. Both are observed in the normal grieving process.

When the dying client seems withdrawn and unapproachable, nurses may mislabel this behavior as depression. To help the nurse distinguish depression from "holding" (Carter, 1989), the nurse assesses the client's response to direct questions such as

- What are you thinking about?
- Whom do you need at this time?

Responses such as "It's hopeless" or "What's the use" may indicate clinical depression, whereas responses such as "I'm figuring things out" or "I'm sorting out some things by myself" may indicate that the client is engaged in "holding."

Awareness   It is widely accepted that clients know they are dying whether they are told or not and that clients dealing with other types of losses have a perceptive awareness. The awareness contexts described by Glaser and Strauss (1965) offer helpful guidelines for the nurse in assessing the client's and others' desire to talk about the actual or perceived loss. Awareness should not be forced. Even though the nurse may feel that open awareness promotes acceptance of the loss, clients in the initial shock and disbelief phase may need to deal with the loss through closed awareness or mutual pretense (Glaser & Strauss, 1965). Thus an accurate assessment of the desired awareness context is imperative: The nurse assesses the client's desire for knowledge and the family's beliefs about how much and what knowledge needs to be shared.

It is important to recognize that grieving clients may appear to accept a loss by making statements such as "It was for the best" while keeping their true feelings repressed. If grief is to be resolved successfully, however, a true state of "developing awareness" must follow. The client who overtly continues to behave as though nothing has happened is at risk for developing delayed or morbid grief reactions (Lindemann, 1944).

Denial   As a defense mechanism, denial is initially beneficial in helping the grieving client deal with the shock of loss. However, the nurse needs to assess the extent and usefulness of this defense mechanism. For example, denial helps the dying client preserve hope, but it becomes dysfunctional when it is used to avoid making decisions that must be made before the client dies.

Research on the maternal bereavement experience in intrauterine fetal death reveals that denial may be used to support hope until the stillborn fetus is delivered. "No matter how overwhelming the information may be that the fetus has died, as long as the fetus remains inside, the mother will use various sources of data to support her hope that the diagnosis is wrong" (Grubb-Phillips, 1988). In the initial stage of grief, denial gives the client and family time to mobilize and bond before confronting the diagnosis, but if denial causes them to refuse health care because "nothing is wrong," it becomes an ineffective way of coping.

"The criteria that most clearly distinguishes healthy forms of defensive process from pathological ones (as in dysfunctional grieving) are the length of time during which they persist and the extent to which they influence . . . mental functioning or come to dominate it completely" (Bowlby, 1980). Information on the length of time that has elapsed since the loss occurred therefore can provide important data for the nurse's assessment.

Imagery and art, which are frequently used to assess the meaning of loss to children, can also be used to assess the meaning of a loss that an adult client is denying. Through verbal descriptions of images (e.g., "It feels like a black cavern"), or through art, the client may be able to explore feelings and fears that he or she may not be able to convey directly.

Social Support   Assessment of the client's social support system is important because of its potentially positive influence on the successful resolution of grief. Some losses may lead to social isolation, placing clients at high risk for dysfunctional grief reactions. For example, survivors of people with AIDS (SOPWAs) often report feeling excluded by the deceased person's family and by health care providers. Characteristic factors that can interfere with successful grieving include the following (Kneisl & Pheifer, 1992):

- Perceived inability to share the loss
- Lack of social recognition of the loss
- Ambivalent relationships prior to the loss
- Traumatic circumstances of the loss

A move, a divorce, or even the death of a pet can cause a person to feel extremely isolated, yet the person experiencing these types of loss does not ordinarily receive the same social support that is offered to the person mourning the death of a loved one. A woman having an abortion or giving up a child for adoption seldom receives the same social support as the mother of a child who died at birth. It is therefore especially imperative that the nurse refrain from placing a value on the client's loss in assessing the need for support.

The painful nature of grief can cause the client to withdraw from a previously established social support system, thereby increasing the feelings of loneliness caused by the loss. A woman who is recently widowed, for example, may refuse invitations involving married couples with whom she had socialized while her husband was alive. The client's needs for social interaction remain similar to those established before the loss. In assessing the social support system, the nurse must therefore identify the frequency of interactions as well as the people who constitute the client's social network. By asking clients to name significant people in their lives, the nurse will have the opportunity to encourage the client to maintain contact with them when he or she experiences the loneliness and isolation of grief.

Families   A well-functioning family usually rallies after the initial shock and disbelief and provides support for each other during all phases of the grieving process. After a loss, the well-functioning family is able to shift roles, levels of responsibility, and ways of communicating. The nurse's assessment of the family patterns of interaction includes the following (Newman, 1993):

- Family structure and usual roles
- Family norms, values, and attitudes
- Level of trust among family members
- Perceptions of relationships with extended family
- Willingness to call on outside supports

The nurse needs to be alert for the negative as well as positive effects the family may have on the grieving client. For example, the dying client may request that someone the family perceives as an outsider be near, and the family may respond with anger to the perceived "intrusion." Similarly, certain family members may express hurt feelings or anger if the client is unresponsive to other family members. Well-meaning family members also may try to shield the client from the pain of grieving. Because no two people grieve alike, the nurse must assess the individual family members' reactions to the loss. It is rare for the family and the client to experience anger, denial, and acceptance in unison. While one member is in denial, another may be angry because "not enough is being done."

A pattern of detrimental changes in behaviors in the relationships with friends and family may lead the nurse to suspect dysfunctional grieving. If their grief becomes dysfunctional, family members may begin missing work or school, getting in trouble with the law, or abusing alcohol or drugs.

Ceremonies   The institutionalization of mourning occurs in the stage of restitution and is an important part of the work of mourning and grieving a loss (Engel, 1964). Culture primarily defines and dictates the rituals of mourning a loss. Through the participation in religious ceremonies such as baptism, confirmation, and Bat or Bar Mitzvah, people joyously celebrate progression to a new stage of life and loss of a former way of being. The funeral ceremony serves many of the same purposes in meeting the needs of the bereaved as people gather to share loss. Through the ceremony, people symbolically express triumph over death and deny the fear of death (Murray & Zentner, 1985).

The nurse's observations of the planning and participation in ceremonies provides assessment data on the importance of the loss to the client. The nurse needs to be aware that as the survivors publically adapt to the loss, this adaptation does not decrease the suffering that the bereaved will continue to feel, but it does move them toward reinvesting emotionally in new relationships.

Nursing Diagnoses

The nursing diagnoses related to loss are **Anticipatory Grieving** and **Dysfunctional Grieving.** The definitions, related factors, and defining characteristics of these diagnoses are presented in the box on page 398.

In addition to these diagnoses, other responses related to loss, grief, and dying may be significant enough to require a nursing diagnosis. The following list provides some examples of NANDA-approved diagnoses with causative statements related to loss, grief, and dying:

- *Altered Family Processes* related to the loss of spouse, child, or parent
- *Altered Sexuality Patterns* related to impaired relationship with or lack of a significant other
- *Anxiety* related to perceived threat to self-concept, health status, socioeconomic status, role functioning, interaction patterns, environment, or death
- *Altered Nutrition: Less Than Body Requirements* related to grieving
- *Ineffective Individual Coping* related to awareness of impending death
- *Ineffective Family Coping* related to role change
- *Powerlessness* related to loss of independence
- *Social Isolation* related to perceived abandonment by friends
- *Spiritual Distress* related to separation from religious ties
- *Sleep Pattern Disturbance* related to fear of death

Expected Outcomes

Goals and expected outcome criteria for the client responding to an actual or perceived loss are based on the subjective and objective data gathered from the assessment and reflect the individual needs of the client. It is important for the nurse to allow the client to set the pace for the grief work. The nurse and client together establish expected outcomes for working through the grief associated with the loss. Nevertheless, the following broad goals for grieving clients are suggested.

The long-term goals for the client experiencing normal grieving are that the client will

- Accept the reality of the loss.

Nursing Diagnoses Related to Loss

■ ■ ■

Anticipatory Grieving

Definition
The state in which an individual experiences responses to an actual or perceived loss of a person, relationship, object, or functional abilities before the loss occurs.

Related Factors
- Effects of actual or potential loss of significant other, health status, social status, or valued object.

Defining Characteristics
- Potential loss of significant object
- Expression of distress at potential loss
- Denial of potential loss
- Guilt
- Anger
- Sorrow
- Choked feelings
- Changes in eating habits
- Alterations in sleep patterns
- Alterations in activity level
- Altered libido
- Altered communication patterns

Dysfunctional Grieving

Definition
The state in which an individual experiences an exaggerated response to an actual or potential loss of person, relationship, object, or functional abilities.

Related Factors
- Effects of actual or perceived loss of significant other, health or social status, or valued object
  - a. People   d. Home
  - b. Possessions   e. Ideals
  - c. Job status   f. Parts and processes of the body

- Absence of anticipatory grieving
- Thwarted grieving in response to a loss
- Effects of multiple losses or crises
- Lack of resolution of previous grieving response
- Ambivalent feelings toward loss
- Changes in lifestyle
- Decreased support system

Defining Characteristics
- Verbal expression of distress at loss
- Expression of unresolved issues
- Crying
- Weight loss
- Amenorrhea
- Changes in
  - a. Sleep patterns   d. Dream patterns
  - b. Activity   e. Libido
  - c. Eating patterns
- Decreased interest in personal appearance
- Interference with life functioning
- Reliving of past experiences
- Difficulty in expressing loss
- Alterations in concentration and/or pursuit of tasks
- Developmental regression
- Hyperactivity
- Fear of future
- Absence of emotion
- Suicidal thoughts
- Social withdrawal
- Labile affect

Notes. From *NANDA Nursing Diagnoses: Definitions and Classification 1992–1993* by North American Nursing Diagnosis Association, 1992, Philadelphia: NANDA; and from *Nursing Diagnosis and Care Planning* (2nd ed.) by B. Taptich, P. Iyer, & D. Bernocchi-Losey, 1994, Philadelphia: Sanders.

- Regain a sense of self-esteem.
- Begin to put the loss into perspective.

The goal for the client who is experiencing anticipatory grieving is to engage in constructive grief work (McFarland & Gerety, 1989). For dysfunctional grieving, the

goals are to engage in normal grieving and resolve the dysfunctional grieving (McFarland & Wasli, 1986).

Caring for dying clients requires the nurse and client to formulate additional goals to meet the client's physical needs and to maintain quality of life. The nurse reassesses the dying client frequently and develops goals with the client to attain and maintain comfort levels, nutritional status, and the desired environment for dying.

Planning and Implementation

Nursing interventions for the grieving client are highly individualized. The nurse's knowledge that the client's grief is affected by many factors, including personality, previous losses, intimacy of the relationship, and personal resources, provides a constant reminder of the necessity for interventions to be based on the specific needs of the individual client experiencing the loss (Carpenito, 1993). However, the following interventions may be appropriate for most clients experiencing a loss. Special interventions for dying clients are discussed on pages 402–405.

Nursing Interventions for Physical Needs

As stated previously, grieving clients may experience related somatic disorders, such as gastrointestinal symptoms, respiratory distress, and somatic pain. The nursing interventions for these clinical manifestations are discussed in the related chapters of this text.

Altered Sensorium On first hearing the news of a loss, clients may collapse, feel faint or dizzy, experience visual disturbances, or become disoriented. Help the client to sit or lie down, and remain near the client throughout this initial phase of shock. Because the client may be unable to hear or to interpret words, do not attempt to convey important information at this time. As the initial shock wears off, begin to assess the client's orientation to time, place, and circumstances. If the client is able to listen and respond appropriately, some limited information may be conveyed. It is important, however, to repeat information frequently. Use simple language that the client can readily comprehend, and ask the client to repeat information back. This allows for clarification and ensures understanding.

Crying When the news of a loss is received, the client or family may collapse in tears and anguish and/or lose control. In this stage of shock and disbelief, crying helps to provide relief from feelings of acute pain and stress. It is at this moment that the nurse needs to convey acceptance of the client's grief reaction, either verbally or nonverbally. There should be no attempt to suppress the crying during this time. When the client cries, remain quietly to offer comfort, rather than leaving the client at the time of greatest need. The silent presence of the nurse communicates caring to the client.

Rest and Sleep Although crying provides emotional relief, it is physically exhausting and can cause daily or even hourly fluctuation in the client's energy level. Ensuring adequate rest becomes a challenge for the nurse. Encourage the client to maintain the regular sleeping pattern as much as possible. Clients may complain of lethargy and want to sleep during the day, but encouraging them to stay awake and engaging them in as much physical activity as possible will help tire them enough to enable them to sleep at night. Many of the gastrointestinal symptoms observed in the grieving client can be reduced by encouraging sleeping, eating, and activity patterns that were part of the client's normal routine before the loss.

Nursing Interventions for Spiritual Needs

Spirituality is at the core of human existence, integrating and transcending the physical, emotional, intellectual, and social dimensions (Landrum et al., 1988). The principles, values, personal philosophy, and meaning of life by which the client has pursued goals and self-actualization, however, may be called into question when the client responds to an actual or perceived loss. Because of a fear of intruding on the personal spiritual beliefs and practices of the client, the nurse often feels at a loss in implementing interventions that would be helpful to the client responding to a loss. The responses to the questions that guided the assessment serve as a basis for meeting the spiritual needs of the client.

Developing a trusting relationship with the client and family helps the nurse overcome initial discomfort in dealing with the spiritual aspects of care, even when the client and nurse have different views. During the initial stages of grief, the nurse is accepting and nonjudgmental when the client expresses a belief that the loss is related to some past misdeed or failure "to do right" for which punishment is being dealt out. Even spiritually healthy clients need time to challenge their beliefs and values before moving on to the next stage of grieving.

In the next stage, as the client becomes aware of the full impact of the loss, spiritual beliefs and rituals provide comfort and help the client to find meaning in the loss. (Not all clients, however, pass through these stages in the sequence described.) The nurse provides spiritual support by listening as the client analyzes beliefs and values, begins to put the loss in perspective, and expresses renewed interest in getting on with life.

When the nurse perceives blocks in the client's grief work that are due to spiritual distress, interventions to help the client remove the barriers to finding spiritual comfort may be needed. For example, providing a client with spiritual comfort may involve role-playing with the client who feels the need to seek forgiveness from someone whom the client cannot confront directly.

Nursing Interventions for Psychosocial Needs

The client experiencing a loss has many psychosocial needs that vary with the type of loss experienced, the client's previous experiences with loss, the age of the client, and numerous other factors. In responding to any of these varied needs, the nurse's primary intervention is therapeutic communication.

Therapeutic Communication   Therapeutic communication with the client experiencing an actual or perceived loss begins with total acceptance of the client's feelings, attitudes, and values related to the loss. When the client does not want to talk, sitting quietly conveys caring and acceptance. If touch is acceptable to the client, it can be used as a nonverbal expression of caring and acceptance. Stiffening or pulling away, however, may indicate that touching is unacceptable to the client. Such clients may be more comfortable with the nurse sitting close to the bedside. Spending time listening to clients, as opposed to interacting with them only to provide physical care, conveys acceptance of their emotional response to loss.

Being an active, nonjudgmental listener is essential to assure clients that their feelings are being accepted and no value judgements are being made. The nurse can acknowledge the client's grief by a nonthreatening statement such as "It must be very difficult for you." If the client is ready to talk about the loss, listening is the most appropriate intervention. Allowing the client to verbalize fears and anxieties when the client chooses to do so is helpful; forcing the client to talk, however, may increase discomfort.

The clouded sensorium and numbness clients experience may cause them to question their mental stability, so assurances that these are normal expressions of grief are important. It may be helpful to encourage the client to identify strengths in dealing with past losses as a way to deal with the current loss. Encourage the client to talk about the loss and the changes it will bring. This provides the opportunity for the client to become aware of the impact of the loss and encourages the client to plan for the necessary changes.

Open-ended and reflective statements are more effective than direct questions in helping the client move through the grieving process. When the client has demonstrated a readiness to move to the awareness or restitution stage, explaining recognized grief reactions is an appropriate intervention.

Involve the client in decision making to give the client a sense of control and to help diminish the feelings of hopelessness and helplessness related to the loss. Help the client make informed decisions by answering the client's questions honestly and directly. For example, a client who asks, "Do I have cancer?" has a right to expect an honest answer to the question.

Nevertheless, it is necessary to keep in mind the contexts of awareness described by Glaser and Strauss (1965) when providing information about the actual or perceived loss. For example, if the client asks, "Am I going to die?" answering "Yes, the doctor says you have about a month to live," is inappropriate. An appropriate reflective response is to ask, "Do you think you are dying?" This allows the client to express thoughts and allows the nurse to assess the client's desired level of awareness. This response expresses the nurse's honest concern without taking away the client's hope. Determining what information to disclose and when to disclose it presents a dilemma for many nurses because of their difficulty in weighing the client's "right to know" against the desire to protect the client. Regardless of the nurse's stance, it is the client who must be allowed to set the pace.

Encourage the client to work on progressing through the tasks of grieving. Gaining an intellectual understanding of the loss and what they can do to help themselves is often empowering for clients.

Denial   The nurse needs to allow and accept the client's intermittent use of denial. If the client's denial is destructive, however, the nurse needs to help the client examine the purpose of the behavior. When the client manifests denial by going from one physician to another or postponing or prematurely terminating treatment, the nurse explores with the client the reasons for the behavior. Rather than criticize or try to talk the client out of it, the nurse might ask what the client expects to be told or what will happen when the client hears the same thing again.

Anger and Guilt   When a client is dealing with a loss, feelings of anger and guilt are normal and need to be expressed if the grief is to be resolved successfully. The client who expresses anger toward the lost person or object near the time of the loss will not likely turn that anger inward at a later time. The nurse understands that anger usually replaces denial and as such represents progression in the grieving process. When family members are upset by the client's anger, it may be helpful to explain to them that anger serves to give the client a sense of control over his or her environment and thereby offset the client's lack of control over the loss (Carpenito, 1993).

It is difficult not to take the client's anger personally. A nurse who reacts defensively to the anger communicates that the client is acceptable only when he or she is "good." Knowing that expressions of anger are normal, however, the nurse might respond by saying "I see you are really upset. I just want to let you know I'm available to talk if you'd like" (Kozier et al., 1995).

Criticizing the client's anger or expressions of guilt creates barriers to communication and may make the client less willing to share feelings related to the loss. For example, well-intentioned remarks such as "At least you're alive" or "You're young; you can have other children," may make the client feel more guilty or increase the anger.

When clients indicate they are moving toward the awareness stage of grief, the nurse can intervene by helping them examine the guilt feelings and consider whether these feelings are realistic. The following is an example:

Client: If I had gone to the doctor earlier, this would not have happened.

Nurse: Did you have any reason to suspect something was wrong?

Client: Not really, but . . .

Nurse: Then how would you have known to go to the doctor earlier?

Even if the client ignored symptoms or engaged in health habits that led to the condition, discussing these factors now is not helpful and may reinforce the client's feelings of guilt.

Grief Related to Loss of Body Image Losses associated with body image include the loss of a body part, weight gain or loss, loss of hair, and other physical effects of illness or treatment. For grief associated with body image, nursing interventions are directed toward minimizing the outward manifestations of the loss. Allowing clients to wear their own clothing, put on make-up, or wear a wig or turban helps to minimize the changes. Helping a woman who has had a mastectomy to be fitted with a temporary prosthesis can help her feel less self-conscious. If the woman has begun to accept the loss of her breast, the nurse can introduce her to a "Reach for Recovery" volunteer, who will talk to her about breast prostheses, clothing, and exercise and provide her with other information to help her resume normal activities.

Social Support Among other factors, an individual's reaction to loss is affected by personal resources, primarily the perception of social support. Grieving is painful and lonely. Lack of a support system has been identified as one of the causative and contributing factors that may delay grief work (Carpenito, 1993). Even if the client is reacting to the loss in an expected manner, feelings of isolation and withdrawal behaviors are often observed. Interventions are focused on helping clients reestablish contact with significant others in their lives to allow them to share their grief. If the client is not making progress in grief work, the nurse may need to intervene by explaining to the client the benefit of sharing their grief with significant others.

The nurse works with the significant others in the client's life to assist them in helping the client achieve the goal of resuming social interaction patterns similar to those established before the loss. Using open-ended questions, reflection, and silence, the nurse facilitates expression of feelings (Buck, 1991). For example, in the case of a 28-year-old woman with no children who is experiencing problems of loss following a hysterectomy, the nurse gives the significant others information about the grief process, what to expect, and how long each stage might last. In the case of body image disturbance after ostomy surgery, the nurse tells the significant others what to expect concerning the care and appearance of the ostomy. The nurse then listens to the significant others' responses, answers questions, and prepares the significant others to be supportive of the client with the ostomy (Buck, 1991).

Because no two people grieve alike, the nurse should promote family cohesiveness by recognizing and supporting the stage of grieving and strengths of each family member. The nurse explains the need to discuss behaviors that interfere with relationships in the family and encourages family members to explore with one another their feelings about the loss, to talk directly to each other, and to listen to each other. The trusting relationship the nurse has built with the client and family helps facilitate the process.

Community Resources Assisting clients and families to seek support from concerned others in their community decreases feelings of loneliness and helplessness in managing the loss. Direct the client to appropriate community resources that provide group support from others who have experienced a similar loss. See Appendix X for appropriate community resources.

Dysfunctional Grieving When a diagnosis of dysfunctional grieving is made, the nurse intervenes to help the client establish a more functional pattern of grieving. Persistent absence of any emotion, inability to cry, or ruminations beyond a period of time culturally established for dealing with the loss may signal a delay in the work of mourning or a delayed grief reaction. The nurse intervenes by providing positive reinforcement of behaviors observed in normal grief reactions. For example, in a trusting relationship, the nurse can intervene simply by stating, "Sometimes crying helps." The nurse can offer support and reassurance that grieving is normal and painful and that the nurse will be available if the client fears losing control.

When the interventions directed toward the physical aspects of normal grief and anticipatory grieving are ineffective in preventing or relieving dysfunctional grieving, interventions directed toward depression may be necessary. Requesting a consultation with a psychiatric-mental health clinical nurse specialist is an appropriate nursing intervention.

Evaluation: Grief Resolution

Resolution of grief related to an actual or perceived loss may require months or years. Evaluation of nursing care for a client diagnosed with grieving, anticipatory grieving, or dysfunctional grieving is measured within the context of the expectations stated in the goals and the outcome criteria. Because the nurse usually encounters the grieving client for a relatively short period of time, establishing small, measurable goals gives the nurse the opportunity to evaluate progress toward meeting the goals. If the feedback indicates that the client is not progressing toward grief resolution, the nurse can reassess and establish new goals with the client.

Special Interventions for Dying Clients

■ ■ ■

The dying client has special needs that are different from those of the client experiencing other types of loss. These needs may range from physical concerns to worries about financial affairs to uncertainty about how to say goodbye to friends and family.

Nurses who recognize their limitations in providing appropriate interventions to the dying client can seek support from nurses who are more experienced or have had special training. In addition, the following discussion provides guidance in meeting the special needs of the dying client.

Physical Needs

Interventions for the dying client require special attention to physical needs. The dying client needs to be kept as comfortable as possible. Nursing measures directed to the physical care of the client are essential: wrinkle-free sheets, bowel and bladder care, prevention of skin breakdown, positioning, turning, mouth care, nutrition and hydration, pain management, and any other aspects with which the client needs assistance.

Not all dying clients experience pain, but most fear it. Open communication during the assessment phase of the nursing process allows the client to express this fear, and the nurse to explain ways to control pain (see Chapter 4). Assure the client or family that all possible methods of managing pain will be used, and address unrealistic fears of addiction by explaining the appropriate use of the medication in relieving the client's pain. If family members want to assist in the client's care, instruct them in the use of therapeutic massage. If they are not comfortable massaging the upper body or trunk, or if the massage is painful for the client, the feet can be massaged. The foot is usually relatively free of pain, and foot massage achieves similar results, promoting increased comfort, touching, and feelings of togetherness.

In addition to promoting physical comfort, nurses caring for dying clients should promote client independence and self-esteem by allowing the client to remain as self-sufficient as possible. For example, if the client cannot perform complete self-care, allow the client to do the things that will maintain self-esteem and dignity, such as washing the face and holding a cup.

Even if the family wants to participate in the physical care of the client, it is important that the client's independence be maintained as much as possible. The role of the

nurse as client advocate may be to gently but firmly encourage the family to allow the client to be as self-sufficient as possible. Explain that clients need to feel some sense of control over the loss and that doing for them what they are themselves capable of doing robs them of their dignity. Moreover, nurses must guard against implying that the family's role is to provide nursing care for the client. Hostility and mistrust of the nursing staff can result if the family perceives they are being relied on to care for the client.

If the client decides to return home to die, the nurse may need to teach the family skills to enable them to care for the client and to discuss the positive and negative aspects of returning home to die. Care by hospice nurses can make the transition easier for the family. The hospice functions on a 24-hour, 7-days-a-week basis; back-up medical, nursing, and counseling services are available. Knowing that symptom control is of vital importance to most clients and their families, hospice nurses assure them that pain-relieving medications will not be withheld.

Spiritual Needs

Throughout the stages of dying, the nurse demonstrates continued acceptance of the client and the client's beliefs. Meeting the client's spiritual needs may take many forms, including involvement by the clergy; however, the nurse should not assume that the client desires contact with clergy.

Clients who do not consider themselves religious often turn to religion as a way to seek spiritual comfort when they are dying. Nurses have a responsibility not to impose their own religious beliefs on clients when they are most vulnerable.

It is appropriate for the nurse to participate in religious practices such as communion or prayer if the client so requests and if the nurse is comfortable with the request. If the client expresses comfort in prayer or the reading of religious material, the nurse arranges the time and privacy for these activities with members of the client's religious group or members of the health care team who wish to participate. The clergy can be a valuable resource to the nurse who needs guidance in meeting the client's specific requests.

Whether through providing direct intervention or arranging access to spiritual care, the nurse ensures that the client's spiritual needs are met with the same care and concern given to physical needs.

Psychosocial Needs

Preventing Social Isolation

As they come to accept the reality of the loss, many clients are inclined to prematurely abandon jobs, hobbies, vacations, and social interests. Although nurses support clients' attempts to adapt to the anticipated loss, they also assist clients in restructuring their lives in a meaningful way. Encourage the client to remain involved in established relationships, particularly the most significant ones, and to maintain or renew meaningful interests and hobbies, which can be therapeutic and contribute to a sense of accomplishment. Encourage the client and family to maintain current roles, personal interests, and lifestyles as long as possible. For example, encourage clients to celebrate birthdays, anniversaries, and other meaningful events.

Discussing subjects that span the past, present, and future allows clients to affirm their lives. Nurses and family members often avoid discussing present or future events because they fear upsetting dying clients by talking about plans in which the client may not be able to participate. The opportunity for communication and sharing may be lost if the nurse or family assumes that talking about the present or future will make the dying client uncomfortable. Clients experience greater feelings of loneliness, isolation, and abandonment when they feel that significant others are excluding them from conversations about topics that are a meaningful part of their lives.

Other interventions to decrease loneliness and social isolation include the following:

- Provide meaningful environmental stimulation.
- Help the family learn how to interact with the dying client.
- Provide information on the client's condition.
- Encourage the family to stay in communication through caring, silence, touch, and telling the client of their love.
- Refer the client and family to appropriate support groups.

Psychosocial Needs of the Client Dying of AIDS

The client with AIDS is especially vulnerable to the development of dysfunctional grieving related to loneliness and social isolation. When fears about caring for dying clients are compounded by fear of AIDS, the nurse may avoid the client and the client may experience an overwhelming loneliness. Developing self-awareness is imperative for the nurse in providing sensitive care to the client and family.

Although AIDS affects all segments of the population, the mortality rate currently is highest in homosexual men. The grief of the single, homosexual, bereaved partner is just as legitimate and as overwhelming as that experienced by married, heterosexual people experiencing a similar loss. During the course of grief work, the homosexual client dying from AIDS and his lover are supported by the nurse in the same way as other clients dealing with loss (Oerlemans-Bunn, 1988).

Life Review and Framing Memories

Talking about the past may be helpful for the dying client. *Life review* is an intervention the nurse uses to encourage the client and family to talk about past accomplishments, pleasures, and hardships. Past recollections of success or of overcoming setbacks offer affirmations of the self. The past represents control that dying clients may feel they are losing. The past is something that cannot be taken away.

Framing memories is another effective technique the nurse can use to encourage the client and family members to review the past and envision the future. The client and family reminisce about a happy experience. The nurse asks the client to give the family members meaningful information to pass on to future generations. The family members, in return, share what the client means to them and their future aspirations.

Visualization and Imagery

If dying clients imagine death negatively, the nurse can help them engage in activities to gain a sense of control. Visualization and imagery can be used to help the client explore and even alter their fears and concerns. For example, if the client's image of death is darkness, the nurse can help the client to imagine lights and soft music in the room or to imagine being surrounded by family and friends, free of pain, with favorite music playing. In addition, clients may benefit from drawing pictures that the nurse can use to facilitate discussions of images of death.

If the client expresses a desire to die at home, the nurse works with the family to achieve that goal. If it is not possible, the nurse helps the client to amend the goal by visualizing the hospital room as a safe, comfortable place to die and by surrounding the client with familiar articles brought from the client's home (Figure 11–1).

Final Wishes and Saying Goodbye

As the client's condition deteriorates, the nurse's knowledge of the client and family's awareness context guides the interventions. For example, if there is an open awareness, the nurse assists the client in exploring the impact the client's death may have on the survivors. It may also be necessary to provide opportunities for clients to express personal preferences about where they want to die and about their preferences for funeral and burial arrangements. If the family feels that this is morbid, the nurse explains that it helps clients to maintain a sense of control when they feel so overwhelmed by their impending death.

The client needs the opportunity to say goodbye to others. The nurse encourages and supports the client and family as they terminate relationships as a necessary part of the grief process. The nurse acknowledges that termination is painful and, if the client or family desires, stays with them during this time. Being present at the moment of death is a fear commonly expressed by family mem-

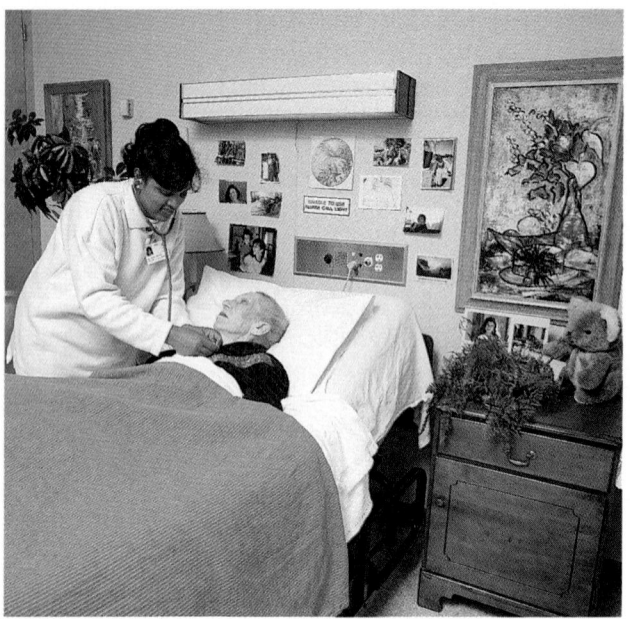

Figure 11–1 The nurse helps the client to visualize the hospital room as a safe, comfortable place to die by surrounding the client with familiar articles brought from the client's home.

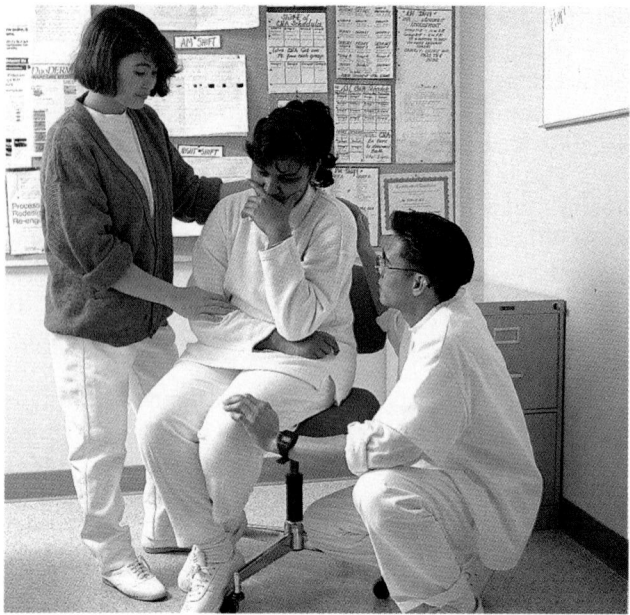

Figure 11–2 Nurses who work with dying clients need support from their colleagues to work through their often overwhelming feelings of grief.

bers, yet dying alone is the greatest fear expressed by clients (Kübler-Ross, 1969, 1978). In recognizing these common fears, the nurse can reduce the possibility of client abandonment as death approaches by encouraging the client and family to participate in support groups that offer help in dealing with these fears.

The nurse also may fear being present at the moment of the client's death. In fact, Kübler-Ross (1969) noted that the nurse's fear of death frequently interferes with the ability to provide support for the dying client and family. Thoughts such as "Please, God, don't let him die on my shift" are common, and they express the nurse's emotional turmoil in dealing with the task. Nurses who have worked through their own feelings about death and dying are more at ease in assisting the dying client toward a peaceful death.

Because a client near death may have an altered sensorium, the nurse stands near the bedside and speaks clearly and distinctly. Clients' levels of consciousness just before death vary; some clients may be alert, whereas others may be drowsy, stuporous, or comatose. Because hearing is thought to be the last sense a dying client loses, the nurse should never whisper or engage in conversation with the family as if the client were not there.

After Death

After the death, the family is encouraged to acknowledge the pain of loss. The nurse's presence and support as the bereaved express their sorrow, anger, or guilt can facilitate

the resolution of grief. It is important not to suppress the pain of grieving with drugs. In allowing for variations in the expression of grief, the nurse is acknowledging acceptance and support of the family's grief reaction as a necessary part of preventing dysfunctional grieving.

The resolution of grieving begins with the acceptance of the loss. Grief work cannot begin until the loss is acknowledged. The nurse can encourage this acknowledgement by maintaining open, honest dialogue and by providing the family with the opportunity to view the body (Carpenito, 1993). After making the body appear as natural and comfortable as possible, the nurse prepares the family for what to expect. As family members realize the finality of the death, they are often comforted by the presence of the nurse who cared for the client during the final days.

Nurses' Grief

If the nurse has developed a close relationship with the client who has died, the nurse may experience powerful feelings of grief. At one time considered unprofessional, crying with families is now recognized as simply an expression of empathy and caring. Sharing grief with the family after the death of a loved one helps both the nurse and family to cope with their feelings related to the loss. In addition, taking time to grieve after the death of a client provides a release that can help prevent the "blunting" of feelings that is often experienced by nurses who care for terminally ill clients.

Health Promotion and Teaching for Clients Experiencing a Loss

▪ ▪ ▪

I.   Provide anticipatory guidance in dealing with an expected or impending loss.
   A.   Encourage both children and adults to discuss expected or impending loss and to express feelings.
   B.   Teach problem-solving skills.
      1.   Define potential changes and problems related to the predicted loss.
      2.   Develop potential strategies to deal with problems.
      3.   List consequences of each strategy.
      4.   Determine a priority of the strategies in terms of usefulness in solving potential problems associated with loss.
   C.   Identify persons who are at risk for potential dysfunctional grieving reactions, such as those who
      1.   Present a brave, stoic front.
      2.   Have a history of multiple losses.
      3.   Are socially isolated.
      4.   Perceive their social network as unsupportive.
      5.   Have a history of dealing ineffectively with loss.

   D.   Teach individuals and families how to support a person dealing with an impending loss.
   E.   Explain what to expect with a loss: sadness, fear, rejection, anger, guilt, loneliness.
   F.   Teach signs of grief resolution:
      1.   Griever no longer lives in past but is future oriented.
      2.   Griever breaks ties with lost object or person. Time varies, but acute stage shows signs of resolving in 6 to 12 months.
      3.   Griever may have painful "waves" of grief years after the loss, especially on the anniversary of the loss.
   G.   Teach signs of exaggerated responses requiring treatment, especially in persons at risk: hallucinations, delusions, isolation, egocentricity, or overt hostility.
II. Provide intervention to persons dealing with loss to reduce potential for dysfunctional loss.
III. Identify agencies that may be helpful to people responding to loss.

Note. From *Nursing Diagnosis: Application to Clinical Practice* by L. Carpenito, 1993, Philadelphia: Lippincott; and from *Nursing Diagnosis and Process in Psychiatric Mental Health Nursing* by G. McFarland & E. Wasli, 1986, Philadelphia: Lippincott.

Nurses working with critically or terminally ill clients should be aware that witnessing clients' deaths and the reactions of grieving family members may reactivate feelings related to an unresolved grief in their own lives. In these cases, nurses may need to reflect on the responses they have had to losses in their own lives. In addition to self-reflection, nurses who work with dying clients also need support from peers and other professionals to work through the often overwhelming feelings that result from dealing with death, grief, and loss (Figure 11–2).

Client and Family Teaching

▪ ▪ ▪

In addition to teaching clients and families to carry out the physical skills that are necessary to the client's care, nurses also provide information on identifying signs of deterioration and additional sources of support. Hospice, home health care agencies, and public health departments provide nursing care services. Families are encour-

aged also to identify friends and other family members who can help out either routinely or occasionally. Discharge planning includes providing the client or family with the information necessary to contact the appropriate support groups listed in Appendix X. General guidelines for teaching clients and families about grief include those suggested in the accompanying box.

Legal and Ethical Issues Related to Loss, Grief, and Dying

▪ ▪ ▪

Right-to-die issues such as those involved in euthanasia, quality of life, advance directives, and living wills are especially important to nurses in effectively upholding the specific care requests of their clients.

Euthanasia

Euthanasia, a word of Greek origin meaning painless, easy, gentle, or good death, is now commonly used to sig-

To My Family, My Physician, My Lawyer
And All Others Whom It May Concern

Death is as much a reality as birth, growth, and
aging—it is the one certainty of life. In anticipation of
decisions that may have to be made about my own
dying and as an expression of my right to refuse
treatment, I _____, being of sound
(print name)
mind, make this statement of my wishes and
instructions concerning treatment.

By means of this document, which I intend to be
legally binding, I direct my physician and other care
providers, my family, and any surrogate designated by
me or appointed by a court, to carry out my wishes. If I
become unable, by reason of physical or mental
incapacity, to make decisions about my medical care, let
this document provide the guidance and authority
needed to make any and all such decisions.

If I am permanently unconscious or there is no
reasonable expectation of my recovery from a seriously
incapacitating or lethal illness or condition, I do not
wish to be kept alive by artificial means. I request that I
be given all care necessary to keep me comfortable and
free of pain, even if pain-relieving medications may
hasten by death, and I direct that no life-sustaining
treatment be provided except as I or my surrogate
specifically authorize.

This request may appear to place a heavy
responsibility upon you, but by making this decision
according to my strong convictions, I intend to ease that
burden. I am acting after careful consideration and with
understanding of the consequences of your carrying out
my wishes. *List optional specific provisions in the
space below. (See other side)*

Figure 11–3   Sample living will. For more information and a
complete document, contact Concern for Dying or the Society for
the Right to Die.

nify a killing that is prompted by some humanitarian motive (Kelly, 1992). There are many arguments in favor of and in opposition to euthanasia most fall into secular or religious categories. In the past, nurses often found themselves at the center of the dilemma. Every experienced clinical nurse can recall the horror of lonely, middle-of-the-night decisions regarding resuscitation of clients in irreversible coma. As a result of having faced this dilemma repeatedly, nurses have been largely responsible for the development of appropriate guidelines and procedures regarding *DNR (do not resuscitate)* orders. Many hospitals

still do not have written guidelines and policies in place, and it is when no such orders exist that the nurse faces a dilemma. Certainly there are situations in which the nurse's role is clear; for example, participating in "slow codes" (in which the nurse does not hurry to alert the emergency team when a terminally ill client who does not have a DNR order stops breathing) is considered malpractice.

Equally perplexing for the nurse are right-to-die issues involving nutrition and hydration. According to Kelly (1992), the American Medical Association (AMA), in a statement titled "Withholding or Withdrawing Life Prolonging Medical Treatment," expresses the view that nutrition and hydration are medical treatments that can be "withheld from a patient in an irreversible coma even when death is not imminent." However, guidelines issued by the American Nurses Association (ANA) Committee on Ethics in 1988 state there are few instances in which it is morally permissible for nurses to withhold or withdraw food and/or fluid from persons in their care (Kelly, 1992).

The natural death laws seek to preserve the notion of voluntary versus involuntary euthanasia. In *voluntary euthanasia*, the competent adult client and a physician, nurse, or both, or an adult friend or relative make the decision to terminate life. *Involuntary euthanasia*, or "mercy killing" is performed without the client's consent (Kelly 1992). In a setting that offers many complex and technologic interventions, it is not likely that the ethical aspects of euthanasia will soon be resolved. However, through the use of advance directives, clients are now taking a much more active role in decisions regarding their own care.

Advance Directives

A general discussion of the terminology involved in advance directive documents is presented here. For an in-depth treatment of this topic, consult a text on ethics and/or legal issues in health care.

Advance directives are legal documents that allow a person to plan for the management of health care and/or financial affairs in the event of incapacity. A **durable power of attorney for health care** (or *health care proxy*) is a legal document written by a competent adult empowering another competent adult to make health care decisions on his or her behalf in the event of incapacitation. The legal authority is limited to decisions about health care. A **living will** is a legal document that formally expresses a person's wishes regarding life-sustaining treatment in the event of terminal illness or permanent unconsciousness (Figure 11–3). It is not a type of durable power of attorney and usually does not designate a substitute decision maker (Singleton et al., 1992).

Although all 50 states have legislation in place recognizing durable power of attorney for health care, only 43 states have living will legislation, and there is no continu-

Applying Research to Nursing Practice: Clarifying Advance Directives

■ ■ ■

In accordance with the Patient Self-Determination Act (PSDA), passed in 1990, all health care institutions that receive any government funding are required to have written policies and procedures concerning the formulation and execution of advance directives. The PSDA requires institutions to ask clients upon admission whether they have an advance directive already prepared and then to provide them with information regarding advance directives, including any applicable state laws and the institution's policies. Public education is a major responsibility defined in the PSDA.

One study (Elpern et al., 1993) reported on the overall knowledge level of and attitudes toward the use of advance directives in planning care for both inpatients and outpatients. The results of the study indicated that of the subjects 77% were familiar with the terms of living will or durable power of attorney for health care, but only about half (52%) understood the true purpose of these forms; moreover, fewer than one-third (29%) had actually prepared an advance directive. Major reasons cited as barriers to completing advance directives included unfamiliarity, misconceptions regarding the purpose of these documents, and procrastination. The majority of the subjects in this study (83%) indicated that they would be comfortable discussing advance directives with their physician or nurse, and 81% would prefer to have their family members also involved. The outpatient setting was the preferred site to receive information. The data for this study was collected before the PSDA was enacted, so it may be expected that a greater number of people are now familiar with advance directives. The need for explanation and client advocacy still exists.

Implications for Nursing

By explaining the purpose and use of advance directives, nurses can act as client advocates to promote client participation in medical decisions. Nurses should clarify written materials, providing explanations in simple terms, and address the client's questions and concerns. This study showed that clients prefer face-to-face discussions with either a physician or a nurse, who should offer to include clients' support systems (family members, significant others) in these discussions.

Critical Thinking in Client Care

1. Which factors may influence clients to prepare an advance directive?

2. What members of the health care team should be included in a discussion about end-of-life decisions?

3. What are the responsibilities of the hospital to ensure that clients receive accurate and compassionate information regarding advance directives?

4. What are some possible reasons that health care providers may hesitate to discuss end-of-life decisions with their clients?

---

ity among these documents from state to state. To further complicate the situation, no state has been able to define the terms *terminal* or *permanently unconscious* to allow for the removal of life-sustaining treatment without going to court for an evidentiary hearing (Singleton et al., 1992). Thus it still often falls to the health care team to interpret the statute.

It is the responsibility of the nurse as client advocate to request and record the client's preference for care and include it in the plan of care. The nurse's documentation of the specific measures acceptable to the client helps communicate these preferences to the other members of the multidisciplinary health care team.

As of December 1991, all facilities that receive Medicare and Medicaid funds are required to provide to all clients written information and counseling regarding advance directives and the institution's policies governing them. The specific terms of this requirement are found in the *Patient Self-Determination Act (PSDA)*. A copy of the signed advance directive must be kept in the client's medical record. Clients do not, however, have to sign an advance directive to be treated at any facility.

Nursing plays a vital role in the successful implementation of this statute (Weber, 1993). The accompanying research box discusses some nursing implications of the Patient Self-Determination Act. In addition, to minimize problems inherent in complying with this legislation, as well as to ensure that clients and their surrogates are aware of their choices, nurses need to

■ Participate in formulating advance directives.

■ Assist in the process of determining client's competence when there is reason to doubt it.

■ Ensure that the client and family have sufficient information on the state statute and the PSDA itself to make any desired decision.

- Recognize that not all clients are ready to formulate decisions.

- Be prepared to act on the client's behalf if necessary.

- Recognize the emotional states of the client's family and help them come to terms with the client's advance directive formulated as a result of the PSDA.

- Ensure that agency administration has provided detailed policy and procedures, as well as thorough and comprehensive education of the people enforcing the statute.

- Facilitate discussions so that the clients and their families recognize that they are involved in a decision-making process, not a death-producing process.

- Ensure that formative, summative, and ongoing evaluation prodedures are in place for implementing and enforcing the PSDA.

- Serve and be active on ethics committees.

- Ensure that no client is discriminated against regarding type or quality of health care for any reason.

- Ensure that whatever the client's decision, it was not coerced—decisions must be strictly voluntary and must reflect the individual's values, desires, and wishes (Weber, 1993).

In all cases, nurses are the ones in intimate contact with clients and are often left with unresolved feelings about the moral, ethical, and legal aspects of their actions. Nurses may agonize for a lifetime over "If only I had known . . ." decisions. Dysfunctional grieving is thus a diagnosis that is not exclusive to clients. Although they do not ease the pain of seeing clients die, advance directives do help nurses to provide clients with a measure of control over the final act of dying.

Applying the Nursing Process

Case Study of a Client Experiencing Grief: Pearl Rogers

Pearl Rogers is a 79-year-old African-American female who is admitted to the Methodist Home Nursing Center. Mrs. Rogers lived with her husband of 58 years until his death 9 months ago. She had one son who died in an auto accident 2 years ago, and she has one daughter who lives nearby. After her husband's death, Mrs. Rogers lived with her daughter until her admission to the Nursing Center. Mrs. Rogers has become increasingly agitated and helpless, complaining constantly of pain. Her daughter states that Mrs. Rogers is chronically constipated, has difficulty sleeping, and has stopped engaging in all social activities, including weekly church services. She cries frequently.

Extensive medical testing prior to her admission to the Nursing Center revealed Mrs. Rogers has arthritis but no other pathologic disorder.

Assessment

When Mrs. Rogers arrives at the Nursing Center, she is admitted by her case manager, Sandy Sutphin. Mrs. Rogers tells Ms. Sutphin, "I'm a sick woman, and no one will listen to me! I can't walk, I'm so weak. My head hurts, and I'm always sick at my stomach. I haven't had a bowel movement in a week, and I never sleep more than 3 hours a night." Ms. Sutphin completes an assessment and finds that Mrs. Rogers has no significant physical problems except impaired mobility related to arthritis.

Diagnoses

Ms. Sutphin makes the following nursing diagnoses for Mrs. Rogers:

- *Dysfunctional Grieving* related to stress of husband's death

- *Sleep Pattern Disturbance* related to grieving

- *Constipation* related to inactivity

Expected Outcomes

The expected outcomes established in the plan of care specify that Mrs. Rogers will

- Engage in normal grief work: work through grief process, discuss reality of losses, use nondestructive coping mechanisms, and discuss positive and negative aspects of the loss.

- Experience adequate and restful sleep: fall asleep 20 to 30 minutes after retiring and awaken feeling rested after 7 to 8 hours of sleep.

- Have a bowel movement with soft formed stools at least every other day.

Planning and Implementation

The following interventions are planned and implemented during care of Mrs. Rogers:

Dysfunctional Grieving Related to Stress of Husband's Death

- Promote trust: Show empathy and caring, demonstrate respect for her culture and values, offer support and reassurance, be honest, engage in active listening.

- During one-to-one interactions, encourage Mrs. Rogers to recognize normal grieving behavior. Assist her in labeling her feelings: anger, fear, loneliness, guilt, isolation.

- Explore previous losses and the ways in which the client has coped.

- Discourage the use of drugs to blunt feelings.
- Encourage Mrs. Rogers to express her feelings of anger. Do not become defensive, and explain to her family that anger helps her feel as though she has some control over her environment, even though she has no control over her loss.
- Encourage Mrs. Rogers to review her relationship with her dead husband.
- Reinforce expressions of behaviors associated with normal grieving.
- Foster an environment in which loss can be placed in a spiritual context: discuss beliefs, philosophy, values; encourage Mrs. Rogers to participate in her spiritual practices.
- Encourage Mrs. Rogers to participate in a grief group that meets at the facility.

Sleep Pattern Disturbance Related to Grief

- Assess Mrs. Rogers' sleep pattern before her husband's death by communicating with her and her daughter.
- Consult with the physical and recreational therapist to help the nursing staff provide afternoon activities for Mrs. Rogers.
- Provide evening care: warm sponge bath; clean, warm bed; night-light; soft music for relaxation; closed door.

Constipation Related to Inactivity

- Provide measures that assist in bowel evacuation: encourage exercise as tolerated, including walks and rocking in a rocking chair. Offer foods that stimulate bowel movements. Offer privacy: Close the door, ensuring that the emergency call bell is within reach, and do not interrupt. Assure Mrs. Rogers that a nurse will be there to help her clean herself if she needs one, and have toilet paper, soap, warm water, and a cloth available to promote her dignity.
- Administer a mild laxative and/or stool softener to Mrs. Rogers, if necessary, but discontinue as soon as possible.

Evaluation

After 4 weeks at the Nursing Center, Mrs. Rogers states, "I don't feel any better, but I know I have to accept my situation." Although Mrs. Rogers states that she doesn't feel better, Ms. Sutphin reports that she is walking the length of the hall, sleeping better, and having regular bowel movements. Mrs. Rogers is also less withdrawn and has openly discussed her feelings related to her husband's death, including her anger at the loss of her son and her husband less than 2 years apart. She has attended the grief group once and has attended chapel services on Sunday for the past 2 weeks. She plays bridge with the other residents 2 or 3 afternoons a week. Her daughter visits her each Saturday and takes her in a wheelchair to the shopping mall.

Critical Thinking in the Nursing Process

1. What common physical manifestations of grief did Mrs. Rogers experience?
2. Write a nursing care plan for Mrs. Rogers for the diagnosis *Social Isolation*.
3. How might Ms. Sutphin involve Mrs. Rogers's daughter in developing and implementing her mother's plan of care?
4. Suppose Mrs. Rogers told Ms. Sutphin that she did not want any help, that she just wanted to be left alone to die. If you were Ms. Sutphin, how would you respond?
5. In addition to the loss of her husband, what other losses has Mrs. Rogers suffered in recent years? How might these multiple losses have affected her grief process?

Bibliography

■ ■ ■

Aerwekh, J. (1994). The truth-tellers: How hospice nurses help patients confront death. *American Journal of Nursing, 94*(2), 30–34.

American Nurses Association. (1976). *Code for nurses.* (1976). Kansas City, MO: ANA.

American Psychiatric Association. (1994). *Diagnostic and statistical manual of mental disorders (DSM-IV™)* Washington, DC: American Psychiatric Association.

Badger, J. (1994). Calming the anxious patient. *American Journal of Nursing, 94*(5), 46–50.

Baumer, J., Wadsworth, J., and Taylor, B. (1988). Family recovery after the death of a child. *Archives of Disease in Childhood, 63,* 942.

Bloom-Feshbach, J., et al. (1987). *The psychology of separation and loss.* San Francisco: Jossey-Bass.

Bowlby, J. (1973). *Attachment and loss: Vol. 2. Separation, anxiety, and anger.* New York: Basic Books.

———(1980). *Attachment and loss: Vol 3. Loss, sadness, and depression.* New York: Basic Books.

Browning, M., and Lewis, E. (1972). *The dying patient: A nursing perspective.* New York: American Journal of Nursing.

Buck, M. (1991). The physical self. In C. Roy and H. Andrews (Eds.). *The Roy Adaptation Model: The definitive statement.* Norwalk, CT: Appleton & Lange.

Bugen, L. (1977). Human grief: A model for prediction and intervention. *American Journal of Orthopsychiatry, 46*(2), 196.

Caplan, G. (1990). Loss, stress, and mental health. *Community Mental Health Journal, 26*(1), 27.

Carpenito, L. (1993). *Nursing diagnosis: Application to clinical practice* (5th ed.). Philadelphia: Lippincott.

Carter, S. (1989). Themes of grief. *Nursing Research, 36*(6), 354.

Castles, M., and Murray, R. (1979). *Dying in an institution: Nurse/patient perspectives.* New York: Appleton-Century-Crofts.

Cody, W. (1991). Grieving a personal loss. *Nursing Science Quarterly, 4*(2), 61.

Collison, C., and Miller, S. (1987). Using images of the future in grief work. *Image: Journal of Nursing Scholarship, 19*(1), 9.

Demi, A. and Miles, M. (1986). Bereavement. *Annual Review of Nursing Research, 4,* 115.

Edwards, B. (1994). When the family can't let go. *American Journal of Nursing, 94*(1), 52–56.

Elpern, E. H., Yellen, S. B., & Burton, L. A. (1993). A preliminary investigation of opinions and behaviors regarding advance directives for medical care. *American Journal of Critical Care, 2*(2), 161–167.

Engel, G. (1964). Grief and grieving. *American Journal of Nursing, 64,* 93.

Epstein, C. (1975). *Nursing the dying patient.* Reston, VA: Reston Publishing.

Freud, S. (1917, 1957). Mourning and melancholia. In J. Strachey & A. Tyson (Eds.). *The complete psychological works of Sigmund Freud* (Vol. 14). London: Hogarth Press.

Furman, E. (1985). Children's patterns in mourning the death of a loved one. *Issues in Comprehensive Pediatric Nursing, 8*(6), 185.

Gifford, B., & Cleary, B. (1990). Supporting the bereaved. *American Journal of Nursing, 90*(2), 49.

Glaser, B. and Strauss, A. (1965). *Awareness of dying.* Chicago: Aldine Publishing.

Gordon, M. (1991). *Manual of nursing diagnosis 1991–1992.* St Louis: Mosby-Year Book.

Granstrom, S. (1985). Spiritual nursing care for oncology patients. *Topics in Clinical Nursing, 7*(1), 39.

Grubb-Phillips, C. (1988). Intrauterine fetal death: The maternal bereavement experience. *Journal of Perinatal Neonatal Nursing, 2*(2), 34.

Gullo, S., and Church, S. (1988). *Loveshock.* New York: Simon and Schuster.

Horsley, G. (1988). Baggage from the past. *American Journal of Nursing 88,* 60.

Kavanaugh, R. (1972). *Facing death.* Kingsport, TN: Kingsport Press, Inc.

Kelly, L. (1992). *The nursing experience: Trends, challenges, and transitions.* New York: McGraw-Hill.

Kim, M., McFarland, G., and McLane, A. (1991). *Pocket guide to nursing diagnoses* (3rd ed.). St Louis: Mosby-Year Book.

Kneisl, C., and Pheifer, W. (1992). HIV/AIDS: A mental health challenge. In H. Wilson & H. Kneisl, (Eds.). *Psychiatric nursing.* Redwood City, CA: Addison-Wesley Nursing.

Kozier, B., Erb, G., Blais, K., & Wilkinson, J. (1995). *Fundamentals of nursing: Concepts, process, and practice* (5th. ed.). Redwood City, CA: Addison-Wesley Nursing.

Kübler-Ross, E. (1969). *On death and dying.* New York: Macmillan.

———(1978). *To live until we say goodbye.* Englewood Cliffs, NJ: Prentice-Hall.

Lake, M., et al. (1987). Evaluation of a perinatal grief support team. *American Journal of Obstetrics and Gynecology, 157*(5), 1203.

Lambert, V., and Lambert, C. (1985). *Psychosocial care of the physically ill* (2nd ed.). Englewood Cliffs, NJ: Prentice Hall.

Landrum, P., Rawlins, R., Beck, C., and Williams, S. (1988). The person as a client. In C. Beck, R. Rawlins, & S. Williams, (Eds.). *Mental health—Psychiatric nursing.* (2nd. ed.). St Louis: Mosby.

Lewis, C. (1961). *A grief observed.* New York: Seabury Press.

Lindemann, E. (1944). Symptomatology and management of acute grief. *American Journal of Psychiatry, 32,* 141.

McFarland, G. and Gerety, E. (1989). Grieving, anticipatory. In M. Kim, G. McFarland, & A. McLane (Eds.), *Pocket guide to nursing diagnosis* (3rd. ed.). St Louis: Mosby.

McFarland, G., and Wasli, E. (1986). *Nursing diagnosis and process in psychiatric mental health nursing.* Philadelphia: Lippincott.

Melges, F. (1982). *Time and the inner future.* New York: Wiley.

Mishkin, B. (1985). *Decisions in Hospice.* Arlington, VA: National Hospice Organization.

Morris, D. (1988). Management of perinatal bereavement. *Archives of Disease in Childhood, 63,* 870.

Murray, R. and Zentner, J. (1985). Crisis intervention: A therapy technique. In *Nursing Concepts for Health Promotion* (3rd. ed.). Englewood Cliffs, NJ: Prentice Hall.

Neeld, E. (1990). *Seven choices: Taking the steps to new life after losing someone you love.* New York: Clarkson N. Potter.

Newman, A. (1993). Loss. In Rawlins, R., Williams, S., and Beck, C. *Mental health-psychiatric nursing.* (3rd. ed.). St Louis: Mosby.

North American Nursing Diagnosis Association. (1992). *NANDA nursing diagnosis: Definitions and classification 1992–1993.* Philadelphia: NANDA.

Null, S. (1989). Nursing care to ease parents' grief. *Maternal Child Nursing, 14,* 84.

Oerlemans-Bunn, M. (1988). On being gay, single, and bereaved. *American Journal of Nursing, 80*(4), 472.

Paquette, M., Neal, M., and Rodemich, C. (1991). *Psychiatric nursing diagnosis care plans for DSM-III-R.* Boston: Jones and Bartlett.

Parks, R. (1972). *Bereavement: Studies of grief in adult life.* London: Tavistock.

Polanyi, M. (1967). *The tacit dimension.* Garden City, NY: Anchor Books.

Reed, P. (1991). Preferences for spiritually related nursing interventions among terminally ill and nonterminally ill hospitalized adults and well adults. *Applied Nursing Research, 4*(3), 122.

Shipes, E. (1987). Sexual functioning following ostomy surgery. *Nursing Clinics of North America, 22*(2), 303.

Singleton, K., Dever, R., & Donner, T. (1992). Durable power of attorney: Nursing implications. *Dimensions of Critical Care Nursing, 11*(1), 41.

Stewart, R. and Eoyang, T. (1988). Grieving. In B. Kozier & G. Erb (Eds.). *Concepts and issues in nursing practice.* Menlo Park, CA: Addison-Wesley Nursing.

Strother, A. (1991). Drawing the line between life and death. *American Journal of Nursing, 91*(4), 24.

Taptich, B., Iyer, P., & Bernocchi-Losey, D. (1994). *Nursing diagnosis and care planning.* (2nd ed.). Philadelphia: Saunders.

Weber, G. (1993). Tips on implementing the Patient Self-Determination Act. *Nursing and Health Care, 14*(2), 86.

Worden, W. (1982). *Grief counseling and grief therapy,* New York: Springer.

Zlsook, S. (1987). *Biophysical aspects of bereavement.* Washington, DC: American Psychiatric Press.

Nutrition and
Metabolic Patterns

Responses to Altered Nutrition

Assessing Clients with Nutritional Disorders

LEARNING OBJECTIVES

After completing this chapter, you will be able to

- Identify the major structures and functions of the mouth, esophagus, stomach, small intestine, liver, gallbladder, and pancreas.
- Describe the processes of carbohydrate, fat, and protein metabolism.
- Describe the functions and sources of nutrients and vitamins.

- Identify interview questions pertinent to assessment of the gastrointestinal tract, the accessory digestive organs, and nutritional status.
- Describe physical assessment techniques used to evaluate digestion and nutritional status.
- Identify manifestations of impairment in gastrointestinal function.
- Describe variations in assessment findings for the older adult.

Nutrition is the process by which the body ingests, absorbs, transports, uses, and eliminates food. The digestive organs that are responsible for these processes are the gastrointestinal tract (also called the alimentary canal) and the accessory digestive organs. The *gastrointestinal tract* consists of the mouth, pharynx, esophagus, stomach, small intestine, and large intestine; the *accessory digestive organs* include the liver, gallbladder, and pancreas (Figure 12–1). This chapter discusses the assessment of all of these organs except the large intestine. Assessment of the large intestine, which is primarily responsible for elimination, is discussed in Chapter 22.

Review of Anatomy and Physiology

■ ■ ■

The Gastrointestinal Tract

The gastrointestinal (GI) tract is a continuous hollow tube. Once foods are ingested into the mouth, they are subjected to a variety of processes that move them and break them down into end products that can be absorbed from the lumen of the small intestine into the blood or lymph. These digestive processes comprise the following:

- The ingestion of food
- The movement of food and wastes
- Secretion of mucus, water, and enzymes
- Mechanical digestion of food
- Chemical digestion of food
- Absorption of digested food

Mouth

The *mouth,* also called the *oral* or *buccal cavity,* is a cavity lined by mucous membranes that is enclosed in front by the lips, on the sides by the cheeks, on top by the palate, and on the bottom by the tongue (Figure 12–2).

The *lips* and *cheeks* are made up of skeletal muscle and are covered externally by skin. Their function in the digestive process is to keep food in the mouth during chewing. The lips have a margin where skin and mucous mem-

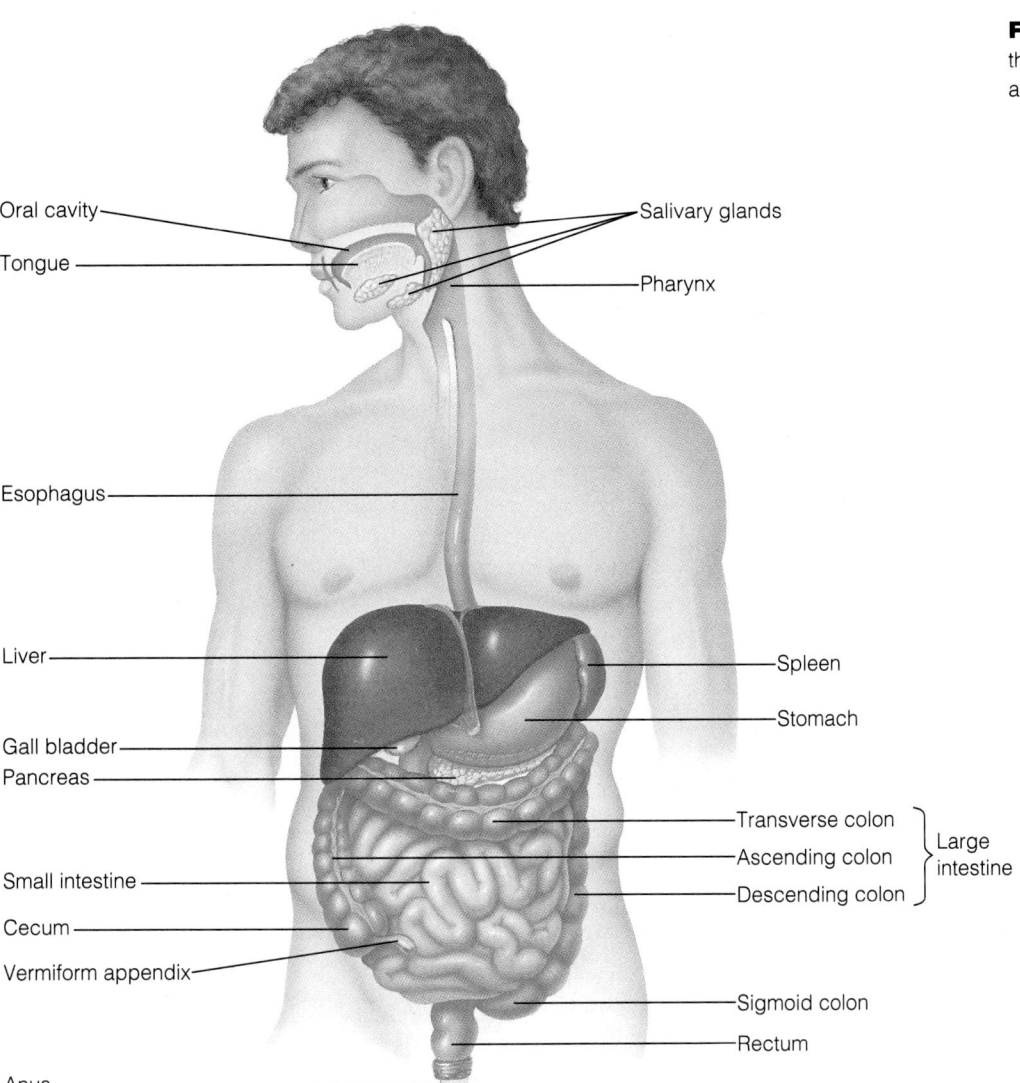

Figure 12–1 Organs of the gastrointestinal tract and accessory digestive organs.

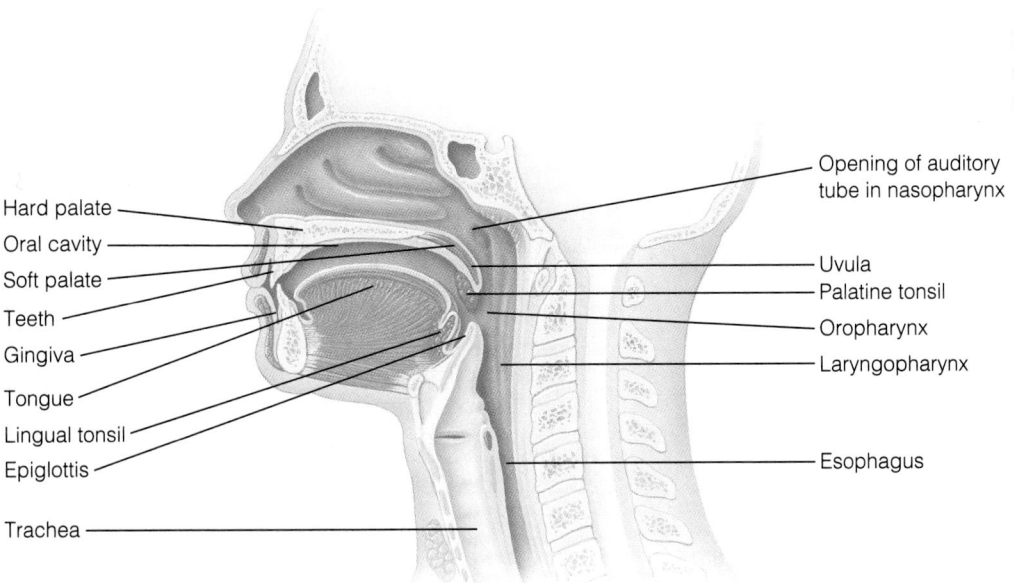

Figure 12–2 Structures of the mouth, the pharynx, and the esophagus.

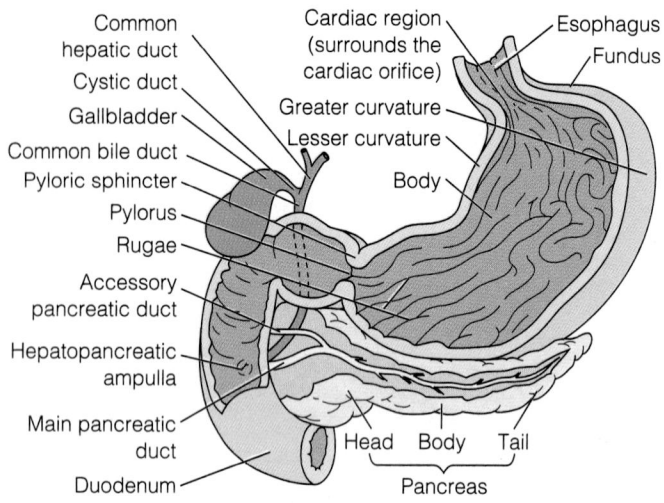

Figure 12–3 The internal anatomic structures of the stomach, including the pancreatic, cystic, and hepatic ducts, the pancreas, and the gallbladder.

brane meet; this area does not contain sweat or sebaceous glands and is prone to drying and cracking unless moistened with saliva.

The *palate* is composed of two regions: the hard palate and the soft palate. The *hard palate* covers bone and provides a hard surface against which the tongue forces food. The *soft palate* is made up primarily of muscle and ends at the back of the mouth as a fold called the *uvula*. When food is swallowed, the soft palate rises as a reflex to close off the oropharynx.

The *tongue,* which is composed of skeletal muscle and connective tissue, is located in the floor of the mouth. The tongue contains mucous and serous glands, taste buds, and papillae. The tongue mixes food with saliva during chewing, forms the food into a mass (called a *bolus*), and initiates swallowing. Some papillae provide surface roughness to facilitate licking and moving food; other papillae house the taste buds.

Saliva moistens food so it can be made into a bolus, dissolves food chemicals so they can be tasted, and provides enzymes (such as *amylase*) that begin the chemical breakdown of starches. Saliva is produced by salivary glands, most of which lie superior or inferior to the mouth and drain into it. The salivary glands include the parotid, the submaxillary, and the sublingual glands.

The *teeth* chew (*masticate*) and grind food to break it down into smaller parts. As the food is masticated, it is mixed with saliva. Adults have 32 permanent teeth. The teeth are embedded in the *gingiva* (gums), with the crown of each tooth visible above the gingiva.

Pharynx

The *pharynx* is made up of the *oropharynx* and the *laryngopharynx* (see Figure 12–2). Both of these structures provide passageways for food, fluids, and air. The pharynx is made of skeletal muscles and is lined with mucous membranes. The skeletal muscles move food to the esophagus via the pharynx through **peristalsis**, alternating waves of contraction and relaxation of involuntary muscle. The mucosa of the pharynx contains mucus-producing glands that provide fluid to facilitate the passage of the bolus of food as it is swallowed.

Esophagus

The *esophagus,* a muscular tube about 10 in. (25 cm) long, serves as a passageway for food from the pharynx to the stomach (see Figures 12–1 and 12–2). The *epiglottis,* a flap of cartilage over the top of the larynx, keeps food out of the larynx during swallowing. The esophagus descends through the thorax and diaphragm, entering the stomach at the *cardiac orifice.* This opening is surrounded by the *gastroesophageal sphincter.* This sphincter, along with the diaphragm, keeps the orifice closed when food is not being swallowed.

For most of its length, the esophagus is lined with stratified squamous epithelium; simple columnar epithelium lines the esophagus where it joins the stomach. The mucosa and submucosa of the esophagus lie in longitudinal folds when the esophagus is empty.

Stomach

The *stomach,* located high on the left side of the abdominal cavity, is connected to the esophagus at the upper end and to the small intestine at the lower end (Figure 12–3). Normally about 10 in. (25 cm) long, the stomach is a distensible organ that can expand to hold up to 4 L of food and fluid. The concave surface of the stomach is called the *lesser curvature;* the convex surface is called the *greater curvature.* The stomach may be divided into regions extending from the esophagus to the small intestine; as shown in Figure 12–3, these are the *cardiac region,* the *fundus,* the *body,* and the *pylorus.* The *pyloric sphincter* controls emptying of the stomach into the duodenal portion of the small intestine. The stomach is a storage reservoir for food, continues the mechanical breakdown of food, begins the process of protein digestion, and mixes the food with gastric juices into a thick fluid called **chyme.**

The stomach is lined with columnar epithelial, mucus-producing cells. This lining has millions of openings leading to gastric glands that produce up to 4 to 5 L of gastric juice each day. The gastric glands contain a variety of secretory cells, including the following:

- *Mucous cells,* which produce an alkaline mucus that clings to the lining of the stomach and provides protection from gastric juice.

- *Zymogenic cells,* which produce pepsinogen (an inactive form of pepsin, a protein-digesting enzyme).

- *Parietal cells,* which secrete hydrochloric acid and intrinsic factor. Hydrochloric acid activates and increases the activity of protein-digesting cells and also is bactericidal. Intrinsic factor is necessary for the absorption of vitamin B_{12} in the small intestine.
- *Enteroendocrine cells,* which secrete gastrin, histamine, endorphins, serotonin, and somatostatin. These hormones or hormonelike substances diffuse into the blood. Of these substances, gastrin is important in regulating secretion and motility of the stomach.

The secretion of gastric juice is under both neural and endocrine control. Stimulation of the parasympathetic vagus nerve increases secretory activity; in contrast, stimulation of sympathetic nerves decreases secretions. The three phases of secretory activity are the cephalic phase, the gastric phase, and the intestinal phase:

- The *cephalic* phase serves as a preparation for digestion and is triggered by the sight, odor, taste, or thought of food. During this initial phase, motor impulses are transmitted via the vagus nerve to the stomach.
- The *gastric phase* begins when food enters the stomach. This phase is initiated by both stomach distention (stimulating stretch receptors) and chemical stimuli from partially digested proteins. Gastrin-secreting cells are stimulated to produce gastrin, which in turn stimulates the gastric glands (especially the parietal cells) to produce more gastric juice. Histamine also stimulates hydrochloric acid secretion.
- The *intestinal phase* is initiated when partially digested food begins to enter the small intestine, stimulating mucous cells of the intestine to release a hormone that promotes continued gastric secretion.

Mechanical digestion is also a function of the stomach. This is accomplished by peristaltic movements that churn and mix the food with the gastric juices to form chyme. Gastric motility is enhanced or retarded by the same factors that affect secretion, namely, distention and the effect of gastrin. After a person eats a normal, well-balanced meal, the stomach empties completely in approximately 4 to 6 hours.

Small Intestine

The *small intestine* begins at the pyloric sphincter and ends at the *ileocecal junction* at the entrance of the large intestine (see Figure 12–1). The small intestine is about 20 ft (6 m) long but only about 1 in. (2.5 cm) in diameter. This long tube hangs in coils in the abdominal cavity, suspended by the mesentery and surrounded by the large intestine. The small intestine has three regions: the duodenum, the jejunum, and the ileum. The *duodenum* begins at the pyloric sphincter and extends around the head of the pancreas for about 10 in. (25 cm). Both pancreatic enzymes and bile from the liver enter the small intestine at

the duodenum. The *jejunum* is the middle region of the small intestine. It extends for about 8 ft (2.4 m). The *ileum,* which is the terminal end of the small intestine, is approximately 12 ft (3.6 m) long and meets the large intestine at the ileocecal valve.

Food is chemically digested, and most of it absorbed, as it moves through the small intestine. Microvilli (tiny projections of the mucosa cells), villi (fingerlike-projections of the mucosa cells), and circular folds (deep folds of the mucosa and submucosa layers) all increase the surface area of the small intestine to enhance absorption of food. Although up to 10 L of food, liquids, and secretions enter the GI tract each day, less than 1 L reaches the large intestine.

Enzymes in the small intestine break down carbohydrates, proteins, lipids, and nucleic acids. Pancreatic amylase acts on starches, converting them to maltose, dextrins, and oligosaccharides; these products are further broken down into monosaccharides by the intestinal enzymes dextrinase, glucoamylase, maltase, sucrase, and lactase. Proteins continue to be broken down into peptides by pancreatic enzymes (trypsin and chymotrypsin) and by intestinal enzymes. Lipids are digested in the small intestine as a result of the actions of the pancreatic lipases. Triglycerides enter as fat globules and are coated by bile salts and emulsified. Nucleic acids are hydrolyzed by pancreatic enzymes and then broken apart by intestinal enzymes. Both pancreatic enzymes and bile are excreted into the duodenum in response to the secretion of secretin and cholecystokinin, which are hormones produced by the intestinal mucosa cells when chyme enters the small intestine.

Nutrients are absorbed through the mucosa of the intestinal villi into the blood or lymph by active transport, facilitated transport, and passive diffusion. Almost all food products and water, as well as vitamins and most electrolytes, are absorbed in the small intestine, leaving only indigestible fibers, some water, and bacteria to enter the large intestine.

The Accessory Digestive Organs

Liver and Gallbladder

The *liver* is the largest gland in the body, weighing about 3 lb (1.4 kg) in the average-sized adult. The liver is located in the right side of the abdomen, inferior to the diaphragm and anterior to the stomach (Figure 12–1). The liver has four lobes: right, left, caudate, and quadrate. A mesentery ligament separates the right and left lobes and suspends the liver from the diaphragm and anterior abdominal wall. The liver is encased in a fibroelastic capsule.

Liver tissue is made up of units called lobules, which are composed of plates of *hepatocytes* (liver cells). Communicating with each lobule are a branch of the hepatic artery, a branch of the hepatic portal vein, and a bile duct.

Sinusoids, which are blood-filled spaces within the lobules, are lined with Kupffer cells. These phagocytic cells remove debris from the blood.

The liver performs many different functions essential to life. For example, it

- Secretes bile.
- Stores fat-soluble vitamins (A, E, D, and K).
- Metabolizes bilirubin.
- Stores blood and releases blood during hemorrhage.
- Synthesizes plasma proteins to maintain plasma oncotic pressure.
- Synthesizes prothrombin, fibrinogen, and factors I, II, VII, IX, and X, which are necessary for blood clotting.
- Synthesizes fats from carbohydrates and proteins to be either used for energy or stored as adipose tissue.
- Synthesizes phospholipids and cholesterol necessary for the production of bile salts, steroid hormones, and plasma membranes.
- Converts amino acids to carbohydrates through deamination.
- Releases glucose during times of hypoglycemia.
- Takes up glucose during times of hyperglycemia and stores it as glycogen or converts it to fat.
- Alters chemicals, foreign molecules, and hormones to make them less toxic.
- Stores copper and releases it as needed.
- Stores iron as ferritin, which is released as needed for the production of red blood cells.

Of these various functions, the liver's digestive function is to produce bile. **Bile** is a greenish, watery solution containing bile salts, cholesterol, bilirubin, electrolytes, water, and phospholipids. These substances are necessary to emulsify and promote the absorption of fats. Liver cells make from 700 to 1200 mL of bile every day. When bile is not needed for digestion, the *sphincter of Oddi* (located at the point at which bile enters the duodenum) is closed, and the bile backs up the cystic duct into the gallbladder for storage.

Bile is concentrated and stored in the *gallbladder,* a small sac cupped in the inferior surface of the liver. When food containing fats enters the duodenum, hormones stimulate the gallbladder to secrete bile into the cystic duct. The cystic duct joins the hepatic duct to form the common bile duct, from which bile enters into the duodenum (Figure 12–3).

Pancreas

The *pancreas,* a gland located between the stomach and small intestine, is the primary enzyme-producing organ of the digestive system. It is a triangular gland extending across the abdomen, with its tail next to the spleen and its head next to the duodenum (see Figure 12–3). The body and tail of the pancreas are retroperitoneal, lying behind the greater curvature of the stomach. The pancreas is actually two organs in one, having both exocrine and endocrine structures and functions. The exocrine portion of the pancreas, through secretory units called *acini,* secretes alkaline pancreatic juice containing many different enzymes. The acini, which are clusters of secretory cells surrounding ducts, drain into the pancreatic duct. The pancreatic duct joins with the common bile duct just before it enters the duodenum (so that pancreatic juice and bile from the liver enter the small intestine together). The pancreas also has endocrine functions (see Chapter 19).

The pancreas produces from 1 to 1.5 L of pancreatic juice every day. Pancreatic juice is clear and has a high bicarbonate content. This alkaline fluid neutralizes the acidic chyme as it enters the duodenum, facilitating a pH that is optimal for intestinal and pancreatic enzyme activity in the small intestine. The secretion of pancreatic juice is controlled by the vagus nerve and the effect of the intestinal hormones secretin and cholecystokinin. Pancreatic juice contains enzymes that can digest all categories of foods: Lipase promotes fat breakdown and absorption; amylase completes starch digestion; and trypsin, chymotrypsin, and carboxypeptidase are responsible for half of all protein digestion. Also present in pancreatic juice are nucleases, which digest nucleic acids.

Metabolism

After nutrients (carbohydrates, fats, and proteins) are ingested, digested, absorbed, and transported across cell membranes, they must be metabolized in order to produce and provide energy to maintain life. **Metabolism** is the complex of biochemical reactions occurring in the body's cells. Metabolic processes are either catabolic or anabolic. **Catabolism** involves the breakdown of complex structures into simpler forms. An example is the breakdown of carbohydrates to produce *adenosine triphosphate (ATP),* an energy molecule that fuels cellular activity. **Anabolism** is a process by which simpler molecules combine to build more complex structures, for example, the bonding of amino acids to form proteins.

The biochemical reactions of metabolism produce water, carbon dioxide, and ATP. Food provides the raw materials for metabolic fuels, whereas ATP mobilizes these fuels for use by cells. The energy value of foods is measured in kilocalories (kcal). A *kilocalorie* is defined as the amount of heat energy needed to raise the temperature of 1 kilogram (kg) of water 1 degree centigrade.

Nutrients

Nutrients are substances in food that are used by the body to promote growth, maintenance, and repair. The categories of nutrients are carbohydrates, proteins, fats, vitamins, minerals, and water.

Carbohydrates

The primary sources of *carbohydrates* (which include sugars and starches) are plant foods. Monosaccharides and disaccharides come from milk, sugar cane, sugar beets, honey, and fruits. Polysaccharide starch is found in grains, legumes, and root vegetables. Following ingestion, digestion, and metabolism, carbohydrates are converted primarily to glucose, which is the molecule that body cells use to make ATP. Glucose is carefully regulated to maintain cellular functions. Excess glucose in the healthy person is converted to glycogen or fat. Glycogen is stored in the liver and muscles; fat is stored as adipose tissue. Carbohydrate use by the body is shown in Figure 12–4, *A*.

Regardless of source, all carbohydrates supply 4 kcal per gram. The minimum necessary daily carbohydrate intake is unknown, but the recommended daily intake is 125 to 175 g, most of which should be complex carbohydrates (such as milk, potatoes, and whole grains). Excess intake of carbohydrates over time can result in obesity, dental caries, and elevated plasma triglycerides. Over extended periods of time, carbohydrate deficiencies lead to tissue wasting from protein breakdown and metabolic acidosis from an excess of ketones as a by-product of fat breakdown.

Proteins

Proteins are classified as either complete or incomplete. Complete proteins are found in animal products, such as eggs, milk, milk products, and meat. They contain the greatest amount of amino acids and meet the body's amino acid requirements for tissue growth and maintenance. Incomplete proteins are found in legumes, nuts, grains, cereals, and vegetables. These sources are low in or lack one or more of the amino acids essential for building complete proteins.

The body uses proteins to build many different structures, including skin keratin, the collagen and elastin in connective tissues, and muscles. They also are used to make enzymes, hemoglobin, plasma proteins, and some hormones. Protein use by the body is shown in Figure 12–4, *B*.

The recommended intake of protein is 0.8 g per kilogram of body weight. Healthy people with adequate caloric intake have an equal rate of protein synthesis and protein breakdown and loss, reflected as nitrogen balance. If the breakdown and loss of proteins exceeds intake, a negative nitrogen balance results. This may be due to starvation, altered physical states (from injury or illness, for example), and altered emotional states (such as depression or anxiety). A positive nitrogen balance, which results when protein intake exceeds breakdown, is normal during growth, tissue repair, and pregnancy. The rate of protein synthesis is affected by anabolic hormones; for example, the adrenal corticosteroids are released in times of stress to increase protein breakdown and conversion of amino acids to glucose. Excessive intake of proteins may lead to obesity, whereas deficits cause weight loss and tissue wasting, edema, and anemia.

Fats (Lipids)

Fats, also called *lipids,* include phospholipids; steroids, such as cholesterol; and neutral fats, more commonly known as triglycerides. Neutral fats are the most abundant fats in the diet. They may be either saturated or unsaturated. Saturated fats are found in animal products (milk and meats) and in some plant products (such as coconut). Unsaturated fats are found in seeds, nuts, and most vegetable oils. Sources of cholesterol include meats, milk products, and egg yolks. Fat use by the body is shown in Figure 12–4, *C*.

Fats are a necessary part of the structure and function of the body. For example:

- Phospholipids are a part of all cell membranes.
- Triglycerides are the major energy source for hepatocytes and skeletal muscle cells.
- Adipose tissue serves as a protection around body organs, as a layer of insulation under the skin, and as a concentrated source of fuel for cellular energy.
- Dietary fats facilitate absorption of fat-soluble vitamins.
- Linoleic acid, an essential fatty acid, helps form prostaglandins, which are regulatory molecules that assist in smooth muscle contraction, maintenance of blood pressure, and control of inflammatory responses.
- Cholesterol is the essential component of bile salts, steroid hormones, and vitamin D.

The recommended intake of fats is less than 30% of the total daily caloric intake. Saturated fats should account for no more than 10% of the total daily caloric intake, and cholesterol intake should not exceed 250 mg per day. When a person consumes more than the body requires, the excess is stored as adipose tissue, increasing the risk of obesity and heart disease. A deficit of fats may cause excessive weight loss and skin lesions.

Vitamins

Vitamins are organic compounds that facilitate the body's use of carbohydrates, proteins, and fats. All of the vitamins except vitamin D and vitamin K must be ingested in foods or taken as supplements. Vitamin D is made by ultraviolet irradiation of cholesterol molecules in the skin, and vitamin K is synthesized by bacteria in the intestine. Vitamins are categorized as either fat soluble or water soluble. The fat-soluble vitamins (A, D, E, and K) bind to

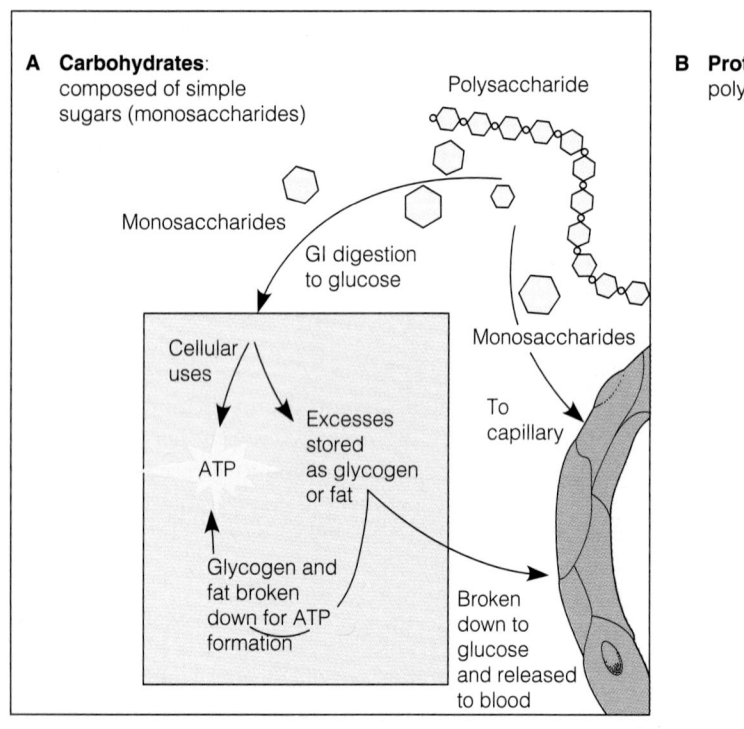

A Carbohydrates: composed of simple sugars (monosaccharides)

Polysaccharide

Monosaccharides

GI digestion to glucose

Monosaccharides

To capillary

Cellular uses

ATP

Excesses stored as glycogen or fat

Glycogen and fat broken down for ATP formation

Broken down to glucose and released to blood

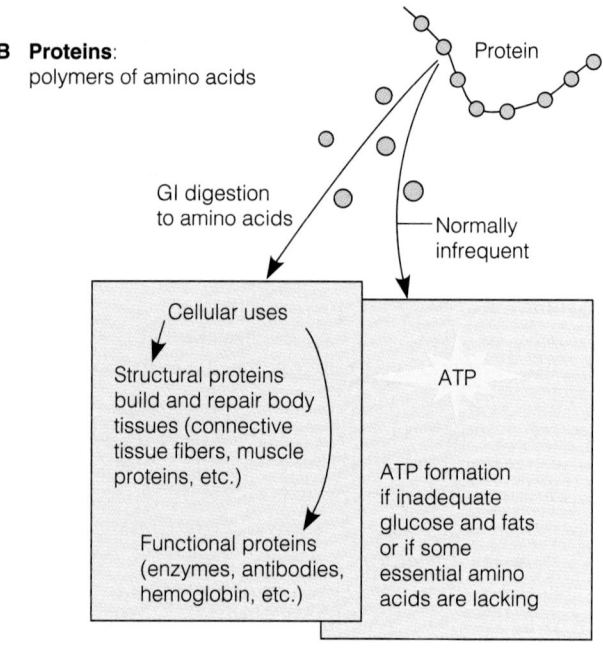

B Proteins: polymers of amino acids

Protein

GI digestion to amino acids

Normally infrequent

Cellular uses

ATP

Structural proteins build and repair body tissues (connective tissue fibers, muscle proteins, etc.)

Functional proteins (enzymes, antibodies, hemoglobin, etc.)

ATP formation if inadequate glucose and fats or if some essential amino acids are lacking

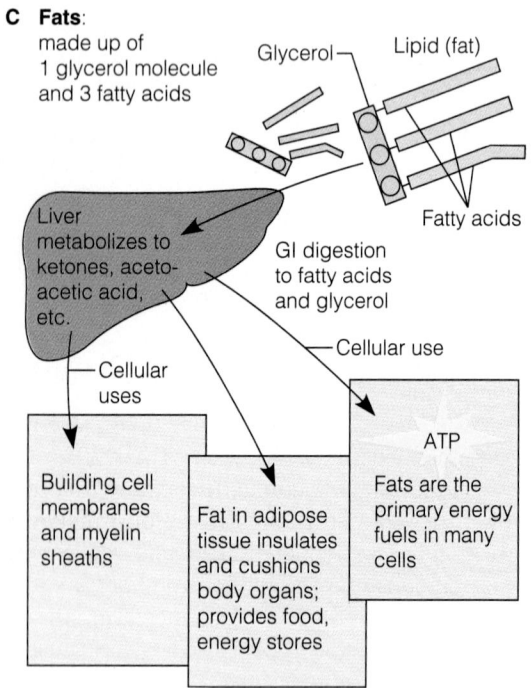

C Fats: made up of 1 glycerol molecule and 3 fatty acids

Glycerol

Lipid (fat)

Fatty acids

Liver metabolizes to ketones, aceto-acetic acid, etc.

GI digestion to fatty acids and glycerol

Cellular use

Cellular uses

ATP

Building cell membranes and myelin sheaths

Fat in adipose tissue insulates and cushions body organs; provides food, energy stores

Fats are the primary energy fuels in many cells

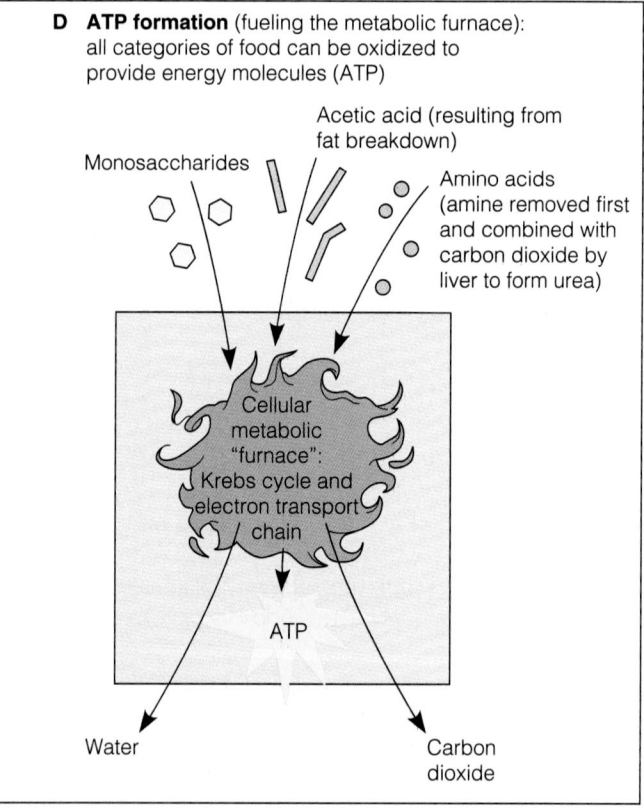

D ATP formation (fueling the metabolic furnace): all categories of food can be oxidized to provide energy molecules (ATP)

Acetic acid (resulting from fat breakdown)

Monosaccharides

Amino acids (amine removed first and combined with carbon dioxide by liver to form urea)

Cellular metabolic "furnace": Krebs cycle and electron transport chain

ATP

Water

Carbon dioxide

Figure 12–4 A schematic overview of nutrient use by body cells, including A, carbohydrates; B, proteins; C, fats; and D, ATP formation.

ingested fats and are absorbed as the fats are absorbed. Water-soluble vitamins (the B complex and C) are absorbed with water in the GI tract (however, vitamin B_{12} must become attached to intrinsic factor to be absorbed). Fat-soluble vitamins are stored in the body, and excesses may cause toxicity; water-soluble vitamins in excess of body requirements are excreted in the urine.

The fat-soluble vitamins are listed below:

- *Vitamin A* (also called *retinol*) is found in fish liver oils, egg yolk, liver, fortified milk, and margarine. Vitamin A is necessary to vision, skin and mucous membrane integrity, normal reproductive function, and cell membrane structure. The recommended daily allowance (RDA) is 5000 IU for men and 4000 IU for women.

- *Vitamin D* (also called the *antirachitic factor*), is formed by the action of sunlight on cholesterol in the skin. Vitamin D is necessary for blood calcium homeostasis, which in turn is essential to normal blood clotting, bone formation, and neuromuscular function. The RDA is 400 IU.

- *Vitamin E* (also called *antisterility factor*) is found in vegetable oils, margarine, whole grains, and dark green leafy vegetables. Vitamin E is believed to be an antioxidant; that is, it helps prevent the oxidation of vitamins A and C in the intestine and decreases the oxidation of unsaturated fatty acids to facilitate cell membrane integrity. The RDA is 30 IU.

- *Vitamin K* (also called the *coagulation vitamin*), is synthesized by coliform bacteria in the large intestine and is found in green leafy vegetables, cabbage, cauliflower, and pork. Vitamin K is essential for the formation of clotting proteins in the liver. The RDA has not been established.

The water-soluble vitamins are as follows:

- *Vitamin B_1* (also called *thiamin*) is found in lean meats, liver, eggs, green leafy vegetables, legumes, and whole grains. This B vitamin is an essential coenzyme for carbohydrate catabolism and use. It is essential for the healthy functioning of the nerves, muscles, and heart. The RDA is 1.5 mg.

- *Vitamin B_2* (also called *riboflavin*) is found in liver, egg whites, whole grains, meat, poultry, and fish; a major source is milk. This B vitamin is involved in the catabolism and use of carbohydrates, fats, and proteins, and the use of other B vitamins. It is also important in the production of adrenal hormones. The RDA is 1.7 mg.

- *Vitamin B_6* (also called *pyridoxine*) is found in meat, poultry, fish, potatoes, tomatoes, sweet potatoes, and spinach. This B vitamin is necessary for amino acid metabolism, formation of antibodies, and formation of hemoglobin. The RDA is 2 mg.

- *Vitamin B_{12}* (also called *cyanocobalamin*) is found in liver, meat, poultry, fish, dairy foods (except butter), and eggs. Vitamin B_{12} is not found in any plant foods, however. It is essential for the production of nucleic acids and of red blood cells in the bone marrow. It also plays an important role in the use of folic acid and carbohydrates and in the healthy functioning of the nervous system. The RDA is 6 micrograms.

- *Vitamin C* (also called *ascorbic acid*) is found in citrus fruits, fresh potatoes, tomatoes, and green leafy vegetables. Vitamin C acts as an antioxidant and a vasoconstrictor. It also serves in the formation of connective tissue, in the conversion of cholesterol to bile salts, in iron absorption and use, and in the conversion of folic acid to its active form. The RDA is 60 mg.

- *Niacin* (also called *nicotinamide*) is found in meat, poultry, fish, liver, peanuts, and green leafy vegetables. Niacin plays an important role in the metabolism of carbohydrates and fats and inhibits cholesterol synthesis. It is important for the health of the integumentary, nervous, and digestive systems, and assists in the manufacture of reproductive hormones. The RDA is 20 mg.

- *Biotin* is found in liver, egg yolk, nuts, and legumes. Biotin is essential for the catabolism of fatty acids and carbohydrates. It also helps dispose of the waste products of protein catabolism. The RDA has not been established.

- *Pantothenic acid* is found in meats, whole grains, egg yolk, liver, yeast, and legumes. Pantothenic acid assists in the synthesis of steroids and the heme of hemoglobin. It is essential for the metabolism of carbohydrates and fats and for the manufacture of reproductive hormones. The RDA is 10 mg.

- *Folic acid* (also called *folacin*) is found in liver, dark green vegetables, lean beef, eggs, veal, and whole grains. Folic acid is also synthesized by bacteria in the intestine. Folic acid is the basis of a coenzyme necessary to the manufacture of nucleic acids and is therefore essential for the formation of red blood cells, growth and development, and the health of the nervous system. The RDA is 0.4 mg.

Minerals

Minerals work with other nutrients in maintaining the structure and function of the body. An adequate supply of calcium, phosphorus, potassium, sulfur, sodium, chloride, and magnesium—as well as other trace elements, such as iron, iodine, copper, and zinc—is necessary to health. Most minerals in the body are found in body fluids or are bound to organic compounds. The best sources of minerals are vegetables, legumes, milk, and some meats. Dietary sources for minerals are discussed in Chapter 5.

Table 12–1   Assessment Findings Due to Malnutrition

Body System	Assessment Findings
Nails	Soft and spoon-shaped in iron deficiency. Splinter hemorrhages in vitamin C deficiency.
Hair	Dry, dull, and scarce in zinc, protein, and linoleic acid deficiencies.
Skin	Flaky and dry in vitamin A, vitamin B, and/or linoleic acid deficiency. Cracks and/or hyperpigmentation in niacin deficiency. Bruising in vitamin C or vitamin K deficiency.
Eyes	Eyes become dry and soft with decrease in vitamin A. Conjunctiva is pale with a decrease in iron, and red with a decrease in riboflavin.
Nervous system	Reflexes are decreased and client may have peripheral neuropathies with thiamine deficiency. Client may be irritable and/or disoriented with thiamine deficiency.
Musculoskeletal system	Muscle wasting is seen with deficits in protein, carbohydrate, and fat metabolism. Calf pain occurs with thiamine deficiency; joint pain may occur with vitamin C deficiency.
Cardiovascular system	Heart size and rate may increase with thiamine deficiency. Diastolic blood pressure may be increased with a high intake of fat. Lowered cardiac output and decreased blood pressure may occur with caloric deficiencies over a long time period.
Respiratory system	Excessive fat can restrict respirations, and excessive fluids can impair gas exchange.
Gastrointestinal system	Cheilosis (sores at corner of mouth) seen in vitamin B-complex deficiencies, especially riboflavin. Stomatitis and spongy, bleeding gums may also be seen in malnutrition.

Assessment of Digestion and Nutritional Status

■ ■ ■

To assess the client's digestive function and nutritional status, the nurse conducts both a health assessment interview (to collect subjective data) and a physical assessment (to collect objective data).

Physical assessment of the integumentary system, nervous system, musculoskeletal system, cardiovascular system, and respiratory system may also reflect the client's nutritional status. Table 12–1 summarizes abnormal nutritional assessment findings related to these body systems.

The Health Assessment Interview

This section provides guidelines for collecting subjective data through a health assessment interview specific to the GI tract, accessory digestive organs, and nutritional status. Interview questions and leading statements for assessing GI function and nutritional status also are provided.

Digestion and Nutrition

A health assessment interview to determine problems with digestion and nutrition may be conducted during a health screening, may focus on a chief complaint (such as nausea or unexplained weight loss), or may be part of a total health assessment. If the client has a health problem involving digestion or nutrition, analyze its onset, characteristics and course, severity, precipitating and relieving factors, and any associated symptoms, noting the timing and circumstances. For example, ask the client:

- Have you had any episodes of indigestion, nausea, vomiting, diarrhea, or constipation? If so, describe the vomitus or stool and anything that makes these problems better or worse.

- What is your usual dietary intake pattern during a 24-hour period?

- Describe what you believe to be a "healthy" diet.

When collecting information about the client's current health status, ask about any changes in weight, appetite, and the ability to taste, chew, or swallow. What is the client's perception of the role of nutrition in maintaining health? Who buys and prepares the food? What medications (prescribed, over-the-counter, or vitamins) is the client currently taking? Does the client consume alcohol (how much and type)? If the client has experienced nausea or vomiting, ask whether the vomitus contains bright red blood, dark (old) blood, bile, or fecal material. If the client is very thin or verbalizes concerns about body size that are incongruent with the ratio of height to weight, ask whether the client induces vomiting or use laxatives to control weight. Ask whether the client has appliances such as braces, bridges, or dentures, and ask the client to describe self-care measures for such appliances, as well as oral hygiene practices and frequency of dental visits.

Ask the client to describe any heartburn, indigestion, abdominal discomfort, or pain. Explore the location of the pain, the type of pain, the time it occurs, associated foods that aggravate or relieve it, and how it is relieved.

Abdominal pain is often referred to other sites (see Figure 4–4 on page 75). For example, a client with a liver disorder may experience pain over the right shoulder (Kehr's sign). Epigastric (middle upper abdominal) pain is experienced in cases of acute gastritis, obstruction of the small intestine, and acute pancreatitis. Pain in the right upper quadrant is associated with cholecystitis. Pain in the left upper quadrant may be related to a gastric ulcer.

The health history should include questions about any prior surgeries or trauma of the GI tract. Explore the past history of any medical condition that may affect the client's ingestion, digestion, and/or metabolism (for example, Crohn's disease, diabetes mellitus, irritable bowel syndrome, peptic ulcers, or pancreatitis). Other areas significant to assessment of the GI system and nutrition are food allergies (especially to milk, which is evidenced as lactose intolerance with abdominal cramping, excessive flatus, and loose stools) and a family history that may provide clues to increased risk for health problems.

Interview Questions

The following interview questions and leading statements are categorized by functional health patterns (Gordon, 1987):

Health Perception–Health Management

- Have you had any illness or surgery that affects your nutrition and digestion (for example, Crohn's disease or other gastrointestinal disorders, diabetes mellitus, cancer, cardiovascular disease, mouth or throat surgery, abdominal surgery)?
- If so, how have these health problems been treated?
- What medications do you take?
- Do you take antacids? If so, when and how much?
- Do you ever have tooth or gum pain that prevents you from eating certain foods?
- When was your last dental examination?
- Describe what you do each day to take care of your teeth.

Nutritional–Metabolic

- List all the foods you ate and fluids you drank in the past 24 hours.
- Describe any special or prescribed diet you now follow or have ever followed.
- Have you noticed any change in your appetite? If so, explain.
- What is your current weight? What do you feel your ideal weight would be? Have you had a recent weight gain or loss? If so, explain.
- Describe your food preferences and dislikes.
- Do you have episodes of nausea or vomiting? If so, do you know what causes them? Describe these episodes.
- Do you have excessive belching or indigestion? Explain.
- Do you have any difficulty swallowing? Explain.
- Do you take any special vitamins or food supplements? Explain.
- Do you drink alcohol? If so, describe your average number and type of drinks each day.

Elimination

- Describe the pattern and consistency of your bowel movements.
- Has there been a recent change in your bowel patterns? Explain.
- Describe any laxatives you use. How often and when do you take them?

Activity–Exercise

- Describe your activities on a typical day.
- What exercise do you get, and how often?
- Who shops for and prepares the foods you eat?
- Do you smoke? What do you smoke? How many per day?

Sleep–Rest

- Do you ever wake up hungry during the night? If so, do you eat? What and how often?
- Do you ever have abdominal discomfort, pain, cramping, or diarrhea that interferes with your sleep or rest?

Cognitive–Perceptual

- Can you describe the type and amount of foods you should eat each day?
- List foods that are high and low in fat and calories.
- List foods that are high and low in nutritional value.
- Describe how you might improve your present diet.
- Rate your ability to taste foods on a scale of 1 to 10 (with 10 being excellent).
- Rate your ability to smell foods on a scale of 1 to 10 (with 10 being excellent).
- Describe any discomfort or pain you have experienced in your mouth or throat. What causes this? What do you do to relieve it?
- Describe any stomach or abdominal pain you have experienced. Is it dull, crampy, achy, burning, colicky? What seems to cause it? What do you do to relieve it?

Self-Perception–Self-Concept

- Are you satisfied with your appearance in terms of your weight?

- Have you been successful in the past in losing or gaining weight? Explain.
- How has the problem you have described made you feel about yourself?
- How has this problem affected how you feel about your life?

Role–Relationship
- Do you usually eat alone or with others?
- If you eat with others, who are they?
- Has there been a recent change in your relationships with others at work, in your family, or in your social activities that has affected your usual eating patterns? (Examples may include divorce, recent move, loss of significant other.)

Sexuality–Reproductive
- Have your health problems altered your usual sexual activities?
- Describe how your nutritional problems have made you feel about yourself as a man or woman.

Coping–Stress
- Do certain events (such as work or daily tasks) affect your enjoyment of food or your appetite? If so, explain.
- Do you ever eat or drink more to help you cope with stressful situations? Explain.
- What do you feel is the most stressful experience you have had with your nutritional problem?
- Who or what will be able to help you cope with stress from this nutritional problem?

Value–Belief
- Do you follow certain food restrictions or a diet based on your religious or cultural beliefs? Explain.
- Are there significant others, practices, or activities that help you cope with your nutritional problem? Explain.
- How do you perceive your future with this health problem?

Guidelines for Assessing the Abdomen

■ ■ ■

Ask the client to empty the bladder before beginning the examination. Assist the client to the dorsal recumbent (supine) position, with a small pillow under the head, a pillow under the knees (if desired), and the arms at the sides of the body. Warm the stethoscope before applying it to the client's skin. Ask the client to point to areas that are painful, and explain that those areas will be examined last. Expose the abdomen from below the breasts to the pubic symphysis, and drape the client's thoracic and genital areas. When you document your findings, specify the location by abdominal quadrant.

General guidelines for abdominal assessment are as follows:

1. Inspect the abdomen under a good light source that is shining across the abdomen. Sit at the right side of the client, and note symmetry, distention, masses, visible peristalsis, and respiratory movements. If masses are detected, ask the client to take a deep breath, which decreases the size of the abdominal cavity and makes any abnormality more visible.

2. Auscultate each quadrant of the abdomen, using the diaphragm of the stethoscope. Listen for bowel sounds, arterial bruits, venous hums, and friction rubs.

3. Percuss several areas within each quadrant of the abdomen, using a systematic path. (For example, always begin in the lower left quadrant, then proceed to the lower right quadrant, upper right quadrant, and upper left quadrant, respectively). The predominant percussion tones for the entire abdomen are tympany and dullness. Tympany is present over gas-filled intestines. Dullness is present over the liver, the spleen, an enlarged kidney, or a full stomach. Percuss for fluid, gaseous distention, and masses.

4. Palpate each quadrant of the abdomen for shape, position, mobility, size, consistency, and tenderness of the major abdominal organs. Begin this part of the assessment with light palpation, and increase the depth of palpation to elicit tenderness or better identify organ size and shape. Deep palpation should be conducted only by nurses with considerable experience. Remember to palpate areas of indicated tenderness last and to use gentle pressure. Palpation may be difficult or impossible if the client exhibits muscle guarding from pain or is ticklish. The gallbladder and the spleen are normally not palpable.

The Physical Assessment

Physical assessment of digestion and nutritional status may be performed as part of a total health assessment, in combination with assessment of the urinary and reproductive systems (problems which may cause clinical manifestations similar to those of the GI system), or alone for clients with known or suspected health problems. The nurse uses the techniques of inspection, auscultation, percussion, and palpation; palpation is the last method used in assessing the abdomen, because pressure on the abdominal wall and contents may interfere with bowel sounds and elicit pain preventing continuation of the examination.

Preparation

The nurse gathers objective data by obtaining **anthropometric measurements** (height, weight, triceps skinfolds, and midarm circumference) and by examining the mouth and abdomen. The equipment necessary for the assessment are a stethoscope, a scale, a tape measure, and skinfold calipers. Prior to the examination, all necessary equipment should be collected and techniques explained to the client to decrease anxiety. The client may be seated during assessment of the mouth but is supine during the abdominal assessment.

The quadrants of the abdomen, with related internal structures, are illustrated in Figure 12–5. General guidelines for assessing the abdomen are provided in the box on page 424.

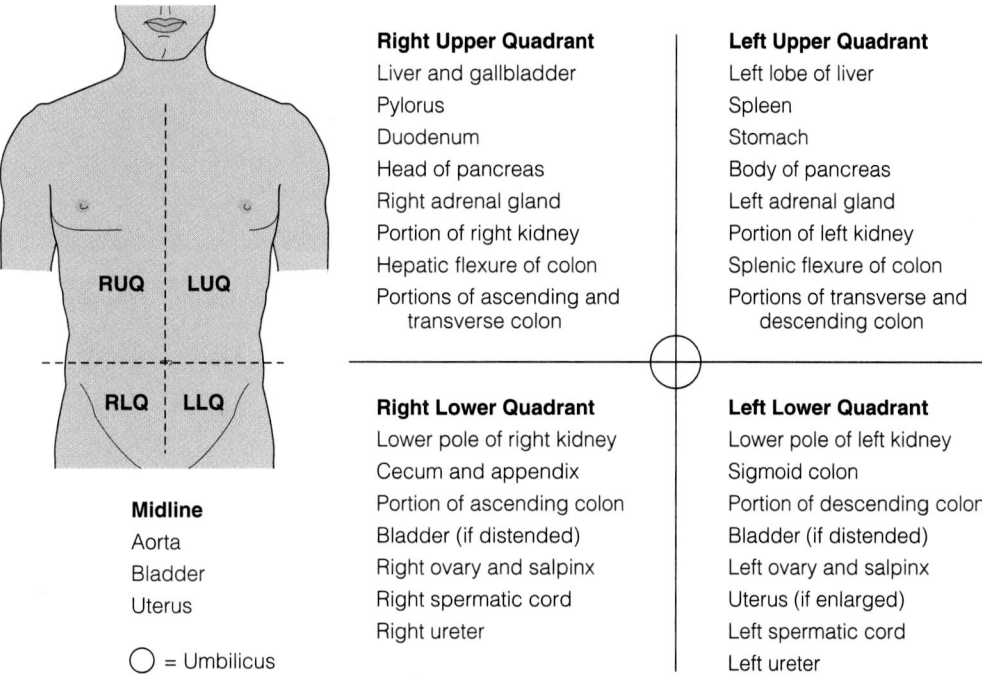

Right Upper Quadrant
Liver and gallbladder
Pylorus
Duodenum
Head of pancreas
Right adrenal gland
Portion of right kidney
Hepatic flexure of colon
Portions of ascending and
    transverse colon

Left Upper Quadrant
Left lobe of liver
Spleen
Stomach
Body of pancreas
Left adrenal gland
Portion of left kidney
Splenic flexure of colon
Portions of transverse and
    descending colon

Right Lower Quadrant
Lower pole of right kidney
Cecum and appendix
Portion of ascending colon
Bladder (if distended)
Right ovary and salpinx
Right spermatic cord
Right ureter

Left Lower Quadrant
Lower pole of left kidney
Sigmoid colon
Portion of descending colon
Bladder (if distended)
Left ovary and salpinx
Uterus (if enlarged)
Left spermatic cord
Left ureter

Midline
Aorta
Bladder
Uterus

◯ = Umbilicus

Figure 12–5   The four quadrants of the abdomen, with anatomic location of organs within each quadrant.

Assessment Technique	Possible Abnormal Findings
Anthropometric Measurements	
■ **Weigh the client.**	
■ **Compare the client's actual weight to ideal body weight (IBW).** Use the table on page 426.	Malnutrition is indicated by a weight 10% to 20% less than ideal body weight. ➤

Height and Weight Tables for Men and Women According to Frame

Height			Weight*		
	Feet	Inches	Small Frame	Medium Frame	Large Frame
Men	5	2	128–134	131–134	138–150
(ages	5	3	130–136	133–143	140–153
25–29)	5	4	132–138	135–145	142–156
	5	5	134–140	137–148	144–160
	5	6	136–142	139–151	146–164
	5	7	138–145	142–154	149–168
	5	8	140–148	145–157	152–172
	5	9	142–151	148–160	155–176
	5	10	144–154	151–163	158–180
	5	11	146–157	154–166	161–184
	6	0	149–160	157–170	164–188
	6	1	152–164	160–174	168–192
	6	2	155–168	164–178	172–197
	6	3	158–172	167–182	176–202
	6	4	162–176	171–187	181–207
Women	4	10	102–111	109–121	118–131
(ages	4	11	103–113	111–123	120–134
25–29)	5	0	104–115	113–126	122–137
	5	1	106–118	115–129	125–140
	5	2	108–121	118–132	128–143
	5	3	111–124	121–135	131–147
	5	4	114–127	124–138	134–151
	5	5	117–130	127–141	137–155
	5	6	120–133	130–144	140–159
	5	7	123–136	133–147	143–163
	5	8	126–139	136–150	146–167
	5	9	129–142	139–153	149–170
	5	10	132–145	142–156	152–173
	5	11	135–148	145–159	155–176
	6	0	138–151	148–162	158–179

* Weight in pounds. Men: allow 5 lb of clothing. Women: allow 3 lb of clothing.

Courtesy of Metropolitan Life Insurance Company, 1983.

■ **Calculate the client's percentage of ideal body weight (%IBW).**

Use this formula:
$$\frac{\text{current weight}}{\text{ideal weight}} \times 100$$

%IBW	%UBW	Nutrition Status
>120	——	Obese
110–120	——	Overweight
80–90	85–95	Mildly undernourished
70–79	75–84	Moderately undernourished
<70	<75	Severely undernourished

Note. From *Understanding Normal and Clinical Nutrition* (p. 47) by
C. Cataldo, S. Rolfes, and E. Whitney, 1991, St. Paul: West Publishing.

A client whose weight is 10% above ideal body weight is considered overweight. A client whose weight is 20% above ideal body weight is considered obese.

Refer to the accompanying table to determine the presence of obesity and/or malnutrition based on percentage of ideal body weight.

| ASSESSMENT TECHNIQUE | POSSIBLE ABNORMAL FINDINGS |

- **Calculate the client's percentage of usual body weight (%UBW).**

Use this formula:

$$\frac{\text{current weight}}{\text{usual weight}} \times 100$$

- **Measure triceps skinfold thickness (TSF).**

Find the midpoint between the client's olecranon and acromion processes. Grasp the skin and fat, and pull it away from the muscle. Apply skinfold calipers for 3 seconds, and record reading (Figure 12–6). Repeat 3 times, and average the 3 readings. Compare the client's reading to the standard values shown in the table below.

Figure 12–6 Measuring triceps skinfold thickness with calipers.

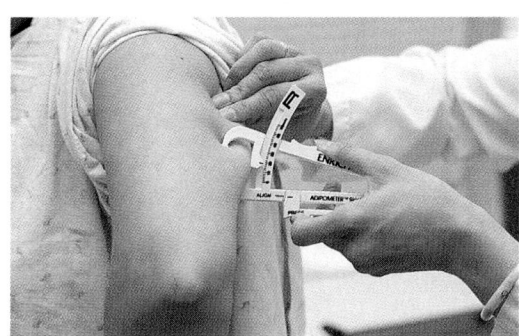

Standard Value

Measurement	Male	Female
Triceps skinfold thickness	12.5 mm	16.5 mm
Midarm circumference	29.3 cm	28.5 cm
Midarm muscle circumference	25.3 cm	23.2 cm

- **Measure midarm circumference (MAC).**

Find the midpoint between the client's olecranon and acromion processes. Wind tape measure around arm (Figure 12–7). Compare the client's reading to the standard values shown in the table above.

Figure 12–7 Measuring midarm circumference with a tape measure.

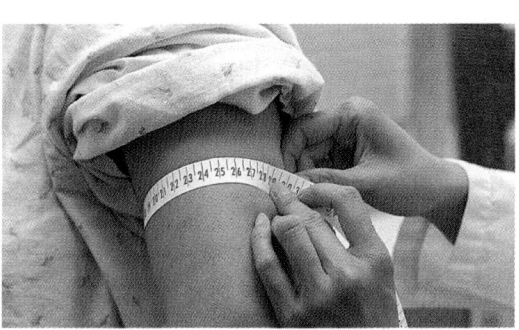

Calculate percentage of usual body weight to determine recent weight change. Use of %IBW may result in overlooking malnutrition in a very obese client. Refer to the table at the bottom of page 426 to determine nutritional status based on %UBW.

Triceps readings are 10% or more below standards in malnutrition and 10% or more above standards in obesity or overnutrition.

MAC decreases with malnutrition and increases with obesity.

➤

ASSESSMENT TECHNIQUE	POSSIBLE ABNORMAL FINDINGS

■ **Calculate Midarm Muscle Circumference (MAMC).**

Use the client's TSF and MAC readings to calculate the client's MAMC.
Use this formula:

MAMC = MAC − (0.314 × TSF)

Compare the result to the standard values shown in the table on page 427.

In mild malnutrition, the MAMC is 90% of the standard; in moderate malnutrition, 60% to 90%. In severe malnutrition (muscle wasting), the MAMC is less than 60% of the standard.

Mouth

Note: Wear gloves!

■ **Inspect and palpate the lips.**

Cheilosis (painful lesions at corners of mouth) is seen with riboflavin and/or niacin deficiency. Cold sores or clear vesicles with a red base are seen in herpes simplex I.

■ **Inspect and palpate the tongue.**

Atrophic smooth glossitis is characterized by a bright red tongue. It is seen in B_{12}, folic acid, and iron deficiencies. Vertical fissures are seen in dehydration. A black, hairy tongue may be seen following antibiotic therapy.

■ **Inspect and palpate the buccal mucosa.**

Leukoplakia (small white patches) may be a sign of a premalignant condition. A reddened, dry, swollen mucosa may be seen in stomatitis. *Candidiases* (white cheesy patches that bleed when scraped) may be seen in immune-suppressed clients receiving antibiotics or chemotherapy and in terminally ill clients.

■ **Inspect and palpate the teeth.**

Cavities and excessive plaque are seen with poor nutrition and/or poor oral hygiene.

■ **Inspect and palpate the gums.**

Swollen, red gums that bleed easily (*gingivitis*) are seen in vitamin C deficiencies and with hormonal changes.

■ **Inspect the throat and tonsils.**

In acute infections, tonsils are red and swollen and may have white spots.

■ **Note the client's breath.**

Sweet, fruity breath is noted in ketoacidosis. Acetone breath may be a sign of uremia. Foul breath may result from liver disease, respiratory infections, and poor oral hygiene.

Abdomen

Ensure that the client has emptied the bladder.
Help the client to lie supine with a small pillow under the knees and the arms at the sides.

■ **Inspect the abdomen.**

See the guidelines in the box on page 424.

Generalized abdominal distention may be seen in gas retention or obesity. Lower abdominal distention is seen in

ASSESSMENT TECHNIQUE	POSSIBLE ABNORMAL FINDINGS

bladder distention, pregnancy, or ovarian mass. General distention and an everted umbilicus is seen with ascites and/or tumors. A *scaphoid* (sunken) *abdomen* is seen in malnutrition or when fat is replaced with muscle. A bluish umbilicus (called *Cullen's sign*) may be seen in intra-abdominal hemorrhage.

- Observe skin integrity.

Striae (whitish-silver stretch marks) are seen in obesity and during or after pregnancy. Spider angiomas may be seen in liver disease.

- Observe venous pattern.

Dilated veins are prominent in cirrhosis of the liver, ascites, portal hypertension, or venocaval obstruction.

- Observe aortic pulsation.

Pulsation is increased in aortic aneurysm.

- **Auscultate the abdomen with the diaphragm of the stethoscope.**

See the guidelines in the box on page 424.

Auscultate before percussing or palpating the abdomen to prevent stimulation of peristalsis and distortion of bowel sounds.

Auscultate bowel sounds in all four quadrants (Figure 12–8). Begin in the lower right quadrant, where bowel sounds are almost always present. Normal bowel sounds (gurgling or clicking) last 5 to 30 minutes.

Borborygmus (hyperactive high-pitched, tinkling, rushing, or growling bowel sounds) is heard in diarrhea or at the onset of bowel obstruction. Bowel sounds may be absent later in bowel obstruction, with an inflamed peritoneum, and/or following surgery of the abdomen. Listen for at least 5 minutes to confirm the absence of bowel sounds.

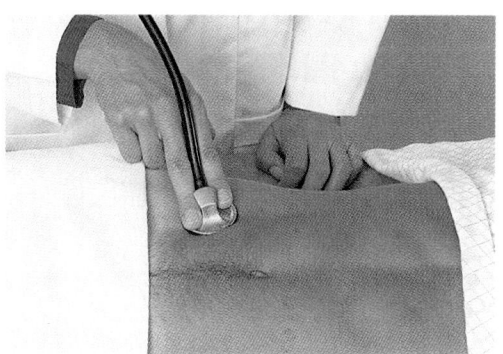

Figure 12–8   Auscultating the abdomen with the diaphragm of the stethoscope.

- **Auscultate the abdomen for vascular sounds with the bell of the stethoscope** (Figure 12–9).

Bruits (blowing sound due to restriction of blood flow through vessels) may be heard over constricted arteries. A bruit over the liver may be heard in hepatic carcinoma. A *venous hum* (continuous medium-pitched sound) may be heard over a cirrhotic liver. *Friction rubs* (rough grating sounds) may be heard over an inflamed liver or spleen.

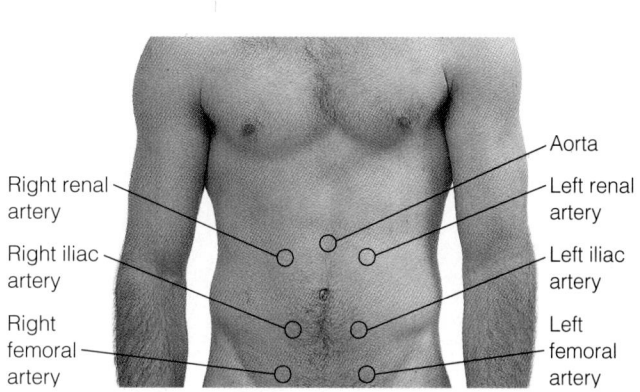

Figure 12–9
Location of placement of the stethoscope for auscultation of arteries of the abdomen.

Right renal artery
Right iliac artery
Right femoral artery
Aorta
Left renal artery
Left iliac artery
Left femoral artery

➤

ASSESSMENT TECHNIQUE	POSSIBLE ABNORMAL FINDINGS

■ **Percuss the abdomen.**

See the guidelines in the box on page 424.
Percuss in all four quadrants (Figure 12–10). Normally, tympany is heard over the stomach and gas-filled bowels.

Dullness is heard instead of tympany when the bowel is displaced with fluid or tumors or filled with a fecal mass.

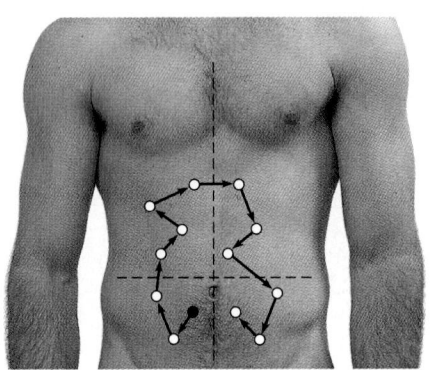

Figure 12–10 Location of sites for systematic percussion of all four quadrants.

■ **Percuss the liver.**

See the accompanying box for guidelines for percussing and palpating the liver.
Note the characteristic dullness of sound over the liver in the midclavicular line (MCL) (Figure 12–11).

In cirrhosis and/or hepatitis, the liver is greater than 6 to 10 cm in the MCL and greater than 4 to 8 cm in the midsternal line (MSL).

Guidelines for Percussing and Palpating the Liver

■   ■   ■

The size of the liver may be determined by percussion and palpation, as follows:

1. Percuss in the right midclavicular line (MCL), beginning below the umbilicus (see Figure 12–11). Begin to percuss over a region of tympany, and move upward. The first dull percussion tone occurs at the lower border of the liver. Determine the upper liver border by beginning percussion over an area of lung resonance (in the MCL) and percussing downward to the first dull tone, usually at the 5th to 7th interspace. Mark each of these locations, and measure the distance from one mark to the other to determine liver size. The normal liver size is 6 to 12 cm in the MCL; however, men have larger livers than women.

2. Conduct bimanual palpation of the liver by placing your left hand under the client at the level of the 11th to 12th ribs and applying upward pressure. Place your right hand below the costal margin, ask the client to take a deep breath, and palpate for the liver border. The liver is not normally palpable in a healthy adult, although it may be in very thin people.

ASSESSMENT TECHNIQUE	POSSIBLE ABNORMAL FINDINGS

Figure 12–11
Anatomic location of the liver, with the midclavicular line (MCL) and midsternal line (MSL) superimposed. The normal liver span is 6 to 12 cm.

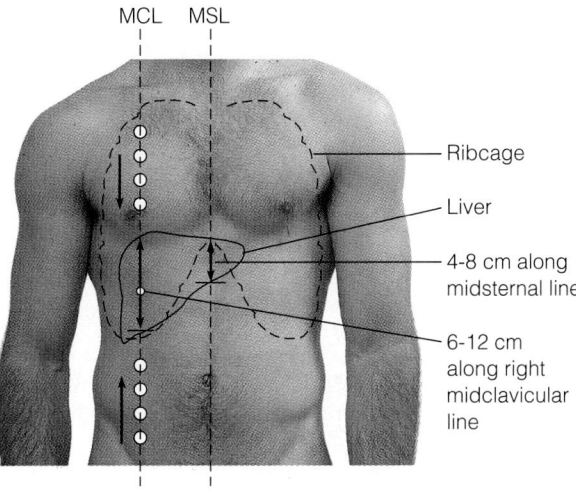

MCL   MSL

Ribcage

Liver

4–8 cm along midsternal line

6–12 cm along right midclavicular line

■ **Percuss the spleen.**

Percuss for dullness posterior to the midaxilliary line at the level of the 6th to 11th rib (Figure 12–12).

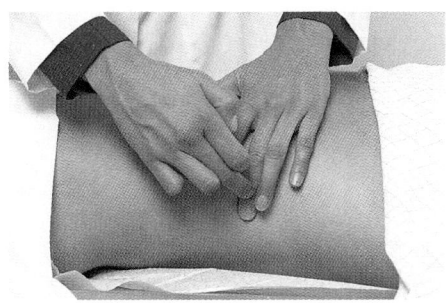

Figure 12–12
Percussing the spleen.

A large area of dullness that extends to the left anterior ancillary line on inspiration is seen in an enlarged spleen in trauma cases, infection, or mononucleosis.

■ **Percuss for shifting dullness** (Figure 12–13).

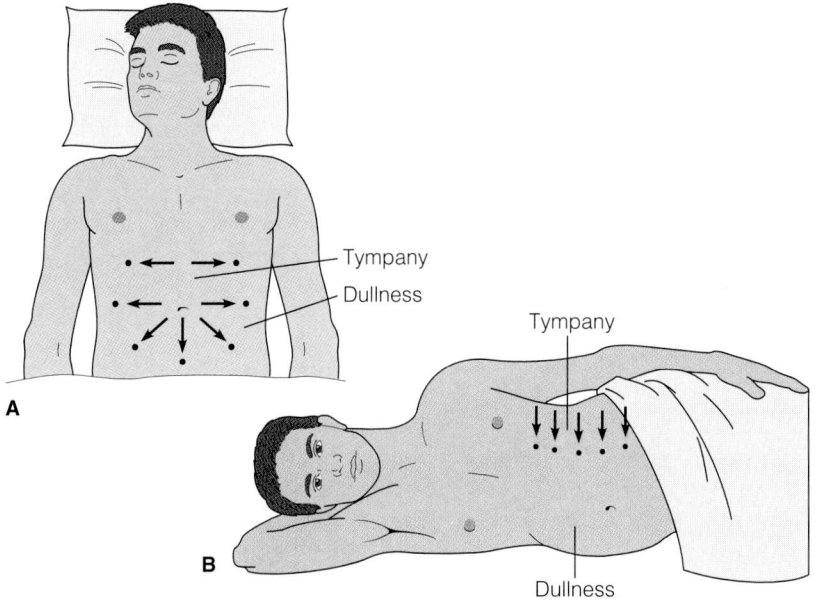

Tympany

Dullness

Tympany

A

B

Dullness

In a client with ascites, the level of dullness increases when the client turns to the side.

Figure 12–13   Percussing for shifting dullness in ascites. *A*, common percussion tones when the client is lying supine; *B*, changes in percussion tones (shifting dullness) when the client turns to the side.

- **Palpate the abdomen in all four quadrants.**

See the guidelines in the box on page 424.

Use a circular motion to move the abdominal wall over underlying structures (Figure 12–14). Feel for masses, and note any tenderness or pain the client may have during this part of the exam. Palpate lightly at first ($\frac{1}{2}$ to $\frac{3}{4}$ in.), then deeply ($1\frac{1}{2}$ to 2 in.) with caution.

Never use deep palpation in a client who has had a renal transplant or has polycystic kidneys.

Normal findings on palpating the abdomen include the aorta, rectus abdominus muscle, uterus, and feces in colon.

Figure 12–14   Light to moderate palpation of the abdomen. *A,* In light palpation, the examiner, keeping the fingers approximated, gently depresses the abdominal wall about 1 cm to assess for large masses, slight tenderness, and muscle guarding. *B,* The examiner performs moderate palpation by using the palm or the side of the hand to depress the abdominal wall to a slightly greater depth than in light palpation. This technique is useful for assessing abdominal organs that move with respiration (such as the liver and the spleen).

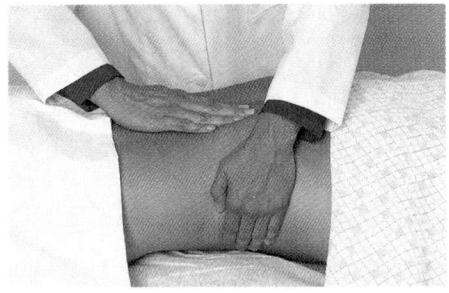

A

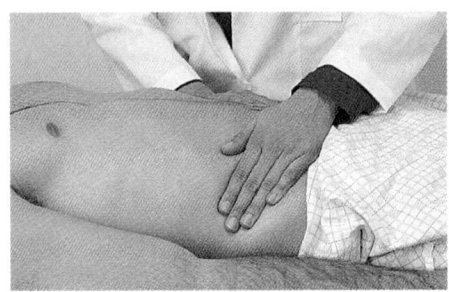

B

If a mass is palpated, ask the client to raise head and shoulders.

- **Check for rebound tenderness.**

Press the fingers into the abdomen slowly.
Release the pressure quickly.

In cases of peritoneal inflammation, palpation causes abdominal pain and involuntary muscle spasms.

Abnormal masses include aortic aneurysms, neoplastic tumors of the colon or uterus, and a distended bladder or distended bowel due to obstruction. A rigid, boardlike abdomen may be palpated in a client with a perforated duodenal ulcer.

A mass in the abdomen may become more prominent with this maneuver. A ventral abdominal wall hernia will also become more prominent with this maneuver. If the mass is no longer palpable, it is deeper in the abdomen.

In peritoneal inflammation, pain occurs when the fingers are withdrawn. Right upper quadrant pain occurs with acute cholecystitis. Upper middle abdominal pain occurs with acute pancreatitis. Right lower quadrant pain occurs with acute appendicitis, and left lower quadrant pain is seen in acute diverticulitis.

ASSESSMENT TECHNIQUE	POSSIBLE ABNORMAL FINDINGS

- **Palpate the liver** (Figure 12–15).

Guidelines for palpation of the liver are listed in the box on page 430.

An enlarged liver with a smooth, tender edge may indicate hepatitis or venous congestion. An enlarged, nontender liver may be felt in malignant condition.

Figure 12–15
Palpating the liver with the bimanual method.

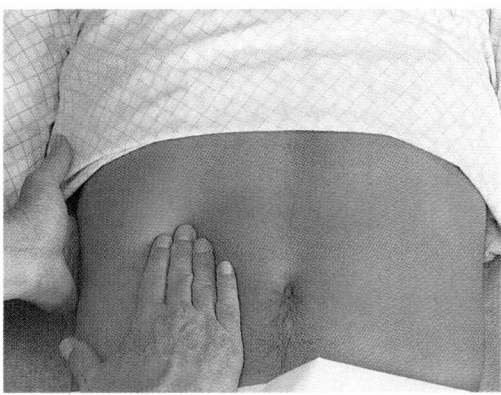

Note whether the client guards the abdomen or reports any sharp pain, especially on inspiration.

The client with inflammation of the gallbladder feels sharp pain on inspiration and stops inspiring. This is called *Murphy's sign*.

Variations in Assessment Findings for the Older Adult

The older adult may be at risk for alterations in nutrition for a variety of reasons. These include decreased ability to identify odors, poor vision, impaired mobility and strength, limited access to food and cooking facilities, decreased socialization, and reduced income. If the older adult becomes too sedentary (because of musculoskeletal problems, for example), caloric intake may exceed requirements, resulting in weight gain. However, the older adult also has had a lifetime of choosing and eating foods and often has a knowledge of proper nutrition.

Several age-related changes in structure and function of the GI system and of nutritional status may occur as a result of aging:

- Anthropometric measurements (midarm circumference and triceps skinfolds) may be inaccurate because of sagging skin, decreased subcutaneous fat, and a reduced muscle mass.

- Loss of teeth may result from periodontal disease and dental caries.

- Decreased salivation increases the risk of oral infections and decreases taste perception.

- The tongue and buccal mucosa may be smoother and thinner because of atrophy.

- Abdominal organs may be easier to palpate as a result of thinning of the abdominal wall.

- The processes of digestion, absorption, peristalsis, and metabolism slow.

- Cellular losses associated with aging often lead to a decrease in muscular tissue and an increase in fatty tissue. Fat is redistributed from the face and extremities to the abdomen and hips.

- Decreased gastric acid secretion may predispose the older client to malabsorption of vitamin B_{12} and calcium.

- The liver decreases in size.

Bibliography

■ ■ ■

Bhaskar, S. N., Lilly, G. E., & Pratt, L. W. (1990). A practical, high-yield mouth exam. *Patient Care, 24*(2), 53–57, 60, 62.

Bishop, C., & Pelchey, S. (1987). Estimation of the mid-upper arm circumference measurement error. *Journal of the American Dietetic Association, 87*(4), 469–473.

Bowman, B. B., & Rosenberg, I. H. (1982). Assessment of nutritional status of the elderly. *American Journal of Clinical Nutrition, 1*(1), 11–22.

Carotenuto, R., & Bullock, J. (1980). *Physical assessment of the gerontologic client.* Philadelphia: F. A. Davis.

Collinsworth, R. (1991). Determining nutritional status of the elderly surgical patient: Steps in the assessment process. *AORN Journal, 54*(3), 622–628, 630–631.

Gordon, M. (1987). *Nursing diagnosis: Process and application.* (2nd ed.). New York: McGraw-Hill.

Holmgren, C. (1992). Abdominal assessment. *RN, 55*(3), 28–34.

Marieb, E. N. (1995). *Human anatomy and physiology* (3rd ed.). Redwood City, CA: Benjamin/Cummings.

Massoni, M. (1990). Nurses GI handbook. *Nursing90, 20*(11), 65–80.

McConnell, E. A. (1991a). Exploring postoperative abdominal discomfort. *Nursing91, 21*(5), 84–86.

McConnell, E. A. (1991b). Investigating abdominal pain. *Nursing91, 2*(11), 111, 113–114.

Rubin-Terrado, M., & Linkenheld, D. (1991). Don't choke on this: A swallowing assessment. *Geriatric Nursing, 12*(6), 288–291.

Smith, C. E. (1988). Assessing bowel sounds: More than just listening. *Nursing88, 18*(2), 42–43.

Waltman, N. L. (1991). Nutritional status, pressure sores and mortality in elderly patients with cancer. *Oncology Nursing Forum, 18*(5), 867–873.

Whitney, E., Cataldo, C., & Rolfes, S. (1991). *Understanding normal and clinical nutrition.* St. Paul: West Pub. Co.

Nursing Care of Clients with Nutritional, Oral, and Esophageal Disorders

LEARNING OBJECTIVES

After completing this chapter, you will be able to

- Describe the pathophysiology of common nutritional, oral, and esophageal disorders.

- Compare and contrast the clinical manifestations of nutritional disorders.

- Discuss the clinical manifestations of disorders of the mouth and esophagus.

- Identify laboratory and diagnostic tests used to diagnose nutritional, oral, and esophageal disorders.

- Discuss nursing implications for the various collaborative treatments prescribed for clients with nutritional, oral, and esophageal disorders.

- Provide appropriate nursing care for a client receiving enteral or parenteral nutrition.

- Use the nursing process as a framework for providing individualized nursing care to clients with nutritional, oral, or esophageal disorders.

Changes related to nutritional disorders and the ingestion of food are major causes for illness and disability. The major nutritional disorders in the world today are obesity and undernutrition (malnutrition). Problems of ingestion include inflammations, infections, mechanical disorders, and neoplasms of the mouth and esophagus.

Clients with nutritional, oral, and esophageal disorders require complex, skilled nursing care. Developmental, so-

ciocultural, psychologic, and physiologic factors may play a role in these disorders. Nursing care is directed toward identifying causative factors, meeting nutritional and physiologic needs, providing client education, and meeting the psychologic needs of clients and families. The complexity of these disorders and the appropriate nursing care demand a holistic approach.

▪▪▪ Nutritional Disorders ▪▪▪

Both obesity and undernutrition may present as either primary illnesses or symptoms of other diseases. Regardless of the cause, both conditions affect various systems

and organs, often leading to serious health consequences, such as hypertension, heart disease, fluid and electrolyte imbalances, resultant disability, and even death.

Health-Related Problems in Obesity

- Arteriosclerosis
- Arthritis
- Atherosclerosis
- Cancers of the breast, uterus, prostate, and colon
- Cardiac enlargement
- Cholecystitis and cholelithiasis
- Chronic renal failure
- Congestive heart failure
- Diabetes mellitus, type II
- Hiatal hernia
- Postoperative complications
- Hypertension
- Impaired pulmonary function
- Low back pain
- Muscle strains and sprains
- Stress incontinence
- Thrombophlebitis
- Varicosities

The Client with Obesity

Obesity is one of the most prevalent, preventable health problems in the United States (Dudek, 1993). Weight gain occurs when energy consumption exceeds energy expenditure. The term **overnutrition (overweight)** designates body weight that is more than the ideal but less than 20% over the ideal. The term **obesity** designates body weight that is more than 20% above the ideal. Obesity may result in grave physiologic and psychologic consequences, such as diabetes mellitus, cardiovascular disease, and depression, and it is associated with an increased morbidity and mortality rate. The term **morbid obesity** is applied to a person who is more than 100% over ideal body weight. Health-related problems associated with obesity are listed in the accompanying box.

Pathophysiology

Obesity occurs when excess calories are stored as fat. The central nervous system plays a significant role in calorie use, eating behaviors, and satiety. However, most experts agree that obesity is due to many factors, including genetic, physiologic, psychologic, environmental, and sociocultural factors.

Many studies demonstrate a strong link between hereditary factors and obesity. A person with one obese parent has a 40% chance of becoming obese; one with two obese parents, an 80% chance. Researchers have, moreover, reported a strong correlation between the weight of adopted children and their biologic parents (Stunkard, Sorensen et al., 1986).

Environmental influences, such as an abundant and readily accessible food supply, fast-food restaurants, advertising, and vending machines, contribute to increased food intake. Sociocultural influences that contribute to obesity include overeating at family meals, rewarding behavior with food, religious and family gatherings that promote food intake, and sedentary life-styles.

Psychopathology

Theorists have speculated that many psychologic factors interact as a person becomes obese and then suffers from obesity. Low self-esteem may precipitate unhealthy eating behaviors, and the resulting weight gain in turn may diminish self-image even further. A person may overeat as a result of anxiety, depression, guilt, or boredom or as a means of getting attention (Dudek, 1993). Social prejudices and discrimination may also foster these negative self-beliefs and behaviors (Wadden & Stunkard, 1985). Some experts characterize overeating as a food addiction and as a coping mechanism for stressful life events. However, it is important to note that researchers have not identified a single psychologic disorder or personality type associated with obesity.

Collaborative Care

Treatment of obesity focuses on changing both eating and exercise habits. A pound of body fat is equivalent to 3500 kcal. To lose 1 pound, therefore, a person must reduce daily caloric intake by 250 kcal for 14 days or increase activity enough to burn the equivalent kcal.

Many people are psychologically well-adjusted to being overweight, and some experts believe that encouraging weight loss in those with no life-threatening health problems may lead to *"yo-yo" dieting* (repeated cycles of weight loss and gain). "Yo-yo" dieting may also result in a metabolic deficiency that makes subsequent weight loss efforts increasingly difficult (Neil & Kushner, 1993). Therefore, it is critical that dieters take any weight loss effort seriously and include plans for long-term maintenance.

Because obesity is due to many factors, the treatment of obesity is far more complex than just reducing the amount of food that is consumed. Treatment is an ongo-

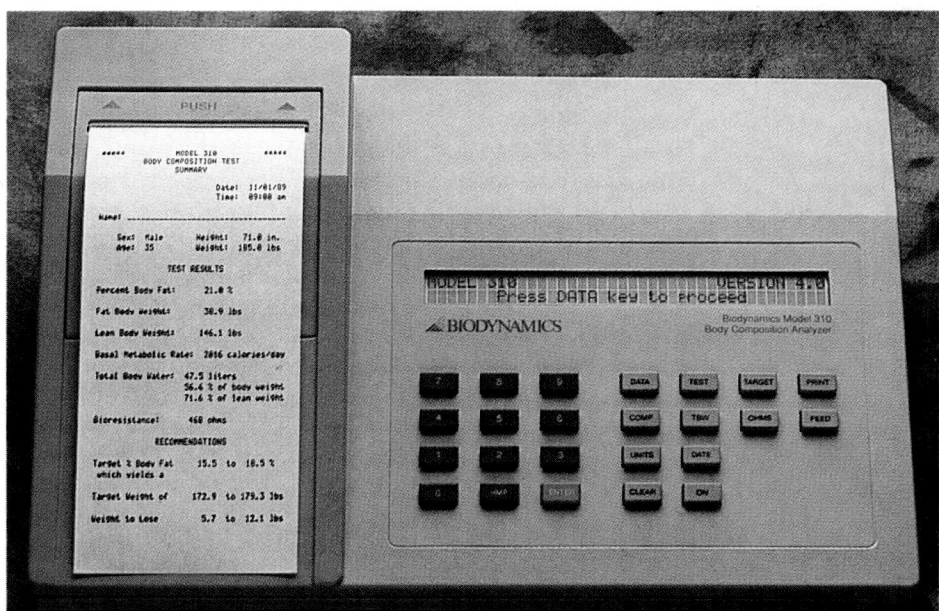

Figure 13–1   Equipment for measuring bioelectrical impedance.

ing process requiring a number of different strategies. Group programs, exercise, dieting, behavior modification, drug therapy, and surgery have all been used in weight control. Most experts recommend an individualized program of exercise, diet, and behavior modification designed to meet the client's specific needs.

Laboratory and Diagnostic Tests

The standard measurements to assess for obesity are height and weight. This information is then compared to height and weight standards that are based on the size of the person's frame (small, medium, or large). However, height and weight are not reliable measurements of *body composition* (the percentages of lean body mass and body fat). A person can be of normal body weight yet have a high percentage of body fat.

Body composition is best determined by measuring **body density** (weight compared to volume). There are three techniques for measuring body density: *Skinfold thickness* is measured with calipers on various body sites, such as the triceps (see Chapter 12). *Underwater weighing* is considered the most accurate way to determine body fat. Generally used as a research tool to obtain an accurate weight, this technique involves submerging the whole body and then measuring the amount of displaced water. **Bioelectrical impedance** is a technique in which the percentage of body fat is analyzed by measuring the electrical resistance of the body and converting it into a measure of body fat (Figure 13–1). In this painless procedure, a low-energy electrical impulse is sent into the body through electrode patches. Males at ideal body weight have 10% to 20% body fat, whereas females at ideal body weight have 20% to 30% body fat.

An important step in treating overweight or obesity is to rule out any physiologic reasons for that condition. The most common concern is to determine whether the person has any underlying endocrine disorder, such as hypothyroidism. For this reason, most health care practitioners order a thyroid profile, including a T_3, T_4, and TSH (see Chapter 20).

Obesity often promotes a number of physiologic consequences. To determine the presence and extent of various sequelae, the following laboratory studies may be ordered:

- *Serum glucose* is measured to determine whether there is coexisting diabetes mellitus.

- *Serum cholesterol* is measured to assess for elevated levels, which may result from a diet that is high in saturated fat.

- A *lipid profile* is ordered; high-density lipoprotein (HDL) levels are reduced in obese clients, whereas low-density lipoprotein (LDL) levels are elevated, because the liver produces LDL in response to the ingestion of a high-fat diet.

- An *electrocardiogram (EKG)* is performed to detect any rate or rhythm disturbances or left ventricular strain. These findings may indicate myocardial infarction or heart enlargement, conditions often associated with morbid obesity.

Exercise Counseling

Exercise is a critical element in any weight loss or maintenance program. Physical activity increases energy consumption and promotes weight loss. Physical activity improves physical fitness, decreases appetite, promotes

Behavioral Change Strategies for the Obese Client

■ ■ ■

Controlling the Environment

- Purchase low-calorie foods.
- Shop from a prepared list and on a full stomach.
- Keep all foods in the kitchen.
- Store all foods in the refrigerator or in the cabinets in opaque containers.
- Prepare exact portions of food to eliminate leftovers.
- Eat all foods in the same place, avoiding the kitchen.
- Avoid eating when watching television or reading.
- Reduce frequency of eating out at restaurants, parties, and picnics.

Controlling Physiologic Responses to Food

- Eat slowly by taking small bites, allowing 20 minutes for a meal.
- Eat a salad or drink a hot beverage before a meal.
- Chew each bite thoroughly and slowly.
- Put eating utensils or food down between bites.
- Concentrate on the eating process; savor the food.
- Stop eating with the first feelings of fullness.

Controlling Psychologic Responses to Food

- Appreciate the aesthetic experience of eating.
- Use attractive dinnerware, and prepare a formal setting for eating.
- Use small plates and cups to make servings of food look larger.
- Concentrate on conversations and socialization during the meal.
- Use nonfood rewards for meeting a goal.
- Acknowledge small successes and improvements in all behavior.
- Substitute other activities for eating (e.g., reading, exercise, hobbies).

self-esteem, and increases the basal metabolic rate. Exercise promotes the utilization of kilocalories while preserving lean body mass and stimulating the loss of body fat. An exercise/activity program should reflect the client's physical condition, interest, life-style, and abilities. Prior to initiating an exercise program, clients should consult their health care providers (Callaway, Foreyt, Nuckolls, & VanIntallie, 1992). After medical clearance, the nurse counsels the client to increase the duration and intensity of activity and to stop exercising and report symptoms if chest pain or shortness of breath occur. An aerobic exercise program of 30 minutes of exercise 3 to 5 days a week promotes weight loss while reducing adipose tissue, increasing lean body mass, and promoting long-term weight control.

Nutritional Counseling

The diet should be low in kilocalories and fat and contain adequate nutrients, minerals, and fiber. The client should eat regular meals with small servings. Most experts recommend a gradual, slow weight loss of no more than 1 to 2 pounds per week. For most individuals, this means a diet of 1000 to 1500 kcal per day. Fewer than 1200 kcal each day may lead to loss of lean tissue and nutritional deficiencies. Additionally, the latest research points to the importance of maintaining a low-fat diet when attempting either weight loss or control (Gabello, 1993). It is important to remember that when restricting kilocaloric intake, the client may tend to overeat if placed in a situation where the opportunity exists. In other words, excessive calorie restrictions can eventually lead to overeating. The best approach is to modify dietary intake without severe restrictions, eating a well-balanced, low-fat diet and developing improved eating habits.

Very low calorie diets (VLCD) are an alternative diet intervention, generally indicated for clients who are more than 35% overweight. This type of program offers a protein-sparing modified fast (400 to 800 kcal/day or less) under close medical supervision. In a typical program, the client observes a 12-week fast, ingesting only a liquid protein supplement. This initial fast is followed by a 12-week refeeding program with nutrition and behavior modification counseling. The client generally experiences a dramatic and rapid weight loss while maintaining lean body mass. This type of program is indicated for short-term use only and requires very close medical supervision (Neil & Kushner, 1993).

Life-Style Counseling

Behavior modification is a critical component of successful weight management. Strategies such as keeping food records, eliminating cues that precipitate eating, and changing the act of eating are often very helpful.

Recording food intake, amount, location of eating, as well as situations that induce eating often help the dieter gain self-control. These strategies are often most effective when used in combination with other behavior-modification approaches.

Researchers have found that most overweight people are stimulated to eat by external cues, such as the prox-

Nursing Implications for Pharmacology: The Client with Obesity

ANOREXIANTS (NONAMPHETAMINES)

Diethylpropion (Tenuate, Tepanil)

Fenfluramine (Pondimin)

These drugs are used on a short-term basis for exogenous obesity. They are thought to inhibit the appetite center in the limbic areas and the hypothalmus and to improve mood. These drugs are used on a very limited basis because of the abuse potential. They are controlled substances and require a prescription.

Nursing Responsibilities

- Encourage the client to participate in a weight-loss program that includes exercise, behavior modification, and a low-calorie, low-fat diet.
- Monitor for excessive central nervous system stimulation, such as nervousness, irritability, or restlessness.

- When medication is discontinued, monitor for drowsiness and fatigue.
- Monitor for tolerance, which can occur 6 to 12 weeks after treatment begins.
- Do not give these drugs during pregnancy.
- Administer on an empty stomach.
- Monitor BP and pulse. Discontinue if hypertension, tachycardia, or angina occurs.

Client and Family Teaching

- Do not take later than 4:00 p.m.
- Remember the key components of a successful weight loss program: exercise, behavior modification, and a low-calorie, low-fat diet.
- Do not take these drugs during pregnancy.

---

imity to food and the time of day. In contrast, hunger and satiety are the cues that regulate eating in adults of normal weight. Strategies to control food cues include keeping food out of view, eliminating snack foods, and eating only in designated areas. See the box on page 438 for a list of behavior-modification strategies.

Changing the act of eating includes developing positive habits for eating, such as making meals last for at least 20 minutes, chewing food slowly, and making mealtimes enjoyable. The key is to modify previous eating habits and food practices.

Other behavior-modification approaches focus on helping individuals examine the factors that affect eating behaviors. Examining the client's life-style, personality, and environment promotes an understanding of eating behaviors and their consequences. The goal is to empower the person who is stimulated to eat to choose activities that are not related to food.

Social support from one's family or friends as well as group programs enhance lasting weight loss. Organizations such as Weight Watchers, Overeaters Anonymous, and Take Off Pounds Sensibly provide social support. Most organized programs require participants to pay a fee, which may enhance compliance. Many participants report greater success in group weight-loss programs because of the peer support they offer.

Pharmacology

Many prescription and over-the-counter drugs have been used to help people lose weight. Drugs may be helpful in

short-term weight loss, but long-term follow-up shows that tolerance, addiction, and side effects may occur.

Prescription medications, such as amphetamines and indirect-acting fenfluramine, are appetite-control agents. Amphetamines indirectly stimulate the sympathetic nervous system through the release of norepinephrine, resulting in hunger suppression (Callaway et al., 1992). Fenfluramine increases the release of serotonin, subsequently depressing the central nervous system. Amphetamines may cause insomnia, irritability, and nervousness, and fenfluramine may cause depression and sedation. These drugs are used with extreme caution in clients with cardiac disease and are contraindicated for children and pregnant or lactating women. The use of these drugs is limited because of the potential for abuse, side effects, and withdrawal symptoms. See the accompanying box for the nursing implications for clients receiving anorexiant drugs as part of therapy for obesity.

Over-the-counter products such as phenylpropanolamine, benzocaine, and bulk-forming agents are commonly used in weight-management efforts. Phenylpropanolamine is an adrenergic agent that suppresses appetite. This product is contraindicated in clients with hypertension, coronary artery disease, diabetes mellitus, and thyroid disease. Benzocaine, a local anesthetic agent, may reduce appetite by numbing the oral cavity, thus impairing taste and sweetness sensation. Methylcellulose and other bulk-forming products may decrease appetite by producing a sensation of fullness. Clients taking these products may experience flatulence or diarrhea and may need to increase fluid intake.

Although the Food and Drug Administration has approved these drugs for short-term weight loss, most clinicians question their usefulness. Use of these products is usually recommended only as an adjunct to therapy and only when traditional therapies have been unsuccessful.

Surgical Interventions

Surgical approaches to obesity include lipectomy, jejunoileal bypass, and gastric partitioning. These procedures have a limited degree of success and are associated with a number of complications. Most of these procedures are reserved for morbidly obese individuals or those who have failed conventional therapy. Prior to these procedures, clients must undergo extensive evaluation and meet specific medical and psychologic criteria.

Lipectomy or removal of adipose tissue has been suggested as a way for clients to lose weight and maintain that loss. **Liposuction,** suctioning of adipose tissue from under the skin, is increasing in popularity to remove fat deposits from under the skin. However, after these procedures fat can be regenerated in affected areas.

Intestinal (jejunoileal) bypass is a surgical procedure in which the jejunum is connected directly to the terminal ileum, bypassing most of the absorptive area of the small intestine. This procedure produces weight loss through malabsorption. Weight loss averages 60 to 100 pounds in the year following surgery. This procedure is rarely performed today because of serious surgical, metabolic, and biochemical complications.

The most commonly used gastric partitioning procedures are the *gastric bypass* and *gastroplasty*. These surgical procedures result in a smaller stomach capacity. Unable to consume normal portions of food, the client stabilizes at 20% to 25% above ideal body weight. Side effects of these procedures include persistent nausea and vomiting, vitamin deficiencies, and gastrointestinal scarring.

Maintaining Weight Loss

Losing weight and maintaining that loss are two separate but related issues. Most experts agree that the majority of dieters regain lost weight within a 2-year period. The potential risks associated with regaining weight make maintenance a critical issue. Dieters should be encouraged to continue exercise, self-monitoring, and treatment support. Long-term weight loss and maintenance mean a life-long commitment to significant life-style changes, including food and eating habits, activity and exercise routines, and behavior modification.

Nursing Care

In planning and implementing nursing care for the overweight or obese client, the nurse considers the client's physiologic and psychologic responses to this disorder. The nurse assesses each client from a holistic framework and identifies individual needs. Nursing diagnoses dis-

cussed in this section focus on nutrition, activity tolerance, management of therapeutic regimen, and self-esteem. A critical pathway for a client participating in a weight-loss program is provided on page 441.

Altered Nutrition: More Than Body Requirements

Although overweight is not always due to overconsumption, there is usually an imbalance of consumption to energy expenditure.

Nursing interventions with rationales follow:

- Assess height, weight, skinfold, and body composition. Assess for the presence of coexisting medical problems, including cardiovascular disease and diabetes mellitus. Assess eating and exercise/activity patterns and factors associated with dietary and exercise habits, as well as prior weight-loss efforts. *This helps determine ideal body weight. Knowledge of coexisting medical problems provides a framework for collaborative nursing care. Knowledge of factors associated with an imbalance of food intake and energy expenditure provide the basis for planning and implementing diet and exercise regimens.*

- Encourage the client to identify the factors that contribute to excess food intake. *Identification of cues to eating helps the client eliminate or reduce these cues.*

- Establish realistic weight-loss goals and exercise/activity objectives. *Small, reasonable goals, such as 1 to 2 pounds per week, increase the likelihood of success.*

- Assess the client's knowledge and provide teaching-learning opportunities regarding well-balanced diet plans. Provide necessary teaching related to diet. *Knowledge empowers the client to participate and make appropriate diet choices.*

- Discuss behavior-modification strategies, such as self-monitoring and environmental management. *Behavior modification, diet, and exercise are critical to promoting successful, long-term weight loss.*

Activity Intolerance

Morbidly obese clients often suffer from activity intolerance related to the difficulty associated with moving. By the time people enter a weight-loss program, they may need a medical evaluation. Additionally, the obese client may benefit from an individualized exercise program developed by an exercise physiologist.

Nursing interventions with rationales follow:

- Assess current activity level and tolerance to that activity. Assess vital signs. *This provides baseline information to plan an activity program and assess response to that activity.*

- After medical clearance, plan with the client a program of regular, gradually increasing exercise. Consider a consultation with an exercise physiologist. *An individualized exercise program promotes activities within the client's physical capabilities.*

Critical Pathway for a Client Participating in a Weight-Loss Program			
Date	**Initial Visit and Initiation of Weight-Loss Program**	**Ongoing Weekly Visits**	**Maintenance Program When Weight Goal Achieved**
Expected length of treatment: 1 week for each ½- to 1-lb weight loss, then maintenance for life			
Outcomes	Client will ■ Verbalize commitment to regular exercise program. ■ Verbalize understanding of dietary plan and behavior modification strategies to change eating habits. ■ Verbalize feelings regarding weight.	Client will ■ Maintain exercise diary and exercise aerobically at least 30 minutes every other day. ■ Maintain diet diary and discuss strategies to reshape eating habits. ■ Lose up to 1 lb each week. ■ Maintain blood pressure in normal range.	Client will ■ Continue aerobic exercise at least 30 minutes every other day. ■ Maintain a low-kilocalorie, low-fat diet. ■ Maintain stable weight, within a 5-lb range.
Tests and treatments	Height and weight Blood pressure Bioelectrical impedance and skinfold Thyroid profile Serum glucose, lipid profile Electrocardiogram	Weight Blood pressure Review laboratory results and any required therapies and goals of weight loss.	Monthly weight and blood pressure measurements by office nurse Follow-up laboratory studies based on any previously detected abnormalities
Psycho-social	Encourage to verbalize feelings regarding weight. Set small, achievable goals. Discuss cues to eating. Explore the possibility of psychological counseling.	Continue encouraging client to discuss feelings about weight. Continue to identify ways to eliminate or reduce eating cues. Discuss feelings regarding weight loss and self-concept. Discuss availability of support systems in weight loss efforts.	Continued use of identified strategies for behavior modification. Continued assistance from support persons.
Diet	Calculate kilocalorie needs. Instruct in low-kilocalorie, low-fat diet. Stress the importance of a well-balanced diet. Instruct client to maintain diet diary.	Assess ability to adhere to low-kilocalorie, low-fat diet and any problems incurred since modifying diet. Assess diet diary for compliance and discuss related problems. Continue strategizing meals and food selection.	Continue low-kilocalorie, low-fat diet. Manage social situations by making low-kilocalorie, low-fat choices. Fully integrate behavior-modification strategies in daily life.
Activity/exercise	Discuss current and past exercise patterns. Explore aerobic exercise interests. Establish contract with client that delineates a regular exercise program, such as walking 30 minutes every other day.	Review the importance of regular aerobic exercise and its relationship to weight loss. Encourage client to maintain exercise diary considering intensity and duration. Explore ways to increase overall level of activity (e.g., stair-walking, parking further away).	Continue aerobic exercise 30 minutes every other day. Client increases duration and intensity of exercise when kilocalorie or fat intake is higher than usual. Client fully integrates increased activity in daily life.

Ineffective Individual Management of Therapeutic Regimen

Most overweight or obese clients experience some difficulty integrating all the components of a weight-loss program into a daily routine. For a weight-loss and weight-maintenance program to be successful, the overweight client must modify dietary intake in a world of daily temptations. There may be many obstacles to exercise, including a busy schedule, activity intolerance, impaired physical mobility, lack of equipment, and the embarrassment of being fat.

Nursing interventions with rationales follow:

- Explore the client's ability and willingness to incorporate changes into daily patterns of diet, exercise, and life-style. *This provides assessment data from which to set realistic goals with the client.*

- Help the client identify behavior-modification strategies and support systems that promote weight loss and maintenance. *Weight loss and maintenance are most successful if the client establishes life-style patterns that promote interest and motivation and thus exercise and diet management. Family and social support is critical to successful adherence to the therapeutic regime.*

- Have the client establish strategies for dealing with "stress" eating or interruptions in the therapeutic regime. *Many dieters express a sense of failure when they overeat or fail to exercise. This sense of failure can lead to further overeating. Identifying positive strategies to deal with these situations promotes a sense of self-acceptance and limits self-punishment through overeating.*

Self-Esteem Disturbance

Although many obese clients may have accepted their weight and body appearance on some level, most overweight and obese individuals verbalize the experience of "fat prejudice" in their family, workplace, or community. Unless one has struggled with a weight problem, it is difficult to fully imagine the experience of being obese. Obese clients report such experiences as being ridiculed at school, being prejudged at work as being slow, and being told that their health problems are due to being "fat." These experiences, coupled with the difficulty of finding attractive clothing or a chair large enough to sit on, can contribute to disturbances in self-esteem. Hospitalized obese clients are often asked to wear the same size gown as a client of average weight, and they may be subject to frequent comments about their physical condition. Many clients report that "fat" jokes or comments contribute to a sense of negative self-worth.

Nursing interventions with rationales follow:

- Encourage the client to verbalize the experience of being overweight, and validate the client's experience. *This provides baseline assessment data that you can use to develop individualized interventions and addresses self-esteem disturbances.*

- Set small goals with the client and offer positive feedback and encouragement. *Small goals provide more opportunities for success. Positive feedback and encouragement provide a comfortable environment in which to develop self-esteem.*

- Explore the possibility of psychologic counseling with the client. *Many clients benefit from psychologic counseling for issues related to self-esteem.*

Other Nursing Diagnoses

Other nursing diagnoses that are appropriate for the obese client include the following:

- *Ineffective Individual Coping* related to sense of personal vulnerability secondary to obesity
- *Fatigue* related to discomfort with activity
- *Impaired Physical Mobility* related to decreased strength and endurance
- *Powerlessness* related to life-style of helplessness

Client and Family Teaching

Obese clients may be hospitalized because of coexisting conditions. However, most long-term treatment for obesity occurs on an outpatient basis. To promote the client's highest level of wellness, tailor the teaching and individualized treatment plan to address coexisting health problems. For example, the overweight client with diabetes needs instruction in a diabetic, calorie-restricted diet. An overweight cardiac client requires an individualized exercise prescription. Give the overweight or obese client information about community or hospital-based programs and resources.

Applying the Nursing Process

Case Study of a Client with Obesity: Sam Elliott

Sam Elliott is a 57-year-old retired electronics manufacturer who has gained 30 pounds since his retirement 2 years ago. The most active thing he does each day is "puttering around" and "walking to the end of the driveway to get the mail." He reports eating juice, oatmeal, muffin, and coffee with cream each day for breakfast. He meets friends at a local coffee shop midmorning for doughnuts and coffee. Lunch is usually a bologna-and-cheese sandwich with chips and a root beer. He usually has cheese, crackers, and wine before a dinner of meat, potatoes, vegetables, and dessert. When discussing his health care provider's recommendations for weight loss, he tells the nurse, "I have never had to diet. I just don't know how to get this weight off."

Assessment

Mr. Elliott's history indicates a weight gain of 30 pounds in the last 2 years. He is 5'10" (178 cm) tall and weighs 201 lb (91.2 kg). His cholesterol level is 240 mg/dL (normal range: 150 to 200 mg/dL) with an HDL of 37 mg/dL (normal values for a male: >45 mg/dL) and an LDL of 180 mg/dL (normal: <130 mg/dL). His BP is 138/90. His fasting blood glucose is normal at 103 mg/dL (normal: 75 to 110 mg/dL). His EKG is read as normal sinus rhythm. His bioelectrical impedance measure indicates 32% body fat. He reports easy fatigue and shortness of breath with activity. His health care provider has advised a weight loss of 30 pounds and a regular exercise program.

Diagnosis

The nurses make the following nursing diagnoses for Mr. Elliott:

- *Altered Nutrition: More Than Body Requirements* related to food intake in excess of energy expenditure manifested by weight more than 20% over ideal for height and frame and sedentary activity level

- *Ineffective Management of Therapeutic Regimen* related to knowledge deficit manifested by statement "I don't know how to get this weight off"

- *Activity Intolerance* related to sedentary life-style manifested by reports of lack of energy and decreased performance

Expected Outcomes

The expected outcomes established in the plan of care specify that Mr. Elliott will

- Lose 1 pound each week.

- Walk 30 minutes 5 days each week.

- Verbalize an understanding of the relationship between weight loss, weight control, and exercise.

- Identify behavior-modification strategies to avoid overeating.

- Identify support systems for behavior modification.

Planning and Implementation

The following nursing interventions are planned and implemented for Mr. Elliott:

- Assess weight and blood pressure once or twice each week before breakfast.

- Discuss current eating habits and strategies to reduce fat and calorie intake.

- Discuss cues that promote eating. Identify strategies to eliminate or reduce eating cues.

- Instruct Mr. Elliott to keep a food diary for the purpose of examining and reshaping eating habits.

- Discuss with Mr. Elliott the role of regular exercise in weight loss and weight control. Instruct Mr. Elliott to maintain an exercise record to keep track of the intensity and duration of activity.

- Discuss life-style and behavior-modification strategies that promote successful weight loss and control.

Evaluation

Two weeks after initiating dietary and exercise modifications, Mr. Elliott has lost 2 pounds and maintained a food diary. He has identified boredom as an appetite stimulant and a cue to eating. In light of that fact, he has started volunteering at the local hospital, where he is working with children. He is walking five times a week for a period of 30 minutes. He reports plans to increase his activity periods to 45 minutes. He verbalizes commitment to a lifelong plan of exercising and eating a low-fat diet. His BP has ranged from 132/76 to 136/84. He reports plans to have the employee health nurse at the hospital check his weight and BP each week and to join Weight Watchers for ongoing support.

Critical Thinking in the Nursing Process

1. What are some of the possible pathophysiologic bases for Mr. Elliott's abnormal cholesterol, HDL, and LDL levels?

2. What is the scientific rationale for reducing both calories and fat when one is attempting weight loss?

3. If Mr. Elliott called and reported worsening shortness of breath and chest pain with walking, how would you respond?

4. What is the physiologic basis for Mr. Elliott's borderline hypertension?

5. Develop a teaching plan for a group of overweight men and women.

6. Identify potential barriers to losing weight and strategies to reduce or eliminate these barriers.

The Client with Undernutrition

■ ■ ■

Undernutrition occurs when there is a less-than-adequate intake, absorption, or utilization of calories, nutrients, or minerals for growth, development, and/or function. Undernutrition is a type of malnutrition. Malnutrition occurs when long-term deficiencies of nutrients or calories result in health problems.

Undernutrition can present as a primary illness or as the result of other conditions, such as cancer, chronic

Conditions Associated with Undernutrition

■ ■ ■

- Acute respiratory failure
- Aging
- AIDS
- Alcoholism
- Burns
- COPD
- Eating disorders
- Gastrointestinal disorders
- Neurologic disorders
- Renal disease
- Short bowel syndrome
- Surgery
- Trauma

Table 13–1	Clinical Findings of Calorie and Nutrient Deficiencies
Deficiency	**Assessment Data**
Calorie	Weakness, listlessness Loss of subcutaneous fat Muscle wasting
Protein	Thin or sparse hair Flaking skin Hepatomegaly
Vitamin A	Night blindness Altered taste and smell Dry, scaling, rough skin
Thiamine	Confusion, apathy Cardiomegaly, dyspnea Muscle cramping and wasting Paresthesia, neuropathy Ataxia
Riboflavin	Cheilosis, stomatitis Neuropathy, glossitis
Vitamin C	Swollen, bleeding gums Delayed wound healing Weakness, depression Easy bruising
Iron	Smooth tongue Listlessness, fatigue Dyspnea

obstructive pulmonary disease (COPD), or renal disease. Undernutrition may also be due to disorders of digestion or absorption or to inadequate intake of protein, calories, vitamins, or minerals. Undernutrition may be present when a client enters the hospital or develop after surgery or serious illness. See the accompanying box for a listing of conditions associated with undernutrition. Regardless of its cause, it affects the client's recovery and prognosis. The nurse conducts an admission and ongoing nutritional assessment and stays alert for signs and symptoms of undernutrition throughout the client's hospital stay. In most acute care settings, registered dietitians work with the multidisciplinary team to identify and treat clients who are at risk for or experience undernutrition. Undernutrition in the hospital can contribute to morbidity and mortality, poor wound healing, and infection (Coats, Morgan, Bartolucci, & Weinsier, 1993). See the box on page 445 for a discussion about older adults and nutritional deficiencies.

Pathophysiology

Undernutrition affects individuals of all ages, cultures, and economic circumstances. Hunger is a worldwide problem, and each day millions go hungry throughout the world, including the United States. Groups at risk for hunger include the young, poor, elderly, homeless, low-income women, and ethnic minorities (Whitney, Cataldo, & Rolfes, 1991). Even when food is plentiful, clients may be undernourished because of poor food choices.

Additionally, illnesses or other problems may lead to undernutrition or an inadequate intake. For example, an inability to chew or swallow may contribute to inadequate intake. Prolonged nausea or vomiting alters food intake, and other gastrointestinal disorders may lead to problems with digestion and absorption. Fad diets or conditions such as obesity, anorexia nervosa, and bulimia may also result in nutritional deficiencies.

Symptoms of undernutrition vary according to the cause, type, and course of development. Physical indicators may include a wasted appearance, dry and brittle hair, and pale mucous membranes. Additionally, there may be a loss of subcutaneous fat, weight loss, peripheral edema, and a sore, smooth tongue. See Table 13-1 for a further description of clinical findings associated with specific nutritional deficiencies. A 10% weight loss for a person at ideal body weight may result in undernutrition. All body systems are affected by undernutrition, and undernourished clients have lower resistance to infection and higher morbidity and mortality rates. Figure 13–2 depicts the systemwide effects of undernutrition.

Kwashiorkor Protein-Energy Undernutrition

Kwashiorkor protein-energy undernutrition, or, as it is also known, *protein-energy malnutrition (PEM),* occurs because of inadequate protein intake or as a result of high-stress situations, such as surgery or massive infection, that deplete protein reserves. Generally, the client with kwashiorkor PEM has normal or above-normal weight for height but decreased serum protein, hemoglobin, and hematocrit levels.

Gerontologic Considerations: Nutrition

■ ■ ■

Older adults are at greater risk for nutritional deficiencies. Physiological age-related changes that contribute to this problem include changes in taste and smell, a higher incidence of gastrointestinal disease, poor oral health, loss of teeth or ill-fitting dentures, anorexia caused by medications used to treat chronic conditions, and functional limitations that impair the ability to shop and cook. Psychosocial issues also contribute to the problem. Older adults living on fixed incomes, many of them at the poverty level, may not be able to afford well-balanced meals. Loss of appetite is a problem commonly seen with depression. Social isolation and loneliness contribute to the problem. Eating is a social event, and older adults who eat alone may not eat as well as those who share meals with companions, and may consume too few, or too many, calories.

Caloric requirements to maintain homeostasis vary and are based on body size, gender, age, and physical activity. In general, older adults have a decreased basal metabolism resulting in decreased caloric needs. To compensate for this deficit, older adults need to decrease their caloric intake, but maintain a diet that meets their nutritional needs.

A thorough assessment should be completed to determine nutritional status. Psychological factors that influence eating habits should be assessed, such as loneliness, isolation, and depression. The client's general appearance should be assessed. A history of the client's diet should be noted, including information about foods and nutrients the client consumes, and

any information on weight loss or gain. Laboratory values, including complete blood count, total protein, and albumin, should be reviewed.

Nutritional deficiencies in older adults has been a problem that has been recognized for many years. The federal government has established locally administered nutrition programs in an effort to reduce the problem. These programs include home-delivered meals to people who are homebound and physically unable to prepare meals, and congregate meals, which are usually offered through senior centers. Congregate meals are inexpensive and provide opportunities for socialization. Nurses should be aware of programs in the area and refer clients to them whenever possible.

Client and Family Teaching

To maintain nutritional status, the older client should be instructed to

- Eat a well-balanced diet.
- Eat fresh fruits and vegetables.
- Shop wisely to get the most value for their money.
- Avoid processed foods.
- Avoid foods high in fat.
- Drink adequate fluids.
- Maintain ideal body weight through physical activity.
- Exercise regularly.

Marasmus Protein-Energy Undernutrition

In **marasmus protein-energy undernutrition,** the intake of kilocalories is inadequate to meet metabolic needs. Subcutaneous fat and muscle mass are depleted, and ketosis occurs as the body attempts to conserve protein. Anemias and electrolyte disturbances may occur as protein-energy deficiencies increase.

Collaborative Care

Treatment of the undernourished client varies according to the cause, type, and severity of nutritional deficiency. The goal of treatment is to restore the client to ideal body weight while replacing and restoring depleted nutrients and minerals. The client's age, severity of undernutrition, and coexisting health problems determine the type and level of intervention. Nutritional treatment may include

oral supplementation, tube feedings, or total parenteral nutrition (TPN).

Laboratory and Diagnostic Tests

As with obesity, the standard measurements to assess for undernutrition are height, weight, and body composition. To determine the type and severity of undernutrition, the following laboratory studies may be ordered:

- *Serum albumin* is measured to assess undernutrition. Clients with protein-calorie undernutrition have decreased levels of serum protein. In adult malnourished clients, the albumin level is below 3.0 mg/dL.
- *Serum cholesterol levels* are measured. Levels may either be decreased or elevated as a result of undernutrition.
- *LDL levels* are measured. Decreased levels occur in either undernutrition or malabsorption.

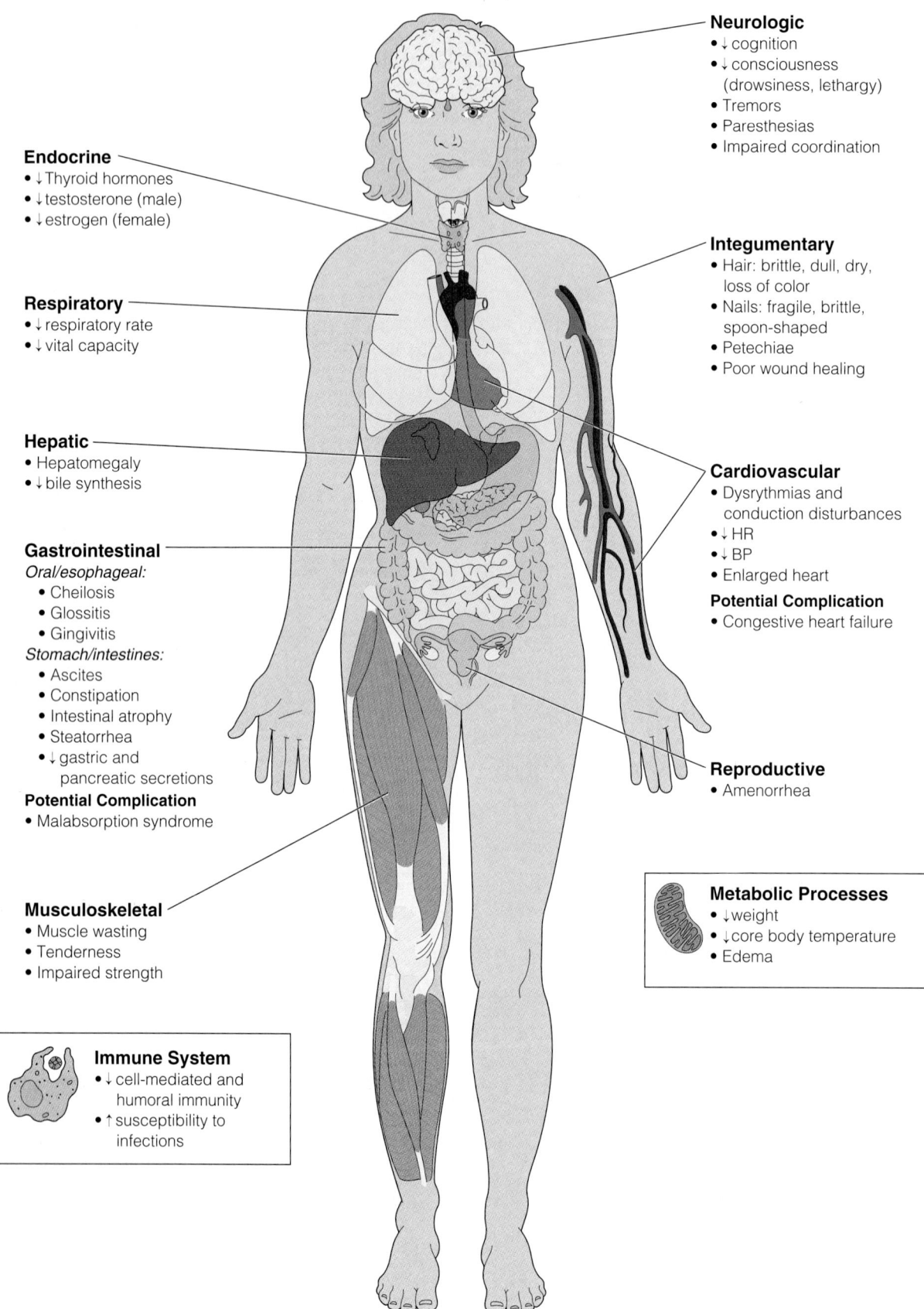

Neurologic
- ↓ cognition
- ↓ consciousness (drowsiness, lethargy)
- Tremors
- Paresthesias
- Impaired coordination

Endocrine
- ↓ Thyroid hormones
- ↓ testosterone (male)
- ↓ estrogen (female)

Respiratory
- ↓ respiratory rate
- ↓ vital capacity

Hepatic
- Hepatomegaly
- ↓ bile synthesis

Gastrointestinal
Oral/esophageal:
- Cheilosis
- Glossitis
- Gingivitis
Stomach/intestines:
- Ascites
- Constipation
- Intestinal atrophy
- Steatorrhea
- ↓ gastric and pancreatic secretions

Potential Complication
- Malabsorption syndrome

Musculoskeletal
- Muscle wasting
- Tenderness
- Impaired strength

Integumentary
- Hair: brittle, dull, dry, loss of color
- Nails: fragile, brittle, spoon-shaped
- Petechiae
- Poor wound healing

Cardiovascular
- Dysrythmias and conduction disturbances
- ↓ HR
- ↓ BP
- Enlarged heart

Potential Complication
- Congestive heart failure

Reproductive
- Amenorrhea

Metabolic Processes
- ↓ weight
- ↓ core body temperature
- Edema

Immune System
- ↓ cell-mediated and humoral immunity
- ↑ susceptibility to infections

Figure 13–2 Multisystem effects of undernutrition.

Table 13–2   Nutrition Characteristics of Selected Protein and Calorie Supplements

Contents per Liter

Product	Protein (g)	Carbohydrate (g)	Fat (g)	Sodium (mg)	Potassium (mg)	Kcal/mL
Compleat Regular	43	130	43	1300	1400	1.07
Isocal	34	135	44	530	1320	1.06
Ensure Liquid and Powder	37	143	37	833	1542	1.06
Travasorb Hepatic Diet	29.4	215.2	14.7	235	882	1.1
TraumaCal Liquid	83	195	69	1200	1400	1.5
Pulmocare Liquid	62	104	92	1292	1708	1.5
Sustacal Liquid	60.4	138	23	1000	2092	1.0

Note. Used with permission from *Drug Facts and Comparisons.* 1995. St Louis: Facts and Comparisons, a Division of J. B. Lippincott Company.

- *Hematocrit levels* are measured. Decreased levels are seen in iron deficiencies and undernutrition.
- *Serum potassium levels* are assessed for evidence of potassium depletion, which commonly occurs in severe cases of undernutrition.

Nutritional Intervention

When the cause, type, and severity of the nutritional deficit is determined, an individualized nutritional program is designed. The goals of therapy are to maintain or restore both body weight and protein stores and to prevent further loss of weight and protein. Total energy, protein, calorie, mineral, vitamin, and trace elements requirements are calculated by a registered dietitian. These calculations should reflect any increased needs due to surgery or illness. In severe acute or chronic undernutrition, food and fluids must be gradually reintroduced to avoid diarrhea and congestive heart failure. Small, around-the-clock feedings are generally tolerated best. Fluid and electrolyte imbalances must be treated, and intravenously administered solutions may be ordered to restore and maintain fluid and electrolyte balance. If an oral diet is ordered, energy- and protein-rich foods or commercially available nutritional supplements (such as Carnation Instant Breakfast, Ensure, and Sustacal) may be indicated. If the client cannot ingest an adequate diet, tube feedings or total parenteral nutrition may be ordered to meet caloric and nutrient needs.

Enteral Feedings

Enteral tube alimentation is commonly known as tube feeding. Its purpose is to meet kilocaloric and protein requirements more completely in clients unable to take adequate nutrition orally. Tube feedings may be used to pro-

vide part or all of a client's nutritional needs. See Table 13-2 for a comparison of some common enteral formulas. Indications for tube feedings include difficulty in swallowing, unresponsiveness, oral or neck surgery or trauma, anorexia, or serious illness. Feedings usually consist of high-kilocalorie or high-protein supplements. Elemental diets that provide nutrients, require limited or no digestion, and have little residue may also be prescribed. Not all supplements are complete diets in terms of meeting nutritional requirements. Therefore, it is critical to assess the nutritional formula in terms of the client's requirements (Rombeau & Caldwell, 1990).

Tube feedings are usually administered through a soft, small-caliber nasogastric or nasoduodenal tube with a weighted mercury tip. They can also be administered through a gastrostomy or jejunostomy tube.

Commercially available products come with instructions for initiating therapy. Some formulas are initially diluted to half strength for the first day of therapy. If tolerated, the formula is given at three-fourths strength on the second day and at full strength thereafter. Some formula manufacturers recommend smaller volumes of full-strength formula with a gradual increase in volume rather than strength. Diarrhea and gastric distress are the most common side effects. Fluid and electrolyte status is monitored carefully, and additional water is administered to meet the client's specific requirements. The volume of feedings is gradually increased, with a maximum feeding of 240 to 360 mL every 2 to 4 hours or 2 liters for a 24-hour period based on the client's caloric needs. Formulas may be administered as a bolus feeding or as a continuous drip feeding regulated by a feeding pump. To avoid aspiration, the nurse elevates the client at least 30 degrees during feeding and for at least 1 hour after feeding.

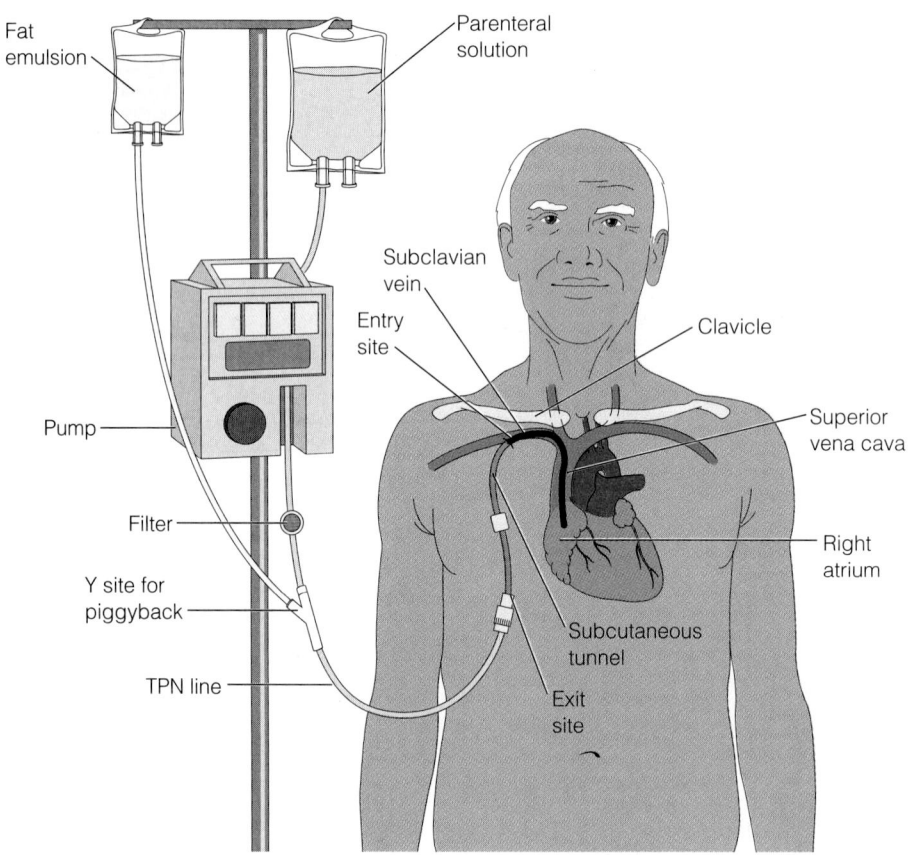

Figure 13–3 Total parenteral nutrition through a catheter in the right subclavial vein.

Fat emulsion

Parenteral solution

Subclavian vein

Entry site

Clavicle

Superior vena cava

Pump

Right atrium

Filter

Y site for piggyback

Subcutaneous tunnel

TPN line

Exit site

Total Parenteral Nutrition

Total parenteral nutrition (TPN), also known as *hyperalimentation,* is a nutritional intervention that permits the intravenous administration of carbohydrates (high concentrations of dextrose), protein (amino acids), electrolytes, vitamins, minerals, and fat emulsions. These solutions are administered intravenously through a central vein, such as the subclavian vein (Figure 13–3).

TPN is initiated when a client's nutritional requirements cannot be met through oral diet, enteral feedings, or peripheral vein infusions. Clients who have undergone major surgery or trauma, or are seriously undernourished are often candidates for TPN. TPN is used for both short- and long-term management of nutritional deficiencies, and many clients are discharged to home with TPN and monitored by home health nurses.

To initiate therapy, the physician inserts the central venous catheter under aseptic conditions. Initially, dextrose or normal saline is infused until there is X-ray confirmation of the location of the catheter tip. A triple-lumen catheter is most commonly used. This type of catheter permits the administration of medications, intralipids, or blood through other lumens. Once the position of the catheter is confirmed, the specially ordered solution can be added to the infusion. Solutions are mixed under a laminar-flow-air hood and under sterile conditions. A

commonly used solution includes 500 mL of 50% dextrose, 500 mL of an 8.5% amino acid solution, electrolytes, minerals, and vitamins. The nurse maintains the sterility of the solution and never adds medication, other than intralipids, to the solution or to the lumen through which the TPN is being administered. Most hospitals have specific policies and procedures for changing the tubing and the dressing at the insertion site as well as for hanging new containers. TPN solutions are always administered with an infusion pump to ensure the correct rate of infusion.

Initially, these hypertonic solutions are administered slowly and gradually increased, according to the physician's order. The type and amount of solution are based on the client's condition and daily weight, blood sugar, hematocrit, electrolytes, and blood chemistries. The nurse maintains accurate intake and output records. Because of the high glucose content of these solutions, many clients receive regular insulin every 6 hours based on finger-stick blood sugars.

The nurse monitors for complications from catheter insertion, such as air embolism, circulatory overload, or collection of air or fluid in the pleural cavity. During the course of therapy, the nurse assesses the client carefully for signs of infection, systemically or at the catheter insertion site. Other possible complications include hyperglycemia, hyperosmolar nonketotic dehydration, and embolism.

Pharmacology

If clients are undernourished, vitamin replacement therapy may be necessary. Either oral or parenteral supplements may be prescribed. Vitamin therapy is usually based on specific nutritional deficiencies (see Table 13–1). The box on page 450 lists the nursing implications of vitamin and mineral therapy for undernourished clients.

Nursing Care

When planning and implementing nursing care for the client with undernutrition, consider the etiology and type of undernutrition along with coexisting health problems. Each client has individual responses to undernutrition and its treatments. The complex effects of nutritional deficiencies on multiple body systems place this client at high risk for a number of other problems. This section addresses problems with nutrition, infections, fluid volume, and skin integrity.

Altered Nutrition: Less Than Body Requirements

The undernourished client experiences *Altered Nutrition: Less Than Body Requirements.* There may be situations when the nurse cannot independently diagnose and treat this condition. However, the nurse plays a critical role in the ongoing assessment of the client, while collaborating with the multidisciplinary team to provide nutritional therapies.

Nursing interventions with rationales follow:

- Gather complete baseline data and ongoing anthropometric measurements, baseline physical indicators, nutritional history, and laboratory findings. *These assessment data provide baseline information to assess the degree and type of undernutrition and the responses to nutritional therapy. Gastrointestinal assessment and oral assessments provide information pertinent to digestion and absorption problems.*

- If oral nutrition intake is offered, provide an environment and nursing measures that encourage eating. Eliminate foul odors, provide oral hygiene before and after meals, make meals appetizing, and offer frequent, small meals as well as foods the client prefers. Consult with the nutrition support team to provide adequate protein, calories, minerals, and vitamins. *Oral hygiene and a pleasant environment make food more appetizing. Small, frequent meals are generally more appealing and less overwhelming to a client with anorexia. Many clients require complicated nutritional therapy such as enteral or parenteral therapy to meet nutritional needs.*

- Provide a rest period before and after meals. *Eating is an energy-consuming activity, and the undernourished client may have decreased physical strength and energy.*

- Assess client's knowledge and provide appropriate teaching regarding nutritional requirements. *A common reason for undernutrition is the client's lack of adequate knowledge regarding nutrition. Education empowers the client to make healthy choices.*

Risk for Infection

Undernourished clients suffer from a much higher rate of infection than well-nourished people. Undernutrition affects many components of the immune system, including the skin, mucous membranes, and lymph tissue and cells. The risk for local or systemic infection is always present.

Nursing interventions with rationales follow:

- Monitor for any temperature elevation from baseline and assess for any signs and symptoms of infection every 4 hours. *Although the baseline temperature may be subnormal in undernourished clients, any elevation from baseline may indicate infection. Signs and symptoms of infection may include chills, malaise, erythema, and leukocytosis. Early detection of infection may prevent complications.*

- Maintain medical asepsis when providing care or surgical asepsis when carrying out procedures. *Hand washing is the best strategy to prevent the spread of pathogens. Sterile technique is required for procedures such as inserting central lines and changing dressings.*

- Assess the client's knowledge and provide appropriate teaching regarding signs and symptoms of infection, good hand-washing technique, and factors that place the client at risk for infection. *Knowledge empowers the client to participate in self-care, thus reducing exposure to infectious pathogens.*

Risk for Fluid Volume Deficit

The client with undernutrition may concurrently experience a fluid volume deficit. Difficulty in swallowing food and fluids or administration of hyperosmolar nutritional solutions may lead to dehydration or electrolyte disturbances.

Nursing interventions with rationales follow:

- Monitor oral mucous membranes, specific gravity of urine, level of consciousness, and laboratory findings every 4 to 8 hours. *Dry mucous membranes may indicate dehydration. An increased specific gravity may also indicate dehydration. Somnolence may indicate dehydration. Dehydration may result in electrolyte disturbances.*

- Weigh the client daily at the same time, on the same scale, and with the same clothing, and monitor intake

Nursing Implications for Pharmacology: The Client with Undernutrition

FAT-SOLUBLE VITAMINS

Vitamin A

Vitamin D (cholecalciferol, ergocalciferol)

Vitamin E (alpha-tocopherol)

Vitamin K (menadione)

The fat-soluble vitamins include vitamin A, vitamin D, vitamin E, and vitamin K. When taken orally, these vitamins are absorbed in the gastrointestinal tract. Vitamins A and D are stored in the liver. It is critical that the client consume the correct amount of the fat-soluble vitamins: All may become toxic if taken in excess amounts.

Nursing Responsibilities

- Monitor client for signs and symptoms of vitamin excesses or deficiencies as well as for adverse effects from vitamin administration.

- Provide a well-balanced diet including whole-grain cereals, protein, and fresh vegetables.

- Monitor dietary intake of fat-soluble vitamins.

- Monitor carefully for hypersensitivity reactions during the administration of parenteral vitamin therapy. Have emergency equipment available during the parenteral administration of vitamin therapy.

- Administer vitamin A with food.

- Do not administer vitamin K intravenously.

Client and Family Teaching

- Instruct regarding the importance of a well-balanced diet. Encourage the intake of a well-balanced diet, and, if indicated, provide lists of foods high in specific vitamins.

- Caution that excessive intake of the vitamins, whether through supplements or in the diet, may result in health problems.

- Instruct regarding the name, dose, purpose, frequency, and effects of the prescribed fat-soluble vitamin.

WATER-SOLUBLE VITAMINS

Vitamin C (ascorbic acid)

Vitamin B complex:
  Thiamine (B_1)
  Riboflavin (B_2)
  Niacin (Nicotinic acid)
  Pyridoxine hydrochloride (B_6)
  Pantothenic acid
  Biotin

These vitamins are used to prevent or treat deficiency problems. If the client's diet is deficient in one vitamin, it is usually deficient in other vitamins as well; therefore, multivitamin preparations are often administered. Most of these vitamins are well absorbed from the gastrointestinal tract. Recommended dosages rarely exceed the recommended daily allowance.

---

and output. *Taking weight daily and recording intake and output help monitor fluid balance.*

- If fluids are ordered, offer them frequently in small amounts, considering the client's preferences. *Clients tolerate frequent, small amounts of fluids best, and frequent drinking promotes adequate intake.*

Risk for Impaired Skin Integrity

Skin integrity depends on adequate nutrition. Pressure areas are at high risk for decreased circulation and therefore breakdown. Impaired skin and impaired immune function place the client at even higher risk for local or systemic infection.

- Assess the skin every 2 hours, and identify coexisting risk factors for skin breakdown. *Baseline and ongoing assessments provide data to evaluate the effectiveness of skin care.*

- Turn and position the client every 2 hours, and encourage passive and active range-of-motion exercises.

These nursing measures reduce pressure and promote oxygenation of cells.

- Keep skin dry and clean, and minimize shearing forces. Keep linens smooth, clean, and dry. Provide therapeutic beds, mattresses, or pads. *These nursing measures promote comfort and reduce the risk of skin breakdown.*

Other Nursing Diagnoses

Other diagnoses that may be appropriate for the client with undernutrition include

- *Knowledge Deficit* about home enteral or parenteral feedings related to unfamiliarity with resources manifested by questions and verbalized lack of understanding

- *Fatigue* related to decreased metabolic energy production manifested by inability to maintain usual routines and irritability

Pharmacology: The Client with Undernutrition (continued)

Nursing Responsibilities

- Monitor the client for signs and symptoms of vitamin excesses or deficiencies and responses to replacement therapy.
- Provide a well-balanced diet including whole-grain cereals, protein, and fresh vegetables.
- Monitor for hypersensitivity reactions from parenteral administration. Have emergency equipment available.

Client and Family Teaching

- Instruct regarding the importance of a balanced diet. Provide lists of foods high in specific vitamins.
- Do not exceed the recommended daily allowances for the specific vitamin.
- Instruct regarding the name, dose, purpose, frequency, and effects of water-soluble vitamins.

MINERALS

Sodium	Copper	Manganese
Potassium	Fluoride	Chromium
Magnesium	Iodine	Selenium
Calcium	Zinc	

Minerals are inorganic chemicals that are vital to a variety of physiologic functions. Also called trace elements, these minerals are part of a balanced diet. Recommended daily allowances have not been established for all mineral substances. The dosage of prescribed minerals depends on the specific deficiency, route of administration, and the client's general health.

Nursing Responsibilities

- Monitor the client for signs and symptoms of mineral excesses or deficiencies.
- Monitor for adverse effects to prescribed minerals.
- Prior to administration, dilute oral mineral preparations.
- Prior to the administration of iodine, assess for history of hypersensitivity to iodine. If the client is hypersensitive, notify the physician.

Client and Family Teaching

- Instruct the client regarding the importance of a well-balanced diet.
- Encourage the client to avoid exceeding the known recommended daily allowances of the mineral.
- Instruct the client to take minerals other than fluoride and zinc with or after meals.

HEMATINICS

Iron	Folic acid	Cyanocobalamin (B_{12})

Chapter 31 discusses nursing responsibilities and client and family teaching regarding these substances.

- *Activity Intolerance* related to generalized weakness manifested by dyspnea and complaints of weakness and fatigue
- *Risk for Altered Oral Mucous Membranes* related to undernutrition/dehydration, intake restrictions, endotracheal or nasogastric tubes, and oral cavity surgery
- *Risk for Self-Care Deficit: Feeding* related to decreased strength and endurance

Client and Family Teaching

Clients with undernutrition may be cared for at home or in the hospital with diet, enteral, or parenteral therapy. Each year, it is more common to see clients managing tube feeding or TPN at home. Teaching varies according to the client's individualized nutritional plan and the client's and family's teaching needs. If home enteral or parenteral feedings are required, the client will have been hospitalized and received teaching prior to discharge. To promote the client's highest level of wellness, the client and family members need to know how to (1) prepare and/or handle solutions, (2) add them to either the feeding tube or central line, (3) manage infusion pumps, (4) care for the feeding tube or central catheter, and (5) recognize and manage problems and complications. Usually the client or family members will practice these skills in the hospital and then receive ongoing care and support from visiting nurses.

Applying the Nursing Process

Case Study of a Client with Undernutrition: Rose Chow

Rose Chow is a 65-year-old widow. Her husband died unexpectedly 3 years ago, and her only child died of congenital heart disease 12 years before. She lives alone and reports that she has a lack of interest in eating and cooking since her husband died. She is active, travels with friends, and enjoys golfing and volunteer work at a local day-care center. She walks or swims 45 minutes each day for exercise. Mrs. Chow reports eating a "good diet" when she is with friends but states, "I'm really not sure what I should be eating." Mrs. Chow reports that lately she has not felt "energetic" and "can't do everything I used be able to do."

Assessment

The admission assessment indicates that Mrs. Chow weighs 95 lb (43.1 kg) and is 5'3" (160 cm) tall. She reports weighing 118 lb (53.5 kg) 5 years ago. Her triceps skinfold thickness measurement is 11 mm (normal values for a female: >13 mm). Physical assessment findings include a wasted look and pale skin. Her temperature is 97 F (36.1 C). Her diagnostic tests reveal the following abnormal findings: serum albumin 29 g/L (normal >35 g/L) and serum cholesterol 130 mg/dL (normal 150 to 200 mg/dL). A medical diagnosis of protein-calorie undernutrition is made, and the nutritional support team recommends a diet of 1500 kcal per day.

Diagnosis

The following nursing diagnoses were made by the nurses caring for Mrs. Chow:

- *Altered Nutrition: Less Than Body Requirements* related to knowledge deficit of daily requirements and anorexia manifested by weight loss of more than 10% of ideal body weight
- *Risk for Infection* related to protein-calorie undernutrition
- *Fatigue* related to decreased metabolic energy production, manifested by complaints of decreased energy and inability to participate in usual activities
- *Risk for Fluid Volume Deficit* related to limited dietary intake

Expected Outcomes

The expected outcomes established in the plan of care specify that Mrs. Chow will

- Gain at least 1 pound per week.
- Verbalize understanding of nutritional requirements and identify strategies to incorporate requirements into daily diet after discharge.
- Remain infection free, evidenced by normal vital signs.
- Verbalize actions to reduce risk of infection as well as signs and symptoms of infection.
- Demonstrate good hand-washing technique.

- Verbalize the relationship of undernutrition to fatigue and establish a routine of rest and activity to modify fatigue.

Planning and Implementation

The following nursing interventions were planned and implemented for Mrs. Chow:

- Weigh daily before breakfast and document, using same scale.
- Discuss high-calorie, high-protein foods and supplements with Mrs. Chow. Provide education related to nutritional requirements, and plan an eating program that meets both calorie, protein, and nutrient needs and reflects her likes, dislikes, and intolerances. Encourage small, frequent meals.
- Consult with the nutritional support team to ensure adequacy of diet and plan the use of supplements, such as Carnation Instant Breakfast or Ensure.
- Accurately record food intake and output.
- Maintain medical and/or surgical asepsis.
- Teach Mrs. Chow hand washing and ways to reduce risks for infection.
- Offer liquids and encourage drinking every hour while she is awake.
- Provide a comfortable environment at mealtime.

Evaluation

Now, on discharge, Mrs. Chow has gained 3 pounds and has discussed her nutritional requirements with the nurse and registered dietitian. She is drinking 2 liters of fluid each day, has normal electrolytes, and has no signs and symptoms of dehydration. She verbalizes feeling "more energetic." She has planned meals with the dietitian and has had a friend purchase the necessary groceries for her at home. She remains afebrile and free of infection. She verbalizes understanding of her nutritional requirements and strategies to meet them at home. She has scheduled follow-up appointments with the dietitian and physician.

Critical Thinking in the Nursing Process

1. What is the pathophysiologic basis for Mrs. Chow's abnormal albumin and cholesterol levels?
2. What is the rationale for having the client drink 2 liters of fluid each day?
3. Mrs. Chow asks, "Can I get better by just taking more vitamins?" What is your response?
4. Design a teaching plan for a client with protein-calorie undernutrition.
5. Develop a teaching plan for a client discharged with tube feedings.

Collaborative Health Care: The Client with Oral Cancer	
Health Care Team	**Client-Centered Goals**
Otorhinolaryngologist	Preoperatively: biopsies lesions, orders CT scans to determine spread of cancer, and with oncologist stages tumor and recommends treatments. During surgical treatment excises tumor and adjacent tissues. May perform a tracheotomy to maintain patent airway. For extensive oral cancer may perform a radical neck dissection. May recommend radiation and/or chemotherapy.
Dietician	Assesses and monitors nutritional needs and intake. Makes recommendations regarding total parenteral nutrition or enteral feedings. Teaches client and family regarding nutrition and diet.
Speech Therapist	Evaluates client for any speech and swallowing difficulties. Provides a "magic slate" or alternate communication methods for immediate postoperative period. Teaches client swallowing techniques if swallowing impairments occur.
Social Worker	Assists client and family with financial concerns. Coordinates discharge referrals for home care and community-based services including speech therapy and dietician. If required, arranges for suction equipment, enteral or parenteral feedings, and psychologic support. May coordinate support services through American Cancer Society including transportation to radiation therapy.
RN and Health Care Team Communications	Reports to surgeon any respiratory difficulty, hemorrhage, signs and symptoms of infection or other complications. Alerts social worker to home care needs including suction equipment, parenteral/enteral feedings, and visiting nurse. Consults with dietician regarding client's tolerance of parenteral/enteral therapies. Informs speech therapist about client's swallowing abilities and effectiveness of communication methods.

Disorders of the Mouth

Inflammations, infections, and neoplastic lesions of the mouth contribute to problems with the ingestion and thus the digestion of food. These disorders may be primary illnesses or associated with a variety of other health problems. Regardless of the cause, appropriate treatment of the underlying factors and associated symptoms is essential.

Disorders of the mouth may be limited to the mouth alone or occur as manifestations of dermatologic or systemic problems. Oral lesions may result from a variety of causes, including infection, mechanical trauma, irritants such as alcohol, and hypersensitivity. Ulcerative lesions in the mouth are often associated with pain, malodorous breath, and blood-tinged saliva.

Although these problems affect many adults, clients are not frequently admitted to acute care facilities for infectious or inflammatory problems of the mouth. Clients with neoplastic disorders of the mouth require some type of surgical intervention and are often hospitalized for postoperative management. See the accompanying Collaborative Health Care box for a discussion of the health care team in the plan of care.

The Client with Stomatitis

The most common inflammatory and infectious disorders of the mouth can be grouped under the classification of *stomatitis*. Clients with this group of conditions may experience pain, difficulty eating, and body image disturbances. Frequently these problems coexist with other conditions such as cancer, dental disease, and acquired immune deficiency syndrome (AIDS).

Pathophysiology

Stomatitis is an inflammation of the oral mucosa. The causes include viral (herpes simplex) or fungal (*Candida albicans*) infections; mechanical trauma, such as cheek biting; and irritants, such as tobacco or chemotherapeutic agents. See the accompanying nursing research box for a further discussion of the relationship of chemotherapy to stomatitis.

The clinical manifestations vary according to the type of stomatitis and are outlined in the box on page 454; acute oral **herpes simplex** is associated with vesicular lesions on the lips and oral mucosa. *Thrush (candidiasis)* is manifested by white, slightly raised patches on the mucous membranes. In cases of mechanical trauma, the nature of the injury determines the extent of abrasions or lacerations. Chemotherapy or chemical irritation may result in generalized redness, swelling, and ulcerations.

Aphthous ulcers (*canker sores*) are a type of stomatitis with an unknown etiology. These ulcers are usually less than 1 cm in diameter and last weeks to months. Aphthous ulcers are extremely painful, shallow erosions of the mucous membranes. They are well circumscribed with a white or yellow center encircled by a red ring.

Applying Research to Nursing Practice
Controlling Stomatitis in Clients
Undergoing Chemotherapy

■ ■ ■

One side effect of chemotherapy is stomatitis. Stomatitis can result in pain, decreased oral intake, and impaired communication. Oral lesions also can contribute to the development of systemic viral or bacterial infections. Factors that contribute to the incidence of stomatitis include the type of tumor, age, pretherapy oral health, the type and dose of the chemotherapeutic agent, and the use of radiation therapy. However, as research indicates (Wujcik, 1992), regular oral hygiene can prevent the onset of stomatitis or minimize its severity.

Implications for Nursing Practice

Nursing interventions should include brushing the client's teeth at least twice a day and flossing daily. Rinsing teeth after brushing and eating can help to establish regular routines of oral hygiene. Topical anesthetics or patient-controlled anesthesia should be used to control pain. To prevent cross-contamination, the nurse wears gloves when coming in contact with mucous membranes. Prevention and early recognition of stomatitis in the cancer client is critical to prevent complications.

Critical Thinking in Client Care

1. What is the pathophysiologic process in immunocompromised clients that places them at high risk for altered oral mucous membranes (see Chapter 8)?

2. Develop a plan of care for oral hygiene in clients who are immunocompromised.

3. Identify dietary interventions for a client experiencing stomatitis to ensure an adequate intake of food and fluids.

4. Design a handout that could be used to instruct caregivers about oral hygiene and nutritional interventions for clients with stomatitis.

Clinical Manifestations of Stomatitis

■ ■ ■

Symptoms vary according to the type of stomatitis.

Oral Herpes Simplex

■ Vesicular lesions on the lips and oral mucosa

Thrush

■ White, slightly raised patches

Other possible symptoms

■ Dry mouth   ■ Ulcerations
■ Swelling   ■ Pain

---

tary oral lesion that is present for more than 1 week and does not respond to therapy must be evaluated for malignancy.

Laboratory and Diagnostic Tests

The laboratory and diagnostic tests performed on clients with stomatitis vary according to the clinical manifestations and the client's history. Direct smears and cultures from lesions may be performed to establish the identity of any causative organisms. *Candida albicans,* herpes simplex, or bacteria may be present. If systemic illness is suspected, a variety of laboratory and diagnostic tests may be ordered, depending on the differential diagnosis.

Pharmacology

Treatment for stomatitis addresses both the symptoms and the cause. General measures include the use of a topical anesthetic, such as 2% viscous lidocaine, as an oral rinse. This solution is not swallowed, because swallowing large amounts can impair the swallowing mechanism. Orabase, a protective paste, may be applied to oral ulcers to promote comfort. Triamcinolone acetonide may be mixed in Orabase to promote healing and used as an oral rinse for its antihistamine effects. Sodium bicarbonate mouthwashes may provide relief and promote cleansing, whereas alcohol-based mouthwashes may cause pain and burning.

Fungal oral infections are most commonly treated with a nystatin oral suspension, and clients are directed to "swish and swallow" the solution. Clotrimazole lozenges are also used to treat oral fungal infections. If the thrush is unresponsive to nystatin, occurs systemically, or involves the gastrointestinal or respiratory mucosa, fluconazole or ketoconazole may be used. Antifungals are usually continued for at least 3 days after symptoms disappear.

Collaborative Care

Often the exact cause of stomatitis is difficult to determine, but the client's history may help establish a diagnosis. The treatment addresses both the underlying cause and coexisting illnesses. Evaluation includes a direct physical examination and, if indicated, cultures, smears, and evaluation for systemic illness. An undiagnosed, soli-

Nursing Implications for Pharmacology: The Client with Stomatitis

TOPICAL ORAL ANESTHETICS

Orajel	Anbesol
Viscous lidocaine	Triamcinolone acetonide

These drugs reduce the pain associated with mucous membrane lesions or stomatitis. They provide temporary relief of pain. Any oral lesion that persists longer than 2 weeks should be evaluated by an oral surgeon.

Nursing Responsibilities

- Instruct the client to seek medical attention for any oral lesion that does not heal within 2 weeks.
- Monitor for local hypersensitivity reactions, and discontinue use if they occur.

Client and Family Teaching

- Apply every 1 to 2 hours as needed.
- Perform oral hygiene after meals and at bedtime.

TOPICAL ANTIFUNGAL AGENTS

Clotrimazole	Nystatin

These products help in the topical treatment of candidiasis. Their effects are primarily local rather than systemic.

Nursing Responsibilities

- Instruct the client to dissolve lozenges in the mouth.
- Instruct the client to rinse mouth with oral suspension for at least 2 minutes and expectorate or swallow as directed.

- These drugs are contraindicated in pregnancy.

Client and Family Teaching

- Take medication as prescribed.
- Do not eat or drink 30 minutes after medication.
- Contact physician if symptoms worsen.
- Perform good oral hygiene after meals and at bedtime; remove dentures at bedtime.

ANTIVIRAL AGENT

Acyclovir (Zovirax)

Acyclovir is useful in the treatment of oral herpes simplex virus. It helps reduce the severity and frequency of infections. It interferes with the DNA synthesis of herpes simplex virus.

Nursing Responsibilities

- Start therapy with acyclovir as soon as herpetic lesions are noted.
- Administer with food or on an empty stomach.

Client and Family Teaching

- The virus remains latent and can recur during stressful events, fever, trauma, sunlight exposure, and treatment with immunosuppressive drugs.
- Take the medication as ordered, and contact the physician if symptoms worsen.

Herpetic lesions may be treated with topical or oral acyclovir. Acyclovir ointment provides comfort and lubrication while limiting the spread of the virus. Acyclovir capsules provide relief by reducing the severity of symptoms and the duration of the lesions.

Bacterial infections are treated with antibiotics based on cultures and smears. Oral penicillin is the treatment of choice if the client is not allergic and the cultured bacteria is sensitive. The accompanying box lists nursing implications for clients receiving medications used to treat stomatitis.

Nursing Care

When caring for the client with stomatitis, the nurse considers the client's responses to the stomatitis as well as any coexisting conditions. The client may be suffering from cancer, AIDS, or other systemic illnesses and undergoing extensive therapy for these problems. Therefore, it is critical to provide client-focused nursing care based on assessment findings. Although the nursing care must be individualized, this section focuses on nursing diagnoses related to problems with mucous membranes and nutrition.

Altered Oral Mucous Membrane

The client with stomatitis suffers from a disruption in the integrity of the oral mucous membranes. Regardless of the cause, the pain and symptoms must be relieved while treating the underlying cause. Oral pain usually results in a reduced oral intake of food and fluids, which can lead to nutritional, fluid, and electrolyte imbalances.

Nursing interventions with rationales follow:

- Assess oral mucous membranes and the character of any lesions, and document findings every 4 to 8 hours. *Baseline and ongoing assessment data provide the basis for evaluation.*

- Help the client to provide (or provide, if the client cannot) thorough mouth care after meals, at bedtime, and every 2 to 4 hours while awake. If the client is unable to tolerate a toothbrush, offer sponge or gauze toothettes. Avoid the use of alcohol-based mouthwashes. *Mouth care promotes hygiene and comfort. Alcohol-based mouthwashes may be irritating to mucous membranes and cause pain and further tissue damage.*

- Assess the client's knowledge and provide teaching regarding condition, mouth care, and treatments. Teach the patient to avoid alcohol, tobacco, and spicy or irritating foods. *Knowledge promotes client participation in the therapeutic plan of care and compliance. Alcohol, tobacco, and hot, spicy rough foods may injure altered mucous membranes.*

Altered Nutrition: Less Than Body Requirements

Oral lesions and pain may result in a limited oral intake, which may in turn lead to nutritional deficiencies. Anorexia and general malaise may also contribute to decreased intake.

Nursing interventions with rationales follow:

- Assess usual and current dietary intake as well as the client's ability to chew and swallow. Monitor weight daily on same scale. Provide appropriate assistive devices such as straws or feeding syringes. *Adequate nutrition is essential for healing. Daily weights provide baseline information regarding adequacy of diet. Use of assistive devices may allow the client to ingest food or fluids but avoid their contact with ulcerations or lesions.*

- Encourage a high-kilocalorie, high-protein diet reflective of the client's likes and dislikes. Offer soft, lukewarm, or cool foods or liquids such as eggnogs, milk shakes, nutritional supplements, popsicles, and puddings frequently in small amounts. Avoid spicy, hot, or irritating foods. Obtain nutritional consultation. *A diet adequate in fluids, nutrients, vitamins, and minerals is essential for healing and prevents nutritional deficiencies. Oral intake may be limited, and enriched foods and liquids enhance nutrition. Hot, spicy, or rough foods may cause further injury to the oral mucosa, resulting in more pain and further limiting oral intake. A nutritional consultation may be required to ensure adequacy of diet or assist in meeting nutritional requirements with supplements.*

Other Nursing Diagnoses

Examples of other nursing diagnoses that may be appropriate for the client with stomatitis include

- *Risk for Fluid Volume Deficit* related to limited oral intake
- *Knowledge Deficit* regarding ongoing care related to unfamiliarity with resources manifested by questions and lack of understanding
- *Pain* related to altered oral mucous membranes

Client and Family Teaching

Clients with stomatitis most frequently require self-care at home. To provide the client's highest level of wellness, focus teaching and discharge planning on meeting the client's individual needs with respect to any underlying health conditions and ongoing treatments such as chemotherapy. Critical components of the teaching plan include diet, oral hygiene, and medication regime. The client and family need to be instructed about nutritional requirements and strategies to provide for the client's individualized needs. If oral medications are prescribed upon discharge, teach the client and family about the type of medication, its route, side effects, frequency of administration, and signs and symptoms to report. It is important that clients receiving antibiotics, antivirals, or antifungals understand the importance of completing the full course of therapy. Instructions for oral care should be clear and easily understood. Clients and their families should understand the signs and symptoms to report as well as the importance of follow-up care.

The Client with Neoplasms of the Mouth

■ ■ ■

Oral cancers and their related treatment are associated with high morbidity and mortality. Approximately 29,600 cases of oral cancer will be diagnosed in 1994 in the United States (American Cancer Society, 1994). Incidence is twice as high in men as in women, and it is seen more often in men over 40. The stage of an oral cancer determines the prognosis, treatment, and degree of disability. Risk factors include smoking, drinking alcohol, and chewing tobacco.

Pathophysiology

Most early cancers of the mouth, lips, tongue, or pharynx present as inflamed areas with irregular, ill-defined borders. See the accompanying box for early signs of oral cancer. More advanced cancers appear as deep ulcers that are fixed to deeper tissues. Early lesions involve the mucosa or submucosa, whereas more advanced tumors may involve the tongue, oropharynx, mandible, or maxilla. Figure 13–4 gives an example of an oral cancer. The most frequent cell type is squamous cell carcinoma.

Early Signs of Oral Cancer

■ ■ ■

Oral Mucous Membranes

- White patches (leukoplakia)
- Red patches (erythroplakia)
- Ulcers
- Masses
- Areas of pigmentation (brownish or black)

Lips

- Fissures
- Ulcers
- Patches of leukoplakia
- Areas of pigmentation

Floor of the Mouth (Under the Tongue)

- Leukoplakia
- Masses
- Areas of ulceration

Tongue

- Masses or lesions
- Areas of pigmentation

Other

- Asymmetry of the head, face, jaws, or neck

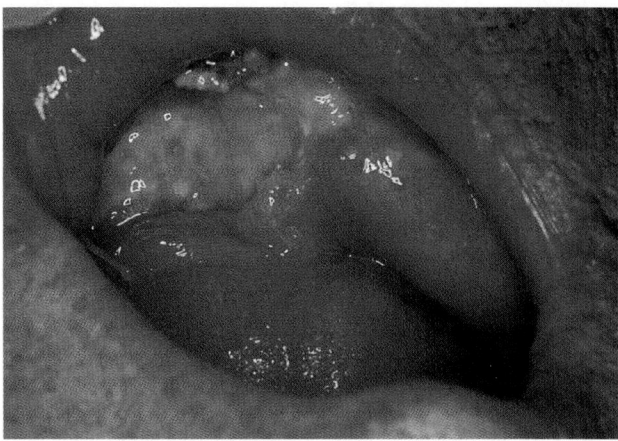

Figure 13–4   Oral cancer.

The earliest symptom of oral cancer is a painless oral ulceration or lesion. Later symptoms vary and may include difficulty in speaking, swallowing, or chewing; swollen lymph nodes; and blood-tinged sputum. Any oral lesion that does not heal or respond to treatment within 1 to 2 weeks should be evaluated for malignancy.

Collaborative Care

The treatment of oral cancer is determined by the staging of the tumor. The first component of therapy is eliminating any causative factors such as chewing tobacco, smoking, or drinking alcohol. A surgeon and oncologist discuss treatment options with the client. Extensive surgery, such as a radical neck resection with chemotherapy and radiation, may be required. If the tumor involves surrounding tissues, then cosmetic effects of surgery are important considerations. Radiation and chemotherapy may be considered based on the staging, client's age, general condition, and preferences.

Laboratory and Diagnostic Tests

Physical examination of the oral mucosa and cervical lymph nodes provides the basis for laboratory and diagnostic tests. A biopsy of the oral lesion allows for direct vi-sualization of cells to determine the presence or absence of cancerous cells. Staging of cancer may require further diagnostic tests such as CT scans or MRI studies.

Pharmacology

Chemotherapy may be indicated depending on the stage of the tumor and the oncologist's recommendations (see Chapter 9). Prescribed chemotherapeutic agents may include methotrexate, bleomycin, cisplatin, cyclophosphamide, doxorubicin, or vincristine.

Radiation Therapy

Radiation therapy may be used preoperatively to "shrink" the tumor or postoperatively to limit the risks of metastasis.

Surgery

Following the biopsy and staging of the tumor, surgery is generally indicated. An advanced or extensive tumor may be considered unresectable. Surgical interventions are based on removal of the lesion while considering cosmetic outcomes. Advanced carcinomas require more extensive excisions or a radical neck resection, which is a potentially disfiguring procedure.

Nursing Care

Nursing management of the client with oral cancer depends on the severity of the cancer, the type of management, and the client's responses to the diagnosis and associated treatments. The mouth provides the mechanism for ingesting food, and the lips are integral to verbal and nonverbal expression. The head and therefore the mouth and lips play significant roles in one's self-perception and body image. The nursing needs of any client with oral cancer are highly individual. Nursing diagnoses discussed in this section consider such problems as airway clearance, nutrition, communication, and body image.

Risk for Ineffective Airway Clearance

The location and the extent of an oral cancer and its excision may compromise the patency of the airway. Swelling of adjacent tissues or an increase in oral secretions, coupled with difficulty swallowing, may contribute to respiratory distress. If extensive surgery is performed, the airway may be maintained by an endotracheal tube or tracheostomy.

Nursing interventions with rationales follow:

- In the initial postoperative period, assess patency of oral airway and respiratory status every hour or according to clinical practice guidelines. *Oxygen is necessary for cell life. Frequent, ongoing assessment helps detect early signs and symptoms of respiratory compromise.*

- Unless contraindicated, place client in Fowler's position, supporting arms, and assist the client to turn, cough, and deep breathe every 2 to 4 hours and as needed. *Fowler's position promotes lung expansion, and turning, coughing, and deep breathing help maintain a patent airway by preventing pooling of secretions.*

- Assess client's knowledge and provide teaching regarding the importance of activity, turning, coughing, and deep breathing. *Client understanding promotes client participation in care.*

- Maintain adequate hydration (2000 to 3000 mL per day unless contraindicated) and maintain humidity of inspired air. *Adequate hydration helps thin and loosen secretions.*

Altered Nutrition: Less Than Body Requirements

The type and extent of surgery may affect the client's ability to take food or fluids orally. Enteral feedings or total parenteral nutrition may be required. If an oral diet is permitted, anorexia or pain may affect intake.

Nursing interventions with rationales follow:

- Monitor weight daily on same scale. Assess daily oral intake for adequacy of protein, kilocalories, and nutrients. *Daily weights and nutritional assessments provide baseline and ongoing information about the adequacy of diet.*

- Offer a soft, bland diet with enriched foods or dietary supplements. Offer small, frequent feedings, making mealtimes pleasant. *The postoperative client generally finds a soft, bland diet most palatable and most easily tolerated. Large meals may be overwhelming, whereas small meals may be accepted and tolerated best.*

- Consider a nutritional consultation to assess diet and plan appropriate supplements. *A registered dietitian can calculate energy requirements and plan an individualized diet plan to meet nutritional requirements.*

Impaired Verbal Communication

Oral surgery can cause problems with communication. If this problem is anticipated, a plan for communication should be established and practiced prior to surgery. Communication between the client and family and staff is essential postoperatively.

Nursing interventions with rationales follow:

- Before surgery, establish and practice a communication plan such as using a magic slate or flash cards or lip reading. *Practicing communication techniques reduces fear and anxiety while promoting communication. Alternative communication strategies promote effective communication.*

- Provide ample time for communication efforts and do not answer for the client. Be alert to the use of nonverbal communication techniques. Use yes/no questions and simple phrases. *Providing adequate time gives clients the opportunity to express ideas and thoughts. Nonverbal communication is natural for the client after oral surgery. Simple yes/no questions are easiest for the client to answer.*

- Provide an emergency call system and always respond promptly. All staff should be aware that the client cannot respond verbally over an intercom system. (It is usually best to leave this information on the intercom.) *Nonverbal clients rely on an emergency call system to summon help. Answering promptly reduces fear and anxiety and maintains the client's safety.*

- If indicated by type of surgery, consult with a speech therapist. *A speech therapist is an expert in promoting or restoring the client's ability to communicate effectively.*

Body Image Disturbance

Radical surgery of the head or neck can seriously affect an individual's body image. An altered speech pattern and any disfigurement can affect an individual's ability to feel attractive or effective in work or social roles. Indeed, clients may defer life-saving surgery so as to postpone disfiguring interventions or therapies.

Nursing interventions with rationales follow:

- Assess the client's coping style, self-perception, and responses to altered appearance or function. *Knowledge of the client's usual and current status helps the nurse plan appropriate care.*

- Encourage the client to verbalize feelings regarding perceived and actual changes. *Nonjudgmental acceptance of the client validates the client's experience.*

- Provide emotional support, encourage self-care, and provide decision-making opportunities. *Self-care promotes self-acceptance and independence. Providing choices empowers the client to participate in care.*

Other Nursing Diagnoses

Other diagnoses for clients with oral surgery include the following:

- *Altered Oral Mucous Membrane* related to oral tumors, radiation, or surgery, manifested by oral lesions, stomatitis, and verbalizations of pain
- *Pain* related to disruption of oral mucous membranes, manifested by complaints of pain
- *Fear* related to perceived lack of control, manifested by verbalizations, restlessness, muscle tension, and feelings of dread
- *Risk for Infection* related to chemotherapy or radiation

Client and Family Teaching

Discharge planning depends on the type of surgery, and associated treatments should be initiated before surgery. The nurse provides individualized teaching to the client and family. To promote the client's maximum level of wellness, nurses should ensure that all clients with oral cancer understand their diagnosis and associated care. Once oral cancer has occurred, the client must be monitored for new lesions or recurrences. Other aspects of discharge teaching relate to diet, nutrition, activity, airway management, pain control, care of incision, and signs and symptoms to report. Depending on the age and condition of client and the availability of support systems, referral to community health care agencies may be an essential component of care.

Applying the Nursing Process

Case Study of a Client with Oral Cancer: Juan Chavez

Juan Chavez is a 44-year-old farmer who is married and has 2 adult children. He and his wife live together on a large farm where they raise fruits and vegetables. Two months ago Juan discovered a bump on his tongue that would not heal. Mr. Chavez tells his admission nurse, Sara Bucklin, "I smoke two packs of cigarettes every day and have for over 20 years. I drink two to four beers every day." He also reports, "The doctor says he will have to remove part of my tongue." Mr. Chavez anxiously asks Ms. Bucklin, "Will I ever look the same? How will I be able to talk?"

Assessment

Mr. Chavez's admission history shows an otherwise healthy individual with a biopsy report positive for squamous cell carcinoma of the tongue. Mr. Chavez reports being anxious and fearful of surgery and its outcomes. He also reports quitting smoking and drinking two weeks ago. He has no enlarged cervical nodes and reports no bloody sputum or saliva. He denies having difficulty swallowing, chewing, or talking. His weight is in the normal range for his height. The surgeon planned wide excision of the oral lesion and temporary placement of a small bore nasogastric tube.

Diagnosis

The nurses caring for Mr. Chavez make the following diagnoses:

- *Risk for Ineffective Airway Clearance* related to oral surgery and increased oral secretions
- *Risk for Altered Nutrition: Less Than Body Requirements* related to NPO status
- *Impaired Verbal Communication* related to surgical disruption of tongue manifested by difficulty in speaking and verbalizing
- *Body Image Disturbance* related to surgical intervention, manifested by verbalization of negative feelings about surgery and potential outcomes

Expected Outcomes

The expected outcomes established in the plan of care specify that Mr. Chavez will

- Maintain a patent airway and remain free of respiratory distress.
- Maintain a stable weight and level of hydration.
- Effectively communicate with staff and family with use of a magic slate and flash cards.
- Verbalize an increased ability to accept changes in body image.

Planning and Implementation

The following interventions are planned and implemented for Mr. Chavez:

- Assess patency of oral airway and respiratory status every hour until stable.
- Maintain semi-Fowler's position supporting arms and encourage Mr. Chavez to turn, cough, and deep breathe every 2 to 4 hours.
- Teach Mr. Chavez the importance of activity, turning, coughing, and deep breathing.
- Monitor weight daily on same scale.
- Consult with registered dietitian to assess energy requirements, and provide enteral feeding based on dietary prescription. Carefully assess Mr. Chavez's response to enteral feedings.

- Prior to surgery practice using a magic slate and flash cards.
- Provide time for communication efforts and do not answer for Mr. Chavez.
- Keep emergency call system in reach at all times and answer light promptly. Make sure all staff are aware that Mr. Chavez cannot respond verbally.
- Each shift, assess Mr. Chavez's coping style, self-perception, and responses to altered appearance and/or function.
- Encourage Mr. Chavez to express feelings regarding perceived and actual changes.
- Provide emotional support, encourage self-care, and provide decision-making opportunities.

Evaluation

Now, at the time of discharge, Mr. Chavez has maintained his weight and has started on a liquid oral diet that includes supplements and enriched liquids. He has maintained a patent airway throughout the hospitalization and is effectively coughing and deep breathing. He did not require suctioning. He has effectively communicated using the magic slate throughout hospital stay, has begun to regain the use of his tongue, and can speak a few words. Although initially distressed about the changes in his appearance, he has begun to verbalize an increased ability to cope with the loss of part of his tongue. He and his wife verbalize understanding of his discharge instructions, including diet, activity, follow-up care, and signs and symptoms to report.

Critical Thinking in the Nursing Process

1. What are the primary prevention interventions for oral cancer?

2. Plan a health education program for young athletes who chew tobacco.

3. Design a support group for clients with oral cancer.

4. Mr. Chavez's wife calls you 2 weeks after discharge. She tells you that he refuses to try to talk and is relying on his magic slate to communicate. What advice would you offer her?

5. Develop a plan of care for Mr. Chavez based on the nursing diagnosis: *Fear* related to surgery.

▪▪▪ Disorders of the Esophagus ▪▪▪

The esophagus plays an essential role in the ingestion of food and liquids. Disorders of the esophagus can be inflammatory, mechanical, or cancerous. The symptoms of esophageal disorders may mimic those of a variety of other illnesses, but regardless of the etiology, early recognition, diagnosis, and intervention are priorities. Figure 13–5 shows the anatomy of the esophagus.

The Client with Gastroesophageal Reflux

▪ ▪ ▪

Gastroesophageal reflux (GER) is the backward flowing of gastric contents into the esophagus. This condition may occur as a result of the incompetence of the lower esophageal sphincter, transient lower esophageal relaxation, and/or increased intragastric pressure. Figure 13–6 shows the mechanisms contributing to reflux esophagitis. Many individuals may never be symptomatic from this disorder. The term **gastroesophageal reflux disease (GERD)** is used when an individual experiences symptoms such as heartburn and indigestion and has tissue damage consistent with reflux.

Pathophysiology

The client with GERD may have an abnormality of the lower gastroesophageal sphincter, delayed gastric emptying, impaired esophageal peristalsis, and/or altered mucosal defenses. Increased abdominal pressures, for instance, due to obesity and bending over, can also contribute to gastroesophageal reflux. Normally, the differences between the negative intrathoracic and the positive intra-abdominal pressure lessens the chance that gastric contents will be forced back into the esophagus. Other factors that contribute to the development of GERD are increased gastric acid and pepsin production, smoking, drinking alcohol and caffeine, eating peppermint and chocolate, fatty meals, obesity, and increased gastric volume.

GERD results in heartburn, most commonly occurring after the client eats a meal or reclines at night. The client may also report regurgitation and difficulty and pain in swallowing. Complications, including esophageal strictures, ulcers, and erosions, may occur. GERD may also cause chest pain, sore throat and hoarseness, as well as respiratory and laryngeal symptoms (Schwinghammer, 1992). The box on page 461 summarizes the major clinical manifestations of GERD.

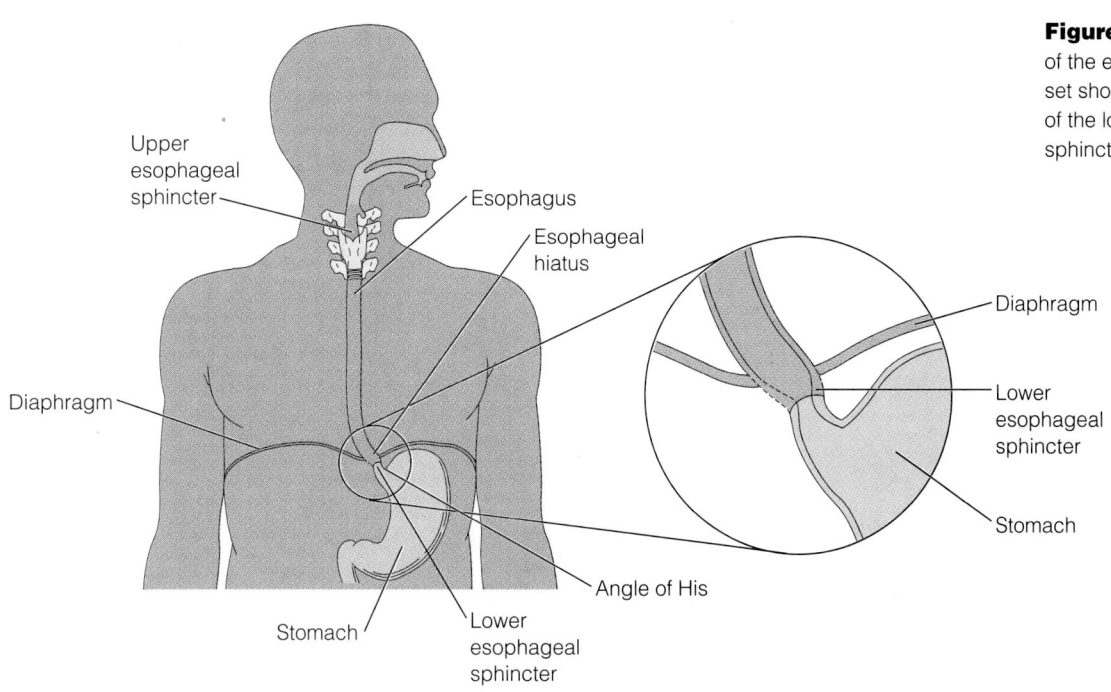

Figure 13–5   Anatomy of the esophagus. The inset shows a cross section of the lower esophageal sphincter (LES).

Upper esophageal sphincter

Esophagus

Esophageal hiatus

Diaphragm

Diaphragm

Lower esophageal sphincter

Stomach

Angle of His

Stomach

Lower esophageal sphincter

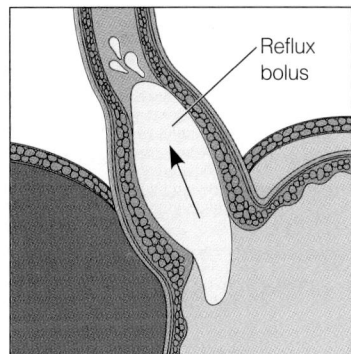

Reflux bolus

Transient lower esophageal sphincter relaxation

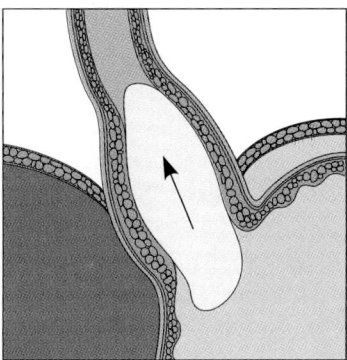

Incompetent lower esophageal sphincter

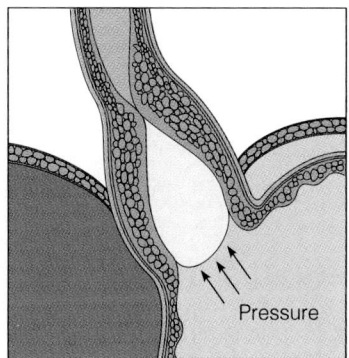

Pressure

Increased intragastric pressure

Figure 13–6 Mechanisms contributing to esophagitis.

Collaborative Care

The critical components of care for GERD are life-style changes, diet modification, and for more severe cases, pharmacologic therapy. Surgery is reserved for clients who develop serious complications. GERD is considered a chronic condition, and clients are asked to limit or eliminate their intake of citrus juices, fatty and spicy foods, coffee, alcohol, chocolate, and peppermint. Additionally, clients are instructed to achieve and maintain ideal body weight, eat smaller meals, refrain from eating for 3 hours before bedtime, and stay upright for 2 hours after meals. Clients are instructed to elevate the head of their bed on 6- to 8-inch blocks. Stopping smoking is a necessary life-style change. Avoiding tight clothing and avoiding bending may help to relieve symptoms. If these measures do not relieve symptoms or if there is evidence of esophageal damage at the time of endoscopy, pharmacologic therapy is required.

Clinical Manifestations of GERD

- Heartburn
- Regurgitation
- Pain after eating
- Dysphagia
- Chest pain
- Belching

Laboratory and Diagnostic Tests

Often the diagnosis of GERD is made by the history of symptoms and predisposing factors. However, if symptoms are unrelieved by changes in life-style and diet, further diagnostic work is ordered.

The following diagnostic tests may be ordered:

- A *barium swallow* is ordered to evaluate the esophagus and rule out cancer or peptic ulcers.

Nursing Implications for Diagnostic Tests: Esophagogastroduodenoscopy (EGD)

■ ■ ■

Preparation of Client

- Ensure that the client has signed the informed consent after receiving an explanation of the procedure and prior to receiving any premedication.
- Clients are NPO for 8 to 10 hours before the procedure.
- Complete the preprocedure checklist according to the hospital policy.
- Remove dentures and eyewear.
- Encourage questions, and provide answers and support.

Client and Family Teaching

- The client will be NPO for 8 to 10 hours before the procedure and until client is fully alert and the swallowing response returns to normal.
- The throat will be anesthetized with a topical anesthetic to allow passage of the endoscope.
- The client is placed in a left lateral decubitus position and sedated with intravenous drugs.
- The procedure is somewhat uncomfortable but takes only 20 to 30 minutes.
- Although the client will be unable to speak, respirations will not be affected.
- The client may experience mild bloating, belching, or flatulence following the procedure.

- **Endoscopy** is performed to permit direct visualization of the esophagus and rule out mass lesions or ulcers. Tissue may also be obtained for biopsy to establish the diagnosis and rule out malignancy. The most commonly performed procedure is an **esophagogastroduodenoscopy (EGD)**. See the accompanying box for nursing care of the client undergoing an EGD.
- A *24-hour ambulatory pH monitoring* may be performed to establish the diagnosis of GERD.
- *Esophageal manometry* measures pressures of the esophageal sphincters and esophageal peristalsis.

Pharmacology

Antacids, such as Mylanta or Maalox, may relieve mild or moderate symptoms by neutralizing stomach acid. Gaviscon, which forms a floating barrier between the gastric contents and the esophageal mucosa when the client is an upright position, may be used.

The histamine$_2$-receptor (H$_2$-receptor) antagonists reduce production of gastric acid and are effective in the treatment of GERD symptoms. When H$_2$-receptor antagonists are used in GERD, they are usually given twice a day or more frequently and for longer periods of time than in ulcer disease. Cimetidine, ranitidine, famotidine, and nizatidine are all approved by the FDA for the treatment of GERD (Feldman & Burton, 1990a; Feldman & Burton, 1990b). Currently, manufacturers are developing over-the-counter formulations of these products.

Omeprazole (Prilosec) is an antisecretory agent that inhibits the hydrogen-potassium-ATP pump, thereby reducing gastric secretions. Clinical trials have demonstrated its effectiveness in esophageal healing as well as in symptom relief. At this time, it is recommended only for short-term use (8 weeks) in GERD with follow-up treatment with an H$_2$-receptor antagonist (Schwinghammer, 1992).

The effectiveness of sucralfate (Carafate) in the treatment of GERD continues to be investigated. Sucralfate is an aluminum sucrose polysulfate that binds with pepsin and bile salts and promotes mucosal blood flow. When used for GERD, 1 g of sucralfate should be dissolved in 1 ounce of warm water. It is usually administered four times a day (Schwinghammer, 1992).

Several other products are being investigated for possible use in the treatment of GERD. Recent clinical trials suggest that most clients should be started on antacids, progressing to H$_2$-receptor antagonists, and then to a trial of omeprazole. See the box on page 463 for a discussion of the nursing implications for clients receiving antacids and H$_2$-receptor antagonists as part of therapy for GERD.

Nursing Care

Nursing diagnoses that are appropriate for the client with GERD include the following:

- *Pain* related to dysphagia and heartburn manifested by verbal complaints of pain and discomfort.
- *Ineffective Management of Therapeutic Regimen* related to complex therapeutic regimen manifested by ineffective nutritional and life-style choices
- *Knowledge Deficit* related to unfamiliarity of resources manifested by questions and lack of understanding

The Client with Hiatal Hernia

■ ■ ■

A **hiatal hernia** or a diaphragmatic hernia occurs when part of the stomach protrudes through the esophageal hiatus of the diaphragm into the mediastinal cavity. This problem may occur in over 40% of the population. However, most individuals are asymptomatic.

Nursing Implications for Pharmacology: The Client with GERD

ANTACIDS

Maalox	Gaviscon	Gelusil	Tums
Mylanta	Aludrox	Riopan	Amphojel

Antacids neutralize gastric acid, thus diminishing the pain from GERD and ulcer disease. These medications are administered orally. Antacid potency is described as acid-neutralizing capacity, that is, the number of milliequivalents of hydrochloric acid that can be neutralized by a volume or weight of antacid.

Nursing Responsibilities

- Monitor for worsening signs and symptoms of gastrointestinal distress, such as indigestion, heartburn, and/or pain.
- Administer on a regular basis, usually 7 times a day: 1 and 3 hours after meals, and at bedtime.
- Monitor for diarrhea or constipation.
- If the antacid is high in sodium, monitor for signs and symptoms of sodium and fluid overload.
- In the presence of renal disease, avoid magnesium-containing antacids.
- In the presence of cardiac problems, avoid antacids high in sodium.

Client and Family Teaching

- Do not administer within 2 hours of other medications. Administer 1 and 3 hours after meals and at bedtime.
- Shake suspensions well prior to administration.
- Chew tablets thoroughly, and follow with 4 to 6 ounces of water.
- Report worsening symptoms, diarrhea, or constipation.
- Do not take the medication for longer than 2 weeks without consulting health care provider.

- Avoid long-term use of calcium carbonate.

H_2-RECEPTOR ANTAGONISTS

Cimetidine (Tagamet)	Ranitidine (Zantac)
Famotidine (Pepcid)	Nizatidine (Axid)

H_2-receptor antagonists are administered either orally or intravenously. They inhibit the secretion of gastric acid by inhibiting histamine action at the H_2-receptor sites in the gastric parietal cells. These drugs are helpful in managing GERD as well as in preventing and treating ulcer disease.

Nursing Responsibilities

- Administer antacids at least 1 hour before or after the administration of histamine H_2 antagonists.
- Monitor elderly or debilitated clients for signs and symptoms of confusion.
- Monitor the client for complaints of abdominal or epigastric pain or gastrointestinal bleeding.
- Monitor CBC.
- Monitor for adverse effects.

Client and Family Teaching

- Avoid the use of alcohol, aspirin, and other non-steroidal anti-inflammatory drugs (NSAIDs).
- Take the full course of therapy as ordered.
- Discontinue smoking because it interferes with the action and effectiveness of the drug.
- Be aware that these preparations can cause drowsiness, and avoid operating hazardous machinery if drowsiness occurs.
- Report worsening symptoms, such as tarry stools, fever, sore throat, fever, or hallucinations.
- Notify the physician if any side effects occur.

Pathophysiology

The causes of hiatal hernias include congenital problems, trauma, and increased intra-abdominal pressure. In clients with a sliding hiatal hernia, part of the stomach and part of the gastroesophageal junction are above the diaphragm. However, in those with a paraesophageal hiatal hernia, part of the stomach moves alongside the esophagus. Figure 13–7 shows the two types of hiatal hernias. Clinical manifestations may include heartburn, substernal discomfort or pain, reflux, and indigestion or a feeling of fullness. (See the box on page 464.) Hiatal hernias may become incarcerated and necrotic, and they may hemorrhage.

Collaborative Care

An EGD and a barium swallow are the two diagnostic tests used to diagnose a hiatal hernia (see the box on page 462). Treatment for most hiatal hernias is based on the symptoms of gastroesophageal reflux. The same medical,

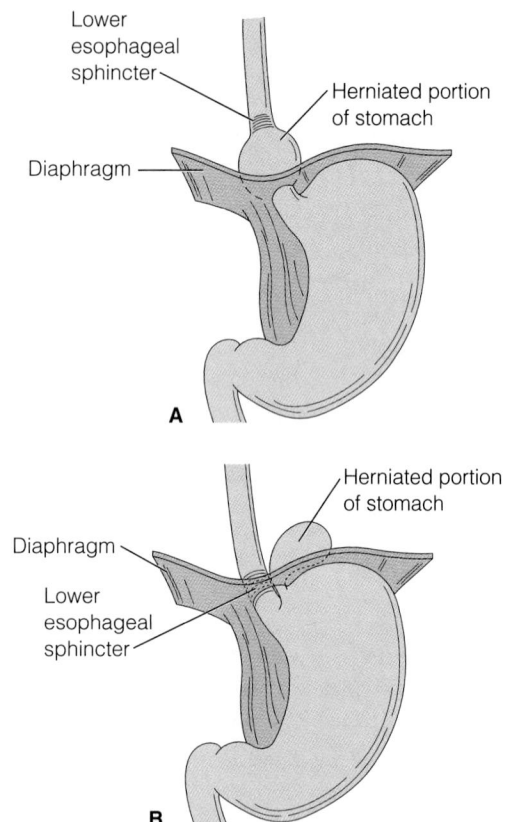

Figure 13–7   Hiatal hernias. *A,* Sliding (direct). *B,* Para-esophageal (indirect or rolling).

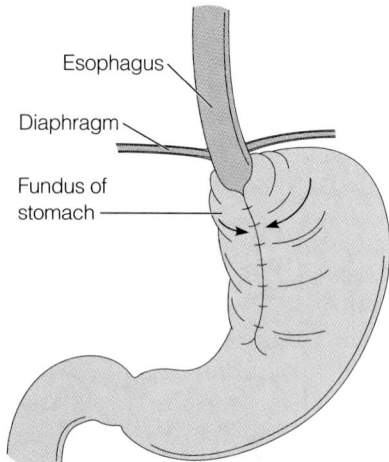

Figure 13–8   Nissen fundoplication to repair a hiatal hernia. The fundus of the stomach is wrapped around the lower esophagus, and the edges are sutured together.

Clinical Manifestations of Hiatal Hernia

■ ■ ■

- Reflux
- Chest pain
- Occult bleeding
- Regurgitation
- Dysphagia
- Belching

The Client with Diffuse Esophageal Spasm

■ ■ ■

Clients with diffuse esophageal spasm experience spastic contractions of the smooth muscle of the esophagus resulting in dysphagia and anginalike pain. Clinical manifestations are included in the accompanying box. Smooth muscle relaxants, including the calcium channel blockers, nitrates, and anticholinergics, are used to decrease the intensity and frequency of spasms.

Clinical Manifestations of Esophageal Spasm

■ ■ ■

- Intermittent esophageal contractions
- Chest pain
- Dysphagia
- Esophageal narrowing
- Spasmodic pain

---

life-style, and pharmacologic interventions used for GER are usually prescribed. If these interventions are not effective or if complications such as incarceration (irreducible hernia) occur, then surgery may be performed.

The most common surgical procedure is a **Nissen fundoplication.** This surgery involves wrapping the fundus of the stomach around the lower esophagus and suturing the fundus to itself. The fundus prevents the gastroesophageal junction from slipping into the thoracic cavity (Figure 13–8). Nursing care for the client undergoing hiatal hernia surgery is similar to that for a client undergoing other abdominal or thoracic surgery (see Chapters 7, 14, and 33).

The Client with Achalasia

■ ■ ■

The client with **achalasia** experiences an absence of peristalsis of the esophagus and a high gastroesophageal sphincter pressure that results in dilation and loss of tone in the esophagus. The cause is unknown.

The client experiences fullness in the chest during meals, chest pain, and nighttime cough. (See the box on page 465.) The client often experiences dysphagia when

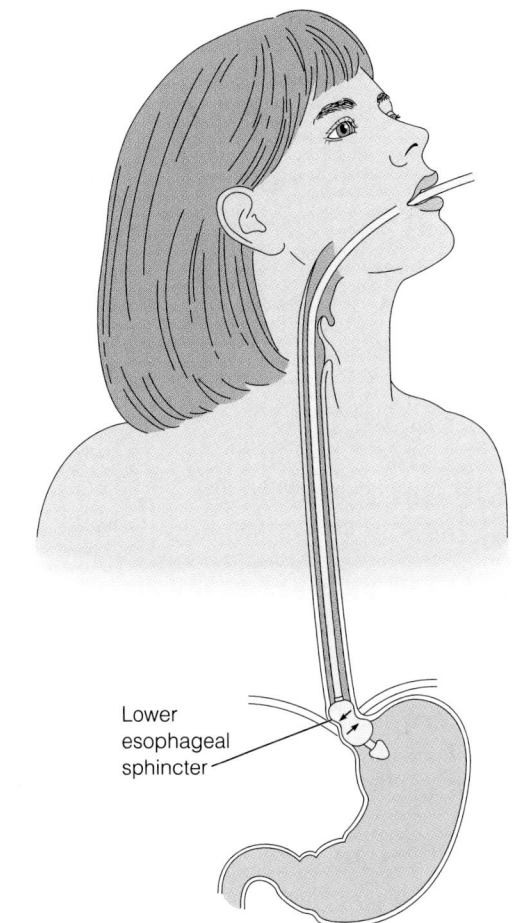

Clinical Manifestations of Achalasia

- Dysphagia
- Regurgitation
- Chest pain
- Weight loss
- Nocturnal cough

---

ingesting either fluids or solids. Initial treatment may include small frequent feedings of soft, warm foods and fluids. The client should avoid hot, spicy foods and alcohol.

Further treatment may include dilation of the lower esophageal sphincter with use of a balloon dilator. This device has an inflatable bag at the end of an esophageal tube. The client swallows the tube, and with the aid of fluoroscopy the physician places the inflatable bag at the diaphragmatic hiatus and inflates and deflates the balloon at designated intervals and pressures (Figure 13–9). The frequency of dilation is based on the severity of the client's condition and the response to this therapy. Some clients require dilation as frequently as every other week, whereas other clients may undergo the procedure once or twice a year or less frequently.

Calcium channel blockers and nitrates may also be used to decrease symptoms of dysphagia. Medications and balloon dilation may be used in combination to treat symptomatic achalasia. A surgical myotomy, or opening, of the esophageal sphincter may be required. Complications of surgery include reflux esophagitis and stricture formation.

Lower esophageal sphincter

Figure 13–9   Balloon dilation of the lower esophageal sphincter.

The Client with Esophageal Diverticulum

There are three types of esophageal diverticula: Zenker's, midesophageal, and epiphrenic. *Zenker's diverticula* are located in the upper esophagus and result in transient episodes of dysphagia. The client who regurgitates undigested food is at risk for pulmonary aspiration. *Midesophageal diverticula* are generally small and may result from scarring of pulmonary tissues. These types of diverticula rarely cause symptoms and are often an incidental finding on an upper gastrointestinal series. *Epiphrenic diverticula* are found near the lower esophageal sphincter. A large diverticulum could result in regurgitation, dysphagia, or obstruction. Treatment of diverticulum varies according to the severity of symptoms. Pulmonary aspiration or regurgitation of food are the usual indications for surgery (Rubenstein & Federman, 1978–1993).

The Client with Esophageal Cancer

Cancer of the esophagus is a relatively uncommon problem in the United States. It is estimated that 10,600 cases of esophageal cancer were diagnosed in the United States in 1990 (Ellis, Levitan, & Lo, 1991). Although the prognosis for cancer of the esophagus is generally poor, recent improvements in detection and treatment have led to an increase in overall survival rates.

Pathophysiology

Two-thirds of esophageal cancers are of the squamous cell type; adenocarcinoma is the second most common cell type. Adenocarcinoma is commonly associated with *Barrett's esophagus* (a premalignant metaplastic condition), which may result from chronic GERD and achalasia.

Clinical Manifestations of Esophageal Cancer

- Dysphagia
- Weight loss
- Regurgitation
- Aspiration pneumonitis
- Pain on swallowing
- Anemia
- GER-like symptoms
- Anorexia
- Persistent cough

Nitrosamines and alcohol have also been associated with esophageal cancer (Ellis, Levitan, & Lo, 1991).

The most common symptom of esophageal carcinoma is dysphagia (difficulty or pain in swallowing). Other symptoms include reflux, weight loss, regurgitation, and blood loss. Symptoms of advanced disease include lymph node enlargement, chronic coughing, hoarseness, hemoptysis (expectoration of blood), and hematemesis (vomiting of blood). The accompanying box summarizes the chief clinical manifestations of esophageal cancer.

Collaborative Care

After diagnosis, esophageal tumors are staged. Diagnostic and staging procedures may include esophagography, bronchoscopy, and computed tomography.

Dysphagia is a very unpleasant symptom, and control of dysphagia is an essential goal of therapy, regardless of the stage of esophageal cancer. Unfortunately, many esophageal cancers are diagnosed after metastasis has occurred. Treatment in this instance is palliative and may involve surgery, radiation therapy, and/or chemotherapy.

Laboratory and Diagnostic Tests

The following laboratory tests may be ordered:

- *Complete blood count (CBC)* is performed to establish the presence or absence of anemia, which may indicate blood loss from the gastrointestinal tract.

- *Liver function tests (SGOT, alkaline phosphatase, and bilirubin)* are performed to rule out liver metastasis.

Diagnostic procedures for esophageal cancer include

- A *barium swallow* to identify any areas of irregular mucosal pattern or narrowing of the lumen. These findings are suggestive of esophageal cancer.

- An *esophagoscopy* to allow direct visualization of the tumor and obtain tissue for histologic examination.

- A *CT scan or MRI study* to identify the presence of tumor outside of the esophagus.

- A *bronchoscopy* in clients with tumors of the upper portion of the esophagus to establish the presence of tumor in the tracheobronchial tree.

Pharmacology

Chemotherapy may be used alone or in combination with radiation therapy and surgery. Cisplatin-based therapy has been used with reports of tumor regression. See Chapter 9 for information on chemotherapy.

Radiation Therapy

If the cell type is squamous cell carcinoma, radiation therapy controls local tumor growth and relieves obstruction and pain. External beam irradiation is most commonly used, but it may be associated with esophageal perforation, hemorrhage, and stricture.

Surgery

Aggressive surgical approaches are usually indicated in early stages of esophageal cancer. If surgery is not curative, it is usually palliative and combined with radiation and/or chemotherapy. An **esophagogastrectomy** is the removal of the esophagus and part of the stomach; the remainder of the stomach takes on the function of the esophagus. The procedure is usually performed through the left chest, transhiatal approach, or through the right chest along with an abdominal incision. The surgical approach depends on the location of the tumor. Cardiovascular complications and dysfunctional gastric emptying are among the most common postoperative problems.

Nursing Care

When planning and providing care for the client with esophageal cancer, the nurse must consider the complexity of an individual's responses to the diagnosis of cancer and provide individualized care. Treatment and symptoms vary according to the stage of the cancer. Therefore, the nurse must identify client-specific needs. Although nursing care may be highly individualized, nursing diagnoses considered in this section address problems with nutrition, respiratory function, and grief.

Altered Nutrition: Less Than Body Requirements

The client diagnosed with esophageal cancer may already be suffering from some degree of undernutrition because of difficulty and pain with swallowing. Following surgical intervention, the client requires TPN or tube feedings to meet nutritional needs. Following an esophagogastrectomy, the client is NPO until the anastomosis has healed sufficiently. If the tumor is inoperable and obstruction occurs, a feeding gastrostomy tube may be inserted. See pags 447–449 for interventions related to enteral and parenteral feedings.

Risk for Ineffective Airway Clearance and Aspiration

Following thoracic and esophageal surgery, the client may experience difficulty swallowing oral or gastrointestinal secretions, placing the client at high risk for aspiration or problems maintaining a patent airway.

Nursing interventions with rationales follow:

- Assess level of consciousness and orientation as well as respiratory status every hour during the initial postoperative period. *Altered consciousness places the client at risk for aspiration. An increased respiratory rate, dyspnea, or diminished breath sounds may be indicators of an aspiration pneumonia.*

- Encourage coughing and deep breathing every 2 to 4 hours and as needed. *These activities assist in the mobilization of secretions.*

- If the client is receiving tube feedings, stop feedings if feelings of fullness or nausea occur and apply suction as needed, positioning the client on the side. *Overdistention of the stomach or delayed gastric emptying may result in regurgitation of stomach contents. Nausea or a feeling of fullness may indicate stomach overdistention. Suctioning and positioning limit the risk of aspiration.*

Anticipatory Grieving

Upon a diagnosis of cancer, the client and family may experience a grief reaction. The pessimistic prognosis associated with esophageal cancer and the disruptions in relationships may result in an intense sense of loss. Chapter 11 discusses care of client experiencing grief and loss.

Other Nursing Diagnoses

Other nursing diagnoses that may be appropriate for the client with esophageal cancer include the following:

- *Pain* related to dysphagia manifested by verbal complaints of pain and limited oral intake

- *Knowledge Deficit* related to unfamiliarity with resources manifested by questions and verbalized lack of understanding regarding discharge care

Client and Family Teaching

Clients with esophageal cancer may be hospitalized for surgery, but the diagnostic evaluation and adjunct therapies are managed on an outpatient basis. To promote the client's highest level of wellness, the nurse tailors discharge planning to the client's individual needs, condition, and prescribed therapies. For example, the client who has undergone surgery must understand both the diagnosis and treatment protocols, including wound care and follow-up care. If the client requires home tube feedings or TPN, the client and family must be able to demonstrate skills required to perform the procedure. Based on the client's needs and prognosis, referral to a community health agency and/or hospice may be appropriate.

> ### Applying the Nursing Process
>
> ## The Client with Esophageal Cancer: George Harvey
>
> George Harvey is a 51-year-old father of two adult children. He is an estate attorney who lives with his wife, Harriet. For the last 3 months, Mr. Harvey has experienced dysphagia and has lost 10 pounds. Recent outpatient testing indicates esophageal cancer, and George is admitted to the hospital for an esophagogastrectomy. On admission, he asks his nurse, Lauren Walsh, "What will happen to my wife if something happens to me? I'm afraid this cancer will get me." He also tells Ms. Walsh that he has eaten very little for the past few weeks.

Assessment

Mr. Harvey's admission assessment indicates a 10-pound weight loss and a 14-week history of dysphagia. His preadmission barium swallow and esophagoscopy indicate esophageal cancer. A biopsy is positive for squamous cell carcinoma. His preoperative laboratory and diagnostic workup, including CBC, chemistry profiles, EKG, and chest X-ray study, are all within normal limits. He is admitted for an esophagogastrectomy, and the oncologist has recommended postoperative chemotherapy and radiation. Mr. Harvey reports that the doctor told him "that will give me the best chance for cure."

Diagnosis

The nursing diagnoses for Mr. Harvey include the following:

- *Altered Nutrition: Less Than Body Requirements* related to dysphagia and NPO status manifested by recent 10-pound weight loss

- *Anticipatory Grieving* related to recent diagnosis of cancer manifested by verbal expressions of distress and potential loss of life

- *Risk for Ineffective Airway Clearance and Aspiration* related to presence of feeding tube and depressed cough

Expected Outcomes

The expected outcomes established in the plan of care specify that Mr. Harvey will

- Maintain his present weight during hospitalization.

- Resume a high-calorie, high-protein diet by time of discharge.

- Verbalize feelings regarding diagnosis and participate in decision making.

- Maintain a patent airway and have no episodes of aspiration.

Planning and Implementation

The following nursing interventions are planned and implemented for Mr. Harvey:

- Weigh Mr. Harvey daily on same scale.

- Administer tube feedings as ordered, keeping the head of the bed elevated and monitoring tolerance.

- Stop Mr. Harvey's feedings if he reports feelings of fullness or nausea, and apply suction as needed, positioning Mr. Harvey on his side.

- Prior to discharge, instruct Mr. Harvey and his wife about the importance of a high-calorie, high-protein diet and strategies for consuming adequate nutrients at home.

- Spend time with Mr. Harvey each shift, and encourage him to verbalize his feelings regarding his diagnosis as well as his perceived losses.

- Encourage Mr. Harvey to participate in decision making.

- Assess Mr. Harvey's level of consciousness and orientation as well as respiratory status every hour during the initial postoperative period.

- Encourage Mr. Harvey to cough and deep breathe every 2 to 4 hours and as needed.

Evaluation

Now, at the time of discharge, Mr. Harvey has gained one-half pound and is taking a high-protein, high-calorie diet. He and his wife have reviewed his diet with the dietitian and are planning on using some dietary supplements at home to meet protein needs. Mr. Harvey has maintained a patent airway and did not aspirate during hospitalization. He and his wife have begun to discuss the meaning of his diagnosis and tell the discharge nurse, "We are going to a support group called 'Coping with Cancer' when George is stronger."

Critical Thinking in the Nursing Process

1. What is the rationale for elevating the head of the bed during tube feedings?

2. Develop a preoperative teaching plan for a client undergoing an esophagogastrectomy.

3. Mr. Harvey calls you just prior to the initial dose of chemotherapy and says, "Everyone tells me that chemotherapy will cause vomiting, and I don't think I can take being sick again." How would you respond?

4. Design interventions to ensure adequate nutrition for individuals diagnosed with or undergoing treatment for esophageal cancer.

Bibliography

■ ■ ■

Alfaro-LeFevre, R., Blicharz, M. E., Flynn, N. M., & Boyer, M. J. (1992). *Drug handbook: A nursing process approach.* Redwood City, CA: Addison-Wesley Nursing.

American Cancer Society. (1994). *Cancer facts & figures—1994.* Atlanta: American Cancer Society.

Bockus, S. (1991). Troubleshooting your tube feedings. *American Journal of Nursing, 91,* 24–29.

Callaway, C. W., Foreyt, J. P., Nuckolls, J. G., & VanItallie, T. B. (1992, September 15). Obesity: A quartet of approaches. *Journal of Patient Care.* pp. 157–164, 171–174, 183–188, 193–199.

Carpenito, L. J. (1993). *Nursing diagnosis: Application to clinical practice* (5th ed.). Philadelphia: Lippincott.

Coats, K. G., Morgan, S. L., Bartolucci, A. A., & Weinsier, R. L. (1993). Hospital-associated malnutrition: A reevaluation 12 years later. *Journal of the American Dietetic Association, 93,* 27–33.

Dudek, S. G. (1993). *Nutrition handbook for nursing practice* (2nd ed.). Philadelphia: Lippincott.

Eastwood, G. L., & Avunduk, C. (1988). *Manual of gastroenterology.* Boston: Little, Brown.

Ellis, F. H., Levitan, N., & Lo, T. C. M. (1991). Cancer of the esophagus. In A. I. Holleb, D. J. Fink, & G. P. Murphy (Eds.), *Clinical oncology* (pp. 254–262). Atlanta: American Cancer Society.

Feldman, M., & Burton, M. E. (1990a). Histamine$_2$-receptor antagonists. *The New England Journal of Medicine, 323,* 1672–1680.

Feldman, M., & Burton, M. E. (1990b). Histamine$_2$-receptor antagonists (Part II). *The New England Journal of Medicine, 323,* 1749–1755.

Gabello, W. J. (1993, March 15). In-office counseling on a shrinking budget of time. *Journal of Patient Care.* pp. 168–177, 181–194.

Gordon, M. (1993). *Manual of nursing diagnoses.* St Louis: Mosby.

Holleb, A. I., Fink, D. J., & Murphy, G. P. (1991). *Clinical oncology.* Atlanta: American Cancer Society.

Keithley, J. K., & Eisenberg, P. (1993). The significance of enteral nutrition in the intensive care unit patient. *Critical Care Nursing Clinics of North America, 5*(1), 23–29.

Kozier, B., Erb, G., Blais, K., Johnson, J. Y., & Temple, J. S. (1993). *Techniques in clinical nursing.* Redwood City, CA: Addison-Wesley Nursing.

Neil, K. M., & Kushner, R. F. (1993). When your obese patient can't lose weight. *Postgraduate Medicine, 93*(2), 155–169.

Newbern, V. B. (1992). Failure to thrive: A growing concern in the elderly. *Journal of Gerontological Nursing, 18*(8), 21–25.

Rex, D. K. (1992). Gastroesophageal reflux disease in adults: Pathophysiology, diagnosis, and management. *The Journal of Family Practice, 35*(6), 673–681.

Rombeau, J. L., & Caldwell, M. D. (1990). *Clinical nutrition: Enteral and tube feeding* (2nd ed.). Philadelphia: Saunders.

Rubenstein, E., & Federman, D. D. (Eds.). (1978–1993). *Scientific American Medicine.* New York: Scientific American.

Schwinghammer, T. L. (1992, October). Focus on drug therapy. *American Druggist.* pp. 34–41.

Stunkard, A. J., Fosh, T. T., Hrubec, Z. (1986). A twin study of human obesity. *Journal of the American Medical Association, 256,* 51–54.

Stunkard, A. J., Sorensen, T. A., Hanis, C., Teasdale, T. W., Chakraborty, R., Schull, W. H., Schulsinger, F. (1986). An adoption study of human obesity. *New England Journal of Medicine, 314,* 193–198.

Tappen, R. M., & Beckerman, A. (1992). The hospitalized frail older adult. *Geriatric Nursing, 13,* 149–152.

Wadden, T. A., & Stunkard, A. J. (1985). Social and psychological consequences of obesity. *Annals of Internal Medicine, 103,* 1062–1067.

Weaver, K. (1991). Reversible malnutrition in AIDS. *American Journal of Nursing, 91,* 25–31.

Whitney, E. N., Cataldo, C. B., & Rolfes, S. R. (1991). *Understanding normal and clinical nutrition.* New York: West.

Wujcik, D. (1992). Current research in side effects of high-dose chemotherapy. *Seminars in Oncology Nursing, 8*(2), 102–112.

Young, C. K., & White, S. (1992). Preparing patients for tube feeding at home. *American Journal of Nursing, 29,* 46–53.

Nursing Care of Clients with Gastric Disorders

LEARNING OBJECTIVES

After completing this chapter, you will be able to

- Describe the pathophysiology of gastric disorders, including gastritis, ulcerative diseases, and cancer of the stomach.
- Relate the manifestations of gastric disorders to the pathophysiologic processes.
- Identify laboratory and diagnostic tests used to diagnose disorders of the stomach.

- Discuss the nursing implications for medications prescribed for the client with a gastric disorder.
- Provide appropriate preoperative and postoperative care for the client who has had gastric surgery.
- Use the nursing process to assess needs, plan and implement individualized care, and evaluate responses for the client with a gastric disorder.

The stomach and upper intestinal tract (duodenum and jejunum) are responsible for the majority of food digestion. When an acute or chronic disease process interferes with the function of this portion of the gastrointestinal (GI) tract, altered nutritional status is a real or potential problem. In addition, the client often experiences symptoms that can interfere with life-style.

Gastritis, peptic ulcer disease, and cancer of the stomach are the major disorders that affect digestion. Nursing roles in the management of these disorders include both acute care for the hospitalized client and teaching to provide the client with the skills and knowledge needed to manage these conditions at home.

The Client with Gastritis

■ ■ ■

Gastritis, inflammation of the stomach lining, results from irritation of the gastric mucosa and is the most prevalent disease affecting the stomach.

The most common form of gastritis, **acute gastritis,** is generally a benign, self-limiting disorder associated with the ingestion of gastric irritants such as aspirin, alcohol, caffeine, or foods contaminated with certain bacteria. Manifestations of acute gastritis may range from asymptomatic to mild heartburn to severe gastric distress, vomiting, and bleeding with **hematemesis** (vomiting blood).

Chronic gastritis is a separate group of disorders characterized by progressive and irreversible changes in the gastric mucosa (Porth, 1994). Chronic gastritis is more common in the elderly, chronic alcoholics, and cigarette smokers. When symptoms of chronic gastritis occur, they are often vague, ranging from a feeling of heaviness in the epigastric region after meals to gnawing, burning, ulcerlike epigastric pain that is unrelieved by antacids.

Pathophysiology

Normally, the stomach is protected from the digestive substances it secretes—namely hydrochloric acid and

Collaborative Health Care: The Client with Ulcer Disease

Health Care Team	Client-Centered Goals
Gastroenterologist or Primary Care Physician	Orders hematocrit and stools for occult blood to assess for bleeding. Orders upper GI series and performs EGD. During endoscopy biopsies tissue to assess for presence of gastric cancer. Makes recommendations regarding treatment of ulcer disease. Orders follow-up diagnostic evaluation to assess healing of ulcer.
Dietician	Instructs client to avoid caffeine-containing beverages, foods that cause distress, and alcohol. Explains the importance of eating in a relaxed environment and the importance of a well-balanced diet.
Psychiatric Nurse Clinician	Assesses client's coping style and level of anxiety. Assists client to identify stressful situations and explores strategies to enhance coping style. Teaches client relaxation techniques and discusses the need for rest and relaxation. Discusses client's use of tobacco products and refers client to quit-smoking program.
RN and Health Care Team Communicators	Reports to physician any evidence of hemorrhage, perforation, or obstruction. Refers client to psychiatric nurse clinician to assist and manage anxiety and stress.

pepsin—by the mucosal barrier (see Figure 14–2 on page 480). When this barrier is disrupted by an acute or chronic irritant, or when the processes that maintain the barrier are altered by disease, the gastric mucosa becomes irritated and inflamed. Lipid-soluble substances such as aspirin and alcohol penetrate the gastric mucosal barrier, leading to irritation and possible inflammation. Bile acids also break down the lipids in the mucosal barrier, increasing the potential for irritation (Porth, 1994). In addition, aspirin and other nonsteroidal anti-inflammatory drugs (NSAIDs) inhibit prostaglandins. Prostaglandins stimulate the production of bicarbonate, which neutralizes hydrochloric acid and increases the thickness of the mucosal barrier (Wilson et al., 1991).

Acute Gastritis

Acute gastritis is characterized by disruption of the mucosal barrier by a local irritant. This disruption allows hydrochloric acid and pepsin to come into contact with the gastric tissue, resulting in irritation, inflammation, and superficial erosions (Andreoli et al., 1990; Wilson et al., 1991). The gastric mucosa rapidly regenerates, generally making acute gastritis a self-limiting disorder, with resolution and healing occurring within several days.

The ingestion of aspirin or other NSAIDS, corticosteroids, alcohol, and caffeine is commonly associated with the development of acute gastritis. Consuming food contaminated with staphylococcus, salmonella, or *Escherichia coli* may result in an abrupt, severe gastritis as bacterial endotoxins attack the gastric mucosa.

Accidental or purposeful ingestion of a corrosive alkali (such as ammonia, lye, Lysol, and other cleaning agents) or acid leads to severe inflammation and possible necrosis of the stomach. Gastric perforation, hemorrhage, and peritonitis are possible results.

Iatrogenic causes of acute gastritis include radiation therapy and administration of chemotherapeutic agents such as cytotoxic drugs and antimetabolites.

The client with acute gastritis may be asymptomatic, have very mild symptoms of **anorexia** (loss of appetite), or report mild epigastric discomfort that is relieved by belching or defecating. Abdominal pain, nausea, and vomiting may be present, as well as evidence of gastric bleeding, such as hematemesis or **melena,** black, tarry stool that contains blood. Corrosive gastritis may present with severe bleeding, signs of shock, and an acute abdomen (severely painful, rigid, boardlike abdomen) if perforation has occurred.

A severe form of acute gastritis, erosive or **stress-induced gastritis,** occurs as a complication of other life-threatening conditions such as shock, severe trauma, major surgery, sepsis, burns, or head injury. Ischemia of the gastric mucosa and the diffusion of acid into gastric mucosal tissues result in multiple superficial erosions of the gastric mucosa. Bleeding, which may be severe, is common in erosive gastritis (Andreoli et al., 1990; Wilson et al., 1991).

Chronic Gastritis

Unrelated to acute gastritis, chronic gastritis is a progressive, irreversible atrophy of the gastric mucosa and glandular tissue of the stomach (Bullock & Rosendahl, 1992; Porth, 1994). Superficial changes in the gastric mucosal epithelium and a decrease in mucus characterize the initial stages. As the disease evolves, glands of the gastric mucosa are disrupted and destroyed. The inflammatory process involves deep portions of the mucosa, which thins and atrophies (Wilson et al., 1991). There appear to be at least two different forms of chronic gastritis, classified as type A and type B.

Type A gastritis, also known as autoimmune atrophic gastritis, occurs most commonly in persons of Northern European heritage (Farinati & DiMario, 1991). This type of gastritis may be triggered by a physical or psychoemotional stressor, although a cause-and-effect relationship is not clear. In autoimmune atrophic gastritis, antibodies to parietal cells and to intrinsic factor are produced. These antibodies destroy gastric mucosal cells, resulting in tissue atrophy and the loss of hydrochloric acid and pepsin secretion. Because intrinsic factor is required for the absorption of vitamin B_{12}, this immune response also results in pernicious anemia (Wilson et al., 1991). For further discussion of pernicious anemia, see Chapter 30.

Type B gastritis or *simple atrophic gastritis* is the more common form of chronic gastritis. Its incidence increases with age, reaching nearly 100% in individuals over the age of 70. Type B gastritis is strongly associated with colonization of the gastric mucosa by *Helicobacter pylori,* a gram-negative spiral bacterium (Wilson et al., 1991). Chronic alcohol use, cigarette smoking, exposure to toxins such as lead, and metabolic conditions such as uremia may also contribute to the development of simple atrophic gastritis. The outermost layer of gastric mucosa thins and atrophies, providing a less effective barrier against the autodigestive properties of hydrochloric acid and pepsin.

Chronic gastritis is often asymptomatic until atrophy is sufficiently advanced to interfere with digestion and gastric emptying. The client may complain of vague gastric distress, epigastric heaviness after meals, or ulcerlike symptoms. In contrast to peptic ulcers, chronic gastritis is not relieved by antacids and does not occur at night.

The client with chronic gastritis may experience not only localized symptoms but also fatigue and other symptoms of anemia. If intrinsic factor is lacking, paresthesias and other neurologic manifestations of vitamin B_{12} deficiency may be present. The accompanying box compares the clinical manifestations of acute and chronic gastritis.

Chronic atrophic gastritis increases the risk of other gastric disorders. It is estimated that 50% of individuals with gastric ulcers also have chronic gastritis. Gastric carcinoma is an additional risk, especially in persons with autoimmune atrophic gastritis. Gastric carcinoma develops in approximately 7% to 10% of people with chronic gastritis (Porth, 1994).

Collaborative Care

Acute gastritis is generally easily diagnosed by the history and clinical presentation and is appropriately treated on an outpatient basis unless severe vomiting or hemorrhage threatens homeostasis. In contrast, the vague symptoms and serious conditions associated with chronic gastritis warrant a more extensive diagnostic workup. Because chronic gastritis is a progressive, irreversible disorder, the client requires lifelong therapy for its management.

Clients with acute and chronic gastritis are generally managed on an outpatient basis. The client is seen in the acute care facility only when nausea, vomiting, and possible diarrhea are severe enough to interfere with normal fluid and electrolyte balance and nutritional status. If hemorrhage results, surgical intervention with a partial gastrectomy, vagotomy, or pyloroplasty may be required.

Clinical Manifestations of Acute and Chronic Gastritis

■ ■ ■

Acute Gastritis

Gastrointestinal
- Anorexia
- Nausea and vomiting
- Hematemesis
- Melena
- Abdominal pain

Systemic
- Possible shock

Chronic Gastritis

Gastrointestinal
- Vague discomfort after eating; may be asymptomatic

Systemic
- Anemia
- Fatigue

These procedures are discussed later in this chapter, in the section on peptic ulcer disease.

Laboratory and Diagnostic Tests

Laboratory tests that may be ordered for the client with gastritis include the following:

- *Gastric analysis* is performed to assess levels of hydrochloric acid secretion. A nasogastric tube is passed into the stomach, and pentagastrin is injected subcutaneously to stimulate gastric secretion of hydrochloric acid. Secretion may be decreased in clients with chronic atrophic gastritis.

- *Serum vitamin B_{12} levels* are measured to evaluate the client with chronic gastritis for possible pernicious anemia. Normal values for vitamin B_{12} are 200 to 1000 pg/mL, with lower levels seen in aging clients. The loss of or damage to parietal cells may lower vitamin B_{12} levels, causing megaloblastic anemia.

- *Hemoglobin, hematocrit, and red blood cell indices* are also used to assess for the presence and type of anemias associated with chronic gastritis. The client with gastritis may develop pernicious anemia because of the destruction of parietal cells or iron-deficiency anemia because of chronic blood loss.

The following diagnostic studies may be ordered for the client with acute or chronic gastritis:

- **Gastroscopy** may be performed to assess the gastric mucosa visually for changes, identify areas of bleeding, and obtain tissue for biopsy. A flexible endoscope is used to identify areas of atrophic gastritis and obtain tissue specimens for histologic examination. Areas of

Nursing Care of the Client Having a Gastroscopy

PREOPERATIVE NURSING CARE

- Assess the client's understanding of the procedure, providing explanation, clarification, and emotional support as needed. Reassure the client that although he or she will remain awake during the procedure, local anesthesia and/or sedation will be administered to minimize discomfort. During the examination, the client may have difficulty swallowing and will be unable to talk; breathing however, will not be affected. A feeling of pressure or fullness in the stomach may be experienced during the procedure. The examination will be performed in an endoscopy room and will require 20 to 30 minutes to complete. *The client who is knowledgeable about the procedure and expected sensations is less anxious and better able to cooperate with instructions.*

- Ensure that a signed consent for the procedure is present in the chart. *Gastroscopy is an invasive procedure requiring informed consent.*

- Instruct the client to abstain from intake of food or fluids for 6 to 12 hours prior to the examination; if the client is hospitalized, ensure NPO status after midnight prior to the procedure. *Withholding food and fluids helps ensure that the stomach will be empty for better visualization and to prevent vomiting upon insertion of the endoscope. If local anesthesia is used, aspiration of stomach contents into the respiratory tract is more likely if vomiting or regurgitation occurs because of loss of the gag and cough reflexes.*

- Remove dentures and check for loose teeth prior to the procedure. Provide for mouth care. Remove eyewear, jewelry, hairpins, and combs. *Although flexible endoscopes are less traumatic to the mouth and teeth than rigid ones, dentures and loose teeth can be dislodged during insertion, posing a risk for aspiration. Glasses, jewelry, and hair ornaments are removed to minimize the risks of loss, interference with accompanying radiologic procedures, and injury.*

POSTOPERATIVE NURSING CARE

- Monitor vital signs, and evaluate the client for evidence of complications: bleeding, abdominal or back pain, dyspnea, dysphagia, or fever. *Gastroscopy is a low-risk procedure, but the tissues of the esophagus and stomach may be traumatized or perforated during the procedure.*

- Withhold all food and fluids until gag and swallow reflexes have returned. Position client in semi-Fowler's position with the head to side to allow drainage of saliva from mouth. Provide an emesis basin and tissues or a washcloth for the client to expectorate into. *Until the gag and swallow reflexes have returned following local anesthesia, the risk of aspiration is high if food or fluids are consumed. The client may not be able to swallow saliva or sense its presence until sensation returns.*

- Inform client that a sore throat, hoarseness, abdominal bloating, belching, and flatulence are common following the procedure. Warm saline gargles or throat lozenges may be used to relieve discomfort. *Trauma to the upper GI tract by the instrumentation and inflation of the stomach with air or carbon dioxide commonly causes the above discomforts in the early postoperative period. The client should notify the physician if any of these symptoms persist.*

- Ensure that the client is not discharged alone before sedation is completely worn off. *Sedation used during the procedure may interfere with balance, coordination, judgment, and reaction time, resulting in an increased risk of injury.*

- Instruct the client to inform the physician immediately if any of the following signs of complications develop: persistent difficulty swallowing; epigastric, substernal, or shoulder pain; vomiting blood or black tarry stools; or fever. *Mucosal trauma, hemorrhage, perforation, and infection are potential complications of gastroscopy. Early identification and intervention are important to a successful outcome.*

---

bleeding may be treated with electro- or laser coagulation or injected with a sclerosing agent. See the accompanying box for nursing care of the client having a gastroscopy.

Pharmacology

Dietary modifications and pharmacologic interventions are the mainstay of gastritis management. The client with acute gastritis is appropriately treated with gastrointestinal tract rest as provided by 6 to 12 hours of NPO status, then slow reintroduction of clear liquids (broth, tea, gelatin, carbonated beverages), followed by ingestion of heavier liquids (cream soups, puddings, milk) and finally a gradual reintroduction of solid food.

Antiemetics such as trimethobenzamide hydrochloride (Tigan) or prochlorperazine (Compazine) and antacids

Procedure 14–1   Gastric Lavage

When it is important to remove or dilute gastric contents rapidly, gastric lavage, the irrigation or washing out of the stomach, may be indicated. In acute poisoning or ingestion of a caustic substance, a large-bore 30- to 36-gauge french Ewald nasogastric tube is inserted, and lavage performed. When gastric hemorrhage occurs, lavage is used to remove blood from the GI tract and stimulate vasoconstriction to slow the bleeding. Because the GI tract is not a sterile area of the body, clean technique is appropriate for use, although the solution used will generally be sterile.

■ Obtain a baseline assessment, including vital signs, abdominal inspection, girth, and bowel sounds. *It is important to have assessment data documented prior to instituting the procedure for comparison.*

■ Explain the procedure to the client, answering questions and clarifying perceptions. Instruct client to report any pain, difficulty breathing, or other problems during the procedure. *A client who is able to understand and cooperate with the procedure will tolerate lavage better. The client may be aware of symptoms associated with complications such as perforation or tube displacement before they are evident to the nurse performing the procedure.*

■ Place the client in semi-Fowler's or Fowler's position. If the client is unable to tolerate elevation of the head of the bed because of hypotension, place the client in the left side-lying position. *Placing the client in the side-lying position or elevating of the head of the bed minimizes the risk of aspiration.*

■ Insert a nasogastric tube (14- to 16-gauge french, unless otherwise indicated) if one is not already in place. Verify tube placement by as- pirating gastric contents and auscultating gastric region while injecting 20 to 30 mL of air. *Proper placement is vital to prevent aspiration or overdistention of the small bowel with irrigating solution.*

Closed System Irrigation

■ Wearing clean gloves, connect bag or bottle of normal saline irrigating solution to nasogastric tube using a Y connector. Attach drainage or suction tube to other arm of connector (Figure 14–1). Empty the

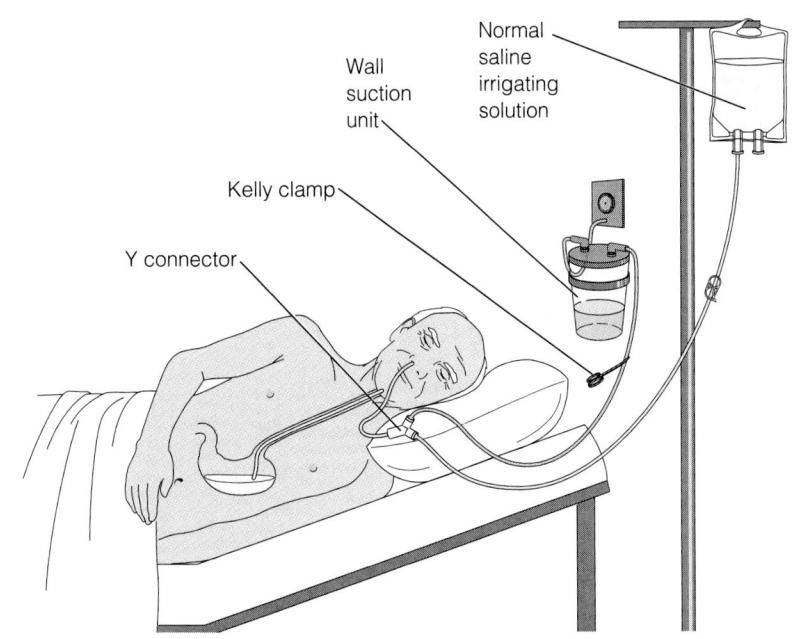

Normal saline irrigating solution

Wall suction unit

Kelly clamp

Y connector

Figure 14–1   The client with a closed system gastric lavage.

---

are used in acute gastritis to control gastric distress and vomiting. Commonly used antacids include aluminum hydroxide (AlternaGEL, Amphojel), magnesium hydroxide (Milk of Magnesia), and combination products such as Maalox and Mylanta.

The client who experiences nausea and vomiting to a degree that threatens fluid and electrolyte balance requires intravenous fluids and replacement of lost electrolytes. When bacterial food contamination is found to be the cause, antibiotic therapy is initiated.

When acute gastritis is the result of the ingestion of a poisonous or corrosive substance (acid or strong alkali), immediate dilution and removal of the substance is indicated. Vomiting is not induced because it might further damage the esophagus and possibly the trachea; instead, **gastric lavage,** washing out of the stomach contents, is performed (Chowdry, 1993). See Procedure 14–1.

With chronic atrophic gastritis, therapy is tailored to the disease characteristics of the individual. If a normal or excessive amount of hydrochloric acid is present in the stomach, clamp drain tube or turn off suction, and allow 50 to 200 mL of solution to run into stomach by gravity. Stop solution and allow to drain or suction out. Repeat until ordered amount has been used or desired results are obtained, for example, absence of further clots and solution returns that are clear or light pink. Measure the amount of the drainage, subtracting the amount of irrigant instilled, to obtain gastric output. *The closed system minimizes the risk of contact with body fluids for the nurse. Measurement of gastric output is important in monitoring fluid balance.*

Intermittent Open System

- Wearing clean gloves and other personal protective equipment as necessary (gown and face protection), empty the stomach using suction or a 50-mL catheter-tip syringe. Measure and discard the as-

pirate. Using the syringe, draw up approximately 50 mL of irrigation solution, and instill it using gentle pressure. Aspirate the nasogastric tube, and discard the solution into a measuring container. Continue this procedure until the desired amount of irrigant or desired results have been obtained. *Manual irrigation with a catheter-tip syringe may be more effective in removing clots from the stomach and nasogastric tube.*

- Continue to monitor the client's vital signs (including temperature), tolerance of the procedure, and other assessment data as lavage is being performed. *The client who requires gastric lavage is often unstable and requires continuous reevaluation. Using solutions at room temperature may cause hypothermia; therefore, the client requires frequent monitoring for temperature and other indications*

of hypothermia, such as lethargy and changes in cardiac rate and rhythm. Because of the increased risk for hypothermia and the danger of severe vasoconstriction and ischemia of the gastric mucosa, iced solutions are no longer recommended.

- If the aspirate has not cleared to light pink or pink-tinged after 20 to 30 minutes of lavage or if the client is unable to tolerate the procedure, notify the physician. *Medical or surgical intervention may be necessary to stop hemorrhage in some instances.*

- On completion of lavage, provide mouth and nares care. Continue to monitor vital signs, abdominal status, and other assessment data.

- Document the procedure, including the amount and type of irrigant used, gastric output character and amount, and the client's condition and tolerance of the procedure.

---

stomach, antacids and histamine$_2$ (H$_2$)-receptor antagonists are used to reduce the amount or effects of hydrochloric acid on the gastric mucosa. Cimetidine (Tagamet), ranitidine (Zantac), famotidine (Pepcid), and nizatidine (Axid) are examples of H$_2$ antagonists. Sucralfate (Carafate), a drug closely related to aluminum hydroxide, may also be used. Although this drug does not neutralize acid or inhibit acid secretion, it works locally to prevent the damaging effects of acid and pepsin on gastric tissue.

The client with autoimmune atrophic gastritis produces little or no hydrochloric acid; therefore, antacids and H$_2$-receptor antagonists are of little use for treatment. Anticholinergic drugs such as glycopyrrolate (Robinul) or propantheline bromide (Pro-Banthine) may be beneficial. Corticosteroids may be used to manage the parietal-cell destruction resulting from the autoimmune response. Vitamin B$_{12}$ injections are necessary when there is no remaining intrinsic factor to allow B$_{12}$ absorption from the GI tract.

Nursing implications for drugs commonly used in managing gastritis are included in the pharmacology box on page 476.

Nursing Care

In planning and implementing nursing care for the client with acute or chronic gastritis, the nurse should consider not only the direct effects of the disorder on the client's gastrointestinal system and nutritional status but also the actual or potential effects on the client's life-style and psychosocial homeostasis. Although the needs of clients with acute and chronic gastritis differ, this section focuses on problems of fluid balance and nutrition.

Fluid Volume Deficit

Nausea, vomiting, and abdominal distress are the primary manifestations of acute gastritis. The risk for fluid and electrolyte imbalance is high because of inadequate intake of food and fluids, and abnormal losses of fluids and electrolytes with vomiting.

Nursing interventions with rationales follow:

- Assess, monitor, and record vital signs every 2 hours (or more frequently) until the client is stable, then every 4 hours. Check for orthostatic hypotension. *Tachycardia, tachypnea, and hypotension, especially orthostatic hypotension, may indicate fluid volume deficit. Elec-*

trolyte imbalances may cause cardiac rhythm disturbances or other vital sign changes; metabolic alkalosis from vomiting and resultant loss of hydrogen ions may lead to depressed respirations.

- Assess, monitor, and record all intake and output carefully, including urine output and specific gravity every 1 to 4 hours as needed. Weigh the client daily. *Hypovolemia from fluid loss results in low output and high specific gravity of urine. Daily weights performed at the same time, on the same scale, and with similar clothing or covering provide an accurate indicator of fluid volume status.*

- Assess and record skin turgor and condition and status of oral mucous membranes frequently. Provide meticulous skin and mouth care frequently. *Skin turgor and condition of mucous membranes are indicators of hydration status. When poorly hydrated, the skin and oral mucous membranes are at high risk for impaired tissue integrity and require particular care.*

- Monitor laboratory values for electrolytes and acid-base balance. Report significant changes or deviations from normal. *Significant changes in electrolyte or acid-base balance affect physical function, including organ systems, mental status, and musculoskeletal function.*

- Administer fluids by mouth or parenteral route as ordered. *Clients may be NPO until vomiting has ceased, with a gradual reintroduction of oral fluids thereafter. Intravenous fluids are used to restore or maintain hydration until adequate oral intake is resumed.*

- Administer antiemetic and other medications as ordered to relieve vomiting and allow restoration of enteral intake. Encourage oral intake of fluids as soon as feasible. *The oral route is preferred for fluid and nutrient intake; medications may be used to allow earlier resumption of feeding.*

- Take measures to assure the safety of clients with orthostatic hypotension: place the signal light within reach, put up the side rails, instruct the client not to ambulate or get up without assistance. *Orthostatic hypotension may lead to syncope and to falls if the client attempts to get up without assistance.*

Altered Nutrition: Less Than Body Requirements

Manifestations of chronic gastritis, including sensations of fullness, pain, or vague epigastric distress, are often associated with eating. Because of this association, the client may become fearful of eating or may gradually reduce food intake to the point that metabolic needs are not met. Associated anorexia also contributes to a lack of intake and high risk for altered nutrition.

Nursing interventions with rationales follow:

- Monitor and record food and fluid intake and any abnormal losses (such as vomiting). *Careful monitoring of food and fluid intake and output can help provide clues for developing a dietary plan to meet the caloric needs of the client.*

- Weigh the client daily at the same time. Monitor nutritional status through the results of laboratory studies such as serum albumin, hemoglobin, hematocrit, and red blood cell indices. *Accurate daily weight and laboratory tests provide data regarding the client's nutritional status and the effectiveness of interventions.*

- Arrange for dietary consultation to determine the client's caloric and nutrient needs and to develop a dietary plan for meeting those needs. Consider client food preferences and tolerences in menu planning. *The client may require increased amounts of protein, certain vitamins, and minerals in the diet because of abnormal losses, needs for tissue healing, and loss of normal gastric mucosa. Clients with chronic gastritis may have specific food intolerances that need to be considered. Food likes and dislikes need to be taken into account to assure consumption of diet provided.*

- Provide nutritional supplements between meals or frequent small feedings as needed. *Many clients with chronic gastritis tolerate small, frequent feedings better than three large meals per day.*

- Maintain tube feedings or parenteral nutrition as ordered. Refer to Chapter 13 for further information on enteral and parenteral feedings.

Other Nursing Diagnoses

Other nursing diagnoses appropriate for the client with acute or chronic gastritis include the following:

- *Pain* related to gastric mucosal irritation by pepsin and hydrochloric acid

- *Knowledge Deficit* related to lack of information regarding aggravating factors and treatment

- *Activity Intolerance* related to associated anemia

Client and Family Teaching

Because the client with acute or chronic gastritis is often managed in the home environment, teaching is a vital component of nursing care. Teaching for the client with acute gastritis focuses on the identification and avoidance of causative factors, the management of acute symptoms, the reintroduction of fluids and foods, and the indicators of the need for further medical intervention (intractable vomiting, signs of dehydration and electrolyte imbalance).

Clients with chronic gastritis must learn to manage their condition on a long-term basis. These clients require information on maintenance of nutritional status, helpful dietary modifications, use of prescribed medications, and

Text continues on page 478

Nursing Implications for Pharmacology: The Client with Gastritis or Peptic Ulcer Disease

ANTIEMETICS

Bismuth subsalicylate (Pepto-Bismol)	Prochlorperazine (Compazine)
Scopolamine (Transderm-Scop)	Thiethylperazine (Torecan)
Dimenhydrinate (Dramamine)	Dronabinol (Marinol)
Cyclizine (Marezine)	Metoclopramide (Reglan)
Meclizine (Antivert)	Trimethobenzamide (Tigan)
Hydroxyzine (Vistaril)	

Antiemetics are used to suppress vomiting and relieve nausea. Some antiemetics, for example, bismuth subsalicylate (Pepto-Bismol), may act directly on gastric mucosa; other antiemetics act centrally on the vomiting center in the brain. Irritation of the gastrointestinal mucosa in acute gastritis can stimulate the vomiting center, as can many other sources of input, such as strong emotions, motion sickness, severe pain, increased intracranial pressure, and chemotherapy drugs. Several classes of drugs act centrally to suppress vomiting, including anticholinergics, such as scopolamine; antihistamines, such as dimenhydrinate and hydroxyzine; phenothiazines, such as prochlorperazine; cannabinoids (marijuana derivatives), including dronabinol; and miscellaneous agents, such as metoclopramide and trimethobenzamide HCl.

Nursing Responsibilities

- Assess for contraindications or allergies to the prescribed medication. The antihistamine and anticholinergic antiemetics are contraindicated for clients with glaucoma because of resulting pupillary dilation. These drugs are used with caution in clients with asthma, GI obstruction, or urinary tract obstruction.

- The oral route is preferred for centrally acting antiemetics (with the exception of scopolamine, which is administered transdermally). Treatment in anticipation of nausea and vomiting (e.g., 1 hour before a meal or treatment) is more effective. Rectal suppositories may be used for clients unable to take oral medication.

- When administering antiemetics parenterally to achieve a more rapid response, make deep intramuscular injections into the ventrogluteal site. Z-track and air-lock techniques may be used to prevent tracking of the drug into subcutaneous tissues. Be alert for more severe side effects when the parenteral route is used (Shlafer, 1993).

- Monitor for adverse effects, such as abdominal pain, constipation, urinary hesitancy or retention, tachycardia, muscle tremor, or involuntary movements.

- Drowsiness is a common side effect of antiemetic therapy. Ensure client safety.

- Centrally acting antiemetics interact with other central nervous system depressants, potentially causing respiratory depression. Monitor the client's respiratory status carefully, especially if the client has also received a narcotic analgesic, ingested alcohol, or taken another drug which depresses the central nervous system.

Client and Family Teaching

- Centrally acting antiemetics may cause drowsiness; therefore, avoid driving or operating hazardous machinery while taking these drugs.

- While using antiemetics, abstain from drinking alcohol or using other drugs that cause sedation, unless they are prescribed by the physician.

- These drugs are not recommended for use during pregnancy. Nonpharmacologic measures to control nausea and vomiting should be employed.

- Using antiemetics to prevent, rather than treat, nausea and vomiting is more effective. Take the medication 30 to 60 minutes before any activity that generally causes nausea, such as eating or traveling.

ANTACIDS

Aluminum hydroxide (Amphojel, AlternaGEL)

Magnesium hydroxide (Milk of Magnesia)

Calcium carbonate (Tums)

Magnesium hydroxide and aluminum hydroxide (Maalox, Mylanta, Gelusil)

Antacids buffer or neutralize gastric acid, generally by a local or nonsystemic action, although some work systemically. Antacids are used in gastritis and peptic ulcer disease to relieve pain and prevent further damage to the gastric mucosa when hyperacidity is present or loss of the mucosal barrier has occurred.

Nursing Responsibilities

- Check for possible interaction of the prescribed antacid with other pharmacologic preparations. Antacids interfere with the absorption of many orally administered drugs; separate administration times by at least 2 hours to avoid this problem.

- Antacids can increase the absorption of oral anticoagulants. Monitor carefully for signs of bleeding.

Pharmacology: The Client with Gastritis or Peptic Ulcer Disease (continued)

- By raising the gastric pH, antacids can cause enteric-coated preparations to dissolve in the stomach rather than the intestine, increasing the risk of gastric irritation. Administer antacids no sooner than 1 hour after enteric-coated preparations such as aspirin and bisacodyl (Dulcolax).

- Monitor for constipation or diarrhea resulting from antacid therapy. Notify the physician should either occur; a different antacid may be prescribed.

- Although the amount of systemic activity of most antacids in small, electrolyte imbalance is a potential complication of therapy. Monitor clients taking high doses of calcium carbonate or aluminum-containing antacids for signs of hypercalcemia. Monitor clients taking magnesium salts for magnesium intoxication, especially elderly clients and those whose renal function is poor.

Client and Family Teaching

- If you have gastritis or suspected ulcer disease, never use sodium bicarbonate as an antacid. It interacts with gastric acid to form large amounts of carbon dioxide, which can stretch and further damage the stomach wall. Sodium bicarbonate can also aggravate hypertension, edema, and congestive heart failure and may cause metabolic alkalosis (Shlafer, 1993).

- Take antacids frequently as prescribed; to work effectively, the antacid must be present in the stomach. Gastric activity will normally eliminate the antacid from the stomach within approximately 2 hours.

- Avoid taking the antacid for approximately 2 hours before and 1 hour after taking other medication.

- Report diarrhea or constipation to the physician. Do not self-treat these conditions, because they may be related to the antacid therapy.

- Continue taking the antacid for the duration prescribed. Pain and gastric discomfort are often relieved early in the course of therapy, but mucosal healing takes 6 to 8 weeks.

H₂-RECEPTOR ANTAGONISTS

Cimetidine (Tagamet)   Famotidine (Pepcid)
Ranitidine (Zantac)   Nizatidine (Axid)

H₂-receptor antagonists or blockers reduce acidity of the stomach environment by blocking the ability of histamine to stimulate acid secretion by the gastric parietal cells. This action reduces both the volume and concentration of hydrochloric acid within the stomach.

Nursing Responsibilities

- Assess the client for conditions that contraindicate H₂-receptor antagonist therapy or require caution and reduced dosages. H₂-receptor antagonists are not recommended for use in pregnancy or lactating mothers. They are contraindicated for clients who have had a previous hypersensitivity reaction to one of the drugs in this class. Reduced dosages are used in clients with renal or hepatic impairment.

- Assess for the concurrent use of drugs having significant interaction with the H₂-receptor antagonists. Cimetidine, a nonspecific H₂-antagonist, interacts with a greater number and variety of drugs than the other H₂-antagonists. Cimetidine inhibits the metabolism of oral anticoagulants, beta blockers (propranolol in particular), benzodiazepines, tricyclic antidepressants, theophylline, antidysrhythmics, phenytoin, calcium channel blockers, cyclosporine, carbamazepine, and narcotic analgesics, increasing their levels and effects (Baer & Williams, 1992).

- Administer cimetidine with meals and at bedtime; other H₂-receptor antagonists have a longer duration of action and may be administered once per day, generally at bedtime. Do not administer antacids within 1 hour before or after histamine-blocking drugs to ensure absorption.

- When administered intravenously, do not mix with other drugs. Administer in 20 to 100 mL of solution over 15 to 30 minutes. Rapid intravenous injection as a bolus may cause cardiac dysrythmias and hypotension (McKenry & Salerno, 1992).

Client and Family Teaching

- Take the drug as directed, even if pain and gastric discomfort are relieved early in the course of therapy.

- Drugs prescribed on a once-a-day schedule should be taken at bedtime. If spaced through the day, take before meals. Avoid taking antacids for 1 hour before and 1 hour after taking H₂-receptor antagonists.

- To promote healing, avoid cigarettes, which increase acid secretion, and gastric mucosal irritants such as alcohol, aspirin, and NSAIDs.

- Long-term use of H₂ antagonists may cause gynecomastia (breast enlargement) and impotence in men, and tenderness of the breasts in women. These effects are reversible when the drug is discontinued (Skidmore-Roth, 1993).

- Report any of the following to the physician: diarrhea, confusion, rash, fatigue, malaise, or bruising. They may indicate an adverse effect.

avoidance of known gastric irritants, such as aspirin, alcohol, and cigarette smoking. Referral to smoking-cessation classes or programs to treat alcohol abuse may be necessary.

Case Study of a Client with Chronic Atrophic Gastritis: Helen Rogers

Helen Rogers is an 81-year-old widow who lives alone. She reports having had a "touchy stomach" all her life but recently has noticed a vague sensation of fullness, nausea, and epigastric discomfort whenever she eats. Initially she thought it was "just heartburn," but because it has continued for several months, she is now concerned that she may have an ulcer or stomach cancer.

Assessment

The history obtained by Carl Havner, the nurse admitting Mrs. Rogers, reveals that she has avoided highly spiced and fatty foods for a number of years because she associates them with nausea and mild abdominal pain. Over the past year, she began experiencing similar symptoms after eating beef or ham, cheese, and vegetables in the cabbage family. Mrs. Rogers reports smoking approximately one pack of cigarettes per day for the past 35 years. She has taken aspirin an average of four times per week for mild osteoarthritis in her hands and hips. Normally an active person, she complains of becoming tired after just a couple of hours of gardening. "I suppose it's my age catching up with me finally," she said. Physical examination reveals the following findings: T, 97.6; BP, 136/62; P, 82; R, 16. Her weight is 110 lb (49.9 kg), down 10 lb (4.5 kg) from her previous visit a year ago. Her skin is pale and slightly cool, and slight epigastric tenderness is noted on palpation of her abdomen. Laboratory studies reveal a red blood cell count of 3.5 million/mm^3, hemoglobin of 9 g/dL, and hematocrit of 24% with increased mean corpuscular volume (MCV). Mrs. Rogers's serum vitamin B_{12} level is 120 pg/mL compared with a normal range of 160 to 950 pg/ml. Gastric secretory studies showed **hypochlorhydria,** a deficiency of hydrochloric acid in the gastric juice. The diagnosis of chronic atrophic gastritis was established on gastroscopy. Mrs. Rogers receives an injection of vitamin B_{12} and is started on an oral antacid every 2 hours while awake. A dietary consultation is arranged, and the physician prescribes Nicoderm patches to help Mrs. Rogers stop smoking.

Diagnosis

The nursing diagnoses established by Mr. Havner include the following:

- *Altered Nutrition: Less Than Body Requirements* related to discomfort associated with food intake
- *Fatigue* related to anemia
- *Knowledge Deficit* related to lack of information about new diagnosis of chronic gastritis
- *Anxiety* related to need to quit smoking

Expected Outcomes

The expected outcomes established in the plan of care specify that Mrs. Rogers will

- Maintain current weight without further loss.
- Demonstrate a gradual increase in activity to her previous normal level.
- Verbalize an understanding of the processes of chronic gastritis and measures to control the symptoms.
- Verbalize modifications of behavior and knowledge of support systems available to assist with smoking cessation.
- Demonstrate a reduction in anxiety.

Planning and Implementation

Mr. Havner plans and implements the following nursing interventions for Mrs. Rogers:

- Weigh daily before breakfast and record.
- Discuss food preferences and intolerances with Mrs. Rogers prior to developing a meal plan. Provide small feedings with high-calorie, between-meal supplements.
- Allow activities as tolerated, providing for rest periods.
- Provide teaching about chronic atrophic gastritis, the prescribed medical regimen (including the need for monthly injections of vitamin B_{12}), and the effects of aspirin, smoking, and alcohol consumption on gastritis.
- Teach Mrs. Rogers techniques to help during the process of withdrawal from nicotine.
- Refer Mrs. Rogers to a local smoking-cessation clinic.

Evaluation

Now, on discharge, Mrs. Rogers has lost no more weight. She is feeling less fatigued and is looking forward to getting out in her garden. She has met with the dietitian to identify foods that she can tolerate and that will meet her caloric needs. By eating three small meals with a snack between each and at bedtime, she is experiencing less *postprandial* (after meal) discomfort and no nausea. She verbalizes an understanding of the need for antacids and monthly injections of vitamin B_{12}, stating, "I'm willing to do almost anything that will allow me to enjoy eating and gardening again!" Having "survived" 3 days of not smoking while hospitalized, she expresses less anxiety and more confidence that she will be able to quit "once and for all." Mr. Havner has set up an appointment for her to meet with a counselor at the smoking-cessation clinic in her area.

Critical Thinking in the Nursing Process

1. Pernicious anemia is often associated with chronic atrophic gastritis. What mechanism causes anemia when vitamin B_{12} is not absorbed? Why are red blood cells decreased in number and larger than normal? What other symptoms are associated with pernicious anemia?

2. How does cigarette smoking contribute to the development of chronic gastritis?

3. Mrs. Rogers says that she understands why she should not take aspirin and asks what would be safe and effective for relief of her arthritic pain. How would you respond?

4. Outline a teaching plan for the client seen on an outpatient basis for acute gastritis resulting from bacteria-contaminated food.

5. Develop a care plan for Mrs. Rogers for the nursing diagnosis *Noncompliance* with prescription to stop smoking.

The Client with Ulcers of the Stomach and Duodenum

■ ■ ■

Peptic ulcer disease, a break in the mucous lining of the gastrointestinal tract where it comes in contact with gastric juice, is a chronic health problem that affects approximately 10% of the population at some point and accounts for 10% of hospital admissions (Burke, 1992; Porth, 1994). Although the incidence of peptic ulcer disease appears to be decreasing in the total population, an increase in its incidence and associated complications is being seen in the elderly (Gilinsky, 1990).

Peptic ulcers occur in any area of the gastrointestinal tract exposed to acid-pepsin secretions, including the esophagus, stomach, or duodenum. Duodenal peptic ulcers are the most prevalent ulcerative condition affecting the upper gastrointestinal tract. They are seen most frequently in middle adulthood (ages 30 to 50 years) and affect men more frequently than women. These ulcers tend to recur in susceptible individuals, with exacerbations often occurring in a seasonal pattern (spring and fall). Ulcer recurrence may be related to physical or psychologic stress, fatigue, or infection; however, there is no clearly identifiable "ulcer personality," as had previously been thought (Wilson et al., 1991).

Although peptic ulcers may occur in the stomach, some **gastric ulcers** are the result of a different mecha-

nism. These ulcers, occurring most often in the lesser curvature and antrum of the stomach, are associated with chronic gastritis and seen more commonly in the older adult. Some authorities consider gastric ulcers to be premalignant lesions.

Stress ulcers represent a third type of ulcerative disease affecting the upper GI tract. These ulcers develop in response to a major physiologic stressor, such as trauma or illness. Common precipitating conditions include major burns, central nervous system trauma or surgery, hypotension, and organ system failure such as respiratory, renal, or liver failure.

The clinical features of peptic, gastric, and stress ulcers are outlined in Table 14–1. This section focuses on the client with peptic ulcer disease, identifying differences in pathophysiology and symptoms for gastric and stress ulcers as indicated.

Pathophysiology

Peptic Ulcer

The innermost layer of the stomach wall, the gastric mucosa, consists of columnar epithelial cells, supported by a middle layer of blood vessels and glands, and a thin outer layer of smooth muscle. The mucosal barrier of the stomach, a thin coating of mucous gel and bicarbonate (Figure 14–2), protects the gastric mucosa. The mucosal barrier is maintained by bicarbonate secreted by the epithelial cells, by mucous gel production stimulated by prostaglandins, and by an adequate blood supply to the mucosa (Andreoli et al., 1990; Chowdry, 1993; Wilson et al., 1991).

An ulcer, or break in the gastrointestinal mucosa, develops when the mucosal barrier is unable to protect the mucosa from damage by hydrochloric acid and pepsin, the gastric digestive juices. Peptic ulcers are the most common form of ulcers affecting the upper gastrointestinal tract.

Peptic ulcer disease (PUD) is the result of an imbalance between acid and pepsin formation and the inability of the mucosal layer to resist the destructive action of these substances.

Several factors can increase the production of gastric acid: (1) increased numbers of acid- and pepsin-producing cells (parietal and chief cells, respectively), (2) increased sensitivity of the parietal cells of the stomach to food and other stimuli such as alcohol and caffeine, (3) excess vagal (parasympathetic or cholinergic) stimulation resulting in increased acid and pepsin production, and (4) lack of inhibition of the production of gastric secretions once food has moved out of the stomach. Figure 14–3 illustrates the pathogenesis of PUD.

An ineffective mucosal barrier may result from an inadequate blood supply to the mucosa, the inability of epi-

Table 14–1   Clinical Features of Ulcers of the Stomach and Duodenum

Type	Risk Factors	Pathophysiology	Clinical Presentation
Peptic	Greater incidence in males Age 30 to 50 Family history Blood group O Alcohol use, aspirin ingestion, cigarette smoking	Impaired mucosal barrier and/or excess hydrochloric acid and pepsin secretion allows erosion of gastric mucosa; ulcers predominantly duodenal (4:1) but may be gastric or esophageal	Chronic, relapsing-remitting disease, often with spring and fall occurrence. Epigastric pain with typical pain-food-relief pattern. Complications include bleeding, perforation, and obstruction.
Gastric	Equal incidence in both sexes Age 60 to 70 Chronic atrophic gastritis	Disruption of mucosal barrier allows erosion of gastric mucosa with normal or low levels of hydrochloric acid. Lesser curvature and antrum of stomach are common sites. Lesions are considered premalignant.	Dull, aching abdominal pain exacerbated by food intake. Vomiting is common.
Stress	Major physiologic stressor: trauma or surgery of central nervous system (Cushing's ulcer); major burn (Curling's ulcer); respiratory or renal failure; shock	Central nervous system stimulation from stress response causes systemic vasoconstriction leading to ischemia of gastric mucosa, tissue acidosis, and formation of multiple superficial erosions. Increased hydrochloric acid production contributes to ulcer formation.	Painless; initial symptom is often upper gastrointestinal bleeding.

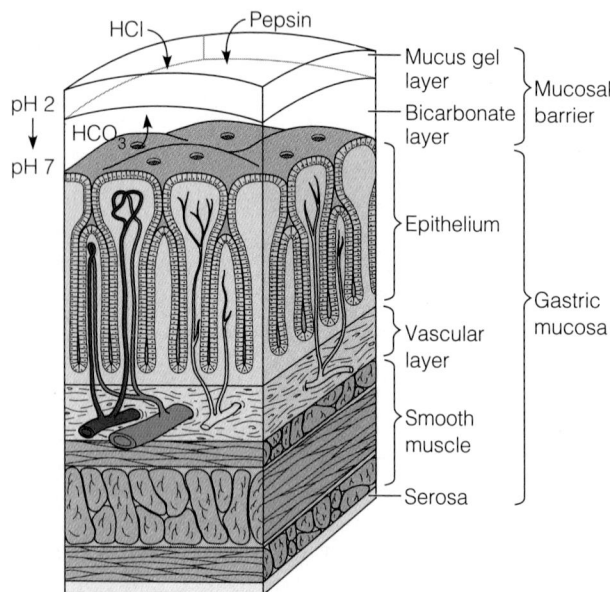

Figure 14–2 The gastric mucosa and mucosal barrier. The mucous gel and bicarbonate of the mucosal barrier protect the gastric mucosa (the epithelial, vascular, and smooth muscle layers) from damage by digestive substances such as hydrochloric acid and pepsin.

thelial cells to secrete sufficient mucus, the reflux of bile or pancreatic enzymes, or the ingestion of substances such as aspirin or alcohol (Porth, 1994).

Recent findings indicate that in up to 90% of people with PUD, *Helicobacter pylori,* a gram-negative bacteria that colonizes the mucus-secreting cells of the stomach and digests the protective mucous layer, may be responsible for the ulcerative process (Glass, 1991; Porth, 1994).

The ulcers of PUD may affect the esophagus, stomach, or duodenum, with the duodenum the most frequently affected by a 4 to 1 ratio over the stomach (Chowdry, 1993). When peptic ulcers occur in the stomach, the lesser curvature and area immediately proximal to the pylorus are most often affected (Figure 14–4). Ulcers may be superficial or deep, affecting all layers of the mucosa. Figure 14–5 illustrates superficial gastric erosions and ulcerations of the upper GI tract.

Peptic ulcer disease tends to be chronic, with spontaneous remissions and exacerbations. Exacerbations of the disease may be associated with trauma, infection, or other physical or psychologic stressors. A stong familial pattern and increased prevalence in people with blood group O suggest a genetic factor in the development of PUD (Bullock & Rosendahl, 1992). Cigarette smoking is a significant risk factor, doubling the risk of PUD (Fina, 1991). Although cigarette smoking does not increase the secretion of gastric acid, it appears to inhibit the secretion of bicarbonate by the pancreas and possibly causes more rapid transit of gastric acid into the duodenum (Wilson et

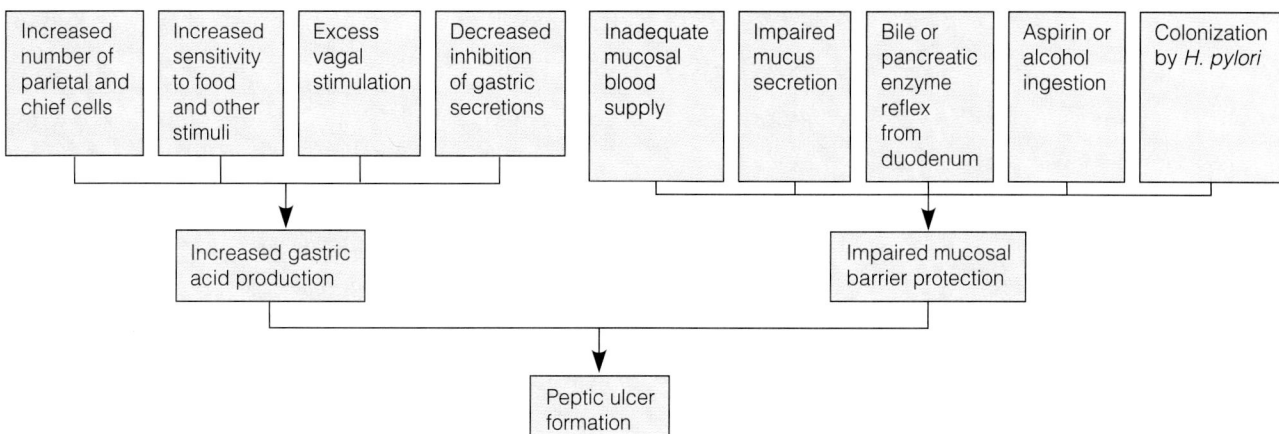

Figure 14–3   The pathogenesis of peptic ulcer disease.

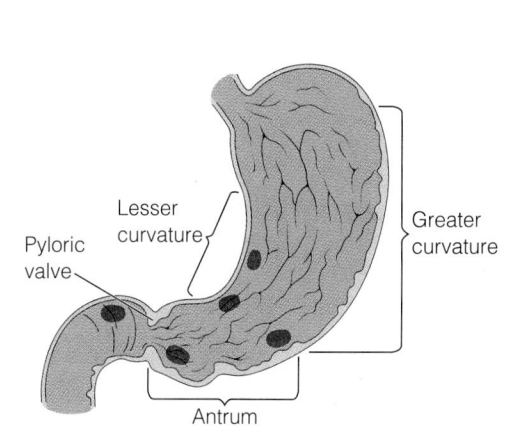

Figure 14–4   Common sites affected by peptic ulcer disease.

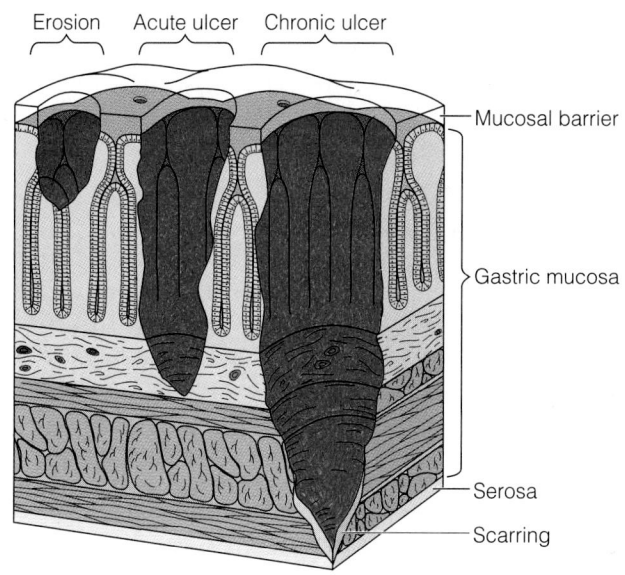

Figure 14–5   Erosion and ulcerations of the upper gastrointestinal tract.

al., 1991). Another significant risk factor, particularly in the older adult, is the use of prescription or nonprescription nonsteroidal anti-inflammatory drugs or NSAIDs, which inhibit prostaglandins (Gilinsky, 1990).

Pain is the classic symptom of peptic ulcer disease. The pain is typically described as gnawing, burning, aching, or hungerlike and is experienced in the epigastric region, sometimes radiating to the back. The pain occurs when the stomach is empty (2 to 3 hours after meals and in the middle of the night) and is relieved by eating with a classic "pain-food-relief" pattern (Bullock & Rosendahl, 1992). The client may complain of heartburn or regurgitation and may vomit.

The clinical presentation of peptic ulcer disease in the older adult is often less clear, with vague and poorly localized discomfort, perhaps chest pain or dysphagia, weight loss, or anemia. In the older adult, a complication

of PUD such as upper GI hemorrhage or perforation of the stomach or duodenum may be the presenting symptom (Gilinsky, 1990).

The complications associated with peptic ulcers include hemorrhage, obstruction, and perforation.

Among people with PUD, 10% to 20% experience bleeding as a result of ulceration and erosion into the blood vessels of the gastric mucosa. In the older adult, bleeding is the most frequent complication seen (Gilinsky, 1990). When small blood vessels are eroded, the blood loss may be slow and insidious, with occult blood in the stool the only initial sign. If bleeding continues, the client becomes anemic and experiences symptoms of weakness, fatigue, dizziness, and orthostatic hypotension. Erosion into a larger vessel can lead to sudden and severe bleeding with hematemesis, melena or **hematochezia** (blood in the stool), and signs of hypovolemic shock.

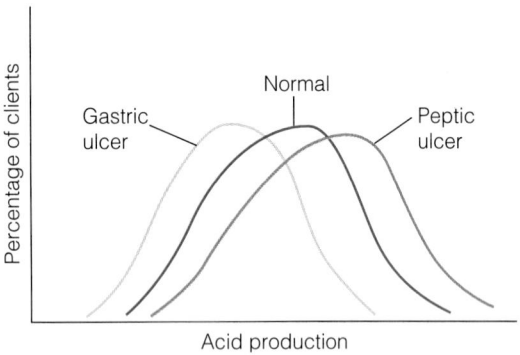

Figure 14–6 A comparison of gastric acid secretion in the normal adult, in gastric ulcer disease, and in peptic ulcer disease. Gastric ulcers may develop with low to normal gastric acid secretion; peptic ulcers are typically associated with high gastric acid secretion.

Obstruction of the upper GI tract may result from edema surrounding the ulcer, smooth muscle spasm, or the formation and contraction of scar tissue. Generally, obstruction is a gradual rather than an acute process. Symptoms include a feeling of epigastric fullness, accentuated ulcer symptoms, and nausea. If the obstruction becomes complete, vomiting occurs. Vomiting leads to the loss of hydrochloric acid, sodium, and potassium, and, if prolonged, to fluid and electrolyte imbalance and metabolic alkalosis.

The most lethal complication of peptic ulcer disease is perforation of the ulcer through the mucosal wall. Five to ten percent of ulcers perforate, with the majority of these being duodenal ulcers. When perforation occurs, gastric or duodenal contents enter the peritoneum, resulting in an inflammatory process and peritonitis. Chemical peritonitis from the hydrochloric acid, pepsin, bile, and pancreatic fluid is immediate; bacterial peritonitis follows within 6 to 12 hours from gastric contaminants entering the normally sterile peritoneal cavity. When an ulcer perforates, the client experiences immediate, severe upper abdominal pain, radiating throughout the abdomen and possibly to the shoulder. The abdomen becomes rigid and boardlike, with absent bowel sounds. Signs of shock may be present, including diaphoresis, tachycardia, and rapid, shallow respirations.

In the older adult, perforation is the second most common complication of PUD. An older adult may not experience pain and the typical acute presentation of perforation and may instead present with mental confusion and other nonspecific symptoms. This atypical presentation may lead to delays in diagnosis and treatment, increasing the associated mortality rate (Gilinsky, 1990).

Gastric Ulcer

Ulcers occurring in the stomach are often associated with gastric gland atrophy and decreased protection of the gas-

tric mucosa by the mucosal barrier rather than with increased secretion of hydrochloric acid. People with chronic gastritis and an inadequate mucosal barrier may develop ulcers while demonstrating normal or low hydrochloric acid secretion (see Figure 14–6). Gastritis is always present in the area surrounding a gastric ulcer. Gastric ulcers are considered to be premalignant lesions because of an associated increased incidence of gastric cancer. It appears, however, that chronic atrophic gastritis and decreased hydrochloric acid secretion—rather than the ulcer lesion itself—are the common factors in this increased risk for gastric cancer.

The lesser curvature and the antrum (the area just proximal to the pylorus) of the stomach are the most common sites for gastric ulcer formation. Gastric ulcers are more common in the older adult, with a higher incidence in people over the age of 60.

The client with a gastric ulcer may complain of dull, aching abdominal pain after eating. Unlike the pain associated with a duodenal ulcer, the discomfort may be exacerbated by food intake, not relieved. Vomiting is more common with gastric ulcers as well (Burke, 1992).

Stress Ulcer

Unlike peptic and gastric ulcers, which tend to be chronic, stress ulcers are an acute condition. These ulcers develop as a secondary result of a major physiologic stressor. People who have experienced a major burn, trauma, or surgery involving the central nervous system, respiratory or renal failure, or shock are especially at risk for stress-ulcer development. When these ulcers follow a major burn, they are called **Curling's ulcers,** after the man who first described them in 1842 (Chowdry, 1993). When stress ulcers occur as a sequela of head injury or central nervous system surgery, they are referred to as **Cushing's ulcers.**

Stress ulcers tend to be multiple and superficial, affecting primarily the fundus of the stomach. Figure 14–7 shows the multiple gastric erosions and small ulcers typical of stress ulceration. The primary mechanisms leading to stress-ulcer formation appear to be ischemia of the gastric mucosa resulting from sympathetic vasoconstriction, and tissue injury due to gastric acid. Although gastric acid secretion may be normal, it appears that these ulcers do not develop in the absence of acid. Cushing's ulcers are often associated with hypersecretion of gastric acid. Maintaining the gastric pH at greater than 3.5 and inhibiting gastric acid secretion with H_2-receptor antagonists help prevent stress ulcers (Porth, 1994; Wilson et al., 1991).

Unlike other ulcers, stress ulcers are not typically associated with pain. Often the initial symptom of stress ulcers is painless gastric bleeding occurring 2 or more days after the initial stressor. Bleeding is typically minimal but may be massive. When hemorrhage occurs, it can be difficult to control, often coming from multiple sites in the gastric mucosa (Bullock & Rosendahl, 1992; Wilson et al., 1991). Because hemorrhage from stress ulcers is associated with a high mortality rate and may be the first and only symptom, prevention is key in the management of this condition.

Zollinger-Ellison Syndrome

Zollinger-Ellison syndrome is peptic ulcer disease caused by a *gastrinoma,* or gastrin-secreting tumor of the pancreas, stomach, or intestines. Gastrinomas may be benign, although 50% to 70% are malignant tumors. Gastrin is a hormone that stimulates the secretion of pepsin and hydrochloric acid. The increased gastrin levels associated with these tumors result in hypersecretion of gastric acid, which in turn causes mucosal ulceration.

The peptic ulcers of Zollinger-Ellison syndrome may affect any portion of the stomach or duodenum, as well as the esophagus or jejunum. Characteristic ulcerlike pain is common. The high levels of hydrochloric acid entering the duodenum may also cause diarrhea and **steatorrhea** (excess fat in the feces), from impaired fat digestion and absorption.

Complications of bleeding and perforation are often seen with Zollinger-Ellison syndrome. Fluid and electrolyte imbalances may also result from persistent diarrhea with resultant losses of potassium and sodium in particular.

Collaborative Care

The management of peptic ulcer disease is directed toward the goals of (1) symptom relief, (2) healing of existing ulcers and preventing complications from those ulcers, and (3) preventing or reducing recurrences of ulcers. Management strategies include behavior modification, pharmacologic therapy, and surgical interventions.

Laboratory and Diagnostic Tests

Routine laboratory tests often are of little use in the diagnosis of peptic ulcer disease. However, the following laboratory tests may be ordered:

- *Complete blood count (CBC)* is performed to assess for the presence of anemia, which may indicate a bleeding ulcer. If anemia is present, hemoglobin levels will be less than 14 g/dL in the male and less than 12 g/dL in the female. The hematocrit will be less than 42% in the male and less than 37% in the female.

- *Stool* is tested for occult blood. The presence of blood in the stool may indicate bleeding from ulcer disease.

- *Gastric analysis* may be performed to determine the basal secretion of gastric acid when the client is fasting and the effect of histamine or pentagastrin stimulation on its secretion. Gastric analysis may help differentiate the cause of ulcer disease. Stomach contents are aspi-

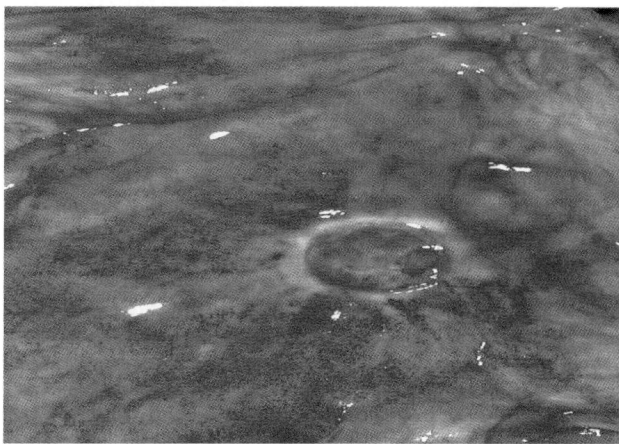

Figure 14–7   Gastric erosions and multiple small ulcers of the gastric mucosa typical of stress ulceration.

rated through a nasogastric tube and analyzed. Elevated levels may indicate the presence of a duodenal or jejunal ulcer; lower than normal levels are seen with gastric ulcers or gastric carcinoma. In Zollinger-Ellison syndrome, levels are very high.

Diagnostic studies performed for the client with ulcer disease include the following:

- *An upper GI X-ray study* can demonstrate the presence of craters and identify deformity of the gastric outlet (pylorus). The upper GI series is 80% to 90% reliable in diagnosing peptic ulcers and is less costly and less invasive than gastroscopy. Small or very superficial ulcers may be missed, however.

- *Gastroscopy* is the definitive tool for diagnosing peptic ulcer disease. In addition to allowing visualization of the esophageal, gastric, and duodenal mucosa and direct inspection of ulcers, it allows tissue to be obtained for biopsy. Nursing care of the client undergoing a gastroscopy is outlined in the box on page 472.

Pharmacology

Several classes or groups of drugs are used in the treatment of peptic ulcer disease. Medications can help achieve the management goals of neutralizing acid, preventing acid secretion, and promoting healing. Used appropriately, pharmaceuticals not only control the symptoms of peptic ulcer disease but also promote healing of existing ulcers and prevent further ulcer formation.

Antacids and H_2-receptor blockers are the mainstays of pharmacologic treatment for peptic ulcer disease:

- *Antacids* act locally to neutralize hydrochloric acid and reduce pepsin activity in the stomach. Used as directed, 1 and 3 hours after meals and at bedtime for a period of 6 weeks or more, antacids promote ulcer healing. Newer, four-per-day, low-dose regimens are proving to be effective as well. Antacids are inexpensive and available without prescription, making them a desirable therapy. The primary drawback of antacid therapy is poor compliance with the prescribed regimen due to (1) the frequent doses required for full effectiveness, and (2) the side effects of diarrhea (common with magnesium-based antacids) and constipation (associated with aluminum-type antacids). Antacids also interfere with the absorption of iron, digoxin, some antibiotics, and other drugs.

- H_2-receptor antagonists or blockers, including cimetidine (Tagamet), famotidine (Pepsid), nizatidine (Axid), and ranitidine (Zantac) act specifically to block H_2 receptors that control the secretion of hydrochloric acid by the parietal cells. These drugs are very effective in reducing gastric acid, thus allowing ulcer healing to occur. Reducing the frequency of administration to once or twice a day increases compliance during the 8-week (or longer) period of therapy required for healing.

Nursing responsibilities related to pharmacologic therapy for gastritis and peptic ulcer disease are outlined in the box on page 476.

Two other drugs may also be used in the treatment of peptic ulcer disease:

- Sucralfate (Carafate) is a mucosal protective agent that also inhibits pepsin secretion and promotes wound healing. Although this drug does not neutralize acid or decrease acid secretions, it acts locally by combining with protein in the stomach to form a substance that coats the ulcer and protects it from acid and pepsin. The dose of sucralfate is 1 g four times a day before meals and at bedtime.

- Bismuth subsalicylate (Pepto-Bismol) or colloidal bismuth subcitrate (CBS) have also been shown to bind with ulcer craters, providing a protective coating. These preparations also inhibit pepsin activity and stimulate healing. Resultant healing rates are comparable to those achieved with H_2-receptor antagonists such as cimetidine or ranitidine (Glass, 1991). In addition to the ulcer-healing properties of these drugs, recent evidence indicates that they have a bactericidal action against Helicobacter pylori, the bacterium that has been implicated in the development of peptic ulcer disease in many individuals (Wilson et al., 1991). Not yet mainstays of ulcer treatment, these drugs hold promise for the future.

In clients with demonstrated colonization of the gastric mucosa by Helicobacter pylori, a new, triple-therapy regimen has been demonstrated effective in healing ulcers and preventing their recurrence. This regimen involves 2 weeks of combination therapy with metronidazole (Flagyl or Protostat), bismuth sulfate (Pepto-Bismol), and either tetracycline or amoxicillin followed by up to 16 weeks of an H_2 antagonist such as cimetidine. Compliance may be a problem because of cost, frequent doses of multiple drugs, and side effects (Feldman et al., 1992).

As with any chronic, relapsing-remissing disorder, lifestyle changes must accompany pharmacologic therapy for maximal effectiveness. Known ulcergenic substances and activities should be avoided, including aspirin and other NSAIDs, alcohol, cigarette smoking, and possibly caffeine. No other specific dietary changes are currently recommended; however, clients with peptic ulcer disease are encouraged to eliminate foods or beverages that cause pain or other symptoms. Stress reduction is beneficial, because increased levels of gastric acid are associated with the stress response.

The client hospitalized with a complication of PUD such as bleeding, gastrointestinal obstruction, or perforation and peritonitis requires additional interventions to restore homeostasis.

In hemorrhage associated with PUD, initial interventions are directed toward restoration and maintenance of adequate circulatory status. Normal saline, lactated Ringer's, or other balanced electrolyte solutions are administered intravenously to restore intravascular volume if signs of shock are present. These signs include tachycardia, hypotension, pallor, and anxiety (see Chapter 6). Whole blood or red blood cell concentrate (packed cells) may be administered to restore hemoglobin and hematocrit levels.

Gastric intubation and saline lavage may be required, depending on the extent of the bleeding. A nasogastric tube is inserted to determine the extent of the bleeding and to evacuate blood and clots from the GI tract. Nursing responsibilities in performing and caring for the client with gastric lavage are outlined in Procedure 14–1 on page 473.

Additional measures used to control hemorrhage may include intravenous or intra-arterial administration of vasopressin (ADH), a potent vasoconstrictive agent. Gastroscopy with direct injection of a clotting or sclerosing agent into the bleeding vessel may be performed. Laser photocoagulation, using light energy, or electrocoagulation, which uses electric current to generate heat, can also be done via gastroscopy to seal bleeding vessels.

In caring for clients having these procedures, the nurse needs to be aware of and monitor for potential complications. Vasopressin may cause signs of impaired tissue perfusion, such as angina or local necrosis, or problems with urination and fluid balance related to its antidiuretic properties. The client having direct treatment of the bleeding site via gastroscopy requires nursing care as outlined in the box on page 472.

The client is kept NPO until bleeding is controlled. Antacids are administered hourly via the nasogastric tube to protect the bleeding ulcer from gastric acid and to prevent acid reflux. H_2-receptor antagonists such as cimetidine, ranitidine, and famotidine are administered intravenously until the client can resume oral intake. Surgical intervention may be necessary if medical measures are ineffective in controlling bleeding. Older adults who experience bleeding as a complication of PUD are more likely to rebleed or require surgery to control the hemorrhage (Gilinsky, 1990).

Repeated inflammation, healing, scarring, edema, and muscle spasm can lead to gastric outlet (pyloric) obstruction. This ulcer complication may also require surgical treatment if conservative management with nasogastric suction and pharmacologic ulcer therapy are not successful in relieving the obstruction.

Gastric or duodenal perforation resulting in contamination of the peritoneum with gastrointestinal contents requires immediate intervention to restore homeostasis and minimize peritonitis. Fluids are administered intravenously to maintain fluid and electrolyte balance. The client is kept NPO with a nasogastric tube connected to suction to remove gastric contents and minimize peritoneal contamination. Placing the client in Fowler's or semi-Fowler's position allows peritoneal contaminants to pool in the pelvis. Antibiotics are administered intravenously to provide aggressive treatment of bacterial infection from intestinal flora. The nurse should prepare the client for probable surgical intervention.

Surgery

When drug therapy and life-style management are not fully successful in controlling the debilitating symptoms or complications of peptic ulcer disease, surgical intervention may be necessary. The client with an acute perforation or massive hemorrhage usually requires emergency surgery to preserve life. Elective surgical procedures are designed to decrease gastric secretions, resect damaged tissue, and promote gastric emptying (Porth, 1994).

Partial gastrectomy with vagotomy, pyloroplasty with vagotomy, and parietal cell or highly selective vagotomy are the most common surgical interventions for PUD (Wilson et al., 1991). Table 14-2 illustrates and outlines the individual surgical procedures most likely to be performed and the advantages and disadvantages of each.

Partial gastrectomy is performed for clients with recurrent or nonhealing gastric ulcers and occasionally for those with acute hemorrhage. This procedure involves removal of a portion of the stomach, usually the distal half to two-thirds. Removal of the entire antrum of the stomach may be termed an **antrectomy.** The antrum, that portion of the stomach just proximal to the pylorus, contains most of the gastrin-producing cells of the stomach. Gastrin is a potent stimulant for gastric acid production; removal of this portion of the stomach removes much of this stimulus.

When partial gastrectomy is performed, the surgeon may construct an anastamosis from the remainder of the stomach directly to the duodenum or proximal jejunum, to facilitate gastric emptying. The **gastroduodenostomy,** or **Billroth I,** and the **gastrojejunostomy,** or **Billroth II,** are commonly used partial gastrectomy procedures. A critical pathway for a client following a partial gastrectomy is provided on page 489.

A **total gastrectomy,** removal of the entire stomach, is rarely performed because of its impact on the digestive processes and nutritional status of the client. Extensive gastric cancer and Zollinger-Ellison syndrome unresponsive to medical management may be indicators for a total gastrectomy. When performing a total gastrectomy, the surgeon constructs an anastamosis from the esophagus to the duodenum or jejunum.

Pyloroplasty, surgical enlargement of the opening between the stomach and duodenum, is a relatively simple procedure used to improve gastric emptying. The Heineke-Mikulicz pyloroplasty procedure, which involves making a small longitudinal incision in the pylorus and resuturing the tissues at a 90-degree angle to the original incision, is most commonly performed.

Vagotomy, severing all or a portion of the vagus nerves to the stomach, is commonly performed in conjunction with either partial gastrectomy or pyloroplasty. Removing vagal stimulation results in significant reduction of acid secretion by the parietal cells. A *truncal vagotomy* eliminates all vagal input to the liver, pancreas, and other viscera along with the gastric innervation. Diarrhea and impaired gastric emptying are common adverse effects of this procedure.

Selective vagotomy and *highly selective* or *parietal cell vagotomy* preserve vagal innervation of other abdominal organs and viscera, while selectively eliminating vagal stimulation of the stomach. Highly selective vagotomy interrupts vagal innervation to the upper portion of the stomach and the parietal cells of the fundus. With this procedure, gastric acid is greatly reduced, but gastric emptying remains normal.

A vagotomy combined with a partial gastrectomy enhances ulcer healing and decreases the rate of recurrence. For the older client and people who are poor surgical risks, vagotomy and pyloroplasty allow healing to occur and reduce factors contributing to ulcer recurrence while allowing the stomach and duodenum to remain intact.

Nursing care of the client who has undergone surgery for peptic ulcer disease is outlined in the box on page 488.

Several long-term complications may be associated with surgical procedures used to treat peptic ulcer disease.

| **Table 14–2** | Surgical Procedures Used for Peptic Ulcer Disease | |

Procedure	Description	Advantages/Disadvantages
Billroth I (Gastroduodenostomy) Duodenal anastomosis Portion of stomach removed Body Duodenum	Removal of the distal half of the stomach with anastamosis to the duodenum. Performed to remove ulcers or other lesions, such as cancer in the antrum. Vagotomy is usually done at the same time.	**Advantages:** Allows resection of damaged mucosa; reduces the number of gastrin- and acid-secreting cells; reduces ulcer recurrence. **Disadvantages:** Decreases size of the stomach reservoir causing problems in absorption and emptying.
Billroth II (Gastrojejunostomy) Portion of stomach removed Duodenal stump Jejunal anastomosis Jejunal loop	Removal of the distal portion of the stomach with anastamosis to the proximal jejunum. The duodenal stump is left intact to allow bile to enter the intestines. Performed in conjunction with a vagotomy for persons with duodenal ulcers or lesions.	**Advantages:** As for Billroth I procedure. **Disadvantages:** As for Billroth I procedure.

Dumping syndrome is the most common problem. It may follow a partial gastrectomy with duodenal or jejunal anastamosis or pyloroplasty. When the pylorus has been resected or bypassed, a hypertonic, undigested food bolus may rapidly enter the duodenum or jejunum. Water is pulled into the lumen of the intestine by the hyperosmolar character of the chyme, resulting in a decrease in blood volume and intestinal dilation. Peristalsis is stimulated, and intestinal motility is increased.

Early symptoms of dumping syndrome occur within 5 to 30 minutes after eating. These symptoms result from intestinal dilation, peristaltic stimulation, and hypovolemia caused by undigested food in the proximal small intestine. Manifestations include nausea with possible vomiting, epigastric pain with cramping and **borborygmi** (loud, hyperactive bowel sounds), and diarrhea. Systemic symptoms from the hypovolemia and reflex sympathetic stimulation include tachycardia, orthostatic hypotension, dizziness, flushing, and diaphoresis.

The entry of hyperosmolar chyme into the jejunum also causes a rapid rise in the blood glucose. This stimulates the release of an excessive amount of insulin, leading to hypoglycemic symptoms 2 to 3 hours after the meal. The pathogenesis and clinical manifestations of dumping syndrome are represented in Figure 14–8 on page 489.

Dumping syndrome is managed primarily by a dietary pattern that delays gastric emptying and allows smaller boluses of undigested food to enter the intestine. Meals

Table 14–2   (continued)

Procedure	Description	Advantages/Disadvantages
Pyloroplasty Pylorus Longitudinal incision **1** **2** Transverse suture **3**	Surgical enlargement of the pylorus or gastric outlet. Performed to improve gastric emptying for clients with obstructive complications or in conjunction with a vagotomy that interferes with gastric emptying.	**Advantages:** Relief of obstruction and improved gastric emptying; relatively simple procedure with low surgical risk. **Disadvantages:** May contribute to dumping syndrome; ulcer recurrence is common.
Vagotomy Esophagus Vagus nerve Truncal — Selective Highly selective (proximal parietal cell) Stomach Duodenum	Severing vagal innervation to the stomach to remove the autonomic stimulus that causes the parietal cells to produce hydrochloric acid. Truncal vagotomy: Severs the entire vagus nerve trunk below the diaphragm. Selective vagotomy: Severs only those vagal fibers innervating the stomach. Highly selective vagotomy: Severs vagal branches serving the upper two-thirds of the stomach, the primary site of acid production.	**Advantages:** Reduces the amount of gastric acid produced. **Disadvantages:** May cause delay in gastric emptying; increased risk of diarrhea and gallstone formation with truncal vagotomy.

should be small and more frequent. Liquids and solids are taken at separate times instead of together during a meal. The amount of proteins and fats in the diet is increased, because they exit the stomach more slowly than carbohydrates. Carbohydrates, especially simple sugars, are reduced. The client is instructed to rest in a recumbent or semirecumbent position for 30 to 60 minutes after meals. Anticholinergics, sedatives, and antispasmodics may be prescribed.

Dumping syndrome is typically self-limiting, lasting 6 to 12 months after surgery; however, a small percentage of persons continue to experience long-term symptoms.

Anemia may be a chronic problem for the client who has undergone a major gastric resection. Iron is absorbed primarily in the duodenum and proximal jejunum; rapid gastric emptying or a gastrojejunostomy may interfere with adequate absorption.

The cells of the stomach produce intrinsic factor, required for the absorption of vitamin B_{12}. Vitamin B_{12} deficiency leads to pernicious anemia. Because of hepatic stores of vitamin B_{12}, symptoms of anemia may not be seen for 1 to 2 years following surgery. Levels should be monitored routinely in clients who have had extensive gastric resections.

Other nutritional problems seen following surgery include folic acid deficiency and decreased absorption of calcium and vitamin D. Poor absorption of nutrients, combined with the inability to eat large meals, puts the

Nursing Care of the Client Having Surgery for Peptic Ulcer Disease

PREOPERATIVE NURSING CARE

- Ensure that a valid signed consent for the procedure is present in the chart. *When surgery is to be performed, it is imperative that the client and family understand the procedure, its potential risks and benefits, and alternatives. A signed consent form specific to the procedure provides documentation that the client or family consents to having the procedure performed.*

- Assess the client's and family's knowledge and understanding of the procedure, clarifying and interpreting as needed. Provide instructions regarding what to expect during the postoperative period, including pain-relief measures, expected tubes (such as a nasogastric tube), intravenous fluids, breathing exercises, and the reintroduction of oral foods and fluids. *The client who is well prepared preoperatively is significantly less anxious and better able to assist in his or her care during the postoperative period. Adequate preparation also decreases the need for narcotic analgesia and enhances the client's recovery postoperatively.*

- Insert a nasogastric tube if ordered preoperatively. *Although it is often inserted in the surgical suite just prior to surgery, the nasogastric tube may be placed preoperatively to remove secretions and empty stomach contents.*

POSTOPERATIVE NURSING CARE

- Provide routine care for the surgical client as outlined in Chapter 7. Monitor vital signs; intake and output, including gastric drainage. Assess for bleeding and other wound complications, and maintain physiologic integrity. Monitor bowel sounds and degree of abdominal distention. Provide appropriate pain-relief and comfort measures, such as position changes. Assess respiratory status, providing abdominal splinting with a blanket or pillow to assist with coughing. *Procedures performed in the treatment of peptic ulcer disease are considered as major abdominal surgery. Care regarding pain relief, maintenance of adequate respiratory function, and prevention of surgical complications is similar to that for clients having other abdominal surgeries.*

- Assess position and patency of nasogastric tube, connecting it to low suction. Gently irrigate with sterile normal saline if tube becomes clogged. *The nasogastric tube will be placed in surgery to avoid disruption of the gastric suture lines and should be well secured. If repositioning or tube replacement is needed, notify the surgeon. Patency must be maintained to keep*

the stomach decompressed, reducing pressure on sutures.

- Assess color, amount, and odor of gastric drainage, noting any changes in these parameters or the presence of clots or bright bleeding. *Initial drainage is bright red. It becomes dark, then clear or greenish-yellow over the first 2 to 3 days. A change in the color, amount, or odor may indicate a complication such as hemorrhage, intestinal obstruction, or infection.*

- Maintain intravenous fluids while nasogastric suction is in place. *The client on nasogastric suction is not only unable to take oral food and fluids but also is losing electrolyte-rich fluid through the nasogastric tube. If replacement fluid and electrolytes are not maintained, the client is at risk for dehydration; imbalances of sodium, potassium, and chloride; and metabolic alkalosis.*

- Provide antacids, H_2-receptor antagonists, and antibiotic therapy as ordered. *These medications may be ordered for the postoperative client, depending on the procedure performed. Antibiotic therapy is a common preventive measure for infection that may result from contamination of the abdominal cavity with gastric contents.*

- Resume oral food and fluids as ordered. Initial feedings are clear liquids, progressing to full liquids and then frequent small feedings of regular foods. Monitor bowel sounds and for abdominal distention frequently during this period. *Oral feedings are reintroduced slowly to minimize trauma to the suture lines by possible gastric distension.*

- Encourage ambulation. *Ambulation stimulates peristalsis.*

- Begin discharge planning and teaching. Consult with a dietitian for diet instructions and menu planning; reinforce teaching. Teach the client about potential postoperative complications, such as abdominal abscess, dumping syndrome, postprandial hypoglycemia, or pernicious anemia. Also, teach the client to recognize signs and symptoms and preventive measures. *The client's gastric capacity is reduced after partial gastrectomy, necessitating a corresponding reduction in meal size. Changes in gastric emptying and reduction in gastric secretions may change the client's tolerance for many foods, requiring slow reintroduction of these foods. Dumping syndrome, postprandial hypoglycemia, and pernicious anemia are possible long-term complications of partial gastrectomy. For most clients, dietary modifications can control both dumping syndrome and postprandial hypoglycemia.*

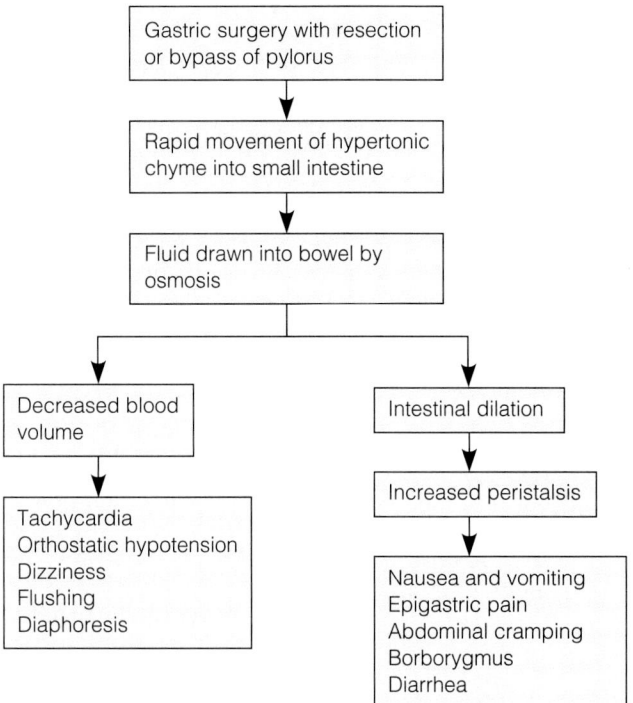

Figure 14–8 Pathogenesis and clinical manifestations of dumping syndrome.

client at risk for weight loss in addition to the more specific nutrient deficiencies. Nearly 50% of clients who undergo gastric surgery experience significant weight loss, primarily because of insufficient calorie intake. Factors contributing to insufficient intake of calories include early satiety (feeling of fullness), decreased stomach size, and altered emptying patterns.

Nursing Care

In planning and implementing nursing care for the client with peptic ulcer disease, nurses need to consider the direct effects of the disorder or its treatment, as well as potential complications. This section focuses on problems of comfort and nutrition, and the potential problems associated with acute bleeding of a peptic ulcer.

Pain

The pain associated with peptic ulcer disease is often predictable and preventable. Pain is typically experienced 2 to 4 hours after eating, as high levels of gastric acid and pepsin irritate the exposed mucosa. Measures to neutralize the acid, minimize its production, or protect the mucosa are often effective in relieving this pain, minimizing the need for analgesics.

Critical Pathway for a Client Following a Partial Gastrectomy			
Date	**Date** _____ **Preoperative**	**Date** _____ **1st Day Postoperative**	**Date** _____ **2nd & 3rd Day Postop**
Expected length of stay: 5 to 7 days			
Daily outcomes	Client ■ Verbalizes understanding of preoperative teaching, including turning, coughing, deep breathing, incentive spirometer, mobilization, nasogastric tube, possible other tubes, and pain management ■ Demonstrates ability to cope. ■ Verbalizes understanding of procedures. ■ Informed consent obtained.	Client will ■ Be afebrile. ■ Have a clean, dry wound with edges that are well approximated and healing by first intention. ■ Recover from anesthesia, as evidenced by: return of vital signs to baseline, awake, alert, and oriented. ■ Demonstrate cooperation with turning, coughing, deep breathing and splinting. ■ Demonstrate ability to use patient-controlled analgesia. ■ Verbalize control of pain. ■ Be up to chair four times. ■ Demonstrate ability to cope.	Client will ■ Be afebrile. ■ Have a clean, dry wound with edges that are well approximated and healing by first intention. ■ Demonstrate cooperation with turning, coughing, deep breathing, and splinting. ■ Ambulate 4 to 6 times. ■ Verbalize control of incisional pain. ■ Demonstrate ability to cope. ■ Verbalize beginning understanding of home care instructions.

➤

Date	Date _____ **Preoperative**	Date _____ **1st Day Postoperative**	Date _____ **2nd & 3rd Day Postop**
Tests and treatments	CBC. Urinalysis. Chest X-ray study. Baseline physical assessment with a focus on respiratory status and gastrointestinal function. Assess and record the description, location, duration, and characteristics of client's pain. Instruct in relaxation and distraction techniques as an adjunct to pain medications.	CBC. Electrolytes. Vital signs and O_2 saturation, neurovascular assessment, dressing and wound drainage assessment q15min × 4; q30min × 4; q1h × 4 and then q4h if stable. Assess respiratory status and gastrointestinal function q4h and prn. Incentive spirometer q2h. Intake and output every shift. Assess patency of nasogastric (NG) tube q2h, noting volume q2h. Report nausea or vomiting. Do not irrigate NG tube. Assess voiding: If unable to void, suggest voiding techniques or catheterize q8h or prn. Assess and record the description, location, duration and characteristics of client's pain q2–4h and prn. Encourage verbalization of pain and discomfort. Reduce or eliminate pain-producing factors and employ distraction or relaxation techniques. Provide back rubs.	Vital signs and dressing and wound drainage assessment q4h. Assess respiratory status and gastrointestinal function q4h. Incentive spirometer q2h until fully ambulatory. Intake and output every shift. Assess patency and output of NG tube q4–8h. Do not irrigate NG tube. Discontinue NG tube when ordered. Assess voiding pattern at every shift. Using sterile asepsis, change dressing: Assess wound healing and wound drainage. Assess and record the description, location, duration and characteristics of client's pain q4h and prn. Reduce or eliminate pain-producing factors, employ distraction or relaxation techniques, and offer back rubs.
Knowledge deficit	Orient to surroundings. Provide simple instructions. Review preoperative preparation, including hospital and surgical routines. Discuss surgery and specific postoperative care: turning, coughing, deep breathing, splinting incision, incentive spirometer, mobilization, possible tubes (e.g., NG nasogastric and intravenous lines), pain management (PCA or prn medications). Include family in teaching.	Reorient to room and postoperative routine. Review plan of care and importance of early mobilization. Review importance of turning, coughing, deep breathing, splinting incision, incentive spirometer, mobilization, possible tubes (e.g., NG tube and intravenous lines), pain management (PCA or prn medications). Include family in teaching.	Reinforce earlier teaching regarding ongoing care. Begin discharge teaching regarding wound care/dressing change. Include family in teaching.

Date	Date _____ Preoperative	Date _____ 1st Day Postoperative	Date _____ 2nd & 3rd Day Postop
Psycho-social	Assess anxiety related to diagnosis and pending surgery. Assess fears of the unknown and surgery. Encourage verbalization of concerns. Offer emotional support. Provide information regarding surgical experience. Provide support to family. Minimize external stimuli (e.g., noise, movement).	Assess level of anxiety. Encourage verbalization of concerns. Provide information. Provide information, ongoing support, and encouragement to client and family.	Encourage verbalization of concerns. Provide information, ongoing support, and encouragement to client and family.
Diet	NPO. Baseline nutritional assessment.	NG tube until return of bowel sounds.	NPO until return of bowel sounds.
Activity	Assess safety needs and provide safety precautions. Activity as tolerated.	Maintain safety precautions. Bathroom privileges with assistance. Assist to chair 4 times.	Maintain safety precautions. Ambulate 4 to 6 times with assistance.
Medications	Administer preoperative medications as ordered.	Administer IM or IV/PCA analgesics and record response. Encourage client to request analgesic or use PCA before pain becomes severe. IV antibiotics and IV fluids. TPN if ordered. IV H_2-receptor antagonists if ordered.	Administer IM or IV/PCA analgesics and record response. Encourage client to request analgesic or use PCA before pain becomes severe. IV antibiotics and IV fluids. TPN if ordered. IV H_2-receptor antagonists if ordered.
Transfer/ discharge plans	Assess potential discharge needs and support system. Establish discharge goals with client and family.	Review progress toward discharge goals with client and significant other. Consult with social service re projected needs for home health care (if any).	Review progress toward discharge goals with client and significant other.

Date	Date _____ 4th Day Postoperative	Date _____ 5th Day Postoperative	Date _____ 6th & 7th Day Postop
Daily outcomes	Client will ■ Be afebrile. ■ Have a clean, dry wound with edges that are well approximated and healing by first intention.	Client will ■ Be afebrile. ■ Have a clean, dry wound with edges that are well approximated and healing by first intention.	Client will ■ Be afebrile. ■ Have a dry, clean wound with edges that are well approximated and healing by first intention.

Date	**Date** _____ **4th Day Postoperative**	**Date** _____ **5th Day Postoperative**	**Date** _____ **6th & 7th Day Postop**
Daily outcomes (cont.)	Client will ■ Tolerate clear liquids without nausea or vomiting. ■ Ambulate independently 4 to 6 times. ■ Verbalize control of incisional pain. ■ Demonstrate ability to cope. ■ Verbalize beginning understanding of home care instructions.	Client will ■ Tolerate ordered diet without nausea or vomiting. ■ Be fully ambulatory. ■ Verbalize control of incisional pain. ■ Demonstrate ability to cope. ■ Verbalize beginning understanding of home care instructions.	Client will ■ Manage pain with non-pharmacologic measures. ■ Be independent in self-care. ■ Be fully ambulatory. ■ Have resumed preadmission urine and bowel elimination pattern and remain free of diarrhea. ■ Verbalize home care instructions. ■ Tolerate ordered diet. ■ Remain free of dumping syndrome and afferent loop syndrome. ■ Demonstrate ability to cope with ongoing stressors.
Tests and treatments	Assess vital signs, dressing, and wound drainage q4h. Incentive spirometer q2h until fully ambulatory. Intake and output at every shift. Assess voiding pattern every shift. Assess respiratory status and gastrointestinal function q4–8h. Using sterile asepsis, change dressing: Assess wound healing and wound drainage. Assess and record description, location, duration, and characteristics of client's pain q4h and prn. Encourage client to employ relaxation techniques.	Assess vital signs, dressing, and wound drainage q4h. Assess respiratory status and gastrointestinal function. Using sterile technique, change dressing and assess wound healing and drainage. Assess and record description, location, duration, and characteristics of client's pain q4h and prn. Encourage client to employ relaxation techniques.	Assess vital signs, dressing, and wound drainage q4h. Assess respiratory status and gastrointestinal function. Remove dressing, and assess wound healing. Assess and record description, location, duration, and characteristics of client's pain q4h and prn. Encourage client to employ relaxation techniques.
Knowledge Deficit	Initiate discharge teaching regarding wound care, diet, and activity. Review written discharge instructions with client and significant other.	Continue discharge teaching regarding wound care, diet, signs and symptoms to report, medications, and activity. Review interventions to minimize recurrence of peptic ulcer disease. Review written discharge instructions with client and significant other.	Complete discharge teaching to include wound care, diet, follow-up care, signs and symptoms to report, activity, and medications: dose frequency, route, food interactions, and side effects. Review strategies to prevent dumping syndrome, the importance of adequate nutrition, and the necessity of

Date	Date _____ **4th Day Postoperative**	Date _____ **5th Day Postoperative**	Date _____ **6th & 7th Day Postop**
Knowledge deficit (*continued*)			follow-up care and laboratory work to monitor for pernicious anemia. Provide client with written discharge instructions.
Psycho-social	Encourage verbalization of concerns. Provide ongoing support and encouragement.	Encourage verbalization of concerns. Provide ongoing support and encouragement.	Encourage verbalization of concerns. Provide ongoing support and encouragement.
Diet	If NG tube is removed and bowel sounds are present, begin ordered diet (clear liquids) as ordered in small amounts. Avoid simple carbohydrates.	Advance to full liquid diet in small amounts throughout the day if tolerated. Visit with dietitian for meal planning at home.	Advance to soft diet if tolerated. Offer small, frequent feedings. Instruct client in the importance of drinking fluids between meals and to chew food well and eat slowly.
Activity	Ambulate independently at least 4 to 6 times per day.	Fully ambulatory.	Fully ambulatory.
Medications	Analgesics as ordered. Intermittent IV device. IV medications as ordered.	Provide PO analgesics. Discontinue intermittent IV device.	PO medications as ordered.
Transfer/ discharge plans	Continue to review progress toward discharge goals.	Finalize discharge plans. Continue to review progress toward discharge goals. Finalize plans for home care if needed.	Complete discharge instructions.

Nursing interventions with rationales follow:

- Assess pain, including location, type, severity, frequency and duration, and its relationship to food intake or other contributing factors. *When assessing pain, you must fully assess each episode and individual, avoiding assumptions about cause and severity. Clients with peptic ulcer disease are vulnerable to complications such as perforation, which may be heralded by sudden, severe epigastric pain. In addition, pain may be totally unrelated to the client's PUD, caused by coronary artery disease, gallbladder disease, or another process.*

- Administer antacids, H_2-receptor antagonists such as cimetidine or ranitidine, or mucosal protective agents such as sucralfate or bismuth sulfate as ordered. Monitor for effectiveness and side effects or adverse reac-

tions. *The pain associated with PUD is generally caused by the effect of gastric juices on exposed mucosal tissue. The above medications act to reduce pain by neutralizing acid, reducing the production of acid, or providing a barrier for the damaged mucosa. Adhering to the prescribed schedule of administration, particularly with antacids and protective agents, is vital to prevent pain and allow healing to occur. Side effects such as diarrhea or constipation may necessitate changing to a different drug in the same class or changing the type of therapy.*

- Provide adjunctive relief measures such as distraction, relaxation (back rub, change in position), and breathing exercises. Teach relaxation, stress-reduction, and life-style management techniques for the client to use. Refer for stress-management counseling or classes as indicated. *Although a clear relationship between stress and PUD has not been established, measures to relieve stress and promote physical and emotional rest help reduce the perception of pain and may reduce ulcer genesis.*

Sleep Pattern Disturbance

Nighttime ulcer pain, which typically occurs between 1:00 and 3:00 a.m., may disrupt the client's sleep cycle and result in inadequate rest. Not only pain but fear of pain may lead to insomnia or other sleep disruptions.

Nursing interventions with rationales follow:

- Administer medications as prescribed, stressing the importance of maintaining the medication schedule at home. *The bedtime dose of antacids or histamine$_2$-receptor blockers minimizes the production or effects of hydrochloric acid during the night. If the client's disease is being managed with antacids, a middle-of-the-night dose may be necessary.*

- Limit food intake after the evening meal, eliminating any bedtime snack. *Eating before bed can stimulate the production of gastric acid and pepsin, increasing the likelihood of nighttime pain.*

- Provide comfort measures such as a back rub, soft music or silence, and sleep aids as needed. *Once the pain associated with PUD has been controlled, the client may need these measures to reduce anxiety and reestablish a normal sleep pattern.*

Altered Nutrition: Less Than Body Requirements

In an attempt to avoid discomfort, the client with peptic ulcer disease may gradually reduce food intake, sometimes jeopardizing nutritional status. Anorexia and early satiety are additional problems associated with PUD.

Nursing interventions with rationales follow:

- Assess the client's current diet, including pattern of food intake, eating schedule, and foods that precipitate pain or are being avoided in anticipation of pain. *The client may be unaware of the extent of changes in the diet, especially if symptoms have persisted for an extended time. Assessment not only increases client awareness but also helps you identify the adequacy of nutrient intake.*

- Arrange consultation with a dietitian to identify a meal plan that minimizes PUD symptoms yet meets the nutritional needs of the client. *Because dietary changes may be long-term, you need to consider the client's normal eating patterns and preferences. Although no specific diet appears to be useful for all clients, foods that increase pain should be avoided. Providing six small meals per day generally helps increase the client's food tolerance and decrease postprandial discomfort.*

- Monitor for complaints of anorexia, fullness, nausea, and vomiting or symptoms of dumping syndrome. Adjust dietary intake or medication schedule as indicated. *Problems with gastric emptying may be associated with PUD or surgical procedures to treat PUD. It is important to monitor symptoms and stress the importance of reporting them, because a change in therapy or food intake may be necessary.*

- Assess and monitor laboratory values for indications of anemia or other specific nutritional deficits. Monitor for therapeutic and side effects of therapeutic measures such as oral replacement of iron. If the client is receiving iron orally, do not administer iron and antacids at the same time; wait at least 1 to 2 hours before giving the second medication. *Clients with PUD may be anemic as a result of poor nutrient absorption or chronic blood loss. Oral iron supplements may cause GI distress, nausea, and vomiting; if these side effects are intolerable, notify the physician for a possible change of therapy. Antacids bind with oral iron preparations, blocking absorption.*

Fluid Volume Deficit

Erosion of a blood vessel with resultant hemorrhage is a significant risk for the client with peptic ulcer disease. The client who experiences an acute bleeding episode is at risk for hypovolemia and fluid volume deficit, which can lead to a decrease in cardiac output and impaired tissue perfusion.

Nursing interventions with rationales follow:

- Monitor and record blood pressure and apical pulse every 15 to 30 minutes until stable; monitor cardiovascular pressure or pulmonary artery pressure (Swan-Ganz pressure monitoring) as indicated. Insert a Foley catheter and monitor urinary output hourly. Weigh daily. *Continuous monitoring of cardiac output parameters is essential in clients with an acute hemorrhage to identify possible shock and intervene at an early stage.*

- Monitor stools and gastric drainage for overt and occult blood. *Assess gastric drainage (vomitus or from a nasogastric tube) to estimate the amount and rapidity of hemorrhage. Drainage is bright red with possible clots in acute hemorrhage; dark red or the color of coffee grounds when blood has been in the stomach for a period of time. Hematochezia, stool containing red blood and clots, is present in acute hemorrhage; melena (black, tarry stool) is an indicator of less acute bleeding. When small vessels are disrupted, bleeding may be slow and not overtly evident. With chronic or slow gastrointestinal bleeding, the risk of a fluid volume deficit is minimal; anemia and activity intolerance are more likely.*

- Maintain intravenous therapy with fluid volume and electrolyte replacement solutions; administer whole blood or packed cells as ordered. *To prevent shock, it is essential to maintain a blood volume and cardiac output sufficient for perfusion of body tissues. Both fluids and electrolytes are lost through vomiting, nasogastric drainage, and diarrhea in an episode of acute bleeding. Whole blood and packed cells replace both blood volume and red blood cells, providing additional oxygen-carrying capacity to meet cell needs.*

- Insert a nasogastric tube and maintain its position and patency; irrigate with sterile normal saline until returns are clear, if ordered. Initially, measure and record gastric output every hour (be sure to subtract the volume of saline irrigant used), then every 4 to 8 hours. *Nasogastric suction is used to remove blood from the gastrointestinal tract, preventing vomiting and possible aspiration. Irrigation with sterile saline solution at room temperature has a vasoconstrictive effect, slowing active bleeding. Iced or refrigerated solution is not recommended because tissue ischemia may result from excess vasoconstriction. The use of water rather than normal saline may result in water intoxication; the solution should be sterile because of the possibility of perforation. Gastric output is replaced milliliter for milliliter with a balanced electrolyte solution to maintain homeostasis.*

- Monitor laboratory data for hemoglobin and hematocrit, serum electrolytes, BUN, and creatinine. Report abnormal findings. *Hemoglobin and hematocrit are lower than normal in clients with acute or chronic GI bleeding, although initial studies may be within normal range in cases of acute hemorrhage, because both cells and fluid components are lost. Loss of fluids and electrolytes with gastric drainage and diarrhea will alter normal levels. Digestion and absorption of blood in the GI tract may result in elevated BUN and creatinine levels.*

- Assess abdomen, including bowel sounds, distention, girth, and tenderness every 4 hours and record findings. *Borborygmi or hyperactive bowel sounds with abdominal tenderness are common in clients with acute GI bleeding. Increased distention, increasing abdominal girth, absent bowel sounds, or extreme tenderness with a rigid, boardlike abdomen may indicate perforation.*

- Maintain client on bed rest with the head of the bed elevated. Ensure client safety. *Loss of blood volume may cause orthostatic hypotension with resultant syncope or dizziness upon standing.*

Other Nursing Diagnoses

Other nursing diagnoses that may be appropriate for the client with peptic ulcer disease include

- *Knowledge Deficit* related to lack of information about disease process and home management
- *Ineffective Breathing Pattern* related to pain and upper abdominal incision

- *Altered Tissue Perfusion* related to blood loss
- *Risk for Injury* related to perforation or hemorrhage
- *Ineffective Individual Coping* related to life stresses

Client and Family Teaching

Because peptic ulcer disease is a chronic, relapsing-remissing disease, the client requires education about both therapeutic and preventive strategies. Prior to discharge, the client needs written and verbal instruction about the medication regimen prescribed, including the importance of continuing therapy even when symptoms are relieved. Information about the relationship between peptic ulcers and factors such as smoking, alcohol intake, and caffeine use needs to be provided. If indicated, refer the client to a smoking-cessation clinic or a program to treat alcohol abuse. It is important for the client to avoid the use of aspirin and other nonsteroidal anti-inflammatory drugs; stress the necessity of reading the labels of over-the-counter medications to identify the presence of aspirin. Teach the client the symptoms that may indicate a complication, such as increased abdominal pain or distention, vomiting, black or tarry stools, light-headedness, or fainting. Reinforce stress- and life-style management techniques that may help prevent exacerbation. Refer the client to resources for stress management, such as classes, counseling, and formal or informal groups.

Applying the Nursing Process

Case Study of a Client with Peptic Ulcer Disease: Sean O'Donnell

Sean O'Donnell is a 47-year-old policeman who lives and works in a metropolitan area. He is married with two children, both of whom are in college. Sean has experienced "heartburn" and abdominal discomfort for years but thought it went along with his job. Last year, after becoming weak, light-headed, and short-of-breath, he was found to be anemic and was diagnosed as having a duodenal ulcer. He was on cimetidine and ferrous sulfate for 3 months before stopping both, saying he had "never felt better in his life." Sean has been admitted to the hospital with active upper GI bleeding.

Assessment

Rachel Clark is Mr. O'Donnell's admitting nurse and case manager. On initial assessment, Ms. Clark finds Mr. O'Donnell to be alert and oriented, though very apprehensive about his condition. His skin is pale and cool; his BP, 136/78; and his pulse, 98. Mr. O'Donnell's abdomen is distended and tender with extremely active bowel sounds. On insertion of a nasogastric tube, 200 mL of bright red blood is obtained. Diagnostic studies done on admission included the following abnormal findings: hemoglobin 8.2 g/dL, and hematocrit 23%. Mr. O'Donnell's bleeding is controlled with cool saline washes, and he receives two units of packed red blood cells as well as intravenous fluids to replace his lost blood volume. Endoscopy showed scarring from multiple previous ulcers, and it is decided that Mr. O'Donnell should be scheduled for a partial gastrectomy with gastrojejunostomy (Billroth II) and selective vagotomy.

Diagnosis
The postoperative nursing diagnoses for Mr. O'Donnell include the following:

- *Fluid Volume Deficit* related to acute bleeding duodenal ulcer
- *Pain* related to surgical incision
- *Ineffective Breathing Pattern* related to upper abdominal incision
- *Risk for Infection* related to potential perioperative contamination of the peritoneal cavity
- *Risk for Altered Nutrition: Less Than Body Requirements* related to risk of postoperative dumping syndrome
- *Knowledge Deficit* related to lack of information about stress-reduction techniques

Expected Outcomes
The expected outcomes established in the plan of care specify that Mr. O'Donnell will

- Regain a normal body fluid balance as evidenced by stable vital signs within the normal range and normal hemoglobin and hematocrit.
- Report a reasonable level of comfort postoperatively.
- Maintain clear breath sounds.
- Remain free of infection.
- Tolerate a diet adequate to maintain ideal weight and meet energy demands.
- Verbalize at least three techniques for reducing perceived stress.

Planning and Implementation
Ms. Clark plans and implements the following interventions for Mr. O'Donnell:

- Monitor vital signs and mental status every 4 hours until stable, then every 8 hours.
- Maintain careful records of intake and output, including urine and gastric outputs every 4 hours.

- Maintain intravenous fluids and blood replacement; replace gastric output with intravenous fluid as ordered.
- Monitor laboratory values including hemoglobin, hematocrit, serum electrolytes, and urine specific gravity, reporting abnormal values to the physician as indicated.
- Assess level of comfort and effectiveness of pain-relief measures frequently; provide analgesia and nonpharmacologic interventions as indicated; teach use of guided imagery, meditation, distraction, and other relaxation techniques.
- Assess and document breath sounds and respiratory pattern every 4 hours.
- Assist with coughing and deep breathing exercises; teach to splint incision with a pillow or folded blanket when coughing. Keep the head of the bed elevated to at least 30 degrees; get out of bed within 12 hours after surgery, then assist to chair or ambulate three to four times per day.
- Monitor temperature, incision, and drainage; assess and record abdominal girth, tenderness, and bowel sounds every shift or more often if needed.
- Administer antibiotics as ordered.
- Monitor and document food and fluid intake. Assess for signs of dumping syndrome, including nausea, weakness, diaphoresis, orthostatic hypotension, and diarrhea.
- Instruct in dietary modifications to avoid premature gastric emptying. Modifications include consuming meals without liquids; waiting 1 to 2 hours after eating before drinking fluids; eating small, frequent meals; increasing dietary protein and fat, decreasing carbohydrates, avoiding concentrated sugars.
- Discuss stress-reduction techniques including exercise, meditation, ventilation, and other methods to reduce stress. Refer to counseling and stress-reduction workshops if needed.

Evaluation
Now, discharged 5 days after surgery, Mr. O'Donnell is able to eat a regular diet in three small meals with between-meal snacks. His hemoglobin and hematocrit levels are just below normal, with other blood values within normal limits. No episodes of dumping syndrome occurred while he was hospitalized, and he is able to verbalize a good understanding of how to detect and prevent it. Mr. O'Donnell is looking forward to time off for recovery but is also anxious to get back to his job. He states that the hardest part of going back to work will be not drinking six to ten cups of coffee a day, as he used to, and "keeping his cool

on the inside" when under stress. Ms. Clark, his case manager, gives him the names of several resources to help with stress management in case he wants help during his recovery period or after returning to work.

Critical Thinking in the Nursing Process

1. Why is the client who has had a gastrojejunostomy at particular risk for developing dumping syndrome?

2. Describe the physiologic cause of the symptoms associated with dumping syndrome: nausea and vomiting, diaphoresis, tachycardia and decreased blood pressure, syncope.

3. What is the rationale for the dietary modifications recommended in dumping syndrome?

4. Develop a diet plan for a client with dumping syndrome that does not increase the client's risk of coronary artery disease.

5. Mr. O'Donnell also had a selective vagotomy. Develop a teaching plan to meet his learning needs in relation to the effects of this surgery.

The Client with Cancer of the Stomach

■ ■ ■

The incidence of gastric cancer is decreasing in the United States, with a current mortality rate of less than 7 per 100,000 persons. In several other countries, however, the incidence remains high. Japan has the highest gastric cancer mortality rate (Chowdry, 1993). In Korea, it is the most common form of cancer and the cause of most cancer deaths (Sawyers & Eaton, 1992). Males are affected more often than females. Other factors correlated with an increased risk include low socioeconomic status, urban residence, and occupations that involve exposure to nitrates. Genetics appear to play a role, as a familial predisposition and an increased incidence in persons with type A blood group is seen (Bullock & Rosendahl, 1992).

A diet high in nitrates, used as food preservatives and present in smoked foods, is known to increase the risk of gastric cancer. Nitrates are converted to nitrites and then to nitrosamine, which is a recognized carcinogen (Bullock & Rosendahl, 1992).

Gastric cancer is also associated with several other conditions affecting the stomach. **Achlorhydria,** a lack of hydrochloric acid secretion, is a known risk factor. Chronic atrophic gastritis and pernicious anemia are also thought to increase the risk of carcinoma. The relationship between gastric ulcers and tumors is less clear; however, an increased cancer rate is seen in persons who have had gastric surgery for ulcerative disease.

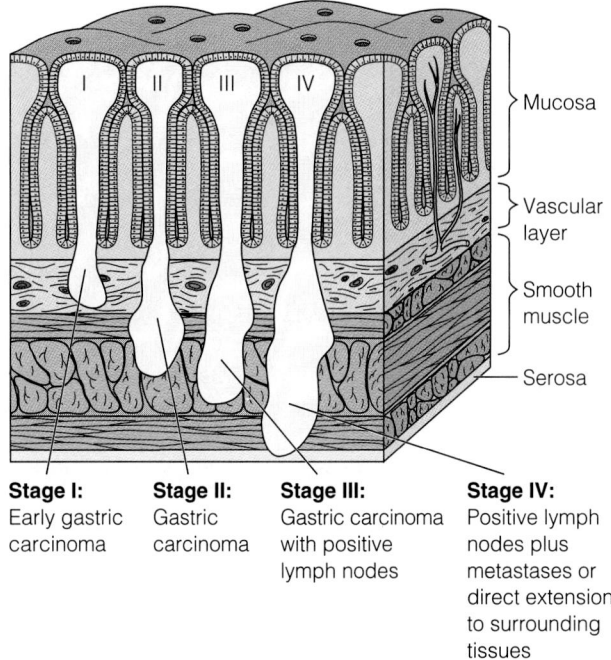

Figure 14–9   Staging of gastric cancer.

Stage I:
Early gastric carcinoma

Stage II:
Gastric carcinoma

Stage III:
Gastric carcinoma with positive lymph nodes

Stage IV:
Positive lymph nodes plus metastases or direct extension to surrounding tissues

Mucosa
Vascular layer
Smooth muscle
Serosa

Pathophysiology

Adenocarcinoma, which involves the mucus-producing cells of the stomach, is the most common form of gastric cancer. These carcinomas may arise anywhere on the mucosal surface of the stomach but are most frequently found in the distal portion. Half of all gastric cancers occur in the antrum or pyloric region (Porth, 1994). When the disease is limited to the mucosa or submucosa, it is called *early gastric carcinoma.* Lesions may spread by direct extension to tissues surrounding the stomach, the liver in particular. Lymph node involvement and metastasis occur early due to the rich blood and lymphatic supply to the stomach. Metastatic lesions are often found in the liver, lungs, ovaries, and peritoneum. Figure 14–9 illustrates the staging of gastric cancer.

Few symptoms are associated with gastric cancer. Unfortunately, the disease is often quite advanced and metastases are usually present at the time of diagnosis. Early symptoms are vague, including feelings of early satiety, anorexia, indigestion, and possibly vomiting. The client may experience ulcerlike pain, typically occurring after meals and unrelieved by antacids. As the disease progresses, weight loss occurs, and the client may be **cachectic** (in very poor health and malnourished) at the time of diagnosis. An abdominal mass may be palpable, and occult blood may be present in the stool, indicating gastrointestinal bleeding.

Nursing Care of the Client with a Gastrostomy Tube

Clients who have had extensive gastric surgery or who require long-term enteral feedings to maintain their nutrition may have a gastrostomy tube inserted.

PROCEDURE

Gastrostomy tubes are surgically placed in the stomach, with the stoma in the epigastric region of the abdomen (see figure below). Immediately following the procedure, the tube may be connected to low suction or plugged. If the client has been receiving tube feedings, these may be reinitiated shortly after tube placement.

NURSING CARE

- Assess tube placement by noting length of tube, aspirating stomach contents, and, if necessary, checking the pH of aspirate to determine gastric or intestinal placement. *Displacement of a gastrostomy tube is rare because of the short length and surgical insertion; however, the tube may slip out of the stomach or be drawn through the pylorus into the duodenum. Recent studies show auscultation to be an ineffective means of determining feeding tube placement (see the nursing research box on page 499).*

- Inspect the skin surrounding the insertion site for healing, redness, swelling, and the presence of any drainage. If drainage is present, note the color, amount, consistency, and odor. *Changes in the insertion site, drainage, or lack of healing may indicate the presence of an infection.*

- Assess the abdomen for distention, bowel sounds, and tenderness *to evaluate functioning of the gastrointestinal tract.*

- Until the stoma is well healed, use sterile technique for dressing changes and site care. Clean technique is appropriate for use once healing is complete. *To minimize the risk of infection, the wound must initially be treated like any other surgical incision. Once healing has occurred, clean technique is acceptable because the gastrointestinal tract is not a sterile body cavity.*

- Wearing clean gloves, remove old dressing. Cleanse the site with antiseptic swabs or soap and water, and rinse as appropriate. For the client with a well-healed stoma, this may be done in the shower with the tube clamped or plugged. Pat dry with 4×4 gauze pads, and allow to air dry. Apply Stomadhesive, karaya, or other protective agents around tube if skin is irritated and requires additional protection. *Gastric acid and other wound drainage is irritating to the skin. Meticulous care is important to maintain the integrity of the skin surrounding the stoma.*

- Redress the wound using a stoma dressing or folded 4×4 gauze pads. *Do not cut gauze pads, because threads may enter the wound, causing irritation and increasing the risk of inflammation.*

- Irrigate the tube with 30 to 50 mL of water, and clean the tube inside and out as indicated or ordered. Soft gastric tubes may require cleaning of the inner lumen with a special brush to maintain patency. *Tube feeding formulas may coat the inside of the gastrostomy tube and eventually cause it to become occluded. Regular irrigation with water and brushing as indicated maintain tube patency.*

- Provide mouth care or remind the client to do so. *When feedings are not being taken orally, the usual stimulus to do mouth care is lost. In addition, salivary fluids may not be as abundant, and oral mucous membranes may become dry and cracked. Maintenance of the integrity of the oral cavity is vital to good health, even when the client is not eating.*

- If the client is to be discharged with a gastrostomy tube, teach the client and family how to care for the tube and feedings. Refer to a home health agency or visiting nurse for support and reinforcement of learning. *Gastrostomy tubes are often in place long-term. When the client and family are able to assume care, independence and self-image are enhanced.*

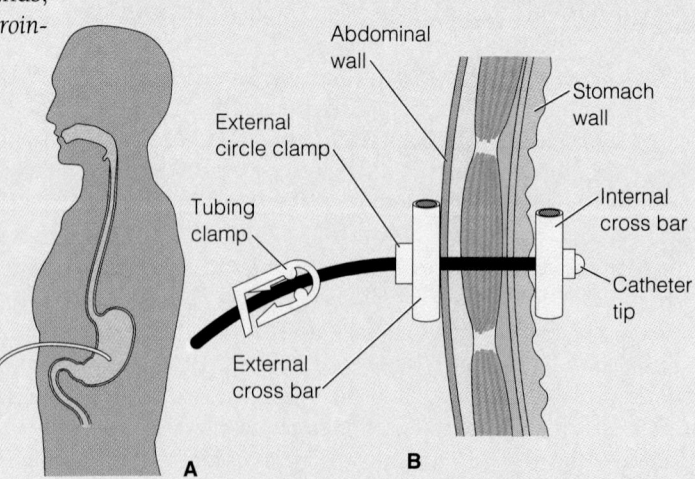

Gastrostomy. *A,* Gastrostomy tube placement. *B,* The tube is fixed against both the abdomen and stomach walls by cross bars.

Applying Research to Nursing Practice
Using Auscultation to Determine Feeding Tube Location

The auscultatory method of determining the location for feeding tubes on initial placement and prior to initiating feeding is commonly recommended in nursing textbooks and is frequently used. The premise is that injecting a small amount of air into the tube will produce a distinctive sound if the tube is correctly located, presumably in the stomach. Sounds produced by tubes located in the esophagus, intestines, and respiratory tract are presumed to be different enough to alert the nurse to the improper location. According to one study, however, experienced clinicians using tape-recorded sounds identified correct nasogastric or nasointestinal feeding tube placement only 34.4% of the time, about what would be expected by chance (Metheny, McSweeney, Wehrle, & Wiersema, 1990). These results suggest that the auscultatory method is ineffective in differentiating tube placement in the stomach from placement in the small intestine. Although only three of the tubes were located in the respiratory tract, the sounds in two of these were thought to indicate gastric placement.

Implications for Nursing

With the advent of small-bore nasogastric and nasointestinal feeding tubes and the increasing use of gastrostomy and jejunostomy feeding tubes, more and more clients are receiving enteral feedings. Nurses need to use alternative methods to auscultation to determine correct initial and continued placement of these tubes. Aspiration of contents and pH testing may prove to be a more effective tool for determining tube placement.

Critical Thinking in Client Care

1. This study investigated differences in auscultatory sounds through small-lumen feeding tubes. Would the sound be more noticeably different with the larger bore tubes used for gastric lavage and drainage?

2. What other methods for determining tube placement are recommended in fundamentals and skills texts?

3. Compare the normal pH of aspirates obtained from the respiratory tract, esophagus, stomach, duodenum, and jejunum.

4. Develop a teaching plan for the client being discharged with a gastrostomy or jejunostomy feeding tube.

Collaborative Care

Several laboratory and diagnostic tests may by used to confirm the diagnosis of gastric cancer. Blood tests will show the presence of anemia, either iron deficiency anemia from chronic blood loss or pernicious anemia. Gastric analysis may reveal a deficiency of hydrochloric acid secretion.

An upper GI X-ray study with barium swallow is useful to identify the presence of lesions, and ultrasound or other radiologic techniques may identify a mass. Gastroscopy with visualization and biopsy of the lesion provides the definitive diagnosis.

When gastric cancer is identified prior to the development of metastasis, surgical intervention with a subtotal radical gastrectomy is the treatment of choice (Porth, 1994). Total gastrectomy with esophagojejunostomy is illustrated in Figure 14–10. Radiation and/or chemotherapy may be used to eliminate any lymphatic or metastatic spread. For the client with more advanced disease, treatment is palliative and may include surgery and chemotherapy. These clients may require a gastrostomy or jejunostomy feeding tube. See the accompanying box for nursing care of the client with a gastrostomy tube.

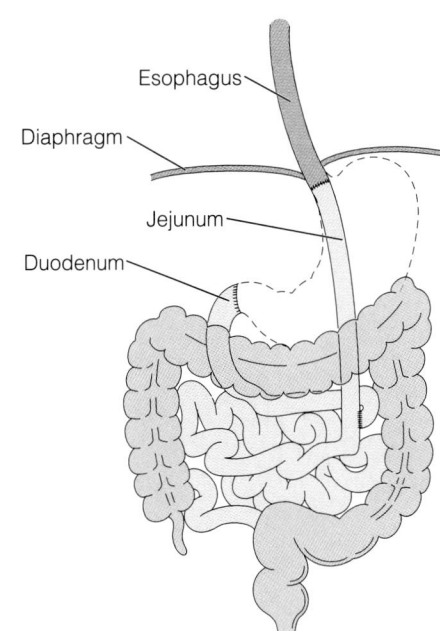

Figure 14–10 Total gastrectomy with esophagojejunostomy.

Because gastric cancer is generally advanced by the time of diagnosis, the prognosis is poor. The 5-year survival rate of all clients treated for gastric carcinoma is 10% (Chowdry, 1993).

Nursing Care

Although the care needs vary according to the individual, nursing diagnoses for the client with gastric carcinoma include the following:

- *Altered Nutrition: Less Than Body Requirements* related to increased metabolic needs and anorexia
- *Impaired Tissue Integrity* (gastric) related to altered cell growth
- *Pain* related to invasive tumor and possible metastasis
- *Anticipatory Grieving* related to diagnosis and prognosis.
- *Body Image Disturbance* related to weight loss.

Bibliography

■ ■ ■

Andreoli, T. E., Carpenter, C. C. J., Plum, F., & Smith, L. H. (1990). *Cecil Essentials of medicine* (2nd ed.). Philadelphia: W. B. Saunders.

Baer, C. L., & Williams, B. R. (1992). *Clinical pharmacology and nursing* (2nd ed.). Springhouse, PA: Springhouse.

Bullock, B. L., & Rosendahl, P. P. (1992). *Pathophysiology: Adaptations and alterations in function* (3rd ed.). Philadelphia: Lippincott.

Burke, S. R. (1992). *Human anatomy and physiology in health and disease* (3rd ed.). Albany, NY: Delmar Publishers.

Burke, M. M., & Walsh, M. B. (1992). *Gerontologic nursing: Care of the frail elderly.* St. Louis: Mosby-Year Book.

Chowdry, P. L. (1993). *Pathophysiology with practical applications.* Dubuque, IA: William C. Brown Publishers.

Cole, G. (Ed.). (1991). *Basic nursing skills and concepts.* St. Louis: Mosby-Year Book.

Corbett, J. V. (1992). *Laboratory tests and diagnostic procedures with nursing diagnoses* (3rd ed.). Norwalk, CT: Appleton & Lange.

Eisenberg, P. (1994). Gastrostomy and jejunostomy tubes. *RN, 57*(11), 54–59.

Farinati, F., & DiMario, F. (1991). Gastric ulcer, epithelial dysplasia, and the development of cancer in the elderly patient. *Geriatric Medicine Today, 10*(3), 25–30.

Feldman, M., Maton, P. N., McCallum, R. W., & McCarthy, D. M. (1992, August 15). Treating ulcers and reflux: What's new? *Patient Care, 26*(13), 53–72.

Fina, M. F. (1991). Recertification notebook: Diagnosis and treatment of duodenal ulcer. *Clinician Reviews, 1*(5): 88.

Gilinsky, N. H. (1990). Peptic ulcer disease in the elderly. *Gastroenterology Clinics of North America, 19*(2): 255–267.

Glass, H. A. (1991). Peptic ulcer disease: Current trends and future directions. *Clinician Reviews, 1* (7), 45–46, 49–50, 53–54, 56.

Lederer, J. R., Marculescu, G. L., Mocnik, B., & Seaby, N. (1993). *Care planning pocket guide: A nursing diagnosis approach* (5th ed.). Redwood City, CA: Addison-Wesley Nursing.

McKenry, L. M., & Solerno, E. (1992). *Mosby's pharmacology in nursing* (18th ed.). St. Louis: Mosby-Year Book.

Memmler, R. L., Cohen, B. J., & Wood, D. L. (1992). *The human body in health and disease* (7th ed.). Philadelphia: Lippincott.

Metheny, N., McSweeney, M., Wehrle, M. A., & Wiersema, L. (1990). Effectiveness of the auscultatory method in predicting feeding tube location. *Nursing Research, 39* (5), 262–267.

Pagana, K. D., & Pagana, T. J. (1992). *Mosby's diagnostic and laboratory test reference.* St. Louis: Mosby-Year Book.

Porth, C. M. (1994). *Pathophysiology: Concepts of altered health states* (4th ed.). Philadelphia: Lippincott.

Sawyers, J. E. & Eaton, L. 1992. Gastric cancer in the Korean American: Cultural implications. *Oncology Nursing Forum, 19* (4): 619–623.

Shlafer, M. (1993). *The nurse, pharmacology, and drug therapy* (2nd ed.). Redwood City, CA: Addison-Wesley Nursing.

Skidmore-Roth, L. (1993). *Mosby's 1993 nursing drug reference.* St. Louis: Mosby-Year Book.

Sparks, S. M., & Taylor, C. M. (1993). *Nursing diagnosis reference manual* (2nd ed.). Springhouse, PA: Springhouse.

Swearingen, P. L. (Ed.). (1991). *Photo atlas of nursing procedures* (2nd ed.). Redwood City, CA: Addison-Wesley Nursing.

Thompson, J. M., McFarland, G. K., Hirsch, J. E., & Tucker, S. M. (1993). *Mosby's clinical nursing* (3rd ed.). St. Louis: Mosby-Year Book.

Tucker, S. M., Canobbio, M. M., Paquette, E. V., & Wells, M. F. (1992). *Patient care standards: Nursing process, diagnosis, and outcome* (5th ed.). St. Louis: Mosby-Year Book.

Wesorick, B. (1990). *Standards of nursing care: A model for clinical practice.* Philadelphia: Lippincott.

Wilson, J. D., Braunwald, E., Isselbacher, K. J., Petersdorf, R. G., Martin, J. B., Fauci, A. S., & Root, R. K. (Eds.). (1991). *Harrison's Principles of internal medicine* (12th ed.). New York: McGraw-Hill.

Nursing Care of Clients with Gallbladder, Liver, and Pancreatic Disorders

LEARNING OBJECTIVES

After completing this chapter, you will be able to

- Describe the pathophysiology of commonly occurring disorders of the gallbladder, liver, and exocrine pancreas.

- Discuss laboratory and diagnostic tests, including client preparation, used to diagnose disorders of the gallbladder, liver, and exocrine pancreas.

- Describe the pathophysiologic basis for assessments of gallbladder, liver, and exocrine pancreatic disorders.

- Discuss nursing implications for dietary and pharmacologic interventions related to the gallbladder, liver, and exocrine pancreas.

- Provide appropriate nursing care for the client who has surgery of the gallbladder, liver, or pancreas.

- Explain the rationale for selected nursing interventions related to care of clients with biliary, hepatic, and exocrine pancreatic disorders.

- Use the nursing process as a framework for providing individualized care to clients with disorders of the gallbladder, liver, or exocrine pancreas.

Gallbladder, liver, and exocrine pancreatic disorders may present as solitary problems or as disorders related to other disease processes. One organ's functioning frequently affects that of another. Duct inflammation or obstruction and changes in the multiple functions of the gallbladder, liver, and exocrine pancreas are some of the problems that can adversely affect a person's health.

Clients who have a gallbladder, liver, or exocrine pancreatic disorder may experience severe pain, altered body image, and a host of metabolic and nutritional disturbances. Nursing care addresses the client's and family's physiologic and psychosocial needs through attention to individualized care planning.

◥◥◥ Gallbladder Disorders ◥◥◥

Alteration in the flow of bile via the hepatic, cystic, or common bile duct is a common disorder. Gallstone formation, called *cholelithiasis,* is the most common cause of the obstruction; it usually leads to inflammation, called *cholecysitis,* and other complications. Other causes of blockage include tumors, discussed later in this section, and abscesses.

Collaborative Health Care: The Client with Hepatitis

Health Care Team	Client-Centered Goals
Primary Care Physician	Completes physical exam and assesses client's history and risk factors for hepatitis. Orders diagnostic tests and establishes etiology of hepatitis. Monitors liver function tests and serologic markers. Determines infection control precautions and discusses with client and family. Orders antiemetics, rest, and diet therapy.
Social Worker	Assists client and family with financial concerns and problems. Refers family to local health department for infection control information. Arranges home care including home health aides to assist with self-care and meal preparation and visiting nurse to assess responses to therapy.
Dietician	Provides a high-carbohydrate, high calorie diet of small frequent feedings. Recommends supplemental vitamins or feedings. Instructs client and family regarding the importance of a well-balanced diet and strategies to improve nutrition.
RN and Health Care Team Communications	Alerts dietician to client's food preferences. Consults with dietician to identify strategies to improve nutritional intake. Obtain orders for antiemetic if nausea or vomiting present. Assesses home situation and discusses home care needs with social worker.

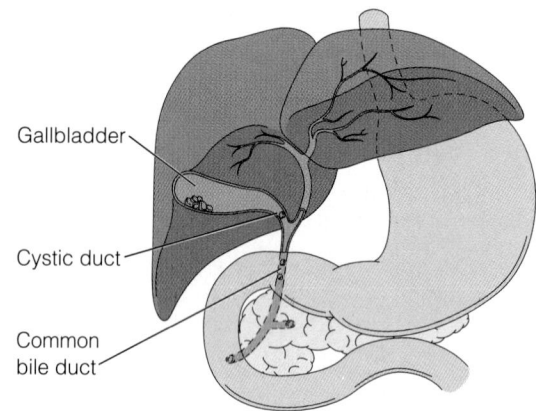

Figure 15–1 Common locations of gallstones.

The Client with Cholelithiasis and Cholecystitis

■ ■ ■

Cholelithiasis is the formation of stones, also called *calculi*, within the gallbladder or biliary duct system. Clients who have gallstones present with a variety of problems, including not only localized inflammation but also systemic symptoms and problems.

Pathophysiology

The pathophysiology of gallstones varies with the type of stone, its location within the ductal system, and whether the problem is acute or chronic. See Figure 15–1 for an illustration of typical locations of gallstones.

Cholelithiasis

Gallstones are made up of bile pigments or hardened cholesterol. Pigment stones are composed of a bilirubin salt, calcium bilirubinate, and are associated with the presence of bacteria in the bile. Cholesterol stones are more common than pigmented stones. Cholesterol stones also contain small amounts of other materials, such as calcium salts and bile pigments. Clients may present with one stone or with multiple stones. Stone formation occurs when the bile crystallizes.

Factors that contribute to stone formation include stasis of the bile in the gallbladder and increased bile concentration. For example, hypercholesterolemia and slower gallbladder emptying are common in the last trimester of pregnancy. The risk factors listed in the box on page 503 also predispose clients to gallstone formation.

Most gallstones are formed in the gallbladder and migrate out of the organ to cause symptoms of either *cholangitis* (duct inflammation) or *choledocolithiasis* (stone in the common bile duct). Although some people with cholelithiasis may be asymptomatic, many have manifestations at some point in the disease process. Manifestations vary according to where the stones are located:

- Stones in the cystic duct cause the gallbladder to distend, resulting in severe, cramplike, colicky pain. Secondary infection combined with severe inflammation and edema results in duct blockage and abdominal pain, nausea, and sometimes vomiting.

- Obstruction of the common bile duct may result in bile reflux into the liver, producing jaundice, pain, possible hepatic damage, pancreatitis (discussed later in this chapter), or sepsis (Gallo & Fontanarosa, 1989).

Factors that Increase the Risk of Gallstone Formation

■ ■ ■

- Family history of gallstones
- Diseases or Conditions
  a. Cirrhosis
  b. Crohn's disease
  c. Hemolytic anemia
  d. Hyperlipidemia
  e. Congenital malformation of biliary ducts
  f. Obesity
- Hyperalimentation
- Race or Ethnicity
  a. Native American
  b. Caucasian
  c. Mexican American
- Female Gender
  a. Multiparity
  b. Use of oral contraceptives

Note. Adapted from *Pathophysiology: Clinical Concepts of Disease Process* by S. A. Price and L. M. Wilson (4th ed.), 1992, St Louis: Mosby-Year Book.

Clinical Manifestations of Cholelithiasis and Cholecystitis

■ ■ ■

Cholelithiasis

- Epigastric pain
- Heartburn
- Right upper abdominal pain (may radiate to subscapular area); pain may be called "biliary colic"
- Jaundice (with obstruction of the common bile duct)
- Intolerance to fat-containing foods

Cholecystitis
The manifestations listed above, plus the following:

- Fever
- High white blood cell count
- Abdominal muscle guarding with rebound tenderness and rigidity (may indicate peritoneal involvement)
- Elevated serum bilirubin
- Elevated alkaline phosphatase
- Elevated serum amylase if pancreatic ducts are involved

Cholecystitis

Cholecystitis is inflammation of the gallbladder. It is most commonly associated with stones in the cystic or common bile duct. About 5% of clients develop acalculous cholecystitis, which may be related to trauma, hyperalimentation, extended fasting, or surgery (Gallo & Fontanarosa, 1989).

Cholecystitis is classified as either acute or chronic. *Acute cholecystitis* is characterized by severe pain radiating from the abdominal right upper quadrant to the midline and posteriorly to the scapular region. Frequently, nausea and vomiting accompany the pain, which may be described as "colicky." This spasmodic pain results from contraction of the ducts and is usually initiated by a high-fat meal. Some patients have a low-grade fever or develop jaundice. The accompanying box compares the clinical manifestations of cholecystitis and cholelithiasis.

Chronic cholecystitis generally has a more moderate presentation; symptoms are not as severe and are more vague compared to those that present with the acute form. Clients complain of long-term intolerance to fatty foods, vague gastric symptoms, or increased flatulence.

Complications of chronic cholecystitis include gallbladder perforation and peritonitis, infection of the biliary system, pancreatitis, blockage from inflammation or a stone that causes an adynamic ileus or intestinal obstruction, fistula formation, and cancer.

Collaborative Care

Care of the client with cholelithiasis and cholecystitis focuses on reducing inflammation and blockage. Results of diagnostic assessments and the client's overall condition indicate whether treatment should be curative or palliative. Treatment options include pharmacologic, surgical, and noninvasive procedures. When stones are found in the gallbladder or ducts, usually surgery is indicated.

Laboratory and Diagnostic Tests
Tests ordered focus on determining the location of stones, the extent of possible complications, and differentiating the problem from other disorders.

The following laboratory tests may be ordered:

- *Complete blood count (CBC),* shows an elevated WBC due to infection and inflammation.
- *Serum amylase and lipase* are measured to determine the presence of pancreatitis.

Examples of High-Fat Foods to Avoid for the Client with Gallstones*

■ ■ ■

- Whole-milk products (e.g., cream, ice cream)
- Doughnuts, deep-fried
- Avocados
- Sausage, bacon
- Gravies with fat, cream
- Most nuts (e.g., pecans, cashews)
- Corn chips and potato chips
- Butter and cooking oils
- Fried foods (e.g., cheeseburgers, hamburgers, french fries)
- Peanut butter
- Chicken pot pie
- Hot dogs
- Whole-cheese products
- Chocolate

*Teach the client to read food labels.

- *Serum bilirubin levels* are measured to ascertain either obstruction in the biliary duct system (elevated direct bilirubin) or hepatic damage (elevated indirect bilirubin).
- Other baseline studies may be ordered, depending on the needs of the individual client. For example, if the client has a preexisting cardiac condition, electrolytes may be monitored; for a client with diabetes, glucose and creatinine levels are checked. These would be especially indicated if surgery is planned.

Diagnostic studies include the following:

- *X-ray study* of the abdomen, called a flat plate, is conducted to visualize stones; this has limited value because most stones are not radiopaque.
- *Oral cholecystogram* is performed in nonacute situations. In this study, an oral dye is used to assess the gallbladder's ability to concentrate and excrete bile.
- Other cholangiograms may employ various techniques, including endoscopic, intravenous, transhepatic, and direct, or operative, techniques (via T-tube, described in the section discussing surgical procedures). Each of these techniques permits detection of stones in the biliary duct system.
- *Ultrasonography* of the gallbladder is used for clients who are not obese. Excess adipose tissue causes poor

visualization of the gallbladder and ducts. Stones and edema or distention of the gallbladder and ducts can be detected with abdominal sonogram.

- *Gallbladder scans,* also called HIDA scans, are done through nuclear medicine techniques to assess acute cholecystitis. These scans are called *cholescintigraphy.*

More than one of the above diagnostic studies may be performed to verify or give further evidence of the presence of stones; therefore, clients frequently need teaching about several procedures.

Pharmacology

The major pharmacologic intervention aimed at curing gallstones involves a relatively new group of agents, oral bile acids, called *dissolvers.* One of these, ursodeoxycholic acid (UDCA), is used for cholesterol stones under 20 mm in diameter. Nurses need to monitor hepatic enzymes and watch for possible diarrhea when this drug is used. Another bile acid agent currently in use is chenodeoxycholic acid (also called chenodiol), which works by decreasing the amount of cholesterol in bile, causing the stones to be more soluble. One problem identified with oral dissolution therapy is the possible recurrence of gallstones (Rowland, Marks, & Torres, 1989).

Both agents are most commonly used for clients who are not experiencing complications from the gallstones and for clients for whom surgery would pose a high risk, such as the elderly or those who may have multiple disorders. Several years of therapy may be needed to ensure that the stones are dissolved and do not recur.

Other pharmacologic agents are used for palliative relief of specific symptoms. If infection is suspected, antibiotics may be prescribed to reduce the bacterial count and the associated inflammation and edema. Some clients experience severe obstructive jaundice that results in an accumulation of bile salts on the skin, producing pruritus (itching). In severe pruritic cases, cholestyramine (Questran), which binds with bile salts, is administered orally to hasten the excretion of bile salts through the feces.

Diet Therapy

Because dietary fat is a stimulus for gallbladder contraction, clients are usually placed on a low-fat diet. Foods to avoid are listed in the accompanying box. Clients who are obese are encouraged to lose weight, particularly if surgery is inevitable. If bile flow is greatly reduced because of obstruction, fat-soluble vitamins—A, D, E, and K—and bile salts may need to be administered. With severe nausea and vomiting, the client may be temporarily NPO. To relieve or prevent abdominal distention, a nasogastric tube may be inserted.

Surgery

The type of surgical procedure performed for the client with gallstones depends on where the stone is located and

Critical Pathway for Client Following Laparoscopic Cholecystectomy		
	Date _____ **Preoperative**	Date _____ **1st 24 hours following surgery**
Expected length of stay: less than 24 hours		
Daily outcomes	Client will ■ Verbalize understanding of preoperative teaching, including turning, coughing, deep breathing, use of incentive spirometer, mobilization, and pain management. ■ Demonstrates ability to cope.	Client will ■ Be afebrile. ■ Have a dry, clean wound with well approximated edges healing by first intention. ■ Manage pain with nonpharmacologic measures or oral medications. ■ Be independent in self-care. ■ Be fully ambulatory. ■ Resume preadmission urine and bowel elimination pattern. ■ Verbalize home care instructions. ■ Tolerate usual diet. ■ Demonstrate ability to cope with ongoing stressors.
Tests and treatments	CBC Urinalysis Baseline physical assessment with a focus on respiratory status and gastrointestinal function Anesthesia consult	Vital signs and O_2 saturation, neurovascular assessment, dressing and wound drainage assessment q15min × 4; q30min × 4; q1h × 4 and then q4h if stable. Assess lung sounds and gastrointestinal function q4h and prn. Intake and output every shift. Assess voiding; if client is unable to void, suggest voiding techniques or catheterize q8h or prn.
Knowledge deficit	Orient to room and surroundings. Include family in teaching. Provide simple, brief instructions. Review preoperative preparation, including hospital and surgical routines. Reinforce preoperative teaching regarding specific postoperative care: turning, coughing, deep breathing, use of incentive spirometer, mobilization, and pain management. Assess understanding of teaching.	Reorient to room and postoperative routine. Include family in teaching. Review plan of care and importance of early mobilization, as well as any activity restrictions. Complete discharge teaching regarding wound care/dressing change, follow-up care, signs and symptoms to report, medications, and diet. Assess understanding of teaching.

the severity of complications. If stones are found only within the gallbladder, a simple **cholecystectomy** (removal of the gallbladder) is performed. Options include either conventional surgical methods or laparoscopic laser surgery. The accompanying Critical Pathway describes the expected nursing care and outcomes for the client undergoing laparoscopic cholecystectomy.

When stones are lodged within the ducts, a cholecystectomy with common bile duct exploration and T-tube insertion may be indicated (Figure 15–2). Inserted after common bile duct exploration, a T-tube maintains patency of the duct and promotes bile passage while the edema decreases. Excess bile is collected in a drainage bag secured below the surgical site. If it is suspected that a

	Date _____ **Preoperative**	Date _____ **1st 24 hours following surgery**
Psycho- social	Assess anxiety related to pending surgery. Assess fears of the unknown and surgery. Encourage verbalization of concerns. Provide emotional support to client and family. Provide information regarding surgical experience. Minimize external stimuli (e.g., noise, movement).	Assess level of anxiety. Encourage verbalization of concerns. Provide emotional support to client and family. Provide information and ongoing support and encouragement.
Diet	NPO Baseline nutritional assessment	Advance to clear liquids; if tolerated, advance to full liquids/soft diet morning following surgery.
Activity	OOB ad lib until premedicated for surgery.	Provide safety precautions. Bathroom privileges with assistance evening after surgery. Begin progressive ambulation to tolerance the morning following surgery until client is fully ambulatory.
Medications	NPO except ordered medications.	IM or PO analgesics Antibiotics if ordered IV fluids until adequate PO intake; intermittent IV device thereafter. Discontinue prior to discharge.
Transfer/ discharge plans	Assess discharge plans and support system.	Probable discharge within 24 hours of surgery. Complete discharge home care teaching when client is fully awake and oriented and before discharge. Provide written discharge instructions.

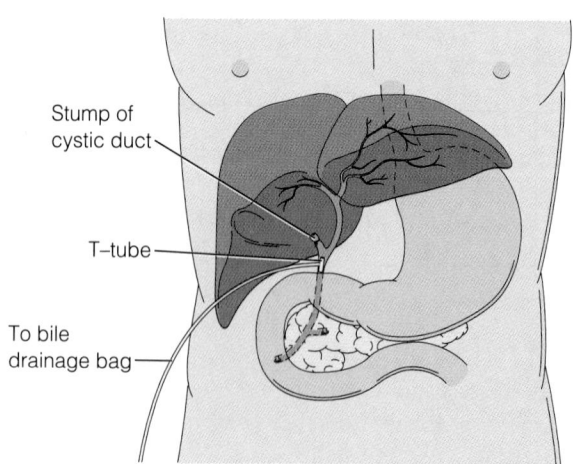

Stump of
cystic duct

T-tube

To bile
drainage bag

Figure 15–2   T-tube placement in the common bile duct. Bile fluid flows with gravity into a drainage collection device below the level of the common bile duct.

stone has been retained following surgery, a postoperative cholangiogram via the T-tube or direct visualization of the duct with an endoscope may be performed. The box on page 507 and Table 15–1 describe nursing care of the client undergoing a cholecystectomy with T-tube placement, and possible postoperative complications and nursing interventions.

For clients who are poor surgical risks, a *cholecystostomy* or *choledochostomy* may be performed. A cholecystostomy permits drainage of the gallbladder; a choledochostomy allows for the removal of stones and placement of a T-tube in the common bile duct.

Treatment Alternatives

Besides the more conventional operative procedures discussed above, clients may opt for lithotripsy or a percutaneous stone dissolution. With *extracorporeal shock wave lithotripsy (ESWL)*, the physician uses ultrasound to align

Nursing Care of the Client with a T-Tube

- Ensure that the T-tube is properly connected to a sterile container; keep the tube below the level of the surgical wound. *This position promotes the flow of bile when the common bile duct is edematous and also prevents the backflow of bile or seepage of caustic bile onto the skin. The tube itself decreases biliary tree pressure.*

- Monitor the drainage from the T-tube for color and consistency; record results as part of output. Normal drainage is as follows: the tube may drain up to 500 mL in the first 24 hours after surgery; the drainage decreases to under 200 mL in 2 to 3 days; thereafter, drainage is minimal. The drainage may be blood tinged initially, changing to green-brown. Report excessive drainage to the physician immediately (after 48 hours, drainage greater than 500 mL is considered excessive). *Stones or edema and inflammation can obstruct ducts below the tube, requiring medical interventions.*

- Place the client in the Fowler's position. *This promotes gravity drainage of bile.*

- Assess the skin for bile leakage during dressing changes. *Bile irritates the skin; it may be necessary to apply protection for the skin with karaya or another barrier product.*

- Teach the client how to manage the tube when turning, ambulating, and performing activities of daily living. *The client must avoid direct pull or traction on the tube while carrying out activities that promote lung expansion.*

- When drainage subsides and stools return to a normal brown color, clamp the T-tube for 1 to 2 hours before and after meals. *Decreasing drainage usually indicates the return of bile flow and decreased edema. Gradually clamping the tube while the operative site heals helps prevent nausea.*

- If indicated, teach the client care of the T-tube, how to clamp it, and signs of infection. *Clients may be discharged home with the tube in place. Reporting early signs of infection facilitates prompt treatment.*

Table 15–1   Possible Postoperative Complications with Nursing Interventions for the Client Having a Cholecystectomy with T-Tube

Complications	Nursing Interventions
Pulmonary: atelectasis, pneumonia	Teach preoperatively and implement postoperatively the use of incentive spirometer, turning, deep breathing and coughing (T, DB, & C) with splinting incision at least every 2 hours; encourage early progressive ambulation. Monitor lung sounds at least every 2 hours.
Cardiovascular: emboli, thrombophlebitis	In addition to the above, teach and implement leg exercises; perform exercises at least every 2 hours while client remains in bed; assess for signs of vascular interruption; check Homans' sign and record.
Wound: dehiscence, infection	Use sterile technique and good hand washing; monitor for early signs of infection, and report promptly. Especially for obese clients: splint wound site during T, DB, & C exercises.
Gastrointestinal: paralytic ileus, peritonitis	Monitor bowel sounds and vital signs at least every 4 hours; expect return of bowel sounds within 48 hours. Implement ambulation and other measures as above to promote return of peristalsis.
Pain	Teach client what to expect postoperatively; remember that perception of pain varies from client to client. Incorporate nonpharmacologic measures of pain relief: distraction, position changes, back rub. Administer analgesics on a schedule rather than waiting until pain becomes severe; decrease doses as tolerated.

---

the stones with the source of shock waves and the computerized lithotripter. Positioning is of prime importance throughout the procedure, which usually takes an hour. Mild sedation may be indicated during the procedure. Postprocedure nursing care includes monitoring for bil-

iary colic that may result from the gallbladder contracting to remove stone fragments, nausea, and transient hematuria (Rowland et al., 1989).

Percutaneous stone dissolution is a treatment option for patients who are at high risk for postsurgical problems.

Using fluoroscopy, the physician positions a catheter via the hepatic biliary system to the point of the stone. Dissolution agents are then instilled. The transhepatic percutaneous catheter may also be inserted to relieve the obstruction and permit bile flow without attempting to dissolve the stone.

Nursing Care

Although clients' responses to cholelithiasis and cholecystitis may vary, some of the more frequent problems include pain; altered nutrition due to nausea, vomiting, and impaired fat metabolism; risk for impaired gas exchange due to altered breathing patterns postcholecystectomy; and risk for infection following surgical or alternative procedures for stone removal. Nursing interventions, such as monitoring for hemorrhage, are similar to those for clients undergoing abdominal surgery.

Pain

The pain associated with cholelithiasis can be severe. Sometimes a combination of interventions is indicated.
Nursing interventions with rationales follow:

- Teach clients to avoid fat in their diets. *Fat initiates gallbladder contractions and is a stimulus for pain.*

- If diet therapy is not effective, administer prescribed medications. *Medications such as dicyclomine HCl (Bentyl) or nitroglycerin are used to decrease spasms and relax smooth muscle. Interventions aimed at decreasing spasm of the biliary tree decrease the stimulus for abdominal pain.*

- If severe pain is unrelieved by other methods or by medications, administer prescribed narcotic analgesia. *The drug of choice both preoperatively and postoperatively is meperidine (Demerol); morphine sulfate is contraindicated as it causes spasms of the sphincter of Oddi.*

- Monitor for temperature elevations every 4 hours, and assist the client to a Fowler's position. *Temperature elevation indicates the presence of infection of inflammation; Fowler's position decreases diaphragmatic pressure on the inflamed area.*

- For clients who have pain associated with pruritus, see the section on nursing care under hepatic disorders.

Risk for Impaired Gas Exchange and Pulmonary Infection

Following a cholecystectomy, clients may have difficulty with effective breathing and gas exchange because of the high abdominal incision. Preoperative teaching and postoperative follow-through is important. Nursing interventions with rationales follow:

- Institute a regimen of turning, deep breathing, and coughing at least every 2 hours; use of an incentive spirometer every hour while awake, and begin early ambulation at least four times daily. *These interventions help prevent accumulation of secretions in the lungs and pneumonia, help expand the lungs to prevent atelectasis, and aid in surfactant production.*

- Provide proper analgesia for the postoperative client. *Nursing interventions, including the judicious use of analgesics and splinting the incisional area enhance the patient's ability to take deep breaths, thus promoting adequate gas exchange.*

Risk for Infection

Infection following a cholecystectomy with T-tube insertion may arise from varying sources. Possible infections are subhepatic abscess, infection of the surgical incision site, peritonitis, and pancreatitis.
Nursing interventions with rationales follow:

- Assess for signs of systemic and localized infection during the immediate postoperative period by monitoring temperature every 4 hours. *The goal is to discover any infectious process as early as possible so that appropriate action can be taken.*

- Assess the wound at least every 4 hours. *Along with carrying out the usual wound assessments, monitor for purulent discharge, which indicates an infectious process.*

- Perform abdominal assessment at least every 4 hours. *Peritonitis is manifested by a rigid abdomen and absence of bowel sounds with pain; report manifestations immediately.*

Nursing interventions to prevent infection are similar to those for other abdominal surgeries; see Chapter 7 for more information. Care of the client with a T-tube is discussed below, under the section on client teaching.

Other Nursing Diagnoses

Examples of other nursing diagnoses related to the client experiencing cholelithiasis and cholecystitis include:

- *Altered Nutrition: Less Than Body Requirements* related to effects of nausea and vomiting (preoperatively or postoperatively) and disruption of bile flow

- *Risk for Fluid Volume Deficit* related to limited intake, effects of nasogastric intubation, and effects of infection

- *Impaired Skin Integrity* related to severe pruritus (preoperatively)

- *Anxiety* related to lack of knowledge about self-care on discharge

- *Diarrhea* related to effects of medications (UDCA and chenodiol)

Client and Family Teaching

Teaching interventions for the client and family vary with their choice of treatment options. Nonsurgical interventions require teaching about medications that dissolve stones, specific procedures, and maintaining a low-fat, low-kcalorie diet if indicated. Teaching needs to include an explanation about the role of bile and the function of the gallbladder in terms that the client and family can understand.

Preoperative teaching is aimed toward preventing or decreasing the possibility of complications after surgery. Prepare the client for what to expect, regarding not only pain and possible nausea but also nursing assessments. Client and family teaching that focuses on self-care methods to prevent specific problems, such as pneumonia, may be more effective than general teaching that does not actively elicit client participation and self-care.

The goal of postoperative teaching is to prepare the client for discharge and home care. Pain control, monitoring for and preventing infection, and T-tube care are included in teaching. Some clients require a T-tube cholangiogram following discharge. See the box on page 507 for care of the client with a T-tube.

Consult a dietitian to review low-fat foods, and include the person preparing foods. Most patients start with a low-fat diet and gradually add fatty foods as tolerated. Follow-up with the physician or community health nurse is part of discharge planning.

Applying the Nursing Process

Case Study of a Client with Cholelithiasis: Joyce Red Wing

Joyce Red Wing is a 44-year-old married mother of three children. A member of the Chickasaw tribe, she is active in tribal activities and works part time as a cook at a community kitchen. Recently Ms. Red Wing has noticed a dull pain in her upper abdomen that gets worse after eating fatty foods; nausea and sometimes vomiting accompany the pain. She had a similar pain after the birth of her last child. Outpatient diagnostic tests indicate that Ms. Red Wing has cholelithiasis. She enters the hospital for an elective cholecystectomy. Her husband accompanies her but soon leaves to care for their children.

Assessment

David Corbin, RN, takes Ms. Red Wing's admission history. It includes intolerance to fatty foods and abdominal pain (described as periodically "colicky") that radiates to her back. Her usual diet consists of fatty foods, particularly tacos or fried bread and biscuits with gravy for breakfast. She reports "not wanting to eat much of anything lately." She states she has never had surgery before and hopes "everything goes well." Physical assessment

findings: T, 100 F (37.7 C); BP, 130/84; P, 88; R, 20. She weighs 130 lb (59 kg), which represents a 5-pound (2.3-kg) weight loss, and is 5 feet, 3 inches (160 cm) tall. With abdominal palpation, pain is elicited on inspiration at the right upper subcostal area, indicating a positive Murphy's sign. She has no jaundice, chills, or signs to indicate complications.

Diagnosis

Mr. Corbin identifies the following nursing diagnoses for Ms. Red Wing:

- *Altered Nutrition: Less Than Body Requirements* related to anorexia and recent weight loss
- *Pain* related to effects of surgery and high abdominal incision
- *Risk for Infection* related to effects of surgery
- *Anxiety* related to lack of information about perioperative experience

Expected Outcomes

The expected outcomes established in the plan of care specify that Ms. Red Wing will:

- Maintain her present weight within 5 lb (2.3 kg) over the next 3 weeks.
- Resume eating habits, selecting foods from a variety of sources and according to her ability to tolerate fatty foods, within 2 weeks of her surgery.
- Verbalize control of pain following surgery and resumption of activities.
- Remain free of infection postoperatively.
- Verbalize a decrease in anxiety before surgery.

Planning and Implementation

Mr. Corbin plans and implements the following interventions for Ms. Red Wing, including her husband as much as possible:

- Teach Ms. Red Wing about the gallbladder and the function of bile.
- Discuss what to expect preoperatively and postoperatively, including ways to prevent pneumonia and the need for postoperative follow-up.
- Initiate turning, deep breathing and coughing, early ambulation, and use of the incentive spirometer with splinting of incision at least every 2 hours during the initial postoperative period.
- Teach Ms. Red Wing aseptic care of her surgical wound.
- Review with Ms. Red Wing specific high-fat foods to avoid and ways to maintain her weight.

- Provide analgesia as appropriate to ensure Ms. Red Wing's comfort and allow her to participate in self-care.

Evaluation

Ms. Red Wing is discharged on the fourth postoperative day. She has no fever or other signs of infection and is able to perform wound care with aseptic technique. She identifies signs of infection and talks about the importance of eating a low-fat diet and keeping her weight stable as well as gradually resuming activities. Ms. Red Wing states that she "is glad it is over, but it wasn't as bad as I thought it would be at first." She has an appointment to see her surgeon in 1 week.

Critical Thinking in the Nursing Process

1. What is the rationale for a low-fat diet with cholelithiasis? Discuss nutritional practices as they relate to the medical problem and Ms. Red Wing's culture.

2. Why would it be important to place Ms. Red Wing in a Fowler's position after surgery?

3. List five interventions for Ms. Red Wing appropriate to home care; be realistic given her family situation.

4. Design a nursing care plan for Ms. Red Wing for the nursing diagnosis: *Fatigue.*

The Client with Cancer of the Gallbladder

■ ■ ■

Gallbladder cancer is rare, primarily affecting people over 65. Women are more likely to develop the disorder. Clients with cancer of the gallbladder complain of intense pain in the right upper quadrant of the abdomen; a mass may be palpated in the region. Jaundice and weight loss usually accompany the pain. Most gallbladder cancers metastasize via the blood, lymph system, or through direct extension; the liver is most commonly affected.

Most cancers of the gallbladder cannot be treated surgically, unless they are found at an early stage incidental to another surgical procedure. Ninety-five percent of clients with primary cancer of the gallbladder die within 1 year. Radical and extensive surgical interventions may be performed, but the prognosis is poor regardless of treatment (Greenberger & Isselbacher, 1991).

▗▗▗ Liver Disorders ▗▗▗

Optimal hepatic function is essential to the body's well-being. Impaired hepatic function has many metabolic consequences because the liver is responsible for:

- The metabolism of protein, carbohydrate, fat, and steroids
- Bile production and excretion
- Mineral and vitamin storage
- Drug and alcohol detoxification
- Fluid volume regulation
- Phagocytosis performed by the Kupffer cells that line the sinusoids

Hepatitis is one of the most common liver disorders.

The Client with Hepatitis

■ ■ ■

Hepatitis is inflammation of the liver. This condition is usually caused by a virus. Other causes include alcohol, toxins (such as a drugs), or cholestasis due to hepatobiliary disease. Acute and chronic forms of hepatitis exist, and both may occur secondary to other types of systemic viral infections, such as from varicella zoster. Cirrhosis,

discussed in the next section, is a sequela to severe hepatocellular damage.

Pathophysiology

Although the underlying pathophysiology of hepatitis varies, the general manifestations are similar. Much depends on the degree of liver damage and the client's concurrent health status. The most common type of acute hepatitis is viral hepatitis; it is discussed in depth following a discussion of the other types of hepatitis.

Alcoholic Hepatitis

Alcoholic hepatitis can result from chronic alcohol abuse or from an acute toxic reaction to alcohol. Only a small percentage of chronic alcoholics develop this type of hepatitis, which results in necrosis of hepatocytes and inflammation of the liver parenchyma with leukocytic infiltration (Lieber & Guadagnini, 1990). Treatment is avoidance of alcohol and support of liver function during recovery. Without ongoing abstinence, progression to cirrhosis is common.

Toxic Hepatitis

The causes of toxic hepatitis are varied and can be idiosyncratic to the individual affected. Potentially hepatotoxic agents include acetaminophen, benzene, carbon tetrachloride, halothane, chloroform, and poisonous mushrooms. Hepatic necrosis results. Toxic hepatitis is treated by removing the offending agent and providing supportive therapy.

Hepatobiliary Hepatitis

Hepatobiliary hepatitis is due to *cholestasis,* the interruption of the normal flow of bile. Cholestasis may result from obstruction of the hepatic duct with stones or inflammation secondary to cholelithiasis. Other agents, such as oral contraceptives and allopurinol (a drug used to lower uric acid levels), also can cause cholestasis. When bile flow is disrupted, inflammation of the liver parenchyma may result. Reestablishing bile flow by removing the stone or other causative agent is the treatment for hepatobiliary hepatitis.

Viral Hepatitis

Acute viral hepatitis has several etiologic agents, the most common of which are hepatitis A virus (HAV) and hepatitis B virus (HBV). Hepatitis A is transmitted by the fecal-oral route, paricularly in conditions of poor hygiene. Contaminated food, water, or shellfish and intimate contact with carriers of the virus are also sources of transmission. Hepatitis B is usually transmitted by parenteral innoculation with contaminated blood or blood products. Health care workers are at risk of acquiring the disease through handling contaminated materials; wearing gloves and following universal precautions can prevent this avenue of transmission. Intimate contact, such as through sexual intercourse or kissing, is another mode of transmission.

Other viral agents include hepatitis C (HCV; previously classified as non-A non-B), which most commonly occurs following transfusions; delta virus, also known as hepatitis D (HDV), which only occurs with HBV; and hepatitis E.

The major pathophysiologic event in viral hepatitis is destruction of hepatocytes with inflammation. The client may have a variety of manifestations stemming from the inflammatory process, edema, and altered blood flow; these include jaundice, right upper abdominal pain, elevated temperature, and malaise. The course of acute viral hepatitis is generally divided into three phases:

1. Preicteric or prodromal—the phase that occurs prior to the onset of jaundice

2. Icteric—the onset of jaundice

3. Posticteric or convalescent—the period following jaundice

The **preicteric phase** mimics influenza, eliciting manifestations of malaise and gastrointestinal complaints, including nausea, vomiting, diarrhea, and anorexia. The client may also complain of headache, fatigue, myalgia,

---

Clinical Manifestations of Acute Hepatitis

Preicteric Phase

- "Flulike" symptoms: malaise, fatigue
- Gastrointestinal: nausea, vomiting, diarrhea, anorexia
- Pain: headache, muscle aches, polyarthritis

Icteric Phase

- Jaundice
- Pruritus
- Lighter-colored stools
- Brown urine
- Decrease in preicteric phase symptoms (e.g., appetite improves; no fever)

Posticteric/Convalescent Phase

- Serum bilirubin and enzymes return to normal levels
- Energy level increases
- Pain subsides
- Gastrointestinal: minimal to absent

---

polyarthritis, and sore throat. Right upper abdominal pain may be elicited upon palpation (Porth, 1994).

The **icteric phase** is heralded by jaundice of the mucous membranes and skin. The jaundice occurs because inflammation of the liver and bile ducts prevents bilirubin from being excreted into the small intestine. As a result, the bilirubin pigment is elevated in the blood, causing yellowing of the skin and mucous membranes. Pruritus may be caused by the deposit of bile salts on the skin. The client frequently has light brown or clay-colored stools because the pigment is not excreted through the normal fecal pathway. Instead, the pigment is excreted by the kidneys, causing the urine to turn brown.

During the icteric phase, the initial prodromal manifestations usually diminish even though the serum bilirubin increases. The client's appetite increases, and the temperature returns to normal; for uncomplicated forms of hepatitis, spontaneous recovery usually begins within 2 weeks of the onset of jaundice (Price & Wilson, 1992).

The **posticteric phase,** or convalescent phase, lasts several weeks. During this time, manifestations gradually improve: Serum enzymes decrease, hepatic pain decreases, and gastrointestinal symptoms and weakness subside. The accompanying box summarizes the clinical manifestations of each phase of hepatitis.

Table 15–2   Comparison of Laboratory Tests for Viral Hepatitis

Hepatitis Type	Antigen	Antibody	Comments
A	Hepatitis A virus (HAV)	anti-HAV	Found in serum and stool early in hepatitis A; found in serum during convalescent phase
B	Hepatitis B surface antigens (HBsAg)	Hepatitis B surface antibody (anti-HB)	HBsAg found in serum, hepatocytes, and body fluids; anti-HBs present after infection as a protective antibody
	Core antigen (HBcAG)	Core antibody (anti-HBc)	Anti-HBc found in serum during and after acute infection
C	Not identified	Anti-HCV	Antibody appears after 1 to 3 months
D	HDAg	Anti-HD	Must have HBV present
E	HEAg	Anti-HEV	Virus detected in stool.

Fulminant Hepatitis

Fulminant hepatitis is a rare sequela of viral hepatitis. It is manifested by clinical signs of hepatic failure, including hepatic encephalopathy (degeneration of mental functions and progressive loss of consciousness). The underlying pathophysiology is widespread necrosis of the functional units of the liver, called the parenchyma; the liver actually shrinks (Dienstag, Wands, & Isselbacher, 1991).

Chronic Hepatitis

Chronic hepatitis can be classified as chronic persistent hepatitis or chronic active hepatitis. Generally, the persistent form is considered benign and results from either HBV or HCV hepatitis infections. The client has low serum transferase levels, but there is no progression of the disease. The client usually does not develop cirrhosis (Wands & Isselbacher, 1991). Manifestations may include malaise, mild fatigue, and hepatomegaly, but the client is otherwise healthy (Koff & Galambos, 1987). Diagnosis is made by liver biopsy, and clients are followed as needed every 6 to 12 months. There is no specific treatment.

The client with chronic active hepatitis frequently progresses to cirrhosis with liver failure; manifestations vary but fatigue is common. Cirrhosis is discussed in the next section. Some cases of chronic active hepatitis result from hepatotoxic drug administration (Price & Wilson, 1992), but most follow infection with the hepatitis B or hepatitis C virus. If chronic active hepatitis is suspected, a liver biopsy is performed in addition to the diagnostic and laboratory tests for acute hepatitis. It is the chronicity of symptoms and long-term abnormal hepatic function test results that distinguish the chronic form of hepatitis from the acute disease.

Collaborative Care

Management of the client with hepatitis focuses on determining the causative agent, providing appropriate treatment and supportive therapies, and teaching methods to prevent further liver damage. Effective management begins with thorough assessment of diagnostic and laboratory data.

Laboratory and Diagnostic Tests

Laboratory test results that are seen in the various types of viral hepatitis are shown in Table 15–2.

Several tests are available to test for hepatitis, including the following laboratory tests:

- *Anti-HAV* is the antibody to HAV and is found from the onset of symptoms and persists throughout the person's life.

- *IgM anti-HAV* is an antibody found in clients with recent infection for up to 6 months after the infection.

- *HBsAg* is the hepatitis B surface antigen; several subtypes have been discovered. Its presence indicates active disease or a carrier state.

- *HBeAg* is an antigen that correlates with HBV activity and replication in serum, as well as with the degree of infectiveness of the serum (Centers for Disease Control [CDC], 1990). The test is used in chronic carriers to assess infectiousness.

- *Anti-HBs,* the antibody to HbsAg, correlates with past infection with and/or immunity to HBV. This antibody may be checked to monitor immune response following HB vaccine.

- *Anti-HBe,* an antibody to HbeAg, is present in chronic carriers of HBV, but there is minimal or no viral replication activity.

- *Anti-HBc-IgM* is an antibody to the HB core antigen and, if present, indicates current infection.

- *HDAg* is the delta antigen and is detectable in early acute infection; its antibody—anti-HDV—is present with current or previous delta virus infection.

- *Anti-HCV* is the antibody to HCV (formerly non-A non-B) and seems to be most accurate in detecting chronic states of hepatitis C (Lee, 1990).

Enzymes reflecting liver function are also commonly measured. The serum levels frequently elevated with hepatitis include the following:

- *Alkaline phosphatase (ALP),* a nonspecific test of liver or bone dysfunction, is frequently elevated in obstructive jaundice or hepatitis.

- *Gamma-glutamyl transferase (GGT)* is a more specific test of liver function than the ALP, but alcohol or hepatotoxic drugs can also cause the GGT to be elevated.

- Two transaminases are elevated in hepatitis: *alanine aminotransferase (ALT),* formerly serum glutamic-pyruvic transaminase (SGPT), and *aspartate aminotransferase (AST),* formerly serum glutamic-oxaloacetic transaminase (SGOT). ALT may be as high as 1000 IU or more in acute hepatitis; the AST is frequently less than the ALT in acute hepatitis (Corbett, 1992). AST levels may increase prior to the onset of jaundice that accompanies acute viral hepatitis.

- *Isoenzymes 4 and 5 of lactic dehydrogenase (LDH)* are specific to liver organ damage.

- Both *conjugated and unconjugated bilirubin levels* may be elevated in viral hepatitis. The increase is due to the liver's inability to break down the pigment from normal red blood cell hemolysis and from obstruction of the hepatobiliary ducts due to inflammation and edema. The serum bilirubin level decreases as the inflammation and edema subside.

- *Prothrombin time* may be prolonged if the liver is not able to manufacture the protein needed for blood coagulation.

Diagnostic studies of liver function may also be conducted; however, serum studies are usually definitive. Occasionally the physician may perform a liver biopsy or liver scan to assist in diagnosis, especially if a mixed etiology is present. Both tests are more commonly done when carcinoma, hepatobiliary disease, or cirrhosis is suspected, and they are discussed in detail under those sections.

Pharmacology

In this section, both preexposure and postexposure pharmacology for the various types of acute hepatitis is discussed. Besides adhering to universal precautions, health care workers can decrease the risk of contracting hepatitis, particularly hepatitis B, through vaccination; nevertheless, only about 30% of health care workers are immunized (Grau, 1991). The CDC (1990) recommendations serve as a basis for this discussion.

Preexposure Prophylaxis

- Hepatitis A clinical illness can be avoided in up to 90% of cases when immune globulin (IG) is given either before exposure or during the early incubation period. People traveling to undeveloped countries, notably rural areas, need to receive IG. Those who remain for prolonged periods should receive IG every 5 months.

- Hepatitis B prophylaxis is recommended for people at risk of developing hepatitis B. Nurses and other health care workers at risk need to be vaccinated. It is recommended that infants receive immunization against hepatitis B to achieve lifelong prophylaxis. See the box on page 514 for a summary of who should receive hepatitis B vaccine.

Postexposure Prophylaxis

- Hepatitis A prophylaxis is obtained with a single dose of IG given as soon after exposure as possible. Indications for IG vary with the degree of probable contact with the hepatitis A virus. For example, IG is recommended for all persons with household or sexual contact with a person known to be infected with hepatitis A. IG is not recommended for hospital personnel who are not exposed to the feces of an infected client.

- Hepatitis B postexposure prophylaxis is indicated for persons exposed to the hepatitis B virus. The usual method of treatment is hepatitis B immune globulin (HBIG) for short-term immunity. HBV vaccine may be given concurrently for long-term immunity, depending on the situation. With perinatal exposure, infants are given both HBIG and the vaccine within 12 hours of birth; following sexual contact, adults are given HBIG and the vaccine within 14 days of sexual contact.

Although vitamin supplementation is usually not necessary during acute viral hepatitis, the client's condition may call for vitamin supplementation. Vitamin K, for example, is administered if the client's prothrombin time is prolonged.

Nursing Care

When implementing care for clients with hepatitis, the nurse is aware of the multiple functions of the liver and the myriad problems which the client may face. The nurse plans care for current problems and observes for potential complications. Clients with acute hepatitis, particularly those with hepatitis B and hepatitis C, are at risk for long-term complications. Client and family teaching about follow-up is important; this is discussed in the next section. Nursing diagnoses discussed in this section focus on risk for infection and on problems with inactivity, nutrition, and body image.

Risk for Infection (Transmission)

One of the most important goals when caring for clients with acute viral hepatitis is preventing the spread of infection.

CDC Recommendations for Preexposure: Hepatitis B Vaccination

■ ■ ■

- *High occupational risk.* Recommended for people exposed to blood and blood products or suspected contaminated body fluids; special note made for those in *training:* nurses, physicians, dentists, laboratory technicians.

- *Developmentally disabled.* Recommended for clients and staff at institutions for the developmentally disabled and for the staffs of nonresidential day care centers that are attended by a known HBV carrier.

- *Hemodialysis clients:* Clients should be vaccinated early in the course of the disease.

- *Homosexual men and sexually active heterosexual people.* Recommended for those who remain sexually active; those who have multiple partners face greater risk. Prostitutes are at high risk.

- *Users of illicit intravenous drugs.* Vaccinate as soon as possible.

- *Household and sexual contacts of HBV carriers.* Sexual contacts at greater risk, but vaccination is recommended for both.

- *Adoptees from high-risk countries.* HBV is endemic in some countries.

- *High-risk populations.* Alaskan Natives, Pacific Islanders, and refugees from endemic countries need vaccination during infancy.

- *Prison inmates.* Drug abuse and homosexual practices put prison inmates at high risk.

- *International travelers.* Recommended for those traveling to areas in which HBV is endemic and who anticipate close contact with the local population or exposure to blood products.

Note. Centers for Disease Control. (1990) Protection against viral hepatitis: Recommendations of the Immunization Practices Advisory Committee (ACIP). *MMWR, 39* (No. RR-2), 1-26.

Nursing interventions with rationales follow:

- Use universal precautions and meticulous hand washing. *Proper aseptic technique can stem transmission of the viruses that cause hepatitis.*

- For clients with either hepatitis A or hepatitis E, use strict isolation, and place the client in a private room if fecal incontinence is present. Clients with hepatitis B

who are bleeding profusely may also require isolation (Dienstag et al., 1991). *The fecal and oral routes are the primary modes of transmission of these two viruses. Hepatitis B is transmitted through blood and other body secretions.*

Activity Intolerance

Fatigue, sometimes accompanied by weakness, is common in clients with hepatitis. Although strict bed rest is rarely indicated, adequate periods of rest and limitation of activities may be necessary.

Nursing interventions with rationales follow:

- Facilitate the client's self-direction of activities as determined by the client's feeling of fatigue. Encourage the client to resume activities gradually. *Participating in and maintaining a specific level of activity depend on the client's motivation, strength, endurance, and level of consciousness.*

- Provide progressive ambulation and simple exercises as part of nursing care. Consult a physical or occupational therapist for specific exercises to build muscle strength. *Complications from immobility can be decreased through preventive interventions; the capacity for activity in the supine position is diminished following periods of bed rest (Carpenito, 1992).*

- Plan nursing care activities that promote rest as well as incorporate safety and fall-prevention techniques. *Rest helps relieve the symptoms of activity intolerance (Carpenito, 1992).*

Altered Nutrition: Less Than Body Requirements

Nutrition is an important aspect of care for clients with acute hepatitis.

Nursing interventions with rationales follow:

- Help clients with acute viral hepatitis select a diet that provides a high kcaloric intake of approximately 16 carbohydrate kcalories per kilogram of ideal body weight (Koff & Galambos, 1987). *Sufficient energy is required for healing; adequate carbohydrate intake can spare protein.*

- Explain that the majority of kcalories need to be consumed in the morning hours. Low-fat diets are sometimes better tolerated. *Many clients with acute hepatitis are nauseated in the afternoon and evening hours (Dienstag et al., 1991). Changes in bilirubin interfere with fat metabolism.*

- If nausea and vomiting persist, intravenous fluid supplementation is ordered. Monitor fluid and electrolytes, and assess for signs of dehydration. Clients may prefer smaller, more frequent meals. *Smaller meals are frequently better tolerated. Prompt assessment of fluid and electrolyte imbalance leads to early treatment and return to homeostasis.*

Body Image Disturbance

Clients who experience jaundice may have an altered body image. Jaundice, combined with rashes and pruritus, may cause the client embarrassment. Nursing measures focus on preventing skin breakdown and improving the client's self-image. These interventions are fully discussed under the section on cirrhosis, page 516.

Other Nursing Diagnoses

Other nursing diagnoses that may apply to clients with acute viral hepatitis include the following:

- *Impaired Physical Mobility* related to muscle weakness and bed rest
- *Knowledge Deficit* related to lack of information about viral hepatitis
- *Pain* related to the effects of arthritis, myalgia, and pruritus
- *Risk for Fluid Volume Deficit* related to anorexia and nausea

Client and Family Teaching

Many clients with acute viral hepatitis are cared for at home. Teaching about the disease and methods to prevent its transmission is therefore imperative. Instruct the client and family in prevention measures, such as not sharing eating utensils or bath towels. If the client requires hospitalization, discuss as part of discharge planning the need to undergo follow-up evaluation and to avoid hepatotoxic substances, such as alcohol and acetaminophen. Explain that until the client's serologic indicators return to normal, sexual and close personal contact with others should be avoided.

Applying the Nursing Process

Case Study of a Client with Hepatitis A: Nathan Johns

Nathan Johns is a developmentally disabled 24-year-old who resides at a group home. He works 20 hours per week at a local restaurant as a janitor. About 4 weeks ago he ate contaminated shellfish. He complained of suddenly getting "the flu" along with abdominal discomfort, which lasted about 10 days. Recently his "skin turned yellow." He visited the clinic, where laboratory tests were performed, revealing elevated liver enzymes and HAV and IgM antibodies. He was diagnosed with hepatitis A.

Assessment

Mr. Johns's history of eating shellfish may be the source of the virus, but transmission from another resident at the group home also needs to be ruled out. When questioned, Mr. Johns indicates that he is not hungry, he is nauseated, weak, and that he has had diarrhea and cannot eat the "fried foods" he likes. He has lost about 12 lb (5.4 kg) in 3 weeks. Abdominal assessment reveals that Mr. Johns has hepatic pain, especially with jarring movement. Mild scleral jaundice is present; there are no skin rashes, and he denies pruritus. Diagnostic tests reveal the following abnormal values: ALT, 1200 U/L; AST, 800 U/L; total serum bilirubin, 3.2 mg/dL; and the presence of antibodies as noted above. Because of his weight loss and potential for dehydration, Mr. Johns is admitted to the hospital.

Diagnosis

Mr. Johns's nurse, Lori Holland, makes the following nursing diagnoses:

- *Activity Intolerance* related to weakness and pain, as manifested by inability to work
- *Diarrhea* related to increased peristalsis, as manifested by frequent stools, up to eight daily
- *Risk for Infection* related to poor hygiene practices
- *Altered Nutrition: Less Than Body Requirements* related to anorexia and nausea

Expected Outcomes

The expected outcomes established in the plan of care specify that Mr. Johns will

- Progressively increase activity with planned rest periods until he reaches preillness activity level.
- Resume normal bowel elimination pattern.
- Avoid transmitting the virus to others in the group home or the restaurant.
- Gain at least $\frac{1}{2}$ to 1 lb per week until he reaches his ideal weight.

Planning and Implementation

Ms. Holland plans the following nursing interventions for Mr. Johns:

- Gradually increase Mr. Johns's participation in activities, especially walking. Walk at least three times a day for 10 minutes, increasing the distance and time as tolerated.
- Resume diet as tolerated—including foods that are high in kcalories, moderate in protein, and low in fat—and adjust as necessary if client experiences nausea. Monitor intake and output and electrolytes if nausea persists.
- Incorporate correct hygiene in care; teach necessary aseptic measures to Mr. Johns and the director of the group home. Teach Mr. Johns and the family about hepatitis A and how it is transmitted; keep information at

his level of comprehension. Consult a community health nurse; testing the other group home residents for hepatitis A may be indicated.

- Monitor and record weight every day; use consistent routine for weighing. Encourage Mr. Johns to eat the majority of kcalories in the morning hours; consult a dietitian to individualize meal plan.

Evaluation

Mr. Johns's symptoms and serum aminotransferase and bilirubin levels decrease significantly. On discharge to the group home, Mr. Johns has gained 5 lb (2.3 kg) and is eating a high-kcalorie, moderate-protein, low-fat diet. Fats may be added as Mr. Johns tolerates them. Both he and the group home director verbalize an understanding of the need for exercise, including a plan to incorporate exercises that rebuild strength and endurance. Specific hygiene measures, especially hand washing, have been discussed and will be reviewed at the group home. A community health nurse is scheduled to assess the group home's environment.

Critical Thinking in the Nursing Process

1. Explain the rationale for the interventions regarding Mr. Johns's diet and activity.

2. Outline the teaching plan to explain hepatitis A to the group director; how would you adapt this to meet Mr. Johns's needs? He functions at the fourth grade level.

3. How does hepatitis A differ from hepatitis B in terms of mode of transmission, treatment, and long-term considerations?

4. List several methods by which nurses can protect themselves from contracting hepatitis B and hepatitis C.

5. Design a nursing care plan for Mr. Johns for the diagnosis: *Risk for Altered Nutrition: Less Than body requirements.*

The Client with Cirrhosis

■ ■ ■

Cirrhosis is a type of chronic liver disease that results in extensive hepatocellular damage; the liver parenchyma is destroyed, regenerates, and eventually becomes scarred and fibrotic until it is no longer able to function (Conn & Atterbury, 1987). Because the liver performs so many functions, cirrhosis and ultimate hepatic failure are systemically devastating and often lead to death.

Pathophysiology

There are several causes of cirrhosis, but the clinical manifestations are usually similar regardless of cause. The manifestations of cirrhosis are the direct result of the liver's inability to detoxify substances, such as medications, alcohol, and hormones; to produce essential proteins, such as clotting factors and albumin; to regulate glucose and bilirubin metabolism; and to serve as a blood volume regulator. Problems that result from faulty liver metabolism and altered blood flow include ascites, esophageal varices, hepatic encephalopathy, splenomegaly, and bacterial peritonitis. Figure 15–3 illustrates the systemwide effects of cirrhosis on the body. Table 15–3 provides specific manifestations and their underlying pathophysiology.

Portal hypertension is abnormally elevated blood pressure within the portal vein. The increased circulatory resistance in the portal vein causes blood to be rerouted to adjoining vessels that normally have a lower blood pressure than the portal vein (McCance & Huether, 1994). This is called *collateral circulation* or *shunting* of blood to collateral vessels. Affected vessels, which are engorged and congested, are located in the esophagus, rectum, and abdomen.

Portal hypertension also contributes to an increased hydrostatic pressure within the vessel lumen. As the pressure within the vessel increases, fluid is forced out of the vessel. This fluid shift contributes to the formation of ascites and esophageal varices (McCance & Huether, 1994).

Splenomegly (enlargement of the spleen) occurs in the client with portal hypertension as a result of the shunting of blood into the splenic vein. Splenomegly can result in hematologic disorders such as anemia, thrombocytopenia, and leukopenia (Porth, 1994).

Ascites is the accumulation of plasma-rich fluid in the abdominal cavity. Although portal hypertension is the primary cause of ascites formation, decreased serum proteins and increased aldosterone also contribute to the fluid accumulation. *Hypoalbuminemia,* low albumin in the blood, causes a decrease in plasma colloidal osmotic pressure. This pressure normally holds fluid in the intravascular compartment; when plasma colloidal osmotic pressure decreases, fluid escapes into extravascular compartments. *Hyperaldosteronism,* an increase in aldosterone, causes sodium and water to be retained, thus contributing to ascites formation and generalized edema, called **anasarca.**

Esophageal varices are enlarged overdistended veins formed within the esophagus when the portal venous system is congested and collateral channels become engorged with venous blood. Clients with esophageal varices are at high risk for bleeding; even high-roughage foods can precipitate hemorrhage. *Thrombocytopenia,* a deficiency in platelets, contributes to the client's high risk for bleeding.

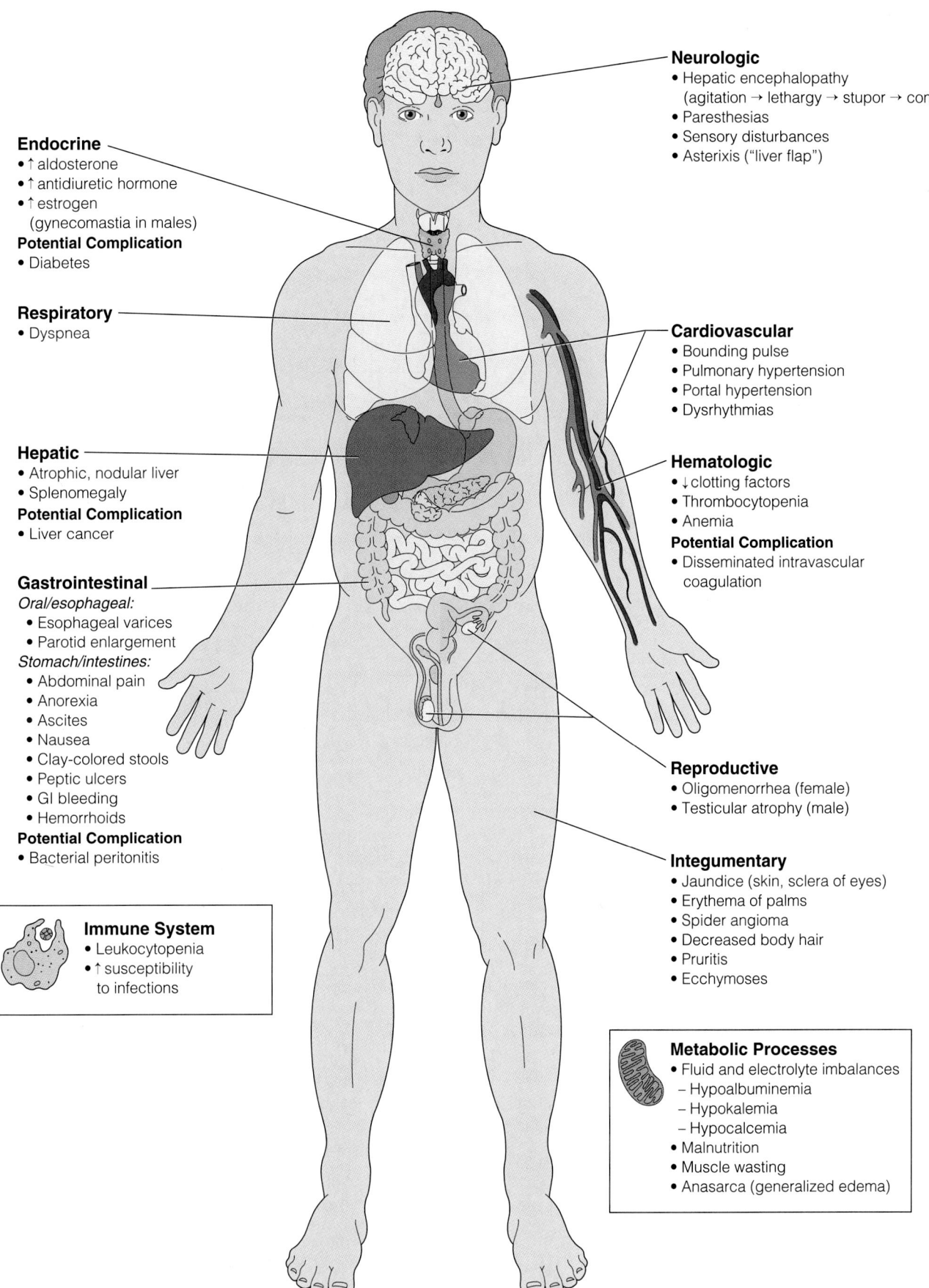

Neurologic
- Hepatic encephalopathy
  (agitation → lethargy → stupor → coma)
- Paresthesias
- Sensory disturbances
- Asterixis ("liver flap")

Endocrine
- ↑ aldosterone
- ↑ antidiuretic hormone
- ↑ estrogen
  (gynecomastia in males)
Potential Complication
- Diabetes

Respiratory
- Dyspnea

Cardiovascular
- Bounding pulse
- Pulmonary hypertension
- Portal hypertension
- Dysrhythmias

Hepatic
- Atrophic, nodular liver
- Splenomegaly
Potential Complication
- Liver cancer

Hematologic
- ↓ clotting factors
- Thrombocytopenia
- Anemia
Potential Complication
- Disseminated intravascular
  coagulation

Gastrointestinal
Oral/esophageal:
- Esophageal varices
- Parotid enlargement
Stomach/intestines:
- Abdominal pain
- Anorexia
- Ascites
- Nausea
- Clay-colored stools
- Peptic ulcers
- GI bleeding
- Hemorrhoids
Potential Complication
- Bacterial peritonitis

Reproductive
- Oligomenorrhea (female)
- Testicular atrophy (male)

Integumentary
- Jaundice (skin, sclera of eyes)
- Erythema of palms
- Spider angioma
- Decreased body hair
- Pruritis
- Ecchymoses

Immune System
- Leukocytopenia
- ↑ susceptibility
  to infections

Metabolic Processes
- Fluid and electrolyte imbalances
  - Hypoalbuminemia
  - Hypokalemia
  - Hypocalcemia
- Malnutrition
- Muscle wasting
- Anasarca (generalized edema)

Figure 15–3 Multisystem effects of cirrhosis.

Table 15–3   Physiologic Responses to Cirrhosis

	Manifestation	**Pathologic Basis**
Gastrointestinal	Parotid enlargement	Unknown; may be linked to poor nutrition
	Esophageal or rectal varices	Portal hypertension; collateral venous circulation develops
	Peptic ulcers	Probably due to shunting of blood into portal system
	Gastritis	Related to alcohol ingestion and portal hypertension, causing venous dilation
Hematologic	Altered coagulation	Decreased production of clotting factors, lack of platelets, increased fibrinolysis
	Anemia	Blood loss, folic acid deficiency, splenic hemolysis secondary to splenomegaly
	Leukopenia	Splenomegaly
Neurologic	Asterixis	Result of metabolic abnormalities; related to high ammonia levels
	Encephalopathy	Toxic levels of metabolites, ammonia
Cardiovascular	Dilation of abdominal wall veins (caput medusae)	Portal hypertension, causing engorgement and dilation
	Peripheral edema	Obstruction of venous flow from lower extremities; hypoproteinemia; hyperaldosteronism
	Bounding pulse	Hyperkinetic circulatory state
	Ascites	Portal hypertension, low albumin levels, low aldosterone levels
Pulmonary	Dyspnea, cyanosis	Ascites prevents expansion of lungs and capillary arteriovenous shunting within the lungs
	Pulmonary hypertension	Portal hypertension
Dermatologic	Spider angiomata and palmar erythema	Hormone imbalance; more commonly occur with alcohol-related cirrhosis
	Jaundice	Hyperbilirubinemia
	Decreased body hair	Hormone imbalance
Endocrine	Gynecomastia	Altered estrogen metabolism
	Oligomenorrhea, infertility	Decreased levels of estradiol and progesterone
	Diabetes mellitus	Unknown; possibly due to decreased hepatic parenchymal function
Nutritional/ Metabolic	Potassium deficiency	Vomiting, diarrhea, hyperaldosteronism, iatrogenic through use of diuretics
	Hyponatremia	Secondary to fluid volume overload
	Hypoalbuminemia	Lack of hepatocellular production of proteins
	Increased risk of liver cancer	Excess regenerative activity
	Malnutrition, muscle wasting	Dietary deficiencies, lack of protein production

Another underlying pathophysiologic process that affects cirrhotic clients is **hepatic encephalopathy,** which is manifested by altered consciousness, mentation, and motor function. The accumulation of toxic substances in the circulation causes the cognitive and motor changes that are characteristic of hepatic encephalopathy. Because of destruction of hepatic parenchyma, proteins cannot be metabolized to urea. Ammonia and other unidentified substances cause the manifestations. *Asterixis,* or liver flap, the flapping tremor of the hands when the arms are extended, is another sign of hepatic encephalopathy. Hepatic encephalopathy has four stages, ranging from the prodromal stage to complete coma; see Table 15–4 for a description of the stages. This process can be reversed, or at least improved, by decreasing the body's nitrogenous waste load. Bleeding in the gastrointestinal tract is a common source of protein and thus, nitrogen, in clients who have portal hypertension.

Laënnec's Cirrhosis

Laënnec's cirrhosis is associated with chronic alcohol abuse. At least 50% of clients with cirrhosis have Laënnec's cirrhosis, also called *portal, alcoholic,* or *nutritional cirrhosis* (Price & Wilson, 1992). Liver destruction and dysfunction follow the stages outlined below, beginning with fatty liver and progressing to full-blown cirrhosis. The process of hepatocyte destruction can be halted and, in some cases, reversed if the client can avoid the offending agent.

Table 15–4   Stages of Hepatic Encephalopathy

Stage	Description	Clinical Manifestations
1: Prodromal	Changes may be subtle in this stage; be aware of and report even seemingly minor changes in personality or mentation.	Agitation Restlessness Inability to concentrate Altered sleep habits Impaired judgment Slurred speech Forgetfulness
2: Impending	Increasingly obvious impairments are present. The client has periods of confusion alternating with alertness.	Lethargy Confusion Disorientation to time Asterixis
3: Stuporous	Severe mental deficits are evident. The client is difficult to rouse.	Incoherence Hyperreflexia Asterixis Muscle twitching
4: Coma	Final stage is deep coma.	Comatose Fetor hepaticus (offensive breath typical of advanced hepatic disease) Positive Babinski's reflex

In early Laënnec's cirrhosis, fatty liver develops in response to repeated liver injury. This initial change in hepatocytes is characterized by the accumulation of fat (Lieber & Guadagnini, 1990). Generally the client has few symptoms, but the liver may be enlarged and tender. If the client abstains from alcohol, the prognosis for hepatic recovery at this stage is good (Podolsky & Isselbacher, 1991).

Continued alcohol abuse leads to alcoholic hepatitis, the next stage of Laënnec's cirrhosis. This stage of cirrhosis is characterized by infiltration of lymphocytes and polymorphonuclear leukocytes into the liver, which produces necrosis, fibrosis, and cholestasis (Lieber & Guadagnini, 1990). Clinical symptoms of hepatic injury are evident but variable and range from anorexia, malaise, weight loss, low-grade fever, and jaundice to more complex manifestations, such as ascites, hemorrhage, and encephalopathy. Malnutrition is a frequent concurrent problem (Podolsky & Isselbacher, 1991). Supportive care and abstinence from alcohol are indicated.

Cardiac Cirrhosis

Cardiac cirrhosis is seen in clients who have chronic right-sided congestive heart failure. This condition results from prolonged elevation of venous pressure and consequent liver congestion and damage. The symptoms reflect the course of right-sided failure and may include ascites formation and dependent peripheral edema. If the right-sided cardiac failure improves, the cirrhosis usually reverses.

Postnecrotic Cirrhosis

Cirrhosis following hepatitis B or C accounts for about 25% of postnecrotic cirrhosis incidence. Many other etiologic agents have been identified, among them infections, as exemplified by toxoplasmosis; metabolic dysfunctions, such as Wilson's disease, a disorder of copper metabolism; and medications, particularly methyldopa, methotrexate, and isoniazid. Other possible causes include cystic fibrosis, diabetes mellitus, and sarcoidosis (Podolsky & Isselbacher, 1991). Postnecrotic cirrhosis related to viral hepatitis B has been identified as a precursor to hepatic carcinoma (Porth, 1994).

Biliary Cirrhosis

Obstruction of the biliary duct system from stones or tumors can result in biliary cirrhosis. Obstructive jaundice usually develops, along with the typical pattern of necrosis with regeneration and hepatic scarring (Conn & Atterbury, 1987).

Collaborative Care

Manifestations in and therapeutic interventions for clients with cirrhosis are similar regardless of the pathophysiologic etiology. Treatment of the client with cirrhosis has a holistic focus, addressing not only the client's biophysical needs but also the psychosocial needs. The importance of including the family in the plan of care cannot be overemphasized, particularly if alcohol abuse is identified as the etiologic agent. The major emphases of treatment include pharmacologic agents to assist in regulating protein metabolism and maintaining fluid and electrolyte balance, and supportive therapies, including treatment of underlying problems, such as malnutrition, anemia, bleeding, encephalopathy, renal failure, and infections.

Laboratory and Diagnostic Tests

A thorough workup is indicated when a client is admitted with symptoms of cirrhosis; the results of the laboratory and diagnostic tests are the basis for treatment and nursing care. Test results reflect the liver's inability to function. The following laboratory tests may be ordered:

- *Serum electrolytes* are measured. Sodium is usually decreased, a reflection of the overload of body water and hemodilution. Sodium below 125 mEq/L is an ominous sign (Adinaro, 1987). Potassium levels may be decreased secondary to diuretic therapy or poor intake associated with malnutrition, or they may be related to

Nursing Implications for Diagnostic Tests: Liver Biopsy

■ ■ ■

Preparation of Client

- Review chart for signed consent form.

- Maintain NPO status as policy directs, usually 4 to 6 hours preprocedure.

- Assess and record prebiopsy baseline vital signs.

- Review prothrombin time (PT) and platelet count; administer vitamin K as prescribed.

- Have the client empty bladder immediately before the test.

- Position the client in the supine position on far right side of bed; turn head to left and extend right arm above head to enhance visualization of the biopsy site.

Client and Family Teaching

- Describe preprodecure events: NPO status, positioning, bladder emptying, local anesthetic used.

- Practice the following breathing pattern during biopsy: Hold breath following expiration to keep diaphragm and liver high and stabilized in the abdominal cavity.

- Actual needle insertion and biopsy time is short, usually only 10 to 15 seconds; needle manipulation may cause some pain or discomfort.

- Direct pressure will be applied immediately after the needle is removed; client is positioned to right side with side rails up.

- Client may feel pain in the right shoulder as the anesthetic loses effect.

- Vital signs are assessed after a surgical procedure to monitor for bleeding.

- Client usually remains NPO for 2 hours and then resumes preprocedure diet.

- Avoid coughing, lifting, or straining for 1 to 2 weeks.

metabolic alkalosis. Low levels of phosphorus and magnesium are not uncommon and are related not only to malnutrition but also to renal excretion of these electrolytes. Respiratory alkalosis from severe ascitic hyperventilation contributes to the hypophosphatemia (Adinaro, 1987).

- *CBC with platelets* is performed. Frequently the results of a low red blood cell count, hemoglobin and hematocrit levels are consistent with anemia. The anemia may be due to active bleeding or malnutrition. Platelets are low from the lack of production; splenomegaly can cause thrombocytopenia (Corbett, 1992). It is not uncommon for a client with cirrhosis to have leukopenia (low total white blood cell count) secondary to splenomegaly.

- *Bilirubin measurements* are collected. In severe cirrhosis with jaundice, both the direct (conjugated) and indirect (unconjugated) bilirubin are elevated. With severe hepatic involvement, unconjugated bilirubin levels over 20 mg have been reported.

- *Total protein, serum albumin, and ammonia levels* are measured to assess protein metabolism. Levels of each protein are low in cirrhosis; low protein levels contribute to the edema. Another serum value that reflects problems with protein metabolism is the serum ammonia level; its elevation signifies that the liver cannot effectively metabolize ammonia to urea for renal excretion.

- *Coagulation studies* are performed and show prolonged bleeding time due to decreased coagulation protein production, fewer platelets, and lack of vitamin K.

- *Serum glucose values* are abnormal because the liver is not able to carry out glucogenesis. A greater incidence of diabetes mellitus has been reported in clients with Laënnec's cirrhosis (Lieber & Guadagnini, 1990). Fat metabolism is also impaired as evidenced by a decreased cholesterol level.

- *Enzyme studies* that measure hepatic function are performed and include ALT, AST, alkaline phosphatase, and gamma-glutamyl transferase (GGT). All may be elevated in cirrhosis, but usually not as severely as in acute hepatitis. The degree of liver damage is not consistently reflected in the abnormal laboratory values. In alcoholic hepatitis, the AST to ALT ratio is usually more than 2:1 (Kools & Bloomer, 1987). GGT has been found helpful in assessing alcohol abuse (Corbett, 1992).

Diagnostic tests may include an ultrasonogram of the liver, a liver biopsy, and, if indicated, esophagoscopy or upper gastrointestinal series to assess for esophageal varices. Results demonstrate the severity of liver damage. Nursing implications for liver biopsy are found in the accompanying box. Figure 15–4 shows the site and position for liver biopsy. If coagulation studies indicate a high degree of risk, the invasive studies are deferred until the values return to a minimum level. For example, if the prothrombin time (PT) is more than 3 seconds over the control, the biopsy is delayed and vitamin K administered to improve the PT.

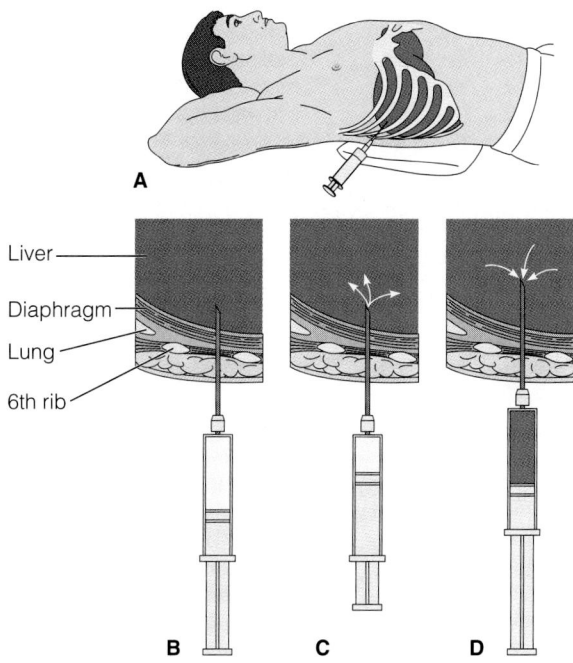

Figure 15–4   Liver biopsy procedure. *A,* Ask the client to exhale completely and then to hold his or her breath. This brings the liver and diaphragm to their highest position. *B,* The physician now inserts the biopsy needle into the liver. *C,* The physician injects approximately 1 mL of saline to clear the needle of blood and tissue. *D,* The physician guides the needle farther into the liver and aspirates a tissue sample. The needle is withdrawn, and pressure is applied to the site. The liver specimen is expelled into formalin to preserve it for laboratory analysis.

Pharmacology

Pharmacologic interventions for the client with cirrhosis depend on the degree of existing complications and the client's response to therapy. One major consideration in therapy for alcoholic cirrhosis is total abstinence from any type of alcohol product. Several groups of drugs are the mainstays of treatment. See the pharmacology box on page 522 for nursing responsibilities and client teaching for these drug categories.

- Diuretics are an important part of therapy, especially if the client has ascites. Mild diuresis helps prevent dehydration and fluid shifts. Spironolactone (Aldactone) is frequently the first drug of choice because it addresses one of the causes of ascites accumulation—the increase of aldosterone. If the client's serum potassium level remains within normal limits, another diuretic, such as furosemide (Lasix), may be added to the regimen (Conn & Atterbury, 1987).

- Medications to reduce the nitrogenous load are another cornerstone of therapy, particularly for clients with high blood ammonia levels. Two commonly administered medications are lactulose and neomycin.

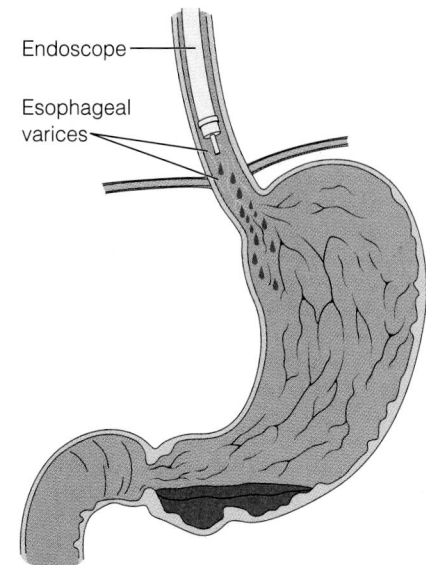

Figure 15–5   Sclerotherapy is one method of treating bleeding esophageal varices. An endoscope is inserted into the esophagus. A sclerosing agent is then injected onto the bleeding varices.

- Vitamin K and other therapies, such as administration of platelets, to promote clotting, may be required.

- Antacids are prescribed as indicated; gastritis is not uncommon. Magaldrate (Riopan) is a frequently prescribed low-sodium antacid.

- Medications that are metabolized by the liver are avoided. Examples include barbiturates, sedatives, hypnotics, and acetaminophen.

Surgical Procedures

The surgical procedures performed vary with the type of cirrhosis. For example, the client with biliary cirrhosis may undergo a surgical procedure that restores patency of the ducts and relieves the obstruction, whereas the client with esophageal varices may have sclerotherapy via an endoscopic procedure (Figure 15–5).

If the client with cirrhosis has severe ascites, paracentesis, which is the aspiration of ascitic fluid from the abdominoperitoneal cavity, may be performed. The goal of this procedure is to decrease the effort of breathing. Generally, paracentesis is reserved for severe ascites, because unless the underlying cause of the fluid formation is corrected, the fluid will reaccumulate. Because ascitic fluid is high in protein, valuable protein is lost from the vascular system into the abdominal cavity. Nursing implications for the client undergoing paracentesis are listed in the box on page 523. Figure 15–6 depicts paracentesis sites and how to position the client.

In addition to the therapeutic effects it offers, paracentesis may be a useful diagnostic tool. In particular, it may be indicated for the cirrhotic client who has a fever of unknown origin or other unexplained symptoms. For this

Nursing Implications for Pharmacology: The Client with Cirrhosis

DIURETICS

Spironolactone (Aldactone)   Furosemide (Lasix)

Spironolactone is a potassium-sparing diuretic that competes with aldosterone. The drug reduces ascites by increasing renal excretion of fluid and decreasing aldosterone levels. Furosemide is a loop diuretic that promotes the excretion of potassium. Drugs may be given in combination if serum potassium level permits.

Nursing Responsibilities

- Assess baseline ECG, serum potassium, BUN, creatinine levels, and hydration status.
- Weigh the client daily.
- Carefully monitor intake and output.
- Monitor for signs of hyperkalemia if the client is on spironolactone alone: bradycardia; widening QRS complex, spiking T waves, or ST segment depression on ECG; diarrhea; and muscle twitching.
- Assess for hyponatremia: thirst, confusion, lethargy, apprehension.

Client and Family Teaching

- Maintain diet, particularly potassium-containing foods, and fluid restrictions as prescribed.
- Report increases in weight or edema.
- Immediately report signs of hyponatremia, hyperkalemia, or hypokalemia (see Chapter 5).
- Expect increased urinary output; take medications in morning hours to avoid nocturia.

LAXATIVES

Lactulose (Cephulac, Chronulac)

Lactulose is a disaccharide laxative that is not absorbed by the gastrointestinal tract. The drug pulls water into the bowel lumen, causing accelerated passage of stool and decreased absorption of intestinal ammonia. Colonic pH decreases, promoting the conversion of ammonia to ammonium ion. The drug may be administered orally or rectally.

Nursing Responsibilities

- Assess bowel sounds and presence of abdominal distention.
- Maintain accurate stool chart.
- Adjust dose to achieve two to three soft stools per day.
- Monitor electrolytes and hydration status.

Client and Family Teaching

- Drink adequate fluids.
- Report diarrhea; if present, decrease dose.
- Some clients become nauseated; stress importance of continuing the medication, using preventive or palliative measures such as drinking effervescent soda or eating crackers with medication.

ANTI-INFECTIVE AGENTS

Neomycin sulfate (Neo Tabs)

Neomycin sulfate is a nonsystemic aminoglycoside that is used to destroy intestinal bacteria and thereby decrease protein in the bowel lumen. The drug may be administered as an oral or rectal preparation.

Nursing Responsibilities

- Prior to administration, assess hearing, renal, and neurologic functions. Drug is ototoxic, nephrotoxic, and neurotoxic.
- Prior to administration, check for previous hypersensitivity reaction.
- Monitor intake and output.
- Monitor BUN and creatinine levels.
- If the client is taking digitalis, monitor levels; oral neomycin interferes with its absorption.

Client and Family Teaching

- Report dizziness, tinnitus (ringing in ears), hearing loss, headaches, tremors, or visual alterations immediately.
- Keep follow-up appointments.
- Maintain fluids; avoid dehydration. (Teach signs of dehydration.)

procedure, the physician may determine that a *peritoneovenous shunt* is indicated. The device used for this procedure, a *LeVeen shunt,* routes fluids from the abdominal cavity to the superior vena cava. See Figure 15–7 for an illustration of a client with a LeVeen shunt.

When the client develops portal hypertension with bleeding varices, a surgical shunt may be indicated. The goal is to relieve pressure within the portal venous system. See Figure 15–8 on page 524 for examples. Surgical anatomical shunts are usually reserved for clients who

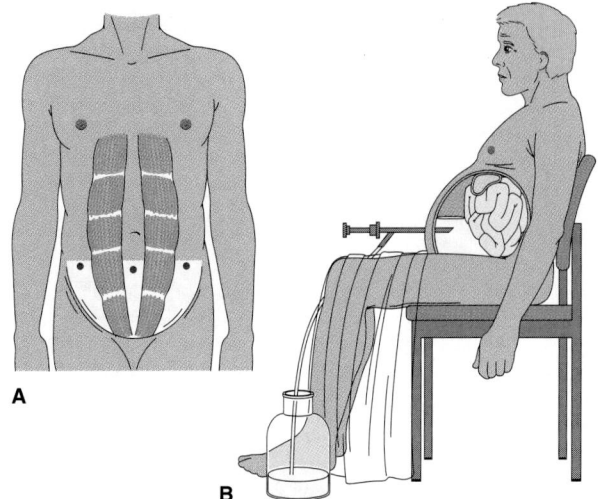

Nursing Implications for Diagnostic Tests: Abdominal Paracentesis

■ ■ ■

Preparation of Client

- Verify that the client has signed an informed consent form.

- Weigh the client prior to paracentesis to assess amount of fluid obtained.

- Assess vital signs for baseline.

- Have client void immediately prior to the test to avoid bladder puncture.

- Position client in a sitting position, either on the side of the bed or in a chair, and support feet.

Client and Family Teaching

- Describe what to expect during and following the paracentesis; blood pressure is monitored during the procedure.

- Following cleansing and local anesthesia, a small incision is made and a needle or trocar is inserted to withdraw fluid. The trocar is connected to tubing and a collection bottle; specimens may be sent to laboratory.

- A small dressing is placed over the puncture site after the needle is withdrawn. There may be some fluid leakage from the site.

- Client may receive salt-poor albumin after the procedure to replace lost protein.

Figure 15–6 Sites and position for paracentesis. *A,* The physician uses the sites indicated for trocar insertion to avoid internal injury. *B,* The client sits comfortably; notice that in this position, the intestines float back and away from the insertion site.

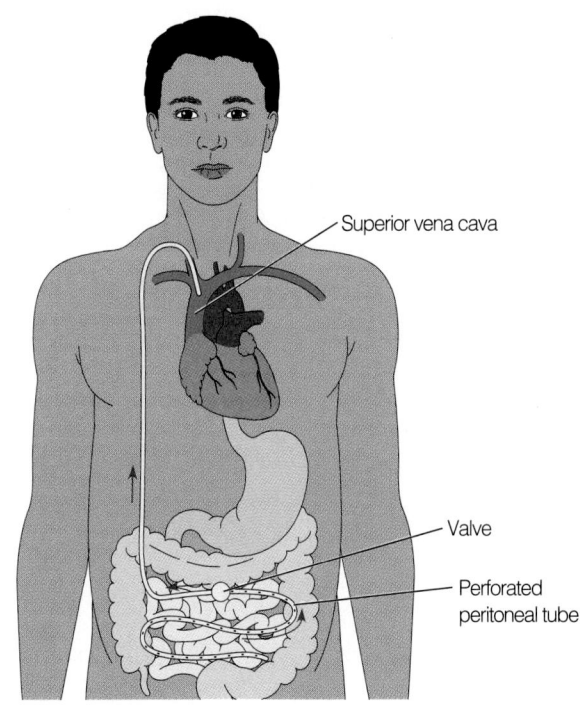

Figure 15–7 LeVeen shunt in position. Fluid is absorbed from the abdominal cavity into a perforated peritoneal tube. It is then recirculated into the general circulation via the superior vena cava.

have bleeding even after a series of endoscopic sclerotherapy injections (Podolsky & Isselbacher, 1991). Initially, an endoscopy is performed to determine the site of bleeding, because it is possible that the source of the bleeding is a gastric lesion rather than an esophageal site. *Transjugular intrahepatic portosystemic shunt (TIPS)* shunts blood from the portal vein to the hepatic vein; this angiographic-type procedure is experimental (Doherty & Carver, 1993).

Liver transplantation is another surgical option for selected clients with cirrhosis. Clients are evaluated for the type of cirrhosis and degree of complications from cirrhosis. The box on page 525 discusses nursing care of the client undergoing liver transplantation.

Nutritional Considerations

Dietary support is an essential part of care for the client with cirrhosis. Dietary needs change as hepatic function fluctuates.

- Sodium intake is restricted to under 2 g/day, and fluids are limited as needed to maintain balance of both fluids and electrolytes. Fluids are most restricted during periods of severe ascites and are often limited to 1500 mL/day. Fluid needs are calculated based on response to diuretic therapy, urinary output, and serum electrolyte values (Mahan & Arlin, 1992).

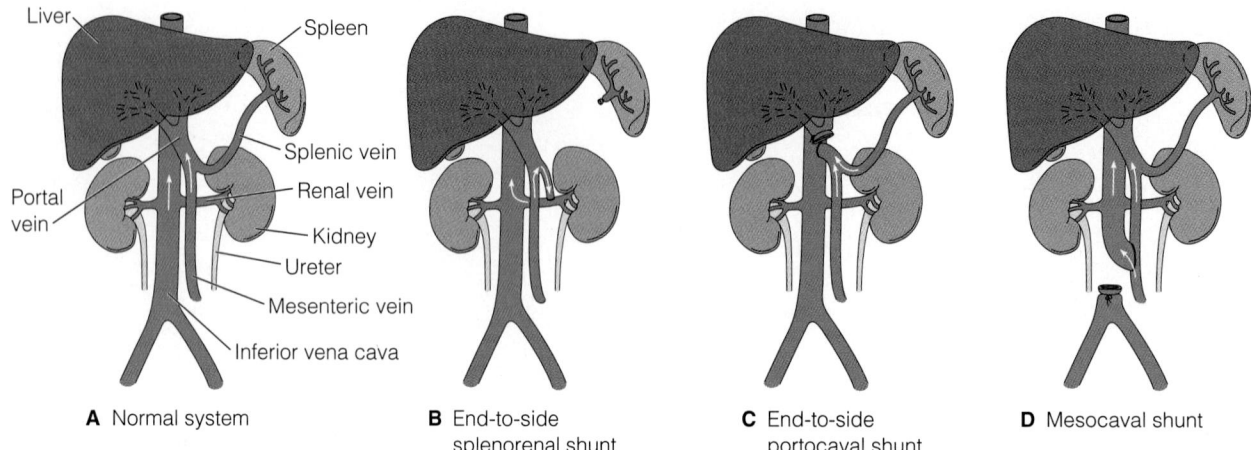

Figure 15–8   Common types of portacaval and portal-systemic shunts. *A,* Normal portal system. *B,* End-to-side splenorenal shunt, which involves removal of the spleen with anastamosis of splenic vein to left renal vein. *C,* End-to-side portacaval shunt, in which the portal vein is anastomosed to the inferior vena cava. *D,* Mesocaval shunt, in which the inferior vena cava is anastomosed to the superior mesenteric vein.

- Dietary protein is adjusted to the client's ability to handle the nitrogenous load. If hepatic encephalopathy is present, protein is restricted. When encephalopathy is absent and serum ammonia levels are stabilizing, protein is returned to the diet in amounts tolerated to avoid altered cognition. The client's needs for high kcalorie, moderate fat intake continue during the healing process. Clients who are NPO may be maintained on total parenteral nutrition.

- Vitamin and mineral supplements are ordered based on laboratory values. The client is often deficient in the B-complex vitamins, particularly thiamin, folate, and B₁₂, and the fat-soluble vitamins, A, D, and E, may need to be administered in a water-soluble form (Mahan & Arlin, 1992). Clients with alcohol-induced cirrhosis are at high risk for magnesium deficiency, which requires supplementation.

Nursing Care

Nursing care of the client with cirrhosis presents many challenges because the hepatic dysfunction affects a multitude of body systems. The nurse is responsible for both the biophysical and psychosocial coordination of the client's care, and many nursing diagnoses may apply. The diagnoses discussed in this section focus on problems with fluid and electrolyte balance, altered thought processes, risk for bleeding, poor oxygenation, and jaundice.

Fluid Volume Excess

Clients with cirrhosis have problems regulating water and salt for several reasons: portal hypertension, hypoalbu-

minemia, and hyperaldosteronism. Esophageal varices and splenomegaly are examples of volume problems (Price & Wilson, 1992). The client may exhibit many of the signs of fluid volume overload and portal hypertension: ascites, peripheral pitting edema, internal hemorrhoids, prominent abdominal wall veins (caput medusae), and splenomegaly, as illustrated in Figure 15–3. Careful monitoring is important because clients are in a tenuous position—the treatment for the ascites can cause further fluid shifts and electrolyte imbalances. Achieving balance is often difficult and challenging.

Nursing interventions with rationales follow:

- Monitor weight daily using a consistent technique. Monitor for fluid shifts: Check jugular vein distention, measure abdominal girth for ascites daily, and check for peripheral edema. Monitor intake and output strictly. *Fluid changes can be quickly ascertained through continued and careful monitoring.*

- Assess client's urine specific gravity. *Specific gravity measures hydration status; an elevation designates dehydration.*

- Provide a diet low in salt (500 to 2000 mg/day) and with restricted fluids. *Sodium causes water retention, which clients with cirrhosis need to avoid.*

- Inspect skin for injury at least every shift. *Edema makes the skin more friable and thus more susceptible to breakdown.*

Altered Thought Processes

Clients with cirrhosis experience altered thought processes, resulting primarily from the accumulation of nitrogenous products and other metabolites, including

Nursing Care of the Client Undergoing Liver Transplantation

PREOPERATIVE CARE

1. Evaluate physical and psychologic status. Physical workup includes history and physical examination, liver size and function assessment, match of donor and recipient ABO compatibility, and screening for HIV and hepatitis B.

2. Determine client's acuity along with need for transplant.

3. Provide in-depth teaching to prepare client and family for transplant.

4. Once a donor liver is located, check client for absence of infection; if no infection is present, client is started on antibiotics in preparation for transplant.

POSTOPERATIVE CARE

1. Client initially is cared for in intensive care unit; all systems monitored, especially neurologic signs of disorientation, which reflect poor hepatic function. Hypertension is treated with hydralazine (Apresoline).

2. Avoid pulmonary problems by implementing appropriate postoperative measures.

3. Monitor renal function carefully; cyclosporin A is nephrotoxic and administration of diuretics and dopamine may be necessary.

4. Administer drugs to prevent rejection, as ordered. These agents include cyclosporin A, corticosteroids, and azathioprine (Imuran). Monitor for infection. The drugs are taken for the client's entire life. Monitoring glucose is indicated with corticosteroid use.

5. Monitor for signs of rejection: increasing temperature (an early sign), discomfort over transplant site, anorexia, decreased bile drainage from Jackson-Pratt drain, arthralgia, abnormal liver function tests.

6. Provide discharge teaching:
   a. Instruct the client in ways to avoid infections, signs of infection, and the need to report all fevers.
   b. Teach client to recognize signs of rejection.
   c. Provide a rationale for medications and schedule. Explain precautions involved with long-term steroid use, such as follow-up with an ophthalmologist. (See Chapter 20 for steroid information.)
   d. Prepare the client for potential changes in body image associated with steroid use and for feelings associated with receiving a liver that has been transplanted from another person.
   e. *Stress the importance of follow-up with the primary caregiver.*

---

mercaptans and phenol (Podolsky & Isselbacher, 1991). Several factors have been identified as precipitators of hepatic encephalopathy (see the box on page 526). Hepatic encephalopathy has four stages ranging from mild confusion to coma, as outlined in Table 15–4.

Nursing interventions with rationales follow:

- Avoid factors that have been identified as precipitating hepatic encephalopathy. *Cautious and judicious use of medications and appropriate monitoring can eliminate iatrogenic causes.*

- Assess neurologic signs and signs of early encephalopathy: changes in handwriting, speech, and development of asterixis. Perform neurologic assessment, which includes assessing the client's level of consciousness. *Early assessment of problems allows for prompt intervention—subtle changes in neurologic functioning are important!*

- If possible, plan to have the same nurses care for client. *Consistent care may contribute to early assessment of neurologic changes and prompt treatment.*

- Provide a low-protein diet as prescribed; teach the family the importance of maintaining diet restrictions. *Nitrogenous by-products from dietary protein increase serum ammonia levels.*

- Administer medications or enemas as ordered to reduce nitrogenous products, especially blood, in the gastrointestinal tract; schedule a regular bowel routine to avoid constipation. Check coagulation studies prior to enema administration. *Reducing the intestinal protein level results in a lower serum ammonia level.*

- Orient the client as possible to surroundings, person, and place; provide simple explanations for nursing interventions. *Modify verbal interactions to client's level of understanding, based on neurologic condition; cognitive*

Factors that Precipitate Hepatic Encephalopathy

■ ■ ■

- High ammonia level
- Constipation
- High-protein diet
- Medications: sedatives, tranquilizers, narcotic analgesics, anesthetics
- Hypoxia
- Gastrointestinal bleeding
- Hypokalemia
- Blood transfusions
- Severe infection
- Hypovolemia
- Surgery

Bleeding Precautions

■ ■ ■

- Prevent constipation.
- Avoid rectal manipulation—no rectal temperatures or enemas.
- Avoid injections; if needed, use small-gauge needle and apply pressure.
- Monitor platelet count, PT, and PTT.
- Assess ecchymotic areas and areas of purpura.
- Apply pressure to areas that are bleeding. After venipuncture, apply direct pressure for at least 5 minutes.
- Use only a soft toothbrush.
- Avoid blowing nose.
- Assess oral cavity for bleeding gums.

abilities relate to the client's physiologic function (Carpenito, 1992).

Risk for Injury: Bleeding

Bleeding is a possible problem for the client with cirrhosis, not only because of the liver's inability to manufacture clotting factors but also because of the threat of hemorrhage from varices. If the liver's ability to produce bile has diminished to the extent that the body's absorption of fat-soluble vitamins is impaired, a deficiency of vitamin K may occur. The liver requires adequate amounts of vitamin K to manufacture coagulation factors II, VII, IX, and X. Splenomegaly contributes to a low platelet count. Nursing interventions are aimed at reducing the risk of injury associated with bleeding.

Interventions and their rationales follow:

- Monitor vital signs for early signs of bleeding. *Increased pulse and decreasing blood pressure may indicate hemorrhage.*

- Institute bleeding precautions. See the accompanying box for specific interventions. *Changes in hepatic function result in increased susceptibility to bleeding; preventive measures can decrease the incidence of active bleeding.*

- Monitor coagulation studies and platelet count. *The results of these studies determine the need to continue bleeding precautions and to administer vitamin K as ordered.*

Clients with bleeding esophageal varices may have specialized nasogastric tubes inserted to provide direct pressure on the varices. See Figure 15–9 for an illustration of one type of tube. Clients who have these tubes inserted are in intensive care units because careful monitoring is required. Nursing interventions for clients with either a Sengstaken-Blakemore or Minnesota nasogastric tube include suctioning to prevent aspiration, releasing balloon pressures as per protocol to avoid tissue damage and possible necrosis, and maintaining pressure at the ordered level to promote hemostasis. The client's nasal area is a pressure point that is checked frequently for signs of tissue damage; the nasal cuff, a small piece of foam material, remains in place to prevent injury. The client's head is elevated at 45 degrees to prevent aspiration of secretions and promote gas exchange.

Risk for Impaired Gas Exchange

Ascites and the client's weakened condition limit lung expansion and potentially impair gas exchange.

Nursing interventions with rationales follow:

- Position client in the high-Fowler's position with feet elevated; assist to chair as tolerated. Avoid supine position when possible. *The sitting position permits full expansion of the lungs and promotes the gravitational shift of fluid and abdominal organs away from the diaphragm.*

- Monitor respirations as needed; obtain oxygen saturation level, if indicated. Monitor arterial blood gases. *Respiratory assessments and arterial blood gas measurements indicate the degree of impaired oxygenation and the presence of respiratory alkalosis, which can occur with hyperventilation.*

- Administer oxygen as indicated and ordered. Oxygen is ordered continually or "as needed," based on the oxygen saturation results; the nurse must then assess when oxygen therapy is needed. *Hypoxia can result*

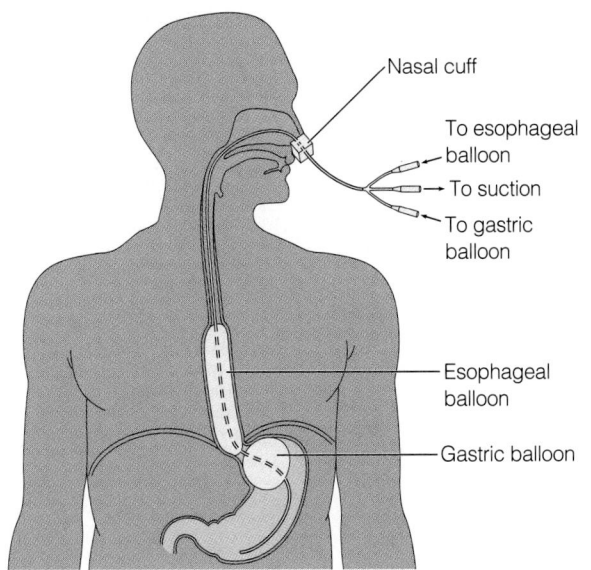

Figure 15–9 Triple-lumen esophageal-nasogastric tube (Seng-staken-Blakemore) tube used to control bleeding esophageal varices.

from inadequate respirations; oxygen administration is one method of enhancing oxygenation.

Impaired Skin Integrity

Severely jaundiced clients who have bile salt deposits on the skin may develop pruritus and resulting loss of skin integrity. Malnutrition, particularly protein deficiency, and edema also impair skin integrity. Nursing interventions focus on decreasing dry skin and pruritus.

Nursing interventions with rationales follow:

- Use warm water rather than hot water when bathing. *Water that is too hot stimulates pruritus (Carpenito, 1992).*

- Initiate measures to prevent dry skin: Apply an emollient or lubricant as needed to keep skin moist, avoid soap or preparations with alcohol, and do not rub the skin. *Dry skin contributes to pruritus.*

- If indicated, protect skin from injury by applying mittens to the client's hands. *Clients with encephalopathy may not understand the need to refrain from scratching.*

- Institute preventive measures: Turn the client at least every 2 hours, use an alternating pressure mattress, and assess skin for breakdown (Fredette, 1984). *Rotating positions relieves pressure and thereby promotes oxygenation of tissues.*

- Administer prescribed antihistamine cautiously. *Decreased hepatic function increases the client's risk for erratic drug reactions and improper drug metabolism.*

Other Nursing Diagnoses

The following nursing diagnoses may also be appropriate for the client with cirrhosis:

- *Activity Intolerance* related to ineffective gas exchange and fatigue

- *Altered Nutrition: Less Than Body Requirements* related to anorexia and to the liver's decreased ability to metabolize fats, protein, and carbohydrates

- *Pain* related to edema and bile salt deposits on skin

- *Ineffective Family Coping* or *Ineffective Individual Coping* related to inability to manage alcohol

- *Risk for Infection* related to altered immune response secondary to low leukocyte count and diminished phagocytosis (see Chapter 8 for nursing interventions pertinent to immunosuppressed clients)

- *Sexual Dysfunction* related to effects of hormone imbalance

- *Knowledge Deficit* about disease process, effects of alcohol (if the predisposing agent), and treatment measures

Client and Family Teaching

Including the family or significant other is a prime consideration when caring for the client with cirrhosis. This is most evident when the etiologic agent is alcohol abuse. Constant reinforcement of explanations for interventions is a necessary part of the teaching plan. Another important aspect of teaching is the team concept; nutritionist, physician, nurses, social worker, and psychologist collaborate with the client and family. Discharge planning is based on the individual needs of the client. For example, the client who has a LeVeen shunt requires information on what symptoms to report immediately to the primary caregiver, such as increasing abdominal girth and feeling of fullness. The nurse coordinates appropriate referrals for home care, including follow-up visits to the community health agencies and, if needed, Alcoholics Anonymous.

Applying the Nursing Process

Case Study of a Client with Laënnec's Cirrhosis: Richard Wright

Richard Wright is a 48-year-old divorced father of two teenagers. Mr. Wright has Laënnec's cirrhosis and is admitted to the community hospital with ascites and malnutrition. He has had three previous hospital stays for treatment of cirrhosis, the most recent stay being 6 months ago.

Assessment

Mr. Wright is lethargic but responds appropriately to verbal stimuli. He complains of "spitting up blood the past week or so" and says, "I just don't feel hungry." He has lost 20 lb (9 kg) since his previous admission. He is jaundiced and has petechiae and ecchymotic areas on his arms and legs. Liz Mowdi, Mr. Wright's nurse, notes 3+ pitting pretibial edema. Abdominal assessment reveals a fluid wave and tight, protuberant abdomen with caput medusae. The liver margin is palpable at 5 cm below the right costal margin; the spleen is enlarged. Assessment of vital signs reveals the following: T, 100 F (37.7 C); BP, 110/70; P, 110; R, 24.

Laboratory test results reveal the following:

WBC: 3700/mm^3 (normal range: 4300/mm^3 to 10,800/mm^3)

RBC: 4.0 million/mm^3 (normal range: 4.6 to 5.9 million/mm^3)

Platelets: 75,000/mm^3 (normal range: 150,000/mm^3 to 350,000/mm^3)

Serum ammonia level: 105 μm/dL (normal range: 35 to 65 μm/dL)

Total bilirubin: 4.9 μg/dL (normal range: 0.1 to 1.0 μg/dL)

Serum sodium: 150 mEq/L (normal range: 135 to 145 mEq/L)

Oxygen saturation per pulse oximeter (O$_2$ sat): 88% (normal range: 96% to 100%)

Potassium, hemoglobin, hematocrit, total protein, and albumin levels are markedly decreased. Enzymes are elevated: AST:ALT ratio is greater than 2:1. Blood urea nitrogen and creatinine levels are marginally elevated.

Evaluation shows bleeding from gastric ulcer, and a diagnosis of alcohol-induced cirrhosis with gastritis is made. Mr. Wright is started on Aldactone, 25 mg orally every 8 hours; Riopan, 30 mL 2 hours after meals and at bedtime; lactulose, 30 mL every hour until the onset of diarrhea, with the dose decreased thereafter to 15 mL three times daily; and a low-protein diet with sodium restricted to 800 mg/day and fluids restricted to 1500 mL/day.

Diagnosis

Ms. Mowdi makes the following nursing diagnoses:

- *Impaired Gas Exchange* related to pressure on the diaphragm and inadequate respiratory pattern as manifested by increased respirations and decreased oxygen saturation
- *Fluid Volume Excess* related to fluid shifts and hypernatremia as manifested by ascites and peripheral edema
- *Altered Nutrition: Less Than Body Requirements* related to anorexia and possible alcohol abuse manifested by weight loss and low serum protein levels

- *Altered Thought Processes* related to effects of altered protein metabolism as manifested by high ammonia levels and lethargy
- *Risk for Injury* (bleeding) related to impaired platelet formation and malnutrition

Expected Outcomes

The expected outcomes established in the plan of care specify that

- Respiration will decrease to 18 per minute; O$_2$ sat will be 95% or greater.
- Abdominal ascites will decrease by 1 to 2 cm per day; peripheral edema will decrease to no more than 1+.
- Mr. Wright will gain 1 lb (0.45 kg) per week; weight gain will not be due to fluid retention. Serum protein levels will return to normal range.
- Mr. Wright will demonstrate an alert level of consciousness, maintaining serum ammonia levels within normal range.
- Mr. Wright will experience no incidents of active bleeding.
- Mr. Wright will verbalize willingness to join a community support group.

Planning and Implementation

Ms. Mowdi plans the following nursing interventions for Mr. Wright:

- Monitor weight consistently each morning before breakfast.
- Prepare a diet high in kcal, low in salt, and low in protein.
- Maintain stool chart and decrease lactulose dose as appropriate.
- Plan consistent nursing care; evaluate for complications, such as increasing hepatic encephalopathy, bleeding, and decreasing renal function.
- Measure abdominal girth every shift at the initiation of diuretic therapy; use consistent measuring technique.
- Institute bleeding precautions.
- Keep head of bed elevated; assist Mr. Wright to chair with legs elevated three times daily as tolerated.
- Incorporate significant others in plan of care; provide a referral to community agencies for discharge follow-up.

Evaluation

After several weeks of supportive therapy, Mr. Wright's ascites resolves, and active gastrointestinal bleeding stops. His serum protein levels return to normal, as do his platelets and other blood values. He does not experience any ecchymosis during his hospitalization. After his edema resolves, he begins to gain weight on his high-kcalorie diet; protein is added as serum ammonia levels return to normal. On discharge, O$_2$ saturation is 96%; respirations are 18. Lactulose will be continued on discharge.

Ms. Mowdi provides both written and verbal information about the medication and the process of cirrhosis, including how to avoid its recurrence. Mr. Wright and his children express interest in Alcoholics Anonymous and Al Anon and are referred to those agencies. With Ms. Mowdi's help, the Wrights make follow-up appointments with a psychiatric social worker and primary caregiver.

Critical Thinking in the Nursing Process

1. Describe the relationships of the development of Mr. Wright's ascites and portal hypertension.

2. How can the nurse present the available community services to Mr. Wright and his family?

3. Outline a day's diet for Mr. Wright that is low in protein, high in kcal, and low in salt.

4. What is the pathophysiologic basis for Mr. Wright's encephalopathy? What are the nursing implications for Mr. Wright's use of lactulose and neomycin?

5. Design a nursing care plan for Mr. Wright for the diagnosis *Ineffective Individual Coping.*

The Client with Cancer of the Liver

■ ■ ■

Primary hepatic cancer is uncommon in the United States, but metastases to the liver from pulmonary, breast, and gastrointestinal cancers are relatively frequent. Primary hepatic cancer is more common in Asia and Africa, where the incidence is as high as 150 per 100,000. This higher incidence is linked to chronic hepatitis B infection (Isselbacher & Wands, 1991). The prognosis for primary hepatic carcinoma is poor; the 6-month survival rate for those unresponsive to therapy is lower than 20%, in part because the disease often is not diagnosed before it reaches an advanced stage. Metastases frequently present in the lungs (Oberfield, Steele, Gollan, & Sherman, 1989).

Pathophysiology

About 90% of primary hepatic cancers arise from the liver's parenchymal cells; the remaining 10% form in the bile duct. Regardless of the type of primary hepatic can-

---

Primary Hepatic Cancer: Etiologic Agents
■ ■ ■

- Chronic hepatitis B infection*
- Chronic cirrhosis, regardless of type
- Vinyl chloride (used in manufacturing plastics, tires)
- Inorganic arsenic
- Mycotoxin aflatoxin
- Nitrosamines
- Hepatocarcinogenic pesticides
- Prolonged androgen therapy
- Contraceptive steroids†

---

*Suspected as the primary carcinogen in up to 80% of the cases of liver cancer worldwide.
†Benign liver masses more commonly occur with the use of oral contraceptives.

---

cer, the progress of the disease is similar. Several etiologic factors have been identified and are listed in the box above. Most primary hepatic cancer in the United States results from alcohol-induced cirrhosis (Oberfield et al., 1989). Definitive diagnosis is made by biopsy. Imaging studies such as MRI, ultrasound, and CT scans can aid in diagnosis, as can tests for serum markers such as alpha-fetoprotein (AFP).

Manifestations of hepatic carcinoma include malaise, painful mass in the right upper quadrant, fullness in the epigastric region, weight loss, anorexia, and fever of unknown origin (see the box below) Clients with alcoholic cirrhosis who stop drinking and then present with ascites

---

Clinical Manifestations of Hepatic Cancer
■ ■ ■

- Malaise
- Anorexia
- Lethargy
- Weight loss
- Fever of unknown origin
- Feeling of fullness in the epigastric region
- Painful mass in the right upper quadrant
- With advanced disease, symptoms of liver failure: prolonged bleeding time, ascites

Applying Research to Nursing Practice
Managing Pain in Older Adults

■ ■ ■

To explore nurses' knowledge of, attitudes toward, and perceived barriers to medication management of cancer pain, researchers examined the responses of 128 oncology nurses and 72 long-term care facility (LTCF) nurses to an 82-item questionnaire (Ryan, Vortherms, & Ward, 1994). Although the oncology nurses demonstrated significantly more knowledge, both groups' attitudes about pain management were consistent, with one exception: LTCF nurses more frequently responded that patients overreport pain. Neither group demonstrated a thorough knowledge of specific opioid side effects, a fact that suggests the need for continued education in this area.

Implications for Nursing

Controlling cancer pain with medications is one of the most important nursing interventions. Because pain is a subjective experience, nurses must respond to client's reports of pain. Oral analgesics, given around-the-clock, are effective tools to manage cancer pain. If one type of oral analgesic is not successful in controlling pain, the nurse needs to consult the physician and obtain orders for another analgesic, using a ladder approach starting with acetaminophen and progressing to opioids. Nurses are in a unique position to advocate for better pain management.

Critical Thinking in Client Care

1. What barriers do you perceive in providing effective pain control?
2. How would you respond to the cancer patient's family member who says, "He doesn't need anymore of that medicine; he'll get hooked"?
3. Are there any normal age-related changes that affect the perception of pain?

or jaundice need to be evaluated for hepatic carcinoma (Edmundson & Craig, 1987). Not uncommonly, clients exhibit signs of hepatic failure, such as ascites, esophageal varices, and splenomegaly.

Collaborative Care

Partial hepatectomy is possible for clients who have single lesions without extrahepatic manifestations. These clients are usually followed with serial AFP tests to assess response to therapy (Isselbacher & Wands, 1991). Liver transplantation is another surgical option for clients who fit the criteria established by the liver transplant center.

Radiation therapy is used for palliative pain management, sometimes with adjunctive chemotherapy. The goal of this therapy is to shrink the size of the tumor, thus decreasing pressure on surrounding organs and reducing pain. Controlling pain is a priority (see the accompanying research box regarding pain management). As a primary therapy, chemotherapeutic agents have shown limited response ratios. Agents used include 5-fluorouracil, methotrexate, and doxorubicin. Direct continuous hepatic arterial infusion with an implanted pump is another method of chemotherapeutic drug delivery that has shown promise in prolonging survival rates (Oberfield et al., 1989).

Extensive nursing support is needed for both the client and the family. Preventive nursing care focused on teaching about etiologic agents is important. Altering alcohol consumption patterns may be an appropriate preventive measure (Foltz, 1988).

Nursing Care

Nursing diagnoses for the client with liver cancer are similar to those for the client with advanced cirrhosis:

- *Risk for Infection* related to altered immune response and malnutrition
- *Risk for Injury* (skin breakdown) related to impaired tissue oxygenation and malnutrition
- *Grieving* related to effects of multiple losses

The Client with Liver Trauma

■ ■ ■

Liver trauma can result from any injury to the abdomen and is frequently seen in combination with injuries to other abdominal organs. Automobile accidents, stab or gunshot wounds, and iatrogenic sources, such as liver biopsy, are among the sources of these injuries (DeBakey & Jordan, 1987).

Pathophysiology

Because the liver is a highly vascular organ, the major pathophysiologic event is hemorrhage. Bleeding can result from both the initial injury and the resulting dysfunction of the hepatic parenchyma, which are unable to produce sufficient amounts of clotting factors. If the ducts are injured, bile leakage may occur, causing peritonitis.

Collaborative Care

Care of the client with hepatic trauma is an emergency situation. Typically, the client enters the health care system via the emergency room, where the goal is treatment of hypovolemic shock. The client is typed and cross-matched for blood products, and intravenous fluids are instituted along with other supportive care.

Surgical intervention is usually indicated to locate the precise area of hemorrhage and to control it; thoracoabdominal or median sternotomy are frequent approaches (DeBakey & Jordan, 1987). Postoperative nursing care is aimed at preventing pulmonary complications, such as atelectasis, and monitoring for and promptly reporting signs of infections.

Nursing Care

Nursing care of the client with liver trauma focuses on fluid management and other supportive care related to shock. Keeping family members informed is an important aspect of care, especially during the period of client instability. Diagnoses include the following:

- *Fluid Volume Deficit* related to effects of severe hemorrhage
- *Risk for Infection* related to pain on respiration
- *Risk for Injury* (bleeding) related to dysfunction of coagulation.

The Client with Hepatic Abscess

■ ■ ■

Hepatic abscesses usually are pyogenic (bacterial) or amebic (protozoal) in origin. Pyogenic abscesses may follow trauma or surgical procedures, including biopsy. Multiple or single abscesses occur most commonly in the right lobe (DeCock & Reynolds, 1987). Amebic abscesses most frequently occur following infestation of the liver by *Entamoeba histolytica*. Amebic infestation is associated with poor hygiene, unsafe sexual practices, or travel in areas where drinking water is contaminated.

Pathophysiology

Following bacterial or amebic invasion of the liver, healthy tissue is destroyed, leaving an area of necrosis, inflammatory exudate, and blood. This damaged region become walled off from the healthy liver tissue. Pyogenic liver abscess may be caused by cholangitis, distant localized infections, or intra-abdominal infections, such as peritonitis or diverticulitis. *Escherichia coli* is the most frequently identified causative organism (DeCock & Reynolds, 1987). The onset of pyogenic abscess is usually sudden, causing the acute onset of such symptoms as fever, malaise, vomiting, hyperbilirubinemia, and pain in the right upper abdomen.

The infection pathway for amebic hepatic abscesses usually is the portal venous circulation from the right colon (Plorde, 1991). Generally, the onset of amebic abscess is insidious.

Collaborative Care

Hepatic abscess is diagnosed through biopsy, hepatic aspirate, serologic and fecal cultures, and CT scan and ultrasound studies. Therapy is based on identifying the causative organism through laboratory cultures.

Pyogenic abscesses are treated with antibiotics to which the causitive organism is sensitive. Pharmacologic agents used for amebic hepatic abscess are the same as those used for intestinal amebic infestation; however, combination therapy is commonly used. Two drugs commonly used in treating amebic liver abscesses are metronidazole (Flagyl) and iodoquinol (Diquinol). Both medications can cause gastrointestinal symptoms. With metronidazole, nurses need to watch for signs of bone marrow suppression.

If the abscess does not respond to combination antibiotic administration, it may be treated with percutaneous aspiration or surgical drainage. In these procedures, a *percutaneous closed-catheter drain* is placed during ultrasound or fluoroscopy.

Nursing Care

A major aspect of nursing care is prevention; teaching clients to avoid contaminated water and foods is especially important. Nursing interventions include teaching hikers to treat water and food handlers to wash hands thoroughly.

Clients who have a hepatic abscess require supportive care to prevent dehydration from the accompanying fever, nausea, vomiting, and anorexia. Careful monitoring of fluid and electrolyte status is indicated, as are comfort measures for abdominal pain. Possible nursing diagnoses include the following:

- *Risk for Fluid Volume Deficit* related to effects of prolonged fever and vomiting
- *Knowledge Deficit* about transmission of amebic abscess
- *Activity Intolerance* related to pain and weakness

◥ ◥ ◥   Exocrine Pancreas Disorders   ◥ ◥ ◥

The pancreas is both an exocrine and an endocrine gland. It is made up of two basic cell types, each having different functions. The exocrine cells produce enzymes that empty through ducts into the small intestine, whereas the endocrine cells produce hormones that enter the bloodstream directly. Disorders of the exocrine pancreas cause changes in the secretion and glandular control of digestive enzymes, whereas disorders of the endocrine pancreas cause changes in the production of hormones necessary for normal carbohydrate, protein, and fat metabolism. Disorders of the exocrine pancreas are discussed in this section of the chapter; diabetes mellitus, a disorder of the endocrine pancreas, is discussed in Chapter 21.

The Client with Pancreatitis

■ ■ ■

Knowledge of the structure and functions of the exocrine pancreas is necessary for understanding how inflammation of this organ affects the client. The exocrine pancreas is composed of lobules made up of acinar cells. The acinar cells secrete digestive enzymes and fluids (pancreatic juices) into ducts that empty into the main pancreatic duct (the duct of Wirsung). The pancreatic duct joins the common bile duct and empties into the duodenum through the ampulla of Vater (in some individuals, however, the main pancreatic duct empties directly into the duodenum). The epithelial lining of the pancreatic ducts secretes water and bicarbonate to modify the composition of the pancreatic secretions. Pancreatic enzymes are secreted primarily in an inactive form and are activated in the intestine, a modification that prevents digestion of pancreatic tissue by its own enzymes (Porth, 1994). The pancreatic enzymes, with related functions, are as follows:

- Proteolytic enzymes, including trypsin, chymotrypsin, carboxypolypeptidase, ribonuclease, and deoxyribonuclease, which break down dietary proteins
- Pancreatic amylase, which breaks down starch
- Lipase, which hydrolyzes neutral fats into glycerol and fatty acids

Inflammatory processes and tumors of the pancreas that result in changes in the secretion and outflow of pancreatic enzymes are serious and potentially life-threatening disorders. Clients with disorders of the exocrine pancreas are often acutely ill and may require lifelong adaptations to chronic changes in enzyme and hormone production. Depending on the cause of the illness, nursing care for clients with pancreatic disorders is provided in hospital and in community settings with interventions designed to meet both short- and long-term physical and psychosocial needs.

Pathophysiology

The pathophysiology of pancreatitis varies according to whether the disorder is acute or chronic in nature.

Acute Pancreatitis

Acute pancreatitis is an inflammatory disorder of the pancreas that results in the self-destruction of the pancreas by its own enzymes through autodigestion. *Acute interstitial pancreatitis*, which involves inflammation and edema of the interstitium, most often occurs secondary to other disease processes. *Acute hemorrhagic pancreatitis*, often a more severe form of acute interstitial pancreatitis, is characterized by inflammation, hemorrhage, and ultimately necrosis of pancreatic tissue.

Acute pancreatitis is more common in middle adults; the incidence is higher in men than in women. Acute pancreatitis is most often associated with gallstones in women and with alcoholism in men. Some clients recover completely, others experience recurring attacks, and still others develop chronic pancreatitis. The mortality and symptoms depend on the degree of severity and the type of pancreatitis: With mild pancreatic edema, mortality is low (5% to 10%); with massive hemorrhagic pancreatitis, the mortality rate ranges from 50% to 80% (Price & Wilson, 1992).

The exact cause of pancreatitis is not known. However, it is believed that several factors can activate pancreatic enzymes, leading to autodigestion of the pancreas and resulting inflammation, edema, and/or hemorrhage. These factors may include any of the following:

- Obstruction by a gallstone results in the movement of bile into the pancreas, causing pancreatic irritation.
- Obstruction of bile ducts raises pressure in these ducts, blocking pancreatic duct outflow. In turn, the continued secretion of pancreatic juices into the obstructed ducts raises pressure within the pancreas.
- Contents of the duodenum (with activated pancreatic enzymes) back up into the pancreatic duct.
- Excess hydrochloric acid (as from chronic alcohol intake) causes spasms of the sphincter of Oddi and the ampulla of Vater, obstructing pancreatic fluid flow.

Other factors that are associated with acute pancreatitis include trauma or surgery, pancreatic tumors, third-trimester pregnancy, infectious agents (viral, bacterial, or parasitic), elevated calcium levels, and hyperlipidemia. Some medications have been linked with this disorder,

Table 15–5   Laboratory Tests in Exocrine Pancreatic Disorders

Test	Normal Value	Significance
Serum amylase	25 to 125 U/L	Indicates the degree of destruction of pancreatic tissue. Increased up to 2.5 times normal early in the acute disease (within the first 6 to 12 hours) but may return to normal after the first 48 hours.
Serum lipase	20 to 180 IU/L	Increased in acute pancreatitis and pseudocyst; elevated values after the first 48 hours that persist for 5 to 7 days are seen in acute pancreatitis. Lipase may remain elevated in pseudocyst.
Urine amylase	4 to 370 U/L/2h	In acute pancreatitis, clearance increases and urine amylase is elevated.
Serum glucose	70 to 110 mg/dL	Indicates injury to pancreatic cells; there may be a transitory increase in serum glucose in acute pancreatitis. Hyperglycemia may be an early symptom of cancer of the pancreas.
Serum bilirubin	0.1 to 1.0 mg/dL	If pancreatitis causes impaired liver function, bilirubin will be mildly increased.
Serum alkaline phosphatase	30 to 120 IU/L	If pancreatitis causes impaired liver function, alkaline phosphatase will be increased. Alkaline phosphatase also increases in common duct obstruction and in metastases of cancer to the liver.
Serum calcium	4.5 to 5.5 mEq/L	When calcium is deposited in fatty necrotic pancreatic tissue, the serum levels are decreased for 7 to 10 days. Decreased serum calcium levels are a sign of severe pancreatitis.
Serum magnesium	1.5 to 2.5 mEq/L	Decreased serum magnesium levels occur with fat necrosis.
White blood cells	4500/mm^3 to 10,000/mm^3	Indicates inflammation or infection when increased; most often this occurs in acute pancreatitis.
Carcinoembryonic antigen levels (CEA)	<2.5 ng/mL	Elevated levels of CEA are found in the blood serum of 70% of all clients with pancreatic cancer. The primary use of CEA is in evaluating the effectiveness of treatment. Levels are also increased in clients with other malignancies, surgeries, renal failure, or inflammations and in clients who smoke.

including thiazide diuretics, estrogen, steroids, salicylates, and nonsteroidal anti-inflammatory drugs (NSAIDs).

Regardless of the related factor, the pathophysiologic process begins with the release of pancreatic enzymes into the pancreatic tissue. The enzymes believed to be most responsible for damage are phospholipase A, which digests cell membrane phospholipids, and elastase, which digests the elastic tissue of blood vessel walls (causing hemorrhage). In hemorrhagic pancreatitis, these enzymes cause fat necrosis of acinar cells and blood vessels; hemorrhage follows necrosis of blood vessels. In response, a large volume of fluid may shift from the circulating blood volume into the retroperitoneal space, the peripancreatic spaces, and the abdominal cavity. This fluid accumulation is often called pancreatic ascites.

The onset of acute pancreatitis is often sudden; the most noticeable manifestation is continuous severe epigastric and abdominal pain. This pain commonly radiates to the back and is relieved somewhat by sitting up and leaning forward. The onset of pain is often related to intake of a fatty meal or excessive alcohol (Smith, 1991).

Other manifestations include nausea and vomiting; abdominal distention and rigidity; decreased bowel sounds;

tachycardia; hypotension; elevated temperature; and cold, clammy skin. Within 24 hours, mild jaundice may appear. Abnormal laboratory data include elevated serum amylase and lipase and hypocalcemia (see Table 15–5). Retroperitoneal bleeding may occur 3 to 6 days after the onset of hemorrhagic pancreatitis; manifestations of bleeding include bruising in the flanks (Turner's sign) or around the umbilicus (Cullen's sign).

Complications of acute pancreatitis include the development of diabetes mellitus, tetany, hypovolemic shock, and pancreatic pseudocyst and abscess formation. Tetany results from hypocalcemia, which follows fat necrosis and the formation of calcium soaps from a combination of fatty acids and calcium (Price & Wilson, 1992). Hypovolemic shock may occur from hemorrhage or from a shift of fluid into the abdomen (see Chapter 6).

A *pancreatic pseudocyst* is a collection of liquid secretions and necrotic products outside the pancreas (in the abdominal cavity) that is enclosed in a layer of inflammatory tissue. Often, the pseudocyst is connected to the pancreas by a pancreatic duct and may increase in size as the destruction of pancreatic tissue continues. A *pancreatic abscess* is a collection of liquid secretions and necrotic

Clinical Manifestations of Chronic Pancreatitis

■ ■ ■

- Upper abdominal pain radiating to the back
- Nausea and vomiting with weight loss
- Flatulence and constipation
- Steatorrhea
- Manifestations of malabsorption
- Manifestations of diabetes mellitus
- Elevated serum and urinary amylase levels
- Elevated serum bilirubin

products located inside the pancreas; this complication, which results from bacterial contamination, is fatal if untreated. These complications usually occur 2 to 3 weeks after the onset of pancreatitis.

Other complications of pancreatitis include cardiac failure, renal failure, pleural effusion, multiple organ failure, adult respiratory distress syndrome, and ascites.

Chronic Pancreatitis

Chronic pancreatitis is a progressive disease that causes normal pancreatic tissue to be replaced by connective tissue. In contrast to acute pancreatitis, in which the client may regain normal function after recovery from the illness, chronic pancreatitis is an irreversible process that leads to pancreatic insufficiency.

There are two types of chronic pancreatitis: chronic calcifying pancreatitis and chronic obstructive pancreatitis. In *chronic calcifying pancreatitis,* calculi form in the pancreatic ducts and block the flow of pancreatic juices. This type, which is the more common type, most often occurs in men as a result of chronic alcohol abuse. In *chronic obstructive pancreatitis,* an obstruction or spasm of the sphincter of Oddi blocks the flow of pancreatic juices; this type of chronic pancreatitis is more common in women with gallstones. Chronic pancreatitis has a higher incidence in people of age 40 to 60.

Chronic pancreatitis may follow an acute pancreatic inflammation or may have no identified cause. The causative factors associated with the chronic form are the same as those associated with acute pancreatitis. In chronic pancreatitis, recurrent episodes of inflammation eventually lead to fibrotic changes in the parenchyma of the pancreas, with loss of both exocrine and endocrine functions. As a result, the client experiences malabsorption from pancreatic insufficiency and diabetes mellitus from the gland's inability to produce insulin.

The client with chronic pancreatitis typically has episodes of upper abdominal pain that radiates to the back. This pain may last for days to weeks, disappear, and then reappear. As the disease progresses, the interval between episodes of pain becomes shorter. Other manifestations include nausea and vomiting, weight loss, flatulence, constipation, and steatorrhea (fatty, frothy, foul-smelling stools caused by a decrease in pancreatic enzyme secretion). See the accompanying clinical manifestations box. As the disease progresses, the client manifests symptoms of malabsorption (discussed in Chapter 23) and diabetes mellitus (discussed in Chapter 21). Serum and urinary amylase and serum bilirubin are elevated.

Collaborative Care

Treatment of the client with acute pancreatitis focuses on eliminating the factors that precipitated the inflammation; decreasing further damage to the pancreas by reducing pancreatic secretions; and providing interventions to relieve pain, prevent or reverse hypovolemia, and treat secondary infections. Treatment for chronic pancreatitis often focuses on managing symptoms and includes pain relief, nutritional support, and pharmacologic replacement of deficient enzymes and hormones. Surgical treatment may be indicated to treat inflammation caused by biliary obstruction or to treat complications, such as pseudocyst and/or abscess.

Laboratory and Diagnostic Tests

The laboratory tests that may be ordered for the client with pancreatitis are summarized in Table 15–5.

Diagnostic studies include the following:

- *Ultrasonography* may be ordered to identify gallstones, a pancreatic mass, or pseudocyst.
- *Computed tomography (CT) scan* may be ordered to identify pancreatic enlargement, fluid collections in or around the pancreas, and perfusion deficits in areas of necrosis.
- *CT scan with vascular enhancement* may be conducted to determine the extent of edema and necrosis or to identify an abscess or pseudocyst.
- *Abdominal X-ray study* may be ordered to determine the presence of gallstones or the presence of fluid in the abdominal cavity.
- *Chest X-ray study* may be ordered to identify pleural effusion or elevation of the diaphragm on the left side.
- *Endoscopic retrograde cholangiopancreatography (ERCP)* may be performed to diagnose chronic pancreatitis and to differentiate inflammation and fibrosis from carcinoma.
- *Percutaneous fine-needle aspiration biopsy* may be performed to differentiate chronic pancreatitis from can-

Nursing Implications for Pharmacology: The Client with Chronic Pancreatitis

PANCREATIC ENZYME REPLACEMENT

Pancrelipase (Cotazym, Ilozyme, Pancrease)

Pancrelipase enhances the digestion of starches and fats in the gastrointestinal tract by supplying an exogenous source of the enzymes protease, amylase, and lipase. The drug promotes nutrition and decreases the number of bowel movements.

Nursing Responsibilities

- Assess the client for allergy to pork protein.
- Monitor frequency and consistency of stools.
- Weigh the client every other day. Record weights.

- Administer the drug with meals; if administered in a form that is not enteric coated, H_2 antagonists or antacids may be administered with meals to prevent destruction of the enzymes by hydrochloric acid.
- Monitor for side effects: rash, hives, respiratory difficulty, hematuria, hyperuricemia, or joint pain.

Client and Family Teaching

- Take the drug with meals or snacks.
- If medicine is enteric coated, do not crush, chew, or mix with alkaline foods (e.g., milk, ice cream).
- Be sure to follow prescribed diet.

---

cer of the pancreas; the cells that are aspirated are examined for malignancy.

Pharmacology

The pharmacologic treatment of acute pancreatitis focuses primarily on relieving pain. Meperidine hydrochloride (Demerol) is usually prescribed because opiate drugs (such as morphine) are more likely to cause spasm of pancreatic duct smooth muscle and the sphincter of Oddi, further obstructing pancreatic juice outflow. Other medications that may be used to relax smooth muscle and decrease pain include nitroglycerine and papaverine. Antibiotics may be administered to prevent or to treat infection. Antacids and H_2 blockers (cimetidine [Tagamet], ranitidine [Zantac]) may be given to neutralize or decrease gastric secretions. Carbonic anhydrase inhibitors (acetazolamide [Diamox]) or antispasmodics (dicyclomine [Bentyl]) may be administered to decrease the volume of pancreatic secretions.

Clients with chronic pancreatitis also require medications for pain but must be closely monitored to prevent drug dependence. Other medications used to treat chronic pancreatitis include pancreatic enzyme supplements (see the accompanying pharmacology box), antiemetics, antacids or H_2 blockers, and (if diabetes mellitus results) insulin.

Dietary Management

The client with severe pancreatitis is given nothing by mouth; instead, a nasogastric tube is inserted and connected to suction, and total parenteral nutrition (TPN) is initiated. These interventions decrease stimulation of the pancreas to slow the production of pancreatic juices (Howard, 1987). Clients who have milder cases of pan-

creatitis may not require nasogastric suction, and they may have intravenous fluids instead of TPN. Oral food and fluids are begun once the serum amylase levels have returned to normal, bowel sounds are present, and pain disappears. The client begins with clear liquids and progresses to a low-fat diet as tolerated.

Surgery

If the pancreatitis is the result of a gallstone lodged in the sphincter of Oddi, an endoscopic transduodenal sphincterotomy may be performed to remove the stone. A cholecystectomy may be performed to remove gallstones; however, this surgery is not performed until the acute pancreatitis has resolved. Surgical resection of all or part of the pancreas may be performed to remove necrotic tissue. If the client has a pseudocyst or abscess, percutaneously inserted tubes may be placed for external drainage.

Nursing Care

The nursing care for the client with acute pancreatitis focuses on managing pain, altered nutrition, and the risk for fluid volume deficit.

Pain

The client with pancreatitis experiences continuous, severe left upper abdominal or epigastric pain that radiates to the back. The pain, which is often accompanied by nausea and vomiting, abdominal tenderness, and muscle guarding, is caused by obstruction of pancreatic ducts, edema and swelling of the pancreas within the pancreatic capsule, and inflammation from autodigestion by pancreatic enzymes.

Nursing interventions with rationales follow:

- Administer prescribed narcotic analgesics (usually, meperidine [Demerol] or Tylenol #3) on a regular schedule. Assess the location, radiation, duration, character, and intensity of the pain. Have the client rate the intensity of the pain on a scale from 1 to 10, with 1 being no pain and 10 the worst possible pain. In addition, assess nonverbal cues of pain: restlessness or holding body rigidly still; tense facial features; clenched fists; rapid, shallow respirations; tachycardia; diaphoresis. *Pain intensity and pain relief must be assessed and reassessed at regular intervals, because pain that has become established and severe is difficult to control (Acute Pain Management Guideline Panel, 1992, p. 5). Unrelieved pain has negative physical and psychologic consequences; for example, pain, anxiety, and restlessness may increase secretion of pancreatic juices.*

- Maintain nothing by mouth (NPO) status and nasogastric tube patency as prescribed. *Gastric secretions stimulate hormones that stimulate pancreatic secretion, aggravating pain. Gastric secretions are minimized by eliminating oral intake and maintaining gastric suction. Nasogastric suction also decreases nausea, vomiting, and intestinal distention.*

- Maintain client on bed rest in a calm, quiet environment. *Decreasing physical movement and mental stimulation decreases metabolic rate and gastrointestinal secretion. This in turn minimizes stimulation of pancreatic secretions and resulting pain.*

- Provide comfort measures:
  a. Provide oral and nasal care every 1 to 2 hours.
  b. Encourage the client to maintain a comfortable position, such as a side-lying position with knees flexed and head elevated 45 degrees.
  c. Encourage the client to relax and use guided imagery to decrease pain.
  d. Provide careful explanations of all procedures and care; listen carefully to the client's concerns and evaluation of pain relief.

  NPO status and medications to relieve pain and to decrease pancreatic secretions may result in dryness and discomfort of the mucous membranes. The presence of a nasogastric tube stimulates mucous secretion and irritates tissues. Inflammation and edema of the pancreas causes pain from stretching of the peritoneum. Sitting up, leaning forward, or lying in a fetal position tends to decrease the pain. In addition to pharmacologic methods (see Chapter 4), the nurse should employ alternative methods of pain relief, take steps to reduce the client's anxiety, and involve the client in self-care.

- Discuss with family and visitors the reason why food should not be taken into the client's room. *The sight of food may stimulate secretory activity of the pancreas through the cephalic phase of digestion.*

Risk for Altered Nutrition: Less Than Body Requirements

In the client with pancreatitis, both the illness itself and its treatment may result in malnutrition. Inflammation increases the client's metabolic demand and frequently causes nausea, vomiting, and diarrhea. In addition, the loss of digestive enzymes directly affects the digestion and use of nutrients. At a time of increased metabolic demand, NPO status and gastric suction further decrease available nutrients.

Nursing interventions with rationales follow:

- Monitor nutritional parameters: serum albumin, serum transferrin, total lymphocyte count, blood urea nitrogen, hematocrit, and hemoglobin. *Serum transferrin (normal value: 205 to 410 mg/dL) and serum albumin (normal value: 4 to 5 g/dL) are decreased in malnutrition and negative nitrogen balance. A low total lymphocyte count is also common with malnutrition. Decreased pancreatic enzymes result in decreased protein catabolism and absorption; decreased transferrin causes inadequate iron absorption and transport, thereby decreasing hematocrit and hemoglobin levels.*

- Weigh the client daily at the same time each day. *Weight can be an indication of nitrogen balance; in malnutrition with negative nitrogen balance, the body is in a catabolic state and loses protein from muscles and other tissues.*

- Maintain stool chart; include frequency, color, odor, and consistency of stools. *Protein and fat metabolism are impaired in pancreatitis; as a result, undigested fats are excreted in the stool. The fat content of stools may increase to 50% to 90% (normally, fat content is about 20%). Steatorrhea indicates impaired digestion and, possibly, an increase in the severity of pancreatitis.*

- Assess the presence and character of bowel sounds. *The return of bowel sounds indicates that the client is regaining bowel motility; nasogastric suction usually is discontinued within 24 to 48 hours thereafter.*

- Administer prescribed intravenous fluids and/or TPN. *When the client is NPO, has increased metabolic need, and is unable to take in food and fluids orally to meet nutritional needs, TPN is essential to supply fluids, electrolytes, and kcal (see Chapter 13).*

- Provide interventions and teaching when oral feeding is resumed:
  a. Provide oral hygiene before and after meals.
  b. Offer small, frequent feedings.
  c. Discuss the type of foods to select to meet nutritional needs and to maintain a high-carbohydrate, low-protein, low-fat diet.
  d. Discuss the type of foods or drinks to avoid: alcohol, coffee, spicy foods, gas-producing foods.
  e. Discuss with the client and family the need to avoid large meals and restrict dietary fats, such as fried foods, whole milk, gravy, meat fat.

Oral hygiene decreases the numbers of microorganisms that can cause foul odor and taste, decreasing the client's appetite. Small, frequent feedings are more easily digested and absorbed. A diet low in protein and fat helps minimize the secretion of pancreatic enzymes, thereby decreasing autodigestion and preventing the return of symptoms. Gastric stimulants, gas-producing foods, fats, or the ingestion of large meals may excessively stimulate the pancreas and cause symptoms to recur.

Risk for Fluid Volume Deficit

The client with acute pancreatitis is at increased risk for fluid volume deficit from NPO status, from continuous nasogastric suction, and from the shift of fluid into the abdominal cavity. The third-spacing of fluid may cause hypovolemic shock with further complications involving cardiovascular function, respiratory function, renal function, and mental status. The nurse is responsible for making baseline assessments and for assessing manifestations that indicate impairments in function.

Nursing interventions with rationales follow:

- Perform cardiovascular assessments at regular intervals, according to client status and the unit's protocol:
  a. Assess cardiac rate and rhythm, or place the client on continuous cardiac monitoring.
  b. Assess blood pressure, or establish continuous hemodynamic pressure monitoring (e.g., central venous pressure or pulmonary capillary wedge pressure).
  c. Assess the rate, rhythm, and quality of peripheral pulses.
  d. Assess skin temperature, moisture, turgor, and color.
  Assessments of heart rate, blood pressure, peripheral pulses, and skin color indicate fluid volume status. Stable values are as follows: cardiac rate less than 100; blood pressure within 10 mm Hg of baseline; central venous pressure from 0 to 8 mm Hg; pulmonary wedge pressure from 8 to 12 mm Hg; cardiac output of approximately 5 liters per minute; and skin that is warm, dry, of good turgor, and of usual color. (See Chapter 6 for a full discussion of nursing interventions for the client in hypovolemic shock.)
- Assess and monitor respiratory function at regular intervals:
  a. Assess rate, rhythm, and patterns of breathing.
  b. Auscultate breath sounds.
  c. Assess symmetry of chest wall and diaphragm movement.
  d. Assess arterial blood gases.
  e. Assess quality, quantity, color, odor, and consistency of sputum.
  Abdominal pain causes shallow respirations and hypoventilation. Hypoventilation and decreased pulmonary blood supply increase the risk of atelectasis and hypercapnia. Abdominal pain predisposes the client to immobility and sup-

pression of coughing; pooling of secretions increases the risk of atelectasis and pneumonia. In addition, the client with acute pancreatitis may develop pleural effusion. The client should maintain a respiratory rate of less than 25 per minute, and blood gases should remain within normal physiologic ranges: PaO_2 greater than 60 mm Hg, $PaCO_2$ less than 35 to 45 mm Hg, pH between 7.35 and 7.45, and base excess between $+2$ and -2.

- Assess and monitor renal function:
  a. Measure urine output hourly. Maintain 8-hour and 24-hour intake and output totals.
  b. Weigh the client daily.
  Urine output of less than 30 mL per hour suggests decreased renal perfusion from hypovolemic shock or from acute renal failure, which is a major complication of acute pancreatitis. The pattern of intake and output and changes in body weight are indicators of hydration status and renal function.
- Assess neurologic function at regular intervals:
  a. Assess mental status, level of consciousness, and behavior.
  b. Assess cranial nerve function.
  c. Assess deep-tendon reflexes.
  Hypotension and hypoxemia may decrease cerebral oxygenation. Manifestations of decreased cerebral oxygenation include changes in mental status, level of consciousness, behavior, cranial nerve function, and deep-tendon reflexes. In addition, the client with acute pancreatitis may experience changes in mental status from alcohol withdrawal.

Other Nursing Diagnoses

Other nursing diagnoses that are appropriate for the client with pancreatitis include the following:

- *Ineffective Breathing Pattern* related to severe abdominal pain, immobility, and anxiety
- *Risk for Infection* related to malnutrition and invasive procedures
- *Impaired Gas Exchange* related to decreased respiratory effort secondary to pain, immobility, and pleural effusion
- *Altered Health Management* related to chronic use of alcohol as a coping mechanism
- *Altered Protection* related to alcohol abuse and inadequate nutrition

Client and Family Teaching

The client with pancreatitis is often acutely ill and, along with family members, needs information about both hospital procedures and self-care at home following discharge. During the acute stage, the client in severe pain and the anxious family require explanations couched in short, simple terms.

When the client and family members are physically and emotionally able to learn, the nurse teaches them about the disease and how to prevent further attacks of inflammation. Topics, individualized to the precipitating factors and specific needs, might include the following:

- Alcohol increases the protein content of pancreatic juice. As a result, stones can form, blocking the ducts in the pancreas and thus preventing pancreatic juice from flowing. Continued intake of alcohol is very likely to cause further inflammation and destruction of pancreatic tissue. Refer the client with an acknowledged problem with alcohol to community agencies, such as Alcoholics Anonymous, or for individual counseling.

- Smoking and stress stimulate the pancreas and should be avoided.

- If pancreatic function has been severely impaired, the client will need to take pancreatic enzymes and perhaps also insulin for diabetes mellitus (see Chapter 21).

- The client should consume foods that are low in fat and avoid crash dieting and binge eating, which can sometimes precipitate attacks. The client also should avoid spicy foods; coffee, tea, or colas; and gas-forming foods (all of which stimulate gastric and pancreatic secretions).

- An abscess may form months after the initial attack; symptoms of infection (a fever of 102 F (38.8 C) or more, pain, rapid pulse, malaise) should therefore be immediately reported.

Further information about pancreatitis may be obtained from local community agencies. In addition, the nurse should provide referrals to a community or home health agency to ensure continuity of care during convalescence at home.

Applying the Nursing Process

Case Study of a Client with Pancreatitis: Rose Schliefer

Rose Schliefer is a 59-year-old wife, mother of three, and grandmother of four. She has been in the hospital for the past 3 months for treatment of acute hemorrhagic pancreatitis and pseudocyst. The pancreatitis was caused by gallstones. Mrs. Schliefer spent 3 weeks in the intensive care unit and then underwent surgery to remove the gallstones and to insert drains into the pseudocyst. Two weeks before discharge she had progressed to a soft, high-carbohydrate, low-protein, low-fat diet; had all drains re-

moved; and had regained enough strength to walk in the hall. Prior to discharge, Mrs. Schliefer was given a referral to a community health agency in the small rural town where she lives.

Assessment

Mrs. Schliefer's husband and two daughters greet the community health nurse, Lee Quinn, at the door. Mrs. Schliefer is resting on the couch in the living room, wearing a housecoat. Ms. Quinn asks Mrs. Schliefer to return to bed so that she can carry out an assessment. Ms. Quinn also asks Mrs. Schliefer's family to be available to discuss Mrs. Schliefer's health care needs so that a nursing care plan can be developed.

On assessment, Ms. Quinn finds that Mrs. Schliefer is thin and appears anxious and tired. Mrs. Schliefer states that she had lost 30 lb (13.6 kg) in the hospital and now weighs only 102 lb (46 kg). She is 66 inches (168 cm) tall. Her vital signs are within normal limits. Mrs. Schliefer has a well-healed upper abdominal scar and two round wounds (from drains) on each side of her abdomen. The wounds are closed but still have scabs. Her skin is cool and dry, and turgor is poor. She is alert and oriented and responds appropriately to questions. Blood glucose levels are normal. Mrs. Schliefer states that her main problems are lack of energy and lack of appetite for the low-fat diet that has been prescribed. Ms. Quinn confers with Mrs. Schliefer's husband and daughters, who express concern about their ability to care for Mrs. Schliefer. They feel that although they have been taught all about the disease and how to provide care, they still are not sure they know exactly what should be done now that Mrs. Schliefer is at home.

Diagnosis

Ms. Quinn, together with Mr. and Mrs. Schliefer and their two daughters, develop a plan of care based on the following nursing diagnoses:

- *Fatigue* related to decreased metabolic energy production

- *Altered Nutrition: Less Than Body Requirements* related to prolonged hospitalization, dietary restrictions, and impaired digestion

- *Self-Care Deficit: Bathing/Hygine* (Level II: requires help of another person, supervision, and teaching) related to decreased strength and endurance

- *Risk for Caregiver Role Strain* related to inexperience with caregiving tasks

Expected Outcomes

The expected outcomes established in the plan of care specify that Mrs. Schliefer, within 1 month, will

- Verbalize causes of fatigue, set priorities for daily and weekly activities, and incorporate a rest period into daily activity.
- Gain 3 to 4 lb.
- Bathe and maintain personal hygiene without assistance.

In addition, family members will verbalize comfort with providing care necessary for Mrs. Schliefer.

Planning and Implementation

Ms. Quinn plans and implements the following interventions for the Schliefer family:

- Explain causes of fatigue: Review effects of pancreatitis, surgery, and acute illness on Mrs. Schliefer's energy levels.
- Identify activities that are most tiring for Mrs. Schliefer. Develop activity goals, incorporating small, incremental steps toward achieving goal. Mrs. Schliefer says that the first thing she wants to do is to cook a meal for the whole family. To reach this goal, she will:
  a. Identify times of fatigue and energy in a 24-hour period and schedule the meal in a peak energy period.
  b. Write a list of actions necessary to preparing the meal and delegate difficult tasks to her husband or daughters.
  c. Ask her daughters to reorganize the kitchen so that she can avoid unnecessary steps.
  d. Plan to prepare the meal no sooner than the fourth week after being home.
- Rest in bed each day from 1:00 to 3:00 p.m.
- Eat six small meals a day at the kitchen table with her husband or other family members and friends.
- Sit and rest quietly for 15 minutes before eating.
- Discuss dietary restrictions and how they can be adapted to the usual foods that are bought and prepared.
- Use shower chair and work toward self-care goals for bathing and hygiene in small steps. Make a list of all steps involved in brushing teeth, combing hair, taking a shower, and applying deodorant; begin with what Mrs. Schliefer can do now and each week add additional steps in the list.
- Discuss with all family members the following, and divide responsibilities:
  a. Physical care (shower, brushing teeth, washing hair)
  b. House cleaning and laundry
  c. Buying groceries and preparing meals
  d. Trips for medical care
- Encourage family discussion of concerns about unknown future and acknowledgement of strengths of this family.

Evaluation

After 1 month of being at home, Mrs. Schliefer and her family have established new routines based on the times when Mrs. Schliefer is most energetic. One big change is that Mrs. Schliefer now fixes lunch because she feels best during midday and because she and her husband can share this time together without interruption. Mrs. Schliefer still rests during the day but can now provide her own shower and hygiene. She has gained only 2 lb but states that she is getting used to the new diet and that "things are even starting to taste good without butter." She also says that sitting quietly before meals is helpful and that she prefers eating six small meals a day. Mr. and Mrs. Schliefer and their daughters agree that their initial worries about Mrs. Schliefer's care have been resolved; now they all know what they must do, and because they love each other and have strong faith that their mother is getting better, the future looks much brighter.

Critical Thinking in the Nursing Process

1. Describe comfort measures for the following responses to pancreatitis: itching, nausea, altered skin integrity from diarrhea.
2. Your client with acute pancreatitis is also an alcoholic. Describe assessments that indicate the beginnings of withdrawal.
3. Discuss the pathophysiologic basis of hypovolemic shock in acute hemorrhagic pancreatitis.
4. Outline a teaching plan that includes specific foods to omit and to include in a high-carbohydrate, low-protein, low-fat diet.
5. Develop a plan of care for the nursing diagnosis *Impaired Home Maintenance Management*.

The Client with Pancreatic Cancer

■ ■ ■

It is estimated that cancer of the pancreas occurs in 3% to 4% of all cancers. An estimated 27,000 new cases occurred in the United States in 1994, and there were 25,900 deaths from cancer of the pancreas (American Cancer Society, 1994). Pancreatic cancer is more common in adults in their 50s to 70s. The incidence is 30% higher in men than in women and 65% higher in African Americans than in Caucasians (American Cancer Society, 1991). Most cancers of the pancreas occur in the exocrine pancreas, are adenocarcinomas, and cause death in 1 to 3 years after diagnosis.

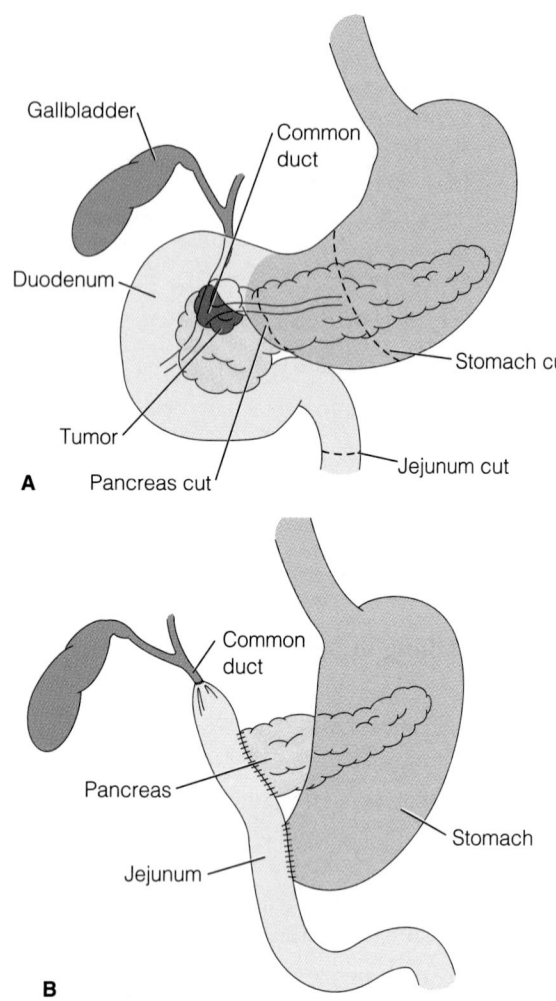

Figure 15–10 Pancreatoduodenectomy (Whipple's procedure): *A,* areas of resection; *B,* appearance following resection.

The major risk factor for cancer of the pancreas is smoking; the incidence is twice as high in smokers as in nonsmokers. Other associated risk factors are exposure to industrial chemicals or environmental toxins, high-fat diet, pancreatitis, and diabetes mellitus.

Cancer of the pancreas has a slow onset, with nonspecific manifestations of anorexia, nausea, weight loss, flatulence, and dull epigastric pain. The pain increases in severity as the tumor grows. Other manifestations depend on the location of the tumor. Cancer of the head of the pancreas, which is the most common site, often obstructs bile flow through the common bile duct and the ampulla of Vater, resulting in jaundice, clay-colored stools, dark urine, and pruritus. Cancer of the body of the pancreas presses on the celiac ganglion, causing pain that increases when the person eats or lies supine. Cancer of the tail of the pancreas often causes no overt symptoms until it has metastasized. Other late manifestations include a palpable abdominal mass and ascites. Because the manifesta-

tions are nonspecific, up to 85% of clients with cancer of the pancreas do not seek health care until the cancer becomes too far advanced for a cure and treatment is only palliative.

The client with early diagnosis of cancer of the head of the pancreas may have a resectable tumor. In this case, a pancreatoduodenectomy (more commonly called Whipple's procedure) is performed to remove the head of the pancreas, the entire duodenum, the distal third of the stomach, a portion of the jejunum, and the lower half of the common bile duct. The common bile duct is then sutured to the end of the jejunum, and the remaining pancreas and stomach are sutured to the side of the jejunum (Figure 15–10). Radiation and chemotherapy are often used in addition to surgery.

Postoperative nursing care of the client undergoing Whipple's procedure is similar to that of the client undergoing intestinal surgery (see Chapter 23). Specific postoperative nursing interventions for the client having Whipple's procedure are outlined in the accompanying box. In most instances, care in the immediate postoperative period is provided in the intensive care unit.

The client with pancreatic cancer has multiple problems requiring nursing care. Chapter 9 provides a discussion of care of the client with cancer; the nursing diagnoses and interventions discussed for the client with pancreatitis are also appropriate for the client with pancreatic cancer.

Bibliography

■ ■ ■

Acute Pain Management Guideline Panel. (1992). *Acute pain management in adults: Operative procedures. Quick reference guide for clinicians.* AHCPR Pub. No. 92-0019. Rockville, MD: Agency for Health Care Policy and Research, Public Health Service, U.S. Department of Health and Human Services.

Adinaro, D. (1987). Liver failure and pancreatitis: Fluid and electrolyte concerns. *Nursing Clinics of North America, 22,* 843–852.

Alfaro-LeFevre, R., Blicharz, M. E., Flynn, N. M., & Boyer, M. J. (1992). *Drug handbook: A nursing process approach.* Redwood City, CA: Addison-Wesley Nursing.

American Cancer Society. (1994). *Cancer facts and figures 1994.* Atlanta: Author.

Anderson, F. D. (1986). The cirrhotic process in the alcoholic. *Critical Care Quarterly, 8*(4), 74–78.

Boring, C. C., Squires, T. S., & Tong, T. (1991). *Cancer statistics 1991.* American Cancer Society. (Pub. No. 91-30M-No. 3033.00-PE).

Brown, B. R. (1989). The patient with an abnormal liver function study. *Current Reviews for Post Anesthesia Care Nurses, 11*(11), 81–88.

Butler, L. (1992). Hepatitis: A nurse's story. *RN, 55*(4), 66–68.

Butler, R. (1994). Managing the complications of cirrhosis. *American Journal of Nursing, 94*(3), 46–49.

Carpenito, L. J. (1992). *Nursing diagnosis: Application to clinical practice* (4th ed.). Philadelphia: J. B. Lippincott.

Centers for Disease Control. (1990). Protection against viral hepatitis: Recommendations of the Immunization Practices Advisory Committee (ACIP). *MMWR, 39*(No. RR-2), 1–26.

Centers for Disease Control. (1991). Hepatitis B virus: A comprehensive strategy for eliminating transmission in the United States

Postoperative Nursing Care of the Client Undergoing Whipple's Procedure

■ ■ ■

■ Maintain the client in semi-Fowler's position. *Semi-Fowler's position facilitates lung expansion and reduces stress on the anastomosis and suture line.*

■ Maintain patency of gastrointestinal suction (usually via a Salem tube, which is a double-lumen gastric decompression tube). Keep suction at low position. If Salem tube drainage is not adequate, obtain a physician order to irrigate, and do so with minimal pressure. Do not reposition nasogastric tube. *Pressure within the operative area from retained secretions increases intraluminal pressure and places stress on the suture line. Forceful irrigations and repositioning of the nasogastric tube may disrupt the suture line.*

■ Administer prescribed medications for pain at regular intervals, assessing the effectiveness of pain relief. *The client's response to narcotic analgesics may be decreased if they have been used prior to surgery. Increased pain may indicate complications such as disruption of suture line, leakage from anastomosis, or peritonitis. Adequate pain management increases resistance to stress, facilitates healing and increases the client's ability to cough, deep breathe, and change position.*

■ Assist client with coughing, deep breathing, and changing position every 1 to 2 hours. Splint incision during coughing and deep breathing. *The location of the incision makes coughing and deep breathing more painful. The prolonged surgical procedure, anes-thesia, location of incision, and immobility increase the risk of retained secretions, atelectasis, and pneumonia. Changing position facilitates drainage of secretions; effective coughing and deep breathing decrease retained secretions.*

■ Monitor the client for complications:
   a. Maintain an accurate rate of flow for intravenous fluids and blood.
   b. Assess skin color, temperature, moisture, and turgor.
   c. Assess peripheral pulses.
   d. Measure urinary output, gastrointestinal output, and drainage from any other tubes; monitor amount and type of wound drainage.
   e. Assess level of consciousness.
   f. Maintain accurate intake and output data.
   g. Take vital signs on a regular basis; immediately report changes (such as elevated temperature; hypotension; weak, thready pulse; increased or difficult respirations).
   h. Monitor results of laboratory tests, especially arterial blood gases, hemoglobin, and hematocrit.

The major complications following Whipple's procedure are hemorrhage, hypovolemic shock, and hepatorenal failure. The assessments listed provide information about the client's status and alert the nurse to abnormal findings that signal the onset of these complications.

through universal childhood vaccination: Recommendations of the Immunization Practices Advisory Committee (ACIP). *MMWR, 40*(No. RR-13), 1–25.

Clark, J. B., Queener, S. F., & Karb, V. B. (1990). *Pharmacological basis of nursing practice.* St. Louis: Mosby.

Conn, H. O., & Atterbury, C. E. (1987). Cirrhosis. In L. Schiff & R. R. Schiff (Eds.), *Diseases of the liver* (pp. 725–864). Philadelphia: J. B. Lippincott.

Corbett, J. V. (1992). *Laboratory tests and diagnostic procedures with nursing diagnoses* (3rd ed.). Norwalk, CT: Appleton & Lange.

DeBakey, M. & Jordan, G. (1987). Liver trauma. In L. Schiff & R. R. Schiff (Eds.), *Diseases of the liver* (pp. 1203–1222). Philadelphia: Lippincott.

DeCock, K. & Reynolds, I. (1987). Hepatic abscess. In L. Schiff & R. R. Schiff (Eds.), *Diseases of the liver* (pp. 1235–1234). Philadelphia: J. B. Lippincott.

Dienstag, J. L., Wands, F. R., & Isselbacher, K. J. (1991). Acute hepatitis. In J. D. Wilson, E. Braunwald, J. K. Isselbacher, R. G. Petersdorf, J. B. Martin, A. S. Fauci, & R. K. Root (Eds.), *Harrison's principles of internal medicine* (12th ed.) (pp. 1322–1337). New York: McGraw-Hill.

Dimango, E. P. (1989). Acute pancreatitis. In W. N. Kelly (Ed.), *Textbook of internal medicine.* Philadelphia: Lippincott.

Doherty, M. M., & Carver, D. K. (1993). New relief for esophageal varices. *American Journal of Nursing, 93*(4), 58–63.

Dolan, J. T. (1991). *Critical care nursing: Clinical management through the nursing process.* Philadelphia: F. A. Davis.

Edmundson, H., & Craig, J. (1987). Liver cancer. In L. Schiff & E. R. Schiff (Eds.), *Diseases of the liver* (pp. 1109–1158). Philadelphia: Lippincott.

Fain, J. A., & Amato-Vealy, E. (1988). Acute pancreatitis: A gastrointestinal emergency. *Critical Care Nurse, 8*(5), 47–63.

Foltz, A. T. (1988). Nutritional factors in the prevention of gastrointestinal cancer. *Seminars in Oncology Nursing, 4,* 239–245.

Fredette, S. L. (1984). When the liver fails. *American Journal of Nursing, 84,* 64–67.

Gallo, U. E., & Fontanarosa, P. B. (1989). Acute cholecystitis. *Emergency Care Quarterly, 5*(3), 84–89.

Given, B. S., & Simmons, S. J. (1979). *Gastroenterology in clinical nursing* (3rd ed.). St Louis: Mosby.

Gordon, M. (1993). *Manual of nursing diagnosis: 1992–1994.* St. Louis: Mosby-Year Book.

Grau, P. A. (1991, March). Are you at risk for Hepatitis B? *Nursing91,* 45–46.

Greenberger, N. J., & Isselbacher, K. J. (1991). Diseases of the gallbladder. In J. D. Wilson, E. Braunwald, J. K. Isselbacher, R. G. Petersdorf, J. B. Martin, A. S. Fauci, & R. K. Root (Eds.), *Harrison's principles of internal medicine* (12th ed.) (pp. 1358–1368). New York: McGraw-Hill.

Heeg, J. M., & Coleman, D. A. (1994). Hepatitis kills. *RN, 55*(4),

60–66.

Howard, J. M. (1987). Treatment of acute pancreatitis. In J. M. Howard et al. (Eds). *Surgical diseases of the pancreas* (pp. 426–449). Philadelphia: Lea & Febiger.

Hyder, S. A., & Barken, J. S. (1990). A new look at acute pancreatitis. *Contemporary Gastro-enterology, 3*(6), 34.

Isselbacher, K. J., & Wands, J. R. (1991). Neoplasms of the liver. In J. D. Wilson, E. Braunwald, J. K. Isselbacher, R. G. Petersdorf, J. B. Martin, A. S. Fauci, & R. K. Root (Eds.), *Harrison's principles of internal medicine* (12th ed.) (pp. 1350–1352). New York: McGraw-Hill.

Jackson, M., & Rhymer, T. (1994). Viral hepatitis: Anatomy of a diagnosis. *American Journal of Nursing, 94*(1), 43–48.

Jeffers, C. (1989). Complications of acute pancreatitis/CE quiz. *Critical Care Nurse, 9*(4), 38–44, 46, 48.

Jurf, J. B., Clements, L., & Lloremte, J. (1990). Cholecystectomy made easier. *American Journal of Nursing, 90*, 38–39.

Kee, J. L. (1991). *Laboratory and diagnostic tests with nursing implications* (3rd ed.). Norwalk, CT: Appleton & Lange.

Kools, A. M., & Bloomer, J. R. (1987). Abnormal liver function tests. *Postgraduate Medicine, 8*(6), 45–51.

Lee, W. M. (1990). Hepatitis up-date: Diagnosis, treatment, and prevention. *Modern Medicine, 58*(9), 46–65.

Lieber, C. S., & Guadagnini, K. S. (1990, February). The spectrum of alcoholic liver disease. *Hospital Practice,* 51–69.

Mahan, L. K., & Arlin, M. (1992). *Krause's food, nutrition & diet therapy.* Philadelphia: W. B. Saunders.

McCance, K. L., & Huether, S. E. (1994). Pathophysiology: *The biologic basis for disease in adults and children* (2nd ed.). St. Louis: Mosby-Year Book.

Oberfield, R. A., Steele, G., Gollan, J. L., & Sherman, D. (1989). Liver cancer. *CA-A Cancer Journal for Clinicians, 39*, 206–218.

Ondrusek, R. (1993). Cholecystectomy: An update. *RN, 56*(1), 28–33.

Plorde, J. J. (1991). Amebiasis. In J. D. Wilson, E. Braunwald, K. J. Isselbacher, R. G. Petersdorf, J. B. Martin, A. S. Fauci, & R. K. Root (Eds.), *Harrison's principles of internal medicine* (12th ed.) (pp. 778–782). New York: McGraw-Hill.

Podolsky, D. K., & Isselbacher, K. J. (1991). Cirrhosis of the liver. In J. D. Wilson, E. Braunwald, K. J. Isselbacher, R. G. Petersdorf, J. B. Martin, A. S. Fauci, & K. R. Root (Eds.), *Harrison's principles of internal medicine* (12th ed.) (pp. 1340–1350). New York: McGraw-Hill.

Porth, C. M. (1994). *Pathophysiology: Concepts of altered health states* (4th ed.). Philadelphia: Lippincott.

Price, S. A., & Wilson, L. M. (1992). *Pathophysiology: Clinical concepts of disease processes* (4th ed.). St. Louis: Mosby-Year Book.

Rowland, G. A., Marks, D. A., & Torres, W. E. (1989). The new gallstone destroyers and dissolvers. *American Journal of Nursing, 89*, 1474–1476.

Ryan, P., Vortherms, R., & Ward, S. (1994). Cancer pain: Knowledge, attitudes of pharmacologic management. *Journal of Gerontologic Nursing, 20*(1), 7–15.

Schmid, R. (1991). Liver transplantation. In J. D. Wilson, E. Braunwald, K. J. Isselbacher, R. G. Petersdorf, J. B. Martin, A. S. Fauci, & K. R. Root (Eds.), *Harrison's principles of internal medicine* (12th ed.) (pp. 1355–1358). New York: McGraw-Hill.

Schoenfield, L. J. (1988). Gallstones. *Clinical symposia, 40*(2), 2–32.

Smith, A. (1991). When the pancreas self-destructs. *American Journal of Nursing, 91*(8), 38–48.

Swearingen, P. L. (1984). *The Addison-Wesley photo-atlas of nursing procedures.* Menlo Park, CA: Addison-Wesley Nursing.

Thompson, C. (1992). Managing acute pancreatitis. *RN, 55*(3), 52–57.

Wands, J. R., & Isselbacher, K. J. (1991). Chronic hepatitis. In J. D. Wilson, E. Braunwald, J. K. Isselbacher, R. G. Petersdorf, J. B. Martin, A. S. Fauci, & R. K. Root (Eds.), *Harrison's principles of internal medicine* (12th ed.) (pp. 1337–1340). New York: McGraw-Hill.

Wilkinson, M. M. (1990). Your role in needle biopsy of the liver. *RN, 35*(8), 62–66.

Responses to Altered Skin Integrity

Assessing Clients with Skin Disorders

● ●

LEARNING OBJECTIVES

After completing this chapter, you will be able to

- Identify the layers and functions of the skin and its associated glands.
- Describe the structure and functions of the hair and nails.
- Discuss factors that influence skin color.
- Identify interview questions pertinent to the assessment of the integumentary system.
- Describe techniques for assessing the integrity and function of the skin, hair, and nails.
- Identify assessment findings that may indicate impairment of the integumentary system.
- Describe normal variations in assessment findings for the dark-skinned client.
- Describe normal variations in assessment findings for the older adult.

The skin and its glands, the hair, and the nails make up the *integumentary system.* The skin provides an external covering for the body, separating the body's organs and tissues from the external environment. It is the largest organ of the body and has many functions. In addition, the integumentary system

- Protects the body from injury from the external environment.
- Provides a barrier to the loss of body fluids and electrolytes.
- Maintains the integrity of the body surface through wound repair.
- Serves as a sense organ for touch, pressure, pain, and temperature.
- Provides a film over the body through the action of glandular secretions, which protects the body from bacterial and fungal invasion.
- Dissipates body heat through the evaporation of sweat.

- Participates in the production of vitamin D.
- Serves as a reservoir for blood.
- Serves as an indicator of emotions and health or illness through color changes.

Review of Anatomy and Physiology

■ ■ ■

The Skin

The *skin* has a surface area of 15 to 20 square feet and weighs about 9 pounds. It has been estimated that each square inch of skin contains 15 feet of blood vessels, 4 yards of nerves, 650 sweat glands, 100 oil glands, 1500 sensory receptors, and over 3 million cells that are constantly dying and being replaced (Marieb, 1995).

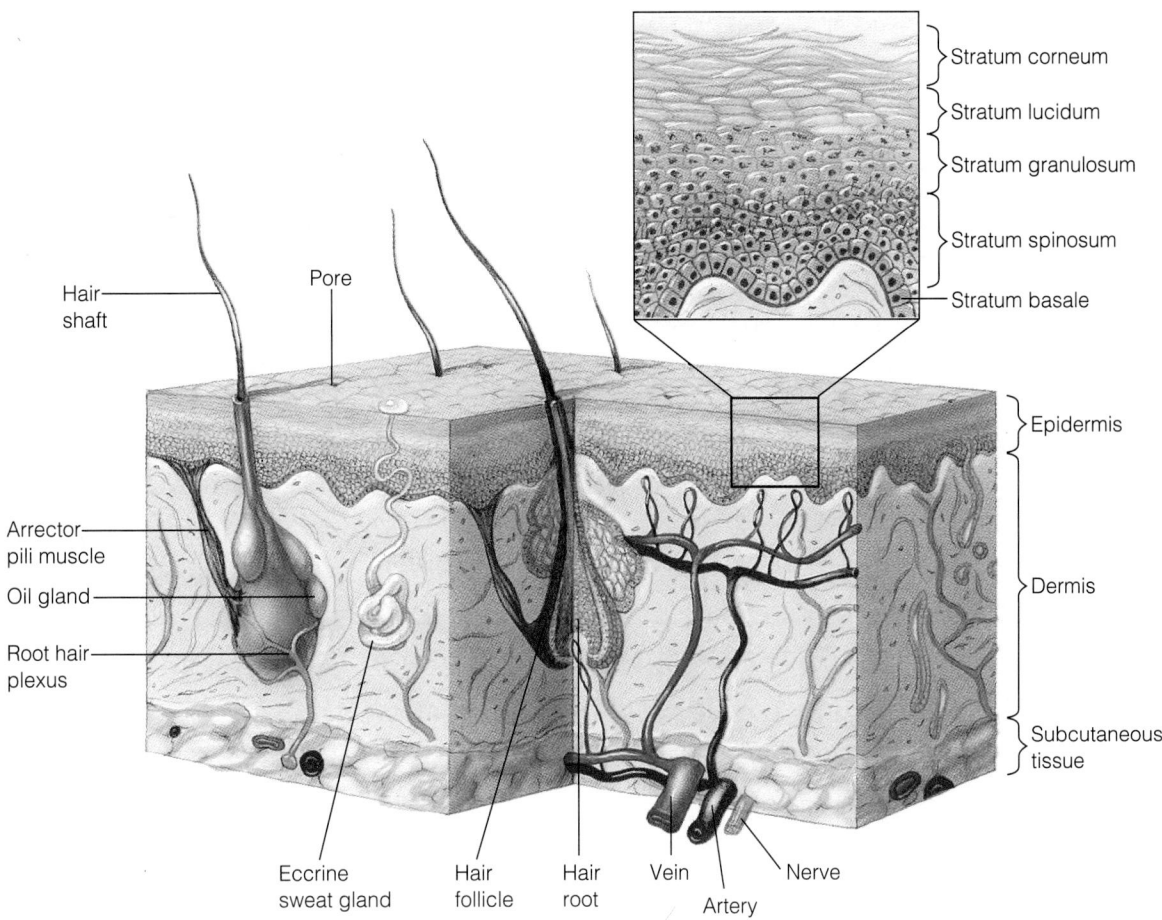

Hair shaft
Pore
Arrector pili muscle
Oil gland
Root hair plexus
Eccrine sweat gland
Hair follicle
Hair root
Vein
Artery
Nerve

Stratum corneum
Stratum lucidum
Stratum granulosum
Stratum spinosum
Stratum basale
Epidermis
Dermis
Subcutaneous tissue

Figure 16–1 Anatomy of the skin.

The skin is composed of two regions: the epidermis and the dermis (Figure 16–1). The *epidermis,* which is the surface or outermost part of the skin, is made up of epithelial cells. The epidermis has either four or five layers, depending on its location; there are five layers over the palms of the hands and the soles of the feet, and four layers over the rest of the body.

The *stratum basale* is the deepest layer of the epidermis. It contains *melanocytes,* cells that produce the pigment *melanin,* and *keratinocytes,* which produce *keratin.* Melanin forms a protective shield to protect the keratinocytes and the nerve endings in the dermis from the damaging effects of ultraviolet light. Melanocyte activity probably accounts for the difference in skin color in humans. Keratin is a fibrous, water-repellent protein that gives the epidermis its tough, protective quality. As keratinocytes mature, they move upward through the epidermal layers, eventually becoming dead cells at the surface of the skin. Millions of these cells are worn off by abrasion each day, but millions are simultaneously produced in the stratum basale.

The next layer of the epidermis is the *stratum spinosum.* Several cells thick, this layer contains abundant Langer-

hans cells that arise from the bone marrow and migrate to the epidermis. Mitosis occurs at this layer, although not as abundantly as in the stratum basale.

The *stratum granulosum* is only two to three cells thick. Langerhans cells are also found here. The cells of the stratum granulosum contain a glycolipid that slows water loss across the epidermis. Keratinization, a thickening of the cells' plasma membranes, begins in the stratum granulosum.

The *stratum lucidum* is present only in areas of thick skin. It is made up of flattened, dead keratinocytes.

The outermost layer of the epidermis, the *stratum corneum,* is also the thickest, making up about 75% of the epidermis's total thickness. It consists of about 20 to 30 sheets of dead cells filled with keratin fragments arranged in "shingles" that flake off as dry skin.

The *dermis* is the second, deeper layer of skin. Made up of a flexible connective tissue, this layer is richly supplied with blood cells, nerve fibers, and lymphatic vessels. Most of the hair follicles, sebaceous glands, and sweat glands are located in the dermis. The dermis consists of a papillary and a reticular layer. The papillary layer contains ridges that indent the overlying epidermis. It also

Table 16–1   Functions of the Skin and Its Appendages

Structure	Functions
Epidermis	Protects tissues from physical, chemical, and biologic damage. Prevents water loss and serves as a water-repellent layer. Stores melanin, which protects tissues from harmful effects of the ultraviolet radiation in sunlight. Converts cholesterol molecules to vitamin D when exposed to sunlight. Contains phagocytes, which prevent bacteria from penetrating the skin.
Dermis	Regulates body temperature by dilating and constricting capillaries. Transmits messages via nerve endings to the central nervous system.
Sebaceous (oil) glands	Secrete sebum, which lubricates skin and hair and plays a role in killing bacteria.
Eccrine sweat glands	Regulate body heat by excretion of perspiration.
Apocrine sweat glands	Unknown.
Hair	Cushions the scalp. Eyelashes and cilia protect the body from foreign particles. Provides insulation in cold weather.
Nails	Protect the fingers and toes, aid in grasping, and allow for various other activities, such as scratching the skin, picking up small items, peeling an orange, and so on.

contains capillaries and receptors for pain and touch. The deeper, reticular layer contains blood vessels, sweat and sebaceous glands, and deep pressure receptors. It also contains dense bundles of collagen fibers. The regions between these bundles form lines of cleavage in the skin. Surgical incisions parallel to these lines of cleavage heal more easily and with less scarring than incisions or traumatic wounds across cleavage lines.

Underlying the skin is a layer of *subcutaneous tissue* called the superficial fascia. It is composed primarily of adipose (fat) tissue. It helps the skin adhere to underlying structures.

The color of the skin is the result of varying levels of pigmentation. Melanin, a yellow-to-brown pigment, is darker and is produced in greater amounts in persons with dark skin color than in those with light skin. Exposure to the sun causes a buildup of melanin and a darkening or tanning of the skin in people with light skin. Carotene, a yellow-to-orange pigment, is found most in areas of the body where the stratum corneum is thickest, such as the palms of the hands. Carotene is more abundant in the skins of persons of Asian ancestry, and together with melanin accounts for their golden skin tone. The epidermis in Caucasian skin has very little melanin and is almost transparent. Thus, the color of the hemoglobin found in red blood cells circulating through the dermis shows through, lending Caucasians a pinkish skin tone.

Skin color is influenced also by emotions and illnesses. **Erythema,** a reddening of the skin, may occur with embarrassment (blushing), fever, hypertension, or inflammation. It may also result from a drug reaction, sunburn, acne rosacea, or other factors. A bluish discoloration of the skin and mucous membranes, called **cyanosis,** results from poor oxygenation of hemoglobin. **Pallor,** or paleness of skin, may occur with shock, fear, or anger or in anemia and hypoxia. **Jaundice** is a yellow-to-orange color visible in the skin and mucous membranes; it is most often the result of a hepatic disorder.

The functions of the skin are summarized in Table 16–1.

Glands of the Skin

The skin has three types of glands: sebaceous (oil) glands, sweat (sudoriferous) glands, and ceruminous glands. Each of these glands has a different function (see Table 16–1).

Sebaceous glands are found all over the body except the palms and soles. These glands secrete an oily substance called *sebum,* which usually is ducted into a hair follicle. Sebum softens and lubricates the skin and hair and also decreases water loss from the skin in low humidity. Sebum also protects the body from infection by killing bacteria. The secretion of sebum is stimulated by hormones, especially androgens. If a sebaceous gland becomes blocked, a pimple or whitehead appears on the surface of the skin; as the material oxidizes and dries, it forms a blackhead. *Acne vulgaris* is an inflammation of the sebaceous glands.

There are two types of *sweat glands:* eccrine and apocrine. *Eccrine sweat glands* are more numerous on the forehead, palms, and soles. The gland itself is located in the dermis; the duct to the skin rises through the epidermis to open in a pore at the surface. Sweat, the secretion of the eccrine glands, is composed mostly of water but also contains sodium, antibodies, small amounts of metabolic wastes, lactic acid, and vitamin C. The production of sweat is regulated by the sympathetic nervous system and serves to maintain normal body temperature. Sweating also occurs in response to emotions. Most *apocrine sweat glands* are located in the axillary, anal, and genital areas. The secretions from apocrine glands are similar to those of sweat glands, but they also contain fatty acids and proteins. Their function is unknown.

Ceruminous glands are modified apocrine sweat glands. Located in the skin of the external ear canal, they secrete yellow-brown waxy *cerumen*. This substance provides a sticky trap for foreign materials.

The Hair

Hair is distributed and scattered all over the body, except the lips, nipples, parts of the external genitals, the palms of the hands, and the soles of the feet. Hair is produced by a hair bulb, and its root is enclosed in a *hair follicle* (Figure 16–2). The exposed part, called the *shaft,* consists mainly of dead cells. Hair follicles extend into the dermis and in some places, such as the scalp, below the dermis. Many factors, including nutrition and hormones, influence hair growth.

Hair in various parts of the body has protective functions: The eyebrows and eyelashes protect the eyes; hair in the nose helps keep foreign materials out of the upper respiratory tract; and the hair on the head protects the scalp from heat loss and sunlight. See Table 16–1 for a summary of the various functions of the hair.

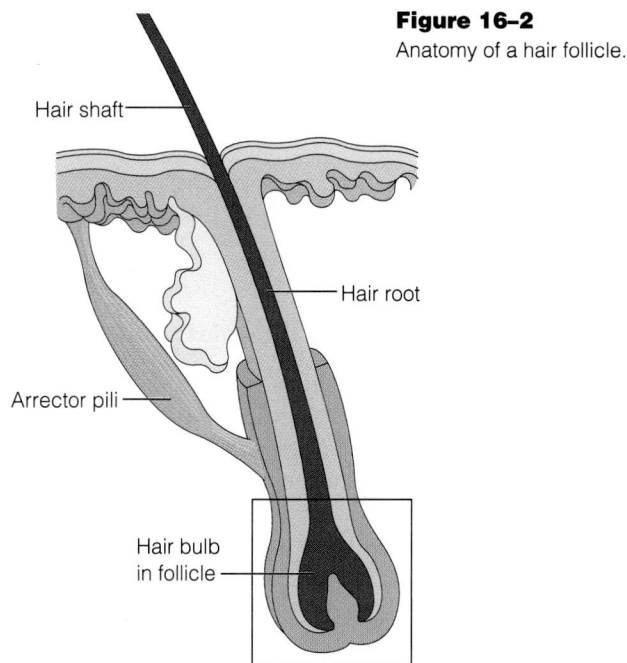

Figure 16–2
Anatomy of a hair follicle.

The Nails

A *nail* is a modified scalelike epidermal structure. Like hair, nails consist mainly of dead cells. They arise from the stratum germinativum of the epidermis. The body of the nail rests on the *nail bed* (Figure 16–3). The *nail matrix* is the active, growing part of the nail. The proximal visible end of the nail has a white crescent, called a *lunula*. The sides of the nail are overlapped by skin, called *nail folds*. The proximal nail fold is thickened and is called the *eponychium* or *cuticle*. Nails form a protective coating over the dorsum of each digit on the fingers and toes.

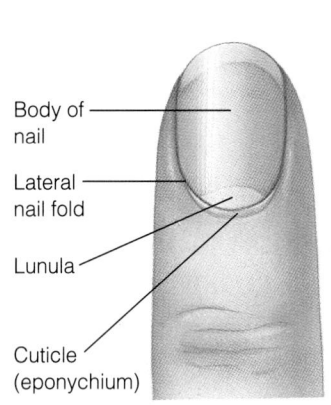

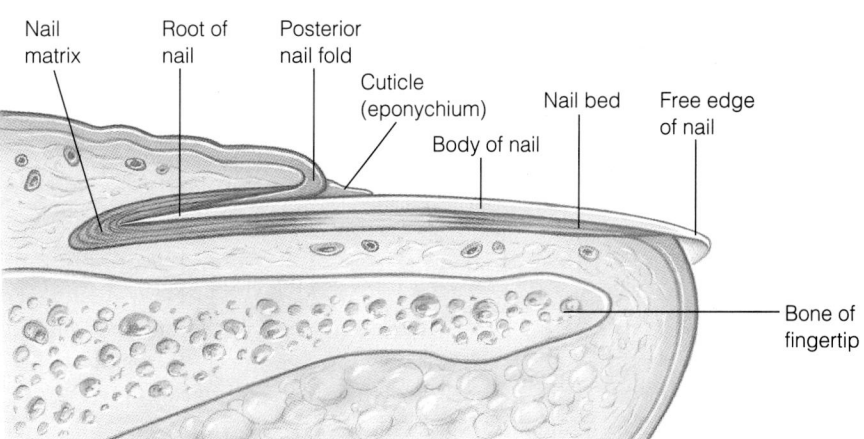

Figure 16–3 Anatomy of a nail.

Assessment of Integumentary Function

■ ■ ■

The function of the integumentary system (skin, glands, hair, and nails) is assessed by both a health assessment interview to collect subjective data and a physical assessment to collect objective data.

The Health Assessment Interview

This section provides guidelines for collecting subjective data through a health assessment interview specific to the functions of the skin and its appendages. Interview questions and leading statements for assessing these structures are also provided.

Overview

A health assessment interview to determine problems with the integumentary system may be conducted as part of a health screening or total health assessment, or it may focus on a chief complaint (such as itching or rash). If the client has a skin problem, the nurse analyzes its onset, characteristics and course, severity, precipitating and relieving factors, and any associated symptoms, noting the timing and circumstances. For example, the nurse may ask the client:

- Describe the type of itching you have experienced.

- When did you first notice a change in this mole?

- Did you change to any different kinds of shampoo or other hair products just before this hair loss began?

The nurse asks about any change in health, rashes, itching, color changes, dryness or oiliness, growth of or changes in warts or moles, and the presence of lesions. Precipitating causes, such as the use of new soaps, skin-care agents, cosmetics, pets, travel, stress, or dietary changes, must also be explored. In assessing hair problems, the nurse asks about any thinning or baldness, excessive hair loss, change in distribution of hair, use of hair-care products, diet, and dieting. In assessing nail problems, the nurse asks about nail splitting or breakage, discoloration, infection, diet, and exposure to chemicals.

The client's medical history is important. Questions focus on previous problems, allergies, and lesions. Skin problems may be manifestations of other disorders, such as cardiovascular disease, endocrine disorders, hepatic disease, and hematologic disorders. Occupational and social history may provide cues to skin problems; the client should be asked about travel, exposure to toxic substances at work, use of alcohol, and responses to stress.

The presence of risk factors for skin cancer should be assessed carefully. These include male gender; age over 50; family history of skin cancer; extended exposure to sunlight; tendency to sunburn; history of sunburn or other skin trauma; light-colored hair or eyes; residence in high altitudes or near the equator; and exposure to radiation, X-rays, coal, tar, or petroleum products.

The risk factors for malignant melanoma also are explored. These include a large number of moles, the presence of atypical moles, a family history of melanoma, prior melanoma, repeated severe sunburns, ease of freckling and sunburning, or inability to tan.

Interview Questions

The following interview questions and leading statements are categorized by functional health patterns.

Health Perception–Health Management

- Describe any skin problems or injuries, nail problems, and/or scalp problems you have had.

- How was this problem treated?

- Describe your current problem.

- Are you taking any medications for this problem? If so, what do you take, and how often?

- Have you recently had any insect bites? Explain.

- Describe any food, drug, plant, or animal allergies that you have.

- Describe how you care for your skin.

Nutritional-Metabolic

- Describe your usual intake of fluids and food over a 24-hour period.

- Have you made any changes in your diet or have you recently introduced new foods into your diet? What are they? When did you eat them?

- How well do your skin cuts or scratches heal? Has there been a recent change in the way you heal?

Elimination

- Is your skin and/or scalp dry or oily?

- Do you perspire heavily?

Activity-Exercise

- Describe your usual activities in a 24-hour period.

- How much sun exposure do you get? Do you use sunscreen or sun-block products?

- Do you bruise easily? Explain.

Sleep-Rest

- How many hours of sleep do you get each night?

- Does itching or sweating wake you at night?

- Are you unable to rest because of a skin problem?

Cognitive-Perceptual

- Do you have any skin pain, including itching, burning, stinging, tingling, achiness, tenderness, or numbness? Explain.

Self-Perception–Self-Concept

- Describe the appearance of your skin, hair, and nails.
- Do you have a rash or open area on your skin? If so, where is it located? What size and shape is it? Is it flat or raised? Do you have any drainage from it? How long have you had the rash or open area? What precipitates or relieves it?
- Describe any changes you have recently noticed in the appearance of a mole (such as changes in color and size, bleeding, or pain).
- Have you recently lost any hair? From where, and how much?
- Have your nails changed in color or shape? Have they become more brittle?
- Has a problem with your skin, scalp, or nails affected how you feel about yourself?
- Has a problem with your skin, scalp, or nails affected how you feel about your normal life?

Role-Relationship

- Is there a history of allergic disorders or skin problems in your family? Describe.

- Has a problem with your skin affected your relationships with others in your family? At work? In social activities? Explain.
- Has a problem with your skin or scalp affected your ability to work? Explain.

Sexuality-Reproductive

- Has a health problem with your skin or scalp interfered with or changed your usual sexual activities? Explain.
- Describe how problems with your skin, scalp, or nails have made you feel about yourself as a man or woman.

Coping-Stress

- Does your skin problem seem to become worse when you experience increased stress? Explain.
- Have health problems with your skin created stress for you? Explain.
- Describe what you do to cope with stress.
- Who or what will be able to help you cope with stress from this skin problem?

Value-Belief

- Are there significant others, practices, or activities that help you cope with this skin problem? Explain.
- How will this health problem affect your future?

The Physical Assessment

Physical assessment of the skin and its appendages may be performed either as part of a total assessment or alone for clients with known or suspected problems.

The physical examination of the skin, hair, and nails is conducted by inspection and palpation. The skin is assessed for color, presence of lesions, temperature, texture, moisture, turgor, and presence of edema. The hair is examined for color, texture, quality, and scalp lesions. The shape, color, contour, and condition of the nails are also determined.

Preparation

The equipment necessary for assessment of the skin includes a ruler (to measure lesions), a flashlight (to illuminate lesions), and disposable rubber gloves to protect the examiner. Prior to the examination, the nurse collects all necessary equipment and explains techniques to the client to decrease anxiety.

The examination should be conducted in a warm, private room. The client removes all clothing and puts on a gown or drape. The areas to be examined should be fully exposed, but the client's modesty is protected by keeping other areas covered. The client may be standing, sitting, or lying down at various times of the examination.

ASSESSMENT TECHNIQUE	POSSIBLE ABNORMAL FINDINGS

Skin

- **Inspect color.**

Pallor and/or cyanosis are seen with exposure to cold and with decreased perfusion and oxygenation. In cyanotic dark-skinned clients, skin loses glow and appears ashen. Cyanosis may be more visible in the mucous membranes and nail beds of these clients. In dark-skinned clients, jaundice may be most apparent in the sclerae of the eyes. Redness, swelling, and pain are seen with various rashes, inflammations, infections, and burns. First-degree burns cause areas of painful erythema and swelling. Red, painful blisters appear in second-degree burns, whereas white or blackened areas are common in third-degree burns. Vitiligo, an abnormal loss of melanin in patches, typically occurs over the face, hands, or groin. Vitiligo is thought to be an autoimmune disorder.

- **Inspect the skin for lesions.**

Pearly-edged nodules with a central ulcer are seen in basal cell carcinoma. Scaly, red, fast-growing papules are seen in squamous cell carcinoma. Dark, asymmetric, multicolored patches (sometimes moles) with irregular edges appear in malignant melanoma. Circular lesions are usually present in ringworm and in tinea versicolor. Grouped vesicles may be seen in contact dermatitis. Linear lesions appear in poison ivy and herpes zoster. **Urticaria** (hives) appears as patches of pale, itchy wheals in an erythematous area. In psoriasis, scaly red patches appear on the scalp, knees, back, and genitals. In herpes zoster, vesicles appear along sensory nerve paths, turn into pustules, and then crust over. Bruises are raised bluish or yellowish vascular lesions. Multiple bruises in various stages of healing are suggestive of abuse. Primary, secondary, and vascular lesions are described and shown in Tables 16–2 through 16–4 on pages 554 through 557.

- **Palpate skin for temperature.**

Skin is warm and red in inflammation and is generally warm with elevated body temperature. Decreased blood flow decreases the skin temperature; this may be generalized, as in shock, or localized, as in arteriosclerosis.

ASSESSMENT TECHNIQUE	POSSIBLE ABNORMAL FINDINGS

- **Palpate skin for texture.**

  Changes in the texture of the skin may indicate irritation or trauma. The skin is soft and smooth in hyperthyroidism and coarse in hypothyroidism.

- **Palpate skin for moisture.**

  Dry skin often is present in the elderly and clients with hypothyroidism. Oily skin is common in adolescents and young adults. Oily skin may be a normal finding, or it may accompany a skin disorder such as acne vulgaris. Excessive perspiration may be associated with shock, fever, increased activity, or anxiety.

- **Palpate skin for turgor.**

  Pinch the client's skin gently over the collarbone. *Tenting*, in which the skin remains pinched for a few moments before resuming its normal position, is common in elderly clients who are thin (Figure 16–4).

  Skin turgor is decreased in dehydration. It is increased in edema and scleroderma.

Figure 16–4 Tenting in an elderly client.

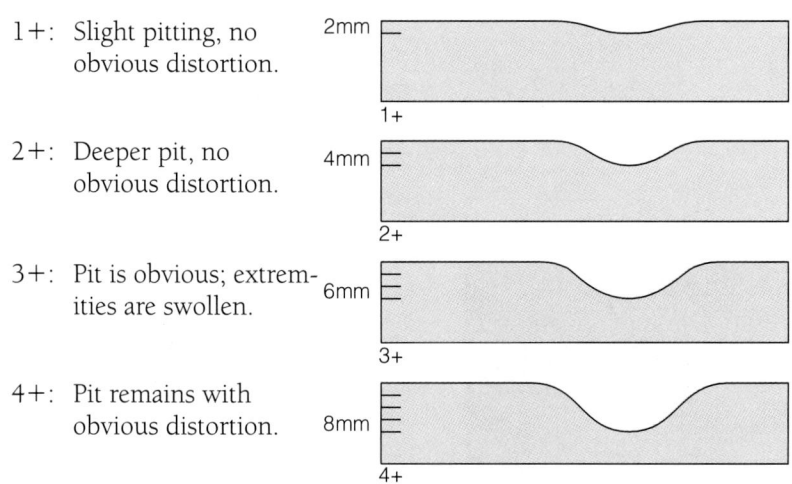

- **Assess skin for edema.**

  Assess **edema** (accumulation of fluid in the body's tissues) by depressing the client's skin over the ankle (Figure 16–5). Record findings as follows:

  Edema is common in cardiovascular disorders, renal failure, and cirrhosis of the liver. It also may be a side effect of certain drugs.

  1+: Slight pitting, no obvious distortion.

  2+: Deeper pit, no obvious distortion.

  3+: Pit is obvious; extremities are swollen.

  4+: Pit remains with obvious distortion.

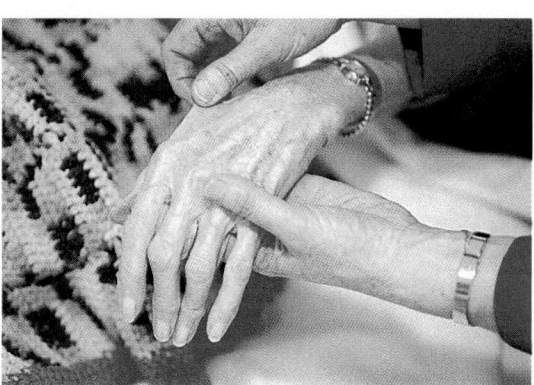

Figure 16–5 Degrees of pitting in edema.

ASSESSMENT TECHNIQUE	POSSIBLE ABNORMAL FINDINGS

Hair

- **Inspect distribution and quality.**

A deviation in the normal hair distribution in the male or female genital area may indicate an endocrine disorder. **Hirsutism** (increased growth of coarse hair, usually on the face and trunk) is seen in Cushing's syndrome, acromegaly, and ovarian dysfunction. **Alopecia** (hair loss) may be related to changes in hormones, chemical or drug treatment, or radiation. In adult males whose hair loss follows the normal male pattern, the cause is usually genetic.

- **Palpate hair for texture.**

Some systemic diseases change the texture of the hair. For instance, hypothyroidism causes the hair to coarsen, whereas hyperthyroidism causes the hair to become fine.

- **Inspect the scalp for lesions.**

With a gloved finger, part the hair at various locations, and inspect the scalp for lesions.

Mild dandruff is normal, but excessive, greasy flakes indicate seborrhea requiring treatment. Hair loss, pustules, and scales appear on the scalp in *tinea capitis* (scalp ringworm). Red, swollen pustules appear around infected hair follicles and are called *furuncles*. Head lice may be seen as oval nits (eggs) adhering to the base of the hair shaft. Head lice are usually accompanied by itching.

Nails

- **Inspect nail curvature.**

Inspect the nails from above and from the sides. The angle of the nail base should be about 160 degrees. Ask the client to hold two symmetric fingers together to assess for clubbing (Figure 16–6).

Clubbing, in which the angle of the nail base is greater than 180 degrees, is seen in respiratory disorders, cardiovascular disorders, cirrhosis of the liver, colitis, and thyroid disease. The nail becomes thick, hard, shiny, and curved at the free end.

Figure 16–6
Assessing clubbing of the nails.

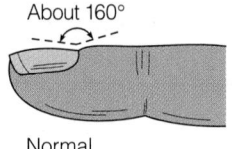 About 160°

Normal

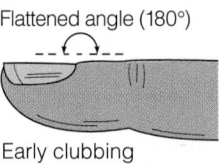 Flattened angle (180°)

Early clubbing

- **Inspect the surface of the nails.**

Figure 16–7   Oncolysis.

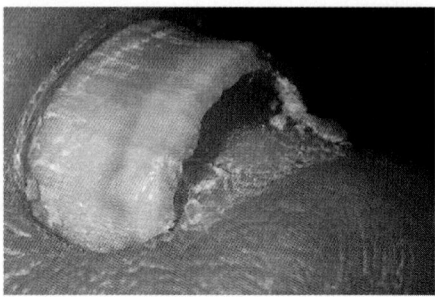

The nail folds become inflamed and swollen and the nail loosens in *paronychia*, an infection of the nails. Inflammation and transverse rippling of the nail is associated with chronic paronychia and/or eczema. The nail plate may separate from the nail bed in trauma, psoriasis, and *Pseudomonas* and *Candida* infections. This separation is called *oncolysis* (Figure 16–7). Nail grooves may be caused by inflammation, by lichen

ASSESSMENT TECHNIQUE	POSSIBLE ABNORMAL FINDINGS

Figure 16–8
Spoon-shaped nails.

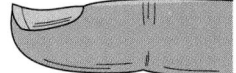

planus or by nail biting. Nail pitting may be seen with psoriasis. A transverse groove (Beau's line) may be seen in trachoma and/or acute diseases. Thin spoon-shaped nails (Figure 16–8) may be seen in anemia.

■ Inspect nail color.

The sudden appearance of a pigmented band may indicate melanoma. However, pigmented bands are normally found in over 90% of African-Americans. Yellowish nails are seen in psoriasis and fungal infections. Dark nails occur with trauma, *Candida* infections, and hyperbilirubinemia. Blackish-green nails are apparent in injury and in *Pseudomonas* infection, which is painless. Red splinter longitudinal hemorrhages may be seen in injury and/or psoriasis.

■ Inspect nail thickness.

Trauma to the nails usually causes thickening. Other causes of thick nails include psoriasis, fungal infections, and decreased peripheral vascular blood supply. Thinning of the nails is seen in nutritional deficiencies.

Variations in Assessment Findings for the Older Adult

A variety of normal skin changes may be apparent in the older adult. Loss of subcutaneous tissue, dermal thinning, and decreased elasticity may cause wrinkles and sagging of the skin. The skin is thinner, and turgor is decreased. Other age-related changes include the following:

■ Dry, itchy skin may result from the reduction of sweat and oil glands.

■ Overall production of melanocytes decreases, while abnormal localized proliferations of melanocytes may occur in specific areas. This localized hyperpigmentation may lead to the development of *senile lentigines,* commonly called "liver spots." These flat, brown macules commonly appear on the arms and hands in areas of sun exposure (Figure 16–9). Keratoses also result from hyperpigmentation. *Seborrheic keratoses* are dark, raised lesions (Figure 16–10). Actinic keratoses are reddish, raised plaques on areas of high sun exposure. They may become malignant.

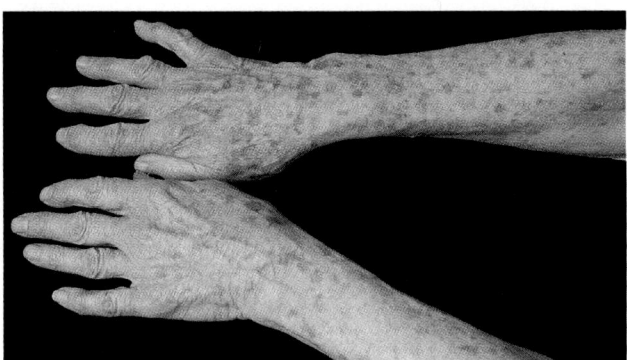

Figure 16–9   Senile lentigines: small, flat, brown, macules called "liver spots."

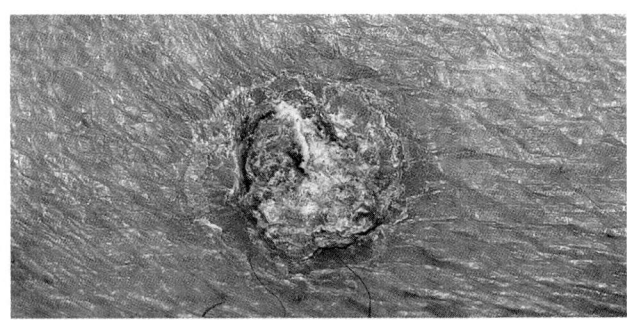

Figure 16–10   Seborrheic keratoses.

- Skin tags, small flaps of excess skin, may also be noted as a normal variation of the aging skin (Figure 16–11).

- Both hair and nail growth decreases with aging. Older men may develop coarse hair in the ears and nose and over the eyebrows. Decreased estrogen levels may cause postmenopausal women to develop dark facial hair over the upper lip and under the chin.

- Hair becomes gray due to a reduction of melanocytes.

- Nails may thicken, yellow, and peel. Some nail thickening may also be due to peripheral vascular disease.

Finally, older clients and others on low incomes are at increased risk for nutritional deficiencies, which often manifest in changes in the skin. Some of the most common of these deficiency-related changes are listed in Table 16–5 on page 557.

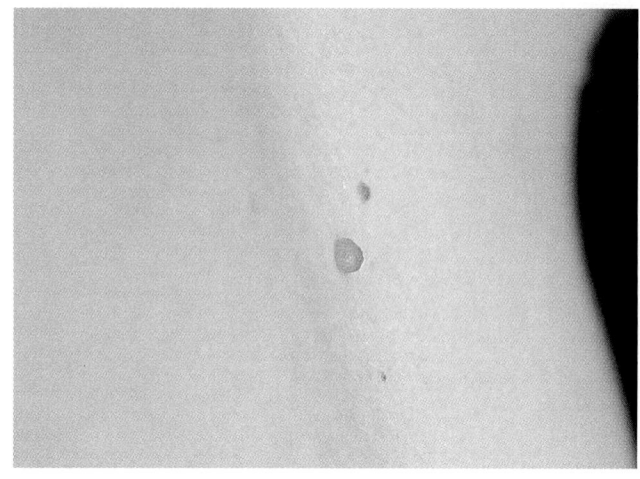

Figure 16–11 Skin tags.

Table 16–2   Primary Skin Lesions

Macule, Patch

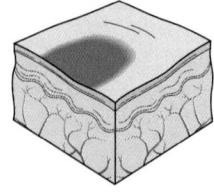

Flat, nonpalpable change in skin color. Macules are smaller than 1 cm, with a circumscribed border, and patches are larger than 1 cm and may have an irregular border.

Examples Macules: freckles, measles, and petechiae. Patches: mongolian spots, port-wine stains, vitiligo, and chloasma.

Papule, Plaque

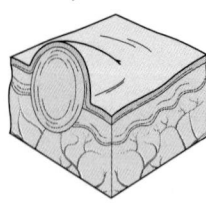

Elevated, solid, palpable mass with circumscribed border. Papules are smaller than 0.5 cm; plaques are groups of papules that form lesions larger than 0.5 cm.

Examples Papules: elevated moles, warts, and lichen planus. Plaques: psoriasis, actinic keratosis, and also lichen planus.

Nodule, Tumor

Elevated, solid, hard or soft palpable mass extending deeper into the dermis than a papule. Nodules have circumscribed borders and are 0.5 to 2 cm; tumors may have irregular borders and are larger than 2 cm.

Examples Nodules: small lipoma, squamous cell carcinoma, fibroma, and intradermal nevi. Tumors: large lipoma, carcinoma, and hemangioma.

Vesicle, Bulla

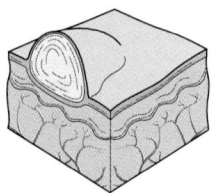

Elevated, fluid-filled, round or oval shaped, palpable mass with thin, translucent walls and circumscribed borders. Vesicles are smaller than 0.5 cm; bullae are larger than 0.5 cm.

Examples Vesicles: herpes simplex/zoster, early chickenpox, poison ivy, and small burn blisters. Bullae: contact dermatitis, friction blisters, and large burn blisters.

Wheal

Elevated, often reddish area with irregular border caused by diffuse fluid in tissues rather than free fluid in a cavity, as in vesicles. Size varies.

Examples Insect bites and hives (extensive wheals).

Pustule

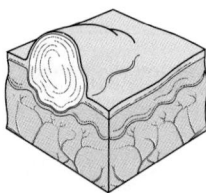

Elevated, pus-filled vesicle or bulla with circumscribed border. Size varies.

Examples Acne, impetigo, and carbuncles (large boils).

Cyst

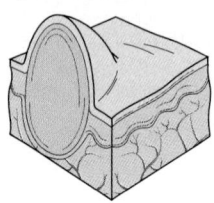

Elevated, encapsulated, fluid-filled or semisolid mass originating in the subcutaneous tissue or dermis, usually 1 cm or larger.

Examples Varieties include sebaceous cysts and epidermoid cysts.

Table 16–3   Secondary Skin Lesions

Atrophy

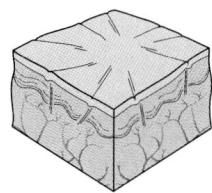

A translucent, dry, paperlike, sometimes wrinkled skin surface resulting from thinning or wasting of the skin due to loss of collagen and elastin.

Examples Striae, aged skin.

Ulcer

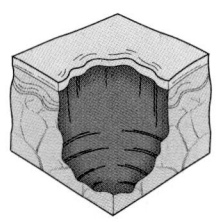

Deep, irregularly shaped area of skin loss extending into the dermis or subcutaneous tissue. May bleed. May leave scar.

Examples Decubitus ulcers (pressure sores), stasis ulcers, chancres.

Erosion

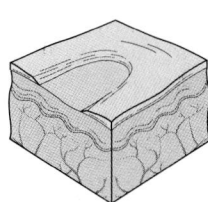

Wearing away of the superficial epidermis causing a moist, shallow depression. Because erosions do not extend into the dermis, they heal without scarring.

Examples Scratch marks, ruptured vesicles.

Fissure

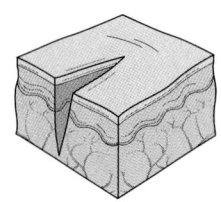

Linear crack with sharp edges, extending into the dermis.

Examples Cracks at the corners of the mouth or in the hands, athlete's foot.

Lichenification

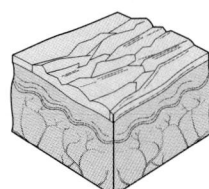

Rough, thickened, hardened area of epidermis resulting from chronic irritation such as scratching or rubbing.

Example Chronic dermatitis.

Scar

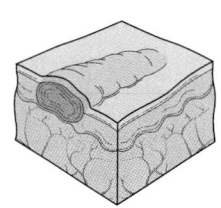

Flat, irregular area of connective tissue left after a lesion or wound has healed. New scars may be red or purple; older scars may be silvery or white.

Examples Healed surgical wound or injury, healed acne.

Scales

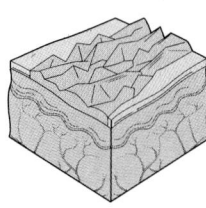

Shedding flakes of greasy, keratinized skin tissue. Color may be white, gray, or silver. Texture may vary from fine to thick.

Examples Dry skin, dandruff, psoriasis, and eczema.

Keloid

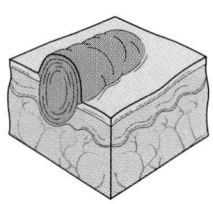

Elevated, irregular, darkened area of excess scar tissue caused by excessive collagen formation during healing. Extends beyond the site of the original injury. Higher incidence in people of African descent.

Examples Keloid from ear-piercing or surgery.

Crust

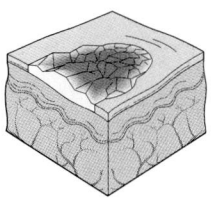

Dry blood, serum, or pus left on the skin surface when vesicles or pustules burst. Can be red-brown, orange, or yellow. Large crusts that adhere to the skin surface are called scabs.

Examples Eczema, impetigo, herpes, or scabs following abrasion.

Table 16–4 Vascular Skin Lesions

Port-Wine Stain

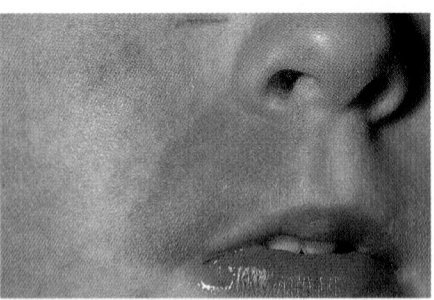

Flat, irregularly shaped lesion ranging in color from pale red to deep purple-red. Color deepens with exertion, emotional response, or exposure to extremes of temperature. It is present at birth and typically does not fade.

Cause A large, flat mass of blood vessels on the skin surface.

Localization/Distribution Most commonly appears on the face and head but may occur elsewhere.

Strawberry Mark

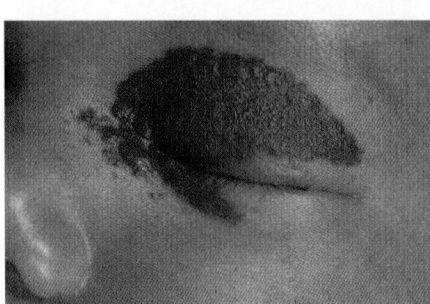

A bright red, raised lesion about 2 to 10 cm in diameter. It does not blanch with pressure. It is usually present at birth or within a few months of birth. Typically, it disappears by age 3. The lesion pictured here is located on the upper and lower lid of the left eye.

Cause A cluster of immature capillaries.

Localization/Distribution Can appear on any part of the body.

Spider Angioma

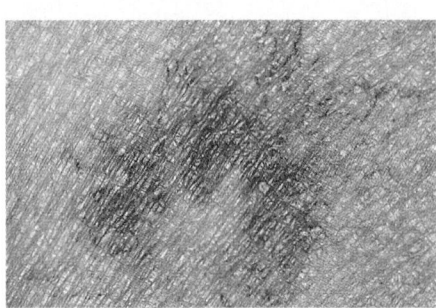

A flat, bright red dot with tiny radiating blood vessels ranging in size from a pinpoint to 2 cm. It blanches with pressure.

Cause A type of telangiectasis (vascular dilatation) caused by elevated estrogen levels, pregnancy, estrogen therapy, vitamin B deficiency, or liver disease, or may not be pathological.

Localization/Distribution Most commonly appear on the upper half of the body.

Venous Star

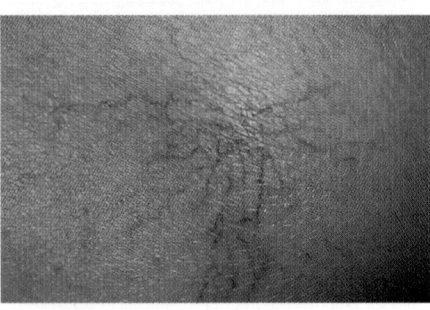

A flat blue lesion with radiating, cascading, or linear veins extending from the center. It ranges in size from 3 to 25 cm.

Cause A type of telangiectasis (vascular dilatation) caused by increased intravenous pressure in superficial veins.

Localization/Distribution Most commonly appear on the anterior chest and the lower legs near varicose veins.

Petechiae

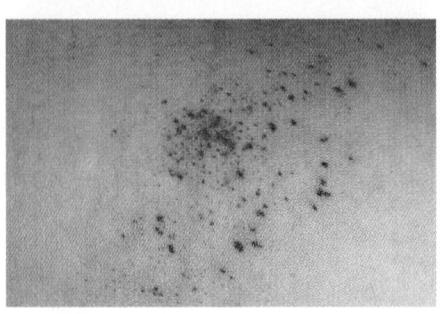

Flat red or purple rounded "freckles" approximately 1 to 3 mm in diameter. Difficult to detect in dark skin. Do not blanch.

Cause Minute hemorrhages resulting from fragile capillaries, petechiae are caused by septicemias, liver disease, or vitamin C or K deficiency. They may also be caused by anticoagulant therapy.

Localization/Distribution Most commonly appear on the dependent surfaces of the body, e.g., back, buttocks. In the client with dark skin, look for them in the oral mucosa and conjunctivae.

Table 16–4   *Continued*

Purpura

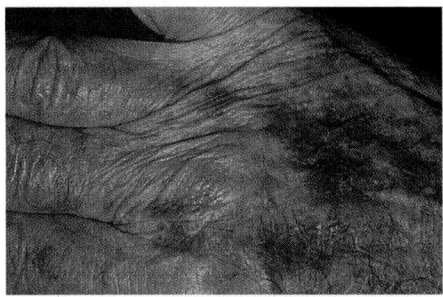

Flat, reddish blue, irregularly shaped extensive patches of varying size.

Cause Bleeding disorders, scurvy, and capillary fragility in the older adult (senile purpura).

Localization/Distribution May appear anywhere on the body, but are most noticeable on the legs, arms, and backs of hands.

Ecchymosis

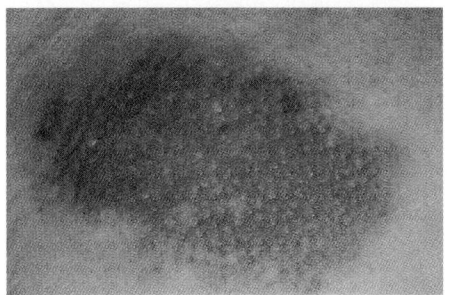

A flat, irregularly shaped lesion of varying size with no pulsation. Does not blanch with pressure. In light skin, it begins as bluish purple mark that changes to greenish yellow. In brown skin, it varies from blue to deep purple. In black skin, it appears as a darkened area.

Cause Release of blood from superficial vessels into surrounding tissue due to trauma, hemophilia, liver disease, or deficiency of vitamin C or K.

Localization/Distribution Occurs anywhere on the body at the site of trauma or pressure.

Hematoma

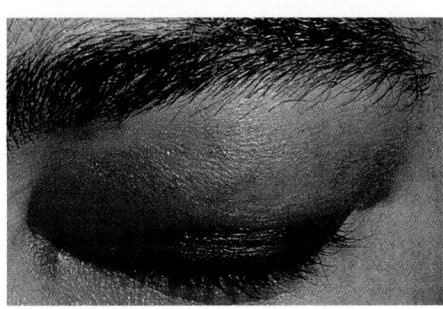

A raised, irregularly shaped lesion similar to an ecchymosis except that it elevates the skin and looks like a swelling.

Cause A leakage of blood into the skin and subcutaneous tissue as a result of trauma or surgical incision.

Localization/Distribution May occur anywhere on the body at the site of trauma, pressure, or surgical incision.

Table 16–5   The Skin as a Mirror of Health

Some nutritional deficiencies are signaled by changes in the skin. Thus, assessment of the skin may provide clues to the client's general health.

Nutrient	Result of Deficiency
Protein	Dry skin, loss of skin color
Essential fats	Patches of baldness, eczema
Vitamin A	Thickened skin that is dry or rough
Vitamin C	Bleeding gums, delayed wound healing
Vitamin B$_6$	Flaky skin, sores in the mouth, cracks at the corners of the mouth
Riboflavin	Oily skin, sores in the mouth, cracks at the corners of the mouth
Niacin	Dark, round spots in areas of the skin exposed to the sun; sores in the mouth and rectum

Bibliography

Collier, M. (1993). Assessing a wound. *Nursing Standard, 7*(20), 3–8, 15–16.
Coulter, J. A. (1991). ABCD's of assessing skin lesions. *Advancing Clinical Care, 6*(6), 18–19.
Cubbin, B. (1991). Trail of a pressure area risk calculator for intensive therapy patients. *Intensive Care Nursing, 7*(1), 40–44.
Duncan, D. J. (1991). Burn-wound management. *Critical Care Nursing Clinics of North America, 3*(2), 199–220.
Ertl, P. (1992). Look beyond the ulcer itself: Assessment of leg ulcers. *Professional Nurse, 7*(4), 258, 260–262.
Flory, C. (1992). Perfecting the art: Skin assessment. *RN, 55*(6), 22–27.
Gilkison, C. (1992). Assessment of patients with acanthosis nigricaus skin lesion for hyperinsulinemia, insulin resistance and diabetes risk. *Nurse Practitioner, 17*(2), 26, 28, 37.
Irwin, M. J. (1991). Assessing color changes for dark skinned patients. *Advancing Clinical Care, 6*(6), 8–11.
Mairis, E. (1992). Four senses for a full skin assessment: Observation and assessment of the skin. *Professional Nurse, 7*(6), 376–378, 380.
Marieb, E. (1995). *Human anatomy and physiology* (3rd ed.). Redwood City, CA: Benjamin Cummings.
McConnell, E. A. (1992). Clinical do's and don'ts: Assessing the skin. *Nursing92, 22*(4), 86.

CHAPTER 17

Nursing Care of Clients with Common Skin Disorders

LEARNING OBJECTIVES

After completing this chapter, you will be able to

- Describe the pathophysiology of common skin disorders, including pruritus, dry skin, and psoriasis.

- Compare and contrast the pathophysiology, collaborative care, and nursing care of clients with infections and infestations of the skin.

- Discuss various inflammatory disorders of the skin, including dermatitis, acne, pemphigus vulgaris, and toxic epidermal necrolysis.

- Compare and contrast the pathophysiology, collaborative care, and nursing care of clients with benign and malignant neoplasms.

- Discuss factors contributing to the development of pressure ulcers.

- Discuss the pathophysiology of selected common disorders of the hair and nails.

- Identify laboratory and diagnostic tests used to diagnose various disorders of the integument.

- Discuss nursing implications for pharmacologic agents used to treat disorders of the integument.

- Discuss surgical options for excision of neoplasms, reconstruction of facial or body structures, and cosmetic procedures.

- Provide client and family teaching appropriate for prevention and self-care of disorders of the integumentary system.

- Use the nursing process to assess needs and to plan and implement care for clients with common disorders of the skin.

The skin encloses the body, providing protection by serving as a barrier between the internal and external environments. It also has both physical and psychosocial functions. Physically, the skin contains the receptors for touch and sensation, helps regulate body temperature, and maintains fluid and electrolyte balance. Psychosocially, the skin provides cues to a person's racial and ethnic background, allows emotional responses, and plays a major role in determining self-concept, roles, and relationships.

There are many different common disorders of the skin and its accessory organs: the hair, nails, and sebaceous

glands. The client with minor or benign disorders is often treated in a physician's office or outpatient setting, but the client with disorders that involve large areas of the body, are chronic, or are malignant may require inpatient care. Nursing care for clients with common skin disorders focuses on health promotion, disease prevention, and health restoration. The nurse assesses client needs and implements collaborative and nursing care to meet a wide variety of physical, emotional, and social responses.

This chapter discusses common disorders of the skin, hair, and nails; Chapter 18 discusses the client with burns.

▝▝▝   **Common Skin Disorders**   ▝▝▝

The disorders discussed in this section of the chapter are those commonly experienced by a large number of people. Although they are considered minor health problems in terms of health care, they may cause major problems for the person experiencing a high level of discomfort/or and chronicity.

Common primary and secondary skin lesions are described and illustrated in Tables 16–2 and 16–3 in the preceding chapter. These terms are used throughout this chapter and in Chapter 18.

The Client with Pruritus

■ ■ ■

Pruritus is a subjective itching sensation producing an urge to scratch. Almost all people at some time in their lives experience the sensation of itching. Pruritus may occur in a small, circumscribed area, or it may involve a widespread area; it may or may not be associated with a rash. Pruritus is not a disorder itself but is rather a manifestation of an underlying irritation or condition. The exact cause of pruritus is not known, but it is believed to result from either stimulation of itch receptors in the skin (although these structures have not been identified) or as a response to the stimulation of skin receptors for pain and touch that the central nervous system interprets as an itch through central summation (Herndon, 1982; Porth, 1994). Almost anything in the internal or external environment can cause pruritus. Insects, animals, plants, fabrics, metals, medications, allergies, and even emotional distress are among the most common causes. Pruritus also may occur as a secondary manifestation of systemic disorders, such as certain types of cancer, diabetes mellitus, hepatic disease, and renal failure.

Although the exact physiology is unknown, it is known that pruritus is triggered by heat and prostaglandins and that it is increased by histamine and morphine.

Pathophysiology

The pathophysiologic response of pruritus to stimulation or irritation follows a similar pathway, regardless of cause. The irritating agent stimulates receptors in the junction between the epidermis and dermis, and may also trigger the release of histamine and other chemical mediators that either further stimulate or mediate the itch response. The response of the person experiencing the itch is to scratch or rub the affected area. This may irritate the skin and cause further inflammation, which in turn sets off a cycle of increasingly intense itching and scratching, called the itch-scratch-itch cycle.

The secondary effects of pruritus include skin excoriation, *erythema* (redness of the skin), *wheals*, changes in pigmentation, and infections. Pruritus that persists may interrupt sleep patterns, because the itching sensation is often more intense at night. Long-term pruritus may be debilitating and increases the risk of infection as excoriation occurs.

Collaborative Care

Management of pruritus focuses on identifying and eliminating the cause. The nurse records the client's subjective description of the extent, location, and times of maximum intensity of the pruritus. A complete assessment, as described in Chapter 16, is essential.

Laboratory and Diagnostic Tests

Pruritus is a subjective experience; therefore, the diagnosis is based on the client's report of an itching sensation. However, the following diagnostic tests may be conducted to identify the causative agent:

- *Culture and sensitivity of skin scrapings* are conducted for microscopic examination to distinguish pruritus from psoriasis, dermatitis, and other disorders.
- *Studies for fungal infections* may be done, especially if the pruritus is reported in the anogenital area, the palms of the hands, or the soles of the feet.
- *Cutaneous patch testing* (see Chapter 8) may be performed if hypersensitivity reactions are the suspected cause.

Pharmacology

If possible, the client discontinues all medications to determine whether the pruritus is due to a drug reaction. Chemically unrelated drugs may be substituted.

Pharmacologic treatments for pruritus include both oral and topical agents. Oral medications include antihistamines, tranquilizers, and antibiotics. Antihistamines have provided relief from pruritus in some clients. Tranquilizers provide sedation, which may in turn relieve the emotional stress associated with pruritus; however, eliminating the stressors produces a more successful result. Systemic antibiotics are used to treat the infection resulting from the scratching and excoriation.

Topical medications that contain corticosteroids are often used to relieve the pruritus and inflammation. Topical medications may also be administered through therapeutic baths or soaks with agents that relieve pruritus, such as cornstarch and baking soda or coal tar concentrates.

Nursing Implications for Pharmacology: Therapeutic Baths

AGENTS USED IN THERAPEUTIC BATHS

Saline or tap water

Antibacterial agents: Potassium permanganate, acetic acid, hexachlorophene

Colloid substances: Oatmeal (Aveeno), cornstarch, sodium bicarbonate

Coal tar derivatives: Balnetar, Zetar, Polytar

Potassium permanganate

Emollients: Alpha-Keri, Lubath, mineral oil

Therapeutic baths have a variety of uses in treating skin disorders. Depending on the agent used, therapeutic baths soothe the skin, lower the skin bacteria count, clean and hydrate the skin, loosen scales, and relieve itching.

Nursing Responsibilities

- Ensure that the bath water is at a comfortable temperature that is neither too hot nor too cool (usually 110 to 115 F [43 to 46 C]).
- Fill the tub one-third to one-half full.
- Mix the agent well with the water.

- Assist the client into and out of the tub to prevent falls.
- Dry the client by blotting with the towel.

Client and Family Teaching

- Use a bath mat in the tub; the medications may cause the tub to become slippery.
- Keep the bathroom warm but adequately ventilated.
- Follow directions carefully for the amount of medication to use in the bath.
- Fill the bath one-third to one-half full of water that is at a comfortable temperature.
- Stay in the bath for 20 to 30 minutes, and immerse the areas to be treated.
- Do not get the bathwater in your eyes.
- Dry by blotting (not rubbing) with the towel.
- If the medications cause staining, use old towels or linens.
- If the itching is not relieved or the skin becomes excessively dry, call your health care provider.

Creams containing a topical anesthetic or antibiotic may also be used. Therapeutic baths are discussed in the accompanying box. Table 17–1 lists types of topical agents commonly used to treat skin disorders.

Nursing Care

Nursing care for the client with pruritus focuses on promoting comfort and decreasing the risk of infection. The following guidelines serve as a base for individualized interventions:

- Administer medications or therapeutic baths as prescribed.
  a. Apply creams and gels by rubbing them into the skin, wearing disposable gloves as appropriate.
  b. Apply pastes and ointments either by hand (wearing gloves as appropriate) or with a wooden tongue depressor.
- Maintain a comfortable room temperature; excessively warm environmental temperatures may increase pruritus.
- Monitor for skin excoriation and manifestations of infection.

- Monitor effects of therapeutic baths and topical medications.

  Nursing diagnoses to consider include the following:

- *Risk for Infection* related to excoriation from scratching with fingernails
- *Powerlessness* related to inability to control pruritus
- *Sleep pattern disturbance* related to nighttime pruritus

Client and Family Teaching

Teaching the client and family focuses on decreasing the pruritus to improve comfort and on decreasing the risk of infection. Most often, the client and family manage pruritus in the home setting; teaching is therefore an important aspect of care.

The client and family should be taught how to take the therapeutic bath and/or how to apply topical medications. Recommend that the nails be trimmed short, the environmental temperatures be slightly cool, and loose clothing be worn. Other suggestions for relieving pruritus and decreasing the risk of infection follow:

- Rub the pruritic area with the surface of the hand rather than scratching with the nails.

Table 17–1	Medications Used to Treat Skin Disorders	
Type	**Use**	**Examples**
Creams	Moisturize the skin	Aquacare Curel Nutraderm
Ointments	Lubricate the skin Retard water loss	Aquaphor Vaseline
Lotions	Moisturize the skin Lubricate the skin	Alpha-Keri Dermassage Lubriderm
Anesthetics	Relieve itching	Xylocaine
Antibiotics	Treat infection	Bacitracin Polysporin Gentamicin Silvadene
Corticosteroids	Suppress inflammation Relieve itching	Dexamethasone Hydrocortisone Clocortolone Desonide

- A brief application of pressure or cold may relieve pruritus.
- Cotton gloves may be worn at night if scratching during sleep causes skin excoriation.
- Distraction or relaxation techniques may prove helpful.
- Wash clothing in a mild detergent and rinse twice; do not use fabric softeners.
- Avoid using perfumes and lotions containing alcohol.
- Apply skin lubricants after a bath to help retain moisture.

The Client with Dry Skin

■ ■ ■

Dry skin, also called **xerosis**, may occur at any age, but it is most often a problem in the older adult (Figure 17–1). In this population, xerosis commonly results from a decrease in the activity of sebaceous and sweat glands, which reduces the skin's lubrication and moisture retention. However, dry skin may occur at any age from exposure to environmental heat and low humidity, sunlight, excessive bathing, and a decreased intake of liquids.

Two types of severe dry skin are xeroderma and ichthyosis. *Xeroderma* is a chronic skin condition characterized by dry, rough skin. *Ichthyosis* is an inherited dermatologic condition in which the skin is dry, fissured, and

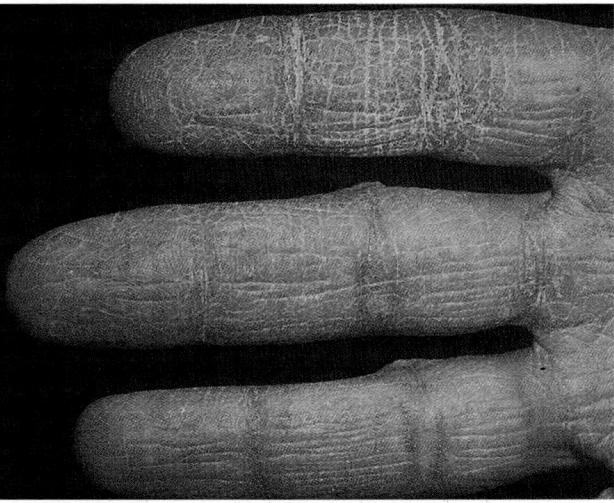

Figure 17–1   Severe xerosis, or dry skin, produces dry, rough skin with visible flaking of the skin surface.

hyperkeratotic; the surface of the skin has the appearance of fish scales.

The primary manifestation of dry skin is pruritus. Other manifestations include visible flaking of surface skin and an observable pattern of fine lines over the area. If the skin has been excessively dry and puritic for a long period, the client may have secondary skin lesions and lichenification (thickening).

Nursing care focuses on teaching the client and family how to reduce the dry skin and relieve the pruritus (see the preceding section). General guidelines for teaching the client and family to reduce dry skin follow:

- Soaps and hot water are drying. Clean the skin with tepid water and either a mild soap or cleansing creams. If soap is used, rinse it off carefully.
- It is not necessary to take a bath every day.
- If bath oils are used, add them to the bath water at the end of the bath (the moist skin is more likely to retain the oil). Use care not to slip in the tub.
- Use a humidifier to humidify the air.
- Apply creams and lotions when the skin is slightly damp after bathing.
- Increase oral intake of fluids.

The Client with Psoriasis

■ ■ ■

Psoriasis is a chronic, noninfectious skin disorder that is characterized by raised, reddened, round circumscribed plaques covered by silvery white scales (Figure 17–2). The size of these lesions varies. The lesions may appear anywhere on the body; however, they are most commonly

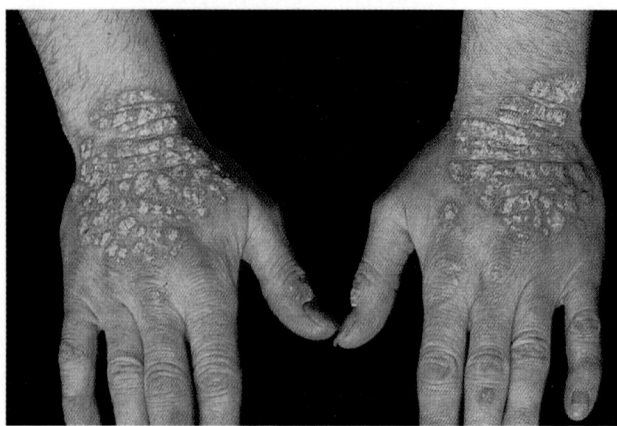

Figure 17–2 The characteristic lesions of psoriasis are raised, red, round plaques covered with thick, silvery scales.

found on the scalp, extensor surfaces of the arms and legs, elbows, knees, sacrum, and around the nails. The characteristic lesions in psoriasis are well-demarcated regions of erythematous plaques that shed thick gray flakes. As with any chronic illness, the skin manifestations may occur and disappear throughout life, with no discernible pattern to the recurrence.

The actual cause is unknown, but some evidence suggests psoriasis may be an autoimmune disorder. Sunlight, stress, seasonal changes, hormone fluctuations, steroid withdrawal, and certain drugs (such as alcohol, corticosteroids, lithium and chloroquine) appear to exacerbate the disorder. About one-third of clients have a family history of psoriasis. Trauma to the skin from such events as surgery, sunburn, or excoriation is also a common precipitating factor; lesions that result from trauma are called *Koebner's reaction* (Porth, 1994).

The disease affects about 1% of the population of the United States (Porth, 1994). The incidence is lower in warm, sunny climates. Onset usually occurs in the 20s, but it may occur at any age. Psoriasis occurs more often in Caucasians. Men and women are affected equally.

Pathophysiology

Normally, the keratinocyte (an epidermal cell making up 95% of the epidermis) migrates from the basal cell to the stratum corneum (the outer skin layer) in about 14 days and is sloughed off 14 days later. Psoriatic skin cells, by contrast, have a shorter cycle of growth, completing the journey to the stratum corneum in only 4 to 7 days, a condition called *hyperkeratosis*. These immature cells produce an abnormal keratin that forms thick, flaky scales at the surface of the skin. The increased cell metabolism stimulates increased vascularity, which contributes to the erythema of the lesions.

Various forms of psoriasis exist:

- *Psoriasis vulgaris* is the most common form of psoriasis. The lesions can be found anywhere on the skin but most commonly involve the skin over the elbows, knees, and scalp. Initially, the lesions are papules that form into erythematous plaques with thick, silvery scales. The plaques bleed when removed (Auspitz sign). The plaques in darker-skinned persons may appear purple. Psoriasis vulgaris requires specialized, long-term management such as that available at a psoriasis treatment center.

- *Guttate (drop-like)* or *eruptive psoriasis* is more common in people with early onset of the disease. The lesions are smaller than those seen in psoriasis vulgaris and usually appear on the upper trunk and extremities. This form may appear a few weeks after a streptococcal respiratory infection and may resolve spontaneously.

- *Pustular psoriasis* is a form of the disease that is manifested by the eruption of pustules and a fever. The pustules are found over the trunk and extremities and may appear on the palms of the hands, the nail beds, and the soles of the feet.

- *Psoriatic erythroderma (exfoliative psoriasis)* affects all body surfaces and is characterized by generalized scaling and erythema without lesions.

- *Psoriasis annularis* is a rare form characterized by annular (ring-shaped) lesions with a clear center.

- *Psoriatic arthritis* is a form of arthritis associated with psoriatic lesions of the skin and nails. The lesions are typically found at the distal interphalangeal joints of the fingers and toes.

Clinical manifestations of psoriasis vary according to the form of the disease, as described above. Pruritus is common over the lesions. If the lesions are located in an intertriginous zone, such as between the toes, under the breasts, or in the perianal region, the psoriatic scales may soften, allowing painful fissures to form.

When psoriasis affects the nails, pitting and a yellow or brown discoloration results. The nail may separate from the nail bed, thicken, and crumble. The involved nails, which are more often fingernails than toenails, are at high risk for infection.

The client may experience physical and psychologic pain from the pruritus and the appearance of the lesions, especially if they are widespread.

Permanent remission of psoriasis is rare. The prognosis depends on the type, extent, and severity of the initial attack. The age of onset is also a factor; early-onset disease is usually more severe.

Collaborative Care

Treatment modalities are based on the type of psoriasis, the extent and location of the lesions, the age of the client, and the degree of disfigurement or disability.

Laboratory and Diagnostic Tests

The diagnosis of psoriasis typically is made by examination of the characteristic type and location of lesions. Other diagnostic studies follow:

- *Skin biopsy* may be done if the client presents with atypical manifestations, or to differentiate psoriasis from other inflammatory or infectious skin disorders.
- *Ultrasonography* may be performed to measure skin thickness; results reveal typical psoriatic changes in the stratum corneum and dermal inflammation (Stiller et al., 1994).

Pharmacology

A variety of different pharmacologic treatments may be prescribed for the client with psoriasis, including topical medications and photochemotherapy. Although there is no cure, treatment decreases the severity and pain of the lesions.

Topical medications are administered to decrease inflammation, prolong the maturity time of keratinocytes, and increase remission time. Corticosteroids, tar preparations, anthralin, and the retinoids are typically used.

Topical corticosteroids decrease inflammation, suppress mitotic activity of psoriatic cells, and delay the movement of keratinocytes to the surface of the skin (thus giving them time to mature and decreasing hyperkeratinosis). The most effective topical corticosteroids are potent preparations that are well absorbed through the skin and are used under an occlusive dressing. Corticosteroids may also be taken systemically or injected directly into the lesions.

Tar preparations suppress mitotic activity and are also anti-inflammatory. Their exact mechanism of action is unknown, but they are effective in removing scales and increasing remission time. Preparations made of coal tar are messy, cause staining, and have an unpleasant odor, but they are an effective form of treatment.

Topical anthralin (dithranol) inhibits the mitotic activity of epidermal cells and is effective in some cases of chronic, localized psoriasis that do not respond to other topical agents. The medication is applied to the plaque patches at bedtime and left in place for 8 to 12 hours. Clients should be tested for sensitivity to the drug before it is used, and it should not be applied to inflamed or open areas of skin.

The retinoids, such as tretinoin (Retin-A) appear to inhibit keratinization. They are applied topically, and erythema and peeling are expected. Beneficial effects usually appear in 2 to 6 weeks.

Photochemotherapy

Photochemotherapy is the preferred treatment modality for severe psoriasis (Porth, 1994). A light-activated form of the drug methotrexate-methoxsalen (8-MOP) is used. This drug is an antimetabolite that inhibits DNA synthesis and thereby prevents cell mitosis, decreasing hyperkeratosis. Exposure to ultraviolet-A (UVA) rays activates 8-MOP; it is administered orally, and the client is exposed to UVA 2 hours later. Treatments are administered 2 to 3 times a week; usually, 10 to 20 total treatments are given over 1 to 2 months. The eyes are covered by dark glasses during the treatment. Treatment causes tanning, and direct sunlight must be avoided for 8 to 12 hours thereafter. If the client exhibits erythema, the treatments are stopped until the redness and swelling resolve.

Photochemotherapy has had a high success rate in achieving remission of psoriasis, but it can accelerate aging of exposed skin, induce cataract development, and alter immune function. The drug may also cause pruritus, erythema, and blisters.

Ultraviolet Light Therapy

Ultraviolet-B (UVB) light is often used to treat psoriasis. UVB light decreases the growth rate of epidermal cells, thereby decreasing hyperkeratosis. Exposure to sunlight provides ultraviolet light, but because the timing and amount are unpredictable, artificial light sources of UVB are more commonly used. Mercury vapor lights or fluorescent UV tubes provide the UVB light; the latter are often arranged in a cabinet so the client can stand and expose psoriatic lesions more easily. These units may be purchased or constructed to be used in the client's home.

The light therapy is administered in gradually increasing exposure times, until the client experiences a mild erythema, like a mild sunburn. Treatments are given daily and are measured in seconds of exposure. The eyes are shielded during the treatment. The erythema response occurs in about 8 hours. Careful assessment is necessary to prevent more severe burning, which could exacerbate the psoriasis.

In clients with extensive psoriasis, UVB treatments may be combined with tar preparations, which increase the photosensitivity of the skin; this is called Goeckerman's treatment.

Nursing Care

The client with psoriasis requires nursing care to meet physical and psychologic responses to the illness. The nursing interventions discussed in this section focus on common problems of the client with psoriasis: impaired skin integrity and body image disturbance. The client also experiences problems with pruritus, which may evolve into chronic pain. (Nursing interventions for pruritus were discussed earlier in the chapter.)

Impaired Skin Integrity

The client with typical psoriatic skin lesions has impaired skin integrity that may range from a few scaly lesions to open, bleeding areas. These lesions increase the risk of infection, which can further compromise healing. In addition, certain treatments (for example, the use of UVA or retinoids) may cause erythema or peeling of the skin, further altering skin integrity.

Nursing interventions with rationales follow:

- Demonstrate methods to reduce injury to the skin when taking therapeutic baths or treatments:
  a. Use warm, not hot, water.
  b. Gently rub lesions with a soft washcloth, using a circular motion.
  c. Dry the skin with a soft towel, using a blotting or patting motion.
  d. Keep the skin lubricated at all times.
  Hot water and dry skin increase pruritus, further stimulating the itch-scratch-itch cycle. Dry skin also causes psoriasis to become worse. Washing or drying the skin with rough linens or pressure may excoriate the skin over the psoriatic lesions.

- Demonstrate application of topical medications:
  a. Apply the medication as prescribed in a thin layer, using hands (gloved, if appropriate), wooden tongue depressors, or a gauze pad.
  b. Avoid getting medications in the eyes, on mucous membranes, or in skinfolds.
  c. Apply a covering (occlusive dressing) over the medicated areas as prescribed, especially when using corticosteroids. Usually, the covering is applied for only 12 hours, often during the evening and night hours. Choose some type of plastic wrap that covers the area well.
  Applying a thin layer of medication more frequently is often more effective than applying a single thick layer of medication. The medications used to treat psoriasis may irritate the eyes and mucous membranes; when applied in skinfolds, they may also cause maceration (skin breakdown due to prolonged exposure to moisture). Topical corticosteroids are often covered with occlusive dressing to increase absorption and thus facilitate treatment. However, constant occlusion may increase the effects of the medications to undesired levels and also increases the risk for infections.

- Teach the client and family the manifestations of infection and how to contact the health care provider if these occur. Teach them to watch for elevated temperature; increased swelling, redness, or pain; increase in drainage; and any change in the color of the drainage. *The client with skin lesions is at high risk for infection, because the skin is the body's first line of defense.*

- Teach the client and family to assess for the complications of treatment: excoriation, increased erythema, increased peeling, blister formation. *The medications or treatments may cause cellular damage through chemical burns or excessive exposure to ultraviolet light. Times and methods of treatment need to be adjusted if these manifestations occur.*

Body Image Disturbance

The obvious skin lesions that accompany psoriasis often cause clients to isolate themselves from social contacts, withdraw from normal roles and responsibilities, and feel helpless or powerless.

Nursing interventions with rationales follow:

- Establish a trusting relationship by expressing acceptance of the client, both verbally and nonverbally. For example, touch the client during social communications, demonstrating that the lesions are not contagious and are not offensive. *One's body image is affected not only by self-perception but also by the responses of others. Nonjudgmental acceptance helps the client adapt to the change in body image. By touching the client during interactions, the nurse demonstrates that acceptance.*

- Encourage the client to verbalize feelings about self-perception in view of the chronic nature of psoriasis and to ask questions about the disease and treatment. *The client adapts to a changed body image through a process of recognition, acceptance, and resolution. Each person responds individually to disfigurement and loss; the nurse assesses the client's perceptions and knowledge base before initiating interventions.*

- Promote social interaction through family involvement in care, referral to support groups of people with psoriasis or other chronic skin conditions, and referral to the National Psoriasis Foundation. *Acceptance by others is critical to acceptance of self. The treatment of psoriasis is lifelong, time consuming, and often unappealing. By becoming involved in care, the family communicates acceptance. Sharing experiences with others who have the same health problem is a source of strength in adjusting to a visible, chronic illness. The National Psoriasis Foundation can provide information about resources and treatments (see Appendix O).*

Other Nursing Diagnoses

The following nursing diagnoses may also be appropriate for the client with psoriasis:

- *Risk for Infection* related to open lesions
- *Anxiety* related to unknown progression of the disease
- *Fatigue* related to interruption of sleep from pruritus
- *Sleep Pattern Disturbance* related to chronic pruritus
- *Social Isolation* related to presence of skin lesions
- *Powerlessness* related to inability to control exacerbations of psoriatic lesions

Client and Family Teaching

Client and family teaching is geared primarily to self-care at home and focuses on treatments and skin care needs. Educate the client about the chronic nature of the disease, factors that may precipitate an exacerbation, and methods

---

General Guidelines for Applying Topical Medications

■ ■ ■

Each time a medication is applied, the skin surface must be clean and dry. Remove the medication from the previous application: Remove creams by washing the skin with tap water; remove ointments by washing the skin first with mineral oil and then with a mild soap and water.

- To apply gels, creams, and pastes: Squeeze about ½ to 1 inch of the gel or cream into the palm of the hand. Rub the hands together until they are covered. Apply gels and creams to the affected areas with long strokes until the skin is thinly covered. Differences from these general guidelines follow:
  a. Corticosteroids are usually applied two to three times a day in small amounts and rubbed directly onto the lesions. Apply the medication after a bath and cover with an occlusive dressing.
  b. Apply medications containing tar in the direction of hair growth. Do not apply these medications to the face, to the genitals, or in skinfolds. If the tar is water based or oil based, it will stain clothing.
  c. Anthralin stains; wear gloves when applying the medication.

- To apply lotions: Shake the bottle of lotion well. Pour a small amount into the palm of the hand, and pat the medication onto the skin. If the lotion is thin, apply it with a gauze pad.

- To apply sprays: Hold the container about 6 inches from the skin, and apply the medication in a short spray.

- To apply medicated shampoo: Rinse out medication from the previous application. Apply the shampoo, massage into the hair and over the scalp carefully, and allow it to remain for the prescribed time. Rinse.

- To apply pastes: Use enough paste on an applicator (such as a wooden tongue depressor) to cover the lesion thinly.

---

to reduce stress. Discuss the nursing interventions for pruritus, dry skin, and specific care for psoriasis. Also provide the following instructions:

- Eat a healthy, well-balanced diet (and, if the client is overweight, one that is also low in calories).
- Avoid cold or hot temperatures.
- Practice relaxation techniques to reduce stress.
- Get adequate rest and regular exercise.
- Expose the skin to sunlight, but avoid sunburn.
- Avoid trauma to the skin; for example, do not scrub off scales, and use only an electric razor.

- Avoid exposure to contagious illnesses, such as influenza and colds.

- Discuss current medications with the physician. Certain drugs (such as indomethacin, lithium, and beta-adrenergic blocking agents) are known to precipitate exacerbations of psoriasis.

Supply written instructions to help the client and family to provide care, and ensure that a resource person is available to answer questions. The accompanying box outlines general guidelines for teaching clients to apply topical medications.

▪▪▪ Infections and Infestations ▪▪▪

The skin's resistance to infections and infestations is provided by protective mechanisms, including skin flora, sebum, and the immune response. Although the skin is normally resistant to infections and infestations, adults of all ages can experience these disorders as a result of a break in the skin surface, a virulent agent, and/or decreased resistance due to a compromised immune system. This section discusses the various skin disorders resulting from bacterial infections, fungal infections, parasitic infestations, and viral infections.

The Client with a Bacterial Infection of the Skin

■ ■ ■

A number of bacteria, or flora, normally inhabit the skin. Most do not cause an infection. However, when a break in the skin allows invasion by pathogenic bacteria, an infection, called a **pyoderma**, may occur. The most common bacterial infections are caused by gram-positive *Staphylococcus aureus* and beta-hemolytic streptococci.

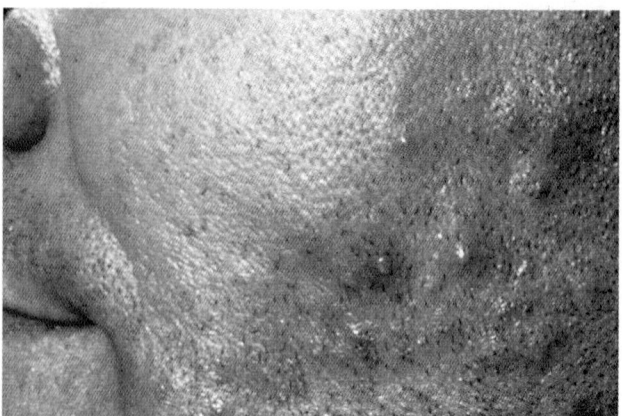

Figure 17–3 The lesions of folliculitis are pustules surrounded by areas of erythema.

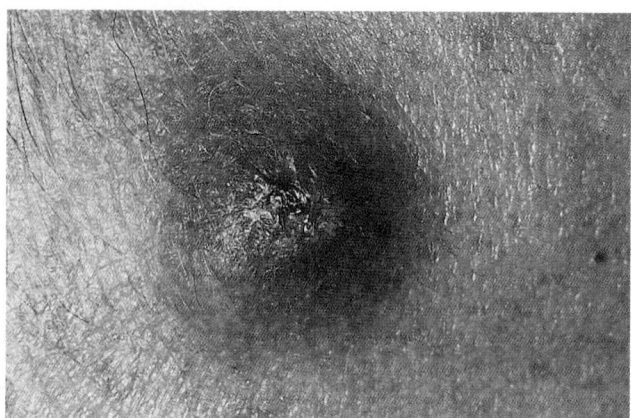

Figure 17–4 A furuncle (or boil) is a deep, firm, red, painful nodule.

Bacterial infections of the skin may be primary or secondary. Primary infections are caused by a single pathogen and arise from normal skin; secondary infections develop in skin that is traumatized or diseased.

Most bacterial infections are treated by a primary care provider, and the client remains at home for care. However, if the infection becomes more serious, inpatient care is required. In addition, nosocomial infections of wounds or open lesions in hospitalized clients are often the result of bacterial infections, especially by methicillin-resistant *Staphylococcus aureus* (MRSA).

Pathophysiology

Bacterial infections of the skin arise from the hair follicle, where bacteria can accumulate and grow and cause a localized infection. However, the bacteria can invade deeper tissues and cause a systemic infection, a potentially life threatening disorder.

There are various types of bacterial infections of the skin, including folliculitis, furuncles, carbuncles, cellulitis, erysipelas, and impetigo.

Folliculitis

Folliculitis is a bacterial infection of the hair follicle, most commonly caused by *Staphylococcus aureus*. The infection begins at the follicle opening and extends down into the follicle. The bacteria release enzymes and chemical agents that cause an inflammation. The lesions appear as pustules surrounded by an area of erythema on the surface of the skin (Figure 17–3). Folliculitis is found most often on the scalp and extremities. It is also often seen on the face of bearded men (called *sycosis barbae*), on the legs of women who shave, and on the eyelids (called a *stye*). Although folliculitis may appear without any apparent cause, contributing factors include poor hygiene, poor nutrition, prolonged skin moisture, and trauma to the skin.

Furuncles

Furuncles, often called boils, are also inflammations of the hair follicle. They often begin as folliculitis, but the infection spreads down the hair shaft, through the wall of the follicle, and into the dermis. The causative organism is commonly *Staphylococcus aureus*. A furuncle is initially a deep, firm, red, painful nodule from 1 to 5 cm in diameter (Figure 17–4). After a few days, the nodule changes into a large, tender cystic nodule. The cysts may drain substantial amounts of purulent drainage.

One or more furuncles may occur on any part of the body that has hair. Contributing factors include poor hygiene, trauma to the skin, areas of excessive moisture (including perspiration), and systemic diseases, such as diabetes mellitus and hematologic malignancies.

Carbuncles

A **carbuncle** is a group of infected hair follicles. The lesion begins as a firm mass located in the subcutaneous tissue and the lower dermis. This mass becomes swollen and painful and has multiple openings to the skin surface.

Carbuncles are most frequently found on the back of the neck, the upper back, and the lateral thighs. In addition to the local manifestations, the client may experience chills, fever, and malaise.

The contributing factors for carbuncles are the same as for furuncles. Both infections are more common in hot, humid climates.

Cellulitis

Cellulitis is a localized infection of the dermis and subcutaneous tissue. Cellulitis can occur following a wound or skin ulcer or as an extension of furuncles or carbuncles. The infection spreads as a result of a substance called spreading factor (hyaluronidase). This factor, which is produced by the causative organism, breaks down the fibrin network and other barriers that normally localize the infection.

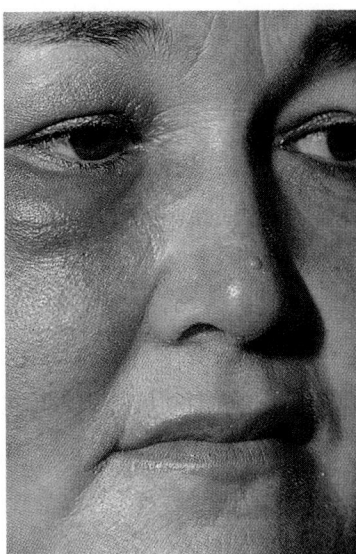

Figure 17–5   Cellulitis is a bacterial infection localized in the dermis and subcutaneous tissue. The involved area is red, swollen, and painful.

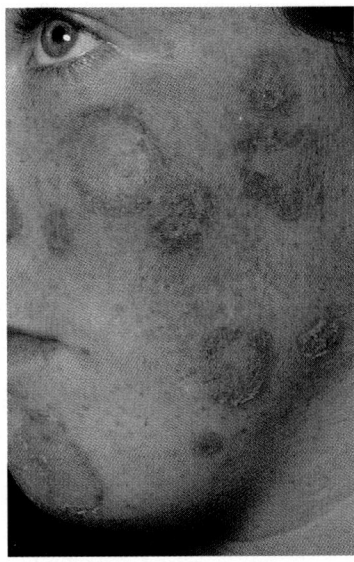

Figure 17–6   Impetigo is characterized by red, macular lesions as well as broken, crusted vesicles.

The area of cellulitis is red, swollen, and painful (Figure 17–5). In some cases, vesicles may form over the area of cellulitis. The client may also experience fever, chills, malaise, headache, and swollen lymph glands.

Erysipelas

Erysipelas is an infection of the skin most often caused by group A streptococci. Chills, fever, and malaise are prodromal symptoms, occurring from 4 hours to 20 days before the skin lesion appears. The initial infection appears as firm, red spots that enlarge and join to form a circumscribed, bright red, raised, hot lesion. Vesicles may form over the surface of the erysipelas lesion. The area usually is painful, itches, and burns.

Erysipelas most commonly appears on the face, the ears, and the lower legs.

Impetigo

Impetigo is an infection of the skin caused by either *Staphylococcus aureus* or beta-hemolytic streptococci. Impetigo typically begins with a vesicle or pustule. This lesion ruptures, leaving an open area that discharges a honey-colored serous liquid that hardens into a crust (Figure 17–6). Within hours, more vesicles form. The pruritus that accompanies the eruptions causes scratching and excoriation, which spreads the infection. This disease occasionally occurs in adults but is much more common in children.

Collaborative Care

The diagnosis of a bacterial infection of the skin is made by assessing the appearance of the lesion and by identify-ing the causative organism. Antibiotics specific to the organism are used in treatment.

Laboratory and Diagnostic Tests

- Culture and sensitivity of the drainage from the lesion may be conducted to identify the organism and to target the most effective antibiotics.

- If the infection is systemic, a blood culture may be conducted to identify a causative organism.

- People who experience repeated bacterial skin infections, or who provide care for others who exhibit infections, may have a culture taken from the external nares to determine whether they are carriers of bacteria (for example, MSRA) and are reinfecting themselves or others.

Pharmacology

The primary treatment for bacterial infections of the skin is an antibiotic specific to the organism. The antibiotic is usually taken systemically and may also be applied topically. Multiple furuncles and carbuncles may be treated with cloxacillin (a penicillinase-resistant penicillin); the cephalosporins also are often effective.

Nursing Care

Nursing care of the client with a bacterial infection of the skin focuses on preventing the spread of infection and restoring normal skin integrity. Most clients provide self-care at home, but the incidence of secondary bacterial infections in the inpatient population is great enough to warrant their inclusion in planning and implementing care.

The nurse assesses the client for any increase in infection, which may be manifested systemically by fever, tachycardia, chills, and malaise. Local manifestations of the spread of the infection include an increase in erythema, the size of the lesion, and drainage. This assessment is especially important for clients who are older, debilitated, or immunosuppressed and for those who have large and/or dirty wounds.

The hospitalized client should be placed on isolation precautions to limit the spread of the organisms to other patients. All health care providers and visitors follow the procedures and protocols of the institution exactly to prevent cross-contamination.

One of the most effective methods to reduce the spread of infection both in and out of the hospital setting is careful hand washing. Health care providers must wash their hands with soap and water before and after client care and between each client contact. All clients, family members, and visitors (both in the home and hospital setting) should be taught the importance of hand washing, but it is even more important for the client with a bacterial infection.

Stress the importance of bathing daily with an antibacterial soap. The client can gently wash off crusts during the bath. Warm compresses may be applied to the lesions two to three times a day to increase comfort and decrease swelling.

Cover draining lesions with a sterile dressing, and handle soiled dressings or linens according to universal precautions. When changing dressings, always wear disposable rubber gloves and masks.

Nursing diagnoses that may be appropriate for the client with a bacterial infection of the skin follow:

- *Body Image Disturbance* related to presence of multiple furuncles on face and neck
- *Pain* related to large area of cellulitis
- *Anxiety* related to repeated infections

Client and Family Teaching

Client and family teaching focuses on facilitating tissue healing and eliminating the infection. Stress the importance of maintaining good nutrition and maintaining cleanliness through careful hand washing and proper handling and disposal of dressings. To prevent the spread of infection in the home, teach the client not to share linens and towels and to wash clothing and linens in hot water.

Teach the client with an infection never to squeeze or try to open a bacterial lesion. To prevent infections, teach the client to clean the skin and keep it dry, especially in hot weather, and to avoid plucking nasal hair or picking the nose.

Also teach the client and family members the importance of taking the full course of prescribed antibiotics on a regular schedule until the prescribed supply is finished.

The Client with a Fungal Infection of the Skin

■ ■ ■

Fungi are free-living plantlike organisms that live in the soil, on animals, and on humans. The fungi that cause superficial skin infections are called **dermatophytes.** In humans, the dermatophytes live on keratin in the stratum corneum, hair, and nails. Fungal disorders are also called *mycoses.*

Fungal infections of the skin are common disorders that most people experience at some time in their lives. The disorders discussed in this section are dermatophyte infections and candidiasis infections.

Pathophysiology

The superficial fungal infections of the skin are called *dermatophytoses* or, more commonly, *ringworm* or *tinea*. The deep fungal infections involve the dermis, epidermis, and subcutaneous tissue.

Fungal infections occur when a susceptible host comes in contact with the organism. The organism may be transmitted by direct contact with animals or other infected persons or by inanimate objects such as combs, pillowcases, towels, and hats. The most important factor in the development of the infection is moisture; the onset and spread of the fungal infection is greatest in areas where moisture content is high, such as within skinfolds, between the toes, and in the mouth. Other factors that increase the risk of a fungal infection include the use of broad-spectrum antibiotics that kill off normal flora and allow the fungi to grow, the presence of diabetes mellitus, immunodeficiencies, nutritional deficiencies, pregnancy, increasing age, and iron deficiency.

Fungal infections of the skin are more common in warm, humid climates. Some tinea infections are gender specific.

Dermatophyte (Tinea) Infections

The dermatophyte (tinea) infections are named by the body part affected:

- *Tinea pedis* is a fungal infection of the soles of the feet, the space between the toes, and/or the toenail (Figure 17–7). More often called *athlete's foot*, this is the most common tinea infection. The lesions vary from mild scaliness to painful fissures with drainage, and they are usually accompanied by pruritus and a foul odor. The

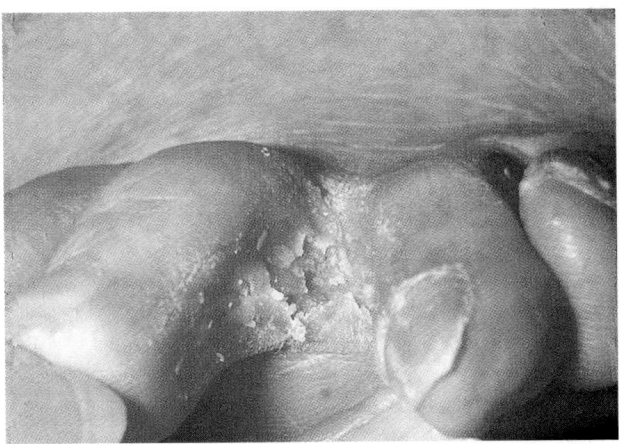

Figure 17–7 Tinea pedis (athlete's foot) is a fungal infection that often occurs between the toes.

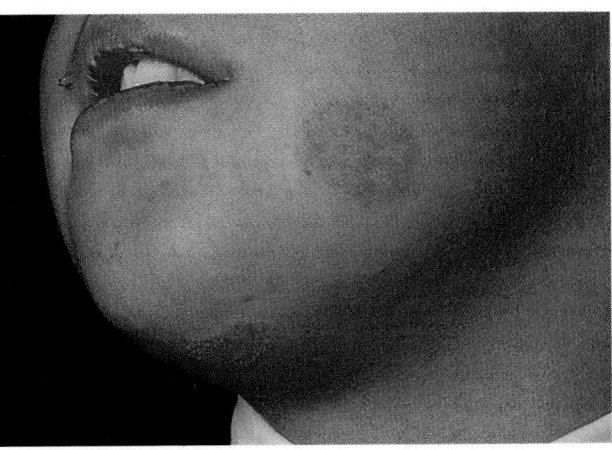

Figure 17–9 Tinea corporis commonly causes large, circular lesions with raised red borders.

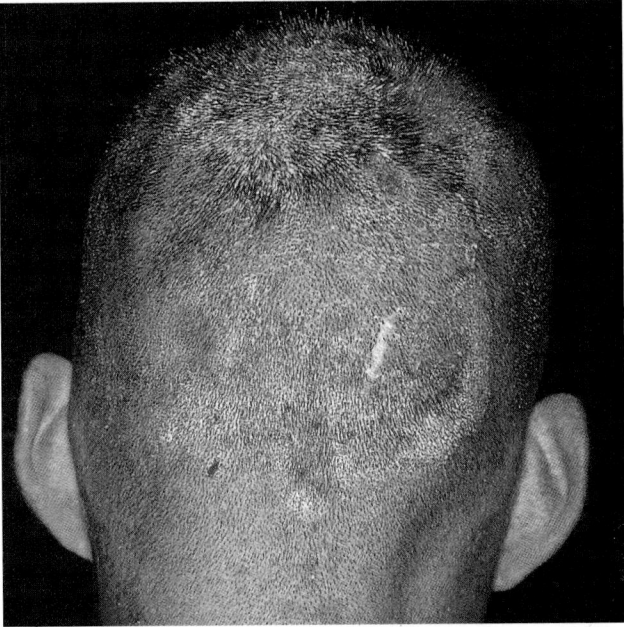

Figure 17–8 Tinea capitis is a fungal infection of the scalp that causes erythema, crusting, and hair loss.

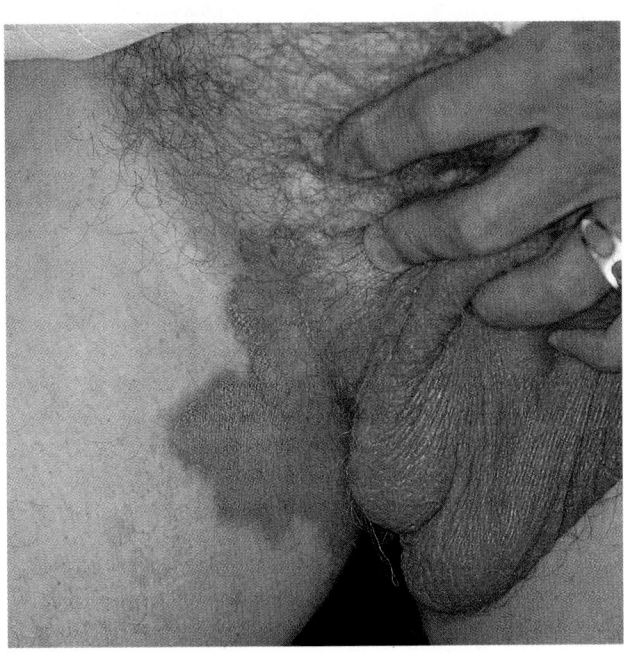

Figure 17–10 Tinea cruris (jock itch) is a fungal infection of the groin and inner thighs.

infection is often chronic, reappearing in hot weather, when perspiring feet are encased in shoes.

- *Tinea capitis* is a fungal infection of the scalp (called ringworm of the scalp). The primary lesions are gray, round, bald spots, often accompanied by erythema and crusting (Figure 17–8). The hair loss is usually temporary. Tinea capitis is seen more often in children than in adults.

- *Tinea corporis* is a fungal infection of the body (called ringworm of the body). It can be caused by several different fungi, and the lesions vary according to the

causative organism. The most common lesions are large circular patches with raised red borders of vesicles, papules, or pustules (Figure 17–9). Pruritus and erythema are also present. This fungal infection can occur at any age, but it affects children primarily.

- *Tinea cruris* is a fungal infection of the groin that may extend to the inner thighs and buttocks (Figure 17–10). Called ringworm of the groin or jock itch, it is often associated with tinea pedis and is more common in people who are physically active, are obese, and/or wear tight underclothing.

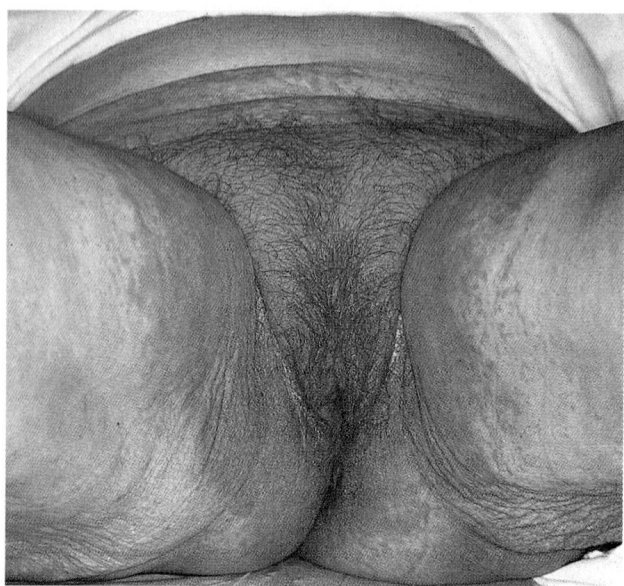

Figure 17–11 *Candida albicans,* a fungus, causes a skin infection characterized by erythema, pustules, and a typical white substance covering the area.

Candidiasis Infections

Candidiasis infections are caused by *Candida albicans,* a yeastlike fungus. This fungus is normally found on mucous membranes, on the skin, in the vagina, and in the gastrointestinal tract. The fungus becomes a pathogen when certain factors encourage its growth:

- A local environment of moisture, warmth, or altered skin integrity
- The administration of systemic antibiotics
- Pregnancy
- The use of birth control pills
- Poor nutrition
- The presence of diabetes mellitus, Cushing's disease, or other chronic debilitating illnesses
- Immunosuppression
- Some malignancies of the blood

Candidiasis affects only the outer layers of the skin and mucous membranes. It occurs in the mouth, vagina, uncircumcised penis, nails, and deep skinfolds.

The first sign of infection is a pustule that extends under the stratum corneum. The pustule has an inflamed base and often burns and itches. As the infection spreads, the accumulation of inflammatory cells and shedding of surface cells produce a white to yellow curdlike substance that covers the infected area (Figure 17–11). Satellite lesions are characteristic of candidiasis; these are maculopapular areas found outside the clearly demarcated border of the original infection. The appearance of the

Table 17–2	Characteristics of Candidiasis Infections by Location
Location	**Characteristics**
Skinfolds (under breasts, in groin, axillae, anus, umbilicus, and between toes or fingers)	Erythematous lesions that are either dry or moist. The lesions have clear borders, and satellite lesions are present.
Nails	Nail bed is red, swollen, and painful.
Mouth (*thrush*)	Mucous membranes are red and may be swollen; surface is covered with white, creamy material. Eroded areas may be present over the tongue and the oral cavity.
Penis (*balanitis*) (glans and shaft)	The penis is covered with small, red, clearly demarcated lesions that are painful and itch. The lesions may be covered with a white plaque.
Vagina	Red mucous membranes contain brighter red, demarcated, oozing lesions. The cervix may be covered with white plaque. A white, cheesy, foul-smelling vaginal discharge is present, accompanied by itching and burning. The vaginal and labial membranes may be swollen; the infection may extend to the anus and groin.

infection differs by location, as summarized in Table 17–2.

Collaborative Care

Fungal infections are primarily diagnosed in outpatient settings and treated at home by the client and family. However, fungal infections may also occur in hospitalized clients and require nursing care. The treatment is the same, regardless of the setting.

Laboratory and Diagnostic Tests

Diagnostic tests are conducted to determine the causative fungi and may include the following:

- Cultures of skin scrapings, nail scrapings, or hairs.
- Microscopic examination of scrapings from the lesions. The scrapings are prepared in a solution of 10% potassium hydroxide (KOH) to reveal more clearly the spores and filaments (hyphae) of each fungus.
- Observation of the skin under ultraviolet light (called a Wood's lamp). The fungal spores fluoresce blue-green.

Nursing Implications for Pharmacology: Antifungal Agents

ANTIFUNGAL AGENTS

Clotrimazole (Lotrimin, Mycelex, Gyne-Lotrimin)

Nystatin (Mycolog, Mycostatin, Nilstat)

Econazole (Spectazole)

Haloprogin (Halotex)

Miconazole (Monistat)

Undecylenic acid (Desenex)

Ketoconazole (Nizoral)

Fluconazole (Diflucan)

Griseofulvin (Fulvicin, Grisactin, Gris-PEG)

Antifungal medications are prepared in a variety of forms, depending on the specific drug: powders, creams, shampoos, suspensions, troches, vaginal suppositories, and oral tablets. Some drugs interfere with the permeability of the fungal cell membrane; others interfere with DNA synthesis. Most of these medications are fungistatic but in large doses they may be fungicidal.

Nursing Responsibilities

- When taking the health history, ask about known hypersensitivity reactions to these agents; document carefully.

- Assess for side effects: skin rash, local irritation, gastrointestinal symptoms (if given PO), and mental status.

- Administer ketoconazole with food to minimize gastrointestinal irritation.

- Shake suspensions well before administration, and ask the client to swish them around the mouth before swallowing.

- Tell the client to allow oral tablets to dissolve in the mouth.

Client and Family Teaching

- Therapy usually continues over a long period of time, but regular use of medications for the recommended period is necessary. Do not miss doses, and complete the full treatment.

- For griseofulvin: Take with meals or foods high in fat (such as ice cream) to avoid stomach upset and help with absorption. Avoid alcohol (which may cause rapid pulse and flushing) and exposure to sunlight (this drug causes increased sensitivity).

- For nystatin: Dissolve lozenges completely in the mouth. Hold suspensions in the mouth and swish throughout the mouth as long as possible before swallowing. Insert intravaginal medication high in the vagina. Continue with intravaginal applications throughout the menses.

- For antifungal shampoo: Use two times a week for 4 weeks, allowing at least 3 days between each shampoo. Wet hair, apply shampoo to produce lather, leave in place for 1 minute, then rinse. Apply shampoo a second time, lather, leave in place for 3 minutes, then rinse thoroughly.

- For topical application: Rub well into the affected areas, but do not get the medication in your eyes.

- For vaginal candidiasis infections: During therapy, refrain from sexual intercourse or advise partner to use a condom.

- Your sexual partner will need to be treated at the same time so that you do not pass the infection back and forth to each other.

Pharmacology

Fungal infections of the skin are treated by topical or systemic antifungal medications. Nursing implications for the antifungal medications are described in the accompanying pharmacology box.

The dermatophyte infections are treated differently, depending on the area of the body involved:

- Tinea capitis is treated by shampooing the hair two to three times a week, applying a topical antifungal to inactivate organisms on the hair, and taking griseofulvin, an antifungal agent, orally.

- Tinea pedis is treated by soaking the feet in Burrow's solution, potassium permanganate solution, or saline solution to remove crusts and scales. Topical antifungals are applied to the infected areas for several weeks.

- Mild cases of tinea cruris are treated with topical medications for 3 to 4 weeks. More severe cases may require oral griseofulvin.

Candidiasis infections are treated, depending on the location, with nystatin (Mycostatin) in powder, tablet, or vaginal suppository form. The antibiotic is effective in controlling the infection. Other medications include the antifungal agents ketoconazole and fluconazole, administered orally.

Nursing Care

Nursing care of the client with a fungal infection may take place in the hospital or may be done through teaching for home care. The interventions discussed for nursing care of the client with a bacterial infection are also appropriate for the client with a fungal infection.

Many people treat themselves with over-the-counter antifungal medications. It is recommended, however, that the person be diagnosed the first time through the health care system; if further symptoms reappear, self-treatment is usually satisfactory.

Client and Family Teaching

The nurse teaches the client and family how to manage care at home, providing the following information:

- Fungal diseases are contagious. Do not share linens or personal items with others.
- Use a clean towel and washcloth each day.
- Carefully dry all skinfolds, including those under the breasts, under the arms, and between the toes.
- Wear clean cotton underclothing each day.
- Fungi grow in moist environments, such as on sweaty feet. To prevent further infections:
  a. Do not wear the same pair of shoes every day.
  b. Wear cotton socks or hose with cotton feet.
  c. Put cotton balls between the toes.
  d. Do not wear rubber- or plastic-soled shoes.
  e. Use talcum powder or an over-the-counter antifungal powder twice a day.
- If you have a vaginal *Candida albicans* infection:
  a. Avoid tight clothing, such as jeans and pantyhose.
  b. Wear cotton or cotton-crotch underwear.
  c. Bathe more frequently, and dry the genital area well.
  d. Have your sexual partner treated at the same time you are so that you don't pass the infection back and forth to each other.

The Client with a Parasitic Infestation of the Skin

■ ■ ■

The skin may be invaded by parasites or insects. These infestations are more common in developing countries but may occur in any geographic area of the world. They affect people of all social classes but are associated with crowded or unsanitary living conditions.

Pathophysiology

Two of the more common parasitic infestations of the skin are caused by mites and lice. These parasites do not normally live on the skin, but infest the skin through contact with an infested person or contact with clothing, linens, or objects infested with the parasites.

Pediculosis

Pediculosis is an infestation with lice. Lice are parasites that live on the blood of an animal or human host. Three types of lice live on human hosts: *Pediculus humanus corporis* (*body lice*), *Pediculus pubis* (*pubic lice*), and *Pediculus humanus capitis* (*head lice*).

All species of lice have a similar life cycle. The first stage is an unhatched egg, called a *nit*, laid by the female louse on a hair shaft. The nit is a small pearl-gray or brown egg visible to the naked eye. The female louse can lay hundreds of nits. The louse within the egg develops, hatches, goes through three moult stages, reaches the adult reproductive stage, and dies; the average life span of the louse is 30 to 50 days (Porth, 1994). The louse is a 2- to 4-mm oval organism with a stylet that pierces the skin; it has an anticoagulant in its saliva that prevents host blood from clotting while it eats.

There are three types of human pediculosis:

- *Pediculosis corporis* is an infestation with body lice. This type of louse infestation is more common in people who do not have access to facilities for bathing or washing clothes, such as the homeless. The lice live in clothing fibers and are transmitted primarily by contact with infested clothing and bed linens. The skin lesions occur at the site of a louse bite; macules appear initially, followed by wheals and papules. Pruritus is common, and scratching often results in linear excoriations. Secondary infections cause hyperpigmentation and scarring. The lesions are most often seen on the shoulders, trunk, and buttocks.
- *Pediculosis pubis* is an infestation with pubic lice (often called crabs). This infestation is spread through sexual activity with someone already infested or by contact with infested clothing or linens. The lice are found in the pubic region and occasionally spread to the axillae or men's beards. The lice cause skin irritation and intense itching.
- *Pediculosis capitis* is an infestation with head lice. This infestation primarily affects Caucasians and is more common in female children. The lice are most often found behind the ears and at the nape of the neck but may also spread to other hairy areas of the body: the eyebrows, pubic area, or beard. The lice are transmitted by contact with an infected person. Manifestations of head lice include pruritus, scratching, and erythema of the scalp. If untreated, the hair appears matted and crusted with a foul-smelling substance.

Scabies

Scabies is a parasitic infestation caused by a mite *(Sarcoptes scabiei).* The pregnant female mite burrows into the skin and lays two to three eggs each day for about a month. The eggs hatch in 3 to 5 days, and the larvae migrate to the surface of the skin but burrow into the skin for food or protection. The larvae develop, and the cycle repeats.

Scabies is an infestation that affects people of all socioeconomic classes. Formerly it was seen most often in times of war or famine, but it has become more common as a result of international travel and sexual promiscuity.

The infestation is found in webs between the fingers, the inner surfaces of the wrist and elbow, the axillae, the female nipple, the penis, the belt line, and the gluteal crease. The lesions are characteristic: a small red-brown burrow, about 2 mm in length, sometimes covered with vesicles. The collection of lesions appears as a rash. Pruritus in response to the mite or its feces is common, especially at night, and excoriations may develop. The excoriations predispose the person to secondary bacterial infections.

Collaborative Care

Parasitic infestations are diagnosed by identifying the organism and are treated with medications that kill the lice or mites.

Laboratory and Diagnostic Tests
When a client exhibits manifestations of pediculosis, the hair shaft and the clothing are examined to identify the lice or the nits. Microscopic examination of the parasite provides a positive diagnosis.

Scabies is diagnosed by skin scrapings and microscopic examination for the mites or their feces.

Pharmacology
Lice are eradicated with agents that kill the parasite. Infestations of the body and pubic area are treated with topical medications that contain gamma benzene hexachloride, malathion (Prioderm lotion), or pyrethrum (RID).

Infestations of the head are treated with shampoos containing lindane, such as Kwell. The shampoo is applied to dry hair and massaged in. A small amount of water is added to produce a lather, and the head is scrubbed for 4 minutes, then rinsed. The treatment may need to be repeated in a week to kill newly hatched lice. A fine-toothed comb can be used to comb the dead nits off the hair shaft. Infestations of the eyebrows are treated by applying a thick covering of petroleum jelly for several days.

Scabies may be eradicated by a single treatment of lindane lotion or Kwell applied to the entire skin surface for 12 hours.

The associated itching is treated with systemic or topical medications, including corticosteroids. Secondary bacterial infections are treated with the appropriate antibiotic.

Nursing Care

The nursing care for clients with a parasite infestation most often focuses on teaching to prevent infestation or to eradicate an existing infestation. For a hospitalized client with pediculosis, isolation procedures are instituted until the client no longer has the infestation.

Nursing diagnoses for the client with a parasitic infestation follow:

- *Anxiety* related to the presence of lice and social embarrassment
- *Risk for Infection* related to pruritus from mites
- *Knowledge Deficit* of transmission of parasites
- *Impaired Skin Integrity* related to excoriation from pruritus

Client and Family Teaching

Client and family teaching is necessary to facilitate treatment at home, to prevent the spread of the infestation, and to dispel the myth that lice infest only people with poor hygiene or in dirty living conditions. Specific information includes the following:

- Wash clothing and linens in soap and hot water, or have them dry-cleaned.
- Ironing the clothes kills any lice eggs.
- Personal care items, such as combs or brushes, may be boiled to kill the parasites.
- All family members and sexual partners must also be treated.
- Avoid using the combs, brushes, or hats of others.
- Lice and mites may infest anyone.

The Client with a Viral Infection of the Skin

Viruses are pathogens that consist of an RNA or DNA core surrounded by a protein coat. They depend on live cells for reproduction and so are classified as intracellular pathogens. The viruses that cause skin lesions invade the keratinocyte, reproduce, and either increase cellular growth or cause cellular death.

An increase in the incidence of viral skin disorders has been attributed to a variety of causes. Some commonly used drugs, such as birth control medications and corticosteroids, are known to have immunosuppressive properties that allow the viruses to multiply. Other drugs, such

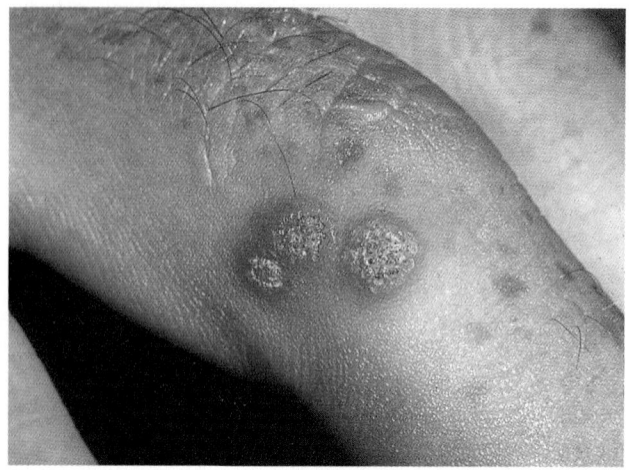

Figure 17–12 The common wart is a lesion of the skin caused by a virus. It commonly appears as a raised, dome-shaped lesion.

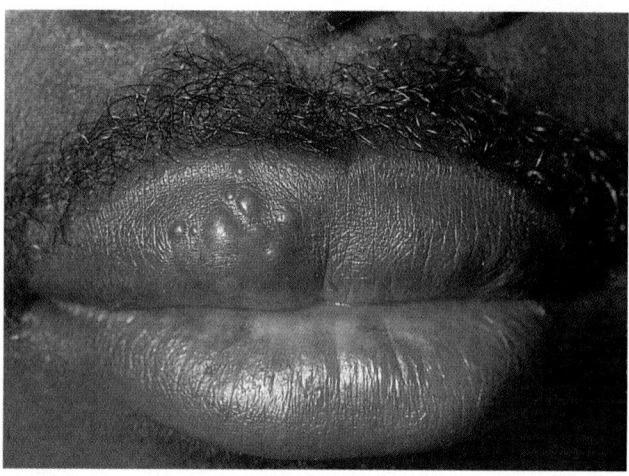

Figure 17–13 Herpes simplex is a viral infection of the skin and mucous membranes. This client has lesions in the early stage, with erythema and vesicles.

as antibiotics, kill off normal skin bacteria that would otherwise serve as defense against viral infections.

Pathophysiology

Viral infections cause many different kinds of skin disorders, including warts, herpes simplex infections, and herpes zoster infections.

Warts

Warts, or *verrucae,* are lesions of the skin caused by the human papillomavirus (HPV). Over 60 types of HPVs are found on the human skin and mucous membranes (Porth, 1994). Warts may be found on nongenital skin or genital skin and mucous membranes. Nongenital warts are benign lesions; genital warts may be precancerous. Warts are transmitted through skin contact.

Wart lesions may be flat, fusiform (tapered at both ends), or round, but most are round and raised and have a rough, gray surface. There are many different types of HPV; location and appearance of the warts depend on the causative HPV. Those most common are described below:

- A *common wart* (verruca vulgaris) may appear anywhere on the skin and mucous membranes of the body; most commonly appear on the fingers. Common warts grow above the skin surface and may be dome-shaped with ragged borders (Figure 17–12).

- *Plantar warts* occur at pressure points on the soles of the feet. The pressure of shoes and walking prevents these warts from growing outward, so they tend to extend deeper beneath the skin surface than do common warts. Plantar warts are often painful.

- A *flat wart* (verruca plana) is a small flat lesion, usually seen on the forehead or dorsum of the hand.

- *Condylomata acuminata,* also called *venereal warts,* occur in moist areas, along the glans of the penis, in the anal region, and on the vulva. They are usually cauliflowerlike in appearance and have a pink or purple color.

Warts resolve spontaneously when immunity to the virus develops. This response may take up to 5 years.

Herpes Simplex

Herpes simplex *(fever blister, cold sore)* virus infections of the skin and mucous membranes are caused by two types of herpesvirus: HSV I and HSV II. Most infections above the waist are caused by HSV I, with herpes simplex lesions most often found on the lips, face, and mouth. (Genital herpes infections, which result from either HSV I or HSV II, are classified as sexually transmitted diseases and are discussed in Chapter 49). The virus may be transmitted by physical contact, oral sex, or kissing.

The infection begins with a burning or tingling sensation, followed by the development of erythema, vesicle formation, and pain (Figure 17–13). The vesicles progress through pustules, ulcers, and crusting until healing occurs in 10 to 14 days.

The initial infection is often severe and accompanied by systemic manifestations, such as fever and sore throat; recurrences are more localized and less severe. The virus lives in nerve ganglia and may cause recurrent lesions in response to sunlight, menstruation, injury, or stress.

Herpes Zoster

Herpes zoster, also called *shingles,* is a viral infection of a dermatome section of the skin caused by varicella zoster, the same herpesvirus that causes chickenpox. The infection is believed to result from reactivation of a varicella virus remaining in the sensory dorsal ganglia after a child-hood infection of chickenpox. When reactivated, the virus travels from the ganglia to the corresponding skin dermatome area.

Herpes zoster affects an estimated 10% to 20% of the population, most often adults over the age of 50. Clients with Hodgkin's disease, certain types of leukemia, and lymphomas are more susceptible to an outbreak of the disease. Herpes zoster is more prevalent in people who are immunocompromised, such as those with HIV infections, those who are receiving radiation therapy or chemotherapy, and those who have had major organ transplants. The appearance of the lesions in people with HIV infections may be one of the first manifestations of immune compromise.

The lesions of herpes zoster are vesicles with an erythematous base. The vesicles appear on the skin area supplied by the neurons of a single or associated group of dorsal root ganglia (although they may occur beyond this area in people who are immunosuppressed). The lesions usually appear unilaterally on the face, trunk, and thorax (Figure 17–14).

New lesions continue to erupt for 3 to 5 days, then crust and dry. Recovery occurs in 2 to 3 weeks. The client experiences severe pain before and during eruption of the lesions. The older adult is especially sensitive to the pain and often experiences more severe outbreaks of herpes zoster lesions.

In most cases, the disease is benign and localized. Complications of herpes zoster include postherpetic neuralgia (a sharp, spasmodic pain along the course of one or more nerves) and visual loss. The neuralgia, described as burning or stabbing, results from inflammation of the root ganglia. This complication occurs in 50% of clients over the age of 60 (Tierney, McPhee, & Papadakis, 1994). Permanent loss of vision may follow occurrence of lesions that arise from the ophthalmic division of the trigeminal nerve.

The disease may disseminate in immunocompromised clients, causing lesions beyond the dermatome, visceral lesions, and encephalitis. This serious complication may cause death.

Collaborative Care

The treatment for viral skin infections focuses on stopping viral replication and treating client responses, such as itching and pain.

Laboratory and Diagnostic Tests
Although diagnosis may be based on manifestations and appearance of the lesions, laboratory tests may be necessary to differentiate herpes zoster from impetigo, contact dermatitis, and herpes simplex. The laboratory tests include the following:

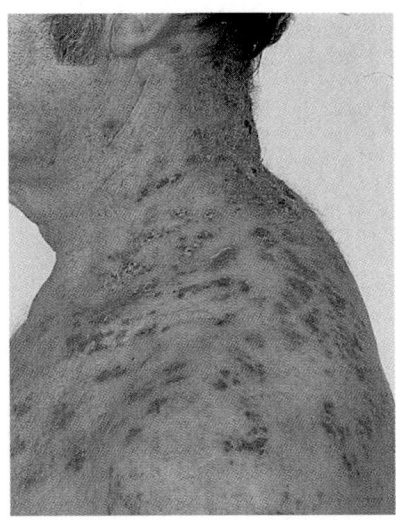

Figure 17–14   Herpes zoster is a viral infection of a dermatome section of the skin. The typical lesions are painful vesicles lying along the path of the nerve.

- A *Tzanck smear* identifies the herpes virus, but it does not distinguish herpes zoster from herpes simplex. This is a microscopic examination of cells from the base of the lesion.

- *Cultures of fluid from the vesicles and antibody tests* are used to make the differential diagnosis of herpesvirus types.

- *Immunofluorescent methods* can identify varicella in skin cells.

Pharmacology
Most viral skin disorders are treated with antiviral medications, and other types of medications are used to relieve pruritus and pain in herpes zoster.

Warts   Depending on their size, location, and any associated discomfort, warts may be treated with medications, cryotherapy, or electrodesiccation and curettage. A common method of wart removal is acid therapy, using a colloidal solution of 16% salicylic acid and 16% lactic acid. The solution is applied to the wart every 12 to 24 hours; the wart disappears in 2 to 3 weeks. Other methods of eradicating warts are cryosurgery, freezing with liquid nitrogen, and electrodesiccation of the wart with an electric current followed by excision of the dead tissue. The treatment of venereal warts is described in Chapter 49.

Herpes Simplex   Herpes simplex lesions are treated with acyclovir (Zovirax), an antifungal agent. Acyclovir shortens the time of symptoms and speeds healing.

Herpes Zoster   The treatment of the client with herpes zoster is aimed at relieving the pain and pruritus and decreasing the severity and length of the illness. Most clients are treated at home, although older adults or those with concomitant illnesses may require hospitalization.

The drug of choice for herpes zoster infections is acyclovir. This antiviral drug interferes with viral synthesis and replication. Although it does not cure herpes infections, it does decrease the severity of the illness and also decreases pain. It may be administered topically, orally, or parenterally. It is more effective if administration begins within the first 1 to 2 days after the first vesicles appear. Acyclovir has little effect on postherpetic neuralgia.

Another antiviral drug that may be prescribed is vidarabine (Ara-A, Vira-A). This drug is given either by intravenous infusion or as an ophthalmic ointment.

Corticosteroids may be used to decrease the inflammatory response and have been effective in some cases, but their use is controversial because they also decrease healing and suppress the immune response (see Chapter 20). Narcotic and nonnarcotic analgesics are prescribed for pain management, and antihistamines may be administered for relief of pruritus.

Clients with eye involvement are treated with topical steroid ophthalmic ointments and mydriatics. Antivirals may sometimes be administered.

Nursing Care

Nursing care of the client with a viral infection is individualized and may be more complex if the client has herpes zoster and other chronic illnesses. This section discusses care of the client with herpes zoster, focusing on the nursing diagnoses of pain, sleep pattern disturbance, and risk for infection.

Pain

The client with herpes zoster often experiences severe pain over the entire dermatome supplied by the affected nerve root. The pain is described as burning, tearing, or stabbing. The client may avoid movement and does not want clothing or bed linens to touch the affected area.

Nursing interventions with rationales follow:

- Assess and monitor the location, duration, and intensity of the pain. *Each person experiences and expresses pain in his or her own manner. Pain tolerance is also individual. Accurate assessment of the client's perception and tolerance of pain is essential in facilitating pain management.*

- Administer prescribed medications regularly, and evaluate their effectiveness. *Delaying or withholding medications may allow the pain to reach an intensity at which the medication is less effective in promoting relief.*

- Use measures to relieve pruritus:
  a. Administer prescribed antipruritic medications.

  b. Apply calamine lotion or wet compresses, if prescribed.
  c. Keep the room temperature cool.
  d. Use a bed cradle to keep sheets off affected areas of the body.

Pruritus is a common problem for clients with herpes zoster; scratching may excoriate the skin and increase the risk for secondary infections. Pruritus may intensify the experience of pain. Lotions and cool, wet compresses are effective in decreasing the itch-scratch-itch cycle. Warmth and touch intensify pruritus.

- Encourage the use of distraction (such as music) or a specific relaxation technique (such as progressive muscle relaxation or deep breathing). *The use of noninvasive methods to relieve pain not only helps the client manage the pain experience but also increases the effectiveness of pain medications.*

Sleep Pattern Disturbance

The pain and pruritus of herpes zoster often interfere with normal sleep patterns; often these responses are more intense at night, probably as a result of decreased distraction.

Nursing interventions with rationales follow:

- Provide appropriate interventions to relieve pain and pruritus (as described above). *Pain and pruritus interfere with normal sleep. Analgesics and noninvasive methods of relief may be necessary before the client prepares for sleep.*

- Maintain a cool environment and avoid heavy bed covering. *Heat and touch intensify pruritus. Pruritus stimulates scratching, which awakens the client. The client may then perceive the pain more acutely. A cycle is established that interferes with sleep.*

Risk for Infection

Clients with herpes zoster have impaired skin integrity and pruritus with scratching and possible excoriation; moreover, they may be immunocompromised. All of these factors contribute to a high risk for secondary bacterial infection. In addition, the client is contagious to others who did not have chickenpox as children.

Nursing interventions with rationales follow:

- Monitor the client for manifestations of infection:
  a. Take and record vital signs every 4 hours, noting increased temperature.
  b. Assess skin lesions for increased erythema, formation of pustules, and/or purulent drainage.
  c. Monitor white blood cell count.
  d. Assess for lymph gland enlargement.

Secondary bacterial infections may occur in any client with impaired skin integrity; if the client is immunocompromised, the risk is even greater. Fever, changes in lesions or drainage, an increased white blood cell count, and lymph gland enlargement are manifestations of an infection.

- Use interventions to decrease the itch-scratch-itch cycle, thereby decreasing the possibility of excoriation (see discussion about nursing care of clients with pruritus and psoriasis, earlier in this chapter). *Excoriation from scratching provides an avenue for bacterial invasion.*

- Institute infection control procedures:
    a. Maintain strict isolation in immunocompromised clients.
    b. Wear gloves and gown if contact with lesions is likely.
    c. Instruct pregnant women to avoid exposure until lesions have crusted over.
    Isolation procedures are instituted for the immunocompromised client to prevent client infection. The nurse wears gloves and gown to prevent spreading the infection to self or others. Pregnant women need to avoid exposure because the herpesvirus can cross the placental barrier.

Other Nursing Diagnoses

Other nursing diagnoses that may be appropriate for the client with herpes zoster follow:

- *Impaired Skin Integrity* related to excoriation secondary to pruritus over herpes zoster lesions

- *Social Isolation* related to imposed isolation procedures

- *Anxiety* related to the presence of lesions and severe pain

- *Fatigue* related to the inability to sleep secondary to constant pruritus and pain from herpetic lesions

- *Self-Care Deficit: Bathing/Hygiene* related to the presence of multiple vesicles over lateral thorax with pain on movement

Client and Family Teaching

Because most clients with viral infections provide self-care at home, the nurse focuses on teaching the client and family how to provide the necessary care. With herpes zoster increasing in incidence in clients who are older or have a serious chronic illness, it may also be necessary for the nurse to make a referral to a community health provider for continued support. The nurse provides the following information and instructions:

- The diseases are usually self-limiting and heal completely. Second occurrences of herpes zoster are rare.

- Do not have social contact with children or pregnant women until crusts have formed over the blistered areas with herpes zoster, as the disease is contagious to people who have not had chickenpox.

- Use pain medications regularly.

- Follow suggestions to help reduce itching, scratching, and pain: Use medications as prescribed, wear lightweight cotton clothing, keep room temperatures cool, wear cotton gloves at night if scratching is a problem, and practice relaxation and distraction activities.

- Report any increase in pain, fever, chills, drainage that smells bad and has pus, or a spread in the blisters to your health care provider.

Applying the Nursing Process

Case Study of a Client with Herpes Zoster: Jesus Rivera

Jesus Rivera is a 34-year-old migrant farm worker who currently lives in temporary housing in a rural area of the southwestern United States. His family members include his wife, Marta, who is 3 months pregnant, and two children, ages 3 and 5. He takes his wife to a medical clinic staffed by volunteer nurses, physicians, and students from a nearby university for a prenatal checkup. The clinic is open only on Saturday and provides care on a sliding fee scale or for free if the family is unable to pay. While Mrs. Rivera is being examined, Mr. Rivera asks the nurse to have someone look at some very painful blisters on his chest that developed about a week ago. He is afraid that exposure to pesticides has caused the sores.

Assessment

Mr. Rivera speaks Spanish and is able to communicate only slightly in English. The initial assessment of Mr. Rivera is performed by Anita Mendez, a student nurse fluent in Spanish. The nurse practitioner supervising Miss Mendez is also able to converse in Spanish.

Mr. Rivera's history reveals problems with lower back pain but no significant past medical illnesses. He is not aware of any allergies and cannot remember having had chickenpox as a child. Two years ago, both children were sick and had blisters on their bodies, and a friend told them it was chickenpox. Mrs. Rivera thinks she had chickenpox as a child.

Because Mr. Rivera has not had any medical care for several years, baseline laboratory tests are ordered to screen for any other illnesses; the complete blood count (CBC), blood chemistry, and urinalysis are all within normal limits.

Mr. Rivera says that he did not feel well for several days before the blisters appeared, having experienced chills and general achiness. He had not taken his temperature because the family does not own a thermometer. Current vital signs are as follows: T, 99 F (37.2 C); BP, 148/88; P, 74; R, 22.

Physical examination of the trunk reveals a bandlike pattern of lesions across the left thorax. Some of the lesions are vesicles filled with serous fluid; others are darker in color and are oozing a light yellow drainage. The skin around the lesions is red and inflamed. Mr. Rivera complains of a severe, burning pain with itching across his chest. Mr. Rivera was diagnosed with herpes zoster.

Diagnosis

Miss Mendez makes the following nursing diagnoses for Mr. Rivera:

- *Risk for Infection* related to open oozing areas on the left thorax
- *Pain* related to the presence of lesions and pruritus
- *Knowledge Deficit* of the cause of the skin disorder and recommended treatment
- *Anxiety* related to need to work in areas of pesticide application
- *Altered Health Maintenance* related to limited access to health care, transitory work conditions, and cultural and language barriers

Expected Outcomes

The expected outcomes established in the plan of care specify that:

- Mr. Rivera's skin lesions will heal without evidence of a secondary infection.
- Mr. Rivera will limit exposure (as much as possible) to his wife and children and to persons with debilitating illnesses to prevent the spread of the virus.
- Mr. Rivera will obtain relief of pain and pruritus with the proper use of medications.
- Mr. Rivera will verbalize an understanding of the disease process and participate in the treatment plan.
- Mr. Rivera will obtain follow-up care.
- Mr. Rivera will make an appointment for a referral for information about occupational hazards.

Planning and Implementation

Miss Mendez implements the following interventions for Mr. Rivera:

- Take cultures of the draining lesions and send them for laboratory analysis.
- Provide verbal and written instructions (in Spanish) for self-care:
  a. Wear a clean cotton undershirt each day.
  b. Trim the fingernails short, and keep the hands clean.
  c. Wash the hands each time the area is touched.
  d. Wash any soiled clothes or linens in hot water and soap.

  e. Don't let other family members use your towels.
  f. Take medications as prescribed for itching and pain. Because these medications may cause drowsiness, do not drink alcohol while taking them.
  g. Take the medicine for your sores every 4 hours. Set the alarm to wake yourself up at night so that you never miss a dose. You will have to take this medicine in this way for 7 days.
  h. As much as possible, do not touch your wife and children until the sores are covered with scabs. Do not have sex with your wife while you have these sores.

- Teach Mr. Rivera how to take care of his skin lesions:
  a. Wear the rubber gloves we give you every time you do this treatment.
  b. Wash the sores and the skin around them very gently with a soft washcloth and a mild soap.
  c. Using your fingers, carefully rub the cream that we give you on the sores.
  d. Do this once every morning after breakfast and once every evening after supper.
  e. Wash your hands carefully before and after each treatment.

- Make a follow-up appointment for Mr. Rivera and his family for the next week.
- Provide Mr. Rivera with the name and phone number of the Occupational Safety and Health Administration (OSHA) and recommend he call for an appointment to discuss his concerns about pesticides.

Evaluation

Both Miss Mendez and the nurse practitioner are at the clinic when Mr. Rivera returns the next Saturday. Mrs. Rivera explains how she has taken care of her husband, and Mr. Rivera is careful to describe how he has followed the nurse's instructions. The skin lesions are dry and crusty, with no new blister formation. Mr. Rivera says he has not called OSHA and is not sure that he will, but he thanks Miss Mendez for the phone number. The nurses make an appointment in 1 month for a prenatal checkup for Mrs. Rivera and for follow-up of Mr. Rivera's herpes zoster. Mr. Rivera promises to return if they are still living close enough to keep the appointment.

Critical Thinking in the Nursing Process

1. Identify barriers to care present in this case study. How may nursing interventions promote health care delivery to disadvantaged populations?

2. Although most cases of herpes zoster are self-limiting, what further assessments and interventions might have been indicated had the lesions shown little improvement over time and/or the pain remained severe?

3. During a detailed health assessment, Mr. Rivera denies any risk factors for HIV exposure. List the risk factors and state current guidelines and policies for assessing a person's HIV status (see Chapter 8).

4. If Mr. Rivera is advised not to work until his lesions heal, the family may face economic and sociocultural hardships. Develop a plan of care for Mr. Rivera for the nursing diagnosis *Altered Role Performance*.

Inflammatory Disorders

Inflammatory skin disorders often do not have a known cause. They are usually localized to the skin and are rarely associated with systemic manifestations. The inflammatory skin disorders discussed in this section include dermatitis, acne, pemphigus, lichen planus, drug eruptions, and toxic epidermal necrolysis.

The Client with Dermatitis

Dermatitis is an inflammation of the skin characterized by erythema and pain or pruritus. Dermatitis may be acute or chronic.

Pathophysiology

In dermatitis, various exogenous and endogenous agents cause an inflammatory response of the skin. Different types of skin eruptions occur, often specific to the causative allergen, infection, or disease. The initial skin responses to these agents or illnesses include erythema, formation of vesicles and scales, and pruritus (Figure 17–15). Subsequently, irritation from scratching promotes edema, a serous discharge, and crusting. Finally, long-term irritation in chronic dermatitis causes the skin to become thickened and leathery (a condition called *lichenification*) and darker in color.

The types of dermatitis discussed here are contact dermatitis, atopic dermatitis, seborrheic dermatitis, and exfoliative dermatitis.

Contact Dermatitis

Contact dermatitis is a type of dermatitis caused by a hypersensitivity response or chemical irritation. The major sources known to cause contact dermatitis are dyes, perfumes, poison plants (ivy, oak, sumac), chemicals, and metals (see the accompanying box). A contact dermatitis that has become more common in the health care field is latex (glove) dermatitis.

Allergic contact dermatitis is a cell-mediated or delayed hypersensitivity to a wide variety of allergens. Sensitizing antigens include microorganisms, plants, chemicals, drugs, metals, or foreign proteins.

On initial contact with the skin, the allergen binds to a carrier protein, forming a sensitizing antigen. The antigen

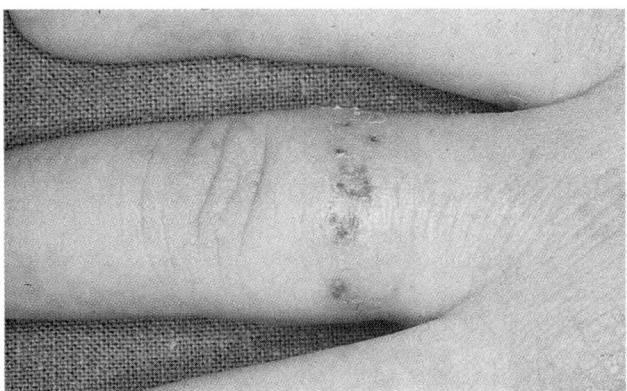

Figure 17–15 Inflammation of the skin, or dermatitis, may be a response to allergens, infections, or chemicals. This client has contact dermatitis resulting from the metal salts in jewelry.

Common Causes of Contact Dermatitis

- Acids
- Alkalis: soaps, detergents, ammonia, lye, household cleaners
- Bromide
- Chlorine
- Cosmetics: perfumes, dyes, oils
- Dusts of lime, arsenic, wood
- Hydrocarbons: crude petroleum, lubricating oil, mineral oil, paraffin, asphalt, tar
- Iodine
- Insecticides
- Fabrics: wool, polyester, dyes, sizing
- Metal salts: calcium chloride, zinc chloride, copper, mercury, nickel, silver
- Plants: ragweed, poison oak, poison sumac, poison ivy, pine
- Coloring agents
- Rubber products
- Soot

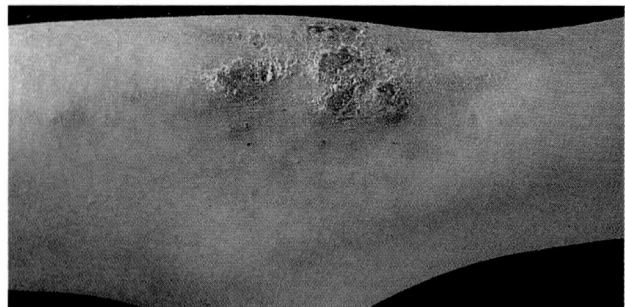

Figure 17–16 Atopic dermatitis, or eczema, causes pruritus, resulting in lichenification, erythema, and scaling.

is processed and carried to the T cells, which in turn become sensitized to the antigen. The first exposure is the sensitizing contact; skin manifestations occur with subsequent exposures. These manifestations include erythema, swelling, and pruritic vesicles in the area of allergen contact. For example, a person who is hypersensitive to metal may have lesions under a ring or watch.

Irritant contact dermatitis is an inflammation of the skin from irritants; it is not a hypersensitivity response. Common sources of irritant contact dermatitis include chemicals (such as acids), soaps, and detergents. The skin lesions are similar to those seen in allergic contact dermatitis.

Atopic Dermatitis

Atopic dermatitis is an inflammatory skin disorder that is also called *eczema*. This is a common skin disorder, affecting 9% to 12% of the population (Schultz-Larson & Hanifin, 1992). The exact cause is unknown, but related factors include depressed cell-mediated immunity, elevated IgE levels, and increased histamine sensitivity. The disorder is seen more often in children, but chronic forms persist throughout life.

Clients with atopic dermatitis have a family history of hypersensitivity reactions, such as dry skin, eczema, asthma, and allergic rhinitis. Although up to one-third of clients with atopic dermatitis also have food allergies, a positive correlation has not been found.

The dermatitis results when mast cells, T lymphocytes, monocytes, and other inflammatory cells are activated and release histamine, lymphokines, and other inflammatory mediators. The immune response interacts with the allergen to create a chronic inflammatory condition.

In the adult form of atopic dermatitis, characteristic lesions include chronic lichenification, erythema, and scaling, the result of pruritus and scratching. The lesions are usually found on the hands, feet, or flexor surfaces of the arms and legs (Figure 17–16). Scratching and excoriation increase the risk of secondary infections, as well as invasion of the skin by viruses such as herpes simplex.

Seborrheic Dermatitis

Seborrheic dermatitis is a common and chronic inflammatory disorder of the skin that involves the scalp, eyebrows, eyelids, ear canals, nasolabial folds, axillae, and trunk. The cause is unknown.

This disorder is seen in all ages, from the very young (called "cradle cap") to the very old. Clients taking methyldopa for hypertension occasionally develop this disorder, and it is a component of Parkinson's disease. Seborrheic dermatitis is also frequently seen in clients with AIDS.

The lesions are yellow or white plaques with scales and crusts. The scales are often yellow or orange and have a greasy appearance. Mild pruritus is also present. Diffuse dandruff with erythema of the scalp often accompanies the skin lesions.

Exfoliative Dermatitis

Exfoliative dermatitis is an inflammatory skin disorder characterized by excessive peeling or shedding of skin. The cause is unknown in about half of all cases, but a preexisting skin disorder (such as psoriasis, atopic dermatitis, contact dermatitis, or seborrheic dermatitis) is found in about 40% of the cases (Tierney et al., 1994). Exfoliative dermatitis is also associated with leukemia and lymphoma.

Both systemic and localized manifestations may appear. Systemic manifestations include weakness, malaise, fever, chills, and weight loss. Scaling, erythema, and pruritus may be localized or involve the entire body (Figure 17–17). In addition to peeling of skin, the client may lose the hair and nails.

Generalized exfoliative dermatitis may cause debility and dehydration. The impairment of skin integrity increases the risk for local and systemic infections.

Collaborative Care

The client with dermatitis is treated primarily with topical medications and therapeutic baths. If the dermatitis is due to hypersensitivity to an allergen, the client avoids exposure to environmental irritants and suspected foods. The client also discontinues as many medications as possible to determine whether the dermatitis is the result of a drug allergy.

Laboratory and Diagnostic Tests

The diagnosis is often based on the manifestations of the disorder. Laboratory and diagnostic tests may include the following:

- *Scratch tests and intradermal tests* are conducted to identify a specific allergen.
- *Serum studies* may find elevated eosinophil and IgE levels in atopic dermatitis.

- *Skin biopsy* may reveal specific changes in inflammatory dermatitis.

Pharmacology

The type of pharmacologic agent used depends on the cause of the dermatitis as well as the severity of the manifestations. Minor cases are treated with antipruritic medications, whereas more severe cases are treated with oral antihistamines, oral and/or topical corticosteroids, and wet dressings. Topical anti-infectives may be prescribed if necessary.

Nursing Care

Nursing care of the client with dermatitis focuses primarily on providing information for self-care at home. However, if the client is hospitalized, the interventions for pruritus and for many of the nursing diagnoses discussed throughout the chapter are appropriate.

Nursing diagnoses for the client with dermatitis are listed below:

- *Anxiety* related to the exacerbation of skin rash and pruritus
- *Body Image Disturbance* related to the presence of skin lesions
- *Hopelessness* related to the inability to control the progression of exfoliative dermatitis
- *Risk for Infection* related to skin excoriation
- *Altered Sexuality Patterns* related to feelings of self-revulsion secondary to skin lesions
- *Impaired Skin Integrity* related to peeling of skin surface
- *Sleep Pattern Disturbance* related to pruritus
- *Social Isolation* related to embarrassment about appearance

Client and Family Teaching

Most forms of dermatitis are chronic, with remissions and exacerbations. The client is responsible for managing skin problems and requires education and support. General guidelines in teaching follow:

- Medications and treatments do not cure the disease; they only relieve the symptoms.
- Dry skin increases pruritus, which stimulates scratching. Scratching may in turn cause excoriation, and excoriation increases the risk of infection.
- It may be necessary to change the diet or environment to avoid contact with allergens.
- When using steroid preparations, apply only a thin layer to slightly damp skin (for example, after taking a bath).

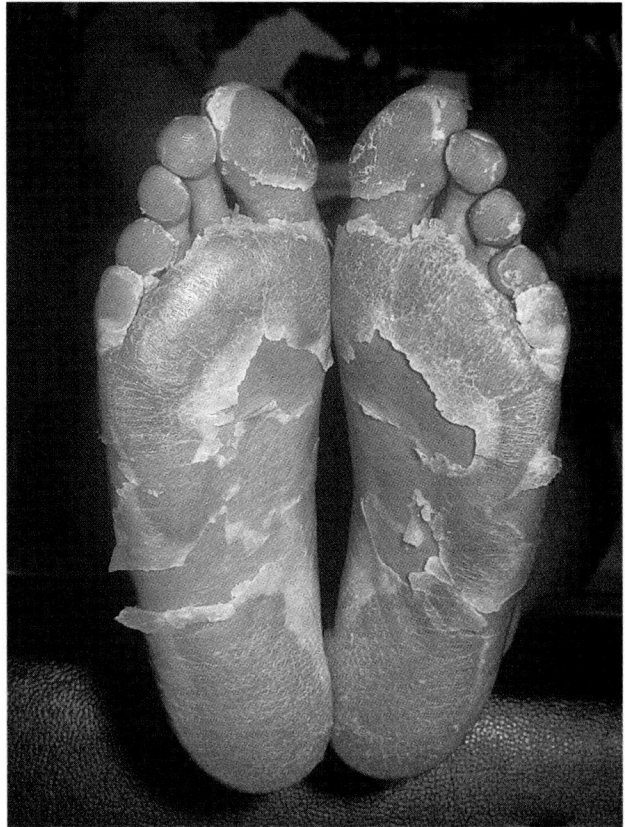

Figure 17–17   Exfoliative dermatitis is an inflammatory skin disorder causing excessive skin peeling.

- If occlusive dressings are necessary, a plastic suit may be used. These garments are manufactured by the Simmons Company, Chattanooga, TN and by Sleep Sauna, Lower Bwynedd, PA.
- When using oral corticosteroids, never abruptly stop taking the medication. Rather, follow instructions to taper the dosage gradually.
- Antihistamines cause drowsiness. When using these medications, avoid alcohol, and use caution when driving or working around machinery.

The Client with Acne

■ ■ ■

Acne is a disorder of the pilosebaceous (hair and sebaceous gland) structure, which opens to the skin surface through a *pore*. The sebaceous glands, which empty directly into the hair follicle, produce *sebum*, a lipid substance. Sebaceous glands are present over the entire skin surface except the soles of the feet and the palms of the hands, but the largest glands are on the face, scalp, and

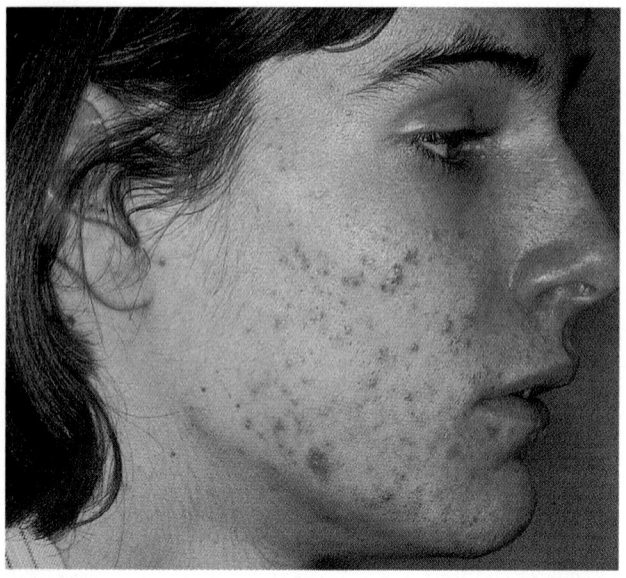
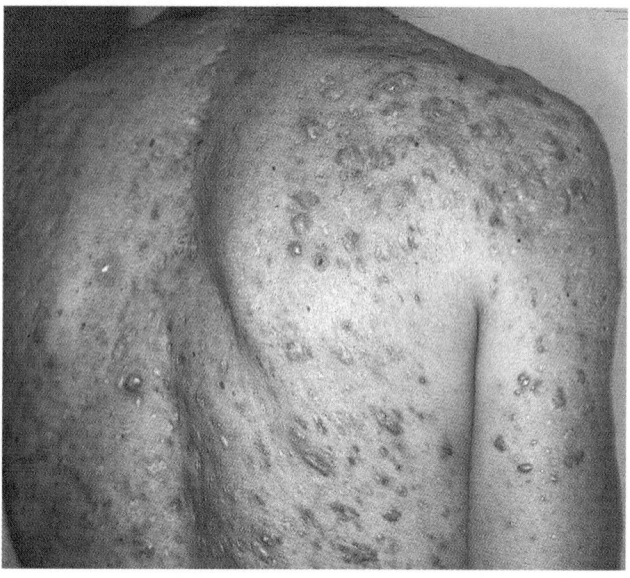

A

B

Figure 17–18   Acne is a disorder of the hair and sebaceous skin structures. *A,* In noninflammatory forms of acne, the characteristic lesions are comedones (pimples). *B,* Inflammatory acne lesions include comedones, erythematous pustules, and cysts. These lesions often leave scars when they heal.

scrotum. Sebum production is a response to direct hormonal stimulation by testicular androgens in men and adrenal and ovarian androgens in women.

Pathophysiology

Acne may be inflammatory or noninflammatory. Noninflammatory acne lesions are primarily comedones, more commonly called pimples, whiteheads, and blackheads. Whiteheads are pale, slightly elevated papules categorized as closed comedones (Figure 17–18, *A*). *Blackheads* are plugs of material that accumulate in the sebaceous glands. They are categorized as open comedones; the color is the result of the movement of melanin into the plug from surrounding epidermal cells. Inflammatory acne lesions include comedones, erythematous pustules, and cysts (Figure 17–18, *B*). Inflammation close to the skin surface results in pustules, whereas deeper inflammation results in cysts. The inflammation is believed to result from irritation from fatty acid constituents of the sebum and from substances produced by *Propionibacterium acnes* bacteria, both of which escape into the dermis when the follicular wall of closed comedones ruptures.

There are several forms of acne, occurring at different periods of the life span. The most common are acne vulgaris, acne rosacea, and acne conglobata.

Acne Vulgaris

Acne vulgaris is the form of acne that is common in adolescents and young to middle adults. Most people experience acne vulgaris at some point in their lives. Although the lesions may persist longer in women, the incidence is greater in men. The actual cause of acne vulgaris is unknown; possible causes include androgenic influence on the sebaceous glands, increased sebum production, and proliferation of the organism *Propionibacterium acnes,* which contains enzymes that break down lipids to produce the irritating fatty acids. Many factors once thought to cause acne vulgaris, including high-fat diets, chocolate, infections, and cosmetics, have been disproved (Porth, 1994).

Mild cases of this type of acne may involve only a few scattered comedones, but severe cases are manifested by multiple lesions of all types. Most acne vulgaris lesions form on the face and neck, but they also occur on the back, chest, and shoulders. The lesions are usually mildly painful and may itch.

The complications of acne vulgaris, especially in severe cases, are formation of cysts, pigment changes in persons with dark skin, severe scarring, and lowered self-concept from the obvious skin eruptions.

Acne Rosacea

Acne rosacea is a chronic type of facial acne that occurs more often in middle and older adults. The cause is unknown.

The lesions of acne rosacea begin with erythema over the cheeks and nose. Other skin lesions may or may not appear. Over years of time, the skin color changes to dark red, and the pores over the area become enlarged (Figure 17–19). The soft tissue of the nose may exhibit *rhino-*

phyma, an irregular bullous thickening that can be treated with plastic surgery.

Acne Conglobata

Acne conglobata is also a chronic type of acne of unknown cause that begins in middle adulthood. This type causes serious skin lesions: Comedones, papules, pustules, nodules, cysts, and scars occur primarily on the back, buttocks, and chest but may occur on other body surfaces. The comedones have multiple openings and a discharge that ranges from serous to purulent with a foul odor.

Collaborative Care

The management of acne is similar, regardless of type. Because acne vulgaris is most common, the discussions of collaborative and nursing care focus on that type.

Treatment is primarily by medications and continues for several weeks. The treatment is based on the type and severity of the lesions. Although dietary restrictions were once believed necessary, clients are now advised to avoid only foods that appear to cause an increase in lesions. Clients are also advised to avoid topical exposure to oils and greases.

Laboratory and Diagnostic Tests

There are no special laboratory and diagnostic tests for acne. The disease is diagnosed by the typical location and appearance of lesions. If the client has pustules, a culture of the drainage is performed to differentiate viral or bacterial dermatitis from acne.

Pharmacology

The treatment of acne is tailored to the individual and is based on the severity of the lesions. For acne with comedones, tretinoin (retinoic acid, Retin-A) or benzoyl peroxide preparations are prescribed. The administration of these vitamin A analogues is discussed in the accompanying pharmacology box. Benzoyl peroxide preparations are found in over-the-counter medications such as Fostex, Acne-Dome, Desquam-X, Benzagel, Clear By Design, and Xerac BP. These products are keratolytic and loosen the comedones. They are effective for many mild cases of acne.

Mild forms of papular inflammatory acne are treated with topical clindamycin (Cleocin T), a bacteriostatic agent that decreases the amount of fatty acids on the skin surface. This medication may be combined with tretinoin therapy.

Moderate forms of papular inflammatory acne are treated with oral or topical antibiotics, such as tetracycline, erythromycin, and minocycline. These antiacne antibiotics are administered for 3 to 4 months; if the client's skin is clear, the dose is lowered gradually to a maintenance dose that will maintain clear skin.

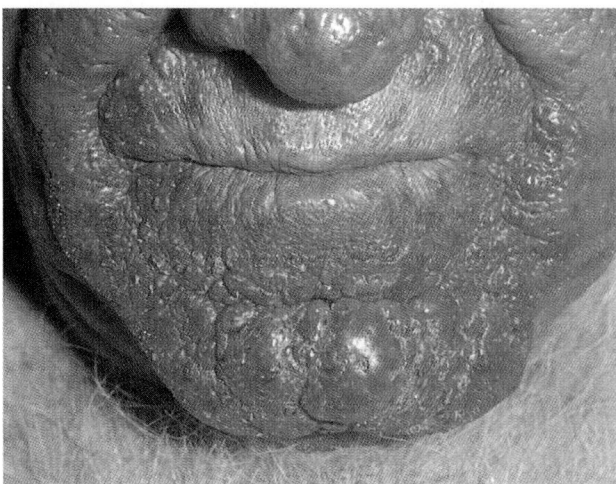

Figure 17–19   Acne rosacea is more common in the middle to older adult. It causes changes in skin color, enlarged pores, and in some cases thickening of the soft tissues of the nose.

Severe forms of papular inflammatory acne are treated with isotretinoin (Accutane). This drug is effective, but has serious side effects. Isotretinoin, with nursing responsibilities, is discussed in the pharmacology box on page 584.

Other pharmacologic agents that may be used to treat acne include estrogens (for women) and corticosteroids. The corticosteroids, which are used for severe cases, are injected into the cysts. This treatment has been effective in temporarily reducing the cysts.

Dermabrasion

Dermabrasion of inactive acne lesions can improve the client's appearance, especially if the scars are flat. The skin is first frozen (and anesthetized) with Freon or ethyl chloride. The lesions are carefully abraded with fine sandpaper or abrasive brushes. Dermabrasion is discussed in greater detail later in this chapter.

Nursing Care

Nursing care is individualized to the client's developmental needs and is conducted primarily through teaching in clinics or the home setting. Regardless of the client's age or gender, it is important to remember that almost all clients with acne are embarrassed by and self-conscious of their appearance. Prior to teaching, the nurse must establish rapport with the client and must clarify beliefs; for example, the client may believe the lesions result from poor hygiene, masturbation, use of cosmetics, eating the wrong types of foods, or lack of sexual activity. It is critical that the nurse teach the client about the causes of and factors involved in acne prior to teaching self-care.

Nursing diagnoses appropriate for the client with acne follow:

Nursing Implications for Pharmacology: Acne Medications

ANTIACNE RETINOIDS

Tretinoin (Retin-A)   Isotretinoin (Accutane)

Tretinoin is a vitamin A derivative classified as an acne agent. This topical agent acts as an irritant to decrease cohesiveness of follicular epithelial cells, thereby decreasing comedone formation while increasing the extrusion of comedones from the skin surface.

Isotretinoin is a vitamin A analogue classified as an acne product. It reduces the size of sebaceous glands, inhibits sebaceous gland differentiation to decrease sebum production, and alters sebum lipid composition.

Nursing Responsibilities

- Administer tretinoin with caution to pregnant women; the effects of absorption on the developing fetus are not clearly defined.

- Isotretinoin is absolutely contraindicated for pregnant women or for women who want to become pregnant. The medication poses a high risk of major deformities in the infant if pregnancy occurs during use, even use that continues only for short periods.

- Do not administer to clients with eczema or to those who are hypersensitive to the sun.

Client and Family Teaching

Tretinoin
- Use the cream in a test area twice at night to test for sensitivity; if no reaction occurs, increase applications gradually to the prescribed frequency.

- A pea-sized amount of the cream is enough to cover the entire face.

- Apply the cream to clean, dry skin.

- Do not apply the cream to the eyes, mouth, angles of the nose, or mucous membranes.

- Wash your face no more than two to three times a day, using a mild soap. Do not use skin preparations (such as after-shave lotion or perfumes) that contain alcohol, menthol, spice, or lime; they may irritate your skin.

- The medication may cause a temporary stinging or warm sensation but should not cause pain.

- The skin where you apply the cream will be mildly red and may peel; if you experience a more severe reaction, consult your health care provider.

- The medication may cause increased sensitivity to sunlight; use sunscreens and wear protective clothing when outdoors.

- Your acne may become worse during the first 2 weeks of treatment; this is an expected response.

Isotretinoin
- Take the pills with food.

- Your acne may become worse during the initial period of treatment; this is an expected response.

- The medication causes dryness of the eyes, so you may have trouble wearing contact lenses during and after treatment.

- Do not take vitamin A supplements; they will increase the effects of the medication.

- Avoid prolonged exposure to sunlight; use sunscreen and protective clothing when in the sun.

- Notify the physician at once if you have abdominal pain, severe diarrhea, rectal bleeding, headache, nausea or vomiting, or visual disturbances.

- Do not drink alcohol while taking this medication (it causes an increase in triglycerides).

- Night vision may become worse; use caution when driving at night.

- Do not donate blood while or for 1 month after taking this medication.

- *(For female clients)* You must use two reliable forms of contraception simultaneously for at least 1 month before, during, and at least 1 month after therapy with this medication. The medication may cause deformities in a baby conceived at this time.

- *Anxiety* about the long-term effects and benefits of antiacne medications

- *Hopelessness* related to the chronicity of acne pustules and cysts on the face

- *Risk for Infection* related to comedones on the back and shoulders

- *Self-Esteem Disturbance* related to cosmetic effects of acne lesions and scarring

Client and Family Teaching

The teaching plan for the client with acne includes general guidelines for skin care and health as well as specific guidelines for care of the acne lesions:

- Wash the skin with a mild soap and water at least twice a day to remove accumulated oils.

- Shampoo the hair often enough to prevent oiliness.

- Eat a regular, well-balanced diet. If a particular food seems to increase the number or severity of the pimples, stop eating that food for about a month. Then gradually start eating the food again to see whether it makes the pimples worse. If it does not, there is no need to eliminate it from your diet.

- Expose the skin to sunlight, but avoid sunburn.

- Get regular exercise and sleep.

- Try to avoid putting your hands on your face.

- Do not squeeze a pimple. Squeezing forces the material of the pimple deeper into the skin and usually causes the pimple to become larger and infected.

- The treatment for acne lasts months, in some cases for the rest of one's life. It is very important to take the medications each day for the prescribed length of time.

The Client with Pemphigus Vulgaris

■ ■ ■

Pemphigus vulgaris is a chronic disorder of the skin and oral mucous membranes characterized by vesicle (blister) formation. The disease is believed to be due to autoantibodies that cause acantholysis, the separation of epidermal cells from one another. The disorder is associated with IgG antibodies and HLA-A10 antigen.

Pemphigus vulgaris is a rare disease with an unknown cause. If untreated, the disease is usually fatal within 2 months to 5 years (Tierney et al., 1994). However, better methods of diagnosis and treatment have improved the prognosis.

The disease occurs in middle and older adults of all races and ethnic backgrounds. Even though the actual cause is unknown, the disorder has been associated with other autoimmune disorders and with the administration of certain drugs, such as penicillamine and captopril.

Pathophysiology

The blisters that form in pemphigus vulgaris usually appear first in the mouth and scalp and then spread in crops or waves to involve large areas of the body, including the face, back, chest, umbilicus, and groin. Blisters in the mouth ulcerate. The blisters form in the epidermis and cause the epidermal cells to separate above the basal layer. These blisters rupture, leaving denuded skin, crusting, and oozing of fluid with a musty (often described as "mousy") smell (Figure 17–20). The lesions are painful. Pressure on a blister causes it to spread to adjacent skin (*Nikolsky's sign*). Secondary bacterial infections are a serious risk and a major cause of death.

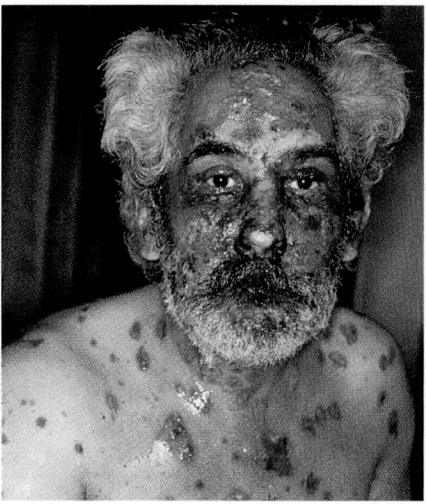

Figure 17–20 Pemphigus vulgaris is a chronic skin disorder characterized by vesicles that ooze fluid and form crusts.

Collaborative Care

The goals of treatment are to control the severity of the disease, to prevent infection and loss of fluids, and to promote healing. Clients who experience severe attacks or secondary infections are usually hospitalized. Although the disease cannot be cured, the manifestations can be controlled.

Laboratory and Diagnostic Tests

Pemphigus vulgaris is diagnosed by clinical manifestations and laboratory and diagnostic tests. These tests may include the following:

- *Immunofluorescence microscopy* is done to identify the presence of IgG antibodies in the epidermis.

- *Indirect immunofluorescence microscopy* uses the patient's serum to detect circulating pemphigus antibodies.

- *Skin biopsy* may be performed to determine the presence of acantholysis.

Pharmacology

Early lesions are treated with highly potent topical corticosteroids. As the disease becomes more severe, systemic corticosteroids or immunosuppressive agents (such as azathioprine or methotrexate) are prescribed. Secondary infections are treated with topical and/or systemic antibiotics.

Plasmapheresis

Plasmapheresis is occasionally used to treat pemphigus. In this procedure, the plasma is selectively removed from whole blood and reinfused into the client. This decreases the serum level of antibodies for a period of time. Plasmapheresis is discussed in greater detail in Chapter 8.

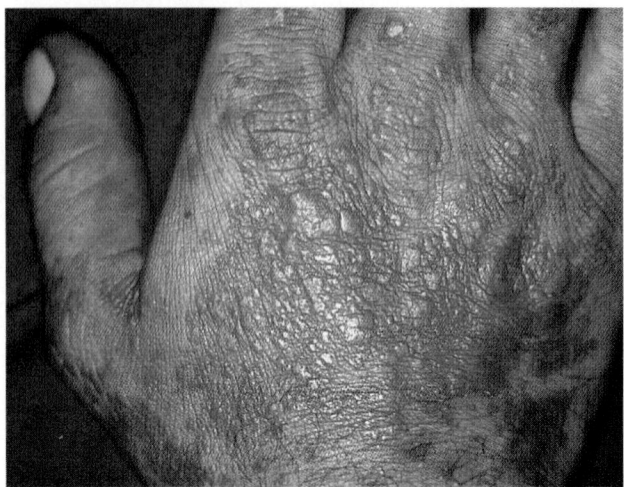

Figure 17–21   These violet-colored lesions are typical of lichen planus, a benign inflammatory disease of the skin and mucous membranes.

Nursing Care

The hospitalized client with pemphigus requires careful assessment of skin lesions and monitoring for manifestations of infection. The nurse provides skin care through bathing and applying dressings to denuded areas, using aseptic technique to prevent infection. The client may be placed on reverse isolation as a protective measure. The nurse monitors the client's hydration status to prevent fluid volume deficit and incorporates pain medications and noninvasive pain management techniques in the plan of care. Oral lesions often make eating difficult; the client requires meticulous oral hygiene and nonirritating foods. The client often is depressed and fearful; establishing a therapeutic relationship is essential, and referrals for counseling may be necessary.

The following nursing diagnoses are appropriate for the client with pemphigus:

- *Body Image Disturbance* related to the presence of large blisters and open skin areas
- *Risk for Fluid Volume Deficit* related to the loss of fluid from open and closed blisters over extensive body areas
- *Risk for Infection* related to open skin lesions
- *Altered Oral Mucous Membrane* related to the presence of pemphigus lesions
- *Impaired Skin Integrity* related to the presence of blisters and open lesions
- *Pain* related to large areas of open skin and blistering

Client and Family Teaching

Teaching the client and family how to provide care at home also involves the same topics: skin care, oral care, diet, pain management, and prevention of infection. In addition, the nurse teaches the client and family how to take prescribed medications. A referral to a home health agency or local health department may be necessary.

The Client with Lichen Planus

■ ■ ■

Lichen planus is a benign inflammatory disorder of the mucous membranes and skin. It has no known cause but has been associated with exposure to drugs or to film processing chemicals (McCance & Huether, 1994). The disease affects adults from 30 to 70 years of age.

The lesions first appear as violet-colored papules, 2 to 10 mm in size, commonly occurring on the wrists, ankles, lower legs, and genitals (Figure 17–21). The lesions are intensely pruritic. Over time, persistent lesions thicken and become dark red, forming hypertrophic lichen planus. Lesions on the oral mucous membranes appear as white lacey rings; lesions may also appear on the mucous membranes of the vaginal area and the penis. The nails become thin and may shed.

Lichen planus lesions are self-limiting but last for an average of 12 to 18 months. The disorder is diagnosed by clinical manifestations. Corticosteroids are used to control the inflammation, and antihistamines are used to control the pruritus. Lesions recur in about 20% of cases (McCance & Huether, 1994).

The Client with Toxic Epidermal Necrolysis

■ ■ ■

Toxic epidermal necrolysis (TEN) is a rare, life-threatening disease in which the epidermis peels off the dermis in sheets, leaving large areas of denuded skin. Conjunctivitis and mucositis of the mouth, upper airway, esophagus, and sometimes the genitourinary tract are often associated with TEN. The client usually requires critical care, often in a burn center.

The incidence of TEN has not been documented, but it is seen more often in men and in people of African descent. The mortality rate ranges from 25% to 100% but is decreasing because of current methods of care (DePew, 1991). The cause of death is almost always sepsis.

About one-third of all cases result from a drug reaction, and another third are associated with a serious concomitant illness, such as cancer or AIDS. In other cases, the disease has no known cause. Drugs that have been associated with TEN are the sulfonamides, barbiturates, NSAIDs, phenytoin, allopurinol, and penicillin.

Pathophysiology

The pathophysiologic process in TEN is not completely understood, but the triggering mechanism is believed to be a hypersensitivity or immune response. TEN begins with a painful, localized erythema of the face and extremities, accompanied by fever, chills, muscle aches, and generalized malaise. A macular rash develops, followed by the formation of large, flaccid blisters over the body surface during the next 24 to 96 hours. The skin begins to slough, leaving the dermal surface exposed. Even in areas without blistering, the skin may peel off in layers (a response called *Nikolsky's sign*). The skin sloughing continues over several days and can expose 95% or more of the dermal surface (Figure 17–22). Other manifestations include conjunctivitis, pharyngitis, stomatitis, and enlargement of lymph glands. Urethral slough is common, causing such painful voiding that the client voluntarily retains urine. The client is often disoriented, may be nearly comatose, and is seriously ill.

The loss of skin leads to fluid and electrolyte imbalances and secondary infections, as well as systemic effects on all other body systems. These complications may cause death. However, if the complications can be prevented, healing by epidermal regeneration occurs in about a month. The long-term complications of TEN include blindness, lacrimal duct occlusion, scarring and contractures, loss of nails, esophageal strictures, and glomerulonephritis.

Collaborative Care

The client is hospitalized and requires rapid diagnosis and treatment. Any suspected drug in use by the client is stopped immediately. Collaborative care involves fluid replacement, correction of electrolyte imbalances, prevention or management of infection, and pain control.

Laboratory and Diagnostic Tests

In the early stages, TEN may be difficult to distinguish from other disorders that cause widespread skin loss. The lesions must be differentiated from those caused by less serious drug reactions, exfoliative dermatitis, pemphigus vulgaris, or an illness with similar manifestations caused by *Staphylococcus* infections in immunosuppressed adults (called *staphylococcal scalded skin syndrome*). A biopsy of the skin lesions is used in making the differential diagnosis.

Pharmacology

Although their use is controversial, systemic corticosteroids have successfully reversed allergic drug reactions, especially if administered early in the course of the disease. However, these drugs also have been associated with an increase in gram-negative infections with no improvement in skin lesions and may actually increase mortality.

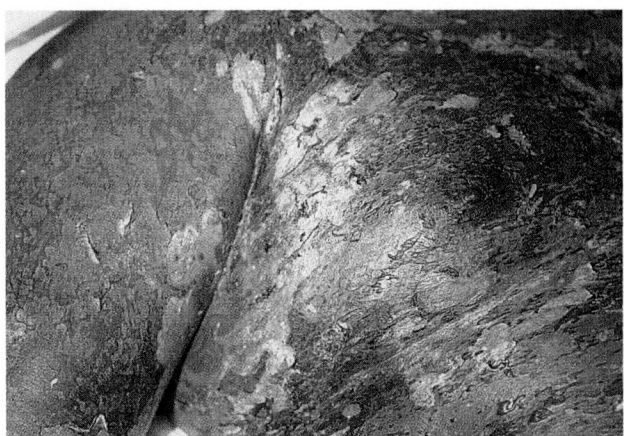

Figure 17–22   Toxic epidermal necrolysis (TEN) is a life-threatening skin disease characterized by the sloughing of large skin surfaces.

Other treatments focus on relieving symptoms and include the administration of intravenous fluids and electrolytes, pain medications, ophthalmic medications, and topical agents to promote reepithelialization of the skin. Topical medications containing sulfa, such as Silvadene, are avoided in skin treatment because they have been implicated as possible causative agents.

Surgery

The denuded areas of skin are often covered with dressings of biologic or synthetic skin. These dressings are applied in the operating room. The biologic dressings are then left uncovered. The following products (further described in Chapter 18) are used to treat clients with partial-thickness noninfected skin loss:

- Pigskin (xenograft) is a biologic dressing that promotes reepithelialization and provides a barrier against fluid loss. Pigskin eventually sloughs off if it is not removed before the body rejects it. Clients are assessed for hypersensitivity, manifested by a temperature spike and rejection of the graft.

- Biobrane is a synthetic, semipermeable silicone membrane impregnated with collagen that has been found to be effective in promoting healing in clients with TEN. If infection develops, the membrane becomes purulent and nonadherent.

- Bacitracin on petrolatum gauze (for example, Xeroform, Aquaphor, Adaptic) has been used in exfoliative disease.

- Hydrogen-absorbing foam dressings may be used to promote reepithelialization.

The extremities may be placed in padded splints to prevent shearing of the dressing with movement. The client should also be placed on an air-fluidized bed to prevent shearing and pressure and to keep the skin dressing dry.

Nursing Care

The client with TEN is usually acutely ill and requires intensive, expert nursing care. The client has multiple problems; those most common include impaired skin integrity, altered oral mucous membranes, risk for infection, risk for fluid volume deficit, and pain. The nursing care for clients with TEN is much like that provided to clients with burns (discussed in Chapter 18).

Impaired Skin Integrity

The client with TEN, who has large areas of denuded skin or of skin that is easily lost through touch or movement, presents a nursing challenge. Nursing care focuses on preventing further damage and on promoting healing of the lesions.

Nursing interventions with rationales follow:

- Monitor the skin every 8 hours to assess the characteristics of current lesions and to identify the spread of lesions to intact skin surfaces. Document the area and extent of body surface area involved, including the color, size, drainage, and odor of lesions. All lesions should be photographed on admission and on discharge to verify skin condition. *The initial assessment of the skin is carefully documented to serve as a base for ongoing assessment and management of lesions.*

- Place the client on an alternating air flow mattress. *The extent of skin involvement requires maximum support with minimal pressure against the skin.*

- Apply protective dressings in collaboration with medical care. *These products provide protective barriers, thereby decreasing the risk of infection, decreasing fluid loss, increasing comfort, and promoting moist healing.*

- Monitor nutritional status:
  a. If possible to do so without traumatizing the skin, take and record the client's weight daily.
  b. Consult with the dietition to determine the client's kcaloric needs and the best method of meeting them. Nasogastric tube feedings or total parenteral nutrition is instituted for most clients.
  c. Review laboratory data for total protein and albumin levels and general chemistry assessments.
  Because of their debilitating illness and sloughing mucous membranes, most clients require nutritional support. Extensive skin loss increases kcaloric and protein requirements for wound healing and tissue repair.

Altered Oral Mucous Membranes

In the client with TEN, extensive erosion of oral mucous membranes results in pain and alterations in the ability to eat and drink.

Nursing interventions with rationales follow:

- Assess the condition of the oral mucous membranes every 4 hours, noting appearance, size, and location of lesions. *Assessments are required to monitor any increase in lesions or signs of healing.*

- Provide oral care every 2 hours while the client is awake, as well as before and after meals if the client is able to eat. To clean the oral mucous membranes, use sponge applicators and a nonirritating solution, such as a 25% solution of hydrogen peroxide in water or 1 teaspoon of sodium bicarbonate in 8 ounces of water; then rinse with water. Petroleum jelly may be used on crusted or bleeding lips. *Oral lesions are painful and increase the risk for infection. Regular cleaning promotes comfort and increases healing of oral lesions.*

- If client is able to eat or drink, ensure that food or fluids are cool or at room temperature, are nonirritating, and are easily swallowed. Liquid protein drinks are often useful. *The client should not be given any oral food or fluid that will further irritate the oral lesions. Food and fluids at cool or tepid temperatures are better tolerated. Liquid protein supplements are more easily swallowed and help meet protein needs.*

Risk for Infection

Sepsis is a major concern in the client with skin loss and altered mucous membrane integrity. Many clients also have additional underlying diseases and compromised immune systems, which make any infection more serious. In addition, invasive procedures such as catheterization, intubation, and insertion of intravenous lines are often used in the treatment of severely ill clients and further increase the risk for infection.

Nursing interventions with rationales follow:

- Maintain reverse isolation precautions. Instruct family members in hand-washing and gowning procedures. Explain the purpose of protective isolation and request that visitors be limited to close friends and family members. *Reverse isolation procedures decrease the risk of infection from the environment. Explaining the purpose of reverse isolation is essential to decrease anxiety and stress in the client and family*

- Monitor for manifestations of infection every 4 hours:
  a. Take and record vital signs, assessing especially for increased temperature, rapid pulse, or increased respiratory rate. Avoid taking the temperature orally, which may increase tissue loss from lesions on mucous membranes; core temperatures are usually monitored in the intensive care unit.
  b. Assess the appearance of lesions for increased inflammation or pain.
  c. Assess drainage for increased amount of purulence.
  d. Monitor laboratory reports for increased white blood cell (WBC) count.

e. Monitor changes in sensorium.

f. Auscultate breath sounds, and review chest X-ray reports.

Infection and sepsis are manifested by increased temperature, pulse, and respiratory rate; changes in lesions and drainage; increased WBC count; and mental confusion or a decreasing level of consciousness. Sloughing of the upper airway membranes increases the risk of ineffective airway clearance and the development of pneumonia.

Risk for Fluid Volume Deficit

The client with TEN loses fluid into blisters and from the large areas of denuded skin. Oral lesions often prevent the client from maintaining an adequate intake of fluids. If septicemia develops, the client becomes hypovolemic (see the discussion of septic shock in Chapter 6).

Nursing interventions with rationales follow:

■ Weigh the client daily, preferably on an automatic bed scale. *Change in body weight is an accurate indicator of fluid status. Avoid sliding the client on and off scales; this may cause further skin trauma.*

■ Record intake and output each 8 hours, noting the pattern of intake compared to output over time. *Intake and output should be approximately equivalent over each 24-hour period. Urinary output should be maintained at 30 to 50 mL per hour.*

■ Monitor for manifestations of fluid imbalance: increased urine specific gravity, increased serum creatinine and blood urea nitrogen (BUN) levels, abnormal serum sodium levels, decreased blood pressure, and increased pulse. *These manifestations are indicative of fluid volume deficit and hypovolemia.*

■ Maintain a warm room temperature; if the client is on a fluidized bed, assess the controls every 4 hours to avoid chilling the client. *Great loss of epidermis impairs the skin's thermoregulatory function. Cold temperatures and shivering increase the client's metabolic rate and can cause further fluid loss from the skin.*

Pain

The exposed nerve endings in the dermal layer cause severe pain in most clients with TEN. Altered mucous membranes cause even more distress.

Nursing interventions with rationales follow:

■ Assess the client's pain using a consistent scale, for example, a scale of 1 to 10, with 10 being the worst possible pain. *Pain is a subjective experience and can be determined only by the person experiencing the pain.*

■ Consult with the physician regarding the use of patient-controlled analgesia (PCA) for intravenous administration of medications. Evaluate the route of pain medication as the client's condition improves. *PCA provides consistent medication for a client who otherwise would require frequent injections. It also allows the client control over the management of pain. Most clients have difficulty swallowing oral pain medications. If the pain is less acute, liquid narcotics may be given orally.*

■ Teach the client noninvasive methods of pain management. *Noninvasive methods of pain management often increase the effectiveness of systemic pain medications. They also enable the client to manage the pain experience.*

Other Nursing Diagnoses

Other nursing diagnoses that are appropriate for the client with TEN follow:

■ *Anxiety* related to unknown progress of skin loss

■ *Fatigue* related to the inability to rest and sleep secondary to pain from denuded areas of skin and mucous membranes

■ *Hopelessness* related to uncertain prognosis and constant pain

■ *Self-Care Deficit: Bathing/Hygiene* related to loss of skin surface with movement

■ *Impaired Swallowing* related to lesions of esophageal mucous membranes

■ *Ineffective Thermoregulation* related to loss of skin surface

■ *Decreased Cardiac Output* related to the loss of fluids from denuded skin areas with resultant hypovolemia

Client and Family Teaching

Ongoing teaching is essential for the client and family throughout hospital care. The client may have been healthy prior to the unexpected and abrupt onset of TEN and, as a result, may respond to the illness and the need for intensive care with emotions that range from depression to anger. The combination of the pain, skin disfigurement, and serious illness elicits anxiety and fear and often leads to a crisis situation for most clients and family members.

While providing care, the nurse explains the treatment plans and goals to the client and family. These plans and goals may be established initially by the health care team, but should then be revised by the client and nurse together as the client's health status improves. The nurse also explains all procedures and addresses any client or family concerns before performing the procedures.

To provide emotional support, the nurse informs family members of the client's condition. It is also helpful to provide a quiet, private place where family members can discuss the client's condition with health care providers and to give the family a list of unit policies and phone numbers so that they can contact care providers. If the client and/or family appears very anxious, referral to a social worker, counselor, or pastor may be beneficial.

Applying the Nursing Process

Case Study of a Client with TEN: Jean Murphy

Jean Murphy is a 68-year-old retired teacher who lives with her husband. Their three children are grown and live in other states. Mrs. Murphy is brought to the emergency department of the local hospital by her husband early in the morning. On admission to the emergency department, Mrs. Murphy is lethargic, and her vital signs are as follows: T, 101.2 F (38.4 C); BP, 92/58; P, 112; R, 32. Her skin is erythematous and is peeling in layers.

Assessment

The nursing staff immediately administers intravenous fluids and oxygen as emergency measures, conducts a physical examination, closely monitors vital signs, draws blood, and sends it to the laboratory. Mr. Murphy helps by providing his wife's medical history. Mrs. Murphy has been undergoing treatment at a university medical center several hours away for recurrent lymphocytic lymphoma and was given chemotherapy with chlorambucil several weeks earlier. A week after receiving the chlorambucil, Mrs. Murphy developed itching, which progressed to a macular rash. She was diagnosed as having erythema multiforme and was treated with hydroxyzine hydrochloride (Atarax) for itching and prednisone for inflammation. Her symptoms improved until 2 days ago, when she became weak and developed spreading redness over her skin and painful sores in her lips and mouth. Mr. Murphy says that he had planned to take his wife back to the university hospital today but that because she was so ill this morning he brought her to the nearest emergency department.

Mr. Murphy adds that his wife had in the past developed an allergy to sulfa after using it to treat a urinary tract infection. A skin rash resulted, but it disappeared after Mrs. Murphy stopped taking the medicine. He is unaware of any other allergies and states that except for the lymphoma his wife has always been healthy. Mr. Murphy states that his wife has made a living will that includes a provision against employing aggressive means to keep her alive, but he wants to discuss this with her and their children before any decisions are made.

Mrs. Murphy's blood gases are as follows:

pH: 7.30 (normal: 7.35 to 7.45)

Pa_{O_2}: 90 mm Hg (normal: 95 to 100 mm Hg)

Pa_{CO_2}: 48 mm Hg (normal: 35 to 45 mm Hg)

HCO_3: 24 mEq/L (normal: 20 to 26 mEq/L)

Her hematocrit is 46% (normal for females: 40% to 48%), and her WBC count is 11,000/mm^3 (normal: 5000/mm^3 to 10,000/mm^3). Her blood urea nitrogen

(BUN) is 28 mg/dL (normal: 10 to 20 mg/dL), and her creatinine is 1.2 mg/dL (normal: 0.7 to 1.4 mg/dL). Other laboratory values are normal. Mrs. Murphy is then transferred to the intensive care burn unit in critical, but currently stable, condition.

Diagnosis

Mrs. Murphy's case manager, Astra Riklin, RN, identifies the following nursing diagnoses for Mrs. Murphy:

- *Fluid Volume Deficit* related to fluid loss from extensive areas of skin loss
- *Ineffective Airway Clearance* related to mucosal sloughing
- *Risk for Infection* related to denuded skin areas
- *Impaired Skin Integrity* related to lesions of TEN
- *Ineffective Thermoregulation* related to skin loss
- *Pain* related to lesions of skin and mucous membranes
- *Anticipatory Grieving* related to presence of life-threatening acute illness

Expected Outcomes

The expected outcomes established in the plan of care specify that Mrs. Murphy will:

- Regain normal vital signs, with resolution of borderline low blood pressure and tachycardia, following adequate fluid administration.
- Maintain a urinary output of 30 to 50 mL per hour.
- Maintain her body weight within 5% of preillness range.
- Demonstrate absence of infection, as evidenced by normal WBC counts, core temperature values, appearance of skin lesions, and clear airways.
- Gain adequate pain relief, as demonstrated by verbal report of comfort and ability to rest and sleep.
- Regain normal skin and mucous membrane integrity.
- Verbalize understanding of and willingness to participate in treatment plan.
- Verbalize concerns and feelings about dealing with this life-threatening illness and hospitalization.

Planning and Implementation

Ms. Riklin implements the following interventions for Mrs. Murphy:

- Administer prescribed fluids through the central line inserted in the emergency department.
- Insert a Foley catheter, and monitor urine output hourly.
- Take and record vital signs, including core temperature, hourly and prn.

- Use a bed with an alternating air mattress and a built-in scale (for daily weights).
- Maintain room and bed temperatures to keep core body temperature between 97 and 99 F (36.1 and 37.2 C).
- Collaborate with the respiratory therapist in assessing breath sounds and arterial blood gases and administering oxygen. The respiratory therapist will teach deep-breathing exercises and the use of incentive spirometry (see Chapter 34).
- Encourage use of PCA pump, and carefully monitor pain relief, respiratory effort, and mental status.
- Assist with the application of Biobrane dressings, and document the condition of skin and mucous membranes at each shift.
- Provide oral care every 2 hours during the client's waking hours.
- Assist the client with meals, recording caloric and fluid intake at each shift.
- Teach family members the importance of hand washing, gloving, and gowning when they come in contact with Mrs. Murphy's open skin.
- Discuss with Mr. and Mrs. Murphy the need to limit visitors to the immediate family and one close friend during this critical stage of care.
- Request a visit from hospital social worker to provide counseling and relaxation techniques.

Evaluation

Mrs. Murphy remains in critical condition for several weeks. She develops pneumonia, which responds to an-tibiotics and respiratory therapy. All her previous medications are discontinued, and the medical team decides against steroid therapy. Mrs. Murphy loses weight and requires nasogastric tube feedings to maintain adequate nutrition. The Biobrane gradually peels away as new epidermis forms. As Mrs. Murphy's condition stabilizes, she is transferred to a medical unit for continued care. When her strength returns, her lymphoma therapy is reevaluated. Mrs. Murphy and her family develop renewed hope as her condition improves but acknowledge that the lymphoma remains a serious health problem.

Critical Thinking in the Nursing Process

1. Consider Mrs. Murphy's admission laboratory results. What do the abnormal arterial blood gases indicate? (Refer to Chapter 5 if necessary.) Describe factors that may have caused this change.

2. If Mrs. Murphy says to you, "I know I'm going to die," what would be your response? Why would you make this response?

3. Mrs. Murphy has strong religious beliefs but expresses concern that this illness is a sign that she has done something very wrong in her life. What could you do to encourage her to call upon her beliefs to help her cope?

4. Develop a plan to teach Mr. and Mrs. Murphy to provide her oral care.

5. Develop a nursing care plan for Mrs. Murphy for the diagnosis *Sleep Pattern Disturbance*.

▪▪▪ Neoplastic Disorders ▪▪▪

The skin is a common site for benign and malignant lesions. Many of these lesions are found on skin surfaces that have undergone long-term exposure to the sun or the environment. The most common benign skin lesions are nevi (moles). Malignant skin tumors are the most common of all cancers. This section of the chapter discusses these and other common benign and malignant skin lesions.

The Client with a Benign Skin Lesion

▪ ▪ ▪

The skin is subject to many different types and kinds of benign skin lesions, including cysts, keloids, nevi, angiomas, skin tags, and keratoses. Although these benign lesions are often considered more of a nuisance than an illness, they do require monitoring for an increase in size that interferes with the skin's appearance or function and for the potential to develop into malignant lesions.

Pathophysiology

Benign skin lesions are common in the adult population. Sun exposure and aging can cause these lesions; occupation, gender, and racial background also influence their incidence to some degree.

Cysts

Cysts of the skin are benign closed sacs in or under the skin surface that are lined with epithelium and contain fluid or a semisolid material. Epidermal inclusion cysts and pilar cysts are the most common types.

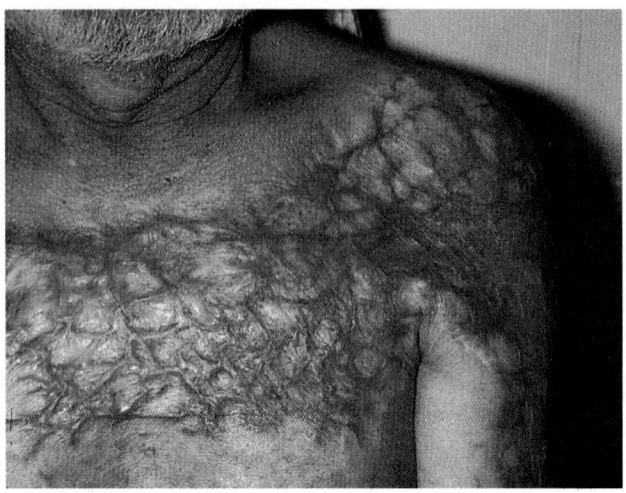

Figure 17–23 Keloids form from the deposit of excessive amounts of collagen during scar formation.

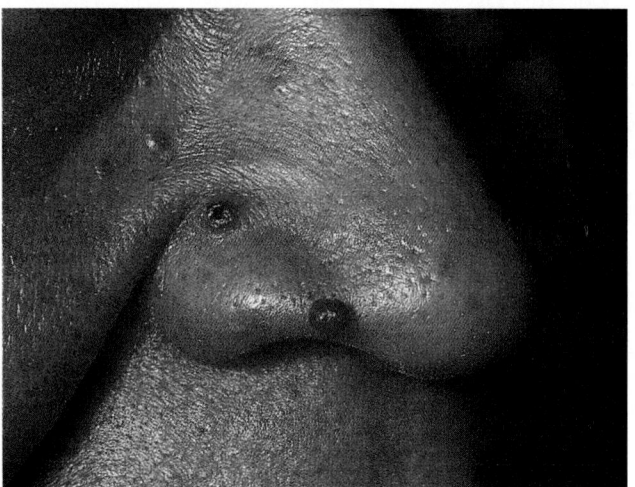

Figure 17–24 Nevi, more commonly called moles, arise from melanocytes and are common in all adults.

Epidermal inclusion cysts may occur anywhere on the body but are most often found on the head and trunk. Although they are painless, they may grow so large that they become irritated by contact with clothing (for example, if located on the back of the neck) or cause obstruction (for example, if located on the nose). The cysts contain a semisolid material composed mainly of keratin; this material has a foul odor. *Pilar cysts* are found on the scalp and originate from sebaceous glands. They are also painless. Both types of cysts rarely require treatment unless they become large and bothersome.

Keloids

Keloids are elevated, irregularly shaped, progressively enlarging scars. They arise from excessive amounts of collagen in the stratum corneum during scar formation in connective tissue repair (McCance & Huether, 1994). These lesions are more common in young adults and appear within one year of the initial trauma.

This abnormal response most often occurs in people of African and Asian descent who sustain burns of the skin; even seemingly minor trauma, however, can result in keloid formation. There is a familial tendency to develop keloids. Other risk factors for keloid formation include excessive tension on a wound and poor alignment of skin edges following accidental or intentional skin trauma. Certain skin surfaces are also more likely to develop keloids: the chin, ears, shoulders, back, and lower legs.

The excessive scar formation is associated with increased metabolic activity of fibroplasts and increased type III collagen. The principal cells of the keloids are myofibroblasts, which have characteristics of both fibroblasts and smooth muscle cells. The swollen appearance of the keloids is the result of an excess of extracellular material.

The keloids first appear as red, firm, rubbery plaques that persist for several months after the initial trauma

(Figure 17–23). Uncontrolled overgrowth over time causes the keloids to extend beyond the original scar. Eventually, the keloid becomes smooth and hyperpigmented.

Nevi

Nevi, more commonly called moles, are flat or raised macules or papules with rounded, well defined borders (Figure 17–24). Nevi arise from melanocytes during early childhood, with the cells initially accumulating at the junction of the dermis and epidermis. Over time, the cluster of cells moves into the dermis, and the lesion becomes visible. Almost all adults have nevi.

Nevi range from flesh colored to black and occasionally contain hair. They can occur on any skin surface of the body and may arise as single lesions or in groups. Some pigmented nevi can transform into malignant lesions; although the average adult has about 20 nevi, only 4 people out of 100,000 develop a malignant melanoma (Porth, 1994). However, it is important to monitor nevi for indicators of transformation: changes in size, thickness, color, bleeding, or itching. If any of these changes occur, the person should seek immediate professional assessment.

Angiomas

Angiomas, also called *hemangiomas,* are benign vascular tumors. They appear in the adult in different forms:

- *Nevus flammeus (port-wine stain)* is a congenital vascular lesion that involves the capillaries. The lesions tend to occur on the upper body or face as macular patches that range from light red to dark purple. These lesions are present at birth and grow proportionately with the child into adulthood.

- *Cherry angiomas* are small, rounded papules that may occur at any age, but they most commonly arise in the

40s and gradually increase in number. The lesions range in color from bright red to purple. These lesions are often found on the trunk.

- *Spider angiomas* are dilated superficial arteries; they are not actually tumors. They are common in pregnant women and in clients with hepatic disease. Spider angiomas occur most often on the face, neck, and upper chest. The lesions are usually small, bright red papules with radiating lines.

- *Telangiectases* are single dilated capillaries or terminal arteries that appear often on the cheeks and nose. These lesions are most common in older adults and result from photoaged skin. The lesions look like broken veins.

- *Venous lakes* are small, flat, blue blood vessels. They are seen on the exposed skin of the older adult: the ears, lips, and backs of the hands.

Skin Tags

Skin tags are soft papules on a pedicle. They can be as small as a pinhead or as large as a pea and are most often found on the front or side of the neck and in the axillae. These lesions have normal skin color and texture.

Keratoses

A **keratosis** is any skin condition in which there is a benign overgrowth and thickening of the cornified epithelium. These lesions most often appear in adults after the fifth decade of life. The most common types of keratoses are seborrheic keratosis and actinic keratosis.

Seborrheic Keratoses   *Seborrheic keratoses* are lesions that appear as superficial flat, smooth or warty-surfaced growths, 5 to 20 mm in diameter, most often on the face and trunk. The lesions may be tan, waxy yellow, dark brown, or flesh colored, and they often appear greasy.

These lesions are most often seen in the older adult and do not appear to be related to damage from sun exposure (Kurban & Kurban, 1993). On rare occasions, the lesions become malignant.

Actinic Keratoses   *Actinic keratosis*, also called *senile* or *solar keratosis*, is an epidermal skin lesion directly related to chronic sun exposure and photodamage (Kurban & Kurban, 1993). The prevalence is highest in people with light-colored skin; these lesions are rare in people with dark skin.

Actinic keratosis may progress to squamous cell carcinoma. Fewer than 1% of early lesions become malignant, but as many as 10% to 20% of those that persist progress to malignancy (Kao, 1990). Because of this tendency, the lesions are classified as premalignant.

The lesions are erythematous rough macules a few millimeters in diameter. They are often shiny but may be scaly; if the scales are removed, the underlying skin bleeds. They occur in multiple patches, primarily on the

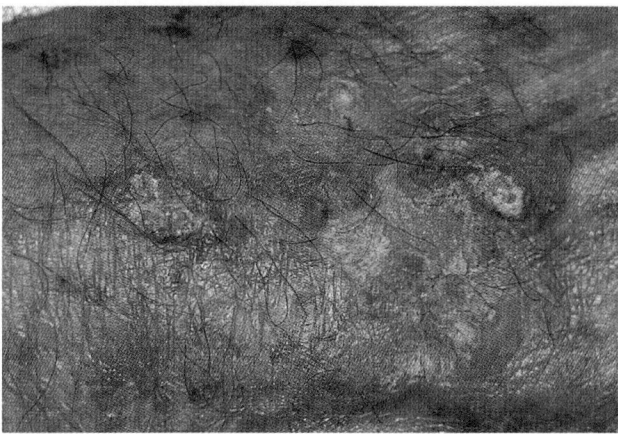

Figure 17-25 The effects of long-term sun exposure are illustrated in this epidermal skin lesion, called actinic keratosis.

face, dorsa of the hands, the forearms, and sometimes on the upper trunk (Figure 17–25). Enlargement or ulceration of the lesions suggests transformation to malignancy.

Collaborative Care

Most benign skin lesions do not require treatment. However, there are certain instances in which excision or treatment with laser surgery or cryosurgery may be necessary. Cysts may enlarge, nevi may change in color or appearance, skin tags may become irritated and bleed, or any of the lesions (especially those located on the face) may cause problems with appearance. In most instances the lesions are removed by excision and are examined to detect any possible malignancy.

Nursing Care

Nursing care for the client with a benign skin lesion consists primarily of health promotion and education. Education to prevent lesions from sun exposure must begin in childhood and continue through the adult years, with emphasis on the need to use sunscreens, avoid direct exposure to the sun, and wear protective clothing when in the sun. If the client has a large lesion that causes embarrassment, referrals for cosmetic coverage or possible surgical removal are appropriate.

It is important to assess all skin surfaces of the older adult carefully during any health care encounter. Benign skin lesions are common in this population, and some of the lesions may become malignant; therefore, early detection and treatment are essential.

Client and Family Teaching

The nurse teaches the client and family with benign skin lesions not only to avoid sun exposure but also to conduct a monthly skin self-examination (for example, the

Nursing Assessment for Skin Cancer

■ ■ ■

Interview Questions

- Have any members of your family ever been treated for skin cancer?
- Have you had a skin cancer removed from any part of your body?
- Have you noticed any change in the size, shape, or color of a mole, wart, birthmark, or scar?
- Do you have any moles, warts, birthmarks, or scars that itch, are painful, have crusting, or bleed?
- In what parts of the country or world have you lived?
- Have you ever been badly sunburned?
- Do you visit tanning salons?
- Are you exposed to any hazardous chemicals in your job?
- Have you been taught how to examine your skin? If so, how do you do this examination? How often?

Physical Assessment

1. Ask the client to remove all clothing and put on an examination gown. Ensure good light; natural, bright light is best for inspection of lesions. The client may sit, stand, or lie down.
2. Inspect and palpate the skin. Stretching the skin tightly during assessment facilitates assessment of nodular and scaly lesions and lesions in the dermis. Assess for:

a. Obvious lesions
b. Visible swellings
c. Alterations in normal contour and borders of nevi
d. Enlarged lymph glands
e. Skin or mucosal discolorations
f. Areas of ulceration, scaling, crusting, or erosion

3. The order of assessment follows:
a. Head and neck: entire scalp, eyelids, external ear, auditory canals, external surface of the nose, internal surface of the nose, the oral cavity, facial skin, the facial glands (parotid, submaxillary, sublingual)
b. Thyroid and neck, including lymph glands
c. Chest and abdomen, with special attention under pendulous breasts, in skinfolds, and in areas covered with hair
d. Back and buttocks, with special attention to the area between the buttocks
e. Extremities, with special attention to the axillae, nail beds, webs between the fingers and toes, and soles of the feet
f. External genitals, with special attention to skinfolds, mucous membranes, and areas covered with hair

4. Measure and record a description of all skin lesions on an anatomic chart. Take photographs (if possible) of any suspicious lesion, and include them in the client's record for future reference.

---

first day of each month). Using a mirror to examine lesions on the back of the body and extremities, the client looks for the following changes:

- A change in color, especially any lesion that becomes darker or variegated in shades of tan, brown, black, red, white, or blue
- A change in size, especially any lesion that becomes larger or spreads out
- A change in shape, especially any lesion that protrudes more from the skin or begins to have an irregular outline
- A change in the appearance of a lesion, especially bleeding, drainage, oozing, ulceration, crusting, scaliness, or development of a mushrooming outward growth
- A change in the consistency, especially any lesion that becomes softer or is more easily irritated

- A change in the skin around a lesion, such as redness, swelling, or leaking of color from a lesion into the surrounding skin
- A change in sensation, such as itching or pain

If any of these changes occur, the client should immediately contact the health care provider for further assessment. Skin assessment is discussed further in the accompanying box.

The Client with Kaposi's Sarcoma

■ ■ ■

Kaposi's sarcoma is a rare malignant skin lesion that formerly occurred primarily in elderly white men. However, homosexual men living in major U.S. metropolitan areas who were infected with AIDS early in the epidemic have been diagnosed with Kaposi's sarcoma. For unknown reasons, the incidence in this population now seems to be decreasing. Kaposi's sarcoma is also endemic in young black men in equatorial Africa, but it is rare in African Americans (Tierney et al., 1994).

The disease is systemic, involving lesions of the lung, gastrointestinal tract, and skin. Skin lesions are red or dark purple nodules or plaques. The management of AIDS-associated Kaposi's sarcoma consists of observation and supportive care. If the lesions cause cosmetic problems or interfere with normal function, they may be treated with cryotherapy, vinblastine, radiation therapy, or laser surgery. Progressive disease is treated with intravenous chemotherapy. See Chapter 8 for a further discussion of Kaposi's sarcoma in the client with AIDS.

The Client with Nonmelanoma Skin Cancer

■ ■ ■

The skin, despite its ability to protect the internal body from external damage, is a fragile organ and is subject to damage from ultraviolet radiation and chemicals. Over time, this damage results in alterations in cellular structure and function, and malignancies of the skin occur. The nonmelanoma skin cancers are basal cell carcinoma and squamous cell carcinoma. Melanoma skin cancer is discussed in the following section.

Overview and Etiology

It is estimated that over 700,000 new cases of nonmelanoma skin cancer occurred in 1994 in the United States; of this number, 2300 deaths will occur (American Cancer Society, 1994). However, 95% to 99% of nonmelanoma skin cancers can be cured if they are detected and treated early. Nonmelanoma skin cancer is the most common malignant neoplasm found in fair-skinned Americans. Of the two types of nonmelanoma skin cancer, basal cell carcinoma is the most common, outnumbering squamous cell carcinoma three to one. Men develop nonmelanoma skin cancer more often than do women, probably because of occupational exposures (National Cancer Institute, 1988). Although nonmelanoma skin cancer may occur at any age, the incidence increases with each decade of life. Adults between the ages of 30 and 60 have the majority of these cancers.

There are multiple etiologic factors involved in the development of nonmelanoma skin cancer, including environmental factors and host factors.

Environmental Factors

The environmental factors implicated in the nonmelanoma skin cancers are ultraviolet radiation, pollutants, chemicals, ionizing radiation, viruses, and physical trauma.

Ultraviolet radiation (UVR) from the sun is believed to be the cause of most nonmelanoma skin cancers. Sunlight contains both short-length rays (UVB) and long-length rays (UVA). UVB rays are absorbed by the top layer of skin and cause sunburn. UVA rays penetrate deeper into the skin layers, causing tissue damage. Both types of rays are believed to cause DNA alterations and also suppress T-cell and B-cell immunity. The amount of ultraviolet radiation reaching the earth is increasing, most likely because industrial chlorofluorocarbons are depleting the normally protective ozone layer surrounding the planet. The U.S. Environmental Protection Agency predicts that for every 1% decrease in the ozone layer, a corresponding 1% to 3% increase in nonmelanoma skin cancer per year will occur (National Institutes of Health Consensus Development Conference, 1991).

Geographic, environmental, and life-style factors affect the amount of exposure to the sun and the risk for nonmelanoma skin cancer. People who live in latitudes close to the equator and those who live at higher altitudes receive greater ultraviolet radiation exposure. The amount of clothing worn, the time of day, and amount of time in the sun also determine the amount of exposure. Exposure to ultraviolet radiation in tanning booths has also been implicated in the development of nonmelanoma skin cancer.

Certain chemicals have long been associated with nonmelanoma skin cancer. In 1775, Percivall Pott reported on squamous cell cancer of the scrotum in chimney sweeps, induced by exposure to soot. Polycyclic aromatic hydrocarbons, found in mixtures of coal, tar, asphalt, soot, and mineral oils, have been linked with skin cancers (Fraser, Hartage, & Tucker, 1991). Psoralens, used in conjunction with UVA for treatment of psoriasis and cutaneous T-cell lymphoma, increase the risk of squamous cell carcinoma.

Other factors associated with nonmelanoma skin cancer are the use of ionizing radiation, viruses, and physical trauma. X-ray therapy for tinea capitis and the use of radium to treat other malignancies are risk factors. Human papillomavirus is implicated in the development of squamous cell carcinoma, as is damage to the skin from burns (Ketcham & Loescher, 1993).

Host Factors

Certain host factors increase the risk of nonmelanoma skin cancer. These include skin pigmentation as well as the presence of premalignant lesions.

Skin pigmentation is an important factor in the development of nonmelanoma skin cancer. The amount of melanin pigment produced by the melanocytes determines a person's skin color; the more melanin, the more the skin is protected from the damage produced by ultraviolet rays. Thus, African Americans, Asian Americans,

Table 17–3   Types and Characteristics of Basal Cell Cancers

Type	Common Location	Manifestation
Nodular	Face, neck, head	Small, firm papule; pearly, white, pink, or flesh-colored; telangiectasis; enlarges; may ulcerate.
Superficial	Trunk, extremities	Papules or plaque that is flat, erythematous, or scaling; pink color; well-defined borders; may have shallow erosions and surface crusting.
Pigmented	Head, neck, face	Dark brown, blue, or black color; border is shiny and well defined.
Morpheaform	Head, neck	Looks like a flat scar; ivory or flesh-colored.
Keratotic	Ear	Small, firm papule; pearly, white, pink, or flesh-colored; may ulcerate.

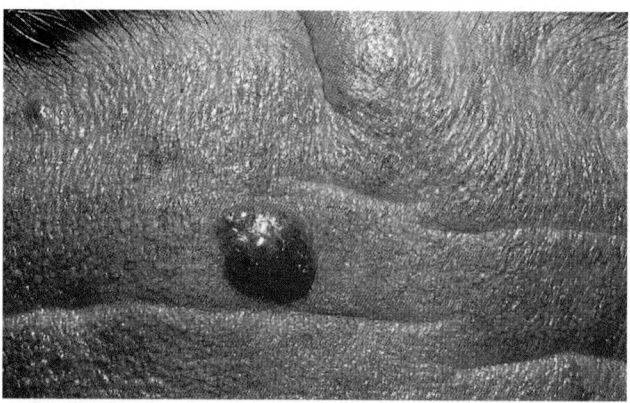

Figure 17–26   A superficial basal cell cancer often is erythematous, has well-defined borders, and ulcerations.

and people of Mediterranean descent have a much lower incidence of nonmelanoma skin cancer than do people who have red hair and fair complexions who tend to freckle or sunburn easily, such as people of Irish, Scandinavian, or English ancestry (Fraser, Hartage, & Tucker, 1991).

Although most people have numerous pigmented lesions on their body, almost all of these are normal. However, a major risk factor in the development of nonmelanoma skin cancer is a change in an existing lesion or the presence of a premalignant lesion, such as actinic keratosis. Other people at risk for the development of squamous cell carcinoma include organ transplant recipients who undergo immunosuppression to prevent rejection (Ketcham & Loescher, 1993).

Pathophysiology

The two nonmelanoma skin cancers, basal cell carcinoma and squamous cell carcinoma, arise from epithelial tissue but have different pathophysiology, classifications, and manifestations.

Basal Cell Carcinoma

Basal cell carcinoma is an epithelial tumor that is believed to originate either from the basal layer of the epidermis or from cells in the surrounding dermal structures. These tumors are characterized by an impaired

ability of the basal cells of the epidermis to mature into keratinocytes, with mitotic division beyond the basal layer. This results in a bulky neoplasm that grows by direct extension and destroys surrounding tissue, including healthy skin, nerves, blood vessels, lymphatic tissue, cartilage, and bone. Basal cell carcinoma is the most common but least aggressive type of skin cancer, rarely metastizing (Vargo, 1991).

Basal cell carcinoma is classified into different types: nodular, superficial, pigmented, morpheaform, and keratotic. These types are described below and are summarized in Table 17–3.

- *Nodular basal cell carcinoma (noduloulcerative)*, the most common type of basal cell cancer, most often appears on the face, neck, and head. The tumor is made up of masses of cells that resemble epidermal basal cells and grow in a bulky, nodular form from lack of keratinization. In early stages, the tumor is a papule that looks like a smooth pimple. It is often pruritic and continues to grow at a steady rate, doubling in size every 6 to 12 months. As the tumor grows, the epidermis thins, but it remains intact. The skin over the tumor is shiny, and either pearly white, pink, or skin colored. Telangiectasis may be visible over the area of the tumor. As the tumor continues to increase in size, the center or periphery may ulcerate, and the tumor develops well-circumscribed borders. It bleeds easily from mild injury (Ketcham & Loescher, 1993; Vargo, 1991).

- *Superficial basal cell carcinoma*, found most often on the trunk and extremities, is the second most common type of basal cell cancer. This tumor is a proliferating tissue that attaches to the undersurface of the epithelium. The tumor is a flat papule or plaque, often erythematous, with well-defined borders. The tumor may ulcerate and be covered with crusts or shallow erosions (Figure 17–26).

- *Pigmented basal cell carcinoma,* found on the head, neck, and face, is less common. This tumor concentrates melanin pigment in the center of the basal cancer cells, giving it a dark brown, blue, or black appearance. The border of the tumor is shiny and well defined.

- *Morpheaform basal cell carcinoma,* the rarest form of basal cell cancer, develops most often on the head and neck. The tumor forms fingerlike projections that extend in any direction along dermal tissue planes. The tumor resembles a flat scar that is ivory or flesh colored. This form is more likely to extend into and destroy adjacent tissue, especially muscle, nerve, and bone. It is often more difficult to diagnose because of its appearance.

- *Keratotic basal cell carcinoma (basosquamous)* is found on the preauricular and postauricular groove. It contains both basal cells and squamoid-appearing cells that keratinize. Its appearance is much like that of nodular basal cell cancer. This type of basal cell cancer tends to recur locally and also is the type most likely to metastasize.

Basal cell carcinomas do tend to recur, but they rarely metastasize. Tumors that are greater than 2 cm in diameter have a high recurrence rate. The recurrence rate of basal cell cancer has been reported to be 33% at 1 year after treatment, 66% within 3 years, and 82% within 5 years (Rowe, Carroll, & Day, 1989). Predisposing factors for metastasis are the size of the tumor and the client's resistance to treatment with surgery or chemotherapy (Vargo, 1991). Even though they rarely metastasize, untreated basal cell carcinomas invade surrounding tissue and may destroy body parts, such as the nose or eyelid.

Squamous Cell Carcinoma

Squamous cell carcinoma is a malignant tumor of the squamous epithelium of the skin or mucous membranes. It occurs most often on areas of skin that are exposed to ultraviolet rays and weather, such as the forehead, helix of the ear, top of the nose, lower lip, and back of the hands. Squamous cell carcinoma may also arise on skin that has been burned or has chronic inflammation. This is a much more aggressive cancer than basal cell cancer, with a faster growth rate and a much greater potential for metastasis if untreated (Ketcham & Loescher, 1993).

The tumors arise when the keratinizing cells of the squamous epithelium proliferate, producing a growth that eventually fills the epidermis and invades the dermal tissue planes. Keratinization of some cells is present, and the formation of keratin "pearls" is common. The keratin formation diminishes as the tumor grows. In addition, with growth of the tumor, the tumor cells increase in number and rate of mitosis, forming odd shapes.

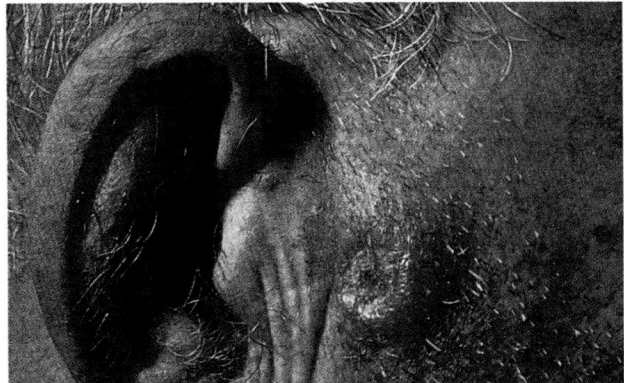

Figure 17–27 As a squamous cell cancer grows, it tends to invade surrounding tissue. It also ulcerates, may bleed, and is painful.

Squamous cell carcinoma begins as a firm papule that is flesh colored or erythematous. The tumor may be crusted with keratin products. As it grows, it may ulcerate, bleed, and become painful. As the tumor extends into the surrounding tissue and becomes a nodule, the area around the nodule becomes indurated (hardened) (Figure 17–27).

Recurrent squamous cell carcinoma can be invasive, increasing the person's risk of metastasis. Invasive squamous cell carcinoma may arise from preexisting skin lesions, such as scars and actinic keratosis, and extend into the dermis; it is then called *intraepidermal squamous cell carcinoma.* This form appears as a slightly raised erythematous plaque with well-defined borders. Metastasis occurs most often via lymphatic tissue. The degree of risk for metastasis depends on the size and depth of penetration of the tumor. Most metastasis occurs within 2 years of the primary tumor diagnosis and lowers the survival rate to 50% at 5 years after diagnosis (Vargo, 1991).

Collaborative Care

Treatment of nonmelanoma skin cancer focuses on removal of all malignant tissue using such methods as surgery, curettage and electrodesiccation, cryotherapy, or radiotherapy. These modalities offer a greater than 90% cure rate. After the malignant tissue is removed, the client should have regular examinations for recurrence. See the box on page 598 on collaborative care for the client with skin cancer.

Laboratory and Diagnostic Tests

Nonmelanoma cancer is diagnosed by microscopic examination of tissue biopsied from the tumor. The biopsies are usually done as office procedures under local anesthesia. The types of biopsy commonly conducted follow:

Collaborative Care: The Client with Skin Cancer

Health Care Team	Client-Centered Goals
Dermatologist, General or Plastic Surgeon	■ Conducts skin assessment
	■ Provides local treatment or biopsies and excises skin lesions
	■ Monitors clients for cancer recurrence
	■ Instructs client regarding strategies to prevent skin cancer
General or Plastic Surgeon	■ Excises large lesions and performs skin grafts or flaps if indicated
	■ May consult with oncologist and recommend radiation or chemotherapy
Visiting Nurse	■ May provide home care services for clients who require dressing changes
	■ Teaches client and family regarding the type of dressing, how to remove and replace with clean dressing
	■ Teaches client and family regarding signs and symptoms to report
RN and Health Care Team Communications	■ Refers client to health care provider for any suspicious skin lesion
	■ Documents the presence of all skin lesions and associated symptoms
	■ Reports signs or symptoms of infection or hemorrhage

■ A shave biopsy, in which the lesion is shaved with a scalpel to the level of the mid-dermis

■ A punch biopsy, in which a circular punch removes a section of tissue in a "cookie cutter" fashion to a level of the reticular dermis or subcutaneous tissue

■ An incisional biopsy, in which a part of the tumor is removed with a scalpel

■ An excisional biopsy, in which the entire tumor is removed and analyzed (Ketcham & Loescher, 1993)

Surgery

Nonmelanoma skin cancers may be removed through surgical excision or through another type of surgical treatment called Mohs micrographic surgery.

Surgical Excision   Both basal cell and squamous cell cancers are excised surgically. The surgery may be minor or major, depending on the size and location of the tumor. Surgery for small tumors is most often performed in the outpatient surgery department or in the surgeon's office. Surgical excision allows rapid healing and yields good cosmetic results, but as does any surgery, carries the risk of infection.

The goal of surgical excision is to remove the tumor completely, so some surrounding tissue is excised along with the tumor. If the tumor is on the face, the incision is made along normal wrinkle or anatomic lines so that the scars will be less obvious. The incision is closed in layers to leave the smallest possible scar. A pressure dressing is usually applied over the incision to provide support.

If a large tumor is removed, a skin graft or skin flap may be performed to cover the excised area. If grafting is necessary, the client is hospitalized.

Mohs Micrographic Surgery   In Mohs micrographic surgery, thin layers of the tumor are horizontally shaved off. A frozen section of the tissue is stained at each level to determine tumor margins. This is the most accurate method of assessing the extent of nonmelanoma skin cancer and the method that conserves the most normal tissue. It is often used in areas such as the nose, the nasolabial fold, the medial canthus, and the ear. Cure rates with Mohs microscopic surgery are at 99% for primary basal cell cancer and 94% for squamous cell carcinoma.

Curettage and Electrodesiccation

Curettage and electrodesiccation are used to treat basal cell cancers that are less than 2 cm in diameter, are superficial, or recur because of poor margin control. It may also be used for primary squamous cell cancers that are less than 1 cm in diameter and have distinct borders. This type of treatment is most successful for tumors that occur on anatomic sites over a fixed underlying surface, such as the ear, chest, and temple.

To conduct the treatment, the physician scrapes away abnormal tissue (curettage) within 1 to 2 mm of the margin and then uses a low-voltage electrode to abrade the tumor base (electrodesiccation). Tumor tissue is much softer and more friable than normal tissue. Therefore, curettage and electrodesiccation is not used for lesions where the dermis is thin (such as the eyelid) or where the tumor extends into the subcutaneous tissue.

Curettage and electrodesiccation provide good cosmetic results and preserve normal tissue. However, healing time is longer, and it is difficult to ensure that all tumor margins have been removed.

Instead of a low-voltage electrode, some physicians use a carbon dioxide laser to vaporize the tumor. When used in conjunction with curettage, this treatment is effective on superficial basal cell carcinomas. Carbon dioxide vaporization results in minimal thermal injury to adjacent cells, less pain, and quicker healing (Vargo, 1991).

Cryosurgery

Cryosurgery is a noninvasive method of treating nonmelanoma skin cancer in which liquid nitrogen is used to freeze and thereby destroy the tumor tissue. The area of the tumor is locally anesthetized; then, liquid nitrogen is applied to the lesion by either a spray or cryoprobes. This causes a quick intensive freezing of the tissue, which is then allowed to thaw slowly. The process is repeated several times before complete tumor necrosis and erosion occur.

Cryosurgery is used for some primary basal cell cancers and for low-risk squamous cell cancers. It is not used to treat cancers on the rim of the ear or the medial canthus. The treatment causes minimal pain, yields good cosmetic results, and can be done on an outpatient basis. However, healing is prolonged; moreover, during healing the wound tends to be edematous and painful, with significant blistering and inflammation. Other possible disadvantages include temporary nerve damage, bleeding, and lack of a specimen for tissue analysis.

Radiation Therapy

Radiation usually is used only for lesions that are inoperable because of their location (such as tumors on the corner of the nose, the eyelid, the canthus, and the lip) or size (between 1 cm and 8 cm). Radiotherapy is also used for clients who are older and of poor surgical risk.

Radiation is painless and can be used to treat areas surrounding the tumor if necessary. However, the treatment is given over a 3- to 4-week period in a clinical facility, does not allow control of tumor margins, and may itself cause skin cancer.

Nursing Care

Nursing care for the client with nonmelanoma skin cancer depends on the treatment employed. Surgical excision is the most common form of treatment; nursing care depends on the extent of the procedure. However, regardless of the type of treatment, the client will have impaired skin integrity, an increased risk for infection, and anxiety about the future following a diagnosis of cancer. Interventions with rationale for the client with any type of skin cancer are discussed in the section on melanoma.

The client who has been treated for a nonmelanoma skin cancer has some degree of impaired skin integrity, increasing the risk for infection. If surgical excision has been conducted, the incision may range from small to large, with possible skin grafting. The client who has had other forms of treatment also has skin impairments, such as inflammation and blisters.

If treatment is conducted in an outpatient setting, teach the client and family specific measures for self-care, including how and when to change dressings, the use of aseptic technique and careful hand washing when caring for the wound, symptoms to report (such as bleeding, fever, or signs of wound infection), and how to protect the operative site against trauma and irritations.

The client who undergoes extensive surgery will require preoperative and postoperative care (see Chapter 7). Nursing care for the client with skin cancer is discussed further in the section on melanoma.

Client and Family Teaching

Client and family teaching is a critical factor in caring for the client with a nonmelanoma skin cancer. The increasing number of people with skin cancer requires that nurses be involved in prevention and early detection. Nurses have the opportunity to teach preventive behaviors in all settings, including the hospital, home, community, school, and clinic.

It is well known that cumulative sun exposure positively correlates with nonmelanoma skin cancers. Many skin cancers can be prevented by limiting exposure to risk factors. Primary prevention behaviors, recommended by the American Cancer Society and the Skin Cancer Foundation (1988) follow:

- Minimize exposure to the sun between the hours of 10 a.m. to 3 p.m., when ultraviolet rays are the strongest.

- Cover up with a wide-brimmed hat, sunglasses, long-sleeved shirt, and long pants made of tightly woven material when you are in the sun.

- Use a waterproof or water-resistant sunscreen with an SPF of 15 or more before every exposure to the sun. Apply sunscreen not only on sunny but also on cloudy days, when ultraviolet rays can penetrate 70% to 80% of the cloud cover. Reapply the sunscreen before the protection time is up. If you are at risk for skin cancer, apply sunscreen daily. See the box on page 600 for information about sunscreens.

- Use sunscreen and protective clothing when you are on or near sand, snow, concrete, or water, which can reflect more than half of the ultraviolet rays onto the skin.

Sunscreen Information

■ ■ ■

Types of Sunscreen

Chemical

Chemical sunscreens absorb ultraviolet light and act as a radiation filter. Examples follow:

- *p*-aminobenzoic acid (PABA)
- Benzophenones
- Anthranilates
- Salicylates

Physical

Physical sunscreens reflect and scatter ultraviolet light. Examples follow:

- Zinc oxide
- Titanium dioxide
- Magnesium silicate
- Ferric chloride
- Kaolin
- Ichthyol

Adverse Reactions Associated with Sunscreens

Adverse reactions associated with sunscreens include contact and photocontact dermatitis. People with previous hypersensitivity reactions to benzocaine, procaine, sulfonamides, or paraphenylenediamine may develop hypersensitivity responses to PABA. People who are also taking systemic thiazide diuretics or sulfonamides may develop eczematous dermatitis.

Sunscreen Ratings

In the United States, the Food and Drug Administration (FDA) rates commercial sunscreens according to their "sun protection factor," or SPF. The SPF value is the ratio of the time required to produce minimal skin redness through a sunscreen product with the time required to produce the same degree of redness without the sunscreen. A person who can tolerate ½ hour of sun without a sunscreen should be able to tolerate 3 hours of sun when a sunscreen of SPF 6 is applied to the skin. SPF values of sunscreens range from 2 to 50.

- Avoid tanning booths; UVA radiation emitted by tanning booths damages the deep skin layers.

Nurses also provide client and family education for early detection of nonmelanoma skin cancer. Numerous brochures describing the types of skin cancers, photographs of lesions, and prevention behaviors are available from the American Cancer Society, health education and support agencies, and pharmaceutical companies that manufacture sunscreen. Most of this literature is free of charge. The addresses for these organizations are listed in Appendix O.

The client or family who is at risk for or has been diagnosed with a skin cancer must be taught how to conduct a self-examination of the skin as well as the importance of conducting the examination on the same day of each month. Family members can help with areas that are hard to examine, such as the ears, scalp, and back.

The Client with Malignant Melanoma

■ ■ ■

Malignant melanoma, also called cutaneous melanoma, is a skin cancer that arises from melanocytes. This serious skin cancer is increasing in incidence each year, with about 32,000 people diagnosed in 1994. Of this number, an estimated 7200 deaths will be due to melanoma (American Cancer Society, 1995).

This disease is over ten times more common in fair-skinned people than in dark-skinned people. As with the nonmelanoma skin cancers, an increase in the incidence of malignant melanoma is believed to be related to the thinning ozone layer and increased exposure to ultraviolet rays. The incidence is highest in Caucasian upper-middle class professionals who work indoors (Porth, 1994). This group of people often had severe sunburn with blistering during childhood and tend to vacation in areas of intense sun exposure. Malignant melanoma is also more common in people who live in sunny climates, burn easily, and patronize tanning parlors. However, malignant melanoma may arise from lesions that are already present or from skin that is normally covered with clothing.

Pathophysiology

Melanocytes are cells that are located at or near the basal layer (the deepest epidermal layer). These cells produce *melanin*, the dark skin pigment. Melanin is made in granules and transferred to keratinocytes, where it accumulates on the superficial side of each keratinocyte and forms a shield of pigment over the nucleus as protection against ultraviolet rays. Malignant melanomas can develop wherever there is pigment, but about one-third of them originate in existing nevi.

Almost all malignant melanomas are more than 6 mm in diameter, are asymmetric, and initially develop within the epidermis over a long period. While they are still confined to the epidermis, the lesions (called malignant melanoma in situ) are flat and relatively benign. However, when they penetrate the dermis, they mingle with blood and lymph vessels and are capable of metastasizing. At this latter stage, the tumors develop a raised or nodular appearance and often have smaller nodules, called satellite lesions, around the periphery (Roses, Gumport, Harris, & Kopf, 1988).

The prognosis for survival for people diagnosed with malignant melanoma is determined by several variables, including tumor thickness, ulceration, metastasis, site, age, and gender. Younger clients and women have a somewhat better chance of survival. Tumors on the hands, feet, and scalp have a poorer prognosis; tumors of the feet and scalp are less visible and may not be diagnosed until they grow into the dermis (Ketcham & Loescher, 1993).

Precursor Lesions

There are three specific precursor lesions for the development of malignant melanoma: dysplastic nevi, congenital nevi, and lentigo maligna. A precursor lesion is also called a premalignant lesion, a name that indicates that the lesion's risk of becoming malignant is greater than normal.

Dysplastic Nevi   Dysplastic nevi are also called atypical moles. Although dysplastic nevi are not present at birth, they appear as normal nevi during childhood and become dysplastic (having abnormal development) after puberty. A client with classic dysplastic nevi has more than 100 nevi, at least one of which is larger than 8 mm in diameter, and at least one has the characteristics of malignant melanoma (asymmetry, irregular border, color variegation, and a diameter greater than 6 mm). A familial tendency to dysplastic nevi increases the risk for the development of malignant melanoma. However, it is not known whether people with dysplastic nevi and no family history of melanoma face a higher risk of melanoma.

Dysplastic nevi most often appear on the face, trunk, and arms but also are seen on the scalp, female breast, groin, and buttocks. The pigmentation of the nevi is irregular, with mixtures of tan, brown, black, red, and pink. An area of lighter pigmentation is surrounded by a papular area of deeper pigmentation (described as a "fried egg appearance"). The borders of the nevi are irregular.

Congenital Nevi   Congenital nevi are present at birth. Some lesions are small; others are large enough to cover an entire body area. Their color can range from brown to black. They are often slightly raised, with an irregular surface and a fairly regular border.

Lentigo Maligna   Lentigo maligna, also called Hutchinson's freckle, is a tan or black patch on the skin that looks like a freckle. It grows slowly, becoming mottled, dark, thick, and nodular. It is usually seen on one side of the face of an older adult who has had a large amount of sun exposure.

Classification

Malignant melanomas are classified into different types. The major types are superficial spreading melanoma,

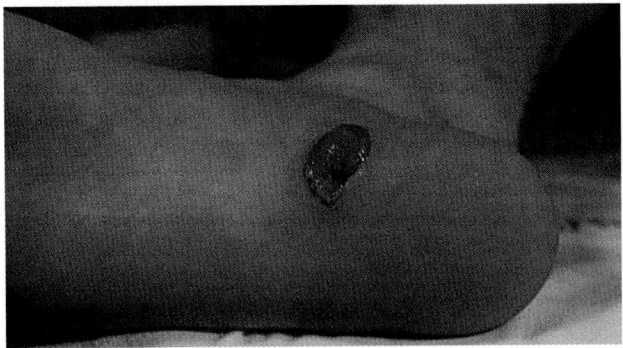

Figure 17–28   Malignant melanoma is a serious skin cancer that arises from melanocytes.

lentigo maligna melanoma, nodular melanoma, and acral lentiginous melanoma. Each of these tumors is characterized by a radial and/or vertical growth phase. During the initial radial phase, which may last from 1 to 25 years (depending on the type), the melanoma grows parallel to the skin surface. During this phase, the tumor rarely metastasizes and is often curable by surgical excision. However, during the vertical growth phase, atypical melanocytes rapidly penetrate into the dermis and subcutaneous tissue, greatly increasing the risk for metastasis and death.

Superficial Spreading Melanoma   Superficial spreading melanoma is the most common type, making up about 70% of malignant melanomas (Porth, 1994). The lesions are usually flat and scaly or crusty and are about 2 cm in diameter. They often arise from a preexisting nevus. This type of melanoma is found on the trunk and back of men and on the legs of women. Superficial spreading melanomas occur more often in women than in men. The median age of occurrence is the 50s.

The radial growth phase lasts from 1 to 5 or more years. When the lesion enters the vertical growth phase, it grows rapidly, and its color changes in color from a mixture of tan, brown, and black to a characteristic red, white, and blue color. The lesion also develops irregular borders and often has raised nodules and ulcerations (Figure 17–28).

Lentigo Maligna Melanoma   Lentigo maligna melanoma often arises from the precursor lesion, lentigo maligna. The lesions are large and tan with different shades of brown. This type of melanoma makes up 4% to 10% of malignant melanomas and is the least serious form (Porth, 1994). It occurs on skin that has had long-term sun exposure, such as the face, neck, and, sometimes, the dorsal surface of the hands and lower extremities. Lentigo maligna melanoma affects women more than men. It is typically diagnosed in people in their 60s and 70s.

Lentigo maligna melanoma is characterized by a proliferation of atypical melanocytes parallel to the basal layer of the epidermis. The radial growth phase may last from 10 to 25 years, with the lesion growing to as large as 10 cm. The lesion becomes malignant as soon as the melanocytes invade the dermis. In the vertical growth phase, raised nodules may appear on the surface of the lesion. The lesion tends to acquire a freckled or mottled appearance.

Nodular Melanoma   Nodular melanoma lesions are raised, dome-shaped blue-black or red nodules on areas of the head, neck, and trunk that may or may not have been exposed to the sun. The lesions may look like a blood blister, or they may ulcerate and bleed. The lesions arise from unaffected skin rather than from a preexisting lesion. This type makes up 15% to 30% of malignant melanomas and is often diagnosed in people in their 50s.

Nodular melanoma has only a vertical growth phase, but it grows aggressively during that phase. However, the absence of a radial growth phase makes this type more difficult to diagnose before it metastasizes.

Acral Lentiginous Melanoma   Acral lentiginous melanoma, also called mucocutaneous melanoma, is less common in people with fair skin and more common in people with dark skin. The lesions progress from tan, brown, or black flat lesions to elevated nodules and are about 3 cm in diameter. The radial phase lasts from 2 to 5 years. They are found on the palms of the hands, soles of the feet, the mucous membranes, and the nailbeds. Acral lentiginous melanoma affects both men and women equally and is most often diagnosed in people in their 50s and 60s.

Collaborative Care

The management of the client with malignant melanoma begins with assessment through identification, diagnosis, and tumor staging. If treatable, the tumor is removed through surgical excision. Malignant melanoma is also treated with chemotherapy, immunotherapy, and radiation therapy.

Assessment

Malignant melanoma is most often found on the trunk of men and on the lower extremities of women. Nevertheless, it is important for the client to have a complete physical examination and total skin assessment. In addition to a visual examination of all skin surfaces, palpation of regional lymph nodes, the liver, and the spleen is essential to assess for metastasis when a melanoma is suspected or found.

A change in the color or size of a nevus is reported in 70% of people diagnosed with a malignant melanoma. The ABCD rule (American Cancer Society, 1994) is used to assess suspicious lesions:

A = asymmetry (one half of the nevus does not match the other half)

B = border irregularity (edges are ragged, blurred, or notched)

C = color variation or dark black color

D = diameter greater than 6 mm (size of a pencil eraser)

Laboratory and Diagnostic Tests

In addition to biopsy of any suspicious lesion, laboratory and diagnostic tests are conducted to determine whether the tumor has metastasized. Because malignant melanoma may metastasize to any organ or tissue of the body, a variety of tests may be conducted.

Laboratory tests include the following:

- *Liver function tests* are done to determine whether the tumor has metastasized to the liver. The combination of an elevated LDH, alkaline phosphatase, and SGOT suggests liver involvement.
- *Complete blood count* is conducted to determine hematologic abnormalities.
- *Serum blood chemistry* tests are conducted to identify electrolyte and mineral abnormalities.

The following diagnostic tests may also be conducted:

- *Biopsy of the lesion* is the only definitive method of diagnosing a malignant melanoma. An excisional biopsy is the diagnostic procedure of choice because this allows the most complete histologic evaluation and microstaging. A shave biopsy should not be performed if melanoma is suspected, because the thickness and depth of the lesion cannot be assessed, making decisions about prognosis and treatment difficult (Lawler, 1991).
- *CT scan of the liver* is conducted if hepatic enzymes are abnormal to determine the extent of liver metastasis more accurately.
- *Chest X-ray* films are taken if the client has respiratory difficulty or hemoptysis, which suggests possible lung metastasis.
- *Bone scan* is performed to determine possible metastatic cause of undetermined bone pain.
- *CT scan or MRI of the brain* is conducted to assess for metastasis if the client has headaches, seizures, or neurologic deficits.
- *Biopsy of tissue from lymph nodes or other skin lesions* are done to identify metastasis.

Staging

The term used to describe the assessment of the level of invasion of a malignant melanoma and the maximum tumor thickness is called *microstaging*. In the Clark system of microstaging, the vertical growth of the lesion is measured from the epidermis to the subcutaneous tissue to determine the level of invasion (Figure 17–29). However, variations in individual skin thicknesses and different anatomic sites can affect the accuracy of the measurement. In the Breslow system, an adaptation of the Clark level of assessment, the vertical thickness is measured from the granular level of the epidermis to the deepest level of tumor invasion (Lawler, 1991). This determination is important, because as the thickness of the melanoma increases, survival rate decreases.

After the thickness and depth of the tumor are determined, a clinical stage is assigned. The traditional three-stage system is still used, although it does not include tumor thickness. The American Joint Committee on Cancer has adopted a four-stage system that includes tumor thickness, level of invasion, lymph node involvement, and evidence of metastasis.

Surgery

Surgical excision is the preferred treatment for malignant melanoma. If a biopsy identifies the lesion as a melanoma, a wide excision is performed that includes the full thickness of the skin and subcutaneous tissue. Because the risk of local recurrence for thin melanomas (those that are less than 0.76 mm) is quite low, margins of 0.5 to 1.0 cm of normal skin are excised around the tumor. Thick tumors require a 1- to 3-cm margin excision because they are at risk for local recurrence or satellite lesions.

Regional lymph nodes are the most common sites for metastasis of malignant melanoma. Standard surgical treatment for clinically suspicious lymph node involvement includes excision of the primary lesions as well as surgical dissection of the involved lymph nodes. Elective lymph node dissection (ELND) in the treatment of localized malignant melanoma remains controversial. Advocates of ELND believe that the procedure benefits clients with intermediate-thickness tumors because approximately 20% of people whose lymph nodes were clinically negative at diagnosis show some metastasis on removal of the nodes. Those opposed to ELND believe the risks associated with the procedure are too high for the 80% of people who have no evidence of metastasis after removal of the nodes.

Surgery also is indicated for palliative management of isolated metastasis. Removal of metastatic tumors in the brain, liver, lung, gastrointestinal tract, or subcutaneous tissue may relieve symptoms and prolong life.

Chemotherapy

Chemotherapy is used to treat metastatic melanoma, but currently available systemic agents are not very effective. However, chemotherapy may be used as an adjunct to other therapy for advanced melanoma that is confined to one limb, for the treatment of melanoma with satellites, or for poor-risk clients. In this treatment, called *isolated limb perfusion*, the client is given a general anesthetic, and

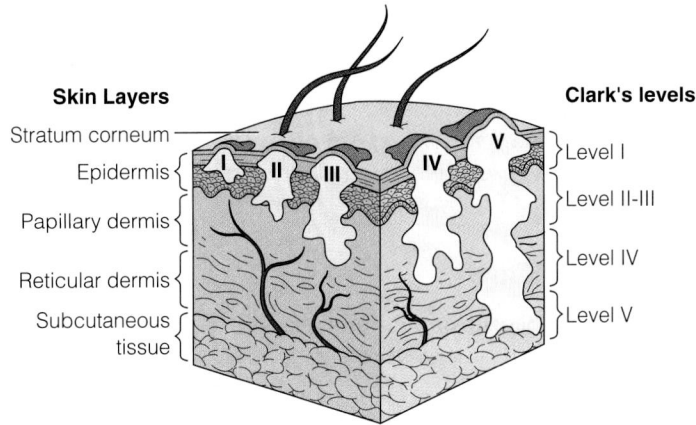

Figure 17–29 Clark's levels for staging measure the invasion of a melanoma from the epidermis to the subcutaneous tissue.

the blood circulation to the affected extremity is controlled mechanically. A chemotherapeutic agent at 39 to 40 C is perfused by means of a pump directly into the area containing the malignant melanoma. Hyperthermia decreases the amount of agent required. The treatment usually continues for an hour. Potential complications include thrombosis, damage to muscle and nerves, and, very rarely, loss of the limb (Lawler, 1991). The use of this treatment remains controversial.

Immunotherapy

Immunotherapy is a relatively new treatment modality for malignant melanoma. The role of the immunologic response initially was recognized because of the numerous spontaneous remissions seen in clients with melanoma—a higher occurrence than with any other adult tumor. In addition, researchers have recently identified tumor-specific antigen-antibodies in clients with melanoma. This also has stimulated an interest in immunotherapeutic interventions for the treatment of malignant melanoma.

Agents such as interferons, interleukins, monoclonal antibodies, Calmette-Guérin bacillus (BCG), levamisole, transfer factors, and tumor vaccines have all shown activity in melanoma, with varying response rates. The effectiveness of these agents, used either alone, in combination with chemotherapy, or in combination with each other, is under investigation. The use of immunotherapy in the treatment of melanoma is still new and requires further investigation.

Radiation Therapy

Traditionally, malignant melanoma was regarded as a radiation-resistant tumor. However, beginning in the 1970s it was found that melanoma responds to higher dose radiation, especially if the tumor is small. Response rates to radiation therapy depend on the site of the tumor, the thickness of the tumor, the type of melanoma, and the client's general health, but may range from 0% to 71% (Ho & Sober, 1990).

Radiation frequently is used for palliation of symptoms resulting from metastasis to the brain, bone, lymph nodes, gastrointestinal tract, skin, or subcutaneous tissue. Liver and lung metastases are not treated with radiation therapy because a loss of organ function may result.

Nursing Care

The nurse has the opportunity to assess the skin of clients requiring care for many different health problems and may be the first person to identify suspicious lesions. Wide excision and the high risk of metastasis from malignant melanoma usually requires inpatient surgical treatment, with the nurse providing care and teaching. Although many different nursing diagnoses may be appropriate, the most common responses are impaired skin integrity, hopelessness, and anxiety.

Impaired Skin Integrity

Impaired skin integrity is a common problem for the client with malignant melanoma. These cancers not only destroy skin layers but also invade body structures. Certain types of tumors may ulcerate prior to diagnosis, and treatment typically involves some type of surgical biopsy and excision. Any open lesion or incision increases the risk for secondary infection.

Nursing interventions with rationales follow:

- Monitor the client every 4 hours for manifestations of infection: fever, tachycardia, malaise, and incisional erythema, swelling, pain, or drainage that increases or becomes purulent. *Intact skin is the first line of defense against infection; impaired skin integrity increases the risk for infection. If infection is present, the client may have both systemic and local manifestations.*

- Keep the incision line clean and dry by changing dressings as necessary. *Moisture increases the risk of infection.*

- Follow principles of medical and surgical asepsis when caring for client's incision. Teach family members and visitors the importance of careful hand washing. Maintain universal precautions if drainage is present. *Careful hand washing is essential in preventing the spread of infection. Aseptic techniques are necessary when caring for any surgical incision to prevent infection. Nurses must use precautions with blood and body fluids to protect themselves from exposure to HIV.*

- Encourage and maintain adequate kcaloric and protein intake in the diet. Suggest a consultation with the dietitian if client does not want to eat. *Adequate kcalories and protein are necessary for proper healing. The client with cancer has increased metabolic needs; if these needs are not met, nutritional problems that impair healing may result.*

Hopelessness

Hopelessness is often described in the literature as a response to the diagnosis of cancer. It is an emotional state in which a person feels that there is no possibility that life will improve. Clients who experience hopelessness are often withdrawn, passive, and apathetic.

The diagnosis of malignant melanoma threatens the quality and quantity of life as the client faces the possibility or reality of metastasis; the possibility that the cancer may recur and cause death; and alterations in self-concept, roles, and relationships. Inspiring hope in clients during this health crisis is a legitimate nursing action.

Nursing interventions with rationales follow:

- Provide an environment that encourages the client to identify and express feelings, concerns, and goals:
  a. To help the client verbalize feelings and concerns, use active listening, ask open-ended questions, and reflect on the client's statements.
  b. Acknowledge and respect the client's feelings of apathy and/or anger as expressions of distress.
  c. Convey an empathetic understanding of the client's fears and concerns.
  d. Provide opportunities for the client to express positive emotions: hope, faith, a sense of purpose, and the will to live.
  e. Explore the client's perceptions, and modify or clarify them if necessary by providing information and correcting misconceptions.
  f. Encourage the client to identify support systems and sources of strength and coping in the past.
  Verbalizing feelings, concerns, and goals allows others to validate or correct them, promotes a therapeutic nurse-client relationship, and fosters feelings of self-worth. Expressing positive emotions and calling on support systems and sources of strength that were effective in coping with past crises help the person resolve the crisis and develop hope.

- Encourage the client to participate actively in self-care as well as in mutual decision making and goal setting. *Meeting self-care needs and making decisions about one's own care increase personal confidence in one's capacity for coping.*

- Encourage the client to focus not only on the present but also on the future: Review past occasions for hope, discuss the client's personal meaning of hope, establish and evaluate short-term goals with the client and family, and encourage them to express hope for the future. *The nurse mobilizes the client's resources to strengthen motivation, hope, and the will to live.*

Anxiety

Anxiety is one of the most common psychosocial responses in clients with cancer. Anxiety increases at the time of diagnosis and remains a constant emotion throughout the course of treatment, regardless of treatment type or setting. Interventions center on helping the client recognize the manifestations of anxiety, determining whether the client wishes to do anything about the anxiety, and facilitating coping strategies (Bulechek & McCloskey, 1992).

Nursing interventions with rationale:

- Provide reassurance and comfort:
  a. Set aside time to sit quietly with the client.
  b. Speak slowly and calmly.
  c. Convey empathetic understanding by touch and supporting present coping mechanisms, such as crying, talking.
  d. Do not make demands or expect the client to make decisions.

  The client with newly diagnosed melanoma is likely to experience anxiety. Anxiety is a feeling aroused by a perceived threat; its intensity depends on the severity of the present situation and the client's ability to handle the threat. Coping behaviors differ from situation to situation and from person to person. Anxiety at moderate to severe levels narrows perceptions and the ability to function.

- Decrease sensory stimuli by using short, simple sentences; focusing on the here and now; and providing concise information. *Higher levels of anxiety result in a focus on the present, inability to concentrate, and difficulty in understanding verbal communications.*

- Provide interventions that decrease anxiety levels and increase coping:
  a. Provide accurate information about the illness, treatment, and expected length of recovery.
  b. Encourage discussion of expected physical changes and ways to minimize disfigurement through cosmetics and clothing.
  c. Include family members in teaching sessions.
  d. Provide the client with strategies for participating in the recovery process.

  Although the prognosis and treatment of melanoma depend on various factors, the prognosis of complete cure is decreased with metastasis. Surgical incisions include excision with wide margins, which may cause disfigurement. Active participation in care provides the client with some control over the future and is often an effective means of coping with anxiety.

Other Nursing Diagnoses

Other nursing diagnoses that may be appropriate for the client with malignant melanoma follow:

- *Body Image Disturbance* related to the surgical removal of malignant melanoma
- *Pain* related to the presence of a surgical incision
- *Anticipatory Grieving* related to diagnosis of cancer and unknown future

- *Risk for Infection* related to the presence of an incision and treatment with immunotherapy
- *Risk for Peripheral Neurovascular Dysfunction* related to treatment of melanoma with isolated limb perfusion
- *Spiritual Distress* related to the inability to accept the diagnosis of cancer
- *Altered Sexuality Patterns* related to perceived lack of attractiveness from scarring secondary to surgical excision of melanoma

Client and Family Teaching

Teaching the client and family experiencing the diagnosis and treatment of malignant melanoma involves two areas: prevention and facilitation of self-care and ongoing self-monitoring. Techniques for avoiding sun exposure and carrying out skin self-examination and general guidelines for wound care were described in the preceding section. Community agencies are listed in Appendix O. Other areas of client and family education are described in this section; they apply to both the client with malignant melanoma and the client with nonmelanoma skin cancer.

The nurse assesses the skin of clients in many different settings and has the opportunity to provide education and early detection. Guidelines for performing nursing assessment of the skin, specific to the detection of a skin cancer, are provided in the box on page 594.

Teaching the client who is at high risk for or who has skin cancer is based on the client's knowledge base, educational background, and anxiety level and readiness to learn. Because the diagnosis of cancer increases anxiety, the nurse may need to present information in a simple format and to repeat it several times. Showing photographs of both normal and cancerous skin lesions may help teach the client and family what to watch for when doing self-examination.

Education for the client and family is specific to the type of treatment. In addition to wound care, clients who have had a lymph node dissection are given instructions in how to protect the extremity from bleeding, trauma, and infection. The nurse describes the manifestations and side effects of chemotherapy and radiation and provides information about how to decrease nausea and vomiting, anorexia, and fatigue. Clients with these forms of treatment also require information about skin care in irradiated skin areas (see Chapter 9).

Clients with malignant melanoma are encouraged to schedule regular medical checkups every 3 months for the first 2 years, every 6 months for the next 5 years, and yearly thereafter. The nurse should emphasize that proper self-care combined with regular medical care can help the client lead a fairly normal life. If assistance for home care is necessary, the nurse provides referrals to a community health agency or a home care agency. In addition, the nurse can refer the client to a local cancer support group if the client believes this will be helpful.

Applying the Nursing Process

Case Study of a Client with Malignant Melanoma: Geoff Sanders

Geoff Sanders, age 69, is retired from the postal service. He has always been an avid participant in outdoor sports: When he was younger he played baseball and tennis, and for the last 10 years he has played golf at least twice a week. He now lives in Connecticut, but as a younger man he lived in Florida for almost 15 years. Mr. Sanders has a variety of warts and moles and rarely paid attention to them. However, after taking a shower one day he noticed that a mole on his left lower leg looked bigger and darker. Mr. Sanders had just seen a public announcement on television about the dangers of changes in moles, and he immediately called his primary HMO physician for an appointment at the dermatology clinic.

Assessment

On arriving at the clinic, Mr. Sanders is interviewed and examined by Tom Hall, a clinical nurse specialist. Following the assessment, Mr. Hall documents the following information.

Mr. Sanders has a family history of skin cancer; his father had several squamous cell carcinomas removed from his face. He has numerous nevi on his body; the one causing concern is located on the medial anterior left leg, 2 inches below the patella. Mr. Sanders states that the mole has been present for years but that he noticed just yesterday that it has become larger and darker. On further questioning, he states that the mole itches sometimes but has never hurt or bled. Mr. Sanders lived in Florida for 15 years and experiences a sunburn early each summer before he tans. The sunburn involves the lower legs because Mr. Sanders wears shorts during his twice-weekly golf game.

A complete skin assessment reveals various freckles, warts, and nevi. With the exception of the nevus that prompted Mr. Sanders to come to the clinic, all lesions appear normal. The nevus in question is raised, 3 cm in diameter, with irregular borders and a nodular surface. It is variegated in color, with various shades of brown. The skin surrounding the nevus is slightly erythematous. Inguinal lymph nodes are not enlarged or painful. A photograph of the lesion is taken with Mr. Sanders's permission.

Following the assessment, Mr. Sanders discusses the lesion with a surgeon, who recommends excision. They discuss the possibility of skin cancer and the importance of early detection and treatment. Mr. Sanders is scheduled for a biopsy of the nevus under a local anesthetic the following morning. Following the biopsy, histologic examination reveals lentigo maligna melanoma. Staging of the tumor reveals that it is a melanoma in situ, with no metastasis to regional lymph nodes. Mr. Sanders undergoes a wide excision of the lesion in inpatient surgery the following afternoon and goes home the day after.

Diagnosis

Mr. Hall identifies the following nursing diagnoses for Mr. Sanders:

- *Impaired Skin Integrity* related to excision of melanoma from the left lower leg
- *Risk for Infection* related to surgical wound on left lower leg
- *Pain* related to wide excision of melanoma on left lower leg
- *Anxiety* related to diagnosis of skin cancer

Expected Outcomes

The outcomes established in the plan of care specify that Mr. Sanders will:

- Demonstrate complete healing of the incision without manifestations of infection.
- Verbalize fears and concerns about his diagnosis.
- Verbalize relief of pain by the time the incision is healed.

Planning and Implementation

The nurses caring for Mr. Sanders implement the following interventions:

- Make the first dressing change, but ensure that Mr. Sanders can safely change the dressing himself prior to discharge the day after surgery.
- On discharge, provide Mr. Sanders with adequate dressings and tape for the first home dressing change; include in discharge instructions necessary information about where to buy supplies and how many dressing supplies will be needed.
- Review and provide written instructions for prescribed systemic antibiotic and pain medication.
- Provide Mr. Sanders with written instructions for dressing change, manifestations of infection, and phone number of clinic; stress importance of calling if any abnormal symptoms occur.
- Discuss diagnosis, positive outlook for treatment of melanoma in situ, and the client's concerns.

- Teach Mr. Sanders to protect the incision from bumps and to protect the site from irritants.
- Stress importance of lifelong regular health care evaluations to identify any recurrence or metastasis.

Evaluation

Mr. Sanders returns to the dermatology clinic 1 week after his surgical incision. By this time his incision is well approximated and shows no signs of infection. He is taking his antibiotic 4 times a day as prescribed and reports that his need for pain medications is decreasing. During his clinic visit the following week, Mr. Hall removes the sutures and assesses the wound as healed. Mr. Sanders completed his antibiotics and no longer requires pain medications. He says he is still "scared to death" about having cancer, but he has decided to join a local cancer support group. He also says he had gotten a list of skin safety rules from the American Cancer Society and will be sure to cover up and use sunscreens when he plays golf. Mr. Sanders makes an appointment for follow-up care in 3 months.

Critical Thinking in the Nursing Process

1. Consider reasons why people who notice a change in a skin lesion put off seeking health care. What can nurses do to effect change?

2. Design a teaching plan for older adults for preventing skin cancers.

3. What would you say to Mr. Sanders if he called the clinic and said that the antibiotics were making him sick and he didn't think he needed them anyway?

4. Design a nursing care plan for Mr. Sanders for the diagnosis *Powerlessness.*

◼◼◼ Skin Trauma ◼◼◼

Trauma to the skin can be intentional (as in the case of surgery) or unintentional. Chemicals, radiation, pressure, or thermal changes cause skin trauma. This section discusses pressure ulcers and frostbite, as well as intentional trauma from cutaneous and plastic surgery or treatment. Thermal injury, or burns, is discussed in Chapter 18.

The Client with a Pressure Ulcer

◼ ◼ ◼

Pressure ulcers are ischemic lesions of the skin and underlying tissue caused by external pressure that impairs the flow of blood and lymph (Porth, 1994, p. 373). The ischemia causes tissue necrosis and eventual ulceration. These ulcers, also called *bed sores* or *decubitus ulcers*, tend to develop over a bony prominence (such as the heels, greater trochanter, sacrum, and ischia), but they may appear on the skin of any part of the body that is subjected to external pressure, friction, or shearing forces.

The incidence of pressure ulcers in hospitals, long-term care facilities, and home settings is high enough to warrant concern for health care providers. The incidence in hospitals has been reported as ranging from 2.7% to 29%, whereas the incidence in long-term care facilities is reported to be around 23% (Agency for Health Care Policy and Research, 1992). Little research has been done to determine the extent of the problem in the home setting. However, with increasing numbers of clients (and especially older adult clients) being cared for in the home, it is probable that the incidence is great enough to warrant plans of care to prevent their occurrence.

Although a pressure ulcer may develop in an adult of any age who has an impairment in mobility, those most at risk are older adults with limited mobility (see the box on page 608), people with quadriplegia, and clients in the critical care setting (Porth, 1994). Other clients who are prone to develop pressure ulcers are clients with fractures of large bones (e.g., hip or femur) or who have undergone orthopedic surgery or sustained spinal cord injury. In addition to deficits in mobility and activity, other contributing factors that increase the risk of pressure ulcer development include incontinence and nutritional deficit. Clients with chronic illnesses, such as renal failure and anemia, and those with edema or infection are also at increased risk.

Pathophysiology

Pressure ulcers develop from external pressure that compresses blood vessels or from friction and shearing forces that tear and injure vessels. Both types of pressure cause traumatic injury and initiate the process of pressure ulcer development.

External pressure that is greater than capillary pressure and arteriolar pressure interrupts blood flow in capillary beds. When pressure is applied to skin over a bony prominence for 2 hours, tissue ischemia and hypoxia from external pressure cause irreversible tissue damage. For example, when the body is in the supine position, the body's weight applies pressure to the sacrum. The same

Gerontologic Considerations: The Client with Pressure Ulcers

■ ■ ■

Older adults are at high risk for developing pressure ulcers because of age-related changes in the integumentary system. Cell renewal slows resulting in skin that has decreased elasticity. The margin between the epidermis and the dermis separates more easily, making the skin more prone to tearing. In addition, thinning subcutaneous tissue provides less cushioning over bony prominences. Water content decreases, and the skin becomes drier. These changes increase the older adult's susceptibility to skin trauma and prolong wound healing.

Chronic conditions associated with immobility and self-care deficit place older adults at risk of developing pressure ulcers. For example, bowel or bladder incontinence can produce regions of wet skin that are prone to infections and breakdown. Furthermore, sensory-perceptual alterations and impaired cognitive functioning may reduce the frequency in which the older adult shifts position when sitting or lying in bed. Finally, undernutrition, which is often seen in older adults, heightens the risk for developing pressure ulcers.

To prevent pressure ulcers, the skin of older adults should be kept clean, dry, and well-hydrated. Moisturizers are recommended to keep the skin free of excessive dryness. Older adults should be taught to avoid bumping into furniture and to wear long skirts or pants to help protect the lower extremities from trauma.

When hospitalized, older adults should have a validated risk assessment for pressure ulcers completed on admission and as often as the tool suggests. A daily systematic skin inspection with particular attention to bony prominences should be completed.

Once pressure ulcers develop in older adults, the treatment is the same as for younger clients. However, there are additional steps that may need to be taken. Because local perfusion to tissues is compromised, steps should be taken to prevent under or over hydration. It is essential that optimal nutritional status be maintained. Also, keep in mind that it is going to take a longer time for the pressure ulcer to heal.

Note. From "The Integumentary System and its Problems in the Elderly" in *Gerontological Nursing* (pp. 148–159) by M. Stanley and P. Beare, eds., 1995, Philadelphia: F. A. Davis.

amount of pressure causes more damage when it is applied to a small area than when it is distributed over a large surface.

Shearing forces result when one tissue layer slides over another. The stretching and bending of blood vessels cause injury and thrombosis. Clients in hospital beds are subject to shearing forces when the head of the bed is elevated and the torso slides down toward the foot of the bed. Pulling the client up in bed also subjects the client to shearing forces. (For this reason, clients are always lifted up in bed). In both cases, friction and moisture cause the skin and superficial fascia to remain fixed to the bed sheet, while the deep fascia and bony skeleton slides in the direction of body movement.

When a person lies or sits in one position for an extended length of time without moving, pressure on the tissue between a bony prominence and the external surface of the body distorts capillaries and interferes with normal blood flow. If the pressure is relieved, blood flow to the area increases, a brief period of reactive hyperemia occurs, and no permanent damage occurs. However, if the pressure continues, platelets aggregate in the endothelial cells surrounding the capillaries and form microthrombi. These microthrombi impede blood flow, resulting in ischemia and hypoxia of tissues. Eventually, the cells and tissues of the immediate area of pressure and of the surrounding area die and become necrotic (McCance & Huether, 1994).

Alterations in the involved tissue depend on the depth of the injury. Injury to superficial layers of skin results in blister formation, whereas injury to deeper structures causes the pressure ulcer area to appear dark reddish-blue. As the tissues die, the ulcer becomes an open wound that may be deep enough to expose the bone. The necrotic tissue elicits an inflammatory response, and the client experiences increases in temperature, pain, and white blood cell count. Secondary bacterial invasion is common. Enzymes from bacteria as well as macrophages dissolve necrotic tissue, resulting in a foul-smelling drainage.

Because of age-related skin changes, the older adult is at increased risk for the development of pressure ulcers. The skin of the older adult has a thicker epidermis, a thinner dermis with decreased vascularity, decreased sebaceous gland activity, and decreased strength and elasticity. As a result, the more fragile and less nourished dermal layer is more prone to shear and friction problems. In addition, the skin of the older adult responds more slowly to inflammation, and wounds heal more slowly; when pressure ulcers occur, they are more difficult to reverse.

Pressure ulcers are graded or staged to classify the degree of damage. The stages, defined by the Panel for the Prediction and Prevention of Pressure Ulcers in Adults as part of the U.S. Department of Health and Human Services (1992) are listed in the accompanying box.

Pressure Ulcer Staging

∎ ∎ ∎

Stage I

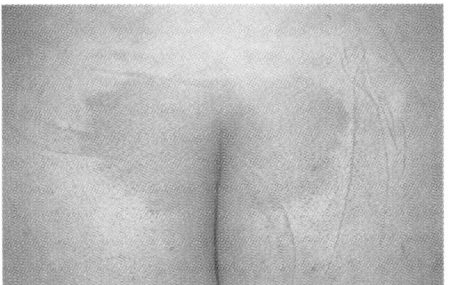

Nonblanchable erythema of intact skin; the heralding lesion of skin ulceration. Identification of stage I pressure ulcers may be difficult in clients with darkly pigmented skin. *Note:* Reactive hyperemia can normally be expected to be present for one-half to three-fourths as long as the pressure occluded blood flow to the area. This should not be confused with stage I pressure ulcer.

Stage II

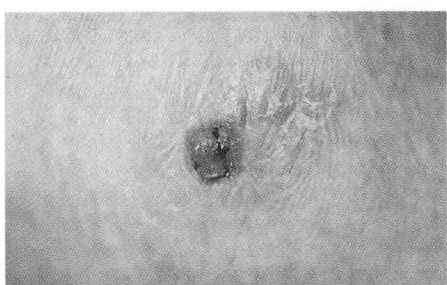

Partial-thickness skin loss involving epidermis and/or dermis. The ulcer is superficial and presents clinically as an abrasion, blister, or shallow crater.

Stage III

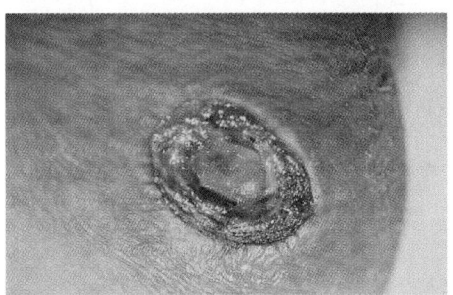

Full-thickness skin loss involving damage or necrosis of subcutaneous tissue that may extend down to, but not through, underlying fascia. The ulcer presents clinically as a deep crater with or without undermining of adjacent tissue.

Stage IV

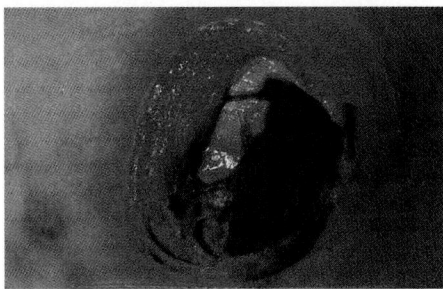

Full-thickness skin loss with extensive destruction, tissue necrosis, or damage to muscle, bone, or supporting structures (for example, tendon or joint capsule). Sinus tracts may also be associated with stage IV ulcers.

Note: When eschar is present, accurate staging of the pressure ulcer is not possible until the eschar has sloughed or the wound has been debrided.

Note. Text is from *Pressure Ulcers in Adults: Prediction and Prevention* by the Agency for Health Care Policy and Research, 1992, Rockville, MD: U.S. Department of Health and Human Services.

Table 17-4   Products Used to Treat Pressure Ulcers

Stage	Product	Purpose
I	Skin Prep	Toughens intact skin and preserves skin integrity.
	Granulex	Prevents skin breakdown, increases blood supply, adds moisture, contains trypsin to aid in removal of necrotic tissue.
	Hydrocolloid dressing (e.g., DuoDerm)	Prevents skin breakdown and promotes healing without the formation of a crust over the ulcer. Is permeable to air and water vapor; prevents the growth of anaerobic organisms.
	Transparent dressing (e.g., Tegaderm)	Prevents skin breakdown; prevents entrance of moisture and bacteria but allows oxygen and moisture vapor permeability.
II	Transparent dressing	Enhances healing (see above).
	Hydrocolloid dressing	Enhances healing (see above). *Note:* If infection is present, these types of dressings are contraindicated. A sterile dressing should be applied instead.
III	Wet-to-dry gauze dressing with sterile normal saline	Allows necrotic material to soften and adhere to the gauze, so that the wound is debrided.
	Hydrocolloid dressing	Enhances healing (see above).
	Proteolytic enzymes (such as Elase)	Proteolytic enzymes serve as a debriding agent in inflamed and infected lesions.
IV	Wet-to-dry gauze dressing with sterile normal saline	Enhances healing (see above). *Note:* Transparent or hydrocolloid dressings or skin barriers are contraindicated.

Collaborative Care

For the client at risk for pressure ulcers, the goal is prevention. Ulcers that are already present require collaborative treatment to promote healing and restore skin integrity.

Laboratory tests are conducted to determine the presence of a secondary infection and to differentiate the cause of the ulcer. If the ulcer is deep and/or appears infected, drainage or biopsied tissue is cultured to determine the causative organism.

Topical and systemic antibiotics specific to the infectious organism are used to eradicate any infection present. Additionally, a variety of topical products is used to promote healing. Examples are listed in Table 17-4.

Surgical debridement may be necessary if the pressure ulcer is deep; if subcutaneous tissues are involved; or if an eschar (a scab or dry crust that forms over skin damaged by burns, infections, or excoriations) has formed over the ulcer, preventing healing by granulation. Large wounds may require skin grafting for complete closure.

Nursing Care

The client with one or more pressure ulcers not only has impaired skin integrity but also is at increased risk for infection, pain, and decreased mobility. Pressure ulcers also prolong treatment for other conditions, increase health care costs, and diminish the client's quality of life. The research box on page 611 discusses the importance of nurs-

ing interventions for preventing and treating pressure ulcers in residents of a nursing home.

The nursing diagnoses appropriate for the client with a pressure ulcer are *Risk for Impaired Skin Integrity* and *Impaired Skin Integrity*. The interventions and rationales discussed below are adapted from the clinical guidelines developed by the Agency for Health Care Policy and Research (1992) in identifying adults at risk and treating those with stage I pressure ulcers.

- Identify at-risk individuals needing prevention and the specific factors placing them at risk.
  a. Assess bed- and chair-bound clients, as well as those who are unable to reposition themselves, for additional risk factors: immobility, incontinence, nutritional factors (such as inadequate dietary intake and impaired nutritional status), and altered level of consciousness.
  b. Assess clients on admission to acute care and rehabilitation hospitals, nursing homes, home care programs, and other health care facilities.
  c. Use a systematic risk assessment by using a validated risk assessment tool.
  d. Document all assessments of risk.
  Individuals at risk for pressure ulcers must be identified so that risk factors can be reduced through intervention. The primary risk factors for pressure ulcers are immobility and limited activity; therefore, clients who cannot reposition themselves or whose activity is limited to bed or chair should be assessed. Use of validated tools ensures system-

atic evaluation of individual risk factors. The client's condition is not static; the client therefore requires periodic reassessment for pressure ulcers. Accurate and complete documentation of all risk assessments ensures continuity of care and may be used as a foundation for the skin care plan.

- Conduct a systematic skin inspection at least once a day, paying particular attention to the bony prominences. *Systematic, comprehensive, and routine skin care may decrease pressure ulcer incidence (although the exact role is unknown). Skin inspection provides data the nurse uses in designing interventions to reduce risk and in evaluating outcomes of those interventions.*

- Clean the skin at the time of soiling and at routine intervals, as frequently as the client's need or preference dictates. Avoid hot water, use a mild cleansing agent, and clean the skin gently, applying as little force and friction as possible. *Metabolic wastes and environmental contaminants accumulate on the skin; these potentially irritating substances should be removed frequently. Feces and urine cause chemical irritation and should be removed as soon as possible. Hot water may cause skin injury. Mild cleansing agents are less likely to remove the skin's natural barrier.*

- Minimize environmental factors leading to skin drying, such as low humidity and exposure to cold. Treat dry skin with moisturizers. *Well-hydrated skin resists mechanical trauma. Hydration decreases as the ambient air temperature decreases, especially when the air humidity is low. Poorly hydrated skin is less pliable, and severe dryness is associated with fissuring and cracking of the stratum corneum. Moisturizers reduce dry skin.*

- Avoid massage over bony prominences. *Although massage has been practiced for years, preliminary evidence now suggests that massage over bony prominences may lead to deep tissue trauma in clients who are at risk for or who have beginning skin manifestations of a pressure ulcer.*

- Minimize skin exposure to moisture due to incontinence, perspiration, or wound drainage. When these sources of moisture cannot be controlled, use underpads or briefs made of materials that absorb moisture and present a quick-drying surface to the skin. Change underpads and briefs frequently. Do not place plastic directly against the skin. *Moisture from incontinence, perspiration, or wound drainage may contain factors that irritate the skin; moisture alone can increase the susceptibility of the skin to injury.*

- To minimize skin injury due to friction and shearing forces, use proper positioning, transferring, and turning techniques. Lubricants (such as cornstarch or creams), protective films (such as transparent dressings and skin sealants), protective dressings (such as hydrocolloids), and protective padding may also re-

---

Applying Research to Nursing Practice Skin Care Strategies in a Skilled Nursing Home Facility

■ ■ ■

Researchers conducted a study to evaluate the effects of strategies to prevent and treat pressure ulcers in a 160-bed skilled nursing home facility (Burd et al., 1994). The strategies were as follows: (1) A set of standardized skin care protocols for preventing and treating pressure ulcers were added to the agency's procedure manual. (2) Flowsheets were placed at the bedside of residents with a pressure ulcer and were used to document turning schedules. (3) A skin care committee was formed to address skin integrity issues on a monthly basis. (4) Ongoing collaboration between nursing and dietary personnel regarding nutritional interventions was initiated. (5) A policy was established requiring the use of a standardized pressure ulcer risk assessment tool. Assessments were conducted quarterly for 1 full year. Findings indicated a significant reduction in the overall prevalence and severity of pressure ulcers.

Implications for Nursing

The older adult is at increased risk for developing pressure ulcers, an ongoing problem in nursing home settings. Pressure ulcers cause pain and limit mobility in nursing home residents and are also a source of financial concern for the facility. Results of this study support the use of pressure ulcer risk assessment, inservice education to heighten awareness of the importance of nursing interventions, and interdisciplinary collaboration to improve dietary interventions.

Critical Thinking in Client Care

1. Describe factors that increase the nursing home resident's risk for developing pressure ulcers.

2. In this study, 86% of the pressure ulcers were found on the lower half of the body (sacrum, toes, heels). Discuss probable reasons for this finding.

3. The care of nursing home residents with pressure ulcers is more costly to the agency than the care for residents who do not have pressure ulcers. List reasons for the increased cost of care.

duce friction injuries. *Shear injury occurs when skin remains stationary and the underlying tissue shifts. This shift diminishes the blood supply to the skin and results in ischemia and tissue damage. Proper positioning, however, can eliminate most shear injuries. Friction injuries to the skin occur when it moves across a coarse surface, such as bed linens. Most friction injuries can be avoided by using appropriate techniques to move clients so that their skin is never dragged across the linens. Any agent that eliminates contact or decreases the friction between the skin and the linens reduces the potential for injury.*

- Assess factors involved in inadequate dietary intake of protein or kcalories. Offer nutritional supplements, and support the client during mealtimes. If dietary intake remains inadequate, consider more aggressive nutritional interventions, such as enteral or parenteral feedings. *The role that nutrition plays in the development of (and to a lesser degree, the healing of) pressure ulcers is not understood, but poor dietary intake of kcalories, protein, and iron has been associated with the development of pressure ulcers.*

- Maintain the client's current level of activity, mobility, and range of motion. *Frequent turning, repositioning, and movement are essential in reducing the risk of pressure ulcers.*

- For the client who is on bed rest or who is immobile, provide interventions against the adverse effects of external mechanical forces of pressure, friction, and shear:
  a. Reposition all at-risk clients at least every 2 hours, using a written schedule for systematic turning and repositioning.
  b. For clients on bed rest, use positioning devices, such as pillows or foam wedges, to protect bony prominences.
  c. For clients who are completely immobile, use devices to totally relieve pressure on the heels (the most common method is to raise the heels off the bed). Do not use donut-type devices.
  d. Avoid placing clients in the side-lying position directly on the trochanter.
  e. Maintain the head of the bed at the lowest degree of elevation consistent with the client's medical condition and other restrictions. Limit the amount of time the head of the bed is elevated.
  f. Use assistive devices, such as a trapeze or bed linen, to move clients in bed who cannot assist during transfers and position changes.
  g. Place any at-risk client on a pressure-reducing device, such as foam, static air, alternating air, gel, or water mattress.

Data indicate that the more spontaneous movements that bedridden, older adult clients make, the lower the incidence of pressure ulcers. Studies reveal that fewer pressure ulcers

develop in at-risk clients who are turned every 2 to 3 hours. Proper positioning can reduce pressure on bony prominences. It is difficult to redistribute pressure under heels; suspending the heels is the best method. Donut cushions are more likely to cause than to prevent pressure ulcers. Shearing forces are exerted on the body when the head of the bed is elevated. Lifting (rather than dragging) is less likely to cause injury from friction. Pressure-reducing devices and beds can decrease the incidence of pressure ulcers.

- For chair-bound clients, use pressure-reducing devices. Consider postural alignment, distribution of weight, balance and stability, and pressure relief when positioning these clients. Avoid uninterrupted sitting in a chair or wheelchair. Reposition the client every hour. Teach clients who can do so to shift their weight every 15 minutes. Use a written plan for positioning, movement, and the use of positioning devices. Do not use donut devices. *Prolonged, uninterrupted mechanical pressure results in tissue breakdown. The client's weight should be shifted at least every hour.*

Other nursing diagnoses that may be appropriate for the client with a pressure ulcer follow:

- *Anxiety* related to pain and loss of skin from pressure ulcer
- *Body Image Disturbance* related to large pressure ulcer
- *Risk for Infection* related to sacral pressure ulcer and fecal incontinence
- *Pain* related to pressure ulcer

See the accompanying box on rehabilitation principles when caring for clients at risk for skin breakdown.

Client and Family Teaching

Client and family teaching for care of a pressure ulcer also focuses on prevention and includes much of the same information presented in the preceding section. Because many clients with pressure ulcers are older or have other serious illnesses, a caregiver may require teaching on such topics as the following:

- Definition and description of pressure ulcers
- Common locations of pressure ulcers
- Risk factors for the development of pressure ulcers
- Skin care
- Ways to avoid injury
- Diet

Depending on the stage of the pressure ulcer, the nurse teaches the client or caregiver how to care for ulcers that are already present: how to change wet-to-dry dressings, apply skin barriers, and avoid injury and infection. Referrals to a home health agency or community health de-

---

Applying Rehabilitation Principles to Medical/Surgical Nursing: Skin Care

■ ■ ■

In many instances, applying rehabilitation principles for skin care early in your client's plan of care can decrease the potential for skin breakdown and decrease the length of stay.

Case Example

Mr. Arthur Berenson is a 60-year-old stockbroker admitted to your unit from the emergency room with a diagnosis of right-sided weakness due to a CVA. His vital signs are stable, and he is alert and talkative. Mr. Berenson is connected to a heart monitor and has been prescribed bedrest and a low sodium diet.

Rehabilitation Principle
Conservation of existing function as well as prevention of further loss of function is a central goal of rehabilitation nursing. Pressure ulcers are a potential threat to any client on bedrest.

Rehabilitation Time Frame
Mr. Berenson will stay in your unit for five days. He is most at risk for skin injury until he is able to get out of bed.

Nursing Diagnosis: Risk for Impaired Skin Integrity
Due to right-sided weakness, Mr. Berenson has decreased mobility and sensation. Consequently, he is at risk for developing pressure ulcers.

Rehabilitation Goals and Interventions

1. Relieve pressure areas at least every 2 hours by turning or repositioning the client in bed or chair. Weight-shifting devices such as arm lifts from a chair will reduce the pressure area on the sacrum. Clients placed on alternating pressure devices should also be repositioned at 2-hour intervals.

Pressure ulcers develop when the pressure exerted on the skin is in excess of capillary pressure (32mm Hg). Over time, insufficient tissue perfusion will cause cell death. Disruptions in capillary circulation of from 1 to 2 hours have been demonstrated to cause irreversible dermal breakdown.

2. Encourage the client to be as mobile as possible. This can be accomplished by encouraging the client to use his stronger left side to exercise his right side while on bedrest. The client should be encouraged to get out of bed as soon as possible. *Any movement, even in bed, will relieve pressure areas and allow for capillary circulation.*

3. Maintain clean and dry skin. This can be accomplished by examining the client's skin during repositioning. Clean soiled areas as soon as they are discovered and remove damp or soiled bedding quickly. *Moisture from sweating or soiling combined with pressure is a factor that predisposes the client to pressure ulcers.*

4. Reduce friction or shearing forces when repositioning the client. This can be accomplished by making sure that the person aiding the client to reposition does not drag the weakened side of the client on the bedding. *Shearing forces irritate the skin and can cause abrasions.*

5. Encourage the client to maintain a balanced diet. If the client is unable to eat solid food, consult the dietician to plan appropriate nourishment. Avoid placing the client on NPO status for more than a 24-hour period. Feeding tubes may be necessary and should be encouraged. *Nutrition greatly influences the skin's condition. Protein, vitamins A, B, and C, zinc, and sulfur are necessary for healthy skin.*

---

partment can help the family through the lengthy healing process. National agencies that can provide information and referral to local agencies are listed in Appendix O.

The Client with Frostbite

■ ■ ■

Frostbite is an injury of the skin from freezing. If the exposure to freezing temperatures is limited, only the skin and subcutaneous tissues become involved. However, as

exposure increases, deeper structures freeze. The skin freezes when the temperature drops to 14 to 24.8 F (-10 to -4 C). Frostbite is most common on exposed or peripheral areas of the body, such as the nose, ears, feet, and hands.

As human tissues freeze, ice crystals form and increase intracellular sodium content. Small blood vessels initially vasoconstrict but then vasodilate and become more permeable, causing cellular and tissue swelling. With continued exposure, vasoconstriction and increased viscosity of the blood cause infarction and necrosis of the affected tissue (McCance & Huether, 1994).

Superficial frostbite causes numbness, itching, and prickling. The skin appears cyanotic, reddened, or white. Deeper frostbite causes stiffness and paresthesias. As the skin and tissues thaw, the skin becomes white or yellow and loses its elasticity. The client experiences burning pain. Edema, blisters, necrosis, and gangrene may appear.

Rapid thawing may significantly decrease tissue necrosis. General guidelines for rewarming areas of frostbite follow:

- If you are outdoors, treat superficial frostbite by applying firm pressure with a warm hand or by placing frostbitten hands in the axillae. If the feet are frostbitten, remove wet footwear, dry the feet, and put on dry footwear. Do not rub the areas with snow.
- In the hospital, rapidly rewarm affected areas in circulating warm water, 104 to 105 F (40 to 40.5 C) for 20 to 30 minutes. Do not rub or massage the areas.

Following rewarming, the client is kept on bedrest with the affected parts elevated. Pain medications and anti-inflammatory agents are administered. Blisters are debrided. Whirlpool therapy may be used to clean the skin and debride necrotic tissue. Recovery from frostbite is usually complete if the involved area has not become necrotic. Necrotic tissue may require amputation.

The Client Undergoing Cutaneous and Plastic Surgery

■ ■ ■

Although many skin disorders are so small and benign that no treatment is necessary, others require some type of surgery of the skin to remove the lesion. Other surgeries and treatments for skin lesions and deformities are used to restore function and change appearance. This section discusses both cutaneous and plastic surgery, as well as other types of treatment modalities used in the care of the client with a skin disorder.

Cutaneous Surgery and Procedures

The basic types of cutaneous surgery described here are excision, electrosurgery, cryosurgery, curettage, and laser surgery. Two nonsurgical procedures, chemical destruction and sclerotherapy, are also discussed. Most of these procedures are performed in the office or outpatient clinic. If needed, a local anesthetic is used.

Excision

Fusiform excision is the removal of a full thickness of the epidermis and dermis, usually with a thin layer of subcutaneous tissue. It is used to remove tissue for biopsies and for complete removal of benign and malignant lesions of the skin. Most fusiform excisions have a length-to-width ratio of 3 to 1.

Excision of small, superficial lesions is performed under a local anesthetic, and care is taken to place the incision in a way that will provide good cosmetic results. The incision line is usually closed with sutures, and the wound is covered with a dry dressing, an occlusive dressing, or a hydrocolloid dressing.

Electrosurgery

Electrosurgery involves the destruction or removal of tissue with high-frequency alternating current. A variety of surgical procedures may be performed, including electrodesiccation (which produces superficial skin destruction), electrocoagulation (which produces deeper tissue destruction), and electrosection (which can cut through skin and tissue). Electrodesiccation is used to remove benign surface lesions, such as skin tags, keratoses, warts, and angiomas. It is also used to produce hemostasis for capillary bleeding. Electrocoagulation is used to remove telangiectases, warts, and superficial nonmelanoma skin cancers. Electrosection is used to make incisions, excise tissue, and perform biopsies.

Cryosurgery

Cryosurgery is the destruction of tissue by cold or freezing with agents such as fluorocarbon sprays, carbon dioxide snow, nitrous oxide, and liquid nitrogen. Cryosurgery is used to treat many skin lesions (for example, keratoses, lentigo maligna, venous lakes, nevi, keloids, and Kaposi's sarcoma). The freezing agents are applied topically to the lesion.

The effects of freezing depend on the degree of freeze. Light freezing causes damage to the epidermis with blistering or crusting that heals without scarring. Deeper freezes, used to treat malignant cells, cause edema, necrosis, and tissue slough. The effects of cryosurgery may not be obvious until 24 hours following the treatment. Postoperatively, infection is prevented by applying a topical antibiotic and keeping the treated areas clean. Healing occurs in 2 to 3 weeks.

Curettage

Curettage is the removal of lesions with a curette (a semisharp cutting instrument). The design of the curette allows it to cut through soft or weak tissue, but not through normal tissue. It is used primarily to remove benign and malignant superficial epidermal lesions. Benign lesions removed by curettage include keratoses, nevi, and angiomas. Nonmelanoma skin lesions are removed by curettage if they are small, well-defined, primary tumors. Curettage is also used to remove specimens of tissue for biopsy.

Following curettage, the wound may be treated with electrodesiccation to destroy any remaining malignant cells and to provide hemostasis. These wounds are not closed; rather, they are left open to heal by second intention. Topical antibiotic ointments and dressings may be used in the postoperative period.

Laser Surgery

Laser surgery is used to treat clients with a wide variety of skin disorders, including port-wine stains, telangiectases, and venous lakes. A laser is an intense light that produces a thermal injury on contact with tissue. The injury causes coagulation, vaporization, excision, and ablation (removal of a growth). Argon, pulsed dye, carbon dioxide, and Nd: YAG lasers are used in cutaneous and plastic surgery. A local anesthetic may be used, although pulsed dye laser causes minimal pain and rarely requires anesthesia.

The response differs by type of laser. Following treatment with the argon laser, the lesion appears from white to black in color, a blister forms, and the skin may peel. The area weeps, and an eschar forms; in 10 to 14 days, the eschar separates, revealing an underlying red area. The redness fades over a period of up to 1 year. However, pulsed dye laser does not result in blistering or weeping; only rarely does it result in eschar.

Chemical Destruction

Chemical destruction is the application of a specific chemical to produce destruction of skin lesions. Chemical destruction is used to treat both benign and premalignant lesions. The chemical is applied to the lesion or is used to cause peeling. After application, the treated area forms a thin crust that sloughs off in about a week.

Sclerotherapy

Sclerotherapy is the removal of benign skin lesions with a sclerosing agent that causes inflammation with fibrosis of tissue. Agents that cause therapeutic sclerosis include aethoxysklerol (Sclerodex) and hypertonic sodium chloride. This type of treatment is used for telangiectases and superficial spider veins of the lower extremities. The solution is injected into the affected veins, causing a reaction that closes the lumen of the vein (Strohecker, Carmody, Hibshman, & Wong, 1991).

Plastic Surgery

Many of the skin disorders discussed in this chapter cause changes in appearance. For example, acne may leave deep pitting scars, nevi and keloids are often disfiguring, and skin cancers may require wide excision and skin grafting. These scars, lesions, and wounds often cause embarrassment and alterations in body image. In addition, the removal of lesions may leave unsightly scars or areas of obviously missing tissue.

Plastic surgery is the alteration, replacement, or restoration of visible portions of the body, performed to correct a structural or cosmetic defect (Glanze, 1990, p. 929). The word *plastic* comes from the Greek word *plastikos*, which means "able to be molded."

Plastic surgery is an ancient art. It was practiced in India over 3000 years ago to repair noses and ear lobes injured in battle. Chinese physicians in the third century reconstructed cleft lips. In 1597, Tasparo Tagliacozzi of Bologna published the first book on plastic surgery, *De Curtorum Chirurgia*. In it, he described nasal reconstruction using flaps of skin from the arm. The Catholic Church, which influenced medicine a great deal at the time, opposed his work.

The techniques of modern plastic surgery developed slowly. The greatest advances did not come until World War II (1939–1945), when horrendous battle wounds motivated surgeons to refine their ability to move tissue from one part of the body to another. More recently, advances in the manufacture of synthetic materials and high-technology instrumentation have led to further advances in skin grafting, implantation of artificial tissues and joints, and procedures requiring microsurgery.

Cosmetic surgery, also called *aesthetic surgery,* is one of two fields within plastic surgery. Cosmetic surgery enhances the attractiveness of normal features. The other field, *reconstructive surgery*, uses similar techniques; however, its purpose is to improve the function or appearance of parts of the body damaged by trauma, disease, or birth defects. Reconstructive surgeries make up approximately 60% of all plastic surgeries performed in the United States.

Many of the plastic surgeries permanently alter body image. To provide the client with a preview of what surgery will accomplish, some surgeons integrate computer imaging into preoperative teaching. The computer projects a photograph of the client's face onto a monitor and uses graphics to demonstrate how the size and or shape of the body part or area will change as a result of the surgery.

There are many different types of plastic surgery; the information in this section provides a background for understanding some of the different types of surgeries as well as the nursing care for common responses to plastic surgery. A case study at the end of this section illustrates the application of the nursing process for the client having plastic surgery.

Skin Grafts and Flaps

Skin grafts and flaps are used to restore function while also maintaining an acceptable appearance. Both of these procedures involve the movement of skin from one part of the body to another part.

A *skin graft* is a surgical method of detaching skin from a donor site and placing it in a recipient site, where it

Figure 17–30 Skin depth of split-thickness and full-thickness grafts.

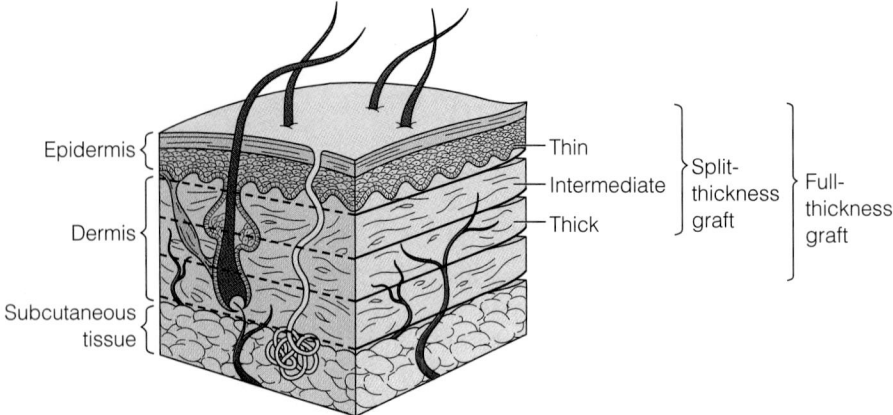

develops a new blood supply from the base of the wound (Meeker & Rothrock, 1991). Skin grafting is an effective way to cover wounds which have a good blood supply, which are not infected, and in which bleeding can be controlled.

Skin grafts may be either split-thickness or full-thickness (Figure 17–30). A split-thickness graft contains epidermis and only a portion of dermis of the donor site. Split-thickness grafts range in thickness from 0.010 inch to greater than 0.015 inch. A common donor site for a skin graft is the anterior thigh. Skin is removed in sheets from the donor site with a dermatome. Donor sites of split-thickness grafts heal by reepithelialization. A *meshed graft* is a type of split-thickness graft that is rolled under a special cutting machine to form a mesh pattern with perforations. The perforations allow drainage of serum and blood from under the graft. After healing, however, the skin has a rough appearance (often referred to as alligator hide).

A full-thickness graft contains both epidermis and dermis. These layers contain the greatest number of skin elements (sweat glands, sebaceous glands, or hair follicles) and are best able to withstand trauma. Areas of thin skin are the best donor sites for full-thickness skin grafts. The donor site must be surgically closed and will scar.

Other types of grafts are composite grafts and cultured epithelial grafts. *Composite grafts* are free grafts and are usually used on the face. They contain skin, subcutaneous tissue, cartilage, or other tissue. *Cultured epithelial grafts* are made from epithelial cells that are cultured in vivo, coalesced into sheets, and then used to cover full-thickness wounds. They are used primarily to treat burns.

A *flap* is a piece of tissue whose free end is moved from a donor site to a recipient site while maintaining a continuous blood supply through its connection at the base or pedicle (Westlake, 1991). Flaps carry their own blood supply and are therefore used to cover recipient sites that have a poor blood supply or have sustained a major tissue loss. They are often used for reconstruction or closure of large wounds. Microsurgical techniques, with anastomo-sis of small blood vessels and nerves, allow reconstruction with *free flaps* (in which the flap is completely removed from its donor site and moved to the recipient site).

Chemical Peeling

Chemical peeling is the application of a chemical to produce a controlled and predictable injury that alters the anatomy of the epidermis and superficial dermis. The result is skin that appears firmer, smoother, and less wrinkled (Forte, Hack, & Jackson, 1993). This form of cosmetic surgery is more useful in people with fair, thin skin with fine wrinkling.

Chemical agents used for peeling include phenol, trichloracetic acid (TCA), and alpha-hydroxy acids (AHA). Phenol, a keratocoagulant, penetrates the epidermis and dermis; regeneration of the epithelium produces the desired results. After treatment, the entire surface of the face except the eyelids is covered with adhesive tape for 1 to 2 days. The adhesive is then removed, and the treated area forms a crust that heals in about a week. TCA has been used for years to obtain the desired effect. A light peel causes mild erythema followed by peeling (as from a mild sunburn) in 3 to 5 days. AHA are organic acids that are used to produce light to moderate peeling to remove acne, fine lines, seborrheic keratosis, warts, and mild scarring. Both TCA and AHA treatments may be repeated weekly. One complication of chemical peeling is bleaching of the skin (due to removal of melanocytes).

Liposuction

Liposuction is a method of changing the contours of the body by aspirating fat from the subcutaneous layer of tissue. This treatment is used to remove excess fat from the buttocks, flanks, abdomen, thighs, upper arms, knees, ankles, and chin. It is not a cure for obesity and should not be used as a substitute for weight loss. The procedure is usually done for younger clients because their skin is more elastic. Liposuction may be performed on either an outpatient or inpatient basis.

To aspirate the fat, a small incision is made close to the area, and a suction cannula or curette is inserted and attached to a suction apparatus. The high vacuum pressure caused by the suction machine causes fat cells to emulsify, and they are aspirated out of the body. Following removal of the fat, a pressure dressing is applied to help the skin conform to the new tissue size.

Dermabrasion

Dermabrasion is a method of removing facial scars, severe acne, and pigment from unwanted tattoos. The area is sprayed with a chemical to cause light freezing and is then abraded with sandpaper or a revolving wire brush to remove the epidermis and a portion of the dermis.

Facial Reconstructive Surgery

Many different reconstructive surgeries may be performed to correct deformities or improve cosmetic appearance. Those discussed here are rhinoplasty, blepharoplasty, and rhytidectomy (face lift). A Critical Pathway for the client undergoing rhinoplasty is provided on page 618.

- A *rhinoplasty* is conducted to improve the appearance of the external nose. The nasal skeleton is reshaped, and the overlying skin and subcutaneous tissue are allowed to redrape over the new framework. A *submucous resection* of the nasal septum is often done at the same time; this surgery resects a segment of the septal cartilage to improve the nasal airway and also to alter the appearance of the nose. This surgery is done through incisions within the nose, so no visible scars remain after healing.

- A *blepharoplasty* is a cosmetic surgery in which loose skin and protruding periorbital fat is removed from the upper and lower eyelids. With aging, the eyelid skin sags, allowing the periorbital fat to bulge; the skin of the upper eyelid can be so lax that it partially obstructs vision. The procedure is performed under local anesthesia, and excess skin and fat are excised. The incision is made in the normal eyelid lines so that scars are not visible after healing.

- A *rhytidectomy,* or facelift, is a cosmetic surgery done to improve appearance by removing excess skin (and sometimes fat) from the face and neck. As one ages, the skin of the face and neck tends to become loose and wrinkled. The procedure is usually performed with local anesthesia. To perform the surgery, bilateral incisions are made from the scalp at the temple, in front of the ear in the natural skin line, around the ear lobe, and to the occipital scalp. The skin is then elevated, fat is removed or suctioned, and excess skin is excised. The incision lines are sutured, and a pressure dressing is applied.

Nursing Care

Nursing care for the client having cutaneous or plastic surgery is highly individualized. It depends on the type of surgery or procedure performed, the type of deficit treated, the reason for the surgery or procedure, the expected results of the treatment, and the response of the client to the lesion or surgery. Although some surgeries, such as skin grafts and flaps, require in-hospital care, many of the surgeries are carried out in the primary care setting, and the client provides self-care at home following or between treatments.

Although a variety of nursing diagnoses may be appropriate for the client having cutaneous or plastic surgery or procedures, the most common are *Impaired Skin Integrity*, *Body Image Disturbance*, and *Pain*.

Impaired Skin Integrity

The client who is having surgery of the skin has impaired skin integrity. Skin grafts and flaps are performed to repair large wounds, and it is necessary to inflict further wounds to collect the graft or flap from a donor site. Excisions and various cosmetic surgeries cause wounds. Skin is traumatized by freezing, chemicals, abrasion, sclerosing agents, electrical currents, and lasers. Although all of these treatment modalities are conducted to remove lesions, improve function, or improve appearance, they first impair the integrity of the skin. These impairments increase the risk for infection, which would further impair the skin integrity and may negate the benefits of surgery.

Nurses provide preoperative care and teaching, intraoperative assistance, and postoperative care and teaching; in each case, care and teaching are specific to the type of surgical treatment and the individual client. In all cases, the nurse provides appropriate preoperative interventions to prepare the client physically and emotionally for surgery and the postoperative period. The interventions described below are appropriate for the client having inpatient skin grafts or flaps:

- Monitor incisions and graft and flap donor and recipient sites for manifestations of infection and necrosis:
  a. Take and record vital signs every 4 hours.
  b. Monitor all wounds for changes in color, consistency, amount, and odor of drainage every 4 to 8 hours.
  c. Monitor wounds for increased swelling, redness, and pain every 4 to 8 hours.
  d. Monitor and document assessment of graft every 4 hours.
  e. Monitor and document temperature, turgor, color, dermal bleeding, and capillary refill of flaps every 4 hours (Westlake, 1991).

When bacterial infection is present, the inflammatory phase of wound healing is prolonged, retarding healing.

Critical Pathway for Client Following Rhinoplasty		
	Date _____ **Preoperative**	Date _____ **1st 24 hours following surgery**
Expected length of stay: less than 24 hours		
Daily Outcomes	Client will ■ Verbalize understanding of preoperative teaching, including turning, coughing, deep breathing, mobilization, and pain management. ■ Demonstrate ability to cope.	Client will ■ Be afebrile. ■ Have a dry, clean dressing. ■ Have nasal packing, splint/cast and mustache dressing intact and in place. ■ Manage pain with nonpharmacologic measures or oral medications. ■ Be independent in self-care. ■ Be fully ambulatory. ■ Verbalize/demonstrate home care instructions. ■ Tolerate usual diet. ■ Demonstrate ability to cope with ongoing stressors.
Tests and treatments	CBC Urinalysis Baseline physical assessment with a focus on respiratory status Anesthesia consultation	Vital signs and O_2 saturation, neurovascular assessment, dressing, edema, and wound drainage assessment q15min × 4; q30min × 4; q1h × 4 and then q4h if stable. Assess for posterior nasal bleeding. Assess lung sounds q4h and prn. Assess voiding—if unable to void, try suggestive voiding techniques or catheterize q8h or prn if unable to void. Cool compresses to nose, eyes, or face to reduce swelling and prevent excessive discoloration.
Knowedge deficit	Orient to room and surroundings. Include family in teaching. Provide simple, brief instructions. Review preoperative preparation, including hospital and surgical routines. Reinforce preoperative teaching regarding specific postoperative care: turning, coughing, deep breathing, mobilization, and pain management. Assess understanding of teaching.	Reorient to room and postoperative routine. Include family in teaching. Review plan of care and importance of early mobilization, as well as any activity restrictions. Complete discharge teaching regarding splint/cast care/dressing change, follow-up care, signs and symptoms to report, medications, and diet. Instruct the client to avoid activities that might result in a blow or pressure on the nose and procedures to follow if bleeding occurs. Instruct client to avoid the Valsalva maneuver and to avoid aspirin and other nonsteroidal medications. Assess understanding of teaching.
Psychosocial	Assess anxiety related to pending surgery. Assess fears of the unknown and surgery. Encourage verbalization of concerns. Provide emotional support to client and family. Provide information regarding surgery. Minimize stimuli (e.g., noise, movement).	Assess level of anxiety. Encourage verbalization of concerns. Provide emotional support to client and family. Provide information and ongoing support and encouragement.

	Date _____ **Preoperative**	**Date _____** **1st 24 hours following surgery**
Diet	NPO	Advance to clear liquids. If tolerated, advance to full liquids/soft diet following surgery.
Activity	OOB ad lib until premedicated for surgery.	Provide safety precautions. Semi-Fowler's position. Bathroom privileges with assistance on evening after surgery. Begin progressive ambulation to tolerance the morning following surgery until fully ambulatory.
Medications	NPO except ordered medications.	IM or PO analgesics. Antibiotics if ordered. IV fluids until adequate PO intake then intermittent IV. Discontinue prior to discharge.
Transfer/discharge plans	Assess discharge plans and support system.	Probable discharge within 24 hours of surgery. Complete discharge home care teaching when client is fully awake and oriented and before discharge. Provide a written copy of discharge instructions.

Critical Pathway for Client Following Rhinoplasty

Increased body temperature and tachycardia are manifestations of infection. The drainage in wounds that become infected is often increased in amount, purulent, thicker, and has a musty or foul odor. Tissue response to infection includes edema, increased erythema, and pain. Grafts and flaps that do not have adequate blood supply will appear black instead of the normal pink-red color.

■ Provide care for the donor site:
   a. Position the client to minimize pressure on the donor site.
   b. Use a bed cradle to keep linens off the area.
   c. If the donor site is left open and a heat lamp is to be applied to the area, place the lamp no closer than 2 feet from the wound.
   d. Avoid moving the body part containing the donor site, if possible.
   e. If the donor site is on the posterior portion of the body, place the client on a special bed (such as a low-pressure or fluidized bed) to decrease pressure and allow air circulation around the donor site.

Minimizing trauma from pressure and movement facilitates healing of the donor site. Leaving the site open to the air and providing heat increase healing. Special beds minimize ischemia and allow donor sites on the posterior side of the body to dry.

■ Encourage a diet high in protein, ascorbic acid, vitamins, and minerals. *An adequate protein intake is necessary to supply amino acids for tissue repair. Vitamin C is necessary for collagen formation and wound strength. Vitamins and minerals contribute to the healing process.*

■ Change dressings as prescribed, or if the frequency is not indicated, as necessary. Determine which dressings are not to be removed during the healing process and which are to be changed, and whether the wound is to be kept dry or moist.
   a. Use aseptic technique and follow universal precautions when changing dressings.
   b. Remove old dressings carefully and gently.
   c. Choose the appropriate dressing materials.

Donor sites may be covered with an adherent gauze dressing that is allowed to dry and remains adherent through the healing process. Aseptic techniques are used to prevent secondary bacterial infections. Universal precautions are used to protect the nurse from HIV infection. Unless care is taken, the removal of adherent old dressings may damage the wound by traumatizing granulation tissue or wound edges. The use of semipermeable transparent dressings provides an environment that optimizes wound healing by promoting collagen synthesis and the formation of granulation tissue; it also increases cell migration and epithelial resur-

facing and prevents the formation of scabs, crusts, and eschar (Krasner, 1992).

Pain

Cutaneous and plastic surgery results in pain. The client having a graft or flap has two wounds; in fact, the donor site may be more painful than the recipient site. Cutaneous surgeries, dermabrasions, and chemical treatments result in blistering, swelling, and loss of epidermal tissue. The client having facial reconstructive surgery has edema. In preoperative teaching, the nurse describes the type of pain the client will experience and discusses measures to help the client manage the pain.

Nursing interventions with rationales follow:

- Administer pain medications on a regular basis, following guidelines for controlling pain in clients having operative procedures (see Chapter 4). *Pain that is established and severe is difficult to control and has negative physical and psychological consequences.*

- Elevate the head of the bed to a 30- to 45-degree angle to decrease edema in clients having facial surgery or treatments. Explain to the client and family that this swelling is expected and will subside. *Clients with facial surgery or treatments often have edema of the face, which may cause the eyes to swell shut. Elevating the head of the bed facilitates venous return from the face to lessen edema.*

- Use alternative pain-relief measures as appropriate and prescribed, such as ice bags or cold compresses. *Cold reduces swelling, acts as a local anesthetic, and decreases pain.*

- Teach the client noninvasive methods of pain relief, such as deep breathing, relaxation, and guided imagery. *Noninvasive methods of pain relief increase the effectiveness of pharmacologic agents and also allow the client some control and self-management of pain.*

Body Image Disturbance

Cosmetic surgery is performed for a variety of reasons in adult clients of all ages. Changes in appearance, especially in a society that values youth and beauty, affect one's self-perception. Lesions or scars, especially of the face, may decrease self-esteem and cause a person to avoid social interactions and relationships. With aging, the skin becomes looser and wrinkles appear; this can be a source of anxiety and despair, especially to the woman who has always prided herself on her youthful appearance. Most clients cite one reason for having plastic surgery: to "feel better about myself" (Pruzinsky, 1993, p. 66).

Nursing interventions with rationales follow:

- Provide preoperative teaching:
  a. Explain that bruising and swelling will be present and that it will be several weeks before these responses to surgery disappear.
  b. Explain that it may take a year for healing to complete and the final results to appear.
  Expectations differ; many people expect immediate results. Knowledge of postoperative responses is necessary for the client to adapt to change. The client may need to make arrangements to take time off from work during the initial healing stage.

- Provide time for the client to verbalize feelings and concerns. Be empathetic, and listen nonjudgmentally. *The nurse provides an environment in which the client is able to verbalize feelings and concerns; this interaction facilitates acceptance of changes in body image.*

- Provide information on the use of cosmetics and apparel to enhance personal appearance. *Knowledgeable use of cosmetics and clothing can make scars much less noticeable. If the client feels better about appearance, body image is improved.*

Other Nursing Diagnoses

Other nursing diagnoses that are appropriate for the client having plastic surgery follow:

- *Impaired Adjustment* related to unresolved feelings about changes in appearance
- *Anxiety* related to lack of knowledge of the results of skin graft
- *Dysfunctional Grieving* related to the inability to accept diagnosis of cancer
- *Risk for Infection* related to open wounds at donor and recipient sites for skin flap
- *Impaired Social Interaction* related to refusal to take part in activities with friends secondary to facial surgery

Client and Family Teaching

The nurse teaches the client and family to provide self-care at home after inpatient and outpatient cutaneous and plastic surgery and procedures. The nurse asks about the client's expectations and stresses that final results will not be seen for several months, providing written instructions about the following:

- Wound care, including application of topical medications and dressing changes. If the client is to return to the office or clinic for removal of tape or pressure dressings, or for dressing changes in the first weeks after surgery, an appointment is made. For some procedures, the wound is left open to the air.

- Specific care for the type of surgery or procedure, such as type of oral care, avoiding blowing the nose, or limiting talking.

- Limitations on physical activity, especially lifting or straining.

- Manifestations of wound infection, such as increased temperature, malaise, changes in the appearance of the wound, or changes in drainage. If any of these manifestations occur, the client should notify the health care provider immediately.

- When to resume bathing or showering, shampooing the hair, and using cosmetics.

- The need to avoid picking at crusts or scabs. If the healing wound itches, the client should contact the health care provider for a topical medication.

- Use of a 15 SPF sunblock when the client is outdoors. This may be prescribed for several months or for the rest of the client's life.

Applying the Nursing Process

Case Study of a Client Undergoing Rhinoplasty: Mary Jane Baker

Mary Jane Baker, 22 years old, has been self-conscious about her nose for as long as she can remember. It is large and irregularly shaped and has a prominent bump. It seemed to Ms. Baker that people always stare at her nose. Her self-consciousness increased after she started working as a receptionist at an advertising agency, where her duties included greeting potential clients each day. She has never become used to people staring at her nose or making remarks. She finally decides to make an appointment with a plastic surgeon to see whether anything can be done to help her.

Assessment

Trish Roberts, RN, the nurse-practitioner in the plastic surgery clinic, conducts a history and physical examination of Ms. Baker and discovers no abnormal findings. After discussing Ms. Baker's feelings about her appearance and her hopes for improvement and determining that her state of health is normal, the surgeon agrees she is a good candidate for a rhinoplasty. Surgery is scheduled for the following week in the clinic.

Ms. Baker's surgery takes approximately 2 hours and was performed under a local anesthetic. The nasal bones and cartilage are sculpted to remove the bump, and the nose is shortened and lifted at the tip. A nasal splint is applied and is to remain in place for 1 week.

Diagnosis

The postoperative nursing diagnoses for Miss Baker follow:

- *Ineffective Airway Clearance* related to obstruction of the nasal passages by packing and swelling

- *Pain* related to surgical manipulation and remodeling of nose

- *Body Image Disturbance* related to ecchymosis, swelling, and nasal splint

- *Anxiety* related to lack of knowledge of final cosmetic outcome of reconstructive surgery

Expected Outcomes

The outcomes established in the plan of care specify that Ms. Baker will within 2 weeks

- Regain normal nasal airway passages.

- Verbalize only slight pain.

- Perform self-care activities necessary for healing.

- Verbalize increased acceptance of appearance.

Planning and Implementation

Ms. Roberts implements the following interventions for Ms. Baker:

- Provide teaching for postoperative safety and self-care during the clinic visit scheduled 2 days before surgery:
  a. Ask a friend to bring you to the clinic and drive you home after surgery.
  b. Do not blow your nose until the physician allows you to do so, even though you will have swelling and drainage.
  c. Use the prescribed medications to relieve pain.
  d. As much as possible, rest in bed with your head elevated on 2 pillows. Apply cold compresses to your nose to help decrease swelling and pain.
  e. Do not jog, go swimming, lift heavy packages, bend over, or engage in sexual activity until your nose has healed.
  f. Call Ms. Roberts at the number provided if you notice increased pain, temperature, or nasal bleeding or drainage.

- Schedule a return visit to the clinic for Ms. Baker each week for the next 2 weeks.

Evaluation

During the first follow-up visit, Ms. Baker's nasal splint is removed. She says that she is having little pain and is taking one to two pain pills each day. She has followed the postoperative instructions. At the second follow-up visit, the swelling and bruising are noticeably decreased. Ms. Baker reports that she can breathe easily through her nose and has no significant pain. She tells Ms. Roberts that she already feels much less embarrassed about her nose and that she is going to have a cosmetic consultant suggest ways to cover up the bruising until full healing takes place.

Critical Thinking in the Nursing Process

1. Consider the implication of the client's expectations of plastic surgery. If the postoperative result does not meet the client's expectations, what might be the emotional response?

2. Does the client's developmental level, age, and gender have an effect on the choice to have cosmetic plastic surgery? Describe differences that might occur.

3. Develop a nursing care plan for Ms. Baker for the diagnosis *Social Isolation*.

▚ ▚ ▚ Hair and Nail Disorders ▚ ▚ ▚

The Client with a Disorder of the Hair

Although hair disorders are not serious threats to health, they may cause embarrassment and a negative body image. Changes in hair growth and pattern occur secondary to other illnesses and treatment for illness and also as a part of the aging process.

The hair grows at various rates. The male beard grows the most rapidly, followed by the hair of the scalp, axillae, thighs, and eyebrows. Normally, an adult's hair grows at a rate of 10 to 12 mm per month; however, the growth rate is influenced by both the person's state of health and the environment (hair grows faster in hot climates, more slowly in cold climates).

Racial and ethnic characteristics and gender influence the amount and type of hair. Caucasians have more facial and body hair than do Asians. People of Mongolian or Native American descent have straight hair, those of African descent have wavy to curly hair, and Caucasians have straight to curly hair. In addition, male hair growth characteristics (such as facial hair and hair on the lower extremities) are normal in certain women of some races and families. Women do not normally become bald.

Pathophysiology

Hair color, growth, and pattern varies from person to person, and is determined largely by genetic inheritance. However, changes do occur. For example, in some instances, hair loss is a trait that recurs in successive generations of males in a family; in other cases, hair loss may be the result of chemotherapy. Excessive facial hair may be a response to certain endocrine disorders or to the loss of estrogen after menopause. These changes may seem minor, but they may create psychosocial problems for the person experiencing the changes.

Hirsutism

Hirsutism, also called *hypertrichosis*, is the appearance of excessive hair in normal and abnormal areas of the body in women. Hirsutism most often occurs in a male distribution (that is, on the upper lip, chin, abdomen, and

chest) in women. The excess hair is primarily the result of an increase in androgen levels (especially testosterone) which may be due to any of the following:

- Familial predisposition (considered normal)
- Polycystic ovary syndrome
- Ovarian, adrenal, or pituitary tumors
- Cushing's syndrome
- Central nervous system disorders
- Medications, such as minoxidil, cyclosporine, phenytoin, certain progestins, and anabolic steroids

The manifestations of hirsutism include increased male pattern hair growth, acne, and menstrual irregularities. If the androgen excess is great, defeminization (a decrease in breast size and loss of normal adipose tissue) and virilization (frontal balding, increased muscle mass, deepening of the voice, and enlargement of the clitoris) may occur. Virilization indicates the presence of an androgen-producing tumor (Tierney et al., 1994).

Alopecia

Alopecia is loss of hair, or baldness (Figure 17–31). Alopecia may result from scarring, various systemic diseases, or genetic predisposition. Scarring from trauma, radiation, and severe bacterial, fungal, or viral infections causes permanent and irreversible hair loss over the scarred area. Systemic diseases that may cause alopecia include systemic lupus erythematosus, thyroid disorders, and pituitary insufficiency. The hair loss from these disorders may be reversible. Hair loss from androgenic causes may also occur in the postmenopausal woman. Alopecia may be drug induced and is a side effect of a variety of medications (see the box on page 623).

Types of alopecia follow:

- *Male pattern baldness* is the most common cause of alopecia in men and is genetically predetermined. The hair loss begins at the temples, with recession of the hairline and baldness of the crown.

- *Female pattern alopecia* begins in women in their 20s and 30s, with progressive thinning and loss of hair over the central part of the scalp. Unlike men, women do not lose hair from the frontal hairline. Many of these women have elevated adrenal androgens.

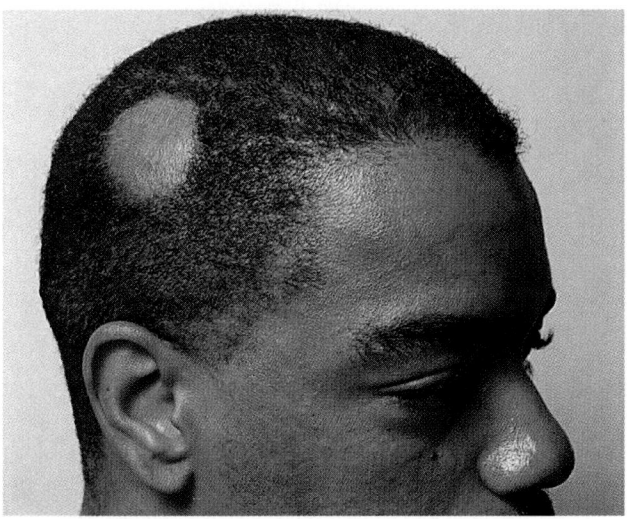

Figure 17–31   Alopecia, or baldness, may be the result of scarring, disease or genetic predisposition.

Medications Causing Alopecia

■ ■ ■

■ Thallium	■ Allopurinol
■ Retinoids	■ Propranolol
■ Anticoagulants	■ Indomethacin
■ Antimitotic agents	■ Amphetamines
■ Antithyroid drugs	■ Salicylates
■ Oral contraceptives	■ Levodopa
■ Trimethadione	■ Gentamicin

Note. Data are from *Current Medical Diagnosis and Treatment* (p. 144) by L. Tierney, Jr., S. McPhee, and M. Papadakis, 1994, Norwalk, CT: Appleton & Lange.

■ *Alopecia areata* is characterized by round or oval bald patches on the scalp as well as on other hairy parts of the body. The cause is unknown. This type of alopecia is usually self-limiting and reverses without treatment, although it often recurs.

■ *Alopecia totalis* is the loss of all hair on the scalp. This rare condition is irreversible.

■ *Alopecia universalis* is the total loss of hair on all parts of the body.

Collaborative Care

Alopecia is diagnosed by assessing the appearance of the hair and hair loss and by assessing the client for other systemic diseases and the use of medications that may cause hair loss. Various treatments are used to restore hair.

The client with hirsutism is examined for hormone levels and indications of other systemic illnesses. Hirsutism is treated by addressing the underlying systemic disorder and stopping medications that may be causing the problem.

Laboratory and Diagnostic Tests

Laboratory and diagnostic tests that may be ordered for the client with hirsutism follow:

■ *Serum testosterone levels* are measured; levels above 200 ng/dL indicate the need for further diagnostic work, including a pelvic examination and tests of ovarian function.

■ *Adrenal CT scan* may be performed to assess for an adrenal tumor.

Pharmacology

Hirsutism is treated with medications specific to the underlying cause. Oral contraceptives containing estrogen decrease ovarian androgen production and decrease free testosterone levels. Dexamethasone may be prescribed for people with high cortisol levels. Ketoconazole inhibits androgen production. Antiandrogenic medications cause congenital abnormalities in male infants and are therefore given only to nonpregnant women, who are cautioned to avoid pregnancy while taking the medications.

Male pattern baldness has been successfully treated with topical minoxidil or Rogaine, a commercial product that contains minoxidil. These drugs, which are vasodilators, stimulate vertex hair growth, probably by stimulating the epithelium of the hair follicle. These agents have been most successful in clients who have a recent onset of alopecia or are less than 50 years old. About 40% of clients treated two times a day for a year will have moderate to dense regrowth of hair at the temples (Tierney et al., 1994).

Surgery

Surgical movement of tissue containing hair is used to restore hair or reduce the size of areas of alopecia. These surgical procedures include punch grafting, scalp reduction, and flaps.

■ Punch grafting of small hair plugs taken from the back or sides of the scalp is an effective means of replacing hair to areas of alopecia. This procedure is done on an outpatient office or clinic at 1- to 2-month intervals.

■ Scalp reduction is done by excising a portion of the affected scalp. In some cases, a tissue expander (such as a silicone balloon) is first implanted under the scalp to enlarge the hair-bearing scalp so that larger areas of alopecia can be removed.

■ Flaps from hair-bearing areas of the scalp can be surgically transplanted from adjacent areas into areas of alopecia. This procedure may be done in stages.

Nursing Care

The client with either hirsutism or alopecia is often self-conscious about appearance and tries a variety of over-the-counter treatments before seeking medical care. Nursing care for the client with hair disorders focuses on teaching the client self-care and providing support during long-term care. Women with hirsutism are taught to use various means of removing unwanted hair, such as shaving, applying depilatories, waxing, or undergoing electrolysis. Women with mild hirsutism may bleach facial hair to make it less obvious. Clients with alopecia may wear hair-pieces or wigs.

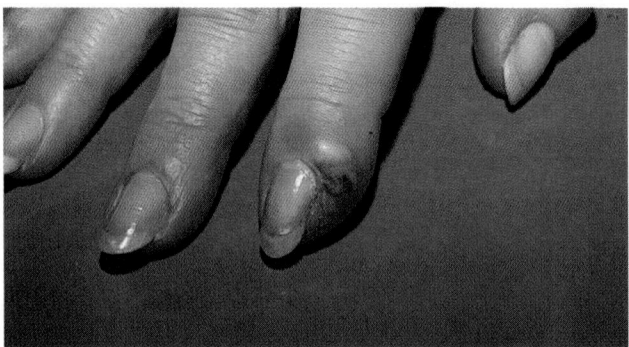

Figure 17–32   A paronychia is an infection of the cuticle of the fingernails or toenails.

The Client with a Disorder of the Nails

■ ■ ■

Nail disorders may be due to systemic diseases, trauma, allergies, or irritants. They may also be congenital or genetic. Nails may be discolored, multicolored, malformed, infected, or separated from underlying tissue.

Pathophysiology

The nail disorders discussed here are separation of the nail, infection, and ingrown toenails.

- *Onycholysis* is the separation of the distal nail plate from the nail bed. It occurs most often in the fingernails. This disorder may result from many different factors, including excessive or prolonged exposure to water, soaps, detergent, alkalies, and industrial keratolytic agents; *Candida* infections; nail hardeners; and thyroid disorders. Prolonged application of false fingernails may also cause this disorder.

- A *paronychia* is an infection of the cuticle of the fingernails or toenails (Figure 17–32). The disorder often follows a minor trauma and secondary infection with staphylococci, streptococci, or *Candida*. The acute form begins with a painful inflammation that may progress to an abscess. The chronic form is seen most often in people who have frequent exposure to water. In the chronic form, the skin around the nail is painful, edematous, and infected. The nail plate may become ridged and discolored.

- An *onychomycosis* is a fungal or dermatophyte infection of the nail plate. The nail plate elevates and becomes yellow or white. Psoriasis infections of the nail plate cause the nails to pit.

- An ingrown toenail (*unguis incarnatus*) results when the edge of the nail plate grows into the soft tissue of the toe. Pain and infection may occur. The infection, if untreated, may spread to the bone. This disorder is es-

pecially dangerous for the person with chronic illnesses such as diabetes mellitus or peripheral vascular disease.

Collaborative Care

The treatment of disorders of the nail vary from pharmacologic treatment to surgical removal. Infections of the nails are treated, depending on the causative agent, with anitfungal or antibiotic medications. If the causative agent is a fungus or chronic dermatologic disorder, treatment is difficult and may not be effective. Persistently painful and/or infected nails are in some cases surgically removed.

Nursing Care

Nursing care of the client with a disorder of the nail focuses on teaching self-care. Clients with nail disorders that are caused by frequent exposure to water are taught to protect the hands or feet by wearing rubber gloves or boots and to keep the nails as clean and dry as possible. Clients with ingrown toenails are cautioned not to cut into the lateral nail bed, but rather to soak the nail twice a day and insert a piece of cotton or gauze under the softened nail until the nail has grown out enough to trim.

Bibliography

■ ■ ■

Agency for Health Care Policy and Research. (1992). *Pressure ulcers in adults: Prediction and prevention.* Rockville, MD: U.S. Department of Health and Human Services.

American Cancer Society. (1994). *Cancer facts & figures—1994.* Atlanta: Author.

Arndt, K. (1991). *Manual of dermatologic therapeutics* (4th ed.). Boston: Little, Brown.

Beahrs, O., Henson, D., Hutter, R., & Kennedy, B. (Eds.). (1992). *Manual for staging cancer: American Joint Committee on Cancer* (4th ed.). Philadelphia: Lippincott.

Berkow, R., & Fleecher, A. (1992). *Merck manual* (16th ed.). Rathway, NJ: Merck.

Birdsall, C., & Gabasan, A. (1993). Preventing complications in severe exfoliative skin diseases. *Dimensions of Critical Care Nursing, 12*(3), 138–148.

Bulechek, G., & McCloskey, J. (1992). *Nursing interventions: Essential nursing treatments* (2nd ed.). Philadelphia: W.B. Saunders.

Burd, C., Olson, B., Langemo, D., Hunter, S., Hanson, D., Osowski, K., & Sauvage, T. (1994). Skin care strategies in a skilled nursing home. *Journal of Gerontological Nursing, 20*(11), 28–34.

Carpenito, L. (1993). *Nursing diagnosis: Application to clinical practice* (5th ed.). Philadelphia: Lippincott.

DePew, C. (1991). Toxic epidermal necrolysis. *Critical Care Nursing Clinics of North America, 3*(21), 256–267.

Devereaux, D. (1990). Diagnosis and management of dysplastic nevus syndrome and early melanoma. *Oncology, 4*(1), 73–80.

DeWitt, S. (1990). Nursing assessment of the skin and dermatologic lesions. *Nursing Clinics of North America, 25*(1), 235–245.

Farber, E., & Nall, L. (1993). Psoriasis: A stress-related disease. *Cutis, 51*(5), 322–326.

Fitzgerald, E., & Kantor, D. (1994). Alleviating the pain of herpes zoster. *Emergency Medicine, 26*(3), 35–39.

Forte, R., Hack, J., & Jackson, I. (1993). Chemical peeling. *Plastic Surgical Nursing, 13*(4), 194–200.

Fraser, M., Hartage, P., & Tucker, M. (1991). Melanoma and nonmelanoma skin cancer: Epidemiology and risk factors. *Seminars in Oncology Nursing, 7*(1), 2–12.

Glanze, W. (Ed.) (1990). *Mosby's medical, nursing, and allied health dictionary.* St. Louis: Mosby.

Goodridge, D. (1993). Pressure ulcer risk assessment tools: What's new for gerontological nurses. *Journal of Gerontological Nursing, 19*(1), 23–27.

Groenwald, S., Frogge, M., Goodman, M., & Yarbo, C. (1993). *Cancer nursing: Principles and practice.* Boston: Jones & Bartlett.

Gurevich, I. (1992). Varicella zoster and herpes simplex virus infections. *Heart & Lung, 21*(1), 85–93.

Herndon, J. (1982). Pruritus. In S. Moschella (Ed.). *Dermatology Update* (pp. 185–196). New York: Elsevier Biomedical.

Hinojosa, R. (1990). Choosing the right pressure relief device. *Plastic Surgical Nursing, 10*(3), 118–125.

Ho, V., & Sober, A. (1990). Therapy for cutaneous melanoma: An update. *Journal of the American Academy of Dermatology, 22,* 159–176.

Hodgson, B., Kizior, R., & Kingdon, R. (1994). *Nurse's drug handbook: 1994.* Philadelphia: W.B. Saunders.

Kao, G. (1990). Precancerous lesions and carcinoma in situ. In E. Farmer & A. Woods (Eds). *Pathology of the skin* (pp. 550–567). East Norwalk, CT: Appleton & Lange.

Ketcham, M., & Loescher, L. (1993). Skin cancers. In S. Groenwald, M. Frogge, M. Goodman, & C. Yarbro. *Cancer nursing: Principles and practice* (3rd ed.) (pp. 1238–1257). Boston: Jones & Bartlett.

Kiely, M. (1987). Type II toxic epidermal necrolysis. *Critical Care Nurse, 7*(2), 26.

Koh, H. (1991). Cutaneous melanoma. *New England Journal of Medicine, 325,* 171–182.

Krasner, D. (1992). Resolving the dressing dilemma: Selecting wound dressings by category. *Plastic Surgical Nursing, 12*(1), 22–27.

Kurban, R., & Kurban, A. (1993). Common skin disorders of aging: Diagnosis and treatment. *Geriatrics, 48*(4), 30–42.

Lawler, P. (1991). Cutaneous malignant melanoma. *Seminars in Oncology Nursing, 7*(1), 26–35.

Litt, J. (1992). Acute skin disorders of summer. *Emergency Medicine 24*(7), 170–172.

McCance, K., & Huether, S. (1994). *Pathophysiology: The biologic basis for disease in adults and children* (2nd ed). St. Louis: Mosby.

Meeker, M., & Rothrock, J. (1991). *Alexander's care of the patient in surgery* (9th ed.). St. Louis: Mosby.

Moncada, G. (1992). The healing wound: Clinical management. *Plastic Surgical Nursing, 12*(2), 56–60.

National Cancer Institute. (1988). *Nonmelanoma skin cancers: Research report.* Bethesda, MD: National Institutes of Health. NIH Pub. No. 88-2977.

National Institutes of Health Consensus Development Conference. (1991). *Sunlight, ultraviolet radiation, and the skin.* Bethesda, MD: National Institutes of Health.

Nicol, N., & Penske, N. (1993). Photodamage: Cause, clinical manifestations, and prevention. *Dermatology Nursing, 5*(4), 263–277, 326.

Orkin, M., Maibach, H., & Dahl, M. (1991). *Dermatology.* Norwalk, CT: Appleton & Lange.

Porth, C. (1994). *Pathophysiology: Concepts of altered health status.* Philadelphia: Lippincott.

Pruzinsky, T. (1993). Psychological factors in cosmetic surgery: Recent developments in patient care. *Plastic Surgical Nursing, 13*(2), 64–71, 119.

Reese, J. (1990). Nursing interventions for wound healing in plastic and reconstructive surgery. *Nursing Clinics of North America, 25*(1), 223–233.

Ritchie, S., & Thompson, P. (1992). Primary bacterial skin infections. *Dermatology Nursing, 4*(4), 261–268.

Roses, D., Gumport, S., Harris M., & Kopf, A. (1988). *The diagnosis and management of common skin cancers.* Atlanta: American Cancer Society.

Rowe, D., Carroll, R., & Day, C. (1989). Long-term recurrence rates in previously untreated (primary) basal cell carcinoma: Implications for patient follow-up. *Journal of Dermatologic Surgery, 15,* 315–328.

Schultz-Larsen, F., & Hanifin, J. (1992). Secular changes in the occurrence of atopic dermatitis. *Acta Dermato-Venereologica Suppl. (Stockholm), 176,* 7–12.

Skin Cancer Foundation. (1988). *Simple guidelines to help protect you from the damaging rays of the sun.* New York: Author.

Somma, S., & Glassman, D. (1991). Malignant melanoma. *Dermatology Nursing, 3*(2), 93–99.

Sowder, L. (1992). Biobrane wound dressing used in treatment of toxic epidermal necrolysis: A case study. *Journal of Burn Care and Rehabilitation, 11*(3), 237–239.

Stiller, M., Gropper, C., Shupack, J., Lizzi, F., Driller, J., & Rorke, M. (1994). Diagnostic ultrasound in dermatology: Current uses and future potential. *Cutis, 53*(1), 44–48.

Strohecker, B., Carmody, P., Hibshman, M., & Wong, R. (1991). Sclerotherapy for telangiectasia. *Plastic Surgical Nursing, 11*(3), 110–112.

Tierney, Jr., L., McPhee, S., & Papadakis, M. (1994). *Current medical diagnosis & treatment* (33rd ed.). Norwalk, CT: Appleton & Lange.

Vander Kam, V., & Achauer, B. (1990). Lasers in plastic surgery: Applications and nursing interventions. *Plastic Surgical Nursing, 10*(3), 107–112.

Vargo, N. (1990). Basal cell carcinoma: Classifications and characteristics. *Dermatology Nursing, 2*(4), 209–214.

Vargo, N. (1991). Basal and squamous cell carcinomas: An overview. *Seminars in Oncology Nursing, 7,* 13–25.

Westlake, C. (1991). Commitment to function: Microsurgical flaps. *Plastic Surgical Nursing, 11*(3), 95–100.

Wingo, P., Tong, T., & Bolden, S. (1995). Cancer Statistics, 1995. *CA: A Cancer Journal for Clinicians, 45*(1), 8–30.

Zalla, M. (1994). Basic cutaneous surgery. *Cutis, 53*(4), 172–186.

CHAPTER 18

Nursing Care of Clients with Burns

LEARNING OBJECTIVES

After completing this chapter, you will be able to

- Describe the prevalence, incidence, and etiology of burn injuries.
- Describe the pathophysiology of major and minor burn injuries.
- Estimate burn wound depth and extent.
- Classify types of burns and causative agents.
- Determine prehospital, intrahospital, and posthospital intervention strategies.

- Identify laboratory and diagnostic tests used to monitor burn therapies.
- Discuss the nursing implications for burn wound management across all phases of care.
- Provide client and family teaching specific to managing burn injury during all phases of care.
- Compare and contrast the advantages and disadvantages of antimicrobial therapies used in burn care.
- Use the nursing process as a framework for developing the standard of care for the burn-injured client.

Burns range in severity from a minor loss of small segments of the outermost layer of the skin to a complex injury involving all body systems. Treatments vary from simple application of a topical antiseptic agent in an outpatient clinic to an invasive, multisystem, interdisciplinary health team approach in the aseptic environment of a burn center.

The Client with a Major Burn

■ ■ ■

A major burn typically involves serious injury to the underlying layers of skin and covers a large body surface area. The American Burn Association has classified burn injuries into three categories—minor, moderate, major—according to their severity (Table 18–1). Major burns involve injuries to the head, hands, feet, perineum, and joints; all inhalation injuries; electrical injuries; extensive burn injuries involving large body surface areas; and injuries to high-risk clients.

Overview

A *burn* is an alteration in skin integrity resulting in tissue loss or damage. A transfer of energy from a source of heat to the human body initiates a sequence of physiologic events that in the most severe cases leads to irreversible tissue destruction.

Etiology

There are four types of burn injury: thermal, chemical, electrical, and radiation. Although all four types can lead to generalized tissue damage and multisystem involvement, the causative agents and priority treatment measures are unique to each (Table 18–2).

Table 18–1   American Burn Association Classification of Burn Injury

Minor Burn Injury	Moderate Burn Injury	Major Burn Injury
Excludes electrical injury, inhalation injury, complicated injuries (such as multiple trauma), and all clients who are considered to be at high risk (such as older adults and those with chronic illnesses)	Excludes electrical injury, inhalation injury, complicated injuries (such as multiple trauma), and all clients who are considered to be at high risk (such as older adults and those with chronic illnesses)	Includes all burns of the hands, face, eyes, ears, feet, and perineum; all electrical injuries, inhalation injuries, multiple trauma injuries, and all clients who are considered to be at high risk
Second-degree burns of less than 15% of the total body surface area in adults	Second-degree burns of 15% to 25% of the total body surface area in adults	Second-degree burns of greater than 25% of the total body surface area in adults
Third-degree burns of less than 2% of the total body surface area not involving special care areas (eyes, ears, face, hands, feet, perineum)	Third-degree burns of less than 10% of the total body surface area not involving special care areas (eyes, ears, face, hands, feet, perineum)	All third-degree burns of 10% or greater of the total body surface area

Note. Burn injuries described in this table (except minor burns) should be treated in a specialized burn center. These criteria have been established by the American Burn Association.

Thermal Burns   Thermal burns result from exposure to dry heat (flames) or moist heat (steam and hot liquids). They are the most common burn injuries and occur predominantly in children and older adults. Direct exposure to the source of heat causes cellular destruction that can result in charring of vascular, bony, muscle, and nervous tissue.

Chemical Burns   Chemical burns are caused by direct skin contact with either acidic or basic agents. More than 25,000 products found in the home or workplace can cause chemical burns. The chemical destroys tissue protein, leading to necrosis. Acids cause coagulation necrosis, whereas bases cause liquification necrosis. The injury progresses as long as the agent is in direct contact with body surfaces (Achauer, 1987; Boswick, 1987; Klein & O'Malley, 1987).

Chemical agents are further classified according to the manner by which they structurally alter proteins. Oxidizing agents, such as household bleach, alter protein configuration through the chemical process of reduction. Corrosives, such as lye, cause extensive protein denaturation. Protoplasmic poisons, such as organic compounds, form salts with proteins, inhibiting calcium and other ions needed for cell viability. The severity of the chemical burn is related to the type of agent, the concentration of the agent, the mechanism of action, the duration of contact, and the amount of body surface area exposed (Achauer, 1987; Boswick, 1987; Klein & O'Malley, 1987). See the box on page 628 for a list of household cleaning agents that may cause burns.

Electrical Burns   The severity of electrical burns depends on the type and duration of current, and amount of voltage. It is particularly difficult to assess the extent of the electrical burn injury, because the destructive processes initiated by the electrical insult persist for weeks beyond the time of the incident. Electricity follows the path of least resistance, which in the human body tends to lie along muscles, bone, blood vessels, and nerves. Necrosis of the tissue results from impaired blood flow, secondary to blood coagulation at the site of the electrical injury. More than 90% of electrical burn wounds that develop gangrene result in amputation (Achauer, 1987; Boswick, 1987; Jepsen, 1992; Martyn, 1990).

Alternating current, as is found in conventional households, produces repeated electrical surges that lead to tetanic muscle contractions. Such sustained muscle contractions inhibit respiratory efforts for the duration of contact and result in respiratory arrest. Direct current, as in injury from a lightning bolt, exposes the body to very high voltage for an instantaneous period of time. High voltage injury usually results in entry and exit wounds. The flash-over effect, a phenomenon unique to lightning injury, actually saves the client from death. It is seen in those instances in which the current travels along the outside of the client's body to the ground, thereby sparing the internal organs from harm (Achauer, 1987; Boswick, 1987; Jepsen, 1992; Martyn, 1990).

Radiation Burns   Radiation burns are usually associated with sunburn or radiation treatment for cancer. These kinds of burns tend to be superficial, involving only the outermost layers of the epidermis. All functions of the skin remain intact. Symptoms are limited to mild systemic reactions: headache, chills, local discomfort,

Table 18–2 Types, Causative Agents, and Priority Treatment Measures for Burns

Type	Causative Agent	Priority Treatment
Thermal	Open flame Steam Hot liquids (water, grease, tar, metal)	Extinguish flame. Flush with cool water. Consult fire department.
Chemical	Acids Strong alkalis	Neutralize or dilute chemical. Remove clothing. Consult Poison Control Center.
Electrical	Direct current Alternating current Lightning	Disconnect source of current. Initiate CPR if necessary. Move to area of safety. Consult electrical experts.
Radiation	Solar (ultraviolet) X-rays Radioactive agents	Shield the skin appropriately. Limit time of exposure. Move the client away from the radiation source. Consult a radiation expert.

Household Cleaning Agents That May Cause Burns

■ ■ ■

- Drain cleaners
- Lye
- Industrial-strength ammonia
- Household ammonia

- Oven cleaners
- Toilet bowl cleaners
- Dishwasher detergents
- Bleach

---

nausea, and vomiting. More extensive exposure to radiation or radioactive substances, as in nuclear power accidents, leads to the same degree of tissue damage and multisystem involvement associated with other types of burns (Bomberger & Dannenfelser, 1984; Dressler, Hozid, & Nathan, 1988).

Epidemiology

An estimated 2 million Americans suffer burn injuries each year, 70,000 to 108,000 of whom require hospitalization. Annually, 12,000 die as a result of burn wound complications. Sixty-eight percent of burns occur in the home, 24% in the workplace. Home burn injuries occur most frequently in the kitchen and bathroom (Achauer, 1987).

Risk Factors

There are two groups who face a high risk for burns and to whom preventive strategies must be targeted: children and seniors. Young children may suffer burns as a result of child abuse, accidental scalding, or playing with matches. Older adults are known to be burn prone and make up 15% of all burn admissions (Staley & Richard, 1993). Sensory awareness can diminish as a result of aging (Richard & Staley, 1994), and many older adults may experience burns from heating pads, stoves, or showering in excessively hot water. Smoking while intoxicated has been associated with fires started in bed linen and upholstered furniture.

Educational programs to alert the public to the need for greater caution to prevent burns in these two age groups can help decrease the incidence of burn injury.

Prevention

Although treatments have improved significantly over the last several decades, there is no cure for burns. Prevention remains the primary goal (DiMola, 1993). With the public's increasing attention to health promotion and disease prevention, the nursing profession currently is well positioned to collaborate with other disciplines to develop initiatives to reduce the number of burn injuries. For example, as client advocates, nurses can alert political leaders to the need to pass legislation aimed at reducing the incidence of burns. Appropriate legislative themes might center around safety in the workplace (e.g., requirements for smoke alarms/sprinkler systems), on the highways (e.g., regulations regarding the transportation of flammable liquids), and in the home (e.g., requirements for safety devices for water heaters and wood-burning stoves, and for self-extinguishing cigarettes) (Boswick, 1987; Hammond, 1993; Rutan, Desai, & Herndon, 1993). As educators, nurses can develop teaching plans for families and communities to heighten awareness of the problem. As researchers, nurses can investigate conditions leading to burn injury and suggest methods to reduce its prevalence. Working together with health care policy makers and community leaders, nurses can join the effort to lower the numbers of burn cases treated annually.

Pathophysiology

The pathophysiologic changes specific to major burn injuries involve all body systems. Extensive loss of skin, the body's protective barrier, can result in massive infection, fluid and electrolyte imbalances, and hypothermia. Often the person inhales the products of combustion; exposure to the heat source in this manner compromises respiratory function. Cardiac dysrhythmias and circulatory failure are common manifestations of serious burn injuries.

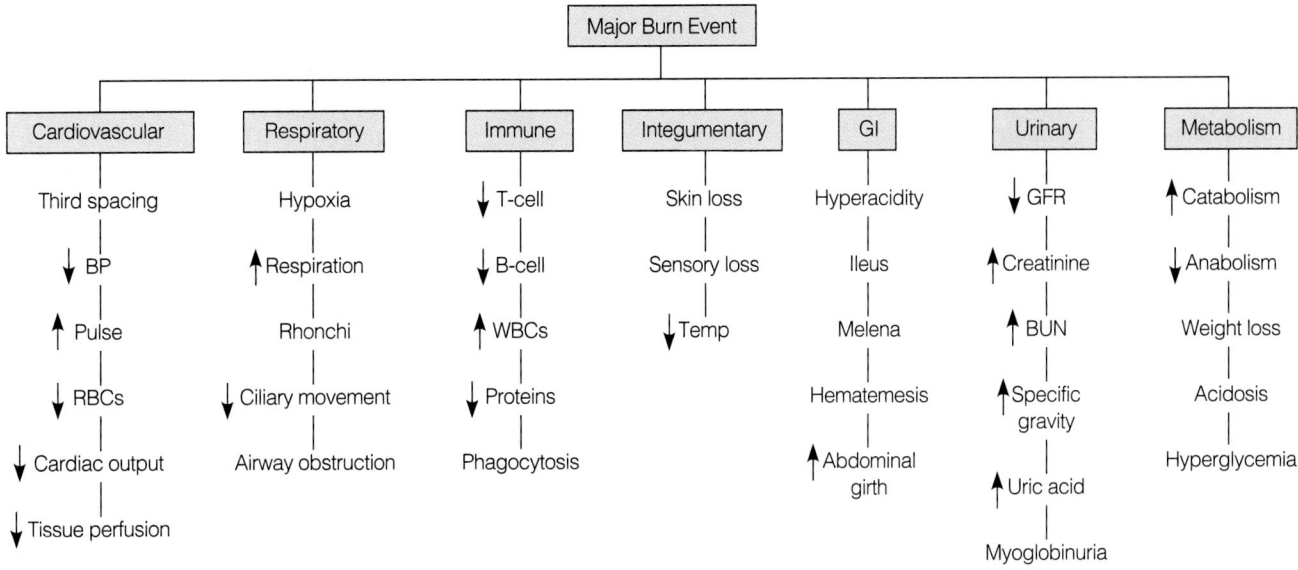

Figure 18–1 Effects of a severe burn on major body systems and metabolism.

A profound catabolic state dramatically increases caloric expenditure and nutritional deficiencies. An alteration in gastrointestinal motility predisposes the client to developing paralytic ileus, and hyperacidity leads to the formation of gastric and duodenal ulcerations. Dehydration slows glomerular filtration rates and renal clearance of toxic wastes and may lead to acute tubular necrosis and renal failure.

Systemic Responses
A major burn can disrupt the physiologic processes of the cardiovascular, immune, integumentary, respiratory, gastrointestinal, and urinary systems. Moreover, overall body metabolism may be profoundly altered. Systemic responses to burns are shown in Figure 18–1 and are discussed in the following sections.

Cardiovascular System Although the pathophysiologic mechanisms of postburn vascular changes and fluid volume shifts are not clearly understood, three processes occur early in the postburn phase: (1) an increase in microvascular permeability at the burn wound site; (2) a generalized impairment of cell wall function, resulting in intracellular edema; and (3) an increase in osmotic pressure of the burned tissue, leading to extensive fluid accumulation (Martyn, 1990). Within minutes of the burn injury, a massive amount of fluid shifts from the intracellular and intravascular compartments into the interstitium, thereby creating a state of hemodynamic instability, called **burn shock.** This shifting is the direct result of a loss of cell wall integrity at the site of injury and in the capillary bed. Fluid leaks from the capillaries into interstitial compartments located at the burn wound site and throughout the body, resulting in a decrease in fluid vol-

ume within the intravascular space. Plasma proteins and sodium escape into the interstitium, enhancing edema formation. Blood pressure falls as cardiac output diminishes. Vasoconstriction results as the vascular system attempts to compensate for fluid loss. Abnormal platelet aggregation and white blood cell (WBC) accumulation result in ischemia in the deeper tissue below the burn, leading to eventual thrombosis. Red blood cells (RBCs) and WBCs remain in the circulation, producing an elevation in erythrocyte and leukocyte counts secondary to hemoconcentration (Achauer, 1987; Boswick, 1987; Burgess, 1991; Richard & Staley, 1994).

The leakage of fluid into the interstitium compromises the lymphatic system, resulting in intravascular hypovolemia and edema at the burn wound site. Edematous body surfaces impair peripheral circulation and result in necrosis of the underlying tissue. During burn shock, potassium ions leave the intracellular compartment, predisposing the client to developing cardiac dysrhythmias. The process of burn shock continues until capillary integrity is restored, usually within 24 hours of the injury (Achauer, 1987; Boswick, 1987; Burgess, 1991; Richard & Staley, 1994).

Burn shock reverses when fluid is reabsorbed from the interstitium into the intravascular compartment. The blood pressure rises as cardiac output increases, and urinary output improves. Diuresis continues from several days to 2 weeks postburn. During this phase, the extra cardiac workload may predispose the elderly client, or the client with cardiovascular disease, to fluid volume overload (Achauer, 1987). Fluid restriction, diuretic therapy, and close monitoring of hemodynamic function are needed to support circulatory function (Martyn, 1990).

Table 18–3   Manifestations of Carbon
Monoxide Poisoning

Level of Carbon Monoxide	Manifestations
10% to 20%	Headache, dizziness, nausea, abdominal pain
21% to 40%	Headache, nausea, drowsiness, dizziness, irritability, confusion, stupor, hypotension, bradycardia, skin color ranging from pale to dark red
41% to 60%	Convulsion, coma, hypotension, tachycardia
> 60%	Death

Fluid replacement and maintenance are the major goals of treatment during the early phases of the burn injury. Even after capillary integrity is restored, fluid losses continue until closure of the burn wound is effected. The client is placed on a fluid maintenance plan over the duration of the acute phase (Achauer, 1987; Boswick, 1987; Burgess, 1991; Richard & Staley, 1994).

Immune System   The function of the immune system is to protect the human body from invasion by foreign microorganisms. The capillary leak that occurs in the early stages of the burn injury continues throughout the burn shock phase and impairs the active components of both the cell-mediated and humoral immune systems (Achauer, 1987; Boswick, 1987; Robins, 1989; Tribett, 1989).

The humoral immune system relies on B cells to produce antibodies or immunoglobulins (see Chapter 8). In the burn client, the serum levels of all immunoglobulins are significantly diminished. Serum protein levels remain persistently low throughout the clinical course until wound closure is effected. A marked decrease in T-cell counts results in a reduction of cytotoxic activity and suppression of the cell-mediated immune system (Achauer, 1987; Boswick, 1987; Robins, 1989; Tribett, 1989).

The compromise in the humoral and cell-mediated immune systems constitutes a state of acquired immunodeficiency, which places the burn client at risk for infection. The period of vulnerability is transient and may last from 1 to 4 weeks following the onset of the burn injury. During this time frame, opportunistic infections can develop and produce death despite aggressive antimicrobial therapy (Achauer, 1987; Boswick, 1987; Robins, 1989; Tribett, 1989).

Integumentary System   The integumentary system functions as a thermoregulator, a synthesizer of vitamin D, an excretory organ, a sensory organ, as well as a barrier against infection. The burn injury impairs the normal physiologic functions of the skin (Achauer, 1987; Boswick, 1987; Burgess, 1991; Richard & Staley, 1994).

Heat transfer to skin is a complex phenomenon. During burning, the temperature of the skin rises in an inverse relation to the distance from the heat source. A thermal gradient hottest at the skin surface is established at the onset of the burn injury. If the microcirculation of the skin remains intact during burning, it cools and protects the deeper portions of the skin and cools the outer surface once the heat source is removed. With extensive burn injury, the integrity of the microcirculation is lost, and the burning process continues even after the heat source is removed (Boswick, 1987).

The overall thickness of the dermis and epidermis varies considerably from one area of the body to another. Similiar temperatures produce different depths of injury to different body parts. For example, in the adult, skin covering the medial aspect of the forearm is thinner and more easily damaged than the skin covering the back of the same person. Skin dissipates heat maximally in areas of greatest vascularization. When heat absorption exceeds the rate of dissipation, cellular temperatures rise, and skin tissue is destroyed (Boswick, 1987; Richard & Staley, 1994).

Respiratory System   Inhalation injury is a frequent and often lethal complication of burns. The injury may range from mild respiratory inflammation to massive pulmonary failure. Exposure to asphyxiants, smoke, and heat initiates the pathophysiologic processes associated with inhalation injury (Achauer, 1987; Boswick, 1987; Cioffi & Rue, 1991; Martyn, 1990; Richard & Staley, 1994).

Carbon monoxide, a common asphyxiant, is a colorless, tasteless, odorless gas that displaces oxygen to bind with hemoglobin, forming carboxyhemoglobin. The resulting decrease in arterial oxyhemoglobin produces tissue hypoxia. Carbon monoxide impairs both oxygen delivery and cellular oxygen use (Achauer, 1987; Boswick, 1987; Cioffi & Rue, 1991; Martyn, 1990; Richard & Staley, 1994). The clinical manifestations of carbon monoxide poisoning range from mild visual impairment to coma and death (Table 18–3).

Smoke poisoning results when toxic gases and particulate matter, the products of incomplete combustion, deposit directly onto the pulmonary mucosa. The composition of the products of combustion depends on the combustible material, the rate at which the temperature increases, and the amount of ambient oxygen present. Irritant gases and particulate matter have a direct cytotoxic effect. The degree of injury is determined by their solubility in water, duration of exposure, and the size of the particulate or aerosol droplet (Cioffi & Rue, 1991).

Inflammation occurs at localized sites within the airway and is manifested as hyperemia. As a result, cells are destroyed and the bronchial cilia are rendered inactive.

Because the mucociliary transport mechanism no longer functions, the client may develop bronchial congestion and infection.

Interstitial pulmonary edema develops secondary to extravasation of fluid from the pulmonary vasculature into the interstitial compartment of the lung tissue. Surfactant is inactivated, and atelectasis and alveolar collapse may result. Sloughing of the damaged and dead lung tissue occasionally produces debris that may lead to complete airway obstruction (Cioffi & Rue, 1991).

Edema damages the upper and lower airways. Exposure to compounds with a high water solubility causes upper airway damage. Lower airway damage is caused by compounds with a lower water solubility and the ability to penetrate more distal areas (Achauer, 1987; Boswick, 1987; Cioffi & Rue, 1991; Richard & Staley, 1994).

Upper airway thermal injury results from the inhalation of heated air. Physical findings include the presence of soot, charring, edema, blisters, and ulcerations along the mucosal lining of the oropharynx and larynx. The resulting edema in the airway peaks within the first 24 to 48 hours of injury (Achauer, 1987; Boswick, 1987; Cioffi & Rue, 1991; Richard & Staley, 1994).

Lower airway thermal injury is a rare occurrence. Because the lower airway is protected by laryngeal reflexes, thermal injury below the vocal cords is seldom seen. However, when it does occur, it is typically associated with the inhalation of steam or explosive gases or the aspiration of hot liquids. The xenon perfusion-ventilation lung scan and flexible bronchoscopy are used to confirm lower airway injury. Both are employed as early diagnostic procedures (Achauer, 1987; Boswick, 1987; Cioffi & Rue, 1991; Richard & Staley, 1994).

Gastrointestinal System   **Curling's ulcer** is an acute ulceration of the stomach or duodenum that forms following the burn injury. Abdominal pain, acidic gastric pH levels, hematemesis, and melanotic stool may indicate the presence of gastric ulcer formation (Achauer, 1987; Boswick, 1987; Richard & Staley, 1994).

A decrease in or absence of bowel sounds is a manifestation of paralytic ileus (adynamic bowel) secondary to burn trauma. The resulting cessation of intestinal motility leads to gastric distention, nausea, vomiting, and hematemesis (Achauer, 1987; Boswick, 1987; Richard & Staley, 1994; Swearingen, Sommers, & Miller, 1988).

Urinary System   During the early stages of the burn injury, massive fluid losses occur. These losses, if unchecked, lead to dehydration, hemoconcentration, and oliguria. Dark brown concentrated urine may indicate myoglobinuria. Acute tubular necrosis and renal failure may develop if fluids are not adequately replaced (Achauer, 1987; Boswick, 1987; Burgess, 1991; Richard & Staley, 1994).

Metabolism   Two distinct phases characterize the body's metabolic response to the burn injury. Lasting over the first 3 days of the injury is the *ebb phase*, which is manifested by decreased oxygen consumption, fluid imbalance, shock, and inadequate circulating volume. These responses protect the body from the initial impact of the injury (Boswick, 1987; Martyn, 1990; Richard & Staley, 1994).

A second phase, the *flow phase,* occurs when adequate burn resuscitation has been accomplished. This phase is characterized by increases in cellular activity and protein catabolism, lipolysis, and gluconeogenesis. The basal metabolic rate (BMR) significantly increases, reaching twice the normal rate. Body weight and heat drop dramatically. Total energy expenditure may exceed 100% of normal BMR. Hypermetabolism persists until after wound closure has been accomplished and may reappear if complications occur (Boswick, 1987; Martyn, 1990).

Stages of Burn Injury

The clinical course of treatment for the burn client is divided into three stages: the emergent/resuscitative stage, the acute stage, and the rehabilitative stage (Burgess, 1991). Although these stages are useful predictors of the clinical needs of the burn client, it is important to recognize that the process of burn injury is dynamic and that in many cases, the clinical stage may not be clearly delineated. Assessment and management of the burn-injured client are ongoing processes that are determined by the clinical picture and last throughout the course of treatment. Figure 18–2 shows the burn client's progression through the health care system during each clinical stage of burn care. During each stage, different groups of nurses, physicians, and allied health care specialists collaborate to manage the client's recovery.

Emergent/Resuscitative Stage   The emergent/resuscitative stage lasts approximately 48 to 72 hours, from the onset of injury through successful fluid resuscitation (Burgess, 1991). During this stage, health care workers estimate the extent of burn injury, institute initial first-aid measures, and implement fluid resuscitation therapies. The client is assessed for shock and evidence of respiratory distress. If indicated, intravenous lines are inserted, and the client may be prophylactically intubated. During this stage, health care workers determine whether the client is to be transported to a burn center for the complex intervention strategies of the professional, interdisciplinary burn team.

Acute Stage   The acute stage begins with diuresis and ends with closure of the burn wound (Burgess, 1991). During this stage, wound care management, nutritional therapies, and measures to control infectious processes are initiated. Hydrotherapy and excision and grafting of full-thickness wounds are performed as soon as possible after injury. Enteral and parenteral nutritional interventions are started early in the treatment plan to address

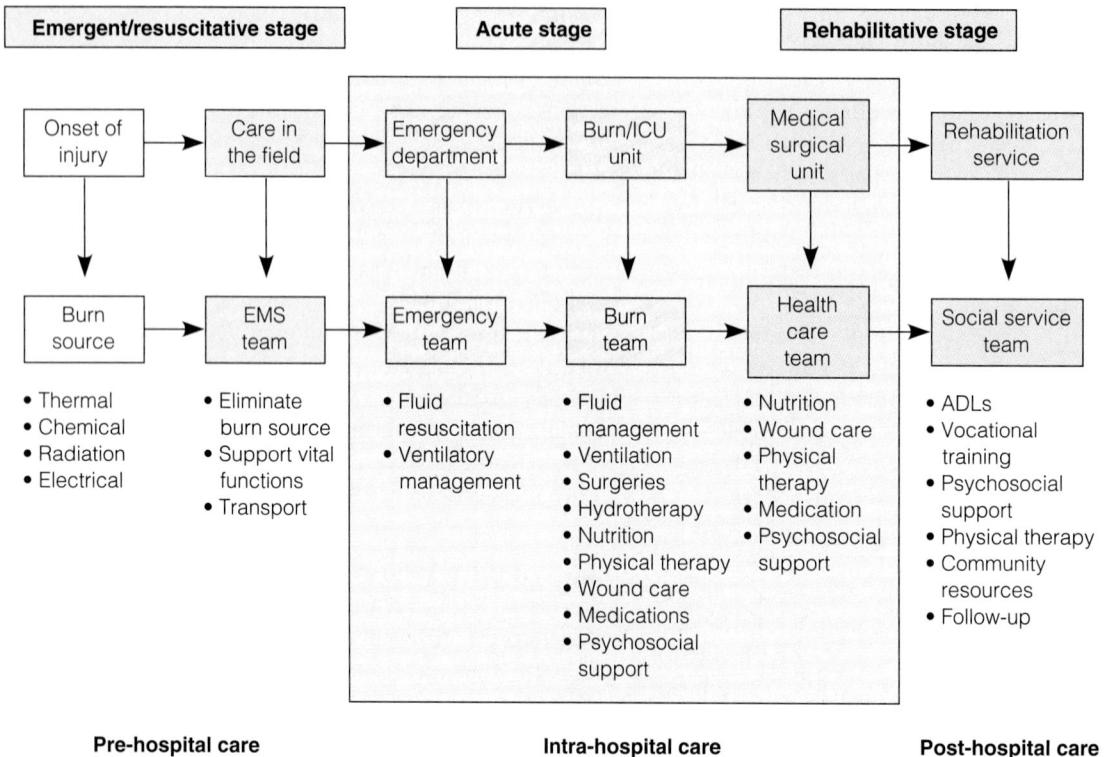

Figure 18–2 The client's progression through the health care system during the emergent, acute, and rehabilitative stages of burn injury.

caloric needs resulting from extensive energy expenditure. Measures to combat infection are implemented during this stage, including the administration of topical and systemic antimicrobial agents. Pain management constitutes a significant segment of the nursing care plan throughout the clinical course of the burn-injured client. The administration of narcotic pharmaceutical agents must precede all invasive procedures to maximize client comfort and to reduce the anxieties associated with wound debridement and intensive physical therapy.

Rehabilitative Stage The rehabilitative stage begins with wound closure and ends when the client returns to the highest level of health restoration (Burgess, 1991). During this stage, the primary focus is the biopsychosocial adjustment of the client, specifically the prevention of contractures and scars and the client's successful resumption of work, family, and social roles through physical, vocational, occupational, and psychosocial rehabilitation. The client is taught to perform range-of-motion (ROM) exercises to enhance mobility and to support injured joints.

Prehospital Care

Treatment at the scene of the injury includes measures to limit the severity of the burn and support vital functions.

Emergency Measures to Limit Burn Severity

Before attempting to remove the client from the source of burn injury, rescuers must ensure their own safety. Depending on the causative agent, rescuers may need to consult with experts to determine the best way to eliminate the source of the injury. Once the safety of the rescuers has been established, all prehospital interventions are aimed at eliminating the heat source, stabilizing the client's condition, identifying the type of burn, preventing heat loss, reducing wound contamination, and preparing for emergency transport (Achauer, 1987; Boswick, 1987; Burgess, 1991; Dressler et al., 1988; Martyn, 1990). Restrictive jewelry and clothing is removed at the scene to prevent circumferential constriction of the torso and extremities.

Thermal Burns If the thermal injury has been caused by dry heat, smother inflamed clothing or lavage with water. Assist the client to initiate a "stop, drop, and roll" maneuver to extinguish the flame and limit the extent of burn (Achauer, 1987). Once the flame has been extinguished, cover the body to prevent hypothermia. If the thermal injury has been caused by moist heat, lavage the area with cool water.

Chemical Burns For chemical burns, immediately remove the clothing, and use a hose or shower to lavage the involved area thoroughly. Unusual chemicals may require consultation with the poison control center for instructions regarding appropriate treatment (Klein & O'Malley, 1987).

Electrical Burns Electrical injuries pose serious potential harm to both rescuer and client. Ensure that the source of electrical current has been disconnected, or move the client to safety using nonconductive devices that can serve as rods to push the client away from the energy source. Monitor the client for cardiopulmonary arrest. If the client is unresponsive, assess for the presence of cardiac and respiratory function. If indicated, begin cardiopulmonary resuscitation (CPR). A spinal cord injury may be present secondary to the forceful contraction of the muscles of the neck and back during exposure to the current. If possible, place the client in a cervical collar and transport the client on a spinal board (Achauer, 1987; Jepsen, 1992; Martyn, 1990).

Radiation Burns Radiation injuries are usually minor and involve only the epidermal layer of skin. Treatment focuses on helping normal body mechanisms promote wound healing. For severe radiation burns, such as those that result from industrial radiation accidents, trained personnel may need to render the area safe for entry prior to rescue. All interventions are aimed at shielding, establishing distance, and limiting the time of exposure to the radioactive source (Bomberger & Dannenfelser, 1984).

Emergency Measures to Support Vital Function

The initial assessment of the client's respiratory and hemodynamic status begins with an evaluation of the client's airway, breathing, and circulation (the ABCs of care). Prehospital care personnel determine the adequacy of ventilation and circulation and institute the following measures as necessary.

Cardiopulmonary Resuscitation If the client has no pulse and is not breathing, begin CPR. Establish an airway, and start mouth-to-mouth breathing and chest compressions. Continue CPR until spontaneous cardiopulmonary function returns or until the emergency management team takes over.

When the emergency team arrives, begin oxygen therapy. Use high-flow oxygen for all suspected cases of inhalation injury. Observe for the cessation of respiration in the client with a history of chronic obstructive pulmonary disease (COPD), and reduce oxygen flow accordingly. If the client is unconscious and carbon monoxide poisoning is suspected, administer 100% oxygen until blood gas measurements are obtained (Boswick, 1987). Agitation, anxiety, and combative behavior may indicate hypoxia. Do not include sedation in the initial treatment.

When available, connect the client to a cardiac monitor and observe for dysrhythmias. Watch for the development of premature ventricular contractions (PVCs), runs of ventricular tachycardia, and ventricular standstill. Treat according to protocol.

Maintaining Ventilation All burn injuries involving the face, neck, or anterior chest require prophylactic intubation. Tracheal intubation is required when edema obstructs the airway. Pulmonary edema, a sequela of inhalation injury, requires mechanical ventilatory management with large tidal volume, positive end expiratory pressure (PEEP), and oxygen concentrations that maintain oxygen saturation levels above 90%.

All burn-injured clients must be frequently assessed for respiratory distress. Signs and symptoms include hoarseness, dyspnea, tachypnea, stridor, cyanosis, wheezing, crackles, poor chest excursion, progressive changes on chest X-ray film, and deteriorating ABGs.

Nursing measures for on-scene airway management include interventions to promote alveolar oxygen exchange. Position the client with the head elevated at greater than 30 degrees, and administer oxygen. Employ frequent nasotracheal suctioning to maintain a patent airway. Auscultate the lungs often on site to monitor respiratory status. Continuous pulse oximetry is used for ongoing assessment of the client's oxygen saturation levels (Achauer, 1987; Cioffi et al. 1991; Martyn, 1990; Rue & Cioffi, 1991).

Maintaining Circulation At the scene of the injury, insert large-bore intravenous lines to begin fluid management. Fluid replacement therapy is necessary in all burn wounds that involve more than 20% of the total body surface area. Many formulae are available to calculate the fluid requirements of the severely burn-injured client. The most commonly used is the Parkland/Baxter formula. Several types of fluids are used to restore fluid volume: colloids, crystalloids, blood, and blood products. See the section on fluid resuscitation on page 637 for a more extensive discussion.

Continuously assess the client's hemodynamic status at the scene by auscultating heart and lung sounds and by observing level of consciousness, cardiac rate and rhythm, blood pressure, and urine output (Achauer, 1987; Boswick, 1987; Burgess, 1991; Martyn, 1987).

Maintaining Body Temperature The client loses heat through open burn-injured areas via evaporation and radiation. At the scene of the injury, use blankets and heavy clothing to maintain body core temperatures at 99.6 to 101 F (37.5 to 38.3 C).

Emergency Department Care

On arriving at the hospital, the client is taken to the emergency department. Prehospital personnel report to the emergency department staff all findings and medical interventions that occurred at the scene of the injury. The nurse obtains a history of the injury, estimates the depth

Table 18–4   Characteristics of Burns, by Depth

Characteristic	First-Degree	Second-Degree	Third-Degree
Skin layers lost	Epidermis	Epidermis and dermis	Epidermis, dermis, and underlying tissues
Skin appearance over burn	Red to gray; may have local edema	Fluid-filled blisters; may appear waxy white with deep partial-thickness burns	Waxy white; dry, leathery, charred
Skin function	Present	Absent	Absent
Pain sensation	Present	Present	Absent
Manifestations at the burn site	Moderate pain; local edema	Severe pain; edema; weeping of fluid	Little pain; edema
Treatment	Regular cleaning Topical agent of choice	Regular cleaning Topical agent of choice May require skin grafting	Regular cleaning Topical agent of choice Skin substitutes Excision of eschar Skin grafting
Scarring	None	Often extensive	Of grafted area
Time to heal	3 to 5 days	1 to several months	Requires skin grafting to heal

and extent of the burn, begins fluid resuscitation, and maintains ventilation according to protocol.

History of the Burn Injury
Once the client arrives at the emergency department (ED), the staff must act quickly to obtain the history of the burn injury, including the time of the injury, the causative agents, the early treatment, the medical history, and the client's age and body weight. In most cases, the client is awake and oriented and able to relate the information during the emergent phase of care. Because changes in sensorium will become evident within the first few hours following a major burn injury, the nurse obtains as much information as is possible immediately on the client's arrival.

Time of Injury   In many cases, the client is admitted to the ED an hour or more after the injury occurred. The time of the burn injury must be documented as precisely as possible at the scene, because all fluid resuscitation calculations are based on the time of the burn injury, not on the time of the client's arrival at the ED.

Identification of the Cause   Because the type of burn injury determines which nursing measures take priority, the nurse must identify the specific causative agent to establish the appropriate plan of care.

First-Aid Treatment   Prior to the arrival of medical personnel, the client or family may have applied home remedies to treat the burn wound. It is important for the nurse to ascertain and document the nature of all home treatment interventions, including the application of neu-

tralizing agents, liquids, and immobilizing devices used to splint associated injuries. Tetanus toxoid is administered early in the treatment plan, often in the field.

Past Medical History   Clients with histories of respiratory, cardiac, renal, metabolic, neurologic, gastrointestinal, or skin diseases; alcohol abuse; or altered immune states require more intense observation.

Age   Older adults tend to require more supportive care.

Medications   Drugs, either prescribed or recreational, taken by the client prior to the burn injury may further complicate the treatment regimen. Drugs that affect any of the major body systems or cause mood alterations will need to be factored into the treatment plan. As part of the early assessment, the nurse obtains and documents blood levels of therapeutic pharmaceutical agents and mood-altering substances.

Body Weight   During the acute and rehabilitative phases of the burn injury, the client will lose as much as 20% of preburn weight. This fact will have significant implications for all clients, especially for those who were underweight or cachectic at the time of the injury.

Classification of Burn Depth
Tissue damage following a burn is determined primarily by two factors: the extent of the burn (the percentage of body surface area involved) and the depth of the burn (the layers of underlying tissue affected). The recognized system for describing a burn injury, developed by the American Burn Association, uses both the extent and depth of burn to classify burns as minor, moderate, or

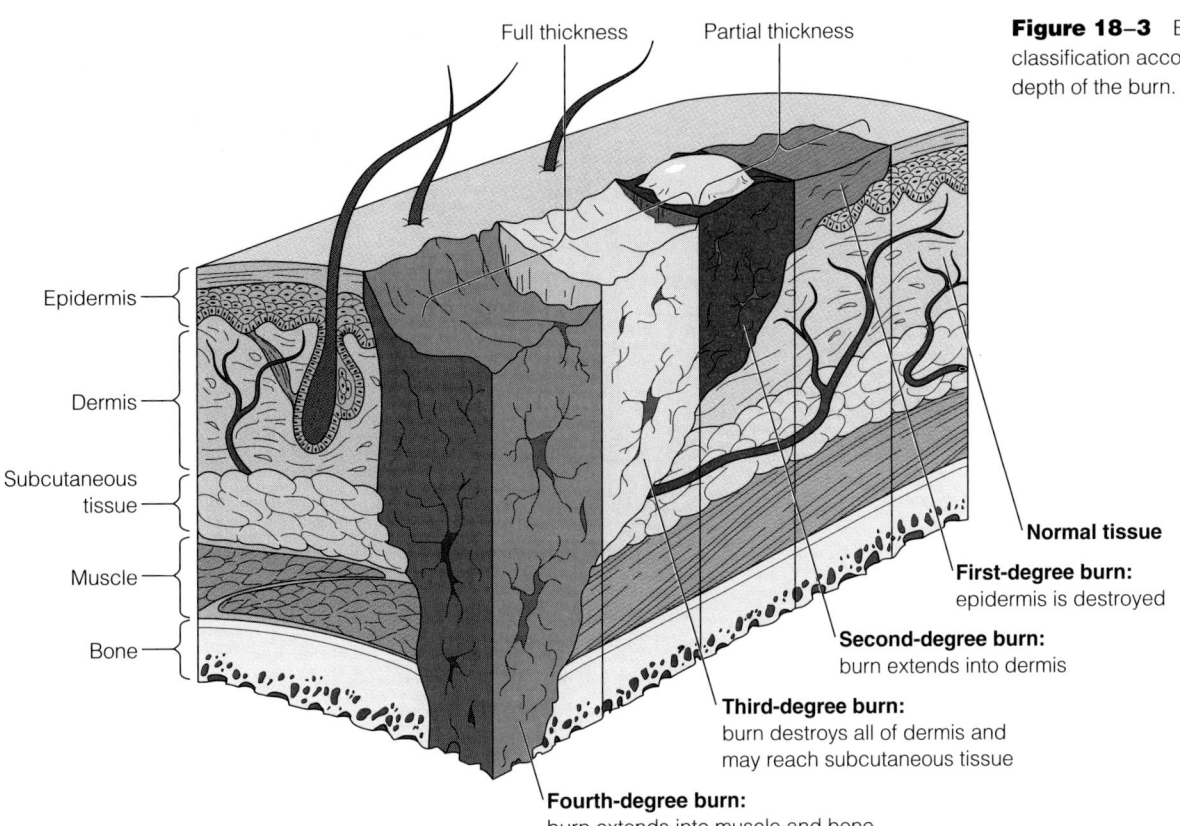

Full thickness

Partial thickness

Figure 18–3 Burn-injury classification according to the depth of the burn.

Epidermis

Dermis

Subcutaneous tissue

Muscle

Bone

Normal tissue

First-degree burn:
epidermis is destroyed

Second-degree burn:
burn extends into dermis

Third-degree burn:
burn destroys all of dermis and
may reach subcutaneous tissue

Fourth-degree burn:
burn extends into muscle and bone

major (see Table 18–1). Formulas for estimating the extent of a burn are discussed on page 636 (Achauer, 1987; Boswick, 1987; Burgess, 1991; Martyn, 1987; Richard & Staley, 1994).

The depth of a burn may be classified in one of four categories: first-degree, second-degree, third-degree, or fourth-degree. Characteristics of burns within each classification are summarized in Table 18–4 and illustrated in Figure 18–3.

First-Degree Burn A first-degree burn involves only the epidermal layer of the skin. Because the skin remains intact, first-degree burns are usually not calculated into estimates of the extent of burn injury. Local pain and erythema are present at the site of the burn, and blisters may form within the first 24 hours. First-degree burns involving large body surface areas may cause chills, headache, pain at the site, nausea, and vomiting. The injury usually heals in 3 to 5 days without scar formation. These kinds of burns are treated with mild analgesics and the application of water-soluble lotions. Causative agents include ultraviolet solar radiation (sunburn) and mild radiation burns associated with cancer treatment.

In older clients, extensive first-degree burns may lead to systemic dehydration secondary to fluid losses into blistered areas and profound nausea and vomiting. Treatment focuses on rehydrating the client with intravenous fluids.

Second-Degree Burn Second-degree burn injuries are subclassified into superficial and deep partial-thickness wounds (Figure 18–4). Superficial injuries involve the epidermal and dermal layers of the skin and are red to pale ivory in color. Fluid-filled blisters form immediately, and the client experiences pain at the site. Healing occurs in 21 to 28 days and, depending on the client's genetic heritage, may or may not be associated with extensive scarring. Generally, darker-pigmented races (people of Asian and African descent) are more susceptible to hypertrophic scarring (Richard & Staley, 1994).

Deep partial-thickness burns involve the destruction of the entire dermal layer. A flat dry blister forms at the site, and pain is either absent or greatly diminished. The surrounding tissue of lesser depth may, however, have intact pain sensors and be sensitive to touch. Healing occurs in 30 days. Because these wounds are associated with extensive scarring, contemporary therapeutic interventions include excision of the wound and skin grafting to effect early wound closure.

Third-Degree Burn Third-degree full-thickness burns involve all layers of the skin and subcutaneous tissues. These burns are white, cherry red, or black (Figure 18–5). Skin loses its elasticity, resulting in a leathery appearance, with progressive restriction of circumferential wounds involving the extremities or torso. Visibly thrombosed superficial blood vessels are evident. Deep blisters

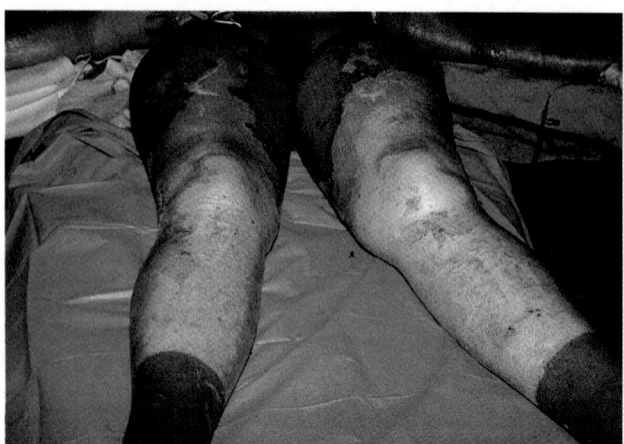

Figure 18–4 Partial-thickness burn injury.

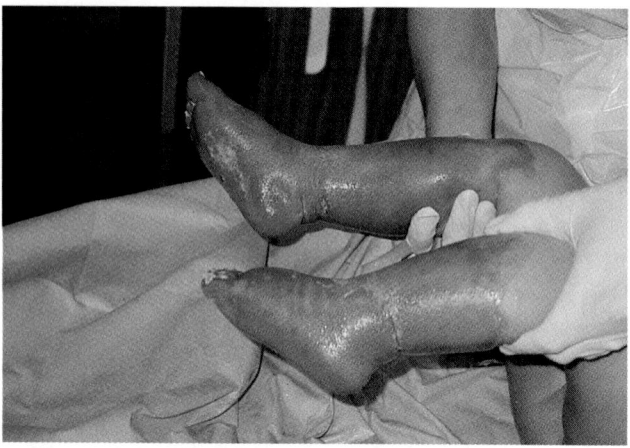

Figure 18–5 Full-thickness burn injury.

may form under dry dehydrated skin. Because all pain sensors have been destroyed, third-degree burns are characteristically painless. Injuries larger than 2 inches in diameter will not heal and will require skin grafting.

Fourth-Degree Burn Fourth-degree burns involve all layers of underlying tissue: bone, muscle, blood vessels, and nerves. These injuries tend to be extensive and to require grafting. Bone tissue that is left exposed invariably dies, leading to a nonhealing wound with potential for infection. One method of treating exposed bone involves drilling holes into the marrow cavity to permit the outgrowth of granulation tissue, which eventually covers the bone. The use of pedicles or flaps to cover exposed bone is also an effective method of treatment. If the joint is exposed, the involved extremity in many cases must be amputated. If exposed joints can be kept moist and free of infection, however, they can sometimes obtain coverage from granulation tissue. Immobilizing the joint with pins or splints may also help promote return of granulation tissue (Richard & Staley, 1994).

Burn Zones Burns have a characteristic skin surface appearance that resembles a bull's-eye, with the most severe burn located centrally and the lesser burns located along the peripheral wound edges. Depending on the intensity of burning, burns consist of one, two, or three concentric three-dimensional zones closely corresponding on the skin surface to areas of first-, second-, or third-degree burns, respectively:

- The outer *zone of erythema* blanches on pressure and heals in 2 to 7 days postburn.
- The medial *zone of stasis* is initially moist, red, and blistered and blanches on pressure. It becomes pale and necrotic on days 3 to 7 postburn.
- The inner *zone of coagulation* immediately appears leathery and coagulated. It merges with the necrotic zone of stasis in 3 to 7 days postburn (Boswick, 1987).

Estimation of Burn Extent

Although many burn injuries are treated in local tertiary care facilities, the American Burn Association has developed guidelines for determining whether the client should be transported to a burn center for interdisciplinary approaches to treatment and rehabilitation. Clients who should be treated at burn centers include those with

- A burn covering 10% or more of body surface and who are less than 10 or greater than 50 years of age.
- A burn covering 20% or more of body surface and who are between the ages of 10 and 50.
- A burn involving the hands, feet, face, eyes, ears, or perineum.
- An inhalation injury.
- An electrical injury.
- Any burn associated with extenuating problems, preexisting illness, fractures, or other trauma (Burgess, 1991).

There are several methods used for determining the extent of injury. The "rule of nines" is a rapid method of estimation used during the prehospital and emergency care phases (Figure 18–6). In this method, the body is divided into five surface areas: head, trunk, arms, legs, and perineum, and percentages are assigned to each body area. For example, a client with burns of the face, anterior right arm, and anterior trunk has burn injury involving 27% of the total body surface area (TBSA) (Achauer, 1987; Martyn, 1990; Richard & Staley, 1994; Rue & Cioffi, 1991).

On the client's admission to the hospital, critical care area, or burn center, more accurate methods for estimating the extent of injury are employed. The Lund and Browder method (Figure 18–7) determines surface area measurements for each body part according to the age of the client (Rue & Cioffi, 1991).

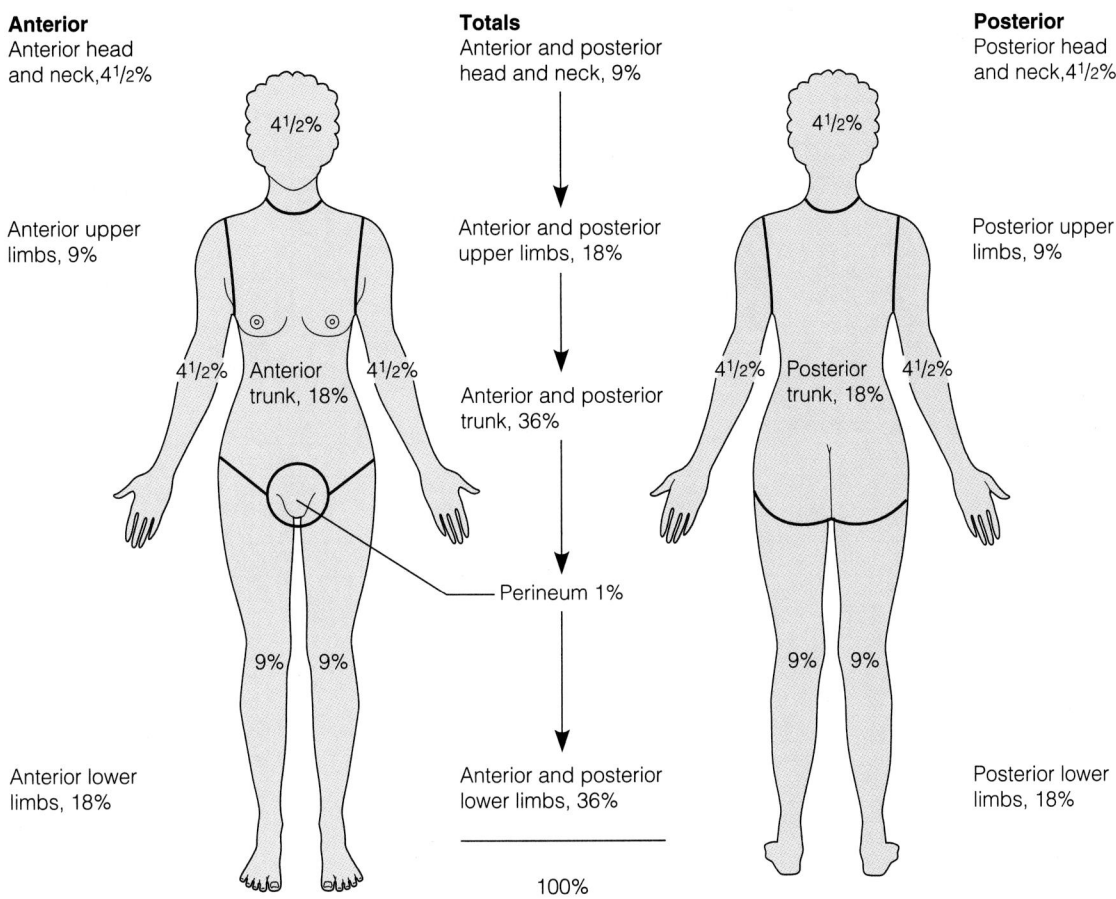

Anterior
Anterior head
and neck, 4 1/2%

Anterior upper
limbs, 9%

4 1/2% | Anterior
trunk, 18% | 4 1/2%

Anterior lower
limbs, 18%

Totals
Anterior and posterior
head and neck, 9%

Anterior and posterior
upper limbs, 18%

Anterior and posterior
trunk, 36%

Perineum 1%

Anterior and posterior
lower limbs, 36%

100%

Posterior
Posterior head
and neck, 4 1/2%

Posterior upper
limbs, 9%

4 1/2% | Posterior
trunk, 18% | 4 1/2%

Posterior lower
limbs, 18%

Figure 18–6   The "rule of nines" is a method of quickly estimating the percentage of TBSA affected by a burn injury. Although useful in emergency care situations, the rule of nines is not accurate for estimating TBSA for adults who are short, obese, or very thin.

Fluid Resuscitation

To counteract the effects of burn shock, **fluid resuscitation** guidelines are used to replace the extensive fluid and electrolyte losses associated with major burn injuries. Fluid replacement is necessary in all burn wounds that involve more than 20% of the TBSA. Colloids, crystalloids, blood, and blood products are used for fluid resuscitation and maintenance.

There are several formulas (such as the Brooke army formula, Evans formula, and hypertonic saline solution) that may be used to replace fluid loss. The Parkland/Baxter formula, however, is the most commonly used (see the box on page 639). Fluids are administered through large-bore central lines at rates sufficient to maintain urine output at 30 to 50 mL/h. Lactated Ringer's solution is the intravenous fluid of choice because it most closely approximates the body's extracellular fluid composition. To calculate the fluid resuscitation rate using the Parkland/Baxter formula, the nurse determines the total amount of intravenous solution to infuse over the first 24 hours postburn. The rate is based on 4 mL/kg per percent of TBSA burned: 50% of the total amount is administered over the first 8 hours postburn, 25% over the second 8 hours postburn, and 25% over the third 8 hours postburn. Over the second 24 hours postburn, the lactated Ringer's solution is discontinued and a colloid (e.g., albumin, plasmanate, or dextran) is infused at a rate of 0.3 to 0.5 mL/kg per percent of TBSA burned, along with dextrose in water titrated to maintain urine output.

Fluid resuscitation rates are adjusted periodically throughout the emergent stage of care. The nurse should be particularly aware of several situations that may warrant the administration of fluids at rates in excess of the calculations needed to maintain adequate urine output: initial underestimation of the burn size, sequestration of fluid into the lung tissue in inhalation injury, electrical injury (which tends to cause more extensive damage than is immediately visible), fourth-degree burns, and inordinately delayed starts of fluid resuscitation.

During the fluid resuscitation stage, the client may require invasive hemodynamic monitoring (see Chapter 28). A pulmonary artery catheter monitors cardiac output, cardiac index, and pulmonary artery wedge pressures. All measurements must be maintained within normal limits to effect adequate fluid resuscitation (Boswick, 1987; Burgess, 1991; Martyn, 1990; Rue & Cioffi, 1991).

Figure 18–7 The Lund and Browder burn assessment chart. This method of estimating TBSA affected by a burn injury is more accurate than the "rule of nines" because it accounts for changes in body surface area across the life span.

Area	Age (years) 0–1	Age (years) 1–4	Age (years) 5–9	Age (years) 10–15	Age (years) Adult	% 1°	% 2°	% 3°	% Total
Head	19	17	13	10	7				
Neck	2	2	2	2	2				
Ant. trunk	13	13	13	13	13				
Post. trunk	13	13	13	13	13				
R. buttock	$2\frac{1}{2}$	$2\frac{1}{2}$	$2\frac{1}{2}$	$2\frac{1}{2}$	$2\frac{1}{2}$				
L. buttock	$2\frac{1}{2}$	$2\frac{1}{2}$	$2\frac{1}{2}$	$2\frac{1}{2}$	$2\frac{1}{2}$				
Genitalia	1	1	1	1	1				
R.U. arm	4	4	4	4	4				
L.U. arm	4	4	4	4	4				
R.L. arm	3	3	3	3	3				
L.L. arm	3	3	3	3	3				
R. hand	$2\frac{1}{2}$	$2\frac{1}{2}$	$2\frac{1}{2}$	$2\frac{1}{2}$	$2\frac{1}{2}$				
L. hand	$2\frac{1}{2}$	$2\frac{1}{2}$	$2\frac{1}{2}$	$2\frac{1}{2}$	$2\frac{1}{2}$				
R. thigh	$5\frac{1}{2}$	$6\frac{1}{2}$	$8\frac{1}{2}$	$8\frac{1}{2}$	$9\frac{1}{2}$				
L. thigh	$5\frac{1}{2}$	$6\frac{1}{2}$	$8\frac{1}{2}$	$8\frac{1}{2}$	$9\frac{1}{2}$				
R. leg	5	5	$5\frac{1}{2}$	6	7				
L. leg	5	5	$5\frac{1}{2}$	6	7				
R. foot	$3\frac{1}{2}$	$3\frac{1}{2}$	$3\frac{1}{2}$	$3\frac{1}{2}$	$3\frac{1}{2}$				
L. foot	$3\frac{1}{2}$	$3\frac{1}{2}$	$3\frac{1}{2}$	$3\frac{1}{2}$	$3\frac{1}{2}$				
					Total				

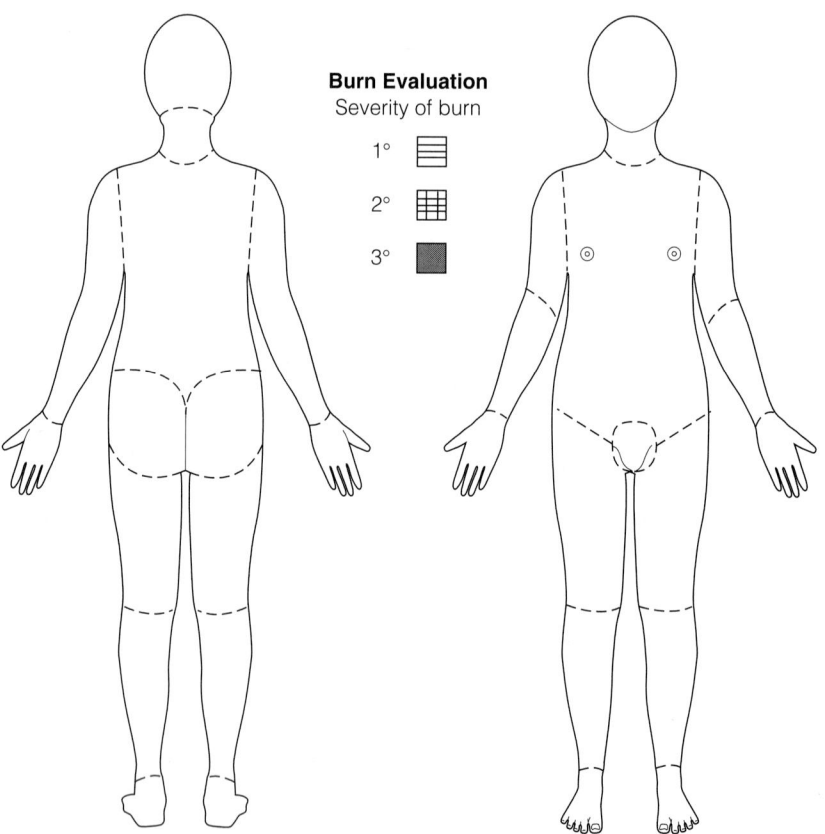

Burn Evaluation
Severity of burn

1°
2°
3°

Ventilatory Management

Upon the client's admission to the ED, several baseline assessments of respiratory status must be obtained: chest X-ray study, ABGs, vital signs, and carboxyhemoglobin levels. Intubation is indicated for all clients with burns of the chest, face, or neck. The primary treatment plan is oriented toward preventing atelectasis and maintaining alveolar oxygen exchange. Airway management is a funda-

Fluid Replacement Guidelines for the First 24 Hours Post Burn

■ ■ ■

Parkland/Baxter Formula

1. Formula: 4 mL × kg body weight × % TBSA burned
2. Fluids: Lactated Ringer's
3. Administration: Give half in the first 8 hours and half over the next 16 hours

Brooke Army Formula

1. Formula: 2 mL × kg body weight × % of total body surface area (TBSA) burned + 2000 mL per 24 hours for maintenance fluid
2. Fluids:
   a. Colloids: 0.5 mL × kg body weight × % TBSA burned (see Chapter 5)
   b. Lactated Ringer's: 1.5 mL × kg body weight × % TBSA burned
   c. 5% dextrose in water for maintenance
3. Administration: Give half in the first 8 hours and half over the next 16 hours

Evans Formula

1. Formula: 2 mL × kg body weight × % TBSA burned
2. Fluids:
   a. Colloids: 1 mL × kg body weight × % TBSA burned (see Chapter 5)
   b. Normal saline: 1 mg × kg body weight × % TBSA burned
   c. 5% dextrose in water for insensible water loss
3. Administration: Give half in the first 8 hours and half over the next 16 hours

Consensus Formula

1. Formula: 2 to 4 mL × kg body weight × % TBSA burned
2. Fluids: Lactated Ringer's
3. Administration: Give half in the first 8 hours and half over the next 16 hours

Winski Formula

1. Formula: 2 mL × kg body weight × % TBSA burned
2. Fluids: Lactated Ringer's and maintenance fluids
3. Administration: Give half in the first 8 hours and half over the next 16 hours

Hypertonic Saline Solution

1. Formula: Solution containing 250 mEq of sodium per liter of solution
2. Fluids: Hypertonic saline with added sodium
3. Administration: Give at a rate to maintain an hourly urinary output of 30 mL (in adults)

---

mental nursing measure in the control of ventilation and includes positioning, respiratory toileting, oxygenation, drug administration, and continuous assessment.

Positioning   Maintain the head of the bed at 30 degrees or greater to maximize the client's ventilatory efforts. Turn the client side to side every 2 hours to prevent hypostatic pneumonia.

Respiratory Toileting   To keep airway passages clear, suction the client frequently, encourage the client to use incentive spirometry hourly, and help the client perform coughing and deep-breathing exercises every 2 hours.

Intubation   In the face of impending airway obstruction, the client will require intubation. Nasotracheal tube placement is the preferred route because it seems to be better tolerated and can be more effectively secured. If the client has suffered nasolabial burns, however, the orotra-cheal route is preferred. Nasotracheal and orotracheal intubation is reserved for short-term ventilatory management. For long-term ventilatory management (i.e., greater than 3 weeks), a tracheostomy is performed.

Oxygenation   Humidification of either room air or oxygen helps prevent the drying of tracheal secretions. Ambient air or oxygen flow is based on ABG results. The client may be placed on a face mask, steam collar, T-piece, mechanical ventilation with PEEP, pressure support ventilation, or high-frequency jet ventilation. The goal of all therapies is to maintain adequate tissue oxygenation with the least amount of inspired oxygen flow necessary.

Drug Administration   Medications used to dilate constricted bronchial passages are administered intravenously and as inhalants to control bronchospasms and wheezing. Mucolytic agents are employed to liquefy tenacious sputum and aid in expectoration.

Continuous Assessment An arterial line is placed in the client with major burn injury for continuous assessment of ABGs. Pulmonary artery pressure catheters also are inserted to measure pulmonary vascular resistance (PVR), pulmonary artery pressure (PAP), pulmonary capillary wedge pressure (PCWP), and mixed venous oxygen saturation (SVO_2). The PVR and PAP rise in the presence of hypoxia. The SVO_2 is the average percentage of hemoglobin bound with oxygen in the venous blood and reflects overall tissue utilization of oxygen. Pulse oximetry, a noninvasive assessment, is used to monitor arterial oxygen saturation levels, especially during routine nursing procedures. Frequent auscultation of lung sounds, documentation of sputum production, observation of signs of respiratory distress, and monitoring of hemodynamic parameters are all priority nursing responsibilities (Cioffi et al., 1991; Eisenberg, 1991; Rue & Cioffi, 1991).

Inpatient Collaborative Care

After stabilization in the emergency department, the client is transferred to the critical care unit or a specialized burn center, where continuous monitoring of laboratory tests, administration of pharmaceutical agents, pain control, wound management, and nutrition support therapies constitute the initial plan of care.

The Burn Team

The burn team (see Figure 18–2) is composed of an interdisciplinary group of health care professionals, who together plan the care and treatment of the burn-injured client during the acute and rehabilitative phases. The burn team consists of the nurse, physician, physical therapist, nutritionist, social worker, and burn technician. The team members meet regularly to discuss client progress and to determine collaboratively the most effective regimen of care (Achauer, 1987; Boswick, 1987).

Nurse Burn nursing is a subspecialty of critical care nursing practice. In addition to the routine procedures performed by the critical care nurse, the burn nurse carries out hydrotherapy, applies skin grafts according to protocol, maintains laminar flow environments, assesses the extent and depth of the burn injury, and calculates fluid replacement. Burn nurses continue their education on an ongoing basis by attending in-service programs and national conferences.

Physician The burn physician is a specially trained medical practitioner who usually serves as the director of the burn unit or center and establishes all treatment protocol. Research-based strategies guide all practice and procedure, and are developed and implemented under the direct supervision of the burn physician.

Physical Therapist The physical therapist works together with the nurse in the burn unit at the bedside. The therapist determines the exercise regimen, which is implemented early in the treatment plan. Splinting, progressive ambulation, active and passive ROM exercises, and the application of pressure support garments are collaboratively included in the plan of care under the guidance and direction of the therapist.

Nutritionist The nutritionist works closely with the nurse and physician to calculate the client's daily caloric needs. The nutritionist collaboratively determines the composition of feeding formulas, taking into consideration all laboratory findings, anthropometric measurements, parenteral therapies, and the changing clinical picture.

Social Worker The social worker meets with the family unit early in the admission process to begin to plan for the rehabilitative phase of care. The social worker assesses the home and social environment and makes referrals to appropriate community resources.

Burn Technician The burn technician is a supportive member of the team who has been specially trained to implement advanced procedures under the direct supervision of the burn nurse. The complex nursing care of the burn-injured client often necessitates 2:1, or higher, nurse-client ratios. The nurse–burn technician dyad is a cost-effective approach to delivering the kind of highly technical, labor-intensive care needed in the burn unit. The burn technician helps maintain the level of care required.

Laboratory and Diagnostic Tests

The following laboratory tests and procedures are ordered early in the treatment phase to evaluate the client's progress and to modify intervention strategies (Cioffi & Rue, 1991; Swearingen et al., 1988):

- *Culture and sensitivity* reports indicate the presence of infection in sputum, blood, urine, and wound tissue.

- *Urinalysis* indicates the adequacy of renal perfusion and the client's nutritional status. In catabolic states, nitrogen is excreted in large amounts into the urine. Nitrogen loss is measured through 24-hour urine collections for total nitrogen, urea nitrogen, and amino acid nitrogen. Myoglobinuria, which manifests as a dark brown, wine-colored urine, signals the development of acute tubular necrosis. Loss of plasma protein and dehydration lead to proteinuria and elevated urine specific gravity. Glycosuria is a transient development following major burn injury that indicates a need to adjust the nutritional program.

- *Hematocrit* is elevated secondary to hemoconcentration and fluid shifts from the intravascular compartment.

- *Hemoglobin* is decreased secondary to hemolysis.

- *Sodium levels* are decreased secondary to massive fluid shifts into the interstitium.

- *Blood urea nitrogen (BUN)* is elevated secondary to dehydration.
- *Potassium levels* initially are elevated during burn shock, as a result of cell lysis and fluid shifts into the extracellular space. Potassium levels decrease after burn shock resolves, as fluid shifts back to intracellular and intravascular compartments.
- *Total protein, albumin, transferrin, prealbumin, retinol binding protein, alpha 1-acid glycoprotein, and C-reactive protein* are indicators of protein synthesis and nutritional status. Because of the fluid shifts that occur during the early stages of the burn injury, they are more useful markers during the rehabilitative phase of care.
- *Creatine phosphokinase (CPK)* is elevated following an electrical burn, secondary to extensive muscle damage.
- *Blood type and crossmatch* are performed on the client's arrival to the unit in case transfusions are required.
- *WBCs* are elevated in the presence of infection and depleted in immunodeficient states.
- *Creatinine* is elevated in the presence of renal insufficiency.
- *Blood glucose* is transiently elevated after major burn injury. Hyperglycemia is treated by adjusting the nutritional program or administering exogenous insulin.

The following diagnostic tests may be ordered:

- *Serial ABGs* indicate the presence of hypoxia and acid-base disturbances and indicate client responses to changes in oxygen therapies. The burn-injured client may demonstrate elevated or lowered pH, decreased P_{CO_2}, decreased P_{O_2}, and low-normal bicarbonate levels.
- *Pulse oximetry* allows continuous assessment of oxygen saturation levels. The burn-injured client may have saturation levels below 95%.
- *Serial chest X-ray studies* document changes within the first 24 to 48 hours that may reflect the presence of atelectasis, pulmonary edema, or acute respiratory disease (ARD).
- *Ventilation-perfusion scan* is performed following the intravenous injection of isotope xenon 133. Serial scintiphotograms are taken to determine pulmonary clearance of the isotope. A complete washout of the isotope occurs in 90 seconds. Delayed pulmonary clearance, (i.e., greater than 90 seconds) indicates lower airway injury.
- *Flexible bronchoscopy* permits direct visualization of the upper airways. The procedure can be performed at the bedside with appropriate administration of conscious sedation. The bronchoscope is inserted into the trachea via the the nose or mouth and advanced to the bronchi. The bronchial passages are observed for evidence of burn injury and presence of mechanical obstruction.

- *Pulmonary function tests* include forced vital capacity (FVC), forced expiratory volume in 1 second (FEV_1), and forced mid-expiratory flow (FEF). All values are decreased in the presence of airway obstruction. The nurse and respiratory therapist assess vital capacity, tidal volume, and minute ventilation frequently at the bedside, to monitor for the development of respiratory distress or failure.
- *Serial electrocardiograms (ECGs)* are necessary to monitor the development of dysrhythmias, especially those associated with hypokalemic and hyperkalemic states.
- *Indirect calorimetry* is used to track the client's basal metabolic rate. The **basal metabolic rate (BMR)**, a function of the body's energy expenditure, depends on the extent of the burn injury. Total energy expenditure (TEE) in the burn-injured client may be elevated to 15% to 100% more than basal metabolic needs.

Pharmacology

Pain Control   Second- and some third-degree burns cause excruciating pain. In the early stages of care, intravenously administered narcotics are the best means of managing pain. Once the client has been stabilized, it is appropriate to administer narcotic agents prior to initiating hydrotherapy or intensive exercising routines. The intramuscular route of administration should be avoided until hemodynamic stability and unimpaired tissue perfusion returns.

As the client enters the rehabilitative stage of care, alternative therapies for pain control may be added to the plan of care. Distraction, self-hypnosis, guided imagery, and relaxation techniques are helpful adjuncts in managing pain. The nurse can help the client engage in these therapies. Allowing the client some control in the treatment process is another important nursing intervention in the effective management of pain. Patient-controlled analgesia (PCA) has been demonstrated to enhance the client's ability to cope with pain. Allowing the client to participate in planning treatment and scheduled procedures gives the client more control over his or her environment and fosters the development of coping strategies (Achauer, 1987; Martyn, 1990; Richard & Staley, 1994). See Chapter 4 for a discussion of strategies for managing pain.

Antimicrobial Agents   Most invasive wound infections are caused by the following organisms: *Pseudomonas aeruginosa, Enterobacter cloacae, Klebsiella, Staphylococcus aureus,* enterococci, and *Candida.* To eliminate infection on the surface of the burn wound, topical antimicrobial therapy is used. There are many antimicrobial agents available. The three most widely used are 0.5% silver nitrate, 1% silver sulfadiazine, and 10% mafenide acetate. The latter two agents are broad-spectrum antibiotics that are supplied in a cream form. Using aseptic technique, the nurse applies the cream directly to the wound or to a

Nursing Implications for Pharmacology: Topical Burn Medications

TOPICAL ANTIMICROBIAL AGENTS

Mafenide acetate (Sulfamylon)

Silver nitrate

Silver sulfadiazine (Silvadene)

The use of topical antimicrobial therapy was first investigated more than 60 years ago. Researchers found that the most effective topical agents are those that (1) act against the major pathogens responsible for causing burn wound infection, (2) achieve levels of concentration sufficient to decrease microbial colonization, (3) are rapidly excreted or metabolized, (4) are nontoxic, and (5) are easy to use and inexpensive (Martyn, 1990).

Mafenide Acetate

Mafenide is a synthetic antibiotic closely related chemically, but not pharmacologically, to the sulfonamides. Although the mechanism of action is unclear, the drug appears to interfere with the metabolism of bacterial cells. Mafenide is a bacteriostatic agent effective against many gram-positive and gram-negative organisms (Martyn, 1990).

For topical administration, mafenide is used in an 8.5% cream in a water-miscible base. Following application, the drug is rapidly diffused through the burn eschar and absorbed systemically.

In the general circulation, mafenide metabolizes to a weak carbonic anhydrase inhibitor known as *p*-carboxybenzenesulfonamide, a substance that impairs the renal mechanisms involved in the buffering of blood. Bicarbonate excretion in the urine increases, and ammonia and chloride excretion decreases. To maintain normal acid-base balance, the pulmonary system effects a compensatory hyperventilatory state. If the compensatory hyperventilation is insufficient, the client develops metabolic acidosis.

Nursing Responsibilities

- Use mafenide with caution in clients with renal or pulmonary disease.

- Approximately 3% to 5% of clients develop a hypersensitivity to mafenide, resulting in a maculopapular rash on the unburned areas. Assess the client for the following:

Pruritus	Urticaria
Facial edema	Blisters
Swelling	Eosinophilia

If hypersensitivity reactions occur, discontinue the drug and administer antihistamines.

- Monitor the client for superinfection within the burn eschar, in the subeschar tissue, or in viable tissue adjacent to the wound.

Client and Family Teaching

- Expect pain or a burning sensation following drug application. Take appropriate measures to control pain before applying the drug.

- Apply the drug to clean, debrided burn wounds once or twice daily. Continue applications until healing is apparent (Martyn, 1990).

- If any signs of allergy develop, discontinue the drug and notify the physician.

- Report any sudden and prolonged increases in respiratory rate.

Silver Nitrate

Silver nitrate is a bacteriostatic agent that inhibits a wide variety of gram-positive and gram-negative organisms. Its antimicrobial effect is due to the actions of silver ions, which markedly alter the microbial cell wall and membrane. Additionally, the drug denatures bacterial protein, thereby inactivating and precipitating the microbes (Martyn, 1990).

Nursing Responsibilities

- Silver nitrate is used as a 0.5% solution in distilled water. Apply the solution to bulky gauze dressings every 2 hours, and provide complete dressing changes twice daily.

mesh gauze pad that is then applied to the wound and changed twice daily. Silver nitrate is applied as a wet dressing, which is changed twice daily and soaked every 2 hours. With each dressing change, the nurse carefully assesses the wound for evidence of healing or signs of infection. The nurse tracks all culture and sensitivity reports, which serve as the basis for the selection of the an-

timicrobial agent. The choice of topical antibiotic is based on the extent of the burn wound, the presence of identified bacterial organisms, and client response.

Prophylactic administration of systemic antimicrobial agents is not recommended. Because the avascular burn-injured tissue cannot maintain therapeutic blood levels of antimicrobial agents, it is difficult to control the growth of

Pharmacology: Topical Burn Medications (continued)

- Silver nitrate has limited penetrating ability and is ineffective if used more than 72 hours following a burn injury.

- At the local tissue level, silver nitrate immediately interacts with chloride ions to form a black silver chloride precipitate that discolors both the burn wound and the adjacent tissues. The discoloration significantly hampers visual inspection of the wound.

- High concentrations of the drug result in cellular toxicity of surrounding healthy tissue.

- Because large amounts of water are systemically absorbed from the dressing site, the client may demonstrate a hypotonic state. Hyponatremia and hypochloremic alkalosis are common manifestations in burn-injured clients treated with silver nitrate (Martyn, 1990).

Client and Family Teaching

- Watch for and report any signs and symptoms of hypotonicity: swelling, weight gain, difficulty in breathing.

- This drug causes a black discoloration on all skin surfaces and dressings with which it comes into contact.

- Because discoloration can conceal evidence of infection, watch for systemic manifestations of infection: fever, malaise, rapid pulse rate, listlessness.

- Saturate the wound dressings every 2 hours with a 0.5% aqueous solution of the drug. Change the dressings completely twice daily.

Silver Sulfadiazine

Silver sulfadiazine, a sulfonamide, is the most commonly used topical agent. The drug acts on the cell membrane and cell wall of susceptible bacteria and binds to cellular DNA. The drug is bactericidal and effective against a wide variety of gram-negative and gram-positive organisms.

Nursing Responsibilities

- Many clients develop a marked leukopenia in response to this drug, which tends to improve spontaneously over the course of therapy. This finding does not contraindicate use of the drug (Boswick, 1987).

- Hypersensitivity to silver sulfadiazine has been reported in a small number of cases. If the client develops hypersensitivity, administer antihistamine, and change the topical agent.

- If sulfa crystals form in the urine, keep the client well hydrated (Boswick, 1987).

- Treatment with this drug can cause systemic uptake of propylene glycol, which results in an elevated serum osmolality and high urine specific gravity in the client who is not dehydrated. These findings tend to create confusion during the fluid resuscitative stage of care. Whenever the serum osmolality and urine specific gravity fail to correlate with a clinical picture that reflects fluid volume overload (elevated CVP/PCWP, rhonchi/wheezing, edema), suspect systemic propylene glycol uptake (Boswick, 1987).

Client and Family Teaching

- Apply the drug to clean, debrided wounds once or twice daily, completely covering the burn wound at all times (Martyn, 1990).

- Continue applying the drug until healing is apparent (Martyn, 1990).

- If any signs of allergy develop, discontinue the drug and notify the physician.

- Watch for evidence of concentrated urine, and notify the physician.

- If not contraindicated, drink large amounts of fluids to prevent sulfa crystals from forming in the urine.

bacteria at the site. Further, the indiscriminate use of systemic agents contributes to the development of resistant strains.

Systemic antimicrobial therapy is, however, indicated in the immediate preoperative and postoperative period associated with excision and autografting. Postoperatively, the therapy is discontinued as soon as the client's hemodynamic status returns to normal, usually within the first 24 hours. In the long-term treatment of identified infectious processes, drug administration is limited to the least amount of time required to eradicate the infection (Boswick, 1987; Duncan & Driscoll, 1991; Martyn, 1990; Walter, 1993; Weber & Tompkins, 1993). See the accompanying box for a discussion of the nursing implications for topical antimicrobial therapy for the burn client.

Table 18–5 Calculating Total Energy Expenditure from Metabolic Cart Measurements

TEE = REE × activity factor × injury factor

REE = Resting energy expenditure (reading from metabolic cart)
TEE = Total energy expenditure

Activity Factors	*Injury Factors*	
1.2 = bedridden patient	1.2	= surgery
1.3 = ambulatory patient	1.35	= trauma
	1.6	= sepsis
	2.1	= burns

Tetanus Prophylaxis If the client's immunization status is in doubt, tetanus toxoid is administered intramuscularly early in the acute phase of care to prevent *Clostridium tetani* infection (Boswick, 1987).

Prevention of Gastric Hyperacidity To prevent Curling's ulcer, an erosion of the gastric and duodenal linings associated with burn injury, hyperacidity must be controlled. A nasogastric tube is placed during the emergent phase of care, and gastric aspirant is obtained hourly. The gastric pH should be assessed and maintained at levels above 5. To control gastric acid secretion during the acute phase of care, histamine H_2 blockers (e.g., cimetidine and ranitidine) can be administered intravenously, either intermittently or as continuous infusions. As soon as bowel sounds become audible, the client is placed on an antacid regimen (Driscoll et al. 1993; Hansbrough & Hansbrough, 1993; Martyn, 1990).

Nutritional Support
A total assessment of the nutritional needs of the burn-injured client is crucial in planning nutritional support therapies to decrease catabolic states. The nurse and nutritionist collaborate to develop the client's dietary plan, carefully evaluating the client's energy needs prior to implementing the selected nutritional therapy.

Energy expenditure depends on the extent of catabolism and the client's physical activity, size, age, and sex. An anthropometric assessment includes measurement of height, weight, and triceps skinfold thickness. Both the nurse and nutritionist perform anthropometric assessments on an ongoing basis to monitor kcal expenditure. These assessments are not always reliable indicators, however; for example, the administration of large amounts of intravenous fluids, the application of bulky immobilizing devices, and the amputation of extremities can account for changes in weight. Additionally, upper arm anthropometry, which indicates fat stores and muscle mass, may be difficult to perform if the burn injury involves the upper extremities.

Recently the **metabolic cart** has been demonstrated to be a more accurate indicator of energy needs. The cart, which can be taken to the bedside, functions on the principle of **indirect calorimetry**, which refers to the calculation of TEE by measuring respiratory gas exchange. Indirect calorimetry is based on the theory that oxygen consumption and carbon dioxide production profile intracellular metabolism. The cart generates estimates of the resting energy expenditure (REE) and the respiratory quotient (RQ), a measurement that represents the ratio of carbon dioxide production (VCO_2) to oxygen consumption (VO_2) (Table 18–5). Indirect calorimetry should be performed at regular intervals and the client's dietary regimen adjusted accordingly (Swearingen et al., 1988).

Enteral Feeding Traditional dietary management based on oral intake seldom meets the kcal requirements necessary to reverse negative nitrogen balance and begin the reparative process. Enteral feedings are therefore instituted within 24 to 48 hours of the burn injury to offset hypermetabolism, improve nitrogen balance, and decrease length of hospital stay. A nasointestinal feeding tube is placed under fluoroscopy, with the tip extending past the pylorus to prevent reflux and aspiration.

To maintain proper tube placement, the nurse monitors and documents the position of the tube. Tube placement is determined by pH-paper or pH-meter measurements. (See the accompanying research box.) Because nasointestinal feeding tubes have very small diameters, they tend to dislodge during vigorous coughing or vomiting episodes. Additionally, such tubes are also prone to clogging and must be frequently flushed to maintain patency, especially after the administration of medications. The nurse auscultates bowel sounds and measures abdominal girth frequently to monitor feeding tolerance.

Gastric secretions may accumulate above the level of the pylorus despite appropriate nasointestinal tube placement. It may be necessary to connect the nasogastric tube to low-intermittent suction to maintain gastric decompression. If aspiration is suspected, the nurse suspends all feedings until tube placement is verified.

A feeding pump can control the continuous infusion of tube feedings. Initial feedings are calculated at one-half the kcal need and advanced at the rate of 10 mL/h until the recommended daily kcal intake is reached. The nurse evaluates the client's tolerance of the feedings and reports any evidence of vomiting, diarrhea, or constipation. The nutritionist can modify the feeding formula to reduce these complications. As the client becomes able to tolerate oral feedings, the tube feeding is slowly titrated off (Carlson & Jordon, 1991).

Parenteral Nutrition Although enteral feeding is the preferred nutritional therapy, it is contraindicated in Curling's ulcer, bowel obstruction, feeding intolerance, pancreatitis, or septic ileus. When the enteral route can-

Applying Research to Nursing Practice: Feeding Tube Placement

■ ■ ■

The nurse is responsible for ensuring that all enteral tubes are correctly positioned. Inaccurate tube placement may lead to pulmonary complications, such as pneumonitis, pleuritis, empyema, sepsis, and aspiration. Small-bore enteral tubes tend to be the most difficult to insert and can be easily displaced during retching, vomiting, violent coughing, or tracheal suctioning. Standard nursing protocol requires that the nurse verify tube placement on initial insertion, prior to all bolus feedings, and once per shift during continuous feedings.

In one study, researchers investigated the use of pH meters in differentiating gastric, intestinal, and inadvertent respiratory placement of feeding tubes (Metheny, Reed, Wiersema, McSweeney, Wehrle, & Clark, 1993). The study sample consisted of 405 aspirates from small-bore nasogastric tubes and 389 aspirates from nasointestinal tubes. The samples were obtained from 605 subjects ranging from age 18 to 94. Although over half of the sample population received gastric acid inhibitors, all clients receiving antacids either orally or by tube within 4 hours of testing were excluded from the study to prevent interference with the measurement of pH values. Aspirates were obtained within 5 minutes of abdominal radiographic imaging, which was used to verify tube placement. Gastric contents were aspirated 1 hour after feedings or medication administration, and the feeding tube was flushed with 20 mL of air to clear all substances prior to each aspiration. Because many of the subjects were confused and frequently removed their own tubes, were transferred to other facilities, or could not be studied for all phases of the investigation, pH-meter readings of the gastric contents, not the clients themselves, were the focus of analysis.

Implications for Nursing

In the severely burn-injured client, continuous enteral feedings are instituted early in the treatment phase to offset hypermetabolism. The continual assessment of feeding tube placement is a priority nursing intervention. The study indicated that whereas pH measurement cannot confirm the initial placement of enteral tubes, pH-metered testing can be an appropriate means to detect manual manipulation or tube migration. Although this study reported only those findings associated with pH-meter measurements, it did point out the differences noted between pH-meter readings and pH-paper readings. The researchers found that pH-meter readings tended to be 0.5 unit higher than pH-paper readings, a finding especially evident in clients receiving acid inhibitors. Moreover, pH-paper readings are based on the use of color charts; differences in the ways people interpret the readings can also affect the accuracy of these measurements.

Critical Thinking in Client Care

1. This study included clients at both ends of the age spectrum. How might differences in gastric motility and gastric acid productivity in the younger versus aged client affect the study's results?

2. How might subjective assessments based on pH-paper measurement differ from objective assessments obtained with pH-meter measurement?

3. Why do pH measurements correlate well with radiographic findings of tube placements?

4. Develop a plan to teach nurses to perform pH-paper and pH-meter gastric measurements using radiographic findings to corroborate tube placement.

not be used, a central venous catheter is inserted via the subclavian or jugular vein for the administration of total parenteral nutrition (TPN). Prior to initiating TPN, the nurse must verify central line placement on chest X-ray film. All risks associated with central lines require astute nursing observation and continuous assessment for catheter contamination, pneumothorax, air embolism, and venous thrombosis.

Cleaning the Wound

As soon as the client's condition stabilizes, the nurse prepares the client for **hydrotherapy**. Depending on the medical protocol, the client may be submersed into a Hubbard tank, hosed over a spray table, showered, or given a bed bath (Figure 18–8). The nurse applies a mild cleaning solution, such as chlorhexidine gluconate (Hibiclens), to the wound site and gently washes the burned area. Because this is a very painful procedure, the client will need appropriate medication. To maintain body temperature, the nurse warms the client using heat shields and warm bathwater. Hydrotherapy remains part of the daily cleaning routine until wound closure is accomplished. See the box on page 646 for the nursing implications for hydrotherapy.

Debriding the Wound

Burned tissue releases chemical mediators that stimulate phagocytosis in an attempt to digest debris that is left by

Nursing Implications for Hydrotherapy: Tubbing

■ ■ ■

The purpose of hydrotherapy is to provide an opportunity for an initial assessment of the wound following a thorough cleansing. Hydrotherapy is also employed daily to remove topical agents and debride the wound. Depending on medical protocol, the client may be submersed in a Hubbard tank (tubbing), hosed over a spray table, showered, or given a bed bath.

Nursing Responsibilities

■ Prepare the client for the tubbing procedure as soon as possible after admission to the burn unit. Prior to transporting the client to the tub room, ensure that the client is hemodynamically stable.

■ Follow strict isolation procedure. Thoroughly disinfect the tub before and after bathing the client.

■ Maintain a warm environment.

■ Explain the entire tubbing process to the client, including the pain that he or she can expect and how it will be managed.

■ Pain management is a primary concern. Prophylactically, administer narcotic analgesia, and make every effort to promote relaxation and comfort.

■ Allow the client to participate in the planning of this daily routine to lower anxiety.

■ Gently lower the client into the tub, completely submersing the burn wound.

■ Wash the burn wound with a mild disinfectant solution, and allow it to soak to soften the eschar.

■ During hydrotherapy, remove eschar with sterile scissors and forceps.

■ Shave the hair on and around the burn wound.

■ Have the client perform ROM exercises during hydrotherapy.

■ To minimize heat loss, pain sensations, and electrolyte depletion, limit the entire procedure to 30 minutes.

Client and Family Teaching

■ Instruct in the importance of performing active ROM exercises during the tubbing procedure.

■ Explain all rationale supporting the implementation of this very uncomfortable procedure.

■ Assure the client that the procedure will be discontinued as soon as the wound shows evidence of healing.

■ Teach the client how to prevent contractures, emphasizing the need for aggressive exercise therapy early in the rehabilitative phase. Help the client understand how hydrotherapy facilitates the exercise routine.

---

decaying necrotic tissue. Necrotic tissue that remains despite phagocytic action retards healing and prolongs inflammation. **Debridement is** the process of removing dead tissue from the wound. Three methods of debridement are employed: mechanical, enzymatic, and surgical.

Mechanical debridement is performed during hydrotherapy by the nurse or therapist. In this procedure, loose necrotic tissue is washed with a washcloth or gauze pad to remove dead skin and separate eschar. Blistered skin is grasped with a dry gauze and gently removed. The edges of blisters or eschar are trimmed with blunt scissors. Wounds should be rubbed sufficiently hard to remove debris yet not cause bleeding. Following debridement, the nurse shaves hair from the burn site. Hair tends to trap debris, foster bacterial growth, and cause pain during debridement procedure.

Enzymatic debridement involves the use of a topical agent to dissolve and remove necrotic tissue. Following hydrotherapy, the nurse applies an enzyme of choice in a thin layer directly to the wound and covers it with one layer of fine mesh gauze. The nurse then applies a topical antimicrobial agent, covers the wound with a bulky wet dressing, and immobilizes the wound with expandable mesh gauze.

Surgical debridement is discussed under the section on surgical management of the burn wound.

Dressing the Wound

Once the wound has been cleaned and debrided, it may be dressed using one of two methods. In the **open method,** the burn wound remains open to air, covered only by a topical antimicrobial agent. This method allows the wound to be easily assessed; however, it can be used only where strict isolation precautions are followed. Topical agents must be frequently reapplied because they tend to rub off onto the bedding.

In the **closed method,** a topical antimicrobial agent is applied to the wound site, which is covered with gauze or a nonadherent dressing and then gently wrapped with a gauze roll bandage (Figure 18–9). With the closed

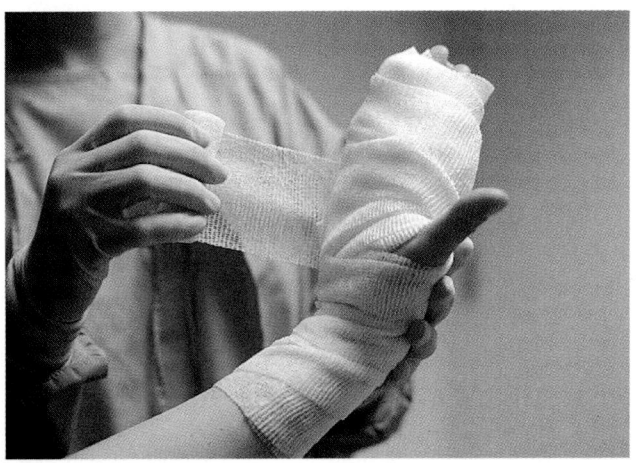

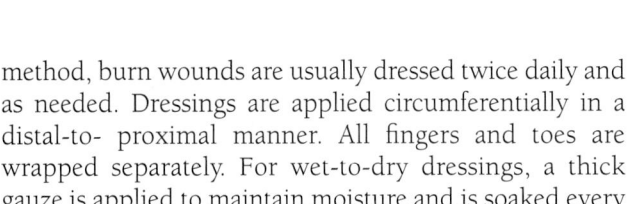

Figure 18–9 Closed method of dressing a burn.

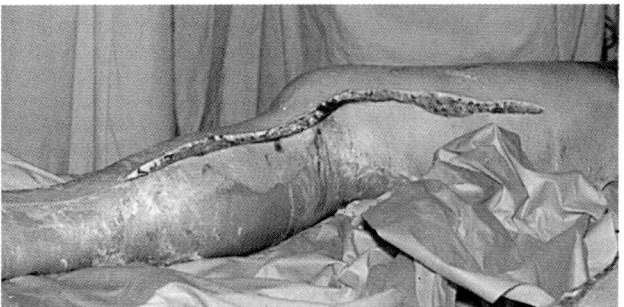

Figure 18–10 Escharotomy. The surgical procedure consists of removing the eschar formed on the skin and underlying tissue following severe burns. The procedure is particularly helpful in restoring circulation to the extremities of clients when scar tissue forms a tight, constrictive band around the circumference of a limb.

method, burn wounds are usually dressed twice daily and as needed. Dressings are applied circumferentially in a distal-to- proximal manner. All fingers and toes are wrapped separately. For wet-to-dry dressings, a thick gauze is applied to maintain moisture and is soaked every 2 hours with the ordered solution.

Surgical Management of the Burn Wound

Three surgical interventions are commonly employed to manage the burn wound: surgical debridement, escharotomy, and autografting.

Surgical Debridement Surgical debridement refers to the process of excising the wound to the level of fascia (fascial excision) or sequentially removing thin slices of the burn wound to the level of viable tissue (sequential excision). Because fascial excision, or **fasciectomy,** sacrifices potentially viable fat and lymphatic tissue, its use is reserved for clients with extensive or fourth-degree burns. The most common technique is electrocautery with cutting and coagulating current capabilities. Sequential excision is performed with the use of a dermatome. Shallow burns and some of moderate depth bleed briskly after one slice. If bleeding does not occur, the procedure is repeated until a viable bed of dermis or subcutaneous fat is reached. Following surgical debridement, the client is returned to the burn unit (Boswick, 1987; Richard & Staley, 1994).

Escharotomy The burn injury results in the formation of necrotic skin and subcutaneous tissue. During the acute stage of the injury, a hard crust (**eschar**) forms, which covers the wound and harbors necrotic tissue. The eschar is characteristically leathery and rigid. When the burn eschar forms circumferentially around the torso or extremities, it acts as a tourniquet, impairing circulation. Left unchecked, the affected body part becomes gangrenous.

To prevent circumferential constriction of the torso or extremity, an **escharotomy** is performed by the physician with a scalpel or by electrocautery (Figure 18–10). A sterile surgical incision is made longitudinally along the extremity or the trunk to release taut skin and allow for expansion caused by edema formation (Achauer, 1987; Richard & Staley, 1994). In the first 24 hours following the procedure, the incision should be gently packed with fine mesh gauze. After 24 hours, the site may be treated with a direct application of silver sulfadiazine. See the box on page 648 for the nursing implications for the client undergoing escharotomy.

Autografting Autografting, a procedure performed in the surgical suite, is used to effect permanent skin coverage. Skin is removed from healthy tissue (donor site) of the burn-injured client and applied to the burn wound (Figures 18–11 and 18–12). After the autograft is applied, the grafted area is immobilized. The site is assessed daily for evidence of adherence. The client resumes ROM exercises 5 days postgraft. As the wound heals, the client may complain of itching, which can be treated with the application of mild lotions.

The nurse assesses the donor site postoperatively for healing and the absence of infection and applies a dressing such as Op-Site directly to the donor site. Op-Site is a biosynthetic transparent dressing that permits frequent direct observation of the wound throughout the healing process. At any sign of infection, the nurse removes synthetic dressings and applies antimicrobial agents.

Cultured epithelial autografting is a new technique in which skin cells are removed from unburned sites on the client's body and are then minced and placed in a culture medium for growth. Over a 5- to 7-day period, the cells expand 50 to 70 times the size of the initial biopsies. The cells are again separated out and placed in a new culture medium for continued growth. With this technique,

---

Nursing Implications for Circumferential Wound Management: Escharotomy

■ ■ ■

When a burn wound totally encircles an extremity, the torso, or the neck, the client is at risk for impaired tissue perfusion of the involved area. To prevent arterial occlusion, a circumferential burn wound may need to be excised. An escharotomy is a lengthwise incision made by the physician along the circumferential burn wound to release tension and permit unobstructed arterial blood flow. The nurse continuously assesses the involved area and notifies the physician of the need to perform this emergent procedure, which is done at the bedside. Because only the dead burn wound tissue is excised, the client experiences very little pain.

Nursing Responsibilities

- For circumferential burn wounds of the extremity, assess the extremity for absence of blood flow:
  a. Using a Doppler ultrasound stethoscope, check hourly for the presence of a pulse.
  b. Assess the extremity hourly for warmth, color, sensation, and capillary refill.
  c. Observe for evidence of numbness or tingling.
- For circumferential burn wounds of the torso, assess for evidence of respiratory distress:
  a. Obtain ABGs as needed.
  b. Auscultate lung sounds hourly.

  c. Observe for evidence of cyanosis, tachypnea, anxiety, or restlessness.
- For circumferential burn wounds of the neck, assess for evidence of respiratory distress. Prepare the client for prophylactic intubation.
- Monitor for excessive blood loss, and transfuse the client if indicated.
- Dress the open wound (escharotomy) with topical antimicrobial agents as ordered.

Client Teaching

- Teach the client the importance of reporting any evidence of impaired circulation: numbness, tingling, blue color to the extremity, absence of sensation.
- Assure the client that the procedure will not be painful and will provide immediate relief.
- Teach the client the importance of protecting the open wound (escharotomy) from infection.
- Explain the rationale supporting prophylactic intubation for burn wounds involving the head and neck.
- Provide assurance that all blood loss will be replaced and that bleeding at the site will be controlled.

---

enough skin can be grown over a period of 3 to 4 weeks to cover an entire human body. The cells are prepared in sheets and attached to petroleum jelly gauze backing, which is applied to the burn wound site. The procedure is conducted in the aseptic environment of the operating room. After 7 to 10 days, the petroleum jelly gauze backing is removed and nonadherent dressings applied to prevent mechanical trauma to the cells.

Burn Wound Closure: Biologic and Biosynthetic Dressings

The terms **biologic dressing** and **biosynthetic dressing** refer to any temporary material that rapidly adheres to the wound bed, promotes healing, and/or prepares the burn wound for permanent autograft coverage. Ideally, these kinds of dressings should be easy to apply and remove, inexpensive, nonantigenic, elastic, able to reduce pain, able to serve as a bacterial barrier, and able to enhance the natural healing process. The dressings are applied to the burn wound as soon as possible. Covering the wound eliminates the loss of water through evaporation, reduces infection, and promotes wound healing. Biologic and

biosynthetic dressings that are currently in use include homograft (allograft), heterograft (xenograft), amnionic membranes, and synthetic materials.

Homograft, or **allograft,** is human skin that has been harvested from cadavers. It is stored in skin banks located throughout the nation. The development of methods to achieve prolonged storage of frozen, viable skin has increased the use of this dressing; however, its short supply and expense still pose problems. It is manufactured as strips that are cut to the pattern of the burn and applied using sterile technique. Under normal circumstances, a homograft is rejected within 14 to 21 days following application.

Heterograft, or **xenograft,** is skin obtained from an animal, usually the pig. The use of this grafting material was first reported in 1880. Although fresh porcine heterograft is available to some centers, frozen heterograft is much more commonly used. Once applied, heterograft appears to undergo early softening and lysis from enzymatic action from the wound. As a result, frequent changes of the heterograft dressing are necessary. Because of the high infection rates associated with this dressing,

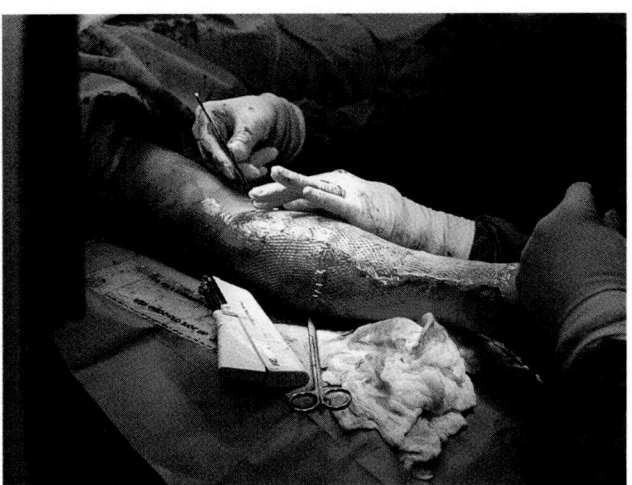
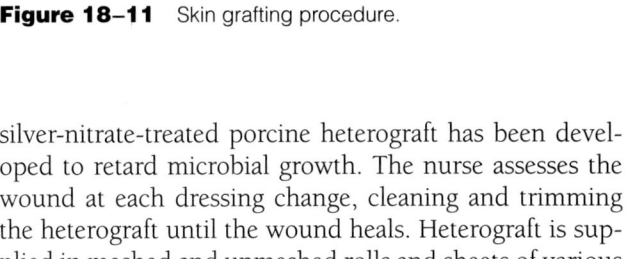

Figure 18–11 Skin grafting procedure.

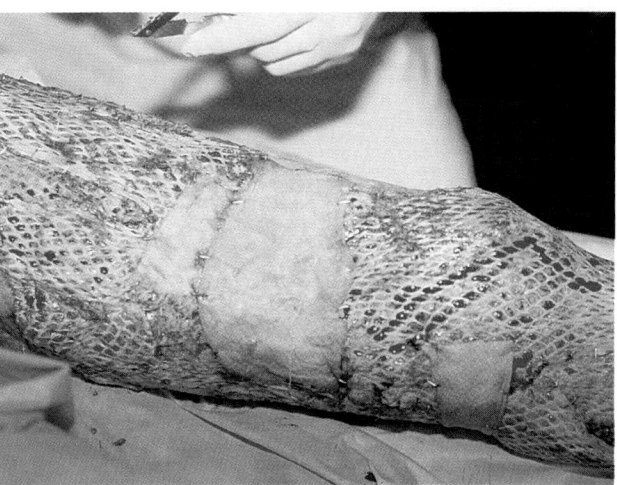

Figure 18–12 Skin graft for burn injury (autograft).

silver-nitrate-treated porcine heterograft has been developed to retard microbial growth. The nurse assesses the wound at each dressing change, cleaning and trimming the heterograft until the wound heals. Heterograft is supplied in meshed and unmeshed rolls and sheets of various sizes.

Amnionic membranes have been used as biologic dressings since 1912. They are readily available and inexpensive. Because they tend to disintegrate within 48 hours after application, frequent dressing changes are necessary. Amnionic membranes are less effective than homograft and heterograft dressings in reducing evaporative loss.

The multiple problems associated with the use of biologic dressings have driven the development of *synthetic materials*. One such material is Biobrane, a composite material consisting of nylon mesh bonded to silicone that has proved successful in the temporary coverage of second- and third-degree burns. Whereas Biobrane adheres well to moderately clean wounds, it cannot adhere to or lower bacterial counts in grossly contaminated wounds. Biobrane dressing is supplied in various sizes, cut to fit the wound site, and secured with tape or steri-strips. It spontaneously separates from the wound when the underlying tissue heals. Hydrocolloid dressings are another type of biosynthetic material. They are occlusive wafers composed of gumlike materials that provide a water-resistant outer layer for coverage of the donor site. They protect healing tissue from excessive drying, liquefy necrotic tissue, and absorb wound drainage (Boswick, 1987; Fowler, Cuzzell, & Papen, 1991).

Preventing Scars, Keloids, and Contractures

In normal healing following a minor burn injury, the newly formed skin closely resembles its neighboring tissue. The epidermis does not thicken or heighten as a scar. However, when a burn injury extends into the dermal

layer of skin, the skin is repaired through scar formation. Two types of excessive scar may develop. A **hypertrophic scar** is an overgrowth of dermal tissue that remains within the boundaries of the wound. A *keloid* is a scar that extends beyond the boundaries of the original wound. During the healing process, the burn scar shrinks and becomes fixed and inelastic, resulting in contracture of the wound. A **contracture** is a permanent shortening of connective tissue. Once a contracture forms, the tissue resists being stretched, and its inelasticity limits body movement. Positioning, splinting, exercise, and constant pressure application help prevent contractures from forming (Richard & Staley, 1994).

Positioning   During the course of therapy, the client must be maintained in positions that prevent contractures from forming. Because flexion is the natural resting position of joints and extremities, early physical therapy includes maintaining **antideformity positions** (Table 18–8).

Splinting   Splints are used to immobilize body parts and prevent contractures of the joints. They are applied and removed according to schedules established by the physical therapist.

Exercise   Early in the acute phase of care, the client's physical therapist prescribes active and passive ROM exercises, which are performed during hydrotherapy and every 2 hours at the bedside. Early ambulation is also part of the plan of care once the client's condition becomes stable.

Support Garments   Applying uniform pressure can prevent or reduce hypertrophic scarring. Tubular support bandages are applied 5 to 7 days postgraft to maintain a tension ranging from 10 to 20 mm Hg to control scarring. The client wears custom-made elastic pressure garments for 6 months to a year postgraft (Figure 18–13).

Table 18–6   Positioning the Client with Burns

Area Burned	Position
Head and neck	To achieve *hyperextension*, place a rolled towel or small soft pillow under the neck or shoulder. To achieve *extension*, use no pillow.
Shoulder/axilla	To achieve *abduction* and *external rotation* of the anterior shoulder, abduct the arm 90 degrees from the side of the trunk. To achieve *flexion* and *interior rotation* of the posterior shoulder, position the arm slightly behind the midline of the body.
Elbow	To achieve *extension* and *supination*, maintain the joint in extended position, palm upward.
Wrist	To achieve *extension*, use a splint to maintain 30 to 45 degrees of extension.
Fingers	To achieve *flexion* and *extension*, use splints.
Legs	To maintain slight *abduction*, place a pillow between the legs; use a trochanter roll to prevent external rotation.
Knee	To achieve *extension*, position the client in the supine position with the knees extended and in the supine position with the feet hanging over the lower end of the mattress; knee splints may also be used; while the client sits in a chair, legs should be elevated and extended.
Ankle	To achieve a *neutral* position, use a padded footboard and ankle splints to avoid inversion and eversion.

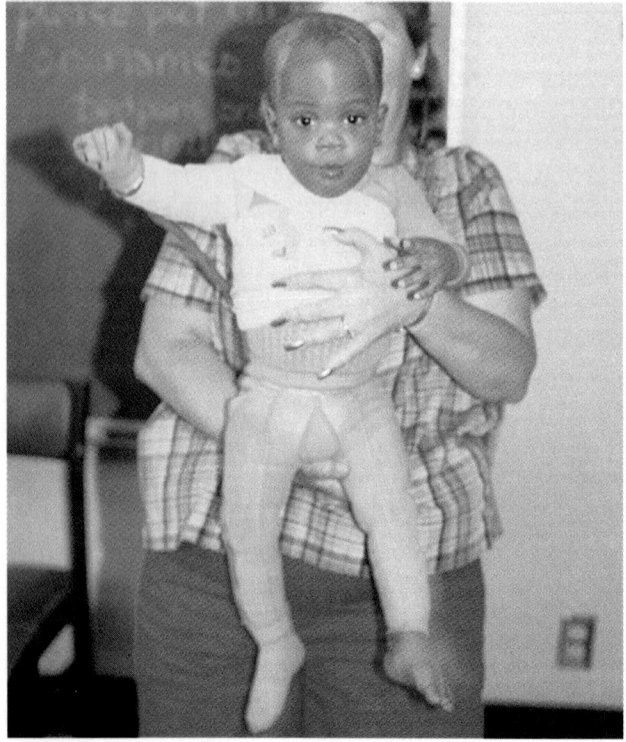

Figure 18–13 Pressure garment worn to prevent hypertrophic scarring following a burn injury.

Nursing Care

The goals of the nursing plan of care for the burn-injured client are to

- Maintain fluid balance.
- Control infection.
- Enhance mobility.
- Reduce pain.
- Preserve coping mechanisms.
- Improve gas exchange.
- Reestablish skin integrity.
- Promote tissue perfusion.
- Restore adequate nutrition.
- Educate the client and family unit in the rehabilitative process.

Table 18–7 lists overall nursing interventions for the emergent, acute, and rehabilitative stages of burn injury. Because the rehabilitative stage is long term, sometimes lasting for years, the client and family unit may experience extensive psychologic reactions ranging from denial to extreme depression.

Impaired Skin Integrity

The burn injury significantly impairs skin integrity. The severity of wounds varies according to the depth of the burn. General treatment measures are designed to restore normal skin function as quickly as possible. Nursing care focuses on assessing and cleaning the wound and controlling infection.

Nursing interventions with rationales follow:

- Estimate the extent and depth of the burn wound. *The severity of the burn injury is the basis for determining which type of dressing is appropriate.*
- Obtain relevant history. *All prehospital therapies must be reported to help prioritize nursing measures specific to care of the skin.*

Table 18–7   Nursing Interventions in Various Stages of Burn Injury

Stage of Burn Injury	Onset	End Point	Nursing Interventions
Emergent/Resuscitative	Occurrence of burn injury	Successful fluid resuscitation	Remove client from heat source. Initiate first aid. Assess extent of burn injury. Prevent hypothermia. Assess for shock. Determine need for intubation. Determine need for intravenous therapy. Follow protocol for fluid resuscitation. Obtain history. Transport to tertiary care facility.
Acute	Diuresis	Wound closure	Begin hydrotherapy. Determine need for excision of burn wound. Control spread of infection. Institute wound care. Start nutrition support. Graft burn wound. Initiate physical therapy. Manage pain.
Rehabilitative	Wound closure	Return to highest level of health restoration	Prevent scar formation. Continue physical therapy. Address psychosocial, cultural, and spiritual needs. Consider occupational therapy. Consider vocational training. Assess home maintenance management.

- Assess for the presence of pain. *The presence or absence of pain at the burn wound site is a critical finding that indicates depth of the injury.*

- Initiate hydrotherapy. *In the hemodynamically stable client, hydrotherapy is instituted early to begin wound debridement and allow assessment of wound appearance.*

- Apply topical antimicrobial agents. *Controlling infection is a priority of care.*

- Dress the burn wound using the open or closed method as ordered. *Maintaining asepsis controls the spread of infection.*

- Apply a biologic or biosynthetic dressing as ordered. *Early coverage of the burn wound reestablishes the skin's protective barrier.*

- Provide special skin care to sensitive body areas.
  a. Clean burns involving the eyes with normal saline or sterile water. If contracture of the eyelid develops, apply drops or ointment to the eye to prevent corneal abrasion.
  b. Gently wipe burns of the lips with saline-soaked pads. Apply an antibiotic ointment as ordered. Assess the mouth frequently, and perform mouth care routinely. If an oral endotracheal tube is in place, reposition it often to prevent pressure sore formation.
  b. Gently debride burns of the nose, and apply mafenide acetate cream. Position nasogastric and nasotracheal tubes to prevent excessive pressure.
  c. Apply mafenide acetate cream to burns of the ear. Gently debride and thoroughly clean the wound with a water spray. Do not cover ears with dressings. Do not use pillows; to reduce pressure to the area, use a foam doughnut instead.
  d. Clean burns of the perineum during hydrotherapy. Assess the area for evidence of infection, and rinse thoroughly after toileting.
  c. Keep exposed bone or tendon in a moist environment until grafting occurs. Soak wet-to-wet dressings frequently and reapply every 4 hours.

- *The eyes, mouth, nose, ears, perineum, and exposed deeper tissues require more intensive treatment therapies.*

Fluid Volume Deficit

In the early stages of the burn injury, managing the client's fluid balance and maintaining hemodynamic stability take priority. Massive fluid losses occur immediately following the injury and continue throughout the first 2 to 5 days. During this period, nursing care focuses on restoring fluid losses and continuously assessing hemodynamic parameters.

Nursing interventions with rationales follow:

■ Assess vital signs frequently. *Vital signs rapidly deteriorate when fluid resuscitation is inadequate.*

■ Follow prescribed formulas for intravenous fluid resuscitation. *Therapy for burn shock is aimed at supporting the client through the period of hypovolemic instability.*

■ Monitor intake and output hourly. Report urine outputs of less than 50 mL/h. *Intake and output measurements indicate the adequacy of fluid resuscitation.*

■ Weigh the client daily. *Body weight is used to calculate fluid requirements.*

■ Monitor hemodynamic status, including CVP and PCWP. *Inadequate fluid resuscitation is manifested by a drop in the central venous pressure and pulmonary capillary wedge pressure.*

■ Test all stools and emesis for the presence of blood. *Occult blood in emesis or stool indicates internal bleeding.*

■ Maintain a heated environment. *Hypothermia leads to shivering and further loss of body fluid through increased energy expenditure and catabolism.*

■ Monitor the client for fluid volume overload. *Older clients and those with underlying cardiac disease may demonstrate symptoms of congestive heart failure during the fluid resuscitation stage.*

Risk for Infection

From the onset of the burn injury, loss of the body's natural barrier to the external environment predisposes the client to developing infection. Nursing measures focus on controlling infectious processes. The nurse obtains daily laboratory tests, maintains nutritional therapies, and applies antimicrobial agents to monitor and prevent the spread of infection, a major complication of the burn injury.

Nursing interventions with rationales follow:

■ Monitor and record body temperature every 2 hours. *Elevated body temperature indicates the presence of infection.*

■ Obtain daily WBC counts. *Leukocyte counts are indicators of immune system function.*

■ Determine tetanus immunization status. *Burn clients are at risk for anaerobic infection caused by* Clostridium tetani.

■ Maintain high kcal intake. *Nutritional support provides the nutrients needed for maintaining the body's defense mechanisms.*

■ Maintain an aseptic environment. *Strict isolation technique deters the development of nosocomial infection.*

■ Culture all wounds and body secretions as ordered. *Culture and sensitivity reports identify the presence of infectious microbes and indicate appropriate antimicrobial therapies.*

■ Observe the client for signs of infection. *Continuous assessment enables the nurse to evaluate intervention strategies.*

Impaired Physical Mobility

As the burn wound heals and new skin tissue forms, the involved area tends to shrink. Contractures form at the site and significantly limit mobility, especially when a joint is involved. Physical therapy therefore plays an important role, beginning in the early stages of treatment. The nurse institutes ambulation and planned exercise regimens as soon as the client's condition stabilizes.

Nursing interventions with rationales follow:

■ Perform active or passive ROM exercises to all joints every 2 hours as ordered. Ambulate when stable. *Regular exercise prevents further loss of motion, restores movement, and improves functional status.*

■ Apply splints as ordered. Maintain antideformity positions, and reposition the client hourly. *Splinting and positioning retard the formation of contractures.*

■ Maintain limbs in functional alignment. *This preserves joint mobility.*

■ Anticipate the need for analgesia. *Administering analgesics promotes the client's comfort during vigorous exercising sessions.*

Altered Nutrition: Less Than Body Requirements

The burn injury initiates a complex series of events that have a profound effect on the body's use of nutrients and expenditure of energy. Daily kcal requirements are determined by the nutritionist, and as soon as possible, enteral feedings are initiated. Duodenal tubes are placed to enhance intestinal absorption and retard gastric reflux. Parenteral nutrition is reserved for those instances in which enteral feedings are contraindicated. Nursing measures focus on assessing feeding tolerance and use of nutrients, preventing gastric ulcer formation, and maintaining adequate bowel evacuation.

Nursing interventions with rationales follow:

■ Maintain nasogastric/nasointestinal tube placement. *Correct tube placement ensures appropriate absorption of nutrients and prevents aspiration.*

■ Maintain enteral/parenteral nutritional support as ordered. Observe and report any evidence of feeding intolerance: diarrhea, vomiting, excessive gastric residue, abdominal distention, absent bowel sounds, and constipation. *The nutritionist, in collaboration with the physician, selects and individualizes the feeding formula according to the client's daily energy expenditure requirements and feeding tolerance. Failure to maintain rates of infusion predisposes the client to continued catabolism and negative nitrogen balance.*

■ Weigh the client daily. *Anthropometric measurements indicate the adequacy of nutritional support therapies.*

- Obtain daily laboratory values for protein, iron, CBC, glucose, and albumin. *Decreased serum values indicate inadequate nutritional intake.*
- Administer antacids and histamine H_2 blockers. Maintain gastric pH above 5. *Lowering gastric acidity retards the development of ulcers.*

Pain

With extensive first-degree and all second-degree burns, the client experiences excruciating pain. Early in the treatment phase, once the client's hemodynamic status becomes stable, narcotic analgesics are administered to minimize discomfort; in addition, these medications are administered prophylactically before the client undergoes any painful procedure. For more persistent or continuous pain, PCA may be appropriate. As the client progresses to the rehabilitative stage, nonnarcotic analgesia and relaxation techniques are prescribed. Nursing measures focus on implementing both pharmaceutical and psychosocial pain-control strategies.

Nursing interventions with rationales follow:

- Assess the client's level of pain. *Pain tolerance is the duration and intensity of pain that the client is able to endure. Pain tolerance differs from one client to the next and may vary in the same client in different situations.*
- Anticipate the need for prophylactic analgesia. Determine whether PCA is appropriate. *The inability to manage pain results in feelings of despair and frustration.*
- Administer narcotic analgesics as ordered. *Nurses' fear of precipitating addiction often makes them reluctant to administer narcotics. During the acute stage of burn injury, however, invasive procedures and exposed neurosensory nerve endings dictate the need for narcotic pharmaceutical agents.*
- Explain to the client all procedures and expected levels of discomfort. *Clients who are prepared for painful procedures and know beforehand the actual sensations they will feel experience less stress.*
- Explore other methods of nonnarcotic pain control. *The use of noninvasive pain-relief measures (e.g., relaxation, massage, distraction) can enhance the therapeutic effects of pain-relief medications.*
- Allow the client to verbalize the pain experience. *Each individual experiences and expresses pain in his or her own manner, using various sociocultural adaptation techniques.*

Powerlessness

Usually, the client with a major burn injury endures a lengthy hospital stay involving many treatments and care protocols that are beyond his or her control. During the early stages, furthermore, much of the care regimen involves excruciating pain. Further still, the foreign environment of the burn unit makes it difficult for the client to relate to the immediate surroundings. For example, the need to control infection in the burn unit requires hospital personnel and family members to don sterile clothing prior to coming to the client's bedside. Family members and nursing personnel appear radically different when they are masked and gowned, and their odd appearance can add to the burn-injured client's sense of alienation.

Decreasing the client's feelings of powerlessness during the emergent and acute stages of burn care often poses a challenge to the nurse. Balancing care protocol with the client's need for control is difficult, but the nurse can best accomplish this objective by maintaining an objective approach and by implementing established psychosocial nursing interventions.

Nursing interventions with rationales follow:

- Allow the client as much control over the surroundings and daily routine as possible. For example, allow the client to choose times of dressing changes. *Powerlessness derives from the belief that one is unable to influence the outcome of a situation.*
- Keep needed items within reach, such as call bell, urinal, water pitcher, and tissues. *This reinforces the client's feelings of control.*
- Allow the client to express feelings. *The nurse can help the client cope by therapeutically listening, by displaying a caring presence, by clarifying misconceptions, and by providing positive feedback.*
- Set short-term, realistic goals. For example, set a goal for the client to ambulate from bedside to chair twice daily. *Small incremental gains are easier to achieve and allow for frequent positive reinforcement.*
- Help the client access supportive mechanisms, such as spiritual/cultural healing, support group consultation, and psychologic intervention. *These resources can enable the client to discover new life meanings and to cope more effectively.*

Other Nursing Diagnoses

Other nursing diagnoses that may be appropriate for the burn-injured client follow:

- *Ineffective Breathing Pattern* related to respiratory distress
- *Altered Tissue Perfusion* related to circumferential burn wound of the extremities/torso
- *Risk for Impaired Home Maintenance Management* related to unavailable support system
- *Risk for Ineffective Individual Coping* related to change in body image
- *Anxiety* related to lack of knowledge
- *Anticipatory Grieving* related to developing awareness of loss
- *Sensory/Perceptual Alterations* related to sensory overload/deprivation, sleep pattern disturbance

Client and Family Teaching

Client and family teaching is an important component of all phases of burn care. As treatment progresses, the nurse encourages family members to assume more responsibility in providing care. From admission to discharge, the nurse teaches the client and family to assess all findings, implement therapies, and evaluate progress.

Rehabilitation Care

Early in the plan of care, explain to the client and family the long-term goals of rehabilitation care: to prevent soft tissue deformity, protect skin grafts, maintain physiologic function, manage scars, and return the client to his or her optimal level of independence. The teaching plan focuses on helping the client and family prevent dehydration, infection, and pain; maintain adequate nutrition and skin integrity; and restore mobility and psychosocial well-being.

Dehydration

Teach the client and family unit how to assess for evidence of fluid volume deficit. Explain the rationale supporting all fluid therapies and emphasize the need to report immediately all signs and symptoms of fluid imbalance: weight loss, oliguria, dry mucous membranes.

Infection

Teach the client and family the rationale supporting asepsis. Instruct them to protect the client from exposure to people with colds or infections and to follow aseptic technique meticulously when caring for the wound. Ensure that the client and family are able to recognize all signs and symptoms of infection: fever, poor wound healing purulent drainage, malaise.

Mobility

Consultation with physical therapy begins early in the treatment plan and continues throughout the long-term rehabilitative process. Explain to the client and family the need for progressive physical activity and help them establish realistic goals. Explain the rationale supporting the use of splints, pressure support garments, and other assistive devices, and demonstrate how to apply them. Ensure that the client and family understand the importance of reporting any evidence of lack of progress.

Nutrition

Identify and answer all questions related to the client's nutritional therapies. Consult with a nutritionist early in the treatment plan and throughout rehabilitation to help the client and family maintain adequate daily kcal intake. Instruct them to report immediately any evidence of malnutrition, such as food intolerance, weight loss, or cachexia.

Pain

Encourage the client and family to express concerns related to pain management. Explain the causes of pain and discomfort and the rationale supporting the use of analgesia. Teach the client and family alternative pain-control therapies, such as guided imagery, relaxation techniques, and diversional activities. Instruct them to report evidence of inadequate pain control: facial grimacing, verbalization of pain, guarding.

Skin Care

Instruct the client and family in the care of the graft and donor sites. Provide the rationale supporting the use of all pressure support garments, emphasizing the need to report any evidence of inadequate wound healing: altered skin integrity, drainage, swelling, redness.

Psychosocial Adaptation

Encourage the client and family to express their fears and concerns, and provide referrals to appropriate community resources. The circumstances surrounding the burn injury are often emotionally charged and challenge the nurse to consider all psychosocial implications. Powerlessness, anger, guilt, anxiety, and feelings of loss are common reactions to burn injury and may be related to ineffective coping mechanisms. The goal of psychosocial nursing care is to promote functional adaptation and to facilitate psychologic adjustment. The burn injury can precipitate dramatic changes in the client's self-concept, role function, value system, and interpersonal relationships. Direct the client and family to occupational therapy, social service, clergy, and/or psychiatric services as appropriate.

Three basic stages of burn recovery have been consistently identified: early, intermediate, and long-term. The duration of each stage varies from client to client and depends on the client's preburn psychologic state, the extent of the injury, and the treatment environment.

In the *early stage of recovery*, the client undergoes intensive critical care. Direct psychologic intervention is generally inappropriate during this stage: rather, interventions are directed toward maintaining the client's family support system and helping family members work through their grief and maintain a sense of calm and hope. The presence of the family alleviates the client's anxiety and agitation and helps the client cope with the sensory overload of the burn unit.

The *intermittent stage of recovery* is characterized by the client's return to a state of physical stability. The client is moved out of the critical care environment, and the procedures associated with wound care become matters of routine. The most common psychologic problems experienced by the burn-injured client during this stage include depression and post-traumatic stress disorder (PTSD). Depression tends to occur in clients whose hospital stays exceed 1 month. Brief psychologic counseling is helpful during this stage and may include treatment with antidepressants, especially when the episodes are severe or associated with suicidal ideation. PTSD is characterized by repeated intrusive memories of the burn injury, which agitate the client and cause the client to avoid situations that provoke these memories. PTSD is brief and self-limiting, seldom occurring beyond hospital discharge. Less severe psychologic difficulties, such as nightmares, anxiety, and regression, may occur but usually subside spontaneously. Behavioral difficulties, such as hostility, noncompliance, and acting out, may also occur. The family can employ behavior modification, limit setting, and the help of support groups to minimize these behaviors.

The *long-term stage of recovery* begins when the client leaves the hospital and returns to the community setting. The first year following discharge is usually the most difficult and is characterized by problems associated with vocational and emotional adjustment. Clients frequently experience depression and anxiety, which typically decrease in intensity after the first year. Problems with self-esteem and diminished quality of life, however, may require more long-term psychologic adjustment. Family support is extremely important during this stage. Community support resources can also help the client adjust successfully. Ongoing psychologic counseling may be necessary for clients with histories of ineffective and dysfunctional coping skills (Richard & Staley, 1994).

Applying the Nursing Process

Case Study of a Client with Major Burn: Craig Howard

Craig Howard, a 39-year-old truck driver, is admitted to the hospital following an accident in which the cab of his truck caught on fire. He was freed from the truck by a passing motorist, who stayed with him until the rescue team arrived and transported him to a local ED. Mr. Howard's wife, Mary, and twin daughters, Jessica and Jane, age 10, have been notified.

Assessment
On his admission to the ED, Mr. Howard is diagnosed with second- and third-degree burns of the anterior chest, arms, and hands. A quick assessment based on the rule of nines estimates the extent of his burn injury at 36% of TBSA. His vital signs are as follows: T, 96.2 F (35.6 C); P, 140; R, 40; BP, 98/60. In the field, the paramedics had inserted a large-bore central line into Mr. Howard's right subclavian vein and started the rapid infusion of lactated Ringer's solution. Mr. Howard is receiving 40% humidified oxygen via face mask. Initial ABGs are as follows: pH, 7.49; PO_2, 60 mm Hg; PCO_2, 32 mm Hg; bicarbonate,

22 mEq/L. Lung sounds indicate inspiratory and expiratory wheezing, and a persistent cough reveals sooty sputum production. A Foley catheter is inserted and initially drains a moderate amount of dark, concentrated urine. A nasogastric tube is connected to low-intermittent suction. Mr. Howard is alert and oriented and complains of severe pain associated with the burn injuries. The burn unit is notified, and Mr. Howard is prepared for transfer.

Diagnosis
On Mr. Howard's arrival to the burn unit, Ana Salazar, RN, assesses Mr. Howard and makes the following prioritized nursing diagnoses:

- *Risk for Ineffective Airway Clearance* related to increasing lung congestion secondary to smoke inhalation
- *Fluid Volume Deficit* related to abnormal fluid loss secondary to burn injury
- *Risk for Altered Tissue Perfusion* related to peripheral constriction secondary to circumferential burn wounds of the arms

Expected Outcomes
The expected outcomes established in Ms. Salazar's plan of care specify that during the emergent phase of care, Mr. Howard will

- Demonstrate a patent airway, as evidenced by clear breath sounds; absence of cyanosis; and vital signs, chest X-ray findings, and ABGs within normal limits.
- Demonstrate adequate fluid volume and electrolyte balance, as evidenced by urine output, vital signs, mental status, and laboratory findings within normal limits.
- Demonstrate adequate tissue perfusion, as evidenced by palpable pulses, warm extremities, normal capillary refill, and absence of paresthesia.

Planning and Implementation
Ms. Salazar plans and implements the following interventions for Mr. Howard during the emergent phase of care:

- Prepare Mr. Howard for prophylactic nasotracheal intubation to maintain airway patency.
- Initiate fluid resuscitation therapy using the Parkland/Baxter formula to calculate intravenous fluid rate for the first 24 hours postburn.
- Assist the physician to perform escharotomies of both upper extremities.

Evaluation
The nurse anesthetist has inserted a nasotracheal tube and connected Mr. Howard to a T-piece delivering 40% oxygen. Vigorous respiratory toileting has significantly improved his ABGs. Bronchodilators have been parenterally administered and mucolytic agents added to his

respiratory treatments. His tracheal secretions have begun to show evidence of clearing.

Hourly urine outputs indicate adequate fluid resuscitation. Urine output has been maintained at 50 mL/h, and color and concentration have improved. CVP readings have been maintained at 6 cm H_2O, and blood pressure has increased to 100/64. The pulse rate has decreased to 100.

To improve tissue perfusion of both arms, the physician has performed bilateral escharotomies and Ms. Salazar has dressed the wounds using sterile procedure. The extremities have demonstrated improved circulation.

Critical Thinking in the Nursing Process

1. Explain the rationale for the immediate insertion of a Foley catheter and nasogastric tube.

2. An escharotomy was performed on both arms. Why was this procedure necessary in Mr. Howard's case?

3. What is the rationale supporting the intravenous administration of narcotics to control Mr. Howard's pain?

4. Explain the purpose of instituting hydrotherapy early in Mr. Howard's treatment plan.

5. Explain the sequence of events that led to a fluid and electrolyte shift during the first 24 to 48 hours after Mr. Howard sustained his injury.

6. One week following Mr. Howard's accident, fluid and electrolyte balance were restored, and infection was controlled. Nevertheless, his condition remained serious. Over the next several months, the treatment plan was aimed at the prevention or early detection of other complications. Identify three of these potential burn complications, and discuss preventive strategies.

The Client with a Minor Burn Wound

■ ■ ■

A minor burn injury is usually treated in an outpatient facility. The goal of therapy is to promote wound healing, eliminate discomfort, maintain mobility, and prevent infection.

Pathophysiology

Minor burn injuries consist of first-degree burns that are not extensive, superficial second-degree burns that involve less than 15% of TBSA, and third-degree burns that involve less than 2% of TBSA, excluding the special care areas (eyes, ears, face, hands, feet, perineum, and joints). Minor burn injuries are not associated with immunosup-

pression, hypermetabolism, or increased susceptibility to infection.

Sunburn

Sunburns result from exposure to ultraviolet light. Such injuries, which tend to be first-degree, are more commonly seen in clients with lighter skin. Proper use of sunscreen and limiting sun exposure to the less hazardous hours of the day (before 10 a.m. and after 3 p.m.) can prevent sunburn. Because the skin remains intact, the symptoms in most cases are mild and are limited to pain, nausea, vomiting, skin redness, chills, and headache. Treatment is performed on an outpatient basis and generally consists of applying mild lotions, increasing liquid intake, administering mild analgesics, and maintaining warmth. Older adults are monitored for evidence of extensive dehydration.

Scald Burn

Minor scald burns result from exposure to moist heat and involve first-degree and superficial second-degree burns of less than 15% of TBSA. The goals of therapy are to prevent wound contamination and to promote healing. The nurse teaches the client to apply antibiotic solutions and light dressings and to maintain adequate nutritional intake. Mild analgesics may be ordered to help the client carry out activities of daily living. Tetanus toxoid is administered as appropriate.

Collaborative Care

At the scene of the injury, small burns may be rinsed with tepid water to reduce pain. Ice packs should be avoided. In the field, the wound should be covered with a clean cloth until appropriate treatment becomes available.

Outpatient treatment follows the same general guidelines as those for major burn injuries. The history and physical examination include the following:

- Assessment of the extent and depth of the burn injury
- Identification of the cause
- Time of the incident
- Previous medical history
- Age of the client
- Body weight
- Medications
- First-aid treatment

In the outpatient facility, the wound may be washed with mild soap and water. Tar and asphalt can be removed with mineral oil, petroleum ointments, or Medisol (a citrus and petroleum distillate with hydrocarbon structure). As with major burns, the tetanus toxoid booster is recommended for all clients whose immunization histories are in doubt. Potent topical chemotherapeutic agents, such as mafenide acetate, silver sulfadiazine, or povidone-iodine, should not be applied to a minor burn wound. Although controversy regarding the care of blisters remains, blisters may be managed in one of three ways: left intact, evacuated, or debrided. Follow-up care for the minor burn injury includes twice daily wound cleansing with application of bland ointment, ROM exercises to affected joints, and weekly clinic appointments until the wound heals completely (Boswick, 1987; Martyn, 1990).

Nursing Care

Although the nurse seldom treats the minor burn in the acute care environment, the burn treatment methods used in the outpatient setting follow the same standard approaches to care. General nursing measures include taking the history, estimating the extent and depth of the injury, cleaning the wound, applying topical agents, dressing the wound, controlling pain, and establishing follow-up care.

History Taking
In gathering client information, the nurse must be alert for any evidence of underlying disease that may complicate the healing process. Histories of chronic illness, substance abuse, or inadequate family support systems may make outpatient treatment inadvisable. The nurse obtains the client's immunization history and administers tetanus toxoid as indicated.

Estimate of Extent/Depth of Wound
In most cases, the rule of nines is an adequate means of determining the extent of the injury. Only first-degree and superficial second-degree burns are treated in the outpatient setting. More extensive injuries require hospitalization.

Wound Cleaning
The nurse cleans the wound according to protocol, which usually consists of washing the area gently with a mild soap and water and patting it dry using sterile technique. The nurse assesses the wound for evidence of infection.

Topical Agents
Only very mild ointments are used to cover the wound and prevent infection. The use of potent topical antimicrobial agents is not recommended.

Wound Dressing
The nurse uses either the open or closed method to dress the wound according to protocol. The nurse explains the dressing technique and teaches the client to follow the prescribed regimen.

Pain Control
The client is encouraged to use mild analgesics during the initial phases of care. As healing progresses, pharmaceutical agents are discontinued, and alternative pain manage-

ment therapies (relaxation, distraction, guided imagery) are employed.

Follow-Up
Depending on the severity of the wound, the client returns for follow-up care within the next 24 hours and weekly thereafter until the wound has healed completely.

Client and Family Teaching

In the outpatient setting, the client and family manage the minor burn wound throughout the rehabilitative process. The client returns to the clinic or doctor's office regularly until the wound has healed completely. In developing and implementing the teaching plan, the nurse supports client and family participation in care.

The nurse teaches the client and family

- To identify and report signs and symptoms of impaired wound healing:
  a. Change in healthy appearance of the wound (altered skin integrity, swelling, blister formation, erythema)
  b. Signs of infection (fever, purulent drainage, foul odor)
  c. Ill-fitting pressure garment (discomfort, numbness, tingling)
- The importance of adequate nutritional intake:
  a. How to identify a change in food tolerance (manifested by diarrhea, weight loss, muscle atrophy)
  b. How to prepare nutritionally balanced meals
  c. How to maintain adequate fluid intake
- Wound care:
  a. Daily cleaning with mild soap and water
  b. Use of sterile technique to change dressings
  c. Correct application of ordered topical agents
- Active ROM exercises:
  a. Exercise of limbs and joints daily as ordered
  b. Gradual increase in endurance
- Pain management:
  a. Use of mild analgesics as ordered
  b. Implementation of alternative pain management therapies

Bibliography

■ ■ ■

Achauer, B. M. (1987). *Management of the burned patient.* Norwalk, CT: Appleton & Lange.

Bomberger, A. S., & Dannenfelser, B. A. (1984). *Radiation and health: Principles and practice in therapy and disaster preparedness.* Rockville, MD: Aspen Publishers.

Boswick, J. A. (1987). *The art and science of burn care.* Rockville, MD: Aspen Publishers.

Burgess, M. C. (1991). Initial management of a patient with extensive burn injury. *Critical Care Nursing Clinics of North America, 3*(2), 165–169.

Carpenito, L. J. (1992). *Nursing diagnosis: Application to clinical practice* (4th ed.). Philadelphia: Lippincott.

Carlson, D. E., & Jordon, B. S. (1991). Implementing nutritional therapy in the thermally injured patient. *Critical Care Clinics of North America, 3*(2), 221–235.

Cioffi, W. G., & Rue, L. W. (1991). Diagnosis and treatment of inhalation injuries. *Critical Care Nursing Clinics of North America, 3*(2), 191–198.

Cioffi, W. G., Rue, L. W., Graves, T. A., McManus, W., Mason, D., & Pruitt, B. (1991). Prophylactic use of high-frequency percussive ventilation in patients with inhalation injury. *Annals of Surgery, 213*(6), 575–582.

DiMola, M. A. (1993). The cutting edge in burn care. *Critical Care Nurse Supplement, 13*(3), 24–26.

Dressler, D. P., Hozid, J. L., & Nathan, P. (1988). *Thermal injury*. St. Louis: Mosby.

Driscoll, D. M., Cioffi, W. G., Molter, N. C., McManus, W., Mason, D., & Pruitt, B. (1993). Intragastric pH measurement. *Journal of Burn Care and Rehabilitation, 14*(5), 517–524.

Duncan, D. J., & Driscoll, D. M. (1991). Burn wound management. *Critical Care Nursing Clinics of North America, 3*(2), 199–220.

Eisenberg, P. G. (1991). Pulmonary complications from enteral nutrition. *Critical Care Nursing Clinics of North America, 3*(4), 641–649.

Everett, R. L., Patterson, D. R., Burns, L., et al. (1993). Adjunctive interventions for pain control: Comparison of hypnosis and ativan: The 1993 clinical research award. *Journal of Burn Care and Rehabilitation, 14*(6), 676–683.

Fowler, E., Cuzzell, J. Z., & Papen J. C. (1991). Healing with hydrocolloid. *American Journal of Nursing, 91*(2), 63–64.

Fuller, F. W., Parrish, M., & Nance, F. C. (1994). A review of the dosimetry of 1% silver sulfadiazine cream in burn wound treatment. *Journal of Burn Care and Rehabilitation, 15*(3), 213–223.

Gianino, S., & St. John, R. E. (1993). Nutrition assessment of a patient in the intensive care unit. *Critical Care Nursing Clinics of North America, 5*(1), 1–16.

Hammond, J. (1993). The status of statewide burn prevention legislation. *Journal of Burn Care and Rehabilitation, 14*(5), 473–475.

Hansbrough, W. B., & Hansbrough, J. F. (1993). Success of immediate intragastric feeding of patients with burns. *Journal of Burn Care and Rehabilitation, 14*(5), 512–516.

Harden, N. G., & Luster, S. H. (1991). Rehabilitation considerations in the care of the acute burn patient. *Critical Care Nursing Clinics of North America, 3*(2), 245–253.

Hu, O. Y., Ho, S. T., Wang, J. J., et al. (1993). Evaluation of gastric emptying in severe burn-injured patients. *Critical Care Medicine, 21*(4), 527–531.

Ireton-Jones, C. S., & Gottschlich, M. M. (1993). The evolution of nutrition support in burns. *Journal of Burn Care and Rehabilitation, 14*(2), 272–280.

Jepsen, D. L. (1992). How to manage a patient with lightning injury. *American Journal of Nursing, 92*(8), 38–42.

Jurgrau, A. (1990). How to spot child abuse. *RN, 53*(10), 26–32.

Klein, D. G., & O'Malley, P. (1987). Topical injury from chemical agents: Initial treatment. *Heart & Lung, 16*(1), 49–54.

Lehman, S. (1993). Nutritional support in the hypermetabolic patient. *Critical Care Nursing Clinics of North America, 5*(1), 97–103.

Martyn, J. A. (1990). *Acute management of the burned patient*. Philadelphia: W. B. Saunders.

McNeal, G. J., Gonzalez, E. W., Petit de Mange, E., & Perez, I. G. (in press). Multiculturally diverse clients. In J. Rothrock (Ed.), *Nursing care planning* (2nd ed.). St. Louis: Mosby.

Metheny, N., Reed, L., Wiersema, L., McSweeney, M., Wehrle, M. A., & Clark, J. (1993). Effectiveness of pH measurements in predicting feeding tube placement: An update. *Nursing Research, 42*(6), 324–331.

Meyer, N. A., Muller, M. J., & Herndon, D. N. (1994). Nutrition support of the healing wound. *New Horizons, 2*(2), 202–214.

Mosley, S. (1988). Inhalation injury: A review of the literature. *Heart & Lung, 17*(1), 3–9.

Richard, R., & Staley M. (1994). *Burn care and rehabilitation: Principles and practice*. Philadelphia: F. A. Davis.

Robins, E. V. (1989). Immunosuppression of the burned patient. *Critical Care Nursing Clinics of North America, 1*(4), 767–774.

Royall, D., Fairholm, L., Peters, W. J., et al. (1994) Continuous measurement of energy expenditure in ventilated burn patients: An analysis. *Critical Care Medicine, 22*(3), 399–406.

Rue, L. W., & Cioffi, W. G. (1991). Resuscitation of thermally injured patients. *Critical Care Nursing Clinics of North America, 3*(2), 181–189.

Rutan, R. L., Desai, M. H., & Herndon, D. N. (1993). Thermal injuries caused by ignition of volatile substances by gas water heater. *Journal of Burn Care and Rehabilitation, 14*(2), 218–220.

Rutherford, K. A. (1989). Principles and application of oximetry. *Critical Care Nursing Clinics of North America, 1*(4), 649–657.

Shenkman, B., & Stechmillar, J. (1987). Patient and family perception of projected functioning after discharge from a burn unit. *Heart & Lung, 16*(5), 490–496.

Shlafer, M., & Marieb, E. N. (1993). *The nurse, pharmacology, and drug therapy* (2nd ed). Redwood, CA: Addison-Wesley Nursing.

Staley, M., & Richard, R. (1993). The elderly patient with burns: Treatment considerations. *Journal of Burn Care and Rehabilitation, 14*(5), 559–565.

Summers, T. M. (1991). Psychosocial support of the burn patient. *Critical Care Nursing Clinics of North America, 3*(2), 237–244.

Sutherland, S. (1988). Burned adolescents' descriptions of their coping strategies. *Heart & Lung, 17*(2), 150–157.

Swearingen, P., Sommers, M. S., & Miller, K. (1988). *Manual of critical care applying nursing diagnoses to adult critical illness*. St. Louis: Mosby.

Tribett, D. (1989). Immune system function: Implications for critical care nursing practice. *Critical Care Nursing Clinics of North America, 1*(4), 725–740.

Walter, P. H. (1993). Burn wound management. *AACN Clinical Issues in Critical Care Nursing, 4*(2), 378–387.

Weber, J. M., & Tompkins, D. M. (1993). Improving survival: Infection control in burns. *AACN Clinical Issues in Critical Care Nursing, 4*(2), 414–423.

Responses to Altered Endocrine Function

Assessing Clients with Endocrine Disorders

LEARNING OBJECTIVES

After completing this chapter, you will be able to

- Explain the endocrine system's role in regulating body functions.
- Identify the major endocrine organs.
- Describe the function of the hormones secreted by the major endocrine organs.

- Identify interview questions pertinent to the assessment of the endocrine system.
- Describe techniques for physical assessment of endocrine function.
- Identify findings that may indicate malfunction of the endocrine system.
- Describe the normal variations in assessment findings for the older adult.

The *endocrine system* is an essential regulator of the body's internal environment. Through hormones secreted by its glands, the endocrine system regulates such varied functions as growth, reproduction, metabolism, fluid and electrolyte balance, and sex differentiation. It also assists the body in adapting to constant alterations in the internal and external environment.

Review of Anatomy and Physiology

▪ ▪ ▪

The major endocrine organs are the pituitary gland, thyroid gland, parathyroid glands, adrenal glands, pancreas, and gonads (reproductive glands). The location of these glands is illustrated in Figure 19–1. Table 19–1 summarizes the role of the endocrine organs and their hormones. Specific information about the gonads is found in Chapters 45 through 48.

The Pituitary Gland

The *pituitary gland* (or *hypophysis*) is located in the skull beneath the hypothalamus of the brain. It often is called the "master gland" because its hormones regulate many different body functions.

The pituitary gland is made up of two parts: the *anterior pituitary* (or *adenohypophysis*) and the *posterior pituitary* (or *neurohypophysis*). The anterior pituitary is made up of glandular tissue, whereas the posterior pituitary is actually an extension of the hypothalamus.

The Anterior Pituitary

The anterior pituitary has several different types of endocrine cells and secretes at least six major hormones (Figure 19–2).

- Somatotropic cells secrete *growth hormone (GH),* also called somatotropin. GH stimulates growth of the body by signaling cells to increase protein production and by stimulating the epiphyseal plates of the long bones.

- Lactotropic cells secrete *prolactin (PRL)*. Prolactin stimulates the production of breast milk.

- Thyrotropic cells secrete *thyroid-stimulating hormone (TSH)*. TSH stimulates the synthesis and release of thyroid hormones from the thyroid gland.

- Corticotropic cells secrete *adrenocorticotropic hormone (ACTH)*. ACTH stimulates release of hormones, especially the glucocorticoids, from the adrenal cortex.

- Gonadotropic cells secrete the gonadotropin hormones, *follicle-stimulating hormone (FSH)* and *luteinizing hormone (LH)*. These hormones stimulate the ovaries and testes (the gonads). In women, FSH stimulates the development of ovarian follicles and induces the secretion of estrogenic female sex hormones. In men, FSH is involved in the development and maturation of sperm. In women, increasing levels of LH work together with FSH to lead to ovulation and the formation of the corpus luteum from an ovarian follicle. In men, LH is called interstitial cell–stimulating hormone (ICSH). This hormone stimulates the interstitial cells of the testes to produce male sex hormones.

The Posterior Pituitary

The posterior pituitary is made up of nervous tissue. Its primary function is to store and release two hormones that are produced in the hypothalamus:

- *Antidiuretic hormone (ADH),* also called vasopressin, inhibits urine production by causing the renal tubules to

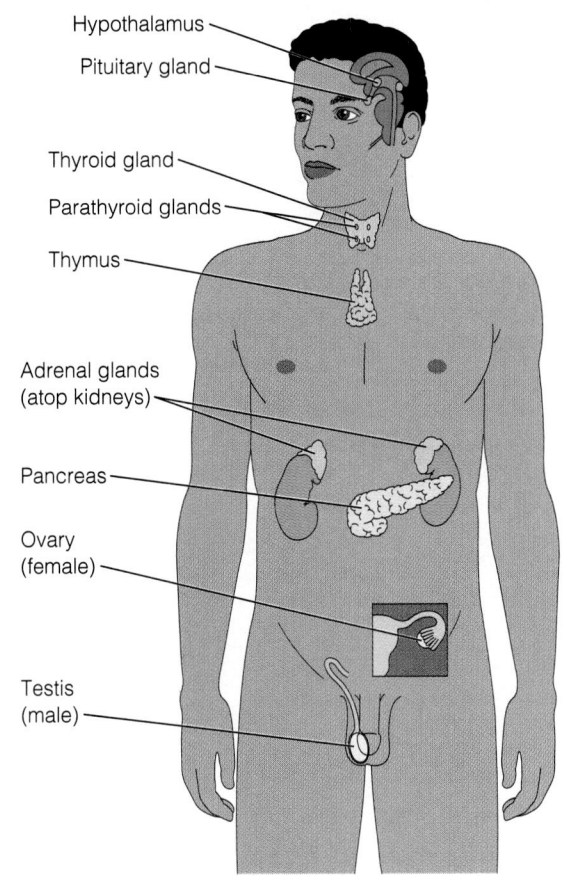

Figure 19–1   Location of the major endocrine glands.

Figure 19–2   Actions of the major hormones of the anterior pituitary.

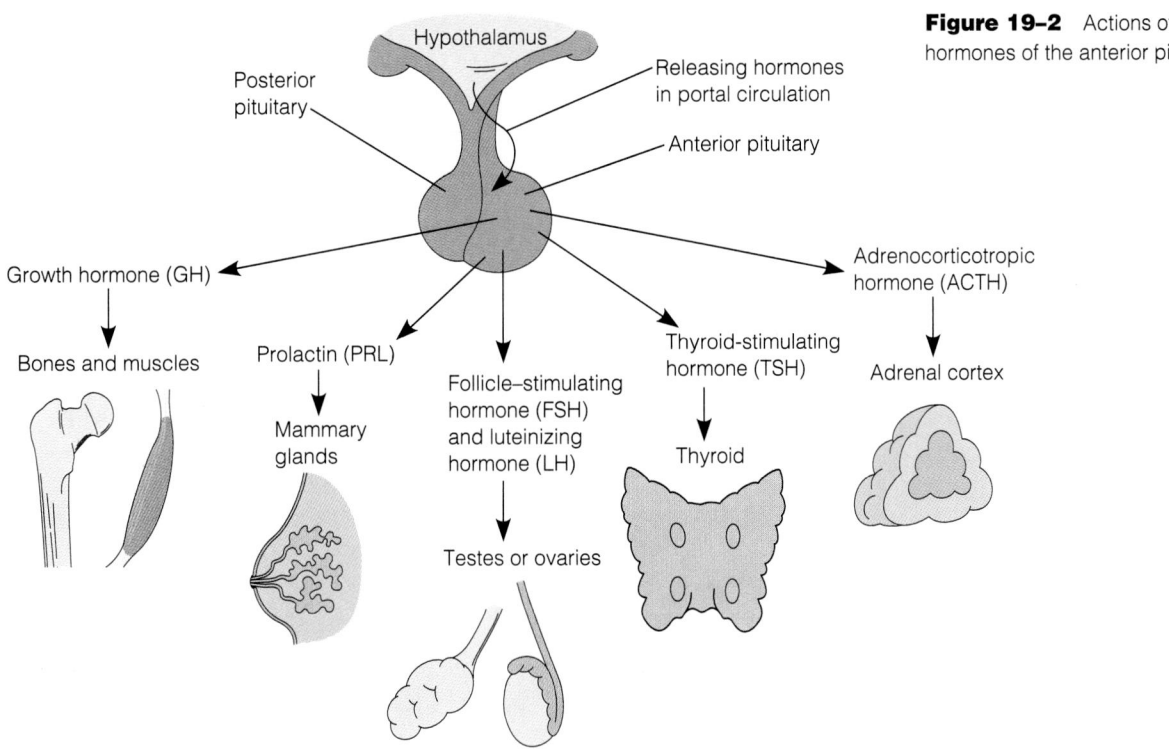

Table 19–1   Organs, Hormones, Functions, and Feedback Mechanisms of the Endocrine System

Endocrine Organ	Hormone Secreted	Target Organ and Feedback Mechanism
Thyroid gland	Thyroid hormone (TH): thyroxine (T$_4$) is the major hormone secreted by the thyroid gland. It is converted to triiodothyronine (T$_3$) at the target tissues.	Maintains metabolic rate and growth and development of all tissues. T$_3$ and T$_4$ are secreted in response to thyroid-stimulating hormone (TSH).
	Calcitonin	Maintains serum calcium levels by decreasing bone resorption and decreasing resorption of calcium in the kidneys whenever levels of plasma calcium are elevated.
Parathyroid gland	Parathyroid hormone (PTH)	Maintains serum calcium levels by stimulating bone resorption and formation and by stimulating kidney resorption of calcium in response to falling levels of plasma calcium.
Adrenal cortex	Mineralocorticoids (e.g., aldosterone)	Promote kidney tubule reabsorption of sodium and water and excretion of potassium in response to elevated levels of potassium and low levels of sodium, thereby increasing blood pressure and blood volume.
	Glucocorticoids (e.g., cortisol)	Help regulate metabolism of carbohydrates, fats, and proteins. Activate anti-inflammatory responses to stressors. Low cortisol levels stimulate hypothalamic secretion of corticotropin-releasing hormone (CRH), which stimulates the anterior pituitary gland to release ACTH, which in turn stimulates the adrenal cortex to secrete cortisol.
	Gonadocorticoids (androgens and small amounts of estrogen and progesterone)	The quantity of sex hormones produced here is small, and the mechanism is not well understood.
Adrenal medulla	Catecholamines (epinephrine and norepinephrine)	Stimulate the heart, constrict blood vessels, inhibit visceral muscles, dilate bronchioles, increase respiration and metabolism, promote hyperglycemia. Secreted in response to physical or psychologic stress.
Anterior pituitary (adenohypophysis)	Growth hormone (GH)	Promotes growth of body tissues by enhancing protein synthesis and promoting use of fat for energy and thus conserving glucose. Release is stimulated by growth hormone releasing hormone (GHRH) in response to low GH levels, hypoglycemia, increased amino acids, low fatty acids, and stress.

reabsorb water from the urine and return it to the circulating blood.

■ *Oxytocin* induces contraction of the smooth muscles in the reproductive organs. In women, oxytocin stimulates the myometrium of the uterus to contract during labor. It also induces milk ejection from the breasts.

The Thyroid Gland

The *thyroid gland*, one of the largest endocrine organs in the body, is located anterior to the upper part of the trachea and just inferior to the larynx. This gland has two lobes connected by a structure called the *isthmus.*

The glandular tissue is made up of follicles filled with a jelly-like colloid substance called thyroglobin, a glycoprotein-iodine complex. Cells within the follicles secrete thyroid hormone (TH), a general name for two similar hormones: *thyroxine (T$_4$)* and *triiodothyronine (T$_3$).* The primary role of thyroid hormones is to increase metabolism; they are also responsible for growth and development in children. The secretion of TH is initiated by the release of TSH by the pituitary gland and is dependent on an adequate supply of iodine.

The thyroid gland also secretes *calcitonin*, a hormone that decreases excessive levels of calcium in the blood by slowing the calcium-releasing activity of bone cells.

The Parathyroid Glands

The *parathyroid glands* (usually four to six in number) are embedded on the posterior surface of the lobes of the thyroid gland. They secrete *parathyroid hormone (PTH)*, or

Table 19–1 (continued)

Endocrine Organ	Hormone Secreted	Target Organ and Feedback Mechanism
	Thyroid-stimulating hormone (TSH)	Promotes the growth and function of thyroid gland. Release is stimulated by thyrotropin-releasing hormone (TRH) and inhibited by increased levels of thyroid hormones.
	Adrenocorticotropic hormone (ACTH)	Stimulates growth and function of adrenal cortex. Secreted in response to corticotropin-releasing hormone (CRH) from the hypothalamus. CRH is released in response to fever, hypoglycemia, and stress. High glucocorticoid levels inhibit ACTH release.
	Follicle-stimulating hormone (FSH)	Stimulates ovary development and egg and sperm production.
	Luteinizing hormone (LH)	Stimulates ovary maturation, ovulation, and progesterone secretion in females.
	Interstitial cell-stimulating hormone (ICSH)	Stimulates testosterone production in males.
		The gonadotropins (FSH, LH, and ICSH) are activated during puberty in response to hypothalamic release of gonadotropin-releasing hormone (GnRH). Rising levels of gonadal hormones suppress the release of FSH and LH.
	Prolactin (PRL)	Stimulates breast milk production in response to hypothalamic release of prolactin-releasing hormone (PRH) when estrogen levels are low. High estrogen levels stimulate hypothalamic release of prolactin-inhibiting hormone (PIH) and in turn inhibit prolactin release.
Posterior pituitary	Antidiuretic hormone (ADH)	Stimulates renal tubules to reabsorb water, thus inhibiting the formation of urine. Released in response to hypothalamic impulses, which are stimulated by decreased blood volume, increased blood osmolarity, low blood pressure, certain drugs, and pain. Proper hydration and alcohol intake inhibits ADH secretion.
	Oxytocin	Promotes contraction of the uterus in pregnancy. Stretching of the uterus and cervix during childbirth stimulates the hypothalamus to manufacture and release oxytocin, which promotes release of stored oxytocin from the posterior pituitary gland. Sucking of the breasts also triggers oxytocin release and the "letdown" reflex in women whose breasts are already producing milk in response to prolactin production.

parathormone. When calcium levels in the plasma fall, PTH secretion increases. PTH also controls phosphate metabolism. It acts primarily by increasing renal excretion of phosphate in the urine, by decreasing the excretion of calcium, and by increasing bone reabsorption to cause the release of calcium from bones. Normal levels of vitamin D are necessary for PTH to exert these effects on bone and kidneys.

The Adrenal Glands

The two *adrenal glands* (also called *suprarenal glands* because of their location above the kidneys) are pyramid-shaped organs that sit on top of the kidneys. Each gland consists of two parts, which are distinct organs: an inner medulla and an outer cortex.

The Adrenal Medulla

The *adrenal medulla* produces two hormones (also called *catecholamines*): *epinephrine* (also called adrenaline) and *norepinephrine* (or noradrenaline). These hormones are similar to substances released also by the sympathetic nervous system and thus are not essential to life. Epinephrine increases blood glucose levels and stimulates the release of ACTH from the pituitary; ACTH in turn stimulates the adrenal cortex to release glucocorticoids. Epinephrine also increases the rate and force of cardiac contractions; constricts blood vessels in the skin, mucous membranes, and the kidneys; and dilates blood vessels in the skeletal muscles, coronary arteries, and pulmonary arteries.

Norepinephrine increases heart rate as well as the force of cardiac contractions. It also vasoconstricts blood vessels throughout the body.

The Adrenal Cortex

The adrenal cortex secretes several different hormones, all of which are corticosteroids. These corticosteroids are classified into two groups: mineralocorticoids and glucocorticoids.

The primary mineralocorticoid, *aldosterone*, is secreted in response to a decrease in blood volume or to hypotension. Aldosterone prompts the distal tubules of the kidneys to release increased amounts of water and sodium back into the circulating blood to increase volume and pressure.

The release of the mineralocorticoids is controlled primarily by an enzyme called *renin*. When a decrease in blood pressure or sodium is detected, specialized kidney cells release renin to act on a substance called *angiotensinogen*, which is manufactured by the liver. Angiotensinogen is modified by renin and other enzymes to become angiotensin, which stimulates the release of aldosterone from the adrenal cortex.

The glucocorticoids include *cortisol* and *cortisone*. These hormones affect carbohydrate metabolism by regulating glucose use in body tissues, mobilizing fatty acids from fatty tissue, and shifting the source of energy for muscle cells from glucose to fatty acids. Glucocorticoids are released in times of stress. An excess of glucocorticoids in the body depresses the inflammatory response and inhibits the effectiveness of the immune system.

The Pancreas

The *pancreas*, located behind the stomach between the spleen and the duodenum, is both an endocrine gland (producing hormones) and an exocrine gland (producing digestive enzymes). The endocrine cells of the pancreas produce hormones that regulate carbohydrate metabolism. They are clustered in bodies called *pancreatic islets* (or islets of Langerhans) scattered throughout the gland. There are at least four different cell types in the pancreatic islets:

- Alpha cells produce *glucagon*, which decreases glucose oxidation and promotes an increase in the blood glucose level by signaling the liver to release glucose from glycogen stores.

- Beta cells produce *insulin*, which facilitates the uptake and use of glucose by cells and prevents an excessive breakdown of glycogen in the liver and muscle. In this way, insulin decreases blood glucose levels. Insulin also facilitates lipid formation, inhibits the breakdown and mobilization of stored fat, and assists in the movement of amino acids into cells to promote protein synthesis. In general, the actions of glucagon and insulin oppose one another, helping to maintain a stable blood glucose level.

- Delta cells secrete *somatostatin*, which inhibits the secretion of glucagon and insulin by the alpha and beta cells.

- F cells secrete *pancreatic polypeptide*, which is believed to inhibit the exocrine activity of the pancreas.

The Gonads

The *gonads* are the testes and ovaries. These organs are the primary source of steroid sex hormones in the body. The hormones of the gonads are important in regulating body growth and promoting the onset of puberty.

In men, *androgens* (primarily *testosterone*) produced by the testes maintain reproductive functioning and secondary sex characteristics. Androgens also promote the production of sperm.

In women, the ovaries secrete *estrogens* and *progesterone* to maintain reproductive functioning and secondary sex characteristics. Progesterone also promotes the growth of the lining of the uterus to prepare for implantation of a fertilized ovum.

The structure and functions of the gonads are discussed fully in Chapter 45.

An Overview of Hormones

Hormones are chemical messengers secreted by the endocrine organs and transported throughout the body, where they exert their action on specific cells called *target cells*. Hormones do not cause reactions directly but rather are regulators of tissue responses. They may produce either generalized or local effects.

Hormones are transported from endocrine gland cells to target cells in the body in one of four ways:

1. Most hormones, including TH, insulin, and others, are released from the endocrine glands into the bloodstream. Some of these require a protein carrier.

2. Some hormones, such as epinephrine, are released from neurons into the bloodstream. This is called the neuroendocrine route.

3. The hypothalamus releases its hormones directly to target cells in the posterior pituitary by nerve cell extension.

4. With the paracrine method, released messengers diffuse through the interstitial fluid. This method of transport involves a number of hormonal peptides that are released throughout various organs and cells and act locally. An example is endorphins, which act to relieve pain.

Hormones act by binding to specific receptor sites located on the surfaces of the target cells. These receptors recognize a specific hormone and translate the message into a cellular response. The receptor sites are structured

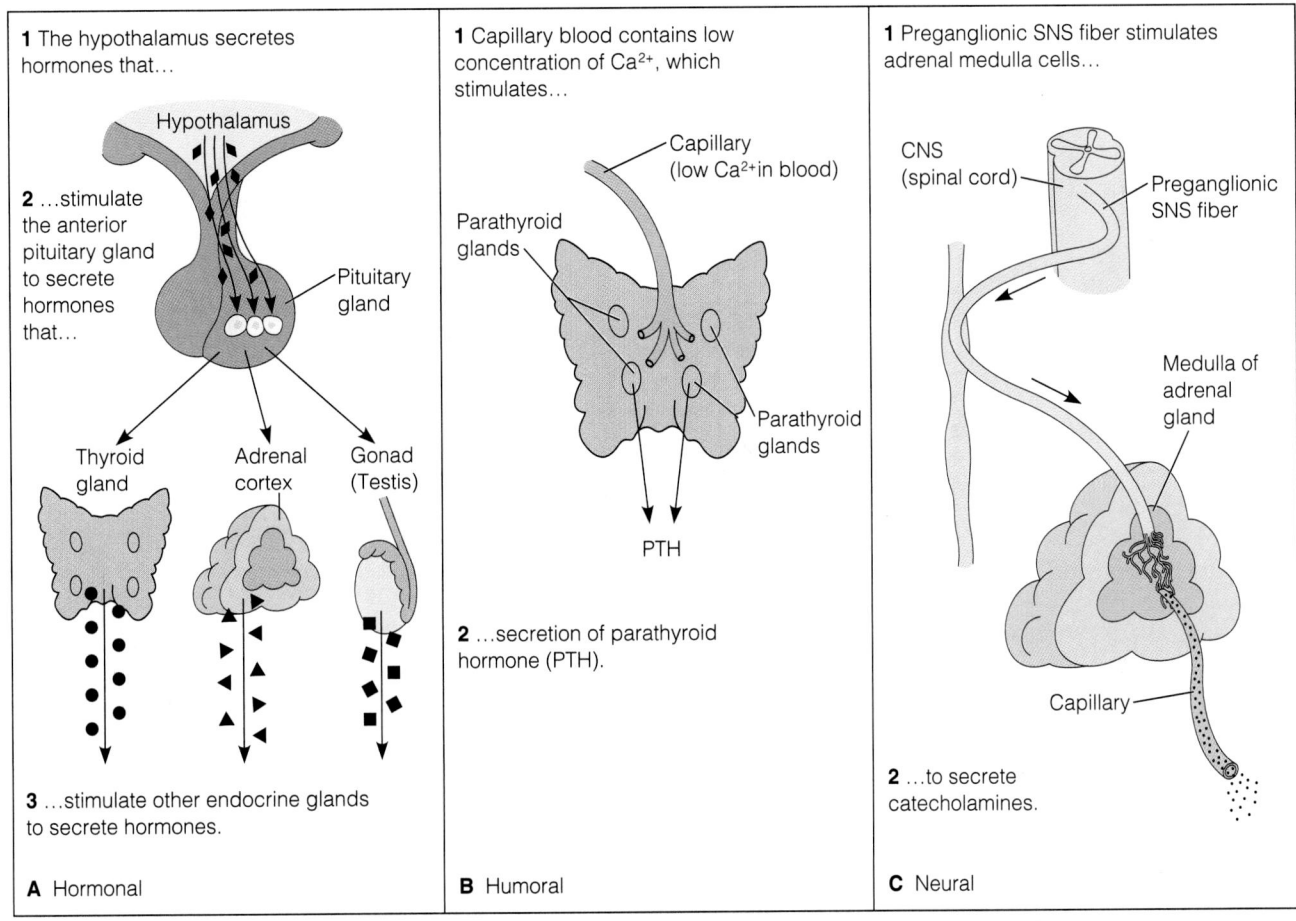

1 The hypothalamus secretes hormones that...

2 ...stimulate the anterior pituitary gland to secrete hormones that...

Hypothalamus

Pituitary gland

Thyroid gland

Adrenal cortex

Gonad (Testis)

3 ...stimulate other endocrine glands to secrete hormones.

A Hormonal

1 Capillary blood contains low concentration of Ca²⁺, which stimulates...

Capillary (low Ca²⁺ in blood)

Parathyroid glands

Parathyroid glands

PTH

2 ...secretion of parathyroid hormone (PTH).

B Humoral

1 Preganglionic SNS fiber stimulates adrenal medulla cells...

CNS (spinal cord)

Preganglionic SNS fiber

Medulla of adrenal gland

Capillary

2 ...to secrete catecholamines.

C Neural

Figure 19–3   Examples of three mechanisms of hormone release: *A*, hormonal; *B*, humoral; *C*, neural.

so that they respond only to a specific hormone; in other words, receptors in the thyroid gland are responsive to TSH but not to LH.

Hormone levels are controlled by the pituitary gland as well as by feedback mechanisms. Although most feedback mechanisms are negative, a few of them are positive in nature.

Negative feedback is controlled much as the thermostat in a house regulates temperature. Sensors in the endocrine system detect changes in hormone levels and adjust hormone secretion to maintain normal body levels. When the sensors detect a decrease in hormone levels, they begin actions to cause an increase in hormone levels; when hormone levels rise above normal, the sensors cause a decrease in hormone production and release. For example, when the hypothalamus or anterior pituitary gland senses increased blood levels of TH, they release hormones causing a reduction in the secretion of TSH, which in turn prompts a decrease in the output of TH by the thyroid gland (Porth, 1994).

Positive feedback mechanisms are initiated when in-

creasing levels of one hormone cause another gland to release a hormone. For example, production of estradiol (a female ovarian hormone) is increased during the follicular stage of the menstrual cycle; this in turn stimulates increased FSH production by the anterior pituitary gland. Estradiol levels continue to increase until the ovarian follicle disappears, eliminating the source of the stimulation for FSH, which then decreases.

Stimuli for hormone release may also be classified as hormonal, humoral, or neural (Figure 19–3):

- In hormonal release, hypothalamic hormones stimulate the anterior pituitary to release hormones. Fluctuations in the serum level of these hormones in turn prompt other endocrine glands to release hormones.

- In humoral release, fluctuations in the serum levels of certain ions and nutrients stimulate specific endocrine glands to release hormones to bring these levels back to normal.

- In neural release, nerve fibers stimulate the release of hormones.

Assessment of Endocrine Function

■ ■ ■

Function of the endocrine glands is assessed both by a health assessment interview to collect subjective data and a physical assessment to collect objective data. Hormones affect all body tissues and organs, and manifestations of dysfunction are often nonspecific, making assessment of endocrine function often more difficult than assessment of other body systems.

The Health Assessment Interview

This section provides guidelines for collecting subjective data through a health assessment interview specific to the functions of the endocrine glands. Interview questions and leading statements for assessing endocrine function are also provided.

Overview

A health assessment interview to determine problems with the endocrine system may be done as part of a health screening or total health assessment, or it may focus on a chief complaint (such as increased urination or changes in energy levels). If the client has a problem with endocrine function, the nurse analyzes its onset, characteristics and course, severity, precipitating and relieving factors, and any associated symptoms, noting the timing and circumstances. For example, the nurse may ask the client:

■ Describe the swelling you noticed in the front of your neck. When did it begin? Have you noticed any changes in your energy level?

■ When did you first notice that your hands and feet were getting larger?

■ Have you noticed that your appetite has increased even though you have lost weight?

The health history includes information about the client's medical history, family history, and social and personal history. The nurse asks the client about any changes in normal growth and development as well as in height and weight. Changes in the size of extremities can often be detected by asking whether the client has had to have rings enlarged or to buy increasingly larger gloves and shoes. Enlargement of the neck may be brought to light by asking whether the client has difficulty finding shirts or blouses with a collar that fits. Other changes that should be explored include difficulty swallowing; increased or decreased thirst, appetite, and/or urination; visual changes; sleep disturbances; altered patterns of hair distribution (such as increased facial hair in women); changes in menstruation; changes in memory or ability to

concentrate; and changes in hair and skin texture. The client should be questioned about any blow to the head, as well as previous hospitalizations, chemotherapy, radiation (especially to the neck), and the use of medications (especially hormones or steroids).

Because many endocrine disorders have a familial tendency, the nurse asks the client about a family history of such diseases as diabetes mellitus, diabetes insipidus, thyroid disorders, hypertension, tumors, autoimmune disorders, and obesity. Women should be asked about problems with pregnancy, menstruation, and/or menopause.

Because the endocrine system often is affected by long-term stress, the nurse also asks about the client's occupational and social history. Questions about the client's satisfaction with his or her occupation, personal relationships, and life-style also should be included. Other areas of assessment include the client's usual means of coping; use of alcohol, smoking, or drugs; diet; exercise patterns; and sleep patterns. Although the client may not recognize changes in behavior, family members may be able to provide important information.

Interview Questions

The following interview questions and leading statements are categorized by functional health patterns:

Health Perception–Health Management

■ Describe your overall state of health. Rate it on a scale of 1 to 10, with 10 being the best health you have had.

■ Describe any endocrine problems you have had (pituitary, thyroid, parathyroid, adrenal, pancreas, ovaries, testes).

■ How was this problem treated? With medications, surgery, hormone replacements, diet?

■ What prescribed and/or over-the-counter medications do you use?

■ Do you smoke tobacco? If so, how much per day, and for how long?

■ Have you ever been tested for high or low blood sugar?

■ Do you drink alcohol? If so, how much and what kind?

■ Describe how you care for your health.

■ When was your last physical examination?

Nutritional-Metabolic

■ Describe your usual dietary intake for a 24-hour period.

■ Describe how much water or fluids you drink in a 24-hour period.

■ Have you noticed that you are thirsty more often than you used to be?

- Has your appetite changed? If so, describe.

- Has your weight changed? If so, by how many pounds? Over what period of time?

- Have you noticed any changes in your energy levels? Explain.

- Have you noticed any change in your ability to tolerate heat or cold?

- Have you had any difficulty swallowing? Explain.

Elimination

- Describe your usual pattern for emptying your bladder in a 24-hour period. Has this changed? If so, describe.

- Have you noticed any changes in the color or odor of your urine? If so, describe.

- Do you have to get up at night to empty your bladder? How often?

- Have you ever had kidney stones? If so, how were they treated?

- Has there been any change in your bowel elimination? Explain.

Activity–Exercise

- Describe your usual activities over a 24-hour period.

- Do certain activities make you short of breath or very tired? Explain.

- Has your ability to care for yourself changed with this endocrine problem? If so, describe.

- Has your energy level decreased or increased? If so, explain.

Sleep–Rest

- On a scale of 1 to 10, with 10 being uninterrupted sleep throughout the night, rate your ability to rest and sleep. Explain your rating.

- Do you feel nervous or unable to rest?

Cognitive–Perceptual

- Do you feel restless, anxious, or confused?

- Have you noticed any hoarseness or changes in your voice?

- Have you noticed any changes in the color or condition of your skin, such as a darker color, changes in the ability to tan, dryness, oiliness, bruises?

- Have you had any heart palpitations?

- Have you had any abdominal pain?

- Have you had headaches, memory loss, changes in sensation, or depression?

- Have you had any pain or stiffness in your muscles and joints?

Self-Perception–Self-Concept

- How do you feel about this health problem?

- How has having this problem made you feel about yourself and the future?

- How do you feel about taking medications for the rest of your life?

Role–Relationship

- Is there a history of any type of endocrine problem in your family? Explain.

- How has this health problem affected others you live with?

- Has having this health problem changed your role and responsibilities in your family? Explain.

- Has having this health problem affected your ability to work? Explain.

Sexuality–Reproductive

- Have you noticed any change in your interest in sexual activities? Explain.

- Have you noticed any change in your ability to have sexual relations? Explain.

- (*For females*) Have you had any change in your menstrual periods? Describe.

- (*For males*) Have you had difficulty achieving and maintaining an erection?

- (*For females*) Have you had any difficulty becoming pregnant?

- (*For males*) Have you had any difficulty fathering a child?

- How many children do you have? What were their weights at birth?

Coping–Stress

- Does stress seem to increase the symptoms of your endocrine problem? If so, in what way?

- What or who helps you most in coping with your health problem?

- Describe what you usually do to cope with stress.

Value–Belief

- Are there significant others, practices, or activities that help you cope with this health problem? Explain.

- How do you perceive the future in regard to living with this health problem?

The Physical Assessment

Physical assessment of the endocrine system may be performed as part of a total health assessment, or it may be done alone for clients with known or suspected problems with endocrine function.

Preparation

The only endocrine organ that can be palpated is the thyroid gland. However, other assessments that provide information about endocrine problems include inspection of the skin, hair and nails, facial appearance, reflexes, and musculoskeletal system. Measurement of height and weight as well as vital signs also provides clues to altered endocrine system function.

The client may sit during the examination. A reflex hammer is used to test deep-tendon reflexes. Prior to the examination, the nurse collects the necessary equipment and explains the techniques to the client to decrease anxiety. Additional techniques for assessing hypocalcemic tetany, a complication of endocrine disorders or surgery, are included in the examination sequence.

ASSESSMENT TECHNIQUE	POSSIBLE ABNORMAL FINDINGS
Skin ■ **Inspect skin color.**	Hyperpigmentation may be seen in clients with Addison's disease or Cushing's syndrome. Hypopigmentation may be seen in diabetes mellitus, hyperthyroidism, or hypothyroidism. A yellowish cast to the skin might indicate hypothyroidism. Purple striae over the abdomen and bruising may be present in the client with Cushing's syndrome.
■ **Palpate the skin.** Assess for texture, moisture, and the presence of lesions.	Rough, dry skin is often seen in clients with hypothyroidism, whereas smooth and flushed skin can be a sign of hyperthyroidism. Lesions on the lower extremities might indicate diabetes mellitus.
Nails and Hair ■ **Assess texture and condition of nails and hair.**	Increased pigmentation of the nails is often seen in clients with Addison's disease. Dry, thick, brittle nails and hair may be apparent in hypothyroidism; thin, brittle nails and thin, soft hair may be apparent in hyperthyroidism. *Hirsutism* (excessive facial, chest, or abdominal hair) may be seen in Cushing's syndrome.
Face ■ **Inspect the symmetry and form of the face.** ■ **Inspect position of eyes.**	Variations of form and structure may indicate growth abnormalities such as acromegaly.

ASSESSMENT TECHNIQUE	POSSIBLE ABNORMAL FINDINGS

Thyroid Gland

■ **Palpate the thyroid gland for size and consistency.**

Stand behind the client, and place your fingers on either side of the trachea below the thyroid cartilage (Figure 19–4). Ask the client to tilt the head to the right. Now ask the client to swallow. As the client swallows, displace the left lobe while palpating the right lobe. Repeat to palpate the left lobe.

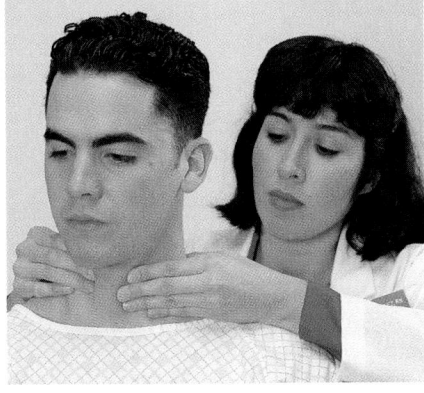

Figure 19–4 Palpating the thyroid gland from behind the client.

Exophthalmos (protruding eyes) may be seen in hyperthyroidism.

The thyroid may be enlarged in clients with Graves' disease or a goiter. Multiple nodules may be seen in metabolic disorders, whereas the presence of only one nodule may indicate a cyst or a benign or malignant tumor. One enlarged nodule suggests malignancy.

Motor Function

■ **Assess the deep-tendon reflexes.**

The deep-tendon reflexes include the following. See Chapter 39 for guidelines on assessment.

- Biceps
- Brachioradialis
- Triceps
- Patellar
- Achilles

Increased reflexes may be seen in hyperthyroidism; decreased reflexes may be seen in hypothyroidism.

Sensory Function

■ **Assess sensory function.**

Test the client's sensitivity to pain, temperature, vibration, light touch, and *stereognosis* (the ability to identify an object merely by touch). Compare symmetric areas on both sides of the body, and compare the distal to the proximal regions of the extremities.

Ask the client to close his or her eyes. To test pain, use the blunt and sharp ends of a new safety pin. Discard the pin after use. To test temperature, use cups or other containers of cold and hot water. To test vibration, use a tuning fork over one of the client's finger or toe joints. To test light touch, use a cotton wisp. To test stereognosis, place in the client's hand a simple, familiar object, such as a rubber band, cotton ball, or button. Ask the client to identify the object.

Peripheral neuropathy and paresthesias may occur in diabetes, hypothyroidism, or acromegaly.

Musculoskeletal Structure

■ **Inspect the size and proportions of the client's body structure.**

Extremely short stature may indicate **dwarfism**, which is caused by insufficient growth hormone. Extremely large bones may indicate **acromegaly**, which is caused by excessive growth hormone.

Hypocalcemic Tetany

■ **Assess for Trousseau's sign.**

Inflate pressure cuff above antecubital space to occlude blood supply to the arm.

Decreased calcium levels cause the client's hand and fingers to contract (carpal spasm).

■ **Assess for Chvostek's sign.**

Tap your finger in front of the client's ear at the angle of the jaw.

Decreased calcium levels cause the client's lateral facial muscles to contract.

Variations in Assessment Findings for the Older Adult

The effects of aging on the endocrine system are more difficult to detect than those on many other body systems. However, endocrine disorders are more common in adults over age 40. Female hormone production decreases with the onset of menopause. In both men and women, anterior pituitary hormone output decreases, which may decrease the body's resistance to infection, alter the body's immune responses, or lead to disease (diabetes, for example).

Age-related changes in the structure and function of the endocrine glands include the following:

- The thyroid gland undergoes some degree of atrophy, fibrosis, and nodularity. Thyroid hormone levels decrease, and hypothyroidism is seen more often in the older adult.

- The adrenal glands lose some weight and become more fibrotic.

- The anterior pituitary gland decreases in size and becomes more fibrotic.

Other normal variations occurring in the older adult, which should not be confused with abnormal endocrine findings, include the following:

- Senile lentigines, which are small, brown, flat macules, may be seen on the forearms and dorsa of the hands.

- Seborrheic keratoses, thickened areas of pigmentation, may be seen on the face and hands.

- Hair growth decreases.

- Nails are often thick, brittle, and yellow.

- Facial skin sags, and bones become more prominent.

- Sensation of touch decreases.

- Deep-tendon reflexes decrease.

- Height decreases.

Age-related changes in the reproductive organs are discussed in Chapter 45.

Bibliography

■ ■ ■

Becker, K. (1990). *Principles and practice of endocrinology and metabolism.* Philadelphia: Lippincott.

Halloran, T. (1990). Nursing responsibilities in endocrine emergencies. *Critical Care Nursing Quarterly, 13*(3), 74–81.

Handerhan, B. (1992). Recognizing adrenal crisis: How to respond to severe steroid withdrawal, *Nursing92, 22*(4), 33.

Hershman, J. (1988). *Endocrine pathophysiology: A patient-oriented approach* (3rd ed.). Philadelphia: Lea & Febinger.

Kessler, C. (1992). An overview of endocrine function and dysfunction. *AACN Clinical Issues in Critical Care Nursing, 3*(2), 289–299.

Krug, L., Haire, J., & Hady, S. (1991). Exercise habits and exercise relapse in persons with non-insulin-dependent diabetes mellitus. *Diabetes Educator, 17*(3), 185–188.

McCargar, L., Tauton, J. & Pare, S. (1991). Benefits of exercise training for men with insulin-dependent diabetes mellitus. *Diabetes Educator, 17*(3), 179–184.

McConnell, E. (1985). Assessing the thyroid. *Nursing85, 15*(5), 60–62.

McGovern, M., & Kuhn, J. (1992). Skin assessment of the elderly client. *Journal of Gerontological Nursing, 18*(4), 39–43.

Port, A. (1992). Thyroid problems: Eighteen questions physicians often ask. *Consultant 32*(8), 71–73, 77–78, 87–88.

Porth, C. (1994). *Pathophysiology: Concepts of altered health states.* Philadelphia: Lippincott.

Sikes, P. J. (1992). Endocrine responses to the stress of critical illness. *Issues in Critical Care Nursing 3*(3), 289–299.

Nursing Care of Clients with Thyroid, Parathyroid, Adrenal, and Pituitary Disorders

LEARNING OBJECTIVES

After completing this chapter, you will be able to

- Describe the pathophysiology of common disorders of the thyroid, parathyroid, adrenal, and pituitary glands.

- Identify laboratory and diagnostic tests used to diagnose disorders of the thyroid, parathyroid, adrenal, and pituitary glands.

- Compare and contrast the manifestations of disorders that result from hyperfunction and hypofunction of the thyroid, parathyroid, adrenal, and pituitary glands.

- Discuss the nursing implications for medications prescribed for the client with disorders of the thyroid and adrenal glands.

- Provide appropriate nursing care for the client in the preoperative and postoperative phases of a subtotal thyroidectomy and an adrenalectomy.

- Use the nursing process as a framework for providing individualized care to clients with disorders of the thyroid, parathyroid, adrenal, and pituitary glands.

The thyroid, parathyroid, adrenal, and pituitary glands are part of the endocrine system. Disorders of the structure and function of these glands alter normal hormone levels and the way body tissues use those hormones. When increases or decreases in hormone production or use occur, individuals experience alterations in health.

Clients with disorders of the glands discussed in this chapter require nursing care for multiple problems. They often face exhausting diagnostic tests, changes in physical appearance and emotional responses, and permanent alterations in life-style. Nursing care is directed toward meeting physiologic needs, providing education, and ensuring psychologic support for the client and family. A holistic approach to the complex needs of clients with these endocrine disorders is an essential component of nursing care. The collaborative care box on page 672 discusses the responsibilities of each health care team member.

Disorders of the Thyroid Gland

Altered thyroid hormone (TH) production or use affects all major organ systems. In the adult, TH changes primarily affect metabolism, cardiovascular function, gastrointestinal function, and neuromuscular function. Thyroid disorders — both hyperthyroidism and hypothyroidism — are among the most common endocrine disorders.

Collaborative Health Care: The Client with Thyroid Disorders

Health Care Team	Client-Centered Goals
Endocrinologist	Responsible for evaluation, treatment, and management of thyroid disorders. Orders diagnostic tests and evaluates results. Prescribes appropriate medication.
General surgeon	For clients requiring surgery, conducts preoperative assessment, performs surgery removing or resecting tumor, manages postoperative course, monitors surgical outcomes following discharge.
Radiologist	Performs radiological procedures used to diagnose thyroid-related problems, such as thyroid scan. If indicated, provides and monitors response to radiation therapy.
Primary care physician	Refers to and consults with endocrinologist.
Dietitian	Provides client with diet that promotes achieving or maintaining ideal body weight. Teaches client and family strategies to maintain a well-balanced diet inclusive of all food groups. Provides snacks appropriate to calorie recommendations.
RN and health care team communications	Reports any adverse effects from medications. Reports any difficulty breathing or speaking, and/or signs and symptoms of hemorrhage following surgery. Advises dietitian regarding client's intake and food preferences. Alerts social worker to any home care needs.

The Client with Hyperthyroidism

■ ■ ■

Hyperthyroidism (also called *thyrotoxicosis*) is an excess of TH in the body. Because the primary effect of TH is to increase the rate of protein, carbohydrate, and fat metabolism in most body tissues, hyperthyroidism affects all major organ systems of the body. The increase in metabolic rate and the alterations in cardiac output, peripheral blood flow, oxygen consumption, and body temperature are similar to those found in increased sympathetic nervous system activity (Porth, 1994).

Complications of untreated hyperthyroidism include cardiac failure, psychiatric disorders, and thyroid crisis (discussed below). Paradoxically, treatment of hyperthyroidism with medications and radioactive iodine may result in hypothyroidism.

Pathophysiology

Hyperthyroidism results from many different factors, including autoimmune reactions (as in Graves' disease), excess secretion of thyroid-stimulating hormone (TSH) by the pituitary gland, thyroiditis, neoplasms (such as toxic multinodular goiter), and an excessive intake of thyroid medications. The most common forms of hyperthyroidism are Graves' disease and toxic multinodular goiter.

The manifestations of hyperthyroidism are the result of increased circulating levels of TH. This hormonal excess increases the person's metabolic rate and heightens the sympathetic nervous system's physiologic response to stimulation. The sensitizing effect of abnormally elevated TH levels increases the cardiac rate and stroke volume. As a result, cardiac output and peripheral blood flow increase. Elevated TH levels also increase the metabolism of carbohydrates, proteins, and lipids. Lipids are depleted, and glucose tolerance decreases. Protein degradation increases, resulting in a negative nitrogen balance. Over time, the hypermetabolic effects of excess TH result in caloric and nutritional deficiencies.

As a result, the client with hyperthyroidism typically has an increased appetite, yet loses weight; sometimes the person may have hypermotile bowels and diarrhea. Additional manifestations related to hypermetabolism include heat intolerance and increased sweating. The client's hair is fine, and the skin is smooth and warm. Emotional lability is common. The systemwide manifestations of hyperthyroidism are shown in Figure 20–1.

Graves' Disease

Graves' disease is the most common form of hyperthyroidism. It is seen seven to ten times more often in women than in men and occurs most frequently in women under age 40. The cause is unknown, but a hereditary link and emotional stress have been suggested.

Graves' disease is generally classified as a multisystem autoimmune disorder that is believed to result from stimulation of the thyroid gland by a long-acting thyroid stimulator (LATS). The presence of LATS in the plasma is probably stimulated by immunoglobulins of the IgG class (called thyroid-stimulating immunoglobulins), but the exact mechanism for the development of the immunoglobulins is not known. This stimulation causes the

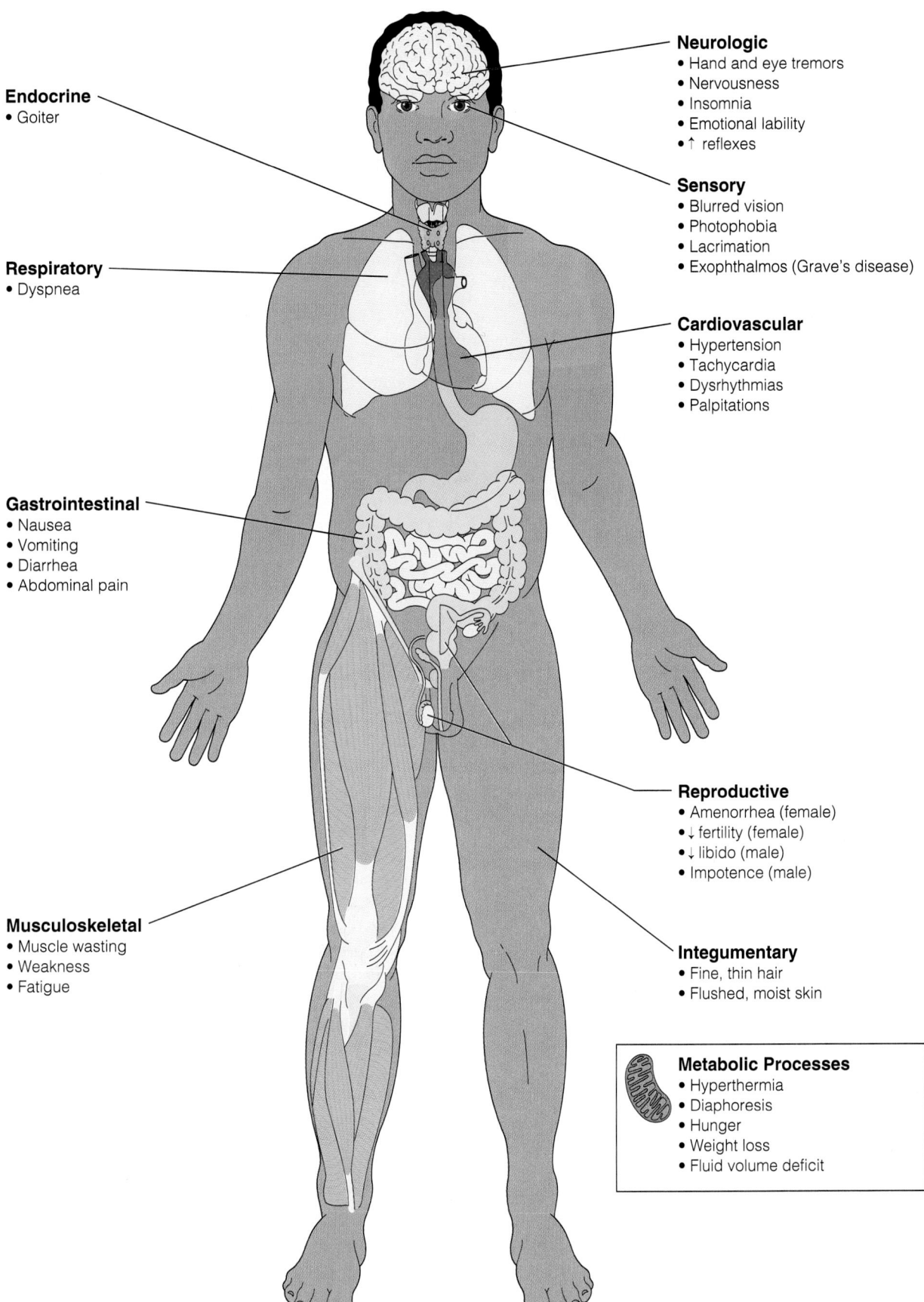

Neurologic
- Hand and eye tremors
- Nervousness
- Insomnia
- Emotional lability
- ↑ reflexes

Sensory
- Blurred vision
- Photophobia
- Lacrimation
- Exophthalmos (Grave's disease)

Cardiovascular
- Hypertension
- Tachycardia
- Dysrhythmias
- Palpitations

Reproductive
- Amenorrhea (female)
- ↓ fertility (female)
- ↓ libido (male)
- Impotence (male)

Integumentary
- Fine, thin hair
- Flushed, moist skin

Metabolic Processes
- Hyperthermia
- Diaphoresis
- Hunger
- Weight loss
- Fluid volume deficit

Endocrine
- Goiter

Respiratory
- Dyspnea

Gastrointestinal
- Nausea
- Vomiting
- Diarrhea
- Abdominal pain

Musculoskeletal
- Muscle wasting
- Weakness
- Fatigue

Figure 20–1   Multisystem effects of hyperthyroidism.

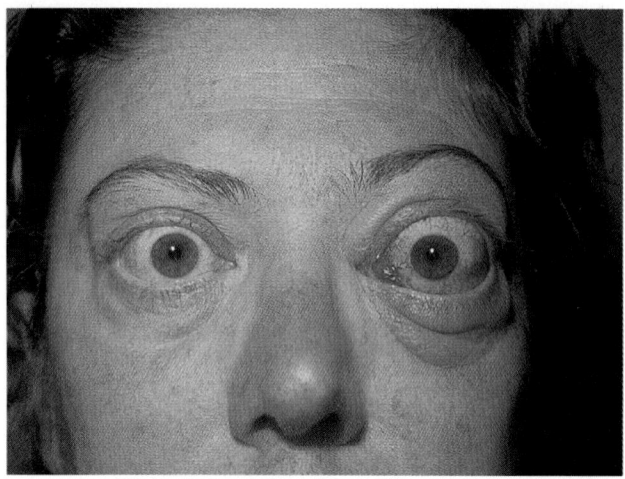

Figure 20–2 Exophthalmos in a client with Graves' disease. The disease causes edema of fat deposits behind the eyes and inflammation of the extraocular muscles. The accumulating pressure forces the eyes outward from their orbits.

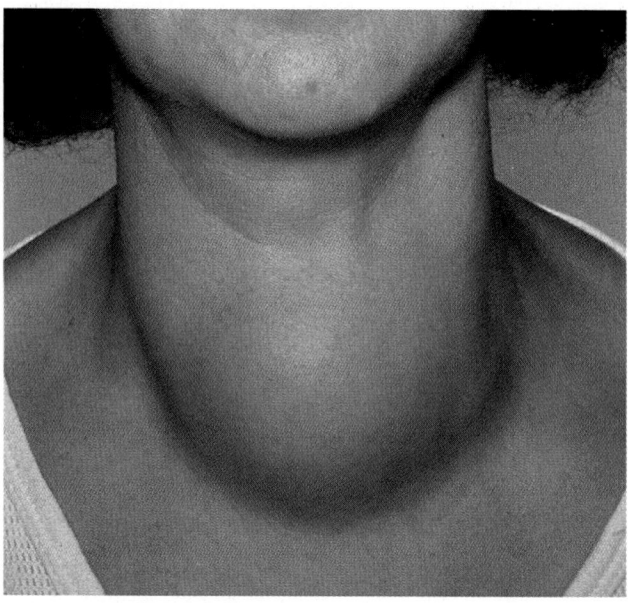

Figure 20–3 Toxic multinodular goiter. The formation and growth of numerous nodules in the thyroid gland cause the characteristic massive enlargement of the neck.

increased production of TH, resulting in the characteristic manifestations of the disease, such as diffuse enlargement of the thyroid gland and exophthalmos.

Exophthalmos, the forward protrusion of the eyeballs occurring in Graves' disease, results from the accumulation of fat deposits and inflammation by-products in the retro-orbital tissues. Often the sclera is visible above the iris. The upper lids are often retracted, and the person has a characteristic unblinking stare (Figure 20–2). Exophthalmos is usually bilateral, but it may involve only one eye. The client may experience blurred vision, eye pain, lacrimation, and photophobia. The inability to close the eyelids completely over the protruding eyeballs increases the risk of corneal dryness, irritation, infection, and ulceration. The treatment of Graves' disease does not reverse these changes in the eyes.

The client with Graves' disease may also have thickening and discoloration of the skin over the pretibial areas, extending from the knee to the foot. This condition, called infiltrative dermopathy, is not common and rarely requires treatment.

Toxic Multinodular Goiter

A simple **goiter** is an enlargement of the thyroid gland. This hypertrophy of the gland can result from excess TSH stimulation (when the amount of circulating TH is deficient), growth-stimulating immunoglobulins, or substances that inhibit TH synthesis. A goiter may be present in hyperthyroidism or hypothyroidism.

Toxic multinodular goiter (Figure 20–3) is characterized by small, discrete, *independently functioning* nodules (palpable deformities) in the thyroid gland tissue that secrete TH. These nodules may be benign or malignant. If TH levels are elevated, manifestations of hyperthyroidism occur. However, they are slower to develop and differ somewhat than those of Graves' disease. The client with this type of hyperthyroidism is usually a woman in her 60s or 70s who has had a goiter for a number of years.

Thyroid Crisis

Thyroid crisis (also called *thyroid storm*) is an extreme state of hyperthyroidism that is rare today because of improved diagnosis and treatment methods (Porth, 1994). When it does occur, those affected are usually people with untreated hyperthyroidism (most often Graves' disease) and people with hyperthyroidism who have experienced a stressor, such as an infection, trauma, untreated diabetic ketoacidosis, or manipulation of the thyroid gland during surgery. Thyroid crisis is a life-threatening condition.

The rapid increase in metabolic rate that results from the excessive TH causes the manifestations of thyroid crisis. The manifestations include hyperthermia, with body temperatures ranging from 102 F (39 C) to 106 F (41 C); tachycardia; systolic hypertension; and gastrointestinal symptoms (abdominal pain, vomiting, diarrhea). Agitation, restlessness, and tremors are common, progressing to confusion, psychosis, delirium, and seizures. The client may become comatose.

Rapid treatment of thyroid crisis is essential to preserve life. Treatment includes relieving respiratory distress, stabilizing cardiovascular function, and reducing TH synthesis and secretion.

Excess TSH Stimulation

Overproduction of TSH by the pituitary usually stimulates the thyroid gland to produce excess TH. The elevation in TSH secretion often results from a pituitary adenoma. This secondary form of hyperthyroidism is rare.

Thyroiditis

Thyroiditis (inflammation of the thyroid gland) is most often the result of a viral infection of the thyroid gland. The symptoms of thyroiditis are those of acute inflammation and the effects of increased TH. Thyroiditis is an acute disorder that may become chronic, resulting in a hypothyroid state as repeated infections destroy gland tissue. See the discussion of Hashimoto's thyroiditis later in this chapter.

Collaborative Care

Treatment of hyperthyroidism focuses on reducing the production of TH by the thyroid gland, thus establishing a euthyroid (normal thyroid) state, and preventing or treating complications. Depending on the client's age and physical status, pharmacologic treatment, radioactive iodine therapy, or surgery may be used.

Laboratory and Diagnostic Tests

Hyperthyroidism is diagnosed according to the manifestations of the specific disorders causing excessive TH, and by laboratory and diagnostic test results. Elevated levels of TH (both T_3 and T_4) and increased radioactive iodine (RAI) uptake are diagnostic criteria of hyperthyroidism. Laboratory findings in hyperthyroidism are shown in Table 20–1.

The following laboratory tests may be ordered:

- *TA test.* Serum thyroid antibodies (TA) are measured to determine whether a thyroid autoimmune disease is causing the client's symptoms. TA is elevated in Graves' disease.

- *TSH test.* Serum thyroid-stimulating hormone (TSH) levels are measured and compared with thyroxine (T_4) levels to differentiate pituitary from thyroid dysfunction. A decreased T_4 level and a normal or increased TSH level can indicate a thyroid disorder. A pituitary disorder is indicated when T_4 and TSH levels are decreased.

- *T_4 test.* Serum thyroxine (T_4) levels are measured to determine TH concentration and to test thyroid gland function. T_4 levels are elevated in hyperthyroidism and in acute thyroiditis.

Table 20–1	Laboratory Findings in Hyperthyroidism	
Test	**Normal Values**	**Findings**
Serum TA	Negative to 1:20	Increased
Serum TSH	2 to 5.4 μU/mL	1. Normal or increased TSH and decreased T_4 suggests thyroid dysfunction. 2. Decreased TSH and T_4 suggests pituitary dysfunction.
Serum T_4	5 to 12 μg/dL	Increased
Serum T_3	80 to 200 ng/dL	Increased
T_3 uptake (T_3RU)	25 to 35 relative percentage	Increased
Thyroid suppression		Increased RAI uptake and T_4 levels

- *T_3 test.* Serum triiodothyronine (T_3) is measured by radioimmunoassay (T_3RIA), which measures bound and free forms of this hormone. This test is effective for the diagnosis of hyperthyroidism (especially T_3 thyrotoxicosis). T_3 levels may also be elevated in thyroiditis.

- *T_3 uptake test.* T_3 uptake (T_3RU) is measured by an in vitro test in which the client's blood is mixed with radioactive T_3; the results are elevated in hyperthyroidism.

Diagnostic studies of the thyroid gland follow:

- *RAI uptake test.* A radioactive iodine (RAI) uptake test (thyroid scan) measures the absorption of ^{131}I or ^{123}I by the thyroid gland. A calculated dose of radioactive iodine is given orally or intravenously, and the thyroid is then scanned (often after 24 hours). The distribution of radioactivity in the gland is recorded (increased uptake of radioactive iodine is seen in hyperthyroidism). In addition, the scan reveals the size and shape of the gland.

- *Thyroid suppression test.* RAI and T_4 levels are measured first. The client then takes TH for 7 to 10 days, after which the tests are repeated. Failure of hormone therapy to suppress RAI and T_4 indicates hyperthyroidism.

Pharmacology

Hyperthyroidism is treated pharmacologically by administering antithyroid medications that reduce TH production. Because these drugs do not affect the release or activity of hormone that is already formed, therapeutic effects may not be seen for several weeks (Loebl, Matejski,

Nursing Implications for Pharmacology: Hyperthyroidism

IODINE SOURCES

Potassium iodide, saturated solution

Potassium iodide (Pima)

Sodium iodine

Large doses of iodine inhibit TH synthesis and release. Iodine also makes the hyperplastic thyroid less vascular prior to surgery and hastens the ability of other antithyroid drugs to reduce natural hormone output.

Nursing Responsibilities

- Assess for hypersensitivity to iodine before giving medication; for example, ask client about allergies to shellfish.
- Dilute liquid iodine sources in chocolate milk, plain milk, or orange juice to disguise bitter taste.
- Have the client drink medication through a straw to prevent discoloration of teeth.
- Monitor for increased bleeding tendencies if the client is also taking anticoagulants; iodine increases their effect.

Client and Family Teaching

- The maximum effect of iodine in large doses usually occurs in 1 to 2 weeks.
- Long-term iodine therapy is not effective in controlling hyperthyroidism.

ANTITHYROID DRUGS

Methimazole (Tapazole)

Propylthiouracil (PTU, Propyl-Thracil)

Antithyroid drugs inhibit TH production. They do not affect already formed hormones; thus, several weeks may elapse before the client experiences therapeutic effects.

Nursing Responsibilities

- Monitor for side effects: pruritus, rash, elevated temperature, (for iodides) swelling of the eyelids, anorexia, loss of taste, changes in menstruation.
- Administer drugs at the same time each day to maintain stable blood levels.
- Monitor for symptoms of hypothyroidism: fatigue, weight gain.

Client and Family Teaching

- Watch for unusual bleeding, nausea, loss of taste, or epigastric pain. Report any such symptoms to the physician.
- If you are also taking anticoagulants, report any signs of bleeding.
- It may take up to 12 weeks before you experience the full effects of the drug. Take the medication regularly and exactly as prescribed.

Spratto, & Woods, 1991). Some commonly prescribed drugs, their actions, and nursing implications are shown in the accompanying pharmacology box.

Radioactive Therapy

Radioactive iodine (^{131}I) concentrates in the thyroid gland. In large doses, radioactive iodine damages or destroys thyroid tissue so that it produces less TH. Radioactive iodine is given orally. Results typically occur in 6 to 8 weeks. In most instances, the client is not hospitalized during treatment and does not require radiation precautions. This type of therapy is contraindicated in pregnant women because radioactive iodine crosses the placenta and can have negative effects on the developing fetal thyroid gland. Because the amount of gland destroyed is not readily controllable, the client may become hypothyroid and require life-long TH replacement.

Surgery

Some hyperthyroid clients have such enlarged thyroid glands that pressure on the esophagus or trachea causes breathing or swallowing problems. In these cases, removal of all or part of the gland is indicated. A subtotal **thyroidectomy** is usually performed. This procedure leaves enough of the gland in place to produce an adequate amount of TH. A total thyroidectomy is performed to treat cancer of the thyroid; the client then requires life-long hormone replacement.

Before surgery, the client should be in as nearly a euthyroid state as possible. Thus, the client may be given antithyroid drugs to reduce hormone levels and iodine preparations to decrease the vascularity and size of the gland (which also reduces the risk of hemorrhage during and after surgery).

Nursing care of the client having a subtotal thyroidectomy is discussed in the accompanying nursing care box.

Nursing Care of the Client Having a Subtotal Thyroidectomy

PREOPERATIVE CARE

- Administer ordered antithyroid medications and iodine preparations, and monitor their effects. *Antithyroid drugs are given before surgery to promote a euthyroid state. Iodine preparations are given to the client before surgery to decrease vascularity of the gland, thereby decreasing the risk of hemorrhage.*

- Teach the client to support the neck by placing both hands behind the neck when sitting up in bed, while moving about, and while coughing. *Placing the hands behind the neck provides support for the suture line.*

- Answer questions, and allow time for the client to verbalize concerns. *Because the incision is made at the base of the throat, clients (especially women) are often concerned about their appearance after surgery. Explain that the scar will eventually be only a thin line and that jewelry or scarves may be used to cover the scar.*

POSTOPERATIVE CARE

- Provide comfort measures: Administer analgesic pain medications as ordered, and monitor their effectiveness; place the client in a semi-Fowler's position after recovery from anesthesia; support head and neck with pillows. *Analgesic medications reduce the perception of pain and reduce physical stress during the postoperative period. Positioning the client in a semi-Fowler's position and supporting the head and neck decrease strain on the suture line.*

- Perform focused assessments to monitor for complications:
  a. *Hemorrhage.* Assess dressing (if present) and the area under the client's neck and shoulders for drainage. Monitor blood pressure and pulse for symptoms of hypovolemic shock. Assess tightness of dressing (if present). *The vascularity of the gland increases the risk of hemorrhage. The location of the incision and the position of the client may cause the drainage to run back and under the client. The danger of hemorrhage is greatest in the first 12 to 24 hours after surgery.*

  b. *Respiratory distress.* Assess respiratory rate, rhythm, depth, and effort. Maintain humidification as ordered. Assist the client with coughing and deep breathing. Have suction equipment, oxygen, and a tracheostomy set available for immediate use. *Respiratory distress may result from hemorrhage and edema, which may compress the trachea; from tetany and laryngeal spasms resulting from decreased hormones due to removal or damage to the parathyroid glands; and from damage to the laryngeal nerve, causing spasms of the vocal cords. Equipment must be immediately available if the client experiences respiratory distress that requires interventions and treatment.*

  c. *Laryngeal nerve damage.* Assess for the ability to speak aloud, noting quality and tone of voice. *The location of the laryngeal nerve increases the risk of damage during thyroid surgery. Although hoarseness may be due to edema or the endotracheal tube used during surgery and will subside, permanent hoarseness or loss of vocal volume is a potential danger.*

  d. *Tetany.* Assess for signs of calcium deficiency, including tingling of toes, fingers, and lips; muscular twitches; positive Chvostek's and Trousseau's signs; and decreased serum calcium levels. Keep calcium gluconate or calcium chloride available for immediate intravenous use, if necessary. *The parathyroid glands are located in and near the thyroid gland; surgery of the thyroid gland may injure or remove parathyroid glands, resulting in hypocalcemia and tetany. Tetany may occur in 1 to 7 days after thyroidectomy.*

A Critical Pathway for the client following thyroidectomy is provided on page 678.

Nursing Care

In planning and implementing nursing care for the client with hyperthyroidism, the nurse considers the client's responses to the systemic effects of the disorder. Although each client may have different needs, nursing diagnoses discussed in this section focus on the most common problems: cardiovascular problems, visual deficits, altered nutrition, and body image disturbance.

Risk for Decreased Cardiac Output

The client with hyperthyroidism is at high risk for alterations in cardiac output. Excess TH directly affects the heart, resulting in increased rate and stroke volume. Increases in the metabolic demands and oxygen requirements of peripheral tissues increase the demands on the heart, and systolic hypertension, angina, arrhythmias, or

text continues on page 679

Critical Pathway for Client Following Thyroidectomy

	Date _____ **1st Day Postoperative**	Date _____ **2nd Day Postoperative**	Date _____ **3rd Day Postoperative**
Expected length of stay: 3 days			
Daily outcomes	Client will ■ Be afebrile. ■ Have clean, dry wound with well-approximated edges healing by first intention. ■ Recover from anesthesia, as evidenced by return of vital signs to baseline, awake, alert, and oriented. ■ Verbalize understanding and demonstrate cooperation with turning, coughing, deep breathing, and splinting. ■ Demonstrate strategies to minimize stress on the suture line. ■ Tolerate ordered diet without nausea and vomiting. ■ Verbalize control of incisional pain. ■ Demonstrate ability to cope.	Client will ■ Be afebrile. ■ Have clean, dry wound with well-approximated edges healing by first intention. ■ Demonstrate cooperation with turning, coughing, deep breathing, and splinting. ■ Tolerate ordered diet without nausea and vomiting. ■ Ambulate 4 times per day. ■ Verbalize control of incisional pain. ■ Demonstrate ability to cope. ■ Verbalize beginning understanding of home care instructions.	Client will ■ Be afebrile. ■ Have a dry, clean wound with well-approximated edges healing by first intention. ■ Manage pain with nonpharmacologic measures. ■ Be independent in self-care. ■ Be fully ambulatory. ■ Have resumed preadmission urine and bowel elimination pattern. ■ Verbalize/demonstrate home care instructions. ■ Verbalize understanding of neck ROM exercises. ■ Tolerate usual diet. ■ Demonstrate/verbalize ability to cope with ongoing stressors.
Assessments, tests, and treatments	CBC. Vital signs and O$_2$ saturation, neurovascular assessment, dressing and wound drainage assessment q15min × 4; q30min × 4; q1h × 4 and then q4h if stable. Assess respiratory status and voice quality q2–4h and prn. Incentive spirometer q2h. Intake and output every shift. Assess voiding. If client is unable to void, try suggestive voiding techniques or catheterize q8h or prn. Keep HOB elevated 30 degrees. Place a small pillow under the head. Monitor for signs and symptoms of hypocalcemia, respiratory distress, hemorrhage, thyroid storm, or laryngeal nerve damage.	Vital signs and dressing and wound drainage assessment q4h. Assess respiratory status and voice quality q4h. Incentive spirometer q2h until fully ambulatory. Intake and output every shift. Assess voiding pattern q shift. Keep the HOB elevated 30 degrees. Keep a small pillow under the head.	Vital signs, dressing and wound drainage assessment q4h. Assess respiratory status and voice quality. Keep the HOB elevated 30 degrees. Keep a small pillow under the head.

	Date _____ 1st Day Postoperative	Date _____ 2nd Day Postoperative	Date _____ 3rd Day Postoperative
Knowledge deficit	Reorient to room and postoperative routine. Include family in teaching. Review plan of care and importance of early mobilization. Begin discharge teaching regarding wound care/dressing change. Instruct regarding the importance of minimizing stress on the suture line, including avoiding quick movements, hyperextension of the neck, and supporting head and neck when moving. Assess understanding of teaching.	Initiate discharge teaching regarding wound care, diet, and activity. Include family in teaching. Review written discharge instructions. Reinforce instructions regarding minimizing stress on the suture line. Instruct client regarding the importance of neck range-of-motion exercises. Demonstrate exercises, providing written instructions. Assess understanding of teaching.	Complete discharge teaching to include wound care, diet, follow-up care, signs and symptoms to report, activity, and medications: name, purpose, dose, frequency, route, dietary interactions, and side effects. Include family in teaching. Provide client with written discharge instructions. Assess understanding of teaching.
Psycho-social	Assess level of anxiety. Encourage verbalization of concerns. Provide information and ongoing support and encouragement to client and family.	Encourage verbalization of concerns. Provide ongoing support and encouragement to client and family.	Encourage verbalization of concerns. Provide ongoing support and encouragement to client and family.
Diet	Clear liquids to regular diet as tolerated.	Regular diet as tolerated.	Regular diet as tolerated.
Activity	Provide safety precautions. Bathroom privileges with assistance. Ambulate 4 times with assistance.	Provide safety precautions. Ambulate independently at least 4 times.	Fully ambulatory.
Medications	IM, IV, or PCA analgesics. IV fluid or intermittent IV device.	PO analgesics. Intermittent IV device.	PO analgesics.
Transfer/discharge plans	Assess discharge needs with client and family. Establish discharge goals with client and family.	Complete discharge plans. Make any appropriate referrals. Continue home care instructions.	Complete discharge instructions.

cardiac failure may occur. The client often has palpitations and shortness of breath and is easily fatigued. The risk of complications is greater in clients who have preexisting cardiovascular disorders.

Nursing interventions with rationales follow:

- Monitor blood pressure, pulse rate and rhythm, respiratory rate, and breath sounds. Assess for peripheral edema, jugular vein distention, and increased activity intolerance. *Increased TH increases cardiac rate, stroke volume, and tissue demand for oxygen, causing stress on the heart. This may result in hypertension, arrhythmias, tachycardia, and congestive heart failure.*

- Provide an environment that is cool and as free of distraction as possible. Decrease stress by explaining interventions and teaching relaxation procedures. *A calm environment that is physically comfortable and psychologically calm can reduce stimuli and stressors. Stress increases circulating catecholamines, which further increase cardiac workload.*

- Balance activity with rest periods. *Rest periods decrease energy expenditure and tissue requirements for oxygen, decreasing demands on the heart by decreasing cardiac workload.*

Sensory-Perceptual Alterations: Visual

Visual changes that occur in clients with hyperthyroidism include difficulty in focusing, diplopia, or visual loss. If the client is unable to close the eyelids because of exophthalmos, the risk of corneal dryness with resultant infection or injury increases. Visual deficits may also result from pressure on the optic nerve from retro-orbital edema and the shortening of eye muscles. Although treatment of hyperthyroidism may stop the progression of eye changes, not all of the symptoms are reversible.

Nursing interventions with rationales follow:

- Monitor visual acuity, photophobia, integrity of the cornea, and lid closure. *Edema behind the eyeball and in the extraocular muscles with forward protrusion of the eyeball may prevent complete eye closure. As a result, the cornea is at risk for dryness, injury, conjunctivitis, and corneal infections. Injury and infection of the cornea can result in further loss of visual acuity.*

- Teach the client measures for protecting the eye from injury and maintaining visual acuity:
  a. Use tinted glasses or shields as protection.
  b. Use artificial tears to moisten the eyes.
  c. Use cool, moist compresses to relieve irritation.
  d. Cover or tape the eyelids shut at night if they do not close.
  e. Sleep with the head of the bed elevated.
  f. Promptly report any pain or changes in vision.
  The measures outlined decrease the risk of injury, provide comfort, decrease periorbital edema that can further compromise vision, and ensure immediate care for problems, thereby minimizing the risk of further visual loss.

Risk for Altered Nutrition: Less Than Body Requirements

The hypermetabolic state that occurs in hyperthyroidism causes gastrointestinal hypermotility, with nausea, vomiting, diarrhea, and abdominal pain. Although the client

may have an increased appetite and eat more than usual, weight loss continues.

Nursing interventions with rationales follow:

- Weigh the client daily (at the same time each day), and record results. *The inability to meet metabolic demands results in loss of body weight. Regular monitoring detects continued weight loss.*

- In collaboration with a dietitian, teach the client the necessity to eat a diet that is high in carbohydrates and protein and includes between-meal snacks. Six small meals a day may be more desirable than three large meals. Caloric intake may need to be increased to 4000 kcal per day if weight loss exceeds 10% to 20% for height and frame. *Increased nutrients as part of a well-balanced diet are necessary to meet metabolic demands. Clients are often better able to increase food intake by eating frequent small meals. A 1-lb weight gain requires approximately 3500 extra kcal (Eschleman, 1991).*

- Monitor nutritional status through results of laboratory data. *Serum albumin, transferrin, and total lymphocyte counts are commonly lower than normal in nutritional deficits. A negative nitrogen balance signifies a catabolic state in which protein is lost and metabolic demands are not being met.*

Body Image Disturbance

The client with hyperthyroidism is at increased risk for disturbances in body image. Physical changes that are common in this disorder include exophthalmos, goiter, tremors, hair loss, increased perspiration, loss of strength, fatigue, weight loss, and changes in sexuality (amenorrhea in women, impotence in men, and increased libido in both men and women). In addition, the client often has mood changes and insomnia and is constantly nervous and anxious. There may even be periods of psychosis. These changes are frightening not only for the client but also for family members.

Nursing interventions with rationales follow:

- Establish a trusting relationship with the client, encouraging the client to verbalize feelings about self and to ask questions about the illness and treatment. Provide reliable information, and clarify misconceptions. *Body image is a person's self-perception, composed of interrelated phenomena of body surface and depth as well as the person's attitudes toward his or her body. Body image changes constantly, but there is a time lag between actual change and the person's perception of the change. The nurse must be aware that during the lag the client may reject both the diagnosis and the education and treatment that is prescribed (Carpenito, 1992).*

- Encourage family members to ask questions about changes they have noticed. Explain the effects of the illness on the client's physical and emotional status.

Feelings must be recognized before they can be adequately dealt with. Family members (including significant others) can be sources of strength and support as the client adapts to the illness, but they must first understand that the client's behavior and changes in appearance are often disease related and can be controlled with treatment.

Other Nursing Diagnoses

Examples of other nursing diagnoses that are appropriate for the client with hyperthyroidism follow:

- *Hyperthermia* related to increased metabolic rate and heat production
- *Activity Intolerance* related to muscle weakness and fatigue
- *Anxiety* related to a knowledge deficit about the effects of hyperthyroidism and the required length of treatment
- *Risk for Fluid Volume Deficit* related to diarrhea and excessive sweating
- *Sleep Pattern Disturbance* related to restlessness secondary to increased metabolic rate

Client and Family Teaching

Clients with hyperthyroidism primarily require self-care at home. Discharge planning focuses on individualizing teaching to the client's needs, depending on the type of treatment prescribed. For example, the client taking oral medications must understand the need for lifelong treatment, the client who has a thyroidectomy requires information about postoperative wound care, and the client having radioactive iodine therapy needs to know the symptoms of hypothyroidism. Depending on the age of the client and the support systems available, referral to community health care agencies may be necessary.

Applying the Nursing Process

Case Study of a Client with Graves' Disease: Juanita Manuel

Juanita Manuel is a 33-year-old mother of four small children. She is a second-year student at the local community college, within one semester of completing the requirements for an associate degree in child care. For the past 3 months, Ms. Manuel has been constantly hungry and has eaten more than usual, but she has still lost 15 lb (6.8 kg). She has repeated bouts of diarrhea and often feels nauseated. Her hands shake, she can feel her heart beating rapidly, and she finds herself laughing or crying for no apparent reason.

After visiting her family physician and having numerous tests, Ms. Manuel is admitted to the hospital for treatment of Graves' disease. Her nurse, Jennifer Booke, enters the room to complete the admission assessment. Noting that Ms. Manuel looks thin and anxious, Ms. Booke asks how she is feeling. Ms. Manuel answers, "Well, I'm scared to death, I'm hungry, and I'm so warm. Do you think you could get me something to eat and turn down the heat?"

Assessment

The admission history for Juanita Manuel indicates that although her appetite has increased, she had recently lost 15 lb (6.8 kg). She states that she has had diarrhea, nausea, palpitations, heat intolerance, and mood changes. Physical assessment findings include the following: T, 101 F (38.3 C); BP, 162/86; P, 110; R, 24. Her skin is moist and warm, her hair thin and fine. She has visible tremors in her hands. Her eyeballs protrude, and she is unable to close her eyelids completely. Her thyroid is enlarged and palpable. Diagnostic tests reveal the following abnormal results: T_3, 350 g/dL (normal range: 80 to 200 ng/dL); T_4, 15.1 μg/dL (normal range: 5 to 12 μg/dL). A thyroid scan demonstrates an enlarged thyroid with increased iodine uptake. After the medical diagnosis of Graves' disease is made, Ms. Manuel is started on the antithyroid medication propylthiouracil, 150 mg orally every 8 hours.

Diagnosis

Ms. Booke makes the following nursing diagnoses:

- *Risk for Altered Nutrition: Less Than Body Requirements* related to weight loss of 15 lb (6.8 kg), with present weight 10% less than normal for height
- *Diarrhea* related to increased peristalsis as evidenced by eight to ten liquid stools per day
- *Risk for Sensory/Perceptual Alterations: Visual* related to an inability to close the eyelids completely
- *Anxiety* related to a lack of knowledge about disease process

Expected Outcomes

The expected outcomes established in the plan of care specify that Ms. Manuel will:

- Gain at least 1 lb (0.45 kg) per week.
- Regain normal bowel elimination patterns.
- Maintain normal vision (with no evidence of corneal damage) and verbalize measures to protect her eyes.
- Verbalize medical treatment and self-care needs.
- Verbalize a decrease in anxiety.

Planning and Implementation

Ms. Booke plans and implements the following nursing interventions for Ms. Manuel:

- Take and record her weight before breakfast daily.

- Discuss adopting a high-kcalorie diet with Ms. Manuel. Identify her food likes and dislikes, as well as foods that increase her diarrhea, before instituting a plan to increase food intake.

- Maintain a stool chart. Note the time, type, and precipitating factors for diarrhea stools. Provide comfort measures for irritated anal area (clean washcloth and soap, nonirritating ointment).

- Teach Ms. Manuel how to apply eye drops (artificial tears).

- Elevate the head of her bed to 45 degrees at night. Tape eye shields over her eyes before sleep.

- Teach Ms. Manuel about Graves' disease, her medication's effects and side effects, and the need for continued medical care.

- Refer Ms. Manuel to a home health agency on discharge.

Evaluation

On discharge, Juanita Manuel has gained 1 lb (0.45 kg) and has discussed her dietary needs with the nurse and her husband. She is no longer having diarrhea. She has safely applied the eye drops and states that she will use the eye shields and elevate the head of her bed at night. Ms. Booke gives Ms. Manuel written and verbal information about Graves' disease and the medication prescribed. Ms. Manuel verbalizes her understanding, stating, "I'll always take my medicine—I never want to feel like that again!" She also says that she feels much less anxious now that she understands what has happened to her body and how she can help control those changes. Ms. Booke makes a referral to a home health agency in Ms. Manuel's community for any further questions and follow-up care.

Critical Thinking in the Nursing Process

1. What is the pathophysiologic basis for Ms. Manuel's abnormal vital signs on admission?

2. What is the rationale for having the client with exophthalmos elevate the head of the bed at night?

3. Suppose Ms. Manuel called two weeks after returning home, saying "This medicine isn't doing any good at all. I think I'll just stop taking it." What would your response be?

4. Outline a teaching plan that could be given to clients for home care following a subtotal thyroidectomy; include specific activities to promote self-care and wellness.

5. Develop a care plan for Ms. Manuel for the nursing diagnosis *Altered Family Processes.*

The Client with Hypothyroidism

Hypothyroidism results when the thyroid gland produces an insufficient amount of TH. Because a decrease in TH levels decreases metabolic rate and heat production, hypothyroidism affects all body systems (Figure 20–4). Hypothyroidism may be either primary or secondary. Primary hypothyroidism (which is the more common) may be caused by congenital defects in the gland, loss of thyroid tissue following treatment for hyperthyroidism with surgery or radiation, antithyroid medications, thyroiditis, or endemic iodine deficiency. Secondary hypothyroidism may result from pituitary TSH deficiency or peripheral resistance to thyroid hormones. Hypothyroidism has a slow onset, with manifestations occurring over months or even years. With treatment, the mental and physical symptoms rapidly reverse in clients of all ages. Unfortunately, the replacement of thyroid hormones may result in hyperthyroidism.

The complications of untreated hypothyroidism include adrenal insufficiency, cardiovascular disorders, and myxedema coma (discussed below).

Pathophysiology

Hypothyroidism is more common in women between ages 30 and 60; the incidence rises after age 50. However, the disorder can occur at any stage of life. Careful evaluation of symptoms is important in the older adult because manifestations of hypothyroidism are often thought to be the result of aging instead of a pathologic process.

The hypothyroid state in adults is sometimes called **myxedema**. The term *myxedema* reflects the characteristic accumulation of nonpitting edema in the connective tissues throughout the body. The edema is the result of water retention in mucoprotein (hydrophilic proteoglycans) deposits in the interstitial spaces. The face of a client with myxedema appears puffy, and the tongue is enlarged (Porth, 1994).

When TH production decreases, the thyroid gland enlarges in a compensatory attempt to produce more hormone. The goiter that results is usually a simple or nontoxic form. People living in certain areas of the world where the soil is deficient in iodine, the substance necessary for TH synthesis and secretion, are more prone to become hypothyroid and develop simple goiter. (Iodine deficiency is discussed below.)

Hypothyroid clients characteristically have the manifestations of goiter, dyspnea, fluid retention and edema, decreased appetite, weight gain, constipation, dry skin, and muscle stiffness. Also, many clients have neurologic changes, anemias, and cardiovascular deficits. Deficient amounts of TH cause abnormalities in lipid metabolism, with elevated serum cholesterol and triglyceride levels. As a result, the client is at increased risk for atherosclerosis and cardiac disorders.

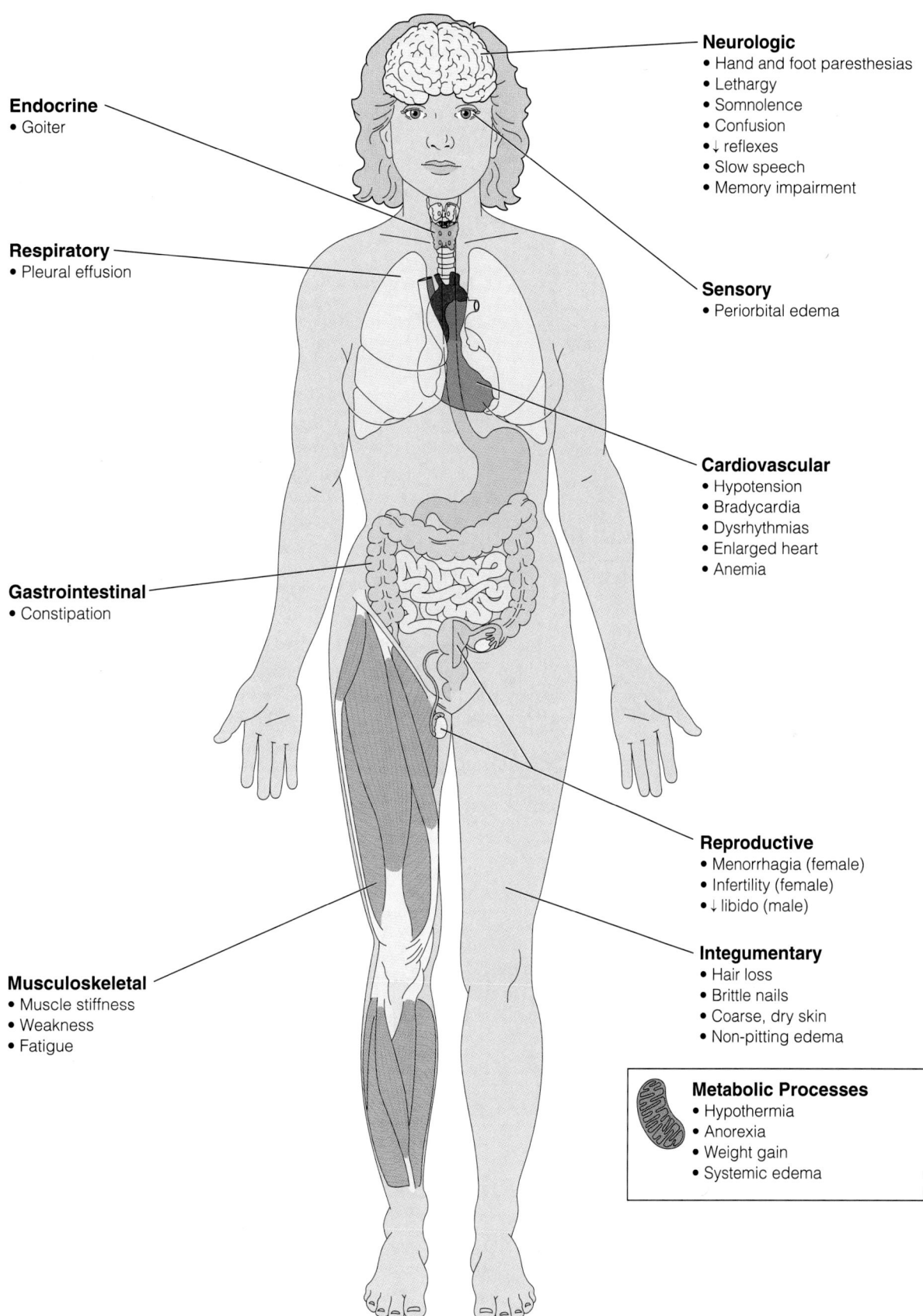

Endocrine
• Goiter

Respiratory
• Pleural effusion

Gastrointestinal
• Constipation

Musculoskeletal
• Muscle stiffness
• Weakness
• Fatigue

Neurologic
• Hand and foot paresthesias
• Lethargy
• Somnolence
• Confusion
• ↓ reflexes
• Slow speech
• Memory impairment

Sensory
• Periorbital edema

Cardiovascular
• Hypotension
• Bradycardia
• Dysrhythmias
• Enlarged heart
• Anemia

Reproductive
• Menorrhagia (female)
• Infertility (female)
• ↓ libido (male)

Integumentary
• Hair loss
• Brittle nails
• Coarse, dry skin
• Non-pitting edema

Metabolic Processes
• Hypothermia
• Anorexia
• Weight gain
• Systemic edema

Figure 20–4   **Multisystem effects of hypothyroidism.**

Table 20–2	Laboratory Findings in Hypothyroid Disorders	
Test	**Normal Values**	**Findings**
Serum TA	None to 1:20	Normal
Serum TSH	2 to 5.4 μU/mL	Increased in primary hypothyroidism
Serum T$_4$	5 to 12 μg/dL	Decreased
Serum T$_3$	80 to 200 ng/dL	Decreased
T$_3$ uptake (T$_3$RU)	25 to 35 relative percentage	Decreased
Thyroid suppression		No change in RAI uptake or T$_4$ levels

Factors that result in decreased TH (in addition to those described) include iodine deficiency and Hashimoto's thyroiditis. A severe state of hypothyroidism is called myxedema coma.

Iodine Deficiency

Iodine is necessary for TH synthesis and secretion. Iodine deficiency may result from certain goitrogenic drugs (which block TH synthesis); lithium carbonate, which is used to treat manic-depressive mental disorders, and antithyroid drugs are examples. Goitrogenic compounds in foods such as turnips, rutabagas, and soybeans may also block TH synthesis if consumed in sufficient quantities. In areas of the world where the soil is deficient in iodine, dietary intake of iodine may be inadequate. However, the use of iodized salt has reduced this risk in the United States.

Hashimoto's Thyroiditis

The most common form of primary hypothyroidism is **Hashimoto's thyroiditis**. In this disease, classified as an autoimmune disorder, antibodies develop that destroy thyroid tissue. Functional thyroid tissue is replaced with fibrous tissue, and TH levels decrease. In addition, decreasing levels of TH prompt the gland to enlarge to compensate, causing a goiter. This disorder is more common in women and has a familial link.

Myxedema Coma

Myxedema coma, or *hypothyroid crisis,* is a serious complication of extreme or prolonged hypothyroidism. It is a life-threatening state characterized by severe metabolic disorders (hyponatremia, hypoglycemia, lactic acidosis), hypothermia, cardiovascular collapse, and coma. Myxedema coma most commonly occurs in the older adult.

Myxedema coma may be precipitated by trauma, infection, failure to take thyroid replacement medications, the use of central nervous system depressants, and exposure to cold temperatures (Porth, 1994). The treatment of myxedema coma addresses the symptoms and involves maintaining a patent airway; maintaining fluid, electrolyte, and acid-base balance; maintaining cardiovascular status; increasing body temperature; and increasing TH levels.

Collaborative Care

The medical treatment of the client with hypothyroidism focuses on diagnosis, prevention or treatment of complications, and replacement of the deficient TH.

Laboratory and Diagnostic Tests

Hypothyroidism is diagnosed by the manifestations and by a decrease in TH, especially T$_4$. TSH concentration often is increased, because the negative hormonal feedback from TH is lost. The same laboratory and diagnostic tests that are used to diagnose hyperthyroidism are also used to diagnose hypothyroidism, with opposite results in most cases (see Table 20–2).

Pharmacology

Hypothyroidism is treated with pharmacologic preparations that replace TH. Drug therapy is initiated with small doses, which are gradually increased. Drugs commonly used to treat hypothyroidism and their nursing implications are shown in the accompanying pharmacology box.

Surgery

If the hypothyroid client has a goiter large enough to cause respiratory difficulties or dysphagia, a subtotal thyroidectomy may be performed. See the nursing care box on page 677.

Nursing Care

In planning and implementing care for clients with hypothyroidism, the nurse takes into account that the disorder affects all organ systems. Although many nursing diagnoses might be valid, this section focuses on client problems with cardiovascular function, elimination, and skin integrity.

Decreased Cardiac Output

A TH deficit causes a reduction in heart rate and stroke volume, resulting in decreased cardiac output. Additionally, there may be an accumulation of fluid in the pericardial sac (from the edema characteristic of hypothyroidism), and coronary artery disease may be present, further compromising cardiac function.

Nursing interventions with rationales follow:

Nursing Implications for Pharmacology: Hypothyroidism

THYROID PREPARATIONS

Levothyroxine sodium (T_4) (Levoid, Levothroid, Synthroid, Synthrox)

Liothyronine sodium (T_3) (Cyronine, Cytomel)

Liotrix (Euthroid, Thyrolar)

Thyroglobulin (Proloid)

Desiccated thyroid

Thyroid preparations increase blood levels of TH, thus raising the client's metabolic rate. As a result, cardiac output, oxygen consumption, and body temperature increase. The dosage depends on the drug chosen and the client's degree of thyroid dysfunction, sensitivity to TH, age, body size, and health. The older adult may require lower doses.

Nursing Responsibilities

- Give 1 hour before meals or 2 hours after meals for best absorption.

- Thyroid preparations potentiate the effect of anticoagulant drugs. If the client is also receiving an anticoagulant, monitor for bruising, bleeding gums, and blood in the urine.

- Thyroid medications potentiate the effect of digitalis. If the client is also receiving a digitalis preparation, monitor for signs of digitalis toxicity.

- Monitor for symptoms of coronary insufficiency: chest pain, dyspnea, tachycardia.

- If the client has insulin-dependent diabetes, monitor the effects of insulin. The effect of the insulin may change as thyroid function increases.

Client and Family Teaching

- Do not substitute brands of drugs or use generic equivalents without the physician's approval.

- The medications must be taken for the rest of one's life.

- Report symptoms of excess thyroid hormone to the physician: excess weight loss, palpitations, leg cramps, nervousness, or insomnia.

- If you have diabetes and use insulin, monitor blood glucose levels closely; the thyroid medications may alter the amount of insulin required.

- Thyroid preparations increase the risk of iodine toxicity. Do not use iodized salt or over-the-counter drugs containing iodine.

- If you are also taking an anticoagulant, report any signs of bleeding.

- Report any changes in menstrual periods.

- Take the thyroid preparation each morning to decrease the possibility of insomnia.

- Closely monitor blood pressure and pulse (older clients).

- Avoid excessive intake of foods that are known to inhibit TH utilization such as turnips, cabbage, carrots, spinach, and peaches.

- Assess blood pressure, rate and rhythm of apical and peripheral pulses, respiratory rate, and breath sounds. *TH deficit results in a reduced heart rate and stroke volume, decreasing peripheral blood flow; this in turn is evidenced by hypotension. Fluid may accumulate in the pericardial sac, restricting cardiac function. Monopolysaccharide deposits in the respiratory system decrease vital capacity and cause hypoventilation.*

- Maintain the environment to avoid chilling; increase room temperature, use additional bed covers, avoid drafts. *Chilling increases metabolic rate and puts increased stress on the heart.*

- Alternate activity with rest periods. Ask the client to report any breathing difficulties, chest pain, heart palpitations, or dizziness. *Activity increases demands on the heart and should be balanced with rest. Symptoms of car-* *diac stress include dyspnea, chest pain, palpitations, and dizziness.*

Constipation

The hypothyroid client is likely to have a reduced appetite and decreased food intake, a diminished activity level because of muscle aches and weakness, and reduced peristalsis to the point that fecal impactions may occur.

Nursing interventions with rationales follow:

- Encourage the client to maintain a liquid intake of up to 2000 mL per day. Discuss the client's preferred liquids and the best times of day to force fluids. If kcal intake is restricted, ensure that liquids have no kcal or are low in kcal. *Sufficient fluid intake is necessary to promote proper stool consistency.*

Applying Research to Nursing Practice
Predicting Pressure Sore Risk

■ ■ ■

The Braden Scale for Predicting Pressure Sore Risk was developed to identify clients who are at increased risk for developing pressure sores. The Braden Scale has six subscales: sensory perception, skin moisture, activity, mobility, friction and shear, and nutritional status. The scale was found to be a highly reliable tool for predicting pressure sore risk when used by registered nurses (Bergstrom, Braden, Laguzza, & Holman, 1987). However, continued research in carefully controlled situations is necessary before the scale is widely adopted.

Implications for Nursing

Clients with endocrine disorders commonly have or are at risk for developing pressure sores, which impair skin integrity. In addition, because the population of acutely ill and elderly clients requiring nursing care is increasing, the need to assess clients' risk of developing pressure sores has become more urgent. Pressure sores are disabling, require increased nursing interventions, and lengthen hospital stay; as a result, health care expenses increase. An accurate assessment tool can benefit clients and nurses and help contain spiraling health care costs.

Critical Thinking in Client Care

1. What specific pathophysiologic processes in clients with disorders of the thyroid or adrenal glands increase the risk of pressure sores?
2. How do alterations in each of the areas identified in the Braden Scale affect skin integrity?
3. What normal physiologic changes in the older adult increase the risk of pressure sores?
4. Describe nursing interventions to prevent an at-risk client from developing pressure sores.

■ Discuss with the client ways to maintain a high-fiber diet. *Diets high in fiber and fluid produce soft stools. Fiber that is not digested absorbs water, which adds bulk to the stool and assists in the movement of fecal material through the intestines.*

■ Encourage activity as tolerated. *Activity influences bowel elimination by improving muscle tone and stimulating peristalsis.*

Risk for Altered Skin Integrity

The client with hypothyroidism is at risk for altered skin integrity related to the accumulation of fluid in the interstitial spaces and to dry, rough skin. Further increasing the risk is decreased peripheral circulation, decreased activity levels, and slow wound healing.

Nursing interventions with rationales follow:

■ Monitor skin surfaces for redness or lesions, especially if the client's activity is greatly reduced. Use a pressure sore risk assessment scale to identify clients at risk. See the accompanying research box. *Hypothyroidism causes dry, rough, edematous skin conditions that increase the risk of skin breakdown.*

■ Provide or teach the immobile client measures to promote optimal circulation:
   a. Use a turning schedule if the client is on bed rest, or teach the client to change position every 2 hours.
   b. Limit the time for sitting in one position; shift weight or lift the body using arm rests every 20 to 30 minutes.
   c. Use pillows, pads, or sheepskin or foam cushions for bed and/or chair.
   d. Teach and implement a schedule of range-of-motion exercises.
   Prolonged pressure, especially in clients with edema and circulatory impairment, can occlude capillaries and cause hypoxic tissue damage.

■ Provide or teach the client measures to maintain skin integrity:
   a. Take baths only as necessary; use warm (not hot) water.
   b. Use gentle motions when washing and drying skin.
   c. Use alcohol-free skin oils and lotions.
   The dry skin and edema common in clients with hypothyroidism increase the risk of skin breakdown. Hot water, rough massage, and alcohol-based preparations may increase skin dryness, further impairing the body's ability to maintain skin integrity.

Other Nursing Diagnoses

Examples of other nursing diagnoses appropriate for the client with hypothyroidism follow:

■ *Altered Thought Processes* related to the effects of nervous system involvement secondary to the hypothyroid state

■ *Risk for Altered Body Temperature* related to TH deficit

■ *Activity Intolerance* related to muscle weakness and fatigue

■ *Impaired Verbal Communication* related to an enlarged tongue and impaired speech patterns

■ *Self-Esteem Disturbance* related to changes in appearance and self-care abilities.

Client and Family Teaching

Clients with hypothyroidism require lifelong care, primarily at home. Client and family teaching focuses on teaching self-care, compliance with prescribed medications, and the need for regular health assessments to promote wellness. The older adult may need referrals to social services or community health services, especially if home support is not available.

Applying the Nursing Process

Case Study of a Client with Hypothyroidism: Jane Lee

Jane Lee is a 60-year-old retired nurse living with her husband and daughter on a farm that has been in the family for four generations. Jane has gained 10 lb (4.5 kg) in the past few months, even though she is rarely hungry and eats much less than normal. She is always cold, tired, and weak—so tired that she has not even been able to help with the chores on the farm or do housework. She is concerned about her appearance and the way she sounds when she talks. Her face is puffy, and her tongue always feels thick. Mrs. Lee's husband, Jim, is concerned, because his wife "can't remember anything these days." Finally, Mr. Lee and their daughter, Kim, convince Jane to make an appointment at a health center in a nearby town.

Assessment

Brian Henning, RN, completes the admission assessment for Mrs. Lee at the health center. He finds that she now weighs 150 lb (68 kg), an increase of 10 lb (4.5 kg) over her weight at her last visit 6 months earlier. Mrs. Lee states that she always feels cold, tired, and weak. She also states that she is constipated, has difficulty remembering things, and looks different. Physical assessment findings included a palpable and bilaterally enlarged thyroid; dry, yellowish skin; nonpitting edema of the face and lower legs; and slow, slurred speech. Diagnostic tests revealed the following abnormal findings: T_3, 56 ng/dL (normal range: 80 to 200 ng/dL); T_4, 3.1 (normal range: 5 to 12 μg/dL); TSH, 6.2 μU/mL (normal range: 2.0 to 5.4 μU/mL). The medical diagnosis of hypothyroidism is made, and Mrs. Lee is started on levothyroxine 0.05 mg daily.

Diagnosis

The nursing diagnoses for Mrs. Lee include the following:

- *Constipation* related to decreased peristalsis, as evidenced by hard, formed stools every 4 days
- *Impaired Verbal Communication* related to changes in speech patterns and enlarged tongue
- *Self-Esteem Disturbance* related to changes in physical appearance and activity intolerance

Expected Outcomes

The expected outcomes established in the plan of care specify that Mrs. Lee will:

- Regain normal bowel elimination patterns, having a soft, formed stool at least every other day.
- Eat a diet high in fiber and in fluids.
- Experience improvement in verbal communication.
- Regain positive self-esteem as medications reduce physical changes and increase activity levels.

Planning and Implementation

In teaching Mrs. Lee to care for herself at home, Mr. Henning plans and implements the following interventions:

- Teach Mrs. Lee how to increase fluids, bulk, and fiber in her diet to help her regain a normal bowel elimination pattern of a soft, formed stool every other day.
- Teach her to take medications as prescribed and not to expect immediate reversal of symptoms affecting speech.
- Assist Mrs. Lee in planning activities around rest periods. Encourage her to allow her husband and daughter to help with housecleaning and cooking.
- Discuss with Mrs. Lee the effects of the disease and the effects of the medications in reversing physical and mental changes.

Evaluation

On her return visit to the health center 2 months later, Mrs. Lee tells Mr. Henning that she is no longer constipated but that she is continuing to drink six glasses of water and eating oatmeal every day. She no longer feels cold, is regaining her normal energy, and even feels well enough to plant her garden. Her speech is clear and easy to understand. As she leaves the examining room, Mrs. Lee says, "It's hard to believe that I have changed so much—now I look and feel like the 'old' me!"

Critical Thinking in the Nursing Process

1. What physical changes that normally occur with aging are similar to the manifestations of hypothyroidism?

2. Describe the factors that put Mrs. Lee's safety at risk. What alterations in her home environment would you suggest to promote safety until the prescribed medication takes effect?

3. The client taking oral thyroid medications may become hyperthyroid. List the signs and symptoms you

would include in a teaching plan to signal this condition.

4. Describe a home-based nursing care plan to promote wellness in Mrs. Lee despite the presence of this chronic illness.

5. Develop a care plan for Mrs. Lee for the nursing diagnosis *Sleep Pattern Disturbance*.

The Client with Cancer of the Thyroid

■ ■ ■

Thyroid cancer is relatively rare, with an estimated rate of 13,000 new cases annually. Thyroid cancer accounts for approximately 0.5% of all cancer deaths (American Cancer Society, 1994). The most consistent risk factor is exposure to ionizing radiation to the head and neck during childhood. For example, many adults in their 50s and 60s received X-ray treatments for colds and sinus infections during childhood.

Thyroid cancer is manifested by a small nodule in the thyroid. If undetected, the tumor may grow and impinge on the esophagus or trachea, causing difficulty in swallowing or breathing. Most people with thyroid cancer do not have elevated thyroid hormone levels.

The diagnosis is made by measuring thyroid hormones, performing thyroid scans, and by biopsy of the nodule. The usual treatment is subtotal or total thyroidectomy. TSH suppression therapy with levothyroxine may be conducted prior to surgery. Radioactive iodine therapy (^{131}I) and chemotherapy are additional therapeutic options. The 5-year survival rate, if the tumor has not metastasized, is 95% (American Cancer Society, 1994). Nursing care for the client with cancer is discussed in Chapter 9.

■ ■ ■ Disorders of the Parathyroid Glands ■ ■ ■

Disorders of the parathyroid glands, hyperparathyroidism and hypoparathyroidism, are not as common as those of the thyroid gland. Hypercalcemia and hypocalcemia (the primary results of alterations in parathyroid function) are discussed in Chapter 5.

The Client with Hyperparathyroidism

■ ■ ■

Hyperparathyroidism is the result of an increase in the secretion of parathyroid hormone (PTH), which regulates normal serum levels of calcium. The increase in PTH affects the kidneys and bones, resulting in the following pathophysiologic changes:

- Increased resorption of calcium and excretion of phosphate by the kidneys, which increases the risk of hypercalcemia and hypophosphatemia

- Increased bicarbonate excretion and decreased acid excretion by the kidneys, which increases the risk of metabolic acidosis and hypokalemia

- Increased release of calcium and phosphorus by bones, with resultant bone decalcification

- Deposits of calcium in soft tissues and the formation of renal calculi

Pathophysiology

Hyperparathyroidism occurs more often in older adults and is two times more common in women. The disorder itself is not common.

There are three types of hyperparathyroidism:

- *Primary hyperparathyroidism* occurs when there is hyperplasia or an adenoma in one of the parathyroid glands. These disorders interrupt the normal regulatory mechanism between serum calcium levels and PTH secretion and increase the absorption of calcium through the gastrointestinal tract.

- *Secondary hyperparathyroidism* is a compensatory response by the parathyroid glands to chronic hypocalcemia. It is characterized by an increased secretion of PTH.

- *Tertiary hyperparathyroidism* results from hyperplasia of the parathyroid glands and a loss of response to serum calcium levels. This disorder is most often seen in clients with chronic renal failure (McCance & Huether, 1994).

Many clients with hyperparathyroidism are asymptomatic. When symptoms occur, they are related to hypercalcemia and various musculoskeletal, renal, and gastrointestinal manifestations. Bone reabsorption results in pathologic fractures, while elevated calcium levels alter neural and muscular activity, leading to muscle weakness and atrophy. Proximal renal tubule function is altered, and metabolic acidosis, renal calculi formation, and polyuria occur.

Manifestations of the effect of hypercalcemia on the gastrointestinal tract include abdominal pain, constipation, anorexia, and peptic ulcer formation. Hypercalcemia also affects the cardiovascular system, causing arrhythmias, hypertension, and increased sensitivity to cardiotonic glycosides (for example, digitalis preparations).

The manifestations of hyperparathyroidism are summarized in the accompanying box.

Collaborative Care

Hyperparathyroidism is diagnosed by excluding all other possible causes of hypercalcemia; by at least a 6-month history of symptoms; by laboratory analysis of levels of calcium, phosphorus, magnesium, bicarbonate, and chloride; and by bone X-ray studies and scans (McCance & Huether, 1994).

The treatment of hyperparathyroidism focuses on decreasing the elevated serum calcium levels. Large amounts of saline fluids are given intravenously. Diuretics, such as furosemide (Lasix), are given orally or intravenously to increase renal excretion of calcium. If calcium levels are to be reduced more rapidly, medications might include oral or intravenous phosphates (which inhibit bone reabsorption and interfere with calcium absorption) and intravenous calcitonin (which directly inhibits bone reabsorption).

The treatment of primary hyperparathyroidism is surgical removal of the parathyroid glands affected by hyperplasia or adenoma. The preoperative and postoperative nursing care of the client having surgery of the parathyroids is essentially the same as that for the client having a thyroidectomy (see the nursing care box on page 677).

Nursing Care

Nursing care of the client with hypercalcemia is discussed in Chapter 5.

Examples of nursing diagnoses that are appropriate for the client with hyperparathyroidism follow:

- *Risk for Injury* related to loss of calcium from bones and potential pathologic fractures
- *Pain* related to the effects of increased parathyroid hormones: muscle weakness, abdominal pain
- *Impaired Physical Mobility* related to muscle weakness and osteoporosis.
- *Risk for Altered Urinary Elimination* related to hypercalcemia and formation of renal calculi
- *Fluid Volume Excess* related to intravenous administration of large amounts of fluids as therapy

The Client with Hyperparathyroidism

Hypoparathyroidism results from abnormally low PTH levels. The most common cause is damage to or removal of the parathyroid glands during thyroidectomy. The lack of circulating PTH causes hypocalcemia and an elevated blood phosphate level.

Clinical Manifestations of Hyperparathyroidism

Musculoskeletal System

- Bone pain (back, joints, shins)
- Pathologic fractures (women)
- Muscle weakness
- Muscle atrophy

Renal Effects

- Renal calculi
- Polyuria
- Polydipsia

Gastrointestinal System

- Abdominal pain
- Peptic ulcers
- Pancreatitis
- Nausea
- Constipation

Cardiovascular System

- Arrhythmias
- Hypertension

Central Nervous System

- Paresthesias
- Depression
- Psychosis

Metabolic Effects

- Acidosis
- Weight loss

Pathophysiology

Reduced levels of PTH result in impaired renal tubular regulation of calcium and phosphate. In addition, decreased activation of vitamin D results in decreased absorption of calcium by the intestines. The low calcium levels cause changes in neuromuscular activity, affecting peripheral motor and sensory nerves. Hypocalcemia lowers the threshold for nerve and muscle excitability; a slight stimulus anywhere along a nerve or muscle fiber initiates an impulse.

The neuromuscular manifestations that result include numbness and tingling around the mouth and in the fingertips, muscle spasms of the hands and feet, convulsions, and laryngeal spasms. **Tetany,** a continuous spasm of muscles, is the primary symptom of hypocalcemia. In severe cases of tetany, death may occur. Nursing assessments for tetany include Chvostek's sign and Trousseau's sign (see Chapter 19). The manifestations of hypoparathyroidism are summarized in the box on page 690.

Clinical Manifestations of Hypoparathyroidism

Musculoskeletal System

- Muscle spasms
- Carpopedal spasms
- Facial grimacing
- Tetany or convulsions

Integumentary System

- Brittle nails
- Dry, scaly skin
- Hair loss

Gastrointestinal System

- Abdominal cramps
- Malabsorption

Cardiovascular System

- Arrhythmias

Central Nervous System

- Paresthesias (lips, hands, feet)
- Hyperactive reflexes
- Psychosis
- Mood disorders (irritability, depression, anxiety)
- Increased intracranial pressure

Collaborative Care

Hypoparathyroidism is diagnosed by low serum calcium levels and high phosphorus levels in the absence of renal failure, an absorption disorder, or a nutritional disorder.

The treatment of hypoparathyroidism focuses on increasing calcium levels. Intravenous calcium is given immediately to reduce tetany. Long-term therapy includes supplemental calcium, increased dietary calcium, and vitamin D therapy.

Nursing Care

Nursing care for the client with hypocalcemia is discussed in Chapter 5.

Examples of nursing diagnoses that are appropriate for the client with hypoparathyroidism follow:

- *Risk for Injury* related to low levels of calcium and risk of tetany
- *Anxiety* related to a lack of knowledge about a diet that is high in calcium and low in phosphorus

Disorders of the Adrenal Gland

Disorders of the adrenal cortex or adrenal medulla result in changes in the production of adrenocorticotropic hormone (ACTH). Hormones of the adrenal cortex are essential to life. They maintain homeostasis in response to stressors. Disorders of the adrenal cortex result in complex physical, psychologic, and metabolic alterations that are potentially life threatening. Hormones of the adrenal medulla are not essential to life, because the sympathetic nervous system produces similar body responses. The disorders that occur are hyperfunction and hypofunction of the adrenal cortex and hyperfunction of the adrenal medulla.

The Client with Adrenal Cortex Hyperfunction

Cushing's syndrome is a chronic disorder in which hyperfunction of the adrenal cortex produces excessive amounts of circulating cortisol or ACTH. This disorder may be classified as primary, secondary, or iatrogenic, depending on the etiologic origin:

- Primary Cushing's syndrome is the result of a benign or malignant adrenal tumor that causes an increased production of cortisol.
- Secondary Cushing's syndrome is the result of one of the following conditions:
  a. A pituitary or hypothalamic disorder that causes increased release of ACTH; this disorder is called Cushing's disease.
  b. An ectopic disorder that produces ACTH (for example, bronchogenic or pancreatic carcinoma); this disorder is called ectopic Cushing's syndrome.
  In either case, the increased ACTH stimulation results in hyperplasia of the adrenal cortex with increased cortisol production.
- Iatrogenic Cushing's syndrome is the result of long-term glucocorticoid therapy (and excess cortisol levels).

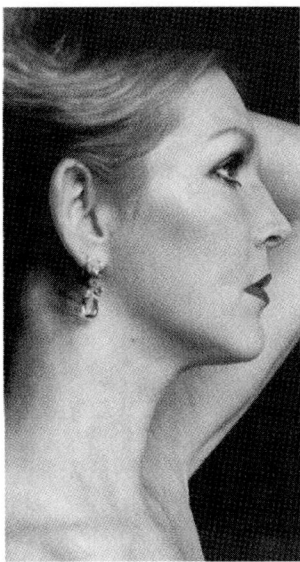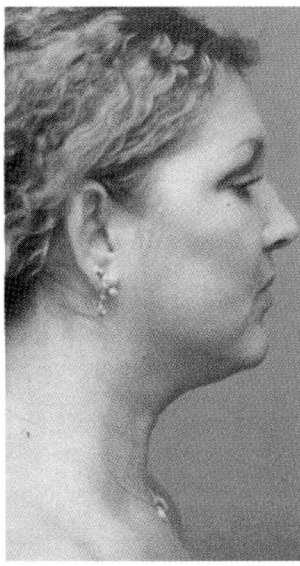

Figure 20–5 A woman before and after developing Cushing's syndrome. In the photo at right, notice the swollen facial features.

Pathophysiology

Both primary and secondary Cushing's syndrome are more common in women, with the average age of onset between 30 and 50 years (Figure 20–5). However, the disorder may occur at any age, especially when it is the result of pharmacologic therapy. Clients who take steroids over long periods of time (for example, for the treatment of arthritis, after an organ transplant, or as an adjunct to chemotherapy) are at increased risk for developing the iatrogenic form of the disorder.

The manifestations of Cushing's syndrome are the result of the ACTH or cortisol excess. Changes in fat metabolism result in fat deposits in the abdominal region, fat pads under the clavicle, a "buffalo hump" over the upper back, and a round "moon" face. Changes in protein metabolism cause muscle weakness and wasting, especially in the extremities. As thinned skin stretches over the abdomen and buttocks, purple striae (stretch marks) appear. Glucose metabolism is altered in the majority of clients, and diabetes mellitus may occur.

Electrolyte imbalances also occur with the increased hormone levels. Changes in calcium absorption result in osteoporosis, compression fractures of the vertebrae, fractures of the ribs, and renal calculi. Hypokalemia and hypertension occur as potassium is lost and sodium is retained. Inhibited immune responses increase the risk of infection, and increased gastric acid secretion increases the risk of peptic ulcers. Emotional changes range from depression to psychosis. In women, increasing androgen levels cause hirsutism (excessive facial hair in particular), acne, and menstrual irregularities. Additional pathophysiology related to specific nursing diagnoses is discussed in

the Nursing Care section. The manifestations and effects of Cushing's syndrome are grouped by body system in the accompanying box.

The complications of Cushing's syndrome, if untreated, include electrolyte imbalances (hyperglycemia, hypernatremia, and hypokalemia), hypertension, and emotional disturbances. If the client undergoes a bilateral adrenalectomy as a treatment for Cushing's syndrome, an acute deficit of cortisol (addisonian crisis) may result.

Clinical Manifestations of Cushing's Syndrome

Musculoskeletal System

- Weakness
- Muscle wasting
- Osteoporosis

Integumentary System

- Thin, easily bruised skin
- Skin infections
- Poor wound healing
- Eccymosis
- Purple striae (around thighs, breasts, abdomen)
- Hirsutism

Central Nervous System

- Emotional lability
- Psychoses

Gastrointestinal System

- Peptic ulcers

Cardiovascular System

- Hypertension

Renal Effects

- Renal calculi
- Polyuria
- Polydipsia
- Glycosuria

Metabolic Effects

- Hypokalemia
- Hypernatremia
- Truncal obesity

Reproductive System

- Oligomenorrhea or amenorrhea
- Impotence
- Decreased libido

Table 20–3   Laboratory Findings in Cushing's Syndrome

	Test	Normal Values	Findings
Serum	Cortisol	8 a.m. to 10 a.m.: 5 to 23 µg/dL	Increased
		4 p.m. to 6 p.m.: 3 to 13 µg/dL	
	Blood urea nitrogen (BUN)	5 to 25 mg/dL	Normal
	Sodium	135 to 145 mEq/L	Increased
	Potassium	3.5 to 5.0 mEq/L	Decreased
	Glucose (serum)	70 to 100 mg/dL	Decreased
Urine	17-KS	Male: 5 to 25 mg/24h	Increased
		Female: 5 to 15 mg/24h > 65: 4 to 8 mg/24h	

Collaborative Care

The treatment of Cushing's syndrome includes pharmacologic treatment, radiation therapy, or surgery, depending on the etiologic origin of the disorder. The most common treatment is surgery.

Laboratory and Diagnostic Tests

Cushing's syndrome is diagnosed through a variety of tests, including serum measurement of cortisol and urine tests for cortisol. Laboratory test findings in Cushing's syndrome are shown in Table 20–3.

The following laboratory tests may be ordered:

- *Measurement of plasma cortisol levels.* If Cushing's disease is present, test results show a loss of the normal diurnal variations of higher levels in the morning and lower levels in the afternoon.

- *Measurement of plasma ACTH levels* to determine the etiologic origin of the syndrome. Normally, plasma ACTH levels are highest from 7 a.m. to 10 a.m. and lowest from 7 p.m. to 10 p.m. In secondary Cushing's syndrome, ACTH is elevated; in primary Cushing's syndrome, ACTH is decreased.

- *24-hour urine tests* (17-ketosteroids and 17-hydroxycorticosteroids) to measure free cortisol and androgens; these hormones are increased in Cushing's syndrome.

- *Measurement of serum potassium, calcium, and glucose levels.* The levels are elevated in Cushing's syndrome.

Diagnostic studies for adrenal cortex function include

- *ACTH suppression test* to identify the cause of the disorder. A synthetic cortisol (dexamethasone) is given to suppress the production of ACTH, and plasma cortisol levels are measured. If an extremely high dose of cortisol is necessary to suppress ACTH, the primary disorder is adrenal cortex hyperplasia. If ACTH is not suppressed with the synthetic cortisol, an adrenal tumor is suspected.

Pharmacology

Cushing's syndrome that results from a pituitary tumor is treated by drugs as an adjunct to surgery or radiation. Pharmacologic treatment is also used for clients with inoperable pituitary or adrenal malignancies. Although the drugs control symptoms, they do not effect a cure. Examples of some commonly prescribed drugs follow:

- Mitotane directly suppresses activity of the adrenal cortex and decreases peripheral metabolism of corticosteroids.

- Metyrapone inhibits cortisol synthesis by the adrenal cortex.

Radiation Therapy

Radiation therapy may be useful in some clients with primary Cushing's syndrome. Local implants of radioactive isotopes or pituitary irradiation are used to destroy the pituitary gland. If the pituitary gland is destroyed by irradiation, lifelong replacement of pituitary hormones is necessary.

Surgery

When Cushing's syndrome is caused by an adrenal cortex tumor, an adrenalectomy may be performed to remove the tumor. Only one adrenal gland is usually involved; however, if an ACTH-producing ectopic tumor is involved, a bilateral adrenalectomy is performed. Lifelong hormone replacement is necessary if both adrenal glands are removed. Nursing care of the client having an adrenalectomy is discussed in the accompanying box.

Surgical removal of the pituitary gland (*hypophysectomy*) is indicated when Cushing's syndrome is the result of a pituitary disorder. The gland is removed either by a transphenoidal route or by a craniotomy. Nursing care for the client having cranial surgery is discussed further in Chapter 40.

Nursing Care

The nurse caring for the client with Cushing's syndrome must take a holistic approach to plan and implement interventions for a wide variety of responses, including problems related to fluid and electrolyte balance, injury, infection, and body image. For additional information about clients with alterations in fluid and electrolyte balance, see Chapter 5.

Nursing Care of the Client Having an Adrenalectomy

PREOPERATIVE CARE

- Request a dietary consultation to discuss with the client about a diet high in vitamins and proteins. If hypokalemia exists, include foods high in potassium. *Glucocorticoid excess increases catabolism. Vitamins and proteins are necessary for tissue repair and wound healing following surgery.*

- Use careful medical and surgical asepsis when providing care and treatments. *Cortisol excess increases the risk of infection.*

- Monitor the results of laboratory tests of electrolytes and glucose levels. *Electrolyte and glucose imbalances are corrected before the client has surgery.*

- Teach the client to turn, cough, and perform deep-breathing exercises. *Although they are important for all surgical clients, these activities are even more important for the client who is at risk for infection. Having the client practice and demonstrate the activities increases postoperative compliance.*

POSTOPERATIVE CARE

- Take and record vital signs, measure intake and output, and monitor electrolytes on a frequent schedule, especially during the first 48 hours after surgery. *Removal of an adrenal gland, especially a bilateral adrenalectomy, results in adrenal insufficiency. Addisonian crisis and hypovolemic shock may occur. Cortisol is often given on the day of surgery and in the postoperative period to replace inadequate hormone levels. Intravenous fluids are also administered.*

- Assess body temperature, WBC levels, and wound drainage. Change dressings using sterile technique. *Impaired wound healing increases the risk of infection in clients with adrenal disorders. Use aseptic technique to decrease this risk.*

Fluid Volume Excess

The excess cortisol secretion associated with Cushing's syndrome results in sodium and water reabsorption, causing fluid volume excess. The client will have weight gain, edema, and hypertension.

Nursing interventions with rationales follow:

- Weigh the client at the same time each day, and record results. *Body weight—provided that the client is weighed on the same scale at the same time each day and in the same clothing—is an accurate indicator of fluid status. One liter of fluid retention corresponds to about 2 lb (0.9 kg) of body weight.*

- Record accurate intake and output on each shift. *An analysis of the intake and output ratio of the previous 24 to 72 hours is necessary for assessing the risk of fluid imbalance.*

- Monitor blood pressure, rate and rhythm of pulse, respiratory rate, and breath sounds. Assess for peripheral edema and jugular vein distention. *Extracellular fluid volume excess resulting from sodium and water retention is manifested by hypertension and a bounding, rapid pulse. In addition, there may be crackles and wheezes, dependent edema, and venous distention.*

- Teach the client and family the reasons for restricting fluid and the importance of limiting fluids if ordered. *Restricting fluid can help decrease the risk of fluid volume excess. Involving the client and family in the plan of care and teaching the rationale for interventions facilitates achieving goals.*

Risk for Injury

The client with Cushing's syndrome is at risk for injury from several causes. Excess cortisol causes increased absorption of calcium and demineralization of bones, resulting in osteoporosis and risk of pathologic fractures. Muscle weakness and fatigue are common, increasing the potential for accidental falls.

Nursing interventions with rationales follow:

- Maintain a safe environment:
  a. Keep unnecessary clutter and equipment out of the way and off the floor.
  b. Ensure adequate lighting, especially at night.
  c. Encourage the client to use assistive devices for ambulation or to ask for help if needed.
  d. If the client wears corrective lenses, be sure they are available and clean.
  e. Encourage the use of nonskid slippers or shoes.
  f. Monitor for signs of fatigue (increased pulse and respirations); plan rest periods.
  An environment that is free of clutter and well lighted decreases the risk of falls and injury. Sensory and motor deficits increase the risk of falls; corrective lenses, assistive devices, and nonslip footwear can decrease this risk. Rest relieves fatigue. To reduce energy expenditure, the nurse should include alternating periods of rest and activity in daily schedules.

Risk for Infection

Elevated cortisol levels impair the immune response and put the client with Cushing's syndrome at increased risk for infection. Increased cortisol also affects protein synthesis, causing delayed wound healing, and inhibits collagen formation, which results in epidermal atrophy, further inhibiting resistance to infection. In addition, impaired blood flow to edematous tissue results in altered cellular nutrition, which increases the potential for infection.

Nursing interventions with rationales follow:

- Place the client in a private room, and limit visitors. *The client with Cushing's syndrome has an impaired immune response, and therefore must avoid exposure to environmental infection.*

- Monitor the client's vital signs and verbalizations of his or her physical state (for example, the client's response to, "How do you feel?") every 4 hours. *Increased body temperature and pulse are systemic indicators of infection. However, because Cushing's syndrome impairs the normal inflammatory response, the usual indicators of inflammation may not be present. A generalized feeling of malaise may be the primary manifestation of infection.*

- Use principles of medical asepsis and sterile asepsis when caring for the client, conducting procedures, or providing wound care. *An impaired immune response increases the risk of infection. Impaired skin and tissues make aseptic techniques even more necessary to decrease this risk. Intact skin is the first line of defense against infection; if invasive procedures are performed or a wound is present, this defense is lost.*

- If wounds are present, assess the color, odor, and consistency of wound drainage. Also assess for increased pain in and around the wound. *Cortisol excess delays wound healing and closure.*

- Teach the client to increase intake of protein and vitamins C and A. *Protein, vitamin C, and vitamin A are necessary to collagen formation; collagen helps support and repair body tissues.*

Body Image Disturbance

The client with Cushing's syndrome has obvious physical changes in appearance. The abnormal fat distribution, moon face, buffalo hump, striae, acne, and facial hair (in women) all contribute to disruptions in the way clients with this disorder perceive themselves.

Nursing interventions with rationales follow:

- Encourage the client to express feelings and to ask questions about the disorder and its treatment. *The loss of one's normal body image may prompt feelings of hopelessness, powerlessness, anger, and depression. Understanding the disease and adapting to changes from that disease are the first steps in regaining control of one's own body.*

- Ask the client to discuss strengths and previous coping strategies. Enlist the support of family or significant others in reaffirming the client's worth. *Disturbances in body image are often accompanied by low self-esteem. Self-esteem derives from one's perception of competence and from appraisals of others.*

- Discuss signs of progress in controlling symptoms; for example, decreased facial edema or increased activity tolerance. *Many of the physical changes from cortisol excess disappear with treatment. The nurse should clearly communicate this fact, because the client may believe changes are permanent.*

Other Nursing Diagnoses

Examples of other nursing diagnoses that are appropriate for the client with Cushing's syndrome follow:

- *Activity Intolerance* related to muscle weakness and fatigue

- *Risk for Impaired Skin Integrity* related to capillary fragility and edema

- *Altered Thought Processes* related to cortisol excess

- *Risk for Decreased Cardiac Output* related to hypokalemia

- *Anxiety* related to lack of knowledge about preoperative and postoperative care for cranial surgery

- *Altered Sexuality Patterns* related to changes in physical appearance and fear of partner's response

Client and Family Teaching

The client with Cushing's syndrome requires education about self-care at home specific to the type of treatment given. Discharge planning focuses on safety measures if fatigue, weakness, and osteoporosis are present; on taking medications as prescribed; and on having regular health assessments to maximize wellness. Clients often require medications for the rest of their lives, and dosage changes are highly likely. Although all clients should have access to information and health resources, the older client may especially require referrals to social services or community health services because of the complexity of the treatment and care required.

Applying the Nursing Process

Case Study of a Client with Cushing's Syndrome: Sara Domico

Sara Domico is a 30-year-old lawyer living in a major metropolitan area. She has never been married, and she shares her life with her cat, Beau, and her parents, who live nearby. Her physician recently diagnosed Ms. Domico as having Cushing's syndrome and admits her to the hospital to identify the cause of her disease. She has been having increased muscle weakness, so much so that she has difficulty climbing the one flight of stairs to her apartment. She has also had difficulty sleeping, irregular menstrual periods, and hypertension. Ms. Domico is especially concerned about her protruding abdomen, round face, development of facial hair, and the numerous bruises that have appeared on her skin.

Assessment

When Ms. Domico arrives at the hospital, she is admitted by her case manager, Ann Sprengel. Ms. Sprengel completes a physical assessment and finds that Ms. Domico has thin lower extremities, an enlarged abdomen, purple striae over the abdomen and buttocks, a round face, and obvious facial hair. Her blood pressure is 160/96. Ms. Domico tells Ms. Sprengel that she is always tired and that sometimes it "just wears me out to walk from the bedroom to the kitchen." Diagnostic tests at 9 a.m. reveal the following abnormal findings:

Glucose: 186 mg/dL (normal range: 70 to 110 mg/dL)

Sodium: 152 mEq/L (normal range: 135 to 145 mEq/L)

Potassium: 3.2 mEq/L (normal range: 3.5 to 5.0 mEq/L)

Calcium: 4.3 mEq/L (normal range: 4.5 to 5.5 mEq/L)

Cortisol: 35 μg/dL (normal for a.m.: 5 to 23 μg/dL)

Following several more days of tests, the health care team determines that Ms. Domico has an adrenal cortex tumor, and an adrenalectomy is scheduled.

Diagnosis

The nursing diagnoses for Ms. Domico include the following:

- *Fluid Volume Excess* related to sodium retention causing edema and hypertension
- *Risk for Injury* related to generalized fatigue and weakness
- *Risk for Infection* related to impaired immune response and edema
- *Body Image Disturbance* related to physical changes secondary to Cushing's syndrome

Expected Outcomes

The expected outcomes established in the plan of care specify that Ms. Domico will

- Regain a normal body fluid balance.
- Remain free of injury.
- Remain free of infection.
- Verbalize understanding of the physical effects of the disease process and realistic expectations of desired changes in her appearance.

Planning and Implementation

Ms. Sprengel plans and implements the following interventions to care for Ms. Domico:

- Weigh her each morning, using the same scale.
- Maintain an accurate record of her intake and output. Discuss fluid restriction and mutually determine the amount of liquid to be included with meals and the amount of liquid to be provided at other times of the day.
- Ensure adequate lighting in the room, and ask Ms. Domico to wear glasses and shoes when she gets out of bed.
- Develop with Ms. Domico a written schedule of rest and activity periods.
- If agreeable, provide her with a private room, and restrict her visitors to her mother and father at this time.
- Use strict medical and surgical asepsis when providing care.
- Provide time for discussion of the disease and treatment; encourage Ms. Domico to verbalize her feelings and to identify successful coping mechanisms used in the past.

Evaluation

Ms. Domico stated that she is "ready to have surgery and start feeling better." She has not fallen or injured herself, and she has remained free of infection. Although edema is still present, she has lost 8 lb (3.6 kg), and her blood pressure is lower. Ms. Domico has openly discussed her concerns about the way she looks and feels; she understands that symptoms will improve following surgery. Ms. Domico has strong religious beliefs and family support, both of which provide strength and help her cope with the effects of the disorder and the need for further treatment.

Critical Thinking in the Nursing Process

1. When Sara Domico was admitted to the hospital, several of her test results were abnormal. Describe the pathophysiologic reason for those results.

2. List the assessments that nurses can make to determine body fluid balance.

3. One of the nursing interventions for this client was to ask her to wear her glasses and shoes when she got out of bed. What is the rationale for this intervention?

4. Develop a teaching plan for Ms. Domico that will help her return to an optimal level of functioning after she returns home.

5. Develop a plan of care for this client for the nursing diagnosis *Fatigue*.

The Client with Adrenal Cortex Hypofunction

▪ ▪ ▪

Adrenal cortex hypofunction may be either primary or secondary:

- Primary adrenal insufficiency is the result of the destruction of the layers of the adrenal cortex. Although the exact cause is unknown, most cases are believed to be an autoimmune disorder resulting in atrophy of the adrenal cortex (Porth, 1994). The most common form of adrenal cortex insufficiency is Addison's disease. Other causes include tuberculosis, septicemia, bilateral adrenalectomy, and infiltrative diseases. With loss of glandular tissue, chronic low levels of cortisol secretion develop.

- Secondary adrenal insufficiency is caused by an ACTH deficit resulting from pituitary tumors, pituitary surgery or irradiation, and the use of exogenous steroids.

Pathophysiology

There are many possible causes of adrenal cortex hypofunction. The most common form of the disorder, Addison's disease, and the most severe form, addisonian crisis, are described in this section.

Addison's Disease

Addison's disease is a condition resulting from failure of adrenal cortex function, with deficits of glucocorticoids, mineralocorticoids, and androgens. It can occur at any age, although it is more common in adults under the age of 60. Like many endocrine disorders, Addison's disease is more common in women.

The risk of developing the disorder is high in clients who are abruptly withdrawn from long-term, high-dose steroid therapy. Other clients at risk are those with tuberculosis or acquired immune deficiency syndrome (AIDS); the pathogens responsible for either disease can infiltrate and destroy adrenal tissue. Finally, anticoagulant drugs may cause adrenal hemorrhage and subsequent adrenal hypofunction.

The onset of Addison's disease is slow; the client experiences symptoms after about 90% of the function of the gland is lost (Schira, 1987). The primary manifestations are the result of elevated ACTH levels and decreased aldosterone and cortisol. (See the accompanying box.) Aldosterone deficiency affects the ability of the distal tubules of the nephron to conserve sodium. Hence, sodium is lost, potassium is retained, extracellular fluid is depleted, and the blood volume is decreased. Postural hypotension and syncope are common, and hypovolemic shock may occur. Hyponatremia causes dizziness, confu-

sion, and neuromuscular irritability. Hyperkalemia causes cardiac arrhythmias.

Cortisol insufficiency also causes decreased hepatic glyconeogenesis with hypoglycemia. The client tolerates stress poorly and experiences lethargy, weakness, anorexia, nausea, and vomiting. The increased ACTH levels stimulate hyperpigmentation in about 98% of clients with Addison's disease (Porth, 1994). In Caucasian clients, the skin looks deeply suntanned or bronzed in both exposed and unexposed areas.

Complications of Addison's disease include addisonian crisis (discussed below) and the onset of other autoimmune endocrine disorders, such as insulin-dependent diabetes mellitus and thyroid disease.

Addisonian Crisis

Addisonian crisis is a serious, life-threatening response to acute adrenal insufficiency. This response can occur in any person with Addison's disease. However, it is most commonly precipitated by major stressors, especially if the disease is poorly controlled. Addisonian crisis may also occur in clients who are abruptly withdrawn from glucocorticoid medications or who have hemorrhage into the adrenal glands from either septicemia or anticoagulant therapy.

The client with addisonian crisis may have any of the symptoms of Addison's disease, but the primary problems are severe hypotension, circulatory collapse, shock, and coma. Treatment of the crisis is rapid intravenous replacement of fluids and glucocorticoids. Fluid balance is usually restored in 4 to 6 hours.

Collaborative Care

The client with Addison's disease requires early diagnosis and treatment. Medical treatment includes cortisol replacement therapy. Unfortunately, this can induce Cushing's syndrome.

Laboratory and Diagnostic Tests

Addison's disease is diagnosed through findings of decreased levels of cortisol, aldosterone, and urinary 17-ketosteroids. Dehydration may result in increased hematocrit and blood urea nitrogen (BUN). Blood glucose levels are decreased, and potassium is increased. A list of laboratory findings in Addison's disease is shown in Table 20–4.

The following laboratory tests may be ordered:

- *Serum cortisol levels.* Cortisol levels are decreased in adrenal insufficiency.

- *Blood glucose levels.* Blood glucose levels are decreased in adrenal insufficiency.

- *Serum sodium levels.* Serum sodium levels are decreased in adrenal insufficiency.

Clinical Manifestations of Addison's Disease

Integumentary System

- Delayed wound healing
- Hyperpigmentation

Cardiovascular System

- Postural hypotension
- Tachycardia
- Arrhythmias

Central Nervous System

- Lethargy
- Emotional lability
- Tremors
- Confusion

Musculoskeletal System

- Weakness
- Joint pain
- Muscle wasting
- Muscle pain

Gastrointestinal System

- Anorexia
- Diarrhea
- Nausea and vomiting

Reproductive System

- Menstrual changes

Metabolic Effects

- Hyperkalemia
- Hypoglycemia
- Hyponatremia

Table 20–4		Laboratory Findings in Addison's Disease	
	Test	**Normal Values**	**Findings**
Serum	Cortisol	8 a.m. to 10 a.m.: 5 to 23 μg/dL	Decreased
		4 p.m. to 6 p.m.: 3 to 13 μg/dL	
	Blood urea nitrogen (BUN)	5 to 25 mg/dL	Increased
	Sodium	135 to 145 mEq/L	Decreased
	Potassium	3.5 to 5.0 mEq/L	Increased
	Glucose (serum)	70 to 100 mg/dL	Decreased
Urine	17-KS	Male: 5 to 25 mg/24h	Low/ Absent
		Female: 5 to 15 mg/24h	
		> 65: 4 to 8 mg/24h	

- *Electrocardiogram (EKG)*. Changes that are characteristic of hyperkalemia include peaked T waves, widening QRS complex, and an increased PR interval.

Pharmacology

The primary medical treatment of Addison's disease is replacement of corticosteroids and mineralocorticoids, accompanied by increased sodium in the diet. Hydrocortisone is given orally to replace cortisol; fludrocortisone (Florinef) is given orally to replace mineralocorticoids. Nursing implications in cortisol replacement are given in the box on page 698.

Nursing Care

The client with Addison's disease requires nursing care for a wide variety of responses to the decrease in cortisol levels. Nursing diagnoses discussed in this section are directed toward problems with fluid and electrolyte balance and compliance with lifelong hormone replacement.

Fluid Volume Deficit

In the client with Addison's disease, fluid volume deficit results from loss of water and sodium, as well as from vomiting and diarrhea. Extracellular fluid volume deficit, decreased cardiac output, hypotension, and hypovolemic shock may occur, especially in crisis situations.

Nursing interventions with rationales follow:

- Monitor intake and output, and assess for signs of dehydration:
  a. Dry mucous membranes
  b. Thirst

- *Serum potassium levels*. Serum potassium levels are increased in adrenal insufficiency.
- *BUN levels*. BUN is increased in adrenal insufficiency.
- *Urinary 17-hydroxycorticoids and 17-ketosteroids (17-KS) levels*. These measure adrenal cortical function and are decreased in adrenal insufficiency.
- *Plasma ACTH levels*. These are increased in primary adrenal insufficiency but decreased in secondary adrenal insufficiency.

Diagnostic studies may include

- *ACTH stimulation test*. Cortisol levels rise with pituitary deficiency but do not rise in primary adrenal insufficiency.
- *CT scans of the head*. These identify any intracranial problem impinging on the pituitary gland.

Nursing Implications for Pharmacology: Addison's Disease

CORTISOL REPLACEMENTS

Cortisone (Cortone, Cortogen)

Hydrocortisone (Cortisol, Hydrocortone, Cortef)

Prednisone (Meticorten, Deltasone, Orasone)

Fludrocortisone acetate (Florinef, F-Cortef)

Dexamethasone (Decadron, Hexadrol, Dexasone)

Prednisolone (Meticortelone)

Methylprednisolone (Medrol, Solu-Medrol)

Adrenocorticosteroids are used for replacement therapy in acute and chronic adrenal insufficiency. These drugs have anti-inflammatory and immunosuppressant effects. They also facilitate coping with stress.

Because corticosteroids are immunosuppressants, their use is contraindicated when an infection is suspected because they mask the signs of infection. Corticosteroids are also contraindicated in many other disorders, including peptic ulcer, Cushing's syndrome, cardiac disease, hyperthyroidism, hypothyroidism, and tuberculosis.

When these drugs are administered in small doses for replacement therapy, side effects are uncommon. Large doses or prolonged therapy may cause a Cushing-like syndrome, with atrophy of the adrenal cortex. Older clients, especially postmenopausal women, are more prone to develop hypertension and osteoporosis when undergoing glucocorticoid therapy. These drugs are used with caution in children and the older adult and are not usually administered to pregnant women.

Nursing Responsibilities

- Establish baseline data, including mental status, neurologic function, vital signs, and weight.
- Identify medications that might interact with corticosteroids: antidiabetic agents, cardiac glycosides, oral contraceptives, anticoagulants.

- Document and report increased blood pressure, edema or weight gain, bleeding or bruising, weakness, or manifestations of Cushing's syndrome.
- Administer oral forms of the drug with food to minimize its ulcerogenic effect.
- Monitor electrolyte levels for increased sodium and decreased potassium.

Client and Family Teaching

- Take medications with food or milk, and report any gastric distress or dark stools.
- Most people need to take the medications for the rest of their lives.
- Consume a diet that is high in potassium, low in sodium, and high in protein.
- Weigh yourself each day at the same time, and report any consistent weight gain, which indicates fluid retention.
- Use safety measures in the home to prevent falls and injuries.
- Corticosteroids may impair the effectiveness of oral contraceptives.
- Take the medication regularly and continuously. *Abruptly discontinuing the medication is dangerous.*
- Obtain a MedicAlert bracelet.
- Monitor for increased stressors (infection, dental work, personal crisis) and increase the dose as indicated by the physician.
- Anticoagulant drugs or insulin may decrease the effectiveness of corticosteroids.
- Report the following to the physician: dizziness on sitting or standing, nausea and vomiting, pain, thirst, feelings of anxiety, malaise, infections.

c. Poor skin turgor
d. Sunken eyeballs
e. Scanty, dark urine
f. Increased urine specific gravity
g. Weight loss
h. Increased hemoconcentration (increased hematocrit and BUN).

Glucocorticoid and mineralocorticoid depletion causes fluid volume deficit. Fluid volume deficit may reach crisis levels

if undetected, causing altered tissue perfusion and hypovolemic shock. Manifestations of dehydration include dry mucous membranes, thirst, poor skin turgor, decreases in urine output and changes in urine concentration and appearance, weight loss, and alterations in blood composition.

- Monitor cardiovascular status: Take and record vital signs, assess character of pulses, and monitor potassium levels. *Fluid volume deficit may lead to hypotension and a rapid, weak, or thready pulse. As aldosterone levels fall, renal excretion of potassium decreases, increasing blood levels of potassium. High serum potassium causes changes in cardiac muscle function, which are reflected in EKG changes.*

- Weigh the client daily at the same time and in the same clothing. *A 2% to 4% weight loss indicates mild dehydration; a 5% to 9% loss indicates moderate dehydration (Carpenito, 1992).*

- Encourage the client to maintain an oral fluid intake of 3000 mL per day to increase salt intake. *Cortisol deficiency increases fluid loss, leading to extracellular fluid volume depletion. Oral fluid replacement is necessary to balance this loss. An increase in dietary sodium can decrease the hyponatremia characteristic of adrenal insufficiency.*

- Teach the client to sit and stand slowly, and provide assistance as necessary. *Extracellular fluid volume deficit causes orthostatic hypotension, dizziness, and possible loss of consciousness. These manifestations increase the risk of injury from falls.*

Risk for Ineffective Management of Therapeutic Regimen

The client with Addison's disease must be taught about the need for lifelong treatment and self-care, including medication, diet, fluid intake, and response to stressors. Changes in life-style are difficult to maintain permanently.

- Teach the client the effects of illness and treatment. Encourage the client to verbalize concerns. *Lack of knowledge about the illness, as well as the possibility of complications from disregarding or altering the treatment, can negatively affect compliance.*

- Include the following in the teaching plan:
  a. Self-administration of steroids
  b. The importance of carrying at all times an emergency kit containing parenteral cortisone and a syringe/needle
  c. Wearing a MedicAlert bracelet containing information about the illness and treatment
  d. Increasing oral fluid intake
  e. Maintaining diet that is high in sodium and low in potassium
  f. Not to skip meals
  g. The necessity of altering the medication dose when experiencing emotional or physical stressors
  h. The importance of continuing health care
  One of the most important components of caring for the client with Addison's disease is teaching both the client and family to provide care. Family stability, an awareness of the serious nature of the disease, and the effectiveness of treatment all promote compliance. The length of treatment and the side effects of medications, however, can discourage compliance.

Other Nursing Diagnoses

Other possible nursing diagnoses for the client with Addison's disease follow:

- *Ineffective Individual Coping* related to emotional lability and intolerance of stress secondary to decreased cortisol levels
- *Activity Intolerance* related to muscle weakness and fatigue
- *Altered Tissue Perfusion* related to fluid volume deficit secondary to decreased cortisol levels
- *Anxiety* related to lack of knowledge about the effects of the disease
- *Risk for Injury* related to dizziness and syncope secondary to postural hypotension.

Client and Family Teaching

The client with Addison's disease provides self-care at home. Education, as described in the Nursing Care section, is critical to ensuring that the client and/or family can safely and knowledgeably provide care and maximize wellness in daily life and in crisis situations. The nurse makes referrals to community health services for information and follow-up health care.

Applying the Nursing Process

Case Study of a Client with Addison's Disease: Don Sardoff

A 51-year-old unemployed salesman, Don Sardoff is brought to the emergency room by his wife, Ellen, at 8 a.m. Mrs. Sardoff tells the emergency room nurse that her husband has not been feeling well for the last week, but that when he got up this morning, he was so weak he couldn't dress himself and didn't know where he was. Mrs. Sardoff also tells the nurse that her husband has been taking a cortisone drug for treatment of his rheumatoid arthritis for the past 2 years but notes, "We didn't have the money to buy it this month."

Assessment

On admission to the emergency room, Mr. Sardoff is dehydrated, with dry oral mucous membranes and tongue, poor skin turgor, and sunken eyeballs. His blood pressure is 94/44, and his pulse is rapid and thready. He is weak, dizzy, and disoriented about time and place. Diagnostic tests reveal the following abnormal findings at 8:30 a.m.:

EKG: widening QRS complex and increased PR interval

Sodium: 129 mEq/L (normal range: 135 to 145 mEq/L)

Glucose: 54 mg/dL (normal range: 70 to 110 mg/dL)

Potassium: 5.3 mEq/L (normal range: 3.5 to 5 mEq/L)

Cortisol: 2 μg/dL (normal for a.m.: 5 to 23 μg/dL)

The medical orders for Mr. Sardoff include intravenous administration of 5% dextrose in normal saline (D_5NS) at 250 mL/h and hydrocortisone (Solu-Cortef) 200 mg. After the fluids and medication are initiated, Mr. Sardoff is moved to an in-hospital medical bed.

Diagnosis

Mr. Sardoff's nurse, Peg Flaherty, develops the following nursing diagnoses:

- *Fluid Volume Deficit* related to hypovolemia secondary to adrenal insufficiency
- *Altered Tissue Perfusion: Peripheral* related to fluid volume deficit
- *Anxiety* related to lack of knowledge about the effects and treatment of adrenal insufficiency

Expected Outcomes

The expected outcomes established in the plan of care specify that Mr. Sardoff will

- Regain normal fluid balance.
- Regain normal peripheral perfusion with blood pressure within normal range.
- Verbalize his knowledge of the causes and effects of adrenal insufficiency.

Planning and Implementation

Ms. Flaherty plans and implements the following interventions in caring for Mr. Sardoff:

- Monitor the client's intake and output carefully.
- Take and record his weight at the same time daily.
- Monitor Mr. Sardoff's blood pressure, pulses, and skin turgor every 2 hours until stable, then 4 times a day.
- Monitor the results of electrolytes, and report abnormal results.
- Discuss with Mr. and Mrs. Sardoff a diet that is high in sodium, low in potassium, and has an increased fluid intake (3000 ml per day). Discuss the types of fluids desired and the best times for intake of increased fluids.
- Assist Mr. Sardoff during activity to prevent falls.
- Implement a teaching plan for Mr. and Mrs. Sardoff; provide verbal and written instructions, and encourage verbal feedback about the causes and effects of the disease, the effects of medications, the effects of not taking long-term cortisone drugs, the diet, and self-care at home.

Evaluation

Following treatment for acute adrenal insufficiency, Mr. Sardoff is no longer dehydrated, and his blood pressure has returned to his normal reading of 132/88. He is alert and oriented and anxious to learn to care for himself at home. Following dietary instructions and teaching for self-care that included his wife, Mr. Sardoff verbalizes an understanding of his illness and the need to take his medication carefully and accurately. Ms. Flaherty has contacted the social service department to arrange for the Sardoffs' church pastor to visit, and Mrs. Sardoff has been given emergency funds from their church to buy medications. The nurse from the community health agency visits before Mr. Sardoff's dismissal from the hospital and reviews the teaching plan with Ms. Flaherty.

Critical Thinking in the Nursing Process

1. Adrenal insufficiency is often diagnosed only when the client becomes seriously ill in response to a stressor. Explain why this statement is or is not true.
2. Describe the physical assessments that are found in the severely dehydrated client.
3. Mr. Sardoff's diagnostic test results were abnormal. Describe the pathophysiologic basis for these abnormal findings.
4. Outline a teaching plan for Mr. Sardoff with specific foods for a high-sodium, low-potassium diet.
5. Develop a plan of care for Mr. Sardoff for the nursing diagnosis *Altered Tissue Perfusion: Peripheral.*

The Client with Hyperfunction of the Adrenal Medulla

■ ■ ■

Because disorders of the adrenal medulla are rare, only the most common disorder, pheochromocytoma, will be discussed. **Pheochromocytomas** are tumors of chromaffin tissues in the adrenal medulla. These tumors, which are usually benign, produce catecholamines (epinephrine or norepinephrine) that stimulate the sympathetic nervous system. Although many organs are affected, the most dangerous effects are peripheral vasoconstriction and increased cardiac rate and contractility with resultant paroxysmal hypertension. Systolic blood pressure may rise to 200 to 300 mm Hg, the diastolic to 150 to 175 mm Hg. Attacks are often precipitated by physical, emotional, or environmental stimuli. This is a life-threatening condition.

A pheochromocytoma is diagnosed by increased catecholamine levels in the blood or urine, by X-ray studies, and by surgical exploration. Surgical removal of the tumor(s) by adrenalectomy is the treatment of choice.

Disorders of the Pituitary Gland

The pituitary gland produces hormones that affect multiple body systems through regulation of endocrine function. Target tissues include the thyroid, adrenal cortex, ovary, uterus, mammary glands, testes, and kidneys. Disorders result from an excess or deficiency of one or more of the pituitary hormones due to a pathologic condition within the gland itself or to hypothalamic dysfunction.

Although disorders of the pituitary cause diverse and serious problems, they are not as common as disorders of other endocrine glands. Hyperpituitarism and hypopituitarism are discussed in this section.

The Client with Disorders of the Anterior Pituitary Gland

■ ■ ■

Hyperfunction of the anterior pituitary gland, which is characterized by excess production and secretion of one or more trophic hormones, is usually the result of a pituitary tumor or pituitary hyperplasia. The most common cause of hyperpituitarism is a benign adenoma. The manifestations result from an excess of growth hormone (GH), prolactin (PRL), or ACTH.

Hypofunction of the anterior pituitary gland results in a deficiency of one or more of the gland's hormones. Conditions causing hypopituitarism include pituitary tumors, surgical removal of the pituitary gland, radiation, and pituitary infarction, infection, or trauma.

Pathophysiology

Growth hormone (also called somatotropin) is produced by cells in the anterior pituitary throughout life. GH is necessary for growth and also contributes to metabolic regulation. GH stimulates all aspects of cartilage growth, and one of its major effects is to stimulate the growth of the epiphyseal cartilage plates of long bones. In addition, other body tissues respond to the metabolic effect of GH with increases in bone width and the growth of visceral and endocrine organs, skeletal and cardiac muscle, skin, and connective tissue. The conditions that result from overstimulation are gigantism and acromegaly (discussed below). The conditions that result from deficient production of GH are growth retardation and short stature.

Hypersecretion of PRL affects sexual function. Women may have irregular or absent menses, difficulty in becoming pregnant, and decreased libido. Men may be impotent and have decreased libido. PRL deficiency in postpartal women causes a failure to lactate.

An excess secretion of ACTH overstimulates the adrenal cortex, which in turn increases secretion of adrenal hormones. The result is Cushing's syndrome. A deficit of TSH causes hypothyroidism.

Gigantism

Gigantism occurs when GH hypersecretion begins before puberty and the closure of the epiphyseal plates. The person becomes abnormally tall, often exceeding 7 ft (213 cm) in height, but body proportions are relatively normal. Most often the result of a tumor, the condition is rare today as a result of improved diagnosis and treatment.

Acromegaly

Acromegaly, which literally means "enlarged extremities," occurs when sustained GH hypersecretion begins during adulthood, most commonly because of pituitary tumors. As a result of constant stimulation, bone and connective tissue continue to grow. The forehead enlarges, the maxilla lengthens, the tongue enlarges, and the voice deepens (Figure 20–6). Overgrowth of bone and soft tissue in the hands and feet causes clients to buy increasingly larger rings, gloves, and shoes (McCance & Huether, 1994).

Other manifestations include peripheral nerve damage from entrapment of nerves, headache, hypertension, congestive heart failure, seizures, and visual disturbances. Impaired glucose tolerance and diabetes may also occur.

Collaborative Care

Acromegaly is treated by surgical removal or irradiation of the pituitary tumor. A transphenoidal or transfrontal surgical procedure is most commonly used (see Chapter 40).

Nursing Care

Clients with anterior pituitary disorders require interventions to help the client cope with physical and emotional changes, as well as to prevent complications involving other organs and functions of the endocrine system. Nursing care for the client having cranial surgery is discussed in Chapter 40.

Nursing diagnoses that are appropriate for the client with hypopituitarism or hyperpituitarism follow:

- *Sexual Dysfunction* related to the effects of excess PRL
- *Activity Intolerance* related to joint pain secondary to GH excess
- *Body Image Disturbance* related to bone overgrowth and tissue changes secondary to GH excess
- *Anxiety* related to an unknown future following surgery
- *Anticipating grieving* related to the knowledge that skeletal changes are irreversible

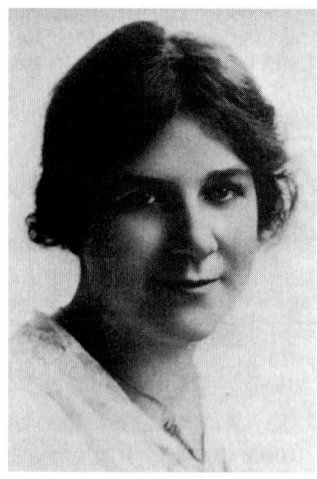 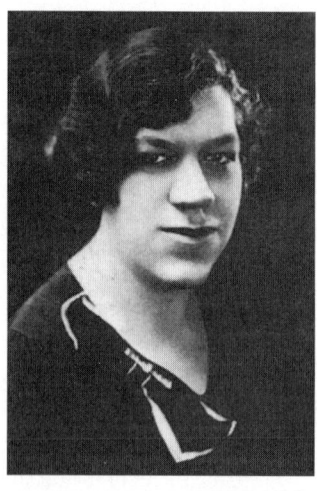 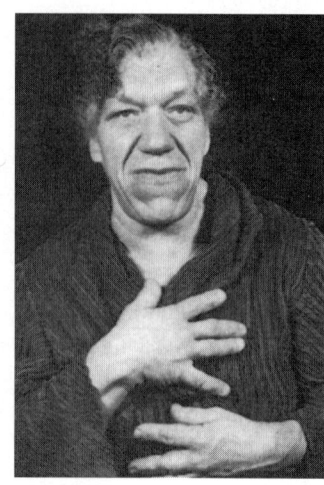

Figure 20–6 Clinical manifestations of acromegaly. Progressive alterations in facial appearance include enlargement of the cheekbones and jaw along with thickening of soft-tissue structures such as the nose, lips, cheeks and the flesh above the brows.

The Client with Disorders of the Posterior Pituitary Gland

■ ■ ■

Disorders of the posterior pituitary are related primarily to excessive or deficient antidiuretic hormone (ADH) secretion. The disorders discussed here are the syndrome of inappropriate ADH secretion and diabetes insipidus.

Pathophysiology

Antidiuretic hormone is secreted in response to serum osmolality, which is monitored by osmoreceptors in the hypothalamus. When a condition of hyperosmolality occurs, ADH secretion increases, and renal water is reabsorbed. Hypoosmolality causes the suppression of ADH, and renal water excretion increases.

Syndrome of Inappropriate ADH Secretion

The **syndrome of inappropriate ADH secretion (SIADH)** is characterized by high levels of ADH in the absence of serum hypoosmolality. This disorder is most often caused by the ectopic production of ADH by malignant tumors (for example, oat cell carcinoma of the lung, pancreatic carcinoma, leukemia, and Hodgkin's disease). A transient form may follow a head injury, pituitary surgery, or the use of medications such as barbiturates, anesthetics, or diuretics.

The manifestations of SIADH occur as a result of water retention, hyponatremia, and serum hypoosmolality. Blood volume expands, but the plasma is diluted. Aldosterone is suppressed; as a result, renal excretion of sodium increases. Water moves from the hypotonic plasma and the interstitial spaces into the cells.

Manifestations of SIADH are usually nonspecific but are related to hyponatremia and water intoxication (see Chapter 5). Brain cells swell, causing neurologic symptoms: headache, changes in level of consciousness, muscle twitches, and seizures. Usually no edema is present, because water is distributed between the intracellular and extracellular spaces.

Diabetes Insipidus

Diabetes insipidus is the result of ADH insufficiency. There are two types:

- *Neurogenic diabetes insipidus* can either result from a disruption of the hypothalamus and pituitary gland (as from trauma, irradiation, or cranial surgery) or be idiopathic.

- *Nephrogenic diabetes insipidus* is a disorder in which the renal tubules are not sensitive to ADH. This may be familial in origin or the result of renal failure.

Diabetes insipidus may result from brain tumors or infections, pituitary surgery, cerebral vascular accidents, and renal and organ failure. It is also a complication of closed-head trauma with increased intracranial pressure.

A deficit of ADH causes excretion of large amounts of dilute urine (polyuria), in some instances as much as 12 L per day. The client has extreme thirst and drinks large volumes of water (polydipsia). If unable to replace the water loss, the client becomes dehydrated and hypernatremic. Even though hyperosmolality is present, the urine is dilute and has a low specific gravity.

If this disorder is caused by cerebral injury, symptoms commonly appear 3 to 6 days after the initial injury and last for 7 to 10 days. If the increased intracranial pressure is relieved, symptoms of diabetes insipidus usually disappear. However, diabetes insipidus may also be a chronic illness requiring lifelong treatment and care.

Collaborative Care

SIADH is treated by correcting underlying causes, treating the hyponatremia with intravenous hypertonic saline, and restricting oral fluids to less than 800 mL per day. Manifestations of the disorder usually resolve within 3 days.

Diabetes insipidus is also treated by correcting underlying causes, if possible. Other medical interventions include administering intravenous hypotonic fluids, increasing oral fluids, replacing ADH hormone, and using vasopressin for neurogenic diabetes insipidus.

Nursing Care

Nursing care for the client with SIADH and diabetes insipidus focuses on client problems with fluid and electrolyte balance, discussed in Chapter 5. Examples of nursing diagnoses that are appropriate for the client with hypopituitarism follow:

- *Fluid Volume Excess* related to the effects of SIADH
- *Fluid Volume Deficit* related to the effects of diabetes insipidus secondary to closed-head injury
- *Risk for Injury* related to altered level of consciousness
- *Risk for Altered Health Maintenance* related to insufficient knowledge of the disease process (diabetes insipidus)
- *Sleep Pattern Disturbance* related to urinary frequency during the night
- *Altered Urinary Elimination* related to excessive urine output

Bibliography

■ ■ ■

Alfaro-LaFevre, R., Blicharz, M. E., Flynn, N. M., & Boyer, M. J. (1992). *Drug handbook: A nursing process approach.* Redwood City, CA: Addison-Wesley Nursing.

American Cancer Society. (1994). *Cancer statistics: 1994.* New York: Author.

Baer, C. L. (1988). Why does this patient have polyuria? *Nursing88, 18*(10), 94–95.

Bergstrom, N., Braden, B. J., Laguzza, A., & Holman, V. (1987). The Braden scale for predicting pressure sore risk. *Nursing Research, 36*(4), 205–210.

Bryce, J. (1994). S.I.A.D.H. *Nursing94, 24*(4), 33.

Caine, R. M., & Bufalino, P. M. (Eds.). (1991). *Applying nursing diagnosis: Nursing care planning guides for adults.* (2nd ed.). Baltimore: Williams & Wilkins.

Camunas, C. (1983, June). Pheochromocytoma. *American Journal of Nursing, (83)* 6, 887–891.

Carpenito, L. J. (1992). *Nursing diagnosis: Applications to clinical practice.* Philadelphia: Lippincott.

Chambers, J. K. (1987). Metabolic bone disorders: Imbalances of calcium and phosphorus. *Nursing Clinics of North America, 22*(4), 861–872.

Corsetti, A., & Buhl, B. (1994). Emergency! Managing thyroid storm. *American Journal of Nursing, 94*(11), 39.

Eschleman, M. M. (1991). *Introductory nutrition and diet therapy* (2nd ed.). Philadelphia: Lippincott.

Giefer, C., & Cassmeyer, V. (1994). The syndrome of primary aldosteronism: A case study. *MEDSURG Nursing, 3*(4), 277–284.

Halloran, T. H. (1990). Nursing responsibilities in endocrine emergencies. *Critical Care Nursing Quarterly, 13*(3), 74–81.

Hart, L. K., Freel, M. I., & Milde, F. K. (1990). Fatigue. *Nursing Clinics of North America, 25*(4), 967–976.

Hartshorn, J., & Hartshorn, E. (1988). Vasopressin in the treatment of diabetes insipidus. *Journal of Neuroscience Nursing, 20*(1), 58–59.

Isley, W. L. (1990). Thyroid disorders. *Critical Care Nursing Quarterly, 13*(3), 39–49.

Kee, J. L. (1991). *Laboratory and diagnostic tests with nursing implications.* (3rd ed.). Norwalk, CT: Appleton & Lange.

Ladenson, P. W. (1991). Treatments for Graves' disease: Letting the thyroid rest. *New England Journal of Medicine, 324,* 989–999.

Lane, G., & Peirce, A. G. (1982). When persistence pays off: Resolving the mystery of unexplained electrolyte imbalance. *Nursing82,* January, 44–47.

Loebl, S., Matejski, M., Spratto, G. R., & Woods, A. L. (1991). *The nurse's drug handbook.* (6th ed.). Albany, NY: Delmar.

McCance, K. L., & Huether, S. E. (1994). *Patho-physiology: The biologic basis for disease in adults and children.* (2nd ed.). St. Louis: Mosby.

Nurse's Clinical Library. (1984). *Endocrine disorders.* Springhouse, PA: Springhouse Corporation.

Porth, C. M. (1994). *Pathophysiology: Concepts of altered health status.* (4th ed.). Philadelphia: Lippincott.

Reasner, C. A. (1990). Adrenal disorders. *Critical Care Nursing Quarterly, 13*(3), 67–73.

Schira, M. G. (1987). Steroid-dependent states and adrenal insufficiency: Fluid and electrolyte disturbances. *Nursing Clinics of North America, 22*(4), 837–841.

Smith, D., & Bumann, R. (1994). Assessing and treating decreased cardiac output. *MEDSURG Nursing, 2*(5), 351–357.

Stuckey, P., & Waters, H. (1988). Oncology alert for the home care nurse: Syndrome of inappropriate antidiuretic hormone. *Home Health Nurse, 6*(6), 26–30.

Swearingen, P. L. (1990). *Manual of nursing therapeutics: Applying nursing diagnoses to medical disorders.* (2nd ed.). St. Louis: Mosby.

Swearingen, P. L. (1992). *Pocket guide to medical-surgical nursing.* St. Louis: Mosby.

Winer, N. (1990). Pheochromocytoma. *Critical Care Nursing Quarterly, 13*(3), 14–22.

Nursing Care of Clients with Diabetes Mellitus

LEARNING OBJECTIVES

After completing this chapter, you will be able to

- Describe the prevalence, incidence, costs, and etiology of diabetes mellitus.

- Describe the pathophysiology of the disease and of acute and long-term complications in people with insulin-dependent and non-insulin-dependent diabetes mellitus.

- Discuss the specific concerns of adults with diabetes mellitus by developmental level.

- Compare and contrast the manifestations and collaborative care of hypoglycemia, diabetic ketoacidosis (DKA), and hyperosmolar nonketotic coma (HNKC).

- Identify the laboratory and diagnostic tests used to diagnose and monitor self-management of diabetes mellitus.

- Discuss the nursing implications for insulin and oral hypoglycemic agents used to treat clients with diabetes mellitus.

- Provide accurate information to clients with diabetes mellitus to facilitate self-management of medications, diet planning, exercise, and foot care.

- Use the nursing process as a framework for providing individualized care in the management of the health needs of clients with diabetes mellitus.

Diabetes mellitus is a common chronic disease of adults. However, depending on the type of diabetes and the age of the client, both client needs and nursing care may vary greatly. Consider the following examples.

Jackie Lewis is a 23-year-old woman who has just graduated from college with a degree in interior design. Diagnosed with diabetes at the age of 15, she takes two injections of insulin each day. Jackie struggles daily with the management of her diabetes, often grabbing a hamburger for lunch and going out for drinks in the evening. She wants to marry and have children, but she wonders what she will do if her children also have diabetes. She also often wonders whether anyone will want to marry her because of her chronic illness.

Cheryl Draheim is a 45-year-old schoolteacher. She developed diabetes at age 34 after an automobile accident

caused such severe abdominal injuries that her pancreas and spleen had to be removed. Cheryl has always been very careful about taking her insulin, following her diet, and exercising regularly. However, she is beginning to notice that her vision is getting worse and that she is having increasing pain in her legs, especially after standing for long periods of time. Cheryl says that sometimes she believes the disease controls her more than she controls it.

Tom Chang is 53 years old. Tom was a sales representative for a tire company for 20 years. Early in his 40s, Tom was diagnosed with non-insulin-dependent diabetes. Although Tom was taught about the disease and the importance of taking his oral medications, following his diet plan, and getting exercise, he rarely did more than take the medication. Five years ago, he was hospitalized for hyperglycemia and started taking insulin. Last year

Tom had a stroke, leaving him unable to walk. He has now been admitted to the hospital for treatment of gangrene of the large toe on his left foot.

Grace Staples is an independent 82-year-old woman who lives alone and happily takes care of her two cats. She is slightly overweight. Last year, during Grace's annual eye examination, eye changes typical for diabetes were found. She was referred to her family doctor, who diagnosed non-insulin-dependent diabetes and started her on oral medications. Grace sticks to her diet, walks a mile every day, and plans to live to be 100.

As illustrated in these examples, **diabetes mellitus (DM)** is not a single disorder but a group of chronic disorders of the endocrine pancreas, all categorized under a broad diagnostic label. The condition is characterized by inappropriate hyperglycemia caused by a relative or absolute deficiency of insulin or by a resistance to the action of insulin (Ratner, 1992). Diabetes mellitus is the most common endocrine disorder, and, although it is one of the oldest identified diseases, the actual cause is still unknown. Research has vastly improved the diagnosis and management of this disease, but as yet no cure has been found.

Clients with diabetes mellitus face lifelong changes in life-style and health status. Nursing care is provided in the clinical setting for the diagnosis of the disease and treatment of complications. A major role of the nurse is that of educator in both hospital and community settings.

The term *diabetes,* or DM, when used throughout the chapter, refers to diabetes mellitus.

Overview of Diabetes Mellitus

■   ■   ■

This overview of diabetes mellitus includes a discussion of the prevalence, incidence, and costs of the disease; its historical background; hormones; and the different types of the disease.

Prevalence, Incidence, and Costs

Diabetes is estimated to affect 12 million people in the United States and perhaps 200 million people worldwide (Ratner, 1992). It is difficult to collect accurate statistics because many people who have diabetes are undiagnosed; it is estimated that there are 4 to 7 million undiagnosed people with diabetes at any one time. According to the American Diabetes Association (1993b), approximately 750,000 people are diagnosed each year. Diabetes as a disease process affects 4% to 6% of the population, making it one of today's most serious chronic diseases (Guthrie & Guthrie, 1991).

There is an increased prevalence of diabetes (especially non-insulin-dependent diabetes) among older adults and

in minority populations (see the box on page 706). When compared with an age-matched European American population, diabetes is 2 times more common in African Americans, 2½ times more common in Hispanic Americans, and 5 times more common in Native Americans (Harris, 1989). Insulin-dependent diabetes mellitus is slightly more common in men, whereas non-insulin-dependent diabetes mellitus is diagnosed more often in women.

Diabetes is the fourth leading cause of death by disease in the United States, primarily because of the widespread cardiovascular effects that result in atherosclerosis, coronary artery disease, and cardiovascular accident (CVA or stroke). People with diabetes are two to four times more likely to have heart disease, and two to six times more likely to have a stroke than people who do not have diabetes. Each year, 150,000 Americans die from complications caused by diabetes (American Diabetes Association, 1993a). Diabetes is also the major cause of newly diagnosed blindness and of nontraumatic amputations in the United States. Complications of diabetes that involve the kidneys are common; 25% of all patients receiving renal dialysis for renal failure have diabetes.

Americans with diabetes use a disproportionate amount of the nation's health care services. They visit outpatient services and physicians' offices more often than people who do not have the disease, and they require more frequent hospitalizations with longer days of in-hospital treatment. The cost of illness and resulting loss of productivity for people with diabetes is estimated to exceed $20 billion per year (American Diabetes Association, 1993a).

Historical Background

Diabetes mellitus has been recognized as a disease for centuries. *Diabetes* derives from a Greek word meaning "to siphon," referring to the increased output of urine. *Mellitus* derives from a Latin word meaning "sweet." The two words together identify the disease as an outpouring of sweet urine.

The development of the microscope increased the knowledge of the physiology of the pancreas and of diabetes mellitus. In the 18th century, Langerhans described the islets of the pancreas that contain the beta cells. Virchow (1821–1902) described lesions of the pancreas. Minkowsky (1858–1931), theorizing that the pancreas was in some way associated with diabetes, removed the pancreas in animals, thereby causing diabetes. However, the internal secretion that was deficient was still unknown.

In 1921, Banting and Best developed techniques for extracting the hormone, which they named *insulin,* from pancreatic tissue and for measuring blood glucose. They also discovered that when injected, insulin produces a

Gerontologic Considerations for Clients with Non-Insulin Dependent Diabetes Mellitus

■ ■ ■

Diabetes mellitus affects 15% to 20% of older adults. Cases often are undiagnosed because the signs and symptoms of diabetes sometimes go unrecognized among the elderly. The presenting symptoms of hyperglycemia may include urinary frequency, nocturia, incontinence, and disturbances in vision. Other general signs and symptoms include: weight loss, weakness, confusion, fatigue, and increased incidents of falls. These signs and symptoms are often mistakenly attributed to the aging process.

A slight increase in fasting blood glucose levels (impaired glucose tolerance) is a common finding in older adults. Older cells lose their sensitivity to glucose; thus, it takes longer for the body to release insulin following a rise in glucose levels. In addition, the pancreas may produce less insulin in older adults. The kidneys reabsorb glucose less well, which may result in glycosuria. About 20% of older adults with impaired glucose tolerance will progress to overt non-insulin dependent diabetes mellitus (NIDDM).

NIDDM is due to alterations in the way insulin is secreted, bound, and used by the body. There is a strong genetic predisposition for this condition. Another etiologic factor of NIDDM is obesity. About three-fourths of older adults with NIDDM are overweight. Regardless of the pathophysiologic mechanism, all older adults with NIDDM will develop insulin resistance. The goal of treatment is to lower blood glucose levels to normal or near normal limits. An obese older adult with NIDDM may be managed with diet, exercise, and weight reduction. In addition, oral hypoglycemic agents may have to be added to control blood glucose levels.

Dietary goals for management of NIDDM in older adults include:

- Achieve and maintain an age-appropriate body weight.

- Provide adequate protein to maintain nitrogen balance.

- Avoid foods high in saturated fat and cholesterol to reduce blood lipids and control calories.

- Avoid high-sodium foods to minimize hypertension and congestive disease.

- Provide adequate calcium to retard osteoporosis.

- Avoid high-sugar foods which interfere with glucose control.

- Increase meal frequency with added snacks to improve carbohydrate tolerance and glucose control.

In order to improve the likelihood of compliance with dietary modifications, the nurse should consider the following with an older adult: dietary preferences, eating habits, motivation, coexisting illnesses, dental health, and food preparation skills. The older adult must be able to follow the prescribed diet in order for it to be useful in controlling glucose levels.

Although exercise will improve glucose tolerance in older adults, it is unclear how effective exercise is in lowering glucose levels. Encourage the older adult with NIDDM to exercise if it can be tolerated. Exercise improves the body's response to insulin and helps burn calories. The overall cardiovascular and musculoskeletal benefits of exercise cannot be underemphasized.

---

dramatic drop in blood glucose. This meant that diabetes was no longer a terminal illness because hyperglycemia could now be controlled.

Since that time, oral hypoglycemic drugs, human insulin products, insulin pumps, home blood glucose monitoring, and transplantation of the pancreas or of pancreatic islet or beta cells have advanced the treatment and care of people with diabetes.

Hormones of the Endocrine Pancreas and Glucose Homeostasis

To understand the pathophysiology, manifestations, complications, and treatment of diabetes mellitus, one must first understand the physiology of the hormones of the endocrine pancreas and the homeostatic mechanisms responsible for maintaining normal blood glucose levels.

Endocrine Pancreas Hormones

The endocrine pancreas produces hormones necessary for the metabolism and cellular utilization of carbohydrates, proteins, and fats. The cells that produce these hormones are clustered in groups of cells called the **islets of Langerhans.** There are three different types of cells in these islets:

- **Alpha cells** produce the hormone *glucagon.* Glucagon stimulates the breakdown of glycogen in the liver, the formation of carbohydrates in the liver, and the breakdown of lipids in the liver and in adipose tissue. The primary function of glucagon is to decrease glucose oxidation and to increase blood glucose levels.

- **Beta cells** secrete the hormone *insulin,* which has many opposite effects. Insulin facilitates the movement of glucose across cell membranes into cells, decreasing

---

Gerontologic Considerations (continued)

■ ■ ■

Oral hypoglycemic agents may be required if diet, exercise, and weight reduction do not control glucose levels. Oral sulfonylureas are the drugs of choice to treat NIDDM in older adults. The major risk of sulfonylurea therapy is hypoglycemia. Consequently, older adults taking these drugs need to be taught the signs and symptoms of hypoglycemia: headache, nervousness, shakiness, and weakness. (The older adult may not feel hungry when hypoglycemic). To counteract drug-induced hypoglycemia, the older adult should eat or drink something containing sugar, such as orange juice or hard candy.

Other medications that the older adult with NIDDM is taking may cause either hypoglycemia or hyperglycemia. Drugs that cause hypoglycemia include: alcohol, dicumarol, salicylates, beta-adrenergic blockers, and sulfonamide antibacterial agents. Drugs that can cause hyperglycemia include: glucocorticosteroids, thiazides, sympathomimetic agents such as epinephrine, amphetamines, and ephedrine. Some of these agents are found in over-the-counter cold remedies. The older adult should inform the primary care provider of all medications that are being taken, including over-the-counter medications.

Diabetes can cause long-term complications such as heart, kidney, eye, and nerve diseases. In order to prevent these complications from occurring, the older adult with NIDDM needs to monitor blood glucose levels and check for signs of complications. Older adults should be taught to do their own glucose testing if possible. A record of the glucose levels needs to be kept. Regular medical care is essential. An annual eye exam is suggested. Visual changes such as blurring, difficulty in reading, or flashing lights should be reported. Any changes in urination and cardiac symptoms should be reported. Blood pressure should be controlled within normal limits. Because leg and foot problems can result in limb amputation, proper foot care is essential. The older adult should wear proper fitting shoes. Medical care must be sought for any sores or cuts on the feet.

The older adult with NIDDM should be taught to report the following signs and symptoms to the primary care provider: high glucose levels (give parameters to follow), any infection, changes in sensorium, changes in sensation, change in warmth or color of the feet or hands, slow healing sore, and prolonged aches and/or pains. Finally, the older adult with NIDDM should wear an identification bracelet or necklace stating that the wearer has diabetes. In a medical emergency, this will ensure that the proper treatment will be obtained.

American Diabetes Association. Standards of Medical Care for Patients with Diabetes Mellitus. *Diabetes Care, 17,* 6, June 1994, pp. 616–623.

U.S. Department of Health and Human Services. *Noninsulin-Dependent Diabetes.* NIH Publication No. 92-241, September 1992.

Yoshikawa, T. T., Cobbs, E. L., Brummel-Smith, K. *Ambulatory Geriatric Care.* St. Louis: Mosby, 1993.

---

blood glucose levels. Insulin prevents the excessive breakdown of glycogen in the liver and in muscle, facilitates lipid formation while inhibiting the breakdown of stored fats, and helps move amino acids into cells for protein synthesis.

■ **Delta cells** produce a substance called *somatostatin,* which is believed to be a neurotransmitter that inhibits the production of both glucagon and insulin.

Glucagon   Glucagon, through *glycogenolysis* (the breakdown of liver glycogen) and *gluconeogenesis* (the formation of glucose from fats and proteins), prevents blood glucose from decreasing below a certain level when the body is fasting or in between meals. The action of glucagon is initiated when blood glucose falls below about 70 mg/dL.

Insulin   After secretion by the beta cells, insulin enters the portal circulation, travels directly to the liver, and is then released into the general circulation. Circulating insulin is rapidly bound to peripheral tissues (especially muscle and fat cells) or is destroyed by the liver or kidneys. Insulin release is regulated by blood glucose; it increases when blood glucose levels increase, and it decreases when blood glucose levels decrease. When a person eats food, insulin levels begin to rise in minutes, peak in 30 to 60 minutes, and return to baseline in 2 to 3 hours.

Insulin facilitates the active transport of glucose into muscle and fat cells, where it is used as an energy source for adenosine triphosphate (ATP) production and for cell functions. Insulin also causes glucose in excess of the amount used by cells to be stored in fat cells, preventing glucose from accumulating in the blood.

Figure 21-1 Regulation (homeostasis) of blood glucose levels by insulin and glucagon. *A,* High blood sugar is lowered by insulin release. *B,* Low blood sugar is raised by glucagon release.

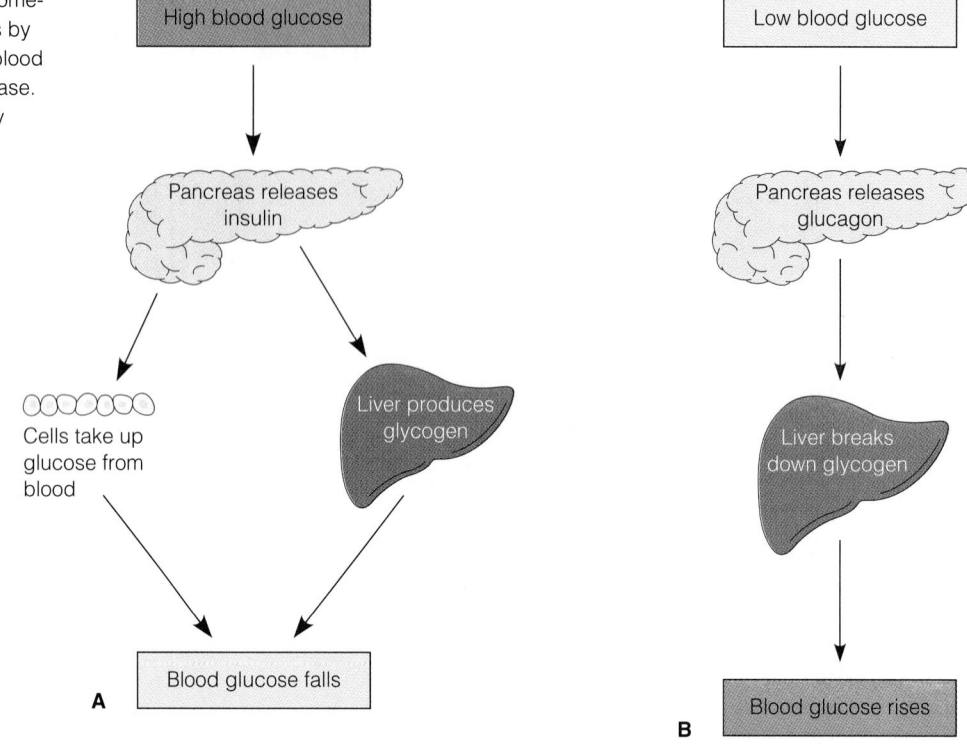

Blood Glucose Homeostasis

All body tissues and organs require a constant supply of glucose; however, not all tissues require insulin for glucose uptake. The brain, the liver, the intestines, and the renal tubules do not require insulin to transfer glucose into their cells. Skeletal muscle, cardiac muscle, and adipose tissue do require insulin for glucose movement into the cells.

Normal blood glucose is maintained in healthy people primarily through the actions of insulin and glucagon. Pancreatic beta cells are stimulated to produce insulin by increased blood glucose levels, but increased plasma levels of amino acids and fatty acids also stimulate insulin release. As cells of cardiac muscle, skeletal muscle, and adipose tissue take up glucose, plasma levels of nutrients decrease, and the stimulus to produce insulin is suppressed. If blood glucose falls, glucagon is released to bring glucose levels up to within normal limits. Epinephrine, growth hormone, thyroxine, and glucocorticoids (often referred to as glucose counterregulatory systems) also stimulate an increase in glucose in times of hypoglycemia, stress, growth, or increased metabolic demand. The regulation of blood glucose levels by insulin and glucagon is illustrated in Figure 21-1.

Definitions of normal blood glucose levels vary in clinical practice, depending on the laboratory that performs the assay. In this chapter, normal blood glucose is defined as 70 to 110 mg/dL.

Types of Diabetes Mellitus

Diabetes mellitus is not a single disease but many disorders that ultimately cause a failure of the beta cells or a decrease in cellular response (sometimes called peripheral resistance) to insulin. The types of diabetes mellitus, described by the National Diabetes Data Group (1979), are as follows:

- Type I, or insulin-dependent diabetes mellitus
- Type II, or non-insulin-dependent diabetes mellitus
- Other types of diabetes (those that occur secondary to other causes, such as injury or disease of the pancreas)
- Gestational diabetes

In addition to these types, disorders of glucose tolerance are included in the classification. The labeling of these types of diabetes mellitus, as well as the characteristics of each type, are subject to change as research is conducted. Table 21-1 lists the classification and characteristics of the different types of diabetes mellitus and related carbohydrate intolerance disorders.

It is important to remember that the type of diabetes that is diagnosed may change during a person's life span. A person may be classified as non-insulin-dependent yet still require insulin, especially in stressful situations (such as physical illness, surgery, or emotional stress). Women diagnosed with gestational diabetes may require treatment following childbirth for either insulin-dependent

Table 21–1	Classification and Characteristics of Types of Diabetes and Related Carbohydrate Intolerance Disorders	
	Classification	**Characteristics**
Diabetes Mellitus (DM)	Type I: Insulin-dependent diabetes mellitus (IDDM)	Onset: any age, but usually before age 30. Rapid onset of symptoms. Client usually is thin to normal weight. Client depends on insulin to sustain life. Frequent complications. Constitutes 10% to 20% of all diabetes cases.
	Type II: Non–insulin-dependent diabetes mellitus (NIDDM) Nonobese NIDDM Obese NIDDM	Onset: any age, but usually after age 35. Slow onset of symptoms. Client often is obese, but weight may be normal. Oral antidiabetic drugs are effective; 20% to 30% of clients may require insulin. Frequent complications. Constitutes 80% to 90% of all diabetes cases.
	Other types of DM	Occur secondary to other conditions or pharmacologic treatment. Pancreatic causes: pancreatitis, pancreatectomy, cystic fibrosis. Hormonal causes: acromegaly, Cushing's syndrome, pheochromocytoma. Drug-induced causes: phenytoin (Dilantin), steroids, estrogen (e.g., oral contraceptives), beta-adrenergic blockers, monoamine oxidase (MAO) inhibitors.
Gestational Diabetes Mellitus (GDM)		Onset: during pregnancy. Increases risk of complications. Treated with diet and insulin as needed to maintain normal blood glucose levels. Increases client's risk of developing diabetes later in life.
Impaired Glucose Tolerance	Impaired glucose tolerance (IGT) (may be nonobese, obese, or associated with other conditions)	Glucose tolerance test results are abnormal, but fasting blood glucose is normal or only slightly elevated. Client rarely has symptoms. Client may revert to normal. Although now normal, client has had elevated blood glucose levels or an abnormal glucose tolerance test.
	Potential abnormality of glucose tolerance (Pot AbGt)	Client is normal at time of glucose testing; has risk factors for DM, such as family history of DM, identical twin with DM, obesity, high-risk ethnic background.

Note. Adapted from "Classification and diagnosis of diabetes mellitus and other categories of glucose intolerance" by the National Diabetes Data Group, 1979, *Diabetes, 28,* pp. 1039–1057.

diabetes or non-insulin-dependent diabetes, or they may require no further treatment.

Although there are various types of diabetes mellitus, the two major types are insulin-dependent diabetes and non-insulin-dependent diabetes.

Pathophysiology

Type I: Insulin-Dependent Diabetes Mellitus (IDDM)

Insulin-dependent diabetes mellitus (IDDM), or *Type I diabetes,* can occur at any age but most commonly occurs before age 30. Formerly called juvenile diabetes, this disorder is characterized by **hyperglycemia** (elevated blood glucose levels), a breakdown of body fats and proteins, and the development of **ketosis,** an accumulation of ketone bodies produced during the oxidation of fatty acids. IDDM is the result of the destruction of the beta cells of the islets of Langerhans in the pancreas. When beta cells are destroyed, insulin is no longer produced. The destruction of the beta cells with the onset of IDDM is believed to result from a combination of three factors: a genetic predisposition, viral or toxic chemical agents, and an autoimmune attack. The disease develops in five stages (Ratner, 1992):

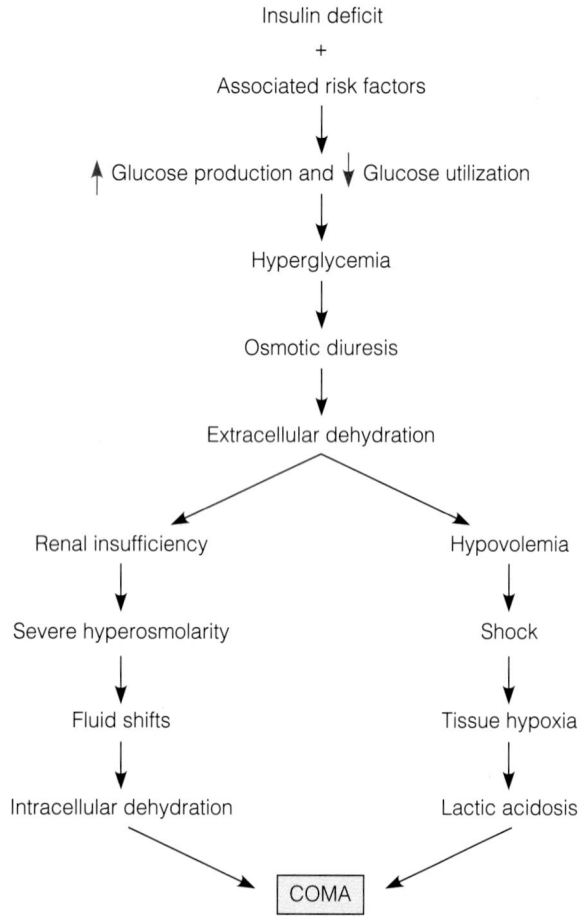

Figure 21–2 Pathophysiologic results of IDDM.

Stage 1: Genetic predisposition

Stage 2: Environmental trigger

Stage 3: Active autoimmunity

Stage 4: Progressive beta cell dysfunction

Stage 5: Overt diabetes mellitus

Although the manifestations of IDDM appear rapidly, the changes that lead to the manifestations may take place over several years.

There is a relationship between the occurrence of IDDM and genetic predisposition. Although the general risk of IDDM ranges from 1 in 400 to 1 in 1000, the children of a person with diabetes have a 1 in 20 to 1 in 50 risk (Raffel & Rotter, 1985). Genetic markers that determine immune responses (specifically, DR3 and DR4 histocompatibility locus antigens chromosome 6) have been found in 95% of people diagnosed with IDDM. Although the presence of these markers does not guarantee that the person will develop IDDM, they do indicate increased susceptibility (Ratner, 1992).

Environmental factors are believed to trigger the development of IDDM. The trigger can be a viral infection (mumps, rubella, or coxsackievirus B4) or a chemical toxin, such as those found in smoked and cured meats. As a result of exposure to the virus or chemical, an abnormal autoimmune response occurs in which antibodies respond to normal islet beta cells as though they were foreign substances, destroying them. The symptoms of IDDM appear when approximately 90% of the beta cells are destroyed. However, manifestations may appear at any time during the loss of beta cells if an acute illness or stress increases the demand for insulin beyond the reserves of the damaged cells. The actual cause and exact sequence of IDDM are not completely understood, but research continues to identify the genetic markers of this disorder and to investigate ways of altering the immune response to prevent or cure IDDM.

Manifestations of IDDM   The manifestations of IDDM are the result of a lack of insulin to transport glucose across the cell membrane into the cells (Figure 21–2). Glucose molecules accumulate in the circulating blood, resulting in hyperglycemia. Hyperglycemia causes serum hyperosmolality, drawing water from the intracellular spaces into the general circulation. The increased blood volume increases renal blood flow, and the hyperglycemia acts as an osmotic diuretic, thereby increasing urine output. This condition is called **polyuria**. When the blood glucose level exceeds the renal threshold for glucose—usually about 180 mg/dL—glucose is excreted in the urine, a condition called **glucosuria**. The decrease in intracellular volume and the increased urinary output cause dehydration. The mouth becomes dry and thirst sensors are activated, causing the person to drink increased amounts of fluid (**polydipsia**).

Because glucose cannot enter the cell without insulin, energy production decreases. This decrease in energy stimulates hunger, and the person eats more food (**polyphagia**). Despite increased food intake, the person loses weight as the body loses water and breaks down proteins and fats in an attempt to restore energy sources. Malaise and fatigue accompany the decrease in energy. Blurring vision is also common, resulting from osmotic effects that cause swelling of the lenses of the eyes.

Thus, the classic manifestations of IDDM are polyuria, polydipsia, and polyphagia, accompanied by weight loss, malaise, and fatigue. Depending on the degree of insulin lack, the manifestations vary from slight to severe. People with IDDM require an exogenous source of insulin to maintain life.

Important research findings about the management of IDDM were reported in 1993. The results of a 10-year Diabetes Control and Complications Trial (DCCT), sponsored by the National Institutes of Health (NIH), have significant implications about the management of IDDM. People in the study who kept their blood glucose levels close to normal by frequent monitoring, several daily insulin injections, and life-style changes that included exercise and a healthier diet reduced by 60% their risk for the development and progression of complications involving the eyes, the kidneys, and the nervous system. (These complications, as well as the components of the management of IDDM, are fully discussed later in the chapter.)

Diabetic Ketoacidosis (DKA)

As the pathophysiology of untreated IDDM continues, the insulin deficit causes fat stores to break down, resulting in continued hyperglycemia and mobilization of fatty acids with a subsequent ketosis (see Figure 21–2). When ketone production by the liver exceeds cellular utilization and renal excretion, ketosis occurs. This results in a form of metabolic acidosis called **diabetic ketoacidosis (DKA)**. The onset of and recovery from DKA is slower than from insulin reaction, with manifestations occurring and progressing over 1 to 2 days (Porth, 1994).

DKA occurs in a person with untreated IDDM, and it also may occur in a person with diagnosed diabetes when energy requirements increase during physical or emotional stress. Stress states initiate the release of gluconeogenic hormones, resulting in the formation of carbohydrates from protein or fat. The individual with IDDM who is sick, has an infection, or who decreases or omits insulin doses is at a greatly increased risk for developing DKA.

DKA involves four metabolic problems:

- Hyperosmolarity from hyperglycemia and dehydration
- Metabolic acidosis from an accumulation of ketoacids
- Extracellular volume depletion from osmotic diuresis
- Electrolyte imbalances from osmotic diuresis (Graves, 1990)

The manifestations of DKA are the result of severe dehydration and acidosis. These manifestations are summarized in the accompanying box. Laboratory findings include the following:

- Blood glucose levels higher than 300 mg/dL
- Plasma pH less than 7.3
- Plasma bicarbonate less than 10 mEq/L
- Presence of serum ketones
- Presence of urine ketones and glucose
- Abnormal levels of serum sodium, potassium, and chloride

Depression of the central nervous system (CNS) from the accumulation of ketones and the resulting acidosis may cause death if left untreated. DKA is a life-threatening medical emergency; it causes 57 deaths per 100,000 people with diabetes each year (American Diabetes Association, 1992a). The treatment of DKA is directed toward lowering hyperglycemia, correcting fluid and electrolyte imbalances, and returning serum pH to normal. These are

---

Clinical Manifestations of Diabetic Ketoacidosis (DKA)

Dehydration (from Hyperglycemia)

- Thirst
- Warm, dry skin with poor turgor
- Dry mucous membranes
- Soft eyeballs
- Weakness
- Malaise
- Rapid, weak pulse
- Hypotension

Metabolic Acidosis (from Ketosis)

- Nausea and vomiting
- Ketone (fruity, alcohol-like) breath odor
- Lethargy
- Coma

Other Manifestations

- Abdominal pain (cause unknown)
- Kussmaul's respirations (increased rate and depth of respirations, with a longer expiration; a compensatory response to prevent a further decrease in pH)

---

accomplished by intravenous administration of fluids and insulin.

Type II: Non-Insulin-Dependent Diabetes Mellitus (NIDDM)

Non-insulin-dependent diabetes mellitus (NIDDM), or *type II diabetes,* is a condition of hyperglycemia that occurs despite the availability of endogenous insulin (Porth, 1994). Formerly called adult-onset or maturity-onset diabetes, NIDDM can occur at any age, but it is usually seen in people over age 35. Heredity plays a role in the transmission of NIDDM. Although there is no identified HLA linkage, the children of a person with NIDDM have a 15% chance of developing NIDDM and a 30% risk of developing one of the glucose intolerances (Raffel & Rotter, 1985). Other risk factors associated with NIDDM are obesity, increasing age, and membership in a high-risk ethnic group. (The prevalence of NIDDM is greater among Hispanic Americans, Native Americans, and African Americans.)

Although the exact cause of NIDDM is unknown, several theories have been suggested. These theories include limited beta cell response to hyperglycemia, peripheral insulin resistance, and insulin-receptor or post-receptor abnormalities. Whatever the cause, there *is* sufficient insulin production to prevent the breakdown of fats with

Factors Associated with Hyperosmolar Nonketotic Coma (HNKC)

■ ■ ■

Therapeutic Agents

- Glucocorticoids
- Diuretics
- Beta-adrenergic blocking agents
- Immunosuppressants
- Chlorpromazine
- Diazoxide

Therapeutic Procedures

- Peritoneal dialysis
- Hemodialysis
- Hyperosmolar alimentation (oral or parenteral)
- Surgery

Acute Illness

- Infection
- Gangrene
- Urinary infection
- Burns
- Gastrointestinal bleeding
- Myocardial infarction
- Pancreatitis
- Stroke

Chronic Illness

- Renal disease
- Cardiac disease
- Hypertension
- Previous stroke
- Alcoholism

Note. Data are from *Physician's Guide to Non-insulin Dependent (Type II) Diabetes: Diagnosis and Treatment* by the American Diabetes Association, 1988, Alexandria, VA: American Diabetes Association.

resultant ketosis; thus, NIDDM is characterized as a nonketotic form of diabetes. However, the amount of insulin available is not sufficient to lower blood glucose levels through the uptake of glucose by muscle and fat cells.

Two subgroups of NIDDM are classified by the presence or absence of obesity. The majority of people with NIDDM are overweight. Obesity, especially of the upper body, decreases the number of available insulin receptor sites in cells of skeletal muscles and adipose tissues, a process called peripheral insulin resistance. In addition, the ability of the beta cells to release insulin in response to increasing glucose levels is impaired. Both insulin resistance and impaired insulin release can be improved with weight loss (Porth, 1994).

People with nonobese NIDDM have a decreased early insulin response to glucose, are usually younger, and have a family history of NIDDM. Those with this type of NIDDM usually respond well to oral hypoglycemic medications.

Manifestations of NIDDM The person with NIDDM experiences a slow onset of manifestations and is often unaware of the presence of the disease until health care is sought for some other problem. The hyperglycemia that accompanies NIDDM is usually not as severe as in IDDM, but similar symptoms occur, especially polyuria and polydipsia. Polyphagia is not often seen, and weight loss is uncommon. Other manifestations are also the result of hyperglycemia: blurred vision, fatigue, paresthesias, and skin infections.

If available insulin decreases, especially in times of physical or emotional stress, the person with NIDDM may develop DKA, but this occurrence is uncommon. The major metabolic complication in NIDDM is hyperosmolar nonketotic coma.

Hyperosmolar Nonketotic Coma Hyperosmolar nonketotic coma (HNKC) is a metabolic problem that occurs in people who have NIDDM. HNKC is characterized by a plasma osmolarity of 340 mOsm/L or greater (the normal range is 280 to 300 mOsm/L), greatly elevated blood glucose levels (over 600 mg/dL and often 1000 to 2000 mg/dL), and altered levels of consciousness. HNKC is a serious, life-threatening medical emergency and has a higher mortality rate than DKA. Mortality is high not only because the metabolic changes are serious but also because people with NIDDM are usually older and have other medical problems that either cause or are caused by HNKC.

The risk factors associated with HNKC include therapeutic agents, therapeutic procedures, acute illness, and chronic illness (see the accompanying box). The precipitating conditions for HNKC are an increased resistance to the effects of insulin and an excessive intake of carbohydrates (Porth, 1994). The manifestations of this disorder may be slow to appear, with onset ranging from 24 hours to 2 weeks. The manifestations are initiated by the hyperglycemia, which causes increased urine output. With increased output, plasma volume decreases and glomerular filtration rate (GFR) drops. As a result, glucose is retained and water is lost. Glucose and sodium accumulate in the blood and increase serum osmolarity.

Serum hyperosmolarity results in severe dehydration, reducing intracellular water in all tissues, including the brain. The person has dry skin and mucous membranes, extreme thirst, and altered levels of consciousness (progressing from lethargy to coma). Neurologic deficits may include hyperthermia, motor and sensory impairment, positive Babinski's sign, and seizures. Treatment is directed toward correcting fluid and electrolyte imbalances, lowering blood glucose levels with insulin, and treating underlying conditions.

Complications of Diabetes Mellitus

The person with diabetes mellitus, regardless of type, is at increased risk for complications involving many different

Table 21–2   DKA, HNKC, and Hypoglycemia Compared

		DKA	HNKC	Hypoglycemia
Diabetes type		IDDM	NIDDM	Both
Onset		Slow	Slow	Rapid
Cause		↓ Insulin	↓ Insulin	↑ Insulin
		Infection	Older age	Omitted meal/snack
				Error in insulin dose
Risk Factors		Surgery	Surgery	Surgery
		Trauma	Trauma	Trauma
		Illness	Illness	Illness
		Omitted insulin	Dehydration	Exercise
		Stress	Medications	Medications
			Dialysis	Lipodystrophy
			Hyperalimentation	Renal failure
				Alcohol intake
Assessments	Skin	Flushed; dry; warm	Flushed; dry; warm	Pallor; moist; cool
	Perspiration	None	None	Profuse
	Urine output	Increased	Increased	Normal
	Breath	Fruity	Normal	Normal
	Vital signs	BP ↓	BP ↓	BP ↓
		P ↑	P ↑	P ↑
		R Kussmaul's	R normal	R normal
	Mental status	Lethargic	Lethargic	Anxious; restless
	Urine output	Increased	Increased	Normal
	Fluid intake	Increased	Increased	Normal
	Gastrointestinal effects	Nausea/vomiting; abdominal pain	Nausea/vomiting; abdominal pain	Hunger
	Level of consciousness	Decreasing	Decreasing	Decreasing
	Energy level	Weak	Weak	Fatigue
	Other	Weight loss	Weight loss	Headache
		Blurred vision	Malaise	Altered vision
			Extreme thirst	Mood changes
			Seizures	Seizures
Laboratory Findings	Blood glucose	> 300 mg/dL	> 600 mg/dL	< 50 mg/dL
	Plasma ketones	Increased	Normal	Normal
	Urine glucose	Increased	Increased	Normal
	Urine ketones	Increased	Normal	Normal
	Serum potassium	Abnormal	Abnormal	Normal
	Serum sodium	Abnormal	Abnormal	Normal
	Serum chloride	Abnormal	Abnormal	Normal
	Plasma pH	> 7.3	Normal	Normal
	Osmolality	< 340 mOsm/L	> 340 mOsm/L	Normal
Treatment		Insulin	Insulin	Glucagon
		Intravenous fluids	Intravenous fluids	Rapid-acting carbohydrate
		Electrolytes	Electrolytes	Intravenous solution of 50% glucose

body systems. Alterations in blood glucose levels, alterations in the vascular system, neuropathies, an increased susceptibility to infection, and periodontal disease are common. In addition, the interaction of several complications can cause problems of the feet. Figure 21–3 illustrates the progression from cardinal signs to acute complications to late multisystem complications for the client with diabetes. A discussion of each of these complications

follows; related collaborative care and nursing care are discussed later in the chapter.

Alterations in Blood Glucose Levels   The discussion below provides additional information about hyperglycemia and hypoglycemia. Table 21–2 shows a comparison of DKA, HNKC, and hypoglycemia.

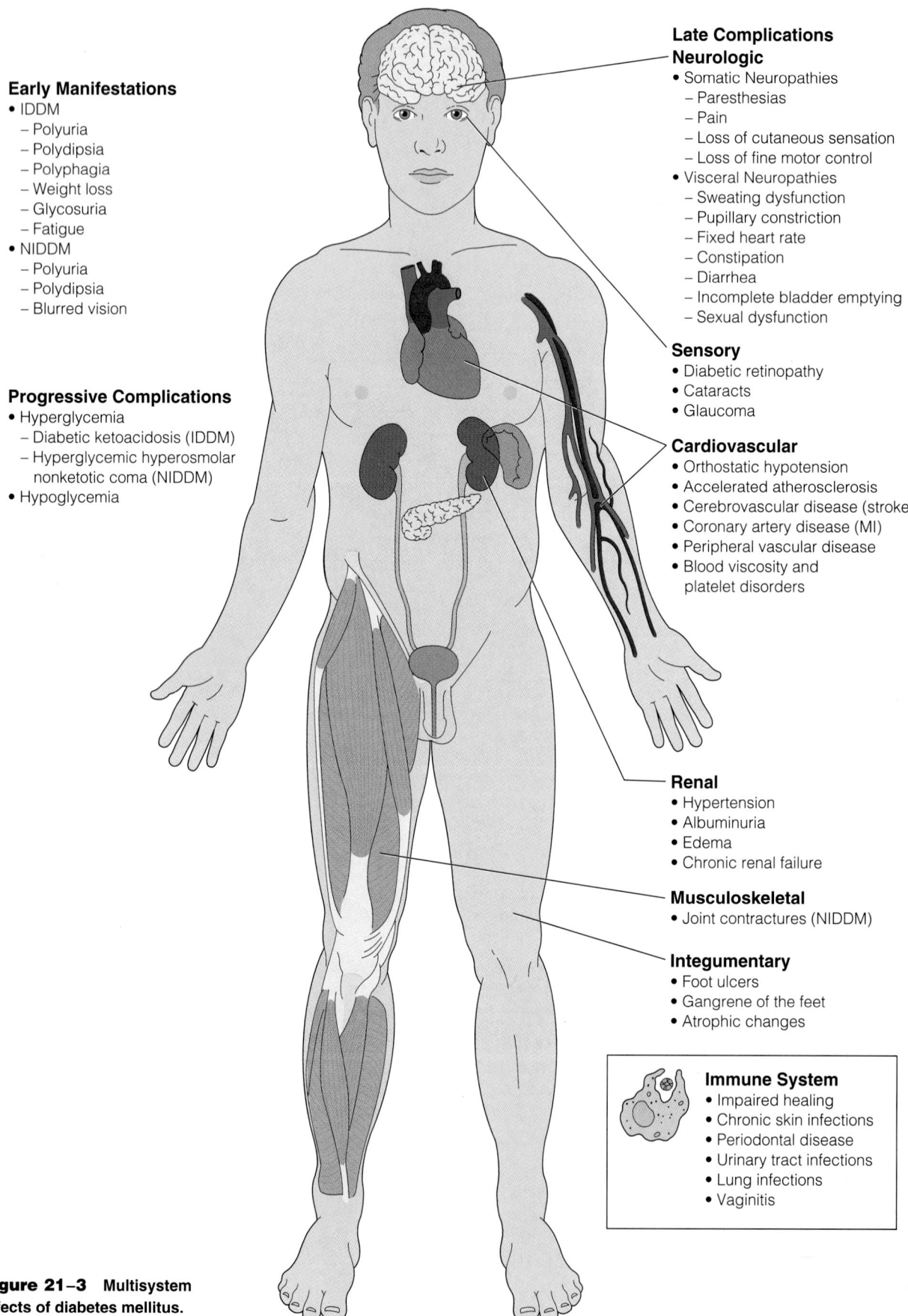

Early Manifestations
- IDDM
  - Polyuria
  - Polydipsia
  - Polyphagia
  - Weight loss
  - Glycosuria
  - Fatigue
- NIDDM
  - Polyuria
  - Polydipsia
  - Blurred vision

Progressive Complications
- Hyperglycemia
  - Diabetic ketoacidosis (IDDM)
  - Hyperglycemic hyperosmolar nonketotic coma (NIDDM)
- Hypoglycemia

Late Complications
Neurologic
- Somatic Neuropathies
  - Paresthesias
  - Pain
  - Loss of cutaneous sensation
  - Loss of fine motor control
- Visceral Neuropathies
  - Sweating dysfunction
  - Pupillary constriction
  - Fixed heart rate
  - Constipation
  - Diarrhea
  - Incomplete bladder emptying
  - Sexual dysfunction

Sensory
- Diabetic retinopathy
- Cataracts
- Glaucoma

Cardiovascular
- Orthostatic hypotension
- Accelerated atherosclerosis
- Cerebrovascular disease (stroke)
- Coronary artery disease (MI)
- Peripheral vascular disease
- Blood viscosity and platelet disorders

Renal
- Hypertension
- Albuminuria
- Edema
- Chronic renal failure

Musculoskeletal
- Joint contractures (NIDDM)

Integumentary
- Foot ulcers
- Gangrene of the feet
- Atrophic changes

Immune System
- Impaired healing
- Chronic skin infections
- Periodontal disease
- Urinary tract infections
- Lung infections
- Vaginitis

Figure 21–3 Multisystem effects of diabetes mellitus.

Hyperglycemia The major problems resulting from hyperglycemia in the person with diabetes are DKA and HNKC. Two other problems are the dawn phenomenon and the Somogyi phenomenon.

The **dawn phenomenon** is a rise in blood glucose between 4 a.m. and 8 a.m. that is not a response to hypoglycemia. This condition occurs in people with both IDDM and NIDDM. The exact cause is unknown but is believed to be related to diurnal variations in growth hormone and/or insulin clearance.

The **Somogyi phenomenon** (named for the scientist who confirmed the finding that low blood glucose levels cause high blood glucose rebound in some individuals) is a morning rise in blood glucose to hyperglycemic levels following an episode of nocturnal hypoglycemia and a counterregulatory hormone response. Although it was at first suggested that this condition is a response to excessive amounts of insulin, this is no longer believed to be true.

The primary consideration for managing morning hyperglycemia is careful self-monitoring of blood glucose levels, regular bedtime snacks, and assessment for manifestations of nocturnal hypoglycemia: tremors, night sweats, nightmares, restlessness, early morning headache, and stomachaches (White & Henry, 1992).

Hypoglycemia **Hypoglycemia** (low blood glucose levels) is common in people with IDDM and occasionally occurs in people with NIDDM who are treated with oral hypoglycemic agents. This condition is often referred to as **insulin reaction** in clients with IDDM. Low blood glucose levels result primarily from a mismatch between insulin intake (due to an error in insulin dose, for example), physical activity, and carbohydrate availability (for example, omitting a meal) (White & Henry, 1992). The intake of alcohol and certain drugs (chloramphenicol, coumadin, monoamine oxidase [MAO] inhibitors, probenecid, salicylates, sulfonamides) can also cause hypoglycemia.

The manifestations of hypoglycemia result from a compensatory autonomic nervous system (ANS) response and from impaired cerebral function due to a decrease in glucose available for use by the brain. The manifestations vary, particularly in older adults. The onset is sudden, and blood glucose is usually less than 50 mg/dL. The manifestations of hypoglycemia are listed in the accompanying box. Severe hypoglycemia may cause death.

People who have IDDM for 4 or 5 years fail to secrete glucagon in response to a decrease in blood glucose. They are then dependent on epinephrine to serve as a counterregulatory response to hypoglycemia. However, this compensatory response can become absent or blunted. The person then develops a syndrome called *hypoglycemia unawareness*. The person does not experience symptoms of hypoglycemia, even though it is present. Because treat-

---

Clinical Manifestations of Hypoglycemia

Manifestations Caused by Responses of the Autonomic Nervous System

- Hunger
- Nausea
- Anxiety
- Pale, cool skin
- Sweating
- Shakiness
- Irritability
- Rapid pulse
- Hypotension

Manifestations Caused by Impaired Cerebral Function

- Strange or unusual feelings
- Headache
- Difficulty in thinking
- Inability to concentrate
- Change in emotional behavior
- Slurred speech
- Blurred vision
- Decreasing levels of consciousness
- Seizures
- Coma

---

ment is not initiated, the person is likely to have episodes of severe hypoglycemia (White & Henry, 1992).

Alterations in the Vascular System Diabetes mellitus can alter the structure and function of the macrocirculation and the microcirculation. These changes accompany both IDDM and NIDDM and are believed to be caused by the pathophysiologic effects of hyperglycemia. The following categories of complications and their implications are summarized in Table 21–3.

Alterations in the Macrocirculation The macrocirculation (the large blood vessels) in people with diabetes undergoes changes due to atherosclerosis; abnormalities in platelets, red blood cells, and clotting factors; and changes in arterial walls. It has been established that atherosclerosis has an increased incidence and earlier age of onset in people with diabetes (although the reason why is unknown); the other factors are suggested as risk factors but have not been proved to be responsible. Other risk factors that contribute to the development of macrovascular disease of diabetes are hypertension, hyperlipidemia, cigarette smoking, and obesity. Alterations in the vascular system increase the risk of the long-term complications of coronary artery disease, cerebral vascular disease, and peripheral vascular disease.

Table 21–3   Implications of the Complications of Diabetes

Complication	Implications
Changes in macrocirculation	Early onset of atherosclerosis Increased risk of coronary artery disease and cerebrovascular accident (CVA) Peripheral vascular insufficiency with claudication, ulcerations, and gangrene of the legs
Changes in microcirculation	Diabetic retinopathy with retinal ischemia and loss of vision Diabetic nephropathy with hypertension, albuminuria, edema, and progressive renal failure (Kimmelstiel-Wilson syndrome)
Somatic neuropathies	Changes in sensation in the feet and hands (paresthesias), such as numbness, tingling, pain, and impaired sense of touch Palsy of cranial nerve III with headache, eye pain, and inability to move the eye up, down, or to the middle Pain or loss of cutaneous sensation over the chest Motor and sensory deficits in the anterior thigh and medial calf Carpal tunnel syndrome with pain and weakness of the hand Compression of the peroneal nerve, resulting in foot drop
Visceral neuropathies	Anhidrosis (absence of sweating) on the hands and feet Increased sweating on the face or trunk Constricted pupils Fixed cardiac rate and postural hypotension Dysphagia, anorexia, heartburn Nausea and vomiting Constipation Diabetic diarrhea Inability to empty the bladder completely, with resulting urinary tract infections Ejaculatory and erection changes. Arousal, orgasm, and vaginal lubrication changes
Periodontal disease	Gingivitis Periodontitis Loss of teeth
Changes in the lower extremities	Arteriosclerosis and occlusion of blood flow Ulcerations Increased infections Gangrene Amputations

Atherosclerotic coronary artery disease is a major risk factor in the development of myocardial infarction in people with diabetes, especially in the middle to older adult with NIDDM (Rifkin, 1988). Myocardial infarction is two times more common in men with diabetes and three times more common in women with diabetes. People with diabetes who have myocardial infarction are more prone to develop congestive heart failure as a complication of the infarction and are also less likely to survive in the period immediately following the infarction (McCance & Huether, 1994). (Myocardial infarction is fully discussed in Chapter 28.)

People with diabetes, especially older adults with NIDDM, are two to six times more likely to have a CVA. Although the exact relationship between diabetes and cerebral vascular disease is unknown, hypertension (a risk factor for CVA) is a common health problem in those who have diabetes. In addition, atherosclerosis of the cerebral vessels develops at an earlier age and is more extensive in people with diabetes (Porth, 1994).

The manifestations of impaired cerebral circulation (see Chapter 41) are often similar to those of hypoglycemia or HNKC: blurred vision, slurred speech, weakness, and dizziness. People with these manifestations have potentially life-threatening health problems and should always have medical attention.

Peripheral vascular disease of the lower extremities accompanies both IDDM and NIDDM, but the incidence is greater in people with NIDDM. Atherosclerosis of vessels in the legs of people with diabetes begins at an earlier age, advances more rapidly, and is equally common in both men and women (McCance & Huether, 1994). Impaired peripheral vascular circulation leads to peripheral vascular insufficiency with intermittent claudication and ulcerations of the lower legs. Occlusion and thrombosis of large vessels and small arteries and arterioles, as well as alterations in neurologic function and infection, result in gangrene (necrosis, or the death of tissue). Gangrene from diabetes is the most common cause of nontraumatic amputations of the lower leg. In people with diabetes, dry gangrene is most common, manifested by cold, dry, shriveled, and black tissues of the toes and feet. The gangrene usually begins in the toes and moves proximally into the foot.

Alterations in the Microcirculation   Alterations in the microcirculation (*microangiopathies*) in the person with diabetes involve structural defects in the basement membrane of smaller blood vessels and capillaries. (The basement membrane is the structure that supports and serves as the boundary around the space occupied by epithelial cells.) These defects cause the capillary basement membrane to thicken, eventually resulting in decreased tissue perfusion. Changes in basement membranes are believed to be due to one or more of the following: the presence of increased amounts of sorbitol (a substance formed as an intermediate step in the conversion of glucose to fructose), the formation of abnormal glycoproteins, or problems in the release of oxygen from hemoglobin (Porth, 1994). The effects of alterations in the microcirculation affect all body tissues but are seen primarily in the eyes and the kidneys.

Diabetic retinopathy is the collective name for the changes in the retina that occur in the person with diabetes. The retinal capillary structure undergoes alterations in blood flow, leading to retinal ischemia and a breakdown in the blood retinal barrier. Diabetic retinopathy is the leading cause of blindness in people between ages 25 and 74.

Retinopathy has three stages:

- Stage I: Nonproliferative retinopathy. This stage is characterized by dilated veins, microaneurysms, edema of the macula, and the presence of exudates.

- Stage II: Preproliferative retinopathy. Retinal ischemia causes infarcts of the nerve fiber layer, with characteristic "cotton wool" patches on the retina. Shunts form between occluded and patent vessels.

- Stage III: Proliferative retinopathy. As fibrous tissue and new vessels form in the retina or optic disc, traction on the vitreous humor may cause hemorrhage or retinal detachment.

As many as 90% of people with diabetes may have manifestations of stage I retinopathy, usually within 5 to 15 years of diagnosis. Only a small percentage progress to stage III. However, if exudate, edema, hemorrhage, or ischemia occurs near the fovea, the person will experience visual impairment at any stage (Herman & Greene, 1992). In addition, the person with diabetes is at increased risk for developing cataracts (opacity of the lens) as a result of increased glucose levels within the lens itself.

Diabetic nephropathy is a disease of the kidneys characterized by the presence of albumin in the urine, hypertension, edema, and progressive renal insufficiency. This disorder is the most common cause of renal failure requiring dialysis or transplantation in the United States. Nephropathy occurs in 30% to 50% of people with diabetes who have had the disease for 15 years or longer (American Diabetes Association, 1991).

Despite research, the exact pathologic origin of diabetic nephropathy is unknown; it has been established, however, that thickening of the basement membrane of the glomeruli eventually impairs renal function. It is suggested that an increased intracellular concentration of glucose supports the formation of abnormal glycoproteins in the basement membrane. The accumulation of these large proteins stimulates *glomerulosclerosis* (fibrosis of the glomerular tissue). Glomerulosclerosis severely impairs the filtering function of the glomerulus, and protein is lost in the urine. *Kimmelstiel-Wilson syndrome* is a type of glomerulosclerosis found only in people with diabetes. In advanced nephropathy, tubular atrophy occurs, and end-stage renal disease results. (Renal failure is discussed in Chapter 26.)

Somatic and Visceral Neuropathies   Somatic and visceral neuropathies are disorders of the peripheral nerves and the autonomic nervous system. In people with diabetes, these disorders are often called **diabetic neuropathies.** Diabetic neuropathies cause one or more of the following problems: sensory and motor impairment, muscle weakness and pain, cranial nerve disorders, impaired vasomotor function, impaired gastrointestinal function, and impaired genitourinary function.

The etiologic origin of diabetic neuropathies involves three pathologic changes: (1) a thickening of the walls of the blood vessels that supply nerves causes a decrease in nutrients, (2) demyelinization of the Schwann cells that surround and insulate nerves slows nerve conduction, and (3) the formation and accumulation of sorbitol within the Schwann cells impairs nerve conduction. The manifestations depend on the locations of the lesions.

Somatic Neuropathies   The *somatic neuropathies* (also called *peripheral neuropathies*) include polyneuropathies and mononeuropathies. *Polyneuropathies,* the most common type of neuropathy associated with diabetes, are bilateral sensory disorders. The manifestations appear first in the toes and feet and progress upward. The fingers and hands may also be involved, but usually only in later stages of the disorder. The manifestations of polyneuropathy depend on the nerve fibers involved.

The person with polyneuropathy commonly has distal *paresthesias* (a subjective feeling of a change in sensation, such as numbness or tingling); pain described as aching, burning, or shooting; and feelings of cold feet. Other manifestations may include impaired pain sensations, temperature, light touch, two-point discrimination, and vibration. There is no specific treatment for polyneuropathy.

Mononeuropathies are isolated peripheral neuropathies that affect a single nerve. Depending on the nerve involved, manifestations may include the following:

- Palsy of the third cranial (oculomotor) nerve, with headache, eye pain, and an inability to move the eye up, down, or medially
- Radiculopathy, with dermatomal pain and loss of cutaneous sensation, most often located in the chest
- Diabetic femoral neuropathy, with motor and sensory deficits (pain, weakness, areflexia) in the anterior thigh and medial calf
- Entrapment or compression of the medial nerve at the wrist, resulting in carpal tunnel syndrome with pain and weakness of the hand; the ulnar nerve at the elbow, with weakness and loss of sensation over the palmar surface of the fourth and fifth fingers; and the peroneal nerve at the head of the fibula, with foot drop

Neuropathies involving the cranial nerves, dermatomes, skeletal muscles, and the femoral nerve often resolve spontaneously in weeks or months, but there is no specific treatment.

Visceral Neuropathies The *visceral neuropathies* (also called *autonomic neuropathies*) cause many different manifestations, depending on the area of the ANS involved. These neuropathies may include the following:

- Sweating dysfunction, with an absence of sweating (*anhydrosis*) on the hands and feet and increased sweating on the face or trunk
- Abnormal pupillary function, most commonly seen as constricted pupils that dilate slowly in the dark
- Cardiovascular dysfunction, resulting in such abnormalities as a fixed cardiac rate that does not change with exercise, postural hypotension, and a failure to increase cardiac output or vascular tone with exercise
- Gastrointestinal dysfunction, with changes in upper gastrointestinal motility (resulting in dysphagia, anorexia, heartburn, nausea, and vomiting) and altered blood glucose control. Constipation is one of the most common gastrointestinal symptoms associated with diabetes, possibly a result of hypomotility of the bowel. Diabetic diarrhea is not as common, but it does occur and is often associated with fecal incontinence during sleep due to a defect in internal sphincter function.

- Genitourinary dysfunction, resulting in changes in bladder function and sexual function. Bladder function changes include an inability to empty the bladder completely, loss of sensation of bladder fullness, and an increased risk of urinary tract infections. Sexual dysfunctions in men include ejaculatory changes and impotence. Sexual dysfunctions in women include changes in arousal patterns, vaginal lubrication, and orgasm. Alterations in sexual function in people with diabetes are the result of both neurologic and vascular changes.

Increased Susceptibility to Infection The person with diabetes has an increased risk of developing infections and developing them often. The exact relationship between infection and the presence of diabetes is not clear, but many of the dysfunctions that result from diabetic complications predispose the person to develop an infection. Vascular and neurologic impairments, hyperglycemia, and altered neutrophil function are believed to be responsible (Porth, 1994).

The person with diabetes may have sensory deficits resulting in inattention to trauma and vascular deficits that decrease circulation to the injured area; as a result, the normal inflammatory response is diminished and healing is slowed. Nephrosclerosis and inadequate bladder emptying with retention of urine predispose the person with diabetes to pyelonephritis and urinary tract infections. Bacterial and fungal infections of the skin, nails, and mucous membranes are common. Tuberculosis is more prevalent in people with diabetes than in the general population.

Periodontal Disease Although periodontal disease does not occur more often in people with diabetes, it does progress more rapidly, especially if the diabetes is poorly controlled. It is believed to be caused by microangiopathy, with changes in vascularization of the gums. As a result, *gingivitis* (inflammation of the gums) and *periodontitis* (inflammation of the bone underlying the gums) are more likely to occur.

Complications Involving the Foot People with diabetes are at high risk for amputation of a lower extremity. Such amputations are about 15 times more common than in people without the disease (American Diabetes Association, 1993a). The high incidence of both amputations and problems with the feet in people with diabetes is the result of angiopathy, neuropathy, and infection.

Vascular changes in the lower extremities of the person with diabetes result in arteriosclerosis. Diabetes-induced arteriosclerosis tends to occur at an earlier age, occurs equally in men and women, is usually bilateral, and progresses more rapidly. The blood vessels most often affected are located below the knee. Blockages form in the large, medium, and small arteries of the lower legs and

Clinical Manifestations of Peripheral Vascular Disease

- Loss of hair on lower leg, feet, and toes
- Atrophic skin changes: shininess and thinning
- Cold feet
- Feet and ankles darker than leg
- Dependent rubor, blanching on elevation
- Thick toenails
- Diminished or absent pulses
- Nocturnal pain
- Pain at rest, relieved by standing or walking
- Intermittent claudication
- Patchy areas of gangrene on feet and toes

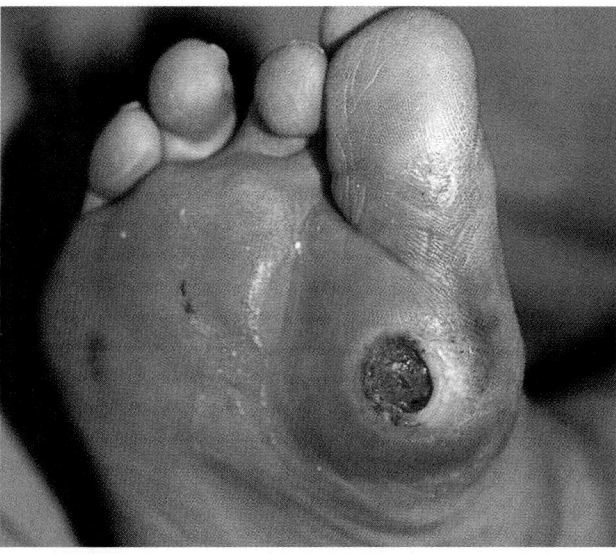

Figure 21–4   Ulceration following trauma in the foot of the person with diabetes.

feet. Multiple occlusions with decreased blood flow result in the manifestations of peripheral vascular disease, listed in the accompanying clinical manifestations box. (Peripheral vascular disease is discussed in Chapter 30.)

Diabetic neuropathy of the foot produces multiple problems. Because the sense of touch and perception of pain is absent, the person with diabetes may have some type of foot trauma without being aware of it. The person thus is at increased risk for trauma to tissues of the feet, leading to ulcer development (Figure 21–4). Infections commonly occur in traumatized or ulcerated tissue.

Although there are many different potential sources of foot trauma in the person with diabetes, the most common ones are cracks and fissures caused by dry skin or infections such as athlete's foot, blisters caused by improperly fitting shoes, pressure from stockings or shoes, ingrown toenails, and direct trauma (cuts, bruises, or burns). It is important to remember that the person with diabetic neuropathy who has lost the perception of pain may not be aware that these injuries have occurred. In addition, when a part of the body loses sensation, the person tends to dissociate from or ignore the part, so that an injury may go unattended for days or weeks. The injury may even be forgotten entirely.

Foot lesions usually begin as a superficial skin ulcer. In time, the ulcer extends deeper into muscles and bone, leading to abscess or osteomyelitis. Gangrene can develop on one or more toes; if untreated, the whole foot eventually becomes gangrenous. (Care of the feet, an essential part of client and family education, is discussed later in the chapter.)

Diabetes Mellitus and the Adult Client

Diabetes can affect men and women at any stage during adulthood, either as a newly diagnosed disease process or as a disease present since childhood or adolescence. The impact of the disease on the adult is discussed here at two developmental levels: diabetes in the young and middle adult, and diabetes in the older adult. (See Chapter 2 for the adult client's developmental stages and tasks, risks for alterations in health, and chronic illness.)

Diabetes in the Young and Middle Adult

Diabetes in the young and middle adult has the potential to disrupt normal physical, emotional, and sociocultural aspects of life and development. Although young and middle adults may have either type of diabetes, IDDM more commonly occurs before age 35, whereas NIDDM occurs more commonly thereafter.

Young and middle adults with diabetes are at risk for developing complications at an earlier age if they do not make necessary life-style changes. Accordingly, teaching healthy behaviors is very important for this age group. Specific topics follow:

- *Diet.* Obesity is a major modifiable risk factor in the development of atherosclerosis, cardiovascular disease, and hypertension. In addition, young adults who are obese may develop a type of non-insulin-dependent diabetes called **maturity-onset diabetes of the young (MODY).** A further important part of dietary management is adding fiber and limiting fat, both of which may help in the management of diabetes. Dietary rec-

Concerns of Young and Middle Adults with Diabetes

■ ■ ■

The Young Adult

- Establishing and maintaining personal relationships
- Life-style changes
- Self-management of the disease
- Fear of independence from family members
- Problems with employment
- Decisions to marry and have children
- Accepting altered self-concept and body image
- Fear of hypoglycemic attacks
- Economic costs of the illness

The Middle Adult

- Loss of roles (work, marriage, relationships)
- Coping with a chronic illness as well as aging
- Life-style changes
- Self-management of the disease
- Fear of complications
- Altered sexuality
- Becoming a burden to significant others
- Economic costs of the illness and of treating complications
- Loss of independence

ommendations for the young and middle adult include decreasing salt intake through careful consideration of the sodium content of foods (especially from fast-food restaurants), decreasing saturated fat intake, and increasing fiber intake. These recommendations should be integrated into the prescribed diet.

- *Cigarette smoking.* If a person starts smoking during adolescence, the habit becomes well established. Nicotine vasoconstricts small blood vessels, increasing the risk of peripheral vascular disease. Smoking is a major risk factor for cardiovascular disease. Through teaching, referrals, and careful follow-up, nurses should strongly encourage clients with diabetes to stop smoking.

- *Exercise.* Exercise helps maintain ideal body weight and cardiovascular health. Moderate exercise is a regular and important part of diabetes management.

In addition to learning to promote their own good health, young and middle adults with diabetes must also learn about the disease itself to prevent further illness. General guidelines for teaching include these topics:

- The pathophysiology of diabetes
- Nutrition, food preparation, and the diabetic diet
- Hypoglycemia and hyperglycemia
- Maintaining a balance among diet, exercise, and medications
- Medication administration (insulin or oral hypoglycemic drugs)
- Foot care
- Self-monitoring for blood glucose levels
- Managing sick days
- Identification, supplies, and emergency contacts
- Support groups and referrals

These topics are discussed later in the chapter. Other concerns of young and middle adults with diabetes are listed in the accompanying box.

Diabetes in the Older Adult

Diabetes is a common chronic illness in the older adult population, affecting 14% of all older men and women (Dellasega, 1990). It is almost ten times as common among people over age 65 as in people from age 20 to 44 (Barrett-Connor, 1989). It is predicted that the number of older adults with diabetes will continue to increase because the incidence of the disease increases with age and because the number of people over 65 is increasing.

Although most older adults with diabetes have NIDDM, the improved survival rates for people with diabetes have resulted in an increased number of older adults with IDDM. The reason is that older adults who have been diagnosed with NIDDM sometimes become insulin dependent late in life. The picture is complicated by the fact that blood glucose levels do increase with age, beginning in the 50s. For this reason, it is more difficult to diagnose diabetes in the older adult; conversely, the older adult may be mistakenly diagnosed with the disease simply for exhibiting essentially normal age-related changes in glucose. The relationship between normal increases in glucose levels and the presence of diabetes is not yet understood.

The older adult with diabetes has multiple and complex health care problems and needs. The normal physiologic changes of aging may mask manifestations of the onset of diabetes and may also increase the potential for complications. Table 21–4 presents common problems in the older adult that make the diagnosis and management of diabetes more difficult. The older adult with diabetes also has a longer recovery period after surgery or serious

Table 21–4	Implications for Nursing Care for the Older Adult with Diabetes
Health Problem/Complication	**Implications for Nursing Care**
Urinary incontinence	Polyuria, a classic manifestation of diabetes, often is ignored. This problem also often leads to social isolation.
Decreased thirst	Polydipsia, a classic manifestation of diabetes, often is ignored. This further increases the risk of dehydration and electrolyte imbalances.
Decreased hunger and weight loss	Polyphagia, a classic manifestation of diabetes, often is ignored. The aging process, medications, depression, or lack of socialization may decrease hunger. Weight loss may be gradual and go unnoticed.
Fatigue	Fatigue is a common symptom of diabetes but may be blamed on increased age.
Hypoglycemia	The older adult may have either very mild manifestations or none at all. As a result, hypoglycemia is often ignored until it causes serious effects.
Peripheral neuropathy	Manifestations may be thought to be due to arthritis, and over-the-counter drugs often are used to self-medicate. The risk of falls increases, as does the risk of gangrene and amputation.
Peripheral vascular disease	May go undetected if the person does not get enough exercise to cause claudication. May also impair abilities to climb stairs and walk.
Diabetic retinopathy	May be undetected if the person has cataracts. Diabetic clients also have an increased incidence of cataracts and glaucoma. Deficits in vision threaten independence, mobility, and social interactions.
Hypertension	Treatment with diuretics may further impair glucose tolerance and result in electrolyte imbalances.
Arthritis	Older adults may believe the pain from arthritis to be more important than the diabetes management. Also, depression from chronic pain as well as inactivity and loss of appetite may interfere with diabetes self-care.
Parkinson's disease	The tremors and rigidity of this disease make self-care involving fine and gross motor skills difficult or impossible.
Medications	Older adults commonly take more than one type of medication and are at increased risk for problems relating to drug interactions.

Note. Data are from "Diabetes Mellitus and the Older Adult" by M. M. Funnell and J. H. Merritt, pp. 505–564, in D. Haire-Joshu, *Management of Diabetes Mellitus: Perspectives of Care across the Life Span,* 1992, St. Louis: Mosby.

illness, often requiring insulin to maintain blood glucose levels.

Older adults have the same basic needs for nursing care and teaching as young and middle adults, but often the nurse must individualize plans to meet clients' specific needs. Consider the following:

- The long-term presence of a chronic illness often interferes with family communication and relationships.
- Dietary restrictions may cause the older adult to avoid social gatherings.
- Low-income older adults may have difficulty affording nutritious foods, may not have access to transportation to purchase foods, or may lack storage space for foods.
- Physical limitations may interfere with food preparation, activities of daily living, foot care, and hygiene. Limited range of motion may make insulin administration and blood glucose testing difficult or impossible.

- Alterations in sexual function may lead to withdrawal from one's partner.
- Older adults usually have lower incomes, but the cost of medical care continues to increase. The person with diabetes faces costs for medications, blood glucose monitoring, visits to the physician, and hospitalization. Even though Medicare pays a part of medical costs, the client is still responsible for part of the expenses.
- Because of cultural background and ethnic origin, the older adult may have a fatalistic acceptance of illness and its complications and/or have little concern for the future. Therefore, the client may be less likely to adhere to recommended management.
- Vision and hearing deficits in older adults require that the nurse adapt teaching materials. If the client's educational level prohibits reading literature and instructions, the nurse must use other teaching methods.

Collaborative Care

Treatment of the client with diabetes focuses on maintaining blood glucose at levels as nearly normal as possible through medications, dietary management, and exercise. Treatment of the acute complications of diabetes (hypoglycemia, DKA, and HNKC) is also included in this section.

Laboratory and Diagnostic Tests

Laboratory and diagnostic tests are conducted for screening purposes to diagnose diabetes, and ongoing laboratory tests are conducted to evaluate the effectiveness of diabetic management. The screening test of choice is a fasting plasma glucose test (American Diabetes Association, 1992b). The criteria for the diagnosis of diabetes in the nonpregnant adult are listed below. Any one criterion is sufficient to establish the medical diagnosis.

1. A random (nonfasting) plasma glucose level greater than 200 mg/dL, together with classic manifestations of polyuria, polydipsia, polyphagia, and weight loss

2. A fasting plasma glucose level above 140 mg/dL on two measurements, regardless of the absence of symptoms

3. A fasting plasma glucose level below 140 mg/dL but accompanied by an abnormal response to two oral glucose tolerance tests, as manifested by a 2-hour plasma glucose greater than 200 mg/dL with an intervening value greater than 200 mg/dL (American Diabetes Association, 1992a; National Diabetes Data Group, 1979)

Screening Tests   The following laboratory and diagnostic tests may be ordered for screening purposes:

- *Serum blood glucose level.* This is a fasting blood sugar (FBS) sample, meaning the client must have nothing by mouth except water for at least 3 hours before the test. Normal levels are 70 to 110 mg/dL for young and middle adults and 70 to 120 mg/dL for older adults.

- *A 2-hour postprandial (feasting) blood glucose level.* If the fasting blood glucose level is slightly elevated, this test is conducted to determine the client's response to a high carbohydrate intake (from a meal or from a measured amount of glucose, usually 75 to 100 g). The normal level for young and middle adults is below 140 mg/dL/2h for serum and below 120 mg/dL/2h for blood. Normal levels for the older adult are below 160 mg/dL/2h for serum and below 140 mg/dL/2h for blood. Smoking may increase the blood glucose level.

- *Glucose tolerance test (GTT).* This test is conducted to diagnose diabetes in people with slightly elevated fasting blood glucose levels or 2-hour feasting levels. This test should not be conducted if the FBS is greater than 200 mg/dL. The peak glucose level for an oral GTT occurs 0.5 to 1 hour after the ingestion of 100 g of glucose, and the blood glucose level should return to normal after 3 hours. The client with diabetes will not return to normal blood glucose levels within this interval. Client preparation and teaching for a glucose tolerance test are described in the accompanying box.

- *Intravenous glucose tolerance test (IV-GTT).* This test is performed if the client cannot eat or is unable to tolerate the oral glucose. The blood glucose should return to normal in 2 hours.

Tests to Monitor Diabetes Management   The following laboratory tests may be used to monitor diabetes management:

- *Fasting blood sugar (FBS).* This test is often ordered, especially if the client is experiencing symptoms of hypoglycemia or hyperglycemia.

- *Glycosylated hemoglobin.* This test is done to determine the average blood glucose level over approximately the previous 4 months. When glucose is elevated or control of glucose is erratic, glucose attaches to the hemoglobin molecule and remains attached for the life of the hemoglobin, which is about 120 days. The normal level depends on the type of assay done, but values above 7% to 9% are considered elevated.

- *Urine glucose and ketone levels.* These are not as accurate in monitoring changes in blood glucose as serum or blood levels. The presence of glucose in the urine indicates hyperglycemia. Most people have a renal threshold for glucose of 180 mg/dL; that is, when the blood glucose exceeds 180 mg/dL, glucose is not reabsorbed by the kidney and spills over into the urine. This number varies highly, however. *Ketonuria* (the presence of ketones in the urine) occurs with the breakdown of fats and is an indicator of DKA; however, fat breakdown and ketonuria also occur in states of less than normal nutrition.

- *Urine test for the presence of protein as albumin (albuminuria).* This test is performed to detect the early onset of nephropathy.

- *24-hour urine test for creatinine clearance.* This test is often conducted to evaluate renal function if albuminuria is present.

- *Serum cholesterol and triglyceride levels.* These are indicators of atherosclerosis and an increased risk of cardiovascular impairments.

- *Serum electrolytes.* Levels are measured in clients who have DKA or HNKC to determine imbalances.

Monitoring Blood Glucose   People with diabetes must monitor their condition daily by testing glucose levels. Two types of tests are available. The first type, long used prior to the development of devices to directly measure blood glucose, is urine testing for glucose and ketones. Urine testing is less commonly used today. The second type, direct measurement of blood glucose, is widely used in all types of health care settings and in the home. The information about these tests provides guidelines for the nurse in performing the tests and in teaching clients to self-monitor their blood glucose at home.

Urine Testing for Ketones and Glucose   Urine testing for glucose and ketones was at one time the only available method for evaluating the management of diabetes. An inexpensive and noninvasive test, it has unpredictable results and cannot be used to detect or measure hypoglycemia. The results are affected by some of the following factors:

- Urine from the urinary bladder does not reflect the blood glucose level at the time of the test.

- The renal threshold for glucose varies from person to person. Also, it is higher in older adults and in adults with renal disease; therefore, false-negative results may be measured even when the blood glucose level is greatly elevated.

- Certain drugs, such as aspirin and some antibiotics, affect the results.

Urine testing should be done in people with IDDM who have unexplained hyperglycemia, during illness, and during pregnancy to monitor for hyperglycemia and ketoacidosis.

To test the urine for ketones:

1. Ask the client to void, discard the urine, and drink a full glass of water.

2. Thirty minutes later, collect a urine sample.

3. For Acidtest tablets: Place the tablet on a white paper towel, place 1 drop of urine on the tablet, and wait 30 seconds. If the tablet turns any shade from lavender to deep purple, the test is positive for ketones.

4. For Ketostix: Dip the reagent stick into the urine sample. Wait 15 seconds, and compare the color of the pad at the end of the stick to an accompanying color chart. Purple is indicative of ketones.

To test the urine for glucose:

1. Follow the same procedure to collect a urine sample.

2. Dip the reagent stick into the urine sample, and wait the time indicated. Compare the color of the pad on the end of the reagent stick with an accompanying color chart. The glucose is expressed as a percentage (for example, ½%, 1%, 2%). Remember that normally no glucose is found in the urine, so the presence of glucose is an abnormal manifestation indicating hyperglycemia.

Nursing Implications for Diagnostic Tests: Oral Glucose Tolerance Test

■ ■ ■

Preparation of Client

- Have the client eat a diet high in carbohydrates for 3 days before the test.

- If possible, discontinue drugs that may interfere with test results for 3 days before the test:
  a. Corticosteroids
  b. Oral contraceptives
  c. Synthetic estrogens
  d. Phenytoin (Dilantin)
  e. Vitamin C
  f. Aspirin
  g. Thiazide diuretics
  h. Nicotinic acid

- Keep the client NPO except for water for 10 hours before the test.

- The client is given a specified amount of glucose (either 75 g or 100 g) as a lemon-flavor or glucola liquid after fasting blood and urine samples are taken.

- Blood and urine samples are taken after the glucose is ingested at 30 minutes, 1 hour, and 2 hours. In some instances the test may continue for up to 5 hours.

- Observe the client for symptoms of hyperglycemia and hypoglycemia.

Client and Family Teaching

- The procedure for the test.

- Foods that are high in carbohydrates.

- For 10 hours before the test and during the test, the following are not allowed: food, tea, coffee, or alcohol. Smoking is not permitted during the test.

- Nausea, weakness, dizziness, and sweating may be experienced during the test; these symptoms often disappear, but report them to the nurse as soon as they occur.

- Limit activity because increased activity may change the test results. (The client may be requested to remain seated during the test.)

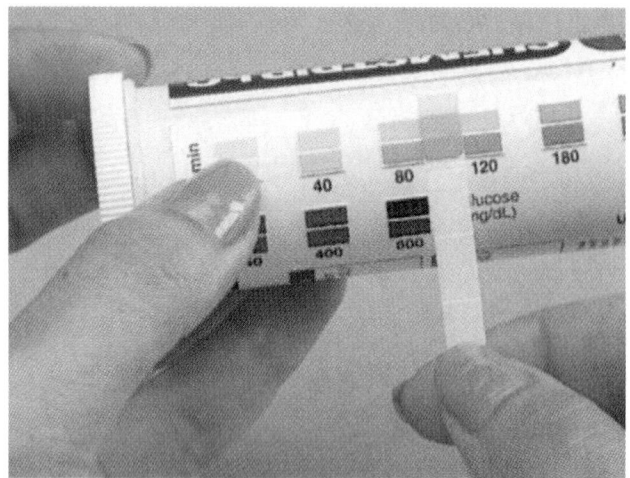

Figure 21–5 Determination of blood glucose levels by visual reading. The color of the strip is compared with the color chart on the side of the container.

Self-Monitoring of Blood Glucose   *Self-monitoring of blood glucose (SMBG)* is a useful method for all people with diabetes to manage their disease. SMBG allows the person with diabetes to monitor and achieve metabolic control and decrease the danger of hypoglycemia. SMBG has been described by some authorities as "the greatest innovation in diabetic care in the last 30 years" (Guthrie & Guthrie, 1991, p. 145).

The American Diabetes Association's 1991 Standards of Medical Care for Patients with Diabetes Mellitus states that all clients must be taught some method of monitoring glycemic control. Clients with IDDM, as well as those with poorly controlled NIDDM, should use blood glucose testing. The timing of SMBG is highly individualized, depending on the person's diagnosis, general disease control, and physical state. Some people may test from four to six times daily, whereas others who have achieved good control may test once daily or weekly. In addition, SMBG is useful when the person is ill, pregnant, or has symptoms of hypoglycemia or hyperglycemia.

Below is a list of equipment needed for SMBG:

- Some type of device to perform a finger-stick for obtaining a drop of blood (such as an Autolet, Penlet, or Soft Touch).
- Chemically impregnated test strips that change color when they come into contact with glucose or that can be read by machine (for example, Glucostix and Chemstrip bG).
- A blood glucose measuring machine (the Glucometer, the Accuchek, or the Ultra, for example) if the most accurate measurement is desired or recommended.

The American Diabetes Association annually publishes in the magazine *Diabetes Forecast* a comprehensive list of currently available blood glucose monitoring machines and strips with approximate prices. Most medical insurance policies cover the cost of these machines.

Usually, the strip is read by comparing its color with a color chart on the side of the container or on an insert (Figure 21–5).

Most blood glucose machines operate by reflecting light from the strip after the strip is inserted. The absorbed or reflected light is picked up by an electric eye, which converts the light to electric current. The current usually appears digitally.

The manufacturer's instructions must be followed carefully. If the timing of the blood on the strip is not exact, or if the strip is overblotted or underblotted, the test will not be accurate. In addition, the machine must be cleaned according to the manufacturer's directions to ensure accuracy. Monitors that use no-wipe technology, thereby improving the accuracy of glucose measurement, are now being marketed. Other monitors are computerized and/or include a memory of previous glucose readings to show a pattern of control.

Pharmacology

The pharmacologic treatment for diabetes mellitus depends on the type of diabetes. People with IDDM must have insulin; those with NIDDM are usually able to control glucose levels with an oral antidiabetic medication, but they may require insulin if control is inadequate.

Insulin   The person with IDDM requires a lifelong exogenous source of the insulin hormone to maintain life. Insulin is not a cure for diabetes; rather, it is a means of controlling hyperglycemia. Insulin is also necessary in other situations, such as the following:

- People with NIDDM who are unable to control glucose levels with oral antidiabetic drugs and/or diet
- People with NIDDM who are experiencing physical stress (such as an infection or surgery) or who are taking corticosteroids
- Women with gestational diabetes who are unable to control glucose with diet
- In the treatment of DKA or HNKC
- People who are receiving high-calorie tube feedings or parenteral nutrition

Nursing implications for administering insulin are given in the accompanying box and further discussion follows below.

Insulin Sources   The sources of insulin are beef, pork, a mixture of beef and pork, and humans. Insulin from beef and pork was used for years, but human insulin is more

Nursing Implications for Pharmacology: Insulin

Nursing Responsibilities

- Discard vials of insulin that have been open for several weeks or whose expiration date has passed.

- Refrigerate extra insulin vials not currently in use, but do not freeze them.

- Store insulin in a cool place, and avoid exposure to temperature extremes or sunlight.

- Store compatible mixtures of insulin for no longer than 1 month at room temperature or 3 months at 36 to 46 F (2 to 8 C).

- Discard any vial with discoloration, clumping, granules, or solid deposits on the sides.

- If breakfast is delayed, also delay the administration of regular insulin.

- Monitor and maintain a record of blood glucose readings 30 minutes before each meal and bedtime (or as prescribed).

- Monitor food intake, and notify the physician if food is not being consumed.

- Monitor electrolytes (especially potassium), blood urea nitrogen (BUN) levels, and creatinine.

- Observe injection sites for manifestations of hypersensitivity, lipodystrophy, and lipoatrophy.

- If symptoms of hypoglycemia occur, confirm by testing blood glucose level, and administer an oral source of a fast-acting carbohydrate, such as juice, milk, or crackers. Hypoglycemic symptoms may vary but commonly include feelings of shakiness, hunger, and/or nervousness accompanied by sweating, tachycardia, or palpitations.

- If symptoms of hyperglycemia occur, confirm by testing blood glucose level, and notify the physician.

Client and Family Teaching

- The manifestations of diabetes mellitus.

- Self-administration of insulin, with a return demonstration:
  a. Wash hands carefully.
  b. Have a vial of insulin, the insulin syringe with needle, and alcohol pads ready to use.
  c. Remove the cover from the needle.
  d. Fill the syringe with an amount of air equal to the number of units of insulin, and insert the needle into the vial.

  e. Push air into the vial, invert the vial, and withdraw the prescribed units of insulin.
  f. Replace the cover over the needle.
  g. Wipe the selected site with alcohol. The injection is less likely to be painful if the alcohol is allowed to dry.
  h. Pinch up a fold of skin, and insert the needle into the tissue at the recommended angle.
  i. Insert the insulin.
  j. Withdraw the needle; if desired, apply firm pressure to the site for a few seconds.
  k. Recap the needle. Many people with diabetes reuse disposable syringes with attached needles without adverse effects. The primary reason for discarding after several uses is that the needle becomes dull and makes the injection painful.

- Follow instructions for mixing insulins (refer to the box on page 729).

- Always keep an extra vial of insulin available.

- Always have a vial of regular insulin available for emergencies.

- Be aware of the signs of hypersensitivity responses, hypoglycemia, and hyperglycemia.

- Keep candy or a sugar source available at all times to treat hypoglycemia, if it occurs.

- Vision may be blurred during the first 6 to 8 weeks of insulin therapy; this is the result of fluid changes in the eye and should clear up in 8 weeks.

- Avoid alcoholic beverages, which may cause hypoglycemia.

- Follow these guidelines for sick days:
  a. Never omit insulin.
  b. Always monitor blood glucose and/or urine ketones at least every 2 to 4 hours.
  c. Always drink plenty of fluids; try to drink at least one glass of water or other calorie-free, caffeine-free liquid each hour.
  d. Get as much rest as possible.
  e. Contact the physician if there is persistent fever, vomiting, shortness of breath, severe pain in the abdomen, dehydration, loss of vision, chest pain, persistent diarrhea, blood glucose levels above 250, or ketones in the urine.

- Establish a plan for rotating injection sites, and observe closely for changes in tissues such as hardness, dimpling, or sunken areas.

Table 21–5 Insulin Preparations

	Type	Trade Names	Onset of Action (h)	Peak Action (h)	Duration of Action (h)

Rapid-Acting	Regular (R)	Regular Iletin I
		Regular Insulin
		Beef Regular Iletin II
		Pork Regular Iletin II
		  Velosin
		    Regular Purified Pork
		Humulin R
		    Novolin R
		    Velosulin
			0.5 to 1	2 to 4	4 to 6

	Crystalline Zinc	Crystalline Zinc	0.5 to 1	2 to 4	4 to 6
	Semilente	Semilente Iletin I Semilente Insulin Semilente Purified Pork	1 to 1.5	4 to 7	12 to 16

Intermediate-Acting	NPH (N)	NPH Iletin I
		NPH Insulin
		Beef NPH Iletin I
		NPH Purified Pork
		  Pork NPH Iletin II
		  Isulatard NPH
		Humulin N
		  Novolin N
		  Insulatard NPH
			1 to 2	8 to 12	18 to 24

	Lente (L)	Lente Insulin I Lente Insulin Lente Iletin II Lente Purified Pork Insulin Humulin L Novolin L	1 to 4	8 to 12	18 to 24
	Globulin Zinc	Globulin Zinc	2 to 4	6 to 10	12 to 18
Long-Acting	Protamine Zinc	Protamine Zinc & Iletin I Protamine Zinc & Iletin II	4 to 8	16 to 18	> 36
	Ultralente	Ultralente Iletin I Ultralente Insulin Ultralente Purified Beef Humulin Ultralente	4 to 8	16 to 18	> 36
	Mixed	Mixtard: 70% N + 30% R Novolin Mix: 70% N + 30% R			

commonly used today. Although all sources are equally effective in controlling blood glucose levels, human insulin is indicated for people who use insulin temporarily, people who are hypersensitive to pork or beef insulin, people who refuse animal products for religious or ethical reasons, pregnant women with diabetes, and those newly diagnosed with IDDM (White & Campbell, 1992).

Human insulins are synthetically derived by either an enzymatic conversion of pork insulin or by recombinant DNA technology from *Escherichia coli* bacteria. The human insulins are structurally identical to natural insulin,

induce less antigen formation, act more predictably, and provide better control of glucose. They are also less likely to cause tissue changes from repeated injections.

Insulin Preparations Insulins are available in rapid-acting, intermediate-acting, and long-acting preparations. The trade names and times of onset, peak, and duration of action are listed in Table 21–5.

Regular insulin is unmodified crystalline insulin. Regular insulin has the most rapid onset and peak of action of all the insulin preparations, but it also has the shortest duration of action. Regular insulin is clear in appearance and is the only type that can be given by the intravenous route; the other types are suspensions and could be harmful if given by this route. Regular insulin is also the type used to treat diabetic ketoacidosis.

NPH (isophane insulin suspension) and protamine zinc insulin (PZI) suspension are preparations in which the insulin has been conjugated with protamine, a large protein. The protamine decreases the solubility of the preparation and thus slows the action, delaying the onset and peak and prolonging the duration of action. These preparations appear cloudy when properly mixed prior to injection. Protamine is a foreign substance and may cause hypersensitivity reactions.

Semilente, lente, and ultralente insulins have altered solubility as a result of a modification of the insulin itself; no foreign proteins are added. Of these insulins, semilente insulin acts most rapidly, whereas ultralente insulin has the longest duration of action. Lente insulin is a mixture of ultralente (70%) and semilente (30%) and is intermediate-acting.

Concentrations of Insulin   Insulin is dispensed in three concentrations: 40 U/mL (U-40), 100 U/mL (U-100), and 500 U/mL (U-500). Each of the basic types of insulin (regular, semilente, NPH, lente, protamine zinc, and ultralente) is available in both U-40 and U-100 concentrations. Only regular insulin is also dispensed in U-500 concentration.

The American Diabetes Association has recommended that U-40 concentrations no longer be used and that U-100 become the universal preparation. In actual practice, U-100 insulin is most commonly used. U-500 insulin is reserved for people who need doses in excess of 200 U per day. These people are said to be insulin resistant, and the larger unit amount of insulin per mL makes administration more manageable.

Insulin Administration   The considerations for administering insulin include routes of administration, syringe and needle selection, preparing the injection, sites of injection, mixing insulins, and insulin regimens.

Routes of Administration. All insulins are given parenterally. Only regular insulin is given by both subcutaneous and intravenous routes; all others are given only subcutaneously. If the intravenous route is not available, regular insulin may also be administered intramuscularly in an emergency situation.

Regular insulin is also used in *continuous subcutaneous insulin infusion (CSII)* devices, often called *insulin pumps.* CSII devices have a small pump that holds a syringe connected to a subcutaneous needle by tubing. The needle is placed in the skin, usually in the abdomen. This device delivers a constant amount of programmed insulin throughout each 24-hour period. It also can be used to deliver a bolus of insulin manually (for example, before meals). The programming of the amount of insulin to be delivered is determined by frequent blood glucose monitoring. There are several different pumps available, and each has rechargeable batteries, a syringe, a programmable computer, and a motor and drive mechanism. Many people with diabetes believe the CSII device allows more normal regulation of blood glucose and provides greater life-style flexibility.

Syringe and Needle Selection. Insulin is administered in sterile, single-use, disposable insulin syringes, calibrated in units per milliliter. This means that in U-100 insulin, there are 100 U of insulin in 1 mL. Syringes for administering U-100 insulin, the most common concentration, can be purchased in either 0.3-mL (30 U), 0.5-mL (50 U), or 1.0-mL (100 U) size. The advantage of the 0.3-mL and 0.5-mL sizes is that the distance between unit markings is greater, making it easier to measure the dose accurately.

Most insulin syringes are manufactured with the needle permanently attached in a 25- to 26-gauge, 0.5-inch size. If this type of syringe is not available, an insulin syringe and a 25-gauge, 0.5-inch or 0.75-inch needle should be used.

Other special injection products are available for people with physical handicaps. These products include automatic injectors and jet spray injectors.

Preparing the Injection. The vial of insulin in use may be kept at room temperature for up to 4 weeks. Stored insulin should be kept in the refrigerator and brought to room temperature prior to administration.

Regular insulin does not require mixing. If the solution is cloudy or discolored, the vial should be discarded. The other types of insulin must be mixed to disperse the particles evenly throughout the solution. Mix the vial by gently rolling it between the hands; vigorous shaking causes bubble formation and frothing, which makes the dose inaccurate. It is critical that no air bubbles remain in the prepared dose, because even a small bubble can displace several units of insulin.

Sites of Injection. Although in theory any area of the body with subcutaneous tissue may be used for injections of insulin, certain sites are recommended (Figure 21–6). The rate of absorption and peak of action of insulin differs according to the site. The site that allows the most rapid absorption is the abdomen, followed by the deltoid muscle, then the thigh, and then the hip.

When administering insulin, gently pinch a fold of skin, and inject the needle at a 90-degree angle. If the person is very thin, a 45-degree angle may be required to avoid injecting into muscle. Do not massage the site after administering the injection, because this may interfere

Figure 21–6 Sites of insulin injection.

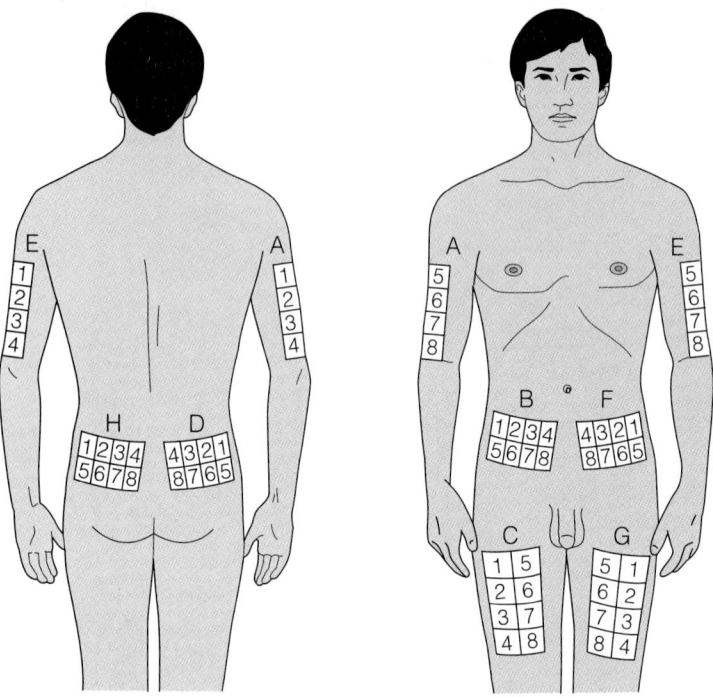

with absorption; pressure, however, may be applied for about 1 minute. Rotation of injection sites is recommended for clients using pork or beef insulin; rotation within sites is recommended for those using human or purified pork insulin. The distance between injections should be about 1 inch (avoiding the area within a 2-inch radius around the umbilicus). Insulin should not be injected into an area which will be exercised (such as the thigh before a vigorous walk) or to which heat will be applied; exercise or heat may increase the rate of absorption and cause a more rapid onset and peak of action.

Lipodystrophy (hypertrophy of subcutaneous tissue) or *lipoatrophy* (atrophy of subcutaneous tissue) may result if the same injection sites are used repeatedly, especially with pork and beef insulins. The use of refrigerated insulin may trigger the development of tissue atrophy or hypertrophy. These problems rarely occur with the use of human insulins. Lipodystrophy and lipoatrophy alter insulin absorption, delaying its onset or retaining the insulin in the tissue for a period of time instead of allowing it to be absorbed into the body. Lipodystrophy usually resolves if the area is unused for a minimum of 6 months.

Mixing Insulins. When a person with diabetes requires more than one type of insulin, mixing is recommended to avoid administering two injections per dose. Two different concentrations are administered because a single dose of intermediate-acting or long-acting insulin rarely provides adequate control of blood glucose levels. The proce-

dure for mixing insulins is described in the box on page 729. Below are some general guidelines:

- Commercially mixed insulins are recommended if the insulin ratio is appropriate for the requirements of the client.

- Only insulins of like concentration should be mixed (for example, regular insulin U-100 with NPH insulin U-100).

- Regular insulin may be mixed with all other types of insulin; it may be injected immediately after mixing or stored for future use.

- NPH insulin and PZI insulin may be mixed only with regular insulin.

- Lente insulin preparations may be mixed with each other; mixing with regular insulin or with PZI and NPH insulin is not recommended.

- Do not mix human and animal insulins.

- Always withdraw regular insulin first to avoid contaminating the regular insulin with intermediate-acting insulin.

Insulin Regimens. The appropriate insulin dosage is individualized by achieving a balance among insulin, diet, and exercise. For most people with diabetes, the timing of insulin action requires two or more injections each day, often a mixture of rapid-acting and intermediate-acting insulins. Timing of the injections depends on blood

Mixing Insulins: 10 Units of Regular and 20 Units of NPH

1. Wash hands.
2. Inspect regular insulin for clarity.
3. Gently rotate NPH insulin to mix well.
4. Wipe off the top of both vials with an alcohol pad.
5. Draw 20 U of air into the syringe, and inject air into the NPH vial (Figure *A*). Withdraw needle.
6. Draw 10 U of air into the syringe, and inject air into the regular vial (Figure *B*).
7. Invert the vial, and withdraw 10 U of regular insulin (Figure *C*). Withdraw the needle.
8. Insert the needle into the NPH vial, and carefully withdraw 20 U of NPH insulin (Figure *D*).
9. Administer the insulin.
10. Wash hands, and properly dispose of the syringe.

A Injecting air into the NPH vial.

B Injecting air into the regular insulin vial.

C Withdrawing regular insulin.

D Withdrawing NPH insulin.

20 Units / 20 U air / NPH insulin / (Cloudy)

10 Units / 10 U air / Regular insulin / (Clear)

Air / Regular insulin / (Clear) / 10 Units regular insulin

Air / NPH insulin / (Cloudy) / 20 Units NPH insulin / 10 Units regular insulin / 30 Units total dosage

---

glucose levels, food consumption, exercise, and types of insulin used. The objective is to avoid daytime hypoglycemia while achieving adequate blood glucose control overnight. Typical insulin regimens are discussed in Table 21–6.

Hypersensitivity Responses When injected, insulin may cause local and systemic hypersensitivity responses. Manifestations of local reactions are a hardening and reddening of the area area that develops over several hours. Local reactions result from a contaminant in the insulin and are more likely to occur when less purified insulin products are used.

Systemic reactions occur rapidly and are characterized by widespread red, intensely pruritic welts. Respiratory difficulty may occur if the respiratory system is involved. Systemic responses are due to an allergy to the insulin itself and are most common with beef insulin. The client can be desensitized by administering small doses of puri-

fied pork or human insulin, followed by progressively larger doses (Lehne, 1990).

Oral Hypoglycemic Agents Oral hypoglycemic agents (also called oral antidiabetic agents) are used to treat people with NIDDM. Nursing implications for this category of drugs are discussed in the pharmacology box on page 731.

Dietary Management

The management of diabetes requires a careful balance between the intake of nutrients, the expenditure of energy, and the dose and timing of insulin or oral hypoglycemic agents. Although everyone has the same need for basic nutrition, the person with diabetes must eat a more structured diet in order to prevent hyperglycemia. The goals for dietary management for adults with diabetes, based on guidelines established by the American Diabetes Association (1992e) are to

Table 21–6   Insulin Regimens

Regimen	Insulin Type*	General Information
One injection per day	NPH or NPH/R before breakfast	One injection is used to cover all meals (see figure at left). This is a simple regimen, but it is often difficult to control FBS levels, and afternoon hypoglycemia may result from increases in NPH.

Regimen	Insulin Type*	General Information
Two injections per day	NPH or NPH/R before breakfast and dinner	This regimen is the least complex of those aiming to mimic normal pancreatic function; the person must have a fairly rigid schedule of food intake and exercise (see figure at left).

Regimen	Insulin Type*	General Information
Three or four injections per day	R before each meal; NPH at dinner or bedtime	This regimen more closely mimics normal pancreatic function; it allows greater choice in mealtimes and exercise (see figure at left). However, each preprandial dose of R must be determined by blood glucose tests.

*Insulin types are abbreviated as follows: NPH = intermediate-acting, R = regular, rapid-acting.

- Restore normal blood glucose and optimal lipid levels to prevent hyperglycemia or hypoglycemia, prevent or delay the onset of long-term complications, and contribute to a normal outcome of pregnancy in women with diabetes.

- Attain and maintain reasonable body weight.

- Stay consistent in the timing of meals and snacks.

- Determine a meal plan appropriate for the person's lifestyle and cultural/ethnic background.

- Manage weight for obese people with NIDDM.

- Improve the overall health of people with diabetes through optimal nutrition.

The plan should consider food preferences, food habits, age, and other medical conditions. The nutrient recommendations for adults with diabetes mellitus are summarized in Table 21–7.

Distribution of Kilocalories   To maintain or attain reasonable weight, the client must control kcal intake.

Nursing Implications for Pharmacology: Oral Hypoglycemic Agents

ORAL HYPOGLYCEMIC AGENTS

Acetohexamide (Dimelor, Dymelor)$_2$

Chlorpropamide (Diabinese, Glucamide)$_2$

Glipizide (Glucotrol)$_1$

Glyburide (DiaBeta, Micronase)$_1$

Tolazamide (Tolamide, Tolinase)$_2$

Tolbutamide (Orinase)$_2$

The drugs listed above are sulfonylureas; they are related to sulfonamides but lack antibacterial action. They are used primarily to treat mild, nonketotic NIDDM usually associated with obesity. These clients cannot control the symptoms by diet alone, but they do not require insulin. The drugs act by stimulating the pancreatic cells to secrete more insulin and by increasing the sensitivity of peripheral tissues to insulin. The most common side effect is hypoglycemia.

The sulfonylureas are divided into two groups: first-generation agents and second-generation agents. The primary difference between the two groups is that maximum effective doses are lower in those agents classified as second generation. In the list above, first-generation agents are identified by the subscript 1, second-generation agents by the subscript 2.

Nursing Responsibilities

- Assess clients taking oral hypoglycemic agents closely for the first 7 days to determine therapeutic response.

- Administer the drug with food.

- Teach the client the importance of maintaining a prescribed diet and exercise program.

- Monitor for hypoglycemia if the client is also taking nonsteroidal anti-inflammatory agents (NSAIDs),

sulfonamide antibiotics, ranitidine, cimetidine, or beta-blockers; these drugs intensify the action of sulfonylureas.

- Monitor for hyperglycemia if the client is also taking calcium channel blockers, oral contraceptives, glucocorticoids, phenothiazines, or thiazide diuretics; these drugs decrease the hypoglycemic responses to sulfonylureas.

- Do not administer these drugs to pregnant or lactating women.

- Assess for side effects: nausea, heartburn, diarrhea, dizziness, fever, headache, jaundice, skin rash, urticaria, photophobia, thrombocytopenia, leukopenia, or anemia.

- If the client is to have a thyroid test, determine whether the drug has been taken; sulfonylureas interfere with the uptake of radioactive iodine.

Client and Family Teaching

- Maintain prescribed diet and exercise regimen.

- You may need insulin if you have surgery, trauma, fever, or infection.

- Follow instructions to monitor blood glucose.

- Report illness or side effects to the physician.

- Undergo periodic laboratory evaluations as prescribed by the physician.

- Avoid alcohol intake, which may cause a reaction involving flushing, palpitations, and nausea.

- The medication interferes with the effectiveness of oral contraceptives; other birth-control measures may be required.

- Mild symptoms of hyperglycemia may appear if a different agent is begun.

The daily kcal allowance for the person with diabetes is usually calculated on the basis of his or her desirable weight (that is, weight at age 25, provided that the person was healthy and not overweight). This number of kcal is then divided among carbohydrates, proteins, and fats. The following guidelines or used to determine kcal needs for adults with diabetes:

1. Calculate basal calories: desirable body weight (lb) × 10.

2. Add activity calories:
   a. Sedentary: desirable body weight (lb) × 3.
   b. Moderate: desirable body weight (lb) × 5.
   c. Strenuous: desirable body weight (lb) × 10.

3. Add calories for indicated weight gain, growth in pregnant women, or lactation:
   a. Pregnancy: Add 300 kcal per day to gain 23 lb in 9 months.
   b. Lactation: Add 500 kcal per day.
   c. To gain 1 lb per week, add 500 kcal per day.

Table 21-7	Nutrient Recommendations for Adults with Diabetes

Nutrient	Recommended Daily Intake
Calories (kcal)	Amount needed to attain and maintain reasonable weight (defined as the weight an individual and health care provider acknowledge as being short-term and long-term achievable and maintainable).
Carbohydrates	Individualized, based on client's individual eating habits, and glucose and lipid goals.
Protein	Approximately 10% to 20% of the daily caloric intake; should be from both animal and vegetable sources.
Saturated fat and cholesterol	Less than 10% of the daily calories should be from saturated fats, with dietary cholesterol limited to 300 mg or less per day.
Fiber	20 to 30 g of dietary fiber each day from a wide variety of food sources.
Sodium	The same as for the general population; no more than 2,400 mg to 3,000 mg per day.
Vitamins and minerals	Sufficient to meet daily requirements.
Alcohol	For people using insulin, up to 2 alcoholic beverages can be ingested with and in addition to the usual meal plan (1 alcoholic beverage equals 12 ounces of beer, 5 ounces of wine, or one and one-half ounces of distilled spirits). Special considerations are important for people with a history of alcohol abuse, those who are pregnant, and those with other medical problems. The alcohol should only be ingested with a meal to decrease the risk of hypoglycemia.

Note. "Nutritional Recommendations and Principles for Individuals with Diabetes Mellitus" by the American Diabetes Association, 1994, *Diabetes Care, 17*(5), 519–522.

4. Subtract calories for indicated weight loss: to lose 1 lb per week, subtract 500 kcal per day. (Friesen, 1991, p. 95)

Obese people often improve their diabetes management with weight loss. Nonobese people with diabetes must have adequate kcal intake to maintain body weight.

Carbohydrates The American Diabetes Association (1994) currently recommends that carbohydrates should be individualized to the client's needs. Carbohydrates contain 4 kcal per gram. This group of nutrients is made up of plant foods (grains, fruits, vegetables), milk, and some dairy products. Carbohydrates can be divided into

simple sugars and complex carbohydrates. Simple sugars are limited because they cause an immediate and rapid increase in blood glucose levels. These high-glycemic foods include sucrose and refined sugars such as honey, molasses, and syrup.

In contrast, complex carbohydrates and starches are digested and absorbed more slowly, so blood glucose levels rise more slowly and are more easily controlled. This group is further divided into high-glycemic foods, such as cereals, root vegetables, and breads; and low-glycemic foods, such as legumes, nuts, and some dairy products. The higher the glycemic index of foods, the more rapidly they will raise the blood sugar during a 2-hour period (Friesen, 1991). Complex carbohydrates, in particular low-glycemic foods that are high in fiber and starch, should make up 90% to 95% of the daily carbohydrate allowance.

Protein The recommended daily protein intake is 10% to 20% of total daily kcal intake. Protein has 4 kcal per gram. Sources of protein should be low in fat, low in saturated fat, and low in cholesterol.

Although this amount of protein is much less than that which most people normally consume in the diet, it is recommended to help prevent or delay renal complications. To help the client accept the decrease in the amount of protein, the nurse may suggest a less severe restriction at diagnosis with a gradual decrease to take place over a period of years.

Fats Dietary fats should be low in both saturated fat and cholesterol. Fats are restricted to less than 10% of the total kcal allowed per day. Fat has 9 kcal per gram. Below are the sources for the different types of fat:

- *Saturated fat.* Sources are animal meats (meat and butter fats, lard, bacon), cocoa butter, coconut oil, palm oil, and hydrogenated oils.

- *Polyunsaturated fat.* Sources are oils of corn, safflower, sunflower, soybean, sesame seed, and cottonseed.

- *Monosaturated fat.* Sources are peanut oil, olive oil, and canola oil.

Within the fat allowance, cholesterol should not exceed 300 mg daily. Limiting fat and cholesterol intake may help prevent or delay the onset of atherosclerosis, a common complication of diabetes.

Intake of Fiber Fiber plays an important role in the dietary management of diabetes. Current evidence suggests that a diet high in fiber, especially soluble fiber, helps improve carbohydrate metabolism, lowers total cholesterol, and lowers low-density lipoprotein (LDL) cholesterol. Soluble fiber is found in dried beans, oats, barley, and in some vegetables and fruits (for example, peas, corn, zucchini, cauliflower, broccoli, prunes, pears, apples, bananas, oranges). Insoluble fiber, which is found in wheat, corn, and in some vegetables and fruits (carrots, brussels sprouts, eggplant, green beans, pears, apples, strawberries), is not as beneficial in reducing blood sugar or lipid levels, but it does facilitate intestinal motility and give a feeling of fullness.

The ideal level of fiber has not been determined, but an intake of 20 to 30 grams per day is recommended. An increase in fiber may cause nausea, diarrhea or constipation, and increased flatulence, especially if the person does not also increase fluid intake. Fiber in the diet should therefore be increased gradually.

Other Dietary Considerations Other dietary considerations include the use of sodium, sweeteners, and alcohol.

Sodium Although the body requires sodium, most people consume much more than is needed each day, especially in processed foods. The recommended daily intake is 1000 mg of sodium per 1000 kcal, not to exceed 3000 mg. The primary concern with sodium is its association with hypertension, a common health problem in people with diabetes. It is suggested that table salt (which is 40% sodium) and processed foods high in sodium be avoided in the diabetes meal plan.

Sweeteners The diet plan for people with diabetes restricts the amount of refined sugars. As a result, many people use noncaloric sweeteners and foods or drinks made with noncaloric sweeteners. Commercially produced nonnutritive sweeteners are approved for use by the Food and Drug Administration (FDA). Although questions have been raised about the safety of these substances in laboratory animal studies, they are considered safe for use by humans. Included in this category of sweeteners are saccharin (Sweet and Low), aspartame (Nutrasweet, Equal), and acesulfame potassium (Sunnette). The nonnutritive sweeteners have negligent amounts of kcal or no kcal and produce very little or no changes in blood glucose levels.

People with diabetes also use nutritive sweeteners, including fructose, sorbitol, and xylitol. The kcal content of these substances is similar to that of table sugar (sucrose), but they cause less elevation in blood glucose. They are often included in foods labeled as "sugar-free." Sorbitol may cause flatulence and diarrhea.

Researchers are continuing to study the safety and effectiveness of the sweeteners. In addition, the FDA recommends that the food industry label products with the amount of each ingredient in milligrams per serving and the number of servings per container. When teaching clients about diet, the nurse should include information about the kcal content of sweeteners and the meaning of such words as *sugar-free* and *dietetic* on labels.

Alcohol Although drinking alcoholic beverages is not encouraged, neither is it totally prohibited for the client with diabetes. Alcohol consumption may potentiate the hypoglycemic effects of insulin and oral agents. The American Diabetes Association recommends that people with diabetes consume no more than two drinks at one time, limited to once or twice a week. Below are guidelines for people who include alcohol in their diet plan:

- The signs of intoxication and hypoglycemia are similar; thus, the person with IDDM is at increased risk for an insulin reaction.

- Two of the first-generation oral hypoglycemic agents (chlorpropamide and tolbutamide) may interact with the alcohol, causing headache, flushing, and nausea.

- Liqueurs, sweet wines, wine coolers, and sweet mixes contain large amounts of carbohydrate.

- Light beer is the recommended alcoholic drink.

- The person with IDDM should consume alcohol with meals and add it to the daily food intake.

- In most instances, the alcohol is substituted for fat in calculating the diet; a drink with 1.5 oz of alcohol is the equivalent of two fat exchanges (90 kcal). (Food exchanges are discussed below.)

Meal Planning Several different systems for meal planning are available to the person with diabetes. These systems include exchange lists, point systems, food groups, and calorie counting. The system most often used is the meal planning exchange list. No matter what system is used, however, it must take into account the person's usual eating habits, diet history, food values, and special needs. Altering foods and meal patterns is often one of the most difficult parts of diabetes management; careful consideration of individualized preferences enhances compliance with the diet.

Calculating the Diabetic Diet Plan The diabetic diet is based on the person's ideal (or reasonable) weight, activity level, age, and occupation. These factors determine the total kcal that the person may consume each day. After the calories have been determined, the proportions of carbohydrates, proteins, and fats are calculated, using the guidelines established by the American Diabetes Association (see Table 21–7).

The distribution of foods throughout the day is based on exchange lists, as shown in Table 21–8. There are six categories of food: milk, vegetables, fruits, breads, meats, and fats. The name and quantity of food that make up one exchange (or serving) are listed; standard household measurements are used. One food portion on the list can be substituted ("exchanged") for another with very little difference in calories or amount of carbohydrates, proteins, and fats. The meal plan prescribes how many exchanges

Table 21–8 Exchange List Examples

	Exchange		Food	Quantity in One Exchange
Milk	One exchange equals 12 g carbohydrate, 8 g protein, trace of fat, and 80 kcal.		Whole milk (delete 2 fat exchanges)	1 cup
			Canned evaporated whole milk	½ cup
			2% fat fortified milk (delete 1 fat exchange)	1 cup
			Skim or nonfat milk	
			Yogurt made from skim milk (plain, unflavored)	1 cup
				1 cup
Vegetable	One exchange equals 5 g carbohydrate, 2 g protein, and 25 kcal.		Asparagus	½ cup
	Raw vegetables from this exchange that may be used as desired include cucumbers, Chinese cabbage, lettuce, dill pickles, and radishes.		Beets	½ cup
			Broccoli	½ cup
			Greens	½ cup
			Summer squash	½ cup
			Tomatoes	½ cup
	One exchange equals 10 g carbohydrate and 40 kcal.		Tomato juice	½ cup
Fruits			Apple	1 small
			Apple juice	⅓ cup
			Apricots, fresh	2 medium
			Banana	½ small
			Grapes	12
			Orange	1 small
			Prunes	2 medium
Breads	One exchange equals 15 g carbohydrate, 2 g protein, and 70 kcal.	Bread	White	1 slice
			Whole wheat	1 slice
			Small bagel	½
			Hamburger bun	½
			Tortilla	1
		Cereal	Unsweetened ready-to-eat	½ cup
			Cooked	½ cup
			Grits, cooked	½ cup
			Rice or barley, cooked	½ cup
			Pasta, cooked (spaghetti, noodles, macaroni)	½ cup
			Popcorn, popped, no added fat	3 cups
			Flour	2½ T

are allowed for each food group per meal and snacks. A sample meal plan is given in Table 21–9 on page 736.

Special Considerations Special considerations for the diet plan include the needs of non-insulin-dependent people, the needs of insulin-dependent people, sick days, and the older adult.

Needs of the Client with NIDDM. The goals of the diet plan for the person with NIDDM are to improve blood glucose levels, improve overall health, prevent or delay complications, and attain or maintain reasonable body weight. Because the majority of these clients are overweight, weight loss is important and facilitates achieving the other goals.

There are no specific guidelines for the NIDDM diet, but in addition to decreasing kcal, it is recommended that the client consume three meals of equal size, evenly spaced approximately 4 to 5 hours apart, with one or two snacks. The person with NIDDM should also decrease fat intake. If the exchange list is difficult to use, calorie counting or designing the diet by grams of fat may be more useful.

Needs of the Client with IDDM. Diet and insulin prescription for the person with IDDM must be integrated for optimal energy metabolism and the prevention of hyperglycemia or hypoglycemia. The goals of the diet plan are to achieve optimal glucose and lipid levels, improve overall health, and maintain reasonable body weight. To

Table 21–8   (continued)

Exchange		Food		Quantity in One Exchange
Breads *(continued)*		Crackers	Graham, 2.5 inches square	3
			Matzoh, 4 inches × 6 inches	2
			Saltines	6
		Dried beans, peas, and lentils	Dried and cooked	½ cup
			Baked beans, no pork, canned	¼ cup
		Starchy vegetables	Corn	⅓ cup
			Corn on the cob	1 small
			Lima beans	½ cup
			Peas	½ cup
			Potato, mashed	½ cup
			Sweet potato	¼ cup
Meats, Cheeses, and Eggs	One exchange of lean meat equals 7 g protein, 3 g fat, and 55 kcal. One exchange of medium-fat meat equals 7 g protein, 5 g fat, and 75 kcal. One exchange of high-fat meat equals 7 g protein, 8 g fat, and 100 kcal. All visible fat should be trimmed off and meat measured after cooking.	Lean Meats	Beef: chuck, flank, round, rump	1 oz
			Pork: whole, center shank	1 oz
			Fish (fresh or frozen)	¼ cup
		Medium-fat meats	Ground beef	1 oz
			Dried beans and peas (delete 1 bread exchange)	½ cup
			Creamed cottage cheese	¼ cup
			Parmesan cheese	3 T
			Egg	1
		High-fat meats	Commercial hamburger, rib roast	1 oz
			Pork, ribs	1 oz
			Cheddar cheese	1 oz
			Frankfurter	1 small
Fats	One exchange equals 5 g fat and 45 kcal.		Margarine (soft, tub, stick)	1 tsp
			Avocado (4 inches in diameter)	⅛
			Peanut oil	1 tsp
			Olives (small)	5
			Spanish peanuts	20
			Bacon, crisp	1 strip
			French dressing	1 T

meet these goals, the following strategies must be implemented:

- Glucose regulation requires correlating eating patterns with insulin onset and peak of action.
- Meals, snacks, and insulin regimens should be based on the person's life-style.
- Meal planning depends on the specific insulin regimen prescribed.
- Snacks are an important consideration in relation to the amount and timing of exercise.
- The diet plan must consider the availability of foods, based on occupational, financial, religious, and ethnic constraints.

- Self-monitoring of blood glucose levels helps the client make adjustments for planned and unplanned changes in routines.

Sick-Day Management   When the person with diabetes is sick or has surgery, blood glucose levels increase, even though food intake decreases. The person often mistakenly alters or omits the insulin dose, causing further problems. The guidelines for dietary management during illness focus on preventing dehydration and providing nutrition for promoting recovery. In general, sick-day management includes the following:

- Monitoring blood glucose at least four times a day throughout an illness.

Table 21–9   Meal Plan Examples: 1800 kcal

		Breakfast	**Lunch**	**Dinner**	**Bedtime**
Exchange Allowances	Milk	1	1	1	
	Vegetable		1	1	
	Fruit	1	1	1	
	Bread	2	2	2	1
	Meat	2	2	2	1
	Fat	2	2	1	1
Food Choices from the Exchange List		1 cup skim milk 2 slices toast ¾ cup strawberries 2 slices bacon 2 tsp margarine	1 cup yogurt 1 cup cooked pasta ½ cup zucchini ½ cup pineapple 2 oz mozzarella cheese 2 T Italian dressing	1 cup skim milk 1 cup mashed potatoes Lettuce salad ½ cup cauliflower ½ cup applesauce 2 oz baked turkey 1 tsp margarine 1 T French dressing	½ small English muffin ½ cup cottage cheese 1 tsp margarine

- Testing urine for ketones if blood glucose is greater than 240 mg/dL.
- Continuing to take the usual insulin dose or oral hypoglycemic agent.
- Sipping 8 to 12 oz of fluid each hour.
- Substituting easily digested liquids or soft foods if solid foods are not tolerated. The substituted liquids and foods should be carbohydrate equivalents, for example, ½ cup sweetened gelatin, ½ cup fruit juice, one Popsicle, ¼ cup sherbet, and ½ cup regular soft drink.
- Calling the physician if the client is unable to eat for more than 24 hours or if vomiting and diarrhea last for more than 6 hours. (Ley & Goldman, 1990)

Diet Plan for the Older Adult   The majority of older adults have NIDDM and should follow the general guidelines for the NIDDM diet plan. However, special considerations for the older adult are important if the diet plan is to be followed:

- Dietary likes and dislikes
- Eating habits
- Who prepares the meals
- Other illnesses
- Age-related changes in taste perception
- Dental health
- Transportation to buy foods
- Available income
- Support persons

Other factors to consider in planning the diet for the older adult include the age-related decline in kcal re-

quirements, decline in physical activity due to age and/or chronic illnesses, and the onset or progression of other chronic illnesses. The older adult who is overweight should reduce kcal intake to ensure weight loss, but at the same time, careful monitoring for malnutrition is necessary. It is possible for the older adult to revert to normal glucose tolerance if ideal body weight is regained. A nursing study of the effect of health beliefs on self-care behaviors and glycemic control in older adults is described in the accompanying research box.

Information Sources   Information about exchange lists and meal planning may be obtained from the American Diabetes Association, the American Dietetic Association, and the International Diabetes Center.

Examples of available resources follow:

- *Family Cookbook*
- *Exchange Lists for Meal Planning*
- *Large-Print Exchange Lists for Meal Planning*
- *Month of Meals Menu Planner*
- *Meal Planning with Mexican Foods*
- *Meal Planning with Jewish Foods*
- *Chinese American Food Practices, Customs, and Holidays*
- *Navajo Food Practices, Customs, and Holidays*
- *Guidelines for the Use of the Exchange Lists for Low-Sodium Meal Planning*
- *Guidelines for the Use of the Exchange Lists for Low-Fat Meal Planning*
- *Convenience Food Facts*
- *Exchanges for All Occasions*

Applying Research to Nursing Practice: Meeting the Needs of the Older Adult with Diabetes

■ ■ ■

A descriptive study of 102 older adults with NIDDM examined the relationships between diabetes-specific health beliefs and adherence to the diabetes regimen and glycemic control (Polly, 1992). The diabetes regimen included taking medications, limiting calories, avoiding sweets, limiting alcohol, eating at regular times, following a meal plan, checking blood glucose, and exercising. Data from the study suggest that glucose control may be associated with the client's perception of the severity of the illness and with barriers to treatment. Those who perceived their illness to be more severe and were more recently diagnosed were more likely to follow prescribed regimens, including medications and diet. Barriers to carrying out prescribed therapy included limited finances and low educational level.

Implications for Nursing

The special needs of the older adult with diabetes is an area that has had minimal attention in nursing research. With an ever-increasing population of older adults and a predicted increase in diabetes with aging, this information is essential. Nurses must not only identify the special needs of the older adult but also know how to teach self-care to improve the client's adherence to the prescribed diabetes regimen. Because the majority of older adults provide self-care in the home or in community settings, nursing histories must include the client's perception of illness and beliefs about personal barriers to achieving optimal health.

Critical Thinking in Client Care

1. In the older adult with diabetes, what normal age-related changes may act as barriers to providing self-care?

2. You are assigned to teach two clients how to use exchange lists to plan their meals. One client has a sixth-grade education, the other a college degree. Describe how your teaching plans would differ.

3. Your 82-year-old client states, "Why should I follow this diet? I'm not going to live much longer anyway." What would be your reply?

4. You are assigned to teach a 70-year-old homeless man about the necessity of decreasing high-sugar foods in his diet. What would your discussion with him include?

■ *Fast Food Facts*
■ *The Joy of Snacks*

Exercise

The third component of diabetes management is a regular exercise program. The benefits of exercise are the same for everyone, with or without diabetes: improved physical fitness, improved emotional state, weight control, and improved work capacity. In people with diabetes, exercise causes glucose reduction by increasing the uptake of glucose by muscle cells, potentially reducing the need for insulin. Exercise also decreases cholesterol and triglycerides, reducing the risk of cardiovascular disorders. People with diabetes should consult their primary health care provider before beginning or changing an exercise program.

It is as important to assess the person's usual life-style before establishing an exercise program as it is before planning a diet. Factors to consider include the client's usual exercise habits, living environment, and community programs. The exercise that the person enjoys most is probably the one that he or she will continue throughout life.

IDDM Exercise Programs   In the person with IDDM, glycemic responses to exercise vary according to the type, intensity, and duration of the exercise. Other factors that influence responses include the timing of exercise in relation to meals and insulin injections, and the time of day of the activity. Unless these factors are integrated into the exercise program, the person with IDDM has an increased risk of hypoglycemia and hyperglycemia. Below are some general guidelines for an IDDM exercise program:

■ People who have frequent hyperglycemia or hypoglycemia should avoid prolonged exercise until glucose control improves.

■ The risk of exercise-induced hypoglycemia is lowest before breakfast, when free-insulin levels tend to be lower than they are before meals later in the day or at bedtime.

■ Low-impact aerobic exercises are encouraged.

■ Exercise should be moderate and regular; brief, intense exercise tends to cause mild hyperglycemia, and prolonged exercise can lead to hypoglycemia.

■ Exercising at a peak insulin action time may lead to hypoglycemia.

- Self-monitoring of blood glucose levels is essential both before and after exercise.
- Food intake may need to be increased to compensate for the activity.
- Fluid intake, especially water, is essential.

Young adults may continue participating in sports with some modifications in diet and insulin dosage. It is recommended that athletes begin training slowly, extend activity over a prolonged period, take a carbohydrate source (such as a drink consisting of 5% to 10% carbohydrate) after about 1 hour of exercise, and monitor blood glucose levels for possible adjustments. In addition, a snack should be available after the activity is completed. It may be necessary to omit the usual regular insulin dose prior to an athletic event; even if the athlete is hyperglycemic at the beginning of the event, blood glucose levels will fall to normal after the first 60 to 90 minutes of exercise.

NIDDM Exercise Programs An exercise program for the person with NIDDM is especially important. The benefits of regular exercise include weight loss in those who are overweight, improved glycemic control, increased well-being, socialization with others, and a reduction of cardiovascular risk factors. A combination of diet, exercise, and weight loss often decreases the need for oral hypoglycemic agents. This decrease is due to an increased sensitivity to insulin, increased kcal expenditure, and increased self-esteem.

Below are some general guidelines for an NIDDM exercise program:

- Before the client begins the program, carefully assess for previously undiagnosed hypertension, neuropathy, retinopathy, nephropathy, and cardiac ischemia.
- Begin the program with mild exercises, and gradually increase intensity and duration.
- Self-monitoring of blood glucose before and after exercise is essential.
- Exercise at least three times a week or every other day, for at least 20 to 30 minutes.
- Include muscle-strengthening and low-impact aerobic exercises in the program.

All people with diabetes should follow the recommendations of the American Diabetes Association when exercising: Use proper footwear, inspect the feet daily and after exercise, avoid exercise in extreme heat or cold, and avoiding exercise during periods of poor glucose control. The American Diabetes Association further recommends that people over age 35 have an exercise-stress electrocardiogram prior to beginning an exercise program.

Surgical Management

Surgical management of diabetes involves replacing or transplanting the pancreas, pancreatic cells, or beta cells.

Although it is still in the investigative stage, many researchers believe that transplantation of the tail of the pancreas is the most promising technique for achieving long-term disease control. Islet cell transplantation has had moderate success, and research is continuing. Other research is being conducted in the use of an internally implanted artificial pancreas, or closed-loop artificial beta cell. This device is still being developed (Guthrie & Guthrie, 1991).

Surgery is a stressor that often alters self-management and glycemic control in people with diabetes. In response to stress, levels of catecholamines, cortisol, glucagon, growth hormones increase, as does insulin resistance. Hyperglycemia occurs, and protein stores are decreased. In addition, diet and activity patterns change, and medication types and dosages vary. As a result, surgical clients who have diabetes are at increased risk for postoperative infection, delayed wound healing, fluid and electrolyte imbalances, hypoglycemia, and DKA.

Preoperatively, all clients should be in the best possible metabolic state. Screening for complications and regular blood glucose monitoring are part of preoperative preparation. Oral hypoglycemic agents may be withheld for 1 or 2 days before surgery, and regular insulin is often administered to the client with NIDDM during the perioperative period (Rifkin, 1988). The client with IDDM follows a carefully prescribed insulin regimen individualized to specific needs.

The insulin regimen in the preoperative, intraoperative, and immediate postoperative periods is individualized and may involve any of the following:

- No intermediate- or long-acting insulin is given the day of surgery; regular insulin is given with intravenous glucose, or
- Half of the usual intermediate- or long-acting insulin is given before surgery and the remaining half is given in the recovery room, or
- The total daily dose of insulin is divided into four equal doses of regular insulin, and one dose is administered subcutaneously every 6 hours. An intravenous solution of 5% dextrose in 0.45% normal saline is administered for fluid replacement, and blood glucose monitoring precedes each insulin dose. (Guthrie & Guthrie, 1991)

The surgical procedure should be scheduled for as early as possible in the morning to minimize the length of fasting. If there is no food intake after surgery, intravenous dextrose should be administered, accompanied by subcutaneous regular insulin every 6 hours. The dose can be adjusted to blood glucose levels. Although kcal intake is decreased postoperatively, stress can increase insulin requirements. Glucose control is also affected postoperatively by nausea and vomiting, anorexia, and gastrointestinal suction.

During the postoperative period, the client with NIDDM may continue to require insulin or may resume oral medications, depending on glucose control. The client with IDDM may require reduced insulin as healing progresses and stress diminishes. Regular blood glucose monitoring is essential, as are assessments for hypoglycemia.

Acute Complications

The acute complications of diabetes are hypoglycemia (insulin reaction), DKA, and HNKC. The pathophysiology and manifestations of these complications have already been discussed; this section discusses the collaborative care.

Treatment of Hypoglycemia (Insulin Reactions)

Hypoglycemia is a potential complication in adults with IDDM or NIDDM. Hypoglycemia occurs when there is too much insulin, too much exercise, or too little food. The most common cause is skipping a meal or eating a less than normal quantity of carbohydrates at a meal. Although hypoglycemia may occur at any time, it most often occurs during exercise, 8 to 24 hours after strenuous exercise, and in the middle of the night. Mild hypoglycemia is usually recognized and self-managed, but severe hypoglycemia requires treatment by health care providers.

Mild Hypoglycemia   When mild hypoglycemia occurs, immediate treatment is necessary. People experiencing hypoglycemia should take about 15 g of a rapid-acting sugar. This amount of sugar is found, for example, in three glucose tablets; ½ cup of fruit juice or regular soda, 8 oz of skim milk, five Life Savers candies, three large marshmallows, or 3 tsp of sugar or honey. Although it was previously suggested that sugar be added to fruit juice, this is no longer recommended. Adding sugar to the fruit sugar already in the juice could cause a rapid rise in blood glucose, with persistent hyperglycemia.

If the manifestations continue, the *15/15 rule* should be followed: Wait 15 minutes, monitor blood glucose, and, if it is low, eat another 15 g of carbohydrate. This procedure can be repeated until blood glucose levels return to normal (Heins & Beebe, 1992; Lumley, 1989). People with diabetes should have some source of carbohydrate readily available at all times so that hypoglycemic symptoms can be quickly reversed. If hypoglycemia occurs more than two or three times a week, the diabetes management plan should be adjusted.

Severe Hypoglycemia   People with diabetes who have severe hypoglycemia are often hospitalized. As established by the American Diabetes Association, the criteria for hospitalization are one or more of the following:

1. Blood glucose is less than 50 mg/dL, and the prompt treatment of hypoglycemia has not resulted in recovery of sensorium.

2. The client has coma, seizures, or altered behavior.

3. The hypoglycemia has been treated, but a responsible adult cannot be with the client for the following 12 hours.

4. The hypoglycemia was caused by a sulfonylurea drug.

If the client is conscious and alert, 10 to 15 g of an oral carbohydrate may be given. If the client has altered levels of consciousness, parenteral glucose or glucagon is administered.

Glucose is administered intravenously as a 50% solution (D50W), usually at a rate of 10 mL over 1 minute by intravenous push, followed by intravenous infusion of 5% dextrose in water (D5W) at 5 to 10 g/h (Gahart, 1993). This is the most rapid method of increasing blood glucose levels.

Glucagon is an antihypoglycemic agent that raises blood glucose by promoting the conversion of hepatic glycogen to glucose. It is used in severe insulin-induced hypoglycemia and may be given in the recommended dose of 1 mg by the subcutaneous, intramuscular, or intravenous route. Glucagon has a short period of action; an oral or intravenous carbohydrate should be administered following the glucagon to prevent a recurrence of hypoglycemia. If the client has been unconscious, glucagon may cause vomiting when consciousness returns.

Treatment of Diabetic Ketoacidosis (DKA)

Diabetic ketoacidosis (DKA) is the most serious metabolic disturbance of people with IDDM. DKA requires immediate medical attention. Admission to the hospital is appropriate when the person has a blood glucose of greater than 250 mg/dL, a decreasing pH, and ketones in the urine.

DKA is treated with fluids (for dehydration), insulin (to reduce hyperglycemia and acidosis), and correction of electrolyte imbalances. It is the nurse's responsibility to administer prescribed fluids and insulin and to monitor the client's response to therapy.

If the client is alert and conscious, fluids may be replaced orally. However, alterations in levels of consciousness, vomiting, and acidosis are common, necessitating intravenous fluid replacement. The initial fluid replacement is accomplished by administering 0.9% saline solution at a rate of 500 to 1000 mL/h. After 2 to 3 hours (or when blood pressure is returning to normal), the administration of 0.45% saline at 200 to 500 mL/h may continue for several more hours. When the blood glucose levels reach 250 mg/dL, dextrose is added to prevent rapid decreases in glucose; hypoglycemia could result in fatal cerebral edema.

Nursing Implications for Pharmacology: Intravenous Insulin

General Guidelines

- Regular insulin may be given undiluted directly into the vein or through a Y-tube or three-way stopcock.
- Insulin is usually diluted in 0.9% saline or 0.45% saline solution for infusion.
- The glass or plastic infusion container and plastic tubing may reduce insulin potency by at least 20% and possibly by up to 80% before the insulin reaches the venous system.

Nursing Responsibilities

- Monitor blood glucose levels hourly.

- Infuse the insulin solution separately from the hydration solution.
- Flush the intravenous tubing with 50 mL of insulin mixed with normal saline solution to saturate binding sites on the tubing before administering the insulin to the client; this step increases the amount of insulin delivered over the first few hours.
- Do not discontinue the intravenous infusion until subcutaneous administration of insulin is resumed.
- Monitor for manifestations of hypoglycemia.
- Ensure that glucagon is readily available as an antidote for insulin overdose.

Regular insulin is used in the management of DKA and may be given by various routes, depending on the severity of the condition. Mild ketosis may be treated with subcutaneous insulin, whereas severe ketosis requires intravenous insulin infusion. Nursing responsibilities for the client receiving intravenous insulin are described in the accompanying box.

The electrolyte imbalance of primary concern is depletion of body stores of potassium. Initially, serum potassium levels may be normal, but they decrease during treatment. In DKA (and from rehydration), the body loses potassium from increased urinary output, acidosis, catabolic state, and vomiting or diarrhea. Potassium replacement is begun early in the course of treatment, usually by adding potassium to the rehydration fluids. Replacement is essential for preventing cardiac arrhythmias secondary to hypokalemia. Cardiac rhythms (through EKGs or cardiac monitoring) and potassium levels must be monitored every 2 to 4 hours.

Treatment of Hyperosmolar Nonketotic Coma (HNKC)

Hyperosmolar nonketotic coma (HNKC) is a serious, life-threatening metabolic condition that occurs in people with NIDDM. The client admitted to the intensive care unit for treatment typically manifests blood glucose levels over 700 mg/dL, increased serum osmolarity, and altered levels of consciousness or seizures. Treatment is similar to that of DKA: correcting fluid and electrolyte imbalances and providing insulin to lower hyperglycemia. In general, treatment modalities include the following:

- Establishing and maintaining adequate ventilation
- Correcting shock with adequate intravenous fluids

- Instituting nasogastric suction if comatose to prevent aspiration
- Maintaining fluid volume with intravenous isotonic or colloid solutions
- Administering potassium intravenously to replace losses
- Administering insulin to reduce blood glucose, usually discontinuing administration when blood glucose levels reach 250 mg/dL (because ketosis is not present, there is no need to continue insulin, as with DKA)

Nursing care for the client with DKA or HNKC includes administering prescribed fluids, insulin, and electrolytes; monitoring fluid status through intake and output, skin turgor, vital signs, and central venous pressure; assessing the level of consciousness; assessing blood glucose levels; and monitoring cardiac activity.

Nursing Care

The responses of the person with diabetes to the illness are often complex and individual and involve multiple body systems. Assessments, planning, and implementation differ for the person with newly diagnosed diabetes, the person with long-term diabetes, and the person with acute complications of diabetes. The plan of care and content of teaching also differ according to the type of diabetes, the person's age, and the person's intellectual, psychological, and social resources. However, nursing care focuses primarily on teaching the client to manage the illness. A Critical Pathway for the client with new-onset type II diabetes is provided on page 741.

Although many different nursing diagnoses are appropriate for the person with diabetes, those discussed in this

text continues on page 745

Critical Pathway for Client with New-Onset Type II Diabetes

	Date _____ Day 1	Date _____ Day 2	Date _____ Day 3
	Expected length of stay: 5 days		
Daily outcomes	Client will ■ Have stable vital signs. ■ Verbalize beginning understanding and importance of diet compliance and regular blood sugar testing. ■ Have episodes of hypo- or hyperglycemia detected early. ■ Verbalize beginning ability to cope with diagnosis.	Client will ■ Have stable vital signs. ■ Verbalize understanding and importance of diet compliance and regular blood sugar testing. ■ Have weight loss of _____ lb. ■ Have episodes of hypo- or hyperglycemia detected early. ■ Demonstrate ability to cope. ■ Verbalize beginning understanding of home care instructions.	Client will ■ Have stable vital signs and unlabored respirations at rest. ■ Verbalize understanding and importance of diet compliance and regular blood sugar testing. ■ Have weight loss of _____ lb. ■ Have episodes of hypo- or hyperglycemia detected early. ■ Demonstrate ability to cope. ■ Verbalize willingness to participate in a regular exercise program. ■ Identify eating behaviors that lead weight gain. ■ Demonstrate ability to self-administer insulin and perform self-monitoring of blood glucose safely and correctly with minimal supervision. ■ Verbalize beginning understanding of home care instructions.
Tests and treatments	CBC. Fasting blood sugar. Glycosylated hemoglobin. Baseline laboratory work. Vital signs q4h if stable. Daily weight. Fingerstick blood sugar ac, hs, & prn; if blood glucose over 240 mg/dL, then obtain serum glucose. Monitor for signs and symptoms of hypo- and hyperglycemia, and implement appropriate protocol if signs or symptoms are present. Intake and output every shift.	Fasting blood sugar. Vital signs q4h if stable. Daily weight. Fingerstick blood sugar ac, hs, & prn. Monitor for signs and symptoms of hypo- and hyperglycemia. Follow appropriate protocol if symptoms occur. Intake and output every shift.	Fasting blood sugar. Vital signs q4h if stable. Daily weight. Fingerstick blood sugar ac, hs, & prn. Monitor for signs and symptoms of hypo- and hyperglycemia. Follow appropriate protocol if symptoms occur. Intake and output every shift.

	Date _____ Day 1	Date _____ Day 2	Date _____ Day 3
Knowledge deficit	Orient to room and hospital routine. Review plan of care. Assess readiness for teaching. Include family in teaching program. Review steps of insulin administration, and provide written instructions sheets. Review steps of self monitoring of blood glucose (SMBG). Consult with diabetes nurse educator. Consult with registered dietitian for instruction in diet and exchange lists. Assess understanding of teaching.	Reorient to room and hospital routine. Review plan of care. Include family in teaching. Review steps of insulin administration and SMBG. Allow client to practice with related equipment. Show client and significant other videotapes related to type II diabetes and self-care practices. Assess understanding of teaching.	Reorient to room and hospital routine. Review plan of care. Include family in teaching. Supervise client in self--administration of insulin and performing SMBG. Have client attend classes on general health care practices and foot care and watch video on identifying and managing hypo- and hyperglycemia and sick day management. Assess understanding of teaching.
Psycho-social	Assess level of anxiety. Encourage verbalization of concerns. Provide information. Provide ongoing support and encouragement.	Assess level of anxiety. Encourage verbalization of concerns. Provide information. Provide ongoing support and encouragement.	Encourage verbalization of concerns. Provide ongoing support and encouragement.
Diet	Daily weight. Dietary consult. ADA diet. Encourage fluid intake of 2000 mL/day. Assess for causes of excessive weight gain. Encourage client to identify activities and food that contribute to excessive intake.	Daily weight. ADA diet. Encourage fluid intake of 2000 mL/day. Encourage client to identify activities and food that contribute to excessive intake. Discuss with client behavior-modification strategies to use instead of eating when watching TV. Identify behavior-modification strategies (e.g., drink 8 oz of water before each meal, eat slowly, and chew thoroughly) to assist in weight loss.	Daily weight. ADA diet. Encourage fluid intake of 2000 mL/day. Encourage client to identify activities and food that contribute to excessive intake. Encourage client to use behavior-modification strategies. Explain the relationship between regular physical exercise and weight loss and control. Encourage client to establish regular exercise program.
Activity	Assess safety needs and provide appropriate precautions. Bathroom privileges. OOB ad lib in room. Provide rest periods.	Maintain safety precautions. OOB ad lib. Encourage rest periods.	Maintain safety precautions. Ambulate ad lib. Encourage rest periods.

	Date _____ **Day 1**	Date _____ **Day 2**	Date _____ **Day 3**
Medications	Regular insulin to scale ac & hs. Oral agents as ordered.	Regular insulin to scale ac & hs. Oral agents as ordered, or NPH insulin per order a.m. & p.m.	Regular insulin to scale ac & hs. Oral agents if ordered, or NPH insulin per order a.m. & p.m.
Transfer/ discharge plans	Establish discharge goals with client and significant others. Consult with social service re: VNA and projected needs for home health care (if any).	Review progress toward discharge goals with client & significant other. Assess need for referrals.	Review progress toward discharge goals with client & significant other. Refer to Diabetic Support group. Refer to diabetic nurse educator for teaching after discharge. Make appropriate referrals.

	Date _____ **Day 4**	Date _____ **Day 5**	
Daily outcomes	Client will ■ Have stable vital signs. ■ Verbalize understanding and importance of diet compliance and regular blood sugar testing. ■ Have weight loss of 1 lb. ■ Verbalize responsibility for weight loss. ■ Have episodes of hypo- or hyperglycemia detected early. ■ Demonstrate ability to cope. ■ Verbalize understanding of home care instructions.	Client will ■ Have stable vital signs. ■ Have a normal blood sugar. ■ Be independent in self-care. ■ Be fully ambulatory. ■ Verbalize responsibility for weight loss. ■ Verbalize plan to exercise 15 to 20 minutes 3 to 4 times/week. ■ Have resumed preadmission urine and bowel elimination pattern. ■ Verbalize/demonstrate home care instructions, including aspects of diabetic care: diet control, SMBG, insulin care and administration, foot care, general health care rules, and signs and symptoms of hypo- and hyperglycemia and management of those problems. ■ Verbalize importance of ongoing medical care. ■ Tolerate ordered diet and have fluid intake of 2000 mL/day. ■ Demonstrate/verbalize ability to cope with ongoing stressors.	

➤

	Date _____ Day 4	Date _____ Day 5
Tests and treatments	Fasting blood sugar. Vital signs q4h if stable. Daily weight. Fingerstick blood sugar ac, hs, & prn. Monitor for symptoms of hypo- and hyperglycemia. Follow appropriate protocol if symptoms occur. D/C intake and output monitoring if stable.	Fasting blood sugar. Vital signs q4h if stable. Daily weight. Fingerstick blood sugar ac, hs, & prn. Monitor for symptoms of hypo- and hyperglycemia. Follow appropriate protocol if symptoms occur.
Knowledge deficit	Include family in teaching. Reinforce earlier teaching regarding ongoing care. Review written discharge instructions with client and significant other. Attend diabetic classes per diabetes nurse educator. Assess understanding of teaching.	Include family in teaching. Reinforce earlier teaching regarding ongoing care. Complete discharge teaching to include diet, follow-up care, symptoms to report, follow-up appointment, activity, and medications: dose, frequency, route, name, purpose, and side effects. Provide client with written discharge instructions specific to management of diabetes. Assess understanding of teaching.
Psycho-social	Encourage verbalization of concerns. Provide support and encouragement to client and family.	Encourage verbalization of concerns. Provide support and encouragement to client and family.
Diet	Daily weight. 1200 calorie ADA diet. Encourage fluid intake of 2000 mL/day. Encourage use of behavior-modification strategies. Encourage establishment of exercise program after discharge.	Daily weight. 1200 calorie ADA diet. Encourage fluid intake of 2000 mL/day. Encourage use of behavior-modification strategies. Encourage establishment of exercise program after discharge.
Activity	Fully ambulatory.	Fully ambulatory.
Medications	Regular insulin to scale ac & hs. Oral agents if ordered, or NPH insulin per order a.m. & p.m.	Regular insulin to scale ac & hs. Oral agents if ordered, or NPH insulin per order a.m. & p.m.
Transfer/discharge plans	Continue to review progress toward discharge goals. Finalize discharge plans.	Finalize plans for home care if needed. Complete discharge teaching.

section address problems with skin integrity, infection, injury, sexuality, coping, and health maintenance.

Altered Skin Integrity

The person with diabetes is at increased risk for altered skin integrity as a result of decreased or absent sensation from neuropathies, decreased tissue perfusion from cardiovascular complications, and infection. In addition, poor vision increases the risk of trauma, and an open lesion is more prone to infection and delayed healing. Altered skin integrity, with resultant gangrene, is especially common in the feet and lower extremities.

Nursing interventions with rationales follow:

- Conduct baseline and ongoing assessments of the feet, including:
  a. Musculoskeletal assessment that includes foot and ankle joint range of motion, bone abnormalities (bunions, hammertoes, overlapping digits), gait patterns, use of assistive devices for walking, and abnormal wear patterns on shoes.
  b. Neurologic assessment that includes sensations of touch and position, pain, and temperature.
  c. Vascular examination that includes assessment of lower-extremity pulses, capillary refill, color and temperature of skin, lesions, and edema.
  d. Assessment of hydration, including dryness or excessive perspiration.
  e. Assessment of lesions, fissures between toes, corns, calluses, plantar warts, ingrown or overgrown toenails, redness over pressure points, blisters, cellulitis, or gangrene.
  People with diabetes are at significant risk for lower-extremity gangrene. Peripheral neuropathies may result in alterations in the perception of pain, loss of deep-tendon reflexes, loss of cutaneous pressure and position sensation, foot drop, changes in the shape of the foot, and changes in bones and joints. Peripheral vascular disease may cause intermittent claudication, absent pulses, delayed venous filling on elevation, dependent rubor, and gangrene. Injuries, lesions, and changes in skin hydration potentiate infections, delayed healing, and tissue loss in the person with diabetes mellitus.

- Teach foot hygiene. Wash the feet daily with lukewarm water and mild hand soap; pat dry, and dry well between the toes. Apply a very thin coat of lubricating cream if dryness is present (but not between the toes). *Proper hygiene decreases the chance of infection. Temperature receptors may be impaired, so the water should always be tested before use. The person with diabetes should never step into a tub of water before testing the temperature.*

- Discuss the importance of not smoking. *Nicotine in tobacco causes vasoconstriction, further decreasing the blood supply to the feet.*

- Discuss the importance of maintaining blood glucose levels through prescribed diet, medication, and exercise. *Hyperglycemia promotes the growth of microorganisms.*

- Conduct foot care teaching sessions as often as necessary. (See the box on page 746.) Include information about proper shoe fit and composition, avoiding clothing or activities that decrease circulation to the feet, foot inspections, the care of toenails, and the importance of obtaining medical care for lesions. If the person has visual deficits, is obese, or cannot reach the feet, teach the caregiver how to inspect and care for the feet. Feet should be inspected daily. *Foot care is a priority in diabetes management to prevent serious problems. Many people with diabetes are unaware of lesions or injury until infection and compromised circulation are far advanced. The hows and whys of each component must be included in teaching. A variety of methods may be used, including demonstration, return demonstration, audiovisual aids, and written lists. If the person is wearing shoes and socks, ask him or her to remove them to practice foot care effectively.*

Risk for Infection

The person with diabetes is at increased risk for infection. The risk of infection is believed to be due to vascular insufficiency that limits the inflammatory response, neurologic abnormalities that limit the awareness of trauma, and a predisposition to bacterial and fungal infections. For example:

- Infections of nails are common in people with diabetes.

- Osteomyelitis is one of the most serious problems of the diabetic foot.

- Chronic gingivitis and pyorrhea are common in people with diabetes, especially if the hyperglycemia is poorly controlled.

- Urinary tract infections are two to four times more common in women with diabetes.

- Tuberculosis is more prevalent in people with diabetes.

- Malignant external otitis occurs in the older adult with diabetes.

- Vaginal yeast infections are common in women with diabetes; both men and women with diabetes are prone to yeast infections of the oral mucous membranes and in skinfolds (especially if the person is obese).

Nursing interventions with rationales follow:

- Use and teach meticulous hand washing. *Hand washing is the single most effective method for preventing the spread of infection.*

A Sample Foot Care Teaching Session

■   ■   ■

Buying and Wearing Shoes and Stockings

- Shoes that allow ½ to ¾ inch of toe room are best; there should be room for toes to spread out and wiggle. The lining and inside stitching should be smooth, and the insole soft. The sole should be flexible and cushion the foot. The heel should fit snugly, and the arch support should give good support.

- Do not wear open-toed shoes, sandals, high heels, or thongs; they increase the risk of trauma.

- Buy shoes late in the afternoon, when feet are at their largest; always buy shoes that feel comfortable and do not need to be "broken in."

- Shoes made of natural fibers (leather, canvas) allow perspiration to escape.

- Check the shoes before each wearing for foreign objects, wrinkled insoles, and cracks that might cause lesions.

- Stockings made of wool or cotton allow perspiration to dry.

- Do not wear garters, knee stockings, or panty hose; they may interfere with circulation.

- Wear insulated boots in the winter.

Inspecting the Feet

- Check the feet daily for red areas, cuts, blisters, corns, calluses, or cracks in the skin. Check between the toes for cracks or reddened areas.

- Check the skin of the feet for dry or damp areas.

- Use a mirror to check each sole and the back of each heel.

- If you are unable to inspect the feet daily, be sure that someone else does so.

Care of Toenails

- Cut the toenails after washing, when they are softer and easier to trim.

- Cut the nails straight across with a clipper, and smooth edges and corners with an emery board.

- Do not use razor blades to trim the toenails.

- If you are unable to see well or to reach the feet easily, have someone else trim the nails. If the nails are very thick or ingrown, if the toes overlap, or if circulation is poor, get professional care.

General Information

- Never go barefoot. Wear slippers when leaving the bed during the night.

- Do not use commercial corn medicines or pads, chemicals (such as boric acid, iodine, or hydrogen peroxide), or over-the-counter cortisone medications on the feet.

- Do not put heating pads, hot water bottles, or ice packs on the feet. If the feet become cold at night, wear socks or use extra blankets.

- Do not allow the feet to become sunburned.

- Do not put tape on the feet.

- Do not sit with the legs crossed at the knees or ankles.

- Monitor for clinical manifestations of infection for clients at high risk: increased temperature, pain, malaise, swelling, redness, discharge, cough. *Early diagnosis and treatment of infections can control their severity and decrease complications. Clients with diabetes who have an infection may require alterations in diet and medications.*

- Discuss the importance of skin care. Keep the skin clean and dry, using lukewarm water and mild soap. *People with diabetes are more prone to develop furuncles and carbuncles; the infection often increases the need for insulin. Clean, intact skin and mucous membranes are the first line of defense against infection.*

- Teach dental health measures:
  a. Obtain a dental examination every 4 to 6 months.
  b. Maintain careful oral hygiene, which includes brushing the teeth with a soft toothbrush and fluoridated toothpaste at least twice a day and flossing as recommended.
  c. Be aware of the symptoms requiring dental care: bad breath, unpleasant taste in the mouth, bleeding, red, or sore gums, and tooth pain.
  d. If dental surgery is necessary, monitor for adjustments in insulin.
  Teach all people with diabetes about proper oral hygiene, the risk of periodontal disease, and the importance of ob-

taining dental care for symptoms of oral or dental problems.

- Teach women with diabetes the symptoms and preventive measures for vaginitis caused by *Candida albicans*:
  a. Symptoms are an odorless, white or yellow cheese-like discharge and itching.
  b. Take preventive measures by maintaining good personal hygiene, wiping front to back after voiding, wearing cotton underwear, avoiding tight jeans and nylon pantyhose, and avoiding douching.
  c. Sexual transmission is unlikely, but discomfort may cause the client to avoid sexual activity.

  Diabetes is a predisposing factor for Candida albicans *vaginitis, the most common form of vaginitis. Poor personal hygiene and wearing clothing that keeps the vaginal area warm and moist increase the risk of vaginitis. The infection may spread to the urinary tract, resulting in urinary tract infections; preventing and treating vaginitis decrease this risk.*

Risk for Injury

The person with diabetes is at risk for injury from multiple factors. Neuropathies may alter sensation, gait, and muscle control. Cataracts or retinopathy may cause visual deficits. Hyperglycemia often causes osmotic changes in the lenses of the eye, resulting in blurred vision. In addition, changes in blood glucose alter levels of consciousness and may cause seizures. The impaired mobility, sensory deficits, and neurologic effects of complications of diabetes increase the risk of accidents, burns, falls, and trauma.

Nursing interventions with rationales follow:

- Assess for the presence of contributing or causative factors that increase the risk of injury: blurred vision, cataracts, decreased adaptation to dark, decreased tactile sensitivity, hypoglycemia, hyperglycemia, hypovolemia, joint immobility, unstable gait. *A knowledge base is necessary to develop an individualized plan of care to meet client needs. The risk of injury increases with the number of factors identified.*

- Reduce environmental hazards in the health care facility, and teach the client about safety in the home and in the community.

In the Health Care Facility
  a. Orient the client to new surroundings on admission.
  b. Keep the bed at the lowest level, and raise the side rails at night if needed.
  c. Keep the floors free of objects.
  d. Use a night light.
  e. Assess the temperature of the bath or shower water before the client uses it.

  f. Instruct the client to wear shoes or slippers when leaving the bed.
  g. Monitor blood glucose levels regularly.
  h. Monitor for side effects of prescribed medications, such as dizziness or drowsiness.

In the Home and Community
  a. Use a night light, preferably one with a soft, nonglare bulb.
  b. Turn the head away when switching on a bright light.
  c. Avoid directly looking into headlights when driving at night.
  d. Test the temperature of the bath or shower water before use.
  e. Conduct a daily foot inspection.
  f. Wear shoes and slippers with nonskid soles.
  g. Do not use throw rugs.
  h. Provide hand grips in the tub and shower and next to the toilet.
  i. Wear a seat belt when driving or riding in a car.

  Strange environments and the presence of hazardous environmental factors increase the risk of falls or other accidents. Glare is often responsible for falls in people with visual deficits. The nurse can reduce factors that increase the risk of injury by implementing care and teaching safe practices during the activities of daily life.

- Monitor for and teach the client and family to recognize and seek care for the manifestations of DKA in the client with IDDM: hyperglycemia, thirst, headaches, nausea and vomiting, increased urine output, ketonuria, dehydration, decreasing level of consciousness. *Blood glucose levels increase if the insulin need is unmet or insufficiently met; the cellular use of fats for fuel results in ketosis. Osmotic diuresis increases urinary output, resulting in thirst and dehydration.*

- Monitor for and teach the client and family to recognize and seek care for the manifestations of HNKC in the client with NIDDM: extreme hyperglycemia, increased urinary output, thirst, dehydration, hypotension, seizures, decreasing level of consciousness. *HNKC in people with NIDDM is a life-threatening condition requiring recognition and treatment.*

- Monitor for and teach the client and family to recognize and treat the manifestations of hypoglycemia: low blood glucose, anxiety, headache, uncoordinated movements, sweating, rapid pulse, drowsiness, visual changes. Severe hypoglycemia causes a decrease in the level of consciousness. *Hypoglycemia may occur in clients with either IDDM or NIDDM. The decrease in blood glucose most often results from too much insulin (insulin shock in people with IDDM), too little food, or too much exercise. The person should carry some form of rapid-acting sugar source at all times.*

■ Recommend that client wear a MedicAlert bracelet or necklace identifying self as a person with diabetes. *In case of sudden, severe illness or accident, a MedicAlert bracelet can allow immediate medical attention for diabetes to be instituted.*

Sexual Dysfunction

Sexuality is a complex and inseparable part of every person. It involves not only physical sexual activities but also people's perception of themselves as male or female, of their roles and relationships, and of their attractiveness and desirability. Changes in sexual function and in sexuality have been identified in both men and women with diabetes.

Alterations in erectile ability occur in approximately 50% of all men with diabetes (Ellenberg, 1971, 1979; Jensen, 1981; Podolsky, 1982; Rubin, 1967). The incidence of impotence increases with the duration of the diabetes and is often associated with peripheral neuropathy. Libido is usually unaffected, even when impotence is present.

Women with diabetes also have alterations in sexual function, although the reason is less clear. Although initially it was believed that women with diabetes experienced difficulty with orgasm, the problems reported by the majority of women involve decreased desire and decreased vaginal lubrication (Ellenberg, 1979; Jensen, 1985). Women with diabetes are also at increased risk for vaginitis and may avoid sexual intercourse in order to avoid pain.

Nursing interventions with rationales follow:

■ Include a sexual history as a part of the initial assessment of the client with diabetes. A specific history form may be used that addresses sexual development, personal and family values, current sexual practices and concerns, and changes desired. Ask a nonthreatening, open-ended question to elicit information, such as, "Tell me about your experience with sexual function since you have been diagnosed with diabetes." *Obtaining accurate information to assess the sexual health of a client is necessary before counseling can begin or referrals can be made. Sexual function is a private matter, and clients rarely share concerns unless the nurse initiates the discussion.*

■ Provide information about the actual and potential physical and emotional effects of diabetes, including erectile dysfunction in men and decreased vaginal lubrication in women. Include the effect of poor control of blood glucose on sexual function as part of any teaching plan. *Clients benefit from basic information about male and female anatomy and the sexual response cycle, and how diabetes can affect this part of the body. Changes in blood glucose levels not only may cause changes in desire and physical response but also may alter sexual responses as a result of depression, anxiety, and fatigue.*

■ Provide counseling or make referrals as appropriate. *The nurse is responsible for knowing about sexuality and sexual health throughout the life span and provides information based on knowledge of the effects of illness and treatment on sexual function. The nurse may make specific suggestions to facilitate positive sexual functioning, referring the client to the appropriate health care provider as necessary for intensive therapy. For example, men who are impotent may regain the ability to have sexual intercourse through penile implants, suction apparatus, or injections of medications (such as yohimbine, an alpha-2 adrenergic blocker) that increase vascular blood flow into the corpus of the penis. Women with decreased vaginal lubrication can decrease painful intercourse by using vaginal lubricants (such as K-Y jelly) or estrogen creams.*

Ineffective Individual Coping

Coping is the process of responding to internal or environmental stressors or potential stressors. When coping responses are ineffective, the stressors exceed the individual's available resources for responding (Hymovich & Hagopian, 1992). The person diagnosed with diabetes is faced with lifelong changes in many parts of his or her life. Diet, exercise habits, and medications must be integrated into the life-style and be carefully controlled. Daily injections may be a reality. Fear of potential complications and of negative effects on the future is common.

If the person is unable to cope successfully with these changes, emotional stress can interfere with glycemic control. In addition, unsuccessful coping often results in noncompliance with prescribed treatment modalities, further impairing glycemic control and increasing the potential for acute and chronic complications. Nursing research about adaptive responses to diabetes is described in the accompanying box.

Nursing interventions with rationales follow:

■ Assess the client's psychosocial resources, including emotional resources, support resources, life-style, and communication skills. *Chronic illness affects all dimensions of a person's life, as well as the lives of family members and significant others. A comprehensive assessment of strengths and weaknesses is the first step in developing an individualized plan of care to facilitate coping.*

■ Explore with the client and family the effects (actual and perceived) of the diagnosis and treatment of diabetes on finances, occupation, energy levels, and relationships. Common frustrations associated with diabetes are the disease itself, the treatment modalities, and the health care system. Effective coping involves maintaining a healthy self-concept and satisfying relationships, emotional balance, and handling emotional stress.

Applying Research to Nursing Practice
Adaptive Responses to Diabetes Mellitus

■ ■ ■

A descriptive study investigated the relationships among the physiologic responses of adults to IDDM, coping patterns, hardiness, and demographic variables (Pollock, 1989). The findings indicated that the people who adapt better to diabetes are those who view the illness as harmful, use a variety of coping strategies, have the personal characteristic of hardiness, and participate in educational programs. The study findings support the thesis that how one perceives one's situation (stress appraisal) and what one does about the situation (coping strategies) are important variables in predicting adaptation to a chronic illness.

Implications for Nursing

As the incidence of diabetes rises and as more clients are taught to provide self-care at home, it becomes more important for nurses to know the most effective ways of encouraging self-care. Too often, nurses focus on teaching clients about the disease and treatment, without first considering how the client accepts the prescribed care and copes with the changes the care brings about. If the nurse first collects information about the client's health values and methods of coping, teaching is likely to be more effective. Although this study included only adults with IDDM, the adult with NIDDM has much the same type of coping demands.

Critical Thinking in Client Care

1. Suppose you were a client with diabetes. Outline your own coping activities, both those that are effective and those that are ineffective.

2. Hardiness is a personal characteristic that reflects commitment, a tendency to appraise demands as challenging rather than threatening, and a sense of control over fate. How may the presence of this characteristic in the person with diabetes facilitate self-care?

3. Can the findings from this study be useful in designing a diabetes education program? Support your answer.

■ Teach constructive problem-solving techniques:
   a. Identify the problem.
   b. Find the cause of the problem.
   c. Determine the options.
   d. List the advantages and disadvantages of each option.
   e. Choose an option, and make a plan.
   Problem-focused behaviors include setting attainable and realistic goals, learning about all aspects of the problem, learning new procedures or skills that increase self-esteem, and reaching out to others for support.

■ Provide information about support groups and resources, such as suppliers of products, journals, books, and cookbooks for people with diabetes. *The resources available vary from client to client. Sharing with others who have similar problems provides opportunities for mutual support and problem solving. Using available resources improves the ability to cope.*

Altered Health Maintenance

Altered health maintenance in the person with diabetes is a state in which the individual experiences, or is at risk for experiencing, a disruption in health because of a lack of knowledge about managing the condition. Teaching for the client, family, and significant others encompasses all aspects of diabetes and treatment modalities. Depending on the situation, nurses may collaborate with other nurses who are certified diabetes educators or diabetes clinical specialists.

The client and nurse should establish goals for teaching/learning, focusing primarily on self-management. Nurses plan and implement programs to teach people with diabetes how their bodies ought to work and how diabetes alters normal functioning. This information is followed by how food, medications, and exercise can be used to improve functioning as well as how to make adjustments as their lives change—for example, when meals are unavoidably delayed or when diarrhea begins. It is critical that both the nurse and the client believe that the person with diabetes is the most important consideration and that the disease is only one small part of that person.

Information about and rationales for all aspects of teaching are included throughout this chapter. The material below summarizes the knowledge and skills needed for self-managing diabetes.

The content of a teaching plan for the person with diabetes includes the following:

■ Information about normal metabolism, diabetes mellitus, and how diabetes changes metabolism

■ Diet plan: how diet helps keep blood glucose in normal range; number of kcal required and why; amount of carbohydrates, proteins, and fats allowed and why; how to calculate the diet, integrating personal food preferences

- Exercise: how it helps lower blood glucose; the importance of a regular program; types of exercise; integrating personal exercise preferences; how to handle increased activity

- Self-monitoring of blood glucose: how to perform the tests accurately, how to care for equipment, what to do for high or low blood glucose

- Medications:
  a. *Insulin*: type, dosage, mixing instructions (if necessary), times of onset and peak actions, how to get and care for equipment, how to give injections, where to give injections
  b. *Oral agents*: type, dosage, side effects, interaction with other drugs

- Signs and symptoms of acute complications of hypoglycemia and hyperglycemia; what to do when they occur

- Hygiene: skin care, dental care, foot care

- Sick days: what to do about food, fluids, and medications

- Support groups and literature available

- Whom to contact for answers to questions
  The American Diabetes Association recommends that teaching be carried out on three levels. The first level focuses on survival skills, with the person learning basic knowledge and skills to be able to provide diabetes management for the first week or two while he or she adjusts to the idea of having the disease. The second level focuses on home management, emphasizing self-reliance and independence in the daily management of diabetes. The third level is aimed at improving life-style, educating clients to individualize self-management of the illness.

Other Nursing Diagnoses

Other nursing diagnoses appropriate for the client with diabetes mellitus follow:

- *Altered Protection* related to age over 60, surgical procedure, and increased stress

- *Anxiety* related to a lack of knowledge about insulin administration

- *Fatigue* related to uncontrolled blood glucose levels

- *Ineffective Management of Therapeutic Regimen* related to increased illness symptoms (increased urination, thirst, hunger, fatigue), occurrence of ketoacidosis and hypoglycemia, and verbalized difficulty with regulating the prescribed treatment

- *Risk for Peripheral Neurovascular Dysfunction* related to arterial insufficiency and peripheral neuropathy

- *Risk for Fluid Volume* deficit related to increased urine output and hyperglycemia

- *Sexual Dysfunction* related to vaginitis and decreased vaginal lubrication (women) or impotence (men)

- *Altered Nutrition: More Than Body Requirements* related to intake in excess of activity expenditures and a lack of knowledge

Client and Family Teaching

Teaching the client and family to self-manage diabetes is a nursing responsibility. Even if a formal teaching plan is developed and implemented by advanced practice nurses, all nurses must be able to reinforce knowledge and answer questions. Teaching is necessary for both the person who is newly diagnosed and for the person who has had diabetes for years. In fact, the latter may need almost as much teaching as the newly diagnosed person (Guthrie & Guthrie, 1991).

For the hospitalized client with diabetes, teaching should begin on admission. Prior to designing the teaching plan, the nurse makes an initial assessment of the client's and family's knowledge and learning needs, outlining past diabetes management practices and identifying physical, emotional, and sociocultural needs. Educational level, preferred learning methods and style, life experiences, and support systems are also assessed.

It is important that the nurse and client mutually establish goals based on the assessment data. It is equally important that family members understand that the responsibility for daily management lies with the client and that the primary role of the family is supportive. The client is the person with the disease, and it is the client who each day must take medications or inject insulin, test blood or urine, calculate and balance foods, exercise, adjust medications, inspect the body for injury, and determine whether and when medical assistance is needed. However, family members require the same knowledge so that they can provide emotional support as well as physical care if necessary.

Below are some general guidelines for teaching:

- Consider the client's priorities. Anxiety about the ability to keep one's job or to have children may be initially more important than knowing how to administer insulin.

- Discuss the effect of metabolic changes on emotions.

- Remember that the illness is only one part of the life and identity of the client.

- Listen to questions and provide information about common myths about diabetes.

- Use language the client understands; avoid clinical terminology.

- Be nonjudgmental.

- Use positive reinforcement.

- Set a goal to have the client adjust to the disease rather than accept the disease.

- Repeat and reinforce information as many times as necessary.

- Use a variety of teaching methods.

- Validate the person's knowledge and skills.

Teaching may have to be adapted to the special needs of the older adult. Because 40% of all people with diabetes are over the age of 65, considering the special needs of this population is essential. Uncontrolled diabetes in the older adult increases the potential for functional loss, social disengagement, and increased morbidity and mortality (Gambert, 1990). Education for self-care allows the older adult to be more actively involved in his or her diabetes management and decreases the potential for acute and long-term complications from the disease. Considerations for teaching the older adult with diabetes include the following:

- Changes in diet may be difficult to implement for many reasons. Favorite foods are difficult to give up. Balanced meals at regular intervals may not have been part of the client's life-style. Purchasing, storing, and preparing foods may be a problem. Dentures may not fit well. Changes in taste sensation often cause the client to increase the use of salt and sugar.

- Exercise of any type may not have been part of the activities of daily living. Exercise must be individualized for any physical limitations imposed by other chronic illnesses, such as arthritis, Parkinson's disease, chronic respiratory diseases, and/or cardiovascular diseases.

- The diagnosis of a chronic illness threatens independence and self-worth. After years of taking care of self, the older adult with diabetes may now have to depend on others for help in meeting self-care needs. This in turn often leads to withdrawal from social interactions with others.

- Money to purchase medications and supplies often must be taken out of a fixed income.

- Visual deficits make insulin administration difficult or impossible. Visual deficits also interfere with blood glucose monitoring, food preparation, exercises, and foot care.

Many different resources providing information on all aspects of self-management are available for the person with diabetes. Educational programs and support groups are available through most hospitals and may also be provided in outpatient settings. Blood glucose screenings are often provided at little or no cost as part of community health promotion activities. Restaurants and airlines now provide diabetic meals on request. The client should be encouraged to explore community resources that provide information about diabetes.

Applying the Nursing Process

Case Study of a Client with Insulin-Dependent Diabetes Mellitus: James Meligrito

James Meligrito is 24 years old. He is a third-year nursing student at a large midwestern university. In addition to going to school full time, Mr. Meligrito also works 20 hours a week as a campus student security guard. His working hours are from 8 p.m. to 12 midnight, five nights a week. He lives with his father, who is also a student. Neither Mr. Meligrito nor his father likes to cook, and they usually eat "whatever is handy." Mr. Meligrito was diagnosed with insulin-dependent diabetes mellitus when he was 12. Although his insulin dosage has varied, he currently takes a total of 32 units of insulin each day, 10 U of NPH and 6 U of regular insulin each morning and evening. He monitors his blood glucose about three times a week. He feels that he is too busy for a regular exercise program and that he gets enough exercise in clinicals and in weekend sports activities. He has not seen a health care provider for over a year.

One day during a 6-hour clinical laboratory in pediatrics, Mr. Meligrito notices that he is urinating frequently, is thirsty, and has blurred vision. He also is very tired but blames all his symptoms on drinking a couple of beers and having had only 4 hours of sleep the night before while studying for an examination, and the stress he has been under lately from school and work. When he remembers that he had forgotten to take his insulin that morning, he realizes he must have hyperglycemia but decides that he will be all right until he gets home in the afternoon. Around noon, he begins having abdominal pain, feels weak, has a rapid pulse, and vomits. When he reports his physical symptoms to his clinical instructor, she sends him immediately to the hospital emergency department, accompanied by another student.

Assessment

As soon as Mr. Meligrito arrives at the emergency room, his blood glucose level is measured; it is 300 mg/dL. Urine samples and additional blood samples are sent to the laboratory for analysis. Blood glucose is 330 mg/dL, urine shows the presence of ketones, electrolytes are normal, and pH is 7.1. His vital signs are as follows: T, 99 F (37.2 C); P, 140; R, 28; BP = 102/52. An intravenous infusion of 1000 mL normal (0.9%) saline with 40 mEq of KCl is started at a rate of 400 mL/h. Intravenous regular insulin at 25 mL/h (5 U/h) is begun. Hourly blood glucose monitoring is initiated. Mr. Meligrito is nauseated and lethargic but remains oriented. Three hours later, he has a blood glucose level of 160, and his pulse and blood pressure are normal. He is dismissed from the emergency department after making an appointment for the next morning with the hospital's diabetes clinical specialist, Carole Traci.

When Mr. Meligrito arrives for his appointment, Ms. Traci asks him to complete a thorough assessment. The completed assessment is used as the basis for developing an individualized teaching plan for Mr. Meligrito. He states that he feels the diabetes is controlling him more than he is controlling it. He also expresses concern about being able to complete school and to reach his goal of becoming a nurse anesthetist.

Diagnosis

Ms. Traci makes the following nursing diagnoses after conducting the assessment:

- *Powerlessness* related to a perceived lack of control of diabetes due to present demands on time
- *Knowledge Deficit* of self-management of diabetes
- *Risk for Altered Role Performance* related to uncertainty about capacity to achieve desired role as registered nurse

Expected Outcomes

The expected outcomes established in the teaching plan developed by Ms. Traci specify that after completing 2 months of weekly meetings of the diabetes education program, Mr. Melegrito will

- Identify those aspects of diabetes that can be controlled and participate in making decisions about self-managing care.
- Explore and clarify his perceptions of his role as a student nurse, verbalizing his ability to meet his expectations.
- Demonstrate an understanding of diabetes self-management through planned medication, diet, exercise, and blood glucose self-monitoring activities.

Planning and Implementation

Ms. Traci plans and implements the following nursing interventions for Mr. Melegrito during the diabetes education program:

- Mutually establish specific and individualized short-term and long-term goals for Mr. Meligrito's self-management of control of blood glucose.
- Provide opportunities for Mr. Meligrito to express his feelings about himself and his illness.
- Explore Mr. Meligrito's perceptions of his own ability to control his illness and his future, and clarify these perceptions by providing information about resources and support groups.
- Facilitate Mr. Meligrito's decision-making abilities in self-managing his prescribed treatment regimen.

- Provide positive reinforcement for increasing involvement in self-care activities.
- Provide relevant learning activities about insulin administration, dietary management, exercise, self-monitoring of blood glucose, and healthy life-style.

Evaluation

After taking an active part in the weekly educational meetings for 2 months, Mr. Meligrito has greatly enhanced his understanding of and compliance with self-management of his diabetes. He states that he finally understands how insulin, food, and exercise affect his body, having previously thought they were "just things I should do when I wanted to." He decides to perform self-management activities one week at a time, rather than think too far into (and thereby feel overwhelmed by) the future. Mr. Meligrito and his father have developed a workable meal schedule and weekly grocery list, and they have begun eating breakfast and dinner together. Mr. Meligrito and a friend have arranged to walk 2 to 3 miles three times a week on a community hiking trail.

To gain a sense of control over his illness, Mr. Meligrito has also worked out a schedule that allows time for school, health care, and himself. He decides to decrease his working hours to 3 days a week. In a diabetes support group, he has met two nurses who have diabetes and has discussed mutual problems with them. He says that knowing that other people with diabetes have made it through nursing school is the best encouragement he could have. He decides to continue attending meetings of the support group and also to attend an advanced diabetes education program to help him learn how to live with the disease.

Critical Thinking in the Nursing Process

1. What is the pathophysiologic basis for the changes in temperature, pulse, respirations, and blood pressure that occurred on Mr. Meligrito's admission to the hospital emergency department?

2. How can smoking and poor self-management of diabetes increase the risk of long-term complications?

3. Is powerlessness a common response to a chronic illness? Why, or why not?

4. Outline a teaching plan for Mr. Meligrito specific to his diet. Consider his age, school demands, and work demands. Calculate his kcal intake based on height of 5 ft, 9 in (175.3 cm) and weight of 155 lb (70 kg). Designate allowed exchanges, and plan one day's menu.

5. Develop a care plan for Mr. Meligrito for the collaborative problem of hypoglycemia.

Bibliography

■ ■ ■

Alfaro-LeFevre, R., Blicharz, M. E., Flynn, N. M., & Boyer, M. J. (1992). *Drug handbook: A nursing process approach.* Redwood City, CA: Addison-Wesley Nursing.

American Diabetes Association. (1990). *Diabetic foot care.* Alexandria, VA: Author.

American Diabetes Association. (1992a). Office guide to diagnosis and classification of diabetes mellitus and other categories of glucose intolerance. *Diabetes Care, 15* (Supplement 2), 4.

American Diabetes Association. (1992b). Screening for diabetes. *Diabetes Care, 15* (Supplement 2), 7–9.

American Diabetes Association. (1992c). Screening for diabetic retinopathy. *Diabetes Care, 15* (Supplement 2), 16–18.

American Diabetes Association. (1992d). Foot care in patients with diabetes mellitus. *Diabetes Care, 15* (Supplement 2), 19–20.

American Diabetes Association. (1992e). Nutritional recommendations and principles for individuals with diabetes mellitus. *Diabetes Care, 15* (Supplement 2), 21–28.

American Diabetes Association. (1993a). *Diabetes facts and figures.* Alexandria, VA: Author.

American Diabetes Association. (1993b). *Diabetes: 1993 vital statistics.* Alexandria, VA: Author.

American Diabetes Association. (1994). Nutritional recommendations and principles for people with diabetes mellitus. *Diabetes Care, 17*(S) 519–522.

Armstrong, N. (1987). Coping with diabetes mellitus. *Nursing Clinics of North America, 22,* 559–568.

Barrett-Connor, E. (1989). Commentary. *Diabetes Spectrum, 2,* 164–166.

Basic facts about diabetes. (1992). Indianapolis: Eli Lilly.

Bertorelli, A. M. (1990). Nutrition counseling: Meeting the needs of ethnic clients with diabetes. *Diabetes Educator, 16*(4), 285–289.

Caine, R. M., & Bufalino, P. M. (Eds.). (1991). *Nursing care planning guides for adults* (2nd ed.). Baltimore: Williams & Wilkins.

Campbell, L. V., Redelman, M. J., Borkman, M., McLay, J. G., & Chisholm, D. J. (1989). Factors in sexual dysfunction in diabetic female volunteer subjects. *Medical Journal of Australia, 151,* 550–552.

Carpenito, L. J. (1992). *Nursing diagnosis: Application to clinical practice.* (4th ed.). Philadelphia: Lippincott.

Christensen, M. H., Funnell, M. M., Ehrlich, M. R., Fellows, E. P., & Floyd, J. C. (1991). How to care for the diabetic foot/CE test. *American Journal of Nursing, 91,* 50–58.

Classification of diabetes: A fresh look for the 1990s? (1990). *Diabetes Care, 13*(11), 1123–1128.

Cox, D. J., & Gonder-Frederick, L. (1992). Major developments in behavioral diabetes research. *Journal of Consulting and Clinical Psychology, 4,* 628–638.

Deakins, D. (1994). Teaching elderly patients about diabetes. *American Journal of Nursing, 94*(4), 38–43.

DeFronzo, R. A., Bonadonna, R. C., & Ferrannini, E. (1992). Pathogenesis of NIDDM: A balanced over-view. *Diabetes Care, 3,* 318–332.

Dellasega, C. (1990). Self-care in the elderly diabetic. *Journal of Gerontological Nursing, 16* (1), 16–20.

Diabetes Update90. (1990). *Nursing90, 20*(10), 49–51.

Edelwich, J., & Brodsky, A. (1986). *Diabetes: Caring for your emotions as well as your health.* Reading, MA: Addison-Wesley.

Elinskas, A. (1993). B-G-T-E-S-T: A basic review. *RN, 56*(6), 49–51.

Eliopoulos, C. (1987). *A guide to the nursing of the aging.* Baltimore: Williams & Wilkins.

Ellenberg, M. (1971). Impotence in diabetes: The neurologic factor. *Annals of Internal Medicine, 75,* 213–219.

Ellenberg, M. (1979). Sex and diabetes: A comparison between men and women. *Diabetes Care, 2*(1), 4–8.

Friesen, J. (1991). Meal plan. In D. W. Guthrie & R. A. Guthrie, *Nursing management of diabetes mellitus* (3rd ed.). (pp. 87–101). New York: Springer.

Gahart, B. L. (1993). *Intravenous medications.* (9th ed.). St. Louis: Mosby.

Gambert, S. (1990). Atypical presentation of diabetes mellitus in the elderly. *Clinics in Geriatric Medicine, 6*(4), 721–729.

Graves, L. (1990). Diabetic ketoacidosis and hyperosmolar hyperglycemic nonketotic coma. *Critical Care Nursing Quarterly, 13*(3), 50–61.

Guthrie, D. W., & Guthrie, R. A. (1991). *Nursing management of diabetes mellitus.* (3rd ed.). New York: Springer.

Harris, J. (1989). Impaired glucose tolerance in the U.S. population. *Diabetes Care, 12*(7), 464–474.

Heins, J., & Beebe, C. (1992). Nutritional management of diabetes mellitus. In D. Haire-Joshu, *Management of diabetes mellitus: Perspectives of care across the life span* (pp. 21–79). St. Louis: Mosby Year Book.

Herman, W. H., & Greene, D. A. (1992). Microvascular complications of diabetes. In D. Haire-Joshu, *Management of diabetes mellitus: Perspectives of care across the life span* (pp. 149–189). St. Louis: Mosby.

Hernandez, C. M. G. (1987). Surgery and diabetes: Minimizing the risks. *American Journal of Nursing, 87,* 788–792.

Hotta, S. S., & Adams, D. (1990). Reassessment of external insulin infusion pumps. *Health Technology Assessment Reports, Number 9.* (DHHS Publication No. AHCPR 91-0030). Rockville, MD: U.S. Department of Health & Human Services.

Hurley, C. C., & Shea, C. A. (1992). Self-efficacy: Strategy for enhancing diabetes self-care. *Diabetes Educator, 18,* 146–150.

Hymovich, D. P., & Hagopian, G. A. (1992). *Chronic illness in children and adults: A psychosocial approach.* Philadelphia: Saunders.

Jensen, S. B. (1981). Diabetic sexual dysfunction: A comparative study of 160 insulin treated diabetic men and women and an age-matched control group. *Archives of Sexual Behavior, 10,* 493–504.

Jensen, S. B. (1985). Sexual relationships in couples with a diabetic partner. *Journal of Sex and Marital Therapy, 11,* 259–270.

Joseph, D. H., Schwartz-Barcott, D., & Patterson, B. (1992). Risk taking among diabetic clients. *Diabetes Educator, 18,* 34–39.

Kee, J. L. (1991). *Laboratory and diagnostic tests with nursing implications.* (3rd ed.). Norwalk, CT: Appleton & Lange.

Kestle, F. (1994). Are you up to date on diabetes medication? *American Journal of Nursing, 94*(7), 48–52.

Kopeski, L. M. (1989). Diabetes and bulimia: A deadly duo. *American Journal of Nursing, 89,* 483–485.

Leedom, L., Feldman, M., Procci, W., & Zeidler, A. (1991). Symptoms of sexual dysfunction and depression in diabetic women. *Journal of Diabetic Complications, 5*(1), 38–41.

Lehne, R. A. (1990). *Pharmacology for nursing care.* Philadelphia: W. B. Saunders.

LeMone, P. (1993). Human sexuality in adults with insulin-dependent diabetes mellitus. *Image: Journal of Nursing Scholarship, 25*(2), 101–105.

LeMone, P. (1994). Responses of the older adult to the effects and management of diabetes mellitus. *MEDSURG Nursing, 3*(2), 122–127.

Ley, B, & Goldman, D. (1990). Sick day management: A partnership in preparation for the expected. *Clinical Diabetes, 8,* 25–30.

Lumley, W. A. (1989). Recognizing and reversing insulin shock. *Nursing89, 9,* 34–41.

Macheca, M. (1993). Diabetic hypoglycemia: How to keep the threat at bay. *American Journal of Nursing, 93*(4), 26–30.

Mackowiak, L., & McCarthy, R. (1989). Managing diabetes on "sick days." *American Journal of Nursing, 89,* 950–951.

Managing your diabetes. (1991). Indianapolis: Eli Lilly.

McCance, K. L., & Huether, S. E. (1994). *Pathophysiology: The biologic basis for disease of adults and children.* (2nd ed.). St. Louis: Mosby.

McFarland, G. K., & McFarlane, E. A. (1993). *Nursing diagnosis and intervention: Planning for patient care.* (2nd ed.). St. Louis: Mosby.

Morrison, J. (1991). Home management of diabetes. *Canadian Nurse, 87*(6), 23–24.

National Diabetes Data Group. (1979). Classification and diagnosis of diabetes mellitus and other categories of glucose intolerance. *Diabetes, 28,* 1039–1057.

National Diabetes Data Group. (1985). *Diabetes in America.* National Institute of Arthritis, Diabetes and Kidney Diseases. (DHHS Publication No. NIH 58–1468). Washington, DC: U.S. Department of Health and Human Services.

Packard, N. J., Haberman, M. R., Woods, N. F., & Yates, B. C. (1991). Demands of illness among chronically ill women. *Western Journal of Nursing Research, 13,* 434–457.

Peyrot, M., & McMurry, J. F. (1985). Psychosocial factors in diabetes control: Adjustment of insulin-treated adults. *Psychosomatic Medicine, 6,* 542–557.

Podolsky, S. (1982). Diagnosis and treatment of sexual dysfunction in the male diabetic. *Medical Clinics of North America, 66,* 1389–1396.

Pollock, S. E. (1989). Adaptive responses to diabetes mellitus. (1989). *Western Journal of Nursing Research, 11*(3), 265–275.

Polly, R. K. (1992). Diabetes health beliefs, self-care behaviors, and glycemic control among older adults with non-insulin-dependent diabetes mellitus. *Diabetes Educator, 18*(4), 321–327.

Porth, C. M. (1994). *Pathophysiology: Concepts of altered health states.* (4th ed.). Philadelphia: Lippincott.

Raffel, L. J., & Rotter, J. I. (1985). The genetics of diabetes. *Clinical Diabetes, 3,* 49–54.

Ratner, R. E. (1992). Overview of diabetes mellitus. In D. Haire-Joshu, *Management of diabetes mellitus: Perspectives of care across the life span* (pp. 3–20). St. Louis: Mosby.

Rifkin, H. (Ed.). (1988). *Physician's guide to type II diabetes (NIDDM) diagnosis and treatment.* New York: American Diabetes Association.

Rubin, A. (1967). Sexual behavior in diabetes mellitus. *Medical Aspects of Human Sexuality, 1*(4), 23–25.

Sinnock, P. (1985). Hospital utilization for diabetes. In National Diabetes Data Group, *Diabetes in America.* (Publication No. 85–1468). Washington, DC: U.S. Government Printing Office.

Sullivan, M. M. (1991). Diabetes instruction of the person with HIV infection. *Diabetes Educator, 17*(2), 92, 96–97.

Wakefield, B., Wakefield, D. S., & Booth, B. M. (1992). Evaluating the validity of blood glucose monitoring strip interpretation by experienced users. *Applied Nursing Research, 5*(1), 13–19.

White, J. R., & Campbell, R. K. (1992). Pharmacologic therapies in the management of diabetes mellitus. In D. Haire-Joshu, *Management of diabetes mellitus: Perspectives of care across the life span* (pp. 119–148). St. Louis: Mosby.

White, N. H., & Henry, D. N. (1992). In D. Haire-Joshu, *Management of diabetes mellitus: Perspectives of care across the life span.* (pp. 249–309). St. Louis: Mosby.

White, N. E., Richter, J. M., & Fry, C. (1992). Coping, social support, and adaptation to chronic illness. *Western Journal of Nursing Research, 14*(2), 211–224.

Elimination
Patterns

Responses to Altered Bowel Elimination

Assessing Clients with Bowel Elimination Disorders

LEARNING OBJECTIVES

After completing this chapter, you will be able to

- Identify the major structures and functions of the small and large intestines.
- Describe the physiologic processes involved in bowel elimination.
- Identify interview questions pertinent to the assessment of bowel elimination.

- Describe physical assessment techniques for bowel function.
- Identify abnormal findings in assessment of bowel function.
- Describe typical variations in assessment findings for the older adult.

▪▪▪ Review of Anatomy and Physiology ▪▪▪

Bowel elimination is the end process in digestion; after foods are eaten and broken down into usable elements, nutrients are absorbed and indigestible materials are eliminated. This chapter focuses on that process. The structure and function of the large intestine, including the rectosigmoid region and the anus, are described, as is the assessment of bowel function.

Although the anatomy and physiology of the small intestine are discussed in Chapter 12, the information is provided in this chapter as a base for understanding health problems that may occur after bowel surgery. In addition, this chapter discusses the function of the small intestine in the absorbtion of digested end products. **Malabsorption** (impaired absorption of nutrients) is discussed fully in Chapter 23.

The Small Intestine

The *small intestine* begins at the pyloric sphincter and ends at the ileocecal junction at the entrance of the large intestine (see Figure 12–1 on page 415). The small intestine is about 20 feet (6 m) long, but only about 1 inch (2.5 cm) in diameter. This long tube hangs in coils in the abdominal cavity, suspended by the mesentery and surrounded by the large intestine.

The small intestine has three regions: the duodenum, the jejunum, and the ileum. The *duodenum* begins at the pyloric sphincter and extends around the head of the pancreas for about 10 inches (25 cm). Both pancreatic enzymes and bile from the liver enter the small intestine at the duodenum. The *jejunum* is the middle region of the small intestine. It extends for about 8 feet (2.4 m). The

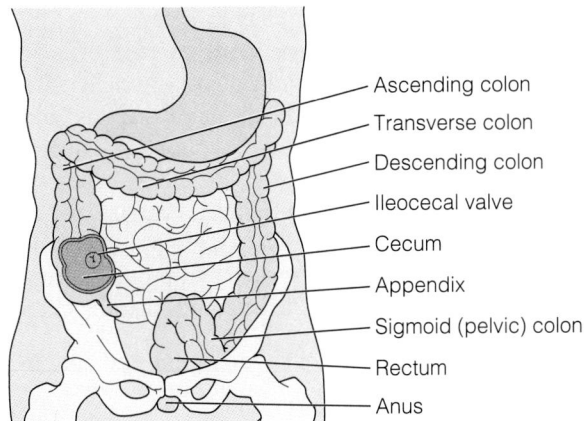

Figure 22-1   Anatomy of the large intestine.

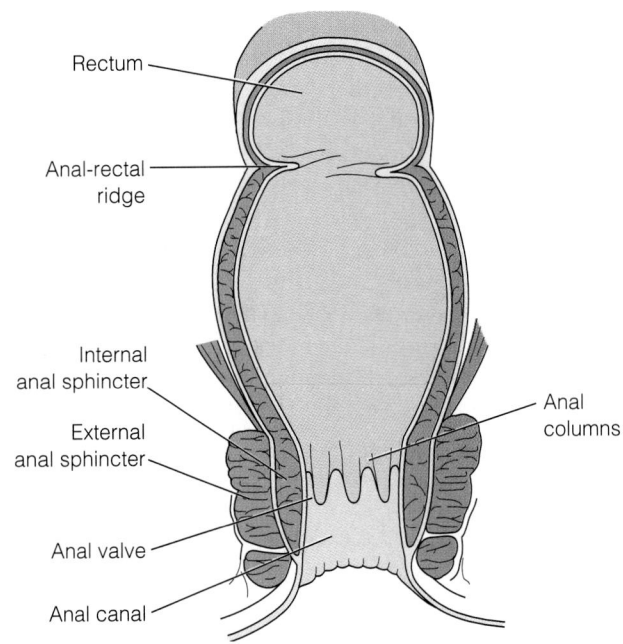

Figure 22-2   Structure of the rectum and anus.

ileum, which is the terminal end of the small intestine, is approximately 12 feet (3.6 m) long and meets the large intestine at the ileocecal valve.

Food is chemically digested and mostly absorbed as it moves through the small intestine. Microvilli (tiny projections of the mucosa cells), villi (fingerlike projections of the mucosa cells), and circular folds (deep folds of the mucosa and submucosa layers) all increase the surface area of the small intestine to enhance absorption of food. Although up to 10 L of food, liquids, and secretions enter the gastrointestinal tract each day, most is digested and absorbed in the small intestine; less than 1 L reaches the large intestine.

Enzymes in the small intestine break down carbohydrates, proteins, lipids, and nucleic acids:

- Pancreatic amylase acts on starches, converting them to maltose, dextrins, and oligosaccharides; these products are further broken down into monosaccharides by the intestinal enzymes dextrinase, glucoamylase, maltase, sucrase, and lactase.
- Proteins are broken down into peptides by the pancreatic enzymes trypsin and chymotrypsin and by intestinal enzymes.
- Lipids are broken down in the small intestine by the pancreatic lipases.
- Triglycerides enter as fat globules, are coated by bile salts, and emulsified.
- Nucleic acids are hydrolyzed by pancreatic enzymes and then broken apart by intestinal enzymes.

Both pancreatic enzymes and bile are excreted into the duodenum in response to the secretion of secretin and cholecystokinin, which are hormones produced by the intestinal mucosa cells when chyme enters the small intestine.

The absorption of nutrients through the mucosa of the intestinal villi into the blood or lymph takes place by active transport, facilitated transport, and passive diffusion. Almost all food products and water, as well as vitamins and most electrolytes, are absorbed in the small intestine, leaving only indigestible fibers, some water, and bacteria to enter the large intestine.

The Large Intestine

The *large intestine,* or *colon,* begins at the *ileocecal valve* and terminates at the *anus* (Figure 22–1). It is about 5 feet (1.5 m) long. The large intestine frames the small intestine on three sides and has several divisions: the cecum, the colon, the appendix, the rectum, and the anal canal.

The first part of the large intestine is the *cecum.* The *appendix* is attached to its surface as an extension. The appendix, a twisted structure in which bacteria can accumulate, may become inflamed.

The *colon* is divided into ascending, transverse, and descending segments. The *ascending colon* extends along the right side of the abdomen to the *hepatic flexure,* where it makes a right-angle turn. The next segment, called the *transverse colon,* crosses the abdomen to the *splenic flexure.* At this juncture, the *descending colon* descends down the left side of the abdomen and ends at the **S**-shaped *sigmoid colon.* The sigmoid colon terminates at the rectum.

The *rectum* is a mucosa-lined tube approximately 12 cm in length (Figure 22–2). The rectum has three *transverse folds* (valves of Houston) that serve to retain feces yet allow flatus to be passed through the anus. The rectum ends at the *anal canal,* which terminates at the anus.

The *anus,* a hairless, dark-skinned area, is the end of the digestive tract. It has both an internal involuntary sphincter and an external voluntary sphincter. The sphincters are usually open only during defecation. The anorectal junction separates the rectum from the anal canal and may be the site of internal **hemorrhoids,** clusters of dilated veins in swollen anal tissue.

The major function of the large intestine is to eliminate undigestible food residue from the body. The large intestine absorbs water, salts, and vitamins that are formed by the food residue and bacteria. The semiliquid chyme that passes through the ileocecal valve is formed into *feces* (*stool*) as it moves through the large intestine. Feces are moved along the intestine by peristalsis, waves of alternating contraction and relaxation. Goblet cells lining the large intestine secrete mucus that facilitates the lubrication and passage of feces.

The *defecation reflex* is initiated when feces enter the rectum and stretch the rectal wall. This spinal cord reflex causes the walls of the sigmoid colon to contract and the anal sphincters to relax. This reflex can be suppressed by voluntary control of the external sphincter. Expulsion of feces is facilitated by closing the glottis and contracting the diaphragm and abdominal muscles to increase intraabdominal pressure; this movement is called *Valsalva's maneuver.* Prolonged suppression of defecation can result in a weakened reflex that may in turn lead to **constipation,** infrequent and often uncomfortable passage of hard, dry stool. Frequent bouts of constipation may lead to the development of external hemorrhoids at the area of the external hemorrhoidal plexus.

Assessment of Bowel Function

■ ■ ■

Bowel function is assessed both by a health assessment interview to collect subjective data and a physical assessment to collect objective data.

The Health Assessment Interview

This section provides guidelines for collecting subjective data through a health assessment interview specific to the bowel function. Interview questions and leading statements for assessing bowel function also are provided.

Overview

Clients may feel embarrassed and hesitant to provide information about bowel elimination patterns. To promote effective rapport with the client, it is important to remain nonjudgmental and obtain less personal information first.

A health assessment interview to determine problems with bowel function may be done as part of a health screening or as part of a total health assessment. Alternatively, it may focus on a chief complaint, such as blood in the stool. The assessment of bowel sounds is a common part of routine assessments. If the client has a health problem involving bowel function, analyze its onset, characteristics and course, severity, precipitating and relieving factors, and any associated symptoms, noting the timing and circumstances. For example, ask the client:

- Can you describe the type of cramping and abdominal pain you are experiencing?

- Have you ever had bleeding from your rectum?

- Have you noticed increased constipation since your surgery?

Begin the interview by inquiring about any medical conditions that may influence the client's bowel elimination pattern, such as a stroke or spinal cord impairment, inflammatory gastrointestinal diseases, endocrine disorders, and allergies. Note any recent travel. Information on the client's psychosocial history is also important. Assess the client's life-style for any patterns of psychologic stress and/or depression, which may alter bowel elimination patterns. Depression may be associated with constipation, whereas **diarrhea** (frequent passage of loose, watery stools) may occur in situations of high stress and anxiety. Explore the client's activities of daily living, including exercise, sleep-rest patterns, and dietary and fluid intake. Changes in activities of daily living can influence bowel elimination patterns.

Determine whether the client has had any lower abdominal pain or rectal pain, which may be associated with a distended colon filled with gas or fluid. Crampy, colicky pains occur with diarrhea and/or constipation. Sudden onset of lower abdominal cramping occurs in obstruction of the colon. Left lower abdominal pain is associated with diverticulitis. Rectal pain may occur with stool retention and/or hemorrhoids.

Ask the client to describe the frequency and character of the stools. Ask about any history of diarrhea, constipation, or bleeding from the rectum, and collect information about the use of laxatives, suppositories, or enemas. Current use of anticholinergic drugs, antihistamines, tranquilizers, or narcotics may cause constipation.

If the client has an *ostomy* (surgical opening into the bowel), ask about skin care problems, consistency of stool, foods that cause problems, the number of times that the client empties the appliance bag each day, and irrigation habits. Finally, explore the client's feelings about the appliance.

To obtain information about the client's nutritional status, ask about changes in weight, appetite, food preferences, food intolerances, special diets, and any cultural or ethnic influences on dietary intake. Ask whether the client is experiencing nausea and vomiting; if so, determine any relation to food intake, and ask the client to describe character of the emesis. In addition, ask about indigestion, the use of antacids, and episodes of diarrhea and its character.

Explore any family history of colon cancer, colitis, gallbladder disease, or malabsorption syndromes, such as lactose intolerance and celiac sprue. Assess the client's risk factors for cancer, including age greater than 50; family member with colon cancer; history of endometrial, ovarian, or breast cancer; and previous diagnoses of colon inflammation, polyps, or cancer.

Interview Questions

The following interview questions and leading statements are categorized by functional health patterns. (See the interview questions in Chapter 12 for additional information specific to nutrition.)

Health Perception–Health Management

- Have you had any illness or surgery that may have affected your bowel elimination patterns, such as gastrointestinal diseases, ulcerative colitis, Crohn's disease, diverticulitis, spastic colon, anal fissures, hemorrhoids, colostomy, or ileostomy?
- How was this condition treated?
- Do you use any medications to control or prevent diarrhea or constipation? Describe.
- Do you use any type of treatment for hemorrhoids? Describe.
- Do you use laxatives, suppositories, or enemas? What type, and how often?

Nutritional-Metabolic

- Do you have any food allergies or food intolerances? Describe them. What type of reaction do you have: indigestion, nausea, vomiting, diarrhea, excessive gas, abdominal pain, other?
- What do you normally eat within a 24-hour period?
- Does your bowel problem prevent you from eating certain foods? Explain.
- (If the client has an ostomy.) Do certain foods cause elimination problems? Explain. Do you have skin irritation around the opening of your stoma?

Elimination

- How often do you have a bowel movement?

- Describe the color and consistency of your stools.
- Have your bowel habits recently changed? Explain.
- Do you have to strain excessively to have a bowel movement?
- Do you ever notice blood in your stools or on the toilet paper after you wipe?
- (If the client has an ostomy.) How often do you irrigate your colostomy? How often do you empty the drainage bag?

Activity-Exercise

- Describe your activities in a typical day. Does your bowel elimination pattern interfere with your activities of daily living? Explain.

Sleep-Rest

- Do the symptoms of your bowel problem (such as frequent stools) interfere with your ability to rest and sleep? Explain.
- Does abdominal cramping interefere with your ability to rest and sleep? Explain.

Cognitive-Perceptual

- Do you have abdominal cramping and/or pain? Where is it located? What brings it on or relieves it?
- Do you have any rectal pain? What brings it on or relieves it?
- Describe the bowel elimination pattern that is normal for you.

Self-Perception–Self-Concept

- Describe how you feel about your bowel function problems.
- How has this problem made you feel about yourself?
- (If the client has an ostomy.) How do you feel about having to wear a drainage bag for stool?

Role-Relationship

- Has this bowel problem affected your role in your family? If so, how?
- Has this bowel problem interfered with your work? Explain.
- Have your relationships with your family, friends, or coworkers changed recently? Explain.

Sexuality-Reproductive

- Has this health problem changed or interfered with your usual sexual activities? Explain.

- Have you noticed any change in your ability to participate in your usual sexual activities? Explain.
- How has this problem affected the way you feel about yourself as a man or woman?

Coping-Stress

- Do you ever feel depressed or extremely anxious? Explain.
- Are there certain events that seem to make your bowel function problems worse? Describe them.
- On a scale of 1 to 10 (with 10 being the most stressful), how would you rate the stress of your daily life?

- What do you feel is the most stressful aspect of your bowel problem?
- Describe what you do to cope with stress.
- Who or what will be able to help you cope with the stress of this health problem?

Value-Belief

- Are there significant others, practices, or activities that help you cope with this health problem? Explain.
- How do you perceive this health problem will affect your future?

The Physical Assessment

Physical assessment of bowel function may be performed as part of a total assessment or alone as a focused assessment. The function of the bowels is assessed through a rectal examination, an anal examination, and examination of the client's stool. A complete assessment also includes inspection of the abdomen and auscultation of bowel sounds. Guidelines for abdominal assessment and assessment of bowel sounds are outlined in Chapter 12.

Preparation

Necessary equipment includes water-soluble lubricant, material for testing the stool, and disposable gloves for the examiner.

Ask the client to empty the bladder before the examination and lie in the supine position. Have the client turn to the left lateral (Sims') position for the rectal examination. The older client or the client with limited mobility may need assistance in assuming this position.

Explain what will occur during the examination, and encourage the client to take deep, regular breaths to increase relaxation. Explain that during the examination, it may feel as though the client is about to have a bowel movement and that sometimes flatus (gas) is passed. Assure the client that this is normal. As always, ensure that the examination area is private and the client is draped properly to prevent unnecessary exposure.

ASSESSMENT TECHNIQUE	POSSIBLE ABNORMAL FINDINGS
- **Inspect the abdomen.**	Retention of flatus (gas) or stool may cause generalized abdominal distention. Malnutrition causes a scaphoid abdomen.
- **Auscultate bowel sounds.** Auscultate in all four quadrants as described in Chapter 12. Normal bowel sounds are gurgling or clicking sounds that last from 5 to 30 seconds.	High-pitched, tinkling, rushing, or growling bowel sounds may be heard in the client who has diarrhea or who is experiencing the onset of a bowel obstruction. Bowel sounds may be absent in later stages of a bowel obstruction or after surgery of the abdominal organs.

ASSESSMENT TECHNIQUE	POSSIBLE ABNORMAL FINDINGS

■ **Inspect the perianal area.**

Ask the client to turn to the left side. Wearing gloves, spread the client's buttocks apart. Observe the area, and ask client to bear down (Valsalva's maneuver.)

Swollen, painful, longitudinal breaks in the anal area may appear in clients with anal fissures. These are caused by the passing of large, hard stools, or diarrhea, which irritates the area. Dilated anal veins appear with hemorrhoids. A red mass may appear with prolapsed internal hemorrhoids. Doughnut-shaped red tissue at the anal area may appear with a prolapsed rectum.

■ **Palpate the anus and rectum.**

Lubricate the gloved index finger and ask the client to bear down. Touch the tip of your finger to the client's anal opening. Flex the index finger, and slowly insert it into the anus, pointing the finger towards the umbilicus (Figure 22–3). Rotate the finger in both directions to palpate any lesions or masses. (The prostate or cervix may also be examined at this time. See Chapter 45).

Movable, soft masses may be *polyps.* Hard, firm, irregular embedded masses may indicate carcinoma.

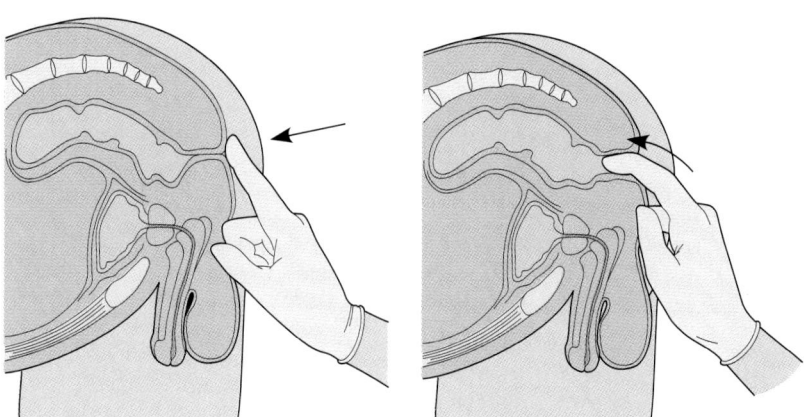

Figure 22–3 Digital examination of the anus and rectum.

■ **Inspect the client's feces.**

Withdraw your finger gently. Inspect any feces on the glove.
Note color and/or presence of blood. Also use gloved fingers to note consistency.

The box on page 764 provides guidelines for assessment of stool characteristics.

■ **Test the feces for occult blood.**

Use a commercial testing kit.

A positive occult blood test requires further testing for colon cancer or gastrointestinal bleeding due to peptic ulcers, ulcerative colitis, or diverticulosis.

■ **Note the odor of the feces.**

Distinctly foul odors may be noted with stools containing blood or extra fat or in cases of colon cancer.

Assessment of Stool Characteristics

■ ■ ■

Inspect feces for color, odor, and consistency after the rectal exam or after defecation. Both hands are gloved.

Color

- Blood *on* the stool results from bleeding from the sigmoid colon, anus, or rectum. Blood *within* the stool indicates bleeding from the colon due to ulcerative colitis, diverticulosis, or tumors. Black, tarry stools, called **melena**, occur with upper gastrointestinal bleeding. Oral iron may turn stools black and mask melena.
- Grayish or whitish stools can result from biliary tract obstruction due to lack of bile in stool.
- Greasy, frothy, yellow stools, called **steatorrhea**, may appear with fat malabsorption.

Odor

- Distinct, foul odors may be noted with stools containing blood or extra fat or in cases of colon cancer.

Consistency

- Hard stools or long, flat stools may result from a spastic colon or bowel obstruction due to a tumor or hemorrhoids. Hard stools may also result from ingestion of oral iron.
- Mucousy, slimy feces may indicate inflammation and occur in irritable bowel syndrome.
- Watery, diarrhea stools appear with malabsorption problems, irritable bowel syndrome, emotional or psychologic stress, ingestion of spoiled foods, or lactose intolerance.

Variations in Assessment Findings for the Older Adult

As the client ages, the large intestine tends to dilate and lengthen because of lack of regular bowel elimination. However, the colon does not atrophy until after the age of 90 years. Precipitating factors leading to decreased bowel elimination in the older adult include lack of bulk in diet, decreased fluid intake, decreased activity, laxative abuse, and avoidance of the need to defecate. Rectal neurons may degenerate in the older client, resulting in relaxation of the perianal area and decreased sphincter control, which may lead to **fecal incontinence**, an involuntary release of feces from the rectum.

Anal sphincter control and tone of the perianal musculature may also decrease, placing the older adult at risk for fecal incontinence and/or rectal prolapse. The older adult is also at risk for constipation because peristalsis, digestive enzymes, and intestinal muscle tone decrease with age. A sedentary life-style and poor dietary and fluid intake can increase the risk of constipation.

Bibliography

■ ■ ■

Gehring, P. E. (1991). Physical assessment begins with a history. *RN, 54* (11), 26–32.

Holm, M. A. (1990). Elimination concerns with acute spinal cord trauma: Assessment and nursing interventions. *Critical Care Nursing Clinics of North America, 2*(3), 385–398.

Marieb, E. N. (1995). *Human anatomy and physiology* (3rd ed.). Redwood City, CA: Benjamin/Cummings.

McShane, R., & McLane, A. M. (1988). Constipation: Impact of etiologic factors. *Journal of Gerontologic Nursing, 14* (4), 31–34, 46–47.

O'Toole, M. T. (1991). Advanced assessment of the abdomen and gastrointestinal problems. *Nursing Clinics of North America, 25* (40), 771–776.

Salvadalnea, G. D. (1991). Enterostomal therapy nursing data base for use with patients with ostomies. *Journal of Enterostomal Nursing, 18* (3), 100–104.

Sims, L., D'Amico, D., Stiesmeyer, J., & Webster, J. (1995). *Health assessment in nursing.* Redwood City, CA: Addison-Wesley Nursing.

Nursing Care of Clients with Bowel Disorders

• •

LEARNING OBJECTIVES

After completing this chapter, you will be able to

- Discuss the pathophysiology, manifestations, and management of bowel absorption and elimination disorders.

- Identify laboratory and diagnostic tests used to diagnose disorders of the small and large bowel.

- Discuss the nursing implications of medications used in managing bowel absorption and elimination disorders.

- Compare and contrast the manifestations and care of clients with ulcerative colitis and Crohn's disease.

- Discuss the care of clients with a colostomy or ileostomy.

- Provide appropriate nursing care for the client in the preoperative and postoperative phases of intestinal surgery.

- Provide appropriate teaching for clients with bowel absorption and elimination disorders and their families.

- Use the nursing process as a framework for providing individualized care to clients with disorders of bowel absorption and elimination.

Alterations in bowel elimination occur in response to inflammations, tumors, infections, obstructions, or changes in structure. In addition, malabsorption within the small intestine can severely impair the client's health, while hernias and anorectal disorders may cause intense pain and may require surgical management.

Clients with the disorders discussed in this chapter often face extensive diagnostic testing, surgical intervention, and permanent alterations in physical appearance and life-style. Nursing care is directed toward meeting the client's physiologic needs, providing emotional support, and educating the client to adapt to changes in life-style.

▖▖▖ Disorders of Intestinal Motility ▖▖▖

Few body functions respond as readily to both internal and external influences as the process of defecation. Factors affecting the gastrointestinal tract directly, such as food intake and bacterial population, affect the number and consistency of stools. Indirect factors, such as psychologic stress or voluntary postponement of defecation, also affect the client's pattern of elimination.

In modern society, "normal" patterns of defecation vary widely. For some clients, two to three stools per day is the usual pattern. Others may normally have as few as three stools per week. It is therefore necessary to evaluate each client's elimination pattern against his or her own normal pattern.

The Client with Diarrhea

■ ■ ■

Diarrhea is an increase in the frequency, volume, and fluid content of the stool. In diarrhea, the water content of feces is increased, usually as a result of either malabsorption or water secretion in the bowel. It is a symptom rather than a primary disorder.

Among the many causes of diarrhea are bacterial toxins, infections and parasitic infestations, malabsorption syndromes, medications, systemic diseases, allergies, and psychogenic factors (e.g., preexamination diarrhea).

Pathophysiology

Excess fecal water can result from the presence of water-soluble molecules in the feces, which causes retention of water in the bowel lumen. This form of diarrhea is known as *osmotic diarrhea*. Some stool softeners and laxatives work on this principle. Lactose intolerance also causes diarrhea by this mechanism. The diarrhea associated with cholera and pathogenic *Escherichia coli* infection is caused by excess secretion of water in the small and large intestines. Unabsorbed dietary fat, some cathartics and other drugs, as well as other factors can also cause *secretory diarrhea*. Diseases that affect the intestinal mucosa, such as regional enteritis (Crohn's disease) and ulcerative colitis, are associated with *exudative diarrhea*. The mucosal inflammation results in the accumulation of plasma, serum proteins, blood, and mucus in the bowel, increasing fecal bulk and fluidity. An alteration in bowel transit time or surface for water absorption can also decrease the amount of water that is normally absorbed from the chyme, leading to diarrhea. Laxatives that increase bowel motility and bowel resection or bypass can lead to diarrhea for this reason (Berkow & Fletcher, 1992; Tierney, McPhee, & Papadakis, 1994).

Just as normal bowel elimination (volume, frequency, and consistency) varies from person to person, the manifestations of diarrhea vary, ranging from several large, watery stools in the course of a day to very frequent small stools containing blood, mucus, or exudate. The manifestations depend on the cause, duration, and severity of the diarrhea, as well as the area of bowel affected and the client's general health.

Even though diarrhea is rarely the primary disorder, it can have devastating results. Water and electrolytes are lost in diarrheal stool. The client can become dehydrated, particularly the very young client, the older client, or the debilitated client who is unable to respond to the thirst reflex. With severe diarrhea, vascular collapse and hypovolemic shock may occur. Potassium and magnesium are lost, potentially leading to hypokalemia and hypomagnesemia. The client may develop metabolic acidosis due to the loss of bicarbonate in the stool. See Chapter 5 for further discussion of the effects of these imbalances.

Collaborative Care

Management of the client with diarrhea focuses on identifying and treating the underlying cause of the diarrhea. It may be necessary to treat the diarrhea itself as well as to provide for client comfort and to prevent complications. The client's history and physical examination often provide enough information to identify the cause of diarrhea. It is important to obtain information about the onset and associated circumstances of the diarrhea.

Laboratory and Diagnostic Tests

When the client's history and physical examination do not reveal the reason for the diarrhea, laboratory and diagnostic testing is done to determine its cause.

The following laboratory tests may be ordered:

- *Stool specimen* is obtained for gross and microscopic examination. The gross examination includes noting the volume and water content of the stool, as well as the presence of any blood, pus, mucus, or excess fat. Microscopic examination is conducted to determine the presence of white blood cells (WBCs), unabsorbed fat, and parasites. WBCs in the stool may indicate a bacterial infection or ulceration of the bowel mucosa. Although the microscopic examination may reveal parasites, ova, or larvae, they may not be continuously present. A series of three stool specimens, spaced 2 to 3 days apart, is obtained when parasitic infection is suspected.

- *Stool culture* is ordered when it has been established that the client has been exposed to an enteric pathogen or has persistent or bloody diarrhea accompanied by fever and/or recent travel out of the country (Chernecky, Krech, & Berger, 1993).

- *Serum electrolytes, serum osmolality, and arterial blood gases* may be ordered to assess for adverse effects of severe or long-standing diarrhea. Increased serum osmolality is an indicator of water loss and dehydration. As noted earlier, the client may have hypokalemia, hypomagnesemia, and metabolic acidosis as a result of diarrhea. The serum sodium may be increased or decreased, depending on the type of diarrhea.

In addition to the above laboratory tests, the following diagnostic tests may be ordered:

- *Sigmoidoscopy* is done to allow direct examination of the bowel mucosa. Stool may also be obtained during sigmoidoscopy for microscopic examination. The preparation and teaching for a client undergoing sigmoidoscopy is outlined in the accompanying box.

Nursing Implications for Diagnostic Tests: Sigmoidoscopy

■ ■ ■

Client Preparation

- Ensure that client or family member signs an informed consent form.
- Check hospital policy on withholding food and fluids. Generally, a light diet is ordered for the evening before the procedure; the client does not have to be NPO. Enemas or rectal suppositories are given immediately before the procedure.

Client and Family Teaching

Before Procedure

- The procedure takes approximately 15 minutes.
- You may be positioned in the knee-chest position (on the left side for the older or debilitated client).
- The scope will be inserted and advanced through the sigmoid colon.
- Air insufflation may be used to help outline structures in the colon.
- Feces may be suctioned.
- A biopsy may be taken. Polyps may be removed.
- Taking deep breaths when you feel discomfort may help you relax.

After Procedure

- Report any abdominal pain, fever, chills, or rectal bleeding.
- If a polyp is removed, avoid heavy lifting for 7 days, and avoid high-fiber foods for 1 to 2 days.

- *Rectal biopsy* may also be performed to assist in the diagnosis. Biopsy is a useful means to identify chronic inflammatory processes, infection, and other causes of diarrhea. For rectal biopsy, the client is given an analgesic medication, and a small section of tissue (which may include the mucosal and muscle layers) is removed and examined for gross microscopic and histologic (cell character) changes.

Both sigmoidoscopy and rectal biopsy are most appropriately performed before any treatment of the diarrhea has been initiated to avoid interference with findings.

Dietary Management

Fluid replacement is of primary importance in the management of the client with diarrhea. If the client is able to

Table 23–1   Foods That May Aggravate Chronic Diarrhea

Foods	Reason
Milk, ice cream, yogurt, soft cheeses, cottage cheese	Contain lactose; not tolerated by clients who are deficient in lactase and cannot digest lactose.
Apple juice, pear juice, grapes, honey, dates, nuts, figs, fruit-flavored soft drinks	Contain fructose; when consumed in large quantities, fructose may not be totally absorbed, resulting in an osmotic draw of fluid into the bowel.
Table sugar	Contains sucrose, which is not tolerated by clients with sucrase deficiency.
Apple juice, pear juice, sugarless gums and mints	May contain sorbitol or mannitol, sugars that are not absorbed and can cause osmotic draw.
Antacids	Magnesium-containing antacids decrease bowel transit time and contain poorly-absorbed salts that can exert an osmotic draw.
Coffee, tea, cola drinks, over-the-counter analgesics	Contain caffeine, which can decrease bowel transit time.

Note. Adapted from "Chronic Diarrhea" by T. Bayless, 1989, January 15, *Hospital Practice*, p. 131.

---

tolerate oral fluids (that is, if the client is not experiencing nausea and vomiting), an oral glucose/balanced electrolyte solution provides the best fluid replacement. Commercial preparations such as Gatorade and other sports drinks are available, as are pediatric solutions (e.g., Pedialyte), which can be used for adults as well as children. A solution of 5 mL (1 teaspoon) each of table salt and baking soda and 4 teaspoons (20 mL) of granulated sugar added with desired flavoring (such as lemon extract or juice) to 1 quart (1 L) of water can be made at home to replace water and electrolytes.

The client should avoid food in the first 24 hours of acute diarrhea to provide bowel rest. After that time, frequent, small, soft feedings can be added. Milk and milk products are added *last,* because the lactose they contain frequently aggravates the diarrhea. The client should avoid raw fruits and vegetables, fried foods, bran, whole-grain cereals, condiments, spices, coffee, and alcoholic beverages during the recovery period.

Clients with chronic diarrhea require a more extensive diagnostic workup to determine the cause of the diarrhea. Once the cause is identified, specific foods may be eliminated from the diet. Foods and nonfood substances that may aggravate diarrhea are outlined in Table 23–1.

Nursing Implications for Pharmacology: Antidiarrheal Preparations

ABSORBANTS AND PROTECTANTS

Kaolin and pectin (Kaopectate, Donnagel-MB)

Charcoal

Bismuth subsalicylate (Pepto-Bismol)

Absorbant preparations act locally in the intestines to bind substances that can cause diarrhea. Absorbants are considered to be safe and are generally available over-the-counter. Their efficacy has not been proved, although bismuth subsalicylate has been demonstrated to be somewhat effective in preventing and managing traveler's diarrhea, usually related to contaminated water supplies. Bismuth salts not only act as an absorbant but also have a protective and antimicrobial effect.

Nursing Responsibilities

- Assess the client for contraindications to antidiarrheal therapy, such as some infections or chronic inflammatory bowel disease, including ulcerative colitis.
- If fever is present, check with physician before administering the medication.
- Administer these medications at least 1 hour before or 2 hours after other oral medications; they may interfere with the absorption of other drugs.
- Observe the client's response to the medication. Constipation is a potential problem.

Client and Family Teaching

- Take the recommended dosage at the onset of diarrhea and after each loose stool.

- Do not take any of these preparations for more than 48 hours. If diarrhea persists, notify the physician.
- Do not give antidiarrheal medications to debilitated older clients without physician supervision.
- Chew bismuth subsalicylate tablets, rather than swallowing them whole, for maximal effectiveness. This medication may cause harmless darkening of the tongue and stool.
- If you are allergic to aspirin, use bismuth subsalicylate with caution; as a general rule, avoid taking aspirin while taking bismuth subsalicylate.

OPIUM AND OPIUM DERIVATIVES

Camphorated tincture of opium (Paregoric)

Tincture of opium (laudanum, opium tincture)

Difenoxin (Motofen)

Diphenoxylate (Lomotil, Lotrol, others)

Loperamide hydrochloride (Imodium)

Opium and its derivatives act on the central nervous system (CNS) to decrease the motility of the ileum and colon, slowing the transit time and promoting more water absorption. They also decrease the sensation of a full rectum and increase anal sphincter tone. Paregoric and tincture of opium have a greater potential for abuse and are prescription drugs subject to controls under the federal Controlled Substance Act of 1970. Difenoxin, diphenoxylate, and loperamide are derivatives of opium with few analgesic, euphoric,

---

The client with chronic diarrhea needs to consume a diet that is high in calories and nutritional value. Vitamin supplements may be necessary, particularly the fat-soluble vitamins (A, D, E, K). Clients with severe chronic diarrhea may require parenteral nutrition. Parenteral nutrition is discussed in Chapter 13.

Pharmacology

Antidiarrheal medications are used sparingly or not at all until the cause of diarrhea has been determined. In diarrhea associated with botulism or bacillary dysentery, administration of an antidiarrheal agent can worsen or prolong the disease by causing retention of the toxin in the bowel. Opium and some of its derivatives, anticholinergics, absorbants, and demulcents are commonly used as antidiarrheal preparations. Specific preparations, their

method of action, and the nursing implications for these medications are outlined in the accompanying pharmacology box.

Once the underlying cause for diarrhea has been established, specific medications may be prescribed; for example, antibiotics may be prescribed if the diarrhea is caused by an infection. Antibiotics are used with caution because they alter the normal bacterial population of the bowel and may actually worsen diarrhea. A balanced electrolyte intravenous solution may be required to replace fluid losses. Intravenous or oral potassium preparations may also be prescribed.

Nursing Care

Nursing care of the client with diarrhea is directed toward identifying the cause, relieving the symptoms, preventing

Pharmacology: Antidiarrheal Preparations (continued)

or abuse-promoting effects and are in more common use today (Shlafer, 1993).

Nursing Responsibilities

- Assess the client for contraindications to antidiarrheal or narcotic medications prior to administering these drugs.
- Administer paregoric undiluted with water.
- Do not administer difenoxin and diphenoxylate to clients receiving monoamine oxidase (MAO) inhibitors; hypertensive crises may occur.
- Observe the client closely for increased effects of other CNS depressants, such as alcohol, narcotic analgesics, or barbiturate sedatives.
- Observe the client for abdominal distention; toxic megacolon may occur if these drugs are administered to the client with ulcerative colitis.

Client and Family Teaching

- Take the medication as recommended at the onset of diarrhea and after each loose stool.
- These drugs may be habit forming; use for no more than 48 hours.
- Avoid the use of alcohol and over-the-counter cold preparations while taking these drugs.
- These preparations may cause drowsiness; avoid driving or operating machinery while taking them.

ANTICHOLINERGICS

Atropine

Belladonna alkaloids (Donnagel, Donnatal)

Anticholinergic medications reduce bowel spasticity and acid secretion in the stomach. They are used to treat only diarrhea that is associated primarily with peptic ulcer disease and irritable bowel syndrome. These are nonspecific drugs; their systemic effects are their major drawback.

Nursing Responsibilities

- Assess the client for contraindications to atropine and other anticholinergic medications: glaucoma, prostatic hypertrophy, and gastrointestinal or genitourinary obstruction.
- Observe the client for side effects, such as eye pain, impaired urination, or constipation.

Client and Family Teaching

- Take only as directed; stop the drug and notify the physician if any of the following side effects occur: eye pain, impaired urination, constipation.
- Do not operate machinery while taking this medication; drowsiness may occur.
- Hard candies help relieve oral dryness associated with these preparations.

---

complications, and, if the cause is infectious, preventing the spread of infection to others.

Diarrhea

The nursing assessment can help identify the cause of the client's diarrhea, as well as early signs of complications. Nursing interventions focus on measures to help the client recover a normal elimination pattern without adverse consequences.

Nursing interventions with rationales follow:

- Explore the client's history, asking specific questions about dietary intake, recent travel out of the country or to wilderness areas, and use of prescription and non-prescription medications. *Without direct questioning, the client may not associate recent activities or medication use with the onset of diarrhea.*

- Carefully delineate the duration and extent of the client's diarrhea and associated symptoms. *Diarrhea is often self-limiting, requiring no medical intervention. If the client has had one or two loose stools without associated symptoms, further observation may be warranted before recommending specific measures.*

- Observe the client's stool for steatorrhea (bulky, foul-smelling stool), and obvious blood, pus, or mucus. Check the stool for occult blood. *Changes in the character of the stool may provide clues to the underlying cause.*

- Monitor and record the frequency and characteristics of bowel movements. *This provides a measure of the effectiveness of treatment.*

- Measure abdominal girth and auscultate bowel sounds every shift as indicated. *These indicate the effectiveness and possible complications of treatment, such as constipation or toxic megacolon.*

■ Administer antidiarrheal medications as prescribed. *Antidiarrheal medications promote comfort and prevent excess fluid loss.*

■ Limit the client's food intake if the diarrhea is acute, reintroducing solid foods slowly, in small amounts. *Limiting food allows the bowel to rest and mucosa to heal in acute diarrhea states.*

Risk for Fluid Volume Deficit

The increased water content of the stool places the client at risk for fluid deficit. Nursing measures are employed to minimize this risk and to prevent possible adverse effects of dehydration.

Nursing interventions with rationales follow:

■ Record intake and output; weigh the client daily; assess the client's skin turgor, mucous membranes, and urine specific gravity every 8 hours. *These assessments help monitor fluid volume status.*

■ Monitor and record vital signs, including orthostatic blood pressures. *If the blood pressure drops more than 10 mm Hg when the client moves from a lying to a sitting position or from a sitting to a standing position, orthostatic hypotension, an indicator of fluid volume deficit, may be present. This is typically accompanied by an increase in pulse rate.*

■ Provide fluid and electrolyte replacement solutions as indicated. Be sure the client has ready access to fluids; assist the debilitated client with fluid intake. *If the client is able to tolerate oral fluids, they should be encouraged to prevent dehydration. The client who is unable to take oral fluid replacement will require intravenous fluids. An intake of 3000 mL per day or more is often needed to replace fluid losses.*

■ Remind the client to seek assistance when getting up. *The client with orthstatic hypotension may become dizzy or lightheaded on rising.*

Risk for Impaired Skin Integrity

Decreased extracellular fluid volume and the irritating effects of diarrheal stool place the client at risk for skin breakdown. Preventive nursing care measures reduce this risk.

Nursing interventions with rationales follow:

■ Provide good skin care. *Poorly hydrated skin is at increased risk for breakdown.*

■ Assist the client with cleaning the perianal area as needed. Use warm water and soft cloths. *These measures will help prevent tissue irritation and trauma.*

■ Apply protective ointment to the perianal area. *Protective ointment or creams help prevent breakdown of affected tissues.*

Other Nursing Diagnoses

Each client has different nursing care needs. Among the other nursing diagnoses that may be applicable for the client with diarrhea are the following:

■ *Activity Intolerance* related to fluid and electrolyte losses

■ *Bowel Incontinence* related to frequent explosive stools

■ *Ineffective Individual Coping* related to chronic diarrhea

■ *Altered Nutrition: Less Than Body Requirements* related to loss of nutrients in diarrhea stool

■ *Low Self-Esteem: Situational* related to frequent bowel movements

Client and Family Teaching

The client with acute or chronic diarrhea must be taught to manage the disorder. Teach the client and family members about causes of acute diarrhea, including infectious disorders, and about food and water safety as preventive measures. For clients planning travel outside the United States or to wilderness areas, teach measures to purify water for drinking and cooking.

Teach the client about the importance of maintaining an adequate fluid intake to replace lost water and electrolytes. Encourage the client to use Gatorade or a similar product (purchased or home-prepared) rather than water for fluid replacement. Teach the client that food intake is not vital or recommended during episodes of acute diarrhea. If an antidiarrheal preparation is used, teach the client the precautions to take and limitations of the drug's use. For the client with chronic diarrhea, provide information on foods to avoid and foods to include to maintain adequate nutritional status.

Teach the client measures to prevent the spread of bacteria. Stress the importance of good hand washing after every bowel movement. In addition, stress the importance of seeking medical intervention if diarrhea continues or recurs.

The Client with Constipation

■ ■ ■

Constipation is defined as the infrequent or difficult passage of stools. In evaluating a client's complaints of constipation, it is important to identify the usual pattern of defecation, stool consistency, and stool bulk. Many clients complain of constipation when they have less than one stool per day, even though the feces may be of normal consistency and they experience no difficulty in expelling the stool. The term *constipation* is appropriately applied

Gerontologic Considerations: The Client with Constipation

▪ ▪ ▪

Although constipation is not a consequence of aging, it is a common gastrointestinal complaint among older adults. Risk factors for developing constipation in older adults include: immobility, medication side effects, poor dentition, depression, dehydration, diabetes, and diseases of the central nervous system such as Parkinson's disease. Laxative abuse and poor bowel habits, common among older adults, also contribute to the development of constipation.

In older adults, constipation and its accompanying complications of gas and impaction are called *presbycolon*. The condition includes three forms of constipation: hypertonic, hypotonic, and habit constipation. Hypotonic constipation is caused by decreased intestinal mobility. This form of presbycolon is seen in patients with diabetes, as a side-effect of laxative abuse, and as a side effect of anti-Parkinson's medications and oral iron therapy. Fecal impaction is common in hypotonic constipation. Digital examination of the rectum reveals soft putty-like stools. Hypertonic constipation is caused by decreased transit time and increased water absorption in the lower intestine. Lower abdominal pain may be a symptom. Stools in patients with hypertonic constipation often are hard and dry. When impaction is present, diarrhea-like stool may leak around the impacted feces. Habit constipation is a result of dietary habits and/or ignoring the urge to defecate. Diets lacking in intake of fiber or bulk can produce this condition.

The most common symptom of presbycolon is the complaint of a change in the normal bowel pattern with a decrease in the number of bowel movements. Evacuation of stool is difficult and may be painful. Other manifestations include: loss of appetite, nausea, irritability, abdominal pain, cramping, abdominal distention, and urinary incontinence. Constipation may be manifested in the individual with dementia as increased irritability and agitation.

Assessment of the client with presbycolon focuses on bowel patterns and uncovering underlying causes. Older adults should be asked about frequency, timing, size and consistency of stools. Dietary patterns and medications should be reviewed to determine their role as contributing factors. In hospitalized and institutionalized older patients, it is essential for the nurse to closely observe and monitor bowel patterns to prevent constipation and fecal impaction.

The goal of managing presbycolon is to improve bowel patterns. Constipation may be managed pharmaceutically with the use of laxatives, suppositories, or enemas. The specific type of medication used depends on the type of constipation. Stimulants such as biscadoyl should be used with care in debilitated older adults to prevent fatigue.

Teaching older adults about presbycolon focuses on prevention. Older adults should be taught about normal elimination patterns, the importance of fiber or bulk in the diet, and the goal of drinking at least 6 glasses of water per day, unless contraindicated. Older adults should be taught that exercise is an important part of bowel programs because it improves intestinal motility. For those who are disabled, turning in bed or shifting weight while chair bound increases gastrointestinal motility. The importance of regular toileting schedules should be emphasized. This includes privacy, toileting at the same time every day in an unhurried manner, and taking advantage of the gastrocolic reflex. The gastrocolic reflex is activated after eating. With a full stomach the internal rectal sphincter is relaxed which makes defecation easier to accomplish without straining. The gastrocolic reflex is generally most pronounced in the morning.

Heitkemper, M. & Carnevali, D. (1993) Gastrointestinal problems. In Carnevali, D. & Patrick, M. Eds. *Nursing Management of the Elderly.* Philadelphia: J. B. Lippincott, 492–497.

Palmer, E. (1976) "Presbycolon" problems in the nursing home. *Journal of the American Medical Association.* 235: 1150.

only when the client has unexplained delay of defecation for several days or if the feces is unusually dry, hard, or difficult to expel (Tierney et al., 1994).

Constipation affects older adults more frequently than younger people. Recent studies indicate that approximately 20% to 35% of people over age 65 report recurrent constipation and laxative use. Although fecal transit in the large intestine slows with aging, the increased incidence of constipation is thought to relate more to impaired general health status, increased number of medications, and decreased physical activity in the older client (Hazzard, Bierman, Blass, Ettinger, & Halter, 1994). The accompanying box discusses constipation in the older adult.

Table 23–2	Selected Causes of Constipation
Factor	**Related Cause**
Activity	Lack of exercise; bed rest
Dietary	Highly refined, low-fiber foods; inadequate fluid intake
Drugs	Antacids containing aluminum or calcium salts; narcotic analgesics; anticholinergics; many antidepressants, tranquilizers, and sedatives; antihypertensives, such as ganglionic blockers, calcium-channel blockers, beta-adrenergic blockers, and diuretics; iron salts
Large bowel	Diverticular disease, inflammatory disease, tumor, obstruction; changes in rectal or anal structure or function
Psychogenic	Voluntary suppression of urge; perceived need to defecate on schedule; depression
Systemic	Advanced age; pregnancy; neurologic conditions (trauma, multiple sclerosis, tumors, cerebrovascular accident, Parkinsonism); endocrine and metabolic disorders (hypothyroidism, hypercalcemia, uremia, porphyria)
Other	Chronic laxative or enema use

Pathophysiology

Acute constipation that is a definite change in pattern for the client suggests an organic process. A change in bowel patterns that persists or becomes more frequent or severe may be due to a tumor or other cause of partial bowel obstruction. Other, more common causes of constipation are listed in Table 23–2. With chronic constipation, functional causes that impair storage, transport, and evacuation mechanisms impede the normal passage of stools.

Psychogenic factors are the most frequent causes of chronic constipation. These factors are related primarily to the client's willingness to respond to the urge to defecate and the client's perception of satisfaction with defecation. Many clients abuse the use of laxatives and enemas to stimulate a bowel movement when they perceive themselves to be constipated. Overuse of these measures can result in real intestinal problems that worsen the client's condition. For example, *cathartic colon* mimics ulcerative colitis in that the normal pouchlike or saccular appearance of the colon is lost. *Melanosis coli* is a brownish-black discoloration of the colon mucosa. Both conditions may be caused by long-term laxative use (Berkow & Fletcher, 1992).

With significant constipation or long-term dependence on laxatives or enemas, the client may develop a *fecal impaction*. Impaction may also occur following barium administration for radiologic exam. The impaction is felt as a rock-hard or puttylike mass of feces in the rectum. The client often experiences an associated full sensation in the rectal area and abdominal cramping. Although constipation with no evacuation of stool may be present, the client may pass watery mucus or liquid stool around the impaction, and complain of diarrhea.

Collaborative Care

Initially, the client's history and response to simple treatment measures are used to evaluate constipation. On examination, the abdomen may appear somewhat distended, and bowel sounds may be reduced. Digital examination of the rectum in the client with an impaction reveals a palpable hard or puttylike fecal mass.

Simple or chronic constipation is best treated with education (a daily bowel movement is not necessary for health), and modification of the client's diet and exercise routines. If the problem is acute or does not resolve, further diagnostic examination may be ordered.

Laboratory and Diagnostic Tests
The following tests and examinations may be ordered:

- *Serum electrolytes and thyroid function tests* may be performed to identify metabolic and endocrine problems that may contribute to constipation.

- *Radiologic examination of the abdomen and bowel* may be ordered. The most commonly ordered examination is a barium enema. In this test, barium is instilled into the large intestine and X-ray films taken to evaluate bowel structure. This test is particularly useful to identify tumors and diverticular disease. Nursing care for the client undergoing a barium enema is described in the accompanying box.

- *Sigmoidoscopy or colonoscopy* may also be performed to evaluate constipation, particularly when the problem is acute and a tumor or obstruction is suspected. Using a flexible sigmoidoscope, the physician can inspect bowel mucosa and structure. Suspicious lesions may be biopsied at the time of the scope. The box on page 774 outlines nursing care for the client having a colonoscopy.

Dietary Management
The recommended diet for bowel elimination is one that is low in refined foods, high in dietary fiber, and contains adequate fluids. Perceived constipation in older adults may be due to inadquate food intake.

Foods that have a high fiber content are recommended. Vegetable fiber is largely indigestible and unabsorbable, increasing stool bulk. Fiber also helps draw water into the fecal mass, softening the stool and making

Nursing Implications for Diagnostic Tests: Barium Enema

Client Preparation

- Ensure that the client or family member signs an informed consent form if required by agency policy.
- Check agency policy on withholding food and fluids. A liquid diet is given the day prior to the procedure; the client will be NPO 8 hours prior to the procedure.
- Administer laxatives, enemas, or suppositories as ordered the evening prior to the procedure. Additional bowel preparation may be ordered for the morning just prior to the procedure. Nursing implications for commonly prescribed bowel preparations are outlined in the box below.

Client and Family Teaching

Before Procedure
- You will be allowed to take nothing by mouth for 8 hours before the enema.

- The procedure takes approximately 1 hour.
- You will be positioned on the left side and then onto back.
- A lubricated enema tip will be inserted into the rectum.
- The sensation is similar to that felt during a tap water enema.
- A fluoroscope will be used to follow the progress of the barium.
- X-ray films will be taken.
- Air insufflation may be used to help outline structures in the colon.
- You will expel the barium in the bathroom.
- Another X-ray film will be taken.

After Procedure
- Following the procedure, a laxative will be given.
- The stools may be white for the next 1 to 2 days.

Nursing Implications for Pharmacology: Cathartics for Bowel Preparation

MAGNESIUM CITRATE

Citrate of magnesia   Citro-Nesia

Citroma

POLYETHYLENE GLYCOL AND ELECTROLYTES

Colyte   GoLYTELY

Magnesium citrate and polyethylene glycol promote bowel evacuation by causing osmotic retention of fluid. The accumulating fluid distends the colon and stimulates peristaltic activity, inducing diarrhea, which rapidly cleans the bowel. Electrolytes are added to some solutions to minimize electrolyte imbalance with their use. These laxatives often are used as a bowel preparation prior to colon X-ray studies or colonoscopy (Shannon, Wilson, & Stang, 1992).

Nursing Responsibilities
Magnesium Citrate

- Administer magnesium citrate on an empty stomach followed by a full glass of water.

- Chill the solution or pour over ice to enhance palatability.
- Give the medication in early evening so as not to interfere with sleep.

Polyethylene Glycol

- Administer 8 ounces of the 1 gallon Colyte solution every 10 minutes.
- Chill the solution to enhance palatability.
- No food should be consumed 3 to 4 hours prior nor within 2 hours of ingesting the solution.
- Give the medication in early evening so as not to interfere with sleep.
- The first bowel movement begins within 1 hour and continues until the stool is clear and free of solid matter.

Client and Family Teaching

- Expect some degree of abdominal cramping.
- Do not use this medication for routine treatment of constipation.

Nursing Implications for Diagnostic Tests: Colonoscopy

■ ■ ■

Client Preparation

- Ensure that the client or family member signs an informed consent form.

- Check agency policy for withholding food and fluids. A liquid diet is often prescribed for 3 days prior to the procedure, and the client is usually NPO for 8 hours just before the procedure.

- Administer or instruct the client in bowel preparation procedures such as taking citrate of magnesia or polyethylene glycol the evening before.

- Sedation is usually ordered before the procedure.

Client and Family Teaching

Before Procedure

- Explain dietary restrictions and their purpose.

- The procedure takes 30 minutes to 1 hour.

- The client may be positioned on left side and then onto back.

- The scope will be inserted and advanced to the cecum.

- Air insufflation may be used to help outline structures in the colon.

- A biopsy may be taken.

- Polyps may be removed.

- Discomfort is minimal.

After Procedure

- Report any abdominal pain, chills, fever, rectal bleeding, or mucopurulent discharge.

- If a polyp has been removed, avoid heavy lifting for 7 days, and avoid high-fiber food for 1 to 2 days.

defecation easier. Raw fruits and vegetables are good sources of dietary fiber, as is cereal bran. Two to three teaspoons of unprocessed bran with meals (sprinkled on fruit or cereal) or up to ¼ cup daily supplies adequate fiber to meet the client's needs.

Fluids are also important to maintain bowel motility and soft stools. The client should drink 6 to 8 glasses of fluid per day.

Pharmacology

Laxative and cathartic preparations to promote stool evacuation were among the earliest drugs. Milder preparations are generally known as *laxatives; cathartics* have a stronger effect. Most laxative preparations are appropriate only for short-term use. Cathartics and enemas interfere with normal bowel reflexes and should not be used for simple constipation. Laxatives should *never* be administered to clients who may have a bowel obstruction or impaction, nor to people with abdominal pain of undetermined origin (Tierney et al., 1994). When the bowel is obstructed, administering laxatives or cathartics may cause serious mechanical damage and perforate the bowel.

The only laxatives that are appropriate and safe for long-term use are bulking agents, such as psyllium seed, calcium polycarbophil, and methylcellulose. These agents act by increasing the bulk of the feces and drawing water into the bowel to soften it. Commonly prescribed laxatives are discussed in the pharmacology box on page 776.

Enemas

Significant or chronic constipation or a fecal impaction may require the administration of an enema. As a general rule, enemas should be used only in acute situations and only on a short-term basis. They may also be prescribed to prepare the bowel for diagnostic testing or examination. The following types of enemas may be prescribed:

- A saline enema using 500 to 2000 mL of warmed physiologic saline solution is the least irritating to the bowel.

- Tap-water enemas use 500 to 1000 mL of water to soften feces and irritate the bowel mucosa, stimulating peristalsis and evacuation.

- Soap-suds enemas consist of a tap-water solution to which soap is added as a further irritant.

- Phosphate enemas (eg, Fleet) use a hypertonic saline solution to draw fluid into the bowel and irritate the mucosa, leading to evacuation.

- Oil retention enemas instill mineral or vegetable oil into the bowel to soften the fecal mass. The instilled oil is retained overnight or for several hours before evacuation.

The repeated use of enemas can lead not only to impaired bowel function, but also to fluid and electrolyte imbalances. Tap-water and phosphate enemas are particularly likely to cause these problems. In acute conditions where there is a risk of bowel obstruction, perforation, ulceration, or other problem, enemas should not be administered until their safe use can be established.

Nursing Care

Nursing care for the client with constipation focuses chiefly on education. Obvious and priority nursing diagnoses include *Constipation* and *Perceived Constipation*.

Constipation

Whether real or perceived, constipation is disruptive to the client's activities of daily living (ADLs) and life satisfaction. As such, it is the primary focus for nursing interventions.

Nursing interventions with rationales follow:

- Assess and document the client's pattern of defecation, including time of day, amount, and stool consistency. *This provides information about the client's bowel habits and the reality of constipation as a physiologic versus perceived problem.*
- Assess the client's diet, fluid intake, and activity pattern. *These provide clues about possible causes of constipation.*
- Evaluate the client for other factors that may contribute to constipation, such as the use of narcotic analgesics, prescribed bed rest, painful hemorrhoids, and perianal surgery. *The client may require a bulk laxative or stool softener while contributing factors are present.*
- Assess abdominal girth and shape, bowel sounds, tenderness, and percussion tone. *The client with constipation may have a distended abdomen, reduced bowel sounds, and some abdominal tenderness.*
- If an impaction is suspected, perform a digital examination of the rectum. *Impacted stool is felt as a hard or puttylike mass in the rectum. Digital removal of the impacted stool may be necessary.*
- Provide additional fluids to maintain an intake of at least 2500 mL per day. *Well-hydrated status facilitates normal bowel elimination.*
- Encourage the client to drink a glass of warm water prior to breakfast. Provide time and privacy following breakfast for bowel elimination. *This helps develop a pattern of natural elimination; the warm water provides mild stimulation of bowel peristalsis.*
- Consult with the dietitian to provide a diet high in natural fiber, if the client can tolerate such a diet. *Natural fiber adds bulk to the stool and has a mild stimulant effect.*
- Provide foods such as natural bran, prunes, or prune juice, if they are not contraindicated. *These foods not only contain fiber but also provide a mild irritant effect on the bowel, stimulating evacuation.*
- Encourage the client to maintain as high an activity level as he or she can tolerate. *Activity stimulates peristalsis and strengthens abdominal muscles, facilitating elimination.*

- If indicated, consult with the primary care provider about the use of bulk laxatives, stool softeners, or other laxatives as needed. *Pharmacologic agents may be needed for prompt relief of acute constipation. Clients with long-term activity or diet restrictions or impaired abdominal muscle strength may need a bulk-forming laxative to maintain normal elimination patterns and prevent constipation.*

Other Nursing Diagnoses

Other nursing diagnoses that may be appropriate for the client with constipation are related to factors that contribute to chronic constipation. Examples follow:

- *Impaired Physical Mobility* related to physical condition
- *Altered Nutrition: Less Than Body Requirements* (fiber) related to lack of information
- *Altered Health Maintenance* related to chronic use of laxatives/cathartics or enemas

Client and Family Teaching

Education can help prevent constipation. The measures to relieve constipation are often the same as those to prevent it.

Teach the client and family about the importance of maintaining a diet high in natural fiber. Foods such as fresh fruits, vegetables, whole-grain products, and bran provide natural fiber. Encourage the client to reduce the consumption of meats and refined foods, which are low in fiber and can be constipating. Emphasize the need to maintain a high fluid intake every day, particularly when hot weather or exercise increases fluid losses. Discuss the relationship between exercise and bowel regularity. Encourage the client to engage in some form of exercise, such as walking daily.

Include information about normal bowel habits, and explain that a daily bowel movement is not the norm for all people. Encourage the client to respond to the urge to defecate when it occurs. Suggest setting aside a time, usually following a meal, for elimination. Discuss the use of laxatives and enemas, and stress that bulk-forming laxatives are the only preparations safe for long-term use. Teach the client that straining to have a bowel movement can lead to hemorrhoid formation and tissue damage. Suggest that the client use abdominal massage to reduce discomfort and promote elimination.

The Client with Irritable Bowel Syndrome

■ ■ ■

Irritable bowel syndrome, also known as *spastic bowel, functional colitis,* or *mucous colitis,* is a motility disorder of the gastrointestinal tract. It is a functional disorder with

Nursing Implications for Pharmacology: Laxatives

BULK-FORMING AGENTS

Bran

Calcium polycarbophil (Fibercon)

Methylcellulose (Citrucel)

Psyllium hydrophilic mucilloid (Metamucil, Effer-Syllium)

Bulk-forming agents are the only laxatives that are safe for long-term use. They contain vegetable fiber, which is not digested or absorbed in the gut. This natural fiber creates bulk and draws water into the intestine, softening the stool mass.

Nursing Responsibilities

- Mix the agent with a full glass of cool liquid just prior to administering to the client.
- Do not administer the agent to clients with possible stool impaction or bowel obstruction.

Client and Family Teaching

- Drink at least 6 to 8 full glasses of nonalcoholic fluid per day. Increasing normal fluid intake by 1 to 2 glasses per day is recommended because adequate hydration is necessary to produce the drug's laxative effect.
- These agents may be mixed with water, milk, or fruit juice.
- Take the drug in the morning or with meals. To reduce the risk of impaction, do not take the drug at bedtime.
- Because of the increased risk of impaction, check with the physician before increasing the amount of dietary fiber, such as bran, while you are taking these agents.

WETTING AGENTS

Docusate (Colace, Surfak, Doxidan, others)

Wetting agents act to reduce stool surface tension and form an emulsion of fat and water, softening the stool. They are used primarily to prevent straining and reduce the discomfort of expelling hard stools.

Nursing Responsibilities

- Administer the agent with ample fluids to promote softening effect.
- Wetting agents may alter the absorption of other drugs. Do not administer the agent within 1 hour of other oral medications.

- Do not attempt to crush or open caplets; a liquid form is available for clients who cannot swallow pills or capsules.

Client and Family Teaching

- Limit the use of this drug to 1 week or less unless otherwise specifically recommended by the physician.
- Take the medication in the morning or evening, but avoid taking it at the same time as other medications.
- Drinking adequate amounts of fluid is necessary to obtain the beneficial effect of the drug. Drink 6 to 8 glasses of nonalcoholic fluid per day.

OSMOTIC AND SALINE LAXATIVES/CATHARTICS

Lactulose (Rhodialose)

Sorbitol

Magnesium hydroxide (Milk of Magnesia)

Magnesium citrate

Polyethylene glycol (Klean-Prep)

Laxatives in this group contain poorly absorbed salts or carbohydrates that remain in the bowel, increasing osmotic pressure and drawing water into the intestine. Stool volume increases, consistency decreases, and peristalsis is stimulated. Many of these agents also have an irritant effect on the bowel, further stimulating peristalsis. They are used to stimulate rapid or complete bowel evacuation to relieve constipation and to prepare the bowel for diagnostic and surgical procedures. They should be limited to acute, short-term use; chronic use may suppress normal bowel reflexes.

Nursing Responsibilities

- Assess the client for possible contraindications to osmotic or saline laxatives, including bowel ulceration or obstruction, dehydration, electrolyte imbalances, cardiac failure (which may be aggravated by the sodium or other salt content), or renal failure.
- Administer the drug with a full glass of liquid, preferably in the morning to avoid sleep disturbance.
- Monitor the client's fluid and electrolyte status: skin turgor; mucous membranes; intake and output; daily weight; and laboratory studies, such as hemoglobin and hematocrit levels, serum osmolality and electrolytes, and urine specific gravity.

Pharmacology: Laxatives (continued)

Client and Family Teaching

- Do not use these agents on a routine basis to treat or prevent constipation.

- Use only as directed. Increase fluid intake to at least 6 to 8 glasses of nonalcoholic fluid per day.

- Notify the physician if adverse effects occur, including abdominal pain, bloody stool, excessive skin or mucous membrane dryness, rapid weight loss, dizziness, or other unusual symptoms.

- These agents work in 3 to 6 hours; take them in the morning to avoid sleep disturbance.

IRRITANT OR STIMULANT LAXATIVES

Bisacodyl (Dulcolax, Bisco-Lax, Carter's Liver Pills, Codylax, others)

Phenolphthalein (Evac-U-Gen, Evac-U-Lax, Feen-A-Mint, Phenolax, others)

Cascara sagrada

Senna (Senna laxative, Fletcher's Castoria)

Castor oil

Stimulant laxatives work by stimulating the motility and secretion of intestinal mucosa. Their use results in watery stool, which is often accompanied by abdominal cramping and pain. They are used to relieve constipation, although they should not be used as the initial treatment. Stimulant laxatives are also used for preparing the bowel for diagnostic testing.

Nursing Responsibilities

- Assess the client for potential contraindications to these laxatives, including abdominal pain and cramping, nausea and vomiting, anal or rectal fissures.

- Administer the laxative on an empty stomach to minimize the effects of food on its dissolution and absorption.

- Do not crush enteric-coated bisacodyl tablets or administer with alkaline products. This may hasten their dissolution in the stomach, leading to gastric distress.

Client and Family Teaching

- Discourage the use of this type of laxative, even in over-the-counter preparations, for the initial or continuing relief of constipation.

- Do not use the laxative for more than 1 week; chronic use can be habit forming and may suppress normal bowel reflexes.

- These laxatives are excreted in breast milk and should not be used by lactating women.

- Phenolphthalein-containing products may discolor the urine pink or red. Report possible hypersensitivity manifestations, such as difficulty breathing, dizziness or lightheadedness, or skin rashes, to the primary care provider, and stop taking the medication.

LUBRICANTS

Mineral oil

Mineral oil is the only lubricant laxative available. It acts by forming an oily coat on the fecal mass, preventing the reabsorption of water, and resulting in softer stool. Problems associated with the use of mineral oil as a laxative include reduced absorption of the fat-soluble vitamins A, D, E, and K; possible damage to the liver and spleen due to systemic absorption; and potential pneumonitis from aspiration of oil droplets into the lungs.

Nursing Responsibilities

- Assess the client for possible contraindications to use of mineral oil, including advanced age, preexisting pulmonary disease, and hemorrhoids or other rectal lesions.

- Do not administer mineral oil concurrently with wetting agents or stool softeners, because these increase the potential for systemic absorption and increase the effects of the mineral oil.

- Administer mineral oil in the evening before bedtime to reduce the effect on the absorption of fat-soluble vitamins and minimize the risk of aspiration.

- Assess the client for manifestations of vitamin deficiency. Monitor the client taking oral anticoagulants concurrently for evidence of increased bleeding, such as bleeding gums, easy bruising, or melena.

Client and Family Teaching

- Long-term use of mineral oil as a laxative is not recommended because of its risks and adverse effects.

- Do not use mineral oil if hemorrhoids or rectal lesions are present; leakage of the oil through the anal sphincter may cause itching and interfere with healing.

- Suck on a lemon or orange slice after taking oral mineral oil to reduce the oily aftertaste.

Clinical Manifestations of Irritable Bowel Syndrome

■ ■ ■

- Abdominal pain
  - May be relieved by defecation
  - May be intermittent and colicky or dull and continuous
- Altered bowel elimination
  - Constipation
  - Diarrhea
  - Mucous stools
- Abdominal bloating and flatulence
- Abdominal tenderness, especially over sigmoid colon
- Possible nausea, vomiting

---

no identifiable organic cause frequently characterized by alternating periods of constipation and diarrhea.

Irritable bowel syndrome is common, affecting up to 20% of people in Western civilization (Porth, 1994). It accounts for one-half of all gastroenterology referrals on initial gastrointestinal complaints. Women are affected to a greater extent than men, by a 3:1 ratio (Berkow & Fletcher, 1992).

Pathophysiology

Although no organic cause or irritable bowel syndrome has been identified, significant factors have been identified in its pathogenesis. Motor activity of both the small and large bowel may be affected by food ingestion, stress, the hormones gastrin and cholecystokinin, and drugs affecting the autonomic nervous system. Small bowel motility is often increased in clients with predominant diarrhea, and decreased in those with constipation. Large bowel pressures may also be altered, with changes in the frequency and strength of contractions. Hypersecretion of colonic mucus is a common feature of the syndrome.

Psychologic stress and food intake are typically associated with manifestations of irritable bowel syndrome. Although it is normal for stress to affect the motor activity of the bowel, clients with irritable bowel syndrome appear to have an exaggerated response. The ingestion of food causes a similar enhanced response. Diet may contribute to the disorder. A low-fiber or low-residue diet is a common predisposing factor. The ingestion of lactose or fructose (fruit sugar) may also precipitate symptoms.

Irritable bowel syndrome is characterized by abdominal pain that often is relieved by defecation and a change in bowel habits (see the accompanying clinical manifestations box). The pain may be either colicky, occurring in spasms, or dull and continuous. Altered patterns of defecation that may be seen include the following:

- A change in the frequency of elimination
- An alteration in stool form, either hard or loose and watery
- A change in the passage of stool, such as straining, urgency, or a sensation of incomplete evacuation
- The passage of mucus (Porth, 1994; Tierney et al., 1994)

The client may also complain of abdominal bloating and excess gas. Other manifestations include nausea, vomiting, and anorexia; fatigue, headache, depression, or anxiety. The abdomen is often tender to palpation, particularly over the sigmoid colon.

Collaborative Care

The diagnosis of irritable bowel syndrome is based on the client's history, the pattern of symptoms and elimination, physical examination, and diagnostic testing. Evaluation is performed to rule out organic disease of the bowel, such as colonic polyps, neoplasms, and inflammatory bowel diseases. Management is directed toward relieving the client's symptoms and reducing or eliminating precipitating factors. Stress reduction measures, exercises, or counseling may benefit the client.

Laboratory and Diagnostic Tests

No diagnostic test or examination is specific for irritable bowel syndrome. The primary purpose of diagnostic testing is to rule out the presence of organic causes for the client's symptoms.

The following laboratory studies may be ordered:

- *Stool examination for occult blood, ova and parasites, and culture for pathologic bacteria* may be performed. A stool smear for WBCs may also be performed; an elevated WBC count may be an indicator of an inflammatory or infectious process.
- *Complete blood count (CBC) and erythrocyte sedimentation rate (ESR)* are performed to assess for possible anemia or infectious/inflammatory processes. The presence of anemia may indicate blood loss and a possible neoplasm, polyps, or other organic problem. An elevated WBC count is often an indicator of bacterial infection, and an elevated ESR is seen with many inflammatory processes.

Diagnostic tests that may be performed follow:

- *Sigmoidoscopy or colonoscopy* may be ordered for visual evaluation of the bowel mucosa, measuring intraluminal pressures, and possible biopsy of suspicious lesions. The expected findings for a client with irritable bowel syndrome are a normal appearance of the bowel with increased mucus, marked spasm, and possible hyperemia (increased redness), but no suspicious lesions. Intraluminal pressures are often increased, and the procedure itself may stimulate manifestations of the syndrome.

- *Radiologic examination* of the gastrointestinal tract with barium contrast media may include a small bowel series (also known as an upper GI series with small bowel follow-through) and barium enema. For the small bowel series, the client is given an oral barium preparation, and the small intestine is examined under fluoroscopy. With irritable bowel syndrome, the entire gastrointestinal tract may demonstrate increased motility. The accompanying box outlines nursing care of the client undergoing a small bowel series. Nursing care of the client having a barium enema is described in the box on page 773.

Dietary Management

No specific diet is recommended for the client with irritable bowel syndrome. Many clients, particularly those in high-risk groups for lactose intolerance (African Americans, Asians, Native Americans), may benefit by reducing their intake of milk and milk products. When excess gas and flatulence is a problem, reducing the intake of gas-forming foods, such as cabbage, apple and grape juices, bananas, nuts, and raisins, may be helpful. Clients who respond adversely to fructose may need to limit their consumption of fruits and berries. Caffeinated drinks, such as coffee, tea, and soft drinks, act as gastrointestinal stimulants; limiting intake of these fluids may also prove beneficial.

Many clients benefit from additional dietary fiber. Adding bran to meals can provide added bulk and water content to the stool, reducing the incidence of both loose diarrheal stools and hard, constipated stools. The client can also increase fiber intake by using a bulk-forming agent such as psyllium (Metamucil, others).

Pharmacology

Although they are not the treatment of choice for this functional condition, medications may be prescribed in specific instances. An anticholinergic drug such as propantheline (Pro-Banthine) may be ordered to inhibit bowel motility by interfering with parasympathetic stimulation of the gastrointestinal tract. In clients with diarrhea, loperamide (Imodium) or diphenoxylate (Lomotil) may be given before meals.

Nursing Implications for Diagnostic Tests: Small Bowel Series

Client Preparation

- Explain the procedure to the client, answering questions and addressing concerns.
- A low-residue diet may be prescribed for 48 hours preceding the examination, and a tap-water enema or cathartic may be administered the evening before.
- The client must avoid food, fluids, and smoking for at least 8 hours before the examination.
- Withhold medications affecting bowel motility for 24 hours prior to examination if possible (unless prescribed as part of the preparation procedure).

Client and Family Teaching

- Although the test is not uncomfortable, it requires several hours to complete. Bring reading material, paperwork, or crafts along to occupy time.
- For a small bowel enema, a weighted tube will be inserted into the small bowel, orally or endoscopically. The barium is then inserted through this tube rather than by drinking.
- Increase intake of fluids for at least 24 hours after the procedure to facilitate evacuation of the barium. A laxative or cathartic may be prescribed.
- Stool will be chalky white for up to 72 hours after the exam. Normal stool color will return on complete evacuation of barium.

Note. Data are from *Laboratory Tests and Diagnostic Procedures* by C. C. Chernecky, R. L. Krech, and B. J. Berger, 1993, Philadelphia: W. B. Saunders; *Diagnostic and Laboratory Test Reference* by K. D. Pagana and T. J. Pagana, 1992, St. Louis: Mosby-Year Book.

If chronic anxiety is identified as a probable precipitating factor, an antianxiety medication, such as alprazolam (Xanax) or chlordiazepoxide (Librium, Lipoxide, SK-Lygen, others) may be prescribed for temporary relief of symptoms. This is a short-term measure only; the client may need referral to counseling to develop coping skills and relaxation techniques.

Depression is also commonly associated with irritable bowel syndrome. In clients for whom this is a problem, an antidepressant agent such as amitriptyline (Amitril, Elavil, others) or doxepin (Sinequan) may be prescribed. These agents have the added benefit in this case of anticholinergic side effects.

Nursing Care

Clients with irritable bowel syndrome are rarely seen in the acute care setting unless the disorder is present as a secondary condition. However, nurses frequently interact with these clients in clinics and other outpatient settings. The primary nursing responsibility is education; providing referrals and counseling are additional nursing responsibilities to clients who have irritable bowel syndrome.

The following nursing diagnoses may be appropriate for this client:

- *Constipation* related to altered gastrointestinal motility
- *Diarrhea* related to altered gastrointestinal motility and excess mucus secretion
- *Anxiety* related to situational stress
- *Ineffective Individual Coping* related to stress

Refer to the previous sections on diarrhea and constipation for selected nursing interventions.

Client and Family Teaching

On initiating teaching for the client with irritable bowel syndrome, emphasize that although no organic disease is present, the client's symptoms are very real. Reinforce that care providers believe the client's complaints and do not discount them as "all in the mind." However, because there is a well-documented relationship between irritable bowel syndrome and stress, anxiety, and depression, it is especially important to discuss these factors. Assist the client to explore any relationship between mental stress and the bowel manifestations. Teach stress- and anxiety-reduction techniques, such as meditation, visualization, exercise, "time out," and progressive relaxation. Refer the client to a counselor or other mental health professional for assistance in dealing with psychologic factors.

Help the client identify possible dietary influences that may contribute to irritable bowel syndrome. Suggest dietary changes, including additional fiber and water intake, which may help alleviate symptoms while maintaining good nutritional status.

Stress to the client that any prescribed medications are generally considered to be temporary measures for managing irritable bowel syndrome. Encourage the client to change exercise and dietary patterns appropriately and

use stress-reduction techniques to gradually eliminate the need for medication.

In teaching the client, emphasize the need for routine follow-up appointments. Stress the importance of notifying the primary care provider if the disease manifestations change, such as blood in the stool, significant constipation or diarrhea, increasing abdominal pain, or weight loss. The manifestations of irritable bowel syndrome may mask symptoms of an organic problem, such as a neoplasm.

The Client with Fecal Incontinence

■   ■   ■

Fecal incontinence, the loss of voluntary control of defecation, occurs less frequently than urinary incontinence but is no less distressing to the client. Multiple factors contribute to fecal incontinence, including both physiologic and psychologic conditions (see the accompanying box). Bowel incontinence is usually considered a manifestation of a disorder rather than a disorder unto itself. Clients often do not reveal fecal incontinence in discussing health concerns. Little information is available about the incidence and prevalence of fecal incontinence. Because many of the etiologic factors are more prevalent in the older adult, older clients are more often affected.

Pathophysiology

To understand the pathophysiology underlying fecal incontinence, it is necessary to understand the normal mechanisms leading to defecation. The rectum is normally empty. When it is distended by the entry of feces from the sigmoid colon, the defecation reflex is stimulated. This reflex causes involuntary relaxation of the internal sphincter and stimulates the urge to defecate. When the external sphincter, which is under both voluntary and autonomic (involuntary) control, relaxes, defecation occurs. Adults normally can override the defecation reflex by voluntary contraction of the external sphincter and pelvic floor muscles. The wall of the rectum gradually relaxes, and the urge to defecate subsides (McCance & Huether, 1994).

The most common causes of fecal incontinence are those that interfere with either sensory or motor control of the rectum and anal sphincters. If the external sphincter is paralyzed as a result of spinal cord injury or disease, defecation occurs automatically when the internal sphincter relaxes with the defecation reflex. If sphincter muscles have been damaged or excessive pelvic floor relaxation has occurred, it may not be possible to override the defecation reflex with voluntary control.

Age-related changes in anal sphincter tone and response to rectal distention increase the risk for fecal incontinence in older adults. Resting and maximal anal sphincter pressures are decreased, particularly in older women. In addition, less rectal distension is needed to produce sustained relaxation of the anal sphincter in older females (Hazzard et al., 1994).

Collaborative Care

The diagnosis of fecal incontinence is based on the client's history. Physical examination of the pelvic floor and anus is performed to determine muscle tone and rule out the presence of a fecal impaction. Disruptions of the sphincter muscle may be palpable on digital exam. *Anorectal manometry* or a rectal motility test may be used to evaluate the functional ability of the sphincter muscles. A small, flexible balloon catheter is introduced into the rectum, and pressures are measured in the rectum, internal, and external sphincters. Normally, rectal dilation causes the internal sphincter to relax and the external sphincter to contract. Sigmoidoscopy also may be performed to provide visual examination of the rectum and anal canal.

Once the cause of fecal incontinence has been identified, management of the disorder is directed toward treating the cause. Medications to relieve diarrhea or constipation may be prescribed. A high-fiber diet, ample fluids, and regular exercise are helpful for many clients. Exercises to improve sphincter and pelvic floor muscle tone (Kegel exercises) may be of long-term benefit. See Chapter 25 for further discussion about Kegel exercises.

A bowel training program is often effective, even for clients who have impaired sensory or motor function. The goal of dietary changes and bowel training is to establish a regular pattern of elimination. The client is taught to establish a regular time of day for elimination, usually 15 to 30 minutes after breakfast. A stimulant, such as a cup of coffee or a rectal suppository, may be given to prompt defecation. In some cases, a phosphate enema may be used to stimulate evacuation. Clients with neurologic incontinence may learn to initiate defecation with digital stimulation of the anal canal using a gloved finger (Way, 1994).

If the above measures are ineffective, a low-residue diet may be prescribed to reduce the frequency of defecation. Residue, the solid material in the large intestine that remains after food is digested, includes indigestible food components (such as fiber) and foods that increase stool volume. A low-residue diet consists of foods that are easily digested and absorbed (Lutz & Przytulski, 1994). Medications such as loperamide often help by both reducing frequency of defecation and enhancing sphincter muscle tone (Berkow & Fletcher, 1992). Biofeedback therapy may be used for mentally alert clients with intact

---

Selected Causes of Fecal Incontinence
■ ■ ■

Neurologic Causes

- Spinal cord injury or disease (tumor, multiple sclerosis)
- Head injury, stroke, or brain tumor
- Degenerative neurologic disease, such as multiple sclerosis, amyotrophic lateral sclerosis (ALS), dementia
- Diabetic neuropathy

Local Trauma

- Obstetric tears
- Anorectal injury
- Anorectal surgery with sphincter damage (hemorrhoidectomy, fistulotomy, dilation of the anal sphincter)

Inflammatory Processes

- Infection
- Radiation

Other Physiologic Causes

- Diarrhea
- Stool impaction
- Pelvic floor relaxation or loss of sphincter tone
- Tumors

Psychologic Causes

- Depression
- Confusion and disorientation

---

sphincter muscles but low muscle tone. With motivation and reinforcement, clients achieve improved sphincter control in response to a stimulus.

When damage to the sphincter or rectal prolapse (protrusion of rectal mucous membrane through the anus) is the cause of fecal incontinence, surgical repair is the treatment of choice. Surgery may also be indicated for the client for whom conservative management measures have not been effective. Permanent colostomy, the creation of an opening from the large bowel on the abdominal wall, is a last-choice option for some clients, but it can be an effective means of controlling fecal output when other measures fail.

Nursing Care

Nursing care for the client with fecal incontinence is supportive. Fecal incontinence can have significant physical and psychologic effects.

The skin of the perianal and perineal region is likely to be irritated by fecal material. This irritation can lead to tissue breakdown and pressure ulcers, particularly in the client who has a neurologic disorder (such as spinal cord injury, dementia, or stroke) that impairs mobility as well.

For the client with intact cognitive abilities, fecal incontinence can be psychologically devastating. The client may become socially isolated from fear of odor or clothing soilage, and the client's self-esteem may suffer from a sense of lost control over body functions. The inability to provide self-care also adversely affects self-esteem.

Bowel Incontinence

Nurses are often responsible for assessing the client with fecal incontinence and instituting bowel training programs. For the institutionalized client, the nurse may be responsible for ensuring a high fiber intake and adequate fluid intake as well.

Nursing interventions with rationales follow:

- Teach caregivers to place the client on a toilet or commode and provide for privacy at a certain time of day. *Placing the client in a normal position to defecate at a consistent time of day stimulates the defecation reflex and helps reestablish a pattern of stool evacuation.*

- If necessary, insert a glycerine or bisacodyl (Dulcolax) suppository 15 to 20 minutes before placing the client on the toilet or commode. *This helps to stimulate evacuation. Once a regular elimination pattern is established, it may be possible to discontinue suppository use.*

- Maintain a caring, nonjudgmental manner in providing care. *This helps the client feel accepted when he or she feels unacceptable.*

- Provide room odor control with deodorizer tablets, sprays, or other devices. *This helps reduce the client's embarrassment when caregivers or visitors enter the room.*

Risk for Impaired Skin Integrity

Good skin care is vital for the client affected by fecal incontinence. Stool contains enzymes and other irritating substances that promote skin breakdown when they are not promptly removed.

Nursing interventions with rationales follow:

- Clean the skin thoroughly with soap and water after each bowel movement. *Toilet tissue may be more irritating to the skin and less effective in removing fecal material.*

- Apply a skin barrier cream or ointment after each bowel movement. *These help protect the skin from irritating substances in the feces.*

- If incontinence pads or briefs are used, check frequently for soiling and change whenever feces is noted. *Although these help protect bedding and clothing from soilage, they can contribute to skin breakdown if they are not checked and changed frequently.*

- If a rectal tube is used to drain feces, check the perianal area frequently for soiling or evidence of skin or anal irritation. *A rectal tube may be useful for a client with continuous drainage of liquid feces but can contribute to relaxation of the anal sphincter and anal ulceration.*

Other Nursing Diagnoses

Additional nursing diagnoses that may be considered for the client with fecal incontinence follow:

- *Body Image Disturbance* related to the inability to control defecation

- *Risk for Caregiver Role Strain* related to the need for frequent removal of fecal material

- *Self-Care Deficit: Toileting* related to neurologic impairment

- *Low Self-Esteem: Situational* related to unpredictable fecal elimination

- *Social Isolation* related to concerns of odor and soiled clothing

Client and Family Teaching

The management of fecal incontinence is a challenging problem for both the client and family caregivers. It is important to stress to clients that incontinence is never normal (i.e., aging alone is not a cause of incontinence) and often is treatable.

Unless contraindicated, teach the client to consume a high-fiber diet and ample fluids throughout the day. Encourage regular exercise as a measure to stimulate bowel peristalsis and regular evacuation. Discuss the daily use of bulk-forming laxatives, such as psyllium seed (Metamucil) to provide stool bulk and reduce the number of small, liquid stools. If a low-residue diet and loperamide are recommended to reduce the number of stools, provide instruction on their use. Teach the client to be alert for possible signs of constipation on this regimen, and discuss appropriate management.

Provide the client and caregivers with instructions for a bowel training program. If digital anal stimulation, suppositories, or enemas are recommended as part of the program, teach appropriate techniques.

Stress the importance of good skin care to the client and caregivers, particularly if neurologic impairment is present. The client with a neurologic disorder may not be able to sense pain or irritation associated with early skin breakdown.

Applying Rehabilitation Principles to Medical/Surgical Nursing: Fecal Incontinence

■ ■ ■

Rehabilitation principles for bowel training programs can be implemented in hospital and community settings. Fecal incontinence is especially problematic when caring for an older, cognitively impaired client.

Case Example

Mrs. Mary Frank is a 72-year-old widow who lives with her daughter and son-in-law. Mrs. Frank has been experiencing episodes of confusion over the last few months. During your home visit, Mrs. Frank's daughter requests information concerning her mother's fecal incontinence. "I can handle my mother's confusion," she states, "but I thought I was through with diapers a long time ago!"

Rehabilitation Principle

Helping clients recover lost function is perhaps the greatest challenge of rehabilitation nursing. Fecal incontinence in an older adult usually occurs due to a loss of voluntary control. This is termed an *uninhibited bowel.*

Rehabilitation Time Frame

Bowel programs can take from several weeks to several months to establish fecal continence. Patience and adherence to a schedule are the key elements.

Nursing Diagnosis: Alteration in Bowel Elimination

During episodes of confusion, Mrs. Frank cannot voluntarily inhibit the need to evacuate her bowels.

Rehabilitation Goals and Interventions

- Determine the client's normal bowel emptying pattern by asking the client or a family member. *Regulation and control of bowel emptying can be facilitated if the pattern or schedule of interventions is closely related to the normal emptying pattern of the client.*

- The client is given a glycerin suppository 30 minutes prior to the normal emptying time and is placed on the toilet or commode to accomplish the squatting position which aids in emptying. *The suppository stimulates the anal reflexes responsible for bowel emptying.*

- Eventually, the interval between the suppository insertion and bowel evacuation will decrease. When the time decreases to approximately 5 minutes, digital stimulation with a lubricated gloved finger can be introduced instead of the suppository. *The digital stimulation will stimulate the anal reflexes and enhance peristalsis and emptying.*

- Over time (several weeks), the need to digitally stimulate will decrease and the client can be placed directly on the toilet or commode. Encourage the client to maintain the daily pattern once regularity and continence has been reestablished. *As the defecation reflex "relearns" the emptying pattern, the squatting position will eventually be enough to stimulate bowel emptying.*

If biofeedback and surgical intervention are proposed interventions for the client, discuss their potential benefits and any associated risks. The accompanying box discusses rehabilitation principles for bowel incontinence.

■ ■ ■   Acute Inflammatory and Infectious Disorders   ■ ■ ■

The gastrointestinal tract is particularly vulnerable to inflammatory and infectious disorders because of its continual exposure to the external environment. Although most pathogens affecting the gastrointestinal tract are ingested in food or water, infection also may be spread by direct contact, possibly by the respiratory route. Pathogens may also be transmitted sexually through anal intercourse, causing infection and disease.

Although it may be the pathogen itself that causes acute disease of the gastrointestinal tract, often a bacterial or other toxin is implicated. With acute inflammatory disorders such as appendicitis and peritonitis, the client's own endogenous or resident bacteria can cause problems in damaged or normally sterile tissue.

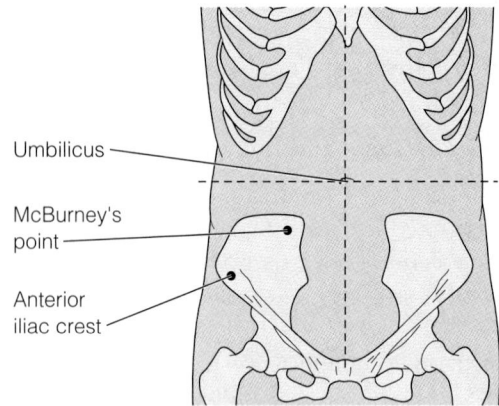

Figure 23–1 McBurney's point, located midway between the umbilicus and the anterior iliac crest in the right lower quadrant. It is the usual site for localized pain and rebound tenderness due to appendicitis.

The Client with Appendicitis

■ ■ ■

Appendicitis, the inflammation of the vermiform appendix, is a common cause of acute abdominal pain and the most common reason for emergency abdominal surgery in the United States. The appendix is a tubelike pouch attached to the cecum just below the ileocecal valve. It is usually located in the right iliac region, at an area designated as McBurney's point (Figure 23–1). The function of the appendix is not fully understood, although it regularly fills and empties with digested food.

Appendicitis can occur at any age, with the incidence rate at 1 to 2 per 1000. It is more common in adolescents and young adults and slightly more common in males than females (Thompson, McFarland, & Hirsch, 1993). Approximately 200,000 appendectomies for acute appendicitis are performed every year in the United States (Way, 1994).

Pathophysiology

Appendicitis can be classified as simple, gangrenous, or perforated, depending on the stage of the process. In *simple appendicitis,* the appendix is inflamed but intact. When areas of tissue necrosis and microscopic perforations are present in the appendix, the disorder is called *gangrenous appendicitis.* With a *perforated appendix,* there is evidence of gross perforation of the appendix and contamination of the peritoneal cavity.

Obstruction of the proximal lumen of the appendix is apparent in approximately two-thirds of acutely inflamed appendices (Way, 1994). The obstruction is often caused by a *fecalith,* or hard mass of feces. Other obstructive causes include a calculus or stone, a foreign body, inflammation, a tumor, parasites (e.g., pinworms), or edema of lymphoid tissue. Following obstruction, the appendix becomes distended with fluid secreted by its mucosa. Pressure within the lumen of the appendix increases, impairing its blood supply and leading to inflammation, edema, ulceration, and infection. Purulent exudate forms, further distending the appendix. Within 24 to 36 hours, tissue necrosis and gangrene results, leading to perforation if treatment is not initiated. Perforation results in bacterial peritonitis, which may remain localized (Tierney et al., 1994; Way, 1994).

Continuous mild generalized or upper abdominal pain is the initial characteristic symptom of acute appendicitis. Over the next 4 hours, the pain intensifies and localizes in the right lower quadrant of the abdomen. It is aggravated by moving, walking, or coughing. On palpation, localized and rebound tenderness are noted at McBurney's point. *Rebound tenderness* is demonstrated by relief of pain with direct palpation of McBurney's point followed by tenderness on release of pressure. Extension or internal rotation of the right hip increases the pain. In addition to pain, the client typically presents with a low-grade temperature, anorexia, nausea, and vomiting.

Pain and local tenderness may be less acute in pregnant women and older adults, delaying the diagnosis (Berkow & Fletcher, 1992). This can present a significant problem in older adults, in whom the course of acute appendicitis is more virulent and the onset of complications occurs earlier (Way, 1994).

Perforation, peritonitis, abscess, and pylephlebitis are possible complications of acute appendicitis. Perforation is manifested by increased pain and a high fever. It can result in a small, localized abscess, local peritonitis, or significant generalized peritonitis. (Peritonitis is discussed in the next section of this chapter.) Pylephlebitis is inflammation of the portal venous system with pus formation. It is a rare but highly lethal complication of appendicitis marked by chills, high fever, jaundice, and hepatomegaly (Tierney et al., 1994; Way, 1994).

A less common disorder is chronic appendicitis, which is characterized by chronic abdominal pain and recurrent acute attacks at intervals of several months or more. Other conditions, such as Crohn's disease and renal disorders, often cause symptoms attributed to chronic appendicitis.

Collaborative Care

Because the acutely inflamed appendix can perforate within 24 hours, it is important to establish the diagnosis rapidly and intiate treatment. Because of this urgency and because the low incidence of morbidity associated with surgical intervention, laboratory and diagnostic testing and preoperative treatment are limited. The client is admitted to the hospital, and intravenous fluids are initiated. Oral food and fluids are withheld until a diagnosis is confirmed. Once the diagnosis is established, an appendectomy is performed.

Laboratory and Diagnostic Tests

Laboratory tests are used along with a physical examination to determine the diagnosis and rule out other possible causes for the client's symptoms. The following laboratory tests may be ordered:

- *WBC count* is measured to indicate the presence of infection. With appendicitis, the total white count is elevated (10,000/mm^3 to 20,000/mm^3), with an increased number of immature WBCs (shift to the left).

- *Urinalysis* is performed to determine whether the urine contains erythrocytes or leukocytes. Although microscopic hematuria or pyuria may be present in acute appendicitis, significant numbers of blood cells or bacteria may indicate a urologic cause for the client's symptoms.

The following diagnostic studies may be ordered:

- *Abdominal X-ray* films are taken with the client in the flat and upright postion. A fecalith or calculus may be noted in the right lower quadrant, or a localized ileus may be demonstrated.

- *Abdominal ultrasound* is the most effective test for establishing the diagnosis of acute appendicitis. In this noninvasive test, high-frequency sound waves are reflected back to a doppler (a device that amplifies sound) by tissue of varying densities to create a computer-generated image. The test requires fewer than 30 minutes to complete. Ultrasound examination has reduced the incidence of exploratory surgery and is particularly useful with clients who have atypical symptoms, such as older adults.

- *Pelvic examination* is generally performed on female clients of childbearing age to rule out a gynecologic disorder or pelvic inflammatory disease (PID).

- *Intravenous pyelogram (IVP)* may be used to differentiate appendicitis from possible urinary tract disease.

Pharmacology

Prior to surgical intervention, intravenous fluids are administered to replenish or maintain vascular volume and prevent electrolyte imbalance. Antibiotic therapy with a third-generation cephalosporin effective against many gram-negative bacteria, such as cefoperazone (Cefobid), cefotaxime (Claforan), ceftazidime (Fortaz), or ceftria-

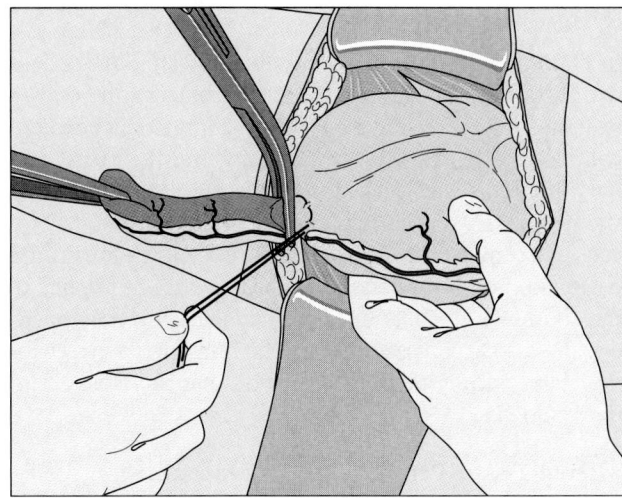

Figure 23–2   Appendectomy. The appendix and cecum are brought through the incision to the surface of the abdomen. The base of the appendix is clamped and ligated; the appendix is then removed.

xone (Rocephin) is initiated prior to surgery. The antibiotic is repeated during surgery and continued for at least 48 hours postoperatively. The nursing implications for cephalosporin antibiotics are included in the pharmacology box in Chapter 8 on page 257. It is important to note that antibiotic therapy alone is not generally used to treat acute appendicitis.

Surgery

The treatment of choice for acute appendicitis is an *appendectomy,* surgical removal of the appendix. An *exploratory laparotomy,* surgical opening of the abdomen to allow direct examination of the organs, may be performed even if the diagnosis cannot be confirmed to rule out appendicitis. In such cases, the appendix is usually removed, even if it is not inflamed, to avoid future risk of appendicitis. A *laparotomy* may also be used to perform an open appendectomy. A small transverse incision is made at McBurney's point; the appendix is isolated and ligated (tied off) to prevent contamination of the site with bowel contents, and then removed (Figure 23–2). Recovery is generally uneventful. Refer to Chapter 7 for further discussion of preoperative and postoperative nursing care.

An appendectomy can also be performed via laparoscopy, using a very small incision and laparoscope. This procedure has several advantages: (1) direct visualization of the appendix allows a definitive diagnosis to be established without laparotomy; (2) postoperative hospitalization is significantly reduced; (3) postoperative complications are reduced; and (4) recovery and resumption of normal activities take place more rapidly (Way, 1994).

Nursing Care

In planning and implementing nursing care of the client with appendicitis, the nurse should consider the client's response to emergency surgery. On admission, the client will be experiencing abdominal pain, and the nurse may have limited time for preoperative teaching before the client is taken to surgery. The client should not receive laxatives or enemas, because these procedures may cause perforation of the appendix. No heat should be applied to the abdomen; this may increase circulation to the appendix and also cause perforation. The nursing diagnoses for the client with appendicitis include *Altered Tissue Perfusion* and *Pain*.

Altered Tissue Perfusion: Gastrointestinal

A primary goal in caring for a client with appendicitis is to prevent complications in both the preoperative and postoperative periods. Perforation and peritonitis are the most likely preoperative complications; postoperative complications include wound infection, abscess, and possible peritonitis.

Nursing interventions with rationales follow:

- Monitor for perforation and peritonitis preoperatively. *A sudden relief of pain as the distended and edematous appendix ruptures, followed by increased generalized pain and abdominal distention, may indicate a perforation.*

- Preoperatively and postoperatively, monitor the client's vital signs, including blood pressure, pulse rate and rhythm, respiratory rate, and temperature. *An elevated pulse rate and rapid shallow breathing can indicate perforation of the appendix with resultant infection and peritonitis. The temperature may be elevated as well, and the blood pressure may fall if sepsis is present.*

- Maintain intravenous fluid replacement preoperatively and until the client is able to drink adequate amounts postoperatively. *Intravenous fluids are administered to maintain proper fluid and electrolyte balance and vascular volume.*

- Assess the client's wound, abdominal girth, and pain status postoperatively. *Swelling of the wound, increased abdominal girth, or an increase in the client's pain level may indicate an infection or peritonitis.*

Pain

The client with appendicitis experiences pain before and after surgery. It is important to remember that pain is a subjective experience, unique to the individual. Although limited analgesia is provided prior to establishing the diagnosis, postoperative pain is controlled by narcotic or nonnarcotic analgesics.

Nursing interventions with rationales follow:

- Assess the client's pain, including its character, location, severity, and duration. Note and report any unex-

pected changes in the client's pain description. *Both preoperatively and postoperatively, careful assessment of the client's pain can provide important clues about the diagnosis and possible complications. For example, postoperative discomfort associated with abdominal distention and flatulence may be aggravated rather than relieved by the use of narcotic analgesics.*

- Administer prescribed pain medications. *Preoperatively, pain medication can be given after a diagnosis is established. Postoperatively, provide analgesics to maintain the client's comfort and enhance mobility.*

- Assess effectiveness of medication ½ hour after administration. *If the client has not experienced the desired effect, the nurse may use other pain-relieving methods or contact the physician.*

- Provide alternative methods of pain relief, including distraction, therapeutic touch, massage, meditation, or visualization. *These techniques can enhance the client's level of comfort and the effectiveness of analgesics.*

Other Nursing Diagnoses

Other nursing diagnoses that may be appropriate for the client with appendicitis follow:

- *Fear* related to unknown diagnosis and possibility of surgery
- *Risk for Infection* related to disruption of bowel integrity
- *Impaired Skin Integrity* related to the presence of abdominal incision

Client and Family Teaching

Preoperative teaching may be limited because of the client's pain and the possibility of emergency surgery. Explain the reason food and fluids are not permitted during this time. If time allows, provide instruction on turning, coughing, and deep breathing, as well as postoperative pain management.

Following an uncomplicated appendectomy, the client is usually dismissed from the health care setting either the day of surgery or the day following surgery. Postoperative teaching includes wound or incision care. Instruct the client to report swelling, redness, drainage, bleeding, or warmth at the operative site to a health care provider. If there is a dressing over the incision, teach the client and/or family members proper hand-washing and dressing change procedures. Instruct the client to report any fever or increased abdominal pain.

Discuss activity following discharge with the client and family. Heavy lifting is to be avoided for 6 weeks to allow healing of the abdominal tissues and muscles. Depending on the surgeon's orders, driving may be allowed within 2 weeks, and clients may return to work within 4 to 6 weeks of surgery. Community health or home health care nurses may be required if the client has preexisting illness or experiences difficulties in performing activities of daily living and self-care.

Case Study of a Client with Acute Appendicitis: Jamie Lynn

Jamie Lynn is a 19-year-old college student majoring in physical therapy. Ms. Lynn arrives at the emergency department at 1:00 a.m. with complaints of general lower abdominal pain that had started the previous evening. By midnight, the pain had become more localized over the right lower quadrant. She reports loss of appetite, nausea, and vomiting.

Assessment

Sue Grady, RN, completes the admission assessment of Ms. Lynn in the emergency department. She finds Ms. Lynn complaining of nausea and severe abdominal pain, stating, "Walking makes my stomach hurt worse." Physical assessment findings include the following: T, 100.2 F (37.8 C); P, 84; R, 16; BP, 110/70. Her skin is warm to the touch. Her abdomen is flat and soft, with marked tenderness over the right lower quadrant. Guarding is present. Her diagnostic tests reveal the following: WBC, $14,000/mm^3$ (normal: 3.5 mm^3 to $11,000/mm^3$); neutrophils, 81.1% (normal: 50% to 75%); lymphocytes, 12.5% (normal: 19% to 48%). The diagnosis of acute appendicitis is made, and Ms. Lynn is transferred directly to surgery, where an appendectomy is performed.

Diagnosis

The nurses caring for Ms. Lynn make the following diagnoses:

- *Altered Skin Integrity* related to abdominal incision
- *Pain* related to surgical intervention
- *Anxiety* related to situational crisis

Expected Outcomes

The expected outcomes established in the plan of care specify that Ms. Lynn will:

- Have normal healing of abdominal incision.
- Verbalize a tolerable level of discomfort.
- Verbalize a decrease in anxiety.
- Return to presurgical activities.

Planning and Implementation

The nurses plan and implement the following nursing interventions for Ms. Lynn:

- Assess Ms. Lynn's level of pain, and provide analgesics as needed.
- Teach Ms. Lynn about the use of analgesia following discharge.
- Teach Ms. Lynn to splint the abdomen when coughing or turning.
- Teach Ms. Lynn to care for the incision at home.
- Discuss activity limitations after discharge, such as refraining from heavy lifting and not driving for 2 weeks to avoid placing excess stress on the incision and healing muscles.
- Instruct Ms. Lynn to report evidence of infection, such as temperature elevation and warmth, redness, or drainage from the incisional site.

Evaluation

On discharge, Ms. Lynn is fully ambulatory. Her appetite has improved, and she is maintaining an adequate fluid intake. Her temperature is normal. The nurse provides Ms. Lynn with written and verbal information on postoperative care following an appendectomy. Ms. Lynn verbalizes an understanding of which activities are allowed following discharge.

Critical Thinking in the Nursing Process

1. What is the pathophysiologic basis for Ms. Lynn's elevated WBC?
2. What is the rationale for having Ms. Lynn splint her abdomen when she coughs or turns in bed?
3. Outline a teaching plan to give to clients for home care following an appendectomy.
4. Develop a care plan for Ms. Lynn for the nursing diagnosis *Anxiety* related to a situational crisis.

The Client with Peritonitis

Peritonitis, inflammation of the peritoneum, is the most significant complication of many acute abdominal disorders. The peritoneum is a double-layered serous membrane lining the walls (parietal peritoneum) and organs (visceral peritoneum) of the abdominal cavity. There is a potential space between the parietal and visceral layers of the peritoneum that contains a small amount of serous fluid. Peritonitis results from contamination of this normally sterile space by infection or a chemical irritant. Penetrating, inflammatory, infectious, or ischemic injuries of the gastrointestinal or genitourinary tracts can lead to peritonitis. Examples include perforation of the appendix, an intestinal diverticulum (discussed later in this chapter), or a peptic ulcer; other causes include acute

---

Clinical Manifestations of Peritonitis

▪ ▪ ▪

Abdominal Effects

- Diffuse or localized abdominal pain
- Abdominal tenderness with rebound
- Boardlike abdominal rigidity
- Diminished or absent bowel sounds
- Abdominal distention
- Anorexia, nausea, and vomiting

Systemic Effects

- Fever
- Malaise
- Tachycardia
- Tachypnea

- Restlessness
- Confusion or disorientation
- Oliguria

Potential Complication

- Shock

---

pancreatitis, salpingitis (inflammation of the uterine tube), traumatic injuries such as gunshot wounds, and contamination during a surgical procedure in which the bowel is nicked by a scalpel or suture.

Peritonitis most commonly follows perforation of the gastrointestinal tract, in which bacteria contaminate the peritoneal cavity. Chemical peritonitis occurs in the period immediately following perforation of a peptic ulcer, in which gastric juices (hydrochloric acid and pepsin) enter the peritoneal cavity, and with acute pancreatitis.

Pathophysiology

Peritonitis is most often the result of a bacterial infection by *Escherichia coli, Klebsiella, Proteus,* and *Pseudomonas* bacteria, which are normally present in the bowel lumen. Normal inflammatory and immune defense mechanisms are activated when bacteria enter the peritoneal space. These defenses can effectively eliminate small numbers of bacteria. When these mechanisms are overwhelmed by massive or continued contamination, however, mast cells release histamine and other vasoactive substances, causing local blood vessels to dilate and capillaries to become more permeable. Polymorphonuclear leukocytes (PMNs, a type of white blood cell) infiltrate the peritoneum to remove the bacteria and foreign matter through phagocytosis. Fibrinogen-rich plasma exudate helps promote bacterial destruction and forms fibrin clots to seal off and

segregate the bacteria. This process may be effective in limiting and localizing the infection, allowing host defenses to eradicate it. Continued contamination, however, leads to generalized inflammation of the peritoneal cavity. *Septicemia,* systemic disease caused by the presence of pathogens or their toxins in the blood, may follow (Way, 1994). The inflammatory process causes a fluid shift into the peritoneal space (third-spacing). Circulating blood volume is depleted, leading to hypovolemia.

The clinical manifestations of peritonitis depend on the severity and extent of the infection, as well as the age and general health of the client. Both abdominal and systemic signs are noted (see the accompanying clinical manifestations box). The client often presents with evidence of an acute abdomen, including diffuse abdominal pain that may localize and intensify near the area of infection. The pain may be severe, and movement may intensify it. The entire abdomen is tender, with guarding or rigidity of abdominal muscles. The acute abdomen is often described as "boardlike." Rebound tenderness is referred to the area of inflammation. Peritoneal inflammation inhibits peristalsis, resulting in a paralytic ileus. (See the section of this chapter on intestinal obstruction for further discussion of paralytic ileus.) Bowel sounds are markedly diminished or absent, and progressive abdominal distention is noted. Pooling of gastrointestinal secretions may lead to nausea and vomiting. Systemic manifestations of peritonitis include fever, malaise, tachycardia and tachypnea, restlessness, and possible disorientation. The client may be oliguric and show signs of dehydration and shock.

The older, chronically debilitated, or immunosuppressed client may present with few of the classic signs of peritonitis. Increased confusion and restlessness, decreased urinary output, and vague abdominal complaints may be the only manifestations present. These clients are at increased risk for delayed diagnosis, contributing to a higher mortality rate.

Complications of peritonitis may be life-threatening and either localized or systemic. Abscess formation is the most frequent sequela. The very defense mechanisms designed to isolate and localize the infection can protect it from immune system responses and systemic antibiotics. Fibrous adhesions in the abdominal cavity are a late complication and may lead to subsequent obstruction.

Without prompt and effective treatment, the client with peritonitis can develop septicemia and septic shock. Fluid loss into the abdominal cavity may also precipitate hypovolemic shock. These potentially lethal complications require immediate, aggressive intervention to prevent multiple organ failure and death. Shock and its management are discussed in depth in Chapter 6.

The client with peritonitis is seriously ill; the overall mortality rate associated with this disease is about 40%. Clients with other medical conditions, older clients, and those with greater bacterial contamination have a higher risk of multiple organ failure and death. Young people with perforated ulcers or appendicitis, those with less extensive bacterial contamination, and those who receive early surgical intervention have mortality rates of less than 10% (Way, 1994).

Collaborative Care

Care of the client with peritonitis focuses on establishing the diagnosis and identifying and treating its cause as well as the peritonitis. Preventing complications is an important aspect of care, requiring aggressive management. Surgical intervention may be required.

Laboratory and Diagnostic Tests

Laboratory and diagnostic tests are used to establish the diagnosis of peritonitis, rule out other disorders, and help identify the precipitating cause. The following laboratory tests may be ordered:

- *White blood cell count* will be elevated to approximately 20,000/mm^3 in peritonitis. A left shift occurs as immature blood cells are released from the bone marrow to combat the infection.
- *Blood cultures* are performed to determine whether *bacteremia* (bacterial invasion of the blood) has occurred. Bacteremia may be an indication of impending *septicemia,* a serious systemic disease that can complicate peritonitis.
- *Arterial blood gases (ABGs)* are measured to assess acid-base balance and respiratory function.
- *Liver and renal function studies* and other laboratory studies may be ordered to evaluate the extent of infection and help guide therapy.

The following diagnostic tests may be ordered:

- *Paracentesis or laparotomy* is performed to obtain peritoneal fluid for analysis (see Chapter 15). The peritoneal fluid is examined for amylase (increased levels are indicative of acute pancreatitis), protein, bacteria, and other abnormal components. Peritoneal fluid analysis is important to establish the diagnosis and underlying cause of acute peritonitis. In peritonitis, the protein content and WBCs are increased in the fluid.
- *X-ray study of the abdomen,* with the client supine and upright, is used to detect intestinal distention, air-fluid levels indicative of ileus or bowel obstruction, and free air under the diaphragm indicative of a gastrointestinal perforation.

Pharmacology

Until the infecting organism has been identified, a broad-spectrum antibiotic effective against commonly impli-

cated organisms in peritonitis is prescribed. Once culture results have been obtained, antibiotic therapy can be modified to the specific organism(s) responsible. Cephalosporin antibiotics (discussed in the box on page 257) are often prescribed if gram-negative enteric bacteria are suspected. Other antibiotics that may be ordered include ampicillin (Omnipen, Polycillin, others), metronidazole (Flagyl, others), clindamycin (Cleocin), or an aminoglycoside antibiotic such as gentamycin (Garamycin) or amikacin (Amikin)(Way, 1994). Nursing implications for these antibiotics are outlined in the pharmacology box in Chapter 8 on page 257.

In addition to antibiotic therapy, the client will likely receive narcotic analgesics and possibly sedatives to promote comfort and rest.

Surgery

If peritonitis is the result of a perforation, gangrenous bowel, or inflamed appendix, a laparotomy will be performed to close the perforation or remove the damaged and inflamed tissue. Surgical treatment also may be used to remove an abscess if one is present.

Peritoneal lavage, the washing out of the peritoneal cavity with copious amounts of warm isotonic fluid, may be done during surgery. This procedure removes gross particulate matter, blood, and fibrin clots and dilutes residual bacteria. In rare instances, peritoneal lavage may be continued for up to 3 days following surgery. The solution is infused into the upper portion of the peritoneal cavity and removed via drains in the pelvic cul-de-sac. Careful attention to the client's fluid and electrolyte status and strict aseptic technique are necessary.

Clients who have had laparotomy for peritonitis often return from surgery with either Penrose or closed drain systems such as a Jackson-Pratt drain. In some cases, the incision may be left unsutured. For the client with severe and long-standing peritonitis, the abdomen may be closed temporarily with polypropylene mesh containing a nylon zipper or Velcro to allow repeated exploration of the abdomen and drainage of infectious sites (Way, 1994).

Intestinal Decompression

The inflammatory process of peritonitis often draws large amounts of fluid into the abdominal cavity and the bowel. In addition, peristaltic activity of the bowel is affected by the inflammation, resulting in **paralytic ileus** (or *ileus*), an impairment in the propulsion or forward movement of bowel contents. Intestinal decompression is initiated to relieve abdominal distention, facilitate closure, and minimize postoperative respiratory problems (Way, 1994). A nasogastric or long intestinal tube is inserted and connected to continuous drainage (Figure 23–3). When prolonged intestinal decompression is anticipated, a gastrostomy may be performed for the client's comfort. Suction is maintained until peristaltic activity resumes and the

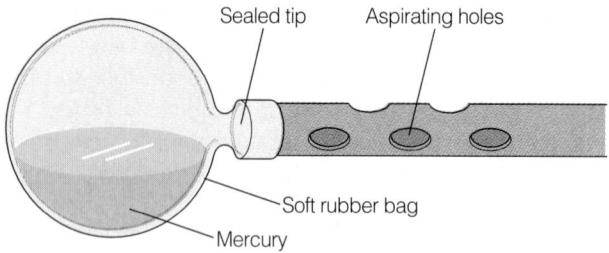

Figure 23–3 Cantor tube used for intestinal decompression. Tubes may be weighted with mercury, causing them to be drawn into the small intestine by peristaltic contractions.

client has audible bowel sounds and is passing flatus. The client remains NPO until intestinal motility has returned and suction is discontinued.

Supportive Care

Additional measures to manage peritonitis focus on correcting fluid, electrolyte, acid-base, and nutritional disorders (Tierney et al., 1994). Intravenous fluids and electrolyte replacements are necessary, as is parenteral nutrition until the client is able to resume oral intake. The client is placed on bed rest in Fowler's position to help localize the infection and facilitate adequate respirations. Oxygen is often prescribed to these clients to facilitate cellular metabolism and healing.

Nursing Care

As noted earlier, peritonitis is a serious illness. Clients require intensive nursing and medical interventions to recover fully. Without aggressive management, the infectious or septic process of peritonitis may lead to multiple organ systems failure. Nursing interventions for these clients address pain; disruptions in fluid balance; altered protection due to the presence of an infection, drains, and possibly repeated surgeries; and anxiety.

Pain

Abdominal distention and the acute inflammatory process contribute to the pain experienced by a client with peritonitis. If surgery has been performed, the client also experiences pain related to disruption of abdominal muscles and other tissues. As with any acutely ill or surgical client, managing the client's pain is necessary to promote healing as well as comfort and to prevent complications from immobility.

Nursing interventions with rationales follow:

- Assess the client's pain, including its location, severity, and type. *A change in the location or type of pain or an increase in its severity may indicate further infection, abscess formation, or other complications of peritonitis. Report these to the primary care provider.*

- Place the client in a Fowler's or semi-Fowler's position with the knees and feet elevated. *This position helps minimize stress on abdominal structures and facilitate respirations, promoting comfort.*

- Once the diagnosis has been established, administer analgesics as ordered on a routine basis or using patient-controlled analgesia (PCA). *Analgesics typically are withheld or minimized to avoid masking symptoms until the diagnosis has been made. Thereafter, routine administration of analgesics helps maintain pain control, facilitating healing and movement.*

- Teach and assist the client to use alternative pain management techniques along with pharmacologic interventions. *Techniques such as meditation, visualization, massage, and progressive relaxation augment analgesics and increase the client's level of comfort.*

- Frequently evaluate the client's response to analgesics. *Decreasing effectiveness of the medication may indicate a complication or extension of the inflammatory process.*

Fluid Volume Deficit

In peritonitis, significant amounts of fluid are drawn into the abdominal cavity and bowel. Much of this fluid may be removed from the body by intestinal decompression with a nasogastric or intestinal tube to suction and drains placed in the abdomen during surgery. If the incision is left unsutured, an additional significant fluid loss is likely.

Nursing interventions with rationales follow:

- Monitor and record the client's intake and output carefully. Urine output is generally measured every 1 to 2 hours; report a urinary output of less than 30 mL per hour to the physician. Gastrointestinal output is measured at least every 4 hours. *Careful assessment of intake and output provides valuable information about the client's fluid volume status. Urinary output of less than 30 mL per hour may indicate hypovolemia and places the client at risk for acute renal failure.*

- Monitor vital signs, including blood pressure, pulse, respirations, venous pressure, cardiac output, and pulmonary artery pressures every hour or as indicated. *These measurements provide important imformation about the client's fluid and vascular volumes as well as cardiovascular status.*

- Weigh the client daily using the same scale and consistent clothing or drapes. *Weight is an accurate reflection of fluid status. Sudden weight gains or losses are usually related to changes in fluid volume.*

- Assess the client's skin turgor, color, temperature, and mucous membranes at least every 8 hours. *These assessments provide additional information about fluid volume; warm, dry skin with poor turgor and dry, shiny mucous membranes indicate dehydration.*

- Measure or estimate fluid losses through abdominal drains and on dressings. *Significant amounts of exudative fluid may be lost.*

- Monitor laboratory values, including hemoglobin and hematocrit, urine specific gravity, serum osmolality, serum electrolytes, and blood gases. Report changes to the physician. *These values provide information about the client's fluid status, as well as electrolyte and acid-base homeostasis.*

- Provide intravenous fluid and electrolyte replacement as ordered. *Gastrointestinal drainage may be replaced milliliter for millileter with a balanced electrolyte solution to compensate for this loss of water and electrolytes. The fluid that would normally be consumed daily, as well as that lost in exudate, must also be replaced while the client is NPO.*

- Provide good skin care and frequent oral hygiene. *Fluid loss increases the risk of skin breakdown and ulceration of mucous membranes.*

Altered Protection

Repeated surgical interventions, an unsutured incision, and/or the presence of drains into the peritoneal cavity interrupt the integrity of the skin and the body's first line of defense against microorganisms. The client's immune defenses also are stressed by the presence of a significant infection. These factors place the client at increased risk for impaired healing and further infection.

Nursing interventions with rationales follow:

- Monitor the client for manifestions of infection, including increased temperature, increased pulse, redness and increased swelling around incisions and drain sites, increased or purulent drainage, and changes in the character of urine output. *Impaired defenses place the client at increased risk for further infection.*

- Obtain cultures of purulent drainage from any site. *Early identification of any additional infection allows appropriate intervention to be instituted.*

- Monitor laboratory work for evidence of immune function, including WBC count and differential, serum protein, and albumin. *Adequate immune function depends to an extent on the bone marrow's ability to produce leukocytes in response to the increased need and on the production of immune globulins, which are present in the protein fraction of the blood.*

- Practice meticulous hand washing on entering and leaving the client's room. *Hand washing reduces transient bacteria on the skin and remains the most important method of controlling infection.*

- Use strict aseptic technique when performing dressing changes and wound or peritoneal irrigations. *The protective barrier of the skin has been interrupted, decreasing the client's ability to resist infection.*

- Maintain fluid balance and adequate nutrition through either enteral or parenteral feedings, as indicated. *Adequate nutrition and fluid balance are necessary for optimal immune system function.*

Anxiety

The severity and potential threat to life associated with peritonitis presents a situational crisis for the client. Anxiety is a common response to a situational crisis for both the client and family.

Nursing interventions with rationales follow:

- Assess the anxiety level of the client and family and their present coping skills. *This provides a basis on which to plan interventions.*

- Present a calm, reassuring manner to both the client and family. Encourage the client and family to express their concerns; listen carefully, and acknowledge their validity. *This helps establish trust.*

- Minimize changes in caregiver assignments. *Consistency of nursing care and care providers helps reduce the client's and family's anxiety. Complex wound care and irrigation procedures are best performed by people who are very familiar with prescribed techniques.*

- Explain all treatments, procedures, tests, and examinations. *An increased understanding of what is being done can reduce the client's anxiety.*

- Reinforce and clarify information provided by physicians. *This improves understanding and promotes acceptance.*

- Teach and assist the client to practice relaxation techniques such as meditation, visualization, and progressive relaxation. *These measures promote positive coping skills and reduce physical manifestations of anxiety.*

Other Nursing Diagnoses

In any client with a potentially critical illness, many nursing diagnoses may be appropriate. Consider the following additional diagnoses for the client with peritonitis:

- *Ineffective Breathing Pattern* related to abdominal pain and distention

- *Risk for Injury* related to multiple invasive procedures and treatments

- *Altered Nutrition: Less Than Body Requirements* related to disruption of gastrointestinal function

- *Altered Oral Mucous Membrane* related to presence of nasogastric tube and lack of oral intake

- *Impaired Tissue Integrity* related to infectious process

Client and Family Teaching

As with any client who has a potentially critical illness, teaching is vital throughout hospitalization and prior to discharge. Initial teaching is limited to explaining any examination or procedure and typical responses or sensations that the client may experience. Provide brief but complete explanations to reduce anxiety and improve cooperation. Alert the client to report any unexpected sensations or responses that might indicate an adverse reaction, such as a hypersensitivity response to medication.

As the client begins to improve, begin teaching home care. Include procedures for wound care, including any dressing changes or irrigations that will be required. Provide verbal and written instructions, and allow the client and family members to practice and demonstrate the procedure prior to discharge. Include information on where to obtain necessary supplies. Discuss the client's medications, including the name and purpose of the drug, along with potential adverse effects and their management.

Describe the signs and symptoms of further infection (redness, heat, swelling, purulent drainage, chills, and fever) and other potential complications. Emphasize the importance of promptly reporting untoward responses to the primary care provider. Reinforce instructions about activity restrictions. Discuss the need to consume a diet with adequate calories and protein to meet the needs of the body for healing and optimal immune function. Provide a referral to home health services for assessment, wound care, and further teaching, as needed.

The Client with a Viral or Bacterial Infection

■ ■ ■

Gastroenteritis is a general term used to denote inflammation and pathologic processes involving the gastrointestinal tract. Gastroenteritis is not a specific disease, but a group of syndromes or a collection of related manifestations. Upper gastrointestinal symptoms such as anorexia, nausea, and vomiting are common. Diarrhea of varying intensity is a nearly universal feature of gastroenteritis, as is abdominal discomfort. Bacterial, viral, and parasitic infections can cause gastroenteritis, as can toxins.

Bacterial and viral infections of the gastrointestinal tract are often termed "food poisoning," because the ingestion of contaminated food is often the route of entry for the microorganism. The term *food poisoning* is most appropriately applied to acute food infections, infection with an enteric pathogen, and disorders caused by the toxins produced by bacteria in food.

Certain viruses can also cause acute gastroenteritis. Diarrhea due to the Norwalk virus occurs year-round in both adults and children. Its prevalence is thought to be second only to that of the common cold, accounting for about 40% of nonbacterial diarrhea (Berkow & Fletcher, 1992).

Pathophysiology

Bacterial or viral infection of the gastrointestinal tract produces inflammation, tissue damage, and clinical manifestations by two primary mechanisms:

- *The production of exotoxins.* A number of bacteria produce and excrete an exotoxin that enters the surrounding environment (gastrointestinal lumen), causing damage and inflammation. Exotoxins in the gastrointestinal tract are often referred to as *enterotoxins*. They impair intestinal absorption and can cause electrolytes and water to be secreted into the bowel in significant amounts, leading to diarrhea and fluid loss (Berkow & Fletcher, 1992). Common bacterial enterotoxins include those produced by *Staphylococcus*, *Clostridium perfringens, Clostridium botulinum,* some strains of *Escherichia coli,* and *Vibrio cholerae.*

- *Invasion and ulceration of the mucosa.* Other bacteria, including some *Shigella, Salmonella,* and *Escherichia coli* species produce tissue damage more directly. They invade the intestinal mucosa of the small bowel or colon, producing microscopic ulceration, bleeding, fluid exudate, and water and electrolyte secretion (Berkow & Fletcher, 1992).

In some cases, the mechanism of injury is unclear. It may be that a combination of direct and toxic damage occurs. The Norwalk virus can cause acute mucosal damage to the jejunum, with fluid and electrolyte secretion.

Although the manifestations of bacterial and viral enteritis vary according to the organism involved, several features are common (see the accompanying clinical manifestations box). Anorexia, nausea, and vomiting are caused by distension of the upper gastrointestinal tract by unabsorbed chyme and excess water. These factors, along with irritation of the bowel mucosa and gas production due to fermentation of undigested food, also lead to abdominal pain and cramping. *Borborygmi,* excessively loud and hyperactive bowel sounds, are another result. The abdomen is typically distended and tender.

Diarrhea is usually predominant with enteritis. Not only is fluid secreted into the bowel lumen, but the unabsorbed chyme and electrolytes also create an osmotic draw of fluid into the bowel. Motility is stimulated, and stools become watery and frequent. It is the loss of fluids and electrolytes through the diarrhea that can lead to the most serious manifestations of enteritis. The client's fluid volume can deplete very rapidly, leading to dehydration and hypovolemia. Orthostatic hypotension may be noted initially, along with an elevated temperature. If the fluid loss continues, hypovolemic shock with a fall in blood pressure, tachycardia, and impaired tissue perfusion may occur.

Electrolyte and acid-base imbalances may lead to multiple problems. The client with extensive vomiting may develop metabolic alkalosis due to the loss of hydrochloric acid from the stomach. When diarrhea predominates, metabolic acidosis is more likely. Potassium is lost in either case, leading to hypokalemia. Hyponatremia may also occur if fluids are replaced without corresponding electrolyte replacement. Headache, cardiac irregularities, changes in respiratory rate and pattern, malaise and weakness, muscle aching, and signs of neuromuscular irritability are the possible manifestations of these disturbances in homeostasis.

Several gastrointestinal infections produce significant and specific effects that need further elaboration. These are discussed below and summarized in Table 23–3.

Traveler's Diarrhea

People traveling to another country frequently develop diarrhea within 2 to 10 days. This is particularly true when travel involves a marked change in climate, sanitation standards, or unusual food and drink. Strains of enterotoxin-producing *Escherichia coli* can often be identified as the etiologic agent in traveler's diarrhea; occasionally, viral infections are implicated. Less frequent causes of traveler's diarrhea include *Salmonella, Shigella, Camylobacter,* and *Entamoeba* (Tierney et al., 1994).

The client with traveler's diarrhea may have up to 10 or more loose stools per day. Abdominal cramping commonly accompanies the diarrhea. Nausea and vomiting occur less frequently; fever is rare. Symptoms usually resolve spontaneously within 2 to 5 days. No long-term sequelae are associated with traveler's diarrhea.

Staphylococcal Food Poisoning

Certain staphylococcal strains of bacteria produce an enterotoxin. When a person consumes food that has been contaminated by the enterotoxin, an acute enteritis with vomiting and diarrhea commonly results.

Certain foods provide an excellent medium for staphylococcal growth when contaminated and left at room temperature. Examples include meats and fish, dairy products (e.g., custards), and bakery products (e.g., cream-filled pastries). The organism itself does not affect the bowel; the toxin it produces, however, impairs intestinal absorption and acts on receptors in the gut, stimulating the medullary center to produce vomiting.

The onset of staphylococcal food poisoning is abrupt, occurring typically within 2 to 8 hours after the person consumes the contaminated food. Nausea and vomiting is severe but usually short-lived. The manifestations typically last for 3 to 6 hours but may continue for up to 24 hours. Abdominal cramping and diarrhea may occur, as can headache and fever. Recovery is usually spontaneous and complete. Although acid-base, electrolyte, and fluid imbalances can result, they are usually minimal. Older adults and people with underlying chronic disease processes are at the highest risk for complications with staphylococcal food poisoning.

Clinical Manifestations of Bacterial or Viral Enteritis

Gastrointestinal Effects

- Anorexia
- Nausea and vomiting
- Abdominal pain and cramping
- Borborygmi
- Diarrhea

General Effects

- Malaise and weakness
- Muscle aches
- Headache
- Dry skin and mucous membranes
- Poor skin turgor
- Orthostatic hypotension
- Tachycardia and possible shock
- Elevated temperature

Botulism

Botulism is a severe, life-threatening form of food poisoning caused by *Clostridium botulinum.* These gram-positive spore-forming anaerobic bacteria grow in improperly preserved foods, such as home-canned vegetables, smoked meats, and vacuum-packed fish. The spores are highly resistant to heat; exposure to moist heat at a temperature of 248 F for 30 minutes is required to kill the bacteria. The bacterial toxin, however, is easily destroyed by heat, at temperatures as low as 176 F.

The incubation time can vary from 18 to 96 hours following ingestion of the bacteria. The toxin is absorbed into the bloodstream from the intestines and produces neuromuscular blockade by blocking the release of acetylcholine, a neurotransmitter, from nerve endings. An abrupt onset of bilateral and symmetric neurologic symptoms occurs. Cranial nerves are often the first affected, followed by descending weakness or paralysis. Visual disturbances, including diplopia (double vision) and loss of accommodation, are common initial symptoms and are often accompanied by dry mouth and dysphagia. Nausea, vomiting, and abdominal cramps may precede neurologic manifestations. Diarrhea is rare with botulism; once the neurologic manifestations occur, constipation is common. As neuromuscular paralysis progresses, respiratory muscles become progressively weaker. Respiratory muscle paralysis may lead to death unless respiratory support

Table 23–3   Selected Bacterial Infections of the Bowel

Disease and Organism	Incubation	Pathogenesis	Manifestations	Management
Traveler's diarrhea: *Escherichia coli*	24 to 72 hours	Enterotoxin causes hypersecretion of the small intestine.	Abrupt onset of diarrhea; vomiting rare	Prophylactic bismuth subsalicylate; anti-diarrheals such as loperamide or diphenoxylate; 3- to 5-day course of norfloxacin, ciprofloxacin, or trimethoprim-sulfamethoxazole
Staphylococcal food poisoning	2 to 8 hours	Enterotoxin impairs intestinal absorption and affects medullary vomiting centers.	Severe nausea and vomiting; abdominal cramping and diarrhea; headache and fever	Fluid and electrolyte replacement as needed
Botulism: *Clostridium botulinum*	1.5 to 8 days	Absorbed enterotoxin produces neuromuscular blockade and progressive paralysis.	Diplopia, loss of pupillary accommodation; pupils fixed and dilated; dry mouth, dysphagia; progressive cephalocaudal weakness and paralysis; GI symptoms minimal; respiratory failure possible complication	Gastric lavage to remove toxin from gut; administration of botulinus antitoxin; respiratory, fluid, and nutritional support
Cholera: *Vibrio cholerae*	1 to 3 days	Enterotoxin affects entire small intestine, causing secretion of water and electrolytes into bowel lumen.	Severe diarrhea with "rice water stool," grey, cloudy, odorless, with no blood or pus; vomiting; thirst, oliguria, muscle cramps, weakness; dehydration and vascular collapse	Oral or intravenous rehydration; possible antimicrobial therapy with ampicillin, tetracycline, trimethoprim-sulfamethoxazole, others
Hemorrhagic colitis: *E. coli*	1 to 3 days	Enterotoxin causes direct mucosal damage in large intestine; also toxic to vascular endothelial cells.	Severe abdominal cramping, watery diarrhea that becomes grossly bloody; fever; possible complications: hemolytic uremic syndrome and thrombotic thrombocytopenic purpura	Supportive care with fluid replacement and bland diet; may require dialysis or plasmapheresis for complications
Salmonellosis: *Salmonella*	8 to 48 hours	Disorder is due to the superficial infection of the GI tract without invasion or the production of toxins.	Diarrhea with abdominal cramping, nausea, and vomiting; low-grade fever, chills, weakness	Treatment of symptoms: trimethoprim-sulfamethoxazole, ampicillin, or ciprofloxacin for the severely ill client
Shigellosis (bacillary dysentery): *Shigella*	1 to 4 days	Local tissue invasion, primarily involving the large intestine and distal ileum; endotoxin causes fluid and electrolyte secretion into bowel lumen.	Watery diarrhea with severe abdominal cramping and tenesmus; lethargy	Fluid and electrolyte replacement; correction of acidosis; antibiotic therapy with trimethoprim-sulfamethoxazole, ciprofloxacin, or ampicillin

is provided. Sensation is not impaired, and the client remains mentally alert.

Cholera

Cholera is an acute diarrheal illness caused by certain strains of *Vibrio cholerae*. Cholera is endemic in parts of Asia, the Middle East, and Africa. Epidemics occur periodically, more recently in South America and sub-Saharan Africa. Cholera is spread by ingestion of water or food contaminated by the feces of infected persons. Children are particularly susceptible to the infection.

The organism causing cholera produces an enterotoxin, enzymes, and other substances that affect the entire small intestine. Water and electrolytes are secreted into the bowel lumen in response to the toxin. The effect of the enzymes and other substances produced by the bacteria is unclear; they may alter the mucous protection of bowel endothelium.

Cholera has an incubation period of 1 to 3 days. The disease itself ranges in severity. In some cases, few or no symptoms are present (but the disease is nonetheless transmissible to others); in other cases, the disease is mild and uncomplicated; in still other cases, it is acute and fulminant. The onset is typically abrupt, with severe, frequent, watery diarrhea. The person may pass up to 1 L of stool per hour and, as a consequence, rapidly develop dehydration and hypotension. Stool is often described as "rice water stool" and characteristically gray and cloudy, with no fecal odor, blood, or pus (Tierney et al., 1994). Vomiting may accompany the diarrhea. Other manifestations of the disease are related to the loss of fluid and electrolytes: thirst, oliguria, muscle cramps, weakness, and significant signs of dehydration. Metabolic acidosis and hypokalemia develop. If untreated, circulatory collapse and acute renal failure may occur.

Recovery from cholera is usually spontaneous, occurring in 3 to 6 days with uncomplicated cases. With prompt and adequate fluid replacement, the fatality rate from cholera is low, less than 1%. However, it may be greater than 50% in untreated severe cases. Some clients become chronic biliary carriers of the bacteria (Berkow & Fletcher, 1992).

Escherichia coli Hemorrhagic Colitis

Most pathologic forms of the common gram-negative *Escherichia coli* bacteria cause little more than common "traveler's diarrhea"; however, some strains produce high levels of a potent enterotoxin in the large intestine after being ingested. This toxin causes direct mucosal damage, has a toxic effect on the endothelial cells of blood vessels in the gastrointestinal tract, and, if absorbed, may also affect other blood vessels, such as those of the kidney.

The most common strain of *E. coli* that produces hemorrhagic colitis is serotype 0157:H7. Outbreaks have occurred throughout the United States and Canada, one of which claimed four lives and affected nearly 500 people in the northwest United States in early 1993. Cattle provide the reservoir for *E. coli* 0157:H7. It is usually spread through undercooked beef (hamburger in particular) and unpasteurized milk. This infection may also be spread by direct contact via the fecal-oral route.

The onset of hemorrhagic colitis is abrupt, with severe abdominal cramping and watery diarrhea. The diarrhea typically becomes grossly bloody within 24 hours. Fever may be present.

Hemolytic uremic syndrome and thrombotic thrombocytopenic purpura are significant complications of *E. coli* hemorrhagic colitis, affecting about 5% of persons with the disease. Older adults over age 59 have the highest risk for developing thrombotic thrombocytopenic purpura (see Chapter 31).

Salmonellosis

Salmonellosis is a form of food poisoning caused by the ingestion of raw or improperly cooked meat, poultry, eggs, and dairy products contaminated with one or more varieties of *Salmonella* bacteria. These bacteria produce superficial infection of the gastrointestinal tract, rarely invading further. They do not produce a toxin.

Symptoms of salmonellosis occur 8 to 48 hours after ingestion of the bacteria. Diarrhea may be violent with abdominal cramping, nausea, and vomiting. A low-grade fever, chills, and weakness may accompany gastrointestinal manifestations.

Shigellosis (Bacillary Dysentery)

Shigellosis, also called bacillary dysentery, is an acute bowel infection caused by microorganisms of the *Shigella* genus. Shigellosis occurs worldwide, accounting for up to 5% to 10% of diarrheal illness in some regions. When shigellosis occurs in epidemic form, the potential for loss of life is high (Figure 23–4 compares the pathogenesis and outcome of cholera to that of shigellosis). Humans are the reservoir for the infection, which is spread directly via the fecal-oral route or indirectly through contaminated food, fomites (such as inanimate objects), and vectors (such as fleas). The incubation period for shigellosis is 1 to 4 days (Berkow & Fletcher, 1992).

Shigella organisms infect primarily the lower intestine, although the distal ileum may be infected in severe cases. They invade the tissue, causing an inflammatory response, and produce an enterotoxin. The result is a watery diarrhea containing blood, mucus, and inflammatory exudate.

The client with shigellosis presents with an abrupt onset of diarrhea, severe abdominal cramping, and *tenesmus,* a sensation of urgent and continuing need to defecate. The stool may initially be formed, but becomes watery and often contains blood and pus as the disease progresses. Lethargy is common; on rare occasions,

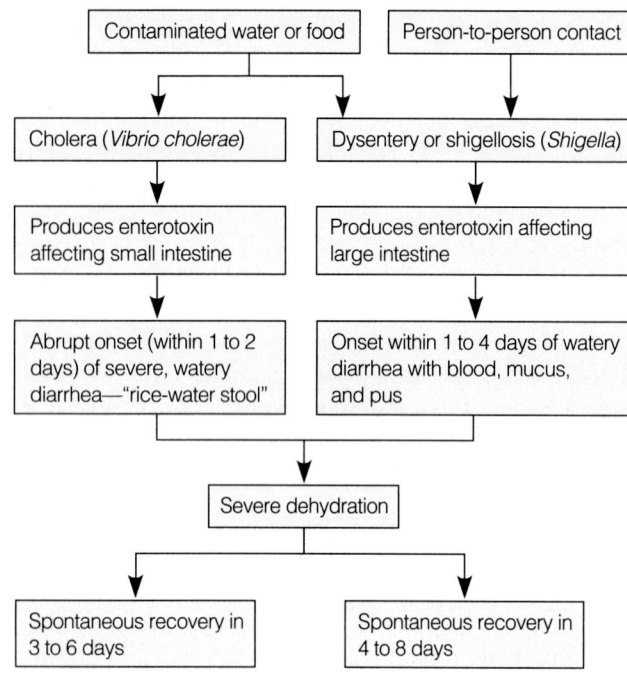

Figure 23–4 Pathogenesis and outcome of cholera and dysentery. Both are potentially epidemic intestinal infections.

shigellosis presents with delirium, convulsions, and coma (Berkow & Fletcher, 1992).

In adults, shigellosis is usually mild and self-limiting, resolving spontaneously in 4 to 8 days. Older adults and clients with debilitating conditions are at particular risk for severe dehydration and electrolyte imbalances leading to circulatory collapse. Secondary infection is also a potential complication of shigellosis in debilitated clients. Acute blood loss can occur from mucosal ulcerations.

Collaborative Care

Identifying the causative agent, managing the client's symptoms, and preventing complications are the primary goals of care for the client with an acute viral or bacterial infection of the gastrointestinal tract. The client's history and presentation provide valuable cues about the etiologic origin and causative agent. Laboratory and diagnostic testing is used to confirm the pathogen present and to evaluate the client's status. In most cases, therapeutic management is supportive, directed toward alleviating symptoms, restoring fluid and electrolyte balance, and maintaining physical function.

Laboratory and Diagnostic Tests
Laboratory and diagnostic testing is used to identify the causative organism when the client's symptoms are severe or do not resolve within about 48 hours. It is also used to assess the client's fluid, electrolyte, and acid-base balance

when symptoms are prolonged. Additionally, these studies are used to identify possible complications.

The following laboratory studies may be ordered:

- *Stool specimen* for culture, ova and parasites, and fecal leukocytes. In most cases of bacterial infection, culture of the feces will reveal the infective organism. However, some bacteria may require as long as 6 weeks for culture, making this test impractical. In some infections, such as botulism, the toxin itself may be isolated from the stool. Specimens obtained late in the course of the disease as the infection is resolving may be negative for an infective organism. Contamination of the stool by urine or treatment with antibiotics, bismuth subsalicylate (Pepto-Bismol), or mineral oil may interfere with the growth of pathogens, altering the results of stool culture. Provide the client with a clean bedpan or collection device to obtain the stool specimen, and instruct the client to avoid mixing the stool with urine or toilet tissue.

- *Gram stain of vomitus* may reveal the presence of staphylococci in staphylococcal food poisoning.

- *Blood culture* may be performed to assess for bacteremia with suspected infection of the gastrointestinal tract.

- *Blood serum* may also be examined for the presence of the suspected toxin, particularly if botulism is suspected.

- *Serum osmolality, serum electrolytes, and arterial blood gases* are used to assess the client's fluid volume status and electrolyte and acid-base balance. Common disruptions associated with infectious diseases causing diarrhea are outlined in Table 23–4.

The primary diagnostic test ordered for the client with a suspected bacterial or viral infection of the gastrointestinal tract is a sigmoidoscopy. Through direct visualization of bowel mucosa using a sigmoidoscope, this examination helps to differentiate ulcerative colitis (discussed later in this chapter) from infectious processes. It cannot, however, take the place of stool cultures, because the lesions associated with some infectious processes are indistinguishable from those of ulcerative colitis (Berkow & Fletcher, 1992). Nursing care of the client undergoing a sigmoidoscopy is included in the box on page 767.

Pharmacology
Most acute infections of the bowel resolve spontaneously, requiring no pharmacologic intervention. However, if the client is severely ill and the symptoms are prolonged, medications may be prescribed.

Antibiotic therapy may be initiated for clients with cholera, salmonellosis, or shigellosis. Trimethoprim-sulfamethoxazole (Septra, Bactrim), ciprofloxacin (Cipro), ampicillin (Ampicin, Omnipen, Polycillin-N, others), or another antibiotic may be prescribed. Stool culture is ob-

Table 23–4	Laboratory Values Associated with Infectious Disorders of the Bowel Causing Diarrhea	
Test	**Normal Value**	**Change with Significant Diarrhea**
Serum osmolality	275 to 295 mOsm/kg	Increased; levels above 320 mOsm/kg H_2O indicate significant dehydration
Serum potassium	3.5 to 5.0 mEq/L	Decreased as a result of loss through stool and vomitus; levels below 2.5 mEq/L indicate critical illness
Serum sodium	136 to 148 mEq/L	Decreased as a result of loss through stool and vomitus; may be significantly low when water has been replaced without corresponding salt replacement; levels below 120 mEq/L may indicate critical illness
Serum chloride	96 to 106 mEq/L	Increased when diarrhea causes sodium loss that is greater than chloride loss; decreased with severe diarrhea and with vomiting; possible critical values are those below 80 mEq/L or above 115 mEq/L
Blood gases		
■ pH	Arterial: 7.35 to 7.45	Decreased in metabolic acidosis, as a possible result of severe diarrhea; increased in metabolic alkalosis, as a possible result of severe vomiting and chloride loss; values below 7.25 or above 7.55 indicate critical illness
■ Pco_2	Arterial: 35 to 45 mm Hg	Typically decreased in metabolic acidosis as the body attempts to eliminate excess acid by "blowing off" CO_2; increased with metabolic alkalosis as the body retains CO_2 in an attempt to normalize pH
■ Bicarbonate	22 to 26 mEq/L	Decreased in metabolic acidosis; increased in metabolic alkalosis
Hematocrit	Males: 40% to 50% Females: 37% to 47%	Increased with dehydration and hypovolemia as a result of concentration of blood cells
Urine specific gravity	1.010 to 1.025	Increased with dehydration and hypovolemia as kidneys attempt to conserve fluid

tained prior to initiating antibiotic therapy; however, therapy may be initiated before the culture results have been obtained. The choice of antibiotic is based on a presumptive diagnosis using the client's history and presenting symptoms.

For infections in which diarrhea predominates, an antidiarrheal drug may be prescribed to promote client comfort and reduce fluid loss. Nursing measures related to the use of antidiarrheal agents are outlined in the box on page 768.

It is vital to remember that antidiarrheal agents are *not* used for clients with symptoms of botulism. In fact, cathartics may be ordered for these clients to facilitate removal of the toxin from the bowel.

Botulism antitoxin is administered as soon as possible to the client with suspected botulism. The antitoxin may be administered on a strong suspicion of bacterial or toxin ingestion, without firm confirmation of the diagnosis. If the toxin is given more than 72 hours after the onset of symptoms, it may yield no benefit (Berkow & Fletcher, 1992). The antitoxin neutralizes circulating toxin; however, it cannot displace the toxin that is already bound to nerve endings, so existing paralysis will not resolve with its administration. Because botulism antitoxin

is a biologic substance made from horse serum, its most frequent adverse effects are anaphylaxis and serum sickness (see the section on hypersensitivity responses in Chapter 8). Sensitivity testing and progressive desensitization is recommended prior to administration of the antitoxin. This may not always be possible because of progression of the client's symptoms. To reduce the risk of anaphylaxis, epinephrine should be given along with the antitoxin (Shlafer, 1993).

Supportive Care

Replacing lost fluids and electrolytes is the primary focus of collaborative care for the client with an infectious process manifest by significant vomiting and/or diarrhea. In most bacterial infections of the bowel, fluid and electrolyte replacement is all that is necessary to provide support until the infection resolves.

Oral rehydration is the preferred route for administering physiologic fluids. An oral glucose-electrolyte solution is often well tolerated in sips, even by the client who is vomiting. Commercial preparations such as Gatorade, All-Sport, and Pedialyte are available. A solution can also be easily prepared by adding 5 mL (1 teaspoon) table salt, 5 mL baking soda, 20 mL (4 teaspoons) granulated sugar, and flavoring (such as lemon extract or juice) to 1 L (1 quart) of water.

Intravenous rehydration is often necessary for the client with severe diarrhea and fluid loss. For some infections, such as cholera, a combination of oral and intravenous fluids may be administered to replace lost fluids and maintain vascular volume. Balanced electrolyte solutions, such as glucose in normal saline, Ringer's solution, and others, are used. Lactated Ringer's solution or another alkalinizing solution may be prescribed if metabolic acidosis is present.

Gastric lavage and catharsis—in effect, "washing out" the stomach and intestines—may be ordered if botulism is suspected and if the food has been recently ingested. This is done to remove unabsorbed toxin from the gastrointestinal tract. The progressive paralysis associated with botulism necessitates close observation of the client for signs of respiratory distress. These clients often require respiratory support with endotracheal intubation or tracheostomy and mechanical ventilation (see Chapters 33 and 34).

Plasmapheresis is another technique that may be used to remove circulating antigen in clients with botulism or hemorrhagic colitis caused by *Escherichia coli*. In plasmapheresis, harmful components in the plasma are removed from the client's blood along with the plasma by passing the blood through a blood cell separator. An equal amount of albumin or human plasma is returned to the client, along with the client's red blood cells (RBCs). This procedure is usually done in a series, rather than as a one-time-only treatment. It is not without risk, and informed consent is required. Potential complications of plasmapheresis include those associated with the placement of intravenous catheters, shifts in fluid balance, and alteration of blood clotting.

The client with acute tubular necrosis and renal failure due to the enterotoxins of certain *Escherichia coli* strains may require dialysis. Acute renal failure significantly impairs the capacity of the kidneys to remove excess fluid, electrolytes, and waste products from the body. Although acute renal failure often resolves spontaneously and renal function resumes, dialysis can be life-saving as a means of removing wastes to prevent severe fluid and electrolyte imbalances and metabolic acidosis. Either hemodialysis or peritoneal dialysis may be used, generally as a temporary measure. Nursing care of the client with acute renal failure and undergoing dialysis is discussed in Chapter 26.

Nursing Care

Few clients with acute infections of the bowel require hospitalization. Nurses are more likely to encounter these clients in outpatient and community settings. Assessment of the client, education, and support of self-care measures are major nursing responsibilities related to these disorders. Diarrhea and fluid volume deficit are priority nursing diagnoses.

Diarrhea

The nursing assessment can help identify the food source and probable organism causing the client's diarrhea, as well as signs of complications. Nursing interventions focus on providing measures to restore a normal elimination pattern and improve the client's comfort. Nursing interventions with rationales for the client with diarrhea are represented earlier in this chapter on page 769.

Other Nursing Diagnoses

Other nursing diagnoses that may be appropriate for the client with an acute bacterial or viral infection of the gastrointestinal tract follow:

- *Activity Intolerance* related to fluid loss and dehydration.
- *Risk for Aspiration* related to impaired swallow reflex (botulism)
- *Fluid Volume Deficit* related to vomiting and diarrhea
- *Altered Nutrition: Less Than Body Requirements* related to inability to retain food
- *Impaired Home Maintenance Management* related to lack of knowledge about safe food preparation and storage practices
- *Inability to Sustain Spontaneous Ventilation* related to respiratory muscle paralysis (botulism)
- *Altered Urinary Elimination* related to effects of enterotoxin on renal function (*Escherichia coli* infections).

Client and Family Teaching

Nurses play a significant part in preventing bacterial and viral infections of the bowel in their roles as educators, community health providers, and advocates for environmental safety.

Teach clients and their families about the importance of maintaining proper food temperatures. Adequate cooking of meat products is vital to prevent disorders such as staphylococcal food poisoning, *Escherichia coli* hemorrhagic colitis, and salmonellosis. Emphasize the importance of not consuming raw meat products, and cooking hamburger in particular to the point that no redness is noted in the meat. The highly pathogenic *Escherichia coli* serotype 0157:H7 is present in the gut of infected animals. Meats from the animal may be contaminated with bowel contents. Although the organism is readily destroyed by heat (for example, on the outside of a steak or roast), the process of grinding hamburger can allow it to become mixed throughout the meat. Thorough cooking will destroy the organism. This pathogen (and others) may also be spread through unpasteurized milk. Discuss the dangers of consuming milk that has not been pasteurized and encourage clients not to drink it.

Dairy products, eggs, and egg products left at room temperature provide a good growth medium for bacteria. Discuss the importance of prompt refrigeration of meats and these products to minimize this risk.

Nonacidic canned foods, such as vegetables, mushrooms, meats, and fish, are potential sources of botulism toxin. The high temperatures required to destroy the bacteria and its spores can be achieved only through pressure canning using appropriate pressures and duration. Emphasize the importance of following directions precisely when home-canning foods. Teach the client to boil home-canned foods for 10 to 15 minutes to destroy any potential toxin. Any food that is discolored or comes from a can or jar that has been punctured, is cracked or bulging, or does not have a tight seal should be destroyed without tasting or touching. Food contaminated with botulism may have *no* unusual odor or color. If the seal is questionable, discard the food.

Many gastrointestinal infections are spread through contaminated water. Encourage clients traveling out of the country to consume only bottled water unless local water supplies are clearly safe. Water purification tablets are available for hikers and campers, and may also be used when traveling abroad.

Teach people who are affected with gastroenteritis the importance of good hand washing. Many of these infections can be spread to others via the fecal-oral route. Washing hands thoroughly with soap and running water for at least 10 seconds after each defecation helps minimize this risk. Clothing and linens contaminated with feces should be washed separately in hot water and detergent.

The Client with a Protozoal Infection of the Bowel

■ ■ ■

Parasites are organisms that live within, upon, or at the expense of other organisms. Parasitic infections are common in developing countries and include both protozoal and helminthic infections (discussed in the next section of this chapter). Parasites that infect the bowel generally enter the gastrointestinal tract through the mouth by the fecal-oral route, although some may be spread by direct contact or through sexual activity.

Of the protozoal infections of the bowel, only giardiasis is common in the United States. Amebiasis is found chiefly in the tropics but exists anywhere sanitation is poor. Cryptosporidiosis, a form of coccidiosis, has been recognized only recently as an important worldwide

cause of sporadic mild diarrhea, traveler's diarrhea, and severe diarrhea in people with acquired immune deficiency syndrome (AIDS) and others who are immunocompromised (Tierney et al., 1994).

Pathophysiology

The most common protozoal infections of the bowel are discussed below and summarized in Table 23–5.

Giardiasis

Giardiasis is a protozoal infection of the upper small intestine caused by *Giardia lamblia*. It is the most common intestinal protozoal pathogen in the United States and occurs worldwide. Although people of all ages may be affected, children have the highest incidence. Humans are the reservoir for *Giardia,* although it may be found in dogs and beavers as well. The disease is spread by the fecal-oral route, usually by contaminated food or water. It is also spread by direct contact (Tierney et al., 1994).

When the cyst form of the organism is ingested, trophozoites emerge in the duodenum and jejunum, attaching themselves to the intestinal mucosa. This disease causes superficial invasion, inflammation, and destruction of the mucosa of the small intestine.

Although many clients with giardiasis are asymptomatic, symptoms may develop after a 1- to 3-week (or longer) incubation period. Manifestations may develop suddenly or insidiously. Diarrhea is a common symptom. Usually mild, manifest by one or several large, loose stools per day, diarrhea may be severe in some cases, with frequent, copious, frothy, malodorous, and greasy stools. Diarrhea may be daily or intermittent, with normal stools on some days. Other manifestations of giardiasis include weight loss and weakness; anorexia, nausea, and vomiting; epigastric pain, abdominal cramping and distention, flatulence, and belching. The client may develop a malabsorption syndrome (discussed later in this chapter).

Amebiasis

Amebiasis (amebic dysentery) is chiefly found in the tropics but exists worldwide and can be found anywhere sanitation is poor. This disease accounts for 40,000 to 100,000 deaths annually throughout the world, but in the United States it tends to be mild and often asymptomatic.

Amebiasis is caused by the protozoon *Entamoeba histolytica.* Several strains of *Entamoeba histolytica* with differing pathogenicity (disease-causing ability) have been identified. Strains found in the tropics tend to be more virulent and pathogenic than those found in temperate climates. This difference probably accounts for the variation in severity of the disease noted around the world. Humans are the host for this parasite, which usually is transmitted through ingestion of fecally contaminated

Table 23–5 Common Protozoal Infections of the Bowel

Disease and Organism	Incubation	Pathogenesis	Manifestations	Management
Giardiasis: *Giardia lamblia*	1 to 3 weeks or more	Trophozoite attaches to mucosa in duodenum and jejunum, causing superficial invasion, inflammation, and tissue destruction.	Diarrhea, mild or severe, daily or intermittent; anorexia, nausea, vomiting; epigastric pain, cramping, distension; flatulence and belching; client may be asymptomatic	Metronidazole, quinacrine, furazolidone
Amebiasis: *Entamoeba histolytica*	2 to 4 weeks	Organisms may reside in large intestine without causing disease or invade colon wall, causing ulceration; may be carried via blood to liver to produce abscess.	Client is most often asymptomatic; diarrhea may be mild, with few semiformed mucus-containing stools per day, or severe, with 10 to 20 blood-streaked liquid stools per day; abdominal cramps and flatulence; colic, tenesmus, vomiting, tenderness; fatigue, weight loss; prostration and toxicity	Metronidazole and diloxanide furoate or iodoquinol; chloroquine for hepatic abscess
Cryptosporidiosis: *Cryptosporidium*	2 to 10 days	Organisms attach to epithelial surface of small bowel (jejunum), causing villous atrophy and mild inflammatory changes; may secrete enterotoxin.	In immunocompetent clients: Asymptomatic to profuse, watery diarrhea of sudden onset, abdominal cramping; malaise, fever; anorexia, nausea, vomiting. In immunodeficient clients: Profuse watery diarrhea with loss of up to 15 to 20 L per day; severe malabsorption, electrolyte imbalance; weight loss; lymphadenopathy	Self-limiting in immunocompetent clients, requiring only supportive care. For immunodeficient clients: spiramycin, zidovudine (AZT), paromomycin (Humatin), octreotide, eflornithine; fluid and electrolyte replacement; parenteral nutrition as needed

food or water. Person-to-person contact is also an important means of its transmission. The parasite enters the intestines, where it may live *commensally* (without harm) without causing disease, or invade the intestinal wall to cause ulceration and inflammation. The cecum, appendix, ascending colon, sigmoid colon, and rectum are most often affected. Ulcers may spread to cause hemorrhage, edema, and mucosal sloughing. The infection may also be carried via the blood to the liver, producing hepatic abscess, and, rarely, to other organs, such as the lungs or brain.

Amebiasis is asymptomatic in most infected people. When manifestations are present, they may range from mild to severe. The client may have abdominal cramps, flatulence, and intermittent diarrhea containing blood and mucus. Severe manifestations of amebic dysentery include frequent watery stools containing blood, mucus, and necrotic tissue; colic, tenesmus, and abdominal tenderness; nausea and vomiting; and fever. With hepatic involvement, the liver may be enlarged and tender to palpation.

Although complications of amebiasis are rare, they may include appendicitis, bowel perforation with peritonitis, and fulminating colitis (Tierney et al., 1994).

Cryptosporidiosis (Coccidiosis)

Cryptosporidium, the organism that causes *cryptosporidiosis*, has been recognized only recently as a significant cause of diarrheal disorders worldwide. It causes sporadic mild diarrhea and traveler's diarrhea in all age groups. In immunocompromised people, particularly those with human immunodeficiency virus (HIV) infection and AIDS, *Cryptosporidium* is responsible for severe diarrhea, malabsorption, and significant weight loss.

This organism is transmitted from other humans or animals by the fecal-oral route. Contaminated water is a frequent source of infection. The organism attaches to bowel epithelium, causing surface damage and inflammation. It does not invade the tissues. It appears that an enterotoxin is secreted, causing the characteristic watery diarrhea of the disease.

Clients who are immunocompetent have a self-limited disease course which may be asymptomatic or marked by watery diarrhea of up to 10 stools per day. A low-grade fever, nausea, vomiting, abdominal cramps, and general malaise may also be present.

Profuse watery diarrhea with loss of significant amounts of fluid and electrolytes, and severe malabsorption with marked weight loss are characteristic of the disease in people with immunodeficiency, AIDS in particular. These clients may have an associated lymphadenopathy as well.

Collaborative Care

The collaborative care of the client with a protozoal infestation of the intestines involves identifying the causative organism, followed by pharmacologic treatment. The following laboratory and diagnostic tests may be ordered:

- *Stool examination* is done to identify the presence of ova and parasites. Many protozoa are shed intermittently rather than continuously, making sequential stool collection (e.g., every other day for a total of three specimens) beneficial in identifying their presence. A freshly collected stool specimen is examined microscopically to identify protozoa, trophozoites (their immature forms), or their cysts. A laxative such as sodium sulfate, sodium phosphate, or bisacodyl may be administered prior to the collection of one of the specimens to increase protozoal shedding and the likelihood of their presence in the stool.

- *Indirect hemagglutination assay (IHA)* is a serologic test to detect antibodies to specific protozoa. Because positive antibody titers may continue for several years following a protozoal infection, this test may not be able to differentiate current from previous infection. A positive IHA test is indicated by a blood titer above 1:128.

- *Sigmoidoscopy* may be performed to examine the bowel mucosa directly, particularly with suspected amebiasis. In addition to allowing visualization of bowel mucosa, a stool or exudative specimen can be collected and examined for trophozoites. If this is anticipated, no pre-procedure bowel preparation is performed to prevent disruption of stool and exudative material in the bowel.

- *Duodenal string test (Entero-Test), duodenal aspiration, or duodenal biopsy* may be ordered for the client with suspected giardiasis if stool specimens have been negative but the client's history and presentation strongly suggest the disease. Duodenal aspirate is stained and microscopically examined for evidence of the protozoa. Small bowel biopsy may also be used to identify infection with *Cryptosporidium*.

Pharmacologic management focuses on providing antiparasitic drugs, such as metronidazole (Flagyl), diloxanide furoate (Entamide), iodoquinol (Yodoxin, Amebaquine), and tinidazole (Fasigyn). Clients are generally treated on an outpatient basis, although those with severe amebic dysentery may be hospitalized to receive intravenous fluids and electrolyte replacements. Nursing responsibilites in caring for clients receiving common antiprotozoal drugs are outlined in the pharmacology box on page 802.

Nursing Care

Nursing care measures for the client with a protozoal infection of the gastrointestinal tract are very similar to those indicated for clients with bacterial or viral infections. *Diarrhea* and *Risk for Fluid Volume Deficit* are priority nursing diagnoses. Refer to the previous sections of this chapter for specific nursing interventions related to these diagnoses.

Client and Family Teaching

Nurses need to teach not only the client and family members but also members of the general public about how parasitic diseases are transmitted and how to avoid spreading the infection. Prevention of amebiasis and giardiasis involves the following:

- Provision of safe water supplies
- Appropriate disposal of human feces
- Safe food storage, handling, and preparation practices
- Adequate hand washing after defecating and before handling food

Teach people living in high-risk areas (tropical climates, areas with untreated water supplies) methods to ensure water safety and to avoid foods that cannot be peeled or cooked. Water may be boiled, filtered, or treated with iodine to eliminate protozoal contamination (Tierney et al., 1994). People also need to be able to recognize signs and symptoms of protozoal infections and know where to obtain treatment.

Emphasize the importance of keeping toilet areas clean and maintaining good personal hygiene. Advise the client to avoid rectal contact during sexual activity. Other household members should also have stool specimens examined for parasites. No drug is safe or effective to prevent protozoal infections of the bowel.

Nursing Implications for Pharmacology: Antiprotozoal Agents

LOCAL (GASTROINTESTINAL) AGENTS

Iodoquinol (Yodoxin, Amebaquine)

Paromomycin (Humatin)

Clients with asymptomatic amebiasis who shed cysts may be treated with a single antiprotozoal agent that is active only in the intestinal lumen. Local agents have the advantage of provoking fewer side effects than systemically active agents. Although these drugs differ in chemical composition, all exert a local amebicidal effect in the intestines and are poorly absorbed when administered orally.

Nursing Responsibilities

- Assess the client for potential contraindications to therapy:
  a. Report to the primary care provider any hypersensitivity to the drug or drug class before administering the drug.
  b. Use iodoquinol with caution in clients who are malnourished or have thyroid disorders; it is contraindicated for people with hepatic or renal impairment, optic neuropathy, or hypersensitivity to iodine (Spencer et al., 1993).
  c. Administer paromomycin with caution to clients with ulcerative bowel lesions because of possible increased absorption of the drug. It is contraindicated for clients who are hypersensitive to aminoglycoside antibiotics, have impaired renal function, or have intestinal obstruction.
- Administer the drug as ordered. Administering doses after meals may help decrease gastrointestinal side effects.
- Observe the client for adverse effects. Gastrointestinal side effects, such as anorexia, nausea, vomiting, abdominal cramping, diarrhea, and increased flatulence, are not uncommon. Report skin rash, visual disturbances, or changes in blood work to the primary care provider.

Client and Family Teaching

- Take the drug as prescribed for the full course of therapy.
- Take with food to reduce gastrointestinal effects.
- Keep follow-up appointments as recommended to evaluate the success of antiprotozoal therapy.
- Report adverse effects to the physician:
  For iodoquinol:
  a. Any change in vision
  b. Numbness, tingling, pain, or other indicators of possible peripheral neuropathy
  c. Chills, fever, dermatitis; development of boils; enlargement of the thyroid gland
  For paromomycin:
  d. A change in urination or character of the urine
  e. Diminished hearing or tinnitus
  f. Rash
  g. Signs of neuropathy
  h. Weight loss, diarrhea, fatty stools indicative of malabsorption
  i. Candidiasis of the mouth or vagina
- Practice good hand washing, particularly after using the toilet, to prevent transmitting the protozoa to others.

SYSTEMIC AGENTS

Metronidazole (Flagyl, Satric, Metzol, others)

Diloxanide furoate (Entamide)

Emetine and dehydroemetine

Quinacrine (Atabrine)

Chloroquine (Aralen, Chlorocan)

Clients with symptomatic protozoal infections are generally treated with a systemic antiprotozoal agent, often in combination with one or more local agents. These drugs range from emetine, a highly toxic drug first used as an amebicide in 1912, to diloxanide, an

The Client with a Helminthic Disorder

■ ■ ■

Helminths are parasitic worms, capable of causing infectious diseases in humans. Helminths are subclassified as round worms (nematodes), flukes (trematodes), or tapeworms (cestodes).

Pathophysiology

Although all helminths can infect humans, the definitive host and intermediate hosts vary with each organism. In nearly all instances of helminthic disorders, the organism enters the body via the gastrointestinal tract through contaminated and inadequately cooked foods. Some of these organisms remain in the intestinal tract of the infected host; others migrate to infect the liver, lungs, or other

Pharmacology: Antiprotozoal Agents (continued)

investigational drug of apparently low toxicity (Spencer et al., 1993). Metronidazole is the most widely used of these antiprotozoal agents and is the drug of choice for treating amebiasis.

Nursing Responsibilities

- Assess the client for possible contraindications to therapy:
  a. Check for a history of hypersensitivity to the prescribed agent or related drugs.
  b. Use emetine and dehydroemetine with extreme caution in the older adult and people with preexisting cardiovascular or renal disease.
  c. Liver dysfunction or blood dyscrasias may contraindicate therapy with metronidazole.
  d. Use chloroquine with caution also in clients with impaired liver function.
- Administer the drug as ordered.
  a. Metronidazole may be administered either orally after meals or as a continuous or intermittent intravenous infusion.
  b. Diloxanide and quinacrine are orally administered medications; give after meals to minimize gastrointestinal side effects.
  c. Emetine is administered by deep intramuscular injection. Clients are hospitalized during therapy because of its toxicity.
  d. Chloroquine may be administered by mouth or by intramuscular injection.
- Observe for possible adverse effects; notify the physician if significant. Gastrointestinal effects are common.
  a. Peripheral neuropathy and other nervous system effects may occur with metronidazole and quinacrine.
  b. Emetine and dehydroemetine may cause severe cardiotoxicity; monitor for dysrhythmias, changes in vital signs, chest pain, or evidence of congestive heart failure.
  c. Chloroquine is toxic to the 8th cranial nerve; both chloroquine and quinacrine may cause retinopathy, affecting vision.
- Monitor the character and number of stools; obtain specimens as ordered to evaluate the effectiveness of therapy.

Client and Family Teaching

- Take the drug as prescribed for the full duration of the prescription.
- Taking oral preparations after meals helps minimize gastrointestinal side effects. Notify the physician if these effects interfere with activities of daily living.
- Do not use alcohol while taking these drugs, metronidazole in particular. An Antabuse-type response with severe headache, flushing, and vomiting may occur.
- Keep all follow-up appointments, including recommended vision examinations.
- Report adverse effects to the physician, including visual changes, hearing loss or tinnitus, dizziness and other nervous system changes, sore throats, fatigue, bruising, or infection.
- Candidiasis of the mouth or vagina may occur with metronidazole therapy. Report symptoms to the physician.
- Metronidazole, chloroquine, and quinacrine may cause a change in urine color to deep yellow (quinacrine) or rust or brown (metronidazole or chloroqine).
- Practice good hand washing, particularly after using the toilet, to prevent transmitting the protozoa to others.

structures. Few helminths are common in the United States; the discussion below focuses on the most common. These as well as other helminths are identified and their effects summarized in Table 23–6.

Ascariasis

The most common of the intestinal helminths is the nematode *Ascaris lumbricoides*. It is estimated to infect 1 bil-

lion people worldwide, primarily in areas of poor sanitation or where human feces is used as fertilizer.

Humans are the host for this infection. Adult worms live in the upper small intestine, producing eggs that are excreted in the feces. The eggs mature in the soil and are ingested in contaminated food and water. After ingestion, they hatch in the intestine, producing motile larvae that migrate through the intestinal wall, entering the lym-

Table 23–6   Selected Helminthic Diseases

	Infection	Host	Area	Pathogenesis	Manifestations
Nematode Infections	Ascariasis	Humans	Worldwide, cosmopolitan; warm, moist climates	Eggs are ingested in fecally contaminated food and drink; motile larvae migrate to lungs and back to small intestine, where they mature to produce more eggs.	Pulmonary: Low-grade fever, cough, blood-tinged sputum, wheezing, dyspnea, substernal chest pain. GI: Ulcerlike epigastric pain, vomiting, abdominal distention
	Enterobiasis (Pinworm infection)	Humans	Worldwide, cosmopolitan	Infect cecum; eggs deposit on perianal skin, organisms may be transmitted to others or reinfect host by oral ingestion.	Nocturnal perianal and perineal pruritus; insomnia, irritability, restlessness
	Hookworm disease	Humans	Tropics and subtropics	Larvae enter through skin or by ingestion and migrate to lungs, up bronchial tree, and down esophagus to mature in upper small bowel, where they attach and suck blood.	Skin: Pruritic dermatitis at site of entry Pulmonary: Dry cough, wheezing, blood-tinged sputum GI: Anorexia, diarrhea, abdominal pain Systemic: Anemia, pallor, cardiac insufficiency
	Strongyloidiasis	Humans, dogs, cats, and primates	Tropics and subtropics; moist areas of southern United States	Larvae enter through skin, migrate to lungs via bloodstream, ascend, and are swallowed to mature and become embedded in mucosa of duodenum and upper jejunum.	Skin: Pruritic dermatitis at site of entry Pulmonary: Dry cough, throat irritation, bronchitis GI: Diarrhea, epigastric abdominal pain, flatulence; anorexia, nausea, vomiting Systemic: Fever, malaise, weakness Hyperinfection: Severe diarrhea, bronchopneumonia, pleural effusion; paralytic ileus

Note. Adapted from *The Merck Manual of Diagnosis and Therapy* (16th ed.) edited by R. Berkow and A. J. Fletcher, 1992, Rahway, NJ: Merck Research Laboratories; *Current Medical Diagnosis and Treatment* (33rd ed.) edited by L. M. Tierney, Jr., S. J. McPhee, and M. A. Papadakis, 1994, Norwalk, CT: Appleton & Lange.

phatic or venous system. The larvae are transmitted to the heart and from there to the lungs. The larvae burrow through alveolar walls, from there migrating up the bronchial tree to the pharynx, then down the esophagus to return to the intestines as adults (Tierney et al., 1994).

Although the infection is an intestinal one, many of the manifestations are pulmonary, caused by the migrating larvae and the inflammatory response they provoke. Low-grade fever, cough productive of blood-tinged sputum, wheezing, and dyspnea are common manifestations. Mild substernal chest pain may be present. Abdominal symptoms may not be present unless the infestation is severe. Epigastric pain, abdominal distention, and, occasionally,

vomiting are the most common gastrointestinal manifestations. Occasionally, bowel obstruction may occur, as can biliary or pancreatic duct obstruction.

Enterobiasis (Pinworm Infection)

Enterobiasis, also called pinworm infection, is caused by *Enterobius vermicularis.* Although adults may be infected, enterobiasis affects children more often. The parasite is transmitted by oral ingestion of contaminated food, drink, or other fomites (any substance that transmits infectious material). Adult worms inhabit the cecum and surrounding bowel. Females migrate to lay their eggs on perianal skin. From there, they may be transmitted to

Table 23–6   (continued)

	Infection	Host	Area	Pathogenesis	Manifestations
	Trichinosis	Pigs; dogs, cats, rats, many wild animals	Temperate areas where pork is consumed	Larvae are ingested in undercooked meat; adult female burrows into mucosa of small intestine to produce larvae that disseminate via blood and lymphatic system to body tissues and become encysted in striated muscle.	GI: Diarrhea, abdominal cramps, malaise Muscle: Fever; muscle pain, tenderness, edema, and spasm Systemic: Periorbital and facial edema, sweating; photophobia and conjunctivitis; manifestations of inflammation in tissues invaded by larvae
Trematode Infections	Trichuriasis	Humans	Tropics and subtropics; uncommon in United States	Larvae are ingested in fecally contaminated food or water; worms mature and attach to mucosa of large intestine.	Most clients are asymptomatic; manifestations include chronic diarrhea, abdominal cramps and distention, flatulence, tenesmus; nausea, vomiting; weight loss
Cestode Infections	Trichuriasis	Humans and pigs	Central and Southeast Asia	Cysts are ingested by eating uncooked water plants, such as water chestnuts or bamboo shoots; mature and live organisms attach to small intestine mucosa.	Nausea, anorexia, upper abdominal pain, diarrhea; later, ascites and facial and extremity edema
	Fasciolopsiasis (intestinal fluke) Tapeworm	Humans; other mammals and fish	Worldwide	Organism is ingested by eating uncooked fish or meat containing embryo cysts, by fecal contamination, or by swallowing infected intermediate hosts, such as arthropods, fleas, or lice; head (scolex) of adult worm attaches in upper small intestine, and eggs form in individual segments.	Large tapeworms: Client often is asymptomatic; infection may cause mild nausea, diarrhea, abdominal pain; anemia, thrombocytopenia, and mild leukopenia Small tapeworms: Client may be asymptomatic; diarrhea, abdominal pain, anorexia, vomiting, weight loss, and irritability

others or back to the infected host. The eggs hatch in the duodenum, and the larvae migrate to the cecal region to mature (Tierney et al., 1994).

When manifestations are present, they include nocturnal perianal and perineal pruritus, insomnia, restlessness, and vague abdominal pain. Other manifestations, such as nausea, vomiting, and diarrhea, may occur but are uncommon.

Hookworm Disease

Hookworm disease is caused by either *Ancylostoma duodenale* or *Necator americanus*. This disease is widespread throughout the tropics, infecting approximately one-fourth of the world's population. It is rarely found outside the tropics. Humans are the only host. Eggs hatch in warm, moist, fecally contaminated soil and enter the body through the skin, usually the bare feet. Transmission can also occur through ingestion of contaminated food. The larvae migrate to the lungs, through the alveoli, and up the bronchial tree to be swallowed. Once in the intestines, they attach to the mucosa of the upper small bowel, where they subsist by sucking blood (Tierney et al., 1994).

Pruritic dermatitis at the site of entry is usually the first manifestation of hookworm disease. As the larvae migrate through the lungs, the client may have a dry cough with blood-tinged sputum, wheezing, and fever. Gastrointestinal manifestations may be absent, or mild, including anorexia, diarrhea, and vague abdominal pain. Anemia resulting from the blood and iron loss can be significant.

Trichinosis

Trichinosis is caused by *Trichinella spiralis,* a roundworm that lives in the intestines of humans, pigs, bears, rats, and many other wild animals. Usually, humans acquire the disease by ingesting inadequately cooked pork that contains encysted larvae. Once ingested, the larvae are liberated by gastric fluid and rapidly mature. The adult female discharges larvae into the mucosa of the small intestine. These larvae migrate via blood and lymphatic tissue to most body tissues, becoming encysted in striated muscle.

Gastrointestinal symptoms of trichinosis include diarrhea, cramps, and malaise. With muscle invasion and inflammation, the client develops fever and muscle pain and tenderness, with edema and spasm. Other manifestations caused by larval dissemination include dyspnea and coughing; dysphagia; photophobia and conjunctivitis; rashes, weakness, and prostration.

Collaborative Care

As with other intestinal infections, the primary means of diagnosing helminthic disorders is examination of the stool for presence of ova and parasites. Enterobiasis is diagnosed by the presence of the parasite's eggs on the perianal skin or on cellulose tape placed over the anus. A CBC may also be ordered when helminthic diseases are suspected. Anemia may be present, particularly with hookworm disease. Eosinophilia (an increased percentage of eosinophils on the WBC differential) is common in helminthic disorders. With trichinosis, serum muscle enzymes such as the creatinine kinase (CK) and aspartate aminotransferase (AST) are typically elevated. Serologic testing for antibodies to the worm may also be performed. Blood, duodenal washings, and cerebrospinal fluid (CSF) may be examined for the presence of the trichinosis larvae. Inflamed muscle may be biopsied.

Ascariasis and enterobiasis are treated effectively with a single oral dose of pyrantel pamoate (Antiminth). Hookworm infection may require a 3-day course of the drug or, for clients with heavy infections, repeated doses every 2 weeks. Pyrantel pamoate is generally a safe drug requiring few precautions. Possible gastrointestinal side effects of vomiting and diarrhea can be minimized by administering after meals. Headache, dizziness, and drowsiness may also occur infrequently. Mebendazole (Vermox) is a good alternative to pyrantel pamoate. It is given as a one-time or three-day course of therapy, depending on the infection. Gastrointestinal side effects may occur, but they are typically mild. Treatment is followed with a stool culture at 2 weeks to evaluate its effectiveness. If necessary, an ad-

ditional course of treatment may be prescribed. Other members of the household are generally also treated.

Trichinosis treatment is generally supportive, because most clients recover spontaneously without long-term effects. The drug of choice in the intestinal phase of the disease is mebendazole for a 13-day course of therapy. Thiabendazole (Mintezol) may be used as an alternative, but has common central nervous system (CNS) side effects, including headache, weakness, vomiting, vertigo, and decreased mental alertness. This drug may also be used to manage the muscle phase of the disease. Clients often need hospitalization during this phase if the infection is severe. Corticosteroids may be used to reduce the inflammation and manage the symptoms (Tierney et al., 1994).

Nursing Care

Although nurses rarely encounter clients with helminthic disorders in the acute care setting, they are not uncommon in outpatient settings, particularly those where recent immigrants or travelers from tropical regions are seen. Because many clients with these disorders are asymptomatic, nurses need to be alert for histories that indicate risk and subtle manifestations of the disorder.

In providing care, take measures to minimize the risk of spreading these infections to other clients. As with all clients, the use of universal precautions is vital. In addition, follow enteric precautions, using gloves and gowns as necessary to prevent fecal contamination of hands and uniforms. On rare occasions, parasites may be present in the client's sputum or vomitus, so handle these secretions with care also. Disinfect toilets, toilet seats, and commodes after use by the client. To the client, emphasize the importance of washing hands after using the toilet and before handling food to prevent reinfection.

The client with a helminthic disorder may feel dirty or be ashamed of the disease, affecting their body image. While teaching the client about measures to prevent future infections, it is important to talk about the prevalence of these disorders. Assure the client that infection can occur despite good health practices when the eggs or larva of the organism are prevalent.

Other nursing diagnoses for consideration include *Diarrhea, Impaired Tissue Integrity,* and *Activity Intolerance.*

Client and Family Teaching

Although helminthic infections are not common in the United States, general health teaching should include measures to prevent infection.

Many of these disorders are acquired by ingesting food that has been fecally contaminated or contains larval forms of the organism. Emphasize the importance of not fertilizing food or grain crops with fecal material, particularly from human origin. Teach clients to cook all meats and fish adequately to destroy possible larvae. In general, pickled or salt-preserved meats and fish are no safer than raw. Smoking, another means of preserving fish and meat, may not achieve temperatures that are high enough to destroy the organisms. Vegetables grown in soil that may be contaminated with eggs or larvae should be peeled or cooked prior to eating.

Emphasize the importance of safe water supplies. Encourage people traveling to areas in which the purity of the water is questionable to drink only bottled water or carry purification tablets. Work with clients who have private water systems to ensure protection of the water from fecal contamination by either humans or animals.

Some helminthic disorders are spread by vectors, such as fleas, ticks, or arthropods, that infest flour and other grain products. Freezing grains prior to storage can destroy these arthropods. Encourage clients to store grain products in containers with tight-fitting lids (e.g., plastic storage containers). Clients should avoid touching the feces of domestic and wild animals. Discuss the importance of flea and tick control on family pets and the need to wash hands thoroughly after petting or touching animals.

Talk to affected clients and their families about measures to prevent spread of the disease in the household. Emphasize the importance of hygiene measures including changing bedding, daily cleaning of toilets with disinfectant, and, of course, hand washing.

▰ ▰ ▰ Chronic Inflammatory Bowel Disease ▰ ▰ ▰

Two inflammatory conditions affecting the bowel fall under the category of chronic inflammatory bowel disease: ulcerative colitis and Crohn's disease. These conditions have a number of similarities linking them. The etiologic origins of both illnesses are unknown, but both have a genetic component with increased incidence in some families and ethnic groups. Both affect primarily young adults between the ages of 15 and 35 years. Both are chronic and recurrent disease processes. Diarrhea is the predominant symptom of each; both may have associated manifestations, such as arthritis.

Despite all the similarities, there are also distinctive differences between ulcerative colitis and Crohn's disease. In ulcerative colitis, the large bowel is primarily affected in a continuous pattern, progressing distally to proximally. With Crohn's disease, a patchy pattern of involvement is seen, affecting primarily the small intestine. Ulcerative colitis shows mainly mucosal involvement; in Crohn's disease, the submucosal layers of the bowel are affected. A comparison of ulcerative colitis and Crohn's disease is found in Table 23–7.

The Client with Ulcerative Colitis

▰ ▰ ▰

Ulcerative colitis is a chronic inflammatory bowel disorder of the mucosa and submucosa of the colon and rectum. It affects primarily the young, with onset typically between the ages of 15 and 40 years. A second, smaller peak in the incidence of ulcerative colitis occurs in people between ages 50 and 70. Its annual incidence is 4 to 12 per 100,000 people. Although found worldwide, it is more common in Western countries (Way, 1994).

The cause of ulcerative colitis is unknown (Hampton & Bryant, 1992). There is a genetic component to the disease, as it occurs more frequently in families with a history of ulcerative colitis, Crohn's disease, and certain types of arthritis. Anticolon antibodies found in the serum of some clients with the disease suggest an autoimmune component to the disorder. Infection, dietary factors (such as ingested chemicals and fiber-poor foods), and environmental factors (such as smoking) may also play a role in development of the disease. Although stress and psychologic factors likely affect the severity of the illness, there is no evidence to support them as causes of ulcerative colitis.

Pathophysiology

Ulcerative colitis begins with inflammation at the base of the crypts of Lieberkühn in the distal large intestine and rectum (Figure 23–5). Initially, microscopic, pinpoint mucosal hemorrhages occur, and eventually crypt abscesses develop. These abscesses penetrate the superficial submucosa and spread laterally, leading to mucosal necrosis and sloughing. The inflammatory process leads to further tissue damage from exudates and the release of inflammatory mediators, such as prostaglandins and other cytokines (see Chapter 8 for further discussion of the inflammatory process). The mucosa becomes red because of vascular congestion, friable (easily broken), and edematous. It bleeds easily, and hemorrhage is common. Edema obscures the submucosal vessels and creates a granular appearance. Pseudopolyps, tonguelike projections of bowel mucosa into the lumen, are commonly found. These polypoid changes represent areas of edematous tissue between areas of ulceration. Chronic inflammation leads to shortening of the colon from fibrosis and loss of haustra (the normal saclike pouches of the colon).

Table 23–7   Characteristics of Ulcerative Colitis and Crohn's Disease

	Characteristic	**Ulcerative Colitis**	**Crohn's Disease**
Clinical	Gender	Equal	Equal
	Age at Onset	15 to 40 years; secondary peak between 50 and 70 years	10 to 30 years
	Course of disease	Typically chronic and intermittent	Slowly progressive, relapsing
	Diarrhea	5 to 30 stools per day with blood and mucus	Common, usually less severe than colitis, with no obvious blood or mucus in stool
	Abdominal pain	Cramping in left lower quadrant; relieved by defecation	Cramping or steady right lower quadrant or periumbilical pain; tenderness and mass noted in right lower quadrant
	Nutritional deficit	Common; involves anemia, hypoalbuminemia, and weight loss	Common and significant: involves anemia, weight loss, and multiple vitamin and mineral deficits
	Constitutional manifestations	Fever rare; may have associated arthritic, skin, or other organ involvement, such as erythema nodosum or uveitis	Fever, malaise, fatigue; may have same associated conditions plus urinary complications
Pathologic	Depth of involvement	Mucosa and submucosa	Transmural
	Portion of bowel involved	Typically rectum and sigmoid colon; may extend to involve entire large bowel	Any portion of GI tract; terminal ileum and ascending colon involvement predominates
	Distribution	Continuous from rectum	Patchy; skip lesions
	Appearance of mucosa	Granular, dull, hyperemic, friable; disease uniform in affected bowel; pseudopolyps may be seen	Cobblestone appearance, with areas of normal tissue surrounded by ulceration and fissures
Complications	Acute	Toxic megacolon, perforation, massive hemorrhage	Obstruction, fistulization, abscess formation, malabsorption
	Long-term	Carcinoma of colon or rectum common	Colon carcinoma in clients with colonic disease

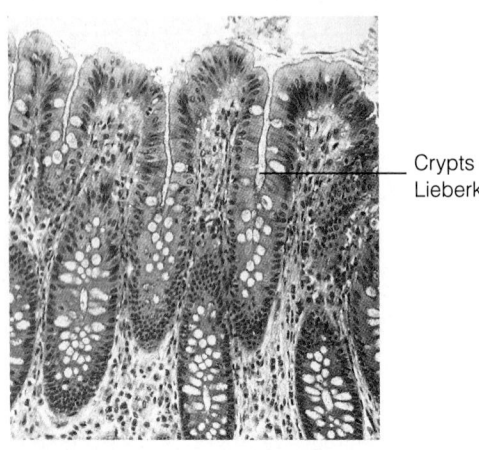

Crypts of Lieberkühn

Figure 23–5 Photomicrograph of the mucosa of the large intestine showing the entrances to the crypts of Lieberkühn. The crypts are the focal points for ulcerative colitis.

The inflammatory process begins at the rectosigmoid area of the anal canal and progresses proximally. In most clients, the disease is confined to the rectum and sigmoid colon. It may progress to involve the entire colon, stopping at the ileocecal junction. Blood, mucus, and pus pool in the lumen of the colon, accounting for the characteristic diarrhea. The extent of colon involvement generally correlates with the severity of the disease.

Chronic intermittent colitis, or recurrent *ulcerative colitis*, is the most common form of the disease. It is characterized by an insidious onset with attacks that last 1 to 3 months occurring at intervals of months to years. Typically, only the distal colon is affected, and few systemic manifestations occur (Price & Wilson, 1992). Diarrhea is the predominant symptom of all types of ulcerative colitis. Stools, which may number up to 30 to 40 per day, contain both blood and mucus. Nocturnal diarrhea may occur. *Chronic ulcerative colitis* can range in severity. Mild cases are characterized by the passage of fewer than four stools per day, intermittent rectal bleeding, mucus passage, and few constitutional symptoms. Severe cases can involve the passage of more than six to ten bloody stools per day, extensive colon involvement, anemia, hypovolemia, and evidence of nutritional impairment. Rectal inflammation causes the client to experience fecal urgency and tenesmus. Left lower quadrant cramping relieved by defecation is common. Other common systemic manifestations include fatigue, anorexia, and weakness.

Approximately 15% of people with ulcerative colitis develop *fulminant colitis,* with involvement of the entire colon, severe bloody diarrhea, acute abdominal pain, and fever. Clients with fulminant disease are at high risk for complications such as toxic megacolon (Porth, 1994).

Clients with severe disease also may have manifestations that are not directly related to inflammation of the colon but are associated with disease activity. A nondeforming arthritis involving one or several joints may occur, as well as other inflammatory conditions such as ankylosing spondylitis, *uveitis* (inflammation of the uvea, the vascular layer of the eye, which may also involve the sclera and cornea), or lesions of the skin and mucous membranes. Some clients develop thromboemboli, with blood vessel obstruction due to clots carried from the site of their formation. Lesions of the liver, gallbladder, and pancreas may also occur, as can pericarditis (Tierney et al., 1994; Way, 1994).

Ulcerative colitis predisposes the client to develop colorectal carcinoma. (Nugent, Haggitt, & Gilpin, 1991). Colorectal carcinoma may appear 5 to 8 years after onset of ulcerative colitis. The risk of cancer in clients with ulcerative colitis is 30% at 35 years after the diagnosis and 49% for clients who were under the age of 15 at the time of diagnosis (Podolsky, 1991).

Complications such as perforation of the colon, toxic megacolon, and massive hemorrhage may occur and necessitate a colectomy (surgical removal of the colon). Of these complications, colonic perforation is the leading cause of death in clients with ulcerative colitis. The risk of perforation increases with the extent and severity of the disease; it is particularly high in clients with toxic megacolon. Severe attacks of toxic megacolon, a condition characterized by acute paralysis of colonic motor function with rapid dilation of the colon to greater than 6 cm, may occur over segments or over all of the colon. Toxic megacolon occurs most often in the transverse segment of the large bowel. Signs and symptoms of this life-threatening complication include elevated temperature, tachycardia, hypotension, dehydration, abdominal tenderness and cramping, electrolyte disturbance, an improvement or reduction in diarrhea (Jagelman, 1992). Massive hemorrhage, uncommon in ulcerative colitis, may also lead to emergency colectomy.

Collaborative Care

Collaborative care for the client with ulcerative colitis begins with establishing the extent and severity of the disease. There is no specific therapy for this disorder; treatment is supportive and includes pharmacologic and dietary measures to decrease inflammation, promote intestinal rest and healing, and reduce intestinal motility. Surgical intervention may be necessary, however, depending on the response to medical therapy and the severity of the disease.

Laboratory and Diagnostic Tests

The diagnosis of ulcerative colitis does not require extensive testing in order to be determined. Sigmoidoscopy, which provides for visual examination of the bowel mucosa, is generally used to establish the diagnosis with clients presenting with a typical history and physical examination findings. Additional laboratory and diagnostic tests are used to evaluate systemic responses to the disease. The following laboratory tests may be ordered:

- *Examination of stool for the presence of blood and mucus and stool cultures* are performed to rule out infectious causes of bowel inflammation and diarrhea.
- *Hemoglobin and hematocrit levels* may be decreased, indicating anemia due to intestinal bleeding.
- *Serum albumin* may be decreased as a result of protein loss from diarrhea and nutritional deficits.
- *Liver function tests* are performed to assess for possible accompanying sclerosing cholangitis (hardened, inflamed bile ducts). Liver enzymes, such as ALT, alkaline phosphatase, AST, GGTP, and LDH will be elevated if sclerosing cholangitis is present, as will the total bilirubin level.

The following diagnostic tests may be ordered:

- *Sigmoidoscopy* is performed to allow visual inspection of the bowel mucosa. Edema, inflammation, mucus and pus, a friable granular appearance, and crypt abscesses may be seen. Nursing implications for the client having a sigmoidoscopy are listed in the box on page 767.
- *Colonoscopy* may also be conducted to visualize changes in the intestinal mucosa beyond the sigmoid colon and help determine the extent of the disease. Endoscopy poses a risk of perforation, particularly if the disease is active and severe. Nursing implications for the client having a colonoscopy are described in the box on page 774.
- *Rectal biopsy,* if performed, indicates inflammatory changes of the intestinal mucosa characteristic of ulcerative colitis.

Nursing Implications for Pharmacology: Chronic Inflammatory Bowel Disease

SULFASALAZINE (AZULFIDINE)

Sulfasalazine is an anti-inflammatory drug used for its local effect on the intestinal mucosa in ulcerative colitis and Crohn's disease. The active part of the drug is 5-aminosalicylic acid, which inhibits prostaglandin production in the bowel. Prostaglandin is an important mediator of the inflammatory process; blocking its production reduces inflammation.

Nursing Responsibilities

- Assess the client for contraindications to sulfasalazine, including pregnancy or a history of hypersensitivity to sulfonamides or salicylates.
- Prior to initiating therapy, assess baseline values for renal function tests (serum creatinine, BUN, urinalysis), liver function tests, and CBC.
- Administer the drug as ordered. Suppositories or retention enemas may be administered at bedtime. Administer oral forms with a full glass of water.
- Have resuscitation equipment available; anaphylactic responses may occur.
- Evaluate the client for therapeutic response, including reduction in the number of stools, reduction in mucus and blood, and improvement in stool consistency.
- Monitor the client for possible adverse responses:
  a. Skin rash, dermatitis, urticaria, or pruritus
  b. Evidence of blood dyscrasias, such as bleeding, easy bruising, fever
  c. Leukopenia, thrombocytopenia, hemolytic anemia, or angranulocytosis
  d. Changes in urinary output or renal function studies
  e. Evidence of hepatitis or myocarditis

Client and Family Teaching

- Take oral preparations after meals to decrease nausea, vomiting, and abdominal discomfort.
- Drink at least 2 quarts of fluid per day to reduce the risk of kidney damage.

- Use sunscreen to prevent burns; this drug increases a person's sensitivity to sun.
- Do not take aspirin, vitamin C, or any other over-the-counter medications containing aspirin or vitamin C without consulting with the primary care provider.
- This medication may interfere with the effectiveness of oral contraceptives; use alternative methods of contraception.
- Notify the primary care provider if signs of an adverse reaction occur, such as skin rash or hives, sore throat or mouth, bleeding gums, joint pain, easy bruising, or fever.

MESALAMINE (ROWASA) AND OLSALAZINE (DIPENTUM)

Mesalamine and olsalazine contain the same active ingredient, 5-aminosalicylic acid, as sulfasalazine, but cause fewer adverse effects. Their mechanism of action is the same as that of sulfasalazine. These drugs are available as suppositories, suspension for enema, or oral tablets.

Nursing Responsibilities

- Assess the client for possible contraindications such as pregnancy, lactation, or hypersensitivity to these drugs or aspirin.
- Administer the drug as ordered. Give daily enemas or suppositories at bedtime. If more than one dose per day is ordered, space doses evenly over the 24-hour period.
- Evaluate the client for desired effects (as for sulfasalazine) and potential adverse effects:
  a. Nausea, diarrhea, abdominal cramps, or flatulence
  b. CNS effects including headache, dizziness, insomnia, weakness, or fatigue
  c. Rash or itching
  d. Flulike symptoms, general malaise

- *Abdominal X-ray studies* performed with or without contrast media are used to demonstrate shortening of the colon; loss of haustra; irregularities in the intestinal mucosa, including polyps and ulcers; or complications such as a dilated colon in toxic megacolon. A barium enema may be performed, but not during acute flare-ups of ulcerative colitis because of the danger of intestinal perforation. Nursing implications for the client

receiving a barium enema are listed in the box on page 773.

Pharmacology

The ultimate goal of care is to terminate acute attacks as quickly as possible and reduce the incidence of relapse. Pharmacologic management is a key component used to achieve this goal. Locally acting and systemic anti-inflam-

Pharmacology: Chronic Inflammatory Bowel Disease (continued)

Client and Family Teaching

- Teach the client the recommended method of administration, including how to insert rectal suppositories or administer a retention enema.
- Shake suspension forms well prior to using.
- Diarrhea is the most common side effect of these drugs. Notify the primary care provider if adverse effects occur.

CORTICOSTEROIDS

Methylprednisolone (Medrol, Solu-Medrol)	Prednisolone (Delta-Cortef)
	Prednisone

Glucocorticoids are hormones normally produced by the cortex of the adrenal glands. These hormones affect the metabolism of carbohydrates, proteins, and fat in the body and are necessary for the stress response. Cortisol, the main glucocorticoid, has potent anti-inflammatory effects. Corticosteroids are used to treat acute episodes of ulcerative colitis. Because of their multiple and significant side effects, they are not used to maintain remission.

Nursing Responsibilities

- Assess the client for conditions that may be adversely affected by corticosteroid administration: peptic ulcer disease, glaucoma or cataracts, diabetes, or psychiatric disorders.
- Obtain baseline vital signs and weight; monitor both routinely while the client remains on corticosteroid therapy. Hypertension and weight gain may result from salt and water retention.
- Monitor intake and output; assess for edema.
- Administer the drug as ordered. For daily or alternate-day dosing, administer corticosteroids in the morning, when physiologic glucocorticoid levels are highest, to reduce adrenal cortisone suppression.
- Administer oral preparations with food to decrease gastrointestinal side effects. Antacids or histamine H_2-receptor blocking agents, such as cimetidine

(Tagamet), may be prescribed while the client is on corticosteroid therapy.
- Monitor the client for desired effects: reduced diarrhea, less blood and mucus in the stool, and less abdominal cramping.
- Monitor the client for adverse effects:
  a. Increased susceptibility to infection and masking of early signs of infection
  b. Hyperglycemia
  c. Hypokalemia, as manifested by muscle weakness, nausea, vomiting, and cardiac rhythm disturbances
  d. Edema, hypertension, and signs of cardiac failure due to fluid overload
  e. Peptic ulcer formation and possible gastrointestinal hemorrhage, as manifested by abdominal pain, black or tarry stools, and signs of bleeding
  f. Changes in mental status, including depression, euphoria, aggression, and behavioral changes
  g. With long-term use, Cushingoid effects, such as abnormal fat deposits in the face (moon faces) and trunk (buffalo hump), muscle wasting and thin extremities, thinning of the skin, and osteoporosis

Client and Family Teaching

- Take the drug as prescribed; do not change the dose or time of day. Do not stop the medication abruptly. The dose will be tapered down gradually when the drug is discontinued.
- Notify the physician if adverse or Cushingoid effects occur.
- Take the medication with food or at mealtimes to decrease the gastrointestinal effects.
- Monitor body weight. If a gain of more than five pounds is noted, notify the physician.
- Moderate salt intake and avoid foods and snacks high in sodium, such as processed meats and potato chips. Increase intake of foods high in potassium, such as fruits, vegetables, and lean meats.
- Carry a card or wear a bracelet or tag at all times identifying corticosteroid use.

matory drugs are the primary medications used to manage ulcerative colitis.

Sulfasalazine (Azulfidine) is a sulfonamide antibiotic that is poorly absorbed from the gastrointestinal tract and acts topically on the colonic mucosa to inhibit the inflammatory process (Hampton & Bryant, 1992). Sulfasalazine may be administered by enema when the colitis is confined to the rectum and sigmoid colon, or orally for more

extensive disease. Mesalamine (Rowasa) and olsalazine are related drugs available as suppositories, as a suspension for administration by enema, or in sustained-release oral tablets. They have the advantage of causing fewer adverse effects than sulfasalazine. Nursing implications for these drugs are outlined in the accompanying pharmacology box.

Table 23–8 Low-Residue Diet

Food Group	Allowed	Avoid
Beverages	Coffee, teas, juices, carbonated beverages; milk limited to 2 cups per day	Alcohol, prune juice
Breads and cereals	Products made from refined flours (white bread, crackers) or finely milled grains (e.g., corn flakes, crisp rice cereal, puffed wheat); cooked cereals without whole grains	Whole-grain breads, rolls, or cereal; breads or rolls with seeds, nuts, or bran
Desserts	Gelatins, tapioca, plain custards, or puddings; angel-food or sponge cake; ice cream or frozen desserts without fruit or nuts	Any desserts containing dried fruits, nuts, seeds, or coconut; rich pastries, pies
Fruits	Fruit juices and strained fruits; cooked or canned apples, apricots, cherries, peaches, pears; bananas	All other raw or cooked fruits
Meats and other protein sources	Roasted, baked, or broiled tender or ground beef, veal, pork, lamb, poultry, or fish; smooth peanut butter; cottage, cream, American, or mild chedder cheeses in small amounts	Tough or spiced meats and those prepared by frying; highly flavored cheeses; nuts
Potatoes, rice, and pasta	Peeled potatoes; white rice; most pasta products	Potato skins, potato chips, or fried potatoes; brown rice; whole-grain pasta products
Sweets	Sugar, honey, jelly, hard candy and gumdrops, plain chocolates	Jam, marmalade; candy made with seeds, nuts, coconut
Vegetables	Vegetable juices and strained vegetables; cooked or canned vegetables	Raw or whole cooked vegetables
Other	Salt, ground seasonings; cream sauce and plain gravy	Chili sauce, horseradish; popcorn, seeds of any kind; whole spices, olives, vinegar

Note. From *Nutrition and Diet Therapy* by C. A. Lutz and K. R. Przytulski, 1994, Philadelphia: F. A. Davis; and *Nutrition and Diet Therapy* (6th ed.) by S. R. Williams, 1989, St. Louis: Times Mirror/Mosby.

For an acute episode, corticosteroids are also used to reduce inflammation. Local or topical forms of the drug are preferred to reduce the incidence of systemic side effects. Hydrocortisone can be administered by enema; if necessary, oral prednisone may be prescribed. Intravenous methylprednisolone is used to terminate an acute, severe attack of ulcerative colitis. Immunosuppression with azathioprine (Imuran) or cyclosprine (Sandimmune) may be used to maintain remission for some clients.

Antidiarrheal agents, such as loperamide and diphenoxylate, may be given to slow gastrointestinal motility and reduce diarrhea. These drugs are safe for use in clients with mild, chronic symptoms, but they are not given during acute attacks because they may precipitate toxic dilation of the colon.

Dietary Management

Dietary management for clients with chronic ulcerative colitis is individualized. Generally, a diet free of milk products, caffeine, and gas-producing or raw fruits and vegetables is recommended. Bulk-forming agents, such as bran, psyllium, or methylcellulose, may be used to decrease diarrhea and relieve rectal symptoms.

During an acute exacerbation of ulcerative colitis, the client is usually kept NPO. Total parenteral nutrition (TPN) is administered to maintain the client's nutritional status. In the presence of less severe symptoms or as the acute episode begins to resolve, an elemental diet such as Ensure, which contains all essential nutrients in a residue-free formula, may be prescribed. These measures are undertaken to reduce intestinal motility and allow the bowel to rest.

Surgery

Surgical removal of the colon effects a cure for the client with ulcerative colitis. For most clients, however, this is not the initial treatment of choice because of its anticipated effects on bowel function, self-image, and social interactions (Tierney et al., 1994). Conservative medical management is preferred, and surgical treatment is used only when the disease resists treatment. Indications for surgical therapy may include frequent exacerbations,

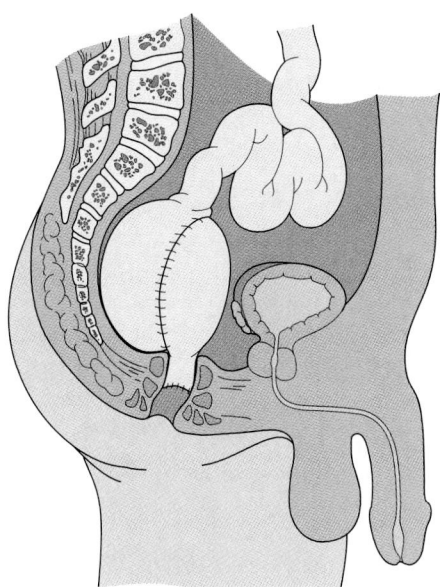

Figure 23–6 Ileoanal anastomosis with reservoir.

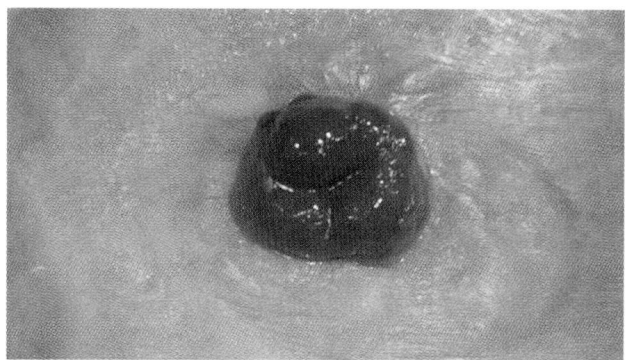

Figure 23–7 A healthy-appearing stoma.

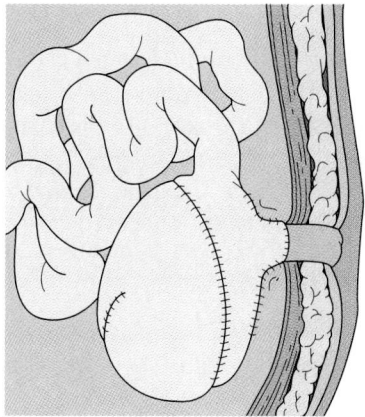

Figure 23–8 Kock's (continent) ileostomy.

chronic continuous symptoms, malnutrition, weakness, and interference with ability to work or enjoy social and sexual activities (Way, 1994). Dependence on corticosteroids to maintain long-term remission is another possible indication for surgery. Acute complications of ulcerative colitis, such as toxic megacolon, perforation, or hemorrhage, may require emergency surgical intervention.

The procedure of choice for most clients having surgery for ulcerative colitis is a *total colectomy with ileoanal anastomosis,* also called a restorative proctocolectomy or ileal pouch-anal anastomosis. In this procedure, the entire colon and rectum are removed; a pouch is formed from the terminal ileum; and the pouch is brought into the pelvis and anastomosed to the anal canal (Figure 23–6). A temporary or loop ileostomy (described below) is generally performed at the same time and is maintained for 2 to 3 months to allow healing of the anal anastomosis. When the anastomosis sites are healed, the ileostomy is closed, and the client has bowel movements through the anus.

Advanced age, obesity, or other factors may preclude an ileoanal anastomosis. For these clients, a permanent ileostomy or continent ileostomy may be used.

An intestinal **ostomy** is a surgically created opening between the intestine and the abdominal wall which allows the passage of fecal material. The surface opening is called a **stoma** (Figure 23–7).

The precise name of the ostomy depends on the location of the stoma. An **ileostomy** is an ostomy made in the ileum of the small intestine. In an ileostomy, the colon is usually completely removed.

The three most common types of ileostomy are total proctocolectomy with permanent ileostomy; Kock's

ileostomy (also called continent ileostomy); and a temporary or loop ileostomy.

Total proctocolectomy with permanent ileostomy involves removal of the colon, the rectum, and the anus. The anal canal is closed, and the end of the terminal ileum is brought to the body surface through the right abdominal wall to form the stoma.

A *Kock's ileostomy,* or *continent ileostomy,* involves construction of an intra-abdominal reservoir from the terminal ileum (Figure 23–8). Stool collects in the internal pouch until the client drains it with a catheter. A nipple valve prevents leakage of stool between catheterizations.

A *temporary* or *loop ileostomy* is often used to eliminate feces and allow tissue healing for 2 to 3 months following an ileoanal anastomosis. A loop of ileum is brought to the body surface to form a stoma and allow stool drainage into an external pouch. When the ileostomy is no longer necessary, a second surgery is performed to close the stoma and repair the bowel, restoring fecal elimination through the anus.

Nursing care of the client with an ileostomy is outlined in the box on page 814. Procedure 23–1 on page 816 describes how to apply one- and two-piece drainable ostomy pouches.

text continues on page 816

Nursing Care of the Client with an Ileostomy

PREOPERATIVE CARE

- Discuss the impending surgery and the client's concerns regarding surgery and the presence of an ileostomy. Listen actively to the client's responses and concerns. *Open discussion and active listening are important means of gaining the client's trust and encouraging expression of physical, psychologic, and social concerns about the surgery.*

- Provide or refer the client to an enterostomal therapist for teaching about the location of the stoma, ostomy care, and options for ostomy appliances. *It is important to begin teaching prior to surgery to facilitate the client's learning and acceptance of the ostomy postoperatively.*

- Advise the client of the availability of a local United Ostomy Association chapter, and provide a referral as necessary or desired. *Local chapters often have members with ostomies who are willing to provide both preoperative and postoperative teaching, listening, and support for clients.*

- Provide preoperative bowel preparation as ordered. *Cathartics, enemas, and preoperative antibiotics are often ordered to reduce the risk of abdominal contamination and infection after surgery.*

POSTOPERATIVE CARE

- Apply an ostomy pouch over the stoma. (Application of one- and two-piece drainable ostomy pouches is described in Procedure 23–1.) *Stool from an ileostomy is expressed continuously or irregularly, and it is liquid in nature; continuous use of a pouch to collect the drainage is therefore necessary.*

- Assess the client frequently for bleeding, stoma viability, and function. In the early postoperative period, small amounts of blood in the pouch are expected. A healthy stoma appears pink or red and moist as a result of mucus production (Figure 23–7). It should protrude approximately 2 cm from the abdominal wall. *Frequent assessment is particularly important in the initial postoperative period to ensure stoma health and monitor for possible complications. A dusky, brown, black, or white stoma indicates circulatory compromise. Other possible stoma complications include retraction (indentation or loss of the external portion of the stoma); or prolapse (outward telescoping of the stoma, that is, an abnormally long stoma).*

- As the stoma starts to function, empty the pouch, explaining the procedure to the client. The initial effluent (drainage) from the ileum is dark green, vis-cid, and usually odorless. The effluent gradually thickens and becomes yellow-brown. Empty the pouch when it is one-third full. Measure the drainage, and include it as output on intake and output records. Rinse the pouch and reapply the clamp. *Emptying the pouch when it is no more than one-third full helps prevent the skin seal from breaking as a result of the weight of the pouch. Because of the potential for excess fluid loss through ileostomy drainage, it is important to include it as fluid output.*

- Assess the peristomal skin. Skin around the stoma should remain clean and pink and free of irritation, rashes, inflammation, or excoriation. *Skin complications may arise from appliance irritation or hypersensitivity, excoriation from a leaking appliance, or Candida albicans, a yeast infection.*

- Protect peristomal skin from enzymes and bile salts in the ileostomy effluent. Using a skin barrier on the pouch is essential. Change the pouch if any sign of leakage occurs or if the client complains of burning or itching skin. *Enzymes and bile salts normally reabsorbed in the large intestine are very irritating to the skin. Excoriation of skin surrounding the stoma not only impairs the client's first line of defense against microorganisms but also can interfere with the ability to achieve a tight skin seal and prevent pouch leakage.*

- Report the following abnormal assessment findings to the physician:
  a. Allergic or contact dermatitis. *A rash may result from contact with fecal drainage or indicate sensitivity to pouch, paste, tape, or sealant.*
  b. Purulent ulcerated areas surrounding the stoma. *Disruption of the protective barrier of the skin allows bacterial entry.*
  c. A red, bumpy, itchy rash or white-coated area. *This is a manifestation of* Candida albicans, *a yeast infection.*
  d. Bulging around the stoma. *This finding may indicate herniation, caused by loops of intestine protruding through the abdominal wall.*

- Apply protective ointments to the perirectal area of clients with newly functioning ileoanal reservoirs and anastomoses. *This helps protect the skin from the initial stools. As stools thicken and become fewer per day, the client experiences less perirectal irritation.*

CLIENT AND FAMILY TEACHING

- While applying the pouch, explain the procedure to the client. *For the client with an ileostomy, teaching is*

Nursing Care of the Client with an Ileostomy (continued)

immediate and ongoing to facilitate acceptance of the ostomy and self-care.

- Teach the client to manage the clamp on the pouch, to empty and rinse it, and to perform pouch changes. *Self-care is vital to the client's independence and self-esteem.*

- Instruct the client to use an electric razor to shave the peristomal hair if necessary. *An electric razor prevents accidental cutting of the stoma with a razor blade.*

- Teach the client to check the stoma and peristomal skin with each pouch change. *Ongoing assessment is important for optimal health and function of the stoma and surrounding skin. Stripping of tape or excessively frequent pouch removal may cause mechanical trauma to peristomal skin. Chronic skin irritation by ileostomy effluent may lead to the development of* pseudoveracous *lesions, or wartlike nodules.*

- Instruct the client to report any abnormal appearance of the stoma or surrounding skin (as noted previously and below) to the physician:
  a. Narrowing of the lumen of the stoma. *This is indicative of stenosis and may interfere with fecal elimination.*
  b. Lacerations or cuts in the stoma. *The stoma contains no nerves, so the client may not experience pain if the stoma undergoes trauma.*
  c. Separation of the stoma from the abdominal surface. *This potential complication may require surgical repair.*

- Emphasize the need to maintain an adequate fluid and salt intake; the client is at increased risk for dehydration and hyponatremia, particularly when the client is active in hot weather, when fluid is lost through perspiration as well as ileostomy effluent. Low-salt diets and diuretic therapy increase the client's risk and should generally be avoided. Water intake should be sufficient to maintain pale urine and an output of at least 1 quart per day. When exercising in hot weather, the client should consume extra water and salt. High-potassium foods, such as bananas and oranges, may also be recommended. *Loss of the reabsorptive surface of the large bowel increases the amount of water and sodium loss in the stool. If the ileostomy is high (more proximal in the ileum), additional potassium losses may also occur.*

- Discuss signs and symptoms of fluid and electrolyte imbalances:
  a. Extreme thirst
  b. Dry skin and oral mucous membrane

  c. Decreased urine output
  d. Weakness, fatigue
  e. Muscle cramps
  f. Abdominal cramps, nausea, vomiting
  g. Shortness of breath
  h. Orthostatic hypotension (feeling faint when suddenly changing positions)

- Discuss dietary concerns with the client. A low-residue diet is recommended initially (Table 23–8 on page 812). Foods that may cause excessive odor or gas are typically avoided as well. *Because food blockage is a potential problem, the client is taught to limit high-fiber foods, chewing them well when they are consumed, and to avoid foods that may cause blockage, such as popcorn, corn, nuts, cucumbers, celery, fresh tomatoes, figs, strawberries, blackberries, and caraway seeds. Symptoms of food blockage include abdominal cramping, swelling of the stoma, and absence of ileostomy output for over 4 to 6 hours.*

- Teach the client self-care measures to relieve food blockage:
  a. Take a warm shower or tub bath. *This can help relax the abdominal muscles.*
  b. Assume a knee-chest position. *The knee-chest position reduces intra-abdominal pressure.*
  c. Drink warm fluids or grape juice if not vomiting. *This provides a mild cathartic effect.*
  d. Massage peristomal area. *Massage may stimulate peristalsis and fecal elimination.*
  e. Remove pouch if the stoma is swollen, and apply a pouch with a larger opening. *If the stoma swells, the pouch may create a mechanical obstruction to output.*

- Notify the physician or enterostomal therapy nurse if
  a. The above measures fail to relieve the obstruction.
  b. Signs of a partial obstruction persist, including high-volume odorous fluid output, abdominal cramps, nausea, and vomiting.
  c. There is no ileostomy output for 4 to 6 hours.
  d. Signs of fluid and electrolyte imbalance occur, such as weakness, dizziness, light-headedness, or headache.

  Should self-care measures not succeed in breaking up a blockage, the client may need an ileostomy lavage, as described in Procedure 23–2 on page 817.

Procedure 23–1 Changing a One-Piece or Two-Piece Drainable Ostomy Pouch

SUPPLIES

- One-piece or two-piece pouch
- Skin barrier paste
- Skin prep
- Clamp
- Deodorant
- Measuring guide
- Adhesive remover wipe
- Skin cleanser
- Washcloths
- Plastic bag

COMMENTS

Explain the procedure to the client and provide for the client's privacy. Follow universal precautions.

PROCEDURE

1. Remove soiled pouch (and the skin barrier flange if the client has a two-piece pouch) by gently pulling on the pouch or flange and pushing on skin. Use an adhesive remover wipe to remove the skin barrier paste.

2. Empty the pouch, discarding it and the flange (if applicable) in a plastic bag. Save the tail closure (clamp). The pouch from a two-piece system may be cleaned out and reused.

3. Cleanse the skin and stoma with warm water and skin cleanser or mild soap. Rinse the skin and stoma, and pat dry.

4. Note the color of the stoma and the condition of the peristomal skin, as discussed in the nursing care box on page 814.

5. If necessary, clip or shave peristomal hair.

6. Use a measuring guide or previous pattern to check size of stoma (Figure 23–9A).
   a. Pre-sized pouch: check to verify that size is correct.
   b. Cut-to-fit pouch or flange: Trace the correct size of the stoma onto the back of the flange, and cut the opening to match the pattern. The opening should be no more than 1/8 inch larger than stoma.

7. Protect the skin that was covered by a wafer, pouch, or tape with an application of skin prep. Allow the skin to dry.

8. Remove the backings from pouch or flange.

9. Apply a bead of skin barrier paste around the base of stoma or around the opening of the pouch or flange. Allow the paste to air-dry for 1 to 2 minutes.

10. Center the pouch or flange over the stoma, and press to adhere (Figure 23–9B).

11. For a two-piece pouch, snap the pouch onto skin barrier flange.

12. Place deodorizing tablets or a few drops of liquid pouch deodorizer (in some cases, antiseptic mouthwash may be used) in the pouch. Apply the clamp.

13. "Picture frame" the pouch with tape to provide extra security.

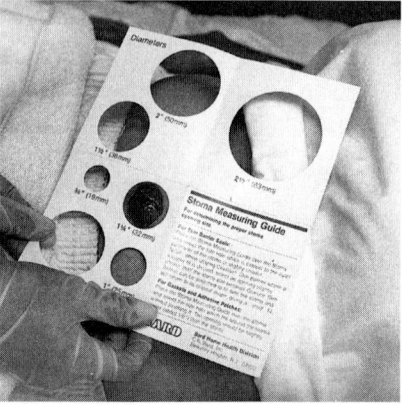
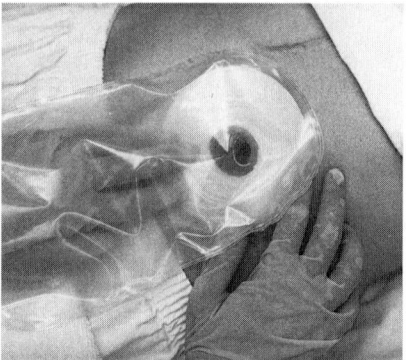

A   B

Figure 23–9 *A,* A guide for measuring the stoma. *B,* Applying the disposable pouch.

Nursing Care

Nursing care of the client with ulcerative colitis is directed at relieving abdominal cramping, providing emotional support, and teaching the client about the illness and special care needs. The priority nursing diagnoses for this client are related to the persistent diarrhea and the potential for body image disturbance due to the disease and prescribed treatments.

Diarrhea

During an acute exacerbation of ulcerative colitis, clients can experience frequent, painful diarrhea. The frequency of defecation and associated abdominal pain and cramping may interfere with the client's ADLs and place the client at risk for fluid volume deficit and impaired skin integrity.

Nursing interventions with rationales follow:

Procedure 23–2 Ileostomy Lavage

SUPPLIES

- Disposable irrigation sleeve
- 60-mL catheter-tipped syringe
- #14 Fr. catheter
- Water-soluble lubricant
- Normal saline for irrigation
- Bedpan
- Clean ostomy pouch

COMMENTS

Explain the procedure to the client and provide for the privacy of the client. Follow universal precautions.

PROCEDURE

1. Remove the pouch. Apply disposable irrigation sleeve.
2. Clamp the bottom of the sleeve, or place it into the bedpan.
3. Gently perform digital examination of stoma to break up any mass proximal to stoma and determine direction of the bowel.
4. Lubricate a #14 Fr. catheter, and insert it into the stoma until blockage is reached. If the catheter does not reach the blockage after 8 to 10 cm, notify the physician. This may indicate a more proximal obstruction.
5. Instill 30 to 50 mL of normal saline.
6. Remove the catheter. Allow it to drain.
7. Repeat the procedure until the mass is removed.
8. When the blockage is removed, remove the irrigation sleeve.
9. Clean peristomal skin.
10. Apply the pouch and clamp.

POSTPROCEDURE

1. Document the procedure, the amount of solution used, consistency of results, and the client's tolerance of the procedure.
2. Discuss dietary concerns at this time to help determine cause of blockage.

- Monitor the appearance and frequency of bowel movements using a stool chart. *The severity of diarrhea often correlates well with the severity of the disease and is an indicator of the need for fluid replacement.*

- Monitor for the presence of blood in stools by testing for occult blood as well as observing for bright red bleeding. *An increase in the amount of blood may indicate the need for blood replacement and/or emergency surgery because of hemorrhage.*

- Assess and document the color, amount, and frequency of diarrhea and, if present, emesis. Maintain accurate intake and output records. *Documentation of fluid loss is needed to monitor adequate fluid replacement.*

- Assess and document vital signs every 4 hours. *Elevated temperature, cardiac rate, and respiratory rate may indicate fluid volume deficit.*

- Record the client's weight daily. *A reduction in weight can indicate dehydration from persistent diarrhea.*

- Assess the client for other indications of fluid deficit: warm, dry skin, poor skin turgor, dry shiny mucous membranes, weakness, lethargy, complaints of thirst. *Thirst is an early symptom of dehydration; other signs are frequently present as well.*

- Administer prescribed anti-inflammatory and antidiarrheal medications as indicated. *Anti-inflammatory medications are important in mediating the severity of the disease and its manifestations. Unless contraindicated by complications, antidiarrheal medications help reduce fluid loss and increase the client's comfort.*

- Maintain fluid intake by mouth or by parenteral means as indicated. *Adequate fluid replacement is vital for the client with ulcerative colitis. If an elemental diet or total parenteral nutrition is prescribed, additional fluids may be necessary to meet the client's needs.*

- Provide good skin care. *The client with a fluid deficit is at increased risk for skin excoriations or breakdown.*

- Assess the perianal area for irritation or denuded skin from the diarrhea. Provide measures to protect the perianal area. Use gentle cleansing agents, such as Periwash or Tucks, or cottonballs saturated with witch hazel. A zinc oxide–based cream, such as Critic Aid, is useful in providing skin protection. *Digestive enzymes in the stool are very corrosive to the skin, increasing the risk of breakdown where skin is exposed to diarrheal stool (Tucker, Canobbio, Paquette, & Wells, 1992).*

Body Image Disturbance

The client with ulcerative colitis may experience frustration at not being able to control, or even predict, fecal elimination, particularly when the disease is severe. Diarrhea can interfere with the ability to complete a task

Role of the Enterostomal Therapy Nurse

■ ■ ■

An enterostomal therapy nurse (ET nurse) is specially trained to care for and teach clients with ostomies, draining wounds, fistulas, urinary and fecal incontinence, and special skin care problems. The ET nurse is an RN, usually with a bachelor's degree in nursing, who has completed a 6- to 8-week program in enterostomal therapy nursing. ET nurses may become certified by passing an examination, which must be repeated every 5 years.

The ET nurse assesses, plans, implements, and evaluates ostomy care for clients on an inpatient and outpatient basis. The ET nurse serves as a consultant for clients with complex wound and drainage problems and participates in educational programs for health care staff and students. The ET nurse also provides emotional support for clients and their family members and usually serves as an advisor to the local United Ostomy Association Support Group.

satisfactorily, maintain employment, take part in social activities, and even meet basic needs such as eating, sleeping, and sexual activity. As a result, the client's body image can suffer. Treatment of ulcerative colitis, be it total colectomy with ileoanal anastomosis, ileostomy, or chronic corticosteroid therapy can also affect the client's view of self.

Nursing interventions with rationales follow:

■ Accept the client's feelings and perception of self. *Negating or denying the reality of the client's perception impairs trust.*

■ Encourage the client to discuss physical changes and their consequences that have affected his or her self-concept. *This demonstrates acceptance and gives the client an opportunity to express the impact of the disease and its treatment on his or her life.*

■ Encourage discussion about concerns regarding the effect of the disease or treatment on close personal relationships. *This demonstrates understanding of the client and the disease and provides an opportunity for the client to express feelings about its impact on relationships and significant others.*

■ Encourage the client to make choices and decisions regarding care. *This increases the client's sense of control.*

■ Discuss possible effects of treatment options openly and honestly. *Open discussion allows the client to make more informed decisions.*

■ Involve the client in care, providing teaching and instruction as needed. *This encourages and facilitates independence and decision making.*

■ Provide care in an accepting, nonjudgmental manner. *Acceptance of the client despite potential embarrassment about odors or diarrhea enhances self-esteem.*

■ Arrange for interaction with other clients or groups of people with ulcerative colitis or ostomies. *The client may feel that no one who has not experienced a similar problem can understand his or her feelings.*

■ Teach coping strategies (odor control, dietary modifications, and so on), and support the client's use of them. *This facilitates healthy adaptation to the disease.*

Other Nursing Diagnoses

Other nursing diagnoses that may be appropriate for the client with ulcerative colitis follow:

■ *Pain* related to disease process

■ *Fluid Volume Deficit* related to multiple diarrhea stools

■ *Altered Sexuality Patterns* related to feelings of loss of control over body functions

■ *Ineffective Individual Coping* related to effect of disease on ADLs and life-style

■ *Knowledge Deficit* of the disease process and its treatment

■ *Social Isolation* related to frequent diarrhea

Client and Family Teaching

Teach the client and family about ulcerative colitis, including the disease process, short- and long-term effects, and the relationship of stress to exacerbations of the illness. Provide information about prescribed medications, including drug names, desired effects, schedules for tapering the doses if ordered (as with corticosteroids), and possible side effects or adverse reactions and their management. Provide verbal and written instructions about the recommended diet, and make a referral to a dietitian as necessary. Emphasize the need to maintain a fluid intake of at least 2 to 3 quarts per day to compensate for additional fluid losses through the stool. Tell the client to drink additional fluid when the weather is very warm, during exercise or strenuous work, or if feverish.

Discuss the increased risk for colorectal cancer and the need for medical follow-up with periodic checkups. Talk about various treatment options and the risks and benefits of each.

If surgical intervention is planned or has been done, provide instruction about the surgery and follow-up care. Contact an enterostomal therapy (ET) nurse (see the accompanying box) to meet with the client and family. Teach the client who has a proctocolectomy with ileostomy how to care for the ileostomy. In addition, provide verbal and written instructions to the client and family about what foods to avoid, how to avoid dehydration, and where to obtain ostomy supplies. Discuss the use of over-the-counter medications, such as enteric-coated and timed-release capsules that may not be absorbed adequately before elimination through the ileostomy. Inform the client of various ostomy support groups in the community, such as the Foundation for Colitis and Ileitis and the United Ostomy Association. Make a community health care agency referral if needed to assist in the care of the client after discharge.

When a colectomy with ileoanal anastomosis and temporary ileostomy has been performed, emphasize to the client that the ileostomy will be eliminated surgically once the anastomoses have healed. After that time, the client will eliminate feces through the anus as before. Five to seven loose bowel movements per day without problems of incontinence usually result from this procedure.

Applying the Nursing Process

Case Study of a Client with Ulcerative Colitis: Cortez Lewis

Cortez Lewis is a 42-year-old real estate agent and mother of three school-age children. She has had ulcerative colitis for 18 years and has been treated with prednisone and sulfasalazine. Over the past 4 months she has been having abdominal pain and cramping and frequent bloody diarrhea stools. During the same period, she has had a weight loss of 20 lb (9 kg), and has had difficulty maintaining her career. Recently, she has developed several lesions of the lower leg identified as erythema nodosum. A recent colonoscopy revealed 25 cm of the rectal sigmoid colon extensively involved. On admission, Mrs. Lewis states "I'm tired of fighting this disease. I am a prisoner in my home because of the diarrhea." She is admitted for a total proctocolectomy and ileostomy.

Assessment

Janet Wheeler, RN, completes the admission assessment for Mrs. Lewis. She finds that Mrs. Lewis now weighs 115 lb (52.2 kg), indicating a recent 20-lb (9-kg) weight loss. She has abdominal cramping, pain, and frequent bloody diarrhea stools. She also has several reddened lesions on her lower legs. Physical assessment findings are as follows: BP, 104/72; T, 98 F (36.6 C); P, 72; R, 20. Her skin is cool and pale. Abnormal laboratory findings include the following: hemoglobin, 7.3 g/dL (normal: 11.7 to 15.7 g/dL); hematocrit, 23.3% (normal: 35% to 47%); WBC, 15,580/mm^3 (normal: 3500/mm^3 to 11,000/mm^3): platelet count, 995,000/mm^3 (normal: 150,000/mm^3 to

450,000/mm^3); serum protein, 4.6 g/dL (normal: 6 to 8 g/dL); serum albumin, 2.4 g/dL (normal: 3.5 to 5 g/dL). Preparation for a total proctocolectomy and ileostomy is begun.

Diagnosis

Ms. Wheeler identifies the following nursing diagnoses for Mrs. Lewis:

- *Risk for Altered Nutrition: Less Than Body Requirements* related to impaired absorption
- *Diarrhea* related to inflammation of bowel
- *Risk for Fluid Volume* deficit related to abnormal fluid loss
- *Risk for Impaired Tissue Integrity* related to drainage from ileostomy
- *Pain* related to surgical intervention
- *Risk for Sexual Dysfunction* related to presence of ileostomy
- *Risk for Self-Esteem Disturbance* related to presence of ileostomy

Expected Outcomes

The expected outcomes established in the plan of care specify that Mrs. Lewis will

- Tolerate prescribed diet.
- Attain an elimination pattern normal for an ileostomy.
- Maintain adequate fluid balance, as demonstrated by physical assessment, vital signs, and laboratory results.
- Perform adequate ostomy care to prevent skin breakdown.
- Report a tolerable level of discomfort.
- Verbalize feelings about sexuality.
- Acknowledge importance of discussing sexual issues with her husband.
- Perform self care of ileostomy.
- Return to work and social activity in 6 weeks following surgery.

Planning and Implementation

The nurses plan and implement the following nursing interventions for Mrs. Lewis:

- Discuss dietary modifications related to presence of ileostomy, including foods to avoid and the need to limit high-fiber foods and to chew them well.
- Instruct Mrs. Lewis about the importance of maintaining a high fluid intake and means to assess its adequacy.
- Teach Mrs. Lewis to empty and change either a one-piece or two-piece ostomy pouch.

- Teach Mrs. Lewis to assess her stoma and peristomal skin with each pouch change.
- Teach Mrs. Lewis the signs and symptoms of dehydration.
- Teach Mrs. Lewis how to manage a food blockage.
- Refer Mrs. Lewis to the local United Ostomy Association.
- Refer Mrs. Lewis to local medical supply companies that sell ostomy appliances.

Evaluation

On discharge, Mrs. Lewis is caring for her ileostomy appliance, demonstrating her ability to empty, rinse, and change the pouch. The ET nurse has given Mrs. Lewis written and verbal instructions on ileostomy care. Mrs. Lewis verbalizes her understanding of the need to avoid high-fiber foods in large quantities, to avoid timed-release medications, and to avoid harsh laxative preparations prior to any radiographic examination (Madda, 1991). The ET nurse has also discussed sexual aspects of having an ileostomy and has given Mrs. Lewis a booklet, "Sex and the Female Ostomate," available through the United Ostomy Association.

Critical Thinking in the Nursing Process

1. Erythema nodosum is a possible extracolonic (outside the bowel) complication of ulcerative colitis. Identify the pathophysiology of erythema nodosum and its physical manifestations.

2. Why is the client with an ileostomy at risk for dehydration? What assessments can Mrs. Lewis use at home to monitor her fluid volume status?

3. Why would Mrs. Lewis's hemoglobin and hematocrit be low on admission? If her hemoglobin had been low but her hematocrit normal on admission, what might be the explanation?

4. Outline a teaching plan that could be given to clients for home care of an ileostomy.

5. Develop a care plan for Mrs. Lewis for the nursing diagnosis *Risk for Impaired Skin Integrity*.

The Client with Crohn's Disease

■ ■ ■

Like ulcerative colitis, **Crohn's disease,** also known as *regional enteritis,* is a chronic, relapsing inflammatory disorder affecting the gastrointestinal tract. It also affects young people primarily, with the peak age of onset between 10 and 30 years. The overall incidence of Crohn's disease is estimated to be from 1 to 7 per 100,000, with a higher incidence among people of Jewish ancestry (Hampton &

Bryant, 1992). At least 10,000 new cases are reported annually (Meize-Grochowski, 1991). Crohn's disease is distributed equally in males and females, and both geographic and ethnic variations are seen. It is more common in urban settings, among residents of the northern United States, and among Ashkenazi Jews (Way, 1994).

Crohn's disease can occur anywhere in the gastrointestinal tract from the mouth to the anus, but it most frequently affects the terminal ileum and right colon. In about 30% of clients with Crohn's disease, only the small bowel is involved, usually the terminal ileum. Another 50% have involvement of both the small and large bowel, often the terminal ileum and adjacent ascending right colon. Only the large bowel is involved in up to 20% of persons with Crohn's. Crohn's disease is a transmural (full-thickness) inflammatory disease of the bowel and can lead to ulceration, strictures, fistula development, and the formation of abscesses (Tierney et al., 1994).

The cause of Crohn's disease is unknown. Several etiologic origins are suspected. Crohn's disease has a familial tendency, suggesting a genetic link. Environmental factors also appear to play a role in its development. Infectious agents and autoimmune processes are possible influences. Like ulcerative colitis, extraintestinal manifestations, such as hepatobiliary disease, uveitis, arthritis, thromboembolism, and vascular disorders are associated with Crohn's disease. Cystitis, renal calculi, and ureteral obstruction may occur as well.

Pathophysiology

Crohn's disease typically begins as a small inflammatory *aphthoid lesion* (shallow ulcers with a white base and elevated margin, similar to a canker sore) of the mucosa and submucosa of the bowel. These initial lesions may regress, or the inflammatory process can progress to involve all layers of the intestinal wall. Deeper ulcerations, granulomatous lesions, and fissures or knifelike clefts that extend deeply into the bowel wall develop. The lumen of the affected bowel assumes a "cobblestone appearance" as fissures and ulcers surround islands of intact mucosa over edematous submucosa. The inflammatory lesions of Crohn's disease are not continuous; rather, they often occur as "skip" lesions with intervening areas of normal-appearing bowel. Some evidence suggests that despite its normal appearance, the entire bowel is affected by this disorder.

As the disease progresses, fibrotic changes in the bowel wall cause it to thicken and lose flexibility, taking on an appearance that has been likened to a rubber hose. The inflammation, edema, and fibrosis can lead to local obstruction, abscess development, and the formation of fistulas between loops of bowel or bowel and other organs (Figure 23–10). Fistulas between loops of bowel are known as enteroenteric fistulas; those that occur between

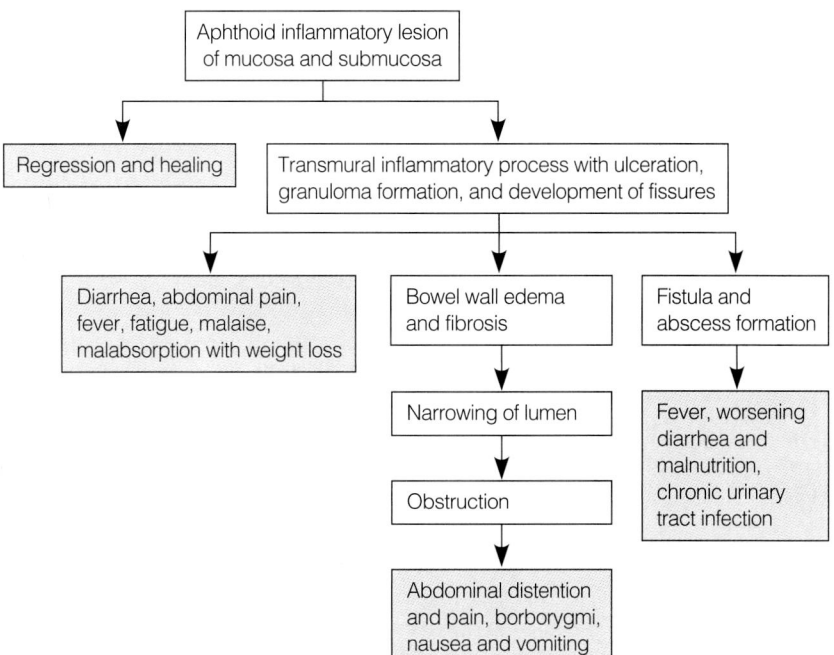

Figure 23–10 The pathologic progression of Crohn's disease.

bowel and bladder are known as enterovesical fistulas; and fistulas that occur between bowel and skin are known as enterocutaneous fistulas. Perineal fistulas are relatively common, originating in the ileum (Porth, 1994).

Depending on the severity of the disease and amount of involvement, malabsorption may occur because the ulcers prevent absorption of nutrients. When the jejunum and ileum are affected, the absorption of multiple nutrients may be impaired, including carbohydrates, proteins, fats, vitamins, and folate (Thompson et al., 1993). Disease in the terminal ileum can lead to vitamin B_{12} malabsorption and bile salt reabsorption. The ulcerations can also result in protein loss as well as chronic, slow blood loss and consequent anemia.

Because the gastrointestinal system involvement possible with Crohn's disease is so diverse, manifestations may vary among clients. About 90% of people with Crohn's disease experience continuous or episodic diarrhea (Way, 1994). Stools are liquid or semiformed and typically do not contain blood, although some clients with involvement of the colon may pass blood. Abdominal pain and tenderness is also common. It may be centered in the right lower quadrant and relieved by defecation. A palpable right lower quadrant mass is often present. Systemic manifestations, such as fever, fatigue, malaise, weight loss, and anemia, are common. Anorectal lesions, such as fissures, ulcers, fistulas, and abscesses, affect a number of clients with Crohn's disease and may occur years before intestinal disease presents (Way, 1994).

Some complications of Crohn's disease, such as intestinal obstruction, abscess, and fistula, are so common that they are considered part of the disease process. For many

clients, the disease initially presents with one of these complications. The client with an intestinal obstruction experiences abdominal distention, cramping pain, and borborygmi. Nausea and vomiting may occur. Fistulas may be asymptomatic, particularly if they occur between loops of small bowel. When fistulization causes an abscess to form, the client develops chills and fever, a tender abdominal mass, and leukocytosis. A fistula between the small bowel and colon may exacerbate diarrhea, weight loss, and malnutrition. When the bladder is involved, recurrent urinary tract infections occur. Perforation of the bowel occurs in 5% of Crohn's disease clients (Podolsky, 1991). Fortunately, hemorrhage is uncommon in Crohn's disease.

The client with colonic Crohn's disease has an increased risk for developing colon cancer. One research study noted a nearly sixfold increase in risk over the general population (Podolsky, 1991).

Collaborative Care

Crohn's disease is a chronic disease process for which there is no specific treatment. Medical therapy is directed toward managing the symptoms and controlling the disease process by using a combination of supportive measures, such as physical rest and stress reduction, pharmacologic agents, and nutritional support. Clients with severe uncomplicated Crohn's disease usually respond well to aggressive medical management, including total parenteral nutrition and bowel rest (Sitzmann, Converse, & Bayless, 1990). Complications of the disease may necessitate surgical intervention.

Laboratory and Diagnostic Tests

Because there is no disease-specific test for Crohn's disease, it is often diagnosed by ruling out other disease processes. The following laboratory tests may be ordered:

- *Culture and occult blood testing* is performed on stool specimens. Culture is performed to rule out an infectious cause for the client's symptoms.

- *Serum albumin* may be decreased because of malabsorption, protein loss through intestinal lesions, and chronic inflammation.

- *CBC* reveals anemia from chronic inflammation, blood loss, and malnutrition; and leukocytosis due to inflammation and possible abscess formation. The sedimentation rate is typically elevated during periods of acute inflammation.

- *Liver function test* results may be altered if pericholangitis (inflammation of the tissues surrounding a bile duct), a possible effect of Crohn's disease, is present. Liver enzymes, such as ALT, alkaline phosphatase, AST, GGTP, and LDH, will be elevated, as will the total bilirubin level.

- Folic acid (normal: 5 to 20 μg/mL) and serum levels of most vitamins, including A, B complex, C, and the fat-soluble vitamins, are decreased as a result of malabsorption.

The following diagnostic tests may be ordered:

- *Radiologic examination with contrast media of the entire gastrointestinal tract,* including an upper GI series with small bowel follow-through and a barium enema. These X-ray films can demonstrate the presence of the ulcerations, strictures, and fistulas characteristic of Crohn's disease.

- *Colonoscopy* is performed to allow visualization and possible biopsy of the colon mucosa. With Crohn's disease, aphthoid ulcers, linear or stellate ulcers, strictures, and segmental involvement with adjoining areas of diseased and normal mucosa are typical (Tierney et al., 1994). Biopsy of bowel mucosa allows microscopic tissue examination that may differentiate Crohn's disease from ulcerative colitis, cancer, and other inflammatory bowel disorders.

As with ulcerative colitis, harsh bowel preparations are not used prior to diagnostic tests for Crohn's disease because they may exacerbate the disease. These clients typically receive a clear liquid diet for 2 to 3 days prior to endoscopic examination.

Pharmacology

The mainstays of pharmacologic management for Crohn's disease are much the same as those for ulcerative colitis. Medications include sulfasalazine and related anti-inflammatory agents; potent anti-inflammatory agents, such as glucocorticoids; and antidiarrheal preparations, including loperamide, diphenoxylate, and codeine. Antidiarrheal medications can significantly reduce the diarrhea associated with Crohn's disease. They may be used more freely for this disorder than for ulcerative colitis because Crohn's disease has no associated risk of toxic megacolon.

Sulfasalazine is a locally active anti-inflammatory agent useful in Crohn's disease limited to the large bowel. The related drugs mesalamine and olsalazine release in the distal small bowel and are more effective in treating ileal inflammation. The active ingredient in these drugs, 5-aminosalicylic acid (5-ASA), has been found to be effective to prevent clinical relapse in Crohn's disease (Prantera, Pallone, Brunetti, Cottone, Miglioli, and the Italian IBD Study Group, 1992). The client is taught to take the oral medication with food to minimize gastrointestinal upset.

Corticosteroids are very effective in suppressing acute clinical signs of Crohn's disease involving either the small or large bowel. Intravenous steroids may be required for the client with severe disease, weight loss, and malnutrition; oral preparations are used for less severe manifestations and longer-term therapy. Many clients are unable to withdraw from steroid therapy without experiencing relapse and may need chronic low-dose therapy (Tierney et al., 1994). The nursing implications for 5-ASA products, including sulfasalazine and others, and corticosteroids are included in the box on page 810.

Mercaptopurine (6-MP, Purinethol) and other immunosuppressive agents such as azathioprine (Imuran) and cyclosporine (Sandimmune) may be used to treat clients who have not responded to other treatments, those requiring chronic steroid therapy, and those with symptomatic fistulas. Use of these drugs allows reduction in corticosteroid doses, helps close fistulas, maintains remission, and facilitates healing of perianal disease. Azathioprine and mercaptopurine require 4 months or more for beneficial effect; cyclosporine may work within days to weeks (Way, 1994). Nursing implications for these drugs are outlined in the pharmacology box in Chapter 8 on page 283.

Although a variety of broad-spectrum antibiotics may be used to prevent and treat infections related to Crohn's disease, metronidazole is generally the antibiotic of choice because of its effectiveness on enterobacteria. It is particularly useful to treat perianal lesions (Berkow & Fletcher, 1992). Refer to the box on page 802 for further discussion of this drug.

In addition to the above agents, the pharmacologic management of Crohn's disease may include the use of antispasmotic drugs such as propantheline (Norpanth, Pro-Banthine) or hyoscyamine (Anaspaz, Cystospaz, Levsin, others). When taken before meals, these drugs may reduce abdominal cramping and discomfort.

Intravenous fluid and electrolyte replacement, as well as vitamin, iron, and folate supplementation may also be prescribed for clients with Crohn's disease.

Dietary Management

A well-balanced diet is recommended for clients with Crohn's disease. Because lactose intolerance is a frequent problem, elimination of milk and milk products may be recommended on a trial basis to determine whether manifestations improve. Many clients show weight gain and improved nutritional status when elemental enteral feedings such as Ensure are added to the diet. If the disease is limited primarily to the colon, increasing the amount of dietary fiber may have a beneficial effect on the diarrhea. However, clients with symptoms of obstruction or small bowel narrowing need a low-roughage diet in which raw fruits and vegetables, popcorn, nuts, and similar foods are eliminated.

Clients in acute exacerbation of the disease or those for whom the disease is difficult to control may not tolerate enteral feedings at all. These clients require short- or long-term total parenteral nutrition (TPN). TPN is discussed in detail in Chapter 13.

Surgery

Generally, surgical intervention in Crohn's disease is limited to people with complications of the disease. Bowel obstruction is the leading indication for surgery. Other complications that may require surgical intervention include perforation, internal or external fistula, abscess, and perianal complications. Resections of the diseased colon may also be performed when medical management is ineffective to eliminate symptoms or the client is dependent on corticosteroids. The disease process tends to recur in other areas following removal of affected bowel segments. There is an increased risk of fistula formation following surgery. Resection of the affected portion of bowel with an end-to-end anastomosis is preferred; total colectomy with ileostomy may be necessary in severe large bowel disease. In one study, the recurrence of Crohn's disease after small bowel resection and ileo-colonic anastomosis was 73% at 1 year and 85% at 3 years (Rutgerts, Geboes, Vantrappen, Beyls, Kerremans, & Hiele, 1990).

Nursing Care

In planning and implementing the nursing care for the client with Crohn's disease, the nurse will need to consider that this disease is a chronic, lifelong illness. Teaching is a major aspect of nursing care. Diarrhea and body image disturbance are significant nursing care problems for the client with Crohn's disease, as they are for the client with ulcerative colitis. Refer to the preceding ulcerative colitis section for appropriate nursing interventions.

The client with Crohn's has a significant risk for altered nutrition, which must be considered a priority diagnosis as well.

Altered Nutrition: Less Than Body Requirements

Crohn's disease is a chronic condition that can significantly alter the bowel's ability to absorb nutrients. In addition, blood and protein-rich fluid may be lost in diarrheal stools. With continuing malabsorption and nutrient losses, multiple nutrient deficits may occur, resulting in impaired growth and development, impaired healing, muscle wasting, bone disease, and electrolyte imbalances.

Nursing interventions with rationales follow:

- Weigh daily and maintain accurate intake, output, and dietary records. *These measures, will help evaluate the effectiveness of interventions.*

- Monitor the results of laboratory studies, including hemoglobin and hematocrit, serum electrolytes, and total serum protein and albumin levels. *These studies provide a measure of the client's nutritional status.*

- Provide the prescribed diet: high-kcal, high-protein, low-fat diet with restricted milk and milk products if lactose intolerance is present. *Calories and protein are important to replace lost nutrients. Fat restriction helps reduce diarrhea and nutrient loss, particularly when significant portions of the terminal ileum have been resected.*

- Provide parenteral nutrition as necessary for the client who is unable to absorb enteral nutrients. *Parenteral nutrition can help reverse nutritional deficits and promote weight gain in the client with acute symptoms.*

- Arrange for dietary consultation. Provide for the client's food preferences as allowed. *These measures can help increase the client's food intake.*

- Administer prescribed nutritional supplements. *These are important to replace losses and bring levels closer to normal more rapidly than dietary means alone can effect.*

- Include family members, the primary food preparer in particular, in teaching and dietary discussions. *Families can reinforce teaching and help the client maintain required restrictions or kcal intake.*

Other Nursing Diagnoses

Other nursing diagnoses that may be appropriate for the client with Crohn's disease follow:

- *Diarrhea* related to inflammation of bowel mucosa
- *Risk for Impaired Skin Integrity* related to perianal manifestations of the disease
- *Activity Intolerance* related to fatigue and malaise
- *Altered Family Processes* related to chronic disease state
- *Risk for Infection* related to fistula and abscess formation

Client and Family Teaching

Like ulcerative colitis, Crohn's disease is a chronic condition for which the client will need to provide day-to-day self-management. For this reason, teaching is a vital component of care. Teach the client and family members about the disease, prescribed medications, and dietary management.

Instruct the client about possible manifestations of disease complications and their appropriate management. Present information on stress management. Provide a written schedule for medications and tapering of corticosteroids if ordered. Explain desired and side effects of prescribed drugs, as well as possible drug toxicities and interactions.

Explain the rationale for restricting milk and milk products in the diet. Provide detailed information about the need to consume a diet of good nutritional value, with any specific restrictions recommended. Discuss the use of nutritional supplements, such as Ensure. Explain possible indications of malabsorption and impaired nutrition along with recommendations for self-treatment and when to seek medical intervention. If the client is to be discharged with a central catheter and home parenteral nutrition, provide written and verbal instructions on catheter care and trouble-shooting as well as TPN administration. Have the client and a family member demonstrate proficiency in catheter care techniques and initiation of feedings.

If surgery is indicated, give preoperative and postoperative instructions for care. Prior to discharge, provide the client with information on the disease and instruction on fistula, ileostomy, or wound care as applicable.

The client should return for practice in central line care, ileostomy care, and care of a wound or fistula. Provide a home care nursing referral to assist in the management and further teaching of ileostomy or fistula care.

◣◣◣ Malabsorption Syndromes ◣◣◣

Malabsorption syndrome is a condition in which nutrients—including carbohydrates, proteins, fats, water, electrolytes, minerals, and vitamins—are ineffectively absorbed by the intestinal mucosa, resulting in their excretion in the stool. Malabsorption syndromes may be caused by multiple bowel disorders.

Diseases of the small intestine are often accompanied by malabsorption. Additionally, many different medical and/or surgical conditions may lead to malabsorption if they affect digestion or the intestinal mucosa. Primary diseases of the small bowel mucosa, such as sprue, regional enteritis (Crohn's disease), and acute infections can lead to malabsorption. It may also result from *maldigestion,* a situation in which chyme is inadequately prepared for absorption. For example, significant gastric resections, pancreatic disorders involving the loss of pancreatic enzyme secretion, and biliary disorders involving reduced bile secretion can result in impaired digestive processes and poorly absorbed chyme. Selected causes of malabsorption and maldigestion are listed in Table 23–9.

Regardless of the cause, malabsorption syndrome is characterized by common manifestations resulting from the impaired absorption of chyme and the nutrients it contains (Table 23–10). Predominant local or gastrointestinal manifestations include anorexia; abdominal bloating; diarrhea with loose, bulky, foul-smelling stools; and steatorrhea (fatty stools). Weight loss, weakness, general malaise, muscle cramps, bone pain, abnormal bleeding, and anemia are frequent systemic manifestations of malabsorption. These manifestations are the result of malnutrition and fluid loss due to poor absorption.

Three common malabsorption disorders in adults are sprue, lactose intolerance, and short bowel syndrome.

The Client with Sprue

■ ■ ■

Sprue is a chronic primary disorder of the small intestine in which the absorption of nutrients, particularly fats, is impaired. The severity of the disease depends on the extent of mucosal involvement in the intestine as well as the duration of the disease. Two major forms of sprue are celiac disease (celiac sprue) and tropical sprue.

Pathophysiology

Although the causes of celiac disease and tropical sprue differ, both are characterized by flattening of the intestinal mucosa with a loss of villi and microvilli. With the loss of villi, the intestine loses absorptive surface, and the production of enzymes, such as disaccharidase and particularly lactase, is reduced.

Celiac Disease
Celiac disease, also known as *celiac sprue* or *nontropical sprue,* is a chronic hereditary disorder characterized by sensitivity to the gliadin fraction of gluten, a cereal protein. Gluten is found in wheat, rye, barley, and oats. It is also used as a filler in many prepared foods and in medications. In the United States, celiac disease affects ap-

Table 23–9	Selected Causes of Malabsorption Syndromes

Cause	Related Factors or Conditions
Impaired absorption by intestinal mucosa	Sprue
	Short bowel syndrome
	Acute enteritis and other bowel infections or infestations
	AIDS-related opportunistic infections and Kaposi's sarcoma
	Celiac disease
	Crohn's disease
	Intestinal ischemia or infarction
	Scleroderma
Impaired digestive processes	Lactose intolerance
	Gastrectomy (Billroth II)
	Chronic pancreatitis, cancer of the pancreas
	Cystic fibrosis
	Biliary obstruction
	Cirrhosis, hepatitis, or liver failure
	Zollinger-Ellison syndrome

Note. Adapted from *The Merck Manual of Diagnosis and Therapy* (16th ed.) edited by R. Berkow and A. J. Fletcher, 1992, Rahway, NJ: Merck Research Laboratories.

Table 23–10	Local and Systemic Manifestations of Malabsorption

Category	Manifestation	Cause
Local (GI)	Diarrhea	Impaired absorption of fluid and electrolytes, leading to excess water in the stool
	Abdominal distention	Gas formation from fermentation of undigested carbohydrates
	Steatorrhea	Impaired fat absorption leading to excess fat in feces
Systemic	Weight loss	Carbohydrate, protein, and fat deficit with kcal wasting
	Weakness and malaise	Kcal deficit, anemia, fluid, and electrolyte losses
	Anemia	Vitamin B_{12}, folic acid, and iron deficits
	Bone pain	Calcium and vitamin D deficits
	Muscle cramps, paresthesias	Protein wasting, vitamin B_{12} and electrolyte deficits
	Easy bruising and bleeding	Vitamin K deficit
	Glossitis, cheilosis	Iron, folic acid, and vitamin B_{12} deficits

proximately 1 in 5000 persons, occurring primarily in whites. It is rare in native Africans and Asians (McCance & Huether, 1994; Berkow & Fletcher, 1992).

The mechanism by which intestinal mucosa is damaged in celiac disease is not entirely clear. Gliadin acts as an antigen (a substance that induces the formation of antibodies that interact specifically with it) in people with celiac disease, prompting the formation of antibodies and immune complexes. These complexes may deposit in the intestinal mucosa, prompting an inflammatory response and loss of villi. Villi, minute projections of the intestinal mucosa into the lumen of the small intestine, absorb fluids and nutrients. The gluten may also damage the villi directly, causing cell loss, inflammation, and edema. With damage, the villi shorten and atrophy, causing the intestinal wall to become smooth and resulting in loss of absorptive surface.

The manifestations of celiac disease may begin during early childhood or as an adult. Local manifestations of celiac disease include abdominal bloating and cramps, diarrhea, and steatorrhea. Systemic manifestations result from the effects of malabsorption and the resulting deficiencies. Anemia is common. Clients with celiac disease are often small in stature, and may have delayed maturity. Other signs of nutrient deficiencies include tetany, vitamin deficiencies, muscle wasting, and even rickets (impaired bone development). When gluten is removed from the diet, the client's manifestations abate.

Tropical Sprue

Tropical sprue is an acquired chronic disease thought to be caused by an infection, either bacterial or viral. Its exact cause is unknown. Tropical sprue occurs chiefly in the Caribbean, south India, and southeast Asia. It may affect clients months to years after exposure. The pathophysiologic changes in bowel mucosa closely resemble those of celiac disease, although gluten intake has no effect on this condition.

Manifestations of tropical sprue include sore tongue, diarrhea, and weight loss. Initially, diarrhea may be explosive and watery; as the disease progresses, stools become fewer in number and more solid with obvious steatorrhea. Folic acid, vitamin B_{12}, and iron deficiencies may occur, resulting in glossitis, stomatitis, dry, rough skin, and anemia.

Collaborative Care

With any malabsorptive disorder, the initial focus of management is to identify the cause. Once this has been determined, specific therapy can be prescribed.

Nursing Implications for Diagnostic Tests: Enteroscopy

■ ■ ■

Client Preparation

- Assess the client's understanding of the procedure, providing explanation, clarification, and emotional support as needed.

- Ensure that an informed consent form has been signed for this invasive procedure.

- Instruct the client to take nothing by mouth for 6 to 12 hours prior to the examination; if the client is hospitalized, ensure NPO status after midnight prior to the procedure.

- Remove dentures and check for loose teeth prior to the procedure. Provide mouth care. Remove eyewear, jewelry, hairpins, and combs.

- Take and record vital signs before the procedure; administer any prescribed premedication.

Postprocedure Care

- Monitor vital signs and evaluate the client for evidence of complications: bleeding, abdominal or back pain, dyspnea, dysphagia, or fever. Observe the client for 2 to 4 hours before discharge or until swallowing reflex is normal.

- Withhold all food and fluids until gag and swallow reflexes have returned. Position client in semi-Fowler's position with the head to the side to allow saliva to drain from the mouth. Provide an emesis basin and tissues or a washcloth in which the client can expectorate.

- Ensure that client is not discharged alone before sedation is completely worn off.

Client and Family Teaching

- Although you will remain awake during the procedure, local anesthesia and/or sedation will be administered to minimize discomfort. During the examination, you may have difficulty swallowing and will be unable to talk; breathing, however, will not be affected.

- The examination will be performed in an endoscopy room and require 20 to 30 minutes to complete.

- Sore throat, hoarseness, abdominal bloating, belching, and flatulence are common following the procedure. Warm saline gargles or throat lozenges may be used to relieve discomfort. Notify the physician if symptoms persist.

- Sedation often results in some amnesia around the time of the examination.

- Notify the physician immediately should any of the following signs of complications develop: persistent difficulty in swallowing; epigastric, substernal, or shoulder pain; vomiting blood; black tarry stools; or fever.

Laboratory and Diagnostic Tests

Laboratory and diagnostic testing are used to make the differential diagnosis for various causes of malabsorption syndromes and to determine the severity of nutrient deficiencies.

The following laboratory tests may be ordered:

- *Fecal fat* is measured to document the presence of steatorrhea. Either a random stool sample or a 24- or 72-hour stool collection is used. The total fat output over a 72-hour period provides the most accurate measurement (Pagana & Pagana, 1992). The client may be placed on a diet of 60 to 100 g fat per day prior to or during the test or may be asked to provide a diet diary. The client avoids suppositories, oily lubricants, and mineral oil laxatives for 3 days prior to and during the exam. The expected result is a fecal fat content of 5 g/24 hours, or less than 50 globules/HPF (high power field) of neutral fat and less than 100 globules/HPF of fatty acids (Chernecky et al., 1993; Pagana & Pagana,

1992). The fat content of stool is increased in many malabsorptive disorders. In celiac disease, it may range from 7 to 50 g/24 hours.

- *The D-xylose absorption test* or *xylose tolerance test* is used to evaluate intestinal absorption. D-xylose is an inert sugar that normally is absorbed easily in the proximal small intestine and is excreted unchanged in the urine. It is not metabolized and does not require pancreatic or biliary secretion for absorption. Measurement of blood and urine levels after administration of a fixed amount of D-xylose provides information about the absorptive ability of the intestine. The expected results in an adult are a blood level of 25 to 40 mg/dL 2 hours after ingestion and excretion in the urine of 80% to 95% of the amount ingested 5 hours after ingestion. The absorption of D-xylose is impaired in celiac disease, tropical sprue, and other malabsorptive disorders such as Crohn's disease. It is not affected by maldigestive disorders.

Table 23–11 Dietary Sources of Gluten

Food Group	Contain Gluten	May Contain Gluten
Cereals, grains, and grain products	Bread, crackers, cereal, and pasta containing wheat, oat, rye, or barley grain or flour	Seasoned rice and potato mixes
Beverages	Malt, Postum, Ovaltine, beers, and ales	Commercial chocolate milk, cocoa, and other beverage mixes, such as instant tea mix, dietary supplements
Desserts	Cakes, cookies, and pastries made with wheat, oat, rye, or barley flour	Commercial ice cream and sherbet
Meats and other protein sources		Meat loaf, cold cuts and prepared meats, breaded meats; cheese products; soy protein meat substitutes; commercial egg products
Fruits and vegetables		Commercial seasoned vegetable mixes or vegetables with sauce; canned baked beans; commercial pie fillings
Miscellaneous		Commercial salad dressings and mayonnaise; ketchup and prepared mustard; gravy, white sauce; nondairy creamer; syrups; commercial pickles

Note. Adapted from *Nutrition and Diet Therapy* by C. A. Lutz and K. R. Przytulski, 1994, Philadelphia: F. A. Davis.

- *Schilling test, or vitamin B_{12} absorption test,* may also be ordered to rule out other causes for malabsorption and anemia. In this test, radioactive or "tagged" vitamin B_{12} is administered orally, and its excretion in the urine is measured. The expected result is that 8% or more of the radioactive B_{12} will be excreted within the first 24 hours. This amount is reduced in people who lack intrinsic factor (e.g., people with pernicious anemia) and in those with intestinal malabsorption.

- *Serum complement levels,* an indicator of inflammatory activity, are often reduced in the client with celiac disease. Removing gluten from the diet causes these levels to rise (Berkow & Fletcher, 1992).

- *Numerous laboratory tests for nutrient deficiencies* may be ordered to evaluate the effects of malabsorption on the client. Serum levels of protein, albumin, cholesterol, electrolytes, and iron may be determined. The hemoglobin, hematocrit, and RBC indices are used to evaluate anemia. Prothrombin time is increased in vitamin K deficiency.

In addition to the preceding laboratory tests, the following diagnostic tests may be ordered:

- *Upper GI series with small bowel follow-through* uses barium as a contrast medium to provide visualization of the esophagus, stomach, and duodenum. Following oral or enteric administration of barium sulfate, fluoroscopy and still films are used to evaluate specific portions of the gastrointestinal tract as the barium outlines the structures (Chernecky et al., 1993). With malabsorption syndromes, and sprue in particular, the typi-cal "feathery" pattern of barium in the small bowel is lost, and the barium may precipitate and clump. Nursing care of the client undergoing an upper gastrointestinal series with small bowel follow-through is similar to that outlined in the box on page 779.

- *Enteroscopy* employs the use of an extra-long fiberoptic endoscope to visualize and biopsy the upper small intestine (Pagana & Pagana, 1992). This procedure permits direct examination of intestinal mucosa as well as collection of a tissue specimen for biopsy. Although this invasive procedure involves risks, including perforation, bleeding, and aspiration of gastric contents, the information it provides is more specific and diagnostic for malabsorptive syndromes than that obtained with other tests. Nursing care of the client undergoing an enteroscopy is included in the box on page 826.

Dietary Management

The client with celiac disease is placed on a gluten-free diet. This treatment is generally successful, as long as the client avoids gluten totally. Gluten is so widely used in prepared foods that this may be no easy task. Consultation with a dietitian and detailed dietary instructions are necessary. Clients need to become very aware of hidden sources of gluten and to analyze dietary labels. Common sources of gluten and foods to be avoided are indicated in Table 23–11.

The prescribed diet is also high in calories and protein to correct nutrient deficits. Fat content is restricted to minimize steatorrhea. Initially, the diet usually is restricted in lactose as well to compensate for the loss of lactase-containing microvilli. Foods containing lactose may be reintroduced once remission has occurred (Tierney et al., 1994).

For tropical sprue, a high-kcal, high-protein, low-fat diet is prescribed.

Pharmacology

Clients with severe nutritional deficits may require vitamin and mineral supplementation as well as iron and folic acid to correct anemia. Vitamin K may be administered parenterally if the prothrombin time is abnormal (Berkow & Fletcher, 1992). In clients whose disease responds poorly to dietary management, corticosteroids may be prescribed. They help reduce the inflammatory response and stimulate the appetite.

Tropical sprue is treated with a combination of folic acid and tetracycline. This regimen is continued for 1 to 2 months. Other nutrient deficiencies are treated as for celiac disease.

Nursing Care

Nursing care needs for the client with sprue and many other malabsorptive disorders are related to the usual effects of the disease on the client. Diarrhea and malnutrition are significant problems and priority foci for nursing intervention.

Diarrhea

Steatorrhea and diarrhea are typically associated with sprue because fat, water, and other nutrients are poorly absorbed, remaining in the bowel to be eliminated in the stool. Diarrhea has the potential to interfere with the client's life-style, ADLs, skin integrity, and fluid and electrolyte balance.

Nursing interventions with rationales follow:

- Assess and document the frequency and character of stools. *Bowel function provides a measure of the severity of the disease and efficacy of treatment. As the condition improves with therapy, stools become less frequent and more normal in color and appearance.*

- Weigh the client daily, monitor intake and output, and assess skin turgor and mucous membranes for indications of fluid balance. *The client with diarrhea is at risk for hypovolemia and dehydration resulting from excess fluid loss in the stool.*

- Assess and document the condition of perianal skin. *Frequent passage of stool may irritate skin and mucous membranes, increasing the risk of breakdown.*

- Encourage increased fluid intake. *Oral fluids are important to replace excess losses.*

- Arrange dietary consultation and a gluten-free, lactose-reduced diet as ordered for celiac disease. *As the intestinal mucosa recovers from the disease process, diarrhea improves.*

Altered Nutrition: Less Than Body Requirements

Sprue often is a chronic condition. With continuing malabsorption, multiple nutrient deficits may occur, resulting in impaired growth and development, impaired healing, muscle wasting, bone disease, and electrolyte imbalances.

Nursing interventions with rationales follow:

- Weigh the client daily and maintain accurate intake, output, and dietary records. *These measures will help evaluate the effectiveness of interventions.*

- Monitor the results of laboratory studies, including hemoglobin and hematocrit, serum electrolytes, total serum protein, and albumin levels. *These studies provide a measure of the client's nutritional status.*

- Provide the prescribed high-kcal, high-protein, low-fat diet restricted in gluten for celiac disease. *Calories and protein are important to replace lost nutrients. Fat restriction helps reduce diarrhea and nutrient loss.*

- Provide parenteral nutrition as necessary for the client who is unable to absorb enteral nutrients. *Parenteral nutrition can help reverse nutritional deficits and promote weight gain in the client with acute symptoms.*

- Arrange for dietary consultation. Provide for the client's food preferences as allowed. *These measures can help increase the client's food intake.*

- Administer prescribed nutritional supplements. *These are important to replace losses and bring levels closer to normal more rapidly than dietary means alone can effect.*

- Include family members, the primary food preparer in particular, in teaching and dietary discussions. *Families can reinforce teaching and help the client maintain required restrictions or kcal intake.*

Other Nursing Diagnoses

Other nursing diagnoses that may be appropriate for the client with sprue follow:

- *Fluid Volume Deficit* related to excess loss of body fluids in diarrhea

- *Anxiety* related to manifestations and treatment of the disorder

- *Risk for Noncompliance* with dietary regimen related to lack of understanding

Client and Family Teaching

Although tropical sprue may be curable with antibiotic and folic acid therapy, the client with celiac disease has a chronic condition that requires continuing dietary management.

Provide the client and family with a detailed list of foods that contain gluten and need to be eliminated from the diet, as well as foods that are allowed. Teach the client how to identify gluten-containing commercial products by reading labels and lists of ingredients. Encourage the client and primary food preparer to purchase and use a gluten-free cookbook.

If corticosteroids have been prescribed for the client, stress the importance of taking the medication as ordered. Emphasize the need to avoid stopping the medication abruptly and to notify all caregivers that a corticosteroid is part of the client's medication regimen. Teach the client to monitor his or her weight frequently. A weight gain of 5 lb (2.3 kg) or more in less than a week is more likely the result of fluid gain, a possible adverse effect of corticosteroids. Other potential effects include decreased resistance to infection, an impaired inflammatory response, and changes in the metabolism of carbohydrates, proteins, and fats.

The Client with Lactose Intolerance

■ ■ ■

For carbohydrates to be absorbed from the small intestine, they first must be broken down into simple sugars, or monosaccharides. Lactose is the primary carbohydrate in milk and milk products. It is a disaccharide, requiring the enzyme lactase for digestion and absorption. Lactase deficiency causes *lactose intolerance,* a common cause of malabsorption.

Lactase deficiency affects up to 90% of Asians and 75% of African Americans and Indians. There is also a high incidence among southern Europeans (Berkow & Fletcher, 1992). Approximately 5% to 15% of the white population is affected. Although lactase deficiency is hereditary in origin in most cases, it may also occur secondarily to conditions affecting the intestinal mucosa, such as the sprue syndromes, regional enteritis, cystic fibrosis, and intestinal infections.

Although the defect causing lactase deficiency and lactose intolerance is genetic, symptoms often do not present until adolescence or early adulthood. Symptoms of lactose intolerance include lower abdominal cramping, pain, and diarrhea following milk ingestion. Undigested lactose ferments in the intestine, forming gases that contribute to bloating and flatus. Lactic and fatty acids produced by this fermentation irritate the bowel, leading to increased motility and abdominal cramping. The undigested lactose produces an osmotic gradient in the intestine, drawing in water which also causes increased motility and diarrhea. The diarrhea associated with lactose intolerance may be explosive (Price & Wilson, 1992).

Collaborative Care

The diagnosis of lactose intolerance is based on the client's history of intolerance to milk and milk products, a lactose breath test, and a lactose tolerance test.

The lactose breath test is a noninvasive test that uses measurements of the expired hydrogen gas (H_2) following administration of 50 g of lactose by mouth. If lactose is broken down and absorbed normally, there is little change in the amount of exhaled H_2 from fasting to post-lactose administration. The client with lactose intolerance shows a significant increase in H_2 exhaled following lactose administration as the sugar ferments in the bowel (Price & Wilson, 1992).

The lactose tolerance test closely resembles glucose tolerance testing. Lactose solution, usually 100 g diluted in 200 mL of water, is administered to the client by mouth. Plasma glucose levels are then measured at 30-, 60-, and 120-minute intervals following the lactose ingestion. If lactose is digested and absorbed normally, a rise of more than 20 mg/dL in the blood glucose is expected. Clients who are lactase deficient will not demonstrate the expected elevation of blood glucose levels.

Placing the client with lactase deficiency on a lactose-free or reduced lactose diet relieves the manifestations of the disorder. Some clients may require total elimination of milk and milk products from the diet. Many are able to tolerate lactose in small amounts. Lactase enzyme preparations are available to improve milk tolerance. Yogurt containing bacterial lactases may be well tolerated. Calcium supplementation is often recommended, particularly for women on a reduced-lactose or lactose-free diet.

Nursing Care

Nursing care for the client with lactose intolerance is directed primarily toward providing education and support. Clients need instruction about the recommended diet. Potential "hidden" sources of lactose include sherbets, desserts made from milk and milk chocolate, sauces and gravies, and cream soups. It is important to emphasize the need to obtain nutrients contained in milk and milk products from other sources. Proteins may be obtained from meats, eggs, legumes, and grains. Other sources of calcium include sardines, oysters, and salmon, as well as plant sources such as beans, cauliflower, rhubarb, and green leafy vegetables (Lutz & Przytulski, 1994).

The Client with Short Bowel Syndrome

■ ■ ■

Resection of significant portions of the small intestine may result in a condition known as *short bowel syndrome.* The severity of the disorder depends on the total amount of bowel resected, as well as the portions of bowel removed. Removal of the proximal portions, including the duodenum, jejunum, and proximal ileum, and distal portion of the ileum are associated with more severe malabsorption and symptoms than resection of midportions of the ileum.

Small bowel may be resected due to cancerous processes, mesenteric thrombosis with bowel infarction, strangulated hernias, Crohn's disease (regional enteritis), trauma, and enteropathy resulting from radiation therapy.

Resection of the small intestine affects the absorption of water, nutrients, vitamins, and minerals. Transit time of ingested foods and fluids is reduced, and digestive processes are impaired. The bowel undergoes an adaptive process in which the remaining villi enlarge and lengthen to increase absorptive surface following resection. For many clients, absorption and bowel function returns to preoperative or near-normal levels. Others have continued significant impairment of digestion and absorption, leading to nutrient deficiencies, weight loss, and diarrhea.

Collaborative Care

Laboratory and diagnostic studies are used primarily to evaluate the severity of nutrient deficiencies. Total serum proteins and albumin are reduced, as are serum levels of folate, iron, vitamins, minerals, and electrolytes. Anemia may be present, as well as a prolonged prothrombin time (indicative of vitamin K deficiency). X-ray studies with barium contrast media, upper and lower gastrointestinal series, are used to estimate the amount of small intestine remaining.

Management of short bowel syndrome focuses on alleviating symptoms. Clients often simply require frequent, small, high-kcal, high-protein feedings. Multivitamin and mineral supplementation is also frequently necessary. Antidiarrheal medications are used to reduce bowel motility, allowing a greater amount of time for nutrient absorption. Some clients are affected by gastric hypersecretion following bowel resection. For these clients, a histamine H_2-receptor antagonist (H_2 blocker) such as cimetidine or ranitidine may be prescribed. Clients with severe manifestations of short bowel syndrome may require intravenous fluid and electrolyte replacement and maintenance with total parenteral nutrition to sustain life.

Nursing Care

Nursing management for the client with short bowel syndrome focuses on the problems of potential fluid volume deficit, altered nutritional status, and diarrhea. Frequent assessment of the client's intake and output, daily weights, skin turgor, and condition of mucous membranes provides valuable information about hydration.

Fluid losses are generally greatest in the initial periods following surgery, warranting the closest attention at that time. It is important to remember however, that the client is at increased risk when other abnormal fluid losses occur through, for example, fever, increased respiratory rate, draining wounds, or excess perspiration.

Document the client's nutritional status, including weight, anthropometric measurements, laboratory values, and kcal intake. Provide nutritional supplementation with enteral feedings as needed. Maintain central lines and total parenteral nutrition, using aseptic technique.

For diarrhea, document the number and character of stools. Administer antidiarrheal medications as ordered. If the client is lactose intolerant, limit intake of milk and milk products. Provide good skin care of the perianal region to prevent breakdown from frequent bowel movements. Refer to the discussion of nursing care for the client with sprue for other measures for altered nutrition and diarrhea.

The client and family affected by this condition require extensive education. Because there is no way to cure or replace the lost bowel at this time, the client must manage the disorder on a day-to-day basis. Provide instructions about the recommended diet and medication regimen. Emphasize the importance of maintaining an adequate fluid intake, particularly in hot weather or during strenuous exercise. Teach the client to monitor his or her weight frequently and report changes. Include teaching about possible manifestations of dehydration and nutrient deficiencies that should be reported to the physician. Referring the client to a dietitian or counselor can help the person cope with what may be a lifelong problem.

▗ ▗ ▗ Neoplastic Disorders ▗ ▗ ▗

Cancer remains the second leading cause of death in the United States, preceded only by heart disease. Although cancer may affect any portion of the digestive tract, the large intestine and rectum are the most common sites. Malignant neoplasms of the lower bowel are the second leading cause of death from cancer (after lung cancer), making this a significant health care concern.

The Client with Polyps

▪ ▪ ▪

A **polyp** is a mass of tissue that arises from the bowel wall and protrudes into the lumen. Polyps may arise in any portion of the bowel, but they occur most often in the sigmoid colon and rectum. They vary considerably in size and may be single or multiple. It is estimated that between 9% and 50% of the general population have polyps, with the incidence increasing with age (Berkow & Fletcher, 1992; Way, 1994). Although most polyps are benign, some have the potential to become malignant.

Pathophysiology

Polyps are identified by their structure and tissue type. Most polyps are adenomas, benign epithelial tumors that are considered premalignant lesions. Less than 10% of these lesions progress to become cancers; however, virtually all colorectal cancers arise from adenomatous polyps (Hazzard et al., 1994). Adenomas may occur in a pedunculated or villous form.

A *pedunculated polyp* is a globelike structure attached to the intestinal wall by a thin, stalklike stem (Figure 23–11). The incidence of this type of polyp increases with age, although it occurs in all age groups and in both sexes. Most are small, 1 cm or less in diameter, although they may be as large as 4 to 5 cm. The malignant potential of these polyps seems to be related to their size. One percent of those under 1 cm in diameter are cancerous, whereas 45% of adenomas larger than 2 cm are cancerous (Price & Wilson, 1992; Way, 1994). These polyps contain a proliferation of glands and are sometimes also called *tubular adenomas.*

A *villous* or *sessile* (broad-based) *polyp* is attached by a broad membranous base. This type of polyp is generally larger than pedunculated or tubular adenomas, usually more than 5 cm. It is less common than the pedunculated type and occurs more frequently as a single lesion. Villous polyps contain a proliferation of villi and have a higher malignant potential than tubular adenomas, estimated at 25% to 40% (Berkow & Fletcher, 1992; Way, 1994). Some adenomatous polyps contain both tubular epithelium and villi and are known as *tubulovillous adenomas.*

Familial polyposis is an uncommon autosomal dominant genetic disorder characterized by hundreds of adenomatous polyps throughout the entire large intestine. Both pedunculated and sessile polyps are seen, usually developing at puberty. The risk of malignancy is almost 100% by age 40 with familial polyposis (Price & Wilson, 1992).

Most polyps are asymptomatic, found coincidentally during routine examination or diagnostic testing. Intermittent painless rectal bleeding, bright or dark red, is the most common presenting complaint. A large polyp may cause abdominal cramping, pain, or manifestations of obstruction. Diarrhea and mucus discharge may be associated with a large villous adenoma.

Collaborative Care

The diagnosis of intestinal polyps is generally based on diagnostic studies such as barium enema, sigmoidoscopy,

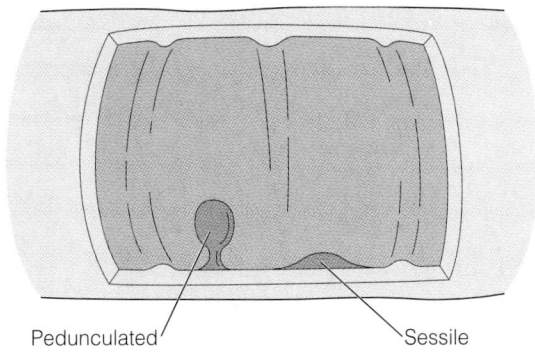

Figure 23–11   Sessile and pedunculated intestinal polyps.

Pedunculated   Sessile

or colonoscopy. A rectal polyp may be palpable on digital examination, but further studies are necessary to determine polyp size and type, to determine the extent of colon involvement, and to assess for malignancy. The following diagnostic studies may be ordered:

- *Barium enema* generally shows the polyp as a rounded filling defect with smooth, sharply defined margins. Very small polyps, less than 0.5 cm, may not be visible on X-ray film. Thorough colon cleansing is vital prior to radiologic examination for polyps (Way, 1994).

- *Colonoscopy* provides the most reliable diagnosis of polyps, allowing visual inspection of the large intestine, biopsy of masses or lesions, and polypectomy. Nursing care of the client undergoing a colonoscopy is included in the box on page 774.

Once identified, polyps are generally removed because of the risk of malignancy. Pedunculated polyps and small sessile or villous lesions may be removed during colonoscopy using an electrocautery snare or hot biopsy forceps passed through the scope. This is a relatively safe procedure, with a less than 2% risk of complications such as perforation or hemorrhage. Large villous adenomas are completely excised and examined histologically for evidence of malignancy. In some cases, the colon segment containing the polyp is resected; a total colectomy with ileorectal anastomosis may be performed for multiple polyps in different anatomic parts of the colon.

Treatment following polypectomy depends on histologic examination of the excised tissue. Because polyps tend to recur, follow-up colonoscopy is recommended at 1 year and 3 years if no further polyps are detected. When the polyp is found to be malignant, follow-up care is determined by the tissue type and degree of invasion. Segmental resection or colectomy may be performed. If malignant changes are early and confined to the polyp, the client may simply be followed closely for further evidence of malignancy.

Risk Factors for Colorectal Cancer

■ ■ ■

- Age over 50 years
- Polyps of the colon and/or rectum
- Cancer elsewhere in the body
- Family history of colorectal cancer
- Ulcerative colitis
- Crohn's disease
- Exposure to radiation
- Immunodeficiency disease
- Dietary influences: high fat and kcal intake, low calcium and fiber intake

---

Nursing Care

Nursing care for the client with polyps focuses on education and assisting the client through diagnostic testing and polyp removal. Polyps are a "silent" disease, with few or no symptoms, but represent a significant risk factor for colorectal cancer. The following nursing diagnoses may be appropriate for the client with polyps:

- *Risk for Noncompliance* with recommended follow-up appointments related to lack of understanding
- *Impaired Tissue Integrity* related to removal of polyps from bowel
- *Risk for Fluid Volume Deficit* related to bowel preparation

It is important to stress the need for follow-up appointments and repeat colonoscopy as ordered. In caring for the client before and after colonoscopy and polypectomy, provide direct care as well as instruction about the procedure, expected sensations during the procedure, and anticipated postoperative care. Cathartics and multiple cleansing enemas may be prescribed prior to barium enema and/or colonoscopy. It is important to observe the client for evidence of fluid and electrolyte imbalance through this prepratory procedure. Use of normal saline enemas rather than tap water help minimize the risk of electrolyte imbalances. Following polypectomy, observe closely for possible complications such as hemorrhage. Instruct the client to report any rectal bleeding, light-headedness, or other indications of possible blood loss.

Client and Family Teaching

Client education should include the significance of polyps and their relationship to colorectal cancer. Discuss symptoms that should be reported to the physician, such as altered bowel elimination (diarrhea or constipation), rectal bleeding, and pain. Stress the importance of ongoing monitoring by the physician, including recommendations for repeat colonoscopy at 1 year and 3 years following polypectomy. Clients with multiple polyps or a family history of colorectal cancer are followed yearly; those with familial polyposis every 6 months. Instructing both the client and family is particularly important when the diagnosis is familial polyposis. These clients need a good understanding of the high risk for cancer. Referral to an enterostomal therapist for discussion about colectomy with ileoanal reservoir may help the client with decisions about treatment options.

The Client with Colorectal Cancer

■ ■ ■

Colorectal cancer, a malignant tumor arising from the epithelial tissues of the colon or rectum, is the second leading cause of cancer deaths in Western countries. In the United States, about 150,000 new cases of colorectal cancer are diagnosed yearly; in 1991, more than 56,000 persons died from this disease, and the 5-year survival rate is less than 50% (Hampton & Bryant, 1992; Way, 1994). Among American-born citizens, the incidence of colorectal cancer is 5% (DeVita, Hellman, & Rosenberg, 1989). It occurs most frequently after the age of 50 years, with a slightly higher incidence in males than females. The incidence continues to rise with increasing age, approximately doubling with each decade over the age of 50 years (Hazzard et al., 1994). One study found a higher incidence of colorectal cancer in African-Americans and later detection in African-American males (Griffin, Liff, Greenberg, & Clark, 1991).

Although the specific cause of colorectal cancer is unknown, a number of risk factors have been identified (see the accompanying box). Genetic factors are strongly linked to the risk for colorectal cancer. Persons with familial adenomatous polyposis have a nearly 100% risk of developing colon cancer (Price & Wilson, 1992). A familial history of colorectal cancer is also associated with an increased risk of the disease. Polyps of the rectum and large intestine also indicate a high risk for colorectal cancer; approximately 25% of clients with five or more adenomatous polyps also have colon cancer at the time of initial colonoscopy (Way, 1994). There is an increased incidence of colon cancer in clients with ulcerative colitis and Crohn's disease, and there is a suggested link between colon cancer and previous cholecystectomy (Hampton & Bryant, 1992). Many malignancies, including cancer of the large intestine, occur more frequently in clients who are immunosuppressed because of impaired immune surveillance of abnormal cells.

Diet also has been implicated as a risk factor for colorectal cancer. The disease is prevalent in economically prosperous countries where people consume high-fat, high-kcal, and highly refined foods that are low in fiber. Red meat and alcohol consumption have been implicated as well. It is thought that this dietary pattern, common in the United States, increases the production and bowel concentration of cholesterol and bile acids, which are converted to carcinogen-promoting compounds by fecal bacteria. Dietary fiber and an increased calcium intake, in contrast, are protective against cancer, although the mechanisms are unclear (Way, 1994).

Pathophysiology

Nearly all malignant colorectal tumors are adenocarcinomas that develop from adenomatous polyps. The incidence of tumors of the right colon is increasing, although the majority still occur in the rectum and sigmoid colon (Figure 23–12). The tumor typically grows undetected, producing few symptoms. By the time symptoms occur, the disease may have spread into deeper layers of the bowel tissue and adjacent organs. Colorectal cancer spreads by direct extension to involve the entire bowel circumference, the submucosa, and outer bowel wall layers. Neighboring structures such as the liver, greater curvature of the stomach, duodenum, small intestine, pancreas, spleen, genitourinary tract, and abdominal wall also may be involved by direct extension. Metastasis to regional lymph nodes is the most common form of tumor spread. This is not always an orderly process; distal nodes may contain cancer cells while regional nodes remain normal (Way, 1994). Cancerous cells from the primary tumor may also spread by way of the lymphatic system or circulatory system to secondary sites such as the liver, lungs, brain, bones, and kidneys. "Seeding" of the tumor to other areas of the peritoneal cavity can occur when the tumor extends through the serosa or during surgical resection.

As noted earlier, bowel cancer often produces no symptoms until it becomes advanced. Because of its slow growth pattern, 5 to 15 years of growth may occur before symptoms present (Way, 1994). The manifestations depend on its location, type and extent, and complications. Bleeding is often the initial manifestation that prompts clients to seek medical care. Other common early symptoms include a change in bowel habits, either diarrhea or constipation. Pain, anorexia, and weight loss are characteristic in advanced disease. A palpable abdominal or rectal mass may be present. Occasionally the client presents with anemia from occult bleeding.

The prognosis of colon cancer depends most on the stage the disease has reached by the time of diagnosis and

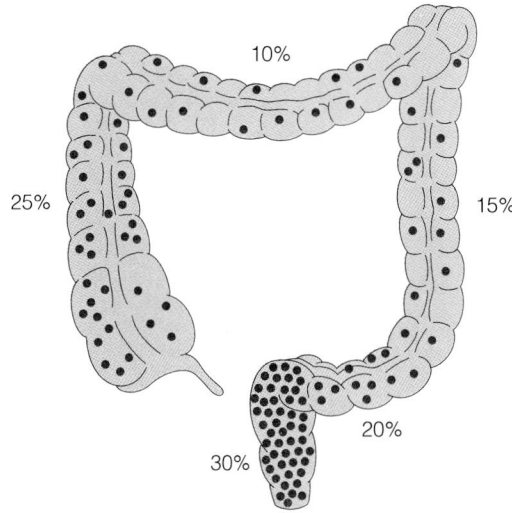

Figure 23–12   The distribution and frequency of cancer of the colon and rectum.

on initial treatment. Overall 5-year survival for colorectal cancer is 57%. The survival rate is poorer in older adults (Hazzard et al., 1994).

Current staging methods primarily use the TNM system, as outlined in Table 23–12. The Dukes Classification System (see the box on page 835) is an older staging system still in use in some facilities.

The primary complications associated with colorectal cancer: (1) bowel obstruction due to narrowing of the bowel lumen by the lesion; (2) perforation of the bowel wall by the tumor, allowing contamination of the peritoneal cavity by bowel contents; and (3) direct extension of the tumor to involve adjacent organs.

Collaborative Care

The focus of collaborative care for the client with colorectal cancer is to establish an accurate diagnosis and disease stage and initiate treatment. Depending on the extent of disease present at the time of diagnosis, a 5-year cure rate of up to 80% to nearly 100% may be achieved. The overall survival rate is 35% to 50%. Colorectal cancer is always treated by surgical intervention, with chemotherapy and radiation therapy used as adjuncts.

Laboratory and Diagnostic Tests
Because colorectal cancer is often a silent disease and treatment at an early stage has a high cure rate, the American Cancer Society recommends routine screening procedures for early detection of the disease. Their recommendations are as follows:

- Annual digital rectal examination for all people over age 40

Table 23–12   The TNM Classification for Colorectal Cancer

Stage	Primary Tumor (T)	Regional Lymph Nodes (N)	Distant Metastasis (M)
	TX—Primary tumor cannot be assessed	NX—Regional lymph node cannot be assessed	MX—Presence of distant metastasis cannot be assessed
	T0—No evidence of primary tumor		
Stage 0	Tis—Carcinoma in situ	N0—No regional lymph node metastasis	M0—No distant metastasis
Stage I	T1—Tumor invades submucosa		
	T2—Tumor invades muscularis propria		
Stage II	T3—Tumor invades through muscularis propria into subserosa or into nonperitonealized pericolic or perirectal tissues		
	T4—Tumor perforates visceral peritoneum or directly invades other organs or structures		
Stage III	Any T	N1—Metastasis in 1 to 3 pericolic or perirectal lymph nodes	
		N2—Metastasis in 4 or more pericolic or perirectal lymph nodes	
		N3—Metastasis in any lymph node along course of a major named vascular trunk	
Stage IV	Any T	Any N	M1—Distant metastasis

- Annual guaiac testing for occult fecal blood for people over age 50
- Flexible sigmoidoscopy every 3 to 5 years for everyone over the age of 50 years

The client with suspected colorectal cancer may undergo extensive diagnostic procedures in addition to physical examination. Laboratory tests, radiographic examinations, and surgical biopsies may be ordered.
The following laboratory tests may be ordered:

- *CBC* is ordered to evaluate anemia. A microcytic anemia, characterized by small RBCs, without apparent cause is generally considered an indication for further diagnostic testing to rule out colorectal cancer.
- *Stool guaiac* is ordered to detect occult blood in the feces, because nearly all colorectal cancers bleed intermittently.
- *Carcinoembryonic antigen (CEA)* is a glycoprotein found in cell membranes of many tissues, including colorectal cancers. This antigen can be detected by radioimmunoassay of the serum or other body fluids and secretions. Because this test is not specific for colorectal cancer and is positive in less than half of clients with localized disease, it is not useful as a screening measure or diagnostic test in a curable stage of the disease. It is

primarily used as a predictor of postoperative prognosis and for detection of recurrence following surgical resection (Way, 1994).

- *Blood chemistry studies* may reveal elevated alkaline phosphatase and bilirubin levels, indicating liver involvement. Other laboratory studies include serum proteins, calcium, and creatinine.

The following diagnostic studies may be ordered:

- *Barium enema* is often used to detect or confirm the presence and location of a tumor. When a contrast medium such as barium is instilled into the lower bowel, cancer appears as either a mass within the bowel lumen, a constriction, or a filling defect. The bowel wall is fixed at the site of the tumor, and the normal mucosal pattern is lost. Although this examination is useful for colon tumors, X-ray studies are unreliable in detecting rectal involvement (Way, 1994). (See the box on page 773 for nursing implications for this test.)
- *Chest X-ray* is obtained to detect tumor metastasis to the lung.
- *Computed tomography (CT) scan,* magnetic resonance imaging (MRI), or ultrasonic examination may be used to assess involvement of other organs by direct extention of the tumor or metastasis.

Dukes Staging Classification for Colorectal Cancer

■ ■ ■

Stage A	Cancer confined to bowel wall
Stage B	Direct penetration of the bowel to involve extrarectal tissue; no lymph node involvement
Stage C	Lymph node involvement
Stage D	Evidence of distant metastases

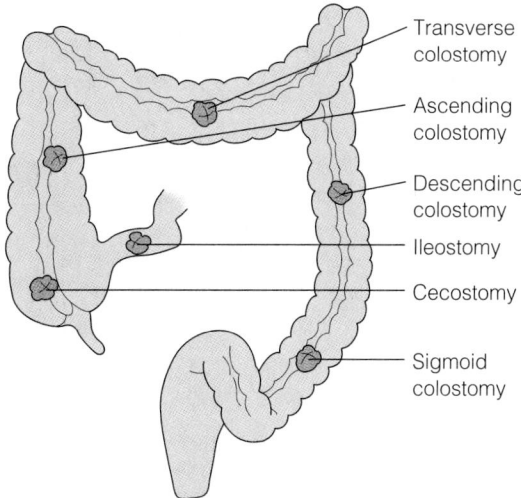

Figure 23–13   Colostomies take the name of the portion of the colon from which they are formed.

■ *Endoscopy (sigmoidoscopy or colonoscopy)* is the primary diagnostic test used to detect and visualize tumors. It also allows tissue collection for biopsy. A flexible sigmoidoscope can detect 50% to 65% of colorectal cancers. Endoscopic examination of the entire colon (colonoscopy) is recommended to locate and biopsy lesions in clients presenting with rectal bleeding. When colonoscopy is performed and the entire colon visualized to the cecum, a barium enema may not be necessary. Tumors typically appear as raised, red, centrally ulcerated, bleeding lesions. This examination is also useful to differentiate cancer from other bowel disease, such as diverticular disease, ulcerative colitis, and Crohn's disease. (See the boxes on pages 767 and 774 for nursing implications for these tests.)

■ *Tissue biopsy* is conducted at the time of endoscopy to confirm cancerous tissue.

Surgery

Surgical resection of the tumor, adjacent colon, and regional lymph nodes is the treatment of choice for colorectal cancer. Options for surgical treatment vary from destruction of the tumor by laser photocoagulation performed during endoscopy to abdominoperineal resection with permanent colostomy. Whenever possible, the anal sphincter is preserved and colostomy avoided (Way, 1994).

Laser photocoagulation uses a very small, intense beam of light to generate heat in tissues toward which it is directed. The heat generated by the laser beam can be used to destroy small tumors. It is also used for palliative surgery of advanced tumors to remove obstruction. Laser photocoagulation can be performed endoscopically and is useful for clients who are unable to tolerate major surgery.

Other surgical treatment options for small, localized tumors include local excision and fulguration. These procedures also may be performed during endoscopy, eliminating the need for abdominal surgery. *Local excision* may be used to remove a disk of rectum containing the tumor in clients with a small, well-differentiated, mobile polypoid lesion. *Fulguration* or electrocoagulation is used to reduce the size of some large tumors for clients who are poor surgical risks. This procedure requires general anesthesia and may need to be repeated at intervals (Way, 1994).

Most clients with colorectal cancer undergo surgical resection of the colon with anastomosis of remaining bowel as a curative procedure. The distribution of regional lymph nodes determines the extent of resection as these may contain metastatic lesions (Way, 1994). Most tumors of the ascending, transverse, descending, and sigmoid colon can be resected.

Tumors of the rectum usually are treated with an abdominoperineal resection in which the sigmoid colon, rectum, and anus are removed through both abdominal and perineal incisions. A permanent sigmoid colostomy is performed to provide for elimination of feces. Nursing care of the client having bowel surgery is outlined in the box on page 836. A Critical Pathway for the client undergoing colon resection is provided on page 837.

Surgical resection of the bowel may be accompanied by a colostomy for diversion of fecal contents. A **colostomy** is an ostomy made in the colon. It may be performed if the bowel is obstructed by the tumor, as a temporary measure to promote healing of anastomoses, or as a permanent means of fecal evacuation when the distal colon and rectum are removed. Colostomies take the name of the portion of the colon from which they are formed: ascending colostomy, transverse colostomy, descending colostomy, and sigmoid colostomy (Figure 23–13).

Nursing Care of the Client Having Bowel Surgery

PREOPERATIVE NURSING CARE

- Ensure that a valid signed consent for the procedure is present in the chart. *It is imperative that the client and/or family understand the procedure along with its potential risks and benefits, as well as alternatives to the proposed procedure. A signed consent form specific to the procedure provides documentation that the client and/or family consent to having the procedure performed.*

- Assess the client's and family's understanding of the procedure, clarifying and interpreting as needed. Provide instructions regarding what to expect during the postoperative period, including pain relief measures; expected tubes, such as a nasogastric tube; intravenous fluids; breathing exercises; and the reintroduction of oral foods and fluids. *The client who is well prepared preoperatively is significantly less anxious and better able to assist in care during the postoperative period. Adequate preparation also decreases the need for narcotic analgesia and enhances the client's recovery.*

- Insert a nasogastric tube if ordered preoperatively. *Although it is often inserted in the surgical suite just prior to surgery, the nasogastric tube may be placed preoperatively to remove secretions and empty stomach contents.*

- Perform bowel preparation procedures as ordered. *Oral and parenteral antibiotics as well as cathartics and enemas may be prescribed preoperatively to clean the bowel and reduce the risk of peritoneal contamination by bowel contents during surgery.*

POSTOPERATIVE NURSING CARE

- Provide routine care for the surgical client. Monitor vital signs and intake and output, including gastric and other drainage from wound drains. Assess for bleeding from abdominal or perineal incision, colostomy, or anus. Evaluate for other wound complications, and maintain physiologic integrity.

- Monitor bowel sounds and degree of abdominal distention. *Surgical manipulation of the bowel disrupts peristalsis, resulting in an initial ileus. Bowel sounds and the passage of flatus indicate a return of peristalsis.*

- Provide for appropriate pain-relief and comfort measures, such as position changes. *The client whose postoperative pain is adequately managed recovers more rapidly and experiences fewer complications.*

- Assess respiratory status, providing abdominal splinting with a blanket or pillow to assist with coughing. *Resection of colorectal cancer with bowel anastomosis or colostomy is a major abdominal surgery. Nursing care to relieve pain, maintain adequate respira-*

tory function, and prevent surgical complications is similar to that for clients having other abdominal surgeries.

- Assess the position and patency of the nasogastric tube, connecting it to low suction. If the tube becomes clogged, gently irrigate with sterile normal saline. *A nasogastric or gastrostomy tube is used postoperatively to provide gastrointestinal decompression and facilitate healing of the anastomosis. Ensuring its patency is important for client comfort and healing.*

- Assess the color, amount, and odor of drainage from surgical drains and the colostomy (if present), noting any changes or the presence of clots or bright bleeding. *Initial drainage may be bright red and then become dark and finally clear or greenish yellow over the first 2 to 3 days. A change in the color, amount, or odor of the drainage may indicate a complication such as hemorrhage, intestinal obstruction, or infection.*

- Alert all personnel caring for the client with an abdominoperineal resection to avoid rectal temperatures, suppositories, or other rectal procedures. *These procedures could disrupt the anal suture line, causing bleeding, infection, or impaired healing.*

- Maintain intravenous fluids while nasogastric suction is in place. *The client on nasogastric suction is unable to take oral food and fluids and, moreover, is losing electrolyte-rich fluid through the nasogastric tube. If replacement fluid and electrolytes are not maintained, the client is at risk for dehydration; sodium, potassium, and chloride imbalance; and metabolic alkalosis.*

- Provide antacids, histamine$_2$-receptor antagonists, and antibiotic therapy as ordered. *The above medications may be ordered for the postoperative client, depending on the procedure performed. Antibiotic therapy is a common measure to prevent infection resulting from contamination of the abdominal cavity with gastric contents.*

- Resume oral food and fluids as ordered. Initial feedings may be clear liquids, progressing to full liquids, and then frequent small feedings of regular foods. Monitor bowel sounds and monitor for abdominal distention frequently during this period. *Oral feedings are reintroduced slowly to minimize abdominal distention and trauma to the suture lines.*

- Encourage ambulation. *This stimulates peristalsis.*

- Begin discharge planning and teaching. Consult with a dietitian for diet instructions and menu planning; reinforce teaching. Teach the client about potential postoperative complications, such as abdominal abscess or bowel obstruction. Teach the client to recognize signs and symptoms of these complications and preventive measures.

Critical Pathway for Client Following Colon Resection

	Date _____ **Preoperative**	Date _____ **1st 24 Hours Postoperative**	Date _____ **2nd to 3rd Day Postoperative**
	Expected length of stay: 6 to 7 days		
Daily outcomes	Client ■ Verbalizes understanding of preoperative teaching, including turning, coughing, deep breathing, incentive spirometer, mobilization, possible tubes (nasogastric tube, IV, Foley catheter, Penrose or other drains, pain management. ■ Demonstrates ability to cope. ■ Verbalizes understanding of procedure.	Client ■ Has stable vital signs. ■ Has a clean, dry wound with well-approximated edges healing by first intention. ■ Recovers from anesthesia, as evidenced by vital signs return to baseline; awake, alert, and oriented. ■ Verbalizes understanding and demonstrates cooperation with turning, coughing, deep breathing and splinting; lungs clear to ausculatation. ■ Demonstrates ability to use patient-controlled analgesia (PCA), if in use. ■ Verbalizes control of incisional pain. ■ Transfers out of bed with assistance 2 to 3 times. ■ Demonstrates ability to cope.	Client ■ Is afebrile. ■ Has clean, dry wound with well-approximated edges healing by first intention. ■ Has active bowel sounds. ■ Tolerates ordered diet without vomiting. ■ Demonstrates cooperation with turning, coughing, deep breathing, and splinting. ■ Ambulates 4 times. ■ Verbalizes control of incisional pain. ■ Verbalizes ability to cope. ■ Verbalizes beginning understanding of home care instructions.
Tests and treatments	CBC Urinalysis Chest X-ray study Baseline physical assessment with a focus on respiratory status and gastrointestinal function Assess and record the description, location, duration, and characteristics of client's pain. Reduce or eliminate pain-producing factors (e.g., fear, anxiety).	CBC Electrolytes Vital signs and O_2 saturation, neurovascular assessment, dressing and wound drainage assessment q15min × 4; q30min × 4; q1h × 4 and then q4h if stable. Assess respiratory status and gastrointestinal function q4h and prn. Incentive spirometer q2h. Intake and output every shift. Assess patency of nasogastric (NG) tube q2h, noting volume q4–8h. Assess Foley catheter or voiding; if unable to void, try suggestive voiding techniques or catheterize q8h or prn. Assess amount, color, and volume of drainage from NG and other drainage tubes.	Vital signs and dressing and wound drainage assessment q4h. Assess respiratory status and gastrointestinal function q4h. Incentive spirometer q2h until fully ambulatory. Intake and output every shift. If still in place, assess patency and output of NG tube q4–8h. Assess voiding pattern every shift. Using sterile asepsis to change dressing: assess wound healing and wound drainage. Assess and record the description, location, duration, and characteristics of pain q4h and prn. Reduce or eliminate pain-producing factors, employ distraction or relaxation techniques, and offer back rubs.

	Date _____ Preoperative	Date _____ 1st 24 Hours Postoperative	Date _____ 2nd to 3rd Day Postoperative
		Assess and record description, location, duration, and characteristics of pain q2–4h and prn. Encourage verbalization of pain and discomfort. Reduce or eliminate pain-producing factors and employ distraction or relaxation techniques. Provide back rubs. Encourage client to request analgesic or use PCA before pain becomes severe.	
Knowledge deficit	Orient to room and surroundings. Provide simple, brief instructions. Review preoperative preparation including hospital and surgical routines. Include family in teaching. Discuss surgery and specific postoperative care: turning, coughing, deep breathing, splinting incision, incentive spirometer, mobilization, possible tubes (NG and intravenous), pain management (PCA, epidural, or prn medications). Instruct regarding distraction techniques (e.g., slow rhythmic breathing and guided imagery) to produce pain relief. Instruct in relaxation techniques (e.g., tensing and relaxing muscle groups and rhythmic breathing). Assess understanding of teaching.	Reorient to room and postoperative routine. Include family in teaching. Review plan of care and importance of early mobilization. Review importance of turning, coughing, deep breathing, splinting incision, incentive spirometer, mobilization, drainage tubes, Foley catheter, and intravenous tubes, pain management (PCA, epidural, or prn medications). Assess understanding of teaching.	Reinforce earlier teaching regarding ongoing care. Include family in teaching. Begin discharge teaching regarding wound care/dressing change. Assess understanding of teaching.
Psycho-social	Assess anxiety related to diagnosis and pending surgery. Assess fears of the unknown and surgery. Encourage verbalization of concerns.	Assess level of anxiety. Encourage verbalization of concerns. Provide information and ongoing support and encouragement to client and family.	Encourage verbalization of concerns. Provide ongoing support and encouragement.

	Date _____ **Preoperative**	Date _____ **1st 24 Hours Postoperative**	Date _____ **2nd to 3rd Day Postoperative**
Psycho-social (continued)	Provide information regarding surgical experience. Minimize external stimuli (e.g., noise, movement).		
Diet	NPO Baseline nutritional and hydration assessment	NG tube until return of bowel sounds NPO	On NG tube removal, clear liquids to tolerance
Activity	Assess safety needs and provide appropriate safety measures. Activity as ordered.	Maintain safety precautions. Assist to chair 2 to 3 times.	Maintain safety precautions. Ambulate 4 times with assistance.
Medications	Preoperative medications as ordered.	IV fluids IV antibiotics Pain medication (PCA, IV, or prn) as ordered.	IV fluids IV antibiotics Convert IV to intermittent IV device as ordered. Pain medication (PCA, IV, or prn) as ordered.
Transfer/ discharge plans	Assess discharge plans and support system. Establish discharge goals with client and family.	Review progress toward discharge goals with client and significant other. Consult with social service re: VNA and projected needs for home health care (if any).	Review progress toward discharge goals with client and significant other. Make appropriate discharge referrals.

	Date _____ **4th Day Postoperative**	Date _____ **5th Day Postoperative**	Date _____ **6th to 7th Day Postoperative**
Daily outcomes	Client ■ Is afebrile. ■ Has a clean, dry wound with well-approximated edges healing by first intention. ■ Tolerates ordered diet without nausea or vomiting. ■ Ambulates 4 to 6 times. ■ Verbalizes control of incisional pain. ■ Verbalizes ability to cope. ■ Verbalizes beginning understanding of home care instructions.	Client ■ Is afebrile. ■ Has a clean, dry wound with well-approximated edges healing by first intention. ■ Tolerates ordered diet without nausea or vomiting. ■ Ambulates 4 to 6 times. ■ Verbalizes control of incisional pain. ■ Verbalizes ability to cope. ■ Verbalizes beginning understanding of home care instructions.	Client ■ Is afebrile. ■ Has a dry, clean wound with well-approximated edges healing by first intention. ■ Manages pain with nonpharmacologic measures and any ordered medications. ■ Is independent in self-care. ■ Is fully ambulatory. ■ Has resumed preadmission urine and bowel elimination pattern. ■ Verbalizes home care instructions. ■ Tolerates usual diet. ■ Verbalizes ability to cope with ongoing stressors.

➤

Critical Pathway for Client Following Colon Resection (continued)

	Date _____ **4th Day Postoperative**	Date _____ **5th Day Postoperative**	Date _____ **6th to 7th Day Postoperative**
Tests and treatments	Vital signs, dressing, and wound drainage assessment q4h. Incentive spirometer q2h until fully ambulatory. Intake and output every shift. Assess voiding pattern every shift. Assess respiratory status and gastrointestinal function q4–8h. Using sterile asepsis to change dressing: assess wound healing and wound drainage. Assess and record description, location, duration, and characteristics of client's pain q4h and prn. Encourage client to use distraction or relaxation techniques.	Vital signs and dressing and wound drainage assessment q4h. Assess respiratory status and gastrointestinal function q4–8h. Remove dressing, and assess wound healing and drainage. Assess and record description, location, duration, and characteristics of client's pain q4h and prn. Encourage client to employ distraction or relaxation techniques.	Vital signs and dressing and wound drainage assessment q4–8h. Assess respiratory status and gastrointestinal function. Assess wound healing. Assess and record description, location, duration, and characteristics of client's pain q4h and prn. Encourage client to employ distraction or relaxation techniques.
Knowledge deficit	Include family in teaching. Initiate discharge teaching regarding wound care, diet, and activity. Review written discharge instructions with client and significant other. Assess understanding of teaching.	Continue discharge teaching regarding wound care, diet, signs and symptoms to report, medications, and activity, including family. Review written discharge instructions with client and significant other. Assess understanding of teaching.	Complete discharge teaching to include wound care, diet, follow-up care, signs and symptoms to report, activity, and medications: name, purpose, dose, frequency, route, dietary interactions, and side effects. Provide client with written discharge instructions. Assess understanding of teaching.
Psycho-social	Encourage verbalization of concerns. Provide ongoing support and encouragement.	Encourage verbalization of concerns. Provide ongoing support and encouragement.	Encourage verbalization of concerns. Provide ongoing support and encouragement.
Diet	If tolerating liquids, advance to full liquids as tolerated.	Advance diet to soft, regular diet to tolerance.	Regular diet as tolerated.
Activity	Ambulate independently at least 4 times. Maintain safety precautions.	Fully ambulatory Maintain safety precautions.	Fully ambulatory
Medications	Provide PO analgesics Intermittent IV device for any IV medications; discontinue when so ordered	Provide PO analgesics	Provide PO analgesics

	Date _____ **4th Day Postoperative**	Date _____ **5th Day Postoperative**	Date _____ **6th to 7th Day Postoperative**
Transfer/ discharge plans	Continue to review progress toward discharge goals.	Finalize discharge plans. Continue to review progress toward discharge goals. Finalize plans for home care if needed.	Complete discharge instructions.

A *sigmoid colostomy* is the most common permanent colostomy performed, particularly for cancer of the rectum. It is usually created during an abdominoperineal resection. This procedure involves the removal of the sigmoid colon, rectum, and anus through abdominal and perineal incisions. The anal canal is closed, and a stoma formed from the proximal sigmoid colon. The stoma is located on the lower left quadrant of the abdomen.

When a *double-barrel colostomy* is performed, two separate stomas are created (Figure 23–14). The distal colon is not removed, but bypassed. The proximal stoma, which is functional, diverts the fecal flow to the abdominal wall. The distal stoma may be located near the proximal stoma or at the end of the midline incision. Also called the mucus fistula, the distal stoma expels mucus from the distal colon. It may be pouched or dressed with a 4- × 4-inch gauge dressing. A double-barrel colostomy may be indicated for cases of trauma, tumor, or inflammation, and it may be temporary or permanent.

An emergency procedure used to relieve an intestinal obstruction or perforation is called a *transverse loop colostomy*. During this procedure, a loop of the transverse colon is brought out from the abdominal wall and suspended over a plastic rod or bridge, which prevents the loop from slipping back into the abdominal cavity. The loop stoma may be opened at the time of surgery or a few days later at the client's bedside. The bridge may be removed in 1 to 2 weeks. Transverse loop colostomies are typically temporary.

In a *Hartmann procedure,* a common temporary colostomy procedure, the distal portion of the colon is left in place and is oversewn for closure. A temporary colostomy may be performed when bowel rest or healing is required, such as following tumor resection or inflammation of the bowel. It also may be performed following traumatic injury to the colon, such as a gunshot wound. Surgical reconnection or anastomosis of the severed portions of the colon is not done immediately because the heavy bacterial colonization of the colon would not allow the anastomosis to heal properly. About 3 to 6 months following a temporary colostomy, the colostomy is closed and a colon anastomosis is performed. Clients with tem-

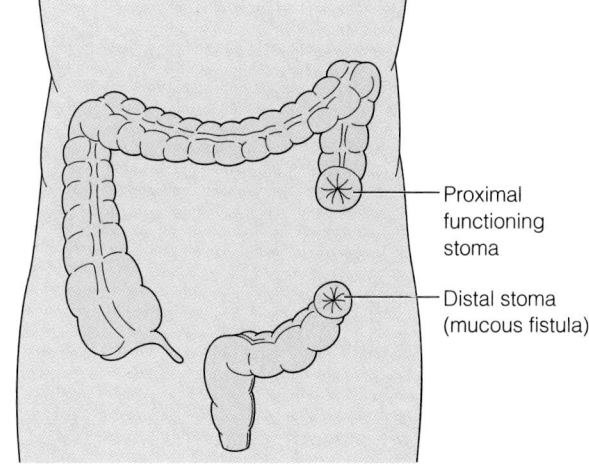

Figure 23–14   A temporary, double-barrel colostomy. The proximal stoma is the functioning stoma, whereas the distal stoma expels mucus from the distal colon.

porary colostomies require the same care as clients with permanent colostomies.

Nursing care of the client with a colostomy is outlined in the box on page 842. Collaborative care for the client with a colostomy is discussed in the box on page 844.

Radiation Therapy
Radiation therapy is often used in addition to surgical resection of bowel tumors. For small rectal cancers, intracavitary, external, or implantation radiation may be employed with or without accompanying surgical excision of the tumor. Preoperative radiation therapy may be administered to clients with large tumors to improve their resectability. When megavoltage radiation therapy is used, possibly in combination with chemotherapy, rectal carcinoma is reduced in size, cells in regional lymphatic tissue are killed, and recurrence is delayed or prevented (Berkow & Fletcher, 1992; Way, 1994). Megavoltage radiation therapy also may be used postoperatively to decrease the risk of recurrence and to reduce pain. Large fixed lesions that are not resectable may be treated to reduce their bulk and slow progression of the cancer.

Nursing Care of the Client with a Colostomy

PREOPERATIVE CARE

- Contact the ET nurse to provide recommendations for stoma location and initial teaching. *The ET nurse is specially trained to work with the client in planning and instituting management of the colostomy. Factors such as the client's weight, preferred style of clothing, and waistline are considered in stoma placement to facilitate long-term comfort and ease of management.*

- Answer the client's questions directly, providing clarification of information as needed. *The client with good preoperative understanding of the procedure and postoperative care is less anxious and better able to cooperate.*

- Provide a referral to an ostomy support group as needed or desired by the client. *Talking with someone else who has an ostomy may help the client become more comfortable with and accepting of the colostomy.*

POSTOPERATIVE CARE

- Assess the location of the stoma and the type of colostomy performed. *Stoma location is an indicator of the section of bowel in which it is located and a predictor of the type of fecal drainage to expect.*

- Assess stoma appearance and surrounding skin condition frequently (see the box on page 814). *Assessment of stoma and skin condition is particularly important in the early postoperative period, when complications are most likely to occur and most treatable.*

- Position a collection bag or drainable pouch over the stoma. *Initial drainage may contain more mucus and serosanguineous fluid than fecal material. As the bowel starts to resume function, drainage becomes fecal in nature. The consistency of drainage depends on the stoma location in the bowel.*

- A descending or sigmoid colostomy may be managed either by use of a drainable pouch or irrigation. *Elimination patterns from a sigmoid colostomy are* similar to the client's normal elimination pattern preoperatively. *Many clients will resume a daily evacuation of stool and not require constant use of a pouch or drainage system. A light pouch may be used for security.*

- If necessary, perform a colostomy irrigation, instilling water into the colon similar to an enema procedure (Procedure 23–3 on page 845). *The water stimulates the colon to empty. The client may irrigate the colon daily or every other day.*

- When a colostomy irrigation is ordered for a client with a double-barrel or loop colostomy, irrigate the proximal stoma. Digital assessment of the bowel direction from the stoma can assist in determining which is the proximal stoma. *The distal bowel carries no fecal contents and does not need irrigation. On occasion, it may be irrigated for cleansing just prior to reanastomosis.*

- Empty a drainable pouch or replace the colostomy bag as needed or when it is no more than one-third full. *If the pouch is allowed to fill, its weight may impair the seal and cause leakage.*

- Clients with ascending or transverse colostomies are not candidates for irrigations. *Only a small portion of the colon is functional, and fecal drainage is generally liquid and constant.*

- Provide stomal and skin care for the client with a colostomy as for the client with an ileostomy, as discussed in the box on page 814. *Good skin and stoma care is important to maintain the skin's integrity and function as the first line of defense against infection.*

- Use caulking agents, such as Stomahesive or karaya paste, and a skin barrier wafer as needed to maintain a secure ostomy pouch. This may be particularly important for the client with a loop colostomy. *The main challenge for a client with a transverse loop colostomy is to maintain a secure ostomy pouch over the plastic bridge.*

Chemotherapy

Chemotherapeutic agents, such as oral levamisole and intravenous fluorouracil (5-FU), are also used postoperatively as adjunctive therapy for colorectal cancer. When combined with radiation therapy, chemotherapy improves local control and survival for clients with stage II and stage III rectal tumors. The benefit for colon cancers is less clear, but chemotherapy may be used to aid in reducing its spread to the liver and preventing recurrence. Leucovorin may also be given with 5-FU to enhance its antitumor effect. Further discussion about chemotherapy and nursing implications is included in Chapter 9.

Nursing Care

In planning and implementing care for the client with colorectal cancer, the nurse needs to consider not only physical care needs but also the client's emotional response to the diagnosis. Because colorectal cancer is often advanced at the time of diagnosis, the prognosis, even

Nursing Care of the Client with a Colostomy (continued)

- A small needle hole high on the colostomy pouch will allow flatus to escape. This hole may be closed with a Band-Aid and opened only while the client is in the bathroom for odor control. *Ostomy bags may "balloon" out, impairing the integrity of the skin seal, if excess gas collects.*

CLIENT AND FAMILY TEACHING

- Prior to discharge, provide written, verbal, and psychomotor instruction on colostomy care, pouch management, skin care, and irrigation for the client. *Whether the colostomy is temporary or permanent, the client will be responsible for its management for a period of time. Good understanding of procedures and care helps ensure the client's ability to provide self-care, as well as enhancing self-esteem and control.*

- Allow ample time for the client (and family, if necessary) to practice changing the pouch, either on the client or a model. *Practice of psychomotor skills improves learning and confidence.*

- If an abdominoperineal resection with removal of the rectum has been performed, emphasize the importance of using no rectal suppositories, rectal temperatures, or enemas. Suggest that the client carry medical identification or a MedicAlert tag or bracelet. *These measures are important to prevent trauma to the tissues when the rectum has been removed.*

- The diet for a client with a colostomy is individualized and may require no alteration from that consumed preoperatively. Dietary teaching should, however, include information on foods that cause stool odor and gas and foods that thicken and loosen stools. Foods that cause these adverse effects on ostomy output are listed below.

Foods That Increase Stool Odor

- Asparagus
- Beans
- Cabbage
- Eggs
- Fish
- Garlic
- Onions
- Some spices

Foods That Increase Intestinal Gas

- Beer
- Broccoli
- Brussels sprouts
- Cabbage
- Carbonated drinks
- Cauliflower
- Corn
- Cucumbers
- Dairy products
- Dried beans
- Onions
- Peas
- Radishes
- Spinach
- String beans

Foods That Thicken Stools

- Applesauce
- Bananas
- Bread
- Cheese
- Yogurt
- Marshmallows
- Pasta
- Pretzels
- Rice
- Tapioca
- Creamy peanut butter

Foods That Loosen Stools

- Chocolate
- Dried beans
- Fried foods
- Greasy foods
- Highly spiced foods
- Leafy green vegetables
- Raw fruits and juices
- Raw vegetables

Foods That Color Stools

- Beets
- Red gelatin

with treatment, may be poor. The client may experience feelings of denial and anger. Extensive abdominal surgery and potentially a colostomy may have occurred or be planned. Moreover, extensive diagnostic tests and the effects of chemotherapy and radiation therapy can leave the client fatigued and discouraged.

Nursing care is aimed at providing emotional support, teaching the client about specific diagnostic procedures, providing preoperative and postoperative care if surgery is indicated, and providing instruction in colostomy care

if a stoma is created. Priority nursing diagnoses for this client include *Pain, Altered Nutrition,* and *Anticipatory Grieving. Risk for Sexual Dysfunction* should be considered as a priority diagnosis if surgery has resulted in formation of a colostomy.

Pain

The client with colorectal cancer may experience pain from a number of sources. Diagnostic examinations and preparatory procedures are often uncomfortable. Nearly

Collaborative Care: The Client with a Colostomy	
Health Care Team	**Client Centered Care**
Gastroenterologist	Consults with primary care physician. May perform endoscopy procedures if indicated.
General surgeon	Conducts preoperative assessment, removes diseased bowel and creates colostomy, manages postoperative course, monitors surgical outcomes following discharge.
Oncologist	For clients with a cancer diagnosis, makes recommendations regarding surgery, radiation, and/or chemotherapy. Monitors responses to therapies.
Enterostomal therapist	Preoperatively, evaluates clients requiring an ostomy to determine stoma placement. Postoperatively, assists client and family to manage ostomy and provides teaching related to stomal care. Obtains appropriate external pouch, teaches skin care, and application and emptying of external pouch.
Social worker	Arranges for purchase of necessary supplies. Coordinates visiting nurse visits to assist with stoma and dressing care. Refers client and family to resources such as the American Cancer Society and stoma support groups.
Dietitian	Makes recommendations regarding nutritional therapies such as total parental nutrition, enteral feedings, vitamins, and minerals. Provides teaching regarding strategies to maintain fluid and electrolyte balance and avoid gas-producing foods.
RN and Health Care Team Communications	Reports abdominal distention, worsening pain, nausea or vomiting, signs and symptoms of hemorrhage or infection to physician. Consults with enterostomal therapist regarding client's progress with teaching and self-care of ostomy. Discusses anticipated home care needs with client. Collaborates with dietitian to provide a well-balanced diet when the client begins eating.

all clients with colorectal cancer undergo a surgical procedure, often involving an abdominal and possibly a perineal incision. When an abdominoperineal resection is performed, the client may experience "phantom" rectal pain. This discomfort is related to severing of nerves during the wide excision of the rectum. Finally, the primary tumor itself and, potentially, metastatic tumors may impinge on nerves and other organs, causing pain. In the early postoperative period, patient-controlled analgesia (PCA) can be very effective in relieving the discomfort, as can routine administration of ordered analgesics. These measures may also be employed along with continuous analgesia delivery (CAD) systems should the tumor be far enough advanced to preclude surgical resection. Nursing care focuses on assessing the adequacy of pain relief, providing supportive measures that will enhance analgesia, and ensuring that pain or the fear of pain does not lead to respiratory complications. See Chapter 4 for more information on caring for clients with pain.

Nursing interventions with rationales follow:

- Assess the client frequently for adequate pain relief. Use subjective and objective information, including

   a. The location, intensity, and character of the pain.

   b. Nonverbal signs, including grimacing; tense body position; apparent dozing; elevated pulse; an increase or decrease in blood pressure; rapid, shallow respirations.

The client may assume that pain is to be expected or tolerated or may fear becoming addicted to analgesic medications. Careful questioning and assessment can provide the nurse with accurate information regarding the client's pain status, allowing better control of discomfort.

- Ask client to rate pain on a scale of 0 to 10 (0 = no pain, 10 = worst pain). Document the level of pain. *Pain is a subjective experience. Clients perceive and respond to pain differently. Religion and ethnic background may affect a client's response to pain.*

- Assess the effectiveness of pain medications ½ hour after administration. Monitor for medication effectiveness and adverse effects. *A dosage adjustment may be required to provide adequate pain relief without harmful effects.*

- Assess the incision for signs of inflammation or swelling; assess drainage catheters and tubes for patency. *Poorly controlled pain or pain that changes may be related to organ distention from an obstructed nasogastric tube or urinary catheter or may indicate the presence of an infection or abscess.*

- Assess the abdomen for distention, tenderness, and bowel sounds. *Intra-abdominal bleeding, peritonitis, or paralytic ileus can cause pain that may be confused with incisional pain.*

- Administer pain medication prior to an activity or procedure. *The analgesic can relieve the client of discomfort, allowing for more comfortable ambulation.*

Procedure 23–3 Colostomy Irrigation

SUPPLIES

- Colostomy irrigation set
- Plastic bag
- Water-based lubricant
- Clean ostomy pouch

COMMENTS

Explain the procedure to the client, and provide for privacy. The client may sit in a chair beside the toilet or commode or on the toilet seat. Position the bed-confined client on the right side with a bedpan in front. Follow universal precautions.

PROCEDURE

1. Close the clamp on the irrigation bag.
2. Fill the irrigation bag with the prescribed amount of warm water (usually 1000 mL).
3. Remove the pouch. Dispose in plastic bag.
4. Attach the irrigation sleeve over stoma using the belt. Place the bottom of sleeve into the toilet, commode, or bedpan. (For a two-piece appliance, snap the irrigation sleeve onto the skin barrier flange.)
5. Open the clamp on the bag, allowing fluid to run through tubing to clear the air. Close the clamp.
6. Lubricate the cone. Insert the cone tip into the stoma and hold it securely to prevent backflow of water.
7. Open the clamp, and allow solution to flow into the colon from a height of no greater than 12 to 18 inches. This usually takes 5 to 10 minutes.
8. Allow irrigation fluid and feces to flow into the toilet or bedpan. Allow about 15 minutes for drainage.
9. Client may then clamp bottom of the sleeve and go about other activities.
10. After approximately 30 to 45 minutes, drain the sleeve and remove.
11. Clean the stoma and peristomal skin.
12. Apply a clean ostomy pouch.

POSTPROCEDURE

1. Wash and dry all equipment before storing. Irrigation sleeves are reusable.
2. Document the amount of solution used, the consistency and amount of results, and the client's tolerance of the procedure.

- Provide nonpharmacologic relief measures, such as positioning, diversional activities, management of environmental stimuli, guided imagery, and teaching the use of relaxation techniques. *These techniques are useful to enhance the effects of analgesia.*

- Splint incision with a pillow, and teach the client how to self-splint incision when coughing and deep breathing *to prevent respiratory complications related to fear of pain.*

Altered Nutrition: Less Than Body Requirements

The client undergoing extensive diagnostic procedures for suspected colorectal cancer is at risk for nutritional deficiencies due to frequent and extensive bowel preparation procedures and liquid diets.

Postoperatively, the client will have nothing by mouth (be NPO) until bowel function resumes. Fluid and electrolyte replacement will be ordered along with possible total parenteral nutrition (see Chapter 13). Adequate kcal and nutrient intake is necessary for healing after surgery. Additionally, if the tumor is advanced, the client's metabolic needs may be increased and the appetite decreased.

Nursing interventions with rationales follow:

- Assess the client's readiness for enteral feedings after surgery or diagnostic procedures using data such as statements of hunger, presence of bowel sounds, passage of flatus, and minimal abdominal distention. Provide a dietary referral for the client as needed. *Peristalsis of the gastrointestinal tract is interrupted by manipulation of the bowel. It is important to ensure that peristalsis has resumed prior to institution of oral feedings.*

- Monitor and document food and fluid intake. *Documentation of kcal intake is essential to meet the client's dietary requirements.*

- Weigh the client daily. *Fluctuation in the client's weight may indicate adequate or inadequate dietary intake.*

- Maintain total parenteral nutrition and central intravenous lines as ordered. *The client who is unable to take food enterally for more than 2 to 3 days requires parenteral nutrition to prevent tissue catabolism and facilitate healing.*

- When oral intake is resumed, develop a meal plan with the client. *Participation by the client allows the nurse to develop a diet that incorporates the food likes and dislikes of the client and meets the demands of the client's schedule and environment.*

Anticipatory Grieving

When a bowel resection is performed for colorectal cancer, the client not only loses part of a major organ but also has to adjust to the diagnosis of cancer. Even if the prognosis for recovery is good, many people perceive cancer as always fatal. Providing support for the client and family during the initial stages of grieving can improve physical recovery as well as psychologic coping and eventual adaptation.

Nursing interventions with rationales follow:

- Work to develop a trusting relationship with the client and family. *This increases the nurse's effectiveness in helping them work through the grieving process.*
- Listen actively to the client and family, encouraging them to express their fears and concerns. Assist the client and family to identify strengths, past experiences, and support systems.
  a. Demonstrate respect for the client's and family's cultural, spiritual, and religious values and beliefs; encourage them to use these resources to cope with losses.
  b. Encourage the client and family to discuss the potential impact of loss on the individual family members, family structure, and family function. Assist family members to share concerns with one another.
  c. Provide referral to cancer support groups, social services, or counseling as appropriate.
  These resources can be employed in working through the grief process.

Risk for Sexual Dysfunction

The client undergoing ostomy surgery is at risk for sexual dysfunction (the loss of or alteration in sexual function). Sexual function may be impaired by the physical disruption of the nerves and blood vessels that supply the genitals. In addition, radiation therapy, chemotherapy, or other medications prescribed after surgery may have physical effects that alter sexual function.

Psychologically, an *ostomate* (client with an ostomy), experiences an altered body image and may develop low self-esteem. The client may feel undesirable and fear rejection. He or she may be concerned about odors or pouch leakage during sexual activity. This emotional stress can also contribute to sexual dysfunction. Self-image changes following an ostomy are addressed in the nursing research study described in the accompanying box.

Nursing interventions with rationales follow:

- Provide opportunities for the client and family to express their feelings about the ostomy. *The nurse can encourage the client to verbalize feelings regarding the ostomy, acknowledging that feelings of anger and depression are normal responses to this change in body function.*

- Provide consistent colostomy care. *An accepting attitude and consistent care that provides a secure appliance and controls odor and leakage instills a sense of confidence in the client.*
- Encourage expression of sexual concerns. Provide privacy and caregivers who have established trust with the client and family and are comfortable in discussions about sexual concerns. *Sexuality is a very private concern to most people. The client and family are not likely to express their concerns openly unless trust has been established.*
- Reassure the client and significant other that physical illness and prescribed interventions usually have a temporary effect on sexuality. *The client and partner may misinterpret an initial decrease in libido as evidence that sexual activity will not be possible or resume following recovery.*
- Refer the client and partner to social services or a family counselor for further interventions. *Clients are often discharged from acute care settings well before concerns about sexual activity surface. Ongoing counseling provides a continuing resource.*
- Arrange for a visit from a member of the United Ostomy Association. *This is a group of people who are coping and living with an ostomy. This personal experience can provide information and support, helping the new ostomate overcome feelings of isolation and rejection.*

Other Nursing Diagnoses

Other nursing diagnoses that may be appropriate for the client with colorectal cancer follow:

- *Altered Skin Integrity* related to surgery and radiation therapy
- *Risk for Ineffective Individual Coping* related to support systems
- *Fear* related to uncertain future following diagnosis of malignancy
- *Body Image Disturbance* related to the presence of an abdominal stoma and altered bowel elimination route
- *Impaired Social Interaction* related to fear of odor and leakage of intestinal drainage
- *Anxiety* related to lack of knowledge of colostomy care routines

Client and Family Teaching

Primary prevention of colorectal cancer is a significant nursing care issue. As nurses interact with adult clients in a variety of settings, they provide education about cancer prevention and early detection of tumors. Teach clients about dietary recommendations provided by the American Cancer Society for the prevention of colorectal cancer.

Applying Research to Nursing Practice: Self-Image Changes in Colostomy Clients

■ ■ ■

The focus of one study was the change in clients' self-concept at 4 weeks and 12 weeks following colostomy surgery (Ramer, 1992). The Acceptance of Disability Modified Scale (ADM) was used to measure *trust,* defined as the client's acceptance of physical changes and willingness to assume self-care. The Ostomy Adjustment Scale (OAS) was used to measure *autonomy,* that is, perceived control, ability to perform self-care, feelings of shame, and knowledge of colostomy care. Finally, the Brief Symptom Inventory (BSI) was used to measure *psychosocial discomfort,* that is, the behavior clients displayed when they were unable to meet developmental tasks. Results showed that the score for trust increased between 4 weeks and 12 weeks after surgery. Scores for men at 12 weeks increased noticeably, whereas scores for women barely changed. Women, however, showed a slight increase in perceived autonomy at 12 weeks, whereas men perceived a slight decrease. This finding is consistent with clinical observations that whereas wives assist their husbands with ostomy care, women provide their own care. The data showed a decrease in psychosocial discomfort between 4 and 12 weeks after surgery. At 4 weeks, the clients experienced obsessive-compulsive behavior in checking pouches frequently. They also experienced depression and anxiety, which had lessened by the 12-week interview.

The author pointed out that nursing research in this area is limited and that nurses' judgment about clients' progress is not based on scientific data. The author concluded that the study did help define trust, autonomy, and psychosocial discomfort as measurable quantities. Further research is needed, in particular, research that focuses on larger groups and on clients of different ethnic backgrounds.

Implications for Nursing
Clients undergoing colostomy surgery face physical mutilation, loss of control over some bodily functions, feelings of grief over that loss, and disturbances in self-concept. Nurses in the clinical setting should observe clients with new colostomies for evidence of trust, autonomy, and psychosocial discomfort. Nursing intervention can influence self-concept changes in a positive direction. Gender may influence self-concept changes: Men tend to rely on their spouses for care, whereas women tend to care for themselves. Long-term follow-up is needed for ostomy clients and may be channeled through local ostomy associations.

Critical Thinking in Client Care

1. Give an example of how an ostomy client deals with the concepts of trust, autonomy, and psychosocial discomfort.

2. Cite nursing interventions that may help a client accept an ostomy.

3. What normal physiologic changes in the older adult can hamper a client's performance of ostomy self-care?

These recommendations include decreasing the amount of fat, refined sugar, and red meats in the diet while increasing intake of dietary fiber. Foods that contain high amounts of fiber include raw fruits and vegetables, legumes, and whole-grain products.

Nurses help educate clients about recommended screening procedures as well as prevention. Stress the importance of regular health examinations, including digital rectal exams. Discuss recommendations for regular guaiac testing of stool after age 40. Stress the noninvasiveness and low cost of this screening measure. Include the importance of seeking medical treatment if blood is noted in or on the stool. Teach clients the warning signs for cancer, including those specific to bowel cancer, such as a change in bowel habits.

When colorectal cancer is suspected or diagnosed, the client and family have multiple teaching/learning needs. The client undergoing diagnostic procedures needs in-struction about the various tests to be performed and preparatory procedures. Teach the client about dietary restrictions, laxatives, enemas, and the restriction of food and fluids prior to the procedure. Discuss any recommended postprocedure care measures and potential adverse effects to watch for.

When surgery is anticipated, instruct the client about routine preoperative care, such as intestinal preparation, oral antibiotics, possible intravenous fluids, and nasogastric tube. Teach coughing, deep breathing, and movement techniques to be used postoperatively. Emphasize the importance of using analgesics in the postoperative period to control pain, reassuring the client that addiction rarely results from analgesic use after surgery. If a colostomy is planned, provide instruction, and refer the client to the enterostomal therapist. If radiation therapy or chemotherapy is prescribed either preoperatively or postoperatively, discuss skin care and management of potential adverse effects with the client. Refer to Chapter 9 for further discussion of teaching needs related to these therapies.

The client with an inoperable tumor has multiple teaching/learning needs as well, although these may differ significantly from those for clients in whom cure is anticipated or possible. Provide information about pain and symptom management. Discuss the hospice philosophy and available services. Provide a referral to a local hospice or home health department.

Applying the Nursing Process

Case Study of a Client with Colorectal Cancer: William Cunningham

William Cunningham is a 65-year-old retired railroad employee who is married and has grown children. For the past 3 months, Mr. Cunningham has noticed small amounts of blood in his stools along with occasional passage of mucus. He has noticed a pressure sensation in the rectum and also a decrease in the caliber of the stools. After noting a palpable mass on digital examination of the rectum, the physician orders a colonoscopy to be performed on an outpatient basis. A large sessile lesion is noted in the rectum and biopsied. The pathology report shows the lesion to be adenocarcinoma. Mr. Cunningham is scheduled for an abdominoperineal resection and sigmoid colostomy.

Assessment
Madonna Hart, RN, completes the admission assessment. The history indicates that Mr. Cunningham has stated that he had recently had a change in bowel habits. He states that he has no pain or other symptoms. Physical assessment findings include the following: BP, 118/78; T, 98.4 F (36.9 C); P, 82; R, 18. He is 5 feet, 10 inches (178 cm) tall and weighs 185 lb (84 kg). There are no abnormal laboratory findings other than the previous pathology report of adenocarcinoma of rectal lesion.

Mr. Cunningham states, "I really don't want a colostomy, but if that is what it takes to keep me well, I'm ready to get it over with."

Diagnosis
Ms. Hart identifies the following nursing diagnoses for Mr. Cunningham:

- *Pain* related to surgical intervention
- *Risk for Impaired Skin Integrity* (peristomal) related to fecal drainage and pouch adhesive.
- *Constipation* and/or *Diarrhea* related to the colostomy
- *Risk for Self-Esteem Disturbance* and *Body Image Disturbance* related to the colostomy

- *Risk for Sexual Dysfunction* related to wide rectal incision and colostomy

Expected Outcomes
The expected outcomes established in the plan of care specify that Mr. Cunningham will

- Report a decrease in the level of pain on a scale of 0 to 10, after receiving pain medication.
- After discharge, continue to report an improvement in comfort level as measured on a pain scale of 0 to 10.
- Perform colostomy care using correct technique.
- Maintain adequate hygiene and grooming measures.
- Demonstrate willingness to discuss changes in sexual function.
- Wear clothing to enhance physical and emotional self-esteem.
- Verbalize understanding of medically imposed restrictions.

Planning and Implementation
Ms. Hart plans and implements the following nursing interventions for Mr. Cunningham:

- Provide analgesia as ordered, evaluating its effectiveness.
- Discuss foods that cause odor and gas.
- Teach colostomy care.
- Teach the colostomy irrigation procedure.
- Maintain consistent nursing personnel assignment to facilitate trust.
- Refer Mr. Cunningham to the local United Ostomy Association.
- Refer Mr. Cunningham to local medical supply companies for ostomy supplies.
- Provide for privacy when teaching and discussing concerns about ostomy.

Evaluation
On discharge, Mr. Cunningham is able to empty and rinse out his colostomy pouch. He is performing daily colostomy irrigations and pouch changes. Ms. Hart has given him verbal and written instructions on colostomy care. He verbalizes understanding of "phantom" rectal pain, and the necessity to avoid rectal temperatures and rectal suppositories. He verbalizes understanding of measuring his stoma before ordering new supplies, carrying an extra pouch with him, avoiding heavy lifting, and the importance of follow-up care. Ms. Hart has referred Mr. Cunningham to a home health agency in his community for any further questions and follow-up care.

Critical Thinking in the Nursing Process

1. What is the pathophysiologic basis for a decrease in the caliber of Mr. Cunningham's stools and the passage of blood and mucus?

2. What is the cause of "phantom" rectal pain?

3. Why is it important to discuss dietary concerns with a client with a colostomy, especially odor- and gas-forming foods?

4. Outline a plan to teach Mr. Cunningham how to irrigate a colostomy.

5. Develop a care plan for Mr. Cunningham for the nursing diagnosis *Body Image Disturbance*.

Structural and Obstructive Disorders

Any portion of the intestines may be affected by a structural or obstructive disorder. When the structural defect is in the bowel wall, structural disorders may directly affect the intestine, as is the case with diverticula. **Hernias** are defects in the abdominal wall that allow intra-abdominal contents (such as loops of bowel) to protrude, with a potential indirect effect on bowel function. Likewise, bowel obstructions may result from disease of the bowel itself or from obstruction of the bowel lumen due to an external source.

The Client with a Hernia

A hernia is a protrusion of an organ or structure through a defect in the muscular wall of the abdomen. Hernias are generally composed of the covering skin and subcutaneous tissues, a peritoneal sac, and the underlying viscera, such as loops of bowel or other internal organs. Hernias may be congenital, caused by a structural closure defect, or acquired. Acquired hernias are associated with weakening of the normal musculature. Precipitating factors include surgery; abrupt increases in intra-abdominal pressure, which may occur during heavy lifting or coughing; and more gradual and prolonged increases in intra-abdominal pressure related to pregnancy, obesity, or ascites.

Pathophysiology

Hernias are classified by the location in which they appear (Figure 23–15). Approximately 75% of hernias occur in the groin. These are known as either inguinal or femoral hernias. Another 10% are ventral or incisional hernias of the abdominal wall, 3% are umbilical hernias. Other types of hernias may include hiatal hernias and diaphragmatic hernias, discussed in other chapters.

Inguinal Hernias

Inguinal hernias are further divided into *indirect* and *direct* inguinal hernias. Indirect inguinal hernias are the most common type and usually affect males. An indirect inguinal hernia is caused by improper closure of the tract that develops as the testes descend into the scrotum before birth. A sac containing peritoneum, intestine, and/or omentum emerges through the inguinal ring and follows the spermatic cord through the inguinal canal. It often descends into the scrotum. Although indirect inguinal hernias are congenital defects, they often do not become apparent until adulthood, when increased intra-abdominal pressure and dilation of the inguinal ring allow abdominal contents to enter the channel.

Direct inguinal hernias are always acquired defects that result from weakness of the posterior inguinal wall. Direct inguinal hernias occur more often in older adults. Femoral hernias are also acquired defects in which a peritoneal sac protrudes through the femoral ring. These hernias usually occur in obese or pregnant women.

Inguinal hernias often produce no symptoms and are discovered during routine physical examination. They may produce a lump, swelling, or bulge in the groin, particularly with lifting or straining. The male client may

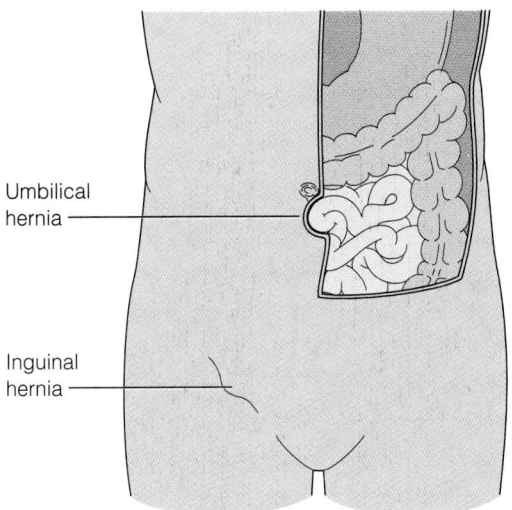

Umbilical hernia

Inguinal hernia

Figure 23–15 Two types of hernia.

experience either sharp pain or a dull ache that radiates into the scrotum. A palpable mass may be present in the groin, although it may be felt only with increased intra-abdominal pressure (as occurs during coughing) and invagination of scrotum toward the inguinal ring.

If a hernia is *reducible*, contents of the sac return to the abdominal cavity either spontaneously as intra-abdominal pressure is reduced (as with lying down) or with manual pressure. Few complications are associated with a reducible hernia. When the contents of a hernia cannot be returned to the abdominal cavity, it is said to be *irreducible* or *incarcerated*. Contents of an incarcerated hernia are trapped, usually by a narrow neck or opening to the hernia. Incarceration increases the risk of complications, including obstruction and strangulation. Obstruction occurs when the lumen of the bowel contained within the hernia becomes occluded, much like the crimping of a hose.

If the blood supply to the hernia contents is compromised, the result is a *strangulated hernia*. This complication can lead to infarction of the affected bowel with severe pain and perforation with contamination of the peritoneal cavity. Manifestations of a strangulated hernia include abdominal pain and distention, nausea, vomiting, tachycardia, and fever.

Umbilical Hernia

Pregnancy and obesity also contribute to the development of umbilical hernias in adults. *Umbilical hernias* may be congenital and evident during infancy, or acquired as the tissue closing the umbilical ring weakens, allowing protrusion of abdominal contents. These hernias are more common in women. Other predisposing factors include multiple pregnancies with prolonged labor, ascites, and large intra-abdominal tumors (Way, 1994).

Umbilical hernias tend to enlarge steadily and contain omentum, although they may also contain small or large bowel. The client may experience sharp pain on coughing or straining or a dull, aching sensation. Strangulation is a common complication of umbilical hernias.

Incisional or Ventral Hernia

Incisional or *ventral hernias* occur at a previous surgical incision site. The cause of this hernia is inadequate healing of the incision. Contributing factors include poor wound closure technique, postoperative wound infection, age or debility, obesity, inadequate nutrition, and excess incisional stress caused by vigorous coughing.

Ventral hernias are often evident when the client pulls to a sitting position from a lying position; they are characterized by a bulge noted at the incisional site. Ventral hernias often are asymptomatic, and the risk of incarceration is low because of the size of the defect.

Collaborative Care

The diagnosis of a hernia is made by a physical examination. The client is examined in a supine and sitting or standing position. A bulge may be seen or felt when the client coughs or bears down. No laboratory or diagnostic testing is usually required, unless bowel obstruction or strangulation is suspected.

The treatment of hernia is generally surgical repair, although the client may be taught to reduce the hernia by lying down and gently pushing against the mass. A binder or truss may be worn to prevent or control the protrusion. The client should not attempt to reduce an incarcerated hernia.

All types of hernia are surgically repaired unless specific contraindications to surgery exist. Surgery is generally well tolerated by people of all ages and carries a much lower risk of complication than do the complications of incarceration, obstruction, and strangulation. Emergency surgery is indicated for a hernia that is incarcerated, painful, or tender (Way, 1994). A *herniorrhaphy* is surgical repair of a hernia. In a herniorrhaphy, the defect that allowed herniation of abdominal contents is closed by suturing or using wire or mesh over the defect. Surgery is scheduled as an elective procedure unless complications occur. If incarceration has occurred or strangulation is suspected, the abdomen is explored at the time of surgery and any infarcted bowel resected. Heavy lifting and heavy manual labor are restricted for approximately 3 weeks after surgery.

Nursing Care

Nurses need to be alert for the possible presence of a hernia, particularly in clients who have multiple risk factors. Should an abnormal bulge be noted in the client's groin, umbilical area, or in an old or new incision, the primary care provider should be notified. The risk of strangulation with any hernia makes *Altered Tissue Perfusion* a high-priority nursing diagnosis.

Herniorrhaphy is generally an uncomplicated procedure, often performed as same-day surgery. The client has few acute nursing care needs apart from preoperative assessment and immediate postoperative care. Operative nursing care is similar to care of a client with an appendectomy.

Risk for Altered Tissue Perfusion: Gastrointestinal

When providing care for a client with a known hernia, the possibility of obstruction and strangulation must be considered throughout nursing assessments. Although it may not be possible to prevent these complications through nursing interventions, rapid identification of the problem allows timely surgical intervention. This not only improves the client's comfort and healing but also may prevent major complications related to infection and peritoneal contamination by bowel contents.

Nursing interventions with rationales follow:

- Assess the client's comfort level, taking particular note of any acute increase in abdominal, groin, perineal, or scrotal pain. *An abrupt increase in the intensity of pain experienced by the client may indicate bowel ischemia due to strangulation.*
- Assess bowel sounds and abdominal distention at least every 8 hours. *A change in bowel sounds—either cessation of sounds or an onset of hyperactive, high-pitched sounds—may indicate obstruction. With obstruction, abdominal girth may increase.*
- Notify the primary care provider if the hernia becomes painful or tender. *These signs may indicate incarceration and increased risk for strangulation.*
- If signs of possible obstruction or strangulation occur, notify the physician, and place the client in a supine position with the hips elevated and knees slightly bent. Keep the client NPO, and begin preparations for surgery. *This position helps relax abdominal muscles and may facilitate reduction of the hernia. Strangulation or obstruction require immediate surgical intervention.*

Other Nursing Diagnoses

Additional nursing diagnoses for the client with a hernia may include the following:

- *Impaired Skin Integrity* related to surgical incision
- *Risk for Urinary Retention* related to surgical manipulation of the groin area
- *Risk for Altered Role Performance* related to postoperative restriction on heavy manual labor

Client and Family Teaching

Most client and family teaching related to hernias is conducted in the course of routine health examinations. Explain why examinations of the groin and abdominal region are included. Teach clients what hernias are and the risk factors for their development. Reassure clients that surgical intervention is generally without complications, even in older adults, and carries a lower risk than not repairing the hernia. Teach clients how to reduce hernias if necessary, and stress the importance of seeking immediate medical intervention if signs of strangulation or obstruction occur. When surgery is planned, instruct the client to notify the physician should he or she develop an upper respiratory infection and cough, because forceful coughing is not recommended postoperatively. Reinforce postoperative teaching about pain management and activity restrictions following surgery.

Applying the Nursing Process

Case Study of a Client with an Inguinal Hernia: Lee Pajer

Lee Pajer is a 25-year-old cattle rancher who developed a "bulge" in the right inguinal area after lifting a cattle head chute. He visits his family physician and is referred for a surgical consultation. The physician and Mr. Pajer decide to proceed with a herniorrhaphy to avoid the possibility of Mr. Pajer's developing an incarcerated hernia.

Assessment

The assessment history for Mr. Pajer is unremarkable. Except for the hernia, he is in excellent health. Physical assessment findings include the following: T, 99.8 F (37.6 C);, P, 68; R, 16; BP, 110/76. There are no abnormal laboratory findings, and he is prepared for same-day surgery.

Diagnosis

Gina Wu, the nurse caring for Mr. Pajer in the same-day surgery unit, identifies the following nursing diagnoses:

- *Pain* related to surgical intervention
- *Knowledge Deficit* related to lack of information about care after discharge
- *Risk for Urinary Retention* (postoperative) related to surgical intervention in groin area

Expected Outcomes

The expected outcomes established in the plan of care specify that Mr. Pajer will

- Report a tolerable level of discomfort.
- Verbalize understanding of care and activity restrictions after discharge.
- Regain normal urinary elimination prior to discharge, voiding in quantities of at least 250 mL without evidence of bladder distention.

Planning and Implementation

Ms. Wu plans and implements the following nursing interventions for Mr. Pajer:

- Give analgesics as needed for pain and discomfort.
- Teach Mr. Pajer to splint the abdomen when turning.
- Teach Mr. Pajer to care for the incision after discharge.
- Teach Mr. Pajer to avoid heavy lifting for 2 to 6 weeks after discharge, depending on surgeon's specific instructions.
- Instruct Mr. Pajer to refrain from driving for 2 weeks to avoid any undue stress on incision.

- Discuss measures to aid in urination and the importance of drinking fluids.

Evaluation

Ms. Wu makes a follow-up phone call the day after surgery. Mr. Pajer reports minimal discomfort and states that he is able to urinate and the incision is doing well, with no evidence of redness, warmth, or swelling. He states that he has an appointment next week with the surgeon to remove the surgical clips.

Critical Thinking in the Nursing Process

1. What is the pathophysiologic basis for difficulty urinating after surgery?

2. Describe the progression from reducible hernia to incarceration, strangulation, and possible peritonitis when these complications of hernia occur.

3. Develop a teaching plan for a client who chooses to use a binder or truss instead of undergoing surgical repair of hernia.

The Client with an Intestinal Obstruction

■ ■ ■

An **intestinal obstruction** occurs when intestinal contents fail to be propelled through the lumen of the bowel. Obstruction is the most common precipitating cause for small bowel surgery.

Pathophysiology

While an obstruction can occur in any portion of the intestinal tract, the small intestine is affected most often; only about 15% of bowel obstructions occur in the large intestine. The ileum of the small intestine is the usual site for obstruction.

Small Bowel Obstruction

In addition to their classification by area of bowel affected, obstructions are further classified as either mechanical or functional. With a *mechanical obstruction,* the bowel lumen is obstructed by a physical barrier, such as scar tissue or a tumor. The obstruction may be partial or complete. *Functional obstruction* occurs when peristalsis fails to propel intestinal contents without mechanical obstruction (Way, 1994).

Adhesions, or bands of scar tissue, are the most common cause of mechanical bowel obstruction, accounting for approximately 60% of small bowel obstructions. In adults, adhesions are usually acquired from abdominal surgery or inflammatory processes. Adhesions generally

produce a *simple obstruction,* or single blockage in one portion of the intestine.

Although the incidence of obstruction due to hernia is decreasing with the focus on their surgical repair, incarcerated hernia still ranks second as a cause of small bowel obstruction. The obstruction produced by an incarcerated hernia is a *closed-loop obstruction,* with two different portions of the bowel lumen obstructed.

Tumors, either intrinsic (of the bowel itself) or extrinsic (of another organ but affecting the bowel because of their size), can progressively occlude the bowel lumen and eventually obstruct it. Other, less common causes of bowel obstruction include intussusception (rare in adults); volvulus, the rotation of loops of bowel about a fixed point; foreign bodies; stricture; and inflammatory bowel disease (Way, 1994).

Both volvulus and an incarcerated hernia can result in a *strangulated obstruction.* In a strangulated obstruction, not only is the lumen of the bowel obstructed, but the blood supply to the affected portion is compromised as well. An incarcerated obstruction indicates necrosis caused by the strangulation.

In a functional obstruction or *paralytic ileus,* peristalsis stops as a result of either neurogenic or muscular impairment. The bowel lumen remains patent, but contents are not propelled forward. Paralytic ileus is a common disorder associated with many intra-abdominal conditions. Gastrointestinal surgery often results in temporary paralytic ileus. It may also result from tissue anoxia or peritoneal irritation due to hemorrhage, peritonitis, or perforation of an organ. Other conditions that can precipitate paralytic ileus include renal colic, spinal cord injuries, uremia, and electrolyte imbalances, hypokalemia in particular. In addition, the effects of some narcotics, anticholinergic drugs, and antidiarrheal medications such as diphenoxylate can produce a functional obstruction.

When obstruction occurs, gas and fluid collect in the bowel proximal to the obstruction, distending its lumen. Swallowed air and gases produced by bacterial fermentation of bowel contents contribute to the gaseous distention. Mediator substances such as bacterial endotoxins and prostaglandins are released, drawing tremendous quantities of extracellular fluid and electrolytes into the bowel lumen and producing further distention. A cycle of intestinal distention; secretion of water, sodium, and potassium; and further reduction in motility occurs. The distention can lead to pressure necrosis of the bowel wall. Large volumes of fluid may be trapped in the intestine, causing symptoms of hypovolemia and possible shock.

The manifestations of a small bowel obstruction vary according to the rapidity with which the obstruction develops and the level of obstruction. The client typically experiences cramping or colicky abdominal pain that may be intermittent or increasing in intensity. Vomiting is common, particularly in high or proximal obstructions, because distention of the lumen stimulates the vomiting center. As bacterial fermentation occurs, vomitus becomes feculent, particularly with a low or distal obstruction. Flatus and feces already present in the lower bowel may be expelled early in the obstructive process, but this expulsion ceases as the obstruction continues.

Early in the course of a mechanical obstruction, borborygmi and high-pitched tinkling bowel sounds are present, reflecting the small bowel's attempts to propel contents past the obstruction. Visible peristaltic waves may be noted in the distended loops of bowel in thin clients. In the later stages, the bowel becomes silent. With a paralytic ileus, bowel sounds are greatly diminished or absent throughout the process. Abdominal distention is minimal with proximal obstructions, but may be pronounced with distal obstruction and paralytic ileus. The abdomen may be tender to palpation as well.

In addition to the abdominal and gastrointestinal manifestations, the client demonstrates signs of fluid and electrolyte imbalance. Dehydration can occur rapidly as extracellular fluid is sequestered in the bowel and vomiting occurs. Although early vital signs may be normal, as dehydration and hypovolemia develop, changes are noted. The client becomes tachycardic and tachypneic, and blood pressure falls. Temperature may be elevated. Urine output drops, and the client may show signs of hypovolemic shock.

Hypovolemia and hypovolemic shock with multiple organ failure is a significant complication of bowel obstruction and can lead to death. Renal insufficiency from hypovolemia can lead to acute renal failure. Pulmonary ventilation can also be impaired as abdominal distention elevates the diaphragm and interferes with respiratory processes.

Strangulation is a threat with bowel obstruction, particularly with a closed-loop obstruction. With obstruction caused by an incarcerated hernia or volvulus, the blood supply to the bowel is impaired as well as the intestinal lumen. Gangrene may rapidly result, causing bleeding into the lumen and peritoneal cavity and eventual perforation. With perforation, bacteria and toxins from the strangulated intestine enter the peritoneum and, potentially, the circulation, resulting in peritonitis and possible septic shock.

The mortality rate for bowel obstruction is 2% to 10% in clients with obstruction of the small bowel. Most deaths occur among older adults. When strangulation occurs, the mortality rate for small bowel obstruction is as low as 8% with early surgical intervention, and up to 20% to 75% if surgery is delayed (McConnell, 1987; Way, 1994).

Large Bowel Obstruction

Obstruction of the large intestine occurs much less frequently than small bowel obstruction, accounting for approximately 15% of all bowel obstructions in adults. Al-

though any portion of the colon may be affected, obstruction usually occurs in the sigmoid segment. Cancer of the bowel is the most common cause; other etiologic factors include volvulus, diverticular disease, inflammatory disorders, and fecal impaction (Way, 1994).

If the ileocecal valve between the small and large intestines is competent, distention proximal to the obstruction is limited to the colon itself. This is known as a *closed-loop obstruction*, and it may result in massive dilation as the ileum continues to empty gas and fluid into the colon. With increasing pressure within the obstructed colon, circulation to the bowel wall is impaired. Gangrene and perforation are potential complications. Approximately 10% to 20% of clients with large bowel obstruction have an incompetent ileocecal valve in which colonic pressure is relieved by reflux into the ileum (Way, 1994).

Constipation and abdominal pain are the most frequent manifestations of a large bowel obstruction. The pain is often deep and cramping; severe, continuous pain may signal bowel ischemia and possible perforation. Vomiting is a late sign, if it occurs at all. The abdomen is distended, with high-pitched, tinkling bowel sounds with rushes and gurgles. On palpation, localized tenderness or a mass may be noted.

Collaborative Care

The management of a client with a bowel obstruction focuses on relieving the obstruction and providing supportive care. Fluid and electrolyte balance is restored, along with intestinal decompression. Surgical intervention may be necessary for a client with a mechanical obstruction or if strangulation is suspected.

Laboratory and Diagnostic Tests

The presence of a bowel obstruction is generally confirmed by the use of plain and bowel contrast X-ray studies. Laboratory testing is done to evaluate the client's response to the obstruction.

The following laboratory tests may be ordered:

- *WBC count* is often elevated. Mild leukocytosis is common due to hemoconcentration from fluid loss and changes within the obstructed bowel lumen that provoke the inflammatory response. With strangulation, leukocytosis is marked.

- *Hemoglobin and hematocrit levels* are elevated, again because of extracellular fluid loss and hemoconcentration.

- *Serum osmolality and electrolyte levels* are altered as a result of extracellular fluid and electrolyte losses from vomiting and sequestering in the bowel lumen. With hypovolemia, the serum osmolality is increased, as is the urine specific gravity. Potassium losses from vomiting may be significant, with resultant hypokalemia.

Chloride is also lost during vomiting, leading to hypochloremia.

- *Arterial blood gases* may reveal a metabolic alkalosis with small bowel obstruction due to the loss of hydrochloric acid from the stomach. With metabolic alkalosis, the arterial blood pH is greater than 7.45, the bicarbonate level is often greater than 26 mEq/L, and the P_{CO_2} is greater than 45 mm Hg.

The following diagnostic examinations may be ordered:

- *Abdominal X-ray study* is used to visualize an intestinal obstruction. In a small bowel obstruction, distended loops of intestine with fluid and gas in the intestine will be present. Free air under the diaphragm indicates a perforation. A distended colon may be visualized with a large bowel obstruction.

- *X-ray with contrast media* is used to confirm the presence of mechanical obstruction and assess the completeness of the obstruction. Meglumine diatrizoate (Gastrografin) is generally used to provide contrast rather than barium when a bowel obstruction is suspected. Unlike barium, meglumine diatrizoate contains iodine; therefore, it is vital to question the client about iodine or seafood hypersensitivity prior to exam. A barium enema is used to confirm the diagnosis of large bowel obstruction and determine its location.

Gastrointestinal Decompression

Ninety percent of partial small bowel obstructions are successfully treated with gastrointestinal decompression using a nasogastric or long intestinal tube. Functional obstructions respond to treatment with bowel rest and intestinal decompression as well. Cantor and Miller-Abbot tubes are intestinal tubes that may be used (see Figure 23–3 on page 790). These tubes may be inserted nasogastrically or via gastrostomy. A balloon or weighted tip draws the tube from the stomach into the intestine and to the area of obstruction via peristalsis. Collected fluid and gas is removed using low suction until persitalsis resumes or the obstruction is relieved.

Surgery

Surgical intervention is required for complete mechanical obstructions as well as for strangulated or incarcerate obstructions of the small intestine. Clients with incomplete mechanical obstruction may also require surgery if the obstruction persists.

Prior to surgery, a nasogastric or intestinal tube is inserted to relieve vomiting and abdominal distention and to prevent aspiration of intestinal contents. Fluid and electrolyte balance must be restored before surgical intervention. Isotonic intravenous fluids, such as normal (physiologic) saline, Ringer's solution, and other balanced electrolyte solutions, are used. Additional electrolytes may be added to the solution to correct low levels. It is particularly important to correct hypokalemia prior to surgery. Acid-base imbalances are also addressed, often using intravenous acidifiers or alkalinizing agents. If strangulation has occurred, the client may require plasma or blood replacement. Intravenous broad-spectrum antibiotics are administered prophylactically (see the section on peritonitis).

The surgical procedure carried out depends on the cause and the location of the obstruction. The incision is usually made at the abdomen to allow wide exposure of the small intestine for identification and removal of any areas of infarcted or gangrenous tissue. If adhesions are the cause of the obstruction, they are removed or lysed. Obstructing tumors are resected, and foreign bodies are removed. Any bowel that appears to be gangrenous is resected, usually followed by an end-to-end anastomosis of remaining intestine. In clients with a large tumor mass or dense adhesions, the area of obstruction may be bypassed by anastomosis of proximal small bowel to small or large intestine distal to the obstruction. Nursing care of the client having bowel surgery is included in the box on page 836.

Surgical intervention is usually required to treat a large intestinal obstruction. The primary goal is to relieve colonic distention and prevent perforation; the secondary goal is to remove the obstructing lesion (Way, 1994). With some obstructing cancers, laser photocoagulation may be used to enlarge the bowel lumen when the client's condition prohibits major surgery or the tumor is advanced. Removal of the obstructing lesion is the preferred treatment. Anastomosis of proximal and distal bowel segments may be accomplished, or a permanent colostomy or ileostomy may be required. (The previous section on bowel cancer discusses these surgical interventions.)

Nursing Care

Nurses may be instrumental in the early identification of intestinal obstructions in older adults, the home-bound client, or the institutionalized client. Early identification and intervention significantly reduces morbidity from bowel obstruction.

In clients with a suspected or confirmed bowel obstruction, frequent assessment for complications such as fluid and electrolyte imbalance, acid-base imbalances, hypovolemic shock, perforation, and peritonitis is necessary. The nurse cares for the client undergoing surgery.

Nursing diagnoses for this client may include *Altered Tissue Perfusion, Fluid Volume Deficit,* and *Pain.*

Fluid Volume Deficit

Because of the large collection of fluid in the bowel proximal to an obstruction, the accompanying vomiting, and nasogastric suction, the client with an intestinal obstruction often experiences a fluid volume deficit. If not corrected promptly, hypovolemic shock, acute renal failure, and multiple organ failure from poor tissue perfusion are potential consequences.

Nursing interventions with rationales follow:

- Monitor vital signs, pulmonary artery pressures, cardiac output, and central venous pressure hourly. *A decrease in blood pressure and an increase in heart and respiratory rate may indicate hypovolemia. Although they are invasive, pulmonary artery pressures, central venous pressure, and cardiac output measurements provide even better means of assessing fluid volume status.*

- Measure urinary output hourly and nasogastric suction volume every 2 to 4 hours. *A urinary output of 30 mL per hour or more usually indicates an adequate glomerular filtration rate (GFR), another indicator of fluid volume. Nasogastric output indicates the volume of fluid lost via the intestinal tract, providing a tool for evaluating fluid replacement needs.*

- Maintain intravenous fluids and blood volume replacement as ordered. The amount of fluid administered is calculated to meet the client's current fluid needs and to replace existing and current losses. *Rapid restoration of blood volume is necessary to maintain blood pressure and tissue and organ perfusion.*

- Measure abdominal girth every 4 to 8 hours. Mark the area to be measured on the client's abdomen. *A reference mark allows consistent, accurate measurements. An increase in abdominal girth indicates increasing intestinal distention.*

- Notify the physician of changes in client's status. *Changes in vital signs, pain, and signs of increasing distention can indicate the need for immediate surgical intervention (Deters, 1987).*

Altered Tissue Perfusion: Gastrointestinal

The same processes causing obstruction of the bowel lumen may reduce or block the blood supply to the bowel wall. The goal is to maintain adequate tissue perfusion and promote normal peristalsis and bowel elimination.

Nursing interventions with rationales follow:

- Monitor blood pressure, rate and rhythm of pulse, and respiratory rate every hour. Assess skin color, temperature, and capillary refill. *Cardiovascular assessment is vital for early detection of hypovolemic shock resulting from sequestering large volumes of fluid in the intestines. Hypovolemia and shock may convert mild bowel ischemia to infarction as the blood supply to the tissue falls.*

- Monitor intake and output hourly. Notify the physician if urine output falls to less than 30 mL per hour. *The urinary output provides a good indicator of the glomerular filtration rate (GFR) and tissue perfusion. A drop in urine output often precedes recognizable changes in vital signs resulting from hypovolemia.*

- Measure the client's temperature at least every 4 hours. *An elevated temperature may be an early indication of sepsis from bowel perforation as a result of gangrene.*

- Assess the client's pain frequently. *A change in the character of the client's pain or a rapid increase in intensity may signal bowel infarction or perforation.*

- Administer nothing by mouth until peristalsis is restored. *Enteral food or fluids may worsen distention and bowel ischemia. They also must be restricted until the possibility of perforation is eliminated or until initial postsurgical healing has occurred.*

Ineffective Breathing Pattern

Significant abdominal distention from a bowel obstruction can cause the diaphragm to flatten, impairing pulmonary ventilation. In addition, surgical disruption of abdominal muscles can lead to shallow respirations as the client attempts to prevent pain. These factors, plus the risk of aspiration of gastrointestinal contents during vomiting, account for a high risk for respiratory complications in the client with a small bowel obstruction.

Nursing interventions with rationales follow:

- Assess the client's respiratory rate, pattern, and lung sounds at least every 2 to 4 hours. *An increasing respiratory rate, shortness of breath, or apparent dyspnea may be early signs of respiratory compromise. Diminished breath sounds, particularly in the bases of the lungs, or crackles are indicative of poor lung expansion and possible impaired ventilation.*

- Monitor arterial blood gas results for indications of respiratory alkalosis or acidosis. *An increased respiratory rate may lead to respiratory alkalosis as excess carbon dioxide is eliminated. Conversely, with further impairment of breathing, respiratory acidosis may develop because of alveolar hypoventilation. Either may be a sign of respiratory compromise or possible infection.*

- Elevate the head of the bed. *Elevating the head of the bed makes breathing easier by reducing the pressure of abdominal distention on the diaphragm.*

- Provide a pillow or folded bath blanket for the client to use in splinting the abdomen while coughing postoperatively. *The ease and effectiveness of coughing is improved when abdominal muscles and incisions are splinted.*

- Maintain the patency of nasogastric or intestinal suction. *This is important to prevent further abdominal distention or aspiration of intestinal contents during vomiting.*

- Assist the client to use incentive spirometry or other assistive devices. *These devices encourage the client to breathe deeply, opening distal airways and preventing atelectasis.*

- Contact respiratory therapy as indicated. *The respiratory therapist may suggest or perform additional measures to maintain the client's pulmonary status.*

- Provide good oral care at least every 4 hours. *Dehydration and the presence of nasogastric suction lead to dry mouth and throat, increasing the risk of bacterial growth. Many respiratory infections are the result of aspirated organisms.*

Other Nursing Diagnoses

Examples of other nursing diagnoses that are appropriate for the client with intestinal obstruction follow:

- *Pain* related to abdominal distention and compromised intestinal blood supply
- *Altered Nutrition: Less Than Body Requirements* related to vomiting
- *Colonic Constipation* related to an obstructive mass
- *Anxiety* related to life-threatening symptoms of intestinal obstruction

Client and Family Teaching

In the acute period, teaching for the client (and family) generally is limited to explaining the client's condition, symptoms, and procedures performed for diagnosis and treatment of the obstruction. Explain the rationale for the nasogastric or intestinal tube and comfort measures to reduce its irritation. Discuss the reasons for surgery and possible results. Prior to surgical intervention, teach the client how to use postoperative pain-relief measures and how to cough, move, and breathe more comfortably with the incision. Postoperatively, provide instructions regarding wound care, activity level after discharge, the return to work, and any other recommended restrictions or procedures. If a temporary colostomy has been created, teach the client and family about its care. Discuss planned reanastamosis. For the client with recurrent obstructions, discuss their cause, early identification of symptoms, and possible preventive measures, if possible.

Teach health-promotion activities, such as increasing dietary intake of fiber, maintaining a moderate to high fluid intake, and exercising daily to help prevent constipation and possible large bowel obstruction, particularly in the older adult.

Applying the Nursing Process

Case Study of a Client with an Intestinal Obstruction: Charles Harrell

Charles Harrell is a 66-year-old retired city official who developed colicky abdominal pain, nausea, and vomiting earlier in the day. After several hours, Mr. Harrell sees his physician. The physician finds Mr. Harrell's abdomen distended with high-pitched bowel sounds and some tinkles present on auscultation, suggestive of obstruction. Mr. Harrell is admitted to the hospital.

Assessment

The admission history for Mr. Harrell indicates that his abdominal pain, nausea, and vomiting started shortly before noon. His medical history includes a radical cystectomy with ileal conduit performed 7 years previously for bladder cancer. He received postoperative radiation therapy as well. He has no other significant medical conditions and no medication allergies. Physical assessment findings are as follows: T, 98.1 F (36.6 c); P, 82; R, 20; BP, 124/80. An ileal conduit pouch is in place in the right lower quadrant. Mr. Harrell's abdomen is distended, with high-pitched bowel sounds.

His laboratory test results show moderate leukocytosis with a WBC of 15,000/mm^3 and a left shift on differential, indicating an inflammatory response. His hemoglobin and hematocrit are both elevated at 19.2 g/dL (normal: 14 to 18 g/dL) and 57% (normal: 42% to 52%), respectively. Serum glucose levels are elevated to 155 mg/dL, probably indicative of a stress response. On urinalysis, the specific gravity is 1.035 (normal: 1.010 to 1.030), indicative of dehydration and increased urine concentration. Other abnormal urinalysis findings included 2+ protein, 10 to 14 WBCs, 4+ bacteria, and nitrate positive, all indicative of urinary tract infection and expected findings with an ileal diversion. Abdominal X-ray findings revealed dilated small bowel loops with visible air-fluid levels indicative of obstruction, and the absence of colonic gas.

The physician diagnoses small bowel obstruction. Because there is no evidence of strangulation, the physician opts for intestinal decompression and supportive care initially, hoping to avoid surgical intervention. A nasointestinal tube is inserted and connected to low intermittent suction. Pain and antiemetic medications are given to increase Mr. Harrell's comfort and prevent possible aspiration. A central intravenous line is inserted for fluid replacement, pressure measurement, and the administration of total parenteral nutrition.

Diagnosis

The nurses caring for Mr. Harrell develop the following nursing diagnoses:

- *Fluid Volume Deficit* related to vomiting and intestinal suction
- *Risk for Altered Nutrition: Less Than Body Requirements* related to NPO status
- *Pain* related to abdominal distention
- *Risk for Altered Tissue Perfusion: Gastrointestinal* related to obstructive process.
- *Anxiety* related to lack of knowledge about disease process and fear of cancer recurrence

Expected Outcomes

The expected outcomes established in the plan of care specify that Mr. Harrell will

- Regain fluid and electrolyte homeostasis, as demonstrated by normal physical assessment findings, normal intake and output, and normal laboratory values.
- Maintain body weight and nutritional status.
- Verbalize increased comfort level, as evidenced by pain rating on a scale of 0 to 10.
- Regain normal bowel function, as evidenced by normal bowel sounds, passage of flatus, and passing soft-formed stool.
- Describe dietary measures to help prevent future small bowel obstructions.
- Verbalize understanding of the disease process and potential complications.

Planning and Implementation

The nurses plan and implement the following nursing interventions for Mr. Harrell:

- Measure abdominal girth every 4 hours.
- Monitor vital signs every 2 hours initially and as needed.
- Record intake and output every 2 hours.
- Maintain patent intestinal tube and low suction.
- Monitor laboratory results, reporting abnormal values to the physician.
- Provide oral and nares care every 4 hours.
- Weigh Mr. Harrell daily.
- Give pain medication as needed.
- Keep head of bed elevated to at least 30 degrees.
- Maintain central line and intravenous fluids and parenteral nutrition as ordered.
- Discuss home dietary management, including the need to monitor fiber intake and chew food well.
- Instruct Mr. Harrell to maintain a fluid intake of 2500 mL per day.
- Encourage follow-up care with physician.

Evaluation

On discharge, Mr. Harrell is ambulating well, tolerating a low-residue diet, and having normal bowel movements. The dietitian has given him verbal and written information on a low-residue diet. He verbalizes understanding of the importance of chewing the food well and drinking plenty of fluids. His nurses have also stressed the importance of follow-up visits with the doctor.

Critical Thinking in the Nursing Process

1. What are Mr. Harrell's risk factors for a bowel obstruction? What is the most likely cause of partial obstruction in his case?

2. Why did the physician choose to initiate total parenteral nutrition immediately?

3. The physician also ordered a serum alkaline phosphatase on admission, which was normal. Why was this test ordered? If the results of this test had been elevated, how might Mr. Harrell's medical care have differed?

4. Develop a care plan for Mr. Harrell for the nursing diagnosis: *Risk for Altered Nutrition: Less Than Body Requirements* related to vomiting and nasogastric suction.

The Client with Diverticular Disease

■ ■ ■

Diverticula are acquired saclike projections of mucosa through the muscular layer of the colon (Figure 23–16). Diverticula may occur anywhere in the gastrointestinal tract, excluding the rectum; the vast majority, however, affect the large intestine, with 90% to 95% occurring in the sigmoid colon.

People in the United States, Australia, the United Kingdom, and France have high and increasing incidence rates of diverticular disease. Both sexes are equally affected. Five percent of people in their 40s have diverticula, and the incidence increases with age, affecting 50% to 65% of those over 80 years of age. Millions of people have diverticular disease, but only one-fifth of those with the disease develop symptoms (Hampton & Bryant, 1992). The disease is uncommon in Africa and Asia.

Cultural factors, diet in particular, are thought to play an important role in the development of diverticula. A diet consisting of highly refined and fiber-deficient foods is believed to be the major factor contributing to the disease. Diverticular disease was essentially unknown before grain milling (which removes two-thirds of the fiber from flour) became prevalent in the early 1900s (Hazzard et al., 1994). Decreased activity levels and postponement of defecation have been suggested as contributing factors. The increasing incidence of diverticula with aging suggests that weakness of the wall of the colon may also contribute to the disease.

Pathophysiology

Diverticula form when increased pressure within the bowel lumen causes herniation of mucosa through defects in the wall of the colon. Clients with diverticular disease often have thickening or hypertrophy of the circular and longitudinal (teniae coli) muscles in the area affected by diverticula. The bowel lumen is narrowed, increasing intraluminal pressure. Deficient dietary fiber and a lack of fecal bulk contribute to this muscle hypertrophy and

Figure 23–16 Diverticula of the colon. Note the herniation of bowel mucosa through a weak point in the bowel wall, primarily where blood vessels penetrate the wall.

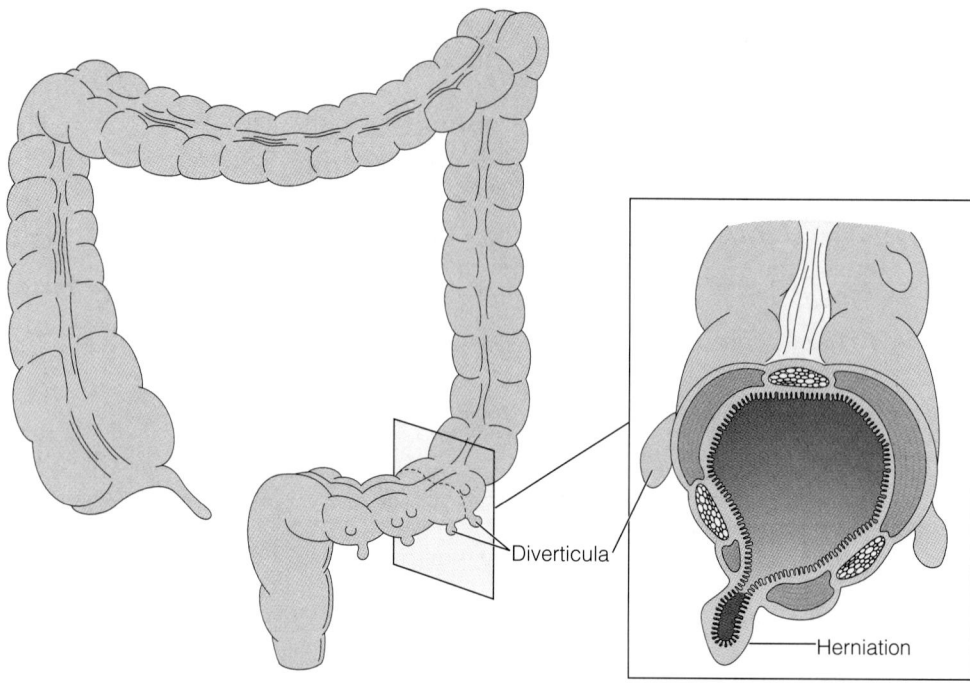

Diverticula

Herniation

narrowing of the bowel. Contraction of the muscles in response to normal stimuli such as meals may occlude the narrowed lumen, further increasing intraluminal pressure. The high pressure causes mucosa to herniate through the muscle wall, forming a diverticulum. Areas where nutrient blood vessels penetrate the circular muscle layer are the most common sites for diverticula formation.

Diverticulosis

Diverticulosis denotes the presence of diverticula. It is estimated that 80% or more of clients with diverticulosis are asymptomatic. When manifestations such as episodic pain (usually left-sided), constipation, and diarrhea do occur, they often can be attributed to irritable bowel syndrome, which commonly accompanies diverticular disease. (Irritable bowel syndrome is discussed earlier in this chapter.) As the disease progresses, the client may experience abdominal cramping, narrow stools (decrease in caliber), increased constipation, occult bleeding in the stools, weakness, and fatigue.

Complications of diverticulosis include hemorrhage and diverticulitis. A diverticulum may bleed, whether it is inflamed or not, possibly as a result of erosion of an adjacent blood vessel. Bleeding may be massive and is often from diverticula proximal to the splenic flexure (Berkow & Fletcher, 1992).

Diverticulitis

Diverticulitis is an inflammation and gross or microscopic perforation of the diverticular mucosa. Diverticuli-

tis affects only one diverticulum, usually in the sigmoid colon. The use of corticosteroids and nonsteroidal anti-inflammatory drugs (NSAIDs) contributes to its development. This complication of diverticular disease is most serious and usually severe in the older adult.

Diverticulitis may occur acutely from perforation due to increased intraluminal pressure, or it may develop gradually from an infection that extends through the wall of the colon to involve surrounding tissues. Infection occurs when undigested food becomes trapped in a diverticulum, impairing mucosal blood supply and allowing bacterial invasion. Perforation results from mucosal ischemia. With microscopic perforation, inflammation is localized. Gross perforation of a diverticulum results in more extensive bacterial contamination and may lead to abscess formation or peritonitis (see the earlier section on peritonitis).

Pain is a common manifestation of diverticulitis. It is usually left-sided and may be mild to severe and either steady or cramping. The client may also experience either constipation or increased frequency of defecation. Depending on the location and severity of the inflammation, nausea, vomiting, and a low-grade fever may occur. On examination, the client may have a distended abdomen, tenderness of the left lower quadrant, and a palpable mass resulting from the inflammatory response.

The older adult may present with less specific signs, complaining of vague abdominal pain. A palpable mass and signs of a large bowel obstruction may be present.

Complications associated with diverticulitis (in addition to peritonitis and abscess formation) include bowel obstruction, fistula formation, and hemorrhage. Severe or repeated episodes of diverticulitis may lead to scarring and fibrosis of the bowel wall, further narrowing the bowel lumen. This predisposes the client to obstruction of the large bowel. Acutely inflamed tissue may adhere to the small bowel, increasing the risk of small bowel obstruction as well. Fistulas may form, usually between the sigmoid colon and the bladder. Urinary tract infection is the usual sign of a *colovesical* fistula. Fistulas may also perforate into the small intestine, ureter, vagina, perineum, or abdominal wall. Bleeding from perforation of a vessel wall can occur with diverticulitis. Although it may be significant, bleeding usually stops spontaneously.

Collaborative Care

Management of the client with diverticular disease varies from no prescribed intervention to surgical resection of affected colon, depending on the severity of the disease and its complications.

Uncomplicated diverticulosis is managed with dietary changes. Acute diverticulitis usually is treated medically with bowel rest and broad-spectrum antibiotic therapy. Recurrent or complicated diverticulitis often requires surgical intervention with resection of the affected bowel segment.

Laboratory and Diagnostic Tests

Although the client's history and physical examination are often strongly suggestive of diverticular disease, diagnostic testing is used to confirm its presence and evaluate its extent.

Laboratory studies do not contribute to establishing the diagnosis of diverticulosis. When diverticulitis is suspected, the following laboratory tests may be ordered:

- *WBC count* may be elevated with a left shift (an increased number of immature WBCs) from the inflammatory response in diverticulitis.

- *Urinalysis* may reveal the presence of RBCs and WBCs along with multiple bacteria if the bladder or a ureter has been perforated by a fistula. Urine culture may be positive as well.

- *Guaiac testing of the stool* often reveals the presence of occult blood.

The following diagnostic studies may be ordered:

- *Barium enema* may be performed to demonstrate the presence of diverticular disease. In addition to illustrating the diverticula, X-ray films can reveal segmental spasm and muscular thickening with a narrowed bowel lumen. Barium enema is contraindicated in early acute diverticulitis because of the risk of barium leakage into the peritoneal cavity.

- *Abdominal X-ray* study can reveal free abdominal air in the presence of diverticulitis and perforation of a diverticulum. When there is a risk of perforation, water-soluble contrast media may be used to illustrate an abscess, fistulas, or narrowing of the bowel lumen.

- *CT scan* is also used in diagnosing diverticulitis. Oral or intravenous contrast media may be administered to enhance the image obtained. This cross-sectional radiologic procedure provides a detailed image helpful in assessing the inflammation and the presence of abscess or fistulas.

- *Ultrasound of the abdomen* may reveal an abscess.

- *Flexible sigmoidoscopy or colonoscopy* is used to detect diverticulosis and assess for strictures or possible bleeding. These procedures are avoided during an acute attack of diverticulitis because they increase the risk of bowel perforation.

- *Intravenous pyelogram (IVP)* may be conducted to rule out a mass on the left ureter or a colovesical fistula.

Pharmacology

Systemic broad-spectrum antibiotics effective against usual bowel flora are prescribed for the client with acute diverticulitis. Oral antibiotics such as cephalexin (Keflex) may be used for the client with mild symptoms who does not require hospitalization. Severe, acute attacks often require that the client be hospitalized and treated with intravenous fluids and third-generation cephalosporin antibiotics such as cefotaxime (Claforan) or ceftazidime (Fortaz). Other antibiotics such as penicillins, aminoglycosides, and metronidazole may be prescribed if peritonitis develops. These antibiotics and their nursing implications are discussed in the box in Chapter 8 on page 257.

Pentazocine (Talwin) may be prescribed for pain relief in the client with diverticulitis. This analgesic results in less increase in colonic pressure than does morphine or meperidine (Demerol).

Although a stool softener such as docusate sodium (Colace) may be prescribed, it is important to note that laxatives (which can further increase intraluminal pressure in the colon) are avoided for the client with diverticular disease.

Dietary Management

Dietary modification is central to the management of diverticular disease. Although it is not known whether dietary changes will prevent the complications of diverticulosis, a high-fiber diet increases stool bulk, decreases intraluminal pressures, and may reduce spasm. A high-residue diet with fiber is recommended (Table 23–13). Bran provides the least expensive fiber supplement and may be added to cereal, soups, salads, or other foods.

Table 23–13	Foods Recommended in a High-Fiber, High-Residue Diet
Food Group	**Recommended Foods**
Cereals and grains	Wheat or oat bran; cooked cereals, such as oatmeal; dry cereals, such as bran buds or flakes, corn flakes, shredded wheat; whole-grain breads or crackers; brown rice; popcorn
Fruits	Unpeeled raw apples, peaches, and pears; blackberries, raspberries, strawberries; oranges
Vegetables	Dried beans (navy, kidney, pinto), lima beans; broccoli; peas; corn; squash; raw vegetables, such as carrots, celery, and tomatoes; potatoes (with skins)

Commercial bulk-forming products, such as psyllium seed (Metamucil) or methylcellulose also may be recommended. These products are discussed in the box on page 776. The client may be advised to avoid foods with small seeds (such as popcorn, caraway seeds, figs, or berries), which could obstruct diverticula.

Bowel rest is prescribed for the client with an acute episode of diverticulitis. The client initially may be NPO with intravenous fluids and possibly total parenteral nutrition. Feeding is resumed gradually. Initially, a clear liquid diet is prescribed with gradual advancement to a soft, low-roughage diet (that is, a diet low in insoluble fiber) with daily added psyllium seed to soften stool and increase its bulk. Among the foods the client should avoid are wheat and corn bran, vegetable and fruit skins, nuts, and dry beans. The high-roughage diet is resumed following full recovery.

Surgery
Approximately 25% of clients with acute diverticulitis require surgical intervention, usually because of generalized peritonitis or an abscess that fails to respond to medical treatment. Hemorrhage that recurs or cannot be controlled may also indicate the need for surgery. Elective surgery may be performed when the client has episodes of recurrent diverticulitis or persistent diverticulitis with continuing pain, tenderness, and a palpable mass.

The affected bowel segment is resected, and if possible an anastomosis of the proximal and distal portions is performed. When an acute infection and diverticulitis are present, a two-stage Hartmann procedure is necessary. A temporary colostomy is created and anastomosis delayed until the inflammation has subsided. A second surgery is performed 2 to 3 months later to create the anastomosis and close the temporary colostomy. Refer to the boxes on pages 836 and 842 for nursing care of the client with bowel surgery and a colostomy.

Nursing Care
Because few clients with diverticulosis have symptoms of the disease, the nurse's role is mainly to educate the client. The nurse's involvement with clients who have diverticular disease may occur at several different levels. Teaching clients in many different settings about the benefits of a high-fiber diet is an important primary prevention for diverticular disease. In such facilities as residential or foster care settings, the nurse can work with dietary staff and care providers to increase the amount of fiber in residents' diets, unless this is contraindicated by a preexisting condition.

Clients with acute diverticulitis, in contrast, are acutely ill and may have multiple nursing care needs. Priority nursing diagnoses include *Impaired Tissue Integrity, Pain,* and *Anxiety* related to the possibility of a significant complication or possible surgery.

Impaired Tissue Integrity: Gastrointestinal
During an acute phase of diverticulitis, the client is at risk for bowel perforation because of inflammation and mucosal ischemia. In addition to maintaining bowel rest and minimizing diagnostic procedures to reduce the risk of perforation, the nurse closely monitors the client for manifestations of perforation, hemorrhage, and/or sepsis.

Nursing interventions with rationales follow:

- Monitor blood pressure, rate and rhythm of pulse, and respiratory rate at least every 4 hours. *An increased pulse and respiratory rate may be early indications of fluid volume deficit due to bleeding or of infection.*

- Take temperature every 4 hours. *Temperature elevation greater than 101 F (38.3 C) may indicate an increase in the severity of the disease process. Little temperature elevation may occur in the older client. A change in behavior or increasing lethargy may be subtle indications of infection in the older adult.*

- Perform an abdominal assessment every 4 to 8 hours or more often as indicated, including measuring abdominal girth, auscultating bowel sounds, and palpating the abdomen for tenderness. *Increasing abdominal distention, a decrease or change in the quality of bowel sounds, and/or increasing tenderness or guarding may indicate spread of the infectious process, peritonitis, or possible hemorrhage. Report significant changes promptly to the physician.*

- Assess for evidence of lower intestinal bleeding by visual examination and guaiac testing of stools for occult blood. *Perforation of a diverticulum may produce either intestinal or intra-abdominal bleeding necessitating immediate treatment such as surgery.*

- Maintain intravenous fluids, total parenteral nutrition, and accurate intake and output records. *During an acute phase of diverticulitis, oral intake is usually elimi-*

nated or restricted. *Intravenous fluids are necessary to maintain proper fluid and electrolyte balance; total parenteral nutrition will maintain the client's nutritional status, facilitating healing and recovery.*

Pain

Pain is a common manifestation of acute diverticulitis. It results from inflammation of the bowel and edema of affected tissues. If surgery is required, postoperative pain is managed through the use of narcotic analgesia.

Nursing interventions with rationales follow:

- Ask the client to rate pain on a scale of 0 to 10 (0 = no pain, 10 = worst pain). Document the level of pain, and note any changes in the location or character of the client's pain. *The perception and response to pain is individual and is affected by past experiences, religion, ethnic background, and many other factors. A change in the character or intensity of the pain may be an early indication of a complication such as perforation or abscess formation.*

- Administer prescribed analgesic, assessing its effectiveness ½ hour after administration. Avoid morphine administration. *If client has not obtained adequate pain relief, further assessment and intervention are necessary. Provide adjunctive medications as prescribed; encourage the client to use other pain-relieving methods, such as relaxation techniques, repositioning, and distraction; and notify the physician if necessary.*

- Maintain bowel rest and total body rest (bed rest with limited activity). *These measures help reduce the inflammation and promote healing, increasing the client's comfort.*

- Reintroduce oral foods and fluids slowly, providing a soft, low-fiber diet with bulk-forming agents. *This allows continued healing of the affected bowel while promoting soft, easily expelled stools.*

Anxiety

The client with acute diverticulitis faces not only hospitalization, but also potential serious complications such as peritonitis and hemorrhage. Surgery with formation of a temporary colostomy may be necessary. Furthermore, episodes of acute diverticulitis are often recurrent, and the client may be aware that similar problems can occur in the future.

Nursing interventions with rationales follow:

- Assess and document the client's level of anxiety. *Severe anxiety or panic states can interfere with the client's ability to respond to instructions and assist with care. Low to moderate anxiety levels enhance learning and compliance with prescribed interventions.*

- Demonstrate empathy and awareness of the perceived threat to the client's health. *It is important that the nurse recognize and respect the client's feelings and perceptions as reality for the client.*

- Attend to the client's physical care needs. *This provides reassurance that these needs will be met and relieves the client from being concerned with them.*

- Spend as much time as possible with the client. *This helps relieve fears of abandonment or that help will not be available if needed. It also enhances trust and provides opportunity for the client to express fears or concerns.*

- Assess the client's level of understanding about his or her condition. *This allows correction of misperceptions that may contribute to anxiety.*

- Encourage supportive family and friends to remain with the client as much as possible. *This provides a supportive environment for the client and also distracts from physical concerns.*

- Assist the client to identify and use appropriate coping mechanisms. *Coping mechanisms provide immediate relief of anxiety while the client adapts to the situation.*

- Involve the client and family members (as appropriate) in care decisions. *This increases the client's sense of control over the situation.*

Other Nursing Diagnoses

Examples of other nursing diagnoses that are appropriate for the client with diverticulitis follow:

- *Knowledge Deficit* related to lack of information about dietary management of diverticulosis

- *Risk for Fluid Volume Deficit* related to inflammatory process and diarrhea

- *Altered Sexuality Patterns* related to feelings of loss of control over body functions.

Client and Family Teaching

As noted earlier, teaching is a primary nursing intervention for the prevention of diverticular disease. Nurses working with groups and individuals in the community should emphasize the importance of a high-fiber diet and its benefits in preventing diverticular disease, bowel cancer, and other disorders. In working with the client with diverticular disease, instruction in the particulars of a high-fiber diet is even more important. Stress the need to maintain this diet for the remainder of the client's life to reduce the incidence of complications associated with diverticula. Discuss means of increasing dietary fiber, and refer the client to a dietitian for further teaching as needed. Provide instruction about the complications of diverticular disease and recognition of their manifestations.

For the client with acute diverticulitis, explain all diagnostic and therapeutic procedures. Discuss oral food and fluid limitations, and explain why a low-residue diet is prescribed initially but contraindicated in the chronic management of diverticular disease. Clients undergoing surgery and the creation of a temporary colostomy will require instruction in home care. Provide instruction and practice in colostomy management, including where to obtain supplies and dietary management. See the box on page 842 for further information about colostomy care. Discuss the planned procedure to reanastomose the colon and revise the colostomy. Referral to community health care agencies may be needed.

Applying the Nursing Process

Case Study of a Client with Diverticulitis: Roseline Ukoha

Roseline Ukoha is a 45-year-old school teacher who is married and has two children. For the past 2 days, Mrs. Ukoha has had intermittent abdominal pain and bloating. The pain increased in severity over the past 9 to 10 hours, and Mrs. Ukoha developed nausea, lower back pain, and discomfort radiating into the perineal region. She reports having had no bowel movement for the past 2 days. The emergency department nurse, Jasmine Sarino, RN, completes her admission assessment.

Assessment

In her nursing history, Ms. Sarino notes that Mrs. Ukoha relates a history of chronic irritable bowel symptoms, including alternating constipation and diarrhea and intermittent abdominal cramping for about the past 10 years. She states that she assumed these manifestations were due to the stress of teaching at the middle-school level and that they never became severe enough to prompt her to seek medical advice. When questioned about her diet, she called it a typical American high-fat, fast-food diet, usually consisting of a sweet roll and coffee for breakfast, a hamburger or sandwich and soft drink for lunch, and a balanced dinner, usually consisting of meat, a vegetable or salad, and potatoes or pasta, "except on pizza night!"

Physical assessment findings are as follows: T, 101 F (38.3 C); P, 92; R, 24; BP, 118/70. Her abdomen is slightly distended and tender to light palpation. Bowel sounds are diminished. Her diagnostic tests reveal the following abnormal results: WBC, 19,900/mm^3 (normal: 3500/mm^3 to 11,000/mm^3) with a left shift and increased immature and mature neutrophils on differential; hemoglobin, 12.8 g/dL (normal: 13.3 to 17.7 g/dL); hematocrit, 37.1% (normal: 40% to 52%). X-ray films of the abdomen show slight to moderate distention of the large and small bowel with suggestion of possible early ileus in the midabdominal area. A small amount of free air is noted in the peritoneal cavity.

The diagnosis of probable diverticulitis with diverticular rupture is made, and Mrs. Ukoha undergoes an emergency laparotomy. A perforated diverticulum is discovered, and the affected portion of the sigmoid colon is resected and a temporary colostomy performed.

Diagnosis

Following surgery, the nurses caring for Mrs. Ukoha identified the following nursing diagnoses:

- *Pain* related to surgical intervention
- *Risk for Fluid Volume Deficit* related to surgical fluid loss and inflammation
- *Impaired Tissue Integrity: Gastrointestinal* related to perforated diverticulum
- *Knowledge Deficit* of dietary management, disease process, and care of the colostomy.

Expected Outcomes

The expected outcomes established in the plan of care specify that Mrs. Ukoha will

- Demonstrate adequate pain relief by self-report, facial expression, and ease of movement postoperatively.
- On discharge, report a comfort level conducive to maintaining activities of daily living.
- Maintain adequate fluid balance while hospitalized, as demonstrated by balanced intake and output, stable weight, good skin turgor and mucous membrane moisture, and laboratory values within the normal range.
- Heal adequately without further evidence of peritonitis.
- Demonstrate appropriate technique in performing colostomy care.
- Verbalize understanding of the relationship between diet and diverticulosis.
- Verbalize understanding of the recommended high-fiber diet and the need to increase physical activity and fluid intake to promote optimal bowel function at home.

Planning and Implementation

The nurses on the surgical unit plan and implement the following nursing interventions for Mrs. Ukoha:

- Assess comfort status frequently, providing analgesics as needed.
- Maintain intravenous infusion until bowel sounds are active and flatus is passed.
- Monitor status and output of nasogastric tube; replace fluid milliliter for milliliter with intravenous solution as ordered.
- Measure intake and output every 4 to 8 hours; weigh Mrs. Ukoha daily.

- Provide mouth and nares care every 2 to 4 hours while nasogastric tube is in place, then every 4 hours until client assumes self-care.
- Assess surgical incision, bowel sounds, and colostomy output at least every 8 hours.
- Measure temperature every 4 hours.
- Provide instruction and dietary consultation for high-fiber diet.
- Teach colostomy care (see the box on page 842) and provide referral to an enterostomal therapist and to the local chapter of United Ostomy Association.
- Discuss sexual aspects of having an ostomy and give booklet "Sex and the Female Ostomate," available through the United Ostomy Association.

Evaluation

On discharge, Mrs. Ukoha's incision is healing well, she is afebrile, and her abdomen is flat and tender only around the surgical site. She is taking food and fluids well and passing formed stool through the colostomy. She was able to perform colostomy care: emptying and rinsing out pouch, performing skin care, and changing her pouch. She verbalizes an understanding of dietary management of diverticulosis and also those foods causing odor and gas. Her nurse, Bob Lyster, provides her with verbal and written instructions on colostomy care. Mrs. Ukoha also verbalizes an understanding that the colostomy is temporary and that she will return to the hospital in 2 to 3 months to have the colostomy closed. She states, "I can deal with this for a few months. I'm just thankful it's not permanent."

Critical Thinking in the Nursing Process

1. Why did the physician choose to perform an immediate colon resection and temporary colostomy?
2. Mrs. Ukoha called 2 days after discharge and said, "I had a small bowel movement of mucus from my rectum. Is this normal, or is something wrong?" What would your response be?
3. How did Mrs. Ukoha's diet before surgery contribute to the development of diverticula and diverticulitis? Did the symptoms of irritable bowel syndrome also contribute? How?
4. Develop a teaching plan to instruct clients with diverticular disease about dietary recommendations.
5. Develop a care plan for Mrs. Ukoha for the nursing diagnosis *Altered Health Maintenance* as evidenced by dietary patterns and history of untreated symptoms.

◾◾◾ Anorectal Disorders ◾◾◾

Anorectal lesions include hemorrhoids, a normal condition common to all adults that may become enlarged and painful; anal fissure; anorectal fistulas; anorectal abscess; and pilonidal disease. Fecal incontinence also may be considered an anorectal disorder.

The Client with Hemorrhoids

◾ ◾ ◾

The anus and anal canal contain two superficial venous plexuses with the hemorrhoidal veins. When pressure on these veins is increased or venous return impeded, they can develop *varices,* or varicosities, becoming weak and distended. This condition is commonly known as **hemorrhoids,** or piles. When asymptomatic, hemorrhoids are considered to be a normal condition found in all adults.

Pathophysiology

Hemorrhoids develop when venous return from the anal canal is impaired. Straining to defecate while in the sitting or squatting position increases venous pressure and is the most common cause of distended hemorrhoids. Pregnancy increases intra-abdominal pressure, raising venous pressure, and is a second important cause of hemorrhoids. Other factors that may contribute to symptomatic hemorrhoids include prolonged sitting, obesity, chronic constipation, and the low-fiber diet common to Western nations.

Hemorrhoids are classed as either internal or external. *Internal* hemorrhoids affect the venous plexus above the mucocutaneous junction of the anus (Figure 23–17). Internal hemorrhoids rarely cause pain, usually presenting with bleeding. Bleeding from internal hemorrhoids is bright red and unmixed with the stool. It can vary in quantity from streaks on toilet tissue to enough to color the water in the toilet. Recurrent bleeding of internal hemorrhoids is occasionally sufficient to result in anemia. Mucus discharge and a feeling of incomplete evacuation of stool also may be manifestations of internal hemorrhoids.

External hemorrhoids affect the inferior hemorrhoidal plexus below the mucocutaneous junction. Bleeding is rare with external hemorrhoids. Anal irritation, a feeling of pressure, and difficulty cleaning the anal region may be manifestations of external hemorrhoids.

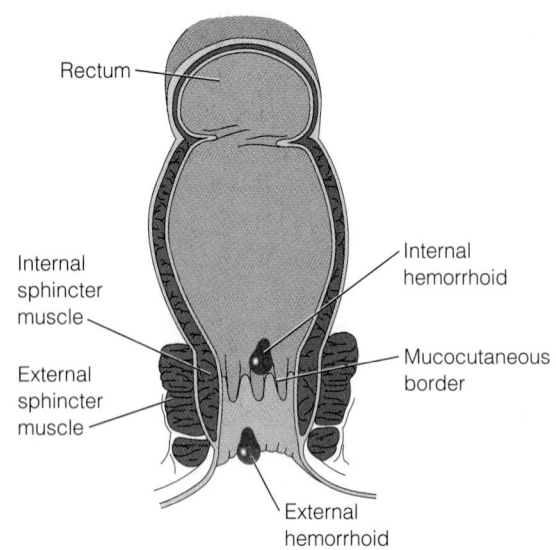

Figure 23–17 The location of internal and external hemorrhoids. Note their relationship to the mucocutaneous border.

As they enlarge, hemorrhoids may prolapse or protrude through the anus. Initially, prolapse occurs only with defecation and the hemorrhoids spontaneously regress back into the anal canal. Eventually, the client may need to manually replace internal hemorrhoids after defecation, or they may become permanently prolapsed and replacement not possible. Symptoms of permanently prolapsed hemorrhoids include mucus discharge and clothing soilage.

"Normal" hemorrhoids are not painful. Pain is associated with ulcerated or thrombosed hemorrhoids, and it can be severe. Prolapsed hemorrhoids may become strangulated as a result of congestion and edema, leading to thrombosis. Hemorrhoidal thrombosis causes extreme pain and may lead to infarction of skin and mucosa overlying the hemorrhoid. Internal hemorrhoids associated with portal hypertension in liver disease may bleed profusely if ruptured. (See Chapter 15 for further discussion of portal hypertension.)

A *thrombosed external hemorrhoid* is a thrombosis of the subcutaneous external hemorrhoidal veins of the anal canal, rather than a true hemorrhoid (Way, 1994). It appears as a painful bluish hematoma beneath the skin and typically occurs following a sudden increase in venous pressure, for example, heavy lifting, coughing, or straining. Pain is significant at onset but gradually subsides. Spontaneous rupture with bleeding may occur. Thrombosed external hemorrhoids resolve spontaneously without intervention.

Collaborative Care

Because hemorrhoids are a normal condition, management is conservative unless complications such as permanent prolapse or thrombosis occur.

Hemorrhoids are diagnosed by the client's history and by examination of the anorectal area. External hemorrhoids can be seen on visual inspection, especially if thrombosed. The client is asked to strain (Valsalva's maneuver) during the examination to detect prolapse. Internal hemorrhoids are usually not palpable or tender on digital examination of the rectum. Anoscopic examination is used to detect and evaluate internal hemorrhoids. For this exam, a speculum or endoscope is introduced into the anus to provide visual inspection of the tissues. Internal hemorrhoids are vascular structures which protrude into the lumen. Additional diagnostic examinations including testing of stool for occult blood, barium enema, and sigmoidoscopy are performed to rule out cancer of the colon or rectum, which may aggravate hemorrhoidal symptoms or produce similar manifestations. If liver disease with portal hypertension is suspected, liver function studies are ordered.

Hemorrhoids that are not permanently prolapsed or acutely thrombosed generally are treated conservatively. A high-fiber diet and increased water intake to increase stool bulk, improve its softness, and reduce straining, is effective for most clients with internal or external hemorrhoids. Bulk-forming laxatives such as psyllium seed (Metamucil) or stool softeners such as docusate sodium (Colace) may be prescribed to improve constipation and reduce straining as well. Suppositories and local ointments such as Preparation H or Nupercaine have an anesthetic and astringent effect, reducing discomfort and irritation of surrounding tissues. They have little or no effect on the hemorrhoid itself. Warm sitz baths, bed rest, and local astringent compresses may be recommended to reduce the swelling of edematous prolapsed hemorrhoids after digital reduction.

Hemorrhoids that are permanently prolapsed, are thrombosed, or produce significant symptoms may be treated more aggressively. *Sclerotherapy* involves the injection of a chemical irritant into tissues surrounding the hemorrhoid to induce inflammation and eventual fibrosis and scarring. It is used to treat recurrent bleeding and early prolapse of internal hemorrhoids. The treatment produces minimal pain. Enlarged or prolapsing hemorrhoids also may be treated with *rubber band ligation*. A rubber band is placed snugly around the hemorrhoidal plexus and surrounding mucosa, causing the tissue to necrose and slough within 7 to 10 days. Treatment is limited to one hemorrhoidal complex at a time, so repeat treatments may be necessary. Pain should be minimal if the band is placed appropriately; persistent pain following band ligation may signal an infection. Bleeding can

---

Perianal Postoperative Care
■ ■ ■

Assessment

- Monitor vital signs every 4 hours for 24 hours.
- Inspect rectal dressing every 2 to 3 hours for 24 hours.
- Check the client for signs of restlessness and thirst.
- Monitor urinary output.

Pain Control

- Assist the client to position of comfort, usually the side-lying position.
- Give analgesic medication as prescribed.
- Keep fresh ice packs over the rectal dressing as ordered by physician.
- Have the client use moist heat (sitz bath) 3 to 4 times per day.
- Ensure that the client uses a flotation pad when sitting.

Elimination

- Give stool softeners as prescribed.
- Give an analgesic before the first postoperative bowel movement or enema if possible.
- When tolerated, encourage oral intake of at least 2000 mL per day.

Client and Family Teaching

- Take sitz bath after each bowel movement for 1 to 2 weeks after surgery.
- Drink at least 2000 mL or 2 quarts of fluid per day.
- Eat adequate dietary fiber, and exercise moderately.
- Take stool softeners as prescribed.
- Report to the physician the following symptoms: rectal bleeding, continued pain on defecation, temperature elevation greater than 101 F (38.3 C), purulent rectal drainage.

---

occur as the hemorrhoid sloughs. Other procedures used to treat hemorrhoids include *cryosurgery*, in which hemorrhoids are necrosed by freezing with a cryoprobe, infrared photocoagulation, or electrocoagulation.

Clients with chronic symptoms, permanent prolapse, chronic bleeding and anemia, or painful thrombosed hemorrhoids may be treated surgically with a *hemorrhoidectomy*. In this procedure, hemorrhoids are surgically excised, leaving normal skin and surrounding tissues. This procedure may use conventional techniques or a laser to remove both internal and external hemorrhoids. Few complications are associated with hemorrhoidectomy.

Nursing Care

Most clients with hemorrhoids are treated in outpatient settings where the primary nursing focus is educational. Nurses also have frequent opportunities to provide teaching about measures to prevent the formation of hemorrhoids.

When a hemorrhoidectomy is performed, the client requires more direct nursing intervention. Postoperative care of the client with perianal surgery is outlined in the accompanying box. Anal packing may be in place for the first 24 hours following the procedure. When it is removed, the client needs close observation for bleeding. Pain is a common postoperative problem. Although the

operative procedure is a minor one, postoperative discomfort can be significant because of rich innervation of the anal region and possible muscle spasms. In addition to systemic analgesics, sitz baths usually are ordered. These not only help promote relaxation and reduce discomfort but also clean the anal area. Use of a rubber ring or donut device minimizes pressure on the surgical site while the client sits in the bath.

The client may remain in the hospital until the first bowel movement is passed after surgery. Stool softeners, adequate fluids, and analgesia before defecation can reduce the client's anxiety and discomfort. Adequate cleaning following defecation, usually with a sitz bath, is vital.

Whether caring for a client with hemorrhoidectomy or for a client for whom hemorrhoids are a secondary problem, the nurse may find the following nursing diagnoses appropriate:

- *Pain* related to inflamed anal tissues
- *Constipation* related to dietary habits and/or delay of defecation
- *Risk for Infection* related to disruption of anal tissue

Client and Family Teaching

Primary prevention of symptomatic hemorrhoids involves education of clients of all ages. When providing general health teaching and education specific to gastrointestinal function, stress the importance of maintaining an adequate intake of dietary fiber, a liberal fluid intake, and regular exercise to maintain stool bulk, softness, and regularity. Discuss the need to respond to the urge to defecate rather than postponing defecation. Provide teaching about the management of constipation, including the use of bulk-forming laxatives. Stress that stool softeners should be used only for short-term relief of symptoms. Discuss the appropriate use of over-the-counter preparations for the relief of minor hemorrhoidal symptoms. If necessary, teach clients how to reduce prolapsed hemorrhoids digitally.

Teach the client the signs of possible hemorrhoidal complications, such as chronic bleeding, prolapse, and thrombosis. Stress the need to seek medical evaluation if symptoms persist. Discuss the link between manifestations of hemorrhoids and colorectal cancer, and urge the client to seek medical intervention for persistent, unresolved, or progressive symptoms.

The Client with an Anorectal Lesion

■ ■ ■

Unlike the rectum, which is relatively insensitive to pain, the anal canal is richly supplied with sensory nerves and highly sensitive to painful stimuli. Lesions of the anorectal area may cause the client significant pain, particularly with defecation. Infection is another potential complication of anorectal lesions because of contamination by fecal bacteria. The superior boundary of the anal canal (the anorectal juncture or pectinate line) contains 8 to 12 anal crypts where anorectal abscesses or fistulas can form.

Pathophysiology and Collaborative Care

Anal Fissure

Anal fissures or ulcers occur when the epithelium of the anal canal over the internal sphincter becomes denuded or abraded. Irritating diarrheal stools and tightening of the anal canal with increased sphincter tension are frequent causes of anal fissures. Other factors that may contribute to their development include childbirth trauma, habitual cathartic use, laceration by a foreign body, and anal intercourse. Chronic inflammation and infection of surrounding tissues accompanies an anal fissure.

Clients with anal fissures typically have periods of exacerbation and remission. Because they occur below the mucocutaneous line, anal fissures are painful. The pain occurs with defecation and may be described as tearing, burning, or cutting. Bright red bleeding is noted with a bowel movement as well. Bleeding is typically minor and

noted on toilet tissue. Because of fear of defecation, the client may experience constipation, which further disrupts normal bowel habits and aggravates symptoms.

The diagnosis of anal fissure is made on gentle digital examination of the anal canal and anoscopy using a small anoscope. Treatment is usually conservative, involving dietary changes to increase fiber intake and stool bulk, increased fluid intake and bulk-forming laxatives. A topical agent such as hydrocortisone cream may be prescribed. Surgical intervention with an internal *sphincterotomy*, an incision into the internal sphincter to increase its diameter, is considered when the fissure does not heal with medical intervention.

Anorectal Abscess

Invasion of the pararectal spaces by pathogenic bacteria can lead to an *anorectal abscess*. Commonly caused by infection that extends from the anal crypt into a pararectal space, the abscess may appear small but often contains a large amount of pus. Multiple pathogens may be present, including *Escherichia coli, Proteus*, streptococci, and staphylococci. Other factors that may contribute to the development of an anorectal abscess include infection of a hair follicle, sebaceous gland, or sweat gland; and abrasions, fissures, or anal trauma. The incidence of anorectal abscess is higher in men.

Pain is the primary manifestation of an anorectal abscess. Sitting or walking may aggravate the pain, but it is unrelated to defecation. External swelling, redness, heat, and tenderness are apparent on examination. With a deeper abscess, swelling may not be visible, but the abscess is palpable on digital examination.

If the abscess either does not drain spontaneously or is not drained surgically, adjacent anatomic spaces will be affected. Systemic sepsis is also a potential complication.

Incision and drainage (I & D) is the treatment of choice for an anorectal abscess because it rarely resolves with antibiotic therapy alone. This treatment often results in a persistent fistula, which is surgically closed after the infection has cleared.

Anorectal Fistula

A *fistula* is a tunnel or tubelike tract with openings at each end. *Anorectal fistulas* have one opening in the anal canal with the other usually found in perianal skin. Most occur spontaneously or as a result of anorectal abscess drainage. Crohn's disease is a predisposing factor to fistula development as well.

The primary manifestation of an anorectal fistula is intermittent or constant drainage or discharge, which may be purulent. This may be accompanied by local itching, tenderness, and pain associated with defecation.

Digital and anoscopic examination with gentle probing of the fistula tract are used to establish the diagnosis. Although some fistulas may heal spontaneously, the treatment of choice is a *fistulotomy*. The primary opening of the fistula is removed, and the tract is opened to allow it to heal by secondary intention, from the inside outward. If the sphincter is involved, a two-stage operation may be done to preserve the muscle and prevent fecal incontinence.

Pilonidal Disease

The client with *pilonidal disease* has an acute abscess or chronic draining sinus in the sacrococcygeal area. Underlying the abscess or sinus is a cyst with granulation tissue, fibrosis, and, often, hair tufts. This disease affects young hirsute (hairy) males most frequently and is probably due to hair entrapment in deep tissues of the sacrococcygeal area; some researchers, however, believe that it is congenital in origin.

The lesion of pilonidal disease is generally asymptomatic unless it becomes acutely infected. Manifestations of acute inflammation accompany infection, including pain, tenderness, redness, heat, and swelling of the affected area. Purulent discharge may be noted from one or more sinuses or openings in the midline.

The preferred treatment option for pilonidal disease is incision and drainage. The sinus tract and underlying cyst are excised and closed by either primary- or secondary-intention healing. The client may be instructed to remove hair from the area routinely by shaving or using a depilatory to prevent further hair entrapment and recurrence of the problem.

Nursing Care

Clients with anorectal disorders are often treated in outpatient settings, and the primary nursing responsibility is education. Teach the client to maintain a high-fiber diet and liberal fluid intake to increase stool bulk and softness and thereby decrease discomfort with defecation. Stress the importance of responding to the urge to defecate to prevent constipation.

Following surgical treatment of any of these disorders, teach the client to keep the perianal region clean and dry. If a dressing is in place, teach the client to avoid soiling it with urine or feces during elimination. Following removal of the dressing, instruct the client to clean the area gently with soap and water following a bowel movement. Discuss the use of sitz baths for cleaning and comfort. Suggest taking an analgesic if necessary prior to defecation, but caution that some analgesics may promote constipation. Teach the client the signs and symptoms of infection or other possible complications to report to the physician. If an antibiotic has been prescribed, provide written and verbal instructions about its use, its desired and possible adverse effects, and their management.

Bibliography

■ ■ ■

American Cancer Society. (1992). *Cancer facts and figures.* Atlanta: Author.

Atkinson, K.G. (1993). The role of surgery in the treatment of inflammatory bowel disease. *Ostomy Quarterly, 30*(2), 52–53.

Bayless, T. M. (1989). Extra-intestinal manifestations of inflammatory bowel disease. *Ostomy Quarterly, 27*(1), 15–17.

Beahrs, O. H., Henson, D. E., Hutter, R., & Kennedy, B. J. (1991). *Manual for staging of cancer* (4th ed.). Philadelphia: Lippincott.

Berkow, R., & Fletcher, A. J. (Eds.). (1992). *The Merck manual,* 16th ed. Rahway, NJ: Merck.

Broadwell, D. C., & Jackson, B. S. (1982). *Principles of ostomy care.* St. Louis: Mosby.

Brown, K. K. (1994, September). Septic shock: How to stop the deadly cascade. *American Journal of Nursing, 94*(9), 20–6.

Bullock, B. L., & Rosendahl, P. P. (1992). *Pathophysiology: Adaptations and alterations in function* (3rd ed.). Philadelphia: Lippincott.

Cerrato, P. (1987). What to tell your patients about dietary fiber. *RN, 50*(1), 63–64.

Chernecky, C. C., Krech, R. L., & Berger, B. J. (1993). *Laboratory tests and diagnostic procedures.* Philadelphia: W. B. Saunders.

Coellen, D. (1989). Understanding diverticular disease. *Journal of Enterostomal Therapy Nursing, 16*(4), 176–180.

Deters, G. E. (1987). Managing complications after abdominal surgery, *RN, 50*(3), 27–32.

DeVita, V., Hellman, S., & Rosenberg, S. A. (1989). *Cancer principles and practice of oncology* (3rd ed.). Philadelphia: Lippincott.

Dittmar, S. S. (1989). *Rehabilitation nursing.* St. Louis: C. V. Mosby.

Doughty, D. B. (1994). What you need to know about inflammatory bowel disease. *American Journal of Nursing, 94*(7), 24–30.

Griffin, P. A., Liff, J. M., Greenberg, R. S., & Clark, W. S. (1991). Adenocarcinomas of the colon and rectum in persons under 40 years old. *Gastroenterology, 100,* 1033–1040.

Gurevich, I. (1994). Your patients don't need diarrhea, too! *RN, 57*(4), 52–55.

Hampton, B. G., & Bryant, R. A. (1992). *Ostomies and continent diversions.* St. Louis: Mosby.

Hazzard, W. R., Bierman, E. L., Blass, J. P., Ettinger, W. H., Jr., & Halter, J. B. (Eds.). (1994). *Principles of geriatric medicine and gerontology* (16th ed.). New York: McGraw-Hill.

Holloway, N. M. (1993). *Nursing the critically ill adult* (4th ed.). Redwood City, CA: Addison-Wesley Nursing.

Hurd, L. B. (1993). A patient's guide to ileoanal reservoir surgery. *Ostomy Quarterly, 30*(2), 56–59.

Jagelman, D. G. (1992). Toxic colitis: Diagnosis and management. *Journal of Enterostomal Therapy, 19*(6), 204–206.

Jess, L. W. (1993). Acute abdominal pain. *Nursing93, 23*(9), 34–42.

Lederer, J. R., Marculescu, G. L., Mocnik, B. & Seaby, N. (1993). *Care planning pocket guide.* Redwood City, CA: Addison-Wesley Nursing.

Lutz, C. A., & Przytulski, K. R. (1994). *Nutrition and diet therapy.* Philadelphia: F. A. Davis.

Madda, M. A. (1991). Helping ostomy patients manage medications. *Nursing91, 21*(3), 47–49.

Marchiondo, K. (1994). When the dx is diverticular disease. *RN, 57*(2), 42–46.

McCance, K. L., & Huether, S. E. (1994). *Pathophysiology: The biologic basis for disease in adults and children* (2nd ed.). St. Louis: Mosby-Year Book.

McConnell, E. A. (1987). Meeting the challenge of intestinal obstruction. *Nursing87, 17*(7), 34.

McConnell, E. (1994). Loosening the grip of intestinal obstructions. *Nursing94, 24*(3), 34–42.

Meissner, J. (1994). Caring for patients with ulcerative colitis. *Nursing94, 24*(7), 54–55.

Meize-Grochowski, A. R. (1991). When the dx is Crohn's disease. *RN, 54*(2), 52–55.

Mihalopoulos, N., Trunnell, E., Ball, K., & Moncur, C. (1994). The psychologic impact of ostomy surgery on persons 50 years and older. *Journal of Wound, Ostomy and Continence Nursing, 21*(4), 149–155.

Nugent, F. W., Haggitt, R. C., & Gilpin, P. A. (1991). Cancer surveillance in ulcerative colitis. *Gastroenterology, 100*(5), 1241–1248.

Pagana, K. D., & Pagana, T. J. (1992). *Diagnostic and laboratory test reference.* St. Louis: Mosby-Year Book.

Paulford-Lecher, N. (1993). Teaching your patient stoma care. *Nursing93, 23*(9), 47–49.

Physicians' desk reference (PDR) (48th ed.). (1994). Montvale, NJ: Medical Economics Data Production Company.

Podolsky, D. K. (1991). Inflammatory bowel disease. *New England Journal of Medicine, 325*(14) 1008–1013.

Porth, C. M. (1994). *Pathophysiology: Concepts of altered health states* (4th ed.). Philadelphia: Lippincott.

Prantera, C., Pallone, P., Brunetti, G., Cottone, M., Miglioli, M., & the Italian IBD Study Group. (1992). Oral 5-aminosalicylic acid (Asacol) in the maintenance treatment of Crohn's disease. *Gastroenterology, 103*(2), 363–368.

Price, S. A. & Wilson, L. M. (1992). *Pathophysiology: Clinical concepts of disease processes* (4th ed.). St. Louis: Mosby-Year Book.

Ramer, L. (1992). Self-image changes with time in the cancer patient with a colostomy after operation. *Journal of Enterostomal Therapy Nursing, 19,* 195–203.

Rutgerts, P., Geboes, K., Vantrappen, G., Beyls, J., Kerremans, R., & Hiele, M. (1990). Predictability of the post-operative course of Crohn's disease. *Gastroenterology, 99,* 956–963.

Shannon, M. T., Wilson, B. A., & Stang, C. L. (1992). *Drugs and nursing implications* (7th ed). Norwalk, CT: Appleton & Lange.

Shlafer, M. (1993). *The nurse, pharmacology, and drug therapy: A prototype approach* (2nd ed.). Redwood City, CA: Addison-Wesley Nursing.

Sitzmann, J. V., Converse, R. L., Jr., & Bayless, T. M. (1990). Favorable response to parenteral nutrition and medical therapy in Crohn's colitis. *Gastroenterology, 99,* 1647–1652.

Skidmore-Roth, L. (1993). *Nursing drug reference.* St. Louis: Mosby-Year Book.

Sparks, S. M. & Taylor, C. M. (1993). *Nursing diagnosis reference manual* (2nd ed.). Springhouse, PA: Springhouse.

Spencer, R. T., Nichols, L. W., Lipkin, G. B., Henderson, H. S., & West, F. M. (1993). *Clinical pharmacology and nursing management* (4th ed.). Philadelphia: Lippincott.

Stanely, M., & Beare, P. G. (1995). *Gerontological nursing.* Philadelphia: F. A. Davis.

Surratt, S., Ryan, A., Hallenbeck, P., Blandon, M., & Sugarbaker, P. (1993). Troubleshooting a sump pump. *American Journal of Nursing, 93*(1), 42–47.

Swartz, B. A. (1994). An 84-year-old woman with abdominal pain. *Clinician Reviews, 4*(9), 85–88, 91–92.

Thompson, J. M., McFarland, G. K., Hirsch, J. E., & Tucker, S. (1993). *Clinical nursing* (3rd ed.). St. Louis: Mosby.

Tierney, L. M., McPhee, S. J., & Papadakis, M. A., (Eds.). (1994). *Current medical diagnosis and treatment,* (33rd ed.). Norwalk, CT: Appleton & Lange.

Tucker, S. M., Canobbio, M. M., Paquette, E. V., & Wells, M. F. (1992). *Patient care standards: Nursing process, diagnosis, and outcome,* St. Louis: Mosby-Year Book.

Way, L. M. (Ed.). (1994). *Current surgical diagnosis and treatment,* (10th ed.). Norwalk, CT: Appleton & Lange.

Responses to Altered Urinary Elimination

Assessing Clients with Urinary Elimination Disorders

LEARNING OBJECTIVES

After completing this chapter, you will be able to

- Identify and describe the structures of the urinary system.
- Describe the functions of the urinary system.
- Explain the role of the urinary system in maintaining homeostasis.
- Identify interview questions pertinent to the assessment of the urinary system.
- Describe techniques for the physical assessment of urinary function.
- Identify manifestations of impairment in the function of the urinary system.
- Describe variations in assessment findings for the older adult.

The functions of the urinary system are to regulate body fluids, to filter metabolic wastes from the bloodstream, to reabsorb needed substances and water into the bloodstream, and to eliminate metabolic wastes and water as urine. Any alteration in the structure or function of the urinary system quickly affects the whole body. In turn, healthy urinary system function depends on the health of other body systems, especially the circulatory, endocrine, and nervous systems.

Review of Anatomy and Physiology

■ ■ ■

The organs of the urinary system are the paired kidneys, the paired ureters, the urinary bladder, and the urethra (Figure 24–1). Each of these structures is essential to the total functioning of the urinary system.

Structures of the Urinary System

The anatomic structures of the urinary system reach from the retroperitoneal space in the lower thoratic region into the pelvis.

Kidneys

The two *kidneys* are located outside the peritoneal cavity and on either side of the vertebral column at the levels of T12 through L3. These highly vascular, bean-shaped organs are approximately 4.5 inches (11.4 cm) long and 2.5 inches (6.4 cm) wide. The lateral surface of the kidney is convex; the medial surface is concave and forms a vertical cleft known as the *hilum*. The ureter, renal artery, renal vein, lymphatic vessels, and nerves enter or exit the kidney at the level of the hilum.

The kidney is supported by three layers of connective tissue: the outer renal fascia, the middle adipose capsule, and the inner renal capsule. The *renal fascia*, made up of dense connective tissue, surrounds the kidney (and the adrenal gland, a discrete organ that sits on top of each

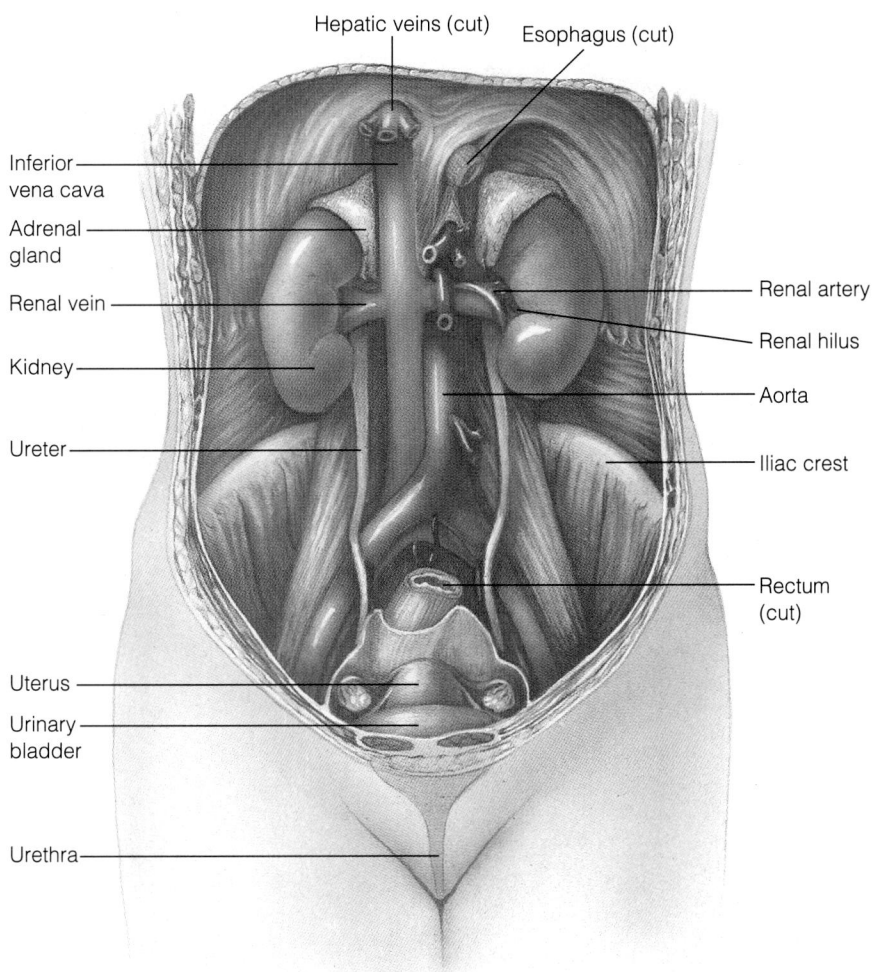

A

Figure 24–1   The urinary system. *A,* Anterior view of the urinary system in a female. *B,* The kidneys are shown in relation to the vertebrae and ribs.

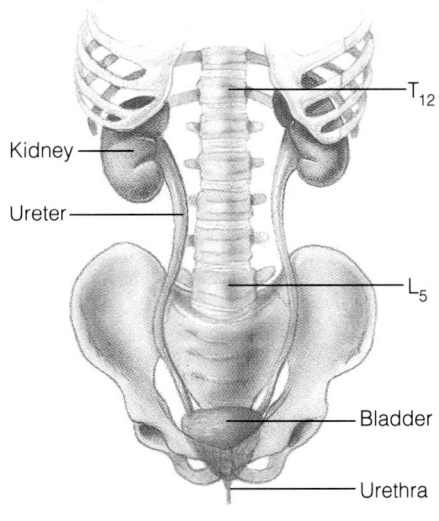

B

kidney) and anchors it to surrounding structures. The middle *adipose capsule* is a fatty mass that holds the kidney in place and also cushions it against trauma. The inner *renal capsule* provides a barrier against infection and helps protect the kidney from trauma.

The functions of the kidney are to

- Balance solute and water transport.
- Excrete metabolic waste products.
- Conserve nutrients.
- Regulate acid-base balance.
- Secrete hormones to help regulate blood pressure, erythrocyte production, and calcium metabolism.
- Form urine.

Figure 24–2   Internal anatomy
of the kidney.

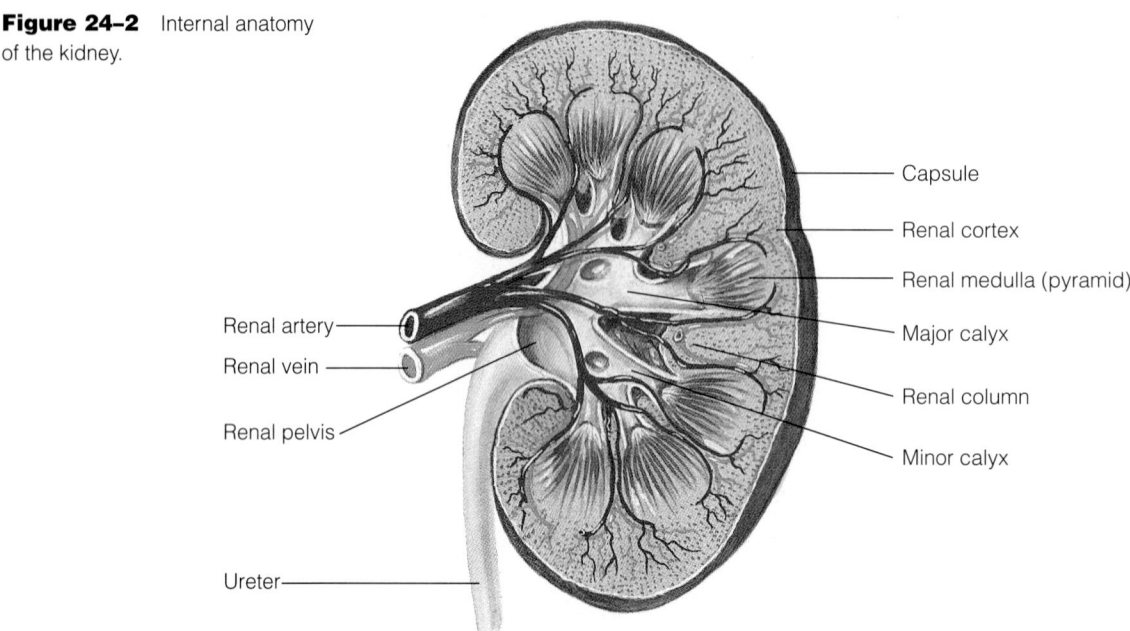

Capsule

Renal cortex

Renal medulla (pyramid)

Major calyx

Renal column

Minor calyx

Renal artery

Renal vein

Renal pelvis

Ureter

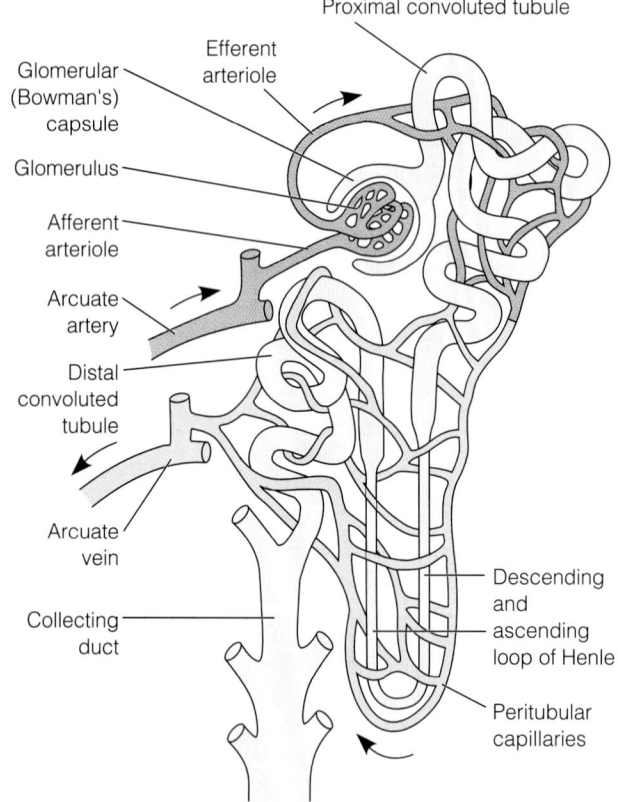

Proximal convoluted tubule

Efferent
arteriole

Glomerular
(Bowman's)
capsule

Glomerulus

Afferent
arteriole

Arcuate
artery

Distal
convoluted
tubule

Arcuate
vein

Collecting
duct

Descending
and
ascending
loop of Henle

Peritubular
capillaries

Figure 24–3   The structure of a nephron, showing the glomerulus within the glomerular capsule.

Internally, each kidney has three distinct regions: the cortex, medulla, and pelvis. The outer region, or *renal cortex*, is light in color and has a granular appearance (Figure 24–2). This region of the kidney contains the *glomeruli,* small clusters of capillaries. The glomeruli bring blood to and carry waste products from the nephrons, the functional units of the kidney.

The *renal medulla* is the region just below the cortex. This area contains cone-shaped tissue masses called *renal pyramids,* which are formed almost entirely of bundles of collecting tubules. Areas of lighter-colored tissue called *renal columns* are actually extensions of the cortex and serve to separate the pyramids. The collecting tubules that make up the pyramids channel urine into the innermost region, the renal pelvis.

Lying just medial to the hilum, the *renal pelvis* is continuous with the ureter leaving the hilum. Branches of the pelvis known as the *major* and *minor calyces* extend toward the medulla and serve to collect urine and empty it into the pelvis. From the pelvis, urine is channeled through the ureter and into the bladder for storage. The walls of the calyces, the renal pelvis, and the ureter contain smooth muscle that moves urine along by peristalsis.

Each kidney contains approximately one million *nephrons,* which process the blood to make urine (Figure 24–3). Each nephron contains a tuft of capillaries called the *glomerulus,* which is completely surrounded by the *glomerular capsule* (or *Bowman's space*). Together, the glomerulus and its surrounding capsule is referred to as the *renal corpuscle.* The endothelium of the glomerulus allows capillaries to be extremely porous. Thus, large amounts of solute-rich fluid pass from the capillaries into the capsule. This fluid, called the *filtrate,* is the raw material of urine. Filtrate leaves the capsule and is channeled into the *proximal convoluted tubule (PCT)* of the nephron. Microvilli on the tubular cells increase the surface area and allow for active reabsorption of some substances from the filtrate. Past the PCT is the U-shaped *loop of Henle,* which consists of both descending and ascending limbs. The descending limb is relatively thin and freely permeable to water, whereas the ascending segment is thick and thereby less permeable. The *distal convoluted tubule (DCT)* receives filtrate from the loop of Henle. Although this segment is structurally similar to the PCT, it lacks microvilli and is more involved with secreting solutes into the filtrate than in reabsorbing substances from it. The collecting tubule receives the newly formed urine from many nephrons and channels urine through the minor and major calyces of the renal pelvis and into the ureter.

Ureters

The *ureters* are bilateral tubes approximately 10 to 12 inches (25 to 30 cm) long. They transport urine from the kidney to the bladder through peristaltic waves originating in the renal pelvis. The wall of the ureter has three layers: an inner epithelial mucosa, a middle layer of smooth muscle, and an outer layer made up of fibrous connective tissue.

Urinary Bladder

The *urinary bladder* is located posterior to the symphysis pubis and serves as a storage site for urine. In males, the bladder lies immediately in front of the rectum; in females, the bladder lies next to the vagina and the uterus. Openings for the ureters and the urethra are located inside the bladder: the *trigone* is the smooth triangular portion of the base of the bladder outlined by these three openings (Figure 24–4).

The layers of the bladder wall (from internal to external) are the epithelial mucosa lining the inside, the connective tissue submucosa, the smooth muscle layer, and the fibrous outer layer. The muscle layer, called the *detrusor muscle,* is made up of fibers arranged in inner and outer longitudinal layers and in a middle circular layer. This arrangement allows the bladder to expand or contract according to the amount of urine it holds.

The size of the bladder varies with the amount of urine it contains. In healthy adults, the bladder holds about 300 to 500 mL of urine before internal pressure rises and signals the need to empty the bladder through *micturition* (also called *urination* or *voiding*). However, the bladder is capable of holding more than twice that amount if necessary. The bladder has an *internal urethral sphincter* that relaxes in response to a full bladder and signals the need to urinate. A second *external urethral sphincter* is formed by skeletal muscle and is under voluntary control.

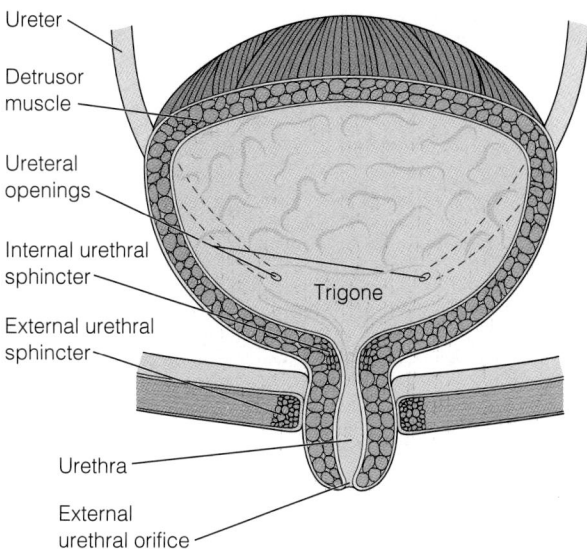

Figure 24–4   Internal view of the urinary bladder and trigone.

Urethra

The *urethra* is a thin-walled muscular tube that channels urine to the outside of the body. It extends from the base of the bladder to the *external urethral orifice* (or *urinary meatus*). In females, the urethra is approximately 1.5 inches (3 to 5 cm) long, and the urinary meatus is located anterior to the vaginal orifice. In males, the urethra is approximately 8 inches (20 cm) long and serves as a channel for semen as well as urine. The prostate gland encircles the urethra at the base of the bladder in males. The male urinary meatus is located at the end of the glans penis.

Formation of Urine

The complex structures of the kidneys process about 180 liters (47 gallons) of blood-derived fluid each day. Of this amount, only 1% is excreted as urine; the rest is returned to the circulation. (The normal characteristics of urine on laboratory analysis are listed in Table 24–1.) Urine formation is accomplished entirely by the nephron through three processes: glomerular filtration, tubular reabsorption, and tubular secretion (Figure 24–5).

Glomerular Filtration

Glomerular filtration is a passive, nonselective process in which fluid and solutes are forced through a membrane by hydrostatic pressure. The amount of fluid filtered from the blood into the capsule per minute is called the **glomerular filtration rate (GFR).** This rate is influenced by three factors: (1) the total surface area available for fil-

Table 24–1 Characteristics of Normal Urine

Color	Pale to deep yellow, clear
Odor	Aromatic
Specific gravity	1.001–1.030
pH	4.5–8.0
Protein	Negative to trace
Glucose	Negative
Ketones	Negative
WBCs	0–5/high power field (hpf)
RBCs	0–5/hpf
Casts	Negative to occasional

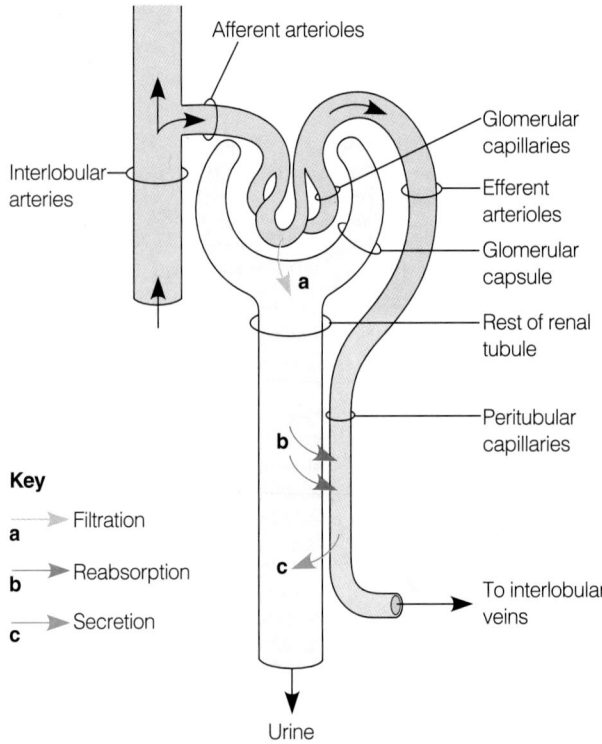

Figure 24–5 Schematic view of the three major mechanisms by which the kidneys adjust to the composition of plasma: *A*, glomerular filtration; *B*, tubular reabsorption; and *C*, tubular secretion.

tration, (2) the permeability of the filtration membrane, and (3) the net filtration pressure.

The glomerulus is a far more efficient filter than most capillary beds because the filtration membrane of the glomerulus is much more permeable to water and solutes than other capillary membranes are. In addition, the glomerular blood pressure is much higher, resulting in higher net filtration pressure.

Net filtration pressure is responsible for the formation of filtrate and is determined by two forces: hydrostatic pressure ("push") and osmotic pressure ("pull"). The glomerular hydrostatic pressure pushes water and solutes across the membrane. This pressure is opposed by the osmotic pressure in the glomerulus (primarily the colloid osmotic pressure of plasma proteins in the glomerular blood) and the capsular hydrostatic pressure exerted by fluids within the glomerular capsule. The difference between these forces determines the net filtration pressure, which is directly proportional to the GFR.

The normal GFR in both kidneys is 120 to 125 mL/min in adults. This rate is held constant under normal conditions by intrinsic controls (or renal autoregulation). Autoregulation is achieved through the control of the diameter of the afferent arterioles by the **myogenic mechanism,** which responds to changes in pressure in the renal blood vessels. An increase in systemic blood pressure causes the renal vessels to constrict, whereas a decline in blood pressure causes the afferent arterioles to dilate. These changes result in adjustments to the glomerular hydrostatic pressure and, indirectly, in the maintenance of the glomerular filtration rate.

Another intrinsic control of the GFR is the result of the **renin-angiotensin mechanism** at work in the kidneys. Special cells known as the *juxtaglomerular apparatus* are located in the distal tubules and respond to slow filtrate

flow by releasing chemicals that cause intense vasodilation of the afferent arterioles. Conversely, an increase in the flow of filtrate results in the promotion of vasoconstriction, decreasing the GFR. Renin release by the juxtaglomerular cells is often triggered by a drop in systemic blood pressure. Renin acts on a plasma globulin known as angiotensinogen to release angiotensin I, which is in turn converted to angiotensin II. As a vasoconstrictor, angiotensin II activates vascular smooth muscle throughout the body, causing systemic blood pressure to rise. Thus, the renin-angiotensin mechanism is a factor in renal autoregulation, even though its main purpose is the control of systemic blood pressure.

Glomerular filtration is also under an extrinsic control mechanism through the sympathetic nervous system. During periods of extreme stress or emergency, stimulation of the sympathetic nervous system causes strong constriction of the afferent arterioles and inhibits the formation of filtrate. The sympathetic nervous system also stimulates the juxtaglomerular cells to release renin, bringing about an increase in systemic blood pressure.

Tubular Reabsorption

Tubular reabsorption, a second major variable in urine formation, is a transepithelial process that begins as the filtrate enters the proximal tubules. In healthy kidneys, virtually all organic nutrients such as glucose and amino acids are reabsorbed. However, the rate and degree of water and ion reabsorption are continuously regulated and adjusted in response to hormonal signals. Reabsorption of substances may be active or passive. Substances reclaimed through active tubular reabsorption are usually moving against electrical and/or chemical gradients. These substances, including glucose, amino acids, lactate, vitamins, and most ions, require an ATP-dependent carrier to be transported into the interstitial space. In passive tubular reabsorption, which encompasses diffusion and osmosis, substances move along their gradient without expenditure of energy.

Tubular Secretion

The final major mechanism in urine formation is tubular secretion, which is essentially reabsorption in reverse. Substances such as hydrogen and potassium ions, creatinine, ammonia, and organic acids move from the blood of the peritubular capillaries into the tubules themselves as filtrate. Thus, the urine is composed of both filtered and secreted substances. Tubular secretion is important for disposing of substances not already in the filtrate, such as medications. This process eliminates undesirable substances that have been reabsorbed by passive processes and rids the body of excessive potassium ions. It is also a vital force in the regulation of blood pH.

Maintaining Normal Composition and Volume of Urine

Maintaining the normal composition and volume of urine involves a *countercurrent exchange system,* also called a *two-solute mechanism.* In this system, fluid flows in opposite directions through the parallel tubes of the loop of Henle and the *vasa recta,* tiny capillaries that run along the loop of Henle. Fluid is exchanged across these parallel membranes in response to a concentration gradient (Figure 24–6). When the filtrate enters the proximal convoluted tubule, its osmolality (at 300 mOsm/kgs) is essentially the same as that of the plasma and the interstitial fluid of the renal cortex. These are the steps in the process:

1. The descending loop of Henle is highly permeable to water and allows chloride and sodium to enter the loop through diffusion. The hyperosmotic interstitium causes water to move out of the descending loop, so that the remaining filtrate becomes increasingly concentrated.

2. The lumen of the ascending loop of Henle is impermeable to water but allows chloride and sodium to move out into the interstitium of the medulla. As a result, the filtrate in the ascending loop becomes hypoosmotic, and the medullary interstitium becomes hyperosmotic.

3. As the filtrate progresses through the ascending limb of the loop of Henle and enters the distal convoluted tubule, sodium and chloride are removed and water is retained. Thus the filtrate becomes more dilute.

4. As the filtrate passes through the deep medullary regions, urea (an end product of protein metabolism and, along with water, the main constituent of urine) begins to diffuse out from the collecting tubules into the interstitial space and establishes a concentration gradient to facilitate water movement.

5. Some urea enters the ascending loop of Henle. Urea entering the vasa recta typically diffuses out again.

The dilution or concentration of urine is largely determined by the action of antidiuretic hormone (ADH), which is secreted by the posterior pituitary gland. ADH causes the pores of the collecting tubules to enlarge, so that increased amounts of water move into the interstitial space. As the end result, water is reabsorbed and urine is more highly concentrated. When ADH is not secreted, the filtrate passes through the system without further water reabsorption, so that the urine is more dilute.

Urine is composed, by volume, of about 95% water and 5% solutes. The largest component of urine by weight is urea. Other solutes normally excreted in the urine include sodium, potassium, phosphate, sulfate, creatinine, uric acid, calcium, magnesium, and bicarbonate.

Clearance of Waste Products

The kidneys are responsible for the excretion of water-soluble waste products and other chemicals or substances from the body. This process is called *renal plasma clearance,* which refers to the ability of the kidneys to clear (cleanse) a given amount of plasma of a particular substance in a given time (usually 1 minute). The kidneys clear 25 to 30 g of urea (a nitrogenous waste product formed in the liver from the breakdown of amino acids) each day. They also clear creatinine (an end product of creatine phosphate, found in skeletal muscle), uric acid (a metabolite of nucleic acid metabolism), and ammonia as well as bacterial toxins and water-soluble drugs. Tests of renal clearance are often used to determine the GFR and glomerular damage.

Renal Hormones

Hormones that are either activated or synthesized by the kidneys include the active form of vitamin D, erythropoietin, and natriuretic hormone.

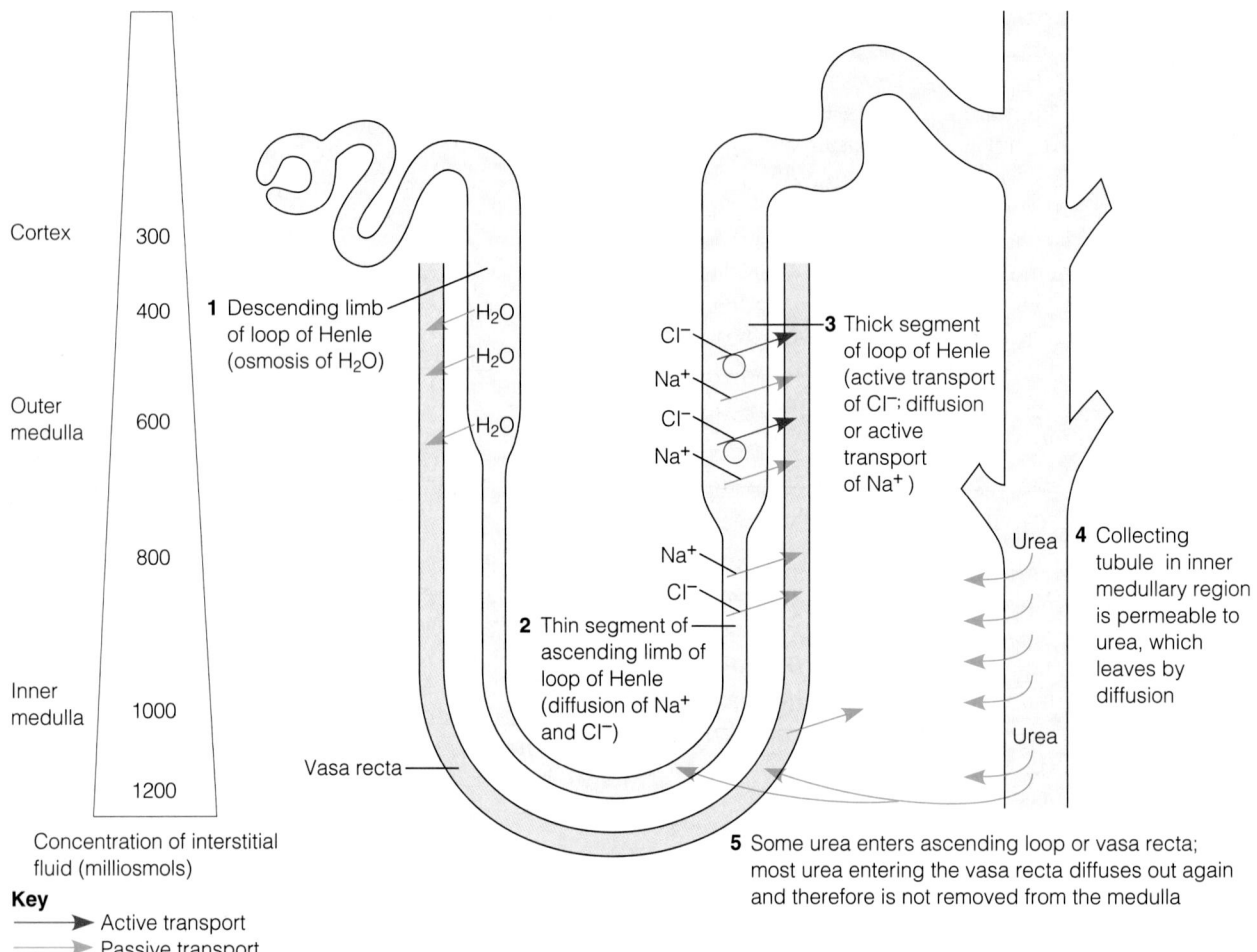

Figure 24–6   The countercurrent exchange system, responsible for establishing and maintaining an osmotic gradient necessary to the composition, volume, and pH of urine.

Vitamin D is necessary for the absorption of calcium and phosphate by the small intestine. In an inactive form, vitamin D enters the body either by dietary intake or through the action of ultraviolet rays on cholesterol in the skin. Activation occurs in two steps, the first in the liver and the second in the kidneys. The renal step is stimulated by parathyroid hormone, which in turn responds to a decreased plasma calcium level.

Erythropoietin stimulates the bone marrow to produce red blood cells in response to tissue hypoxia. The stimulus for the production of erythropoietin by the kidneys is decreased oxygen delivery to kidney cells.

Natriuretic hormone is released from the right atria of the heart in response to increased volume and stretch, as occurs in increased extracellular volume. This hormone inhibits ADH secretion, so that the collecting tubules are less porous and a large amount of dilute urine is produced.

Assessment of Urinary System Function

■   ■   ■

Nurses assess functions of the urinary system and overall health status during both the health assessment interview to collect subjective data and the physical assessment to collect objective data.

The Health Assessment Interview

This section provides guidelines for collecting subjective data through a health assessment interview specific to urinary elimination. You might assess problems with urinary elimination as part of the total health assessment, or you may conduct a focused interview if the client has problems specific to the urinary system. Interview questions and leading statements for assessing urinary elimination are provided.

Overview

If you identify a problem with urinary elimination, analyze its onset, characteristics and course, severity, precipitating and relieving factors, and any associated symptoms, noting the timing and circumstances. For example, you may ask the following questions:

- Do you experience any burning when you urinate?

- Do you have difficulty starting to urinate?

- When did you first notice that you were unable to control the loss of urine from your bladder?

Current urinary status should include such information about

- Color, odor, and amount of urine

- Difficulty initiating a stream of urine

- Frequency of urination

- Painful urination (**dysuria**)

- Excessive urination at night (**nocturia**)

- Blood in the urine (**hematuria**)

- Voiding scant amounts of urine (**oliguria**)

- Voiding excessive amounts of urine (**polyuria**)

- Discharge

- Flank pain

You should explore further any abnormalities you identify in the client's current urinary status. Focus questions on changes in patterns of urination, changes in the urine, and pain.

You can assess changes in patterns of urination by asking the client:

- How many times a day do you urinate? Do you feel that you empty your bladder each time?

- How many times do you get up at night to urinate? Do you feel you empty your bladder each time?

- Do you experience a very strong desire to urinate and feel that you just can't wait?

- Do you have any burning or pain while you urinate?

- Have you noticed that you urinate small amounts of dark, strong-smelling urine?

Changes in the urine that should be explored include the presence of hematuria or a cloudy appearance of the urine. If the client has noticed blood, explore the use of medications (such as anticoagulants or dye-containing drugs) and other bleeding problems. Women may not understand that blood in the toilet after urination is normal during menstruation. Cloudy, foul-smelling urine often indicates infection and signals **pyuria (bacteriuria)**; ask the client about temperature elevations, chills, and gen-

eral malaise. Cloudy urine in men may result from retrograde ejaculation.

If the client reports pain, explore its location, duration, and intensity. Kidney pain is experienced in the back and the costovertebral angle (the angle between the lower ribs and adjacent vertebrae) and may spread toward the umbilicus. Renal colic is severe, sharp, stabbing, and excruciating; often it is felt in the flank, bladder, urethra, testes, or ovaries. Bladder and urethral pain is usually dull and continuous but may be experienced as spasms. The client with a distended bladder experiences constant pain that is increased by any pressure over the bladder.

Information concerning surgeries or other treatment of previous urinary problems is essential to the health history, as is a family history of altered structure or function. A family history of renal problems may be the first clue to abnormalities in the client's urinary function. You need to explore information regarding family occurrence of end-stage renal disease, renal calculi, and frequent infections as well as related problems such as hypertension and diabetes mellitus.

Questions about life-style, diet, and work history should explore cigarette smoking, exposure to toxic chemicals, usual fluid intake, type of fluid intake, and self-care measures to replace fluids lost during work or physical activity in hot temperatures.

Interview Questions

The following interview questions and leading statements are categorized by functional health patterns

Health Perception–Health Management

- Have you ever had a bladder or kidney disease, injury, or surgery? Describe.

- How was this problem treated?

- Describe your usual intake of fluids and food for a 24-hour period. What type of fluids do you drink?

- Describe the current problem you are having with urinary elimination.

- Are you taking any medications for this problem? If so, what are you taking and how often?

- Are you taking medications for any other health problem? Explain.

- For women: Describe how you care for yourself in terms of urinary elimination (for example, hygiene and direction of wiping after voiding).

- What do you do to care for yourself if you believe you have a urinary infection?

- If you have had a surgical alteration of urine flow (such as an ileal conduit), describe how you care for yourself (what skin and appliance care do you provide, how often do you empty the bag?).

- Have you ever been taught to begin the flow of your urine by using the Credé maneuver or any other method? Explain.
- Have you worn or do you now wear an incontinence pad, external catheter, or indwelling catheter? Explain.
- Have you ever done self-catheterization? If so, why and how often?

Nutritional-Metabolic

- Do you limit the amount of salt in your diet? Explain.
- How much coffee, tea, or alcohol do you drink in a 24-hour period?
- Have you ever restricted your fluid intake? Explain.
- Do you ever have swelling of any part of your body? Describe.

Elimination

- How many times a day do you urinate? Do you have to get up at night to urinate? Has there been a change in your usual pattern of urination?
- Do you experience a sudden urge to urinate?
- Has there been a recent increase or decrease in the amount of urine you eliminate with each voiding?
- Has there been a recent change in the color or odor of your urine?
- Have you ever had problems controlling urination when you laugh, sneeze, or cough?
- Is it difficult for you to start or maintain the flow of urine?
- Have you ever had difficulty controlling urination when you are sleeping?
- Do you have any discharge from your urethra? Describe.

Activity-Exercise

- Do your urinary problems interfere with your usual activities of daily living (such as walking, cleaning house, shopping, driving, socializing)? Explain.
- Have you ever been taught to do Kegel exercises to tone bladder muscles? If so, how often do you practice these?
- Describe your energy level. Has there been a recent change? Explain.

Sleep-Rest

- Does a problem with urinary elimination interfere with your ability to rest or sleep? Explain.
- Has there been a recent change in the number of times you wake up to urinate during the night? Explain.

Cognitive-Perceptual

- Do you have any pain or burning with urination? Explain.
- Have you experienced any tenderness or pain over the lower sides of your back or severe pain that spreads to your lower abdomen? If so, describe its location, intensity, aggravating factors, and duration.

Self-Perception–Self-Concept

- How has this problem with your urinary elimination affected how you feel about yourself?
- How has this problem with your urinary elimination affected how you feel about your normal life?
- If appropriate: How do you feel about wearing incontinence pads? using an external catheter? having an indwelling catheter? having a urinary diversion?

Role-Relationship

- Is there a history of bladder or kidney problems in your family? If so, describe.
- Has your urinary elimination problem affected your role in your family? If so, how?
- Has your problem with urinary elimination affected your interactions with your family? with friends? at work? in social activities?
- Has a urinary elimination problem affected your ability to work? Explain.

Sexuality-Reproductive

- Has your problem with urinary elimination affected your usual sexual activities? Explain.
- Describe how having this health problem has made you feel about yourself as a man or a woman.

Coping-Stress

- Have you experienced increased stress because of this problem with urinary elimination? Explain.
- Have you noticed an increase in urination when you experience stress?
- What do you feel is the most stressful time you have had with this urinary problem?
- Describe what you do to cope with stress.
- Who or what will be able to help you cope with stress caused by this problem with urinary elimination?

Value-Belief

- Are there significant others, practices, or activities that help you cope with this health problem? Explain.
- How do you perceive the future with this problem?

The Physical Assessment

Physical assessment of the urinary system may be performed as part of a total health assessment, as part of an abdominal assessment, or as part of the back examination (for the kidneys). For clients with known or suspected problems of this system, urinary assessment requires using the techniques of inspection, palpation, percussion, and auscultation. Auscultation should be performed immediately after inspection because percussion or palpation may increase bowel motility and interfere with sound transmission during auscultation.

The equipment necessary to assess the urinary system is a urine specimen cup and disposable gloves. At the beginning of the assessment, the client may be sitting or lying supine. Prior to the examination, collect all necessary equipment and explain the techniques to the client to decrease anxiety.

Before beginning the assessment, ask the client to provide you with a clean-catch urine specimen and give the client a specimen cup. Assess the specimen for color, odor, and clarity before you send it to the laboratory.

Because the examination involves exposure of the genital area, provide the client with a gown and drape the client appropriately to minimize exposure.

Guidelines for percussion and palpation of the kidneys are outlined in the box on page 880.

Assessment Technique	Possible Abnormal Findings
■ Inspect the skin and mucous membranes. Note color, turgor, and excretions.	Pallor of the skin and mucous membranes may indicate kidney disease with resultant anemia. Decreased turgor of the skin may indicate dehydration. Edema may indicate fluid volume excess. Either change may indicate renal insufficiency with either excess fluid loss or retention. An accumulation of uric acid crystals, called *uremic frost*, may be seen on the skin of the client with untreated renal failure.
■ Inspect the abdomen. Help the client to a supine position. Note size, symmetry, any masses or lumps, swelling, prominent veins, distention, glistening, or skin tightness.	Enlargements or asymmetry may indicate a hernia or superficial mass. Prominent veins may indicate renal dysfunction. Distention, glistening, or skin tightness may be associated with fluid retention. *Ascites* is an accumulation of fluid in the peritoneal cavity.
■ Inspect the urinary meatus. (This technique is not part of a routine assessment, but it is an important component in clients with health problems of the urinary system.) Help the male client to a sitting or standing position. Compress the tip of the glans penis with your gloved hand to open the urinary meatus (Figure 24–7). Assist the female client to the dorsal lithotomy position. Spread the labia with your gloved hand to expose the urinary meatus.	Increased redness, swelling, or discharge may indicate infection or sexually transmitted disease. Ulceration may indicate a sexually transmitted disease. In male clients, a deviation of the meatus from the midline may suggest a congenital defect.

➤

Guidelines for Physical Assessment of the Kidneys

■ ■ ■

Percussion of the Kidneys

Percussion of the kidneys helps assess pain or tenderness. Assist the client to a sitting position, and stand behind the client. For indirect percussion, place the palm of your nondominant hand over the costovertebral angle (see Figure A). Strike this area with the ulnar surface of your dominant hand, curled into a fist (see Figure B). For direct percussion, also strike the area over the costovertebral angle with the ulnar surface of your dominant hand, curled into a fist. Repeat the technique for the other kidney.

You should do percussion of the kidneys with only enough force so the client feels a gentle thud. Percussion is usually done at the end of the assessment.

Palpation of the Kidneys

Although the technique of palpation of the kidneys is outlined here, this technique is best performed by an advanced practitioner, because it involves deep palpation. In addition, the kidneys are difficult to palpate.

Assist the client to the supine position and stand at the right side of the client. To palpate the left kidney, reach across the client and place your left hand under the client's left flank with your palm upward. Elevate the left flank with your fingers, displacing the kidney upward. Ask the client to take a deep breath and use the palmer surface of your right hand to palpate the kidney (see Figure C). Repeat the technique for the right kidney.

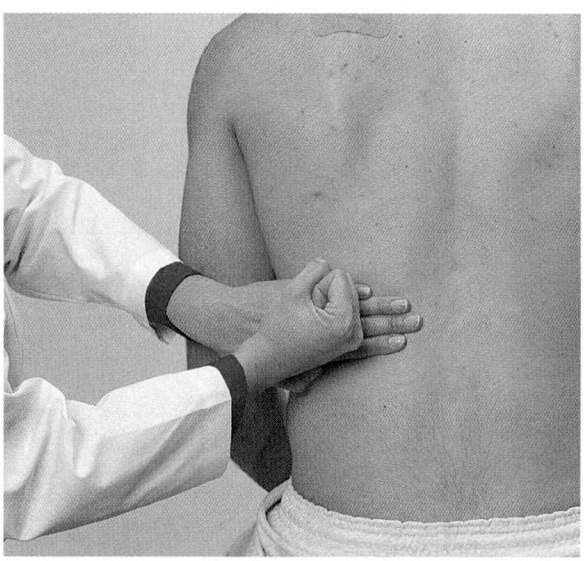

B   Percussing the kidney.

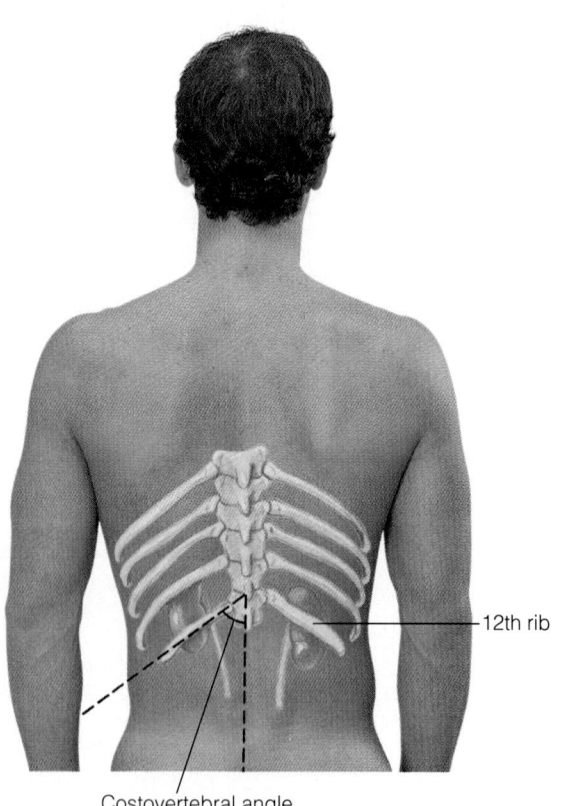

—12th rib

Costovertebral angle

A   Location of the kidneys and the costovertebral angle.

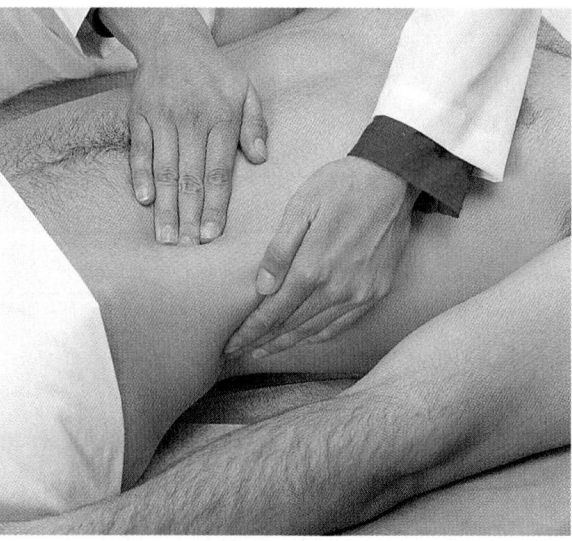

C   Palpating the left kidney.

ASSESSMENT TECHNIQUE	POSSIBLE ABNORMAL FINDINGS

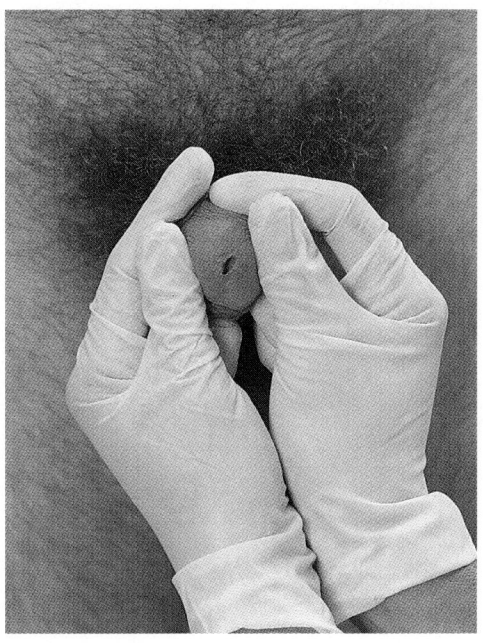

Figure 24–7 Inspecting the urinary meatus of the male.

■ **Auscultate the renal arteries.**
Help the client to a supine position.
Place the bell of the stethoscope lightly in the areas of the renal arteries, located in the left and right upper abdominal quadrants.

Systolic bruits (whooshing sounds) may indicate renal artery stenosis.

■ **Percuss the kidneys for tenderness or pain.**
See the box on page 880 for guidelines for percussion of the kidneys.

Tenderness and pain elicited on percussion of the costovertebral angle suggest glomerulonephritis or glomerulonephrosis.

■ **Palpate the kidneys.**
See the box on page 880 for guidelines for palpation of the kidneys.

A mass or lump may indicate a tumor or cyst.
Tenderness or pain on palpation may suggest an inflammatory process.
A soft kidney that feels spongy may indicate chronic renal disease.
Bilaterally enlarged kidneys may suggest polycystic kidney disease.
Unequal kidney size may indicate hydronephrosis.

■ **Percuss the bladder for tone and position.**
Help the client to a supine position.

A dull percussion tone over the bladder of a client who has just urinated may indicate urinary retention.

■ **Palpate the bladder for distention.**
Gently palpate over the symphysis pubis and abdomen.

A distended bladder may be palpated at any point from the symphysis pubis to the umbilicus and is felt as a firm, rounded organ.

Variations in Assessment Findings for the Older Adult

There is a progressive decline in kidney function with age. The bladder shrinks, having less than half the capacity of the bladder of a young adult. Nocturia, frequency, and urgency are common symptoms related to two physiologic changes associated with the aging process: a decrease in bladder capacity and tone, and a diminished response to vasopressin, a hormone with an antidiuretic effect. However, urinary incontinence is not a normal aspect of aging. Changes in the kidneys associated with aging affect urine formation; a decrease in renal blood flow, often from arteriosclerosis, can result in a decrease in the size and number of nephrons. By age 70, the rate of filtrate formation in the older adult is half that of the middle adult.

These variations in assessment findings are common in the older adult:

- The desire to urinate is often delayed, and the bladder does not empty as well, leading to retention and increased residual urine.

- Urinary retention is often a problem in men with prostate enlargement.

- Stress incontinence is often a problem in postmenopausal women because the urethra loses tone and tends to atrophy along with genital structures.

- Glucose is not as well absorbed, contributing to an increased amount of glucose in the urine.

Bibliography

■ ■ ■

Andresen, G. (1989). A fresh look at assessing the elderly. *RN, 33*(6), 28–40.

Baer, C. (1989). Assessing flank pain. *Nursing, 19*(10), 75–77.

Braverman, B. (1990). Eliciting assessment data from a patient who is difficult to interview. *Nursing Clinics of North America, 25*(4), 743–750.

Kain, C. (1990). The older adult: A comparative assessment. *Nursing Clinics of North America, 25*(4), 833–848.

Lindsey, M. (1989). Abdominal assessment. *Orthopaedic Nursing, 8*(4), 34–38.

Marieb, E. N. (1995). *Human anatomy and physiology* (3rd ed.). Redwood City, CA: Benjamin/Cummings.

McConnell, E. (1988). Seeing your patient as a mosaic. *Nursing, 18*(12), 50–51.

O'Toole, M. (1990). Advanced assessment of the abdomen and gastrointestinal problems. *Nursing Clinics of North America, 25*(4), 771–776.

Swartz, M. (1989). *Textbook of physical diagnosis: History and examination*. Philadelphia: Saunders.

Nursing Care of Clients with Urinary Tract Disorders

LEARNING OBJECTIVES

On completion of this chapter, you will be able to

- Describe the pathophysiology of commonly occurring disorders of the urinary tract, including infection, calculi, tumors, urinary retention, neurogenic bladder, and urinary incontinence.
- Identify laboratory and diagnostic tests used to diagnose disorders affecting the urinary tract.

- Compare and contrast the manifestations of common disorders of the urinary tract.
- Discuss the nursing implications of medications prescribed for the client with a urinary tract disorder.
- Provide appropriate nursing care for the client having surgery of the urinary tract.
- Use the nursing process as a framework for providing individualized care to clients with disorders of the urinary tract.

Disorders of the urinary tract may result from a variety of health alterations affecting the tract directly or indirectly. These include congenital malformations, infections, obstructions, trauma, tumors, and neurologic conditions. Any portion of the tract—from the kidney through the urethra—can be affected, with serious or even life-threatening consequences if the problem is diagnosed incorrectly or left untreated. Diseases or infections of the kidney may impair renal function directly. Diseases or infections of the **urinary drainage system** (the ureters, urinary bladder, and urethra) may spread to the kidneys or obstruct urine flow. In either case, destruction of nephrons and impaired renal function may result.

When caring for the client with any of the urinary tract disorders discussed in this chapter, the nurse needs to consider a client's modesty in voiding, possible difficulty in discussing the genitals, embarrassment about being exposed for examination and testing, and fear of changes in body image or function. These psychosocial issues may interfere with the client's willingness to seek help, discuss the treatment plan, and learn about preventive measures.

Nursing interventions for the client with a urinary tract disorder are directed toward (1) prevention through asepsis, health teaching, and early detection and (2) management of the disorder through health teaching and nursing care.

The Client with a Urinary Tract Infection

■ ■ ■

Infections of the urinary tract are the second most prevalent bacterial disease (Porth, 1994). Ten to twenty percent of adult females are affected by lower urinary tract infections (McCance & Huether, 1994). Adult males have a much lower incidence. Urinary tract infections occur 50 times more frequently in women between the ages of 20 and 50 than in men of the same age. With increasing age, this ratio decreases as the incidence of urinary tract infection (UTI) increases in both men and women (Berkow &

Fletcher, 1992). Unfortunately, *nosocomial* infections (infections acquired during hospitalization) are among the most common of urinary tract infections.

An infectious process can lead to inflammation of any portion of the urinary tract. Urinary tract infections are broadly classified according to the region and primary site affected. *Lower urinary tract infections* include **urethritis**, inflammation of the urethra; *prostatitis,* inflammation of the prostate gland (discussed in Chapter 46); and **cystitis**, inflammation of the urinary bladder. The most common *upper urinary tract infection* is **pyelonephritis**, an inflammation affecting the kidney and renal pelvis. Clinical manifestations may be unreliable indicators of the site affected. In addition, diagnostic tests to differentiate upper and lower UTI are invasive, expensive, and not readily available. Fortunately, identifying the exact site of the infection is often not necessary for appropriate clinical management (Gillenwater et al., 1987).

Pathophysiology

The urinary tract is normally sterile above the urethra. Adequate urine volume, a free flow from the kidneys through the urinary meatus, and complete bladder emptying are the most important mechanisms maintaining sterility. Other normal defenses for preventing infection include acid urine, peristaltic activity of the ureters, a competent ureterovesical junction, and bacteriostatic properties of the bladder and urethral cells. In males, a long urethra and the antibacterial effect of zinc in prostatic fluid are also important.

Pathogens enter the urinary tract by one of two routes: by *ascending* from the mucous membranes of the perineal area into the lower urinary tract; or *hematogenously,* from the blood. The ascending route is the most common source of UTI. Gram-negative bacteria, which commonly reside in the intestinal tract, are often responsible; *Escherichia coli* is the infective organism in 80% to 90% of first-time infections (Berkow & Fletcher, 1992; Tierney et al., 1994). Other common gram-negative pathogens causing UTI include *Proteus, Klebsiella, Enterobacter,* and *Pseudomonas.* Less common causes are gram-positive bacteria such as *Staphylococcus* and fungi. Hematogenous spread of infection to the urinary tract is rare. Infections introduced in this manner are usually associated with previous damage or scarring of the urinary tract. Bacteria introduced into the urinary tract may result in asymptomatic bacteriuria or in an inflammatory response with manifestations of UTI.

Clients can be predisposed to UTI by a variety of factors, some of which (e.g., the short urethra of the female) cannot be changed. Congenital or acquired factors contributing to the risk of infection include urinary tract obstruction by tumors or calculi, structural abnormalities such as strictures, impaired bladder innervation, bowel

incontinence, and chronic diseases such as diabetes mellitus. Prostatic hypertrophy and bacterial prostatitis are risk factors among males. Lack of a normally protective mucosal enzyme, possible decreased levels of cervicovaginal antibodies to enterobacteria, and use of a diaphragm increase the risk among females. Instrumentation of the urinary tract (e.g., catheterization or cystoscopy) is a major risk factor for UTI (Porth, 1994). Even when performed under strict aseptic conditions, catheterization can result in bladder infection. The placement of the catheter prevents the flushing action of voiding, and bacteria may ascend to the bladder either through the catheter lumen or via exudate between the urethral mucosa and the catheter.

An increased incidence of UTI is seen in older clients. The greatest degree of increase is seen in men as the ratio of female to male UTI changes from 50:1 to less than 5:1. An increased risk of urinary stasis, chronic disease states (such as diabetes mellitus), and an impaired immune response contribute to the higher incidence of UTI in the older adult. In men, the prostate typically hypertrophies with aging, potentially resulting in urinary retention as the urethra narrows. Prostatic secretions are lessened, diminishing their protective, antibacterial effect. In older women, loss of tissue elasticity and weakening of perineal muscles often contribute to the development of a cystocele or rectocele. Resulting changes in bladder and urethral position increase the risk of incomplete bladder emptying.

Cystitis

Cystitis, inflammation of the urinary bladder, is the most common form of urinary tract infection. Although cystitis may be noninfectious—resulting from exposure to radiation, chemotherapeutic agents, or a metabolic disorder—most commonly a bacterial infection causes the inflammatory process. Inflammation causes the bladder mucosa to become hyperemic (red) and may lead to diffuse hemorrhage or pus formation. This inflammatory process causes the classic manifestations associated with cystitis. (See the accompanying clinical manifestations box.) Typical presenting symptoms of cystitis include *dysuria* (painful or difficult urination), urinary frequency and **urgency** (a sudden, compelling need to urinate), and nocturia (voiding two or more times at night). In addition, the urine may have a foul odor and appear cloudy (pyuria) or bloody (hematuria) because of mucus, excess white cells in the urine, and bleeding of the bladder wall (Bullock & Rosendahl, 1992). The client may also experience suprapubic pain and tenderness.

Older clients may not exhibit the classic symptoms of cystitis. Instead, they often present with nonspecific manifestations such as nocturia, incontinence, confusion, behavior change, lethargy, anorexia, or "just not feeling right" (Millette-Petit, 1988). Fever may be present; how-

---

Clinical Manifestations of Cystitis

- Dysuria
- Frequency
- Urgency
- Nocturia
- Pyuria
- Hematuria
- Suprapubic discomfort

---

ever, hypothermia also may signal sepsis in an older adult (Schoemick et al., 1991).

Cystitis occurs most frequently in adult females, usually because of colonization of the bladder by bacteria normally found in the lower gastrointestinal tract. These bacteria gain entry by ascending the short, straight female urethra (Burke, 1992; Memmler et al., 1992). Additional risk factors that contribute to the higher incidence of infection among adult females include the proximity of the urinary meatus to the vagina and anus, and tissue trauma and potential contamination during sexual intercourse. Poor personal hygiene practices and voluntary urinary retention also contribute to the risk of bacterial contamination of the bladder.

Although the bacteriostatic effect of prostatic fluid and a longer urethra provide an effective barrier to bladder infection for the adult male, the prostatic hypertrophy commonly associated with aging increases the risk of cystitis for elderly males. The enlarged prostate may impede urine flow, leading to incomplete bladder emptying and urinary stasis. Bacteria are not completely flushed with voiding, allowing multiplication and potential infection.

Although cystitis is generally uncomplicated and often resolves spontaneously, sequelae can occur. The infection can ascend to involve the kidneys. Severe or prolonged infection may lead to sloughing of bladder mucosa and ulcer formation. Gangrenous cystitis with necrosis of the bladder wall can complicate the most severe infections (McCance & Huether, 1994).

Pyelonephritis

Pyelonephritis is an inflammatory disorder affecting the renal pelvis and *parenchyma,* the functional portion of the kidney tissue. Acute pyelonephritis is a bacterial infection of the kidney; chronic pyelonephritis is associated with nonbacterial infections and noninfectious processes that may be metabolic, chemical, or immunologic in origin.

The ascending route from the lower urinary tract is the most common pathway for infection of the kidney (Memmler et al., 1992). Asymptomatic bacteriuria or cystitis can lead to acute pyelonephritis. Risk factors include pregnancy (because of slowed ureteral peristalsis), urinary tract obstruction, and congenital malformation. Uri-

nary tract trauma, scarring, calculi (stones), kidney disorders such as polycystic or hypertensive kidney disease, and chronic diseases such as diabetes may also contribute to pyelonephritis. **Vesicoureteral reflux,** a condition in which urine moves from the bladder back toward the kidney, is a common risk factor in children who develop pyelonephritis and is also seen in adults when bladder outflow is obstructed (Porth, 1994).

The infection develops in patchy or scattered foci, spreading from the renal pelvis to the cortex. The pelvis, calyces, and medulla of the kidney are primarily affected, with white blood cell infiltration and inflammation. The kidney becomes grossly edematous. Localized abscesses may develop in the medulla and spread to the renal cortex. Tissue destruction from the inflammatory process can occur in the renal parenchyma, primarily affecting the tubules. With healing, scar tissue replaces the lesions of acute pyelonephritis, and affected tubules atrophy.

As with cystitis, *E. Coli* is the organism responsible for 85% of the cases of acute pyelonephritis. Other organisms commonly found include *Proteus* and *Klebsiella,* bacteria that normally inhabit the intestinal tract.

The client with acute pyelonephritis demonstrates manifestations associated with an acute inflammatory response. The onset is typically rapid, with chills and fever, malaise, and vomiting, as well as the more localized manifestations of flank pain, costovertebral tenderness, urinary frequency, and dysuria. (See the accompanying clinical manifestations box.) In addition, symptoms of cystitis

---

Clinical Manifestations of Acute Pyelonephritis

Urinary

- Urinary frequency
- Dysuria
- Pyuria
- Hematuria
- Bacteriuria
- Leukocyte casts in urine
- Flank pain
- Costovertebral tenderness

Gastrointestinal

- Vomiting
- Diarrhea

Cardiovascular

- Tachypnea

Hematologic

- Leukocytosis

Musculoskeletal

- Muscle tenderness

Metabolic Processes

- Acute onset fever
- Shaking chills
- Malaise

may be present. In older clients, acute pyelonephritis may be manifested by a change in behavior, an acute confusional state, incontinence, or a general deterioration in condition.

Chronic pyelonephritis, unlike the acute form, appears to result from an autoimmune process (see Chapter 8) leading to inflammation of the kidney. Chronic, recurrent, or nonbacterial infections may contribute to its development; these infections may in turn result from the inflammation and scarring associated with chronic pyelonephritis. With chronic pyelonephritis, fibrosis and scarring lead to dilation of the renal pelvis and calyces, and gradual destruction of the tubules. Chronic renal failure and end-stage renal disease may develop as a result of chronic pyelonephritis.

The client with chronic pyelonephritis may be asymptomatic or have few manifestations of the disease. Mild symptoms of pyelonephritis, including frequency, dysuria, and flank pain, may be present. Hypertension can develop as the renal parenchyma is destroyed.

Collaborative Care

Treatment of the client with a urinary tract infection is focused on eradicating the causative organism, preventing relapse or reinfection, and identifying and correcting any contributing factors. Pharmacologic treatment with antibiotics and urinary anti-infectives is commonly used. Surgical interventions to correct contributing factors may be employed.

Laboratory and Diagnostic Tests

Laboratory testing for the client presenting with manifestations of a UTI includes urine studies and a complete blood count (CBC).

The following laboratory tests may be ordered:

- *Urinalysis* is performed to assess for the presence of blood cells and bacteria in the urine. A bacteria count greater than 100,000 (10^5) per milliliter is indicative of infection.

  The preferred method of obtaining a specimen is using the midstream clean-catch procedure. If necessary, urine may be obtained via straight catheterization or "mini-cath," using strict aseptic technique. This technique is less desirable, however, because of the association of infection with urinary tract instrumentation.

- A *Gram's stain of urine* is obtained for tentative identification of the infecting organism by shape and characteristic (gram positive or negative). Rapid identification of the probable pathogen allows timely therapy.

- *Urine culture and sensitivity* tests are necessary for definitive identification of the infecting organism and the

most effective antibiotic. Culture requires 24 to 72 hours for organism growth and identification in the laboratory (Pagana & Pagana, 1992).

- A *white blood cell (WBC) count* is performed with differential identification of the types of WBCs. An infectious process elevates the total WBC. An acute bacterial infection generally causes an increase in the relative proportion of neutrophils to other types of WBCs on differential examination (Kee, 1991; Pagana & Pagana, 1992).

In men and in adult females with recurrent infections or infections resistant to treatment, a more extensive diagnostic workup may be prescribed to rule out structural abnormalities and other contributing factors. These tests may include the following:

- *Intravenous pyelography (IVP)*, also known as *excretory urography*, is used to visualize the kidneys, ureters, and bladder for evaluation of structure and excretory function. As the kidneys clear an intravenously injected contrast medium from the blood, the radiologist can identify the size and shape of the kidneys, their calices and pelvises, the ureters, and the bladder. IVP permits detection of structural or functional abnormalities that may contribute to UTI (Kee, 1991; Pagana & Pagana, 1992).

- *Voiding cystourethrography* involves instilling contrast medium into the bladder, then taking X-ray films to assess the bladder and urethra when filled and during the voiding process. This study allows assessment of the bladder for structural or functional abnormalities, as well as the urethra for strictures. The risk of hypersensitivity reaction to the contrast dye is less than with an IVP.

- *Cystoscopy*, direct visualization of the urethra and bladder through an endoscope, is a valuable diagnostic and therapeutic tool. Cystoscopy is used to diagnose conditions that may contribute to UTI such as prostatic hypertrophy, urethral strictures, bladder calculi, tumors, polyps or diverticula, and congenital abnormalities. During the procedure, biopsy tissue may be obtained, lesions resected, calculi removed, or strictures dilated. A ureteral catheter may be inserted into the renal pelvis for pyelography during cystoscopy.

- Manual pelvic or prostate examination are performed to assess structural changes of the genitourinary tract, such as prostatic enlargement, cystocele, or rectocele, that may be contributing to UTI.

A more complete description of urinary diagnostic procedures and related nursing implications are included in the accompanying box.

Nursing Implications of Diagnostic Studies: The Client with UTI

Intravenous Pyelography

Preparation of the Client

- Assess client knowledge of procedure, clarifying purpose and explaining preparation and procedure.
- Ask the client about, and check the medical record for, any history of allergy to seafood (which is high in iodine content), iodine preparations, or radiologic contrast media. Notify the physician or radiologist if any of these allergies are known.
- Ensure that a signed consent form for the procedure is in the client's chart.
- Assess renal and fluid status. The dye used is nephrotoxic and may worsen renal function, particularly in clients who are older, dehydrated, or have compromised renal status (Pagana & Pagana, 1992).
- Prepare the client for the procedure as specified by radiology department. Preparation may include a bowel-preparation routine and restricted food and fluids for 8 to 12 hours before the test because gas, feces, or barium in the intestinal tract can interfere with visualization of the kidneys, ureters, and bladder, invalidating the procedure. Schedule any ordered barium studies to follow IVP.
- After completion of the study, monitor vital signs and urinary output. Observe and report possible signs of delayed reaction to the contrast media such as dyspnea, tachycardia, itching, hives, or flushing. Check the injection site for redness, pain, warmth. Apply warm packs to the site if indicated.

Client and Family Teaching

- This examination uses X-rays to show the structures of the kidney, ureters, and bladder by injecting a dye that is rapidly excreted in the urine. The test takes about 30 minutes.
- You may have to observe some food and fluid restrictions before the test.
- As the dye is injected, you may feel a transient flushing or burning sensation, along with possible nausea and a metallic taste.
- A rash, difficulty breathing, rapid heart rate, or hives may signal an allergic reaction to the dye. Notify the physician immediately if these occur.
- Increase fluid intake after the test is completed.

Voiding Cystourethrography

Preparation of the Client

- Assess client knowledge and understanding of the procedure. Provide additional instruction as indicated.
- Make sure there is a signed consent form in the client's chart.
- Ask the client about, and check the chart for, indications of allergy to seafood, iodine preparations, or X-ray contrast media. Notify the physician if noted; however, because the dye is not injected, allergic reactions are rare, and allergy does not contraindicate proceeding with the examination.
- Restrict diet to clear liquids on the morning of the exam, or follow the food and fluid restrictions recommended by radiology department.
- Insert indwelling catheter if ordered.

Client and Family Teaching

- First the bladder is filled with dye solution. Then X-rays are taken of the filled bladder and of the bladder and urethra during urination.
- You remain awake during the procedure and should have little or no discomfort. The procedure takes approximately 30 to 45 minutes to complete.
- After the procedure, drink fluids to rapidly dilute remaining contrast medium and reduce burning on urination.
- Report to the physician any signs of infection, such as frequency, urgency, painful urination, cloudy or bloody urine, or malodorous urine.

Cystoscopy

Preparation of the Client

- Assess client knowledge and understanding of the procedure and its purpose. Provide information as needed, referring the client to the physician if necessary for clarification.
- Make sure there is a properly signed consent form in the client's chart.
- Follow preprocedure guidelines as specified by the physician. If general anesthesia will be used, food and fluids are restricted for 8 to 12 hours prior to the procedure. If local anesthesia is used, fasting is not required.

➤

Diagnostic Studies: The Client with UTI (continued)

■ ■ ■

- Assist the client with bowel preparation as ordered, administering laxatives and/or enemas. Record results.

- Administer preprocedure sedation and other medications as ordered.

Client and Family Teaching

- The procedure is performed in a special cystoscopy room. Local or general anesthesia is used. You may feel some pressure or the sensation of needing to urinate as the scope is inserted through the urethra into the bladder. The procedure takes approximately 30 to 45 minutes.

- You may need to observe some food or fluid restrictions prior to the procedure.

- You may feel dizzy or faint if you stand immediately after the procedure. Don't attempt to stand up without assistance.

- Burning on urination for a day or two after the procedure is considered normal.

- Bloody urine for more than three voidings after the procedure, the onset of bright bleeding, low urine output, abdominal or flank pain, and chills or fever may indicate a complication. Notify the physician immediately about any of these symptoms.

- Warm sitz baths, analgesic agents, and antispasmodic medications may relieve discomfort after the procedure.

- Increase fluid intake to decrease pain and difficulty voiding and reduce the risk of infection.

- Laxatives and/or cathartics are prescribed after the procedure to prevent constipation and straining, which may cause bleeding in the lower urinary tract.

Pharmacology

Traditional or conventional treatment of UTI involves 7 to 10 days administration of oral antimicrobial therapy. Although many drugs are effective in treating UTI, the ideal drug is concentrated in the urine, has minimal adverse effects, and is low in cost. The most commonly used antimicrobials are the sulfonamides, amoxicillin, co-trimoxazole (TMP-SMZ, Bactrim, Septra), and tetracycline. Because all of these drugs are effective against the usual infecting organisms, culture of the urine and sensitivity tests are not always necessary before starting therapy (Todd, 1990).

Conventional antimicrobial therapy is associated with a high rate of side effects, including gastrointestinal distress and superinfections, such as candidiasis of the mouth or vagina. Poor compliance to the treatment and a relatively high failure rate as evidenced by recurrent infection are additional problems with conventional antimicrobial treatment regimens. For the reasons noted above, single-dose antibiotic therapy or a short, 3-day course is often prescribed by physicians for infections of the lower urinary tract. Drugs such as amoxicillin or sulfamethoxazole-trimethoprim may be prescribed for single-dose or short-term therapy. The advantages of this regimen include reduced cost, increased compliance, and a lower rate of side effects (Gillenwater et al., 1987). Single-dose therapy is not used for clients with recurrent infections, manifestations of upper urinary tract infection, or contributing risk factors such as structural abnormalities or chronic disease.

The client with acute pyelonephritis is at risk for bacteremia. This client may require hospitalization and initial treatment with intravenous antibiotics when the infection is severe or nausea and vomiting are present. If the client is severely ill, parenteral ampicillin or a cephalosporin and an aminoglycoside are often prescribed initially. Clients with less severe symptoms are usually treated with one of the antibiotics often used for lower UTI, with the course of therapy lasting 14 to 21 days.

The outcome of pharmacologic treatment of UTI is determined by follow-up urinalysis and culture. *Cure,* as evidenced by absence of pathogens in the urine, is the desired outcome of therapy. **Persistence** is the continued presence of significant numbers of bacteria in the urine after 48 hours of antimicrobial therapy. A **relapse** is diagnosed when the client develops another UTI due to the same strain of bacteria within 1 to 2 weeks after treatment; **reinfection** indicates development of a second UTI with a new strain of bacteria following therapy.

Urinary anti-infectives are used most often for resistant or recurrent urinary tract infections rather than acute, uncomplicated infections. These drugs do not achieve effective plasma concentrations at recommended doses but do reach effective concentrations in the urine. Therapy may be prolonged, lasting 2 weeks to 6 or 12 months, to ensure complete eradication of the infecting organism and prevent relapse or reinfection.

Drugs commonly used in the treatment of urinary tract infections, and their nursing implications, are summarized in the accompanying pharmacology box.

Nursing Implications for Pharmacology: The Client with UTI

SULFONAMIDES

Sulfisoxazole (Gantrisin)

Sulfamethoxazole (Gantanol)

Co-trimoxazole (TMP-SMZ, Bactrim, Septra)

The sulfonamides are among the most effective and least expensive drugs used in the treatment of UTI. They are considered to be the drug of choice for acute, recurrent, or chronic urinary tract infections when there is no evidence of obstruction or bacteremia (Malseed & Harrigan, 1989). These drugs are effective administered alone but may be administered as a combination product with tetracycline or a urinary analgesic.

Nursing Responsibilities

- Assess for history of allergies to sulfonamides or structurally related drugs such as salicylates or thiazide diuretics. Discontinue the drug and notify the physician if you note any signs of allergy such as rash.
- Administer medication on an empty stomach, 1 hour before or 2 hours after meals, with a full glass of water.
- Monitor intake and output.
- Assess the client for signs of bone marrow depression such as bruising, bleeding, fever, and other signs of systemic infection.
- If the client is also taking oral anticoagulants (warfarin, Coumadin), assess for signs of excessive anticoagulation, such as increased bruising, bleeding gums, or joint pain.
- If the client is also receiving phenytoin, monitor for toxicity.
- Diabetic clients receiving oral hypoglycemic agents and sulfonamides are at increased risk of hypoglycemia and need close monitoring for hypoglycemic manifestations.
- In older clients, impaired renal function increases the risk of crystalluria. Monitor closely.

Client and Family Teaching

- Take all ordered doses and complete the course of therapy. If you miss a dose, take it as soon as you can.
- Drink at least eight full glasses of water per day and avoid cranberry juice or other food or drink that

contributes to urine acidity. *Sulfonamides are poorly soluble in urine and may crystallize in the renal tubules if the urine output falls or the pH becomes too acidic* (Shlafer, 1993).

- Sulfonamides potentiate the effect of anticoagulants. If you are also taking an anticoagulant, report any signs of bleeding.
- Sulfonamides increase risk of hypoglycemia. If you are taking an oral hypoglycemic, monitor blood glucose closely.
- Sulfonamides increase the risk of phenytoin toxicity. If you are taking phenytoin, report any symptoms to the physician.
- Don't take sulfonamides if you are pregnant or breast-feeding.
- Use sunscreen and avoid sunbathing while on sulfonamides because of increased photosensitivity and risk of burns.
- Sulfonamides may cause the urine to turn orange. This discoloration is harmless and will resolve when drug is discontinued.

URINARY ANTI-INFECTIVES

Methenamine (Mandelamine; Hiprex)

Nalidixic acid (NegGram)

Nitrofurantoin (Furadantin; Macrodantin)

Trimethoprim (Proloprim, Trimpex)

The agents classed as urinary anti-infectives are most often used prophylactically for clients with chronic UTI to prevent recurrence. They are also used when the client is unable to tolerate sulfonamides, penicillin, or tetracycline because of allergy or other adverse reactions.

Nursing Responsibilities

- These drugs work best if the client is adequately hydrated (producing at least 1500 mL of urine per 24 hours) but are less effective when overdiluted by excess urine output. Ensure adequate intake of fluids, approximately 1500 to 2000 mL per day, but do not overhydrate with fluids.
- Administer these drugs with meals to minimize potential GI side effects, such as nausea, gastric upset, and abdominal cramping.
- These drugs are relatively contraindicated for use in clients with renal or hepatic impairment. Check

➤

Pharmacology: The Client with UTI (continued)

laboratory results before administering for indicators of compromised renal function, including an elevated creatinine or blood urea nitrogen (BUN). Elevated bilirubin, alanine aminotransferase (ALT or SGPT), aspartate aminotransferase (AST or SGOT), and lactic dehydrogenase (LDH) levels may reflect impaired liver function.

- Use with caution in older or chronically ill clients. Monitor closely for adverse effects and side effects.

- These drugs should not be used in pregnant women because of possible adverse effects on the fetus. Verify that female clients of child-bearing age are not pregnant before administering.

- Methenamine is not effective unless the urine is acidic. Check urine pH before administering; if greater than 5, administer urinary acidifier.

- Nalidixic acid interacts with oral anticoagulants, oral hypoglycemics, and anti-inflammatory drugs. Dosages may need to be lowered to avoid toxicity.

- CNS side effects of headache, malaise, vertigo, syncope, confusion, and peripheral neuropathy may necessitate discontinuation of nalidixic acid. Notify the physician if the client develops CNS effects.

- Monitor the client taking nitrofurantoin for an acute or chronic pulmonary reaction during therapy. This may occur within 3 weeks after initiation of therapy or after 6 months of drug administration. Manifestations include dyspnea, cough, chills, fever, and chest pain. Discontinue the drug and notify the physician.

- Nitrofurantoin may cause peripheral neuropathy, especially in older clients and adult diabetics. Notify the physician if symptoms develop.

- If administering nitrofurantoin in oral suspension form, have the client rinse the mouth thoroughly after administration, because it may stain the teeth.

- If the client taking trimethoprim is also taking phenytoin or another hydantoin anticonvulsant, monitor for signs of toxicity such as sedation, ataxia, and increased blood levels. Phenytoin doses may need to be reduced.

Client and Family Teaching

- Long-term therapy with these drugs is common, and it's important to take them even if you're feeling better. Try to develop a pattern, such as taking the drug with meals, to remember to take them.

- While taking these drugs, you should drink at least eight glasses of water or fluid per day.

- Taking these drugs with meals or food minimizes potential gastric effects; however, avoid milk products because they may interfere with absorption.

- These drugs shouldn't be taken during pregnancy. Contact your physician before attempting to become pregnant.

- If you are taking methenamine, maintain urine acidity by drinking two glasses of cranberry juice per day. Avoid milk and milk products, other fruit juices, and sodium bicarbonate, which raise the pH of the urine.

- Watch out for side effects if you are taking nalidixic acid along with an oral anticoagulant, oral hypoglycemic, or anti-inflammatory drug. Notify the physician if any of these occur: bleeding gums, easy bruising, low blood sugar, or fluid retention.

- Nalidixic acid may cause side effects such as headache, fatigue or malaise, visual disturbances, dizziness, numbness and tingling of extremities, or confusion. If these occur, stop taking the drug and notify the physician.

- Nalidixic acid increases photosensitivity. Use sunscreen and avoid excessive exposure to the sun.

- If you are taking nitrofurantoin, notify the physician if you have respiratory symptoms such as chest pain, difficulty breathing, cough, chills, and fever. If respiratory symptoms occur at any point during therapy, the drug may be discontinued.

- If you are taking nitrofurantoin and develop numbness and tingling or weakness of the extremities discontinue the drug and notify the physician.

- If you are taking nitrofurantoin in oral suspension form, rinse your mouth thoroughly after taking each dose to avoid staining the teeth.

- Nitrofurantoin turns the urine brown. This discoloration is not harmful and subsides when the drug is discontinued.

- If you are taking trimethoprim and develop a rash or pruritus, you may need to discontinue the drug. Notify the physician if symptoms develop.

- If you are taking trimethoprim along with phenytoin (Dilantin) or a related anticonvulsant, symptoms of toxicity such as sedation or a staggering gait may indicate toxicity. Notify the physician.

Pharmacology: The Client with UTI (continued)

URINARY ANALGESIC

Phenazopyridine (Pyridium)

Phenazopyridine is a urinary tract analgesic that may be used to provide symptomatic relief of the pain, burning, frequency, and urgency associated with UTI during the first 24 to 48 hours of therapy. Its use is somewhat controversial, because it does not treat the cause and may delay effective treatment in the client with recurrent UTI who saves a dose or two "for the next time" (Malseed & Harrigan, 1989).

Nursing Responsibilities

- Phenazopyridine stains the urine reddish orange. Do not mistake this discoloration for hematuria.
- Yellow-tinged sclera or skin may indicate reduced excretion and possible toxicity. Discontinue the drug and notify the physician.

- This drug is contraindicated for use in clients with renal insufficiency or failure; ensure that renal function is adequate before administering.

Client and Family Teaching

- Protect your clothing, because the discolored urine stains clothing.
- Obtain prompt diagnosis and treatment for urinary tract infection. Avoid taking phenazopyridine before you seek medical help if your symptoms recur.
- This drug may not be effective for more than 24 to 48 hours. Do not continue using it beyond that time. If symptoms continue, notify the physician.
- If you notice a yellow tinge to your skin or eyes, stop taking the drug and notify the physician.
- Taking the drug after meals minimizes gastric upset.

Surgery

Surgical intervention may be indicated for the client with recurrent UTI if diagnostic testing indicates the presence of calculi, structural anomalies, or strictures that contribute to the risk of infection. Table 25–1 lists major causes of urinary tract obstruction that may contribute to UTI. Common procedures used to relieve obstruction or correct defects are summarized in Table 25–2.

Stones, or calculi, in the renal pelvis or in the bladder are an irritant and provide a matrix for the growth of bacteria. Treatment may include surgical removal of a large calculus from the renal pelvis or cystoscopic removal of bladder calculi. *Percutaneous ultrasonic pyelolithotomy* or *extracorporeal shock wave lithotripsy (ESWL)* (described in Table 25–2) may be used rather than surgical intervention for renal calculi. Nursing management of the client having a cystoscopy is included in the box on page 887. Management of the client undergoing surgery or lithotripsy for stone removal is covered later in this chapter.

A **ureteroplasty,** surgical repair of a ureter, may be indicated for the client with a structural abnormality or stricture of a ureter. This may be combined with a ureteral reimplantation for the client with vesicoureteral reflux. After these surgeries, the client will have an indwelling urinary catheter (Foley or suprapubic) and a **ureteral stent** (a thin catheter inserted into the ureter to provide for urine flow and ureteral support) in place for 3 to 5

days. Care of the client with a ureteral stent is outlined in the box on page 893.

Nursing Care

In planning and implementing nursing care for the client with a urinary tract infection, the nurse considers the client's general health status, abilities for self-care, and risk factors that may contribute to UTI. Nursing diagnoses discussed in this section focus on problems with client comfort, urinary elimination, and teaching/learning needs.

Pain

Pain is a common manifestation of both lower and upper UTI. Urinary tract pain is caused primarily by distention and increased pressure within the tract. The severity of the pain experienced is related to the *rate* at which inflammation and distention develop, not their degree.

In cystitis, the inflammatory response leads to a feeling of fullness; a dull, constant suprapubic pain; and possibly low back pain. The inflamed bladder wall and urethra cause dysuria, pain, and burning on urination. Bladder spasms may be present, causing periodic, severe, stabbing discomfort.

The pain associated with pyelonephritis is typically a steady, dull pain localized to the outer abdomen, flank, or

Table 25–1	Major Causes of Urinary Tract Obstruction by Location
Location	**Obstructive Process**
Kidney pelvis	Calculi Polycystic kidney disease Infection and scarring
Ureters	Calculi Scarring and stricture Congenital defects or strictures External processes such as pregnancy, tumors, lymph node enlargement
Bladder	Neurogenic bladder Tumors Calculi and other foreign bodies
Urethra	Benign prostatic hypertrophy Tumors Scarring and stricture Trauma

Table 25–2	Procedures Used to Correct Urinary Tract Obstruction or Deformity
Procedure	**Description**
Extracorporeal shock-wave lithotripsy (ESWL)	Use of externally generated shock waves to fragment renal calculi for noninvasive elimination
Nephrolithotomy	Incision into the kidney parenchyma to remove calculi
Percutaneous nephrostomy	Insertion of an endoscope through a small flank incision into the renal pelvis, usually for removal or crushing (with laser or ultrasound) of calculi
Pyelolithotomy	Incision into the kidney pelvis to remove calculi
Transurethral basket lithotomy	Use of a basket catheter inserted through urethra via a cystoscope and/or ureteroscope to remove a calculus
Ureteroplasty	Surgical repair of a ureter

costovertebral angle region. Urologic pain rarely is experienced in the central abdominal region.

Pain associated with UTI should subside within 24 to 48 hours after the initiation of antibiotic therapy.

Nursing interventions with rationales follow.

- Assess pain parameters: timing, quality, intensity, location, duration, and aggravating and alleviating factors. *A change in the nature, location, or intensity of the pain could indicate an extension of the infectious process or presence of additional disease.*

- Provide comfort measures. Nonpharmacologic relief measures include warm sitz baths, warm packs or heating pads, balanced rest and activity. Systemic analgesics, urinary analgesics, or antispasmodic medication may be administered as ordered. *Warmth relaxes muscles, relieves spasms, and increases local blood supply. Because pain can stimulate a stress response and delay healing, it should be relieved when possible.*

- Increase fluid intake unless contraindicated by therapeutic regimen. *Increased fluid dilutes urine, lessening irritation of the inflamed bladder and urethral mucosa.*

Altered Patterns of Urinary Elimination

The client with a urinary tract infection often experiences dysuria, frequency, urgency, and nocturia related to the inflammatory changes in bladder and urethral mucosa. In addition, urine may be blood-tinged, cloudy, and mal-

odorous. These manifestations generally abate within 24 to 48 hours after therapy is initiated.

Nursing interventions with rationales follow.

- Monitor urinary output and color, clarity, and character of urine, including odor. *If the client is not taking a drug that causes discoloration of the urine, the urine should return to normal clear yellow within 48 hours. If it does not, further disease may be present that requires investigation.*

- Provide for easy access to a bedpan, urinal, commode, or bathroom. Make sure that lighting is adequate and that pathways are free of obstacles. *Frequency, urgency, and nocturia increase the risk of urinary incontinence and of injury due to falls.*

- Teach the client to avoid caffeinated drinks, including coffee, tea, cola, and alcoholic beverages. *Caffeine can increase bladder spasms and mucosal irritation.*

Knowledge Deficit

The client with a urinary tract infection is at an increased risk for future UTI and needs to understand the disease process, risk factors, methods of preventing recurrent infection, diagnostic procedures, and home care.

Nursing interventions with rationales follow.

- Assess the client's level of knowledge about the disease process, risk factors, and preventive measures. *Clients may not have received prior instruction regarding UTI or may have misunderstandings about the causes of UTI and its contributing factors.*

Nursing Care of the Client with a Ureteral Stent

Ureteral stents (small, specialized catheters) are used to maintain patency and promote healing of the ureters (see the accompanying figure). A stent may be a temporary measure used during and after a surgical procedure, or it may be used for longer periods in clients with ureteral obstruction due to tumors, strictures, or other causes.

Stents may be positioned during surgery or cystoscopy. They are generally made of a biocompatible, nontoxic material such as silicone or polyurethane, with side drainage holes placed along the length of the stent. Stents are generally radiopaque for easy radi-

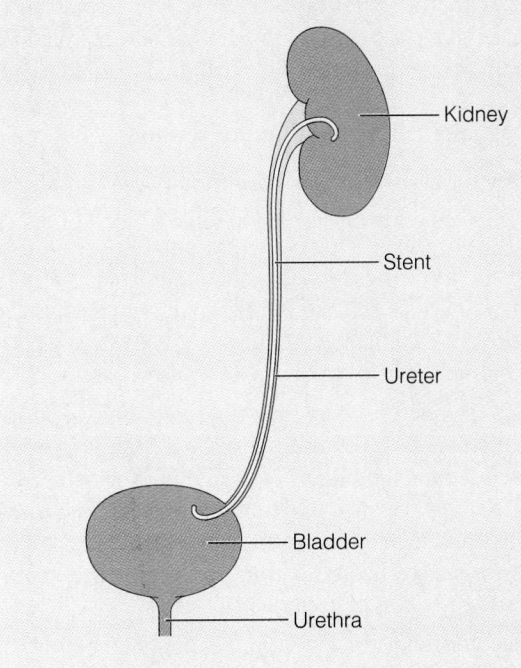

ographic identification. One or both ends of the stent may be pigtail or J-shaped to prevent migration of the stent.

- Label all drainage tubes including stents for easy identification. Attach each catheter and stent to a separate closed drainage system. *Careful labeling facilitates close monitoring of output from all sources and reservoirs. Maintaining separate drainage systems minimizes the risk of urinary tract infection.*

- If the stent has been brought to the surface, secure it and maintain its position. *The stent is usually placed in the renal pelvis, and it is important to secure it well to prevent trauma to the kidney, inadvertent removal of the stent, and ureter obstruction.*

- Monitor urine output, including color, consistency, and odor. Monitor for signs of infection or bleeding: fever, tachycardia, pain, hematuria, and cloudy or malodorous urine. *The stent facilitates urine flow but may become obstructed because of bleeding, calculi, or sediment. Obstruction may result in hydronephrosis and damage to the kidney. The stent itself is a foreign body in the urinary tract and can increase the risk of UTI.*

- Maintain the client's fluid intake, encouraging fluids that acidify urine, such as apple and cranberry juice. *The stent can precipitate calculus formation as well as UTI. Increasing fluid intake and acidifying the urine help prevent these complications.*

- For an indwelling stent, teach the client and family about the need for regular follow-up care, to monitor for and prevent complications such as UTI and calculi. *The client with an indwelling stent may tend to forget that the stent is in place and become lax in compliance with follow-up and preventive measures.*

- Teach the client to follow the treatment regimen prescribed by the primary care provider. *Symptoms are largely relieved within 24 to 48 hours after antibiotic therapy is initiated; however, this may not be adequate time to eliminate bacteria from the urinary tract. It is important to complete the prescribed regime to prevent recurrent infections and resistant bacteria.*

- Teach measures to prevent future UTI:
  a. Empty bladder at least every 2 to 4 hours while awake, avoid voluntary urinary retention.
  b. Maintain intake of 2 to 2.5 quarts or 8 to 10 glasses of fluid per day.

For women:
Cleanse perineal area front to back after voiding and defecating.
Void before and after sexual intercourse.
Avoid bubble baths, feminine hygiene sprays, and douches.
Wear cotton briefs; avoid nylon.

Keeping urine dilute and voiding regularly flush bacteria out of the bladder and urethra. The proximity of the female urethral meatus to the vagina and anus increases the risk of bacterial contamination, especially during intercourse. Bubble baths, feminine hygiene sprays, synthetic fibers and

Applying Research to Nursing Practice: Clean Intermittent Self-Catheterization

■ ■ ■

Bladder retention, often caused by neurologic disease or injury such as spinal cord damage, can frequently be effectively managed with clean intermittent self-catheterization (Wyndaele & Maes, 1990). This technique is effective in preserving normal kidney function in the majority of clients. In addition, clients using proper technique have a lower incidence of urinary tract infection than those using other methods to manage urinary retention. Clean intermittent catheterization also provides good continence, especially when combined with a mild fluid restriction of 1.5 to 2.5 liters per day and pharmacologic therapy to inhibit detrusor contraction as needed. When self-catheterization is used over a long term, urethral complications such as strictures and fistulas are not uncommon, probably because of the repeated trauma to the urethra.

Implications for Nursing

Clients with urinary retention can be effectively managed using clean intermittent catheterization. The responsibility for teaching will likely fall on the nurse. It is important for the client not only to demonstrate a safe technique but also to identify frequency of catheterization, measures to prevent and identify infection, and possible complications.

Critical Thinking in Client Care

1. How do the rates of infection for clean intermittent catheterization compare with those for an indwelling catheter?

2. Why is sterile technique used for catheterization in hospitalized clients and clean technique used for self-catheterization?

3. What measures might be effective in reducing the risk of urethral trauma in the client who requires long-term self-catheterization?

4. Develop a teaching plan for a paraplegic client who will manage neurogenic bladder with self-catheterization.

tion of the specimen by external cells and bacteria. Ninety percent of urethral bacteria are cleared in the first 10 mL of voided urine; a midstream specimen thus accurately reflects the status of the urine in the bladder.

- Unless contraindicated, teach the client measures to maintain acidic urine, e.g., drink two glasses of cranberry juice per day; take ascorbic acid (vitamin C); avoid excess intake of milk and milk products, other fruit juices, and sodium bicarbonate (baking soda). Acidity of the urine (pH of 5 or less) inhibits bacterial growth.

Noncompliance

Once the manifestations of UTI are relieved, the client is less motivated to continue the prescribed therapeutic regimen and comply with follow-up instructions. Noncompliance can lead to continued bacteriuria and recurrent infection with the potential for chronic pyelonephritis and damage to renal parenchyma. Ultimately, renal failure may result from repeated UTI with renal damage and scarring.

Nursing interventions with rationales follow.

- Collaborate with the client to mutually develop a plan for taking medications, such as taking them with meals (unless contraindicated) or setting out all doses for the day in the morning. Missed doses of antibiotic can result in subtherapeutic blood levels and reduced effectiveness. Taking medication in association with a regular daily activity such as meals helps clients to remember doses.

- Instruct the client to complete the full course of antibiotic therapy even though symptoms resolve rapidly. Although the manifestations of UTI resolve within 1 to 2 days of therapy, significant bacteriuria may still be present. It is important to maintain therapeutic blood levels of medication to prevent relapse and the development of antibiotic-resistant strains of bacteria.

- Instruct the client to keep appointments for follow-up and urine culture. Follow-up urine culture, scheduled 1 to 3 days after single-dose therapy and 7 to 14 days after conventional therapy, is vital to ensure complete eradication of bacteria and prevent relapse or recurrence.

Other Nursing Diagnoses

The following nursing diagnoses may also be appropriate for the client with a urinary tract infection:

- Activity Intolerance related to malaise and fatigue associated with infection
- Hyperthermia related to infectious process
- Risk for infection related to unresolved risk factors
- Sleep Pattern Disturbance related to pain and nocturia
- Anxiety related to potential long-term effects of infectious process

douches may dry and irritate perineal tissues, thus promoting bacterial growth.

- Teach the client how to obtain a midstream clean-catch urine specimen. Adequate cleansing of the urinary meatus and perineal area is important to prevent contamina-

Client and Family Teaching

Because both upper and lower urinary tract infections are usually managed on an outpatient basis, teaching becomes the most important nursing intervention.

Clients and their families need to understand the risk factors that contribute to the infectious process. They need instruction in how to minimize or eliminate these factors through increased fluid intake, regular elimination, and personal hygiene measures. Clients should be able to identify the early manifestations of UTI and state the importance of seeking medical intervention promptly.

Like many infectious processes, urinary tract infection often occurs when the immune defenses of the host are less than optimal. Physical and psychosocial stressors, such as lack of adequate rest, poor nutrition, and high levels of emotional stress, are often implicated. Clients need to be aware of the role of stressors in the development of infection to determine if life-style changes may reduce the risk of future UTI.

It is important for the client and family to understand the importance of completing the prescribed treatment and keeping follow-up appointments. Failure to do so contributes significantly to unresolved and recurrent infections.

The client with an indwelling urinary catheter is at continued risk for UTI. This risk can be minimized by the use of alternatives to the catheter if possible. For the client with problems of urinary incontinence, preferred alternatives to catheterization include scheduled toileting, incontinence pads or diapers, and external catheters if possible. Urinary retention is better managed by teaching the client or a family member to perform straight catheterization every 3 to 4 hours using clean technique. (See the box on page 894 for the application of research to nursing practice.) If no alternative to an indwelling catheter is feasible, clients and their families need to be taught appropriate care measures related to meatal cleansing, managing and emptying the collection chamber, maintaining a closed system, and bladder irrigation or flushing if ordered. For these clients, maintenance of adequate immune and urinary function becomes very important in preventing upper urinary tract infections.

Applying the Nursing Process

Case Study of a Client with Cystitis: Miija Waisanen

Miija Waisanen is a 25-year-old second-year nursing student. She was recently married, and she and her husband live in an apartment near the college she attends. Ms. Waisanen has never been pregnant, and she is using a diaphragm for birth control. She presents at the local urgent care clinic complaining of low back pain, frequency, urgency, and burning on urination that began the day before.

Assessment

Patrice Ramiros, RN, admits Ms. Waisanen to the clinic and prepares her to see the nurse practitioner. In her assessment, Ms. Ramiros notes that Ms. Waisanen denies having had similar symptoms in the past or ever having been diagnosed with a urinary tract infection. Ms. Waisanen describes her pain as a constant, dull ache that doesn't change with movement. She feels the need to urinate almost constantly but experiences difficulty in starting her stream, and burning pain and cramping when voiding. She reports getting up four times the night before to urinate. She denies painful intercourse and states that she could not be pregnant because her last menstrual period began only 2 weeks ago. Ms. Ramiros makes these findings: BP: 112/68; P: 90 and regular. Ms. Waisanen is afebrile. On examination, Ms. Ramiros notes suprapubic tenderness but no flank or costovertebral angle tenderness. A clean-catch urine specimen showed hematuria, multiple WBCs, and a bacteria count greater than 10^5 per milliliter.

The nurse practitioner performs a pelvic examination and finds no evidence of vaginitis, cervicitis, or pregnancy. She prescribes amoxicillin 3 g orally as a single dose, and aspirin or acetaminophen gr x po every 4 hours as needed for pain. Ms. Waisanen is instructed to return to the clinic within 24 to 72 hours for a follow-up urine culture, or sooner if her symptoms do not improve.

Diagnosis

Ms. Ramiros develops the following nursing diagnoses for Ms. Waisanen:

- *Pain* related to infection and inflammatory process in the urinary tract
- *Altered Patterns of Urinary Elimination* related to inflammatory process as evidenced by frequency, urgency, nocturia, and dysuria
- *Knowledge Deficit* related to lack of information about risk factors for UTI

Expected Outcomes

The expected outcomes for the plan of care are that Ms. Waisanen will

- Report relief of low back pain and burning on urination.
- Regain a normal voiding pattern as evidenced by absence of frequency, urgency, nocturia, and abnormal urine characteristics.

- Verbalize understanding of the disease process, related risk factors, follow-up instructions, and symptoms of recurrence indicating the need for medical attention.

Planning and Implementation

Ms. Ramiros plans and implements the following interventions for Ms. Waisanen prior to her discharge from the urgent care clinic:

- Assess Ms. Waisanen's level of knowledge and understanding regarding UTI and associated risk factors.
- Instruct Ms. Waisanen in measures to relieve her discomfort: warm sitz baths, a heating pad on low heat applied to her lower back or abdomen, rest, increased fluid intake, avoidance of caffeinated beverages, and aspirin or acetaminophen as prescribed.
- Advise Ms. Waisanen to refrain from sexual intercourse until infection and inflammation have cleared to avoid further irritation of inflamed tissues.
- Discuss the possible relationship between use of a diaphragm for birth control and UTI in women.
- Implement a teaching plan for Ms. Waisanen covering dietary and hygiene practices to prevent UTI, symptoms indicating the need for further intervention, and the risks of undertreatment.

Evaluation

Six months later, Ms. Waisanen has rotated through the urgent care clinic for clinical experience in community health nursing. Ms. Ramiros asks how she was doing. Ms. Waisanen reports that her symptoms and urine cleared within about 18 hours after taking the amoxicillin and she has had no further problems. She has seen her women's health care nurse practitioner to change her birth control method to oral contraceptives, increased her intake of fluid and vitamin C, and no longer puts off urinating "until she has time to go!"

Critical Thinking in the Nursing Process

1. What physiologic and psychosocial factors put Ms. Waisanen at risk for developing a urinary tract infection?
2. Compare and contrast the benefits and drawbacks to single-dose therapy versus conventional therapy for UTI.
3. Differentiating an upper and lower urinary tract infection by symptoms can be difficult. Why was it appropriate for the nurse practitioner to use single-dose therapy with the advice to return if symptoms did not clear?
4. Develop a care plan for Ms. Waisanen for the nursing diagnosis *Altered Health Maintenance.*

The Client with Urinary Calculi

■ ■ ■

The most common cause of urologic obstruction is **urolithiasis,** the development of stones within the urinary tract. The term **nephrolithiasis** indicates stone formation within the kidney. The stone formed is called a **calculus.** Stones or **calculi** may develop and cause obstruction at any point within the urinary tract (Figure 25–1); however, in the United States and other industrialized countries, renal or kidney stones are the most common.

Calculi are masses of crystals composed of materials normally excreted in the urine. The majority (75% to 80%) are composed of calcium; sturvite stones, composed of magnesium ammonium phosphate, occur less frequently (15%) and are associated with recurrent or chronic UTI. The remainder of stones are made up of uric acid or cystine (McCance & Huether, 1994; Porth, 1994).

Urolithiasis affects 0.1% to 1% of the population, with up to 720,000 people in the United States afflicted every year (Berkow & Fletcher, 1992; Tierney et al., 1994). In the United States, the incidence varies by region, with the highest frequency in southern and midwestern states. Males are affected more often than females by a 4:1 ratio, although sturvite stones, associated with recurrent or chronic UTI, are more likely to affect women. Calculi are more common among whites than blacks. Most people affected are in young or middle adulthood.

Although the majority of stones are idiopathic (having no demonstrable cause), a number of risk factors are implicated. The greatest risk factor for stone formation is a prior personal or family history of urinary calculi. A genetic predisposition toward the accumulation of certain mineral substances in the urine or a congenital lack of protective factors may explain the familial link. Urine is thought to normally contain substances that inhibit the formation of stones. An endogenous compound called *nephrocalcin,* which inhibits stone formation, has recently been identified. Other identified risk factors include dehydration with resultant increased urine concentration, immobility, and excess dietary intake of calcium, oxalate, or proteins. Gout, hyperparathyroidism, and urinary stasis or repeated infections also contribute to calculus formation (Bullock & Rosendahl, 1992; Porth, 1994).

Pathophysiology

Urolithiasis involves the precipitation of a poorly soluble salt around an organic matrix or mucoprotein to form a crystalline structure. When the concentration of the salt in the urine is very high, that is, when the urine is supersaturated, the stimulus required to initiate crystallization or precipitation is minimal. Ingestion of a meal high in the involved mineral or decreased fluid intake, as occurs during sleep, allow the concentration to increase to the point where precipitation occurs and stones are formed and grow. When fluid intake is adequate, no stone growth occurs (Gillenwater et al., 1987). Lithiasis is also affected by the acidity or alkalinity of the urine and the presence or absence of calculus-inhibiting compounds in the urine.

The majority (75% to 90%) of kidney stones are composed of calcium oxalate or calcium phosphate. These stones are generally associated with high concentrations of calcium in the blood or urine (Bullock & Rosendahl, 1992; Porth 1994). The types of renal calculi, associated risk factors, and recommended dietary modifications are listed in Table 25–3.

The symptoms caused by urinary calculi vary with their size and location. Clinical manifestations are due to the obstruction of urine flow and resulting distention, and to tissue trauma caused by movement of the rough-edged, crystalline stone.

Clients with renal calculi affecting the kidney calices and pelvis may have few symptoms. If the stone has gradually or partially obstructed urinary flow, a dull, aching flank pain may be present, but renal calculi often are silent, without symptoms. Bladder calculi may cause few symptoms other than dull suprapubic pain with exercise or after voiding.

Renal colic, an acute, severe, intermittent pain in the flank and upper outer abdominal quadrant on the affected side, is generally associated with acute obstruction

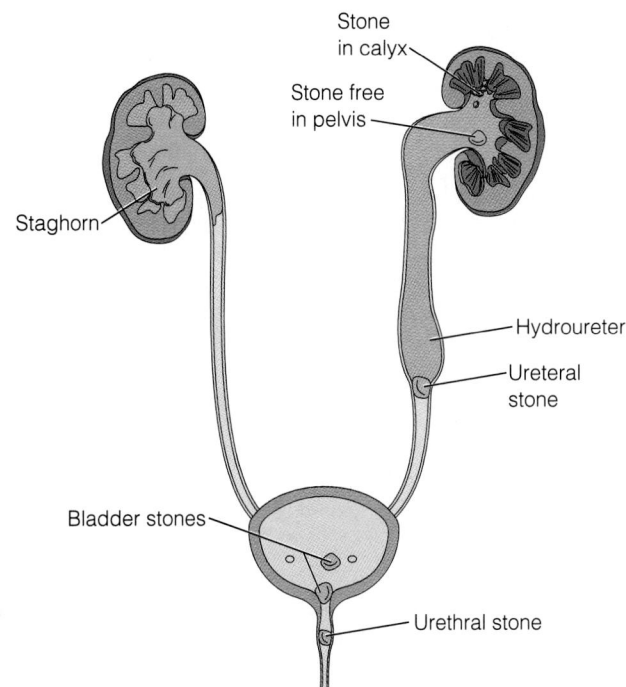

Figure 25–1   Development and location of calculi within the urinary tract.

of a ureter and resulting ureteral spasm. The pain of renal colic may radiate to the suprapubic region, groin, and external genitals (the scrotum or labia). The severity of the pain often causes a sympathetic response with associated nausea, vomiting, pallor, and cool, clammy skin.

Table 25–3   Risk Factors and Interventions for Renal Calculi

Stone Type and Incidence	Risk Factors	Management
Calcium phosphate and/or oxalate 75%–90%	Hypercalciuria and hypercalcemia: hyperparathyroidism, immobility, bone disease, vitamin D intoxication, multiple myeloma, renal tubular acidosis, prolonged steroid intake Alkaline urine Dehydration Inflammatory bowel disease	Pharmacology: Thiazide diuretics, phosphates, calcium-binding agents Dietary: Acid ash diet, limit foods high in calcium and oxalate Other: Increase hydration, exercise
Sturvite 15%–20%	UTIs, especially *Proteus* infections	Pharmacology: Antibiotic therapy for UTI Dietary: Acid ash diet Other: Surgical intervention or lithotripsy to remove stone
Uric acid 5%–10%	Gout, increased purine intake, acid urine	Pharmacology: Allopurinol Dietary: Alkaline ash and low purine diet Other: Increase hydration
Cystine (uncommon)	Genetic defect, acid urine	Pharmacology: Penicillamine, sodium bicarbonate Dietary: Alkaline ash diet Other: Increase hydration

Manifestations of UTI, including chills and fever, frequency, urgency, and dysuria, may accompany urinary calculi at any level. Trauma to the urinary tract by the calculi may cause gross or microscopic hematuria. Gross hematuria is often the only sign of bladder stones.

Obstruction of the urinary tract from renal calculi may impede the outflow of urine at any point from the calyces of the kidney to the distal urethra. If the obstruction develops slowly, the client may experience few or no symptoms. The client with rapidly developing obstruction may experience severe manifestations. Obstruction is a risk factor for infection, and, if unrelieved, may lead to kidney damage and destruction. Ultimately, renal failure and uremia is a potential result of an obstructed urinary tract. Table 25–1 lists the common causes of obstruction by location within the urinary tract.

The degree of obstruction, its location, and the duration of impaired urine flow determine the extent of the effects on renal function. The kidneys continue to produce urine during an obstructive process. Impaired urine outflow causes urinary stasis, increased pressure and distention of the urinary tract behind the obstruction. **Hydronephrosis** and **hydroureter**, distention of the ureter with urine, are possible results.

When the obstruction is unilateral and develops slowly, the client may experience no symptoms related to hydronephrosis or hydroureter. When symptoms are present, they are often mild, limited to vague abdominal, back, or flank pain. An acute obstruction causes rapid distention of proximal structures and is frequently associated with severe pain. The pain may be localized to the flank region or radiate to the genitals.

The urinary stasis associated with partial or complete obstruction increases the client's risk of infection. Either upper or lower urinary tract infection with its associated clinical manifestations may result.

Collaborative Care

Management of the client with renal calculi is directed toward relief of acute manifestations, destruction or removal of stones, and prevention of further stone formation.

Laboratory and Diagnostic Tests

The following laboratory tests may be ordered:

- *Urinalysis* is useful in the diagnosis of renal calculi. Hematuria, either gross or microscopic, is generally present. Tests may also reveal WBCs and crystal fragments. The urine pH is helpful in identifying the type of stone.

- *Urine calcium,* which measures the amount of calcium excreted during a 24-hour period, may be helpful in identifying possible causes of calculus formation. Lev-

els are elevated in hyperparathyroidism, Cushing's syndrome, and osteoporosis, all of which may contribute to lithiasis (Pagana & Pagana, 1992).

- *Urine uric acid* studies measure the excretion of uric acid over 24 hours. Uric acid levels may be elevated in clients with gout and those at risk for forming uric acid calculi (Pagana & Pagana, 1992).

- *Urine oxalate excretion,* another 24-hour study, may help to differentiate calcium oxalate from calcium phosphate stones.

- *Urine culture* may be ordered to determine if infection (UTI) is a contributing factor to calculus formation.

- *Serum calcium,* normally 9.0 to 10.5 mg/dL in the adult, may be elevated, causing increased urinary excretion of calcium and possible precipitation as calculi.

- *Serum phosphorus,* normally 2.5 to 4.5 mg/dL in adults, may be lower than normal when serum calcium is elevated and calcium phosphate stones are formed.

- *Serum uric acid* levels provide another indicator of excess production of uric acid and the potential for the formation of uric acid stones.

- *Chemical analysis* of any stones passed in the urine is valuable in suggesting measures to prevent further lithiasis. Retrieval of stones is often a nursing responsibility. All urine is strained and may be saved. Any visible stones or sediment are sent for analysis.

Nursing responsibilities in the collection of a 24-hour urine specimen are outlined in the accompanying box.

The following diagnostic studies may be ordered for renal lithiasis:

- *KUB* (kidneys, ureters, and bladder) is a flat-plate X-ray study of the lower abdomen. This is a simple X-ray film, completed in a few minutes and requiring no special preparation. Calculi can be identified by opacities in the kidneys, ureters, and bladder.

- *Intravenous pylography* is used to visualize the kidneys, ureters, and bladder after injection of a contrast medium. This study allows visualization of calculi and any resultant obstruction, hydroureter, or hydronephrosis.

- *Retrograde pyelography* uses a contrast medium instilled into the ureter(s) before X-ray films of the ureter(s) and bladder are obtained. This test is useful when IVP is contraindicated or provides poor visualization bilaterally (Pagana & Pagana, 1992).

- *Renal ultrasonography* is a noninvasive test that uses reflected sound waves to allow visualization of the kidneys. Calculi in the kidney parenchyma or pelvis, as well as hydronephrosis resulting from obstruction, may be visualized.

- *Computed tomography* (*CT scan*) of the kidney, with or without the use of contrast medium, uses X-rays directed at the kidney from many angles to provide a computer-generated photograph that shows calculi, ureteral obstruction, and other renal disorders.

- *Magnetic resonance imaging* (*MRI*) is a noninvasive diagnostic study that uses strong magnetic fields and radio waves to create images reflecting the proton (hydrogen) density of body tissues. High-resolution images of normal and abnormal body tissues are produced. Urinary tract calculi, obstructions, and other disorders such as tumors can be clearly identified through this technique.

- *Cystoscopy* is used to visualize and possibly remove calculi from the urinary bladder and distal ureters.

Nursing implications for the diagnostic studies used in urolithiasis are included in the box on page 900.

Pharmacology

Treatment of an acute episode of renal colic is directed at pain relief. Narcotic analgesics, either morphine sulfate or meperidine hydrochloride, are used to provide analgesia and moderate the ureteral spasms. Initially, these are often administered intravenously to ensure prompt absorption and a rapid onset of action. Indomethacin, a nonsteroidal anti-inflammatory drug (NSAID), in suppository form, has been found helpful in reducing the amount of narcotic analgesia required for acute renal colic (*Emergency Medicine* 1990).

Drugs with anticholinergic activity such as atropine, oxybutynin chloride (Ditropan), methantheline bromide (Banthine), or propantheline bromide (Pro-Banthine) may be used adjunctively to help relieve ureteral spasm. It is important to remember that these drugs may inhibit micturition (urination). Urinary output and bladder emptying must be monitored carefully in clients receiving these drugs.

After analysis of the calculus composition, various medications may be prescribed to inhibit or prevent further lithiasis. A thiazide diuretic, frequently prescribed for calcium calculi, acts to reduce urinary calcium excretion and is very effective in preventing further stones. See Table 25–3 for other preparations related to types of stones. Nursing responsibilities focus on teaching the client about the prescribed medication, its importance in preventing further stone formation, and potential adverse effects.

Dietary Intervention

Modification of the client's diet is often prescribed to change the character of the urine and prevent further lithiasis.

Increased fluid intake of 2½ to 3 liters per day is a common recommendation, regardless of stone composi-

---

Nursing Implications for Diagnostic Tests: 24-Hour Urine Specimen Collection

■ ■ ■

Preparation of the Client

- Check whether any modifications in diet or medication regimen have been ordered during the collection period. Notify the appropriate individuals and departments.

- Obtain a specimen container with preservative (if indicated). Label the container with the client's identifying data, the name of test, the time started, and the time of completion.

- Obtain a clean commode, bedpan, or urine-collection device for the toilet and place it in the client's room.

- Post notices—on the client's chart, in the Kardex file, on the door, over the client's bed, and over the toilet—alerting all personnel that all urine is to be saved.

- When collection is to begin, have the client completely empty the bladder and discard this urine.

- Save all urine produced during the 24-hour period in a container, refrigerating it or keeping it on ice as indicated.

- When the collection period is to end, have client empty the bladder completely and save this specimen as part of the total. Take the full specimen with requisition to the lab for analysis.

- Chart appropriately.

Client and Family Teaching

- This test requires you to collect all the urine you void over 24 hours. The test results will tell us more about your stones.

- You may have to follow some dietary or medication modifications.

- Urinate (and save your urine) before you move your bowels; do not discard any toilet tissue in the urine container.

---

tion. A fluid intake to ensure the production of approximately 2 to 2½ liters of urine a day prevents the stone-forming salts from becoming concentrated enough to precipitate. Fluid intake should be spaced throughout the day and evening. Some authorities recommend that clients drink one to two glasses of water at night to prevent concentration of urine during sleep (Gillenwater et al., 1987).

Nursing Implications for Diagnostic Tests: The Client with Urolithiasis

■ ■ ■

Retrograde Pyelography

Preparation of the Client

- This procedure is invasive; ensure that informed consent is obtained beforehand.

- Check for allergies to iodine, X-ray contrast dye, and seafood. An allergy does not necessarily contraindicate this examination, because the dye is not intravenously injected and rarely causes a hypersensitivity reaction.

- Prepare the client as ordered. The client may be on NPO status after midnight if general anesthesia is to be used or allowed clear liquids if local anesthesia is planned. Sedation may be ordered for 1 hour prior to the procedure.

- Assist the client with bowel preparation as needed. Laxatives or enemas may be ordered. Record results.

Client and Family Teaching

- This procedure is performed to identify possible kidney stones.

- You will be placed in stirrups. If local anesthesia is used, you may experience a sensation of pressure and the need to urinate as the cystoscope is inserted.

- The test takes approximately 1 hour to complete.

- Indications of an allergic reaction to the contrast dye include rash, urticaria (hives), flushing, or difficulty breathing.

- Urine is usually pink-tinged following the examination; if it becomes bright red or clots are present, notify the physician.

- Increased fluid intake after the examination dilutes the dye and decreases discomfort with voiding. Medications may be needed if bladder spasms occur.

Renal Ultrasound

Preparation of the Client

- No special preparation is indicated; however, barium in the bowel may interfere with results. If both studies are ordered, the renal ultrasound should be scheduled first.

Client and Family Teaching

- This test requires no exposure to radiation, and you should feel no discomfort.

- Food, fluids, and ordered medications are not restricted prior to this test.

- The test takes approximately 30 to 60 minutes to complete. During this time, you need to remain relatively still.

- A conductive paste or gel (which may feel cold) is applied to the back and flank area to allow for sound wave transmission. Then a transducer is passed over the skin, producing pictures of the reflected sound waves.

Recommended dietary changes include reduced intake of the primary substance composing the calculi. For calcium stones, dietary calcium and vitamin-D enriched foods are limited. Limiting vitamin D inhibits the absorption of calcium from the GI tract. Calcium stones may be either a calcium phosphate salt, calcium oxalate, or a combination of both; therefore, phosphorus and/or oxalate may also be limited in the diet.

The client with uric acid stones requires a diet low in purines. Organ meats, sardines, and other high-purine foods are eliminated from the diet. Foods with moderate levels of purines, such as red and white meats and some seafoods, are limited.

In addition to limiting the foods implicated in stone formation, the diet is modified to maintain a urinary pH that does not promote lithiasis. Uric acid and cystine stones form most readily in acid urine. Dietary measures to control these stones include increased amounts of alkaline ash foods, which alkalinize or raise the pH of the urine. Because alkaline urine promotes calcium stones and urinary tract infections, for these conditions the diet is modified toward acid ash foods, which lower the urinary pH. Acid and alkaline ash foods as well as those high in various stone components are summarized in Table 25–4.

Surgery

Stones that are too large (greater than 5 mm in diameter) to be passed spontaneously may require surgical intervention. Other indicators for surgery include stones associated with bacteriuria or infection, impaired renal function, or persistent symptoms such as pain, nausea, and

---

Diagnostic Tests: The Client with Urolithiasis (continued)

▪ ▪ ▪

Computed Tomography (CT Scan) of the Kidney

Preparation of the Client
- Ensure that the client or family has signed an informed consent form.
- Check for allergies to iodine, X-ray contrast dye, and seafood. Inform the radiology department if such an allergy exists.
- Prepare the client as ordered. Clients may be placed on NPO status for 4 hours prior to examination; laxatives and/or enemas may be ordered to prevent interference by gas, fecal material, or retained barium.

Client and Family Teaching
- The test requires 30 to 60 minutes to complete, and you must lie still during the procedure.
- You lie flat on your back during the test while a doughnut-shaped scanner revolves around your body. This can cause a sensation of claustrophobia. The machine emits loud clicking sounds as it rotates.
- The radiology technician is not in the room with you, but you can communicate through an intercom system at all times.
- If contrast medium is used, you may experience a flushing sensation and nausea as it is injected.

Magnetic Resonance Imaging (MRI) of the Kidney

Preparation of the Client
- Obtain informed consent for the procedure if required.
- Assess the client for contraindications to the examination, including pregnancy, confusion, and the presence of any external or internal metal objects such as monitor electrodes, infusion pumps, or pacemakers.
- Remove all metal objects such as dental bridges and jewelry, including watches, rings, hair pins, and hair clips.
- No food or fluid restrictions apply prior to MRI.

Client and Family Teaching
- MRI does not require the use of radiation, sedation, or restriction of food, fluids, or activities before or after the procedure. It takes approximately 30 to 90 minutes to complete.
- During the procedure, you need to lie very still on a platform that slides into the doughnut-shaped magnetic apparatus.
- The procedure may cause a claustrophobic sensation, and the machine is noisy.
- The only discomfort associated with this examination is the requirement to remain still on a hard surface throughout the test. You may feel some tingling in teeth with metal fillings (Pagana & Pagana, 1992).

---

vomiting (Mackety, 1990). Today, there are a variety of surgical and nonsurgical interventions for stone removal.

Bladder stones may be removed transurethrally by passing an instrument via the cystoscope to crush the stones. The remaining stone fragments are then irrigated out of the bladder using an acid solution to counteract the alkalinity that precipitated stone formation.

The transurethral uroscopic approach is often used to remove calculi from the ureters. A ureteral catheter may be passed via the cystoscope to drain urine proximal to the stone and dilate the ureter, allowing the stone to pass spontaneously. A *basket catheter* passed through the cystoscope may be used to snare a stone from the distal ureter. For stones in the mid or proximal ureter, a stone basket passed through the ureteroscope may allow removal of a lodged calculus. Laser technology allows disintegration of a ureteral stone via the ureteroscope. Stone fragments are then irrigated out.

Stones in the renal pelvis or calices may require **percutaneous nephrostomy** for removal (Figure 25–2). For this procedure, a small incision is made in the flank to allow insertion of an nephroscope for visualizing the renal pelvis. Forceps or a basket device may then be used to remove stones, or lithotripsy may be performed to crush the calculi.

Lithotripsy, or crushing of renal calculi, may be performed either by the percutaneous ultrasonic or laser technique, or by extracorporeal shock wave technology. *Percutaneous ultrasonic* or *laser lithotripsy* is surgical removal of kidney stones using a nephroscope inserted through a small incision in the portion of the kidney or ureter in which the stone is lodged. If attempts to retrieve

Table 25-4	Examples of Food and Fluids for Teaching Clients with Urolithiasis
Acid ash foods	Cheese, cranberries, eggs, grapes, meat and poultry, plums and prunes, tomatoes, whole grains
Alkaline ash foods	Green vegetables, fruit (except acid ash fruits as noted above), legumes, milk and milk products, rhubarb
Foods high in calcium	Beans and lentils, chocolate and cocoa, dried fruits, canned or smoked fish except tuna, flour, milk and milk products
Foods high in oxalate	Asparagus, beer and colas, beets, cabbage, celery, chocolate and cocoa, fruits, green beans, nuts, tea, tomatoes
Purine-rich foods	Goose, organ meats, sardines and herring, venison; moderate in beef, chicken, crab, pork, salmon, veal

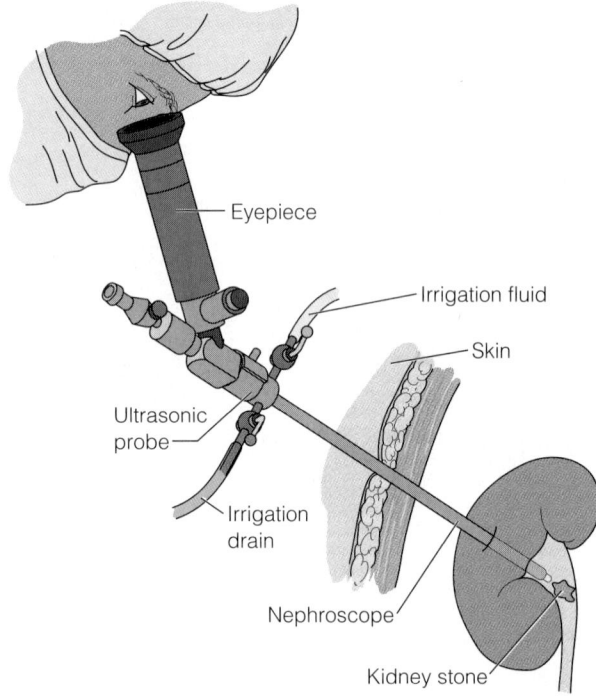

Figure 25-2 Percutaneous nephrostomy. A nephroscope is inserted percutaneously into the renal pelvis, and the stone is removed using a basket device or forceps.

the stone by basket or forceps are unsuccessful, either high-frequency sound waves or laser beams are used to break up the stone. Continuous irrigation and suction are used to remove the fragments.

The newest procedure for destruction and removal of renal stones is **extracorporeal shock-wave lithotripsy (ESWL).** ESWL (also called transcutaneous shock-wave lithotripsy) is a noninvasive technique for fragmenting kidney stones using shock waves generated outside the body. Acoustic shock waves are aimed under fluoroscopic guidance at the stone (Figure 25–3). These shock waves travel through soft tissue without inflicting damage but shatter the stone as its greater density stops their progress. The stone is pulverized into fragments small enough to be eliminated in the urine. The accompanying box outlines nursing care for clients having percutaneous ultrasonic or extracorporeal shock-wave lithotripsy.

On rare occasions it is not possible to remove calculi using one of the preceding techniques and surgical intervention is required. **Ureterolithotomy** involves an incision in the affected ureter to remove a calculus. **Pyelolithotomy** is direct visualization and removal of a stone from the kidney pelvis. A **staghorn calculus**, which invades the calices and renal parenchyma, may require a **nephrolithotomy** for removal. If the renal damage has been severe, a partial or total **nephrectomy** (removal of the kidney) may be necessary. These surgical procedures require a large flank incision and an extended recovery

period because of the location of the incision and the disruption of muscle tissue. See Chapter 7 for care of the surgical client.

Nursing Care

Nursing care for the client with urolithiasis is directed at providing for comfort during acute renal colic, assisting with diagnostic procedures, ensuring adequate urinary output, and teaching the client information necessary to prevent future stone formation.

Pain

Pain is the primary outward manifestation of urolithiasis, particularly when a stone lodges within a ureter, causing acute obstruction and distention. Invasive and noninvasive procedures to remove or crush stones are also painful for many clients. In clients requiring a nephrolithotomy or nephrectomy, the extensive surgical incision can be particularly painful.

Nursing interventions with rationales follow.

- For all complaints of pain, assess the intensity, quality, location, timing, aggravating and relieving factors, and associated symptoms. *The type of pain experienced often provides valuable clues as to its cause. It is important to assess each complaint of pain to ensure appropriate intervention.*

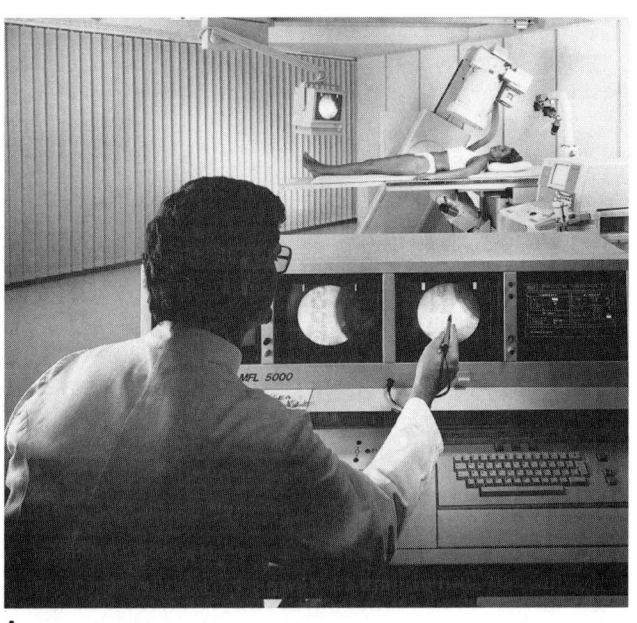

A

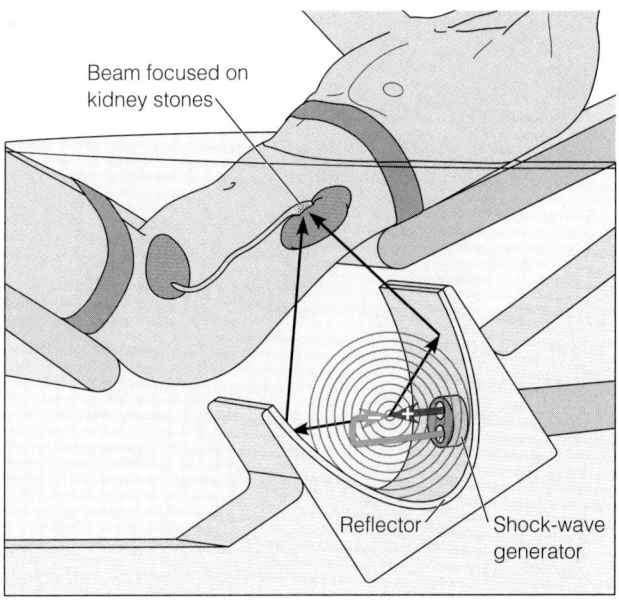

B

Figure 25–3   Extracorporeal shock-wave lithotripsy. Acoustic shock waves generated by the shock-wave generator travel through soft tissue to shatter the renal stone into fragments, which are then eliminated in the urine. *A,* A shock-wave generator that does not require water immersion. *B,* An illustration of water immersion lithotripsy procedure.

Nursing Care of the Client Having Lithotripsy

PREOPERATIVE CARE

- Assess the client's knowledge about the procedure, providing information as needed. *Anxiety is reduced, and recovery is enhanced and hastened when the client is fully prepared for surgery.*

- Follow directions from the radiology department, physician, or anesthetist for withholding food and fluids and for bowel preparation prior to surgery. *Percutaneous ultrasonic and extracorporeal transcutaneous shock-wave lithotripsy usually require epidural or general anesthesia. The presence of fecal material in the bowel may impede fluoroscopic visualization of the kidney.*

POSTOPERATIVE CARE

- In the initial period, monitor vital signs frequently. *Hemorrhage and resulting shock are possible complications of surgery, because the kidney is a highly vascular organ. Bleeding may be internal or retroperitoneal and difficult to detect; therefore, it is vital to monitor blood pressure and pulse rates.*

- Monitor urine output for amount, color, and clarity. *Urine is often bright red initially, but the amount of*

bleeding should diminish during the first 2 to 3 days after surgery. Cloudy urine may indicate the presence of an infection.

- Maintain placement and patency of urinary catheters. Anchor ureteral catheters or nephrostomy tubes securely. Irrigate gently if ordered. *A kinked or plugged catheter may result in hydroureter, hydronephrosis, and kidney damage. Decreased urinary output and flank pain are possible symptoms of obstructed urine flow. Excessive force in irrigation may cause bleeding.*

- Prepare for discharge by teaching the client to care for the indwelling catheter, urine-collection device, and incision site. Teach the client about signs and symptoms to report: drainage of urine from incision for more than 4 days, symptoms of infection, pain, bright hematuria. *Many clients are discharged with dressings and catheters in place. The client and family need necessary information to provide self-care.*

- Teach the client about measures to reduce the risk of further lithiasis. *Many clients have repeated episodes of lithiasis and renal colic. Prevention of stone formation is important to preserve renal function.*

- Administer pain-relief measures as prescribed. *Pain is controlled more effectively by administering prescribed analgesics on a regular basis than by waiting until the client reports pain. In clients with ureteral colic, administration of ordered NSAIDs or antispasmodic medication on a routine schedule may significantly reduce the need for narcotic analgesia.*

- Unless contraindicated, increase fluid intake and encourage ambulation in the client with ureteral colic. *Increased fluids and ambulation increase urinary output, facilitating movement of the calculus through the ureter and decreasing pain.*

- Use nonpharmacologic measures such as positioning, moist heat, relaxation techniques, guided imagery, and diversion as adjunctive therapy for pain relief. *Although the pain of ureteral colic rarely can be fully managed with nonpharmacologic measures alone, use of these measures can enhance the effectiveness of analgesic agents and other prescribed treatment.*

- For the client who has had surgery, monitor urinary output, catheters, incision, and wound drainage. *Pain may be a symptom of proximal distention due to a blocked catheter. Infection or hematoma at the surgical site can significantly increase perceived pain.*

Altered Patterns of Urinary Elimination

Obstruction of the urinary tract is the primary problem associated with urolithiasis and may ultimately result in stasis, infection, or irreversible renal damage.

Nursing interventions with rationales follow.

- Monitor urinary output for quantity, pattern, and presence of stones. Measure all urine. If the client is catheterized, measure hourly. Document the presence of hematuria, dysuria, frequency, urgency, and pyuria. Strain all urine for stones, saving any recovered stones for laboratory analysis. *The amount of urine output is an indicator of possible urinary tract obstruction and adequacy of hydration. Hematuria, gross or microscopic, is often associated with calculi and with procedures for stone removal such as cystoscopy, nephrostomy, or lithotripsy. A change in the degree of hematuria may indicate stone passage or a complication. Dysuria, frequency, urgency, and cloudy urine are symptoms of urinary tract infection, which is often associated with urolithiasis. Antibiotic therapy may be required. Analysis of stones recovered from the urine can provide direction for prevention of further stone formation.*

- Maintain patency and integrity of all catheter systems in place. Secure catheters well, label as indicated, and use sterile technique for all ordered irrigations or other procedures. *A kinked or plugged catheter, particularly a ureteral catheter or nephrostomy tube, may damage the urinary system. Prevention of hydroureter or hydronephrosis is vital to the preservation of renal function. Labeling catheters can prevent mistakes, such as inappropriate irrigation or clamping. Any catheter increases the risk of infection; aseptic technique in all procedures minimizes this risk.*

Knowledge Deficit

The client admitted with urolithiasis has multiple learning needs. These include information about the disease and its possible consequences, any diagnostic or therapeutic procedures performed, and management strategies to prevent future stone formation.

Nursing interventions with rationales follow.

- Assess the client's level of understanding and previous learning. *Having the client relate information to previously learned material enhances retention and understanding.*

- Present all material in a manner appropriate to the client's knowledge base, developmental and educational level, and current needs. *Learning is an active process that requires participation by the client. Tailoring teaching to the individual increases the client's involvement.*

- Teach the client about all diagnostic and therapeutic procedures. *Knowing what to expect reduces anxiety, enhances compliance, and shortens the recovery period.*

- If client is to be discharged prior to stone passage, teach client to
  a. Collect and strain all urine, saving any stones.
  b. Report stone passage to the physician and bring the stone in for analysis.
  c. Observe the amount and character of urine, reporting any changes to physician.
  Clients whose pain can be managed with oral analgesic agents are appropriate candidates for outpatient management. The client needs to know the procedures and rationale for collecting the calculus and indicators of complications, such as reduced urine output and cloudy or bloody urine.

- Instruct client in measures to prevent further urolithiasis.
  a. Increase fluid intake to 2500 to 3500 mL per day.
  b. Follow recommended dietary guidelines.
  c. Maintain activity at a level that will prevent urinary stasis and bone resorption.
  d. Take medications as prescribed by physician. *The risk of recurrent calculus formation is approximately 50%; however, this risk can be reduced by following measures to prevent conditions favoring stone formation.*

- Teach the client and family about the relationship between urinary calculi and urinary tract infection, emphasizing the symptoms of UTI, measures to prevent UTI, and the need to seek medical help if UTI occurs. *Urinary tract infection in the client prone to calculi requires prompt treatment to prevent further urolithiasis.*

Other Nursing Diagnoses

The following nursing diagnoses may also be appropriate for the client with urinary calculi:

- *Anxiety* related to anticipation of severe pain and lack of knowledge about disease process
- *Risk for Infection* related to urinary stasis and presence of foreign body within the urinary tract
- *Noncompliance* with prescribed medical regimen related to lack of understanding
- *Risk for Impaired Skin Integrity* related to presence of nephrostomy tube and skin contact with urine.
- *Urinary Retention* related to obstruction of urinary tract by stones.

Client and Family Teaching

Because a history of lithiasis increases the risk of stone formation, teaching is an essential component of nursing care. The client and family need to know what factors increase the risk of stone formation and what they can do to minimize this risk. Emphasize the importance of preventing further lithiasis by following fluid intake and dietary recommendations and taking medication as prescribed. The client and family also need to understand the relationship between urolithiasis and urinary tract infection. Have them verbalize their knowledge of how to prevent, recognize, and manage UTI.

When the client is discharged with dressings, a nephrostomy tube, or a catheter, both the client and family need to know how to change dressings and manage the drainage systems. Teach sterile technique for dressing changes as well as principles of wound and skin assessment. Emphasize the importance of maintaining tube and catheter patency. Teach how to empty drainage bags and assess urine output, and make sure they know when to contact the physician.

Applying the Nursing Process

Case Study of a Client with Urinary Calculi: Richard Leton

Richard Leton is a 44-year-old male who owns a small business. He is admitted to the medical unit from the emergency department after awakening at 4:00 a.m. with severe right-sided pain. The CBC is normal, and urinalysis reveals microscopic hematuria, but no protein or bacteria. An IVP study shows partial obstruction of the right ureter by a 4 to 5 mm stone.

Stephen Phillips, the nurse admitting Mr. Leton to his room, notes that Mr. Leton appears pale, diaphoretic, and very anxious. He complains of nausea and asks for an emesis basin. Mr. Phillips notes from the emergency record that Mr. Leton received 4 mg of morphine sulphate shortly after admission to the ED, approximately 2½ hours previously. He denies pain upon being taken to his room but says, "I'm scared to death that it'll come back— that was the worst pain I have *ever* had. Like a knife going from my right side into my groin. I couldn't even move, it hurt so bad."

Assessment

Mr. Leton's history reveals no previous episodes of similar pain. He has never been told that he had a stone or blood in his urine. He says, however, that he thinks his father was treated for a kidney stone "a long time ago." Mr. Leton felt well until awakening during the night with the pain. On questioning, he reveals that he has been working under a deadline to complete a heavy construction project and that he probably hasn't been drinking enough fluids "considering how hot it's been." Physical assessment findings include T: 100.4 F (38.0 C) PO; BP: 160/86; P: 98; R: 24. His color is pale to ashen, skin cool and moist. His abdomen is firm with moderate tenderness in the right upper outer quadrant. The admitting physician orders an intravenous infusion of 5% dextrose in ½ normal saline at 200 mL per hour until nausea is relieved, then encourage fluids PO to at least 3000 mL/24 hr; morphine sulfate (MS) 2 to 10 mg intravenously prn severe pain; indomethacin (Indocin) 50 mg per rectal suppository q8h; promethazine (Phenergan) 25 mg PO or per suppository q6h prn nausea; activity to tolerance; and straining of all urine, sending any recovered stones for analysis.

Diagnosis

Mr. Phillips develops the following nursing diagnoses for Mr. Leton:

- *Anxiety* related to anticipation of recurrent severe pain
- *Risk for Altered Nutrition: Less Than Body Requirements* related to nausea
- *Pain,* acute, related to presence of calculus in right ureter
- *Altered Patterns of Urinary Elimination* related to partial obstruction of ureter by calculus
- *Knowledge Deficit* related to lack of information about disease process, contributing factors, and management

Expected Outcomes

The expected outcomes for the plan of care are that Mr. Leton will

- Demonstrate relief of anxiety by relaxed facial expression, vital signs within normal range for him, and ability to rest when not disturbed.

- Be able to consume at least 50% of diet and 100% of ordered fluids without experiencing nausea or vomiting.

- Request analgesic agents at onset of pain rather than waiting until pain peaks.

- Maintain urine output of 2500 mL per day with no signs of infection or obstruction, such as increased pain, dysuria, pyuria, or hematuria.

- Relate an understanding of the process of urolithiasis and contributing factors.

- Verbalize dietary, fluid intake, and other measures to reduce risk of future stone formation.

Planning and Implementation

Mr. Phillips plans the following nursing interventions to be implemented for Mr. Leton:

- Explain all procedures and tests.

- Reassure Mr. Leton that he is receiving medication to prevent further episodes of pain and that additional medication is available should colic pain recur.

- Administer ordered antiemetic and analgesic medications as needed.

- Provide food and fluids in small quantities until nausea is relieved.

- Assess the effectiveness of the prescribed analgesic agents and their side effects, especially nausea.

- Assess Mr. Leton frequently for outward manifestations of pain such as tense facial expression, increased blood pressure, and rigid body posturing.

- Maintain IV as ordered until Mr. Leton is able to ingest at least 200 mL of fluid per hour while awake.

- Measure and strain all urine. Assess voided urine for color, clarity, and odor.

- Teach Mr. Leton and his family about urolithiasis and its risk factors, especially as they relate to Mr. Leton.

- Teach Mr. Leton and his family about the importance of maintaining a high fluid intake, especially when working outdoors in hot weather; the prescribed dietary modifications and their rationale; the prescribed medications and their effects and side effects; ways to identify and prevent urinary tract infection; and symptoms that indicate he should seek medical treatment.

Evaluation

Mr. Leton has passed the obstructing stone the evening after his admission and is discharged the following day. On discharge, he has no pain or nausea, his urine is clear and pale yellow, and urinalysis is normal. Laboratory analysis shows that the calculus was composed of calcium. Mr. Leton is able to state the importance of continuing a high fluid intake. He verbalizes that he would cut back on his intake of foods high in calcium, such as milk and milk products, and that he would increase his intake of acid ash foods. He is able to list cranberry juice, whole grains, meat, plums, and prunes as foods to include in his diet. He states, "You'd better believe I'll follow my diet, drink my fluids, and make sure I don't get an infection. I hope to never feel pain like that again!"

Critical Thinking in the Nursing Process

1. What factors contributed to the onset and timing of Mr. Leton's ureteral colic?

2. What is the rationale for administering indomethacin, an NSAID, to a client with ureteral colic?

3. Why did Mr. Phillips include a nursing intervention to assess for a relationship between Mr. Leton's nausea, his pain, and the ordered analgesic agent?

4. Develop a care plan for a client undergoing transcutaneous shock wave lithotripsy and identify teaching needs for that client and family.

The Client with a Tumor of the Urinary Tract

■ ■ ■

The majority of tumors affecting the urinary tract arise from epithelial tissue. Transitional epithelium lines the entire tract from the renal pelvis through the urethra; therefore, tumors may occur in any portion of the tract. By far the most common site for tumor formation is the urinary bladder.

Tumors affecting the urinary tract may lead to obstruction and resultant renal failure, hemorrhage, and the invasion and inflammation of surrounding tissues. Tissue destruction may cause fistulas to form, allowing urine to leak into the pelvis, vagina, or bowel.

Pathophysiology

Bladder cancer is diagnosed in approximately 50,000 people in the United States yearly, making it the fifth most common malignancy. It is the tenth leading cause of cancer deaths, claiming more than 10,000 people annually (Centers for Disease Control, 1993; McCance & Huether, 1994; Porth, 1994). In contrast, ureteral tumors account for less than 1% of all genitourinary tract lesions. The incidence varies with geographic location. People living in heavily industrialized states experience higher rates of urinary tract cancers than those living in agricultural states; further, people living in northern regions have a higher risk than those living in southern regions.

Tumors of the urinary tract occur most frequently in people over the age of 50. They are diagnosed in men two to four times more often than in women. Many clients with bladder cancer have more than one tumor present at the time of diagnosis.

Two major factors are implicated in the development of bladder cancer: the presence of carcinogens in the urine and chronic inflammation or infection of bladder mucosa.

Occupational and life-style risk factors are implicated in the formation of urinary tract neoplasms. Cigarette smoke, from both active and passive inhalation, is a significant risk factor and may account for as much as half of the incidence of bladder tumors among men and a third among women (Porth, 1994). Also implicated are the chemicals and dyes used in the plastics, rubber, and cable industries; substances in the work environment of textile workers, leather finishers, spray painters, hair dressers, and petroleum workers; and the chronic use of phenacetin-containing analgesic agents. Carcinogenic breakdown products of these chemicals and from cigarette smoke are excreted in the urine and stored in the bladder, possibly causing a local influence on abnormal cell development.

Squamous cell carcinoma of the urinary tract occurs less frequently than transitional epithelial cell tumors. Chronic infection, especially with *Schistosoma haematobium,* a parasite common in Egypt, and calculi of the urinary tract are associated with an increased risk for squamous cell carcinoma.

Urinary tract tumors begin as nonspecific cellular alterations that develop into either flat or papillary lesions. These lesions may be either superficial or invasive. Papillary lesions or papillomas account for approximately 70% of bladder tumors and are characterized by a polyplike structure attached by a stalk to the bladder mucosa (Figure 25–4). Papillomas are generally superficial noninvasive tumors and are associated with a good prognosis for full recovery. They frequently recur, with 20% of recur-

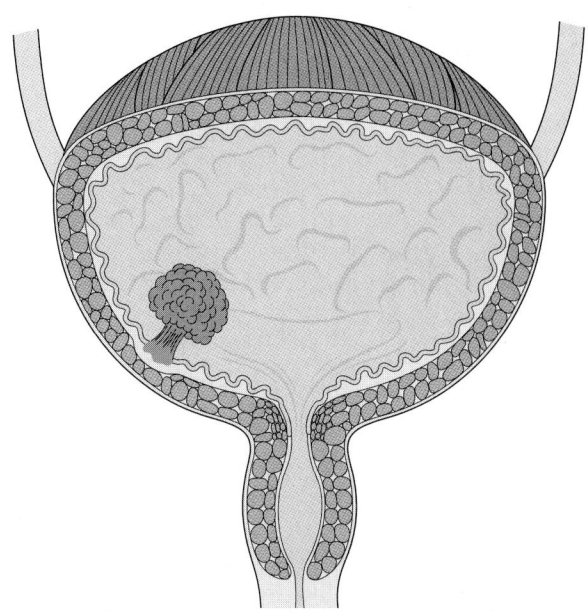

Figure 25–4   A papillary transitional cell carcinoma of the urinary bladder with minimal invasion of the bladder wall.

rent tumors becoming invasive (Way, 1994). Nonpapillary flat tumors lacking well-defined structures are less common than papillary lesions but tend to be more invasive and are associated with a poorer prognosis (McCance & Huether, 1994). Table 25–5 gives the staging of bladder tumors. Malignant tumors of the ureter are much less frequent than those of the bladder. They are also usually transitional cell tumors, which may be either invasive or noninvasive. When metastasis occurs, the pelvic lymph nodes, lungs, bones, and liver are most commonly involved. See Chapter 9 for a more complete discussion of neoplastic disease.

Table 25–5	Bladder Tumor Staging		
Depth of Involvement	**Conventional Stage**	**TNM (Tumor, Node, Metastasis) Stage**	**Tumor Involvement**
Superficial	O	T_a	Limited to the bladder mucosa
	A	T_1	Involvement of the bladder mucosa and submucosal layers
Invasive	B_1	T_2	Invasion of superficial muscle of bladder wall
	B_2	T_{3a}	Deep muscle invasion
	C	T_{3b}	Involvement of perivesicular fat
	D_1	$T_{3-4}N_+$	Regional (pelvic) lymph node involvement
	D_2	$T_{3-4}M_1$	Metastasis to distant lymph nodes or organs

Painless hematuria is the presenting sign in 75% of urinary tract tumors. Hematuria may be gross or microscopic and is often intermittent, causing delay in seeking treatment (Porth, 1994). Inflammation surrounding the tumor occasionally causes manifestations of a urinary tract infection, including frequency, urgency, and dysuria. Ureteral tumors may cause colicky pain from obstruction. Tumors of the urinary tract typically cause few outward signs and may not be discovered until obstructed urine flow causes renal failure or a fistula develops.

Collaborative Care

Treatment of the client with a tumor of the urinary tract focuses on removal or destruction of the cancerous tissue, prevention of further invasion or metastasis, and maintenance of renal and urinary function.

Laboratory and Diagnostic Tests

The following laboratory tests may be ordered for the client with a suspected tumor of the urinary tract:

- *Urinalysis* is performed to assess for the presence of blood cells in the urine. Gross or microscopic hematuria is often the first indicator of a neoplasm in the urinary tract.

- *Urine cytology* is the microscopic examination of cells within the urine for abnormalities. Abnormal cells may include tumor or pretumor cells. Correlation of cell abnormalities with clinical data can help differentiate the diagnosis of a urinary tract neoplasm from infection or other diseases affecting the urinary tract (Chernecky et al., 1993).

The following diagnostic studies may be used to help detect tumors:

- *Intravenous pyelography* is used to evaluate the structure and function of the kidneys, ureters, and bladder. IVP may reveal a rigid deformity of the bladder wall, obstruction of urine flow at the point of the tumor, or bladder filling or emptying defects.

- *Renal ultrasound* (kidney ultrasonography) is a noninvasive test that can reveal the presence of tumors or hydronephrosis resulting from obstruction. The echoes of high-frequency sound waves are used to create a three-dimensional picture of the kidney on an oscilloscope. No dye is required, and the client is not exposed to radiation. Thus, this test is useful when the client is allergic to radiographic dyes or X-ray exposure is contraindicated.

- *Computed tomography* (CT scan) of the kidney is useful to detect variations of tissue density as occur with tumors. CT may be done with or without contrast dye. CT is used to detect minor differences between tissues

and tissue boundaries. These differences are indistinguishable using standard X-ray techniques (Chernecky et al., 1993).

- *Cystoscopy* allows direct visualization, assessment, and biopsy of identified lesions of the urethra and bladder using a lighted scope inserted through the urethra. Cystoscopy provides the definitive diagnosis of bladder tumors.

- *Ureteroscopy*, visualization of the ureters with an endoscope inserted transurethrally, is used when a tumor is suspected to involve the upper portion of the tract.

Pharmacology

Chemotherapy is rarely the primary treatment used for tumors of the urinary tract, but it is used as adjunctive therapy. Systemic agents that may be used include cyclophosphamide, doxorubicin (Adriamycin), or a combination regimen of cisplatin, methotrexate, and vinblastine.

Thiotepa, an alkylating agent, is instilled into the bladder as a topical treatment for recurrent superficial lesions. Before it is instilled, the client is dehydrated for 8 to 12 hours. Then 30 to 60 mL of thiotepa solution is instilled via catheter and allowed to remain in the bladder for 2 hours. During that time, it is important for the client to change positions approximately every 15 minutes to ensure contact of the solution with all areas of the bladder mucosa.

Radiation Therapy

Radiation is another adjunctive therapy used in the treatment of urinary tumors. Although radiation alone is not curative, it can reduce tumor size prior to surgery and is used as palliative treatment for inoperable tumors and clients who cannot tolerate surgery. (See Chapter 9.)

Surgery

A number of surgical procedures, ranging from simple resection of noninvasive tumors to removal of the bladder and surrounding structures, are used to treat urinary tract tumors. Indications for each procedure and specific nursing implications are outlined in Table 25–6.

Transurethral tumor resection may be performed by excision, *fulguration* (destruction of tissue using electric sparks generated by high-frequency current) or *laser photocoagulation* (use of light energy to destroy abnormal tissue). Laser surgery carries the lowest risk of bleeding and perforation of the bladder wall.

A total or radical **cystectomy** involves complete surgical removal of the bladder and adjacent muscles and tissues. See the accompanying Critical Pathway. In men, the prostate and seminal vessels are also removed, resulting in impotence. In women, a total hysterectomy and bilateral salpingo-oophorectomy (removal of the uterus, uter-

Text continues on page 914

Table 25–6   Procedures Used to Treat Bladder Tumors

Procedure	Indications	Nursing Implications
Transurethral resection of bladder tumor	Diagnosis and treatment of superficial bladder tumors having low rate of recurrence; control of bleeding	Maintain continuous bladder irrigation postoperatively; monitor for excessive bleeding; ensure catheter patency. Increase fluids to 2500–3000 mL per day. Give stool softeners to prevent straining.
Partial cystectomy	Resection of solitary, isolated tumor at stage B or C not involving trigone	Maintain patency of urethral and/or suprapubic catheter to make sure suture lines are free of pressure; monitor for excess bleeding.
Complete or radical cystectomy	Removal of large, invasive tumors; involvement of trigone	Permanent urinary diversion is required. Maintain patency and position of stents; urethral catheter may be in place to drain pelvic cavity.

Critical Pathway for Client Following Cystectomy with Ileal Conduit

	Date ——— **Preoperative**	Date ——— **1st 24 Hours Postoperative**	Date ——— **2nd–3rd Day Postoperative**
	Expected length of stay: 6 to 7 days		
Daily outcomes	Client verbalizes understanding of preoperative teaching, including: turning, coughing, deep breathing, incentive spirometer, mobilization, possible tubes (nasogastric tube, IV, Foley catheter, penrose or other drains), urostomy, and pain management. Client demonstrates ability to cope. Client verbalizes understanding of procedure. Obtain informed consent.	Client will ■ Have stable vital signs. ■ Have a clean, dry wound with edges well-approximated, healing by first intention. ■ Recover from anesthesia as evidenced by VS return to baseline, awake, alert, and oriented. ■ Verbalize understanding of and demonstrate cooperation with turning, coughing, deep breathing and splinting, lungs clear to auscultation. 　■ Have urine output > 30mL/hr and patent urostomy. ■ Verbalize understanding of PCA/epidural if in use. ■ Verbalize control of incisional pain. ■ Transfer out of bed with assistance 2–3 times. ■ Demonstrate ability to cope.	Client will ■ Be afebrile. ■ Have a clean, dry wound with edges well-approximated, healing by first intention. ■ Will have active bowel sounds. ■ Tolerate ordered diet without vomiting. ■ Have urine output > 30mL/hr and patent urostomy. ■ Demonstrate cooperation with turning, coughing, deep breathing and splinting. ■ Ambulate 4 times. ■ Verbalize control of incisional pain. ■ Verbalize ability to cope. ■ Verbalize beginning understanding of home care instructions.

Critical Pathway for Client Following Cystectomy with Ileal Conduit (continued)

	Date _____ Preoperative	Date _____ 1st 24 Hours Postoperative	Date _____ 2nd–3rd Day Postoperative
Tests and treatments	CBC Urinalysis Chest X-ray Baseline physical assessment, with a focus on respiratory status and gastrointestinal function Assess and record the description, location, duration, and characteristics of client's pain. Reduce or eliminate pain-producing factors, e.g., fear, anxiety.	CBC Electrolytes Vital signs and O_2 saturation, neurovascular assessment, dressing and wound drainage assessment q15min × 4; q30min × 4; q1h × 4 and then q4 hr if stable. Assess respiratory status and gastrointestinal function q4h and prn. Incentive spirometer q2h. Intake and output every shift. Assess patency of NG tube q2h, noting volume q4–8h. Assess urinary output from urostomy q1–2h and prn. Assess amount, color, and volume of drainage from NG and other drainage tubes. Assess and record the description, location, duration, and characteristics of client's pain q2–4h and prn. Encourage verbalization of pain and discomfort. Reduce or eliminate pain-producing factors and employ distraction or relaxation techniques. Provide back rubs. Encourage client to request analgesic or use PCA (if in use) before pain becomes severe. Assess effectiveness of pain-relief measures. Assess stoma for edema, cyanosis, and bleeding. Assess peristomal skin for erythema, integrity, or irritation. Assess appliance for proper fit.	Vital signs and dressing and wound drainage assessment q4h. Assess respiratory status and gastrointestinal function q4h. Incentive spirometer q2h until fully ambulatory. Intake and output every shift. If still in place, assess patency and output of NG tube q4–8h. Assess urinary output q2–4h. Using sterile asepsis change dressing: assess wound healing and wound drainage. Assess and record the description, location, duration, and characteristics of client's pain q4h and prn. Reduce or eliminate pain-producing factors, employ distraction or relaxation techniques, and offer back rubs. Assess effectiveness of pain-relief measures. Assess appliance for proper fit.

	Date _____ **Preoperative**	**Date _____** **1st 24 Hours Postoperative**	**Date _____** **2nd–3rd Day Postoperative**
Knowledge deficit	Orient to room and surroundings. Provide simple, brief instructions. Review preoperative preparation including hospital and surgical routines. Include family in teaching. Discuss surgery and specific postoperative care: turning, coughing, deep breathing, splinting incision, incentive spirometer, mobilization, possible tubes (NG and intravenous), pain management (PCA, epidural, or prn medications). Instruct regarding distraction techniques, e.g., slow rhythmic breathing and guided imagery, to produce pain relief. Instruct in relaxation techniques, e.g., tensing and relaxing muscle groups and rhythmic breathing. Assess understanding of teaching.	Reorient to room and postoperative routine. Include family in teaching. Review plan of care and importance of early mobilization. Review importance of turning, coughing, deep breathing, splinting incision, incentive spirometer, mobilization, drainage tubes, and intravenous pain management (PCA, epidural, or prn medications). Assess understanding of teaching.	Reinforce earlier teaching regarding ongoing care. Include family in teaching. Begin discharge teaching regarding wound care/dressing change and care of stoma and skin, including application of an appliance, signs and symptoms of urinary tract infection. Assess understanding of teaching.
Psycho-social	Assess anxiety related to diagnosis and pending surgery. Assess fears of the unknown and surgery. Encourage verbalization of concerns. Provide information regarding surgical experience. Minimize external stimuli (e.g., noise, movement). Offer emotional support.	Assess level of anxiety. Encourage verbalization of concerns. Provide information and ongoing support and encouragement to client and family. Offer emotional support.	Encourage verbalization of concerns. Provide ongoing support and encouragement. Offer emotional support.
Diet	NPO Baseline nutritional and hydration assessment	NG tube until return of bowel sounds NPO	When NG tube is removed, begin clear liquids to tolerance
Activity	Assess safety needs and provide appropriate measures. Activity as ordered.	Maintain safety precautions. Assist to chair 2–3 times.	Maintain safety precautions. Ambulate 4 times with assistance.

Critical Pathway for Client Following Cystectomy with Ileal Conduit (continued)

	Date _____ **Preoperative**	Date _____ **1st 24 Hours Postoperative**	Date _____ **2nd–3rd Day Postoperative**
Medications	Preoperative medications as ordered	IV fluids IV antibiotics Pain medication (PCA, IV, or prn) as ordered	IV fluids IV antibiotics When ordered convert IV to intermittent IV device Pain medication (PCA, IV, or prn) as ordered
Transfer/ discharge plans	Assess potential discharge needs and support system. Establish discharge goals with client and family.	Review progress toward discharge goals with client and family. Consult with social service re: VNA and projected needs for home health care (if any).	Review progress toward discharge goals with client and significant other. Make appropriate discharge referrals.

	Date _____ **4th Day Postoperative**	Date _____ **5th Day Postoperative**	Date _____ **6th–7th Day Postoperative**
Daily outcomes	Client will ■ Be afebrile. ■ Have a clean, dry wound with edges well-approximated, healing by first intention. ■ Tolerate ordered diet without nausea or vomiting. ■ Maintain urine output > 30mL/hr and patent urostomy. ■ Ambulate 4–6 times. ■ Verbalize control of incisional pain. ■ Verbalize ability to cope. ■ Verbalize beginning understanding of home care instructions.	Client will ■ Be afebrile. ■ Have a clean, dry wound with edges well-approximated, healing by first intention. ■ Tolerate ordered diet without nausea or vomiting. ■ Maintain urine output > 30mL/hr and patent urostomy. ■ Ambulate 4–6 times. ■ Verbalize control of incisional pain. ■ Verbalize ability to cope. ■ Verbalize beginning understanding of home care instructions.	Client is afebrile. Client has a dry, clean wound with edges well-approximated, healing by first intention. Peristomal skin remains intact and without redness. Client manages pain with nonpharmacologic measures and any ordered medications. Client is independent in self-care. Client is fully ambulatory. Client has resumed preadmission bowel elimination pattern. Client has a patent urostomy, and urine remains free of signs of infection. Client verbalizes home care instructions. Client tolerates usual diet. Client verbalizes ability to cope with ongoing stressors.

	Date _____ **4th Day Postoperative**	Date _____ **5th Day Postoperative**	Date _____ **6th–7th Day Postoperative**
Tests and treatments	Vital signs and dressing and wound drainage assessment q4h. Incentive spirometer q2h until fully ambulatory. Intake and output every shift. Assess urinary output q4h and prn. Assess respiratory status and gastrointestinal function q4–8h. Using sterile asepsis change dressing: assess wound healing and wound drainage. Assess and record description, location, duration, and characteristics of client's pain q4h and prn. Encourage client to employ distraction or relaxation techniques. Continue teaching related to stoma care, including care of stoma, peristomal skin, and application of appliance.	Vital signs and dressing and wound drainage assessment q4h. Assess respiratory status and gastrointestinal function q4–8h. Assess urinary output q4h and prn. Remove dressing and assess wound healing and drainage. Assess and record description, location, duration, and characteristics of client's pain q4h and prn. Encourage client to employ distraction or relaxation techniques. Continue teaching related to stoma care, including care of stoma, peristomal skin, and application of appliance.	Vital signs and dressing and wound drainage assessment q4–8h. Assess respiratory status and gastrointestinal function. Assess wound healing. Assess urinary output. Assess and record description, location, duration, and characteristics of client's pain q4h and prn. Encourage client to employ distraction or relaxation techniques. Continue teaching related to stoma care, including care of stoma, peristomal skin, and application of appliance.
Knowledge deficit	Include family in teaching. Initiate discharge teaching regarding wound care, diet, and activity. Continue teaching related to stoma care, including care of stoma, peristomal skin, and application of appliance. Review written discharge instructions with client and significant other. Assess understanding of teaching.	Continue discharge teaching, including family, regarding wound care, diet, signs and symptoms to report, medications, and activity. Continue teaching related to stoma care, including care of stoma, peristomal skin, and application of appliance. Review written discharge instructions with client and family. Assess understanding of teaching.	Complete discharge teaching to include wound care, diet, follow-up care, signs and symptoms to report, activity, and medications: name, purpose, dose, frequency, route, dietary interactions, and side effects. Provide client with written discharge instructions. Assess understanding of teaching.
Psycho-social	Encourage verbalization of concerns. Provide ongoing support and encouragement.	Encourage verbalization of concerns. Provide ongoing support and encouragement.	Encourage verbalization of concerns. Provide ongoing support and encouragement.
Diet	If tolerating clear liquids, advance to full liquids as tolerated.	Advance diet to soft, regular diet to tolerance.	Regular diet as tolerated.

➤

Critical Pathway for Client Following Cystectomy with Ileal Conduit (continued)

	Date _____ **4th Day Postoperative**	Date _____ **5th Day Postoperative**	Date _____ **6th–7th Day Postoperative**
Activity	Ambulate independently at least 4 times. Maintain safety precautions.	Fully ambulatory Maintain safety precautions.	Fully ambulatory
Medications	Provide PO analgesics Intermittent IV device for any IV medications; D/C when so ordered	Provide PO analgesics	Provide PO analgesics
Transfer/ discharge plans	Continue to review progress toward discharge goals.	Finalize discharge plans. Continue to review progress toward discharge goals. Finalize plans for home care if needed.	Complete discharge instructions.

ine tubes, and ovaries) accompanies the procedure, resulting in sterility. At the time of surgery, a **urinary diversion** is also created to provide for urine collection and drainage. The most common urinary diversion is the ileal conduit (Figure 25–5); however, continent urinary diversions are increasing in popularity for clients who have the desire and ability to care for them (Figure 25–6). Table

25–7 describes the most frequently used urinary diversion techniques. The collaborative care box on page 916 lists the health team members and their respective roles in the care of the client undergoing a cystectomy.

Surgical procedures to remove tumors involving other portions of the urinary tract vary according to the site and stage of the tumor. When the distal ureter is involved, the

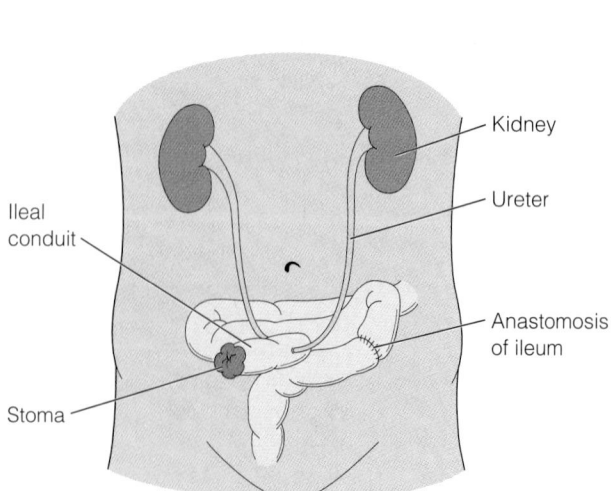

Figure 25–5 Ileal conduit. A segment of ileum is separated from the small intestine and formed into a tubular pouch with the open end brought to the skin surface to form a stoma. The ureters are connected to the pouch.

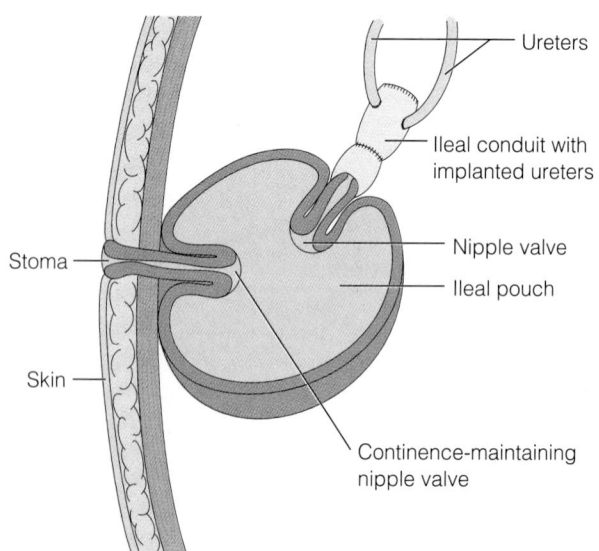

Figure 25–6 A continent urinary diversion. A segment of ileum is separated from the small intestine and formed into a pouch. Nipple valves are formed at each end of the pouch by intussuscepting tissue backward into the reservoir to prevent leakage.

Table 25–7   Urinary Diversion Procedures

Procedure	Description	Nursing Considerations
Cutaneous ureterostomy	One or both ureters are excised from bladder and brought to the surface of skin, with creation of individual or combined stomas.	Continuous urine drainage necessitates wearing appliance; small stoma may make tight seal difficult and increase skin contact with urine. Direct access from skin to kidney increases risk of infection.
Ileal conduit	Portion of ileum is isolated from small intestine, leaving vascular, lymphatic, and neural connections intact; ileum is formed into pouch with open end brought to surface to form stoma; ureters are inserted into pouch.	Most common urinary diversion. Continuous urine drainage necessitates appliance. Postoperative edema may interfere with urine output. Risk of infection is less than for cutaneous ureterostomy, but potential for reflux is high. Good skin care vital because of constant contact with urine.
Colon conduit	As for ileal conduit using a portion of sigmoid colon rather than small intestine.	As for ileal conduit. Edema may be more of a problem; reflux less of a problem.
Ureterosigmoidostomy	Ureters are inserted into the sigmoid colon; urine empties into rectum and is expelled with defecation and passage of flatus.	Seldom performed because of risks of infection (chronic pyelonephritis) and electrolyte imbalance resulting from reabsorption of urine electrolytes. Anal skin irritation and urine leakage are common problems.
Continent internal ileal reservoir or continent ileal bladder conduit (Kock's pouch)	Pouch is created as for ileal conduit but nipple valves are formed by intussuscepting tissue backward into a reservoir to connect pouch to the skin and the ureters to the pouch; filling pressure closes valves, preventing leakage and reflux.	Drainage collection device not necessary. Client must be willing and able to perform clean intermittent self-catheterization every 2 to 4 hours. Continence valve mechanism may fail, requiring surgery for revision.
Indiana continent urinary reservoir	A portion of the terminal ileum, ascending colon, and cecum is isolated from the bowel with vascular and neural connections intact. Reservoir is formed from colon and cecum; portion of the ileum is brought to the surface to form nipple valve and stoma or is attached to urethral stump.	As for Kock's pouch. Client must be able and motivated to manage self-catheterization. Reservoir may absorb urea and electrolytes, resulting in imbalances. Significant portion of bowel is required to form pouch and stoma.
Ileocystoplasty or Camey procedure	Section of the ileum is isolated and formed into U shape. Ureters are implanted in upper portion of the U. Urethra is anastamosed to central section.	Appropriate for men only because urethra is removed with cystectomy in women. Allows client to void by relaxing pelvic muscles and using Valsalva maneuver.

tumor may be resected and the ureter implanted into the opposite ureter to provide for drainage. A proximal ureteral tumor necessitates removal of the ureter and kidney on the affected side.

The box on page 917 describes nursing care of the client undergoing tumor resection and a urinary diversion.

Nursing Care

The client who undergoes treatment for a tumor of the urinary tract has many nursing care needs because of alterations in the functional health patterns of elimination,

health perception/management, cognitive/perceptual, self-perception/self-concept, role/relationship, and coping/stress tolerance. This section focuses on the client's needs for urinary elimination, risk for impairment of skin integrity, change in body image or self-perception, and risk for infection.

Altered Patterns of Urinary Elimination
Whether the client has undergone a transurethral resection of bladder tumors or a radical cystectomy with urinary diversion, urinary elimination is altered at least temporarily.

Nursing interventions with rationales follow.

Collaborative Care: The Client Requiring a Cystectomy

Health Care Team	Client-Centered Care
Urologist	Orders diagnostic tests including IVP, performs cystoscopy and biopsies tumor, and presents surgical options to the client. Removes cancerous bladder, manages postoperative care.
Oncologist	Makes recommendations regarding chemotherapy and/or radiation therapy if necessary, and monitors treatments.
Primary care physician	Assesses client with urinary or other symptoms, refers to the urologist, and/or manages medical care throughout hospitalization and following discharge.
Enterostomal therapist	Preoperatively, discusses the type of urinary diversion and selection of site for the stoma, obtains appropriate external pouch, teaches skin care and application and emptying of external pouch, or teaches catheterization of continent internal ileal reservoir.
Dietitian	Assesses and monitors nutritional needs and intake. Discusses approaches to maintain fluid and electrolyte balance. Teaches client about avoiding gas-producing foods.
Mental health clinical nurse specialist	Assists in preparing for the psychological impact of the diagnosis of cancer and impending surgery. Helps to promote confidence in social situations.
Home care coordinator and/or social worker	Arranges for purchase of necessary supplies and assists with dressing and stoma care. Assists client and family with financial concerns and problems. Consults with agencies such as the American Cancer Society for supplies, transportation, and other resources.
RN and Health Care Team Communications	Notifies physician of urine output when less than 30cc/hr, signs and symptoms of infection, wound dehiscence, small bowel obstruction, or gangrene of stoma. Collaborates with enterostomal therapist to teach stoma care. Discusses home care needs with social worker. Provides dietitian with list of food likes and dislikes and assists with meal planning.

- Monitor urinary output from all catheters, stents, and tubes for amount, color, and clarity hourly for the first 24 hours postoperatively, then every 4 to 8 hours. *Output of less than 30 mL per hour may indicate low vascular volume, renal insufficiency, or impaired patency of drainage system. A change in color or clarity may be indicative of complications such as hemorrhage or infection.*

- Label all catheters, stents, and their drainage containers. Maintain separate closed gravity drainage systems for each. *Clear identification of each tube can prevent errors in irrigation and calculation of outputs. Using separate closed systems minimizes the risk and extent of potential bacterial contamination and resultant infection.*

- Secure ureteral catheters and stents with tape; prevent kinking or occlusion by the client; maintain gravity flow by keeping drainage bag below level of kidneys. *Impaired urine flow through ureteral stents results in retention of urine, which may cause distention within the renal pelvis and hydronephrosis, with resultant renal damage. Impaired catheter patency may also cause bladder or reservoir distention and pressure on suture lines.*

- Encourage intake of 3000 mL per day. *Increased fluid intake with resulting high urinary output keeps the diversion flushed, reducing the risk of infection. Diluted urine is less irritating to the skin surrounding the stoma site. Electrolyte reabsorption from reservoirs may increase risk of calculi; high fluid intake and urine output reduce this risk.*

- Monitor urine output closely for first 24 hours after removal of any stents or ureteral catheters. *Edema or stricture of ureters may impede output.*

- Encourage client activity to tolerance. *Ambulation promotes drainage of urine from reservoirs and helps prevent calcium loss from bones, which could precipitate calculus formation.*

Risk for Impaired Skin Integrity

The skin surrounding the stoma site of a ureterostomy or ileal conduit is at risk for irritation and breakdown. Because urine is acidic and contains high concentrations of electrolytes, it has a corrosive effect on skin. In addition, adhesives and sealants used to prevent pouch leakage may irritate the skin.

Nursing interventions with rationales follow.

- Assess the skin surrounding the stoma for redness, excoriation, or signs of breakdown. Assess for leakage of urine from any catheters, stents, or drains. Keep the skin clean and dry. Change wet dressings. *Intact skin is the first line of defense against infection. Impaired skin integrity may lead to local or systemic infection and impede healing.*

Nursing Care of the Client Having Bladder Tumor Surgery

PREOPERATIVE CARE

- Assess the client's knowledge of the proposed surgery and its long-term implications, clarifying misunderstandings and discussing concerns. *Clients having surgery for cancer of the urinary tract are trying to cope with diagnosis of cancer and may not fully understand the surgery and its potential effects. Open discussion can facilitate postoperative recovery and adjustment.*

- Begin teaching about postoperative tubes and drains, self-care of stoma, and control of drainage and odor. *Physiologic and psychologic stressors in the postoperative period may interfere with learning. A basic understanding of what to expect in the way of tubes, drains, and procedures to prevent complications reduces stress in the immediately postoperative period. Beginning teaching prior to surgery can enhance recall and postoperative learning.*

- Assist the enterostomal therapist or physician in identifying stoma site(s), avoiding folds of skin, bones, scar tissue, and the waistline or belt area. Be sure to consider the client's occupation and style of clothing. The site should be visible to the client and accessible for manipulation. *Stoma placement is a vital component of the client's postoperative adjustment and ability to provide self-care. Care is taken to place the stoma away from areas of constant irritation by clothing or movement. It should be located so that the client can cover and disguise the collecting device, maintain the seal to prevent leakage, and effectively cleanse and maintain the site.*

- Perform bowel-preparation activities as ordered by physician. *Bowel preparation is done to prevent fecal contamination of the peritoneal cavity and to decompress the bowel during surgery.*

POSTOPERATIVE CARE

- Monitor intake and urinary output carefully, assessing output every hour for the first 24 hours, then every 4 hours or as ordered. Call the physician if urine output is less than 30 mL per hour. *Tissue edema and bleeding may interfere with urinary output from stoma, catheters, or drains. Maintenance of urine outflow is vital to prevent hydronephrosis and possible renal damage. A urine output of at least 30 mL per hour is necessary for effective renal function.*

- Assess color and consistency of urine. Expect pink or bright red urine fading to pink and then clearing by the third postoperative day. Clients with urinary diversions using a portion of bowel may have cloudy urine due to production of mucus by the bowel mucosa. *Bright red blood in the urine from a urinary diversion may indicate hemorrhage and the need for further surgery. Excessive cloudiness or malodorous urine may indicate infection.*

- Assess the size, color, and condition of the stoma and surrounding skin every 2 hours for the first 24 hours, then every 4 hours for 48 to 72 hours. Expect the stoma to appear bright red and slightly edematous initially. Slight bleeding when the site is cleansed is normal. *Compromised circulation results in a stoma that appears pale, gray, or cyanotic or that blanches when touched. Other complications, such as infection or inadequate healing, may be evidenced by a change in the appearance of the stoma or incision* (Cavas & Makay, 1991).

- Irrigate the ileal diversion catheter with 30 to 60 mL of normal saline every 4 hours or as ordered by the physician. *Mucus produced by the bowel wall may accumulate in the newly devised reservoir or obstruct catheters.*

- Monitor serum electrolyte values, acid-base balance, and renal function tests such as BUN and serum creatinine. *Reabsorption of electrolytes from reservoirs created by portions of bowel may result in electrolyte imbalance and metabolic acidosis. Optimal renal function is necessary for the client to maintain a normal state of homeostasis.*

- Teach the client and family about stoma and urinary diversion care, including odor management, skin care, increased fluid intake, pouch application and leakage prevention, self-catheterization for clients with continent reservoirs, and signs of infection and other complications. *The ability to provide self-care is a significant factor in the client's adjustment to a changed body image. Teaching family members facilitates their acceptance and adjustment. The family also needs this knowledge in case illness or disability interferes with the client's self-care capacity.*

Procedure 25–1 Urinary Stoma Care

When it is necessary to change the urine-collection device for a client with a urinary stoma, use the following procedure:

- Gather all supplies needed: A clean, disposable pouch; a liquid skin barrier or barrier ring; 4-by-4 gauze squares; a stoma guide; adhesive solvent; clean gloves; and a clean washcloth.
- Assess the client's knowledge, learning needs, and ability and willingness to assist with the procedure. Explain the procedure as needed.
- Wash hands and put on clean gloves.

- Remove the old pouch, pulling gently away from skin. Warm water or adhesive solvent may be used to loosen the seal if necessary.
- Assess the stoma. Normally the stoma is bright red and appears moist. Dark purple, black, or very pale stoma color should be reported to the physician. A small amount of bleeding with cleansing is normal, especially in the immediate postoperative period.
- Prevent urine flow during cleaning process by placing a rolled gauze square or tampon over the stoma opening.
- Cleanse the skin around the stoma with soap and water, rinse, and pat or air dry.

- Use the stoma guide to determine the correct size for the bag opening and/or protective ring seal. Trim the bag or seal as needed.
- Apply the skin barrier; allow to dry.
- Apply the bag with an opening no more than 1 to 2 mm wider than outside of stoma. Allow no wrinkles or creases where the bag contacts the skin.
- Connect the bag to the urine-collection device. Dispose of the old pouch, supplies used, and gloves appropriately. Wash hands.
- Chart procedure, including the appearance of the stoma and the response of the client.

- Ensure gravity drainage of urine-collection device or empty bag every 2 hours. *Overfilling of the collection bag may damage the seal, allowing leakage and contact of urine with skin.*

- Change urine-collection appliance as needed, removing any mucus from stoma. See the accompanying procedure box for care of a urinary drainage stoma. *Meticulous care and protection of skin surrounding stoma can maintain integrity and prevent breakdown.*

Body Image Disturbance

The client who has a tumor of the urinary tract is at risk for body image disturbance. If a radical cystectomy and urinary diversion have been performed, the client is likely to have an abdominal stoma. If so, the client needs to provide for urine elimination either by wearing a collection device or by catheterizing the stoma regularly. Removal of the prostate and seminal vesicles or the uterus and ovaries leaves the client sterile. If radiation or chemotherapy is planned as adjunctive therapy, the client may experience hair loss, stomatitis, nausea and vomiting, or other disturbing side effects of therapy.

Nursing interventions with rationales follow.

- Use therapeutic communication techniques, actively listening and responding to the client's and family's concerns. *Clients need to know that their feelings and con-*

cerns are respected and valued. Denial, anger, guilt, bargaining, or depression are part of the grieving process and normal for a client undergoing a significant change in body image.

- Recognize and accept behaviors that indicate the use of coping mechanisms, encouraging the use of adaptive mechanisms. *The client may initially use defensive coping mechanisms such as denial, minimization, and dissociation from the immediate situation to reduce anxiety and maintain psychologic integrity. Adaptive mechanisms include learning as much as possible about the surgery and its effects, practicing procedures, setting realistic goals, and rehearsing various alternative outcomes.*

- Encourage the client to look at, touch, and care for the stoma and appliance as soon as possible. Allow the client to proceed gradually, providing support and encouragement. *Accepting the stoma as part of the self is vital to adapting to the changed body image and is indicated by a willingness to provide self-care.*

- Discuss client and family concerns about returning to usual activities, perceived changes in relationships with family and friends, and resumption of sexual relations. Initiate referral to support group or provide for contact with someone who has successfully adjusted to a urinary diversion. *Clients and families may be reluctant to initiate discussion on topics of concern. An atmosphere of openness and acceptance facilitates expression of concerns and anxieties related to the change in the client's body image.*

Risk for Infection

Diagnostic instrumentation procedures, surgical manipulation, and disruption of the normal urinary tract defense mechanisms increase the risk of ascending urinary tract infection in the client having surgery for tumor. When an ileal conduit or artificial bladder is created using bowel tissue, the normal bacteriostatic activity of bladder mucosa is no longer present. In addition, the peristaltic action of the ureters may be disrupted, and the uretero-vesicle junction no longer prevents reflux of urine. Adjunctive chemotherapy or radiation treatments may inhibit normal immune function and further increase the risk of infection.

Nursing interventions with rationales follow.

- Maintain separate closed drainage systems, keeping drainage bags lower than the kidney, and prevent loops or kinks in drainage tubing, which impede urine flow. *Although urine is sterile when it leaves the kidney, bacteria grow rapidly in urine. Prevention of urine reflux is essential to preventing UTI.*

- Monitor for signs of infection: elevated temperature, cloudy or foul-smelling urine, hematuria, general malaise, back or abdominal pain, and nausea and vomiting. *Infection undermines the healing process. Early detection and treatment help prevent long-term consequences such as chronic pyelonephritis.*

- Teach the client and family the signs and symptoms of infection and self-care measures to prevent UTI. *The client with a cystectomy and ileal diversion, urostomy, or continent reservoir is at risk of UTI for life because of impaired urinary defense mechanisms. Use of clean or aseptic technique in providing care, increasing fluid intake, and using measures to acidify urine minimize this risk to a certain degree but do not eliminate it.*

Other Nursing Diagnoses

The following nursing diagnoses may also apply to the client who has had surgery for removal of a tumor of the urinary tract:

- *Anxiety* related to an uncertain prognosis and unknown effects on life-style and relationships
- *Activity Intolerance* related to major surgery and adjunctive cancer therapy
- *Ineffective Individual or Family Coping* related to presence of stoma and appliance
- *Anticipatory grieving* related to diagnosis of cancer
- *Altered Health Maintenance* related to urinary diversion
- *Knowledge Deficit* regarding care of stoma and appli-

ance, self-catheterization techniques, and signs of infection.

- *Pain* related to surgical incisions
- *Self-Care Deficit* in toileting related to lack of knowledge regarding care of stoma and appliance or self-catheterization techniques
- *Altered Patterns of Sexuality* related to presence of stoma and surgical impotence or sterility

Client and Family Teaching

The need for individual and family teaching for the client who has had surgery for removal of a urinary tract tumor is significant. For many clients, surgery means a lifelong change in urinary elimination. Even the client who has undergone transurethral excision of bladder tumors requires follow-up cystoscopy on a regular basis and needs to be alert for signs of tumor recurrence.

The client who has had a urinary diversion procedure needs teaching about the care of the stoma and surrounding skin, prevention of urine reflux and infection, signs and symptoms of UTI and renal calculi, and, in some cases, self-catheterization using clean technique.

Applying the Nursing Process

Case Study of a Client with a Bladder Tumor: Ben Hussain

Ben Hussain is a 61-year-old man who is employed as an automobile salesman. He is married and has five children, all of whom are grown and away from home. One week ago, Mr. Hussain became alarmed when his urine became bright red. Even though he had no other symptoms, he called his physician. The physician has ordered a urinalysis and urine cytology study, which reveals gross hematuria and the presence of poorly differentiated abnormal cells. Cystoscopy and tissue biopsy confirm a stage C tumor involving the bladder trigone. He is admitted to the hospital for a radical cystectomy and ileal diversion.

Assessment

Mr. Hussain's admission history, obtained by Tara Mills, his primary nurse, indicates that he has lost 10 to 15 pounds over the last few months. He has smoked two to three packs of cigarettes per day for 40 years, but he cut back to a pack a day about a year ago. He says he didn't think he could ever quit smoking entirely. He drinks five to six cups of coffee daily and consumes a moderate amount of alcohol, averaging three to four drinks a day. Mr. Hussain says that he is "a little nervous about surgery and what they're going to find." Ms. Mills notes that he fidgets and talks rapidly throughout their interview. He also expresses concern about how he will handle the pain after surgery, because he has never been hospitalized before his cystoscopy. Physical assessment findings include BP: 154/86; P: 84; R: 18; T: 98.2 F (36.7 C) PO. Physical assessment findings of integumentary, neuromuscular, and cardiac systems are all within normal limits. Scattered expiratory crackles are noted on ausculation of lung fields. Bowel sounds are very active; Mr. Hussain explains that he began taking his bowel-preparation laxative the day before admission. Slight tenderness is noted in the suprapubic region. Mr. Hussain's urine is clear and bright pink. Findings of CBC and chemistry screening studies are all within normal limits. Surgery is planned for 9:00 a.m. the following day.

Diagnosis

Ms. Mills identifies the following nursing diagnoses for Mr. Hussain:

- *Anxiety* related to undetermined extent of disease and fear of pain
- *Knowledge Deficit* related to lack of information regarding ileal diversion
- *Alteration in Urinary Elimination* related to cystectomy and ileal diversion
- *Risk for Impaired Gas Exchange* related to smoking history and effects of anesthesia

Expected Outcomes

The expected outcomes of the plan of care for Mr. Hussain are that he will

- Verbalize a decrease in feelings of anxiety.
- Demonstrate appropriate postoperative pain relief by relaxed facial expression, ability to move in bed, and vital signs within normal individual range.
- Be able to care for ileostomy stoma, surrounding skin, and collection appliance prior to discharge from hospital.
- Maintain a normal urine output with acceptable color and clarity and no signs of infection.
- Maintain adequate gas exchange as evidenced by good skin color, O_2 saturation greater than 95%, and clear lung sounds upon auscultation.

Planning and Implementation

Ms. Mills plans and implements the following nursing interventions for Mr. Hussain:

- Spend as much time as possible with Mr. Hussain and his family preoperatively, answering questions fully and encouraging expression of fears.

- Ask that all consultants, specialists, and technicians fully explain their role and answer questions for Mr. and Mrs. Hussain.
- Provide written as well as verbal explanations when feasible.
- Administer ordered postoperative analgesic agents on a regular basis for the first 48 to 72 hours. Monitor for outward signs of unrelieved pain.
- Explain all procedures related to stoma and appliance care as they are being performed.
- Encourage Mr. and Mrs. Hussain to look at stoma and touch it when ready.
- Teach Mr. and Mrs. Hussain how to care for the stoma, surrounding skin, and appliance, emphasizing techniques to prevent skin irritation and urinary tract infection.
- Monitor urine for output, color, clarity, and consistency every hour for first 24 hours, then every 4 hours for 24 hours, then every 8 hours. Report output of less than 30 mL per hour, evidence of bright bleeding, excessively cloudy or malodorous urine.
- Assist Mr. Hussain to use an incentive spirometer every hour while awake. Ambulate as soon as possible. Assess lung sounds every 4 hours, reporting increased crackles or diminished breath sounds.
- Refer Mr. and Mrs. Hussain to local stoma group on discharge.

Evaluation

On discharge, Mr. Hussain is not yet fully able to care for his ileal diversion, but he has participated in cleaning the stoma and surrounding skin several times. His wife is able to demonstrate emptying the drainage bag and changing the appliance, cutting the opening to fit. His urine is pale yellow and slightly cloudy. Mr. Hussain is ambulating independently and using oxycodone (Percocet) twice a day for pain relief. His lungs are clear, and he is very proud of having "survived" 7 days without a cigarette. He says, "Now I'm going to shoot for 7 weeks, then 7 months, then 7 years without a smoke!" A home health referral is made to continue teaching Mr. Hussain to care for his diversion and appliance.

Critical Thinking in the Nursing Process

1. How does cigarette smoking contribute to the increased risk of urinary tract tumors?
2. Suppose Mr. Hussain had become confused, disoriented, and tremorous and had begun to experience visual hallucinations 2 to 3 days postoperatively. What would you suspect the cause to be? What would be the appropriate response?

3. Outline a plan for teaching continuing care to clients following an ileal diversion.

4. Develop a care plan for Mr. Hussain for the nursing diagnosis *Altered Patterns of Sexuality.*

The Client with Urinary Retention

■ ■ ■

Normal bladder emptying may be disrupted by mechanical obstruction of the bladder outlet or by a functional problem. When the bladder cannot eliminate urine, it becomes overdistended. The overdistention leads to poor contractility of the detrusor muscle and an inability to urinate.

Benign prostatic hypertrophy (BPH) is a common cause of *urinary retention.* Difficulty initiating and maintaining urine flow is often the presenting complaint in men with BPH. Acute inflammation associated with infection or trauma of the bladder, urethra, or vulvovaginal tissues may also interfere with the ability to urinate. Scarring associated with repeated urinary tract infection can lead to urethral stricture and a mechanical obstruction. Bladder calculi may also be obstructive, leading to urinary retention.

Surgery, particularly abdominal or pelvic surgery, may disrupt the function of the detrusor muscle, leading to the retention of urine. In addition, medications may interfere with detrusor muscle function. Anticholinergic medications such as atropine, glycopyrrolate (Robinul), propantheline bromide (Pro-Banthine), scopolamine hydrochloride (Transderm-Scōp), and others may cause acute urinary retention and bladder distention (Shlafer, 1993). Many other drug groups also have anticholinergic side effects and may cause urinary retention. Among these are antianxiety agents including diazepam (Valium), antidepressant and tricyclic drugs such as imipramine (Tofranil), antiparkinsonian drugs including benztropine mesylate (Cogentin) and trihexyphenidyl (Artane), antipsychotic agents such as chlorpromazine (Thorazine) and haloperidol (Haldol), and some sedative/hypnotic drugs. In addition, antihistamines common in over-the-counter cough, cold, allergy, and sleep-promoting drugs have anticholinergic effects and may interfere with bladder emptying. Diphenhydramine (Benadryl) is an example of a nonprescription antihistamine (Shlafer, 1993).

Voluntary urinary retention (particularly common among nurses!) may lead to overfilling of the bladder and a loss of detrusor muscle tone.

The client with urinary retention is unable to empty the bladder completely. Overflow voiding or incontinence may occur, with 25 to 50 mL of urine eliminated at frequent intervals. Assessment reveals a firm, distended bladder that may be displaced to one side of midline.

For the client with a mechanical obstruction to urine flow, removing or repairing the obstruction is the preferred method for treating urinary retention. The client with BPH may require a resection of the prostate gland; the client with bladder calculi, removal of the stones and measures to prevent their formation.

Placement of an indwelling urinary catheter or intermittent straight catheterization following surgery can prevent overdistention of the bladder and subsequent problems of urinary retention. Cholinergic medications such as bethanechol chloride (Urecholine), which promote detrusor muscle contraction and bladder emptying, may be used. Substituting a different medication with no anticholinergic side effects may be useful for the client with urinary retention related to medication use.

Nursing measures to promote urination can be helpful for the client with urinary retention. Placing the client in normal voiding position and providing for privacy are essential. Additional measures include running water, placing the client's hands in warm water, pouring warm water over the perineum, or taking a warm sitz bath.

The Client with a Neurogenic Bladder

■ ■ ■

The act of urination is reflexive, under control of the autonomic nervous system. In adults, however, higher cerebral control is normally used to maintain continence. The neurologic connections influencing normal bladder filling, the perception of fullness and the need to void, and voluntary bladder emptying are complex. Diseases or trauma to the central or peripheral nervous systems may interfere with normal mechanisms, resulting in a **neurogenic bladder.**

Pathophysiology

A simple reflex arc exists between the bladder and the spinal cord at levels S2 through S4. The stimulus of more than 400 mL of urine in the bladder results in reflex contraction of the detrusor muscle and bladder emptying unless voluntary control (cerebral input) is used to supress it (Wilson et al., 1991).

When central nervous system input to the bladder is disrupted above the sacral spinal cord segment, the typical result is a **spastic (hyperreflexic) neurogenic bladder.** Both sensory and voluntary control of urination are interrupted partially or totally, while the sacral reflex arc remains intact. The stimuli generated by filling of the bladder result in frequent spontaneous contraction of the detrusor muscle and involuntary bladder emptying (Porth, 1994). The most common cause of a spastic bladder is spinal cord injury superior to the sacral segment. Additional causes include cerebral vascular accidents, Alzheimer's disease, multiple sclerosis, and other central nervous system lesions (Porth, 1994; Wilson et al., 1991).

Damage to the sacral spinal cord at the level of the reflex arc, the cauda equina, or the sacral nerve roots results in *bladder atony* or a **flaccid neurogenic bladder.** The perception of bladder fullness is lost, and the bladder becomes overdistended, with weak and ineffective detrusor muscle contractions. Flaccid neurogenic bladder is also seen with myelomeningocele and during the spinal shock phase of a spinal cord injury above the sacral region. During the spinal shock phase, all reflex activity below the level of spinal cord injury is suppressed (Andreoli et al., 1990; Porth, 1994).

Peripheral neuropathies may also cause some degree of hyporeflexia of the bladder. Sensory or motor innervation may be selectively interrupted, or both may be affected. Clients may lose the sensation of bladder fullness and the urge to urinate but retain the ability to control detrusor muscle contraction and the external sphincter. Diabetes mellitus is the most common cause of peripheral bladder neuropathy. Other causes include multiple sclerosis, uremia, hypothyroidism, chronic alcoholism, and prolonged overdistention of the bladder (Porth, 1994; Wilson et al., 1991).

Collaborative Care

In general, the conditions that lead to neurogenic bladder are irreversible. Management is directed at maintaining continence and avoiding complications associated with either overfilling or incomplete emptying of the bladder. Because self-care is the goal, teaching is a primary intervention for the health care team.

Laboratory and Diagnostic Tests

The following laboratory and diagnostic tests may be ordered for the client with a neurogenic bladder:

- *Urine culture* to determine if a urinary tract infection is present. UTI is common when the bladder does not empty normally, and it may interfere with the client's ability to implement management techniques effectively.

- *Urinalysis* and *serum BUN* and *creatinine* to evaluate the renal function of the client. Ascending infection from the bladder or hydronephrosis resulting from bladder overfilling may damage the kidneys and impair their function. If damage has occurred, blood cells or protein may be present in the urine, and the serum BUN and creatinine may be elevated.

- *Postvoiding catheterization* to measure residual urine. After voiding, the bladder normally contains less than 50 mL of urine. Amounts greater than 50 mL may indicate ineffective detrusor muscle contractions, common in neurogenic bladder.

- *Cystometrography* to evaluate the filling pattern of the bladder. Cystometrography allows evaluation of the tone and function of the detrusor muscle. In addition, the type of neurogenic bladder dysfunction can be determined as spastic, flaccid, sensory, or motor (Chernecky et al., 1993).

Pharmacology

Medications may be employed in the management of the client with neurogenic bladder to increase or decrease the contractility of the detrusor muscle, increase or decrease the tone of the internal sphincter, or to relax the external urethral sphincter.

Bethanechol, a parasympathomimetic or cholinergic drug, simulates contraction of the detrusor muscle in flaccid neurogenic bladder. This drug is most effective in management of short-term conditions of urinary retention as may occur following surgery or childbirth. It may also be useful when combined with bladder-training techniques to promote complete emptying of a neurogenic bladder.

Anticholinesterase drugs such as neostigmine (Prostigmin) and pyridostigmine (Mestinon) also may be used to increase the tone of the detrusor muscle. These medications work by inhibiting the destruction of acetylcholine, increasing its availability to receptor sites.

Anticholinergic medications (parasympathetic blockers) such as propantheline bromide (Pro-Banthine), dicyclomine (Bentyl), flavoxate hydrochloride (Urispas), and oxybutynin relax the detrusor muscle and contract the internal sphincter, thereby increasing bladder capacity. Anticholinergics are beneficial in treating the client with a hyperreflexive or spastic neurogenic bladder. See the accompanying pharmacology box for the nursing implications of drugs used to modify detrusor muscle activity.

The internal sphincter is innervated by alpha-receptors of the sympathetic (adrenergic) nervous system. Alpha-adrenergic stimulants such as phenylephrine hydrochloride (Neo-Synephrine) and imipramine can increase internal sphincter tone, thus inhibiting voiding. Alpha-receptor blocking agents such as phenoxybenzamine (Dibenzyline) decrease internal sphincter tone, thereby promoting urination.

In clients with spinal cord injury, multiple sclerosis, or another condition resulting in muscle spasticity, skeletal muscle relaxants such as baclofen (Lioresal) or dantrolene sodium (Datrium) may be useful to control spastic neurogenic bladder (Porth, 1994; Shlafer, 1993).

Nursing Implications for Pharmacology: The Client with Neurogenic Bladder

MEDICATIONS USED TO STIMULATE DETRUSOR MUSCLE CONTRACTION

Cholinergic Drugs

Bethanechol chloride (Urocholine)

Bethanechol stimulates the parasympathetic nervous system, increasing detrusor muscle tone and producing a contraction strong enough to initiate micturition. It is used primarily in the treatment of acute postoperative and postpartum urinary retention and for neurogenic bladder atony with urinary retention.

Nursing Responsibilities

- Assess the client for possible contraindications for bethanechol, including known hypersensitivity, hyperthyroidism, peptic ulcer disease, asthma, significant bradycardia or hypotension, coronary artery disease, epilepsy, and parkinsonism. Do not administer to clients having undergone recent gastrointestinal or bladder surgery or clients with possible obstruction of the gastrointestinal or urinary tract.
- Administer oral preparations on an empty stomach to minimize the risk of nausea and vomiting.
- Parenteral bethanechol is administered subcutaneously.
- Observe for desired effect on urine elimination. Following oral administration, effects are usually noted within 30 to 60 minutes; subcutaneous doses achieve an effect within 5 to 15 minutes following injection.
- Assess the client for possible adverse responses, including malaise, headache, abdominal cramping, nausea, hypotension with reflex tachycardia, wheezing, and dyspnea.
- Atropine is the specific antidote for bethanechol overdose or toxicity. It should be kept on hand when this drug is administered subcutaneously.

Client and Family Teaching

- Take the medication 1 hour before or 2 hours after meals.
- Use caution when rising from a recumbent or sitting position; you may feel dizzy or lightheaded.

Anticholinesterase Agents

Neostigmine (Prostigmin)

Pyridostigmine (Mestinon)

Anticholinesterase agents work by inhibiting the action of cholinesterase (the enzyme responsible for acetylcholine breakdown), thus keeping more neurotransmitter at the neuromuscular junction and facilitating the transmission of impulses. These drugs are used primarily in the treatment of myasthenia gravis, a disease of progressive muscle weakness, but they are also useful in the treatment of urinary retention because they stimulate contraction of the detrusor muscle.

Nursing Responsibilities

- Assess the client for possible contraindications to the medication, as noted for bethanechol. Anticholinesterase drugs are contraindicated for clients with peritonitis or mechanical obstruction of the intestinal or urinary tracts.
- Keep atropine available as an antidote when administering anticholinesterase agents.
- When used for urinary retention, administer neostigmine 0.5 mg subcutaneously or intramuscularly. Repeat doses every 3 hours for a total of at least five injections.
- If the client does not urinate within 1 hour of the first injection, catheterization should be performed to empty the bladder.
- Assess the client for desired and possible adverse effects including allergic responses or anaphylaxis; mental status changes; cardiac dysrhythmias, hypotension; increased respiratory secretions, dyspnea, and respiratory depression; abdominal cramping, nausea, and vomiting; muscle cramps; and urinary frequency.

Client and Family Teaching

- Use the medication as prescribed; do not alter the dose unless recommended by the physician.
- Report any adverse effects promptly.

Pharmacology: The Client with Neurogenic Bladder (continued)

MEDICATIONS USED TO RELAX DETRUSOR MUSCLE AND CONTRACT INTERNAL SPHINCTER

Anticholinergic Agents

Propantheline bromide (Pro-Banthine)

Dicyclomine (Bentyl)

Flavoxate hydrochloride (Urispas)

Oxybutynin (Ditropan)

Anticholinergic drugs inhibit the response to acetylcholine, resulting in smooth-muscle relaxation. Through indirect stimulation of the sympathetic nervous system, these drugs increase contraction of the internal sphincter. The combination of detrusor relaxation and internal sphincter contraction serves to increase the bladder capacity of clients with spastic or hyperreflexive neurogenic bladder.

Nursing Responsibilities

- Assess for possible contraindications to therapy. These drugs should not be adminstered to clients with glaucoma, obstruction of the gastrointestinal or urinary tract, severe ulcerative colitis or toxic megacolon, unstable cardiovascular status, or myasthenia gravis.

- These drugs may delay the absorption of other medications administered at the same time. Observe closely for increased effect if the client is also taking another anticholinergic agent, narcotic analgesic, antidysrhythmic medication, antihistamine, phenothiazine, tricyclic antidepressant, or other psychoactive drug.

- Observe for the desired effect of increased bladder capacity with decreased incontinence and spasm.

- Assess for possible adverse effects, including dry mouth, decreased sweating, visual disturbances, urinary hesitancy or retention, dysrhythmias, mental status changes, and gastrointestinal disturbances.

Client and Family Teaching

- These drugs may cause drowsiness or blurred vision. Use caution when driving, operating machinery, or performing other tasks requiring mental acuity.

- Hard candies may be helpful to relieve dry mouth associated with these drugs.

- These drugs can decrease perspiration; use caution in hot weather to avoid heat prostration.

Dietary Intervention

In addition to taking medications, the client may modify diet to prevent infection and urolithiasis, complications common in clients with spinal cord injury and neurogenic bladder. A moderate to high fluid intake and a diet that acidifies the urine are helpful. Cranberry juice is widely used to maintain urine acidity. See Table 25–4 for additional acid ash foods to be included in the diet and alkaline ash foods to be avoided or minimized. The timing of fluid intake may be regulated to promote continence.

Physical Methods

The method employed to provide for bladder emptying and urinary continence varies according to the type of neurogenic bladder.

In clients with a spastic neurogenic bladder, techniques that stimulate reflex voiding and promote complete emptying of the bladder are used. These techniques include identification and use of trigger points, for example, stroking or pinching the abdomen, inner thigh, or glans penis. Pulling pubic hairs, tapping the suprapubic

region, or inserting a gloved finger into the rectum and gently stretching the anal sphincter can also stimulate urination.

Complete bladder emptying is facilitated by the *Credé method,* applying pressure to the suprapubic region with the fingers of one or both hands. Applying manual pressure to the abdomen and using the Valsalva maneuver (bearing down while holding one's breath) also promote bladder emptying for the client with a spastic or flaccid bladder. Care must be exercised when executing or teaching these maneuvers, because voiding maneuvers that increase lower abdominal and bladder pressure can stimulate *autonomic dysreflexia* in clients with spinal cord injuries. This response is a medical emergency in which the blood pressure rises to potentially fatal levels because of stimulation of the sympathetic nervous system. See Chapter 41 for a complete discussion of autonomic dysreflexia.

The client with a flaccid bladder may require catheterization to achieve complete bladder emptying. An indwelling catheter may be used during the initial period, but intermittent catheterization is preferred. The client

Applying Rehabilitation Principles to Medical-Surgical Nursing: Bladder Training

■ ■ ■

Bladder incontinence is a problem facing many clients in a medical-surgical setting. Rehabilitation principles utilized in bladder training can decrease the incidence of bladder incontinence.

Case Example

Ms. Cheryl Moss is a 23-year-old college student. Two years ago, she was involved in an auto accident, resulting in a complete transection of her spinal cord at C7. Ms. Moss is admitted to your unit for pneumonia. She is alert and oriented. Her vital signs are stable. She refuses an indwelling foley catheter because she states that she is on a bladder program.

Rehabilitation Principle
Conservation of existing function is a central goal of rehabilitation nursing. Alterations in bladder elimination can lead to further complications for a hospitalized client.

Rehabilitation Time Frame
Bladder training programs can take weeks to accomplish. Ms. Moss's hospitalization could force her to begin her bladder training program all over if the schedule of her current program is not maintained.

Nursing Diagnosis: Alteration in Bladder Elimination
Due to her spinal cord injury, Ms. Moss has a form of *neurogenic bladder* called a reflex neurogenic bladder. That is, despite her spinal cord damage, her emptying reflex is still intact. As Ms. Moss's primary nurse, you will need to maintain her bladder program.

Rehabilitation Goals and Interventions
1. Encourage the client to explain her individual bladder program. *Asking the client to actively participate in her plan of care facilitates the client's self-esteem and sense of control.*

2. Remove any indwelling foley catheter in the absence of spinal shock. *Once spinal shock has resolved, the client has spinal reflexes below the level of injury. The micturition reflex is present for Ms. Moss.*

3. Place client on a bedpan or commode every few hours. (Initially, this may be every two hours; then the time between voids can be increased.) When the client is on the commode, stimulate the micturition reflex by suprapubic tapping, stroking the inner thigh or gently pulling the pubic hair. *As the program progresses, improving bladder tone will allow for an increase in the time between voids. Suprapubic tapping, inner thigh stroking, and/or the gentle pulling of the pubic hair will stimulate the micturition reflex which will enhance bladder tone and stimulate emptying.*

4. When voiding has ended, perform a straight catheterization to remove residual urine. *Straight catheterization for residual urine completely empties the bladder. This prevents urinary stasis and also aids the maintenance of bladder function. When the residual urine volume decreases to below 100 cc, the time between straight catheterizations can be increased.*

5. Eventually the straight catheterization may not be necessary, as the bladder will empty effectively with only reflex stimulation.

who is able carries out clean intermittent self-catheterization every 3 to 4 hours to prevent overdistention of the bladder. See the procedure box "Client Self-Catheterization," page 1784, in Chapter 41.

Surgery

When clients with neurogenic bladder cannot effectively manage urination by using the preceding methods, surgical intervention may be necessary.

Rhizotomy, or destruction of the nerve supply to the detrusor muscle or the external sphincter, may be used for clients with hyperreflexia or spasticity. Urinary diversion is another surgical technique used when conservative management fails. See Table 25–7 for a summary of urinary diversion techniques and the box on bladder tumor

surgery (page 917) for nursing care of the client undergoing a urinary diversion.

Implantation of an artificial sphincter may be useful for some clients with neurogenic bladder. In addition, surgical techniques to innervate a flaccid neurogenic bladder are in the process of being developed (Porth, 1994).

Nursing Care

Nursing care of the client with a neurogenic bladder is directed toward promoting urinary drainage and continence, preventing complications, and teaching the client and family members self-care techniques. See the accompanying rehabilitation box.

Although each client has individual nursing care needs, examples of nursing diagnoses appropriate for the client with a neurogenic bladder include

- *Altered Urinary Elimination* related to impaired bladder innervation
- *Knowledge Deficit* related to lack of information about techniques to facilitate urination and bladder emptying
- *Self-Care Deficit* in toileting related to neurologic injury
- *Risk for Impaired Skin Integrity* related to urinary incontinence
- *Risk for Infection* related to impaired urination reflex

The Client with Urinary Incontinence

■ ■ ■

The most common manifestation of impaired bladder control is **urinary incontinence,** or involuntary urination. Incontinence can have significant impact on the client, leading to physical problems such as skin breakdown, infection, and rashes. Psychosocial consequences include embarrassment, isolation and withdrawal, feelings of worthlessness and helplessness, and depression.

Urinary incontinence is especially common among older clients; however, incontinence is not a normal consequence of aging. It is not a disease but rather a generally treatable symptom having many causes. The actual prevalence of urinary incontinence is nearly impossible to determine. Embarrassment and the availability of products to protect clothing and prevent detection contribute to clients' not seeking evaluation of and treatment for incontinence.

Pathophysiology

Approximately 10 million people in the United States have some degree of urinary incontinence. The estimated cost of managing incontinence is $10 billion yearly. In the long-term care, foster care, and home-bound populations, the incidence is about 50% (Burke & Walsh, 1992; Newman, 1994; Wold, 1993).

Urinary continence cannot be achieved unless the bladder is able to expand and contract and the sphincters are able to maintain a urethral pressure higher than that in the bladder. Incontinence results when the pressure within the urinary bladder exceeds the urethral resistance, allowing urine to escape. Any condition causing higher than normal bladder pressures or reduced urethral resistance can potentially result in incontinence. Relaxation of the pelvic musculature, disruption of cerebral and nervous system control, and disturbances of the bladder and its musculature are common contributing factors.

Incontinence may be an acute, self-limited disorder, or it may be chronic. The causes may be congenital or acquired, reversible or irreversible. Congenital disorders associated with incontinence include *epispadias* (a congenital absence of the upper wall of the urethra), and *meningomyelocele* (a neural tube defect in which a portion of the spinal cord and its surrounding meninges protrude through the vertebral column). Traumatic injury to the central nervous system or spinal cord, cerebrovascular accident, and chronic neurologic disorders such as multiple sclerosis and Parkinson's disease are examples of acquired, irreversible causes of incontinence. Acquired reversible causes include acute confusion, use of medications such as diuretics or sedatives, prostatic enlargement, vaginal and urethral atrophy, urinary tract infection, and fecal impaction (Burke & Walsh, 1992).

Incontinence is commonly categorized by the anatomic or physiologic dysfunction as stress incontinence, urge incontinence, overflow incontinence, reflex incontinence, and functional incontinence. Table 25-8 summarizes each type with its physiologic cause and associated factors.

A number of factors increase the incidence of incontinence in older clients. Aging decreases sensation and control of the bladder muscles. Hormone levels fall, resulting in atrophy of vaginal and urethral tissue. Abdominal muscle tone is generally reduced. In addition, a number of chronic diseases associated with incontinence, including cerebrovascular accident (stroke), Parkinson's disease, diabetes, and Alzheimer's disease and other dementias, are more prevalent in older populations. Also, older clients are more likely to be taking medications that contribute to incontinence. Drugs associated with urinary retention and resultant incontinence include certain antihypertensives, antiparkinsonian medications, antihistamines, anticholinergics, antispasmodics, and some sedatives and antianxiety agents.

Incontinence is also associated with multiple functional impairments. As a condition, it is associated with an increased risk for falls, fractures, pressure ulcers, urinary tract infection, and depression. It contributes to the stress of caregivers, who perceive their tasks as difficult, tiring, emotionally upsetting, and financially burdensome (Newman, 1994).

As stated before, however, incontinence is not a normal consequence of aging and should be investigated in the older clients as well as in younger people. See the nursing research box on page 928 for the application of research to nursing practice.

Collaborative Care

Although many people believe that urinary incontinence is something the client needs to learn to live with, in most cases incontinence can be cured or ameliorated. The box on page 928 outlines general principles of treatment de-

Table 25–8   Categories of Urinary Incontinence

	Description	Pathophysiology	Contributing Factors
Stress	Loss of urine associated with increased intra-abdominal pressure as occurs when sneezing, coughing, lifting. Quantity of urine lost is usually small.	Relaxation of pelvic musculature and weakness of urethra and surrounding muscles and tissues leads to decreased urethral resistance	■ Multiple pregnancies ■ Decreased estrogen levels ■ Short urethra, change in angle between bladder and urethra ■ Weakness of abdominal wall ■ Prostate surgery ■ Increased intra-abdominal pressure due to tumor, ascites, obesity
Urge	Inability to inhibit urine flow long enough to reach toilet after urge sensation	Hypertonic or overactive detrusor muscle leads to increased pressure within bladder and inability to inhibit voiding	■ Decreased bladder capacity ■ Bladder irritation from UTI, tumor, stones; irritants such as caffeine and alcohol ■ CNS disorders or spinal cord lesions
Overflow	Inability to empty bladder, resulting in overdistention and frequent loss of small amounts of urine	Outlet obstruction or lack of normal detrusor activity leads to overfilling of bladder and increased pressure	■ Spinal cord injuries below S2 ■ Diabetic neuropathy ■ Prostatic hypertrophy ■ Fecal impaction ■ Drugs, especially those with anticholinergic effect
Reflex	Involuntary loss of moderate volume of urine without stimulus or warning; may occur day or night	Abnormal spinal cord activity causing detrusor hyperreflexia in the absence of perceived sensation; increases bladder pressure	■ Spinal cord lesion or trauma above S2 ■ Neurologic disorders such as Parkinson's disease, multiple sclerosis, Alzheimer's disease ■ Cerebrovascular accident
Functional	Incontinence resulting from physical, environmental, or psychosocial causes	Ability to respond to the need to urinate is impaired	■ Confusion or dementia ■ Physical disability or impaired mobility ■ Diuretic therapy or sedation ■ Depression ■ Regression

veloped at a National Institutes of Health consensus-development conference.

Management of the client with incontinence is directed at identifying the cause and correcting it if possible. If it is not practical or possible to correct the underlying disorder, the client may be able to learn techniques to manage urine output effectively.

Evaluation of the client with incontinence begins with a complete history, including the duration, frequency, volume, and associated circumstances of incontinence. A voiding diary (Figure 25–7) is often used to provide detailed information. The client history also includes information regarding chronic or acute illnesses, previous surgeries, and current use of medications, both prescription and over-the-counter.

Physical assessment of the client with incontinence includes abdominal, rectal, and pelvic assessment as well as evaluation of mental and neurologic status, mobility, and dexterity. Findings often associated with incontinence in women include weak abdominal and pelvic muscle tone, cystocele or urethrocele, and atrophic vaginitis. In men, an enlarged prostate gland is the physical finding most commonly associated with incontinence.

Laboratory and Diagnostic Tests
Laboratory studies ordered to evaluate the client with urinary incontinence include the following:

■ *Urinalysis* and *urine culture* using a clean-catch specimen are used to rule out infection and other acute causes of incontinence.

■ *Serum creatinine* is one test used to assess renal function as a possible cause of incontinence. Unless renal

Applying Research to Nursing Practice: Knowledge, Attitudes, and Management of Urinary Incontinence in Long-Term Care Settings

Caregivers in long-term care settings often passively accept urinary incontinence despite evidence that specific techniques and care practices can be successful in controlling incontinence in the majority of clients. One study (Freundl & Dugan, 1992) looks at the attitudes, knowledge, and institutional culture in selected long-term care settings related to the management of urinary incontinence. Although nurses at all levels (nursing assistants, practical nurses, and registered nurses) were found to have a generally positive attitude toward clients with urinary incontinence, their knowledge of clinical interventions and nursing research was found to be weak. Few clients had written plans for incontinence management, and more than half of the agencies surveyed used indwelling catheters for incontinence in some clients, despite well-published data on their hazards. Nurses with more knowledge about incontinence management perceived greater job satisfaction.

Implications for Nursing

Approximately 60% to 70% of nursing home and long-term care clients have some degree of urinary incontinence. The associated costs are very high; these include laundry, incontinence pads or briefs, infections resulting from catheterization, skin and tissue break-

down, continued institutionalization, and the psychologic and emotional toll on the client and caregivers. Although interventions for incontinence are labor intensive, the reduced cost of clean-up and a more positive, helping attitude of caregivers are benefits beyond the direct benefit to the client. Provision of more educational opportunities for nurses through basic education programs, inservice trainings, and self-study can also help reduce this cost. For these interventions to be fully successful, institutions need to support the shifting of costs to allow labor-intensive programs.

Critical Thinking in Client Care

1. Why is a higher level of knowledge about urinary incontinence associated with more job satisfaction in nurses in long-term care?

2. How could stress, urge, functional, and total incontinence be differentiated in a long-term care client with dementia?

3. What nursing interventions would be specific to each of the above types of incontinence?

4. How would you teach nursing assistants about urinary incontinence management in long-term care?

---

function is impaired, the serum creatinine is normal in most clients with chronic urinary incontinence.

- *Blood urea nitrogen (BUN)* is also used to rule out underlying renal disease as the cause of incontinence.

- *Blood glucose* may be ordered to screen for diabetes which can interfere with neurologic control of the bladder and the perception of bladder fullness.

When further diagnostic evaluation is indicated, the following examinations may be ordered:

- *Measurement of postvoiding residual urine* is the simplest and least expensive of the specialized tests for incontinence. It is used to determine how completely the bladder is emptied with voiding. Less than 50 mL of residual urine is expected; clients having 100 mL or

---

Principles of Urinary Incontinence Treatment

- Evaluation and treatment must be considered for all persons with urinary incontinence.

- Evaluation of the anatomy and of the function of urine storage and emptying guides treatment decisions.

- Treatment decisions are also influenced by the personality, environment, expectations, and clinical status of the individual.

- The client must have adequate information to make an educated choice among treatment options.

- Therapy plans should include strategies to deal with environmental factors in the community or institution.

- Accessible public toilets must be made available in adequate numbers (*Reaching a consensus*, 1989).

Figure 25–7 A sample voiding diary. Courtesy of Oregon Health Sciences University.

DATE ___4/15/96___

Please complete this chart prior to your visit. Choose a 24-hour period when it is convenient for you to measure and record the following: the amount of fluid you void (urinate), the amount of fluid you drink and type of beverage, the time, when leakage episodes occur, whether or not you have an urge to void just prior to leaking, and the activity you are doing when you leak or need to void. For example:

Void Amount (oz.)	Fluid Intake Amount (oz.)	Time	Leak?	Urge prior to leak?	Activity
6 oz.	8 oz. coffee	7:00 AM	–	–	awakening
–	–	7:20 AM	yes	yes	washing

VOIDING DIARY

DIARY.URO

Void Amount (oz.)	Fluid Intake Amount (oz.)	Time	Leak?	Urge prior to leak?	Activity
14 oz.		6:23 am	yes	yes	Awakening
~~14 oz~~ 8 oz.	14 oz. coffee	6:35			
		8:05	yes	yes	reading
	16 oz. coffee	8:30			
10 oz.		9:10	yes	yes	watch TV
10 oz.		9:30	"	"	"
12 oz.	8 oz. water	10:17	"	"	"
6 oz.		11:40	yes	yes	washing dishes
8 oz.	12 oz. coke	2:12 pm	yes	yes	Lunch
	16 oz. water	6:30			Dinner
10 oz.		8:00	yes	yes	Laundry
6 oz.		9:55	yes	yes	folding clothes
	8 oz. water	11:25			Bed time
6 oz.		1:30 am	–	yes	sleeping
8 oz.	–	5:05	–	yes	sleeping
5 oz.		6:30	–	yes	Awakening
	TOTAL				

more of residual urine are generally referred for further testing.

- *Cystometrography* is used to assess the neuromuscular function of the bladder by evaluating detrusor muscle function and tone, the pressure within the bladder, and the filling pattern of the bladder. Sterile water or saline is instilled into the bladder, and the client is asked to describe sensations and feelings of the urge to void. Bladder pressure and volume are recorded on a graph. When the bladder is full, the client voids, and intravesical pressure is noted during voiding.

  Normally, the urge to void is experienced at 150 to 450 mL, and the perception of bladder fullness at 300 to 500 mL (Chernecky et al., 1993).

- *Uroflowmetry* is a noninvasive test used to evaluate voiding patterns. The uroflowmeter, contained in a funnel, measures the rate of urine flow, the continuous flow time, and the total voiding time.

- *Intravenous pyelography* may be ordered to detect ureteral, bladder, and urethral abnormalities, such as malformations or strictures contributing to incontinence.

- *Cystoscopy* allows visualization of the urethra and bladder and identification of possible causes of incontinence, such as an enlarged prostate or a tumor interfering with bladder filling.

- *Ultrasonography* of the kidneys and bladder may allow

Nursing Implications for Diagnostic Tests: The Client with Urinary Incontinence

■ ■ ■

Postvoiding Residual Volume

Preparation of the Client

- Instruct the client to notify the nurse the next time the urge to void (urinate) is felt.

- Have the client void into a bedpan, commode, or measuring device on the toilet. Instruct the client to empty the bladder as completely as possible. Provide for privacy to avoid "shy-bladder" syndrome.

- Immediately after voiding, catheterize the client using aseptic technique and a straight catheter. Drain the bladder completely to determine the amount of residual urine present.

- Record and report findings including time; amount voided; amount obtained on catheterization; color, clarity, and odor of urine; and any other significant data.

Client and Family Teaching

- This test is used to determine how completely you empty your bladder with voiding.

- Residual urine (urine left in the bladder after urination) increases the risks of urinary infection due to urine stagnation and incontinence due to overflow.

- This test, because it is invasive, poses a slight risk of infection. Report symptoms of frequency, urgency, pain on urination, nocturia, and cloudy, bloody, or malodorous urine.

Cystometrogram (CMG)

Preparation of the Client

- Verify the presence of a signed consent for the test.

- Check for presence of UTI as indicated by urinalysis or physical signs; infection may interfere with the test results.

- No food or fluid restriction is required for this test.

Client and Family Teaching

- This test evaluates bladder capacity, and the motor (contraction) and sensory functions of the bladder.

- You will be given privacy during the procedure so that you won't be unnecessarily exposed.

- Don't strain to void during the test; straining may invalidate the results.

- You will be asked to describe your sensations as the bladder is filled, including the first urge to void, the sensation of being unable to delay urination any longer, and any others such as pain, sweating, or nausea.

- The test requires about 45 minutes to complete.

- Report persistent hematuria or signs of infection to the physician.

- A warm tub or sitz bath may help to relieve discomfort after testing.

Uroflowmetry

Preparation of the Client

- Withhold medications that may interfere with test results.

Client and Family Teaching

- This is a rapid, simple test to measure and record the volume of urine voided per second.

- Privacy is provided during testing. Male clients void while standing; females, while sitting.

- You will urinate into a funnel.

- Drugs affecting bladder and sphincter tone, client movement during testing, and straining during voiding may invalidate test results.

- Increase your fluid intake and don't urinate for several hours prior to the test to ensure a full bladder and a strong urge to void during testing.

- No discomfort or risk is associated with this test.

---

identification of abnormal tissue densities or obstructions causing incontinence.

Nursing implications for the specialized studies for urinary incontinence are outlined in the box above.

Pharmacology

Drugs are not considered the treatment of choice in most cases of chronic urinary incontinence, but several classes of drugs may be useful.

Clients with urge incontinence may be treated with preparations that increase bladder capacity. Drugs used to inhibit detrusor muscle contractions and increase bladder capacity include anticholinergics such as propantheline; direct smooth-muscle relaxants such as oxybutynin, flavoxate, and dicyclomine; calcium-channel blockers such as verapamil (Calan) and nifedipine (Procardia); and tricyclic antidepressants, especially imipramine. The anticholinergic effects of many of these drugs may cause the

Nursing Care of the Client Having Surgery for Stress Incontinence

PREOPERATIVE CARE

- Assess the client's knowledge and understanding of the procedure. Provide instruction and clarification as needed. *Knowledge and understanding increase the client's ability to cooperate with postoperative care procedures.*

- Teach the client about the use of analgesia, deep breathing, and movement after surgery. The client should also avoid straining and the Valsalva maneuver postoperatively. *Adequate levels of analgesia promote movement and healing. The risk of respiratory complications postoperatively is minimized by deep breathing techniques, use of incentive spirometry, and movement. Straining and increased abdominal pressure during the Valsalva maneuver may place excessive stress on suture lines and interfere with healing.*

- Make sure there is a signed consent in the client's chart, and carry out preoperative procedures as ordered.

POSTOPERATIVE CARE

- Assess client status on a routine and frequent basis. *Early detection of surgical complications allows for immediate intervention and minimizes long-term effects. Bright red urine, excessive vaginal drainage, or incisional bleeding may indicate hemorrhage.*

- Monitor urinary output for quantity, color, and clarity. *Expect urine to be pink initially, gradually clearing. Instrumentation of the urinary tract increases the potential for UTI; cloudy urine may be an early sign.*

- Maintain stability and patency of urinary catheters (suprapubic, urethral, or both). *Catheter patency and adequate renal function are vital to prevent complications. Bladder decompression eliminates pressure on suture lines. Catheters should be taped in position to avoid movement, pulling, and resultant pressure on surgical incisions.*

- Have the client move and walk as soon as possible. *Early mobility helps prevent respiratory and vascular complications, such as pneumonia and thromboembolism.*

- After the catheter is removed, monitor urine output carefully. *Difficulty voiding is common following catheter removal. Early intervention to prevent bladder distention is important.*

- If the client is to be discharged with a urethral or suprapubic catheter in place, teach proper care to the client and family members as needed. *Appropriate self-care minimizes complications. Recognizing the signs of possible complications, such as UTI, leads to early intervention.*

---

client to experience dry mouth and eyes, constipation, and confusion. Drugs with anticholinergic effects are also contraindicated for the client with glaucoma. Urinary retention is another potential side effect that must be considered when these drugs are used.

Clients with stress incontinence may find drugs causing smooth-muscle contraction of the bladder neck useful. Phenylpropanolamine (Triaminic), a commonly used decongestant, is the most effective preparation used. Pseudoephedrine (Sudafed) and ephedrine (Marax) are also used for this purpose.

When incontinence is associated with postmenopausal atrophic vaginitis, estrogen therapy may be effective. Both systemic estrogens and local creams are used.

Surgery

Surgical techniques are used most often in the treatment of stress incontinence associated with cystocele or ure-

throcele and overflow incontinence associated with an enlarged prostate gland.

Suspension of the bladder neck, a technique that brings the angle between the bladder and urethra closer to normal, is effective in treating stress incontinence associated with urethrocele in 80% to 95% of clients. The procedure used may involve a suprapubic abdominal incision, a vaginal approach, or the use of endoscopic instruments. Care of the client with a bladder neck suspension is outlined in the accompanying box.

Prostatectomy, using either the transurethral or suprapubic approach, is indicated for the client who is experiencing overflow incontinence as a result of an enlarged prostate gland and urethral obstruction. Care of the client with a prostatectomy is outlined in Chapter 46.

Other surgical procedures of potential benefit in the treatment of incontinence include implantation of an artificial sphincter, formation of a urethral sling to elevate and compress the urethra, and augmentation of the bladder with bowel segments to increase bladder capacity.

Nursing Care

In planning nursing care for the client with urinary incontinence, the nurse should consider the client's mental and neurologic status, mobility, and motivation. Behavioral techniques can be very effective in treating incontinence, but they require long-term commitment by the client as well as the physical and mental capability to implement them.

Nursing care and routine modifications can be effective in restoring continence fully or partially even in the institutionalized client. Scheduled toileting, bladder training, and prompted voiding combined with reinforcing techniques such as praise can reduce the need for diapers, incontinence pads, and indwelling catheters.

Although each client has individual needs, the nursing diagnoses discussed in this section focus on knowledge deficit, self-care deficit in toileting, and social isolation.

Knowledge Deficit

Many clients assume urinary incontinence to be a normal consequence of aging and something to "learn to live with." In reality, exercises to strengthen pelvic floor muscles, dietary modifications, and bladder-training programs can be very effective in restoring and maintaining continence.

Nursing interventions with rationales follow.

- Instruct the client to keep a voiding diary. Teach the client to record the the time and amount of all fluid intake and urinary output, status at the time of voiding (dry or wet; minimal, moderate, or large amount) and of arising from sleep, and any other significant factors. *Voiding diaries provide valuable information for diagnosing and treating incontinence.*

- Teach exercises to strengthen pelvic floor muscles, including *Kegel exercises* (see the accompanying box). Instruct the client to consciously tighten the pelvic muscles when the need to void is perceived and to relax the abdomen while walking to the bathroom. *Improved pelvic muscle strength helps clients retain urine and prevents stress incontinence by increasing the urethral pressure. Exercises also decrease abnormal detrusor muscle contractions, decreasing pressure within the bladder.*

- With the help of the client's voiding diary, instruct the client in dietary and fluid intake modifications to reduce stress and urge incontinence. Among these are limiting the consumption of caffeine, alcohol, citrus juices, and artificial sweeteners; limiting fluid intake to 1.5 to 2 liters per day; and limiting evening fluid intake. *Caffeine, alcohol, and citrus juices are bladder irri-*

Pelvic Floor (Kegel) Exercises

■ ■ ■

- Identify the pelvic muscles using the following techniques:
   a. Stop the flow of urine during voiding and hold for a few seconds.
   b. Tighten the muscles at the orifice of the vagina around a gloved finger or tampon.
   c. Tighten the muscles around the anus as though resisting fecal passage.

- Perform exercises by tightening pelvic muscles, holding for 10 seconds, and relaxing for 10 to 15 seconds. Continue the sequence (tighten, hold, relax) for ten repetitions.

- Keep abdominal muscles and breathing relaxed while performing exercises.

- Initially, exercises should be performed twice per day, working up to four times a day.

- Encourage the client to exercise at a specific time each day or in conjunction with another daily activity (such as bathing, watching the news, or preparing for bed). It's important to establish a habitual routine because these exercises should be continued for life.

- Assistive devices, such as vaginal cones and biofeedback, may be useful for clients who have difficulty identifying appropriate muscle groups.

---

tants and tend to promote detrusor instability, increasing the risk of urge incontinence. Artificial sweeteners may also irritate the bladder. Fluid intake of 1.5 to 2 liters per day is adequate for health maintenance in most clients; excess fluid intake may increase stress incontinence if bathroom facilities are not readily available.

- Teach the client to minimize stress and urge incontinence by voiding on schedule. If the bulk of fluid is consumed in the morning hours, voiding every 1 to 2 hours may prevent involuntary loss of urine. *Emptying the bladder before the urge to void is experienced minimizes the risk that bladder pressure will exceed urethral pressure.*

Self-Care Deficit: Toileting

In the institutionalized older adult, functional incontinence may be the predominant problem. Mobility limitations, impaired vision, dementias, lack of access to facilities and privacy, and tight staffing patterns all increase the possibility of incontinence in previously continent people. In clients with functional incontinence, the primary problem is not with the genitourinary tract or pelvic structures, but an outside factor that interferes with the ability to respond normally to the urge to void. An immobilized client may wet the bed if a call bell is not within reach; a client with Alzheimer's disease may experience an urge to void but be unable to interpret the meaning of the sensation and respond by seeking a bathroom. For these clients, self-care deficit in toileting is a primary problem.

Nursing interventions with rationales follow.

- Assess the client's physical and mental capabilities and limitations, usual pattern of voiding, and ability to assist in toileting activities. *A thorough assessment allows you to plan interventions that address the client's specific needs and that encourage independence to the highest possible degree.*

- Provide assistive devices as needed to facilitate independence, such as raised toilet seats, grab bars, a bedside commode, or night lights. *Promoting the highest degree of independence possible in toileting activities bolsters the client's self-concept and helps the client maintain a positive body image.*

- Plan a toileting schedule based on the client's normal patterns of elimination to achieve approximately 300 mL of urine output with each bladder emptying. *Allowing the bladder to fill to a point at which the urge to void is experienced and then emptying it completely helps maintain normal bladder capacity and bacteriostatic functions.*

- Position the client for ease of voiding—sitting for females, standing for males—and provide for privacy. Avoid the use of bedpans and catheters if at all possible. *Normal positioning, usual toileting facilities, and privacy enhance the client's ability to void on schedule and empty the bladder completely.*

- Adjust fluid intake so that the client consumes the majority of fluids during those times of day that the client is most able to remain continent. Assist with toileting activities. *Unless fluids are restricted, maintain a fluid intake of at least 1.5 to 2 liters per day to assure adequate hydration and urinary function.*

- Help the client choose clothing that is easily removed, e.g., loose-fitting pants with a fly for male clients, elastic-waisted pants or loose dresses with loose-fitting undergarments for female clients. Velcro and zipper fasteners may be easier to use than snaps and buttons. *Clothing that is difficult to remove may increase the risk of urge incontinence in the client with mobility problems or impaired dexterity.*

Social Isolation

The client with any form of urinary incontinence is at risk for social isolation due to embarrassment, fear of not having ready access to a bathroom, body odor, or other fac-

tors. Social isolation, in turn, can increase problems of incontinence, because normal cues and relationships are lost, and the need to remain dry and "acceptable" is less strongly felt.

Nursing interventions with rationales follow.

- Assess reasons for and extent of social isolation. Discuss previous social interaction patterns with the client and client expectations for socialization. *To ensure an accurate assessment, it is vital to verify your perceptions of the client's degree of social isolation and its possible causes with the client or significant other.*

- According to the client's ability and readiness to learn, provide the client with information about the isolation and its contributing factors. *The client who is socially isolated as a result of urinary incontinence may not be aware of the extent to which the isolation is self-imposed and interfering with relationships.*

- Refer the client for urologic examination and evaluation of incontinence. *Clients who assume that urinary incontinence is a normal part of the aging may not be aware of behavioral, dietary, pharmacologic, and surgical options for treatment.*

- Explore alternative coping strategies with client, significant other, staff, and other health team members. *Protective pads or shields, good perineal hygiene, scheduled voiding, and clothing that does not interfere with toileting can enhance not only continence but also the client's self-esteem, and willingness to socialize.*

Other Nursing Diagnoses

The following nursing diagnoses may also apply to the client with urinary incontinence:

- *Altered Patterns of Urinary Elimination*
- *Functional Urinary Incontinence* related to impaired physical mobility
- *Risk for Impaired Skin Integrity* related to incontinence
- *Body Image Disturbance* related to incontinence

Client and Family Teaching

Because urinary incontinence is a contributing factor in the institutionalization of many older people, client and family teaching can have a significant impact on maintaining the independence of the client in the community. The areas of greatest teaching need are the possible causes of incontinence, the need for assessment, and the methods for treating and controlling incontinence.

Other teaching/learning needs for the client with urinary incontinence include the management of fluid intake, perineal care to minimize the risk of skin breakdown, and available products for clothing protection.

Case Study of a Client with Urinary Incontinence: Anna Giovanni

Anna Giovanni, a 76-year-old retired school teacher, lives in an urban retirement complex. She has been widowed for 10 years and lives alone. Her three grown children and their families live in the same metropolitan area. Mrs. Giovanni's eldest daughter expresses concern that her mother seems increasingly reluctant to leave the apartment to visit friends and family. She reports that the odor of urine is strong throughout her mother's apartment and that her mother's bed is often wet. She states that she worried about needing to place her mother in a nursing home if she cannot continue to live independently.

Assessment

Jane Oberle, a nurse practitioner, examines Mrs. Giovanni. In talking with Ms. Oberle, Mrs. Giovanni admits that she has problems with urine leakage with a strong urge to void when laughing, coughing, and on hearing the sound of running water. At night, her urge to void is so strong that she is often unable to reach the bathroom in time. Mrs. Giovanni denies a history of UTIs, any neurologic disorders, or difficulty with her bowels. She had a hysterectomy at age 52 and was on estrogen-replacement therapy for approximately 10 years afterward, but she discontinued therapy because "it was such a nuisance." Mrs. Giovanni has been taking digoxin 0.125 mg daily, furosemide 40 mg twice daily, and potassium chloride 20 mEq three times daily for mild congestive heart failure.

Physical assessment reveals a moderate cystourethrocele and atrophy of the vaginal and vulvar tissues. A moderate perineal dermatitis is noted. Pelvic floor strength is weak. Urinalysis is within normal limits, and postvoiding residual urine is 5 mL.

Analysis of Mrs. Giovanni's voiding diary shows a moderate consumption of tea and juices throughout the day, nine daytime voidings and four night voidings with an average volume of about 250 mL per void. She notices urine leakage most often in the late afternoon and at night. Based on Mrs. Giovanni's history, physical assessment, and voiding diary, Ms. Oberle diagnoses Anna's problem as stress incontinence with an urgency component and decides to try a conservative approach before referring Mrs. Giovanni for further testing and possible cystourethrocele repair. She prescribes estrogen cream and a barrier cream to treat Mrs. Giovanni's vulvitis.

Diagnosis

Ms. Oberle identifies these nursing diagnoses for Mrs. Giovanni:

- *Stress Incontinence* related to weak pelvic floor musculature and tissue atrophy

- *Urge Incontinence* related to possible bladder irritation due to intake of caffeine and citrus juices
- *Impaired Skin Integrity* related to constant contact of urine with perineal tissues
- *Ineffective Individual Coping* related to inability to control urine leakage

Expected Outcomes

The expected outcomes of the plan of care are that Mrs. Giovanni will

- Remain dry between voidings and at night.
- Demonstrate improved perineal muscle strength.
- Regain and maintain perineal skin integrity.
- Return to her previous level of social activity.

Planning and Implementation

Ms. Oberle and the clinic staff plan and implement the following interventions with Mrs. Giovanni and her daughter:

- Teach Mrs. Giovanni how to identify pelvic floor muscles and how to perform Kegel exercises to improve strength.
- Switch Mrs. Giovanni to decaffeinated tea and noncitrus fruit juices (grape, apple, and cranberry).
- Encourage her to minimize fluid intake after her evening meal.
- Change afternoon dose of furosemide from 9:00 p.m. to 4:00 p.m.
- Have Mrs. Giovanni void by the clock, gradually increasing intervals from every 45 to 60 minutes to every 2 to 2½ hours. Instruct her to maintain shorter voiding intervals for 2 to 3 hours after furosemide doses.
- Teach Mrs. Giovanni to cleanse the perineal area thoroughly, wiping front to back, after each voiding or incident of urine leakage.
- Introduce Mrs. Giovanni and her daughter to commercial products available for clothing and furniture protection, encouraging them to experiment until they find the most appropriate and helpful product.
- Provide a commode to keep at her bedside at night and adequate lighting to prevent injury.
- Schedule follow-up visits and evaluations to provide reinforcement of teaching and encouragement to continue exercise and dietary program.

Evaluation

Three months after her initial evaluation, Mrs. Giovanni states that she is doing very well, experiencing occasional leakage of small amounts of urine, primarily when sneezing, coughing, or laughing. She finds a minipad adequate for protection and is often able to remain dry all day. She has had no further problems with enuresis since changing her evening furosemide dose to an earlier hour and limiting her fluids after dinner. She still voids nine or ten times during the day, on average, but only once at night. She is able to make it to the bathroom and no longer needs the bedside commode. Her perineal tissue is intact, and she demonstrates improved muscle strength. Anna's daughter says her mother is beginning to resume her normal social activities. Her daughter is no longer worried about her mother's ability to care for herself independently.

Critical Thinking in the Nursing Process

1. What factors in Mrs. Giovanni's past medical history and current medication regimen contributed to her problem with nighttime incontinence? Why?

2. What is the rationale for including an intervention to teach Mrs. Giovanni about perineal cleansing as part of her care plan?

3. Outline a plan for teaching Mrs. Giovanni about uroflowmetry and cystometrography.

4. Develop a care plan for Mrs. Giovanni for the nursing diagnosis *Self-Esteem Disturbance* related to urinary incontinence.

Bibliography

■ ■ ■

Andreoli, T. E., Carpenter, C. C. J., Plum, F., Smith, L. H. (1990). *Cecil essentials of medicine* (2nd ed.). Philadelphia: Saunders.

Berkow, R., & Fletcher, A. J. (Eds.). (1992). *The Merck manual of diagnosis and therapy* (16th ed.). Rahway, NJ: Merck Research Laboratories.

Birchenall, J. M., & Streight, M. E. (1993). *Care of the older adult* (3rd ed.). Philadelphia: Lippincott.

Bullock, B. L., & Rosendahl, P. P. (1992). *Pathophysiology: Adaptations and alterations in function* (3rd ed.). Philadelphia: Lippincott.

Burke, M. M., & Walsh, M. B. (1992). *Gerontologic nursing: Care of the frail elderly*. St. Louis: Mosby-Year Book.

Burke, S. R. (1992). *Human anatomy and physiology in health and disease* (3rd ed.). Albany, NY: Delmar.

Cavas, M., & Makay, S. (1991). The Indiana pouch: A continent urinary diversion system. *AORN Journal, 54*(3), 494–497, 499, 501–506, 508+.

Centers for Disease Control. (1993, August 31). Advance report of final mortality statistics, 1991. *Monthly Vital Statistics Report, 42* (Suppl.) (2).

Chernecky, C. C., Krech, R. L., & Berger, B. J. (1993). *Laboratory tests and diagnostic procedures*. Philadelphia: Saunders.

Clinical laboratory tests: Values and implications. (1991). Springhouse, PA: Springhouse.

Denson, C. E. (1990). Ureteral stents: Indications, placement procedures, patient care. *AORN Journal, 51*(5), 1293–1295, 1297–1298, 1300–1302, 1304+.

Faller, N., & Lawrence, K. (1994, January). Obtaining a urine specimen from a conduit urostomy. *American Journal of Nursing, 94*(1), 37.

Flynn, L., Cell, P., & Luisi, E. (1994). Effectiveness of pelvic muscle exercises in reducing urine incontinence among community residing elders. *Journal of Gerontological Nursing, 20*(5), 23–27.

Freundl, M., & Dugan, J. (1992). Urinary incontinence in the elderly: Knowledge and attitude of long-term care staff. *Geriatric Nursing, 13*(2), 70–75.

Foxman, B. (1990). Recurring urinary tract infection: Incidence and risk factors. *American Journal of Public Health, 80*(3), 331–333.

Gillenwater, J. Y., Grayhack, J. T., Howards, S. S., & Duckett, J. W. (1987). *Adult and pediatric urology* (Vol. 1). Chicago: Year Book.

Kee, J. L. (1991). *Laboratory and diagnostic tests with nursing implications* (3rd ed.). Norwalk, CT: Appleton & Lange.

Kuula, V. (1990). Stoma care: Eye of the beholder. *Nursing Times, 86*(48), 57, 59–60.

Lederer, J. R., Marculescu, G. L., Mocnik, B., & Seaby, N. (1993). *Care planning pocket guide: A nursing diagnosis approach* (5th ed.). Redwood City, CA: Addison-Wesley Nursing.

Mackety, C. J. (1990). Lasers in urology. *Nursing Clinics of North America, 25*(3), 697–709.

Malseed, R. T., & Harrigan, G. S. (1989). *Textbook of pharmacology and nursing care using the nursing process*. Philadelphia: Lippincott.

McCance, K. L., & Huether, S. E. (1994). *Pathophysiology: The biologic basis for disease in adults and children* (2nd ed.). St. Louis: Mosby-Year Book.

Memmler, R. L., Cohen, B. J., & Wood, D. L. (1992). *The human body in health and disease* (7th ed.). Philadelphia: Lippincott.

Miller, B. F., & Keane, C. B. (1987). *Encyclopedia and dictionary of medicine, nursing, and allied health* (4th ed.). Philadelphia: Saunders.

Millette-Petit, J. M. (1988). Urinary tract infections in older adults. *The Nurse Practitioner, 13*(12); 21–24, 29.

Newman, D. K. (1994, August). Strategies for managing urinary incontinence in homebound patients. *Advance for Nurse Practitioners, 2*(8), 11–14.

Newman, D. K., Lynch, K., Smith, D. A., & Cell, P. (1991). Restoring Urinary Continence. *American Journal of Nursing, 91*(1), 28–34.

Pagana, K. D., & Pagana, T. J. (1992). *Mosby's diagnostic and laboratory test reference*. St. Louis: Mosby-Year Book.

Physicians' desk reference (48th ed.). (1994). Montvale, NJ: Medical Economics Data Production Company.

Porth, C. M. (1994). *Pathophysiology: Concepts of altered health states* (4th ed.). Philadelphia: Lippincott.

Price, S. A., & Wilson, L. M. (1992). *Pathophysiology: Clinical concepts of disease processes* (4th ed.). St. Louis: Mosby-Year Book.

Rauscher, J., Farber, R. D., & Parra, R. O. (1991). Camey procedure: A continent urinary diversion technique. *AORN Journal, 54*(1), 34, 36–37, 39–41, 44.

Reaching a consensus on incontinence. (1989). *Geriatric Nursing, 10*(2), 78–80.

Schoemick, L., Katz, P., & Beam, T. (1991). The many guises of infection. *Geriatric Nursing, 12*(5); 223–224.

Shlafer, M. (1993). *The nurse, pharmacology, and drug therapy: A prototype approach* (2nd ed.). Redwood City, CA: Addison-Wesley.

Skach, W., Daley, C. L., & Forsmark, C. E. (1988). *Handbook of medical treatment* (18th ed.). Greenbrae, CA: Jones Medical Publications.

Smith, D. B., & Babaian, R. J. (1989). Patient adjustment to an ileal conduit after radical cystecomy. *Journal of Enterostomal Therapy, 16*(6), 244–246.

Stopping acute ureteral colic at the source. (1990). *Emergency Medicine, 22*(9), 104, 107.

Tierney, L. M., Jr., McPhee, S. J., & Papadakis, M. A. (Eds.). (1994). *Current medical diagnosis and treatment* (33rd ed.). Norwalk, CT: Appleton & Lange.

Tisher, C. C., & Wilcox, C. S. (Eds.). (1993). *Nephrology for the house officer* (2nd ed.). Baltimore: Williams & Wilkins.

Todd, B. (1990). Treating UTIs. *Geriatric nursing, 11*(2), 95–96.

Tucker, S. M., Canobbio, M. M., Paquette, E. V., & Wells, M. F. (1992). *Patient care standards: Nursing process, diagnosis, and outcomes* (5th ed.). St. Louis: Mosby-Year Book.

Tulloch, G. J. (1989). The incontinency taboo. *Geriatric Nursing, 10*(1), 19.

Way, L. W. (Ed.). (1994). *Current surgical diagnosis and treatment* (10th ed.). Norwalk, CT: Appleton & Lange.

Wells, T. (1990). Conquering incontinence. *Geriatric Nursing, 11*(3), 133–135.

Wesorick, B. (1990). *Standards of nursing care: A model for clinical practice*. Philadelphia: Lippincott.

Wilson, J. D., Braunwald, E., Isselbacher, K. J., Petersdorf, R. G., Martin, J. B., Fauci, A. S., & Root, R. K. (Eds.). (1991). *Harrison's principles of internal medicine* (12th ed.). New York: McGraw-Hill.

Wold, G. (1993). *Basic geriatric nursing*. St. Louis: Mosby-Year Book.

Wyndaele, J., & Maes, D. (1990). Clean intermittent self-catheterization: A 12-year followup. *The Journal of Urology, 143*(5), 906–908.

Yurick, A. G., Spier, B. E., Robb, S. S., & Ebert, N. J. (1989). *The aged person and the nursing process* (3rd ed.). Norwalk, CT: Appleton & Lange.

Nursing Care of Clients with Kidney Disorders

LEARNING OBJECTIVES

After completing this chapter, you will be able to

- Describe the pathophysiology of commonly occurring disorders of the kidneys.
- Relate manifestations of renal disease to the pathophysiologic mechanism involved.
- Discuss laboratory and diagnostic tests used to diagnose disorders of the kidneys.
- Discuss the nursing implications for medications prescribed for the client with a renal disorder.

- Identify specific dietary modifications prescribed for clients with renal disorders.
- Compare and contrast peritoneal dialysis and hemodialysis as therapies for renal failure.
- Discuss the nursing implications for a client undergoing dialysis.
- Provide appropriate nursing care for the client who has had a nephrectomy, renal transplant, or other surgery involving the kidney.
- Use the nursing process to plan and provide individualized care to clients with renal disorders.

The internal environment of the body normally remains in a relatively constant or *homeostatic* state. The kidneys help maintain homeostasis by regulating the composition and volume of extracellular fluid. The kidneys excrete excess water and solutes and are also able to conserve water and solute constituents when deficits occur. In addition, they are involved in regulating acid-base balance and excreting metabolic wastes. The long-term regulation of blood pressure is also a key function of the kidneys.

Renal function can be affected by primary diseases and by disorders that are secondary to systemic diseases, such as diabetes mellitus and systemic lupus erythematosus. In North America, more than 20 million people are affected by kidney and urinary tract diseases. Every year, approximately one in every 10,000 people in the United States develops end-stage renal disease (ESRD), the final phase of chronic renal failure in which little or no kidney function remains. Chronic renal disease accounts for about

80,000 deaths per year and is a major cause of lost work time and wages. Ironically, the increased prevalence of chronic renal disease in recent years is partially related to the success of dialysis and transplantation (Porth, 1994; Price & Wilson, 1992).

Two metabolically produced substances are routinely used to evaluate renal function. *Urea* is the end product of protein metabolism. It is created by the breakdown and metabolism of both dietary and body proteins. *Creatinine* is also a metabolic by-product, produced in relatively constant quantities by the muscles. Both of these substances are eliminated from the body by the kidneys via filtration and tubular secretion; neither are reabsorbed in the tubule. For this reason, blood levels of these substances, measured as the *blood urea nitrogen (BUN)* and *serum creatinine,* are effective indicators of renal function. Changes in BUN and serum creatinine levels will be noted throughout this chapter when disorders affecting renal function are discussed. Normally, a 10:1 to 15:1 ratio exists between the BUN and serum creatinine, i.e., the BUN level is normally about ten times greater than the serum creatinine level. In renal disease, the BUN rises at a higher rate than the serum creatinine; for this reason, the BUN/creatinine ratio is also a valuable tool in evaluating renal function (Chernecky et al., 1993).

Age-Related Changes in Kidney Function

■ ■ ■

Glomeruli in the renal cortex are lost with aging, reducing kidney mass. Because of their large functional reserve, however, renal function remains adequate unless additional stressors affect the renal system. The *glomerular filtration rate (GFR),* or amount of filtrate made by the kidneys per minute, declines as a result of other age-related factors affecting the renovascular system. Among these factors are arteriosclerosis, a smaller renal vascular bed, and decreased cardiac output. By age 90, the GFR may be less than half of what it was at age 20 (Wold, 1993). In the older adult with impaired renal function, the BUN rises, but serum creatinine levels often remain within normal limits because reduced muscle mass results in the production of less creatinine. For this reason, serum creatinine is a less effective indicator of renal function in older clients (Kee, 1992). The creatinine clearance (the rate at which creatinine is removed from the body), which does decline with aging, is a more sensitive indicator of the glomerular filtration rate (Brookbank, 1990).

Changes in renal function common in the older adult have implications for nursing. The kidneys become less able to concentrate urine and compensate for increased or decreased salt intake. When combined with a diminished response to antidiuretic hormone (ADH) and a diminished thirst response, both common in aging, this decreased urine concentrating ability puts the older adult at higher risk for dehydration. Potassium excretion may be decreased because of lower aldosterone levels. As a result, shifts in fluid and electrolyte balance are more frequent and potentially critical in the older client, indicating a need for careful assessment.

Decreased GFR in the older adult also reduces the clearance of drugs excreted through the kidneys. This reduced clearance prolongs the half-life of drugs and may necessitate lower drug dosages and longer dosing intervals. Common medications affected by decreased GFR include (Kee, 1992)

■ Cardiac drugs: digoxin, procainamide

■ Antibiotics: aminoglycosides, tetracyclines, cephalosporins

■ Histamine H_2 antagonists: cimetidine

■ Antidiabetic agents: chlorpropamide

It is especially important to monitor the administration and effects of drugs that are toxic to the renal tubules and associated with acute renal failure when providing care to older adults. The aminoglycosides, tetracycline, and the cephalosporin antibiotics are also part of this group.

Age-related changes in renal function and related nursing implications are summarized in Table 26–1.

The Client with a Congenital Kidney Malformation

■ ■ ■

Congenital kidney disorders include abnormalities in form and function. If function is not affected, congenital malformations may be detected only coincidentally. Malformations include agenesis, hypoplasia, alterations in kidney position, and horseshoe kidney.

Agenesis, organ absence, and *hypoplasia,* underdevelopment of the kidney, typically affect only one of these paired organs. Renal function remains normal unless the unaffected kidney is compromised. An abnormal kidney position affects the ureters and urine flow, with the potential result of urinary stasis and increased risk of infection and lithiasis, or stone formation (see Chapter 25).

One in every 500 to 1000 people has horseshoe kidney, making it one of the most common renal malformations. Failure of the embryonic kidneys to ascend normally can result in a single, horseshoe-shaped organ. The two kidneys are fused at either the upper or lower pole (usually the lower). This malformation does not typically affect renal function; however, because the ureters cross the fused poles, the client is at increased risk for developing *hydronephrosis,* or distention of the renal pelvis and calyces with urine. Recurrent infections and renal calculi are also common in clients with horseshoe kidney.

Renal ultrasonography and intravenous pyelography are used to diagnose horseshoe kidney. Correction of the abnormality is rarely indicated, although surgical resection of the isthmus (connection between the kidneys) may be performed to relieve ureteral obstruction or allow access to the abdominal aorta, which lies behind it.

The nursing care needs of clients with horseshoe kidney or other congenital malformations are primarily related to teaching. Because abnormal kidney shape or position increases the client's risk of infection and stone formation, teach the client to maintain an ample fluid intake of at least 2500 mL per day. Emphasize the importance of avoiding dehydration by increasing fluids during hot weather and/or strenuous exercise. Teach hygiene measures such as perineal cleansing and voiding before and after intercourse to help prevent infection. Clients

Table 26-1 Nursing Implications of Age-Related Changes in Kidney Function

Functional Change	Effect	Implications
Decreased glomerular filtration rate (GFR)	Decreased clearance of drugs excreted primarily through the kidneys. Results in increased drug half-life and blood levels, and higher risk of drug toxicity.	Monitor client carefully for signs of toxicity, especially when administering the following: digoxin, aminoglycoside antibiotics, tetracycline, vancomycin, chlorpropamide, procainamide, cimetidine, and cephalosporin antibiotics.
Decreased number of functional nephrons; lower levels of aldosterone; increased resistance to ADH	Decreased ability to conserve water and sodium; impaired potassium excretion; and decreased hydrogen ion excretion, resulting in reduced ability of the kidney to compensate for acidosis.	Monitor the client for dehydration and hyponatremia; maintain a fluid intake of 1500 to 2500 mL/day unless contraindicated; monitor for hyperkalemia, especially if taking a potassium-sparing diuretic, heparin, angiotensin-converting enzyme (ACE) inhibitor, beta-blocker, or NSAID; increased risk for acidosis in clients with impaired respiratory function or metabolic causes.
Reduced numbers of functional nephrons	Decreased renal reserve with increased risk of decompensation.	Avoid administering nephrotoxic drugs if possible; monitor urine output and blood chemistries regularly for early identification of renal failure.

need to recognize early signs and symptoms of urinary tract infection and seek treatment promptly to prevent infection of the kidney.

The Client with Polycystic Kidney Disease

■ ■ ■

A variety of congenital functional disorders of the kidneys can be identified, usually in childhood or adolescence. **Polycystic kidney disease,** a hereditary disease characterized by cyst formation and massive kidney enlargement, affects both children and adults. This disease has infantile and childhood forms, both of which are distinctly different from adult polycystic kidney disease (Price & Wilson, 1992; Wilson et al., 1991).

Pathophysiology

Adult polycystic kidney disease is relatively common, affecting 1 in every 500 to 1000 people (Berkow & Fletcher, 1992; Price & Wilson, 1992). An autosomal dominant disorder, it accounts for approximately 10% of clients with end-stage renal disease who require dialysis

or seek kidney transplantation. Individuals affected by polycystic kidney disease often develop cysts elsewhere in the body, including the liver, spleen, pancreas, and other organs. Nine to ten percent of people affected also experience subarachnoid brain hemorrhage from a form of congenital intracranial aneurysm. There is also an increased incidence of incompetent or "floppy" cardiac valves in people with polycystic kidney disease.

Renal cysts are fluid-filled sacs affecting the nephron, the functional unit of the kidneys. They develop in the tubular epithelium of the nephron, filling with accumulated glomerular filtrate or secreted solutes and fluid. The cysts may range in size from microscopic to several centimeters in diameter and occur bilaterally, affecting the renal cortex and medulla. As the cysts fill, enlarge, and multiply, the kidneys also enlarge. Renal blood vessels and nephrons are compressed and obstructed, and functional tissue is destroyed (Figure 26-1) (Porth, 1994; Tisher & Wilcox, 1993).

Polycystic kidney disease is a slowly progressive disorder, with symptoms usually presenting in the thirties or forties. Common manifestations include flank pain, microscopic or gross *hematuria* (blood in the urine), *proteinuria* (abnormal proteins in the urine), and polyuria and nocturia, as the concentrating ability of the kidney is impaired. Urinary tract infection and renal calculi are com-

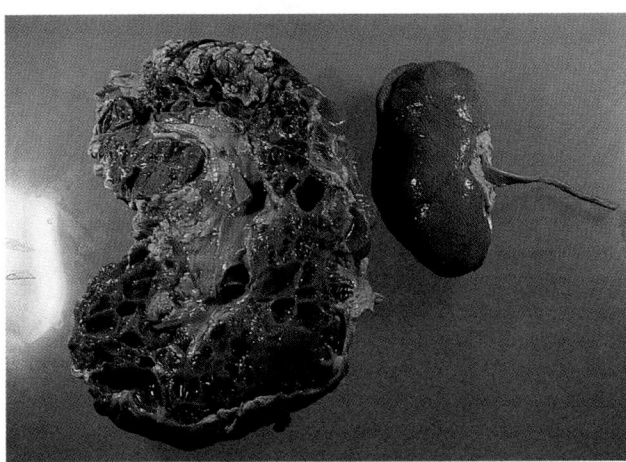

Figure 26–1   Polycystic kidneys. The functional tissue of the kidneys is gradually destroyed and replaced with fluid-filled cysts.

mon, as cysts interfere with normal urine drainage. Most clients develop hypertension from disruption of renal vessels. The kidneys become palpable, enlarged, and knobby. Symptoms of renal insufficiency and chronic renal failure typically occur in the fifties and sixties.

Collaborative Care

The following diagnostic procedures are useful to confirm polycystic kidney disease and determine its extent:

- *Renal ultrasonography* is a noninvasive diagnostic examination that uses reflected sound waves to visualize kidney structures. Lack of exposure to radiation and contrast media are distinct advantages of sonography. It is used to determine kidney size and to identify, locate, and differentiate renal masses such as cysts, tumors, and calculi. Renal ultrasound is the diagnostic procedure of choice for polycystic kidney disease.

- *Intravenous pyelography* (IVP), also known as excretory urography, is used to visualize the kidneys, ureters, and bladder for evaluation of structure and excretory function. As the kidneys clear an intravenously injected contrast medium from the blood, it is possible to identify their size and shape, the calyces and pelvis, the ureters, and the bladder. Cysts may be detected and sized, as well as the extent of kidney involvement noted.

- *Computed tomography* (CT scan) of the kidney uses X-rays passed through the kidneys at many angles to create a detailed picture. The picture produced reflects the different densities and composition of tissues. Computed tomography may be used with or without

contrast media. Kidney computed tomography is most useful for detecting and differentiating renal mass lesions such as cystic disease or tumors.

Nursing management of the client having a kidney ultrasound or CT scan is outlined in the box on page 940. Care of the client having an IVP is detailed in Chapter 25.

Management of adult polycystic kidney disease is largely supportive. Care is taken to avoid further renal damage by nephrotoxic substances, urinary tract infection, obstruction, or hypertension. A fluid intake of 2000 to 2500 mL per day is encouraged to help prevent UTI and lithiasis. Hypertension associated with polycystic disease is generally controllable using sympathetic alpha- or beta-antagonists or calcium-channel blockers (Tisher & Wilcox, 1993) (see Chapter 30). Ultimately, clients with polycystic kidney disease require hemodialysis or kidney transplantation. Although clients are often over the age of 50 years before transplantation is necessary, they are typically good candidates because of the absence of associated systemic disease (Tierney et al., 1994).

Nursing Care

Although each client has individual nursing care needs, the following nursing diagnoses may be appropriate for the client with polycystic kidney disease:

- *Fluid Volume Excess* related to impaired renal function
- *Anticipatory Grieving* related to potential loss of kidney function
- *Knowledge Deficit* related to lack of information regarding measures to help maintain kidney function
- *Ineffective Individual Coping* related to the potential for transmitting an inherited disorder to offspring

Client and Family Teaching

The client with polycystic kidney disease needs education about measures to help maintain optimal renal function and about the implications of the disease itself. Teach the client to maintain an ample fluid intake of approximately 2500 mL per day. Include additional information about preventing urinary tract infection, such as hygiene measures. Discuss early manifestations of UTI, and stress the importance of seeking intervention to prevent further kidney damage. Instruct the client to avoid medications that are potentially toxic to the kidneys and to check with the primary care provider before taking any new drug.

Because adult polycystic kidney disease is an autosomal dominant disorder, discuss genetic counseling and screening of family members for evidence of the disease. This is particularly important if renal transplantation is contemplated and family members are potential donors.

Nursing Implications of Diagnostic Studies: The Client with Polycystic Kidney Disease

■ ■ ■

Renal Ultrasonography

Preparation of the Client
- This test does not require informed consent or any special client preparation.
- Explain the procedure to the client, answering any questions.
- After the procedure, wash the client's back to remove the conductive gel.

Client and Family Teaching
- The procedure takes approximately 20 minutes to complete. No discomfort is associated with it, but the conductive gel will feel cold.

Computed Tomography (CT) of the Kidney

Preparation of the Client
- Explain the procedure to the client, answering any questions. Emphasize the client's need to remain still during the procedure.
- If the client is claustrophobic, premedication with an antianxiety medication may be necessary.
- Ask the client about allergies to iodine, iodated dye, or shellfish if contrast media will be used. If the client indicates a possible allergy, inform the radiologist.
- If contrast media will be injected, the client should be on NPO status for 4 hours prior to the examination.
- Remove any radiopaque objects such as jewelry or snaps prior to the procedure.
- Encourage fluids after the procedure to promote elimination of the dye.
- Observe the client closely for signs of delayed reaction to the contrast media such as dyspnea, tachycardia, rash, or hives. Notify the physician if a reaction occurs.

Client and Family Teaching
- The procedure takes less than 30 minutes to complete, but you will need to remain very still during the procedure.
- The scanner is an encircling tubelike device that makes loud clicking sounds.
- Although the procedure is not painful, you have to lie still on a hard table. Injection of the dye may cause flushing, warmth, and mild nausea.

The Client with Hydronephrosis

■ ■ ■

Hydronephrosis, abnormal dilation of the renal pelvis and calyces, can result from obstructive processes affecting the urinary tract. Congenital malformations, strictures, stones, tumors, and *vesicoureteral reflux* (backflow of urine from the bladder to the ureters) are all possible causes of hydronephrosis. The obstruction and/or impaired urine flow increases pressure in and dilation of the renal pelvis. If the pressure is unrelieved, damage to the collecting tubules, proximal tubules, and glomeruli results in gradual loss of renal function.

Acute hydronephrosis typically causes colicky pain on the affected side. The pain may radiate to the groin area. Chronic hydronephrosis with gradual dilation of renal structures is characterized by intermittent episodes of dull, aching flank discomfort. When hydronephrosis is significant, a palpable mass may be felt in the flank region. Hematuria and signs of a urinary tract infection, such as pyuria, fever, and discomfort, may be present.

Clients with hydronephrosis occasionally experience gastrointestinal symptoms such as nausea, vomiting, and abdominal pain. See the accompanying clinical manifestations box.

A number of diagnostic tests are useful to confirm hydronephrosis and identify the cause. Renal ultrasonography is particularly useful as a noninvasive study. Intravenous pyelography is also used to identify the degree of renal function and dilation, as well as the location of any obstruction. A CT scan may also be used to provide detailed pictures of the affected kidney and other structures. Cystoscopy is ordered to assess anatomic deformities such as strictures.

Prompt treatment of hydronephrosis is necessary to preserve renal function. Immediate treatment involves reestablishing urine drainage from the affected kidney. Drainage may be achieved using a percutaneous nephrostomy tube, a ureteral stent (see Chapter 25), or an indwelling catheter. In some cases, urinary diversion surgery may be required to establish urine drainage from the affected kidney. Urinary diversion is discussed in further detail in Chapter 25.

Clinical Manifestations of Acute and Chronic Hydronephrosis

■ ■ ■

Acute

- Acute, colicky pain; may radiate into groin
- Hematuria, pyuria
- Fever
- Nausea, vomiting, abdominal pain

Chronic

- Intermittent, dull, aching flank pain
- Hematuria, pyuria
- Fever
- Palpable flank mass

Nursing care is directed toward preventing hydronephrosis and ensuring urinary drainage in the client being treated for the disorder. Monitoring intake, urination, and bladder emptying helps ensure early detection of impaired urine outflow. Although monitoring urine output is important for all clients, it is vital for clients with risk factors for hydronephrosis. Risk factors include pelvic or abdominal tumors, urinary calculi, adhesions and scarring from previous surgeries, or neurologic defects that may impede bladder emptying. Ensuring adequate urinary output and flow is also vital in the client with a ureteral stent, nephrostomy, or surgical intervention for hydronephrosis. Catheters and drainage tubes should be clearly labeled, and output should be measured separately. Prevent kinking or obstruction; irrigate tubes only as ordered by the physician.

The following nursing diagnoses are appropriate for the client with hydronephrosis:

- *Altered Urinary Elimination* related to obstruction of outflow from kidney
- *Pain* related to dilation of the ureter and renal pelvis
- *Risk for Infection* related to urinary stasis

The teaching needs of the client with hydronephrosis are primarily related to prescribed diagnostic and treatment measures. Explain all diagnostic tests, including the purpose of each, expected sensations, and client responsibilities during the test. If surgical intervention is indicated, provide additional information to the client and family to make sure they understand the procedure and expected results. Explain all tubes and care measures in language appropriate for the client. If a urinary diversion is performed, teach the client and family about required care and precautions to prevent skin breakdown or infection (see Chapter 25).

The Client with a Disorder of the Glomerulus

■ ■ ■

Disorders and diseases involving the glomerulus are the leading cause of chronic renal failure in the United States. They are the underlying disease process for half of those people needing dialysis and result in 12,000 deaths per year (Porth, 1994).

Glomerular disorders may be either primary, involving mainly the kidney, or secondary to a multisystem disease or hereditary condition. Primary glomerular disease is often immunologic or idiopathic in origin. Diabetes mellitus, systemic lupus erythematosus, and Goodpasture's syndrome are frequently implicated in secondary glomerular disorders (Bullock & Rosendahl, 1992; Wilson et al., 1991).

Pathophysiology

In glomerular disease, both the structure and function of the glomerulus are affected, disrupting glomerular filtration. The capillary membrane becomes more permeable to plasma proteins and blood cells. This increased permeability in the glomerulus results in the signs and symptoms common to glomerular disorders: hematuria, proteinuria, a reduced GFR leading to **azotemia** (increased blood levels of nitrogenous waste products), and hypertension. Glomerular involvement may be diffuse, involving all glomeruli, or focal, involving some glomeruli while others remain essentially normal (Porth, 1994; Wilson et al., 1991).

Both hematuria and proteinuria are the result of a damaged glomerular capillary membrane, which allows blood cells and proteins to escape from the vascular compartment into the filtrate. Hematuria may be either gross or microscopic. Proteinuria is considered to be the most important indicator of glomerular injury, because it increases progressively with increased glomerular damage.

As the GFR falls, the filtration and elimination of nitrogenous wastes, including urea, decreases, resulting in azotemia. *Oliguria,* a urine output of less than 400 mL in 24 hours, may also result from the decreased GFR. Loss of plasma proteins in the urine causes *hypoalbuminemia* (low levels of albumin in the blood). Hypoalbuminemia reduces the *oncotic pressure* (osmotic pressure created by plasma proteins) within the blood vessels, leading to edema. Sodium and water retention further contribute to edema. Hypertension in the client with glomerular disease is caused by fluid retention and disruption of the renin-angiotensin system, a key regulator of blood pressure (Porth, 1994). Figure 26–2 summarizes the pathogenesis of glomerulonephritis.

The major primary glomerular disorders include acute

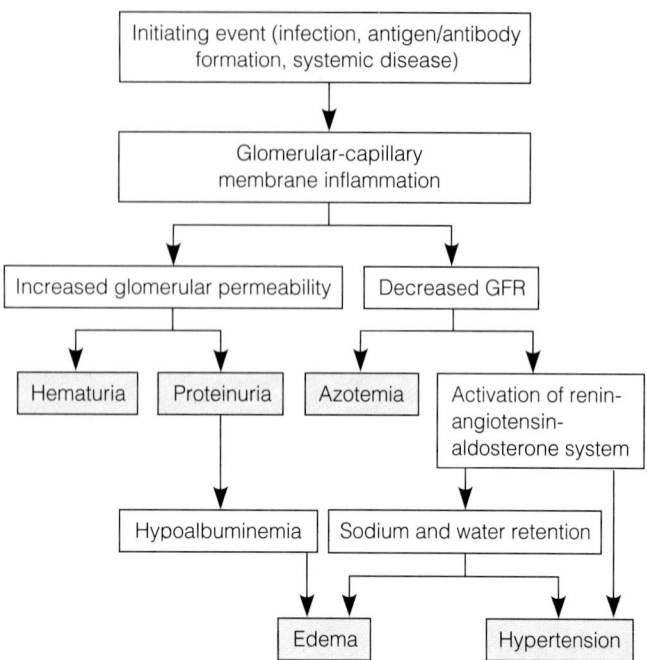

Figure 26–2 The pathogenesis of glomerulonephritis.

Clinical Manifestations of Acute Glomerulonephritis

- Hematuria, cocoa-colored urine
- Proteinuria
- Salt and water retention
- Edema, periorbital and facial, dependent
- Hypertension
- Azotemia
- Fatigue
- Anorexia, nausea, and vomiting
- Headache

glomerulonephritis, rapidly progressive glomerulonephritis, chronic glomerulonephritis, and nephrotic syndrome. Diabetic nephropathy and lupus nephritis are the most common secondary forms of glomerular disease.

Acute Glomerulonephritis

Glomerulonephritis is the inflammation of the capillary loops of the glomeruli. Acute glomerulonephritis can result from systemic diseases such as systemic lupus erythematosus or primary glomerular diseases, but acute poststreptococcal glomerulonephritis is the predominant form. Infection of the pharynx or skin with *group A beta-hemolytic streptococcus* is the common precipitating factor for this disorder. Staphylococcal or viral infections, such as hepatitis B, mumps, or varicella (chickenpox), can lead to a similar postinfectious acute glomerulonephritis. This is primarily a disease of childhood, but it can affect adults.

In acute glomerulonephritis, circulating antigen-antibody immune complexes formed during the primary infection are trapped in the glomerular membrane. These cause an inflammatory response, activating the complement system and stimulating the release of vasoactive substances and inflammatory mediators. Local edema and inflammatory cell proliferation damage the capillary endothelium and basement membrane and increase the porosity or "leakiness" of the glomerular capillaries. This porosity allows plasma proteins and blood cells to escape into the urine (Porth, 1994; Price & Wilson, 1992). Renal involvement is diffuse, spread throughout the kidneys.

Acute glomerulonephritis is characterized by the abrupt onset of hematuria and proteinuria, salt and water retention, and evidence of azotemia occurring 10 to 14 days after the initial infection. The urine often appears cocoa- or coffee-colored. Salt and water retention leads to increased extracellular fluid volume, hypertension, and edema. The edema is primarily noted in the face, particularly the periorbital area. Dependent edema, affecting the hands and upper extremities in particular, may also be noted. Other manifestations may include fatigue, anorexia, nausea and vomiting, and headache. See the accompanying clinical manifestations box.

The older adult may show less characteristic manifestations. Nausea, malaise, arthralgias, and proteinuria are common manifestations; hypertension and edema are seen less often. Pulmonary infiltrates may occur early in the disorder, often due to worsening of a preexisting condition such as heart failure (Abrams & Berkow, 1990).

The prognosis for adults with acute glomerulonephritis is less favorable than it is for children. The symptoms may subside spontaneously within 10 to 14 days, and 50% or more affected adults recover completely. In the remainder, impaired renal function is persistent, with continued proteinuria and/or hematuria, or progressive, ultimately leading to chronic glomerulonephritis or renal failure (Price & Wilson, 1992; Wilson et al., 1991).

Rapidly Progressive Glomerulonephritis

Most clients with acute glomerulonephritis have a period of azotemia and oliguria followed by a spontaneous diuresis and normalizing of the GFR. Some clients, however, develop renal failure, which begins abruptly and rarely resolves spontaneously. These clients are said to have rapidly progressive glomerulonephritis (Wilson et al., 1991).

This form of glomerulonephritis may be either idiopathic or secondary to an acute or subacute infectious disease or a multisystem disease such as vasculitis, systemic lupus erythematosus, or Goodpasture's syndrome. It affects people of all ages, with a higher incidence in males than females.

Glomerular cell proliferation and the formation of crescent-shaped structures that occlude the glomerular capsule are characteristic of rapidly progressive glomerulonephritis. Typically, more than 70% of the glomeruli are involved, resulting in a rapid decline in GFR. Up to 50% of clients require maintenance dialysis within 6 months; approximately 90% eventually develop renal failure and require dialysis or a kidney transplant (Porth, 1994; Wilson et al., 1991).

Clients with rapidly progressive glomerulonephritis typically present with complaints of weakness, nausea, and vomiting. Some may relate a history of a flulike illness preceding the onset of the glomerulonephritis. Other symptoms include oliguria and abdominal or flank pain. Moderate hypertension may develop. On urinalysis, hematuria and massive proteinuria are noted (Wilson et al., 1991).

Chronic Glomerulonephritis

Chronic glomerulonephritis is typically the end stage of other glomerular disorders such as rapidly progressive glomerulonephritis, lupus nephritis, or diabetic nephropathy. In many cases, however, no previous glomerular disease has been recognized.

Slow, progressive destruction of the glomeruli with resulting impairment of renal function is characteristic of chronic glomerulonephritis. The kidneys decrease in size symmetrically, and their surfaces become granular or roughened. Eventually, entire nephrons are lost.

Symptoms develop insidiously, and the disease is often not recognized until signs of renal failure are evident. Chronic glomerulonephritis may also be diagnosed when hypertension, urine abnormalities, and impaired renal function are found coincidentally in the course of a routine physical examination or treatment for an unrelated disorder. Viral or bacterial infectious diseases can exacerbate the glomerulonephritis, prompting the diagnosis to be made.

The course of chronic glomerulonephritis is variable, with years to decades elapsing from the time of the diagnosis to the development of end-stage renal failure (Wilson et al., 1991).

Nephrotic Syndrome

Massive proteinuria, hypoalbuminemia, hyperlipidemia, and edema characterize the **nephrotic syndrome.** A number of disorders can affect the glomerular capillary

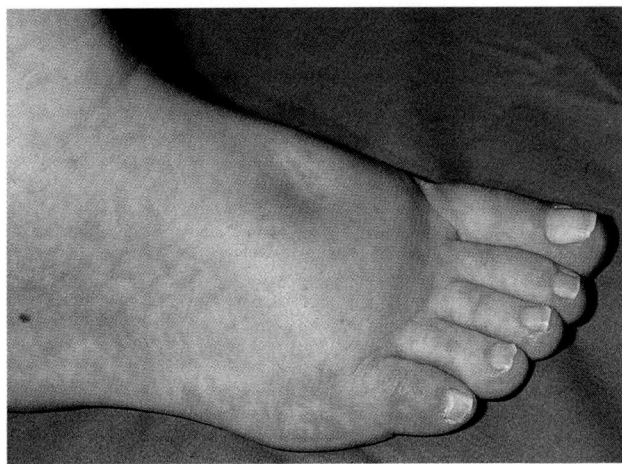

Figure 26–3   *Severe pitting edema in a client with nephrotic syndrome.*

membrane, changing its porosity and allowing plasma proteins to escape into the urine. In the adult, nephrotic syndrome is usually secondary to a systemic disease such as lupus erythematosus or diabetes mellitus. Other precipitating factors include endocarditis, hepatitis B and other infectious processes, exposure to heavy metals such as gold and mercury, certain drugs such as captopril and penicillamine, and some neoplasms including melanoma and lung or colon cancer. Primary or idiopathic nephrotic syndrome is seen more often in children, although it may also affect adults, older adults in particular.

With the loss of plasma proteins in the urine and resulting hypoalbuminemia, the oncotic pressure of the plasma decreases, and fluid shifts from the intravascular to the interstitial spaces, leading to the edema characteristic of nephrotic syndrome. Salt and water retention, possibly due to activation of the renin-angiotensin system, also contribute to the edema. Edema may be severe, affecting the face and periorbital area as well as dependent tissues (Figure 26–3).

The decreased plasma oncotic pressure also stimulates lipoprotein synthesis in the liver, resulting in hyperlipidemia.

Thromboemboli (mobilized blood clots) are a relatively common complication of nephrotic syndrome. Peripheral veins and arteries, pulmonary arteries, and renal veins may be occluded. Manifestations of peripheral arterial occlusion or pulmonary embolism or infarction may be seen. When renal venous thrombosis occurs, the client may experience flank or groin pain on one or both sides, gross hematuria, and a reduced GFR (Wilson et al., 1991).

Nephrotic syndrome usually resolves without long-term consequence in children. The prognosis for adults is less optimistic. Less than 50% of adults experience spontaneous complete remission. Many have persistent proteinuria and may demonstrate progressive renal impairment. As many as 30% of adults with nephrotic syndrome develop end-stage renal failure (Wilson et al., 1991).

Goodpasture's Syndrome

Goodpasture's syndrome is characterized by glomerulonephritis and pulmonary hemorrhage resulting from immune-complex damage to the glomerular and alveolar basement membranes. The etiology of this uncommon syndrome is unknown, although it is thought to be autoimmune in origin. It most often affects young men between the ages of 18 and 35 years, although it can occur at any age and affect women as well.

Although the glomeruli may be nearly normal in appearance and function in Goodpasture's syndrome, extensive cell proliferation and crescent formation characteristic of rapidly progressive glomerulonephritis are more common. Urinary manifestations include hematuria, proteinuria, and edema formation. Rapid progression to renal failure is not uncommon.

Damage to the alveolar membrane of the lungs in Goodpasture's syndrome can result in pulmonary hemorrhage, which may be mild or life-threatening. Cough, shortness of breath, and *hemoptysis* (bloody sputum) are early respiratory manifestations. Repeated incidents of pulmonary hemorrhage may occur, or the client may experience long-term remission of pulmonary effects (Bullock & Rosendahl, 1992; Wilson et al., 1991).

Diabetic Nephropathy

Diabetic nephropathy, kidney disease common in the later stages of diabetes mellitus, is the underlying pathophysiologic process in approximately 35% of people hospitalized for end-stage renal disease (Tisher & Wilcox, 1993). Fifty to sixty percent of insulin-dependent diabetic clients and 5% to 30% of noninsulin-dependent diabetic clients develop clinical nephropathy (Porth, 1994; Price & Wilson, 1992).

Initial evidence of microproteinuria indicating renal damage is typically demonstrated within 10 to 15 years after the onset of diabetes, progressing to overt proteinuria and nephropathy within 15 to 20 years of the initial diagnosis.

The most characteristic lesion of diabetic nephropathy is glomerulosclerosis and thickening of the glomerular basement membrane. Arteriosclerosis, a common feature of long-term diabetes, contributes to the disease, as do nephritis and tubular lesions. *Pyelonephritis,* inflammation of the kidney, is also implicated in the development of diabetic nephropathy (Price & Wilson, 1992; Tisher & Wilcox, 1993; Wilson et al., 1991). A further discussion is found in Chapter 21.

Lupus Nephritis

Systemic lupus erythematosus (SLE) is an inflammatory autoimmune disorder affecting the connective tissue of the body. On biopsy, up to 95% of clients with SLE show evidence of **lupus nephritis,** inflammatory lesions involving the supportive tissues of the glomerulus. Between 35% and 50% of clients with SLE demonstrate manifestations of nephritis (Tisher & Wilcox, 1993; Wilson et al., 1991).

A number of different patterns of nephron damage are seen in lupus nephritis, involving either the thin membrane supporting the capillary loops of the glomerulus or the glomerular capillary wall itself. The renal tubule may also be affected.

Clinical manifestations of lupus nephritis range from microscopic hematuria to massive proteinuria. Its progession may be slow and chronic or *fulminant,* with a sudden onset and the rapid development of renal failure. The management and prognosis vary with the type of renal lesion. Corticosteroids are used in conjunction with cytotoxic agents such as intravenous cyclophosphamide (Cytoxan) or azathioprine (Imuran) to reduce the inflammatory process and slow the progression of the nephritis.

Approximately 85% of clients with minimal or mild lesions survive for at least 10 years, whereas 35% of clients with diffuse proliferative lupus nephritis die within 5 years (Tisher & Wilcox, 1993; Wilson et al., 1991). Improved management of the underlying disease, dialysis, and renal transplantation have significantly improved the prognosis in recent years (Wilson et al., 1991).

Collaborative Care

Care of the client with glomerulonephritis, whether acute or chronic, primary or secondary, focuses on identification and treatment of the underlying disease process and preservation of kidney function. For most glomerular disorders, there is no specific treatment that achieves cure. Care is supportive, with the goals of maintaining renal function, preventing complications, and supporting the healing process.

Laboratory and Diagnostic Tests

Laboratory and diagnostic testing are valuable to identify the cause of glomerulonephritis and evaluate kidney function.

The following laboratory studies may be ordered to help identify the underlying cause or etiology:

- *Throat* or *skin cultures* to determine the presence of an infection by group A beta-hemolytic streptococci. Although poststreptococcal glomerulonephritis typically follows the acute infection by 1 to 2 weeks, cultures may be obtained to identify the continued presence of organisms and direct treatment of the infection.

- *Antibody response tests* for streptococcal **exoenzymes** (bacterial enzymes that stimulate the immune response implicated in acute poststreptococcal glomerulonephritis). The most common antibody response test is the antistreptolysin O, or ASO titer. The ASO titer is typically elevated in pharyngeal infection but not necessarily in skin infection. Other titers such as antistreptokinase (ASK) or antideoxyribonuclease B (ADNAase B) may be useful to identify cutaneous infection.

- The *erythrocyte sedimentation rate* is a general indicator of inflammatory response. It may be elevated in acute poststreptococcal glomerulonephritis and in lupus nephritis.

- Because lupus nephritis may be the presenting symptom of SLE, *serum antinuclear antibody* (ANA) levels may be drawn. Antinuclear antibodies are antibodies to one's own DNA and other material in the cell nucleus. The highest titers are seen in SLE, although they may be elevated in other autoimmune disorders such as rheumatoid arthritis and myasthenia gravis (Chernecky et al., 1993).

The following laboratory tests may be ordered to evaluate kidney function in clients with glomerular disorders:

- *Blood urea nitrogen (BUN)* is a measurement of the nitrogen portion of urea, a product formed in the liver from protein metabolism. It is freely filtered in the glomerulus and excreted in the urine. The BUN is primarily used as an indicator of kidney function because most renal diseases interfere with its excretion and cause blood levels to rise. However, it is important to remember that increased protein catabolism (destruction), which may occur with GI bleeding or tissue breakdown, can also raise the BUN. The normal BUN in the adult is 5 to 20 mg/dL or 1.8 to 6.5 mmol/L. The older adult may have slightly higher levels. Levels up to 50 mg/dL or 17.7 mmol/L indicate mild azotemia, and levels higher than 100 mg/dL or 35.7 mmol/L indicate severe renal impairment.

- *Serum creatinine* measures the amount of creatinine in the blood. Creatinine is the metabolic end product of creatine-phosphate, used in skeletal muscle contraction. It is produced in relatively constant amounts, according to the amount of muscle mass, and is excreted entirely by the kidneys. These factors make the serum creatinine a good indicator of kidney function. The normal serum creatinine for an adult female is 0.5 to 1.1 mg/dL, and 0.5 to 1.2 mg/dL for an adult male. Normal values are lower in the older adult because of decreased muscle mass. Levels of greater than 4 mg/dL indicate serious impairment of renal function.

- *Urine creatinine* is another indicator of renal function

and the GFR in particular. When kidney function is impaired, urine creatinine levels are decreased from the normal of 600 to 1800 mg/24 hours in the adult female and 800 to 2000 mg/24 hours in the male.

- *Creatinine clearance,* a very specific indicator of renal function, is used to evaluate the GFR. The clearance, or amount of blood cleared of creatinine in 1 minute, depends on the amount and pressure of blood being filtered and the filtering ability of the glomeruli. Normal levels for the adult male are 97 to 137 mL/minute and 88 to 128 mL/minute for the adult female. Levels decline with aging because of the normal decrease in GFR in the older adult. Most primary kidney disorders such as glomerulonephritis affect the filtering ability of the glomeruli and thus decrease creatinine clearance.

- *Serum electrolytes,* in particular sodium, potassium, calcium, and phosphate, are evaluated because disruptions in kidney function alter their excretion. Even though sodium retention often occurs with kidney disease, serum levels of sodium may be lower than normal because of dilution with excess water. Potassium levels are often higher than normal, as are phosphate levels. Hypocalcemia results from the reciprocal effect of the elevated serum phosphate. Monitoring the serum electrolytes is particularly important to prevent the complications associated with high or low blood levels.

- *Urinalysis* often reveals the presence of red blood cells and abnormal proteins in the urine of clients with a glomerular disorder. These substances are normally too large to escape the glomerular capillaries and enter the filtrate; therefore, they are not present in normal urine. Glomerular disorders increase the porosity of glomerular capillaries, allowing blood cells and proteins into the urine. A 24-hour urine specimen is used to determine the amount of protein in the urine. A normal level of urinary protein is 50 to 80 mg/24 hours; in glomerular disorders, it may be significantly elevated.

Table 26–2 summarizes the changes in laboratory studies associated with renal disease.

Diagnostic tests used to evaluate the client with glomerular disease may include the following:

- An *abdominal X-ray,* commonly known as the *KUB* (kidney, ureter, bladder), can show enlargement of the kidneys, which may occur with acute glomerulonephritis, or the bilateral small kidneys typical of end-stage chronic glomerulonephritis. Although other studies provide more information, X-ray studies can be a valuable initial tool in the diagnosis of kidney disorders.

- The *kidney scan* is a nuclear medicine procedure that allows visualization of the kidney after intravenous

Table 26–2   Changes in Laboratory Values Associated with Kidney Disease

Test	Normal Value	Value in Renal Disease
Blood urea nitrogen (BUN)	5–20 mg/dL Slightly higher in older adult	20–50 mg/dL or higher
Creatinine, serum	Female: 0.5–1.1 mg/dL Male: 0.6–1.2 mg/dL Slightly lower in older adult	Elevated; levels > 4 mg/dL indicate severe impairment of renal function
Creatinine clearance	Female: 88–128 mL/min Male: 97–137 mL/min Values decline in older adult	Reduced renal reserve: 32.5–90.0 mL/min Renal insufficiency: 6.5–32.5 mL/min Renal failure: < 6.5 mL/min
Serum albumin	3.2–5 g/dL; 3.2–4.8 g/dL in older adult	Decreased in nephrotic syndrome
Serum electrolytes	Potassium: 3.5–5.0 mEq/L Sodium: 136–145 mEq/L Calcium: 4.5–5.5 mEq/L or 8.2–10.5 mg/dL Phosphorus: 3.0–4.5 mg/dL Slightly lower in older adult	Increased in renal insufficiency Decreased in nephrotic syndrome Decreased in renal failure Increased in renal failure
Red blood cell count	Female: 4.0–5.5 million/mm³ Male: 4.5–6.2 million/mm³	Decreased in chronic renal failure
Urine creatinine	Female: 600–1800 mg/24 hours Male: 800–2000 mg/24 hours	Decreased in disorders of impaired renal function
Urine protein	Resting: 50–80 mg/24 hours Ambulatory: < 150–250 mg/24 hours	Increased in disorders of impaired renal function
Urine red blood cells	< 2–3/HPF; no RBC casts	Present in glomerular disorders

administration of a radioisotope. The distribution of radioactivity is mapped, and the time of uptake, transit, and excretion can be plotted for each kidney (Pagana & Pagana, 1992). This plot is compared with a normal or standarized plot to evaluate the function of each kidney individually. In glomerular diseases, the uptake and excretion of the radioactive material are delayed.

- *Biopsy* allows microscopic examination of kidney tissue and is the most reliable diagnostic procedure for glomerular disorders. The examination can help differentiate various types of glomerulonephritis, determine the prognosis, and guide treatment. Renal biopsy is usually performed percutaneously, by inserting a biopsy needle through the skin into the kidney to obtain a tissue sample. Ultrasonography or fluoroscopy may be used to guide needle placement. Open or surgical biopsy, which involves an incision and an operative procedure, may also be done.

The nursing implications for laboratory and diagnostic studies used to evaluate glomerular disorders are included in the accompanying box.

Pharmacology

Although there are no drugs available to cure glomerular disorders, medications are used to treat underlying disorders and manage the symptoms.

Penicillin or other broad-spectrum antibiotics may be prescribed for the client with poststreptococcal glomerulonephritis. The purpose of antibiotic therapy is to eradicate any remaining bacteria, which may prolong the immune response and glomerular inflammation. Care is taken to avoid nephrotoxic antibiotics, such as the aminoglycoside antibiotics, streptomycin, and some cephalosporins.

Antihypertensives may be prescribed to maintain the blood pressure within normal levels. Diuretics, both thiazide and loop type, angiotensin-converting-enzyme (ACE) inhibitors, beta- or alpha-adrenergic blocking agents, and calcium channel blockers can be used for the hypertensive client with a glomerular disorder. Blood pressure management is important because systemic and renal hypertension are associated with a poorer prognosis and more rapid kidney deterioration in clients with glomerular disorders.

Clients with an acute inflammatory process such as rapidly progressive glomerulonephritis, Goodpasture's syndrome, or exacerbation of systemic lupus erythematosus, may be placed on corticosteroids and cytotoxic agents to mediate the inflammatory process. Large doses of methylprednisolone (Solu-Medrol) administered intravenously on a weekly or monthly basis are used for the client with rapidly progressive glomerulonephritis (Berkow & Fletcher, 1992). Daily or alternate-day oral

Nursing Implications of Laboratory and Diagnostic Studies: The Client with Glomerular Disease

■ ■ ■

Creatinine Clearance

Preparation of the Client

- Obtain a 24-hour urine specimen container without preservative.

- Instruct the client to begin the specimen collection at the designated time by voiding and discarding this initial specimen. Collect all urine voided for the next 24 hours, emptying the bladder at the end of the collection time and saving the specimen. Do not discard toilet paper in the specimen container.

- Instruct the client to void and save the specimen prior to defecating to prevent contamination or loss of urine.

- Refrigerate or keep the urine specimen on ice during the collection period.

- Post signs in the client's room and bathroom indicating the hours of urine collection to prevent inadvertent discarding of the urine.

- Collect or have laboratory personnel collect a venous blood sample during the 24-hour urine collection period.

- Note the client's name, age, weight, and height on the laboratory requisition.

Client and Family Teaching

- Generally, no special diet is required during the test, although you may have to avoid cooked meat, tea, coffee, or drugs during the test (Pagana & Pagana, 1992).

- Follow instructions for 24-hour specimen collection if the test is being done on an outpatient basis.

Kidney Scan (Renal Scan)

Preparation of the Client

- Informed consent is required for this invasive procedure. Provide preprocedure teaching and answer questions as needed.

- Make sure that the client is well hydrated prior to the procedure. Have the client drink two to three glasses of water before the procedure if indicated.

- Obtain the client's weight (used in calculating the amount of radioisotope to be injected).

- Have the client void prior to the procedure.

- After the procedure, have the client increase fluid intake to promote excretion of the radioisotope.

- No special radioactivity precautions are indicated, although the client should be instructed to flush the toilet immediately after voiding and to wash hands thoroughly.

- Because of the slight potential for harm to a developing fetus, pregnant personnel should not be assigned to care for clients during the first 24 hours after this procedure.

Client and Family Teaching

- Increase fluid intake before and after the renal scan.

- No special diet or other preparation is required.

- The test takes 1 to 4 hours.

- No anesthesia is required, and you will experience no pain or discomfort other than that associated with remaining still for a period of time.

Renal Biopsy

Preparation of the Client

- Informed consent is required for a kidney biopsy. Ensure that the physician has obtained consent. Answer questions and provide additional information as needed.

- Maintain NPO status from midnight before the procedure.

- Note the client's hemoglobin and hematocrit levels prior to the procedure.

- If the procedure is to be performed at the client's bedside, obtain a biopsy tray and other necessary supplies.

- Following the procedure, apply a pressure dressing and position the client supine to help maintain pressure on the biopsy site.

- Monitor the client closely for evidence of bleeding during the first 24 hours after the procedure:
  a. Check vital signs frequently. Notify the physician if the client develops tachycardia, hypotension, or other signs of shock.
  b. Monitor the biopsy site for bleeding.
  c. Check hemoglobin and hematocrit levels, comparing with preprocedure values.

➤

Diagnostic Studies: The Client with Glomerular Disease (continued)

■ ■ ■

d. Observe the client for other signs of hemorrhage such as complaints of flank or back pain, shoulder pain (caused by diaphragmatic irritation if hemorrhage occurs), pallor, lightheadedness.

e. Monitor urine output for quantity and degree of hematuria. Initial hematuria should clear within 24 hours.

■ Monitor for other potential complications such as inadvertent penetration of the liver or bowel. Observe for signs and symptoms of abdominal pain, guarding, and decreased bowel sounds.

■ Encourage fluids during the initial postprocedure period.

Client and Family Teaching

■ No sedation is given during the procedure. Local anesthesia is used at the injection site. The procedure may be uncomfortable but should not be painful.

■ When the needle is inserted, you will be instructed not to breathe to prevent kidney motion.

■ The entire procedure takes approximately 10 minutes.

■ Avoid coughing during the first 24 hours after the procedure. Strenuous activity such as heavy lifting may be prohibited for approximately 2 weeks after the procedure.

■ Report any signs and symptoms of complications, such as hemorrhage or urinary tract infection, to the physician (Pagana & Pagana, 1992).

---

prednisone is prescribed for Goodpasture's syndrome, lupus nephritis, and other glomerular disorders, depending on biopsy results. Using a cytotoxic agent such as cyclosphosphamide or cyclosporine (Sandimmune) along with corticosteroid therapy provides good suppression of the immune response while allowing lower dosages of corticosteroids. Lower dosages reduce the side effects of steroid therapy. Chlorambucil (Leukeran), another chemotherapeutic agent, may be used in the management of nephrotic syndrome.

Although corticosteroids are helpful in the management of some glomerular disorders, they have not been shown to be effective in all types. Their use in poststreptococcal glomerulonephritis may actually worsen the condition. Nursing implications for the use of cytotoxic agents are outlined in the accompanying box. Corticosteroids are discussed in Chapter 8.

Other Therapies

Plasmapheresis, the removal of harmful components in the plasma, may be used to treat rapidly progressive glomerulonephritis and Goodpasture's syndrome. The glomerular-damaging antibodies are removed from the client's blood along with the plasma by passing the blood through a blood cell separator. An equal amount of albumin or human plasma is returned to the client along with the client's RBCs. This procedure is usually done in a series, rather than as a one-time only treatment. It is not without risk, and informed consent is required. Potential complications of plasmapheresis include those associated with the placement of IV catheters, shifts in fluid balance, and alteration of blood clotting.

When edema is significant or the client is hypertensive, sodium intake may be restricted. Dietary proteins may be increased if a significant amount of protein is being lost in the urine. However, if azotemia is present, dietary protein is restricted. When proteins are restricted, those included in the diet should be complete proteins, primarily. Complete proteins are those that supply all of the essential amino acids required for growth and tissue maintenance. Complete and incomplete proteins are compared in Table 26–3.

The client who experiences renal failure as a result of a glomerular disorder may require dialysis to restore fluid and electrolyte balance and remove waste products from the body. Dialysis procedures and related nursing care are explained in the discussion of the client with chronic renal failure later in this chapter.

Nursing Care

Nursing care for the client with a glomerular disorder is directed at providing supportive care and monitoring renal function and fluid volume status. The client who is receiving corticosteroids and cytotoxic agents has an increased risk for infection, which needs to be addressed in nursing care. Both manifestations of the disorders and prescribed therapies can interfere with a client's ability to maintain usual roles and responsibilities.

Nursing Implications for Pharmacology: The Client with a Glomerular Disorder

CYTOTOXIC AGENTS

Azathioprine (Imuran)

Cyclophosphamide (Cytoxan)

Cyclosporine (Sandimmune)

Certain drugs that are identified as cytotoxic or antineoplastic agents are effective as immunosuppressive agents. They act by decreasing the proliferation of cells within the immune system. Glomerular disorders with an autoimmune component—some forms of acute glomerulonephritis (*not* including poststreptococcal), rapidly progressive glomerulonephritis, nephrosis, Goodpasture's syndrome, and lupus nephritis—may respond to suppression of the immune system. These medications are also used to prevent rejection of a transplanted kidney. Usually they are administered concurrently with corticosteroid therapy, allowing lower doses of both preparations.

Nursing Responsibilities

- Monitor the client's blood count, with particular attention to the white blood cell (WBC) and platelet counts. Notify the physician if WBCs fall below 4000 or platelets below 75,000.
- Monitor renal and liver function studies, including the creatinine, BUN, creatinine clearance, and liver enzymes. Report any abnormal levels to the physician.
- Administer the drug as ordered. Oral preparations should be administered with food to minimize gastrointestinal effects. Antacids may be ordered.
- Increase fluids to maintain good hydration and urinary output.

- Monitor intake and output.
- Monitor for signs of abnormal bleeding: bleeding gums, bruising, petechiae, joint pain, hematuria, and black or tarry stools.
- Use meticulous hand washing and other appropriate measures to protect the client from infection. Assess for signs of infection.
- Pulmonary fibrosis is a potential adverse effect of cyclophosphamines. Therefore, monitor respiratory function using pulmonary function studies and clinical signs of dyspnea or cough.

Client and Family Teaching

- Avoid large crowds and situations where exposure to infection is probable.
- Report signs of infection, such as chills, fever, sore throat, fatigue, or malaise, to the physician.
- Use contraceptive measures to prevent pregnancy while on immunosuppressive therapy, because these drugs cause birth defects.
- Avoid the use of aspirin or ibuprofen while taking these drugs. Report any signs of bleeding to the physician.
- Females may stop having periods while taking cyclophosphamide. The menses will resume after the drug is discontinued.
- If you are taking cyclophosphamide, report coughing or difficulty breathing to the physician.

Fluid Volume Excess

Fluid volume excess and resultant edema are common manifestations of glomerular disorders. When excess blood proteins are lost in the urine, the oncotic pressure of the plasma falls, and fluid shifts into the interstitial spaces. The body responds to this fluid shift by retaining sodium and water to maintain the intravascular volume, resulting in a fluid volume excess.

Nursing interventions with rationales follow.

- Monitor the client's vital signs, including blood pressure, apical pulse, respirations, and breath sounds, at least every 4 hours. Record and report any significant changes. *Fluid volume excess increases the workload of the*

Table 26–3   Complete and Incomplete Protein Sources

	Complete Proteins	**Incomplete Proteins**
Definition	Foods that provide the essential amino acids needed for growth and tissue maintenance	Foods that lack one or more essential amino acids or that have them in inadequate proportions
Examples	Milk, eggs, cheese, meats, poultry, and fish	Vegetables, breads, cereals and grains, legumes, seeds, and nuts

heart and the blood pressure. Tachycardia may be present. Associated electrolyte imbalances can result in cardiac rhythm disturbances. Increased pressure in the pulmonary vascular system can lead to pulmonary edema, tachypnea, dyspnea, and crackles or rales in the lungs.

- Record the fluid intake and output every 4 to 8 hours, or more frequently as indicated. *Accurate intake and output records aid in determining fluid volume status.*

- Weigh the client daily at the same time of day, on the same scale and with the same amount of clothing. *Accurate weight measurements provide a good assessment of fluid volume status and treatment effectiveness.*

- Assess for the presence, location, and degree of edema. *Edema associated with renal disorders often affects low-pressure tissues such as the face and periorbital region as well as the upper extremities.*

- Monitor the serum electrolytes, hemoglobin and hematocrit, blood urea nitrogen, and creatinine. *Changes in serum electrolytes are often associated with altered fluid balance and renal disorders and may result in complications such as cardiac rhythm disturbances or other manifestations of electrolyte imbalance. Low hemoglobin and hematocrit may be due to the increased intravascular volume. BUN and creatinine provide information about the functional ability of the kidneys.*

- Maintain fluid restriction as ordered, offering ice chips (in limited and measured amounts) and frequent mouth care to relieve thirst. Develop a schedule for oral intake with the client. *Clients with severe edema and hypertension may be placed on a strict fluid restriction. Dry mucous membranes in the mouth contribute to the thirst response. Providing ice chips and frequent mouth care to keep the mouth moist can help relieve thirst while maintaining the integrity of oral tissues. Including the client in planning oral intake increases the client's sense of control and compliance with the regimen.*

- Carefully monitor and regulate intravenous infusions, including any fluid used for dilution of medications as intake. *Significant "hidden" fluid intake can occur if the client is receiving multiple intravenous medications.*

- Arrange for consultation with a dietitian to plan the diet when sodium is restricted and proteins are either restricted or increased. *Including the client and dietitian in planning increases the client's sense of control and compliance with the dietary regime. The glomerular disorder may reduce appetite, and providing foods that are appealing to the client can help maintain adequate nutrition.*

- Administer prescribed medications such as thiazide and loop diuretics, monitoring for desired and adverse effects. *Diuretic therapy can be beneficial in reducing the fluid volume. Because clients with glomerular disorders respond variably to diuretics, it is important to assess the client's output and edema status. Diuretics can exacerbate*

electrolyte imbalances and the muscle weakness often experienced by clients with glomerular disorders.

- Provide frequent position changes and good skin care. *Tissue perfusion may be altered by the presence of edema, increasing the risk of skin breakdown.*

Fatigue

Fatigue is a common manifestation of glomerular disorders. Anemia, loss of plasma proteins, headache, anorexia, and nausea compound this fatigue. The client's ability to maintain usual routines may be impaired. Both physical and mental activities can be affected.

Nursing interventions with rationales follow.

- Assess and document the client's energy level. *As the glomerular dysfunction improves, the client's fatigue begins to resolve, and energy increases.*

- Provide for adequate rest and energy conservation through activity and procedure scheduling. Prevent unnecessary fatigue. *Providing adequate rest and avoiding unnecessary energy expenditures reduce fatigue and improve the client's ability to tolerate and cope with required treatments and activities.*

- Assist the client with ADLs as needed. *The goal is to conserve the client's limited energy reserves.*

- Educate the client and family about the relationship between fatigue and the disease process. *Understanding the nature of the disease and the cause of fatigue helps the client and family to cope with reduced energy and comply with prescribed rest.*

- Reduce the client's energy demands by scheduling more frequent, small meals and short periods of activity. Limit the number of visitors and visit length. *Small, frequent meals reduce the amount of energy needed for eating and digestion. Limiting the number of visitors and the length of visits helps conserve energy. In addition, nurses can assist the fatigued client who may be reluctant to ask visitors to leave.*

- Provide a diet with complete proteins and adequate calories, iron, and minerals. *A well-balanced, nutritionally sound diet is important for maintaining nutritional status and preventing anemia.*

- Assist the client to cope with reduced energy by providing support, understanding, and active listening.

Altered Protection

Physiologic stress resulting from the glomerular disorder and the use of anti-inflammatory and cytotoxic drugs can depress the body's immune system. Immune system depression increases the client's risk for infection. The anti-inflammatory effect of corticosteroids may concurrently mask early signs and manifestations of infection.

Nursing interventions with rationales follow.

- Monitor and record the client's vital signs, including temperature and mental status, every 4 hours. *Temperature elevation can indicate the presence of an infection but may be moderated by anti-inflammatory medications. An elevated pulse rate, increasing lethargy, or confusion may be the initial signs of infection.*

- Assess the client frequently for other signs of infection such as purulent wound drainage, productive cough, adventitious breath sounds, and red or inflamed lesions. Monitor for manifestations of urinary tract infection such as dysuria, frequency and urgency, and cloudy, foul-smelling urine. *Frequent assessment for evidence of infection is important when the client's susceptibility is increased and therapy may mask the usual signs.*

- Monitor the CBC, paying particular attention to the WBC and differential. *An elevated WBC and differential shift to the left (more immature WBCs in the blood than normal) may be early indications of infection.*

- Use good hand-washing technique and protect the client from cross-infection by providing a private room and restricting ill visitors. *Clients with decreased resistance to infection need increased protection.*

- Avoid or minimize invasive procedures. *Maintenance of the protective skin barrier is especially important in the client with altered immune status.*

- If the client requires catheterization, use intermittent straight catheterization or maintain a closed drainage system for an indwelling catheter. Prevent reflux of urine from the drainage system to the bladder or the bladder to the kidneys by ensuring a patent, gravity system. *The urinary tract is a frequent portal of infection, particularly in the hospitalized or institutionalized client. Maintaining strict asepsis during catheterization is vital. Intermittent catheterization is associated with a lower risk of UTI than an indwelling catheter.*

- Provide support and education to the client and family. *Measures to prevent infection will be ongoing throughout the course of anti-inflammatory and cytotoxic therapy.*

Altered Role Performance

The clinical manifestations of glomerular disorders and prescribed therapies can affect the client's ability to maintain usual roles and activities. Fatigue and muscle weakness may limit physical and social activities. For some disorders, bed rest or very limited activity is prescribed to minimize the degree of proteinuria. If azotemia is present, associated malaise, nausea, and changes in mental status can interfere with the client's roles. Facial and periorbital edema affect the self-esteem of the client and may lead to isolation.

Nursing interventions with rationales follow.

- Support the client's dignity and individuality, establish-

ing a strong therapeutic relationship. *It is important to gain the client's trust and confidence.*

- Encourage self-care and participation in decision making. *Increased autonomy helps to restore self-confidence and reduce powerlessness.*

- Provide for time to encourage verbalization of thoughts and feelings; listen actively, acknowledging and accepting the client's fears and concerns. *Adequate time and active listening encourage the client to express concerns and identify how the disease or treatments are affecting daily life. Acceptance helps the client deal with the effects of the illness and treatments as well as the associated losses.*

- Support the client's ability to cope, helping the client identify personal strengths. *This support helps the client gain confidence.*

- Whenever possible, enlist the support of family, other clients, and friends. *These people can provide physical, psychologic, emotional, and social support.*

- Discuss the effect of the disease and treatments on the client's roles and relationships, helping the client and family to identify potential changes in roles, relationships, and life-style. Work with the client and family to develop a plan for alternative behaviors and relationships, encouraging the client to maintain usual roles as much as possible within the limitations of the illness. *Developing a plan helps reduce the strain of accommodating to role changes. The plan also helps the client and family maintain a sense of dignity and control.*

- Provide accurate and optimistic information regarding the disorder and the client's limitations. *The client and family need accurate information to plan for the future.*

- Evaluate the need for additional support and social services for the client and family. Provide referrals as indicated to social services and support groups. *Depending on client and family strengths, the severity of the disorder, the prescribed treatments, and the prognosis, the client and family may need ongoing social support services to facilitate coping and adaptation.*

Other Nursing Diagnoses

The following nursing diagnoses may be appropriate for the client with a glomerular disorder:

- *Activity Intolerance* related to reduced energy
- *Body Image Disturbance* related to facial and periorbital edema
- *Anticipatory Grieving* related to progressive loss of renal function
- *Impaired Home Maintenance Management* related to fatigue and other disease manifestations
- *Risk for Noncompliance* with prescribed treatments related to side effects and lack of understanding

Client and Family Teaching

Disorders of the glomerulus may be self-limiting or progressive. In either case, the course is lengthy, ranging from a number of weeks to years. Self-management is essential, and the key to self-management is a good understanding of the disorder and treatment regimen.

The client and family need information about the disease process and prognosis. Knowledge about the prescribed treatment, including activity and diet restrictions, is essential. Information about the use and potential effects, both beneficial and adverse, of all medications is necessary for home management. The risks, manifestations, prevention, and management of complications such as edema and infection should be well understood. Because the client and family may be monitoring kidney status to a certain extent themselves, they require teaching about the signs, symptoms, and implications of improving or declining renal function.

| Applying the Nursing Process |

Case Study of a Client with Acute Glomerulonephritis: Jung–Lin Chang

Jung–Lin Chang is a 23-year-old graduate student in biology. He goes to the university health center when he notices that his urine is brown and foamy. The physician admits him to the infirmary and orders a throat culture, ASO titer, CBC, BUN, serum creatinine, and urinalysis.

Assessment

Connie King, the nurse admitting Mr. Chang to the infirmary, notes that his history is essentially negative for past kidney or urinary problems. On questioning, he relates having had a "pretty bad" sore throat a couple of weeks before admission. However, it was during midterms, so he took a few antibiotics he had left from a previous bout of strep throat, increased his fluids, and did not see a doctor. The sore throat resolved after approximately 5 days, and he felt well until noticing the change in his urine. He admits that his eyes seemed a little puffy, but he thought the puffiness was due to lack of sleep and fatigue. He has eaten little the past 2 days but didn't think much about it because his food intake is pretty irregular most of the time.

On physical assessment, Ms. King notes the following: BP: 136/90; P: 98; R: 18; and T: 98.8 F (37.1C) PO. Mr. Chang's weight is 165 pounds (75 Kg), up from his normal of 160 (72.5 Kg). He has moderate periorbital edema and edema of his hands and fingers.

The lab results show a negative throat culture but high ASO titer. His CBC is essentially normal. The BUN is 42

mg/dL and the serum creatinine 2.1 mg/dL, indicating azotemia. His urinalysis reveals the presence of protein, red blood cells, and RBC casts. A subsequent assessment of protein in a 24-hour urine sample shows 1025 mg of protein, compared to the normal of 30 to 150 mg/24 hours.

The physician makes a diagnosis of acute poststreptococcal glomerulonephritis and places Mr. Chang on bed rest with bathroom privileges. He orders fluid restriction (1200 mL/day) and a diet with restricted sodium and protein.

Diagnosis

Ms. King develops the following nursing diagnoses for Mr. Chang:

- *Fluid Volume Excess* related to plasma protein deficit and sodium and water retention
- *Risk for Altered Nutrition: Less Than Body Requirements* related to anorexia
- *Anxiety* related to prescribed activity restriction
- *Knowledge Deficit* related to lack of information about glomerulonephritis

Expected Outcomes

The expected outcomes for the plan of care are that Mr. Chang will

- Maintain a blood pressure within normal limits.
- Return to his usual weight with no evidence of edema.
- Consume adequate calories following the prescribed dietary limitations.
- Verbalize a reduction in anxiety regarding his ability to continue with his program of study.
- Demonstrate an understanding of acute glomerulonephritis and his prescribed management regimen.

Planning and Implementation

Ms. King plans the following nursing interventions to be implemented for Mr. Chang:

- Monitor and record vital signs every 4 hours. Notify the physician of significant changes.
- Record intake and output every 8 hours.
- Schedule fluids to allow 650 mL on the day shift, 450 mL on the evening shift, and 100 mL on the night shift.
- Weigh Mr. Chang daily.
- Arrange for dietary consultation to plan a diet that includes preferred foods as allowed.
- Provide small meals with high-carbohydrate between-meal snacks.

- Encourage Mr. Chang to talk about his condition and its potential effects.
- Help Mr. Chang with problem solving and exploring options for maintaining his studies.
- Enlist Mr. Chang's friends and family to listen and provide support.
- Teach Mr. Chang and his family about acute glomerulonephritis and his prescribed management regimen.
- Instruct in the appropriate use of antibiotics.

Evaluation

Mr. Chang is released from the infirmary after 4 days. He decides to return to his parents' home for the 6 to 12 weeks of convalescence prescribed by his doctor. He is able to take incompletes in his courses, which he then finishes through a program of self-study while convalescing.

Mr. Chang's renal function gradually returns to normal with no further azotemia and minimal proteinuria after 4 months. He gradually regains the weight he lost because of anorexia and slight nausea during the initial period of his illness. Mr. Chang verbalizes an understanding of the relationship between the episode of strep throat, his inappropriate use of antibiotics, and the glomerulonephritis. He says, "I may not always remember to take every pill on time in the future, but I sure won't save them for the next time again!"

Critical Thinking in the Nursing Process

1. How did Mr. Chang's use of "a few" previously prescribed antibiotics to treat his sore throat affect his risk for developing poststreptococcal glomerulonephritis?
2. What additional risk factors did Mr. Chang have for developing glomerulonephritis?
3. What caused his urine to become brown and foamy?
4. The presentation (initial manifestations) of acute poststreptococcal glomerulonephritis and rapidly progressive glomerulonephritis are very similar. What diagnostic test would the physician use to make the differential diagnosis? Develop a plan of care for a client undergoing this examination.

The Client with a Vascular Disorder of the Kidney

■ ■ ■

Renal function is absolutely dependent on an adequate supply of blood. It not only supports renal cell metabolism but is also vital to the function of the kidney and the nephron in particular. The kidney can regulate fluid, electrolyte, and acid-base balance and serve as a major organ of excretion only when its blood supply is sufficient. Vascular disorders, therefore, can have significant impact on renal function.

Hypertension and Renal Function

Hypertension, a sustained elevation of the systemic blood pressure, can be both the result and the cause of kidney disease.

Long-standing hypertension damages the walls of the arterioles and accelerates the process of atherosclerosis. The organs most often damaged are the heart, brain, kidneys, eyes, and major blood vessels (Andreoli et al., 1990; Price & Wilson, 1992). In the kidney, this vessel damage results in benign **nephrosclerosis,** a thickening and narrowing of intrarenal blood vessels. The afferent arterioles are primarily affected, causing ischemic injury to the glomeruli and tubules (Wilson et al., 1991).

Malignant hypertension is a rapidly progressive form of hypertension that may develop in clients with untreated primary hypertension. The diastolic pressure is in excess of 120 mm Hg and may be as high as 150 to 170 mm Hg. Although malignant hypertension affects less than 1% of hypertensive clients, it is more common in African-Americans than in people of European ancestry (Berkow & Fletcher, 1992). Untreated, malignant hypertension causes a rapid decline in renal function due to vessel changes, renal ischemia, and infarction.

Approximately 5% to 10% of hypertensive clients have secondary hypertension. *Secondary hypertension* is actually a manifestation of an underlying disease. Renal vascular disease and diseases of the renal parenchyma, such as diabetic nephropathy, are commonly associated with secondary hypertension.

Management of hypertension to maintain the blood pressure within normal limits is important to prevent renal damage. Although hypertension is secondary to renal disease, adequate control can slow the decline in renal function. Hypertension and its management is discussed in depth in Chapter 30.

Renal Artery Occlusion

Renal arteries can be occluded by either a primary process affecting the renal vessels or by emboli, clots, or other foreign material. *Acute renal artery thrombosis,* formation of a blood clot in the renal artery, may be secondary to severe abdominal trauma or vessel trauma from surgery or angiography. Aneurysms of the aorta or renal arteries can contribute to thrombosis as well. Severe aortic or renal artery atherosclerosis can also precipitate renal artery thrombosis, particularly when the cardiac output is reduced (as in heart failure or vascular volume depletion). Emboli from the left side of the heart can travel via the aorta to occlude the renal artery. These emboli may be formed as a result of atrial fibrillation (irregular and uncoordinated contraction of the atria of the heart) or following myocardial infarction. Other sources of emboli are vegetative growths on heart valves associated with bacterial endocarditis or fatty plaque released from aortic walls.

Renal arterial occlusion may be asymptomatic when the process of occlusion is slow and the affected vessels are small. Acute occlusion with resultant ischemia and infarction typically causes severe localized flank pain of sudden onset, nausea and vomiting, fever, and hypertension. Hematuria and oliguria may occur. In the older client, the new onset of hypertension or worsening of previously controlled hypertension may signal renal artery thrombosis.

Laboratory studies reveal leukocytosis, an elevated WBC, and elevated levels of renal enzymes, including aspartate transaminase (AST) and lactic dehydrogenase (LDH). These enzymes are normally present in renal cells and are released into the circulation when cells become necrotic and die. In cases of bilateral arterial occlusion and infarction, renal function deteriorates rapidly, leading to acute renal failure (Andreoli et al., 1990; Wilson et al., 1991).

Surgical intervention to restore circulation to the affected kidney may be indicated for clients with acute occlusion. More conservative medical management using anticoagulant therapy, hypertension control, and supportive treatment is more commonly employed.

Renal Vein Occlusion

Occlusion of renal veins results from thrombus formation. The direct cause is often not evident. In adults, renal vein thrombosis occurs most commonly in association with nephrotic syndrome. Other predisposing factors include pregnancy, the use of oral contraceptives, and the presence of certain tumors.

A gradual or acute deterioration of renal function may be the only manifestation of renal vein occlusion. In some instances, the thrombus breaks loose, resulting in a pulmonary embolism. Visualization of the thrombus through renal venography is required to make a definitive diagnosis.

Thrombolytics such as streptokinase or tPA, pharmacologic preparations used to dissolve or break up a thrombus or clot, or anticoagulant therapy are employed to treat renal vein occlusion. Anticoagulants such as heparin and warfarin prevent further pulmonary emboli and often improve renal function.

Renal Artery Stenosis

Renal artery stenosis, or narrowing, is a leading cause of secondary hypertension, accounting for 2% to 5% of all cases of hypertension (Wilson et al., 1991). It can affect one or both kidneys.

The process leading to stenosis may be distinctly different in men and women. Atherosclerotic processes leading to gradual occlusion of the artery lumen by plaque are the primary cause in men. *Fibromuscular dysplasia,* structural abnormalities involving the intimal, medial, or adventitial layers of the arterial wall, is the most common cause of renal artery stenosis in younger women.

Renal artery stenosis is suspected when hypertension develops in people under the age of 30 or in those over 50 years old with no prior history of high blood pressure. Other clinical features of renal artery stenosis include an epigastric bruit and other manifestations of vascular insufficiency. The captopril test for renin activity and renal angiography are used to confirm the diagnosis. In the captopril test for renin activity, captopril, an ACE inhibitor drug that prevents the conversion of angiotensin I to angiotensin II, is administered. Clients with renovascular hypertension demonstrate higher levels of renin activity following captopril administration than those with essential or primary hypertension (Wilson et al., 1991). In renal angiography, radiopaque contrast dye is injected into the renal arteries, permitting visualization of renal blood vessels.

Restoration of blood flow to the affected kidney is the definitive treatment for renal artery stenosis. Percutaneous transluminal angioplasty to dilate the stenotic vessel is the preferred treatment. This procedure, in which a balloon-tipped catheter is inserted via the femoral artery and aorta to dilate the renal artery, is generally effective and much less invasive than surgical revascularization of the kidney. It provides immediate symptom relief in 90% of clients with fibromuscular dysplasia. One year after treatment, the cure rate remains at 60%. Some clients require a bypass graft of the renal artery. A section of saphenous vein or hypogastric artery is grafted from the aorta to the renal artery distal to the stenosis. Although blood pressure may not return to normal following treatment, its medical management is typically facilitated by these procedures.

The Client with Kidney Trauma

■ ■ ■

The kidneys are relatively well protected by the rib cage and back muscles but may be subject to trauma either from blunt force or from a penetrating injury. Many renal injuries heal uneventfully, but prompt diagnosis and immediate treatment can be life-saving in the event of major damage.

Pathophysiology

Blunt force is the most common cause of kidney injury. Falls, motor vehicle accidents, and sports injuries can all result in kidney damage. The injury may be minor, resulting in a renal contusion or small hematoma, or more serious, involving laceration or other damage. The kidney may fragment or "shatter," leading to significant blood loss and urine extravasation. Tearing of the renal artery or vein may cause rapid hemorrhage, leading to shock and possible death.

Gunshot wounds, knife wounds, impalement injuries, and fractured ribs can result in penetrating damage to a kidney. Minor penetrating injuries may involve laceration of the capsule or renal cortex. Laceration or destruction of the renal parenchyma or vascular supply is considered a major injury. Renal artery, renal vein, and renal pelvis lacerations are critical forms of trauma.

The primary manifestations of renal trauma are hematuria (gross or microscopic), flank or abdominal pain, and oliguria or anuria. There may be localized swelling, tenderness, or ecchymoses in the flank region. Retroperitoneal bleeding from the kidney may cause Turner's sign, a bluish discoloration of the flank (Beachley & Farrar, 1993). Signs of shock may be present, including hypotension, tachycardia, tachypnea, cool and pale skin, and alterations to consciousness.

Collaborative Care

Hemoglobin and hematocrit levels fall in significant renal injury with hemorrhage. Hematuria is typically noted on urinalysis. Significant renal trauma causes levels of aspartate aminotransferase (AST, formerly known as SGOT) to rise within 12 hours following the injury. Abdominal ultrasonography is a noninvasive diagnostic technique used to identify bleeding and damage to the kidney. The CT scan is more valuable in providing a definitive diagnosis, especially when combined with intravenous pyelography to allow visualization of renal structures. Renal arteriography is used when major injury is suspected and surgical intervention is anticipated.

Treatment of minor injuries to the kidney is generally conservative, including bed rest and observation. In these injuries, bleeding is typically minor and self-limiting. The immediate treatment for major or critical trauma is focused on the control of hemorrhage and treatment or prevention of shock. Surgical intervention or percutaneous arterial embolization during angiography may be required to stop the bleeding. Major lacerations may require surgical exploration with possible repair, partial nephrectomy, or total nephrectomy of the affected kidney.

Nursing Care

Although each client has individual nursing care needs, the following nursing diagnoses may be applicable to the client with renal trauma:

- *Decreased Cardiac Output* related to hemorrhage
- *Pain* related to significant trauma

- *Altered Urinary Elimination* related to kidney damage
- *Risk for Infection* related to contamination of the abdominal cavity

The Client with a Neoplastic Disorder of the Kidney

■ ■ ■

Tumors involving the kidney may be either benign or malignant, primary or metastatic. Benign renal tumors are infrequent and are often found only on autopsy. Primary malignant neoplasms account for about 2% of adult cancers and approximately 10,000 deaths per year. Renal cell carcinoma is the most common primary tumor. Another primary tumor is a tumor of the renal pelvis. Metastatic lesions of the kidney are associated with lung and breast cancer, melanoma, and malignant lymphoma (Bullock & Rosendahl, 1992; Porth, 1994; Wilson et al., 1991).

Pathophysiology

Approximately 85% of all primary renal tumors are renal cell carcinomas. These tumors arise in the epithelium of the proximal convoluted tubules. Males are affected more than females by a 2:1 ratio. The highest incidence is seen in people over the age of 55 years. Smoking has been identified as an environmental risk factor; the chronic irritation associated with renal calculi may also contribute.

Renal tumors are often silent, with few clinical manifestations. The classic triad of symptoms, gross hematuria, flank pain, and a palpable abdominal mass, is seen in only about 10% of people with renal cell carcinoma. Hematuria, often microscopic, is the most consistent manifestation. Systemic manifestations include fever without evidence of infection, fatigue, and weight loss. Laboratory findings may include either anemia or polycythemia along with an elevated sedimentation rate. See the accompanying clinical manifestations box.

Clinical Manifestations of Renal Tumors

■ ■ ■

- Microscopic or gross hematuria
- Flank pain
- Palpable abdominal mass
- Fever
- Fatigue
- Weight loss
- Anemia or polycythemia

Table 26–4   Renal Cell Cancer Staging

Stage	Extent of Tumor	Prognosis
I	Confined to the kidney capsule	60% to 75% 5-year survival
II	Invasion through the capsule but confined to local fascia	47% to 65% 5-year survival
III	Regional lymph node, ipsilateral renal vein, or inferior vena cava involvement	25% to 50% 5-year survival if regional nodes uninvolved; 5% to 15% if involved
IV	Distant metastases	Less than 5% 5-year survival

Source Bullock & Rosendahl, 1992; Wilson et al., 1991

Renal cell tumors metastasize most commonly to the lungs, mediastinum, bone, lymph nodes, liver, and central nervous system. The tumor may produce hormones or hormonelike substances, including parathyroid hormone, prostaglandins, prolactin, renin, gonadotropins, and glucocorticoids. These substances can cause additional manifestations such as hypercalcemia, hypertension, and hyperglycemia. The progression and behavior of renal cell carcinomas are unpredictable (Bullock & Rosendahl, 1992; Wilson et al., 1991). Table 26–4 outlines the staging and prognosis for renal cell cancers.

Collaborative Care

Hematuria is often the only presenting manifestation of a renal tumor; its presence is typically confirmed through diagnostic testing. Renal ultrasonography often provides the first diagnostic evidence of a kidney tumor. It is particularly beneficial in differentiating cystic kidney disease from renal neoplasms when a renal mass has been identified. CT is used to provide information about the tumor density, local extension of the tumor, and regional lymph node or vascular involvement. Other diagnostic studies that may be used include intravenous pyelography and MRI. Renal angiography, aortography, and inferior venacavography may be employed to determine the extent of vascular involvement prior to surgical intervention. Chest X-ray, bone scan, and liver function studies are done prior to intervention to evaluate the potential spread of tumor to other sites (Berkow & Fletcher, 1992; Wilson et al., 1991).

Radical nephrectomy is the treatment of choice for tumors of the kidney. In a radical nephrectomy, the adrenal gland, perirenal fat, upper ureter, and fascia surrounding the kidney, as well as the entire kidney itself, are removed. Regional lymph nodes may also be removed. If metastases are present at the time of diagnosis, nephrectomy seems to be of little use unless the tumor mass is causing problems such as pain or bleeding. Clients with metastatic disease are typically treated with a regime of combination chemotherapy. Radiation therapy may also be employed for bone or lung lesions (Wilson et al., 1991). See the ac-

companying collaborative care box for a client having a nephrectomy.

Nursing care for the client undergoing kidney surgery is summarized in the box beginning on page 958, and the Critical Pathway beginning on page 959.

Nursing Care

The client with renal carcinoma has nursing care needs related to both the diagnosis of cancer and to the surgical intervention. The incisions used to access the kidney, which are high on the abdomen, back, or flank, disrupt large muscles (Figure 26–4). As a result, the client may experience significant pain in the initial postoperative period, and the risk for respiratory complications is high. The need to protect the remaining kidney from damage is heightened. Psychologically, the client may grieve the loss of a major organ and the diagnosis of cancer.

Pain

The size and location of the incision used for a radical nephrectomy make pain management a challenge. Costal blocks and patient-controlled analgesia (PCA) can be effective in relieving the discomfort, as can administration of ordered analgesics. Nursing care focuses on assessing the adequacy of pain relief, providing supportive measures to enhance analgesia, and ensuring that pain or the fear of pain does not lead to respiratory complications.

Nursing interventions with rationales follow.

- Assess the client frequently for adequate pain relief. Use subjective and objective information including
  a. The location, intensity, and character of the pain.
  b. Nonverbal signs including grimacing, tense body position, apparent dozing, elevated pulse, an increase or decrease in blood pressure, and rapid, shallow respirations.

  The client may assume that pain is to be expected or tolerated or may fear becoming addicted to analgesic medications. Careful questioning and assessment can provide information regarding the client's pain status, allowing better control of discomfort.

Text continues on page 964

Collaborative Care for the Client Having a Nephrectomy

Health Care Team	Client-Centered Care
Urologist	Assesses client's urological status and orders diagnostic tests including IVP, CT scans, and laboratory tests. Performs the surgical removal of the kidney, adrenal gland, lymph nodes, and surrounding fat and fasci.
Radiology oncologist	Manages irradiation preoperatively to reduce the size of the kidney and postoperatively in collaboration with the oncologist as adjunct therapy if necessary.
Oncologist	Orders chemotherapy postoperatively if necessary, monitors for infection, thrombocytopenia, renal toxicity, and other side effects.
Primary care physician	May discover the renal tumor as a palpable mass, assesses client with hematuria for general symptoms of a malignancy. Refers client to a urologist and/or manages medical care following discharge.
Mental health clinical nurse specialist	Helps the client deal with the possible diagnosis of cancer and issues with body image.
Social worker	May coordinate support services through the American Cancer Society. Arranges for home health aides to provide assistance during recovery phase. Arranges for visiting nurse to assess wound healing and perform dressing changes.
RN and health care team communications	Reports to surgeon any signs and symptoms of complications such as fluid and electrolyte disturbances, wound infection, adrenal insufficiency, hemorrhage, or abdominal distention. Alerts social worker to any home care needs.

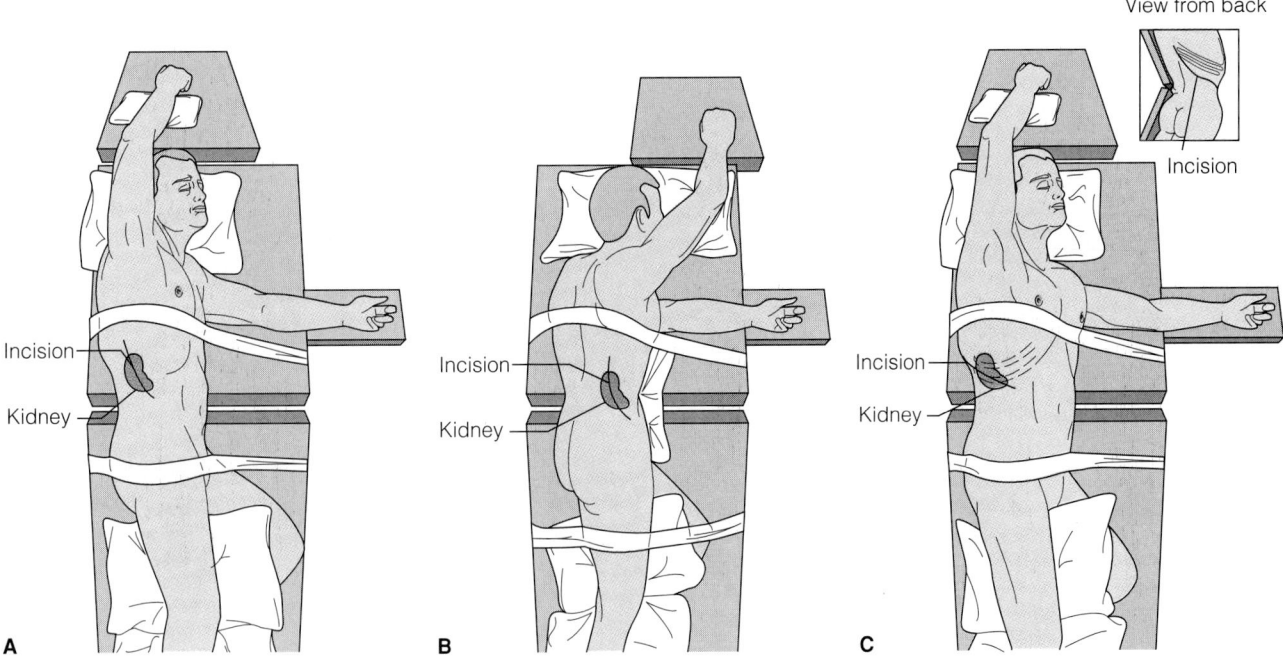

Figure 26–4   Incisions used for kidney surgery. *A,* Flank. *B,* Lumbar. *C,* Thoracoabdominal.

Nursing Care of the Client Having a Partial or Total Nephrectomy

PREOPERATIVE CARE

- Assess the client's knowledge and understanding of the procedure to be performed, its purpose, and the expected results. *To give truly informed consent, clients need to have a good understanding of the purpose, potential risks and benefits, and possible alternative treatments.*

- Document a full nursing assessment prior to surgery. *This assessment provides baseline data for comparison during the postoperative period.*

- Monitor laboratory results, reporting any abnormal findings to the physician. *The presence of bacteriuria, abnormalities in blood clotting studies, or other significant changes may affect the surgical plan.*

- Teach the client and family about the planned procedure and postoperative care including:
  a. The location of the incision
  b. Any anticipated tubes, stents, or drains
  c. Postoperative routines such as spirometry, coughing, turning
  d. Pain management
  The well-prepared client is less anxious and better able to cooperate with postoperative care, shortening the recovery period.

- Prepare the client for surgery as ordered, including any bowel or skin preparation and premedication.

POSTOPERATIVE CARE

- Provide routine postsurgical care as described in Chapter 7.

- Perform and document additional assessments and procedures related to kidney surgery.
  a. Urine color, amount, and character; presence of any hematuria, pyuria, or sediment; any oliguria or anuria. *The removal of one kidney makes it critical to assure and preserve the function of the remaining kidney.*
  b. The placement, status, and drainage from any ureteral catheters, stents, nephrostomy tubes, or drains. Label each clearly. Maintain gravity drainage; irrigate only as ordered by the physician. *Maintaining the patency of all drainage tubes is vital to prevent accumulation of fluids and possible hydronephrosis. Bright bleeding or unexpected drainage may indicate a surgical complication.*
  c. Status of the incision, including its site and the presence of any redness, swelling, bleeding, or

drainage of urine. *These signs could indicate hemorrhage, infection, or other surgical complication.*

- Ensure adequate pain management with patient-controlled analgesia or administration of analgesics as ordered. *The incisions used in kidney surgery (see Figure 26–6) often disrupt major abdominal, flank, or back muscles. Adequate analgesia is necessary for the client to move freely, cough, and breathe deeply.*

- Monitor respiratory status frequently, including oxygen saturation readings, respiratory rate and depth, and lung sounds. Assist the client to turn, use the spirometer, and cough as ordered, splinting the incision as needed. *The upper abdominal location of the incision puts the client at risk for respiratory complications, including pneumonia and atelectasis.*

- Monitor vital signs, urinary output, and level of consciousness frequently. *It is important to promptly identify any decrease in cardiac output due to fluid volume depletion because it may jeopardize blood flow to the remaining kidney.*

- Assess for potential complications of surgery, including infection, paralytic ileus, thrombosis, or embolism. *Early detection and intervention can prevent serious or long-term consequences.*

- Support the client's grieving process and adjustment to the loss of a kidney. *The client has lost a major organ, resulting in a body image change and grief response. When nephrectomy is performed for the diagnosis of cancer, the client may also be grieving the loss of health and potential loss of life.*

- Provide instruction to the client and family about postoperative procedures and home-care measures, including symptoms that should be reported to the physician. Include the following in addition to any instructions specific to the individual client:
  a. The importance of measures to prevent damage to the remaining kidney, including prevention of UTI, calculus formation, and trauma. See Chapter 25 for measures to prevent UTI and calculus formation. *The client is at increased risk for renal failure if the remaining kidney is damaged by infection, stones, or trauma.*
  b. Maintain a fluid intake of 2000 to 2500 mL per day. *This is an important measure to prevent dehydration and maintain good urine flow.*
  c. The client should gradually increase exercise to tolerance, avoiding heavy lifting for a year after

Nursing Care of the Client Having a Partial or Total Nephrectomy (continued)

surgery. Participation in contact sports is not recommended after nephrectomy to reduce the risk of injury to the remaining kidney. *Lifting is avoided to allow full healing and scar formation in disrupted tissues. Trauma to the remaining kidney would seriously jeopardize renal function.*

d. Care of the incision and any remaining drainage tubes, catheters, or stents. *This routine postoperative instruction is vital to support the client's ability to provide self-care.*

e. Prescribed medications, including their purpose, dose, scheduling, and potential side effects.

f. Signs and symptoms that should be reported to the physician. Among these are signs of urinary tract infection (dysuria, frequency, urgency, nocturia, cloudy, malodorous urine) or systemic infection (elevated temperature, general symptoms), redness, swelling, pain, or drainage from the incision or any catheter or drain tube site. *Prompt treatment of any postoperative infection is vital to allow continued healing and prevent compromise of the remaining kidney.*

Critical Pathway for Client Following Nephrectomy

	Date _____ Preoperative	Date _____ 1st 24 Hours Postoperative	Date _____ 2nd–3rd Day Postoperative
Expected length of stay 6–7 days			
Daily outcomes	Client verbalizes understanding of preoperative teaching including: turning, coughing, deep breathing, incentive spirometer, mobilization, possible tubes (NG tube, IV, Foley catheter, Penrose or other drains, pain management [epidural or PCA]). Client demonstrates ability to cope. Client verbalizes understanding of procedure. Obtain informed consent.	Client will ■ Have stable vital signs. ■ Have a clean, dry wound with edges well-approximated, healing by first intention. ■ Recover from anesthesia as evidenced by: VS return to baseline, awake, alert, and oriented. ■ Verbalize understanding and demonstrate cooperation with turning, coughing, deep breathing, and splinting; lungs clear to auscultation. ■ Have urine output > 30 mL/hr. ■ Demonstrate ability to use PCA if in use. ■ Remain free of nausea and vomiting. ■ Verbalize control of incisional pain with ordered medications and nonpharmacologic measures. ■ Transfer out of bed with assistance 2 times. ■ Demonstrate ability to cope.	Client will ■ Have stable vital signs. ■ Have a clean, dry wound with edges well-approximated, healing by first intention. ■ Have a urine output > 30 mL/hr. ■ Have active bowel sounds. ■ Tolerate ordered diet without nausea or vomiting. ■ Demonstrate cooperation with turning, coughing, deep breathing, and splinting. ■ Have lungs clear to auscultation. ■ Ambulate 4 times each day. ■ Verbalize control of incisional pain with ordered medications and nonpharmacologic methods. ■ Demonstrate ability to cope. ■ Verbalize/demonstrate beginning understanding of home care instructions.

	Critical Pathway for Client Following Nephrectomy (continued)		
	Date _____ **Preoperative**	**Date _____** **1st 24 Hours Postoperative**	**Date _____** **2nd–3rd Day Postoperative**
Tests and treatments	CBC, electrolytes Chemistry profile Urinalysis Chest X-ray Baseline physical assessment, with a focus on respiratory status and gastrointestinal and urinary function	CBC Electrolytes Vital signs and O_2 saturation, neurovascular assessment, dressing and wound drainage assessment q15min × 4; q30min × 4; q1h × 4 and then q4h if stable Assess respiratory status and gastrointestinal function q4h and prn. Assess patency of Foley catheter and urine output q1h × 24 hours. Report urine output < 30 mL/hr. Strict intake and output Incentive spirometer q2h Intake and output every shift Assess patency of NG tube q2h, noting volume, color, and character of drainage. Assess and record the description, location, duration, and characteristics of client's pain q2–4h and prn. Encourage verbalization of pain and discomfort. Reduce or eliminate pain-producing factors and employ distraction or relaxation techniques. Provide back rubs. Encourage client to request analgesic or use PCA before pain becomes severe.	Vital signs and dressing and wound drainage assessment q4h Assess respiratory status and gastrointestinal function q4h. Incentive spirometer q2h until fully ambulatory Strict intake and output every q2–4h If still in place, assess patency and output of NG tube q4–8h. Assess Foley catheter and urine output q2–4h and prn. Report urine output < 30 mL/hr. Using sterile asepsis change dressing: assess wound healing and wound drainage. Assess and record the description, location, duration, and characteristics of client's pain q4h and prn. Reduce or eliminate pain-producing factors, employ distraction or relaxation techniques, and offer back rubs.

	Date _____ **Preoperative**	Date _____ **1st 24 Hours Postoperative**	Date _____ **2nd–3rd Day Postoperative**
Knowledge deficit	Orient to room and surroundings. Provide simple, brief instructions. Review preoperative preparation including hospital and surgical routines. Include family in teaching. Discuss surgery and specific postoperative care: turning, coughing, deep breathing, splinting incision, incentive spirometer, mobilization, possible tubes (NG and intravenous), pain management (PCA, epidural, or prn medications). Instruct regarding distraction techniques, e.g., slow, rhythmic breathing and guided imagery, to produce pain relief. Instruct in relaxation techniques, e.g., tensing and relaxing muscle groups and rhythmic breathing. Assess understanding of teaching.	Reorient to room and postoperative routine. Include family in teaching. Review plan of care and importance of early mobilization. Review importance of turning, coughing, deep breathing, splinting incision, incentive spirometer, mobilization, drainage tubes, Foley catheter, and intravenous, pain management (PCA, epidural, or prn medications). Assess understanding of teaching.	Reinforce earlier teaching regarding ongoing care. Include family in teaching. Begin discharge teaching regarding activity level and wound care. Assess understanding of teaching.
Psycho-social	Assess anxiety related to diagnosis and pending surgery. Assess fears of the unknown and surgery. Offer emotional support. Encourage verbalization of concerns. Provide information regarding surgical experience. Minimize external stimuli (e.g., noise, movement).	Assess client's and family's level of anxiety. Encourage verbalization of concerns. Offer emotional support. Provide information and ongoing support and encouragement to client and family.	Encourage verbalization of concerns. Provide ongoing support and encouragement to client and family. Offer emotional support.
Diet	NPO Baseline nutritional and hydration assessment	NG tube until return of bowel sounds NPO	When NG tube removed, begin clear liquids to tolerance.
Activity	Assess safety needs and provide appropriate measures. Activity as ordered	Maintain safety precautions. Assist to chair 2 times.	Maintain safety precautions. Ambulate 4 times with assistance.

➤

Critical Pathway for Client Following Nephrectomy (continued)

	Date _____ **Preoperative**	Date _____ **1st 24 Hours Postoperative**	Date _____ **2nd–3rd Day Postoperative**
Medications	Preoperative medications as ordered	IV fluids IV antibiotics Pain medication (epidural, PCA, IV, or prn) as ordered Assess effectiveness of analgesics.	IV fluids IV antibiotics if ordered When ordered convert IV to intermittent IV device. Pain medication (epidural, PCA, IV, or prn) as ordered Assess effectiveness of analgesics.
Transfer/ discharge plans	Assess potential discharge needs and support system. Establish discharge goals with client and family.	Review progress toward discharge goals with client and family. Consult with social service re: VNA and projected needs for home health care (if any).	Review progress toward discharge goals with client and family. Make appropriate discharge referrals.

	Date _____ **4th Day Postoperative**	Date _____ **5th Day Postoperative**	Date _____ **6th–7th Day Postoperative**
Daily outcomes	Client will ■ Be afebrile with stable vital signs. ■ Be alert and oriented. ■ Have a clean, dry wound with edges well-approximated, healing by first intention. ■ Maintain urine output > 30 mL/hr. ■ Have lungs clear to auscultation. ■ Tolerate ordered diet without nausea or vomiting. ■ Ambulate 4–6 times. ■ Verbalize control of incisional pain with ordered medications and nonpharmacologic measures. ■ Demonstrate ability to cope. ■ Verbalize/demonstrate beginning understanding of home care instructions.	Client will ■ Be afebrile with stable vital signs. ■ Be alert and oriented. ■ Have a clean, dry wound with edges well-approximated, healing by first intention. ■ Maintain urine output > 30 mL/hr. ■ Tolerate ordered diet without nausea or vomiting. ■ Ambulate 4–6 times. ■ Verbalize control of incisional pain with ordered medications and nonpharmacologic measures. ■ Demonstrate ability to cope. ■ Verbalize/demonstrate beginning understanding of home care instructions.	Client will ■ Be afebrile with stable vital signs. ■ Be alert and oriented. ■ Have a dry, clean wound with edges well-approximated, healing by first intention. ■ Maintain urine output > 30 mL/hr. ■ Manage pain with nonpharmacologic measures and any ordered medications. ■ Be independent in self-care. ■ Be fully ambulatory. ■ Have resumed preadmission urine and bowel elimination pattern. ■ Verbalize home care instructions. ■ Tolerate usual diet. ■ Demonstrate ability to cope with ongoing stressors.

	Date _____ **4th Day Postoperative**	Date _____ **5th Day Postoperative**	Date _____ **6th–7th Day Postoperative**
Tests and treatments	Vital signs and dressing and wound drainage assessment q4h Incentive spirometer q2h until fully ambulatory Measure intake and output every shift. D/C Foley catheter and assess voiding pattern every q2–4h and prn. Assess respiratory status and gastrointestinal function q4–8h and prn. Using sterile asepsis, change dressing; assess wound healing and wound drainage. Assess and record description, location, duration, and characteristics of client's pain q4h and prn. Encourage client to employ distraction or relaxation techniques.	Vital signs and dressing and wound drainage assessment q4h Assess respiratory status and gastrointestinal function q4–8h. Measure intake and output every shift and monitor urine output q4h and prn. Report urine output < 30 mL/hr. Remove dressing and assess wound healing and drainage. Assess and record description, location, duration, and characteristics of client's pain q4h and prn. Encourage client to employ distraction or relaxation techniques.	Vital signs and dressing and wound drainage assessment q4–8h Assess respiratory status and gastrointestinal function. Intake and output Report urine output < 30 mL/hr. Assess wound healing. Assess and record description, location, duration, and characteristics of client's pain q4h and prn. Encourage client to employ distraction or relaxation techniques.
Knowledge deficit	Include family in teaching. Initiate discharge teaching regarding wound care, diet, and activity. Review written discharge instructions with client and family. Assess understanding of teaching.	Continue discharge teaching, including family, about wound care, diet, signs and symptoms to report, medications, and activity. Review written discharge instructions with client and family. Assess understanding of teaching.	Complete discharge teaching to include wound care, diet, follow-up care, signs and symptoms to report, activity, and medications: name, purpose, dose, frequency, route, dietary interactions, and side effects. Provide client with written discharge instructions. Assess understanding of teaching.
Psycho-social	Encourage verbalization of concerns. Offer emotional support. Provide ongoing support and encouragement.	Encourage verbalization of concerns. Offer emotional support. Provide ongoing support and encouragement.	Encourage verbalization of concerns. Offer emotional support. Provide ongoing support and encouragement.

➤

	Date _____ 4th Day Postoperative	Date _____ 5th Day Postoperative	Date _____ 6th–7th Day Postoperative
Diet	If tolerating clear liquids, advance to full liquids as tolerated.	Advance diet to soft, regular diet to tolerance. Encourage fluids.	Regular diet as tolerated. Encourage fluids.
Activity	Ambulate independently at least 4 times. Maintain safety precautions.	Fully ambulatory Maintain safety precautions.	Fully ambulatory
Medications	Provide PO or PCA analgesics, D/C epidural. Assess effectiveness of analgesics. Intermittent IV device for any IV medications; D/C when so ordered	D/C PCA Provide PO analgesics. Assess effectiveness of analgesics.	Provide PO analgesics. Assess effectiveness of analgesics.
Transfer/discharge plans	Continue to review progress toward discharge goals.	Finalize discharge plans. Continue to review progress toward discharge goals. Make appropriate discharge referrals. Finalize plans for home care if needed.	Complete discharge instructions.

Critical Pathway for Client Following Nephrectomy (continued)

- Assess the incision for signs of inflammation or swelling and the drainage catheters and tubes for patency. *An obstructed catheter can lead to hydronephrosis, hematoma, or abscess, increasing incisional pain.*

- Assess the abdomen for distention, tenderness, and bowel sounds. *Intraabdominal bleeding, peritonitis, or paralytic ileus can cause pain that may be confused with incisional pain.*

- Monitor for medication effectiveness and adverse effects. *A dosage adjustment may be required to provide adequate pain relief without harmful effects.*

- Provide nonpharmacologic relief measures. Include positioning, diversional activities, management of environmental stimuli, guided imagery, and teaching the use of relaxation techniques. *These can enhance the effects of analgesia.*

- Splint the incision with a pillow and teach the client how to self-splint the incision during coughing and deep breathing. *Splinting helps prevent respiratory complications related to fear of pain.*

Ineffective Breathing Pattern

The location of the incision combined with the respiratory depressant effects of narcotic analgesics puts the postsurgical nephrectomy client at risk for respiratory complications. Active nursing intervention is important to maintain adequate ventilation.

Nursing interventions with rationales follow.

- Position the client to allow optimal respiratory excursion, using semi-Fowler's position and side-lying positions as allowed and tolerated. *Lung expansion is improved in semi-Fowler's and Fowler's positions. If not contraindicated, lying on the operative side splints the incision and may improve lung expansion as well.*

- Assess respiratory status frequently, including respiratory rate and depth, cough, lung sounds, oxygen saturation, and temperature. *Early identification and intervention can prevent major respiratory complications.*

- Change the client's position frequently, ambulate as soon as possible. *These measures promote lung expansion and the movement of mucus out of airways.*

- Encourage frequent (every 1 to 2 hours) deep breathing, use of the spirometer, and coughing. Help the client splint the incision. *These measures promote alveolar ventilation and gas exchange.*

- Administer analgesic agents regularly and assess degree of pain relief and sedation. *Adequate pain management allows the client to move and breathe easily but does not overly sedate the client.*

Risk for Altered Urinary Elimination

Surgical intervention involving the urinary tract puts the client at risk for alterations in renal function and urine elimination. In addition, the presence of only one remaining functional kidney dictates extra caution in the maintenance of renal circulation, a sterile urinary tract, and free urine flow.

Nursing interventions with rationales follow.

- Monitor vital signs and urinary output every 1 to 2 hours in the initial postoperative period, then every 4 hours. Maintain central venous pressure within normal limits. *Hypovolemia due to hemorrhage, diuresis, or fluid sequestering (third-spacing) reduces the blood flow to the kidney and increases the risk of renal ischemia with possible acute tubular necrosis and acute renal failure.*

- Frequently assess the amount and character of drainage on surgical dressings and from drainage tubes, stents, and catheters. Measure and record output from each drain or catheter separately. *Frequent and accurate assessment of the character and amount of drainage helps to identify excess bleeding, abnormal fluid loss, infection, or other potential surgical complications.*

- Monitor drains and tubes for kinking, twisting, or tension. Do not clamp any tubes. Irrigate carefully and only with a physician's order. Notify the physician immediately if any tube becomes dislodged. *It is vital to maintain the patency of drains, particularly any affecting the remaining kidney, to prevent excess pressure of hydronephrosis.*

- Maintain fluid intake with intravenous fluids until oral intake is resumed. Encourage a fluid intake of 2000 to 2500 mL per day as soon as the client is able to tolerate oral liquids. *A liberal fluid intake prevents dehydration, helps to dilute any nephrotoxic substances, and promotes good urinary output.*

- Use strict aseptic technique in caring for all urinary catheters, tubes, stents, and drains as well as the surgical incision. *Asepsis is vital to prevent infection and possible compromise of the remaining kidney.*

- After removal of indwelling urethral catheter, assess frequently for signs of urinary retention. Notify the physician if the client is unable to void within 4 to 6 hours or if manifestions of retention (distended bladder, discomfort, urinary dribbling) occur earlier. *Relief of urinary retention is vital to prevent stasis and the possible complications of infection and hydronephrosis of the remaining kidney.*

- Monitor urinalysis results, renal function studies including the BUN and serum creatinine, and serum electrolytes. Report abnormal findings to the physician. *Changes in these values may indicate early acute renal failure; prompt intervention is necessary to preserve renal function.*

Anticipatory Grieving

The client having a radical nephrectomy for renal cancer not only loses a major organ but also has to adjust to the diagnosis of cancer. Although the prognosis for recovery may be good, many people perceive cancer as always fatal. Providing support for the client and family during the initial stages of grieving can improve physical recovery as well as psychologic coping and eventual adaptation.

Nursing interventions with rationales follow.

- Work to develop a trusting relationship with the client and family. *Trust increases the nurse's effectiveness in helping them work through the process of grieving.*

- Listen actively to the client and family, encouraging them to express their fears and concerns. *As they begin to express their concerns, they can begin to deal more effectively with them.*

- Assist the client and family to identify strengths, past experiences, and support systems. *These resources can be employed in working through the grieving process.*

- Demonstrate respect for the client's and family's cultural, spiritual, and religious values and beliefs; encourage them to use these resources to cope with losses. *The client's value and belief systems can provide a structure and form for dealing with the grieving process.*

- Encourage the client and family to discuss the potential impact of loss on the individual and the family structure and function. Assist family members to share concerns with one another. *Sharing of fears and concerns among family members promotes involvement and support of the entire family unit so that the individual is not left to cope alone.*

- Provide referral to cancer support groups, social services, or counseling as appropriate. *Support groups and counseling services provide the client and family with additional resources for coping.*

Other Nursing Diagnoses

The following nursing diagnoses may also apply to the client with renal cancer:

- *Impaired Home Maintenance Management* related to medical and surgical interventions

- *Knowledge Deficit* related to lack of information about the diagnosis and treatment
- *Impaired Skin Integrity* related to surgical incision

Client and Family Teaching

If renal cancer was detected at an early stage and cure is considered to be likely following radical nephrectomy, teaching centers on the protection for the remaining kidney. The client needs to know measures to prevent infection, renal calculi, hydronephrosis, and trauma. Teach the client to maintain a fluid intake of 2000 to 2500 mL per day, increasing the amount during hot weather or strenuous exercise. Instruct the client to urinate when the urge is experienced, and before and after sexual intercourse.

Teach proper cleansing of the perineal area. Identify the signs and symptoms of urinary tract infection, stressing the importance of early and appropriate evaluation and intervention by a physician or other primary care provider. For clients who have a history of renal calculi, provide instruction in any recommended dietary modifications to prevent further nephrolithiasis. If the client is an older adult male, teach about prostatic hypertrophy, a major cause of urinary tract obstruction, including its signs and symptoms and the importance of routine screening examinations. Stress the importance of minimizing the risk of trauma to the remaining kidney; contact sports such as football or hockey should be avoided. Encourage the client and family to implement measures to prevent motor vehicle accidents and falls, which could damage the kidney.

▪▪▪ Renal Failure ▪▪▪

Renal failure is a condition in which the kidneys are unable to remove accumulated metabolites from the blood, resulting in altered fluid, electrolyte, and acid-base balance. The cause may be a primary kidney disorder, or renal failure may be secondary to a systemic disease or other urologic defects. Renal failure may be either acute or chronic. **Acute renal failure** has an abrupt onset and with prompt intervention is often reversible. **Chronic renal failure** is a silent disease, developing slowly and insidiously, with few symptoms until the kidneys are severely damaged and unable to meet the excretory needs of the body. Both forms of renal failure are characterized by azotemia (Bullock & Rosendahl, 1992; Porth, 1994).

Renal failure is costly. In 1990, approximately 45,000 clients enrolled into a federal program for treatment of end-stage renal disease (ESRD) at a cost of $35,000 per

Table 26–5 Major Causes of Acute Renal Failure

	Cause	Examples
Prerenal failure	Hypovolemia	Skin, GI, or renal volume loss; hemorrhage; ECF sequestration
	Cardiovascular failure	Impaired cardiac output due to infarct, tamponade; vascular pooling due to anaphylaxis, sepsis, drugs
Intrarenal failure	Vascular disease	Vasculitis, malignant hypertension, thrombotic thrombocytopenic purpura; scleroderma; arterial and/or venous occlusion
	Glomerulonephritis	Immune-complex disease; antiglomerular basement membrane disease
	Interstitial nephritis	Drugs, hypercalcemia; infections, idiopathic
	Acute tubular necrosis	
	Post-ischemic	Conditions identified for prerenal failure
	Pigment-induced (hemoglobinemia; myoglobinemia)	Hemolysis; muscle cell breakdown (trauma, muscle disease, coma, heat stroke, severe exercise, potassium or phosphate depletion)
	Toxin-induced	Antibiotics, contrast media, anesthetic agents, heavy metals, organic solvents
	Pregnancy-related	Septic abortion, uterine hemorrhage, eclampsia
Postrenal failure	Extrarenal obstruction	Urethral obstruction; bladder, pelvic, prostatic or retroperitoneal neoplasms; prostatism, surgical accident, medication, calculi, pus, blood clots
	Intrarenal obstruction	Crystals (uric acid, oxalic acid, sulfonamides, methotrexate)
	Bladder rupture	Trauma

Source Wilson et al., 1991

person. More than 167,000 clients with ESRD are currently receiving therapy. It is estimated that by the year 2000, the cost will total more than $10 billion, with 300,000 patients enrolled. The cost is also measured in lives and life-style. A 45-year-old client with ESRD has a life expectancy of about 6 years compared with a life expectancy of more than 31 years for someone of the same age who is well (US Renal Data System, 1993). Although many clients report satisfaction with their quality of life, often clients on dialysis are unable to work, and the family structure may disintegrate under the strain of treatment.

The Client with Acute Renal Failure

■ ■ ■

Acute renal failure (ARF) is a relatively common syndrome characterized by a rapid decline in renal function. Approximately 5% of all hospitalized clients develop ARF; the incidence jumps to as much as 20% in critical and special care units (Price & Wilson, 1992; Wilson et al., 1991). Approximately 60% of all instances of ARF are related to surgery or trauma; the remainder are caused by medical or obstetric conditions. *Iatrogenic* causes, those resulting from treatment by a physician, can be identified for half of the cases seen in hospitalized clients (Wyngaarden et al., 1992). Examples of iatrogenic causes of ARF include nephrotoxic medications, radiologic contrast dye, and shock following surgical intervention for any reason. ARF occurs more frequently in older clients because initiating events such as hypotension, major surgeries, radiologic procedures, and treatment with nephrotoxic drugs are most likely to affect older adults. Preexisting renal insufficiency related to the aging process also puts the older adult at increased risk for ARF (Abrams & Berkow, 1990).

At least 10,000 people in the United States are affected by ARF every year. The mortality rate is high, up to 90%. This high death rate is more closely attributable to the populations at greatest risk for ARF—older clients, the critically ill, and those on life-support systems—than to the disorder itself (Porth, 1994; Wilson et al., 1991).

Acute renal failure is generally recognized by a fall in urine output and rising BUN and/or serum creatinine levels. Although oliguria is common, the urine output may exceed 400 mL per day. This form of ARF is known as *nonoliguric* or *high-output failure*. It is being recognized with increasing frequency, particularly in older adults.

The most common causes of acute renal failure are ischemia (hypoperfusion) and nephrotoxins. The kidney is particularly vulnerable to both because of the amount of blood that passes through it. A fall in blood pressure or volume can cause ischemia of kidney tissues. When nephrotoxins are present in the blood, the exposure of renal tissue to the toxins is great.

Etiologic factors for ARF are commonly divided into the categories of prerenal, intrarenal, and postrenal. Table 26–5 on page 966 summarizes the causes of acute renal failure.

Prerenal Factors

Prerenal causes of ARF are those affecting renal blood flow and perfusion. They include any condition that reduces the renal perfusion pressure, leading to a decreased glomerular filtration rate and azotemia. Prerenal causes account for 40% to 80% of acute renal failure (Wilson et al., 1991). Extracellular fluid losses (e.g., due to hemorrhage or dehydration), decreased cardiac output, and severe vasoconstriction can all lead to renal ischemia. When recognized promptly and treated appropriately, prerenal ARF is readily reversible. If it is not recognized or is inadequately treated, ischemic acute tubular necrosis and intrarenal failure may result.

Intrarenal Factors

Intrarenal failure is characterized by acute damage to the renal parenchyma and nephrons. Intrarenal causes can be further subdivided into those related to kidney diseases and those marked by acute tubular necrosis.

In acute glomerulonephritis, glomerular inflammation can reduce renal blood flow and cause ARF. Vascular disorders affecting the kidney, such as *vasculitis* (inflammation of the blood vessels), malignant hypertension, and arterial or venous occlusion, can damage nephrons sufficiently to result in acute renal failure.

Nephrons are especially susceptible to injury from either ischemia or exposure to a nephrotoxic agent. Nephron damage can lead to **acute tubular necrosis (ATN),** a syndrome of abrupt and progressive decline in tubular and glomerular function. Prolonged ischemia is the most common cause of ATN. When ischemia and nephrotoxin exposure occur concurrently, the risk for ATN and tubular dysfunction is especially high.

The aminoglycoside antibiotics and radiologic contrast media are nephrotoxins commonly associated with acute tubular necrosis and ARF. Other drugs that have been identified as potential nephrotoxins include cephalosporin antibiotics, penicillin, tetracycline, streptomycin, and amphotericin when used in high doses; phenylbutazone and other nonsteroidal anti-inflammatory drugs (NSAIDs); angiotensin-converting enzyme (ACE) inhibitors; and phenytoin, sulfonamides, and cisplatin. Heavy metals such as mercury and gold, and some common chemicals, such as ethylene glycol (antifreeze) and carbon tetrachloride, are also nephrotoxic (Price & Wilson, 1992; Wyngaarden et al., 1992).

Nursing Implications for Pharmacology: Nephrotoxic Drugs

AMINOGLYCOSIDE ANTIBIOTICS

Amikacin (Amikin)

Gentamicin (Garamycin)

Kanamycin (Kantrex, Klebcil)

Neomycin (selected otic and topical preparations)

Streptomycin

Tobramycin (Nebcin, Tobrex)

Hospitalized clients often experience nephrotoxicity caused by aminoglycoside antibiotics. Nephrotoxicity is generally related to the dose and duration of therapy with these drugs. When a high therapeutic blood level is sustained for 5 to 10 days, the risk may be significant. The drug accumulates in tubular cells, eventually killing them. This leads to decreased glomerular filtration and reduced excretion of the drug and metabolic wastes. Older clients, dehydrated clients, clients with impaired renal function, and those receiving other nephrotoxic drugs are most susceptible to ATN as a result of aminoglycoside therapy.

Nursing Responsibilities

■ Monitor and record intake and output, daily weight, skin turgor, and other assessment data related to fluid balance as indicated.

■ Monitor serum levels of the medication; report levels outside the therapeutic range for the drug being administered.

■ Maintain the client's fluid intake at between 2000 and 2500 mL per day unless contraindicated.

■ If the client is receiving diuretic therapy, assess fluid balance and medication levels frequently.

■ Alert the physician if the client is receiving other nephrotoxic drugs.

■ Report manifestations of renal failure immediately, including oliguria, a fixed urine specific gravity, hypertension, edema, and changes in renal function studies such as the BUN, creatinine, and serum electrolytes.

Client and Family Teaching

■ Instruct the client to maintain a fluid intake of 2 to 3 quarts per day while on aminoglycoside therapy.

■ Teach the client the early signs of renal impairment, such as a decrease in urine output, sudden weight gain, headache, and puffy eyes or extremities, and stress the importance of reporting them to the physician.

■ Emphasize the importance of taking the medication as prescribed, never doubling or increasing the frequency of doses.

The risk for ATN is higher when nephrotoxic drugs are prescribed for older clients or clients with preexisting renal insufficiency, and when they are used in combination with other nephrotoxic agents. Dehydration also increases the risk because of increased concentrations of the toxin in the nephrons. The accompanying pharmacology box lists nursing implications for the care of clients taking once class of nephrotoxic drugs.

Myoglobin is a pigmented substance that acts as the oxygen reservoir for muscle fibers, much as hemoglobin does for the blood. The release of either myoglobin or hemoglobin, considered *endogenous nephrotoxins*, in large amounts into the circulation may trigger ATN. Trauma is the usual cause of myoglobin release, although it may also occur with heat stroke, overstrenuous exercise, muscle ischemia, prolonged seizure activity, and sepsis. Severe hemolytic transfusion reactions are the usual cause of hemoglobin release (Price & Wilson, 1992; Wilson et al., 1991).

Postrenal Factors

Obstructive causes of acute renal failure are classified as postrenal. Any condition that prevents the excretion of urine can lead to postrenal ARF. Benign prostatic hypertrophy is the most common precipitating factor. Others include renal or urinary tract calculi and tumors. See Chapter 25 for further discussion of urinary tract obstruction.

Pathophysiology

Acute renal failure results from the interaction of tubular and vascular events. Ischemia is the primary cause of ATN. When allowed to continue for more than 2 hours, ischemia leads to severe and irreversible damage to the kidney tubules with patchy cellular necrosis and sloughing. The GFR is significantly reduced as a result of (1) ischemia, (2) activation of the renin-angiotensin system, and (3) tubular obstruction by cellular debris, which raises the pressure in the glomerular capsule. Figure 26–5 illustrates the pathogenesis of ARF arising from vascular and tubular causes.

Nephrotoxins destroy the tubular cells by both direct and indirect effects. As tubular cells are damaged and lost through necrosis and sloughing, the tubule becomes more permeable. This increased permeability results in filtrate reabsorption, further reducing the ability of the nephron to eliminate wastes (Bullock & Rosendahl, 1992; Wilson et al., 1991).

Regardless of the cause, acute renal failure follows a course characterized by three phases: initiation, maintenance, and recovery. The maintenance phase is further defined by the oliguric period and the diuretic period.

The *initiation phase* begins with the onset of the event causing tubular necrosis, e.g., hemorrhage leading to reduced blood volume and renal perfusion. If ARF is recognized and intervention begun to eliminate the initiating event during this phase, the prognosis is good. The initiation phase ends when tubular injury occurs. This phase of ARF has few manifestations; in fact, it is often identified only after manifestations of later phases have occurred.

The *maintenance phase* of ARF begins within hours of the initiating event and lasts from several hours to 6 to 8 weeks. This phase of ARF is characterized by persistent reduction in GFR and tubular necrosis. Necrotic endothelial cells are sloughed, leading to increased tubular permeability to filtrate and tubular obstruction (Wyngaarden et al., 1992). As a result, oliguria is usually present during the initial portion of the maintenance phase. This is often called the *oliguric period,* although as many as 40% of clients in the maintenance phase of ARF are not oliguric.

The kidney cannot efficiently eliminate metabolic wastes, water, electrolytes, and acids from the body during the maintenance phase of ARF. Azotemia, fluid retention, electrolyte imbalances, and metabolic acidosis develop. The severity of these abnormalities is greater in the oliguric client than in the nonoliguric one; consequently, the nonoliguric client has a better prognosis.

During the maintenance phase, salt and water retention lead to edema and put the client at risk for heart failure and pulmonary edema. Impaired renal elimination of potassium results in hyperkalemia. When the serum potassium level is greater than 6.0 to 6.5 mEq/L, manifestations related to its effect on neuromuscular function are typically seen. These include muscle weakness, nausea and diarrhea, and, most significantly, electrocardiographic changes and possible cardiac arrest. Other electrolyte imbalances include hyperphosphatemia and hypocalcemia. Metabolic acidosis is the result of inadequate elimination of hydrogen ions by the kidneys.

The client in ARF may be anemic because of suppressed erythropoietin secretion and a shorter RBC life. Immune function is also impaired, resulting in a high rate of infectious complications. Infection is the leading cause

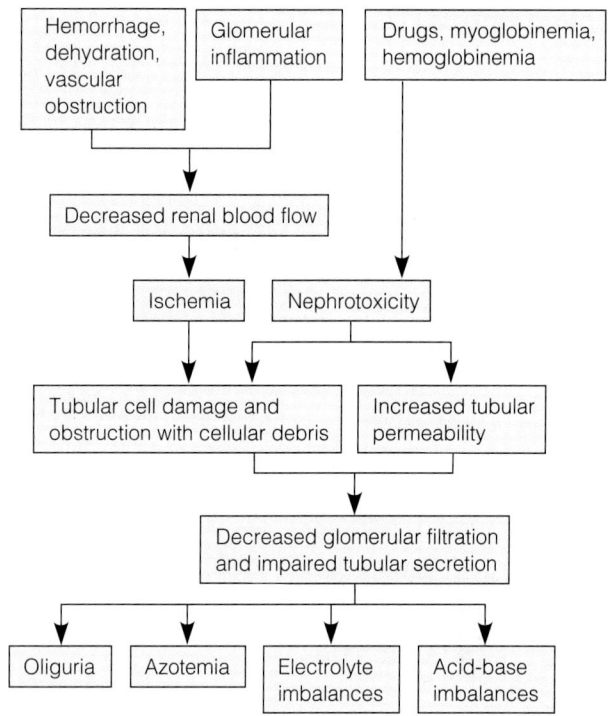

Figure 26–5 The pathogenesis of vascular and tubular causes of acute renal failure.

of death in clients with ARF. Other complications of ARF include

- Hypertension
- Neurologic manifestations, such as confusion, disorientation, agitation or lethargy, hyperreflexia, and possible seizures or coma
- Gastrointestinal manifestations including anorexia, nausea, vomiting, ileus, and hemorrhage (Wilson et al., 1991; Wyngaarden et al., 1992)

The end of the maintenance phase of ARF in oliguric clients is marked by a progressive increase in urine volume, the *diuretic period.* Damaged tubules are repaired through a process of cellular regeneration and healing. Diuresis indicates that the nephrons have recovered sufficiently to permit urine excretion. Renal function is not yet normal, and levels of serum creatinine, BUN, potassium, and phosphate remain high and may continue to rise in spite of increasing urine output.

The third or *recovery phase* of ARF begins when the GFR and tubular function have recovered to the extent that BUN and serum creatinine levels no longer continue to rise. Renal function improves rapidly during the first 5 to 25 days of the recovery phase. Renal healing and functional improvement continue for up to 1 year (Wilson et al., 1991).

Collaborative Care

Prevention of acute renal failure is a goal in the care of all clients, especially those in high-risk groups. Maintaining an adequate vascular volume, cardiac output, and blood pressure is vital to preserving kidney perfusion. Nephrotoxic drugs are avoided if possible. When it is necessary to use a nephrotoxic drug or substance, the risk of ARF can be reduced by using the minimum effective dose, ensuring adequate hydration, and eliminating other known nephrotoxins from the medication regimen.

The goals of care for the client with acute renal failure are to (1) identify and correct the underlying cause if possible, (2) prevent additional injury to the kidneys, (3) restore the urine output and elimination of metabolic waste products, and (4) compensate for the renal impairment until the kidneys regain their function (Wyngaarden et al., 1992).

Careful examination of the client's history and physical assessment can provide clues about the underlying condition precipitating renal failure. Impaired perfusion for as little as 30 minutes may cause significant renal ischemia. It is especially important to exclude urinary obstruction as a cause of ARF in the older adult, particularly prostatic hypertrophy or carcinoma in men and gynecologic malignancy in women (Abrams & Berkow, 1990).

Fluid and electrolyte balance is a key component in the management of a client with either oliguric or nonoliguric ARF. Fluid and electrolyte management remains an important consideration in the diuretic period, when renal function is beginning to return.

Laboratory and Diagnostic Tests

Laboratory and diagnostic testing is performed to identify the cause of acute renal failure and to monitor the effects of the failure on homeostasis.

The following laboratory tests may be ordered for the client with suspected or confirmed acute renal failure:

- *Urinalysis* may reveal the following abnormal findings in acute renal failure.
  a. A fixed specific gravity of 1.010 (equal to the specific gravity of plasma) as the tubules lose the ability to concentrate the filtrate.
  b. The presence of abnormal protein if glomerular damage is the cause of ARF.
  c. The presence of various cells. Microscopic examination of the urine sediment may show red blood cells, indicating glomerumlar dysfunction; white blood cells, indicating an inflammatory process; and renal tubular epithelial cells, indicating ATN.
  d. Cell casts. *Casts* are protein and cellular debris molded in the shape of the tubular lumen. In acute renal failure, RBC, WBC, and renal tubular epithelial casts may be observed. Brownish pigmented

casts together with positive tests for occult blood in the absence of hematuria are indicative of either hemoglobinuria or myoglobinuria (Wilson et al., 1991).

- *Serum creatinine* and *BUN* are determined to evaluate renal function and the presence of azotemia. In acute renal failure, a progressive daily rise in levels of both occurs, with serum creatinine increasing by 1 to 2 mg/dL/day and BUN by 10 to 15 mg/dL/day (Berkow & Fletcher, 1992). Levels tend to increase more slowly in the client with nonoliguric failure. These values may continue to increase even after the onset of diuresis in the client with oliguric ARF. The onset of recovery is marked by a halt in the rise of the serum creatinine and BUN.

- *Serum electrolytes* are monitored to evaluate the fluid and electrolyte status of the client in ARF. The serum potassium rises at a moderate rate and is often used as an indicator of the need to institute dialysis. Hyponatremia is often present, indicative of the water excess associated with ARF.

- *Arterial blood gases* generally show a metabolic acidosis due to the kidneys' inability to adequately eliminate metabolic wastes and hydrogen ions.

- The *complete blood count* demonstrates reduced RBCs and moderate anemia, with a hematocrit of 25% to 30% (Berkow & Fletcher, 1992). ARF reduces secretion of erythropoietin, the hormone that stimulates RBC production. Iron and folate absorption may also be impaired, further contributing to anemia.

Laboratory findings associated with kidney disease are summarized in Table 26–2.

The following diagnostic tests may be performed to evaluate the client with acute renal failure:

- *Bladder catheterization* is performed to rule out urethral obstruction as a cause of renal failure and to obtain a urine specimen for culture. The presence of a urinary tract infection is suggestive of a postrenal cause for ARF.

- *Renal ultrasonography* is useful to identify obstructive causes of renal failure. It is also used to differentiate acute renal failure from end-stage chronic renal failure. In acute renal failure, the kidneys may be enlarged, whereas they typically appear small and shrunken in chronic renal failure.

- *Computed tomography* provides another means of evaluating kidney size and locating possible urinary tract obstructions. Although CT is most useful when performed with radiographic contrast media, these agents are used with extreme caution in the client with ARF because of their potential nephrotoxicity.

- Other radiologic studies such as *intravenous pyelography (IVP), retrograde pyelography,* or *antegrade pyelography* may also be employed to evaluate the structure and function of the kidneys. Retrograde pyelography, which utilizes contrast material injected into the ureters, and antegrade pyelography, in which the contrast medium is injected percutaneously into the renal pelvis, are preferred because they have fewer nephrotoxic effects than IVP does.

- A *renal biopsy* may be necessary when other diagnostic studies do not provide a clear differentiation between acute and chronic renal failure. Microscopic examination of kidney tissue can provide the definitive diagnosis. See the box outlining the nursing implications of laboratory and diagnostic studies, page 947.

Pharmacology

The primary focus in the pharmacologic management of acute renal failure is to restore and maintain renal perfusion and to eliminate drugs that are directly nephrotoxic from the treatment regimen.

The client who is hypotensive receives intravenous fluids and blood volume expanders to restore renal perfusion. Dopamine (Intropin), administered intravenously in low doses, is useful to increase renal blood flow. Dopamine is a sympathetic neurotransmitter that acts as a cardiac stimulant and dilates the blood vessels of the mesentery and kidneys when administered in low therapeutic doses (Shlafer, 1993).

If restoration of renal blood flow does not improve urinary output, a potent loop diuretic such as furosemide (Lasix) or an osmotic diuretic such as mannitol may be administered along with fluid resuscitation. The purpose of this therapy is twofold. First, if nephrotoxins are present, the combination of fluids and potent diuretics may, in effect, "wash out" the nephrons, reducing the toxin concentration. Second, ARF morbidity and mortality are lower in nonoliguric clients, and it is believed that the early establishment of urine flow may prevent oliguria (Wilson et al., 1991). Furosemide may be continued during the course of ARF if it is effective in maintaining the urine output (Wyngaarden et al., 1992).

All drugs that are either directly nephrotoxic or that may interfere with renal perfusion (such as potent vasoconstrictors) are discontinued. NSAIDs, nephrotoxic antibiotics, and other potentially harmful drugs are avoided during the course of acute renal failure and throughout the recovery phase (Wyngaarden et al., 1992).

The client in acute renal failure has an increased risk of gastrointestinal bleeding, probably related to the stress response and impaired platelet function. Histamine H_2-receptor antagonists, such as cimetidine (Tagamet) or ranitidine (Zantac), are often administered to the client in ARF to prevent gastrointesinal hemorrhage.

Hyperkalemia is a constant feature of ARF and may require active intervention as well as restriction of potassium intake. Serum levels of greater than 6.5 mEq/L require intervention to prevent the cardiac disturbances associated with hyperkalemia. A potassium-binding exchange resin such as sodium polystyrene sulfonate (Kayexalate, SPS Suspension) may be administered either orally or by enema. This agent acts to remove potassium from the body by exchanging sodium for potassium, primarily in the large intestine. When administered orally, it is often combined with sorbitol to prevent constipation. If it is administered rectally, it is given as a retention enema, allowed to remain in the bowel for approximately 30 to 60 minutes, and then irrigated out using a tap-water enema. Calcium chloride, bicarbonate, and insulin and glucose may be administered intravenously as well to reduce serum potassium levels (Wilson et al., 1991).

Aluminum hydroxide (AlternaGEL, Amphojel, Nephrox) is an antacid used to control hyperphosphatemia in renal failure. It acts by binding with phosphates in the gastrointestinal tract, which are then excreted in the feces.

Because many medications are eliminated from the body primarily by the kidney, drug dosages may need to be adjusted. Doses within the normal or recommended range can result in potentially toxic blood levels, because their elimination is slowed and half-life prolonged. Nursing implications for medications commonly prescribed for the client in ARF are summarized in the pharmacology box on page 972. NSAIDs are discussed in Chapter 4 and antihypertensives are discussed in Chapter 30.

Conservative Therapy

Many of the consequences and manifestations of acute renal failure can be managed conservatively; that is, by fluid and dietary management.

Fluid Restriction   Once any impairment of renal perfusion is corrected and vascular volume is restored, fluid intake is generally restricted. The allowed daily intake is calculated by allowing 500 mL for insensible losses (respiration, perspiration, bowel losses) and adding the amount excreted as urine during the previous 24 hours. For example, if a client with ARF excretes 325 mL of urine in 24 hours, the client is allowed a fluid intake (including oral and intravenous fluids) of 825 mL for the next 24 hours. Fluid balance is carefully monitored, using an accurate daily weight and the serum sodium as the primary indicators.

Dietary Management   Renal insufficiency and the underlying disease process increase the rate of *catabolism,* the breakdown of body proteins, and decrease the rate of *anabolism,* body tissue repair. The client with ARF

Text continues on page 974

Nursing Implications for Pharmacology: The Client in Acute Renal Failure

LOOP DIURETICS

Bumetanide (Bumex)

Ethacrynic acid (Edecrin)

Furosemide (Lasix)

The loop diuretics, named for their primary site of action in the loop of Henle, are also called *high-ceiling diuretics*, meaning that the response increases with increasing doses. These are highly effective diuretics used in early ARF with the hope of reestablishing urine flow and converting oliguric renal failure to nonoliguric renal failure. Loop diuretics may be administered along with intravenous dopamine to promote renal blood flow. In ATN due to a nephrotoxin, loop diuretics are used to stimulate urine output and clear the toxin from the nephrons more rapidly. Loop diuretics cause potassium wasting, which is generally not a concern because renal failure impairs normal potassium elimination.

Nursing Responsibilities

- Assess the client's weight and vital signs to obtain baseline data before administering loop diuretics.
- Monitor and record intake and output, daily weight (or more frequently as ordered), vital signs, skin turgor, and other indicators of fluid volume status frequently while client is receiving loop diuretics.
- Assess for orthostatic hypotension, because these potent diuretics can lead to hypovolemia.
- Monitor laboratory results, especially serum electrolyte, glucose, BUN, and creatinine levels.
- Administer by mouth or, if ordered, by intravenous route:
  a. Furosemide undiluted at a rate of no more than 20 mg per minute
  b. Ethacrynic acid 50 mg diluted with 50 mL of normal saline at a rate of no more than 10 mg per minute
  c. Bumetanide by direct intravenous injection over at least 1 minute or diluted in lactated Ringer's solution, normal saline, or 5% dextrose in water for infusion
- Assess therapeutic response. Urinary output typically increases within 3 to 5 minutes after intravenous administration.

- Monitor the client's hearing and complaints of adverse manifestations such as tinnitus. The high doses of loop diuretics used in ARF increase the risk of ototoxicity, especially with ethacrynic acid. These effects may be reversible if they are detected early and the drug is discontinued.
- Avoid administering these drugs concurrently with other ototoxic agents, such as aminoglycoside antibiotics and cisplatin.

Client and Family Teaching

- Unless contraindicated, maintain a fluid intake of 2 to 3 quarts per day.
- Rise slowly from lying or sitting positions, because a fall in blood pressure may cause light-headedness.
- Take the medication in the morning to avoid interference with sleep. If it is ordered more than once per day, take the last dose with the evening meal.
- Taking the medication with food or milk will help prevent gastric distress.
- Nonsteroidal anti-inflammatory drugs (especially ibuprofen, indomethacin, and sulindac) interfere with the effectiveness of loop diuretics and should be avoided (Shlafer, 1993).

OSMOTIC DIURETICS

Mannitol (Osmitrol, Isotol)

Urea (Ureaphil)

The osmotic diuretics have a distinctly different mechanism of action than other diuretics. These agents act by increasing the osmotic draw in the blood and urine. In the blood, the effect is to pull extracellular water into the vascular system, increasing the GFR. These substances are then freely filtered in the glomerulus and increase the osmotic draw of the urine, inhibiting water diffusion from the tubule of the nephron. The effect is to increase urine volume and flow. In addition, osmotic diuretics dilute waste products in the urine, decreasing the risk of renal damage due to excess concentrations (Spencer et al., 1993).

Nursing Responsibilities

- Assess the client's ability to excrete urine before administration. Osmotic diuretics are used in early re-

Pharmacology: The Client in Acute Renal Failure (continued)

nal failure to maintain urine output but are contraindicated in the anuric client. A test dose may be administered; urine output of 30 mL per hour following administration of the test dose shows an adequate response to allow further administration.

- Do not administer these diuretics to clients who have impaired heart function, are in congestive heart failure, or are severely dehydrated. Because they increase vascular volume, they may worsen heart failure. These drugs are not effective unless extracellular volume is adequate.

- Administer mannitol solution intravenously, diluting before use if indicated. Check solutions of concentrations greater than 15% for crystallization. Crystals may be dissolved by warming the solution slightly. Always administer solutions of concentrations greater than 15% through a filter to prevent crystals from being infused. Infuse solutions of 15% to 25% concentration over 30 to 90 minutes.

- Administer urea intravenously, diluting in 100 mL of 5% or 10% dextrose in water for every 30 g of urea. Administer solution no faster than 4 mL per minute through a filter.

- Monitor vital signs, breath sounds, and urinary output while the client is receiving the drug.

- Discontinue the drug if the client develops signs of heart failure or pulmonary edema, or if renal function continues to decline.

Client and Family Teaching

- Report symptoms such as shortness of breath, headache, chest pain, or dizziness immediately.

ELECTROLYTES AND ELECTROLYTE MODIFIERS

Calcium chloride

Calcium gluconate

Sodium bicarbonate

Sodium polystyrene sulfonate (Kayexalate)

Renal failure impairs the elimination of body wastes, including the excretion of potassium, phosphate, and hydrogen ions. To correct resulting electrolyte imbalances, other electrolyte solutions or electrolyte modifiers may be administered. Calcium

chloride or gluconate and sodium bicarbonate are administered intravenously in the initial management of hyperkalemia. Calcium is also administered to correct hypocalcemia and reduce hyperphosphatemia (calcium and phosphate have a reciprocal relationship in the body; as the level of one rises, the level of the other falls). Sodium bicarbonate helps correct acidosis and move potassium back into the intracellular space. Sodium polystyrene sulfonate is not used to replace an electrolyte but to remove excess potassium from the body by exchanging sodium for potassium in the large intestine.

Nursing Responsibilities

- Assess the client's serum electrolyte levels prior to and during therapy with these agents. Report rapid shifts or adverse responses to the physician.

- Administer as appropriate:
  a. Intravenous calcium choride at less than 1 mL per minute; intravenous calcium gluconate at 0.5 mL per minute. Administer into a large vein through a small-bore needle; take precautions to avoid infiltration because extravasation of intravenous solution will result in tissue necrosis.
  b. Intravenous sodium bicarbonate infusion over 4 to 8 hours; oral tablets as prescribed.
  c. Sodium polystyrene sulfonate as an oral solution mixed with sorbitol to prevent constipation, or as a retention enema mixed with warm water. Leave in the bowel for 30 to 60 minutes; irrigate using a small tap-water enema.

- Monitor for evidence of adverse reactions, such as cardiac irregularities, electrolyte imbalances, and metabolic alkalosis.

Client and Family Teaching

- Intravenous calcium administration may make you light-headed; remain recumbent for at least 30 minutes after administration.

- Sodium bicarbonate tablets should be chewed and followed with 8 ounces of water. Do not take with milk.

- Retain the sodium polystyrene sulfonate enema as long as possible.

therefore needs an adequate intake of nutrients and calories to prevent catabolism. Proteins are limited to 0.7 to 1.0 g per kilogram of body weight per day to minimize the degree of azotemia. Dietary proteins should be complete, containing all the essential amino acids. Carbohydrates are increased to maintain adequate calorie intake and provide a protein-sparing effect.

Parenteral nutrition providing amino acids, concentrated carbohydrates, and fats may be instituted in the client who cannot consume an adequate diet because of the gastrointestinal effects of the ARF or underlying disease process. The disadvantages of parenteral nutrition in the client with ARF are the high volume of fluid it introduces into the system and the risk it poses for infection through the venous line.

Supportive Therapy

The client in ARF who cannot be managed conservatively and develops manifestations of uremia with encephalopathy or pericarditis, severe fluid overload, hyperkalemia, or metabolic acidosis may require supportive therapy such as dialysis.

Dialysis   Dialysis is the diffusion of solute molecules across a semipermeable membrane from an area of higher concentration to one of lower concentration. Dialysis procedures are used to remove excess fluid and metabolic waste products in the client with renal failure. Many clients with acute renal failure, particularly those who are nonoliguric, can be managed without dialysis. However, early institution of dialysis can simplify management and reduce the rate of complications (Andreoli et al., 1990; Wilson et al., 1991; Wyngaarden et al., 1992). Dialysis may also be used to rapidly remove nephrotoxins in clients with ARF caused by nephrotoxic damage to renal tubules.

Either **hemodialysis,** a procedure in which blood passes by an artificial semipermeable membrane outside the body, or **peritoneal dialysis,** which uses the peritoneum surrounding the adominal cavity as the dialyzing membrane, may be employed for the client with ARF. These procedures and their associated nursing implications are discussed in depth in the section on chronic renal failure later in this chapter.

Continuous Arteriovenous Hemofiltration   Continuous arteriovenous hemofiltration (CAVH),

also known as *continuous arteriovenous ultrafiltration,* is a form of hemodialysis that may be used for the client in acute renal failure. During this procedure, blood from an artery is heparinized and passed through an extracorporeal filter. This filtering process allows water and solutes such as electrolyes, urea, creatinine, uric acid, and glucose to drain into a collection device. The blood is then rediluted with a balanced water, electrolyte, and nutrient solution and returned to the circulation via a vein (Figure 26–6).

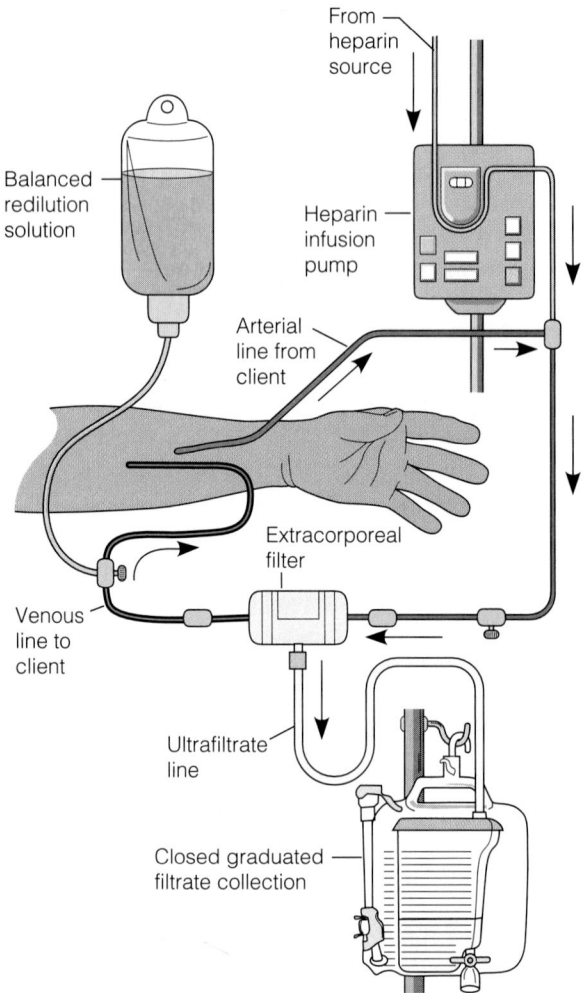

Figure 26–6   Continuous arteriovenous hemofiltration (CAVH).

CAVH mimics the function of the glomerulus in that the arterial pressure of the blood is the primary force driving excess fluid and waste products out of the plasma. The replacement solution added to the blood before its return to the body approximates the reabsorptive function of the renal tubule. CAVH is slower than hemodialysis, both in removing excess fluid and changing electrolyte concentrations. This slower process makes it particularly useful for the client in ARF who has other significant medical conditions and may not tolerate rapid changes in extracellular fluid composition. It may also be used in combination with hemodialysis for selected clients (Berkow & Fletcher, 1992; Price, 1989; Thompson et al., 1993).

CAVH is typically performed in an intensive care unit or specialized nephrology unit. An arteriovenous shunt or fistula in the forearm provides an ideal vascular access site for CAVH. However, because CAVH is often a temporary measure, the femoral artery may be used for arterial access and the femoral vein for the venous return line. This arrangement allows the use of a short tube to and from the filtering unit, minimizing resistance to flow. The subclavian or jugular veins are also appropriate for venous return sites.

Strict aseptic technique is vital in caring for the vascular access sites to minimize the risk of infection. Other risks associated with CAVH include bleeding due to heparin administration and thrombus formation with potential limb loss (Price, 1989). Systemic risks include either hypervolemia or hypovolemia, depending on the rate of fluid removal and replacement, and complications related to the immobility imposed by continuous vascular access.

Nursing Care

The client with acute renal failure has numerous nursing care needs. Often these needs are related not only to the renal failure but also to the underlying condition that precipitated it. This section focuses on nursing care related to fluid volume alterations, changes in appetite and nutrition, and the learning needs of the client.

Fluid Volume Excess

In cases of acute renal failure, the kidneys are often unable to excrete adequate amounts of fluid to maintain a normal extracellular fluid balance. Fluid retention is greater in clients with oliguric renal failure than those with nonoliguric failure. Rapid weight gain and the presence of edema signal excess fluid. In addition to demonstrating the visible signs of volume overload, the client may develop congestive heart failure and pulmonary edema. In the older adult or in the severely debilitated client, this complex can present a significant management problem.

Nursing interventions with rationales follow.

- Assess and document intake and output hourly. *Accurate intake and output records help guide therapy, especially fluid restriction, and make informed decisions regarding dialysis treatment.*

- Weigh the client at the same time each day or more frequently, as ordered. Use the same scale and have the client wear the same amount of clothing or drapes to ensure accuracy. *Changes in fluid volume status are readily reflected in the client's weight, which may provide a more accurate assessment of fluid volume status than intake and output records.*

- Monitor and record vital signs at least every 4 hours. *Increased blood pressure, tachycardia, and tachypnea may indicate increasing hypervolemia.*

- Frequently assess breath sounds for the presence of crackles (rales) and heart sounds for the presence of an S_3 or S_4 gallop. Assess the degree of peripheral edema and distention of neck veins. *The client with a fluid vol-*ume excess is at increased risk for developing congestive heart failure and pulmonary edema.*

- If not contraindicated by other factors, place the client in semi-Fowler's position. *This position enhances cardiac and respiratory function.*

- Monitor serum electrolytes; report abnormal results and signs and symptoms of electrolyte imbalance. *The client with ARF is at particular risk for the following electrolyte imbalances because of water retention and impaired renal function:*
  a. *Hyperkalemia due to impaired excretion of potassium. Manifestations include irritability, nausea, diarrhea, abdominal cramping, cardiac dysrhythmias, and ECG changes.*
  b. *Hyponatremia due to water retention. Manifestations include nausea, vomiting, and headache, with possible CNS manifestations of lethargy, confusion, seizures, and coma.*
  c. *Hyperphosphatemia due to decreased excretion of phosphate in the urine. Manifestations are the same as those associated with hypocalcemia: hyperreflexia, paresthesias, and possible tetany.*

- Restrict fluids as prescribed. Provide frequent mouth care and encourage the use of hard candies to decrease the thirst response. If the client uses ice chips to relieve thirst, measure the water content and include the amount as intake. *Fluid restriction is important to minimize fluid retention and the complications associated with fluid volume excess, especially in the client being managed without dialysis.*

- Administer medications with meals. *Taking oral medications between meals involves consuming liquids that the client might not otherwise ingest.*

- Turn the client frequently and provide good skin care. *Edema decreases tissue perfusion and increases the risk of skin breakdown, especially in the older or debilitated client.*

- Administer diuretics as ordered and monitor the client's response. *Diuretics may promote urination in the client with ARF.*

Altered Nutrition: Less Than Body Requirements

The client in acute renal failure is at risk for nutritional deficits due to the manifestations of renal failure and the dietary restrictions prescribed in the treatment of ARF. Further, the underlying disease process leading to ARF often contributes to the client's poor nutritional status. The body's increased metabolic needs during ARF compound the problem of inadequate intake.

Nursing interventions with rationales follow.

- Monitor and document food intake, including both the amount and type of food consumed. *This information helps guide decisions about supplements ordered, if any.*

- Weigh at the same time daily, documenting weight accurately. *In the client experiencing renal failure, weight gain usually reflects fluid retention. The client's weight may remain stable or even increase even though tissue mass is being lost.*

- Arrange for consultation with a dietitian to plan a diet that meets the therapeutic requirements and takes the client's food preferences into account. *Diets restricted in protein, salt, and potassium may be unpalatable for the client. Including preferred foods to the extent possible increases intake.*

- Engage the client in planning daily menus. *This participation increases the client's sense of control and autonomy.*

- Allow the client's family to prepare meals within the dietary restrictions and encourage family members to eat with the client. *Familiar foods and social interaction encourage eating and heighten the client's enjoyment of meals.*

- Provide frequent, small meals or between-meal snacks. *These measures promote food intake in the fatigued or anorectic client.*

- Administer antiemetic agents as ordered and provide mouth care prior to meals. *Nausea and a metallic taste in the mouth, both common manifestations of uremia, can decrease food intake.*

- Administer and monitor parenteral nutrition as ordered for the client who is unable to eat or tolerate enteral nutrition. *Preventing or slowing tissue catabolism is an important component of care for the client with ARF. It is important to remember, however, that the presence of intravenous lines and the administration of parenteral nutrition may increase the client's risk for infection. Monitor sites carefully for signs of infection or inflammation.*

Knowledge Deficit

The client who experiences acute renal failure has multiple learning needs. These include information about ARF, diagnostic and laboratory studies, management strategies, and implications for the recovery period.

Nursing interventions with rationales follow.

- Assess the client's level of anxiety and ability to comprehend instruction. Tailor information and presentation to the client's developmental level and physical, mental, and emotional status. *The client with ARF may be critically ill or have manifestations of uremia that hinder the ability to learn. It is important to present information in a timely fashion, but during the initial stages of ARF it may be necessary to limit information to immediately pertinent concerns.*

- Assess the client's knowledge and understanding. *To enhance understanding and retention, relate information presented to previous learning.*

- Teach the client about diagnostic tests and therapeutic procedures. *Teaching reduces the client's anxiety and improves understanding and cooperation.*

- Teach the client about dietary and fluid restrictions. *These measures may be continued after discharge.*

- If the client is discharged prior to the end of the maintenance phase of ARF, instruct the client about the signs and symptoms of complications, such as fluid volume excess, CHF, and hyperkalemia during the oliguric phase and fluid volume deficit during diuresis and the recovery phase. *As kidney function returns, urine output increases, but the concentrating ability of the nephrons remains impaired. Impaired concentrating ability increases the risk of excess fluid loss, possible dehydration, orthostatic hypotension, and other symptoms.*

- Teach the client how to monitor weight, blood pressure, and pulse. *These are important means of assessing fluid status.*

- Instruct the client to avoid nephrotoxic drugs and chemicals during the recovery period of acute renal failure. *Recovery of renal function requires up to 1 year. During this period, the nephron remains vulnerable to damage from nephrotoxins. Avoiding known toxins such as NSAIDs, some antibiotics, radiologic contrast media, and heavy metals is important throughout the recovery period. Because the nephrotoxicity of some materials increases when they are taken in conjunction with alcohol, discourage the use of alcohol.*

Other Nursing Diagnoses

The following nursing diagnoses may also be applicable for the client with ARF:

- *Activity Intolerance* related to anemia
- *Risk for Infection* related to invasive procedures
- *Risk for Noncompliance* with dietary and fluid restriction related to alterations in taste and thirst
- *Self-Care Deficit* related to the effects of illness
- *Sensory/Perceptual Alteration: Gustatory* related to uremia
- *Altered Thought Processes* related to excess metabolic wastes in the blood

Client and Family Teaching

Often the client and family are in a state of crisis or critical illness when renal failure occurs. This state of crisis can limit the client's ability to learn and retain information. Teaching during the initial stages may be limited to necessary information about diagnostic and therapeutic procedures, such as a fluid restriction and dialysis.

During this initial period, it is important to include the family in all teaching. Teaching helps them understand what is happening, what symptoms the client is experiencing, and why particular therapies are used. When the client is able to learn and understand more about ARF, the family can be valuable in reinforcing teaching.

Because the healing phase of ARF is prolonged, lasting up to 1 year, teaching needs prior to discharge include: avoiding exposure to nephrotoxins, particularly those in over-the-counter or commercial products; preventing infection and other major stressors that can slow healing; monitoring weight, blood pressure, and pulse; recognizing signs and symptoms of relapse; observing any continuing dietary restrictions; and recognizing when to contact the physician.

Applying the Nursing Process

Case Study of a Client with Acute Renal Failure: Judy Devak

Judy Devak is driving home late one evening when she loses control of her car trying to avoid hitting a deer in the road. Her car strikes a tree and rolls into a deep ditch beside the road, out of sight of passing cars. The accident is not discovered until 2 hours later. On arrival at the accident scene, the paramedics find Ms. Devak hypotensive: BP: 90/60; P: 120; and R: 24. She is alert and in severe pain, with a fractured right femur. After immobilizing Ms. Devak's neck and back and extricating her from the car, they apply a traction splint to her leg and transport her to the local hospital.

Assessment

Katie Leaper, RN, obtains a nursing history from Ms. Devak on her admission to the intensive care unit. Ms. Devak indicates that she has always been healthy, having experienced only the usual colds and flus, and chickenpox as a child. She has never been in the hospital before this and knows of no allergies to medications. Ms. Devak denies taking any prescription or nonprescription drugs currently. Physical assessment findings include BP: 124/68; P: 100; R: 18; T: 97.4 F (36.3 C) po. Ms. Devak's skin is pale, cool, and dry, with multiple scrapes, minor abrasions, and bruises of her face and upper and lower extremities. A linear bruise is noted on her abdomen from the seat belt, and her chest is tender where the shoulder strap crossed it. Lung sounds are clear, heart tones are normal, and her abdomen is tender but soft to palpation. Alignment of Ms. Devak's right leg is being maintained with skeletal traction. One unit of whole blood is infused prior to admission to the ICU, and she is receiving a second unit. An indwelling urinary catheter and a nasogastric tube are in place.

During the first few hours after Ms. Devak's admission, Ms. Leaper notes that Ms. Devak's hourly output has dropped from 55 mL to 45 mL to 28 mL of clear yellow urine. The physician orders a 500-mL intravenous fluid challenge, STAT urinalysis, BUN, and serum creatinine. The fluid challenge elicits only a slight increase in urine output. Urinalysis results show a specific gravity of 1.010 and the presence of WBCs, red and white cell casts, and tubular epithelial cells in the sediment. Ms. Devak's BUN is 28 mg/dL; her serum creatinine, 1.5 mg/dL. The physician makes a diagnosis of probable acute renal failure and orders a nephrology consultation. In addition, the physician places her on aluminum hydroxide, 10 mL every 2 hours per nasogastric tube, and ranitidine 50 mg intravenously every 8 hours.

Diagnosis

Ms. Leaper identifies the following nursing diagnoses for Judy Devak:

- *Pain,* acute, related to injuries sustained in accident
- *Anxiety* related to being in the intensive care unit
- *Fluid Volume Excess* related to impaired renal function
- *Impaired Physical Mobility* related to skeletal traction
- *Altered Protection* related to injuries and invasive procedures

Expected Outcomes

The expected outcomes for Ms. Devak's plan of care are that she will

- Report adequate pain control.
- Relate a reduction in anxiety.
- Maintain weight and vital signs within normal range.
- Maintain skin integrity.
- Demonstrate appropriate use of the trapeze to adjust her position in bed while maintaining body alignment.
- Remain free of signs and symptoms of infection, bleeding, or respiratory distress.

Planning and Implementation

The following nursing interventions are planned and implemented for Ms. Devak in the intensive care unit:

- Maintain patient-controlled analgesia with prescribed analgesic.
- Assess frequently for pain control and adverse responses to analgesic agents.
- Encourage Ms. Devak to express her thoughts, feelings, and fears about her condition and about being in the intensive care unit.
- Explain all procedures to Ms. Devak, using brief, easily understood statements.

- Assess and document vital signs and heart and lung sounds at least every 4 hours.

- Weigh Ms. Devak every 12 hours, using the same scale and with Ms. Devak in clothing of similar weight.

- Document hourly intake and output.

- Maintain fluid restriction, making sure to include diluent for all intravenous medications as intake.

- Provide mouth care every 3 to 4 hours; allow frequent rinsing of mouth and ice chips as ordered.

- Keep linens clean, dry and smooth; massage bony prominences frequently and use skin protectors on heels and elbows.

- Assist Ms. Devak to change upper body position slightly at least every 2 hours; teach her the use of the overhead trapeze.

- Monitor frequently for evidence of infection, bleeding, or respiratory distress, including elevated temperature, signs of inflammation, increase in the girth of the right thigh, changes in vital signs, dyspnea, or chest pain.

Evaluation

After just over 3 days of oliguria, Ms. Devak's urine output has begun to increase. By the end of the fourth day she is excreting about 60 to 80 mL/hour of urine. Although her BUN, serum creatinine, and potassium levels remain high, they never reach a critical point, and dialysis is not required. She is transferred from the ICU on the 5th day after admission. When Ms. Devak is able to begin eating, she is placed on a low-potassium diet, restricted to 50 g of protein. Her renal function gradually improves. By discharge, results of her renal function studies, including BUN and serum creatinine, are nearly normal. Ms. Devak is able to verbalize her understanding of the need to avoid nephrotoxic substances such as NSAIDs until approved by her physician.

Critical Thinking in the Nursing Process

1. What was the most likely specific precipitating factor for Ms. Devak's acute renal failure? Did anything else contribute to her risk?

2. Why did the physician prescribe aluminum hydroxide and ranitidine? Consider both the acute renal failure and Ms. Devak's placement in the intensive care unit.

3. Why was it especially important to include frequent assessment for adverse responses to the prescribed analgesia in Ms. Devak's care plan? Identify common adverse responses to narcotic analgesics.

4. Ms. Devak is at risk for respiratory distress related to potential fluid volume excess. How does her fractured femur further contribute to risk for respiratory distress?

5. Develop a care plan for Ms. Devak for the nursing diagnosis *Diversional Activity Deficit.*

The Client with Chronic Renal Failure

■ ■ ■

Although the kidneys have a remarkable capacity to recover from acute injury, many long-standing conditions can lead to progressive destruction of the renal parenchyma. The functional capacity of entire nephrons is lost and renal mass is reduced, leading to progressive deterioration of glomerular filtration, tubular secretion, and reabsorption. This process, which may progress slowly for a number of years without being recognized, is known as *chronic renal failure (CRF)*. Eventually, the kidneys are unable to excrete metabolic wastes and regulate fluid and electrolyte balance adequately, and the client is said to have *end-stage renal disease (ESRD)*, the final stage of CRF.

End-stage renal disease is increasing in incidence in all age groups, with a particularly sharp increase in people over the age of 74 years noted between 1980 and 1990. See the accompanying box for a discussion of CRF in the older adult. The incidence rates of ESRD among Native Americans and African-Americans is three to four times higher than among Caucasians (US Renal Data System, 1993).

Conditions causing chronic renal failure typically involve diffuse, bilateral disease of the kidneys leading to progressive destruction and scarring of the entire nephron (Price & Wilson, 1993). As indicated in Figure 26–7, diabetic nephropathy and hypertension, followed closely by glomerulonephritis, are the leading causes of CRF in the United States. Among African-Americans, hypertension predominates as a cause of CRF, accounting for 37.7% of cases (US Renal Data System, 1993).

The course of chronic renal failure is quite variable, progressing at a rate ranging from months to many years. In the early stage, known as **renal impairment** or *decreased renal reserve*, unaffected nephrons compensate for the lost nephrons, and the client remains free of symptoms with normal BUN and serum creatinine levels. As the disease progresses and kidney function is further reduced, azotemia and some manifestations of **renal insufficiency** may be seen. Any further insult to the kidneys at this stage (such as infection, dehydration, exposure to nephrotoxins, or a urinary tract obstruction) can lead to a further reduction in function and precipitate the onset of end-stage renal failure, or overt uremia. Clients often do not present for medical treatment until they reach **end-stage renal disease.** This stage is characterized by a GFR of less than 10% of normal. At this stage, serum creatinine

Gerontologic Considerations: The Client with Chronic Renal Failure

The human kidney changes structurally and functionally with age. Structurally, the number of nephron units decreases. Progressive functional changes occur in the glomeruli and tubules. The glomerular filtration rate (GRF) decreases, which results in a decreased renal clearance of drugs. Urine-concentrating ability decreases due to changes in tubular function. The sodium-conserving ability of the kidney also decreases, and renal compensation of acid-base imbalances takes longer to occur. Many chronic diseases common in older adults further decrease renal function.

Normally, these age-related changes do not result in kidney dysfunction in the older adult. Because older adults have reduced muscle mass, they produce less creatinine, a by-product of muscle function. Thus, serum creatinine levels may not rise despite decreased renal function. Likewise, BUN may also appear to be within normal limits even though kidney function diminishes. Kidney dysfunction may occur, however, when the older adult develops various diseases or places unusual physiologic demands on the kidneys.

Chronic renal failure may occur secondary to other age-related diseases including: atherosclerosis, pros-

tatic hypertrophy, renal-vascular hypertension, drug-related renal insufficiency, and diabetic nephropathy. When renal failure develops (a period of many months or years), the older adult may experience few symptoms until little renal function remains. The manifestations associated with chronic renal failure are related to the buildup of metabolic wastes and are usually nonspecific. Manifestations may include: changes in urine output, peripheral edema, weakness and fatigue, irritability, memory loss, and confusion. Sometimes these symptoms are mistaken as a consequence of the normal aging process. At other times, they may be falsely attributed to problems in other organ systems (for example, worsening heart failure due to the inability of the kidney to excrete sodium and water, or acute confusion result from uremia). Once a diagnosis of chronic renal failure is established, a definitive cause should be identified. Potentially reversible causes, such as urinary tract obstruction or nephrotoxic medications, should be corrected. Chronic renal failure may progress to end-stage renal disease in the older adult. Both dialysis and kidney transplantation are treatment options. Prognosis will depend on the underlying problem, complications, and the client's overall health.

Carnevali, D., & Patrick, M. (1993). *Nursing Management for the Elderly.* (3rd ed.). Philadelphia: J. B. Lippincott. Stanley, M., Beare, P. G. (Eds.). (1995). *Gerontological Nursing.* Philadelphia: F. A. Davis Company.

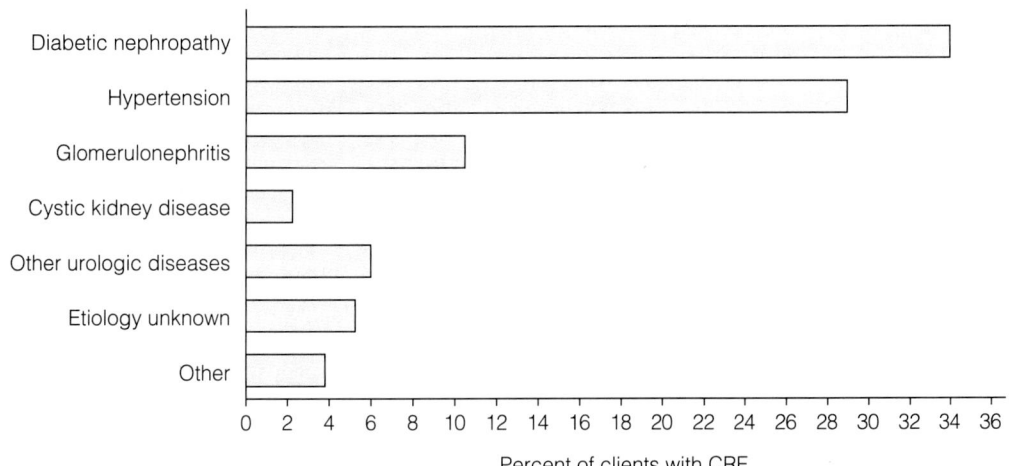

Figure 26–7 The most common causes of chronic renal failure (US Renal Data System, 1993).

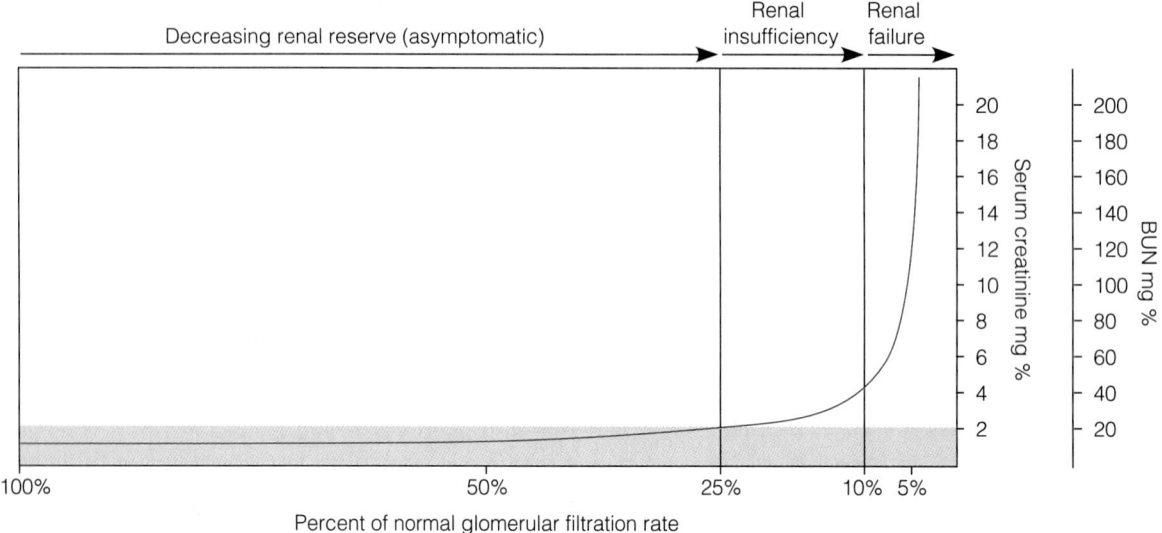

Figure 26–8   The relationship of renal function to BUN and serum creatinine values through the course of chronic renal failure.

and BUN levels rise sharply (Figure 26–8), the client becomes oliguric, and manifestations of uremia are seen (Porth, 1994; Price & Wilson, 1992; Wilson et al., 1991). Table 26–6 summarizes the stages of chronic renal failure.

Pathophysiology

The pathophysiologic process of chronic renal failure appears to be one of gradual loss of entire nephron units. In the early stages, as nephrons are destroyed, the remaining nephrons hypertrophy. Glomerular capillary flow and pressure increase in these nephrons, and more solute par-

ticles are filtered to compensate for the lost renal mass. This increased demand predisposes the remaining nephrons to glomerular sclerosis (scarring), resulting in their eventual destruction (Wilson et al., 1991). Table 26–7 outlines the pathologic processes that lead to nephron destruction and end-stage renal disease for some common causes of chronic renal failure.

Chronic renal failure is not usually identified until the final, uremic stage is reached. **Uremia,** which literally means "urine in the blood," is the term used for the syndrome or group of symptoms associated with end-stage renal failure. In uremia, fluid and electrolyte balance is al-

Table 26–6	Stages of Chronic Renal Failure	
Stage	**Features**	**Clinical Manifestations**
I Decreased renal reserve	GFR > 25% of normal; creatinine clearance 32.5 to 130 mL/min; serum creatinine and BUN within normal limits	None; detected only by careful testing of GFR or a prolonged urine concentration test
II Renal insufficiency	More than 75% of functioning renal parenchyma destroyed; GFR < 25% of normal; creatinine clearance 10 to 30 mL/min; slight fluctuating rise in serum creatinine and BUN	Few symptoms; may have nocturia and polyuria, usually in response to a stressor such as an infection, CHF, or dehydration
III End-stage renal failure or uremia	90% or more of nephrons are destroyed; GFR < 10% of normal; creatinine clearance 5 to 10 mL/min; sharp rises in serum creatinine and BUN; fixed urine specific gravity of 1.010	Oliguria; uremic manifestations

Table 26–7 Major Causes of Chronic Renal Failure

	Cause	Examples
Metabolic	Diabetic nephropathy	Changes in the glomerular basement membrane, chronic pyelonephritis, and ischemia lead to sclerosis of the glomerulus and gradual destruction of the nephron
Inflammatory	Chronic glomerulonephritis	Bilateral inflammatory process of the glomeruli leading to ischemia, nephron loss, and shrinkage of the kidney
Vascular	Hypertensive nephrosclerosis	Long-standing hypertension leads to renal arteriosclerosis and ischemia resulting in glomerular destruction and tubular atrophy
Infectious	Chronic pyelonephritis	Chronic infection commonly associated with an obstructive or neurologic process and vesicoureteral reflux leading to reflux nephropathy (renal scarring, atrophy, and dilated calyces)
Connective tissue disorders	Systemic lupus erythematosus	Basement membrane damage by circulating immune complexes leading to focal, local, or diffuse glomerulonephritis
Congenital	Polycystic kidney disease	Multiple bilateral cysts gradually destroy normal renal tissue by compression

tered, the regulatory and endocrine functions of the kidney are impaired, and accumulated metabolic waste products affect essentially every other organ system (Porth, 1994; Wyngaarden et al., 1992).

Early manifestations of uremia include nausea, apathy, weakness, and fatigue, symptoms that are easily attributable to a viral infection or influenza. As the condition progresses, the client may experience frequent vomiting, increasing weakness, lethargy, and confusion (Porth, 1994). The multisystem effects of uremia are illustrated in Figure 26–9.

Fluid and Electrolyte Effects

With the loss of functional kidney tissue, the ability to regulate fluid, electrolyte, and acid-base balance is impaired.

In the early stages of chronic renal failure, impaired filtration and reabsorption lead to proteinuria, hematuria, and the inability to concentrate urine. Salt and water are poorly conserved, and the client is susceptible to dehydration. Polyuria, nocturia, and a fixed specific gravity of 1.008 to 1.012 are common (Porth, 1994; Wilson et al., 1991). As the GFR decreases and renal function deteriorates further, sodium and water retention are common, necessitating salt and water restrictions.

Hyperkalemia is an indication of advancing renal failure. Manifestations of hyperkalemia, such as muscle weakness, paresthesias, and ECG changes, are not typically seen until the GFR is less than 5 mL/min. Phosphate excretion is also impaired, leading to hyperphosphatemia and hypocalcemia. Calcium absorption is reduced because of impaired activation of vitamin D, further con-

tributing to hypocalcemia. High serum magnesium levels are also seen with advancing renal failure, making it important to avoid the administration of magnesium-containing antacids.

As renal failure advances, hydrogen-ion excretion and the production of buffers are impaired, resulting in metabolic acidosis. The client in metabolic acidosis demonstrates increased respiratory rate and depth (Kussmaul's respirations) and may have fruity breath. Although metabolic acidosis is often asymptomatic, other possible manifestations include general malaise, weakness, headache, nausea and vomiting, and abdominal pain (see Chapter 5).

Cardiovascular and Hematologic Effects

Cardiovascular disease is a common cause of death in clients with end-stage renal disease (Andreoli et al., 1990; Bullock & Rosendahl, 1992). The increased incidence of cardiovasular disease in ESRD results from accelerated atherosclerosis. Hypertension, hyperlipidemia, and glucose intolerance all contribute to the process. Cerebral and peripheral vascular manifestations of the atherosclerotic process are also seen.

Systemic hypertension is the most common complication of ESRD. The primary factor leading to the hypertensive state is fluid volume expansion; increased renin production may also contribute (Porth, 1994; Wyngaarden et al., 1992).

Increased extracellular fluid volume also puts the client at risk for edema and congestive heart failure. Pulmonary edema may result from the congestive heart failure. Increased permeability of the alveolar capillary

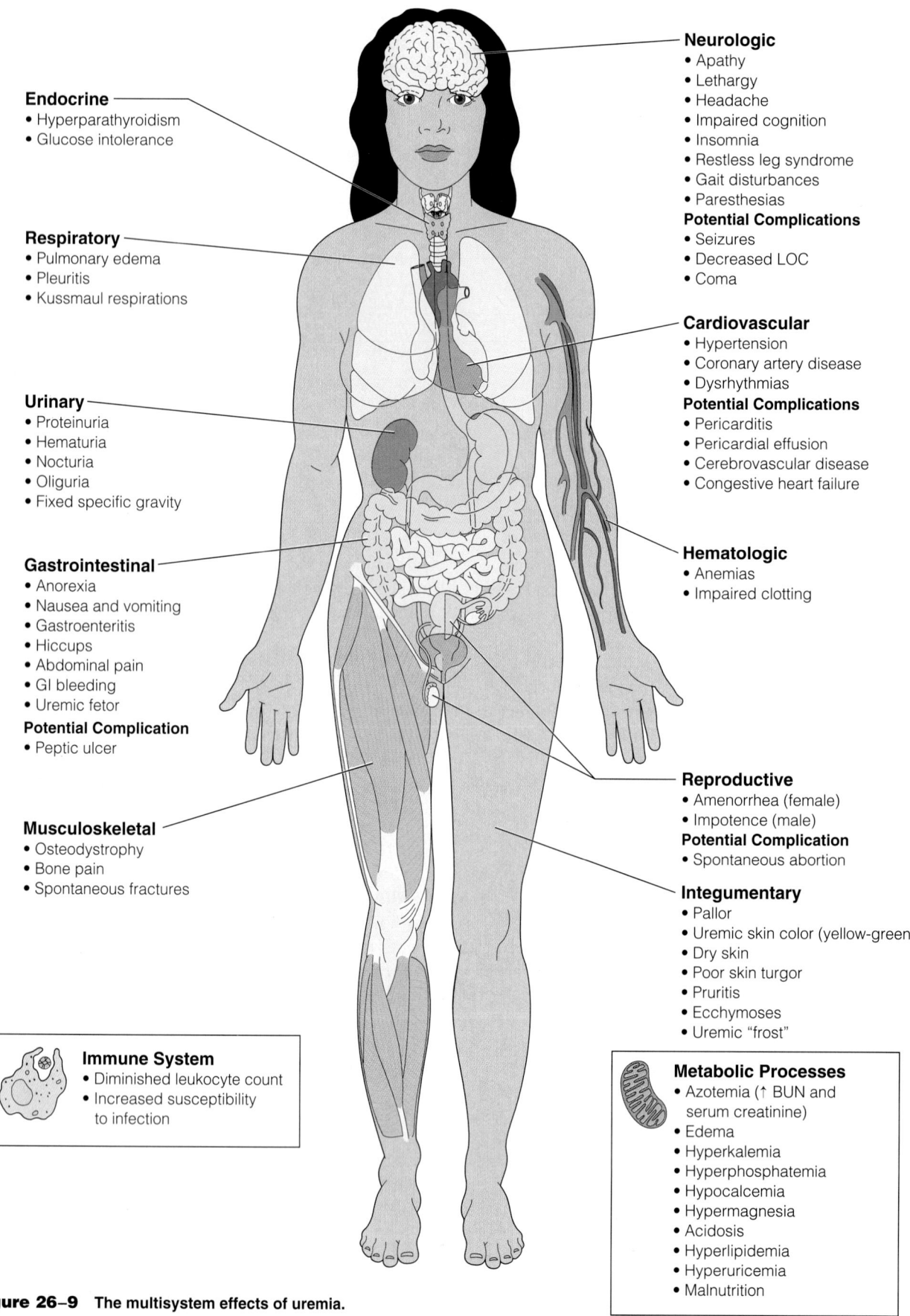

Endocrine
- Hyperparathyroidism
- Glucose intolerance

Respiratory
- Pulmonary edema
- Pleuritis
- Kussmaul respirations

Urinary
- Proteinuria
- Hematuria
- Nocturia
- Oliguria
- Fixed specific gravity

Gastrointestinal
- Anorexia
- Nausea and vomiting
- Gastroenteritis
- Hiccups
- Abdominal pain
- GI bleeding
- Uremic fetor
Potential Complication
- Peptic ulcer

Musculoskeletal
- Osteodystrophy
- Bone pain
- Spontaneous fractures

Immune System
- Diminished leukocyte count
- Increased susceptibility
  to infection

Neurologic
- Apathy
- Lethargy
- Headache
- Impaired cognition
- Insomnia
- Restless leg syndrome
- Gait disturbances
- Paresthesias
Potential Complications
- Seizures
- Decreased LOC
- Coma

Cardiovascular
- Hypertension
- Coronary artery disease
- Dysrhythmias
Potential Complications
- Pericarditis
- Pericardial effusion
- Cerebrovascular disease
- Congestive heart failure

Hematologic
- Anemias
- Impaired clotting

Reproductive
- Amenorrhea (female)
- Impotence (male)
Potential Complication
- Spontaneous abortion

Integumentary
- Pallor
- Uremic skin color (yellow-green)
- Dry skin
- Poor skin turgor
- Pruritis
- Ecchymoses
- Uremic "frost"

Metabolic Processes
- Azotemia (↑ BUN and
  serum creatinine)
- Edema
- Hyperkalemia
- Hyperphosphatemia
- Hypocalcemia
- Hypermagnesia
- Acidosis
- Hyperlipidemia
- Hyperuricemia
- Malnutrition

Figure 26–9   The multisystem effects of uremia.

membrane also contributes to the development of pulmonary edema.

Retained metabolic toxins can irritate the pericardial sac and cause an inflammatory response, leading to signs of pericarditis and the risk of cardiac tamponade. *Cardiac tamponade* occurs when fluid collecting in the pericardial sac interferes with ventricular filling and cardiac output. Once a common complication of uremia, pericarditis is less frequently seen when dialysis is initiated early.

Anemia is common in the uremic client. Multiple factors contribute to the anemia, including decreased erythropoietin production by the kidneys, folate and iron deficiencies, shortened RBC life, and blood loss through ulcerations in the GI tract. Platelet function is also altered in uremia, resulting in bleeding tendencies. The risk for infection is increased because white blood cell function is impaired (Bullock & Rosendahl, 1992; Porth, 1994).

Respiratory Effects

The uremic client is susceptible to respiratory infections because of altered immune function and difficulty clearing secretions. Increased extracellular fluid volume and the deposition of metabolic wastes in pulmonary tissue increase the risk of pulmonary edema, respiratory distress syndrome, and pleural effusions.

Gastrointestinal Effects

Anorexia, nausea, and vomiting are the most common early symptoms of uremia (Wilson et al., 1991; Wyngaarden et al., 1992). Hiccups also are commonly experienced. Gastroenteritis is frequent. Ulcerations may affect any level of the GI tract and contribute to an increased risk of GI bleeding. Peptic ulcer disease is particularly common in uremic clients. Many clients experience *uremic fetor,* a urinelike breath odor, which is often associated with a metallic taste in the mouth. These unpleasant sensations can further contribute to the client's anorexia.

Neurologic Effects

Alterations in both the central and peripheral nervous systems are evident in uremia. CNS manifestations occur early and include changes in mentation, difficulty concentrating, fatigue, and insomnia. Psychotic symptoms, seizures, and coma are associated with advanced uremic encephalopathy.

Peripheral neuropathy is also common in advanced uremia. Both the sensory and motor tracts are involved. The lower limbs are initally affected. "Restless leg syndrome," sensations of crawling or creeping, prickling, or itching of the lower legs accompanied by frequent leg movement, increases when the client is at rest. Paresthesia and sensory loss typically occur in a "stocking-glove" pattern. As uremia progresses, motor function is also impaired, resulting in muscle weakness, decreased deep tendon reflexes, and gait disturbances.

Musculoskeletal Effects

The hypocalcemia associated with uremia stimulates the secretion of parathyroid hormone. Parathyroid hormone causes the resorption of calcium from the bone as the body attempts to normalize the blood calcium levels. This bone resorption, combined with decreased vitamin D synthesis and decreased calcium absorption from the GI tract, leads to *osteodystrophy,* abnormal bone development, also known as renal rickets. Osteodystrophy is characterized by *osteomalacia,* softening of the bones, and *osteoporosis,* decreased bone mass. These changes cause bone tenderness and pain, and may precipitate the development of bone cysts. The client is at increased risk for spontaneous fractures (Bullock & Rosendahl, 1992; Porth, 1994).

Endocrine and Metabolic Effects

Accumulated waste products of protein metabolism are the primary factor involved in all of the effects and manifestations of uremia. The serum creatinine and BUN levels are significantly elevated. Uric acid levels are increased, contibuting to an increased risk of gout.

The tissues develop resistance to the effects of insulin in the uremic state, resulting in glucose intolerance. High blood triglyceride levels and lower-than-normal levels of high-density lipoproteins contribute to the accelerated atherosclerotic process seen in uremia.

Reproductive function is affected by uremia. Pregnancies are rarely carried to term, and menstrual irregularities are common. Reduced testosterone levels, low sperm counts, and impotence affect the male client with end-stage renal disease.

Dermatologic Effects

Anemia and retained pigmented metabolites cause the skin of the uremic client to appear pale and have a yellowish hue. Dry skin with poor turgor, a result of dehydration and atrophy of the sweat glands, is common. Bruising and excoriations are frequently seen. Metabolic wastes not eliminated by the kidneys may be deposited in the skin, contributing to itching or pruritus. In advanced uremia, high levels of urea in the sweat may result in *uremic frost,* crystallized deposits of urea on the skin.

Collaborative Care

Conservative management strategies are often effective for the client with chronic renal failure, even when the GFR is as low as 10 mL/min (Andreoli et al., 1990). The ultimate management goals are to

- Slow or prevent further deterioration of renal function
- Correct fluid and electrolyte imbalances
- Reduce or prevent symptoms of uremia while maintaining adequate nutrition (Tisher & Wilcox, 1993)

Fluid and electrolyte regulation and dietary management are key in the conservative management of chronic renal failure. Medications may be prescribed to facilitate management and improve the client's overall health status. Care is taken, however, to avoid any agents that may further damage the kidneys. When conservative management no longer ameliorates the symptoms of uremia, measures such as dialysis or kidney transplantation are necessary to replace or compensate for the lost kidney function.

Laboratory and Diagnostic Tests

Laboratory and diagnostic testing is used both to identify the presence of chronic renal failure and to monitor kidney function. A number of tests may be performed to determine the underlying renal disorder. Once the diagnosis is established, renal function is monitored primarily through laboratory testing.

The following laboratory tests may be ordered for the client with chronic renal failure:

- *Urinalysis* is done to determine the specific gravity of the urine and the presence of abnormal urine components. In the client with chronic renal failure, the specific gravity is often fixed at approximately 1.010, equivalent to that of the blood plasma. This fixed specific gravity is a result of the inability of the nephron tubules to reabsorb electrolytes and other filtrate components and to concentrate the urine. Abnormal proteins, blood cells, and cellular casts may also be noted in the urine.

- *Urine culture* is ordered to identify the presence of any urinary tract infection that may hasten the progress of chronic renal failure.

- *BUN* and *serum creatinine* are obtained to evaluate kidney function in eliminating nitrogenous waste products. Levels of both are monitored to assess the progress of renal failure. A BUN of 20 to 50 mg/dL signals mild azotemia; levels greater than 100 mg/dL indicate severe renal impairment. Uremic symptoms are seen when the BUN is around 200 mg/dL or higher. Serum creatinine levels of greater than 4 mg/dL indicate serious renal impairment.

- *The creatinine clearance* is an indicator of the glomerular filtration rate and functional capacity of the kidneys. In the earliest stage of chronic renal failure (decreased renal reserve), the GFR is more than 25% of normal and the creatinine clearance 32.5 to 130 mL/min. As the disease progresses and the stage of renal insufficiency is reached, the GFR is reduced to less than 25% of normal and the creatinine clearance to 10 to 30 mL/min. End-stage renal failure is characterized by a GFR of less than 10% of normal and a creatinine clearance of 5 to 10 mL/min or less. Nursing implica-

tions for the creatinine clearance test are outlined in the box on page 947.

- *Serum electrolytes* are monitored throughout the course of chronic renal failure as indicators of renal function. The values are also used to guide therapy. The serum sodium level may be low because of water retention, or it may be within normal limits. Potassium levels are elevated to a moderate degree, usually less than 6.5 mEq/L. The serum phosphate level is elevated, and the calcium level is decreased. Metabolic acidosis is present with a low blood pH, low plasma CO_2, and low bicarbonate levels.

- The *complete blood count* reveals moderately severe anemia with a hematocrit of 20% to 30% and a low hemoglobin level. The number of red blood cells and platelets is reduced.

The following diagnostic studies may be ordered for the client with chronic renal failure:

- *Renal ultrasonography* is performed to determine the size of the kidneys. In chronic renal failure, a significant decrease in size is noted as nephrons are destroyed and kidney mass is reduced. An ultrasound study showing kidneys of normal or increased size is more suggestive of an acute process affecting the kidneys than of chronic renal failure. Preparation of the client and nursing implications for renal ultrasonography are outlined in the box on page 940.

- *Biopsy* of the kidney may be performed to determine the underlying disease process if the cause of chronic renal failure is unclear. It is also used to differentiate acute from chronic failure. Kidney biopsy is sometimes an operative procedure requiring anesthesia and an incision. Needle biopsy performed percutaneously is sometimes used. The box on page 947 outlines the nursing care for a client having a renal biopsy.

Pharmacology

A number of factors need to be considered in administering medications to the client with chronic renal failure. Most medications are excreted primarily by the kidney. This fact is a major consideration whenever drug therapy is considered for the client in chronic renal failure. Drug absorption may be decreased if phosphate-binding agents are administered concurrently. Plasma protein levels can be significantly reduced by urinary protein loss, resulting in manifestations of toxicity when highly protein-bound drugs are administered. In addition, any agent that has the potential to affect the kidneys adversely and hasten the decline in renal function is avoided or used with extreme caution.

Diuretics, furosemide, or other loop diuretics, may be prescribed. They are useful for reducing the volume of extracellular fluid, particularly in the client who has difficulty restricting sodium intake. In addition, diuretic therapy can reduce hypertension and cause potassium wasting, lowering serum potassium levels.

Other antihypertensive agents are often employed to maintain the blood pressure within normal levels and slow the progress of renal failure. Angiotensin-converting enzyme (ACE) inhibitors are preferred for hypertension management. Other antihypertensive agents may also be prescribed, including central and peripheral sympathetic blocking agents such as minoxidil (Loniten) or clonidine (Catapres).

Other pharmacologic preparations may be used to manage the electrolyte imbalances and acidosis accompanying renal failure. Sodium bicarbonate or calcium carbonate are used to correct mild acidosis. High serum phosphate levels are managed using a combination of phosphate-binding agents and calcium supplements to reduce dietary phosphate absorption. A typical regimen for phosphate management is the use of aluminum hydroxide in combination with calcium carbonate (Tums). Complications such as encephalopathy and osteodystrophy are associated with the long-term administration of large doses of aluminum-containing preparations. Combining their use with calcium preparations allows lower doses while maintaining acceptable serum phosphate levels. When the serum phosphate is within normal limits, vitamin D supplements may be added to maintain a normal serum calcium.

If the serum potassium rises to dangerously high levels, therapy to reduce it may be necessary. Sodium polystyrene sulfonate, a potassium-exchange resin, can be administered either by mouth or per rectum as an enema. Acute hyperkalemia may require the intravenous administration of a combination of bicarbonate, insulin, and glucose to promote the movement of potassium into the cells.

Folic acid and iron supplements are useful to combat the anemia associated with chronic renal failure. A multiple vitamin preparation is also often prescribed, because anorexia, nausea, and dietary restrictions may limit nutrient intake.

Dietary and Fluid Management

As renal function declines, the kidneys lose the ability to adjust excretion rates for varying rates of water and solute intake. In addition, the elimination of metabolic wastes is impaired, and the accumulation of these wastes in the body leads to the development of uremic symptoms. Although some renal function remains, dietary modifications are an important aspect of conservative management. Regulating the intake of fluids, proteins, and other substances normally eliminated in the urine can be effective in slowing or preventing the development of uremia and other complications of chronic renal failure.

Water and sodium intake is regulated to maintain the extracellular fluid volume at normal levels. Water intake is matched to the client's output. Typically, 500 mL per day is allowed for insensible losses through the skin and lungs. The client is then allowed to consume as much additional fluid as the total urine output for the previous day. If additional fluid is being lost because of vomiting or diarrhea, allowances need to be made in the intake. Many clients with end-stage renal disease are hyponatremic, so only a moderate salt restriction is indicated. A diet restricting sodium to 3g or a "no added salt" diet may be prescribed. The client is weighed daily and blood pressure is monitored frequently to assess fluid balance. The client is taught to notify the physician of any weight gain in excess of 5 pounds over a 2-day period (Tisher & Wilcox, 1993).

Potassium intake is also carefully regulated to avoid serum levels that put the client at risk for lethal cardiac rhythm disruptions. The client is cautioned to avoid the use of salt substitutes, which typically contain high levels of potassium chloride. Foods high in phosphorus, such as milk, may be restricted as well.

Increasing BUN levels signal worsening of the symptoms of uremia. Because urea is a by-product of protein metabolism, regulation of protein intake is indicated for the client in renal failure. A protein intake of 0.6 g/kg of body weight, or approximately 40 g/day for an average male client, is usually adequate to provide the amino acids necessary for tissue repair and maintain the BUN within acceptable limits. Complete proteins containing all essential amino acids are emphasized. When dietary proteins are restricted, carbohydrate intake is increased to meet energy needs and prevent tissue breakdown.

Supportive and Surgical Therapy

Ideally, the period of conservative management is used to educate the client and family and to explore options for the long-term management of chronic renal failure. When conservative management strategies are no longer effective to maintain fluid and electrolyte balance and prevent uremia, dialysis or renal transplantation need to be considered.

A number of considerations affect the client's choice for long-term treatment. Hemodialysis and peritoneal dialysis each have advantages and disadvantages. Establishing an arteriovenous fistula for vascular access during hemodialysis may take several months. Planning ahead to develop the access during the conservative management period can ease the transition to dialysis when it becomes necessary. Established access is not a consideration for the client who will undergo peritoneal dialysis. The peritoneal catheter can be placed and treatment initiated as soon as the client's condition so warrants. When dialysis will be performed at home, initiation of teaching during the conservative management period can result in more effective learning. If a family member is to be prepared as

---

Applying Research to Nursing Practice: CPR Preferences

■ ■ ■

The question of cardiopulmonary resuscitation (CPR) is often not broached until the client is in the late stages of renal disease, confused, and unable to make an informed decision. Family members or the physician may then need to make the decision, and they are seldom aware of the client's desires. The question of CPR is of particular importance in clients on dialysis who have high frequency of heart disease and sudden death.

One set of researchers (Quintana et al., 1991) interviewed all the clients on a dialysis unit about their preferences. Care was taken to ensure that clients understood cardiac arrest, CPR, and the consequences of each. Clients were also encouraged to involve family members and their religious group in the decision.

Results of the research showed that one-third of the clients decided to decline CPR when given the choice. On the whole, individuals declining were those with severe medical disability; the presence of diabetes mellitus was a related factor of lower significance. No significant difference was seen between clients on hemodialysis versus peritoneal dialysis, in terms of age, or in the duration of dialysis.

Implications for Nursing

Health care workers, including nurses, are often reluctant to ask clients about their preferences for CPR when death is not imminent, yet the client is best able to make an informed decision at that time. This study showed that with appropriate preparation and interviewing techniques, the question could be addressed without causing undue stress for the client or family. Some clients expressed relief that their wishes had been made known. Although the risk for coronary artery disease and sudden death are higher in the client on dialysis, health care teams should not be afraid to ask any client about their wishes regarding CPR.

Critical Thinking in Client Care

1. How would you best approach clients to ask about their desires regarding CPR?

2. Would the type and severity of their health condition make a difference in your approach?

3. How would you explain sudden cardiac arrest and CPR to clients when trying to elicit their wishes?

4. If the client's values regarding CPR differ from your own, how can you resolve the conflict?

---

a dialysis helper, training should begin prior to the onset of uremic symptoms.

If transplantation is considered, tissue typing and identification of family members who might be a good match can be done prior to the onset of end-stage failure. To make an informed decision, both the client and the potential donor need to be aware of the risks, benefits, and options available. If the decision to transplant is made early, dialysis treatment can potentially be avoided. The age of the client, the presence of related health problems, the availability of a donor, and personal preference all influence the client's choice of dialysis, transplant, or no further treatment (Porth, 1994; Wilson et al., 1991).

Dialysis   In dialysis, blood is separated from a dialysis solution by a semipermeable membrane. An artificial membrane is used in hemodialysis; the peritoneum serves as the membrane in peritoneal dialysis. Solutes and water move across the membrane, driven by a concentration gradient and, in hemodialysis and ultrafiltration procedures, by a hydrostatic pressure gradient. Dialysis compensates for the kidneys' inability to eliminate excess water and solutes. However, dialysis cannot compensate for

the kidneys' inability to produce erythropoietin. Thus, anemia is a continuing problem for the client receiving dialysis.

Dialysis is indicated by the presence of severe fluid and electrolyte imbalances such as fluid overload, hyperkalemia, and acidosis. It is also indicated by the presence of uremic manifestations and in clients whose renal function is 5% or less of normal (Andreloi et al., 1990).

Approximately 30,000 people begin dialysis every year in the United States, with an average maintenance cost of $25,000 to $30,000 per year for hemodialysis. For the client who is not a candidate for renal transplantation or who has had a transplant failure, dialysis is life sustaining (Porth, 1994).

The most common therapies for CRF in the United States are hemodialysis performed in an outpatient dialysis center, followed by renal transplantation. Both hemodialysis and peritoneal dialysis can be performed in the home setting, but only a small portion of clients use home hemodialysis. Peritoneal dialysis, by contrast, is typically performed by the client in the home. As the morbidity and mortality for each are comparable, factors such as the client's desire and ability to manage home care, work situations, and proximity to a dialysis center become the primary factors influencing the decision for hemodialysis or peritoneal dialysis (Andreoli et al., 1990; US Renal Data System, 1993).

The morbity and mortality rates for clients on long-term dialysis are higher than those for the general population. Many clients have other severe diseases along with end-stage renal disease. Infection and cardiovascular disease are common causes of illness and death. Clients with diabetes have the poorest prognosis. Survival rates are improving, with a 1-year survival rate of nearly 80% for all clients on dialysis therapy. In the 20-to-44-year-old group, the yearly survival rate is more than 90%; it falls to approximately 60% in people over the age of 75 years (US Renal Data System, 1993).

The decision to initiate dialysis is not an easy one. Like insulin therapy for the diabetic, dialysis manages the symptoms of end-stage renal disease but does not cure it. Dialysis requires a day-in, day-out commitment on the part of the client and is a constant factor in the client's life, requiring thinking and planning ahead at all times. Early evaluation and intervention by a mental health professional help the client make decisions and cope with the stresses of treatment. See the accompanying nursing re-

search box. Clients on dialysis may not be able to maintain employment. Many families fall apart with the day-to-day stress. Even with dialysis, the client may experience constant flulike symptoms, never feeling truly well. Clients on hemodialysis may feel helpless because of their dependence on others for treatment. On the other hand, home peritoneal dialysis is a continuing burden on the client to maintain the therapy. In the end, the client may choose to discontinue treatment, preferring death over continued dialysis (Flaherty & O'Brien, 1992; Rydholm & Pauling, 1991).

Hemodialysis   Hemodialysis uses the principles of diffusion and ultrafiltration to remove electrolytes, waste products, and excess water from the body. Blood is taken from the client via a vascular access and pumped to the dialyzing membrane unit (Figure 26–10), where it moves past an artificial semipermeable membrane of cellulose acetate or a similar substance. A solution of approximately the same composition as normal extracellular fluid, the dialysate, is warmed to body temperature and passed along the other side of the membrane. All solute molecules smaller than blood cells and plasma proteins are able to move freely across the membrane by diffusion.

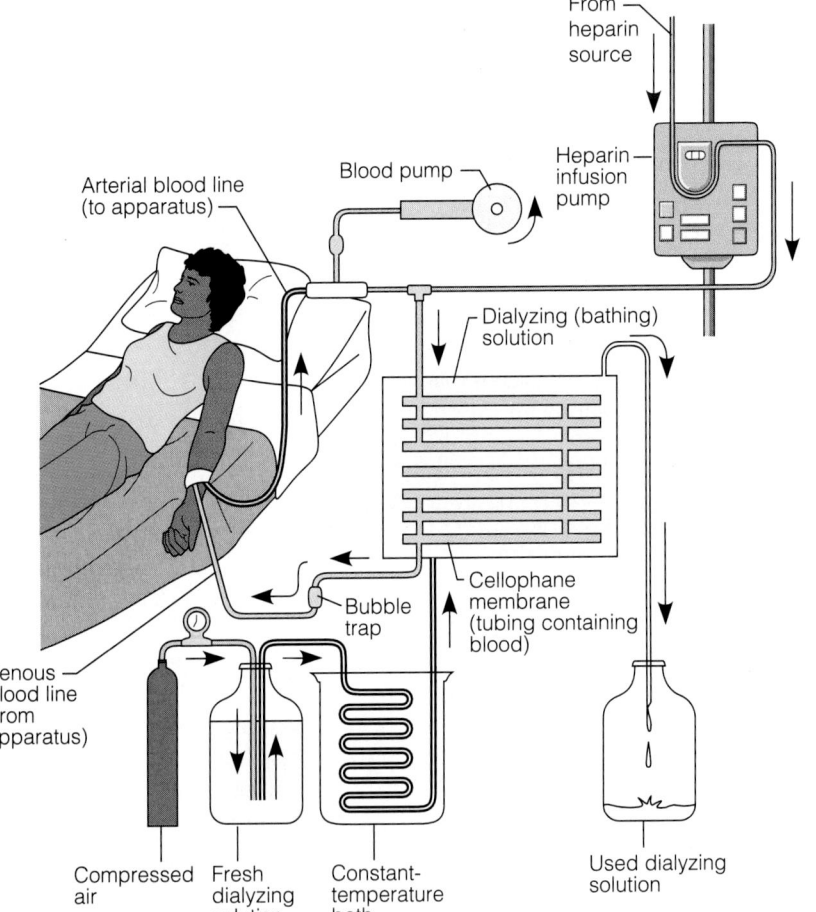

Figure 26–10   A hemodialysis system.

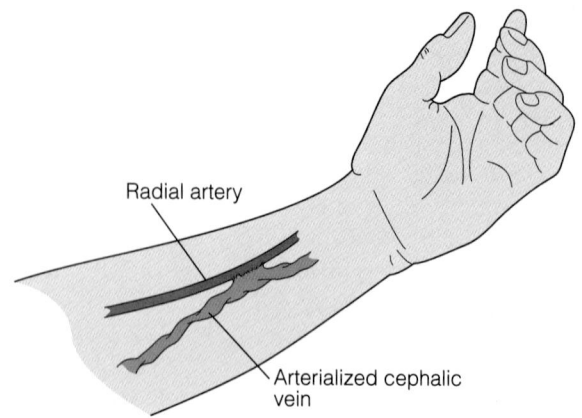

Radial artery

Arterialized cephalic vein

Figure 26–11   An arteriovenous fistula.

The direction of flow for any substance is determined by the concentration of that substance in either the blood or dialysate. Electrolytes and waste products such as urea and creatinine diffuse through the membrane into the dialysate. If it is necessary to add something to the blood, such as bicarbonate to correct acidosis, it can be added to the dialysate to diffuse across the membrane into the blood. Excess water is removed from the blood by creating a higher hydrostatic pressure on the side of the membrane in contact with blood than on the side in contact with dialysate, a process known as **ultrafiltration.**

Acute or temporary vascular access for hemodialysis may be gained using a subclavian or internal jugular venous catheter. An *arteriovenous (AV) fistula* (Figure 26–11) is the most commonly used long-term vascular access. In preparation for fistula formation, the nondominant arm is not used for venipuncture or blood pressure measurement during the early stages of chronic renal failure. The fistula is created by surgical anastomosis of an artery and vein, most often the radial artery and cephalic vein. It takes approximately 1 month for the fistula to mature so that it can be used for taking and replacing blood during dialysis. On assessment, a functional AV fistula has a palpable pulsation and a bruit on auscultation (Tisher & Wilcox, 1993). Venipunctures and blood pressures are avoided on the arm with the fistula.

Clients typically undergo two or three sessions of hemodialysis per week for a total of 9 to 12 hours. Factors such as the client's remaining renal function, diet, and general health determine how much dialysis is necessary (Wilson et al., 1991).

Both systemic and fistula problems may occur as complications in the client on hemodialysis. Systemic complications can occur during or after the dialysis procedure and include the following:

- Hypotension is the most frequent complication during hemodialysis. It is related to many factors, including

changes in serum osmolality, rapid removal of fluid from the vascular compartment, vasodilation, and others. For clients with intermittent excess water weight gain, hemofiltration or ultrafiltration may be used in combination with hemodialysis, reducing the risk of rapid fluid shifts (see page 974).

- Bleeding is a risk because of both altered platelet function associated with uremia and the use of heparin during the dialysis procedure. Hemorrhage may be manifest as subdural hematoma, GI bleeding, or bleeding in other internal structures.

- Infection can be either local, affecting the AV fistula, or systemic. *Staphylococcus aureus* septicemia is commonly associated with contamination of the fistula. Clients on chronic hemodialysis have higher rates of hepatitis B, hepatitis C, cytomegalovirus, and HIV infection than the general population. Multiple blood transfusions, immune system depression, and underlying disease processes all contribute.

- Dialysis dementia is a progressive, potentially fatal neurologic complication that may affect clients on long-term hemodialysis. Aluminum has been implicated in its development, either as a dialysate contaminant or as aluminum hydroxide used to bind phosphate.

Anemia and other systemic manifestations seen in the client on dialysis may be related to end-stage renal disease rather than complications of the dialysis.

Localized AV fistula problems can also occur. Infection and clotting or thrombosis are the most common shunt problems. Aneurysms may also develop. Both infection and thrombosis can lead to systemic manifestations such as septicemia and embolization. These local complications may cause the fistula to fail, necessitating development of a new site. The psychologic impact of AV fistula failure is significant, often resulting in depression and an altered self-concept (Wilson et al., 1991).

The accompanying box outlines nursing care considerations for the client undergoing hemodialysis.

Peritoneal Dialysis   In peritoneal dialysis, the highly vascular peritoneal membrane serves as the dialyzing surface (Figure 26–12). The warmed sterile dialysate is instilled into the peritoneal cavity via a permanent indwelling catheter. Metabolic waste products and excess electrolytes diffuse into the dialysate while it remains in the abdomen. Water diffusion is controlled using dextrose as an osmotic agent to draw it into the dialysate. The fluid is then drained by gravity out of the peritoneal cavity into a sterile bag (Porth, 1990; Wilson et al., 1991).

Peritoneal dialysis was developed before hemodialysis as a method for treating renal failure but is currently used by only about 10% of people who require long-term dialysis in the United States. In Canada, approximately 21%

Nursing Care of the Client Undergoing Hemodialysis

PREDIALYSIS CARE

- Perform and document assessment of the client's vital signs, including orthostatic blood pressures (lying and sitting), apical pulse, respirations, and lung sounds. *These data provide baseline information and help assess the client's ability to tolerate the dialysis procedure. Hypertension may indicate excess extracellular fluid. The client who is hypotensive may not tolerate rapid fluid volume changes during dialysis. Abnormal heart sounds, such as gallops or murmurs, and changes in heart rate or rhythm are possible indicators of fluid overload or electrolyte imbalance. Fluid overload may also lead to dyspnea, tachypnea, and rales or crackles in the lungs.*

- Note the client's weight. *Weight changes provide an indicator of fluid volume status.*

- Assess the vascular access site for patency (a palpable pulsation or vibration and an audible bruit) and signs of inflammation. *Infection and thrombus formation with possible loss of vascular access are the most common problems affecting the access site in hemodialysis clients.*

- Make sure the extremity with the vascular access site (or the nondominant arm, if a site has not been permanently established) is not used for blood pressure measurement or venipuncture. *These procedures may damage vessels and lead to failure of the AV fistula.*

POSTDIALYSIS CARE

- Assess the client's vital signs, weight, and vascular access site and record your findings. *Rapid fluid and solute removal during the dialysis procedure may lead to orthostatic hypotension, changes in cardiac status, and weight loss.*

- Monitor the client's BUN, serum creatinine, serum electrolyte, and hematocrit levels between dialysis treatments. *These values help determine the adequacy of the treatment, the need for fluid and diet restrictions, and the timing of future dialysis sessions. The anemia associated with renal failure does not improve with dialysis, and iron and folate supplements or periodic blood transfusions may be needed.*

- Assess for signs of dialysis disequilibrium syndrome, including headache, nausea and vomiting, altered level of consciousness, and hypertension. *Rapid changes in the blood urea levels and pH, and electrolyte shifts during dialysis may lead to the development of cerebral edema, causing signs of increased intracranial pressure.*

- Assess and intervene for other possible adverse responses to dialysis therapy, such as dehydration, nausea and vomiting, muscle cramps, or seizure activity. *Excess fluid removal and rapid changes in electrolyte status can lead to a fall in blood pressure, nausea, vomiting, and seizure activity.*

- Assess for evidence of bleeding at the access site or elsewhere. Use universal precautions at all times. *Renal failure and heparinization during dialysis increase the client's risk for bleeding. Increased exposure to blood and blood products increase the risk for hepatitis B or C or other blood-borne diseases.*

- If the client received a transfusion during dialysis treatment, monitor for signs and symptoms of transfusion reaction, such as chills and fever; dyspnea; chest, back, or arm pain; and urticaria or itching. *The client who receives multiple transfusions (common in clients with CRF) is at increased risk for transfusion reaction. Close monitoring during and after the transfusion is important for early identification of adverse reactions.*

- Provide psychologic support to the client and family. Listen actively. Address the client's concerns and accept responses such as anger, depression, and noncompliance. Reinforce client and family strengths in coping with end-stage renal disease and hemodialysis. *The loss of organ function, even after a chronic or prolonged course, results in grieving. The client may feel hopeless or helpless and resent dependence on a machine. The nurse can help the client and family work through these responses and focus on positive aspects of living.*

- Help the client and family access social services and counseling as indicated. *Clients with a chronic disease process such as CRF may need additional support services to help them adapt to their condition.*

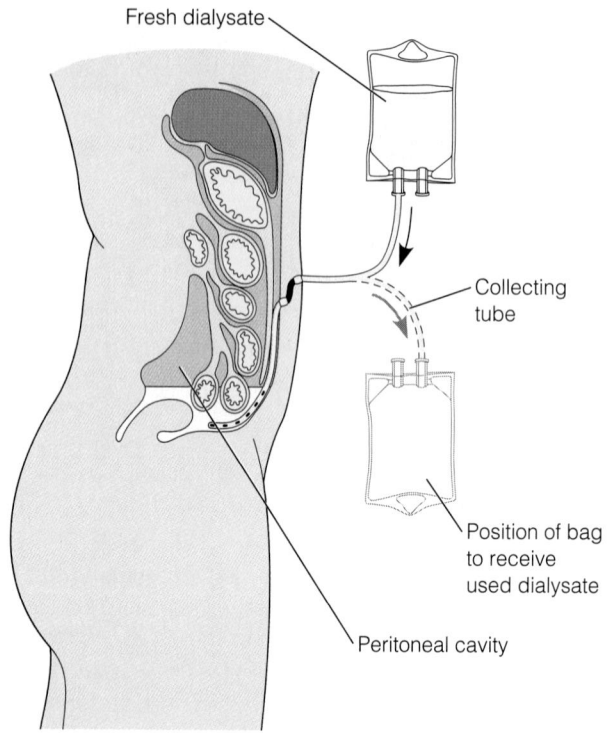

Fresh dialysate

Collecting tube

Position of bag to receive used dialysate

Peritoneal cavity

Figure 26–12   Peritoneal dialysis.

of clients with end-stage renal disease are treated with peritoneal dialysis. Seventy percent of older adult clients with CRF in the United Kingdom were on peritoneal dialysis in 1989. In third-world countries, peritoneal dialysis is used for 85% to 90% of CRF clients (Ismail et al., 1993; Tisher & Wilcox, 1993; US Renal Data System, 1993).

Continuous ambulatory peritoneal dialysis (CAPD) is the most common form of peritoneal dialysis used today. Two liters of dialysate are instilled into the peritoneal cavity, and the catheter is sealed. The client can then continue normal daily activities, emptying the peritoneal cavity and replacing the dialysate every 4 to 6 hours. No special equipment is needed. A variation of CAPD is continuous cyclic peritoneal dialysis (CCPD). CPPD uses a delivery device during nighttime hours and a continuous dwell during the day. CAPD can be performed anywhere, and CCPD allows for home treatment at night, leaving the client free during the day.

Peritoneal dialysis has several advantages over hemodialysis. Heparinization and the vascular complications associated with an AV fistula are avoided. This is particularly advantageous for the diabetic client. The clearance of metabolic wastes is slower but more continuous, avoiding rapid fluctuations in extracellular fluid composition and associated symptoms. More liberal intake of fluids and nutrients is often allowed for the client

on CAPD. The diabetic client can maintain good blood glucose control by adding insulin to the dialysate. The client is better able to self-manage the treatment regimen, reducing feelings of helplessness (Haas, 1993; Rydholm & Pauling, 1991; Wilson et al., 1991).

The major disadvantages of peritoneal dialysis include lower efficiency of metabolite removal and risk of infection (peritonitis). Glucose in the dialysate can be absorbed into the bloodstream, necessitating a reduction in dietary calories. Serum triglyceride levels increase with peritoneal dialysis. Finally, the presence of an indwelling peritoneal catheter may cause a body image disturbance for some clients (Tisher & Wilcox, 1993).

The accompanying box outlines nursing care of the client having peritoneal dialysis.

Renal Transplantation   Renal transplantation, the surgical insertion of a functioning kidney, has become the treatment of choice for many clients with end-stage renal disease (Porth, 1994). Kidneys are the solid organ most commonly transplanted, and to date kidney transplantation is the most successful of transplantation procedures. The first kidney transplantation was performed in 1954; the donor and recipient were identical twins (Cunningham & Smith, 1990). Although the success of kidney transplants cannot necessarily be measured in terms of survival time versus that for dialysis, it certainly can be measured in terms of quality of life. The transplant client is no longer tethered to a dialysis catheter, machine, or center. Dietary and fluid restrictions are reduced, and the client's body image is one of increased "wholeness." The need to remain on immunosuppressive therapy, which has its own risks, tempers these positive aspects to a degree.

Most transplanted kidneys are harvested from cadavers. Related living donors account for the remainder, about 30% in the United States. Even when immunosuppressive drugs are used, the success for well-matched living-donor transplants is superior to that for cadaver organ transplants, with a 1-year transplant survival of 90% compared to 80% for cadaver transplants.

One key to transplant success is obtaining an organ with tissue antigens that are as close to the client's as possible. Close tissue matching probably accounts for the better outcome with related donors. Living relatives with normal kidneys who are in good physical health and have the same ABO blood group as the recipient may serve as donors. Predonation counseling is vital for volunteer donors to ensure they understand the risks involved. Kidney donation involves major surgery, and there is always the risk of trauma or renal disease damaging the remaining kidney at some future time. If transplantation fails, the psychologic impact on the donor can be significant. Nursing care of the client undergoing kidney surgery is summarized in the box on page 958.

Nursing Care of the Client Undergoing Peritoneal Dialysis

PREDIALYSIS CARE

- Assess and document vital signs including temperature, orthostatic blood pressures (lying and standing), apical pulse, respirations, and lung sounds. *These data provide baseline information and help assess the client's ability to tolerate the dialysis procedure. Hypertension, abnormal heart or lung sounds, or dyspnea may indicate excess extracellular fluid. A client with poor respiratory status may not tolerate the peritoneal dialysis procedure well. Obtaining a baseline temperature is vital, because infection is the most common complication of peritoneal dialysis.*

- Weigh the client daily or between dialysis runs as indicated. *Weight is an accurate indicator of fluid volume status.*

- Note the client's BUN, serum electrolyte, creatinine, pH, and hematocrit levels prior to the initiation of peritoneal dialysis and periodically during the procedure. *These values are used to assess the efficacy of treatment.*

- Measure the client's abdominal girth and record. *Baseline data allow future comparison.*

- Maintain fluid and dietary restrictions as ordered. *Following these restrictions helps to prevent hypervolemia and control azotemia.*

- Prior to catheter insertion, have the client empty the bladder. *An empty bladder is vital to prevent inadvertent puncture.*

- Warm the prescribed dialysate solution to body temperature (98.6 F or 37 C) using a warm water bath or heating pad on low setting. *Dialysate is warmed to prevent hypothermia.*

- Explain all procedures and expected sensations to the client. *Knowledge helps reduce the client's anxiety and elicit cooperation.*

INTRADIALYSIS CARE

- Use strict aseptic technique at all times during the dialysis procedure and when caring for the peritoneal catheter. *Peritonitis is common in clients undergoing peritoneal dialysis but can be prevented by the use of sterile technique.*

- Add prescribed medications to the dialysate solution; prime the tubing with solution and connect it to the peritoneal catheter, taping the connections securely and avoiding kinks. *These measures allow the dialysate to flow freely into the abdominal cavity and prevent leaking or contamination.*

- Instill the dialysate into the abdominal cavity, usually over a period of approximately 10 minutes. Clamp tubing and allow the dialysate to remain in the abdomen during the prescribed dwell period. Be sure drainage tubing is clamped at all times during the instillation and dwell periods. *Dialysate should flow freely into the abdomen if the peritoneal catheter is patent. Dialysis, the exchange of solutes and water between the blood and dialysate, occurs across the peritoneal membrane during the dwell period.*

- During the instillation and dwell periods, observe the client closely for signs of respiratory distress, manifested by dyspnea, tachypnea, or rales. Placing the client in Fowler's or semi-Fowler's position and slowing the rate of instillation slightly may relieve respiratory distress associated with overly rapid filling or overfilling. *Respiratory embarrassment may result from overly rapid filling or overfilling of the abdomen or from a diaphragmatic defect that allows fluid to enter the thoracic cavity.*

- After the prescribed dwell time, open drainage tubing clamps and allow the dialysate to drain by gravity into a sterile container. Observe the dialysate for clarity and any evidence of blood, feces, odor, or cloudiness. *The presence of blood or feces in the dialysate may indicate organ or bowel perforation; cloudy or malodorous dialysate may indicate an infection.*

- Accurately record the amount and type of dialysate instilled, including any added medications, the dwell time, and the amount and character of the drainage. *This record provides a measure of the effectiveness of the treatment in removing excess fluid from the client. When more dialysate drains than has been instilled, the client has a net loss of fluid. If less dialysate is returned than has been instilled, the client has a net fluid gain.*

- Monitor the client's laboratory values, including BUN, serum electrolyte, and creatinine levels. *These values are used to assess the effectiveness of peritoneal dialysis.*

- Trouble-shoot for possible problems during dialysis.
  a. Overly slow instillation of dialysate. Increase the container height from the client's abdomen and

Nursing Care of the Client Undergoing Peritoneal Dialysis (continued)

reposition the client. Check the tubing and catheter for kinks. Check the abdominal dressing for wetness, indicating leakage around the catheter. *Slow dialysate flow may be related to a partially obstructed tube or catheter.*

b. Excess dwell time. *Prolonged dwell time may lead to water depletion or hyperglycemia.*

c. Poor dialysate drainage can result from the same problems causing slow instillation; use the same interventions (Thompson et al., 1993). *Tubing or catheter obstruction can also interfere with dialysate drainage.*

POSTDIALYSIS CARE

- Assess and record vital signs, including temperature. *Accurate assessment is important to determine any adverse effects of treatment, including infection.*

- Time meals to correspond with outflow times. *Consuming meals while the abdomen is empty of dialysate enhances intake and reduces nausea.*

- Maintain fluid and dietary restrictions as prescribed. Administer stool softeners and laxatives as needed. *These measures may be necessary to prevent constipation.*

- Teach the client and family about the peritoneal dialysis procedure. *Many clients elect to use continuous ambulatory peritoneal dialysis (CAPD) to manage end-stage renal disease and prevent uremia.*

When a cadaver kidney is used, human leukocyte antigen (HLA) matching is also closely related to the success of the transplant. HLA is the major factor determining the compatibility of donor and recipient tissue in transplantation. Cadaver kidneys are obtained from people who meet the criteria for brain death, are less than 65 years old, and are free of systemic disease, malignancy, or infection, including HIV and hepatitis B or C. Kidneys are removed before or immediately after cardiac arrest and preserved through the use of simple hypothermia or a technique called continuous hypothermic pulsatile perfusion. When simple hypothermia is used, the kidney is transplanted within 24 to 48 hours. Continuous pulsatile perfusion allows the kidney to be stored up to 3 days before transplantation.

Recipients who are in good general health except for primary kidney disease and between the ages of 5 and 50 years have the best prognosis for transplant success. Retinopathy due to uncontrolled hypertension or diabetes often stabilizes or improves with kidney transplantation; transplantation prior to end-stage renal disease may be recommended. The system used to allocate cadaver kidneys for transplantation is outlined in the accompanying box.

Care is taken to preserve the quality of the donor kidney when nephrectomy is done for kidney donation. The donor kidney is generally placed in the lower abdominal cavity (iliac fossa) of the recipient, and anastomosis of the renal artery, vein, and ureter is performed (Figure 26–13). The renal artery of the donor kidney is connected to the hypogastric artery, and the renal vein to the iliac vein. The ureter is connected to one of the recipient's ureters or directly to the bladder, using a tunnel technique to prevent reflux (Way, 1994).

Unless the donor and recipient are identical twins, the presence of foreign tissue in the body stimulates a normal immune response to reject the transplanted organ. This rejection response is minimized with the use of immunosuppressive drugs. Corticosteroids are generally used in combination with azathioprine and/or cyclosporine to achieve immunosuppression (Harasyko, 1989; Tisher & Wilcox, 1993). These drugs act by suppressing a portion of the immune system and the inflammatory response. Consequently, clients receiving immunosuppresive therapy are at increased risk of developing infections and neoplasms. The nursing implications of immunosuppressive therapy are indicated in the box on page 949. The pre- and postoperative care of the client undergoing renal transplantation is outlined in the box on page 994.

Corticosteroids such as prednisone and methylprednisolone are used for both maintenance immunosuppression and for treatment of acute rejection episodes. Side effects of long-term corticosteroid administration include impaired wound healing, emotional disturbances, osteoporosis, and cushingoid effects on glucose, protein, and fat metabolism.

How Cadaver Kidneys Are Allocated to Clients with ESRD

■ ■ ■

The *ANNA Journal* (Harris & DeLone, 1992) describes the allocation process of kidneys harvested from cadavers. Nearly 19,000 people were on a waiting list for a cadaver kidney in 1991; only 9400 people received one in 1990. The scarcity of this resource leads to questions about how kidneys are allocated—who receives a kidney and who does not. Past inequities in the allocation process (e.g., more men than women, more Caucasians than people of color, more rich than poor, and more young than old) led to the development of the United Network for Organ Sharing (UNOS) in 1986. UNOS has developed policies for the distribution of kidneys as well as other transplanted organs such as hearts, livers, lungs, and pancreata.

UNOS maintains national, regional, and local lists of clients awaiting transplants. When a kidney becomes available for transplantation, it is registered with the UNOS computer. Its human leukocyte antigens (HLA) are compared with those of registered clients. When the available kidney and a potential recipient have six antigens in common, the match is said to be "perfect." Because of the likelihood of a good outcome in this instance, a candidate with a perfect match and compatible blood type gets priority for the kidney, regardless of region or geographic area. If no perfectly matched recipient is available, a point system is used to allocate the kidney locally. Points are awarded based on the degree of antigen match, length of time on the waiting list, and a screening crossmatch. The screening crossmatch combines donor cells and recipient serum in a test for reactivity. If donor cells are attacked by recipient antibodies, the transplant will likely not occur. Pediatric clients under the age of 10 years receive additional points. Another consideration is the size of the donor kidney and the recipient; e.g., a pediatric kidney may not be appropriate for a large male adult.

The point scale and UNOS allocation system together with standardized fees and Medicare coverage for transplantation have done much to ensure equitable access to available kidneys. Still, controversy exists. Clients with available resources for travel may register in several different regions for an organ. Up to 10% of clients receiving a transplant in any center may be foreign nationals competing with U.S. citizens for scarce organ resources. A transplant center can accept or reject a candidate for transplant who has lost a kidney because of noncompliance.

As long as the demand for kidneys exceeds the supply of donor organs, it is likely that controversy will exist regarding their allocation. Nurses can help by identifying potential donors and initiating contact with the transplant coordinator. In addition, nurses can teach clients and the public about the system used to help ensure fair distribution of organs.

Azathioprine inhibits both cellular and humoral immunity. Because this drug is rapidly metabolized by the liver, the dose may not need to be altered in the presence of renal failure. Bone marrow suppression, abnormalities of liver function, and alopecia are the primary significant adverse effects for azathioprine.

The primary effect of cyclosporine is on cellular immunity, the helper T cells in particular. Among its many adverse effects, which include hepatotoxicity and hirsutism, nephrotoxicity is the primary concern for the renal transplant client.

Even with the use of immunosuppressive drugs, the transplanted kidney can be rejected at any time following surgery. *Hyperacute rejection* occurs within minutes to hours after the graft; *accelerated rejection* occurs within 2 to 4 days. Both almost inevitably result in graft failure and necessitate its removal. Fortunately, these rejection episodes are rare. *Acute rejection,* the most common and treatable form, occurs during the first 3 months after the transplant. The clinical manifestations of acute rejection

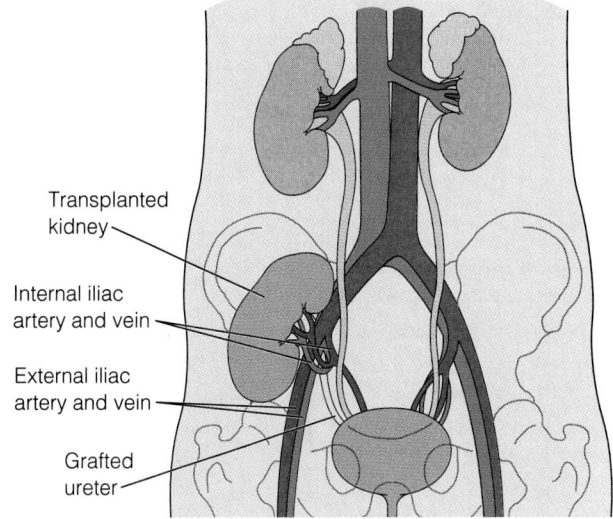

Figure 26–13   Placement of a transplanted kidney in the iliac fossa with anastomosis to the hypogastric artery off the internal iliac artery, iliac vein, and bladder.

Nursing Care of the Client with a Renal Transplant

PREOPERATIVE CARE

- Assess the client's knowledge and feelings about the procedure, answering questions and clarifying information as needed. Listen to and address concerns regarding surgery, the source of the organ to be transplanted, and possible complications. *Addressing concerns and reducing anxiety before surgery are two ways of improving postsurgical outcome.*

- Perform and document a complete nursing history and physical assessment. *The history and assessment provide baseline data for comparison after surgery.*

- Continue dialysis treatments as ordered. *Dialysis is necessary to manage fluid and electrolyte balance and prevent uremia prior to surgery.*

- Administer immunosuppressive medications as ordered prior to surgery. *Immunosuppression is initiated before transplantation to prevent hyperacute or accelerated rejection episodes.*

POSTOPERATIVE CARE

- Provide routine postoperative care as outlined in Chapter 7.

- Maintain patency of indwelling urinary catheter and measure urinary output every 30 to 60 minutes initially. *Careful measurement and recording of the urine output are important to assess fluid balance and function of the transplanted kidney. Acute tubular necrosis (ATN) is a common complication during the immediate postoperative period, usually resulting from tissue ischemia during the period between organ harvest (removal from the donor) and transplantation. It may be*

heralded by the onset of oliguria. Catheter patency is vital to keep the bladder decompressed and prevent pressure on delicate suture lines.

- Monitor vital signs, arterial pressure, and pulmonary wedge pressures closely. *Diuresis may occur immediately after transplantation. The resulting hypovolemia can jeopardize perfusion of the transplanted kidney, precipitating acute tubular necrosis.*

- Maintain adequate fluid replacement, generally calculated to replace the urinary output over the previous 30 or 60 minutes, milliliter for milliliter. *Fluid replacement is vital to maintain vascular volume and prevent dehydration.*

- Administer loop and/or osmotic diuretics such as furosemide or mannitol, as ordered. *These drugs may be used to promote diuresis in the immediate postoperative period.*

- Maintain a closed urinary drainage system. *A closed system helps prevent infection in the immunosuppressed client.*

- Remove the catheter within 2 to 3 days or as ordered. Encourage the client to void every 1 to 2 hours and assess frequently for signs of urinary retention following catheter removal. *The client's bladder may have atrophied prior to surgery, allowing it to hold only small volumes. Urinary retention places stress on suture lines and increases the risk of infection.*

- Monitor electrolytes and urinary function tests. *These tests provide a means of monitoring graft status. Hypokalemia, common after renal transplantation because of diuresis and the use of diuretics, may lead to cardiac dysrhythmias. Hyperkalemia may be indicative of graft dysfunction. Insulin, glucose, and bicarbonate*

include fever, swelling and tenderness over the graft site, and a marked decrease in urine output. Acute rejection is managed using increased doses of immunosuppressive drugs until the response abates. *Chronic rejection* is another major cause of graft loss. The presenting manifestations associated with chronic rejection—progressive azotemia, proteinuria, and hypertension—are evidence of progressive renal failure (Harasyko, 1989; Tisher & Wilcox, 1993; Wilson et al., 1991). The types of rejection processes are summarized in Table 26–8.

In addition to rejection, other complications are associated with renal transplantation. Hypertension may be the result of rejection processes, renal artery stenosis, or

renal vasoconstriction. Many clients develop glomerular lesions and may have manifestations of nephrosis. Preexisting hyperparathyroidism and altered calcium metabolism can lead to aseptic necrosis of the femur head (Wilson et al., 1991).

Long-term immunosuppression is associated with complications as well. Infection is a continuing threat. The client may experience bacterial and viral infections, as well as fungal infections of the blood, lungs, and central nervous system. Tumors are also common, with carcinoma in situ of the cervix, lymphomas, and skin cancers most prevalent. The risk of congenital anomalies is increased in infants whose mothers have undergone im-

Nursing Care of the Client with a Renal Transplant (continued)

may be administered intravenously as an emergency measure to reduce the serum potassium, or hyperkalemia can be treated with dialysis or a potassium-exchange resin.

- Monitor for possible complications:
  a. Hemorrhage from an anastomosis can be either acute or insidious. Indicators include swelling of the operative site, increased abdominal girth, and signs of shock, including changes in vital signs and level of consciousness. *Hemorrhage may indicate failure of the anastomosis and constitutes a surgical emergency.*
  b. Failure of the ureteral anastomosis results in urine leakage into the peritoneal cavity and may be marked by abdominal swelling and tenderness, and decreased urine output. *Failure of the ureteral anastomosis also requires surgical intervention.*
  c. Renal artery thrombosis is characterized by the abrupt onset of hypertension and reduced GFR. *Renal artery thrombosis can result in transplant failure.*
  d. Infection due to immunosuppression is an immediate and continuing risk. The inflammatory response is blunted by corticosteroid use, and infection may not significantly elevate the client's temperature. Monitor for other signs such as a change in level of consciousness, cloudy or malodorous urine, or purulent drainage from the incision. *Prevention and prompt treatment of infections is particularly important in the immunosuppressed client.*
- Provide teaching for the client and family, being sure to include the following:

  a. The use and side effects of prescribed medications, including any antihypertensive medications, immunosuppressive agents, prophylactic antibiotics, and others as ordered. *The client needs a good understanding of medications to perform self-care.*
  b. Monitoring of vital signs and weight. *These are indicators of fluid volume status.*
  c. The manifestations of organ rejection, such as swelling and tenderness over the graft site, fever, joint aching, weight gain, and decreased urinary output. *Make sure the client understands the need to report these signs and symptoms to the physician. Prompt recognition and treatment of organ rejection episodes usually allow preservation of the transplant.*
  d. Any prescribed dietary changes. These may include restricted carbohydrate and increased protein, and sodium restriction due to the effects of corticosteroid therapy. *Chronic corticosteroid therapy may cause cushingoid effects with weight gain, fat redistribution, hyperglycemia, and sodium and water retention. Dietary restrictions may be prescribed to minimize these effects.*
- Provide psychologic support to the client and family, who may be anxious about the outcome of surgery. Address concerns and provide information as needed. *The client knows that success is not guaranteed. In addition, the client has likely been managing a chronic disease independently for a long period and is used to having a degree of control. Providing requested information and allowing the client as much control as possible will relieve anxiety and enhance recovery.* (*Cunninham & Smith, 1990; Harasyko, 1989*).

Table 26–8   Renal Transplant Rejection

Type	Cause	Presentation	Treatment
Hyperacute: Within hours of transplantation	Preexisting antibodies to donor antigens	Kidney appears blue and flaccid; urine output ceases	The transplant cannot be saved and the kidney is removed; prevent by cross-matching before surgery
Acute: Days to months after transplantation	Immune response to foreign tissue	Sharp decline in kidney function; possible fever, graft tenderness and/or swelling	Increase immunosuppression using steroids, monoclonal antibodies
Chronic: Months to years after transplantation	Unclear; may be antibody immune response to foreign tissue	Gradual deterioration of kidney function; possible proteinuria	None; loss of graft will occur requiring retransplantation or dialysis

munosuppressive therapy. Corticosteroid use may lead to bone problems, gastrointestinal disorders such as peptic ulcer disease, and cataract formation (Harasyko, 1989).

Nursing Care

Whether the client with end-stage renal disease is facing long-term dialysis or renal transplantation, a number of nursing care needs can be identified. As for any client with a chronic disease, problems with self-esteem, role performance, and home maintenance management may be significant.

This section focuses on the client's nursing care needs related to the altered renal function, nutritional deficits due to dietary restrictions and uremic manifestations, increased risk for infection, and changes in body image.

Altered Tissue Perfusion: Renal

Capillaries are an integral part of the nephron. As nephrons are destroyed, the perfusion of the kidney declines progressively. When renal perfusion and nephron function decreases, the ability of the kidney to maintain fluid and electrolyte balance and eliminate waste products from the body is impaired.

Nursing interventions with rationales follow.

- Regularly monitor intake and output, vital signs including orthostatic blood pressures, and weight. *These assessments are important to identify changes in fluid volume status.*

- Restrict fluids as ordered, usually to 500 mL per day plus an amount equivalent to the previous 24-hour urinary output unless the client is undergoing dialysis. *As renal function declines, the client's ability to eliminate excess fluid is impaired.*

- Monitor respiratory status, including lung sounds, at least every 8 hours. *Fluid volume overload may result in congestive heart failure and possible pulmonary edema.*

- Monitor laboratory results for BUN, serum creatinine, pH, electrolytes, and CBC. *As renal function declines, progressive azotemia with increasing BUN and serum creatinine is seen. The client develops metabolic acidosis as the kidney loses its ability to eliminate hydrogen ions and conserve bicarbonate. Hyponatremia, hyperkalemia, hyperphosphatemia, and hypocalcemia are associated with renal failure. The RBC count, hemoglobin, and hematocrit are lower than normal because erythropoietin is unavailable to stimulate cell production in the bone marrow.*

- Assess the client for evidence of electrolyte imbalances, including cardiac dysrhythmias and other ECG changes, muscle tremors and possible tetany, and Kussmaul's respirations. *Manifestations of electrolyte imbalance may indicate the need for intervention.*

- Administer aluminum hydroxide gel, calcium carbonate, sodium bicarbonate, and sodium polystyrene sul-

fonate as prescribed. *These medications may be prescribed to treat electrolyte and acid-base imbalances.*

- Monitor the client carefully for desired and adverse effects of all medications administered. *Impaired renal function increases the risk for toxic effects, because drugs are not eliminated efficiently.*

- Monitor blood pressure carefully and administer antihypertensive medications as ordered. *Hypertension management is an important component in slowing the progression of chronic renal failure.*

- Time activities and procedures to allow for periods of rest. *The anemia associated with chronic renal failure may cause significant fatigue for the client.*

Altered Nutrition: Less Than Body Requirements

Anorexia, nausea, and vomiting are manifestations associated with chronic renal failure and uremia. The client often has a metallic taste and bad breath, which also diminish appetite. A diet restricted in protein, sodium, and possibly phosphate compounds these problems, and the client may not eat enough to meet metabolic needs. The catabolic state, the breakdown of body proteins to meet energy needs, exacerbates azotemia and uremia.

Nursing interventions with rationales follow.

- Monitor food intake as well as any episodes of vomiting. *Careful monitoring helps determine the adequacy of intake.*

- Weigh the client daily before breakfast. *This timing provides the most accurate measurement. Remember that a gain of 2 pounds or more over a 24-hour period is more likely to reflect fluid retention than a gain in body mass.*

- Administer antiemetic agents 30 to 60 minutes before eating. *Antiemetics reduce nausea and the risk of vomiting with food intake.*

- Provide mouth care just prior to meals. *Mouth care improves taste and stimulates the appetite.*

- Serve small meals and provide between-meal snacks. *These measures improve food intake.*

- Arrange for a dietary consultation, and provide preferred foods to the extent possible. Involve the client in determining daily menus. Encourage family members to bring the client food as dietary restrictions allow. *The client is more likely to eat favorite foods.*

- Monitor laboratory values related to nutritional status including electrolytes, serum albumin, and BUN. *Changes in values may indicate either improving or declining nutritional status.*

- If the client requires parenteral nutrition, administer as prescribed. *Parenteral nutrition may be necessary to prevent catabolism and increasing azotemia in the client with renal failure.*

- Monitor the client's blood glucose level routinely during parenteral nutrition. *Glucose is a major component of parenteral nutrition solutions; the client may become hyperglycemic during their administration.*

- For the client on parenteral nutrition, use strict aseptic technique when handling the solution and the venous access site. *Parenteral nutrition formulas are an excellent medium for organism growth. In addition, the client in renal failure is at increased risk for infection due to suppression of the immune system.*

Risk for Infection

Chronic renal failure affects the immune system and leukocyte function, increasing the client's susceptibility to infection. When the client is on hemodialysis or peritoneal dialysis, invasive devices add to this risk. The client who has undergone renal transplantation will remain on immunosuppressive therapy for life, further depressing the immune system and increasing the risk for infection.

Nursing interventions with rationales follow.

- Use universal precautions and good hand-washing technique at all times. *Hand washing is a primary means of preventing the transfer of organisms to the client. The client who is on hemodialysis or has had multiple blood transfusions to treat the anemia associated with chronic renal failure is at an increased risk for hepatitis B, hepatitis C, and HIV infection.*

- Use strict aseptic technique when handling ports, catheters, and incisions. *Aseptic technique is vital to reduce the risk of introducing an infectious organism.*

- Monitor the client's temperature and vital signs at least every 4 hours. *Even a modest temperature elevation or increased pulse rate may indicate an infection in the immunosuppressed client.*

- Monitor the client's WBC count and differential. *An elevated WBC count may indicate a bacterial infection; depressed WBC counts are associated with viral infections. A differential shift to the left (more immature WBCs being released from the bone marrow into the blood) is another indicator of infection.*

- Culture urine, peritoneal dialysis fluid, and other drainage as indicated. *Culture is used to determine the presence of pathogens.*

- Provide good oral hygiene at least every 4 hours. *Poor food intake, restricted fluid intake, and immunosuppressive therapy may lead to oral lesions, a possible entry site for bacteria.*

- Provide good respiratory hygiene including position changes, coughing, and deep breathing. *These measures decrease the risk of retained respiratory secretions and resultant infection.*

- Restrict visits from obviously ill family members. Educate the client and family about the risk for infection and measures to reduce the spread of infection. *The client's resistance to infection is impaired, necessitating extra caution in preventing unnecessary exposures.*

Body Image Disturbance

Having a chronic disease and impaired kidney function can cause changes in the client's body image. The client undergoing hemodialysis has an arteriovenous fistula or shunt; the client undergoing peritoneal dialysis, a permanent peritoneal catheter. The client with a transplanted kidney has a visible scar and may feel that the organ is "foreign." All of these affect the client's body image.

Nursing interventions with rationales follow.

- Involve the client in care activities including dialysis, meal planning, and care of the catheter, port, or incision to the extent possible. *Client involvement improves acceptance and stimulates discussion about the effect on the client's life.*

- Encourage the client to express feelings and concerns, accepting the client's perceptions and feelings without criticism. *Self-expression enhances the client's self-worth and acceptance.*

- Involve the client in decision making when readiness is indicated or apparent; encourage self-care. *Increased autonomy enhances the client's sense of control, independence, and self-worth.*

- Support positive gains, but do not support denial. *The client may have difficulty accepting the renal failure, but it is important for the client to adapt to the loss.*

- Work with the client to develop and achieve realistic goals. *Realistic goals allow the client to see progress.*

- Provide positive reinforcement and feedback. *These measures support the client's growth and adaptation.*

- Reinforce effective coping strategies. *Reinforcement helps the client develop positive versus negative strategies for coping.*

- Facilitate contact with a support group or other community members affected by renal failure. *The client benefits by providing and receiving support in a group of people going through similar circumstances.*

- Provide referral to mental health counseling. *Counseling can help the client develop effective coping and adaptation strategies.*

Other Nursing Diagnoses

Although each client has individual nursing care needs, the following nursing diagnoses may be appropriate for the client with chronic renal failure:

- *Fluid Volume Excess* related to impaired renal function

- *Activity Intolerance* related to anemia and other uremic effects

- *Altered Family Processes* related to debilitating illness and treatment regimen

- *Altered Skin Integrity* related to uremic effects
- *Altered Thought Processes* related to effects of uremia on the central nervous system
- *Knowledge Deficit* related to lack of information about the disease and its proposed management

Client and Family Teaching

Chronic renal failure and ESRD are long-term processes that require client management. No matter what treatment option is chosen (hemodialysis, peritoneal dialysis, or renal transplantation), the client and family must implement its day-to-day management. Early teaching focuses on the nature of the kidney disease and renal failure. The client also needs to monitor weight, vital signs, and temperature.

All clients with chronic renal failure must observe some dietary and fluid restrictions. Involve the client, a dietitian, and the family member usually responsible for cooking in the educational process. Participation can improve compliance with the prescribed diet and increase nutritional intake. Teaching should also include strategies to relieve thirst yet observe fluid restrictions.

The client on hemodialysis needs to know how to assess and protect the fistula or shunt. If hemodialysis is to be performed at home, the dialysis helper needs formal training. It is vital to teach catheter care and the dialysis procedure to the client who will perform CAPD. If possible, also teach a family member or significant other, in case the client is ever unable to perform the procedure independently. When a renal transplantation has been done, the client and family members need teaching about the medications the client will take, adverse effects and their management, infection prevention, and the signs and symptoms of organ rejection.

Both the National Kidney Foundation and the National Association of Patients on Hemodialysis and Transplantation may be able to provide support and educational materials for the client with ESRD. Their addresses are listed in Appendix B. Local and state chapters of these organizations can provide additional support.

Applying the Nursing Process

Case Study of a Client with End-Stage Renal Disease: Walter Cohen

Walter Cohen, 45 years old, is the print shop manager at a local community college. He is married; he and his wife have no children. He has been an insulin-dependent diabetic since the age of 20. He was first diagnosed with diabetic nephropathy 10 years ago. Despite blood pressure control with antihypertensive medications and frequent blood glucose monitoring with insulin coverage, he developed overt proteinuria 5 years ago and has now progressed to end-stage renal disease. He enters the nephrology unit for temporary hemodialysis to relieve uremic symptoms. While he is there, a CAPD catheter will be inserted. Walter's desire to continue working is the primary factor in his choice of CAPD over hemodialysis.

Assessment

Richard Gonzalez, Mr. Cohen's assigned care manager, obtains his initial nursing assessment. Mr. Cohen indicates that his diabetes had been difficult to control since its onset. He has experienced numerous hypoglycemic episodes and has been hospitalized "four or five times" for ketoacidosis. Over the past 5 years or so he has developed symptoms of peripheral neuropathy and increasing retinopathy. Even though he knew that his nephropathy would likely result in renal failure and the need for dialysis, he attributed his lack of appetite, nausea, vomiting, and fatigue over the past month to "a touch of the flu." His weight remained stable, so he didn't worry about not eating much.

Physical assessment findings included BP: 178/100; P: 96; R: 20; T: 97.8 F (36.5 C) po. His skin is cool and dry, with minor excorations noted on his forearms and lower legs. Mr. Gonzalez notes that Mr. Cohen has a fetid breath odor. A few fine rales are noted in lung field bases bilaterally. Auscultation of the heart reveals a soft S_3 gallop at the apex. Both lower extremities have 3+ pitting edema to just below the knees; his hands also appear edematous. Abdominal assessment is essentially normal, with hypoactive bowel sounds. Mr. Cohen's urinalysis shows a specific gravity of 1.011, gross proteinuria, and multiple cell casts. CBC results are RBC: 2.9 mill/mm^3; hemoglobin: 9.4 g/dL; hematocrit: 28%. Blood chemistry abnormalities include BUN: 198 mg/dL; creatinine: 18.5 mg/dL; sodium: 125 mEq/L; potassium: 5.7 mEq/L; calcium: 7.1 mg/dL; phosphate: 6.8 mg/dL. Mr. Cohen is to have a temporary jugular venous catheter placed for hemodialysis the following day. The peritoneal catheter will be inserted later in the week.

Diagnosis

Mr. Gonzalez identifies the following nursing diagnoses for Mr. Cohen:

- *Fluid Volume Excess* related to inability of the kidneys to regulate extracellular fluid volume
- *Altered Nutrition: Less Than Body Requirements* related to effects of uremia
- *Impaired Skin Integrity* of lower extremities related to dry skin and itching
- *Risk for Infection* related to invasive catheters and impaired immune function

- *Ineffective Individual Therapeutic Regimen Management* related to multiple complications of diabetes

Expected Outcomes

The identified expected outcomes for Mr. Cohen's plan of care are that he will

- Adhere to the prescribed fluid restriction of 750 mL per day.
- Demonstrate a reduction in excess extracellular fluid by a weight reduction, decreased peripheral edema, clear lung sounds, and normal heart sounds.
- Consume and retain 100% of prescribed diet, including snacks.
- Demonstrate healing of skin lesions on lower extremities.
- Remain free of further skin lesions or breakdown.
- Remain free of signs of infection.
- Demonstrate appropriate technique in performing catheter care and CAPD.
- Develop a plan for integrating CAPD into his health regimen and work schedule.

Planning and Implementation

The following nursing interventions are planned and implemented for Mr. Cohen:

- Space fluids, allowing 350 mL during the day shift, 250 mL during the evening shift, and 100 mL during the night shift.
- Provide mouth care at least every 4 hours and before every meal.
- Keep hard candy and ice chips at the bedside, and include ice consumed as fluid intake.
- Weigh Mr. Cohen daily before breakfast; monitor vital signs, including heart and lung sounds, every 4 hours.
- Document intake and output every 4 hours.
- Arrange a dietary consultation to discover food preferences.
- Administer prescribed antiemetic agent 1 hour before meals.
- Monitor food intake, noting percentage and types of food consumed.
- Clean lesions on lower extremities every 8 hours and assess healing.
- Assess skin every 8 hours and provide good skin care, providing lotion or other moisturizers to ease dryness.
- Practice good hand washing, taking particular care not to transmit organisms from other clients.
- Teach CAPD procedure and peritoneal catheter care.
- Help Mr. Cohen identify his strengths in health regimen management.
- Work with Mr. Cohen to identify ways to perform CAPD at work and home.

Evaluation

Mr. Cohen was hospitalized for 2 weeks, undergoing four hemodialysis sessions to reduce his uremic symptoms. An arteriovenous fistula has been created in his left arm in case he should need further hemodialysis in the future. He begins peritoneal dialysis the 2nd week, and by discharge he is able to manage the catheter care and dialysis runs with the help of his wife. His heart and lung sounds are normal, and he has minimal peripheral edema on discharge. The excoriations on his legs have healed. His temperature is normal, and no evidence of infection is noted. Mr. Cohen remains anorectic and slightly nauseated but is eating most of his prescribed diet and snacks. He has lost 10 pounds with the removal of excess fluid by dialysis, but his weight remains stable during the second week. Mr. Cohen and his wife have been introduced to another client who has been on CAPD for several years and promises to help them with problem solving. They have been referred to the local chapter of the National Kidney Foundation and the home health department for follow-up and continued teaching.

Critical Thinking in the Nursing Process

1. How does diabetes mellitus damage the kidneys and lead to end-stage renal disease? Why is this a more significant problem for diabetics who are insulin-dependent than for those who are not (see Chapter 21)?

2. Why do high levels of urea in the blood often cause alterations in thinking and level of consciousness? What manifestations of encephalopathy would you expect the client to demonstrate?

3. Mr. Cohen indicates that he had experienced episodes of hyperglycemia and hypoglycemia in the past. Identify the signs and symptoms of each, and list appropriate nursing interventions.

4. How might Mr. Cohen's insulin dosage and diet need to be altered with the institution of peritoneal dialysis? Why?

5. Develop a care plan for Mr. Cohen for the nursing diagnosis *Body Image Disturbance*.

Bibliography

■ ■ ■

Abrams, W. B., & Berkow, R. (Eds.). (1990). *The Merck manual of geriatrics.* Rahway, NJ: Merck, Sharp, & Dohme Research Laboratories.

Andreoli, T. E., Carpenter, C. C. J., Plum, F., & Smith, L. H., Jr. (1990). *Cecil essentials of medicine* (2nd ed.) Philadelphia: Saunders.

Beachley, M., & Farrar, J. (1993, November). Abdominal trauma: Putting the pieces together. *American Journal of Nursing, 93*(11), 26–35.

Berkow, R., & Fletcher, A. J. (Eds.). (1992). *The Merck manual of diagnosis and therapy* (16th ed.). Rahway, NJ: Merck Research Laboratories.

Brookbank, J. W. (1990). *The biology of aging.* New York: Harper & Row.

Bullock, B. L. & Rosendahl, P. P. (1992). *Pathophysiology: Adaptations and alterations in function* (3rd ed.). Philadelphia: Lippincott.

Carpenito, L. J. (1995). *Nursing care plans and documentation: Nursing diagnoses and collaborative problems.* (2nd ed.). Philadelphia: Lippincott.

Chernecky, C. C., Krech, R. L., & Berger, B. J. (1993). *Laboratory tests and diagnostic procedures.* Philadelphia: Saunders.

Cunningham, N., & Smith, S. L. (1990). Postoperative care of the renal transplant patient. *Critical Care Nurse, 10*(9), 74–81.

Dunn, S. A. (1993). How to care for the dialysis patient. *American Journal of Nursing, 93*(6), 26–33.

Flaherty, Sr. M. J., & O'Brien, M. E. (1992, August). Family styles of coping in end-stage renal disease. *ANNA Journal, 19,* 345–350.

Haas, L. B. (1993, March). Chronic complications of diabetes mellitus. *Nursing Clinics of North America, 28,* 71–83.

Handerhan, B. (1991). Understanding acute tubular necrosis. *Nursing, 21*(1), 20–21, 23.

Harasyko, C. (1989, December). Kidney transplantation. *Nursing Clinics of North America, 24,* 851–863.

Harris, J. S., & DeLone, P. A. (1992). Allocation of cadaver kidneys. *ANNA Journal, 19*(1), 47–49.

Hauser, M. L., Williams, J., Strong, M., Ganza, M., & Hathaway, D. (1991). Predicted and actual quality of life changes following renal transplantation. *ANNA Journal, 18,* 295–296, 299–304.

Ismail, N., Hakim, R. M., Oreopoulos, D. G., & Patrikarea, A. (1993). Renal replacement therapies in the elderly: Part 1. Hemodialysis and chronic peritoneal dialysis. *American Journal of Kidney Diseases, 22*(6), 759–782.

Kee, C. C. (1992). Age-related changes in the renal system: Causes, consequences, and nursing implications. *Geriatric Nursing, 13,* 80–83.

Kee, J. L., & Hayes, E. R. (1993). *Pharmacology: A nursing process approach.* Philadelphia: Saunders.

Lawyer, L. A., & Velasco, A. (1989). Continuous arteriovenous hemodialysis in the ICU. *Critical Care Nurse, 9*(1), 29–32, 34–35, 38–41.

Lederer, J. R., Marculescu, G. L., Mocnik, B., & Seaby, N. (1993). *Care planning pocket guide: A nursing diagnosis approach* (5th ed.). Redwood City, CA: Addison-Wesley Nursing.

Martinez, N. C. (1993). Diabetes and minority populations. *Nursing Clinics of North America, 28,* 87–95.

McNatt, G. (1992). Testimony: Controversies in organ donation. *ANNA Journal, 19*(4), 341–43+.

Pagana, K. D., & Pagana, T. J. (1992). *Mosby's diagnostic and laboratory test reference.* St. Louis: Mosby-Year Book.

Porth, C. M. (1994). *Pathophysiology: Concepts of altered health states* (4th ed.). Philadelphia: Lippincott.

Price, C. A. (1989). Continuous arteriovenous ultrafiltration: A monitoring guide for ICU nurses. *Critical Care Nurse, 9*(1), 12–24, 17–19.

Price, S. A., & Wilson, L. M. (1992). *Pathophysiology: Clinical concepts of disease processes* (4th ed.). St. Louis: Mosby-Year Book.

Quintana, B. J., Nevarez, M., Rogers, K., Murata, G. H., & Tzamaloukas, A. H. (1991). Reaction of patients on chronic dialysis to discussions about cardiopulmonary resuscitation. *ANNA Journal, 18,* 29–32.

Ritz, E., & Fliser, D. (1993). Hypertension and the kidney: An overview. *American Journal of Kidney Diseases, 21*(6), Suppl. 3, 3–9.

Rydholm, L., & Pauling, J. (1991, April). Contrasting feelings of helplessness in peritoneal and hemodialysis patients: A pilot study. *ANNA Journal, 18,* 183-4, 186+.

Salvetti, A., Giovannetti, R., Arrighi, P., Arzilli, F., & Palla, R. (1993). What effect does blood pressure control have on the progression toward renal failure? *American Journal of Kidney Diseases, 21*(6), Suppl. 3, 10–15.

Shlafer, M. (1993). *The nurse, pharmacology, and drug therapy: A prototype approach* (2nd ed.). Redwood City, CA: Addison-Wesley Nursing.

Skidmore-Roth, L. (1993). *Mosby's nursing drug reference.* St. Louis: Mosby-Year Book.

Sparks, S. M., & Taylor, C. M. (1993). *Nursing diagnosis reference manual* (2nd ed.). Springhouse, PA: Springhouse Corporation.

Spencer, R. T., Nichols, L. W., Lipkin, G. B., Henderson, H. S., & West, F. M. (1993). *Clinical pharmacology and nursing management* (4th ed.). Philadelphia: Lippincott.

Thompson, J. M., McFarland, G. K., Hirsch, J. E., & Tucker, S. M. (1993). *Mosby's clinical nursing* (3rd ed.). St. Louis: Mosby-Year Book.

Tierney, L. M., McPhee, S. J., & Papadakis, M. A. (Eds.). (1994). *Current medical diagnosis and treatment* (33rd ed.). Norwalk, CT: Appleton & Lange.

Tisher, C. C., & Wilcox, C. S. (Eds.). (1993). *Nephrology for the house officer* (2nd ed.). Baltimore: Williams & Wilkins.

Tucker, S. M., Canobbio, M. M., Paquette, E. V., & Wells, M. F. (1992). *Patient care standards: Nursing process, diagnosis, and outcome* (5th ed.). St. Louis: Mosby-Year Book.

US Renal Data System. (1993, October). USRDS 1993 Annual Report. *American Journal of Kidney Diseases, 22*(4), Suppl. 2, 30–68.

Way, L. W. (Ed.). (1994). *Current surgical diagnosis and treatment* (10th ed.). Norwalk, CT: Appleton & Lange.

Wild, J. (1992). Dialysis without tears. *Nursing Times, 88*(18), 50–51.

Wilson, J. D., Braunwald, E., Isselbacher, K. J., Petersdorf, R. G., Martin, J. B., Fauci, A. S., & Root, R. K. (Eds.). (1991). *Harrison's principles of internal medicine* (12th ed.). New York: McGraw-Hill.

Wold, G. (1993). *Basic geriatric nursing.* St. Louis: Mosby-Year Book.

Wyngaarden, J. B., Smith, L. H., & Bennett, J. C. (Eds.). (1992). *Cecil textbook of medicine* (19th ed.). Philadelphia: Saunders.

Activity and Exercise Patterns

Responses to Altered Cardiac Function

Assessing Clients with Cardiac Disorders

⌐ ⌐

LEARNING OBJECTIVES

After completing this chapter, you will be able to

- Identify the major structures and great vessels of the heart.
- Trace the circulation of blood through the heart and coronary vessels.
- Describe the structure and function of cardiac muscle.
- Name and locate the elements of the heart's conduction system.
- Define cardiac output and explain the influence of various factors in its regulation.

- Identify interview questions pertinent to cardiac assessment.
- Describe physical assessment techniques for cardiac function.
- Identify the normal heart sounds and relate them to the corresponding events in the cardiac cycle.
- Identify manifestations of impairment that may indicate cardiac malfunction.
- Describe normal variations in assessment findings for the older adult.

The heart, a muscular pump, beats an average of 70 times per minute, or once every 0.86 seconds, every minute of a person's life. This continuous pumping moves blood through the body, nourishing and removing wastes from tissue cells. Deficits in the structure or function of the heart thus affect all body tissues. Changes in cardiac rate, rhythm, or output may limit almost all human functions, including self-care, mobility, and the ability to maintain fluid volume status, respirations, tissue perfusion, and comfort. Cardiac changes may also affect self-concept, sexuality, and role performance. Assessing the structures and functions of the heart is therefore necessary to promote wellness and to restore and maintain health.

Review of Anatomy and Physiology

The heart, a hollow, cone-shaped organ approximately the size of an adult's fist, weighs less than 1 lb. It is located within the mediastinum of the thoracic cavity, between the vertebral column and the sternum, and is flanked laterally by the lungs. Two-thirds of the heart mass lies to the left of the sternum; the upper *base* lies beneath the second rib, and the pointed *apex* is approximate with the fifth intercostal space, midpoint to the clavicle (Figure 27–1).

Coverings of the Heart

The heart is covered by a double layer of fibroserous membrane, the *pericardium* (Figure 27–2). The peri-

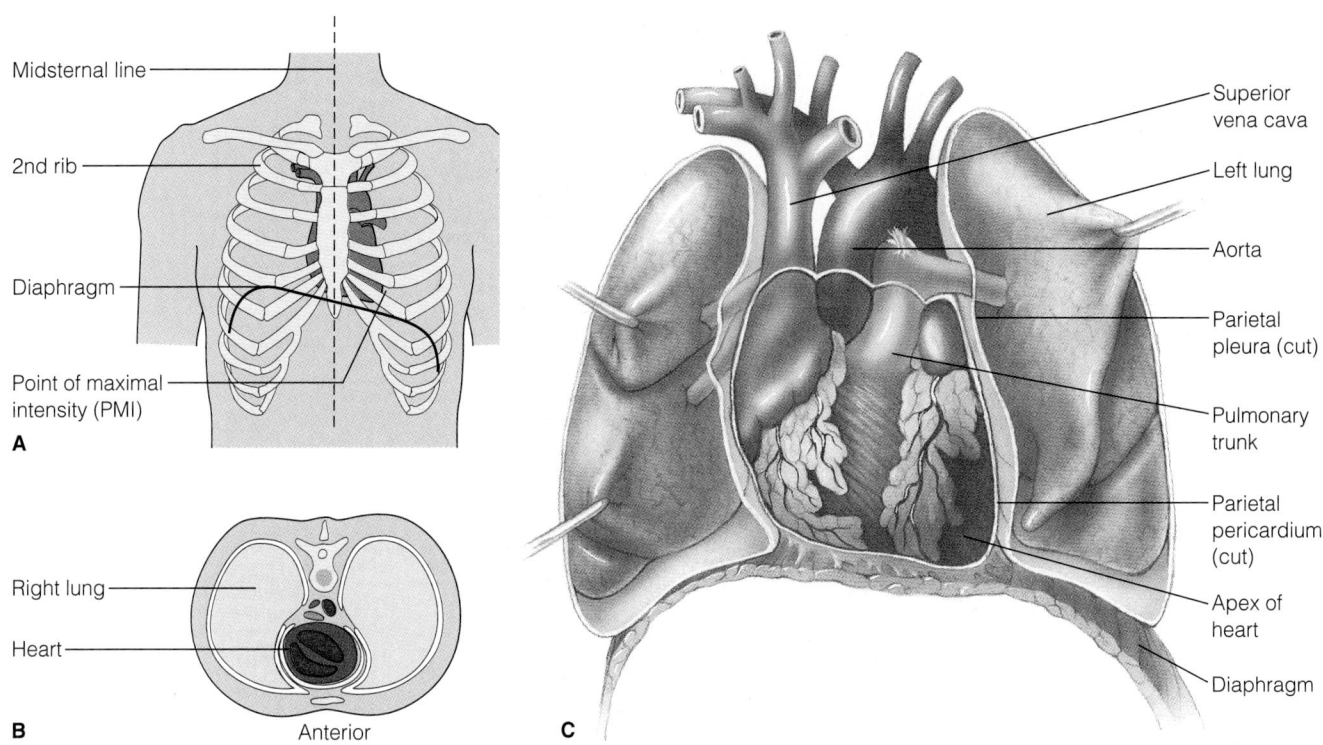

Figure 27–1   Location of the heart in the mediastinum of the thorax. *A,* Relationship of the heart to the sternum, ribs, and diaphragm. *B,* Cross-sectional view showing relative position of the heart in the thorax. *C,* Relationship of the heart and great vessels to the lungs.

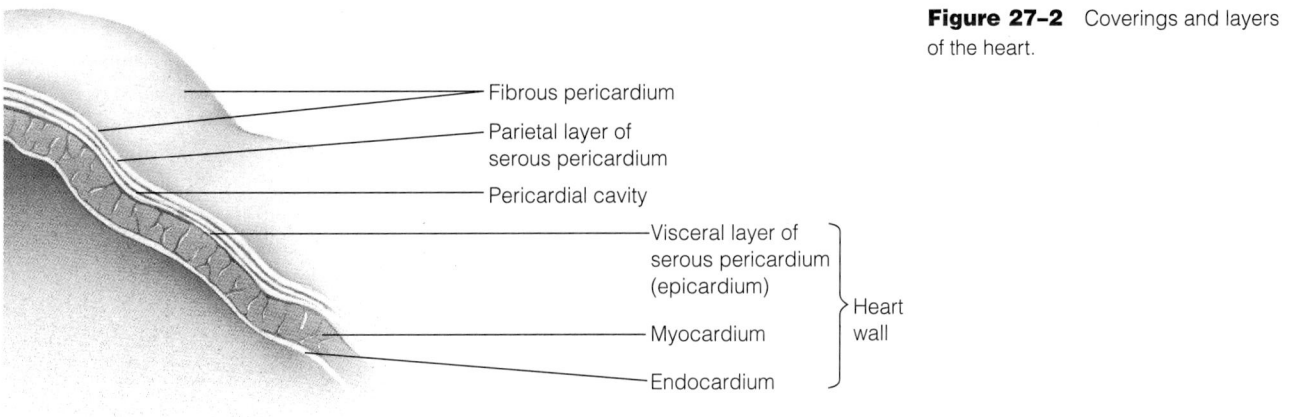

Figure 27–2   Coverings and layers of the heart.

cardium encases the heart and anchors it to surrounding structures, forming the *pericardial sac.* The snug fit of the pericardium prevents the heart from overfilling with blood. The *parietal pericardium* is the outermost layer. The *visceral pericardium* (or epicardium) adheres to the heart surface. Between the visceral and parietal layers of the pericardium is a small space called the *pericardial cavity.* A serous lubricating fluid produced in this space acts to cushion the heart as it beats.

Layers of the Heart Wall

The heart wall is composed of three layers of tissue: the epicardium, the myocardium, and the endocardium (Figure 27–2). The outermost *epicardium* is the same structure as the visceral pericardium. The middle layer of the heart wall, the *myocardium,* is composed of specialized cardiac muscle cells (*myofibrils*) that provide the bulk of contractile heart muscle. The innermost layer, the

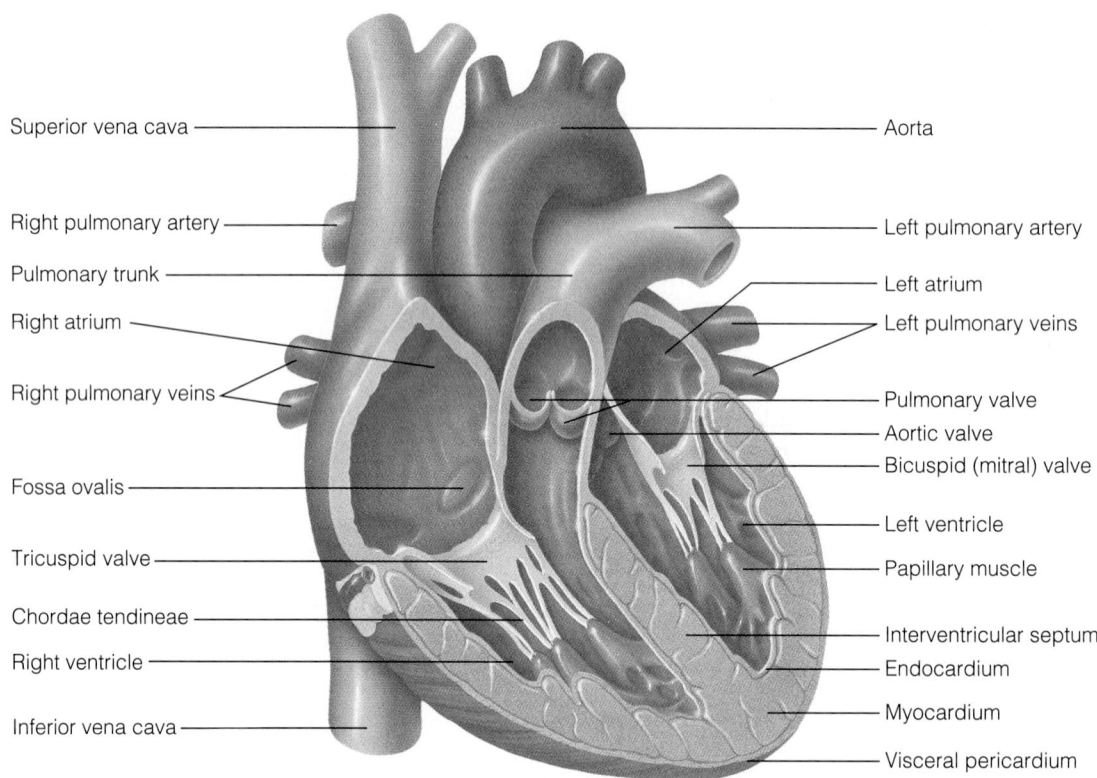

Figure 27–3 The internal anatomy of the heart, frontal section.

endocardium, is a sheath of endothelium that lines the inside of the heart's chambers and great vessels.

Chambers and Valves of the Heart

The heart has four hollow chambers, two upper *atria* and two lower *ventricles.* They are separated longitudinally by the *interventricular septum* (Figure 27–3).

The right atrium receives deoxygenated blood from the veins of the body: The superior vena cava returns blood from the body area above the diaphragm, the inferior vena cava returns blood from the body below the diaphragm, and the coronary sinus drains blood from the heart. The left atrium receives freshly oxygenated blood from the lungs through the pulmonary veins.

The right ventricle receives deoxygenated blood from the right atrium and pumps it through the pulmonary artery to the lungs for oxygenation. The left ventricle receives the freshly oxygenated blood from the left atrium and pumps it out the aorta to the arterial circulation.

Each of the heart's chambers is separated by a valve which allows unidirectional blood flow to the next chamber or great vessel (Figure 27–3). The atria are separated from the ventricles by the two *atrioventricular (AV) valves;* the *tricuspid valve* is on the right side, and the *bicuspid* or *mitral valve* is on the left. The flaps of each of these valves are anchored to the papillary muscles of the ventricles by

the *chordae tendineae.* These structures control the movement of the AV valves to prevent backflow of blood.

The ventricles are connected to their great vessels by the *semilunar valves.* On the right, the *pulmonary valve* joins the right ventricle with the pulmonary artery. On the left, the *aortic valve* joins the left ventricle to the aorta.

Closure of the AV valves at the onset of contraction produces the *first heart sound,* or S_1 (characterized by the syllable "lub"); closure of the semilunar valves at the onset of relaxation produces the *second heart sound,* or S_2 (characterized by the syllable "dup").

Systemic and Coronary Circulation

Because each side of the heart both receives and ejects blood, the heart is often described as a double pump. *Pulmonary circulation* begins with the right heart. Deoxygenated blood from the venous system enters the right atrium through two large veins, the *superior* and *inferior venae cavae,* and is transported to the lungs via the *pulmonary artery* and its branches (Figure 27–4). After an exchange of oxygen and carbon dioxide takes place in the capillaries of the lungs, oxygen-rich blood returns to the left atrium through several *pulmonary veins.* Blood is then pumped out of the left ventricle through the *aorta* and its major branches to supply all body tissues. This second circuit of blood flow is called the *systemic circulation.*

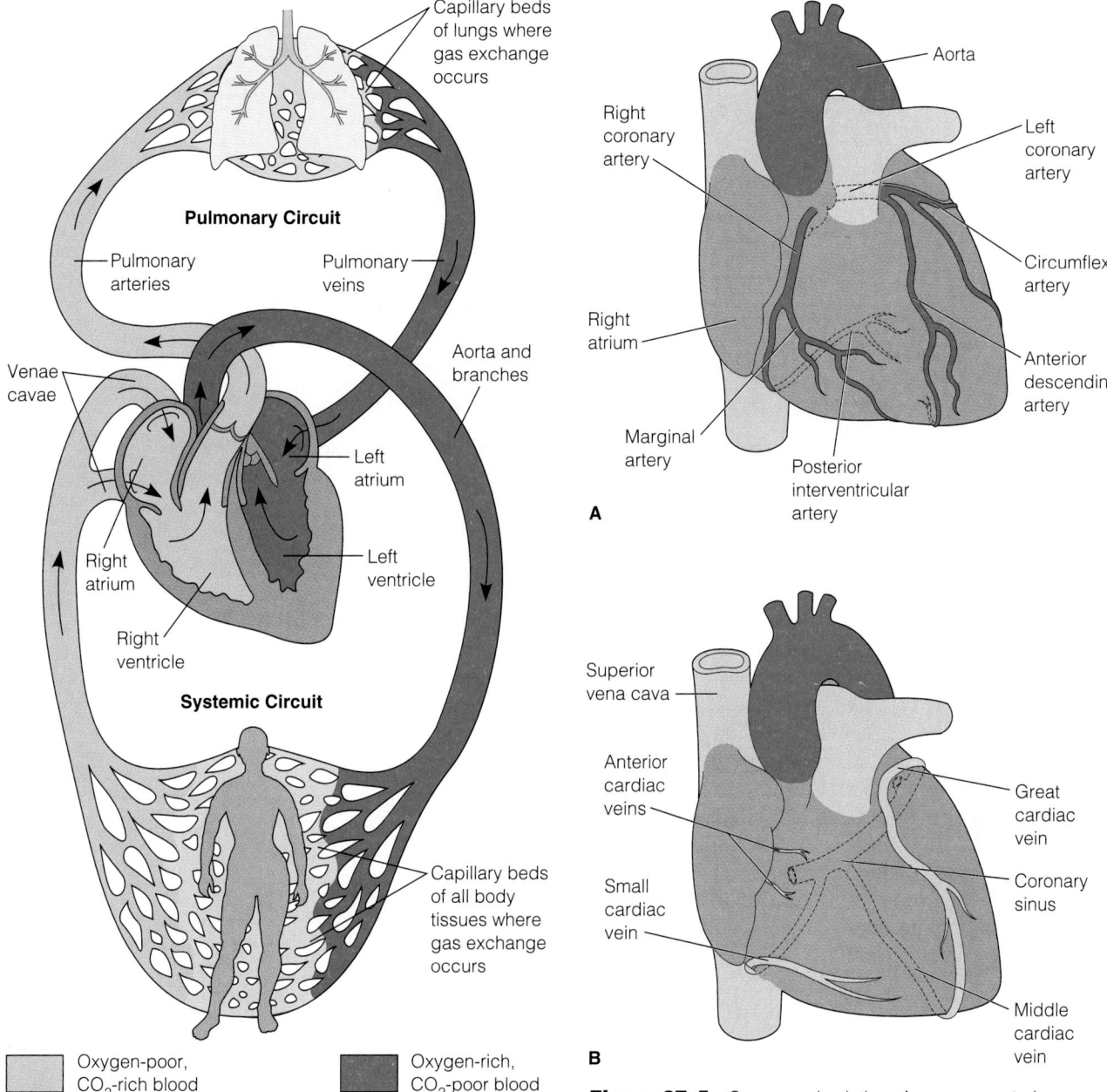

Pulmonary Circuit

Capillary beds of lungs where gas exchange occurs

Pulmonary arteries

Pulmonary veins

Venae cavae

Aorta and branches

Left atrium

Right atrium

Left ventricle

Right ventricle

Systemic Circuit

Capillary beds of all body tissues where gas exchange occurs

Oxygen-poor, CO_2-rich blood

Oxygen-rich, CO_2-poor blood

Figure 27–4 Pulmonary and systemic circulation. The left side of the heart pumps oxygenated blood into the arteries. Deoxygenated blood returns via the venous system into the right side of the heart.

A

Right coronary artery

Aorta

Left coronary artery

Right atrium

Circumflex artery

Anterior descending artery

Marginal artery

Posterior interventricular artery

B

Superior vena cava

Anterior cardiac veins

Great cardiac vein

Small cardiac vein

Coronary sinus

Middle cardiac vein

Figure 27–5 Coronary circulation. *A*, coronary arteries; *B*, coronary veins.

While this continuous circulation of blood through the heart meets the oxygen needs of the body, the heart muscle itself is supplied by its own network of vessels through the *coronary circulation*. The *left* and *right coronary arteries* originate at the base of the aorta and branch out to encircle the myocardium (Figure 27–5, *A*). While ventricular contraction causes blood to be delivered through the pulmonary and systemic circuits as described above, it is during ventricular relaxation that the coronary arteries fill

with oxygen-rich blood. Then, after the blood perfuses the heart muscle, the *cardiac veins* drain the blood into the *coronary sinus*, which empties into the right atrium of the heart (Figure 27–5, *B*).

The Cardiac Cycle and Cardiac Output

The contraction and relaxation of the heart constitutes one heartbeat and is called the *cardiac cycle* (Figure 27–6). Ventricular filling is followed by *ventricular systole*,

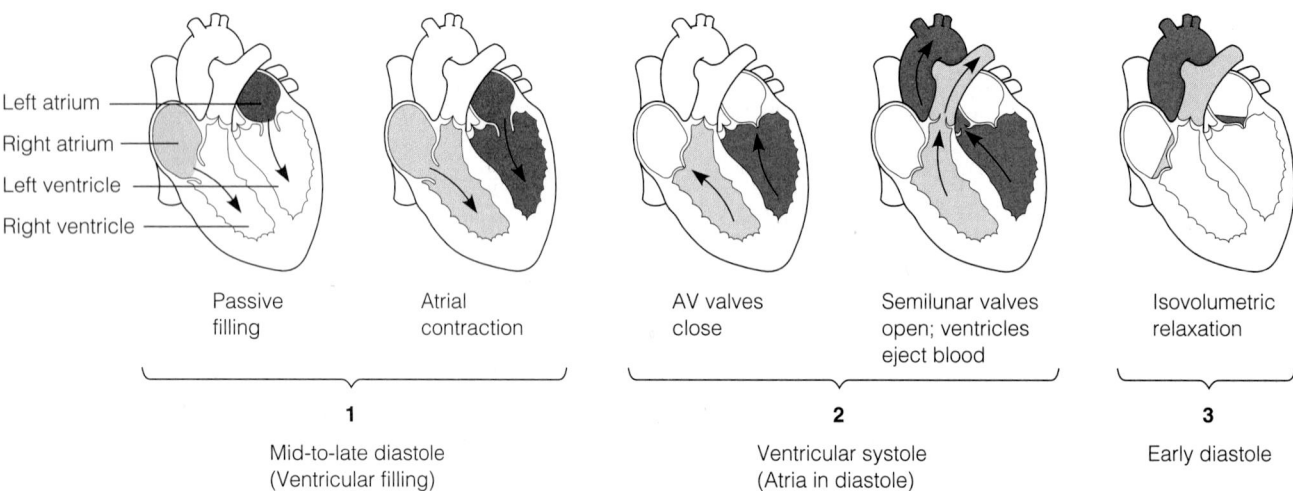

Passive filling	Atrial contraction	AV valves close	Semilunar valves open; ventricles eject blood	Isovolumetric relaxation

1
Mid-to-late diastole
(Ventricular filling)

2
Ventricular systole
(Atria in diastole)

3
Early diastole

Figure 27–6 The cardiac cycle is composed of three events: ventricular filling in mid-to-late distole (1), ventricular systole (2), and isovolumetric relaxation in early diastole (3).

a phase during which the ventricles contract and eject blood into the pulmonary and systemic circuits. Systole is followed by a relaxation phase known as *diastole,* during which the ventricles refill, the atria contract, and the myocardium is perfused. Normally, the complete cardiac cycle occurs about 70 to 80 times per minute. Its frequency is reflected in measurements of the *heart rate (HR).*

With each contraction, a certain volume of blood, called the **stroke volume (SV),** is ejected from the heart. Stroke volume ranges from 60 to 100 mL/beat and averages about 70 mL/beat in an adult. The **cardiac output (CO)** is the amount of blood pumped by the ventricles into the pulmonary and systemic circulations in 1 minute. Multiplying the stroke volume by the heart rate determines the cardiac output:

$$CO = HR \times SV$$

The average adult cardiac output ranges from 4 to 8 liters per minute (L/min). *Ejection fraction (EF)* is the percentage of total blood in the ventricle at the end of the diastole ejected from the heart with each beat. The normal ejection fraction ranges from 50% to 70%.

Cardiac output is an indicator of how well the heart is functioning as a pump: If the heart is unable to pump effectively, cardiac output and tissue perfusion will be decreased. Body tissues that do not receive enough blood and oxygen (carried in the blood on hemoglobin) become **ischemic** (deprived of oxygen). If the tissues do not receive enough blood flow to maintain the functions of the cells, the cells will die. Tissue cell death is called **necrosis.**

Determinants of Cardiac Output

A number of factors influence cardiac output. These include activity level, metabolic rate, physiologic and psychologic stress responses, age, and body size. In addition,

cardiac output is determined by the interaction of four major factors: heart rate, preload, afterload, and contractility. Changes in each of these variables influence cardiac output intrinsically, and each also can be manipulated to affect cardiac output. The ability of the heart to respond to the body's changing need for cardiac output is called **cardiac reserve.**

Heart Rate *Heart rate* is affected by both direct and indirect autonomic nervous system stimulation. Direct stimulation is accomplished through the innervation of the heart muscle by sympathetic and parasympathetic nerves. The sympathetic nervous system increases the heart rate, whereas the parasympathetic *vagal tone* slows the heart rate. Reflex regulation of heart rate in response to systemic blood pressure also occurs through activation of sensory receptors known as baroreceptors or pressure receptors located in the carotid sinus, aortic arch, venae cavae, and pulmonary veins.

If heart rate increases, cardiac output will increase, even if there is no change in stroke volume. However, very rapid heart rates decrease the amount of time available for ventricular filling during diastole. Cardiac output then falls because decreased filling time decreases stroke volume. Coronary artery perfusion also suffers in this situation because the coronary arteries fill primarily during diastole. Bradycardia also decreases cardiac output if stroke volume stays the same, because the number of cardiac cycles is decreased.

Heart rate can be manipulated by stimulating or reducing autonomic nervous system control of the heart through fluids, drugs, mechanical devices, or other clinical treatments.

Preload *Preload* is the amount of cardiac muscle fiber tension, or stretch, that exists at the end of diastole, just before contraction of the ventricles. Preload is influenced by venous return and the compliance of the ventricles. It is related to the total volume of blood in the ventricles: The greater the volume, the greater the stretch of the cardiac muscle fibers, and the greater the force with which the fibers contract to accomplish emptying. This principle is called *Starling's law of the heart.*

There is a physiologic limit to this mechanism. Just as continuous overstretching of a rubber band causes the band to relax and lose its ability to recoil, overstretching of the cardiac muscle fibers eventually results in ineffective contraction. Disorders such as renal disease and congestive heart failure result in salt and water retention and increased preload. Vasoconstriction also increases venous return and preload.

Too little circulating blood volume results in a decreased venous return and therefore a decreased preload. A decreased preload decreases stroke volume and thus cardiac output. Decreased preload may result from hemorrhage or maldistribution of blood volume, such as occurs in third-spacing (see Chapter 5).

Interventions to decrease preload include use of diuretics and vasodilators, phlebotomy, and rotating tourniquets. Measures to increase preload include vasopressors and volume infusion.

Afterload   *Afterload* is the force the ventricles must overcome to eject their blood volume. It is thus the pressure in the arterial system ahead of the ventricles. The right ventricle must generate enough tension to open the pulmonary valve and eject its volume into the low-pressure pulmonary arteries. Right ventricle afterload is thus measured as pulmonary vascular resistance (PVR). The left ventricle, in contrast, ejects its load by overcoming the pressure behind the aortic valve. Afterload of the left ventricle is measured as systemic vascular resistance (SVR). Arterial pressures are much higher than pulmonary pressures; thus, the left ventricle has to work much harder than the right ventricle.

Alterations in vascular tone affect afterload and ventricular work. As the pulmonary or arterial blood pressure increases (e.g., through vasoconstriction), PVR and/or SVR increases, and the work of the ventricles increases. As workload increases, consumption of myocardial oxygen also increases. This increased oxygen demand cannot be met effectively by a compromised heart, and a vicious cycle ensues. By contrast, a very low afterload decreases the forward flow of blood into the systemic circulation and the coronary arteries.

Measures to decrease afterload include vasodilators, diuretics, and other drugs. Vasopressors are used to increase afterload.

Contractility   *Contractility* is the inherent capability of the cardiac muscle fibers to shorten. Poor contractility of the heart muscle reduces the forward flow of blood from the heart, increases the ventricular pressures from accumulation of blood volume, and reduces cardiac output. Increased contractility may overtax the heart.

The methods to increase or decrease contractility are pharmacologic. Beta-blockers, calcium channel blockers, and other agents decrease contractility, whereas calcium gluconate, glucagon, and other agents increase contractility.

Clinical Indicators of Cardiac Output

For many clients who are critically ill, invasive hemodynamic monitoring catheters are used to measure cardiac output in quantifiable numbers. However, advanced technology is not the only means of identifying and assessing compromised blood flow. Because cardiac output perfuses the body's tissues, clinical indicators of low cardiac output may be manifested by changes in organ function that result from compromised blood flow. For example, a decrease in blood flow to the brain presents as a change in level of consciousness. Other clinical manifestations of decreased cardiac output are discussed in Chapters 6 and 28.

Cardiac Index

Cardiac index (CI) is the cardiac output adjusted for the client's body size, also called the client's *body surface area (BSA)*. Because it takes into account the client's BSA, the cardiac index provides more meaningful data regarding the heart's ability to perfuse the tissues and therefore is a more accurate indicator of the effectiveness of the circulation.

BSA is stated in square meters (m^2), and cardiac index is calculated as CO divided by BSA. Cardiac measurements are considered adequate when they fall within the range of 2.5 to 4.2 $L/min/m^2$. For example, two clients are determined to have a cardiac output of 4 L/min. This parameter is within normal limits. However, one client is 5 feet, 2 inches (157 cm) tall and weighs 120 lb (54.5 kg), with a BSA of 1.54 m^2. This client's cardiac index is 4 ÷ 1.54, or 2.6 $L/min/m^2$. The second client is 6 feet, 2 inches (188 cm) tall and weighs 280 lb (81.7 kg), with a BSA of 2.52 m^2. This client's cardiac index is 4 ÷ 2.52, or 1.6 $L/min/m^2$. The cardiac index results show that the same cardiac output of 4 L/min is adequate for the first client but grossly inadequate for the second client.

The Conduction System of the Heart

The cardiac cycle is perpetuated by a complex electrical circuit commonly known as the *intrinsic conduction system* of the heart. Cardiac muscle cells possess an inherent characteristic of self-excitation, which enables them to initiate and transmit impulses independent of a stimulus. However, specialized areas of myocardial cells typically exert a controlling influence in this electrical pathway.

Figure 27–7   The intrinsic conduction system of the heart.

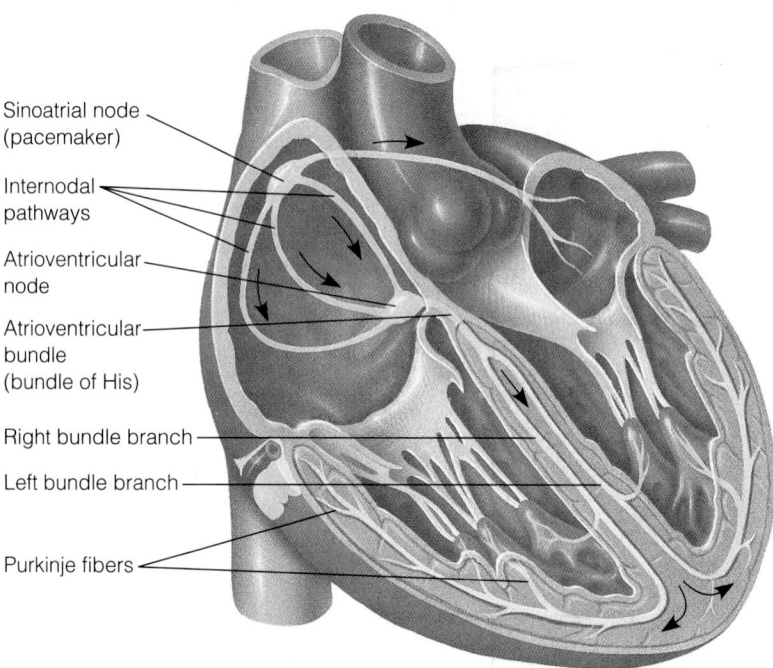

Sinoatrial node (pacemaker)

Internodal pathways

Atrioventricular node

Atrioventricular bundle (bundle of His)

Right bundle branch

Left bundle branch

Purkinje fibers

One of these specialized areas is the *sinoatrial (SA) node,* located at the junction of the superior vena cava and right atrium (Figure 27–7). The SA node acts as the normal "pacemaker" of the heart, usually generating an impulse 60 to 100 times per minute. This impulse travels across the atria via *internodal pathways* to the *atrioventricular (AV) node,* which is located in the floor of the interatrial septum. The very small junctional fibers of the AV node slow the velocity of the impulse, slightly delaying its transmission to the ventricles. It then passes through the *bundle of His* at the atrioventricular junction and continues down the interventricular septum through the *right and left bundle branches* and out to the *Purkinje fibers* in the ventricular muscle walls.

This path of electrical transmission produces a series of changes in ion concentration across the membrane of each cardiac muscle cell. The electrical stimulus increases the permeability of the cell membrane, creating an *action potential* (electrical potential). The result is an exchange of sodium, potassium, and calcium ions across the cell membrane, which changes the intracellular electrical charge to a positive state. This process of *depolarization* results in myocardial contraction. As the ion exchange reverses and the cell returns to its resting state of electronegativity, the cell is *repolarized,* and cardiac muscle relaxes. The cellular action potential serves as the basis for *electrocardiography (ECG),* the recording of the electrical impulses that immediately precede contraction of the heart muscle.

Cardiac conduction and electrocardiography are discussed in greater detail in Chapter 28.

Assessment of Cardiac Function

Cardiac function is assessed both by a health assessment interview to collect subjective data and a physical assessment to collect objective data.

The Health Assessment Interview

This section provides guidelines for collecting subjective data through a health assessment interview specific to cardiac function. Interview questions and leading statements for assessing cardiac function are also provided.

Overview

A health assessment interview to determine problems with cardiac function may be conducted as part of a health screening or as part of a total health assessment, or it may focus on a chief complaint (such as chest pain). If the client has a problem with cardiac function, analyze its onset, characteristics, course, severity, precipitating and relieving factors, and any associated symptoms, noting the timing and circumstances. For example, ask the client:

- Describe the location of the chest pain you experienced. Did it move up to your jaw or into your left arm?
- What type of activity brings on your chest pain?
- Have you noticed any changes in your energy level, or have you felt light-headed during the times your heart is racing?

The interview begins with an exploration of the client's chief complaint (for example, chest pain, palpitations, or shortness of breath). Describe the client's symptoms in terms of location, quality or character, timing, setting or precipitating factors, severity, aggravating and relieving factors, and associated symptoms (Table 27–1).

Explore the history of the client for heart disorders such as angina, heart attack, congestive heart failure (CHF), hypertension (HTN), and valvular disease. Ask the client about previous heart surgery or illnesses, such as rheumatic fever, scarlet fever, or recurrent streptococcal throat infections. The history should also explore the presence and treatment of other chronic illnesses such as diabetes mellitus, bleeding disorders, or endocrine disorders. Review the client's family history for incidence of coronary artery disease (CAD), HTN, stroke, hyperlipidemia, diabetes, congenital heart disease, or sudden death.

Ask the client about past or present occurrence of various cardiac symptoms, such as chest pain, shortness of breath, difficulty breathing, cough, palpitations, fatigue, light-headedness or dizziness, fainting, heart murmur, blood clots, or swelling. Because cardiac function affects all other body systems, a full history may need to explore other related systems, such as respiratory function and/or peripheral vascular function.

Review the client's personal habits and nutritional history, including body weight; eating patterns; dietary intake of fats, salt, fluids; dietary restrictions; hypersensitivities or intolerances to food or medication; and the use of caffeine and alcohol. If the client uses tobacco products, ask about type (cigarettes, pipe, cigars, snuff), duration, amount, and efforts to quit. If the client uses street drugs, ask about type, method of intake (e.g., inhaled or injected), duration of use, and efforts to quit. Include questions about the client's activity level and tolerance, recreational activities, and relaxation habits. Assess the client's sleep patterns for interruptions in sleep due to dyspnea, cough, discomfort, urination, or stress. Ask how many pillows the client uses when sleeping.

Also consider psychosocial factors that may affect the client's stress level: What is the client's marital status, family composition, and role within the family? Have there been any changes? What is the client's occupation, level of education, and socioeconomic level? Are resources for support available? What is the client's emotional disposition and personality type? How does the client perceive his or her state of health or illness, and how able is the client to comply with treatment?

Interview Questions

The following interview questions and leading statements are categorized by functional health patterns.

Table 27–1   Assessing Chest Pain

Characteristic	Examples
Location	Substernal, precordial, jaw, back Localized or diffuse Radiation to neck, jaw, shoulder, arm
Character/quality	Pressure; tightness; crushing, burning, or aching quality; heaviness; dullness; "heartburn" or indigestion
Timing: onset, duration, and frequency	Onset: Sudden or gradual? Duration: How many minutes does the pain last? Frequency: Is the pain continuous or periodic?
Setting/precipitating factors	Awake, at rest, sleep interrupted? With activity? With eating, exertion, exercise, elimination, emotional upset?
Intensity/severity	Can range from 0 (no pain) to 10 (worst pain ever felt)
Aggravating factors	Activity, breathing, temperature
Relieving factors	Medication (nitroglycerine, antacid), rest; there may be no relieving factors
Associated symptoms	Fatigue, shortness of breath, palpitations, nausea and vomiting, sweating, anxiety, light-headedness or dizziness

Health Perception–Health Management

- Have you ever had any cardiovascular problems (such as angina, heart attack, high blood pressure, or valvular disease)? If so, describe these problems.

- How were these problems treated (diet, medications, surgery, exercise)?

- Do you have a history of rheumatic fever, scarlet fever, or strep throat infections? Describe.

- Have you ever had tests to evaluate the function of your heart (such as electrocardiograms, stress tests, cardiac catheterization)? Describe.

- What medications are you currently taking (aspirin, blood pressure medications, beta-blockers, calcium channel blockers, digitalis, diuretics, anticoagulants, others)? How often do you take them?

- Do you smoke or chew tobacco? If so, how much and for how long?

- Do you drink alcohol? If so, what type, how much, and for how long?

- Are you able to manage your activities of daily living and work independently? Describe.

Nutritional-Metabolic

- Describe your usual diet in a 24-hour period. How often do you eat eggs or fatty foods?

- Have you had a recent weight gain or loss? Explain.

- How much salt do you use on and in your food?

- How often do you eat out? What do you usually order?

Elimination

- Have you had any changes in your normal bowel or bladder elimination? Explain.

- Has a heart problem interfered with your normal bowel or bladder elimination? Explain.

Activity-Exercise

- Describe your normal activity and exercise in a 24-hour period.

- Has there been a change in your ability, energy level, or strength to perform your usual activities of daily living (such as bathing, cooking, walking, driving, shopping, socializing)? Explain.

- Do you have shortness of breath with certain activities? If so, what are they? How long do the breathing problems last? What do you do to relieve them?

- Do you feel tired during the day? When? What do you do when you feel tired?

- Have you noticed any changes of color of your skin? For example, has it become flushed, dusky, or pale?

- Have you had any swelling in your feet or legs? Where and how much? Do resting and putting your feet up relieve it?

- Describe any cough you have had. Is it a dry or a congested cough? If you cough up mucus, what color is it? How long have you had the cough?

- Have you ever experienced numbness or tingling, dizziness or light-headedness, or palpitations? Describe.

- Have you ever or do you now need to use oxygen?

Sleep-Rest

- How long do you sleep each night? Do you feel rested after sleeping?

- Does your cardiovascular problem interfere with your rest and sleep? Describe.

- Do you ever feel short of breath when you are resting or sleeping? Does this feeling wake you up if you are asleep?

- How many pillows do you sleep on?

Cognitive-Perceptual

- Describe any chest pain you have experienced. When did it occur? Where was the pain located (below the breastbone, in the arm or neck)? On a scale of from 0 to 10 (with 10 being the worst pain possible), rate the pain and describe it (for example, burning, crushing, stabbing, squeezing, pressing, heavy, tight).

- What were you doing when the pain began? Were you engaging in an activity, or were you at rest)? Did it begin gradually or suddenly? How long did it last?

- Did you have any other symptoms with the pain, such as nausea and/or vomiting, sweating, racing heart, pale skin color, palpitations?

- What made the pain worse? What did you do to try to relieve the pain? Did this help?

- Do you have any leg pain when you walk or exercise? How far can you walk before the pain begins? Does resting relieve the pain?

Self-Perception–Self-Concept

- Has a problem with cardiovascular function affected how you feel about yourself? Explain.

- Has a problem with cardiovascular function affected how you feel about your normal life?

- Are you able to do what you feel is important for yourself and for others who are important to you?

Role-Relationship

- Do you have a family history of high blood pressure, coronary artery disease, high cholesterol, obesity, or diabetes?

- Has a problem with cardiovascular function affected your role in the family? Explain.

- Has a problem with cardiovascular function affected your interactions with others in your family, with friends, at work, or in social activities?

- Has a problem with cardiovascular function affected your ability to work? Explain.

Sexuality-Reproductive

- Have your usual sexual activities been altered by cardiovascular problems? Explain.

- Do you ever have chest pain during sexual activity? How long does the pain last? What do you do?

- Describe how having cardiovascular problems has made you feel about yourself as a man or woman.

- Have you ever been given information on how to alter the pace of and use less strenuous positions during sexual activity? If so, do you use the information?

Coping-Stress

- How stressful do you view your life-style on a scale of from 0 to 10 (with 10 being extremely stressful)?
- What factors seem to cause the most worry or stress for you?
- How often do you feel stressed during the day?
- Do you have chest pain or shortness of breath when you feel stressed?
- Describe what you do to cope with stress.
- Who or what will be able to help you cope with stress from this health problem?

Value-Belief

- What is most important to you in your life?
- Are there significant others, practices, or activities that help you cope with impairments from this health problem? Explain.
- Do you restrict or eat certain foods based on your religious and or cultural beliefs and background?
- How do you perceive the future with this health problem?

The Physical Assessment

Physical assessment of cardiac function may be performed either as part of a total assessment or alone for clients with suspected or known problems with cardiac function. The heart is assessed through inspection, palpation, and auscultation over the *precordium* (the area of the chest wall overlying the heart).

Cardiac Function: Preparation

The equipment necessary to conduct an examination of the heart includes a stethoscope with a diaphragm and a bell, a good light source, and a ruler. Prior to the examination, collect all the equipment, and explain the examination to the client to decrease anxiety. A quiet environment is essential to hear and assess heart sounds accurately.

The client may sit or lie in the supine position. Movements over the precordium may be more easily seen with tangential lighting (in which the light is directed at a right angle to the area being observed, producing shadows). The following types of movements are assessed:

- *Apical impulse:* A normal, visible pulsation (*thrust*) in the area of the midclavicular line in the left fifth intercostal space. It can be seen on inspection in about half of the adult population.
- *Retraction:* A pulling in of the tissue of the precordium; a slight retraction just medial to the midclavicular line at the area of the apical impulse is normal and is more likely to be visible in thin clients.
- *Lift:* A more sustained thrust than normal.
- *Heave:* An excessive thrust.

ASSESSMENT TECHNIQUE	POSSIBLE ABNORMAL FINDINGS
■ Palpate the precordium. First using palmar surface and then repeating with finger pads, palpate the precordium for symmetry of movement and the apical impulse for location, size, amplitude, and duration. The sequence for palpation is shown in Figure 27–8. *Note:* To locate the apical impulse, ask the client to assume a left lateral recumbent position. Simultaneous palpation of the carotid pulse may also be helpful. The apical impulse is not palpable in all clients.	An enlarged or displaced heart is associated with an apical impulse lateral to the midclavicular line (MCL) or below the fifth left intercostal space (ICS). Increased size, amplitude, and duration of the point of maximal impulse (PMI) are associated with left ventricular volume overload (increased preload) in conditions such as HTN and aortic stenosis,

ASSESSMENT TECHNIQUE	POSSIBLE ABNORMAL FINDINGS

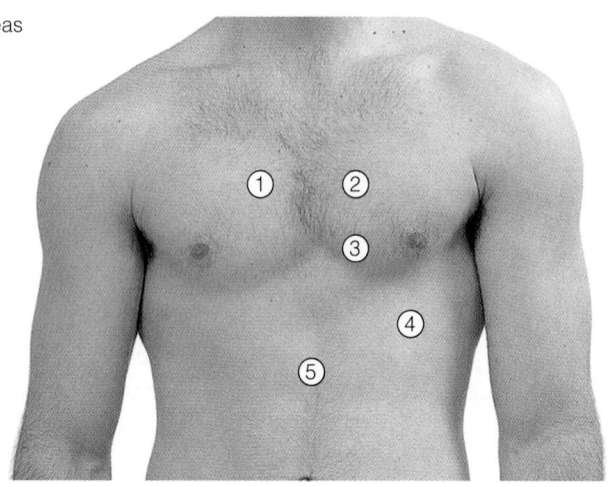

Figure 27–8 Areas for inspection and palpation of the precordium, indicating the sequence for palpation.

and in pressure overload (increased afterload) in conditions such as aortic or mitral regurgitation. Increased amplitude alone may occur with hyperkinetic states, such as anxiety, hyperthyroidism, and anemia. Decreased amplitude is associated with a dilated heart in cardiomyopathy. Displacement alone may also occur with dextrocardia, diaphragmatic hernia, gastric distention, or chronic lung disease. A *thrill* (a palpable vibration over the precordium or an artery) may accompany severe valve stenosis.

- Palpate for the presence of other pulsations or movements.

A marked increase in amplitude of the PMI at the right ventricular area occurs with right ventricular volume overload in atrial septal defect. An increase in amplitude and duration occurs with right ventricular pressure overload in pulmonic stenosis and pulmonary hypertension. A lift or heave may also be seen in these conditions (and in chronic lung disease). A palpable thrill in this area occurs with ventricular septal defect.

- Palpate the subxiphoid area with the index and middle finger.

Right ventricular enlargement may produce a downward pulsation against the fingertips. An accentuated pulsation at the pulmonary area may be present in hyperkinetic states. A prominent pulsation reflects increased flow or dilation of the pulmonary artery. A thrill may be associated with aortic or pulmonary stenosis, pulmonary HTN, or atrial septal defect. Increased pulsation at the aortic area may suggest aortic aneurysm. A thrill occurs with aortic stenosis. A palpable second heart sound (S_2) may be noted with systemic HTN.

Heart Sounds

- **Auscultate heart rate.**

A heart rate exceeding 100 beats per minute (BPM) is called **tachycardia.** A heart rate less than 60 BPM is **bradycardia.**

- **Simultaneously palpate the radial pulse while listening to the apical pulse.**

If the radial pulse falls behind the apical rate, a *pulse deficit* exists, indicating weak, ineffective contractions of the left ventricle.

ASSESSMENT TECHNIQUE	POSSIBLE ABNORMAL FINDINGS

Auscultate heart rhythm.

Dysrhythmias (abnormal heart rate or rhythm) may be regular or irregular in rhythm; their rates may be slow or fast. Irregular rhythms may occur in a pattern (e.g., an early beat every second beat, called *bigeminy*), sporadically, or with frequency and disorganization (e.g., atrial fibrillation). A pattern of gradual increase and decrease in heart rate that is within normal heart rate and that correlates with inspiration and expiration is called *sinus arrhythmia.*

- **Identify S$_1$ (first heart sound) and note its intensity.**

  See guidelines for cardiac auscultation in the box on page 1017. At each auscultatory area, listen for several cardiac cycles. See Figure 27–9 for auscultation areas.

An accentuated S$_1$ occurs with tachycardia, states in which cardiac output is high (fever, anxiety, exercise, anemia, hyperthyroidism), complete heart block, and mitral stenosis. A diminished S$_1$ occurs with first-degree heart block, mitral regurgitation, CHF, coronary artery disease, and pulmonary or systemic HTN. The intensity is also decreased with obesity, emphysema, and pericardial effusion. Varying intensity of S$_1$ occurs with complete heart block and grossly irregular rhythms.

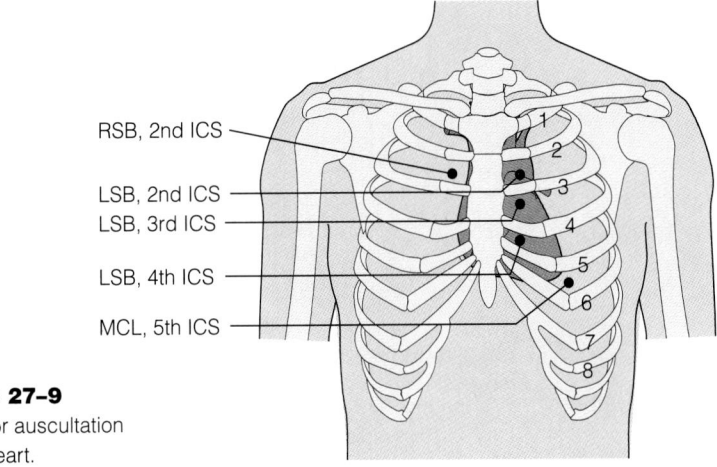

RSB, 2nd ICS
LSB, 2nd ICS
LSB, 3rd ICS
LSB, 4th ICS
MCL, 5th ICS

Figure 27–9
Areas for auscultation
of the heart.

- **Listen for splitting of S$_1$.**

Abnormal splitting of S$_1$ may be heard with right bundle branch block and premature ventricular contractions.

- **Identify S$_2$ (second heart sound) and note its intensity.**

An accentuated S$_2$ may be heard with HTN, exercise, excitement, and conditions of pulmonary HTN such as mitral stenosis, CHF, and cor pulmonale. A diminished S$_2$ occurs with aortic stenosis, a fall in systolic blood pressure (shock), pulmonary stenosis, and increased anterioposterior chest diameter.

- **Listen for splitting of S$_2$.**

Wide splitting of S$_2$ is associated with delayed emptying of the right ventricle resulting in delayed pulmonary valve closure (e.g., mitral regurgitation, pulmonary stenosis, and right bundle branch block). Fixed splitting occurs when right ventricular output is greater

ASSESSMENT TECHNIQUE	POSSIBLE ABNORMAL FINDINGS
	than left ventricular output and pulmonary valve closure is delayed (e.g., with atrial septal defect and right ventricular failure). Paradoxical splitting occurs when closure of the aortic valve is delayed (e.g., left bundle branch block).
■ **Identify the presence of extra heart sounds in systole.**	*Ejection sounds* (or *clicks*) result from the opening of deformed semilunar valves (e.g., aortic and pulmonary stenosis). A midsystolic click is heard with mitral valve prolapse (MVP).
■ **Identify the presence of extra heart sounds in diastole.**	An *opening snap* results from the opening sound of a stenotic mitral valve. A *pathologic* S_3 (a third heart sound that immediately follows S_2), or *ventricular gallop,* results from myocardial failure and ventricular volume overload (e.g., CHF, mitral or tricuspid regurgitation). An S_4 (a fourth heart sound that immediately precedes S_1), or *atrial gallop,* results from increased resistance to ventricular filling after atrial contraction (e.g., HTN, CAD, aortic stenosis, and cardiomyopathy). A less common right-sided S_4 occurs with pulmonary HTN and pulmonary stenosis. A combined S_3 and S_4 is called a *summation gallop* and occurs with severe CHF.
■ **Identify the presence of extra heart sounds in both systole and diastole.**	A *pericardial friction rub* results from inflammation of the pericardial sac, as with pericarditis.
■ **Identify any murmurs.** Note location, timing, presence during systole or diastole, and intensity. Use the following scale to grade murmurs: I = Barely heard II = Quietly heard III = Clearly heard IV = Loud V = Very loud VI = Loudest; may be heard with stethoscope off the chest. A thrill may accompany murmurs of grade IV to grade VI. Also note pitch (low, medium, high), and quality (harsh, blowing, or musical). Also note pattern/shape, crescendo, decrescendo, and radiation/transmission (to axilla, neck).	**Murmurs** are sounds made by turbulent blood flow through the heart. Midsystolic murmurs are heard with semilunar valve disease (e.g., aortic and pulmonary stenosis) and with hypertrophic cardiomyopathy. Pansystolic (holosystolic) murmurs are heard with AV valve disease (e.g., mitral and tricuspid regurgitation, ventricular septal defect). A late systolic murmur is heard with MVP. Early diastolic murmurs occur with regurgitant flow across incompetent semilunar valves (e.g., aortic regurgitation). Middiastolic and presystolic murmurs, such as with mitral stenosis, occur with turbulent flow across the AV valves. Continuous murmurs throughout systole and all or part of diastole occur with patent ductus arteriosus.

Guidelines for Cardiac Auscultation

■ ■ ■

1. Locate the major auscultatory areas on the precordium (see Figure 27–9).

2. Choose a sequence of listening. Either begin from the apex and move upward along the sternal border to the base, or begin at the base and move downward to the apex. One suggested sequence is shown in Figure 27–9.

3. Listen first with the client in the sitting or supine position. Then ask the client to lie on the left side, and focus on the apex. Lastly, ask the client to sit up and lean forward. These position changes bring the heart closer to the chest wall and enhance auscultation. Carry out the following steps when the client assumes each of these positions:

   a. First, auscultate each area with the diaphragm of the stethoscope to listen for high-pitched sounds: S_1, S_2, murmurs, pericardial friction rubs.

   b. Next, auscultate each area with the bell of the stethoscope to listen for lower-pitched sounds: S_3, S_4, murmurs.

   c. Listen for the effect of respirations on each sound; while the client is sitting up and leaning forward, ask the client to exhale and hold the breath while you listen to heart sounds.

Variations in Assessment Findings for the Older Adult

The normal heart functions quietly and efficiently throughout the life span, adapting to changing body needs. With the continuous demand for work, however, special anatomic and functional changes develop as one ages. Anatomic and functional changes within the cardiovascular and other systems over the life span produce variations in cardiac assessment findings for the older adult client. Age-related changes include thickening and hardening in the valves (especially the mitral valve), a decrease in cardiac reserve, and fibrosis of the conduction system. These changes may precipitate such cardiac disorders as valvular incompetence, CHF, dysrhythmias, and myocardial infarction. Changes in assessment findings that result from aging include the following:

- The apical impulse may be difficult to locate because anterioposterior chest diameter increases with age.

- The range of heart rate may increase to 100 or more beats per minute, with a propensity for tachycardia if the client has been sedentary.

- Premature beats are more common, as well as the development of other chronic dysrhythmias.

- The presence of an S_4 is not uncommon, possibly reflecting changes in compliance with the left ventricle.

- Murmurs are possibly due to aortic valve sclerosis and mitral regurgitation.

- Arteriosclerosis of the coronary arteries with angina is more likely.

Bibliography

■ ■ ■

Aherns, T. (1993). Changing perspectives in the assessment of oxygenation. *Critical Care Nurse, 13*(4), 78–83.

Anardi, D. (1991). Assessment of right heart function. *Journal of Cardiovascular Nursing, 6*(1), 12–33.

Bennett, A., & Sauer, H. (1991). Special considerations in cardiovascular assessment of the aged. *Nurse Practitioner Forum, 2*(1), 55–60.

Canobbio, M. M. (1990). *Cardiovascular disorders.* St. Louis: Mosby.

Carpenter, K. (1993). A comprehensive review of cyanosis. *Critical Care Nurse, 13*(4), 66–72.

Criscitiello, M. (1990). Fine-tuning the cardiovascular exam. *Patient Care, 24*(11), 51–54, 57, 60–61.

Fitzgerald, M. (1991). The physical exam. *RN, 54*(11), 34–39.

Gawlinski, A., & Jensen, G.A. (1991). The complications of cardiovascular aging. *American Journal of Nursing, 91*(11), 26–32.

Gehring, P. (1991). Physical assessment begins with a history. *RN, 54*(11), 26–32.

Hurst, J. W. (1992). The importance of the initial cardiovascular examination. *Heart Disease and Stroke, 1*(3), 105–106.

Kernicki, J. (1993). Differentiating chest pain: Advanced assessment techniques. *Dimensions of Critical Care Nursing, 12*(2), 66–76, 78–80.

Marieb, E. N. (1995). *Human anatomy and physiology.* (3rd ed.). Redwood City, CA: Benjamin/Cummings.

McGovern, M., & Kuhn, J. (1992). Cardiac assessment of the elderly client. *Journal of Gerontological Nursing, 18*(8), 40–44.

Merkley, K. (1994). Assessing chest pain. *RN, 57*(6), 58–63.

Morton, L. Y. (1991). Cardiac assessment. *RN, 54*(12), 28–35.

Ronan, J. A. (1992a). Cardiac auscultation: The first and second heart sounds. *Heart Disease and Stroke, 1*(3), 113–116.

Ronan, J. A. (1992b). Cardiac auscultation: The third and fourth heart sounds. *Heart Disease and Stroke, 1*(5), 267–270.

Rossi, L., & Leary, E. (1992). Evaluating the patient with coronary artery disease. *Nursing Clinics of North America, 27*(1), 171–188.

Silverman, M. E. (1992). The value of examining the patient in the upright position. *Heart Disease and Stroke, 1*(4), 168–169.

Smith, C. (1991). Assessment under pressure: When your patient says "my chest hurts." *Nursing91, 21*(11), 66–70.

Urban, N. (1993). Integrating the hemodynamic profile with clinical assessment. *AACN Clinical Issues in Critical Care Nursing, 4*(1), 161–179.

Yacone-Morton, L. (1991). Perfecting the art: Cardiac assessment. *RN, 54*(12), 28–35.

Yacone-Morton, L. (1992). Performing a rapid assessment of the heart. *Nursing92, 22*(2), 32C–32D.

CHAPTER 28

Nursing Care of Clients with Cardiac Disorders

LEARNING OBJECTIVES

After completing this chapter, you will be able to

- Discuss the mechanical and electrical properties of the heart.

- Compare and contrast the pathophysiology and clinical manifestations of common cardiac disorders, including dysrhythmias, coronary artery disease, congestive heart failure, structural disorders, and inflammatory disorders.

- Identify common laboratory and diagnostic tests appropriate for clients with cardiac disorders.

- Discuss the indications for and management of clients with hemodynamic monitoring.

- Discuss nursing implications for pharmacologic agents prescribed for clients with cardiac disorders.

- Describe the following special care procedures for clients with specific functional, structural, and inflammatory disorders of the heart: pacemakers, automatic implantable cardioverter-defibrillators (AICDs), interventional techniques, and ventricular assist devices.

- Discuss common cardiac surgeries, including coronary artery bypass grafting (CABG), valve repair and replacement, and cardiac transplantation, and describe the nursing care appropriate for the preoperative and postoperative client.

- Use the nursing process as a framework for providing individualized nursing care for clients with cardiac disorders.

- Provide appropriate teaching for clients with cardiac disorders and their families.

Cardiovascular disease (CVD) is the leading cause of death and disability in the United States. Nineteen million people suffer from some form of heart disease: Approximately 7 million people have *coronary heart disease (CHD),* and about 500,000 die from it each year. The economic costs of CVD, both direct and indirect, to the nation is estimated at $189 billion dollars annually (National Heart, Lung, and Blood Institute [NHLBI], 1994).

On an encouraging note, however, the incidence of new CVD cases per year is decreasing. Public education efforts aimed at reducing fat intake, increasing exercise, and lowering stress levels have made people more aware of risk factors associated with the development of CVD. The mortality rate from heart disease peaked in 1963 at over 200 people per 100,000; by 1992, that rate had dropped to just over 100 people per 100,000 (NHLBI, 1994).

Alterations in the usual flow of impulses through the heart's conduction system, impaired blood flow to the myocardium, and structural changes in the heart muscle itself influence the heart's ability to fulfill its major purpose: to pump enough blood to meet the body's demand for oxygen and nutrients. Disruptions in cardiac function affect the functioning of other organ systems, potentially leading to organ system failure and death.

Nurses must be knowledgeable about heart disease and its causes to educate and care for clients appropriately. This chapter provides the beginning nurse with the tools necessary to assess, plan, implement, and evaluate care for the client with cardiac disease.

◾◾◾ **Cardiac Rhythm Disorders** ◾◾◾

The Client with a Cardiac Dysrhythmia

◾ ◾ ◾

Contraction of the heart muscle is a mechanical event that occurs only after the myocardial cells have been electrically stimulated. Electrical stimulation in the normal heart produces a synchronized, rhythmic contraction of the heart muscle that enables the heart to propel blood into the vascular system. Alterations in cardiac rhythm can affect this synchronized activity and the heart's ability to pump blood to body tissues effectively.

A cardiac **dysrhythmia** is a disturbance or irregularity in the electrical system of the heart. Cardiac dysrhythmias may be benign or have lethal consequences. Prompt recognition and quick action for a client with a lethal dysrhythmia can be life-saving.

There are many reasons why dysrhythmias develop. They are not always pathologic; some alterations in cardiac rhythm occur in response to known events such as exercise or fear. For example, a rapid heart rate that occurs as a result of exercise, fever, or excitement is a normal response to the body's demand for oxygen or to stimulation of the sympathetic nervous system. Slow heart rates also may be physiologically normal. *Athletic heart syndrome,* which results from the effects of long-term training on the heart muscle, allows the heart to beat more slowly and forcefully while maintaining cardiac output and tissue perfusion. Many athletes have a heart rate of less than 60 beats per minute (BPM).

Regardless of its origin, any dysrhythmia can significantly affect cardiac performance, depending on the state of the myocardium. The client's response to the altered cardiac rhythm is key in determining the urgency and type of treatment needed.

Physiology

Cardiac muscle is unique. Unlike skeletal muscle tissue, cardiac muscle can generate an electrical impulse and contraction independent of the nervous system.

Conduction Pathways

Electrical activity of the heart is normally controlled by the *cardiac conduction system,* a network of specialized cells and conduction pathways that initiate and spread the electrical impulses that cause the heart to beat (see Figure 27.7 on page 1008). *Pacemaker cells* spontaneously generate an electrical impulse at a variety of regular rates that are faster than those from other types of heart tissue. Specialized conduction tissue transmits this impulse more rapidly than other cardiac tissue. *Myocardial muscle*

cells contract in response to that impulse. Electrical stimulation of the heart muscle through the cardiac conduction system *always* precedes mechanical contraction.

Pacemaker cells are located throughout the heart muscle. The primary pacemaker of the heart is the *sinoatrial (SA)* or *sinus node.* It normally initiates the electrical impulse that is conducted throughout the heart and results in ventricular contraction. The SA node usually fires at a regular rate of 60 to 100 BPM, the "normal" heart rate.

The impulse generated by the sinus node spreads throughout the atria via the *interatrial pathways.* The conduction fibers narrow through the *atrioventricular (AV) node,* resulting in a normal delay in the conduction of the impulse. This delay allows atrial contraction to deliver an extra bolus of blood to the ventricles before systole begins. This is often called the **atrial kick.** The AV node also controls the number of impulses reaching the ventricles, preventing extremely rapid heart rates. From the AV node, the impulse travels into the ventricular conduction pathways: down the *Bundle of His,* the right and left *bundle branches,* and to the *Purkinje fibers,* which terminate in the ventricular muscle. The heart's response to electrical stimulation is mechanical contraction, or systole.

If the normal pacemaker fails, secondary pacemaker sites located in the AV nodal tissue (whose intrinsic rate is 40 to 60 BPM), and the Purkinje fibers (whose intrinsic rate is 15 to 40 BPM) will take over as the heart's pacemaker, at their slower rate. This provides an escape or back-up mechanism for electrical stimulation of the heart.

Electrophysiologic Properties

Four unique properties of cardiac cells allow the heart to function effectively. The first three properties are electrical phenomena; the fourth is the cardiac muscle's mechanical response to electrical stimulation.

- *Automaticity* is the ability of the pacemaker cells to initiate an electrical impulse spontaneously. Pacemaker cells initiating the fastest rate supersede slower pacemaker cells. The SA node normally generates impulses at the most rapid rate, making it the dominant pacemaker. Injury, disease, age, medication, or stimulation of the autonomic nervous system can affect the pacemaker function of the SA node. Myocardial muscle cells, in contrast, do not possess this electrophysiologic property.

- *Excitability* is the capacity of the myocardial working cells to respond to electrical impulses generated by the pacemaker cells.

- *Conductivity* is the ability to transmit an impulse from cell to cell. When one cell is stimulated, the impulse

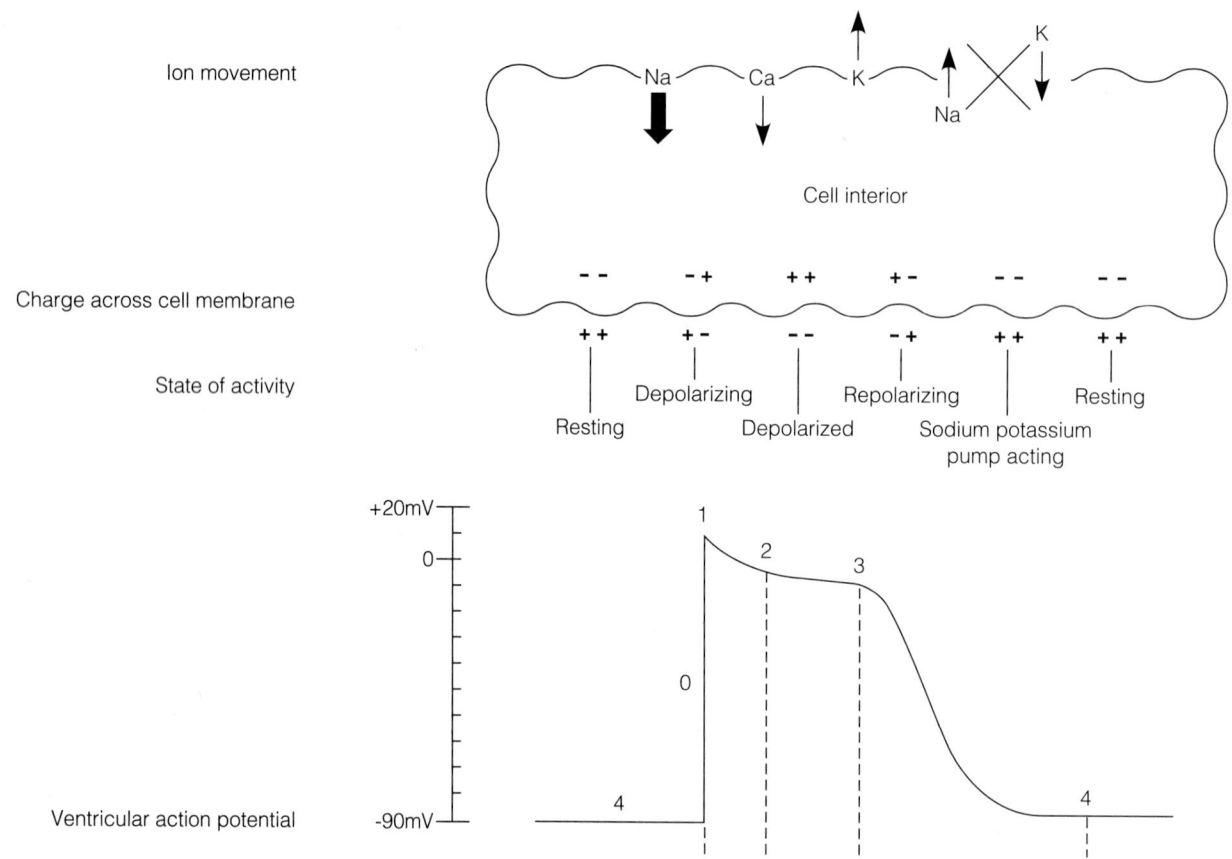

Ion movement

Charge across cell membrane

State of activity

Resting   Depolarizing   Repolarizing   Resting

Resting   Depolarized   Sodium potassium
pump acting

Ventricular action potential

Figure 28–1 Action potential of a cardiac cell. In the resting state (phase 4), the cell membrane is polarized; the membrane's interior has a negative charge compared to that of the extracellular fluid outside the membrane. On depolarization and generation of an action potential (phase 0), sodium ions diffuse rapidly into the cell across the cell membrane and calcium channels open. In the fully depolarized state (phase 1), the membrane's interior has a net positive charge compared to that of the exterior. During the plateau period (phase 2), calcium moves across the membrane into the cell and membrane permeability to potassium decreases, prolonging the action potential. During phase 3, calcium channels close and the sodium-potassium pump removes sodium from the cell's interior, and the membrane interior becomes progressively more negative until the resting potential state is reached.

rapidly spreads throughout the heart muscle, first through the atria and then through the ventricles.

- *Contractility* is the natural ability of the myocardial fibers to shorten in response to an electrical stimulus. The advancing wavefront of electrical stimulation changes the electrical potential of the cardiac cells, causing the muscle to contract in a synchronized fashion. The *all-or-nothing principle* refers to the fact that in the heart, stimulation of one muscle fiber causes the entire muscle mass to contract to its fullest extent as one unit (Guyton, 1991). Therefore, the impulse generated by the SA node rapidly depolarizes the atria, causing atrial contraction; the atrial impulse is conducted to the ventricular muscle fibers, which depolarize and cause ventricular contraction. Contractility is affected by drugs, fluid volume status, electrolyte concentration, acid-base balance, the availability of

oxygen, and the amount of functional myocardial tissue.

The Action Potential

The electrical impulse generated by pacemaker cells is caused by the movement of ions across cell membranes (Figure 28–1). This electrical activity, called the *action potential,* produces the waveforms represented on ECG strips.

In the resting state, positive and negative ions are aligned on either side of the cardiac cell membrane, producing a relatively negative intracellular charge and positive extracellular charge. In this state, the cell is said to be *polarized.* The negative resting membrane potential is maintained at about −90 millivolts (mV) by the sodium-potassium pump in the cell membrane.

The change in the electrical charge across the cell membrane from a negative toward a positive state is called *depolarization*. When the resting cell is stimulated by an electrical charge, either from a neighboring cell or via a spontaneous event, the permeability of the cell membrane is altered, allowing sodium ions to enter the cell rapidly through openings in the cell membrane called *fast sodium channels. Slow calcium-sodium channels* also open at this time allowing calcium into the cell. The addition of these positively charged ions to intracellular fluid changes the normally negative membrane potential to a slightly positive potential of +20 to +30 mV. Membrane permeability to potassium is drastically reduced during this phase.

As the cell becomes more positive, it reaches a point called the *threshold potential*. Once the threshold potential is reached, an action potential is generated. The resulting wavefront depolarizes cardiac muscle cells. The action potential causes a chemical reaction of calcium within the cell, which, in turn, causes actin and myosin filaments to slide together, producing cardiac muscle contraction. As soon as the heart muscle is completely depolarized, repolarization begins.

Repolarization is the process that returns the cell to the polarized state and prepares it to receive the next impulse, beginning the cycle again. During *rapid repolarization*, fast sodium channels close abruptly, and the cell begins to regain its negative charge. During the *plateau phase*, muscle contraction is prolonged as slow calcium-sodium channels remain open and calcium and sodium ions continue to leak across the membrane. Closure of the slow calcium-sodium channels allows the sodium-potassium pump to restore ion concentration to its normal resting levels. The cell membrane is then polarized, ready for the cycle to start again. Each heartbeat represents one cardiac cycle, with one depolarization and repolarization cycle and one systole and diastole.

Normally, only pacemaker cells demonstrate automativity. Pacemaker cells differ slightly from other cardiac muscle cells in that their resting potential is much less negative (−70 to −50 mV). The threshold potential of the SA and AV nodes also is lower than that of other myocardial cells. Their higher potentials are a result of a constant leakage of sodium and potassium ions into the cell, making it highly unstable.

Myocardial cells have a unique protective feature called the **refractory period,** a stage of resistance to stimulation. This property ensures that continuous electrical stimulation does not result in cardiac spasms or tetany. During the *absolute refractory period,* no matter how strongly the myocardial cell is stimulated, another depolarization will not occur. It is followed by the *relative refractory period,* during which a greater-than-normal stimulus is necessary to generate another action potential. The *supernormal period* follows; a mild stimulus during this time will cause the cell to depolarize. Many cardiac dysrhythmias are triggered during the relative refractory and supernormal periods.

Electrocardiography

Electrocardiography is the graphic recording of the heart's electrical activity detected and recorded through electrodes placed on the surface of the body. Electrical activity is demonstrated as a series of waveforms on an *oscilloscope* (visual display), a strip recorder (graphic record), or both. The *electrocardiogram (ECG)* is a hard-copy graphic record of this activity. ECG waveforms and patterns are examined to detect dysrhythmias as well as myocardial damage or enlargement, the effects of drugs, and electrolyte imbalances. The normal ECG waveform consists of a P wave, a QRS complex, and T wave, which represent one cardiac depolarization and repolarization cycle.

Electrocardiography may be used on a continual or intermittent basis, depending on the client's needs.

The Electrocardiogram (ECG)   A graphic representation of cardiac electrical activity is obtained by applying *electrodes* to the client's skin at specific points. Electrodes detect the magnitude and direction of the electrical currents produced in the heart and are attached to the electrocardiograph by an insulated wire called a *lead*. The electrocardiograph converts the electrical impulses it receives into a series of waveforms on the oscilloscope or graphic printout. The placement of electrodes on different parts of the body allows different views of the heart's electrical activity, much like turning the head while holding a camera provides different views of the scenery.

Both bipolar and unipolar leads may be used in recording the ECG. Two electrodes of opposite polarity (negative and positive) form a *bipolar lead.* In a *unipolar lead,* one positive electrode and a negative reference point at the center of the heart are used. The electrical potential between the two monitoring points is graphically recorded as a *waveform,* or "picture" of the heart's electrical activity.

The heart can be viewed from two different dimensions, the *frontal plane* and the *horizontal plane* (Figure 28–2). Each dimension provides a unique perspective of the heart muscle. The frontal plane is an imaginary "cut" through the body that views the heart from top to bottom (superior-inferior) and side to side (right-left). The perspective of the heart from the frontal plane is analogous to a paper doll cut-out. Information about the inferior and lateral walls of the heart can be ascertained from this viewpoint. The horizontal plane is a cross-sectional view of the heart from front to back (anterior-posterior) and side to side (right-left). Information regarding the anterior, septal, and lateral walls of the heart, as well as the posterior wall, are obtained from this view.

Figure 28–2 Planes of the heart. *A*, the frontal plane. *B*, the horizontal plane.

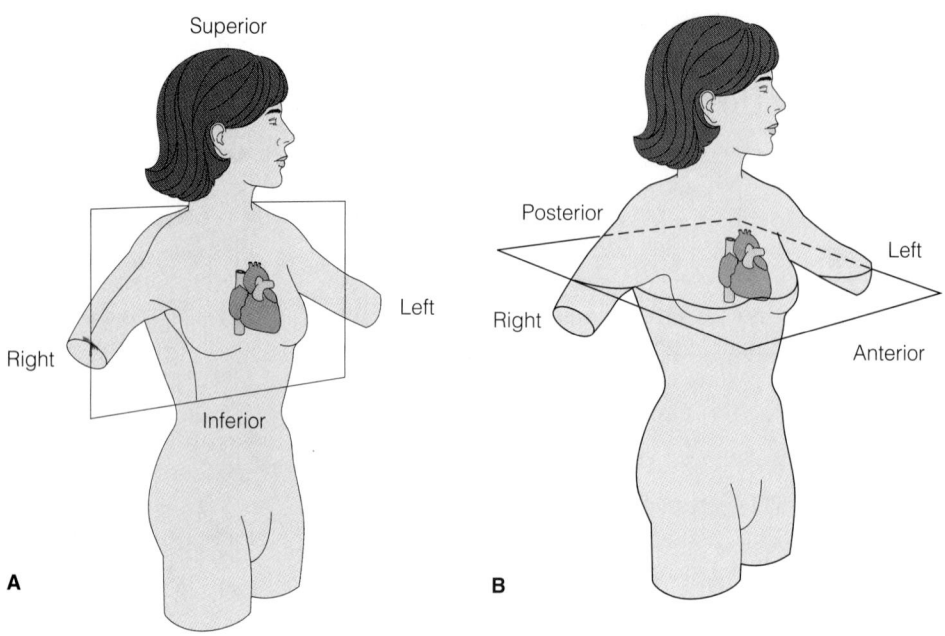

Figure 28–3 Leads of the 12-lead ECG. *A*, bipolar limb leads I, II, III. *B*, Unipolar limb leads aV$_R$, aV$_L$, aV$_F$. *C*, unipolar precordial leads V$_1$ to V$_6$.

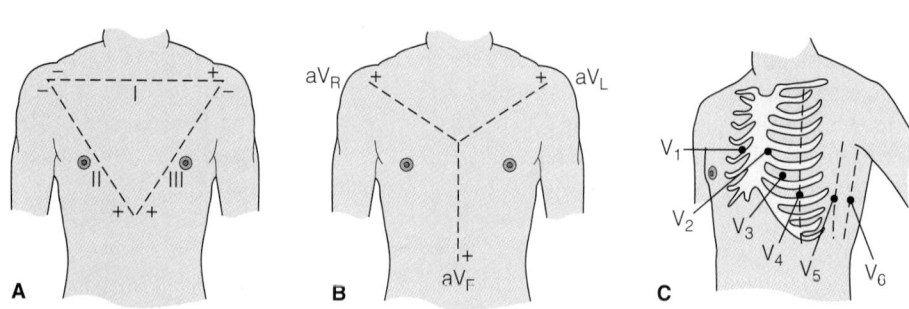

A standard 12-lead ECG consists of a simultaneous recording of 6 *limb leads* and 6 *precordial leads* (Figure 28–3). The limb leads provide information about the heart in the frontal plane and include 3 bipolar leads (I, II, III) and 3 unipolar leads (aV$_R$, aV$_L$, and aV$_F$). The three bipolar limb leads measure electrical activity between a negative lead on one extremity and a positive lead on another. The three unipolar limb leads (called the *augmented leads*) measure the electrical activity between a single positive electrode on one limb (the right arm [R], left arm [L], or left leg [F for *foot*]), and the center of the heart.

The precordial leads, also known as *chest leads* or *V leads*, view the heart in the horizontal plane and consist of 6 unipolar leads (V$_1$, V$_2$, V$_3$, V$_4$, V$_5$, and V$_6$), which measure electrical activity between the center of the heart and a positive electrode located on the chest wall.

The waveforms depicted on the ECG illustrate the direction of the electrical current flow in relation to the positive electrode. Current flowing toward the positive pole produces an upward (positive) waveform; current flowing away from the positive pole produces a downward (nega-

tive) waveform; and current flowing perpendicular to the positive pole produces a *biphasic* (both positive and negative) waveform. The absence of current flow is represented by a straight line, called the *isoelectric line*.

ECG waveforms are recorded by a heated stylus on special heat-sensitive paper. The paper is marked at standard intervals that represent time on the horizontal axis and voltage and amplitude on the vertical axis (Figure 28–4). Each small box is 1 square mm. The normal recording speed of the standard ECG is 25 mm/second, so each small box represents 0.04 seconds. Five small boxes horizontally and vertically make one large box, equivalent to 0.20 seconds. Five large boxes represent 1 full second. Measured vertically, each small box represents 0.1 millivolt (mV).

The cardiac cycle is depicted as a series of waveforms, the P, Q, R, S, and T waves (Figure 28–5). The *P wave* represents atrial depolarization and contraction. The impulse is from the sinus node. The P wave precedes the QRS complex and is normally smooth, round, and upright. P waves may be absent when the SA node is not acting as

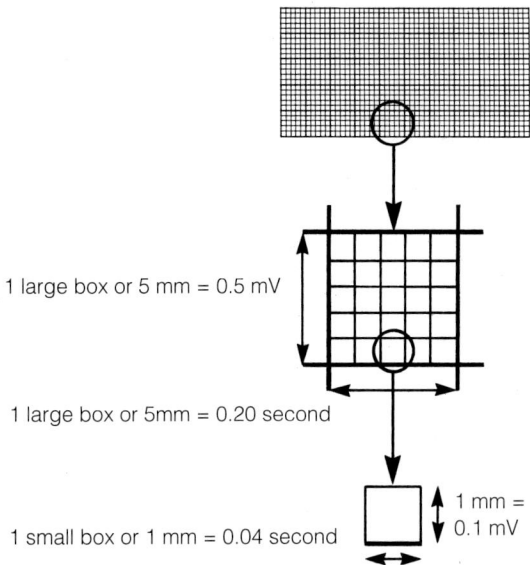

Figure 28–4   Time and voltage measurements on ECG paper at a recording speed of 25 mm/second.

1 large box or 5 mm = 0.5 mV

1 large box or 5mm = 0.20 second

1 small box or 1 mm = 0.04 second

1 mm = 0.1 mV

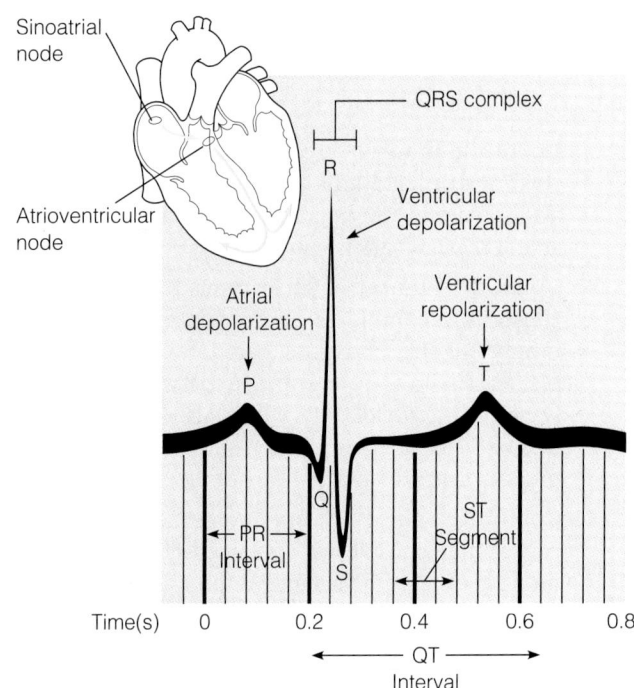

Figure 28–5   Normal ECG waveform and intervals.

the pacemaker. Atrial repolarization occurs during the period of ventricular depolarization and usually is not seen on the ECG.

The *PR interval* represents the time during which the sinus impulse travels to the AV node and into the bundle branches. This interval is measured from beginning of P wave to beginning of QRS complex. If no Q wave is present, the beginning of the R wave is used. The PR interval is normally 0.12 to 0.20 seconds (in the client over age 65, up to 0.24 seconds is considered normal). PR intervals greater than 0.20 seconds signal a delay in conduction from the SA node to the ventricles.

The *QRS complex* represents ventricular depolarization and contraction. The QRS complex consists of three separate waves: The Q wave is the first negative deflection, the R wave is the positive or upright deflection, and the S wave is the first negative deflection *after* the R wave. Not all QRS complexes have all three waves; nonetheless, the complex is called a QRS complex. The normal duration of a QRS complex is from 0.06 to 0.10 seconds. QRS complexes greater than 0.10 seconds in width indicate problems in the transmission of the impulse through the ventricular conduction system.

The *ST segment* signifies the beginning of ventricular repolarization. The ST segment should be isoelectric. It is the period from the end of the QRS complex to the beginning of the T wave. The ST segment is considered abnormal when it is displaced (elevated or depressed) from the isoelectric line.

The *T wave* represents ventricular repolarization. It normally has a smooth, rounded shape that is usually less

than 10 mm tall. It usually points in the same direction as the QRS complex. Abnormalities of the T wave may indicate myocardial ischemia or injury, or electrolyte imbalances.

The *QT interval* is measured from the beginning of the QRS complex to the end of the T wave and represents the total time for ventricular depolarization and repolarization. Normal duration varies with gender, age, and heart rate; usually, it is 0.32 sec to 0.44 seconds long. Prolonged QT intervals indicate an increase in the relative refractory period and a greater risk of dysrhythmias. Shortened QT intervals may result from medications or electrolyte imbalances.

The *U wave* is not normally seen but is thought to signify repolarization of the terminal Purkinje fibers. If present, the U wave follows the same direction as the T wave. It is most commonly seen in hypokalemia.

ECG Rhythm Analysis   Interpreting an ECG strip is a skill that takes practice to learn and master. Many methods are used to analyze ECGs. One sequence of steps in evaluating an ECG strip is listed below. What is most important is to choose one method and use it consistently.

■ *Step 1: Determine rate.* Assess the rate of both the atrial and ventricular beats. Use P waves to determine the atrial rate and R waves for the ventricular rate. There are several approaches to determine the heart rate (see the box on page 1024). *Tachycardia* is a heart rate above 100 BPM, and *bradycardia* is a heart rate below 60 BPM.

■ *Step 2: Determine regularity.* The regularity of the rhythm is the consistency with which the P waves or

Using the ECG to Calculate Heart Rate

■ ■ ■

- Count the number of complexes in a 6-second rhythm strip, and multiply by 10. This provides an estimate of the rate and is particularly valuable if rhythms are irregular.

- Count the number of small boxes between two consecutive complexes, and divide by 1500 (the number of small boxes in 1 minute). For example, small boxes are counted between two R waves; 1500 divided by 19 equals a ventricular rate of 79 BPM. This method provides the most precise measurement of heart rate.

- Count the number of large boxes between two consecutive complexes, and divide by 300 (the number of large boxes in 1 minute). For example, 6 large boxes are noted between two R waves; 300 divided by 6 equals a ventricular rate of 50 BPM. The rate can be calculated rapidly by memorizing the following sequence: 300, 150, 100, 75, 60, 50, 43, where one large box between complexes equals a rate of 300; two, a rate of 150; three, a rate of 100; and so on.

QRS waves occur. In a *regular* rhythm, all waves occur at a consistent rate. The regularity of the rhythm can be determined by using either ECG *calipers* (a measuring device) or paper and pencil. Place one caliper point on the peak of the P wave for atrial rhythm determination or the R wave for ventricular rhythm. Adjust the other point to the peak of the next wave, P to P or R to R (Figure 28–6). Keeping the calipers set at this distance, measure the interval between consecutive waves. The rhythm is considered regular if all caliper points fall on succeeding wave peaks. Alternately, position a strip of blank paper on top of the ECG strip, marking the peaks of two or three consecutive waves. Then move the paper along the strip to the next group of waves. Wave peaks that vary by more than one to three small boxes (depending on the rate) are considered irregular. Irregular rhythms may be called *irregularly irregular* (if there is no pattern to the complex intervals) or *regularly irregular* (if a consistent pattern to the irregularity can be identified).

- *Step 3: Assess P wave morphology.* The presence or absence of P waves helps determine whether the rhythm originates from the sinus node. All the P waves should look alike in size and shape (*morphology*). If P waves are not present or if they differ in shape, the rhythm may not originate in the sinus node.

- *Step 4: Assess P to QRS relationship.* Determine the relationship between the P waves and the QRS complex. There should be one P wave for every QRS complex since the stimulus for normal ventricular contraction originates in the sinus node.

- *Step 5: Determine interval durations.* To evaluate impulse transmission through the cardiac conduction system, measure the PR interval, QRS complex, and the QT interval. To determine the duration of any interval, count the number of small boxes from the beginning of the interval to the end, and multiply by 0.04 seconds. Then determine whether the resulting duration is considered normal for the interval that is being measured. For example, a PR interval that is 3½ small boxes wide is 0.14 seconds long. This is within the expected duration of 0.12 to 0.20 seconds. This interval should normally be consistent; that is, it should not vary from beat to beat. A PR interval of greater than 0.20 seconds or one that varies from beat to beat is abnormal.

The duration of the QRS complex is normally between 0.06 and 0.10 seconds. A QRS complex of greater than 0.12 seconds signifies a delay in ventricular conduction. A wide QRS interval does not necessarily mean that the rhythm did not originate in the sinus node, if each QRS is preceded by a P wave.

The QT interval is normally 0.32 to 0.44 seconds, but this varies inversely with the heart rate. The faster the heart rate, the shorter the QT interval. As a general rule, the QT interval should be no more than half the previous R-R interval. A prolonged QT interval lengthens the relative refractory period of the heart.

- *Step 6: Identify abnormalities.* Note the presence and frequency of ectopic (extra) beats, deviation of the ST segment above or below the baseline, and abnormalities in waveform shape and duration. Using the data collected by a consistent method, the nurse should have enough information to interpret the ECG tracing. Interpretation of complex dysrhythmias, however, requires advanced skills and knowledge in *arrhythmogenic mechanisms* (mechanisms predisposing to dysrhythmia) and ectopic presentations.

Pathophysiology

Disturbances in the electrical activity of the heart can affect its ability to contract in a synchronized manner and provide an effective cardiac output. Dysrhythmias may be triggered by internal or external processes. Internal causes of dysrhythmias include alterations in the cellular environment (e.g., due to hypoxia, electrolyte disturbances, or acidosis.) Dysrhythmias also result from disease processes affecting the myocardium. See the box on page 1026 for a discussion of dysrhythmias and the older adult.

Often, the source of the dysrhythmia is an extracardiac

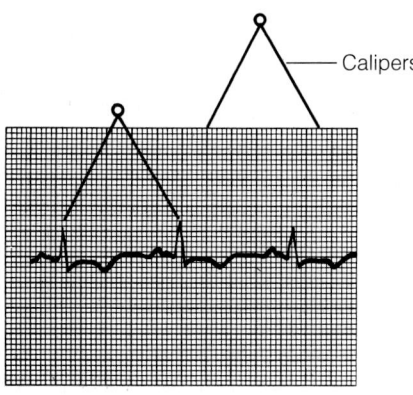

Figure 28-6 Using calipers to measure distances between and assess regularity of ECG waveforms.

event. Exercise, pain, anxiety, anemia, and hypovolemia can cause tachycardia; treating the cause relieves the tachycardia. Pharmacologic therapy can both alleviate dysrhythmias and cause them. Drugs that may cause dysrhythmias are called *proarrhythmic*.

Dysrhythmias are categorized by two major mechanisms: alterations in impulse formation and alterations in conductivity. Abnormalities of impulse formation include changes in rate and rhythm and the development of ectopic beats. This category primarily includes *tachydysrhythmias* (rapid heart rates), *bradydysrhythmias* (slow heart rates), and ectopic rhythms. Impulse formation abnormalities result from a change in the automaticity of cardiac cells. Impulse formation abnormalities are characterized by an abnormal increase or decrease in the initiation of impulses or by *aberrant* (abnormal) impulses that originate outside normal conduction pathways. Impulses originating outside normal conduction pathways are called **ectopic beats.** Under certain conditions, any cardiac muscle cell can initiate an action potential and take over as an ectopic pacemaker. Ectopic beats interrupt the normal conduction sequence; depending on the site of the abnormal impulse, they may be of little consequence to the client or pose a significant threat.

Alterations in conductivity result from a failure or delay in impulse transmission. They result in varying degrees of **heart block,** a block in the normal conduction pathways. Heart block alters normal conduction and can lead to dysrhythmias. Myocardial injury can cause an obstruction or delay in impulse conduction. Bundle branch blocks are common in acute myocardial infarction. Another cause of dysrhythmias is the *reentry* phenomenon, a phenomenon of normal and slow conduction. The impulse is delayed in one area of the heart but conducted normally through the rest. The muscle that has been depolarized by the normally conducted impulse is repolar-

ized by the time the impulse traveling through the area of slow conduction reaches these cells and thus initiates another wave of depolarization (Conover, 1994). The result is a dysrhythmia that propagates itself. Many dysrhythmias are considered to be the result of the reentry mechanism.

Cardiac rhythms are classified according to the site of impulse formation or the site and degree of conduction block. *Supraventricular rhythms* include all rhythms in which the site of impulse formation is above the ventricles. These rhythms usually produce a QRS complex within the normal range. Sinus rhythms, atrial rhythms, and junctional rhythms are all supraventricular rhythms. *Ventricular rhythms* originate in the ventricles and may prove fatal if left untreated. The *AV conduction blocks* result from a defect in impulse transmission from the atria to the ventricles. The major normal and abnormal cardiac rhythms are illustrated and their ECG features summarized in Table 28–1 on page 1027.

Supraventricular Rhythms

Normal Sinus Rhythm   Normal sinus rhythm (NSR) is the normal heart rhythm, in which impulses originate in the SA node and travel through normal conduction pathways without delay. All waveforms are of normal configuration, look alike, and are of a consistent (fixed) duration. The rate is between 60 and 100 BPM.

Sinus Node Dysrhythmias   Sinus node dysrhythmias may occur as a normal compensatory response (e.g., to exercise) or because of an abnormality of automaticity. In all these rhythms, as in NSR, the initiating impulse is from the sinus node. They differ, however, in rate or in irregularity in rhythm. The sinus dysrhythmias include sinus arrhythmia, sinus tachycardia, and sinus bradycardia.

Sinus Arrhythmia   Sinus arrhythmia is a sinus rhythm in which the rate varies during the inspiratory and expiratory phases of respiration, resulting in an irregular rhythm. The rate increases during inspiration and decreases with expiration. Sinus arrhythmia is very common in the very young and the very old. It can be caused by an increase in vagal tone, by digitalis toxicity, or by morphine administration.

Sinus Tachycardia   Sinus tachycardia has all of the ECG characteristics of NSR, except that the rate is greater than 100 BPM. Tachycardia is a normal compensatory response to changes in the internal environment that results in enhanced automaticity. Sympathetic nervous system stimulation or blocked vagal (parasympathetic) activity increases the heart rate. Tachycardia is a normal response to any condition or event that increases the body's demand for oxygen and nutrients, such as exercise or hypoxia. In the client on bed rest, tachycardia is an ominous sign. Sinus tachycardia may be an early warning sign of

Gerontologic Considerations: Care of the Older Adult with a Cardiac Dysrhythmia

■ ■ ■

The process of aging affects the cells and receptors of cardiac muscle, the cardiac conduction system, and the vascular system. These changes affect normal cardiac function. "Abnormal" assessment findings in the older adult may therefore be indicative of normal aging or of disease processes.

Several studies have shown that certain dysrhythmias are common in older adults (Campbell, Caird, & Jackson, 1974; Fleg & Kennedy, 1982; Wajngarten et at., 1990). Older clients without cardiac disease have an increased prevalence of ectopic beats, tachydysrhythmias, and conduction problems (Fleg & Kennedy, 1982). Fibrosis of the bundle branches is the most common cause of chronic atrioventricular block in clients over 65 (Bharati & Lev, 1992). Heart rate variability and the incidence of sinus dysrhythmia normally declines with age because of decreased responsiveness to autonomic stimulation and a decline in the number of pacemaker cells. Maximum heart rate (as with exercise) also declines with normal aging (Lakatta, 1994). A prolonged PR interval is so common that cardiologists have suggested redefining the "normal" limits of the PR interval to 0.22 to 0.24 seconds for clients 65 years and older (Gerstenblith & Lakatta, 1990). Congestive heart failure and valvular disease are common causes of atrial fibrillation in older adults. An increased incidence of both ventricular and supraventricular dysrhythmias in healthy older adults without detrimental effects is common. In this population, ventricular and supraventricular dysrhythmias

are often asymptomatic and do not affect the person's functioning. Healthy older adults are more apt to experience ectopic beats, including short runs of ventricular tachycardia, during exercise than their younger counterparts; these dysrhythmias do not impact cardiac morbidity or mortality (Lakatta, 1994).

Physiologic changes affect the older cardiac client in many ways. Blood flow to the kidneys, liver, and gastrointestinal tracts is decreased. Renal function may be compromised because of glomerular cell loss. These changes have implications for fluid balance and drug excretion. Hypoperfusion of the gastrointestinal tract decreases the absorption and distribution of drugs. A decrease in the production of gastric acid increases the pH of the stomach, which also affects drug absorption. Decreased liver function affects the metabolism of certain drugs and the liver's ability to filter out toxins. Muscle mass and protein stores are decreased, creating a relative increase in adipose tissue. Many drugs are bound to protein or stored in fat tissue, increasing the risk of drug toxicities (Gawlinski & Jensen, 1991).

In caring for the older adult with a dysrhythmia, the nurse needs to be aware of the often atypical presentation of disease states in this population. Preventing injury from falls (resulting from decreased cardiac output) or drug toxicity and preventing complications from common problems affecting the older adult, such as impaired skin integrity, infection, and malnutrition are particularly important nursing interventions for older clients (Gawlinski & Jensen, 1991).

---

cardiac dysfunction, such as heart failure. Sinus tachycardia is detrimental in clients with cardiac disease because it increases cardiac work and oxygen use.

Common causes of sinus tachycardia include exercise, excitement, anxiety, pain, fever, hypoxia, hypovolemia, anemia, hyperthyroidism, myocardial infarction, heart failure, cardiogenic shock, pulmonary embolism, caffeine intake, and the use of certain drugs, such as atropine, epinephrine (Adrenalin), or isoproterenol (Isuprel).

Clinical manifestations of sinus tachycardia include a rapid pulse rate. The client may complain of feeling that the heart is "racing" and experience shortness of breath and dizziness. In the client with heart disease, sinus tachycardia may precipitate chest pain.

Sinus Bradycardia Sinus bradycardia has all of the ECG characteristics of NSR, but the rate is less than 60 BPM.

Sinus bradycardia may result from increased vagal activity or from depressed automaticity caused by injury or ischemia to the sinus node. Sinus bradycardia may be normal in some clients (e.g., clients with athletic heart syndrome). The heart rate is also normally slowed during sleep because the parasympathetic nervous system is dominant at this time. Causes of sinus bradycardia include athletic heart syndrome, increased vagal tone, pain, increased intracranial pressure, sinus node disease, acute myocardial infarction (especially with inferior wall damage), hypothermia, acidosis, and certain drugs.

Clients with sinus bradycardia may be asymptomatic; it is important to assess the client before treating the rhythm. Manifestations of decreased cardiac output, such as decreased level of consciousness, syncope (faintness), or hypotension, indicate that the client is not tolerating the rhythm and requires intervention.

Table 28–1   ECG Characteristics of Selected Cardiac Rhythms and Dysrhythmias

Rhythm/ECG Appearance	ECG Characteristics	Management
Supraventricular Rhythms		
Normal sinus rhythm (NSR)	Rate: 60 to 100 BPM Rhythm: Regular P:QRS: 1:1 PR interval: 0.12 to 0.20 sec QRS complex: 0.6 to 0.10 sec	None; normal heart rhythm.
Sinus arrhythmia	Rate: 60 to 100 BPM Rhythm: Irregular, varying with respirations P:QRS: 1:1 PR interval: 0.12 to 0.20 sec QRS complex: 0.6 to 0.10 sec	Generally none; considered a normal rhythm in the very young and very old.
Sinus tachycardia	Rate: 101 to 150 BPM Rhythm: Regular P:QRS: 1:1 (With very fast rates, P wave may be hidden in preceding T wave) PR interval: 0.12 to 0.20 sec QRS complex: 0.6 to 0.10 sec	Treated only if the client is experiencing symptoms or is at risk for myocardial damage. Treat underlying cause (e.g., hypovolemia, fever, pain). Beta-blockers or verapamil may be used.
Sinus bradycardia	Rate: < 60 BPM Rhythm: Regular P:QRS: 1:1 PR interval: 0.12 to 0.20 sec QRS complex: 0.6 to 0.10 sec	Treated only if the client is experiencing symptoms. Intravenous atropine and/or pacemaker therapy may be used.
Premature atrial contractions (PAC)	Rate: Variable Rhythm: Irregular, with normal rhythm interrupted by early beats arising in the atria P:QRS: 1:1 PR interval: 0.12 to 0.20 sec, but may be prolonged QRS complex: 0.6 to 0.10 sec	Usually require no treatment. Advise client to reduce alcohol and caffeine intake, to reduce stress, and to stop smoking.
Paroxysmal supraventricular tachycardia (PSVT)	Rate: 100 to 280 BPM (usually 150 to 200 BPM) Rhythm: Regular P:QRS: P waves often not identifiable PR interval: Not measured QRS complex: 0.6 to 0.10 sec	Treat if client is experiencing symptoms. Treatment may include vagal maneuvers (Valsalva, carotid sinus massage); oxygen therapy; adenosine, verapamil, procainamide, propranolol, and esmolol; and synchronized cardioversion.

►

Table 28–1 ECG Characteristics of Selected Cardiac Rhythms and Dysrhythmias (continued)

Rhythm/ECG Appearance	ECG Characteristics	Management
Atrial flutter 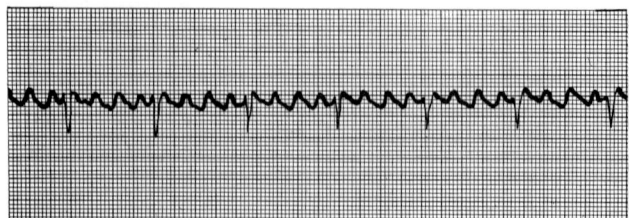	Rate: Atrial 240 to 360 BPM; ventricular rate depends on degree of AV block and usually is < 150 BPM Rhythm: Atrial regular; ventricular usually regular P:QRS: 2:1, 4:1, 6:1; may vary PR interval: Not measured QRS complex: 0.6 to 0.10 sec	Synchronized cardioversion; verapamil or esmolol, followed by digitalis and quinidine.
Atrial fibrillation 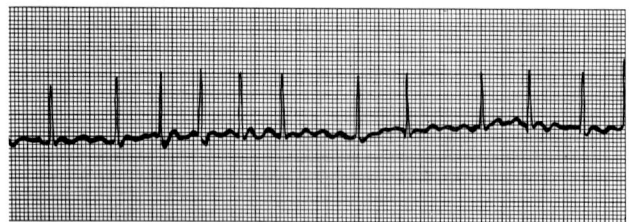	Rate: Atrial 300 to 600 BPM (too rapid to count); ventricular 100 to 180 BPM in untreated clients Rhythm: Irregularly irregular P:QRS: Variable PR interval: Not measured QRS complex: 0.06 to 0.10 sec	Synchronized cardioversion; medications to reduce ventricular response rate: digoxin, verapamil, propranolol; anticoagulant therapy to reduce risk of clot formation and stroke.
Junctional escape rhythm 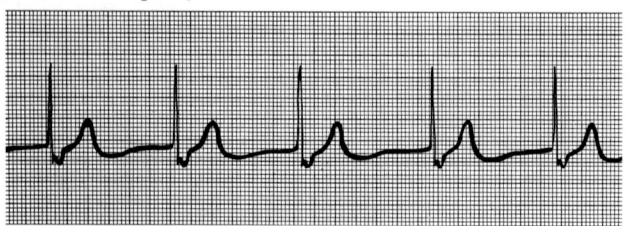	Rate: 40 to 60 BPM; junctional tachycardia 60 to 140 BPM Rhythm: Regular P:QRS: P waves may be absent, inverted and immediately preceding or succeeding QRS complex, or hidden in QRS complex PR interval: < 0.10 sec if P wave is prior to QRS complex QRS complex: 0.06 to 0.10 sec	Treat cause if client is experiencing symptoms.

Ventricular Rhythms

Rhythm/ECG Appearance	ECG Characteristics	Management
Premature ventricular contractions (PVC) 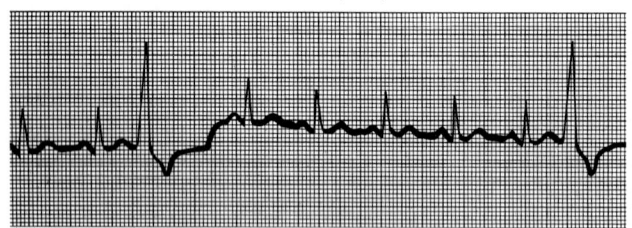	Rate: Variable Rhythm: Irregular, with PVC interrupting underlying rhythm and followed by a compensatory pause P:QRS: No P wave noted before PVC PR interval: Absent with PVC QRS complex: Wide (> 0.12 sec) and bizarre in appearance; differs from normal QRS complex	Treat if client is experiencing symptoms. Advise against stimulant use (caffeine, nicotine). Drug therapy includes intravenous lidocaine, procainamide, quinidine, propranolol, phenytoin, bretylium.
Ventricular tachycardia (VT or V tach) 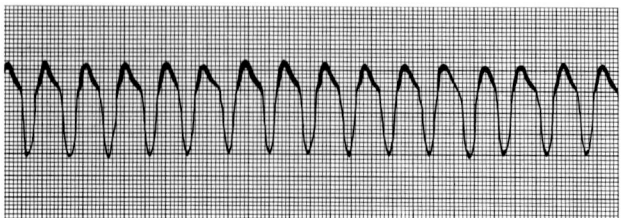	Rate: 100 to 250 BPM Rhythm: Regular P:QRS: P waves usually not identifiable PR interval: Not measured QRS complex: 0.12 sec or greater; bizarre shape	Treat if VT is sustained or if the client is experiencing symptoms. Treatment includes intravenous lidocaine and/or immediate defibrillation if the client is unconscious or unstable.

Table 28–1   (continued)

Rhythm/ECG Appearance	ECG Characteristics	Management
Ventricular fibrillation (VF, V fib)	Rate: Too rapid to count Rhythm: Grossly irregular P:QRS: No identifiable P waves PR interval: None QRS: Bizarre, varying in shape and direction	Immediate defibrillation.
Atrioventricular Conduction Blocks		
First-degree AV block	Rate: Usually 60 to 100 BPM Rhythm: Regular P:QRS: 1:1 PR interval: > 0.21 sec QRS complex: 0.06 to 0.10 sec	None required.
Second-degree AV block, type I (Mobitz I, Wenckebach)	Rate: 60 to 100 BPM Rhythm: Atrial regular; ventricular irregular P:QRS: 1:1 until P wave blocked with no subsequent QRS complex PR interval: Progressively lengthens in a regular pattern QRS complex: 0.06 to 0.10 sec; sudden absence of QRS complex	Monitoring and observation; Atropine if client is experiencing symptoms.
Second-degree AV block, type II (Mobitz II)	Rate: Atrial 60 to 100 BPM; Ventricular < 60 BPM Rhythm: Atrial regular; ventricular irregular P:QRS: Typically 2:1, may vary PR interval: Constant PR interval for each conducted QRS complex QRS complex: 0.06 to 0.10 sec	Atropine or isoproterenol; pacemaker therapy.
Third-degree AV block (Complete heart block)	Rate: Atrial 60 to 100 BPM; ventricular 15 to 60 BPM Rhythm: Atrial regular; ventricular regular P:QRS: No relationship between P waves and QRS complexes; independent rhythms PR interval: Not measured QRS complex: 0.06 to 0.10 sec if junctional escape rhythm; > 0.12 sec if ventricular escape rhythm	Immediate pacemaker therapy.

Sick Sinus Syndrome (Sinus Nodal Disease)   *Sick sinus syndrome (SSS)* results from sinus node disease or dysfunction that causes problems with impulse formation, transmission, and conduction. Sick sinus syndrome has many causes, including direct injury to sinus tissue during surgery, ischemic injury or infarct, fibrosis of conduction fibers that is associated with aging, and such drugs as digitalis, beta-blockers, and calcium channel blockers (Lounsbury & Frye, 1992).

ECG characteristics indicative of SSS include one or more of the following:

- Pathologic sinus bradycardia or sinus arrhythmia
- Sinus pauses or sinus arrest
- A predisposition toward developing **paroxysmal** supraventricular tachycardia (that is, supraventricular tachycardia with abrupt onset and termination).
- The development of a *bradycardia-tachycardia syndrome,* a combination of bradycardia alternating with tachydysrhythmia (most frequently atrial fibrillation)

Clinical manifestations may include a slow or variable heart rate and manifestations related to decreased cerebral and cardiovascular perfusion, such as a decreased level of consciousness, dizziness, syncope, memory loss, disorientation, hypotension, or fatigue.

Atrial and Supraventricular Dysrhythmias   When the conduction impulse originates in the atrial tissue outside the sinus node, the resulting rhythm is classified as an atrial or supraventricular rhythm. In these dysrhythmias, an ectopic pacemaker takes over, or overrides, the SA node. They may also occur when the SA node fails; an *escape rhythm* develops as a fail-safe mechanism to maintain the heart rate. There are a number of atrial and supraventricular dysrhythmias. The most common are premature atrial contractions, paroxysmal supraventricular tachycardia, atrial flutter, and atrial fibrillation. All of these rhythms may be paroxysmal.

Premature Atrial Contractions   A *premature atrial contraction (PAC)* is an ectopic atrial beat that occurs earlier than the next expected sinus beat. The mechanism of action is enhanced automaticity or a reentry phenomenon. PACs can occur in healthy persons as a result of excessive alcohol, caffeine, or nicotine intake, stress, or fatigue. Strong emotions also can precipitate PACs through the release of catecholamine. PACs may occur without an obvious cause and are common in the elderly (Fleg & Kennedy, 1982; Wajngarten, Grupi, Belloti, Da Luz, Azul, & Pileggi, 1990). Although PACs are not in themselves threats to the client's welfare, they are warnings of atrial irritability, and their presence frequently indicates or precipitates a more serious dysrhythmia. Other conditions that may cause PACs include myocardial infarction, heart failure, pericarditis, valvular disorders, hypoxemia, pul-

monary embolism, digitalis toxicity, hypokalemia, hypomagnesemia, and metabolic alkalosis.

The ECG tracing shows an interruption of the underlying rhythm with a premature complex that looks similar but is not identical to the underlying beats. The ectopic impulse of the PAC is usually conducted normally, resulting in the depolarization of the cardiac muscle and a normal QRS complex. Because the impulse comes from above the ventricles, it follows the normal conduction pathway through the ventricles, and the QRS complexes are narrow (unless there is a conduction delay within the ventricles). The P wave of PAC has a shape different from that of the normal P wave because its impulse comes from a site other than the sinus node. A *noncompensatory pause* usually follows a PAC as this ectopic beat resets the SA node rhythm. In some instances, the ectopic impulse may not be conducted to the rest of the cells; the result is a lone P wave without a QRS complex, or a *nonconducted PAC.*

Few manifestations are associated with PACs. If they occur frequently, the client may complain of palpitations or a fluttering sensation in the chest. Occasional to frequent early beats are noted on auscultating or palpating the pulse.

Paroxysmal Supraventricular Tachycardia   *Paroxysmal supraventricular tachycardia (PSVT)* is tachycardia of sudden onset and termination initiated by a reentry loop in or around the AV node; that is, an impulse reenters the same section of tissue over and over, causing multiple depolarizations.

PSVT may be caused by stimulation of the sympathetic nervous system and by hypermetabolic states, such as fever, sepsis, stress, and hyperthyroidism. Clients with heart disease, such as ischemic heart disease, myocardial infarction, rheumatic heart disease, myocarditis, cardiomyopathy, acute pericarditis, and Wolff-Parkinson-White (WPW) syndrome also are susceptible (Lounsbury & Fyre, 1992). Premature atrial or ventricular beats may also precipitate PSVT.

Clinical manifestations of PSVT are those of decreased cardiac output because of the rapid heart rate, inadequate ventricular filling time, and decreased coronary artery perfusion. These include complaints of palpitations and a "racing" heart, anxiety, dizziness, dyspnea, anginal pain, diaphoresis, extreme fatigue, and polyuria (urine output may reach up to 3 liters in the first few hours after PSVT onset).

Atrial Flutter   *Atrial flutter* is a rapid and regular atrial rhythm thought to result from an intra-atrial reentry mechanism. Causes include stimulation of the sympathetic nervous system through anxiety, caffeine and alcohol intake; thyrotoxicosis; coronary artery disease or myocardial infarction; pulmonary embolism; and abnormal conduction syndromes, such as Wolff-Parkinson-White

(WPW) syndrome. Older persons with rheumatic heart disease and/or valvular disease are especially vulnerable.

Clients with atrial flutter may be asymptomatic or complain of palpitations or a fluttering sensation in the chest or throat. If the ventricular rate is rapid, manifestations of decreased cardiac output, such as a decline in level of consciousness, hypotension, decreased urinary output, and cool, clammy skin, may be noted. Clients in atrial flutter may lose the benefit of the atria's contribution to cardiac output (atrial kick) because of inadequate atrial filling and contraction.

ECG characteristics include a "sawtooth" or "picket fence" appearance of the P waves, which are labeled flutter (F) waves. The atrial rate is very rapid, usually around 300 BPM. As a protective mechanism, many impulses are blocked at the AV node, and the ventricular rate is rarely greater than 150 to 170 BPM. Atrial flutter can usually be differentiated from atrial fibrillation by the regularity of the rhythm: The conduction of the ectopic impulses through the AV node is usually even, for example, 2 impulses to 1 QRS complex (2:1), 4 impulses to 1 QRS complex (4:1), or 6 impulses to 1 QRS complex (6:1). A constant conduction ratio results in a regular ventricular rhythm; the ventricular rhythm can be irregular if the conduction ratio varies. The ventricular rate usually ranges from 150 to 170 BPM in 2:1 conduction and 60 to 75 BPM for lower conduction ratios. The T wave is usually not identifiable because of an overriding F wave, and some F waves may be hidden in the QRS complex.

Atrial Fibrillation   *Atrial fibrillation* is chaotic ectopic atrial activity causing the atria to quiver, presenting as fibrillatory (f) waves instead of atrial contractions. It is believed that atrial reentry is the electrophysiologic mechanism for this ectopic activity. Extremely rapid atrial impulses bombard the AV node, resulting in an irregularly irregular ventricular response pattern. Atrial fibrillation may occur suddenly and recur, or it may persist as a chronic rhythm disturbance. Atrial fibrillation is commonly seen in clients with congestive heart failure mitral valve disease, rheumatic heart disease, coronary disease, hypertension, hyperthyroidism, and thyrotoxicosis.

Clinical manifestations of atrial fibrillation are related to the rate of the ventricular response. The client may have manifestations of decreased cardiac output and impaired tissue perfusion from loss of the atrial kick.

The specific ECG characteristics of atrial fibrillation include an irregularly irregular rhythm and the absence of identifiable P waves. The atrial rate is so rapid that it is not measurable. The ventricular rate varies.

The client with atrial fibrillation is at high risk for thromboemboli formation. Embolization of organ systems is a constant threat; the incidence of stroke is high.

Junctional Dysrhythmias   Rhythms that originate in AV nodal tissue are termed *junctional.* The AV junction is composed of the AV node and the bundle of His, which branches into the right and left bundle branches. An impulse arising from the AV junction may be a normal response to the failure of the higher pacemakers, as in a *junctional escape rhythm,* or it may be the result of abnormal mechanisms, such as altered automaticity. When the impulse arises from the AV junction, it may or may not be conducted back up to the atria. This conduction against the normal flow or pattern is termed *retrograde* conduction. The resulting retrograde atrial wave, called a P′ wave, may be located before, during, or after the QRS complex, depending on the rapidity of conduction. The P′ wave is inverted in some ECG leads because the impulse moves from the AV node up to the atria instead of from the SA node down toward the AV node. In addition, the P′R interval is shorter than normal (less than 0.12 sec). The QRS complex is typically narrow.

Causes of junctional rhythm may include digitalis toxicity, a quinidine reaction, or an overdose of beta-blockers or calcium channel blockers. Other causes of junctional rhythm are hypoxemia, hyperkalemia, increased vagal tone or damage to the AV node, myocardial infarction, and congestive heart failure. Clinically, the loss of synchronized atrial contraction and the atrial kick may affect cardiac output. In junctional tachycardia, the client may present with manifestations of decreased cardiac output and decreased myocardial tissue perfusion leading to ischemia; signs of heart failure may follow.

Premature junctional contractions (PJCs), as all premature complexes, occur before the next expected beat of the underlying rhythm. Isolated PJCs may be found in healthy people and are insignificant. *Junctional tachycardia* is a junctional rhythm with a rate greater than 60 BPM. The ventricular rate is usually less than 140 BPM. The mechanism of junctional tachycardia is due to enhanced automaticity. Both rhythms are most commonly associated with digitalis toxicity, hypoxia, ischemia, or electrolyte imbalances.

Ventricular Dysrhythmias

Ventricular dysrhythmias originate in the ventricles. Because the ventricles pump blood into the pulmonary and systemic vasculature, any disturbance in their rhythm can affect cardiac output and tissue perfusion. A wide and bizarre QRS complex (greater than 0.12 sec) is a characteristic feature of ventricular dysrhythmias. This occurs because the ventricular ectopic impulse begins and travels from outside the normal conduction pathway. Other characteristics include a P wave with no relationship to the QRS complex, an increased amplitude of the QRS complex, an abnormal ST segment, and a T wave that has an opposite deflection from that of the QRS complex.

Premature Ventricular Contractions   *Premature ventricular contractions (PVCs)* are ectopic ventricular beats that occur before the next expected beat of the underlying rhythm. They usually do not reset the atrial rhythm and are followed by a full compensatory pause. PVCs may be of no significance in people without cardiac disease. Frequent, recurrent, or multifocal PVCs indicate myocardial irritability and may precipitate lethal dysrhythmias. PVCs result from either enhanced automaticity or a reentry phenomenon. They may be triggered by anxiety or stress; tobacco, alcohol, or caffeine use; hypoxia, acidosis, and electrolyte imbalances; sympathomimetic drugs; ischemic heart disease, coronary artery disease, myocardial infarction, and congestive heart failure; mechanical stimulation of the heart (e.g., the insertion of a cardiac catheter); or reperfusion after thrombolytic therapy. The incidence of PVCs is greatest after damage to the myocardium from ischemia, infarction, hypertrophy, or infection. Ventricular dysrhythmias also are common in the older adult, though not always clinically significant in this population (Fleg & Kennedy, 1982; Wajngarten et al., 1990).

PVCs may be isolated events or demonstrate significant patterns. When the ventricular impulse is initiated from one ectopic site all PVCs look the same and are called *unifocal* PVCs; *multifocal* PVCs are initiated from different ectopic sites and therefore appear different on the ECG. *Ventricular bigeminy* is the presence of one PVC noted every other beat; a PVC noted every third beat is called *ventricular trigeminy*. Two PVCs in a row are called a *couplet* or *paired PVCs*; three PVCs in a row are called a *triplet* or a *salvo* and is a short run of *ventricular tachycardia*. The shape of consecutive PVCs may be all of the same shape (*monomorphic*) or of varying shapes (*polymorphic*).

The frequency and patterns of PVCs can provide indications of increasing irritability of the myocardium. The following are considered warning signs:

- PVCs that occur within the first 4 hours of a myocardial infarction

- Frequent PVCs of six or more per minute

- Couplets or triplets

- Multifocal PVCs

- R-on-T phenomenon (PVCs falling on the T wave)

Manifestations of PVCs depend on their frequency and on concomitant factors. In people without heart disease, isolated PVCs usually have minimal or no consequences and do not require treatment. Clients may complain of feeling their hearts "skip a beat" or of palpitations. By contrast, PVCs in clients with preexisting heart disease may indicate an abnormality of electrophysiologic mechanisms that may lead to lethal dysrhythmias and cardiac arrest. Any PVC is considered potentially lethal for clients suffering from ischemia or myocardial infarction.

Ventricular Tachycardia   *Ventricular tachycardia (VT; V tach)* is a rapid ventricular rhythm disturbance that is defined as three or more consecutive PVCs. VT may present in short bursts, or "runs," or it may persist for a long period of time (*sustained ventricular tachycardia*). The rate is greater than 100 BPM, and the rhythm is usually regular. The most common electrophysiologic mechanism responsible for VT is reentry. Factors that may predispose the client to VT include PVCs, myocardial ischemia and infarction, high levels of circulating catecholamines, sympathomimetic drugs, a prolonged QT interval, exercise, electrolyte disorders, rheumatic and valvular heart disease, cardiomyopathies, anorexia nervosa, antidysrhythmic therapy, digitalis toxicity, and reperfusion therapy.

Nonsustained VT may occur paroxysmally and convert back to an effective rhythm spontaneously. The client may experience a sensation of fluttering in the chest or complain of palpitations and brief shortness of breath. Clients in sustained VT may have manifestations of ineffective cardiac output and hemodynamic instability, including severe hypotension, a weak or nonpalpable pulse, and loss of consciousness. Allowed to continue, VT can rapidly deteriorate into ventricular fibrillation at any time. Sustained ventricular tachycardia is a medical emergency that requires immediate intervention to preserve life.

Ventricular Fibrillation   *Ventricular fibrillation (VF; V fib)* is defined as extremely rapid, chaotic ventricular ectopy causing the ventricles to quiver and cease contracting; the heart does not pump. This is known as **cardiac arrest;** it is a medical emergency requiring immediate intervention with cardiopulmonary resuscitation (CPR) measures. Death will follow the onset of VF within 4 minutes if the rhythm is not recognized and terminated, with a return to a perfusing rhythm.

VF is most commonly triggered by severe myocardial ischemia or infarction and occurs without warning 50% of the time (Conover, 1994). It is the terminal event in many disease processes or traumatic conditions. VF may be precipitated by a single PVC or result from the deterioration of VT. Other causes of VF include digitalis toxicity, reperfusion therapy, antidysrhythmic drugs, hypokalemia and hyperkalemia, hypothermia, metabolic acidosis, mechanical stimulation (as with the insertion of cardiac catheters or pacing wires), and electric shock.

Clinically, the loss of ventricular contraction translates as the absence of a pulse. The client loses consciousness and stops breathing as perfusion ceases. The ECG shows grossly irregular, bizarre complexes with no discernable rate or rhythm.

Atrioventricular Conduction Blocks

Conduction defects that cause delayed or blocked transmission of sinus impulse through the AV node are called *atrioventricular (AV) conduction blocks*. Delays in conduction may result from injured or diseased tissue in the SA node or the AV nodal area, or from an increase in vagal tone. AV conduction blocks vary in clinical severity from benign to severe. All conduction blocks are monitored for progression to a higher degree of block and more serious conduction problems.

First-Degree AV Block *First-degree AV block* is a benign conduction delay that poses no immediate threat to the client and requires no treatment. There are no clinical manifestations except a prolonged PR interval. Myocardial infarction is the most common cause of first degree block. Other causes include digitalis therapy or toxicity, complications from cardiac surgery, chronic heart disease, or drug effects. The ECG tracing features all of the characteristics of NSR, except that PR interval is greater than 0.20 seconds.

Second-Degree AV Block—Type I *Second-degree AV Block—Type I,* also known as *Mobitz I or Wenckebach,* is characterized by a repeating pattern in which PR intervals progressively lengthen until one QRS complex is not conducted, or *dropped.* The nonconduction of the P wave is due to a complete block of the atrial impulse at the AV node. Second-degree block may be caused by myocardial infarction, an electrolyte imbalance, drug toxicity (digitalis, procainamide, quinidine, propranolol, or verapamil), acute rheumatic infections, or myocarditis. Clinical manifestations are usually absent, unless the heart rate slows and compromises cardiac output.

Second-Degree AV Block—Type II *Second-degree AV block—Type II,* also called *Mobitz II,* demonstrates a combination of conduction defects: a complete block of the SA impulse down one bundle branch and an intermittent block of the impulse down the other branch. Type II heart block is usually seen in clients with coronary artery disease and anterior wall myocardial infarction. Other names for this block are *high-grade AV block* and *advanced AV block.*

The conduction disturbance results in nonconducted impulses that usually occur in a regular manner, most commonly with a P:QRS ratio of 2:1. This dysrhythmia presents with a consistent PR interval for each conducted QRS complex. The QRS complex may be normal or have a bundle branch block configuration (see the section below), depending on the location of the block. The manifestations of type II heart block depend on the ventricular rate; cardiac output decreases as ventricular rate slows.

Third-Degree AV Block *Third-degree AV block (complete heart block)* occurs when atrial impulses are completely blocked at the AV node and therefore cannot conduct to the ventricles. Total dissociation of the atrial and ventricular impulses results, with two completely independent rhythms. The ventricular impulse is an escape mechanism from either the junctional fibers (with a rate of 40 to 60 BPM) or a ventricular pacemaker with an inherent rate of 15 to 40 BPM. The width of the QRS complex depends on the location of the escape pacemaker. The further away from the conduction pathway, the further the ectopic impulse has to travel to depolarize the ventricles, and the wider the QRS complex.

Third-degree block can be caused by ischemia or damage to the AV node and is frequently associated with an inferior or anteroseptal myocardial infarction. Other causes include degenerative conduction system disease, damage to the conduction system during cardiac surgery, acute myocarditis, increased vagal tone, digitalis or propranolol toxicity; or electrolyte imbalances. Clinical manifestations are those associated with significant bradycardia and low cardiac output, such as light-headedness, confusion, and syncopal episodes (*Stokes-Adams attacks*). On auscultation, the S_1 heart sound varies in intensity because of the lack of coordination between atrial and ventricular contractions.

Third-degree AV block is life-threatening and requires immediate intervention to maintain an adequate cardiac output.

Bundle Branch Blocks

In *bundle branch blocks,* the right or left bundle branch fails to conduct impulses (Holloway, 1993). As a result, the impulse is conducted more slowly than normal through the ventricles. The appearance of a bundle branch block on the ECG varies according to whether the right or left bundle is affected, but the QRS is prolonged (> 0.12 sec) in either case. Typically, the client with bundle branch block has no clinical manifestations unless it is also associated with an atrioventricular block.

Collaborative Care

Treating the client with a cardiac dysrhythmia requires astute observations and often rapid treatment decisions. Recognizing lethal dysrhythmias is a matter of life and death. Collaboration of the nurse and physician is vital in providing comprehensive, high-quality, holistic care to these clients. Major goals of care include identifying the dysrhythmia, evaluating its effect on the client's physical and psychosocial well-being, and treating underlying causes which may involve correcting fluid and electrolyte or acid-base imbalances; treating hypoxia, pain, or anxiety; administering antidysrhythmic medications; and mechanical and surgical interventions.

Laboratory and Diagnostic Tests

There are no specific laboratory tests to document the presence of dysrhythmias. They may, however, indicate the presence of hypoxia, electrolyte imbalances, acid-base imbalances, or abnormal drug levels and thereby help pinpoint the cause of dysrhythmia.

Diagnostic tests include the electrocardiogram, cardiac monitoring, and electrophysiology studies.

Indications for Cardiac Monitoring

■ ■ ■

- Perioperative monitoring of heart rate and rhythm
- Detection and identification of dysrhythmias
- Monitoring the effects of cardiac and noncardiac diseases on the heart
- Monitoring clients experiencing or at risk for life-threatening conditions:
  a. Major trauma (especially cardiac trauma)
  b. Dissecting aneurysm
  c. Acute myocardial infarction
  d. Shock
  e. Other emergency conditions
- Evaluating the client's response to interventions:
  a. Pharmacologic therapies
  b. Postdiagnostic procedures
  c. Stress testing
  d. Electrophysiology studies
  e. Nonsurgical ablative techniques
  f. Percutaneous transluminal coronary angioplasty or cardiac catheterization
- Evaluating the client's response to surgical interventions:
  a. Surgical ablative techniques
  b. Pacemaker function
  c. Functioning of an automatic implantable cardioverter-defibrillator

---

Electrocardiogram The 12-lead ECG may be necessary for accurate diagnosis of the dysrhythmia. It also provides information about underlying causes of dysrhythmias, such as myocardial infarction or other myocardial disease. The ECG may also be used intermittently to monitor the effects of dysrhythmia treatment.

Cardiac Monitoring Cardiac monitoring allows continuous observation of the client's cardiac rhythm and is used in many different circumstances (see the accompanying box). Different types of ECG monitoring are employed for different situations.

Continuous Cardiac Monitoring Continuous monitoring of a client's cardiac rhythm is provided by a bedside and central monitoring station. Electrodes placed on the client's chest are attached to monitor cables connected to the bedside monitor. The client's heart rate and rhythm is visually displayed on a bedside monitor connected to a

central monitoring station. Central monitor stations allow simultaneous monitoring of multiple clients and privacy for the client. Alarms, found on both bedside and central monitors, are used to warn of potential problems such as very rapid or very slow heart rates. Alarm limits are preset by the nurse for the individual client. Procedure 28–1 describes how to place a client on cardiac monitoring.

Portable Cardiac Monitoring Distance ECG monitoring *(telemetry)* is another type of continuous monitoring frequently used on medical-surgical or cardiac units. Chest electrodes are connected to portable transmitters worn around the neck or waist; the client's cardiac rhythm is transmitted electronically to a central monitoring station for continuous monitoring. Telemetry allows the client the freedom to get out of bed and walk around while being monitored.

Frequently, clients may complain of palpitations or other heart symptoms but do not exhibit signs or symptoms during evaluation (e.g., in the hospital or in the doctor's office). Monitoring the heart rhythm outside the hospital or clinic setting is accomplished through *ambulatory* or *Holter monitoring*. The Holter monitor is used diagnostically to identify dysrhythmias that occur intermittently, to detect silent ischemia, to monitor the effects of medical and surgical therapy, and to assess pacemaker function. Electrodes are applied and the leads attached to the portable telemetry monitor. The client is able to leave the hospital because the telemetry unit records and stores all electrical activity. Clients requiring Holter monitoring are instructed to leave the electrode pads in place during the test, record any cardiac symptoms or events in a journal (such as chest pain, palpitations, syncope) and are told when to return to the clinic. After the prescribed time period, usually 48 to 72 hours, the client returns and the monitor is removed. Diary entries are compared to the recorded heart rhythms to identify the effects of dysrhythmias.

Electrophysiology Studies Cardiac *electrophysiology studies (EPSs)* provide useful information about the cardiac conduction system. EPS is used to analyze components of the heart's electrical system, identify sites of ectopic stimulation, and evaluate the effectiveness of treatment (Darling, 1994). EPS can be used as a diagnostic study or a therapeutic intervention.

In the electrophysiology laboratory, electrode catheters are guided by fluoroscopy into the heart through the femoral or brachial vein. The catheters document normal electrical activity and aberrant activity, locating the site of abnormal activity. Once the site has been located, appropriate treatment can be determined.

As a therapeutic intervention, the electrode catheter may be used to treat certain tachydysrhythmias by *overdrive pacing* (stimulating the client's heart rate to a rate faster than that of the tachydysrhythmia) in an attempt to

Procedure 28–1   Initiating Cardiac Monitoring

SUPPLIES

- Bedside monitor or telemetry unit with fresh battery
- Electrodes—self-adherent, pre-gelled, disposable
- Lead wires
- Monitor cable
- Razor, soap, and water
- Washcloth and towel
- Alcohol prep pads
- Dry gauze pads or ECG prep pads

BEFORE THE PROCEDURE

Explain to the client the reason for continuous ECG monitoring. Reassure the client that any changes in heart rhythm can be noted and immediate treatment initiated if necessary. Explain that loose or disconnected lead wires, poor electrode contact, excessive movement, electrical interference, or equipment malfunction may trigger alarms and alert the staff, allowing the problem to be corrected. Reassure the client he or she may move about, within activity restrictions, while on the monitor. Explain the skin preparation procedure. Provide for privacy, and drape the client appropriately.

PROCEDURE

1. Follow universal precautions.
2. Wash hands.
3. Check equipment for damage (i.e., fraying, bent, or broken wires). Connect lead wires to cable, and secure the connections.
4. Select electrode sites on the chest wall. The selection will depend on the lead to be monitored, the condition of the skin, and any incisions or catheters present.
5. If the chest is excessively hairy, shave a 4-by-4 inch area for each electrode.
6. Clean sites with soap and water, and dry thoroughly. Alcohol may be used to remove skin oils; allow the skin to dry for 60 seconds after use.
7. Gently abrade the site by rubbing with a dry gauze pad or ECG prep pad to remove dead skin cells, debris, and residue.
8. Open the electrode package; peel the backing from the electrode, and check to ensure that the center of the pad is moist with conductive gel.
9. Apply electrode pads to the client, pressing firmly to ensure contact.
10. Attach leads and position the cable with sufficient slack for the client's comfort. Place the telemetry unit (if used) in the client's gown pouch or pocket.
11. Assess the ECG tracing on the monitor, adjusting settings as needed.
12. Set ECG monitor alarm limits for the client, typically at 20 BPM higher and lower than the baseline rate. Turn alarms on, and leave on at all times. Assess the client immediately if an alarm is triggered.
13. Time and date pads with every change.
14. Wash hands.

AFTER THE PROCEDURE

Monitor the client periodically for comfort. Assess electrode and lead wire connections as needed. Remove and apply new pads every 24 to 48 hours or whenever the pad becomes dislodged or nonadherent. Clean gel residue from previous site, and document skin condition under the pads. Choose an alternative site if the skin appears irritated or blistered. ECG strips are documented according to unit policy and/or physician's order, as well as with changes in the cardiac rhythm or the client's condition (especially with complaints of chest pain, decreased level of consciousness, or changes in vital signs). Note on each ECG strip the date, time, client identification, monitor lead, duration of PR and QT intervals, and rhythm interpretation.

---

break the dysrhythmia's cycle, or to perform *ablative therapy* to destroy the ectopic site (Darling, 1994). See the section on ablative techniques following this discussion for further information.

Preparation and postprocedure care of the client undergoing EPS is similar to that of the client having a cardiac catheterization (see the box on page 1065). The client is provided with explanations of the procedure and sensations he or she is likely to experience. The client remains awake during the procedure but is given antianxiety medications or sedatives to reduce apprehension.

Many clients are afraid they will "fail the test" and need reassurance.

Intravenous heparin is given during the procedure. After the EP study is completed, the client is monitored according to routine protocols, which typically include maintaining bed rest for 4 to 6 hours and monitoring the involved limb for hematoma formation, bleeding, the presence of pulses, and signs of decreased tissue perfusion or thromboembolism. The client remains in the hospital for at least 24 hours postoperatively to monitor for complications.

Nursing Implications for Pharmacology: Antidysrhythmic Drugs

CLASS I DRUGS: FAST SODIUM CHANNEL BLOCKERS

Class IA

Quinidine (Cardioquin, Quinidex, Quinaglute, Duraquin)

Procainamide (Pronestyl, Procan SR, Pronestyl-SR)

Disopyramide (Norpace, Norpace CR)

Moricizine (Ethmozine)

Class IA, or quinidine-like, drugs inhibit fast sodium channels, decreasing the flow of sodium into the cell and prolonging the action potential. This results in depressed ventricular depolarization and automaticity and a prolonged refractory period. These drugs may be used to treat symptomatic or frequent PVCs, to treat supraventricular or ventricular tachycardias, and to prevent ventricular fibrillation.

Class IB

Lidocaine (Xylocaine)   Tocainide (Tonocard)

Mexiletine (Mexitil)   Phenytoin (Dilantin)

Class IB, or lidocaine-like, drugs decrease the refractory period but have little effect on automaticity. Drugs in this class are used primarily in treating ventricular dysrhythmias, including PVCs and ventricular tachycardia. They are also used to prevent ventricular fibrillation.

Class IC

Flecainide (Tambocor)   Propafenone (Rythmol)

Encainide (Enkaid)   Aprindine

Class IC drugs decrease automaticity and conduction through the AV node and ventricles; however, they also have significant *prodysrhythmic* (dysrhythmia-causing) effects. For this reason, they are used primarily to treat life-threatening ventricular tachycardia or fibrillation. They may also be employed when the client is experiencing supraventricular tachycardia that does not respond to other therapies.

CLASS II DRUGS: BETA-BLOCKERS

Esmolol (Brevibloc)

Propranolol (Inderal, Betachron, Ipran)

Acebutolol (Sectral)

Class II drugs are beta-blockers that decrease automaticity and conduction through the AV node. They also reduce the heart rate and myocardial contractility. They are used to treat supraventricular tachycardia and may help prevent ventricular fibrillation. These drugs may cause bronchospasm and are contraindicated for clients with asthma, chronic obstructive pulmonary disease (COPD), or other restrictive or obstructive lung diseases.

CLASS III DRUGS: POTASSIUM CHANNEL BLOCKERS

Sotalol (Betapace)   Bretylium (Bretylol)

Amiodarone   N-Acetylprocainamide
(Cordarone)   (NAPA)

Class III drugs, potassium channel blockers, prolong repolarization and the refractory period and decrease intraventricular conduction. Drugs in this class are used primarily to treat ventricular tachycardia and

---

Pharmacology

The goal of pharmacologic therapy is to suppress dysrhythmia formation. No drug has been found to be completely effective. Antidysrhythmic drugs may be used on a short-term basis for acute treatment of dysrhythmias or on a long-term basis to manage chronic conditions. The overall goal of therapy is to maintain an effective cardiac output by stabilizing cardiac rhythm.

Many different classes of drugs are used to treat cardiac dysrhythmias. They are divided according to their effects on the cardiac action potential. Most antidysrhythmic agents are class I drugs, or fast sodium channel blockers. This class is further divided into subclasses A, B, and C.

Class II drugs are beta-blockers, which decrease automaticity and conduction through the AV node. Class III agents are potassium channel blockers, and class IV are calcium channel blockers. Adenosine, a potassium channel opener, and digoxin fall into Class V. Digoxin, discussed later in the section on congestive heart failure, has electrophysiologic properties in addition to its effect on myocardial contraction. It slows conduction through the AV node and is a drug of choice to control chronic atrial fibrillation. The accompanying pharmacology box identifies common antidysrhythmic drugs within each class as well as nursing implications in caring for the client receiving an antidysrhythmic drug.

Pharmacology: Antidysrhythmic Drugs (continued)

ventricular fibrillation. Amiodarone may also be used for supraventricular tachycardias.

CLASS IV DRUGS: CALCIUM CHANNEL BLOCKERS

Verapamil (Calan, Isoptin, Verelan)

Diltiazem (Cardizem, Dilacor XR)

Calcium channel blockers block the flow of calcium into the cell, decreasing automaticity and conduction. They are used to manage supraventricular tachycardias. Like the beta-blockers, calcium channel blockers reduce myocardial contractility.

CLASS V DRUGS

Adenosine (Adenocard)   Digoxin

Class V drugs decrease conduction through the AV node and are used to treat supraventricular tachycardias.

Nursing Responsibilities

- Obtain baseline data, including vital signs, assessment of the cardiac rhythm (including rate, PR and QT intervals, and QRS duration), and physical assessment (especially cardiac, neurologic, and respiratory status).

- Assess the client's medication regimen to identify medications that may interfere with antidysrhythmic therapy.

- Monitor ECG to evaluate the effectiveness of therapy in stabilizing the dysrhythmia. Also assess for possible dysrhythmias precipitated by therapy.

- Observe for manifestations of drug toxicity, and notify the physician immediately should they occur:
  a. Procainimide—signs of heart failure and decreased cardiac output; prolonged PR interval, widening of the QRS complex; skin rash, myalgias or arthralgias, flulike symptoms
  b. Disopyramide—urinary retention, congestive heart failure, ocular pain
  c. Lidocaine—changes in neurologic status, such as agitation, confusion, dizziness, nervousness
  d. Amiodarone—pulmonary fibrosis (increasing dyspnea, cough) or hepatic dysfunction (changes in liver function tests, jaundice)
  e. Digoxin—anorexia, nausea, vomiting; blurred or double vision; yellow-green halos; new-onset dysrhythmias

- Use an infusion pump to administer intravenous infusions. Monitor the dose and assess its appropriateness (in mg/min or μg/kg/min).

Client and Family Teaching

- Take the drug exactly as prescribed. Do not skip or double doses. Check with your physician if a dose is missed.

- Take your pulse and record the rate daily before rising. Count the pulse for 1 full minute. Bring the record with you to each office or clinic appointment.

- Report the following to the physician: irregular pulse rate or rhythm, dizziness, eye pain, changes in vision, skin rashes, wheezing or other respiratory problems, changes in behavior.

Drugs that affect the autonomic nervous system are also used to treat dysrhythmias. Sympathomimetics, such as epinephrine, stimulate the heart, increasing both heart rate and contractility. Parasympatholytics (anticholinergic agents), such as atropine, are used to decrease vagal tone and speed up the heart rate. Magnesium sulfate is an unclassified drug that has been shown to be safe and effective in treating ventricular tachycardias (Horner, 1992).

It is important to remember that all antidysrhythmic drugs can also precipitate dysrhythmias, although the exact triggering mechanisms are unknown (Imperial, 1993). Nursing care includes identifying clients at high risk for developing dysrhythmias and close monitoring of all clients receiving cardiac drugs.

Countershock

Countershock is used to interrupt cardiac rhythms that compromise cardiac output and the client's welfare. Delivery of a direct current charge causes all cells of the heart to depolarize at the same time. This simultaneous depolarization may halt the offending rhythm and allow the sinus node to recover control of impulse formation. There are two types of countershock therapy: synchronized cardioversion and defibrillation.

Procedure 28–2   Elective Synchronized Cardioversion

SUPPLIES

- Cardioverter-defibrillator with an ECG cable and monitor
- Conductive gel pads or paste
- Dry gauze pads
- Emergency drug kit with lidocaine, epinephrine, bretylium, procainamide, and sodium bicarbonate
- Emergency resuscitation equipment, including oxygen tubing, flow meter, oxygen supply, and bag-valve mask device (e.g., Ambu-Bag)

PREPROCEDURE

Explain to the client that the purpose of the procedure is to restore an effective cardiac rhythm. Describe the procedure in simple, nonthreatening terms. Advise the client that he or she may feel some discomfort with each countershock but that a sedative will be given to minimize the discomfort. Witness the client's signature on an informed consent form for this procedure. Document the client's preprocedure rhythm on an ECG strip. Ensure a patent intravenous access site for emergency drug administration. Keep the client NPO for the specified period prior to the procedure (8 to 12 hours). Assess acid-base and electrolyte levels (especially potassium, magnesium, and calcium) and digitalis level if appropriate. Report any abnormalities to the physician prior to the procedure. Document vital signs, level of consciousness, and peripheral pulses for baseline data. Administer the pre-

scribed sedative, and provide for client safety. Remove any medication patches from the client's chest and all metallic objects. Remove dentures if they do not fit well; some physicians, however, prefer that dentures be left in place to facilitate airway management. Place the client in a supine position, and provide for privacy.

PROCEDURE

1. Follow universal precautions.
2. Wash hands.
3. Turn on the cardioverter-defibrillator and ECG monitor.
4. Connect the client's ECG cable to the cardioverter unit. Select a lead with prominent R waves for monitoring.
5. Set the cardioverter unit to "synchronize" mode. Observe the ECG waveform on the monitor for indications of synchronization, such as a flashing bold line or a blip. Many units also display the message "synchronized mode" on the monitor.
6. Place conductive pads on the client's chest below the right clavicle to the right of the sternum and in the midaxillary line on the left. If using conductive paste, spread it evenly on the defibrillator paddles.
7. Turn on the ECG recording strip for a continuous printout during the procedure.
8. **Charge the paddles to the prescribed energy dose.** The machine will beep to indicate that the selected energy level has been reached and that the paddles are ready for discharge.

9. The paddles are applied firmly to the chest over the conductive pads by the physician.
10. If the client is using oxygen, turn it off and remove it.
11. Ensure that no one is touching the client or the bed prior to discharge of the electrical shock.
12. The buttons on the paddles are depressed simultaneously and held in the depressed position until the shock is delivered. There may be a slight delay as the machine synchronizes with the R wave.
13. Assess the client's status and ECG rhythm. Assure a patent airway and the presence of a pulse.
14. The procedure may be repeated if unsuccessful. The energy level is usually increased with each attempt.
15. Remove the conductive pads. Using the dry gauze pad, clean paste from the client's chest and the paddles.
16. Wash hands.

POSTPROCEDURE

Assess the client for a return of consciousness from the sedative or cardioversion. Evaluate neurologic, cardiovascular, and respiratory status after the procedure. Assess for possible complications, including emboli (especially cerebral), respiratory depression, and dysrhythmias. Document the postcardioversion rhythm strip. Assess the client's skin for burns. Document the procedure and the client's response in the medical record.

Synchronized Cardioversion   *Synchronized cardioversion* involves the delivery of a direct electrical current synchronized with the client's rhythm. This synchronization of the shock with the client's QRS complex protects the heart's vulnerable period during repolarization, when a shock can precipitate ventricular fibrillation. Cardioversion is usually performed as an elective procedure to treat supraventricular tachycardia, atrial fibrillation, atrial flutter, or even a hemodynamically stable ventricular tachy-cardia.

The nurse assists the physician performing cardiover-sion by preparing the client before the procedure; obtain-ing any laboratory tests ordered; obtaining and docu-menting ECG strips prior to, during, and after treatment; setting up the equipment; and monitoring the client's re-sponse. Procedure 28–2 describes the synchronized car-dioversion procedure.

Clients in atrial fibrillation who are cardioverted are at high risk for thromboembolism. Loss of atrial contraction during atrial fibrillation causes blood to pool in the atria, increasing the risk of clot formation. If the cardioversion is successful and the atria begin to contract, clots may be dislodged from the atrial wall and embolize to the pul-monary or systemic circulation. If possible, the client is treated with anticoagulants for at least 3 weeks before car-dioversion is attempted.

Defibrillation   Unlike the carefully synchronized car-dioversion procedure, *defibrillation* is an emergency treat-ment that delivers a direct current charge without regard to the cardiac cycle. The client in ventricular fibrillation should be immediately defibrillated as soon as the dys-rhythmia is recognized. Early defibrillation has been shown to improve survival of clients experiencing VF (American Heart Association [AHA], 1994).

Defibrillation can be delivered by external or internal paddles. Conductive gel pads or paste is applied, and ex-ternal paddles are placed on the chest wall at the apex and base of the heart (Figure 28–7). Internal paddles are placed directly on the heart to deliver the shock and may be used in the operating room, emergency room, or criti-cal care units. Internal defibrillation is performed only by a physician, but external defibrillation may be performed by any health care provider who has been trained in the procedure. Nurses in critical care units are trained in this technique and may defibrillate clients in emergency situ-ations. See Procedure 28–3 on page 1040.

Pacemaker Therapy

A **pacemaker** is a pulse generator used to provide an elec-trical stimulus to the heart when the heart fails to gener-ate or conduct its own at a rate that can maintain an ade-quate cardiac output. The pacemaker is connected to one or more electrodes passed intravenously into the heart or sutured directly to the epicardium. The electrodes sense the intrinsic electrical activity of the heart and provide an electrical stimulus when necessary (pacing).

Pacemakers are a mainstay in treating transient and permanent conduction defects. They are indicated in the treatment of both bradydysrhythmias and tachydysrhyth-mias, temporary problems of conduction (such as those that occur after cardiac surgery), or as a long-term inter-vention for conditions such as AV block.

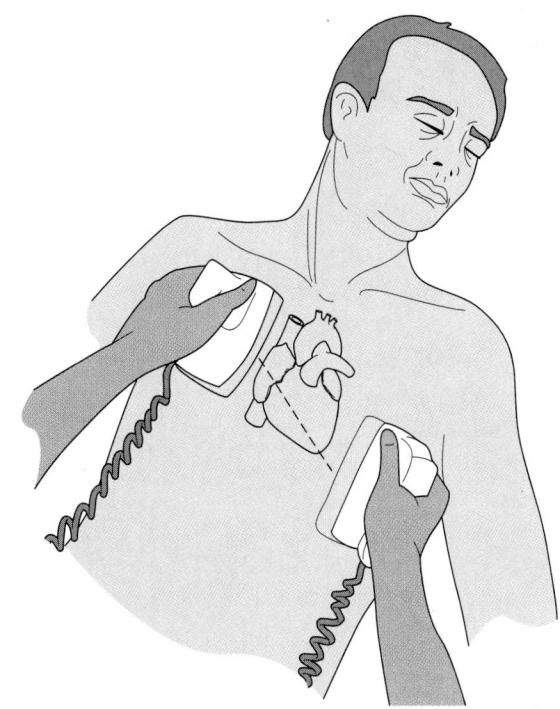

Figure 28–7   Placement of paddles for defibrillation.

Temporary pacemakers are devices that temporarily take over the electrical stimulation of the heart. Tempo-rary pacing is accomplished by attaching an external pacemaker box to an electrode threaded intravenously into the right ventricle, to temporary pacing wires im-planted during cardiac surgery, or via external conductive pads placed on the chest wall for emergency pacing.

Permanent pacemaker electrodes may be sewn directly onto the heart (*epicardial* placement) or passed transve-nously into the heart (*endocardial* placement). Epicardial pacemakers are attached to an internal pulse generator placed in a subcutaneous pocket either in the subclavian space or abdominal wall (Figure 28–8). This approach re-quires that the heart be surgically exposed. Placement of a transvenous (endocardial) pacemaker requires only local anesthesia. The pacemaker leads are positioned in the right heart via the cephalic, subclavian, or jugular vein (Figure 28–9). A subcutaneous pocket is formed under the clavicle for placement of the pulse generator (Haskin, 1989).

Pacemakers are programmed to stimulate either the atria, the ventricles, or both. *Sensing* describes the pace-maker's ability to detect the heart's own beats. When the pacemaker senses a heart rate within preprogrammed limits, it provides no electrical stimuli. *Pacing* is the pace-maker's ability to initiate electrical activity to stimulate the heart to contract. Pacing occurs when the client's heart rate falls below the pacemaker's programmed rate.

Procedure 28–3 Emergency External Defibrillation

SUPPLIES

- Cardioverter-defibrillator with ECG cable and monitor
- Conductive gel pads or paste
- Dry gauze pads
- Emergency cart with drug kit including lidocaine, epinephrine, bretylium, procainamide, sodium bicarbonate, pacemaker, and airway management equipment
- Emergency resuscitation equipment: oxygen tubing, flow meter, oxygen supply, and bag-valve mask device (e.g., Ambu-Bag)

PREPROCEDURE

Verify the presence of a lethal dysrhythmia, such as pulseless VT, VF, or asystole. Initiate the cardiac arrest (code) procedure, and begin CPR until the emergency cart and defibrillator are brought to the bedside. Place the client in the supine position on a firm surface. Reverify the client's rhythm.

PROCEDURE

1. Turn on the defibrillator, and set it in defibrillation mode.
2. Turn ECG recording on for a continuous printout of events during the procedure.
3. Set the energy level and charge the paddles according to advanced cardiac life support (ACLS) protocols. Initial defibrillation is usually performed at 200 joules.
4. Place conductive pads on the client's chest, or spread conductive paste evenly on the paddles.
5. Position the paddles, holding them firmly on the chest wall.
6. **Ensure that no one is touching the client or the bed. State, "All clear."**
7. Depress the button on each paddle simultaneously to discharge the energy.
8. Evaluate the cardiac rhythm and the presence of a pulse after each defibrillation attempt.

9. If the first attempt is unsuccessful, repeat the procedure, increasing the energy level to 300 joules and 360 joules for successive attempts. Reapply conductive paste as necessary.
10. If unsuccessful after three defibrillation attempts, implement ACLS protocols.

POSTPROCEDURE

If the dysrhythmia is successfully converted, evaluate and support the client's neurologic, cardiovascular, and respiratory status. Monitor and titrate any intravenous infusions initiated during the procedure as ordered. Maintain ventilatory support as needed. Evaluate the client's skin for the presence of burns. Obtain blood for laboratory studies as ordered. Monitor vital signs and ECG continuously. Transfer the client to the intensive care unit (ICU) as indicated. Provide support and information to the client and family.

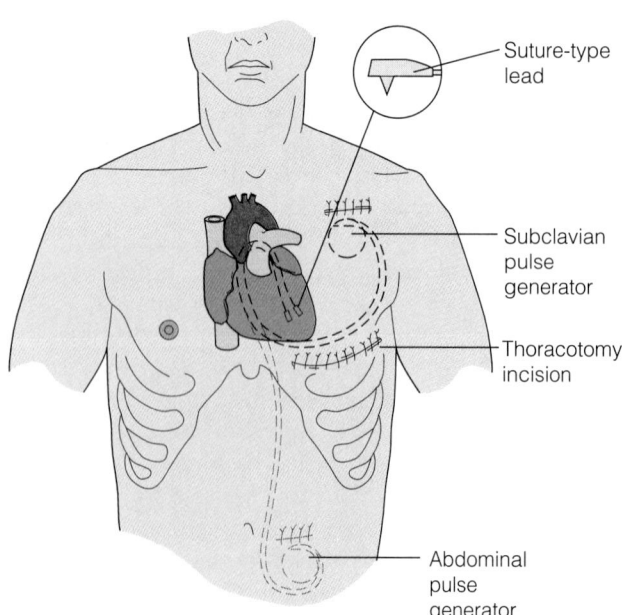

Figure 28–8 Placement of a permanent epicardial pacemaker. The pulse generator may be located in subcutaneous pockets in the subclavian or abdominal regions.

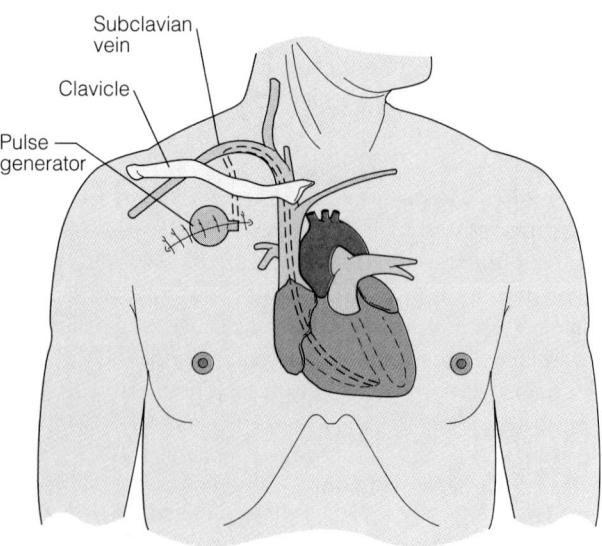

Figure 28–9 Placement of a permanent transvenous (endocardial) pacemaker into the right ventricle via the subclavian vein.

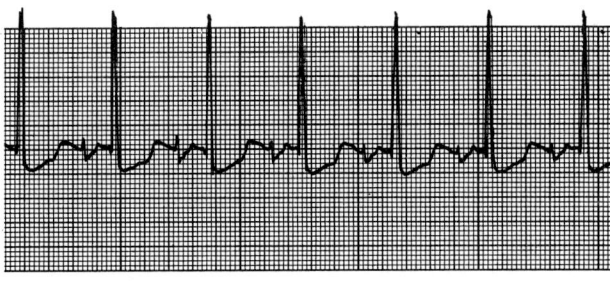

A

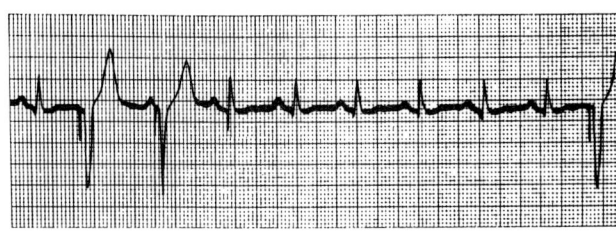

B

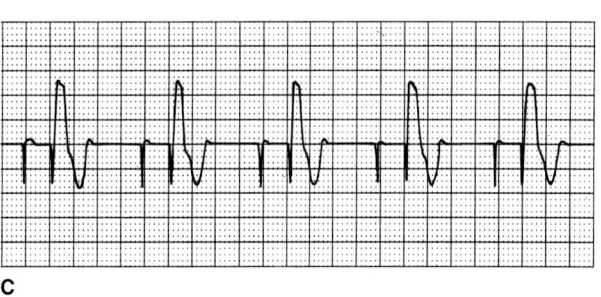

C

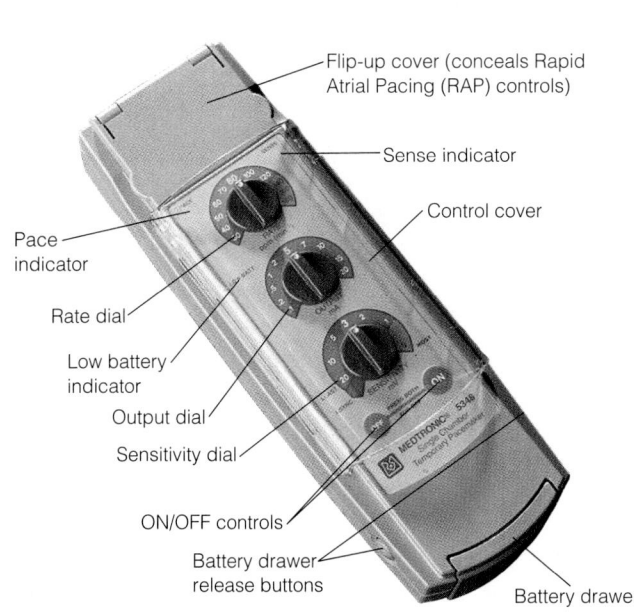

Flip-up cover (conceals Rapid
Atrial Pacing (RAP) controls)

Sense indicator

Control cover

Pace
indicator

Rate dial

Low battery
indicator

Output dial

Sensitivity dial

ON/OFF controls

Battery drawer
release buttons

Battery drawer

Figure 28–10 Programmable settings on a temporary
pacemaker.

Figure 28–11 Pacing artifacts. *A,* Atrial pacing and ventricular sensing. Note the pacer spike preceding the P wave.
B, Ventricular demand pacing. Note the absence of pacer
spikes when the client's natural rhythm predominates. *C,* Atrial
and ventricular pacing. Note the pacer spikes preceding both
P waves and QRS complexes.

Atrial pacing is used for clients with sinus node dysfunction who have reliable conduction through and below the AV node. Atrial stimulation sends the impulse
down the normal conduction pathway to stimulate the
ventricles. *Ventricular pacing* stimulates only the ventricles
to produce a contraction and is often used for AV conduction blocks. *Atrioventricular sequential pacing* stimulates both chambers of the heart in sequence. The benefit
of AV pacing is that it imitates the normal sequence of
atrial contraction followed by ventricular contraction and
preserves the atrial contribution to cardiac output.

Pacemakers are programmed by rate, sensitivity, voltage output, and special functions (Figure 28–10). The
rate control simply directs the pacemaker to fire at the set
rate. The *sensitivity control* allows the pacemaker to be set
either on demand, so that it does not compete with the
heart but fires only when it senses failure of the heart's intrinsic rate, or in *asynchronous* mode. In this setting, the
pacemaker fires at a fixed rate regardless of the client's
own beats. The *output control* regulates the amount of energy used to stimulate the heart muscle. Generally, the
output control is set at the lowest possible setting to provide *capture,* the contraction of the heart due to the pacer
stimulus. Newer rhythm control devices can be programmed to provide for more complex client needs.

Pacing is detected on the ECG strip by the presence of
pacing artifact (Figure 28–11). A sharp spike is noted before the P wave with atrial pacing, and before the QRS

complex with ventricular pacing. Pacing spikes are seen
before both the P wave and QRS complex in AV sequential pacing. Capture is noted if there is a contraction of the
chamber immediately following the pacer spike. Problems in sensing, pacing, and capture are noted in Table
28–2.

Care of the client with a temporary or permanent pacemaker focuses on monitoring for pacemaker malfunctioning, maintaining safety (see the box on page 1044), and
preventing infection and postoperative complications.
Postoperative nursing care for the client after a pacemaker
implant is outlined in the box on page 1046.

Other Therapies

In addition to pharmacologic interventions and pacemaker insertion, other therapeutic measures may be employed to treat dysrhythmias. For clients with supraventricular tachycardias, vagal maneuvers that stimulate the
parasympathetic nervous system may be used to slow the
heart rate. These maneuvers include *carotid sinus massage*

Text continues on page 1044

Table 28–2   Potential Pacemaker Problems and Strategies for Correction

Sample ECG Appearance

UNDERSENSING

Device fails to detect existing cardiac depolarizations, therefore competes with the native rhythms.

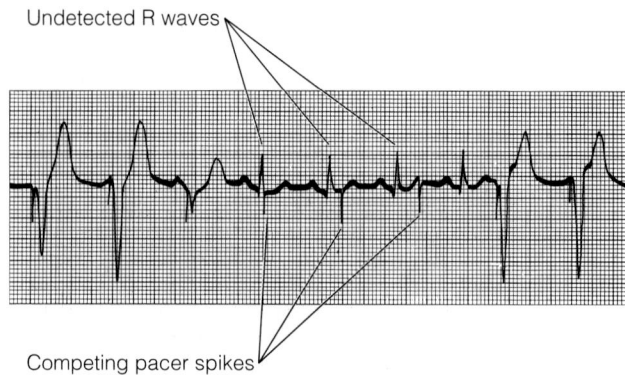

Undetected R waves

Competing pacer spikes

OVERSENSING

Device detects noncardiac electrical events and interprets them as cardiac depolarizations, therefore is wrongly inhibited from pacing.

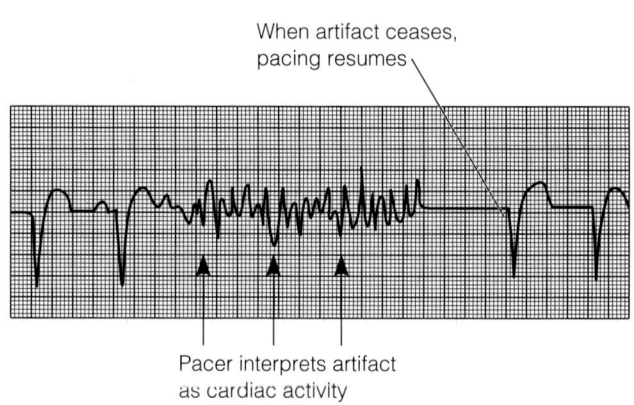

When artifact ceases, pacing resumes

Pacer interprets artifact as cardiac activity and fails to fire

NONCAPTURE

Device emits stimuli which fail to depolarize the myocardium.

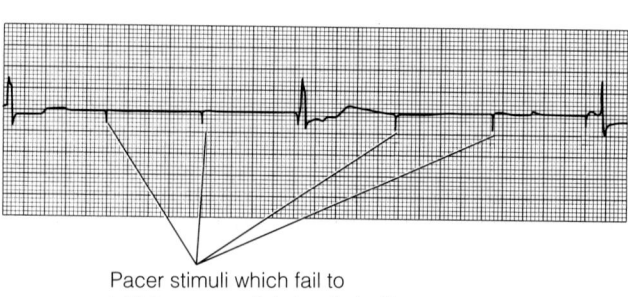

Pacer stimuli which fail to initiate myocardial depolarization

Note: From "Cardiac Rhythm Control Devices" (p. 92) by C. L. Witherell, 1994, *Critical Care Nursing Clinics of North America, 6*(1).

Table 28–2 (continued)

Some Possible Clinical Consequences	Some Possible Causes	Corrective Measures
Competition with a native rhythm. Stimulation of dysrhythmias ("R-on-T").	Lead disconnected from pacer or from viable myocardium.	Check connection of lead to pacer.
	Sensitivity set too low.	Increase sensitivity (turn sensing control to a SMALLER number).
	Lead fracture.	Reposition or change lead.
	Low battery.	Change battery.
Pacemaker-dependent clients receive no stimuli from the pacemaker, producing a pause in rhythm and reduction in cardiac output.	Electrical potential caused by noncardiac muscle contraction (especially pectorals) is detected and misinterpreted by the device.	Decrease sensitivity (turn sensing control to a LARGER number).
	Sensitivity set too high.	
	Interference from electrical sources (ungrounded equipment, short circuits) is detected and misinterpreted by the device.	Remove all ungrounded electrical equipment or have it evaluated by hospital engineers.
Pacemaker-dependent clients receive no stimuli from the pacemaker, producing a pause in rhythm and reduction in cardiac output.	Lead disconnected from pacer or from viable myocardium.	Check connection of lead to pacer.
	Output set too low in the noncaptured chamber.	Increase output in the noncaptured chamber.
	Lead fracture.	Reposition or change lead.
	High pacing threshold due to medication or metabolic changes.	Alter medication regimen, correct metabolic changes.
	Low battery.	Change battery.

Maintaining Safety for Clients with External Pacemakers

■ ■ ■

- Ensure that all electrical equipment has a three-wire grounded plug; do not use adapters or extension cords.

- Do not allow the client to use ungrounded electrical equipment, such as hair dryers, curling irons, or plug-in razors.

- Encourage the use of battery-powered equipment.

- Remove any damaged electrical equipment from the client's unit, including equipment that
  a. Has been abused (e.g., has been dropped or in which liquid has been spilled).
  b. From which anyone has received a shock.
  c. Has frayed, worn, or otherwise damaged electrical cords or plugs.
  d. Has other evidence of impaired function, such as a hot smell during use or control knobs that are loose or do not consistently produce the expected response.

- Wear plastic or rubber gloves when handling pacer electrodes or wires.

- Insulate pacemaker terminals and pacing wires with nonconductive, moistureproof material.

- Test the pacemaker battery prior to use.

- Keep a spare pacemaker, cable, batteries, and battery tester available at all times.

- Immediately report any apparent deviation from expected pacemaker function.

Note. Adapted from "Electrical Hazards in the Cardiac Care Unit" (p. 811) by G. Bashein and S. A. Stephen, in *Cardiac Nursing* (2nd ed.) by S. G. Underhill, S. L. Woods, E. S. S. Froelicher, and C. J. Halpenny (Eds.), 1989, Philadelphia: Lippincott.

and the *Valsalva maneuver.* Carotid sinus massage is performed only by a physician with the client on continuous cardiac monitoring. The Valsalva maneuver, forced exhalation against a closed glottis (e.g., bearing down) increases intrathoracic pressure and vagal tone, slowing the pulse rate.

Cardiac mapping and ablative therapy are used by the cardiologist or the cardiac surgeon to locate and destroy the effects of an ectopic impulse. These diagnostic and therapeutic measures can be performed in the cardiac catheterization laboratory or the operating suite. *Cardiac mapping* is a technique used to identify the site of earliest impulse formation in the atria or the ventricles. Intracardiac and extracardiac catheter electrodes and computer technology are used to pinpoint the ectopic site on a map of the heart. These same catheters can be used to deliver the ablative intervention.

Ablative therapy is the destruction, removal, or isolation of the ectopic focus. It can be performed using a variety of techniques: cryoablation, radiofrequency ablation, direct current ablation, or laser ablation.

- In *cryoablation,* a cooled nitrous oxide probe is applied directly to freeze and destroy the ectopic site.

- In *radiofrequency ablation,* low-power, high-frequency alternating current is used to deliver phased amounts of energy to destroy the ectopic site.

- In *direct current ablation,* a localized electric shock is used to destroy the ectopic site.

- In *laser ablation,* pulsed laser energy is used to destroy electrically active tissue.

Radiofrequency ablation is the most effective catheter ablation method (Finkelmeier, 1994).

Anticoagulants, such as aspirin or warfarin sodium, may be started after ablative procedures to decrease the possibility of clot formation at the ablation site.

Surgery

Surgical intervention may be used either to cure the dysrhythmia, as in surgical ablative or resection techniques, or to control symptoms, as in the surgical insertion of a pacemaker or automatic implantable cardioverter-defibrillator (AICD).

Surgical ablative techniques are used most often for clients whose dysrhythmias arise from infarcted tissue. Cardiac mapping is performed to locate the ectopic site, and a *cryoprobe* of liquid nitrogen is then applied to destroy the electrically active tissue. Alternatively, the ectopic tissue may be surgically excised.

Automatic Implantable Cardioverter-Defibrillator (AICD)

Sudden cardiac death from dysrhythmias affects more than 450,000 people a year in the United States (Moser, Crawford, & Thomas, 1993). The *automatic implantable cardioverter-defibrillator (AICD)* is a device that recognizes life-threatening changes in the client's cardiac rhythm and automatically delivers an electric shock to convert the dysrhythmia back into a normal rhythm. The AICD has pacing and sensing electrodes placed on or within the myocardium. The electrodes are attached to the cardioverter-defibrillator device, which is placed in an abdominal pocket. The AICD is used for clients with recurrent ventricular tachycardia that remains unresponsive to pharmacologic therapy or ablative techniques. It is also used for people who have survived sudden cardiac death due to a tachydysrhythmia not associated with an acute myocardial infarction. Surgery is required to implant the device, although nonsurgical approaches are being investigated (Moser et al., 1993).

The AICD is programmed to sense a change in heart rate or rhythm. When it detects a potentially lethal rhythm, it shocks the heart to convert the rhythm. The device can be programmed or reprogrammed at the bedside as necessary. The lithium-powered battery must be surgically replaced every 5 years.

The AICD is turned off for about 7 days postoperatively to allow the electrodes to adhere to the heart muscle. It may also be temporarily turned off if it needs reprogramming or if it malfunctions. During these times the client is at risk for dysrhythmias and may need external defibrillation or cardioversion.

Nursing care of the AICD client includes both preimplant and postimplant education. Postoperative care is similar to that for the client who has undergone pacemaker implant (see the box on page 1046).

Nursing Care

Caring for the client with cardiac dysrhythmias requires the ability to recognize and identify dysrhythmias and familiarity with appropriate interventions. Nursing care centers around reducing the effects of the dysrhythmia on cardiac output, monitoring the client's response to therapy, and client teaching. The urgency of intervention depends on how well the client tolerates the dysrhythmia and its potential adverse effects.

It is vital to assess the client before treating any suspected dysrhythmia. What appears to be ventricular tachycardia on the monitor may be a client tapping the electrode pad or brushing the teeth. Apparent asystole on the monitor may be a sleeping client whose electrode patch has come loose. Similarly, a heart rate of 52 BPM may be normal for some clients and not affect their functioning at all.

Decreased Cardiac Output

Dysrhythmias can potentially cause a decrease in cardiac output. Tachycardia reduces diastolic filling time, affecting cardiac output and coronary artery perfusion. The loss of atrial kick from the presence of junctional rhythms, atrial fibrillation, or AV blocks also decreases ventricular filling and may adversely affect clients with severe heart disease. Bradycardias decrease cardiac output if the stroke volume does not increase to compensate for the low heart rate. In ventricular fibrillation, the loss of ventricular contractions results in the absence of cardiac output.

Selected nursing interventions with rationales follow:

- Assess the client for clinical manifestations of decreased cardiac output: decreased level of consciousness; tachycardia; tachypnea; hypotension; diaphoresis; decreased urine output; cool, clammy, mottled skin; pallor or cyanosis; decreased peripheral pulses. *Clinical manifestations of decreased cardiac output may be subtle at first. The earliest sign may be a neurologic change. Early identification of decreased cardiac output can facilitate aggressive treatment and correction of the underlying cause, preventing further deterioration.*

- Monitor ECG rhythm and post ECG strip every shift and when rhythm changes occur. *Documentation of the ECG rhythms helps evaluate the client's status, provides a record for treatment rationales, and monitors progression of the disease state.*

- Assess vital signs every 15 minutes during acute dysrhythmic episodes and during cardiac drug infusions. *Vital signs provide an objective record of the client's response and tolerance of the dysrhythmia. Cardiac drugs can adversely affect both heart rate and blood pressure, causing further decline in cardiac output.*

- Assess serum electrolyte levels, especially potassium, calcium, and magnesium, and digitalis and antiarrhythmic drug levels as ordered. Report abnormal values. *The cardiac action potential depends on a normal electrolyte balance. Imbalances affect cardiac depolarization and repolarization and may cause dysrhythmias. Assessing serum levels of antidysrhythmic drugs is important to prevent toxicity and subsequent dysrhythmias. Clients with renal or hepatic dysfunction are at high risk for toxicity, as are older adults.*

- Assess clients with sinus tachycardia for underlying causes. *Sinus tachycardia is frequently a compensatory response to the body's demand for oxygen. Assess the client for signs of hypovolemia, pain, fever, anemia, or anxiety. Provide interventions appropriate to the cause.*

- Be prepared to administer antidysrhythmic medications by the appropriate route, depending on the cause of the dysrhythmia and how well the client tolerates the dysrhythmia. *Emergency drugs should always be readily available, especially on units with high-risk clients. Bradycardias are often treated with atropine; tachydysrhythmias may be treated with digitalis, adenosine, or verapamil. Premature ventricular contractions or ventricular tachycardia are treated initially with lidocaine. Epinephrine is used for cardiac arrest.*

- If appropriate, instruct the client to perform the Valsalva maneuver (bear down as if straining or coughing) for supraventricular tachycardia or ventricular tachycardia without angina. *Vagal maneuvers stimulate the parasympathetic system and may terminate some dysrhythmias. The Valsalva maneuver is contraindicated for clients experiencing chest pain with the dysrhythmia.*

Nursing Care of the Client Having a Permanent Pacemaker Implant

PREOPERATIVE CARE

- Assess the client and family's knowledge and understanding of the procedure, clarifying and elaborating on existing knowledge as needed. *The client may need the pacemaker for an acute or chronic condition. Fears must be dealt with in a constructive and supportive manner. Emotional and informational support helps the client develop a realistic outlook and accept pacer therapy.*

- Position ECG monitor electrodes away from potential incision sites. *This helps prevent skin breakdown before surgery.*

- Teach postoperative exercises, including range-of-motion (ROM) exercises for the affected side, coughing and deep breathing, and turning. *ROM exercises of the affected arm and shoulder prevent stiffness and impaired function following pacemaker insertion. Turning, coughing, and deep-breathing exercises help prevent postoperative complications.*

- Prepare the client for surgery: Verify that informed consent for the procedure has been obtained; document any allergies; obtain ordered laboratory studies; keep the client NPO after midnight; insert an intravenous line; provide a surgical scrub to the area if ordered; and administer prescribed preoperative medications. *Depending on the type of pacemaker, routine preoperative protocols may vary. Local anesthesia is used for insertion of permanent transvenous (endocardial) pacemakers, whereas general anesthesia and a thoracotomy is necessary for epicardial pacemakers.*

POSTOPERATIVE CARE

- Monitor vital signs, including temperature, per postoperative protocols. *Assessment of vital signs provides important information about the hemodynamic status of the client. The temperature is monitored to assess for possible signs of infection.*

- Obtain a chest X-ray as ordered. *A postoperative chest X-ray is used to determine the location of electrodes and detect possible complications, such as pneumothorax or pleural effusion.*

- Administer analgesia and position the client for comfort. In the initial postoperative period, restrict movement of the affected arm and shoulder. *Restricted movement minimizes pain, but the client will have some discomfort following the procedure.*

- Assist the client to perform gentle ROM exercises at least three times daily, beginning 24 hours after transvenous pacemaker implantation. *Initial activity restriction allows the leads to become anchored and helps prevent dislodging.*

- Keep the incision clean and dry, assessing for redness, swelling, warmth, approximation of wound edges, and drainage. *Manifestations of a wound infection should be reported.*

- Monitor pacemaker function with cardiac monitoring or intermittent ECGs. *This is important to evaluate pacemaker function.*

- Report any of the following pacemaker problems to the physician:
  a. Failure to pace. *This may indicate battery depletion, damage or dislodgement of pacer wires, or inappropriate sensing.*
  b. Failure to capture (the pacemaker stimulus is not followed by ventricular depolarization). *The electrical output of the pacemaker may not be adequate, or the lead may be dislodged.*
  c. Improper sensing (the pacemaker is firing or not firing, regardless of the intrinsic rate). *This places the client at risk for decreased cardiac output and dysrhythmias caused by the pacemaker.*
  d. Runaway pacemaker (a pacemaker firing at a rapid rate). *This may by due to generator malfunction or problems with sensing.*

- Be prepared to assist the physician with cardioversion. Prepare the client according to hospital protocol. *Elective or emergency cardioversion is a treatment of choice for certain dysrhythmias. Be sure to provide explanations of the procedure to the client to alleviate anxiety. Make sure emergency equipment is at hand.*

- On recognizing ventricular fibrillation, begin emergency procedures. Call for help. Begin CPR until a defibrillator is available. Initiate ACLS protocols. The client should be defibrillated as soon as a trained provider is available. Assist the code team as needed. *The ultimate cause of decreased cardiac output is cessation of effective ventricular contractions. Immediate resuscitation is required. Prepare for the ever-present possibility of cardiac arrest by reviewing emergency procedures on a routine basis.*

- After a cardiac arrest, transfer the client to critical care. Perform and document a complete head-to-toe assessment; obtain laboratory tests, 12-lead ECG, and a chest X-ray as ordered; maintain supplemental oxygen

Nursing Care of the Client Having a Permanent Pacemaker Implant

e. Hiccups. *If the lead is positioned near the diaphragm, the diaphragm can be stimulated, causing hiccups. Hiccups may occur in extremely thin clients or may indicate a medical emergency resulting from the perforation of the right ventricle by the pacing electrode tip.*

- Assess for possible dysrhythmias and administer antidysrhythmic medications as indicated. *Until the catheter is "seated" or adheres to the myocardium, its movement may cause myocardial irritability and dysrhythmias. Two to three days must elapse for fibrotic tissue to develop.*

- Document the date of pacemaker insertion, the model and type, and settings. *This is important for future reference.*

- Assess for and report immediately signs of potential complications, including myocardial perforation, cardiac tamponade (see the later section of this chapter), pneumothorax or hemothorax, emboli, skin breakdown, bleeding, infection, endocarditis, or poor wound healing. *Early identification of complications allows for aggressive intervention.*

- Provide the client with a pacemaker identification card including the manufacturer's name, model number, mode of operation, rate parameters, and expected battery life. *This card provides a reference for the client and future health care providers.*

CLIENT AND FAMILY TEACHING

- Provide appropriate teaching for the client and family members in the following topics:
  a. The placement of the pacemaker generator and electrodes in relation to the heart.
  b. How the pacemaker works and the rate at which it is set.
  c. The usual battery replacement procedure. Most pacemakers use batteries that last 6 to 12 years.

Replacement requires a short hospital stay to open the subcutaneous pocket and replace the battery.
  d. How to take and record the pulse rate. Instruct to assess the pulse daily before arising and notify the physician if it is 5 beats per minute or more slower than the preset pacemaker rate.
  e. Postoperative care of the site and signs of infection. Bruising may be present following surgery.
  f. Prescribed medications, their action, potential side effects, dose, route, and scheduling.

- Report signs of pacemaker malfunction to the physician, which may include dizziness, fainting, fatigue, weakness, chest pain, or palpitations.

- Restrict activity as ordered. Usually, restrictions are limited to contact sports, which may damage the generator site. Heavy lifting is avoided for 2 months following the implant.

- Resume sexual activity as recommended by the physician. Avoid positions that cause pressure on the site.

- Avoid tight-fitting clothing over the pacemaker site to reduce irritation and potential skin breakdown.

- Carry the pacemaker identification card at all times, and wear a MedicAlert bracelet or tag.

- Notify all care providers of the presence of a pacemaker.

- Do not hold or use certain electrical devices over the pacemaker site, including household appliances or tools, garage door openers, antitheft devices, or burglar alarms. Pacemakers will set off airport security detectors; notify security officials of its presence.

- Maintain follow-up care with the physician as recommended.

---

or ventilator settings; maintain patency of intravenous lines; and monitor infusions, cardiac rhythm, and vital signs. *The postresuscitative period is a critical one, and the client needs careful monitoring. Physical assessment after cardiac arrest allows comparison of the client's condition with prearrest status and identification of CPR-related injuries (Sommers, 1991). Correcting electrolyte disturbances, hypoxia, and acid-base imbalances is important to prevent another dysrhythmic episode and further deterioration of the client's condition. Intravenous access is crucial*

to maintain the infusion of antidysrhythmic drugs, sedatives, and pain medication. Hemodynamic monitoring is usually instituted if not already in place. The 12-lead ECG documents postarrest myocardial injury. A chest X-ray can yield information about pulmonary status and injuries to the thoracic cage.

- Notify the client's family of significant changes in the client's condition or cardiac arrest, providing up-to-date information. Prepare family members before they see the client by explaining interventions that may have been implemented (such as invasive tubes, a ventilator, or additional equipment) since the last visit. *Concern for the family and significant others is part of holistic nursing. Family members are under the same stressors as the client. Many researchers have studied the needs of family members and found that one of the most important needs was information about their loved one's condition. Both clients and families appreciate honest communication and compassionate care. Preparing the family for critical changes in the client's condition and plan of care helps them to cope with a difficult situation.*

Other Nursing Diagnoses

Other nursing diagnoses that may apply to the client experiencing cardiac dysrhythmias follow:

- *Altered Tissue Perfusion* related to decreased cardiac output secondary to altered rate, rhythm, or conduction
- *Pain* (chest pain) related to decreased perfusion of the coronary arteries secondary to tachycardia
- *Risk for Infection* related to invasive procedures and alteration of primary host defenses
- *Activity Intolerance* related to imbalance of oxygen supply to demand
- *Risk for Altered Sexuality Patterns* related to fear of precipitating dysrhythmias or injuring partner (especially for AICD clients)
- *Fear* or *Anxiety* related to actual or perceived threat of death
- *Ineffective Individual Coping* related to change in health status
- *Knowledge Deficit* of availability of community resources

Client and Family Teaching

Dysrhythmias have a significant physical and psychologic impact on the client and all family members. Many of these clients and their families are under a great deal of stress from frequent hospitalizations, experimentation with therapies, frustration, and the fear of sudden cardiac death. A major teaching effort focuses on coping strategies and life-style changes, as well as specific management of prescribed therapies. Both the client and the family need to be involved in all aspects of teaching regarding dysrhythmia management.

Clients with pacemaker implants require comprehensive teaching about the normal functioning of the pacemaker, taking their own pulse, signs of infection and potential malfunction of the pacemaker, resumption of and any limitations to activities of daily living, and safety issues (see the box on page 1046).

Topics to be covered in teaching clients with an AICD are similar to those for people with pacemakers. In addition, in some states driving is prohibited for clients with AICDs; address the impact of this restraint on the client's life-style. Discuss the client's fear of shocking a significant other during close contact or sexual activity, explaining that if a shock occurs, the partner may feel a slight buzz or tingling but should not be harmed. Inform the client that magnetic interference can deactivate the AICD device and should be avoided (Moser et al., 1993). Referrals to support groups are especially helpful for clients and families with AICDs.

Discuss with the client ways to control risk factors for developing dysrhythmias. Teach the client about proper self-administration of antidysrhythmic drugs, including both their desired and their potential adverse or toxic effects. Teach the client the signs of a recurrence or deterioration of the client's condition. Address changes in life-style, and provide any special instructions regarding diagnostic testing or implanted devices. Stress the importance of follow-up visits with the cardiologist, and schedule them, if possible. Encourage the client and family to attend peer support groups for their specific condition. One of the most helpful and important pieces of information is a referral to the AHA or the American Red Cross to learn CPR. This information helps give the family a sense of control and preparedness in case of a cardiac emergency.

Applying the Nursing Process

Case Study of a Client with Supraventricular Tachycardia: Elisa Vasquez

Elisa Vasquez, 53 years old, was admitted 36 hours ago to the coronary care unit from the emergency department after complaining of palpitations, light-headedness, and shortness of breath. Her history reveals a diagnosis of rheumatic fever at age 12, with subsequent rheumatic heart disease and mitral stenosis. An intravenous line is in place and she is receiving supplemental oxygen. Marcia Lewin, RN, is assigned to Ms. Vasquez.

Assessment

Ms. Lewin's assessment reveals that Ms. Vasquez is experiencing moderate anxiety. Her cardiac rhythm shows supraventricular tachycardia with a rate of 154. Other vital signs are recorded as follows: BP, 95/60; R, 26; T, 98.8 F (37.1 C). Peripheral pulses are weak but equal, mucous membranes pale pink, and her skin cool and dry. Fine crackles are auscultated in both lung bases. Heart sounds reveal a loud S_1 gallop and a diastolic murmur. Ms. Vasquez is still complaining of palpitations and tells Ms.

Lewin, "I feel so nervous and weak and dizzy." Ms. Vasquez's cardiologist is notified and orders 2.5 mg of verapamil to be given slowly via intravenous push and tells Ms. Lewin to prepare to assist with synchronized cardioversion if drug therapy does not control the ventricular rate.

Diagnosis

Based upon the assessment findings, Ms. Lewin formulates the following nursing diagnoses for Ms. Vasquez:

- *Decreased Cardiac Output* related to ineffective ventricular filling and the loss of atrial kick
- *Altered Tissue Perfusion: Cerebral/Cardiopulmonary/Peripheral* related to decreased cardiac output
- *Anxiety* and *Fear* related to unknown outcome of altered health state
- *Knowledge Deficit* in pharmacologic and synchronized cardioversion procedure

Expected Outcomes

The expected outcomes established for the plan of care specify that during the immediate phase of treatment, Ms. Vasquez will

- Maintain adequate cardiac output and tissue perfusion.
- Have a controlled ventricular rate with stable vital signs.
- Verbalize a reduction in anxiety.
- Verbalize an understanding of the rationale for the treatment measures to control the heart rate.

Planning and Implementation

Ms. Lewin plans and implements the following selected nursing interventions for Ms. Vasquez:

- Administer oxygen per nasal cannula at 4 L/min.
- Explain the necessity of rapidly reducing the heart rate to maintain hemodynamic stability. Explain the cardioversion procedure and encourage questions.
- Encourage Ms. Vasquez to verbalize her fears and concerns. Answer her questions honestly, and correct any misconceptions regarding the disease process, therapeutic interventions, or prognosis.
- Follow the unit protocol for elective synchronized cardioversion.
- Administer diazepam as ordered to induce amnesia before cardioversion.
- Document the client's vital signs, level of consciousness, and peripheral pulses for baseline assessment data.
- Assist the physician with the procedure.

- Continuously monitor ECG for changes in cardiac rate, rhythm, and conduction. Assess vital signs and associated symptoms with changes in ECG. Report findings to physician.
- Maintain in the unit a supply of emergency cardiac drugs and equipment; lidocaine, epinephrine, verapamil, procainamide, bretylium, atropine, isoproterenol, neosynephrine, the defibrillator, pacemaker, and intubation tray. In the case of a cardiac event, administer appropriate drugs and procedures as prescribed per unit protocol.
- Assess for return of consciousness from sedative or cardioversion attempt. Evaluate neurologic, cardiovascular, and respiratory status after the procedure.
- Document postcardioversion rhythm strip. Assess the client's skin for burns. Document the procedure and the client's response to this intervention.

Evaluation

Ms. Vasquez's cardiologist, Dr. Mullins, assesses her after receiving an update from Ms. Lewin. Ms. Vasquez's heart rate is 158, and her BP is 92/65 at this time. Dr. Mullins performs carotid sinus massage in an attempt to slow the heart rate; the ventricular rate slows to 126 for 2 minutes, revealing atrial flutter waves, and then returns to a rate of 150. Dr. Mullins briefly explains to Ms. Vasquez the treatment options, including the use of synchronized cardioversion. Ms. Vasquez asks a few questions and then agrees to undergo the procedure if the drug therapy does not work.

Intravenous verapamil lowers the heart rate to 138 for a short period of time, after which it increases to 164 with BP of 82/64. Ms. Vasquez is lightly sedated and immediate synchronized cardioversion is performed. Cardioversion is successful after one countershock, converting Ms. Vasquez to a sinus rhythm of 96 BPM with BP 112/60.

Ms. Vasquez is sleepy from the sedation but recovers without incident from the procedure. She states that she feels "much better," and her vital signs return to her normal levels. Physical assessment after the procedure is within normal limits for Ms. Vasquez; no skin burns are noted from the cardioversion. Her cardiac rhythm remains NSR with a rate of 86 to 92 for the remainder of her hospital stay. Dr. Mullins places Ms. Vasquez on digoxin and furosemide to treat manifestations of mild congestive heart failure. These drugs are continued after discharge.

Critical Thinking in the Nursing Process

1. What is the scientific basis for using carotid massage to treat clients with tachydysrhythmias? Was this an appropriate maneuver in the case of Ms. Vasquez?
2. What other treatment options might the physician have used to treat Ms. Vasquez's supraventricular

tachycardia if she had been asymptomatic with stable vital signs?

3. Develop a teaching plan for Ms. Vasquez related to her prescriptions for digoxin and furosemide.

The Client with Sudden Cardiac Death

■ ■ ■

Sudden cardiac death is defined as death occurring within 1 hour of the onset of cardiovascular symptoms. It usually is caused by ventricular fibrillation and cardiac arrest. Cardiac arrest is a clinical condition resulting in complete cessation of effective circulation. Nearly half of cardiac arrest victims die before reaching the hospital; only 25% to 30% of these out-of-hospital cardiac arrest victims survive (Main, 1995).

Almost 50% of all deaths due to coronary heart disease are attributed to sudden cardiac death (Lounsbury & Frye, 1992; Main, 1995). Ventricular fibrillation causes most of these deaths (75%). Only 20% of sudden cardiac death is due to *asystole,* or cardiac standstill, and 5% is associated with pulseless electrical activity or cardiac electrical activity without effective muscle contraction (Greene, 1990). Sudden cardiac death can result from cardiac or noncardiac causes (i.e., electrocution), but the majority of victims have coronary artery disease and a history of myocardial infarction (Crawford & Spence, 1995; Main, 1995; Pillion, 1995). The rate for recurrence of sudden cardiac death is 30% within 1 year (Greene, 1990). Selected cardiac and noncardiac causes of sudden cardiac death are listed in the accompanying box.

Risk factors for sudden cardiac death are those associated with coronary artery disease (see the next section of this chapter). In addition, clients with frequent ectopic ventricular beats (PVCs), bursts of VT, left ventricular hypertrophy, ischemia, acute myocardial infarction, or electrolyte disturbances are at risk. The threat of sudden cardiac death also is higher in clients with psychologic stress, advanced age, hypertension, and diabetes.

Pathophysiology

The mechanism of ventricular fibrillation is not yet known, but various theories have been proposed to explain its generation. PVCs are thought to predispose clients to the development of VT or VF. Abnormalities of myocardial structure or function also contribute. Structural abnormalities include myocardial infarction, hypertrophy, myopathy, and electrical anomalies. Functional deviations are caused by such factors as ischemia followed by reperfusion, alterations in homeostasis, neurophysiologic interactions (e.g., autonomic nervous system and hormone interactions), and toxic effects. The interac-

---

Selected Causes of Sudden Cardiac Death

■ ■ ■

Cardiac Causes

- Coronary artery disease
- Left ventricular dysfunction
- Cardiomyopathy
- Primary electrical disorder
- Acute myocarditis
- Dissecting or ruptured aortic or ventricular aneurysm
- Congenital heart disease
- Cardiac drug toxicity
- Antidysrhythmic drugs

Noncardiac Causes

- Pulmonary hypertension
- Pulmonary embolism
- Cerebral hemorrhage
- Autonomic dysfunction
- Choking
- Electrical shock
- Electrolyte imbalances
- Acid-base imbalances

---

tions of the two result in myocardial instability and may precipitate fatal dysrhythmias.

Collaborative Care

The goal of collaborative care is to restore the cardiac output to perfuse the body tissues and organs. Cardiopulmonary resuscitation (CPR) is a mechanical attempt to maintain tissue perfusion and oxygenation using oral resuscitation and external cardiac compressions. All health care providers need to be proficient in CPR or basic cardiac life support (BCLS). Advanced treatment of cardiac arrest victims, in the form of advanced cardiac life support (ACLS), incorporates electrical and drug therapies in addition to mechanical compressions.

Cardiopulmonary Resuscitation

Effective CPR must be instituted within 2 to 4 minutes of cardiac arrest to prevent permanent neurologic damage and ischemic injury to other organs. Cardiopulmonary resuscitation should be performed according to standard AHA guidelines and hospital protocol. A review of CPR procedures is provided in the accompanying box.

Cardiopulmonary Resuscitation

▦ ▦ ▦

1. Assess the client for responsiveness; shake the client and shout.

2. Call for help. Dial 911 (if outside the health care facility) or initiate the institutional code or cardiac arrest procedure.

3. Check for breathing; look and listen. Inspect the client's chest for rise and fall with respirations; listen and feel for air movement through the nose or mouth.

4. Open the airway using the head-tilt, chin-lift maneuvers. Simultaneously press down on the client's forehead with one hand while lifting the chin upward with the other (part *A* of the accompanying figure).

5. Reassess the client for breathing.

6. If the client is not breathing, begin rescue breathing using a pocket mask, mouth shield, or bag-valve mask (see part *B* of the figure). Administer two full breaths.

7. Check the carotid artery for the presence of a pulse.

8. If a pulse is present, continue rescue breathing until help arrives or the client resumes spontaneous respirations. Recheck the carotid pulse every 12 breaths.

9. If no pulse is present, initiate external cardiac compressions. Place the client on a firm surface. Position the hands as follows:
   a. Locate the lower margin of the rib cage with the middle and index fingers of the hand closer to the client's legs.
   b. Move the fingers up the rib margin to locate the sternal notch.
   c. Place the heel of the hand nearer the client's head on the lower half of the sternum (part *C* of the figure), taking care to avoid positioning the hand directly over the xiphoid process.
   d. Then place the first hand in a parallel position over the second hand with the fingers either extended or interlocked.

10. Initiate cardiac compressions, pressing straight down to depress the sternum 1.5 to 2 inches, keeping the elbows locked and positioning the shoulders directly over the hands (part *D* of the figure). Release pressure completely between compressions but do not lift the hands from the chest.

11. Compress the chest at a rate of 80 to 100 times per minute (one-and-two-and . . .).

a. With one-rescuer CPR, provide 2 breaths after each 15 compressions. Assess the pulse after 4 complete cycles of 15 compressions and 2 breaths; continue CPR until help arrives.

b. With two-rescuer CPR, provide 1 breath after every 5 compressions. Assess the pulse every minute for 5 to 10 seconds. If no pulse is present, continue CPR until help arrives.

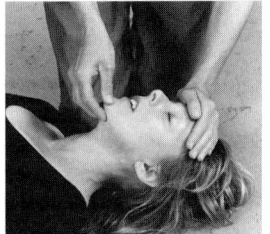

A

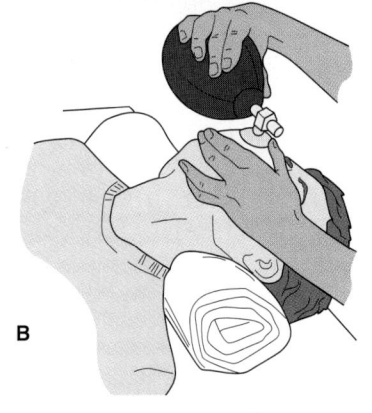

B

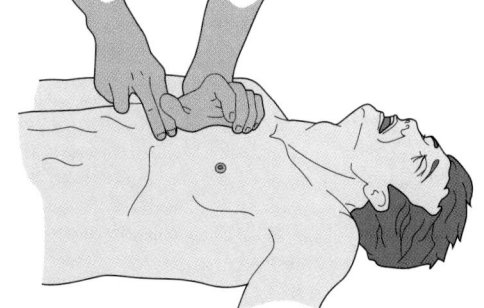

C

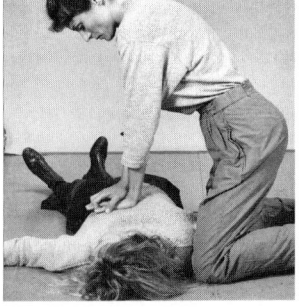

D

A, Head-tilt, chin-lift maneuver. *B,* Using a bag-valve mask. *C,* Placement of hands on lower portion of sternum above the xiphoid process. *D,* Arm, hand, and shoulder position for cardiac massage.

The nurse who witnesses the onset of ventricular fibrillation may administer a *precordial thump,* a sharp blow to the midsternum, in an attempt to jolt the heart out of a lethal dysrhythmia. Immediate defibrillation is the treatment of choice for unstable ventricular rhythms.

CPR carries a high risk for both cardiac and noncardiac trauma. CPR-related complications include injuries to the skin, thorax, upper airway, abdomen, lungs, heart, and great vessels. These complications can be minimized by adhering to accepted CPR techniques (Sommers, 1991).

Defibrillation

Because most instances of sudden cardiac death result from ventricular fibrillation, immediate defibrillation can be a life-saving procedure. Advanced cardiac life support (ACLS) protocols are followed. The procedure for defibrillation is outlined on page 1040.

Pharmacology

Drugs are used to manage the client in cardiac arrest and help stabilize the rhythm once it has been restored. Oxygen is always provided for clients in cardiac arrest. Epinephrine (Adrenalin), a catecholamine, is a first-line drug given to help restore a reperfusing rhythm and blood pressure. Lidocaine, bretylium, and procainamide are used to manage ventricular dysrhythmias. Procainamide also may be used to treat supraventricular dysrhythmias. Calcium channel blockers, beta-blockers, and digitalis glycosides are used to decrease heart rate and conduction time. Dopamine, dobutamine, and norepinephrine are used primarily to control blood pressure.

Nursing Care

Nursing care of the client experiencing sudden cardiac death requires prompt recognition of the event and immediate initiation of CPR and ACLS protocols. As noted before, early defibrillation of unstable VT and VF is the most important key to survival of cardiac arrest victims (Main, 1995). Important concepts of emergency cardiac care follow (AHA, 1994; Main, 1995).

- Treat the client, not the monitor. Recognize signs and symptoms of cardiac compromise early.
- Activate the emergency medical services system (i.e., call a code or call 911).
- Begin and continue basic cardiac life support principles throughout the resuscitation effort.
- Continually assess the effectiveness of emergency interventions.
- Defibrillate pulseless VT or VF as soon as possible.
- Initiate ACLS protocols early.

The family is not forgotten during the resuscitation period. If the family is in the hospital, they are usually offered a private consultation room in which to await the outcome. If the client's family is away from the hospital, they are notified that their family member is not doing well and asked to come to the hospital as soon as possible. The situation is presented in a careful manner to prevent the family from racing to the hospital and precipitating an automobile accident. Pastoral care or the family's choice of spiritual support is offered to help the family through this difficult time. The admission of family members during a resuscitation effort is a controversial issue that is being evaluated in hospitals across the nation (Eichhorn, Meyers, & Guzzetta, 1995).

After the client has been successfully resuscitated, the nurse works with the medical team to stabilize the client. Intravenous drug infusions such as lidocaine, bretylium, or dopamine may be used in the initial postresuscitation period to prevent further dysrhythmic episodes and to maintain an adequate blood pressure and/or heart rate. Depending on the cause of the dysrhythmic event, further electrophysiologic evaluation of the client may be indicated to determine future treatment.

If the client does not survive the arrest, the nurse is responsible for providing postmortem care of the body. Hospital policy dictates the special care of the body after death. The nurse also provides emotional and spiritual support to the family.

Nursing diagnoses that may be appropriate for the client experiencing sudden cardiac death include the following:

- *Altered Tissue Perfusion: Cerebral* related to ineffective cardiac output
- *Inability to Sustain Spontaneous Ventilation* related to cardiac arrest
- *Spiritual Distress* related to unexplained sudden cardiac death
- *Altered Thought Processes* related to compromised cerebral circulation
- *Fear* related to risk for future episodes of sudden cardiac death

Client and Family Teaching

Following an episode of sudden cardiac death in which resuscitation efforts are successful, the need for teaching both the client and family is great. The client who has experienced cardiac arrest is at higher risk for subsequent episodes and needs information to make informed decisions.

If the cause of cardiac arrest is determined, teaching focuses on reducing risk factors for future episodes. For example, if cardiac arrest was precipitated by a myocardial infarction, the client needs to know how to reduce the risk of future myocardial infarction. When the precipitating cause of cardiac arrest is less clear, the client may need to be taught about diagnostic studies to identify the cause, as well as possible interventions. Discussion about the risks and benefits of an AICD may be appropriate. Stress the importance to the client of carrying a card at all times listing all medications and the name of the client's health care provider.

In all cases, the client and family need to be taught to recognize early manifestations or warning signs of cardiac arrest. All family members should become proficient in performing CPR.

Nurses can have an impact on death rates from cardiac arrest through community teaching as well. Survival rates from sudden cardiac death have been shown to improve in such cities as Seattle, Washington, where a significant portion of the population is trained in CPR and early response by EMS agencies is stressed. Work with community groups and individuals can help create a population of people able to perform effective CPR.

Special Focus: Advance Directives and the Do-Not-Resuscitate Order

Most, if not all, hospitals have formal policies and procedures regarding the resuscitation of clients who suffer a cardiac or respiratory arrest. *Advance directives* are measures that focus on the client's right to self-determination, that is, the client's right to make treatment decisions and to be responsible for the outcomes of those decisions. The living will and the durable power of attorney for healthcare are two forms of advance directives available to clients. Both of these forms enable the client to state their wishes for medical treatments in end-of-life decisions. Nurses can assist clients to understand the purpose of advance directives (see the box on page 407 in Chapter 11).

Many health care settings use a classification system to determine the extent of resuscitative measures that will be employed for clients that suffer a cardiac or respiratory arrest:

- Full code: The client will receive all resuscitative measures necessary to revive the client: CPR, respiratory, and pharmacologic support.

- Partial code: This description varies with the institution. It may involve full resuscitative measures but require a daily assessment of code status, or it may limit the therapeutic measures that will be used in a code situation. In some institutions, partial code allows all resuscitative measures except CPR or intubation (that is, pharmacologic means only).

- No code: The third classification may limit resuscitative measures as noted above or prescribe a *do-not-resuscitate (DNR)* order.

- Comfort care: Some institutions have a fourth class that allows the discontinuation of all therapeutic measures except for pain and comfort measures (Flynn, 1993).

Clients are usually considered a full code on admission to the hospital, unless there is a preexisting DNR order in the client's record or the presence of an advance directive. Without a written DNR order, the nurse is obligated to begin resuscitation measures if indicated by the client's condition. The nurse caring for critically ill clients is often faced with the ethical dilemma of whether to initiate resuscitative efforts should the need arise (Flynn, 1993). Nurses should be aware of the policies and procedures regarding code status and advance directives in their institutions.

Caring for clients with DNR orders does *not* mean withdrawing care. The nursing staff still provides an optimal level of care to these clients and their families. Health care providers still collaborate to design a plan of care individualized to the client. The team approach, encouraging discussion of these issues between health care providers and the clients and families, favors information sharing and compassionate care planning (Marsden, 1993). More information on DNRs, advance directives, and care of the family experiencing a loss is provided in Chapter 11.

Disorders of Myocardial Perfusion

The Client with Coronary Artery Disease

Coronary artery disease (CAD), or *atherosclerotic heart disease (ASHD),* affects nearly 7 million people in the United States and causes about 500,000 deaths each year (AHA, 1992). CAD is a generic term that refers to the ef-

fects of the accumulation of atherosclerotic plaque in the coronary arteries that obstructs blood flow to the myocardium. Clients with CAD may be asymptomatic, or the disease may progress from a partial obstruction of blood flow manifested as chest pain (*angina pectoris*) to complete obstruction of coronary blood flow causing the destruction of cardiac muscle (*myocardial infarction*) and possible death. Many risk factors predisposing to CAD can be

Applying Research to Nursing Practice: The Framingham Heart Study

■ ■ ■

The Framingham Heart Study (FHS) is an ongoing, significant clinical research study that has provided data about cardiovascular disease for almost 40 years. The study was initiated in 1948 with an original study group of 5,209 participants in the town of Framingham, Massachusetts. Every 2 years, this original group is evaluated for cardiovascular "events" via their medical history, physical findings, and diagnostic testing. Children of the original group have also been studied as part of the Framingham Offspring Study. It was in reports of the Framingham study that the term "risk factor" first appeared (Cunningham, 1992).

Implications for Nursing

The data collected from both the Framingham Heart Study and the Framingham Offspring Study provide a rich database from which to tailor therapeutic approaches to the care of clients with heart disease. A major application of these research findings to practice is in primary preventive education, for example, through community cardiovascular health programs. As noted in the text, although research shows that increased public awareness of cardiovascular risk factors has lowered morbidity and mortality from heart disease, heart disease still remains the number-one killer in the United States. Education about the effects of lifestyle on the cardiovascular system must begin in the elementary school years and be reinforced throughout the formative years. When healthy choices become habit, cardiac disease will be reduced.

A second application of these findings is in collaborative treatment. Nurses should keep up-to-date on the latest strategies for medical treatment so that they can provide accurate rationales to the clients and formulate effective nursing treatment plans that will complement the physician's efforts. The result is better communication among all parties, a sense of collegiality and teamwork, and positive client outcomes.

Critical Thinking in Client Care

1. What kinds of strategies can be employed in the elementary school setting to teach cardiovascular health in a fun, informative manner?

2. Which health care providers should be included in a multidisciplinary effort to encourage clients to modify their life-styles?

3. What changes do you need to make in your life-style to role model heart healthy living?

---

controlled by the client through life-style modification. In fact, since the increase in public awareness of risk factors related to the development of CAD, mortality rates have declined by about 50%. Nevertheless, CAD continues to present a major community health problem. The nurse is in a prime position to encourage and support the client to make positive life-style changes through education and the promotion of healthy living practices. Individual choices can and do affect health.

The highest incidence of CAD is found in the Western world, mainly in white males age 45 and older. Both men and women are affected by coronary artery disease; in women, however, the onset of CAD is about 10 years later because of the heart-protective effects of estrogen. After menopause, women's risk is equal to that of men. White men have a higher incidence of CAD than nonwhite men, but nonwhite women have a higher incidence than white women.

The causes of atherosclerosis are not known, but certain risk factors have been linked with the development of atherosclerotic plaques. The Framingham Heart Study (Ho, Pinsky, Kannel, & Levy, 1993) has provided vital research into the relationship between risk factors and the development of heart disease (see the accompanying research box).

Risk factors for CAD are frequently classified into categories that reflect the person's ability to change his or her risk (Table 28–3). Age, for example, is a nonmodifiable risk factor. Over 50% of heart attack victims are 65 or older; 80% of deaths due to myocardial infarction occur in this age group. Gender, race, and family history of heart disease are other nonmodifiable risk factors linked with the development of CAD. Men are affected by CAD at an earlier age than women. African-Americans have a higher incidence of hypertension, which contributes to more rapid development of atherosclerosis.

Modifiable risk factors consist of pathologic conditions that predispose the client to developing CAD and factors related to life-style. Behavioral or life-style factors can be controlled or completely eliminated. Reduction of these risk behaviors has been shown to reduce the risk of CAD significantly.

Cigarette smoking is a modifiable risk factor and a primary cause of CAD in the United States. It is responsible for more deaths from CAD than from lung cancer or pulmonary disease (Newton & Froelicher, 1995). The male

Table 28–3   Risk Factors for Coronary Artery Disease

Nonmodifiable	Modifiable	
	Pathophysiologic Factors	Life-Style Factors
Age	Hypertension	Cigarette smoking
Gender	Diabetes mellitus	Obesity
Race/ethnic background	Hyperlipidemia	Physical inactivity
Heredity	Women only: premature menopause	Personality type
		Women only: use of oral contraceptives

cigarette smoker has three times the risk of developing heart disease than the nonsmoker; the female who smokes has up to four times the risk (Newton & Froelicher, 1995). Smoking prevalence is higher in blacks than whites, and more young Hispanics smoke than young blacks or whites (Fuentes & Haynie, 1992). For both men and women who stop smoking, the risk of mortality from cardiac disease is cut in half (Newton & Froelicher, 1995). A few years after smoking is discontinued, the CAD risk for women decreases to that of nonsmokers (Rosenberg, Palmer, & Shapiro, 1990). Cigarette smoking contributes to CAD by several mechanisms. The carbon monoxide produced may damage the blood vessel lining, promoting cholesterol deposition (McGill, 1988). Also, nicotine is a stimulant that causes the coronary vessels to vasoconstrict, reducing blood flow to the heart; additionally, sympathetic stimulation causes catecholamine release, increasing the work and oxygen demand of the heart by increasing the blood pressure and heart rate (Miller & Froelicher, 1995).

Obesity (body weight greater than 30% over ideal body weight) and the distribution of fat in the abdominal area have been shown to increase the risk of cardiac disease. A waist-to-hip ratio greater than 1:1 is significant. A person who stores fat primarily in the abdominal area, a typical pattern for men, is said to have an "apple" (*android*) shape. Women are more likely to store fat in the hips and thighs, a "pear" (*gynoid*) shape. Android obesity is associated with high insulin levels, high triglycerides, low high-density lipoprotein (HDL) levels, hypertension, and an increased risk of CAD (Margolis & Goldschmidt-Clermont, 1993). Hispanics have a higher prevalence of obesity than whites or blacks (Fuentes & Haynie, 1992).

Physical inactivity, or a sedentary life-style, is associated with higher risk. Physical activity seems to protect against

the development of coronary disease. Research data indicate that people who maintain a regular program of physical activity are less prone to developing CAD than sedentary people (Margolis & Goldschmidt-Clermont, 1993). Cardiovascular benefits of exercise include increased availability of oxygen to the heart muscle, decreased oxygen demand and cardiac workload, and increased myocardial function and electrical stability (Newton & Froelicher, 1995). Other positive effects of regular physical activity include a decrease in blood pressure, blood lipids, insulin levels, platelet aggregation, and weight.

Personality type has been linked with the development of CAD. Type A personalities (that is, aggressive, time-oriented personalities) have increased stress levels and a higher risk of CAD. Type B personalities are more relaxed and easygoing. However, a recent study indicates that although type A personalities have a higher incidence of heart attacks than type B personalities, people with type A personalities are more apt to work harder in cardiac rehabilitation programs and thus do better than type B people.

Two risk factors that are unique to women include *premature menopause* and the use of *oral contraceptives*. Premature menopause is associated with low levels of estrogen, which seems to have a protective effect on the heart, an increase in low-density lipoprotein (LDL) levels, and a decrease in HDL levels (Margolis & Goldschmidt-Clermont, 1993). Natural menopause before age 35 increases the risk of myocardial infarction within the next 10 years by 280%. Surgically induced menopause (bilateral oophorectomy) before age 35 increases the risk by 720% (Dougherty, 1992). Estrogen replacement therapy may reduce these risks. The use of oral contraceptives is also associated with high triglyceride and LDL levels, a decrease in HDL levels, and glucose intolerance (Dougherty, 1992).

Educating women about their CAD risk factors is a high priority in cardiovascular health promotion. Many women do not realize that their risk for CAD is just as high as men's risk. Most cardiovascular research studies in the past have been performed on white males; therefore, the results of the studies can be applied only to that population. Other research studies have shown that women are less likely to receive the benefit of diagnostic procedures and cardiac surgery (Dougherty, 1992). Table 28–4 gives an overview of the benefits of cardiovascular risk reduction.

Conditions that contribute to the development of CAD include hypertension, diabetes mellitus, and hyperlipidemia. Although these conditions are not a matter of choice, they are considered modifiable risk factors because they can usually be controlled through medication, weight control, and diet.

Hypertension is classifed as a systolic blood pressure greater than 140 mm Hg or a diastolic blood pressure greater than 90 mm Hg. More than 60 million people in the United States have hypertension; the incidence in

Table 28–4 Benefits of Reducing Cardiovascular Risk

Intervention	Estimated Reduction in Risk of Heart Attack
Quitting smoking	50% to 70% lower risk within 5 years
Lowering total cholesterol	2% to 3% decline in risk for each 1% reduction in total cholesterol
Raising HDL cholesterol	2% to 4% decline in risk for each 1% increase in HDL cholesterol
Controlling high blood pressure	2% to 3% decline in risk for each 1 mm/Hg reduction in diastolic blood pressure
Exercise	45% lower risk for those who maintain an active life-style
Maintaining ideal body weight	35% to 55% lower risk than those who are obese (30% above ideal body weight)
Estrogen replacement (in postmenopausal women)	44% lower risk
Mild to moderate alcohol consumption (one to two drinks per day)	25% to 45% lower risk than non-drinkers
Low-dose aspirin therapy	33% lower risk

Note: From "Coronary Artery Disease" (p. 11) by S. Margolis and P. J. Goldschmidt-Clermont, 1993, *The Johns Hopkins White Papers,* Baltimore: The Johns Hopkins Medical Institutions.

Table 28–5 Classification of Serum Cholesterol Values*

	Total Cholesterol (mg/dL)	LDL Cholesterol (mg/dL)
Desirable	Under 200	Under 130
Borderline High	200 to 239	130 to 159
High	240 or higher	160 or higher

*As defined by the National Blood, Lung, and Heart Institute's National Cholesterol Education Program.

African-Americans is higher than in whites (Fuentes & Haynie, 1992). Controlling blood pressure decreases the risk of cardiac disease, stroke, and renal failure (Newton & Froelicher, 1995).

Diabetes mellitus contributes to CAD in several ways. The disease is associated with a greater incidence of high blood lipids, high blood pressure, and obesity—all risk factors in their own right. In addition, the disease affects both small and large blood vessels, contributing to the process of atherosclerosis. Hyperglycemia, altered platelet function, and elevated fibrinogen levels are also thought to play a role. In women, diabetes seems to negate the protective effects of estrogen (Margolis & Goldschmidt-Clermont, 1993).

Hyperlipidemia is an abnormal level of blood lipids and lipoproteins. Table 28–5 lists desirable and high-risk levels for total serum cholesterol and LDL cholesterol. Lipoproteins carry cholesterol in the blood. LDL is the primary carrier of cholesterol. High levels of LDL (some-times called "bad" cholesterol) promote atherosclerosis because LDL deposits cholesterol on the artery walls. In contrast, HDL helps clear cholesterol from the arteries, transporting it to the liver for excretion. HDL is considered "good" cholesterol, because HDL levels above 35 mg/dL appear to reduce the risk of CAD. HDL levels can be raised by exercise, weight loss (if the person is overweight), quitting smoking, and estrogen replacement therapy. Triglycerides, compounds of fatty acids that are bound to glycerol and used for fat storage by the body, are carried on very-low-density lipoprotein (VLDL) molecules. Elevated triglyceride levels also contribute to the development of CAD. Increases in the total cholesterol and LDL significantly increase the risk of CAD.

Pathophysiology

The most common cause of reduced coronary blood flow is coronary atherosclerosis, a type of arteriosclerosis (see Chapter 30). **Atherosclerosis** is a progressive disease characterized by the formation of *atheromas,* or plaques, affecting the intimal and medial layers of large and medium-sized arteries (see Pathophysiology Illustrated on pages 1058–1059). Atherosclerosis is initiated by an unknown precipitating factor that causes lipoproteins and fibrous tissue to accumulate in the arterial wall. Although the precise mechanisms are unknown, the most accepted theory is that the disease begins with an injury or inflammation to endothelial cells that line the artery. A closely related theory suggests that the atheroma begins with a mural thrombus (a clot in the arterial wall) from endothelial injury. Damage to the endothelium promotes adhesion and aggregation of platelets and attracts leukocytes to the area.

At the injury site, *atherogenic* (atherosclerosis-promoting or atherosclerosis-causing) lipoproteins collect in the intimal lining of the artery. Macrophages are recruited to the injured site as part of the normal process of inflammation. Contact with platelets, cholesterol, and other blood components stimulates smooth muscle cells and connective tissue within the vessel wall to proliferate abnormally. Although blood flow is not affected at this stage, this early lesion may be apparent as a yellowish fatty streak on the inner lining of the artery. Progression of the process depends on mechanical factors that encourage thickening of the intimal wall and an abnormal accumulation of blood lipids to the intimal layer of the vessel (Stary et al., 1994). Fibrous plaque develops as smooth muscle cells enlarge, collagen fibers accumulate, and cholesterol builds up. This lesion is white and elevated, protruding into the arterial lumen and fixed to the inner wall of the tunica intima. It may invade the muscular tunica media as well (McCance & Huether, 1994). As the plaque develops, it not only gradually occludes the vessel lumen but also impairs the vessel's ability to dilate in response to increased oxygen demands. Fibrous plaque lesions often develop at arterial bifurcations or curves or in areas of narrowing. As the plaque expands, it can produce severe stenosis or total occlusion of the artery.

The final stage of the process is the development of *atheromas,* complex lesions consisting of lipids, fibrous tissue, collagen, calcium, cellular debris, and capillaries. These calcified lesions can ulcerate or rupture, stimulating thrombosis. The vessel lumen may be rapidly occluded by the thrombus, or it may embolize to occlude a distal vessel.

Plaque formation may be *eccentric,* located in a specific, asymmetric region of the vessel wall, or *concentric,* involving the entire vessel circumference (Jensen, 1995). Clinical manifestations of the process usually do not appear until about 75% of the arterial lumen has been occluded (Selwyn & Braunwald, 1994).

The major manifestations and complications of CAD are the disorders discussed in the succeeding sections, angina pectoris and myocardial infarction.

Collaborative Care

Care of the client with coronary artery disease focuses on aggressive management of risk factors to slow the atherosclerotic process and reduce the risk of complications. Until the client experiences manifestations of atherosclerotic arterial narrowing, the diagnosis often is presumptive, based on the client's history, physical examination, and the presence of risk factors.

Laboratory and Diagnostic Tests

Laboratory testing is used to confirm the presence of risk factors such as an abnormal blood lipid profile (elevated triglyceride and LDL levels and decreased HDL levels).

- *Total serum cholesterol* is elevated in clients with hyperlipidemia. Elevated levels are associated with an increased risk of atherosclerosis (see Table 28-5 on page 1056). For the most accurate results, clients should maintain a consistent dietary level of cholesterol for 3 weeks prior to the test and fast (except for water) for 12 to 14 hours immediately preceding the test. Alcohol should be avoided for 24 hours before the test. Many medications (e.g., hormones, phenytoin, thiazide diuretics, sulfonamides, captopril, and others) can affect the results; if possible, they too should be avoided for 24 hours before the test.

- *Lipid profile* provides more information than the total serum cholesterol, identifying triglyceride, HDL, and LDL levels as well as the total serum cholesterol. With this test, the ratio of HDL to total cholesterol can be determined. The ratio should be at least 1:5; 1:3 is an ideal ratio (Pagana & Pagana, 1995). Client preparation for a lipid profile is the same as for the total serum cholesterol test.

Risk Factor Management

Conservative management for the client with coronary atherosclerosis focuses on modifying risk factors, including diet, smoking, control of contributing conditions, exercise, and stress.

Diet   A low-fat, low-cholesterol diet is suggested to help control cholesterol levels and promote weight reduction. The fat content of the typical American diet is greater than 40%. The American Heart Association currently recommends a balanced diet that derives less than 30% of total daily kcal intake from fat, 55% from carbohydrates (preferably complex carbohydrates), and 15% from proteins. Dietary cholesterol should be limited to less than 300 mg per day. Limiting sodium intake to less than 3000 mg per day is also recommended.

Research shows that lowering serum LDL levels slows or reverses the progression of CAD and the risk of such complications as myocardial infarction. The greatest benefits are seen in clients who have other risk factors, such as smoking or hypertension. Increasing HDL levels, which can be accomplished through weight reduction and exercise, also reduces the risk of CAD.

The greatest benefit in reducing cholesterol levels is seen when total fat intake and saturated fats are reduced in the diet. Much saturated fat is found in whole-milk products and in red meats. Eating nonfat dairy products, fish, and poultry as primary protein sources can achieve a significant reduction in cholesterol. Monounsaturated fats, found in olive, canola, and peanut oils, may significantly lower LDL and cholesterol levels. Certain cold-water fish, such as tuna, salmon, and mackerel, contain high levels of omega-3 fatty acids, which actually help decrease serum triglycerides, total serum cholesterol, and blood pressure (Lutz & Przytulski, 1994).

Text continues on page 1060

Coronary Artery Disease

Most cases of coronary artery disease are due to *athero-sclerosis*, occlusion of the coronary arteries by fibrous, fatty plaque. Coronary artery disease is manifested by the development of *angina pectoris* and/or *myocardial infarction*. Risk factors for coronary artery disease include age (over 50 years), heredity, smoking, obesity, high serum cholesterol levels, hypertension, and diabetes mellitus. Other factors, such as stress and lack of exercise, also contribute to the risk of CAD.

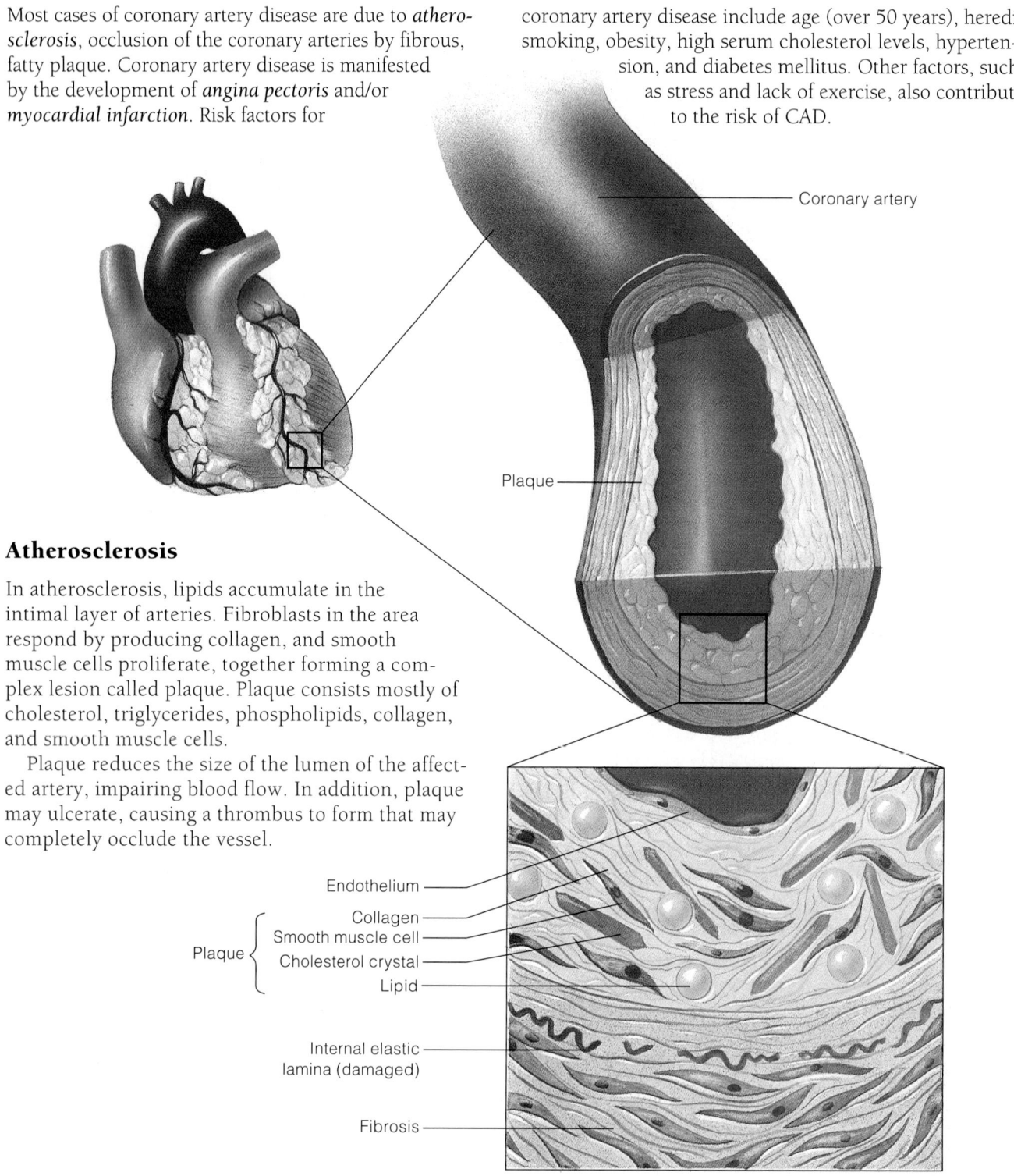

Coronary artery

Plaque

Atherosclerosis

In atherosclerosis, lipids accumulate in the intimal layer of arteries. Fibroblasts in the area respond by producing collagen, and smooth muscle cells proliferate, together forming a complex lesion called plaque. Plaque consists mostly of cholesterol, triglycerides, phospholipids, collagen, and smooth muscle cells.

Plaque reduces the size of the lumen of the affected artery, impairing blood flow. In addition, plaque may ulcerate, causing a thrombus to form that may completely occlude the vessel.

Endothelium

Collagen

Smooth muscle cell

Cholesterol crystal

Plaque

Lipid

Internal elastic lamina (damaged)

Fibrosis

Angina Pectoris

Angina is characterized by episodes of chest pain, usually precipitated by exercise and relieved by rest. When myocardial oxygen needs are greater than partially occluded vessels can supply, myocardial cells become ischemic and shift to anaerobic metabolism. Anaerobic metabolism produces lactic acid that stimulates nerve endings in the muscle, causing pain. The pain subsides when the oxygen supply again meets myocardial demand.

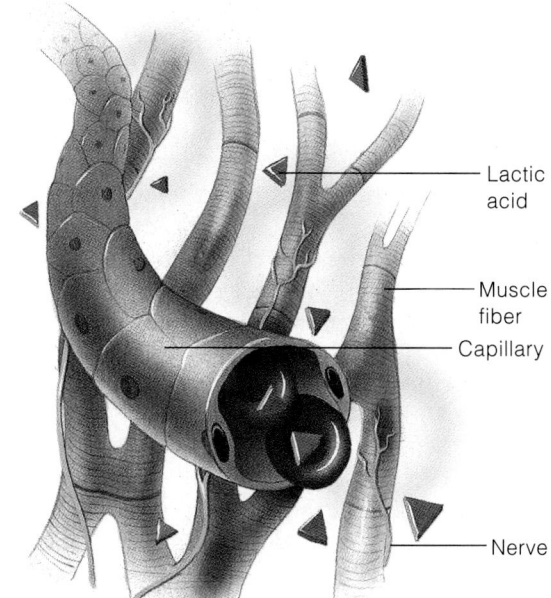

Lactic acid

Muscle fiber

Capillary

Nerve

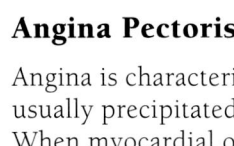

Myocardial Infarction

Myocardial infarction occurs when complete obstruction of a coronary artery interrupts blood supply to an area of myocardium. Affected tissue becomes ischemic and eventually dies (infarcts) if the blood supply is not restored. The necrotic area is bordered by an area of injured or damaged tissue, which is in turn surrounded by an area of ischemic tissue.

As myocardial cells die, they lyse and release various cardiac isoenzymes into the circulation. Elevated serum levels of creatinine kinase (CK) and lactic dehydrogenase (LDH) are specific indicators of myocardial infarction.

Capillary

Muscle fiber

Potassium

Creatinine kinase isoenzyme (CK)

Lactic dehydrogenase isoenzyme (LDH)

Smoking Cigarette smokers are three to six times as likely as nonsmokers to suffer a heart attack. Smoking cessation has an almost immediate benefit on the client's cardiovascular status: People who quit reduce their risk by 50%, regardless of how long they smoked before quitting. Nicotine is a stimulant that increases myocardial oxygen consumption. Smoking also robs the hemoglobin of oxygen-binding sites, because carbon monoxide binds with the hemoglobin instead of oxygen. Smoking decreases HDL levels, increases LDL levels, and increases blood viscosity through its effects on platelets, fibrinogen, and the hematocrit. These effects promote plaque development and thrombosis in narrowed arteries.

Hypertension Although hypertension often cannot be prevented or cured, it can be controlled. It is vital to control hypertension, particularly in clients with CAD, because the effects of hypertension on the blood vessels promote atherosclerosis. Maintaining the blood pressure at less than 140/90 mm Hg prevents these effects. Management strategies include reduction of sodium intake, regular exercise, stress management, and medications. The treatment of hypertension is discussed in Chapter 30.

Diabetes Clients with diabetes have an increased risk of CAD because diabetes accelerates the process of atherosclerosis. It is particularly important for the diabetic client to maintain an appropriate weight, reduce fat intake, and exercise to control the progress of CAD. Because hyperglycemia also appears to contribute to atherosclerosis, it is particularly important for the diabetic to manage blood glucose levels consistently.

Pharmacology

Drug therapy for the client with coronary atherosclerosis is indicated when diet and risk factor reduction is not enough to lower cholesterol levels, as is often the case in familial hyperlipidemias.

Clients at high risk for cardiovascular complications of CAD are often started on prophylactic low-dose aspirin therapy. A dose of 325 mg every other day is common. The benefits of aspirin in lowering the risk of coronary heart disease are thought to be equal to or greater than cholesterol reduction (Tierney, McPhee, & Papadakis, 1994). Aspirin is contraindicated, however, for clients who have a history of sensitivity to the drug, bleeding disorders, or peptic ulcer disease.

Oral estrogen replacement for postmenopausal women reduces LDL levels and increases HDL levels, providing a protective effect.

Drugs used to treat hyperlipidemia act specifically by lowering LDL levels. These drugs do not replace dietary and other cholesterol-lowering measures; they are used in addition to them. Drug therapy is recommended for clients with LDL cholesterol levels greater than 190 mg/dL or levels greater than 160 mg/dL with two or more

other risk factors present. For the most part, pharmacologic treatment of hyperlipidemia is not inexpensive; the cost may be more than $100 per month (Tierney et al., 1994).

Niacin or nicotinic acid (Niacor, Nicobid, Nicolar) has been shown to reduce the incidence of and mortality from coronary artery disease. It acts by reducing the production of very-low-density lipoproteins (VLDLs), thereby lowering LDL levels and raising HDL levels. Flushing, or "hot flashes," and pruritus are common side effects of niacin therapy. Taking one aspirin tablet prior to each dose can minimize this effect. Niacin has also been associated with hepatitis and exacerbations of gout and peptic ulcer disease.

Bile-acid-binding resins such as cholestyramine (Questran) and colestipol (Colestid) act by binding bile acids in the intestine. Cholesterol is a major component of bile acids. When bound with these drugs in the intestine, bile acids cannot be reabsorbed and are eliminated in the feces, gradually lowering serum cholesterol levels. These agents may have gastrointestinal side effects, such as constipation, gas, and abdominal cramping. They also may interfere with the absorption of the fat-soluble vitamins, A, D, E, and K.

Cholesterol-synthesis inhibitors such as lovastatin (Mevacor), pravastatin (Pravachol), and simvastatin (Zocor) inhibit cholesterol synthesis in the liver through enzyme inhibition. They are very effective in lowering LDL levels and also cause some increase in HDL levels. Headache and gastrointestinal effects are the most common side effects of these drugs. Clients may also develop myalgias (muscle aches) or skin rashes. Liver function tests and muscle enzymes are monitored during therapy to assess for possible toxic effects.

Nursing Care

Nursing care for the client with coronary artery disease centers around teaching and providing support for risk factor modification to slow the progress of the disease. The following nursing diagnoses may be appropriate for the client with CAD:

- *Altered Nutrition: More Than Body Requirements* related to excess kcal and fat intake
- *Altered Tissue Perfusion: Cardiac* related to atherosclerotic processes
- *Health-Seeking Behaviors:* risk factor management
- *Decisional Conflict* regarding integration of risk factor management strategies into life-style related to perceived need for changes in curent life-style

Client and Family Teaching

Encourage clients with CAD to participate in some form of cardiac rehabilitation program. Formal programs provide comprehensive assessment of, interventions for, and teaching of clients with cardiac disease. Monitored exercise and information about risk factors help clients begin to reduce their risk for progressive atherosclerosis and CAD.

Strongly encourage the client to stop all forms of tobacco use. Discuss the effects of smoking on the body and the benefits of quitting. In one-on-one counseling sessions, help the client identify specific sources of psychosocial and physical support. Resource materials to help clients stop smoking are available from the American Heart Association, the American Lung Association, and the American Cancer Society. Refer the client to a structured program for smoking cessation to increase the likelihood of success in quitting.

Discuss American Heart Association dietary recommendations with the client, emphasizing the role of diet in heart disease. Encourage the client to assess food intake and patterns of eating to help identify areas that can be improved. Provide guidance regarding the client's specific food choices with "healthy" alternatives. Refer the client to a clinical dietitian for diet planning and further teaching. Encourage the client to make dietary changes gradually but progressively. Advise the client to avoid drastic changes in eating patterns, because they have a tendency to cause frustration and discourage the client from maintaining a healthy diet over the long term. There are many cookbooks that offer low-fat recipes to encourage healthier eating, and the American Heart Association and the American Cancer Society offer recipe pamphlets and other information on low-fat eating.

A diet high in fat and calories and physical inactivity are major contributors to obesity and the development of CAD. Other factors include a family history of obesity and the presence of diabetes. Encourage the client to assess dietary intake and eating patterns and physical activity level to identify risk factors he or she can modify. Provide a dietary referral, and discuss different diet options. Encourage the client to maintain a well-balanced low-fat diet and avoid fad diets for weight loss. Advise the client that liquid diets should be used only under medical supervision.

Physically inactive people are at greater risk of developing heart disease than people who exercise regularly. Regular exercise improves cardiorespiratory function, reduces blood pressure, and promotes weight loss. Discuss the physical and psychosocial benefits of regular exercise. Help the client identify favorite forms of exercise or physical activity. Encourage the client to schedule exercise periods of 20 to 30 minutes of continuous aerobic activity (i.e., running, bicycling, swimming) at least three times a week. Walking provides many benefits and is an easily accessible and low-cost form of exercise. Encourage the client to identify an "exercise buddy" to help maintain motivation. Provide information about manifestations of exercise intolerance, and discuss what the client should do if these are noted.

Stress is a normal part of every person's life. The manner in which one reacts to the stressors has a significant impact on the physiologic and adverse effects of stress on the body. The goal is to manage the stress in one's life to a functional level. Individualize stress-management techniques to the client's preferences. Relaxation techniques, for example, may range from physical exercise to biofeedback to meditation. Provide descriptive information about various techniques, and help the client identify strategies with which he or she is most comfortable. In addition to setting aside time to "relax" every day, encourage the client to evaluate *how* he or she reacts to stressful situations. It is important to emphasize that relaxation techniques require practice. Personality typing characterizes typical behavior patterns and may offer the client an insight into his or her specific style of behavior. Recognizing these behavior patterns provides a starting point toward changing the behaviors so that the person can begin to react to stress in a "healthier" way.

General information regarding life-style changes can be presented to community or religious groups, in the school system (grades K through 12), or through the print media. These are areas in which nurses can be especially influential in educating the public and enhancing nursing's image as primary health care providers.

The Client with Angina Pectoris

■ ■ ■

Angina pectoris is chest pain resulting from a reduction in coronary blood flow, which causes a temporary imbalance between myocardial blood supply and demand. The reduction in coronary blood flow results in *myocardial ischemia* that is temporary and reversible. *Ischemia,* a deficiency of blood to a body part, may be due to the constriction or obstruction of a blood vessel. It causes cells to be deprived of oxygen and nutrients needed for metabolic processes. Cellular waste products build up in the tissue. The return of adequate circulation provides the nutrients the cells need and clears the waste products. Reduced blood flow lasting for more than 30 minutes causes irreversible damage to cardiac cells *(necrosis).*

Pathophysiology

Reduction in coronary blood flow can be caused by the atherosclerotic process, a thromboembolic event, or any condition that severely impacts oxygen supply or demand. Obstruction of a coronary artery reduces blood flow to the region of the heart normally supplied by that vessel. Cellular processes are compromised when the cells are deprived of oxygen. Reduced oxygen causes cells to switch from aerobic metabolism (a very efficient process that requires oxygen) to anaerobic metabolism (a very

---

Clinical Manifestations of Angina Pectoris

▪ ▪ ▪

- Chest pain: Substernal or precordial (across the chest wall); may radiate to neck, arms, shoulders, or jaw
- Quality: Tight, squeezing, constricting, or heavy sensation; may also be described as burning, aching, choking, dull, or constant
- Associated manifestations: Dyspnea, pallor, tachycardia, anxiety and fear
- Precipitating factors: Exercise or activity, strong emotion, stress, cold, heavy meal
- Relieving factors: Rest, position change; nitroglycerine

---

inefficient process that occurs in the absence of oxygen). Anaerobic metabolism causes lactic acid to build up in the cells. It also affects cell membrane permeability, releasing substances such as histamine, kinins, and specific enzymes that stimulate terminal nerve fibers in the cardiac muscle and send pain impulses to the central nervous system (Guyton, 1991). The pain radiates to the upper body because the heart shares the same dermatome as this region.

Hypermetabolic conditions such as anemia, exercise, thyrotoxicosis, substance abuse of stimulants (i.e., cocaine), hyperthyroidism, and emotional stress can increase myocardial oxygen demand, precipitating angina. Congestive heart failure, congenital heart defects, pulmonary hypertension, left ventricular hypertrophy, and cardiomyopathy can cause a decrease in blood and oxygen supply to the myocardium, leading to anginal attacks.

Myocardial ischemia that does not produce pain is called *silent ischemia.* Silent ischemia is a phenomenon that may affect up to 70% to 75% of all clients with ischemia (Jensen, 1995; Miller, 1993). Clients with silent myocardial ischemia have the same risk for significant coronary events as do clients with symptomatic ischemia; the difference is that the clients with silent ischemia do not experience the typical warning sign of angina and therefore may not be aware of their risk.

Coronary artery spasm is another cause of acute coronary occlusion. The exact mechanism of coronary artery spasm is unknown. It can occur suddenly, affecting normal coronary arteries. It may cause ischemia or, if prolonged, myocardial infarction.

Three types of angina have been identified:

- *Stable angina:* This is the most common and predictable form of angina. It occurs with a known

amount of activity or stress. There is no change in the cause, amount, or duration of the pain. Stable angina is relieved by rest and nitrates.

- *Unstable angina:* Angina that occurs with increasing frequency, severity, and duration is called unstable angina. Pain is unpredictable and occurs with decreasing levels of activity or stress and may occur at rest. Clients with unstable angina are at risk for myocardial infarction.
- *Prinzmetal's (variant) angina:* Prinzmetal's angina is an atypical form that occurs without an identified precipitating cause, usually at the same time each day, often waking the client from sleep. It is caused by coronary artery spasm with or without an atherosclerotic lesion.

The cardinal manifestation of angina is chest pain. The pain typically is precipitated by an identifiable event, such as physical activity, strong emotion, stress, eating a heavy meal, or exposure to cold. The classic sequence of angina is activity-pain, rest-relief. The client may describe the pain as a tight, squeezing, heavy pressure, or constricting sensation. It characteristically begins beneath the sternum and may radiate to the jaw, neck, or arm. Anginal pain usually lasts less than 15 minutes and is relieved by rest. Additional manifestations of angina include dyspnea, pallor, tachycardia, and great anxiety and fear. The manifestations of angina are summarized in the accompanying box.

Progression of the disease is marked by a change from stable angina to an unpredictable pattern (unstable angina). This change may herald an impending myocardial infarction.

Collaborative Care

Acute care of the client with angina focuses on relieving pain and preventing ischemic progression to infarction. Long-term management is directed at the causes of impaired blood supply to the myocardium. As for the client with CAD, risk factor management is a vital component of care for the client with angina (see the preceding section of this chapter).

Laboratory and Diagnostic Tests

The diagnosis of angina pectoris is based on the client's past medical history and family history, a comprehensive description of the characteristics of the chest pain, and physical assessment findings. Laboratory tests may confirm the presence of risk factors, such as an abnormal blood lipid profile (elevated triglyceride level and LDL and decreased HDLs) and an elevated blood glucose level. Diagnostic tests can reveal much information about the overall functioning of the heart.

Common diagnostic tests to assess the extent and location of the coronary heart disease and angina include electrocardiography, stress testing, nuclear medicine studies, echocardiography (ultrasound), angiography, and cardiac catheterization.

Electrocardiography   A resting ECG may be normal in clients with angina, or it may show nonspecific changes in the ST segment and T wave or signs of an old myocardial infarction. Characteristic ECG changes are seen during anginal episodes. During periods of ischemia, the ST segment is depressed or downsloping, and the T wave may flatten or invert (Figure 28–12). These changes reverse when ischemia is relieved.

Stress Electrocardiography (Exercise Stress Tests)
Stress electrocardiography uses ECGs to monitor the client's response to increased cardiac workload during progressive, dynamic exercise (on a motorized treadmill or stationary bicycle). This test may also be called exercise electrocardiography, exercise tolerance testing, graded exercise testing, or treadmill testing. It is used as a tool to diagnose angina and to identify clients at risk. As the body exercises, the demand for oxygen to the working muscles is increased. The heart normally responds to the increased demand by increasing cardiac output and oxygen delivery. This increased workload may precipitate signs of myocardial ischemia in the client with coronary artery disease.

The client's ECG, heart rate, and blood pressure are monitored continuously during testing. The client is instructed to report any chest pain or adverse responses immediately; the test can be stopped at any time at the client's request. The test is terminated when the client's predicted maximal or submaximal heart rate is reached, if depression of the ST segment is greater than 3 mm, or at the client's request because of fatigue or other symptoms. The test is considered "positive" if it must be discontinued because of myocardial ischemia or other significant problems, such as hypotension or dysrhythmias, before the predicted heart rate is achieved (Crawford & Spence, 1995).

Cardiac Radionuclear Scan   Radionuclear scanning is a safe, noninvasive technique to evaluate myocardial perfusion and left ventricular function. Thallium-201 or a technetium-based radiocompound is injected intravenously, and the heart is scanned with a radiation detector. Ischemic or infarcted cells of the myocardium do not take up the substance normally, appearing as a "cold spot" on the scan. If the ischemia is transient, these spots gradually fill in, indicating the reversibility of the process. With severe ischemia or a myocardial infarction, these areas may remain devoid of radioactivity.

Left ventricular function can also be evaluated with radionuclear scanning. Whereas the *ejection fraction,* or portion of blood ejected from the left ventricle during systole, normally increases during exercise, it may actually decrease in clients with coronary disease and stress-induced ischemia.

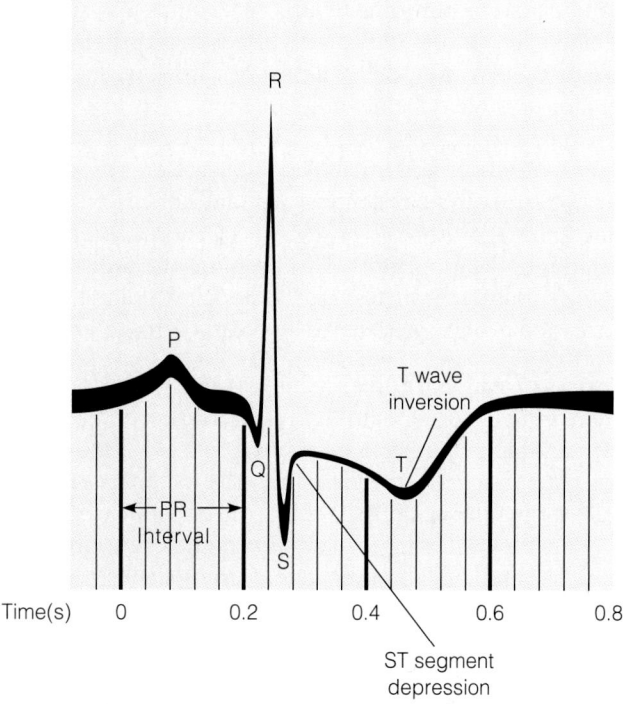

Figure 28–12 ECG changes during an episode of angina. Note the T wave inversion and ST segment depression, which are characteristic of myocardial ischemia.

The amount of radioisotope injected is very small; no special radiation precautions are required during or after the scan. The client is encouraged to consume liberal amounts of fluid afterward to facilitate elimination of the substance from the body.

Pharmacologic stress testing is used in clients who are physically unable to exercise, such as clients with orthopedic problems, peripheral vascular disease, or neurologic deficits (Crawford & Spence, 1995). Vasodilators such as dipyridamole (Persantine) and adenosine (Adenocard) are used to induce the same ischemic changes in the diseased heart, as in exercise-induced ischemia. Coronary arteries that are not affected by atherosclerosis dilate in response to the drugs, thus increasing blood flow to already well-perfused tissue. This causes a reduction in blood flow to ischemic muscle, called *myocardial steal syndrome* (Crawford & Spence, 1995). Pharmacologic stress testing also uses thallium-201. The client receives a dipyridamole infusion before the thallium-201, and the heart is scanned as discussed above.

Echocardiography   Echocardiography is a noninvasive test that uses ultrasound to evaluate heart structure and function. High-frequency sound waves emitted from a transducer are reflected off of heart structures back to the transducer as echoes. These echoes are displayed on an oscilloscope. Echocardiography is usually done transthoracically, that is, with the transducer held to the chest wall. It may be performed with the client at rest, during supine exercise, or immediately following upright exercise to evaluate movement of the myocardial wall and assess for possible ischemia or infarction.

Transesophageal echocardiography (TEE) uses ultrasound to identify abnormal blood flow patterns as well as cardiac structures. In contrast to transthoracic echocardiography, the probe is on the tip of an endoscope inserted into the esophagus. This positions the probe close to the posterior heart (especially the left atrium and the aorta) and avoids interference by breasts, ribs, or lungs.

Coronary Angiography *Coronary angiography* is considered the "gold standard" for the evaluation of the coronary arteries. A catheter introduced into the femoral or brachial artery is threaded into the coronary artery, guided by a fluoroscope. Dye is injected into each coronary opening, allowing visualization of the main coronary branches and any abnormalities, such as stenosis or obstruction. Narrowing of the vessel lumen by more than 50% is considered significant; most lesions that produce symptoms involve more than 70% narrowing. Vessel obstructions are noted on a coronary artery "map" that provides a guide for tracking disease progression and for elective treatment with angioplasty or cardiac surgery. During angiogram, the drug ergonovine maleate may be injected to induce coronary artery spasm and diagnose Prinzmetal's angina. Nursing care of the client undergoing a coronary angiogram or cardiac catheterization (discussed below) is summarized in the accompanying box.

Cardiac Catheterization *Cardiac catheterization* is an invasive procedure used to evaluate cardiac pressures, ventricular function, and the patency of the coronary arteries. The catheter is inserted in the same manner as in coronary angiography. The catheter is threaded into either the right or the left side of the heart, where pressures in each cardiac chamber, pulmonary artery, and/or aorta may be measured and blood samples withdrawn for analysis of oxygen content. Contrast dye is injected to evaluate ventricular size and contractility and cardiac output and ejection fraction.

Pharmacology

Drugs may be employed in both acute and long-term care of the client with angina. The goal of pharmacologic treatment is to reduce oxygen demand and increase oxygen supply to the myocardium. The three main classes of drugs used in the treatment of angina are nitrates, beta-blockers, and calcium channel blockers.

Nitrates Nitrates, including nitroglycerin and longer-acting nitrate preparations, are used in both the acute and long-term management of angina.

Sublingual nitroglycerin is the drug of choice to treat acute anginal attacks. It acts within 1 to 2 minutes, decreasing myocardial work and oxygen demand through venous and arterial dilation, which in turn reduces preload and afterload. It may also improve myocardial oxygen supply by dilating collateral blood vessels and reducing stenosis. Rapid-acting nitroglycerin is also available as a buccal spray in a metered system. For some clients, this may be easier to handle than small nitroglycerin tablets (Tierney et al., 1994).

Longer-acting nitroglycerin preparations are available as oral tablets, ointment, or transdermal patches. In these forms, nitroglycerin is used to prevent attacks of angina, not to treat an acute attack. The primary problem with long-term nitrate use is the development of *tolerance*, a decreasing effect from the same dose of medication. Although tolerance occurs to some degree in most clients, it can be limited by a dosage schedule that allows the client to be free of nitrates for at least 8 to 10 hours daily (Tierney et al., 1994). This nitrate-free period is usually scheduled at night, when the client is less likely to experience angina.

Headache is a common side effect of nitrate therapy and may limit its usefulness for the client. Nausea, dizziness, and hypotension are also common effects of therapy.

Beta-Blockers Beta-blockers, including propranolol, metoprolol, nadolol, and atenolol, are considered first-line drugs to treat chronic angina. They block the cardiac-stimulating effects of norepinephrine and epinephrine, preventing anginal attacks by reducing heart rate, myocardial contractility, and blood pressure, thus reducing myocardial oxygen demand. Beta-blockers may be used alone or in conjunction with other medications to treat angina.

It is important to remember that beta-blockers are contraindicated for use in clients with heart failure, significant bradycardia, or AV conduction blocks. They are also contraindicated for clients with asthma or severe COPD (see Chapter 34) because they may cause severe bronchospasm in these clients. Beta-blockers are not used to treat Prinzmetal's or vasospastic angina because they may make it worse.

Calcium Channel Blockers Calcium channel blockers both reduce myocardial oxygen demand and increase myocardial blood and oxygen supply. These drugs, which include verapamil, diltiazem, and nifedipine, lower the blood pressure, reduce myocardial contractility, and, in some cases, lower the heart rate, decreasing myocardial oxygen demand. They are also potent coronary vasodilators, effectively increasing oxygen supply. Like beta-blockers, calcium channel blockers act too slowly to be effective in treating an acute attack of angina; they are used for long-term prophylaxis. Because they may actually increase ischemia and mortality in clients with heart failure or left ventricular dysfunction, these drugs are not usually prescribed in the initial treatment of angina. They are used with care in clients with cardiac dysrhythmias, heart failure, or hypotension.

Nursing Care of the Client Having a Coronary Angiogram or Cardiac Catheterization

PREPROCEDURE CARE

- Assess the client's knowledge and understanding of the procedure, as well as that of family members. Provide additional information to clarify as needed. *The client with a thorough understanding of the procedure to be performed has a lower anxiety level and is able to cooperate better during the procedure.*

- Ensure that the client has signed an informed consent for the procedure. *This is an invasive procedure that carries a slight risk of mortality or morbidity. The client should have a clear understanding of the risks and alternatives prior to consenting to the procedure.*

- Instruct the client to fast for at least 8 hours prior to the procedure. In some instances, fluids may be allowed until 4 hours prior to the procedure; check with the physician or institutional protocol. *Fasting and fluid restriction decrease gastric contents, reducing the risk of nausea and vomiting during the procedure.*

- Administer routine cardiac medications with a small sip of water prior to the procedure unless contraindicated. *It may be important to continue the client's routine medications to avoid cardiac compromise or dysrhythmias during the procedure.*

- Assess the client for hypersensitivity to iodine, radiographic dyes, or seafood. *An iodine-based radiographic dye is typically used for an angiogram. The client with known hypersensitivities to these substances is at risk for anaphylaxis and requires an alternative dye or special precautions.*

- Record baseline assessment data, including height and weight, blood pressure, pulse, respirations, and temperature. Assess peripheral pulses, and record their equality and amplitude; mark their locations. *This data provides a baseline for determining significant changes after the procedure. Marking pulse points prior to the procedure facilitates their assessment after the procedure.*

- Explain to the client that he or she will remain awake during the procedure, which takes 1 to 2 hours to complete. The client may experience a momentary sensation of warmth (a "hot flash") and a metallic taste as the dye is injected. These sensations, as well as a rapid pulse or a few "skipped beats," are common and expected during the procedure. *To allay fears and anxiety, it is important to inform the client about what to expect during the procedure.*

- Ask the client to void prior to going to the cardiac catheterization laboratory. *This promotes the client's comfort.*

- Provide additional preprocedure care as indicated, including sedation and ensuring the presence of a patent intravenous catheter. *The intravenous catheter is vital to ensure rapid venous access for medications should they be necessary.*

POSTPROCEDURE CARE

- Monitor the client's vital signs as ordered, usually every 15 minutes during the first hour, every 30 minutes during the next hour, and every 2 to 4 hours thereafter. *Assessing vital signs enables the nurse to assess how well the client tolerated the procedure and to detect possible complications.*

- Maintain the client on bed rest for 6 to 8 hours after the procedure. *Bed rest is prescribed to allow the arterial access site to seal, reducing the risk of bleeding.*

- Keep a pressure dressing in place over arterial access sites. Check frequently for bleeding (if the access site is in the groin, check for bleeding under the buttocks). *Arteries are high-pressure systems. The risk for significant bleeding after an invasive procedure is high.*

- Immobilize the affected extremity in an extended position. *This helps reduce the risk of bleeding or thrombus formation.*

- Frequently assess pulses, color, sensation, and capillary refill distal to the access site. *A hematoma or thrombus may form in the vessel, occluding it and impairing circulation to the affected extremity. Early detection of this potential complication is vital to preserve the extremity.*

- Unless contraindicated, encourage the client to consume liberal amounts of fluids. *A high fluid intake promotes excretion of the radiographic dye from the body, reducing the risk of toxicity (particularly to the kidneys).*

- Assess for chest pain and monitor the client's ECG rhythm following the procedure. *The procedure may increase myocardial irritability and the risk of dysrhythmias postoperatively.*

The nursing implications of antianginal medications are summarized in the pharmacology box on page 1066. **Aspirin**   The client with angina, particularly unstable angina, is at risk for myocardial infarction because of significant narrowing of the coronary arteries. Low-dose aspirin (162 to 325 mg per day or 325 mg every other day) is often prescribed to reduce the risk of platelet aggregation and thrombus formation, which could cause a

Text continues on page 1068

Nursing Implications for Pharmacology: Antianginal Medications

ORGANIC NITRATES

Nitroglycerin (Nitropaste, Nitro-Dur, Nitro-Bid, Nitrol, Transderm-Nitro, Nitrogard, Nitrodisc, Tridil)

Isosorbide dinitrate (Isordil)

Isosorbide mononitrate (Ismo)

Amyl nitrite

Nitrates act by dilating both arterial and venous vessels, depending on the dosage of the medication. Coronary artery vasodilation increases coronary blood flow and myocardial oxygen supply. Venous dilation allows blood to pool in the periphery, reducing the venous return to the right side of the heart. This reduces preload and cardiac work. Arterial dilation reduces vascular resistance and afterload, also reducing cardiac work by reducing the force needed for ejection. Sublingual nitroglycerin (NTG) tablets are used to prevent the onset of angina (when taken prophylactically before activity) and to treat acute anginal pain. Nitrates in short -and long-acting forms are administered by various routes: by inhalation (amyl nitrate), intravenously, sublingually, by chewable tablets, by buccal spray, by oral tablets or sustained-release tablets, or topically as pastes, ointments, or transdermal discs.

Nursing Responsibilities

- Review the client's medication history to identify the type and dosage of antianginal medication the client normally takes.

- Dilute intravenous nitroglycerin before infusion; use only glass bottles for the mixture. Nitroglycerin adheres to PVC tubing, affecting the amount of drug that reaches the client; therefore, use non-PVC infusion tubing. If PVC infusion sets are used, the client may require an increased dosage to attain therapeutic effects. Monitor vital signs continuously during the infusion.

- Wear gloves when administering nitroglycerin ointment to the client to prevent absorbing the ointment through your skin. Measure dose carefully and spread evenly in a 2-by-3 inch area.

- Remove nitroglycerin patches or ointment at night to help prevent the client from developing tolerance to the drug.

- Help the client identify events that precipitate anginal attacks.

- Provide the client with information and community resources on quitting smoking.

Client and Family Teaching

- Only the sublingual, buccal, and spray forms of nitrates should be used to prevent or treat acute anginal attacks.

- If the first nitrate dose does not relieve the angina within 5 minutes, take a second dose. After 5 minutes more, a third dose may be taken if needed. Be sure to wait for 5 minutes between each dose. If a third dose does not relieve the pain or if the pain continues for 20 minutes or longer, seek medical assistance immediately.

- In case of an anginal attack, sit down and rest. Carry your nitroglycerin tablets with you. Let the sublingual nitroglycerin tablet dissolve under the tongue or between the upper lip and gum. Do not eat, drink, or smoke until the tablet is completely dissolved.

- Keep sublingual tablets in their original amber glass bottle to protect them from heat, light, and moisture. Every 6 months, have your prescription refilled by the pharmacist and throw away any unused tablets. A burning or tingling sensation may not be a reliable indicator of potency because newer drug preparations may not cause this effect (also, clients with impaired sensation, e.g., older adults, may not notice this sensation) (Shlafer, 1993).

- Rotate sites for the application of ointment or transdermal patches. Apply to a hairless area; spread ointment evenly without rubbing or massaging. Remove the old patch or residual ointment before applying a fresh dose.

- If you are on long-acting oral nitrate therapy, keep a supply of immediate-acting nitrates in case of an acute anginal attack.

- Investigate smoking cessation programs.

BETA-BLOCKERS

Atenolol (Tenormin)

Metoprolol (Lopressor)

Propranolol (Inderal)

Nadolol (Corgard)

Beta-blockers decrease cardiac workload by blocking beta receptors on the heart muscle, thereby decreasing heart rate and contractility and, in turn, myocardial oxygen consumption and blood pressure. Beta-blockers also reduce *reflex tachycardia*, a response that may occur with other antianginal agents, in which decreased cardiac output stimulates the sympa-

Pharmacology: Antianginal Medications (continued)

thetic nervous system, increasing the heart rate. Beta-blockers are frequently prescribed as antianginal and antihypertensive agents.

Nursing Responsibilities

- Obtain and record heart rate and blood pressure before administering the medication. Withhold the medication if the heart rate drops below 50 BPM or if the blood pressure is below prescribed parameters. Report these findings to the physician.

- Assess the client for possible contraindications to therapy, including heart failure, bradycardia, AV block, asthma, or COPD.

- Discontinuing these drugs suddenly, after long-term therapy, can cause heart rate, contractility, and blood pressure to increase, leading to a fatal dysrhythmia, myocardial infarction, or stroke. Withdraw beta-blocker therapy gradually while substituting another antianginal drug.

Client Teaching

- Beta-blockers do not work immediately; therefore, keep a supply of fast-acting nitrates on hand for acute anginal attacks.

- Do not suddenly stop taking this medication. Confer with your cardiologist to discuss discontinuing this medication.

- Take and record your pulse rate daily. Do not take the medication and notify your cardiologist if your heart rate is below 50 BPM. Have your blood pressure checked frequently also.

- Report to your physician a slow or irregular pulse, swelling or weight gain, or difficulty breathing.

CALCIUM CHANNEL BLOCKERS

Nifedipine (Adalat, Procardia)

Diltiazem (Cardizem)

Verapamil (Isoptin, Calan)

Bepridil (Vascor)

Felodipine (Plendil)

Isradipine (DynaCirc)

Nicardipine (Cardene)

Nimodipine (Nimotop)

Calcium channel blockers are used primarily to control angina, hypertension, and dysrhythmias in the cardiac client. By blocking the entry of calcium into the cell, these drugs reduce cardiac contractility, slow the heart rate and conduction, and cause vasodilation. Calcium channel blockers increase myocardial oxygen supply by dilating the coronary arteries and increasing blood flow. They decrease the workload of the heart by lowering vascular resistance and oxygen demand. Calcium channel blockers are often prescribed for clients with coronary artery spasm (Prinzmetal's angina).

Nursing Responsibilities

- Do not mix verapamil in any solution containing sodium bicarbonate. When administering verapamil via intravenous push, administer over 2 to 3 minutes.

- Obtain and record blood pressure and heart rate before administering the drug. Note prescribed parameters that dictate withholding the drug. Usually, the drug is withheld if the heart rate is below 50 BPM. Notify the physician if it becomes necessary to withhold the drug.

- The nifedipine capsule may be punctured and the drug administered by extracting the liquid with a syringe and squirting the dose under the client's tongue (discard the needle first!).

- Be cautious when administering a calcium channel blocker with other cardiac depressants, such as digitalis or beta-blockers. Concomitant administration with nitrates may cause excessive vasodilation.

- Manifestations of calcium channel blocker toxicity include nausea, generalized weakness, signs of decreased cardiac output, hypotension, bradycardia, and AV block. Report these findings immediately. Administer intravenous calcium chloride as an antidote. Maintain intravenous access, and infuse the medication slowly. Do not infuse large volumes of fluid to treat hypotension caused by toxicity: Fluid will overload the compromised heart, and heart failure will ensue.

Client Teaching

- Take your pulse rate before taking the drug. Do not take the drug and notify physician if your heart rate drops below 50 BPM.

- For acute attacks of angina, keep a fresh supply (less than 6 months old) of immediate-acting nitrate form (e.g., sublingual nitroglycerin tablets). Calcium channel blockers will not work fast enough to relieve an acute attack.

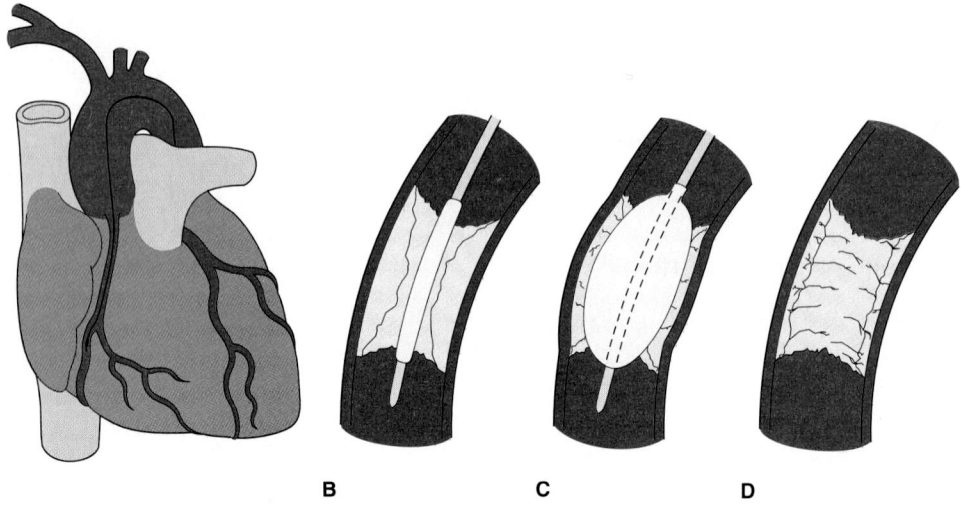

Figure 28-13 PTCA. *A,* The balloon catheter is threaded into the affected coronary artery. *B,* The balloon is positioned across the area of obstruction. *C,* The balloon is then inflated, flattening the plaque against the arterial wall, *D.*

A   B   C   D

myocardial infarction (see the next section of this chapter).

Revascularization Procedures

Several techniques may be used to reopen an occluded coronary artery and restore blood flow and oxygen to ischemic tissue. Nonsurgical techniques include transluminal coronary angioplasty, laser angioplasty, coronary atherectomy, and intracoronary stents. Coronary artery bypass grafting (CABG) is a surgical procedure that may be employed.

Percutaneous Transluminal Coronary Angioplasty

Percutaneous transluminal coronary angioplasty (PTCA) is an invasive procedure that attempts to increase the lumen of the narrowed coronary artery by decreasing the size of the plaque projecting into the lumen. Balloon angioplasty does not remove the plaque from the arterial wall; rather, it widens the coronary lumen by rupturing the plaque, thereby creating channels to increase blood flow. In 1991, over 300,000 PTCAs were performed in the United States (Margolis & Goldschmidt-Clermont, 1993). The overall success rate for PTCA is 61% to 91% (Kadota, 1989). Among clients whose coronary lumen was widened to at least 50%, 90% noted a reduction in anginal symptoms (Margolis & Goldschmidt-Clermont, 1993).

PTCA is performed in the cardiac catheterization laboratory; the client is prepared as for a cardiac catheterization (see the box on page 1065). Under local anesthesia, an incision is made in the femoral artery in the groin. With the help of fluoroscopy, a hollow balloon-tipped catheter is guided into the obstructed coronary artery. Once the catheter enters the artery, it is positioned across the obstructive lesion (Figure 28-13). The balloon is inflated in a step-by-step fashion for about 30 seconds to 2 minutes. The duration of balloon inflation depends on the client's manifestations, ECG evidence of ischemia, and the amount of luminal dilation achieved (Kadota, 1989). The goal of PTCA is to reduce the obstruction to less than 50% of the arterial lumen (Crawford & Spence, 1995).

Complications following PTCA include hematoma at the catheter introduction site, pseudoaneurysm, embolism, hypersensitivity to contrast dye, dysrhythmias, bleeding, and *restenosis,* or reocclusion of the treated vessel (Shaffer & Ruiz, 1992). About 25% to 35% of clients experience restenosis in the first 3 to 6 months after PTCA (Kadota, 1989). Clients undergoing PTCA are also prepared for potential emergency coronary bypass surgery in case reduced blood flow during balloon inflation causes an infarction; this occurs in 1% to 2% of clients. Bypass surgery may also be needed if there is total closure of the artery immediately after PTCA (Margolis & Goldschmidt-Clermont, 1993). An informed consent is obtained for both procedures at the same time.

Nursing care of the client undergoing PTCA includes both preprocedure and postprocedure education, monitoring of the site and distal extremities for potential hematoma or circulatory compromise, and prevention of other complications. The box on page 1070 outlines the nursing care of the client having a PTCA.

Other Nonsurgical Revascularization Techniques

In addition to PTCA, other methods may be used to revascularize the myocardium without surgery. All of these methods are performed in the cardiac catheterization laboratory.

- *Laser angioplasty* uses pulsed laser energy to vaporize plaque and reopen blocked arteries.

- *Coronary atherectomy* involves widening of the artery lumen by removing atherosclerotic plaque. The directional atherectomy catheter is a device that shaves the plaque off the vessel walls by means of a rotary cutting head, retaining the fragments in the device's housing and removing them from the vessel (Speroni, Fiske, Frank, & Morrissey, 1992).

- *Intracoronary stents* are used to prop or support the arterial wall. Stents are used after PTCA to keep the ves-

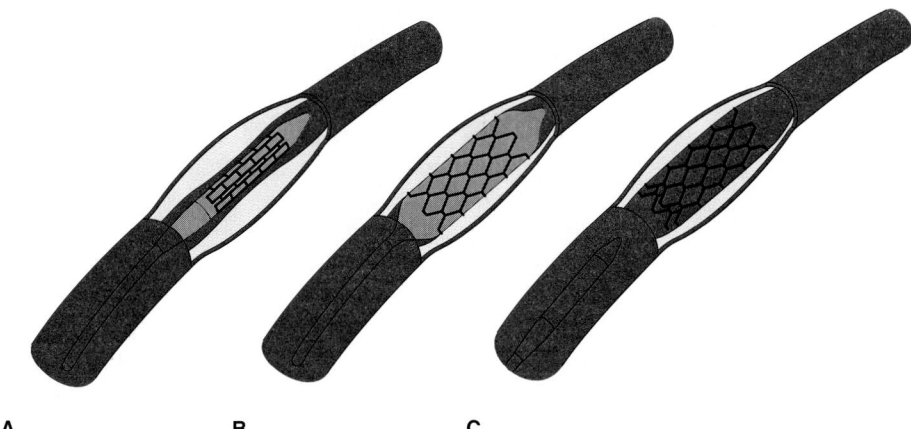

Figure 28-14   Placement of the balloon expandable intra-coronary stent. *A,* The stainless steel stent is fitted over a balloon-tipped catheter. *B,* The stent is positioned along the blockage and expanded. *C,* The balloon is deflated and removed, leaving the stent in place.

A   B   C

sel patent and reduce the rate of restenosis. The stent is placed over a balloon catheter and remains in the artery as a prop after the balloon is deflated. Endothelial cells will completely line the inner wall of the stent to produce a smooth inner lining. Anticoagulant and antiplatelet medications are given to reduce the risk of thrombus formation at the site. Intravascular stents under investigation include a heat-sensitive stent that expands from the warmth of the blood after placement, a self-expanding stainless steel tubular mesh stent, and a balloon-expandable stainless steel coil stent, which fits over the balloon catheter and is expanded into place when the balloon is inflated (Figure 28–14). Early reports indicate favorable results from these devices in the initial clinical studies (Bevans & McLimore, 1992).

Coronary Artery Bypass Grafting (CABG)   Surgical treatment of coronary artery disease involves revascularization of the myocardium using an extracardiac vein or arterial graft to "bypass," or bridge, the coronary artery obstruction and provide blood to the ischemic portion of the heart. The internal mammary artery in the chest and the saphenous vein from the leg are the most popular vessels used for cardiac bypass grafts.

About 407,000 bypass surgeries were performed in the United States in 1991; three times as many men as women underwent bypass surgery during this time (Margolis & Goldschmidt-Clermont, 1993). Coronary artery bypass grafting (CABG) is indicated for clients who have more than one vessel that is critically occluded (that is, occluded by more than 75%) or clients who have one affected vessel but who are at high risk for reocclusion after PTCA (Margolis & Goldschmidt-Clermont, 1993). Clients with evidence of CAD and exercise-induced ischemia, left ventricular dysfunction, chronic angina refractory to medical treatment, or severe restrictions affecting

quality of life may also be surgical candidates (Gregersen & McGregor, 1989).

Preoperatively, laboratory testing is used to evaulate the client's hematologic and blood chemistry status, as well as the function of major organ systems. A coagulation profile is included. The client's blood will be typed and crossmatched so that blood can be available during or after cardiac surgery.

A median sternotomy is used to gain access to the heart. The heart is usually stopped during surgery to make it easier to work on. The *cardiopulmonary bypass (CPB) pump* or *heart-lung machine,* is used to maintain perfusion to the rest of the organs during open-heart surgery. Venous blood is removed from the body through a cannula placed in the right atrium or the superior and inferior venae cavae. Blood then circulates through the CPB pump, where it is oxygenated, its temperature regulated, and filtered. Oxygenated blood is returned to the body through a cannula in the ascending aorta (Figure 28–15 on page 1072) (Bell & Diffee, 1991; Weiland & Walker, 1986). Cardiopulmonary bypass enables the surgeons to operate on a quiet heart and a relatively bloodless field. Hypothermia can be maintained to reduce the metabolic rate and decrease oxygen demand during surgery.

The internal mammary artery (IMA) is preferred for bypass grafting because arterial grafts last longer than vein grafts. Internal mammary grafts do not seem to be as affected by atherosclerotic buildup as vein grafts, reducing the rate of reoperation. The proximal end of the IMA remains attached to the subclavian artery. The distal end is excised and *anastomosed,* or grafted, to the coronary artery distal to the obstruction (Figure 28–16 on page 1072). The still innervated IMA can respond to autonomic nervous stimulation; its intact blood supply promotes faster healing (Jansen & McFadden, 1986).

In contrast, the saphenous vein is considered a "free graft" because it is excised from its normal attachments in the leg before being used as a graft. More than one leg

Nursing Care of the Client Having a PTCA

PREPROCEDURE CARE

- Assess the client's knowledge of the PTCA procedure and expectations of treatment. *This allows the nurse to tailor the information to the client's needs and gives the nurse a chance to clarify any misconceptions. Providing information relevant to the client's needs promotes learning.*

- Describe the cardiac catheterization laboratory and the PTCA procedure, including preoperative preparation:
  a. Food and fluids are withheld after midnight prior to the procedure. *This decreases the potential for nausea and vomiting with narcotic administration.*
  b. The client will be awake during the procedure, although a mild sedative is given. *Sedation is administered to decrease client anxiety.*
  c. Heparin, aspirin, and or dipyridamole may be administered prior to the procedure. *These drugs are given to decrease clot formation and platelet adhesion.*
  d. Intravenous nitroglycerin and a calcium channel blocker may be given during the procedure. *These medications are given for chest pain and to dilate the coronary arteries.*

- Describe sensations that the client may feel during the procedure, including flushing or warmth and a possible metallic taste in the mouth as the contrast dye is injected, and possibly a pressure sensation or chest pain during balloon inflation. *Knowledge of the reasons for unusual sensations may lower anxiety during the procedure and improve client outcomes.*

- Inform the client that he or she will be asked to take deep breaths throughout the procedure, and to cough after the injection of the dye. *The coronary arteries are more visible during inspiration because the diaphragm is lower. Coughing increases intrathoracic pressure and helps force the dye out of the coronary arteries.*

- Describe the recovery phase and expected plan of care after PTCA:
  a. Recovery in the cardiac care unit.
  b. Continuous ECG and vital sign monitoring.
  c. Periodic assessment of peripheral circulatory status and PTCA site.
  d. The need to maintain complete bed rest for 8 to 10 hours and to keep the PTCA leg straight.
  e. Expected transfer plans.
  f. Possibility of emergency bypass surgery.

  Continuous monitoring is required to evaluate the client's recovery from the PTCA procedure. Restenosis and other possible complications may necessitate frequent monitoring and assessments. The PTCA leg must be kept straight and bed rest maintained to permit healing of the site without disruption. All PTCA clients require preoperative instructions for coronary bypass surgery because it may be required in case of severe complications during the PTCA procedure.

POSTPROCEDURE CARE

- Complete a head-to-toe assessment. Note any complaints of chest pain, signs of decreased cardiac output, or signs of myocardial infarction. *The assessment provides baseline data and allows the nurse to*

---

incision may be made to access the saphenous vein, depending on the number of vessels to be bypassed and the condition of the vein. The excised vein is flushed with a cold heparinized saline solution and evaluated for patency. The vein is then reversed so that its valves do not interfere with blood flow. It is anastomosed to the aorta and the coronary artery, distal to the occlusion (Figure 28–16). This provides a bridge or conduit for blood flow past the obstruction.

The IMA may be used to bypass one or two obstructive lesions; however, many clients require a total of three, four, five, or even six bypasses. Saphenous vein grafts may be used in conjunction with the IMA. When both grafts are used, the IMA is used to revascularize the left coronary artery because of the greater oxygen demand of the left ventricle; saphenous vein grafts bypass the remaining blockages.

Once the grafting procedure has been completed, cardiopulmonary bypass is discontinued and the client is rewarmed. This rewarming stimulates the heart to resume beating. Temporary pacing wires are sutured in place and passed through the client's chest wall to be available should the need for temporary pacing arise. Chest tubes are placed in the pleural area and mediastinum to drain blood and to reestablish negative pressure in the thoracic cavity. The sternum is closed using heavy wires and bone wax, the skin is closed with sutures or staples, and sterile dressings are applied over the sternal and leg incisions.

Nursing Care of the Client Having a PTCA (continued)

identify signs of cardiac decompensation from possible complications.

- Monitor vital signs and cardiac rhythm continuously. Obtain a 12-lead ECG if signs of ischemia develop, and notify physician. *ECG waveform changes may indicate ischemia or restenosis of the affected vessel. Restenosis is a common complication of PTCA. The physician should be notified of all complications.*

- Administer heparin, nitrates, aspirin, dipyridamole, and calcium channel blockers as ordered. Maintain intravenous nitroglycerin infusion. *These drugs decrease oxygen demand and increase oxygen supply by dilating the coronary arteries and systemic vasculature. They also decrease platelet aggregation, reducing the risk of thrombus formation. (See the pharmacology box on page 1066). Intravenous nitroglycerin keeps coronary arteries dilated and decreases the potential for reocclusion of the artery.*

- Monitor for chest pain. *Chest pain may indicate ischemia and possible myocardial infarction.*

- Maintain the client on complete bed rest for 8 to 10 hours with the head of the bed below 30 degrees. Keep the leg straight on the affected side. Keep a 5-lb sandbag over the PTCA site for 6 to 8 hours. Assess insertion site with each check of vital signs. *A large puncture wound occurs at the insertion site. Bed rest and immobilization of the leg is necessary to allow the wound to close. The sandbag helps maintain a pressure dressing over the site. The PTCA site must be checked for signs of bleeding, hematoma formation, or pseudoaneurysm. Pseudoaneurysm occurs as a result of inadequate hemostasis after removal of the catheter. Hip*

flexion is limited to reduce the risk of thrombus formation at the site.

- Assess and record vital signs, distal pulses, color, movement, sensation, and temperature of the affected leg, as well as the condition of the insertion site dressing, every 15 minutes for the first hour, every 30 minutes for the next hour, every hour for the next 8 hours, then every 4 hours. *A clot may form at the site, reducing perfusion of the affected leg. Check the dressing for signs of excessive bleeding and the site for hematoma formation.*

- Closely monitor intake and output and laboratory values, including serum electrolytes, blood urea nitrogen (BUN), creatinine, complete blood count (CBC), partial thromboplastin time (PTT), and cardiac enzymes. Report abnormal results to the physician. *Contrast dye causes osmotic diuresis (which may last from 6 to 8 hours after PTCA) and may cause renal damage and a hypersensitivity reaction. Electrolyte abnormalities increase the risk of dysrhythmias. Cardiac enzymes are monitored for indications of possible myocardial damage during the procedure. The PTT monitors the effectiveness of heparin therapy.*

- Be alert for signs of bradycardia, light-headedness, hypotension, diaphoresis, and loss of consciousness during sheath removal in the postprocedure period. Keep atropine at bedside during sheath removal. *Bradycardia and the other signs may occur during sheath removal because of a vasovagal reaction. Atropine is an anticholinergic that decreases vagal tone and increases heart rate.*

Following surgery, the client usually arrives in the cardiac recovery area with the following equipment and invasive lines: a ventilator; central venous line, pulmonary artery catheter, peripheral venous line, and intra-arterial line; ECG electrode patches; temporary pacing wires and an external pacemaker; chest tubes; pulse oximeter; Foley catheter; and nasogastric tube.

Transmyocardial Laser Revascularization   A new development in the field of myocardial revascularization is a surgical technique called *transmyocardial laser revascularization (TMLR)*. In this technique, tiny holes are "drilled" by a laser into the myocardial muscle itself to provide collateral blood flow to ischemic muscle. Clients

whose coronary artery obstructions are too diffuse to bypass adequately are candidates for this new surgical treatment (SoRelle, 1994). Nursing care after this surgery follows the guidelines for any cardiac surgery client.

Nursing Care

The focus of nursing care for clients with angina is much the same as the focus of collaborative care: to reduce myocardial oxygen demands and improve the blood and oxygen supply. Clients with angina are frequently treated in community settings; the primary nursing care focus is education. High-priority nursing problems for the client with angina include altered cardiac tissue perfusion and

Figure 28–15 A diagrammatic representation of cardiopulmonary bypass. A cannula in the superior and inferior venae cavae removes venous blood, which is then pumped through an oxygenator and heat exchanger. After filtering, oxygenated blood is returned to the ascending aorta.

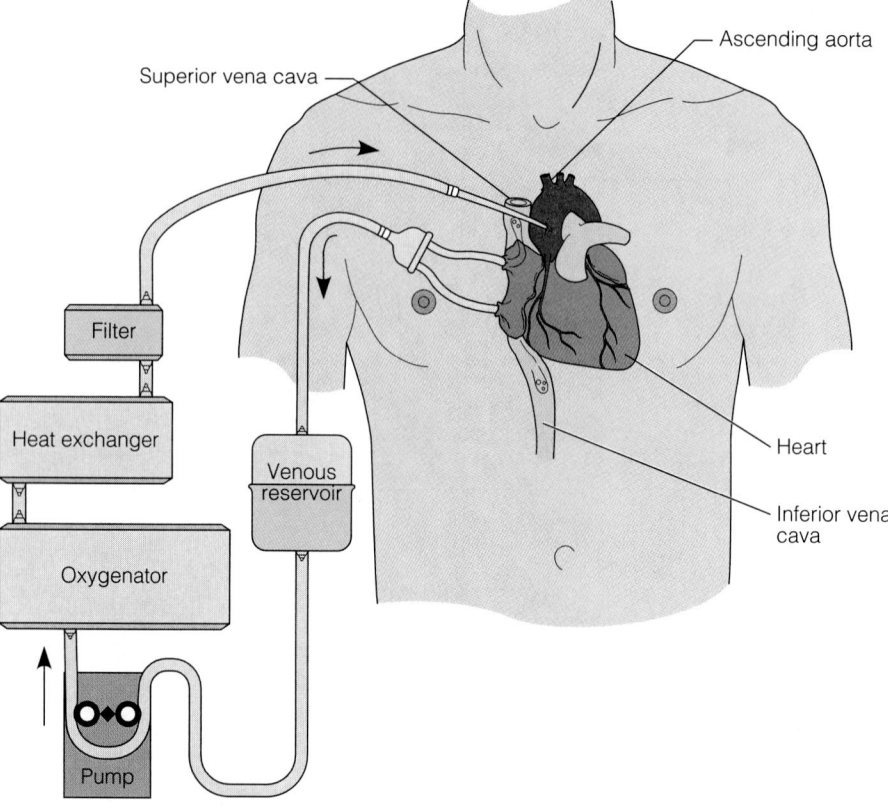

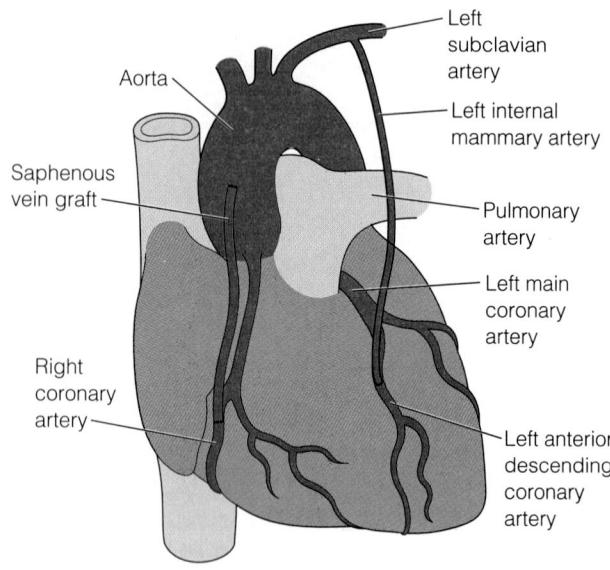

Figure 28–16 Coronary artery bypass grafting using the internal mammary artery and a saphenous vein graft.

ineffective management of the prescribed therapeutic regimen. These problems are addressed below.

The client who undergoes surgical revascularization of the myocardium has special care needs related to open heart surgery. Preoperatively, education is a major nursing focus. Topics to be addressed preoperatively and the roles played by members of the health care team in providing collaborative care are outlined in the accompanying boxes.

Major nursing care goals for the postoperative cardiac surgery client include maintaining hemodynamic stability and cardiac output, monitoring and managing complications, and assisting the client and the family through the recovery process. Nurses need to be sensitive to the needs of the family during this stressful event.

The cardiac surgery client typically spends 2 to 3 days in the cardiac recovery or intensive care unit (ICU), during which the risk of complications is high. These may include altered body temperature; cardiac dysfunction; cardiac tamponade; altered fluid, electrolyte, and acid-base status; pulmonary dysfunction; bleeding complications; dysrhythmias; infection; and pain (especially after the use of the IMA). After recovery, the client is transferred to a cardiac floor and prepared for discharge. The total length of stay after cardiac surgery is about 7 to 10 days. Postoperative nursing care of the client having cardiac surgery is described in the box on page 1074. A Critical Pathway for the client following coronary bypass surgery is provided on page 1079.

Altered Tissue Perfusion: Cardiac

The client with angina experiences pain as a result of impaired blood flow and oxygen supply to the myocardium. Nursing interventions can be instrumental in preventing

Preparing for Cardiac Surgery: Preoperative Teaching Topics for the Client and Family

- Tubes, drains, and general appearance
- Monitoring equipment
  a. Cardiac monitor
  b. Hemodynamic monitoring
- Respiratory support
  a. Ventilator
  b. Endotracheal tube
  c. Suctioning
  d. Communication while intubated
- Incisions and dressings
- Sensory stimuli
  a. Noise and alarms

b. Return of awareness and hearing before the ability to respond
  c. Pain
  d. Sedation and analgesia
- Activity progression
  a. Gentle leg exercises
  b. Antiemboli hose
- Diet progression
- Respiratory exercises
  a. Coughing, deep breathing
  b. Incentive spirometry
- Visiting Hours

Note: Modified from "Management of a Patient Undergoing Myocardial Revascularization: Coronary Artery Bypass Graft Surgery" (p. 253) by J. A. Shinn, 1989, *Nursing Clinics of North America, 27*(1).

Collaborative Care: The Client Undergoing Coronary Bypass Graft Surgery

Health Care Team	Client-Centered Care
Cardiac surgeon	Conducts preoperative assessment, including physical examination. Evaluates results of cardiac catheterization and makes recommendations regarding effectiveness of surgery. Performs surgery, manages postoperative course, stabilizes hemodynamic status, monitors respiratory status, monitors surgical outcomes following discharge.
Cardiologist	Serves as referring physician or as a consultant for nonsurgical cardiac problems, such as dysrhythmias. May perform cardiac catheterization.
Physical therapist	Recommends or provides physical rehabilitation consistent with cardiac rehabilitation program. Provides teaching regarding exercise program following discharge.
Cardiac rehabilitation nurse	May provide cardiac teaching throughout perioperative period. Responsible for coordinating cardiac rehabilitation following discharge. May coordinate referral to smoking cessation program.
Dietitian	Encourages client to eat well-balanced diet following surgery. Provides teaching regarding low-fat, low-cholesterol diet. Helps client identify strategies to incorporate diet into life-style.
Respiratory therapist	Assesses and monitors respiratory status and provides respiratory care. May monitor and provide ventilatory care, perform arterial blood gas (ABG) studies, and administer respiratory therapy.
Registered nurse in charge of health care team communications	Reports changes in postoperative hemodynamic status and respiratory status. Reports signs and symptoms of cardiac tamponade, fluid and electrolyte imbalances, hemothorax, or pneumothorax to physician. Also reports to dysrhythmias, sternal wound infections, and postpericardiotomy syndrome. Provides cardiac rehabilitation nurse information regarding client's and family responses to teaching. Collaborates with physical therapist to promote mobility and self-care. Alerts social worker to specific home care needs.

ischemia and shortening the duration of pain the client experiences.

Selected nursing interventions with rationales follow:

- Assess the location, severity, and quality of the client's pain. Ask the client to rate the pain on a scale of 0 to 10 (0 = no pain, 10 = the most severe pain). *Assessment helps the nurse differentiate anginal pain from other causes of pain. Assessment is particularly important in the client who has had surgery, because the client's pain may be assumed to be incisional pain rather than related to cardiac ischemia.*

Text continues on page 1078

Postoperative Nursing Care of Clients Having Coronary Artery Bypass Grafting

■ ■ ■

Decreased Cardiac Output

The client recovering from CABG surgery is at high risk for decreased cardiac output for a number of reasons:

- Bleeding and fluid loss leading to hypovolemia
- Depression of myocardial function from drugs, anesthesia, hypothermia, surgical manipulation, and preexisting damage
- Dysrhythmias
- Increased peripheral vascular resistance
- *Cardiac tamponade,* compression of the heart due to collected blood or fluid in the pericardium

Selected nursing interventions with rationales follow:

- Monitor vital signs and hemodynamic measurements every 15 minutes. Note trends in vital signs (e.g., decreasing BP, increasing heart rate), and report significant changes to the physician. *Hypothermia and bradycardia are expected in the immediate postoperative period. As the client warms, the heart rate should increase to the normal range. Tachycardia may indicate pain, anxiety, recovery from anesthesia, or fluid deficits. Hypothermia causes vasoconstriction and an increased BP, which can potentially disrupt fresh suture lines of anastomoses, causing bleeding and graft failure. Hypotension may be an indicator of low cardiac output. Pulmonary artery pressures (PAP), pulmonary artery wedge pressure (PAWP), cardiac output, and oxygen saturation are other parameters to assess and document for the client with a pulmonary artery catheter in place. These invasive hemodynamic monitors are discussed further in the section on heart failure.*
- Auscultate heart and breath sounds on admission and at least every 4 hours. *Changes in heart sounds may indicate impaired myocardial function. A ventricular gallop, or S_3, is an early sign of congestive heart failure; an S_4 may be present because of decreased ventricular compliance. Muffled heart sounds may be an early indication of cardiac tamponade. Breath sounds are assessed frequently to detect early signs of heart failure (crackles or rales).*
- Assess the client's skin color and temperature, peripheral pulses, and level of consciousness with vital signs. *Pale, mottled, or cyanotic coloring, cool and clammy skin, and diminished pulse amplitude are indicators of decreased cardiac output.*

- Monitor and document cardiac rhythm. *Dysrhythmias may interfere with cardiac filling and contractility, decreasing the cardiac output.*
- Measure and record intake and output hourly. Report output of under 30 mL/h for 2 consecutive hours. *These measurements provide valuable information about the client's fluid volume status. Because the glomerular filtration rate depends on an adequate cardiac output, the urinary output provides an early indication of decreased cardiac output.*
- Record chest tube output hourly. Monitor for a decrease in hemoglobin and hematocrit values. *Chest tube output and the hemoglobin and hematocrit are indicators of bleeding and blood volume. A sudden decrease in chest tube output may signal cardiac tamponade. Large amounts of blood loss through the chest tubes may indicate bleeding from anastomoses or impaired coagulation. This needs to be reported to the surgeon immediately.*
- Administer intravenous fluids, fluid boluses, and blood transfusions as ordered. *Fluid and blood replacement is necessary to ensure an adequate circulating blood volume and oxygen-carrying capacity.*
- Administer medications as ordered. *Medications that may be prescribed in the immediate postoperative period to maintain the cardiac output include inotropic drugs (e.g., dopamine, dobutamine, digitalis) to increase the force of myocardial contractions; vasodilators (e.g., nitroprusside or nitroglycerin) to decrease vascular resistance and afterload; and antidysrhythmics to manage rhythm disturbances affecting cardiac output.*
- Keep a temporary pacer box at the bedside, and initiate pacing as indicated. *Temporary pacing may be needed to maintain the cardiac output with some dysrhythmias, such as high-level AV blocks.*
- Assess for signs of cardiac tamponade: increased heart rate, decreased BP, decreased urine output, increased central venous pressure, a sudden decrease in chest tube output, muffled/distant heart sounds, diminished peripheral pulses. **Notify physician immediately.** *Cardiac tamponade is a life-threatening complication that may occur in both the early and late postoperative period. Cardiac tamponade interferes with ventricular filling and pumping, decreasing cardiac output. Untreated, cardiac tamponade will lead to cardiac arrest and the possible death of the client.*

Postoperative Nursing Care of Clients Having Coronary Artery Bypass Grafting (continued)

■ ■ ■

Hypothermia

The client is cooled to a moderate hypothermic range (82 to 92 F or 28 to 33.5 C) during surgery to decrease tissue demands for oxygen and protect vital organs from ischemic damage. The client is rewarmed on completion of the surgery; however, clients often remain hypothermic on admission to the recovery area. Gradual rewarming is necessary to prevent peripheral vasodilation and hypotension ("rewarming shock").

Selected nursing interventions with rationales follow:

- Monitor and document core temperature in the immediate postoperative period. Use the same site (tympanic membrane, pulmonary artery, bladder) for consistent measurements. *Oral and rectal temperatures are not reliable measures of core temperature in the first 8 hours after surgery (Howie, 1991).*

- Institute rewarming methods if the client's temperature is below 96.8 F (36 C). *Temperatures below 96.8 F (36 C) may cause shivering, resulting in increased oxygen demand and consumption. Hypothermia may also lead to hypoxia, metabolic acidosis, vasoconstriction and increased cardiac workload, alterations in clotting mechanisms, and cardiac dysrhythmias.*

- Institute rewarming as needed, using warmed intravenous fluids or blood transfusions; warm cotton blankets wrapped around the client's head, extremities, and torso; fluid-filled or warm-air-filled thermal blankets; warm inspired gases; warm ambient air; and radiant heat lamps or lights. *These decrease conductive and radiant heat losses after surgery and promote comfort. Radiant heat lamps or lights promote heat gain as well. Peripheral vasoconstriction, which is common in postoperative clients, may limit the effectiveness of some interventions.*

- Monitor vital signs and oxygen saturation. *Rewarming causes peripheral vasodilation, resulting in changes in blood volume distribution. This may lead to hypotension, compromising tissue perfusion.*

- Administer meperidine, thorazine, morphine sulfate, or diazepam as ordered. *These drugs may be used to treat shivering.*

Pain

The client who has had a CABG experiences postoperative pain in both the chest wall and the leg from which the saphenous vein was harvested. The client

with an IMA graft may complain of more pain on one side of the chest than the other (usually the left, because the left IMA is used most frequently) because of stretching during dissection of the IMA graft from the chest wall. Chest tube sites are also uncomfortable. The leg from which the saphenous vein graft was obtained is usually incised from groin to ankle, often causing more pain than the chest incision.

Selected nursing interventions with rationales follow:

- Instruct the client to report pain promptly, including its location and character. Document intensity, using a rating scale of 0 to 10. Assess the client for verbal and nonverbal indicators of pain. Validate pain cues with the client. *Pain is a subjective experience that differs with each individual. Incisional pain is expected after cardiac surgery; however, some clients also experience anginal pain caused by a perioperative myocardial infarction. Pain characteristics help differentiate incisional chest pain from pain caused by angina or a myocardial infarction. Pain scales are useful to evaluate the effectiveness of interventions. Pain is expressed in many ways, depending on the client's culture and learned experiences. Validation of pain cues with the client is important.*

- Monitor and document vital signs. *Pain stimulates the sympathetic nervous system, increasing the heart rate, respiratory rate, and blood pressure. Clients with severe cardiac dysfunction may exhibit decreases in heart rate and blood pressure.*

- Administer prescribed analgesics on a scheduled basis for the first 24 to 48 hours after surgery. *Research data show that administering analgesics on a scheduled basis in the immediate postoperative period reduces complications from sympathetic stimulation and allows faster recovery (Edwards, 1990). The pain experience causes muscle tension and vasoconstriction, impairing circulation and tissue perfusion, slowing wound healing, and increasing cardiac work.*

- Premedicate the client 30 minutes before activities or planned procedures. *Premedication and the subsequent reduction of pain allows the client to participate and cooperate with the plan of care.*

Ineffective Breathing Pattern/Impaired Gas Exchange

Atelectasis is the most common pulmonary complication after cardiac surgery (McCauley & Brest, 1985).

➤

Postoperative Nursing Care of Clients Having Coronary Artery Bypass Grafting (continued)

■ ■ ■

Breathing and gas exchange may also be affected by blood loss and decreased oxygen-carrying capacity and decreased ventilation and lung expansion from postoperative pain. Phrenic nerve paralysis is a potential complication of myocardial cooling or surgical injury to the phrenic nerve which may also contribute to ventilatory problems.

Selected nursing interventions with rationales follow:

■ Evaluate respiratory rate, depth, effort, and symmetry of chest wall expansion frequently. *Changes in the client's respiratory rate, depth, and effort may be caused by pain, anxiety, fever, fluid volume excess, surgical injury, narcotics and anesthesia, and altered blood levels of oxygen and carbon dioxide. Decreased chest expansion or asymmetry of movement may indicate accumulated secretions, fluid overload, pneumothorax, phrenic nerve paralysis, or displacement of the endotracheal tube (ETT) and needs to be evaluated further.*

■ Auscultate breath sounds, noting any diminished or adventitious sounds. *Left lower lobe atelectasis is common after cardiac surgery and usually resolves with good pulmonary hygiene, including use of the incentive spirometer and deep breathing. Crackles or rhonchi may indicate fluid excess or infection.*

■ Assess skin and mucous membranes for color. *Color is an indicator of the oxygen-carrying capacity and status of the blood. Pallor indicates low hemoglobin and impaired oxygen-carrying capacity; cyanosis or dusky coloring is a late sign of hypoxemia.*

■ Note ETT placement on the chest X-ray. Mark the tube at the client's lips, and secure it in place. Insert an oral airway. *The chest X-ray is used to document correct placement of the ETT above the bifurcation to the right and left mainstem bronchus. Marking its placement externally at the lips provides a baseline for evaluating ETT movement. The ETT is firmly secured in place to prevent slippage or inadvertent removal. Because the ETT can become obstructed when the client bites down, an oral airway is used in conjunction with an ETT.*

■ Maintain ventilator settings as ordered. Obtain and monitor arterial blood gases (ABGs). Record pulse oximetry readings every hour. *Mechanical ventilation promotes optimal lung expansion and oxygenation in the immediate postoperative period. The ABGs and pulse oximetry readings allow monitoring of oxygenation and acid-base balance.*

■ Prepare the client for ventilator weaning and extubation, as appropriate. Decrease narcotic analgesics, as ordered. Elevate the head of the bed, and place the client in Fowler's position. *The client is ventilated in the early postoperative period until the effects of anesthesia wear off and respiratory muscle strength returns. The client is weaned from the ventilator and extubed as soon as possible to reduce complications associated with mechanical ventilation and intubation. Explain the process of weaning and extubation to reassure the client and promote cooperation. Narcotic analgesics may be decreased during the weaning period because they may depress respirations and therefore interfere with weaning. Elevating the head of the bed and placing the client in Fowler's position facilitates lung expansion and respiratory function.*

■ Suction the client as needed. Hyperoxygenate before, during, and after suctioning, and hyperventilate during the procedure. *Suctioning irritates the pulmonary tree and may promote the production of secretions, therefore it should not be done routinely but performed only when indicated. Hyperoxygenation and hyperventilation have been shown to decrease the hypoxic effects of suctioning.*

■ After extubation, teach the client how to use the incentive spirometer, and encourage its use every 2 hours. Encourage deep breathing, but advise the client to avoid vigorous coughing. Teach the client how to use a "cough pillow" to help splint chest and decrease pain. While the client remains on bed rest, turn the client every 2 hours. Dangle the client on postoperative day 1. *These strategies improve respiratory function and help prevent complications. Vigorous coughing is discouraged because it may excessively increase intrathoracic pressure and cause sternal instability.*

Risk for Infection

Following an open chest procedure, the client is at risk for infection of the sternum that may progress to involve the mediastinum. Clients with IMA grafts, diabetic clients, older adults, and the malnourished are especially at risk: harvesting of the IMA interrupts the blood supply to the relatively avascular sternum, and these clients have decreased immune responses and impaired healing.

Selected nursing interventions with rationales follow:

Postoperative Nursing Care of Clients Having Coronary Artery Bypass Grafting (continued)

- Assess the sternal wound every shift. Document the presence of redness, warmth, swelling, and/or drainage from the site. Note approximation of the wound edges. *These assessments allow the nurse to evaluate the progress of wound healing.*

- Maintain a sterile dressing for the first 48 hours after surgery. After 48 hours, leave the incision open to the air. Use Steri-strips as needed to maintain approximation of the wound edges. *The sterile dressing prevents contamination of the wound from the environment. Leaving the incision open to the air after 48 hours promotes healing.*

- Report to the physician any signs of wound infection: swollen, reddened area that is hot and painful to the touch; any drainage from the wound; areas that are not healing, or healed areas that reopen. *These findings are indications of infection or poor healing that require further evaluation and interventions.*

- Obtain a culture of wound drainage as ordered. *Identifying the infective organism allows the health care team to implement appropriate antibiotic therapy.*

- Collaborate with the dietitian to facilitate adequate nutritional and fluid intake. *Good nutritional status is vital to the healing process and optimal immune function.*

Risk for Altered Tissue Perfusion (Cardiac Dysrhythmias)

Postoperatively, the client who has had a CABG is at risk for dysrhythmias. Altered homeostasis, underlying cardiac disease, and myocardial irritation due to ischemia, surgical manipulation, pacing wires, and invasive catheters all contribute to the increased risk for dysrhythmias. Other contributing factors include pain, anemia, hypovolemia, altered temperature, gastric distention, and drugs.

Selected nursing interventions with rationales follow:

- Monitor the rhythm continuously; document the cardiac rhythm every shift and any changes as they occur. Obtain a 12-lead ECG, and notify the physician of any abnormal findings. *Continuous monitoring allows for early identification and treatment of dysrhythmias.*

- Monitor and document vital signs. Assess for manifestations of decreased cardiac output. Investigate reports of chest pain immediately. *Assessment of the client is important to determine the effects of the dysrhythmia and the urgency of intervention.*

- Monitor serum electrolyte values including potassium, calcium, and magnesium levels. *Imbalances in these particular electrolytes adversely affect cardiac rhythm and contractility. Many factors in the postoperative period (e.g., diuresis and bleeding) can alter fluid and electrolyte status. Electrolyte replacement may terminate certain dysrhythmias.*

- Administer antidysrhythmic drugs as indicated. *On many cardiac recovery units, the nurse may administer certain antidysrhythmic agents by protocol when needed to ensure rapid intervention.*

- Initiate temporary pacing as indicated. *Temporary pacing (using either temporary pacing wires or transcutaneous pacing) may be necessary to treat heart blocks or override a complex tachydysrhythmia. A transvenous pacemaker may be necessary if temporary pacing wires are not placed in surgery.*

- Maintain intravenous access. *Maintaining a patent intravenous access is imperative to administer emergency drugs and fluids.*

Altered Thought Processes

Many factors can influence neuropsychologic functioning after CABG (Mravinac, 1991). Postcardiotomy delirium (also called ICU psychosis) may be a direct result of the length of cardiopulmonary bypass, the client's age, any presurgery organic brain dysfunction, the severity of illness, or decreased cardiac output. Other culprits are sensory overload and deprivation and sleep disturbances from the ICU environment and routines. This problem may present on the client's recovery from anesthesia and usually resolves after the client is transferred from the ICU (McCauley & Brest, 1985).

Selected nursing interventions with rationales follow:

- Reorient the client frequently during recovery from anesthesia. State that surgery is over and that the client is in the recovery room or ICU. *Frequent reorientation provides emotional support and reality checks for the client.*

- Explain all procedures to the client before performing them. Speak in a clear, calm voice. Encourage questions, and give honest answers. *These are important measures to provide information, decrease anxiety, and establish trust.*

Postoperative Nursing Care of Clients Having Coronary Artery Bypass Grafting (continued)

■ ■ ■

- Secure all intravenous lines and invasive catheters/tubes (e.g., ETT, Foley catheter, nasogastric tube). *Disoriented clients may tug or pull at invasive equipment, disrupting them and increasing the risk of injury.*

- Note the client's verbal responses to questions. Correct misconceptions immediately (e.g., "Mr. Snow, look at all the special equipment in this room. Does this room look like your bedroom at home?"). *Helping the client recognize differences in the hospital environment offers a basis that the client can use for continual reality checks.*

- Maintain a calendar and clock in the room where the client can easily see them. *This provides current information regarding day, date, and time.*

- Involve family members in keeping the client oriented. Place familiar objects and photographs in the room. Encourage the family to visit. *The family can assist the client by discussing current events and family information and reorienting the client as needed.*

- Allow the client to participate in own care and make decisions where appropriate. *This allows the client to maintain some sense of power and control over his or her life and enables the client to take an active role in recovery.*

- Report signs of hallucinations, delusions, depression, or agitation. *These may indicate progressive deterioration of the client's mental state.*

- Administer sedatives cautiously. *Mild sedation may help to prevent client injury. Some sedatives may, however, have adverse effects on the central nervous system of older adult clients.*

- Reevaluate the client's neurologic status every shift. *This allows the nurse to evaluate the effectiveness of the interventions.*

Other Nursing Diagnoses

Other diagnoses that may be appropriate for the client after cardiac surgery include the following:

- *Fluid Volume Deficit* related to fluid shifts secondary to cardiopulmonary bypass
- *Impaired Skin Integrity* related to surgical procedure and immobility
- *Risk for Infection* related to invasive lines and surgical incisions
- *Ineffective Family Coping* related to lack of information regarding client's status and fear of the unknown
- *Knowledge Deficit* regarding cardiac rehabilitation program

---

- If the client has a prescription for nitroglycerin, keep the medication at the client's bedside so that it may be taken at the onset of pain. *Anginal pain is indicative of myocardial ischemia. It is important to treat it immediately to restore adequate blood flow and oxygen to the heart muscle.*

- Start oxygen at 4 to 6 L/min per nasal cannula unless contraindicated by chronic pulmonary disease. *Supplemental oxygen reduces myocardial hypoxia.*

- Space activities to allow the client to rest between them. *Activity increases cardiac work and may precipitate angina. Spacing of activities allows the heart to recover.*

- Teach the client about the use of prescribed medications to maintain myocardial perfusion and reduce cardiac work. Emphasize that long-acting nitrates, beta-blockers, and calcium channel blockers are used to prevent anginal attacks, not to treat an acute attack. *It is important for the client to understand the purpose and precautions associated with prescribed medications to maintain optimal perfusion of the heart.*

- Instruct the client to take a sublingual nitroglycerin tablet before engaging in activities that precipitate angina (e.g., climbing stairs, sexual intercourse). *This prophylactic dose of nitroglycerin helps maintain cardiac perfusion when increased work is anticipated, preventing ischemia and chest pain.*

- Encourage the client to undertake risk factor management strategies, such as losing weight, making dietary changes (reducing fat, cholesterol, and kcal intake), reducing stress, and others as indicated. *Risk factor management is vital to slow or reverse the process of atherosclerosis in the coronary arteries and preserve myocardial perfusion.*

- Discuss exercise with the client, encouraging the client to implement and maintain a progressive exercise program under the supervision of his or her primary care

Text continues on page 1083

Critical Pathway for Client Following Coronary Bypass Surgery

	Date _____ **Preoperative**	Date _____ **1st 12–24 hours postoperative**	Date _____ **2nd Day postoperative**
	Expected length of stay: 5 to 6 days		
Daily outcomes	The client ■ Verbalizes understanding of preoperative teaching including: ventilator, turn, cough, deep breath TCDC, mobilization, O₂ therapy, chest tubes, IV therapy, Foley catheter, telemetry, pain management. ■ Demonstrates ability to cope. ■ Verbalizes understanding of procedures. ■ Obtain informed consent.	The client: ■ Has stable hemodynamic measurements. ■ Maintains adequate cardiac output. ■ Has equal and bilateral peripheral pulses. ■ Maintains urine output above 30 mL/h. ■ Responds adequately to diuretic therapy. ■ Maintains an effective breathing pattern. ■ Has patent chest tubes. ■ Recovers from anesthesia, as evidenced by return of vital signs to baseline and responsiveness to stimuli. ■ Has a clean wound with well-approximated edges healing by first intention. When extubated, the client ■ Demonstrates an effective breathing pattern. ■ Verbalizes understanding and demonstrates cooperation with turning, deep breathing, coughing, and splinting. ■ Verbalizes understanding and demonstrates cooperation with sternotomy precautions. ■ Verbalizes control of incisional pain with ordered medications. ■ Demonstrates ability to cope.	The client ■ Has stable vital signs and stable cardiac rhythm and is awake, alert, and oriented. ■ Maintains an adequate cardiac output and effective breathing pattern. ■ Maintains urine output above 30 mL/h. ■ Responds appropriately to diuretics. ■ Has a clean wound with well-approximated edges healing by first intention. ■ Demonstrates cooperation with turning, deep breathing, and splinting. ■ Has patent chest tubes (if not removed). ■ Tolerates ordered diet without nausea and vomiting. ■ Demonstrates cooperation with sternotomy precautions. ■ Verbalizes control of incisional pain. ■ Ambulates 2 to 3 times/day as tolerated. ■ Demonstrates ability to cope. ■ Tolerates activity free of signs of cardiac compromise.
Assessments, tests, and treatments	CBC, urinalysis ECG, Chest X-ray Type and crossmatch Baseline physical assessment with focus on respiratory and renal status. Preoperative O₂ saturation.	Vital signs and O₂ saturation, neurovascular assessment, and dressing assessment per guideline for care. Ventilator care and weaning per protocol. ABGs prn.	Vital signs and O₂ saturation, neurovascular assessment, dressing assessment q2–4h and prn. Intake and output q4–8h. Foley catheter. Hemoglobin and hematocrit.

➤

Critical Pathway for Client Following Coronary Bypass Surgery (continued)

	Date _____ Preoperative	Date _____ 1st 12–24 hours postoperative	Date _____ 2nd Day postoperative
Assessments, tests, and treatments (*continued*)		Telemetry monitoring. Hemodynamic monitoring per guidelines for care. Initiate weaning protocol when ABGs stable, then initiate oxygen via face mask. Maintain PO_2 above 90%. Chest tubes to 10 to 20 cm of H_2O pressure. Foley catheter to constant drainage. Assess peripheral pulses q1–2h and prn. ACE wraps to lower legs; remove and replace q shift. Intake and output qh. Transfuse as ordered. Portable chest X-ray, ECG, CBC, serum potassium (K^+) on admission to unit. Hemoglobin and hematocrit. Maintain sterile dressing; reinforce prn. D/C arterial line before transfer to stepdown unit.	Prothrombin time. Incentive spirometer q2h. O_2 as indicated. Assess calves for redness, tenderness, swelling, heat, and edema every shift. ACE wraps: Remove and replace every shift. Maintain dry, sterile dressing; reinforce prn. Assess wound and change dressing per physician's order. Telemetry. Weight. Epicardial wire care per protocol. Hemoglobin and hematocrit. Serum K^+.
Knowledge deficit	Orient to room and surroundings. Provide simple, brief instructions. Preoperative teaching including hospital and surgical routines, including ventilator, TCDB, mobilization, O_2 therapy, chest tubes, IV therapy, Foley catheter, telemetry, pain management.	Orient client and family to room and postoperative routine. Include family in teaching. Review plan of care. When client is extubated, review importance of deep breathing, coughing, splinting incision, incentive spirometer, mobilization, management of drainage tubes and intravenous lines, sternotomy precautions, and pain management. Prepare for transfer to stepdown unit. Assess understanding of teaching.	Review importance of early progressive exercise. Review plan of care with client and family. Reinforce sternotomy precautions and safety measures. Assess understanding of teaching.

	Date _____ **Preoperative**	Date _____ **1st 12–24 hours postoperative**	Date _____ **2nd Day postoperative**
Diet	Baseline nutritional and hydration assessment.	NPO	If clear liquids are tolerated, advance to full to American Heart Association (AHA) diet as tolerated.
Activity	Assess safety needs and provide appropriate measures.	Bed rest and sternotomy precautions Turn, cough, and deep breathe q2h. ROM exercises every shift Assess safety needs and maintain appropriate precautions.	Maintain safety and sternotomy precautions. TCDB q1–2h. Assist out of bed 2 to 3 times. Begin ambulation per physical therapy protocol.
Psycho-social	Assess potential for postoperative confusion. Assess anxiety regarding impending surgery. Assess fear of unknown and surgery. Offer emotional support. Encourage verbalization of concerns. Provide information regarding surgical experience. Include family teaching and provide support. Minimize external stimuli (noise and movement)	Assess level of anxiety. Provide information and ongoing support and encouragement to client and family.	Assess level of anxiety. Encourage verbalization of concerns. Provide information and ongoing support and encouragement to client and family.
Medications	Preoperative medications as ordered per anesthesia.	Analgesics as ordered. IV antibiotics. IV fluids per protocol. IV KCl and magnesium as ordered. Vasoactive IV medications as ordered/per protocol. Diuretics as ordered. Routine medications as ordered.	Analgesics as ordered. Stool softener. Initiate aspirin therapy (81 mg/day). Subcutaneous (SQ) heparin. IV fluid per protocol. IV KCl as ordered. Diuretics as ordered. Routine medications as ordered.
Transfer/ discharge plan	Assess potential discharge needs and support system. Establish discharge goals with client and family.	Home assessment, if not previously completed. Consult with social service regarding projected needs for home health care, including home health aides, visiting nurse, physical and occupational therapist. Establish discharge objectives with client and family.	Review with client and significant others discharge objectives regarding activity and home care. Consult and collaborate with cardiac rehabilitation and physical therapy. Complete discharge planning.

➤

Critical Pathway for Client Following Coronary Bypass Surgery (continued)

	Date _____ 3rd Day postoperative	Date _____ 4th Day postoperative	
Daily outcomes	The client ■ Is afebrile with stable vital signs. ■ Has stable cardiac rhythm. ■ Has lungs clear to auscultation. ■ Has a clean wound with well-approximated edges healing by first intention. ■ Has stable vital signs. ■ Demonstrates cooperation with turning, deep breathing, and splinting. ■ Tolerates ordered diet without nausea and vomiting. ■ Demonstrates cooperation with sternotomy precautions. ■ Verbalizes control of incisional pain. ■ Ambulates 50 to 100 feet three or four times. ■ Demonstrates ability to cope. ■ Tolerates activity without signs of cardiac compromise.	The client ■ Is afebrile, has stable vital signs and stable cardiac rhythm, and is awake, alert, and oriented. ■ Has a clean wound with well-approximated edges healing by first intention. ■ Demonstrates cooperation with turning, deep breathing, coughing, and splinting. ■ Tolerates ordered diet without nausea and vomiting. ■ Demonstrates cooperation with sternotomy precautions. ■ Verbalizes control of incisional pain. ■ Ambulates 150 to 200 feet four times. ■ Demonstrates ability to cope. ■ Tolerates activity without evidence of cardiac compromise.	
Assessments, tests, and treatments	Vital signs and O_2 saturation, neurovascular assessment, dressing assessment q4h. Intake and output every shift. Remove chest dressings and paint incisions with povidone-iodine twice daily. Rewrap ACEs on legs twice daily and prn. Incentive spirometer q2h. O_2 as indicated. Assess calves for redness, tenderness, swelling, heat, and edema every shift. TED stockings: remove and replace every shift and prn. D/C chest tubes. Telemetry. Weight. Epicardial wire care per protocol. D/C Foley catheter, and assess voiding.	Vital signs and O_2 sat q4h and prn Head-to-toe assessment. Change dressings daily and prn. Assess wound healing. TED stockings: Remove and replace every shift Assess calves for redness, tenderness, swelling, heat, and edema every shift. Intake and output every shift; assess urine output; notify physician of imbalance. Weight: Notify physician of weight gain. Epicardial wire care. D/C oxygen if O_2 saturation above 92%. ECG/CXR. Serum K^+ and CBC. D/C telemetry if indicated.	

	Date _____ **3rd Day postoperative**	Date _____ **4th Day postoperative**	
	D/C oxygen when O$_2$ saturation rises above 92%. Serum K$^+$.		
Knowledge deficit	Review plan of care. Include family in teaching. Initiate discharge teaching regarding wound care, home exercise program, and diet. Provide cardiac teaching. Assess understanding of teaching.	Review plan of care. Include family in teaching. Continue discharge teaching regarding wound care, activity, and diet. Assess understanding of teaching. Provide cardiac teaching; include family.	
Diet	AHA diet as tolerated. Encourage high-fiber diet rich in vitamin C. Dietary consult for dietary instruction.	AHA diet as tolerated. Encourage high-fiber diet rich in vitamin C.	
Activity	Maintain safety and sternotomy precautions. TCDB q2h. Assist out of bed 2 to 3 times. Begin ambulation per physical therapy protocol (50 to 100 feet).	Encourage self-care. Ambulate 150 to 200 feet 4 times daily.	
Psycho-social	Assess level of anxiety. Encourage verbalization of concerns. Provide information and ongoing support and encouragement to client and family.	Encourage verbalization of concerns. Provide ongoing support and encouragement to client and family.	
Medications	Oral analgesics. Stool softener. Diuretics as ordered. Aspirin therapy. SQ heparin. Intermittent IV device. Routine medications as ordered.	Analgesics PO. Stool softener. Aspirin therapy. SQ heparin (D/C per order). Routine medications as ordered. D/C intermittent IV device if client is off telemetry. Warfarin therapy if ordered.	
Transfer/discharge plan	Review with client and significant others progress toward discharge objectives. Collaborate with physical therapist. Make appropriate referrals.	Review with client and significant others discharge objectives regarding activity and home care. Collaborate with cardiac rehabilitation and physical therapy departments.	

Critical Pathway for Client Following Coronary Bypass Surgery (continued)

	Date _____ 5th Day postoperative	Date _____ 6th Day postoperative (Discharge Day)	
Daily outcomes	The client ■ Is afebrile, has stable vital signs and stable cardiac rhythm, and is awake, alert and oriented. ■ Has a clean wound with well-approximated edges healing by first intention. ■ Demonstrates cooperation with turning, coughing, deep breathing, and splinting. ■ Tolerates ordered diet without nausea and vomiting. ■ Verbalizes control of incisional pain. ■ Ambulates 150 to 300 feet four times. ■ Tolerates activities without evidence of intolerance. ■ Demonstrates ability to cope.	The client ■ Is afebrile. ■ Is alert and oriented. ■ Has a dry, clean wound with well-approximated edges healing by first intention. ■ Has stable vital signs and stable rhythm pattern. ■ Manages pain with non-pharmacologic measures and ordered medications. ■ Is independent in self-care. ■ Ambulates 300 to 500 feet four times daily. ■ Has resumed preadmission urine and bowel elimination pattern. ■ Verbalizes/demonstrates home care instructions. ■ Tolerates AHA diet. ■ Demonstrates ability to cope with ongoing stressors.	
Assessments, tests, and treatments	Vital signs q4h. Head-to-toe assessment. Remove dressings. Assess wound healing. Hemoglobin and hematocrit. Weight. D/C epicardial pacing wires.	Vital signs every shift. Head-to-toe assessment. Assess wounds. Weight. Assess pacing wire site.	
Knowledge deficit	Review plan of care with client and family. Continue discharge teaching regarding wound care, activity, and diet. Review safety measures for transfers and ambulation for home care. Assess understanding of teaching.	Provide discharge teaching for client and/or significant other, including wound care, activity level and exercise program, safety measures, diet, signs and symptoms to report, follow-up care and physician's appointment, cardiac rehabilitation medications; name, purpose, dose, frequency, route, dietary interactions, and side effects, and home care arrangements. Assess understanding of teaching	

	Date _____ **5th Day postoperative**	**Date** _____ **6th Day postoperative** **(Discharge Day)**	
Diet	AHA diet as tolerated. Encourage high-fiber diet rich in vitamin C.	AHA diet as tolerated. Encourage high-fiber diet rich in vitamin C.	
Activity	Ambulate 150 to 300 feet 4 times daily, and carry out stair climbing per physical therapy regimen. Shower.	Ambulate 300 to 500 feet 4 times daily. Shower.	
Psycho-social	Encourage verbalization of concerns. Provide ongoing support and encouragement to client and family.	Encourage verbalization of concerns. Provide ongoing support and encouragement to client and family.	
Medications	Analgesics (PO). Stool softener. Laxative if no BM in 3 days. Aspirin or warfarin therapy as ordered. Routine medications as ordered.	Analgesics (PO). Stool softener. SQ heparin. Aspirin or warfarin therapy as ordered. Routine medications as ordered.	
Transfer/ discharge plan	Review with client and significant others discharge objectives regarding activity and home care. Collaborate with cardiac rehabilitation and physical therapy departments. Complete referrals for home health care, including home health aides, visiting nurse, physical therapy, and cardiac rehabilitation.	Discharge with referrals for home health care and cardiac rehabilitation.	

provider. _Exercise is important not only to slow the atherosclerotic process but also to develop collateral circulation to the heart muscle._

- Refer the client who smokes to a smoking cessation program. _Nicotine causes vasoconstriction and increases the heart rate, decreasing myocardial perfusion and increasing cardiac workload._

Risk for Ineffective Individual Management of Therapeutic Regimen

Denial may be strong in the client with angina pectoris. Because many people think of the heart as the locus of life itself, problems such as angina remind people of their mortality, an uncomfortable fact. Denial may cause some clients to "forget" to take prescribed medications or to attempt activities that they know will precipitate anginal attacks. Other clients, by contrast, may become "cardiac cripples," fearing to participate in any activities because of anticipated chest pain. Their inactivity may actually hasten the atherosclerotic process and inhibit collateral circulation development, worsening angina.

Selected nursing interventions with rationales follow:

- Assess the client's knowledge and understanding of the pathophysiologic processes involved in angina. *Assessment allows the nurse to tailor teaching and interventions to the needs of the client.*

- Provide teaching about angina and atherosclerosis as needed. *This can help the client understand that angina is a manageable disease and that pain can usually be controlled and the disease progress slowed.*

- Provide written and verbal instructions about prescribed medications and their use. *Written instructions reinforce teaching and are available to the client for future reference.*

- Stress the importance of taking chest pains seriously while maintaining a positive attitude. *Although it is vital for the client to recognize the significance of chest pain and deal with it appropriately, it is also important that the client maintain a positive outlook.*

- Refer the client to a cardiac rehabilitation program or other organized activities and support groups for clients with coronary artery disease. *Programs such as these help the client develop strategies for risk factor management, maintain a program of supervised activity, and gain coping skills.*

Other Nursing Diagnoses

Other nursing diagnoses that may be appropriate for the client with angina follow:

- *Risk for Decreased Cardiac Output* related to myocardial ischemia
- *Altered Role Performance* related to activity-induced chest pain
- *Risk for Altered Sexuality Patterns* related to fear of chest pain
- *Activity Intolerance* related to impaired coronary blood flow
- *Anticipatory Grieving* related to perceived mortality

Client and Family Teaching

Many clients with stable angina can manage their pain effectively, continuing to live active and productive lives. The client needs to understand the disease and the processes that cause chest pain. Emphasize the relationship between the pain and the reduction in blood flow to the heart muscle. Discuss the use of prescribed medica-

tions. Teach the client to take nitroglycerin prophylactically, before activities that tend to cause chest pain. Instruct the client to take a tablet at the first indication of pain rather than waiting to see whether the pain develops. Emphasize the importance of seeking immediate medical assistance if three nitroglycerin tablets over 15 to 20 minutes do not relieve the pain. Instruct the client not to call the physician but to call 911 or go to the emergency department immediately.

Teach the client how to safely store medications, nitroglycerin in particular. Because this is an unstable compound, tell the client to store it in a cool, dry, dark place and to keep no more than a 6-month supply on hand. Tell the client to always carry a few tablets but not the whole supply, because body warmth (which is transmitted through a shirt or pants pocket) causes the tablets to deteriorate more rapidly. If a nitroglycerin patch or ointment is prescribed, teach the client how to apply it. Explain the rationale for removing the patch or ointment at night.

Stress the importance of not discontinuing medications abruptly, particularly the beta-blockers. Review their possible adverse effects with the client, and instruct the client when to notify the physician.

As noted previously, teach the client about the relationship between modifiable risk factors and angina. See the previous section on coronary artery disease for further teaching strategies related to risk factors.

Preoperative teaching for the client undergoing cardiac surgery includes general surgical information (e.g., instruction about postoperative breathing and leg exercises), as well as specifics related to the planned cardiac surgery. See Chapter 7 to review care of the client having surgery. When providing postoperative teaching, reinforce instructions about respiratory care, activity, and pain management. Clients recovering from CABG surgery experience pain and discomfort from both the chest wall injuries and the leg incision(s). In addition, the client is reluctant to breathe deeply and turn. Encourage the client and reinforce the importance of being an active participant in rehabilitation. Predischarge teaching covers any prescribed medications, the manifestations of sternal or leg infection, pain management, diet, and activity. Discuss posthospital cardiac rehabilitation. See the sections on myocardial infarction for further discussion of cardiac rehabilitation.

Applying the Nursing Process

Case Study of a Client After Coronary Artery Bypass Surgery, Cardiac Rehabilitation Phase: John Clements

Six weeks ago, John Clements, 50 years old, was discharged from the hospital after undergoing an emergency triple bypass surgery. Despite the emergency nature of his surgery, his postoperative recovery course was uneventful, and he was discharged 7 days after admission. He has returned to the clinic for a postoperative stress test and to discuss plans for the outpatient phase of the cardiac rehabilitation program with the cardiac rehab nurse. Anne Wagner, a cardiac clinical nurse specialist and the program coordinator, meets Mr. Clements in the clinic to obtain specific information regarding his medical status: a medical history, especially cardiovascular history, risk factor analysis, and information regarding life-style and health habits. Mr. Clements has just come from his physician's office for his 6-week postoperative physical exam.

Assessment

Mr. Clements's medical history reveals significant CAD, an anterior wall myocardial infarction that led to the emergent triple bypass, and hyperlipidemia. Current medications include Cardizem, Isordil, Ecotrin, and Transderm-Nitro 5. The ECG reveals a sinus rhythm with some flattening of the ST segment and T wave. His resting heart rate is 68, and blood pressure is 136/84.

Risk factor assessment shows a family history of CAD. Mr. Clements does not smoke and uses alcohol occasionally in social situations; he enjoys "good Southern-style cooking" and watching TV. Mr. Clements states that the only regular exercise he used to get was an evening of dancing with his wife and friends about once a month, "But I get short of breath walking around the block now, so I guess I can't go dancing anymore!"

Mr. Clements owns his own contracting business and states that he typically works about 50 to 60 hours per week. His partner has been running the business since Mr. Clements's illness. Mrs. Clements does the bookkeeping for the business. Mr. Clements tells Ms. Wagner, "I don't know what this program is supposed to do for me. I have got to get back to work! You just can't sit around in my business—you have to make sure that the work is getting done on time, and you have to check on supplies and equipment and the like. But I feel like a weakling—I need to get my energy back!"

Diagnosis

Based on the assessment data, Ms. Wagner formulates the following nursing diagnoses with Mr. Clements:

- *Activity Intolerance* related to general weakness and fatigue
- *Knowledge Deficit* regarding the cardiac rehabilitation program
- *Altered Role Performance* related to health crisis

Expected Outcomes

Mr. Clements and Ms. Wagner mutually agree that he will

- Verbalize an understanding of the definition and components of a structured cardiac rehabilitation program.
- Verbalize a desire to make life-style changes.
- Identify resources available in the community to assist with life-style changes.
- Participate in the structured activity program without suffering any complications.
- Verbalize an increase in energy after 6 weeks on the program.
- Accept the reality of the temporary change in his usual work responsibilities.

Planning and Implementation

Ms. Wagner plans and implements the following nursing interventions based on the expected outcomes for Mr. Clements:

- Define the purpose of cardiac rehabilitation, and identify the components of a cardiac rehabilitation program.
- Provide information regarding the specific topics included in the "heart health" classes of the cardiac rehabilitation program: basic knowledge of the heart and the coronary artery disease process; the prescription for exercise and activity; the emphasis on life-style modifications, with a focus on nutrition counseling and stress management techniques; emotional reactions to CAD; sexual activity; the use of cardiac medications; and self-responsibility for health.
- Plan an individualized, comprehensive exercise program (including aerobic exercises, flexibility exercises, and muscular strength and endurance training) based on Mr. Clements's stress test results, physical examination, and interview.
- Encourage Mr. Clements to schedule rest periods before and after activity/exercise.
- Review with Mr. Clements the signs and symptoms of overexertion.
- Provide information regarding community and hospital resources for emotional and educational support.
- Emphasize the role of personal responsibility in maintaining optimal health.
- Help Mr. Clements identify strategies for dealing with his concerns about his role in his business.

Evaluation

After the initial information and interview session, Mr. Clements decides to "give the program a try." Ms. Wagner and the exercise physiologist plan an individualized activity and exercise program to meet Mr. Clements's needs, and the registered dietitian provides dietary counseling. Ms. Wagner places special emphasis on stress management strategies. Mr. Clements is able to list manifestations of overexertion and states that despite his desire to get back to full-time work, he realizes the need for gradual activity progression.

After the first 6 weeks, Mr. Clements has reported a significant increase in energy and strength. "I am feeling much stronger lately, and I have been sleeping better. Mary and I have been taking evening walks around the neighborhood, and I find myself looking forward to the exercise! My chest soreness is also gone." He has completed the 12-week cardiac rehabilitation program, and another stress test has been performed. His test results indicate that his cardiac function is adequate. Mr. Clements has joined the local Mended Hearts support group sponsored by the American Heart Association and states that he has continued to incorporate "heart-healthy" considerations into his daily routines.

Critical Thinking in the Nursing Process

1. Develop a personalized risk factor reduction plan for Mr. Clements.

2. How might the concept of denial affect the ability of Mr. Clements to (a) accept the need for cardiac rehabilitation, (b) comply with the proposed life-style changes, and (c) make permanent adjustments to his daily life?

3. How does spousal support influence a client's compliance with a structured cardiac rehabilitation program?

4. Mr. Clements tells you that since the surgery, his wife has been afraid that sexual activity will induce another heart attack. How would you respond to these concerns?

The Client with Acute Myocardial Infarction

∎ ∎ ∎

An acute **myocardial infarction (MI)**, necrosis (death) of cells in an area of cardiac muscle, is a life-threatening event: If circulation to the affected cardiac muscle is not restored in a timely manner, loss of functional myocardium affects the heart's ability to maintain an effective cardiac output and may ultimately result in cardiogenic shock and death.

Heart disease continues to be the leading cause of death in the United States; of the major heart diseases, myocardial infarction or *heart attack,* and other forms of chronic ischemic heart disease cause the majority of deaths. In 1992, almost 230,000 people in the United States died from acute MI. Another 246,000 people died as a result of old MI and other forms of chronic ischemic heart disease that same year (Centers for Disease Control

[CDC], 1994). See the accompanying box for a discussion of older people and MI.

The majority of deaths from MI occur in the initial period following the onset of manifestations; approximately 60% occur within the first hour, and 40% prior to hospitalization. Heightening public awareness of the importance of seeking immediate medical assistance and providing training in cardiopulmonary resuscitation (CPR) techniques are vital components in the effort to decrease deaths due to MI.

Myocardial infarction rarely occurs in clients who have no preexisting coronary artery disease. While no specific cause has been identified, the risk factors for MI are those for coronary artery disease: age, gender, heredity, race; smoking, obesity, hyperlipidemia, hypertension, diabetes, stress, sedentary life-style, and personality type. See the previous section of this chapter on coronary artery disease for further discussion of these risk factors.

Pathophysiology

Myocardial infarction occurs when a coronary artery becomes critically occluded, blocking blood flow to a portion of cardiac muscle for a prolonged period of time. This coronary occlusion and myocardial ischemia is usually caused by a thrombus (clot) developing at a site of arterial narrowing. The coronary artery may also be occluded by ulceration and rupture of atherosclerotic plaque or by prolonged vasospasm. Ulceration or rupture of atherosclerotic plaque stimulates platelet aggregation, platelet-thrombus formation, and changes in vasomotor tone in the region; as a result, a clot forms and the vessel becomes occluded (McCance & Huether, 1994).

Cellular injury occurs when the cells are denied adequate oxygen and nutrients. When ischemia is prolonged, lasting more than 20 to 45 minutes, irreversible hypoxemic damage causes cellular death and tissue necrosis. The infarcted or necrotic tissue ceases to contract. Intracellular enzymes are released through damaged cell membranes into interstitial spaces. Infarcted tissue is identified by a zone of necrosis surrounded by a zone of ischemia (Jensen, 1995). Tissue in this ischemic area is potentially viable; restoration of blood flow minimizes the amount of tissue lost. Vasospasm may occur, however, further impairing blood flow and increasing the ischemic zone and the risk of further necrosis.

At the center of the infarcted zone is an area of nonviable cells. The subendocardium suffers the initial damage, within 20 minutes of injury, because this area is the most susceptible to changes in coronary blood flow. The damage progresses to the epicardium within 1 to 6 hours (Jensen, 1995). Necrotic cells no longer function metabolically, nor do they produce or conduct electrical energy or participate in mechanical contraction. This results in decreased myocardial contractility, which decreases stroke volume, cardiac output, blood pressure, and tissue perfusion.

Collateral vessels are accessory pathways connected to the smaller arteries in the coronary system. When a larger artery is compromised, these collateral vessels dilate to maintain blood flow to the cardiac muscle. The degree of collateral circulation in the heart helps determine the amount of myocardial damage from ischemia. Acute occlusion of a coronary artery without any collateral flow results in massive tissue damage and possible death. Progressive narrowing of the larger coronary arteries allows collateral vessels to develop and enlarge, meeting the demand for blood flow. Good collateral circulation can diminish the size of the infarction.

Myocardial infarction usually affects the left ventricle of the heart because it is the major "workhorse" of the heart; its muscle mass is greater, as are its oxygen demands.

MIs are described according to the areas of the heart that have been damaged. The area of tissue damage is related to the coronary artery that has been occluded. Left ventricular damage is caused by occlusion of the left anterior descending (LAD) artery, decreasing blood flow to the *anterior wall* and part of the interventricular septum; occlusion of the left circumflex artery (LCA) causes *lateral wall* damage. *Right ventricular wall, inferior wall,* and *posterior wall* infarcts involve occlusions of the right coronary artery (RCA) and posterior descending artery (PDA). The most devastating occlusion is that of the left main coronary artery, which causes ischemia of the entire left ventricle, resulting in a grave prognosis. Identification of the infarct site is important to predict possible complications and determine appropriate therapy.

MIs are further classified as either *transmural* or *subendocardial*. A transmural infarction involves all layers of the cardiac tissue. A subendocardial infarction involves only the inner half of the endocardial layer of the heart: It does not progress through the myocardium and epicardium.

MIs may also be classified by the ECG changes they produce. The classic ECG change associated with an MI is development of a Q wave. MIs producing this change may be called *Q-wave infarction.* Those with a nonclassic pattern may be termed *non-Q-wave infarction.* This differentiation does not indicate the extent of myocardial damage (Jensen, 1995), so Q-wave and non-Q-wave infarctions are not synonymous with transmural and subendocardial infarctions. Non-Q wave infarctions are more common in older adults and women (Jensen, 1995). They produce smaller elevations in cardiac enzyme levels and less myocardial dysfunction than Q-wave MIs, but they have a higher incidence of late complications of reinfarction and postinfarction angina (Jensen, 1995).

Pain is a classic manifestation of MI. Other manifestations result from or depend on compensatory mechanisms, the degree of collateral circulation, the location of the infarct, and the amount of muscle damaged.

Chest pain due to MI is more severe than anginal pain. However, it is not the quality and radiation of the chest pain that distinguishes MI from angina, but its duration, the presence of other signs and symptoms, and its continuous nature. The onset of pain is sudden and usually is not associated with activity. In fact, most MIs occur in the early morning. Clients with a history of angina may experience an increased frequency of attacks in the days or weeks prior to an MI. Chest pain is often described as crushing and severe; the client may call it a pressure, heavy, or squeezing sensation, or complain of chest tightness or burning. The pain begins in the center of the chest (in the substernal region), and may radiate to the shoulders, neck, jaw, or arms. It lasts more than 15 to 20 minutes and is not relieved by rest or nitroglycerin.

Gerontologic Considerations: Care of the Older Client with an MI

■ ■ ■

Older people may not present with the typical signs and symptoms of MI. Often, they seek treatment for vague complaints of difficulty breathing, confusion, fainting, dizziness, abdominal pain, or cough. Many older adults who suffer an MI do not complain of chest pain; the prevalence of silent ischemia is greater in older adults (Wenger, 1994). When these clients do present to the emergency room or clinic with vague manifestations and a history of cardiovascular problems, an MI should be suspected.

Older adults comprise up to one-half of all the clients undergoing invasive diagnostic testing, cardiovascular procedures, and cardiac rehabilitation. This population faces higher risks of significant complications and death from MI (Wenger, 1994). Treatment of the elderly client follows the standards discussed earlier. Overall, thrombolytic therapy has been demonstrated to increase older adults' survival after MI (Wenger, 1994). Although the risks of bleeding increase with age, stroke risk is not higher in this population. Interventional and surgical therapies have also proved beneficial in older clients with MI. In older clients who experience symptoms and for whom interventional techniques are indicated and appropriate, PTCA is preferred over CABG surgery; in clients whose lesions are not suitable for PTCA, CABG still offers a favorable prognosis (Wenger, 1994).

Clinical Manifestations of Myocardial Infarction

■ ■ ■

Cardiovascular System

- Chest pain
- Tachycardia
- Possible alteration in blood pressure
- Diminished peripheral pulses
- Dysrhythmias
- Signs of left heart failure
- Diaphoresis
- Cool, mottled skin

Respiratory System

- Tachypnea
- Dyspnea
- Shortness of breath

Neurologic Effects

- Decreased level of consciousness
- Anxiety
- Feeling of impending doom

Gastrointestinal System

- Nausea and vomiting

Laboratory and Diagnostic Changes

- Electrocardiography changes
- Elevated cardiac enzyme levels
- Elevated temperature
- Leukocytosis

Compensatory mechanisms are responsible for many of the other symptoms seen with MI. Stimulation of the sympathetic nervous system causes anxiety, tachycardia, and vasoconstriction. This results in cool, clammy, mottled skin. Pain and blood chemistry changes stimulate the respiratory center, causing tachypnea. The client often experiences a sense of impending doom and death. Tissue necrosis causes an inflammatory reaction that increases the white blood cell count and elevates the temperature. Serum cardiac enzyme levels rise as enzymes are released from necrotic cardiac cells.

Other manifestations may vary, depending on the location and amount of infarcted tissue. The client may de-velop hypertension or hypotension and signs of heart failure. Irritation of the vagus nerve may produce nausea and vomiting, bradycardia, and hypotension. Hiccuping may occur because of diaphagmatic irritation. If a large amount of muscle is damaged, the first sign of MI may be sudden death. Typical signs and symptoms of MI are listed in the accompanying clinical manifestations box.

Cocaine-Induced MI

In recent years, acute myocardial infarction associated with cocaine intoxication has been reported. The effect of cocaine on the heart is not exactly known, but it is spec-ulated that cocaine induces MI by (1) causing intense sympathetic stimulation, severely increasing oxygen de-mands in excess of supply; (2) increasing platelet aggre-gation, predisposing the person to thrombus formation; or (3) inducing coronary artery spasm (Coniglio, 1991). The client with cocaine-induced MI may present with an altered level of consciousness, confusion and restlessness, seizure activity, tachycardia, hypotension, increased res-piratory rate, and respiratory crackles.

Complications

Several complications may occur with an MI. The risk of complications is related to the size and location of in-farcted tissue.

Dysrhythmias Dysrhythmias are the most frequent complication of MI. Clients experiencing inferior wall MIs may develop symptomatic bradycardia or heart blocks (second-degree or Mobitz Type I). Anterior wall infarctions are associated with an increased risk for bun-dle branch blocks, Mobitz Type II AV blocks, and ventric-ular ectopy. Sinus tachycardia is also common. It may be precipitated by adrenergic stimulation or by decreased cardiac output due to hypovolemia or pump failure. Pre-mature atrial contractions (PACs) and atrial fibrillation may occur as well. Because infarcted tissue is arrhythmo-genic, the risk of dysrhythmias increases. Premature ven-tricular contractions (PVCs) are common following an MI, particularly in the first few hours. Frequent PVCs (more than 6 per minute), couplets, short bursts of ven-tricular tachycardia, and early PVCs (R on T wave) are treated with lidocaine to reduce the risk of ventricular fi-brillation. The risk of ventricular fibrillation is greatest the first hour after MI; it is a frequent cause of sudden cardiac death associated with acute MI. Its incidence declines with time. Ventricular tachycardia may also occur, neces-sitating pharmacologic treatment or electrical cardiover-sion. If a condition pathway is affected by the infarct, nor-mal patterns of electrical conduction may be affected. Any degree of AV block may occur following MI. First-degree and Mobitz I (Wenckebach) blocks are most common, al-though up to 5% of clients with inferior infarctions de-velop complete heart block (Tierney et al., 1994).

Pump Failure   Myocardial infarction reduces myocardial contractility, ventricular wall motion, and compliance. The loss of myocardial contractility and altered filling may produce heart failure. The risk of heart failure is greatest when large portions of the left ventricle are affected. It may be more severe with an anterior infarction (McCance & Huether, 1994). With loss of 20% to 30% of the left ventricular muscle mass, the client may develop manifestations of left-sided heart failure, including dyspnea, fatigue, weakness, and respiratory crackles on auscultation. Clients with inferior or right ventricular MI may develop right-sided heart failure with manifestations such as neck vein distention and peripheral edema. Hemodynamic monitoring is often initiated for clients with evidence of heart failure. Heart failure and its manifestations are discussed in greater depth later in this chapter.

As a result of pump failure or hypovolemia, clients may become hypotensive after an acute MI and demonstrate signs of impaired tissue perfusion, such as low urinary output, decreased level of consciousness, and cool, clammy skin. Diaphoresis, vomiting, decreased venous tone, and medications contribute to the risk of relative hypovolemia and decreased cardiac output. *Cardiogenic shock,* impaired tissue perfusion due to pump failure, results when functioning myocardial muscle mass decreases by more than 40%. The heart is unable to pump enough blood to meet the needs of the body and maintain organ function. The low cardiac output that occurs in cardiogenic shock may also affect perfusion of the coronary arteries and myocardium, further increasing tissue damage. Mortality from cardiogenic shock is 80% to 90% (Price & Wilson, 1992), despite the use of sophisticated technology. See Chapter 6 for a more extensive discussion of cardiogenic shock.

Infarct Extension   Approximately 10% of clients experience extension or reinfarction in the area of the original infarction during the first 10 to 14 days after an MI. *Extension* of the MI is characterized by increased myocardial necrosis from continued blood flow impairment and ongoing injury. *Expansion* of the MI is described as a permanent expansion of the infarcted area from thinning and dilation of the muscle. Infarct extension and expansion may be manifested by continuing chest pain, hemodynamic compromise, and worsening heart failure (Cochrane, 1995).

Structural Defects   The scar tissue that replaces necrotic muscle is thinner than the ventricular muscle mass. This structural defect can lead to such complications as ventricular aneurysm, rupture of the interventricular septum or papillary muscle, and myocardial rupture. A *ventricular aneurysm* is an outpouching of the ventricular wall. It may develop when a large section of the ventricle is replaced by scar tissue. Because it does not contract during systole, stroke volume decreases. Blood may

pool within the aneurysm, causing clots to form (Porth, 1994). Ischemia of the papillary muscle or chordae tendineae may cause structural damage leading to *papillary muscle dysfunction* or *rupture.* Damage to these structures produces valvular dysfunction, usually affecting the mitral valve and causing *regurgitation,* a backflow of blood into the atria during systole. The interventricular septum may perforate or rupture due to ischemia and infarction of this tissue. Myocardial rupture usually occurs between days 7 and 10 after MI, when the injured tissue is soft and weak. It is an often fatal complication of MI (Porth, 1994).

Pericarditis   Necrotic myocardial tissue precipitates an inflammatory response. *Pericarditis,* inflammation of the pericardial tissue surrounding the heart, may complicate an MI, usually within 2 to 3 days. Chest pain is also associated with pericarditis, but the pain is sharp and stabbing, aggravated by movement or deep breathing. A pericardial rub may be noted on auscultation of heart sounds. *Dressler's syndrome* is a complex of manifestations associated with pericarditis, pleuritis, and pneumonitis; it is characterized by fever, chest pain, and dyspnea. It develops within days or weeks following the infarction and may spontaneously resolve or recur over several months, causing the client great discomfort and distress. Dressler's syndrome is thought to be a hypersensitivity response to necrotic tissue or an autoimmune disorder (Porth, 1994).

Collaborative Care

Treatment goals for the MI client are to relieve the chest pain, maintain cardiovascular stability, decrease cardiac workload, and prevent complications. Risk factor control is a major goal of long-term management of the client who has had an MI.

Rapid assessment and early diagnosis is important for timely initiation of treatment. "Time is muscle" is a medical truism for the client suffering from acute MI. Research data have shown that the speed with which blood flow is restored to the myocardium is crucial to improving the client's chance of survival (Bahr, 1994; National Institutes of Health [NIH], 1993). The evolution of an MI is a dynamic process: the quicker the artery is reopened, whether by medical or surgical intervention or a spontaneous event, the greater the amount of myocardial muscle that can be salvaged. The American Heart Association (AHA) recommends definitive treatment be initiated within 1 hour of arrival at the emergency center (NIH, 1993).

The major problem interfering with timely reperfusion is delay in seeking medical care when the client first becomes aware of chest discomfort or other cardiac symptoms. Between 26% and 44% of clients with symptoms of chest discomfort or pain wait more than 4 hours before

Applying Research to Nursing Practice:
Factors Influencing Treatment Delay in Patients Experiencing Chest Pain

■ ■ ■

Delay in seeking treatment significantly affects the mortality and morbidity of clients experiencing symptoms of cardiac compromise. Research findings indicate that the sooner clients seek treatment after the onset of symptoms the greater the degree of myocardial salvage (NIH, 1993). However, a great number of clients with acute MI do not receive prompt treatment of these symptoms because they delay seeking medical care; death occurs within 1 hour in over 50% of acute MI cases (AHA, 1992). In one study, researchers used the Health Belief Model as a framework for their study of variables associated with treatment delay in clients experiencing cardiac symptomatology (Reilly, Dracup, & Dattolo, 1995).

These researchers were interested in which internal and/or external motivators affected the client's decision to seek medical care. Seventy-seven subjects with a diagnosis of suspected or confirmed MI made up the sample. The study sample consisted of mainly white (82%) males (71%) with a mean age of 58.6 (± 11.7) years; ages ranged from 35 to 80. Data were collected via a client questionnaire and chart review.

In this study, 60% of the sample delayed seeking treatment for longer than 3 hours. The median delay for the entire sample was 5 hours. Findings revealed that (1) clients over the age of 60 were more likely to delay treatment than younger clients, (2) the presence of family members increased the delay time, possibly because of a "shared denial" of the seriousness of the symptoms, and (3) the client's interpretation of the symptoms as not serious added to the delay.

Implications for Nursing
Efforts to educate the public in the seriousness of cardiac symptomatology must be continued and expanded. Programs should emphasize the warning signs of myocardial ischemia and infarction, the nega-

tive consequences of delay in seeking treatment, and the benefits associated with early treatment of acute MI, and how and when to access the emergency response system.

Nurses should recognize clients over age 60 as high-risk clients. This age group may need extra attention and reinforcement of emergency information. Teaching that is individualized to the client's cardiac history and other existing disease processes may help the client to distinguish manifestations that require treatment from those that are associated with chronic problems. The client's refusal to acknowledge the warnings of cardiac disease was shown to correlate with treatment delay. Therefore, every opportunity must be taken to educate the public to make appropriate decisions during a potential cardiac event. Including the family in this teaching is encouraged. This data showed that clients who had family members present during the cardiac event delayed an average of 9 hours, compared to a 2-hour delay for clients who were alone during the experience.

Critical Thinking in Client Care

1. In what settings, other than the hospital, can nurses provide cardiac education classes to the public?

2. How does the concept of denial affect the client's decision to seek medical care?

3. How does the Health Belief Model offer a framework for the purposes of this study?

4. What is the extent of the emergency response system in your area, and how is it accessed?

5. What is the average length of time from activation of the system to arrival at the emergency center? How does this affect the overall onset-to-treatment goal of 60 minutes?

seeking treatment (NIH, 1993). Clinical trials indicate that mortality from acute MI is significantly reduced when thrombolytic therapy is initiated within 4 hours after the onset of symptoms (Gruppo Italiano per lo Studio Della Streptochinasi nell' Infarcto Miocardico [GISSI], 1986; ISIS Steering Committee, 1987; NIH, 1993; Timm, Ross, McKendall, Braunwald, Williams, & the TIMI Investigators, 1991). Many factors may be cited as reasons

for treatment delay, including advanced age, the client's perception of the seriousness of symptoms, denial, access to medical care, the availability of an emergency response system, and in-hospital delays (see the accompanying research box). Immediate evaluation of the client who presents to the emergency center with manifestations of myocardial infarction is essential to early diagnosis and treatment.

Table 28–6   Cardiac Enzymes and Isoenzymes

Enzyme	Normal Level	Primary Tissue Location	Significance of Elevation	Changes Occurring with MI		
				Appears	Peaks	Duration
CK (CPK)	Male: 12 to 80 U/L Female: 10 to 70 U/L	Cardiac muscle, skeletal muscle, brain	Injury to muscle cells	3 to 6 hours	12 to 24 hours	24 to 48 hours
CK-MB	0% to 3% of total CK	Cardiac muscle	MI, cardiac ischemia, myocarditis, cardiac contusion, defibrillation	4 to 8 hours	18 to 24 hours	72 hours
LDH	45 to 90 U/L	Heart, liver, kidneys, skeletal muscle, brain, RBCs, lungs	MI; pulmonary, liver, renal, RBC, or skeletal muscle disease; CVA; intestinal ischemia; others	24 to 72 hours	3 to 4 days	10 to 14 days
LDH_1	20% to 30% of total LDH	Heart, blood vessels, RBCs	MI, anemias, renal infarction, hepatitis, testicular cancer	12 to 24 hours	48 hours	10 to 14 days
LDH_1:LDH_2 Ratio	Less than 1 (LDH_2 greater than LDH_1)		Ratio greater than 1 strongly indicative of MI	12 to 24 hours	48 hours	

Laboratory and Diagnostic Tests

In addition to the history and physical examination, laboratory and diagnostic testing is used to establish the diagnosis of acute MI.

Laboratory Tests   The principal laboratory tests that are ordered for the client with a suspected MI are *Cardiac enzyme studies*. As cardiac cells die, their contents are released into the bloodstream. The enzymes most specific for diagnosis of MI are the serum creatine kinase (CK; also called creatinine phosphokinase, or CPK) and lactic dehydrogenase (LDH). *Creatine kinase* is an important enzyme for cellular function found principally in cardiac and skeletal muscle and the brain. CK levels rise rapidly with damage to these tissues, appearing in the serum 4 to 6 hours after an MI, peaking within 12 to 24 hours, and then declining over the next 48 to 72 hours. The CK level correlates well with the size of the infarction; the greater the amount of infarcted tissue, the higher the serum level of CK. Three organ-specific subsets of CK called *isoenzymes* are identified. *CK-MB* (also called MB-bands) is the cardiac muscle fraction of CK and considered the most sensitive indicator of MI. CK-BB is found in brain cells, and CK-MM is a component of skeletal muscle cells. Elevated CK alone is not specific for MI; elevated CK-MB greater than 5% is considered a positive indicator of MI

(Olbrych, 1993). CK-MB levels do not normally rise with chest pain from angina or causes other than MI.

Lactic dehydrogenase is also found in many body tissues. Serum LDH levels rise within 24 to 72 hours of an MI, peaking in 3 to 4 days and then declining. It returns to normal levels in 10 to 14 days. Its late peak makes the LDH particularly valuable to diagnose MI when treatment is delayed (Pagana & Pagana, 1995). LDH also has organ-specific isoenzymes, numbered as LDH_{1-5}. Of these isoenzymes, LDH_1 is the most specific to myocardial damage. Serum LDH_2 levels are normally higher than other LDH subsets; when LDH_1 is greater than LDH_2, a "flipped" LDH pattern is said to exist. This pattern is found in 80% of all acute MI clients within 12 to 48 hours after the onset of MI (Olbrych, 1993). Table 28–6 lists normal levels for the cardiac enzymes and isoenzymes with changes typical of MI.

Cardiac enzyme levels are ordered on admission, with *serial enzymes* measured for 3 succeeding days. Serial enzymes are helpful when the diagnosis is not clear and to evaluate the extent of myocardial damage.

Other laboratory tests which may be ordered include the following:

- *Complete blood count (CBC)* shows a rise in the white blood cell (WBC) count because of the presence of

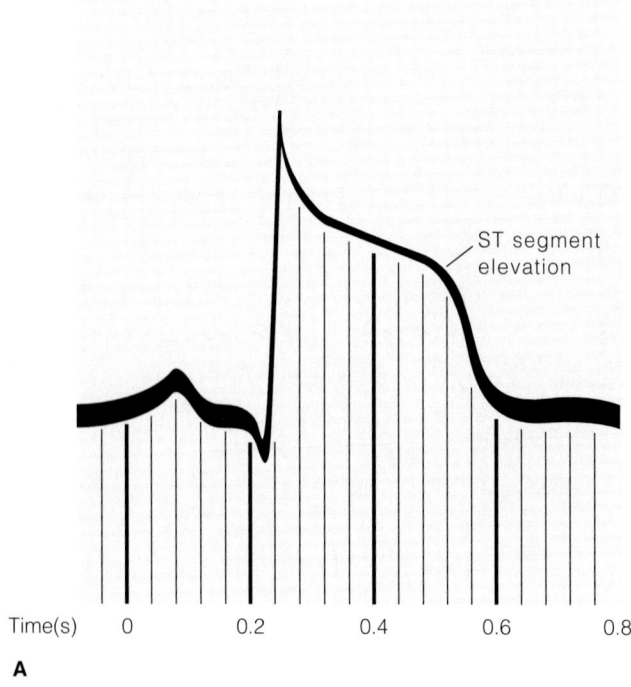

A

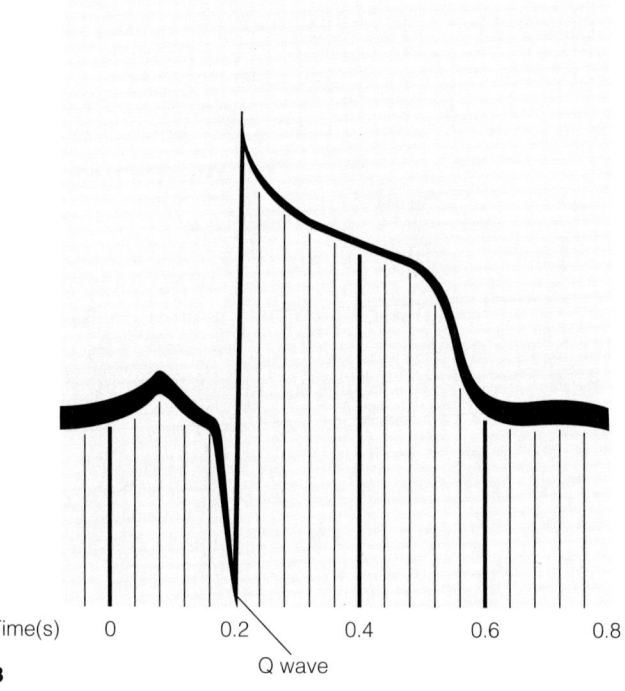

B

Figure 28-17 ECG changes characteristic of MI. *A*, ST segment elevation characteristic of myocardial injury.

B, Clinically significant Q wave characteristic of acute myocardial infarction.

inflammation of the injured myocardial tissue. The erythrocyte sedimentation rate (ESR) also rises because of inflammation.

- *Arterial blood gases (ABGs)* are ordered to assess blood oxygen levels and acid-base balance.

- *Coagulation profile* is performed to evaluate clotting mechanisms. This may be done to identify abnormalities in clotting that may have precipitated thrombus formation and MI and as a baseline prior to initiation of anticoagulant therapy.

- *Lipid profile* may be ordered to confirm the presence of elevated cholesterol and triglyceride levels.

Diagnostic Tests Electrocardiography, echocardiography, and myocardial nuclear scans are the most common diagnostic tests performed for the client with a suspected MI. With the exception of the ECG, the timing of these tests depends on the client's immediate condition. Hemodynamic monitoring may also be initiated in the unstable client following MI.

Electrocardiographic Changes Ischemic or necrotic cardiac cells do not respond normally to electrical stimulation. This causes a change in the usual waveforms. Ischemic changes in the heart are seen as a depression of the ST segment or inversion of the T wave (see Figure 28–12 on page 1063). ST elevation is indicative of myocardial injury. Significant Q wave development (Figure

28–17) confirms a diagnosis of acute infarction; however, 30% to 50% of clients with confirmed MI do not develop Q waves. The location of myocardial damage can be identified on the 12-lead ECG, because electrical activity is recorded using different leads.

Characteristic changes in the ECG with an acute MI include the following:

- Inversion of the T wave

- Depression or elevation of the ST segment

- Formation of a Q wave

Echocardiography Echocardiography is a noninvasive diagnostic test using ultrasound to evaluate cardiac structures and left ventricular function. Images are produced as ultrasound waves strike cardiac structures and are reflected back through a transducer. Echocardiography can be performed at the client's bedside and is useful to diagnose and manage MI and its complications, such as ventricular aneurysm and papillary muscle rupture.

Cardiac Radionuclear Scans Myocardial perfusion imaging scans are nuclear scans used to detect changes in coronary blood flow and myocardial tissue. Nuclear studies use the radioisotopes thallium-201 and technetium-99m pyrophosphate or pertechnetate.

- *Thallium-201* is used to detect myocardial perfusion problems. This isotope collects in normally perfused myocardium; because ischemic areas are not able to take up the isotope, they appear blue or as "cold" spots when the heart is scanned for radioactivity.

- *Technetium-99m pyrophosphate* is another commonly used radioisotope to identify damaged tissue. In contrast to thallium-201, this isotope accumulates in ischemic tissue and appears red, or "hot." Both of these tests assist the physician in pinpointing the location and extent of damage from acute or previous MIs.

- *Technetium pertechnetate* is used to measure the portion of blood ejected from the ventricle during systole and evaluate myocardial function. MI decreases myocardial contractility and the ventricular ejection fraction.

Hemodynamic Monitoring   Hemodynamic monitoring may be initiated for the client who experiences significant alterations in cardiac output and hemodynamic status following MI. These invasive procedures are described in the heart failure section of this chapter.

Medical Management

The client with a suspected or confirmed MI is monitored continuously from his or her entry into the medical system. The client is cared for in the intensive coronary care unit for the first 24 to 48 hours, after which less intensive monitoring (e.g., telemetry) may be required. An intravenous line is established to allow rapid administration of emergency medications.

Bed rest is prescribed initially to reduce the cardiac workload. Most clients can use a bedside commode unless their condition is unstable; studies have shown the bedside commode to be less stressful than using a bedpan. After 48 to 72 hours, activities are gradually increased if the client tolerates them. A quiet, calm environment with limited outside stimuli, such as television and telephone, is preferred. Visitors are limited to close family members for short periods of time. Oxygen is administered by nasal cannula at 2 to 5 L/min to improve oxygenation of the myocardium and other tissues.

A liquid diet is often prescribed for the first 24 hours to reduce gastric distention and myocardial work. Once the client's condition has stabilized, a low-fat, low-cholesterol, reduced-sodium diet is allowed. Sodium restrictions may be lifted after 2 to 3 days if the client has no evidence of heart failure. Small, frequent feedings are often recommended. Drinks containing caffeine and very hot and cold foods may also be limited.

Pharmacology

Drug therapy can help reduce oxygen demand and increase oxygen supply. Thrombolytic agents, analgesics, and antidysrhythmic agents are among the principal classes of drugs used.

Thrombolytic Therapy   *Thrombolytic agents,* drugs that dissolve or break up blood clots, are first-line drugs used

to treat acute MI. These drugs activate the fibrinolytic system to lyse or destroy the clot, restoring blood flow to the obstructed artery. Early administration of thrombolytics (within the first 6 hours of MI onset) has been shown to limit infarct size, reduce heart damage, and improve the chances of survival (Margolis & Goldschmidt-Clermont, 1993). Activation of the fibrinolytic system can cause multiple complications; approximately 0.5% to 5% of clients receiving thrombolytic therapy experience serious bleeding complications. Not every client is a candidate for thrombolytic therapy; for example, it is contraindicated in clients with known bleeding disorders, history of cerebrovascular disease, uncontrolled hypertension, pregnancy, or recent trauma or surgery of the head or spine (Tierney et al., 1994).

Three thrombolytic agents are commonly used today. Among the three, little difference in effectiveness has been demonstrated; there are, however, big differences in cost. Streptokinase is a biologic agent derived from group C *Streptococcus* organisms. It is the least expensive of the drugs, costing approximately $125 per dose. The primary drawback to streptokinase therapy is that it may produce severe hypersensitivity reactions, including anaphylaxis. For this reason, streptokinase should not be used for clients who have received it previously. Streptokinase is administered by intravenous infusion. Anisoylated plasminogen streptokinase activator complex (APSAC) is a related drug that can be administered by bolus over 2 to 5 minutes. While it has many of the same adverse effects as streptokinase, it is considerably more expensive. Tissue plasminogen activator (t-PA) may be more effective in reestablishing myocardial perfusion, especially if the onset of pain occurred more than 3 hours previously. Because of its high cost (it is the most expensive of the three, costing approximately $2800 per dose), t-PA is often reserved for clients who have previously received streptokinase. Nursing care of the client receiving thrombolytic agents is outlined in the box on page 1096.

Analgesia   Pain relief is an important part of treatment for the client with an acute MI. Pain causes sympathetic nervous system stimulation, increasing the heart rate and blood pressure and, in turn, myocardial workload. If nitroglycerin is unsuccessful in relieving chest pain, intravenous narcotic analgesics are usually administered. Morphine sulfate is the drug of choice for pain and sedation. Following an initial intravenous dose of 4 to 8 mg, small doses (2 to 4 mg) may be repeated intravenously every 15 minutes until pain is relieved. Hydromorphone (Dilaudid) or meperidine (Demerol) are alternatives to morphine. It is important to assess the client frequently for pain relief and possible adverse effects of analgesia, such as excessive sedation. Antianxiety agents, such as diazepam (Valium) may also be administered to promote rest.

Nursing Care of the Client Receiving Thrombolytic Therapy

Thrombolytic therapy is now a standard of care for all clients with an acute MI of less than 6 hours' duration. The sooner thrombolytic therapy is instituted, the better the outcome. The client receiving thrombolytic therapy is at high risk for injury from bleeding; strict monitoring and prompt intervention for bleeding problems is vital. Thrombolytic agents may also be used to treat massive pulmonary embolism and are being used experimentally for embolic stroke.

PREINFUSION CARE

- Obtain a medical history, and perform a physical assessment of the client. *Clients presenting to the emergency center with complaints of chest pain and other signs and symptoms suspicious of an acute MI are potential candidates for thrombolytic therapy. Information obtained from the history and physical assessment enables the health care team to determine whether thrombolytic therapy is appropriate. The standard in most emergency centers is to initiate thrombolytic therapy within 30 minutes of the client's arrival.*

- Evaluate the client for contraindications to thrombolytic therapy by checking for a history of chest pain greater than 6 hours' in duration, recent surgery or trauma (including prolonged CPR), bleeding disorders or any active bleeding, cerebral vascular accident, neurosurgery within the last 2 months, gastrointestinal ulcers, diabetic hemor-

rhagic retinopathy, and uncontrolled hypertension. *Thrombolytic agents dissolve clots and therefore may precipitate intracranial, internal, or peripheral bleeding.*

- Identify any recent streptococcal infection or the use of streptokinase within the last 6 months. *Streptokinase is a bacterial protein produced by group C beta-hemolytic streptococci and causes antibodies to be formed. The client may experience a hypersensitivity reaction if preformed antibodies to streptokinase are present.*

- Inform the client of the purpose of the therapy. Discuss the risk of bleeding and the need to keep the extremity immobile during and after the infusion. *Minimal movement of the extremity is necessary to prevent bleeding from the infusion site.*

DURING THE INFUSION

- Assess vital signs and the infusion site for signs of hematoma formation or bleeding every 15 minutes for the first hour, every 30 minutes for the next 2 hours, and then once every hour until the intravenous catheter is discontinued. Assess pulses, color, sensation, and temperature of both extremities with each vital sign check. Record all observations. *Vital signs and the site are frequently assessed to detect possible complications.*

- Remind the client to keep the extremity still and straight. Do not elevate head of bed above 15 de-

Antidysrhythmics   Dysrhythmias are a frequent complication of myocardial infarction, particularly in the first 12 to 24 hours. Antidysrhythmic medications are used as needed to treat dysrhythmias, or prophylactically to prevent their development. Because ventricular dysrhythmias are common, with approximately 5% of hospitalized clients developing ventricular fibrillation, lidocaine is frequently prescribed in the first 1 to 2 days following MI. Symptomatic bradycardia (bradycardia with associated hypotension and other signs of low cardiac output) is treated with intravenous atropine, 0.5 to 1 mg. Intravenous verapamil or the short-acting beta-blocker esmolol (Brevibloc) may be ordered to treat atrial fibrillation or other supraventricular tachydysrhythmias. Other antidysrhythmic medications that may be used are in the box on page 1036.

Other Medications   Beta-blockers such as propranolol (Inderal), atenolol (Tenormin), and metoprolol (Lopressor) have been shown to improve survival rates following

MI. These drugs decrease the heart rate, reducing cardiac work and myocardial oxygen demand. Initial doses are given intravenously to shorten the duration of chest pain due to ischemia and reduce the risk of ventricular fibrillation. Long-term therapy may be continued, particularly in clients at high risk, to reduce the risk of reinfarction and sudden death.

Clients with continued or recurrent ischemia after myocardial infarction may also be treated with vasodilators to reduce afterload and myocardial work. Intravenous nitroglycerin has a rapid onset of action and short duration of effect; it may be administered for the first 24 to 48 hours. Intravenous nitroglycerin is a peripheral and arterial vasodilator that reduces the cardiac workload. It dilates coronary arteries and collateral channels in the heart, increasing coronary blood flow to save myocardial tissue at risk. Nitrates may, however, cause reflex tachycardia or excessive hypotension, so close monitoring is necessary while they are being administered.

Nursing Care of the Client Receiving Thrombolytic Therapy (continued)

grees. *Immobilization of the extremity helps prevent trauma to the infusion site and reduces the risk of bleeding from the site. Streptokinase can cause significant hypotension; keeping the bed flat helps maintain cerebral perfusion.*

- Maintain continuous cardiac monitoring during the infusion. Have antidysrhythmic medications, such as lidocaine, and the emergency cart readily available for treatment of significant or potentially fatal dysrhythmias. *Ventricular dysrhythmias commonly occur with reperfusion of the ischemic myocardium.*

POSTINFUSION CARE

- Assess vital signs, distal pulses, and infusion site frequently as needed. *The client remains at high risk for bleeding following thrombolytic therapy.*

- Evaluate the client's response to therapy: normalization of ST segment, relief of chest pain, reperfusion dysrhythmias, early peaking of the CK and CK-MB band. *These are signs that the clot has been dissolved and the myocardium is being reperfused.*

- Maintain the client on bed rest for 6 hours. Keep the head of the bed at or below 15 degrees. Reinforce the need to keep the extremity straight and immobile. Avoid any injections for 24 hours after catheter removal. *Precautions such as these are important to prevent bleeding and stabilize the client.*

- Assess puncture sites for manifestations of bleeding. On removal of the catheter, hold direct pressure over the site for at least 30 minutes. Apply a pressure dressing to any venous or arterial sites if needed. Perform routine care in a gentle manner to avoid undue bruising or injury to the client. *Thrombolytic therapy disrupts the normal coagulation process. Peripheral bleeding may occur at puncture sites, and there may not be sufficient fibrin to form a clot. Direct or indirect pressure may be needed to control the bleeding.*

- Assess body fluids, including urine, vomitus, and feces, for evidence of bleeding; check neurologic status for changes in level of consciousness and manifestations of increased intracranial pressure, which may indicate intracranial bleeding. Assess any surgical sites for bleeding. Obtain and monitor hemoglobin and hematocrit levels, prothrombin time (PT), and partial thromboplastin time (PTT). *These provide additional means of assessing for bleeding.*

- Administer platelet-modifying drugs (e.g., aspirin, dipyridamole) as ordered. *Platelet inhibitors decrease platelet aggregation and adhesion and are used to prevent reocclusion of the artery.*

- Monitor for and report any manifestations of reocclusion, including changes in the ST segment, chest pain, or dysrhythmias. *Early recognition of reocclusion is vital to save myocardial tissue.*

Calcium channel blockers, diltiazem (Cardizem) or verapamil (Calan, Isoptin), may prevent reinfarction and ischemia in clients with non-Q-wave infarctions. These drugs are used primarily when ischemia does not respond to beta-blocker therapy or when the client is hypertensive. Their use following acute MI is controversial; several studies have indicated that calcium channel blockers may be dangerous when used in the early or later post-MI period. Recent research also suggests an increased risk of MI when calcium channel blockers are used to treat hypertension. See the box on page 1036 for nursing implications of nitrate, beta-blocker, or calcium channel blocker therapy.

Anticoagulants and antiplatelet medications such as aspirin and dipyridamole (Persantine) may be used to decrease clot formation at the plaque site. They are used to maintain patency of the coronary arteries after interventional procedures. An initial intravenous bolus of heparin is generally followed by a continuous infusion or intermittent subcutaneous injections.

Clients with pump failure and hypotension may receive intravenous dopamine, a vasopressor. At low doses (less than 5 μg/kg/min), it improves blood flow to the kidneys, preventing renal ischemia and possible acute renal failure (see Chapter 26). With increasing doses, dopamine increases myocardial contractility and causes vasoconstriction, improving blood pressure and cardiac output.

Antilipemic agents are used for the client with hyperlipidemia. A stool softener such as docusate sodium is prescribed to maintain normal bowel function and reduce straining. Some of the more commonly prescribed drugs, their actions, and nursing implications are presented in the pharmacology box on page 1098.

Revascularization Procedures

For some clients, thrombolytic therapy may be followed by immediate percutaneous transluminal coronary angioplasty (PTCA). More often, cardiac catheterization and PTCA are performed 5 to 10 days after MI. Early revascu-

Nursing Implications for Pharmacology: The Client with Myocardial Infarction

NARCOTIC ANALGESIC

Morphine sulfate (MSO₄)

Morphine is used to treat the pain associated with the effects of ischemia on the myocardium. Morphine is the drug of choice for acute pain relief in MI for several reasons: It stimulates opiate receptors, promoting analgesia and altering the client's perception of pain. Morphine decreases sympathetic nervous system stimulation, decreasing the client's anxiety and myocardial oxygen demand. Morphine has both venodilator and arterial dilator effects, decreasing myocardial oxygen use by reducing preload and afterload. Morphine also reduces respiratory rate and depth.

Nursing Responsibilities

- Assess and record vital signs.
- Evaluate client for relief of pain. Document pain before and after drug administration via a pain rating scale (0 to 10). Administer small increments of morphine (2 to 4 µg intravenous push as ordered) to control pain as needed.
- Monitor the client's respiratory rate and depth. Withhold morphine if the respiratory rate falls below 12 per minute or if respirations are shallow. Obtain ABGs as needed. Encourage the client to turn, cough, and take deep breaths.
- Assess the client for signs of morphine overdose: excessive sedation, pinpoint pupils, and respiratory depression. Administer naloxone as ordered. Provide cardiopulmonary assistance if needed.

- Maintain the client's safety during morphine administration. Keep side rails up, and monitor the client for excessive sedation.
- Monitor fluid balance. Assess the client for bladder distention, and encourage urination at least every 4 hours. Encourage the client to ingest adequate amounts of fluid and fiber.

Client and Family Teaching

- Instruct the client to call for pain medication before the pain gets severe.
- Ease the client's fears of addiction by emphasizing that routine and proper use of morphine rarely causes dependence or addiction (Shlafer, 1993).
- Report the following side effects to the nursing staff: constipation, urinary retention, flushing, skin rash, or behavioral changes.

INJECTABLE ANTICOAGULANT THERAPY

Heparin sodium

The most common cause of acute MI is coronary thrombosis. Anticoagulant, thrombolytic, and antiplatelet drugs are used for clients with an MI to stop, slow, or prevent thrombosis or to dissolve existing clots. Injectable heparin interferes with coagulation and prevents microthrombi from depositing in the vasculature. Heparin is often given as an infusion (especially with thrombolytic therapy) or as a subcutaneous bolus injection. Thrombolytic agents cause lysis of the clot. Antiplatelet agents (platelet inhibitors) decrease platelet aggregation and platelet adherence.

---

larization has been shown to benefit clients with multiple-vessel coronary artery disease and those with evidence of ischemia that continues after MI or thrombolytic therapy. In some cases, CABG surgery may be performed. The choice of procedure depends on the client's age and immediate condition, the time elapsed from the onset of manifestations, and the extent of myocardial disease and damage. These procedures and related nursing care are covered in more depth in the section on angina.

Other Invasive Procedures

For clients with large MIs and evidence of pump failure, invasive devices may be employed to temporarily take over the function of the heart, allowing the injured my-

ocardium to heal. The intra-aortic balloon pump is a widely used device to augment cardiac output. Ventricular assist devices are indicated for clients requiring more artificial support than can be provided by the intra-aortic balloon pump alone.

Intra-Aortic Balloon Pump The *intra-aortic balloon pump (IABP),* also called intra-aortic balloon counterpulsation, is a mechanical circulatory support device that may be used after cardiac surgery or for clients with cardiogenic shock after an MI. IABP temporarily supports the heart's function, allowing the heart gradually to recover by decreasing myocardial workload and oxygen demand and increasing perfusion of the coronary arteries.

Pharmacology: The Client with Myocardial Infarction (continued)

Nursing Responsibilities

- Obtain CBC and coagulation studies for baseline values.
- Monitor PTT per protocol. Maintain PTT at 1.5 to 2 times the control time for heparin therapy.
- Double-check heparin concentration and dosage before administering. Use infusion pumps to administer heparin or thrombolytic infusions.
- Rotate subcutaneous injection sites of heparin, using lower abdominal fat pads (the preferred site). Do not aspirate before injection. Apply gentle pressure for 1 minute after subcutaneous administration.
- Do not mix heparin with other drugs.
- Monitor client for signs and symptoms of bleeding and bruising throughout the therapy. Assess vital signs frequently. Perform guaiac testing of all stools. Evaluate any venous or arterial puncture sites for hematoma or bleeding. Avoid tissue trauma to client by using gentle means when providing nursing care.
- Be prepared to administer blood products if necessary.
- Have protamine sulfate available for heparin toxicity as ordered. Administer via slow intravenous push if needed, and monitor blood pressure.
- Avoid parenteral injections during therapy.
- Explain to the client the purpose of the specific therapy.

Client and Family Teaching

- Immediately report to the nursing staff any bruising

or bleeding from puncture sites; nosebleeds; blood in the stool, urine, or sputum; or pain at the intravenous site.
- Use a soft toothbrush (foam-tipped, if possible) when brushing teeth to avoid injuring gums. Use care when shaving with razors.

STOOL SOFTENERS

Docusate sodium (Colace)

Docusate calcium (Surfak)

Stool softeners are used to assist the MI client to maintain normal bowel elimination and avoid the Valsalva maneuver produced by straining during defecation. The Valsalva maneuver stimulates the vagus nerve and can precipitate an extreme slowing of the heart rate and a lethal dysrhythmia.

Nursing Responsibilities

- The sodium content in docusate sodium may exacerbate heart failure, hypertension, or peripheral edema. Monitor the client closely during therapy.
- Allow the client to use a bedside commode rather than a bedpan; this decreases straining and allows for a more effective use of abdominal and rectal muscles for defecation.

Client and Family Teaching

- Do not strain during defecation.
- Drink 6 to 8 glasses of fluids (water, juice, milk) per day. Increase fiber intake.

A catheter with a 30- to 40-mL balloon is introduced into the aorta, usually via the femoral artery. The balloon catheter is connected to a console that regulates the inflation and deflation of the balloon. The IABP catheter inflates during diastole, increasing perfusion of the coronary and renal arteries, and deflates during systole, decreasing afterload and cardiac workload (Figure 28–18). The inflation-deflation series is triggered by the client's ECG pattern. During the most acute period, the balloon inflates and deflates with each heart beat (1:1 ratio), thus providing maximal assistance to the heart. As the client's condition improves, the IABP is weaned to inflate-deflate at varying intervals (e.g., 1:2, 1:4, 1:8). This provides a continually decreasing amount of support as

the heart muscle recovers its normal functioning. When the client no longer requires mechanical assistance, the IABP catheter is removed.

Ventricular Assist Devices   The use of *ventricular assist devices (VADs)* to aid the failing heart has become more commonplace with advances in technology. The goal of mechanical assistance is to allow the heart to "rest" and recover normal functioning. Whereas the IABP can supplement the cardiac output by approximately 10% to 15%, the VAD temporarily takes partial or complete control of the heart's function, depending on the type of device used (Holloway, 1993). VADs may be used as temporary or complete assist in clients experiencing acute MI

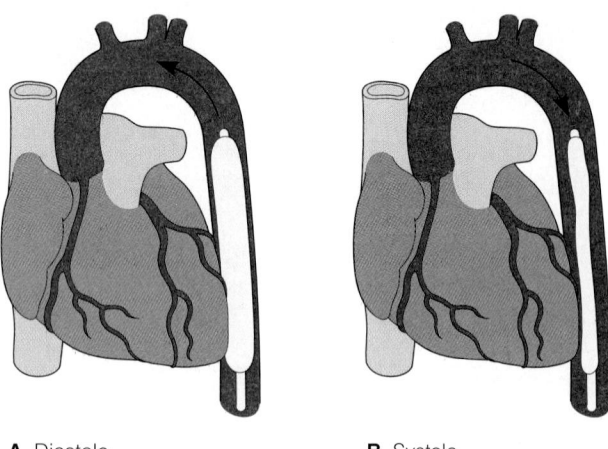

A Diastole   **B** Systole

Figure 28–18 The intra-aortic balloon pump. *A,* When inflated during diastole, the balloon supports cerebral and coronary artery perfusion. *B,* When the balloon is deflated during systole, cardiac output is unimpeded.

and pump failure when IABP and pharmacologic treatments fail to maintain an adequate cardiac output to perfuse all organs and tissues. Clients with infarction of more than 40% of the myocardium and cardiogenic shock often cannot be weaned from VAD; its use is reserved for clients with a reasonable chance of recovery or those awaiting transplant. Following acute MI, approximately 30% to 50% of clients requiring VAD are able to be weaned from the device (Holloway, 1993). Nursing care for the client with VAD is supportive, provided in the cardiac recovery unit, intensive care unit, or critical care unit.

Cardiac Rehabilitation

Cardiac rehabilitation is the return to an optimal level of physical, psychologic, and social health through a planned program of activity and exercises, psychologic support, and client education (King & Froelicher, 1989). Cardiac rehabilitation consists of four phases, beginning with the client's admission to the hospital. Phase I occurs in the coronary care or cardiac surgery intensive care unit and addresses the acute phase of the illness. Phase II encompasses the balance of the hospital stay and encourages progressive activity. Phase III is the home recovery period. This period entails self-monitored progressive activity. The goal of phase IV is long-term conditioning, usually in a structured and supervised setting (King & Froelicher, 1989). The formal part of the program varies in length; a typical program lasts about 12 weeks. Cardiac rehabilitation is appropriate for all clients with CAD.

The components of the formal outpatient program for cardiac rehabilitation should be discussed with the client. These components include education in the anatomy and physiology of the heart and CAD, exercise, emotional adjustment to MI, resumption of work and sexual activity, heart-healthy life-styles, and CPR instruction. Discussion

of risk factors and risk factor modification are especially important. An individualized cardiac rehabilitation program, which includes activity and exercise prescriptions, nutrition and diet counseling, sexual counseling, smoking cessation, and psychologic support, can then be planned to address the client's specific risks and prevent future complications. Participation in a supervised cardiac rehabilitation program has been correlated with significant effects on self-care behaviors and quality of life issues (Conn, Taylor, & Casey, 1992). Clients should be strongly encouraged to attend regularly to gain the most benefit.

Activity after an MI is progressive, and limitations may be quantified by the number of metabolic equivalents (METs) allowed. METs reflect the amount of oxygen consumed per unit of body weight during the resting state. Cardiac workload, or energy expenditure, can be measured in METs (Table 28–7). As the workload increases, so does the metabolic rate and the oxygen demand. The intensity of activity usually progresses from 1.5 to 2.0 METs in the acute phase of illness to 2.0 to 3.0 METs (self-care activities) during hospital recovery and 3.5 to 4.0 METs (light housework/hobbies) by discharge. During this period, clients should be instructed in how to take their own pulse as an indicator of overexertion (King & Froelicher, 1989). Manifestations of excess energy expenditure include a heart rate greater than 120 BPM, chest pain, shortness of breath, irregular pulse, or signs of decreased cardiac output, such as light-headedness or dizziness. Activities should be discontinued if these are noted.

Issues surrounding return to work are discussed and recommendations from the physician are reviewed. Factors affecting the client's ability and/or desire to return to work include the client's physiologic and psychologic health status, financial need, and the client's age (Newton & Froelicher, 1989). Male clients returning to work within 4 months after MI have been shown to have better psychologic outcomes than male clients who did not return to work (Rost & Smith, 1992).

The accompanying box describes the application of rehabilitation principles to care of the client with MI.

Nursing Care

Nursing care for the client with an acute MI includes focuses on decreasing the chest pain, minimizing the size of the infarction, and preventing potential complications. Psychosocial support of the client who has had an MI is especially important, because it often is a debilitating event. For many other clients, an MI brings them face-to-face with their own mortality for the first time.

Pain

Chest pain occurs when the oxygen supply to the heart muscle does not meet the demand. Myocardial ischemia

Table 28–7	Metabolic Equivalents (METs) of Various Activities

Very Light Activity		Light Activity		Moderate to Heavy Activity	Very Heavy Activity	
1 MET	**2 METs**	**3 METs**	**4 METs**	**6 METs**	**8 METs**	**10+ METs**
Resting	Self-care activities	Light housework	Gardening	Shoveling snow	Swimming	Swimming, crawl stroke
Eating		Driving	Ballroom dancing	Tennis	Cross-country skiing or running	Walking uphill, 5 mph
Handwork		Slow walking on level ground	Golf	Walking on level ground, 5 mph	Walking on level ground, 5 to 6 mph	
Reading			Walking on level ground, 4 mph			

Note. Adapted from "Cardiac Rehabilitation: Activity and Exercise Program" (p. 743) by S. C. King and E. S. S. Froelicher, in *Cardiac Nursing* (2nd ed.) by S. G. Underhill, S. L. Woods, E. S. S. Froelicher, and C. J. Halpenny (Eds.), 1989, Philadelphia: Lippincott.

Applying Rehabilitation Principles to Medical/Surgical Nursing: Myocardial Infarction

■ ■ ■

A client who has survived a myocardial infarction may have difficulties performing self-care activities of daily living (ADLs). Rehabilitation nurses view the client's participation in these activities as an important part of the recovery process.

Mr. John Richie, a 52-year-old married man with three grown children is admitted to your unit from the cardiac care unit after experiencing a myocardial infarction. He is not currently experiencing chest pain. Mr. Richie is on telemetry, and his vital signs are stable.

Rehabilitation Principle

Teaching the client to recover control of ADLs fosters the client's sense of self-esteem and ultimately speeds recovery from an MI.

Rehabilitation Time Frame

Most clients who experience an MI will be in the hospital for approximately 5 to 7 days. It is important to stress teaching throughout this period.

Nursing Diagnosis: Activity Intolerance

Clients who have a recent MI often find it difficult to perform many ADLs because of pain and fatigue resulting from decreased oxygenation to the heart muscle and from heart muscle damage. Myocardial healing begins early, but it takes approximately 6 to 8 weeks to complete. Rehabilitation strategies such as using adaptive devices, exercising, and pacing activities can help the client regain control over ADLs while the heart recovers.

Rehabilitation Goals and Interventions

1. Teach the client to avoid extremes of heat and cold and to avoid walking against the wind. *Extremes of heat and cold and walking against the wind cause an increase in respiratory effort and can decrease the amount of oxygen reaching the heart muscle, causing pain.*

2. Teach the client to alternate activity with frequent rest periods and to increase activities gradually. *Frequent rest periods allow for proper oxygenation of the heart muscle.*

3. Avoid activities that tense the muscles, such as lifting, carrying, and performing isometric exercises. *When muscles tense, they increase the need for oxygen, thereby increasing myocardial work.*

4. Instruct the client in the use of adaptive devices, such as a long-handled shoe horn, elastic laces, sock holders, grab extenders, and wheeled carts. *Adaptive devices reduce the muscle tensing that can occur with bending, lifting, reaching, and carrying while allowing the client to perform activities.*

5. Teach the client to avoid eating large meals and exercising immediately after a meal. *Large meals and exercise immediately following a meal increase the body's oxygen requirements. By eating smaller meals and resting between meals, a client can minimize pain and fatigue.*

and infarction cause pain, as does reperfusion of an is-chemic area following thrombolytic therapy or emergent PTCA.

Selected nursing interventions and rationales follow:

- Assess the client for verbal and nonverbal signs of pain. Document characteristics and the intensity of the client's pain, rating on a scale of 0 to 10. Accept verbal reports of pain. If the client exhibits nonverbal indicators of pain, confirm the meaning of these indicators with the client. *Frequent monitoring of the client for chest pain facilitates early intervention to reduce the risk of further damage. Pain is a subjective experience; the expression of pain may vary with the location and intensity of the pain, the client's previous experiences, and cultural and social background. The use of pain scales provides an objective measurement of the pain and a means to assess reduction in or relief of the pain.*

- Assess and document vital signs. *Changes in vital signs alert the nurse to changes in physiologic status and may provide clues about unreported pain.*

- Administer oxygen at 2 to 5 L/min per nasal cannula. *Supplemental oxygen increases oxygen supply to the my-ocardium, decreasing ischemia and pain.*

- Provide for physical and psychologic rest. Provide information and emotional support. *Rest decreases cardiac workload and stimulation of the sympathetic nervous system, promoting the client's comfort. Information and emotional support are important in decreasing anxiety and promoting psychologic rest.*

- Titrate intravenous nitroglycerin as ordered to relieve chest pain, maintaining the systolic blood pressure at greater than 100 mm Hg. *Nitroglycerin is frequently administered via a continuous infusion that may be titrated for complaints of chest pain. Nitroglycerin decreases chest pain by dilating coronary vessels, including collateral channels. It also dilates peripheral vessels, decreasing preload and afterload.*

- Administer 2 to 4 mg morphine by intravenous push for chest pain unrelieved by nitroglycerin. *Morphine sulfate is administered for pain not relieved by the nitro-glycerin alone; it has many advantages for the MI client: It decreases pain and anxiety, acts as a venodilator, and decreases respiratory rate. The reduction in preload and stimulation of the sympathetic nervous system lowers myocardial workload and oxygen consumption.*

- Administer other medications, such as beta-blockers and calcium channel blockers, as ordered. *These drugs help increase oxygen supply and decrease demand. Beta-blockers and calcium channel blockers decrease myocardial oxygen demand by decreasing heart rate, contractility, and afterload. Calcium channel blockers are especially useful for chest pain due to coronary vasospasm.*

- Reassess the client for relief of chest pain. Use a pain scale to assess pain. *Evaluation of the effectiveness of medications and interventions for pain relief are important to quality of care.*

Altered Tissue Perfusion

Damage to the heart muscle affects the pumping effectiveness of the ventricles. The manifestations of decreased tissue perfusion depend on the location and amount of damage. Anterior wall infarcts have a greater effect on the ventricle's ability to pump than do right ventricular infarcts. Infarcted muscle also predisposes the client to cardiac dysrhythmias, which can also affect the delivery of blood and oxygen to the tissues.

Selected nursing interventions and rationales follow:

- Assess and document vital signs. Report increases in heart rate and changes in heart rhythm, blood pressure, and respiratory rate. *Decreased cardiac output activates compensatory mechanisms that may cause increased heart rate and vasoconstriction, increasing cardiac workload.*

- Assess the client for changes in level of consciousness; decreased urine output; moist, cool, pale, mottled or cyanotic skin; dusky or cyanotic mucous membranes and nail beds; diminished to absent peripheral pulses; delayed capillary refill. *These are manifestations of decreased tissue perfusion. A change in level of consciousness is often the first manifestation of altered perfusion because brain tissue and cerebral function depends on a continuous supply of oxygen.*

- Auscultate heart and breath sounds. Note the presence of abnormal heart sounds (e.g., an S_3 or S_4 gallop or murmur) or adventitious sounds in the lungs. *Abnormal heart sounds or adventitious lung sounds may indicate impaired cardiac function, which may put the client at further risk for decreased tissue perfusion.*

- Monitor the client's ECG rhythm continuously. Obtain a 12-lead ECG to assess the client's complaints of chest pain. Report marked changes to the physician. *Dysrhythmias can further impair cardiac output and tissue perfusion. Continued or unrelieved chest pain may indicate further mycoardial ischemia and extension of the infarct; an ECG during episodes of chest pain provides a valuable diagnostic tool to assess myocardial perfusion.*

- Monitor oxygen saturation levels with pulse oximetry. Administer oxygen as ordered. Obtain and assess ABGs as indicated. *Pulse oximetry provides a means of continuously assessing gas exchange, tissue perfusion, and the effectiveness of oxygen administration. ABGs provide a more precise measurement of blood oxygen levels and allow assessment of acid-base balance.*

- Administer antidysrhythmic medications as needed. *Dysrhythmias affect tissue perfusion by altering cardiac output. Alterations in heart rate affect ventricular filling time and the number of cardiac cycles. Dysrhythmias affecting the coordination of atrial and ventricular activity affect stroke volume and effective contractions. The absence of effective ventricular contractions (i.e., ventricular fibrillation) halts perfusion of all tissues, necessitating emergency measures.*

- Obtain serial CK, LDH, and isoenzymes as ordered. *Levels of cardiac enzymes and isoenzymes correlate with the amount of myocardial damage.*

- Anticipate the need to insert invasive hemodynamic monitoring catheters. *These catheters facilitate management of the client with MI. They provide a means of assessing pressure measurements in the systemic and pulmonary arteries, the relationship between oxygen supply and demand, cardiac output, and cardiac index. They also serve as a means of evaluating the effectiveness of interventions.*

- Administer medications to improve cardiac output and tissue perfusion as ordered. These may include drugs to strengthen myocardial contraction (e.g., digoxin, dopamine, dobutamine), and drugs to reduce myocardial workload such as intravenous nitroglycerin, diuretics, and vasodilators. Continuously evaluate the client's response to these interventions. *Drugs that increase the force of contraction increase cardiac output while those that decrease cardiac work make it easier for the heart to pump, thereby increasing cardiac output and tissue perfusion.*

Ineffective Individual Coping

Normal coping mechanisms can help a person deal with a life-threatening event or with acute changes in health. However, certain coping mechanisms may be detrimental to restoring the client's health, particularly if the client relies on them for a prolonged period. Denial, for example, is a common coping mechanism among post-MI clients. In the initial stages, denial can benefit the client by lowering anxiety; a client who continues in denial, however, is less likely to comply with necessary treatment (Lowery, 1991).

Selected nursing interventions and rationales follow:

- Establish an environment of caring and trust. Encourage the client to express feelings. *Establishing a trusting nurse-client relationship provides a safe environment for the client to discuss feelings of helplessness, powerlessness, anxiety, and hopelessness. The nurse may then be able to provide additional resources to meet the client's needs.*

- Accept the use of denial as a coping mechanism, but do not reinforce its use. *Denial may initially help the client by diminishing the psychological threat to health, thereby decreasing anxiety. However, its prolonged use can interfere with the client's acceptance of reality and cooperation, possibly delaying treatment and hindering recovery.*

- Note the presence of aggressive behaviors, hostility, or anger. Document any incidence of failure to comply with treatments. *These signs can indicate anxiety and denial.*

- Help the client identify positive coping skills used in the past (e.g., problem-solving skills, verbalization of feelings, asking for help, prayer). Reinforce the use of positive coping behaviors. *Coping behaviors that have been successful in the past can help the client deal with the current situation. These familiar methods can decrease the client's feelings of powerlessness.*

- Provide opportunities for the client to make decisions about the plan of care, as possible. *This promotes the client's self-confidence and feelings of independence. Participating in care planning gives the client a sense of control and the opportunity to use positive coping skills.*

- Provide privacy for the client and significant other to share their questions and concerns. *Privacy allows the client and partner the opportunity to share their feelings and fears, offer support and encouragement to one another, relieve anxiety, and establish effective coping methods.*

Fear

The fear of death and disability can be a paralyzing emotion that adversely affects the client's recovery from acute MI.

Selected nursing interventions and rationales follow:

- Identify the client's level of fear. Note both verbal and nonverbal signs of fear. *This information enables the nurse to identify appropriate interventions. Clients may not voice concerns, so paying attention to nonverbal indicators is important. Controlling the fear helps decrease sympathetic nervous system responses and catecholamine release that may increase the sense of fear and anxiety.*

- Acknowledge the client's perception of the situation. Allow the client to verbalize concerns. *The sudden change in health status brings on anxiety and fear of the unknown. Verbalizing these fears may help the client cope with the changes and allow the health care team to provide information and correct misconceptions.*

- Encourage the client to ask questions, and provide consistent, factual answers. Repeat information as needed. *Accurate and consistent information can reduce fear. Honest explanations can help strengthen the client-nurse relationship and help the client develop realistic expectations. Anxiety and fear decrease the client's ability to concentrate and retain information; therefore, information may need to be repeated.*

- Recognize opportunities for client independence. Encourage self-care. Allow the client to make decisions regarding the plan of care. *This promotes personal responsibility for health and allows the client to have some* control over the situation. *Clients' confidence increases as their dependence decreases.*

- Administer antianxiety or hypnotic medications as ordered. *These medications are used to promote rest and relaxation and decrease feelings of anxiety, which may act as barriers to restoration of health.*

- Teach the client nonpharmacologic methods of stress reduction (e.g., relaxation methods, mental imagery, music therapy, breathing exercises, meditation, massage). *Stress management techniques may help reduce tension and anxiety, provide the client with a sense of control, and enhance coping skills.*

Other Nursing Diagnoses

Other nursing diagnoses that may be appropriate for the client who has experienced an acute MI include the following:

- *Risk for Decreased Cardiac Output* related to loss of ventricular myocardium

- *Risk for Injury* related to impaired coagulation processes secondary to thrombolytic and anticoagulant therapy

- *Risk for Injury* related to cardiac dysrhythmias

- *Altered Sexuality Patterns* related to fear of precipitating another MI or death

- *Ineffective Breathing Pattern* related to anxiety, pain, and fear

- *Altered Role Performance* related to situational health crisis

- *Knowledge Deficit* regarding disease process and treatment rationales.

Client and Family Teaching

Teaching begins with admission to the coronary care unit and continues through transfer to the medical unit after the client is stabilized, and after discharge into the convalescent period. The emphasis for teaching is on the *realistic application* of the information (e.g., life-style modifications).

Assessing the client's readiness to learn is an important first step. The client in strong denial may not believe that the information being taught has any relevance. Evaluate the client's ability to learn, assessing the client's physiologic and psychologic health status, beliefs regarding personal responsibility for health, and expectations of the health care system. Also assess the client's developmental level and ability to perform psychomotor skills, cognitive function, learning disabilities, existing knowledge base, and the influence of previous learning experiences (Whitman, 1992).

Describe the normal anatomy and physiology of the heart, and identify the specific area of heart damage.

Heart models or other visual media are beneficial for this discussion. Also explain the disease process and implications of MI, as well as the purposes and side effects of the medications the client is taking. Encourage the client to ask questions, and reinforce the information is provided. Written materials are helpful adjuncts to teaching; the client can refer to the written information as needed.

Emphasize the importance of complying with the medical regimen and keeping follow-up appointments. One week after the client is discharged and periodically thereafter during the recovery period, follow up by telephone to offer reassurance, additional information, and clarifications. Provide the client with telephone numbers and addresses of resource personnel who are available to respond to questions and concerns after the client's discharge. These may include nurses, dietitians, exercise physiologists, physical therapists, psychologists, pharmacists, and social workers.

Provide information about community resources, such as the local chapter of the American Heart Association. In addition, the client with CAD, particularly one with continued dysrhythmias, is at high risk for sudden cardiac death; therefore encourage family members to learn CPR in the event of an emergency, and provide information about other community agencies that offer CPR classes. These community resources are listed in the client's local phone book.

Applying the Nursing Process

Case Study of a Client with Acute Myocardial Infarction: Betty Williams

Betty Williams, a 62-year-old psychologist is admitted to the emergency department with complaints of severe substernal chest pain. Mrs. Williams states that she began feeling the pain after eating lunch about 4 hours ago. She had initially attributed the pain to indigestion. She described the pain, which radiates to her jaw and left arm, as "like someone sitting on my chest." It is accompanied by a "choking feeling," severe shortness of breath, and diaphoresis. The pain is unrelieved by rest, antacids, or three sublingual nitroglycerin tablets (gr 1/150).

The emergency room staff start central and peripheral intravenous lines and begin to administer oxygen per nasal cannula at 2L/min. They obtain a 12-lead ECG and the following labwork: cardiac enzymes and isoenzymes, ABGs, CBC, and a chemistry panel. Morphine sulfate is successful at relieving Mrs. Williams's pain.

Mrs. Williams's medical history includes a diagnosis of adult-onset diabetes, angina, and hypertension. She has a 45-year history of cigarette smoking, averaging 1½ to 2 packs per day. Her family history reveals that Mrs. Williams's father died at age 42 of MI, and her paternal grandfather died at age 65 of MI. Mrs. Williams is taking the following medications: tolbutamide (Orinase), hydrochlorothiazide, and isosorbide (Isordil).

The client history, initial assessment data, and ECG results point toward an acute anterior wall MI. Mrs. Williams has no contraindications to thrombolytic therapy and is deemed a good candidate. Intravenous alteplase (t-PA, Activase) is administered by bolus followed by intravenous infusions of alteplase and heparin. She is transferred to the coronary care unit (CCU).

Assessment
Dan Morales, RN, is assigned as Mrs. Williams's primary care nurse. He helps her get settled into the room and then performs a head-to-toe assessment. Mrs. Williams is alert and oriented to person, place, and time. Vital signs are as follows: P, 118; BP, 172/92; R, 24 with adequate depth; temperature 99.6 (37.5 C). Auscultation reveals an S_4 and fine crackles in the bases of both lungs. The ECG shows sinus tachycardia with occasional PVCs and evidence of an evolving anterior MI. Her skin is cool and slightly diaphoretic. Capillary refill time is less than 3 seconds, and peripheral pulses are strong and equal. Her nail beds are pink.

A triple-lumen central line is in place. Nitroglycerin is infusing at 200 μg/min in the distal lumen; the alteplase infusion is in the middle lumen; and a heparin infusion is in the proximal lumen. The peripheral intravenous line is being maintained with an infusion of 5% dextrose in 1/4 normal saline solution at 50 mL/h. Mrs. Williams states, "The pain is better since the nurse in the ER gave me a shot. But it has been going away and then coming back again. I would rate it a 4 right now, but who knows when it will come back? It was terrible before. The doctor told me that this drug I'm getting will quickly open up the artery that is blocked. I hope it works! Do many people get this drug?"

Diagnosis
Based upon the assessment findings, Mr. Morales formulates the following individualized nursing diagnoses:

- *Pain* (chest pain) related to imbalance between oxygen supply and demand
- *Anxiety* and *Fear* related to change in health status
- *Altered Protection* related to the risk of bleeding secondary to thrombolytic therapy
- *Risk for Injury* related to altered cardiac rate and rhythm
- *Knowledge Deficit* regarding myocardial infarction disease process and the use of thrombolytic therapy

Expected Outcomes
The expected outcomes during the initial phase of treatment are related to the administration of thrombolytic agents to restore perfusion to the heart muscle. Identified outcomes specify that Mrs. Williams will:

- Verbalize a reduction in chest pain to a tolerable level.
- Verbalize a reduction of anxiety and fear.
- Exhibit no signs of internal or external bleeding.
- Demonstrate an adequate cardiac output during reperfusion therapy.
- Discuss the development of atherosclerotic plaques and the use of thrombolytic agents to restore blood flow.

Planning and Implementation
The following interventions are planned and implemented during the acute phase of Mrs. Williams's hospitalization with respect to thrombolytic therapy:

- Instruct Mrs. Williams to alert the nurse for any complaints of chest pain. Monitor and evaluate Mrs. Williams's complaints of chest pain using a scale of 0 to 10. Titrate intravenous nitroglycerin infusion for chest pain; withhold medication if systolic BP drops below 100 mm Hg. Administer morphine intravenously in increments of 2 to 4 mg for chest pain unrelieved by nitroglycerin infusion.
- Encourage Mrs. Williams to verbalize her fears and concerns. Answer questions honestly, and correct any misconceptions regarding the disease process, therapeutic interventions, or prognosis.
- Assess Mrs. Williams's knowledge of how atherosclerotic plaques develop and occlude the coronary arteries. Explain that the purpose of the thrombolytic agent used (tPA) is to dissolve the fresh clot and reperfuse the heart muscle, thus limiting heart damage.
- Explain the need for frequent monitoring of vital signs and signs of bleeding problems during and after therapy. Discuss posttherapy care related to risk factor modification to prevent future problems.
- Titrate heparin drip to keep PTT at 1½ to 2 times the control time as ordered.
- Assess for manifestations of internal or intracranial bleeding: Note complaints of back or abdominal pain, headache, decreased level of consciousness, dizziness, bloody secretions or excretions, or pallor. Perform guaiac testing on all stools, urine, and vomitus. Notify physician immediately of any abnormal findings.
- Monitor Mrs. Williams for signs of reperfusion: decreased chest pain, return of ST segment to baseline, reperfusion dysrhythmias (e.g., PVCs, bradycardia, and heart block).
- Continuously monitor ECG for changes in cardiac rate, rhythm, and conduction. Assess vital signs and associated symptoms with changes in ECG. Note

hypotension, dizziness, vertigo, light-headedness, syncope, or palpitations. Report findings to physician.

- Maintain a supply of emergency cardiac drugs and equipment (i.e., lidocaine, epinephrine, verapamil, procainamide, bretylium, atropine, isoproterenol, phenylephrine, the defibrillator, pacemaker, intubation tray) in the unit. In the case of a cardiac event, administer appropriate drugs and procedures as prescribed per unit protocol.

Evaluation

After the initial morphine dose, Mrs. Williams notes a reduction in her chest pain from a pain rating of 8 to 4. The nitroglycerin infusion and thrombolytic therapy further reduce her pain to 2. The nitroglycerin infusion is gradually discontinued (weaned) after 24 hours. As her pain subsides, Mrs. Williams states that she feels "much better now that the pain is gone. I was afraid it would just get worse." She is able to describe a basic understanding of plaque formation and the resulting obstruction to blood flow. Mrs. Williams agrees that it is important to "quickly open up the artery" so that myocardial damage will be limited. No indication of bleeding problems are noted.

Evidence of reperfusion is noted: Chest pain has been relieved; the ECG shows that the ST segment is returning to baseline; there has been an early peaking of CK levels; and there has been an increase in PVCs but no significant dysrhythmias. Mrs. Williams remains in CCU for 2 days and is transferred to the floor.

Critical Thinking in the Nursing Process

1. How would the initial plan of care have changed if Mrs. Williams were not a candidate for thrombolytic therapy?

2. Two days after her initial therapy, Mrs. Williams complains of palpitations. You notice frequent PVCs on the ECG monitor. What do you do?

3. What topics of health promotion would you choose to teach Mrs. Williams before discharge?

4. Mrs. Williams states, "I have been smoking for over 45 years, and I am not going to stop now! Besides, it calms me down when I am feeling anxious." How would you respond to this statement?

▪ ▪ ▪   Heart Failure   ▪ ▪ ▪

Heart failure, the inability of the heart to pump adequate blood to meet the metabolic demands of the body, is the end result of many conditions. Frequently, it is a long-term outcome of myocardial infarction when left ventricular damage is extensive enough to impair cardiac output. Other diseases of the heart may cause heart failure as well, including cardiomyopathies, valve disorders, and inflammatory conditions (e.g., bacterial endocarditis). Heart failure can also result from excessive demands placed on a normal heart. It may present as an acute condition (e.g., pulmonary edema or cardiogenic shock) or as a chronic condition, congestive heart failure. Congestive heart failure and pulmonary edema are discussed below; cardiogenic shock is discussed in Chapter 6.

The Client with Congestive Heart Failure

▪ ▪ ▪

One of the fastest growing cardiovascular health problems in the United States is **congestive heart failure (CHF).** CHF is basically an affliction of the older adult and is the number-one cause of hospital admissions for those over 65 years of age (see the accompanying box). In a country whose population is aging, the impact of CHF

is significant in terms of health care dollars and quality of life.

Heart failure is defined as the inability of the heart to function as a pump to meet the needs of the body. Cardiac output falls, leading to decreased tissue perfusion. The body initially adjusts to reduced cardiac output by activating inherent compensatory mechanisms to restore adequate perfusion. These normal mechanisms may result in vascular congestion—hence the term *congestive heart failure.* As these mechanisms are exhausted, heart failure ensues, with increased morbidity and mortality.

Heart failure may result from any condition that (1) increases cardiac workload beyond its limits, (2) produces structural or functional alterations in the myocardium that interfere with its ability to contract normally, or (3) obstructs or interferes with pumping capacity (Laurent-Bopp, 1995b). The most common cause of chronic heart failure in European-Americans is impaired left ventricular function secondary to coronary artery disease (specifically, ischemic heart disease). Hypertension is the leading cause of CHF in African-Americans (Bourassa et al., 1993). Table 28–8 lists disorders that can precipitate heart failure.

Estimates of the number of people suffering from CHF in the United States range from 2.5 million to over 4 million. Data from the Framingham Heart Study indicate that the incidence of CHF increases significantly with age; its

---

Gerontologic Considerations: Care of the Older Adult Client with CHF

∎ ∎ ∎

Age-related changes in cardiovascular function and life-style habits may contribute to the development of CHF in the older adult. Systolic blood pressure is often elevated because of decreased elastin and increased collagen deposition in the aorta. As a result, left ventricular work increases, as does its muscle mass to generate enough force to eject blood. Changes in cardiac valve structure and function are more common in the older adult, especially calcific aortic stenosis. These may also reduce the efficiency of cardiac function and increase its workload.

Maximal heart rate, cardiac reserve, and tolerance to exercise or stress are generally decreased in older adults (Lakatta, 1994; Massie & Wolfe, 1993). These changes affect the development of and response to CHF. Aging affects diastolic function as well. Left ventricular compliance may be decreased, affecting cardiac filling. Cardiac conditioning in the older adult should be encouraged, because increased aerobic capacity is associated with a decrease in arterial stiffness, improved stroke volume and cardiac output, and enhanced oxygen consumption (Lakatta, 1994).

Older clients may not present with typical manifestations of CHF and are likely to have other conditions that may obscure the diagnosis, such as chronic pulmonary disease or peripheral vascular disease. Many older clients need dosage adjustments of medications because of changes in renal and liver function. Also, older adults have a greater potential for injury due to falls because of their response to fluid volume and electrolyte changes from diuretics.

Table 28–8   Selected Causes of Heart Failure

Increased Cardiac Workload				Altered Function	Filling Disorders
Excess Volume Load	**Excess Pressure Load**	**Increased Metabolic Demand**	**Acute Conditions**		
Volume overload	Hypertension	Anemias	Acute hypertensive crisis	Cardiomyopathy	Valve stenosis (mitral or tricuspid)
Valve regurgitation	Aortic stenosis	Thyrotoxicosis		Myocarditis	Cardiac tamponade
Left-to-right shunts	Hypertrophic cardiomyopathy	Pregnancy	Aortic valve rupture	Rheumatic fever	Restrictive pericarditis
	Coarctation of the aorta	Fever	Massive pulmonary embolism	Ischemia	
		Physical, emotional, or environmental stressors		Infarction	
				Dysrhythmias	
				Toxic disorders	
				Infiltrative disorders	

---

prevalence also increases with age, affecting approximately 2.5% of the population over 45 years of age (Bourassa et al., 1993). Survival statistics for clients after diagnosis of CHF are grim: an average of 1.7 years for men and 3.2 years for women. Five-year survival rates average 25% and 38% for men and women respectively (Ho et al., 1993). In addition to age, other risk factors have been identified for heart failure. These include hypertension, diabetes mellitus, cigarette smoking, obesity, and atrial fibrillation.

Physiology

The mechanical pumping action of cardiac muscle propels the blood it receives to the pulmonary and vascular systems for reoxygenation and delivery to the tissues. *Cardiac output (CO)* is defined as the amount of blood pumped from the ventricles in 1 minute. Cardiac output is an important parameter used to assess general cardiac performance, especially left ventricular function. The heart regulates cardiac output according to the oxygen needs of the body: As oxygen demand increases, oxygen supply must also increase to maintain cellular function. Damage to the cardiac pump, regardless of the cause, eventually causes cardiac output to fall and tissue perfusion to decrease. Decreased tissue perfusion ultimately leads to cell death and organ dysfunction.

Cardiac output is a product of heart rate and stroke volume. Effective cardiac output depends on functional muscle mass and the ability of the ventricles to work together. During systole, the ventricles eject blood into the pulmonary and systemic circulation. *Stroke volume* is the volume of blood ejected with each heartbeat; it is determined by preload, afterload, and myocardial contractility. The *ejection fraction (EF)* is the percentage of blood in the ventricle at the end of diastole (end-diastolic volume) that is ejected during systole. A normal ejection fraction is approximately 60%. *Cardiac reserve* is the ability of the heart to increase CO and blood pressure to meet metabolic demand. Ventricles that are structurally or functionally compromised have little to no cardiac reserve to rely on in times of metabolic stress.

Heart rate affects cardiac output by controlling the number of times blood is ejected from the ventricles in a minute. It is directly and indirectly influenced by the autonomic nervous system, catecholamines, and thyroid hormones. Any internal or external event that activates the body's stress response, such as hypovolemia or fear, stimulates the sympathetic nervous system, increasing the heart rate and its contractility. Elevated heart rates increase cardiac output; however, very rapid heart rates shorten the period for ventricular filling (diastole), reducing stroke volume and cardiac output. On the other hand, if the heart rate is too slow, cardiac output may be reduced simply because the number of cardiac cycles is reduced.

Preload is the amount of cardiac muscle fiber tension (stretch) at the end of diastole. The Frank-Starling law of the heart states that contractile force of the ventricle is related to the amount of stretch in the muscle fibers (within a physiologic limit). Preload is usually defined as the volume of blood in the ventricles at end-diastole. The blood in the ventricles exerts pressure on the ventricle walls, stretching the muscle fibers; the greater the blood volume, the greater force with which the ventricle contracts to propel the blood into the circulation. Overstretching the muscle fibers past their physiologic limit results in an ineffective contraction. End-diastolic volume (EDV) depends on the amount of blood returning to the ventricles (*venous return*), and the distensibility or stiffness of the ventricles (*ventricular compliance*).

Afterload is the amount of force the ventricle must develop to eject blood into the circulation. This force must be great enough to overcome arterial pressures on the other side of the pulmonic and aortic valves. The right ventricle must generate enough tension to open the pul-

monary valve and eject its volume into the pulmonary artery. The left ventricle ejects its volume into the systemic circulation by overcoming the arterial resistance behind the aortic valve. Increased systemic vascular resistance increases afterload, impairing ventricular emptying and increasing myocardial work.

Contractility is defined as the natural ability of the cardiac muscle fibers to shorten during systole. Contractility cannot be directly measured, but it can be estimated clinically and calculated from other hemodynamic measurements. Contractility is necessary to overcome afterload and eject blood during systole. Alterations in contractility affect cardiac output. Poor contractility reduces the forward flow of blood from the ventricle, decreasing stroke volume.

Pathophysiology

In the early stages of heart failure, compensatory mechanisms are activated to maintain the cardiac output. The primary compensatory mechanisms employed are (1) the Frank-Starling mechanism; (2) neuroendocrine responses including activation of the sympathetic nervous system and the renin-angiotensin system; and (3) myocardial hypertrophy. These mechanisms and their effects are summarized in Table 28–9.

Decreased cardiac output initially stimulates the aortic baroreceptors, which in turn stimulate the sympathetic nervous system (SNS). SNS stimulation produces both cardiac and vascular responses through the release of norepinephrine. Norepinephrine increases heart rate and contractility by stimulating cardiac beta receptors. Cardiac output improves as both heart rate and stroke volume increase. Norepinephrine also causes arterial and venous vasoconstriction, increasing venous return to the heart. Increased venous return increases ventricular filling and myocardial stretch, increasing the force of contraction; this is known as the *Frank-Starling mechanism.* Blood flow is redistributed to the brain and the heart to maintain perfusion of these vital organs.

A fall in cardiac output and a resulting decrease in renal perfusion cause renin to be released from the kidneys. Activation of the renin-angiotensin system produces additional vasoconstriction and stimulates the adrenal cortex to produce aldosterone and the posterior pituitary to release antidiuretic hormone (ADH). Aldosterone stimulates sodium reabsorption in renal tubules, promoting water retention. ADH acts on the distal tubule to inhibit water excretion and causes vasoconstriction. The effect of these hormones is significant vasoconstriction and salt and water retention, with a resulting increase in vascular volume. Increased ventricular filling increases the force of contraction, improving cardiac output. The increased vascular volume and venous return also increase atrial pressures, stimulating the release of an additional hor-

Table 28–9	Compensatory Mechanisms Activated in Heart Failure		
Mechanism	**Pathophysiology**	**Effect on Body Systems**	**Complications**
Frank-Starling mechanism	The greater the stretch of cardiac muscle fibers, the greater the force of contraction.	Increased contractile force leading to increased CO	Increased myocardial oxygen demand
Neuroendocrine response	Decreased CO causes sympathetic nervous system stimulation and catecholamine release.	Increased HR, BP, and contractility Increased vascular resistance Increased venous return	Tachycardia with decreased filling time and decreased CO Increased vascular resistance Increased myocardial work and oxygen demand
	Decreased CO and decreased renal perfusion stimulate renin-angiotensin system.	Vasoconstriction and increased BP	Increased myocardial work Renal vasoconstriction and decreased renal perfusion
	Angiotensin stimulates aldosterone release from adrenal cortex.	Salt and water retention by the kidneys Increased vascular volume	Increased preload and afterload Pulmonary congestion
	ADH is released from posterior pituitary.	Water excretion inhibited	Fluid retention and increased preload and afterload Pulmonary congestion
	Atrial natriuretic factor is released.	Increased sodium excretion Diuresis	
	Blood flow is redistributed to vital organs (heart and brain).	Decreased perfusion of other organ systems Decreased perfusion of skin and muscles	Renal failure Anaerobic metabolism and lactic acidosis
Ventricular hypertrophy	Increased cardiac workload causes myocardial muscle to hypertrophy and ventricles to dilate.	Increased contractile force to maintain CO	Increased myocardial oxygen demand Cellular enlargement

mone, *atrial natriuretic factor (ANF)* or *atriopeptin*. ANF balances the effects of the other hormones to a certain extent, promoting sodium and water excretion and inhibiting the release of norepinephrine, renin, and ADH. This hormone is thought to be a natural preventive aid that delays severe cardiac decompensation (Guyton, 1991).

Ventricular remodeling occurs as the heart chambers and myocardium adapt to fluid and pressure increases. The chambers dilate to accommodate excess fluid volume resulting from increased vascular volume and incomplete emptying. Initially, this additional stretch causes more effective contractions. *Ventricular hypertrophy* occurs as existing cardiac muscle cells enlarge, increasing their contractile elements (actin and myosin) and force of contraction.

Although all of these responses may help in the short-term regulation of cardiac output, it is now recognized that they hasten the deterioration of cardiac function (Garg, Packer, Pitt, & Yusuf, 1993). The onset of heart failure is heralded by the loss of effective compensation. The mechanisms involved in the progression of heart failure are the very mechanisms that initially maintained circulatory stability.

The rapid heart rate shortens diastolic filling time, compromises coronary artery perfusion, and increased myocardial oxygen demand. Resulting ischemia further impairs cardiac output. Beta-receptors in the heart become less sensitive to continued SNS stimulation, resulting in decreasing heart rate and contractility. As the beta-receptors become less sensitive, norepinephrine stores in the cardiac muscle become depleted (Laurent-Bopp, 1995b). In contrast, alpha-receptors on peripheral blood vessels become increasingly sensitive to persistent stimulation, promoting vasoconstriction and increasing afterload and cardiac work.

Initially, ventricular hypertrophy and dilation increase cardiac output, but chronic distention causes the ventricular wall eventually to thin and degenerate. The purpose of hypertrophy is thus defeated. In addition, chronic overloading of the dilated ventricle eventually stretches the fibers beyond the optimal point for effective contraction. The ventricles continue to dilate to accommodate

Classifications of Heart Failure

■ ■ ■

- *Backward versus forward failure. Backward failure* refers to the accumulation of blood in the ventricle, atrium, and venous system (pulmonary or systemic) from incomplete ventricular emptying or difficulty filling. *Forward failure* is the heart's inability to eject enough volume to maintain a normal cardiac output. Both result in high atrial and venous pressures, sodium and water retention, and interstitial edema.

- *High-output versus low-output failure.* Clients in hypermetabolic states (e.g., thyrotoxicosis, hyperthyroidism, anemia, or pregnancy) require increased cardiac output to maintain blood flow and oxygen to the tissues. If the increased blood flow cannot meet the oxygen demands of the tissues, compensatory mechanisms are activated to further increase cardiac output, which in turn further increases oxygen demand. Thus, even though cardiac output is high, the heart is unable to meet increased oxygen demands; this condition is known as *high-output failure. Low-output failure* is classic heart failure caused by the failure of the heart to pump adequately; it produces the manifestations of decreased cardiac output. Low-output failure occurs in ischemic heart disease, hypertension, cardiomyopathy, and valvular heart disease.

- *Acute versus chronic failure. Acute failure* is the abrupt onset of a myocardial injury (such as a massive MI) resulting in suddenly decreased cardiac function and signs of decreased cardiac output. *Chronic failure* is a progressive deterioration of the heart muscle due to cardiomyopathies, valvular disease, or a previous MI.

- *Systolic versus diastolic failure. Systolic failure* occurs when the ventricle fails to contract adequately to eject a sufficient blood volume into the arterial system. Systolic function is affected when the loss of myocardial cells resulting from ischemia progresses to muscle necrosis, as from an MI. The manifestations of systolic failure are those of decreased cardiac output. *Diastolic failure* results when the heart cannot completely relax in diastole, disrupting normal filling patterns. Early passive diastolic filling is decreased, and the heart depends more on the late contribution of atrial contraction to preload. Diastolic dysfunction results from increased ventricular stiffness due to hypertrophic and cellular changes and impaired relaxation of the heart muscle (Massie & Wolfe, 1993).

---

the excess fluid, but the heart loses the ability to contract forcefully. The heart muscle may eventually become so large that the coronary blood supply is inadequate, causing ischemia.

Chronic distension exhausts atrial stores of ANF. The effects of norepinephrine, renin, and ADH prevail, and the renin-angiotensin pathway is continually stimulated. This mechanism ultimately raises the hemodynamic stress on the heart by increasing both preload and afterload. As the heart function deteriorates, less blood is delivered to the tissues and to the heart itself. Ischemia and necrosis of the myocardium further weakens the already failing heart, and the cycle repeats.

In normal hearts, cardiac reserve can increase cardiac output by 300% to 400%; in well-trained athletes, it can increase by up to 600% (Guyton, 1991). Clients with CHF have minimal to no cardiac reserve. At rest, they may be unaffected; however, any stressor (e.g., exercise, illness) taxes their ability to meet the demand for oxygen and nutrients. Manifestations of activity intolerance when the person is at rest indicate a critical level of cardiac decompensation.

Heart failure is commonly classified according to the pathology causing its clinical manifestations. Classifications include left-sided versus right-sided failure, systolic versus diastolic failure, backward versus forward failure, high-output versus low-output failure, and acute versus chronic failure (Braunwald, 1994a). The manifestations of the disease in terms of left versus right heart failure are discussed below; see the accompanying box for a brief description of the other classifications.

Left-Sided Heart Failure

Although either side of the heart can fail, the left ventricle is affected more often than the right because of its high workload and oxygen demand. Left-sided heart failure results from ventricular muscle damage or overloading. As left ventricular function deteriorates, cardiac output falls. Left ventricular and atrial end-diastolic pressures increase because the heart fails to eject blood volumes fully during systole. These increased pressures impair filling, resulting in congestion and increased pressures in the pulmonary vascular system. Increased pressures in this normally low-pressure system promote the movement of fluid from the

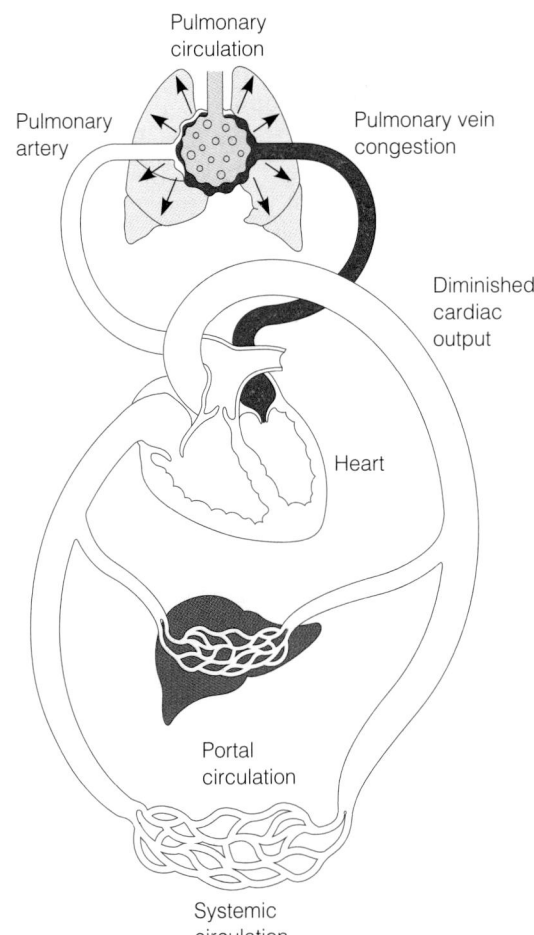

Pulmonary
circulation

Pulmonary
artery

Pulmonary vein
congestion

Diminished
cardiac
output

Heart

Portal
circulation

Systemic
circulation

Figure 28–19 The hemodynamic effects of left-sided heart failure.

Clinical Manifestations of Left-Sided Heart Failure

- Dyspnea
- Shortness of breath
- Crackles (rales) in the bases of both lungs
- Orthopnea
- Dry, hacking cough
- Tachycardia
- S₃ gallop

- Palpitations
- Pallor
- Decreased urine output
- Activity intolerance
- Fatigue
- Weakness

---

blood vessels into interstitial tissues and the alveoli (Figure 28–19).

The manifestations of left-sided heart failure result from pulmonary congestion and decreased cardiac output. Fatigue and activity intolerance are common early manifestations of left ventricular failure. Dizziness and syncope are additional manifestations of decreased cardiac output. Pulmonary congestion causes dyspnea, shortness of breath, and cough. The client may also develop *orthopnea*, difficulty breathing while lying down, prompting the client to sleep propped up on two or three pillows or in a recliner. Cyanosis from impaired gas exchange may be noted. On auscultation of the lungs, inspiratory crackles (rales) and wheezes may be heard in lung bases. An S₃ gallop may be present, reflecting the heart's attempts to fill an already distended ventricle. Manifestations of left-sided heart failure are summarized in the accompanying box.

Right-Sided Heart Failure

Primary right-sided heart failure is caused by pulmonary hypertension *(cor pulmonale)* or right ventricular infarc-

tion; however, the most common cause of right ventricular failure is left ventricular failure. Increased pressures in the pulmonary vasculature or right ventricular muscle damage impair the right venticle's ability to pump blood into the pulmonary circulation. The right ventricle and atrium become distended, and blood accumulates in the systemic venous system. Increased venous pressures cause abdominal organs to become congested and peripheral tissue edema to develop (Figure 28–20).

Dependent tissues tend to be most affected because of the effects of gravity; edema develops in the feet and legs of an upright client, in the sacrum of one who is reclining. The liver may become engorged, causing right upper quadrant pain; anorexia and nausea may result as the blood vessels of the gastrointestinal tract become congested. Increased central venous pressure causes the jugular veins to become distended and visible even when the client is standing. Manifestations of right-sided heart failure are summarized in the box on page 1112.

Biventricular Failure

As noted previously, the most common cause of right ventricular failure is left ventricular failure. When both ventricles fail to function adequately, a state of *biventricular failure* exists. The client with biventricular failure has manifestations of both right- and left-sided heart failure. In addition, the client may experience *paroxysmal nocturnal dyspnea (PND)*, a frightening condition in which the client awakens at night acutely short of breath. PND occurs when edema fluid that has accumulated during the day is reabsorbed into the circulation at night, causing fluid overload and pulmonary congestion. The client in severe heart failure may be dyspneic at rest as well as with activity, signifying little or no cardiac reserve. Both an S₃ and an S₄ gallop may be heard on auscultation.

The compensatory mechanisms initiated in heart failure can lead to complications in other body systems.

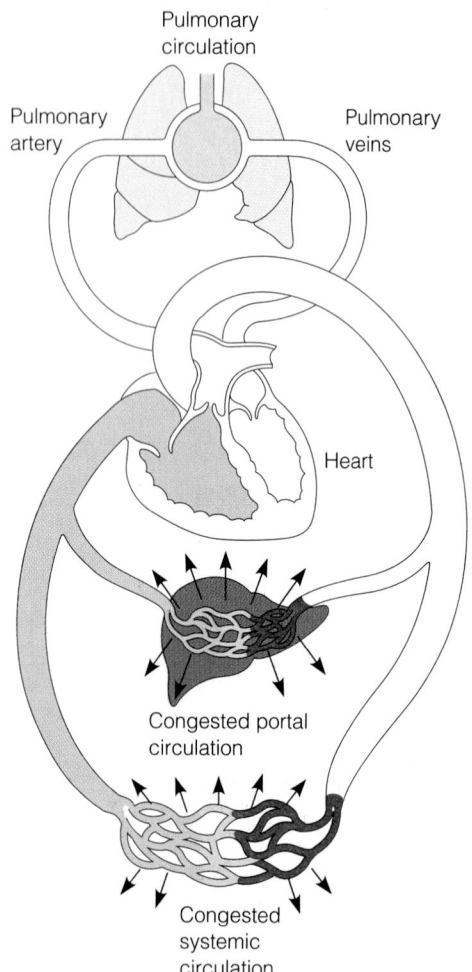

Pulmonary
circulation

Pulmonary
artery

Pulmonary
veins

Heart

Congested portal
circulation

Congested
systemic
circulation

Figure 28–20 The hemodynamic effects of right-sided heart failure.

Clinical Manifestations of Right-Sided Heart Failure

- Elevated central venous pressure
- Jugular venous distention (JVD)
- Peripheral edema
- Liver enlargement and tenderness
- Ascites
- Nausea

- Anorexia
- Abdominal distention
- Nocturia
- Hepatojugular reflux
- Splenomegaly
- Fatigue

Congestive hepatomegaly and splenomegaly caused by engorgement of the portal venous system results in increased abdominal pressure, ascites, and gastrointestinal problems. With prolonged right-sided heart failure, liver function may be impaired. Gastrointestinal congestion may interfere with digestion and absorption (Porth, 1994). Myocardial distention can precipitate dysrhythmias, futher impairing cardiac output. The risk of sudden cardiac death is high. Pleural effusions and other pulmonary problems may ensue. Major complications of severe cardiac decompensation are cardiogenic shock (described in Chapter 6) and acute pulmonary edema, a medical emergency described in the next section of this chapter.

Collaborative Care

The main goals for care of the client with congestive heart failure are to reduce cardiac workload, improve cardiac pumping ability, and control fluid retention. Treatment strategies have changed over the last few decades. Thirty

to 50 years ago, physicians focused on managing excess fluid accumulated in the client's lungs and/or tissues. Today, the focus has shifted toward improving activity tolerance and decreasing mortality and morbidity. The realization that naturally activated compensatory mechanisms may be of more harm than benefit to the client's overall state forms the foundation of new treatment protocols.

Laboratory and Diagnostic Tests

Diagnosis of CHF is based on a multitude of physical and diagnostic findings; it is not based on one single finding or test. Evaluating the client's history, presenting manifestations, and diagnostic testing help validate the diagnosis.

Laboratory tests that may be performed include the following:

- *Serum electrolytes* are measured to evaluate fluid and electrolyte status. In CHF, serum osmolarity may be decreased because of fluid retention. Sodium, potassium, and chloride levels provide a baseline for evaluating the effects of therapy, such as diuretic therapy.

- *Liver function tests* are performed to determine whether hepatomegaly has caused liver dysfunction. Elevated liver enzymes (including ALT, AST, and LDH) and serum bilirubin, coagulation abnormalities, and decreased albumin levels may indicate liver impairment.

- *ABG analysis* is ordered to evaluate gas exchange. Impaired gas exchange may cause decreased oxygen levels (PO_2). Increased respiratory rate may cause carbon dioxide levels (PCO_2) to fall; as heart failure progresses and gas exchange is further impaired, carbon dioxide accumulates, and PCO_2 levels rise.

The following diagnostic tests may be performed:

- *Chest X-ray* may show pulmonary vascular congestion and cardiomegaly if the heart has hypertrophied or dilated.

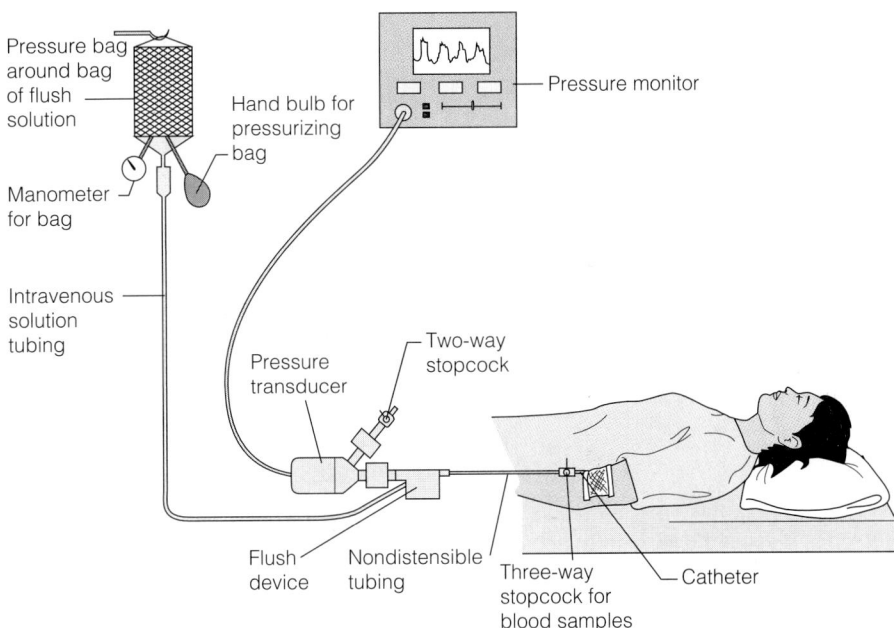

Figure 28–21   A hemodynamic monitoring set-up.

- *Echocardiography* allows evaluation of left ventricular function, as well as providing evidence of ventricular dilation and hypertrophy.
- *Electrocardiography* is used to identify ECG changes associated with ventricular enlargement and to detect dysrhythmias, myocardial ischemia, or infarction.

Hemodynamic Monitoring

Hemodynamics is defined as the study of the forces involved in blood circulation (Thomas, 1994). Hemodynamic monitoring is used to assess cardiovascular function in the critically ill or unstable client. It is indicated when standard vital sign measurements are not adequate to evaluate acute changes in cardiovascular status. The main goals of invasive hemodynamic monitoring are to evaluate cardiac function, the condition of the circulatory system, and the client's response to interventions.

Hemodynamic parameters include heart rate, arterial blood pressure, central venous pressure, pulmonary pressures, and cardiac output. *Direct* hemodynamic parameters are obtained straight from the monitoring device; examples of these parameters are the heart rate and various pressures such as arterial and venous pressures. *Derived* hemodynamic parameters are calculated using the direct hemodynamic data; they include such measurements as the cardiac index, mean arterial blood pressure (MAP), and stroke volume (SV). Invasive hemodynamic monitoring is routinely used in the critical care units and sometimes in other areas of the hospital (i.e., emergency department, surgery suites).

Hemodynamic monitoring systems measure the pressure within the vessel and convert this signal into an electrical waveform that is amplified and displayed (Gardner & Hujcs, 1993). The electrical signal may be graphically recorded on pressure graph paper and displayed numerically on the monitor. System components include an invasive catheter threaded into an artery or vein connected to a transducer by stiff, high-pressure tubing. The *pressure transducer* translates pressure measurements into an electrical signal that is in turn relayed to the monitor. Additional components of the pressure monitoring system include stopcocks and a continuous flush system with normal saline or heparinized saline and an infusion pressure bag to keep clots from forming in the catheter. Figure 28–21 illustrates a pressure transducer and typical hemodynamic monitoring system.

Leveling the transducer is important to ensure accurate pressure readings. The point used as a constant reference for central line monitoring is the level of the right atrium. It is located by intersecting two imaginary lines: one drawn down the lateral chest wall from the client's 4th intercostal space at the lateral margin of the sternum, the other line at midchest level (the midaxillary line, in most clients). Once located, this junction is marked with ink or tape and used consistently for pressure readings.

Hemodynamic pressure monitoring may be used to measure peripheral arterial pressures, or central pressures, such as central venous pressure (CVP) or pulmonary artery pressures (PAP). The client may have more than one invasive monitoring line at a time; indeed, the more critical the client's condition, the more complex the monitoring. Although the information obtained from invasive monitoring lines is valuable, the procedure is not without risk. The box on page 1114 indicates nursing care of the client undergoing hemodynamic monitoring, and the box on page 1115 lists potential complications of central pressure monitoring.

Nursing Care of the Client Undergoing Hemodynamic Monitoring

- Calibrate and level the monitoring system at least once a shift using the right atrium as a constant reference level. Relevel the transducer after a change in position. Mark the right atrial position on the chest wall, and use this as a reference point for all readings. *Accurate measurements record the pressure within the vessel without interference from atmospheric or hydrostatic pressures. Calibration ensures that pressures are correctly recorded. Marking the right atrial level provides a consistent reference point for all caregivers to use.*

- Measure all pressures between breaths. *This ensures that intrathoracic pressure does not influence pressure readings.*

- Maintain 300 mm Hg of pressure on the flush solution at all times. *This ensures a continuous flow of flush solution through the pressure tubing and catheter to prevent clot formation and catheter occlusion.*

- Monitor pressure trends rather than individual readings. *Individual readings may be affected by situational factors and may not reflect the true status of the client. Monitoring trends in pressure readings along with clinical observations provides a better overall picture of the client's status.*

- Obtain a chest X-ray before infusing intravenous fluid into any newly placed central line. *The chest X-ray verifies the location of the catheter and helps prevent pulmonary complications of incorrect catheter placement such as pneumothorax.*

- Set alarm limits for monitored hemodynamic variables. Turn alarms on. *Alarms provide warning of hemodynamic instability. Always investigate the meaning of the alarms. They may be temporarily silenced to change tubing or draw blood but should never be turned off.*

- Use aseptic technique during catheter insertion and site care. *Aseptic technique is important to prevent infection.*

- Assess and document the appearance of the insertion site at least every shift; observe for signs of infiltration, infection, or phlebitis. *Frequent assessment allows early detection and prompt treatment of complications.*

- Change intravenous solutions every 24 hours, site dressing every 48 hours, and tubing to the insertion site every 72 hours. Label solution, tubing, and dressing with date and time of change and nurse's initials. *These measures help prevent infection.*

- Thoroughly flush stopcock ports with flush solution after drawing blood samples from the pressure line. *Flushing prevents colonization of bacteria and occlusion of the catheter.*

- Assess the pulse and perfusion distal to the monitoring site. *Frequent assessment is vital to ensure perfusion of the distal extremity.*

- When discontinuing the pressure line, apply manual pressure to the insertion site as soon as the catheter tip is out. Hold pressure for 5 to 15 minutes or until the bleeding stops. *This is particularly important for arterial lines to prevent bleeding and hematoma formation.*

- Secure all connections and stopcocks. *This is done to prevent disconnection of the invasive line and potential hemorrhage.*

- Be sure that electrical equipment is grounded, intact, and operating as expected. *This is important to prevent electrical injury.*

- Loosely restrain the affected extremity if the client is unable to refrain from pulling on the catheter or connections. *Restraints may be necessary to prevent injury from accidental or intentional disconnection or discontinuation of invasive lines (i.e., if the client has dementia or is agitated or delusional).*

- Keep tubing free of kinks and tension. *This prevents the catheter from becoming clotted or inadvertently dislodged.*

Intra-Arterial Pressure Monitoring A common procedure in intensive and coronary care units is intra-arterial pressure monitoring. An indwelling arterial line, commonly called an *art line* or an *A line*, allows direct and continuous monitoring of systolic, diastolic, and mean arterial blood pressure and provides easy access for arterial blood sampling. Arterial lines are used to assess blood volume, monitor the effects of vasoactive drugs, and to obtain frequent arterial blood gas determinations. Because the invasive catheter is inserted directly into the artery, it offers immediate access for blood gas measurements and serum laboratory testing.

Arterial blood pressure is produced by the delivery of blood from the left ventricle to the systemic circulation. The mean arterial pressure (MAP) is determined by the amount of blood flow through the vessels and the elastic-

---

Potential Complications of Central Catheters

■ ■ ■

- Bleeding
- Hematoma
- Pneumothorax
- Hemothorax
- Arterial puncture
- Dysrhythmias
- Venospasm
- Infection
- Air embolism
- Thromboembolism
- Brachial nerve injury
- Thoracic duct injury

---

ity of those vessels (MAP = CO × SVR). It is a valuable parameter because it depicts the *driving pressure,* or *perfusion pressure,* an indicator of tissue perfusion. Mean arterial pressures of 70 to 90 mm Hg are desirable. Perfusion to vital organs is severely jeopardized at MAPs of 50 or less; MAPs greater than 105 mm Hg may indicate hypertension or a vasoconstrictive state.

Central Venous Pressure Monitoring Central venous pressure (CVP) is a reflection of blood volume and venous return. CVP also reflects right heart filling pressures and is elevated in right-sided heart failure. CVP is monitored for clients who require accurate monitoring of fluid volume status. To measure CVP, an intravenous catheter is inserted in the internal jugular or subclavian vein. The distal tip of the catheter is positioned in the superior vena cava just above the right atrium. CVP may be measured in either centimeters of water (cm H_2O) or in millimeters of mercury (mm Hg). A water manometer is a plastic or glass tube with calibrated markings attached between a central catheter and the intravenous fluid bag. Pressure in the client's venous system causes fluid in the manometer to rise or fall. The CVP is recorded by noting the fluid level in the manometer. If the central line is connected to a pressure transducer, venous pressure is converted to an electrical signal and the waveform displayed on the monitor. Pressure readings are displayed digitally in mm Hg.

The normal range for CVP is 2 to 8 cm H_2O or 2 to 6 mm Hg, but CVP varies in individual clients. Hypovolemia and shock decrease the CVP; fluid overload, vasoconstrictive states, and cardiac tamponade increase CVP. Clients with significant hemodynamic instability and who need acccurate assessment of left ventricular function typically require a pulmonary artery catheter.

Pulmonary Artery Pressure Monitoring The pulmonary artery (PA) catheter is a flow-directed, balloon-tipped catheter first used in the early 1970s. PA catheters are often called *Swan-Ganz catheters,* after the physicians

who developed them. The PA catheter is used to evaluate left ventricular performance and overall cardiac function. The PA catheter is inserted into a central vein, usually the internal jugular or subclavian vein, and threaded into the right atrium. A small balloon at the tip of the catheter allows the catheter to be drawn into the right ventricle and from there into the pulmonary artery. The inflated balloon carries the catheter forward until the balloon wedges in a small branch of pulmonary vasculature. Once in place, the balloon is deflated, and multiple lumens of the catheter allow measurement of different pressures, including right atrial pressure, pulmonary artery pressures, and pulmonary wedge pressures. The normal PA pressure is around 25/10 mm Hg; normal mean pulmonary artery pressure is about 15 mm Hg. Pulmonary artery pressure is increased in left-sided heart failure.

Inflation of the balloon effectively blocks pressure from behind the balloon and allows measurement of pressures generated by the left ventricle. This is known as pulmonary artery wedge pressure (PAWP or PWP) and is used to assess left ventricular function. Cardiac output can also be measured with the PA catheter using a technique called *thermodilution.* Cardiac output and the *cardiac index* (cardiac output adjusted for body size), are used to assess the heart's ability to meet the body's oxygen demands.

Pharmacology

Clients with CHF typically receive multiple medications to reduce cardiac work and improve cardiac function. The main drug classes used to treat CHF are the angiotensin-converting enzyme (ACE) inhibitors, diuretics, inotropic medications (including the digitalis glycosides, sympathomimetic agents, and phosphodiesteras inhibitors), direct vasodilators, beta-blockers, and other antidysrhythmic drugs. Beta-blockers and other antidysrhythmic drugs are discussed in the box on page 1036. Nursing implications for the other medications are discussed in the pharmacology box on page 1116.

ACE inhibitors and beta-blockers are the newest treatments being evaluated for their efficacy in CHF clients. They interfere with the neurohormonal mechanisms of sympathetic activation and the renin-angiotensin system.

ACE inhibitors interrupt the conversion of angiotensin I to angiotensin II, a powerful vasoconstrictor, by inhibiting the enzyme that mediates the conversion (angiotensin-converting enzyme). Angiotensin II causes intense vasoconstriction, increasing afterload and ventricular wall stress and increasing preload and ventricular dilation. It also stimulates aldosterone and ADH production, causing fluid retention. ACE inhibitors block this renin-angiotensin system activity, decreasing cardiac work and increasing cardiac output. They have been shown to benefit the client in CHF by reducing its progression and the clinical manifestations of heart failure, thus reducing the

Text continues on page 1118

Nursing Implications for Pharmacology: The Client with Congestive Heart Failure

POSITIVE INOTROPIC AGENTS

Digitalis Glycosides

Digoxin (Lanoxin)   Digitoxin (Crystodigin)

Digitalis improves myocardial contractility by interfering with ATPase in the myocardial cell membrane and increasing the amount of calcium available for contraction. The increased force of contraction enables the heart to empty more completely, increasing stroke volume and cardiac output. Improved cardiac output improves renal perfusion, decreasing renin secretion. This results in decreased preload and afterload, reducing cardiac work. Digitalis also exerts electrophysiologic effects on the heart by slowing conduction through the AV node. This decreases the heart rate and reduces oxygen consumption.

Nursing Responsibilities

- Assess the apical pulse before administering digitalis. Withhold the drug if heart rate is below 60 BPM and/or the client has manifestations of decreased cardiac output. Notify physician of this occurrence. Record apical rate on medication sheet for every dose.

- Evaluate ECG for scooped (spoon-shaped) ST segment, AV block, bradycardia, and new-onset dysrhythmias (especially PVCs and atrial tachycardias).

- Assess potassium, magnesium, calcium, and serum digoxin levels before administering the medication. Note that even if the digitalis blood level is in the "normal" range, hypokalemia can precipitate digitalis toxicity.

- Note that clients with renal insufficiency or renal failure should have lower doses of digitalis. Older adults also require lower doses of digoxin because they have less muscle mass and decreased renal function.

- Be alert to signs and symptoms of digitalis toxicity: anorexia, nausea, vomiting, abdominal pain, weakness, vision changes (diplopia, blurred vision, yellow-green or white halos seen around objects), and new-onset dysrhythmias.

- Be prepared to administer Digoxin Immune Fab (Digibind) for digoxin toxicity.

- Instruct the client in the proper technique for monitoring pulse rate.

Client and Family Teaching

- Take your pulse rate before each dose of digoxin. Do not take the digoxin if your pulse rate is below 60 or if you are experiencing any of the following: weakness, fatigue, light-headedness, dizziness, shortness of breath, or chest pain. Notify your physician immediately.

- Notify the physician if you are experiencing any of the following manifestations of digitalis toxicity: palpitations, weakness, loss of appetite, nausea, vomiting, abdominal pain, blurred or colored vision, double vision.

- Avoid the use of antacids and laxatives; they decrease the absorption of digoxin.

- Notify your physician immediately if you experience any of the following manifestations of potassium deficiency: weakness, lethargy, thirst, depression, muscle cramps, or vomiting.

- Incorporate foods high in potassium into your diet: fresh orange or tomato juice, bananas, raisins, dates, figs, prunes, apricots, spinach, cauliflower, and potatoes.

Sympathomimetic Agents

Dopamine (Inotropin)   Dobutamine (Dobutrex)

Sympathomimetic agents directly stimulate the heart to improve the force of contraction. Dobutamine is preferred in the management of heart failure because it does not increase the heart rate as much as dopamine, and it also has a mild vasodilatory effect. These drugs are given as an intravenous infusion and may be titrated to obtain their maximal effects.

Phosphodiesterase Inhibitors

Amrinone (Inocor)   Milrinone (Primacor)

Phosphodiesterase inhibitors are used in the treatment of acute heart failure to increase myocardial contractility and cause vasodilation. The net effects are an increase in cardiac output and a decrease in afterload.

Nursing Responsibilities

- Use an infusion pump to administer these agents, and monitor hemodynamic parameters carefully.

- These drugs are frequently adjusted to maintain an effective blood pressure and heart rate. Avoid discontinuing these agents abruptly.

Pharmacology: The Client with Congestive Heart Failure (continued)

- Change solutions and tubing every 24 hours.

- Amrinone is given in an intravenous push bolus over 2 to 3 minutes, followed by an infusion of 5 to 10 μg/kg/min.

- Amrinone may be infused full strength or diluted in a solution of normal saline or half-strength saline. Do not mix this drug with dextrose solutions. After dilution, amrinone may be piggybacked into a line containing a dextrose solution.

- Monitor hepatic function and platelet counts; amrinone may cause hepatotoxicity and thrombocytopenia.

Client and Family Teaching

- Notify the nursing staff if you experience abdominal pain or notice a skin rash or bruising.

VASODILATORS

Hydralazine (Apresoline)   Prazosin (Minipress)

Phentolamine (Regitine)   Nitroprusside (Nipride)

These vasodilating agents reduce afterload and thus reduce the work of the heart.

ANGIOTENSIN-CONVERTING ENZYME (ACE) INHIBITORS

Enalapril maleate   Lisinopril (Prinivil,
(Vasotec)   Zestril)

Captopril (Capoten)

ACE inhibitors have been shown to prevent acute coronary events and reduce mortality in CHF (Fara, 1992). Vasodilator action occurs when this agent blocks the conversion of angiotensin I to angiotensin II, and the aldosterone formation. The result is decreased cardiac workload and reduced edema and sodium retention. Given in early stages of CHF, ACE inhibitors help to prevent ventricular remodeling and further deterioration of the failing myocardium (Fara, 1992).

Nursing Responsibilities

- When administering these agents intravenously, use an infusion pump, and monitor hemodynamic parameters carefully.

- These drugs are adjusted frequently to maintain an effective blood pressure and heart rate. Avoid discontinuing these agents abruptly.

- Change solutions and tubing every 24 hours.

- Monitor the client's total fluid volume status. Administering vasodilators to a hypovolemic client will result in possibly severe hypotension.

- Protect nitroprusside from light. After the drug has been mixed in solution, cover the IV bag completely with an opaque covering (e.g., foil). Discard the solution and remix a new solution every 24 hours.

- Be alert for signs of nitroprusside toxicity: profound hypotension, reflex tachycardia, cyanide poisoning, metabolic acidosis, neurologic symptoms, cherry-red skin coloration, and increasing blood pressure despite high doses of nitroprusside. Obtain thiocyanate levels for clients on prolonged nitroprusside therapy. If cyanide poisoning occurs, turn off the infusion, administer oxygen, and notify the physician.

- Administer captopril 1 hour before meals.

Client and Family Teaching

- Take your drugs at a consistent time every day to ensure a stable blood level.

- Monitor your blood pressure and weight daily. Home blood pressure monitoring kits are available.

- Do not stop taking your drugs, even if you "feel fine," without consulting your physician. Keep your follow-up medical appointments.

- Avoid making sudden position changes; for example, rise from bed slowly.

- ACE inhibitor therapy: Report any signs of easy bruising and bleeding, sore throat, or fever, weight gain of 2 lb or more per day, edema, dizziness, or skin rash. Immediately report swelling of the face, lips, or eyelids, itching, or breathing problems.

- Avoid taking over-the-counter (OTC) medications, alcohol, and smoking.

DIURETICS

Hydrochlorothiazide   Spironolactone (Aldac-
(Hydrodiuril)   tone)

Chlorothiazide (Diuril)   Triamterene (Dyrenium)

Furosemide (Lasix)   Amiloride (Midamor)

Ethacrynic acid (Edecrin)   Acetazolamide
(Diamox)

Bumetanide (Bumex)

Pharmacology: The Client with Congestive Heart Failure (continued)

Diuretics act on different portions of the kidney tubule to inhibit the reabsorption of sodium and water and promote their excretion. With the exception of the potassium-sparing diuretics—spironolactone, triamterene, and amiloride—diuretics also promote potassium excretion, increasing the risk of hypokalemia.

Nursing Responsibilities

- Obtain baseline assessment data including weight and vital signs for comparison and evaluation of the effects of therapy.
- Monitor total fluid volume status: blood pressure, intake & output, body weight, skin turgor, edema.
- Assess the client for manifestations of volume depletion, particularly with loop diuretics (furosemide, ethacrynic acid, and bumetanide): dizziness, orthostatic hypotension, tachycardia, muscle cramping.
- Obtain and evaluate serum electrolyte levels daily to monitor for hyponatremia, hypokalemia, and hypochloremia. Notify the physician of abnormal values. Replace electrolytes as indicated. Severe depletion requires the use of intravenous replacement therapy. Hyperkalemia is a potential risk with potassium-sparing diuretics. It is treated by discontinuing the diuretic and administering glucose and regular insulin, sodium bicarbonate, or an exchange ion resin (e.g., Kayexalate).
- Assess client for manifestations of CHF.
- Consult the physician if the client is receiving both a potassium-sparing diuretic and potassium supplements.
- Evaluate renal function by assessing urine output, BUN, creatinine, and total protein levels.
- Provide information on foods high in sodium and potassium. Enlist the aid of the dietitian to evaluate the client's dietary patterns and suggest modifications. Provide sodium-restricted diet.
- Administer intravenous furosemide slowly, at a rate no greater than 20 mg/minute. Evaluate client for signs of ototoxicity. Do not administer this drug or ethacrynic acid concurrently with aminoglycoside antibiotics, such as gentamycin, which are also ototoxic.
- Discuss the potential side effects of the specific therapy with the client. Emphasize the importance of taking the medication and keeping follow-up appointments.

Client and Family Teaching

- Report the following signs and symptoms: severe abdominal pain, jaundice, dark urine, abnormal bleeding or bruising, flulike symptoms, signs of hypokalemia (see the section on digoxin), hyponatremia, and dehydration (thirst, salt craving, dizziness, weakness, irregular and rapid pulse) and any other side effects noted with the medication.
- Monitor your blood pressure, pulse, and weight daily. Report changes in your weight of 2 lb or more per day.
- Completely dissolve potassium supplements in water or juice before taking.
- Avoid making sudden position changes. You may experience dizziness, light-headedness, or feelings of faintness.
- Drink at least 6 to 8 glasses of water per day.
- Take your diuretic at times that will be the least disruptive to your life-style. Take your medications with meals to decrease gastrointestinal symptoms.
- Avoid the use of antacids and laxatives.
- Unless you are taking a potassium-sparing diuretic, integrate foods rich in potassium into your diet (see section on digoxin). Limit the use of sodium.

number and frequency of hospital admissions, decreasing mortality rates, and preventing cardiac complications (Eichhorn, 1992; Poole-Wilson, 1993).

For most symptomatic clients with CHF, ACE inhibitor therapy is combined with diuretic therapy. Diuretics provide prompt relief of symptoms related to fluid retention in CHF. They may, however, cause significant electrolyte imbalances and prompt a neurohormonal response from rapid fluid loss. Clients with severe heart failure are often treated with a loop, or high-ceiling, diuretic such as furosemide (Lasix), bumetanide (Bumex), or ethacrynic acid (Edecrin). These drugs have a rapid onset of action, inhibiting chloride reabsorption in the ascending loop of Henle, resulting in sodium and water excretion. Their major drawback is their efficacy in promoting diuresis; loss of vascular volume can stimulate the SNS. Thiazide diuretics may be used for clients with less severe manifestations of CHF. These agents promote fluid excretion by blocking sodium reabsorption in the terminal loop of Henle and the distal tubule.

Once considered the mainstay of therapy for CHF, the digitalis glycosides are now used more judiciously (Tierney et al., 1994). Digitalis exerts a *positive inotropic effect* on the heart, increasing the strength of myocardial contraction by increasing the intracellular calcium concentrations. Digitalis also decreases SA node automaticity and slows conduction through the AV node, increasing ventricular filling time.

Digitalis has a narrow therapeutic index; in other words, therapeutic levels are very close to toxic levels. Early manifestations of digitalis toxicity include anorexia, nausea and vomiting, headache, alterations in vision, and confusion. A number of cardiac dysrhythmias are also associated with digitalis toxicity, including sinus arrest, supraventricular and ventricular tachycardias, and high levels of AV block. Low serum potassium levels increase the risk of digitalis toxicity, as do low magnesium and high calcium levels. Older adults are at particular risk for digitalis toxicity.

Digitalis levels may be affected by a number of other drugs. Cholestyramine, some broad-spectrum oral antibiotics, antacids, and kaolin-pectin mixtures may interfere with its absorption. Quinidine, verapamil, amiodarone, and propafenone increase serum digitalis levels.

Vasodilators relax the smooth muscle of the blood vessels and dilate them. Arterial dilation reduces peripheral vascular resistance and decreases afterload, reducing myocardial work. Venous dilation causes pooling of blood, reducing preload. Pulmonary vascular relaxation reduces pulmonary capillary pressure, allowing fluid to be reabsorbed from interstitial tissues and the alveoli. In addition to the ACE inhibitors already discussed, vasodilators include the nitrates, hydralazine, and prazosin, an alpha-adrenergic blocker.

Nitrates produce both arterial and venous vasodilation and may be administered either intravenously or orally. Sodium nitroprusside is an intravenous nitrate and is a potent vasodilator that may be used to treat acute heart failure. It can produce excessive hypotension and is often combined with dopamine or dobutamine to manage this effect. Isosorbide or nitroglycerin ointment are nitrates that may be employed for long-term management of the client with CHF.

Oral hydralazine is a potent direct arterial vasodilator that markedly increases cardiac output, but its use is often limited because of its side effects, such as gastrointestinal distress, headaches, tachycardia, low blood pressure, and a drug-induced lupus syndrome (see Chapter 38). Prazosin, an alpha-adrenergic blocker, also produces arterial vasodilation. Its long-term effects on CHF have not yet been determined.

The use of beta-blockers, once contraindicated in CHF, is still a controversial therapy. They are negative inotropes; that is, they decrease contractile force. Nonetheless, beta-blockers in CHF clients improve cardiac function by inhibiting SNS activity. This circumvents the long-term deleterious effects of sympathetic stimulation (Eichhorn, 1992). Because beta-blockers may actually worsen cardiac failure, they are used in very low doses and with extreme caution. The combination of ACE inhibitors and beta-blockers has been noted to improve client outcomes; the combination of ACE inhibitors and direct vasodilators has been shown to decrease morbidity and mortality (Ho et al., 1993).

Clients with moderate to severe heart failure are likely to develop dysrhythmias. Although PVCs are common and may be frequent in clients with CHF, they are often not associated with an increased risk of ventricular tachycardia and fibrillation. For this reason, and because many antidysrhythmic medications depress left ventricular function, PVCs are frequently left untreated in clients with CHF. Nonsustained ventricular tachycardia is associated with a poor prognosis and may be treated. Amiodarone is the drug of choice.

Diet and Activity

Clients in heart failure are generally put on a diet restricted in sodium to minimize sodium and water retention. An intake of 1.5 to 2 g of sodium per day, a moderate restriction, is recommended. Activity may be restricted to bed rest during acute episodes of heart failure to reduce cardiac workload and allow the heart to recompensate. Prolonged bed rest, however, has not been shown to be beneficial in changing the long-term outcome of CHF (Tierney et al., 1994).

Surgery

In the end stage of chronic heart failure, medical therapy alone is insufficient to manage the disease. Treating the underlying cause of the CHF surgically can be attempted if the cause is related to valvular problems, such as aortic stenosis or mitral regurgitation (discussed later in this chapter). Surgical alternatives that may improve quality of life include two main options: a new therapy called dynamic cardiomyoplasty, which attempts to improve function in the existing heart, and cardiac transplantation. Early reports of the dynamic cardiomyoplasty procedure are encouraging.

Dynamic Cardiomyoplasty *Dynamic cardiomyoplasty* involves wrapping a skeletal muscle graft around the heart to lend support to the failing myocardium (Figure 28–22). The grafted skeletal muscle is stimulated in synchrony with the heart muscle, providing a more forceful contraction and increasing cardiac output. The ultimate purpose of dynamic cardiomyoplasty is to improve the

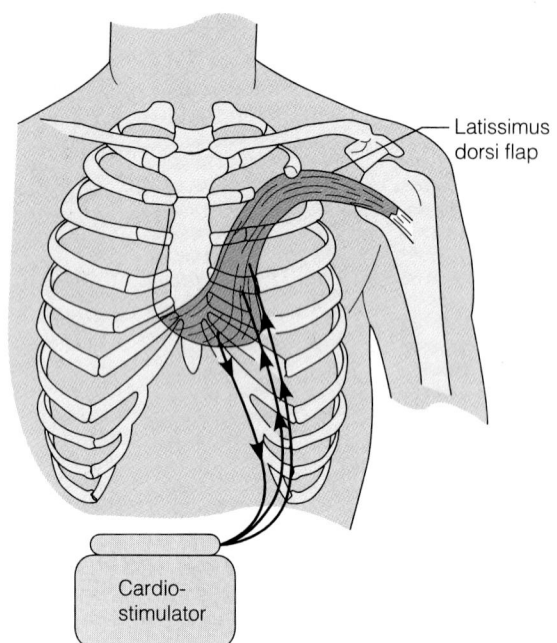

Figure 28–22 Dynamic cardiomyoplasty. The latissimus dorsi muscle is wrapped around the ventricle to provide additional contractile support. *Note.* From "Dynamic Cardiomyoplasty and Its Use in Patients with Chronic Heart Failure" (p. 629) by J. M. Dimengo, 1993, *Critical Care Nursing Clinics of North America, 5*(4).

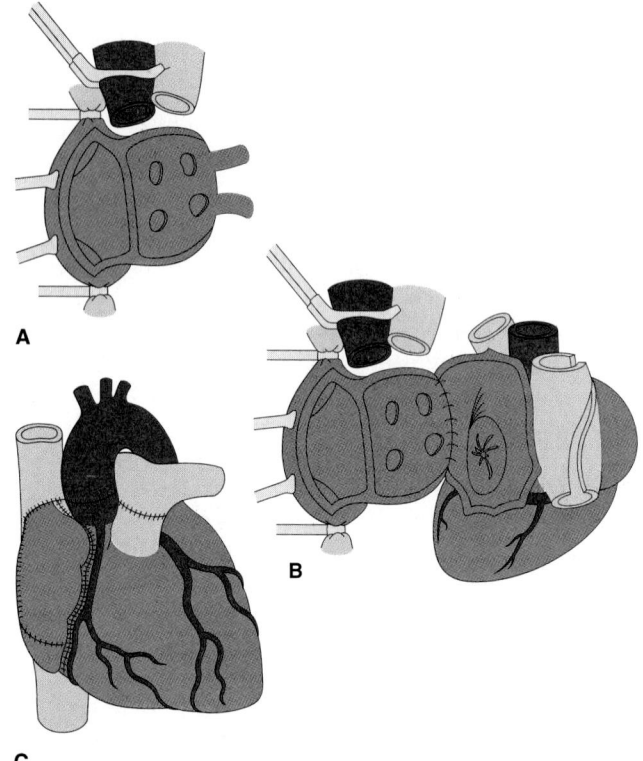

Figure 28–23 Cardiac transplantation. *A,* The heart is removed, leaving the posterior walls of the atria intact. The donor heart is anastomosed to the atria, *B,* and the great vessel, *C.*

client's quality of life by reversing the effects and progression of heart failure (Dimengo, 1993).

Skeletal muscle fibers do not have the innate ability to perform as cardiac fibers and are subject to fatigue. The muscle is conditioned over a period of 10 to 12 weeks using a cardiomyostimulator (an implantable pacemaker device). This process of gradual electrical stimulation is called pulse train stimulation (Dimengo, 1993).

Surgically, two incisions are required to complete this procedure. A thoracotomy incision is made to dissect the latissimus dorsi muscle and bring it through to the mediastinum in place of the second or third rib. A mediastinal incision is made to access and wrap the heart. Cardiostimulator pacing electrodes are inserted into the skeletal muscle, and the sensing electrode is placed on the epicardium. The pericardial sac is reclosed around the skeletal wrap for additional support. The cardiostimulator is then placed in a subcutaneous abdominal pocket beneath the incision. Stimulation of the muscle wrap begins after about 2 weeks to allow for muscle flap recovery and the formation of collateral circulation and muscle-heart adhesions (Dimengo, 1993; Stewart, Hicks, Leflar, Kaempf, Bove, & DiMarzio, 1993).

Clients considered for this treatment are put through a vigorous evaluation that includes physical, emotional,

and psychosocial assessments. The client and family are provided with education and emotional support throughout the perioperative course. Because the transplanted muscle does not provide immediate support to the failing heart, the client requires close monitoring postoperatively. Nursing care is similar to that of clients undergoing open heart surgery (see the box on page 1074).

Cardiac Transplantation   No longer considered experimental surgery, *cardiac transplantation* provides another option for end-stage heart disease (ESHD). There are two types of transplant techniques for ESHD. In *orthotopic* transplantation, the client's diseased heart is removed and replaced with a donor heart (Figure 28–23). *Heterotopic* transplantation, also known as a "piggyback heart," involves leaving the native heart in place, placing the donor heart in the right chest, and connecting the two hearts together. The client then has two functioning hearts, although most of the work is performed by the donor heart. Indications for the heterotopic procedure include pulmonary hypertension, donor-recipient weight mismatch, and the use of suboptimal hearts in emergency situations (Thompson, 1995). Although cardiac transplantation is a good treatment option for many clients with end-stage heart disease, its availability is limited by cost and the availability of donor hearts. Ventricular assist devices are often used as a bridge to transplantation. Transplanted organs typically are obtained from young accident victims with no evidence of cardiac trauma.

Nursing care of the heart transplant client is similar to the care of any cardiac surgery client (see the earlier section of this chapter on cardiac surgery). Infection and rejection are major postoperative concerns. These are the chief causes of mortality in transplant clients (Gamberg & Walton, 1990). Immunosuppressive therapy is necessary to prevent rejection of the transplanted organ, even when the tissue match is good (see Chapter 8). Although immunosuppressive medications help prevent organ rejection, they also leave the client with impaired defenses against infection. The donor heart is also denervated during the transplant procedure. Lack of innervation by the autonomic nervous system affects the client's response to position changes, stress, exercise, and certain drugs.

Nursing Care

CHF impacts the client's quality of life, interfering with such day-to-day activities as self-care and role performance. Reducing the oxygen demand of the heart is a major nursing care goal. This includes providing both physical and psychologic rest, as well as administering and monitoring multiple drugs prescribed to reduce cardiac work, improve contractility, and manage symptoms. Caring for the client after any needed surgical correction of the underlying cause of CHF is outlined in the section on care of the cardiac surgery client.

Decreased Cardiac Output

As the heart fails as a pump, stroke volume and tissue perfusion decrease.

Selected nursing interventions with rationales follow:

- Monitor and record vital signs as indicated. *Decreased cardiac output stimulates the SNS to increase the heart rate in an attempt to restore CO. Tachycardia at rest is common. Diastolic blood pressure may initially be elevated because of vasoconstriction; in late stages, compensatory mechanisms fail, and BP falls.*

- Auscultate heart and breath sounds regularly. S_1 and S_2 *may be diminished if cardiac function is poor. A ventricular gallop* (S_3) *is an early sign of CHF; atrial gallop* (S_4) *may also be present. Crackles are often heard in the lung bases in CHF; increasing crackles, dyspnea, and shortness of breath are indicative of worsening failure.*

- Note and report manifestations of decreased cardiac output: changes in mentation; decreased urine output; cool, clammy skin; diminished pulses; pale or cyanotic coloring; dysrhythmias. *These are manifestations of decreased tissue perfusion to organ systems.*

- Administer supplemental oxygen as needed. *This improves oxygenation of the blood, decreasing the effects of hypoxia and ischemia.*

- Administer prescribed medications as ordered. *Pharmacologic preparations are used to decrease the cardiac workload and increase the effectiveness of contractions.*

- Encourage the client to rest, explaining the rationale for bed rest. Keep the head of the bed elevated to reduce the work of breathing. Provide a bedside commode, and assist the client with personal needs. Instruct client to avoid the Valsalva maneuver: Avoid straining, use the bedside commode rather than the bedpan, and avoid isometric exercises. *These measures reduce cardiac workload.*

- Promote psychologic rest and decrease anxiety. Maintain a quiet environment, allow the client to express fears and feelings, and explain the reasons for medical and nursing management. *These measures also decrease oxygen consumption and improve cardiac function.*

Fluid Volume Excess

As cardiac output falls, normal compensatory mechanisms cause salt and water retention, increasing blood volume. This increased fluid volume places additional stress on the already failing ventricles, making them work harder to move the fluid load.

Selected nursing interventions with rationales follow:

- Assess the client's respiratory status, including respiratory rate, effort, any shortness of breath, dyspnea, cough, orthopnea, or paroxysmal nocturnal dyspnea (PND). Auscultate lung sounds at least every 4 hours. *Declining respiratory status is an indicator of worsening left heart failure. Notify the physician of significant changes in condition.*

- Immediately notify the physician if the client develops air hunger, an overwhelming sense of impending doom or panic, tachypnea, the need to sit straight up in bed, or a cough productive of large amounts of pink, frothy sputum. *Acute pulmonary edema, a medical emergency, can develop rapidly, necessitating immediate intervention to preserve life.*

- Monitor and record intake and output. Notify the physician if urine output drops to less than 30 mL/h. *It is important to monitor fluid status carefully during treatment of CHF. Diuretics may reduce circulating volume, producing hypovolemia despite persistent peripheral edema. A drop in urinary output may indicate significantly reduced cardiac output and renal ischemia.*

- Weigh the client daily. *Weight provides an objective measure of fluid status; 1 liter of fluid is equal to 1 lb of weight.*

- Record abdominal girth every shift. Note complaints of a loss of appetite, abdominal discomfort, or nausea.

Venous congestion leads to ascites and may effect gastrointestinal function.

■ Maintain bed rest, with the head of bed elevated to 45 degrees. *Elevating the head of the bed reduces venous return to the heart, decreasing its work. It also improves lung expansion.*

■ Assess for other manifestations of fluid volume excess, including jugular venous distention, peripheral edema (with or without pitting), and cardiac rhythm changes. *These may be signs of progressive worsening of the client's condition.*

■ Monitor and record hemodynamic parameters. Note changes in pulmonary artery pressures and systemic vascular resistance and decreases in cardiac output and BP. *Hemodynamic measurements provide a means to monitor the client's condition and response to treatment closely.*

■ Administer diuretics and other medications as ordered. *Diuretics increase sodium and water excretion.*

■ Restrict fluids as ordered. Encourage the client to participate in choosing the time and type of fluid consumed, scheduling the majority of intake during the morning and afternoon. Offer ice chips and frequent mouth care; provide hard candies if allowed. *Involving the client increases his or her sense of control. Ice chips, hard candies, and mouth care relieve dry mouth and thirst and promote comfort.*

Activity Intolerance

Clients with CHF have little or no cardiac reserve to meet increased oxygen demands. As the disease progresses and cardiac function becomes more compromised, activity intolerance occurs with lower levels of exertion. The client's low cardiac output and inability to participate in activities may hinder self-care practices.

Selected nursing interventions with rationales follow:

■ Assess vital signs and cardiac rhythm before and after the client engages in activity. Tachycardia, dysrhythmias, changes in blood pressure, diaphoresis, pallor, or complaints of increasing dyspnea, chest pain, excessive fatigue, or palpitations indicate activity intolerance; teach the client to rest if these manifestations are noted. *The failing heart is unable to increase cardiac output to meet the increase in oxygen demands that occurs with activity. Assessing the client's response to activities provides a measure of cardiac function.*

■ Assess the client for signs of decreasing activity tolerance. *This may signal decreasing cardiac function rather than overexertion.*

■ Organize nursing care to allow for rest periods. *Periods of activity should be grouped together as much as possible to allow the client adequate time to "recharge."*

■ Assist client as needed with self-care activities. Encourage the client to perform ADLs independently within prescribed limits. *Assisting the client with ADLs helps meet the client's care needs while reducing the client's cardiac workload. Involving the client promotes a sense of control and reduces helplessness.*

■ Plan and implement progressive activity plan. Employ passive and active ROM exercises as appropriate. Consult with physical therapist on activity plan. *Progressive activity slowly increases the client's exercise capacity by strengthening and improving cardiac function without strain. Progressive activity also helps prevent skeletal muscle atrophy. ROM exercises prevent complications of immobility in bedridden or severely compromised clients.*

■ Provide written and verbal information about activity after discharge. *Written information provides the client with a reference for important information. Verbal information allows clarification and validation of the material.*

Knowledge Deficit: Low-Sodium Diet

Diet is an important part of care of the client with CHF to maintain optimal function and manage fluid retention.

Selected nursing interventions and rationales follow:

■ Teach the client the rationale for sodium restrictions. *Understanding fosters compliance with the prescribed diet.*

■ Consult with dietitian to plan and teach the client about a low-sodium and, if necessary for weight control, low-kcal diet. Provide a list of high-sodium, high-fat, high-cholesterol foods to avoid. Provide materials from the American Heart Association. *Dietary planning and teaching increases the client's sense of control and participation in management of the disease. Food lists are beneficial memory aids.*

■ Teach the client how to read food labels for nutrition information. *Many processed foods contain "hidden" sodium, which the client can identify by carefully reading labels.*

■ Assist the client to construct a 2-day meal plan choosing foods low in sodium. *This allows the nurse to assess the client's learning, clarify misunderstandings, and provide reinforcement.*

■ Encourage the client to eat small, frequent meals rather than three heavy meals per day. *Small, frequent meals provide continuing energy resources and decrease the work required to digest a large meal.*

Other Nursing Diagnoses

Other nursing diagnoses that may be appropriate for the CHF client follow:

■ *Risk for Impaired Gas Exchange* related to alveolar fluid congestion

■ *Risk for Impaired Skin Integrity* related to edema

Activity Guidelines for the CHF Client After Discharge
■ ■ ■

- Perform as many activities as independently as you can.
- Space your meals and activities.
  a. Eat six small meals a day.
  b. Allow time during the day for periods of rest and relaxation.
- Perform all activities at a comfortable pace.
  a. If you get tired during any activity, stop what you are doing and rest for 15 minutes.
  b. Resume activity only if you feel up to it.
- Stop any activity that causes you to have chest pain, shortness of breath, dizziness, feelings of faintness, excessive weakness, or sweating. Rest. Notify your physician if your activity tolerance changes and if symptoms continue after you rest.
- Avoid straining. Do not lift heavy objects. Eat a high-fiber diet and drink plenty of water to prevent constipation. Use laxatives or stool softeners, as approved by your physician, to avoid constipation and straining during bowel movements.
- Begin a graded exercise program. Walking is good exercise that does not require any special equip-

ment (except a good pair of walking shoes). Plan to walk twice a day at a comfortable, slow pace for the first couple of weeks at home, and then gradually increase the distance and pace you walk. Enjoy the weather, scenery, and your significant other. Below is a suggested schedule—but progress at your own speed. Take your time. Aim for walking at least 3 times per week (every other day).

Week 1	200 to 400 ft (1/4 mile)	Twice a day, slow leisurely pace
Week 2	1/4 mile	15 min, minimum of 3 times per week
Weeks 2 to 3	1/2 mile	30 min, minimum of 3 times per week
Weeks 3 to 4	1 mile	30 min, minimum of 3 times per week
Weeks 4 to 5	1 1/2 mile	30 min, minimum of 3 times per week
Weeks 5 to 6	2 miles	40 min, minimum of 3 times per week

- *Altered Role Performance* related to change in health status
- *Risk for Injury* (thromboembolism) related to blood pooling in the atria secondary to atrial fibrillation
- *Altered Tissue Perfusion* related to an ineffective cardiac pump
- *Knowledge Deficit* regarding pharmacologic therapy

Client and Family Teaching

There are many opportunities to educate the client and family affected by CHF. To enlist the client as an active participant in rehabilitation, be sure to provide explanations regarding the disease process and the effects on the client's life. These will help the client to understand the rationale for the treatments. It is very important that the client be able to list the warning signals of cardiac decompensation that require physician notification. The CHF client is on a multiple drug regimen and should be monitored closely for adverse effects. Stress the importance of the medications in managing CHF. Providing information regarding each specific medication is vital to encourage compliance.

Life-style changes are important, although they may be the most difficult to achieve. Diet therapy is an essential component of teaching. Sodium and fluid intake may be restricted to reduce fluid buildup. Give the client practical suggestions for reducing salt intake. The American Heart Association has written materials and recipes that may make the adjustment to a low-sodium diet easier to tolerate for most clients.

Encourage exercise within prescribed limits to strengthen the heart muscle and improve aerobic capacity (Ho et al., 1993). Instruct the client to keep regular follow-up appointments with the cardiologist to monitor progression of the disease and the effects of therapy. The accompanying box provides activity guidelines for the CHF client after discharge.

Discharge considerations include the possible need for assistance at home with shopping, transportation, personal needs, and housekeeping responsibilities. Scheduled visits with a home health nurse may be beneficial. Referrals to community agencies, such as local cardiac rehabilitation programs, heart support groups, or the AHA, can provide the client with additional materials and psychosocial support.

Applying the Nursing Process

Case Study of a Client with Congestive Heart Failure: Arthur Jackson

One year ago, Arthur Jackson, a 67-year-old retired construction worker, suffered an anterior wall MI and underwent subsequent coronary artery bypass surgery. On discharge, he was started on a drug therapy regimen that consisted of digoxin, furosemide, coumadin, and a potassium chloride supplement. He has now been admitted to the medical intensive care unit (MICU) after complaining of severe shortness of breath, hemoptysis, and loss of appetite for one week. He is diagnosed with CHF.

Assessment

When Mr. Jackson is settled into his room in the MICU, his nurse, Myumi Takashi, notices that he prefers to sit in the bedside recliner in high Fowler's position. He states, "Lately, this is the only way I feel fairly comfortable." Mr. Jackson states that he has not been able to work in his garden without getting short of breath. He also complains of his shoes and belt being too tight.

When Ms. Takashi questions him about his medical regimen, Mr. Jackson insists that he takes his medications regularly. He states that he normally works in his garden for light exercise. In his diet history, Mr. Jackson notes a fondness for bacon and Chinese food and sheepishly admits to snacking between meals "even though I need to lose weight."

Ms. Takashi obtains vital signs as follows: BP, 95/72 mm Hg; HR, 124 and irregular; R, 28 and labored; T, 97.5 F (36.5 C). She connects Mr. Jackson to the cardiac monitor, noting that he is in atrial fibrillation. An S_3 is noted on auscultation of the heart, and the cardiac impulse is to the left of the midclavicular line. Auscultation of the chest reveals crackles and diminished breath sounds in the bases of both lungs. Mr. Jackson also has significant jugular venous distention, 3+ pitting edema of his ankles and feet, and abdominal distention. His liver size is within normal limits on percussion. His skin is cool and diaphoretic. The chest X-ray shows cardiomegaly and pulmonary infiltrates.

Diagnosis

Ms. Takashi identifies the following nursing diagnoses for Mr. Jackson:

- *Fluid Volume Excess* related to impaired cardiac pump and salt and water retention
- *Activity Intolerance* related to imbalance between oxygen supply and demand
- *Risk for Altered Tissue Perfusion: Cerebral* related to atrial fibrillation and possible thrombus formation
- *Knowledge Deficit* regarding diet and fluid restrictions

Expected Outcomes

The expected outcomes specify that Mr. Jackson will

- Demonstrate a loss of excess fluid by weight loss and decreases in edema, jugular venous distention, and abdominal distention.
- Achieve improved activity tolerance.
- Acknowledge the risk of developing emboli and verbalize the precautions that must be taken to prevent it.
- Verbalize understanding of diet and fluid restrictions.

Planning and Implementation

Ms. Takashi plans and implements the following selected nursing interventions for Mr. Jackson:

- Monitor vital signs and hemodynamic status hourly. Administer and monitor the effects of prescribed diuretics and vasodilators.
- Weigh the client daily. Record strict intake and output.
- Enforce fluid restriction of 1500 mL over 24 hours, allowing 600 mL during the day, 600 mL during the evening, and 300 mL at night.
- Document skin assessment every shift. Note and record amount and location of peripheral edema.
- Auscultate breath and heart sounds every 4 hours and as necessary.
- Administer oxygen per nasal cannula at 2 L/min. Apply pulse oximeter and monitor continuously. Notify physician for pulse oximetry readings below 94%.
- Keep the head of the bed in high-Fowler's position to maintain client's comfort.
- Obtain laboratory work as ordered. Notify the physician of significant changes in values.
- Administer medications as ordered. Notify the physician and withhold digoxin if manifestations of digitalis toxicity or cardiac instability are noted.
- Teach Mr. Jackson about all medications and how to take and record his pulse daily. Provide information about anticoagulant therapy and signs of bleeding.
- Design an activity plan with Mr. Jackson that incorporates preferred activities and scheduled rest periods throughout the day.
- Instruct Mr. Jackson on a sodium-restricted diet. Allow him to make choices for meals within allowed limits.
- Consult dietitian to assist Mr. and Mrs. Jackson in planning a low-sodium diet.

Evaluation

Mr. Jackson remains in the MICU 3 days, after which he is transferred to the floor. He has lost 8 pounds during his MICU stay and states that it is much easier to breathe and that his shoes fit better. At night, he is able to sleep in bed with only 1 pillow under his head. His peripheral edema also has resolved. Mr. Jackson reports an increase in appetite, although he verbalizes the need to control his intake of sodium, sugar, and fats. Mr. and Mrs. Jackson have met with the dietitian, who has helped them develop a realistic eating plan to limit those foods. The dietitian has also provided a list of foods that contain large amounts of sodium. Mr. Jackson is relieved to know that he can still enjoy Chinese food that is prepared without monosodium glutamate (MSG) or added salt. Ms. Takashi and the physical therapist have designed a progressive activity plan with Mr. Jackson for both in-hospital and at-home activity. Mr. Jackson's atrial fibrillation is a chronic condition. His knowledge of digoxin and coumadin has been assessed and reinforced. Ms. Takashi confirms that Mr. Jackson knows how to take his pulse correctly and can list signs of digoxin toxicity and excessive bleeding.

Mr. Jackson is discharged 8 days after his admission. Upon follow-up with his cardiologist, Mr. Jackson reports no lingering problems. He has increased his exercise tolerance and states that he and his wife often go for short walks in the neighborhood.

Critical Thinking in the Nursing Process

1. How does Mr. Jackson's age impact decisions about appropriate drug therapy?

2. Mr. Jackson tells you, "Talk to my wife about my medications—she's Tarzan and I'm Jane now." How would you respond?

3. Design an exercise plan for Mr. Jackson to prevent deconditioning and conserve energy.

4. Mr. Jackson tells you, "Sometimes I forget whether I have taken my aspirin, so I'll take another just to be sure. After all, they are only baby aspirin. One or two extra a day shouldn't hurt, right?" What is your response?

5. Mr. Jackson is admitted to the neurologic intermediate care floor 6 months later after suffering a cerebral vascular accident (CVA). What is the probable cause of his stroke?

The Client with Pulmonary Edema

■ ■ ■

Pulmonary edema is an abnormal accumulation of fluid in the interstitial tissue and alveoli of the lung. Pulmonary edema may originate from either cardiac or noncardiac causes. Cardiac causes include myocardial infarction, acute volume overload, and valvular disease. *Cardiogenic pulmonary edema* is a sign of severe cardiac decompensation. Noncardiac causes of pulmonary edema include pri-

---

Clinical Manifestations of Pulmonary Edema

■ ■ ■

Respiratory System

- Tachypnea
- Labored respirations
- Dyspnea
- Orthopnea
- Paroxysmal nocturnal dyspnea
- Cough productive of frothy, pink sputum
- Crackles, wheezes

Cardiovascular System

- Tachycardia
- Hypotension
- Cyanosis
- Cool, clammy skin
- Hypoxemia
- Ventricular gallop

Neurologic Effects

- Restlessness
- Anxiety
- Feeling of impending doom

---

mary pulmonary disorders, such as adult respiratory distress syndrome (ARDS), trauma, sepsis, drug overdose, or neurologic sequelae. The onset of pulmonary edema can be gradual or rapid, progressing to severe respiratory distress. Pulmonary edema is a medical emergency: The client is "drowning" as a result of fluid in the alveolar and pulmonary spaces and must be treated immediately.

Pathophysiology

In cardiogenic pulmonary edema, left ventricular contractility is inadequate to eject all of the blood that enters it; the result is a sharp rise in end-diastolic volume and pressures and pulmonary vascular pressures. Increased hydrostatic pressure in pulmonary capillaries exceeds the osmotic pressure of the blood, allowing fluid to escape. This fluid congests interstitial tissues and enters the alveoli, increasing lung stiffness, impairing lung expansion, and interfering with gas exchange (Porth, 1994).

The client with acute pulmonary edema usually presents with classic manifestations of the disorder (see the accompanying box). Dyspnea and shortness of breath are acute and severe; the client usually remains seated, because the client cannot breathe effectively when lying down. The client is highly anxious. Cyanosis is present, and the skin is cool and clammy. A productive cough with pink, frothy sputum is also present. If cerebral hypoxia occurs, the client may be confused or lethargic. On auscultation of the chest, crackles are heard throughout the lung fields. As the condition worsens, breathing becomes more labored and lung sounds harsher.

As noted earlier, pulmonary edema is a medical emergency. Without rapid and effective intervention, severe tissue hypoxia will lead to organ system failure and death.

Collaborative Care

The primary treatment goals for the client with acute pulmonary edema are to reduce excess fluid, particularly in the pulmonary system, and to improve gas exchange. Placing the client in an upright sitting position with the legs dangling helps reduce venous return by trapping some excess fluid in the lower extremities. This position also facilitates breathing.

Although the presentation of acute pulmonary edema is typically classic, laboratory and diagnostic studies may be done to evaluate its severity, effects, and possible causes. Arterial blood gases are drawn to assess the client's respiratory and acid-base status. Oxygen tension is usually reduced. Carbon dioxide levels may also be lower than normal because of rapid respirations. As the condition progresses, these levels rise, and the client develops respiratory acidosis. A pulse oximeter is placed on the client for continuous monitoring of oxygen saturation levels. The chest X-ray shows pulmonary vascular congestion and alveolar edema. The heart may or may not be enlarged, depending on preexisting heart failure. Hemodynamic monitoring is instituted. In cardiogenic pulmonary edema, the pulmonary artery wedge pressure (PAWP) is elevated, usually over 25 mm Hg (Tierney et al., 1994). Cardiac output may be decreased.

Oxygen therapy is instituted for the client in acute pulmonary edema to maintain the partial pressure of oxygen (PO_2) at greater than 60 mm Hg. A mask is used initially; continuous positive airway pressure (CPAP) may be applied to increase alveolar pressures and gas exchange while decreasing the diffusion of fluid into the alveoli. If this is not effective in maintaining blood oxygen levels, the client may be intubated and placed on a mechanical ventilator (see Chapter 34 for further information about positive-pressure and mechanical ventilation).

Morphine sulfate is a drug of choice for treating acute pulmonary edema. It is initially administered intravenously for optimal effect. Morphine not only relieves anxiety and improves the efficacy of breathing but also is a venous vasodilator. As such, it reduces venous return and lowers left atrial pressure. Although morphine is very effective for clients with cardiogenic pulmonary edema, it should not be used when pulmonary edema is neurologic in origin or narcotic induced.

Potent loop diuretics such as furosemide or bumetanide are administered intravenously to promote rapid diuresis. Furosemide is also a venous dilator, reducing venous return to the heart. Vasodilators such as intravenous nitroprusside or intravenous or sublingual nitroglycerin may be administered to improve cardiac output by reducing afterload. Dopamine or dobutamine may be given to clients with low cardiac output and hypotension. Intravenous aminophylline may be used cautiously to reduce bronchospasm and decrease wheezing.

Nursing Care

Nursing care of the client with acute pulmonary edema focuses on relieving the pulmonary effects of the disorder. Interventions are directed toward improving oxygenation, reducing fluid volume, and providing emotional support.

The nurse often plays a key role in recognizing early manifestations of pulmonary edema and initiating treatment. As with many critical conditions, emergent care is directed toward the ABCs: airway, breathing, and circulation.

Ensure airway patency; assess the effectiveness of respiratory efforts and airway clearance. Encourage the client to cough up secretions; provide nasotracheal suctioning if necessary. Have emergency equipment readily available in case of respiratory arrest. Be prepared to assist with intubation and initiation of mechanical ventilation.

Frequently assess the client's respiratory status, including respiratory rate, effort, use of accessory muscles, sputum characteristics, and skin color. Auscultate the chest for crackles and other adventitious sounds. Place the client in high-Fowler's position with the legs dangling to facilitate breathing and decrease venous return. Administer oxygen as ordered by mask, CPAP mask, or ventilator.

Monitor vital signs and hemodynamic status frequently. Maintain cardiac monitor to detect dysrhythmias. Assess heart sounds for possible S_3, S_4, or murmurs. Initiate an intravenous line for medication administration. Administer morphine, diuretics, vasodilators, bronchodilators, and positive inotropic medications (e.g., digoxin) as ordered. Insert an indwelling catheter for accurate measurement of urinary output; record output hourly. Keep accurate intake and output records. Restrict fluids as ordered. Monitor pulse oximetry, arterial blood gases, and other laboratory studies as indicated.

Be prepared to initiate rotating tourniquets if ordered. Place a blood pressure cuff on each of three extremities, and inflate the cuff to the level of diastolic pressure. This reduces venous return, decreasing pulmonary pressures and improving gas exchange. Every 15 minutes, release one cuff and place it on the uncuffed extremity, using a systematic, clockwise rotation. Do not deflate all the cuffs at the same time.

Finally, provide emotional support for the client and family members. Acute pulmonary edema is a very frightening experience for everyone. Explain all procedures and the reasons to the client and family members. Maintain close contact with the client and family, providing re-assurance that recovery from acute pulmonary edema is often as dramatic as its onset. Answer questions, and provide accurate information in a caring manner.

Consider the following nursing diagnoses for the client with acute pulmonary edema:

- *Ineffective Airway Clearance* related to large amounts of fluid and sputum
- *Ineffective Breathing Pattern* related to anxiety
- *Impaired Gas Exchange* related to alveolar and pulmonary interstitial edema
- *Fluid Volume Excess* related to mechanisms to maintain cardiac output
- *Anxiety* related to difficulty breathing
- *Risk for Inability to Sustain Spontaneous Ventilation* related to increased work of breathing

Client and Family Teaching

During the acute period, teaching of the client and the client's family focuses on care measures being performed and their purpose. Keep information brief and to the point. Use short sentences and a reassuring tone to decrease anxiety.

Once the acute episode of pulmonary edema has resolved, teaching is directed toward its underlying cause and prevention of future episodes. If pulmonary edema followed an acute MI, include information to be provided to the client following an MI as well as information appropriate for the client with CHF. Review the client and family teaching sections of these disorders for further information.

▚ ▚ ▚   Disorders of Cardiac Structure   ▚ ▚ ▚

The Client with Valvular Heart Disease

▪ ▪ ▪

Proper functioning of the heart valves is necessary to ensure one-way blood flow through the heart and vascular system. **Valvular heart disease** interferes with blood flow to and from the heart. Acquired valvular disorders can result from an acute condition, such as endocarditis or calcium deposition, or from chronic conditions, such as rheumatic heart disease. Rheumatic heart disease is the most common cause of valvular disease, especially in older adults (Angelini, Basso, Grassi, Casarotto, & Thiene, 1994). Valve disorders frequently occur after a myocardial infarction, which can cause torn, ischemic, or nonfunctional valve leaflets (e.g., through damage to papillary muscles). Congenital heart defects may affect the heart valves, often showing no manifestations until adulthood. Changes in the heart that occur with normal aging also may predispose the person to valvular disease.

Pathophysiology

Valvular heart disease occurs as two major types of disorders: **stenosis** and **regurgitation**. Stenosis occurs when valve leaflets fuse together and are unable to open or close fully. The valve opening narrows and becomes rigid. Scarring of the valves from endocarditis or infarction, and calcium deposits can result in stenosis. Stenotic valves impede the forward flow of blood, decreasing cardiac output because of impairment in either ventricular filling or ejec-

tion and stroke volume. Because stenotic valves also do not fully close, some backflow of blood occurs through the narrowed opening when it should be fully closed.

Regurgitant valves (also called *insufficient* or *incompetent* valves) do not close completely. This allows regurgitation, or backflow of blood, through the incompletely closed valve into the area it just left. Regurgitation can result from deformity or erosion of valve cusps caused by the vegetative lesions of bacterial endocarditis, by scarring or tearing from myocardial infarction, or by cardiac dilation. As the heart enlarges, the valve *annulus* (the supporting ring of the valve) is stretched; the valve edges no longer meet each other and therefore no longer close completely.

With valvular disease, hemodynamic changes occur both in front of and behind the affected valve. Blood volume and pressures are reduced in front of the valve, becuase flow is impeded through a stenotic valve and backflow occurs through a regurgitant valve. Behind the diseased valve, by contrast, volumes and pressures are characteristically increased. These hemodynamic changes may result in pulmonary complications or heart failure. Heart muscle remodeling (hypertrophy) may result from higher pressures and volume or from the heart's attempts to maintain cardiac output.

Stenosis increases the work of the cardiac chamber behind the affected valve as the heart attempts to move blood through the narrowed opening. Excess blood volume behind regurgitant valves causes dilation of the chamber. In mitral stenosis, for example, the left atrium hypertrophies to enable it to generate a pressure high

Table 28–10   Characteristics of Heart Murmurs

Murmur	Cardiac Cycle Timing	Auscultation Site	Configuration of Sound	Continuity
Aortic stenosis	Midsystolic	Right sternal border (RSB) 2nd intercostal space (ICS)		Crescendo-decrescendo, continuous
Pulmonary stenosis	Midsystolic	Left sternal boarder (LSB), 2nd to 3rd ICS		Crescendo-decrescendo, continuous
Mitral regurgitation	Systole	Apex		Holosystolic (occurs throughout systole), continuous
Tricuspid regurgitation	Systole	4th ICS, LSB		Holosystolic, continuous
Mitral stenosis	Diastole	Apical		Rumble that increases in sound towards the end, continuous
Tricuspid stenosis	Diastole	Lower LSB		Rumble that increases in sound towards the end, continuous
Aortic regurgitation	Diastole (early)	3rd ICS, LSB		Decrescendo, continuous
Pulmonic regurgitation	Diastole (early)	3rd ICS, LSB		Decrescendo, continuous

enough to open and deliver its volume through the narrowed and rigid mitral valve. Not all of the volume can be delivered before the valve closes; as a result, the "leftover" blood accumulates in the left atrium, and this chamber dilates to accommodate the excess volume.

Eventually, cardiac output falls as the effectiveness of these compensatory mechanisms declines, the normal balance of oxygen supply and demand is upset, and the heart begins to fail. Increases in muscle mass and size increase myocardial oxygen consumption. The heart may enlarge beyond the capacity of its blood supply, causing ischemia and chest pain. Eventually, necrosis and loss of functional muscle occurs. Contractile force decreases, as

does stroke volume and cardiac output. High pressures on the left side of the heart may be reflected backward into the pulmonary system, causing pulmonary edema, pulmonary hypertension, and, eventually, right ventricular failure.

When the blood volume is forced through the narrowed opening of the damaged valve or regurgitated from a higher pressure area through an incompetent valve, a jet stream effect may occur, much like water spurting out of a hose whose opening has been partially occluded. The physical force of this jet stream may damage the endocardium of the receiving chamber and possibly result in infective endocarditis (Kaye, 1994; Trausch, 1988).

The left side of the heart is subjected to higher amounts of hemodynamic stress and is the most frequent site of valve damage. Pulmonary valve disease is the least common of the valvular disorders. Valvular disorders interfere with the smooth flow of blood through the heart. The flow becomes turbulent as blood moves or attempts to move through damaged valves; the result is a murmur, one of the characteristic manifestations of valvular disease. Table 28–10 describes the murmurs associated with various types of valvular disorders.

Mitral Stenosis

Mitral stenosis is a narrowing of the mitral valve that obstructs blood flow from the left atrium into the left ventricle during diastole. Mitral stenosis is usually associated with rheumatic heart disease; although rare, it may also result from congenital anomalies. It is found more frequently in females (66%) than in males (Braunwald, 1994b). Mitral stenosis is the leading cardiac cause of death during pregnancy, with reported mortality rates as high as 5% (Flynn & Quinn, 1994).

In rheumatic heart disease affecting the mitral valve, fibrosis and calcification of the valve leaflets begin during the inflammatory process, causing the leaflets to thicken and narrow. As the valve leaflets adhere to each other, the chordae tendineae also fuse, thicken, and shorten. Valve cusps become stiff, and the orifice narrows. This narrowing of the valve opening obstructs the forward flow of blood from the left atrium into the left ventricle. As calcium is deposited in and on the valve, the leaflets become more rigid and narrow the opening further. Calcium deposition may also lead to thromboemboli.

The narrowed mitral opening forces the left atrium to generate higher pressure to deliver its volume to the left ventricle; to accomplish this task, the left atrium hypertrophies. The left atrium also dilates, because obstructed blood flow causes excess atrial volume. As the resistance to blood flow increases, high atrial pressures are reflected back into the pulmonary circuit, increasing pulmonary pressures (Figure 28–24). Pulmonary hypertension increases the workload of the right ventricle, causing it also to dilate and hypertrophy. Eventually, right-sided heart failure occurs. Because the right ventricle is unable to deliver its total volume to the pulmonary system, filling of the left ventricle—and thus cardiac output—decreases.

The client with mitral stenosis may be asymptomatic or severely impaired. Clinical manifestations depend on the cardiac output and pulmonary vascular pressures. Dyspnea on exertion (DOE) is typically the earliest manifestation. Others include cough, hemoptysis, frequent pulmonary infections such as bronchitis and pneumonia, paroxysmal nocturnal dyspnea, orthopnea, weakness, fatigue, and palpitations. As the degree of stenosis increases, manifestations become more severe. Signs of sys-

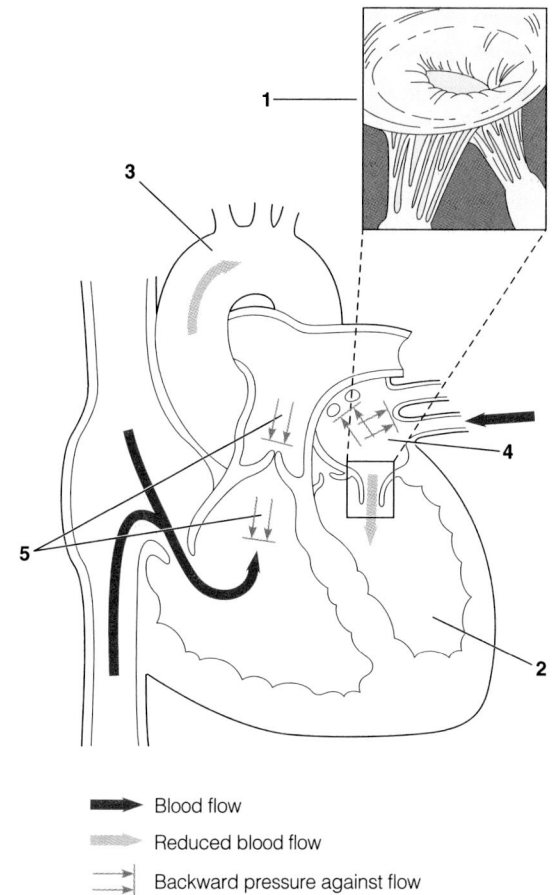

Blood flow

Reduced blood flow

Backward pressure against flow

Figure 28–24 Mitral stenosis. Narrowing of the mitral valve orifice (1), reduces blood volume to left ventricle (2), reducing cardiac output (3). Rising pressure in the left atrium (4) causes left atrial hypertrophy and pulmonary congestion. Pressure reflected backward through pulmonary arteries (5), causes hypertrophy of the right ventricle and right atrium. Right-sided heart failure may result.

temic venous congestion such as jugular venous distension, hepatomegaly, ascites, and peripheral edema result from pulmonary hypertension and right ventricular failure. In severe mitral stenosis, cyanosis of the face and extremities may be noted. Chest pain is rare but may be associated with pulmonary hypertension or coronary atherosclerosis (Braunwald, 1994b).

Atrial dysrhythmias, particularly atrial fibrillation, are commonly associated with mitral stenosis because of chronic atrial distention. The onset of permanent atrial fibrillation often marks the onset of significant manifestations (Braunwald, 1994b). Thrombi may form in the left atrium and subsequently embolize to the brain, coronary arteries, kidney, spleen, and extremities—potentially devastating complications.

Women with mitral stenosis may be asymptomatic until they become pregnant. The heart tries to compensate

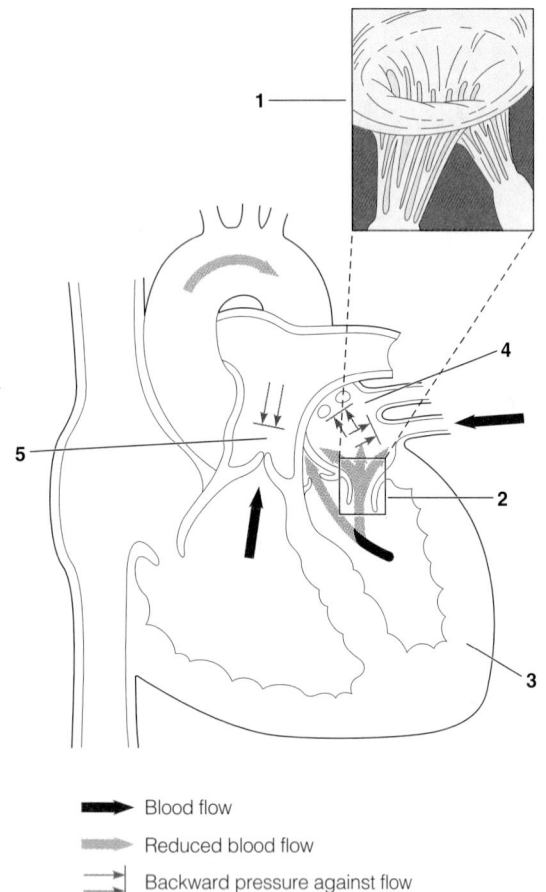

Blood flow

Reduced blood flow

Backward pressure against flow

Figure 28–25   Mitral regurgitation. The mitral valve fails to close (1), causing regurgitation of blood during systole from the left ventricle to the left atrium (2). Cardiac output falls; to compensate, the left ventricle hypertrophies (3). Rising left atrial pressure (4) causes left atrial hypertrophy and pulmonary congestion. Elevated pulmonary artery pressure (5) causes slight enlargement of the right ventricle. Right-sided heart failure may result.

for increased circulating volume (30% more in pregnancy) by increasing cardiac output. However, the extra volume increases left atrial pressures, and tachycardia further reduces stroke volume and cardiac output, increasing pulmonary pressures. Sudden pulmonary edema and heart failure threaten the lives of the mother and fetus. Percutaneous balloon valvuloplasty of the mitral valve during pregnancy has been reported as a successful intervention (Flynn & Quinn, 1994).

On auscultation, a loud S_1, a split S_2, and a mitral opening snap may be heard. The opening snap occurs as the left ventricular pressure falls below that of the atrium. A diastolic murmur characterized as a low-pitched, rumbling, crescendo-decrescendo (heard best with the bell of the stethoscope) in the apical region may be accompanied by a palpable thrill. With advanced mitral stenosis, crackles may be noted in the lungs.

Mitral Regurgitation

Mitral regurgitation or *insufficiency* allows blood to flow back into the left atrium during systole because the valve does not close fully. Rheumatic heart disease is a common cause of mitral regurgitation. Men are more frequently afflicted with this disorder than women. Older women may develop mitral regurgitation because of degenerative calcification of the mitral annulus (Braunwald, 1994b). Any process that dilates the mitral annulus or affects the structures supporting the valve, the papillary muscle or chordae tendineae may cause mitral regurgitation; examples include left ventricular hypertrophy and MI. Other causes include congenital defects and mitral valve prolapse.

In mitral regurgitation, only a portion of the blood is ejected into the systemic circulation during systole, and the rest returned to the left atrium through the deformed valve. This is added to the pulmonary venous return in the left atrium (Figure 28–25). As the left atrium dilates to accommodate this extra volume, the posterior valve leaflet is pulled further away from the valve opening, worsening the defect. The left ventricle also dilates to compensate for increased preload and low cardiac output; this aggravates the problem.

Clients with mitral regurgitation may remain asymptomatic or complain of manifestations such as fatigue, weakness, exertional dyspnea, and orthopnea. In severe or acute mitral regurgitation, manifestations of left-sided heart failure may be present, including pulmonary congestion and edema. With high pulmonary pressures, evidence of right-sided heart failure may be present.

The murmur of mitral regurgitation is usually loud, high-pitched, rumbling, and holosystolic (occurring throughout systole). It is often accompanied by a palpable thrill and is heard most clearly at the cardiac apex. It may be characterized as "cooing" or "sea gull-like" or have a musical quality (Braunwald, 1994b).

Mitral Valve Prolapse

Mitral valve prolapse (MVP) is a form of mitral insufficiency that occurs when one or both mitral valve cusps fall into the left atrium during ventricular systole. Mitral valve prolapse syndrome (MVPS) is commonly found in young women between ages 14 and 30; its incidence declines with age. MVP may be an isolated finding of unknown cause in an otherwise healthy person, or it can result from acute or chronic rheumatic damage, ischemic heart disease, post mitral valvulotomy, or cardiomyopathy (Braunwald, 1994b). Most people with MVP have a benign form of the disorder that does not affect their mortality rates. Approximately 0.01% to 0.02% of people with MVP present with thickened mitral leaflets and a significant risk of possible morbidity and sudden death.

Excess collagen tissue in the valve leaflets and elongated cordae tendineae impair closure of the mitral valve, allowing them to billow into the left atrium during systole. A portion of ventricular blood volume regurgitates into the left atrium (Figure 28–26).

Most clients with MVP are asymptomatic. A midsystolic ejection click or murmur may be the only manifestation. With massive prolapse of the valve or rupture of the chordae tendineae, the client presents with evidence of severe mitral regurgitation and complaints of anginal-type chest pain, palpitations, fatigue, syncope, shortness of breath, headache, exercise intolerance, anxiety, and dizziness (Anderson, 1987; Scordo, 1992; Utz, Whitmire, & Grass, 1993). Sleep disorders and panic attacks have also been linked with MVPS (Anderson, 1987; Scordo, 1992).

In addition to the characteristic midsystolic click, clients with MVP may have a high-pitched late systolic murmur, sometimes described as a "whoop" or "honk," due to the regurgitation of blood through the valve (Braunwald, 1994b).

As with all clients with valvular disease, clients with MVP have an increased risk of bacterial endocarditis, five times that of the general public (Utz et al., 1993). Progressive worsening of the regurgitation can lead to congestive heart failure. Embolic complications from thrombi located on prolapsed valve leaflets may cause transient ischemic attacks (TIA), although the incidence is less than 4% (Anderson, 1987). Sudden cardiac death has also been reported as fatal complication.

Aortic Stenosis

Aortic stenosis obstructs blood flow from the left ventricle into the aorta during systole. Aortic stenosis develops in about 25% of clients suffering from chronic valve problems and is more common in males (80%) than females (Braunwald, 1994b). The cause of aortic stenosis may be unknown, or it may result from a congenital anomaly, rheumatic damage, or degenerative changes. When rheumatic heart disease is the cause, aortic stenosis is often accompanied by a concurrent mitral valve deformity (Braunwald, 1994b). Rheumatic heart disease causes destruction of the leaflets, with fibrosis and calcification causing rigidity and scarring. The older adult may develop idiopathic calcific aortic stenosis from degenerative changes associated with the aging process. The constant "wear and tear" on the valve leaflets, cusps, and annulus subjects the valve to fibrosis and calcification. Idiopathic calcific stenosis generally has mild effects and does not impair cardiac output.

As aortic stenosis progresses, the valve annulus decreases in size, causing the left ventricle to work harder to eject its volume through the narrowed opening into the systemic circulation. As a compensatory mechanism, the ventricles hypertrophy to maintain an adequate cardiac output (Figure 28–27). Left ventricular compliance is also decreased. Because of the extra work, the myocardial oxygen consumption increases. The increased oxygen consumption can precipitate myocardial ischemia. Coro-

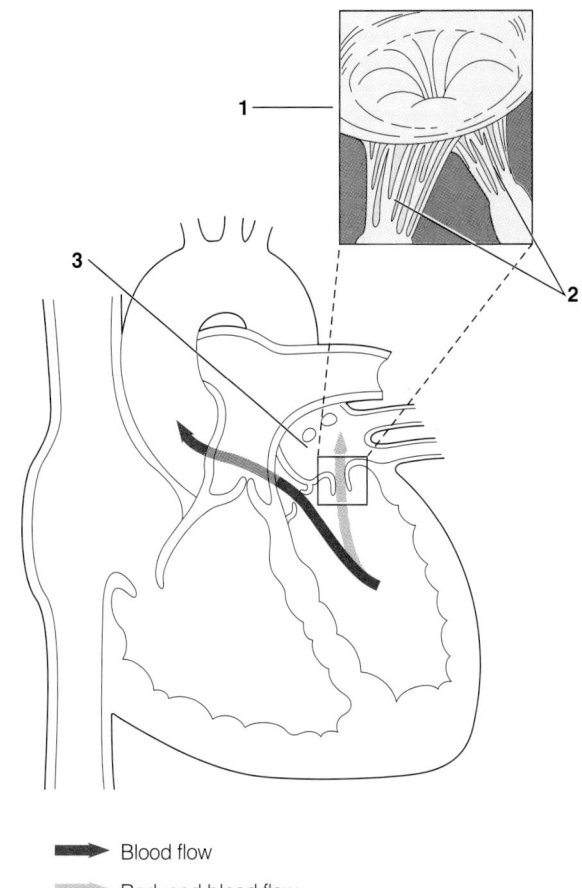

Blood flow

Reduced blood flow

Figure 28–26   Mitral valve prolapse. Excess tissue in the valve leaflets (1) and elongated cordae tendineae (2) impair closure of mitral valve during systole. Some ventricular blood regurgitates into the left atrium (3).

nary blood flow may also be diminished in aortic stenosis. As left ventricular end-diastolic pressure increases because of impaired ventricular output, left atrial pressures increase as well. These pressures are reflected back to the pulmonary vascular system; pulmonary vascular congestion and pulmonary edema may result.

Clients with aortic stenosis may be asymptomatic for many years because the heart is able to compensate. As the disease progresses and compensation fails, usually between age 50 and 70 years, obstructed cardiac output causes manifestations of low cardiac output and high intracardiac pressures. Dyspnea on exertion, angina pectoris, and exertional syncope are the classic manifestations of aortic stenosis. Pulse pressure, an indicator of stroke volume, narrows to 30 mm Hg or less. Hemodynamic monitors show an increase in left atrial pressure and pulmonary artery wedge pressure as well as a decrease in stoke volume and cardiac output.

Auscultation of the heart discloses a harsh systolic murmur in the second intercostal space to the right of the sternum. This crescendo-decrescendo murmur is

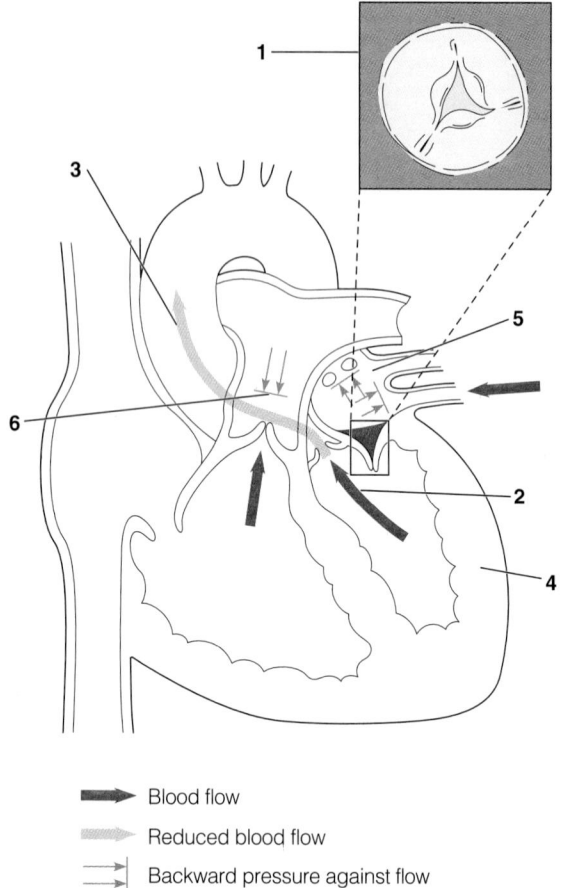

Figure 28–27 Aortic stenosis. Fibrosis and calcification narrow the aortic valve orifice (1), decrease the ejection fraction from left ventricle during systole (2), and decrease cardiac output (3). As a compensatory mechanism, the left ventricle hypertrophies (4). Incomplete emptying of left atrium (5) causes backward pressure through pulmonary veins and pulmonary hypertension. Elevated pulmonary artery pressure (6) causes right ventricular strain.

Blood flow

Reduced blood flow

Backward pressure against flow

produced by the turbulence of the blood entering the aorta through the narrowed aortic valve opening. A palpable thrill is often noted. The murmur may radiate up to the carotid arteries. Ventricular hypertrophy causes the cardiac impulse to be displaced to the left of the chest. As the condition progresses in severity, S_3 and S_4 heart sounds may be noted. An S_3 is a sign of heart failure, and an S_4 is due to a reduction in left ventricular compliance with hypertrophy.

Other manifestations of the progression of aortic stenosis are those of low cardiac output and decreased tissue perfusion, left ventricular failure, and in late stages of the disease, pulmonary hypertension and right ventricular failure. Untreated, symptomatic aortic stenosis has a poor prognosis. Sudden cardiac death occurs in 10% to 20% of clients suffering from this disorder (Braunwald, 1994b).

Aortic Regurgitation

Aortic regurgitation, also called *aortic insufficiency,* allows blood to flow back into the left ventricle from the aorta during diastole. It is found more commonly in males (75%) in its "pure" form; in females, aortic regurgitation is commonly associated with concomitant mitral valve disease. Most cases (67%) of aortic regurgitation result from rheumatic heart disease (Braunwald, 1994b). It may occur secondary to congenital disease, infective endocarditis, blunt chest trauma, aortic aneurysm, syphilis, Marfan syndrome, chronic hypertension, and other disorders.

In aortic regurgitation, the damage from thickened and contracted valve cusps, scarring, fibrosis, and calcification impedes complete closure of the valve. Diseases such as chronic hypertension and aortic aneurysm may dilate and stretch the aortic valve opening, increasing the degree of regurgitation.

With aortic regurgitation, the left ventricle experiences volume overload as blood from the aorta is added to blood received from the atrium during diastole. The ventricle dilates to accommodate the extra volume. Additional stretch of muscle fibers results in a more forceful contraction. This increased contractile strength and decreased afterload from lower blood volumes in the aorta contribute to a high stroke volume (Figure 28–28). The stroke volume in these clients may be twice that of a normal client to meet the demands of the body (LeDoux, 1995). In later stages of the disease, the muscle cells hypertrophy to compensate for increases in cardiac work and afterload, compromising cardiac output and increasing regurgitation. Unlike many other valve disorders, aortic regurgitation shows an advantageous response to exercise. Exercise-induced tachycardia lessens the severity of the regurgitation by decreasing diastolic filling time. Vasodilation from exercising muscle decreases afterload (LeDoux, 1995).

Eventually, high left-ventricular pressures increase the workload of the left atrium and increase left atrial pressure. This pressure is passively transmitted to the pulmonary vessels and eventually to the right side of the heart, causing pulmonary congestion and, possibly, right-sided heart failure. Acute aortic regurgitation from traumatic injury or infective endocarditis causes a rapid decline in hemodynamic status from acute heart failure and pulmonary edema, because compensatory mechanisms of hypertrophy and dilation do not have time to develop.

The client with aortic regurgitation may not exhibit clinical manifestations of the disorder for many years, even with severe disease. People with mild to moderate disease (usually over age 30) may complain of persistent palpitations from the hyperdynamic heartbeat, especially in a recumbent or left-lying position. The heartbeat is visible as a throbbing pulse noted in the arteries of the neck; sometimes the force of the contraction causes a characteristic head bob (Musset's sign) and shakes the whole body (Braunwald, 1994b). Other findings include dizziness, exercise intolerance, and angina.

Fatigue, exertional dyspnea, orthopnea, paroxysmal nocturnal dyspnea, and angina pectoris are common complaints connected with diminished cardiac function. Anginal pain is thought to result from either excessive cardiac workload and decreased coronary perfusion or the hyperdynamic state of the myocardium (Braunwald, 1994b). Unlike CAD, angina often occurs at night and may not respond to conventional therapy.

Hemodynamic changes in aortic regurgitation include high systolic and low diastolic pressures, resulting in a widened pulse pressure. The waveform of the arterial pressure has a rapid upstroke and quickly collapsing downstroke. This is known as a "water-hammer" pulse and results from the force of the rapid and early delivery of the stroke volume into the aorta.

The murmur of aortic regurgitation is heard in diastole as blood flows back into the left ventricle from the aorta. It is described as a "blowing," high-pitched sound heard most clearly at the third left intercostal space. The duration of the murmur is related to the severity of the disease. It may be associated with a diastolic thrill and ventricular heave. Heart failure produces an S_3, and an S_4 will be heard as ventricular compliance diminishes. Because the heart is enlarged, the apical impulse is displaced to the left.

The development of heart failure in a client with aortic regurgitation is an ominous sign. Signs of right-sided heart failure appear in the late stages of this disease. If the disorder is not corrected through surgery, death occurs, on average, within 5 years after the onset of anginal pain and 2 years after manifestations of heart failure become evident (LeDoux, 1995).

Tricuspid Stenosis

Tricuspid stenosis obstructs blood flow from the right atrium to the right ventricle. It affects females more than males and develops primarily as a result of rheumatic damage. Clients with tricuspid stenosis are frequently also affected by mitral stenosis.

In tricuspid stenosis, fibrosed, retracted valve cusps and fused leaflets narrow the valve orifice and prevent complete closure. The stenosed valve opening allows a fraction of blood volume to regurgitate back into the right atrium. The right atrium enlarges in response to the increased pressure needed to force blood through the narrowed valve into the right ventricle. This increased right atrial pressure is reflected backward into the systemic circulation. The amount of blood delivered to the right ventricle is reduced, decreasing the blood volume delivered to the pulmonary system and left heart. Stroke volume, cardiac output, and tissue perfusion are reduced.

Initial manifestations of tricuspid stenosis are usually those of associated mitral stenosis, which commonly pro-

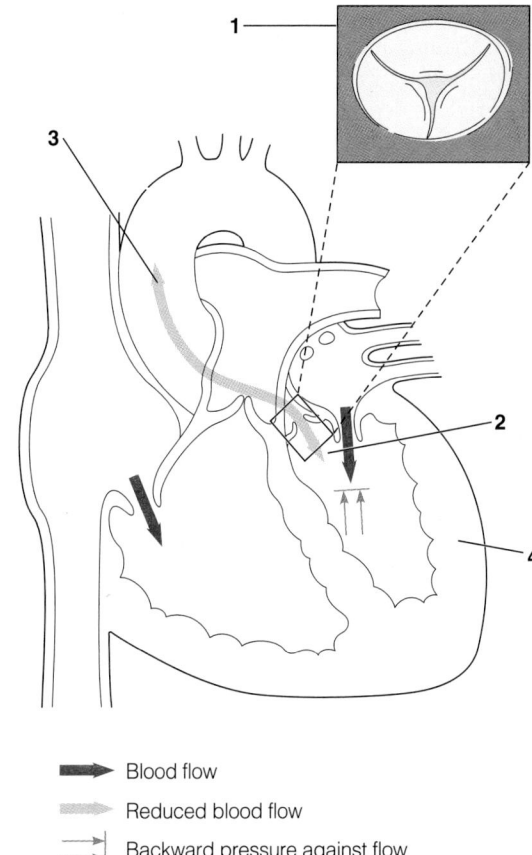

Blood flow
Reduced blood flow
Backward pressure against flow

Figure 28–28   Aortic regurgitation. The cusps of the aortic valve widen and fail to close during diastole (1). Blood regurgitates from the aorta into the left ventricle (2) adding to left ventricular blood volume and decreasing cardiac output (3). The left ventricle eventually dilates and hypertrophies (4) in response to the increase in blood volume and workload.

gresses faster because of higher left-sided pressures. Manifestations of tricuspid stenosis are those of systemic congestion and right-sided heart failure and include increased central venous pressure, jugular venous distention, ascites, hepatomegaly, and peripheral edema. Low cardiac output may initially present as fatigue and weakness. The low-pitched, rumbling diastolic murmur of tricuspid stenosis is most clearly heard in the fourth intercostal space at the left sternal border or over the xiphoid process. The murmur of mitral stenosis may be also audible.

Tricuspid Regurgitation

Tricuspid regurgitation usually occurs secondarily to right ventricular dilation. Stretching distorts the valve and its supporting structures, preventing complete valve closure. Left ventricular failure is the most common cause of right ventricular overload; pulmonary hypertension is another cause. The valve may also be damaged by rheumatic heart disease, infective endocarditis, inferior MI, trauma, or other conditions.

Tricuspid regurgitation allows blood to flow back into the right atrium during systole, increasing right atrial pressures. Increased right atrial pressure causes manifestations of right-sided heart failure, including systemic venous congestion and low cardiac output. Atrial fibrillation due to the atrial distention is common. The retrograde flow of blood over the deformed tricuspid valve causes a high-pitched, blowing systolic murmur heard over the tricuspid or xiphoid area.

Pulmonic Valve Disorders

Pulmonic stenosis obstructs blood flow from the right ventricle into the pulmonary system. Congenital disease is the primary cause, although pulmonic stenosis may be secondary to rheumatic heart disease or cancer. In pulmonic stenosis, the right ventricle hypertrophies to generate the increased pressure needed to pump blood into the pulmonary system. The right atrium also hypertrophies to overcome the high pressures generated in the right ventricle. Right-sided heart failure occurs when the ventricle can no longer generate adequate pressure to force blood past the narrowed valve opening.

Clients with pulmonic stenosis are typically asymptomatic unless the disease is severe. Dyspnea on exertion and fatigue are early signs. As the condition progresses, right-sided heart failure develops, with its associated manifestations of peripheral edema, ascites, hepatomegaly, and increased venous pressures. The turbulence created as blood is forced through the narrowed valve generates a harsh, systolic crescendo-decrescendo murmur heard in the pulmonic area, the second left intercostal space.

Pulmonic regurgitation is more common than pulmonary stenosis. It occurs as a complication of pulmonary hypertension, which stretches and dilates the pulmonary orifice, causing incomplete valve closure. Infective endocarditis, pulmonary artery aneurysm, and syphilis are other causes of acquired pulmonic regurgitation.

Incomplete valve closure allows blood to flow back into the right ventricle during diastole, decreasing blood flow to the pulmonary circuit. The extra blood adds to the end-diastolic volume of the right ventricle. When the ventricle is no longer able to compensate for the increased volume, right-sided heart failure ensues. The murmur of pulmonic regurgitation is a high-pitched, decrescendo, blowing sound heard along the left sternal border during diastole.

Collaborative Care

Valvular disease may remain asymptomatic for many years. The initial indication often is an audible heart murmur that is identified during a routine physical examination. Asymptomatic clients and those with mild manifestations often require no therapy other than close observation for signs of disease progression and prophylactic therapy to prevent infection of the diseased heart. Manifestations of congestive heart failure are treated conservatively, with diet and medications (see the preceding section on heart failure). When medical management no longer controls the client's disease, surgical intervention is considered.

Laboratory and Diagnostic Tests

Many diagnostic tests are used to assist in the diagnosis of valvular disease.

- *Cardiac catheterization* is used to assess contractility and to determine the pressure gradients across the heart valves, in the heart chambers, and in the pulmonary system.
- *Chest X-ray* reveals enlargement of the heart chambers and great vessels and dilation of the pulmonary vasculature. Calcification of the valve leaflets and annular openings may be visible on chest X-ray film.
- *Electrocardiography* is another useful tool that indicates atrial and ventricular hypertrophy, conduction defects, and dysrhythmias associated with valvular disease.
- *Echocardiography* is used routinely to diagnose valvular disease. Thickened valve leaflets, vegetations or growths on valve leaflets, myocardial functional ability, estimations of pressure gradients across the valves and pulmonary artery pressures, and chamber size can be ascertained with this diagnostic tool.

Pharmacology

As noted earlier, clients with symptomatic valvular disease often require therapy to manage the manifestations of heart failure. Digitalis glycosides are employed to increase the force of myocardial contraction and maintain cardiac output. Diuretics and vasodilators (such as ACE inhibitors) are used to reduce preload and afterload.

In clients with valvular disorders, atrial distention often causes atrial fibrillation. Digitalis and class I or III antidysrhythmic agents (such as quinidine, procainamide, or amiodarone) may be used to treat atrial fibrillation or slow the ventricular response rate to this disordered rhythm (see the preceding section on dysrhythmias for further discussion of atrial fibrillation). Anticoagulant therapy is added to prevent clot and embolus formation, a common complication of atrial fibrillation as blood pools in the noncontracting atria. Nursing implications for anticoagulant therapy are found in the box on page 1098.

The client with damaged valves is at increased risk for infective endocarditis because altered blood flow through the heart and valve deformities allows bacterial colonization. Antibiotics are prescribed prophylactically prior to any dental work, invasive procedures, or surgery to minimize the risk of *bacteremia* (bacteria in the blood) and subsequent endocarditis.

Percutaneous Balloon Valvuloplasty

Clients whose stenotic valve disease can no longer be managed with medical therapy may be treated with *percutaneous balloon valvuloplasty*. This nonsurgical invasive technique may be indicated for clients who refuse surgery or for older adults at high risk for surgical complications. It is also used as a "bridge to surgery" for clients with severe compromise of the left heart (Braunwald, 1994b). The procedure is performed in the cardiac catheterization laboratory. A balloon catheter similar to that used in angioplasty procedures (PTCA) is inserted into the femoral vein or artery. With guidance provided by a fluoroscope, the catheter is advanced to the stenotic mitral, aortic, or pulmonic valve. The catheter is positioned with the balloon straddling the stenotic valve. The balloon is then inflated for approximately 90 seconds to divide the fused leaflets and enlarge the valve orifice (Figure 28–29). Although the success rate of this procedure is high, the rate of restenosis is unknown at this time. Complications following balloon valvuloplasty include systemic embolization (1%) and perforation of the myocardium (2%) (Braunwald, 1994b). Nursing care of the client with a balloon valvuloplasty is similar to that of the client following PTCA (see the box on page 1070).

Surgery

Surgery to repair or replace the diseased valve provides definitive treatment for valvular disease. The goal of surgery is to restore normal valve function, alleviate the clinical manifestations, and prevent complications and death. Ideally, diseased valves are repaired or replaced before cardiac and pulmonary functions have been severely compromised. Repair of the diseased valve is the preferred option because its incidence of surgical mortality and the risk of complications are lower than those of valve replacement.

Reconstructive Surgery   Several different reconstructive procedures are available to repair diseased valves:

- *Open commissurotomy,* surgical division of fused valve leaflets, is performed to open stenotic valves. Fused commissures (junctions between valve leaflets or cusps) are incised, and localized calcium deposits are debrided if necessary (Way, 1994).

- *Valvuloplasty* is a general term for reconstruction or repair of a heart valve. Methods include "patching" the perforated portion of the leaflet, resecting excess tissue, debriding vegetations or calcification, and other techniques. Valvuloplasty may be employed for regurgitant mitral and tricuspid valves, mitral valve prolapse, and aortic stenosis (with or without commissurotomy).

- *Annuloplasty* is the repair of a narrowed or an enlarged or dilated valve annulus, the supporting ring of the

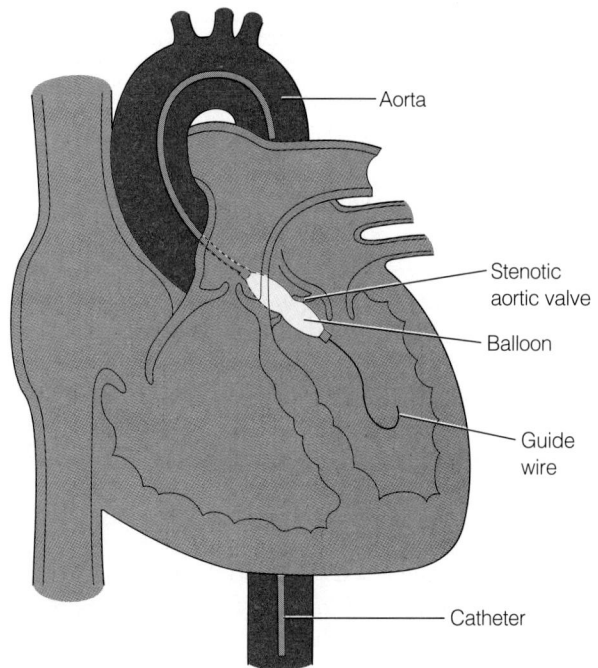

Figure 28–29   Balloon valvuloplasty. The balloon catheter is guided into position straddling the stenosed valve. The balloon is then inflated to increase the size of the valve opening.

valve. A prosthetic ring may be used to resize the opening, or stitches and purse-string sutures may be used to reduce and gather excess tissue. Annuloplasty may be indicated for either stenotic or regurgitant valves.

Valve Replacement   Valve replacement is indicated for clients who are experiencing manifestations, preferably before evidence of critical dysfunction of the left heart develops. The overall survival rate for clients undergoing valve replacement is 60% at 10 years (Braunwald, 1994b). Currently, approximately 50% of clients needing valve repair or replacement are over age 65; aortic stenosis is the most common valve disorder requiring surgery in older adults (Angelini et al., 1994).

Many different prosthetic heart valves are available, including mechanical and biologic tissue valves. The ideal prosthetic valve is one that most closely mimics the function of a normal heart valve, interfering little with normal cardiac hemodynamics. It also does not promote clot development, does not damage blood cells, is durable, is easy to insert, and does not promote the development of endocarditis (Whitman, 1987). The choice of valve depends on the client's age, underlying condition, desire to have children (because some types of prosthetic valves require long-term anticoagulation therapy), and the surgeon's experience and expertise in the specific techniques. All prosthetic valves obstruct the outflow tract to some degree (Whitman, 1987); the bileaflet designs offer the

Table 28–11	Advantages and Disadvantages of Prosthetic Cardiac Valves		
Category	**Types**	**Advantages**	**Disadvantages**
Mechanical valves	Ball-and-cage Single leaflet Bileaflet	Durability Good hemodynamics	Lifetime anticoagulation Audible click Mechanical failure Hemolysis Infections are harder to treat
Biologic tissue valves	Porcine heterograft Bovine heterograft Human aortic homograft	Nonthrombogenic No long-term anticoagulation Good hemodynamics Quiet Infections are easier to treat	Prone to deterioration Frequent replacement is required

least turbulence. The advantages and disadvantages of biologic and mechanical valves are listed in Table 28–11.

Biologic tissue valves include valves excised from a pig (porcine heterograft), made of calf pericardium (bovine heterograft), or from a human cadaver (homograft). The major advantages of biologic valves is that they allow for a more normal hemodynamic flow and are less likely to cause thrombus formation. Their major disadvantage is that they are prone to the same deterioration from fibrosis and calcification as the native valve. Repeat replacement surgery is required in 30% of clients by 10 years after the initial procedure, and 50% by 15 years (Braunwald, 1994b). Tissue valves are used for women in their childbearing years and older adults because they do not require long-term anticoagulation.

Mechanical prosthetic valves have the major advantage of long-term durability. These valves are frequently placed in clients with a life expectancy of more than 10 years. Their major disadvantage is the need for lifetime anticoagulation to prevent the development of clots on the valve.

Mechanical valves employ a variety of designs (Figure 28–30). They include a caged-ball valve, tilting-disc valve, and caged-disc valve. The tilting-disc valve designs, the most common prosthesis used today, have a lower profile than the caged-ball types, allowing blood to flow through the valve with less obstruction. The St. Jude bileaflet design has demonstrated superior hemodynamics and low potential for stimulating clot formation (Whitman, 1987). Both biologic and mechanical valves predispose the client to developing emboli and increase the risk of endocarditis, although the incidence of these complications is fairly low.

Nursing Care

Nursing priorities for the client with valvular disease focus on maintaining an effective cardiac output, managing manifestations of the disorder, providing information and teaching about the disease process and its medical and surgical management, and preventing complications. Nursing care of the client undergoing valve surgery is similar to that of the client having other types of open heart surgery, with increased attention to anticoagulation and preventing endocarditis.

Decreased Cardiac Output

With the possible exception of mitral prolapse, nearly all valve disorders impair ventricular filling and/or emptying, causing the cardiac output to fall. Obstructed flow from the atria to the ventricles in atrioventricular valve stenosis (mitral or tricuspid stenosis) impairs ventricular filling and increases atrial pressures. Regurgitation of these valves causes a portion of the blood in the ventricle to escape back into the atria during systole, also decreasing cardiac output. Stenosis of the semilunar valves obstructs ventricular outflow to the great vessels; regurgitation allows blood to flow back into the ventricles, creating higher filling pressures. The ventricles dilate and hypertrophy to accommodate the problem; however, when these changes can no longer compensate for demand, heart failure develops.

Selected nursing interventions with rationales follow:

- Monitor and record vital signs and hemodynamic parameters, reporting alterations from the baseline. *Declining systolic blood pressure and increasing pulse may indicate decreased cardiac output. Increasing pulmonary artery and pulmonary wedge pressures may also indicate decreased cardiac output. As stroke volume declines, so does cardiac output.*

- Assess for clinical manifestations of decreased cardiac output every shift, or more frequently if indicated. Be alert for the following: changes in level of consciousness; jugular venous distention; respiratory crackles and dyspnea; decreased urine output; cool, clammy,

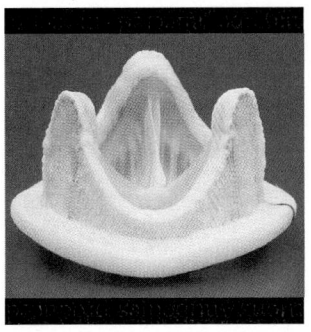
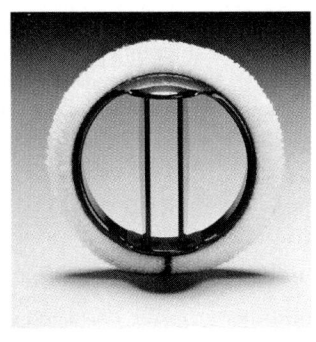
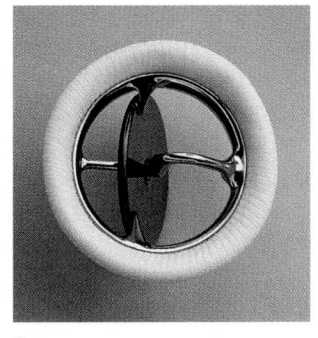
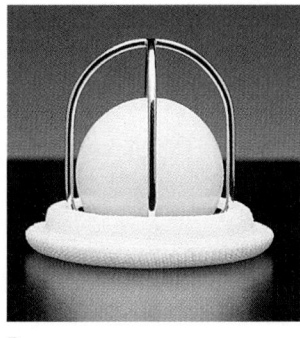

A   **B**   **C**   **D**

Figure 28–30   Prosthetic heart valves. *A*, Carpentier-Edwards porcine xenograft. *B*, St. Jude Medical valve. *C*, Medtronic Hall prosthetic valve. *D*, Starr-Edwards prosthetic valve.

mottled skin; peripheral edema; and decreased peripheral pulses and capillary refill. Notify the physician of significant changes. *Decreased cardiac output impairs tissue and organ perfusion, producing clinical manifestations.*

■ Monitor intake and output; weigh the client daily, reporting any gain of 3 to 5 lb within 24 hours. *Fluid retention is a compensatory mechanism that is activated when cardiac output is decreased; 1 pound of fluid is equal to 2.2 liters of fluid retained.*

■ Maintain fluid restriction as ordered. *Fluid intake may be restricted in the client with valvular disease to minimize cardiac workload and pressures within the heart and pulmonary circuit.*

■ Elevate the head of the bed, and administer supplemental oxygen as ordered. *These measures facilitate effective ventilation of the lungs and improve oxygenation.*

■ Monitor pulse oximetry continually and arterial blood gases as ordered. *Pulse oximetry and ABGs allow assessment of oxygenation.*

■ Ensure the client's physical, emotional, and mental rest. *Physical and psychologic rest decreases the cardiac workload.*

■ Administer prescribed medications aimed at reducing cardiac workload. *Diuretics, ACE inhibitors, and direct vasodilators are often prescribed to reduce or redistribute excess fluid volume and thus lessen the load on the heart.*

Activity Intolerance

In valvular disease, the alteration in blood flow through the heart impairs the delivery of oxygen and nutrients to the tissues. As the heart muscle fails and loses its ability to compensate for changed patterns of blood flow, tissue perfusion is compromised even further. Dyspnea on exertion is often an early manifestation of valvular disease.

Selected nursing interventions with rationales follow:

■ Obtain vital signs before and during activities. *Baseline data provide a means of comparison to assess the client's*

tolerance of the activity. A change in baseline heart rate of more than 20 BPM, a decline or increase in systolic BP of 20 mm Hg or more, and complaints of dyspnea, shortness of breath, excessive fatigue, chest pain, diaphoresis, dizziness, or syncope may indicate poor tolerance of the level of activity.

■ Encourage the client to increase the amount of activity/self-care gradually as tolerated. Ensure adequate rest periods, uninterrupted sleep cycles, and adequate nutritional intake. *Developing activity tolerance is a progressive process. Progressive activity prevents sudden stress on the heart. Encouraging the client to manage self-care needs and activities of daily living may help increase the client's self confidence and sense of power. Adequate rest and nutrition aid the healing process, decrease fatigue, and increase the amount of energy reserve.*

■ Provide assistance as needed. Suggest the client use a shower chair, sit down while brushing hair or teeth, and so on. *Energy saving techniques reduce energy expenditure and help to maintain oxygen supply and demand in balance.*

■ Consult with physical therapist for in-bed exercises and a progressive activity plan of care. *In-bed exercises may help the client build up strength.*

■ Discuss with the client and family methods to decrease energy requirements at home. *Information provides the client with practical ways to deal with activity limitations and empowers the client to make choices applicable to client's home situation.*

Risk for Infection

Damaged and deformed valve leaflets and turbulent blood flow through the cardiac chambers significantly increase the risk of infective endocarditis. Invasive diagnostic and monitoring lines (e.g., cardiac catheterization, hemodynamic monitoring) and disruption of the skin with surgery may also increase the risk of infection.

Selected nursing interventions with rationales follow:

- Maintain aseptic technique for all invasive procedures. *The body's protective mechanisms are breached during invasive procedures, creating opportunities for bacteria to enter. Aseptic technique reduces this risk.*

- Record temperature every 4 hours. Notify physician if the client's temperature exceeds 100.5 F (38.5 C). *An elevated temperature may be an early indication of infection.*

- Assess wounds and catheter sites for redness, swelling, warmth, pain, or evidence of drainage. *These are signs of inflammation and may signal an infection.*

- Administer antibiotics as ordered. Ensure that client receives the full course. *Antibiotics are used to prevent infection and eradicate the causative organism in a documented infection. The full course of antibiotics should be given to prevent organisms from becoming resistant to the drugs.*

- Monitor WBC counts, and notify physician of counts below 5,000/mm^3 or above 10,000/mm^3. *A high WBC count may indicate a bacterial infection; a low WBC count may indicate an impaired immune response and increased susceptibility to infection.*

Altered Protection

Many clients with valve disease require anticoagulant therapy. It may be prescribed for clients with chronic atrial fibrillation, for those with a history of emboli, or for those who have undergone valve replacement surgery. Although chronic anticoagulant therapy decreases the risk of clots and emboli, it puts the client at increased risk for bleeding and hemorrhage.

Selected nursing interventions with rationales follow:

- Perform guaiac testing on all stools and vomitus; test urine and sputum for occult blood every shift. *These tests allow early detection of blood that may not be visible.*

- Caution client about the concomitant use of aspirin or other nonsteroidal anti-inflammatory drugs (NSAIDs). *Encourage the client to read ingredient labels on over-the-counter drugs; many contain aspirin. Aspirin and other NSAIDs interfere with the clotting process and may potentiate the effects of the anticoagulant therapy.*

- Teach the client to modify personal hygiene habits to prevent bleeding; for example, advise the client to use a soft-bristled toothbrush or sponge-tipped applicators, to use an electric razor, and to clean fragile skin gently. *These methods help decrease the risk of skin nicks and cuts or prolonged bleeding from the gums.*

- Monitor the hemoglobin and hematocrit levels for signs of bleeding. Monitor platelet counts as ordered, and notify the physician if the count drops below 50,000/mm^3. *Low hemoglobin and hematocrit levels are indicative of blood loss. Platelet counts below 50,000/mm^3 significantly increase the risk of bleeding episodes.*

Other Nursing Diagnoses

Additional diagnoses that may apply to the client with valvular heart disease include:

- *Risk for Fluid Volume Excess* related to increased sodium and fluid retention

- *Sleep Pattern Disturbance* related to environmental noise in the ICU

- *Anxiety* related to a change in health status

- *Altered Tissue Perfusion* related to systemic emboli

- *Knowledge Deficit* regarding preventive measures against endocarditis

- *Risk for Noncompliance* with pharmacologic regimen related to lack of understanding

Client and Family Teaching

Prevention of rheumatic heart disease is a key element in preventing cardiac valve disorders. Rheumatic heart disease results from rheumatic fever (see the section on inflammatory cardiac conditions, which follows), an immune process that occurs as a sequela to hemolytic streptococcal infection of the pharynx (strep throat). Early treatment of strep throat usually prevents rheumatic fever. Nurses can be instrumental in teaching individual clients, families, and communities about the importance of timely and effective treatment of strep throat. Emphasize the importance of completing the full prescription of antibiotics to prevent development of resistant bacteria.

For the client with valvular disease, explain all tests and procedures, including corrective surgery, to increase the client and family's understanding and decrease anxiety. Discuss management of the client's manifestations, including any activity restrictions or life-style changes necessitated by valve disease. Teach the client to schedule rest periods to prevent fatigue. Instruct the client about diet restrictions to control manifestations of heart failure; arrange a consultation with the dietitian for teaching and menu planning. Provide information about prescribed medications, including their purpose, desired and possible adverse effects, scheduling, and possible interactions with other drugs. Provide referrals to community resources for the client and family prior to discharge. Emphasize the importance of keeping follow-up appointments to monitor the disease and therapeutic interventions. Teach the client about the importance of notifying all health care providers about the valve disease or surgery so that antibiotics can be initiated prophylactically before any procedure that might allow bacterial invasion.

Alert the client and family to manifestations that should be immediately reported to the health care provider. Increasing severity of manifestations, particularly signs of increasing heart failure and pulmonary edema, need to be reported to allow modification of the client's treatment regimen or timely surgical intervention to repair or replace the diseased valve. Evidence of transient ischemic attacks or other embolic events need to be reported as well so that anticoagulation therapy can be adjusted. It is also important for the client to notify the physician of any evidence of excess bleeding, such as joint pain, easy bruising, black and tarry stools, bleeding gums, or blood in the urine or sputum.

Applying the Nursing Process

Case Study of a Client with Mitral Valve Prolapse Syndrome: Julie Snow

Julie Snow, a 22-year-old college student, makes an appointment at the college health clinic for a physical examination after experiencing palpitations, fatigue, and a headache following a week of midterm examinations. Ms. Snow tells Lakisha Johnson, the nurse practitioner, "I'm scared that something is wrong with me."

Over the last few months, Ms. Snow has noted occasional bouts of palpitations that she describes as "feeling like my heart is doing flip-flops." Rarely, these palpitations have been associated with brief episodes (lasting less than 10 seconds) of a sharp, stabbing pain in her chest. She initially had attributed the symptoms to stress associated with school, but she has become increasingly concerned because the "attacks" have become more frequent. Ms. Snow states that she has "always been healthy." She denies any past or concurrent medical problems. When discussing her health habits, Ms. Snow tells the nurse that she does not smoke, uses alcohol socially, and exercises, albeit intermittently. Ms. Snow states that she has been drinking a lot of coffee and cola and eating a lot of "junk food" lately. She blames her recent study habits for her poor diet.

Assessment

Ms. Johnson performs a physical assessment and documents the following findings: Height, 5 feet, 6 inches (168 cm); weight, 140 lb (63.6 kg); T, 99.3; BP, 118/64; P, 82; R, 18. Ms. Snow is slightly anxious but in no acute distress. Auscultation of the heart reveals a systolic click followed by a soft crescendo murmur graded II/VI. Repeat validation of the click-murmur is performed by having the client stand during chest auscultation. Apical impulse is noted at the 5th intercostal space, midclavicular line. The lungs are clear to auscultation. The review of the remaining systems reveals no other abnormalities. An ECG reveals sinus rhythm with occasional PACs. Based on the client's admission history, clinical manifestations, and physical assessment findings, Ms. Johnson suspects mitral valve prolapse syndrome (MVPS). After consultation,

the clinic physician makes a medical diagnosis of MVPS. No medications are ordered at this time.

Diagnosis

Ms. Johnson makes the following nursing diagnoses:

- *Knowledge Deficit* regarding the disease process and symptom management
- *Anxiety* related to fear of valvular disease and implications for changes in life-style
- *Powerlessness* related to the occurrence of symptoms
- *Risk of Infection* (endocarditis) related to alteration in normal valve function

Expected Outcomes

The expected outcomes specify that Ms. Snow will

- Verbalize an understanding of MVPS and the rationale for its management.
- Verbalize an understanding that people with MVPS can live normal lives and the rationale for any necessary life-style changes.
- Discuss methods that decrease or relieve the occurrence of MVPS symptoms.
- Acknowledge the risk of developing endocarditis and identify the precautions to prevent it.

Planning and Implementation

Ms. Johnson plans and implements the following nursing interventions for Ms. Snow:

- Consult with and refer Ms. Snow to a local cardiologist for continued monitoring and follow-up.
- Identify Ms. Snow's degree of existing knowledge about the heart. Provide information in language appropriate to her cognitive level, and use audiovisual aids as appropriate.
- Teach Ms. Snow about MVPS: Include the anatomy and physiology of the heart valves and their function, common manifestations of MVPS, and rationale for management. Discuss manifestations of progressive mitral regurgitation, the need to notify her cardiologist should these manifestations appear, and rationale for yearly follow-up care with her cardiologist.
- Allow Ms. Snow to verbalize her feelings and share her concerns about MVPS. Encourage her to attend a MVPS support group meeting of other students affected by MVPS.
- Discuss the prognosis of MVPS with Ms. Snow, emphasizing that most clients live normal lives through diet and life-style management. Discuss rationale for life-style changes that help to decrease or relieve the MVPS symptoms (diet, fluid intake, exercise, use of over-the-counter drugs).

- Instruct Ms. Snow to keep a weekly record of her symptoms and the frequency of their occurrence for 1 month. This information can help the health care provider better monitor her condition and the methods used to relieve the symptoms.

- Discuss the following nonpharmacologic methods that Ms. Snow can use to manage symptoms: aerobic exercise with warm-up and cool-down periods; maintenance of adequate fluid intake, especially during hot weather or exercise; relaxation techniques, such as meditation, deep-breathing exercises, music therapy, yoga, guided imagery, heat therapy, or progressive muscle relaxation to be performed daily; avoidance of caffeine and crash dieting; forming healthy eating habits.

- Help Ms. Snow develop an individualized management plan.

- Teach Ms. Snow how infective endocarditis may develop on the prolapsed valve and about the prophylactic use of antibiotics to prevent it. Encourage Ms. Snow to notify her dentist and other health care providers of her valve disease **before** undergoing any invasive procedure (such as any dental work, endoscopy, cystoscopy, sigmoidoscopy, and so on).

Evaluation

After a series of educational sessions at the college health clinic, Ms. Snow is able to verbalize her understanding of MVPS by explaining the function of the heart valves, listing the common manifestations of MVPS, and describing indications of deteriorating heart function. She states that she will report these manifestations to her cardiologist should they occur. She is also given a booklet on MVPS for additional reading. She also verbalizes her understanding of the risk of endocarditis by stating that she will notify her doctors of her MVPS so that she can be given antibiotics before any invasive procedure. Ms Snow has been attending a monthly MVPS support group (led by a cardiology clinical nurse specialist) on campus and states, "I am so glad to know that there are other college students with MVPS! It has really helped me to know that I am not alone." The weekly symptom frequency log has pointed out a pattern of symptoms that is associated with late-night study habits, specifically the ingestion of large amounts of coffee and cola. Ms. Snow has modified her caffeine intake and increased her fluids, thus relieving her symptoms. In addition, Ms. Snow has joined several of her support group friends in a relaxation music therapy class. Ms. Snow states that she realizes that she has "the ability to control my life through the choices I make."

Critical Thinking in the Nursing Process

1. Develop an action plan for Ms. Snow that outlines specific activities she can use to manage manifestations of MVPS.

2. What is the physiologic basis for encouraging MVPS clients who are experiencing manifestations of the disorder to include regular exercise in their health habits?

3. How does the support of family, friends, and other MVPS sufferers assist MVPS clients in managing their condition?

4. What manifestations would Ms. Snow present with that would indicate a progressive worsening of her mitral regurgitation?

The Client with Cardiomyopathy

■ ■ ■

Cardiomyopathy is a primary abnormality of the heart muscle that affects its structural or functional characteristics. Cardiomyopathies affect both systolic and diastolic functions and are a significant factor in the development of heart failure. Primary, or "true," cardiomyopathies are idiopathic; their cause is unknown. Secondary cardiomyopathies that occur as a result of other disease processes are not classified as "true" cardiomyopathies; examples include *ischemic cardiomyopathy, alcoholic cardiomyopathy, viral cardiomyopathy,* and *peripartum cardiomyopathy* (Laurent-Bopp, 1995a). This book focuses on the primary cardiomyopathies, a heterogenous group of primary myocardial disorders (Wynne & Braunwald, 1994). Over 10,000 deaths a year, or an estimated 1% of cardiac deaths in the United States, have been attributed to cardiomyopathies (Laurent-Bopp, 1989; Porth, 1994). In the United States, the overall incidence of cardiomyopathies ranges from 0.7 to 7.5 cases per 100,000 people (Laurent-Bopp, 1995a).

Pathophysiology

Because the cause of primary cardiomyopathy is unknown, these disorders are categorized according to their pathophysiology and clinical presentation into three groups: dilated, hypertrophic, and restrictive (Wynne & Braunwald, 1995). A comparison of the causes of cardiomyopathies, their pathophysiologic features, clinical manifestations, and collaborative care is provided in Table 28–12.

Dilated Cardiomyopathy

Formerly known as *congestive cardiomyopathy, dilated cardiomyopathy* is the most common type of the cardiomyopathies. Its prevalence has increased over the last 20 years (Garg et al., 1993). In dilated cardiomyopathy, heart chambers are dilated, and the ventricular contraction is impaired. Both end-diastolic and end-systolic volumes are increased, and the left ventricular ejection fraction is

Table 28–12   Comparison of Cardiomyopathy Classifications

	Dilated	**Hypertrophic**	**Restrictive**
Causes	Usually idiopathic; may be secondary to chronic alcoholism or myocarditis	Hereditary; may be secondary to chronic hypertension	Usually secondary to amyloidosis, radiation, or myocardial fibrosis
Pathophysiology	Scarring and atrophy of myocardial cells Thickening of ventricular wall Dilation of heart chambers Impaired ventricular pumping Increased end-diastolic and end-systolic volumes Mural thrombi common	Hypertrophy of ventricular muscle mass Small left ventricular volume Septal hypertrophy may obstruct left ventricular outflow Left atrial dilation	Excess rigidity of ventricular walls restricts filling Myocardial contractility remains relatively normal
Clinical Manifestations	Heart failure Cardiomegaly Dysrhythmias S_3 and S_4 gallop; murmur of mitral regurgitation	Dyspnea Anginal pain Syncope Left ventricular hypertrophy Dysrhythmias Loud S_4 Sudden death	Dyspnea Fatigue Right-sided heart failure Mild to moderate cardiomegaly S_3 and S_4 Mitral regurgitation murmur
Management	Management of CHF Control dysrhythmias	Beta-blockers Calcium channel blockers Antidysrhythmic agents Surgical excision of part of the ventricular septum	Management of CHF Exercise restriction

substantially reduced, resulting in decreased cardiac output. Dilatation of the left ventricle is prominent; left ventricular hypertrophy is usually minimal. The right ventricle also may be enlarged. Microscopic myocardial cell scarring and atrophy is evident (Porth, 1994). The cause of dilated cardiomyopathy is unknown, although conditions such as alcohol and cocaine abuse, chemotherapeutic agents, pregnancy, and systemic hypertension may contribute to its development.

Manifestations of dilated cardiomyopathy develop gradually. Heart failure often becomes evident years after the onset of dilation and pump failure. The client presents with right-sided and left-sided heart failure, dyspnea on exertion, orthopnea, paroxysmal nocturnal dyspnea, weakness, fatigue, and signs of systemic vascular congestion such as peripheral edema and ascites. Auscultation commonly reveals an S_3 and an S_4 and murmurs related to atrioventricular valve regurgitation. Dysrhythmias are common, including supraventricular tachycardias, atrial fibrillation, and complex ventricular tachycardias. If dysrhythmias remain untreated, the client faces a risk of sudden cardiac death (Porth, 1994). Mural thrombi (blood clots in the heart wall) may form in the left ventricular apex and embolize to other parts of the body.

The prognosis of dilated cardiomyopathy is grim; most clients get progressively worse and die within 2 years of the onset of symptoms (Wynne & Braunwald, 1994); 75% of clients die within 5 years (Laurent-Bopp, 1995a).

Hypertrophic Cardiomyopathy

Hypertrophic cardiomyopathy is characterized by decreased compliance of the left ventricle and hypertrophy of the ventricular muscle mass, resulting in impaired ventricular filling, small end-diastolic volumes, and low cardiac output. Over half of all the cases of hypertrophic cardiomyopathy are genetically transmitted (Wynne & Braunwald, 1994). This disorder is found most commonly in males in their 20s and 30s (Finkelmeier, 1995).

The pattern of left ventricular hypertrophy is unique in that the muscle may not hypertrophy "equally." In a majority of clients, the interventricular septum, especially the upper portion, demonstrates a greater increase in mass than the free wall of the left ventricle (Wynne & Braunwald, 1994). The enlarged upper septum narrows the passageway of blood into the aorta, impairing ventricular outflow. For this reason, this disorder is also known as *idiopathic hypertrophic subaortic stenosis (IHSS)* or *hypertrophic obstructive cardiomyopathy (HOCM)*.

Clinical manifestations of hypertrophic cardiomyopathy may be absent for many years. Typically, manifestations are associated with an increase in oxygen demand and consequent increased ventricular contractility and may present suddenly during or after physical activity; in children and young adults, sudden cardiac death may be the first sign of the disorder (Wynne & Braunwald, 1994). Indeed, hypertrophic cardiomyopathy is cited as the most common cause of sudden cardiac death in young athletes (Laurent-Bopp, 1995a). It is hypothesized that the mechanism for sudden cardiac death is due to ventricular dysrhythmias or hemodynamic factors. Predictors of sudden cardiac death in this population include age of less than 30 years, a family history of sudden death, syncopal episodes, severe ventricular hypertrophy, and evidence of lethal ventricular dysrhythmias noted via ambulatory ECG monitoring (Wynne & Braunwald, 1994).

The most frequent manifestations of hypertrophic cardiomyopathy include dyspnea (90% of clients), angina pectoris (70% to 80%), and syncope (20%) (Finkelmeier, 1995). Angina may result from ischemia due to the overgrowth of the ventricular muscle relative to the available blood supply, coronary artery abnormalities, or decreased coronary artery perfusion. Syncope may occur when the outflow tract obstruction severely decreases cardiac output and blood flow to the brain. Ventricular dysrhythmias are common; atrial fibrillation is noted in 10% of clients (Laurent-Bopp, 1995a). Other clinical manifestations of hypertrophic cardiomyopathy include fatigue, dizziness, and palpitations. A harsh, crescendo-decrescendo systolic murmur of variable intensity heard best at the lower left sternal border and apex is characteristic in hypertrophic cardiomyopathy. A brisk carotid pulse, a double apical

impulse, and a fourth heart sound (S_4) may also be noted on auscultation.

Restrictive Cardiomyopathy

The least common form of cardiomyopathy, *restrictive cardiomyopathy* is characterized by rigidity of the ventricular walls that impair diastolic filling. Causes of restrictive cardiomyopathy include endomyocardial fibrosis, which causes severe endocardial fibrosis, and infiltrative processes, such as amyloidosis. Fibrosis of the myocardium and endocardium causes excessive stiffness and rigidity of the ventricles. Decreased ventricular compliance impairs filling, resulting in decreased ventricular size, elevated end-diastolic pressures, and decreased cardiac output. Contractility is unaffected, and the ejection fraction is normal.

The manifestations of restrictive cardiomyopathy are those of biventricular failure and decreased tissue perfusion. Dyspnea on exertion and exercise intolerance are common complaints. Jugular venous pressure is elevated, and S_3 and S_4 are common. The prognosis for restrictive cardiomyopathy is poor. Most clients die within 3 years and the systemic nature of the underlying disease process precludes effective treatment.

Collaborative Care

Unless an underlying treatable cause can be identified, little can be done to treat either dilated or restrictive cardiomyopathies. Management of these disorders focuses on minimizing manifestations of heart failure and treating dysrhythmias. Refer to the sections of this chapter on heart failure and dysrhythmias for specific management strategies. Goals for the client with hypertrophic cardiomyopathy are aimed at reducing contractility and preventing sudden cardiac death. All clients should be restricted from strenuous physical exertion, which may precipitate dysrhythmias and/or sudden cardiac death. Dietary and sodium restrictions may help diminish the manifestations.

Laboratory and Diagnostic Tests

Diagnosis begins with a history and physical assessment of the client to rule out known causes of heart failure. Other tests may include the following:

- *Electrocardiography* is used to detect enlargement of the heart and the presence of dysrhythmias.
- *Echocardiography* is employed to assess chamber size and thickness, ventricular wall motion, valvular function, and systolic and diastolic function of the heart.
- *Chest X-ray* may reveal **cardiomegaly,** enlargement of the heart. The lung fields are assessed for pulmonary congestion and edema.

- *Hemodynamic studies* are used to assess cardiac output and pressures in the cardiac chambers and pulmonary vascular system.
- *Nuclear scans* help discern changes in ventricular volume and mass and identify defects in myocardial perfusion.
- *Cardiac catheterization* is employed to evaluate coronary perfusion, the cardiac chambers, valves, and great vessels for function and structure, pressure relationships, and cardiac output.
- *Endomyocardial biopsy* involves inserting a transvenous *bioptome* into the ventricle and extracting a piece of the myocardium for examination. The cells are examined for pathologic evidence of infiltration, fibrosis, or inflammation.

Pharmacology

Pharmacologic management of the client with dilated cardiomyopathy and restrictive cardiomyopathy follows the regimen for clients with congestive heart failure and includes vasodilators, diuretics, ACE inhibitors, and cardiac glycosides (see the pharmacology box on page 1116). ACE inhibitors such as captopril, enalapril, and benazepril have been found to improve survival in clients with dilated cardiomyopathy (Wynne & Braunwald, 1994). Beta-blockers may also be employed for selected clients with dilated cardiomyopathy. Anticoagulants are indicated for all clients because of the risk for systemic embolization. Antidysrhythmic agents are used to manage dysrhythmias in all types of cardiomyopathy.

Beta-blockers are the drugs of choice to reduce anginal symptoms and syncopal episodes for clients with hypertrophic cardiomyopathy. The negative inotropic effects of beta-blockers and calcium channel blockers decrease the myocardial contractility, decreasing obstruction of the outflow tract; drugs that cause vasodilation or increased contractility are contraindicated. Beta-blockers also decrease heart rate and increase ventricular compliance, increasing diastolic filling time and increasing cardiac output. Amiodarone has been used to treat ventricular dysrhythmias in clients with hypertrophic cardiomyopathy with good results (Laurent-Bopp, 1995a).

Surgery

Without definitive treatment, clients with cardiomyopathy develop end-stage heart failure. Surgical procedures may be used to treat symptoms and prevent sudden cardiac death. Cardiac transplant is the definitive treatment for dilated cardiomyopathy; without transplant, survival time is limited. Ventricular assist devices may be used in the interim to maintain the client until a donor heart becomes available. Transplantation is not a viable option for clients with restrictive cardiomyopathy, because transplantation does not eradicate the underlying disease process that caused the infiltration or fibrosis, and the transplanted organ will eventually be affected as well (Finkelmeier, 1995). Refer to the section on surgical treatment of CHF for further information about cardiac transplantation and other surgical interventions for the failing heart. Obstructive hypertrophic cardiomyopathy may be surgically treated by resecting excess muscle away from the aortic valve outflow tract. The septum is incised (*myotomy*), and tissue may be removed (*myectomy*). This procedure may ease the manifestations of the disorder, but because its mortality rate is 5%, it is limited to clients with severe symptoms (Wynne & Braunwald, 1994).

Other invasive interventions that may be employed for the client with cardiomyopathy include dual-chamber pacing and the automatic implantable cardioverter-defibrillator (AICD) to prevent sudden death.

Nursing Care

Care of the client with dilated and restrictive cardiomyopathy focuses on easing the manifestations, much like that of the client with congestive heart failure. Nursing goals are to prevent complications, assist the client to conserve energy while encouraging self-care, and support the client and the family's coping skills. Refer to the section on nursing care of the client with congestive heart failure for detailed nursing diagnoses and suggested interventions. The client with hypertrophic cardiomyopathy requires care similar to that for the client with myocardial ischemia; vasodilating agents are not used, however. If surgical intervention is performed, nursing care is similar to that for any client undergoing open heart surgery or cardiac transplant.

Nursing diagnoses that may be appropriate for the client with cardiomyoapathy follow:

- *Decreased Cardiac Output* related to impaired left ventricular filling, contractility, or outflow obstruction
- *Fatigue* related to decreased cardiac output
- *Ineffective Breathing Pattern* related to heart failure
- *Anxiety or Fear* related to possibility of sudden cardiac death
- *Altered Role Performance* related to decreasing cardiac function
- *Anticipatory Grieving* related to poor prognosis

Client and Family Teaching

Client and family teaching focuses on self-care measures such as activity restrictions, dietary changes, and pharmacologic measures to reduce symptoms and/or prevent complications. To make informed decisions about care, the client and family members must understand the disease process, its ultimate outcome, and treatment options. Clients who are undergoing invasive procedures for diagnosis or treatment of cardiomyopathy require preoperative and postoperative teaching specific to the procedure being performed. Instructions provided to the client undergoing myotomy or myectomy are those for any client undergoing open heart surgery. If cardiac transplantation is an option, provide information about the procedure and initiate teaching preoperatively. Emphasize the need for lifetime immunosuppression to prevent rejection of the transplanted organ. Stress the risks of infection postoperatively related to continued immunosuppression. Teach the client and family to recognize manifestations of organ rejection and report them promptly to the physician.

▚ ▚ ▚   Inflammatory Cardiac Disorders   ▚ ▚ ▚

Any layer of cardiac tissue—the endocardium, myocardium, or pericardium—can be affected by an inflammatory process, resulting in damage to the heart valves, heart muscle, or pericardial lining. Manifestations of inflammation may range from very mild to life-threatening. In recent years, especially with the increasing numbers of homeless people, the incidence of inflammatory heart disease due to rheumatic fever has been rising. This section discusses the causes and current management of rheumatic heart disease, endocarditis, myocarditis, and pericarditis.

The Client with Rheumatic Fever and Rheumatic Heart Disease

▪ ▪ ▪

Rheumatic fever is a systemic inflammatory disease caused by an abnormal immune response to infection by group A beta-hemolytic streptococci (Porth, 1994). The peak incidence of rheumatic fever is between ages 5 and 15; although it is rare after age 40, it may affect people of any age. Rheumatic fever is a self-limiting disorder; cardiac involvement is its most significant effect and occurs in about half of all clients. Rheumatic fever is the most common cause of valvular heart damage (Guyton, 1991; LeDoux, 1995).

Worldwide, rheumatic fever affects 15 to 20 million people (Stollerman, 1994). Risk factors for the development and spread of streptococcal infections include environmental and economic factors, such as damp weather, crowded living conditions, malnutrition, immunodeficiency, and poor access to health care (Stollerman, 1994). The risk of developing rheumatic fever as a result of a streptococcal infection is only about 3%. In the United States, mortality attributed to rheumatic fever has steadily decreased with the availability of better treatments and economic conditions; however, rheumatic fever outbreaks are still reported (Stollerman, 1994). Recent outbreaks are tied to pharyngitis caused by new strains of group A beta-hemolytic streptococci (Porth, 1994).

Pathophysiology

The pathogenesis of rheumatic fever is unknown, but it is thought to result from either a self-directed (autoimmune) injury or a hyperallergenic reaction to the *Streptococcus* bacteria. Toxins produced by the bacteria may precipitate a hypersensitivity reaction. Antibodies produced to attack the invading bacteria (the antigen) appear to cross-react with connective tissues of the heart, blood vessels, joints, and subcutaneous tissues, initiating an intense inflammatory response in the acute stage. The antibodies may remain in the serum for up to 6 months following the initiating event (Guyton, 1991). See Chapter 8 for further discussion of the immune system and the inflammatory response.

Any layer of the heart may be affected in acute rheumatic fever; usually all three are involved (Porth, 1994). In acute *carditis,* valve structures become red and swollen, and small vegetative lesions develop on the leaflets. As the inflammatory process abates, fibrous scarring occurs, causing deformity. Myocarditis and pericarditis associated with rheumatic fever are generally mild and reversible, with no long-term sequela. The long-term effects of the disease are caused by endocardial and valve involvement.

Rheumatic heart disease (RHD) is a chronic condition of slowly progressive valvular deformity that may follow acute or repeated attacks of rheumatic fever. Valve leaflets become rigid and deformed; commissures fuse, and the chordae tendineae also become fibrotic and shortened. The result is stenosis or regurgitation of the valve: A narrowed fused valve obstructs forward blood flow, or the valve fails to close properly, allowing blood to flow back through it. Valves on the left side of the heart are most often affected; the mitral valve is most frequently involved.

Manifestations of rheumatic fever typically follow the initial streptococcal infection by about 2 to 3 weeks. Fever and migratory joint pain are often initial manifestations. The knees, ankles, hips, and elbows are common sites of swelling and inflammation; in the adult, a single joint may be involved. *Erythema marginatum* is a temporary nonpruritic skin rash characterized by red, circumscribed lesions with blanched centers usually found on the trunk and proximal extremities. A mild to severe chorea ranging from an inability to concentrate to involuntary muscle spasms also may be present in rheumatic fever, although it is rare in adults.

Cardiac involvement is indicated by complaints of precordial chest discomfort, tachycardia, or evidence of heart failure. A pericardial friction rub, S_3 or S_4, or a heart murmur of mitral or aortic regurgitation may be noted on auscultation. The client may also have manifestations of cardiomegaly or pericardial effusion (see the section on pericarditis later in this chapter). About 50% of clients suffering from rheumatic fever develop some form of rheumatic heart disease.

Collaborative Care

The overall management goals for the client with rheumatic heart disease focus on treating the primary infection, managing its manifestations, and preventing complications and recurrences of the disease. In clients with acute carditis, treatment is directed at decreasing myocardial work. Strict bed rest is prescribed in the acute phase. After about 4 to 5 weeks, the client's activity levels are gradually increased. The client's response to all therapeutic interventions is documented. Treatment of chronic rheumatic heart disease is similar to treatment of valvular disorders.

Laboratory and Diagnostic Tests

In addition to the history and physical examination, a number of laboratory and diagnostic tests may be ordered for the client with suspected rheumatic fever. These tests and values indicative of rheumatic fever with cardiac involvement are outlined in Table 28–13. Several are also described below.

- *Complete blood count (CBC)* and *erythrocyte sedimentation rate (ESR)* provide an indication of the inflammatory process that occurs in rheumatic fever. The white blood cell count is elevated, and a slight decrease in the red blood cell count (due to the inflammatory inhibition of erythropoiesis) is noted. The erythrocyte sedimentation rate, a general indicator of inflammatory response, is elevated.

- *C-reactive protein (CRP)* is used to evaluate the severity and progression of inflammatory conditions. A positive CRP indicates an active inflammatory process.

- *Antistreptolysin titer (ASO) titer* is a streptococcal antibody test that rises within 2 months of the disease's onset and is found in 95% of all clients affected (Stollerman, 1994).

Pharmacology

Treatment during the acute phase of rheumatic fever is aimed at eliminating the streptococcal infection and managing the initial symptoms. Penicillin is the antibiotic of

Table 28–13	Laboratory and Diagnostic Tests in Rheumatic Heart Disease
Test	**Values Characteristic of Rheumatic Heart Disease**
White blood cell count (WBC)	Above 10,000/mm^3
Red blood cell count (RBC)	Below 4 million/mm^3
Erythrocyte sedimentation rate (ESR)	Above 20 mm/h
C-reactive protein	Positive
Antistreptolysin (ASO) titer	Above 250 IU/mL
Throat culture	Positive for group A beta-hemolytic streptococci
Cardiac enzymes	Elevated in severe carditis
ECG changes	May have prolonged PR interval
Chest X-ray	May show enlarged heart with myocarditis or CHF
Echocardiogram	May show valvular damage, enlarged chamber size, decreased ventricular function, or pericardial effusion
Cardiac catheterization	May show valvular damage and decreased ventricular function

choice to treat group A streptococci (Stollerman, 1994). Antibiotic coverage is prescribed for at least 10 days. Erythromycin or clindamycin is used if the client is allergic to penicillin. Antibiotic therapy is continued prophylactically for an extended period of time to prevent recurrences; a minimum of 5 years is the current recommendation (Stollerman, 1994). Recurrences after 5 years or age 25 are rare (Tierney et al., 1994). Penicillin G, 1.2 million units injected intramuscularly every 4 weeks, is the prophylaxis of choice. Oral penicillin, amoxicillin, sulfadiazine, or erythromycin may also be used.

Joint pain and fever are treated with salicylates (e.g., aspirin); corticosteroids may be used for severe pain due to inflammation or carditis. See Chapter 8 for further information about the use of these anti-inflammatory medications.

Nursing Care

Nursing interventions for the client with RHD are tailored to the client's manifestations and focus on providing supportive care and preventing complications. Teaching to prevent future recurrences of this disease is an extremely important nursing action. Nursing management begins with an assessment of the client's complaints and a physical examination. *Pain* and *Activity Intolerance* are priority nursing diagnoses for the client with rheumatic fever and RHD.

Pain

Joint pain due to the acute inflammatory process is a common manifestation of rheumatic fever. Unless pain and inflammation are controlled, they may interfere with rest and healing.

Nursing interventions with rationales follow:

- Administer anti-inflammatory agents as ordered. Report promptly any manifestations of aspirin toxicity, including tinnitus, vomiting, and gastrointestinal bleeding. Administer aspirin with food, milk, or antacids to minimize gastric irritation. *Joint pain and fever may be treated with anti-inflammatory agents such as aspirin or steroids. Steroids are given primarily in cases of severe carditis. As the steroid is tapered off, aspirin is added to prevent the occurrence of rebound rheumatic activity (Stollerman, 1994). When aspirin is used for its anti-inflammatory effect, doses may be high, and it is administered around the clock on a routine basis (e.g., every 4 hours).*

- Place a bed cradle at foot of bed. Provide warm, moist compresses for local pain relief. *A bed cradle and the direct application of moist heat may aid in relieving the pain associated with inflamed joints by relieving the pressure of the linen on the joints and reducing inflammation.*

- Auscultate heart sounds every shift and as necessary. Notify the physician if a pericardial friction rub or a new murmur appears. *A friction rub may be produced as the inflamed pericardial surfaces rub against each other. This also stimulates pain receptors, and may increase the client's discomfort.*

Activity Intolerance

The client with acute carditis or RHD may experience significant cardiac dysfunction; the heart cannot supply enough oxygen to meet the body's demand. Manifestations of fatigue, weakness, and dyspnea on exertion may result.

Selected nursing interventions with rationales follow:

- Explain the importance of bed rest to the client, and enforce bed rest as ordered. *Bed rest is usually enforced for at least the first 2 weeks to decrease the stress on the heart. Explaining the rationale for bed rest fosters the client's cooperation with the plan of care.*

- Allow visits from friends and family members. Encourage the use of diversional activities, such as reading books or magazines, playing cards or board games,

watching television, listening to radio or favorite music cassettes, and so on. *Diversionary activities help the client on bed rest pass the time.*

- Allow the client to increase activity gradually and monitor the client's vital signs and complaints during activity. Consult a physical therapist for input into plan of care. *Gradual activity progression is encouraged as the acute signs and symptoms resolve. Client tolerance to activity is closely monitored and adjustments made as needed. The physical therapist may be consulted to assist in the client's care.*

Other Nursing Diagnoses

Examples of other nursing diagnoses appropriate for the client with rheumatic heart disease follow:

- *Diversional Activity Deficit* related to enforced bed rest
- *Risk for Infection* related to deformed valve structures
- *Risk for Decreased Cardiac Output* related to impaired valve function
- *Risk for Noncompliance* related to boredom
- *Knowledge Deficit* regarding the treatment regimen
- *Ineffective Individual Coping* related to anxiety and prolonged hospitalization

Client and Family Teaching

Client and family education is vital to the promotion of good health and the prevention of recurrences and further tissue damage. Rheumatic fever is preventable. Prompt identification and treatment of streptococcal throat infections helps decrease the spread of this pathogen and the risk of subsequent rheumatic fever. Characteristics of streptococcal sore throat include a red, fiery-looking throat, pain upon swallowing, enlarged and tender cervical lymph nodes, fever in the range of 101 to 104 F (38.3 to 40.0 C), and headache. Emphasize the importance of finishing the complete course of medication to eradicate the pathogen.

Secondary prevention is aimed at preventing a recurrence of the disorder. Emphasize the importance of continuing the antibiotic prophylaxis as prescribed. Teach the client with chronic RHD about the importance of additional antibiotic prophylaxis for any invasive procedure (e.g., dental care, endoscopy, or surgery) to prevent bacterial endocarditis. Pamphlets on endocarditis prevention are available from the American Heart Association and are helpful reminders to clients and their family members. Preventive dental care and good oral hygiene help discourage gingival infections, which can lead to recurrence of the disease.

Encourage appropriate life-style changes, and provide assistance as needed. Instruct the client with rheumatic carditis in restricting sodium in the diet to prevent fluid

Table 28–14   Classifications of Infective Endocarditis

	Acute Infective Endocarditis	Subacute Infective Endocarditis
Onset	Sudden	Gradual
Usual organism	*Staphylococcus aureus*	*Streptococcus viridans,* enterococci, gram-negative and gram-positive bacilli, fungi, yeasts
Risk factors	Usually occurs in previously normal heart; intravenous drug use, infected intravenous sites	Usually occurs in damaged or deformed hearts; dental work, invasive procedures, and infections
Pathologic process	Rapid valve destruction	Valve destruction leading to regurgitation; embolization of friable vegetations
Presentation	Abrupt onset with spiking fever and chills; manifestations of heart failure	Gradual onset of febrile illness with cough, dyspnea, arthralgias, abdominal pain

overload, which can increase the workload of the heart. A high-carbohydrate, high-protein diet is usually recommended to provide energy for healing and to combat weakness and fatigue. Teach the client and family to recognize early manifestations of congestive heart failure. Medication instruction should include proper dosage, route, signs of adverse or allergic reactions, and possible drug interactions. Assess the need for a visiting home health nurse, and provide information as needed.

The Client with Infective Endocarditis

■ ■ ■

Endocarditis, inflammation of the endocardium, may involve any portion of the endothelial lining of the heart but usually affects the valves. Endocarditis is usually infective in nature, rather than inflammatory. Infective endocarditis most often occurs in clients with underlying cardiac disease. Lesions develop on deformed valves, on valve prostheses, or in areas of tissue damage because of congential deformities or ischemic disease. The disease also occurs in intravenous drug users. The left side of the heart, the mitral valve in particular, is the most common site of involvement; in intravenous drug users, the right side, the tricuspid valve in particular, is often involved. A portal of entry for organisms into the bloodstream is the other necessary element for infective endocarditis to occur. Intravenous drug use provides a means of entry for bacteria. Bacteria may also enter through oral lesions or during dental work; as a result of invasive procedures, such as the insertion of intravenous lines, surgery, or urinary catheterization; or in the course of infectious processes such as urinary tract or upper respiratory infection.

Endocarditis is frequently classified by the acuity of onset and its disease course (see Table 28–14). *Acute in-fective endocarditis* has an abrupt onset and is a rapidly progressive, severe disease. Although almost any organism can cause infective endocarditis, its onset is more abrupt and course more destructive with virulent organisms such as *Staphylococcus aureus. S. aureus* is the usual infective organism in acute endocarditis. In contrast, *subacute infective endocarditis* has a more gradual onset, although the incubation period may be short. Systemic manifestations often predominate in subacute endocarditis. It is more likely to occur in clients with preexisting heart disease. *Streptococcus viridans,* enterococci, other gram-negative and gram-positive bacilli, yeasts, and fungi tend to cause the subacute forms of endocarditis. (Porth, 1994).

Prosthetic valve endocarditis (PVE) may occur in clients who have had a mechanical or tissue valve replacement. This infection may occur either early in the postoperative period (within the first 2 months following surgery) or late. Its overall incidence is 10% to 20% in these clients (Kaye, 1994). Early prosthetic valve endocarditis has a high mortality rate (60%) because of the difficulty in eradicating microorganisms from the prosthesis (Christopherson & Froelicher, 1989). The mortality rate in late-onset PVE, by contrast, is 20% to 40% (Kaye, 1994). The incidence of PVE has not been found to vary significantly in mechanical versus biologic prostheses (Seifert, 1987; Whitman, 1987).

Pathophysiology

In infective endocarditis, the initial lesion is a sterile platelet-fibrin vegetation formed on damaged endothelium. In the acute form of infective endocarditis, these lesions develop on healthy valve structures, although the mechanism is unknown (Trausch, 1988). The subacute form usually develops on already damaged valves or in endocardial tissue that has been damaged by abnormal pressures or blood flow within the heart.

Clinical Manifestations of Infective Endocarditis

· · ·

Cardiac Effects

- Murmur

Respiratory System

- Cough
- Shortness of breath

Gastrointestinal System

- Anorexia
- Abdominal pain

Hematologic Effects

- Anemia
- Splenomegaly

Systemic Effects

- Fever and chills
- Migratory arthralgias
- General malaise
- Diaphoresis

Skin

- Petechiae
- Osler's nodes
- Splinter hemorrhages
- Janeway lesions

Eyes

- Roth's spots

immune response to infection. A temperature above 101.5 F (39.4 C) and flulike symptoms are usual in all forms of endocarditis. The client may have a cough, shortness of breath, and complain of joint pain. Acute staphylococcal endocarditis presents with a sudden onset and more severe clinical manifestations, including a high fever.

Cardiac murmurs are present in 90% of persons with infective endocarditis. A change in an existing murmur or the detection of a new murmur is strongly suggestive of endocarditis. Embolic complications may involve any organ system, particularly the lungs, cerebral vasculature, renal system, and the skin and mucous membranes. Splenomegaly is common in chronic disease.

Peripheral manifestations of infective endocarditis may result from microemboli in the vasculature or from circulating immune complexes. These manifestations include the following:

- *Petechiae,* small, purplish-red, hemorrhagic spots mainly found on the trunk, conjunctiva, and mucous membranes
- *Splinter hemorrhages,* hemorrhagic streaks found under the fingernails or toenails
- *Osler's nodes,* small, reddened, painful raised growths noted on the finger pads and toe pads
- *Janeway lesions,* small, nontender, purplish-red macular lesions found on the palms of the hands and soles of the feet
- *Roth's spots,* small, whitish spots (cotton-wool spots) noted upon retinal examination

The accompanying box summarizes the clinical manifestations of infective endocarditis.

Complications commonly associated with infective endocarditis include congestive heart failure, multiorgan infarctions from embolization of vegetative fragments, abscess, and mycotic aneurysms that form from infiltration of the arterial wall by organisms. Without treatment, endocarditis is almost universally fatal; fortunately, antibiotic therapy is usually effective to treat this disease.

Collaborative Care

Prevention is a key component in infective endocarditis care; education of clients at high risk for the disease is essential. Educating the public about the risks of intravenous drug use, including endocarditis, can also help reduce the incidence of this frightening disease. For the client with infective endocarditis, the priorities of management are to establish a timely diagnosis, eradicate the infecting organism using antibiotic therapy, and minimize valve damage and other adverse consequences of the disease.

These vegetations provide a site for colonization of organisms that have invaded the blood. The vegetation enlarges as more platelets and fibrin are attracted to the area of injury and cover the infecting organism; this covering "protects" the bacteria from quick removal by immune system defenses such as phagocytosis by neutrophils, antibodies, and complement. Vegetations may be singular or multiple; they expand while loosely attached to edges of the valve. Friable vegetations can break or shear off, embolizing and traveling through the bloodstream to other organ systems. When they lodge in small vessels, they may cause hemorrhages, infarcts, or abscesses. Ultimately, the vegetations scar and deform the valves and generate turbulence of the circulating blood flow. The normal functioning of the heart valves is affected either from the obstruction of forward blood flow or from incomplete closure of the valve during systole.

The clinical manifestations of infective endocarditis result from direct effects of the vegetative growths and the

Table 28–15   Antibiotic Prophylaxis for Infective Endocarditis

Indications for Prophylaxis	Selected Procedures for Which Prophylaxis Is Recommended	Suggested Antibiotics
Prosthetic valves	Dental procedures in which bleeding is likely, including cleaning	Amoxicillin
Previous episode(s) of infective endocarditis	Most surgeries	Erythromycin
Rheumatic heart disease	Bronchoscopy	Ampicillin
Hypertrophic cardiomyopathy	Cystoscopy	Clindamycin
Mitral valve prolapse with regurgitation and murmur	Urinary catheterization when infection is present	Vancomycin
Sclerotic aortic valve	Incision and drainage of infected tissue	(*Note:* choice of antibiotic depends on procedure)
Most congenital heart malformations	Vaginal delivery if infection is present	

Laboratory and Diagnostic Tests

There are no definitive tests for infective endocarditis, but laboratory and diagnostic data may suggest the diagnosis. Laboratory testing may include the following:

- *CBC* typically shows a normocytic, normochromic anemia in subacute endocarditis. White blood cell counts may be elevated in acute infective endocarditis; however, in subacute forms, the white blood cell and differential counts may be within the normal limits. The ESR is elevated because of the inflammatory response to infection.

- *Serologic immune testing* reveals positive rheumatoid factor in 50% of clients with an infective endocarditis of at least 6 weeks' duration. Most clients display circulating antigen-antibody complexes (Kaye, 1994).

- *Blood cultures* are positive for bacteremia or fungemia in more than 95% of clients with infective endocarditis (Kaye, 1994). In addition to helping establish the diagnosis, identifying the organism allows antibiotic therapy to be specifically tailored to include those drugs to which the organism is most sensitive.

- *Urine testing* usually reveals an elevated serum creatinine, proteinuria, and/or hematuria. These results indicate renal damage due to microemboli and, possibly, circulating immune complexes.

Diagnostic tests that may help confirm the diagnosis of infective endocarditis include echocardiography, which can identify vegetations in clients with infective endocarditis (Kaye, 1994). Echocardiography also allows non-invasive assessment of valve function and is often used to determine whether surgery is necessary. *Transesophageal echocardiography* provides a more sensitive picture of mitral valve lesions and vegetations (Tierney et al., 1994).

Pharmacology

As noted before, prevention of endocarditis in clients at high risk is an important component of care. For clients with preexisting heart disease or damage, antibiotics are commonly prescribed prior to high-risk procedures. Guidelines for antibiotic prophylaxis are provided in Table 28–15.

Antibiotic therapy is the mainstay of treatment for infective endocarditis and is effective in treating the disease in most cases. The goal of therapy is to eradicate the infecting organism from the blood and vegetative lesions in the heart. The fibrin covering that protects colonies of organisms from the client's immune system also protects them from antibiotic therapy. Therefore, an extended course of multiple intravenous antibiotics is required.

Following blood cultures, antibiotic therapy is initiated with drugs known to be effective against the most common infecting organisms: staphylococci, streptococci, and enterococci. The initial regimen may include nafcillin or oxacillin, penicillin or ampicillin, and gentamicin. Once the organism has been identified, therapy is tailored to that organism. Streptococcal and enterococcal infections are treated with a combination of penicillin and streptomycin or gentamicin. If the client is hypersensitive to penicillin, cefazolin or vancomycin may be used. Staphyloccoal infections are treated with nafcillin or oxacillin; cephalothin or vancomycin may be used if the client is hypersensitive to penicillin. Intravenous drug therapy is continued for 2 to 4 weeks, depending on the specific antibiotic or combination of antibiotics used and the results of repeat blood cultures.

The client with prosthetic valve endocarditis requires a longer period of therapy, usually 6 weeks. Combination drug treatment using vancomycin, rifampin, and gentamicin is employed to treat these resistant infections.

Surgery

Some clients with infective endocarditis require surgical intervention to

- Replace severely damaged valves.
- Remove large vegetations at risk for embolization
- Remove a valve that is a continuing source of infection that does not respond to antibiotic therapy.

The most common indication for surgery is valvular regurgitation that causes heart failure and does not respond to medical therapy. When the infection has not responded to antibiotic therapy within 7 to 10 days, the infected valve may be replaced to facilitate eradication of the organism. Clients with fungal endocarditis usually require surgical intervention (Tierney et al., 1994). More information on valve replacement surgery is provided in the section on valve disorders.

Nursing Care

Nursing care of the client with infective endocarditis focuses on managing its manifestations, administering antibiotics, and educating the client and family members. Any organ system may be affected by complications of infective endocarditis; preventing and identifying these complications promptly if they occur is also a nursing priority. Selected nursing diagnoses in this section relate to the presence of an infectious process and potential embolic complications.

Risk for Altered Body Temperature

Fever is a common presenting complaint in the client with infective endocarditis. It may be acutely elevated and accompanied by chills, particularly with acute infective endocarditis. The inflammatory process initiates a cycle of events that affects the regulation of temperature and causes discomfort.

Selected nursing interventions with rationales follow:

- Record the client's temperature every 2 to 4 hours. Notify physician if the temperature rises above 101.5 F (39.4 C). Assess the client for complaints of discomfort. *Fever is usually low grade (below 101.5 F [39.4 C]) in clients with infective endocarditis; higher temperatures may cause discomfort. Most clients regain normal body temperature within 1 week after antibiotic therapy is initiated; continuing temperature elevation may indicate a need to modify the treatment regimen.*
- Obtain blood cultures as ordered, before giving the first dose of antibiotics. Explain to the client the procedure and rationale for the test. *Blood cultures identify the causative organism in 95% of the cases and thus facilitate the initiation of specific drug regimens to eliminate the cause. Initial blood cultures must be obtained before antibi-*

otic therapy is started to obtain an adequate number of organisms to culture and identify. Follow-up cultures are used to assess the effectiveness of therapy.

- Administer anti-inflammatory or antipyretic agents as prescribed. *Fever may be treated with the administration of anti-inflammatory agents, such as aspirin, or antipyretic medications, such as acetaminophen.*
- Administer antibiotics as ordered; obtain peak and trough drug levels as indicated. *Intravenous antibiotics are given for 2 to 6 weeks to eradicate the pathogen. Peak and trough levels are used to evaluate the appropriateness of the prescribed dose in maintaining a therapeutic blood level.*

Risk for Altered Tissue Perfusion

Potential embolization of vegetative lesions can threaten vascular and organ tissue perfusion. Vegetations from the left heart may lodge in arterioles or capillaries of the brain, kidneys, or peripheral tissues, causing infarction or abscess. If the embolism is large, the client may demonstrate manifestations of a stroke or transient ischemic attack, renal failure, or tissue ischemia. Emboli from the right side of the heart become entrapped in the pulmonary vasculature, and the client may have evidence of a pulmonary embolism.

Selected nursing intervention with rationales follow:

- Assess for and document any manifestations of decreased perfusion to major organ systems:
  a. Neurologic system: changes in level of consciousness, complaints of numbness or tingling in extremities, hemiplegia, visual disturbances, or manifestations of cerebral vascular accident
  b. Renal system: decreased urine output, hematuria, elevated BUN or creatinine
  c. Pulmonary system: dyspnea, hemoptysis, shortness of breath, diminished breath sounds, restlessness, sudden chest or shoulder pain
  d. Cardiovascular: complaints of chest pain radiating to jaw or arms, tachycardia, anxiety, tachypnea, hypotension

  All major organ systems, tissues, and the microcirculation are at risk for embolization by vegetations that may break off if subjected to turbulent blood flow (Handerhan, 1991). Embolization is suspected when manifestations of organ dysfunction are evident. The most common embolic site is the brain, causing neurologic dysfunction in up to 31% of clients (Trausch, 1988). Intravenous drug users have a high risk of pulmonary emboli as a result of right-sided endocardial fragments.

- Assess and document skin color and temperature, quality of peripheral pulses, and capillary refill. *Assessment of peripheral tissue perfusion is important to reduce the risk of tissue necrosis and possible extremity loss.*

Teaching Plan: Preventing Infective Endocarditis

■ ■ ■

- Instruct the client and family about the function of the heart valves and the effects of endocarditis on heart function. Include a simple definition of endocarditis, and explain why the client is at risk for its development or recurrence. Have the client repeat manifestations of endocarditis that should be reported to the physician. *Information, in simple terms, provided to both the client and family helps them understand the disease and the reasons for interventions or life-style changes that they may be required to make. Understanding increases compliance. Recognition of manifestations facilitates early diagnosis and prevention of complications.*

- Stress the importance of notifying care providers of valve disease, heart murmur, or valve replacement before undergoing invasive procedures. *Invasive procedures provide a portal of entry for bacteria. Clients with a history of valve disease are at risk for the development or recurrence of endocarditis.*

- Encourage good dental hygiene and mouth care and regular dental checkups. Teach the client how to prevent bleeding from the gums and avoid developing mouth ulcers (e.g., gentle toothbrushing, ensuring that dentures fit properly, and avoiding toothpicks, dental floss, and high-flow water devices).

The oropharynx harbors streptococci, which are common causes of endocarditis. Bleeding gums offer an opportunity for bacteria to enter the bloodstream.

- Encourage the client to avoid people with upper respiratory infections. *Streptococci are normal pathogens in the upper respiratory tract; exposure to people with upper respiratory infections may increase the risk of infection.*

- Explain the indications, actions, proper administration, and major side effects of anticoagulant therapy. Be sure to have the client list manifestations of bleeding and notify the physician immediately should these occur. *Clients with valve disease or a prosthetic valve following infective endocarditis may require continued anticoagulation therapy to prevent thrombi and emboli. They must have good knowledge of the reasons for anticoagulation, the implications of stopping medication, and manifestations of excessive bleeding.*

- Describe the manifestations of heart failure. *Evidence of heart failure may indicate the need to replace diseased valves or modify the client's medication regimen to manage its effect.*

Other Nursing Diagnoses

Examples of other nursing diagnoses appropriate for the client with infective endocarditis follow:

- *Knowledge Deficit* regarding measures to prevent recurrence of disease
- *Activity Intolerance* related to altered cardiac blood flow and the presence of infection
- *Altered Protection* related to deformed valve structures
- *Risk for Decreased Cardiac Output* related to incompetent cardiac valves
- *Altered Nutrition: Less Than Body Requirements* related to hypermetabolic infective process and tissue needs for healing
- *Diversional Activity Deficit* related to activity restrictions

Client and Family Teaching

The client with infective endocarditis needs education and support throughout the course of the disease, as well as teaching to prevent future recurrences. In basic terms, teach the client what is happening in the heart and the reasons for the disease manifestations. Emphasize that infective endocarditis, although serious and frightening, can usually be treated effectively with intravenous antibiotics. Stress the importance of promptly reporting any unusual manifestation, such as a change in vision, sudden pain, or weakness, so that interventions to control complications can be promptly implemented. Explain the rationale for all treatments and procedures, including activity restrictions, to the client and family to reduce anxiety and enhance cooperation.

Client and family education is also extremely important to prevent recurrences of infective endocarditis. The accompanying box outlines a teaching plan for clients at risk.

Clients who contract infective endocarditis as a result of intravenous drug use require additional teaching about the risks associated with the intravenous injection of drugs. Refer the client and family members or significant others as appropriate to a drug or substance abuse treatment program or facility. Provide follow-up care to ensure that the client complies with the referral and treatment plan.

Educational materials on infective endocarditis are available to consumers from the American Heart Association.

The Client with Myocarditis

■ ■ ■

Myocarditis is an inflammatory disorder of the heart muscle that may be initiated by infection (viral, bacterial, protozoal), an immunologic response, or the effects of radiation, chemical poisons, drugs, or burns (Thomas, 1994; Wynne & Braunwald, 1994). In the United States, myocarditis is usually infectious, caused by a Coxsackie B enterovirus infection (Wynne & Braunwald, 1994). Bacterial infections, much less common, may involve *Staphylococcus, Streptococcus,* and *Diphtheria* pathogens; parasitic infections may be caused by *Trypanosoma cruzi* and *toxoplasmosis.*

Myocarditis may occur at any age, and it is more common in men than women. Immunosuppressed clients are at risk. Several factors that alter immune response—such as malnutrition, alcohol use, immunosuppressive drug therapy (steroids, transplant antirejection drugs), ionizing radiation, stress, and advanced age—may predispose the client to the risk of myocarditis. Myocarditis is a common complication of rheumatic fever and pericarditis. It may occur as an acute or chronic disease. Clients suffering from acute viral myocarditis typically recover without consequences; however, recurrences may cause the disorder to become chronic (Wynne & Braunwald, 1994).

Pathophysiology

The basic mechanism of myocardial injury in myocarditis is an inflammatory process that causes local or diffuse swelling and damage to the cells of the myocardium. Infectious agents infiltrate interstitial tissues, forming abscesses. Autoimmune injury may occur when the immune system destroys not only the invading pathogen but also myocardial cells. The extent of damage to cardiac muscle ultimately determines the long-term outcome of the disease. Although many cases resolve spontaneously, severe disease may cause progressive deterioration in heart function and develop into dilated cardiomyopathy (Tierney et al., 1994).

Clinical manifestations depend on the degree of myocardial damage and resulting compensation. The client may be asymptomatic. Nonspecific manifestations of inflammation present as fever, fatigue, general malaise, dyspnea, palpitations, and arthralgias. Often the client presents with a history of a nonspecific febrile illness or upper respiratory infection and manifestations of heart failure, including tachycardia, dysrhythmias, and a gallop with an S_3 and S_4. A systolic murmur, cardiomegaly, and transient ECG abnormalities may be noted (Underhill & McGregor, 1989; Wynne & Braunwald, 1994).

Collaborative Care

Care for the client with myocarditis is directed toward establishing an accurate diagnosis and treating the inflammatory process to prevent further damage to the myocardium.

In addition to the client's history and physical examination, laborabory and diagnostic studies may be ordered to help diagnose myocarditis. Serologic testing to identify viral antigen or antibodies to specific antigens is useful. Studies of serum immunoglobulins can also help determine the stage of the disease; immunoglobulin G antibody titers peak after the first month (Porth, 1994). Echocardiography is used to evaluate cardiac function and rule out other disease processes. Myocardial biopsy provides the definitive diagnosis of myocarditis; patchy cell necrosis and the inflammatory process can be identified in tissue samples.

Once the infecting organism has been identified, antimicrobial therapy is instituted. Immunosupressive therapy with corticosteroids or other immunosuppressive agents (see Chapter 8) may be initiated to minimize the inflammatory response, particularly in clients with chronic myocarditis. Repeated myocardial biopsies are used to evaluate the client's response to therapy. Treatment of the client with myocarditis may include antipyretic medications for fever, antidysrhythmic agents as needed to treat dysrhythmias, anticoagulation therapy to prevent emboli, and digoxin to manage manifestations of heart failure.

Bed rest and activity restrictions are required during the acute inflammatory process to reduce myocardial work. Oxygen is administered to increase oxygen supply in clients with signs of cardiac dysfunction.

Nursing Care

Nursing care is directed at decreasing myocardial work and increasing oxygen supply. Clients are encouraged to maintain strict bed rest to reduce physical activity. Emotional rest also is indicated, because anxiety increases myocardial oxygen demand. Hemodynamic and electrocardiographic parameters are followed closely, especially during the acute phase of the illness. Clients experiencing congestive heart failure follow the typical treatment regimen of diuretic and positive inotropic therapy and diet modifications. Consider the following nursing diagnoses for the client with myocarditis:

- *Activity Intolerance* related to impaired cardiac muscle function
- *Decreased Cardiac Output* related to inflammatory process involving heart muscle
- *Fatigue* related to the inflammatory process and inadequate cardiac output
- *Anxiety* related to possible long-term consequences of the disorder
- *Fluid Volume Excess* related to compensatory mechanisms for decreased cardiac output

Client and Family Teaching

Explain all procedures, tests, and treatments, and provide information regarding the client's progress to decrease anxiety and cardiac workload. Teach the client and family members about early manifestations of heart failure to report to the physician for appropriate intervention. Stress the importance of following the prescribed treatment regimen, including activity restrictions, any recommended dietary modifications (such as a low-sodium diet if signs of heart failure are present), and medications. Emphasize that although most clients recover fully from myocarditis, adherence to the treatment plan can reduce the risk of significant long-term consequences, such as cardiomyopathy.

The Client with Pericarditis

■ ■ ■

The pericardium is the outermost layer of the heart. It is a two-layered membranous sac with a thin layer of serous fluid (normally no more than 30 to 50 mL) separating the layers. Its role is to protect and cushion the heart and the great vessels; it functions as a barrier to infectious processes in adjacent structures, prevents displacement of the myocardium and blood vessels, and prevents sudden distention of the heart (Braunwald, 1994c).

Pericarditis is the inflammation of the pericardium. Pericarditis may develop as a primary disorder or secondarily to another disease affecting the heart or surrounding structures or to a disorder with systemic effects. Some possible causes of pericarditis are listed in the accompanying box. Acute pericarditis is usually viral in origin and affects men (usually under the age of 50) more frequently than women (Tierney et al., 1994). Pericarditis is a frequent complication of uremia, affecting 40% to 50% of clients with end-stage renal disease. Post–myocardial infarction pericarditis and postcardiotomy (following open heart surgery) pericarditis are common forms of the disease.

Possible Causes of Pericarditis

■ ■ ■

Infectious Causes

- Viruses
- Bacteria
- Tuberculosis
- Fungi
- Syphilis
- Parasites

Noninfectious Causes

- Myocardial and pericardial injury
- Uremia
- Neoplasms
- Radiation
- Trauma or surgery
- Myxedema
- Autoimmune disorders
- Rheumatic fever
- Connective tissue diseases
- Prescription and non-prescription drugs
- Postcardiac injury

Pathophysiology

Pericardial tissue damage triggers an inflammatory response. Inflammatory mediators released from the injured tissue cause vasodilation, hyperemia, and edema. Capillary permeability increases, allowing plasma proteins, including fibrinogen, to escape into the pericardial space. White blood cells amass at the site of injury to destroy the causative agent. Exudate is formed, usually fibrinous or serofibrinous (a mixture of serous fluid and fibrinous exudate). In some cases, the exudate may contain red blood cells or, if infectious, purulent material. The inflammatory process may resolve without long-term consequences, or scar tissue and adhesions may form between the pericardial layers (Porth, 1994).

Fibrosis and scarring of the pericardium may restrict the heart's ability to function effectively. Pericardial effusions result from the production of a serous or purulent exudate (depending on the causative agent) and may plague the client on a recurrent basis. Chronic inflammation causes the pericardium to become rigid.

Classic manifestations of acute pericarditis include chest pain, a pericardial friction rub, and fever. Chest pain with an abrupt onset is the most frequent manifestation of pericarditis. It is caused by inflammation of nerve fibers in the lower parietal pericardium and diaphragmatic pleura. It is usually sharp and may radiate to the back or neck. The client may characterize the pain as steady or intermittent. Because the pain can mimic myocardial ischemia, careful assessment is necessary to rule out myocardial infarction. Pericardial pain is aggravated by

Clinical Manifestations of Cardiac Tamponade

- Paradoxical pulse
- Narrowing pulse pressure
- Tachycardia
- Weak peripheral pulses
- Distant, muffled heart sounds
- Jugular venous distention
- High central venous pressure
- Change in level of consciousness
- Low urine output
- Cool, mottled skin
- Hypotension
- Sudden decrease in chest tube drainage (after cardiac surgery)

respiratory movements (i.e., deep inspiration and/or coughing), changes in body position, or swallowing (Goldman & Braunwald, 1994). The client characteristically assumes an upright position and leans forward, which moves the heart away from the diaphragmatic side of the lung pleura and lessens the client's discomfort (Goldman & Braunwald, 1994).

Although not always present, a *pericardial friction rub* is the most characteristic sign of pericarditis. Heard most clearly in the left lower sternal border with the client sitting up or leaning forward, a pericardial friction rub is a leathery, grating sound produced by the inflamed pericardial layers rubbing against the chest wall or pleura. The rub is usually heard on expiration and may be constant, or it may disappear and then reappear hours later. In the event of a large pericardial effusion, heart sounds may be muffled.

A low-grade fever (below 100 F [38.4 C]) is often present because of the inflammatory process. Dyspnea is a common manifestation, as is tachycardia.

Pericardial effusion, cardiac tamponade, and constrictive pericarditis are possible complications of acute pericarditis. An acute pericardial effusion that develops rapidly may lead to cardiac tamponade, a potentially fatal complication that constitutes a medical emergency.

Pericardial Effusion

A *pericardial effusion* is an abnormal collection of fluid between the pericardial layers that threatens normal cardiac function. The fluid may consist of pus, blood, serum, lymph, or a combination (Thomas, 1994). The manifes-

tations of a pericardial effusion depend on the rate at which the fluid collects. Although the normal amount of fluid in the pericardium ranges from about 30 to 50 mL, the relative elasticity of the sac enables it to adjust to a gradual accumulation of fluid. Over a period of time, the pericardial sac may accommodate a buildup of up to 2 liters of fluid without immediate adverse effects (Braunwald, 1994c). Conversely, a rapid buildup of pericardial fluid (as little as 100 mL) does not allow the sac to stretch and can compress the heart, interfering with myocardial function. This compression of the heart is known as cardiac tamponade. Slowly developing pericardial effusion is often painless and has few manifestations. Heart sounds may be distant or muffled. The client may have a cough or mild dyspnea.

Cardiac Tamponade

Cardiac tamponade is a medical emergency that proves fatal if it is not aggressively treated. Cardiac tamponade may result from pericardial effusion, trauma, cardiac rupture, or hemorrhage. Rapid collection of fluid in the pericardial sac interferes with ventricular filling and pumping, causing a critical reduction in cardiac output.

Classic manifestations of cardiac tamponade result from rising intracardiac pressures, decreased diastolic filling time, and decreased cardiac output. A hallmark of cardiac tamponade is a paradoxical pulse, or *pulsus paradoxus,* in which the pulse markedly decreases in amplitude during inspiration. Intrathoracic pressure normally drops during inspiration, enhancing venous return to the right heart. This draws more blood into the right side of the heart than the left, causing the interventricular septum to bulge slightly into the left ventricle. When ventricular filling is impaired by fluid collected within the pericardial sac, this bulging of the interventricular septum causes cardiac output to fall during the inspiratory phase of the respiratory cycle. On palpation of the carotid or femoral artery, the pulse is either diminished or absent during inspiration in pulsus paradoxus. A drop in systolic blood pressure of more than 10 mm Hg during inspirations also indicates pulsus paradoxus.

Other clinical manifestations of cardiac tamponade include muffled heart sounds, dyspnea and tachypnea, tachycardia, and a narrowed pulse pressure. Clinical manifestations of cardiac tamponade are listed in the accompanying box.

Chronic Constrictive Pericarditis

Chronic pericardial inflammation can lead to the formation of scar tissue between the pericardial layers. This scar tissue eventually contracts, restricting diastolic filling and causing chronically elevated venous pressures. Constrictive pericarditis may follow viral infection, radiation therapy, or heart surgery. Usual manifestations of constrictive pericarditis include progressive dyspnea, fatigue, and weakness. Ascites is a common development; peripheral edema may also be present. Neck vein distention is often prominent and may be particularly noticeable during inspiration, a finding known as *Kussmaul's sign.* This occurs because the right atrium is unable to dilate to accommodate increased venous return during inspiration.

Collaborative Care

Management of the client with pericarditis focuses on identifying the cause of inflammation if possible, reducing the inflammatory response, relieving the client's symptoms, and preventing complications. It is vital that the health care team monitor the client closely for early manifestations of cardiac tamponade so that it can be treated promptly.

Laboratory and Diagnositic Tests

The diagnosis of acute pericarditis is often established by the client's clinical presentation. There are no specific laboratory tests to diagnose pericarditis, but tests are often performed to differentiate pericarditis from myocardial infarction. Leukocytosis (elevated WBC count) and an elevated erythrocyte sedimentation rate of more than 20 mm/h indicate an acute inflammatory process. Cardiac enzymes may also be slightly elevated because the inflammatory process extends to involve the epicardial surface of the heart. Cardiac enzymes are typically much less elevated in pericarditis than in myocardial infarction, however. Serologic studies and antibody titers may also be ordered to identify a causative organism if one is present.

The following diagnostic tests may be conducted:

- *Electrocardiography* is used to identify typical changes associated with pericarditis and help differentiate this disorder from a myocardial infarction. Acute pericarditis often produces diffuse ST segment elevation in all leads, which resolves more quickly than that associated with acute MI and is not associated with other changes in the QRS complex or T wave that are typically seen in MI. In the event of a large pericardial effusion, the QRS voltage may be decreased across the leads. Atrial dysrhythmias may also be noted in acute pericarditis.

- *Echocardiography* is used to assess the presence and location of any pericardial effusions, as well as heart motion and the extent of restriction.

- *Hemodynamic monitoring* may be employed for the client with acute pericarditis or pericardial effusion to assess pressures and cardiac output. Elevations in pulmonary artery pressures and right and left heart pressures may indicate impaired filling due to pericardial effusion or constrictive pericarditis.

- *Chest X-ray* may show cardiac enlargement if a pericardial effusion is present.

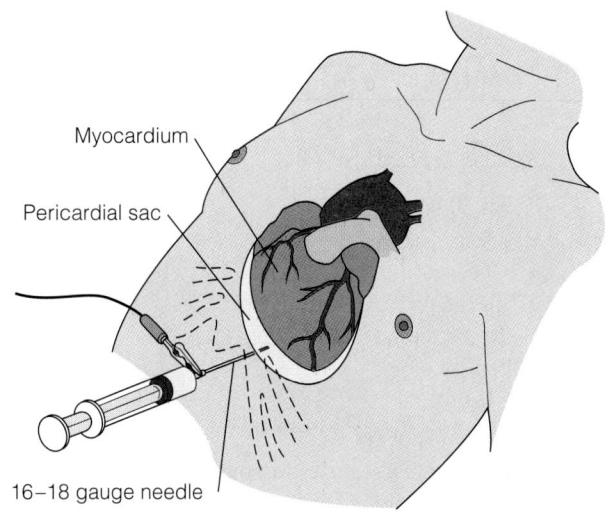

Figure 28–31   Pericardiocentesis.

- *Computed tomography (CT scan)* or *magnetic resonance imaging (MRI)* may also be used to identify pericardial effusions or the pericardial thickening characteristic of constrictive pericarditis.

Pharmacology

Pharmacologic management of the client with pericarditis usually addresses the manifestations of the disorder. Aspirin and acetaminophen may be used to reduce fever. Nonsteroidal anti-inflammatory drugs (NSAIDs) are used to reduce the inflammatory process and promote comfort. In severe cases or with recurrent pericarditis, the client may require corticosteroids to suppress the inflammatory response.

Pericardiocentesis

Pericardiocentesis is a procedure used to remove fluid from the pericardial sac for diagnostic or therapeutic purposes (Figure 28–31). The physician inserts a large (16- to 18-gauge) needle to the left of the xiphoid process into the pericardial sac and withdraws excess fluid. The needle is attached to an electrocardiographic monitoring lead to enable the physician to determine whether the needle is touching the epicardial surface; this helps prevent piercing the myocardium. Pericardiocentesis may be performed as an emergency procedure for the client with cardiac tamponade. Nursing implications for the client undergoing pericardiocentesis are outlined in the box on page 1156.

Surgery

For clients with recurrent pericarditis or recurrent pericardial effusion, a rectangular piece of the pericardium, or "window," may be excised to allow collected fluid to drain

Nursing Implications for Pericardiocentesis

Before the Procedure

- Gather all supplies:
  a. Pericardiocentesis tray
  b. ECG machine and electrode patches
  c. Emergency cart with defibrillator
  d. Chest tube bottle/drainage kit
  e. Towel
  f. Dressing kit
  g. Culture bottles (if indicated)
- Reinforce the physician's explanation of the procedure to the client to reduce anxiety. Answer any questions the client may have about the procedure or the associated care. Provide emotional support.
- Ensure that the client has signed an informed consent.
- Provide for the client's privacy.
- Obtain and document baseline vital signs.
- Ensure that the portable ECG monitor and the emergency cart is charged and operational; turn it on, and place it at the bedside.
- Place the ECG electrodes on the client and connect to the monitor; obtain a baseline rhythm strip for comparison during and after the procedure.
- Connect the precordial ECG lead to the hub of the aspiration needle using an alligator clamp. Observe the ST segment for elevation and the ECG monitor for signs of myocardial irritability (PVCs) during the procedure; these indicate that the needle is touching the myocardium and should be withdrawn slightly.
- Administer oxygen as ordered.

Procedure

- Follow universal precautions.
- Position the client at a 45- to 60-degree angle. Place a dry towel under the rib cage to catch leakage of blood or fluid.
- Assist the physician with the aspiration.
- If a chest tube is inserted during the procedure, ensure that the site is covered with an occlusive dressing and that the chest tube drainage device is secure (see Chapter 34 for more information about chest tubes).
- Monitor for and notify the physician of changes in cardiac rhythm, blood pressure, heart rate, level of consciousness, and urine output. These may indicate cardiac complications.
- Monitor central venous pressure (CVP) and blood pressure closely. As the effusion is relieved, CVP will decrease, and BP will increase.

After the Procedure

- Document the procedure and the client's response to and tolerance of the procedure.
- Continue to monitor the client's vital signs and cardiac rhythm frequently (i.e., every 15 min during the first hour, every 30 min during the next hour, every hour for the next 24 hours).
- Record the total amount of fluid removed as output on the intake and output record.
- If indicated, send a sample of the aspirated fluid for culture and sensitivity and laboratory analysis.
- Assess heart and breath sounds.

into the pleural space. The client with constrictive pericarditis may require a partial or total *pericardiectomy,* removal of part or all of the pericardium, to relieve the compression of the heart and allow it to fill adequately. Surgical resection of the pericardium is recommended in the early stages of constrictive pericarditis; clients with advanced disease have the highest mortality risk, which ranges from 7% to 15% (Braunwald, 1994c).

Nursing Care

Nursing care for the client with pericarditis generally is supportive. Although it is uncomfortable and causes anxiety, acute pericarditis is usually a self-limiting process that will resolve with or without treatment. However, close observation of the client is important to detect early manifestations of increasing effusion or cardiac tamponade. Priority nursing diagnoses for the client with acute pericarditis are related to providing comfort, reducing the risk for tamponade, and facilitating activity restrictions imposed by the acute inflammatory process.

Pain

Inflamed pericardial layers rubbing against each other and the lung pleura stimulate phrenic nerve pain fibers in the lower portion of the parietal pericardium. Pain is usually acute in onset and may be severe until the inflammatory process is resolved.

Nursing interventions with rationales follow:

- Assess the client's complaints of chest pain using a rating scale of 0 to 10 and noting the quality and radiation of the pain. Ask the client about factors that aggravate or relieve the pain. Note nonverbal cues of pain (grimacing, guarding behaviors), and validate them with the client. *Any complaint of chest pain should be assessed to determine its cause. Clients with acute pericarditis typically complain of severe pain that may radiate to the neck or back and is aggravated by movement, coughing, or deep breathing. The pain scale allows the nurse to evaluate the intensity of the client's pain before and after treatment and thereby measure objectively the effectiveness of medication or other interventions.*

- Auscultate heart sounds every 4 hours. *Auscultation of the heart may reveal a pericardial friction rub indicating pericardial inflammation. This often correlates with the location and severity of the pain, although absense of a friction rub does not mean that the client is (or should be) pain free.*

- Administer NSAIDs on a regular basis as prescribed with food. Document effectiveness within 1 hour after administration. *NSAIDs are the drugs of choice to reduce fever, inflammation, and pericardial pain. They are most effective when administered around the clock on a consistent basis. Administering the medications with food helps decrease potential gastrointestinal discomforts.*

- Provide supportive measures: Maintain a quiet, calm environment, and provide position changes, back rubs, heat/cold therapy, diversional activity, and emotional support. *Supportive interventions can enhance the effects of the medication. These measures may decrease the client's perception of pain and convey a sense of caring.*

Ineffective Breathing Pattern

Respiratory movement intensifies pericardial pain. The client, in an effort to decrease the pain, often breathes shallowly to minimize chest movement. Pulmonary complications may arise as a result.

Nursing interventions with rationales follow:

- Assess and document the client's respiratory rate and effort, and auscultate breath sounds every 4 hours. Note and report the presence of adventitious sounds or areas of diminished breath sounds. *Pain associated with respiratory movement may cause the client to increase respiratory rate and effort to compensate for decreased respiratory depth. Breath sounds are monitored for signs of congestion or atelectasis, which may result from decreased ventilation of peripheral alveoli.*

- Assess the client for depth of respirations every 2 hours. Help the client breathe deeply and use the incentive spirometer. Provide pain medication for the client at least 30 minutes before respiratory therapy treatments, as needed. *Deep breathing and the incentive spirometer help ensure adequate alveolar ventilation and prevent atelectasis. Providing analgesia prior to painful treatments promotes comfort and facilitates the client's participation.*

- Administer oxygen as needed. *Supplementary oxygen promotes optimal gas exchange and tissue oxygenation.*

- Elevate head of the bed to Fowler's or high-Fowler's position. Assist the client to assume a position of comfort. *Appropriate positioning reduces the work of breathing and decreases chest pain due to pericarditis.*

Risk for Decreased Cardiac Output

The acute inflammatory process of pericarditis carries the risk of significant pericardial effusion and cardiac tamponade. This potentially fatal complication can also occur in clients with a chronic pericardial effusion if the amount of collected fluid exceeds the pericardial sac's ability to expand. The client with constrictive pericarditis is at risk for decreased cardiac output because of restricted cardiac filling.

Nursing interventions with rationales follow:

- Assess and document vital signs every hour during acute inflammatory processes. *Frequent assessment allows early identification of manifestations of decreased cardiac output, such as tachycardia, hypotension, or changes in pulse pressure.*

- Assess heart sounds and peripheral pulses, and observe for neck vein distention and pulsus paradoxus every hour. Notify the physician of the presence of distant, muffled heart sounds, new murmurs or extra heart sounds, decreasing quality of peripheral pulses, and distended neck veins. *Acute pericardial effusion interferes with normal cardiac filling and pumping, causing signs of venous congestion and decreased cardiac output. The heart is enveloped as the amount of fluid increases in the pericardial sac; as a result, heart sounds diminish. Alterations in systolic blood pressure of more than 10 mm Hg on inspiration signify an abnormal response to changes in intrathoracic pressure.*

- Observe and document changes in trends of hemodynamic parameters and rhythm disturbances. Notify physician of changes. *Compression of the heart interferes with venous return, increasing CVP and right atrial pressures; dysrhythmias may also occur.*

- Document and notify physician of other signs of decreased cardiac output: changes in level of consciousness; decreased urine output; cold, clammy, mottled skin; delayed capillary refill; and weak peripheral pulses. *These signs of decreased organ and tissue perfusion indicate a significant drop in cardiac output.*

- Ensure that at least one intravenous access line is established, and maintain its patency. *The precarious nature of the client with an acute cardiac tamponade necessitates the establishment and maintenance of intravenous access lines (preferably with a large-bore catheter) to restore fluid volume and administer emergency drugs to support the circulation.*

- If emergency pericardiocentesis and/or surgery is needed to evacuate pericardial fluid, prepare the client for the procedure, providing appropriate explanations and reassurance. Observe the client during the pericardiocentesis procedure for adverse effects. *Excess fluid amassed around the heart must be evacuated as soon as possible to prevent further compromise of cardiac output and death. Emotional support and explanations reduce the client's and family's anxiety and promote a caring atmosphere.*

Activity Intolerance

In chronic constrictive pericarditis, pericardial adhesions and scarring cause the pericardium to become rigid, restricting heart filling and movement. Restricted filling and ineffective cardiac contraction decrease the cardiac output. The client is uanable to compensate for increased metabolic demands by increasing cardiac output, and cardiac reserve falls significantly.

Nursing interventions with rationales follow:

- Assess and document the client's vital signs, cardiac rhythm, skin color, and temperature before and after activity. Also note any subjective complaints of fatigue, shortness of breath, chest pain, palpitations, or other evidence of activity intolerance. *Changes in these parameters from baseline help determine the client's response to increased cardiac work. Activity intolerance is manifested by an increase in heart rate, respirations, and respiratory effort, by a decrease in blood pressure, and by dysrhythmias. Pallor or cyanosis and cool, clammy, mottled skin are signs of decreased tissue perfusion. Complaints of weakness, shortness of breath, fatigue, dizziness, or palpitations are further evidence of activity intolerance.*

- Collaborate with the client and the physical therapist to develop a realistic, progressive activity plan. Monitor the client's response. Encourage the client to perform ADLs independently, but provide assistance as needed. *Client involvement in the planning process increases the likelihood of success and the client's sense of self-esteem and control. Promoting self-care activities gives the client additional control and independence and enhances self-image. Any activity that causes a significant increase in heart rate (of more than 20 BPM over resting HR) should be stopped and reassessed for intensity (Muirhead, 1989).*

- Plan interventions and care activities to allow the client uninterrupted rest and sleeping periods. *This supports the healing process and restoration of physical and emotional health.*

Other Nursing Diagnoses

Other nursing diagnoses that may be applicable to the client with pericarditis follow:

- *Knowledge Deficit* regarding pericardiocentesis procedure
- *Fear* related to chest pain
- *Self-Care Deficit* related to pain and decreased activity tolerance

Client and Family Teaching

During the period of acute inflammation and care, teaching of the client and family is related primarily to diagnostic and treatment procedures, activity restrictions, and explanation of the inflammatory process and how it relates to the manifestations experienced by the client. This teaching is vital to reduce anxiety and promote cooperation. Explain the rationale for frequent assessment of the client, providing reassurance that cardiac tamponade is an infrequent complication of acute pericarditis and is readily treatable when detected early. If pericardiocentesis is required, explain the procedure in simple terms to the client and family, answering questions and clarifying information as needed to reduce fear.

On discharge, stress the importance of continuing anti-inflammatory medications as ordered. Teach the client about prescribed medications, including dose, desired and possible adverse effects, and interactions with other drugs or food. Instruct the client to take anti-inflammatory medications with food, milk, or antacids to minimize gastric distress, and to notify the physician if unable to tolerate the drug. Tell clients taking NSAIDs to monitor their weight at least weekly, because these drugs may cause fluid retention. Encourage the client to maintain a fluid intake of at least 2500 mL per day to minimize the risk of renal toxicity. Advise the client to avoid aspirin while taking other NSAIDs because it may interfere with their activity. Instruct the client to avoid over-the-counter preparations containing aspirin, as well.

If any activity restriction is ordered, teach the client about specific measures to maintain this restriction. Emphasize that activity will be gradually increased once the inflammatory process has resolved.

The client may be at risk for recurrence of pericarditis. Teach the client and family members about manifestations that may indicate recurrent pericarditis, and stress the importance of reporting these manifestations promptly to the physician.

Bibliography

■ ■ ■

American Association of Critical-Care Nurses (AACN). (1993). Evaluation of the effects of heparinized and nonheparinized flush solution on the patency of arterial pressure monitoring lines: The AACN thunder project. *American Journal of Critical Care, 2*(1), 3–15.

American College of Cardiology/American Heart Association (ACC/AHA). (1990). ACC/AHA guidelines for the early management of patients with acute myocardial infarction. *Circulation, 82*(2), 664–707.

American Heart Association (AHA). (1992). *1993 Heart & stroke facts statistics.* Dallas: Author.

American Heart Association (AHA). (1993). *Women and heart disease.* Dallas: Author.

American Heart Association (AHA). (1994). *Textbook of advanced cardiac life support.* Dallas: Author.

Anderson, U. K. (1987). Mitral valve prolapse: A diagnosis for primary nursing intervention. *Journal of Cardiovascular Nursing, 1*(3), 41–51.

Angelini, A., Basso, C., Grassi, G., Casarotto, D., & Thiene, G. (1994). Surgical pathology of valve disease in the elderly. *Aging/Clinical and Experimental Research, 6*(4), 225–237.

Aragon, D., & Martin, M. (1993, September). What you should know about thrombolytic therapy for acute MI. *American Journal of Nursing, 93*(9), 24–31.

Baas, L.S. (1991). Acute pericarditis. In P. L. Swearingen and J. H. Keen (Eds.), *Manual of critical care* (2nd ed.) (pp. 124–128). St. Louis: Mosby.

Bahr, R. D. (1994). Reducing time to therapy in AMI patients: The new paradigm. *American Journal of Emergency Medicine, 12*(4), 501–503.

Bashein, G., & Stephen, S.A. (1989). Electrical hazards in the cardiac care unit. In S. G. Underhill, S. L. Woods, E. S. S. Froelicher, & C. J. Halpenny (Eds.), *Cardiac nursing* (2nd ed.) (pp. 805–812). Philadelphia: Lippincott.

Baxendale, L. M. (1992, March). Pathophysiology of coronary artery disease. *Nursing Clinics of North America, 27*(1), 143–152.

Beattie, S. (1993). CABG surgery: The second time around. *American Journal of Nursing, 93*(8), 42–45.

Bell, P. E., & Diffee, G. T. (1991). Cardiopulmonary bypass: Principles, nursing implications. *AORN Journal, 53*(6), 1480–1496.

Berg, J. (1990). Assessing for pericarditis in the end-stage renal disease patient. *Dimensions of Critical Care Nursing, 9*(5), 266–271.

Berkow, R., & Fletcher, A. J. (Eds.). (1992). *The Merck manual of diagnosis and therapy* (16th ed.). Rahway, NJ: Merck Research Laboratories.

Bevans, M., & McLimore, E. (1992). Intracoronary stents: A new approach to coronary artery dilatation. *Journal of Cardiovascular Nursing, 7*(1), 34–49.

Bharati, S., & Lev, M. (1992). The pathologic changes in the conduction system beyond the age of ninety. *American Heart Journal, 124*(2), 486–496.

Bourassa, M.G., Gurné, O., Bangdiwala, S. I., Ghali, J. K., Young, J. B., Rousseasu, M., Johnstone, D. E., & Yusuf, S. (1993). Natural history and patterns of current practice in heart failure. *JACC, 22*(4-Supplement A), 14A–19A.

Brannon, F. J., Geyer, M. J., Foley, M. W., & Wolf, S. L. (1988). *Cardiac rehabilitation: Basic theory and application.* Philadelphia: F. A. Davis.

Braunwald, E. (1994a). Heart failure. In K. J. Isselbacher, E. Braunwald, J. D. Wilson, J. B. Martin, A. S. Fauci, & D. L. Kasper (Eds.), *Harrison's principles of internal medicine* (13th ed.) (pp. 998–1008). New York: McGraw-Hill.

Braunwald, E. (1994b). Valvular heart disease. In K. J. Isselbacher, E. Braunwald, J. D. Wilson, J. B. Martin, A. S. Fauci, & D. L. Kasper (Eds.), *Harrison's principles of internal medicine* (13th ed.) (pp. 1052–1065). New York: McGraw-Hill.

Braunwald, E. (1994c). Pericardial disease. In K. J. Isselbacher, E. Braunwald, J. D. Wilson, J. B. Martin, A. S. Fauci, & D. L. Kasper (Eds.), *Harrison's principles of internal medicine* (13th ed.) (pp. 1094–1101). New York: McGraw-Hill.

Bubien, R. S., Knotts, S. M., McLaughlin, S., & George, P. (1993, July). Radiofrequency ablation: What you need to know. *American Journal of Nursing, 93*(7), 30–37.

Bumgarner, L. I. (1992). Diagnostic uses of epicardial electrodes after cardiac surgery. *Progress in Cardiovascular Nursing, 7*(4), 21–24.

Burroughs Wellcome Co. (1994). *Neurohormonal activation—completing the picture of chronic heart failure* [Brochure]. Research Triangle Park, NC: Author.

Byers, J. F., & Goshorn, J. (1995, February). How to manage diuretic therapy. *American Journal of Nursing, 95*(2), 38–44.

Cameron, D. E., Trexler, S., & Cousar, C.D. (1994). Preoperative assessment. In W. A. Baumgartner, S. G. Owens, D. E. Cameron, & B. A. Reitz (Eds.), *The Johns Hopkins manual of cardiac surgical care* (pp. 5–26). St. Louis: Mosby.

Campbell, A., Caird, F. I., Jackson, T. F. M. (1974). Prevalence of abnormalities of electrocardiogram in old people. *British Heart Journal, 36,* 1005–1011.

Centers for Disease Control. (1991). *MMWR CDC Surveillance Summary, 40,* 1–24.

Centers for Disease Control. (1994, December 8). Advance report of final mortality statistics, 1992. *Monthly Vital Statistics Report, 43*(6), Supplement, 1–76.

Chernecky, C. C., Krech, R. L., and Berger, B. J. (1993). *Laboratory tests and diagnostic procedures.* Philadelphia: W. B. Saunders.

Christopherson, D. J., & Froelicher, E. S. S. (1989). Infective endocarditis. In S. G. Underhill, S. L. Woods, E. S. S. Froelicher, & C. J. Halpenny (Eds.), *Cardiac nursing* (2nd ed.) (pp. 934–943). Philadelphia: Lippincott.

Cochrane, B. B. (1995). Complications of acute myocardial infarction. In S. L. Woods, E. S. Froelicher, C. J. Halpenny, & S. U. Motzer (Eds.), *Cardiac nursing* (3rd ed.) (pp. 496–505). Philadelphia: Lippincott.

Coller, B. S. (1994). Current concepts of thrombosis. *Journal of Invasive Cardiology, 6*(8), 277–284.

Collins, M. A. (1994, March). When your patient has an implantable cardioverter defibrillator. *American Journal of Nursing, 94*(3), 34–39.

Coniglio, K. (1991). Cocaine-induced acute myocardial infarction. *Critical Care Nurse, 11*(2), 16–22.

Conn, V. S., Taylor, S. G., & Casey, B. (1992). Cardiac rehabilitation program participation and outcomes after myocardial infarction. *Rehabilitation Nursing, 17*(2), 58–62.

Conover, M. B. (1994). *Pocket guide to electrocardiography* (3rd ed.). St. Louis: Mosby.

Cowan, M. J. (1989). Pathogenesis of atherosclerosis. In S. G. Underhill, S. L. Woods, E. S. S. Froelicher, & C. J. Halpenny (Eds.), *Cardiac nursing* (2nd ed.) (pp. 184–193). Philadelphia: Lippincott.

Cox, J. K., Boineau, J. P., Schuessler, R. B., Ferguson, T. B., Cain, M. E., Lindsay, B. D., Corr, P. B., Kater, K. M., & Lappas, D. G. (1991). Operations for atrial fibrillation. *Clinical Cardiology, 14,* 827–834.

Crawford, M. V., & Spence, M. I. (1995). *Commonsense approach to coronary care* (6th ed.). St. Louis: Mosby.

Cunningham, S. (1992, March). The epidemiologic basis of coronary disease prevention. *Nursing Clinics of North America, 27*(1), 153–170.

Cuny, J., & Enger, E. L. (1993). Medical management of chronic heart failure: Direct-acting vasodilators and diuretic agents. *Critical Care Nursing Clinics of North America, 5*(4), 575–587.

Daily, E. K. , & Schroeder, J. P. (1989). *Techniques in bedside hemodynamic monitoring* (4th ed.). St. Louis: C. V. Mosby.

Darling, E. J. (1994). Overview of cardiac electrophysiology testing. *Critical Care Nursing Clinics of North America, 6*(1), 1–13.

Dennison, R.D. (1990). Understanding the four determinants of cardiac output. *Nursing90, 20*(7), 34–41.

Dimengo, J. M. (1993). Dynamic cardiomyoplasty and its use in patients with chronic heart failure. *Critical Care Nursing Clinics of North America, 5*(4), 627–634.

Doenges, M. E., Moorhouse, M. F., & Geissler, A. C. (1993). *Nursing care plans: Guidelines for planning and documenting patient care* (3rd ed.). Philadelphia: F. A. Davis.

Dougherty, A. H. (1992). Heart disease in women: An equal opportunity killer. *Houston Heart Bulletin, 12*(2).

Drew, B. (1992). Using cardiac leads: The right way. *Nursing92, 22*(5), 50–54.

Edwards, W. T. (1990). Optimizing opioid treatment of postoperative pain. *Journal of Pain and Symptom Management, 5*(1), 524–526.

Eichhorn, E. J. (1992). The paradox of *β*-adrenergic blockade for the management of congestive heart failure. *The American Journal of Medicine, 92*(5), 527–538.

Eichhorn, D. J. , Meyers, T. A. , & Guzzetta, C. E. (1995). Family presence during resuscitation: It is time to open the door. *Capsules and Comments in Critical Care Nursing, 3*(1), 8–13.

Elpern, E. H., Yellen, S. B., & Burton, L. A. (1993). A preliminary investigation of opinions and behaviors regarding advance directives for medical care. *American Journal of Critical Care, 2*(2), 161–167.

Estes, M. E. (1985). Management of the cardiac tamponade patient: A nursing framework. *Critical Care Nurse, 5*(5), 17–26.

Evans, S. A. (1993). The economics of cardiac surgery. *AACN Clinical Issues in Critical Care Nursing, 4*(2), 340–348.

Fair, J. M., & Burke, L. E. (1995). Cholesterol education. In S. L. Woods, E. S. S. Froelicher, C. J. Halpenny, & S. U. Motzer (Eds.), *Cardiac Nursing* (3rd ed.) (pp. 735–747). Philadelphia: Lippincott.

Finkelmeier, B. A. (1994). Ablative therapy in the treatment of tachyarrhythmias. *Critical Care Nursing Clinics of North America, 6*(1), 103–110.

Finkelmeier, B. A. (1995). *Cardiothoracic surgical nursing.* Philadelphia: Lippincott.

Fleg, J. L. (1986). Alterations in cardiovascular structure and function with advancing age. *American Journal of Cardiology, 57,* 33C–44C.

Fleg, J. L., & Kennedy, H. L. (1982). Cardiac arrhythmias in a healthy elderly population: Detection by 24-hour ambulatory electrocardiography. *Chest, 81*(3), 302–307.

Fleury, J. (1992, March). Long-term management of the patient with stable angina. *Nursing Clinics of North America, 27*(1), 201–230.

Flynn, J. B. (1993). Advanced cardiac life support. In J. B. Flynn & N. P. Bruce (Eds.), *Introduction to critical care skills* (pp. 235–260). St.Louis: Mosby.

Flynn, D. P., & Quinn, J. R. (1994). Mitral valvuloplasty for mitral stenosis during pregnancy: A case study. *Cardiovascular Nursing, 30*(3), 17–20.

Frantz, R. A., & Ferrell-Torry, A. (1993). Physical impairments in the elderly population. *Nursing Clinics of North America, 28*(2), 363–371.

Froelicher, E. S. S., & King, S. C. (1989). Exercise testing. In S. G. Underhill, S. L. Woods, E. S. S. Froelicher, & C. J. Halpenny (Eds.), *Cardiac nursing* (2nd ed.) (pp. 418–430). Philadelphia: Lippincott.

Fuentes, F., & Haynie, M. P. (1992). The practice of cardiovascular disease prevention. *Houston Heart Bulletin, 12*(1).

Futterman, L. G., & Lemberg, L. (1995). New indications for dual chamber pacing: hypertrophic and dilated cardiomyopathy. *American Journal of Critical Care, 4*(1), 82–87.

Gamberg, P., & Walton, K. (1990). Heart transplantation. In K. M. Sigardson-Poor & L. M. Haggerty, *Nursing care of the transplant recipient*. Philadelphia: W. B. Saunders.

Gardner, P. E., & Bridges, E. J. (1995). Hemodynamic monitoring. In S. L. Woods, E. S. S. Froelicher, C. J. Halpenny, & S. U. Motzer (Eds.), *Cardiac Nursing* (3rd ed.), (pp. 424–458). Philadelphia: Lippincott.

Gardner, R. M., & Hujcs, M. (1993). Fundamentals of physiologic monitoring. *AACN Clinical Issues in Critical Care Nursing, 4*(1), 11–24.

Garg, R., Packer, M., Pitt, B., & Yusuf, S. (1993). Heart failure in the 1990s: Evolution of a major public health problem in cardiovascular medicine. *JACC, 22*(4-Supplement A), 3A–5A.

Gawlinski, A., & Jensen, G. A. (1991). The complications of cardiovascular aging. *American Journal of Nursing, 91*(11), 26–31.

Gerstenblith, G., & Lakatta, E. G. (1990). Disorders of the heart. In W. R. Hazzard, R. Andres, E. L. Bierman, & J. P. Blass (Eds.). *Principles of geriatric medicine and gerontology* (2nd ed.) (pp. 466–475). New York: McGraw-Hill.

Gibson, R. K. (1991). Beta-receptor regulation: Dynamics of density and function throughout the cardiac cycle. *Journal of Cardiovascular Nursing, 5*(4), 49–56.

Goldman, L., & Braunwald, E. (1994). Chest discomfort and palpitation. In K. J. Isselbacher, E. Braunwald, J. D. Wilson, J. B. Martin, A.

S. Fauci, and D. L. Kasper (Eds.), *Harrison's principles of internal medicine* (13th ed.) (pp. 55–60). New York: McGraw-Hill.

Greene, H. L. (1990). Sudden arrhythmic cardiac death—mechanisms, resuscitation, and classification: The Seattle perspective. *American Journal of Cardiology, 65,* 4B.

Gregersen, R. A., & McGregor, M. S. (1989). Cardiac surgery. In S. G. Underhill, S. L. Woods, E. S. S. Froelicher, & C. J. Halpenny (Eds.), *Cardiac nursing* (2nd ed.) (pp. 537–560). Philadelphia: Lippincott.

Gruppo Italiano per lo Studio Della Streptochinasi nell' Infarcto Miocardico (GISSI). (1986). Effectiveness of intravenous thrombolytic treatment in acute myocardial infarction. *Lancet, 1,* 397–401.

Guidelines for cardiopulmonary resuscitation and emergency cardiac care. (1992). *Journal of the American Medical Association, 268*(16).

Gulanick, M., Klopp, A., Galanes, S., Gradisher, D., & Puzas, M. K. (1994). *Nursing care plans: Nursing diagnosis and intervention* (3rd ed.). St. Louis: Mosby.

Guyton, A. C. (1991). *Textbook of medical physiology* (8th ed.). Philadelphia: W. B. Saunders.

Handerhan, B. (1991). Staying alert for endocarditis. *Nursing91, 21*(7), 14–15.

Haskin, J. B. (1989). Pacemakers. In S. G. Underhill, S. L. Woods, E. S. S. Froelicher, & C. J. Halpenny (Eds.), *Cardiac nursing* (2nd ed.) (pp. 766–804). Philadelphia: Lippincott.

Henneman, E. A., & Cardin, S. (1992). Need for information: Interventions for practice. *Critical Care Nursing Clinics of North America, 4*(4), 615–621.

Hicks, S. L. (1994). Standing guard against silent ischemia and infarction. *Nursing94, 24*(1), 35–39.

Hine, L. K., Laird, N., Hewitt, P., & Chalmers, T. C. (1989). Meta-analytic evidence against prophylactic use of lidocaine in acute myocardial infarction. *Archives of Internal Medicine, 149*(12), 2694–2698.

Ho, K. K. L., Pinsky, J., Kannel, W. B., & Levy, D. (1993). The epidemiology of heart failure: The Framingham study. *JACC, 22*(4-Supplement A), 6A–13A.

Holloway, N. M. (1993). *Nursing the critically ill adult* (4th ed.). Redwood City, CA: Addison-Wesley Nursing.

Honan, M. B., Harrell, F. E., Reimer, K. A., Califf, R. M., Mark, D. B., Pryor, D. B., Hlatky, M. A. (1990). Cardiac rupture, mortality and the timing of thrombolytic therapy: A meta-analysis. *Journal of the American College of Cardiology, 16*(2), 359–367.

Horner, S. M. (1992). Efficacy of intravenous magnesium in acute myocardial infarction in reducing arrhythmias and mortality: Meta-analysis of magnesium in acute myocardial infarction. *Circulation, 86*(3), 774–779.

Howie, J. N. (1991). Hypothermia and rewarming after cardiac operation. *Focus on Critical Care, 18*(5), 414–418.

Huszar, R. J. (1994). *Basic dysrhythmia: Interpretation and management* (2nd ed.). St. Louis: Mosby Lifeline.

Imperial, F. A. (1993). Antiarrhythmic drugs. In *Deciphering difficult ECGs*. Springhouse, PA: Springhouse.

ISIS Steering Committee. (1987). Intravenous streptokinase given within 0–4 hours of onset of myocardial infarction reduced mortality in ISIS-2. *Lancet, 1,* 502.

Jansen, K. J., & McFadden, P. M. (1986). Postoperative nursing management in patients undergoing myocardial revascularization with the internal mammary artery bypass. *Heart & Lung, 15*(1), 48–54.

Jensen, S. K. (1995). Pathophysiology of myocardial ischemia and infarction. In S. L. Woods, E. S. S. Froelicher, C. J. Halpenny, & S. U. Motzer (Eds.), *Cardiac Nursing* (3rd ed.) (pp. 212–225). Philadelphia: Lippincott.

Kadota, L. T. (1989). Angioplasty. In S. G. Underhill, S. L. Woods, E. S. S. Froelicher, & C. J. Halpenny (Eds.), *Cardiac nursing* (2nd ed.) (pp. 532–536). Philadelphia: Lippincott.

Kahn, J. K. (1993). Caring for patients after coronary artery bypass surgery: Follow-up tips for primary care physicians. *Postgraduate Medicine, 93*(4).

Kaye, D. (1994). Infective endocarditis. In K. J. Isselbacher, E. Braunwald, J. D. Wilson, J. B. Martin, A. S. Fauci, & D. L. Kasper (Eds.), *Harrison's principles of internal medicine* (13th ed.) (pp. 520–525). New York: McGraw-Hill.

King, S. C., & Froelicher, E. S. S. (1989). Cardiac rehabilitation: Activity and exercise program. In S. G. Underhill, S. L. Woods, E. S. S. Froelicher, & C. J. Halpenny (Eds.), *Cardiac nursing* (2nd ed.) (pp. 739–756). Philadelphia: Lippincott.

Lakatta, E. G. (1994). Cardiovascular reserve capacity in healthy older humans. *Aging/ Clinical and Experimental Research, 6*(4), 213–223.

Laurent-Bopp, D. (1989). Cardiomyopathies and myocarditis. In S. G. Underhill, S. L. Woods, E. S. S. Froelicher, & C. J. Halpenny (Eds.), *Cardiac nursing* (2nd ed.) (pp. 924–933). Philadelphia: Lippincott.

Laurent-Bopp, D. (1995a). Cardiomyopathies and myocarditis. In S. L. Woods, E. S. S. Froelicher, C. J. Halpenny, & S. U. Motzer (Eds.), *Cardiac nursing* (3rd ed.) (pp. 842–851). Philadelphia: Lippincott.

Laurent-Bopp, D. (1995b). Heart failure. In S. L. Woods, E. S. S. Froelicher, C. J. Halpenny, & S. U. Motzer (Eds.), *Cardiac nursing* (3rd ed.) (pp. 555–571). Philadelphia: Lippincott.

LeDoux, D. (1995). Acquired valvular heart disease. In S. L. Woods, E. S. S. Froelicher, C. J. Halpenny, & S. U. Motzer (Eds.), *Cardiac Nursing* (3rd ed.) (pp. 798–819). Philadelphia: Lippincott.

Letterer, R. A., Carew, B., Reid, M., & Woods, P. (1992). Learning to live with congestive heart failure. *Nursing92, 21*(5), 34–42.

Lough, M. E., & Love, M. L. (1994). Cardiovascular diagnostic procedures. In L. A. Thelan, J. K. Davie, L. D. Urden, & M. E. Lough (Eds.). *Critical care nursing: Diagnosis and management* (2nd ed.) (pp. 182–276). St. Louis: Mosby.

Lounsbury, P., & Frye, S. J. (1992). *Cardiac rhythm disorders: A nursing process approach.* (2nd ed.). St. Louis: Mosby-Year Book.

Lowery, B. J. (1991). Psychological stress, denial and myocardial infarction outcomes. *Image, 23,* 51–55.

Lutz, C. A., & Przytulski, K. R. (1994). *Nutrition and diet therapy.* Philadelphia: F. A. Davis.

Main, C. C. (1995). Sudden cardiac death and cardiac arrest. In S. L. Woods, E. S. S. Froelicher, C. J. Halpenny, & S. U. Motzer (Eds.), *Cardiac nursing* (3rd ed.) (pp. 594–617). Philadelphia: Lippincott.

Margolis, S., & Goldschmidt-Clermont, P. J. (1993). Coronary artery disease. *The Johns Hopkins White Papers.* Baltimore: The Johns Hopkins Medical Institutions.

Marsden, C. (1993). "Do not resuscitate" orders and end-of-life care planning. *American Journal of Critical Care, 2*(2), 177–179.

Massie, B. W., & Wolfe, C. L. (1993). Heart failure. In F. H. Messerli (Ed.), *Cardiovascular disease in the elderly* (3rd ed.) (pp. 91–120). Philadelphia: Lippincott.

McCance, K. L., & Huether, S. E. (1994). *Pathophysiology: The biologic basis for disease in adults and children* (2nd ed.). St. Louis: Mosby-Year Book.

McCauley, K. M., & Brest, A. N. (1985). *McGoon's cardiac surgery: An interprofessional approach to patient care.* Philadelphia: F. A. Davis.

McGill, H. C. (1988). The cardiovascular pathology of smoking. *American Heart Journal, 115,* 250.

McKenna, M. (1992, March). Management of the patient undergoing myocardial revascularization: Percutaneous transluminal coronary angioplasty. *Nursing Clinics of North America, 27*(1), 231–242.

McKinley, M. G. (1993). Electrocardiographic monitoring. In R. L. Boggs, and M. Woolridge-King (Eds.), *AACN procedure manual for critical care* (3rd ed.) (pp. 234–244). Philadelphia: W. B. Saunders.

Miller, K. M. (1993). Nursing strategies for patients with silent myocardial ischemia. *Dimensions of Critical Care Nursing, 12*(5), 256–262.

Miller, N. H., & Froelicher, E. S. S. (1995). Smoking cessation: A planned approach to managing patients with coronary heart disease. In S. L. Woods, E. S. S. Froelicher, C. J. Halpenny, & S. U. Motzer (Eds.), *Cardiac nursing* (3rd ed.) (pp. 725–734). Philadelphia: Lippincott.

Moritz, D. J., & Ostfeld, A. M. C. (1990). The epidemiology and demography of aging. In W. R. Hazzard, R. Andres, E. L. Bierman, & J. P. Blass (Eds.), *Principles of geriatric medicine and gerontology* (2nd ed.) (pp. 146–156). New York: McGraw-Hill.

Moser, D. K. (1993). Pharmacologic management of heart failure: Neurohormonal agents. *Critical Care Nursing Clinics of North America, 5*(4), 599–608.

Moser, S. A., Crawford, D., & Thomas, A. (1993). Updated care guidelines for patients with automatic implantable cardioverter defibrillators. *Critical Care Nurse, 13*(2), 62–71.

Mravinac, C. M. (1991). Neurologic dysfunctions following cardiac surgery. *Critical Care Nursing Clinics of North America, 3*(4), 691–698.

Muirhead, J. (1988). Constrictive pericarditis. *Progress in Cardiovascular Nursing, 3*(4), 122–127.

Muirhead, J. (1989). Pericardial disease. In S. G. Underhill, S. L. Woods, E. S. S. Froelicher, & C. J. Halpenny (Eds.), *Cardiac nursing* (2nd ed.) (pp. 913–923). Philadelphia: Lippincott.

Murphy, T. G. (1993, December). Digoxin toxicity: Ventricular dysrhythmias to watch for. *American Journal of Nursing, 93*(12), 37–41.

Murphy, T. G., & Bennett, E. J. (1992). Low-tech, high-touch perfusion assessment. *American Journal of Nursing, 92*(5), 36–46.

Myerburg, R. J., Kessler, K. M., Bassett, A. L., et al. (1989). A biological approach to sudden cardiac death: Structure, function and cause. *American Journal of Cardiology, 63,* 1512–1516.

Myerburg, R. J., Kessler, K. M., & Castellanos, A. (1991). Pathophysiology of sudden cardiac death. *PACE: Pacing Clinics in Electrophysiology, 14,* 935–943.

National Institutes of Health & National Heart, Lung, and Blood Institute. (1993). *Emergency department: Rapid identification and treatment of patients with acute myocardial infarction.* Washington, D.C. : U.S. Department of Health and Human Services.

National Heart, Lung, and Blood Institute (NHLBI). (1994). *National Heart, Lung, and Blood Institute (NHLBI) fact book 1993.* (1994). Washington, D.C.: U.S. Department of Health and Human Services.

Neufeld, J. R. (1989). Diagnosis of myocardial ischemia and infarction. In S. G. Underhill, S. L. Woods, E. S. S. Froelicher, & C. J. Halpenny (Eds.), *Cardiac nursing* (2nd ed.) (pp. 483–487). Philadelphia: Lippincott.

Newton, K. M., & Froelicher, E. S. S. (1989). Life-style adjustments. In S. G. Underhill, S. L. Woods, E. S. S. Froelicher, & C. J. Halpenny (Eds.), *Cardiac nursing* (2nd ed.) (pp. 715–738). Philadelphia: Lippincott.

Newton, K. M., & Froelicher, E. S. S. (1995). Coronary heart disease risk factors. In S. L. Woods, E. S. Froelicher, C. J. Halpenny, & S. U. Motzer (Eds.), *Cardiac nursing* (3rd ed.), (pp. 200–211). Philadelphia: Lippincott.

Olbrych, D. D. (1993). Interpreting C. P. K. & L. D. H. results. *Nursing93, 23*(1), 48–49.

O'Neal, P. V. (1994, May). How to spot early signs of cardiogenic shock. *American Journal of Nursing, 94*(5), 36–41.

Pagana, K. D., & Pagana, T. J. (1995). *Mosby's diagnostic and laboratory test reference* (2nd ed.). St. Louis: Mosby-Year Book.

Pillion, J. M. (1991). Care of the cardiac patient. In M. R. Kinney, D. R. Packa, K. G. Andreoli, & D. P. Zipes (Eds.), *Comprehensive cardiac care* (7th ed.), (pp. 270–326). St. Louis: Mosby-Year Book.

Poole-Wilson, P.A. (1993). Relation of pathophysiologic mechanisms to outcome in heart failure. *JACC, 22*(4-Supplement A),

Porth, C. M. (1994). *Pathophysiology: Concepts of altered health states* (4th ed.). Philadelphia: Lippincott.

Price, S. A. & Wilson, L. M. (1992). *Pathophysiology: Clinical concepts of disease processes* (4th ed.). St. Louis: Mosby-Year Book.

Rankin, S. H. (1992, March). Psychosocial adjustments of coronary artery disease patients and their spouses: Nursing implications. *Nursing Clinics of North America, 27*(1), 271–284.

Rosenberg, L., Palmer, J. R., & Shapiro, S. (1990). Decline in the risk of myocardial infarction among women who stop smoking. *New England Journal of Medicine, 322,* 213–217.

Rossi, L., & Leary, E. (1992, March). Evaluating the patient with coronary artery disease. *Nursing Clinics of North America, 27*(1), 171–188.

Rost, K., & Smith, G. R. (1992). Return to work after an initial myocardial infarction and subsequent emotional distress. *Archives of Internal Medicine, 152,* 381–385.

Sandler, R. L. (1994, December). Clinical snapshot: Atrial fibrillation. *American Journal of Nursing, 94*(12), 26–27.

Schakenbach, L. H. (1987). Physiologic dynamics of acquired valvular disease. *Journal of Cardiovascular Nursing, 1*(3), 1–17.

Scordo, K. A. (1992). Helping your patient cope with mitral valve prolapse syndrome. *Nursing92, 22* (10), 34–40.

Scordo, K. A. (1994). Mitral valve prolapse syndrome: Women as second class citizens. *Capsules and Comments in Critical Care Nursing, 2*(1), 1–6.

Seidl, A., Bullough, B., Haughey, B., Scherer, Y., Rhodes, M., & Brown, G. (1991). Understanding the effects of a myocardial infarction on sexual functioning: A basis for sexual counseling. *Rehabilitation Nursing, 16*(5), 255–264.

Seifert, P. C. (1987). Surgery for acquired valvular heart disease. *Journal of Cardiovascular Nursing, 1*(3), 26–40.

Selwyn, A. P., & Braunwald, E. (1994). Ischemic heart disease. In K. J. Isselbacher, E. Braunwald, J. D. Wilson, J. B. Martin, A. S. Fauci, & D. L. Kasper (Eds.), *Harrison's principles of internal medicine* (13th ed.) (pp. 1077–1085). New York: McGraw-Hill.

Shaffer, R. B., & Ruiz, A. M. (1992). Assessing complications of P.T.C.A. *Nursing92, 22*(10), 41–45.

Shinn, J. A. (1992). Management of a patient undergoing myocardial revascularization: Coronary artery bypass graft surgery. *Nursing Clinics of North America, 27*(1), 243–255.

Shlafer, M. (1993). *The nurse, pharmacology, and drug therapy: A prototype approach* (2nd ed.). Redwood City, CA: Addison-Wesley Nursing.

Shurig, L. (1993). Pacemakers. In J. B. Flynn & N. P. Bruce (Eds.), *Introduction to critical care skills* (pp. 138–160). St.Louis: Mosby.

Solack, S. D. (1989). Pathophysiology of myocardial ischemia and infarction. In S. G. Underhill, S. L. Woods, E. S. S. Froelicher, & C. J. Halpenny (Eds.), *Cardiac nursing* (2nd ed.) (pp. 207–219). Philadelphia: Lippincott.

Solomon, J. (1991). Managing a failing heart. *RN, 54*(8), 46–50.

Sommers, M. S. (1991). Potential for injury: Trauma after cardiopulmonary resuscitation. *Heart & Lung, 20*(2/3), 287–295.

SoRelle, R. (1994, January 28). Heart bypass alternative seen. *Houston Chronicle,* pp. 1, 12A.

Speroni, R., Fiske, J., Frank, D., & Morrissey, A. (1992). Coronary atherectomy: Overview and implications for nursing. *Journal of Cardiovascular Nursing, 7*(1), 25–33.

Stary, H. C., Chandler, A. B., Galgov, S., Guyton, J. R., Insull, W., Rosenfeld, M. E., Schaffer, S. A., Schwartz, C. J., Wagner, W. D., & Wissler, R. W. (1994). A definition of initial, fatty streak, and intermediate lesions of atherosclerosis. *Circulation, 89,* 2462–2478.

Stewart, J. V., Hicks, S. L., Leflar, K. M., Kaempf, G., Bove, L. A., & DiMarzio, D. (1993). Cardiomyoplasty: Treatment of the failing heart using the skeletal muscle wrap. *Journal of Cardiovascular Nursing, 7*(2), 23–31.

Stollerman, G. H. (1994). Rheumatic fever. In K. J. Isselbacher, E. Braunwald, J. D. Wilson, J. B. Martin, A. S. Fauci, & D. L. Kasper (Eds.), *Harrison's principles of internal medicine* (13th ed.) (pp. 1046–1051). New York: McGraw-Hill.

Stovsky, B. (1992, March). Nursing interventions for risk factor reduction. *Nursing Clinics of North America, 27*(1), 257–270.

Strimike, C. L. (1995, January). Caring for a patient with an intracoronary stent. *American Journal of Nursing, 95*(1), 40–46.

Swearingen, P. L. (Ed.) (1992). *Pocket guide to medical-surgical nursing.* St. Louis: Mosby.

Swearingen, P. L., & Keen, N. H. (Eds.). (1991). *Manual of critical care: Applying nursing diagnoses to adult critical illness.* St. Louis: Mosby-Year Book.

Thomas, C.L. (Ed). (1994). *Taber's cyclopedic medical dictionary* (17th ed.). Philadelphia: F. A. Davis.

Thompson, C. J. (1995). Denervation of the transplanted heart: Nursing implications for patient care. *Critical Care Nursing Quarterly, 17*(4), 1–14.

Tierney, L. M., Jr., McPhee, S. J., and Papadakis, M. A. (Eds.). (1994). *Current medical diagnosis and treatment* (33rd ed.). Norwalk, CT: Appleton & Lange.

Timm, T. C., Ross, R., McKendall, G. R., Braunwald, E., Williams, D. O., & the TIMI Investigators. (1991). Left ventricular function and early cardiac events as a function of time to treatment with t-PA: A report from TIMI II [abstract]. *Circulation, 84*(4 Suppl 2), 2–230.

Trausch, P. A. (1988). Infective endocarditis: Nursing care and prevention. *Progress in Cardiovascular Nursing, 3*(2), 45–53.

Tumer, N., Houck, W. T., & Roberts, J. (1990). Effect of age on upregulation of the cardiac adrenergic beta receptors. *Journal of Gerontology: Biological Sciences, 45*(2), B48–51.

Underhill, S. G., & McGregor, M. S. (1989) Acquired valvular heart disease. In S. G. Underhill, S. L. Woods, E. S. S. Froelicher, & C. J. Halpenny (Eds.). *Cardiac nursing* (2nd ed.) (pp. 881–882). Philadelphia: Lippincott.

Underhill, S. G., & Stephen, S. A. (1989). Coronary heart disease risk factors. In S. G. Underhill, S. L. Woods, E. S. S. Froelicher, & C. J. Halpenny (Eds.). *Cardiac nursing* (2nd ed.) (pp. 194–206). Philadelphia: Lippincott.

Utz, S. W., Whitmire, V. M., & Grass, S. (1993). Perspectives of the person with mitral valve prolapse syndrome: A study of self-care needs derived from a health deviation. *Progress in Cardiovascular Nursing, 8*(1), 31–39.

Wajngarten, M., Grupi C., Belloti, G. M., Da Luz P. L., Azul L. G., & Pileggi, F. (1990). Frequency and significance of cardiac rhythm disturbances in healthy elderly individuals. *The Journal of Electrocardiography, 23*(2), 171–176.

Walker, C. B. (1993). Precordial shock. In R. L. Boggs, and M. Woolridge-King (Eds.). *AACN procedure manual for critical care* (3rd ed.) (pp. 251–261). Philadelphia: W. B. Saunders.

Way, L. W. (Ed.). (1994). *Current surgical diagnosis and treatment* (10th ed.) Norwalk, CT: Appleton & Lange.

Weaver, W. D., Cerqueira, M., Hallstrom, A. P., Litwin, P. E., Martin, J. S., Kudenchuk, P. J., & Eisenberg, M. S. (for the Myocardial Infarction Triage and Intervention Project Group). (1993). Prehospital-initiated vs hospital-initiated thrombolytic therapy: The Myocardial Infarction Triage and Intervention Trial. *Journal of the American Medical Association, 270*(10), 1211–1216.

Weiland, A. P., & Walker, W. E. (1986). Physiologic principles and clinical sequelae of cardiopulmonary bypass. *Heart & Lung, 15*(1), 34–39.

Wenger, N. K. (1994). The elderly patient with coronary heart disease: Contemporary practices and future challenges. *Aging/Clinical and Experimental Research, 6*(4), 209–212.

Whitman, G. R. (1987). Prosthetic cardiac valves. *Progress in Cardiovascular Nursing, 2*(4), 116–124.

Whitman, N. I. (1992). Assessment of the learner. In N. I. Whitman, B. A. Graham, C. J. Gleit, & M. D. Boyd (Eds.), *Teaching in nursing practice: A professional model* (2nd ed.) (pp. 133–152). Norwalk, CT: Appleton & Lange.

Wilson, R. F. (1992). *Critical care manual: Applied physiology and principles of therapy.* Philadelphia: F. A. Davis.

Wingate, S. (1987). Rehabilitation of the patient with valvular heart disease. *Journal of Cardiovascular Nursing, 1*(3), 52–64.

Witherell, C. L. (1994). Cardiac rhythm control devices. *Critical Care Nursing Clinics of North America, 6*(1), 85–101.

Woods, S. L., & Underhill, S. L. (1989). Myocardial ischemia and infarction. In S. G. Underhill, S. L. Woods, E. S. S. Froelicher, & C. J. Halpenny (Eds.), *Cardiac nursing* (2nd ed.) (pp. 488–508). Philadelphia: Lippincott.

Wynne, J., & Braunwald, E. (1994). The cardiomyopathies and myocarditides. In K. J. Isselbacher, E. Braunwald, J. D. Wilson, J. B. Martin, A. S. Fauci, & D. L. Kasper (Eds.), *Harrison's principles of internal medicine* (13th ed.) (pp. 1088–1093). New York: McGraw-Hill.

Responses to Altered Peripheral Tissue Perfusion

Assessing Clients with Peripheral Vascular and Lymphatic Disorders

LEARNING OBJECTIVES

After completing this chapter, you will be able to

- Identify and describe the structures and functions of the arterial and venous networks of the peripheral vascular system.
- Describe the physiologic dynamics of blood flow, peripheral resistance, and blood pressure.
- Identify and describe the major factors influencing arterial blood pressure.
- Identify and describe the structures and functions of the lymphatic system.

- Identify interview questions pertinent to the assessment of the peripheral vascular and lymphatic systems.
- Describe physical assessment techniques for peripheral vascular and lymphatic function.
- Identify manifestations of impairment in the function of the peripheral vascular and lymphatic systems.
- Describe variations in assessment findings for the older adult.

Review of Anatomy and Physiology

■ ■ ■

As the heart ejects blood with each beat, a closed system of blood vessels transports oxygenated blood to all body organs and tissues and then returns it to the heart for re-oxygenation in the lungs. This branching network of vessels is called the *peripheral vascular system*. Systemic circulation is made possible by the vessels of the peripheral vascular system: the arteries, veins, and capillaries.

Arterial and Venous Networks

The two main components of the peripheral vascular system are the arterial network and the venous network. The *arterial network* begins with the major *arteries* that branch from the aorta. All of the major arteries of the systemic circulation are illustrated in Figure 29–1. These major arteries branch into successively smaller arteries, which in turn subdivide into the smallest of the arterial vessels, called *arterioles*. The smallest arterioles feed into beds of hairlike *capillaries* within the body's organs and tissues.

In the capillary beds, oxygen and nutrients are exchanged for metabolic wastes, and deoxygenated blood begins its journey back to the heart through *venules*, the

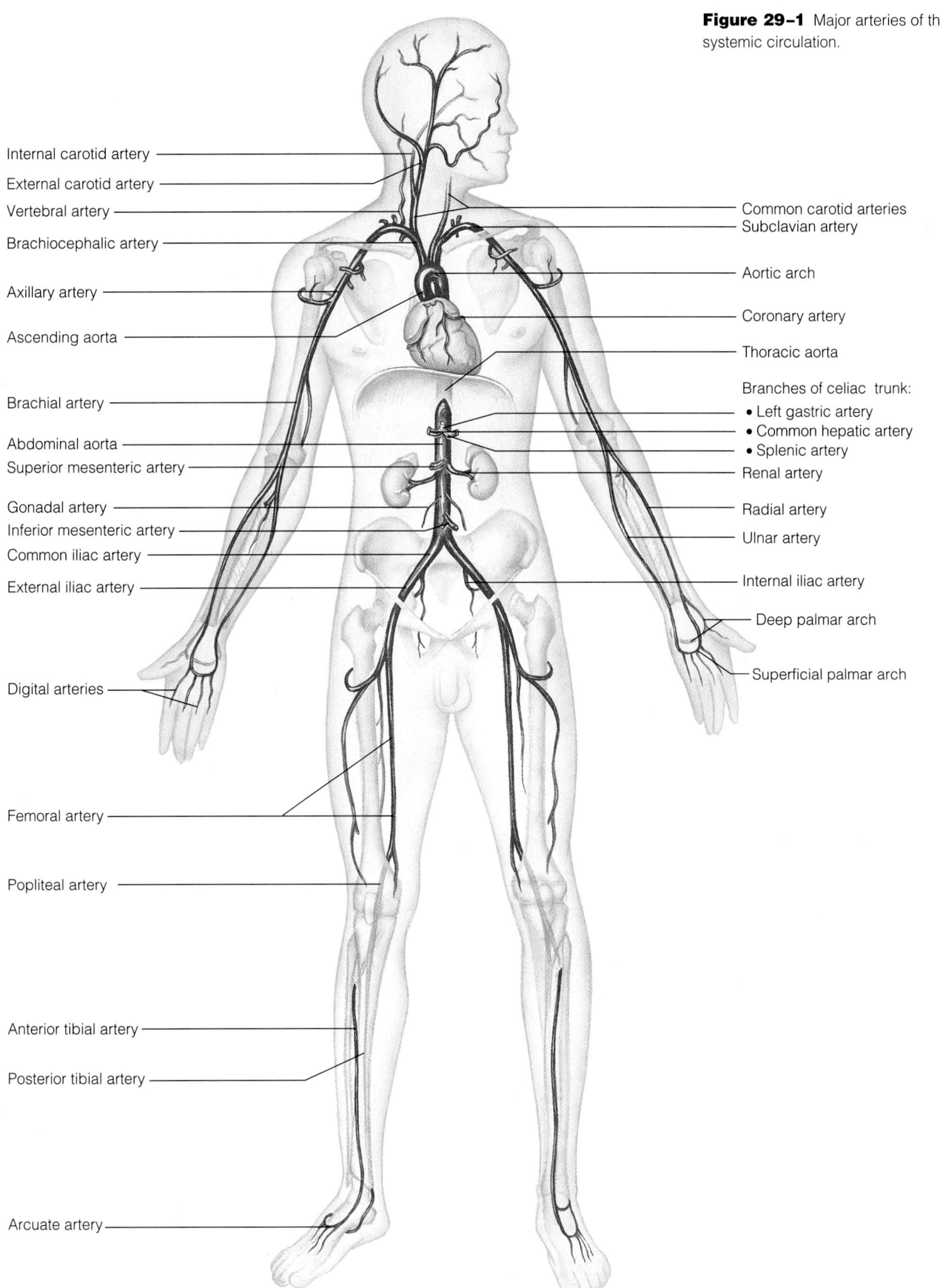

Figure 29–1 Major arteries of the systemic circulation.

Internal carotid artery

External carotid artery

Vertebral artery

Brachiocephalic artery

Axillary artery

Ascending aorta

Brachial artery

Abdominal aorta

Superior mesenteric artery

Gonadal artery

Inferior mesenteric artery

Common iliac artery

External iliac artery

Digital arteries

Femoral artery

Popliteal artery

Anterior tibial artery

Posterior tibial artery

Arcuate artery

Common carotid arteries

Subclavian artery

Aortic arch

Coronary artery

Thoracic aorta

Branches of celiac trunk:
• Left gastric artery
• Common hepatic artery
• Splenic artery

Renal artery

Radial artery

Ulnar artery

Internal iliac artery

Deep palmar arch

Superficial palmar arch

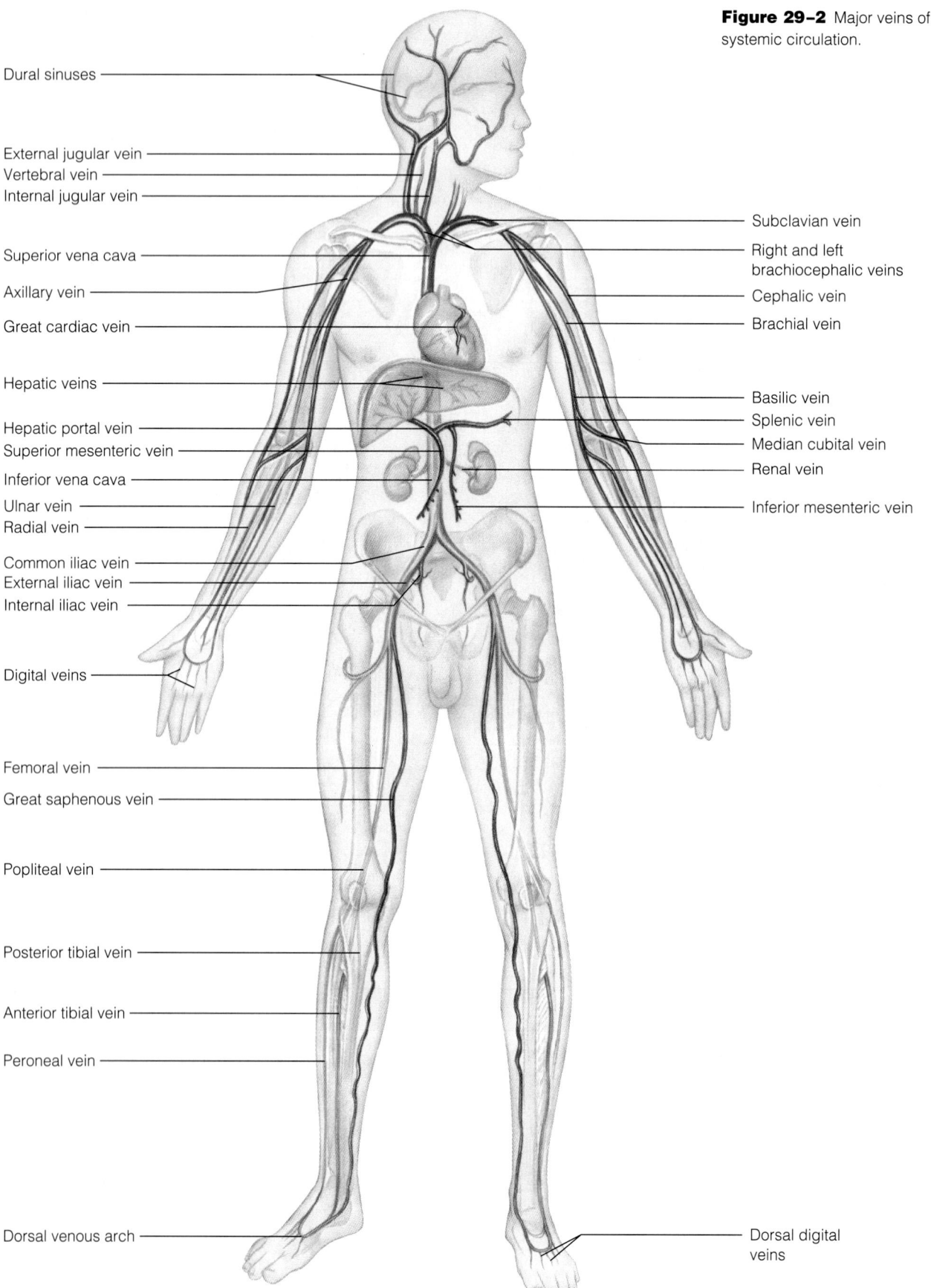

Figure 29-2 Major veins of the systemic circulation.

Dural sinuses

External jugular vein
Vertebral vein
Internal jugular vein

Superior vena cava

Axillary vein

Great cardiac vein

Hepatic veins

Hepatic portal vein
Superior mesenteric vein

Inferior vena cava

Ulnar vein
Radial vein

Common iliac vein
External iliac vein
Internal iliac vein

Digital veins

Femoral vein

Great saphenous vein

Popliteal vein

Posterior tibial vein

Anterior tibial vein

Peroneal vein

Dorsal venous arch

Subclavian vein

Right and left
brachiocephalic veins

Cephalic vein

Brachial vein

Basilic vein
Splenic vein
Median cubital vein
Renal vein

Inferior mesenteric vein

Dorsal digital
veins

smallest of the *venous network*. Venules join the smallest of *veins*, which in turn join larger and larger veins. The blood transported by the veins empties into the superior and inferior venae cavae entering the right side of the heart. All of the major veins of the systemic circulation are shown in Figure 29–2.

Structure of Blood Vessels

The structure of blood vessels reflects their different functions within the circulatory system (Figure 29–3). Except for the very smallest vessels, blood vessel walls have three layers: the tunica intima, the tunica media, and the tunica adventitia. The *tunica intima* is the innermost layer and is made up of simple squamous epithelium (the endothelium); this provides a slick surface to facilitate the flow of blood. The middle layer, or *tunica media*, of arteries is made up of smooth muscle and is thicker than the tunica media of veins. This makes arteries more elastic than veins and allows the arteries to alternately expand and recoil as the heart contracts and relaxes with each beat, producing a pressure wave which can be felt as a **pulse** over an artery. The smaller arterioles are less elastic than arteries but contain more smooth muscle, which promotes their constriction (narrowing) and dilation (widening). In fact, it is arterioles rather than arteries that exert the major control over arterial blood pressure. The *tunica adventitia*, or outermost layer, is made up of connective tissue and serves to protect and anchor the vessel. Veins have a thicker tuica adventitia than do arteries.

Blood in the veins travels at a much lower pressure than blood in the arteries. Thus, veins have thinner walls, a larger lumen, and greater capacity, and many are supplied with *valves* that facilitate the flow of blood against gravity back to the heart (Figure 29–3). Additional support is given to this venous return by the "milking" action of skeletal muscle contraction (called the *muscular pump*). When skeletal muscles contract against veins, the valves proximal to the contraction open, and blood is propelled toward the heart. The abdominal and thoracic pressure changes that occur with breathing (called the *respiratory pump*) also propel blood toward the heart.

The tiny capillaries, which connect the arterioles and venules, contain only one thin layer of tunica intima that is permeable to the gases and molecules exchanged between blood and tissue cells. Capillaries typically are found in interwoven networks. They serve to filter and shunt blood from terminal arterioles to postcapillary venules.

Physiology of Arterial Circulation

The physiology of arterial circulation is based on the dynamics among blood flow, peripheral vascular resistance, and blood pressure. **Blood flow** refers to the volume of blood transported in a vessel, in an organ, or throughout the entire circulation over a given period of time.

Peripheral vascular resistance (PVR) refers to the opposing forces or impedance to blood flow as the arterial channels become more and more distant from the heart. Peripheral vascular resistance is determined by three factors:

- *Blood viscosity:* The greater the viscosity, or thickness, of the blood, the greater its resistance to moving and flowing.

- *The length of the vessel:* The longer the vessel, the greater the resistance to blood flow.

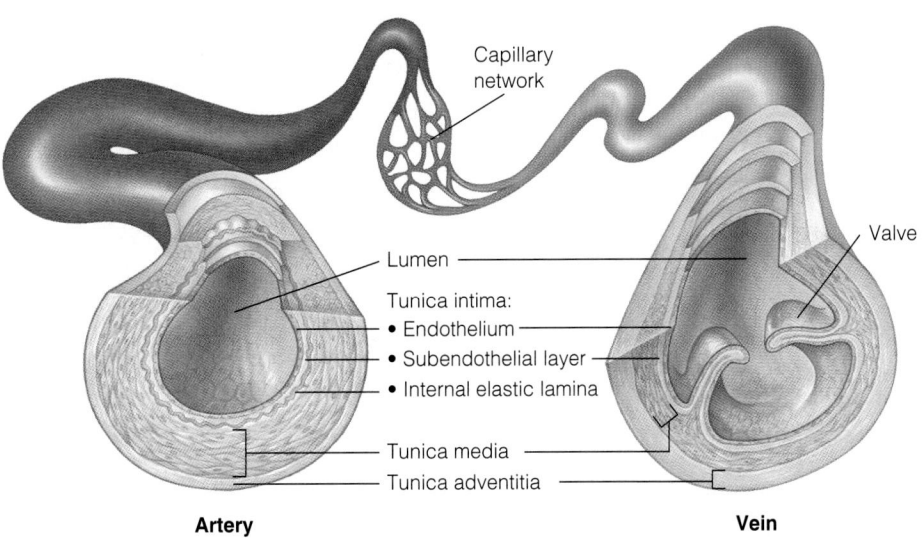

Figure 29–3 Structure of arteries, veins, and capillaries. Capillaries are composed of only a fine tunica intima. Notice that the tunica media is thicker in arteries than in veins.

■ *The diameter of the vessel:* The smaller the diameter of a vessel, the greater the friction against the walls of the vessel and, thus, the greater the impedance to blood flow.

Blood pressure (BP) is the force exerted against the walls of the arteries by the blood as it is pumped from the heart. It is most accurately referred to as *mean arterial pressure (MAP)*. The highest pressure exerted against the arterial walls at the peak of ventricular contraction (*systole*) is called the **systolic blood pressure.** The lowest pressure exerted during ventricular relaxation (*diastole*) is the **diastolic blood pressure.**

Mean arterial blood pressure is regulated mainly by cardiac output (CO) and peripheral vascular resistance (PVR), as represented in this formula: MAP = CO × PVR.

Factors Influencing Arterial Blood Pressure

Blood flow, peripheral vascular resistance, and blood pressure are in turn influenced by various factors. The sympathetic nervous system exerts a major effect on pe-ripheral resistance by causing vasoconstriction of the arterioles, thereby increasing blood pressure. Parasympathetic stimulation causes vasodilation of the arterioles, resulting in lowering of blood pressure. Baroreceptors and chemoreceptors located in the aortic arch, carotid sinus, and other large vessels are sensitive to pressure and chemical changes and cause reflex sympathetic stimulation, resulting in vasoconstriction, increased heart rate, and increased blood pressure.

The kidneys help maintain blood pressure by the excretion or conservation of salt and water. When blood pressure decreases, the kidneys initiate the renin-angiotensin mechanism, which stimulates vasoconstriction and the release of the hormone aldosterone from the adrenal cortex, which increases sodium ion reabsorption and water retention. In addition, pituitary release of antidiuretic hormone (ADH) promotes renal reabsorption of water. The net result is an increase in blood volume and a consequent increase in cardiac output and blood pressure.

Temperatures may also affect peripheral resistance: Cold causes vasoconstriction, whereas warmth produces

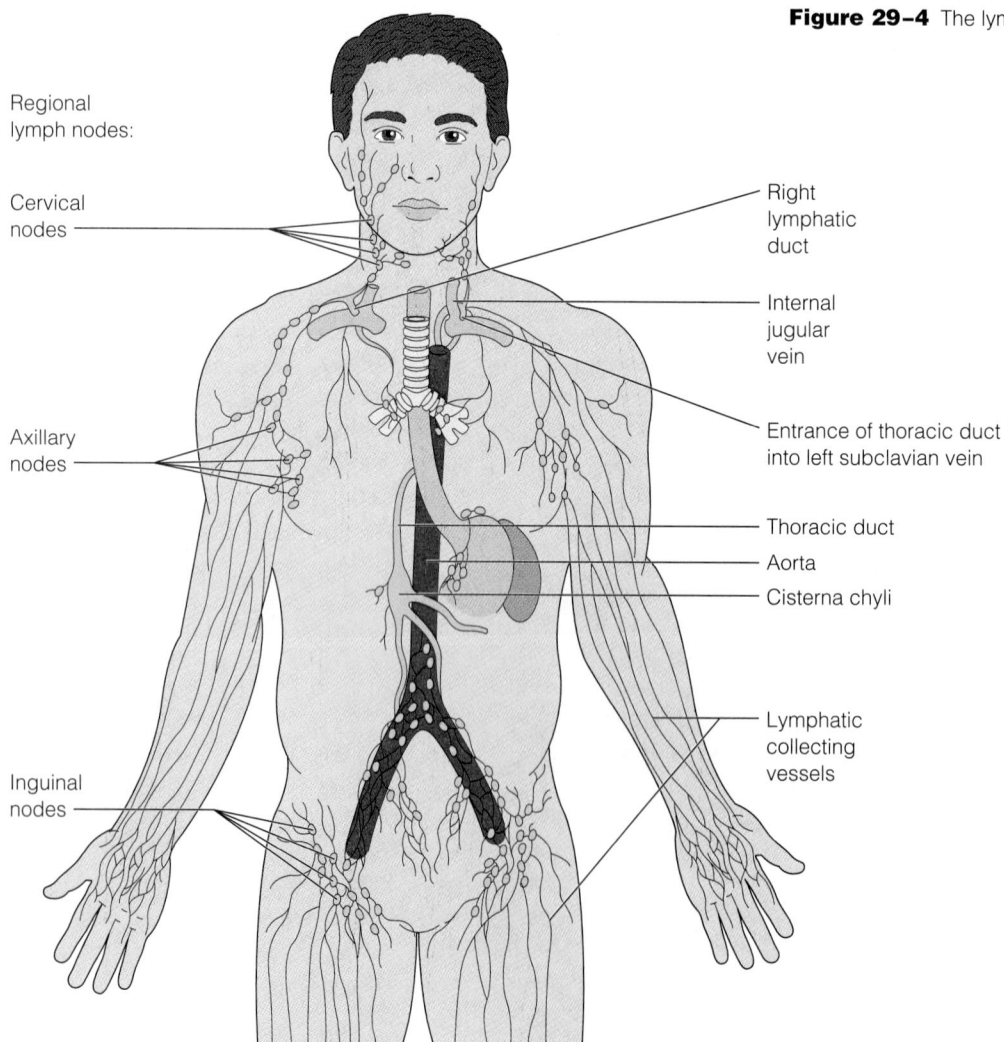

Figure 29–4 The lymphatic system.

Regional lymph nodes:

Cervical nodes

Axillary nodes

Inguinal nodes

Right lymphatic duct

Internal jugular vein

Entrance of thoracic duct into left subclavian vein

Thoracic duct

Aorta

Cisterna chyli

Lymphatic collecting vessels

vasodilation. Many chemicals, hormones, and drugs influence blood pressure by affecting cardiac output and/or peripheral vascular resistance. For example, epinephrine causes vasoconstriction and increased heart rate; prostaglandins modulate changes in blood vessel diameter and blood viscosity; endothelin, a chemical released by the inner lining of vessels, is a potent vasoconstrictor; nicotine causes vasoconstriction; and alcohol and histamine cause vasodilation.

Dietary factors, such as intake of salt, saturated fats, and cholesterol, elevate blood pressure by affecting blood volume and vessel diameter. Blood pressure may also be affected by race, gender, age, weight, time of day, position, exercise, and emotional state. These factors influence the arterial pressure; systemic venous pressure, though it is much lower, is also influenced by such factors as blood volume, venous tone, and right atrial pressure.

The Lymphatic System

The *lymphatic system* helps the heart and peripheral vasculature maintain adequate circulation. Its structures include the lymphatic vessels and several lymphoid organs (Figure 29–4). The lymphatic vessels, or *lymphatics,* form a network around the arterial and venous channels and interweave at the capillary beds. Their function is to collect and drain excess tissue fluid, called *lymph,* that "leaks" from the cardiovascular system and accumulates at the venous end of the capillary bed. The lymphatics return this fluid to the heart through a one-way system of lymphatic venules and veins that eventually drain into the *right lymphatic duct* and *left thoracic duct,* both of which empty into their respective subclavian veins. Lymphatics are a low-pressure system without a pump; their transportation of fluid is dependent on the rhythmic contraction of their smooth muscle and the muscular and respiratory pumps that assist venous circulation.

The organs of the lymphatic system are the lymph nodes, the spleen, the thymus, the tonsils, and the Peyer's patches of the small intestine (see Figure 8–3 on page 219). *Lymph nodes* are small aggregates of specialized cells that assist the body's immune system by removing foreign material, infectious organisms, and tumor cells from lymph. Lymph nodes are distributed along the lymphatic vessels, forming clusters in certain body regions such as the neck, axilla, and groin (Figure 29–4). The *spleen,* the largest lymphoid organ, is located in the upper left quadrant of the abdomen under the thorax. The main function of the spleen is to filter the blood by breaking down old red blood cells and storing or releasing to the liver their by-products (such as iron). The spleen also synthesizes lymphocytes, stores platelets for blood clotting, and serves as a reservoir of blood. The *thymus* gland is located in the lower throat and is most active in childhood, producing hormones (such as *thymosin*) that facilitate the immune action of lymphocytes. The *tonsils* of the pharynx

and *Peyer's patches* of the small intestine are lymphoid organs that protect the upper respiratory and digestive tracts from foreign pathogens.

Assessment of Peripheral Vascular and Lymphatic Function

■ ■ ■

Function of the peripheral vascular and lymphatic systems is assessed both by a health assessment interview to collect subjective data and a physical assessment to collect objective data.

The Health Assessment Interview

This section provides guidelines for collecting subjective data through a health assessment interview specific to the functions of the peripheral vascular system and the lymphatic system. Interview questions and leading statements for assessing peripheral vascular and lymphatic function also are provided.

The Peripheral Vascular System

The health assessment of the peripheral vascular system may focus on the client's chief complaint (such as swelling or pain in the legs), or it may be a part of a full cardiovascular assessment. If a chief complaint exists, analyze its onset, characteristics and course, severity, precipitating and relieving factors, and any associated symptoms, noting the timing and circumstances. For example, ask the client:

- Does the leg pain occur only with activities such as walking, or does it also occur during rest?
- Do your ankles swell at the end of the day, after sitting for prolonged periods, or after sleeping all night?
- Does temperature or the position of your body affect the symptoms?

Next, explore the client's medical and family history for any incidence of cardiovascular disorders, such as heart disease, arteriosclerosis, peripheral vascular disease (PVD), stroke, hypertension (HTN), hyperlipidemia (elevated fat in blood) and blood clots, or other chronic illnesses (e.g., diabetes). Ask questions about past surgery of the heart or blood vessels or tests to evaluate their function and about any medications that affect circulation or blood pressure.

The assessment interview continues with a review of symptoms. Question the client about past or present pain, burning, numbness, or tingling in the limbs or digits; leg fatigue or cramps; changes in skin color or temperature, texture of hair, ulcers or skin irritation, varicose veins, phlebitis (inflamed veins) or edema (swelling). Explore the client's nutritional history for intake of protein, vitamins and minerals, salt, fats, and fluid. Quantify any consumption of caffeine and alcohol and history of smoking (in pack years) or other tobacco use. Assess the client's activity level for exercise habits and tolerance.

It is important to consider socioeconomic factors that may precipitate or aggravate circulatory problems (e.g., inadequate clothing, shoes, or shelter) and occupational factors, such as prolonged standing or sitting or exposure to temperature extremes. Also assess psychosocial factors that may impact the client's stress level and emotional state.

The Lymphatic System

The health assessment of the lymphatic system includes a review of specific lymphatic findings, such as lymph node enlargement or swollen glands, as well as other more general complaints related to infection or impaired immunity, such as fever, fatigue, or weight loss. If a health problem exists, analyze its onset, characteristics, severity, and precipitating and relieving factors, noting the timing and circumstances. For example, ask the client:

- Did you notice that the glands in your neck became swollen after an infection?
- Have you noticed increased fatigue or weakness?
- Have you ever been exposed to radiation?

Explore the client's history for chronic illnesses (e.g., cardiovascular disease, renal disease, cancer, tuberculosis, HIV infection), predisposing factors (e.g., surgery, trauma, infection, blood transfusions, intravenous drug use), and environmental exposure (e.g., radiation, toxic chemicals, travel-related infectious disease). Review the family history for any incidence of cancer, anemia, or blood dyscrasias. Ask the client about past or present bleeding (e.g., from the nose, gums, or mouth; from vomiting; from the rectum; bruising) and associated symptoms (e.g., pallor, dizziness, fatigue, difficulty breathing); lymph node changes (e.g., enlargement, pain or tenderness, itching, warmth); swelling of extremities; and recurrent irritations or infections. Lastly, an assessment of the client's socioeconomic status, life-style, intravenous drug use, and sexual practices may be significant in determining risk for diseases associated with impaired lymphatic function.

Interview Questions

The following interview questions and leading statements are categorized by functional health patterns:

Health Perception–Health Management

- Describe any problems you have with circulation (for example, heart disease, hardening of the arteries, high blood pressure, stroke, blood clots, increased cholesterol).
- Have you ever been diagnosed with vascular or heart problems? If so, how were they treated?
- Have you ever had swollen glands? If so, describe them.
- What medicines do you take now?
- Do you now or have you ever smoked? When? How much?

Nutritional-Metabolic

- What types of food do you usually eat?
- Describe how much salt you use.
- Describe what kind of fats you eat.
- How much fluid do you drink each day?
- Do you drink liquids with caffeine (for example, coffee, tea, colas)? If so, how much each day?
- Do you drink alcoholic beverages? If so, how much?
- Have you noticed any changes in the color, temperature, or appearance of your hands or feet? If so, describe the changes.
- Have you noticed loss of hair on your lower legs or feet?
- Do the veins in your legs bulge? Have you ever worn support stockings?
- Do your feet ever swell or your shoes feel tight? When? What relieves the swelling?
- Have you noticed any skin changes or sores on your legs? If so, describe the changes.

Activity-Exercise

- Describe your activities during a usual day.
- Do you exercise regularly? If so, describe what you do.
- Has your activity level or exercise routine increased or decreased? If so, explain.
- Do you have leg pain when you walk? If so, how far do you walk before you feel pain? Describe the pain. What relieves it?
- Do you feel tired? If so, describe the feeling.

Sleep-Rest

- How much rest do you get each day?
- How much sleep do you get each day?
- Does leg pain or cramps ever wake you at night? If so, describe how the pain feels and what you do.

Cognitive-Perceptual

- Do you have any of these sensations in your legs or feet: pain, cramps, burning, numbness, or tingling?

- If you have these sensations, when do they occur? How long do they last? What relieves them?

Self-Perception–Self-Concept

- How has this health problem affected how you feel about yourself?
- How has this health problem affected how you feel about your normal life?
- How has this health problem affected how you feel about the future?

Role-Relationship

- Has this health problem affected your role in the family? If so, how?
- Has this health problem affected your work? If so, describe how.

Sexuality-Reproductive

- Has there been a change in your sexual activities since you have had this health problem? If so, describe.
- Describe how having this health problem has made you feel about yourself as a man or woman.

Coping-Stress

- Has your health problem affected your ability to handle the stress in your life? If so, explain.
- Describe what you do to cope with stress.
- Describe people that help you when you have stress.

Value-Belief

- How do you perceive the future with this problem?
- Describe those parts of your life that help you get through problems such as this.

The Physical Assessment

The Peripheral Vascular System: Preparation

The physical assessment of the peripheral vascular system can be performed as part of the full cardiovascular assessment or alone for clients who have known or suspected peripheral vascular disease or who are at risk for circulatory complications (e.g., clients who have undergone surgery or are immobile). The techniques used to assess the peripheral vascular system include auscultation of blood pressure, palpation of the major pulse points of the body (Figure 29–5), and inspection of the skin for such changes as edema, ulcerations, or alterations in color and temperature. Recommended equipment for this assessment includes a stethoscope, a tape measure, and a metric ruler. The client may be assessed in the supine, sitting, and standing positions. The box on page 1170 reviews guidelines for blood pressure measurement.

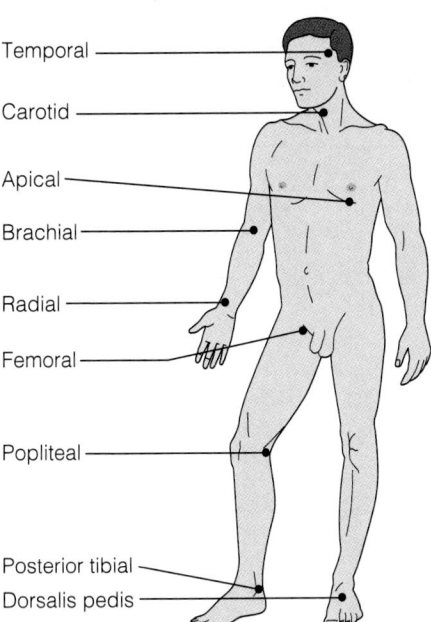

Temporal

Carotid

Apical

Brachial

Radial

Femoral

Popliteal

Posterior tibial

Dorsalis pedis

Figure 29–5 Body sites at which peripheral pulses are most easily palpated.

Guidelines for Blood Pressure Measurement

■ ■ ■

Review of Korotkoff's Sounds

The first sound heard is the systolic pressure; at least two consecutive sounds should be clear. If the sound disappears and then is heard again 10 to 15 mm later, an auscultatory gap is present; this may be a normal variant, or it may be associated with hypertension. The first diastolic sound is heard as a muffling of the Korotkoff sound and is considered the best approximation of the true diastolic pressure. The second diastolic sound is the level at which sounds are no longer heard.

The American Heart Association recommends documenting all three readings when measuring blood pressure, for example, 120/72/64. If only two readings are documented, the systolic and the second diastolic pressure are taken, for example, 120/64.

Technique Reminders

- Choose a cuff of an appropriate size: The cuff should snugly cover two-thirds of the upper arm, and the bladder should completely encircle the arm. The bladder should be centered over the brachial artery, with the lower edge 2 to 3 cm above the antecubital space.
- The client's arm should be slightly flexed and supported (on a table or by the examiner) at heart level.
- To determine how high to inflate the cuff, palpate the brachial pulse, and inflate the cuff to the point on the manometer at which the pulse is no longer felt; then, add 30 mm Hg to this reading, and use the sum as the target for inflation. Wait 15 seconds before reinflating the cuff to auscultate the BP.
- To recheck a BP, wait at least 30 seconds before attempting another inflation.
- Always inflate the cuff completely, then deflate it. Once deflation begins, allow it to continue; do not try to reinflate the cuff if the first systolic sound is not heard or if the cuff inadvertently deflates.
- The bell of the stethoscope more effectively transmits the low-pitched sounds of BP.

Sources of Error

- Falsely high readings can occur if the cuff is too small, too loose, or if the client supports his or her own arm.
- Falsely low readings can occur if a standard cuff is used on a client with thin arms.

- Inadequate inflation may result in underestimation of the systolic pressure or overestimation of the diastolic pressure if an auscultatory gap is present.
- Rapid deflation and repeated or slow inflations (causing venous congestion) can lead to underestimation of the systolic BP and overestimation of the diastolic BP.

Factors Altering Blood Pressure

- A change from the horizontal to upright position causes a slight decrease (5 to 10 mm) in systolic BP; the diastolic BP remains unchanged or rises slightly.
- BP taken in the arm is lower when the client is standing.
- If the BP is taken with the client in the lateral recumbent position, a lower BP reading may be obtained in both arms; this is especially apparent in the right arm with the client in the left lateral position.
- Factors that increase BP include exercise, caffeine, cold environment, eating a large meal, painful stimuli, and emotions.
- Factors that lower BP include sleep (by 20 mm Hg) and very fast, slow, or irregular heart rates.
- BP tends to be higher in taller or heavier clients.

Alternative Methods of Blood Pressure Measurement

- The palpatory method may be necessary if severe hypotension is present and the BP is inaudible. Palpate the brachial pulse, and inflate the cuff 30 mm above the point where the pulse disappears; deflate the cuff, and note the point on the manometer where the pulse becomes palpable again. Record this as the palpatory systolic BP.
- Leg BP measurement may be needed when there is injury of the arms or to rule out coarctation of the aorta or aortic insufficiency when arm diastolic BP is over 90 mm Hg. Place the client in the prone or supine position with the leg slightly flexed. Place a large leg cuff on the thigh with the bladder centered over the popliteal artery. Place the bell of the stethoscope over the popliteal space. Normal leg systolic BP is higher than arm BP; diastolic BP should be equal to or lower than arm BP. Abnormally low leg BP occurs with aortic insufficiency and coarctation of the aorta.

ASSESSMENT TECHNIQUE	POSSIBLE ABNORMAL FINDINGS
■ **Auscultate blood pressure in each arm with the client seated.**	Consistent BP readings over 140/90 in adults under age 40 is considered **hypertension (HTN)**. BP under 90/60 is considered **hypotension**. An *auscultatory gap*—a silent interval between the systolic and diastolic BP—may be a normal variation, or it may be associated with systolic HTN or a drop in diastolic BP due to aortic stenosis. Korotkoff's sounds (see the box on page 1170) may be heard down to zero with cardiac valve replacements, hyperkinetic states, thyrotoxicosis, severe anemia, and following vigorous exercise. The diastolic BP may be obscured by the sounds of aortic regurgitation. A difference of over 10 mm Hg between arms suggests arterial compression on the side of the lower reading, aortic dissection, or coarctation of the aorta.
■ **Auscultate blood pressure in each arm with the client standing.** If orthostatic changes occur, measure the BP with the client supine, legs dangling, and again with the client standing, 1 to 3 minutes apart.	A decrease in systolic BP of over 10 to 15 mm Hg and a drop in diastolic BP on standing is called **orthostatic hypotension**. Causes include antihypertensive medications, volume depletion, peripheral neurovascular disease, prolonged bed rest, and aging.
■ **Observe the pulse pressure.** The **pulse pressure** is the difference between the systolic and diastolic BP. For example, if the BP is 140/80, the pulse pressure is 60. A normal pulse pressure is one-third the systolic measurement.	A widened pulse pressure with an elevated systolic BP occurs with exercise, arteriosclerosis, severe anemia, thyrotoxicosis, and increased intracranial pressure. A narrowed pulse pressure with a decreased systolic BP occurs with shock, cardiac failure, and pulmonary embolus.
■ **Inspect the skin for color.**	Pallor reflects constriction of peripheral blood flow (e.g., due to syncope or shock) or decreased circulating oxyhemoglobin (e.g., due to anemia). Central cyanosis (blue hue) of the lips, earlobes, oral mucosa, and tongue suggests chronic cardiopulmonary disease. (See the box on page 1181 for abnormal findings associated with peripheral vascular and lymphatic assessment.)
■ **Palpate the temporal arteries.**	Redness, swelling, nodularity, and variations in pulse amplitude may occur with temporal arteritis.

ASSESSMENT TECHNIQUE	POSSIBLE ABNORMAL FINDINGS

■ **Inspect and palpate the carotid arteries.**

Note: You may evaluate the following characteristics over any peripheral pulse site; however, many are easier to evaluate at the carotid arteries. Make sure to document your findings for each specific site.
Note symmetry and the pulse rate and rhythm.

Note volume and amplitude of pulse. Remember to describe all pulses as increased, normal, diminished, or absent. Scales ranging from 0 to 4+ are sometimes used as follows:
0 = Absent
1+ = Diminished
2+ = Normal
3+ = Increased
4+ = Bounding.
Pulse waveforms are shown in the accompanying box.

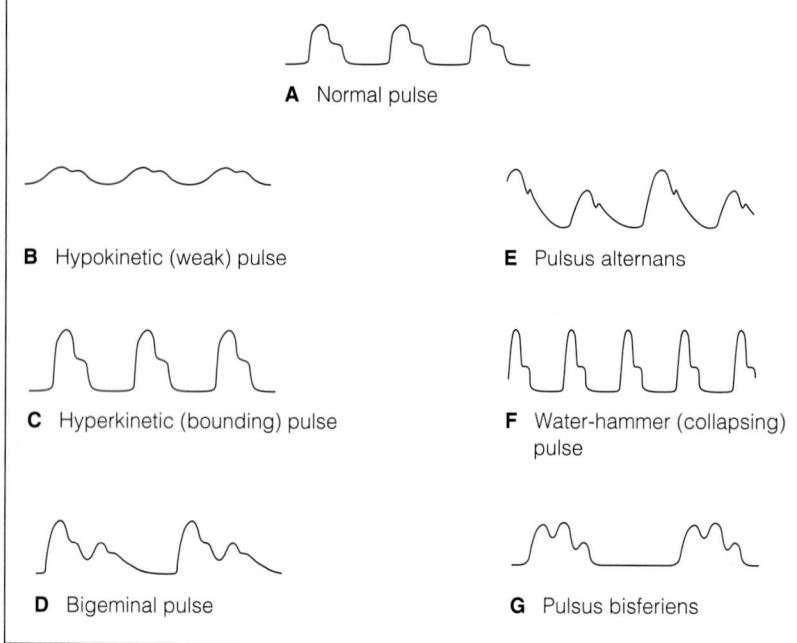

A Normal pulse

B Hypokinetic (weak) pulse

C Hyperkinetic (bounding) pulse

D Bigeminal pulse

E Pulsus alternans

F Water-hammer (collapsing) pulse

G Pulsus bisferiens

A unilateral pulsating bulge is seen with a tortuous or kinked carotid artery.
Alterations in pulse rate or rhythm are due to cardiac dysrhythmias.
An *absent pulse* indicates arterial occlusion.

A *hypokinetic pulse* (weak pulse) is associated with decreased stroke volume (Figure *B*). This may be due to congestive heart failure (CHF), aortic stenosis, or hypovolemia; to increased peripheral resistance, which may result from cold temperatures; or to arterial narrowing, commonly found with atherosclerosis.
A *hyperkinetic pulse* (bounding pulse) occurs with increased stroke volume and/or decreased peripheral resistance (Figure *C*). This may result from states in which cardiac output is high or from aortic regurgitation. It also may occur with anemia, hyperthyroidism, bradycardia, or reduced compliance, as with atherosclerosis.
A *bigeminal pulse* is marked by decreased amplitude of every second beat (Figure *D*). This may be due to premature contractions (usually ventricular).
Pulsus alternans is a regular pulse with alternating strong and weak beats (Figure *E*). This may be due to left ventricular failure and severe HTN.
The *water-hammer pulse* (collapsing pulse) has a greater than normal amplitude with a sharp rise and fall (Figure *F*). It occurs with aortic insufficiency.
Pulsus bisferiens has two main peaks in amplitude ("double beat") and occurs with combined aortic stenosis and regurgitation, pericardial effusion, and constructive pericarditis (Figure *G*).

ASSESSMENT TECHNIQUE	POSSIBLE ABNORMAL FINDINGS
Note any variance with respiration.	*Pulsus paradoxus* is a pulse in which the amplitude is diminished or absent during inspiration and exaggerated during expiration. Pulsus paradoxus occurs with cardiac tamponade, constrictive pericarditis, and severe chronic lung disease. A finding of pulsus paradoxus should be auscultated: Slowly deflate the cuff to the point on the manometer at which the first systolic sounds (first reading) are audible. As the client inhales, the sounds may disappear. Continue to deflate the cuff until systolic sounds are audible again and persist throughout respiration (second reading). Continue to deflate until diastole is reached. A difference of more than 10 mm Hg between the two systolic readings is abnormal. An example recording of pulsus paradoxus is 150–120/80.
Note any *thrills* (palpable fine vibrations).	A palpable thrill over the carotid artery suggests arterial narrowing, as with atherosclerosis.
■ **Auscultate the carotid arteries.** Use the bell of the stethoscope.	A murmuring or blowing sound heard over stenosed peripheral vessels is known as a *bruit*. A bruit heard over the middle to upper carotid artery is suggestive of atherosclerosis.
■ **Inspect and palpate the internal and external jugular veins for venous pressure.** The box on page 1176 provides guidelines for assessing jugular venous pressure.	An increase in jugular venous pressure over 3 cm and located above the sternal angle reflects increased right atrial pressure. This occurs with right ventricular failure or, less commonly, with constrictive pericarditis, tricuspid stenosis, and superior venae cavae obstruction.
■ **If venous pressure is elevated, assess the hepatojugular reflex.** To assess the hepatojugular reflex, compress the liver (in the right upper abdominal quadrant) with the palm of the hand for 30 to 60 seconds while observing the jugular veins.	A decrease in venous pressure reflects reduced left ventricular output or blood volume. Unilateral neck vein distention suggests local compression or anatomic anomaly. A rise in the column of neck vein distention over 1 cm with liver compression indicates right heart failure.
■ **Inspect and palpate the arms.** Note size and symmetry, skin color, and temperature.	Unilateral swelling with venous prominence occurs with venous obstruction. Extreme localized pallor of the fingers is seen with Raynaud's disease. Cyanosis of the nailbeds reflects chronic cardiopulmonary disease. Cold temperature of the hands and fingers occurs with vasoconstriction.

ASSESSMENT TECHNIQUE	POSSIBLE ABNORMAL FINDINGS

Assessment of Jugular Venous Pressure

■ ■ ■

When a client with normal venous pressure lies in the supine position, full neck veins are normally visible, but as the head of the bed is elevated, the pulsations disappear. In the client with greatly elevated venous pressure, visible pulsations of the jugular vein are present even in the upright position. To conduct the inspection:

1. Remove clothing from the client's neck and chest. Elevate the head of the bed 30 to 45 degrees, and turn the client's head to the opposite side. Shine a light tangentially across the neck to increase shadows. If the external jugular veins are distended, they will be visible vertically between the mandible and outer clavicle.

2. If jugular distention is present, assess the jugular venous pressure (JVP) by measuring from the highest point of visible distention to the sternal angle (the point at which the clavicles meet) on both sides of the neck (see the accompanying figure). Bilateral measurements above 3 cm are considered elevated and indicate increased venous pressure; distention on only one side may indicate obstruction.

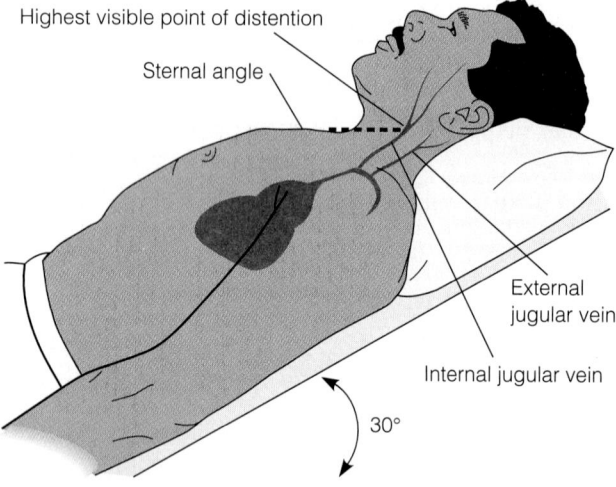

Highest visible point of distention

Sternal angle

External jugular vein

Internal jugular vein

30°

Assessment of the highest point of jugular vein distention.

ASSESSMENT TECHNIQUE	POSSIBLE ABNORMAL FINDINGS
■ **Palpate the nail beds for capillary refill.** Apply pressure to the client's fingertips. Watch for blanching of the nail beds. Now release the pressure. Note the time it takes for **capillary refill**, indicated by the return of pink color on release of the pressure.	Capillary refill that takes more than 2 seconds reflects circulatory compromise, such as hypovolemia.
■ **Assess venous pattern and pressure.** Elevate one of the client's arms over the head for a few seconds. Now slowly lower the arm. Observe the filling of the client's hand veins.	Distention of hand veins at elevations over 9 cm above heart level reflects an increase in systemic venous pressure.
■ **Palpate the radial and brachial pulses.** Count the pulse rate at the radial pulse.	Alterations in pulse rate or rhythm are due to cardiac arrhythmias. A pulse rate over 100 beats per minute (BPM) is *tachycardia;* a pulse rate below 60 BPM is *bradycardia.*
Note the rhythm. (If irregular, palpate the radial pulse while auscultating the apical pulse.)	A *pulse deficit* (slower radial rate than apical) occurs with arrhythmias and CHF. Irregularities of rhythm produce early beats and pauses (skipped beats) in the pulse, which may be regular in pattern, sporadic, or grossly irregular.
Note the volume and amplitude.	Diminished or absent radial pulses may be due to thromboangitis obliterans (Buerger's disease) or acute arterial occlusion. A weak and thready pulse, often with tachycardia, reflects decreased cardiac output. A bounding pulse occurs with hyperkinetic states and atherosclerosis.
Note symmetry.	Unequal pulses between extremities suggest arterial narrowing or obstruction on one side.
Note variance with respiration.	In *sinus dysrhythmia* (a normal variant), the pulse rate increases with inspiration and decreases with expiration.
■ **If arterial insufficiency is suspected, palpate the ulnar pulse and perform the Allen test:** a. Have the client make a tight fist. b. Compress both the radial and ulnar arteries. c. Have the client open the hand to a slightly flexed position. d. Observe for pallor. e. Release the ulnar artery and observe for the return of pink color within 3 to 5 seconds. f. Repeat the procedure on the radial artery.	The normal ulnar artery may or may not have a palpable pulse. Persistent pallor with the Allen test suggests ulnar artery occlusion.
■ **Inspect and palpate the abdominal aorta.** Note size, width, and any visible pulsations or bulging.	A pulsatile mass in the upper abdomen is suggestive of an *aortic aneurysm,* particularly in the older adult. An aorta greater than 2.5 to 3 cm in width reflects pathologic dilation, most likely due to arteriosclerosis.

ASSESSMENT TECHNIQUE	POSSIBLE ABNORMAL FINDINGS

- **Auscultate the epigastrium and each abdominal quadrant.**

Use the bell of the stethoscope (Figure 29–6).

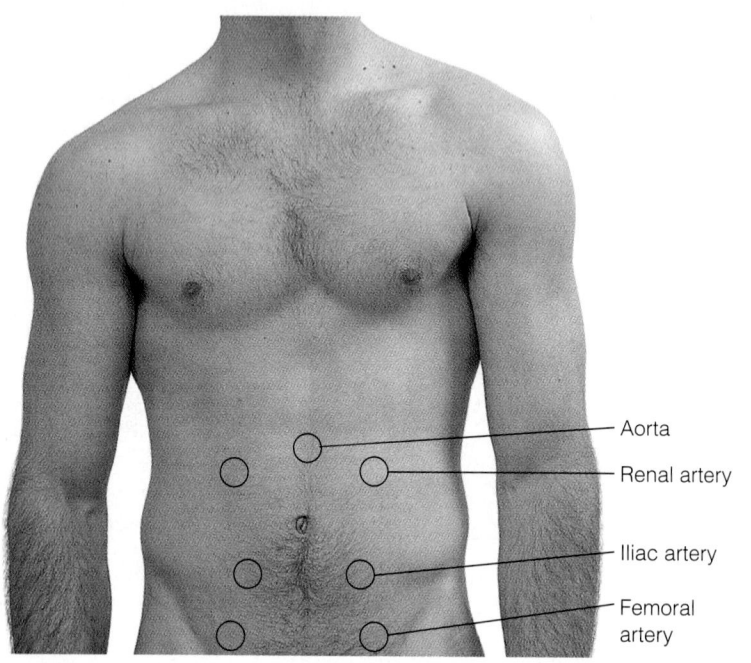

Aorta

Renal artery

Iliac artery

Femoral artery

Figure 29–6 Auscultation sites of the abdominal aorta and its branches.

- **Inspect and palpate each leg.**

Note size, shape, and symmetry; arterial pattern; skin color, temperature, and texture; hair pattern; pigmentation; rashes; ulcers, sensation; and capillary refill.

Abdominal bruits reflect turbulent blood flow associated with partial arterial occlusion. A bruit heard over the aorta is suggestive of an aneurysm. A bruit heard over the epigastrium and radiating laterally, especially with HTN, suggests renal artery stenosis. Bruits heard in the lower abdominal quadrants suggest partial occlusion of the iliac arteries.

Chronic arterial insufficiency may be due to arteriosclerosis or autonomic dysfunction, or to acute occlusion resulting from thrombosis, embolus, or aneurysm.

Signs of arterial disruption include pallor, dependent rubor (dusky redness); cool to cold temperature; and atrophic changes, such as hair loss with shiny and smooth texture, thickened nails, sensory loss, slow capillary refill, and muscle atrophy.

Ulcers characterized by symmetric margins, a deep base, black or necrotic tissue, and absence of bleeding may occur at pressure points on or between the toes, on the heel, on the lateral malleolar or tibial area, over the metatarsal heads, or along the side or sole of the foot. Gangrene due to complete arterial occlusion presents as black, dry, hard skin; pregangrenous color changes include deep cyanosis and purple-black discoloration. (See the box on page 1181.)

ASSESSMENT TECHNIQUE	POSSIBLE ABNORMAL FINDINGS
■ **With the client supine, assess the venous pattern of the legs. Repeat with the client standing.**	Signs of venous insufficiency include swelling, thickened skin, cyanosis, stasis dermatitis (brown pigmentation, erythema, and scaling), and superficial ankle ulcers located predominantly at the medial malleolus with uneven margins, ruddy granulation tissue, and bleeding. Varicose veins appear as dilated, tortuous, and thickened veins, which are more prominent in a dependent position. (See the box on page 1181.)
■ **Palpate the femoral, popliteal, posterior tibial, and dorsalis pedis pulses for volume, amplitude, and symmetry.**	Diminished or absent leg pulses suggest partial or complete arterial occlusion of the proximal vessel and are often due to arteriosclerosis obliterans. Increased and widened femoral and popliteal pulsations suggest aneurysm. Absence of a posterior tibial pulse with signs and symptoms of arterial insufficiency is usually due to acute occlusion by thrombosis or embolus. Diminished or absent pedal pulses are often due to popliteal occlusion associated with diabetes mellitus.
■ **If pulses are diminished, observe for postural color changes.** Elevate both legs 60 degrees, and observe the color of the soles of the feet.	Extensive pallor on elevation is suggestive of arterial insufficiency.
Have the client sit and dangle the legs; note the return of color to the feet.	Rubor (dusky redness) of the toes and feet along with delayed venous return (over 45 seconds) suggests arterial insufficiency.
■ **If arterial insufficiency is suspected, auscultate the femoral arteries.**	Femoral bruits are suggestive of arterial narrowing due to arteriosclerosis.
■ **Inspect and palpate the calves.**	Redness, warmth, swelling, tenderness, and cords along a superficial vein suggest *thrombophlebitis* or *deep vein thrombosis (DVT)*.
■ **If DVT is suspected, check for Homans' sign.** Dorsiflex the client's foot while holding the knee flat or slightly flexed (Figure 29–7).	Calf pain with dorsiflexion of the foot (positive Homans' sign) may further suggest thrombosis. (*Note:* The reliability of Homans' sign is questionable. Some studies have shown significant false positive and false negative results.)

ASSESSMENT TECHNIQUE	POSSIBLE ABNORMAL FINDINGS

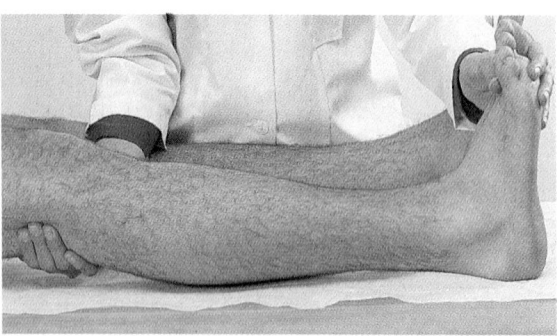

Figure 29–7 Dorsiflexing the foot to check for Homans' sign.

■ **Inspect and palpate for edema.**

Use your thumb to compress the dorsum of the client's foot, around the ankles, and along the tibia (Figure 29–8). A depression in the skin that does not immediately refill is referred to as pitting.

Edema can be graded on a scale of from 1+ to 4+ (Figure 29–8, B):

1+: No visible change in the leg; slight pitting.
2+: No marked change in the shape of the leg; pitting slightly deeper.
3+: Leg is visibly swollen; pitting is deep.
4+: Leg is very swollen; pitting is very deep.

■ **If discrepancy is apparent, measure the leg circumference.**

Leg circumference is measured at the forefoot, above the ankle, at the calf, and mid-thigh.

Edema may be caused by disease of the cardiovascular system such as CHF; by renal, hepatic, or lymphatic problems; or by infection. Venous distention suggests venous insufficiency or incompetence. Lower leg or ankle edema suggests DVT of the calf; edema of the entire leg suggests iliofemoral thrombosis.

Difference in leg circumference over 1 cm above the ankle or over 2 cm at the calf is abnormal.

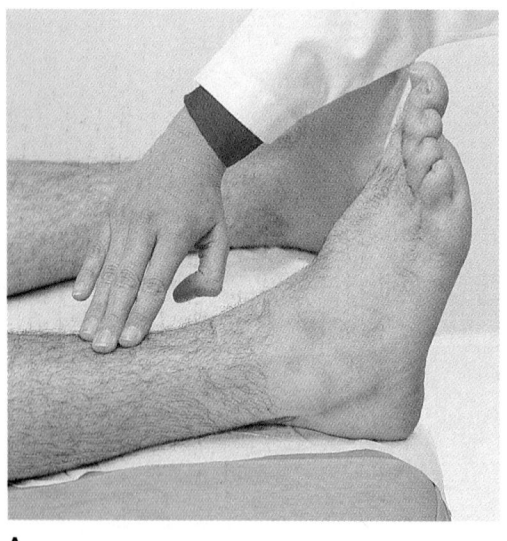

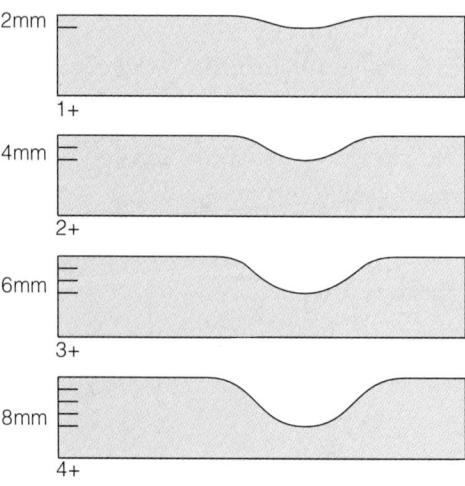

A   B

Figure 29–8 Evaluation of edema. *A,* Palpating for edema over the tibia. *B,* Four-point scale for grading edema.

Abnormal Findings Associated with Peripheral Vascular and Lymphatic Assessment

■ ■ ■

- *Pallor* is an absence of color of the skin. The degree of pallor depends on the client's normal skin color and health status. Dark skin may appear ashen or have a yellowish tinge.

- *Cyanosis* is a bluish discoloration of the skin and mucous membranes in people with light skin. In people with dark skin, cyanosis may be difficult to observe. Inspect the nail beds and conjunctiva.

- *Edema* is an abnormal accumulation of fluid in the interstitial spaces of body tissues. It is often most apparent in the lower extremities.

- *Varicose veins* are tortuous and dilated veins that have incompetent valves. The saphenous veins of the legs are most commonly affected.

- *Enlarged lymph nodes* result from infection or malignancy.

- *Atrophic changes* are changes in size or activity of body tissues as the result of pathology or injury. Decreased blood flow and oxygenation of the lower extremities often cause atrophic changes of loss of hair, thickened toe nails, changes in pigmentation, and ulcerations.

- *Gangrene* is the necrosis (or death) of tissue, most often the result of loss of blood supply and infection. Gangrene often begins in the most distal of the tissues of the extremities.

- *Pressure ulcers,* also called decubitus ulcers or bed sores, are the result of ischemia and hypoxia of tissue following prolonged pressure. These ulcers often are located over bony prominences. If untreated, the tissue changes proceed from red skin to deep, craterlike ulcers.

The Physical Assessment

The Lymphatic System: Preparation

Physical assessment of the lymphatic system is usually integrated into the assessment of other body systems. For example, the tonsils are observed with the pharynx during the head and neck assessment; the regional lymph nodes are evaluated with corresponding body regions (e.g., occipital, auricular, and cervical nodes are evaluated with assessment of the head and neck, axillary nodes with assessment of the breast or thorax, epitrochlear node with assessment of the peripheral vascular exam of the arms, and inguinal nodes with assessment of the abdomen); the spleen can be palpated during the abdominal assessment. The techniques of inspection and palpation are used for the lymphatic examination and may be aided by use of a tape measure and metric ruler.

ASSESSMENT TECHNIQUE	POSSIBLE ABNORMAL FINDINGS

■ **Inspect the extremities and the regional lymph nodes.**

Note any edema, erythema, red streaks, or skin lesions.

Lymphangitis (inflammation of a lymphatic vessel) may produce a red streak with induration (hardness) following the course of the lymphatic collecting duct; infected skin lesions may be present, particularly between the digits. *Lymphedema* (swelling due to lymphatic obstruction) occurs with congenital lymphatic anomaly (Milroy's disease) or with trauma to the regional lymphatic ducts from surgery or metastasis (e.g., arm lymphedema after radical mastectomy with axillary node removal). Edema of lymphatic origin is usually not pitting, and the skin may be thickened; one example is the taut swelling of the face and body that occurs with *myxedema*, which is associated with hypothyroidism.

■ **Palpate the regional lymph nodes of the head and neck, axillae, arms, and groin.**

Use firm, circular movements of the finger pads and note the following:

Size

Shape

Symmetry

Consistency

Delineation

Mobility

Tenderness

Sensation

Condition of overlying skin

Lymphadenopathy refers to the enlargement of lymph nodes (over 1 cm) with or without tenderness. It may be caused by inflammation, infection, or malignancy of the nodes or the regions drained by the nodes. Lymph node enlargement with tenderness suggests inflammation (*lymphadenitis*). With bacterial infection, the nodes may be warm and matted with localized swelling. Malignant or metastatic nodes may be hard, indicating lymphoma; rubbery, indicating Hodgkin's disease; or fixed to adjacent structures. Usually they are not tender. Ear infections and scalp and facial

ASSESSMENT TECHNIQUE	POSSIBLE ABNORMAL FINDINGS

lesions, such as acne, may cause enlargement of the preauricular and cervical nodes. Anterior cervical nodes are enlarged and infected with streptococcal pharyngitis and mononucleosis. Lymphadenitis of the cervical and submandibular nodes occurs with herpes simplex lesions. Brain tumors may metastasize to the occipital nodes.

Enlargement of supraclavicular nodes, especially the left, is highly suggestive of metastatic disease from abdominal and thoracic cancer. Axillary lymphadenopathy is associated with breast cancer. Lesions of the genitals may produce enlargement of the inguinal nodes. Persistent generalized lymphadenopathy is associated with acquired immune deficiency syndrome (AIDS) and AIDS-related complex (ARC).

■ **Palpate for the spleen.**

Palpate in the upper left quadrant of the abdomen (Figure 29–9).

A palpable spleen in the left upper abdominal quadrant of an adult may indicate abnormal enlargement (splenomegaly) and may be associated with cancer, blood dyscrasias, and viral infection, such as mononucleosis.

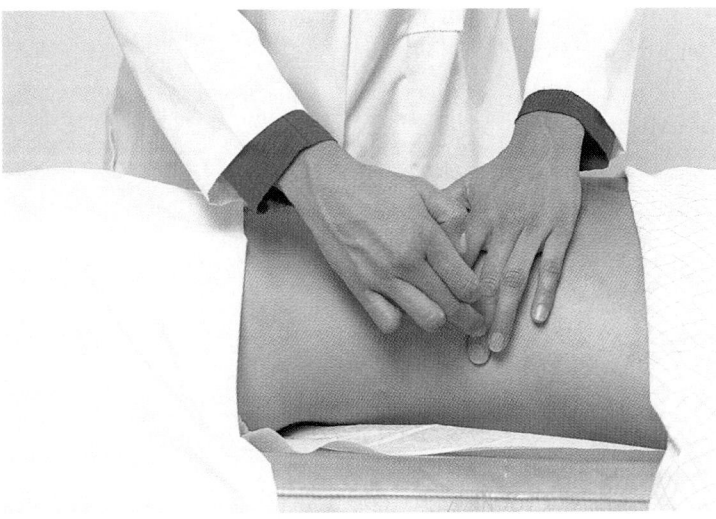

Figure 29–9 Palpating the spleen.

■ **Percuss for splenic dullness.**

Percuss in the lowest left intercostal space (ICS) at the anterior axillary line or in the ninth to tenth ICS at the midaxillary line.

A dull percussion note in the lowest left ICS at the anterior axillary line or below the tenth rib at the midaxillary line suggests splenic enlargement.

Variations in Assessment Findings for the Older Adult

The aging process produces anatomic and functional changes within the peripheral vascular and lymphatic systems. Vascular resistance is affected by changes in the blood vessels that interfere with the exchange of oxygen and nutrients. Aging arteries demonstrate increased rigidity, thinning, redistribution, and the development of arteriosclerosis (hardening of the arterial wall). The aorta and large arteries lose elasticity and often become dilated and tortuous; intra-aortic systolic pressure may rise. Baroreceptor sensitivity decreases, leading to alterations in blood pressure with position changes. As total peripheral vascular resistance increases and blood flow decreases with age, the person is at risk for stroke, renal insufficiency, blood clots, and ischemia of the extremities. Veins become dilated and stretched, and valvular changes impede venous return to the heart, predisposing the older adult to chronic venous insufficiency. The lymphatic system shows a decline in the production and responsiveness of the specific lymphocytes (B and T cells) that mediate the immune response.

Other variations in assessment findings that are common in the older adult include the following:

- Systolic hypertension and orthostatic hypotension are more common.

- As arteries lengthen and become tortuous with aging, they may be more palpable and feel rigid.

- Pulsations may diminish or disappear, and the brachial artery may appear as a snakelike pulsation.

- The skin may become thinner and dryer with scant hair pattern, and nail growth may slow.

- Distal leg pulses (e.g., popliteal and dorsalis pedis pulses) may be less palpable.

- Dilated veins, varicosities, and edema may become more prominent in dependent positions (especially of the lower extremities) as venous competence diminishes.

- Buckling or kinking of the left innominate artery may be seen as a pulsating mass or give the appearance of elevated jugular venous pressure in the neck.

- Progressive arteriosclerosis may result in audible carotid bruits.

- A decrease in the number and size of lymph nodes, along with fibrotic and fatty composition, may result in impaired immunity with more frequent infections.

Bibliography

■ ■ ■

Blank, C. A., & Irwin, G. H. (1990). Peripheral vascular disorders: Assessment and intervention. *Nursing Clinics of North America, 25*(4), 777–794.

Bright, L. D., & Georgi, S. (1992). Peripheral vascular disease: Is it arterial or venous? *American Journal of Nursing, 92*(9), 34–43.

Canobbio, M. M. (1990). *Cardiovascular disorders.* St. Louis: Mosby.

Fellows, E., & Jocz, A. M. (1991). Lower extremity arterial disease. *Nursing91, 21*(8), 34–41.

Gehring, P. (1991). Physical assessment begins with a history. *RN, 54*(11), 26–32.

Handerhan, B. (1987). How to measure jugular venous distention. *Nursing87, 17*(9), 48–49.

Hill, M., & Grim, C. M. (1991). How to take a precise blood pressure. *American Journal of Nursing, 91,* 38–42.

Iyriboz, Y., & Hearon, C. (1992). Blood pressure measurement at rest and during exercise. *Journal of Cardiopulmonary Rehabilitation, 12*(4), 277–287.

Kuhn, J. K., & McGovern, M. (1992). Peripheral vascular assessment of the elderly client. *Journal of Gerontological Nursing, 18*(12), 35–38.

Marieb, E. N. (1995). *Human anatomy and physiology* (3rd ed.). Redwood City, CA: Benjamin/Cummings.

Phoenix, J. (1990). Low blood pressure. *Nursing90, 20*(11), 34–39.

Reckling, J. B., & Neuberger, G. B. (1987). Understanding immune system dysfunction. *Nursing87, 17*(9), 34–38.

Nursing Care of Clients with Peripheral Vascular and Lymphatic Disorders

LEARNING OBJECTIVES

After completing this chapter, you will be able to

- Describe the pathophysiology of commonly occurring peripheral vascular and lymphatic disorders.
- Identify laboratory and diagnostic tests used to identify and assess peripheral vascular and lymphatic disorders.
- Explain the nursing implications of the medications prescribed for treating clients with peripheral vascular and lymphatic disorders.

- Describe the pre- and postoperative care of clients having surgery for the treatment of an aortic aneurysm.
- Provide client and family teaching that contributes to the promotion and maintenance of health in clients with common peripheral vascular and lymphatic disorders.
- Use the nursing process as a framework for providing individualized care to clients with peripheral vascular and lymphatic disorders.

Clients with disorders of the peripheral vascular and lymphatic systems require nursing care centered on relieving pain, improving the circulation of peripheral blood or lymphatic fluid, preventing tissue damage, and promoting healing. In addition, the effects of prolonged bed rest and other therapies may produce emotional, social, and economic stressors that impair the client's long-term health and create situational crises that affect the client's family. For these reasons, the nurse should adopt a holistic approach to caring for the client with peripheral vascular and lymphatic disorders.

The major processes that interfere with the normal flow of peripheral blood (the part of the circulatory system found in the extremities) and lymphatic fluid include constriction, obstruction, inflammation, and vasospasm. These conditions result in disorders of blood pressure regulation, peripheral artery function, aortic structure, venous circulation, and lymphatic circulation.

▗▗▗ Disorders of Blood Pressure Regulation ▗▗▗

Blood moves through the circulatory system in waves, creating pressures that are affected by cardiac output, blood volume, and peripheral vascular resistance. *Peripheral vascular resistance* is the resistance the blood meets as it flows through the arteries. This resistance is, in turn, affected by vessel length, vessel diameter, blood viscosity, and vessel compliance. The systolic and diastolic pressures, measures of the maximum and minimum pressure exerted by the blood against the arterial wall, average 120/80 mm Hg. These values vary with age, gender, race, body weight, physical activity, medications, and health state.

The Client with Hypertension

■ ■ ■

Essential hypertension is a disorder characterized by blood pressure that persistently exceeds 140/90 mm Hg. Almost 60 million people in the United States have elevated blood pressure or report being told by a health care provider that they have high blood pressure. Essential hypertension occurs primarily in people between the ages of 25 and 55. It is reported as being responsible for over 30,000 deaths each year and is often called the "silent killer," because individuals have no manifestations of illness prior to sudden death. Although there is greater awareness of the causes and effects of hypertension, only about 20% of the people with this disorder have satisfactory blood pressure control (Tierney, McPhee, & Papadakis, 1995). About 20% of all adults develop hypertension; more than 90% of those have essential hypertension, with no identified cause.

The rate of occurrence is greater among African-Americans (20% to 30%) than among Caucasian Americans (10% to 15%). Essential hypertension is found equally in all parts of the United States, although the incidence may appear higher in certain locations (such as metropolitan areas) where ethnicity may be a factor. Essential hypertension affects people of all income groups, having great financial effects because of the conditions that result from the persistent increase in blood pressure: cerebrovascular accident (stroke), coronary artery disease, and chronic renal failure.

The criteria for recognition and diagnosis of essential hypertension in people 18 years and older were established in 1993 by the National Institutes of Health Subcommittee on the Diagnosis, Evaluation, and Treatment of High Blood Pressure. The subcommittee defined hypertension as a systolic blood pressure of 140 mm Hg or higher and a diastolic blood pressure of 90 mm Hg or higher when two or more blood pressure measurements are averaged on two or more subsequent visits (Porth, 1994). The committee also indicated that the exception to these parameters is a client systolic blood pressure of 210 mm Hg or higher and/or a diastolic blood pressure of 120 mm Hg or higher, although normally a single event of elevated blood pressure should not warrant a diagnosis of hypertension. Categories of hypertension are:

Stage 1 (mild)	140–150/90–99
Stage 2 (moderate)	160–179/100–109
Stage 3 (severe)	180–209/110–119
Stage 4 (very severe)	>210/120

Blood pressure measurements should be taken when the client has had an opportunity to rest for at least 5 minutes and has neither consumed caffeinated beverages nor smoked for at least 30 minutes prior to the blood pressure measurement (Porth, 1994). Many clients with hypertension use portable home devices to monitor their blood pressure daily; such devices have been found to yield blood pressures that are lower than those recorded in the doctor's office, in a clinic setting, or in a hospital setting. Interestingly, these lower readings are often found to be more reliable as an estimator of the client's prognosis (Massie, 1995).

Pathophysiology

The pathophysiology of essential hypertension (also known as *primary hypertension*) remain unknown in about 95% of cases (Massie, 1995). Despite the fact that no definitive cause can be identified, researchers agree that several factors contribute to essential hypertension (see the accompanying box):

- *Family history.* Studies show that the likelihood of developing essential hypertension is twice as high for individuals with a positive family history as it is for individuals with a negative family history. When obesity is added to a genetic predisposition, the risk of developing essential hypertension increases to four times that of clients without these risk factors (Porth, 1994). Although it is not clear how heredity and family history are related to the development of the disease, these factors are known to create enough of a risk so that affected clients are strongly recommended to have ongoing blood pressure screening beginning in the second decade of life.

- *Age.* Aging changes the sensitivity to fluid within the artery (i.e., baroreceptivity) and the ability of the arteries to accommodate varying amounts of blood (i.e.,

---

Factors Causing Hypertension

■ ■ ■

Modifiable Factors

- High sodium intake
- Obesity
- Excess alcohol consumption
- Low potassium intake
- Smoking
- Stress

Nonmodifiable Factors

- Family history
- Age
- Race

compliance). Because of these changes, the arteries of older clients become more rigid, thereby increasing the pressure of blood against the vessel wall. Blood pressure continues to increase gradually through the adult years, and, although this gradual increase affects individuals differently, aging often results in elevated systolic levels in older adults. Older adults who experience even isolated events of elevated blood pressure are more likely to die from cerebrovascular accident (stroke) than their age cohorts without hypertensive episodes (Porth, 1994). It is uncommon to find true essential hypertension occurring before the age of 20.

- *Race.* Essential hypertension is more common and more severe in African Americans than in people of other ethnic backgrounds. Even though the reasons for the increased incidence of essential hypertension in African Americans are not understood, some studies have recently shown that hypertensive African Americans have lower levels of renin than hypertensive Caucasians. The relationship between renin production and hypertension in African Americans is a topic of ongoing research.

- *High salt intake.* The correlation between increased salt intake and hypertension has been under investigation for many years. The consumption of sodium was implicated in hypertension when researchers noted that primitive tribes from various parts of the world who consumed very little sodium (some less than 1 milliequivalent of sodium daily) suffered little or no hypertension, whereas people in industrialized societies who ate between 10–20 milliequivalents of sodium daily had a higher incidence. It is known that salt holds fluid within the vessels, thereby increasing volume, but it is not understood exactly how salt consumption contributes to the development of the disease or why it is a factor for some clients but not others. Increased sodium consumption does not cause hypertension in normotensive clients, nor does the reduction of sodium intake guarantee reduced blood pressure in all hypertensive clients. Ongoing research regarding this issue is discussed later in this chapter.

- *Obesity.* The association between obesity and hypertension has been recognized for many years. Recent studies, however, suggest that the distribution of fat in the body is a more accurate indicator than the actual extent of obesity. Once again, the specific mechanism by which obesity influences blood pressure is not known. Researchers suspect that the increased metabolic needs of adipose tissue, the increased workload of the heart as a result of obesity, and the general eating habits of most obese clients work together to prevent adequate blood flow from reaching all areas of the enlarged body mass (Porth, 1994).

- *Excess alcohol consumption.* The relationship between alcohol consumption and the development of hypertension was established as far back as 1977, when researchers studied 84,000 clients in the Oakland–San Francisco area. This research demonstrated that the regular consumption of three or more drinks a day increased the risk of hypertension. When alcohol consumption was decreased or discontinued, there was a corresponding drop in systolic blood pressure. Some studies suggest that about 10% of hypertensive people have alcohol-related hypertension.

- *Mineral intake levels.* Current research is focused not only on the role of sodium but also on the relationship between potassium and sodium and their combined influence on blood pressure. Diets high in sodium are often low in potassium, and vice versa. Even though a diet high in potassium increases the elimination of sodium from the body, high-potassium diets did not influence the blood pressure of normotensive clients in the studies (Porth, 1994). As a result, the more common dietary recommendation is to substitute high-potassium and low-sodium foods for high-sodium and low-potassium foods.

- *Smoking.* In recent years, the relationship between levels of plasma norepinephrine (elevated by smoking) and hypertension has been well documented. The goal of ongoing research is to clarify the long-term effects of smoking on blood pressure (Massie, 1995).

- *Stress.* Although the relationship between physical and emotional stress and the constriction of blood vessels has been clearly established, there is still considerable doubt about the link between stress and essential hypertension. During the early course of the disease, hypertensive events often occur on an irregular and transient basis. However, even clients with well-established essential hypertension often have wide fluctuations in blood pressure, believed to be the result of changes in their activity levels and/or stress levels. Several meditative techniques, such as biofeedback, relaxation, and yoga, have been used to control blood pressure, but these techniques are not effective in every client. As a result, the usefulness of these therapies in producing long-term resolution of hypertension is still under investigation.

Other factors implicated in the development of essential hypertension include hyperactivity of the sympathetic nervous system, a defect in the renal excretion of sodium, and alterations in the intracellular concentrations of sodium and calcium (Tierney et al., 1995).

The client with mild-to-moderate essential hypertension commonly does not experience any manifestations, other than increased blood pressure readings, for years. The increase in blood pressure is initially transient but eventually becomes permanent. When symptoms do appear, they are usually vague, consisting primarily of suboccipital headaches occurring during the morning hours and subsiding during the day. As hypertension increases, clients may experience sleepiness, headache, confusion, nausea and vomiting, and visual disturbances. Examination of the retina of the eye may reveal narrowed arterioles, hemorrhages, exudates, and papilledema (swelling of the optic nerve).

Uncontrolled moderate and severe essential hypertension may lead to cardiovascular complications, including ventricular hypertrophy, myocardial ischemia, congestive heart failure, cerebrovascular accident due to thrombosis or hemorrhage, damage to the retina, renal insufficiency, aortic dissection, and sudden death. A severe increase in any form of essential hypertension (called *malignant hypertension*) may cause damage to the brain, kidneys, retina, and myocardium.

Collaborative Care

The management of clients with hypertension focuses on reducing the blood pressure to more normal levels of less than 140 mm Hg systolic and 90 mm Hg diastolic and the subsequent relief of symptoms. Emphasis is placed on client adherence to the plan of care so as to avoid the serious consequences of noncompliance (i.e., stroke, cardiac failure, and chronic renal failure). Several individualized treatment modalities are chosen to decrease total peripheral resistance and improve vascular compliance. Both pharmacologic and nonpharmacologic collaborative approaches may be used, depending on the client's age, type of hypertension, seriousness of the condition, and prognosis. There is no cure for hypertension.

Laboratory and Diagnostic Tests

The laboratory and diagnostic tests conducted for the client with hypertension are aimed at the detection of disorders causing secondary hypertension (discussed later in this section). There are no specific tests for essential hypertension.

Conservative Therapy

A conservative approach to reducing essential hypertension (depending on the severity of the condition) is often the treatment of choice. Conservative management is recommended for clients with mild-to-moderate hypertension, for clients with a family history of cardiovascular complications of hypertension, and for clients with multiple risk factors for coronary artery disease (Tierney et al., 1995). Conservative management includes dietary modifications, changes in alcohol and cigarette use, increased physical activity, and stress reduction. These management strategies are discussed below and summarized in the accompanying box.

Managing Diet The dietary modifications recommended for clients with hypertension are focused on reducing the amount of sodium and fat in the diet. Food habits are often among the most difficult behaviors to

---

Conservative Management of Hypertension
■ ■ ■

Dietary Modifications

- Reduce sodium and fat intake.
- Avoid canned, processed, snack, and fast foods.
- Season foods with herbs instead of salt.
- Limit carbonated beverages.
- Drink adequate amounts of water.

Reduce Alcohol Consumption

- Limit daily intake to no more than 1 ounce of alcohol.

Stop Smoking

- Use resources available through hospital or community groups.

Establish Regular, Daily Exercise Habits

- Aerobic exercise (swimming, walking) is best.

Minimize Stress Whenever Possible

- Focus on relaxation strategies.
- Incorporate stress management into the daily schedule.

---

change because they become internalized over time. Clients should avoid foods high in sodium, such as processed foods, canned fruits and vegetables, carbonated beverages, snack foods, and fast foods (see Chapter 5). These foods are high not only in sodium but often in fats as well, thereby contributing to weight gain. High-sodium, high-fat foods should be replaced with foods higher in potassium and lower in fat (such as fresh asparagus, oranges, bananas, freshly cooked meats, whole grains, and fresh vegetables). Hospital dietary departments work closely with clients and their families to teach them the specifics of their sodium restrictions and provide clients with lists of foods low in sodium and fat and high in potassium.

In addition, clients are taught to season foods with herbs and spices rather than salt. In secondary hypertension, additional dietary restrictions may be necessary because of an underlying disease. For example, clients with certain types of underlying renal disease may have to limit their protein intake temporarily. Regardless of the etiology of the hypertension, the nurse has a responsibility to reinforce dietary teaching and to make appropriate dietary referrals as needed.

Restricting Alcohol and Cigarette Use   Because of the relationship between alcohol consumption and hypertension, clients are cautioned to limit intake of alcohol. This limit, set in 1993 by the Joint National Committee on Detection, Evaluation, and Treatment of High Blood Pressure, is equal to 1 ounce per day. Although the withdrawal from alcohol may increase the client's blood pressure, this effect is usually temporary and diminishes as the withdrawal period lengthens.

Despite the lack of substantial data linking smoking to hypertension, there is a definitive link between smoking and heart disease. Further, because both smoking and hypertension increase the risk of heart disease, clients are strongly urged to quit. A relationship has also recently been noted between smoking and the effectiveness of the drug propranolol (Inderal), often prescribed for hypertension. Recent studies found that smokers using propranolol as a part of a blood pressure treatment plan needed more medication to control blood pressure than their nonsmoking, hypertensive counterparts. A variety of resource groups are available for clients who choose nonpharmacologic smoking-cessation methods.

Increasing Physical Activity   A sedentary life-style is a well-known risk for cardiovascular disease. Regular exercise (such as walking, cycling, jogging, or swimming) not only decreases blood pressure but contributes to weight loss, stress reduction, and feelings of overall well-being. Exercise also serves as a motivator; as clients realize the benefits of regular exercise, they become increasingly confident in their ability to control other risk factors such as obesity, smoking, and stress-related issues. Isometric exercise, however, can raise blood pressure severely and should be avoided unless approved by the physician.

Reducing Stress   The vasoconstricting effects of stress are well documented. Many individuals are unaware of the amount of stress they experience each day and of the effects of stress on physiologic well-being. Regular, moderate exercise is the treatment of choice for reducing stress in the hypertensive client. The relaxation response, whereby individuals are taught to focus on relaxing both mind and body, has also proven to lower blood pressure, yet insufficient clinical trials are available to suggest it be included as a universal, non-pharmacologic treatment for hypertension. While the calming effects of stress reduction techniques such as biofeedback, therapeutic touch, yoga, and meditation cannot be denied, their treatment value for the general hypertensive population continues to be unclear.

Pharmacology

For many years, researchers have been searching for the ideal antihypertensive drug; that is, a drug that would use a physiologic method to lower blood pressure, have no long-term toxic or unpleasant side effects, could be prescribed as a daily medication, would not require complex dosing formulas and trial periods, decrease the number of hypertension-related serious illnesses and deaths, and be moderately priced (Massie, 1995). Although no such single agent has been found, significant progress has been made, and drug treatment plans can be tailored to the needs of clients. Current pharmacologic treatment of hypertension involves the use of one or more of the following categories of drugs: diuretics, beta-adrenergic blockers, centrally acting sympatholytics, vasodilators, angiotensin-converting enzyme (ACE) inhibitors, and calcium channel blockers.

For more than 20 years, the management of blood pressure was implemented in phases, or steps (Figure 30–1). If nonpharmacologic treatment of modifiable risk factors (step 1) produced insufficient results, medication therapy would begin (steps 2, etc.). Clients were initially started on a diuretic or a beta-blocking agent, and, if results were inadequate, other drugs were added. In about 80% of the clients with whom this approach was used (and who adhered to the plan), successful results were obtained. It was direct and relatively inexpensive. However, with the advent of new agents and continued research about the long-term effects of this treatment methodology, the stepped care approach has become somewhat controversial. In fact, it has been found that the long-term use of certain agents produces unfavorable changes in the clients' plasma lipid levels and insulin sensitivity. Researchers found that clients who could not be treated effectively with a particular single agent did respond more favorably to a different single agent without the need for combination therapy (Massie, 1995).

As the research continues, studies show that therapy with low-dose diuretic agents and beta-adrenergic blockers continues to lower blood pressure while also decreasing the risk of cardiac events (such as cardiac failure or stroke). Although newer agents (such as ACE inhibitors and calcium channel blockers) effectively lower blood pressure, they have a shorter history of use, and they cannot yet be claimed to reduce the risk of coronary events. Researchers are hopeful that future longitudinal studies of new drugs will yield positive results. Nursing implications for the administration of the antihypertensive drugs (other than diuretics) are outlined in the pharmacology box on page 1191.

Thiazide diuretics, such as hydrochlorothiazide (HydroDIURIL), are the most widely used category of medications to control hypertension. In major clinical studies, single therapy with diuretics was shown to control blood pressure in approximately 50% of the clients and to be the most effective agents in reducing hypertension-linked morbidity and mortality related to coronary artery disease (Massie, 1995). Diuretics relieve hypertension primarily by preventing the tubular reabsorption of sodium, thereby decreasing volume and increasing cardiac output.

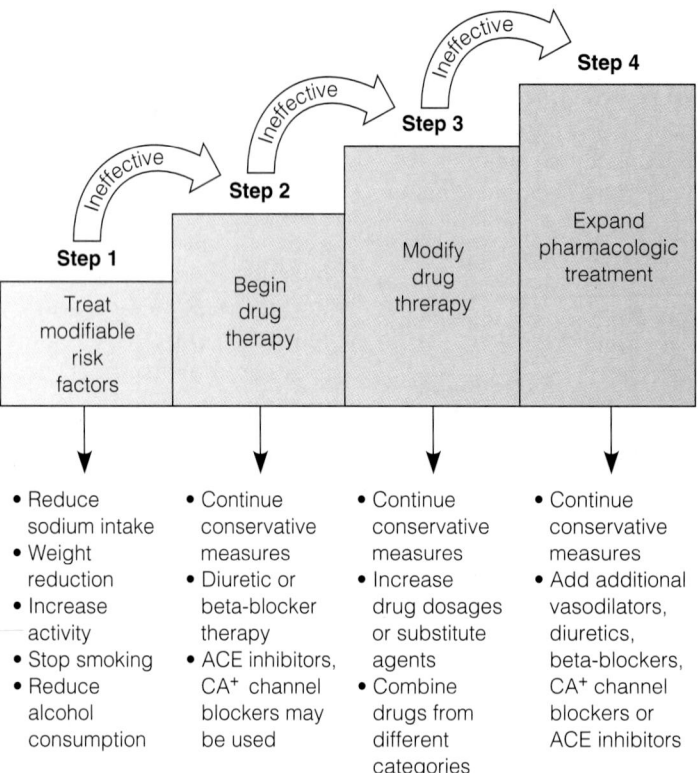

Figure 30–1 Stepped-care approach to the treatment of hypertension.

The heart's increased output increases renal perfusion and, in turn, sodium and water excretion. As less sodium and water are retained and the plasma volume falls, peripheral-vascular resistance decreases, thereby lowering blood pressure readings, especially systolic readings.

Compared to the next two most commonly used antihypertensive medications (i.e., beta-blockers and ACE inhibitors), diuretics are more potent in clients who are obese, older, of African-American ancestry and in groups of clients who have increased plasma volume or low plasma renin activity (Massie, 1995). Because the severity of the hypertension dictates the dosage of medication required to maintain control, side effects and adverse effects are most commonly dose related. In addition to hypokalemia, side effects include increased levels of blood glucose, triglycerides, uric acid, low-density lipoproteins, and plasma insulin. Further information about diuretics is found in Chapter 5 and Chapter 26.

In summary, the pharmacologic treatment of mild-to-moderate hypertension commonly begins with a single antihypertensive agent and incorporates the use of additional medications if initial treatment is not adequate. By combining agents, varying routes of administration, and/or substituting one type of agent for another, treatment goals can be achieved and the serious complications of uncontrolled blood pressure can often be avoided. Treatment of hypertensive crises relies on swift diagnosis and accurate pharmacologic intervention to stabilize the

client and to limit hypertension-related morbidity and mortality. In either situation, the nurse must be ready to implement nursing care protocols that support medical therapy and minimize the effects of hypertensive trauma to the client.

Nursing Care

Nursing care of clients with hypertension depends upon the severity of the condition and the specific needs of each person. Clients with mild-to-moderate hypertension receive care focused on improving cardiac output, decreasing intravascular fluid volume, modifying specific aspects of their nutritional intake, and maintaining health. Although many different nursing diagnoses may be appropriate for the client with hypertension, this discussion centers around the most common: *Decreased Cardiac Output, Fluid Volume Excess, Altered Nutrition: More Than Body Requirements,* and *Altered Heath Maintenance.*

Decreased Cardiac Output

Clients with hypertension have multiple, interconnected problems related to the relationships between plasma volume, peripheral vascular resistance, and cardiac output. As the amount of sodium ingested by the client increases, the amount of water being retained by the body increases. These excesses lead to increased plasma volume and a corresponding increase in peripheral vascular resistance.

Text continues on page 1194

Nursing Implications for Pharmacology: Antihypertensive Drug Therapy

Various groups of medications with distinct sites of action are used to treat the client with hypertension. Diuretics (discussed on page 1189) and drugs that inhibit the renin-angiotensin system reduce circulating blood volume. Beta-blockers reduce cardiac output. Centrally acting sympatholytics and vasodilators reduce peripheral resistance. Calcium channel blockers produce vasodilation. There is no one primary antihypertensive drug used to treat hypertension; rather a combination of drugs or a trial with a different category of antihypertensives is often used.

BETA-ADRENERGIC BLOCKING AGENTS

acebutolol (Sectral)

atenolol (Tenormin)

betaxolol (Kerlone)

labetalol (Normodyne)

metoprolol tartrate (Lopressor)

nadolol (Corgard)

penbutolol (Levatol)

pindolol (Visken)

propranolol hydrochloride (Inderal)

timolol (Blocadren)

Beta-adrenergic blockers are the second most common group of drugs used to control hypertension. Beta-blockers reduce blood pressure by preventing stimulation of the beta receptors in the heart by epinephrine and norepinephrine, thereby decreasing heart rate and cardiac output. Beta-blockers also interfere with the release of renin by the kidneys to decrease the renin-angiotensin mechanism. The side effects of all beta-blockers include bronchospasm, fatigue, sleep disturbances, nightmares, bradycardia, heart block, worsening of congestive heart failure, gastrointestinal disturbances, impotence, and increased triglyceride levels.

Nursing Responsibilities

- Check the client's past medical history carefully; beta-blockers are contraindicated in clients with selected cardiac and chronic health disorders.
- Use, if possible, a cardiac monitor when initiating therapy.
- Assess blood pressure and apical pulse before administration; notify the health care provider if these vital signs are not within established parameters.

- Monitor for manifestations of congestive heart failure (dyspnea, peripheral edema, weight gain, crackles and wheezes, decreased urinary output, jugular vein distention).
- Monitor peripheral circulation, noting warmth, color of skin, and quality of pulses.
- Monitor for manifestations of hypotension if client is also taking a diuretic and for manifestations of hypoglycemia if client is taking insulin or an oral antidiabetic agent.
- Monitor for manifestations of hypertension if client is also taking NSAIDs or cimetidine.
- Carefully monitor responses of the older client.

Client and Family Teaching

- Take blood pressure and pulse as taught at the same time each day.
- Change position (lying to sitting and sitting to standing) slowly to prevent dizziness and possible falls.
- Report side effects to your primary health care provider; the medication may cause fatigue, lethargy, and impotence.
- Check blood glucose levels and blood pressure more frequently if you are also taking insulin, an oral antidiabetic medicine, an over-the-counter NSAID, or medication to treat peptic ulcers, such as cimetidine (Tagamet).
- Do not take over-the-counter cold medications or nasal decongestants.
- Restrict sodium and alcohol as recommended.
- Do not stop taking the medication until you discuss doing so with your health care provider.

CENTRALLY ACTING SYMPATHOLYTICS

Clonidine (Catapres)

Guanabenz (Wytensin)

Guanfacine (Tenex)

Methyldopa (Aldomet)

The centrally acting sympatholytics stimulate the alpha$_2$ receptors in the central nervous system to inhibit the sympathetic cardioaccelerator and vasoconstrictor centers. They also decrease sympathetic outflow from the central nervous system. These actions lower the arterial pressure. These drugs may be administered in combination with a diuretic.

➤

Pharmacology: Antihypertensive Drug Therapy (continued)

Nursing Responsibilities

- Administer PO; tablets may be crushed. They do not need to be given with food unless gastrointestinal upset occurs.

- Administer IV infusion of methyldopa over 30 to 60 minutes by piggyback, diluted in 50 or 100 mL of 5% dextrose.

- Do not administer methyldopa subcutaneously or intramuscularly because absorption is unpredictable.

- Apply transdermal systems (e.g., clonidine) to dry, hairless area of intact skin on the chest or upper arm. Assess for rash, which indicates allergy, at area of application.

- Do not administer sympatholytics to pregnant or lactating women.

- Monitor laboratory data; some drugs in this category increase values of AST, ALT, alkaline phosphatase, bilirubin, BUN, creatine, potassium, sodium, and uric acid; they may also prolong prothrombin time.

- Obtain baseline blood pressure, pulse, and weight.

- Monitor blood pressure and pulse before administration.

- Assess client for peripheral edema (hands and feet if ambulatory, sacrum if on bed rest).

- Assess for and report side effects: dry mouth, drowsiness, constipation, dizziness, postural hypotension, nausea.

Client and Family Teaching

- Relieve dry mouth by sipping water or chewing sugarless gum.

- Treat nausea by eating unsalted crackers, noncola beverages, or dry toast.

- Change position (lying to sitting and sitting to standing) slowly to prevent dizziness and possible falls.

- Do not suddenly discontinue medication or skip doses; this could cause serious hypertension.

- Some of the drugs cause the urine to become darker.

- Report mental depression or decreased mental acuity to your health care provider.

- Side effects (such as dry mouth, nausea, and dizziness) tend to diminish over time.

- Do not drive a car if the medications cause drowsiness.

VASODILATORS

Hydralazine (Apresoline)

Minoxidil (Loniten)

Vasodilators reduce blood pressure by relaxing vascular smooth muscle (especially in the arterioles), thereby decreasing peripheral vascular resistance. These drugs are usually prescribed in combination with a diuretic or a beta-blocker, especially if the client's hypertension is difficult to control or resistant to other therapies.

Nursing Responsibilities

- Administer PO with meals or food; tablets may be crushed.

- Carefully monitor response of mother and newborn if used as therapy.

- Assess blood pressure and pulse before administration of drug.

- Assess for peripheral edema.

- Monitor pattern of bowel movements.

- Monitor client for manifestations of congestive heart failure, fluid retention, and angina.

Client and Family Teaching

- Change position (lying to sitting and sitting to standing) slowly to prevent dizziness and possible falls.

- Eat dry toast or unsalted crackers to relieve nausea.

- Report muscle, joint aches, and fever to your health care provider.

- Tearing and nasal congestion may occur.

- Headache, palpitations, and rapid pulse may occur but should be gone in about 10 days.

- Do not discontinue the medication without the approval of your health care provider.

- If you are taking hydralazine, report black, tarry stools or red blood in the stools to your primary health care provider.

Pharmacology: Antihypertensive Drug Therapy (continued)

ALPHA-ADRENERGIC BLOCKERS

Doxazosin (Cardura)

Prazosin (Minipress)

Terazosin (Hytrin)

Alpha-adrenergic blocking agents decrease vasomotor tone to cause vasodilatation and thus reduce blood pressure; they also decrease the level of low-density and very low density lipoproteins. However, reflex stimulation of the heart as a result of the vasodilatation causes tachycardia and palpitations. The drugs also produce many unwanted side effects. For these reasons, the drugs are primarily used to control acute hypertensive states.

The one drug from this category that is used consistently is prazosin (Minipress), which is often used in combination with a diuretic and a beta-blocker.

Nursing Responsibilities

- Maintain safety when the client is changing positions, because this drug causes severe hypotension.

- Give the first dose at bedtime to minimize risk of fainting (called "first-dose syncope"). If the first dose is given in the daytime (or if the dose is increased) the client should remain recumbent for 3 to 4 hours.

- Assess blood pressure and apical pulse immediately before each dose and every 15 to 30 minutes thereafter until stabilized.

Client and Family Teaching

- Drink sips of water or chew sugarless gum to relieve dry mouth.

- Eat dry toast or unsalted crackers to relieve nausea.

- You may experience nasal congestion.

- Do not expect a full therapeutic effect for 3 to 4 weeks.

- Change position (lying to sitting and sitting to standing) slowly to prevent dizziness and possible falls.

- Do not discontinue the medication without consulting your primary health care provider.

CALCIUM CHANNEL BLOCKERS

Amlodipine (Norvasc)

Diltiazem (Cardizem)

Nicardipine (Cardene)

Nifedipine (Procardia)

Verapamil (Isoptin)

The calcium channel blockers inhibit the flow of calcium ions across the cell membrane of vascular tissue and cardiac cells. This category of antihypertensives relaxes arterial smooth muscle to lower peripheral resistance through vasodilatation. The drugs are effective as single-agent therapy in 60% of clients (Tierney et al., 1995).

Nursing Responsibilities

- If these drugs are administered parenterally, maintain cardiac monitoring and have emergency equipment available.

- Assess blood pressure and apical pulse as baseline data and before administration. Notify health care provider if values are not within established parameters.

- Monitor frequency and consistency of stools.

- Assess lungs for crackles and wheezes.

- Monitor intake and output.

- Assess extremities for peripheral edema.

- Teach the client and family how to take blood pressure and pulse accurately.

Client and Family Teaching

- Take blood pressure and pulse as taught each day.

- Change position (lying to sitting and sitting to standing) slowly to prevent dizziness and possible falls.

- Drink six to eight glasses of water each day, and increase fiber in diet.

- Maintain sodium-restricted diet as prescribed.

- Do not abruptly stop taking medications.

- Report respiratory difficulty or chest pain to your primary health care provider.

ANGIOTENSIN-CONVERTING ENZYME (ACE) INHIBITOR

Benazepril (Lotensin)

Captopril (Capoten)

Enalapril (Vasotec)

➤

Pharmacology: Antihypertensive Drug Therapy (continued)

Fosinopril (Monopril)

Ramipril (Altace)

The ACE inhibitors inhibit the renin-angiotensin-aldosterone mechanism, but they also stimulate vasodilation and (in some clients) reduce sympathetic nervous system activity. These drugs have relatively few side effects in clients with essential hypertension. They are often used in combination with a diuretic or calcium channel blocker.

Nursing Responsibilities

- Administer PO 1 hour before meals to increase absorption; tablets may be crushed.

- Do not administer to pregnant or lactating women.

- Monitor laboratory data for increased potassium, AST, ALT, alkaline phosphatase, bilirubin, BUN, and creatinine values and for decreased sodium values.

- Take blood pressure immediately before giving each dose in addition to monitoring it regularly.

- If the client is hypotensive, maintain recumbent position with legs elevated.

- If the client has renal disease, monitor urine protein with dipstick method on first voiding of the day on a regular basis.

- Monitor skin for rash and hives.

- Assess for peripheral edema.

Client and Family Teaching

- Report peripheral edema, signs of infection, or difficulty breathing to your health care provider.

- Change position (lying to sitting and sitting to standing) slowly to prevent dizziness and possible falls.

- Do not skip doses or stop taking drugs; this could cause a serious rebound in blood pressure.

As the heart becomes increasingly incapable of handling the excess fluid load, there eventually is a decreased stroke volume and a subsequent decrease in the overall cardiac output.

Because the heart is not pumping as much blood with each stroke, the amount of blood perfusing the kidneys is also diminished, thereby triggering the renin-angiotensin-aldosterone mechanism. As a result, the body produces increased amounts of aldosterone, causing vasoconstriction and retention of excessive amounts of sodium and water. This cycle of events continues until blood pressure rises to abnormal levels and the client seeks intervention for complaints of headache, blurred vision, confusion, palpitations, peripheral edema, and/or fatigue.

Nursing interventions with rationales follow:

- Monitor and record level of consciousness, heart rate and rhythm, respirations and blood pressure every 4 hours and more often, if needed. *The early detection of the manifestations of decreased cardiac output, such as cerebral hypoxia, shortness of breath, and increased blood pressure, allows the nurse to act promptly to minimize the damaging effects of inadequate blood flow. Proper documentation keeps members of the health team informed of the client's status.*

- Accurately measure intake and output and record findings. *The balance between intake and output is closely re-lated to the ability of the heart to pump sufficient amounts of blood to perfuse the kidneys adequately, thus allowing them to produce adequate amounts of urine. Increased intake accompanied by decreased output is a sign of poor cardiac output, possible impending cardiac failure, and/or potential kidney failure.*

- Weigh the client daily, before breakfast, having the client wear similar clothing each day. *Weight changes related to increased fluid retention are not uncommon in clients with decreased cardiac output and corresponding decreased renal perfusion. Weighing clients at the same time each day under similar conditions increases the accuracy of measurements and minimizes inconsistency.*

- Teach the client and family ways of decreasing the workload of the heart. *Discuss the reason for the fatigue that commonly accompanies decreased cardiac output and explain ways to modify daily activities and incorporate periods of rest. Help clients assess life-style issues, such as stress, physical activity, and family demands, to help them identify areas needing improvement. Emphasize the importance of conserving energy by balancing rest with activity, setting priorities, and planning effectively.*

Fluid Volume Excess

Clients with hypertension retain excess fluids in the intravascular space because of increased sodium intake, decreased cardiac output, and a compromised renin-angiotensin-aldosterone regulatory mechanism. Because of these changes, clients present with varying degrees of the following symptoms: elevated blood pressure, weight gain, decreased urinary output, altered laboratory values, increased heart rate, headache, and the effects of decreased cerebral perfusion (i.e., confusion, restlessness, altered mood or personality).

Nursing interventions with rationales follow:

- Carefully monitor intake and output daily and routinely throughout the shift. *Excess retained fluids cause an imbalance between the client's fluid intake and output. Because the imbalance may not be realized for the first 24 hours following admission, close observation of input and output is necessary throughout the hospital stay. When intake exceeds output, fluid retention or overload is suspected.*

- Monitor laboratory values, such as blood urea nitrogen, urine specific gravity, creatinine, electrolytes, and hematocrit and hemoglobin. *The decreased renal perfusion found in many hypertensive clients disrupts the body's overall fluid balance and is frequently demonstrated by changes in laboratory values. Changes in the blood urea nitrogen, urine specific gravity, and creatinine indicate changes in renal function, whereas changes in hematocrit and hemoglobin are reflective of fluid status.*

- Assess for signs of fluid retention, such as dependent or sacral edema and/or ascites. *The decreased activity levels of hospitalized patients may contribute to the collection of fluid in dependent areas of the body, such as the extremities (especially the feet), the sacrum and, if portal circulation is affected, the abdomen. Encourage clients to ambulate as often as possible within treatment guidelines, increase self-care activities, and adhere to therapies designed to reduce fluid retention and promote the excretion of wastes.*

- Collaborate with dietary services to provide information for the client and family on how to reduce sodium intake. *Be sure clients understand the relationship between sodium intake and fluid retention. This knowledge helps clients understand and take control of their disease. In addition, provide opportunities for clients to choose low-sodium foods from simulated menus to support their ability to make correct choices independently. Support client efforts and explain that changes in life-style (e.g., dietary habits and exercise) may take time; patience and perseverance are needed to succeed.*

- Teach clients the importance of adhering to treatment plans such as dietary restrictions and medication schedules. *Providing clients and their families with information to promote health and minimize illness encourages them to participate more fully in their care. In addition, it removes feelings of fear and powerlessness because clients learn how to take control of modifiable factors that contribute to their disease.*

Altered Nutrition: More Than Body Requirements

The relationship between obesity, excess sodium intake, alcohol intake, and hypertension is well documented. All of these factors are modifiable by clients who are motivated to take responsibility for their disease and make appropriate life-style changes. Clients classified as overweight weigh 10% over their ideal weight for height and frame; clients classified as obese weigh 20% or more over their ideal weight for height and frame. In addition, most clients report undesirable eating habits, a sedentary life-style, and intake that exceeds metabolic demands.

Nursing interventions with rationales follow.

- Assess for causative or contributing factors for excess weight. *When gathering subjective data, ask clients about changes in taste, smell, or feelings of satiety. Determine if drug-nutrient interactions are occurring with medications prescribed for clients. Discuss how medications can influence dietary intake and explain how scheduling medications at different times or taking medications in different ways may decrease the effects of these interactions while still promoting treatment goals. Inquire about diversional activities, exercise levels, and previous weight-related issues (such as participation in weight-reduction programs or crash diets) to determine a history of weight problems and to identify avenues for further exploration. Encourage clients to consult their physician before beginning any exercise program.*

- Collaborate with dietary services to provide information to clients and families about low-fat diets. *Permanent weight loss begins with the identification of factors that contribute to weight gain, such as excessive fat in the diet, inappropriate portion sizes, and inadequate exercise. Teaching clients ways to reduce fat in the diet assists them in preparing and eating healthier meals while also helping motivate them to take control of modifiable disease factors.*

- Mutually determine with the client a realistic target weight and have client weigh in regularly. *Setting goals for weight loss helps the client formalize the process and provides motivation for continued progress. For clients who have been overweight or obese for a long time, setting realistic goals may be more difficult, because they may be striving for unreasonable young adulthood weights. Encourage clients to plan for small, continuous incremental weight loss to provide proof of their ability to lose weight and to ensure permanent weight reduction. As the client increases exercise levels and continues to adhere to dietary limitations, weight loss will accelerate.*

- Explore feasibility of referring client to approved weight-loss programs. *Although entering a weight-loss program is an important first step, the ability to follow through ultimately makes the difference. Several organizations, such as Weight Watchers, Overeaters Anonymous, and Diet Workshop, offer balanced weight-reduction programs. The support and reinforcement provided through organized weight-loss programs are often very beneficial to clients as they strive to control their hypertension.*

Altered Health Maintenance

Clients with altered health maintenance are those who have a disruption in health because of unhealthy life-style behaviors or who lack the knowledge to manage a known condition. The modifiable factors of hypertension include diet, activity, alcohol use, smoking, and stress-related components. The client's willingness to comply with treatment plans and to take responsibility for changing unhealthy life-style habits is central to the effectiveness of the overall treatment plan.

Regardless of the types of medications used to manage the client's hypertension, lack of adherence to nonpharmacologic treatment strategies prevents clients from establishing good control of the disease and, ultimately, places the client at risk for developing the long-term complications of uncontrolled hypertension. Because the goal of the interventions for this diagnosis are self-care and independent functioning, the education of the client and the family is instrumental in helping clients make necessary changes to ensure and promote good health.

Nursing interventions with rationales follow:

- Assist client and family in identifying unhealthy behaviors that contribute to altered health. *If clients intend to work at controlling their hypertension, they must be willing to acknowledge those life-style behaviors that contribute to their disease and be amenable to adjusting them. Because the goal is adherence to therapy, the nurse's ability to explore current and potential health behaviors with clients and family is an important factor in determining the willingness of clients to maintain their own health. It is also important for families to understand that their support and encouragement are necessary if the client is to realize a high level of wellness.*

- Assist clients in developing a realistic health maintenance plan. *Preparing a health maintenance plan for clients does little to encourage clients to assume responsibility for their own health. However, nurses can be instrumental in guiding clients and family in the development of realistic goals related to the management of modifiable risk factors such as smoking, exercise, diet, and stress. By encouraging clients to use established parameters to develop their own health maintenance plan, the nurse demonstrates trust and respect for the client's knowledge base and fosters independence and self-accountability.*

- Help clients and family identify strengths and weaknesses in maintaining health. *Once a health maintenance plan has been developed, it must be implemented to determine its true usefulness. The nurse should encourage clients to discuss areas of the plan that are working well and areas that present difficulty for the client. Through open communication, clients discover the nurse's willingness to assist*

them in finding and using a realistic plan that produces positive results.

Other Nursing Diagnoses

The following nursing diagnoses may also be appropriate for the client with hypertension:

- *Activity Intolerance* related to exertional fatigue secondary to decreased cardiac output
- *Ineffective Individual Coping* related to necessary life-style changes
- *Anxiety* related to continuing episodes of severe hypertension
- *Fatigue* related to side effects of antihypertensive medication
- *Knowledge Deficit* related to the relationship of alterations in life-style and management of hypertension

Client and Family Teaching

When planning and implementing nursing care for clients with hypertension, nurses need to recognize that, without considerable education and mutually established goals, clients will be unable to adhere to the plan of care. As a result, the disease will remain out of control, placing the client at risk for developing the serious complications of cardiac failure, stroke, and renal failure. The care of clients with hypertension is primarily managed on an outpatient basis with regular visits to the primary care provider's office or hypertension clinic to monitor the course of therapy. The accompanying box lists topics for client and family teaching.

Having hypertension may mean the client must cope with changes in activities of daily living. The decreased cardiac output that accompanies hypertension often produces fatigue and may require clients to modify their approach to activities of daily living. If shortness of breath is an issue, clients should be taught to perform tasks in small steps whenever possible. If walking or climbing stairs becomes difficult, clients should rest and resume an appropriate level of activity when they are rested. If clients begin to experience headache, blurred vision, palpitations, and/or light-headedness, they should be instructed to sit down, loosen tight garments or collars, and rest until symptoms subside. As prescribed antihypertensive medications take effect and life-style changes are implemented, clients often find they are better able to cope with the decreased energy levels they once experienced.

Activity and exercise, through a gradual conditioning of muscles and blood vessels, lower blood pressure by decreasing peripheral vascular resistance and gradually increasing cardiac output. As the heart's ability to pump efficiently increases, kidney perfusion increases and intravascular volume falls, further diminishing vascular

---

Client and Family Teaching Focus for Hypertension

■ ■ ■

Coping with Changes in Activities of Daily Living

- Allow ample time for the activities of daily living.
- Rest when you are fatigued, and incorporate rest periods into your daily schedule.
- Allow yourself to move more slowly during daily activities.

Improving Levels of Activity and Exercise

- Gradually increase daily activity.
- Develop a realistic exercise program.
- Avoid lifting or straining.

Managing Stress

- Make a list of stressors.
- Explore relaxation options.
- Integrate relaxation techniques into your daily schedule.

Monitoring Wellness

- Follow prescribed treatment.
- Make and keep health care appointments.
- Have follow-up laboratory tests.
- Ask questions about treatment that seems to be ineffective.

---

resistance and lowering blood pressure. Clients should be taught to develop a realistic, regular exercise program, discuss it with their primary health care provider, and stick to it. Exercise not only increases stamina and endurance but also provides diversion and helps to manage obesity. Several aerobic exercise options, such as brisk walking, jogging, swimming, and cycling are appropriate; the client's choice is determined by current health status, age, and motivation. Isometric activities (such as weight lifting) should be avoided without physician approval because they increase intrathoracic pressure and diminish cardiac output.

Many clients with hypertension manifest a variety of stress-related behaviors that must be recognized and addressed if treatment goals are to be met. Stress-reduction methods include meditation, relaxation, deep breathing, and various forms of aerobic exercise. The nurse's role includes assessing the client's understanding of the impact of stress on blood pressure and helping the client determine which methods of stress reduction are most appropriate. Prior to initiating an exercise program, clients should be taught to consult their physician to be sure there are no contraindications. Another valuable stress-reduction nursing intervention relates to teaching clients ways of diffusing anger and hostility, emotions that intensify vasoconstriction in the body. By teaching ways of channeling detrimental behaviors into more positive responses, the nurse can be instrumental in helping clients cope with modifiable behaviors and minimize the harmful effects of stress on blood pressure.

Clients and family members should be taught the importance of frequent follow-up appointments to ensure the plan of care is effective and progressing smoothly. For clients using a nonpharmacologic treatment plan, return appointments may be set for 3-month intervals to assess overall wellness. Clients are encouraged to keep all appointments, even if progress is slow or if they have been unable to adhere to the plan. The continued support of health professionals is very important in motivating clients to continue working toward the management of hypertension. During follow-up visits, the client's blood pressure is recorded, and specific laboratory work (such as serum creatinine, BUN, and/or serum electrolytes) may be ordered to determine the progress of the disease and the effectiveness of antihypertensive medications.

Care of the Older Adult

In recent years, the study of the relationship between aging and elevated blood pressure has produced some interesting results. Not only is the prevalence of hypertension in the older adult greater than researchers originally suspected, but, contrary to previous thinking, the need to control blood pressure was found to be as important in the older adult as it is in the rest of the general population. Depending on the values used (i.e., 160 mm Hg or 140 mm Hg systolic and 95 mm Hg or 90 mm Hg diastolic), 44% to 63% of older Caucasian Americans and 60% to 76% of older African Americans in the United States have been found to be hypertensive (Porth, 1994).

Results from the Framingham study show that the number of cardiovascular deaths linked to isolated systolic hypertension were two to five times greater among older populations than they were in the normotensive general population. In addition, stroke was two to three times more common in the older population than it was in the rest of the population whose blood pressure was not elevated (Porth, 1994). The primary reasons for these findings seem to be related to two important changes in blood vessel structure associated with the normal aging process: decreased compliance associated with arteriosclerosis and decreased baroreceptivity. The stiffening of the blood vessels in older adults decreases the ability of the vessels to expand and contract with varying amounts of blood, thereby increasing peripheral vascular resistance and decreasing renal blood flow.

The findings of the 1985 Working Group on Hypertension in the Elderly indicated that the norms for blood pressure in older clients should be the same as the norms for the general adult population, and that the means for determining elevations in systolic and/or diastolic blood pressure in older adults should be the same as the means used in younger adults. To obtain accurate blood pressure readings for older clients, slightly different procedures may be required. A simple procedure known as *Osler's maneuver* has been shown to be effective in differentiating pseudohypertension associated with sclerotic changes in the blood vessels from actual hypertension in the older population. When performing the procedure, the clinician inflates the blood pressure cuff above the client's usual systolic pressure level and carefully palpates the radial or brachial artery. If either vessel remains clearly palpable (in spite of pulselessness), the client is said to be *Osler-positive;* if the vessel is not palpable, the artery has collapsed and the client is said to be *Osler-negative.*

Additional findings related to blood pressure in older clients include auscultatory gap and orthostatic hypotension. It should be noted that an auscultatory gap may be a normal finding in a large segment of the older adult population. As a result, clinicians are advised to inflate the cuff and palpate the artery prior to auscultation of systolic blood pressure in the older client and to deflate the cuff very slowly during auscultation to avoid missing the first of the Korotkoff sounds.

Many individuals experience a transient light-headedness associated with standing that is related to a reflexive but temporary fall in blood pressure. Because the aging process often diminishes these reflexes and because antihypertensive medications can produce side effects of transient orthostatic hypotension, clinicians should allow a 2- to 5-minute standing interval to pass before measuring blood pressure in older clients. In addition, blood pressure should be measured while the older client is sitting as well as standing to obtain a more accurate frame of reference for their actual pressures. These procedures should be used both in the detection and in the follow-up care of older hypertensive clients.

Applying the Nursing Process

Case Study of a Client with Hypertension: Margaret Spezia

Margaret Spezia is a married, 49-year-old Italian-American woman whose 10 pregnancies resulted in eight living children, currently ranging in ages from 3 years to 18 years. For the past 2 months, Mrs. Spezia has been experiencing frequent headaches, dizziness, occasional blurring of vision, and fatigue. She originally came to the nurse practitioner's clinic 2 months ago for her annual physical examination, where her sitting blood pressure was found to be 146/98. At that time, Mrs. Spezia was instructed to reduce her cholesterol intake, to avoid salty foods, and not to add any salt to her foods either at the table or during cooking. An exercise program of short, daily walks was also suggested to increase her activity level and to reduce stress. She now returns to the clinic for follow-up of her blood pressure management.

Assessment

Upon entering her room to complete the admission database and physical assessment, Lisa Christos, RN, notices that Mrs. Spezia seems restless and upset. After introducing herself, Ms. Christos says, "You look upset about something? Is everything OK?" Mrs. Spezia responds, "Well, my head seems to be throbbing, and I feel sort of dizzy. I've felt this way before, but I always just thought I was overdoing it and not getting enough rest. You know, raising eight children is a lot of work and gets pretty expensive. I didn't want us to get behind in our bills, so I recently started working part-time in a local department store. I thought the work might also help relieve some of my stress, but I'm not so sure that's really happening. Now that I'm not getting any better, I'm worried that I'll lose my job and that my husband won't be able to manage the children by himself. I really need to go home, but first, I want to get rid of this awful headache. Would you please get me a couple of aspirin or something to relieve this headache?"

Mrs. Spezia's admission history indicates a steady increase in weight over the past 18 years. There is no known family history of hypertension. Physical findings include the following: height: 5′ 3″ (160 cm); weight: 225 lb (102 kg); T, 99 F (37.2 C); P, 100 (radial, at rest); R, 16; BP, 180/115 (lying), 170/110 (sitting), 165/105 (standing). There is an average 10-point discrepancy between the systolic blood pressure readings in the right arm and those in the left arm and an average 6-point difference in the diastolic pressures in the right versus left arms, with lower readings in the left arm. Her skin is cool to the touch, and capillary refill times are 4 seconds in the right hand and 3 seconds in the left hand. Diagnostic laboratory tests reveal a total cholesterol of 245 mg/dL (normal range for adults is < 200 mg/dL). All other blood and urine laboratory studies are within normal limits. Following the analysis of the data, Mrs. Spezia is started on captopril (Capoten), 25 mg by mouth twice daily; diuretic therapy (spironolactone [Aldactone], 25 mg by mouth daily), and placed on a low-cholesterol, no-added-salt diet.

Diagnosis

The following nursing diagnoses were made for Mrs. Spezia:

- *Fatigue* related to effects of hypertension and stresses of daily life
- *Altered Nutrition: More Than Body Requirements* related to excessive food intake
- *Altered Health Maintenance* related to inability to modify detrimental life-style behaviors
- *Knowledge Deficit* related to effects of prescribed therapies

Expected Outcomes

The expected outcomes established in the plan of care specify that Mrs. Spezia will

- Reduce blood pressure readings to less than 150 systolic and 90 diastolic before returning for her clinic visit next week.
- Incorporate in her diet low-sodium and low-fat foods from a list provided.
- Develop a plan for regular exercise.
- Verbalize how prescribed medications, dietary restrictions, exercise, and follow-up visits will work to help her control her hypertension.

Planning and Implementation

The following nursing interventions are planned and implemented for Mrs. Spezia:

- Teach Mrs. Spezia to take her own blood pressure and to take it before each dose of antihypertensive medication. Teach her to withhold medications and report values lower than 90 mm Hg systolic or 60 mm Hg diastolic to the clinic.
- Teach Mrs. Spezia the name, dose, action, and side effects of her antihypertensive medications.
- Teach Mrs. Spezia to walk for 15 minutes each day this week, and to investigate participation in swimming classes at the local YWCA.
- Teach Mrs. Spezia methods for establishing a realistic weight-loss goal.
- Make a referral for consultation with a dietitian to ensure that Mrs. Spezia understands fat and sodium restrictions.
- Teach Mrs. Spezia how to perform stress-reducing techniques daily.

Evaluation

Mrs. Spezia returns to the clinic 1 week later. Her average systolic pressure is 142 mm Hg, and her average diastolic pressure is 88 mm Hg. She has lost 1.5 lb. She states that her oldest daughter is encouraging her to join a weight-reduction program. Mrs. Spezia is walking at a local mall each day, averaging 20 minutes per day. Mrs. Spezia and Ms. Christos review the schedule for taking her antihypertensive medications and diuretics. In addition, Mrs. Spezia says that she has met with the dietitian and that they discussed ways to replace the sodium in her diet with herbs and spices, which do not add fat or sodium. Alice Gunnerman, the dietitian, has given Mrs. Spezia a list of low-fat, low-sodium foods and has recommended cookbooks that can help her modify her cooking. Mrs. Spezia verbalizes the importance of taking her medications as ordered, reducing the sodium in her diet, and changing life-style behaviors such as overeating, inactivity, and unhealthy responses to stress. Mrs. Spezia says to Ms. Christos, "I just can't believe how much better I feel already. My headaches are gone, and I've actually lost some weight—and I feel motivated to keep going. If I had only known how much better I could feel! I don't expect I'll ever go back to my old habits again; it's just not worth it! Thank you very much for your help."

Critical Thinking in the Nursing Process

1. Identify the factors that contributed to Mrs. Spezia's hypertension. Which were modifiable and which were not?

2. What is the rationale for reducing sodium and fat in Mrs. Spezia's diet?

3. Suppose your client with hypertension is homeless and has no source of income. How would you conduct teaching to ensure your client followed your recommendations to manage hypertension? What would you do if the client did not follow them?

4. Discuss the role of stress in the severity of hypertension. What factors in Mrs. Spezia's life contribute to her stress level?

5. Develop a plan of care for Mrs. Spezia for the diagnosis: *Self-Esteem Disturbance* related to obesity and chronic illness.

The Client with Secondary Hypertension

■ ■ ■

Secondary hypertension is elevated blood pressure resulting from some underlying process. The most common causes of secondary hypertension include estrogen use, renal disease, vascular disease, endocrine disorders, coarctation of the aorta, stress, and pregnancy.

- *Estrogen use.* Uninterrupted, long-term use of oral contraceptives is the most identifiable estrogen-related cause of secondary hypertension. Approximately 5% of women using oral contraceptives develop hypertension but become normotensive within 6 months after discontinuing the medication. Women whose blood pressure does not return to normal are generally over 35 years of age and smoke cigarettes, factors that automatically place them at greater risk for developing long-term hypertension (Porth, 1994).

- *Renal disease.* Any disease that affects (a) the functional portion of the kidney (e.g., the renal parenchyma), (b) the ability of the kidney to produce and maintain enzymatic balance (balance of the renin-angiotensin-aldosterone system), or (c) the arteries that supply the kidney with blood (e.g., renal artery stenosis) will cause hypertension (Porth, 1994). The renin-angiotensin-aldosterone mechanism, which governs vasoconstriction, plays a critical role in blood pressure regulation.

- *Endocrine disorders.* The incidence of hypertension secondary to endocrine disorders is small, contributing only about 0.5% of all cases. Lesions of the adrenal medulla or the adrenal cortex (Cushing's syndrome and primary aldosteronism) can result in hypertension. An adrenal medullary tumor known as pheochromocytoma, a rare tumor of the adrenal medulla, causes persistent or intermittent hypertension (Porth, 1994).

- *Coarctation of the aorta.* Coarctation of the aorta, a congenital heart disease, is a rare condition in which the aortic arch narrows as the arch exits the heart. It is rarely discovered in adults, but, if found, causes hypertension secondary to left ventricular failure or cerebral hemorrhage (Massie, 1995).

- *Pregnancy.* About 10% of all pregnant women are classified as hypertensive. In some women, the hypertension predates pregnancy, and in others the elevated levels are a direct response to the pregnancy. Criteria for determining hypertension in pregnancy are a systolic pressure increase of 30 mm Hg or more or a diastolic pressure increase of 15 mm Hg or more when compared with the average of at least two values obtained before 20 weeks gestation (Porth, 1994). Regardless of the etiology, hypertension in pregnancy is one of the most common causes of maternal and fetal morbidity and mortality and requires careful perinatal management.

Clients with secondary hypertension have varying patterns of hypertension. Clients with pheochromocytoma often have attacks of hypertension that last for minutes to hours, accompanied by anxiety, palpitations, diaphoresis, pallor, and nausea and vomiting. Primary aldosteronism may cause not only hypertension, but also weakness,

paresthesias, polyuria, and nocturia (see Chapter 20). Clients with renal involvement often have hematuria during periods of severe hypertension.

The following laboratory and diagnostic tests may be ordered to diagnose secondary hypertension:

- *Hemoglobin* is measured to detect anemia or polycythemia.

- *Renal function studies* and *complete urinalysis* are done to identify any renal causes of hypertension. Findings of hematuria, proteinuria, and casts indicate renal disease.

- *Serum potassium* is decreased in the client with hyperaldosteronism.

- *Fasting blood sugar,* if increased, may indicate the presence of diabetes mellitus (which increases peripheral vascular disease) or a pheochromocytoma.

- *Plasma lipids* are increased in atherosclerosis, which increases the risk of hypertension.

- *Electrocardiography* and *echocardiography* are performed to assess left ventricular hypertrophy, a complication of long-term hypertension.

- *Renal studies,* including *intravenous pyelography, renal ultrasonography, renal arteriography,* and *CT* or *MRI* may be conducted for clients with suspected secondary hypertension.

Collaborative and nursing care for the client with secondary hypertension is the same as that for the client with essential hypertension, discussed in the previous section. However, the underlying process causing the hypertension also requires medical and nursing interventions.

The Client with a Hypertensive Crisis

■ ■ ■

Some clients with hypertension may, for reasons not clearly understood, experience rapid, significant elevations in systolic and/or diastolic pressures. These elevations require immediate treatment (within 1 hour) to preserve organ function and life. Most hypertensive emergencies, occur in clients who suddenly stop taking their medications or who are poorly controlled by the medication they do take. The nature of the onset of the crisis and the degree of elevation of the blood pressure indicate the seriousness of the problem and direct the protocols for treatment.

In hypertensive *urgencies,* clients often present with a systolic pressure greater than 240 mm Hg and a diastolic pressure greater than 120 mm Hg. At least a partial reduction in pressure is necessary within a few hours to prevent cardiac, renal, and vascular damage. In hypertensive *emergencies,* clients' diastolic pressure is greater than 130 mm Hg, and blood pressure must be significantly reduced within 1 hour to prevent serious morbidity and mortality. Characteristics of hypertensive emergencies are listed in the accompanying box.

Malignant hypertension is an example of a hypertensive emergency (Massie, 1995). A small number of people who have existing secondary hypertension occasionally develop an accelerated and potentially fatal form of hypertension known as malignant hypertension (Porth, 1994). Clients with malignant hypertension have a diastolic pressure greater than 130 mm Hg and are most often younger clients, African-American men, pregnant women with mild to moderate preeclampsia, or clients with collagen and/or renal disease. Malignant hypertension must be rapidly diagnosed and aggressively (yet carefully) treated to prevent encephalopathy and irreversible renal and cardiac failure (Massie, 1995). Intense spasms of the cerebral arteries may create an encephalopathy that causes cerebral edema, manifested by such symptoms as headache, confusion, swelling of the optic nerve (papilledema), blurred vision, restlessness, and motor and sensory deficits (Porth, 1994). Untreated encephalopathy may cause death.

Clinical Manifestations of Hypertensive Emergencies

■ Rapid onset
■ Systolic pressure > 240 mm Hg
■ Diastolic pressure > 130 mm Hg

The goal of care in hypertensive emergencies is to reduce the client's blood pressure substantially in the shortest time possible. Careful monitoring of blood urea nitrogen, serum creatinine, calcium, and total protein levels can be instrumental in establishing a prognosis for recovery (Porth, 1994). The pharmacologic treatment for malignant hypertension includes the parenteral administration of a rapidly acting antihypertensive, such as the potent vasodilator sodium nitroprusside (Nipride). Other medications that may be used are outlined in Table 30-1. Management also includes the treatment of any underlying or coexisting cardiac, renal, and cerebral conditions.

Table 30–1   Intravenous Drugs Used to Treat Hypertensive Emergencies

Type	Name	Onset	Duration	Nursing Tips
Vasodilator	Nipride	seconds	3 to 5 min	■ Most effective drug ■ Easy to titrate
Vasodilator	Nitroglycerin	2 to 5 min	3 to 5 min	■ Tolerances may develop
Vasodilator	Diazoxide (Hyperstat)	1 to 2 min	4 to 24 hr	■ Avoided in clients with coronary artery disease ■ Used with beta-blockers and diuretics ■ Painful if it enters tissues
Vasodilator	Hydralazine (Apresoline)	10 to 30 min	2 to 6 hr	■ Avoided in clients with coronary artery disease
Beta/alpha blocker	Labetalol (Trandate)	5 to 10 min	3 to 6 hr	■ Avoided in clients with congestive heart failure and asthma
Beta-blocker	Esmolol (Brevibloc)	1 to 2 min	10 to 30 min	■ Avoided in clients with congestive heart failure and asthma
ACE inhibitor	Enalaprilat (Vasotec)	15 min	6 hr or more	■ Watch for hypotension
Diuretic	Furosemide (Lasix)	15 min	4 hr	■ Watch for hypotension ■ Watch for hypokalemia
Calcium channel blocker	Nicardipene (Cardene)	1 to 5 min	3 to 6 hr	■ Watch for signs of myocardial ischemia

▪ ▪ ▪ Disorders of the Peripheral Arteries ▪ ▪ ▪

Disorders that interrupt or impede peripheral blood flow are directly related to one or more of the following three mechanisms: (1) vessel compression, (2) vasospasm, and (3) structural defects in the vessel wall. In addition, the presence of thrombi or emboli inside the vessel(s) interrupts peripheral blood flow. The interference in peripheral arterial circulation limits the availability of oxygen and nutrients needed for cellular health and creates an unfavorable vascular environment that may lead to the development of harmful or irreparable conditions.

This section of the chapter discusses disorders of the peripheral arteries: peripheral arteriosclerosis, arterial embolism or thrombus, Buerger's disease, and Raynaud's disease.

The Client with Peripheral Arteriosclerosis

▪ ▪ ▪

Arteriosclerosis is the most common chronic arterial disorder, characterized by thickening, loss of elasticity, and calcification of arterial walls. *Atherosclerosis* is a form of arteriosclerosis in which the thickening and hardening of the arteries are the result of deposits of fat and fibrin. In the peripheral circulation, these pathologic changes result in a decreased blood supply to tissues, called *peripheral vascular disease* (PVD). The manifestations are most commonly seen in the lower extremities.

Pathophysiology

Arteriosclerosis and atherosclerosis are extensively discussed in Chapter 28; this discussion focuses on the effects of these disorders in the peripheral vascular system. The pathologic effects of arteriosclerosis of the peripheral vascular system are most evident in two areas of the body: the abdominal aorta and the lower extremities. The changes involve both the intima and the media of the arteries. The condition is often accompanied by perivascular inflammation and calcified plaques in the media.

As peripheral arteries thicken and harden because of plaque deposits, the lumen of the vessel becomes progressively smaller. In addition, plaque tends to form at bifurcations of branch arteries. As a result, blood flow to the lower extremities is decreased, and tissue hypoxia or anoxia results. If the occlusion develops slowly, collateral circulation often develops, but it is usually not sufficient to supply tissue needs, especially in situations of increased metabolic demands. Manifestations do not usually begin until 60% or more of the blood supply to the tissues is occluded (McCance & Huether, 1993).

The femoral arteries, the common iliac arteries, and the abdominal aorta are the most frequent sites of plaque deposits compromising peripheral circulation. Arteriosclerosis in the abdominal aorta leads to the development of aneurysms as plaque development erodes the vessel wall.

Peripheral arterial disease is more common in people over the age of 50 and is seen in men more than in women. Risk factors for the development of this disorder include a diet high in fat, hypertension, diabetes mellitus, smoking, obesity, and stress (see Chapter 28).

Pain is the primary manifestation of peripheral arterial arteriosclerosis and arterial occlusion. One type of pain, called **intermittent claudication**, is usually described as a cramping or aching sensation in the calves of the legs, the thighs, and the buttocks. The pain is often accompanied by weakness and limping. It is experienced during periods of activity, such as periods of walking, and is relieved by rest.

Rest pain, in contrast, occurs during periods of inactivity. It is often described as a burning sensation in the lower legs. Rest pain increases when the legs are elevated and decreases when the legs are dependent (e.g., hanging over the side of the bed). Clients often complain that the legs feel cold or numb in addition to being painful.

The skin is pale when the legs are elevated but often assumes a dark red color (called *dependent rubor*) when the legs are dependent. The skin is often thin and shiny, with areas of discoloration and hair loss. The toenails may be thickened. In addition, there are often areas of skin breakdown, which may lead to ulcerations or gangrene.

Peripheral pulses may be decreased or absent to palpation. A bruit may be heard over large affected arteries, such as the femoral artery and the abdominal aorta.

The complications of peripheral arteriosclerosis include gangrene and amputation of one or both lower extremities, rupture of abdominal aortic aneurysms, and death from infection or hemorrhage.

Collaborative Care

Management of the client with peripheral arteriosclerosis centers around maintaining or improving the blood supply to tissues and providing symptomatic care.

Laboratory and Diagnostic Tests

The laboratory and diagnostic studies for occlusive disorders of arterial circulation are primarily imaging and arteriographic studies. Because interruption of arterial flow has little effect on laboratory values, few of these tests are performed.

The following diagnostic tests may be ordered:

- *Renal function studies* may be performed to detect potential dysfunction secondary to the interruption of arterial blood flow to the kidneys.

- *Transcutaneous oximetry* evaluates oxygenation of tissues.

- *Digital subtraction angiography (DSA)* is a computerized radiologic examination that allows visualization of specific areas of arteries.

- *Angiography* is conducted to evaluate the extent of arteriosclerosis and occlusion. A contrast medium is injected into the vascular system, and vessels are visualized. This test is done if surgery is being considered. See Chapter 28 for a more detailed discussion of this procedure.

- In a *Doppler ultrasonic flow study,* an electronic stethoscope amplifies the sound of the blood flowing through arteries, even when no sounds are heard through a stethoscope. The instrument also can be used to measure blood pressure in the arteries of the lower extremities. In clients with peripheral vascular disease, the blood pressure in the legs is often lower than the pressure in the arms. Color Doppler is now available to demonstrate the pattern and direction of blood flow within the vessel (Tierney et al., 1995).

- *Oscillometry* measures the volume of the pulse at different locations along the extremity.

- *Plethysmography* illustrates the changes in the pulse with each heartbeat.

- A *lumbar sympathetic nerve block* evaluates peripheral circulation. Following injection of a local anesthetic into the sympathetic nerves that supply the legs, temperature in the legs is measured. If blood flow is normal, blocking sympathetic stimulation produces vasodilation and increased tissue temperature. However, because stenotic vessels do not dilate, no temperature change occurs in the client with peripheral vascular disease.

Pharmacology

Many clients with peripheral arterial disease also have coronary artery disease and take medications such as beta-blockers and vasodilators (see the box on page 1191). These same medications are sometimes prescribed to decrease pain and improve functional abilities. Analgesics may also be prescribed not only to relieve pain but also to allow exercise, which improves circulation.

Because of the risk for inflammation and blood clot formation, low doses of aspirin are recommended for all clients with severe peripheral vascular disease (Tierney et al., 1994).

Conservative Therapy

The client is encouraged to maintain a program of daily walking for fixed periods to improve the development of collateral circulation and function. The client should walk to the point of experiencing claudication pain, then take a 3-minute rest.

Weight reduction may make activity less painful. The client must stop smoking. The nicotine in cigarettes causes vasospasm, further decreasing blood supply to the extremities.

Surgery

Surgery may be performed for clients with peripheral arterial disorders if intermittent claudication becomes worse or significantly interferes with the client's physical activities. Surgery is also indicated if the client has rest pain or pregangrenous or gangrenous lesions on the foot. The following types of surgery may be performed:

- A *lumbar sympathectomy* may be performed if the client has ischemic or pregangrenous lesions on the foot. In this surgery, the sympathetic ganglia are excised or injected with a 6% solution of phenol. Blocking the sympathetic ganglia improves peripheral blood flow.

- An *arterial graft,* using a section of the client's great saphenous vein or a graft made of synthetic material, may be performed to bypass an occluded section of an artery.

- A *thromboendarterectomy* involves removal of the central occluding core of the artery; this may be successful if only a small segment of the artery is occluded.

- *Endovascular surgery* is used to treat more distal lesions. This may be accomplished by balloon angioplasty to dilate the narrow or occluded areas, mechanical atherectomy to remove an occluding plaque from the arterial lumen, or laser or thermal angioplasty to vaporize the occluding material (Tierney et al., 1995).

Nursing Care

Clients with arterial arteriosclerosis have many different health care problems. The pain that accompanies this condition interferes with the activities of daily living, and the ability to walk may be severely diminished. The possibility of losing a lower extremity is a frightening prospect for the client. The research box on page 1204 summarizes clients' concerns about peripheral arterial occlusive disease. Nursing diagnoses discussed in this section are *Altered Peripheral Tissue Perfusion, Pain,* and *Impaired Skin Integrity.*

Altered Peripheral Tissue Perfusion

The interruption in the flow of arterial blood to the lower extremities causes abnormalities in the exchange of gases and nutrients at the capillary (cellular) level. Oxygen and nutrient deprivation compromises tissue integrity. As a result, clients experience pain and are at risk for ulcerations and gangrene. Clients with arterial disorders experience

Applying Research to Nursing Practice: Concerns of Clients with Peripheral Arterial Occlusive Disease

■ ■ ■

Peripheral arterial occlusive disease affects an estimated 2.4 million people in the United States. This disease affects people of all ages but is more common among older adults. Older clients are at increased risk for disability, loss of independence, and even death. This study was conducted to identify the general well-being of clients with arterial occlusive disease so that more comprehensive nursing care could be implemented (Crosby, Ventura, Frainier, & Wu, 1993). The researchers measured the general well-being of 170 clients with this disorder treated at a Veterans Affairs Medical Center. The researchers used an instrument previously employed by the Rand Corporation to measure well-being with healthy individuals, and they also asked open-ended questions. The results demonstrate a lower mean score than was found with previously studied healthy subjects. General well-being scores were lower in clients with increased circulatory impairment. The concerns identified by the open-ended questions included fear of increased pain, lack of mobility, and fear of amputation.

Implications for Nursing

Nurses may assign a lower priority to the concerns of clients with chronic disorders such as peripheral arterial occlusive disease than to those of clients with more acute disorders. However, because these clients rely on

teaching to achieve wellness and self-management of illness at home, client teaching and support are essential, especially for older clients. Nursing interventions to help these clients maintain independence, manage pain, and reduce anxiety are critical factors in reducing health care costs and facilitating optimal health in the older adult.

Critical Thinking in Client Care

1. Teaching about leg and foot care is an important intervention for the older adult with peripheral arterial occlusive disease. What normal changes of aging (such as decreased visual acuity) might require you to adapt a teaching plan?

2. Accept or reject the following statement: Decreased mobility means decreased independence. What aspects of independent living are threatened if this statement is true?

3. You are providing immediate postoperative care to a client who has had abdominal surgery and also has peripheral arterial occlusive disease. How will the latter affect the assessments you make?

4. While making a home visit, your client tells you he is very worried that his leg might be amputated. How would you respond?

pain when extremities are in an elevated rather than a dependent position. Gravity assists arterial flow to the dependent extremity, increasing tissue perfusion and relieving pain.

Nursing interventions with rationales follow:

■ Assess the extremities for peripheral pulses, pain, color, temperature, and capillary refill times at least every 4 hours and as needed. If pulses cannot be palpated, use an electronic ultrasound device (Doppler) to locate pulses. *Baseline information about the location and quality of peripheral pulses (including femoral, popliteal, posterior tibial, and pedal), level of client pain, color and temperature of the extremities, and capillary refill times should be established. Frequent follow-up is necessary to detect changes in the status of arterial blood flow, which may indicate worsening of the client's condition.*

■ Teach the client the importance of keeping extremities in a dependent position. *Because the arterial circulation*

is impaired, blood carrying essential oxygen and nutrients is unable to reach the distal portions of the extremity. When the extremities are in a dependent position, gravity helps arterial blood reach distal areas.

■ Keep extremities warm using lightweight blankets, socks, and slippers. Do not use electric heating pads or hot water bottles to warm extremities. *Keep extremities warm to conserve heat, prevent vasospasm, and promote arterial flow. Avoid electric heating pads and hot water bottles because of the possibility of burns. Many clients experience peripheral sensory changes associated with decreased arterial flow, and they may receive burns because they cannot feel the degree of heat produced by the apparatus. Heavy blankets may increase vessel compression.*

■ Encourage the client to change position at least every hour and to avoid leg crossing. *Changing position hourly promotes blood flow, thereby enhancing arterial perfusion of the extremity and decreasing pain. Improved blood flow also results in warmer, less cyanotic extremities with shorter capillary refill times. Leg crossing is avoided because of its compressive effects upon an already compromised peripheral-arterial system.*

- Provide meticulous leg and foot care daily, using mild soaps and moisturizing lotions. *Proper skin care helps prevent drying and cracking, thereby minimizing the chances of skin breakdown and infection. Decreased arterial circulation causes wounds to heal more slowly; proactive nursing measures like good foot and leg care prevent problems before they begin.*

Pain

The pain of arterial occlusive disease is related to interrupted arterial flow, which deprives cells of necessary oxygen and nutrients and results in tissue hypoxia and, if left untreated, tissue necrosis. Severe and cramplike pain generally follows exercise early in the disease process. Rest initially produces relief, but as the disease progresses, the amount of exercise needed to generate pain decreases until clients experience severe pain even at rest. The pain begins to wake clients during sleep, limit the client's activities, and alter the client's sense of well-being. These events are signals that the occlusion is becoming extensive and requires immediate medical attention if ulceration and gangrene are to be avoided.

Nursing interventions with rationales follow:

- Assess client's level of pain in extremities using a scale of 0 to 10 (0 = no pain; 10 = severe pain) at least every 4 hours and more often if needed. *Frequent assessment of the level of pain allows the nurse to adjust the plan of care to include interventions that reduce pain and are tailored to the degree of pain experienced by the client. By using a scale of 0 to 10, the nurse demonstrates sensitivity and awareness of the subjective nature of pain while obtaining valuable objective data.*

- Evaluate bilateral peripheral pulses at least every 4 hours and more often if needed. *Changes in the degree of arterial obstruction are manifested by changes in the client's level of pain: the pain increases as the vessel becomes more occluded. The amount of occlusion of the vessel is commonly reflected by the quality of the peripheral pulses; changes in the intensity, location, or quality of peripheral pulses frequently indicate worsening of the client's condition.*

- Keep the client's extremities warm, using socks, slippers, or light blankets. *Cooling causes vasoconstriction and increases pain. Because the vessel is already occluded, factors that further limit peripheral blood flow should be avoided. Warming the extremities enhances arterial flow and contributes to more effective collateral blood flow by promoting vasodilation.*

- Teach the client methods for reducing stress and relieving pain. *Stress produces vasoconstriction in the body.*

Measures should be taken to avoid vasoconstriction and promote vasodilation, especially in clients in whom hypertension is a factor. There are many nonpharmacologic techniques that clients may use to relieve stress and minimize pain. Among these are relaxation, meditation, guided imagery, and avoiding exposure to cold. Presurgical exercise should be limited in most clients with arterial occlusion because of the risk of increased blood pressure on the vessel wall; postoperatively, gradual exercise regimens are ordered as the client's condition improves and arterial circulation is restored.

Impaired Skin Integrity

The skin of clients with arterial arteriosclerosis is at risk for breakdown as a result of the cellular depletion of oxygen and nutrients. Cyanosis is evident when the amount of oxygenated hemoglobin is reduced. Additional skin changes resulting from impaired arterial flow include scaliness, dryness, atrophy, dry and brittle nails, and, if the worst eventual change is realized, ulcerations and gangrene.

Nursing interventions with rationales follow:

- Assess the skin of the extremities at least once each shift and more often if needed. Document findings and changes with each assessment. *Reduced arterial blood flow often produces sensory changes in the extremities of clients with peripheral-vascular disorders. Because of these sensory changes, clients may be unaware of accidental injury to the extremity. The prolonged healing time of the tissues caused by poor arterial flow increases the client's risk of developing infections that might be avoided with daily inspection. In addition, changes in skin condition may signal worsening of the client's condition and should be reported for further assessment and intervention.*

- Provide meticulous daily skin care, being sure to keep skin clean, dry, and supple. *Intact skin is the body's first defense against invasion by bacteria and other harmful microorganisms. Once the skin is broken, the warm, moist, dark tissues of the injured extremity provide an excellent medium for the growth of microorganisms. Keeping the skin clean, dry, and supple decreases the risk of breakdown.*

- Apply a bed cradle. *The bed cradle is a metal support on which bed linens are suspended over the client's legs. Bed cradles prevent the bed linens from placing pressure on extremities whose tissue integrity is already compromised. Relief of pressure on the extremities is important to enhance peripheral circulation (especially capillary blood flow) and promote vascular integrity.*

Other Nursing Diagnoses

The following nursing diagnoses may also be appropriate for the client with peripheral arteriosclerosis:

- *Risk for Infection* related to ulcerated areas on feet

- *Altered Family Processes* related to loss of income and inability to work secondary to severe intermittent claudication
- *Impaired Physical Mobility* related to intermittent claudication and fatigue
- *Hopelessness* related to long-term chronic nature of illness and pain
- *Sleep Pattern Disturbance* related to rest pain

Client and Family Teaching

Clients are given information about conservative measures that will help them manage their conditions. Teaching includes information related to stress reduction, smoking cessation, medications, and methods to keep the extremities warm. If available, a list of resources such as support groups, public health services, and other community agencies should be provided for all clients.

Clients and their family members also are taught about care of the legs and feet. A teaching outline is included in the accompanying box.

Care of the Older Adult

With aging, the blood vessels thicken and become less compliant. These changes reduce the delivery of oxygen to the tissues and impair the removal of carbon dioxide and waste products from the tissues. When normal changes of aging are combined with the high likelihood of some degree of arteriosclerosis, the risk of peripheral vascular disease is high.

The older client with peripheral arteriosclerosis requires the same teaching as do clients of any age. However, visual deficits may make it more difficult for the older adult to provide careful and safe foot care. Long-standing smoking habits are difficult to break, and the client who lives alone may resist walking. For these reasons, it is often helpful to have a community health or home health nurse make periodic visits and to encourage the client to join a support group for stopping smoking, changing eating habits, and taking part in regular activity.

The Client with Arterial Thrombus or Embolism

■ ■ ■

Arterial thrombus or embolism occurs most often as a complication of another disease process. Regardless of cause, both emboli and thrombi often result in occlusion. The manifestations depend on the artery involved, the tissue supplied by the occluded artery, and the degree to which collateral circulation is established.

Pathophysiology

This section discusses arterial thrombus and embolism of the peripheral vascular system.

Arterial Thrombosis

A **thrombus** (also known as a blood clot) is an aggregation of blood (and other) cells that adheres to the vessel wall. Acute arterial thrombi often follow the development of atherosclerotic changes in the vessel wall and exacerbate the occlusive effects of atherosclerosis. Sudden or complete occlusion of arterial blood flow in a narrow segment of the vessel may occur in clients whose vessels are already severely damaged by ulcerations, atherosclerotic erosion, and other disorders causing narrowing or irregularity of the arterial lumen. Occasionally, inflammation of the arterial wall leads to the development of arterial thrombosis, as does polycythemia, dehydration, and repeated arterial punctures (Tierney et al., 1995).

The effects of occlusion of arterial blood flow are primarily the same, regardless of the etiology. Because of this, symptoms of arterial thrombosis are essentially the same as those for arterial emboli, resulting in pain in the region of the affected vessel, possible numbness, pallor, mottling, muscle spasm, lack of pulse distal to the blockage, and possible paralysis. See the accompanying manifestations box.

Clients with arterial thrombosis often develop some collateral circulation to compensate for the loss of arterial flow. However, because it takes time for sufficient collateral circulation to develop, the loss of flow threatens the integrity of tissues in the involved areas of the body. Depending on the area of involvement, occlusion may create serious conditions that can result in permanent vascular and/or limb damage. When arterial flow is interrupted, clients are at risk for developing tissue necrosis and gangrene (Tierney et al., 1995).

Arterial Embolism

The occlusion of blood flow by a foreign object other than a blood clot within the vessel is known as **embolism.** Blood clots that dislodge from the vessel wall and move throughout the system are known as **thromboemboli.** Other emboli may be any matter that has formed a bolus and moves through the circulatory system, such as an accumulation of air bubbles, bacteria, fat, amniotic fluid, or cancer cells. Regardless of its composition, the embolus eventually becomes lodged in a vessel that is too small to accommodate its passage. Emboli tend to lodge in areas of the arterial lumen narrowed by atherosclerotic plaque and at arterial bifurcations.

Acute arterial emboli (also known as systemic emboli) generally originate in the left side of the heart. Arterial emboli are most commonly associated with myocardial infarction, valvular disease of the heart, left-sided heart

Leg and Foot Care for the Client with Peripheral Arteriosclerosis

■ ■ ■

1. Keep the legs and feet clean, dry, and comfortable.
   - Wash the legs and feet each day in warm water, using a mild soap.
   - Dry the feet carefully with a soft towel; do not rub, and be sure to dry between the toes.
   - Apply a lotion that does not contain alcohol to dry, scaly skin.
   - Use powder on the feet and between the toes.
   - Buy shoes in the afternoon (when feet are largest); never buy shoes that are uncomfortable. Be sure the toes have adequate room.
   - Wear a clean pair of cotton socks each day.

2. Prevent accidents and injuries to the feet.
   - Always wear shoes or slippers when getting out of bed.
   - Walk on level ground and avoid crowds, if possible.
   - Do not go barefoot.
   - Look at your legs and feet each day; use a mirror to examine the backs of your legs and the bottoms of your feet.

   - Have a professional foot care provider trim toenails and care for corns, calluses, ingrown toenails, or athlete's foot.
   - Always check the temperature of the water before stepping into the tub.
   - Do not get the legs or tops of the feet sunburned.
   - Report any problems with your legs or feet to your health care provider. This includes increased pain, cuts, bruises, blistering, redness, or open areas.

3. Improve blood supply to the legs and feet
   - Do not sit with the legs crossed.
   - Do not wear garters or knee stockings.
   - Do not go swimming in cold water.
   - Do not smoke cigarettes or inhale passive smoke.
   - Walk until you experience pain, stop for 3 minutes, then resume walking as long as you can tolerate it. Do this eight times a day.
   - Take medications as prescribed.

---

failure, atrial fibrillation, or infectious diseases of the heart (McCance & Huether, 1993).

Clients with acute arterial embolism initially complain of pain (either sudden or insidious in onset) and numbness, coldness, and tingling if an extremity is involved. The pain worsens as the occlusion becomes more extensive. Upon assessment, the examiner often cannot palpate a pulse in the areas distal to the blockage; notes coldness, pallor, or mottling of the affected extremity; and may detect neuromuscular effects, such as muscle weakness, spasms, or paralysis. There may be a line of demarcation, with pallor or cyanosis and cooler skin temperature distal to the occlusion. See the manifestations box on page 1208. If the embolism is left untreated, necrosis of the skin (and deeper tissues) and eventual gangrene occur as a result of the interruption in arterial blood flow (Tierney et al., 1995).

Collaborative Care

Arterial thrombosis is usually managed with medical therapy, whereas an embolism requires immediate surgical intervention. In either case, the focus is on relieving

Clinical Manifestations of Arterial Thrombosis

■ ■ ■

- Pain in the region of the affected vessel
- Numbness in the affected extremity
- Pallor or mottling of the skin in the affected extremity
- Muscle spasms
- Pulselessness distal to the blockage
- Possible paralysis

the arterial obstruction and preserving the involved extremity.

Laboratory and Diagnostic Tests

Laboratory and diagnostic tests are conducted to determine any underlying cause for thrombosis or embolism, and to confirm the presence of the obstruction.

> ### Clinical Manifestations of
> ### Arterial Embolism
> • • •
>
> - Pain in the extremity (sudden or insidious)
> - Numbness in the extremity
> - Coldness of the extremity
> - Tingling in the extremity
> - Pulselessness distal to the blockage
> - Pallor or mottling of the extremity
> - Muscle weakness
> - Muscle spasms
> - Paralysis
> - A line of demarcation; with pallor, cyanosis, and cooler skin distal to the blockage

The following laboratory tests may be ordered:

- *Cardiac enzyme studies* determine if the client has had a myocardial infarction.
- *Blood cultures* identify the organism responsible for an infection.

The following diagnostic tests may be ordered:

- *Electrocardiography* identifies changes typical of a myocardial infarction.
- *Arteriography* or *MRI* may be performed either during or after surgery for an acute embolism. (An extremity may have more than one embolism.)
- *Echocardiography* identifies the source of an embolism.

Pharmacology

If there is no tissue necrosis present, arterial thrombosis or embolism may be treated with thrombolytic therapy using streptokinase, urokinase, or tissue plasminogen activator (t-PA) (see Chapter 28). Lysis of the thrombus or embolus is achieved in 50% to 80% of the cases (Tierney et al., 1994). This therapy can not be used if the client is bleeding, has had recent surgery, has uncontrolled hypertension, or is pregnant. Arterial embolism may also be treated with intravenous heparin as an anticoagulant.

Surgery

The surgical treatment of acute arterial embolus involves an emergency *embolectomy* to prevent gangrene and to ensure adequate arterial blood flow to adjacent structures. In most cases, this means surgical incision within 4 to 6 hours after the embolic episode. Surgeries that take place after this time frame have been successful if the vessel and surrounding tissues remain viable.

To expedite the procedure when the embolus is in an extremity, local anesthesia may be used. Once the embolus is removed, the vessel is thoroughly explored for the presence of additional emboli and thrombi using a special balloon-tipped catheter known as a Fogarty catheter. If the embolus is located in the mesenteric area, emergency laparoscopic surgery is required. Clients whose surgery is delayed for more than 12 hours following the occlusion are at a much higher risk of developing acute respiratory distress syndrome or acute renal failure (or both) than their counterparts who have surgery within 4 to 6 hours following the insult (Tierney et al., 1995). Nursing care of the client following an embolectomy is discussed next.

Nursing Care

Nursing care for the client with arterial thrombosis or embolism is essentially the same as for the client with an arterial obstruction due to arteriosclerosis. The nursing diagnoses discussed in this section apply to the client who has undergone embolectomy or arterial reconstruction: *Anxiety, Altered Peripheral Tissue Perfusion,* and *Altered Protection.*

Anxiety

The level of anxiety experienced by clients with arterial occlusive disorders depends upon the severity and nature of the disease process. Clients with peripheral arterial occlusive disorders may be very anxious, particularly if an embolic episode is the cause for hospitalization. The rapid and intense nature of preoperative activities commonly leaves clients feeling overwhelmed and anxious about the outcome. Clients may complain of physiologic, emotional, and cognitive manifestations of anxiety, such as trembling, palpitations, restlessness, dry mouth, helplessness, inability to relax, irritability, forgetfulness, and lack of awareness of their surroundings. Nursing measures should focus on gaining the client's trust and minimizing the effects of anxiety so as to decrease surgical risk and increase the client's chances for an uneventful surgery and recovery.

Nursing interventions with rationales follow:

- Assess the level of anxiety at least once each shift and more often as needed. Intervene to reduce the client's current level of anxiety. *Assessing the client's current anxiety level helps the nurse determine both the intensity of the client's anxiety and the client's ability to control it. Nursing interventions are difficult to implement until the client's anxiety is controlled. Frequent assessments of anxiety provide continuously updated information that helps the nurse choose interventions that correspond to the assessed level of anxiety.*

- Provide opportunities for clients to verbalize anxiety; offer reassurance and support. *Clients often volunteer information about their fears and anxieties if the nurse demonstrates a caring approach. By staying with clients, supporting their current coping mechanisms, and allowing them to verbalize their feelings freely, the nurse demonstrates sensitivity and respect for the individual. It is important for the nurse to be aware of the urgency of matters but to convey a calm, organized, and professional (yet compassionate) presence so as to facilitate essential nursing interventions.*

- Implement measures to decrease sensory stimuli. Speak slowly and clearly to anxious clients, avoid unnecessary interruptions in client statements, give concise directions, focus on the here and now, and attempt to diffuse anxiety by involving the client in some other simple task. *Clients who are anxious often need assistance in controlling the stimuli in their environment so they can focus on reducing their own anxiety. This requires support from people in positions of control, such as the nurse, and careful direction regarding the necessary steps in the client's care. Nurses should be careful not to condescend to clients during the implementation of anxiety-reducing interventions, because condescension effectively reverses any progress the client may have made in controlling anxiety and destroys the trusting relationship between nurse and client.*

Altered Peripheral Tissue Perfusion

The client who has had arterial reconstruction has already experienced decreased peripheral tissue perfusion and is at risk for further impairment after surgery because of thrombosis of the graft or edema in the area of embolism removal.

Nursing interventions with rationales follow:

- Monitor the lower extremities for perfusion, comparing them bilaterally.
  a. Take lower extremity pulses every 2 to 4 hours, using the Doppler stethoscope if necessary.
  b. Assess the temperature and color of the skin every 2 to 4 hours.
  c. Assess capillary refill time of toenails every 2 to 4 hours.
  d. Be alert to complaints of pain, especially if it is unrelieved by medications.
  The graft provides an area for thrombosis formation following surgery. During the first 12 hours following surgery, spasms of the affected artery may cause pulselessness and cyanosis; pulse and normal color should return after that time. Sudden severe foot and toe pain indicates graft occlusion. Notify the surgeon immediately of any change in circulatory status.

- Maintain intravenous fluid replacement as prescribed. *An adequate circulating blood volume is necessary to maintain perfusion of the extremities.*

- Discourage activities such as raising the knee gatch, placing pillows under the knees, or positioning the

client so that there is 90-degree hip flexion. *These activities may further impede peripheral blood flow.*

- Provide measures to promote tissue perfusion.
  a. Maintain the knee of the operated leg in a slightly flexed position.
  b. Elevate the foot of the bed 15 degrees if the lower extremity is edematous.
  c. Encourage the client to perform active ankle and leg exercises every 1 to 2 hours when awake.
  d. Place a bed cradle over the lower half of the bed.
  e. Keep the client and the environment warm.
  Sharply flexing the knee may impede blood flow to the distal part of the extremity. Elevating the leg 15 degrees facilitates venous return without altering arterial flow. Active exercises help prevent venous stasis. The use of a bed cradle prevents pressure on the operative area. Keeping the client warm prevents vasoconstriction.

Altered Protection

The anticoagulant therapy used to prevent postsurgical formation of thrombi in peripheral arteries increases the risk for bleeding. The client most commonly receives heparin parenterally immediately after surgery and then progresses to oral warfarin (Coumadin). The nurse is responsible for monitoring the client's status and reporting any signs of hemorrhage.

Nursing interventions with rationales follow:

- Assess for and report the following manifestations of unusual bleeding:
  a. Excessive bloody drainage from the incision site
  b. Continuous oozing from injection sites
  c. Bleeding from the gums
  d. Bleeding from the nose
  e. Hematuria
  f. Petechiae, purpura, ecchymoses
  Anticoagulants interfere with the clotting cascade; abnormal bleeding may result.

- Monitor laboratory values for activated partial thromboplastin time (APTT) if the client is receiving heparin parenterally and prothrombin time (PT) if the client is taking anticoagulants orally. Report values over target therapeutic range. *Both times are prolonged by anticoagulant therapy. The therapeutic range is from 1.5 to 2 times normal.*

- Monitor the older adult even more carefully. *The older client may be more susceptible to anticoagulants and may therefore require a lower maintenance dose.*

Other Nursing Diagnoses

The following nursing diagnoses may also be appropriate for clients experiencing arterial occlusive disorders:

- *Impaired Physical Mobility* related to pain secondary to arterial occlusion

- *Activity Intolerance* related to generalized weakness secondary to surgery
- *Diversional Activity Deficit* related to prolonged immobility
- *Ineffective Individual Coping* related to perception of current health problem or crisis
- *Risk for Injury* related to diminished arterial blood flow and resulting gangrene
- *Risk for Infection* related to presence of surgical incision

Client and Family Teaching

Client and family teaching for the client with arterial thrombosis or embolism depends on the type of care needed to resolve the health problem. For clients having surgery, preoperative teaching includes the nature of the preoperative, intraoperative, and postoperative courses of therapy. Surgical clients need information about expected postoperative interventions, such as anticoagulant medications, activity restrictions, dietary modifications, strategies for reducing atherosclerotic progress and hypertension, and stress reduction. In addition, prior to discharge, clients are taught about the signs and symptoms of postoperative wound infection and disease-related signs and symptoms to report to their physician. General pre- and postoperative care is discussed in Chapter 7.

Clients who are treated by medical management are given information about conservative measures to promote peripheral circulation and maintain tissue integrity. The general measures described for the care of the client with arteriosclerosis are also appropriate for clients with arterial thrombosis or embolism.

Applying the Nursing Process

Case Study of a Client with an Arterial Embolism: Joseph Ridle

Joseph Ridle is a 53-year-old, married man with three children, ages 20, 17, and 14. He is a stock analyst for a large, competitive financial planning institution and works an average of 9 hours daily. He has a long-standing history of hypertension that is currently controlled by medication (a diuretic and beta-blocking agent), dietary sodium and fat restrictions, and daily exercise. For the past week, Mr. Ridle has noticed a mild, intermittent pain in his right leg, but he believed it was caused by a recent overly rigorous exercise session. Mr. Ridle also notices that the pain seems to go away if he rests. After 2 weeks of pain, Mr. Ridle visits his physician and is admitted to the hospital for diagnosis and treatment. Russel Reed, RN, is assigned to admit and care for Mr. Ridle.

Assessment

Mr. Ridle's admission history provides the following information: height: 6'1" (185 cm); weight: 230 lb (124 kg). He has a 12-year history of mild hypertension that is currently under control, and he has had no previous hospitalizations nor surgeries. For the past 14 days, Mr. Ridle has experienced intermittent right leg pain that subsides when he rests. When questioned, he indicates that he has experienced brief episodes of tingling in the right leg three times in the past week and has noticed that his right foot is always cold and his right leg seems to be strangely bluish in color. Physical assessment findings include: diminished peripheral pulses in the right leg with a right pedal pulse audible only by Doppler; BP: 138/78; cold, pale right extremity with capillary refill time of 8 seconds. All other capillary refill times are 3 seconds or less. The toes on his right leg are markedly cyanotic and there is a delayed response to light sensory stimuli of the right leg. The skin on his right leg is dry, scaly, and cracked in two small areas near the right great toe. Diagnostic studies include a contrast CT and arteriography, both of which reveal a large embolus in the right femoral artery occluding arterial circulation to the right leg. Mr. Ridle is scheduled for an immediate embolectomy.

Diagnosis

Mr. Reed makes the following nursing diagnoses for Mr. Ridle:

- *Impaired Peripheral Tissue Perfusion* related to obstructed arterial blood flow
- *Pain* related to tissue hypoxia
- *Anxiety* related to uncertainty about hospitalization and surgery
- *Risk for Injury* related to diminished arterial blood flow and consequent gangrene

Expected Outcomes

The expected outcomes of the plan of care are that, following surgery, Mr. Ridle will

- Have strong bilateral peripheral pulses by the day of discharge.
- Verbalize relief from pain within 4 days after surgery.
- Use appropriate techniques to cope with need for surgery and hospitalization.
- Adhere to collaborative plan of care to prevent occurrence of gangrene.

Planning and Implementation

Mr. Reed plans and implements the following interventions as part of Mr. Ridle's nursing care:

- Assess peripheral pulses; skin color, temperature, and integrity; and pedal capillary refill times every 2 to 4 hours and as needed.

- Place the right leg in a neutral position and use a bed cradle over the lower body. Cover the bed cradle with blankets to keep Mr. Ridle warm. If the leg appears edematous, elevate the entire leg no more than 15 degrees.

- Assess level of pain using a 0 to 10 scale (0 = no pain, 10 = severe pain). Encourage Mr. Ridle to use nonpharmacologic therapies to relieve pain such as relaxation, imagery, and listening to favorite music.

- Change Mr. Ridle's position at least every 2 hours to enhance collateral circulation. Encourage him to increase ambulation gradually each day and to incorporate daily exercise into his life-style after discharge.

- Provide opportunities for Mr. Ridle and his family to verbalize anxieties about hospitalization and surgical experience. Spend time with them and use open-ended communication to elicit responses.

- Teach Mr. Ridle and his family about the relationship between adhering to the collaborative plan of care and attaining wellness. Encourage questions and use available teaching aids to explain difficult concepts.

- Teach Mr. Ridle and his family about medications and dressing changes, which may be required following discharge.

Evaluation

Following surgery, Mr. Ridle has experienced an uneventful recovery and voices his eagerness to continue complying with the established plan of care once he goes home. By the day of discharge, peripheral pulses in both legs are equally strong, and the color and temperature in the right leg has progressed from cyanotic and cold (on admission) to pink and warm. The two small cracked areas of skin near the right great toe have healed well. The anticoagulation therapy that would be part of the discharge plan for Mr. Ridle has been carefully explained in terms of the dosage and scheduling and written instructions have been provided. Mr. Ridle says that he became very frightened when surgery was first mentioned, but he feels much calmer now that it is over and has gone well.

Critical Thinking in the Nursing Process

1. Which of the factors that interrupt peripheral vascular circulation were responsible for Mr. Ridle's problem? What life-style habits contributed to his health problem?

2. How would the plan of care have changed if the graft had become occluded after surgery?

3. What would be your response if Mr. Ridle tells you that he is afraid to walk now that he has had surgery? Why would you respond this way?

4. Develop a care plan for Mr. Ridle for the diagnosis *Risk for Infection.*

The Client with Buerger's Disease

■ ■ ■

Buerger's disease (also called *thromboangiitis obliterans*) is an occlusive vascular disease in which the small and medium-sized peripheral arteries become inflamed, spastic, and thrombotic. This disease may affect either the upper or lower extremities but more commonly affects a leg or a foot. The exact etiology is unknown. Table 30–2 compares Buerger's disease and Raynaud's disease (discussed in the following section).

Buerger's disease occurs predominantly (95%) in men who smoke and are under the age of 40. Cigarette smoking has been identified as the single, more significant, causative agent. Research studies continue to explore the possibilities of a tobacco allergy or some other type of autoimmune response to tobacco in clients with Buerger's disease (Berkow & Fletcher, 1992).

The disease has an intermittent course with dramatic exacerbations and marked remissions; there may be periods of time (lasting weeks, months, or years) when the disease is dormant. As the disease progresses, the collateral vessels become more extensively involved, making subsequent episodes more intense and longer. These prolonged periods of tissue hypoxia increase the client's likelihood of developing tissue ulceration and gangrene.

Pathophysiology

The changes in the arterial wall in Buerger's disease are in the adventitia, with inflammation and thrombosis. The thrombi contain small abscesses, but the arterial wall does not become necrotic. Vasospasms are common and contribute to the obstruction of blood flow.

Many of the clinical findings in Buerger's disease mimic those in other arterial occlusive disorders: intermittent claudication, numbness, diminished sensation, and, in later stages, ulceration and gangrene. Pain in the involved extremity is the major manifestation, with the client experiencing cramping pain in the instep of the foot or the calves of the legs that is relieved by rest (intermittent claudication), or rest pain in the fingers and toes. Smoking, cold ambient temperature, and emotional distress often trigger burning pain.

On examination, the involved digits and/or extremities are painful, pale in color, and cool or cold to the touch. The skin may be shiny and thin, and the nails are often thick and malformed because of chronic deprivation of oxygen and nutrients to the tissues. It is common to find that distal pulses (such as the dorsalis pedis, posterior tibial, ulnar, or radial) are either difficult to locate or absent, even when a Doppler device is used. As in other arterial occlusive diseases, changes in posture produce changes in the color or temperature of the extremity, but the inten-

Table 30–2 Comparison of Raynaud's Disease and Buerger's Disease

Topic	Raynaud's	Buerger's
Etiology	■ none known ■ possible genetic predisposition	■ cigarette smoking most probable single cause ■ possible tobacco allergy ■ possible autoimmune response ■ conclusive findings about cause pending
Incidence/course of the disease	■ onset commonly between 15 and 45 years of age ■ occurs more often in young women than men ■ becomes progressively worse over time	■ occurs predominantly in men under 40 ■ not found in nonsmokers ■ worsens in severity and duration of attacks over time ■ intermittent course with dramatic exacerbations and remissions
Triggering stimuli	■ emotional events producing stress ■ exposure of extremities to cold temperatures	■ cigarette smoking
Assessment findings	■ usually found in hands ■ pain becomes more severe and prolonged as disease progresses ■ "blue-white-red" changes in color of hands with accompanying changes in skin temperature	■ intermittent claudication ■ numbness or diminished sensation ■ ulceration and gangrene in later stages ■ small, red, tender vascular cords in affected extremities ■ cool skin temperature and pale color ■ shiny, thin skin and white, malformed nails in affected extremities ■ distal pulses difficult to find or absent ■ trophic changes to nail beds
Management	■ have client keep hands warm and injury free ■ have client avoid stressful emotional events ■ emphasize smoking cessation ■ administer medications when indicated ■ provide surgical intervention in some cases	■ have client stop smoking (crucial) ■ have client perform Buerger's exercises ■ have client protect extremities from cold injury ■ provide bedrest if claudication is present ■ teach stress management ■ use dependent positioning of extremities

sity of the rubor is much more noticeable, and the digits of the affected extremity may not be equally affected.

Ulcerations may be present around the nail beds of the fingers or toes, reflecting seriously impaired distal circulation. When trophic changes result in gangrene, amputation may be necessary to prevent the spread of necrosis. In some clients, there may be a coexisting history of Raynaud's phenomenon (Tierney et al., 1995).

Collaborative Care

The collaborative care of clients with Buerger's disease focuses on the relief of symptoms, the prevention of necrosis, and in advanced cases the treatment of gangrene. As with other arterial occlusive diseases, the restoration and maintenance of peripheral blood flow are the most important priorities. However, because there is no known underlying cause of Buerger's disease, treatment focuses on the client's manifestations and the pathophysiologic effects of the disease process. Medical care varies according

to the severity of the disease process and centers on the conservative or surgical treatment of the effects of the inflammatory process on the vessels.

Laboratory and Diagnostic Tests

There are no specific laboratory tests diagnostic of Buerger's disease. Buerger's disease is primarily diagnosed by evaluating the client's history and manifestations to determine the extent of the disease. Doppler studies are commonly used to determine the exact locations and extent of the disease. Angiography, contrast-enhanced computer tomography, and magnetic resonance imaging may also be used (as in the diagnosis of other arterial occlusive disorders) but are often unnecessary.

Conservative Therapy

The one most important component of the conservative management of Buerger's disease is to insist the client stop smoking cigarettes. Clients should be thoroughly informed about the severe vasoconstricting effects of nicotine and about the relationship between smoking and occurrence of this disease. In clients who refuse to stop smoking, the disease will not only persist but also extend to other vessels. The corresponding attacks become increasingly intense and last much longer, thereby significantly raising the client's chances of developing ulcerations and gangrene, both of which eventually require surgical intervention (Porth, 1994).

Additional conservative measures have the goal of preventing vasoconstriction, improving peripheral blood flow, and avoiding the complications of chronic ischemia. These measures are similar to those used for other arterial occlusive disorders: keeping extremities warm, managing stress, keeping the extremities in a dependent position, protecting the extremities from injury (thermal, chemical and/or physiologic), and (in the absence of rest pain) taking daily exercise. If rest pain is present, complete bed rest is necessary.

Buerger-Allen exercises may also significantly improve peripheral-vascular circulation in the conservative management of thromboangiitis obliterans. The exercises involve raising and lowering the extremities, with each of five repetitions taking about 2 minutes. The client elevates the legs from a horizontal position to a 45-degree angle, then lowers them to a dependent position. The positional changes cause the arteries of the legs to refill by gravity. The exercises also work on the premise that the speed of the blood moving through the vessels (whose positions have quickly changed from horizontal to dependent) causes the most distal arterioles to receive more blood, thereby increasing the oxygenation and nutrition of cells. The exercises are most useful in clients who have not developed gangrenous lesions of the extremities and are often repeated between three and four times daily.

Pharmacology

The pharmacologic treatment of Buerger's disease is limited. Medications such as antibiotics, corticosteroids, vasodilators, and anticoagulants produce few benefits and are not widely used. Treatment with calcium channel blocking agents such as diltiazem (Cardizem) and verapamil (Isoptin) or, more recently, pentoxifylline (Trental) has proved to provide some relief of vasoconstriction and the corresponding intermittent claudication (Berkow & Fletcher, 1992).

Surgery

If conservative and pharmacologic approaches to the treatment of inflammatory disorders of arterial circulation prove ineffective, a sympathectomy or arterial bypass graft may be performed. Arterial bypass grafts are seldom used for smaller vessels but may prove useful in some clients experiencing aortic involvement. Sympathectomy involves the removal of a portion of the sympathetic branch of the autonomic nervous system or the removal of the periarterial sheath (as in a periarterial sympathectomy). Removing portions of the nerves prevents the painful effects of arterial vasospasm. The surgery may or may not be effective in relieving intermittent claudication depending on the extent of the disease and the client's willingness to adhere to other conservative treatment strategies, especially smoking cessation. Sympathectomy may also be effective in the establishment of improved collateral circulation and is helpful in promoting wound healing in the event of amputation (Berkow & Fletcher, 1992; Tierney et al., 1995).

Amputation is necessary if irreversible damage to the arterial bed has occurred and resulting irreparable gangrene is present (amputation is discussed in Chapter 37). Regardless of the etiology, the factors that establish the need for amputation are the same, namely the irreversible interruption of arterial blood flow with subsequent tissue necrosis (i.e., gangrene). Amputation may involve only portions of digits or portions of limbs, as the preservation of healthy tissue is a priority in clients with arterial inflammatory disorders. Although it is highly unusual for a client's entire hand to be amputated because of gangrenous involvement, below-the-knee amputation is sometimes performed for clients with gangrene affecting large portions of the lower leg or with intractable foot pain (Tierney et al., 1995). The prognosis for clients who undergo amputation is generally good if the client adheres to prescribed treatments (both pharmacologic and conservative) and if the client carries through with meticulous foot care after discharge (Tierney et al., 1995).

Nursing Care

The nursing care of clients with Buerger's disease is very similar to the care of clients with other arterial occlusive diseases because the results of impaired arterial blood flow are the same. Sufficient amounts of arterial blood bearing oxygen and nutrients do not reach tissues at the cellular level, producing painful, ruborous, cold extremities or digits. For this reason, nursing care focuses on restoring arterial circulation and preventing prolonged tissue hypoxia. In addition, postsurgical care is necessary if amputation has occurred. It is important to note that episodes of arterial inflammation may be unpredictable, and the care of clients with this disorder is somewhat different from the care required by more chronic, progressive disorders of arterial occlusion. Applicable nursing diagnoses include *Altered Peripheral Tissue Perfusion, Pain, Impaired Physical Mobility,* and *Risk for Injury.*

Altered Peripheral Tissue Perfusion

As discussed earlier in this chapter, occluded arterial circulation prevents nutrients and oxygen from reaching the tissues. The inflammation of the arteries produces vasospasm and vasoconstriction, which obliterate the flow of arterial blood to the most distal arterioles, thereby creating episodes of prolonged tissue hypoxia. If adequate circulation is not restored, gangrene will result.

Nursing interventions with rationales follow:

- Assess peripheral pulses, capillary refill, and temperature and color of digits and extremities every shift and more often if changes occur. *An initial assessment of pulses, capillary refill, color and temperature of digits and extremities provides baseline data for future comparison. Changes in these parameters often reflect changes in the degree of extremity involvement and should be documented and reported.*

- Teach clients and families about the importance of smoking cessation. *Nicotine is a potent vasoconstrictor that exacerbates peripheral-vascular disorders, especially disorders of arterial circulation. The apparently direct relationship between smoking and vasoconstriction and vasospasm in Buerger's disease makes smoking cessation crucial. Clients should be referred to smoking-cessation classes and be encouraged to discuss alternative methods of nicotine withdrawal with physicians.*

- Promote activities that improve arterial circulation. *Life-style habits that contribute to vasoconstriction should be discouraged and replaced with activities that enhance arterial blood flow. A variety of nonpharmacologic interventions, such as keeping hands warm and free of injury, and decreasing stress, promote arterial circulation. Clients with altered sensation should use gloves/socks rather than electric or other thermal devices to avoid burns.*

Pain

The pain of intermittent claudication in clients with Buerger's disease is caused by the vasoconstriction and vasospasm secondary to the inflammation of the arteries. Although the pain may be the same as in clients with arteriosclerosis, the nursing interventions used may vary slightly.

Nursing interventions with rationales follow:

- Assess the client's experience of pain every shift and as needed. *Careful assessment of the client's pain level helps the nurse schedule activities during periods of painlessness. It is important to compare the client's verbal complaints of pain (subjective data) with physical signs (objective data) to determine consistency. Be aware that a client's verbal description of the pain may vary widely from the objective signs of pain assessed by the nurse.*

- Place affected extremities in a dependent position, and change position every 2 hours or more often if needed. *Gravity enhances the flow of blood to dependent extremities. In addition, changes in position enhance the development of collateral circulation, which increases the arterial perfusion of affected extremities and decreases pain.*

- Help clients make life-style changes that reduce pain. *Because smoking is a major cause of vasospasm and vasoconstriction in Buerger's disease, clients should be taught about strategies to stop smoking and help with nicotine withdrawal. Hypertensive clients should be taught about the relationship between hypertension and the pain of arterial occlusive disease.*

- Provide time for the client to discuss issues related to the experience of pain. *Expressing concerns about pain often reduces anxiety, thereby reducing the client's response to episodes of pain. For clients who focus on their pain, limit the time spent discussing pain and devote time to other events in the client's life that may influence the perceptions of pain. It may be helpful to ask the client to keep a journal of precipitating and alleviating factors.*

Impaired Physical Mobility

Client mobility is limited by the pain or discomfort of the occlusive disorder both during acute episodes of Buerger's disease and in later stages of vascular involvement. In the absence of rest pain, clients should be encouraged to perform exercises that promote collateral circulation and circulation in affected vessels. During attacks of acute pain, clients should be encouraged to rest with their extremities in a dependent position. Clients whose upper torso is involved should rest in a supine or low Fowler's position to enhance perfusion. For clients with rest pain, bed rest is necessary, and diversional activities should be provided to encourage compliance. Bed rest is particularly difficult for clients who are accustomed to an active life-style. A thoughtful, organized, and skillful approach is necessary to encourage compliance with activity restrictions.

Nursing interventions with rationales follow:

- Explain the pathophysiologic basis for rest. *Clients are more likely to follow the plan of care if they feel involved in its development. Understanding the relationship between the disease process and rest increases compliance. These explanations also encourage the client to accept the disease process and become accountable for participation in the plan of care.*

- Provide diversional activities. *Diversional activities help avoid the boredom that can accompany prolonged periods of bed rest. Clients should be encouraged to practice relaxation techniques and develop interests in reading, crossword puzzles, and other sedentary activities. As long as business does not contribute to stress (and corresponding vasoconstriction), some clients may work on their computers and conduct business from the bedside.*

- Encourage clients to follow the collaborative plan of care. *Adherence to conservative and pharmacologic treatment strategies promotes recovery and a general sense of well-being. Participation in care gives clients an increased sense of control, which promotes recovery.*

- Encourage clients to turn every 2 hours and perform progressive range-of-motion exercises (from passive to active) at least every shift and more often as desired. *The effects of prolonged bed rest are well documented. Preventing muscle atrophy and joint contracture is a priority for clients restricted to bed rest. Changing position at least every 2 hours promotes collateral circulation and prevents skin breakdown.*

Risk for Injury

The changes in peripheral perfusion that accompany Buerger's disease cause significant tissue hypoxia, which, if left untreated, leads to the formation of gangrene. Clients who do not seek care early in the course of the disease are at increased risk for the development of gangrene, as are clients who refuse to stop smoking or otherwise fail to comply with conservative treatment. Education is a key in the treatment of this potential problem and can help avoid irreversible tissue necrosis and amputation.

Nursing interventions with rationales follow:

- Inspect extremities every shift and more often if changes in color, sensitivity, or skin continuity are apparent. *Frequent inspection of the hands and feet alerts the nurse to changes in the color, temperature, and sensitivity of affected areas. Increasing cyanosis, coldness to the touch, and decreasing sensitivity of the affected areas are signs that the disease may be worsening. Care should be taken to perform assessments during periods of vascular constriction and during their absence so that progressive comparisons may be made. Nurses should inspect the skin for reddened areas, blisters, abrasions, and lacerations, being especially careful to monitor clients with decreased sensitivity.*

- Teach clients the importance of meticulous foot care. *Clients should be taught the principles of good foot care for use at home. In addition to the concepts of asepsis and inspection, clients should also be taught to wear warm, soft cotton socks to protect their feet and to break in new shoes slowly so as to avoid blisters. Shoes or slippers should be worn at all times to avoid breaks in the skin that may lead to infections, which heal slowly and may precipitate the formation of ulcerations or gangrene.*

Other Nursing Diagnoses

The following nursing diagnoses are also appropriate for the client with arterial insufficiency secondary to Buerger's disease:

- *Activity Intolerance* related to severe pain in lower extremities
- *Noncompliance* related to failure to stop smoking cigarettes
- *Anxiety* related to possible surgery and related consequences

- *Risk for Peripheral Neurovascular Dysfunction* related to progressive tissue hypoxia
- *Risk for Impaired Skin Integrity* related to decreased oxygenation of tissues secondary to vasospasm and arterial occlusion

Client and Family Teaching

Teaching clients with Buerger's disease, and for their families, centers on adherence to the collaborative plan of care. The importance of smoking cessation cannot be overemphasized. In addition, the necessity of reducing stress, carrying out daily foot care, and seeking health care follow-up regularly should be emphasized.

Applying the Nursing Process

Case Study of a Client with Buerger's Disease: John Kirvis

John Kirvis, a 34-year-old computer programmer, is married and has two children, ages 6 and 12. His wife, Erin, is a preschool teacher. Mr. Kirvis has smoked over two packs of cigarettes a day for 20 years and, over the past month, has noticed the onset of leg cramps when he climbs the two flights of stairs to his office each day. The cramps have become so painful over the last week that he has to stop to rest about every 50 feet or so and must use the elevator instead of climbing the stairs. Mr. Kirvis makes an appointment with his primary health care physician and tells her, "I just can't understand why this has gotten so much worse so fast. Just the other day I noticed blood on my sock, and when I took it off, there was a big open blister on my heel. I never even felt any pain." Following a series of ultrasound tests, Mr. Kirvis is diagnosed with Buerger's disease and referred to the nurse practitioner for care and teaching.

Assessment

The nurse practitioner at the office, Janice VanAndel, RN, GNP, reviews the physician's admission history and notes that Mr. Kirvis has a long history of cigarette smoking and a recent history of increasingly painful leg cramps. During the course of the admission interview, Ms. VanAndel determines that the course of Mr. Kirvis's intermittent claudication has progressed over the last 7 days to the point that he must rest frequently when walking. On physical assessment, Ms. VanAndel finds weak peripheral pulses in the right leg and absent pedal and posterior tibial pulses in the left foot. The third, fourth, and fifth toes of the left foot have lost some feeling and are pale. The right foot is pink and warm, whereas the left foot is cool to the touch. The skin on the left leg is shiny and thin with no hair below the knee, whereas the right leg has a moderate amount of evenly distributed brown hair.

Diagnosis

Ms. VanAndel makes the nursing diagnoses for Mr. Kirvis:

- *Impaired Peripheral Tissue Perfusion* related to insufficient arterial circulation in the left foot
- *Pain* related to tissue hypoxia
- *Peripheral Neurovascular Dysfunction* related to decreased oxygenation of tissue
- *Anxiety* related to uncertainty and lack of information about disease process

Expected Outcomes

The expected outcomes for the plan of care are that Mr. Kirvis will, by the time of his next appointment in 1 week

- Have a capillary refill time of less than 15 seconds in the left foot.
- State factors that increase pain and take action to modify behavior accordingly.
- Enroll in a smoking-cessation program.
- Verbalize a decrease in anxiety.

Planning and Implementation

The following interventions are planned and implemented for Mr. Kirvis:

- Assess peripheral pulses, capillary refill times, and color and temperature of skin bilaterally to obtain baseline data.
- Assess level of pain both at rest and during activity using a scale of 0 to 10 (0 = no pain; 10 = severe pain) and mutually determine with Mr. Kirvis the most effective methods of managing pain.
- Teach Mr. Kirvis and his wife the importance of remaining on bed rest for the next week.
- Teach Mr. Kirvis how to perform Buerger-Allen exercises, and ask him to do them three times each day.
- Teach Mr. Kirvis about the importance of smoking cessation and good foot care in the management of his disease and prevention of gangrene.
- Provide time for Mr. Kirvis to discuss issues that contribute to anxiety.
- Encourage Mr. Kirvis and his wife to ask questions about his disease and their role in managing it.

Evaluation

Because of his pain, Mr. Kirvis has remained on bed rest for a week. By the time he returns for his office appointment, Mr. Kirvis has not smoked for 6 days and is convinced he can continue his nonsmoking behavior. How-

ever, his wife Erin (who is also a smoker) indicates that she really wants to quit, too, and suggests that they both enroll in a local hospital's smoking-cessation program. Mr. Kirvis agrees, stating that they could both probably help each other if they felt the urge to smoke again. The cessation of smoking has made a noticeable difference in the physical signs of the disease for Mr. Kirvis. After 2 weeks, he was able to walk without pain. The capillary refill time in his left foot has improved to 10 seconds. The last three toes on his left foot are still pale but were warmer. Although Mr. Kirvis understands the unpredictable nature of Buerger's disease, he seems sincere in his desire to control whatever factors he can to limit the progression of his disease. No medications are prescribed at this time, but Ms. VanAndel gives Mr. Kirvis written instructions about daily foot care and inspection, and signs and symptoms to report.

Critical Thinking in the Nursing Process

1. You take Mr. Kirvis's blood pressure and it is 180/100. What do you do next?
2. Describe the similarities and differences between Buerger's disease and arteriosclerosis.
3. Explain the pathophysiologic basis of Mr. Kirvis's leg pain. Why did it worsen over time?
4. After a month, Mr. Kirvis tells you that he is having an awful time quitting smoking. Does this statement support a nursing diagnosis of *Noncompliance*? Why or why not?
5. Develop a plan of care for Mr. Kirvis for the diagnosis: *Chronic Pain*.

The Client with Raynaud's Disease

■ ■ ■

Raynaud's disease is a condition in which the digital arteries respond excessively to vasospastic stimuli (Tierney et al., 1995). This disease is diagnosed after 3 years of intermittent attacks of ischemia of the fingers, toes, ears, or nose following exposure to cold or stress; during this time the condition is called **Raynaud's phenomenon.** However, Raynaud's phenomenon is a secondary response to other physical, emotional, or environmental conditions, whereas Raynaud's disease is a primary disorder of unknown cause.

Raynaud's disease is primarily a disease of young women, occurring almost always in women between the ages of 15 and 45. Genetic predisposition may have some part in this disease, although the actual cause is unknown.

Pathophysiology

Raynaud's phenomenon and Raynaud's disease are both characterized by spasms of the small arteries in the digits. The arterial spasms limit arterial blood flow to the fingers and, on occasion, the toes. The vasospasm may occur unilaterally in only one or two digits (more common in Raynaud's phenomenon) or bilaterally in all digits.

Raynaud's phenomenon occurs in response to a variety of illness and conditions, including collagen vascular disease (scleroderma), pulmonary hypertension, thoracic outlet syndrome, serum sickness, and myxedema (McCance & Huether, 1993). The manifestations may also occur secondary to long-term exposure to cold or to work-related vibration.

The manifestations of Raynaud's disease and Raynaud's phenomenon are essentially the same and occur intermittently. Raynaud's disease has been referred to as the blue-white-red disease because the digits turn blue initially because of diminished arterial circulation caused by the vasospasm, then white as the circulation is more severely limited, and finally very red as the fingers are warmed and the spasm resolves. A similar pattern occurs in clients with Raynaud's phenomenon, although the underlying stimuli are different and the extent of involvement is less pronounced. There may be some sensory changes during attacks, including numbness, stiffness, decreased sensation, and aching pain.

The attacks tend to become more frequent and prolonged over time. With repeated attacks (and resultant decrease in oxygenation), the fingertips thicken and the nails become brittle. Ulceration and gangrene are serious complications that rarely occur.

Collaborative Care

There are no laboratory tests for Raynaud's disease or Raynaud's phenomenon. The disease is diagnosed by the manifestations and is confirmed by an arteriogram.

Treatment focuses on keeping the hands warmed and free from injury, as wounds heal slowly and infections may be difficult to manage because of poor arterial circulation. Life-style behaviors that exacerbate vasoconstriction should be stopped, such as smoking and unprotected exposure to the cold. Underlying diseases are treated. If the condition is severe and conservative treatment is not successful, a sympathectomy may be performed.

Conservative Therapy

In Raynaud's phenomenon and Raynaud's disease, similar conservative therapies are used. Clients are instructed to keep their hands warm. Clients should wear gloves when they go outside in cold weather and kitchen gloves when they handle cold items (for instance, when preparing and serving cold foods and cleaning the refrigerator). Clients

are also taught to avoid injury to their hands. Sometimes attacks may be stopped by swinging the arms back and forth; this action increases perfusion pressure in the small arteries by centrifugal force.

Additional conservative measures include learning new (or better) methods of stress relief and smoking cessation. Several methods are available to help clients find ways of coping with the tensions and worries of everyday life, e.g., exercise, relaxation techniques, massage therapy, hobbies, aroma therapy, and counseling. Clients should be encouraged to find a stress-relief method that works well for them and incorporate it into their daily schedule.

Regardless of the client's disorder, life-style habits that contribute to vascular health are taught and encouraged, such as reducing fat in the diet, increasing activity level, maintaining normal body weight, stopping smoking, and managing stress effectively.

Pharmacology

Vasodilators are sometimes prescribed for clients with Raynaud's phenomena and Raynaud's disease. For clients with peripheral vasoconstriction who have no significant organic disease of the vessels and who do not respond to conservative measures, vasodilators may be used to provide some relief. Some clients with Raynaud's phenomenon may get relief by taking low doses of nifedipine (Procardia). Transdermal nitroglycerine (or longer-acting oral nitrates) helps some clients by decreasing the amount of time necessary for the hands to become normothermic following an attack (Tierney et al., 1995). Analgesics are prescribed for pain.

Nursing Care

Nursing care of the client with Raynaud's phenomenon or Raynaud's disease is primarily educative and supportive. The major teaching topic is protection of the hands from exposure to cold and trauma. The nursing care previously outlined for clients with arteriosclerosis and occlusive arterial disorders is also appropriate for clients with these disorders.

The following nursing diagnoses are appropriate for the client with Raynaud's phenomenon or Raynaud's disease:

- *Altered Peripheral Tissue Perfusion* related to decreased blood flow to fingers
- *Risk for Impaired Skin Integrity* related to decreased oxygenation secondary to long-term arterial spasms
- *Chronic Pain* related to inability to control vasospasms in digits
- *Self-Esteem Disturbance* related to presence of chronic illness

⬛⬛⬛ Disorders of the Aorta and Its Branches ⬛⬛⬛

The structure and function of the aorta and its branches are primarily affected by occlusions, aneurysms, and inflammations. These disorders may be long-term and debilitating (as with arterial occlusive or vasospastic diseases) or may be acute and life-threatening (as with a dissecting abdominal aortic aneurysm). Occlusive and vasospastic disorders were discussed previously; this section focuses on aortic aneurysms and aortitis.

The Client with an Aneurysm

⬛ ⬛ ⬛

An **aneurysm** is an abnormal dilation of a blood vessel, commonly at a site of a weakness or a tear in the vessel wall. Aneurysms most commonly occur in the aorta and peripheral arteries, because of the high pressure of blood flow through these vessels. The majority of arterial aneurysms are caused by arteriosclerosis or atherosclerosis; trauma is the second most common cause. Aneurysms of the thoracic ascending aorta commonly cause intracardiac disorders, discussed in Chapter 28. Aneurysms of the thoracic transverse arch may cause cerebral disorders, discussed in Chapter 41.

Arterial aneurysms are most common in men over 50 years of age, the large majority of whom are asymptomatic at the time of diagnosis. It has been noted, however, that hypertension is a major contributing factor in the development of certain types of aortic aneurysms.

Aneurysms are commonly classified according to their location, size, pathologic features, and causative factors. In one method, aneurysms are described according to shape and extent of vessel involvement. *Saccular aneurysms* are shaped like small out-pouchings (sacs) on a portion of the vessel wall. *Circumferential aneurysms* are more invasive and involve the entire diameter of the vessel (McCance & Huether, 1993). Here are some examples of types of aneurysms:

- A *berry aneurysm* is generally small (less than 2 cm in diameter), involves only a portion of the vessel, and is often found in the circle of Willis in the cerebral circulation. Berry aneurysms are examples of saccular aneurysms and are most probably caused by a congenital abnormality in the media of the arterial wall (McCance & Huether, 1993).

- *Fusiform aneurysms* are very large aneurysms and most commonly involve the entire circumference of the vessel. They generally grow slowly but progressively, and their length and diameter vary considerably from client to client (Porth, 1994). In some clients, fusiform aneurysms cover the majority of the ascending aorta as well a large portion of the abdominal aorta.

- *Dissecting aneurysms* are unlike other aneurysms because they are not the result of atherosclerotic damage to the vessel wall. Rather, they occur when blood leaking from the vessel (commonly the aorta) invades or dissects the layers of the vascular wall, often resulting in a saccular collection of blood. Dissecting aneurysms are, with rare exceptions, the result of a break or tear in one of the two inner layers of the arterial wall (Tierney et al., 1995). Aortic dissections are discussed further in the pathophysiology section.

Aneurysms are also commonly categorized as either *true aneurysms*, or *false aneurysms*. True aneurysms are the result of the slow weakening of the arterial wall caused by the long-term, eroding effects of atherosclerosis and hypertension. True aneurysms affect all three layers of the vessel wall, and most are fusiform and circumferential. False aneurysms are also known as traumatic aneurysms or pseudoaneurysms, and most are caused by a traumatic break in the vascular wall rather than a pathologic weakening of the vessel wall (McCance & Huether, 1993).

The following pathophysiology section discusses etiology and manifestations of aneurysms by their location on the aorta or its branches. These manifestations, and those for a dissecting aneurysm, are outlined in Table 30–3.

Pathophysiology

Aneurysms of the different segments of the aorta and its branches have various causes and manifestations. If symptomatic, clients' complaints reflect the effects of the pressure of the aneurysm on adjacent anatomic structures. A discussion of dissecting aortic aneurysms is also included.

Thoracic Aortic Aneurysms

Thoracic aortic aneurysms, which make up only about 10% of all aortic aneurysms, are most often the result of arteriosclerosis and hypertension, which weaken the aortic wall (Tierney et al., 1994). Other causes include trauma, coarctation of the aorta, tertiary syphilis, fungal infections, and Marfan's disease. The syphilis spirochete can invade and weaken aortic smooth muscles, resulting in an aneurysm as long as 20 years after the primary infection. Marfan's syndrome causes fragmentation of the elastic fibers of the aortic media, weakening the vessel wall.

The manifestations experienced by clients with thoracic aneurysms vary according to the location, size, and rate of growth of the aneurysm. However, general manifestations include ptosis (drooping) of the eyelid and absence of sweating on the affected side (called *Horner's syndrome*), deviation of the trachea, edema of the head and neck, unequal blood pressures in the upper extremities,

Table 30–3	Characteristic Manifestations of Aortic Aneurysms

Location of Aneurysm	Symptoms
Thoracic aorta	<ul><li>pain in back, neck, and substernal areas</li><li>dyspnea, stridor, or brassy cough if pressing on the trachea</li><li>hoarseness and dysphagia if pressing on esophagus or laryngeal nerve</li><li>may be asymptomatic; first sign may be rupture</li></ul>
Superior vena cava	<ul><li>distended neck veins</li><li>edema of the face and neck</li><li>possible aortic regurgitation</li></ul>
Abdominal aorta	<ul><li>pulsating abdominal mass</li><li>calcification within aneurysm detected on X-ray</li><li>mild midabdominal or lumbar pain to severe abdominal and back pain</li><li>peripheral emboli</li><li>cool, cyanotic extremities if renal, iliac, or mesenteric arteries are affected</li><li>possible claudication depending on which additional vessels are affected</li></ul>
Dissecting aneurysms	<ul><li>abrupt, extreme, ripping or tearing pain in area of the aneurysm</li><li>blood pressure may be mildly or markedly elevated at first</li><li>blood pressure and radial pulses may become unobtainable as disorder progresses</li><li>possible syncope, hemiplegia, or paralysis of lower extremities</li><li>possible heart failure</li></ul>

distended neck veins, and pain in the substernal area, back, or neck. Most clients with a dissecting aortic aneurysm have a history of hypertension or Marfan's syndrome and commonly complain of severe chest pain that radiates to the back.

Aneurysms of the ascending aortic arch typically cause angina. Aneurysms of the transverse aortic arch often cause dysphagia, dyspnea, hoarseness, confusion, and dizziness. Aneurysms of the thoracic aorta tend to enlarge progressively and may rupture, causing death.

Abdominal Aortic Aneurysms

Abdominal aortic aneurysms are associated with arteriosclerotic occlusive disease and hypertension. Other causative factors are believed to be smoking and increasing age. Most abdominal aortic aneurysms are found in adults over age 70. The vast majority of abdominal aortic aneurysms (over 90%) develop below the renal arteries, most commonly at the branching of the abdominal aorta.

Most clients with abdominal aneurysms are asymptomatic, but on examination have a pulsating mass in the mid and upper abdomen and a bruit over the mass. However, in clients who do complain of pain, the most common site is in the midabdominal or lower back area. The degree of pain is commonly indicative of the severity (and urgency) of the problem. The intensity may range from mild discomfort to severe pain, and the pain may be either constant or intermittent. Pain may be an indication of an impending rupture.

A complication of an abdominal aortic aneurysm may be the formation of emboli (from the sluggish blood flow within the aneurysm) that travel to the lower extremities. The aneurysm may also rupture and lead to death due to hemorrhage and hypovolemic shock. Rupture results in death before hospitalization in up to one-half of all clients, and others die before surgical intervention. Only 10% to 20% of all clients survive rupture of an abdominal aortic aneurysm (Tierney et al., 1994).

Popliteal and Femoral Aneurysms

The cause of most popliteal and femoral aneurysms is arteriosclerosis. Most occur in men. They may be the result of trauma and are often bilateral.

Popliteal aneurysms may be asymptomatic, with a pulsating mass present in the popliteal fossa (behind the knee) found on examination. Manifestations, if any, are usually the result of decreased blood flow to the lower extremity and include intermittent claudication, rest pain, and numbness. Thrombosis and embolism are complications; resultant gangrene often necessitates amputation.

A femoral aneurysm usually is detected as a pulsating mass in the femoral area. The manifestations are the result of occlusion and are similar to those of popliteal aneurysms. Femoral aneurysms may rupture.

Aortic Dissections

Dissection is a major complication of an aortic aneurysm. Although this complication may occur with any aneurysm, it is more common in thoracic aneurysms close to the aortic valve, where the blood is ejected forcefully from the left ventricle. Blood is forced between the layers of the aneurysm, creating a blood-filled cavity that expands along the length of the aorta.

Conditions that weaken or cause degenerative changes in the elastic and smooth muscles of the aortic wall layers increase the risk for dissection. In most cases, the client also has hypertension. Other factors implicated in dissection include Marfan's syndrome, pregnancy, congenital defects of the aortic valve, coarctation of the aorta, and cardiac catheterization or surgery (Porth, 1994).

Dissection of the thoracic aortic walls increases along the length of the vessel, moving toward the heart and into the descending aorta. As the aorta expands, pressure may prevent the aortic valve from closing or may occlude the branches of the aorta. A dissection of an aneurysm of the abdominal aorta may extend into the renal, iliac, or femoral arteries.

The primary manifestation of a dissecting aneurysm is sudden, excruciating pain. The pain, often described as a ripping or tearing sensation, is usually over the area of dissection. Thoracic dissections cause pain in the anterior chest, whereas abdominal dissections commonly cause back pain. Although the blood pressure may initially be increased, it rapidly decreases and is often inaudible as the dissection occludes blood flow. Peripheral pulses are absent for the same reason.

Depending on the area of the dissection, complications include hemiplegia and paralysis of the lower extremities. The mortality rate is high, with more than 20% of untreated clients dying within the first 24 hours, and 90% of all clients dying within 3 weeks (Tierney et al., 1994). Death is the result of rupture of the aorta.

Collaborative Care

Most aneurysms are asymptomatic, detected through a routine physical examination. If a mass is detected, it must be differentiated from a neoplasm or a cyst. Treatment depends on the size of the aneurysm. Small, asymptomatic aneurysms are often not treated; large aneurysms at risk for rupture require surgery. Members and goals of the collaborative health care team are outlined in the accompanying box.

Laboratory and Diagnostic Tests

Laboratory and diagnostic tests are conducted to support the diagnosis and to determine the size and location of the aneurysm.

The following laboratory tests may be ordered:

- *Cardiac enzyme levels* may be measured to determine if a myocardial infarction has occurred.

- *Renal function studies* may be conducted if the aneurysm is pressing on the kidneys.

- *Hemoglobin* and *hematocrit* levels are measured if leakage of blood from the aneurysm is suspected.

The following diagnostic tests may be ordered:

- A *chest X-ray* film is used to visualize a thoracic aortic aneurysm.

- *Transesophageal echocardiography* may be used to detect the specific location and extent of a thoracic aneurysm and to visualize a dissecting aneurysm.

- *Aortography* supports the diagnosis and identifies the precise size and location of the aneurysm. However, fibrin and thrombosis within the aneurysm may obscure the true size of the aneurysm.

- *Abdominal ultrasonography* is most often used to diagnose abdominal aortic aneurysms.

- *Contrast-enhanced CT* or *MRI* give precise measurements of aneurysm size.

Pharmacology

Clients with aortic aneurysms may initially be treated with antihypertensive medications (given either orally or intravenously, depending on the urgency of treatment),

---

Collaborative Care: The Client with a Femoral Bypass Graft

Health Care Team	Client-Centered Goals
Vascular surgeon	Assesses type and severity of ischemia. Orders diagnostic tests, performs surgery to bypass arterial occlusion on clients with severe rest pain or threatened loss of limb.
Primary care physician	Treats symptoms conservatively, may initiate drug therapy, refers client to vascular surgeon or manages care following discharge.
Radiologist	Performs or assists with invasive and noninvasive diagnostic tests such as arteriograms.
Physical therapist	Recommends or provides physical rehabilitation program. Instructs clients regarding Buerger-Allen exercises. Provides teaching regarding exercise program following discharge.
Dietitian	Assesses client's and family's knowledge of low-fat, low-cholesterol diet. Teaches client and family necessary dietary modifications.
RN and Health Care Team Communications	Reports to physician any changes in the neurovascular integrity of the extremity. Reports signs and symptoms of bleeding, swelling, and infection. Consults with dietitian to ensure adequate dietary intake of a well-balanced diet to promote healing. Discusses client's rehabilitation potential with physical therapist and collaborates to maximize potential for self-care. Reports any home care needs to social worker.

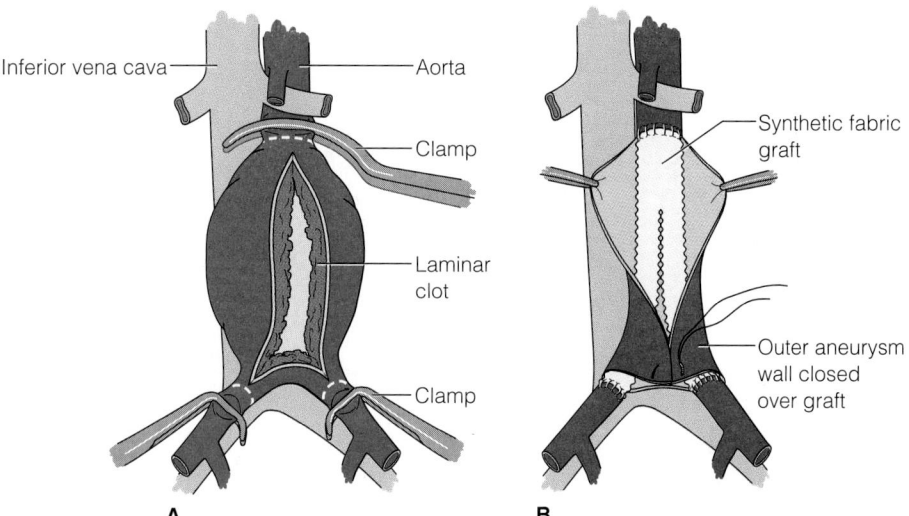

Figure 30–2   Repair of an abdominal aortic aneurysm. *A,* The aneurysm is exposed and clamped below the left renal vein and the iliac arteries. Note the extensive clotting within the aneurysm wall. *B,* A synthetic graft is used to replace the aneurysm. The aneurysm is stripped of clotting, and the arterial wall is sutured around the graft.

and/or beta-adrenergic blocking agents to lower blood pressure and to control the rate and rhythm of the heartbeat. In dissecting aortic aneurysm, pharmacologic agents are often used to stabilize blood pressure and regulate the heartbeat before diagnostic studies are completed. Desirable systolic pressure readings should be around 100 mm Hg and may be achieved by the intravenous administration of sodium nitroprusside (Nipride) in a 5% solution of dextrose and water; the rate of administration (which controls the rate at which the blood pressure falls) is regulated in response to frequent monitoring of blood pressure. Simultaneously, an intravenous infusion of propranolol (Inderal) is administered over a 5-minute period until the heart rate is maintained at 60 beats per minute. If the use of beta-blockers is contraindicated, intravenous reserpine (Serpasil) may be substituted (Tierney et al., 1995).

Following surgical correction of an aneurysm, anticoagulation therapy and prophylactic antibiotic therapy may be initiated. Clients who have undergone vascular surgery are initially placed on continuous heparin therapy for at least a week and gradually switched to warfarin prior to discharge from the hospital. Following convalescence, many clients are maintained indefinitely on warfarin therapy, whereas others are placed on life-long, low-dose aspirin therapy to help prevent recurrence of occlusive disorders. In some clients, prophylactic, broad-spectrum antibiotic therapy may be started before surgery and continued for up to 72 hours postoperatively. If signs of wound infection are noticed during the first 24 to 48 hours postoperatively, the wound is cultured, and additional organism-specific antibiotics may be ordered.

Surgery

All clients with aortic aneurysms that are tender or enlarging or who present with additional symptoms require surgery. The surgical risk status of the client must be considered before surgery; in some situations (e.g., aortic aneurysm rupture, femoral or popliteal aneurysms, acute arterial thrombosis) immediate surgical intervention is necessary to preserve life.

The surgical repair of most aortic aneurysms involves excising the aneurysm and replacing it with a synthetic fabric graft, a procedure known as *aneurysmectomy* (Figure 30–2). Thoracic aneurysmectomies are more difficult to perform than aneurysmectomies of the abdominal aorta because there is a greater risk of rupture owing to the increased pressure in the thoracic aorta. Nursing care of the client having surgery on the aorta is outlined in the box on page 1222, and a Critical Pathway for the client having a femoral bypass graft is outlined on pages 1224–1227.

Nursing Care

The nursing care of clients with an aneurysm of the aorta or its branches centers on the assessment of tissue perfusion and measures to maintain blood flow, relieve pain, and decrease anxiety. Because the majority of clients with an aneurysm are asymptomatic, nursing care is most often required during surgical repair or treatment of an expanding or ruptured aneurysm. Nursing care for the client having surgery was described in the previous section.

Clients are often highly anxious because of the urgent nature of their disorder. The nurse must manage the anxiety levels of both the client and family members to be able to address the client's physiologic needs in an expeditious manner. Every effort must be made to keep clients calm and prevent any additional stress, which might exacerbate hypertension.

Nursing diagnoses with interventions and rationales that have been described throughout this chapter are also appropriate for the client with an aortic aneurysm: *Anxiety, Pain, Altered Tissue Perfusion,* and *Altered Protection.* The

Nursing Care of the Client Having Surgery of the Aorta

PREOPERATIVE NURSING CARE

- Ensure that a valid signed consent for the procedure is in the chart. *The client and/or family must understand the procedure to be done along with its potential risks and benefits. A signed consent form documents that the client or family consent to having the specific procedure performed.*

- Provide preoperative care and teaching as time permits. *Surgery of the aorta is often an emergency situation, conducted to repair a dissecting aortic aneurysm or to remove thrombi or an embolism that is occluding blood flow to organs or extremities. The condition of the client and the urgency of the procedure dictate the amount of care and teaching that can be accomplished. However, if time permits, all usual preoperative care, as discussed in Chapter 7, is completed.*

- Implement interventions to reduce fear and anxiety:
  a. Orient the client and family to the intensive care unit, if appropriate.
  b. Describe and explain the reason for all equipment and tubes, such as cardiac monitors, ventilators, nasogastric tubes, urinary catheters, intravenous lines and fluids, and intra-arterial lines.
  c. Explain all diagnostic tests.
  d. Explain what to expect following surgery (sights, sounds, frequency of taking vital signs, dressings, pain relief measures, method of communicating if the client is to be on a ventilator).
  e. Allow time for the client and family to ask questions and verbalize fears.

These explanations allow the client and family to maintain a sense of control.

- Monitor for and report manifestations of impending rupture, expansion, or dissection of the aneurysm.
  a. Take and compare blood pressure in both upper and lower extremities.
  b. Monitor laboratory results: hemoglobin, hematocrit, red blood cell levels.
  c. Assess peripheral pulses.
  d. Assess for increase in pain.
  e. Assess for increasing size of pulsating mass.
  f. Assess for decrease in motor function or sensation in the lower extremities.

If an aneurysm is expanding or dissecting, blood pressure in the thigh will continue to be lower in comparison to that in the arm. If an aneurysm is leaking blood, hemoglobin, hematocrit, and red blood cell levels will decrease. Expansion, dissection, or rupture result in loss of peripheral pulses. An increase in pain or in the size of the mass, and a decrease in motor function or sensation indicates dissection or an increase in aneurysm size.

- Implement interventions to decrease the risk of rupture of the aneurysm.
  a. Maintain bed rest.
  b. Do not elevate the client's legs, cross the client's legs, or use the knee gatch.
  c. Encourage measures to reduce stress.
  d. Encourage the client to avoid straining (as during a bowel movement) or holding the breath while moving.
  e. Administer antihypertensives if prescribed.

Activity, stress, and the Valsalva maneuver increase blood pressure, increasing the risk for rupture of the aneurysm. Elevating, crossing, and putting pressure on the legs restrict peripheral blood flow and increase pressure on the site of the aneurysm. Antihypertensives may be ordered to reduce pressure in the dilated vessel.

- Assess for and report manifestations of arterial thrombosis or embolism: absent peripheral pulses; pale or cyanotic extremities; coolness in the skin of the extremities; diffuse abdominal pain; or an increase in groin, lumbar, or lower extremity pain. *The client with an aortic aneurysm is at risk for developing an arterial thrombus or embolism. The manifestations listed are indicators of these complications.*

POSTOPERATIVE NURSING CARE

- Monitor for and report manifestations of leakage at the graft site.
  a. Ecchymoses of the scrotum, perineum, or penis
  b. New or expanding hematoma at the incision site
  c. Increased abdominal girth
  d. Decreasing or absent peripheral pulses
  e. Decreased motor function or sensation in the extremities
  f. Decreasing blood pressure and increasing pulse
  g. Decreasing hematocrit, hemoglobin, and red blood cell levels
  h. Increasing pain in the abdomen, pelvic or lumbar regions, or groin
  i. Decreasing urinary output (less than 30 mL/hour)
  j. Decreasing CVP, pulmonary artery pressure, or pulmonary artery wedge pressure

Nursing Care of the Client Having Surgery of the Aorta (continued)

These manifestations may signal leakage at the graft site with resultant hemorrhage. Pain may indicate pressure from an expanding hematoma, bowel ischemia due to embolism or hypovolemia, and decreased renal perfusion due to prolonged aortic clamp time or hypovolemia.

- Implement interventions to prevent hypovolemic shock.
  a. Maintain fluid replacement as prescribed.
  b. Administer blood or fluid expanders as prescribed.
  c. Monitor vital signs, skin color and temperature, and level of consciousness.

Hypovolemic shock is a potential complication due to blood loss during surgery, third-spacing, inadequate fluid replacement, and/or hemorrhage if graft separation or leakage occurs.

- Monitor and report manifestations of lower extremity embolism: pain and numbness in lower extremities, decreasing pulses, and skin that is pale, cool, or cyanotic. *Although pulses are usually absent for 4 to 12 hours as a result of vasospasm, this combination of manifestations indicates lower extremity embolism from a clot at the surgical site.*

- Monitor for and report manifestations of bowel ischemia or gangrene: occult or fresh blood in stools, diarrhea, abdominal pain, and abdominal distention. *Bowel ischemia may be a complication of decreased blood supply to the bowel due to ligature of the inferior mesenteric artery during surgery, hypovolemia, or embolism.*

- Monitor for and report manifestations of impaired renal function: urinary output less than 30 mL per hour, fixed specific gravity, increasing BUN and serum creatinine levels. *Impaired renal function may*

be a complication as a result of hypovolemia and clamping of the aorta during the surgical graft procedure.

- Monitor for and report manifestations of spinal cord ischemia: weakness in the lower extremities and paraplegia. *Obstructed perfusion of the spinal cord may cause spinal cord ischemia.*

- Provide general and specific postoperative care (see Chapter 7):
  a. Monitor patency and status of the chest tube drainage if the client has had thoracic surgery (see Chapter 34).
  b. Monitor temperature, vital signs, and ECG findings.
  c. Assess dressings for signs of bleeding.
  d. Assess incision site for signs of infection.
  e. Encourage coughing and deep breathing every 2 hours if client is not on a ventilator.
  f. Assess abdomen for the return of bowel sounds.
  g. Assess lower extremities for manifestations of thrombophlebitis.
  h. Turn the client every 2 hours.
  I. Administer pain medications on a regular basis.
  j. Administer prescribed antibiotics, anticoagulants, and antihypertensives.

Surgery to repair a thoracic aneurysm requires opening of the chest wall. Sepsis is indicated by increased temperature, increased pulse, and decreased blood pressure. ECG changes may indicate hypovolemia or may be the result of coexisting cardiac disease. Other interventions listed are necessary to prevent pulmonary complications, detect graft leakage, identify wound infection, prevent venous stasis, maintain the client as free of pain as possible, prevent infection, decrease the risk of thrombosis, and prevent hypertension.

following nursing diagnoses may also be appropriate for the client with an aneurysm of the aorta and its branches:

- *Activity Intolerance* related to intermittent claudication
- *Decreased Cardiac Output* related to restriction of cardiac contraction secondary to expanding thoracic aortic aneurysm
- *Fear* related to unknown outcome of surgery for dissecting aneurysm
- *Risk for Infection* related to presence of large abdominal incision

- *Self-Care Deficit: Bathing* related to presence of chest tubes
- *Sexual Dysfunction* related to prolonged reduction of blood flow through the internal iliac arteries during aneurysm repair
- *Altered Thought Processes* related to ischemia secondary to impairment of cerebral blood flow by thoracic aneurysm
- *Altered Renal Tissue Perfusion* related to hypovolemia following rupture of aneurysm

Text continues on page 1227

	Critical Pathway for Client Following Femoral Bypass Graft	
	Date _____ **Preoperative**	**Date _____** **1st 24 hours postoperative**
	Expected length of stay: 3 to 4 days	
Daily outcomes	Client will ■ Verbalize understanding of preoperative teaching including: TCDB, IV therapy, mobilization, O$_2$, PCA/epidural for pain managment. ■ Demonstrate ability to cope. ■ Verbalize understanding of procedure. ■ Obtain informed consent.	Client will ■ Maintain adequate circulation to affected extremity as evidenced by capillary refill less than 3 seconds; pink, warm extremity; palpable distal pulses; and adequate sensation and motion (or pulses by Doppler). ■ Have clean, dry dressing. ■ Recover from anesthesia as evidenced by VS return to baseline, awake, alert, and oriented. ■ Verbalize understanding and demonstrate cooperation with turning, deep breathing, coughing, and splinting. ■ Tolerate ordered diet without nausea and vomiting. ■ Verbalize control of incisional pain with ordered medications or epidural analgesia. ■ Demonstrate cooperation with measures to prevent compromising blood flow. ■ Demonstrate ability to cope.
Assessments, tests, and treatments	CBC, urinalysis, CXR, EKG Baseline physical assessment with focus on respiratory, cardiovascular, and renal function.	Vital signs and O$_2$ saturation, neurovascular assessment, dressing and wound drainage assessment q15min × 4; q30min × 4; q1h × 4 and then q4h if stable Peripheral CSM assessment q1h Report diminished or absent pulse stat. Report signs or symptoms of diminished peripheral blood flow immediately. Monitor for compartment syndrome or nerve damage. Head-to-toe assessment q4h and prn Incentive spirometer q2h Intake and output every shift Assess voiding—if client cannot void, try suggestive voiding techniques or catheterize q8h or prn. Minimize stressful situations. Maintain comfortable room temperature and avoid chilling. Assess coping status of client and family. Provide ongoing emotional support to client and family.

	Date _____ **Preoperative**	**Date** _____ **1st 24 hours postoperative**
Knowledge deficit	Orient to room and surroundings. Provide simple/brief instructions. Preoperative teaching to include: TCDB, IV therapy, mobilization, O$_2$, PCA/epidural for pain management.	Orient to room and surroundings. Provide simple, brief instructions. Include family in teaching. Review specific postoperative care: turning, coughing, deep breathing, incentive spirometer, mobilization, intravenous pain management (epidural, PCA or prn medications). Instruct client not to compromise blood flow, e.g., crossing legs or flexing hips at 90 degrees for prolonged periods. Assess understanding of teaching.
Psycho-social	Assess anxiety regarding impending surgery. Assess fear of unknown and surgery. Offer emotional support. Encourage verbalization of concerns. Provide information regarding surgical experience. Minimize external stimuli (noise, movement).	Assess level of anxiety. Provide information and ongoing support and encouragement to client and family.
Diet	NPO Baseline nutritional and hydration assessment	Clear to ordered diet, as tolerated.
Activity	Assess potential safety needs and provide appropriate safety measures.	Assess safety needs and provide appropriate precautions. Do not use bed gatch. Bed rest until AM then ambulate with assistance Active foot and leg exercises q1–2h while awake Bed cradle over lower extremities
Medications	Preoperative medications per anesthesiologist IV fluids	Epidural, IM, or IV/PCA analgesics IV antibiotics if ordered IV fluids Routine meds as ordered
Transfer/discharge plans	Assess potential discharge needs and support system. Establish discharge goals with client and family.	Establish discharge goals with client and family. Determine possible discharge needs and support system with client and significant others. Begin home care instructions.

➤

Critical Pathway for Client Following Femoral Bypass Graft (continued)		
	Date _____ **48 hours postoperative**	**Date _____** **3–4 days postoperative**
Daily outcomes	Client will ■ Maintain adequate circulation to affected extremity as evidenced by capillary refill less than 3 seconds; pink, warm extremity; palpable distal pulses; and adequate sensation and motion (or pulses by Doppler). ■ Have stable vital signs. ■ Have clean, dry wound with edges well-approximated, healing by first intention. ■ Demonstrate cooperation with turning, deep breathing, coughing, and splinting. ■ Tolerate ordered diet without nausea and vomiting. ■ Ambulate 4 times per day in hallway. ■ Verbalize control of incisional pain with ordered medications. ■ Verbalize beginning ability to cope with changes in body image. ■ Demonstrate ability to cope. ■ Verbalize/demonstrate beginning understanding of home care instructions.	Client is afebrile with stable vital signs. Client has adequate and stable circulation to affected extremity. Client has clean, dry wound with edges well-approximated, healing by first intention. Client manages pain with oral medications and nonpharmacologic measures. Client is independent in self-care. Client is fully ambulatory. Client has resumed preadmission urine and bowel elimination pattern. Client verbalizes home care instructions. Client tolerates ordered diet. Client demonstrates ability to cope with ongoing stressors. Client verbalizes/demonstrates knowledge of discharge instructions and home care routines including strategies to enhance circulation and prevent worsening arteriosclerosis.
Assessments, tests, and treatments	Vital signs and dressing and wound drainage assessment q4h Peripheral CSM assessment q1–2h and prn Report diminished or absent pulse stat. Report signs or symptoms of diminished peripheral blood flow immediately. Monitor for compartment syndrome or nerve damage. Head to toe assessment q4h Incentive spirometer q2h until fully ambulatory. Intake and output every shift Assess voiding pattern every shift. Assess wound and change dressing BID. Minimize stressful situations. Maintain comfortable room temperature and avoid chilling. Assess coping status of client and family. Provide ongoing emotional support to client and family.	Vital signs and dressing, and wound drainage assessment q4–8h Peripheral CSM assessment q2–4h and prn Report absent or diminished pulse stat. Report signs or symptoms of diminished peripheral blood flow immediately. Monitor for compartment syndrome or nerve damage. Head to toe assessment q4–8h Assess wounds and apply dry sterile dressing every day and prn. Minimize stressful situations. Maintain comfortable room temperature and avoid chilling. Assess coping status of client and family. Provide ongoing emotional support to client and family.

	Date _____ 48 hours postoperative	Date _____ 3–4 days postoperative
Knowledge deficit	Review plan of care and importance of early mobilization. Include family in teaching. Begin discharge teaching regarding wound care/dressing change, diet, and activity. Review written discharge instructions with client and family. Review precautions to minimize the compromise of blood flow. Assess understanding of teaching.	Complete discharge teaching to include wound care, diet, follow-up care, signs and symptoms to report, activity, and medication: name, purpose, dose, frequency, route, food interactions, and side effects. Include family in teaching. Provide client with written discharge instructions. Assess understanding of teaching.
Psycho-social	Assess level of anxiety. Encourage verbalization of concerns. Provide ongoing support and encouragement to client and family.	Assess level of anxiety. Encourage verbalization of concerns. Provide ongoing support and encouragement to client and family.
Diet	Diet as ordered or low-salt, low-fat, and low-cholesterol diet to tolerance Dietary consult for teaching	Diet as ordered or low-salt, low-fat, and low-cholesterol diet to tolerance Provide client written copy of diet.
Activity	Maintain safety precautions. Fully ambulatory in room No prolonged sitting Walk in hall 4 to 6 times per day Active foot and leg exercises q1–2h while awake Bed cradle over lower extremities	Maintain safety precautions. Fully ambulatory Active foot and leg exercises q1–2h while awake Bed cradle over lower extremities
Medications	D/C epidural PO, IM, or IV/PCA analgesics IV antibiotics if ordered Intermittent IV device Routine meds as ordered	PO analgesics D/C IV device Routine meds as ordered
Transfer/ discharge plans	Review progress toward discharge goals. Finalize discharge plans. Make referrals for home care.	Complete discharge instructions Finalize any arrangements for home care.

Client and Family Teaching

Teaching for clients with a small aneurysm and their families focuses on controlling hypertension by diet, reducing stress, limiting alcohol intake, stopping smoking, and understanding the medication regimen. The client should understand that the control of hypertension may slow progression of the size of the aneurysm and that compliance with treatment is very important.

Postoperative client and family teaching includes information on preventing infection, caring for the surgical wound, taking medications to control blood pressure and prevent blood clotting, and recognizing manifestations of

complications. Teach the client the importance of regular rest periods and ways to prevent constipation and straining at stool (such as increasing fluid and fiber in the diet). The client is also taught the importance of avoiding prolonged sitting, lifting heavy objects, taking part in strenuous exercise, and having sexual intercourse for the prescribed time after surgery (usually 6 to 12 weeks). Information about control of hypertension is important for the surgical client as well as the client treated conservatively.

Verbal instruction and written guidelines are provided, as is information about return appointments. The client has experienced a major surgical procedure and often requires additional care after discharge, and referrals to a home health agency or community health service may be necessary. Referrals are especially important for older adults and their caregivers, who may require additional assistance with the complex care needs.

The Client with Aortitis

■ ■ ■

Aortitis is an inflammation of the aorta, primarily involving the aortic arch. At one time, aortitis was a common complication of syphilis, but this form is rarely seen to-

day. The most common type is the result of *Takayasu's disease* (also called pulseless disease), a chronic inflammation and stenosis of the aortic arch and its branches. This disorder occurs most frequently in young women of Asian descent.

The manifestations depend on the vessels involved but include attacks of transient cerebral ischemia (see Chapter 41), visual disturbances, and absent pulses in the arms. Angiography provides diagnosis and determines the extent of involvement. Clients in the early stages of aortitis may be treated with steroids, which reverse the vascular stenosis. Bypass arterial grafts are necessary for clients with advanced disease.

▗ ▗ ▗ Disorders of Venous Circulation ▗ ▗ ▗

Disorders of the venous system fall into two primary categories: (a) occlusive venous disorders and (b) disorders related to the ineffective return of venous blood to the heart. The healthy venous system relies on changes in pressures within the abdomen and thorax and effective peripheral muscle-pumping action to force blood to return to the heart. When these mechanisms are altered, venous circulation is impaired, thereby contributing to disease processes associated with the prolonged inertia of venous blood.

Because pressure is lower and blood flow is slower in the venous system than in the arterial system, blood can pool in the veins. The result can be disorders arising from the stagnation of blood in the venous bed, such as thrombosis, venous inflammation, and chronic venous insufficiency (Porth, 1994). This section of the chapter focuses on three of the most common disorders of venous circulation: thrombophlebitis, chronic venous insufficiency, and varicose veins.

The Client with Thrombophlebitis

■ ■ ■

Thrombophlebitis is a condition in which a blood clot (thrombus) forms on the wall of a vein and partially or completely occludes the flow of venous blood back to the heart. The wall of the vein becomes inflamed in response to the clot as a foreign object.

Thrombophlebitis, also known as *venous thrombosis*, is primarily associated with the slow movement of blood through the system. Although thrombi can form in either the arteries or veins, the slower movement of blood in the

venous system makes platelet aggregation (i.e., clotting) more likely there. When sluggish flow is compounded by the prolonged inactivity that may accompany chronic disease or old age, the opportunities for thrombi formation increase dramatically.

A large number of factors are associated with thrombophlebitis; these are outlined in the accompanying box. There is an increased incidence in people with impaired cardiac function, older clients, women who use oral contraceptives, surgical clients, clients who are immobilized, and people with certain cancers. The major complications of thrombophlebitis are chronic venous insufficiency and pulmonary embolism.

Pathophysiology

Three pathologic factors are associated with thrombophlebitis. Called *Virchow's triad*, these factors are stasis of blood, increased blood coagulability, and injury to the vessel wall. Two of these three factors must be present for thrombi to form in the vein.

Trauma to the endothelial lining of the vein brings subendothelial tissues in contact with platelets, which then aggregate, especially if venous stasis is present. The deposit of fibrin, leukocytes, and erythrocytes into the platelet clump causes a thrombus. Initially the thrombus floats within the vein. Within 7 to 10 days, it adheres to the vein wall, but a portion may still float in the lumen of the vessel. Pieces of this "tail" may break loose and travel through the circulation as emboli. At this point, the inflammation begins. Fibroplasts eventually invade the thrombus, scarring the vein wall and destroying venal valves. Although the vein may regain patency, the valves do not regain function, and directional flow is not reestablished (Tierney et al., 1994).

Factors Associated with Thrombophlebitis

- Bed rest
- Intravenous catheters
- Immobilization, e.g., because of fractured hip, spinal cord injury, joint replacement, CVA, casts, splints, or traction
- Obesity
- Myocardial infarction
- Congestive heart failure
- Cancer of the breast, pancreas, prostate, or ovary
- Multiple sclerosis
- Oral contraceptive use, especially in women who smoke
- Pregnancy
- Childbirth
- Surgery in clients over age 40
- Altered coagulability states

Deep veins as well as superficial veins can be affected by thrombophlebitis (Figure 30–3). In *deep vein thrombosis* (DVT), the thrombi form primarily in the lower extremities and may result in complications of pulmonary embolism and chronic venous insufficiency. In *superficial vein thrombosis* (SVT), the thrombi form primarily in the upper extremities. The incidence of SVT is increasing and seems to be most closely associated with trauma to the veins associated with the increased use of catheters in the subclavian vein (Porth, 1994; Tierney et al., 1995). Manifestations of these disorders are listed in the box on page 1230.

Deep Vein Thrombosis

The deep veins of the legs, primarily in the calf, provide the most hospitable environment for the formation of thrombi in the lower extremities. In approximately 80% of clients with deep vein thromboses, the calf vessels are the site of origination; in nearly 10% of that 80% the clotting disorder eventually extends to the popliteal and femoral veins (Tierney et al., 1995). In some clients, a diagnosis of pulmonary embolism may be the first indication of deep vein thrombosis (Goldstone, 1994; Tierney et al., 1995).

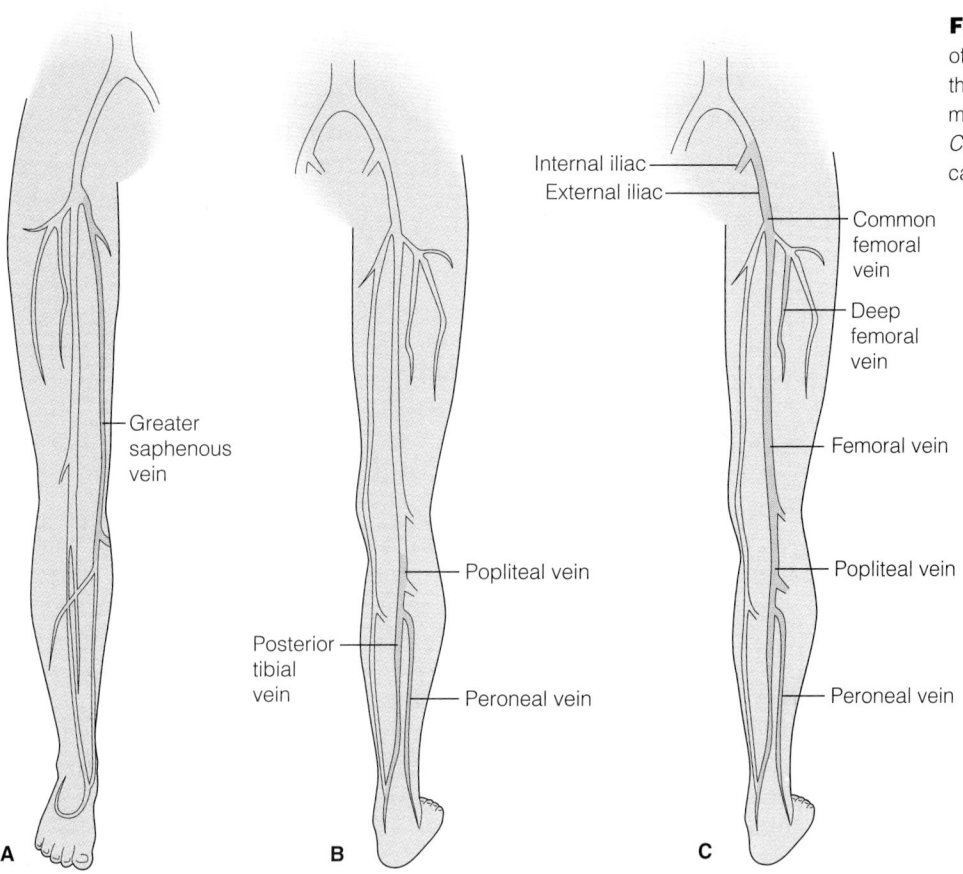

Figure 30–3 Common locations of venous thrombosis. *A,* Superficial thrombophlebitis. *B,* The most common sites of deep thrombophlebitis. *C,* Deep thrombophlebitis from the calf to the iliac veins.

Clinical Manifestations of Thrombophlebitis of the Lower Extremities

■ ■ ■

Deep Vein Thrombophlebitis (Thrombosis)

- Dull, aching pain in affected extremity, especially when walking
- Severe pain, especially when walking
- Cyanosis of the affected extremity
- Slightly elevated temperature
- General malaise

Superficial Vein Thrombophlebitis (Thrombosis)

- Dull, aching pain over the affected vein
- Marked redness along the course of the vein
- Increased warmth over the area of inflammation
- Palpable cordlike structure

The clinical manifestations of thrombophlebitis primarily reflect the inflammatory process affecting the wall of the vein. While the clot is in the formative stage, the clients may notice no symptoms. As the process continues, clients complain of a vague tightness or a dull, aching pain in the affected extremity, particularly upon walking. Once the inflammatory process is well underway, clients complain of severe pain and tenderness in the affected extremity as well as an inability to walk without pain. The skin on the affected extremity may be discolored (cyanotic). The affected extremity may be larger in diameter than the unaffected extremity, and there is usually pronounced tenderness over the affected areas. Clients may also display slight elevations in body temperature and complain of generalized malaise.

Although a positive *Homan's sign* (pain in the calf when the foot is dorsiflexed) was long considered a classic manifestation, this is no longer true. This sign is not specific to DVT and can be elicited by any condition of the calf. In addition, there is a risk of detaching the thrombus from the vein wall as the calf muscles contract.

Superficial Vein Thrombophlebitis

Thrombi form in the superficial veins of the arm just as they do in the deep veins of the legs, but the causative factors may vary slightly. In superficial veins, the primary causative factor is trauma to the venous wall commonly associated with the use of venous catheters, repeated venous punctures, or the use of strong intravenous solutions that produce an inflammatory response in the vessel

wall (Porth, 1994; Tierney et al., 1995). Research continues regarding the reasons for the catheter-induced inflammatory process; it is hypothesized that the use of plastic rather than steel catheters increases the risk (Tierney et al., 1995).

Superficial venous thrombi are also found in pregnant or postpartum women, but there is no known etiologic factor. The coexistence of superficial venous thrombi in clients with underlying Buerger's disease may be related to a disruption in venous circulation as a consequence of the vasospastic interruption in arterial circulation.

The clinical manifestations associated with superficial and deep venous thrombi are similar. See the accompanying box.

The presence of edema, chills, and high fever suggests complications of the inflammatory process, and more immediate attention is required.

Collaborative Care

Thrombophlebitis must be differentiated from cellulitis, calf muscle strain, contusion, and lymphatic obstruction. Following diagnosis, the collaborative care of clients with thrombophlebitis focuses on the treatment of the inflammatory process, prevention of further clotting or extension of the disease, and restoration of venous blood flow. The medical care of the client includes the use of medications to prevent the extension of existing disease, to treat underlying inflammation or infection, and to dissolve existing clots.

Laboratory and Diagnostic Tests

The history and physical examination are not as helpful for diagnosing thrombophlebitis as they are for diagnosing arterial occlusions.

The following laboratory tests may be ordered:

- *Blood cultures* may be conducted in clients with superficial venous thrombosis to rule out the possibility of staphylococcal infection.
- *White cell counts* and *erythrocyte sedimentation rates* may be increased, reflecting the ongoing inflammatory processes in the body.

The following diagnostic tests may be ordered:

- *Ascending phlebography* (also known as ascending venous venography) is a test that involves the injection of a contrast medium into the veins of the leg to assess the location and extent of thrombophlebitis. This test may also show how well the thrombus is adhered to the vessel wall; this information can be helpful in determining both the likelihood of embolization of the thrombus and the direction of future treatment. Although invasive, expensive, and uncomfortable, ascending phlebography is considered the most accurate diagnostic tool for thrombophlebitis and is especially useful in clients in whom calf vein thrombosis is strongly suspected (Goldstone, 1994; Tierney et al., 1995). In a small percentage of clients (less than 5%), performance of the test may create or aggravate a thrombotic condition.

- *Doppler ultrasound* devices deflect sound waves off the vessel wall to determine venous incompetence, obstruction, or occlusion. Hand-held Doppler devices are most effective when used on the larger veins of the lower extremities. This is a simple, noninvasive way to screen clients with suspected venous thrombosis or to determine the extension of existing vein thrombosis.

- *Plethysmography* is a noninvasive diagnostic test used to measure changes in the volume of fluid passing through a vessel, in this case the veins. It is easy to perform and is often used in conjunction with Doppler ultrasonography. Plethysmography is most valuable in the diagnosis of thromboses of the larger or more superficial veins because changes in the flow of blood through these vessels are more easily detected.

- *Radioactive fibrinogen* studies and *venous pressure* measurement tests, although not commonly performed, may be necessary for some clients.

Conservative Therapy

The conservative plan of care for clients with superficial venous thrombosis focuses on the relief of symptoms and the reversal of the inflammatory process. The application of warm, moist compresses over the affected area and the use of anti-inflammatory agents are usually sufficient to give most clients relief. Some clients may require antibiotic therapy either as a therapeutic or a prophylactic measure. Clients who experience a rapid progression or extension of superficial venous thrombophlebitis may be placed on anticoagulants (Berkow & Fletcher, 1992).

Clients with deep vein thromboses usually follow a more rigorous plan of care. Anticoagulation therapy is initiated, and clients are placed on strict bed rest until the symptoms of tenderness and edema resolve. Clients with thrombosis of the calf usually require between 5 and 7 days of bed rest, whereas clients with occlusions of the femoral or popliteal veins may require 10 to 14 days of bed rest.

The client's legs should be elevated, with the knees slightly flexed, above the level of the heart to promote venous return and discourage venous pooling. Elastic antiembolism stockings (TEDS) or pneumatic compression devices are also frequently ordered to stimulate the muscle-pumping mechanism that promotes the return of blood to the heart. When permitted, clients begin taking short walks on the unit, being careful to avoid periods of standing or sitting that may contribute to venous stasis. As the client's condition improves, gradual increases in daily ambulation are encouraged.

Whenever possible, prevention is key. Pneumatic stockings may be ordered as a preventive measure for postoperative clients who must remain immobile for long periods or for clients who cannot tolerate anticoagulants. Clients on bed rest should do leg exercises and begin to ambulate as soon as possible to minimize the effects of the prolonged stasis of venous blood. Clients should be taught not to cross their legs, to wear loose-fitting garments on their legs, and to incorporate exercise into their daily schedule (Tierney et al., 1995).

Pharmacology

The four categories of medications used most commonly in the treatment of clients with thrombophlebitis are anti-inflammatory agents, anticoagulants, thrombolytics, and antibiotics. The medication plan is tailored to each client's individual needs, and not every client requires the use of all categories of medication. Anti-inflammatory therapy is most useful in clients with superficial thrombophlebitis. Clients with deep vein thrombophlebitis usually require some type of anticoagulation therapy. Antibiotic therapy may be used either as a prophylactic or a therapeutic measure in clients whose inflammatory response is caused by infection. In addition, recent studies of clients with deep vein thrombophlebitis indicate that the concurrent use of thrombolytic agents and anticoagulation therapy help dissolve existing thrombi while simultaneously preventing the development of new thrombi (Berkow & Fletcher, 1992). Clients who require analgesics should avoid the use of aspirin or other agents that interrupt platelet aggregation because they may intensify the effects of anticoagulants.

Anti-inflammatory Agents   Nonsteroidal anti-inflammatory agents such as indomethacin [Indocin] or naproxen [Naprosyn] are used to interrupt the inflammatory process occurring in the veins. When used in conjunction with warm, moist compresses, these agents bring symptomatic relief to most clients with superficial venous thrombophlebitis (Berkow & Fletcher, 1992).

Anticoagulants   Clients with deep vein thromboses are most commonly placed on continuous intravenous anticoagulation therapy (heparin sodium) as soon as contraindications to its use are ruled out. For example, clients who have had neurosurgery and extensive orthopedic surgery are usually ineligible to receive anticoagulants because of the risk of hemorrhage. The heparin solution should be administered using an infusion pump, and the accuracy of the delivered dose should be checked every hour.

The dosage is calculated daily on the basis of the results of the activated partial thromboplastin time (APTT). A desirable dosage is achieved when the activated partial thromboplastin time (APTT) is 1.5 to 2 times the normal APTT value. If the client's APTT is less than twice the control, the heparin dosage is usually increased. If the APTT is more than twice the control, the heparin dosage is decreased. Following 7 to 14 days of heparinization, clients are gradually switched to an oral anticoagulant, usually warfarin. During this process, the administration of heparin and warfarin overlaps. As the amount of heparin being given decreases, the amount of warfarin increases, making careful assessment of laboratory results imperative. Effective anticoagulation with warfarin requires the client's prothrombin time to exceed the normal value by 1.5 to 2.5 times (Berkow & Fletcher, 1992).

Once this level is achieved, the intravenous administration of heparin may be discontinued and a maintenance dose of warfarin is established to keep the prothrombin times sufficiently increased to prevent future thrombosis. Regular follow-up is necessary to be sure prothrombin times remain within the desirable range for anticoagulation. Most clients with a single occurrence of phlebitis remain on oral anticoagulation therapy for 2 to 4 months, whereas clients who experience complications (e.g., pulmonary embolism) often require 6 months or more of oral anticoagulation therapy.

Heparin may also be administered subcutaneously and has been found to be equally effective for treating venous thombosis as intravenously administered heparin. If heparin is administered subcutaneously, expensive daily monitoring of the APTT is not required. As a result, outpatient treatment may be possible, depending on the extent of the illness. Although subcutaneous heparin injections are more expensive than heparin infusions, the costs balance out because fewer blood tests are needed, and outpatient care is an option (Abrams, 1995; Tierney et al., 1995).

Thrombolytics   Thrombolytic agents dissolve blood clots in the body by imitating natural enzymatic processes. Examples of thrombolytic medications are streptokinase (Streptase), urokinase (Abbokinase), alteplase (Activase), and anistreplase (Eminase). The use of thrombolytic agents has been shown to destroy venous thrombi that are less than 72 hours old more rapidly and efficiently than heparin therapy while also preventing additional damage to venous valves. However, the side effect of hemorrhage is more common with thrombolytics than with conventional heparinization.

Over the past several years, the simultaneous use of traditional anticoagulant therapy and thrombolytics has received much attention because of the favorable outcomes it has produced. Research studies continue in an effort to determine whether the theoretical advantages of thrombolytics will be consistently proven in the clinical arena (Abrams, 1995; Goldstone, 1994).

Antibiotics   The use of antibiotic therapy in the treatment of thrombophlebitis is limited to the specific treatment of identified infections. Some clients with superficial vein thrombophlebitis develop bacteremia, often

caused by *Staphylococcus*. If blood cultures prove to be positive, antibiotic therapy must be started to prevent the development of systemic sepsis. For most clients, 7 to 10 days of antibiotic therapy eradicates the problem, but clients with complications (such as endocarditis) must often continue antibiotics for 4 to 6 weeks (Berkow & Fletcher, 1992; Tierney et al., 1995).

Surgery

Most clients with thrombophlebitis are effectively treated with conservative and pharmacologic measures. However, in a small segment of the population, surgery is necessary either to remove the thrombus or to control the potential spread of thrombi throughout the system. A venous thrombectomy with insertion of a vena cava filter may be performed for this group.

Venous thrombectomy is performed when thrombi have lodged in the femoral vein and excision of the clots is required to prevent pulmonary embolism or to prevent gangrene. Successful removal of the thrombi improves the venous circulation rapidly, but the longevity of this effect is variable. Despite the fact that thrombectomy has proved successful for clients who initiate therapy within 24 hours after the onset of symptoms, about 66% of the clients who undergo venous thrombectomy suffer a recurrence of the occlusion, making the long-term value of the operation questionable (Goldstone, 1994).

Some clients who suffer from venous thrombosis are not eligible for anticoagulation therapy yet are at considerable risk of developing potentially fatal pulmonary emboli. For many years, permanent surgical interruption of the blood flow through the inferior vena cava was the only option to prevent recurrence of pulmonary emboli in this client group. Recent advances in surgical techniques now permit the insertion of filtering devices into the inferior vena cava via the femoral or jugular vein. These devices are designed to capture venous thrombi while maintaining adequate vena caval flow and patency (Figure 30–4). The most commonly used device is the Greenfield filter because it is associated with a 97% success rate in preventing the recurrence of pulmonary emboli and maintains vena caval flow and patency. The major advantages of the newer surgery over the ligation of the vena cava is the significantly reduced incidence of postoperative complications and the preservation of blood flow and patency of the inferior vena cava (Goldstone, 1994).

Nursing Care

Nursing care for the client with thrombophlebitis addresses the client's responses to the illness, primarily in the areas of pain management, clarification about the disease process and medication therapy, and education about interventions required to reduce inflammation and prevent complications. Knowledge about the causes of

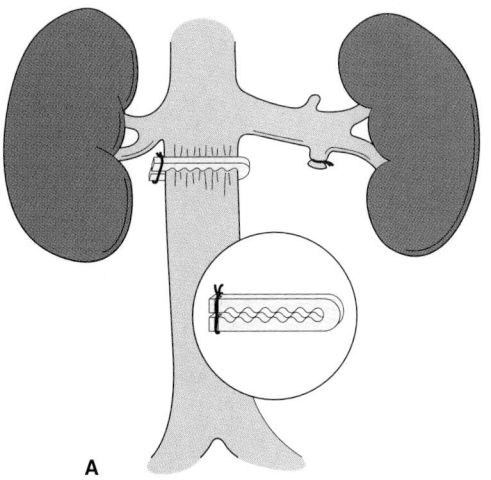
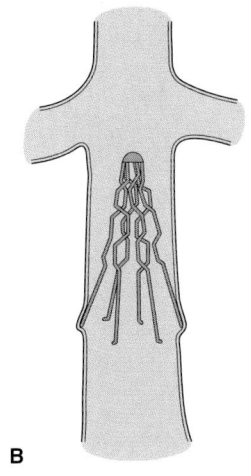
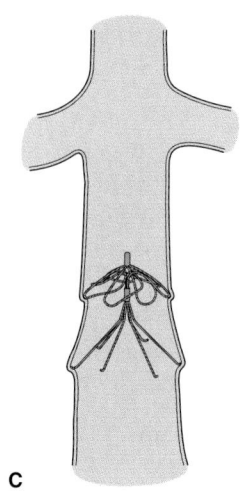

Figure 30–4   Surgical devices used to trap large pulmonary emboli. *A,* Miles serrated caval clip placed distal to renal veins. *B,* Greenfield filter. *C,* Nitinol filter.

venous thrombosis should be provided, even for clients who have not yet developed a problem. Prevention is an important strategy, especially for the categories of most susceptible clients. Every effort should be made to implement interventions that will ensure adequate venous return to the heart in all hospitalized clients. The nursing diagnoses discussed in this section are *Pain, Altered Peripheral Tissue Perfusion, Impaired Physical Mobility* and *Risk for Impaired Skin Integrity.*

Pain

Unlike the pain of clients with arterial occlusive disorders, the pain experienced by these clients is not induced by exercise or relieved by gravity. Instead, the pain is the result of the inflammation of the vein caused by the thrombotic process. Nursing care incorporates measures to reduce vessel inflammation with the goal of reducing the client's pain.

Nursing interventions with rationales follow:

- Assess the client's level of pain on a regular basis, using a scale of 0 to 10 (0 = no pain; 10 = severe pain). *The inflammatory process causes swelling and pain in the affected extremity. Ongoing assessments provide information about the effectiveness of pharmacologic and conservative therapies designed to minimize inflammation and reduce pain. Increased pain may indicate worsening or extension of the problem and should be reported at once.*

- Measure the diameter of the calf and thigh of the affected extremity on admission and daily thereafter. Report increases promptly. *As the inflammatory process increases in the vessel, the body compensates by bringing reserve fluids to the area, causing edema of the affected ex-*

tremity. Measurement upon admission and daily provides a baseline for determining the efficacy of ordered therapies.

- Apply warm, moist heat to affected extremity at least four times daily, using warm, moist compresses or an aqua-K pad. *The application of warm, moist compresses or the use of an aqua-K pad dilates the vessels and promotes the removal of excess fluids via the arterial and venous circulation. The dilation of the vessels improves circulation and reduces the resistance to blood flow from within the vein, thereby reducing pain. As the edema subsides, so does the compression of veins by surrounding tissues, thereby reducing pain.*

- Maintain bed rest and teach the client the rationale for it. *Because the goal of care is to reduce inflammation and pain, ambulatory activities should be restricted. The use of the leg muscles during walking exacerbates the inflammatory process. The body tries to protect the inflamed vein by producing extra fluids. The resulting edema increases venous compression and pain. Despite activity restrictions, care must be taken to maintain adequate circulation and prevent the complications associated with prolonged bed rest, such as venous stasis, pressure sores, constipation, and boredom.*

Altered Peripheral Tissue Perfusion

As thrombi develop, they decrease the size of the venous lumen and obstruct blood flow. In addition, the thrombus formation triggers an inflammatory response and resultant compensatory mechanisms such as swelling and pain. These combined factors have a significant effect on blood flow and tissue perfusion.

Nursing interventions with rationales follow:

- Assess peripheral pulses, skin integrity, capillary refill times, and color of the extremities at least once each shift. Report changes promptly. *Assessment of the circulatory status of both extremities allows the nurse to compare findings between the affected and unaffected limbs. Adverse changes in pulses, skin integrity, capillary refill, or color of the affected extremity can signal worsening of the condition and possible complications.*

- Elevate extremities at all times, keeping knees slightly flexed and legs above the level of the heart. *Elevation of the extremities promotes venous return and reduces peripheral edema. The knees should be kept slightly flexed to prevent contractures and to encourage muscle relaxation.*

- Maintain use of ordered antiembolic stockings, removing them for short periods (30 to 60 minutes) during daily hygiene. *Antiembolic stockings (also known as compression stockings or TEDS) exert a continuous, even pressure on the extremity and promote the return of venous blood to the heart. Promoting venous return is especially important for clients who are required to maintain bed rest as part of their therapeutic plan. As the inflammatory process resolves, edema subsides, and the client may be allowed to ambulate for short periods before discharge. Clients should be instructed in the correct application of antiembolism stockings and to continue their use as prescribed by the physician, even after discharge.*

- Administer and monitor the effectiveness of analgesics, anticoagulants, thrombolytics, and antibiotics. *The effectiveness of the pharmacologic plan of care can be monitored by evaluating its effect. Laboratory values (such as APTT or PTT) should be checked daily before the administration of anticoagulants or (for continuous intravenous medication) at the beginning of the shift to ensure correct dosages are delivered. Abnormal laboratory results should be reported to the physician promptly so that dosages may be adjusted in a timely manner.*

- Encourage position changes every 2 hours while the client is awake. *The edema accompanying venous congestion and inflammation promotes the development of chronic venous insufficiency. Position changes not only reduce edema but also promote joint movement and prevent skin breakdown.*

Impaired Physical Mobility

The client with venous thrombi requires prolonged bed rest. Unfortunately, bed rest is associated with many problems, including constipation, joint stiffening, muscle atrophy, and boredom. The goals of nursing care include maintaining the range of motion of joints, minimizing muscle atrophy, and reducing boredom.

Nursing intervention with rationales follow:

- Encourage active or perform passive range-of-motion exercises at least once each shift. *One of the effects of prolonged immobility is joint stiffening and, if no action is taken, eventual contractures. Range-of-motion exercises promote joint flexibility, preserve joint function, and prevent contractures. This intervention is especially important when medically imposed limitations affect usual daily activities.*

- Encourage client to turn, cough, and breathe deeply at least four times during each shift while awake. *Prolonged immobility can lead to stagnation of respiratory secretions and the development of respiratory complications, such as atelectasis or pneumonia. Turning, coughing, and deep breathing facilitate the expulsion of secretions from the respiratory tract and enhance the oxygenation of blood by promoting effective alveolar gas exchange.*

- Encourage the client to increase intake of fluids and dietary fiber. *Extended bed rest often causes constipation as a consequence of insufficient exercise and decreased gastrointestinal motility. Increasing fluid intake and fiber consumption lessens the constipating effects of bed rest.*

- Provide progressive ambulation within ordered guidelines. *In collaboration with the physical therapy department, the nurse should encourage daily increases in ambulation, which improves circulation and increases stamina and endurance.*

Risk for Impaired Skin Integrity

The impaired peripheral circulation of clients with thrombophlebitis deprives tissues of nutrients and oxygen. The most distal portions of the leg and foot are at highest risk because blood pools in this area. In addition, the poor muscle-pumping action of the edematous tissues and the presence of damaged venous valves impede flow of venous blood back to the heart. As a result, the tissues of the lower leg and foot of the affected extremity are susceptible to infection and ulceration.

Nursing interventions with rationales follow:

- Assess the skin of the affected lower leg and foot at least once every shift and more often if adverse changes occur. *The initial assessment and subsequent daily assessments of the skin help the nurse determine the presence of injuries or breakdown. Daily assessment allows early intervention to minimize the effects of skin breakdown. Clients should be taught the importance of daily skin and foot assessment both while hospitalized and following discharge.*

- Use mild soaps, solutions, and lotions to clean the affected leg and foot daily. *The importance of daily hygiene cannot be overemphasized, especially if an inflammatory process is already underway. Small cracks in the skin or around nail beds permit the entrance of bacteria or other microorganisms. If not swiftly controlled, infections can lead to the development of ulcerations and venous gangrene. Caustic or harsh soaps or solutions can dry and crack the skin, allowing additional opportunities for infec-*

tion. Daily washing with mild soaps or solutions minimizes the presence of potentially harmful microorganisms. Lotions that do not contain alcohol or perfume should also be carefully applied daily to moisten the skin and prevent cracking. Be certain to teach clients to avoid brisk massage during washing or during the application of lotions.

- Use egg crate mattresses or sheepskin on the bed as needed. *The inflammatory process and the presence of edema in clients with thrombophlebitis cause pain in the affected extremity. The swollen tissues exert pressure on areas of the leg and foot, especially bony prominences in direct contact with the surface of the bed. Egg crate mattresses and sheepskin distribute the weight of the leg more equally and prevent skin breakdown and discomfort.*

Other Nursing Diagnoses

The following nursing diagnoses are also applicable to clients with thrombophlebitis:

- *Activity Intolerance* related to diminished stamina and endurance secondary to prolonged bed rest

- *Diversional Activity Deficit* related to lack of environmental stimulation secondary to medically imposed bed rest

- *Ineffective Individual Coping* related to hospitalization and mandated activity restrictions

- *Anxiety* related to unexpected hospitalization and related concerns

Client and Family Teaching

Teaching clients and their families with thrombophlebitis centers on adherence to prescribed collaborative therapy and prevention of complications, especially future thrombotic episodes. A thorough explanation of the disease process should be given and repeated as necessary. Provide information about the course of treatment, including descriptions of laboratory tests and their purposes, medications being administered (including side effects that should be reported), the rationale for heat application, required bed rest and activity restrictions, measures to prevent future episodes of illness, and the importance of follow-up visits. Because clients may be surprised by the need for hospitalization, take time to talk with clients about the anxieties that may accompany this interruption in everyday life.

Clients requiring surgical intervention should be thoroughly informed before surgery about the nature and extent of surgery, the risks involved, the prognosis for improvement, and their role in the recovery and prevention of future bouts of illness. Explicit information should be given regarding the use of anticoagulants and thrombolytics. Effective client and family teaching reduces anxiety and promotes adherence to the plan of care.

Applying the Nursing Process

Case Study of a Client with Deep Vein Thrombosis: Opal Hipps

Mrs. Opal Hipps is a 75-year-old, widowed mother of six who lives alone with her dog, Chester, in her three-bedroom house in the suburbs. She retired from her job as a postal clerk 10 years ago and finds herself spending a lot of time sitting around home reading and watching television. Over the past week she has noticed that she is unable to walk as well because of a vague aching pain in her right leg. She has ignored the pain, thinking it was probably just another sign of old age, but last night she noticed a much more severe pain in her right calf. When she looked at her right lower leg, it seemed larger than the other leg. As she rubbed some lotion on her leg at bedtime, she noticed it was becoming very tender to the touch. After seeing her physician and undergoing Doppler ultrasound studies, Mrs. Hipps is admitted to the hospital with confirmed diagnosis of deep vein thrombosis in the right leg. She is placed on bed rest, and a continuous intravenous heparin solution is to be started using an infusion pump. Michael Cookson is the nurse assigned to admit and care for Mrs. Hipps.

Assessment

While reviewing the medical history, Mr. Cookson notices that Mrs. Hipps was admitted 14 months ago for repair of a fractured femur. Mrs. Hipps tells Mr. Cookson that she is not really afraid of being in the hospital but says, "That business about the blood clot really has me worried." She also tells Mr. Cookson that she is worried about who will take care of her dog while she is in the hospital, since all her children are grown and live out of town. Physical findings include: height, 5'2" (157 cm); weight, 149 lb (68 kg); T, 99.2 F (37.3 C); vital signs within normal limits otherwise. The skin on her left leg is warm, pink, and supple and has good turgor. The skin on her right calf is warm, reddish in color, and dry. The right calf is painful to palpation. The femoral and popliteal pulses are strong bilaterally, but the right pedal and posterior tibial pulses are difficult to locate, and the diameter of the right calf is 0.5 inch (1.27 cm) larger than that of the left.

Diagnosis

Mr. Cookson makes the following nursing diagnosis for Mrs. Hipps:

- *Pain* related to interruption of venous blood flow and inflammation in the right leg

- *Anxiety* related to unexpected hospitalization and uncertainty about the seriousness of her illness

- *Altered Peripheral Tissue Perfusion* related to decreased venous circulation in the right leg

- *Risk for Constipation* related to prolonged immobility
- *Risk for Impaired Skin Integrity* related to pooling of venous blood in the right leg

Expected Outcomes

The expected outcomes of the plan of care are that Mrs. Hipps will

- State that the pain in her right leg is relieved by the day of discharge.
- Verbalize reduced anxiety by the second day of her hospitalization.
- Have a reduction in the diameter of the right leg by 0.25 inch (0.64 cm) by the fifth day of hospitalization
- Have a soft, formed stool at least every 2 days during her hospitalization
- Show no signs of skin breakdown in the right foot throughout the hospital stay

Planning and Implementation

The following interventions are planned and implemented for Mrs. Hipps:

- Elevate her legs, with knees slightly flexed, throughout the hospital stay.
- Apply warm, moist compresses to her right leg (using a 2-hour-on, 2-hour-off schedule) around the clock.
- Administer ordered analgesics and evaluate their effectiveness each shift.
- Provide time to sit and talk with Mrs. Hipps about her understanding of her illness and the need for hospitalization.
- Arrange for assistance from a friend or neighbor in caring for Mrs. Hipps's dog.
- Apply antiembolism stockings and remove for 30 minutes each shift.
- Monitor effectiveness of anticoagulation therapy; check APTT values daily when heparin is used and PTT values daily during oral administration of warfarin.
- Encourage Mrs. Hipps to drink more fluids and incorporate more grains, cereals, fruits, and vegetables in her diet.
- Assist with progressive ambulation when approved by the physician.
- Inspect and compare bilateral skin assessment findings each shift.

Evaluation

Ten days after Mrs. Hipps was admitted, the pain in her right leg has subsided and the diameter of her right calf is equal to that of her left calf. Mrs. Hipps admits to Mr. Cookson that her fears really have to do with a cousin who had once been hospitalized for something similar and had his leg amputated. After talking about her condition and the steps she can take to prevent its recurrence, she is much less anxious. Before she is discharged, Mr. Cookson reviews the discharge instructions regarding the antiembolism stockings, daily walking plan, daily warfarin schedule, and scheduled follow-up appointment. Her neighbor, Kate, came to pick her up, and as Mr. Cookson was helping Mrs. Hipps into the car he saw Kate hand Mrs. Hipps a small brown dog and heard Kate say, "I brought Chester because I knew you'd be worried about him. I took good care of him for you, but he's missed you, too." Mrs. Hipps smiled, hugged Chester, and said she would call the number Mr. Cookson had given her if she had any questions.

Critical Thinking in the Nursing Process

1. Describe the pathophysiologic reasons for the pain in Mrs. Hipps's right leg.
2. What would be your response to Mrs. Hipps if she tells you she does not have the money to buy the prescribed anticoagulant when she goes home?
3. How would you change your teaching plan if Mrs. Hipps lived alone and had difficulty caring for herself?
4. Design a plan of care for Mrs. Hipps for the diagnosis: *Activity Intolerance.*

The Client with Chronic Venous Insufficiency

■ ■ ■

Chronic venous insufficiency is a disorder involving the stasis of blood in the lower extremities as a result of obstruction and reflux of venous valves. It is characterized by lower leg edema and dermatologic changes of the lower leg and foot caused by the prolonged interruption in venous circulation to the area.

Chronic venous insufficiency is often associated with changes in venous circulation that result from thrombophlebitis and valvular incompetence. In addition, the preexistence or coexistence of varicose veins, or the presence of abnormal, tumorous obstruction of the pelvic veins can often be found in clients with chronic venous insufficiency (Tierney et al., 1995).

Pathophysiology

When the incompetence of the venous valves is profound, the muscle-pumping action produced during activity is insufficient to propel blood back to the heart, so blood collects and stagnates in the lower leg. The increased collection of blood in the lower leg is reflected by

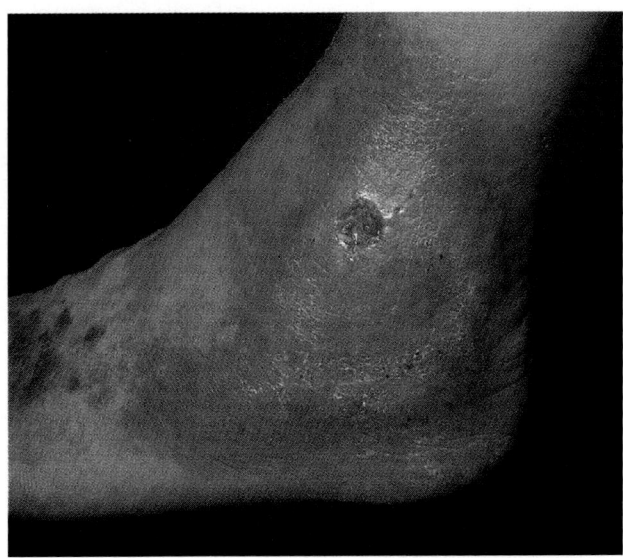

Figure 30–5   Chronic venous insufficiency. Note the discoloration of the ankle and the stasis ulcer.

Clinical Manifestations of Chronic Venous Insufficiency

- Lower leg edema
- Discoloration of the skin of the lower leg and foot
- Hardness of subcutaneous tissues
- Stasis ulcers over the ankle, most often medial

venous pressures in the client's calf that are substantially elevated during ambulation. The increased pressure distends the thin-walled veins, and valves are unable to close completely. This allows the backflow (reflux) of blood in the veins.

Clinical manifestations of chronic venous insufficiency include lower leg edema, discoloration of the skin of the lower leg and foot, fibrosis of subcutaneous tissues, and the eventual development of recurrent stasis ulcers of the lower leg and foot that heal poorly (Figure 30–5) (Porth, 1994). In some clients, the edema of the lower leg becomes so profound that it progresses upward to the knee in the affected extremity. See the accompanying manifestations box.

As the congestion of blood in the lower limb worsens and the peripheral venous circulation continues to slow down, the body's ability to provide sufficient oxygen and nutrients to the cells rapidly diminishes. Eventually, there is so little oxygen and nutrients that cells begin to die, causing the formation of venous *stasis ulcers*. In an attempt to heal the stasis ulcer, the body increases the supply of oxygen, nutrients, and metabolic energy to the diseased area. However, because the venous circulation is impaired by congested tissues, the extra oxygen and nutrients do not reach the diseased tissues. As a result, the condition worsens and, over time, the ulcers enlarge. The congested venous circulation also prevents the blood from delivering naturally occurring biochemicals from the immune system to the diseased tissues, thereby interfering with the normal inflammatory responses of the body and predisposing the client to wound infection (McCance & Huether, 1993).

In most clients, areas around the stasis ulcers appear shiny, atrophic, and cyanotic, and there is a brownish pigmentation to the skin. Some clients also present with other dermatologic changes such as eczema or stasis dermatitis. Scar tissue commonly forms over a fibrous base, causing the affected area of the leg to feel hard and somewhat leathery to the touch, but even the slightest trauma to the area can produce serious tissue breakdown (Tierney et al., 1995).

Collaborative Care

The collaborative care of the client with venous insufficiency centers on relieving symptoms, promoting adequate venous circulation, and preventing the development or extension of tissue injury. Conservative and pharmacologic treatment is instituted to meet these goals.

Laboratory and Diagnostic Tests

Diagnosis of venous insufficiency is most commonly made based on clinical findings, including interview data, family history, past medical history, and physical examination. Because a history of acute thrombophlebitis is often found in clients with varicosities or chronic venous insufficiency, a thorough examination of the client's past medical history and careful questioning of the client regarding any occurrences of thrombophlebitis is important. There are no specific laboratory or diagnostic tests that provide definite diagnosis of chronic venous insufficiency.

Conservative Therapy

Conservative management of venous insufficiency focuses on reducing edema and treating ulcerations. Bed rest, with the legs and feet elevated above heart level, is a fundamental component of care. Clients are advised to avoid long periods of standing and to wear elastic supports from the ankle to the knee while awake if edema is present.

Pharmacology

Medications administered to clients with chronic venous insufficiency include topical agents to treat the client's dermatologic conditions, such as infection, eczema, or tissue inflammation. Systemic antibiotics are organism-specific and are used only if there is evidence of systemic infection.

If stasis dermatitis has developed, the wound is classified as either acute or subsiding/chronic. Treatments of acute weeping dermatitis include wet compresses with boric acid, Burow's solution, or isotonic saline four times daily, for 1-hour intervals. Following the wet compress, topical ointments (such as 0.5% hydrocortisone cream) are applied. If the stasis dermatitis is subsiding or is chronic, the client may continue use of the hydrocortisone cream until no further improvement is noted. Other treatments include the topical application of zinc oxide ointment (3%), or broad-spectrum antifungal agents such as clotrimazole (Lotrimin) cream (1%) or miconazole (Monistat) cream (2%) (Tierney et al., 1995). Clients who have already developed ulcerations are usually treated with saline compresses to promote healing the wound or to help prepare the site for a skin graft. Once the ulcer is healed, the client must wear a heavy elastic stocking to promote adequate venous return and to prevent the recurrence of ulceration.

Other Therapies

The ulcer may be treated by using a semirigid boot applied to the foot and lower leg. This device may be made of Unna's paste or Gauzetex bandage. Bony prominences must be well padded. The boot must be changed every 1 to 2 weeks, depending on the amount of drainage from the ulcer. This device often allows ambulatory treatment.

A very large, chronic ulcer may require surgery. In this case, all of the incompetent veins are ligated, the ulcer is excised, and the area is covered with a skin graft (see Chapter 17).

Nursing Care

Nursing care for the client with chronic venous insufficiency is primarily educative and supportive. Client teaching includes the following recommendations:

- Elevate the legs while resting and during sleep.
- Walk as much as possible, but avoid sitting or standing for long periods of time.
- When sitting, do not cross your legs or sit so that you put pressure on the back of the knees (such as sitting on the side of the bed).
- Do not wear anything that pinches your legs (such as knee-high hose, garters, or girdles).
- Wear elastic hose as prescribed. The elastic hose should be tighter over the feet than they are at the top of the leg. Be sure the tops of the elastic hose do not cut into your legs. Put on the hose after you have had your legs elevated.
- Keep the skin on your feet and legs clean, soft, and dry.
- Follow guidelines for care of the legs and feet (on page 1207).

The following nursing diagnoses may apply to the client with chronic venous insufficiency:

- *Anxiety* related to inability to control chronic disease
- *Body Image Disturbance* related to edema and stasis ulcers on lower leg
- *Risk for Infection* related to ulcerations
- *Impaired Physical Mobility* related to pain and edema in lower legs
- *Impaired Skin Integrity* related to presence of stasis ulcers

The Client with Varicose Veins

■ ■ ■

Varicose veins are irregular, tortuous veins with incompetent valves. Varicosities may develop in veins anywhere in the body (and may be called by other names, such as hemorrhoids in the rectum and varices in the esophagus), but they occur most commonly in the lower extremities. The leg vein most often affected by varicosities is the long saphenous vein, but the short saphenous vein may also be affected (Figure 30–6). Varicose veins are a common disorder, occurring in one out of about every five people in the world. They are more common in women over the age of 35; there is often a familial tendency to develop them. Researchers have found that over 50% of all people over the age of 50 develop varicose veins, possibly owing to the decrease in regular exercise demonstrated by this group in tandem with other factors that contribute to venous stasis. Studies also suggest that the propensity for varicose veins to develop in women rather than in men may be related to the venous stasis that occurs during pregnancy. People who stand for long periods at work are also prone to develop varicose veins; this group includes waiters, beauticians, salespersons, and nurses.

Varicose veins are caused by one or more of the following: severe damage or trauma to a saphenous vein, prolonged venous distention, and the effects of gravity produced by long periods of standing. They may be primary (with no involvement of deep veins) or secondary (caused by the obstruction of deep veins).

Pathophysiology

The major factor leading to the formation of varicose veins is sustained stretching of the vascular wall because of long-standing increased intravenous pressure. As the

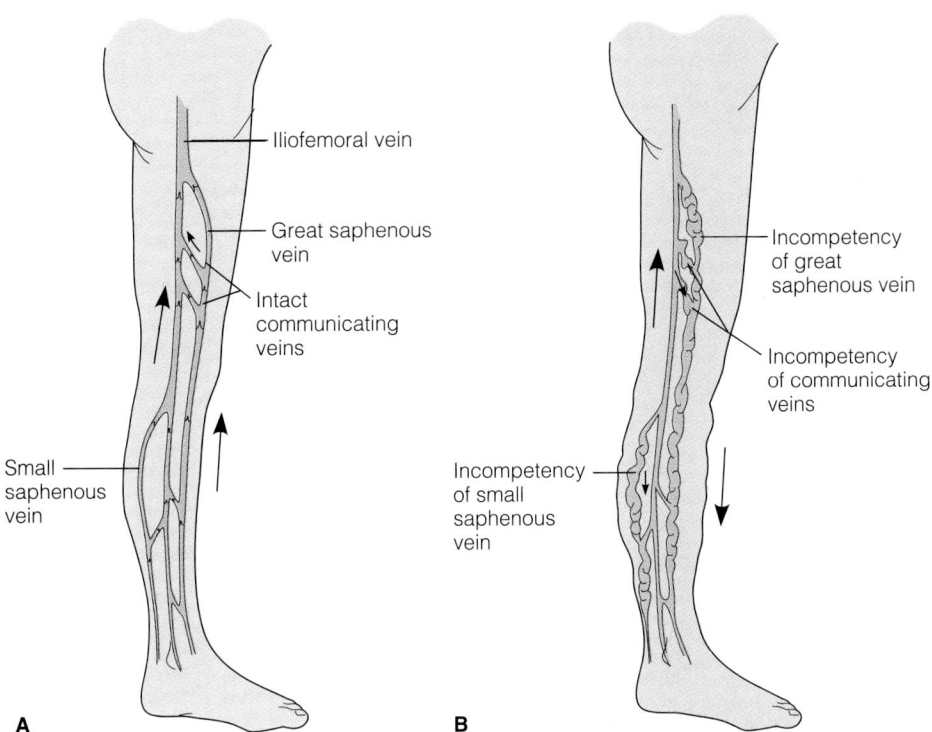

Figure 30-6 A comparison of *A,* normal venous structure and *B,* varicose veins resulting from incompetent valves.

Iliofemoral vein

Great saphenous vein

Intact communicating veins

Small saphenous vein

A

Incompetency of great saphenous vein

Incompetency of communicating veins

Incompetency of small saphenous vein

B

vessels stretch, the valves cannot close properly and become incompetent. The erect position produces a twofold negative effect on the veins. When the client is standing, the veins in the legs resemble vertical columns and must withstand the full force of venous blood pressure. Prolonged standing, the force of gravity, the lack of lower limb exercise, and incompetent venous valves all weaken the muscle-pumping mechanism, and the return of venous blood to the heart diminishes. As the person continues to stand for long periods of time, the amount of blood that collects in the veins increases, the vessel wall continues to stretch, and the valves within the veins become increasingly incompetent. Most varicosities occur in the deep veins of the legs and are caused by obesity, thrombophlebitis, congenital arteriovenous malformations, or sustained pressure on abdominal veins (as in pregnancy and/or the presence of abdominal tumors) (Porth, 1994).

Although some clients are asymptomatic, most complain of one or more of the following manifestations: severe aching leg pain, leg fatigue, leg heaviness, itching, or feelings of heat in the legs. The level of valvular incompetence does not seem to be correlated with the number or extent of symptoms, although the menstrual cycle tends to cause symptoms to worsen, suggesting possible correlations with hormonal variables in women. On assessment, there are obvious dilated veins beneath the skin of the upper and lower leg. If the varicose veins are long-standing, there may be thinning and brown discoloration of the skin above the ankles. See the accompanying manifestations box.

The complications of varicose veins include venous insufficiency and stasis ulcers. Chronic stasis dermatitis may also occur. In addition, thrombophlebitis may develop in the varicose veins, especially in pregnant or postpartal clients, postoperative clients, or clients taking oral contraceptives. The thrombophlebitis increases the risk of pulmonary embolism.

Collaborative Care

Management of varicose veins is by conservative care and by surgery. However, clients must know that surgery of one area does not prevent the development of varicosities in other veins.

Clinical Manifestations of Varicose Veins

- Severe, aching pain in the leg
- Leg fatigue
- Leg heaviness
- Itching over the affected leg (stasis dermatitis)
- Feelings of heat in the leg
- Visibly dilated veins
- Thin, discolored skin above the ankles
- Stasis ulcers

Laboratory and Diagnostic Tests

There are no specific laboratory tests used to diagnose varicose veins. The following diagnostic tests may be ordered:

- The tourniquet test assists in confirming the presence of varicose veins. While supine, the client raises the leg to empty the veins, and a tourniquet is applied to the upper thigh of the leg. The client is asked to stand and the tourniquet is released. The subsequent rate and extent of the blood flow provide valuable information regarding the location of the incompetent valves. This information can guide the treatment plan. The veins of the leg will distend rapidly if only the superficial veins are affected.

- The deeper veins are assessed in a different way. A tourniquet is applied to the leg while the client is standing and the veins are filling. If the distention of the superficial veins (which would naturally follow application of the tourniquet) does not disappear when the client is asked to walk, the deep vein valves are probably affected (Porth, 1994).

- *Doppler ultrasonic flow tests* and *angiographic studies* with instillation of contrast media may be done to confirm the presence of varicose veins or to determine the extent of involvement.

- *Plethysmography* may give valuable information about blood volume within a particular vessel or group of vessels. Such information may be very useful in designing a treatment plan specific to the client's needs.

Conservative Therapy

Although there is no real cure for varicose veins, several conservative measures may be taken to improve venous circulation and relieve the pressure on venous tissues. Properly fitted antiembolism (elastic) stockings are commonly prescribed and work to compress veins, thereby propelling blood back to the heart. They are intended to augment the muscle pumping action of the legs, and in clients with varicosities, they help diminish pain, feelings of leg heaviness, and leg fatigue.

A second important conservative intervention is walking. Clients are taught the importance of regular, daily walking and the adverse effects of sitting and standing. Clients are also taught the benefits of elevating their legs for specified periods of time throughout each day. Elevation of the legs promotes venous return, prevents venous stasis, and decreases leg heaviness and leg fatigue. The importance of these noninvasive therapies in managing the disorder cannot be overemphasized. They are the core of treatment for most clients with uncomplicated varicose veins (Goldstone, 1994; Tierney et al., 1995).

Pharmacology

No medications are customarily prescribed to treat varicose veins. Clients may be instructed by their primary health care providers to take mild, over-the-counter analgesics to relieve the pain or discomfort associated with varicose veins.

Surgery

Two surgical techniques are generally used in the treatment of varicose veins: *compression sclerotherapy* and *vein stripping*. Although surgery may alleviate the major symptoms of the disease, there is no real cure for varicose veins.

Compression Sclerotherapy The use of compression sclerotherapy in clients with primary varicose veins is becoming more common. This procedure involves the injection of an irritating agent into collapsed superficial veins. The irritating substances cause the vessel to harden, permanently closing off the lumen and causing blood to be re-routed through healthy vessels whose valves are not compromised (Porth, 1994). Sclerotherapy is often done for cosmetic reasons, but the physiologic benefits of fibrosing incompetent superficial veins cannot be ignored.

Vein Stripping Surgical intervention for the treatment of secondary varicose veins is usually necessary only in a small segment of the population. Surgical treatment includes the removal of the varicose veins and the ligation of branches of the varicose vein that are also incompetent, a procedure commonly known as vein stripping.

Clients with deep venous insufficiency often undergo surgery only if the severity of the disorder warrants immediate action or if conservative measures prove ineffective in relieving major symptoms of the disease. There are six primary reasons why surgical intervention may be undertaken, including (1) severe symptoms, (2) very large varicose veins, even if the client has no symptoms, (3) episodes of superficial phlebitis, (4) rupture of a varicose vein resulting in hemorrhage, (5) the development of ulcerations caused by venous stasis resulting from varicose veins, and (6) cosmetic reasons (Goldstone, 1994).

On the evening before surgery, the surgeon marks all incompetent superficial and perforating varicose veins with a permanent ink marker. Under either regional or general anesthesia, the greater saphenous vein is removed and the connected smaller tributaries that have not naturally clotted off are tied off. The surgeon may make several small incisions in the client's leg to ensure that the incompetent tributaries that communicate with larger vessels are sufficiently ligated. For clients with less extensive disease or clients seeking cosmetic improvement, surgery may involve only the removal of the lesser saphenous vein through an incision in the popliteal fossa (Goldstone, 1994).

Postoperative care includes the application of pressure bandages for a minimum of 6 weeks, elevation of the extremities to minimize postoperative edema, and gradually increasing amounts of ambulation. It is important to stress to the client and family that sitting and standing are forbidden during the recovery period. These activities are gradually reintroduced at appropriate times in the recuperative process (Goldstone, 1994).

Nursing Care

The nursing care of clients with varicose veins centers on restoring venous circulation, relieving symptoms, preventing complications, and promoting behaviors that minimize symptoms. Emphasis is placed on the importance of the nurse's role in health teaching to manage the symptoms of varicose veins, particularly because there is no cure for the disease. The nursing care of clients who have undergone surgery for the correction of varicose veins includes interventions related to assessing and promoting wound healing and preventing infection. This section focuses on the nursing diagnoses of *Pain, Altered Peripheral Tissue Perfusion, Risk for Impaired Skin Integrity,* and *Risk for Peripheral Neurovascular Dysfunction.*

Pain

The pain experienced by clients with varicose veins relates to the prolonged interruption in the return of venous blood to the heart and subsequent pooling of venous blood in the extremity. The client's pain is a result of the tissue deprivation of oxygen and nutrients because of excessive venous congestion in the lower limbs. In chronic venous insufficiency, cells begin to die (and ulcerations form) when tissues are deprived of necessary oxygen and nutrients over a protracted period of time.

Nursing interventions with rationales follow:

- Assess the client's pain. *Pain assessment helps the nurse design a plan of care that takes into account the times of day when the client experiences the most pain. Interventions may be organized to avoid times when pain levels are high, thereby encouraging the client to adhere to the plan of care and demonstrating the nurse's sensitivity to the client's input. Pain assessments also indicate if the condition is worsening and if treatment modalities are effective.*

- Teach and reinforce methods for relieving pain that do not involve the use of analgesic agents. *The benefit of relaxation, imagery, deep breathing, distraction, and other methods are well documented and encourage clients to take responsibility for their own pain. When used in concert with pharmacologic agents, these pain-relief measures give the client a variety of options for controlling pain, and foster independence.*

- Encourage the client to discuss possible relationships between episodes of pain and life stressors. *The effect of emotional and environmental factors on a person's level of pain is well established. Clients should be given the opportunity to discuss life stressors with the nurse and discover relationships between the exacerbation of pain and the occurrence of stressful life situations. As clients learn which* situations increase their pain, they may also recognize methods for controlling it.

- Collaborate with the client to establish a plan of pain control. *As clients learn about their options for controlling their own pain, they discover that they really are in charge of their own pain. As the nurse continues to work with the client to control the pain, a trusting relationship is formed that encourages open communication. The nurse's willingness to spend time with the client in developing this plan demonstrates the nurse's sensitivity to the client's situation and fosters mutual respect.*

- Regularly evaluate the effectiveness of interventions used to minimize pain. *Most clients are willing to adhere to a plan of care that will produce results, in this case, the relief of pain. By monitoring the effects of pain-relief interventions, the nurse is able to modify the plan of care as needed, communicate outcomes of interventions to the physician and other health team members, and nurture a sense of mutual respect with the client.*

Altered Peripheral Tissue Perfusion

In clients with varicose veins and venous stasis, tissues do not receive sufficient nutrients and oxygen because of an interruption in capillary blood supply due to incompetent venous valves. Venous blood accumulates in the distal portions of the lower extremities, and flow of venous blood back to the heart is impaired. The goal is to improve venous circulation in order to restore capillary blood flow and promote normal tissue nutrition and tissue respiration.

Nursing interventions with rationales follow:

- Assess peripheral pulses, capillary refill time, skin temperature, and degree of edema. *The survival of cells and tissues depends on adequate perfusion. Assessment of perfusion helps the nurse determine the level of cell survival and the projected extent of the disorder.*

- Teach the client to apply properly fitted supportive or antiembolic stockings and to remove stockings each day for 30 to 60 minutes. *Antiembolic stockings exert pressure on the veins of the lower extremities and thus promote the return of venous blood to the heart. If the client is ambulatory, the stockings enhance the blood-pumping action of the muscles. Because elastic stockings can inhibit the flow of blood through small superficial vessels, they should be removed at least once each day for no less than 30 minutes. At that time, the skin should be inspected and cleaned.*

- Teach the client to exercise the extremities at regular intervals. *Exercise stimulates circulation and promotes the normal flow of blood through the vascular system. Range-of-motion exercises should be carried out regularly in addition to Buerger-Allen exercises to promote venous return. Walking is excellent exercise and should be encouraged.*

- Teach the client how to position the legs to promote tissue perfusion. *For clients with venous disorders, af-*

fected extremities are elevated to reduce tissue congestion and to promote the return of venous blood to the heart. By promoting the return of venous blood to the heart, elevation of the extremities also increases renal perfusion, which in turn promotes elimination of excess fluids and decreases peripheral edema. Unless proscribed, the legs should be kept above the level of the heart during sleep.

Risk for Impaired Skin Integrity

The domino effect created by the improper delivery of oxygen and nutrients to the tissues of the lower extremities impairs the normal functioning of skin cells. Because blood is not circulating efficiently through the veins, the cellular needs of tissues are barely being met, and localized skin breakdown may occur. The stagnation of venous blood in the lower extremities may be compounded if bed rest is part of the client's treatment plan; these factors place the client at an even higher risk for skin breakdown.

Nursing interventions with rationales follow:

- Assess the skin on the lower extremities for warmth, erythema, moisture, and signs of breakdown as part of an initial examination. *Data obtained during inspection of the skin provide information about the adequacy of peripheral circulation and the effects of the disease on the skin. Assessment is especially important in clients who are experiencing an interruption in the normal flow of blood to the periphery and in clients who have already developed ulcerations because of poor peripheral circulation. Regular assessment of the skin helps the nurse detect problems early, avert episodes of breakdown, and establish a plan of skin care for clients with existing ulcerations.*

- Teach clients about daily skin hygiene. *The tissues of clients with peripheral vascular disorders are at increased risk of breakdown because blood flow is impaired. Washing the extremities not only removes potentially harmful microorganisms but also stimulates circulation. Vigorous rubbing should be avoided, and gentle soaps or bathing lotions should be used to keep the skin soft, moist, and supple. Prevention of skin breakdown should be emphasized in client teaching.*

- Teach the client to protect the extremities from external forces that may cause breakdown. *Shearing forces can contribute significantly to episodes of skin breakdown. Measures to avoid shearing forces include moving slowly in bed, avoiding the use of stiffly starched sheets and bedclothing, and using heel and elbow protectors. An egg crate mattress or similar device may be used to protect bony prominences from the effects of prolonged pressure. Changing position every hour while awake minimizes circulatory stasis.*

- Encourage adequate nutrition and fluid intake. *Healthy skin tissues cannot develop unless the necessary nutrients and fluids are present. Diets high in protein, carbohydrates,* and vitamins and minerals promote the growth and maintenance of normal skin cells, provide energy, and help prevent skin breakdown. Adequate hydration serves many purposes: it maintains proper fluid and electrolyte balance, promotes normal skin turgor, and prevents dehydration, which can lead to skin breakdown. When nutritional deficits are compounded by poor venous circulation, ulcerations may form and grow.*

Risk for Peripheral Neurovascular Dysfunction

The risk for impaired peripheral neurovascular functioning is high in clients with chronic venous insufficiency. Because varicose veins commonly precede the development of chronic venous insufficiency, clients with severe varicosities are also at greater risk for disruption in circulation or sensation in an extremity.

Nursing interventions with rationales follow:

- Assess circulation, sensation, and motion in the lower extremities. *Disruption in the flow of venous blood back to the heart creates congestion in the tissues of the lower extremities. If congestion is prolonged or extensive, it may interfere with sensory and motor function of the affected extremity. The potential for nerve and muscle involvement is especially high in clients with venous stasis ulcers. Whenever blood supply is altered, the resulting effects on tissues and other structures may warrant additional medical and nursing intervention.*

- Teach the client to avoid flexing the affected extremity and to maintain positions that promote effective neurovascular function. *Flexion of the extremities reduces venous circulation and increases the risk for adverse changes in neurovascular function. Clients with edema of the lower extremities should elevate the limb above the level of the heart (especially during sleep) to promote the return of venous blood to the heart and to discourage fluid retention.*

- Teach the client and family to report any signs of neurovascular dysfunction, such as numbness, coldness, pain, or tingling of an extremity. *Early recognition of the manifestations of neurovascular dysfunction facilitates rapid intervention to prevent complications. Clients who have undergone surgical repair of either varicose veins or chronic venous stasis ulcers must be carefully assessed for interruptions in neurovascular function and must be instructed to promptly report signs and symptoms of abnormalities to their physician. In clients who have not undergone surgery, careful daily assessment should be encouraged to avert the potential complications of skin breakdown, infection, and nerve damage.*

- Teach clients about the importance of maintaining safety and adhering to the plan of care. *Issues of safety should be reinforced with clients to prevent further injury to already compromised tissues. The correct technique for applying antiembolism stockings should be carefully taught to help clients avoid further impairment in peripheral circula-*

tion. Emphasis should also be placed on teaching clients how to prevent further injury by using safety precautions in daily living and by reporting signs or symptoms of impending complications. Failure to follow the plan of care may cause the client's condition to worsen and may lead to additional or extended hospitalization and more extensive treatment measures.

Other Nursing Diagnoses

These nursing diagnoses may also be appropriate for the client with varicose veins:

- *Risk for Infection* related to disruption in the continuity of the skin
- *Impaired Home Health Maintenance* related to prescribed postural limitations
- *Anxiety* related to possible need for surgery

Client and Family Teaching

Most clients with varicose veins provide self-care at home. Because of the chronic nature of varicose veins, the nurse must pay particular attention to client and family teaching. The nurse must assume the responsibility for ensuring that the client and family understand interventions that must be implemented daily. Because there is no cure for varicose veins, emphasis is placed on teaching clients how to adapt their daily living to accommodate the prescribed health regimen. For example, clients are taught the importance of including regular walks in their everyday schedule, the correct technique for applying antiembolism stockings, and the necessity of elevating their legs for specified periods of time throughout the day.

For some clients, incorporation of these interventions may not present a problem, but others need assistance to accomplish the desired outcome of client adherence. Above all, clients should be encouraged to ask questions, report abnormal findings to their physician, attend all follow-up visits, and take appropriate actions to prevent the development of complications.

Care of the Older Adult

Disorders of venous stasis are common after the fifth decade of life. As people age, they lose mobility and experience changes in other aspects of daily living.

An important part of the treatment plan for clients with varicose veins is increasing ambulation and avoiding prolonged periods of standing. Safety when walking is an important issue for older clients, and the nurse needs to assess stability and suggest the use of walkers and quadcanes as needed. In addition, clients holding jobs that require prolonged standing need to consider strategies for minimizing standing and for incorporating activity into the job. The goals are to foster acceptance of interventions

to prevent the condition from worsening and to avoid the onset of complications.

Clients recovering from surgery and clients with stasis ulcers requiring daily treatments may need additional assistance with home-based care. The nurse should initiate referral to the social service department prior to the client's discharge to make arrangements for necessary care and meals if the client is to return home. In some instances, temporary placement in extended care facilities is arranged until the client is sufficiently recovered to return home. In other cases, arrangements for visiting nurse services or home health aide services may be more conducive to the well-being of the client.

Applying the Nursing Process

Case Study of a Client with Varicose Veins: Olga Kacznik

Olga Kacznik is a 59-year-old mother of three children (ages 30, 26, and 19) who lives with her husband in a second-floor apartment in a small Southern town. Mrs. Kacznik is a full-time bank teller and has recently celebrated her tenth year with the bank. Prior to her employment by the bank, she was a cashier at a local supermarket. Over the past 8 years, Mrs. Kacznik has noticed an increased feeling of heaviness in her legs and a burning pain in her right leg. Her right foot becomes swollen by the middle of the day. She has visited her doctor in the past and was given an elastic stocking, which she was told to wear at all times, except during sleep. Because it is difficult to apply, she hasn't been wearing the stocking, nor has she increased her walking as the doctor prescribed. Mrs. Kacznik hadn't paid much attention to her symptoms until yesterday, when she took her shoe off to remove a pebble and noticed that her foot was very swollen and the veins on her right calf were dark blue and seemed to stick out.

After an appointment with her doctor, Mrs. Kacznik has outpatient Doppler flow studies and bilateral angiographic tests of her legs. Two days later, her doctor calls to tell her that she may need surgery to repair a large varicose vein in her right leg but that first he wants to try nonsurgical treatment. He schedules an appointment with a clinic specializing in the care of peripheral vascular problems in a nearby city. At the clinic, Scott Daniels, RN, CNS, takes the initial history, conducts the physical assessment, and develops a plan of care for Mrs. Kacznik.

Assessment

During the history, Mr. Daniels notes a maternal family history of varicose veins. The only time Mrs. Kacznik has been hospitalized in the past was for childbirth and two episodes of thrombophlebitis, one last year and one just 2 months ago. Mrs. Kacznik tells Mr. Daniels that her doctor had once told her to "wear some sort of elastic support stocking, but that made me look like an old woman, so I decided not to use it." When Mr. Daniels questions her about the episodes of thrombophlebitis, Mrs. Kacznik indicates that she was only in the hospital for a few days and that the pain she feels now is nothing like the pain she felt with the "clots in my leg."

Mrs. Kacznik is anxious but alert and oriented to her surroundings. Physical findings include: height: 5′6″ (168 cm); weight: 185 lb (84 kg); vital signs stable and within normal limits. Peripheral pulses are palpable with the exception of the dorsalis pedis and posterior tibial pulse on the right foot. Capillary refill time in Mrs. Kacznik's fingers is less than 3 seconds; in the left foot, 4 seconds; and unobtainable in the right foot. The right leg presents with 3+ pitting edema; the left leg, with only 1+ nonpitting edema. Both legs are warm to the touch, but the right leg feels slightly cooler than the left. On a scale of 1 to 10, Mrs. Kacznik rates the pain in her right leg as a 6.

Diagnosis

Mr. Daniels makes the following nursing diagnoses for Mrs. Kacznik:

- *Pain* related to insufficient tissue oxygenation and nutrition secondary to venous stasis
- *Altered Peripheral Tissue Perfusion* related to interruption of venous blood flow
- *Anxiety* related to uncertain outcome of conservative care and possible need for surgery
- *Altered Nutrition: More Than Body Requirements* related to excessive food consumption and insufficient energy expenditure

Expected Outcomes

The expected outcomes of the plan of care are that Mrs. Kacznik will

- Verbalize a decrease in the level of pain in her right leg within 1 week.
- Have less edema in her right leg within 1 week.
- Improve venous circulation in her right leg as manifested by decreased edema and decreased capillary refill time.
- State that her anxiety is reduced.
- Verbalize a willingness to join a weight-loss program.

Planning and Implementation

The following interventions are implemented for Mrs. Kacznik to meet the expected outcomes:

- Assess peripheral pulses, capillary refill time, level of edema, and skin temperature of lower extremities as a baseline and on each subsequent clinic visit.
- Ask Mrs. Kacznik to keep a log of her pain experiences, using a scale of 0 to 10 (0 = no pain; 10 = severe pain) and noting related activities.
- Discuss with Mrs. Kacznik the importance of elevating her legs above the level of the heart while sitting during the day and while asleep.
- Measure both legs for thigh-high antiembolism stockings; teach Mrs. Kacznik to apply stockings using inside-out toe-first application method and to remove the stockings for an hour each morning and evening. Have Mrs. Kacznik demonstrate her ability to put on these stockings.
- Provide time for Mrs. Kacznik to discuss her fears and concerns about her condition and the possibility of surgery.
- Discuss the relationship between stress, obesity, and varicose veins. Encourage questions.
- Provide information about reputable weight-loss programs such as Weight Watchers, Diet Workshop, and Overeaters Anonymous; encourage Mrs. Kacznik to visit such a program and decide if it would be helpful in a weight-loss program.

Evaluation

Mrs. Kacznik returns to the clinic the following week. Her capillary refill time in the right leg has not quite reached the 5-second mark, but it has decreased. The 3+ pitting edema in Mrs. Kacznik's right leg has decreased to 1+. Mrs. Kacznik has been applying her antiembolism stocking with little trouble and is able to verbalize the importance of elevating her legs for short intervals throughout the day as well as at night. Although Mrs. Kacznik has not yet decided whether to join a weight-loss program, she says her family is encouraging her to do so. An appointment is made for a return visit the following week.

Critical Thinking in the Nursing Process

1. Describe the major factors that contributed to the development of Mrs. Kacznik's varicose veins.

2. Although Mrs. Kacznik is supposed to stay home from work for at least 2 weeks, what if she tells you she must go to work? How would this information change your teaching?

3. How would you recommend a weight-loss program in such a way that the client does not feel belittled?

4. Design a plan of care for the nursing diagnosis *Chronic Pain.* Include noninvasive methods of pain management.

Table 30–4	A Comparison of Arterial and Venous Leg Ulcers	
Factor	**Arterial Ulcers**	**Venous Ulcers**
Location	Toes, feet, shin	Over inner ankle, sometimes over outer ankle
Ulcer appearance	Deep, pale	Superficial, pink
Skin appearance	Normal to atrophic Pallor on elevation Rubor on dependency	Brown discoloration Stasis dermatitis Cyanosis on dependency
Skin temperature	Cool	Normal
Edema	Absent to mild	Present to extreme
Pain	Usually severe Intermittent claudication Rest pain	Usually mild Aching pain
Gangrene	May occur	Does not occur
Pulses	Decreased or absent	Normal

The Client with Leg Ulcers

■ ■ ■

Ulcers of the lower extremity are the result of either chronic arterial insufficiency or chronic venous insufficiency. Although both of these conditions have been discussed in this chapter, this section compares the characteristics of leg ulcers. Table 30–4 summarizes the differences.

Regardless of the cause, the nursing care focus is to improve peripheral blood flow so that tissue integrity is maintained. Nursing diagnoses that are appropriate for the client with leg ulcers, regardless of cause, include:

- *Altered Peripheral Tissue Perfusion* related to decreased blood flow to the lower extremities
- *Impaired Skin Integrity* related to decreased blood flow
- *Risk for Infection* related to open ulcer on the foot or leg
- *Activity Intolerance* related to pain

■ ■ ■ Disorders of the Lymphatic System ■ ■ ■

The lymphatic system is a unique part of the vascular system and is generally responsible for returning fluids to the bloodstream from other tissues in the body. It has its own vessels (lymphatic veins and venules) and is a pumpless system with one-way valves that return fluids to the heart. Lymphatic fluid flow is maintained by contraction of lymph vessels, muscle contraction, respirations, and gravity. Interruptions in lymph flow result primarily in edema.

tion; this condition is rare. Obstruction of the lymph vessels from surgical removal of lymph nodes (as is done in a radical mastectomy), scarring of lymph nodes following radiation, or invasion of lymph nodes by tumor may cause *secondary lymphedema.*

Clients who live in or visit the tropics may develop secondary lymphedema following infestation of the lymphatic vessels by filaria, a nematode worm. This is a chronic condition, more commonly involving the lower extremities, called *elephantiasis.*

Pathophysiology

The obstruction of lymph drainage prevents protein molecules from returning to the circulation from the interstitial fluid. The protein molecules accumulate in the interstitial spaces, increasing interstitial osmotic pressure so that fluid accumulates in the soft tissues of the arms or legs.

The Client with Lymphedema

■ ■ ■

Lymphedema is a primary or secondary disorder that results from inflammation, obstruction, or removal of lymphatic vessels. It is characterized by edema of the extremities from an accumulation of lymph. Most cases of primary lymphedema (also called *lymphedema praecox*) begin in adolescent females after the onset of menstrua-

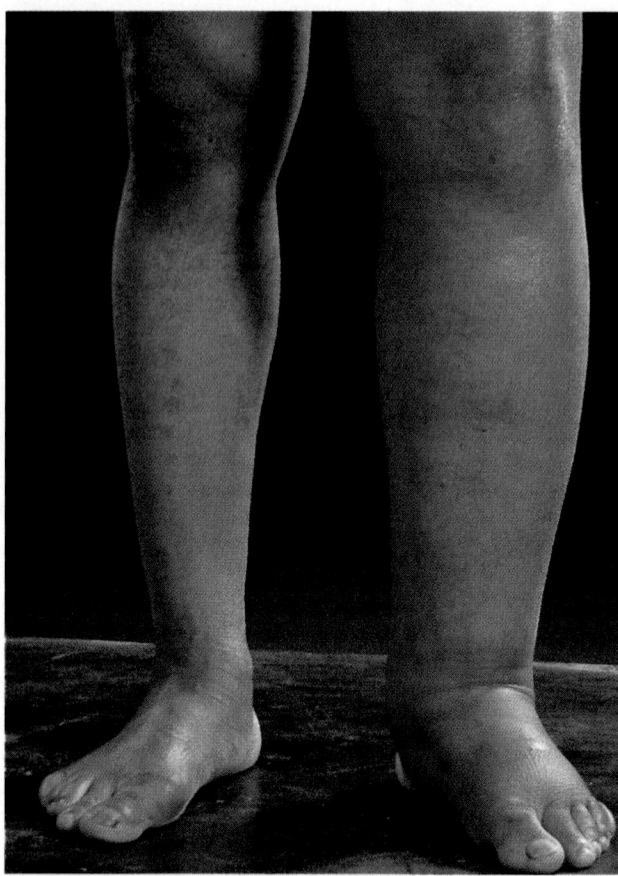

Figure 30–7 Severe lymphedema of the lower extremity.

Clients have swelling in one or both extremities. As the condition progresses, the client complains of increased heaviness and a hardening of the subcutaneous tissues of the affected extremity. Clients do not experience pain but state that their symptoms worsen in warm weather and (if the legs are affected) after standing for long periods. The edema causes a characteristic mound on the posterior surface (dorsum) of the affected extremity. Although the edema found during the early course of the disease is commonly soft and pitting, prolonged edema causes the tissues to become resistant to pressure. Hardened or fibrotic subcutaneous tissues are unresponsive to treatment. The edema often causes massive swelling of the involved extremities (Figure 30–7).

If the affected extremity becomes infected, both *lymphangitis* (inflammation of the lymphatic channels) and *cellulitis* (inflammation of connective or cellular tissue) may occur. The manifestations of lymphangitis include pain at the site of injury, redness of the skin, fever and chills, and a red streak on the skin extending toward the lymph nodes. The lymph nodes are very often enlarged and painful.

Collaborative Care

The collaborative care of clients with disorders of the lymphatic system focuses on relieving edema, maintaining skin integrity in the affected extremity, and preventing or treating infection. It is important to differentiate lymphedema from peripheral venous occlusive disorders, such as chronic venous insufficiency. In clients with lymphedema, the prognosis is variable. They may realize only minimal relief of edema with progressive disability due to the excessive weight and awkwardness of the affected extremity.

Laboratory and Diagnostic Tests

Laboratory and diagnostic tests are conducted to identify organisms responsible for lymphangitis and to determine if the lymphatics are obstructed.

The following laboratory tests may be ordered:

- *White blood counts* (WBC) are increased if an infection is present.
- *Blood cultures* may be conducted to determine the organism causing infection.
- *Cultures of wound drainage* may be conducted to identify the organism causing infection.

The following diagnostic tests may be ordered:

- *Lymphangiography* involves obtaining X-ray films after the injection of organic and radiopaque dyes. The initial injection of organic dyes into the surface of the skin allows enough lymphatic fluid to escape from the vessel to permit the injection of radiopaque contrast media. Once the radiopaque fluid is injected into the lymphatic vessel, the lymphatic vessels can be visualized to detect the causes of chronically swollen lower extremities. Although less frequently performed than angiography or venography, lymphangiography is also useful in the identification of abnormal lymph nodes in the peritoneal area and in the evaluation of clients with lymphomas. Health professionals should be aware that the contrast media used in lymphangiographic studies may produce temporary respiratory symptoms when it reaches the lungs. As a preventive measure, clients with existing respiratory problems should have pulmonary function tests performed prior to lymphangiography. If the findings are significantly abnormal, the test is canceled to prevent further pulmonary disability.
- *Lymphoscintigraphy* involves the interdigital injection of a radioactive substance, followed by X-ray studies to determine the normalcy of the transport of lymphatic fluid. In clients with edema due to venous disorders, lymphatic transport is normal, whereas clients with lymphedema demonstrate abnormal patterns of lymph fluid distribution and transport. The major advantages

of this procedure are that it is relatively simple, involves no adverse side effects, and is cost-efficient because it can be done on an outpatient basis.

Conservative Therapy

Initial treatment of lymphangitis involves the application of moist heat, and (when possible) the elevation and immobilization of the affected extremity. Wounds that are draining or have been surgically incised require meticulous care. As the primary pharmacologic treatment (discussed below) becomes increasingly effective, the condition abates and wound healing progresses more rapidly.

The treatment of lymphedema is often difficult because conservative therapies may not produce the desired effects. However, most clients benefit to some degree from one or more conservative measures. The goals of these measures are to move as much of the fluid as possible out of the interstitium, to maintain normal lymphatic circulation, and to prevent skin breakdown on the affected extremity. These are the measures:

- Elevate the extremity, especially during sleep.
- Use elastic stockings, elastic bandages, or pneumatic pressure devices.
- Provide meticulous skin hygiene.
- Remain on bed rest.
- Restrict dietary sodium.

Pharmacology

The pharmacologic treatment of disorders of the lymphatic system varies according to their cause and type. For clients with an infectious process (as in cellulitis or lymphangitis), organism-specific antibiotic therapy is initiated. Penicillin G is often a therapy of choice in the treatment of lymphatic disorders caused by a streptococcal infection. Erythromycin may be substituted in clients who are allergic to penicillin. Anthelmintic (destructive to worms), antifungal, analgesic, and diuretic therapy may also be used as appropriate (Goldstone, 1994; Tierney et al., 1995).

Surgery

Conservative measures are insufficient in a small portion of clients with disorders of the lymphatic system. In such cases, surgical intervention is necessary to (a) restore functioning to the affected extremity, (b) reduce pain, (c) treat recurrent episodes of cellulitis and lymphangitis, (d) remove lymphosarcomas, or (e) improve the appearance of the affected extremity. Surgical procedures involve the replacement of damaged lymphatic vessels with healthy lymphatic vessels or the removal of skin and lymphedematous subcutaneous tissues and subsequent extensive skin grafting over surgically incised sites. Only about 25% of clients who receive surgical treatment actually experience long-term effective relief of their lymphedema. Research continues for new and better ways of alleviating lymphatic circulation problems; new surgical trials are currently underway in the areas of microlymphatic bypass grafting and lymphatic/venous anastomoses (Goldstone, 1994).

Nursing Care

The nursing care of clients with disorders of the lymphatic system focuses on relieving edema, promoting skin integrity, preventing infection, and establishing effective coping mechanisms as the client adjusts to changes in body image. The nurse teaches the client about the disease process and the importance of meticulous hygiene and skin care to prevent infection. Issues related to the client's altered mobility status, dietary sodium intake, and diuretic therapy should also be addressed as part of the therapeutic approach to reducing edema and promoting more normal lymphatic function. The nursing diagnoses discussed in this section are *Impaired Tissue Integrity, Fluid Volume Excess,* and *Risk for Impaired Skin Integrity.*

Impaired Tissue Integrity

The ineffective flow of fluid in the lymphatic vessels causes fluid to collect in the interstitial spaces of the subcutaneous tissue. The subsequent edema compresses tissues and damages them. The tissues become fibrotic and predisposed to skin breakdown and infection.

Nursing interventions with rationales follow:

- Apply well-fitting elastic stockings or intermittent pneumatic pressure devices according to the prescribed schedule. Remove these devices for at least 1 hour every 8 hours or according to institution protocol. *Elastic stockings and/or pneumatic pressure devices force lymphatic fluid back into the vascular spaces, where it will be transported back to the heart for future circulation. Adherence to the ordered protocol for application and removal helps prevent additional edema and allows for inspection and hygiene of underlying skin.*

- Elevate the extremities while the client is seated and especially at bedtime. *Elevation of the extremities diminishes venous congestion in the affected extremity. This therapy is most useful in clients with lymphangitis but may be of some value during the early course of disease in clients with lymphedema. Nonetheless, elevation of the extremity promotes venous return, facilitates normal tissue perfusion, and helps eliminate the accumulation of excess fluids in the interstitial spaces of the affected extremity.*

- Restrict sodium intake according to prescribed parameters and increase fluid consumption. *Sodium causes fluids to be retained in the interstitial spaces. Limiting sodium helps decrease the amount of fluids held in the interstitial spaces of the subcutaneous tissues, thereby decreasing edema. Diuretic therapy in combination with sodium restriction and increased oral fluid consumption aids in the elimination of excess fluids in the body and decreases peripheral edema.*

- Teach the client the importance of adherence to therapeutic interventions. *Teaching the client about the plan of care decreases anxiety about treatment modalities, decreases fear of the unknown, and encourages the client to participate in self-care. In addition, teaching sessions give the nurse time to develop trust and rapport with the client and demonstrate caring and respect, which increase the likelihood of client adherence to the plan of care.*

Fluid Volume Excess

The normal production and circulation of lymphatic fluid depends on a lymphatic system that is free from obstruction, destruction, or congenital malformation. When the lymphatic regulatory mechanisms are interrupted (as in lymphedema), the client develops fluid volume excess in the subcutaneous tissues of the interstitial spaces of the affected extremity.

Nursing interventions with rationales follow:

- Restrict dietary sodium and help the client choose foods that are low in sodium. *Sodium causes water to be retained in the extracellular space. Restricting dietary sodium helps prevent the accumulation of additional fluids in the interstitial spaces, especially in clients in whom the normal circulation of extracellular fluids is already impaired. In clients with a malfunctioning lymphatic system, controlling edema of the extremity is the central goal of the collaborative plan of care and necessary for the restoration of health.*

- Measure and record intake and output at least every 8 hours. *Because the lymphatic system is malfunctioning, fluids normally reabsorbed into the bloodstream at the venous end of the circulatory loop accumulate in the interstitial spaces. Monitoring intake and output helps the nurse determine how much fluid is being held in the interstitial spaces versus how much fluid is being processed normally through the kidneys and ultimately excreted in urine. Records of intake and output also allow the nurse to monitor the effects of sodium restriction and diuretic therapy, which are often components of the collaborative plan of care.*

- Assess the extremity daily for increased edema; measure the girth of the extremity according to institutional protocols. *The size of the affected extremity is measured at least daily to determine the effectiveness of ordered interventions and the progression of the disease process. In addition, assessment allows the nurse to inspect the skin of the affected extremity, which is at risk for breakdown secondary to the prolonged swelling and stretching of the skin.*

- Weigh the client at the same time daily and report significant changes. *The rapid accumulation of fluids in the interstitial spaces may be reflected by a change in the client's weight. To ensure consistency, weigh the client at the same time each day in the same type of clothing. Weighing the client daily helps the nurse monitor the effects of diuretic therapy and allows early detection of fluid balance problems.*

Risk for Impaired Skin Integrity

Because certain types of lymphatic dysfunction are closely associated with the presence of cellulitis, the risk of skin breakdown is high in these clients. Tissues are vulnerable to both interior and exterior processes, making meticulous skin care an essential component of the nursing plan of care. In all clients with impaired lymphatic function, the swelling and stretching of the skin associated with the collection of fluids in the interstitial spaces increase the risk for skin breakdown.

- Inspect the skin on the affected extremity at least once each shift and document findings. *Antiembolic stockings and intermittent pressure devices should be removed at least once each shift to inspect the underlying skin for evidence of redness, irritation, dryness, or breakdown. Breaks in the skin surface allow microbial invasion, which can lead to potentially dangerous infections if not detected and managed early. Assessment findings should be documented daily to provide a baseline for the ongoing evaluation of skin condition.*

- Use preventive skin care devices according to ordered or institutional protocols. *The collection of fluid in the affected extremity makes the limb heavy. Because of this increased weight, the surfaces of the limb that come in contact with the bed are under greater pressure. Protective devices such as egg crate foam, sheepskin, pillows, or padding help prevent the compression of tissues that come in contact with the bed, thereby promoting effective circulation and minimizing the potential for skin breakdown.*

- Keep client's skin clean and dry, especially in interdigital spaces. Monitor at least every 4 hours. *The edema of the limb can become so profound that it may be difficult to clean the interdigital spaces. The dark, moist interdigital spaces are an excellent environment for the growth of bacteria. Clean, dry, skin is less likely to break or become infected.*

- Teach the client and family how to prevent skin breakdown. *Educating the client about skin care measures to prevent breakdown fosters client independence, encourages client participation in the plan of care, and promotes client self-esteem. The nurse should provide ample time for teaching and questions and encourage the hospitalized client to perform skin care. Having the client demonstrate skin care techniques before discharge allows the client to review what was learned and lets the nurse evaluate the effectiveness of client teaching.*

Altered Body Image

The accumulation of fluids in the extremities of clients with lymphatic disorders can produce changes in body image related to the disproportionate size of the affected extremity. During early stages of the disease, conservative measures may significantly reduce the edema, and therefore the size, of the affected limb. However, in later stages of the disease, collaborative interventions may become less effective or ineffective, causing more permanent disfigurement. Mobility may become difficult, and clients may develop an increasingly negative self-perception that interferes with healthful functioning.

■ Encourage discussions about the client's usual coping patterns and level of self-esteem. *Knowledge of the client's existing coping patterns and behaviors help the nurse assess the client's ability to cope with the current situation. The nurse uses this knowledge to help the client explore new or different methods of effective coping. This exchange also gives the client the opportunity to voice feelings related to actual or perceived changes in body image.*

■ Accept the client's perception of self and of the impact of the changes in appearance. *Nonjudgmental acceptance of the client's view of self and of the effects of changes in appearance builds trust and promotes rapport with the client. Without trust, the client is less likely to adhere to the collaborative plan of care or to take an active role in the management of the current health situation. In addition, nonjudgmental listening promotes mutual respect and demonstrates caring and compassion.*

■ Encourage the client to participate actively in self-care. *Many clients initially have difficulty viewing or touching the affected body part. Gentle encouragement and support from the nurse help clients become responsible for their own activities of daily living, such as hygiene, grooming, and dressing. If the degree of edema in the affected extremity prevents the client from performing certain aspects of care (such as nail care), the nurse should encourage brainstorming to develop acceptable alternative methods.*

Other Nursing Diagnoses

The following nursing diagnoses may also be appropriate for clients with disorders of the lymphatic system:

■ *Pain* related to stretching of skin and tissue compression secondary to lymphedema

■ *Hygiene Self-Care Deficit* related to limb enlargement secondary to lymphedema

■ *Impaired Physical Mobility* related to changes in leg size and contour

Client and Family Teaching

Education for the client and family focuses on the reduction of edema, dietary restrictions, medications, and the importance of prevention of future episodes of illness. While hospitalized, clients are often taught to use intermittent pressure devices or to apply well-fitted elastic stockings to prevent the collection of fluid in the interstitial spaces of the lower legs. Emphasize the importance of maintaining constant pressure (via the elastic stockings) to the affected extremity for the majority of the client's waking hours, and stress the need to remove the stockings while sleeping. The client is also taught to remove the stockings at least once during the day to inspect the skin surface for signs of breakdown or cracking.

Teaching also includes the need for meticulous skin care to promote skin integrity, prevent skin breakdown, and minimize the risk for infection. Elevation of the affected extremity may be prescribed, and clients should be assisted in developing a schedule that allows implementation of ordered interventions but interferes as little as possible with daily schedules. The nurse also provides information about the nature and use of diuretics and the relationship between activity restriction, dietary sodium restriction, and diuretic therapy. If the client is taking a potassium-losing diuretic, provide a list of sources of dietary potassium (see Chapter 5).

Provide the client and family with information about contacts for questions, and make referrals as needed. Clients with a chronic disorder that limits mobility often face long years of self-management and may require additional assistance with health care management, meals, and housework.

Applying the Nursing Process

Case Study of a Client with Lymphedema: Brittany Yonkman

Brittany Yonkman is a 23-year-old single Caucasian woman who works as the host in a busy new restaurant. When she was 15, she began to notice that her right foot would occasionally become puffy and her ankle would swell, especially after a long day at school and after playing volleyball with her high school team. At age 19 she began to experience bouts of swelling that prevented her from wearing some of her favorite shoes, but she never told anyone in her family about her problem. She moved away from home after high school, and she enjoys her second-story walk-up apartment and her busy work and social life. Today Mrs. Yonkman has noticed an increased swelling and uncomfortable heaviness in her right leg and is becoming increasingly concerned. She has noticed a general sense of fatigue but attributes it to a very busy life.

As she dresses after her morning shower, she notices that she is having difficulty fitting her jeans over her right leg. The neighborhood clinic is open today, so Ms. Yonkman makes an appointment. The doctor at the neighborhood clinic orders lymphoscintigraphy and a complete blood count, and Ms. Yonkman is diagnosed with probable cellulitis and lymphedema of the right leg. She is admitted to a local hospital for additional diagnostic testing and treatment. Ke'ala Eustaquio, RN, is the nurse assigned to care for Ms. Yonkman.

Assessment

Ms. Eustaquio completes an admission history and physical assessment. She finds that Ms. Yonkman is an alert, oriented woman; height: 5'8" (173 cm); weight: 128 lb (58 kg); vital signs stable and within normal limits. Ms. Eustaquio notes that the right leg is visibly larger than the left leg and that there is soft, 3+, nonpitting edema in the right leg only. Both extremities are dry and warm to the touch, and the pedal pulses in both feet are present, although the pulse in the right foot is more difficult to find because of the edema. Ms. Eustaquio notes that Ms. Yonkman seems very nervous and has verbalized concerns about losing her job if she has to stay in the hospital for very long. Ms. Yonkman also refers to her affected leg as "ugly" and states that she doesn't ever want her friends to see her like this.

The doctor's orders for Ms. Yonkman are:

- Bed rest with legs elevated
- Antiembolism stockings to be worn continuously while she is awake and removed at bedtime
- Blood cultures × 3
- Regular diet with no added salt
- Furosemide (Lasix) 40 mg daily
- Strict intake and output measurement
- Acetaminophen 650 mg q4–6h prn for pain

The results of Ms. Yonkman's lymphoscintigraphy are positive, but the CBC and blood cultures are both negative, and cellulitis is ruled out.

Diagnosis

Ms. Eustaquio makes the following diagnoses for Ms. Yonkman:

- *Impaired Tissue Integrity* related to stasis of lymphatic fluid
- *Fluid Volume Excess* related to compromised regulatory system
- *Anxiety* related to unexpected hospitalization
- *Body Image Disturbance* related to disproportionate size of the right leg

Expected Outcomes

The expected outcomes for the plan of care are that, by discharge, Ms. Yonkman will

- Have decreased edema in the right leg.
- Verbalize reduced anxiety related to the current hospitalization.
- State at least two positive coping strategies.
- Discuss self-management of her lymphedema, including diet planning to reduce sodium intake, actions and side effects of prescribed medications, and skin care to maintain skin integrity and prevent infection.

Planning and Implementation

Ms. Eustaquio plans and implements the following interventions for Ms. Yonkman:

- Assess degree of edema of right leg every 8 hours by degree of pitting and by measuring calf and thigh circumference. Document findings.
- Apply thigh-length elastic antiembolism stockings to both legs during all waking hours; remove stockings at bedtime.
- Remove stockings once each shift to inspect and provide care to underlying skin.
- Elevate the foot of bed 15 cm or according to physician orders or institution protocols.
- Measure intake and output on each shift; compare 24-hour totals, and report significant changes in fluid balance.
- Teach Ms. Yonkman the reasons for a no-added salt diet. Assist in menu selection of foods low in sodium and foods high in potassium.
- Evaluate her response to diuretic therapy. Monitor electrolyte levels and report abnormal levels, especially of potassium.
- Encourage Ms. Yonkman to discuss her fears regarding her hospital stay. Provide time for Ms. Yonkman to express her feelings about the disease process and to explore her usual methods of coping.
- Provide verbal and written instructions about skin care and prevention of infection prior to discharge.

Evaluation

Four days after Ms. Yonkman's admission to the hospital, her physician writes an order for her discharge to home. Her right leg has decreased in size, the nonpitting edema is reduced to 1+, she has adjusted well to the use of the antiembolism stockings, and she can apply and remove them without too much difficulty. The skin on her right leg is moist, smooth, and supple, and she is able to fit her jeans over her leg with no difficulty. Ms. Yonkman has successfully chosen from a regular menu foods that are low in sodium and has correctly described the relationship between lowering sodium intake and taking diuretics. Ms. Eustaquio and Ms. Yonkman have talked about Ms. Yonkman's perceptions of herself with this disfigurement. Ms. Eustaquio has given Ms. Yonkman written instructions regarding skin care, medication therapy, dietary restrictions, and the importance of the continued use of the antiembolism stocking. Ms. Yonkman makes a follow-up appointment before leaving the hospital, thanks Ms. Eustaquio, and assures her that she will do "whatever it takes to stay out of here."

Critical Thinking in the Nursing Process

1. Compare and contrast the pathophysiology of lymphedema and chronic venous insufficiency.

2. Describe how the plan of care would be different for a client who is homeless. Consider needs for medication, elevation of the legs, special diet, and hygiene.

3. Develop a teaching plan for Ms. Yonkman that includes interventions to reduce edema, promote skin integrity, prevent infection, and minimize negative self-image.

4. Design a nursing care plan for Ms. Yonkman for the diagnosis *Impaired Social Interaction*.

Bibliography

■ ■ ■

Abrams, A. (1995). *Clinical drug therapy: Rationales for nursing practice* (4th ed.). Philadelphia: Lippincott.

Berkow, R. & Fletcher, A. (Eds.). (1992). *The Merck manual of diagnosis and therapy.* (16th ed.). Rathway, NJ: Merck Research Laboratories.

Bright, L. D., & Georgi, S. (1994). How to protect your patient from DVT. *American Journal of Nursing, 94*(12), 28.

Brunwald, E. (1992). *Heart disease: A textbook of cardiovascular medicine* (4th ed.). Philadelphia: Saunders.

Capasso, V., & Cote, K. (1993). The management of patients undergoing arterial reconstructive surgery. *MEDSURG Nursing, 2*(1), 11–20.

Carpenito, L. J. (1995). *Nursing care plans and documentation: Nursing diagnoses and collaborative problems* (2nd ed.). Philadelphia: Lippincott.

Carpenito, L. J. (1992). *Nursing diagnosis: Application to clinical practice* (4th ed.). Philadelphia: Lippincott.

Carrol, P., & Ciani, J. (1993). Deep vein thrombosis. *Orthopaedic Nursing, 12*(4), 6.

Crosby, R., Ventura, M., Frainier, M., & Wu, Y. (1993). Well-being and concerns of patients with peripheral arterial occlusive disease. *Journal of Vascular Nursing, 11*(1), 4–11.

Deglin, J., & Vallerand, A. (1993). *Davis's drug guide for nurses* (4th ed.). Philadelphia: F. A. Davis.

Dziechiuch, J. (1994). Decision making of patients with arterial occlusive disease who are threatened with limb loss. *Journal of Vascular Nursing, 12*(1), 6–9.

Goldstone, J. (1994). Veins and lymphatics. In L. Way (Ed.). *Current surgical diagnosis and treatment* (10th ed.) (pp. 783–809). Norwalk, CT: Appleton & Lange.

U. S. Department of Health and Human Services. (1993) *The fifth report of the Joint National Committee on detection, evaluation, and treatment of high blood pressure.* (NIH Publication). Washington, DC: U. S. Government Printing Office.

Kayser, S. (1994). New drugs 1994: trapidil, torsemide. *Progress in Cardiovascular Nursing, 9*(3), 38–40.

MacDermott, B., & Deglin, J. (1994). *Understanding basic pharmacology: Practical approaches for effective application.* Philadelphia: F. A. Davis.

Massie, B. (1995). Systemic hypertension. In L. Tierney, S. McPhee, & M. Papadikis (Eds.). *Current medical diagnosis and treatment* (34th ed.). Norwalk, CT: Appleton & Lange.

McCance, K., & Huether, S. (1993). *Pathophysiology: The biologic basis for disease in adults and children* (2nd ed.). St. Louis: Mosby.

Nash, C., & Jensen, P. (1994). When your surgical patient has hypertension. *American Journal of Nursing, 94*(12), 38–45.

Patterson, C., & Faux, S. (1993). Uncertainty and appraisal in patients diagnosed with abdominal aortic aneurysms. *Canadian Journal of Cardiovascular Nursing, 4*(1), 4–10.

Porth, C. (1994). *Pathophysiology: Concepts of altered health states* (4th ed.). Philadelphia: Lippincott.

Soloman, J. (1994). Hypertension: New drug therapies. *RN, 57*(1), 26–33.

Sparks, S., & Taylor, C. (1993). *Nursing diagnosis reference manual* (2nd ed.). Springhouse, PA: Springhouse.

Thompson, J., McFarland, G., Hirsch, J., & Tucker, S. (1993). *Mosby's clinical nursing* (3rd ed.). St. Louis: Mosby.

Tierney, L., McPhee, S., & Papadakis, M. (Eds.)(1994). *Current medical diagnosis and treatment* (33rd ed.). Norwalk, CT: Appleton & Lange.

Tierney, L., McPhee, S., & Papadakis, M. (Eds.) (1995). *Current medical diagnosis and treatment* (34th ed.). Norwalk, CT: Appleton & Lange.

Weiner, B. (1993). Thrombolytic agents in critical care. *Critical Care Nursing Clinics of North America, 5*(2), 355–366.

Williams, B., & Baer, C. (1994). *Essentials of clinical pharmacology in nursing* (2nd ed.). Springhouse, PA: Springhouse.

Williams, S. (1993). *Nutrition and diet therapy* (7th ed.). St. Louis: Mosby.

CHAPTER 31

Nursing Care of Clients with Hematologic Disorders

LEARNING OBJECTIVES

After completing this chapter, you will be able to

- Describe the pathophysiology of common hematologic disorders.

- Identify laboratory and diagnostic tests used to diagnose hematologic disorders.

- Discuss nursing implications for medications prescribed for the client with hematologic disorders.

- Discuss nursing implications for bone marrow transplantation, chemotherapy, and radiation for the client with a hematologic disorder.

- Compare and contrast bleeding disorders.

- Describe the major types of leukemia and the most common treatment modalities and nursing interventions.

- Differentiate Hodgkin's disease from non-Hodgkin's lymphomas.

- Use the nursing process as a framework for providing individualized care to clients with hematologic disorders.

Clients who have diseases associated with blood and blood-forming organs experience health problems that range from minor disruptions in daily activities to major physiologic life-threatening crises. Clients with hematologic disorders require emotional support as well as nursing care for problems involving many of the major body systems.

Blood serves as a medium of exchange between the external environment and the body's cells. Blood is made up of plasma, solids (including proteins, inorganic compounds and elements, and organic constituents), red blood cells, several types of white blood cells, and fragments of cells (called platelets or thrombocytes).

The hematopoietic (blood-forming) system is composed of both the bone marrow (myeloid) tissues, where blood cells form, and the lymphoid tissues of the lymph nodes, where white blood cells mature and circulate. All of the blood cells originate from cells in the bone marrow called *stem cells*, or hemocytoblasts. Hormonal regulating mechanisms cause stem cells to differentiate into families of parent cells, each of which gives rise to one of the formed elements of the blood (red blood cells, platelets, and several kinds of white cells). The origin of the cellular components of blood is illustrated in Figure 31–1.

This chapter focuses on alterations in health that result from changes in red cells, white cells, platelets, and clotting factors. An overview of each type of blood cell is provided prior to the discussion of the related pathophysiologies to serve as the basis for understanding the effects of, responses to, and care of clients with hematologic disorders.

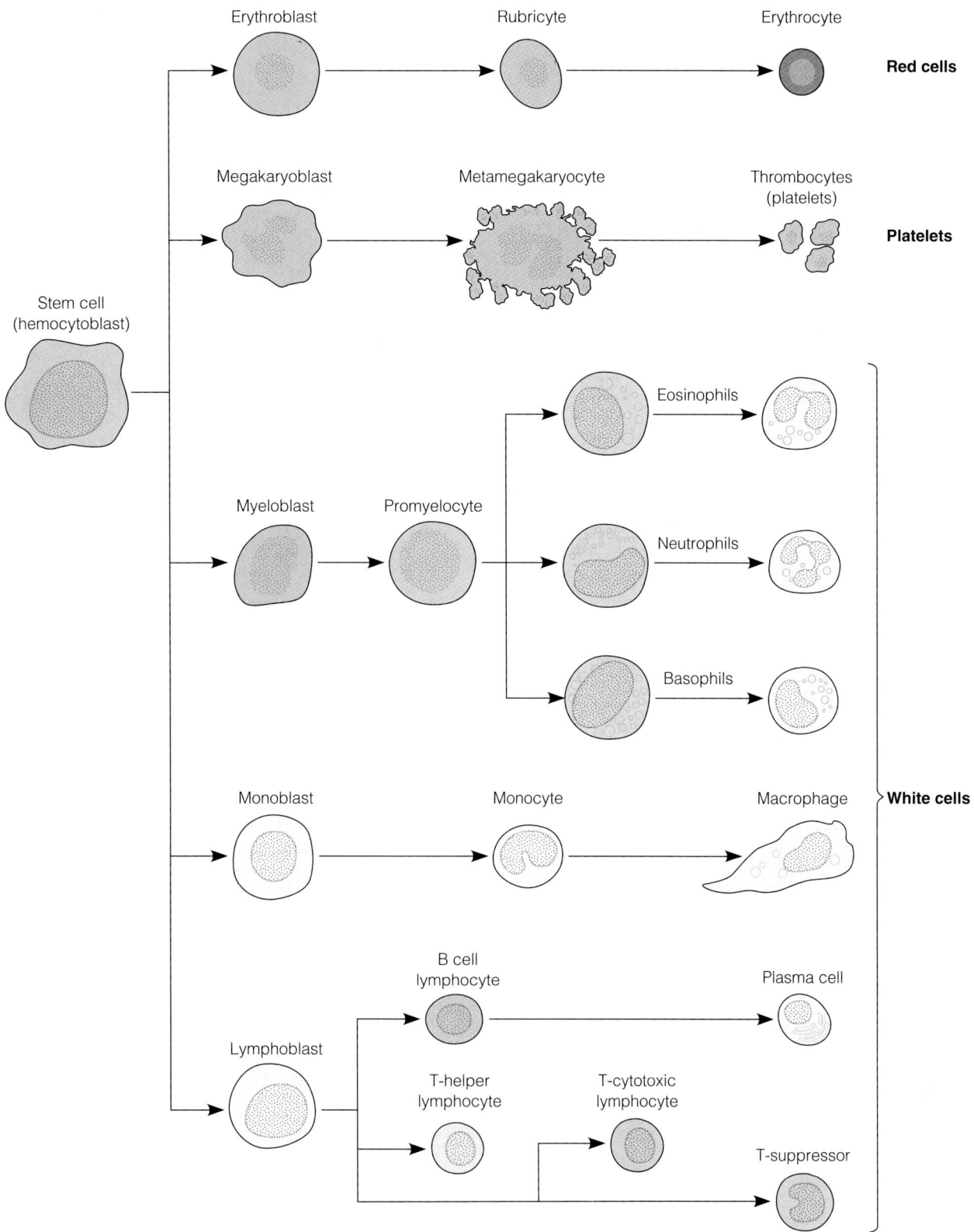

Figure 31–1   The formation of blood components from stem cells. Hormonal regulation and other metabolic factors govern the differentiation of stem cells into blasts. Each of the five kinds of blasts is committed to producing one type of mature blood cell component. Erythroblasts, for example, can differentiate only into RBCs; megakaryoblasts can differentiate only into platelets.

Red blood cells (RBCs) and the hemoglobin molecules within them are necessary for the transport of oxygen to body tissues. In addition, hemoglobin binds with some forms of carbon dioxide and carries it to the lungs for excretion. Alterations in the number of RBCs, alterations in the size and shape of the RBCs, or alterations in the amount of hemoglobin or its molecular structure may adversely affect a client's health. The following overview discusses the characteristics of RBCs and hemoglobin and the process of RBC production and destruction.

Overview of Red Blood Cells

■ ■ ■

A red blood cell (also called an erythrocyte) is shaped like a biconcave disk (Figure 31–2). The RBC's shape increases the cell's surface area for the diffusion of oxygen and also allows the cell to change in volume and shape without disrupting its membrane. RBCs are the most common type of blood cell.

Hemoglobin is the oxygen-carrying protein within RBCs and is composed of two pairs of polypeptide chains designated α_1, α_2 and β_1, β_2 (Figure 31–3). Each of the four polypeptide chains is attached to a heme unit. An atom of iron within each heme unit binds with oxygen. Hemoglobin molecules are synthesized within the RBC; the rate of synthesis depends on the availability of iron (Porth, 1994).

Laboratory values for red blood cells are defined as follows:

- Red blood cell count: The number of circulating RBCs in 1 mm^3 of whole blood

- Reticulocyte count: The number of immature RBCs in 1 mm^3 of blood

- Hemoglobin (Hgb): The amount of hemoglobin in 1 mm^3 of blood

- Hematocrit (Hct): The packed volume of RBCs in 1 mm^3 of blood, expressed as a percentage

- Mean corpuscular volume (MCV): The average volume of individual RBCs

- Mean corpuscular hemoglobin (MCH): A measure of RBC weight, reflecting the amount of hemoglobin and the RBC count

- Mean corpuscular hemoglobin concentration: A measure reflecting the relationship between the amount of hemoglobin in an RBC and the volume of the cell containing it

As Table 31–1 shows, normal RBC laboratory values often differ by gender.

Red blood cells may also be analyzed by studying the size, color, and shape of stained cells. RBCs may be of normal size (normocytic), smaller than normal (microcytic), or larger than normal (macrocytic); they may be of normal color (normochromic) or have decreased color (hypochromic).

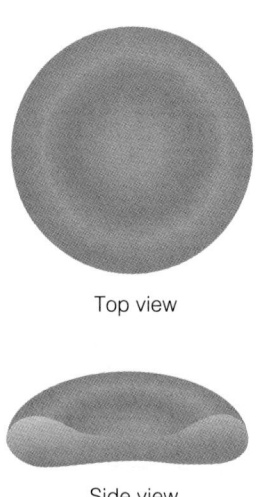

Figure 31–2   Top and side view of a red blood cell (erythrocyte). Note the distinctive concave shape.

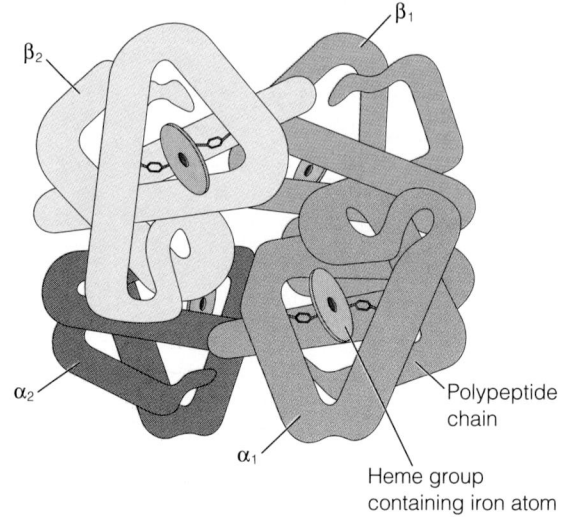

Figure 31–3   The hemoglobin molecule within RBCs. The molecule is composed of the protein globin, which is formed from four subunits designated α_1, α_2 and β_1, β_2. A heme group is nested within the folds of each protein subunit. Hemoglobin's oxygen-carrying ability is due to an iron atom (red dot) located at the center of each heme group.

Table 31-1	Normal Laboratory Values: Red Blood Cells and Platelets

Laboratory Test	Normal Value
Red Blood Cell (RBC) Count	
Men	4.2 to 5.4 million/mm^3
Women	3.6 to 5.0 million/mm^3
Reticulocytes	1.0%–1.5% of total RBC
Hemoglobin (Hgb)	
Men	14 to 16.5 g/dL
Women	12 to 15 g/dL
Hematocrit (Hct)	
Men	40% to 50%
Women	37% to 47%
Mean corpuscular volume (MCV)	85 to 100 fL/cell
Mean corpuscular hemoglobin concentration (MCHC)	31 to 35 g/dL
Mean corpuscular hemoglobin (MCH)	27 to 34 pg/cell
Platelet count	250,000 to 400,000/mm^3

Production and Regulation of Red Blood Cells

The production of RBCs is called *erythropoiesis* (Figure 31–4). In the adult, erythropoiesis occurs in the bone marrow of the vertebrae, sternum, ribs, and pelvis. RBC formation begins in the bone marrow and ends within the circulating blood. *Erythroblasts* forming within the bone marrow contain numerous ribosomes that synthesize hemoglobin, which accumulates within the erythroblast cytoplasm. Next, the erythroblasts differentiate into *normoblasts*. The nucleus and most of the organelles are ejected, eventually causing normoblasts to collapse inward and assume the characteristic biconcave shape of

RBCs. The cells emerge in the circulation as *reticulocytes,* which fully mature in about 48 hours. The complete sequence from stem cell to RBC takes from 3 to 5 days.

The stimulus for RBC production is tissue hypoxia. The hormone *erythropoietin* is released by the kidneys in response to hypoxia and stimulates the bone marrow to produce RBCs. However, the process takes about 5 days for RBC production to reach a maximum. Because RBCs are released into the circulation as reticulocytes, there is a higher percentage of these RBC precursors than of mature red blood cells during periods when RBC production is rising.

Destruction of Red Blood Cells

RBCs have a life span of about 120 days. Old or damaged RBCs are lysed (destroyed) by phagocytes located in the spleen, liver, bone marrow, and lymph nodes. The process of RBC destruction is called *hemolysis.* The phagocytes save and reuse amino acids and iron from the heme units in the lysed RBCs. Most of the heme unit is converted to *bilirubin,* an orange-yellow pigment that is removed from the blood by the liver and excreted in the bile.

During disease processes characterized by heightened hemolysis or suppressed liver function, bilirubin may accumulate in the serum to the extent that the affected individual's skin and sclera assume a yellowish appearance. This condition is called *jaundice.*

The Client with Anemia

■ ■ ■

Anemia is a condition in which the hemoglobin content of the blood is insufficient to satisfy bodily demands. The condition usually is due to a decrease in the number of circulating RBCs. However, insufficient or defective

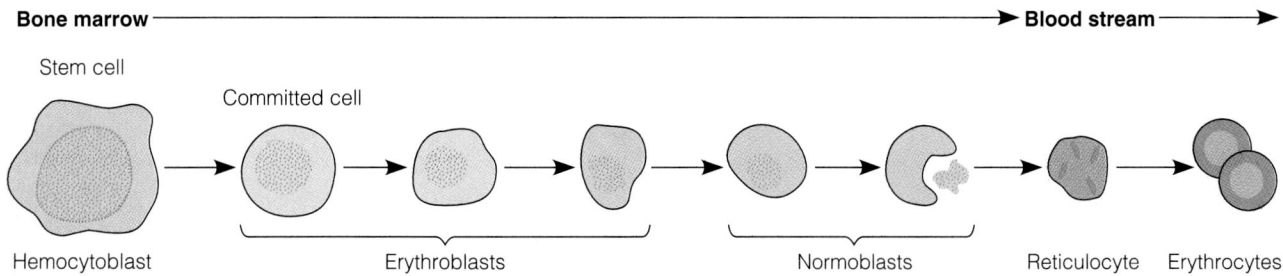

Figure 31-4   Erythropoiesis. RBCs begin forming within the bone marrow as erythroblasts. These mature into normoblasts, which eventually eject their nucleus and organelles to form reticu-

locytes. The reticulocytes mature within the blood or spleen and become erythrocytes.

Table 31–2 Causes of Anemia

Cause	Source
Blood loss	Trauma Conditions causing internal bleeding Complications of pregnancy Blood donation
Increased hemolysis	Chemical of physical agents Autoimmune reactions Hereditary cell membrane disorders ■ G6PD deficiency ■ PK deficiency Splenomegaly and hypersplenism Chronic liver disease Chronic infections Chronic imflammatory diseases
Depressed RBC or hemoglobin production	Iron-related disorders ■ Dietary iron deficiency ■ Iron overloading ■ Impaired iron metabolism Disorders of RBC DNA synthesis ■ Vitamin B_{12} malabsorption or deficit ■ Folic acid malabsorption or deficit Renal failure Endocrine failure ■ Myxedema ■ Addison's disease Hereditary disorders
Defective hemoglobin synthesis	Sickle cell anemias Thalassemias Methoglobinemias
Bone marrow failure	Myeloproliferative leukemias Red cell aplasia Metastatic tumors Chemical and physical agents Bone marrow infections

---

Classification of Selected Anemias

■ ■ ■

Nutritional Anemias

- Iron deficiency anemia
- Vitamin B_{12} anemia
- Folic acid deficiency anemia

Hemolytic Anemias

- Sickle cell anemia
- Thalassemia
- Acquired hemolytic anemia
- Glucose-6-phosphate dehydrogenase anemia

Bone Marrow Depression Anemia

- Aplastic anemia

---

hemoglobin within RBCs may also cause anemia. Decreased numbers of circulating RBCs may result from an inadequate rate of RBC production, accelerated hemolysis, or from high numbers of reticulocytes in the blood. Depending on the severity of the RBC deficit, anemia may affect all major organ systems.

Pathophysiology

Anemias can result from a host of different pathophysiologic mechanisms, the most important of which are summarized in Table 31–2. Regardless of the cause, every form of anemia reduces the oxygen-carrying capacity of the blood, producing generalized tissue hypoxia. The body's attempt to compensate for the resulting oxygen deficit gives rise to the most common manifestations of anemia. As tissue oxygenation decreases, the heart rate and the respiratory rate rise. Tissue hypoxia may cause angina, fatigue, dyspnea on exertion, and night cramps. As another means of compensating for decreased oxygenation, blood is redistributed from the skin and mucous membranes to internal organs, resulting in pallor of the skin, mucous membranes, nail beds, and conjunctiva. In addition, blood viscosity may decrease, causing a systolic murmur, and increased erythropoietin activity may cause bone pain.

Other manifestations specific to the condition causing the anemia are discussed in the following section. The severity of the manifestations of anemia depends on the cause and severity of the underlying disorder. For example, rapid loss of blood causes immediate symptoms, whereas the person with slowly developing anemia may exhibit no symptoms until the condition is well advanced. The manifestations of several kinds of anemia are summarized in Figure 31–5.

Anemia is categorized according to its cause. This chapter discusses the broadest categories of anemia: nutritional anemias, hemolytic anemias, and anemias resulting from bone marrow depression. (See the accompanying box.) The pathophysiology of specific anemias within these categories is then discussed.

Nutritional Anemias

Nutritional anemias result from nutrient deficiencies that disrupt erythropoiesis or hemoglobin synthesis. The nutrient deficiency may be related to dietary factors, mal-

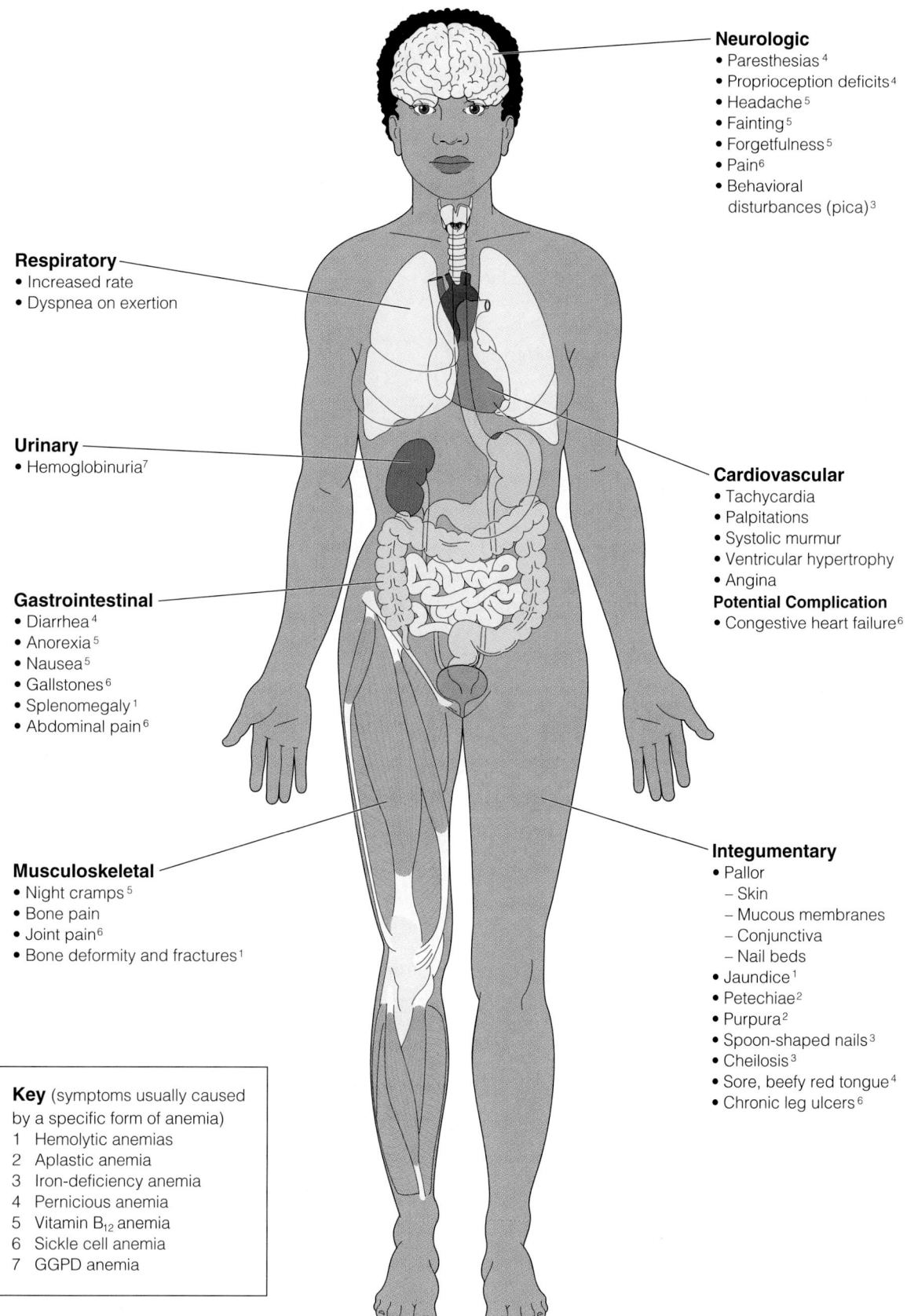

Neurologic
- Paresthesias[4]
- Proprioception deficits[4]
- Headache[5]
- Fainting[5]
- Forgetfulness[5]
- Pain[6]
- Behavioral disturbances (pica)[3]

Respiratory
- Increased rate
- Dyspnea on exertion

Urinary
- Hemoglobinuria[7]

Cardiovascular
- Tachycardia
- Palpitations
- Systolic murmur
- Ventricular hypertrophy
- Angina

Potential Complication
- Congestive heart failure[6]

Gastrointestinal
- Diarrhea[4]
- Anorexia[5]
- Nausea[5]
- Gallstones[6]
- Splenomegaly[1]
- Abdominal pain[6]

Musculoskeletal
- Night cramps[5]
- Bone pain
- Joint pain[6]
- Bone deformity and fractures[1]

Integumentary
- Pallor
  – Skin
  – Mucous membranes
  – Conjunctiva
  – Nail beds
- Jaundice[1]
- Petechiae[2]
- Purpura[2]
- Spoon-shaped nails[3]
- Cheilosis[3]
- Sore, beefy red tongue[4]
- Chronic leg ulcers[6]

Key (symptoms usually caused by a specific form of anemia)
1. Hemolytic anemias
2. Aplastic anemia
3. Iron-deficiency anemia
4. Pernicious anemia
5. Vitamin B_{12} anemia
6. Sickle cell anemia
7. GGPD anemia

Figure 31–5 **Multisystem effects of anemia.**

absorption disorders, or the body's heightened need for the nutrient. The most common types of nutritional anemias are iron deficiency anemia, vitamin B_{12} anemia, and folic acid deficiency anemia. Vitamin B_{12} and folic acid anemias are sometimes called *megaloblastic anemia,* because both are characterized by the presence of enlarged nucleated RBCs called megaloblasts.

Iron Deficiency Anemia   **Iron deficiency anemia** is a condition in which the supply of iron is inadequate for optimal formation of red blood cells. It is the most common type of anemia. As noted earlier, the body cannot synthesize hemoglobin without iron. Iron deficiency anemia results in fewer numbers of RBCs, microcytic RBCs, and hypochromic RBCs; moreover, it causes *poikilocytosis* (malformed cells).

The most common cause of iron deficiency anemia in adults is excessive iron loss due to bleeding. Menstrual blood loss is the most common source of iron-loss-related anemia in adult females. Women also may experience anemia during pregnancy and lactation because of a heightened metabolic need for iron.

Other causes of iron deficiency anemia include inadequate dietary intake of iron (less than 1 mg/day), malabsorption following total or partial gastrectomy, chronic diarrhea, and various malabsorption syndromes (see Chapter 23). The causes of iron deficiency anemia are summarized in the accompanying box.

Iron deficiency anemia is particularly common in older adults. Chronic, occult (hidden) blood loss may occur from disorders such as bleeding ulcers, gastrointestinal inflammation, hemorrhoids, and cancer. However, inadequate dietary intake of iron also contributes to anemia in the older adult. Inaccessibility of transportation (which may limit access to fresh foods) is one factor contributing to the problem of poor dietary iron intake among all adults, especially among those with limited or fixed incomes.

Assessment findings include the general manifestations of anemia described earlier. In addition, clients with chronic iron deficiency may develop brittle, spoonshaped nails; *cheilosis* (cracks at the corners of the mouth); a smooth, sore tongue; and *pica* (a craving to eat unusual substances, such as clay or starch).

The primary form of treatment for iron deficiency anemia is to increase the number and amount of iron-rich foods in the client's diet or to administer oral or parenteral iron preparations.

Vitamin B_{12} Deficiency Anemia   Vitamin B_{12} is necessary for the synthesis of DNA. A deficiency of this vitamin impairs cellular division and maturation, especially in rapidly proliferating red blood cells. **Vitamin B_{12} deficiency** produces an anemia in which the RBCs are macrocytic, have thin membranes, and are oval rather than concave in shape. These abnormal RBCs are unusu-

---

Causes of Iron Deficiency Anemia

■ ■ ■

- ■ Dietary deficiencies
- ■ Decreased absorption
  - a. Partial or total gastrectomy
  - b. Chronic diarrhea
  - c. Malabsorption syndromes
- ■ Increased metabolic requirements
  - a. Pregnancy
  - b. Lactation
- ■ Blood loss
  - a. Gastrointestinal bleeding (especially due to ulcers or chronic aspirin use)
  - b. Menstrual losses
- ■ Chronic hemoglobinuria

---

ally fragile and thus have a shortened life span. Vitamin B_{12} deficiency anemia can occur when the amount of the vitamin in the diet is inadequate or, more commonly, when insufficient amounts are absorbed from the gastrointestinal tract.

Anemia caused by failure to absorb dietary vitamin B_{12} is called **pernicious anemia.** This form of anemia results from a lack of *intrinsic factor,* a substance secreted by the gastric mucosa. Intrinsic factor binds with dietary vitamin B_{12} and travels with it to the ileum, where the vitamin is absorbed. In the absence of intrinsic factor, dietary vitamin B_{12} cannot be absorbed into the body.

A vitamin B_{12} deficiency may also result from other malabsorption conditions and dietary factors. Vitamin B_{12} malabsorption can result from loss of the pancreas or ileum, from chronic gastritis, or following surgical procedures, such as gastrectomy. Dietary deficiencies of vitamin B_{12} are rare, usually occurring only among strict vegetarians.

As noted, a vitamin B_{12} deficit interferes with the maturation of red blood cells. Great numbers of large, immature RBCs pass into the circulation. These cells are fragile and incapable of carrying oxygen in adequate amounts. Laboratory examination therefore shows an increased MCV but a normal MCHC.

Individuals with vitamin B_{12} deficiency anemia gradually develop manifestations as bodily stores of the vitamin are depleted. The client may demonstrate pallor or slight jaundice and complain of weakness. Clients with pernicious anemia may develop a smooth, sore, beefy red tongue and diarrhea. Because vitamin B_{12} is important for proper neurologic functioning, the client may also experience *paresthesias* (altered sensations, such as numbness or

---

Causes of Folic Acid Deficiency Anemia

■ ■ ■

- Inadequate dietary intake
  At risk:
  a. Older adults
  b. Alcoholics
  c. Clients receiving total parenteral nutrition
- Increased metabolic requirements
  At risk:
  a. Pregnant women
  b. Infants
  c. Teenagers
  d. Clients undergoing hemodialysis
  e. Clients with forms of hemolytic anemia
- Folic acid malabsorption and impaired metabolism
  a. Celiac sprue
  b. Jejunitis
  c. Drug-induced malabsorption due to chemotherapeutic agents, folate antagonists (methotrexate, pentamidine), or anticonvulsants
  d. Alcoholism

---

tingling) in the extremities and have problems with *proprioception* (the sense of one's position in space). These manifestations may progress to difficulties in maintaining balance as a result of spinal cord damage.

Clients with anemia resulting from insufficient dietary intake of vitamin B_{12} are instructed to increase their intake of foods containing this vitamin, such as meats, eggs, and dairy products. In addition, vitamin B_{12} supplements may be ordered for severe cases of anemia or for clients who are vegetarians. Parenteral replacement of vitamin B_{12} is required for clients with malabsorption disorders or who lack intrinsic factor. Parenteral replacement therapy must be continued for life to prevent recurring anemia.

Folic Acid Deficiency Anemia   Folic acid is absorbed from the intestines and is found in green leafy vegetables, fruits, cereals, and meats. Like vitamin B_{12}, folic acid is required for DNA synthesis and the normal maturation of red blood cells. Folic acid deficiency produces an anemia characterized by fragile, megaloblastic cells.

Folic acid deficiency anemia is more likely to occur among people who are chronically undernourished. This group includes older adults, alcoholics, and the drug addicted. Alcoholics are especially at risk because alcohol suppresses the metabolism of folate, from which folic acid is formed. People receiving total parenteral nutrition (TPN) also are at risk of folate deficiency.

Clients with increased metabolic requirements also may develop folic acid deficiency anemia. In this group, pregnant women are most at risk. Infants and teenagers can develop temporary folic acid deficiencies during periods of rapid body growth. Clients undergoing hemodialysis and clients with certain hemolytic anemias (see the discussion later in this chapter) also may develop folic acid deficiency anemia.

An additional group of causes of folic acid deficiency anemia includes malabsorption and impaired metabolism of the nutrient. Malabsorption disorders known to trigger folic acid deficiency anemia include celiac sprue (a hereditary gastrointestinal disorder characterized by the inability to metabolize amino acids found in gluten) and jejunitis. Clients taking certain medications, such as methotrexate or various chemotherapeutic agents, are also at risk. The causes of folic acid deficiency anemia are summarized in the accompanying box.

The manifestations develop gradually as bodily stores of folic acid are depleted. Assessment findings may include pallor, progressive weakness and fatigue, shortness of breath, and cardiac palpitations. Gastrointestinal manifestations are similar to but usually more severe than those associated with vitamin B_{12} anemia; glossitis, cheilosis, and diarrhea are common. The neurologic impairment seen in vitamin B_{12} deficiency anemia (paresthesias and altered proprioception) are not found in folic acid deficiency and thus help to differentiate the two conditions. However, folic acid and vitamin B_{12} anemias are sometimes coexistent, complicating the diagnosis.

Among the undernourished, adding foods containing folic acid to the client's diet usually is sufficient to eliminate the condition. For clients experiencing malabsorption or impaired folic acid metabolism, however, oral folic acid supplements are necessary. The duration of folate replacement therapy varies according to the cause of the deficiency. Clients with malabsorption-related folate deficiency or with long-term heightened metabolic demand for folic acid may need to take oral supplements indefinitely.

Hemolytic Anemias

Hemolytic anemias are characterized by the premature destruction of RBCs, usually accompanied by retention in the plasma of iron and other by-products of RBC destruction. The breakdown of RBCs may occur within the circulatory system or as a result of phagocytosis by cells of the reticuloendothelial system. In response to this process, the bone marrow increases its hematopoietic activity, resulting in increased numbers of reticulocytes in the circulating blood. Most forms of hemolytic anemia are characterized by the prevalence of normocytic and normochromic RBCs.

There are many different causes of hemolytic anemias. The condition may arise from disorders within the RBC

Causes of Hemolytic Anemia

■ ■ ■

Intrinsic

- RBC cell-membrane defects
- Hemoglobin structure defects (e.g., sickle cell anemia, thalassemia)
- Inherited enzyme defects (e.g., G6PD deficiency)

Extrinsic

- Drugs
- Chemicals
- Toxins and venoms
- Bacterial and other infections
- Trauma
- Mechanical factors (prosthetic heart valves)
- Burns

itself (intrinsic causes) or originate from factors outside the RBC. Disorders within the RBC include cell membrane defects, defects in hemoglobin structure and function, and inherited enzyme deficiencies. Disorders outside the RBC that cause hemolytic anemia include drugs, bacterial and other toxins, and trauma. (See the accompanying box.) The forms of hemolytic anemia discussed in this section are sickle cell anemia, thalassemia, acquired hemolytic anemia, and glucose-6-phosphate dehydrogenase anemia.

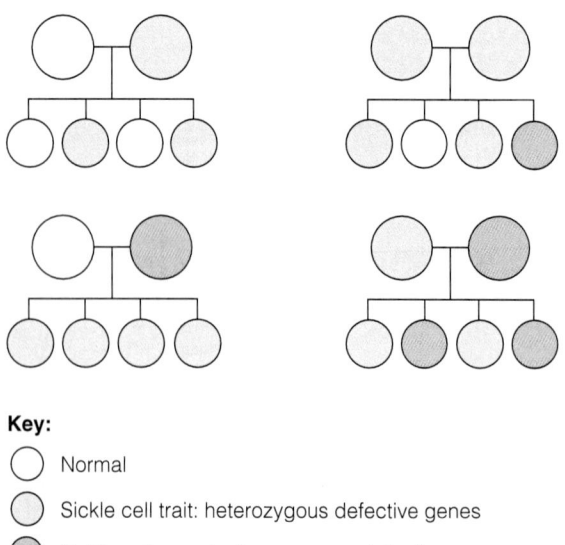

Key:

○ Normal

◔ Sickle cell trait: heterozygous defective genes

◉ Sickle cell anemia: homozygous defective genes

Figure 31–6   Inheritance pattern for sickle cell anemia.

Sickle Cell Anemia   **Sickle cell anemia** is a hereditary, chronic form of hemolytic anemia. It is characterized by episodes in which RBCs become abnormally crescent shaped. The disorder is caused by an autosomal genetic defect that results in the synthesis of an abnormal form of hemoglobin (hemoglobin S) within the red blood cells. This disorder usually causes death between 20 and 40 years of age due to multisystem organ failure.

The disease is most common among people of African descent. The inheritance pattern for sickle cell anemia is shown in Figure 31–6. Approximately 8% of African Americans are heterozygous for sickle cell anemia; that is, they have inherited one abnormal gene from one of their parents. These individuals are said to have *sickle cell trait.* They are likely to remain asymptomatic unless they are stressed by conditions causing severe hypoxia. Another 1% of African Americans are homozygous for the disorder; that is, they have inherited a defective gene from both parents. These individuals are at risk of developing the manifestations of sickle cell anemia. They are especially likely to experience **sickle cell crisis**, the severe episodes of fever and intense pain that are the hallmark of this disorder.

The genetic defect responsible for sickle cell anemia produces a mutation in the beta chain of the hemoglobin molecule, causing an abnormal structure. During conditions causing decreased oxygen tension in the plasma, the hemoglobin S within the RBCs causes them to elongate, become rigid, and assume a crescent or sickle shape. As a result, the sickled cells tend to clump together and obstruct capillary blood flow, causing ischemia and possible infarction of surrounding tissue.

As normal oxygen tension is restored, the sickled RBCs tend to resume their normal shape; that is, they "unsickle." Repeated episodes of sickling and unsickling weaken the RBC cell membranes. The weakened RBCs are hemolyzed and removed. Consequently, the normal life span of RBCs is greatly reduced in sickle cell anemia, increasing the demands on the bone marrow for RBC replacement. Conditions likely to trigger a sickling event include hypoxia, low environmental or body temperature, excessive exercise, anesthesia, dehydration, infections, or acidosis.

The acute and chronic manifestations of sickle cell anemia arise from repeated episodes of RBC sickling. The event is marked by the abrupt onset of intense pain, usually in the abdominal region, but the chest, back, and joints of the extremities may also be affected. On rare occasions, sickle cell crisis may localize in the central nervous system, causing seizures or stroke. This type of sickle cell crisis can be rapidly fatal.

Apart from sickling crises, clients with sickle cell anemia are likely to present with the classic manifestations of anemia. Because of damage to the spleen and hematopoi-

Pathophysiology Illustrated
Sickle Cell Anemia

Hemoglobin S and Red Blood Cell Sickling

Sickle cell anemia is caused by an inherited autosomal recessive defect in (Hb) synthesis. Sickle cell hemoglobin (Hb S) differs from normal hemoglobin only in the substitution of the amino acid valine for glutamine in both beta chains of the hemoglobin molecule.

When Hb S is oxygenated, it has the same globular shape as normal hemoglobin. However, when Hb S off-loads oxygen, it loses its solubility in the intracellular fluid and crystallizes into rod-like structures. Clusters of rods form polymers (long chains) that bend the erythrocyte into the characteristic crescent shape of the sickle cell.

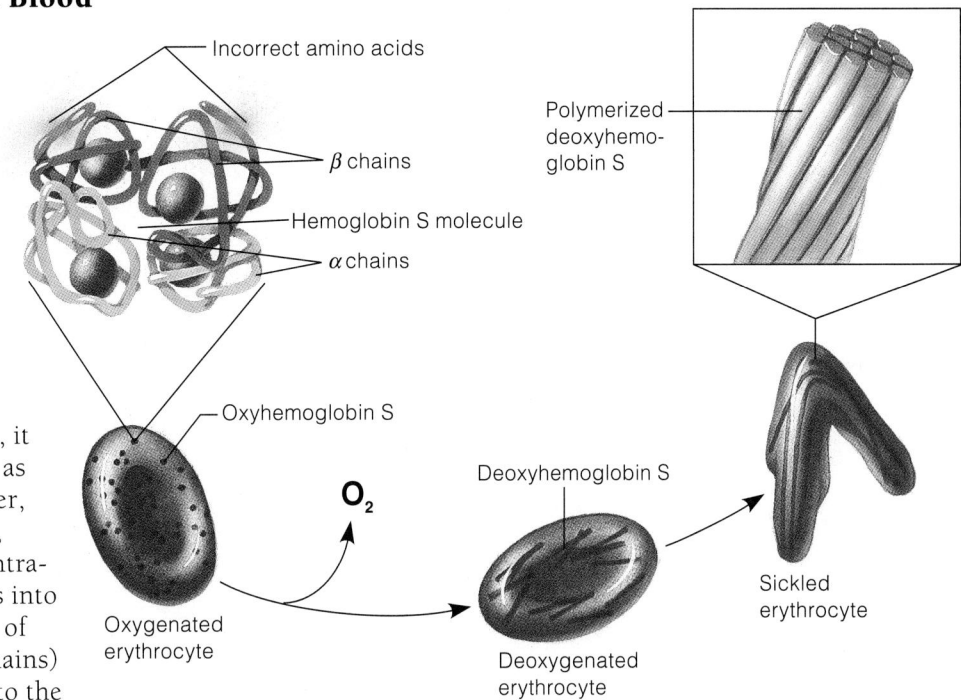

Incorrect amino acids

β chains

Hemoglobin S molecule

α chains

Polymerized deoxyhemoglobin S

Oxyhemoglobin S

Oxygenated erythrocyte

O₂

Deoxyhemoglobin S

Deoxygenated erythrocyte

Sickled erythrocyte

The Sickle Cell Disease Process

Sickle cell disease is characterized by episodes of acute painful crises. Sickling crises are triggered by conditions that cause high tissue oxygen demands or that alter cellular pH. As a sickle cell crisis begins, sickled erythrocytes adhere to capillary walls and to each other, obstructing blood flow and causing cellular hypoxia. The crisis accelerates as tissue hypoxia and acidic metabolic waste products cause further sickling and cell damage.

Sickle cell crises cause microinfarcts in joints and organs, and repeated crises slowly destroy organs and tissues. The spleen and kidneys are especially prone to sickling damage.

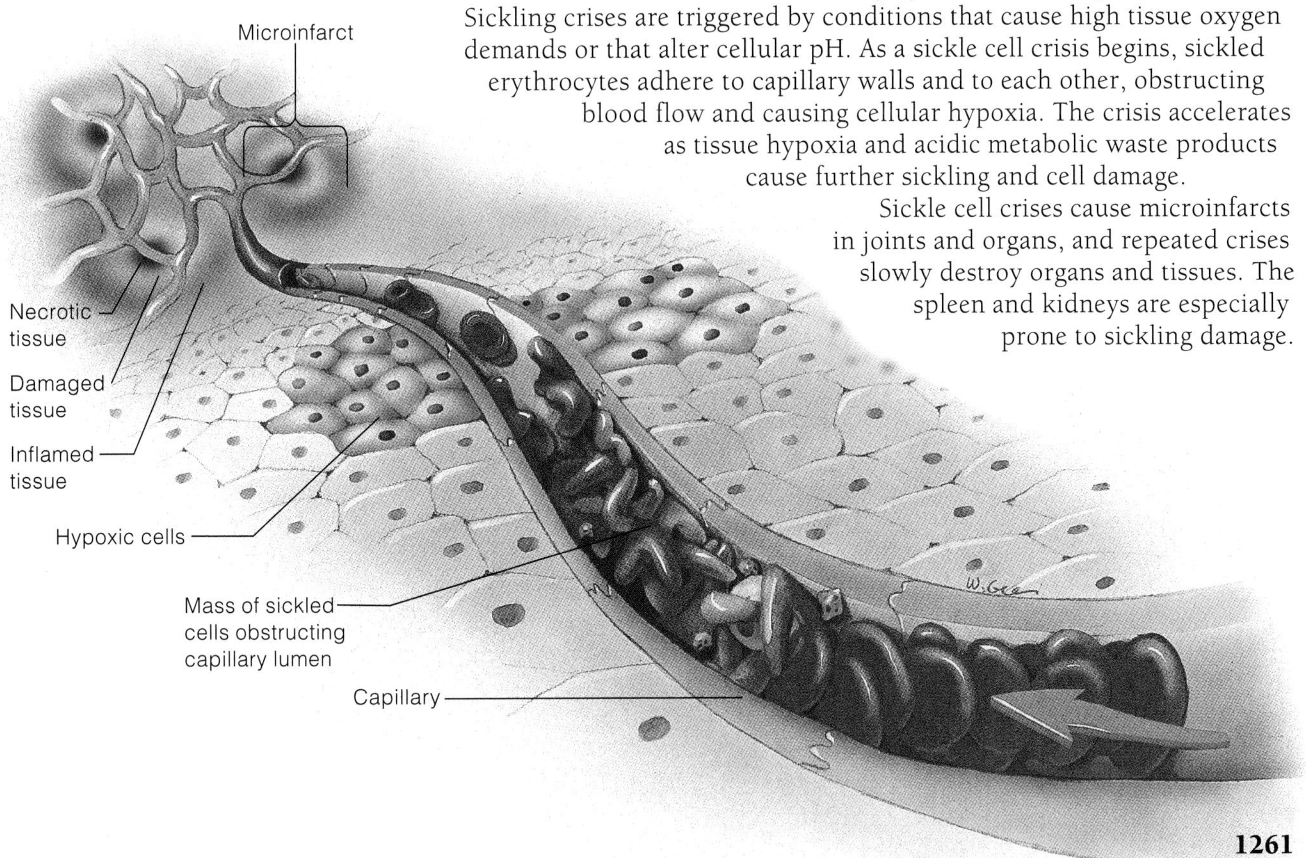

Microinfarct

Necrotic tissue

Damaged tissue

Inflamed tissue

Hypoxic cells

Mass of sickled cells obstructing capillary lumen

Capillary

Systemic Manifestations and Complications of Sickle Cell Anemia

■ ■ ■

Heart

- Heart murmurs
- Congestive heart failure

Genitourinary System

- Reduced urine concentration
- Hematuria
- Hyperuricemia
- Priapism

Liver and Gallbladder

- Hepatomegaly
- Hyperbilirubinemia
- Jaundice
- Hepatic abscesses and fibrosis
- Gallstones

Skeletal System

- Bone marrow aplasia
- Aseptic necrosis (particularly of the head of the femur)
- Osteomyelitis

Skin

- Ulcers (particularly in the lower extremities)

Eyes

- Vitreous hemorrhage
- Retinal detachment

electrophoresis, a test that determines the presence of hemoglobin S. (Electrophoresis can identify a specific protein by tracing its unique pattern of movement as a charged particle in an electric field.) The client with sickle cell anemia has a decreased hematocrit level as well as sickled cells on the smear.

There is no cure for this disease; treatment is primarily supportive. For clients who are experiencing a painful sickle cell crisis, treatment includes rest, oxygen, and analgesics for pain. Hydration therapy is essential to improve blood flow, reduce pain, and prevent renal damage. Treatment of precipitating factors, such as infections, may be undertaken. Folic acid supplements may be given daily to meet the increased metabolic demands of the bone marrow. Blood transfusions may be necessary for those undergoing surgery or for pregnant women. Genetic studies and counseling are recommended for people at risk for sickle cell anemia.

A Critical Pathway for the client with sickle cell crisis is provided on page 1264.

Thalassemia Thalassemia is an inherited disorder of hemoglobin synthesis in which either the alpha or beta chains of the hemoglobin molecule are missing or defective. The disease is characterized by deficient hemoglobin production and the development of fragile hypochromic, microcytic RBCs called *target cells* because of their distinctive "bull's-eye" appearance.

Thalassemia occurs most commonly in certain populations. People of Mediterranean descent (southern Italy and Greece) are more likely to have beta-defect thalassemias (often called *Cooley's anemia* or Mediterranean anemia). People of Asian ancestry, especially those from Thailand, the Philippines, and China, more commonly have alpha-defect thalassemia. Africans and African Americans can have both alpha- and beta-defect thalassemia. As with sickle cell anemia, the person with either form of thalassemia either may be heterozygous for the defect and have mild symptoms or may be homozygous for the trait and have more serious symptoms.

The manifestations of thalassemia depend on the severity of the resulting anemia, which in turn depends on the type of genetic defect producing the condition. People with mild thalassemia and essentially normal hemoglobin may have few if any symptoms.

People with severe forms of the disorder may have such pronounced symptoms that blood transfusions are needed to sustain life. Manifestations of thalassemia include enlargement of the liver and spleen from increased red cell destruction. Fractures of the long bones, ribs, and vertebrae may follow bone marrow expansion and thinning (as a result of increased hematopoiesis). The accumulation of iron in the heart, liver, and pancreas following repeated transfusions for treatment may eventually cause failure of these organs.

etic compartment, children with sickle cell anemia usually exhibit delayed growth and development. In adults, multiple infarcts can damage the anatomy and impair the physiology of nearly every organ system. The heart and lungs are most commonly affected, but the liver, skeleton, skin, and eyes also may become damaged over time from repeated infarctions. The chronic, organ-system-related complications of sickle cell anemia are listed in the accompanying box.

Sickle cell anemia is usually diagnosed during childhood. A definitive diagnosis can be made by *hemoglobin*

The disease is most often diagnosed during infancy or childhood. The adult with thalassemia usually has the milder form, although some children with more severe forms of thalassemia may live into their 20s. Genetic studies and counseling are recommended for people at risk for this illness.

Acquired Hemolytic Anemia   Acquired hemolytic anemia results from factors outside of the RBC that cause hemolysis. Causes of acquired hemolytic anemias include the following:

- Mechanical trauma of RBCs produced by prosthetic heart valves, severe burns, hemodialysis, or radiation
- Antibody reactions following infection by bacteria or protozoa
- Immune-system-mediated responses, such as transfusion reactions
- Drugs, toxins, chemical agents, or venoms

The manifestations of acquired hemolytic anemia depend on the degree of hemolysis as well as on how well the body responds in restoring destroyed RBCs. Commonly, the spleen enlarges as it removes large numbers of RBCs that are defective or have been destroyed. If heme-unit breakdown exceeds the ability of the liver to conjugate and excrete bilirubin, the client becomes jaundiced. If the condition is severe, bone marrow expands, and the bones become deformed or even may develop pathologic fractures. Cardiovascular and respiratory manifestations similar to those produced by other anemias may occur; their severity depends on the degree of anemia and deficiency of tissue oxygenation.

Acquired hemolytic anemias are diagnosed by the clinical manifestations, bone marrow studies, and blood tests. Treatment depends on the cause and may include blood transfusions, fluid and electrolyte replacements, removal of the spleen, and/or folate and steroid therapy.

Glucose-6-Phosphate Dehydrogenase Anemia   Glucose-6-phosphate dehydrogenase (G6PD) anemia is caused by a hereditary defect in RBC metabolism. The disorder is relatively common in people of African and Mediterranean descent. The defective gene is located on the X chromosome and therefore affects more males than females. There are many different variations of this genetic defect.

G6PD is an enzyme that is the initial catalyst in glycolysis, the process in which an RBC derives cellular energy. A defect in the action of G6PD causes direct oxidation of hemoglobin, which damages the RBC. Hemolysis usually occurs only after the susceptive person is exposed to stressors that increase the metabolic demands on RBCs. Stressors include certain drugs (aspirin, antimalarial drugs, sulfonamides, or vitamin K derivatives). The G6PD deficiency hinders the necessary compensating increase in glucose metabolism and results in cellular damage. The

damaged RBCs are destroyed over a period of 7 to 12 days.

The people exposed to a stressor that triggers G6PD anemia usually exhibit no symptoms initially. However, several days later the person may develop pallor, jaundice, hemoglobinuria (hemoglobin in the urine), and an elevated reticulocyte count. As new RBCs develop, counts return to normal.

Diagnosis is made by quantitative assay of G6PD levels. Treatment includes removing the causative agent and maintaining adequate hydration during an episode of hemolysis. Clients susceptible to G6PD anemia should be taught about drugs that may precipitate damage to the RBCs and to monitor for signs of anemia following a fever.

Bone Marrow Depression Anemia (Aplastic Anemia)

Bone marrow depression anemia, commonly called **aplastic anemia,** is a condition in which the bone marrow fails to produce RBCs. The underlying cause of aplastic anemia is unknown in two-thirds of the cases; in those circumstances, the disorder is referred to as idiopathic aplastic anemia. Aplastic anemia may also follow injury to the stem cells in bone marrow following exposure to radiation or certain chemical substances. Benzene, arsenic, nitrogen mustard, certain antibiotics (especially chloramphenicol), and chemotherapeutic drugs can cause aplastic anemia. Aplastic anemia may also develop concurrently with infections and is associated with mononucleosis, hepatitis C, and other viral illnesses (Porth, 1994). Anemia results as the bone marrow fails to replace RBCs that have reached the end of their life and are destroyed. The cells that remain in the blood are normochromic and normocytic.

People with aplastic anemia usually have *pancytopenia;* that is, they have decreased numbers of red blood cells, white cells, and platelets. The clinical manifestations of aplastic anemia may occur at any age, and they vary with the severity of the pancytopenia. The onset of the illness may be gradual or sudden, causing severe manifestations. Signs and symptoms include fatigue, pallor of the skin and mucous membranes, progressive weakness, exertional dyspnea, headache, and ultimately tachycardia and congestive heart failure. Platelet deficiency may cause bleeding problems. A deficiency of white blood cells increases the risk of infection. The diagnosis of aplastic anemia is based on an examination of bone marrow and the presence of pancytopenia.

Primary treatment modalities include removing the causative agent, if known, and using blood transfusion therapy. Transfusion therapy may be discontinued as soon as the client's bone marrow begins to produce red blood cells. Even after the cause has been eliminated, complete recovery may take months. Bone marrow transplant from siblings who have a close tissue match is the treatment of choice for some individuals.

Text continues on page 1268

Critical Pathway for Client with Sickle Cell Crisis

	Date _____ Day 1	Date _____ Day 2	Date _____ Days 3 to 4
	Expected length of stay: 6 to 8 days		
Daily outcomes	Client ■ Has stable vital signs. ■ Has an intake of 3000 mL/day. ■ Remains free of nausea and vomiting. ■ Verbalizes understanding of ongoing care. ■ Verbalizes control of pain and understanding of pain relief measures. ■ Demonstrates ability to cope with current hospitalization. ■ Has intact skin. ■ Maintains urine output above 30 mL/h.	Client ■ Has stable vital signs. ■ Has an intake of 3000 mL/day. ■ Remains free of nausea and vomiting. ■ Verbalizes understanding of ongoing care. ■ Verbalizes control of pain and understanding of pain relief measures. ■ Demonstrates ability to cope with current hospitalization. ■ Has intact skin. ■ Maintains urine output above 30 mL/h.	Client ■ Has stable vital signs. ■ Has an intake of 3000 mL/day. ■ Verbalizes understanding of ongoing care. ■ Verbalizes control of pain and understanding of pain relief measures. ■ Demonstrates ability to cope with current hospitalization and verbalizes ability to cope with chronic illness. ■ Verbalizes/demonstrates beginning understanding of home care instructions. ■ Has intact skin. ■ Maintains urine output above 30 mL/h.
Assessments, tests, and treatments	CBC with differential Chemistry profile Urinalysis Folic acid Reticulocyte count Chest X-ray film Vital signs q4h if stable Intake and output every shift Assess pallor, fatigue, and dyspnea on exertion. Assess pain: location, type, and severity. O$_2$ at 2 L/m. Transfuse as ordered. Pulse oximeter q4h and prn. Provide quiet, restful environment with dimmed lights. Protect client from exposure to infection. Pain management techniques, including massage, heat, relaxation, and guided imagery.	Vital signs q4h if stable Intake and output every shift O$_2$ at 2 L/m Pulse oximeter q4h and prn Assess pallor, fatigue, and DOE. Assess pain: location, type, and severity. Provide quiet, restful environment with dimmed lights. Protect from exposure to infection. Pain management techniques, including massage, heat, relaxation, and guided imagery.	CBC Routine vital signs Intake and output every shift O$_2$ at 2 L/m Pulse oximeter q4h and prn Assess pallor, fatigue, and DOE. Assess pain: location, type, and severity. Transfuse as ordered. Provide quiet, restful environment with dimmed lights. Protect from exposure to infection. Pain management techniques, including massage, heat, relaxation, and guided imagery.

	Date _____ **Day 1**	**Date _____** **Day 2**	**Date _____** **Days 3 to 4**
Knowledge deficit	Orient to room and hospital routine. Review plan of care. Include family in teaching. Assess understanding of teaching.	Review plan of care. Include family in teaching. Assess understanding of teaching.	Reinforce earlier teaching regarding ongoing care. Begin discharge teaching regarding rest, activity, and diet. Include family in teaching. Assess understanding of teaching.
Psycho-social	Assess level of anxiety. Encourage verbalization of concerns. Provide information. Provide ongoing support and encouragement.	Assess level of anxiety. Encourage verbalization of concerns. Provide information. Provide ongoing support and encouragement.	Encourage verbalization of concerns. Provide ongoing support and encouragement.
Diet	Regular diet: Encourage foods high in folic acid, iron, protein, minerals, and vitamins. Offer oral fluids qh.	Regular diet: Encourage foods high in folic acid, iron, protein, minerals, and vitamins. Offer oral fluids qh.	Regular diet: Encourage foods high in folic acid, iron, protein, minerals, and vitamins. Offer oral fluids qh.
Activity	Assess safety needs and provide appropriate precautions. Activity to tolerance, encouraging change of position. Provide rest periods. Encourage ROM exercises to unaffected joints.	Maintain safety precautions. Activity to tolerance, encouraging change of position. Provide rest periods. Encourage ROM exercises to unaffected joints.	Maintain safety precautions. Up ad lib to tolerance. Encourage rest periods. Encourage ROM exercises to unaffected joints.
Medications	IV fluids as ordered. IV antibiotics as ordered. Folic acid 1 mg PO qd. Colace 100 mg b.i.d. Motrin or Toradol as ordered. Narcotic analgesic via PCA q15min bolus $\times$ 24h. Antipyretics as ordered.	IV fluids as ordered. IV antibiotics as ordered. Folic acid 1 mg PO qd. Colace 100 mg b.i.d. Motrin or Toradol as ordered. Narcotic analgesic via PCA q20min bolus $\times$ 24h. Antipyretics as ordered.	IV fluids as ordered. IV antibiotics as ordered. Folic acid 1 mg PO qd. Colace 100 mg b.i.d. Motrin or Toradol as ordered. Narcotic analgesic via PCA q30min bolus $\times$ 24h. Narcotic analgesic via PCA q60min bolus $\times$ 24h. Antipyretics as ordered.
Transfer/ discharge plans	Establish discharge goals with client and significant other. Consult with social service re: VNA and projected needs for home health care (if any).	Review progress toward discharge goals with client and significant other.	Review progress toward discharge goals with client and significant other. Make appropriate referrals.

➤

	Critical Pathway for Client with Sickle Cell Crisis (continued)		
	Date _____ Day 5	Date _____ Day 6	Date _____ Days 7 to 8
Daily outcomes	Client ■ Has stable vital signs. ■ Has an intake of 3000 mL/day. ■ Verbalizes understanding of ongoing care. ■ Demonstrates ability to cope with current hospitalization and chronic nature of illness. ■ Verbalizes/demonstrates beginning understanding of home care instructions. ■ Has intact skin. ■ Maintains urine output above 30 mL/h.	Client ■ Has stable vital signs. ■ Has an intake of 3000 mL/day. ■ Verbalizes understanding of ongoing care. ■ Demonstrates ability to cope with current hospitalization and chronic nature of illness. ■ Verbalizes/demonstrates beginning understanding of home care instructions. ■ Has intact skin. ■ Maintains urine output above 30 mL/h. ■ Verbalizes willingness to follow treatment plan. ■ Verbalizes understanding of precipitating factors.	Client ■ Is afebrile and has stable vital signs. ■ Is independent in self-care. ■ Is fully ambulatory. ■ Has resumed preadmission urine and bowel elimination pattern. ■ Verbalizes/demonstrates home care instructions. ■ Tolerates ordered diet and has an intake of 3000 mL/day. ■ Demonstrates ability to cope with ongoing stressors. ■ Has intact skin. ■ Maintains urine output above 30 mL/h. ■ Identifies support system. ■ Verbalizes understanding of precipitating factors and plans to follow recommendations to prevent future episodes of sickle cell crisis.
Assessments, tests, and treatments	CBC Routine vital signs Discuss need to eat 3 to 4 regularly scheduled meals. Intake and output Assess pallor, fatigue, and DOE. Assess pain: location, type, and severity. O$_2$ at 2 L/m until pulse oximeter is above 93% on room air. Provide quiet, restful environment with dimmed lights. Protect client from exposure to infection. Pain management techniques, including massage, heat, relaxation, and guided imagery.	Routine vital signs Intake and output Assess pallor, fatigue, and DOE. Assess pain: location, type, and severity. O$_2$ at 2 L/m until pulse oximeter is above 93% on room air. Provide quiet, restful environment with dimmed lights. Protect client from exposure to infection. Pain management techniques, including massage, heat, relaxation, and guided imagery.	Routine vital signs CBC Protect from exposure to infection. Pain management techniques, including massage, heat, relaxation, and guided imagery.

	Date ——— **Day 5**	Date ——— **Day 6**	Date ——— **Days 7 to 8**
Knowledge deficit	Reinforce earlier teaching regarding ongoing care. Review written discharge instructions with client and significant other, including signs and symptoms requiring follow-up. Review the importance of avoiding infections, strenuous activity, stress, smoking, inadequate hydration, and exposure to cold. Include family in teaching. Assess understanding of teaching.	Reinforce earlier teaching regarding ongoing care. Include family in teaching. Assess understanding of teaching. Provide client with written discharge instructions.	Reinforce earlier teaching regarding ongoing care. Complete discharge teaching to include diet, follow-up care, signs and symptoms to report, activity, and medications: name, purpose, dose, frequency, route, food interactions, and side effects. Include family in teaching. Assess understanding of teaching. Provide client with written discharge instructions.
Psychosocial	Encourage verbalization of concerns. Provide ongoing support and encouragement.	Encourage verbalization of concerns. Provide ongoing support and encouragement.	Encourage verbalization of concerns. Provide ongoing support and encouragement.
Diet	Regular diet: Encourage foods high in folic acid, iron, protein, minerals, and vitamins. Encourage fluid intake of 3000 mL/day.	Regular diet: Encourage foods high in folic acid, iron, protein, minerals, and vitamins. Encourage fluid intake of 3000 mL/day.	Regular diet: Encourage foods high in folic acid, iron, protein, minerals, and vitamins. Encourage fluid intake of 3000 mL/day.
Activity	Self-care Fully ambulatory	Self-care Fully ambulatory	Self-care Fully ambulatory
Medications	D/C IV if PO intake is above 2000 mL/day. Folic acid 1 mg PO qd. Colace 100 mg b.i.d. Motrin or Toradol as ordered. Oral antibiotic as ordered. Narcotic analgesic via PCA: no bolus. Begin oral analgesic.	Folic acid 1 mg PO qd. Colace 100 mg b.i.d. Motrin or Toradol as ordered. Oral antibiotic as ordered. Taper narcotic analgesic via PCA: no bolus. Continue oral analgesic.	Folic acid 1 mg PO qd. Colace 100 mg b.i.d. Motrin or Toradol. Oral antibiotic as ordered. D/C PCA. Oral analgesics.
Transfer/ discharge plans	Continue to review progress toward discharge goals. Finalize discharge plans.	Finalize plans for home care if needed. Complete discharge teaching. Discuss referral to support group.	Finalize plans for home care if needed. Complete discharge teaching.

The author gratefully acknowledges Emily Dasch at the Medical College Hospitals in Toledo, Ohio, for her assistance in developing this pathway.

Collaborative Care

Treatment of the client with anemia is directed toward ensuring adequate tissue oxygenation. Individual treatment modalities are determined by the underlying cause of the disorder. Common treatments for clients with anemia include pharmacologic therapy, dietary modifications, blood replacement therapy, or supportive interventions. See the accompanying collaborative health care box on the client with sickle cell anemia.

Laboratory and Diagnostic Tests

When anemia is suspected, the following laboratory and diagnostic tests may be ordered:

- *Complete blood count (CBC)* is conducted to detect the abnormalities that are characteristic of many types of anemias.

- *Iron levels and total iron-binding capacity tests* are performed to detect abnormal values characteristic of iron deficiency anemia. If iron deficiency anemia is present, the serum iron concentration will be low, and the total iron-binding capacity will be elevated.

- *Serum ferritin* will be low as a result of a depletion of the total iron reserves available for hemoglobin synthesis. Ferritin is an iron-storage protein. It is produced by the liver, spleen, and bone marrow, and it is also released by tumor cells and inflamed tissues. Ferritin mobilizes stored iron from tissues when metabolic requirements are greater than dietary sources and stores excess iron to help prevent damage from excess iron in the blood.

- *Hemoglobin electrophoresis* may be performed if sickle cell anemia is suspected. A distinction between sickle cell trait and sickle cell anemia can be made with this test.

- *Hematocrit and blood smear studies* are conducted. The client with sickle cell anemia will demonstrate a low hematocrit.

- *Sickle-cell screening test* is conducted to determine the presence of hemoglobin S.

- *Schilling's test* (a test involving the ingestion of radioactive vitamin B_{12}) may be performed to determine the cause of vitamin B_{12} deficiency. If the client has pernicious anemia, radioactivity will be present in the measured 24-hour urine sample. If the problem is the result of an ileal or pancreatic defect, administration of supplemented digestive enzymes during the test will increase absorption of the radioactive vitamin B_{12} and decrease urine radioactivity.

- *Bone marrow examination* may be performed to assist in diagnosing aplastic anemia. In aplastic anemia, findings will demonstrate a severe decrease in normal marrow elements and their replacement by fat cells. Nursing implications for care of the client having a bone marrow study are described in the accompanying box.

- *Quantitative assay of G6PD* may be performed to confirm a diagnosis of glucose-6-phosphate dehydrogenase deficiency.

Pharmacology

The pharmacologic treatment of anemia is determined by the cause. Corticosteroid therapy and/or androgen therapy may be indicated for the client diagnosed with aplastic anemia. If other treatment modalities are unsuccessful, immunosuppressive therapy may be initiated. Iron deficiency anemia is treated by iron replacement therapy.

Collaborative Health Care: The Client with Sickle Cell Anemia

Health Care Team	Client-Centered Goals
Hematologist	Orders diagnostic evaluation including hemoglobin electrophoresis. Recommends that client avoid dehydration and hypoxia. Prescribes folic acid therapy. Monitors client's general health and assists client to manage minor crises at home. Manages more severe crises in the hospital with IV fluids, antibiotics (if indicated), and pain medications.
Social Worker	Assesses adequacy of support system and ability to manage chronic illness. Suggests resources to assist client and family to manage the chronic nature of illness. Refers client and family to support groups and suggests learning relaxation response and breathing exercises.
Dietitian	Provides teaching regarding the importance of a well-balanced diet rich in vitamins and minerals. Teaches strategies to ensure adequate fluid intake and to avoid dehydration. Discusses the importance of limiting alcohol intake.
RN and Health Care Team Communication	Reports signs and symptoms of infection, worsening pain, or stressful situations that contribute to current crisis to physician. Discusses strategies to manage stress with psychiatric nurse clinician or social worker. Provides members of the health care team with strategies to ensure quiet, restful environment and uninterrupted periods of rest. Identifies home care needs and discusses with social worker.

Nursing Implications for Diagnostic Tests: Bone Marrow Studies

■   ■   ■

Bone marrow studies are performed on specimens obtained by either aspiration or biopsy. The preferred site for a bone marrow aspiration is the posterior iliac crest; the sternum may also be used. The procedure is performed by inserting a needle into the middle of the bone and drawing out a sample of the blood in the marrow. A bone marrow biopsy is performed by making a small incision over the bone and screwing a core biopsy instrument into the bone to obtain a specimen. Bone marrow studies are used to diagnose leukemias, metastatic neoplasms, lymphoma, aplastic anemia, and Hodgkin's disease.

Preparation of the Client

- Assess for alterations in blood clotting.
- Explain the purpose and procedure of the test.
- Take and record vital signs.
- Ask the client to void.
- Provide privacy.
- Position the client in a supine position if the aspiration is to be obtained from the sternum or anterior iliac crest; position the client in the prone position if the posterior iliac crest is to be used.
- Assist the client in remaining still during the procedure.

After the Procedure

- Apply pressure to the puncture site for 5 to 10 minutes.
- Assess vital signs, and compare results to preprocedure readings.
- Apply a dressing to the puncture site, and monitor for bleeding and infection for 24 hours.

Client and Family Teaching

- The procedure (either aspiration or biopsy) takes about 20 minutes.
- A sedative may be given prior to the procedure.
- It is important to remain very still during the procedure to prevent accidental injury.
- Although the area will be anesthetized with a local anesthetic, the insertion of the needle will be painful for a short time. Taking deep breaths may make this part of the procedure less painful.
- The site of the aspiration may ache for a day or two.
- Report any unusual bleeding immediately.

Supplemental iron may be administered orally or intramuscularly. Vitamin B_{12} is given subcutaneously or intramuscularly to clients diagnosed with absorption disorders and those lacking intrinsic factor. Folic acid is administered orally or intramuscularly to the client with a folic acid deficiency or sickle cell anemia to meet the increased demands of the bone marrow. Nursing implications for the care of clients receiving iron, vitamin B_{12}, and folic acid are found in the pharmacology box on page 1270.

Dietary Modifications

Dietary modifications are indicated for the client with a nutritional deficiency anemia, such as iron deficiency anemia, vitamin B_{12} deficiency anemia, or folic acid deficiency anemia. Dietary sources of iron include red meats and organ meats. Dietary sources of vitamin B_{12} include liver, milk, most fish, and whole eggs or egg yolk. Fresh, dark green leafy vegetables are sources of folic acid. Selected sources of dietary iron, vitamin B_{12}, and folic acid are outlined in the box on page 1271.

Blood Transfusion Therapy

Blood transfusions may be indicated for clients with anemias resulting from a major blood loss, such as from trauma or major surgery, and are often used to treat severe anemia regardless of cause. Blood transfusions are fully discussed in Chapter 10.

Nursing Care

When caring for clients with various types of anemia, the nurse must consider client responses to a decrease in circulating oxygen and tissue oxygenation. Nursing diagnoses discussed in this section focus on problems resulting from activity intolerance, altered oral mucous membranes, and self-care deficits. The client with anemia is also at risk for insufficient cardiac output.

Nursing Implications for Pharmacology: The Client with Anemia

IRON SOURCES

Ferrous sulfate (Feosol, Fer-in-sol)

Ferrous gluconate (Fergon, Ferralet, Fertinic)

Iron dextran injection

Iron polysaccharide

Iron preparations are normally taken by mouth and are absorbed from the gastrointestinal tract. They are effective only in the treatment of anemias resulting from iron deficiency. When absorbed, iron combines with transferrin. This complex then is transported to the bone marrow and incorporated into hemoglobin.

Nursing Responsibilities

- Prior to administering the medication, assess for the use of drugs that might interact with iron (e.g., antacids, allopurinol, chloramphenicol, tetracyclines, vitamin E), evidence of gastrointestinal bleeding, and manifestations of anemia.

- Administer iron preparations with orange juice to enhance absorption.

- If using an elixir, administer it through a straw to prevent staining of teeth.

- Monitor for manifestations of iron toxicity: nausea, diarrhea, or constipation; symptoms of anaphylactic shock (extreme cases).

- Monitor hemoglobin and reticulocyte counts.

- If the client is also taking tetracyclines, schedule the dose of iron 2 hours before tetracycline (iron reduces the absorption of tetracycline).

Client and Family Teaching

- Gastrointestinal side effects may be decreased by taking iron with food (but not milk, which decreases absorption).

- Stools may be dark green or black, but this is harmless.

- Increase fluids and fiber in diet to decrease constipation.

VITAMIN B$_{12}$ SOURCES

Cyanocobalamin (Kaybovite [oral], Anacobin [parenteral], Bedoz)

Cyanocobalamin is used to treat Vitamin B$_{12}$ deficiencies or malabsorption and pernicious anemia. It is rapidly absorbed when administered orally or by injec-

tion, and it is stored in the liver. Intrinsic factor is necessary for absorption from the gastrointestinal tract.

Nursing Responsibilities

- Do not expose crystalline injection to light.

- Assess if client is taking other drugs that might interfere with response of cyanocobalamin: chloramphenicol decreases effectiveness, as does cimetidine, colchicine, and timed-release potassium.

- Do not mix cyanocobalamin in a syringe with other medications.

- Administer parenteral doses intramuscularly or deep subcutaneously to decrease local irritation.

- Monitor hemoglobin, RBC counts, reticulocyte counts, and potassium levels.

Client and Family Teaching

- The burning sensation that may occur with injection is temporary.

- Avoid alcohol, which interferes with absorption.

- If used to treat pernicious anemia, the medication must be taken for life.

FOLIC ACID SOURCES

Folic acid (Folvite, novofolacid)

Folic acid is necessary for normal red blood cell production and synthesis of nucleoproteins. Synthetic folic acid is absorbed from the gastrointestinal tract and stored in the liver. It is used to treat folic acid deficiency and megaloblastic or macrocytic anemia.

Nursing Responsibilities

- Prior to administering the medication, assess for concomitant use of drugs that alter its effectiveness: corticosteroids, methotrexate, oral contraceptives, phenytoin, sulfonamides.

- Do not mix folic acid with other medications in the same syringe.

- Monitor the client for possible hypersensitivity response of skin rash.

Client and Family Teaching

- Large doses of folic acid may cause the urine to become darker yellow.

- Excess alcohol intake increases folic acid requirements.

Sources of Dietary Iron, Folic Acid, and Vitamin B$_{12}$

Sources of Heme Iron

- Beef
- Chicken
- Egg yolk
- Clams, oysters
- Pork loin
- Turkey
- Veal

Sources of Nonheme Iron

- Bran flakes
- Brown rice
- Whole-grain breads
- Dried beans
- Dried fruits
- Greens
- Oatmeal

Iron from the diet comes from two sources. Heme iron makes up about one-half of the iron from animal sources. Nonheme iron makes up the other half of iron from animal sources and all the iron from plants, legumes, and nuts. Heme iron promotes the absorption of nonheme iron from other foods when both forms are consumed at the same time. The absorption of nonheme iron is also enhanced by vitamin C and inhibited by tea and coffee.

Sources of Folic Acid

- Green leafy vegetables
- Broccoli
- Organ meats
- Eggs
- Wheat germ
- Asparagus
- Liver
- Milk
- Yeast
- Kidney beans

Sources of Vitamin B$_{12}$

- Liver
- Fresh shrimp and oysters
- Eggs
- Milk
- Kidney
- Meats (muscle)
- Cheese

Activity Intolerance

The client with anemia experiences weakness and shortness of breath on exertion. These symptoms are associated with decreased levels of oxygen in circulation secondary to below-normal hemoglobin levels. As a result, the client may be unable to carry out activities of daily living—including those associated with self-care, home life, job performance, and social roles—without becoming dyspneic or experiencing changes in heart rate and rhythm. The client with anemia may experience weakness, fatigue, and/or vertigo during even normal activities of daily living.

Nursing interventions with rationales follow:

- Help the client and family identify ways to perform activities in a slower manner, in an alternative manner, or with assistance. *Modifying the approach to a particular activity may delay the development of cardiac and respiratory symptoms and activity-related fatigue. Alternative methods of task performance (e.g., sitting rather than standing when performing hygiene care and kitchen tasks) may reduce oxygen demands. Helping the client perform an activity will allow the client to conserve energy and experience fewer adverse symptoms.*

- Help the client and family establish priorities in tasks to be done. *Because family members may have to assume responsibility for tasks that the client is not able to perform, the success of the plan will depend on mutually established goals.*

- Help the client and family develop a schedule of activity for the client that alternates exercise with periods of rest throughout the day. *Rest periods will decrease oxygen use, thereby reducing strain on the heart and lungs, and allow the client to regain homeostasis before continuing with the activity.*

- Encourage the client to sleep 8 to 10 hours at night. *Rest decreases oxygen requirements and stress on the heart and lungs. By getting adequate rest, the client increases his or her chance of successfully completing the next morning's tasks.*

- Monitor the client's vital signs before and after each activity. *Comparison of preactivity and postactivity vital signs facilitates evaluation of activity tolerance.*

- Discontinue activity if any of the following occurs:
  a. Complaints of chest pain, breathlessness, or vertigo
  b. Palpitations or excessive increase in pulse rate that

does not return to normal within four minutes of resting

c. Decreased heart rate
d. Excessive increase in respiratory rate
e. Decreased respiratory rate
f. Decreased systolic blood pressure

These changes signify potential cardiac decompensation, which may be associated with insufficient oxygenation. To compensate for impaired oxygen-carrying capacity, the client needs to decrease the activity in intensity, duration, or frequency.

- Instruct the client not to smoke. *Smoking vasoconstricts blood vessels, further increasing cardiac workload and impairing tissue oxygenation.*

Altered Oral Mucous Membrane

Glossitis and cheilosis are associated with the nutritional deficiencies of iron, folate, and vitamin B_{12}. The tongue and lips become very red, and there may be fissures or cracks at the corners of the mouth.

Nursing interventions with rationales follow:

- Monitor the condition of the lips and tongue daily. *A worsening of glossitis and cheilosis places the client at risk for bleeding and infection and may indicate the need for medical intervention. If these areas cause pain and discomfort with eating, the client may decrease oral intake, further worsening the nutritional deficiency.*

- Use a mouthwash of saline, salt water, or half-strength peroxide and water to rinse the mouth every 2 to 4 hours. *This will clean and soothe the oral mucous membranes.*

- Provide frequent oral hygiene (after each meal and at bedtime) with a soft bristle toothbrush or sponge. *Removing food debris from painful fissures promotes comfort. A soft toothbrush is less likely to cause irritation or bleeding of the oral mucosa. Keeping the oral cavity clean also minimizes the risk of infection if the oral mucosa is not intact.*

- Instruct client not to use alcohol-based mouthwashes. *Alcohol is drying and will aggravate cracking of the mucous membranes.*

- Apply a petroleum-based lubricating jelly or ointment to the lips after oral care. *A lubricating ointment helps to retain moisture, facilitate healing, and protect the lips from other drying agents.*

- Instruct the client to avoid hot, spicy, or acidic foods. *Hot, spicy, or acidic foods may be irritating and drying to the mucous membranes.*

- Encourage the client to eat soft, cool, bland foods. *Foods that are soothing to the mucous membranes promote client comfort. The client is more apt to maintain adequate food and fluid intake if he or she does not experience pain when eating. Minimizing oral pain may also encourage compliance with oral care routines.*

- Encourage the client to eat daily four to six small meals with high protein and vitamin content. *The client whose oral mucous membranes are not intact may have difficulty eating and may better tolerate small, frequent meals. Increasing the nutritional adequacy of the meals will promote healing of the mucous membranes.*

Risk for Decreased Cardiac Output

The client with anemia is at risk for alterations in cardiac output. The heart pumps harder or faster to compensate for a decreased oxygen supply. This response can cause tachycardia, palpitations, dysrhythmias, chest pain, and eventual heart failure.

The body's inability to meet oxygen demands may also cause an increased respiratory rate and shortness of breath.

Nursing interventions with rationales follow:

- Monitor vital signs, including breath sounds, respiratory rate and effectiveness, and rate and rhythm of pulse. *In the client with anemia, the heart may pump harder or more rapidly in an attempt to compensate for the decrease in tissue oxygenation. This increase in cardiac activity can place stress on the heart, resulting in alterations in blood pressure, pulse rate and rhythm, and ability to pump. Respiratory rate may also increase as a compensatory mechanism to increase the delivery of oxygen to tissues. This contributes to dyspnea and orthopnea.*

- Assess for pallor, cyanosis, and dependent edema. *In clients with anemia, the blood vessels in the skin constrict, allowing blood to be shunted to vital organs. This compensating mechanism may cause pallor. Cyanosis, especially of the lips and nail beds, indicates venous distention and inadequate oxygenation of blood. Dependent edema occurs in response to right ventricular failure.*

- Stop activity for signs of decreased cardiac output. *When the client with anemia experiences signs of decreased cardiac output, current activity must be stopped so that the client can rest. Cessation of activity will decrease oxygen requirements and help alleviate cardiac strain.*

- Report signs of decreased cardiac output to the physician. *Signs of decreased cardiac output must be reported to the physician so that treatment orders can be adjusted. The client may require medical treatment for cardiac failure or a transfusion to improve oxygen-carrying capacity. The nurse's collaborative role in monitoring and reporting changes in client status to the physician is critical in securing appropriate treatment for the client in a timely manner and thus minimizing associated complications.*

Self-Care Deficit

In clients with anemia, energy expenditures necessary to perform activities of daily living (ADLs) may cause oxygen demands to exceed supply. For this reason, it is difficult for these clients to maintain self-care.

Nursing interventions with rationales follow:

- Determine with the client the significance of the inability to carry out self-care. *Dependence on others to carry out activities of daily living may signify a loss of control. As a result, the client may feel a loss of self-esteem.*

- Assist the client to perform ADLs, such as bathing, grooming, and eating. *Providing assistance decreases the client's energy expenditures and tissue requirements for oxygen, thereby decreasing cardiac workload.*

- Instruct the client and significant others in the importance of taking regular rest periods prior to performing such activities as dressing. *Rest reduces oxygen demand and cardiac workload. The person who is able to perform self-care in activities of daily living maintains independence, self-esteem, and morale.*

Other Nursing Diagnoses

Other nursing diagnoses that are appropriate for the client with anemia follow:

- *Anxiety* related to the effects of chronic illness
- *Altered Health Maintenance* related to the inability to independently care for self
- *Impaired Home Maintenance* management related to the inability to care independently for self and family
- *Risk for Injury* related to weakness secondary to decreased oxygen level
- *Pain* in the bones and sternum secondary to the attempt to increase the rate of RBC production
- *Risk for Impaired Tissue Integrity* related to decreased circulating oxygen or to impaired tissue oxygenation and increased skin fragility secondary to malnutrition

Client and Family Teaching

Clients with anemia of any type need guidance in home maintenance management. Clients with hereditary anemias, such as sickle cell anemia, must be educated about the inheritance patterns of the disorder, symptoms of crisis, and manifestations that signal the need to seek medical help. Referrals for counseling to facilitate decisions about pregnancy may be necessary. Clients with anemias resulting from dietary insufficiencies need instruction regarding proper dietary intake and prescribed medications.

Applying the Nursing Process

Case Study of a Client with Folic Acid Deficiency Anemia: Sheri Matthews

Sheri Matthews is a 76-year-old widow who lives alone. She states to her physician's nurse, Lisa Apana, RN, that she liked to cook when her husband was alive but that now preparing an entire meal just for herself seems senseless. Mrs. Matthews also tells Ms. Apana that a typical day's menu includes nothing for breakfast, a bologna sandwich and a cup of coffee for lunch, and a hot dog or two, a few cookies, and a glass of milk for dinner.

Assessment

The history for Mrs. Matthews indicates that she has lost 20 lb (9 kg) since her husband died 8 months ago. Physical assessment findings are as follows: T, 98.8 F (37.1 C); BP, 90/52; P, 110; R, 22. Her skin is warm, pale, and dry. She states that she sometimes has heart palpitations and always feels weak. Her diagnostic tests reveal the following abnormal results: macrocytosis, decreased reticulocyte count, abnormal platelets, and serum folate less than 4 mg/mL. The Schilling test and a therapeutic trial of vitamin B_{12} injections are instituted to distinguish between folic acid deficiency anemia and pernicious anemia. Results indicate the presence of folic acid deficiency anemia, and Mrs. Matthews is started on an oral folic acid supplement and is provided with dietary instruction about foods containing folic acid.

Diagnosis

Ms. Apana makes the following nursing diagnoses:

- *Activity Intolerance* related to weakness secondary to decreased tissue perfusion
- *Altered Nutrition: Less Than Body Requirements* related to lack of motivation to cook and an inadequate understanding of nutritional needs, as manifested by weight loss of 20 lb, and identified folic acid deficiency
- *Knowledge Deficit* about a well-balanced diet and foods containing folic acid

Expected Outcomes

The expected outcomes established in the plan of care specify that Mrs. Matthews will

- Gain at least 1 lb (0.45 kg) per week.
- Return to prior level of physical energy.
- Consume foods appropriate to achieving a balanced diet, including foods containing folic acid.
- Verbalize the importance of taking folic acid supplements and eating a balanced diet.

Planning and Implementation

Ms. Apana plans and implements the following interventions for Mrs. Matthews:

- Take and record her weight daily before breakfast.
- Discuss foods required for a well-balanced diet, as well as those that are sources of folic acid. Include in the dietary plan foods that Mrs. Matthews likes and that are easy and quick to prepare.

- Discuss the importance of taking the prescribed folic acid supplement. Advise Mrs. Matthews to continue taking it even after she begins to feel better.
- Help Mrs. Matthews develop a daily schedule of activities to ensure that she has adequate rest to complete the necessary cooking tasks.

Evaluation

Mrs. Matthews has gained 1 lb (0.45 kg) during the first week of therapy. She also has discussed proper dietary intake. She states that she feels better able to prepare hot meals when she schedules a rest period before and after her lunch. In addition, Ms. Apana has given her written and verbal information about her prescribed medication and diet. Mrs. Matthews verbalizes understanding, stating, "I will take my medicine and continue it until the doctor tells me to stop. I will also eat a well-balanced diet—making sure to include foods containing folic acid." Ms. Apana also makes a referral to a home health agency in the community to determine whether Mrs. Matthews is able to participate in the local "Meals on Wheels" program.

Critical Thinking in the Nursing Process

1. What is the pathophysiologic basis for Mrs. Matthew's abnormal vital signs during her initial assessment?

2. Design a week's menu that includes foods high in folic acid.

3. Why was Mrs. Matthews placed on a folic acid supplement in addition to dietary modifications?

4. Why is the older adult at increased risk for developing folic acid deficiency anemia? Consider physiologic, economic, and social factors.

5. Design a nursing care plan for Mrs. Matthews for *Risk for Injury* at her home.

The Client with Polycythemia

■ ■ ■

Polycythemia is a condition characterized by an excessive number of circulating red blood cells, as evidenced by an abnormally high total RBC mass.

Pathophysiology

The disorder has primary and secondary forms.

Primary Polycythemia

Primary polycythemia, also called *polycythemia vera (PV)* or *erythremia,* is a neoplastic stem cell disorder characterized by the overproduction of RBCs and, to a lesser extent, certain white blood cell elements. (For this reason,

---

Causes of Polycythemias

■ ■ ■

Primary Polycythemia (Polycythemia Vera)

- Idiopathic

Secondary Polycythemia

Abnormal Erythropoietin Secretion

- Erythropoietin-secreting tumors
  a. Renal cell carcinoma
  b. Hepatocelluar carcinoma
  c. Cerebellar hemangioblastoma
  d. Uterine leiomyomas
  e. Ovarian carcinoma
  f. Pheochromocytoma
- Renal diseases
  a. Cysts
  b. Hydronephrosis
  c. Parenchymal disease
  d. Renal transplantation
  e. Nephrotic syndrome
  f. Long-term hemodialysis
- Cushing's syndrome

Prolonged Hypoxemia

- High altitude
- Chronic lung disease
- Hypoventilation due to obesity
- Cardiovascular right-to-left shunting
- Hemoglobinopathies
- "Smoker's erythrocytosis"
- Familial (2,3-DPG) erythrocytosis

Note. Adapted from "Polycythemia: Evaluation and Management" by W. G. Hocking and D. W. Golde, 1989, *Blood Review,* 3(59).

PV sometimes is classified as a *myeloproliferative disorder.*) The condition is relatively rare but is most common in Caucasian men of European Jewish ancestry. PV has a gradual onset, usually beginning between the ages of 40 and 60. Its cause has not been established, but it seems to occur when erythroid stem cells develop a hypersensitivity to erythropoietin, the hormone that stimulates RBC production.

PV begins without symptoms, and clients are often diagnosed during routine blood tests. The manifestations that do finally appear are related to hypervolemia; for example, clients may complain of headaches, dizziness, tinnitus, and blurred vision, and many clients may present with hypertension. Thrombosis and platelet dysfunction may lead to bruising, gastrointestinal bleeding and ulcers, epistaxis, severe pruritus, and foot pain. The condition also triggers hypermetabolism, which may be manifested by weight loss and sweating.

Clients with symptomatic PV often present with cyanosis and **plethora** (engorged or distended blood vessels). Distended retinal veins are a common finding. Most clients with PV develop splenomegaly, a manifestation that helps differentiate the disorder from secondary polycythemia. Late complications of PV are related to splenomegaly and fibrosis of the bone marrow.

Without treatment, up to half of clients with PV die within 18 months of the onset of the disorder (McCance & Huether, 1993). With effective therapy, however, clients often survive as long as 12 years from the time of diagnosis. Vascular complications are the usual cause of death in clients with PV.

Secondary Polycythemia

Secondary polycythemia, or *erythrocytosis,* is excess erythropoiesis that arises as a response to either an abnormal increase in the secretion of erythropoietin or to prolonged hypoxemia. Secondary polycythemia is the most common form of polycythemia.

Abnormally high levels of erythropoietin can result from erythropoietin-secreting tumors. Secondary polycythemia also may occur as a consequence of Cushing's syndrome (see Chapter 20) as well as from a host of renal disorders that stimulate erythropoietin release. Clients undergoing long-term hemodialysis also may develop the disorder.

Abnormally high levels of erythropoietin may also be due to hypoxemia caused by prolonged exposure to high altitudes or systemic disorders that adversely affect oxygenation, including chronic lung diseases and congenital heart defects. The condition also may arise from a number of genetic defects that result in abnormal forms of hemoglobin. Finally, the morbidly obese and long-term smokers can develop forms of secondary polycythemia. The causes of primary and secondary polycythemia are summarized in the accompanying box.

The manifestations of secondary polycythemia are the same as those of primary polycythemia, with an important exception: the absence of splenomegaly. Early symptoms may be masked or overshadowed by the manifestations of the underlying disorder causing secondary polycythemia. The clinical manifestations of primary and secondary polycythemia are summarized in the accompanying box.

Collaborative Care

For PV, laboratory tests usually reveal below-normal erythropoietin levels, and bone marrow studies show hyperplasia of all hematopoietic elements. For secondary

---

Clinical Manifestations of Polycythemias

- Hypertension
- Headache
- Tinnitus
- Blurred vision
- Dusky cyanosis: dark redness of the lips, feet, ears, fingernails, and mucous membranes
- Plethora
- Splenomegaly (polycythemia vera)
- Severe pruritus
- Pain (especially in the fingers and toes)
- Weight loss
- Night sweats
- Epistaxis
- Gastrointestinal bleeding
- Intermittent claudication
- Symptoms from thrombosis within various organs

---

polycythemia, in contrast, erythropoietin levels usually are elevated. Bone marrow studies for secondary polycythemia usually reveal only red stem cell hyperplasia.

The treatment of polycythemia focuses on reducing blood viscosity and volume and relieving symptoms. Phlebotomy, which is accomplished by removing 300 to 500 mL of blood through a vein, can be performed repeatedly to keep blood volume and viscosity within normal levels. For PV, radioactive phosphorus or chemotherapeutic agents such as melphalan or chlorambucil can be used to suppress marrow function but may increase the risk of developing leukemia (discussed in the next section). Systemic symptoms, such as pruritus, may be relieved by antihistamines or phenothiazines.

Nursing Care

Nursing care focuses on teaching the client and family the importance of maintaining adequate hydration and taking measures to prevent blood stasis: elevating the lower extremities when sitting, using support stockings, and following and complying with medical therapy. To smokers, emphasize the importance of smoking cessation. Advise the client to report any abnormal bleeding immediately. In addition, monitor the platelet count and CBC prior to and during myelosuppressive chemotherapy.

Examples of nursing diagnoses appropriate for the client with polycythemia follow:

- *Anxiety* related to lack of knowledge about the disease process and treatment
- *Impaired Gas Exchange* (hypoxia) related to hyperviscosity of blood
- *Pain* (headache) related to hypervolemia and hyperviscosity of blood
- *Fluid Volume Deficit* related to increase in red blood cells, hypermetabolism, and night sweats

- *Risk for Infection* related to treatment-induced myelosuppression

In addition, the client with polycythemia faces the following potential complication:

- *Potential Complication: Hemorrhage* related to capillary distention and hypercongestion of tissues and organs

▜ ▜ ▜ Platelet and Coagulation Disorders ▜ ▜ ▜

Disorders of platelets and coagulation affect *hemostasis,* the stoppage of bleeding. Through hemostasis, a series of complex events involving platelets and activation of the clotting mechanism maintains a relatively steady state of blood volume, blood pressure, and blood flow through injured blood vessels. An understanding of platelets and coagulation is necessary to understand the body's response to these disorders.

Overview of Platelets and Hemostasis

▪ ▪ ▪

Platelets

Platelets are formed elements found in the blood. They are small fragments of cytoplasm without nuclei that contain many granules. Platelets are formed in the bone marrow as pinched-off portions of large cells called megakaryocytes (Figure 31–1). There are about 250,000 to 400,000 platelets in each milliliter of blood. The production of platelets is controlled by a substance called thrombopoietin. The source of thrombopoietin is not known, but the number of platelets in production and in the circulation appears to control its release (Porth, 1994). Platelets live approximately 10 days in the circulating blood.

Normally, from 30% to 40% of the platelets that are produced in the bone marrow are stored in the spleen before being released into the circulation. However, when the spleen is enlarged, it may hold up to 80% of the platelets, greatly decreasing the number available for coagulation (Porth, 1994). An excess of platelets is *thrombocytosis.* A deficit of platelets is *thrombocytopenia.*

Hemostasis

Hemostasis, or blood clotting, is a complex process initiated within the body to stop bleeding. However, it may become a health problem when it occurs without the need to stop bleeding or when the clotting is not adequate to stop bleeding. There are five stages in hemostasis: (1) vessel spasm, (2) formation of the platelet plug, (3) development of an insoluble fibrin clot, (4) clot retraction, and (5) clot dissolution (Porth, 1994, pp. 312–315).

Vessel Spasm

When a blood vessel is damaged, a substance called thromboxane A_2 is released from platelets and contributes to vessel spasm. This spasm, which lasts for more than a minute, constricts the vessel and reduces blood flow.

Formation of the Platelet Plug

Platelets are attracted to the damaged vessel wall and change in form from smooth disks to spiny spheres. They form the platelet plug by adhering to the vessel wall and to one another (Figure 31–7). Adhesion is made possible by platelet receptor sites and von Willebrand's factor. Aggregation of platelets is made possible by agents such as adenosine diphosphate (a compound), thrombin (an enzyme), and thromboxane A_2, which stimulate the formation of a meshwork as bridges of fibrinogen attach platelets to each other. The plug is cemented together by fibrin, which is converted from fibrinogen by thrombin released by the platelets (Figure 31–8). The plug is now stable. People who have defective receptor sites or lack von Willebrand's factor do not form normal platelet plugs and have bleeding problems.

Blood Coagulation

Coagulation is a process in which fibrin strands form to create a meshwork that cements the blood components together to form an insoluble clot. The process may involve dozens of different biochemical processes, and two different clotting pathways (Figure 31–9). The *intrinsic pathway* is activated by injury to vessels; the *extrinsic pathway* is activated by blood leaking out of the vessel into the tissues. However, in either case the final outcome is the formation of the fibrin clot. Each of the substances that promotes clotting is activated in a specific sequence; the activation of one coagulation factor activates another in turn. Table 31–3 lists the known factors, their origin, and their function or pathway. Abnormal clotting occurs when there is a deficiency in one or more of the factors or when abnormal physiologic conditions cause inappropriate activation of any of the factors.

Clot Retraction

After the clot is stabilized (i.e., after about 30 minutes), the platelets trapped within the clot begin to contract, much like muscle cells. The platelet contraction squeezes the fibrin strands, pulling the broken portions of the ruptured blood vessel closer together. At the same time, growth factors released from within the platelets stimulate cell division and tissue repair in the damaged vessel.

Clot Dissolution

A process called **fibrinolysis** removes the clot after tissue repair has occurred. Without this process, the body's blood vessels would gradually become obstructed by clots. Plasminogen incorporated within the clot is transformed into plasmin by chemical signals released from surrounding tissue and from within the clot itself. Plasmin, an enzyme, dissolves the clot's fibrin strands as well as certain coagulation factors. Fibrinolysis begins within a few days of clot formation and continues until the clot is dissolved.

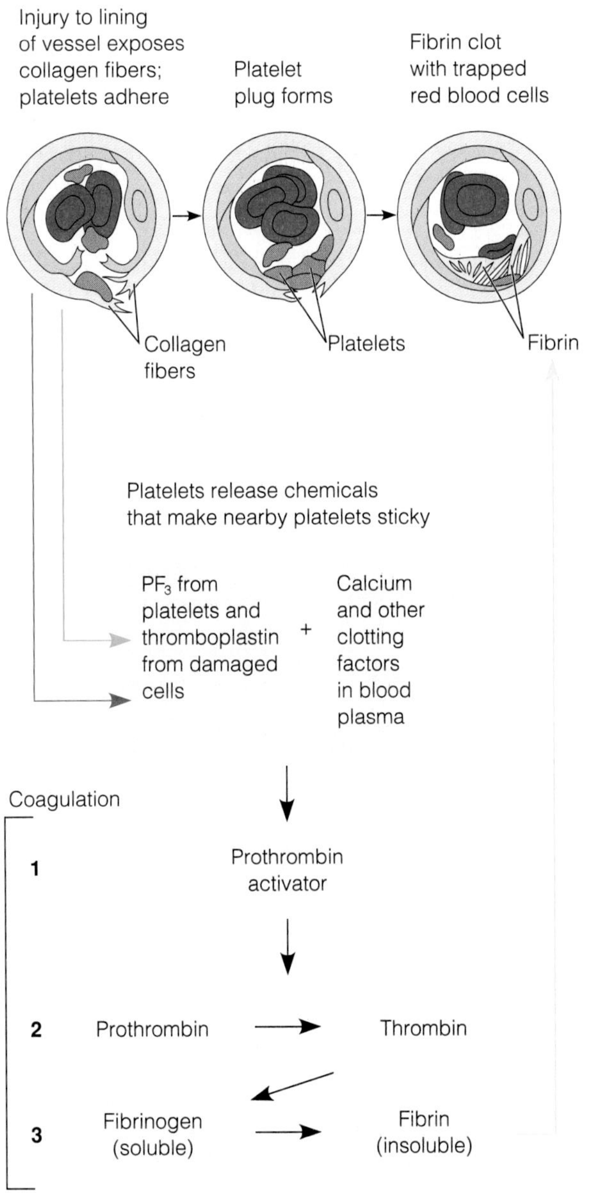

Injury to lining of vessel exposes collagen fibers; platelets adhere

Platelet plug forms

Fibrin clot with trapped red blood cells

Collagen fibers

Platelets

Fibrin

Platelets release chemicals that make nearby platelets sticky

PF₃ from platelets and thromboplastin from damaged cells

+

Calcium and other clotting factors in blood plasma

Coagulation

1 Prothrombin activator

2 Prothrombin → Thrombin

3 Fibrinogen (soluble) → Fibrin (insoluble)

Figure 31–7   Platelet plug formation and blood clotting. The flow diagram beneath the blood vessel cross sections encapsulates the events leading to the formation of a fibrin clot. PF₃ (blue arrow) released from damaged tissue combines with other clotting factors to release prothrombin activator, the first step of coagulation. Second, prothrombin is converted into thrombin. Finally, thrombin transforms soluble fibrinogen into insoluble fibrin (yellow arrow), the substance that forms clots.

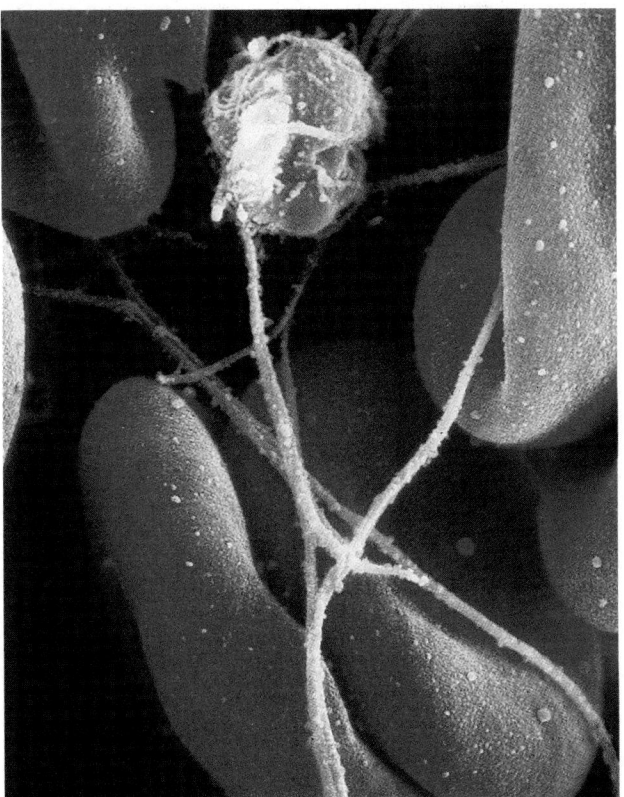

Figure 31–8   Scanning electron micrograph of a RBC trapped in a fibrin mesh. The spherical gray object at top is a platelet.

Intrinsic Pathway

Figure 31–9 Flow diagram of factor activation leading to clot formation. Clotting may be mediated by chemical factors in either of two independent pathways: the longer intrinsic pathway and the "short-cut" extrinsic pathway. Both pathways eventually activate factor X, which begins the series of events leading to clot formation. Once factor X is activated, four sequential steps occur: (1) Factor X combines with other factors to form prothrombin activator; (2) prothrombin activator transforms prothrombin into thrombin; (3) thrombin transforms fibrinogen into long fibrin strands; and (4) thrombin also activates factor XIII, which draws the fibrin strands together into a dense meshwork. The complete process of clot formation occurs within 3 to 6 minutes after blood vessel damage.

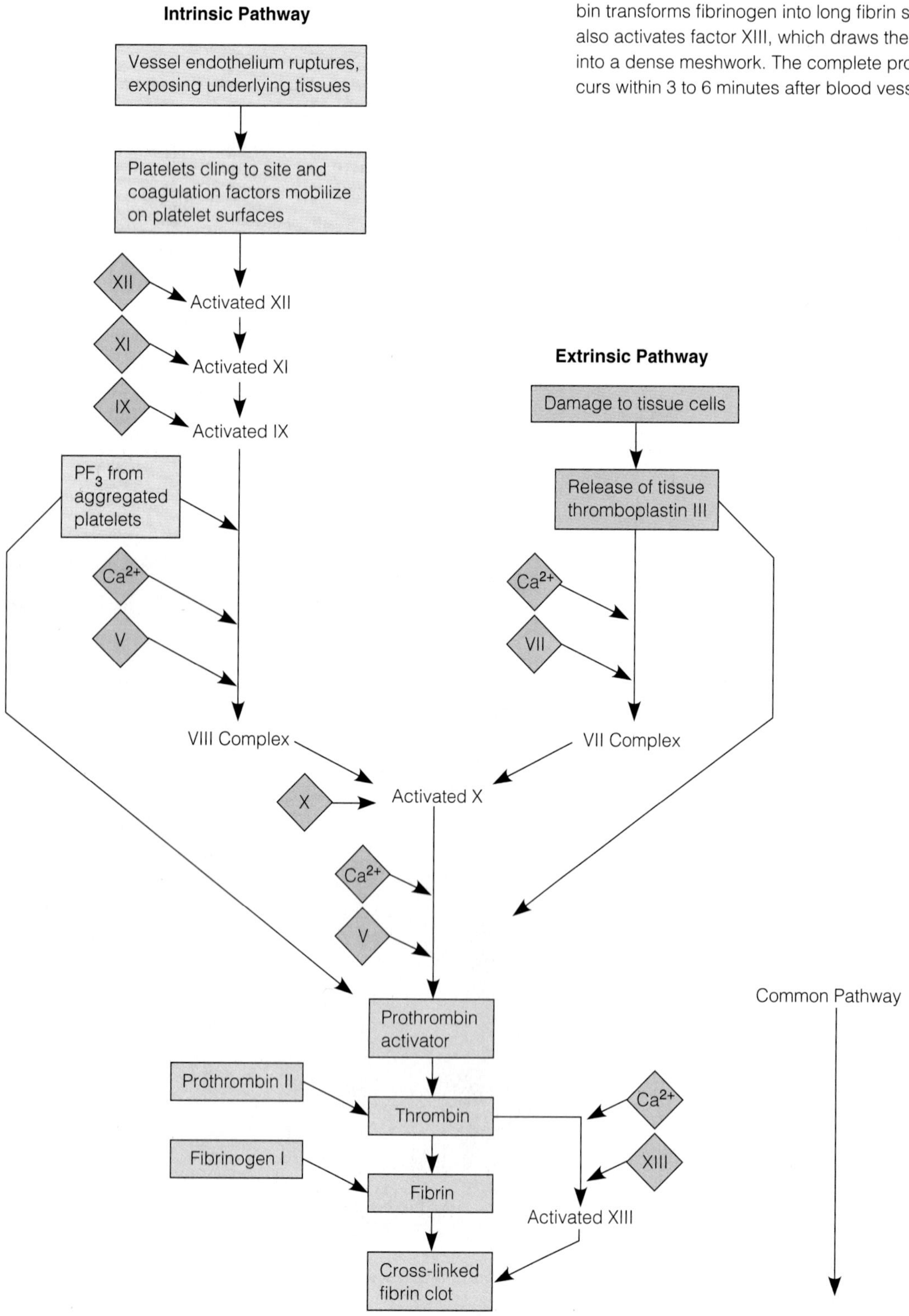

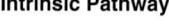

Vessel endothelium ruptures, exposing underlying tissues

Platelets cling to site and coagulation factors mobilize on platelet surfaces

XII → Activated XII

XI → Activated XI

IX → Activated IX

PF$_3$ from aggregated platelets

Ca^{2+}

V

VIII Complex

Extrinsic Pathway

Damage to tissue cells

Release of tissue thromboplastin III

Ca^{2+}

VII

VII Complex

X → Activated X

Ca^{2+}

V

Common Pathway

Prothrombin activator

Prothrombin II

Thrombin

Ca^{2+}

XIII

Fibrinogen I

Fibrin

Activated XIII

Cross-linked fibrin clot

Table 31–3	Blood Coagulation Factors		
Factors	**Name**	**Origin**	**Function or Pathway**
I	Fibrinogen	Liver	Converted to fibrin strands
II	Prothrombin	Liver	Converted to thrombin
III	Thromboplastin	Damaged tissue	Catalyzes conversion of thrombin
IV	Calcium ions	Skeletal compartment	Needed for all steps of coagulation
V	Proaccelerin	Liver and platelets	Extrinsic/intrinsic pathways
VII	Serum prothrombin conversion accelerator	Liver	Extrinsic pathway
VIII	Antihemophilic factor	Liver	Intrinsic pathway
IX	Plasma prothrombin component	Liver	Intrinsic pathway
X	Stuart factor	Liver	Extrinsic/intrinsic pathways
XI	Plasma prothrombin antecedent	Liver	Intrinsic pathway
XII	Hageman factor	Unknown	Intrinsic pathway
XIII	Fibrin stabilizing factor	Unknown	Cross-links fibrin strands to form insoluble clot

The Client with Thrombocytopenia

■ ■ ■

Thrombocytopenia is a platelet count of less than 100,000 platelets per milliliter of blood. This disorder is the most common cause of abnormal bleeding. As the number of circulating platelets continues to decrease, falling below 10,000/mL to 20,000/mL, hemorrhage from minor trauma as well as spontaneous internal or external bleeding is likely. If the platelet count falls below 10,000/mL, serious bleeding results and may be fatal if it occurs in the brain, gastrointestinal tract, or lungs.

Pathophysiology

There are two types of thrombocytopenia: primary idiopathic thrombocytopenia purpura and secondary (or acquired) thrombocytopenia.

Idiopathic Thrombocytopenia Purpura

Idiopathic thrombocytopenia purpura (ITP) is an acute or chronic condition in which the destruction of platelets is greatly accelerated. It is believed that the body's immune system destroys the platelets; ITP is therefore categorized as an autoimmune disorder. Acute ITP is most common in children and young adults and is often preceded by a viral infection. Chronic ITP is most common in women between the ages of 20 and 50 and has no known precipitating factors.

In ITP, the platelets become coated with antibodies as a result of the autoimmune response mediated by B lymphocytes (see Chapter 8). Although the platelets function normally, the spleen reacts to them as "foreign" and destroys the altered platelets after only 1 to 3 days of circulation.

The manifestations of ITP are the result of the escape of blood into the tissues and most often involve the skin and mucous membranes. The client has *purpura* (hemorrhage into the tissues evidenced by bruises), *ecchymoses* (flat or raised areas of discoloration of the skin or mucous membranes caused by subcutaneous bleeding), and *petechiae* (small, flat, purple, or red spots on the skin or mucous membranes caused by minute hemorrhages into the dermis or submucous layer). These signs of ITP are most often seen on the anterior thorax, arms, and neck. Other common types of bleeding are epistaxis, menorrhagia (prolonged and heavy menstrual periods), hematuria, and gastrointestinal bleeding. Spontaneous bleeding of cerebral vessels is rare but does occur.

Secondary Thrombocytopenia

Secondary thrombocytopenia (also called *thrombocytopathia*) is a condition in which there is a defect in platelet production. The platelet production defect is caused by drug hypersensitivities, viral infections, bacterial infections, some autoimmune disorders, and bone marrow disorders. The disorders and drugs that may cause secondary thrombocytopenia are listed in the box on page 1280.

Causes of Secondary Thrombocytopenia

■ ■ ■

Diseases

- Vitamin B$_{12}$ anemia
- Folic acid anemia
- Aplastic anemia
- Leukemia
- Alcoholism
- DIC
- Infectious mononucleosis
- Viral infections
- AIDS

Drugs

- Thiazide diuretics
- Aspirin
- Ibuprofen
- Indomethacin
- Naproxen
- Sulfonamides
- Quinidine
- Cimetidine
- Digitalis
- Furosemide
- Heparin
- Morphine

Treatments

- Radiation therapy
- Chemotherapy

Collaborative Care

The diagnosis of thrombocytopenia is based on manifestations, diagnostic test results, and a thorough client history. The management of the disorder includes removing the causative agent or treating the underlying disease.

Laboratory and Diagnostic Tests

The following laboratory tests may be ordered:

- *CBC* may demonstrate decreased hemoglobin and hematocrit if bleeding is present.
- *Platelet count* is decreased.
- *Bleeding time measurements* evaluate the platelet and vascular response to injury by estimating the integrity of the primary hemostatic plug. The bleeding time is prolonged in thrombocytopenia. A normal bleeding time is 2 to 9 minutes.

The following diagnostic test may be ordered:

- *Bone marrow examination* may reveal decreased platelets and increased megakaryocytes.

Pharmacology

Corticosteroids, such as prednisone, are administered to suppress the immune response and decrease the number of antibodies targeted for the platelets. Although the exact

mechanism of action is not well understood, the corticosteroids also reduce bleeding time.

Platelet Transfusion

Platelet transfusions may be necessary if platelet production has been impaired and the client is bleeding. Platelets are prepared from fresh whole blood; one unit contains 30 to 60 mL of platelet concentrate. The expected increase in platelets after the administration of one unit is 10,000 per microliter.

Surgery

A splenectomy (surgical removal of the spleen) may be necessary if the client does not recover following pharmacologic treatment. The rationale for removal of the spleen is that this organ is the site of platelet destruction and antibody production. This surgery often effects a remission or even cures the disorder.

Nursing Care

Nursing care for the client with thrombocytopenia focuses primarily on the risk for the injury as a result of bleeding. This diagnosis, with related nursing interventions and rationale, is fully discussed in the section describing nursing care for the client with leukemia. Other diagnoses that are appropriate for the client with thrombocytopenia are listed below:

- *Fatigue* related to anemia secondary to bleeding.
- *Anxiety* related to cause of multiple purpura and ecchymoses.
- *Risk for Infection* related to surgical removal of spleen.

The client and the family also require information about the causative factors of secondary thrombocytopenia and medications (both prescription and over-the-counter) that may interfere with platelet function. See the accompanying box.

The Client with Disseminated Intravascular Coagulation

■ ■ ■

Disseminated intravascular coagulation (DIC) is a disorder of hemostasis that occurs as a complication of other disorders or alterations in physical status. DIC is a complex and life-threatening disorder characterized by the simultaneous occurrence of blood clotting and hemorrhage in the vascular system.

Many different conditions can precipitate the onset of DIC, including disease processes, trauma, infections, and obstetric complications. The most significant of these

---

Medications that May Interfere with Platelet Function

■ ■ ■

Over-the-Counter Medications

- Alka-Seltzer
- Anacin
- Aspirin
- Bufferin
- Coricidin "D"
- Doan's Pills
- Excedrin
- Midol
- 4-Way Cold Tablets
- Os-Cal-Gesic
- Pepto-Bismol
- Sine-Off
- Triaminicin
- Trigesic
- Vanquish

Prescription Medications

- Bufferin with codeine No. 3
- Darvon compound
- Equagesic
- Fiorinal
- Norgesic
- Percodan
- Talwin
- Trilisate
- Zorprin

Note. Adapted from *Cancer Chemotherapy: A Nursing Process Approach* (pp. 59–60) by M. Burke, G. Wilkes, D. Berg, C. Bean, and K. Ingwersen, 1991, Boston: Jones and Bartlett.

Conditions that May Cause Disseminated Intravascular Coagulation

■ ■ ■

Widespread Tissue Damage

- Trauma
  a. Burns
  b. Head injuries
  c. Gunshot wounds
  d. Frostbite
- Obstetric complications
  a. Septic abortion
  b. Retained dead fetus
  c. Abruptio placentae
  d. Amniotic fluid embolus
- Neoplasms
  a. Acute promyelocitic leukemia
  b. Metastatic cancers

Hemolysis

- Hemotoxins
- Drugs
- Hemolytic transfusion reactions
- Hemolytic uremic syndrome
- Acute pancreatitis

Hypotension

- Hypovolemic shock
- Septic shock

Hypoxia and Circulatory Stasis

- Sickle cell crisis
- Myocardial infarction
- Pulmonary embolism
- Adult respiratory distress syndrome
- Near drowning in fresh water
- Cardiac arrest
- Respiratory arrest

Metabolic Acidosis

- Aspirin poisoning

---

conditions are shock with arterial hypotension, decreased oxygen in the circulating blood, stasis of capillary blood flow, and acidemia (Bell, 1992). Conditions that may precipitate DIC are listed in the accompanying box.

DIC is estimated to occur in one of every 900 to 2400 adult admissions to large, urban hospitals. It produces a mortality rate of from 50% to 80% (Bell, 1992).

Pathophysiology

DIC is a complex pathophysiologic process that is associated primarily with endothelial damage, release of tissue factors, and an excessive release of thrombin. The process of DIC may be initiated when either the intrinsic or the extrinsic clotting cascade is activated. Normally, blood clotting is restricted to a local area; however, if the stimulus to clot is great, the mechanisms that control the spread of clotting (blood flow and clotting inhibitors, especially antithrombin III) are overcome, and widespread clotting occurs (Tierney, McPhee, & Papadakis, 1994). The sequence of the major events in DIC follows. These events are illustrated in Figure 31–10.

1. Widespread formation of tiny blood clots occurs within the microcirculation of all body organs.
2. The fibrinolytic pathway is activated, promoting the dissolution of the clots that have been formed.
3. The amount of thrombin that enters the systemic circulation greatly exceeds that of clotting inhibitors to regulate it.

Figure 31–10 The process of disseminated intravascular coagulation (DIC). Endothelial cell injury or the release of tissue factors may cause widespread activation of either the intrinsic or extrinsic clotting pathways (or both). As a result, numerous microthrombi form throughout the vasculature, causing ischemic tissue damage. Simultaneously, the rapid consumption of clotting factors by the coagulation pathways and fibrinolytic mechanisms triggers widespread bleeding.

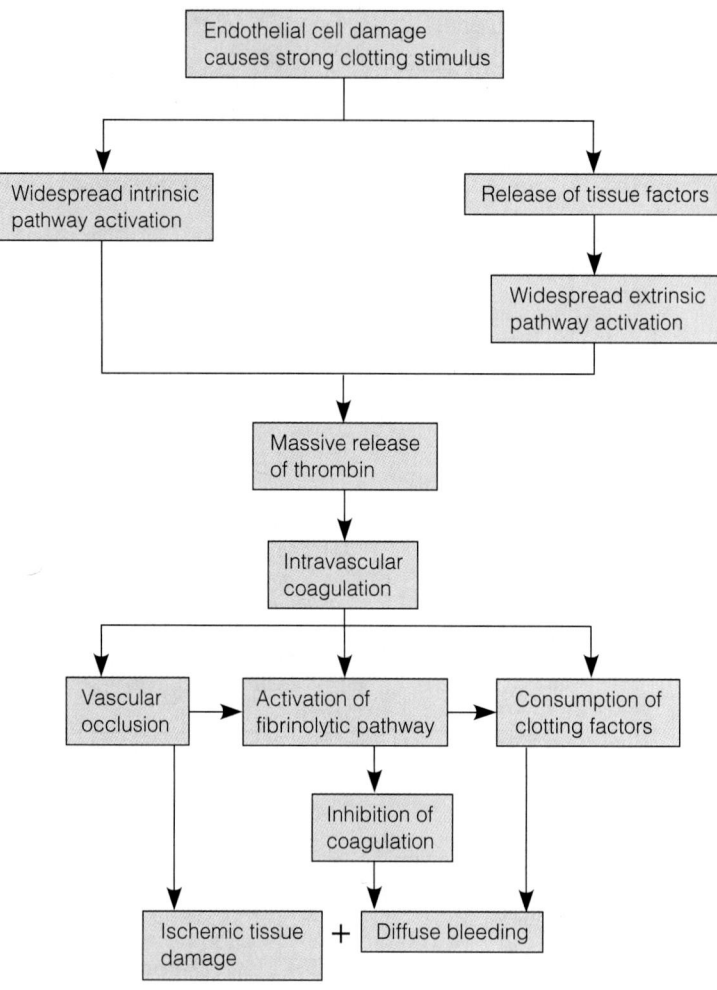

4. The deposit of thrombin decreases blood flow to organs, which may eventually cause tissue ischemia, infarction, and necrosis.

5. The excessive amounts of thrombin also activate platelet aggregation (causing thrombocytopenia with an increased risk of bleeding) and the fibrinolytic pathway (causing bleeding).

6. Plasma begins to break down fibrin before a stable clot is formed.

7. Fibrin degradation products, which are potent anticoagulants, are released and further increase bleeding.

8. Clotting factors are depleted, the ability to form clots is lost, and hemorrhage occurs.

Thus, the client with DIC has both clotting and hemorrhage within the circulatory system at the same time.

The clinical manifestations of DIC are the result of both clotting and bleeding, although bleeding is more obvious. The bleeding ranges from oozing blood following an injection to frank hemorrhage from every body orifice.

The responses of the body to DIC are listed in the accompanying box.

Collaborative Care

Treatment of DIC is directed toward correcting the primary disease process, stopping the bleeding, and preventing further activation of clotting mechanisms. If the underlying disease can be eliminated and liver function is intact, the liver can restore coagulation factors in 24 to 48 hours (Bell, 1992).

Laboratory and Diagnostic Tests

Although there is no one laboratory test that can be used to diagnose DIC, the following tests may be ordered and yield these findings:

- *Bleeding time* is increased.
- *Platelet count* is decreased.
- *Plasma fibrinogen levels* are decreased.
- *Fibrin degradation products (FDP)* or *fibrin split products (FSP)* are increased.

Clinical Manifestations of Disseminated Intravascular Coagulation

Integumentary System

- Purpura
- Ecchymosis
- Petechiae
- Cyanosis of extremities
- Bleeding from wounds
- Gangrene

Gastrointestinal System

- Occult blood in vomitus or stool
- Gastrointestinal hemorrhage
- Abdominal distention

Respiratory System

- Increased respiratory rate
- Decreased breath sounds

Cardiovascular System

- Adult respiratory distress syndrome
- Tachycardia
- Hypotension

Urinary System

- Hematuria
- Oliguria
- Anuria
- Renal failure

Central Nervous System

- Increased intra-cranial pressure
- Anxiety
- Confusion
- Stupor
- Coma
- Seizures

Other

- Malaise
- Weakness

- *Prothrombin time (PT)* is increased. Prothrombin time is an indicator of the activity of prothrombin, fibrinogen, and factors V, VII, and X in the extrinsic clotting sequence. An increased PT indicates less than normal values for one or more of the factors involved in the thromboplastin system.
- *Partial thromboplastin time (PTT)* is increased. The PTT is a general test of the entire clotting mechanism that detects deficiencies of all plasma clotting factors except platelets and factors VII and XIII. The normal PTT is 60 to 90 seconds. An activated partial thromboplastin time (APTT) is a variation of this test in which activators are added to the test reagent; an APTT provides a narrower range of values. The normal APTT is 26 to 42 seconds.
- *Analysis of clotting factors* reveals a decrease in factors II, V, VII, and X.

Pharmacology and Other Therapies

Although the anticoagulant drug heparin has been used in the treatment of DIC, its use in all situations is controversial. When clotting threatens tissue or organ function, heparin is indicated. However, it is contraindicated in septic shock or in any situation of active bleeding. Cryoprecipitate may be given for uncontrollable hemorrhage. Other therapies used include fluid replacement, blood replacement, and oxygen therapy.

Nursing Care

Clients with DIC often have multiple organ system failure, either as a precipitating factor or as a result of the condition itself. They are cared for in an intensive care unit. Nursing diagnoses discussed in this section focus on problems resulting from altered tissue perfusion, impaired gas exchange, pain, and fear. Collaborative problems for which the nurse monitors include potential hemorrhage and shock, as well as potential thrombosis.

Altered Tissue Perfusion

Because of the tiny blood clots forming throughout the microcirculation, the client with DIC has altered tissue perfusion to multiple body areas. Additionally, the bleeding that results from the consumption of clotting factors negatively alters the blood flow to these same areas.

Nursing interventions with rationales follow:

- Assess the client's extremities for pulses, warmth, and capillary refill. Assess level of consciousness and mental status. *Monitoring of central and peripheral tissue perfusion can facilitate early detection of impairment.*
- Promptly report to the physician changes in mental status, extremities, gastrointestinal function, and urinary output. *Changes must be promptly reported to facilitate timely intervention. Alteration in mentation can indicate cerebral ischemia and call for an adjustment in the medical plan. An extremity that has become pale, cold, and pulseless has arterial impairment and requires prompt medical intervention. Decreased bowel sounds and bleeding from the gastrointestinal tract may signify mesenteric occlusion, a surgical emergency. A decrease in urinary output may signify renal artery thrombosis; renal failure may develop if there is no intervention.*
- Carefully turn client from side to side every 2 hours. *Changes in position help relieve pressure points and facili-*

tate circulation. *Changing the client's position also gives the nurse the opportunity to assess for the development of any new areas of purpura, pallor, or bleeding.*

- Discourage client from crossing the legs, and do not use the knee gatch on the bed. *These positions can increase pressure on areas that are already compromised. Pressure necrosis can result in areas of unrelieved pressure and impaired circulation.*

- Minimize the use of adhesive tape on the skin. *Care must be taken to avoid further trauma to the skin. Paper tape is preferable to adhesive tape because it is gentler to the skin, minimizing tissue and vascular trauma that may lead to bleeding. Montgomery strap devices may also be used to minimize repeated removal and reapplication of tape.*

Also see interventions listed below for the nursing diagnosis *Pain*.

Impaired Gas Exchange

Microclots in the pulmonary vasculature are likely to interfere with gas exchange in the client with DIC. Initially, the client may compensate by hyperventilating to improve oxygenation; however, in later stages this is no longer adequate.

Nursing interventions with rationales follow:

- Administer oxygen as ordered. *Providing supplemental oxygen may decrease pulmonary and cardiac workload, relieving the signs of dyspnea.*

- Position client in a semi-Fowler's or high-Fowler's position. *Elevating the head of the bed allows for improved aeration of the lungs and better diaphragmatic excursion.*

- Maintain bed rest. *Bed rest reduces oxygen demands and maximizes oxygen utilization by facilitating effective gas exchange.*

- Encourage deep breathing and effective coughing. *Oxygenation can be improved by increasing the depth of respiratory effort. Movement of secretions out of the airways increases the surface available for gas exchange, thus improving oxygenation.*

- If the client is unable to cough effectively, careful nasotracheal suctioning may be instituted. *For effective gas exchange to occur, secretions must be removed from the airways. However, care must be used to minimize suction-induced hypoxia. Additionally, the nurse must be careful to avoid traumatizing tissues that are prone to bleed easily.*

- Monitor pulse oximetry and arterial blood gas results, and report abnormal results to the physician. *Decreases in pulse oximetry and arterial blood gas results that signify increasing respiratory impairment must be reported so that the physician can make adjustments in the ordered oxygen delivery.*

- Take measures to reduce pain and fear. *Control of pain is likely to decrease respiratory rate and effort, leading to better oxygenation. Reducing fear may also alleviate some of the associated respiratory distress.*

Pain

Pain may result from lack of appropriate blood flow to body tissues. Although attention must be directed at improving tissue perfusion itself (e.g., when the client develops an arterial occlusion or a compartment compression syndrome), comfort measures can also be helpful to the client.

Nursing interventions with rationales follow:

- Handle extremities gently. *Minimizing trauma reduces further injury and pain.*

- Use a pain chart to monitor the client's pain as well as the effectiveness of analgesics. *Monitoring pain and response to medication facilitates identification of an appropriate and effective treatment plan.*

- Notify the physician promptly if any new pain or sudden increase in pain occurs, especially pain that is accompanied by changes in assessment findings. *New or increased complaints of pain in the client with DIC may signify increased circulatory impairment; such impairment should be evaluated by the physician. Extremities that become painful as well as pale, cyanotic, or cold may have become occluded by arterial clots. Prompt medical intervention is necessary to save the extremity. Acute abdominal pain may signify mesenteric occlusion, which is a surgical emergency.*

- Apply cool compresses to painful joints. *Application of cold decreases painful impulses by initiating the gate-control mechanism, inhibiting the dorsal horn of the spinal cord. This area of the spinal cord is responsible for transmission of pain messages, and such inhibition can reduce the sensation of pain.*

- Evaluate the client's respiratory and circulatory status before administering pharmacologic methods of pain control. *The client with DIC is prone to circulatory and respiratory impairment. The additive effect of narcotics in the client with hypotension and respiratory distress may result in a medical crisis. Narcotics should be administered judiciously and in small amounts.*

Fear

A client with a serious complication or illness such as DIC may face a poor prognosis and therefore may experience fear.

Nursing interventions with rationales follow:

- Allow client and family to verbalize concerns. *This helps the client and family identify their concerns and frame questions.*

- Answer questions truthfully. *Providing truthful answers to the client and family facilitates the development of a therapeutic nurse-client relationship. Providing truthful answers to questions posed by the client and family allows them the greatest opportunity to set priorities as they plan for an uncertain future.*

- Identify coping strategies that the client and family may be able to use. *Helping the client and family identify effective coping methods used in the past may provide them with the necessary skills to manage the current crisis.*

- Provide emotional support to the client and family. *The presence of a caring nurse may help reduce the fear and anxiety that the client and family experience in a crisis.*

- Maintain a calm environment. *The client gains a sense of relief to see that the staff is in control of the situation. The client is better able to rest in a calm and quiet environment.*

- Respond promptly when the client calls for help. *Responding to the client's expressed needs helps develop a trusting relationship. The client is more apt to feel secure in knowing that assistance and the nurse's physical presence are at hand.*

- Instruct the client in relaxation techniques. *Relaxation techniques can reduce muscle tension and other signs of anxiety. Gaining control over bodily responses can help clients gain a sense of control over their own future.*

Other Nursing Diagnoses

Other nursing diagnoses that are appropriate for the client with DIC follow:

- *Impaired Skin Integrity* related to skin fragility and multiple bleeding sites
- *Altered Oral Mucous Membrane* related to multiple bleeding sites
- *Altered Nutrition: Less Than Body Requirements* related to increased metabolic needs and difficulty eating

The Client with Hemophilia

■ ■ ■

Hemophilia is a group of hereditary clotting factor disorders characterized by a prolonged coagulation time that results in persistent and sometimes severe bleeding. Hemophilia is a sex-linked recessive disorder most often found in males; however, in about one-third of newly diagnosed cases there is no family history of hemophilia (Porth, 1994). Although often considered a disease of children, hemophilia may be diagnosed in adults. In addition, the improved methods of treatment have greatly prolonged the survival rate, and there are many adults alive who have had the disease for years.

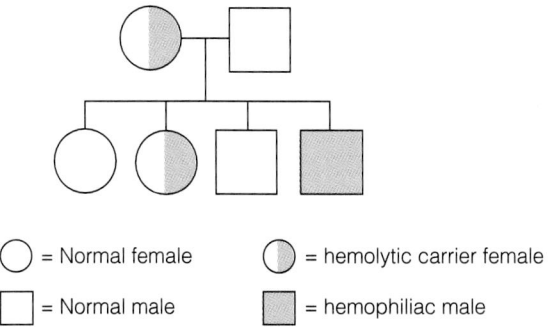

○ = Normal female   ◐ = hemolytic carrier female
□ = Normal male   ■ = hemophiliac male

Figure 31–11   Genogram showing inheritance pattern of hemophilia A and B. Both clotting disorders are X-linked recessive characteristics. Females may be carriers, but only males develop these disorders.

Pathophysiology

There are two major types of hemophilia, each with a deficiency or absence of a specific clotting factor. **Hemophilia A** (also called *classic hemophilia*), accounting for about 80% of cases, is a condition caused by a deficiency in factor VIII. **Hemophilia B** (also called *Christmas disease*), accounting for about 20% of cases, is caused by a deficiency in factor IX. Despite the difference in clotting factor deficits, hemophilia A and B are clinically identical. Hemophilia is transmitted from mother to son as an X-linked recessive characteristic (Figure 31–11). It is uncommon for females to develop the disorder, but they may become carriers.

von Willebrand's disease, another type of hemophilia, is a common hereditary bleeding disorder that is most often diagnosed in adults. It is the result of a deficiency of von Willebrand (vW) factor and is often accompanied by a deficiency of factor VIII and platelet dysfunction. This clotting disorder affects men and women equally. von Willebrand's disease is often diagnosed when surgery or a dental extraction causes prolonged bleeding. A comparison of the types of hemophilia is found in Table 31–4.

People with hemophilia form platelet plugs at the site of bleeding, but the clotting factor deficit impairs the coagulation response and the capacity to form a stable clot. The clinical manifestations of hemophilia are those of bleeding. The extent of bleeding is related to the severity of the factor deficit and of the injury that caused the bleeding. When the factor activity level is greater than 5%, bleeding usually is the result of trauma or surgery. However, if the factor activity level falls below 1%, spontaneous bleeding into the joints (hemarthrosis) and deep

Table 31–4 Comparison of the Types of Hemophilia

Type/Name	Deficiency	Characteristics	Treatment
Hemophilia A (Classic hemophilia)	Factor VIII	Transmitted by females; occurs primarily in males; bleeding time normal; coagulation time prolonged	Factor VII concentrate or cryoprecipitate
Hemophilia B	Factor IX	Transmitted by females; occurs primarily in males; bleeding time normal; coagulation time prolonged	Factor IX (Christmas disease concentrate)
von Willebrand's disease	vW factor Factor VIII	Occurs in both females and males; bleeding time and coagulation time are both prolonged	Cryoprecipitate and DDAVP

tissues may occur (Price & Wilson, 1992). The hemarthrosis often causes joint deformity and disability (most often involving the elbows, hips, knees, and ankles). Deformity and disability are likely in adults who did not receive adequate clotting factor replacement in childhood (Mills, 1992).

The manifestations of hemophilia include one or more of the following:

- Subcutaneous ecchymoses and hematomas (a hematoma is a collection of blood that is trapped in the skin tissues or a body organ)
- Bleeding from the gums
- Gastrointestinal bleeding, evidenced as hematemesis (vomiting blood), occult blood in the stools, gastric pain, or abdominal pain
- Urinary tract bleeding, evidenced by hematuria (blood in the urine)
- Pain or paralysis resulting from the pressure of hematomas on nerves
- Hemarthrosis

In addition, the person with hemophilia may have slow oozing of blood from minor cuts. The onset of bleeding may be delayed for several hours, or even days, after an injury.

Collaborative Care

The treatment of the client with hemophilia focuses on preventing and/or treating bleeding, primarily by replacing deficient clotting factors. Treatment for each type of disorder depends on the clotting defect and the severity of the illness.

The care of the client with hemophilia is complicated by the high incidence of acquired immune deficiency syndrome (AIDS) in people with hemophilia who were treated with HIV-contaminated blood products between 1978 and 1985. Today, routine testing of all blood, better screening of blood donors, and advanced methods for processing clotting factors have decreased the risk of developing AIDS from human blood and blood products (Mills, 1992).

Laboratory and Diagnostic Tests

The following laboratory tests may be ordered:

- *Serum platelet levels* are measured and are usually normal.
- *Blood studies such as APTT, bleeding time, and prothrombin time* are performed as screening criteria to detect deficiencies in some clotting factors and platelet variations. APTT is increased in all types of hemophilia. Prothrombin time is unaffected in these disorders but may be measured to rule out other disorders. Bleeding time is prolonged in von Willebrand's disease but normal in hemophilia A and B.
- *Factor assays* are conducted; factor VIII is decreased in hemophilia and von Willebrand's disease, and factor IX is decreased in hemophilia B.

Pharmacology

People with hemophilia A and B require replacement of the deficient clotting factors for maintenance, as a prophylactic measure before surgery and dental procedures, and to control bleeding. The client may be given clotting factors in the form of fresh-frozen plasma, cryoprecipitates, or concentrates. The dose depends on the severity of the clotting factor deficiency, the severity of manifestations, and the client's weight. Factor levels are measured on a regular basis to determine whether the treatment is adequate (Mills, 1992). Clotting factors are often self-administered and may be taken either on a regular or intermittent schedule.

Fresh-frozen plasma provides the replacement of all clotting factors (including both factor VIII and factor IX) except platelets. In the case of undiagnosed bleeding, fresh-frozen plasma may be administered intravenously until a definitive diagnosis is made.

People with hemophilia A are most often treated with a freeze-dried concentrate of factor VIII, which is classified as an antihemophilic factor. This concentrate is derived from fresh-frozen plasma and is pasteurized or purified to destroy pathogens. The concentrate has various names (Monoclate-P, Hemofil M, Koāte-HS) and is given intravenously.

Another preparation that may be administered to people with hemophilia A is cryoprecipitate, which is prepared from fresh-frozen plasma and contains factor VIII in concentrated form. Before testing blood products for infectious disease, cryoprecipitate prepared from multiple blood donors carried the danger of transmitting blood-borne diseases. Cryoprecipitate is now safer but should be processed from a small number of tested contributors. This medication is also given intravenously.

People with hemophilia B are given a freeze-dried concentrate of factor IX (Konÿne-HT, Proplex SX-T, Proplex) intravenously. Cryoprecipitate cannot be used to treat hemophilia B because it does not contain factor IX.

von Willebrand's disease may be treated with regular intravenous administration of cryoprecipitate, which does contain the vW factor. People with mild von Willebrand's disease may use intravenous desmopressin (DDAVP). This agent encourages the body to release vW factor.

Nursing Care

In planning nursing care for the client with hemophilia, the nurse must consider the individual's response to possible or occurring complications. Although each client has individualized needs, common nursing diagnoses focus on minimizing the risk of skin impairment and injury and on decreasing the occurrence of bleeding complications in the client with hemophilia.

Because the client must learn self-care measures that are carried on throughout life, there is a risk of ineffective management of the therapeutic regimen, which calls for an emphasis on teaching.

Risk for Impaired Skin Integrity

Because the client with hemophilia is prone to bleeding, injury prevention and skin protection are major nursing concerns. Nursing interventions include teaching the client and family safety measures that must be undertaken at home to minimize injury.

Nursing interventions with rationales follow:

- Use safety measures in personal care. For example, use an electric razor rather than a razor blade to shave. *Use*

of an electric razor minimizes the opportunity to develop superficial cuts that may result in bleeding.

- Avoid activities that place the client at risk, including contact sports, minimize physical exertion associated with job performance, and eliminate safety hazards in the home. *To minimize the risk of bleeding, the client needs to avoid the risk of injury. Activities that are safe for the person who does not have hemophilia may be inappropriate for the client with a coagulation problem. The client should learn to substitute safe activities for those that would place him at risk for bleeding injury.*

- Avoid intramuscular injections, rectal temperatures, and enemas. *These can pose a risk of tissue and vascular trauma, which can precipitate bleeding.*

- Monitor for signs of bleeding, including hematomas, ecchymoses, and purpura, as well as surface oozing or bleeding. *Bleeding may occur under the skin as well as at the surface. Early identification will facilitate control of bleeding.*

- If surface bleeding occurs, provide interventions to control blood loss: Apply gentle pressure until bleeding stops; apply ice; apply a topical hemostatic agent, such as absorbable gelatin sponge, microfibrillar collagen hemostat, or topical thrombin. *Direct pressure is a means of occluding bleeding vessels. Ice, which is a vasoconstrictor, may facilitate the stoppage of bleeding. Topical hemostatic agents help control capillary bleeding.*

- Notify the physician at the first sign of bleeding. *Prompt intervention decreases the risk of hemorrhage. The administration of factor replacement may prevent further bleeding and the complication of hypovolemia.*

Risk for Ineffective Management of Therapeutic Regimen

Clients with bleeding disorders need to take an active role in controlling their disorders and preventing complications. This role may necessitate frequent visits to the physician or clinic. Additionally, clients themselves need to learn how to administer medically ordered treatments and to protect themselves from complications. Because these activities must be adopted for life, clients may have difficulty following specific treatment regimens. Clients may resent having to undertake life-style changes that are not required of others.

Nursing interventions with rationales follow:

- Assess the client's knowledge of disorder and the related treatments. *The nurse must have an understanding of the client's previous learning in order to determine what additional information is required. A client who exhibits noncompliance may lack knowledge or may have made a conscious decision not to follow the recommendations of the health care provider.*

- Provide information about the bleeding disorder and

the ordered home medications and treatments. *Instruction must be individualized to the client's learning needs.*

■ Provide emotional support to the client, and express confidence in the client's self-care abilities. *Clients need support in order to incorporate a care regimen into their life-styles.*

■ Provide opportunities for the client to learn and practice administering clotting factors and topical hemostatic agents under supervision. *Clients will gain confidence in self-care regimens as they gradually assume responsibility for their implementation under supervision. This also allows clients to ask questions and explore alternatives.*

Other Nursing Diagnoses

Other nursing diagnoses that are appropriate for the client with a bleeding disorder follow:

■ *Activity Intolerance* related to weakness and fatigue

■ *Body Image Disturbance* related to the presence of purpura, ecchymoses, and hematomas

■ *Risk for Injury* related to bleeding tendencies

■ *Anxiety* related to knowledge deficit about care of bleeding at home

■ *Powerlessness* related to presence of chronic medical condition

Potential complications that may occur in the client with a bleeding or coagulation disorder include the following:

■ *Decreased Cardiac Output* related to insufficient fluid volume secondary to bleeding

■ *Fluid Volume Deficit* related to losses from bleeding

Client and Family Teaching

Clients with bleeding disorders require information regarding the prevention of bleeding, care at home, and the administration of prescribed medications. Teaching is directed at preparing the client and family for home care. The client should be taught to

■ Recognize the manifestations of internal bleeding: pallor, weakness, restlessness, headache, disorientation, pain, swelling. These manifestations require emergency medical care and should be reported immediately.

■ Apply cold packs and immobilize the joint for up to 24 to 48 hours if hemarthrosis occurs.

■ Request a prescription for medications if pain is severe. Do not take aspirin, which increases the risk of continued bleeding.

■ Ensure that the home environment is safe. For example, pad sharp edges of furniture, leave on a light at night, do not use scatter rugs, and wear gloves when working in the house or yard.

■ Use only electric razors.

■ Wear a MedicAlert bracelet in case of accident.

■ Practice good dental hygiene to decrease potential tooth decay and extractions. If dental procedures are necessary, discuss the need for prophylactic factor administration with the dentist and physician.

■ Follow safer-sex practices if the client is HIV-positive or has active AIDS.

■ Prepare and administer the intravenous medications.

Applying the Nursing Process

Case Study of a Client with Hemophilia: Jermiel Cruise

Jermiel Cruise is a 20-year-old student at the community college. He is admitted to the emergency department with a nosebleed that began when he fell during a touch football game. It has continued to bleed for over an hour.

Assessment

Mr. Cruise states that he has hemophilia and realizes that playing contact sports presents special risks to him. He adds that he has "not had problems lately and just wanted to join in the game for a little while." The emergency room staff quickly implements interventions to stop the bleeding. An icebag and manual pressure are applied. The emergency room physician orders factor VIII cryoprecipitate to be administered. Physical assessment findings include the following: T, 97.2 F (36.2 C); BP, 118/64; R, 18. Mr. Cruise's skin is pale but warm. Laboratory tests reveal the following: a prolonged APTT and a normal bleeding time and PT. Following treatment, Mr. Cruise's bleeding subsides.

Diagnosis

The nurses caring for Mr. Cruise make the following nursing diagnoses:

■ *Risk for Aspiration* related to uncontrolled nosebleed

■ *Noncompliance* with activity limitations

The nurses also considered the following potential complications:

■ *Potential Complication: Hypovolemic Shock* related to fluid losses associated with uncontrolled nosebleed

■ *Potential Complication: Hemorrhage* related to uncontrolled nosebleed secondary to insufficient clotting factors

Expected Outcomes

The expected outcomes established in the plan of care specify that Mr. Cruise will

- Exhibit no further signs of bleeding.
- Maintain vital signs within his usual range.
- Exhibit no signs of aspiration of blood.
- Verbalize leisure time activities in which he can safely participate.
- Verbalize self-care measures to control bleeding.

Planning and Implementation

The following nursing interventions are planned and implemented for Mr. Cruise while he is in the emergency department:

- Monitor Mr. Cruise for further signs of bleeding.
- Monitor vital signs.
- Auscultate breath sounds.
- Review with Mr. Cruise local interventions that may help stop bleeding.
- Review with Mr. Cruise the importance of seeking prompt medical attention if bleeding should occur.
- Instruct Mr. Cruise in the importance of wearing a MedicAlert bracelet identifying him as a hemophiliac.
- Discuss with Mr. Cruise alternative noncontact sports and leisure activities.

Evaluation

On discharge from the emergency department, Mr. Cruise exhibits no signs of bleeding, shock, or aspiration. He is able to verbalize interventions to help stop local bleeding and states further that he will seek prompt medical attention if bleeding should occur. Mr. Cruise agrees to stop at a local drug store on the way home to order a MedicAlert bracelet. In addition, Mr. Cruise verbalizes an understanding of the importance of avoiding contact sports and has identified swimming and golf as alternative leisure activities that he might enjoy.

Critical Thinking in the Nursing Process

1. What is the pathophysiologic basis for the bleeding that occurs in hemophilia A and B?
2. What was Mr. Cruise's priority nursing diagnosis? Why?
3. Why is family planning a special consideration with a client who has hemophilia?
4. Outline a plan to teach the family of a client diagnosed with hemophilia how to administer an intravenous infusion.
5. Develop a care plan for Mr. Cruise for the nursing diagnosis *Risk for Self-Esteem Disturbance*. Consider Mr. Cruise's age and developmental level in creating the plan.

▪▪▪ Lymphoproliferative Disorders ▪▪▪

Lymphoproliferative disorders are localized and systemic disorders of the white blood cells and lymphoid tissue. The lymphoproliferative diseases discussed in this section are the leukemias, the malignant lymphomas (Hodgkin's disease and non-Hodgkin's lymphoma), multiple myeloma, and infectious mononucleosis. An overview of white blood cells and lymphoid tissues precedes discussion of the diseases.

Overview of White Blood Cells

▪ ▪ ▪

White blood cells (WBCs), also called leukocytes, are a part of the body's defense against microorganisms. On average, there are 5000 to 10,000 WBCs per cubic millimeter of blood, with leukocytes accounting for about 1% of total blood volume (Marieb, 1992). *Leukocytosis* is a condition in which the WBC count is higher than normal; *leukopenia* is a condition in which the WBC count is lower than normal. Abnormally high or low numbers of leuko-cytes place a person at greater risk for pathologic conditions.

WBCs originate in the bone marrow from multipotential hemopoietic stem cells, which are capable of producing mature lymph and blood cells through a process of differentiation (Figure 31–1). There are two types of WBCs: granular leukocytes and nongranular leukocytes.

The granular leukocytes have cytoplasmic granules and are commonly called *granulocytes*. Granulocytes are divided into three types:

- *Neutrophils* make up 60% to 70% of the total number of WBCs. They have nuclei that are divided into three to five lobes and are often referred to as polymor-phonuclear (PMN) leukocytes. Neutrophils are the first cells to arrive at a site of inflammation, and they increase in number during an inflammation. During this increase, immature forms of WBCs (called band cells or stab cells) are released from bone marrow. Neutrophils have a life span of only about 10 hours and are constantly being replaced in the body.

Table 31–5   Normal Laboratory Values: White Blood Cells

Laboratory Test	Value
WBC count	5000 to 10,000/mm^3
Differential WBC count	
Neutrophils	3000 to 7000/mm^3
Eosinophils	50 to 400/mm^3
Basophils	25 to 200/mm^3
Lymphocytes	1000 to 4000/mm^3
Monocytes	100 to 600/mm^3

- *Eosinophils* make up 1% to 3% of the total number of WBCs and increase during hypersensitivity responses and during infestations with parasites.

- *Basophils* make up 0.3% to 0.5% of the total WBCs and are believed to be a part of the hypersensitivity and stress responses.

The nongranular WBCs are divided into two groups: monocytes and lymphocytes.

- *Monocytes* are the second type of WBC to arrive at a site of inflammation (after neutrophils), but they become the predominant WBC within 48 hours. Monocytes are the largest of the WBCs and make up approximately 3% to 8% of the total WBC count. They are phagocytic cells and are often called *macrophages*. Monocytes are active in chronic inflammation and are also involved in the immune response.

- *Lymphocytes* make up 20% to 30% of the WBC count. Lymphocytes are of two types: B cells and T cells. B cells are involved in antibody formation, whereas T cells take part in the cell-mediated immunity process. Plasma cells (which arise from B cells) are lymphoid or lymphocyte-like cells found in the bone marrow and connective tissue; they also are involved in immune reactions.

Alterations in normal WBC counts include the following:

- **Agranulocytosis:** a decrease in granulocytes; also called granulocytopenia. This condition of seriously reduced neutrophils (less than 500/mm^3) and very low total granulocyte count is most often the result of interference with white cell formation in the bone marrow or increased cell destruction in the circulating blood. Chemotherapy commonly used to treat cancers can cause bone marrow suppression, as can other pharmacologic agents. The reduction in neutrophils greatly increases the risk of infection and is often manifested by ulcerations of the oral mucosa.

- **Neutropenia:** a condition associated with a reduction in the number of circulating neutrophils, usually less than 200/mm^3. This condition occurs during prolonged infection, as a result of hematologic disorders, during starvation, and in autoimmune disorders (such as rheumatoid arthritis).

- **Lymphocytopenia:** a condition of fewer than normal lymphocytes. It may result from serious illness (such as congestive heart failure or aplastic anemia), cancers (such as Hodgkin's disease), AIDS, and chemotherapy or radiation.

Normal laboratory values for WBCs are outlined in Table 31–5.

Overview of Lymphoid Tissues

■ ■ ■

The lymphatic system of the body is made up of lymphatic tissues. These tissues are the lymphatic vessels, the lymph nodes, the spleen, and the thymus. Lymph is body fluid that originates as excess fluid from the capillaries and is returned to the circulation. Lymph nodes are located along the course of the lymphatic channels. The purpose of the lymph nodes is to filter bacteria and other debris from the lymph before it is returned to the bloodstream. Within the lymphatic system, collecting trunks drain lymph from a specific part of the body. When a cancer is present in the body, cancer cells are filtered and retained by the lymph nodes for a period of time.

Lymphadenopathy is swelling and enlargement of the lymph nodes. This abnormal condition may occur in response to infections, inflammation, or cancers. It is characteristic of certain lymphoproliferative disorders, including Hodgkin's disease and non-Hodgkin's lymphomas.

The Client with Acute Infectious Mononucleosis

■ ■ ■

Acute infectious mononucleosis is an infection of B lymphocytes (also called B cells), most commonly caused by the Epstein-Barr virus (EBV). This disease is usually benign and self-limiting. It affects young adults between the ages of 15 and 30. Although the mode of transmission is not completely understood, evidence suggests that saliva from an infected person is the main mode of transfer. As a result, acute infectious mononucleosis is often called the "kissing disease."

When the virus enters the body, unaffected B cells produce antibodies against the virus, with T lymphocytes (also called T cells) helping in the B-cell response by directly attacking the virus. The proliferation of B and T cells, as well as the removal of dead and damaged leukocytes, is responsible for the swelling of lymphoid tissues. The incubation period is about 30 to 50 days (McCance & Huether, 1994).

The manifestations begin with headache, malaise, and fatigue. Most clients with infectious mononucleosis have fever, sore throat, and enlargement and pain in the cervical lymph nodes lasting from 7 to 20 days. The severity of these manifestations varies from person to person. The lymph node involvement may be generalized, and enlargement of the spleen occurs in about half of all people with the illness.

Laboratory findings include an increase in lymphocytes and monocytes, and about one-fifth of the cells are atypical in form. The leukocyte count varies: In the first week of the infection, it is usually normal or even low, but as the person enters the second week, the WBC count increases and remains elevated for 4 to 8 weeks. Platelet counts are often low during the illness.

Recovery occurs in 2 to 3 weeks. However, debility and lethargy may last for up to 3 months. The treatment includes bed rest and analgesic agents to alleviate the symptoms.

The Client with Multiple Myeloma

■ ■ ■

Multiple myeloma is a malignant disorder of plasma cells in which immature cells proliferate in the bone marrow, lymph nodes, spleen, and kidneys. Bone pain, pathologic fractures, and renal problems can occur as a result of the bone destruction.

Pathophysiology

The etiologic origin of multiple myeloma has not been established, but possible causes include genetic predisposition, oncogenic virus, inflammatory stimuli, and chronic antigenic stimulation. Multiple myeloma occurs more often among males, and the incidence among African Americans is approximately twice that of European Americans. In addition, the incidence increases with age, and the disease rarely occurs before age 40.

The manifestations of multiple myeloma are due to changes in bone that occur as a result of the neoplastic process. Plasma cell proliferation suppresses normal marrow components, resulting in bone lesions visible on X-ray examination. Impaired immunoglobulin production suppresses the development of normal immunoglobulins needed to prevent infections.

The disease develops slowly. The earliest symptom usually is diffuse back pain. With progression of the disease, the pain may increase in severity and become more localized. Pathologic fractures occur as the bone marrow is replaced by tumors. As antibody formation decreases, the client becomes more susceptible to infections. Spinal cord compression may cause neurologic manifestations. In addition, bone destruction may cause hypercalcemia, leading to renal failure, anorexia, confusion, and coma. *Bence Jones protein* (a protein found almost exclusively in the urine of people with multiple myeloma) can damage renal tubules.

Collaborative Care

Laboratory and diagnostic tests include the following:

- *Radiographic studies of bone* may reveal punched-out bone lesions.
- *Bone marrow aspiration* findings include an abnormal number of immature plasma cells.
- *CBC* shows moderate to severe anemia.
- *Urine samples* exhibit the presence of Bence Jones protein and hypercalciuria. The absence of Bence Jones protein does not exclude a diagnosis of multiple myeloma, but its presence almost invariably confirms it.

There is no cure for multiple myeloma and, therefore, treatment is primarily palliative.

In the palliative treatment of the client with multiple myeloma, chemotherapy, radiation therapy, and pharmacology are used to decrease the tumor size and lessen bone pain. Melphalan (Alkeran), cyclophosphamide (Cytoxan), and steroids are most commonly used as chemotherapeutic agents. These therapies can prolong life for 1 to 3 years.

Pain is controlled with analgesics. Blood transfusions are used in treating anemia, and infections are controlled with antibiotics. Braces or splints may be indicated when there is spinal involvement. The client must remain mobile to prevent fractures, bone demineralization, osteoporosis, and hypercalcemia.

Nursing Care

Nursing care of the client with multiple myeloma is similar to the care of the client with cancer and care of the client with chronic pain. See the nursing care discussion in Chapters 4 and 9 for additional information. Nursing diagnoses discussed in this section focus on problems resulting from chronic pain, impaired mobility, the risk for injury, and the risk for infection.

Chronic Pain

The client with multiple myeloma probably had a period of chronic back pain prior to diagnosis of the myeloma. As the immature plasma cells saturate the bone marrow and invade the bony structure, the client experiences pain. Pathologic fractures are also a common and reoccurring problem. Although the client may have learned some methods of coping with chronic pain, the nurse can provide additional pain relief measures.

Nursing interventions with rationales follow:

- Assess pain, including onset, duration, precipitating factors, and effective measures of relief. *Identifying the causes of pain and precipitating factors can help the nurse determine effective measures of pain relief.*

- Determine which position allows greatest comfort, and help the client assume this position. *The client is the best judge of which position minimizes pain and allows relief. A client who is weak and uncomfortable is likely to need assistance with periodic repositioning.*

- Support the client with pillows. *Because of bony infiltrate, the client may have painful bony prominences and be unable to remain positioned without the support of many pillows.*

- Provide for uninterrupted periods of rest. *The client will need adequate rest to obtain relief of pain and to restore emotional equilibrium.*

- Teach the client to use nonpharmacologic methods of pain control, including relaxation or guided imagery. *A combination of pharmacologic and nonpharmacologic methods may be necessary to allow the client to cope with chronic pain, especially bone pain.*

- Teach the client how to take ordered analgesics. Involve the family as needed to ensure that the client's pain is relieved. *The client must be taught that analgesics are most effective when taken before the pain becomes too severe.*

- Report unrelieved pain to the physician. *The client or family may need to discuss alternative medications with the physician if pain remains unrelieved. The addition of other medications, including sedatives and hypnotics, or a switch to another analgesic or narcotic may be indicated.*

Impaired Physical Mobility

Painful bony infiltrates may limit the client's mobility. A client who has experienced a fracture may wear a brace or splint to protect the extremity after the cast is removed. In addition, persistent weakness associated with bone pain and with anemia limits the client's ability to participate fully in usual activities.

Nursing interventions with rationales follow:

- Gently hold the client's extremities when repositioning. *Extremities become weakened from lack of use, and infiltration of the bone marrow by plasma cells places the client at risk for pathologic fractures.*

- Provide a change of position every 2 hours or more frequently, if needed. *Because of weakness, the client will need assistance with repositioning. Bony prominences may place the client at risk for impairment in skin integrity, and turning may be needed more frequently than every 2 hours.*

- Provide a trapeze to assist in repositioning. *The client may be able to assist with repositioning if provided with better leverage. Furthermore, the ability to participate in self-care can improve the client's self-image.*

Risk for Injury

Because of bone involvement, the client with multiple myeloma is always at risk for pathologic fractures. These fractures may occur in the long or short bones of the extremities or in the vertebral column. Preventing injury is therefore essential.

Nursing interventions with rationales follow:

- Place needed items close at hand for the client. *By straining to obtain objects out of reach, the client who is weak and unable to move independently increases the risk of falling or sustaining other injury.*

- Provide safety measures to prevent falls from bed: Place the bed in a low position, use side rails, and place the call bell within reach. *Safety measures are necessary to prevent inadvertent injury. A secure environment minimizes risk to the client and helps prevent falls.*

- Provide safety measures to prevent injury when the client is ambulatory: Ensure that the pathway is clear, remove scatter rugs, and provide adequate lighting, a nonslippery floor, and nonskid soles on shoes. *Weight-bearing through walking promotes bone repair. However, safety measures must be taken to prevent falls. Providing an unobstructed pathway and a firm surface underfoot minimizes the chance of falling.*

Risk for Infection

When plasma cells occupy the majority of bone marrow space, white blood cells are not produced in adequate amounts. Additionally, both chemotherapy and radiation treatment for cancer results in neutropenia. The decrease in white cells and antibody production places the client at increased risk for infection.

Nursing interventions with rationales follow:

- Ensure that all people coming in contact with the client wash hands meticulously. *Meticulous hand washing can decrease the number of pathogens carried on the hands. Minimizing the client's exposure to pathogens decreases the risk of infection.*

- Restrict visitors with colds, flu, or other infections. *The client with neutropenia is deficient in normal defenses against common pathogens, whether bacterial, viral, or fungal. Minimizing the client's exposure to these pathogens helps decrease the risk of infection.*

- Provide careful and thorough hygiene care daily. *Decreasing the number of normal flora as well as other pathogens on the skin decreases the risk of infection. Additionally, providing hygiene care presents an opportunity to assess the client for indications of infection and institute early treatment.*

- Provide a high-protein, high-vitamin diet. *Improving nutritional status facilitates the production of blood cells and antibodies necessary to maintain homeostasis and resist infection.*

- Provide oral hygiene after every meal. *Oral mucous membranes are especially prone to breakdown and infection. Decreasing the amount of food debris in the oral cavity decreases the chance of infection and minimizes irritation to damaged membranes. If the oral mucous membranes are in good condition, the client is more likely to eat an adequate diet.*

- Use strict aseptic technique for invasive procedures. *The client with neutropenia is especially prone to infection. Minimizing the entry of pathogens when performing invasive procedures is especially important in the client who is unable to mount a defense against infection.*

- Assess vital signs every 4 hours. Report abnormal findings to the physician. *Fever, tachycardia, tachypnea, or hypotension can indicate infections. Early detection of manifestations of infection facilitates early treatment and may prevent the development of sepsis.*

- Monitor levels of neutrophils to detect any increasing risk of infection. *Neutrophils provide the first line of defense against infection. As the levels of neutrophils decrease, the risk of infection increases. Levels under 2000/mm³ signify an increased risk, and levels under 500/mm³ indicate a severe risk of infection.*

- Institute protective isolation if the neutrophil count drops under 500/mm³. *A neutrophil count under 500/mm³ places the client at severe risk of infection. Extra protection against pathogens of all types helps prevent exposure to potential sources of infection.*

- Restrict fresh flowers and plants from the client's room. *Insects found on fresh flowers and plants may harbor microorganisms that could cause infection.*

- Restrict the use of raw fruits and vegetables. Also, ensure that fruits and vegetables are washed well prior to cooking. *Avoiding raw fruits and vegetables and washing all fruits and vegetables prior to cooking will help to decrease the number of pathogens to which the client is exposed.*

Other Nursing Diagnoses

Other nursing diagnoses that are appropriate for the client with multiple myeloma follow:

- *Activity Intolerance* related to the effects of chronic anemia and persistent pain
- *Anxiety* related to knowledge deficit of disease, treatment, side effects of treatment modalities, and home care

- *Anticipatory Grieving* related to diagnosis of cancer with no cure
- *Fatigue* related to the effects of chronic anemia and chemotherapy treatments
- *Altered Nutrition: Less Than Body Requirements* related to the inability to prepare meals and to increased nutritional needs
- *Fluid Volume Excess* related to renal impairment

Client and Family Teaching

Individuals with multiple myeloma must be taught about home maintenance management. The client and family must learn about signs and symptoms that signify complications and the need to seek medical help. These complications include pathologic fractures, including vertebral compression fractures and fractures of long bone. The disease and its treatment carry the risk of infection and sepsis, so teaching in this area should be ongoing. As the client's status deteriorates, the family may wish to consider hospice care for emotional support as well as for client care.

The Client with Leukemia

■ ■ ■

Leukemia (literally, "white blood") is a group of chronic malignant conditions of white blood cells and white blood cell precursors. In leukemia, the usual ratio of red to white blood cells is reversed. Leukemias are characterized by the replacement of bone marrow with malignant immature white blood cells, the appearance of abnormal immature WBCs in the peripheral circulation, and general infiltration of these cells into the liver, spleen, and lymph nodes throughout the body (Porth, 1994).

Although leukemia is often associated with children, it is diagnosed in many more adults each year. In 1993, 26,700 cases were diagnosed in adults, as compared to 2,600 cases in children (American Cancer Society, 1994). Acute leukemia ranks 20th as a cause of cancer-related death among people of all age groups, with 18,600 deaths in 1993. The incidence of acute leukemia is equal in men and women but increases after age 50. The highest incidence of leukemia is found in the United States, Canada, Sweden, and New Zealand (McCance & Huether, 1993).

The leukemias are named according to the predominant type of abnormal cell involved (lymphocytic or myelogenous) and according to the acuity or chronicity of the condition. The most common types of leukemia in adults are acute granulocytic leukemia (a subtype of acute myelogenous leukemia) and chronic lymphocytic leukemia (discussed later in this section). Acute leukemia is a condition characterized by undifferentiated or poorly

Table 31–6	FAB Classification of Acute Leukemia
Acute Lymphocytic Leukemia	L1—Common childhood leukemia L2—Adult ALL L3—Rare subtype

Acute Myelogenous Leukemia	Granulocytic
	  M1—Myeloblastic leukemia without maturation
	  M2—Myeloblastic leukemia with maturation
	  M3—Hypergranular promyelocytic leukemia
	
	Monocytic
	  M4—Myelomonocytic leukemia
	  M5—Monocytic leukemia
	
	Erythroid
	  M6—Erythroleukemia

differentiated blast cells and has a rapidly fatal course (often 2 to 4 months) if untreated. In chronic leukemia, the leukemic cell is well differentiated, and the prospects for survival are better—even if the condition is untreated. Myelocytic leukemias involve the bone marrow and interfere with the maturation of all types of blood cells, including granulocytes, RBCs, and thrombocytes. In summary, the types of leukemia are as follows:

- Acute lymphocytic leukemia (ALL)
- Chronic lymphocytic leukemia (CLL)
- Acute myelogenous leukemia (AML)
- Chronic myelogenous leukemia (CML)

This general system of classification of leukemias does not differentiate the subtypes of acute leukemias. A French-American-British (FAB) system for classifying the acute lymphoid and myeloid forms of leukemia has been developed (Table 31–6). In this system, the types of acute lymphocytic leukemias are distinguished by cytologic (cellular) features and by the degree of heterogeneity of the leukemic cell population. Acute myeloid leukemias are divided into subtypes by the degree of cell maturation and the direction of differentiation along one or more cell lines. The FAB classification system is being further developed to better diagnose and classify leukemias through the use of monoclonal antibodies to differentiate types of WBCs. (Monoclonal antibodies are produced by a process of fusing an antibody-producing spleen cell from an animal with a malignant myeloma cell.)

Although the exact cause of leukemia is unknown, predisposing factors have been identified. These factors include exposure to chemical agents such as benzene (found in gasoline), genetic factors such as alterations in chromosomes, viruses (especially retrovirus HTVL-1), immune disorders, certain antineoplastic drugs, and exposure to large amounts of radiation. The incidence of leukemia is increased in people that have been treated with radiation or chemotherapy, people living near sites of radiation testing, survivors of atomic bombing sites, radiologists, and people with Down syndrome or other genetic abnormalities.

Without treatment, leukemia is invariably fatal, usually resulting from complications of leukemic cell infiltration of bone marrow or vital organs. With treatment, prognosis varies. The 5-year survival rate is 37% (American Cancer Society, 1994). The types, pathology, manifestations, and treatment modalities for the major leukemias are outlined in Table 31–7.

Pathophysiology

In leukemia, the bone marrow becomes almost totally filled with immature and undifferentiated leukocytes, or "blast" cells, referred to as leukemic cells. The leukemic cells proliferate rapidly and have a prolonged life span. However, they are not able to perform the functions of mature WBCs, so they are ineffective in reducing inflammation or infection or serving as immune cells. It is believed that leukemia begins when a single stem cell undergoes a malignant transformation, begins to proliferate and replaces normal hematopoietic elements in the marrow. Because erythrocyte- and platelet-producing cells are crowded out, severe anemia, splenomegaly, and bleeding difficulties result.

Leukemic cells leave the bone marrow and travel through the circulatory system, crossing the blood–brain barrier and infiltrating other body tissues such as the central nervous system, testes, skin, and gastrointestinal tract as well as the reticuloendothelial system (lymph nodes, liver, and spleen). Death most commonly occurs as a result of internal hemorrhage and infections.

In general, the manifestations of leukemia (regardless of type) are the result of anemia, infection, and increased bleeding. The manifestations of anemia include pallor, fatigue, tachycardia, malaise, lethargy, and dyspnea. Infection, resulting from neutropenia, is manifested by fever, night sweats, oral and pharyngeal ulcerations, sinusitis, bronchitis, pneumonia, cystitis, abscesses of the peritonsillar and perianal areas, skin and nail infections, and septicemia. Increased bleeding, a result of thrombocytopenia, causes bruising; petechiae; hematomas; bleeding from the nose, gums, or bladder; and overt or occult gastrointestinal bleeding, pulmonary bleeding, retinal or scleral hemorrhage, and subarachnoid hemorrhage. The clinical manifestations of leukemia are summarized in the accompanying box.

Other manifestations are the result of leukemic cell infiltration, an increase in metabolism, and destruction of

Table 31–7	Major Types of Leukemia		
Type	**Pathology**	**Manifestations**	**Treatment**
Acute myelogenous leukemia (AML)	Affects the hematopoietic stem cells of monocyte, granulocyte, erythrocyte, and platelet cell lines	Risk of infection, weakness, fatigue, bleeding, liver pain, spleen pain, headache, lymphadenopathy, vomiting, bone pain	Chemotherapy, administration of blood products, bone marrow transplant
Chronic myelogenous leukemia (CML)	Affects myeloid stem cells, but more normal cells are present than in AML	Same as AML, but less severe; also leukocytosis, splenomegaly	Same as AML
Acute lymphocytic leukemia (ALL)	Malignant proliferation of lymphocytes	Leukopenia, anemia, thrombocytopenia, low platelets, low erythrocytes	Chemotherapy
Chronic lymphocytic leukemia (CLL)	Same as ALL, but is often mild	Often none; enlarged lymph glands, anemia, risk of infection	Chemotherapy if disease is severe

large numbers of leukocytes as a part of the disease or as the result of treatment. Infiltration of the liver, spleen, lymph nodes, and bone marrow causes pain in the involved areas. Infiltration of the meninges may cause increased intracranial pressure, manifested by headache, alterations in the level of consciousness, cranial nerve impairment, nausea, and vomiting. Infiltration of the kidneys may result in decreased renal function, with decreased urinary output and increased blood urea nitrogen and creatinine. The increase in metabolism is manifested by heat intolerance, weight loss, dyspnea on exertion, and tachycardia. The destruction of large numbers of WBCs results in the release of substantial amounts of uric acid into the circulating blood as a by-product; uric acid crystals may form in the renal tubules, causing renal insufficiency.

Acute Myelogenous Leukemia

Acute myelogenous leukemia (AML), also called acute nonlymphoblastic leukemia, is characterized by uncontrolled proliferation of myeloblasts (the precursors of granulocytes) and hyperplasia of the bone marrow and spleen. AML accounts for most of the acute leukemias seen in adults. More than half of clients who receive treatment achieve complete remission. Approximately 20% of clients achieve 5-year disease-free survival (Price & Wilson, 1992).

Clinical manifestations of AML are the result of neutropenia and thrombocytopenia. The reduced number of neutrophils results in recurrent severe infections, such as pneumonia, septicemia, perirectal abscesses, and ulcerations of the mucous membranes. A reduction in the number of platelets causes bleeding; the client experiences purpura, petechiae, and ecchymoses from bleeding into

Clinical Manifestations of Leukemia

Integumentary System

- Conjunctival pallor
- Circumoral pallor
- Petechiae
- Ecchymosis
- Lesions

Neurologic System

- Headache
- Papilledema
- Seizures
- Coma

Cardiovascular System

- Tachycardia
- Palpitations
- Orthostatic hypotension
- Murmurs
- Bruits
- Hemorrhage

Respiratory System

- Dyspnea on exertion

Gastrointestinal System

- Anorexia
- Nausea
- Oral lesions
- Bleeding gums
- Occult blood in stools
- Constipation/diarrhea
- Abdominal pain
- Weight loss
- Hepatomegaly

the skin, epistaxis (nosebleeds), hematomas, hematuria, and gastrointestinal bleeding. In addition, bone infarctions or subperiosteal infiltrates of leukemic cells may cause bone pain. Anemia is a late manifestation (because of the 120-day life span of the RBCs) and causes fatigue, headaches, pallor, and dyspnea on exertion. Death is usually the result of infection or hemorrhage.

Bone marrow aspiration usually identifies a proliferation of immature WBCs. The client's blood count will show thrombocytopenia and normocytic, normochromic anemia.

The initial goal of treatment is to eliminate the leukemic stem cells so that normal cells are replenished. Chemotherapy is the primary form of therapy and can result in remissions lasting a year or more. Chemotherapeutic agents commonly used in the treatment of AML include a combination of daunorubicin or doxorubicin, cytarabine, and oral thioguanine; or if these fail to produce remission, a combination of cyclophosphamide, vincristine, prednisone, or methotrexate may be used. Bone marrow transplant is also an important treatment modality.

Chronic Myelogenous Leukemia
Chronic myelogenous leukemia (CML) is characterized by an abnormal proliferation of all of the bone marrow elements. Although CML is a disorder of white cell maturation, most of the cells are mature and functional. In 85% of the cases, a chromosome abnormality called the *Philadelphia chromosome* is present. The Philadelphia chromosome is a translocation of chromosome 22 to chromosome 9. The disease has a slow onset.

This type of leukemia constitutes approximately 20% of adult leukemias and is usually found in clients over age 50. The incidence of the disease is higher in men. Causative agents for CML include ionizing radiation and chemical exposure.

People with CML are often asymptomatic in the early stages and, in fact, are often diagnosed when they have routine examinations and blood tests. The manifestations are the result of a hypermetabolic state: fatigue, weight loss, sweating, and heat intolerance. Leukocytosis (an abnormal increase in circulating WBCs) is always present. The spleen is enlarged in 90% of cases, causing early satiety and feelings of abdominal fullness. Chromosomal analysis of peripheral blood or bone marrow showing the Philadelphia chromosome and low leukocyte levels confirm CML in clients with typical clinical changes. As the disease progresses, the production of myeloblasts greatly increases (this stage is referred to as blast transformation). This condition is indicative of the crisis stage of the illness, and death may result in weeks to months.

Treatment is directed at controlling the disease with chemotherapy. Chemotherapeutic agents commonly used in treatment of CML include busulfan, melphalan, and hydroxyurea. More aggressive treatment modalities include intensive intravenous chemotherapy and autologous bone marrow transplant. The disease may progress to the acute form. Treatment is then the same as that for acute myelogenous leukemia, but at this point the disease is likely to resist treatment. Clients with CML generally live 3 to 5 years; infection or hemorrhage is the typical cause of death.

Acute Lymphocytic Leukemia
Acute lymphocytic leukemia (ALL) involves an abnormal growth of lymphoblasts in the bone marrow and in the lymph nodes and spleen. This type is the most common form of childhood leukemia, although it also occurs in adults.

The onset of ALL is usually rapid. Primitive lymphocytes proliferate in bone marrow and peripheral tissue and crowd the growth of normal cells. Normal hematopoiesis is suppressed, and malignant cell growth leads to thrombocytopenia, leukopenia, and anemia. The client experiences infections, bleeding, and anemia. Bone pain resulting from rapid generation of marrow elements, lymphadenopathy, and liver enlargement are also common. Central nervous system involvement causes headaches, visual disturbances, vomiting, and seizures.

The diagnosis of ALL is made through a complete blood count, differential WBC count, platelet count, and bone marrow examination. The WBC count is elevated with lymphocytosis, whereas the RBC and platelet counts are decreased. Bone marrow studies reveal a hypercellular marrow with growth of lymphoblasts.

Treatment focuses on eliminating the leukemic stem cells with chemotherapy or bone marrow transplant. Drugs commonly used in the treatment of ALL include vincristine and/or prednisone with intrathecal (in the spinal fluid) administration of methotrexate or cytarabine or intravenous administration of asparaginase, daunorubicin, and doxorubicin. Maintenance therapy may require mercaptopurine and methotrexate. Intrathecal chemotherapy and cranial radiation are helpful in preventing central nervous system relapse. Bone marrow transplant is also utilized in the treatment of ALL. If treated, individuals with acute lymphocytic leukemia may survive 5 years or longer.

Chronic Lymphocytic Leukemia
Chronic lymphocytic leukemia (CLL) is characterized by a proliferation and accumulation of small, abnormal, mature lymphocytes in the bone marrow, peripheral blood, and body tissues. The abnormal cells are usually lymphocytes; their proliferation results in a depressed immune response. The disease occurs more commonly in adults, especially in older adults (median age 60); the incidence in men is twice as high as in women (Price & Wil-

Table 31–8   Diagnostic Findings by Type of Leukemia

Test	AML	CML	ALL	CLL
RBC count	Low	Low	Low	Low
Hemoglobin	Low	Low	Low	
Hematocrit	Low	Low	Low	Low
Platelet count	Very low	High early, low late	Low	Low
WBC count	Varies	Increased	Varies	Increased
Myeloblasts	Present			
Neutrophils	Decreased	Increased	Decreased	Normal
Lymphocytes		Normal		Increased
Monocytes		Normal/low		
Blasts	Present	Present (crisis)	Present	
Philadelphia chromosomes		Present		
Bone marrow	Hypercellular		Hypercellular	
Myeloblasts	Present			
Lymphoblasts			Present	
Lymphocytes				Present
Potassium	Decreased	Increased	Increased	
Magnesium			Decreased	

son, 1992). CLL is the least common type of the major leukemia groups.

CLL also has a slow onset and is often diagnosed during a routine physical examination or workups for other medical conditions. If symptoms are present, they usually consist of vague complaints of weakness or malaise. Possible clinical findings include anemia, infection, and enlargement of lymph nodes, the spleen, and the liver. As in other leukemias, bone marrow hyperplasia is present. Erythrocyte and platelet counts are reduced. Leukocyte counts may either be elevated or reduced, but abnormal cells are always present.

Often, years may elapse before treatment becomes necessary. When severe symptoms do appear, chemotherapeutic agents such as chlorambucil with steroids may be administered. Radiation to areas of lymphocytic infiltration may also provide local relief. Survival of this disease averages approximately 7 years.

Collaborative Care

Treatment of the client with leukemia focuses on achieving remission and relieving symptoms. The methods of treatment may include chemotherapy, radiation therapy, and bone marrow transplantation. Although a cure for leukemia has not been found, success in managing the disease to maintain remission is increasing, and people with leukemia are living longer and more comfortable

lives. (A person in remission has no clinical manifestations, and the bone marrow and blood tests are normal.)

Laboratory and Diagnostic Tests

The following laboratory tests may be ordered. (Diagnostic findings for the different types of leukemia are outlined in Table 31–8).

- *CBC* is conducted to measure hemoglobin and hematocrit levels and red and white blood cell counts. A differential red and white blood cell examination assesses cellular morphology (size and shape), number, and distribution.

- *Platelets* are measured to identify changes that alter the clotting process and reflect bone marrow response to the disease. Platelets are decreased in AML and ALL, are normal to increased in CML, and are normal to mildly decreased in CLL.

- *Serum electrolytes* may be abnormal (especially potassium).

Diagnostic tests may include the following:

- *Bone marrow examination* is conducted to gain information about the general cellularity of the marrow, type of erythropoiesis, and maturity of erythropoietic and leukopoietic cells (Byrne, Saxton, Pelikan, & Nugent, 1986). The bone marrow is hypercellular in AML, ALL, and CML; myeloblasts are present in AML, lymphoblasts are present in ALL, and lymphocytes are present in CML.

Chemotherapy

Systemic chemotherapy is used to eradicate leukemic cells and produce remission. Chemotherapy interferes with the division of frequently dividing cells in the bone marrow. In the process, stem cells (whose generation time lasts 6 to 24 hours) may be temporarily injured, resulting in bone marrow depression. The bone marrow is then temporarily unable to replace used blood cell elements, especially the neutrophils and platelets. Chemotherapy does not affect circulating mature blood cells because they are no longer dividing.

All blood cells have a fixed life span (WBCs: 6 hours, RBCs: 120 days, platelets: 10 days), so the effect of chemotherapy in lowering the blood counts occurs a predictable time after the administration of a chemotherapeutic agent—usually 7 to 14 days, depending on the specific drug. The lowest blood count after administration of chemotherapy is called the nadir. The amount of bone marrow depression is also influenced by the following factors:

- *Age.* Increasing age reduces functional bone marrow reserves, so recovery may be delayed.

- *Drug dose.* Bone marrow suppression increases as higher doses of the chemotherapeutic agents are given.

- *Nutritional state.* The ability to repair normal stem cells damaged by chemotherapy may be impaired by protein-calorie malnutrition.

- *Ability to metabolize the drug.* Drug metabolism is impaired by renal or hepatic dysfunction.

- *Prior treatment.* Prior chemotherapy or radiation to sites of bone marrow production can cause bone marrow atrophy and decrease bone marrow reserves.

- *Bone marrow reserves.* Bone marrow reserves may be limited by significant alcohol abuse, which causes fatty marrow, and by invasion of the bone marrow by tumor cells.

Various chemotherapeutic agents are used to treat leukemia. The choice of drug, drug sequence, and drug combination is determined by the oncology specialist. Chemotherapeutic agents used include alkylating agents, antitumor antibiotics, antimetabolites, plant alkaloids, and miscellaneous agents. These classifications, with drugs within each classification, are listed in Table 31–9.

A combination of agents is most often used in treating leukemia. By combining agents, drug resistance is reduced, toxicity from high doses of single agents is reduced, and cell growth is interrupted at various stages of the cell cycle. The improved therapeutic effects of combination chemotherapy are the result of the complementary action of the drugs to provide maximum cell kill. In addi-

Table 31–9	Classification and Drug Names of Chemotherapeutic Agents Used to Treat Leukemia
Alkylating Agents	Busulfan (Myleran)
	Carboplatin (Paraplatin)
	Carmustine (BiCNU)
	Chlorambucil (Leukeran)
	Cisplatin/*cis*-platinum (Platinol)
	Cyclophosphamide (Cytoxan)
	Dacarbazine/DTIC (DTIC-Dome)
	Ifosfamide (IFEX)
	Lomustine/CCNU (CeeNU)
	Mechlorethamine hydrochloride/nitrogen mustard (Mustargen)
	Melphalan (Alkeran)
	Streptozocin (Zonosar)
	Triethylenethiophosphoramide (Thiotepa)
	Uracil mustard (Uracil)
Plant Alkaloids	Vinblastine sulfate (Velban)
	Vincristine sulfate (Oncovin)
	Vindesine sulfate (Eldisine)
Antitumor Antibiotics	Bleomycin sulfate (Blenoxane)
	Dactinomycin/actinomycin D (Cosmegen)
	Daunorubicin hydrochloride (Cerubidine)
	Doxorubicin hydrochloride (Adriamycin)
	Mitomycin (Mutamycin)
	Mitoxantrone hydrochloride
	Plicamycin/mithramycin (Mithracin)
	Procarbazine hydrochloride (Matulane)
Antimetabolites	Cytarabine/ara-C/cytosine arabinoside (Cytosar-U)
	Floxuridine (FUDR)
	Fluorouracil/5-fluorouracil/5-FU (Adrucil)
	Hydroxyurea (Hydrea)
Miscellaneous	Amasacrine/m-AMSA (Amsidyl)
	Asparaginase/L-asparaginase (Elspar)
	Erwinia asparaginase/porton asparaginase
	Etoposide/VP-16 (VePesid)
	Interferon alfa-2a (Roferon-A)
	Interferon alfa-2b (Intron A)
	Levamisole (Ergamisol)
	Teniposide/VM-26 (Vumon)

Note. Data are from *Drug Handbook: A Nursing Process Approach* by R. Alfaro-LeFevre, M. Blicharz, N. Flynn, and M. Boyer, 1992, Redwood City, CA: Addison-Wesley Nursing.

tion, the toxicities of the individual drugs often differ, so that administration of nearly fully tolerated drugs may be given without severe toxicity. Cancer treatment with chemotherapy is discussed in detail in Chapter 9.

Radiation Therapy

When radiation therapy is used, the target for radiation damage is the DNA in the cell. Cellular death is mitotically linked; that is, the cell can function, but it cannot survive division. Cells with high mitotic rates, such as bone marrow cells, and cancer cells, such as leukemic cells, respond quickly to radiation treatment (and are called radiosensitive cells). Although normal cells are affected, they are better able to recover from the damage caused by the radiation than are cancer cells. The types of delivery, effects, and toxicities of radiation are discussed in greater detail in Chapter 9.

Bone Marrow Transplantation

Advances in the technology of bone marrow transplantation (BMT) have increased the treatment of the leukemias when used in conjunction with chemotherapy or radiation. There are two major categories of BMT. In *allogenic BMT,* the bone marrow of a healthy donor is infused into the client with the illness; in *autologous BMT,* the client is infused with his or her own bone marrow.

Allogenic BMT   Allogenic BMT has been used to treat leukemias for almost two decades and has also been useful in treating thalassemia and aplastic anemia. In preparation for an allogenic BMT, high doses of chemotherapy and/or total body irradiation are given prior to the BMT procedure. Then new marrow from a donor (often a sibling with an identical tissue type) is infused through a central venous line.

A disorder peculiar to allogenic BMT is *graft-versus-host disease.* In this disorder, which occurs in 25% to 60% of all clients receiving an allogenic BMT, the immune response of the donated bone marrow sees the recipient's body tissue as foreign. Consequently, T lymphocytes in the donated marrow attack the liver, skin, and gastrointestinal tract, causing skin rashes progressing to desquamation (loss of skin), diarrhea, gastrointestinal bleeding, and liver damage. The disorder is treated with antibiotics and steroids. If these medications do not work, thalidomide and immunotoxin (Xomazyme) may be used (Wilke, Coyle, & Shapiro, 1990).

Autologous BMT   Autologous BMT uses a client's own bone marrow to treat the toxic effects of antineoplastic drugs or radiation (and therefore is often called *bone marrow rescue*). The procedure is used only in malignant diseases, usually when the disease is in remission. The phases of autologous BMT are as follows:

First phase: Screening, complete physical examination, and education.

Second phase: About 1 L of bone marrow is aspirated from the client (usually from the iliac crests) using multiple large-bore needle sites. The bone marrow is usually frozen and stored for use after treatment.

Third phase: During this immunosuppressive phase, lethal doses of chemotherapy or radiation are given to the client to destroy the immune system, to destroy malignant cells, and to prepare space in the bone marrow for new cells. This treatment is given over a period of 4 to 8 days.

Fourth phase: The filtered bone marrow is thawed and infused intravenously through a central line.

Fifth phase: In this phase, called engraftment, the infused marrow cells slowly become a part of the client's bone marrow, the neutrophil count increases, and normal hematopoiesis takes place.

During autologous BMT, the client is hospitalized in a private room for at least 6 to 8 weeks. The major stressor is perhaps the proximity to death resulting from the immunosuppression. Complications that may occur are malnutrition, infection, and bleeding.

Studies are being done to examine the potential role of different combination chemotherapies and different rates of radiation exposure in causing immunosuppression, the separation of stem cells from other marrow components so that reinfused cells are concentrated, and harvesting of stem cells from the peripheral blood. Other promising technologies include the use of interferon before or after grafting for its antileukemic effect, the use of growth factors (such as erythropoietin) to stimulate rapid recovery of the bone marrow, the use of bone-seeking radioisotopes to deliver high doses of radiation to the marrow without harming normal tissue, and the use of monoclonal antibodies attached to radioactive isotopes or chemotherapy directed at target malignant cells (Thomas, 1988).

Colony Stimulating Factors

Colony stimulating factors (CSFs), also called hematopoietic growth factors, are a set of glycoprotein factors that stimulate hemopoiesis of all major types of cells produced in the bone marrow. The factors work by attaching to receptors on the membranes of target cells and setting into action the processes involved in the differentiation, maturation, or proliferation of the cells. The primary use of CSFs at present is to reduce the depth and length of postchemotherapy nadirs (Burke, Wilkes, Berg, Bean, & Ingwersen, 1991).

Nursing Care

In planning and implementing care for the client with leukemia, the nurse must consider the chronic and life-threatening nature of the disease as well as the toxic effects of treatment. Although each client will have different needs, common nursing diagnoses focus on the risk for infection, altered nutrition, altered oral mucous membranes, the risk for injury (bleeding), and grieving.

Risk for Infection

In the client with leukemia, changes in white blood cells impair the immune response. This decreases the client's resistance to infection. The client may have either increased production of immature, nonfunctioning cells or decreased numbers of WBCs. In addition, chemotherapy or radiation used as treatment depresses bone marrow function, increasing the risk for infection.

Nursing interventions and rationales follow:

- Institute measures to prevent exposure to known or potential sources of infection:
  a. If prescribed, maintain protective isolation.
  b. Ensure that all people who are in contact with the client maintain meticulous hand washing.
  c. Provide careful and thorough hygiene daily.
  d. Restrict visitors with colds, flu, or infections.
  e. Provide oral hygiene after every meal.
  f. Avoid invasive procedures that may provide a portal of entry for infection, including injections, intravenous catheters, catheterizations, and rectal and vaginal procedures. If invasive procedures are essential, use strict aseptic technique, and monitor sites carefully postprocedure.
  g. Monitor for manifestations of infection: elevated body temperature, chills, throat pain, cough, chest pain, burning on urination, purulent drainage, and itching and burning in vaginal or rectal areas.

  These precautions minimize the client's exposure to bacterial, viral, and fungal pathogens or detect early changes so that treatment may be instituted. The client is at risk for infection as a result of WBC immaturity; infection is the major cause of death in clients with leukemia (Carpenito, 1995). Mucous membranes are especially susceptible to breakdown and infection as a result of tissue damage from chemotherapy or radiation.

- Monitor vital signs and oxygenation every 4 hours. Assess for temperature spikes with chilling, tachypnea, tachycardia, restlessness, change in PaO_2, and hypotension. *Although body temperature is usually elevated in infection, clients with leukemia may have altered responses, and sepsis may be present before abnormal vital signs appear. The manifestations described are indicative of sepsis; hypotension is usually a late symptom of sepsis.*

- Monitor decreasing levels of neutrophils (measured in mm^3) to detect risk for infection:
  2000 to 2500: no risk
  1000 to 2000: minimal risk
  500 to 1000: moderate risk
  Below 500: severe risk
  WBCs (especially neutrophils) are the first line of defense against infection. As levels decrease, the risk for infection increases.

- Explain the reasons for precautions and restrictions, and explain that decreased measures are usually temporary. *Client and family understanding increases compliance and thereby lowers the risk of infection.*

Altered Nutrition: Less Than Body Requirements

The client with leukemia may have difficulty meeting nutritional requirements as a result of increased metabolism, fatigue, loss of appetite from radiation, nausea and vomiting from chemotherapy, or oral mucous membrane breakdown and infection that makes chewing and swallowing difficult and/or painful.

Nursing interventions with rationales follow:

- Evaluate weight loss over time to determine degree of malnutrition. A weight that is 10% to 20% below ideal for height and weight indicates malnutrition. The percentage of change can be calculated as follows:

$$\% \text{ weight change} = \frac{\text{usual weight} - \text{actual weight}}{\text{usual weight}} \times 100$$

The body requires a minimum level of nutrients for health and growth. Inability to meet metabolic requirements results in weight loss and a decrease in the body's ability to repair itself. Cancer increases metabolic needs, and the client with cancer has nutritional problems that are related to both the disease and its treatment.

- Provide interventions to eliminate causative or contributing factors to inadequate food and fluid intake:
  a. Perform oral hygiene before and after meals; use a soft toothbrush or sponges as necessary.
  b. Use a solution of hydrogen peroxide and water to swish out mouth. Use either equal parts of hydrogen peroxide and water or one part hydrogen peroxide to three parts water.
  c. Provide liquids with different textures and tastes.
  d. Increase liquid intake with meals.
  e. Avoid intake of milk and milk products, which makes mucus more tenacious.
  f. Have the client assume a sitting position when eating.
  g. Ensure that the environment is clean and odor-free.
  h. Provide medications for pain or nausea 30 minutes before meals, if prescribed.
  i. Provide rest periods before meals.
  j. Offer small, frequent meals six times a day; a bland, high-kcal diet may be better tolerated.
  k. Use commercial supplements, such as Ensure.
  l. Avoid painful or unpleasant procedures immediately before or after meals. (See rationale below.)

- Increase food tolerance by suggesting that the client:
  a. Eat dry foods when arising.
  b. Eat salty foods, if permitted.
  c. Avoid very sweet, rich, or greasy foods.
  d. Eat small amounts of food more frequently.
  People with leukemia must deal not only with the metabolic effects of the disease on their nutritional status but also with

the effects of treatment. Anorexia, nausea and vomiting, diarrhea, stomatitis, taste changes, and dysphagia make eating difficult at a time when good nutrition is most important. Nutritional interventions decrease morbidity and mortality of cancer by preventing weight loss, increasing the body's response to treatment, minimizing treatment side effects, and improving quality of life. Although measures to improve nutritional status vary from client to client, any or all of these measures may be useful. Small, frequent meals are often better tolerated, especially high-protein, high-kcal foods. Overactivity increases metabolism and may reduce metabolic reserves.

Altered Oral Mucous Membranes

Stomatitis, the inflammation and ulceration of the mucous membranes of the mouth, is common in the client with leukemia. The client with leukemia is at increased risk for altered oral mucous membranes as a result of the disease-related decrease in the resistance to infection and the use of chemotherapy as treatment. A nursing approach to reducing the incidence of stomatitis in clients undergoing chemotherapy or radiation is described in the accompanying research box.

Nursing interventions with rationales follow:

- Monitor all areas of the mouth daily for mucosal breakdown: buccal region, gums, sublingual area, and the throat. Ask whether the client has a burning feeling in the mouth, and assess for swelling or lesions on the oral mucosa. *Breakdown of the oral mucous membranes increases the risk of infection and bleeding, causes pain and discomfort with eating and swallowing, and may cause swelling great enough to obstruct the airway.*

- Culture any lesions of the oral mucosa. *Herpes simplex virus and* Candida *(yeast) are both more common in clients with neutropenia. Herpes lesions are usually red,*

Applying Research to Nursing Practice: Reducing the Incidence of Stomatitis Using a Quality Assessment and Improvement Approach

Stomatitis occurs in approximately 40% of clients with cancer who receive chemotherapy or head/neck radiation. This side effect alters the client's quality of life and may affect the course of treatment. The purpose of one study was to determine whether quality assessment of specific interventions to decrease the incidence of stomatitis in clients receiving chemotherapy would prove effective (Graham, Pecoraro, Ventura, & Meyer, 1993). The setting for the study was an oncology unit in a Veterans Administration medical center.

Clients who were hospitalized for treatment of cancer on the oncology unit (ranging from 30 to 76 per month) had a prechemotherapy oral assessment. They then were given a soft toothbrush and a sterile saline solution with verbal and written instructions to rinse and gargle with the saline after every meal and at bedtime. Clients with dentures were asked to keep them clean and to refrain from wearing them for 8 hours daily. All clients were taught specific foods and fluids to avoid. Each client was then assessed using an oral assessment guide. The incidence of stomatitis was then plotted, and a marked decrease was noted in the number of clients who developed stomatitis over a 26-month period.

Implications for Nursing

Stomatitis causes many problems for clients, including pain, altered oral mucous membranes, alterations in nutrition, and noncompliance. Nurses can develop and monitor interventions to prevent or diminish the intensity of these responses through such activities as teaching, developing intervention protocols, using standard assessment tools, implementing quality assessment programs, and analyzing trends in data across time. The results of this study demonstrate that nurses can help lower the incidence of chemotherapy-induced stomatitis.

Critical Thinking in Client Care

1. Describe the rationale for rinsing the mouth with saline after eating and at bedtime.

2. Why would saline be preferable to an alcohol-based mouthwash in rinsing the mouth?

3. How could stomatitis interfere with compliance with treatment for cancer?

4. Discuss the relationship between an increased risk for infection and an increased risk for stomatitis in the client who has a hematologic malignancy or is receiving chemotherapy.

raised, *fluid-filled lesions; Candida causes a white-colored coating and areas of white plaque.*

- Ensure that clients rinse the mouth with saline or the mixture of hydrogen peroxide and water described above every 2 to 4 hours. Apply petroleum jelly to the lips whenever necessary to prevent dryness and cracking. *These agents help prevent infection and also increase comfort when infections are present.*

- Encourage use of soft-bristle toothbrush or sponge to clean the teeth and gums. *Toothbrushes with hard bristles may abrade inflamed mucosa, causing bleeding and increasing the risk of infection.*

- Administer medications as prescribed to treat infections or relieve pain. *Topical antifungal agents such as nystatin may be prescribed to treat Candida infections. Topical anesthetics such as lidocaine may be prescribed to relieve comfort and facilitate good oral care.*

- Teach the client to avoid alcohol-based mouthwashes, citrus fruit juices, spicy foods, foods that are either very hot or very cold, alcohol, and crusty foods. Teach the client to eat bland, cool foods and drink cool liquids at least every 2 hours. *Avoidance of mucosa-traumatizing foods and liquids increases comfort; bland, cool foods and liquids cause the least pain. Intake of adequate fluids is necessary to prevent dehydration.*

Risk for Injury: Bleeding

Bleeding is the second most common cause of death in clients with leukemia. As platelet counts (measured in mm^3) decrease, the risk of bleeding increases as follows:

Above 100,000: no risk

50,000 to 100,000: minimal risk

20,000 to 50,000: moderate risk

Below 20,000: severe risk

Nursing interventions with rationales follow:

- Assess all body systems every shift for manifestations of bleeding:
  a. Skin and mucous membranes for petechiae, ecchymoses, and hematoma formation
  b. Gums, nasal membranes, and conjunctiva for bleeding
  c. Any vomitus for bright red or coffee-ground color
  d. Hematuria (blood in the urine)
  e. Vaginal bleeding
  f. Rectal bleeding or tarry stools
  g. Prolonged bleeding from puncture sites
  h. Changes in neurologic status: headache, visual changes, alterations in mental status, decreasing level of consciousness, seizures
  i. Changes in gastrointestinal status: epigastric pain, absence of bowel sounds, increasing abdominal girth, abdominal rigidity

In addition, monitor vital signs every 4 hours as well as platelet counts. *The early assessment of bleeding is necessary to prevent serious blood loss. Internal hemorrhage may be manifested by tachycardia, hypotension, pallor, and diaphoresis. Bleeding into the lungs may cause dyspnea; bleeding into the abdomen causes increased girth, pain, and a rigid, boardlike abdomen. Intracranial bleeding may be manifested by alterations in mental status and level of consciousness as well as by respiratory changes.*

- Avoid the following invasive procedures, if possible:
  a. Use of rectal suppositories and taking rectal temperatures
  b. Use of vaginal douches, suppositories, or tampons
  c. Urinary catheterizations
  d. Parenteral injections
  Diagnostic procedures such as biopsy or lumbar puncture should not be done if the platelet count is less than 50,000. *Invasive procedures can cause tissue trauma and bleeding. Procedures that use large bore-needles should be delayed until the platelet count is increased.*

- Apply pressure to puncture sites for 3 to 5 minutes; apply pressure to arterial blood gas sites for 15 to 20 minutes. *Pressure prevents prolonged bleeding by prompting hemostasis and clot formation.*

- Use soft toothbrushes or sponges for oral hygiene. *These help prevent trauma to oral mucosa, which is at risk of bleeding.*

- Teach the client to avoid the following:
  a. Picking crusts from the nose
  b. Blowing the nose forcefully
  c. Straining to have a bowel movement
  d. Forceful coughing, sneezing, and blowing the nose
  These activities increase the risk of external and internal bleeding.

Anticipatory Grieving

The diagnosis of cancer of any type causes the client and significant others to experience an actual or perceived loss. The diagnosis of a life-threatening illness produces many losses: loss of function, loss of independence, change in appearance, loss of friends, loss of self-esteem, and loss of self. Grieving is the emotional response to those losses. The adaptive process of mourning a loss and resolving grief is called grief work; grief work cannot begin until a loss is acknowledged (Carpenito, 1995). A detailed discussion of grief and loss appears in Chapter 11.

Nursing interventions with rationales follow:

- Assess the roles of the client and family and the ways in which they managed stressful situations prior to diagnosis. Discuss the following issues:
  a. Have the client and family experienced loss?
  b. Have dietary and sleep patterns changed?
  c. Have activities of daily living continued?

d. Have social contacts been maintained?

In addition, assess coping strategies as well as their effectiveness, and determine sources of strength for the client and family; their reactions to changing roles resulting from diagnosis of cancer; spiritual, social, and economic status; usual life-style; and cultural or ethnic factors that affect grief reactions. *Grieving is a normal response to a real or potential loss that begins at the time of diagnosis. The timing, duration, and intensity of grief and the responses to grief may differ among family members. Share information on diagnosis, role change, and physical loss among all family members to build the foundation for mutual understanding and trust.*

■ Use therapeutic communication skills to allow open discussion of losses as well as permission to grieve. *Encouraging the client and family to talk about the meaning of the loss helps to decrease some of the anxiety associated with loss. This in turn allows the client and family to examine the current situation and compare it with past situations that they have coped with successfully.*

■ Identify agencies that may help in resolving grief, and make referrals as indicated. Consider self-help groups, cancer support groups, widow-to-widow groups, single-parent groups, and bereavement groups. *Participating in support groups consisting of others who are anticipating or have experienced a similar loss can decrease the client's feelings of isolation.*

Other Nursing Diagnoses

Other nursing diagnoses that are appropriate for the client with leukemia follow:

■ *Activity Intolerance* related to weakness

■ *Body Image Disturbance* related to alopecia and weight loss

■ *Risk for Impaired Skin Integrity* related to immobility secondary to weakness

■ *Risk for Injury* related to weakness secondary to anemia

■ *Ineffective Individual Coping* related to diagnosis and prognosis of leukemia

■ *Fear* related to prognosis of leukemia

■ *Knowledge Deficit* regarding disease process, self-care, nutritional needs, and medical treatment

■ *Pain* secondary to hepatosplenomegaly

■ *Powerlessness* related to the inability to halt progression of disease process

■ *Self-Care Deficit: Total* related to weakness

■ *Altered Sexuality Patterns* related to weakness and depression associated with chronic illness

In addition, the following potential complications may be applicable to the client with leukemia:

■ *Potential Complication: Hemorrhage* secondary to bleeding due to thrombocytopenia

■ *Potential Complication: Sepsis* secondary to neutropenia following chemotherapy

Client and Family Teaching

Client and family teaching for home care after treatment for leukemia focuses on encouraging self-care, providing information about the disease and the treatment, preventing infection and injury, and promoting nutrition. Teaching topics for each of these areas are presented below.

Encouraging Self-Care

■ Take a daily bath or shower; be sure to clean the vaginal/perianal area carefully.

■ Clean the teeth at least daily with a soft-bristle toothbrush; avoid flossing.

■ Inspect the skin and mucous membranes daily for signs of bleeding or infection.

■ Balance activity with rest.

Providing Information about the Disease and Treatment

■ Explain the pathophysiology of the illness, the function of bone marrow, and the potential complications of leukemia.

■ Explain that cancer is a chronic illness that in most cases can be cured or controlled.

■ Discuss chemotherapy, radiation, and/or bone marrow transplantation: how it is conducted, where it is conducted, who administers the treatment, and its effects (positive and negative).

■ Provide client with information about community resources that offer support to people living with leukemia.

Preventing Infection and Injury

■ Use careful hand-washing practices.

■ Avoid bacteria in the diet: raw fruits and vegetables, fried foods in restaurants.

■ Avoid crowds, and avoid people who are ill.

■ Maintain dental health.

■ Do not take immunizations.

■ Report the following to the health care provider: elevated body temperature, chills, burning on urination, foul-smelling urine, vaginal or rectal discharge, skin lesions.

■ Avoid contact sports or strenuous exercise if platelet count is less than 50,000/mm^3.

- Use an electric or battery-powered razor rather than razor blades for shaving.

- Do not use rectal thermometers, rectal or vaginal suppositories, vaginal tampons, or enemas.

- Increase fiber in the diet, and take a mild stool softener (if needed) to prevent straining to have a bowel movement.

- Do not take over-the-counter or prescription drugs that interfere with platelet function. (See the box on page 1281.)

- Report any bleeding (nosebleeds, rectal bleeding, vomiting blood, excessive menstrual periods, blood in the urine, bleeding gums, bruises, or collections of blood under the skin) or changes in behavior to the health care provider.

Promoting Nutrition

- Eat several small, bland meals each day.

- Drink several glasses of water each day.

- Report any continued weight loss, loss of appetite, or inability to eat for 24 hours.

- Discuss dietary needs with the dietitian.

The client and family may require assistance with physical care, finances, and transportation after the client is dismissed from the hospital. Care of the client with leukemia is ongoing and demanding. Nursing care plans for home care must include referrals to social services, support groups, home care services if needed, and other agencies that can provide needed services (such as local chapters of the American Cancer Society, which can provide, for example, hospital beds and transportation for outpatient cancer treatment). Equally important to the client and family are honest communication, optimism, and hope.

Applying the Nursing Process

Case Study of a Client with Acute Myelogenous Leukemia: Catherine Cole

Catherine Cole is a 37-year-old secretary who was born in England and moved to North America when she was 25. She lives with her husband, Ray, and teenaged daughter, Amy, in an apartment in a large metropolitan area. About 2 months ago, Mrs. Cole began to tire easily, have fever and night sweats several times a week, exhibit pallor, and experience increased bruising and heavier menstrual periods. She goes to her primary care physician, who conducts blood tests that show abnormal findings. The physician admits Mrs. Cole to the hospital for a bone marrow biopsy.

Assessment

Mary Losapio, RN, conducts the admission history and physical assessment for Mrs. Cole. The data from these sources show the following:

Height: 5 feet, 4 inches (156 cm)

Weight: 106 lb (48.1 kg)

Vital signs: T, 100 F; P, 102; R, 22; BP, 130/82

Skin and mucous membranes: Numerous petechiae scattered over trunk and arms; ecchymotic areas on lower right arm and right calf. Oral mucosa is red, with several small ulcerations in the buccal areas.

Reason for admission: "I'm so tired, and I have these bruises all over me. I'm so afraid of what they will find when they do the bone marrow examination. I don't know what we will do if I have cancer."

In addition, the results of the laboratory tests reveal a decreased number of RBCs as well as a decreased hemoglobin and hematocrit. The WBC is high, with myeloblasts present. The platelet count is very low. Mrs. Cole appears tired and anxious. As she speaks, she clutches her husband's hand and then begins to cry. The tentative medical diagnosis for Mrs. Cole is acute myelogenous leukemia.

Diagnosis

Ms. Losapio formulates the following nursing diagnoses for Mrs. Cole:

- *Risk for Infection* related to alterations in the production of WBCs and antibodies

- *Risk for Injury* related to increased bleeding tendencies secondary to reduced platelets

- *Altered Oral Mucous Membrane* secondary to anemia and reduced platelets

- *Fatigue* related to decreased oxygen availability secondary to anemia

- *Anxiety* related to fear of leukemia diagnosis

Expected Outcomes

The expected outcomes established in the plan of care specify that Mrs. Cole will

- Be free of nosocomial infections.

- Be free of significant loss of blood.

- Have intact oral mucous membranes.

- Manage self-care activities despite fatigue.

- Alternate activity/exercise periods with rest periods.

- Verbalize a decrease in anxiety.

Planning and Implementation

Ms. Losapio implements the following nursing interventions for Mrs. Cole:

- If available, move Mrs. Cole to a private room.
- Limit visitors to Mrs. Cole's husband and daughter for the present.
- Ensure meticulous hand washing by the staff, family, and client. Post a sign over the washbasin in the room as a reminder, and discuss with Mrs. Cole and her family the importance of this step.
- Take and record vital signs every 4 hours.
- Do not perform invasive procedures or medications unless absolutely necessary.
- Monitor Mrs. Cole every 4 hours for signs of bleeding: Assess skin, oral mucosa, gastrointestinal tract, body fluids, and menstrual pad count.
- Teach Mrs. Cole to perform oral hygiene every 2 to 4 hours, using a soft-bristle toothbrush or a sponge.
- Ask the dietitian to identify with Mrs. Cole foods that she likes to eat but that also avoid injury to her oral mucosa. Discuss with her the need to avoid foods that are very hot, cold, or cause pain when eaten.
- Encourage Mrs. Cole to be as independent as possible in providing self-care and in moving around in her room; however, emphasize the need to alternate activity with rest.
- Teach the client and her family about the bone marrow biopsy. Allow time for them to ask questions and verbalize fears. Ask the oncology nurse specialist to visit as soon as possible.

Evaluation

The bone marrow biopsy is done that afternoon, and the physician confirms the diagnosis with Mrs. Cole and her family the next day. Understandably, Mrs. Cole is at first very upset, but as the physician and the oncology nurse discuss treatment plans and the possibility of remission, she becomes calmer. She decides to have chemotherapy done on an outpatient basis. During her hospital stay, Mrs. Cole has shown no evidence of infection or further bleeding. She has provided her own oral hygiene and bath and tells Ms. Losapio that her mouth feels better, although it is still painful. During routine assessment, Mrs. Cole remarks, "You know, I was so scared when I came here, but I think I am a little less so now. Sometimes not knowing what is wrong is worse than knowing."

Critical Thinking in the Nursing Process

1. Describe how alterations in WBCs can increase a person's susceptibility to infection.
2. List sources of potential infection for the hospitalized client.
3. What is the rationale for having the client do her own oral and physical hygiene?

4. Outline a teaching plan for this client and her family for home care to prevent infection.
5. Develop a care plan for Mrs. Cole for the nursing diagnosis *Activity Intolerance.*

The Client with Malignant Lymphoma

■ ■ ■

A **malignant lymphoma** is a neoplastic tumor affecting the lymphoid tissue. The disease is characterized by a proliferation of lymphocytes and progressive, painless enlargement of the lymph nodes. These neoplasms affect the cells of the immune system, with malignancies occurring in lymphoid tissue, usually the lymph nodes and the spleen.

Pathophysiology

Lymphocytes originate from stem cells in bone marrow and are responsible for the body's immune defense system. Rapid proliferation of abnormal lymphocytes leads to immune system suppression, rendering the person more susceptible to infectious processes. The lymphomas discussed in this section are Hodgkin's disease and non-Hodgkin's lymphomas.

Hodgkin's Disease

Hodgkin's disease is a lymphatic cancer, occurring most often in adults in their late 20s and after the mid-40s. It is responsible for about 14% of all the malignant lymphomas (Belcher, 1992). The exact cause of Hodgkin's disease is unknown, but it appears to be associated with infections from Epstein-Barr virus and to have genetic factors. Hodgkin's disease is one of the most curable of all cancers. If diagnosed early, as many as 60% to 90% of people with localized manifestations have the possibility of living out a normal life span (Porth, 1994). Hodgkin's disease is believed to begin within one lymph node (usually in the neck); if untreated, it spreads throughout the lymphatic system to nodes throughout the body. The disease may also be found in the spleen, liver, vertebrae, ureters, and bronchi. Hodgkin's disease is characterized by painless, progressive enlargement of the lymph nodes, the spleen, and other lymphoid tissues. The malignant cells may attack nearly any area of the body, producing a variety of symptoms. A characteristic of Hodgkin's disease is the presence of *Reed-Sternberg cells*. These cells secrete interleukin-1, which causes proliferation of T lymphocytes and fibroblasts, both of which are found in the client with Hodgkin's disease (Belcher, 1992).

The most frequently found clinical symptom is the presence of one or more painlessly enlarged lymph nodes.

Clinical Manifestations of Hodgkin's Disease

■ ■ ■

- One or more enlarged but painless lymph nodes
- Fever   ■ Fatigue
- Night sweats   ■ Malaise
- Weight loss   ■ Pruritus

Other common findings include persistent fever, night sweats, fatigue, weight loss, malaise, pruritus, and anemia. If the disease if allowed to progress, edema of the face and neck, jaundice, nerve pain, enlargement of retroperitoneal nodes, and nodular infiltration of the spleen, liver, and bones may also occur. See the accompanying clinical manifestations box.

The severity of the disease is determined through staging. Typically, the Ann Arbor staging system is used to assess the microscopic appearance of the lymph nodes, the extent and severity of the disease, and to estimate the prognosis. The Ann Arbor staging system is as follows:

Stage 1: Involvement of a single lymph node region or a single extranodal site.

Stage 2: Involvement of two or more lymph node regions on the same side of the diaphragm, or localized involvement of an extranodal site and one or more lymph node regions on the same side of the diaphragm.

Stage 3: Involvement of lymph node regions on both sides of the diaphragm and possibly of a single extranodal site on the spleen, or both.

Stage 4: Diffuse or disseminated disease of one or more extralymphatic organs or tissues with or without associated lymph node involvement; the extranodal site is identified as H (hepatic), L (lung), P (pleura), M (marrow), D (dermal), or O (osseous).

Another staging system, the Rye classification system, classifies Hodgkin's disease into four subtypes:

- *Lymphocyte-predominant,* in which lymphocytes diffusely infiltrate the abnormal lymph nodes. This type is found in 5% to 10% of clients with Hodgkin's disease. The prognosis for clients with this subtype is a 5-year survival rate of 90%.

- *Nodular sclerosis,* in which bands of collagen divide the cellular infiltrate into discrete islands and give the lymph nodes a nodular appearance. This subtype, occurring in 30% to 60% of the cases, is seen most often in young women. At diagnosis, the disease is often localized in the cervical nodes and the mediastinum. The 5-year survival rate is high.

- *Mixed cellularity,* in which the nodes contain eosinophils, normal lymphocytes, and Reed-Sternberg cells. This subtype makes up about 33% of all cases. The 5-year survival rate is 50% to 60%.

- *Lymphocyte-depleted,* in which the Reed-Sternberg cells predominate and mature lymphocytes are almost totally absent in affected lymph nodes. This subtype is seen most often in the older adult. The 5-year survival rate is less than 50%.

In Hodgkin's disease, the presence or absence of systemic symptoms is indicated by either an A (no systemic symptoms) or B (systemic symptoms of fever, night sweats, weight loss).

Non-Hodgkin's Lymphoma

Malignant disorders that originate from lymphoid tissues but are not diagnosed as Hodgkin's disease are classified as **non-Hodgkin's lymphoma (NHL).** There are several types of non-Hodgkin's lymphoma, including follicular small cleaved-cell lymphoma, diffuse large-cell lymphoma, and immunoblastic lymphoma. Most of the non-Hodgkin's lymphomas occur in older adults. The cause of these lymphomas has not been identified, but viral infections and exposure to ionizing radiation and toxic chemicals are suspected in at least some cases. In addition, NHL is associated with immunosuppressive therapy for organ transplants and AIDS.

Like Hodgkin's disease, non-Hodgkin's lymphoma often begins with one node and spreads through the lymphatic system. However, some types of non-Hodgkin's lymphoma involve unusual areas, such as the bones, the central nervous system, and the gastrointestinal tract.

The most common early manifestation of NHL is an enlarged lymph node. However, many other manifestations may occur. Gastrointestinal involvement may cause jaundice, abdominal cramping, bloody diarrhea, or bowel obstruction. Ureteral obstruction may cause hydronephrosis. Compression of the spinal cord may impair neurologic function. Late in the disease, hemolytic anemia may appear.

Diagnosis is determined from biopsy of a suspicious mass or node, and the same staging system is used as for Hodgkin's disease. Prognosis for a client with non-Hodgkin's lymphoma can range from excellent to poor, depending on the cell type identified. However, the prognosis is generally poorer than that for clients with Hodgkin's disease. Because NHL originates within lymphoid tissue, it often is widely distributed in nodes, bone marrow, or the blood by the time a diagnosis is made.

Collaborative Care

Chemotherapy and radiation therapy, either alone or in combination, are the primary forms of treatment for Hodgkin's and non-Hodgkin's lymphomas. Occasionally, surgical intervention is carried out. Treatment is determined by disease type and stage of the disease process.

Laboratory and Diagnostic Tests

The following laboratory tests may be ordered:

- *CBC* is conducted. Findings for the client with Hodgkin's disease typically include mild normochromic, normocytic anemia; hemolytic anemia (advanced disease); decreased lymphocytes; increased eosinophils; increased platelet count; and an elevated erythrocyte sedimentation rate. Abnormal findings are often not seen in the client with non-Hodgkin's lymphoma until late in the disease, when a marked reduction in all blood elements may be found (pancytopenia).

- *Blood chemistry studies* are often performed. Clients with Hodgkin's disease often have elevated serum alkaline phosphatase (from bone and liver involvement) and hypercalcemia (from bone involvement and decreased blood proteins).

Diagnostic studies used to diagnose Hodgkin's disease and non-Hodgkin's lymphoma include the following:

- *Chest X-ray study* or *lung computed tomography (CT) scan* may be taken to identify lung or pleural involvement.

- *Abdominal CT scan* may be taken to identify the presence of abnormal or enlarged nodes.

- *Bone marrow biopsy* may be performed to identify abnormal cells.

- *Lymph node biopsy* of the largest, most central enlarged lymph node is conducted. A biopsy is used to establish the diagnosis for both Hodgkin's disease and non-Hodgkin's lymphoma. The presence of Reed-Sternberg cells confirms the diagnosis of Hodgkin's disease.

- *Lymphangiography* (X-ray imaging of the lymph glands and lymphatic vessels after injection of a contrast medium) is performed to detect the extent of lymph node involvement.

- *Bone scans* may be conducted to identify bone involvement in non-Hodgkin's lymphoma.

- *Bone marrow, liver, and spleen biopsies* may also be conducted to identify or exclude further organ involvement.

Radiation Therapy

Radiation therapy is used to treat both Hodgkin's disease and non-Hodgkin's lymphoma. Radiation therapy can effect a cure in most clients with either stage 1 or stage 2 Hodgkin's disease, and some with stage 3 Hodgkin's disease (Belcher, 1992). Therapy usually involves extensive external radiation of the involved lymph node region. If the disease is advanced, total nodal irradiation may be done (Figure 31–12). Men who have radiation therapy of

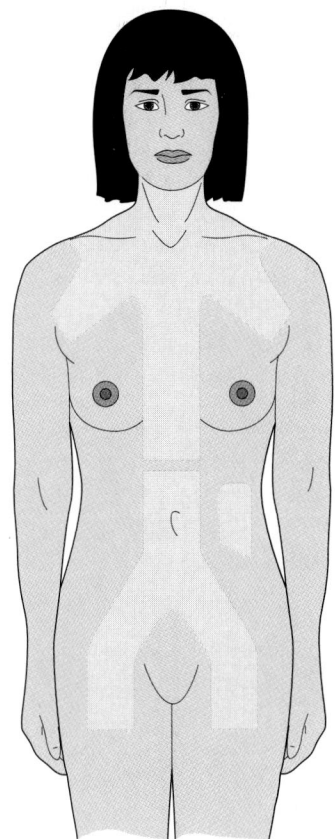

Figure 31–12   Areas of total nodal irradiation in non-Hodgkin's lymphoma.

the abdominal and pelvic regions will become permanently sterile. The goal of radiation therapy in non-Hodgkin's lymphoma is to control the disease in the area where it is evidenced; many lymphomas are highly responsive to radiation and have a high remission rate. In many cases, radiation therapy is used in conjunction with chemotherapy.

Chemotherapy

Single-agent or combination chemotherapy is also used to treat both Hodgkin's disease and non-Hodgkin's lymphoma. Single-agent chemotherapy is used most often in older adults and in clients who have had heavy radiation therapy with myelosuppression and cannot tolerate combined chemotherapy. Combination chemotherapy, with the MOPP regimen (nitrogen mustard, vincristine, procarbazine, and prednisone) has produced a high response rate and a durable remission in clients with Hodgkin's disease. Chemotherapy is the primary treatment for disseminated non-Hodgkin's lymphoma. The choice of drug combination depends on the stage of the disease as well as the client's age and general condition.

Surgery

In Hodgkin's disease, surgery is conducted primarily to obtain biopsy specimens or to obtain tissue for staging. A therapeutic splenectomy (surgical removal of the spleen) may be performed in clients with Hodgkin's disease or non-Hodgkin's lymphoma if the spleen is enlarged, to reduce the size of the radiation field needed to carry out radiation therapy, or to allow the client to undergo more extensive chemotherapy (Belcher, 1992).

Nursing Care

Nursing care of the client with malignant lymphoma involves providing both physical and emotional support throughout the course of treatment. Although nursing interventions must be designed to meet individualized needs, common nursing diagnoses focus on problems with altered comfort, fatigue, altered nutrition, and altered body image.

Altered Protection

The client with a malignant lymphoma may experience manifestations of altered protection for a variety of reasons, including pruritus, nausea, and vomiting. Pruritus and night sweats are manifestations of the illness. The night sweats are often the result of fever; the cause of pruritus is unknown. Nausea and vomiting are common side effects of chemotherapy. Regardless of the cause, these manifestations bring about altered protection.

Nursing interventions with rationales follow:

- Assess the onset, sites, precipitating factors, and methods of relieving pruritus. *Pruritus is aggravated by excessive warmth, excessive dryness, rough fabrics, fatigue, and stress.*

- Provide and teach client and family interventions to enhance comfort and relieve itching: use cool water and a mild soap to bathe; blot (rather than rub) dry skin; apply plain cornstarch or nonperfumed lotion or powder to the skin unless contraindicated; use lightweight blankets and clothing; maintain adequate humidity and a cool room temperature; wash bedding and clothes in mild detergent, and put them through second rinse cycle. *These interventions facilitate the relief of pruritus by reducing or eliminating mechanical and chemical irritation.*

- Assess factors that precipitate nausea and/or vomiting, the frequency and type of vomiting, and relief measures used by the client. *Nausea and vomiting are symptoms of some cancers and are also common side effects of chemotherapy. Interventions to prevent or relieve nausea and/or vomiting must be individualized.*

- Use ordered antiemetics before chemotherapy is started. *Administering the ordered antiemetic before the activity that is known to cause nausea and vomiting allows*

adequate time for drug absorption, maximizing its effectiveness.

- Provide teaching to prevent or relieve nausea and vomiting:
  a. Eat soda crackers and suck on hard candy.
  b. Eat cold or room-temperature foods.
  c. Eat soft, bland foods.
  d. Avoid unpleasant odors, and get fresh air.
  e. Do not eat immediately before chemotherapy.
  f. Use distraction or progressive muscle relaxation when nauseated.
  g. Do not eat for several hours if vomiting occurs. Resume oral intake with clear liquids or ice, and progress to bland foods.

Crackers and hard candy often relieve queasiness. Foods that are hot, warm, salty, sweet, or have strong odors often increase nausea. Alternative methods of relieving nausea may be effective.

Fatigue

General malaise and fatigue are side effects of chemotherapy and anemia. The physical and psychologic stress of dealing with a chronic, debilitating disease and its treatment may cause fatigue. In addition, malaise and fatigue may signify progressive involvement of the disease, including a buildup of toxic waste products.

Nursing interventions with rationales follow:

- Assess the client's subjective experience of malaise (a vague feeling of body weakness or discomfort) and fatigue (a pervasive, drained feeling that cannot be eliminated). *Both malaise and fatigue are subjective experiences with physiologic, situational, and psychologic components.*

- Allow the client to verbalize feelings regarding the impact of the disease and fatigue on life-style. *Discussion of feelings helps the client to feel valued. Clarifying values may assist the client in identifying life-style priorities.*

- Encourage enjoyable but quiet activities, such as reading, listening to music, or doing puzzles. *Enjoyable activities are thought to decrease fatigue. These quiet activities will help to conserve energy yet also yield a sense of accomplishment.*

- Assist the client to establish priorities, and include rest periods or naps when scheduling daily activities. *This will give the client control over which activities are performed and help maintain self-esteem. Energy-enhancing activities generate increased levels of perceived energy and decreased levels of fatigue.*

- Help the client determine how to delegate some responsibilities to family members. *The client is more apt to have adequate time to rest if some activities are delegated to others. The client can also maintain a role in the family by being involved in family decision making.*

- Assist the client in the use of energy-saving equipment. *Performing tasks with less exertion and in less time will help conserve the client's energy.*

- Encourage a diet high in carbohydrates and fluids. *A high-carbohydrate diet slows the depletion of muscle glycogen stores, while an increased intake of fluids promotes the excretion of call destruction end-products that may cause malaise and fatigue (Piper, 1993).*

Altered Nutrition: Less Than Body Requirements

In the client with a malignant lymphoma, chemotherapy and/or radiation, increased metabolic effect of the cancer, depression in response to the diagnosis of cancer, or disease progression to the gastrointestinal tract may contribute to nutritional deficits. One or more of these factors may result in anorexia, fatigue, nausea and vomiting, diarrhea, and a feeling of fullness. The client may be either unable or unwilling to eat, and the nutritional deficit continues and, perhaps, worsens. Nursing interventions with rationales for this nursing diagnosis were fully discussed in the preceding section on the care of the client with leukemia and are also appropriate for the client with a malignant lymphoma. A brief summary follows:

- Provide small feedings of high-kcal, high-protein foods and fluids. *This increases nutritional intake.*

- Assist the client with oral care, general hygiene, and environmental control of temperature, appearance, and odors. *These measures enhance appetite.*

- Identify and provide foods the client prefers. *This promotes and increases nutritional intake.*

- Place the client in a sitting position during and immediately after meals. *This helps decrease early feelings of fullness.*

Body Image Disturbance

The diagnosis of cancer is often devastating to the sense of trust in and the perception of one's body. Radiation and chemotherapy bring about changes in the appearance and function of the body (for example, loss of hair and loss of sexual or reproductive function), further altering the client's perception of body image. There is no one typical response to this diagnosis. Reactions may include any of the following (Carpenito, 1995).

- Refusal to touch or look at a body part
- Refusal to look in a mirror
- Unwillingness to discuss a limitation, deformity, or disfigurement
- Refusal to accept rehabilitation efforts
- Inappropriate attempts to direct own treatment
- Increasing dependence on others
- Signs of grieving: weeping, despair, anger
- Refusal to participate in self-care
- Displaying hostility toward the healthy
- Withdrawal from social contacts

Nursing interventions with rationales follow:

- Assess body image perception by collecting subjective data through the following questions (Carpenito, 1995):
  a. What do you like the most about your body?
  b. What do you like the least about your body?
  c. Before you were sick, how did you feel about people who were sick or disabled?
  d. What do you understand to be your health problem?
  e. What limitations do you think will result from your illness or your treatment?
  f. How do you feel about this illness?
  g. Has the illness changed the way you believe others will respond to you?
  Body image is a person's mental idea of his or her body. It is based on past and present experiences and is made up of the interrelated components of one's actual body and the emotional responses to that body. Body image changes constantly. There is often a time lag between the actual body change and the change in body image; during this time, the client may reject both the diagnosis and the teaching and treatment prescribed (Carpenito, 1995).

- Assess the client for risk of developing alopecia. *Chemotherapeutic agents attack rapidly dividing normal and abnormal cells. The cells and tissues responsible for hair growth have a rapid division rate and are sensitive to chemotherapy. Hair loss usually begins 1 to 2 weeks after chemotherapy is initiated and reaches maximum loss 1 to 2 months later.*

- Provide interventions to enable client to cope with alopecia:
  a. Encourage verbalization of feelings.
  b. Teach the client the effects of chemotherapy on hair follicles, the potential for change in color and texture of hair that regrows, and the potential for regrowth of hair.
  c. Discuss various methods that can be used during periods of hair loss and regrowth: wigs, scarves, hats, caps.
  d. Encourage the client to wear his or her own clothes during hospitalization and at home.
  e. If eyelashes and eyebrows are lost, teach methods of protecting the eyes, such as eyeglasses and caps with wide brims.
  f. Teach proper scalp care: Use baby shampoo or mild soap, use soft brush, always use a sunscreen, and use mineral oil to reduce itching.
  g. Encourage participation in support groups.
  Alopecia may range from thinning of hair to a total hair

loss. Regrowth depends on the schedule of treatments and doses; however, regrowth of hair usually begins 2 to 3 months after treatment ends. New hair may be softer, more curly, and slightly different in color. Client teaching and emotional support helps the client anticipate hair loss, talk about its potential effect on body image, and learn self-care techniques. Resources are available to provide financial assistance for the purchase of wigs, including local American Cancer Society chapters and insurance plans. Support groups are often effective in helping the client deal with the loss and altered body image.

- Provide interventions to enable the client to cope with actual or potential sexual dysfunction or sterility:
  a. Assess the client's knowledge of the effects of the illness and the treatment of the illness on sexuality and reproduction.
  b. Encourage the client and significant others to verbalize their concerns.
  c. Provide information and clarify misconceptions.
  d. Explore realistic alternatives; for example, if a male client is having radiation that will cause permanent sterility, discuss the possibility of storing sperm in a sperm bank.
  e. Provide referrals for counseling if necessary.
  Clients with cancer often experience some form of sexual alteration as the result of the disease and the effects of radiation and chemotherapy. The reproductive tissues are made up of rapidly dividing cells, and damage from cancer treatment may cause temporary or permanent sterility, changes in menstruation, and changes in libido (sexual desire). Any or all of these changes bring about alterations in body image.

Other Nursing Diagnoses

Other nursing diagnoses that are appropriate for the client with malignant lymphomas follow:

- *Impaired Skin Integrity* related to excoriation from scratching
- *Ineffective Breathing Pattern* related to disease progression to lungs and mediastinum
- *Anxiety* related to knowledge deficit of illness, treatment, and side effects of treatment modalities
- *Hopelessness* related to diagnosis of terminal illness
- *Risk for Infection* related to impaired immune response and effects of chemotherapy and radiation therapy

Client and Family Teaching

When providing client and family teaching, include information about the illness, the treatment, and the side effects of the treatment modalities. Topics that are appropriate for the client with leukemia are also appropriate for the client with a malignant lymphoma. In addition, teach the client and family to

- Care for the skin and avoid scratching to decrease the risk of altered skin integrity and infection.
- Report symptoms of vertebral compression, such as decreased sensation or strength in lower extremities.
- Use alternative methods of pain relief as often as possible; bone, nerve, and abdominal pain are chronic.
- Use respiratory therapy if symptoms of lymph node enlargement of the mediastinum or involvement of the lungs and pleurae occur.
- Plan activities of daily living to ensure adequate rest and exercise.
- Eat a well-balanced diet.

In addition, refer clients and family members to the local chapter of the American Cancer Society for information, financial assistance, and counseling. Clients with malignant lymphomas may obtain a list of state and local agencies that offer information about the disease and financial assistance from the Leukemia Society of America.

| **Applying the Nursing Process** |

Case Study of a Client with Hodgkin's Disease: Albin Quito

Albin Quito, age 28, is the nurse manager of a thoracic intensive care unit in a large teaching hospital. Lately he has noticed that he is more tired than usual, often wakes up at night covered with sweat, seems to be itching a lot, and just does not feel well. He had thought that his symptoms were due to a touch of the influenza that has been going around and also to his unusually busy work schedule. However, yesterday morning Albin looked in the mirror after his shower and noticed a large swollen area on the right side of his neck. He called and made an appointment with his primary health provider in his HMO. At that appointment, a large cervical lymph node was found, and blood was drawn. A biopsy of the node and a CT scan of the chest were scheduled on an outpatient basis.

Assessment

When Mr. Quito arrives at the outpatient clinic to discuss the findings from the biopsy of the lymph node, he is first interviewed and assessed by David Herzog, the nurse in charge of the clinic. Mr. Herzog finds that Mr. Quito's physical findings are normal, with the exception of the enlarged node, which is not painful on palpation. However, when Mr. Quito is weighed, he tells Mr. Herzog that he has lost 7 lb (3.2 kg) in the past 2 months. In reviewing the results of the blood studies, Mr. Herzog notes that findings include mild anemia and an increased neutrophil count. The results of the lymph node biopsy reveal the presence of Reed-Sternberg cells. The clinic physician and Mr. Herzog tell Mr. Quito that the findings indicate stage 1-B (lymphocyte-predominant) Hodgkin's disease but that the prognosis is very good. Following a discussion of treatment options, Mr. Quito decides to undergo radiation therapy.

Diagnosis

Mr. Herzog makes the following diagnoses:

- *Anxiety* related to the diagnosis of a malignant disorder and effects of treatment on job performance
- *Risk for Infection* related to impaired immunologic function
- *Fatigue* related to the effects of the cancer, which will be increased by radiation therapy

Expected Outcomes

The expected outcomes established in the plan of care specify that Mr. Quito will

- Verbalize a decrease in anxiety.
- Remain free of infection.
- Use methods to preserve energy.

Planning and Implementation

The following nursing interventions are planned and implemented for Mr. Quito at this point in his treatment:

- Encourage Mr. Quito to discuss with the unit supervisor the possibility of time off from work during his course of treatment.
- Encourage Mr. Quito to join a support group for people with cancer.
- Provide Mr. Quito with information about the illness and the radiation therapy.
- Reinforce Mr. Quito's knowledge of activities to decrease the risk of infection.
- Discuss with Mr. Quito methods to decrease fatigue and maintain energy:
  a. Take a 1- to 2-hour nap once or twice a day; this often increases ability to have a restful night's sleep.
  b. Do not overexert self during weekends.
  c. Maintain a well-balanced diet.

Evaluation

When Mr. Quito returns the following week to begin his radiation treatments, he brings his friend Nancy to meet Mr. Herzog and asks him to discuss his treatment with her. Mr. Quito says, "I am still really scared, but being able to talk about this with Nancy will help a lot." Mr. Quito has made arrangements to take 6 months off from work, with the full understanding that his job will be held for him. He states that he will have some problems with money but is working them out. He also says he feels that taking a nap is silly but that he will do so to maintain his energy level. Both Mr. Quito and Nancy state that they be-

lieve Mr. Quito will be cured and that they both plan to be active members in the cancer support group—even after Mr. Quito recovers.

Critical Thinking in the Nursing Process

1. Discuss the rationale for treating Hodgkin's disease with radiation or chemotherapy.

2. Design a teaching plan to teach Mr. Quito how to prevent infection while he is at home.

3. What effect does the diagnosis of cancer have on the developmental level of a young adult?

4. Develop a care plan for Mr. Quito for the diagnosis *Altered Role Performance*.

Bibliography

■ ■ ■

Acevedo, M. (1992). Blood dyscrasias: Polycythemia, idiopathic thrombocytopenic purpura, and thrombotic thrombocytopenic purpura. *Journal of Intravenous Nursing, 15*(1), 52–57.

Alfaro-Lefevre, R., Blicharz, M. E., Flynn, N. M., & Boyer, M. J. (1992). *Drug handbook: A nursing process approach.* Redwood City, CA: Addison-Wesley Nursing.

American Cancer Society. (1994). *Cancer facts and figures—1994.* Atlanta: Author.

Arena, F. P. (1991). Update on acute lymphocytic leukemia. *Hospital Medicine, 27*(3), 33–36, 41–42, 44.

Bailes, B. K. (1992). Disseminated intravascular coagulation. *AORN Journal, 55*(2), 517–529.

Belcher, A. E. (1992). *Cancer nursing.* St. Louis: Mosby.

Bell, T. N. (1990). Disseminated intravascular coagulation and shock: Multisystem crisis in the critically ill. *Critical Care Nursing Clinics of North America, 2*, 255–268.

Bell, T. N. (1992). Coagulation and disseminated intravascular coagulation. In V. Huddleston (Ed.), *Multisystem organ failure: Pathophysiology and clinical implications* (pp. 57–81). St. Louis: Mosby-Year Book.

Binkley, L. S., & Whittaker, A. (1992). Erythropoietin use in the critical care setting. *AACN Clinical Issues in Critical Care Nursing, 3*(3), 640–651.

Burke, M., Wilkes, G., Berg, D., Bean, C., & Ingwersen, K. (1991). *Cancer chemotherapy: A nursing process approach.* Boston: Jones and Bartlett.

Byrne, C. J., Saxton, D., Pelikan, P., & Nugent, P. (1986). *Laboratory tests: Implications for nursing care* (2nd ed.). Menlo Park, CA: Addison-Wesley Nursing.

Carpenito, L. J. (1995). *Nursing diagnosis: Application to clinical practice* (6th ed.). Philadelphia: Lippincott.

Carpenito, L. J. (1995). *Nursing care plans and documentation: Nursing diagnoses and collaborative problems* (2nd ed.). Philadelphia: Lippincott.

Esposito, M. W. (1992). Thalassemias: Simple screening for hereditary anemias. *Nurse Practitioner, 17*(2), 50, 53–54.

Estey, E.H., & Freireich, E. J. (1991). Therapy for acute myelogenous leukemia. *Hematology, 14*, 1–33.

Fryback, P. B., & Reinert, B. R. (1993). Facilitating health in people with terminal diagnoses by encouraging a sense of control. *MEDSURG Nursing, 2*(3), 197–201.

Gawkikowski, J. (1992). White cells at war. *American Journal of Nursing, 92*(3), 444–451.

Graham, K. M., Pecoraro, D. A., Ventura, M., & Meyer, C. C. (1993). Reducing the incidence of stomatitis using a quality assessment and improvement approach. *Cancer Nursing, 16*(2), 117–122.

Hartshorn, J., Lamborn, M., & Noll, M. L. (1993). *Introduction to critical care nursing.* Philadelphia: W. B. Saunders.

Huddleston, V. B. (1992). *Multisystem organ failure: Pathophysiology and clinical implications.* St. Louis: Mosby-Year Book.

Huston, C. (1994). Emergency! Disseminated intravascular coagulation. *American Journal of Nursing, 94*(8), 51.

Iron deficiency in the elderly. (1990). *Emergency Medicine, 22*(14), 48, 51.

Kurtz, A. (1993). Disseminated intravascular coagulation with leukemia patients. *Cancer Nursing, 16,* 456–463.

Leach, M. (1991). Anemia—nursing care and intervention. *Professional Nurse, 6*(8), 454–456.

Loebl, S., Spratto, G. R., Woods, A. L., & Matejski, M. (1991). *The nurse's drug handbook* (6th ed.). Albany, NY: Delmar.

Marieb, E. N. (1992). *Human anatomy and physiology* (2nd ed.). Redwood City, CA: Benjamin/Cummings.

Massey, J. (1992). Patient's progress: Pilgrimage through harrowing treatment for Hodgkin's lymphoma. *Nursing Times, 88*(24), 44–46.

McCance, K., & Huether, S. (1994). *Pathophysiology: The biologic basis for disease in adults and children* (2nd ed.). St. Louis: Mosby.

McFarland, G. K., & McFarlane, E. A. (1993). *Nursing diagnosis and intervention: Planning for patient care* (2nd ed.). St. Louis: Mosby.

McNally, J., Somerville, E., Miaskowski, C., & Rostad, M. (1991). *Guidelines for oncology nursing practice.* Philadelphia: W. B. Saunders.

Mills, D. (1992). When blood won't clot. *RN, 55*(11), 28–33.

National Cancer Institute. (1990). *What you need to know about non-Hodgkin's lymphomas.* (NIH Pub. No. 90-1567). Bethesda, MD: Author.

National Hemophilia Foundation. (1991). *What you should know about hemophilia.* New York: Author.

Piper, B. F. (1993). Fatigue. In V. Carrieri-Kohlman, A. Lindsey, & C. West. *Pathophysiological phenomena in nursing* (2nd ed.), (pp. 279–302). Philadelphia: W. B. Saunders.

Poleman, C., & Peckenpaugh, N. J. (1991). *Nutrition essentials and diet therapy* (6th ed.). Philadelphia: W. B. Saunders.

Porth, C. (1994). *Pathophysiology: Concepts of altered health states* (4th ed.). Philadelphia: Lippincott.

Price, S., & Wilson, L. (1992). *Pathophysiology: Clinical concepts of disease processes* (4th ed.). St. Louis: Mosby.

Ready, N., Freeman, N. J., & Carbelho, A. (1992). Treatment choices in chronic myelogenous leukemia. *Hospital Practice, 27*(9A), 95–98, 101.

Scott, R. B. (1993). Common blood disorders: A primary care approach. *Geriatrics, 48*(4), 72–76, 79–80.

Simonson, G. M. (1988). Caring for the patient with acute myelocytic leukemia. *American Journal of Nursing, 88*(3), 307–310.

Sorenson, J. T., Gerald, K., Bodensteiner, D., & Holmes, F. F. (1993). Effect of age of survival in acute leukemia. *Cancer, 72*(5), 1602–1606.

Thomas, E. D. (1988). The future of marrow transplantation. *Seminars in Oncology Nursing, 4*(1), 74–78.

Tierney, L., Jr., McPhee, S., & Papadakis, M. (1994). *Current medical diagnosis & treatment.* Norwalk, CT: Appleton & Lange.

Timmerman, P. R. (1993). Intravenous immunoglobulin in oncology nursing practice. *Oncology Nursing Forum, 20*(1), 69–75.

Ulrich, S. P., Canale, S. W., and Wendell, S. A. (1994). *Medical-surgical nursing care planning guides* (3rd ed.). Philadelphia: W. B. Saunders.

Urban, L. D., Davie, J. K., & Thelan, L. A. (1992). *Essentials of critical care nursing.* St. Louis: Mosby.

Wilke, T., Coyle, K., & Shapiro, D. (1990). Bone marrow transplant: Today and tomorrow. *American Journal of Nursing, 90*(5), 48–58.

Wilson, S., & Morse, J. M. (1991). Living with a wife undergoing chemotherapy. *Image: Journal of Nursing Scholarship, 23*(2), 78–84.

Woods, N. F., Yates, B. C., & Primono, J. (1989). Supporting families during chronic illness. *Image: Journal of Nursing Scholarship, 21*(1), 46–50.

Workman, M. L., Ellerhorst-Ryan, J., and Hargrave-Koertge, V. (1993). *Nursing care of the immunocompromised patient.* Philadelphia: W. B. Saunders.

UNIT
TEN

Responses to Altered Respiratory Function

CHAPTER 32
Assessing Clients with Respiratory Disorders

CHAPTER 33
**Nursing Care of Clients with Upper
Respiratory Disorders**

CHAPTER 34
**Nursing Care of Clients with Lower
Respiratory Disorders**

Assessing Clients with Respiratory Disorders

LEARNING OBJECTIVES

After completing this chapter, you will be able to

- Identify the structures of the upper and lower respiratory system.
- Describe the functions of the upper and lower respiratory organs.
- Explain the mechanics of respiration.
- Identify the location of the lobes of the lungs in relation to the major landmarks of the thorax.
- Identify interview questions pertinent to the assessment of the respiratory system.
- Describe physical assessment techniques for respiratory function.
- Identify manifestations of impairment in the function of the respiratory system.
- Describe normal variations in assessment findings for the older adult.

The respiratory system functions primarily to provide the cells of the body with oxygen and to eliminate carbon dioxide, formed as a waste product of cellular metabolism. There are several events in this process, called respiration. These are:

- Pulmonary ventilation (commonly called breathing): Air is moved into and out of the lungs.

- External respiration: Exchange of oxygen and carbon dioxide occurs between the alveoli and the blood.

- Gas transport: Oxygen and carbon dioxide are transported to and from the lungs and the cells of the body via the blood.

- Internal respiration: Exchange of oxygen and carbon dioxide is made between the blood and the cells (Marieb, 1995).

Review of Anatomy and Physiology

Although the system functions as a whole, this unit contains separate chapters dealing with the upper respiratory system (the nose, pharynx, larynx, and trachea) and the lower respiratory system (the lungs).

The Upper Respiratory System

The upper respiratory system serves as a passageway for air to move into the lungs and carbon dioxide to move out to the external environment (Figure 32–1). As air moves through these structures, it is cleaned, humidified, and warmed.

The Nose

The *nose* is the external opening of the respiratory system. The external nose is given structure by the nasal, frontal,

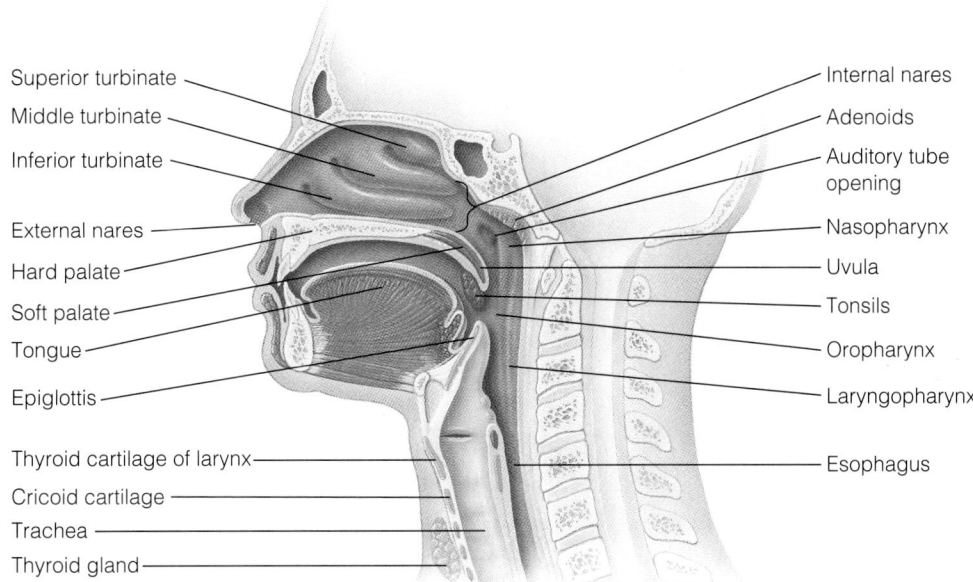

Figure 32–1 The upper respiratory system.

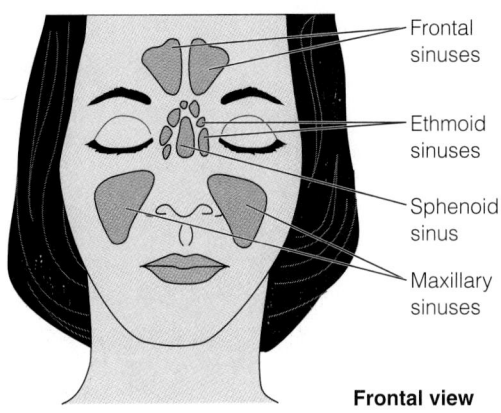
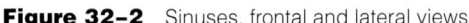
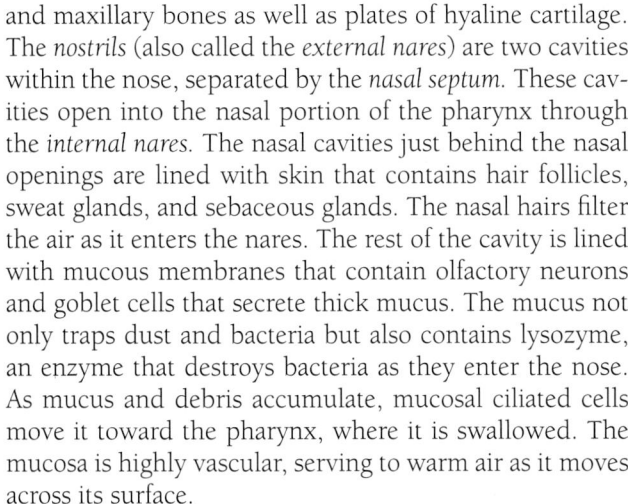

Frontal view

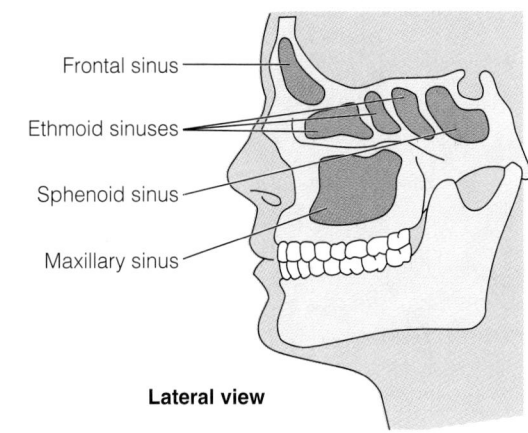

Lateral view

Figure 32–2 Sinuses, frontal and lateral views.

and maxillary bones as well as plates of hyaline cartilage. The *nostrils* (also called the *external nares*) are two cavities within the nose, separated by the *nasal septum.* These cavities open into the nasal portion of the pharynx through the *internal nares.* The nasal cavities just behind the nasal openings are lined with skin that contains hair follicles, sweat glands, and sebaceous glands. The nasal hairs filter the air as it enters the nares. The rest of the cavity is lined with mucous membranes that contain olfactory neurons and goblet cells that secrete thick mucus. The mucus not only traps dust and bacteria but also contains lysozyme, an enzyme that destroys bacteria as they enter the nose. As mucus and debris accumulate, mucosal ciliated cells move it toward the pharynx, where it is swallowed. The mucosa is highly vascular, serving to warm air as it moves across its surface.

Three structures project outward from the lateral wall of each nasal cavity: the *superior, middle,* and *inferior*

turbinates. The turbinates cause air entering the nose to become turbulent and also increase the surface area of mucosa exposed to the air. As air moves through this area, heavier particles of debris drop out and are trapped in the mucosa of the turbinates.

The Sinuses
The nasal cavity is surrounded by *paranasal sinuses* (Figure 32–2). These openings are located in the frontal, sphenoid, ethmoid, and maxillary bones. Sinuses lighten the skull, assist in speech, and produce mucus that drains into the nasal cavities and further facilities the trapping of debris.

The Pharynx
The *pharynx* (commonly called the *throat*), a funnel-shaped passageway about 5 in (13 cm) long, extends from the base of the skull to the level of the C6 vertebra. The

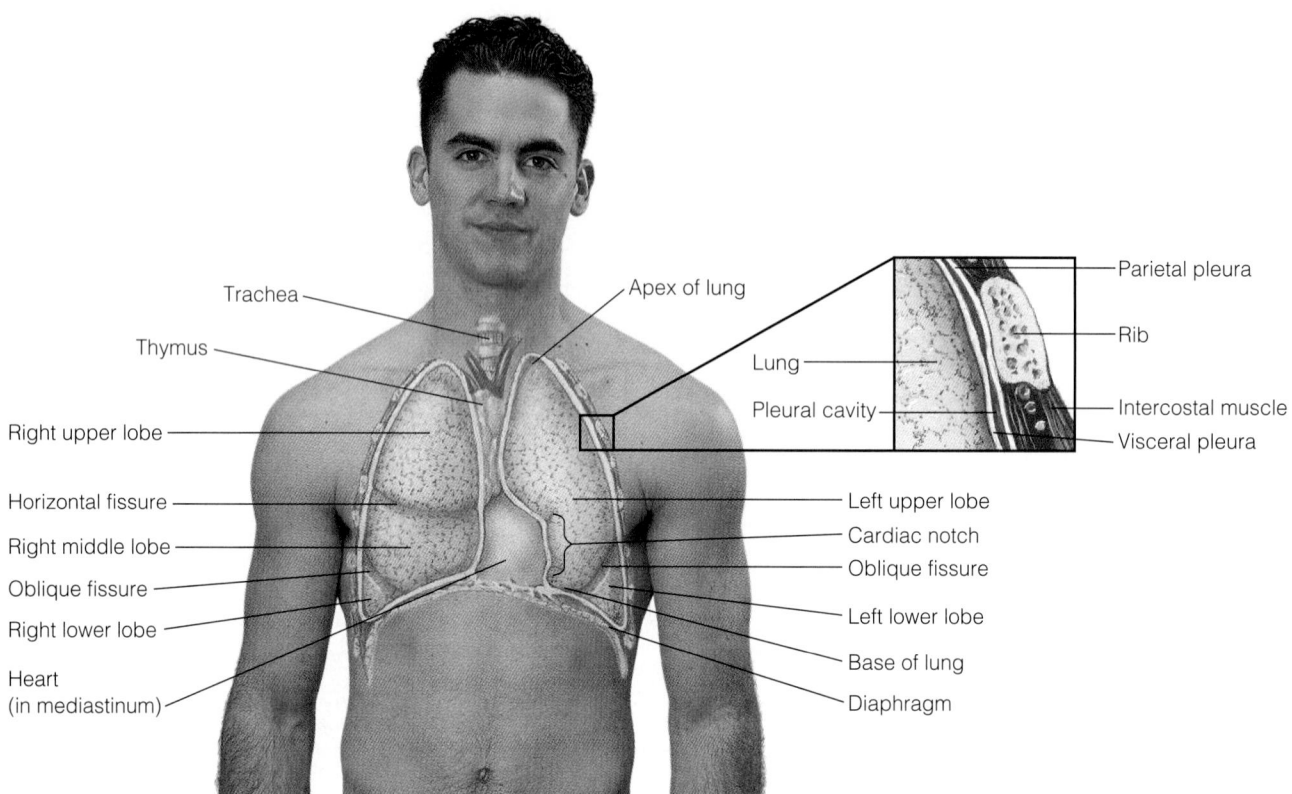

Figure 32–3   The lower respiratory system, showing the location of the lungs, the mediastinum, and layers of visceral and parietal pleura.

pharynx serves as a passageway for both air and food. It is divided into three regions: the nasopharynx, the oropharynx, and the laryngopharynx.

The *nasopharynx* serves only as a passageway for air. Located beneath the sphenoid bone and above the level of the soft palate, the nasopharynx is continuous with the nasal cavities. This segment is lined with ciliated epithelium, which continues to move debris from the nasal cavities to the pharynx. Masses of lymphoid tissue (the *tonsils* and *adenoids*) are located in the mucosa high in the posterior wall; these tissues trap and destroy infectious agents entering with the air. The auditory (eustachian) tubes also open into the nasopharynx, connecting it with the middle ear.

The *oropharynx* lies behind the oral cavity and extends from the soft palate to the level of the hyoid bone. It serves as a passageway for both air and food. Food is prevented from entering the nasopharynx during swallowing by an upward rise of the soft palate. The oropharynx is lined with stratified squamous epithelium that protects it from the friction of food and damage from the chemicals found in food and fluids.

The *laryngopharynx* extends from the hyoid bone to the larynx. It is also lined with stratified squamous epithelium, and serves as a passageway for both food and air. Air does not move into the lungs while food is being swallowed and moved into the esophagus.

The Larynx

The *larynx* (also called the *voicebox*) is about 2 in (5 cm) long. It opens superiorly at the laryngopharynx and is continuous inferiorly with the trachea. The larynx provides an airway and routes air and food into the proper passageway. As long as air is moving through the larynx, its inlet is open; however, the inlet closes during swallowing. The larynx also contains the *vocal cords*, necessary for voice production.

The larynx is framed by cartilages, connected by ligaments and membranes. The *thyroid* cartilage is formed by the fusion of two cartilages; the fusion point is visible as the Adam's apple. The *cricoid* cartilage lies below the thyroid cartilage; other pairs of cartilages form the walls of the larynx. The *epiglottis,* also a cartilage, is covered with mucosa that contains taste buds. This structure normally projects upward to the base of the tongue; however, during swallowing, the larynx moves upward and the epiglottis tips to cover the opening to the larynx. If anything other than air enters the larynx, a cough reflex is initiated to expel the foreign substance before it can enter the lungs. This protective reflex does not work if the person is unconscious.

The Trachea

The *trachea* (or *windpipe*) begins at the inferior larynx and descends anteriorly to the esophagus to enter the medi-

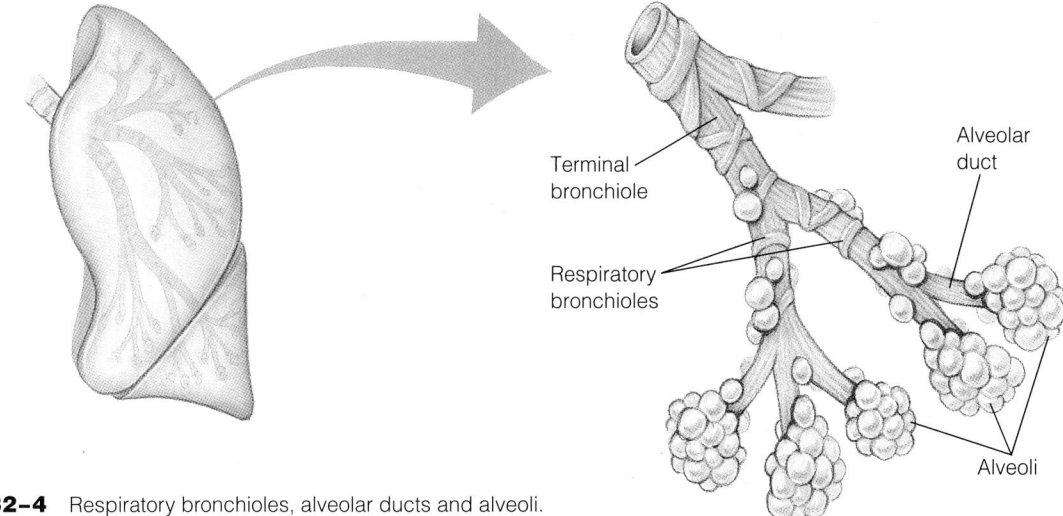

Figure 32–4   Respiratory bronchioles, alveolar ducts and alveoli.

astinum, where it divides to become the right and left primary bronchi of the lungs. The trachea is about 4 to 5 in (12 to 15 cm) long and 1 in (2.5 cm) in diameter. It contains 16 to 20 **C**-shaped rings of cartilage joined by connective tissue. The mucosa lining the trachea is composed of pseudostratified ciliated columnar epithelium containing seromucous glands that produce thick mucus. Dust and debris in the inspired air are trapped in this mucus, moved toward the throat by the cilia, and then either swallowed or coughed out through the mouth.

The Lower Respiratory System

The lower respiratory system includes the lungs and the bronchi (Figures 32–3 and 32–4).

The Lungs

The center of the thoracic cavity is filled by the *mediastinum,* which contains the heart, great blood vessels, bronchi, trachea, and esophagus. The mediastinum is flanked on either side by the *lungs* (see Figure 32–3). Each lung is suspended in its own pleural cavity, with the anterior, lateral, and posterior lung surfaces lying close to the ribs. The *hilus,* located on the mediastinal surface of each lung, is the area where blood vessels of the pulmonary and circulatory systems enter and exit the lungs. The primary bronchus also enters in this area. The *apex* of each lung lies just below the clavicle, whereas the *base* of each lung rests on the diaphragm. The lungs are composed of elastic connective tissue, called *stroma,* and are soft and spongy.

The two lungs differ in size and shape. The left lung is smaller and has two lobes, whereas the right lung has three lobes. Each of the lung lobes contains a different number of bronchopulmonary segments. These segments are separated by connective tissue. There are eight segments in the left lung and ten segments in the right lung.

The vascular system of the lungs is composed of the pulmonary arteries, which deliver blood to the lungs for oxygenation, and the pulmonary veins, which deliver oxygenated blood to the heart. Within the lungs, the pulmonary arteries branch into a pulmonary capillary network that surrounds the avleoli. Lung tissue receives its blood supply from the bronchial arteries and drains by the bronchial and pulmonary veins.

The Pleura

The *pleura* is a double-layered membrane that covers the lungs and the inside of the thoracic cavities (see Figure 32–3). The *parietal pleura* lines the thoracic wall and mediastinum. It is continous with the *visceral pleura,* which covers the external lung surfaces. The pleura produces *pleural fluid,* a serous fluid that lubricates the pleura, allowing the lungs to move easily over the thoracic wall during breathing. The two layers of the pleura also cling tightly together and hold the lungs to the thoracic wall. The structure of the pleura creates a slightly negative pressure in the pleural space (which is actually a potential rather than an actual space), necessary for lung function.

The Bronchi and Alveoli

The trachea divides into *right* and *left primary bronchi.* These main bronchi subdivide into the secondary (lobar) bronchi, then branch into the tertiary (segmental) bronchi, and then into smaller and smaller bronchioles, ending in the terminal bronchioles, which are extremely small (see Figure 32–4). These branching passageways collectively are called the *bronchial* or *respiratory tree.* From the terminal bronchioles, air moves into air sacs (called *respiratory bronchioles*), which further branch into *alveolar ducts* that lead to *alveolar sacs* and then to the tiny *alveoli.* During inspiration, air enters the lungs through the primary bronchus and then moves through the increasingly smaller passageways of the lungs to the alveoli,

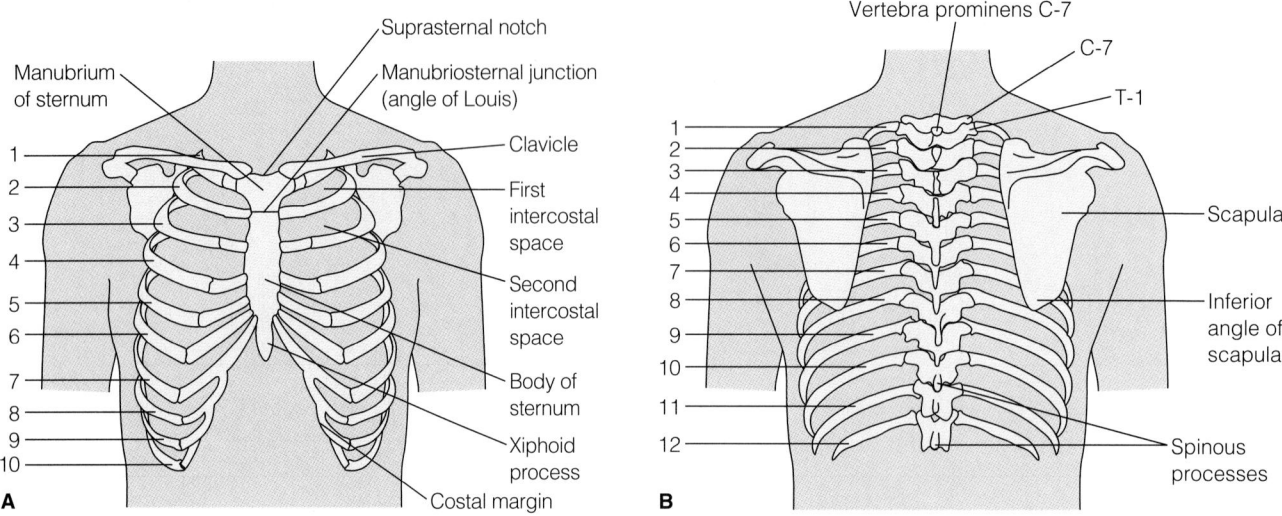

Figure 32–5 *A,* Anterior rib cage, showing intercostal spaces. *B,* Posterior rib cage.

where oxygen and carbon dioxide exchange occurs in the process of external respiration. During expiration, the carbon dioxide is expelled.

Alveoli cluster around the alveolar sacs, which open into a common chamber called the *atrium.* There are millions of alveoli in each lung, providing an enormous surface for gas exchange. Alveoli have extremely thin walls, composed of a single layer of squamous epithelial cells over a very thin basement membrane. The external surface of the alveoli are covered with pulmonary capillaries. The alveolar and capillary walls form the *respiratory membrane.* Gas exchange across the respiratory membrane occurs by simple diffusion. The alveolar walls also contain cells that secrete a surfactant-containing fluid, necessary for maintaining a moist surface and reducing the surface tension of the alveolar fluid to help prevent collapse of the lungs.

The Rib Cage and Intercostal Muscles

The lungs are protected by the bones of the rib cage and the intercostal muscles. There are 12 pairs of *ribs,* which all articulate with the thoracic vertebrae posteriorly (Figure 32–5). Anteriorly, the first 7 ribs articulate with the body of the sternum. The 8th, 9th, and 10th ribs articulate with the cartilage immediately above the ribs. The 11th and 12th ribs are called floating ribs, because they are unattached.

The *sternum* has three parts: the manubrium, the body, and the xiphoid process. The junction between the manubrium and the body of the sternum is called the *manubriosternal junction* or the *angle of Louis.* The depression above the manubrium is called the *suprasternal notch.*

The spaces between the ribs are called the *intercostal spaces.* Each intercostal space is named for the rib imme-

diately above it (for example, the space between the 3rd and 4th ribs is designated as the third intercostal space). The *intercostal muscles* between the ribs, along with the diaphragm, are called the *inspiratory muscles.*

Mechanics of Respiration

Pulmonary ventilation, the movement of air into and out of the lungs (or breathing), is dependent on volume changes within the thoracic cavity. A change in the volume of air in the thoracic cavity leads to a change in the air pressure within the cavity. Because gases always flow along their pressure gradients, a change in pressure results in gases flowing into or out of the lungs to equalize the pressure.

The pressures that normally are present in the thoracic cavity are the intrapulmonary pressure and the intrapleural pressure. The *intrapulmonary pressure* is the pressure within the alveoli of the lungs. The acts of ventilation (inhalation and exhalation) cause this pressure to rise and fall constantly. The *intrapleural pressure* is the pressure within the pleural space. It also rises and falls with the acts of ventilation, but it is always less than (or negative to) the intrapulmonary pressure. Intrapulmonary and intrapleural pressures are necessary not only to expand and contract the lungs, but also to prevent their collapse.

Pulmonary ventilation has two phases: *inspiration,* during which air flows into the lungs, and *expiration,* during which gases flow out of the lungs. The two phases make up a single breath, and normally occur from 12 to 20 times each minute. A single inspiration lasts for about 1 to 1.5 seconds, whereas an expiration lasts for about 2 to 3 seconds.

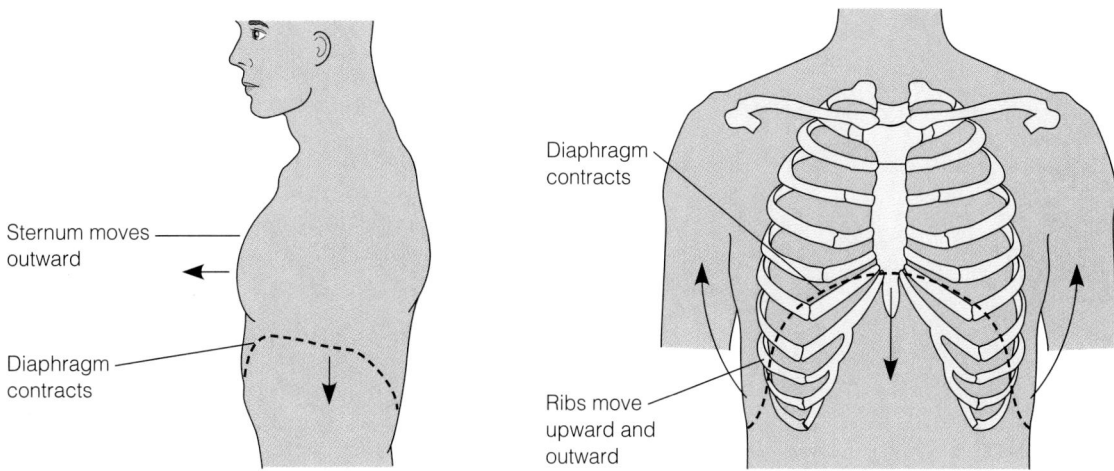

Figure 32–6   Respiratory inspiration: lateral and anterior views. Note the volume expansion of the thorax as the diaphragm flattens.

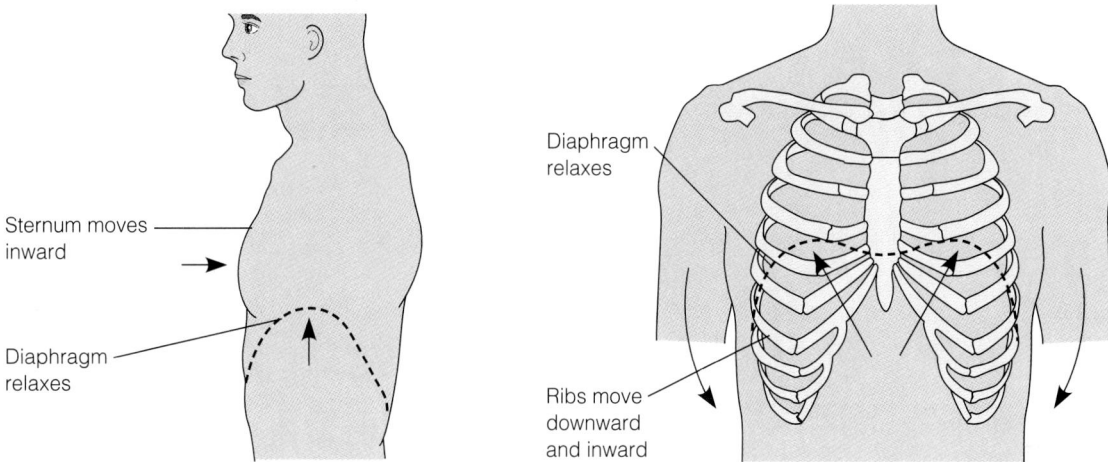

Figure 32–7   Respiratory expiration: lateral and anterior views.

During inspiration, the diaphragm contracts and flattens out to increase the vertical diameter of the thoracic cavity (Figure 32–6). The external intercostal muscles contract, elevating the rib cage and moving the sternum forward to expand the lateral and anteroposterior diameter of the thoracic cavity, decreasing intrapleural pressure. The lungs stretch and the intrapulmonary volume increases, decreasing intrapulmonary pressure slightly below atmospheric pressure. Air rushes into the lungs as a result of this pressure gradient until the intrapulmonary and atmospheric pressures equalize.

Expiration is primarily a passive process that occurs as a result of the elasticity of the lungs (Figure 32–7). The inspiratory muscles relax, the diaphragm rises, the ribs descend, and the lungs recoil. Both the thoracic and intrapulmonary pressures increase, compressing the alveoli. The intrapulmonary pressure rises to a level greater than atmospheric pressure, and gases flow out of the lungs.

Factors Affecting Respiration

The rate and depth of breathing (or respiration) is controlled by respiratory centers in the medulla oblongata and pons of the brain and by chemoreceptors located in the medulla and in the carotid and aortic bodies. The centers and chemoreceptors respond to changes in the concentration of oxygen, carbon dioxide, and hydrogen ions in arterial blood. For example, when carbon dioxide concentration increases or the pH decreases, the respiratory rate increases.

In addition, respiration is affected by respiratory passageway resistance, lung compliance, lung elasticity, and alveolar surface tension forces:

■   Respiratory passageway resistance is created by the friction encountered as gases move along the respiratory passageways, by constriction of the passageways (especially the larger bronchioles), by accumulations

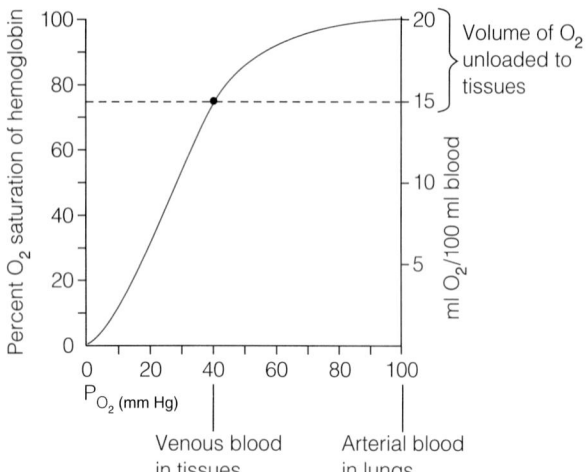

Figure 32–8   Oxygen-hemoglobin dissociation curve. The percent O_2 saturation of hemoglobin and total blood oxygen volume are shown for different oxygen partial pressures (P_{O_2}). Arterial blood in the lungs is almost completely saturated. During one pass through the body, about 25% of hemoglobin-bound oxygen is unloaded to the tissues. Thus, venous blood is still about 75% saturated with oxygen. The steep portion of the curve shows that hemoglobin readily off-loads or on-loads oxygen at P_{O_2} levels below about 50 mm Hg.

of mucus or infectious material, and by tumors. As resistance increases, gas flow decreases.

- Lung compliance is the distensibility of the lungs. It depends on the elasticity of the lung tissue and the flexibility of the rib cage. Compliance is decreased by factors that increase the elasticity of the lungs, block the respiratory passageways, or interfere with movement of the rib cage.

- Lung elasticity is essential for lung distention during inspiration and lung recoil during expiration. Decreased elasticity from disease such as emphysema impairs respiration.

- A liquid film composed mostly of water covers the alveolar walls. At any gas-liquid boundary, the molecules of liquid are more strongly attracted to each other than to gas molecules. This produces a state of tension, called *surface tension,* that draws the liquid molecules even more closely together. The water content of the alveolar film acts to compact the alveoli and aid in the lungs' recoil during expiration. In fact, if the alveolar film were pure water, the alveoli would collapse between breaths. *Surfactant,* a lipoprotein produced by the alveolar cells, interferes with this adhesiveness of the water molecules, reducing surface tension, and facilitating expansion of the lungs. If there is insufficient surfactant, the surface tension forces can become great enough to collapse the alveoli between breaths, requiring tremendous energy to reinflate the lungs for inspiration (Marieb, 1995).

Respiratory Volume and Capacity

Respiratory volume and capacity are affected by sex, age, weight, and health status.

- *Tidal volume (TV)* is the amount of air (approximately 500 mL) moved in and out of the lungs with each normal, quiet breath.

- *Inspiratory reserve volume (IRV)* is the amount of air (approximately 2100 to 3100 mL) that can be inhaled forcibly over the *tidal volume.*

- *Expiratory reserve volume (ERV)* is the approximately 1000 mL of air that can be forced out over the tidal volume.

- The *residual volume* is the volume of air (approximately 1100 mL) that remains in the lungs after a forced expiration.

- *Vital capacity* refers to the sum of TV + IRV + ERV and is approximately 4500 mL in the healthy client.

- About 150 mL of air never reaches the alveoli (the amount remaining in the passageways) and is referred to as *anatomical dead space volume.*

Oxygen and Carbon Dioxide Transport

Oxygen Transport and Unloading

Oxgyen is carried in the blood either bound to hemoglobin or dissolved in the plasma. However, because oxygen is not very soluble in water, almost all of the oxygen that enters the blood from the respiratory system is carried to the cells of the body by hemoglobin. This combination of hemoglobin and oxygen is called *oxyhemoglobin.*

Each hemoglobin molecule is made of four polypeptide chains, with each chain bound to an iron-containing heme group. The iron groups are the binding sites for oxygen; as a result, each hemoglobin molecule can bind with four molecules of oxygen.

Oxygen binding is rapid and reversible. It is affected by temperature, blood pH, partial pressure of oxygen (P_{O_2}), partial pressure of carbon dioxide (P_{CO_2}), and serum concentration of an organic chemical called 2,3-DPG. All of these factors interact to ensure adequate delivery of oxygen to the cells.

The relative saturation of hemoglobin depends on the P_{O_2} of the blood, as illustrated in the oxygen-hemoglobin dissociation curve (Figure 32–8).

- Under normal conditions, the hemoglobin in arterial blood is 97.4% saturated with oxygen. Hemoglobin is almost fully saturated at a P_{O_2} of 70 mm Hg. As arterial blood flows through the capillaries, oxygen is unloaded, so that the oxygen saturation of hemoglobin in venous blood is 75%.

- The affinity of oxygen and hemoglobin decreases as the temperature of body tissues increases above normal. As a result, less oxygen binds with hemoglobin, and oxygen unloading is enhanced. Conversely, as the body is chilled, oxygen unloading is inhibited.

- The oxygen-hemoglobin bond is weakened by increased hydrogen ion concentrations. As blood becomes more acidotic, oxygen unloading to the tissues is enhanced. The same process occurs when the partial pressure of carbon dioxide increases because this decreases the pH.

- The organic chemical 2,3-DPG is formed in red blood cells and enhances the release of oxygen from hemoglobin by binding to it during times of increased metabolism (as when body temperature increases). This binding alters the structure of hemoglobin so that oxygen unloading is facilitated.

Carbon Dioxide Transport

Active cells produce about 200 mL of carbon dioxide each minute; this amount is exactly the same as that excreted by the lungs each minute (Marieb, 1995). Excretion of carbon dioxide from the body requires transport by the blood from the cells to the lungs. Carbon dioxide is transported in three forms: dissolved in plasma, bound to hemoglobin, and as bicarbonate ions in the plasma (the largest amount is in this form).

The amount of carbon dioxide transported in the blood is strongly influenced by the oxygenation of the blood. When the PO_2 decreases, with a corresponding decrease in oxygen saturation, increased amounts of carbon dioxide can be carried in the blood. Carbon dioxide entering the systemic circulation from the cells causes more oxygen to dissociate from hemoglobin, in turn allowing more carbon dioxide to combine with hemoglobin and more bicarbonate ions to be generated. This situation is reversed in the pulmonary circulation, where the uptake of oxygen facilitates the release of carbon dioxide.

Assessment of Respiratory Function

∎ ∎ ∎

The nurse assesses the respiratory system both during a health assessment interview to collect subjective data and a physical assessment to collect objective data.

The Health Assessment Interview

This section provides guidelines for collecting subjective data through a health assessment interview specific to the function of the respiratory system. Interview questions and leading statements for assessing respiratory function are also provided.

Overview

A health assessment interview to determine problems of the respiratory system may be done as part of a health screening or as part of a total health assessment. Alternatively, the interview may focus on a chief complaint (such as difficulty breathing). If the client has a problem of any part of the respiratory system, the nurse analyzes its onset, characteristics and course, severity, precipitating and relieving factors, and any associated symptoms, noting the timing and circumstances. For example, the nurse may ask the client the following:

- Describe the problems you have with your breathing. Is your breathing more difficult if you lie flat? Is it painful to breathe in or out?

- When did you first notice that your cough was becoming a problem? Do you cough up mucus? What color is the mucus?

- Have you had nosebleeds in the past?

During the interview, the nurse should carefully observe the client for difficulty in breathing, pausing to breathe in the middle of a sentence, hoarseness, changes in voice quality, and cough.

Questions are asked about present health status, medical history, family health history, and risk factors for illness. These areas of the client's health status include information about the nose, throat, and lungs.

To determine present health status, the nurse asks if the client has had any pain in the nose, throat, or chest. Information about cough includes what type of cough, when it occurs, and how it is relieved. The client should describe any sputum associated with the cough. Is the client experiencing any **dyspnea** (difficult or labored breathing)? How is the dyspnea associated with activity levels and time of day? Is the client having chest pain? How is this related to activity and time of day? The severity, type, and location of the pain should be noted. Problems with swallowing, smelling, or taste should be explored. Questions should also be asked about nosebleeds and nasal or sinus stuffiness or pain. The client is also asked about current medication use, aerosols or inhalants, and oxygen use.

Past medical history is documented by asking questions about a history of allergies, asthma, bronchitis, emphysema, pneumonia, tuberculosis, or congestive heart failure. Other questions include a history of surgery or trauma to the respiratory structures as well as a history of other chronic illnesses, such as cancer, kidney disease, and heart disease. If the client has a health problem involving the respiratory system, the nurse asks about medications that are used to relieve nasal congestion, cough, dyspnea, or chest pain. A family history of allergies, tuberculosis, emphysema, and cancer should be documented.

The client's personal life-style, environment, and occupation may provide clues to risk factors for actual or potential health problems. The client is questioned about a history of smoking and/or exposure to environmental chemicals (including smog), dust, vapors, animals, coal dust, asbestos, fumes, or pollens. Other risk factors include a sedentary life-style and obesity. The client should also be asked about use of alcohol and use of substances that are injected (such as heroin) or inhaled (such as cocaine or marijuana).

Interview Questions

The following interview questions and leading statements are categorized by functional health patterns.

Health Perception–Health Management

- Describe any respiratory problems (such as allergies, asthma, emphysema, bronchitis, frequent colds or flu, pneumonia, tuberculosis), injury, or surgeries you have had.

- How was this problem treated? (medications, breathing treatments, oxygen, environmental control of allergens, other)

- Do you use oxygen for your respiratory problem? How and when do you use it? What flow rate do you use?

- Do you smoke tobacco? If so, what type, how much, and for how long?

- Is your respiratory problem worse during any one season of the year? Explain.

- Do you do anything to decrease environmental irritants at home or at work? (masks, dust control)

- When was your last chest X-ray and tuberculosis skin test?

- Have you ever had an influenza immunization? When?

Nutritional-Metabolic

- Describe your usual dietary intake for a 24-hour period.

- Has your appetite changed since you have had this respiratory problem? Explain.

- Has there been a recent change in your weight? Explain.

- Is it difficult for you to eat because of your breathing problem? Does it help to eat smaller, more frequent meals?

- Are your eating habits affected by loss of appetite? Fatigue? Feeling full? Difficulty breathing? Explain.

Elimination

- Has having this health problem made it more difficult for you to have a bowel movement?

- (For women) Do you ever have problems holding your urine when you cough?

Activity-Exercise

- Describe your usual activities for a 24-hour period.

- Do you become short of breath or very tired with certain activities? Explain.

- How many flights of stairs can you climb before you begin to have difficulty breathing?

- Are your activities interrupted by frequent coughing? If so, describe the frequency and type of cough.

- Do you cough up phlegm or mucus? If so, describe its amount, color, odor, and the presence of blood.

- Has your ability to care for yourself changed with this respiratory problem? Explain.

- What type of exercise do you usually do? Has this changed? Describe.

- Has your energy level decreased since you have had this respiratory problem? If so, how has it affected your usual activities of daily living?

- Do you work or do hobbies in an area where you are exposed to paints, glues, dust, pollen, fumes, or chemicals that might irritate your respiratory tract?

- Do certain foods, pollens, dust, or animals seem to increase your difficulty with breathing? Explain.

Sleep-Rest

- Does having this respiratory problem interfere with your ability to rest or sleep? Explain.

- Do you need more than one pillow to breathe easily when you sleep at night?

- Do you ever awaken with a cough? Explain.

Cognitive-Perceptual

- Do you ever have sinus pain? Chest pain? Describe how severe it is on a scale of 0 to 10, with 10 being the most severe pain. Describe when and where you feel the pain, how often you have it, what makes it worse, and what you do to relieve it.

- Are there times when you feel faint, confused, anxious, or restless? Describe.

- Do you understand how to use the medications, inhalers, or oxygen prescribed for your respiratory problem?

Self-Perception–Self-Concept

- How do you feel about having this health problem?

- How has this problem affected how you feel about yourself and the future?

- How do you feel about having to use oxygen?

Role-Relationship

- Is there a history of lung disease in your family? Explain.

- How has your respiratory problem affected those you live with?

- Has your respiratory problem changed your role and responsibilities in your family? With friends? At work? In social activities? Explain.

- Has this respiratory problem interfered with your work? Explain.

Sexuality-Reproductive

- Has this health problem interfered in any way with your usual sexual activities? Explain.

- Is your problem with breathing made worse by sexual activities? Explain.

- Describe how having this health problem has made you feel about yourself as a man (woman).

Coping-Stress

- Do your problems with breathing seem to get worse when you feel stressed? Explain.

- What do you usually do to cope with stress?

- What do you find to be most helpful in coping with your respiratory problem?

- Who or what will be able to help you cope with stress from this health problem?

Value-Belief

- Are there significant others, practices, or activities that help you cope with this breathing problem? Explain.

- How do you perceive the future with this health problem?

The Physical Assessment

Physical assessment of the respiratory system may be performed as part of a total assessment, or alone for a client with known or suspected problems. The respiratory system is assessed through inspection, palpation, percussion, and auscultation of the nose, throat, thorax, and lungs. In addition, the client's level of consciousness and the color of the lips, nail beds, nose, ears, and tongue should be noted for signs of respiratory distress.

Preparation

The equipment needed to assess the respiratory system includes a tongue blade, penlight, nasal speculum, metric ruler, marking pen, and stethoscope with diaphragm. The room should be warm and well lighted. The client is asked to remove all clothing above the waist; female clients should be given a gown to wear during the examination. The examination is conducted with the client in the sitting position. Prior to the examination, all necessary equipment should be collected and the techniques explained to the client to decrease anxiety.

There are three different types of normal breath sounds: vesicular, bronchovesicular, and bronchial. Assessment of these sounds is discussed in Table 32–1.

Table 32–1 Normal Breath Sounds

Type of Breath Sound	Characteristics
Vesicular	■ Soft, low-pitched, gentle sounds
	■ Heard over all areas of the lungs except the major bronchi
	■ Have a 3:1 ratio for inspiration and expiration, with inspiration lasting longer than expiration
Bronchovesicular	■ Medium pitch and intensity of sounds
	■ Have a 1:1 ratio, with inspiration and expiration being equal in duration
	■ Heard anteriorly over the primary bronchus on each side of the sternum, and posteriorly between the scapulae
Bronchial	■ Loud, high-pitched sounds
	■ Gap between inspiration and expiration
	■ Have a 2:3 ratio for inspiration and expiration, with expiration longer than inspiration
	■ Heard over the manubrium

ASSESSMENT TECHNIQUE	POSSIBLE ABNORMAL FINDINGS

Nose

■ **Inspect the nose for changes in size, shape, or color.**

The nose may be asymmetrical as a result of previous surgery or trauma. The skin around the nostrils may be red and swollen in allergies.

■ **Inspect the nasal cavity.**

Use an otoscope with a broad, short speculum. Gently insert the speculum into each of the nares and assess the condition of the mucous membranes and the turbinates.

The septum may be deviated. Perforation of the septum may occur with chronic cocaine abuse. Red mucosa indicates infection. Purulent drainage indicates nasal or sinus infection. Watery nasal drainage often indicates allergy. Pale turbinates indicate allergy. Polyps on the turbinates are seen in chronic allergies.

■ **Assess ability to smell.**

Ask the client to breathe through one nostril while pressing the other one closed. Ask the client to close his or her eyes. Place a substance with an aromatic odor under the client's nose (use ground coffee or alcohol) and ask the client to identify the odor. Test each nostril separately. This test is usually done only if the client has problems with the sense of smell.

Changes in the ability to smell may be the result of damage to the olfactory nerve or to chronic inflammation of the nose. Zinc deficiency may also cause a loss of the sense of smell.

Thorax

■ **Assess respiratory rate.**

Count the client's respirations. It is a good idea to count while you perform some other assessment, so that the client is unaware that you are counting his or her respirations. Awareness may alter the client's natural respiratory rate.

Tachypnea is an abnormally rapid respiratory rate. Tachypnea is seen in **atelectasis** (collapse of lung tissue following obstruction of the bronchus or bronchioles), pneumonia, asthma, pleural effusion, pneumothorax, and congestive heart failure. Damage to the brain stem from a stroke or head injury may result in either tachypnea or **bradypnea**, an abnormally low respiratory rate.

ASSESSMENT TECHNIQUE	POSSIBLE ABNORMAL FINDINGS

Bradypnea also is seen with some circulation disorders, lung disorders, as a side effect of some medications, and as a response to pain, as from a fractured rib. **Apnea,** cessation of breathing lasting from a few seconds to a few minutes, may also occur following a stroke or head trauma, as a side effect of some medications, or following airway obstruction.

■ **Inspect the anteroposterior diameter of the chest.**
The anteroposterior diameter of the chest should be less than the transverse diameter. Normal ratios vary from 1:2 to 5:7.

The anteroposterior diameter is equal to the transverse diameter in *barrel chest,* which typically occurs with emphysema.

■ **Inspect for intercostal retraction.**

Retraction of intercostal spaces may be seen in asthma. Bulging of intercostal spaces may be seen in pneumothorax.

■ **Inspect and palpate for chest expansion.**
Place your hands with the fingers spread apart palm down on the client's posterolateral chest. Gently press the skin between your thumbs (Figure 32–9). Ask the client to breathe deeply. As the client inhales, watch your hands for symmetry of movement.

Thoracic expansion is decreased on the affected side in atelectasis, pneumonia, pneumothorax, and pleural effusion. Bilateral chest expansion is decreased in emphysema.

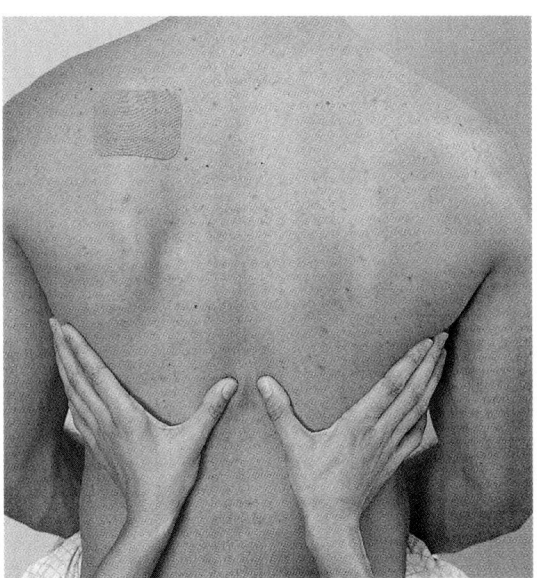

Figure 32–9 Palpating for chest expansion.

■ **Gently palpate the trachea.**
Check for location and position.

The trachea shifts to the unaffected side in pleural effusion and pneumothorax and shifts to the affected side in atelectasis.

■ **Palpate for tactile fremitus.**
Ask the client to say "ninety-nine" as you palpate at three different levels for a vibratory sensation called *tactile fremitus,* which occurs as sound waves from the larynx travel through patent bronchi and lungs to the chest wall.

Tactile fremitus is decreased in atelectasis, emphysema, asthma, pleural effusion, and pneumothorax. It is increased in pneumonia if the bronchus is patent.

Assessment Technique	Possible Abnormal Findings

■ **Percuss the lungs for dullness.**
Percuss over shoulder apices and over anterior, posterior, and lateral intercostal spaces (Figure 32–10).

Figure 32–10
Sequence for lung percussion.

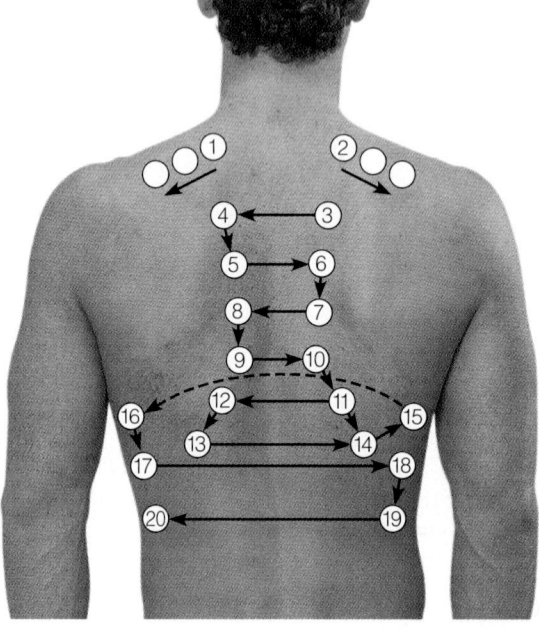

Dullness is heard in clients with atelectasis, lobar pneumonia, and pleural effusion. Hyperresonance is heard in those with chronic asthma and pneumothorax.

■ **Percuss the posterior chest for diaphragmatic excursion.**
Systematic percussion of the posterior chest from a level of lung resonance to the level of diaphragmatic dullness reveals diaphragmatic excursion, a measurement of the level of the diaphragm. First percuss downward over the posterior thorax while the client exhales fully and holds the breath. Mark the spot at which the sound changes from resonant to dull. Then ask the client to inhale and hold the breath while you percuss downward again to note the descent of the diaphragm. Again mark the spot where the sound changes. Measure the difference, which normally varies from about 3 to 5 cm (Figure 32–11).

Diaphragmatic excursion is decreased in emphysema, on the affected side in pleural effusion, and in pneumothorax. A high level of dullness or a lack of excursion may indicate atelectasis or pleural effusion.

Figure 32–11
Measuring diaphragmatic excursion.

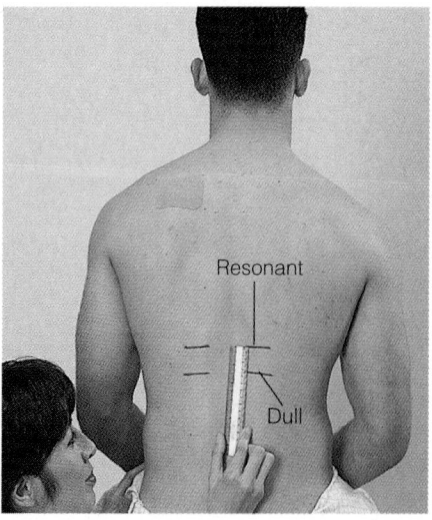

| ASSESSMENT TECHNIQUE | POSSIBLE ABNORMAL FINDINGS |

- **Auscultate the lungs.**
Auscultate for breath sounds with the diaphragm of the stethoscope by having the client take slow deep breaths through the mouth. Listen over anterior, posterior, and lateral intercostal spaces (Figure 32–12).

Figure 32–12
Sequence for lung auscultation.

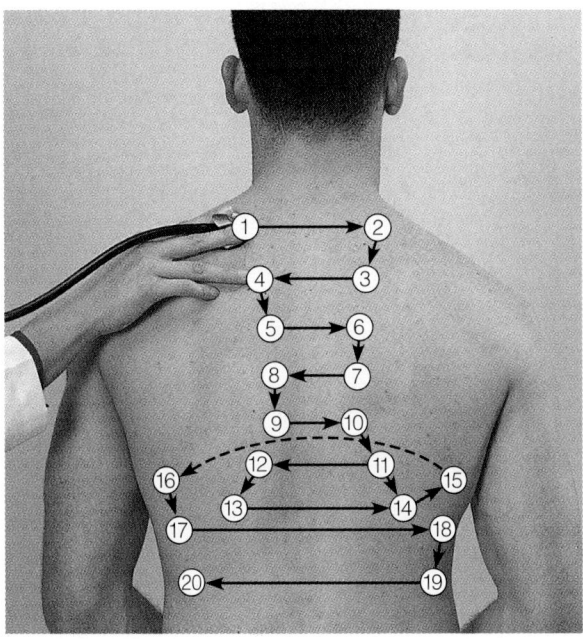

- **Auscultate for crackles, wheezes, and friction rubs.**
Use the diaphragm of the stethoscope to auscultate for crackles and/or wheezes (adventitious sounds). If heard, ask the client to cough and note if adventitious sound is cleared.

- **Auscultate voice sounds.**
Auscultate for voice sounds where any abnormal breath sound is noted by having client say "ninety-nine" (bronchophony); whisper "one, two, three" (whispered pectoriloquy); and say "ee" (egophony). Normally, these sounds are heard by the examiner, but are muffled.

Bronchial breath sounds (expiration > inspiration) and bronchovesicular breath sounds (inspiration = expiration) are heard over lungs filled with fluid or solid tissue. Breath sounds are decreased over atelectasis, emphysema, asthma, pleural effusion, and pneumothorax. Breath sounds are increased over lobar pneumonia. Breath sounds are absent over collapsed lung, pleural effusion, and primary bronchus obstruction.

Crackles (short, discrete, crackling or bubbling sounds; also called rales) may be noted in pneumonia, bronchitis, and congestive heart failure. *Wheezes* (continuous, musical sounds) may be heard in clients with bronchitis, emphysema, and asthma. A *friction rub* is a loud, dry, creaking sound that indicates pleural inflammation.

Voice sounds are decreased or absent over areas of atelectasis, asthma, pleural effusion, and pneumothorax. Voice sounds are increased and clearer over lobar pneumonia.

Variations in Assessment Findings for the Older Adult

Normal age-related variations of the thorax and lungs may be noted in the older adult. The thoracic spine may show an increased curvature (*kyphosis*). The anteroposterior diameter of the thorax may be increased, causing a barrel chest. Changes within the lungs themselves include loss of elastic recoil, stiffening of the chest wall, and

changes in gas exchange. Other age-related changes include the following:

- The sense of smell often decreases.

- Vital capacity decreases and residual volumes increase as the thorax becomes more rigid and the lungs become less elastic. These changes decrease cough effectiveness.

- The protective cilia of the respiratory tract also become less effective. Therefore, the older client is at a higher risk for respiratory infections than is the younger client.

- A decrease in Po_2 and a decreased ventilatory reserve increase the risk for exercise intolerance.

- Decreased response to increases in Pco_2 or decreased Po_2 mean that the older adult, when subjected to stress from illness or increased metabolic demand, is at high risk for tissue **hypoxia** (insufficient supply of oxygen to the tissues).

- As many older adults have smoked for years, the risk of chronic pulmonary diseases is high.

Bibliography

■ ■ ■

Ahrens, T. (1993). Changing perspectives in the assessment of oxygenation. *Critical Care Nurse, 13*(4), 78–83.

Ahrens, T. (1993). Respiratory monitoring in critical care. *AACN Clinical Issues in Critical Care Nursing, 4*(1), 56–65.

Carpenter, K. (1993). A comprehensive review of cyanosis. *Critical Care Nurse, 13*(4), 66–72.

Finesilver, C. (1992). Respiratory assessment. *RN, 55*(2), 22–30.

Gift, A. G. (1989). A dyspnea assessment guide. *Critical Care Nurse, 9*(8), 79, 82–84, 86–88.

Kuhn, J., & McGovern, M. (1992). Respiratory assessment of the elderly. *Journal of Gerontological Nursing, 18*(5), 4–43.

Marieb, E. A. (1995). *Human anatomy and physiology* (3rd ed.). Redwood City, CA: Benjamin/Cummings.

Merkley, K. (1994). Assessing chest pain. *RN, 57*(6), 58–63.

Roberts, S. L. (1990). High permeability pulmonary edema. *Heart & Lung, 19*(3), 287–300.

Stiesmeyer, J. (1993). A four-step approach to pulmonary assessment. *American Journal of Nursing, 93*(8), 22–28, 31.

Stiesmeyer, J. (1991). Assessing the lungs. *Nursing91, 21*(11), 32 C–D, 32F.

Nursing Care of Clients with Upper Respiratory Disorders

LEARNING OBJECTIVES

After completing this chapter, you will be able to

- Describe the pathophysiology of common disorders affecting the upper respiratory tract, relating their manifestations to the pathophysiologic process.
- Identify laboratory and diagnostic tests used to diagnose upper respiratory disorders.
- Discuss the nursing implications for pharmacologic interventions and other treatments prescribed for clients

with upper respiratory disorders.
- Provide care for clients having surgery involving the upper respiratory system.
- Identify nursing care needs for the client with an endotracheal tube or tracheostomy.
- Use the nursing process to assess client needs, plan and implement individualized care, and evaluate responses for the client with an upper respiratory disorder.

Upper respiratory disorders include those of the nose, paranasal sinuses, tonsils, adenoids, larynx, and pharynx. They cover a broad spectrum, from very minor conditions such as the common cold to life-threatening conditions such as laryngeal obstruction. Individuals with upper respiratory disorders may experience a variety of problems, such as alterations in breathing patterns, pain, fear, or alterations in communication and body image.

A patent upper airway is necessary for effective breathing. Acute and even life-threatening problems occur as

clients experience disturbances in airway clearance and patency. When breathing is compromised because of swelling, bleeding, or accumulation of secretions, the client may become frightened and anxious. Nursing care is directed toward airway management, pain control, symptom relief, maintenance of effective communication, and psychologic support for both the client and family.

◤◤◤ Infectious or Inflammatory Disorders ◤◤◤

The upper respiratory tract is vulnerable to a variety of infectious and inflammatory processes because of its constant exposure to the environment. Although most upper respiratory infections and inflammations are minor ill-

nesses, complications may result. In the frail older adult, the risk of serious problems following an upper respiratory infection can be significant.

The Client with Rhinitis

∎ ∎ ∎

Rhinitis, inflammation of the nasal cavities, is the most common upper respiratory disorder. Both acute and chronic forms of rhinitis are seen. *Acute viral rhinitis* is more generally known as the common cold. Colds are highly contagious and are prevalent in schools and work environments. The incidence of acute viral rhinitis peaks during September and late January, coinciding with the opening of schools, as well as toward the end of April. Most adults experience two to four colds each year. Chronic rhinitis has several different forms. *Allergic rhinitis,* commonly known as hay fever, is the result of a sensitivity reaction to allergens such as plant pollens. It tends to be seasonal in incidence. The etiology of *vasomotor rhinitis* is unknown; no allergen can be identified, but it produces manifestations similar to those of allergic rhinitis. *Atrophic rhinitis* is a form of chronic rhinitis characterized by changes in the mucous membrane of the nasal cavities.

Pathophysiology

Inflammatory changes in the mucous membrane of the nasopharyngeal cavity produce the characteristic manifestations of rhinitis, no matter what the cause.

Acute Viral Rhinitis

More than 200 strains of virus can produce manifestations of rhinitis, including 110 or more rhinovirus strains, adenoviruses, parainfluenza viruses, enteroviruses, coronaviruses, and respiratory syncytial virus (Rubenstein & Federman, 1994). In a small number of cases (10%), more than one virus may be present simultaneously. Viruses causing acute rhinitis spread by aerosolized droplet nuclei during sneezing or coughing or by direct contact. Infected clients are highly contagious, shedding virus for a few days *prior* to and *after* the appearance of symptoms.

Secretions of viscous mucus from the upper respiratory tract trap invading organisms, preventing their penetration into more vulnerable areas. Local immunologic defenses, such as secretory IgA antibodies in respiratory secretions, then attempt to inactivate the antigen, producing a local inflammatory response and the typical manifestations of acute rhinitis. The mucous membranes of the nasal passages swell and become hyperemic, appearing red (erythematous) and *boggy* (swollen) on inspection. Clear, watery secretions are produced, causing **coryza** or *rhinorrhea,* profuse nasal discharge. Swollen mucous membranes, local vasodilation, and secretions cause nasal congestion. Sneezing and coughing are common. Systemic manifestations of acute viral rhinitis include low-grade fever, headache, malaise, and muscle aches. The

client is usually symptomatic for a few days up to 2 weeks. Although acute viral rhinitis is typically mild and self-limited, its effects on the immune defenses of the upper respiratory tract can predispose the client to more serious bacterial infections, such as sinusitis or otitis media.

Allergic Rhinitis

Allergic or seasonal rhinitis results from a hypersensitivity reaction to allergens such as plant pollens. Episodes are generally seasonal, corresponding with high pollen or mold counts. Chronic or perennial allergic rhinitis may be seen in clients who are allergic to dust, animal dander, and certain foods such as strawberries or seafood. Both acute and chronic allergic rhinitis result from an IgE-mediated hypersensitivity response in which histamine and other vasoactive mediators such as bradykinin, serotonin, eosinophil chemotactic factor, leukotrienes, and prostaglandins are released. Histamine is a potent vasodilator that increases capillary permeability. Vasodilation and increased capillary permeability cause the mucous membranes to become congested and swollen, leading to nasal irritation and congestion, sneezing, and rhinorrhea (watery nasal discharge), as well as itchy, watery eyes. The nasal turbinates appear pale (gray to dull red), boggy, and swollen on inspection. Indeed, the posterior ends of the turbinates may become so swollen that they obstruct sinus drainage, causing sinus congestion and a frontal or generalized headache. Nasal polyps may be evident. Frequent blowing of the nose may cause the skin around the nose and upper lip to become red and irritated. With perennial allergic rhinitis, increased congestion may cause postnasal drip or be sufficient to cause snoring.

Vasomotor Rhinitis

Vasomotor rhinitis is a chronic form of rhinitis characterized by intermittent episodes of vascular engorgement of the nasal mucosa. It is not allergic in origin; its cause is unknown. Vasomotor rhinitis is characterized by periods of remission and exacerbation. Low humidity of the environment aggravates the condition. In vasomotor rhinitis, an unknown trigger causes an autonomic imbalance with increased parasympathetic tone of the nasal mucosa (Wilson et al., 1991). This results in local vasodilation with nasal congestion, sneezing, and watery rhinorrhea. Nasal mucosa appears bright red or purplish (Berkow & Fletcher, 1992).

Atrophic Rhinitis

Atrophic rhinitis is a chronic form of rhinitis characterized by atrophy and sclerosis of the nasal mucous membrane. Its cause is unknown, although it may be associated with bacterial infection, surgical resection of the turbinates, and granulomatous diseases (Wilson et al., 1991). Clients with atrophic rhinitis develop nasal obstruction with crusting of mucous membranes and a foul odor. The client's sense of smell may be impaired, a condition known as *anosmia.* Tissue necrosis may occur, causing recurrent **epistaxis,** or nosebleeds.

Collaborative Care

Because most acute forms of rhinitis are self-limiting, the client is encouraged to provide self-care. Medical intervention is usually necessary only when complications such as sinusitis or otitis media ensue. Chronic rhinitis rarely interferes with the client's life or ability to maintain ADLs; management is usually symptomatic unless the condition is severe.

Treatment of viral rhinitis (the common cold) focuses on symptomatic relief of fever, runny nose, and nasal congestion. Getting adequate rest, maintaining fluid intake, and preventing chilling help relieve general manifestations such as fever, malaise, and muscle ache. Clients should be instructed to cover the mouth and nose with tissue when coughing or sneezing, and to dispose of soiled tissues properly. Additionally, avoiding crowds helps prevent the spread of infection to others.

Treatment of allergic rhinitis (hay fever) is similar to that of viral rhinitis, with the addition of identification of precipitating allergens. Immunotherapy may be helpful in controlling symptoms caused by pollens.

Laboratory and Diagnostic Tests

Diagnosis of acute viral rhinitis is usually based on the client's history and physical assessment. Laboratory and diagnostic testing is rarely required to establish the diagnosis or monitor the client's progress. If a complication such as a bacterial infection is suspected, a white blood count may be ordered to assess for leukocytosis (an elevated WBC). Cultures of purulent discharge may also be done in this case.

Clients with chronic or severe recurrent allergic rhinitis may undergo skin testing to identify allergens. In this test, known allergens are either applied to the skin followed by a skin prick to expose underlying tissues or injected intradermally. The exposed area is then assessed for evidence of a hypersensitivity response. Once the allergens precipitating a hypersensitivity reaction have been identified, the client is better able to avoid these allergens. Clients who experience a severe response may also undergo immunotherapy.

Pharmacology

No pharmacologic interventions have been proven successful in treating acute viral rhinitis. Mild decongestants such as pseudoephedrine may help relieve the manifestations of coryza and nasal congestion. Warm salt water gargles or throat lozenges may soothe a sore throat. Clients should be encouraged to avoid using aspirin or acetaminophen for mild cold symptoms, because these medications appear to increase nasal manifestations and viral shedding. They may also suppress antibody formation, prolonging the course of the illness (Rubenstein & Federman, 1994).

Decongestants may also help relieve manifestations of allergic rhinitis. Antihistamines are specific to the allergic mechanism, and may also be recommended. Antihistamines such as brompheniramine, chlorpheniramine, and clemastine are available in nonprescription forms. Long-acting nonsedating antihistamines are available by prescription, including astemizole, loratadine, and terfenadine. The box on page 1332 outlines nursing implications of and client teaching about the use of decongestants and common antihistamine preparations.

Drug therapy in clients with allergic rhinitis may include the use of nasally inhaled steroids or inhaled cromolyn, a mast cell stabilizer, if antihistamine or decongestant therapy is not effective.

Immunotherapy, also called hyposensitization or desensitization, may be prescribed for clients with severe allergic rhinitis. An extract of the allergen is injected in gradually increasing doses, causing the client to develop IgG antibodies to the allergen. These antibodies appear to block the allergic IgE-mediated response.

Nursing Care

The primary nursing role in caring for clients with acute or chronic rhinitis is educational. Self-care is appropriate for most clients with rhinitis; unless the problem is recurrent or a complication occurs, medical evaluation and treatment are rarely required.

Acute viral or allergic rhinitis may interfere with the client's ability to maintain usual work and recreational activities. The client with a cold need not necessarily interrupt the normal schedule of daily activities; if the client feels well enough to continue usual activities, it is appropriate to do so. Care should be taken to avoid spreading pathogens to others. Additional rest during the acute phase of illness may contribute to the client's sense of well-being. Additional fluid intake and a well-balanced diet help support the immune response, hastening recovery.

The following nursing diagnoses may be appropriate for the client with acute or chronic rhinitis:

- *Altered Tissue Perfusion* related to inflammatory process of the nasal mucosa
- *Altered Role Performance* related to manifestations of acute rhinitis

Client and Family Teaching

Because rhinitis is appropriately treated by the client, teaching is a vital part of nursing care. Instruction in the

Nursing Implications for Pharmacology: Decongestants and Antihistamines

DECONGESTANTS

Phenylephrine (Neo-Synephrine, others)

Phenylpropanolamine (Comtrex, Ornade, Triaminic, others)

Pseudoephedrine (Sudafed, Actifed, others)

Most decongestant preparations have *sympathomimetic* qualities that cause vasoconstriction, which reduces the inflammation and edema of nasal mucosa and relieves nasal congestion. They are very effective when applied topically (by nasal spray) because of their rapid onset of action. However, the duration of their effect is short, followed by vasodilation and rebound congestion. Because of their rapid effect and short duration, these preparations are habit-forming. Chronic use may lead to *rhinitis medicamentosa*, a rebound phenomenon of drug-induced nasal irritation and inflammation (Shlafer, 1993).

Nursing Responsibilities

- Assess the client for conditions that may contraindicate the use of decongestants, including hypertension or chronic heart disease. These drugs stimulate the sympathetic nervous system, increasing peripheral vascular resistance, blood pressure, and heart rate.

- Evaluate the client's medication regimen for medications that may interact with decongestant preparations such as antihypertensive medications and monoamine oxidase (MAO) inhibitors.

Client and Family Teaching

- Do not use more than the recommended dose.

- Check with the physician before taking these medications if you are taking any prescription medications or are being treated for high blood pressure or heart disease.

- Use for limited periods of time only. Nasal sprays should be used for no more than 2 to 3 days.

- Increase fluid intake to relieve mouth dryness.

- These medications may cause nervousness, shakiness, or difficulty sleeping. Discontinue their use if these effects occur.

ANTIHISTAMINES

Brompheniramine (Dimetane, others)

Chlorpheniramine (Chlor-Trimeton, others)

Clemastine (Tavist)

Dexchlorpheniramine (Dexchlor, others)

Triprolidine (Actidil, Myidil)

Nonsedating

Astemizole (Hismanal)

Loratadine (Claritin)

Terfenadine (Seldane)

Antihistamines are widely available in both prescription and nonprescription forms. They are frequently combined with decongestants in over-the-counter cold and allergy preparations. Antihistamines relieve the systemic effects of histamine and dry respiratory secretions through an anticholinergic effect. Most antihistamines cause drowsiness; the nonsedating antihistamines listed are available in prescription form only at this time.

Nursing Responsibilities

- Before administering or recommending these drugs, assess the client for possible contraindications to antihistamines, including the following:
  a. Acute asthma or lower respiratory disease that may be aggravated by drying of secretions
  b. Hypersensitivity to antihistamines
  c. Glaucoma (increased intraocular pressure)
  d. Impaired gastrointestinal motility or obstruction, which may be worsened by anticholinergic effects
  e. Prostatic hypertrophy or other urinary tract obstruction
  f. Heart disease

- For clients who must remain alert while on antihistamine therapy, recommend nonsedating forms.

Client and Family Teaching

- Do not drive or operate machinery while taking over-the-counter or prescription forms of antihistamines known to be sedating.

- Stop the drug and notify the physician immediately if you experience confusion, excessive sedation, chest tightness, wheezing, bleeding, or easy bruising while you are taking antihistamines.

- Do not use alcohol or other CNS depressants while taking antihistamines.

- Hard candy, gum, ice chips, and liquids help relieve mouth dryness caused by antihistamines.

use of disposable tissues to cover the mouth and nose while coughing or sneezing helps prevent airborne spread of the virus. The nose should be blown with both nostrils open to prevent infected matter from being forced into the auditory tubes. Frequent hand washing, especially after coughing or sneezing, is an important measure to limit viral transmission. Clients can limit the incidence of rhinitis by avoiding exposure to crowds or to known allergens. Teach the client that although becoming chilled or going out in the rain does not cause colds, they are more likely to occur during periods of physical or psychologic stress. Maintenance of good general health and stress-reduction activities support the immune system and help prevent acute viral rhinitis (see the accompanying research box).

Most clients can use over-the-counter preparations for symptomatic relief and to enhance feelings of wellness. Because of the sedative effect of antihistamines, the client taking them should be instructed to avoid driving or working with heavy machinery. Clients should be taught to limit their use of nasal decongestants to every 4 hours for only a few days at a time to prevent rebound effect. Suggest that clients avoid using aspirin or acetaminophen unless needed to relieve muscle aches and promote rest, because these medications may actually prolong acute viral rhinitis.

Help the client with allergic rhinitis identify possible allergens and strategies to avoid contacting them. Discuss the possible benefits of skin testing to identify allergens and, if necessary, immunotherapy to reduce the allergic response.

The Client with Influenza

■ ■ ■

Influenza, or *flu,* is a highly contagious viral respiratory disease characterized by coryza, fever, cough, and constitutional manifestations such as headache and malaise. Influenza usually occurs in epidemics or pandemics, although sporadic cases do occur. Yearly outbreaks of influenza affect about 48 million Americans each winter, accounting for about 3.9 million hospitalizations and 20,000 deaths. Those at increased risk include children under 5 years of age and adults over 65, especially those in nursing homes and those with chronic cardiac or pulmonary problems. Eighty to ninety percent of all influenza-related deaths occur in older adults (Ward, 1992).

Pathophysiology

Influenza is caused by orthomyxoviruses and transmitted by airborne droplet and direct contact. Three major strains of virus have been identified: type A, type B, and

---

Applying Research to Nursing Practice: Meeting the Needs of the Older Adult

■ ■ ■

A volunteer population of healthy older adults are participating in a 3-year study to determine the effects of moderate exercise on the incidence of respiratory tract infections. Participants walk for 30 to 35 minutes at least three times a week, with 10-minute warm-up and cool-down sessions. Stress levels as perceived by the study participants are considered an additional variable, because previous studies have shown an increased incidence of upper respiratory infections in people who have high levels of stress. After just 1 year of the study, 79% of the subjects report reduced stress and fewer symptoms of respiratory infections. Preliminary data also indicate that the majority of the volunteers are maintaining the low incidence of upper and lower respiratory infections into the second year of the study, with some subjects demonstrating an even lower rate of infection (Karper & Boschen, 1993).

Implications for Nursing

Nurses can play an important role in educating older adults about the beneficial effects of regular moderate exercise such as walking. The client is likely not only to reduce the incidence of respiratory infections but also to realize other beneficial effects, such as improved cardiac and respiratory function, and improved musculoskeletal strength, endurance, and flexibility.

Critical Thinking in Client Care

1. How does the level of stress being experienced by a client affect susceptibility to infection of the upper respiratory tract?

2. Why is regular exercise beneficial in reducing a person's perceived level of stress?

3. Plan an exercise program to meet the needs of a mixed group of older adults living in a rural area of the Pacific Northwest. Consider probable access to facilities, weather (usually cool and rainy), age range, and possible gender differences.

---

type C. Type A and type B influenza viruses are responsible for periodic epidemics and may cause significant morbidity and mortality. Type C is more likely to be endemic, causing periodic minor illness. Surface characteristics of the virus change continuously, resulting in new strains

---

Clinical Manifestations of Influenza

Respiratory Manifestations

- Coryza
- Cough, initially dry becoming productive
- Substernal burning
- Sore throat

Systemic Manifestations

- Fever and chills
- Malaise
- Muscle aches
- Fatigue

---

that are named according to the strain, geographic origin, and year (e.g., A/Taiwan/89).

The incubation period for influenza is short, usually only 1 to 4 days. Infection produces one of three syndromes: uncomplicated nasopharyngeal inflammation, viral upper respiratory infection followed by bacterial infection, or viral pneumonia. The onset is rapid; the client may develop profound malaise in as little as 1 to 2 minutes (Porth, 1994). Inflammation of the respiratory tract leads to necrosis and shedding of serous and ciliated cells. This allows extracellular fluid to escape, producing rhinorrhea. With recovery, serous cells are replaced more rapidly than ciliated cells; the client must cough and blow the nose to clear mucus from the sinuses and respiratory tract (Porth, 1994).

Manifestations of influenza include abrupt onset of chills and fever, malaise, muscle aches, and headache. Respiratory manifestations develop, including dry, nonproductive cough, sore throat, substernal burning, and coryza (see the accompanying box). Acute manifestations subside within 2 to 3 days, although fever may last as long as a week. The cough may be severe and productive. Along with fatigue and weakness, the cough can persist for days or several weeks.

The respiratory epithelial necrosis produced by influenza predisposes the client to secondary bacterial infections. Sinusitis and otitis media are frequent complications of influenza. Clients at high risk, such as the older adult and people with chronic cardiac or pulmonary disease, may experience complications such as viral or bacterial pneumonia or tracheobronchitis. Tracheobronchitis, inflammation of the trachea and bronchi, is not considered a serious health risk, but manifestations may persist for up to 3 weeks.

Influenza is clearly linked to an increased risk for pneumonia, particularly in older clients. Changes in respiratory function associated with aging, including decreased effectiveness of cough and increased residual lung volume, pose little risk in the healthy older adult but greatly increase the risk for pneumonia when influenza is also present (Hazzard et al., 1994). Viral pneumonia is a serious complication that may be fatal. It typically develops within 48 hours of the onset of influenza, often in clients with preexisting cardiac valvular or pulmonary disease. Influenza pneumonia progresses rapidly and can cause hypoxemia and death within a few days (Porth, 1994). Bacterial pneumonia is more likely to occur in older at-risk adults but also may affect otherwise healthy adults. It usually presents as a relapse of influenza, with a productive cough and radiographic evidence of pneumonia. See Chapter 34 for further discussion of pneumonias.

Reye's syndrome is a rare but potentially fatal complication of influenza. Although it is more likely to affect children, it also has been identified in older adults. Its onset is usually within 2 to 3 weeks after the onset of influenza, and it has a 30% mortality rate. Hepatic failure and encephalopathy develop rapidly in clients with Reye's syndrome.

Collaborative Care

Prevention of influenza by active immunization of at-risk populations is an important aspect of care. Immunization with polyvalent (containing antigens of several viral strains) influenza virus vaccine is about 85% effective in preventing influenza infection for several months to a year (Tierney et al., 1994). Annual immunization is recommended for at-risk clients, including people over the age of 65, residents of nursing homes, adults and children with chronic disorders of the cardiopulmonary system or other chronic metabolic diseases such as diabetes, and health care workers who have frequent contact with high-risk clients. Additionally, family members of at-risk clients should be vaccinated to decrease the client's risk of exposure. The vaccine should be given in the fall, prior to the annual winter outbreak. Medical treatment of influenza focuses on establishing an accurate diagnosis, providing symptomatic relief, and preventing complications.

Laboratory and Diagnostic Tests

The diagnosis of influenza is based on client history, clinical findings, and knowledge of influenza outbreak in the community. A chest X-ray and white blood cell count (WBC) may be done to rule out complications such as pneumonia. The WBC is commonly decreased in influenza; bacterial infections usually cause an increased WBC.

Pharmacology

Yearly immunization with influenza vaccine is the single most important measure to prevent or minimize manifestation of influenza. Although the vaccine is readily available and inexpensive, only about 30% of at-risk clients are vaccinated each year. Many may fear a reaction from the vaccine, although the vaccines are highly purified and reactions are rare. Because the vaccine is produced in eggs, it should not be administered to people with hypersensitivity to egg protein. Among the more serious adverse reactions are anaphylaxis and *Guillain-Barré syndrome,* an acute neurologic disorder characterized by muscle weakness and distal sensory loss. About 5% of those vaccinated may experience nonserious symptoms of low-grade fever, malaise, or myalgia for up to 24 hours after vaccination.

Amantadine (Symmetrel) may be used for prophylaxis in people who have not been vaccinated but have been exposed to the virus. If the drug is administered before or within 48 hours of exposure, it is presumed to inhibit virus shedding and acts to prevent or decrease the symptoms of influenza. If possible, unvaccinated individuals should receive the vaccine along with amantadine; it can then be discontinued in 2 to 3 weeks. When immunization is not possible, amantadine must be taken daily for the duration of the influenza outbreak.

Over-the-counter analgesics such as aspirin, acetaminophen, or NSAIDs provide symptomatic relief of fever and muscle ache. Antitussives may decrease cough, promoting rest. Antibiotics are not indicated unless secondary bacterial infection occurs.

Nursing Care

Although the manifestations of influenza are distressing, most affected clients provide self-care and do not contact a health care provider. Recommendations to rest in bed during the acute phase of the illness and limit activities until recovery are appropriate for clients with influenza.

Clients with significant manifestations or complications of influenza may require hospitalization for respiratory support and management. For these clients, nursing care focuses on maintaining airway clearance, breathing patterns, and adequate rest.

Ineffective Breathing Pattern

Muscle aches, malaise, and elevated temperature may increase the client's respiratory rate and alter the depth of respirations, decreasing effective ventilation of alveoli. Shallow respirations also increase the risk of *atelectasis,* lack of ventilation of an area of lung.

Nursing interventions with rationales follow.

- Monitor respiratory rate and pattern for changes from baseline. *Tachypnea and/or rapid, shallow respirations may result from fever and muscle ache.*

- Monitor for changes in pulse rate. *Fever may result in tachycardia.*

- Pace activities to provide for periods of rest. *Tachypnea is fatiguing because of the increased work of breathing; fatigue, in turn, can compromise breathing by causing more shallow, rapid respirations.*

- Elevate the head of the bed. *The upright position maximizes optimal lung excursion and reduces the work of breathing by lowering the diaphragm, moving abdominal contents downward, creating less resistance to diaphragmatic excursion, and slightly decreasing venous return.*

Ineffective Airway Clearance

Swelling and congestion of mucous membranes, extracellular fluid exudate, and impaired ciliary action due to cell damage increase the risk of impaired airway clearance in the client with influenza. The older adult is at particular risk because of normally reduced ciliary activity and increased lung compliance.

Nursing interventions with rationales follow.

- Monitor the effectiveness of the client's cough and ability to remove airway secretions. *Fatigue and general malaise may impair the client's ability to cough effectively and mobilize secretions.*

- Maintain adequate hydration. Assess mucous membranes and skin turgor for evidence of dehydration. *Fever and decreased oral intake of fluids may cause dehydration and increased viscosity of secretions. Thick, viscous secretions are more difficult to expectorate.*

- Increase the humidity of inspired air with a bedside humidifier. *Increasing the water content of inhaled air helps loosen thick secretions and soothe mucous membranes.*

- Teach the client how to cough effectively. Administer analgesic medications as ordered. *The huff or cascade technique of coughing increases the effectiveness of the cough and spares energy (see Chapter 34 for client teaching of this technique). Relieving muscle ache increases the client's ability to cough effectively.*

Sleep Pattern Disturbance

Airway congestion, malaise, muscle aches, and persistent cough may interfere with the client's ability to rest, increasing fatigue and prolonging recovery.

Nursing interventions with rationales follow:

- Assess the client's sleep patterns using subjective and objective information. *The client may appear to be sleeping but not achieving normal sleep patterns because of manifestations of influenza. Both subjective and objective data are important to assess the client's sleep accurately.*

- Place the client in a semi-Fowler's or Fowler's position for sleep. *Elevating the head of the bed decreases the work of breathing and may allow the client to rest more comfortably.*

**Applying Research to Nursing Practice:
Self-Care Activities of Older Adults with
Colds and Influenza**

■ ■ ■

Researchers have investigated the self-care activities of older adults related to preventing common colds and influenza, identifying their manifestations and complications, and treating them (Conn, 1991). The researchers found participants most likely to use strategies such as dressing warmly, ensuring adequate nutrition, and taking vitamins. Interestingly, few subjects reported avoiding others who are ill as a prevention strategy. Only 38% of the participants reported getting a vaccination to prevent influenza, with most citing previous side effects from the vaccine or good general health as reasons for not seeking immunization (Conn, 1991).

The majority of the subjects identified symptoms accurately and reported activities consistent with professional advice for self-care and symptom management, including decreasing activities and increasing fluid intake. Older adults commonly use medications to treat both colds and influenza. Few participants in the study were aware of the potential hazards associated with colds and influenza, with only 22 of 160 subjects identifying pneumonia as a possible consequence. Only one person related dehydration as a potential hazard.

Implications for Nursing

The population at highest risk for serious sequelae from colds or influenza is older adults. Nurses can have a positive influence on client outcomes by teaching appropriate prevention strategies and symptom management. It is important to include information about possible adverse consequenses and indicators for medical attention when teaching self-care.

Critical Thinking in Client Care

1. Identify five common reasons clients give for not getting an influenza immunization.

2. For each reason given, identify at least one nursing strategy to encourage at-risk clients to seek immunization.

3. What additional measures can nurses take to reduce the risk of an influenza epidemic in their communities?

- Provide antipyretic and analgesic medications at bedtime or shortly before. *These medications promote comfort by reducing fever and alleviating muscle aches.*

- If necessary, request a cough suppressant medication for night time use. *Cough suppressants are not recommended during the day because coughing promotes airway clearance. They may, however, be necessary at night to allow the client to rest.*

Other Nursing Diagnoses

The following nursing diagnoses may also be appropriate for the client with influenza:

- *Hyperthermia* related to infectious process

- *Activity Intolerance* related to physical discomfort, malaise, and fatigue

- *Self-Care Deficit* related to malaise, fever, and immobility

- *Risk for Impaired Gas Exchange* related to potential complication of bacterial pneumonia

Client and Family Teaching

Teaching of clients and families about influenza focuses on prevention. Stress the importance of yearly influenza vaccination for clients in high risk groups and their families. Teach clients how the disease is spread, including measures for reducing the risk of contracting influenza, such as avoiding crowds and people who are ill (see the accompanying research box).

Encourage clients with influenza to provide appropriate self-care measures. Encourage rest during the acute, febrile phase of the illness. Stress the importance of maintaining adequate hydration to ensure airway clearance. Discuss appropriate use of over-the-counter medications for relief of manifestations. Teach the client about hygiene measures such as using disposable tissues and frequent hand washing to reduce the spread of the disease.

Teach clients about possible complications of influenza and manifestations of these complications. Emphasize that although uncomplicated influenza is appropriately managed at home, manifestations of complications should be promptly reported to the physician.

The Client with Sinusitis

■ ■ ■

Sinusitis is an inflammation of the mucous membranes of one or more of the sinuses (see Figure 32–2 on page 1315). Sinusitis is a common condition that usually follows an upper respiratory infection such as acute viral rhinitis or influenza. Common causative organisms include streptococci, *S. pneumoniae*, *Haemophilus influenzae,* and staphylococci. The risk of sinusitis is increased in immunosuppressed clients such as people taking immunosuppressive drugs or people with HIV infection. Sinusitis is common in clients who have AIDS and may be particularly difficult to resolve in these clients.

Pathophysiology

Sinusitis occurs when nasal mucous membranes swell or other disorders obstruct sinus openings, impairing drainage. Mucus secretions collect in the sinus cavity, serving as a medium for bacterial growth. The nasal and sinus mucous membranes are continuous; therefore bacteria generally spread to the sinuses via the opening into the nasal turbinates. The inflammatory response provoked by bacterial invasion draws serum and leukocytes to the area to combat the infection, increasing swelling and pressure.

Any process that impairs drainage from the sinuses may precipitate sinusitis. These include nasal polyps, deviated septum, rhinitis, tooth abscess, or swimming or diving trauma. In hospitalized clients, sinusitis may develop following prolonged nasotracheal intubation (Wilson et al., 1991). Usually more than one sinus is infected. The frontal and maxillary sinuses are usually involved in adults.

Sinusitis may be acute or chronic. Chronic sinusitis results from nontreatment or inadequate treatment of the acute phase. With continued infection, bacteria can become walled off and produce chronic inflammation. Over time, mucous membranes become thickened. Fungal infections may cause chronic infections, especially in immunosuppressed clients. Other factors that may contribute to chronic sinusitis are smoking, a history of allergy, and habitual use of nasal sprays or inhalants.

General manifestations of sinusitis are pain and tenderness across the infected sinuses, headache, fever, and malaise. The pain usually increases with leaning forward. When the maxillary sinuses are involved, pain and pressure are experienced over the cheek. The pain may be referred to the upper teeth. Frontal sinusitis causes pain and tenderness across the lower forehead. Infection of the ethmoid sinus produces retro-orbital pain and pain over the high lateral aspect of the nose. Sphenoid sinusitis, the rarest form, may produce pain in the occiput, vertex, or middle of the head. The nasal mucous membrane is red and swollen in clients with sinusitis. Purulent drainage may be noted at the meatus to the middle turbinate.

The client with acute sinusitis often looks sick. Additional manifestations include nasal congestion, purulent nasal discharge, bad breath, fever, malaise, and fatigue. In acute sinusitis, the pain is usually constant and severe. In chronic sinusitis, the pain is described as dull and may be constant or intermittent. Purulent nasal discharge may be the only symptom of chronic sinusitis.

Symptoms of sinusitis may worsen for 3 to 4 hours after awakening and then become less severe in the afternoon and evening as secretions drain. Headache may change in intensity and in position as the sinuses drain. Purulent nasal discharge blocks the nose. Swallowed secretions cause the throat to become sore and inflamed and may cause nausea or vomiting. The nasal mucosa is reddened and edematous.

Complications are generally the result of spread of the infection to surrounding structures. These include periorbital abscess or cellulitis, cavernous sinus thrombosis, meningitis, brain abscess or sepsis. Edema of the auditory tube may result in hearing loss. Potential complications of sinusitis are listed in the accompanying box.

Collaborative Care

Treatment of sinusitis is directed toward drainage of the obstructed sinuses, control of infection, relief of pain, and prevention of complications.

Laboratory and Diagnostic Tests

Laboratory and diagnostic tests are used in addition to clinical evidence to make the diagnosis of sinusitis. The white blood count is elevated, indicating bacterial infection. Drainage cultures may be obtained to identify the organism involved, although obtaining a culture specimen uncontaminated by nasal flora is difficult.

Diagnostic tests include transillumination and radiologic examination of the sinuses.

Potential Complications of Sinusitis

■ ■ ■

Local Complications

- Orbital cellulitis
- Subperiosteal abscess
- Orbital abscess
- Cavernous sinus thrombosis
- Mucocele
- Osteomyelitis

Intracranial Complications

- Meningitis
- Epidural abscess
- Subdural abscess
- Brain abscess
- Venous sinus thrombosis

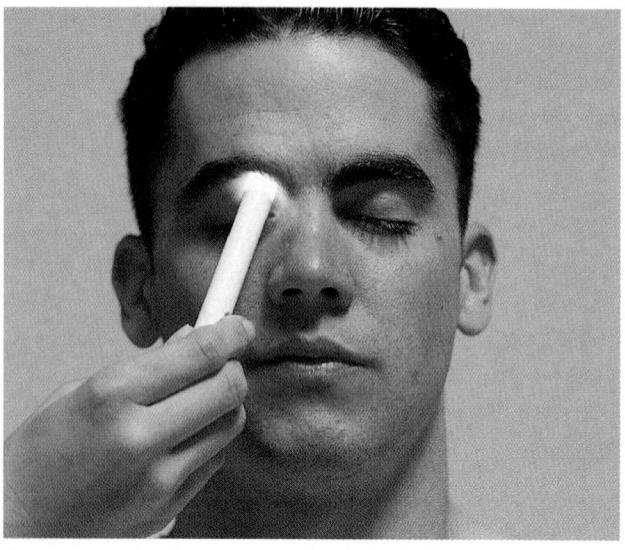
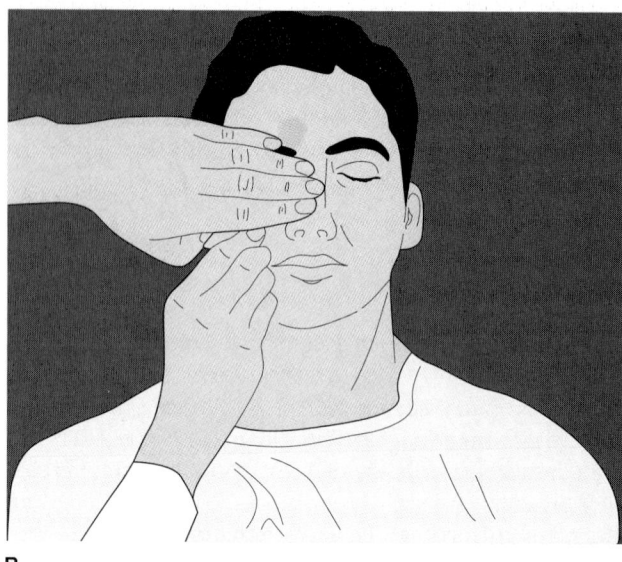

A

B

Figure 33–1 Transillumination of the frontal sinuses. *A,* The penlight is held against the upper eye orbit with the light directed upward. *B,* When the light source is covered and the room darkened, a red glow is seen over the frontal sinus.

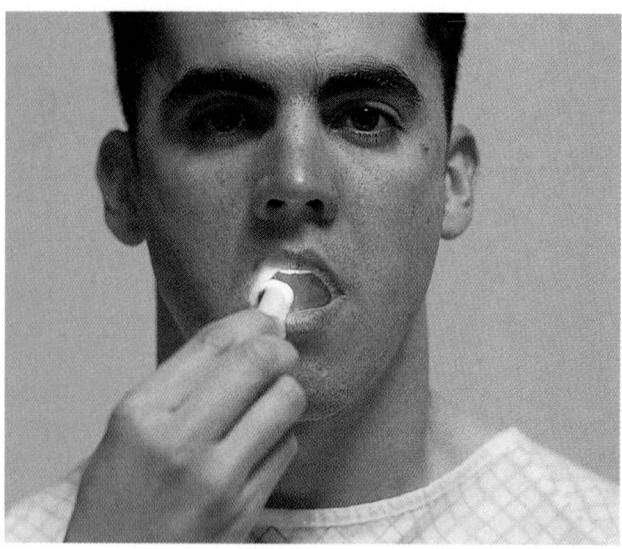
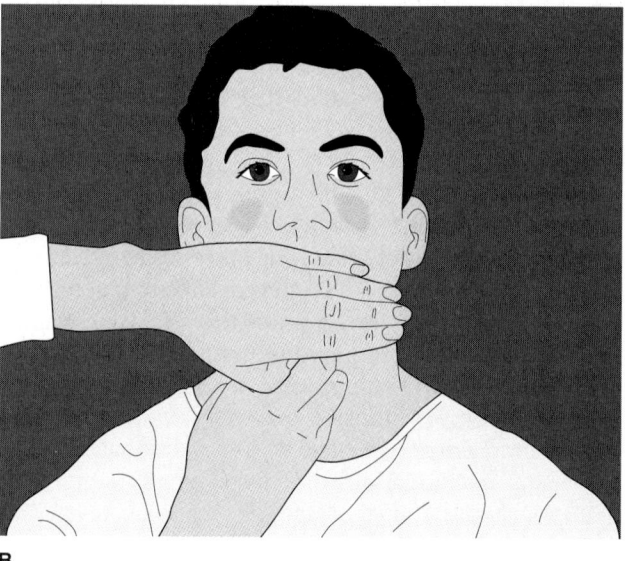

A

B

Figure 33–2 Transillumination of the maxillary sinuses. *A,* A clean penlight is held against the roof of the mouth with the light directed up toward the eyes. *B,* When the light source is covered and the room darkened, a red glow is seen over the maxillary sinuses.

Transillumination of the sinuses is performed by darkening the room and using a penlight to illuminate the sinuses. The frontal sinuses are illuminated by holding a penlight under the superior orbital ridge of the eye and covering the light with the hand. A red glow should be seen over the frontal sinus area (Figure 33–1). To illuminate the maxillary sinuses, the penlight is placed in the client's mouth against first one side of the hard palate and then the other. A red glow is seen under the eyes (Figure 33–2). The affected sinus appears darker than the others.

Variations in soft tissue thickness and examination technique make interpretation of transillumination difficult, however.

Radiologic tests may include either conventional X-rays of the sinuses or CT scan. Sinuses are normally translucent because they are filled with air; affected sinuses appear cloudy or opaque. A visible fluid or fluid/air level may be noted. CT scans are a more sensitive means of detecting inflammatory changes of sinusitis and have replaced X-rays for diagnosis of sinusitis in many centers.

Pharmacology

Once a culture of drainage has been obtained, broad-spectrum antibiotics such as ampicillin and amoxicillin are prescribed. Amoxicillin penetrates the sinuses better, so it is the drug of first choice (Tierney et al., 1994). Alternative drugs for clients who are allergic to penicillin include trimethoprim-sulfamethoxazole (Bactrim, Septra), cephalexin (Keflex), cefuroxime (Ceftin), and cefaclor (Ceclor). Antibiotic therapy is continued for a full 2-week course; occasionally a longer course is prescribed to prevent relapse. If the client's sinusitis does not respond to treatment with oral antibiotics, hospitalization and intravenous antibiotic therapy may be required. See the pharmacology box on page 257 of Chapter 8 for nursing care related to antibiotic therapy.

Oral or topical (in the form of nasal sprays) decongestants such as pseudoephedrine or phenylephrine are also prescribed to reduce mucosal edema and promote sinus drainage. Antihistamines may decrease nasal congestion and facilitate sinus drainage but also tend to increase the viscosity of secretions and hinder drainage. For this reason, they may not be as effective as decongestants. Saline nose drops or sprays promote sinus drainage, as does inhalation of warm steam. Topical nasal steroids may be used after antibiotic therapy has been initiated, in the later stages of treating subacute or chronic sinusitis, and for prophylaxis of recurrent problems. They may also be used in the postoperative phase of endoscopic sinus surgery.

Topical drug administration is best accomplished by tilting the client's head backward and to the side on which the drops are to be instilled. The client may need to remain in position for five minutes to allow the drops to reach the posterior nares. Systemic mucolytic agents such as guaifenesin may be useful to liquefy secretions, promoting sinus drainage. Aerobic exercise also promotes mucus flow and may be recommended.

Surgery

Clients who do not respond to pharmacologic measures and who experience persistent facial pain, headache, or nasal congestion may require surgical intervention.

Antral irrigation, also known as antral puncture and lavage, can be performed in the physician's office under local anesthesia. A large 16-gauge needle is inserted under the inferior turbinate of the nose into the maxillary sinus on the affected side. Saline solution is instilled to irrigate the area and wash out the sinus of purulent exudate. The client is placed in a sitting position with the head forward and mouth open to allow drainage of the solution through the nose and mouth. A culture of the exudate may be obtained to determine appropriate antibiotic therapy.

Endoscopic sinus surgery is rapidly replacing conventional surgical techniques for chronic sinusitis. Detailed evaluation of the sinuses, usually by CT scan, precedes endoscopic surgery. Under local or general anesthesia, a fiberoptic nasal endoscope is inserted to visualize the opening to the sinus. If obstruction of the opening is seen, it can be removed, restoring patency and drainage (Rubenstein & Federman, 1994). This surgery is more effective for local disease and for removing anatomic obstructions (Way, 1994). Clients who have endoscopic sinus surgery usually do not require nasal packing postoperatively. Instead, frequent nasal cleaning and irrigation with normal saline are performed. Clients are more comfortable when little or no packing is used. Postoperative administration of nasal steroid sprays speeds healing.

The *Caldwell-Luc* procedure may be used for clients with maxillary sinusitis. It is performed under local or general anesthesia. An incision is made under the upper lip into the maxillary sinus, and diseased mucous membrane and periosteum are removed. An opening between the maxillary sinus and lateral nasal wall, a "nasal antral window," is created to increase aeration of the sinus and promote drainage into the nasal cavity. The area is packed with gauze for 24 to 48 hours postoperatively. The gauze packing obstructs nasal breathing while it is in place. As the maxillary sinus heals, the exposed bone is covered by mucosa. The client may experience numbness of the upper lip and teeth for up to several months after the procedure because some of the nerves supplying these structures are traumatized. Chewing may be impaired on the affected side. Only liquids are given for the first 24 hours, followed by a soft diet. The client should not wear dentures until the incision heals and should avoid the Valsalva maneuver (no blowing the nose, coughing, or straining at stool) for about 2 weeks after the packing has been removed to prevent bleeding.

In *external sphenoethmoidectomy,* a surgical incision is made along the side of the nose from the middle of the eyebrow to open and remove diseased tissue from the sphenoid or ethmoid sinuses. Nasal polyps may also be removed using this approach. The client has ethmoid and nasal packing inserted as well as an eye pressure patch to decrease periorbital edema. Care is similar to that required after the Caldwell-Luc procedure.

Nursing Care

The client with sinusitis is often acutely uncomfortable. Obstructed and congested sinuses cause pain and pressure that increase when the client changes position and leans forward. Unless the infection is unresponsive to medical therapy, the client is usually treated at home. Education of these clients is a key nursing role. When the client is hospitalized for intravenous antibiotic therapy or sinus surgery, *Pain* and *Altered Nutrition* are priority nursing diagnoses.

Pain

Although sinus surgery is relatively minor, the client experiences discomfort from the incision as well as post operative swelling. Nasal packing, if used, contributes to the client's discomfort.

Nursing interventions with rationales follow.

- Assess the client's pain using a scale of 0 to 10. Administer mild analgesics as ordered. *Relief of pain promotes a feeling of well-being and enhances recovery.*

- Apply ice packs to the nose. *Cold compresses reduce swelling, control bleeding, and provide local analgesia.*

- Elevate the head of the bed to a Fowler's or high-Fowler's position for 24 to 48 hours after surgery. *Elevation of the operative site minimizes tissue swelling and promotes comfort. Elevation of the head of the bed also promotes optimal lung expansion.*

Altered Nutrition: Less Than Body Requirements

Postoperatively, the client may experience numbness in the upper teeth because sensory nerves have been interrupted by the mucosal incision. The sense of smell, a stimulus for appetite, is diminished by the nasal packing. Also, the client may fear choking while eating.

Nursing interventions with rationales follow.

- Provide clear liquid diet progressing to soft foods as tolerated. High-calorie dietary supplements may be used. *A progressive diet is used to assess the client's ability to swallow without choking and allays client fears. Foods high in calories and nutritional value provide for metabolic and healing requirements.*

- Monitor intake and output, as well as daily weight. *This information allows assessment of overall fluid balance. Daily weight is also an indicator of the adequacy of dietary intake.*

- Elevate the head of the bed while the client is eating. *This position facilitates swallowing and minimizes risk of aspiration.*

Other Nursing Diagnoses

The following nursing diagnoses may also be appropriate for the client with sinusitis:

- *Ineffective Airway Clearance* related to surgery, swelling, and nasal packing

- *Risk for Infection* related to surgery

- *Sleep Pattern Disturbance* related to pain, altered breathing pattern, and sleeping with the head of the bed elevated

Client and Family Teaching

Teaching for clients with sinusitis and their families focuses on following through with appropriate treatment and promoting comfort.

Stress the importance of completing the entire course of prescribed antibiotics. Discuss the need for a prolonged course of therapy to achieve levels of antibiotic in the sinuses adequate to eliminate bacteria. Teach the client about the prescribed antibiotic and assist in developing a schedule that helps the client remember to take all doses. Because the course of therapy is prolonged, it is important to discuss the possibility of superinfections such as vaginitis or oral thrush and their management. Unless contraindicated, suggest that the client consume 8 ounces of yogurt containing live bacterial cultures daily while on antibiotics.

Discuss the use of systemic or topical decongestants to promote sinus drainage. Unless the physician has recommended antihistamines for the client, discourage their use. Instruct the client to maintain a liberal fluid intake to reduce the viscosity of mucus drainage. Teach the client how to use a humidifier or steam inhalation. Encourage the client to sleep with the head of the bed elevated to a 45-degree angle and on the unaffected side to promote drainage of affected sinuses. A warm, moist pack may be applied to the area of pain and tenderness to promote comfort.

Instruct the client to notify the physician if manifestations of sinusitis do not improve with therapy or if signs of a complication develop, such as increased pain, and redness and swelling of skin on the side of the nose or around the eyes.

Following sinus surgery, the client and family are provided with instructions to prevent postoperative bleeding, such as avoiding blowing the nose for 7 to 10 days and avoiding strenuous activity such as heavy lifting for about 2 weeks. The client is instructed to begin using saline nasal sprays after about 3 to 5 days postoperatively in order to keep the nasal mucosa moist. The client is instructed to make a return appointment with the surgeon for postoperative evaluation and care.

The Client with Pharyngitis or Tonsillitis

■ ■ ■

Pharyngitis, acute inflammation of the pharynx, is one of the most commonly identified clinical problems. Although it is usually viral in origin, pharyngitis may also be caused by bacterial infection. *Group A beta-hemolytic streptococcus* (strep throat) is the most common cause of bacterial pharyngitis. Other bacteria that may cause pharyngitis include *Neisseria gonorrheae,* a gram negative diplococcus seen in clients who engage in orogenital sex, *Mycoplasma,* and *Chlamydia trachomatis.*

Tonsillitis is an acute inflammation of the palatine tonsils. Although it is sometimes viral in origin, tonsillitis is usually due to streptococcal infection. The incidence of streptococcal infections is greatest between late fall and spring, especially in cold climates. Viral tonsillitis may occur in epidemics in people living in crowded conditions, such as military recruits.

Pathophysiology

Pharyngitis and tonsillitis are contagious and spread by droplet nuclei. Incubation varies from a few hours to several days, depending on the organism. Viral infections are communicable for 2 to 3 days. Symptoms usually resolve within 3 to 10 days after onset.

Although certain clinical features of pharyngitis are more suggestive of viral infection and others are suggestive of bacterial infection, it is not possible to distinguish between these infections on a clinical basis alone.

Acute pharyngitis causes pain and fever. The pain may vary from a scratchy sore throat to one so painful that swallowing is difficult. Streptococcal pharyngitis is usually marked by an abrupt onset, with fever of 101 F (38.3 C) or higher, severe sore throat with dysphagia, malaise, and often arthralgias and myalgias. Anterior lymph nodes are often enlarged and tender. Exudate may be seen on the pharynx and tonsils. In contrast, the onset of viral pharyngitis is often gradual, with manifestations of low-grade fever, sore throat, mild hoarseness, headache, and rhinorrhea. The pharyngeal membranes appear mildly red with vascular congestion. Infectious mononucleosis, another viral infection, may initially also present with manifestations of pharyngitis. Mononucleosis is characterized by marked lymphadenopathy and often associated hepatosplenomegaly.

In tonsillitis, the tonsils appear bright red and edematous. White exudate is present on the tonsils; pressing on a tonsil may produce purulent drainage. The uvula may also be reddened and swollen. Cervical lymph nodes are usually tender and enlarged.

The client with tonsillitis complains of a sore throat, difficulty swallowing, general malaise, fever, and otalgia (pain referred to the ear). Manifestations are often more severe in adolescents and adults than in children. Infection may extend via the auditory tubes, causing acute otitis media. This may lead to further damage such as spontaneous rupture of the eardrums and mastoiditis. The infection may also chronically infect the middle ear, resulting in deafness. See Chapter 44 for further discussion of otitis media and other disorders of the middle ear.

Peritonsillar abscess, or *quinsy,* is a potential complication of tonsillitis. It usually results from group A beta-hemolytic streptococcus infection extending from the tonsils to the surrounding tissue. It is one of the more commonly seen abscesses of the head and neck. The abscess causes pus formation behind the tonsil with marked swelling and asymmetric deviation of the uvula. The degree of swelling may make it difficult for the client to swallow anything other than liquids. The client may exhibit thickening of the voice, drooling, and a tonic contraction of the muscles of mastication, called *trismus.*

Rare (1% to 3%) but serious complications of streptococcal pharyngitis and tonsillitis include acute glomerulonephritis and rheumatic fever, abnormal immune responses to the bacterial infection. Acute glomerulonephritis generally presents with sudden onset of hematuria, proteinuria, and less commonly, hypertension and edema within 7 to 10 days after the acute infection. Rheumatic fever typically presents 3 to 5 weeks after acute infection with fever, painful or swollen joints, rash, and cardiac murmur. Other complications of bacterial infection include sinusitis, otitis media, mastoiditis, and cervical adenitis.

Collaborative Care

Acute pharyngitis, whether viral or bacterial in origin, is usually a self-limiting process. However, because of the possibility of serious complications associated with streptococcal sore throat, an effort is usually made to establish an accurate diagnosis and treat bacterial pharyngitis.

Clients with manifestations suggestive of streptococcal pharyngitis usually undergo a throat swab. The swab may be examined for streptococcus antigen using the latex agglutination (LA) antigen test or enzyme immunoassay (ELISA) testing. These tests allow rapid identification of the antigen (in as little as 10 minutes for the LA test) but are not highly sensitive. When the test is positive, treatment for strep throat is initiated. If the test is negative, the swab is cultured to ensure that streptococcus organisms are not present. Even throat cultures are not always accurate, with approximately 10% false negative and 20% false positive results.

A complete blood count (CBC) may be done on severely ill clients or to rule out other causes of pharyngitis. The white blood cell count (WBC) is usually normal or low in viral infections and elevated in bacterial infections. Nasal swabs or blood cultures may also assist in accurate diagnosis.

Antipyretics and mild analgesics such as aspirin or acetaminophen are useful in providing symptomatic relief for clients with pharyngitis or tonsillitis. Penicillin is the drug of choice for group A streptococci. If the client is allergic to penicillin, erythromycin or tetracycline may be used. Antibiotic therapy is continued for at least 10 days. The client is not considered contagious after 24 hours of antibiotic therapy.

A peritonsillar abscess may be drained by needle aspiration or by incision and drainage. The area is first sprayed with a topical anesthetic such as cetacaine and then injected with a local anesthetic. The procedure is best performed with the client in a sitting position that enables expectoration of the blood and pus. Incision and drainage of a peritonsillar abscess is followed by tonsillectomy. This may be performed immediately, or 6 weeks after incision and drainage.

Surgical removal of the tonsils is controversial and is not usually performed unless the client fails to respond to medical therapy. Tonsillectomy is indicated for recurrent or chronic infections that have not responded to antibiotic therapy, hypertrophy of the tonsils with risk of airway obstruction, peritonsillar abscess, repeated attacks of purulent otitis media, and tonsil malignancy. A tonsillectomy may be done under local or general anesthesia. The most common surgical procedure to remove tonsils is dissection and snare. Laser surgery has been tried, but it prolongs anesthesia time. The most significant postoperative complication of tonsillectomy is hemorrhage.

Nursing Care

The treatment plan for the client with acute uncomplicated pharyngitis focuses on adequate rest and relief of manifestations, and can usually be implemented by the client at home. A liquid or soft diet is useful when swallowing is difficult. The client is encouraged to drink increased amounts of fluids, especially during the febrile stage. Warm saline gargles, moist inhalations, and application of an ice collar are soothing to the sore throat.

Following tonsillectomy, the nurse ensures a patent airway by positioning the client with the head toward the side for drainage of secretions from the mouth and pharynx. The airway is not removed until the client demonstrates the ability to swallow and the presence of a gag reflex. Application of an ice collar reduces swelling and provides a mild analgesic effect. If the client hemorrhages, it is necessary for the surgeon to ligate or suture the bleeding vessel. If there is no bleeding, the client is allowed water and cracked ice as desired. Warm saline mouth washes are helpful in managing thick oral secretions that may be present. A liquid or semiliquid diet is given for several days.

The following nursing diagnoses may be appropriate for the client with pharyngitis or tonsillitis:

- *Hyperthermia* related to the presence of an infection
- *Pain* related to inflamed pharyngeal tissues
- *Risk for Fluid Volume Deficit* related to fever and sore throat
- *Ineffective Airway Clearance* related to pain and surgery
- *Impaired Swallowing* related to pain and surgical intervention

Client and Family Teaching

Clients with pharyngitis or tonsillitis are managed conservatively. Stress the importance of completing the full 10 days of antibiotic therapy. Suggest that the client use warm saline gargles or throat lozenges for symptomatic relief. Provide instruction regarding the signs and symptoms of possible complications of streptococcal infection such as glomerulonephritis or rheumatic fever. Teach clients to monitor their temperature in the morning and evening until convalescence is complete to ensure that the infection has not spread to deeper tissues. Because the disease is contagious, instruct the client in the proper use and disposal of tissues and the need for frequent hand washing to contain the infection.

For the client who has had a peritonsillar abscess drainage or tonsillectomy, provide instructions about prescribed mouth and throat care postoperatively. Instruct the client to avoid aspirin for analgesia to reduce the risk of postoperative bleeding. Discuss the manifestations of bleeding that should be reported to the physician; delayed hemorrhage may occur for up to 1 week post surgery.

Applying the Nursing Process

Case Study of a Client with Peritonsillar Abscess: Monica Wunderman

Monica Wunderman is a 27-year-old woman who has been recently treated for tonsillitis caused by infection by group A streptococcus. She presents to the emergency room 10 days later appearing acutely ill. She states that her throat is so sore that she has difficulty swallowing even liquids. Barbara Ironhorse, the ER nurse, completes an assessment of Ms. Wunderman.

Assessment

T, 102 F (38.8 C). On inspection of her mouth, an acutely swollen and reddened area of the soft palate is observed, half-occluding the orifice from the mouth into the pharynx. Yellow exudate is present. A CBC reveals an elevated WBC of 16,000 per mm^3. A diagnosis of peritonsillar abscess is made. Needle aspiration of the abscess is performed.

Diagnosis

The following nursing diagnoses are made by Ms. Ironhorse for Ms. Wunderman:

- *Pain* related to swelling
- *Risk for Ineffective Airway Clearance* related to pain and swelling
- *Fluid Volume Deficit* related to fever and difficulty in swallowing fluids

Expected Outcomes

The expected outcomes for the plan of care are that Ms. Wunderman will

- Experience minimal or no pain.
- Maintain a patent airway as demonstrated by normal respiratory rate and rhythm.
- Maintain optimal fluid intake as evidenced by ability to consume fluids and semiliquid foods, appearance of moist mucous membranes, normal skin turgor, and a decrease in temperature.

Planning and Implementation

Ms. Ironhorse plans and implements the following interventions in teaching Ms. Wunderman to care for herself at home:

- Teach Ms. Wunderman that ice-cold fluids may be easier to drink than hot or room-temperature beverages and may provide a local analgesic effect. Instruct her to avoid citrus juices, hot or spicy foods, and rough-textured foods for 1 week.
- Teach pain-reduction strategies such as applying an ice collar as desired and gargling with warm saline or mouthwash solution every 1 to 2 hours for the first 24 to 48 hours after aspiration of the abscess.
- Instruct Ms. Wunderman to monitor her temperature in the morning and evening and to report an elevation to her physician.
- Instruct her to take medications as prescribed.

Evaluation

When Ms. Ironhorse contacts Ms. Wunderman by telephone 2 days after her visit to the emergency room, she reports complete relief of symptoms. She is afebrile, taking fluids without difficulty and has had no alteration in breathing status. She has not experienced any pain.

Critical Thinking in the Nursing Process

1. Describe common symptoms in clients with infectious or inflammatory diseases of the upper airway and discuss methods of symptom relief.
2. Describe common pharmacologic interventions for these clients.
3. What themes of nursing diagnoses emerge for these clients?

The Client with Acute Epiglottitis

■ ■ ■

Epiglottitis, inflammation of the epiglottis, is an uncommon disorder in adults but is being recognized more frequently (Rubenstein & Federman, 1994). Epiglottitis may be either viral or bacterial; its onset and course are slower in adults than in children because of the larger airway diameter in the adult. The supraglottic structures as

well as the epiglottis are usually involved in adults, with more significant edema than inflammation. Clients with acute epiglottitis often present with *odynophagia*, painful swallowing of food, as well as manifestations of pharyngitis. The epiglottis appears red, swollen, and edematous.

Acute epiglottitis is a medical emergency; clients require constant monitoring for signs of respiratory distress. Nasotracheal intubation may be required to ensure airway patency. The client is hospitalized and intravenous antibiotic therapy is initiated. Ceftizoxime (Cefizox), or cefuroxime (Ceftin) may be prescribed. Dexamethasone, a systemic corticosteroid, is also administered to suppress the inflammatory response and rapidly reduce inflammation and swelling of the epiglottis.

Nursing care for the client with acute epiglottitis focuses on monitoring and maintaining airway patency. The client requires constant observation for signs of airway obstruction, including nasal flaring, restlessness, stridor, use of accessory muscles, and decreased oxygen saturation measurements. Oropharyngeal and nasopharyngeal airways are avoided. Instrumentation of the airway can provoke spasm and total airway obstruction, although the risk is less in the adult than in the child. The nurse must be prepared for emergency intubation of the client at any time. Epiglottitis is a frightening condition for both the client and the nurse. Maintaining a calm, reassuring manner is an essential nursing role.

The Client with Laryngitis

■ ■ ■

Laryngitis, inflammation of the larynx, is a common disorder that may occur in isolation or in combination with other infectious or inflammatory disorders of the upper respiratory tract. It is commonly associated with viral infections of the upper respiratory tract such as influenza. It may also occur in clients with bronchitis, pneumonia, or other respiratory infections. Excessive use of the voice, sudden changes in temperature or exposure to dust, irritating fumes, smoke, or other pollutants can also cause acute or chronic laryngitis. It is more common in the winter and in colder climates.

In laryngitis, the mucous membrane lining the larynx becomes inflamed; this may be accompanied by edema of the vocal cords. The primary manifestation of laryngitis is a change in the voice. Hoarseness or *aphonia*, complete loss of the voice, may occur. Clients complain of a sore, scratchy throat and may have a dry, harsh cough.

There is no specific treatment for viral laryngitis. If precipitating factors can be identified such as overuse of the voice and exposure to irritants, these should be eliminated. The client is instructed to rest the voice and abstain from using tobacco or alcohol, which are chemical irritants. Treatment may also include inhaling steam or spraying the throat with antiseptic solutions. Identification and control or removal of irritants is helpful in preventing further attacks.

Impaired verbal communication is the priority nursing problem for clients with laryngitis. The meaning of messages is conveyed not only by the words used but also by the tone and loudness of voice. Instruct the client to rest the voice as much as possible. Encourage the client to speak in short sentences or to use alternate methods of communication, such as writing. Resting the voice hastens recovery and decreases throat discomfort. Instruct the client to use soothing throat lozenges, sprays, or other comfort measures such as gargling with a warm antiseptic solution. Help the client identify potential irritants, such as fumes, chemicals, or cold temperature, so that the client can avoid or eliminate them to prevent further bouts of laryngitis.

The Client with Diphtheria

■ ■ ■

Diphtheria is an acute, contagious disease caused by the bacterium *Corynebacterium diphtheriae,* a small aerobic pathogen. Once the leading cause of death in children, this disease is now rare, although there has been a recent resurgence, particularly in alcoholic populations (Tierney et al., 1994). The disease is spread though droplet nuclei and by contamination of articles such as eating utensils. Asymptomatic carriers can be a major factor in the spread of this infection, especially in industrialized countries. Clients who have recovered from this disease may harbor bacteria in their throats for up to 4 weeks. Diphtheria is easily spread in areas where sanitation is poor, living conditions are crowded, and access to health care is limited. Immunization is readily available, and infants and children are usually immunized against diphtheria, pertussis, and tetanus concurrently. The mortality rate from diphtheria is 10 times lower in clients who are immunized.

The most distinctive feature of diphtheria is the development of a pseudomembrane covering the posterior pharynx and sometimes extending into the trachea. Toxins released by the organism inflame the mucosal surfaces of the pharynx. Exudate from inflamed tissues forms a thick, grayish, rubbery pseudomembrane. This pseudomembrane adheres to the inflamed, eroded surfaces and interferes with eating, drinking, and breathing. The airway may be obstructed during the acute phase, necessitating tracheostomy to maintain respirations. The toxins are also particularly harmful to the heart and central nervous system and may result in myocarditis and paralysis of cranial or peripheral nerves.

Clients with diphtheria present with fever, malaise, sore throat, and malodorous breath. In severe cases, the neck may be warm and swollen because of enlarged lymph glands. The client may quickly develop manifestations of airway obstruction, such as stridor and cyanosis. The severity of manifestations depends on the site of the lesion. Clients with anterior nasal lesions may present with few manifestations but may become chronic carriers of the disease. Tonsillar diphtheria is not in itself life-threatening; however, it can rapidly progress to more serious forms.

The diagnosis of diphtheria is confirmed by a throat culture. Gram-stain or immunofluorescent antibody stains may also be used.

The goals of care for clients with diphtheria are to prevent disease transmission, treat the infection, neutralize the toxins, and provide respiratory support. Strict isolation procedures are instituted, and all contacts are screened and immunized. Booster shots should be given to those people who were immunized 5 or more years previously. Contacts who were never immunized are treated with immunization and antibiotics.

Diphtheria antitoxin is administered to neutralize free toxin and prevent further toxin production. The diphtheria antitoxin is derived from horses; a skin test for sensitivity to horse serum should precede immunization. The client is observed closely for anaphylaxis during antitoxin administration. Antibiotics such as penicillin or erythromycin are administered to eliminate the organism.

Clients with diphtheria require intensive nursing care. The client is placed on bed rest and monitored closely for evidence of airway obstruction, cardiac manifestations, and CNS complications. Nutrition and fluid balance may also be affected in the client with diphtheria because of difficulty swallowing. The client is positioned upright and may be able to swallow only liquids during the acute phase of the disease. Suction equipment, emergency intubation equipment, and tracheostomy trays should be kept at the client's bedside.

Preventing further cases of diphtheria is often a nursing responsibility as well. All symptomatic clients are isolated and treated until two throat cultures are negative for the bacterium. Nasopharyngeal and throat cultures are also obtained from all close contacts of the client with diphtheria. Asymptomatic carriers of the disease are confined to their home until at least 3 days of antibiotic therapy has been completed. All contacts of the client, including hospital personnel, receive a diphtheria immunization update using tetanus and diphtheria toxoids (Td).

The client with diphtheria may be gravely ill. The need for strict hospital isolation adds to the stress for both client and family. A thorough explanation of the need for isolation as well as assistance in identifying contacts for screening is an important nursing function. Preventive immunization is encouraged.

Upper Respiratory Trauma or Obstruction

The Client with Epistaxis

The nose has a rich blood supply, receiving major arterial vessels from both the internal and external carotid artery systems (Wilson et al., 1991). **Epistaxis,** or nosebleed, may be precipitated by a number of factors. Trauma (picking the nose or blunt trauma) can cause epistaxis, as can drying of nasal mucous membranes, local or systemic infection, substance abuse (e.g., cocaine), arteriosclerosis, or hypertension. Epistaxis may also be indicative of a bleeding disorder associated with acute leukemia, thrombocytopenia, aplastic anemia, or severe liver disease. Likewise, treatment with anticoagulant or antiplatelet medication may cause nosebleed. In adults, men are affected by nosebleeds more than women.

Pathophysiology

Ninety percent of all nosebleeds are anterior in origin, arising from Kiesselbach's area, a rich vascular plexus in the anterior nasal septum. Because of their location, these vessels are susceptible to trauma from nose picking, drying, and infection. Posterior epistaxis may also be caused by trauma but is more often secondary to systemic disorders such as blood dyscrasias, hypertension, or diabetes. In posterior epistaxis, bleeding is from the terminal branches of the sphenopalatine and internal maxillary arteries (Way, 1994). Posterior epistaxis tends to be more severe and occurs more frequently in the older adult.

Collaborative Care

The goal of treatment for epistaxis is to identify the source of bleeding and to control it.

Anterior bleeding can usually be managed by simple first-aid measures, such as applying pressure (pinching the nose toward the septum) for 5 to 10 minutes and applying ice packs to the nose and forehead to cause vasoconstriction. The client is placed in a sitting position to decrease blood flow to the head and reduce venous pressure. Having the client lean forward reduces drainage of blood backward into the nasopharynx and lessens the likelihood that the client will swallow blood. The client is instructed to spit out the blood to allow better estimation of the amount of bleeding and to prevent nausea and vomiting as a result of swallowed blood.

If applying pressure does not control the bleeding, pharmacologic interventions, nasal packing, or surgery may be necessary.

Pharmacology

Topical vasoconstrictors such as cocaine (0.5%), phenylephrine (Neo-Synephrine) (1:1000), or adrenaline (1:1000) may be useful in managing anterior bleeding. These medications may be applied by nasal spray or on a cotton swab held against the bleeding site. Chemical cauterization of the bleeding vessel may be accomplished using agents such as silver nitrate or Gelfoam. A topical anesthetic such as cetacaine spray, lidocaine, or cocaine may be used to prepare the client for nasal packing. If posterior nasal packing is required, the client is placed on prophylactic antibiotic therapy to prevent sinusitis or possible toxic shock syndrome.

Nasal Packing

If bleeding cannot be controlled with pressure and pharmacologic interventions, the nasal cavity may be packed with 1/4-inch petroleum gauze. For an anterior pack, several feet of packing are placed carefully and systematically along the floor of the nasal cavity and then into the vault of the nose. Anterior nasal packs using petroleum gauze are usually left in place for 24 to 72 hours. If epistaxis is caused by a bleeding disorder, the packing may be left in place for 4 to 5 days while therapy is instituted to correct the disorder.

Posterior nosebleeds are more difficult to control, requiring both anterior and posterior packing. Insertion of a posterior nasal pack is uncomfortable and frightening to the client. A small, red rubber catheter is passed through the nose into the oropharynx and out the mouth (Figure 33–3). Strings or umbilical tape are tied to a sterile gaúze pack that is then tied to the oral end of the catheter. The catheter is then withdrawn through the nose, positioning the pack behind the soft palate in the nasopharynx. The positioning strings of the pack protruding from the nose are tied to a rolled gauze or bolus beneath the nose to keep the pack in position. An additional string comes out through the mouth and is taped to the cheek. This string is used to remove the pack. Posterior packs are usually left in place for 2 to 5 days. A loose anterior nasal pack may also be inserted. A gauze pad is positioned under the nostrils to absorb any drainage. The anterior nasal pack remains in place for 4 to 5 days.

The client with posterior nasal packing is hospitalized because of potential respiratory complications. Hypoxemia is common; supplementary oxygen is administered. Narcotic analgesics are prescribed to manage the discomfort associated with posterior nasal packing. Clients with posterior nasal packing may develop hypertension; dysrhythmias or acute myocardial infarction may occur in clients with severe cardiovascular disease. Toxic shock

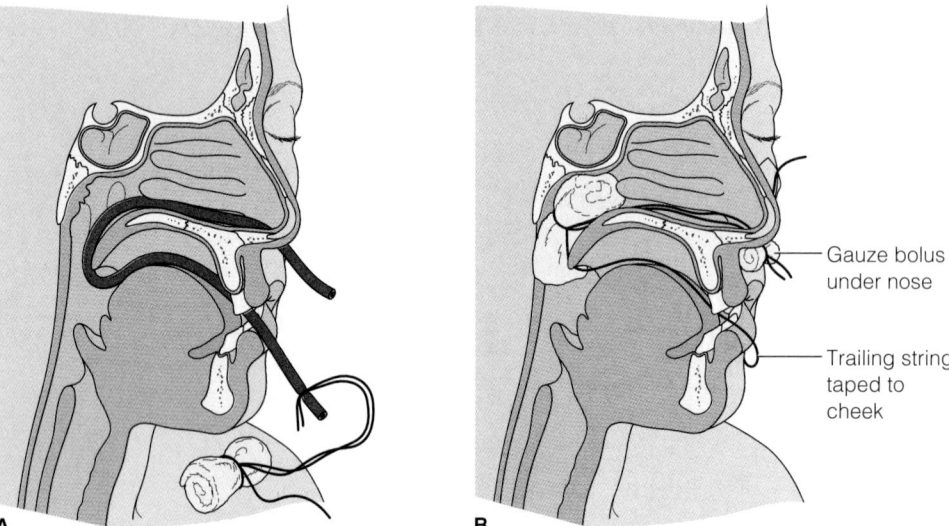

Figure 33–3 Posterior nasal packing. *A,* A rubber catheter is inserted through the nose and out the mouth and attached to the packing. *B,* The catheter is withdrawn through the nose to position the packing in the posterior nasopharynx. Ties exiting through the nose and mouth are used to stabilize the packing in position and remove it when it is no longer needed.

syndrome is another potential complication of posterior nasal packing. The pack may also occlude the auditory tube, resulting in ear discomfort or possible otitis media. Oral and nasal dryness can be minimized by use of a high-humidity face tent. Nursing care of the client with nasal packing is outlined in the box on page 1347.

A Foley catheter or inflatable nasal balloons may be used as an alternative to posterior nasal packing for effective tamponade. The catheter or nasal balloon is inserted through the nose into the nasopharynx, inflated, and left in place for 2 to 3 days.

Surgery

Chemical or surgical cautery procedures may be used to sclerose the involved vessels in the anterior aspect of the nose. The resulting scab must be left undisturbed until the mucosa has healed, or further bleeding may occur.

Surgical intervention is often preferred to posterior nasal packing for clients with posterior bleeding, and surgery is necessary when posterior packing fails to control hemorrhage. The Caldwell-Luc approach involves an incision in the gum above the incisor to access the maxillary sinus and the artery that supplies the area. The artery is then ligated with a suture or a metal clip. Nasal packing is inserted and left in place for at least 24 hours, during which time the client is monitored for bleeding.

Nursing Care

Nosebleeds can be frightening for the client, particularly when they occur spontaneously, without preceding trauma. Nurses provide care for clients with epistaxis in outpatient and emergency settings, and may care for hospitalized clients with nasal packing. Support, reassurance, and education are important roles for nurses caring for clients with epistaxis. Priority nursing diagnoses include *Anxiety* and *Risk for Aspiration.*

Anxiety

The amount of blood lost in a nosebleed can be frightening to the client. The sensation of blood draining down the client's throat and the inability to breathe through the nose contribute to the client's anxiety. If epistaxis has occurred spontaneously, the client may fear that it is indicative of a major health problem such as high blood pressure.

Nursing interventions with rationales follow:

- Maintain an attitude of calm reassurance. *By remaining calm and confident, the nurse reassures the client that the nosebleed is not a life-threatening episode.*

- Have the client pinch the nares together at the bridge of the nose. *Ninety percent of nosebleeds are anterior in origin; in most cases direct pressure stops the bleeding. Having the client place pressure on the nose provides a focus for the client and helps restore a sense of control, reducing anxiety.*

- Encourage the client to breathe slowly and deeply through the mouth. *Controlled mouth breathing maintains lung ventilation and reduces the client's anxiety.*

- Provide a basin and tissues for the client to use. Encourage the client to expectorate blood, not swallow it.

Nursing Care of the Client with Nasal Packing

NURSING RESPONSIBILITIES

- Monitor vital signs and respiratory rate or pattern for changes from baseline. *Clients with nasal packing are at risk for respiratory compromise and hypoxemia. Increased heart and respiratory rates may be early signs of respiratory compromise.*

- Inspect the client's mouth and notify the physician if the packing has slipped into the oropharynx. *Misplacement of nasal packing can result in upper airway obstruction.*

- Monitor pulse oximetry readings frequently. Administer supplementary oxygen as ordered. *Clients with posterior nasal packing may develop hypoxemia, compromising tissue oxygenation.*

- Elevate the head of the bed. *Elevating the head of the bed facilitates ventilation.*

- Encourage deep, slow breathing through the mouth. *The client needs psychologic support, reassurance, and teaching to reduce anxiety and fear associated with being unable to breathe through the nose.*

- Check for blood at the back of the throat and monitor for frequent swallowing. *Visible blood or frequent swallowing could indicate posterior bleeding.*

- Monitor for hematemesis. *Bleeding from the posterior portion of the nose often drains down the nasopharynx and is swallowed by the client. Hematemesis may indicate swallowed blood and continued bleeding.*

- Apply cold compresses to nose. *An ice or cold compress decreases pain and promotes vasoconstriction, decreasing bleeding and swelling.*

- Provide for rest. *Rest reduces the metabolic demands of the body and is important for the client with posterior nasal packing who may experience hypoxemia.*

- Ensure adequate oral fluid intake. *Fluid intake is important to maintain adequate fluid balance and decrease dryness of oral mucous membranes because of mouth breathing.*

- Provide frequent oral hygiene. Use a bedside humidifier. *These are important measures to reduce drying of oral mucous membranes and promote the client's comfort.*

These measures give the client greater control and reduce the fear of choking on blood.

- Assess the client with nasal packing frequently for adequate oxygenation. Maintain supplemental oxygen as ordered. *Cerebral hypoxia produces a sense of apprehension and fear.*

Risk for Aspiration

The highly anxious client who has blood draining into the nasopharynx is at risk for aspiration of blood into the trachea. When nasal packing is in place, the client is unable to breathe through the nose, increasing the risk of aspiration when food or fluids are consumed.

Nursing interventions with rationales follow:

- Place the client in an upright position with the head forward. Provide a basin for the client to expectorate blood. *These measures minimize the amount of blood draining down the nasopharynx and swallowed by the client, reducing the risk of aspiration and minimizing nausea from swallowed blood. Vomiting of swallowed blood increases the risk of aspiration.*

- Apply ice or a cold compress to the nose. *Cold causes vasoconstriction, reducing bleeding.*

- Position the client with nasal packing with the head elevated and on the side when asleep. *This position reduces the risk of aspiration of oral secretions.*

Other Nursing Diagnoses

The following nursing diagnoses may also be appropriate for the client with epistaxis:

- *Ineffective Airway Clearance* related to the presence of blood in nasopharynx

- *Ineffective Breathing Pattern* related to fear

- *Risk for Infection* related to posterior nasal packing and occlusion of auditory tube

Client and Family Teaching

Following an episode of epistaxis, client and family teaching focuses on measures to prevent further bleeding. The client is advised to avoid strenuous exercise for several days or weeks, depending on the severity of the nosebleed and its treatment. Clients are instructed not to blow the nose or engage in activities such as heavy lifting or bending that could increase pressure and dislodge the crust. The client is cautioned to sneeze with the mouth open to avoid increasing pressure in nasal vessels.

> ### Clinical Manifestations of Nasal Fracture
>
> ■ ■ ■
>
> - Epistaxis
> - Deformity or displacement to one side
> - Crepitus
> - Periorbital edema and ecchymosis
> - Instability of nasal bridge

Clients with anterior nasal bleeding may be instructed to use petroleum jelly, a water-soluble lubricant, or bacitracin ointment to lubricate nasal mucosa and reduce the risk of spontaneous bleeding. Use of a humidifier or vaporizer may also be recommended to minimize dryness of the mucous membranes. Clients are instructed to eliminate activities that can cause future nosebleeds, such as blowing the nose forcefully or picking the nose. When epistaxis has occurred spontaneously, encourage the client to seek medical evaluation for any possible underlying problem, such as hypertension or a bleeding disorder.

The Client with Nasal Trauma

■ ■ ■

The nose is the most commonly broken bone of the face. A nasal fracture (broken nose) usually results from a sports injury or from trauma related to violence or motor vehicle accidents. Soft tissue trauma commonly accompanies nasal fracture.

Pathophysiology

One or both sides of the nose may be fractured. A *unilateral fracture* involves only one side of the nose and is associated with little displacement or cosmetic deformity. It is usually not serious, but deviation of the septum and swelling can cause airway obstruction. *Bilateral fractures* are more common, with displacement of both nasal bones to one side or depression of the bones. Bilateral fractures cause the nose to appear flattened, or deviated with an **S** or **C** configuration. *Complex fractures* may also involve the septum, ascending processes of the maxilla, and frontal bones of the face.

Soft-tissue trauma commonly accompanies nasal fracture. Torn mucous membrane causes epistaxis. Soft-tissue hematomas (black eye) are also frequent. Swelling develops rapidly following the injury and may obscure the fracture. Gentle palpation may reveal bony crepitus. Sep-

tal hematoma may develop, increasing the risk for infection. The manifestations of nasal fracture are listed in the accompanying box.

Septal hematoma and abscess formation, perforation or deviation of the septum, and leakage of cerebrospinal fluid (CSF) may complicate nasal fractures. Septal hematoma usually causes complete and bilateral nasal obstruction and increases the risk of staphylococcal abscess if the hematoma is left undrained. Abscess can lead to necrosis of septal cartilage and *saddle nose deformity*. Deviation of the nasal septum causes varying degrees of nasal obstruction, often requiring reconstructive surgery (see the next section of this chapter). Perforations are usually not serious and do not usually require repair unless obstruction or external deformity occur (Way, 1994).

The client with a nasal fracture may also have fractures of other facial bones, particularly when facial trauma is severe. Fractures in the nasoethmoidal or frontal region may result in disruption of the dura, causing CSF leakage or rhinorrhea. CSF rhinorrhea is suspected when the client presents with watery nasal drainage that tests positive for glucose.

Collaborative Care

The major goals of therapy for clients with nasal fractures are to maintain a patent airway and prevent deformity. Respirations are closely monitored. Ideally, reduction of the fracture is achieved early, before significant edema develops. Nasal fractures heal rapidly. Simple reductions may be accomplished in the emergency room under local anesthesia. An external plaster of Paris or metal splint may be applied for 7 to 10 days to maintain proper alignment until healing takes place. The splints are padded to prevent skin breakdown. Ice may be gently applied to the face and nose to control edema and bleeding. Nasal packing may be used to control epistaxis.

Laboratory and Diagnostic Tests

Radiologic examination of the head and face is performed to identify the fracture and assess for other facial fractures. Direct examination of the intranasal cavity using a nasal speculum is important to rule out septal hematoma. If a CSF leak is suspected, additional diagnostic tests may be performed, including a CT scan or instillation of a radiopaque substance or fluorescein dye into the intrathecal or lumbar subarachnoid space to confirm the leakage and identify its site of origin.

Pharmacology

Mild analgesics are prescribed to manage pain. Antibiotics are prescribed for clients who develop septal hematoma to reduce the risk of abscess formation, even after drainage of the hematoma.

Surgery

Clients with complex nasal fractures, fractures that do not heal in normal alignment, or persistent CSF leakage may require surgical repair of the fracture or realignment of the nasal bones. Rhinoplasty with concurrent septoplasty is the most common procedure performed for clients with nasal fracture.

Rhinoplasty is surgical reconstruction of the nose. It is done to relieve airway obstruction and repair visible deformity of the nose following fracture. If excessive edema is present after nasal fracture, surgery is delayed for 7 to 10 days to allow swelling to subside. Using an intranasal incision, the nasal skin is lifted and the framework of the nose reshaped by removing, rearranging, or augmenting bone or cartilage. The skin is then repositioned over the reconstructed frame (Way, 1994). Prosthetic implants may assist in reshaping the nose. Either local or general anesthesia may be used; hospitalization is often not required. Following surgery, nasal packing is left in place for up to 72 hours to minimize bleeding and provide tissue support. A plastic splint is molded to the shape of the nose and is removed in 3 to 5 days. The splint provides protection for the reshaped nose and helps to control the swelling. Most swelling and bruising subside within 10 to 14 days; normal sensation returns within several months following surgery. Rhinoplasty is generally a safe and effective procedure with few complications (Way, 1994).

Small defects in the cribriform plate, fovea ethmoidalis, or sphenoid sinus associated with persistent CSF leakage may also require surgical repair. Either an external incision or an endoscopic approach may be used. The defect is repaired using either a tissue graft from the client or fibrin glue, a gelatinous substance composed of calcium chloride and topical thrombin added to cryoprecipitate. The graft or glue is held in place with an absorbable packing. Large defects may require craniotomy for repair (Way, 1994).

Nursing Care

Nursing care for clients with nasal fracture focuses on control of pain, bleeding, and swelling. Airway management is a priority of care. Because many nasal fractures are managed on an outpatient basis, education is also a vital nursing function.

Ineffective Airway Clearance

In the period immediately following nasal trauma and fracture, the airway is at risk for obstruction by bleeding and edema. If the fracture is malpositioned during healing, resulting deformity can also impair nasal airway clearance.

Nursing interventions with rationales follow:

- Monitor airway patency. *Edema and bleeding may obstruct the airway, leading to signs of respiratory distress such as tachypnea, dyspnea, shortness of breath, tachycardia, and use of accessory muscles.*

- Have suction equipment available. *Airway patency is a priority; suctioning of the oropharynx may be required if the client is unable to expectorate secretions and maintain a clear airway. Suctioning of the nasopharynx is avoided to prevent additional tissue trauma.*

- Monitor for effectiveness of cough and ability to remove airway secretions. *Pain, edema, and nasal bleeding may weaken the client's ability to cough effectively.*

- Maintain adequate hydration. Assess mucous membranes and skin turgor for evidence of dehydration. *Decreased oral intake of fluids or active bleeding may cause dehydration and increase the viscosity of secretions. Thick, viscous secretions are more difficult to expectorate.*

Risk for Infection

The client with a nasal fracture is at increased risk for infection for several reasons. The nasal mucosa is a natural barrier to infection, and trauma in the region creates opportunities for invasion by pathogens. Septal hematoma is strongly associated with abscess formation and staphylococcal infection. A CSF leak is indicative of disruption of the dura, increasing the risk of ascending infection and meningitis.

Nursing interventions with rationales follow.

- Assess the client for potential CSF leakage. *Clear fluid dripping from the ear or nose may indicate CSF leakage. If noted, test drainage for glucose; CSF will test positive for glucose on a dextrostrip.*

- Avoid suctioning if possible. *Suctioning catheters could introduce microorganisms and cause further trauma to tissues.*

- Monitor vital signs every 4 hours. *A rise in temperature may indicate infection.*

- Administer antibiotics as ordered. *Antibiotics are prescribed for clients with septal hematoma to prevent abscess formation; although their prophylactic use is controversial, they may be prescribed for clients with CSF leak to prevent cerebral infection.*

Other Nursing Diagnoses

The following diagnoses may also be appropriate for the client with nasal fracture:

- *Body Image Disturbance* related to edema and bruising of soft tissues around nose

- *Ineffective Breathing Pattern* related to swelling and obstruction of nasal passages

Client and Family Teaching

When a nasal fracture is suspected, it is important for the client to seek medical evaluation and treatment as soon as possible. Encourage the client to elevate the head of the bed with blocks and apply ice or cold packs to the nose for 20 minutes four times a day to reduce swelling. Inform the client that although swelling may subside in several days, bruising may persist for several weeks. Reassure the client with significant swelling that it is difficult to determine the final cosmetic outcome following nasal fracture until swelling has subsided. If indicated by delayed reduction of the fracture or resulting malformation, discuss rhinoplasty and its potential benefits with the client.

Clients who have CSF leakage following nasal fracture are placed on bed rest in a semi-Fowler's or Fowler's position. Fluids may be restricted to reduce intracranial pressure and CSF leakage; with the client, explore ways to distribute allowed fluids throughout the day. Instruct the client to avoid straining, blowing the nose, sneezing, or vigorous coughing until such activity is allowed by the physician (Way, 1994). Discuss manifestations of infection, including stiff neck, headache, and fever. Instruct the client to contact the physician immediately if these manifestations occur.

Applying the Nursing Process

Case Study of a Client with Nasal Trauma: Clifton Kavanaugh

Clifton Kavanaugh is a 36-year-old mailman who sustained a nasal fracture when he was hit in the face by a baseball. He is admitted to the emergency room accompanied by a friend.

Assessment

Mr. Kavanaugh presents with an obvious deformity of the nose. The nose is swollen, bloody, and deviated to one side. He has slight bleeding from his nose. Mr. Kavanaugh complains of pain that he rates as a 6 on a scale of 0 to 10. Vital signs are BP, 132/70; P, 120 and regular; R, 22; T, 98.6 F (37 C) axillary.

Mr. Kavanaugh is breathing through his mouth and holding an ice compress to his nose. On palpation, there is evidence of bony crepitus and edema. There is no evidence of CSF leak from either nose or ears. X-ray studies confirm a nasal fracture.

Diagnosis

Ruth McCracken, Mr. Kavanaugh's nurse, develops the following nursing diagnoses:

- *Pain* related to nasal fracture

- *Ineffective Breathing Pattern* related to nasal swelling and bleeding
- *Anxiety* related to pain and need for emergency care
- *Body Image Disturbance* related to nasal deformity

Expected Outcomes

The expected outcomes for the plan of care are that Mr. Kavanaugh will

- Verbalize relief of pain.
- Maintain a patent airway and normalize his breathing pattern.
- Demonstrate reduced anxiety.
- Verbalize concern over a change in body image.

Planning and Implementation

Ms. McCracken plans and implements the following interventions in caring for Mr. Kavanaugh:

- Administer analgesics as ordered.
- Apply ice compress to nose.
- Inspect back of throat for evidence of bleeding.
- Monitor vital signs every hour.
- Encourage deep, slow breathing through the mouth.
- Provide frequent oral hygiene.
- Discuss client concerns regarding injury.
- Assist the physician in the application of a nasal splint.
- Discuss the risks and benefits of various intervention options.

Evaluation

Following treatment, Mr. Kavanaugh reports a decrease in pain from a level of 6 to a level of 2 on a scale of 0 to 10. He appears more relaxed, as evidenced by absence of facial grimace and relaxed posture. His respirations are nonlabored at 18. The nasal splint is intact. Mr. Kavanaugh is able to look in a mirror and state with a laugh, "I look like a raccoon." He is admitted to the hospital for rhinoplasty.

Critical Thinking in the Nursing Process

1. A client with nasal trauma becomes extremely panicky while in the emergency department because of blood draining down his throat. How would you intervene to reduce this client's anxiety without employing nasal suction? Why is it important to avoid suctioning the nasopharynx in the client with nasal trauma?

2. Develop a plan of care for the client with a leak of CSF from a nasal fracture.

3. Compare and contrast immediate versus delayed rhinoplasty for the client with nasal fracture.

The Client with a Deviated Nasal Septum

■ ■ ■

The nasal septum normally divides the nose into two equal parts. Deviation of the nasal septum may be a congenital condition; however, it is usually the result of trauma. On inspection, the septal cartilage bulges or deviates to one side, creating partial or total obstruction of the nares. Mild deviation from midline is generally asymptomatic. In some clients, obstruction of air passage through one side causes noisy breathing during waking hours and snoring during sleep. Major deviations may cause pain because of sinus obstruction or infection. They may also cause nosebleeds due to dryness of the nasal mucosa. Occasionally, the defect may be severe enough to cause cosmetic deformity.

Surgical intervention is indicated for septal deviation that causes significant manifestations or that adversely affects the client's self-concept and body image. Either a submucous resection (SMR) or a septoplasty may be performed under local anesthesia to correct the defect. *Septoplasty* involves incising one side of the septum, elevating the mucous membrane, and removing or straightening the deviated portion of septal cartilage. In a *submucous resection,* bone and cartilage are removed. In both procedures, packing is applied to both sides of the nose to prevent bleeding and to keep the septal mucosa in midline position.

Nursing care for clients with a deviated nasal septum includes informing them about the risks and benefits of surgical intervention and indications for it. Nurses also care for clients following surgical intervention. Nursing care is similar to that provided for clients undergoing rhinoplasty (see the previous section of this chapter on nasal fracture). It is also important to remember that septal deviation may impede the movement of air through one side of the nose; nurses must consider this possibility when inserting nasogastric tubes or suctioning clients with septal deviation. The following nursing diagnoses may be appropriate:

- *Ineffective Airway Clearance* (upper respiratory) related to unilateral obstruction of nasal passage

- *Self-Esteem Disturbance* related to disfigurement due to septal deviation

Following a septoplasty or submucous resection, the client and family require instructions for home care. Ice packs applied to the nose may relieve discomfort and reduce swelling. Elevating the head of the bed on blocks decreases local edema. The client is instructed not to blow the nose for 48 hours after the packing is removed to prevent bleeding. Vigorous coughing or straining at stool may initiate bleeding and should be avoided. The client is encouraged to perform frequent oral care and increase fluid intake to promote comfort and decrease oral dryness due to mouth breathing. The client will have discoloration around the eyes and nose for several days.

The Client with Laryngeal Obstruction

■ ■ ■

Laryngeal obstruction is a life-threatening emergency. The larynx is the narrowest portion of the upper airway; it may be partially or fully obstructed by aspirated food or foreign objects, or because of laryngospasm or edema due to inflammation, injury, or anaphylaxis. Anything that occludes the larynx may obstruct the airway. The most common cause of obstruction in adults is ingested meat that lodges in the airway (the so-called café coronary). Risk factors for food aspiration include ingesting large boluses of food and chewing them insufficiently, consuming alcohol to excess, and wearing dentures (Way, 1994). A foreign body in the larynx causes pain, laryngospasm, dyspnea, and inspiratory stridor. Aspirated foreign bodies may pass through the larynx into the trachea and lungs, causing pneumonitis.

Laryngospasm may result from repeated or traumatic attempts at intubation, chemical irritation, or hypocalcemia. An acute type I hypersensitivity response may cause anaphylaxis and the release of inflammatory mediators that can lead to angioedema of the upper airways and severe laryngeal edema.

The most common manifestations of laryngeal obstruction are coughing, choking, gagging, obvious difficulty in breathing with use of accessory muscles, and inspiratory stridor. As the airway is obstructed, signs of asphyxia become apparent. Respirations are labored and noisy with wheezing and stridor. The client may become cyanotic. Respiratory arrest and death may result if intervention is not initiated promptly.

The goal of therapy is to maintain an open airway. If airway obstruction is partial and the client is able to cough and move air in and out of the lungs, radiologic and laryngoscopic examination may be performed to locate the foreign body. An endotracheal tube may be inserted to provide for the passage of air through the larynx in spasm or the edematous larynx. For the client in anaphylaxis, epinephrine may be administered to reduce laryngeal edema and relieve obstruction.

When airway obstruction is complete, the Heimlich maneuver is performed immediately to clear the obstruction. Using the heel of the hand, the person performing the maneuver delivers four blows to the back of the choking person, between the shoulder blades, then administers four thrusts to the upper abdomen or lower chest.

These moves are continued until the obstruction is relieved or more definitive care can be given. Endotracheal intubation may be attempted. If intubation is unsuccessful, an immediate cricothyrotomy or tracheotomy must be performed to open the airway.

The priority of nursing care for the client with laryngeal obstruction is restoring a patent airway to prevent cerebral anoxia and death. This is a medical emergency requiring immediate intervention. Clients at risk for laryngeal obstruction (e.g., newly extubated clients and clients receiving medications that pose a high risk of anaphylaxis, such as intravenous antibiotics or radiologic dyes) should be monitored closely for manifestations of obstruction, including dyspnea, nasal flaring, tachypnea, anxiety, wheezing, and stridor. Suction the client's airway as needed; small aspirated foreign bodies might possibly be removed by suctioning. If obstruction is complete, initiate a code procedure and perform the Heimlich maneuver until the obstruction is relieved or the emergency response team arrives. The nurse should be prepared to assist with emergency intubation or tracheotomy as needed.

Client and family teaching focuses on preventing laryngeal obstruction and teaching early intervention techniques. Everyone should be aware of the risk factors for adult aspiration. Clients who wear dentures should be cautioned to take small bites, chewing each carefully before swallowing. Discuss the relationship between excess alcohol intake and food aspiration. Nurses also need to be active in promoting training of the general public in CPR and the Heimlich maneuver. The more people who are adequately trained in emergency procedures, the more likely it is that emergency procedures will be initiated in a timely manner. Clients with a known risk for anaphylaxis, such as people with a previous anaphylactic response and those allergic to bee venom, should wear a medi-alert tag and carry a bee-sting kit to allow early intervention to prevent severe laryngeal edema and spasm.

The Client with Laryngeal Trauma

■ ■ ■

Trauma to the larynx can occur in motor vehicle accidents or assaults (e.g., blows to the neck or attempted strangulation). The cause can also be iatrogenic, as with traumatic endotracheal intubation or tracheotomy. Trauma may result in thyroid and/or cricoid cartilage fractures with loss of airway patency. Soft-tissue injuries can cause swelling that impairs the airway further. The client with laryngeal trauma may demonstrate subcutaneous emphysema or crepitus, a change in voice character, dysphagia and pain with swallowing, inspiratory stridor, hemoptysis, and a cough (Way, 1994).

CT scanning is used to identify laryngeal fractures; however, emergency treatment may be initiated prior to diagnostic procedures to ensure airway patency and preserve life. Soft-tissue injuries may be managed conservatively with bedside humidifier, intravenous fluids, antibiotics, and corticosteroids to reduce edema. More severe injuries require endotracheal intubation or immediate tracheostomy.

As with laryngeal obstruction, the priority of nursing care in laryngeal trauma is airway maintenance. Clients are monitored closely for evidence of airway obstruction; emergency procedures need to be initiated in the event of obstruction. The nurse also provides emotional support, reassurance, and teaching for the client to reduce anxiety.

The Client with Sleep Apnea/Hypopnea Syndrome (SAHS)

■ ■ ■

Sleep apnea syndromes are the most commonly diagnosed conditions in sleep disorder centers. **Sleep apnea** is defined as the absence of airflow through the upper airways for 10 or more seconds. Clients with sleep apnea syndrome experience 30 or more apneic episodes during a 7-hour sleep period (Porth, 1994). Hypopnea is partial closure of the upper airway that reduces airflow by at least 50% for at least 10 seconds (Bootzin, Lahmeyer, & Lilie, 1994). Sleep apnea syndrome occurs most frequently in men and in the obese (Picwickian syndrome). Its incidence increases with age, with the greatest prevalence in clients between 50 and 80 years of age. An increasing incidence is also seen in older women, particularly those over the age of 70 years (Hazzard et al., 1994). The mean incidence of sleep apnea among older people overall is 37% (Bootzin et al., 1994); however, many older adults with sleep apnea are asymptomatic. Enlarged tonsils and the use of alcohol or sedatives before sleep may also contribute to sleep apnea.

Pathophysiology

Three forms of sleep apnea are recognized: obstructive, central, and mixed. During episodes of obstructive sleep apnea, transient obstruction of the upper airway impedes airflow, although ventilatory effort continues. In central sleep apnea, the ventilatory drive is inhibited, and no effort to breathe is observed during the apneic episode. Mixed sleep apnea has both central and obstructive components, usually beginning as central with later development of obstructive apnea. Obstructive sleep apnea is by far the most common form and the one discussed in this section.

During sleep, the tone of all skeletal muscles except the diaphragm is decreased. The most significant decrease in muscle tone occurs during REM (rapid-eye-movement) sleep (Porth, 1994). The loss of normal pharyngeal muscle tone permits the pharynx to collapse during inspiration as pressure within the airways becomes negative in relation to atmospheric pressure. The tongue is also pulled against the posterior pharyngeal wall by gravity during sleep, causing further obstruction. Obesity or skeletal or soft-tissue changes that decrease inspiratory tone, such as a relatively large tongue in a relatively small oropharynx, contribute to the problem (Bootzin et al., 1994). Airflow obstruction causes the client's PO_2 levels, oxygen saturation levels, and pH to fall, and PCO_2 levels to rise. Cardiac dysrhythmias may also occur. Clients with obstructive sleep apnea experience severely fragmented sleep because of repeated awakening to make breathing possible.

Common manifestations of obstructive sleep apnea include cyclical loud snoring, frequent awakening at night with daytime sleepiness, headache, and irritability (see the accompanying box). Fragmented sleep patterns may lead to other systemic problems. Both systemic and pulmonary hypertension are common. Hypercapnia results in a morning headache. Irritability and impotence may also result from disrupted sleep patterns. Clients may demonstrate personality changes, impaired memory, and inability to concentrate (Tierney et al., 1994).

Collaborative Care

The goal of care is to reduce airway obstruction, prevent apneic episodes, and provide psychologic support to clients with sleep apnea syndrome. For clients in whom obesity is a contributing factor, weight loss and strict avoidance of alcohol and hypnotic medications are the initial treatments. Sustained weight loss may cure obstructive sleep apnea.

Laboratory and Diagnostic Tests

The diagnosis of obstructive sleep apnea is based on studies performed in a sleep laboratory. *Polysomnography,* an overnight sleep study, consists of several studies, such as:

- *EEG* to identify sleep stages
- *EKG* to detect dysrhythmias
- *Airflow monitoring, electromyography,* and *esophageal manometry* to assess respiratory effort and airway patency
- Measurement of oxygen saturations by *oximetry* or *transcutaneous oxygen monitoring* (Porth, 1994).

In addition to sleep testing, the client's RBC and hemoglobin levels are measured to assess for erythrocytosis. Thyroid function studies are also obtained to rule out hypothyroidism as a cause of the client's manifestations.

Clinical Manifestations of Sleep Apnea

- Loud, cyclic snoring
- Cessation of breathing during sleep
- Restlessness
- Thrashing extremities during sleep
- Daytime fatigue and sleepiness
- Morning headache
- Personality changes
- Intellectual impairment
- Depression
- Impotence
- Systemic and/or pulmonary hypertension
- Erythrocytosis

Contributing Factors

- Obesity
- Age
- Male gender

Medical Management

Weight loss and maintenance of an optimal weight are often the first interventions prescribed for clients with obstructive sleep apnea. Although weight reduction is often sufficient to cure the disorder, maintaining an optimal weight is difficult.

Respiratory stimulants, such as progesterone and theophylline, have had limited success in treatment, primarily in clients with central sleep apnea. Protriptyline (Vivactil), a tricyclic antidepressant, has been effective for some clients. Hypnotics are avoided in clients with sleep apnea, because they aggravate both the apnea and daytime somnolence. Elimination of alcohol from the client's diet is also necessary.

Continuous positive airway pressure (CPAP) therapy is the treatment of choice for obstructive sleep apnea. The client wears a tightly fitting nasal mask (Figure 33–4). An air compressor blows air into the back of the throat at a positive air pressure between 2 and 20 cm H_2O, depending on individual requirements. This positive pressure prevents the airway from becoming occluded. Nasal airways can become dry and irritated because of continuous airflow with CPAP, so the use of an inline humidifier or a room humidifier is helpful. Currently, at least six nasal CPAP systems designed for home use are commercially available. A newer device, the BiPaP ventilator, administers higher pressures during inhalation and lower

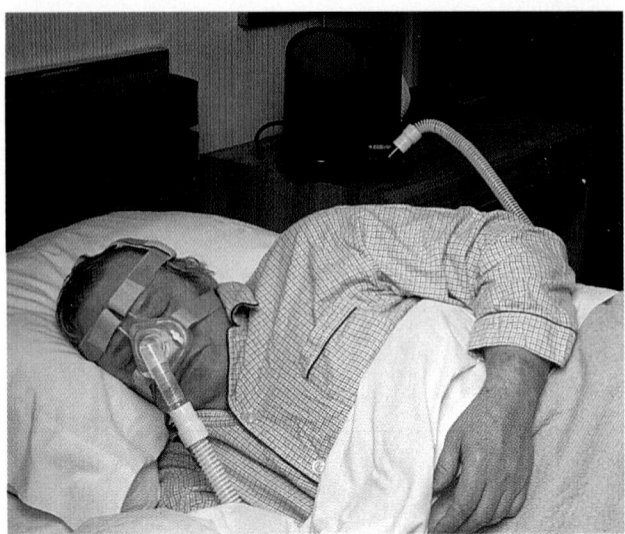

Figure 33-4   A client using a nasal mask and CPAP for treatment of sleep apnea.

Nursing Care

Most clients with sleep apnea syndrome are treated in the home setting. Nursing care focuses on teaching the client and family about the use of respiratory equipment, as well as strategies to decrease factors such as obesity and alcohol intake that aggravate the condition. The following nursing diagnoses are appropriate for clients with sleep apnea syndrome:

- *Sleep Pattern Disturbance* related to repeated apneic episodes
- *Activity Intolerance* related to interrupted sleep patterns
- *Ineffective Breathing Pattern* related to obstruction of upper airway during sleep
- *Impaired Gas Exchange* related to altered lung ventilation during obstructive episodes
- *Risk for Injury* related to daytime somnolence and altered judgment
- *Risk for Sexual Dysfunction* related to impotence resulting from sleep apnea

Client and Family Teaching

Effective management of sleep apnea syndrome depends on the client's willingness to participate in care. Discuss the relationship of obesity to the syndrome and provide instruction and referral as needed for weight loss. Suggest programs such as Weight Watchers to provide additional support. Also discuss the relationship of alcohol and sedative use to sleep apnea. If the client has difficulty eliminating alcohol use, provide referral to a support system such as Alcoholics Anonymous.

When CPAP is prescribed to manage obstructive sleep apnea syndrome, provide instruction in its use. Emphasize the importance of using the CPAP machine continuously at night. Discuss ways to reduce airway dryness, including supplemental humidity and an adequate fluid intake to maintain moist mucous membranes.

If a support group for people with sleep apnea syndrome is available in the local area, refer the client and family to the group.

pressures during expiration, allowing the client to exhale against less resistance.

Oxygen therapy during sleep may also be prescribed for clients with sleep apnea to reduce the severity of oxygen desaturation and hypoxemia that occur during apneic episodes. Oxygen therapy may, however, increase the duration of apnea. Mechanical devices to prevent occlusion of the pharynx by holding the jaw forward are also being tested (Tierney et al., 1994).

Surgery

Tonsillectomy and adenoidectomy may be indicated to relieve upper airway obstruction in some clients. Excision of obstructive tissue from the soft palate, uvula, and posterior lateral pharyngeal wall may be accomplished by *uvulopalatopharyngoplasty (UPPP)*. Although only about 50% of these surgeries are successful in treating sleep apnea, UPPP is useful in selected cases. In severe cases, tracheostomy may also be performed to bypass the area of obstruction.

Upper Respiratory Tumors and Neoplasms

Although tumors of the upper respiratory tract are relatively uncommon, they have the potential to impair the upper airways and interfere with breathing and ventilation of the lungs. Of the upper respiratory tract structures, the larynx is affected by abnormal growths most often.

The Client with Nasal Polyps

Nasal polyps are benign grapelike growths of edematous mucous membrane lining the nose or paranasal sinuses. Polyps are considered neither neoplastic growths nor premalignant. They do, however, have the potential to interfere with the movement of air through nasal passages. They usually occur in clients who have chronic allergic rhinitis or asthma. Clients are often unaware of the polyps.

Pathophysiology

Chronic irritation and swelling of the mucous membranes from allergic rhinitis cause slow polyp formation. Polyps form in areas of dependent mucous membrane, presenting as pale, edematous masses covered with mucous membrane. They are usually bilateral and have a stemlike base, making them fairly moveable. Once present, polyps can continue to enlarge, eventually reaching a size larger than a grape. Large polyps protrude into the nose and may cause nasal obstruction, rhinorrhea, and loss of the sense of smell. Clients with nasal polyps may also develop manifestations of sinusitis and a nasal tone to the voice. Asthmatics who have nasal polyps may have an associated allergy to aspirin of which they are not aware. This syndrome is called Samter's triad (Wilson et al., 1991).

Collaborative Care

When polyps occur in conjunction with an acute upper respiratory infection, they may regress spontaneously with resolution of the infection. Clients with chronic nasal polyps may have few manifestations. When symptomatic, polyps may be managed with topical corticosteroid nasal sprays or low-dose oral corticosteroids to shrink the edematous polyps and manage allergic manifestations. However, once corticosteroid therapy is discontinued, polyps continue to enlarge.

In many clients, surgery is required to restore normal breathing. Surgical removal of polyps (*polypectomy*) is usually done in the physician's office under local anesthesia using lidocaine with epinephrine. The vasoconstrictive properties of epinephrine help control bleeding during the procedure. A wire snare is used to clip the polyps from their stemlike base. Bleeding sites are cauterized, and nasal packing is inserted. An antibacterial ointment such as bacitracin may be applied to the packing to assist healing and to facilitate its removal in 24 to 36 hours. An intranasal splint is sometimes used to prevent formation of adhesions. Alternatively, laser surgery may be used to remove polyps. Healing is more rapid following laser intervention, and the risk of hemorrhage is reduced. Because polyps tend to recur, repeated surgeries may be necessary. With recurrent polyposis, more extensive surgery may be performed such as sinusotomy with removal of polyps from the ethmoid, sphenoid, and maxillary sinuses, or ethmoidectomy.

Nursing Care

Nursing care of the client with nasal polyps focuses on providing symptomatic relief and providing instruction in postoperative management.

Ineffective Breathing Pattern

The client with nasal polyps may have obstructed nasal airflow both prior to and immediately following surgical intervention because of the polyps themselves and postoperative nasal packing.

Nursing interventions with rationales follow.

- Monitor respiratory rate or pattern for changes from baseline. *Tachypnea and/or rapid, shallow respirations may indicate airway obstruction or infection.*
- Pace activities to provide for periods of rest. *Fatigue can further compromise breathing by causing more shallow, rapid respirations.*
- Elevate the head of the bed. *The upright position decreases swelling and maximizes lung excursion.*

Risk for Injury

Although the risk is low, the client is monitored for possible postoperative hemorrhage following polypectomy.

Nursing interventions with rationales follow.

- Monitor for changes in pulse rate. *Tachycardia may be indicative of postoperative hemorrhage or anxiety.*
- Monitor for hemorrhage. *The client is instructed to check for excessive blood on the nasal dressing and to look in the back of the throat for the presence of bloody drainage. Repeated swallowing may indicate bleeding. Emesis of bright red blood should be reported promptly.*
- Teach the client measures to prevent postoperative hemorrhage, including these:
  a. Apply ice or cold compresses to the nose to decrease swelling, promote comfort, and prevent bleeding. *Cold causes vasoconstriction, reducing the risk of bleeding.*
  b. Avoid blowing the nose for 24 to 48 hours after nasal packing is removed. *Blowing the nose may disrupt clots or crusts over the surgical site, allowing bleeding to occur.*
  c. Avoid straining at stool, vigorous coughing, and strenuous exercise. *These activities increase the pressure within the vessels of the nose and may increase the risk or postoperative bleeding.*

Client and Family Teaching

Provide postoperative care instructions for the client following a polypectomy. Discuss the manifestations of possible bleeding. If posterior bleeding occurs, the client may swallow frequently and note blood at the back of the throat. Swallowed blood may cause nausea and vomiting. The client is encouraged to rest for 2 to 3 days after surgery to reduce the risk of bleeding. The client must breathe through the mouth while the nasal packing is in place. Adequate fluid intake and frequent mouth care help prevent dryness. Encourage the client with allergic rhinitis to undergo hypersensitivity testing so as to reduce the exposure to allergens and the recurrence of polyps.

The Client with a Benign Laryngeal Tumor

■ ■ ■

Benign tumors of the larynx include papillomas, nodules, and polyps. Papillomas are small wartlike growths that are believed to be of viral origin. Polyps and nodules may develop on the vocal cords of the larynx, particularly in clients who chronically shout, project, or vocalize in an abnormally high or low tone, abusing the voice. In adults, vocal cord nodules are often referred to as "singer's nodules"; cheerleaders and public speakers may also develop them. Nodules occur as paired lesions at the junction of the anterior one-third and posterior two-thirds of the free edges of the vocal cords. Voice abuse also contributes to the development of vocal cord polyps, as does cigarette smoking and chronic irritation from industrial pollutants. Hoarseness and a breathy voice quality are manifestations of benign vocal cord tumors.

Benign laryngeal tumors may resolve with correction of the underlying problem, such as voice training with a speech therapist or smoking cessation. An inhaled steroid spray may be used for vocal cord polyps. Nodules or polyps that do not resolve with conservative therapy may require surgical excision, which is usually performed via laryngoscopy, using microforceps or a laser. A biopsy of the tumor is performed to rule out laryngeal carcinoma.

Nurses can be instrumental in early identification and treatment of laryngeal disorders by emphasizing the need for clients with new chronic hoarseness to seek treatment. Nursing care for the client with a benign tumor of the larynx focuses on maintaining a patent airway and teaching the client about the disorder and strategies to prevent its recurrence. The client is observed closely in the immediate postoperative period for signs of airway obstruction, such as labored breathing or inspiratory stridor. Cold packs may be applied to the neck area to reduce the risk of swelling. Because of the risk of aspiration, no food or fluids are allowed until the client's cough and gag reflexes have returned.

Client and family teaching emphasizes management of contributing factors. Stress the importance of not yelling or screaming. Refer clients, particularly singers, to a speech therapist for voice training. Emphasize the need

---

Risk Factors for Cancer of the Larynx

■ ■ ■

- Prolonged use of alcohol*
- Prolonged use of tobacco*
- Vocal straining
- Chronic laryngitis

- Exposure to chemicals
- Exposure to radiation
- Exposure to toxins
- Family predisposition

---

*Major risk factors

---

for the client to keep the voice within its normal range to reduce vocal cord stress. Talk to the client about smoking cessation, particularly if the client is also a singer. Discuss the relationship of industrial pollutants to laryngeal tumors and help the client explore ways of reducing exposure to pollutants.

The Client with Laryngeal Carcinoma

■ ■ ■

Squamous cell carcinoma is the most common malignancy of the larynx. Cancer of the larynx accounts for 1% to 3% of all cancers. If detected early, it is potentially curable, especially if the cancer is limited to the vocal cords. Men are affected more often than women by a 9:1 ratio (Way, 1994), but the incidence in women has increased markedly over the years. The disease usually presents in older clients, 60 to 70 years of age. The two major risk factors for laryngeal carcinoma are prolonged use of alcohol and tobacco. Other risk factors include vocal straining, chronic laryngitis, exposure to chemicals, toxins or radiation, and family predisposition (see the accompanying box).

Pathophysiology

Changes in the laryngeal mucosa occur over time as it is continually subjected to noxious irritants such as cigarette smoke. White, patchy precancerous lesions known as *leukoplakia* appear. Red, velvety patches, called *erythroplakia*, are thought to represent a later stage of carcinoma development. Biopsies of both leukoplakia and erythroplakia are obtained to rule out carcinoma in situ or invasive carcinoma. Laryngeal cancer spreads by both direct invasion of surrounding tissues and metastasis. It may

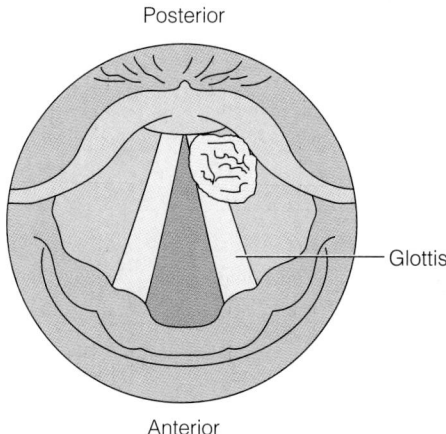

Posterior

Glottis

Anterior

Figure 33–5 Cancer of the larynx. Most lesions form along the edges of the glottis.

Clinical Manifestations of Cancer of the Larynx

- Hoarseness
- Change in the voice
- Painful swallowing
- Dyspnea
- Foul breath
- Palpable lump in neck
- Earache

---

metastasize to the lungs; however, metastases of other cancers to the larynx are rare.

Laryngeal cancer may occur in any of the three areas of the larynx, the glottis, the supraglottis, and the subglottis. Manifestations vary according to site of the lesion.

Lesions of the true vocal cords or glottis occur more frequently than cancers of other regions of the larynx (Figure 33–5). Fortunately, these cancers tend to be well-differentiated and slow-growing. Metastasis occurs late in the course of the disease because of a limited lymphatic supply. The most notable manifestation of glottic cancer is hoarseness, or a change in the voice because the tumor prevents complete closure of the glottis during speech.

The supraglottic area includes the epiglottis, aryepiglottic folds, arytenoid muscles and cartilage, and false vocal cords. Lymphatic supply to this region of the larynx is rich; tumors often invade locally and metastasize to lymph nodes early. Manifestations may not be noted until the tumor is relatively large, because it does not usually affect the voice or breathing in the early stages. Manifestations of supraglottic cancer include painful swallowing, especially noticeable with hot liquids or citrus juices; a sore throat; or a feeling of a lump in the throat. Later manifestations include dyspnea, foul breath, and a palpable lump in the neck. Tumors in this area may also cause pain that radiates to the ear by way of the glossopharyngeal and vagus nerves. Many clients have palpable jugular lymph nodes at the time of presentation. The tumor may spread locally to involve the base of the tongue and the hypopharynx (Way, 1994).

The subglottic area is located below the vocal cords and terminates at the first tracheal ring. Subglottic tumors are the least common laryngeal cancers and often do not have early manifestations. They cause manifestations of airway obstruction as the tumor enlarges and may metastasize rapidly to lymphatics.

Clinical manifestations of laryngeal cancer are listed in the accompanying box.

Collaborative Care

Treatment of laryngeal tumors varies with the extent of the cancer. Early diagnosis and surgical intervention are important aspects of care because with early diagnosis and treatment, as many as 80% to 90% of small cord lesions may be cured. Left untreated, 90% of clients die within 3 years.

A complete history and physical assessment provide cues about the client's risk for laryngeal cancer and early manifestations of the disease. Does the client's occupation involve frequent speaking or singing? Is there a family history of cancer? Does the client smoke or drink alcohol? If so, how much and for what period of time? Although it is important to be sensitive to the fact that clients may be reluctant to admit to these behaviors, it is also important to ascertain an accurate history. Precise therapy is determined by staging of the cancer. Guidelines developed by the American Joint Commission for Cancer (1977) are widely used. The TNM guidelines include tumor size and location (T), number of nodes found (N), and presence or absence of metastases (M) (Table 33–1). See Chapter 9 for further discussion of cancer staging.

Laboratory and Diagnostic Tests

Clients with complaints of persistent hoarseness, a change in voice quality, painful or difficult swallowing, or a lump in the throat should be promptly evaluated by direct or indirect laryngoscopy. Suspicious lesions are biopsied to rule out laryngeal cancer. Other diagnostic tests used to assess laryngeal cancer include X-ray studies of the head, neck, and chest as well as CT or MRI scan. A

Table 33–1   Staging of Laryngeal Tumors

Stage		T-Categories of Laryngeal Tumors			N Categories	M Categories
		Supraglottis	**Glottis**	**Subglottis**		
Stage I	T_1	Confined to site of origin with normal mobility	Confined to glottis with normal mobility	Confined to subglottic region	N_0 - No clinically positive nodes	M_0 - No known distant metastasis
Stage II	T_2	Involves adjacent supraglottic site or glottis without fixation	Supra- and/or subglottic extension with normal or impaired mobility	Extension to vocal cords with normal or impaired cord mobility	N_0 - No clinically positive nodes	M_0 - No known distant metastasis
Stage III	T_3	Limited to larynx with fixation and/or extension to involve postcarotid area, medial wall of pyriform sinus or pre-epiglottic space	Confined to larynx with cord fixation	Confined to larynx with cord fixation	N_0 - No clinically positive nodes; or N_1 - Single clinically positive node on side of tumor not more than 3 mm diameter	M_0 - No known distant metastasis
Stage IV	T_4	Massive tumor extending beyond larynx to involve oropharynx, soft tissues of neck, or destruction of thyroid cartilage	Massive tumor with thyroid cartilage destruction and/or extension beyond the confines of the larynx	Massive tumor with thyroid cartilage destruction and/or extension beyond the confines of the larynx	N_2 - Single or multiple clinically positive node(s) on side of tumor not more than 6 cm diameter; or N_3 - Massive nodes on same side, opposite side, or both sides of neck	M_0 - No known distant metastasis; M_1 - Distant metastasis present

Adapted from Baker, H. W., Vikram, B., Farr, H. W., Bosi, G. J., Shah, J. P., Feghali, J., Schmincke, A., & Muir, C. S. (1983). *Cancer of the head and neck.* New York: American Cancer Society.

Table 33–2   Therapeutic Management of Laryngeal Cancer

Extent of Disease	Stage	Usual Treatment
Limited	T_1 or T_2, N_0 or N_1	Surgery or radiation therapy
Advanced	T_3 or T_4, N_2 or N_3	Surgery plus radiation therapy; may employ chemotherapy
Metastatic	M_1	Palliative surgery and/or radiation therapy; combination chemotherapy

Adapted from Rubenstein, E., & Federman, D. D. (1994). *Scientific American Medicine.* New York: Scientific American.

needle biopsy of enlarged lymph nodes helps confirm the diagnosis. A barium swallow may be performed to evaluate swallowing ability as well as possible extension of the tumor into the esophagus.

Chemotherapy

Chemotherapy may be used as adjunctive therapy for laryngeal cancer, but is not the treatment of choice (see Table 33–2). Clinical investigations of its palliative or therapeutic benefits continue. It may be used to prevent the development and growth of micrometastases that may be present at the time of diagnosis of a primary tumor. It may also be used as adjunct therapy before radiation therapy or surgery.

Chemotherapeutic drugs that have been used include methotrexate (Mexate), 5-fluorouracil, vincristine sulfate (Oncovin), cisplatin (Platinol), and bleomycin sulfate (Blenoxane). A multiple-drug treatment regimen may be employed to maximize therapeutic effects.

Radiation

Radiation therapy is often the treatment of choice for early laryngeal cancer. Radiation disrupts the DNA of the cell, causing it to die. External radiation may be used, or implants of iridium seeds can be placed into hollow plastic needles that are inserted directly into or near the tumor site during surgery to deliver radiation. Radiation therapy is extremely effective for treating glottic cancer, resulting in cure rates of up to 96%, especially if the tumor is limited to the true vocal cord. Radiation therapy preserves the voice; however, radiation therapy using 5000 to 7000 rads over several weeks may ultimately result in a change to the tone or timbre of the voice.

Radiation therapy may be used alone in the early stages of laryngeal cancer or when the client refuses or is not a candidate for surgical intervention. It is often combined with surgical resection of the tumor or a portion of the larynx. In advanced cancer, it may be used following laryngectomy to treat cervical lymph nodes.

Surgery

The type of surgical approach used is based on site, size, and degree of tumor invasion of the larynx. The goals of surgical intervention are to remove the tumor, maintain airway patency, and provide for optimal cosmetic appearance.

Carcinoma in situ and vocal cord polyps may be vaporized via microlaryngoscopy using a CO_2 laser under microscope guidance. The cure rate for early tumors using this method is equal to that achievable with cordotomy or radiation therapy. This surgery may be performed on an outpatient basis. It does not cause mechanical trauma to the vocal cords and thus is associated with less pain, swelling, and hoarseness. The client is able to resume activities and speaking within days (Smalley, 1990).

With early cancers of the vocal cord where the cord is fully mobile and the lesion can be fully exposed, *cordotomy*, limited removal of the tumor from the vocal cord, or *cordectomy*, removal of the affected vocal cord, may be employed. These surgeries may be performed using the oral route and a laryngoscope. Nd:YAG or CO_2 lasers are often employed for excision of localized tumors.

The voice is preserved after cordotomy or cordectomy, although total voice rest is prescribed with only whispering allowed for at least a week following surgery. A tracheostomy is usually performed at the time of surgery to ensure airway patency immediately following surgery when edema of the affected tissues could impair it. The tracheostomy tube is removed within 2 to 3 days after surgery when there is little or no danger of airway impairment because of edema. Following cordotomy and subsequent removal of the tracheostomy tube, the client is able to eat, breathe, and speak normally, although the voice may remain hoarse.

Laryngectomy, removal of the larynx, may be necessary for some clients. A *partial laryngectomy* (hemilaryngectomy, vertical partial laryngectomy) may be employed for tumors localized to a portion of the larynx with limited metastasis to regional lymph nodes. In a partial la-

ryngectomy, one-half or more of the larynx is removed through a vertical midneck incision. Although there may be minor changes, the voice is generally well preserved after this surgery. A cuffed tracheostomy tube may be inserted for airway management in the early postoperative period. It is usually removed in 5 to 7 days as postoperative swelling subsides, and the stoma is allowed to close. As with cordotomy, the client is able to resume normal speaking, breathing, and swallowing following a partial laryngectomy.

Supraglottic (horizontal) laryngectomy is performed via a midneck horizontal incision to remove cancers located above the true vocal cords. The superior portion of the larynx is removed from the false vocal cords up to the epiglottis and including, perhaps, a portion of the base of the tongue. Because the true vocal cords remain intact, voice is preserved. Again, a cuffed tracheostomy tube is inserted to ensure airway patency following surgery. When the tracheostomy tube is removed, the client must be monitored closely for aspiration because the epiglottis, which normally closes off the airway during swallowing, has been surgically removed. Enteral tube feedings or parenteral nutrition may be required for several weeks after surgery. The client is taught swallowing techniques to avoid aspiration but may eventually require a total laryngectomy with permanent tracheostomy to protect the lower airway if repeated episodes of aspiration occur.

A *total laryngectomy* is required for cancers that extend beyond the vocal cords. The entire larynx is removed, along with the epiglottis, thyroid cartilage, several tracheal rings, and the hyoid bone. Because the trachea and the esophagus are permanently separated by this surgery (Figure 33–6), there is no risk of aspiration during swallowing. Normal speech is lost, and a permanent tracheostomy is created in a total laryngectomy. The tracheostomy tube inserted during surgery may be left in place for several weeks and then removed, leaving a natural stoma, or it may be left in place permanently. See the collaborative care box on page 1360.

If cervical lymph nodes are found to be cancerous but no evidence of distal metastasis is present, a *radical neck dissection* may be performed along with total laryngectomy on the same side of the neck as the lesion. In a radical neck dissection, tissue is removed from the lower edge of the mandible down to the clavicle, including cervical lymph nodes, the sternocleidomastoid muscle, internal jugular vein, cranial nerve XI (spinal accessory), and submaxillary salivary gland. Extensive tissue dissection may be necessary, resulting in significant deformity and necessitating skin grafts or flaps to close the wound. Hemovac drains are placed in the wound during surgery to prevent hematoma and extensive edema formation. After surgery, the client may have difficulty lifting and turning the head because of muscle loss. Resection of the spinal accessory nerve causes the shoulder on the affected

Collaborative Care: The Client Requiring a Laryngectomy

Health Care Team	Client-Centered Care
Otorhinolaryngologist	Performs laryngoscopy with biopsy to confirm cancer diagnosis. Removes epiglottis, thyroid, cartilage, larynx, several tracheal rings, and hyoid bond. May perform radical neck dissection, leaving the client with a permanent tracheostomy.
Speech therapist or language pathologist	Provides alternative methods, such as a magic slate or communication board, for communication during postoperative period. Assesses and provides interventions to assist with swallowing and speech during recovery. May teach esophageal speech or provide electronic devices for communication.
Social worker	Arranges for suction, oxygen, and tube feeding equipment in the home for time of discharge. Completes referral for visiting nurse, respiratory therapy, and speech therapy at home. May help client and family cope with anxiety, fear, anger, depression, stress, and altered body image. Refers to American Cancer Society for needed assistance. Refers client to support group such as "Lost Cord."
Dietitian	Plans enteral tube feeding or total parenteral nutrition. Assists client in planning adequate nutritional intake when oral diet is permitted. Teaches client and family well-balanced diet high in vitamins and minerals, taking into account the client's decreased sense of taste and smell.
Respiratory therapist	Administers humidified oxygen via mist collar, assists with oral and tracheal suction, performs chest physical therapy, performs ABGs.
RN and Health Care Team Communications	Reports dyspnea, shortness of breath, hemorrhage, restlessness, apprehension, or labored breathing. Discusses any changes in patency of tracheostomy tube or nasogastric tube. Collaborates with speech therapist to ensure that communication is maintained. Discusses need for suction and oxygen equipment with social worker. Refers coping problems to social worker.

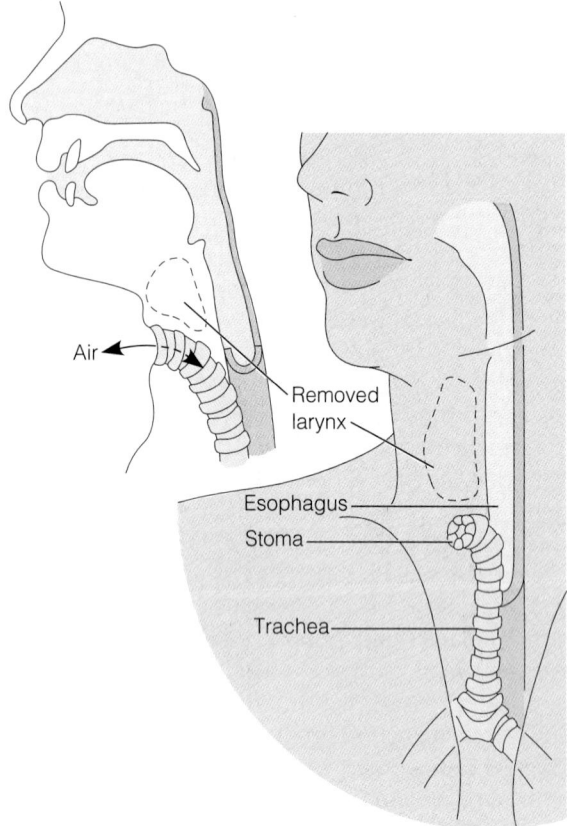

Figure 33–6 Following a total laryngectomy, the client has a permanent tracheostomy. No connection between the trachea and esophagus remains.

side to drop. Postoperative neck exercises can help to reduce the degree of shoulder drop and to increase range of motion on the affected side.

Speech Rehabilitation

Various techniques may be employed to restore oral communication after a total laryngectomy. Some clients are successful at learning esophageal speech or using a battery-powered speech generator ("artificial larynx").

Esophageal speech is a method of creating sound and forming words by swallowing air, holding it in the upper esophagus, and then expelling it in a controlled belch (Figure 33–7). The pharyngoesophageal segment vibrates with the belch, creating sound. The client uses muscles of the mouth and tongue which are normally involved in speech to control the sound and form words. This form of speech takes practice, and many clients are unable to resume fluent speech.

Several speech generators are available for the laryngectomy client. One type is held to the neck and creates vibrations that are transmitted to the neck and into the mouth (Figure 33–8). As the client silently forms words with his mouth, the transmitted vibrations are formed into words. Another device delivers a tone into the mouth via a plastic tube inserted into the corner of the roof of the

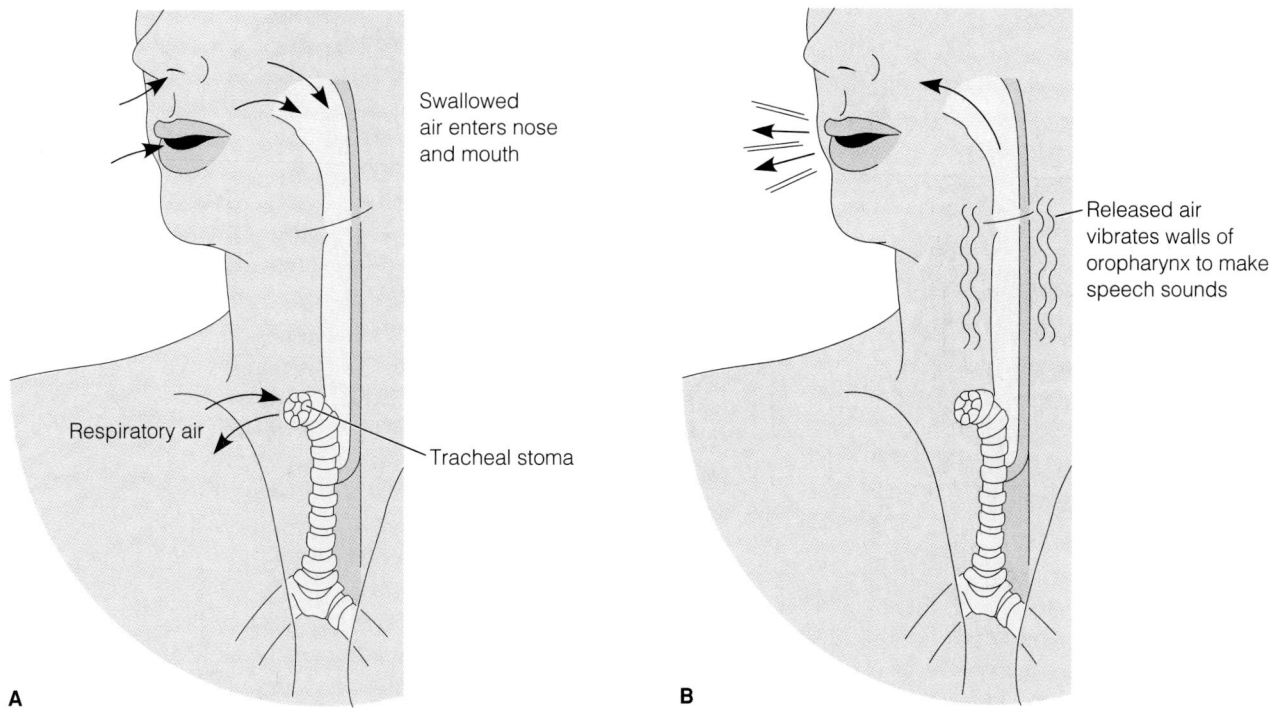

Figure 33–7 Esophageal speech. *A,* The client swallows a small amount of air into the upper esophagus. *B,* The client expels air in a modified belch to vibrate the oropharynx and produce speech.

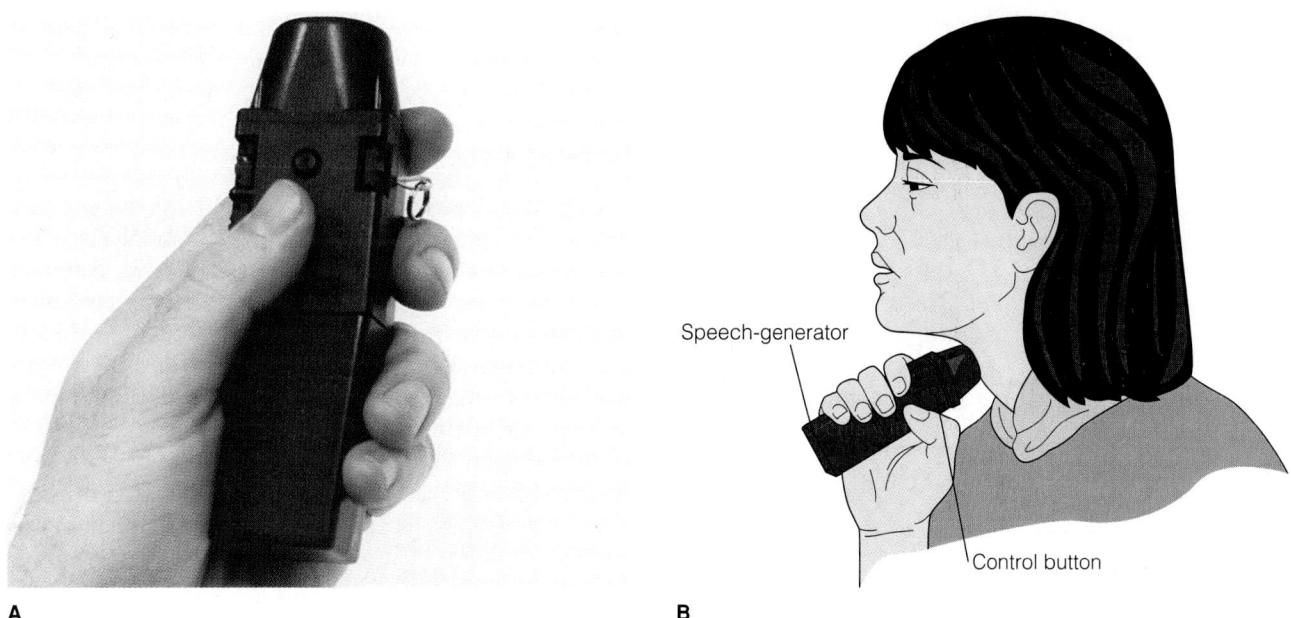

Figure 33–8 *A,* Denrick speech generator. *B,* The client holds the vibrating tip of the device against the throat and articulates with the mouth to form words.

mouth (Figure 33–9). The lips, tongue, and mouth muscles are then used to form the sound into words.

A newer surgical procedure, the *tracheoesophageal puncture (TEP),* is also available to restore speech. A small fistula is created between the posterior tracheal wall and the anterior esophagus and fitted with a valved silicone prosthesis (Figure 33–10). When the client occludes the tube with the finger after inhaling, air is forced through the prosthesis into the esophagus and hypopharynx, creating vibration and sound. The client uses the tongue, lips, teeth, and palate to articulate the words. The one-way valve prevents aspiration from the esophagus into the trachea. An external appliance, a tracheostoma valve, may be worn so that clients do not have to use their hands to

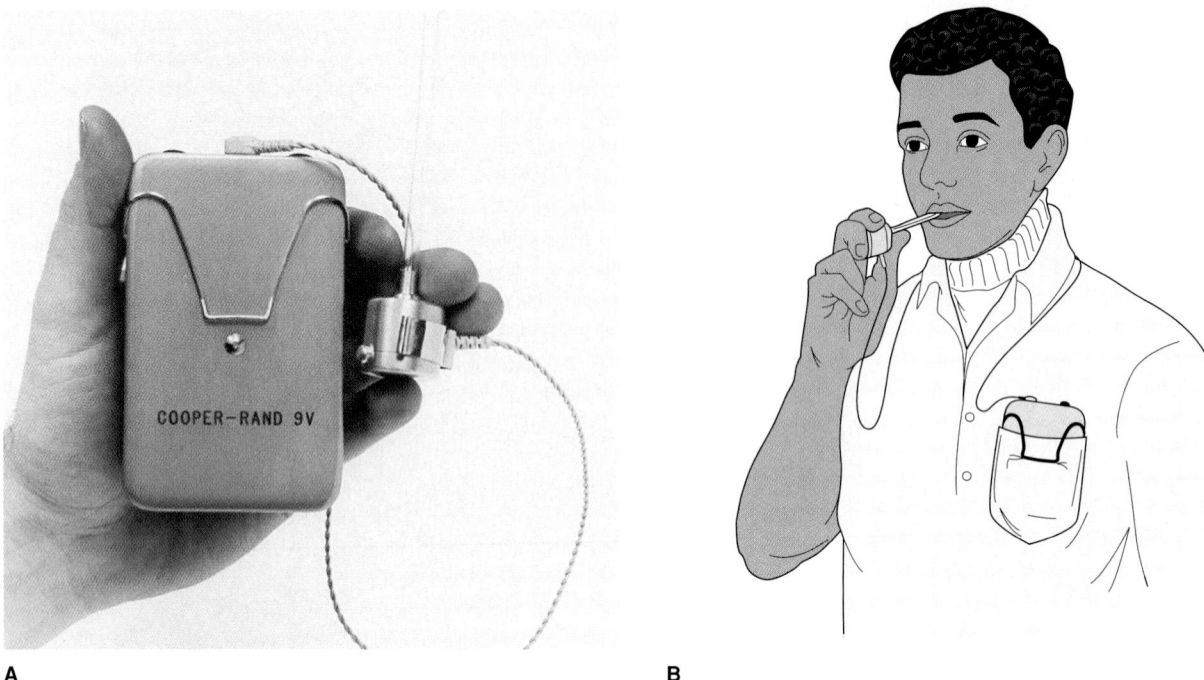

A   B

Figure 33-9 *A*, Cooper-Rand electronic speech aid. *B*, A plastic tube on the handpiece produces an audible tone. The client holds the tube against the roof of the mouth when forming words.

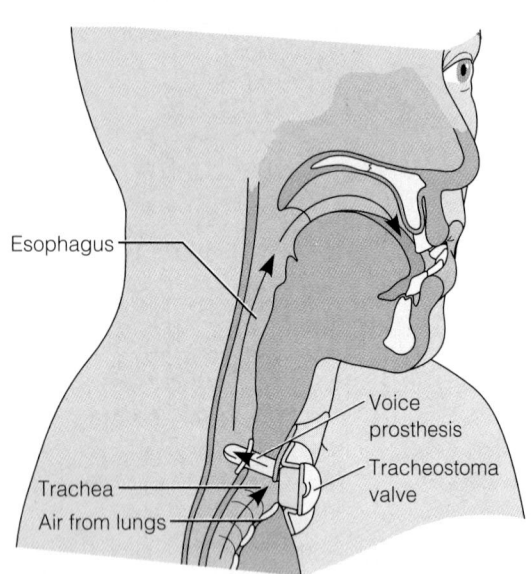

Esophagus

Voice prosthesis

Tracheostoma valve

Trachea

Air from lungs

Figure 33-10 The tracheoesophageal prosthesis allows air from the trachea to be diverted through the prosthesis into the esophagus and oropharynx, producing speech when the tracheostomy stoma is occluded. A one-way valve prevents food from entering the trachea.

occlude the stoma. This device covers the entire laryngostoma and closes during exhalation, forcing air directly into the voice prosthesis. Clients are taught how to remove and clean the prosthesis. Not all postlaryngectomy clients are candidates for this device, because its use requires motivation and manual dexterity.

Nursing Care

The client with laryngeal cancer has multiple nursing care needs. The risk for impaired verbal communication exists, whether or not a total laryngectomy is planned. Clients may experience dysphagia that interferes with swallowing and nutrition prior to the initiation of therapy; radiation, chemotherapy, or surgery also may interfere with nutrition. The diagnosis of cancer is frightening for most clients, no matter what the potential for cure is with treatment. Problems related to communication, nutrition, and anticipatory grieving are included in this section; nursing diagnoses specific to the client undergoing a laryngectomy are included in the accompanying box. A Critical Pathway for a client having a laryngectomy appears on page 1367.

Impaired Verbal Communication

Removal of the larynx with permanent tracheostomy results in voice loss. Prior to surgery, it is important to discuss alternative methods of communication, both short and long-term, with the client and family members. The client ultimately determines the type of surgical procedure performed; some clients may choose to forgo laryngectomy to avoid voice loss when the chance for long-term success and cancer cure is minimal.

Nursing Care of the Client Having a Total Laryngectomy

PREOPERATIVE CARE

Knowledge Deficit: Laryngeal Cancer and Laryngectomy

- Assess the client's and family's knowledge and understanding of the diagnosis and proposed surgery. *Assessment provides a basis for planning interventions to clarify information and expand knowledge.*

- Assess the client's and family's level of anxiety related to the diagnosis and proposed surgery. *High and extreme levels of anxiety interfere with the ability to learn. Interventions to lower anxiety for both the client and family may be vital prior to implementing a teaching plan.*

- Reinforce and clarify information provided by the client's physician about the extent of the client's cancer, the proposed surgical procedure, and the potential for disease cure. *The diagnosis of cancer causes fear in many clients, who often see it as a "death sentence." Reinforcement of the likelihood of a disease cure following surgery and therapy may be important for the client to enter surgery with a positive outlook about its outcome.*

- Without frightening the client or family members, emphasize that total laryngectomy results in a loss of speech and that the client will breathe through a permanent stoma in the neck. *Although clients and family members may verbalize an understanding of the loss of speech following surgery, they may believe that verbal communication will still be possible through the stoma.*

- Point out that surgery will affect the client's sense of taste and smell, and eating in the initial postoperative period. Reassure the client that nutritional and fluid needs will be met with intravenous or enteral feedings until the client is able to resume eating. *The client may not be prepared for the effect of surgery on taste and smell, and therefore the enjoyment of food.*

Impaired Verbal Communication

- Assess the importance of verbal communication to the client's self-concept, occupation, and life-style. *Assessment provides vital information about the client's potential for adapting to the loss of normal verbal communication postoperatively. If the ability to speak is central to the client's occupation (e.g., elementary school teacher, singer) or self-concept (e.g., a politician or attorney), the difficulty of adapting to a total laryngectomy will be great. For these clients, surgical intervention may mean a loss of employment or career.*

- Before surgery, refer the client and family to a speech therapist if a referral has not been made. *Presurgical evaluation allows the speech therapist to initiate teaching about alternative communication strategies.*

- After surgery, reinforce the speech therapist's teaching about alternative communication strategies. *Anxiety or information overload may impair the client's ability to grasp teaching. Reinforcing information facilitates learning.*

- Teach the client how to use a magic slate, alphabet board or other communication board (such as a picture board for people who cannot read), eye signals, or hand signals to communicate with care providers and family members postoperatively. *Early teaching gives the client a chance to practice these communication techniques prior to surgery. Teaching esophageal speech or the use of an electronic speech generator is often delayed until the postoperative period. People who can still speak have difficulty using these techniques and may become discouraged about their potential for verbal communication postoperatively.*

- Maintain a positive attitude about the client's ability to communicate postoperatively, but do not promote unrealistic expectations. *Not all clients are able to use all alternative methods of verbal communication after the laryngectomy. Some clients do not master any technique and remain nonverbal.*

- Following consultation with the client, family members, and the speech therapist, arrange a visit by a rehabilitated laryngectomy client who has mastered an alternative form of verbal communication and has a positive attitude about rehabilitation. *Many clients and their families find that they are better able to communicate their fears with someone who has gone through the same experience they are facing.*

POSTOPERATIVE CARE

Ineffective Airway Clearance

- Monitor respiratory status every 1 to 2 hours and assess airway patency:
  a. Monitor rate and pattern of breathing.
  b. Auscultate lungs for rhonchi as evidence of accumulation of secretions.
  c. Assess for occlusion of the airway because of retained secretions or local edema.
  Ineffective clearing of secretions can impair gas exchange, increase the work of breathing, and result in complications such as pneumonia.

Nursing Care of the Client Having a Total Laryngectomy (continued)

- Monitor oxygen saturation levels and arterial blood gases (ABGs) as needed. *Oxygen saturation levels and ABGs provide evidence of the adequacy of ventilation and gas exchange.*

- Encourage deep breathing and coughing. *Deep breathing helps ensure adequate ventilation of lower airways; coughing helps to move secretions out of airways.*

- Elevate the head of the bed. *The upright position enhances effective ventilation of the lungs.*

- Maintain humidification of inspired gases. *In clients with a tracheostomy, inspired air is no longer humidified as it passes through the upper airways. Proper humidification is necessary to teep secretions loose enough so that coughing or suctioning can remove them.*

- Maintain an adequate fluid intake (initially intravenously, then orally). *Adequate hydration keeps secretions liquid and mucous membranes moist.*

- Perform tracheal suctioning using sterile technique as needed. *The client may be weakened from the effects of surgery and radiation therapy. Impaired nutritional status leads to muscle fatigue and resultant inability to cough effectively. Suctioning via the tracheostomy may be necessary to maintain airway patency.*

- Instill 3 to 5 ml of sterile normal saline into the tracheostomy prior to suctioning. *Normal saline helps to loosen respiratory secretions and to stimulate coughing, facilitating airway clearance with suctioning.*

- Perform tracheostomy care as needed. *The tracheostomy tube must be cleaned periodically to prevent accumulation of secretions and potential occlusion of the airway. See the procedure on page 1366.*

- Encourage the client to move from the bed as soon as allowed after surgery. *Activity increases lung ventilation and helps to clear secretions, helping prevent atelectasis.*

- Teach the client to protect the stoma from particulate matter in the air with a gauze square or other stoma protector. *The client with a permanent tracheostomy no longer has the protective mechanisms of the upper airway that prevent foreign material from entering the lungs.*

Pain

- Assess the client's level of pain, using a scale of 0 to 10. *The pain-rating scale provides an objective means of assessing and recording the client's subjective reports of pain.*

- Provide analgesia as ordered to maintain a level of comfort that allows the client to cough and move as needed. *Pain control is more effective when analgesia is administered to maintain comfort rather than to treat pain.*

- Elevate the head of the bed at all times. *Elevation reduces edema and swelling of the neck, reducing pain.*

- Teach the client to support the head when moving in bed. *Additional head support reduces the strain on muscles in the operative area.*

Nursing interventions with rationales follow:

- Assess the client prior to surgery for additional obstacles to communication. *The client's communication may be impaired by hearing loss, illiteracy, or weakness associated with the disease process, altering the ability to engage in alternative communication strategies.*

- Prior to surgery, introduce the client to nonverbal means of communication such as pencil and paper, magic slate, or an alphabet board. Encourage the client to practice using each method and to choose the most acceptable one. *Having the client determine a means of communication prior to surgery helps to alleviate anxiety and increases the sense of control.*

- Arrange for the client to consult a speech therapist about alternate forms of oral communication prior to surgery if possible. *The client may be a candidate for esophageal speech, voice prosthesis, or electrolarynx. Determining a means of long-term communication prior to surgery helps to relieve the client's fear of inability to communicate and may guide the choice of a surgical procedure.*

- Place the call bell at hand. *Knowing that help is readily available enhances feelings of security and decreases anxiety.*

- Assess the client frequently. *The presence of a caring nurse helps to decrease anxiety and promotes communication.*

Altered Nutrition: Less Than Body Requirements

Large laryngeal tumors often place pressure on the esophagus and may cause dysphagia (difficulty swallowing) or odynophagia (painful swallowing). In either case, the client may experience difficulty eating to the extent that nutrition is impaired. Additionally, cancer often produces

Nursing Care of the Client Having a Total Laryngectomy (continued)

- Assist and encourage the client to use adjunctive pain-relief measures such as progressive relaxation, meditation, and visualization. *These measures facilitate muscle relaxation and augment pain relief provided by analgesics.*

Anxiety

- Assess the client's level of anxiety following surgery. *Although anxiety may be difficult to assess in the initial period following surgery, this assessment is particularly important before teaching is initiated. Extreme anxiety interferes with learning.*

- Place the call light within easy reach at all times; answer the call light promptly. *The client who is unable to speak or call out needs the reassurance that help is within reach at all times.*

- Encourage family members to remain with the client whenever possible. *Supportive family presence helps reassure the client that he or she will not be left alone or helpless.*

- Spend as much time as possible with the client. When leaving the client's room, specify the time when you will return. *These measures help establish trust and relieve anxiety.*

- Encourage the client and family members to express their fears and anxieties. *Expression of fears helps the client and family members deal with them objectively and to support one another.*

Impaired Swallowing

- Maintain intravenous fluids and/or enteral feedings until the client is able to consume adequate amounts of food and fluids orally. *It is important to maintain the client's nutritional and fluid balance until normal eating can be resumed.*

- When the client is able to resume oral intake, begin with soft foods, not liquids. *Soft foods are easier for the client to handle and swallow initially. As recovery progresses, the client will begin to consume viscous liquids and, eventually, a normal diet.*

- Reassure the client with a total laryngectomy that choking is not possible, because there is no connection between the esophagus and trachea. *Clients often fear that swallowing will result in choking and they will be unable to cough effectively.*

- Teach the client to initiate a swallow by placing a small amount of food on the back of the tongue, flex the head forward, and then think "Swallow." *Swallowing is no longer an automatic function and needs to be relearned.*

- Provide for privacy during initial attempts at eating. *Clients may be embarrassed to eat in front of others until they regain confidence in eating. Privacy also reduces distractions, allowing clients to concentrate on swallowing.*

a hypermetabolic state, increasing the client's calorie requirements. If surgery is performed, difficulty swallowing and a fear of aspiration in the early postoperative period also interfere with eating. Enteral or parenteral feedings are usually needed initially to meet the client's nutritional needs. After a total laryngectomy, the client initially loses the senses of taste and smell. Although the client may partially recover the sense of taste, the client may complain that eating no longer holds pleasure.

Nursing interventions with rationales follow:

- Assess the client's nutritional status using height and weight charts, reported weight loss, and anthropometric measurements such as skin folds. *A thorough assessment of the client's nutritional status is important in planning to meet current and anticipated calorie needs.*

- Evaluate the client's current and preferred eating habits and foods, as well as the client's understanding of nu-

trition. *This evaluation provides additional information about nutrition as well as a basis for future planning.*

- Monitor the client's fluid intake and output and food consumption. *It may be difficult for the client to realize that pain or fatigue, rather than a feeling of fullness, is prompting the decision to stop eating.*

- Weigh the client daily. *The daily weight is an easily determined, accurate measure of the client's day-to-day nutritional status.*

- Refer the client to a dietitian for further evaluation, planning, and education. *A professional can identify the client's nutritional needs and help the client plan a diet that will meet them.*

- Encourage the client with dysphagia or odynophagia to experiment with foods of different textures and temperatures. *The client may find that very cold foods or foods of a soft texture are easier to swallow than others.*

Text continues on page 1373

Procedure 33–1   Providing Tracheostomy Care

GATHER ALL SUPPLIES

- Sterile basins or disposable tracheostomy cleaning kit
- Sterile suction catheter and glove kit
- Cleaning solutions, e.g., hydrogen peroxide and sterile normal saline
- Sterile 4×4 gauze dressings (not cotton-filled) or precut dressing
- Sterile cotton-tipped applicators
- Cotton twill ties
- Scissors
- Nonsterile exam gloves

Before the Procedure

Provide for privacy. Explain the procedure to the client. Provide for a means of communication by the client, e.g., eye blinking or raising a finger to indicate distress. If the client's condition permits, provide a pencil and paper or magic slate for questions. Place the client in semi-Fowler's or Fowler's position to facilitate lung ventilation. Assess the client's lung sounds; suction the tracheostomy using sterile technique as needed.

Use Universal Precautions

- Wearing a clean disposable glove, remove the tracheostomy dressing. Dispose of the glove and dressing.
- Open sterile supplies, pouring hydrogen peroxide and normal saline into separate containers. Don sterile gloves.
- Using sterile applicators or gauze dressings moistened with normal saline, clean around the incision, using each applicator or gauze dressing only once. Hydrogen peroxide may be used to remove crusted secretions; thoroughly rinse the area with gauze moistened with normal saline afterward to prevent skin irritation from hydrogen peroxide.

- If the tracheostomy tube has an inner cannula that can be removed for cleaning, remove the tube and place it in the hydrogen peroxide. Cleanse the flange of the outer cannula in the same manner as the incision.
- Clean the inner cannula using a small brush, pipe cleaners (provided in the tracheostomy care kit), or cotton-tipped applicators.
- Rinse the inner cannula thoroughly in normal saline. Tap it gently against the inner aspect of the sterile bowl to remove excess liquid.
- Suction the outer cannula using sterile technique.
- Replace the inner cannula into the tracheostomy tube.
- Replace the dressing, using either a commercially prepared tracheostomy dressing or an opened gauze 4×4 refolded into a V shape (see the accompanying figure). Do not cut the dressing or use a cotton-filled dressing to prevent aspiration of foreign material into the respiratory tract.
- Apply clean tracheostomy ties using either the one- or two-strip method.

One-Strip Method
a. Cut a length of twill tape 2.5 times the length needed to go around the client's neck from one tube flange to the other.
b. Thread one end of the tape through one flange of the tracheostomy tube. Bring the other end around the back of the client's neck, then thread it through the other flange and back around the back of the neck to meet the first end. Tie the loose ends securely using a square knot and allowing one or two fingers' breadth of slack be-

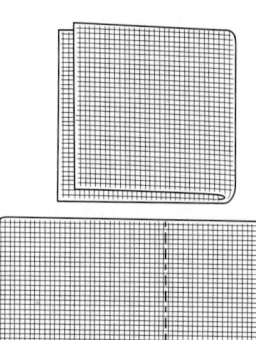
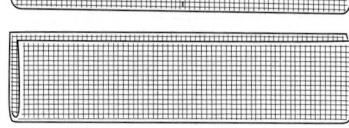
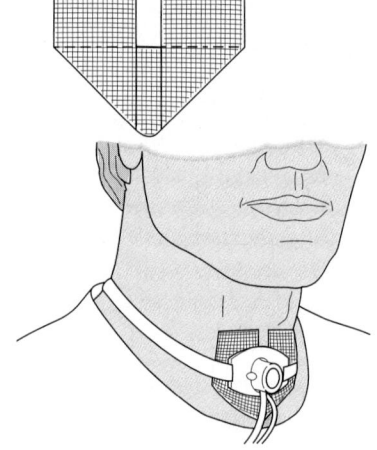

Steps of folding a gauze 4X4 into a tracheostomy dressing.

tween the tie and the client's neck.

Two-Strip Method
a. Cut a length of twill tape equal to about 1.5 times the distance from flange to flange under the client's neck. Divide this into two unequal pieces (approximately 1/3, 2/3).
b. Make a small slit approximately 2 to 3 cm from one end of each piece. Thread the end of the tape with the slit through the flange,

Procedure 33–1 (continued)

then thread the other end of the tape through the slit to secure it. Repeat with the other portion of tape.

c. Position the longer tape behind the client's neck and tie the free ends of tape securely, using a square knot and allowing a small amount of slack as before.

- Once the clean ties are secured, remove the old ties.
- Pad and tape the knot to reduce skin irritation.

After the Procedure

Assess the client's breathing and tolerance of the procedure. Dispose of supplies and used solutions. Wash hands. Chart the procedure and any observations made during the procedure such as amount, color, and consistency of sputum and appearance of the incision.

Critical Pathway for Client Following Laryngectomy

	Date _____ Preoperative	Date _____ 1st 24 hours Postoperative	Date _____ 2nd Postoperative day
	Expected length of stay: 7 days		
Daily outcomes	Client verbalizes understanding of preoperative teaching including: turning, deep breathing, coughing, mobilization, oxygen therapy, suctioning and stoma care, possible tubes (nasogastric or gastrostomy tube, IV, Foley catheter, drains), pain management, and possible transfer to ICU following surgery. Client communicates using an alternate mode of communication. Client demonstrates ability to cope. Client verbalizes understanding of procedure. Obtain informed consent.	Client will ■ Maintain a patent airway and an effective breathing pattern and cough. ■ Recover from anesthesia as evidenced by return of vital signs to baseline and responses to stimuli. ■ Have a stable cardiac rhythm. ■ Have a clean wound with edges well-approximated, healing by first intention. ■ Communicate needs to staff with minimal frustration. ■ Communicate understanding and demonstrate cooperation with turning, deep breathing, and splinting. ■ Communicate control of incisional pain with ordered medications. ■ Demonstrate ability to cope.	Client will ■ Have stable vital signs, stable cardiac rhythm, and be awake, alert, and oriented. ■ Maintain a patent airway and an effective pattern and cough. ■ Maintain urine output >30 mL/h. ■ Remain free of fluid overload or deficit. ■ Have a clean wound with edges well-approximated, healing by first intention. ■ Communicate needs to staff with minimal frustration. ■ Demonstrate cooperation with turning, deep breathing, and splinting. ■ Verbalize control of incisional pain. ■ Ambulate 2 to 3 times/day as tolerated. ■ Demonstrate ability to cope.
Assessments, tests, and treatments	CBC, serum chemistries Urinalysis Chest X-ray Coagulation studies	Vital signs and O_2 saturation, neurovascular assessment, and dressing and wound drainage assessment q15min x4, q30min x4, then q1h and prn	Vital signs and O_2 saturation, neurovascular assessment, dressing and wound drainage assessment q2–4h and prn Respiratory assessment q1–2h

	Date _____ Preoperative	Date _____ 1st 24 hours Postoperative	Date _____ 2nd Postoperative day
Assessments, tests, and treatments *continued*	Type and cross match for designated number of units Baseline physical assessment	Respiratory assessment to include breath sounds, respiratory rate and quality, effectiveness of cough, and color and consistency of secretions ABGs prn Respiratory therapy consultation EKG monitoring Elevate head of bed at least 30 degrees Head-to-toe assessment q4h Tracheostomy care per clinical protocol Suction as needed Turn, cough, and deep breathe q1–2h and prn Oxygen via humidified mist collar; maintain $P_{O_2} > 90$ Small bore NG tube or gastrostomy tube to low continuous suction Foley catheter to closed drainage Assess calves for redness, tenderness, swelling, heat, edema q4h TED stockings: remove and replace every shift Head-to-toe assessment q4h and prn Intake and output q2–4h Hemoglobin and hematocrit Maintain sterile dressing; reinforce prn Mouth care q2h and prn while awake	Tracheostomy care per clinical protocol Suction as needed Intake and output q4–8h D/C Foley catheter and assess voiding Elevate head of bed 30 degrees O_2 via humidified mist collar Assess calves for redness, tenderness, swelling, heat, edema every shift Head-to-toe assessment q4h TED stockings: remove and replace every shift Head-to-toe assessment q4h and prn Maintain dry, sterile dressing; reinforce prn. Assess wound and change dressing per MD order. Intake and output Mouth care q2h and prn while awake
Communication	Listen carefully and provide adequate time for communication. Explore use of word cards, magic slate, or portable computer to enhance communication. Speech therapy consultation.	Listen carefully and provide adequate time for communication. Observe nonverbal communication. Use alternative methods for communication as determined preoperatively. Answer call bell immediately and in person.	Listen carefully and provide adequate time for communication. Observe nonverbal communication. Use alternative methods for communication as determined preoperatively. Answer call bell immediately and in person.

Critical Pathway for Client Following Laryngectomy (continued)

	Date _____ **Preoperative**	Date _____ **1st 24 hours Postoperative**	Date _____ **2nd Postoperative day**
Communi- cation *continued*		Anticipate needs. Speech therapy consultation	Encourage client and family to express feelings regarding changes in body image and function. Anticipate needs. Collaborate with speech therapy.
Knowledge deficit	Orient to room and surroundings. Provide simple, brief instructions. Review preoperative preparation including hospital and surgical routines. Include family in teaching. Discuss surgery and specific postoperative care. Instruct in relaxation techniques. Assess understanding of all teaching.	Orient client and family to room and postoperative routine. Include family in teaching. Review plan of care. Review importance of deep breathing, coughing, incentive spirometer, mobilization, and any drainage tubes, intravenous, and pain management. Assess understanding of teaching. Assess level of anxiety and offer emotional support.	Review importance of early progressive exercise. Review plan of care with client and family. Reinforce safety measures. Assess understanding of teaching. Assess level of anxiety and offer emotional support.
Diet	NPO Baseline nutritional and hydration assessment	NPO Nutritional consultation	NPO Dietary consultation for nutritional assessment
Activity	Assess safety needs and provide appropriate measures. Activity as ordered	Bed rest Turn, cough, and deep breathe q1–2h Range-of-motion exercises each shift Assess safety needs and maintain appropriate precautions.	Maintain safety precautions. TCDB q2h Assist out of bed 2 to 3 times. Begin ambulation (25 to 50 ft).
Medications	Preoperative medications as ordered	Analgesics as ordered IV antibiotics IV fluids per order	Analgesics as ordered Stool softener IV fluids per order
Transfer/ discharge plan	Assess potential discharge needs and support system. Establish discharge goals with client and family.	Home assessment if not previously completed Consult with social service regarding projected needs for home health care; including home health aides, visiting nurse, and speech therapy. Establish discharge objectives with client and family.	Review with client and significant others discharge objectives regarding activity and home care. Consult and collaborate with speech therapy. Complete discharge planning.

➤

Critical Pathway for Client Following Laryngectomy (continued)

	Date _____ **3rd Postoperative day**	Date _____ **4th Postoperative day**	Date _____ **5th to 6th Postoperative day**
Daily outcomes	Client will ■ Be afebrile with stable vital signs. ■ Have a patent airway and an effective breathing pattern and cough. ■ Have lungs clear to auscultation. ■ Have a clean wound with edges well-approximated, healing by first intention. ■ Have stable vital signs. ■ Communicate needs to staff with minimal frustration. ■ Demonstrate cooperation with turning, deep breathing, and splinting. ■ Verbalize control of incisional pain. ■ Ambulate 50 to 100 ft bid. ■ Demonstrate ability to cope.	Client will ■ Be afebrile, have stable vital signs, and be awake, alert, and oriented. ■ Have a patent airway, lungs clear to auscultation, and an effective cough. ■ Have a clean wound with edges well-approximated, healing by first intention. ■ Communicate needs with minimal frustration. ■ Communicate satisfaction with alternative means of communication. ■ Demonstrate cooperation with turning, deep breathing, and splinting. ■ Tolerate feedings without nausea and vomiting. ■ Verbalize control of incisional pain. ■ Ambulate 150 to 200 ft qid. ■ Demonstrate ability to cope. ■ Tolerate activities without evidence of fatigue or pain.	Client will ■ Be afebrile, have stable vital signs, and be awake, alert, and oriented. ■ Have a patent airway, lungs clear to auscultation, and an effective cough. ■ Have a clean wound with edges well-approximated, healing by first intention. ■ Communicate needs with minimal frustration. ■ Communicate satisfaction with alternative means of communication. ■ Demonstrate cooperation with turning, deep breathing, and splinting. ■ Tolerate feedings without nausea and vomiting. ■ Verbalize control of incisional pain. ■ Ambulate 150 to 300 ft qid. ■ Demonstrate ability to cope.
Assessments, tests, and treatments	Vital signs and O_2 saturation, neurovascular assessment, dressing assessment q4h Respiratory assessment q1–2h Tracheostomy care per protocol Suction as needed Air or O_2 via mist collar Intake and output every shift Change dressing and assess wound healing bid Assess calves for redness, tenderness, swelling, heat, edema every shift TED stockings: remove and replace every shift day and prn. Head-to-toe assessment q4h and prn Weight D/C oxygen when O_2 saturation >92% Mouth care q2h and prn while awake	Vital signs and O_2 saturation q4h and prn Respiratory assessment q2–4h and prn Tracheostomy care per protocol Head-to-toe assessment each shift Change dressings each day and prn. Assess wound healing bid. TED stockings: remove and replace every shift. Assess calves for redness, tenderness, swelling, heat, edema every shift. Intake and output each shift Weight D/C oxygen if O_2 saturation >92% Mouth care q2h and prn while awake	Vital signs q4h and prn Respiratory assessment q4h and prn Tracheostomy care per protocol Head-to-toe assessment each shift Remove dressings. Assess wound healing bid. CBC, electrolytes, glucose, serum protein and albumin Intake and output Weight Mouth care q2h and prn while awake

	Date _____ 3rd Postoperative day	Date _____ 4th Postoperative day	Date _____ 5th to 6th Postoperative day
Communi- cation	Listen carefully and provide adequate time for communi-cation. Observe nonverbal communi-cation. Use alternative methods for communication as deter-mined preoperatively. Answer call bell immediately and in person. Encourage client and family to express feelings regarding changes in body image and function. Anticipate needs. Collaborate with speech therapy.	Listen carefully and provide adequate time for communi-cation. Observe nonverbal communi-cation. Use alternative methods for communication as deter-mined preoperatively. Answer call bell immediately and in person. Anticipate needs.	Listen carefully and provide adequate time for communi-cation. Observe nonverbal communi-cation. Use alternative methods for communication as determined preoperatively. Answer call bell immediately and in person. Anticipate needs.
Knowledge deficit	Review plan of care. Include family in teaching. Initiate discharge teaching re-garding wound care and tracheostomy care. Assess understanding of teaching. Assess level of anxiety and offer emotional support.	Review plan of care. Include family in teaching. Continue discharge teaching regarding wound care, tracheostomy care, activity, and diet. Assess understanding of teaching. Offer emotional support.	Review plan of care with cli-ent and family. Continue discharge teaching regarding wound care, tracheostomy care, activity, and diet. Instruct client and family re: home tube feedings. Assess understanding of teaching. Offer emotional support.
Diet	NPO	NG/GT feedings as ordered	NG/GT feedings as ordered
Activity	Maintain safety precautions. TCDB q2h Assist out of bed 2 to 3 times. Begin ambulation (50 to 100 ft) bid	Encourage self-care. Ambulate 150 to 200 ft qid.	Ambulate 150 to 300 ft qid. Shower
Medications	Analgesics as ordered Stool softener IV fluids per order	Analgesics as ordered Stool softener D/C Intermittent IV device	Analgesics as ordered Stool softener
Transfer/ discharge plan	Review with client and signifi-cant others progress toward discharge objectives. Collaborate with speech ther-apy. Make appropriate referrals for discharge care.	Review with client and signifi-cant others discharge objec-tives regarding activity and home care. Arrange visit from laryngecto-my support group.	Review with client and fami-ly discharge objectives regard-ing activity and home care. Complete referrals for home health care; including home health aides, visiting nurse, and speech therapy. Refer to any appropriate support ser-vices such as American Cancer Society.

➤

Critical Pathway for Client Following Laryngectomy (continued)

	Date _____ 7th Postoperative day— Discharge Day
Daily outcomes	Client is afebrile. Client is alert and oriented. Client has a patent airway, lungs clear to auscultation, and an effective cough. Client has a dry, clean wound with edges well-approximated, healing by first intention. Client has stable vital signs. Client manages pain with non-pharmacologic measures and ordered medications. Client communicates needs with minimal frustration. Client and family communicate satisfaction for alternative means of communication. Client is independent in self-care. Client ambulates 300 to 500 feet qid. Client has resumed preadmission urine and bowel elimination pattern. Client verbalizes/demonstrates home care instructions. Client and/or family demonstrates tracheostomy care safely and correctly. Client tolerates ordered feedings. Client and family demonstrate ability to safely and correctly administer tube feedings. Client demonstrates ability to cope with ongoing stressors.
Assessments, tests, and treatments	Vital signs q shift Respiratory assessment q4hr and prn. Tracheostomy care per clinical protocol. Head-to-toe assessment Assess wounds Weight Mouth care q2h and prn while awake

	Date _____ **7th Postoperative day—** **Discharge day**
Communi- cation	Listen carefully and provide adequate time for communication. Observe nonverbal communication. Use alternative methods for communication. Answer call bell immediately and in person. Anticipate needs.
Knowledge deficit	Patient and/or significant other verbalizes understanding of discharge teaching including wound care, tracheostomy care, activity, safety measures, diet, signs and symptoms to report, follow-up care and MD appointment, postoperative treatment, medications: name, purpose, dose, frequency, route, dietary interactions, and side effects, and home care arrangements. Assess understanding of teaching. Offer emotional support.
Diet	NG/GT feedings as ordered
Activity	Ambulate 300 to 500 ft qid. Shower
Medications	Analgesics as ordered Stool softener
Transfer/ discharge plan	Discharge with referrals for home health care and speech therapy.

- Encourage the client to eat frequent, small meals rather than three large meals per day. *The client who has difficulty swallowing is likely to consume more if food is offered in small quantities throughout the day.*

- Recommend liquid supplements such as Ensure for clients who are not meeting their calorie needs. Provide information about where to obtain nutritional supplements. *Liquid dietary supplements provide balanced nutrition as well as additional calories and are an effective way of increasing the client's intake. They are available without prescription in major supermarkets.*

- Provide mouth care prior to meals and supplemental feedings. For the client with stomatitis or esophagitis related to radiation or chemotherapy, provide a topical

Applying Research to Nursing Practice: Measuring Quality of Life After Laryngectomy

■ ■ ■

Quality-of-life (QOL) dimensions were compared after laryngectomy in clients with advanced cancer. The researchers asked 20 clients and 20 health care professionals to identify important QOL items and to rank and rate them on a vertical visual analog scale. Health care professionals ranked impaired communication and self-image/self-esteem as the two most important QOL dimensions. Clients, however, ranked physical consequences of surgery, such as tracheal mucous production and interference with social activities, as the two most important items (Mohide, Archibald, Tew, Young, and Haines, 1992). The results indicate that the priorities of health care workers do not correlate well with client priorities.

Implications for Nursing

These findings are relevant to nurses caring for clients and to nurse researchers developing QOL measures. Additionally, they indicate that nurses may not provide the kind of preoperative teaching and postoperative psychologic support and reassurance that the client with a laryngectomy needs. The nurse must be sure to identify the client's concerns rather than focusing on the nurse's perception of the client's concerns.

Critical Thinking in Client Care

1. Why do you think that clients identify tracheal mucous production and interference with social activities as their primary concerns after a laryngectomy?

2. What interventions can the nurse provide to address these concerns?

3. Identify social support systems that can help the postlaryngectomy client deal with the concerns identified in this study.

anesthetic such as viscous lidocaine before eating. *The client with cancerous tissue or inflammation related to therapeutic measures may complain of bad breath or a foul taste in the mouth, which suppresses appetite. Inflamed mucosa may make eating uncomfortable. A topical anesthetic may relieve this discomfort and thus promote food intake.*

- If the client has problems with nausea as a result of therapy or cancer, provide an antiemetic 30 minutes before eating. *The nauseated client has difficulty eating; an antiemetic can relieve this nausea and make eating possible.*

- Suggest institution of enteral (tube) feeding via nasogastric or gastrostomy tube for the client who is unable to consume enough food to maintain weight and nutritional status orally. *Both cancer and surgery increase calorie needs. Supplemental enteral feedings may be necessary to prevent catabolism and a negative nitrogen balance.*

- Postoperatively, place the laryngectomy client in a semi-Fowler's or Fowler's position. *Elevating the head of the bed facilitates swallowing of oral secretions and helps prevent regurgitation of tube feedings.*

- Prior to initiation of feeding, have the client begin performing mouth rinses. *Rinsing not only helps clean the mouth but also allows the client to begin practicing the use of tongue and cheek muscles to control fluid in the mouth.*

- Refer the client to a physical therapist for rehabilitation following laryngectomy. *Because of surgical changes in the relationship of the trachea, esophagus, and oropharynx, the client needs to relearn swallowing techniques before eating.*

- Reinforce instructions for swallowing. *Reinforcement promotes learning.*

Anticipatory Grieving

The client with laryngeal cancer faces not only the diagnosis of cancer, which is often perceived as a death sentence, but also the prospect of mutilating surgery. If a laryngectomy is necessary to treat the tumor, the client grieves the loss of both a body part and an important function, speech. Speech is a vital aspect of social interaction and is often necessary for one's career (see the accompanying research box). It also enables people to express their needs when they cannot meet them themselves. The loss of speech, therefore, represents a major loss. In addition, the presence of a tracheal stoma after surgery changes the manner in which the client breathes. If radical neck dissection is necessary because lymph nodes are involved, the loss of neck musculature and function also alters the client's self-concept and ability to cope with changes.

Nursing interventions with rationales follow:

- Provide opportunities for the client and family members to express feelings of grief, anger, or fear about the diagnosis of cancer, the impending surgery, and the anticipated loss of speech. *The client with laryngeal cancer who requires a total laryngectomy needs the opportunity (and may need permission) to grieve for anticipated losses. Upon diagnosis of cancer, the client may begin to grieve for unfulfilled plans and expectations, even though a cure may be anticipated. Additionally, laryngectomy causes a major change in the client's body image, because a vital body part is lost and a stoma is created. The client also grieves the loss of the ability to speak. This loss can have a significant impact on the client's occupation and social interaction.*

■ Provide a calm, supportive environment with adequate privacy and emotional support for the client and family members as they work through the grieving process. *It is important for the client and family to know that their feelings of loss are real and accepted by caregivers.*

■ Help the client and family discuss the potential impact of the loss on family structure and function. *Discussion helps family members to understand each other's feelings and to support one another.*

■ Refer the client and family for additional psychologic or spiritual counseling as appropriate. *When the client and family are having difficulty dealing with the diagnosis and proposed treatment plan, counseling may be necessary to prevent a sense of defeat and hopelessness.*

■ Help the client and family identify additional resources for coping, such as strategies they have used in the past to deal with crises. *This exercise helps the client and family identify strengths they can use to deal with the present situation.*

Other Nursing Diagnoses

The following nursing diagnoses may also be appropriate for the client facing laryngeal cancer or a laryngectomy:

■ *Ineffective Breathing Pattern* related to anxiety and fatigue

■ *Body Image Disturbance* related to change in appearance following laryngectomy and radical neck dissection

■ *Pain* related to pressure of the tumor on surrounding tissues

■ *Fear* related to the diagnosis of cancer and potential loss of the ability to speak

■ *Ineffective Individual Coping* related to situational crisis

■ *Sensory-Perceptual Alterations: Gustatory and Olfactory* related to changed breathing pattern and interrupted innervation

■ *Risk for Ineffective Airway Clearance* related to neck breathing and loss of upper airway protection

Client and Family Teaching

In the community, nurses can be instrumental in teaching about the risk factors and early warning signs of laryngeal cancer, facilitating its early recognition and treatment.

When laryngeal cancer has been diagnosed, the client and family may be very concerned about issues regarding body image, impaired communication, and fear of dying. The nurse provides information and clarification of treatment options, discussing the risks and benefits of each. Stress the importance of early intervention to reduce the risk of local spread and metastasis. If a total laryngectomy is the treatment of choice, discuss options for communication after surgery. Present the options realistically. Clients with limited manual dexterity may be unable to manipulate the tracheoesophageal puncture device for speech; only about 30% of clients are able to master esophageal speech. Encourage the client to try using the speech generator prior to surgery to reduce the frustration of trying to use it during the recovery period.

Teach the client undergoing radiation therapy about the treatments, the care of the skin and secretions during therapy, and the expected side effects of therapy. Provide instruction about techniques to manage adverse effects (see Chapter 9 for further discussion about radiation therapy and its effects).

In the postoperative period, teaching about tracheostomy stoma care and prevention of respiratory infection is important. Instruct the client and family members how to care for the tracheostomy and provide the opportunity for redemonstration of techniques. The client uses clean technique rather than sterile technique in providing stoma care. Once the stoma is fully healed, the client may be able to do without the tracheostomy tube. Clients also need teaching about the following:

■ The client should use a humidifier or vaporizer in the home to add humidity to inspired air, a normal function of the upper respiratory tract.

■ The client should increase fluid intake to maintain mucosal moisture and loosen secretions.

■ The client needs to shield the stoma with a stoma guard, such as a gauze square on a tie around the neck, to prevent particulate matter from entering the lower respiratory tract.

■ Secretions coming in contact with the skin surrounding the stoma should be removed promptly to prevent irritation and skin breakdown.

■ Although water sports are contraindicated for the client with a permanent tracheostomy, the client may participate in all other activities. Lifting may be more difficult because of the inability to hold the breath (the Valsalva maneuver).

■ The client can shower or bathe (without submerging the neck or head) normally, providing protection for the stoma with a cupped hand or washcloth.

Before surgery, it is probably not wise to teach the client undergoing a laryngectomy about potential complications, but they need to be addressed postoperatively if they occur. These potential complications include risk of injury to the auditory or facial nerve with possible loss of hearing and facial expression on the affected side. Damage to the spinal accessory nerve may cause shoulder drop on the affected side.

Both the client and family need emotional and motivational support through this trying time. Provide referral to local support groups such as a laryngectomy club or lost cord club (see Appendix B for a list of possible community resources). Encourage the client to discontinue the use of cigarettes and alcohol. Discuss ways to achieve optimal nutrition. If the client and family are having difficulty adjusting to the diagnosis of cancer and the effects of treatment, provide referral to counseling.

Applying the Nursing Process

Case Study of a Client with Total Laryngectomy: David Tom

David Tom is a 61-year-old accountant who lives in a rural area. He is divorced and has two children who are grown and live away from home. He has smoked two packs of cigarettes daily since high school. He drinks three or four cocktails every evening. He enjoys fishing and hunting. Mr. Tom was recently diagnosed with cancer of the larynx. His chief complaints were sore throat and hoarseness that persisted for a few months. He has been admitted to the surgical care unit from the ICU 3 days post total laryngectomy.

Assessment
Mr. Tom's vital signs are stable: BP, 146/84; P, 92 and regular; R, 18; T, 100 F (37.7 C) per rectum. He has a tracheostomy tube sutured in place. A tracheostomy collar delivers humidified oxygen at 28%. Pulse oximetry is 92%. He has a nasogastric tube in place with continuous tube feeding. Two Hemovac wound drains are present in the right neck area. A moderate amount of edema is present in the right facial and submandibular area. Mr. Tom is ambulatory within the room.

Diagnosis
Dana Brown, RN, admits Mr. Tom to the surgical unit and develops the following nursing diagnoses:

- *Risk for Ineffective Airway Clearance* related to postoperative edema
- *Risk for Ineffective Breathing Pattern* related to pain and anxiety
- *Body Image Disturbance* related to total laryngectomy and presence of tracheostomy stoma
- *Impaired Verbal Communication* related to total laryngectomy

- *Pain* related to surgical procedure
- *Risk for Altered Nutrition: Less Than Body Requirements* related to difficulty eating after surgery

Expected Outcomes
The expected outcomes for the plan of care are that Mr. Tom will

- Maintain effective airway clearance.
- Maintain effective breathing pattern.
- Communicate in writing his feelings about changes in his body appearance.
- Demonstrate interest in receiving information regarding various communication devices.
- Communicate relief of pain.
- Maintain appropriate body weight, intake, and output.
- Communicate and demonstrate self-care activities.

Planning and Implementation
The following interventions are planned and implemented for Mr. Tom:

- Assess respiratory rate and rhythm every 2 hours.
- Auscultate lungs for normal and abnormal breath sounds.
- Assess effectiveness of cough.
- Monitor quantity, color, and odor of secretions.
- During each shift, schedule time to sit with Mr. Tom and discuss his concerns and feelings.
- Perform a thorough pain assessment every 2 to 3 hours and administer analgesics as ordered.
- Explore nonpharmacologic methods of pain relief.
- Provide written information as requested.
- Monitor intake and output as well as daily weight.
- Arrange for a dietary consultation to determine caloric requirements.
- Monitor laboratory values such as electrolytes, protein, serum albumin, glucose, and CBC.
- Assist Mr. Tom with ADLs and encourage his active involvement.

Evaluation
Mr. Tom reports in writing that his pain is adequately controlled. His respiratory status is stable as evidenced by vital signs and respiratory rate and rhythm within normal limits. Mr. Tom is tolerating tube feedings well and expresses a desire to begin oral feedings. The dietitian has visited and assisted in planning to begin oral feedings. Intake and output are stable, as is his weight. Mr. Tom has been receptive to receiving written materials regarding follow-up care and exploration of various modalities of speech. He has participated in his morning care and has ambulated in his room several times.

Critical Thinking in the Nursing Process

1. Compare and contrast the various methods to allow speech that are available to clients with total laryngectomy.

2. Develop a plan of care for Mr. Tom for the nursing diagnosis *Body Image Disturbance*.

3. Discuss nursing interventions to provide wound care for the client with laryngectomy and radical neck dissection.

4. List strategies to optimize ventilation.

Bibliography

■ ■ ■

Berkow, R., & Fletcher, A. J. (Eds.). (1992). *The Merck manual of diagnosis and therapy* (16th ed.). Rahway, NJ: Merck Research Laboratories.

Blitzer, A., & Lawson, W. (1991). The Caldwell-Luc procedure in 1991. *Otolaryngology: Head Neck Surgery, 105*(5), 717–722.

Bootzin, R., Lahmeyer, H., & Lilie, J. (Eds.). (1994). *Integrated approach to sleep management.* NJ: Cahners Healthcare Communications.

Brown, K. (1994). Head and neck cancer: After the surgery. *Critical Care Choices 94*, 10–20.

Carpenito, L. (1993). *Nursing Diagnosis: Application to clinical practice.* (5th ed.). Philadelphia: Lippincott.

Christianson, D. (1994, November). Caring for a patient who has an implanted venous port. *American Journal of Nursing, 94*(11), 40–44.

Conn, V. (1991). Self-care actions taken by older adults for influenza and colds. *Nursing Research, 40*(3), 176–181.

El-Silimy, O. (1993). Endonasal endoscopy and posterior espistaxis. *Rhinology, 31*(3), 119–120.

Foster, J. (1992). Intensive care of the patient with cancer after reconstructive surgery. *Focus on Critical Care, 19*(2), 122–127.

Gerchufsky, M. (1995, March). Understanding upper respiratory infections. *ADVANCE for Nurse Practitioners, 3*(3), 25–27.

Godfrey, N. (1994). Sagittal section septoplasty: An intrinsically stabilized septoplasty. *Plastic and Reconstructive Surgery, 93*(1), 188–196.

Harris A., & Komray, R. (1993). Cost-effective management of pharyngocutaneous fistulas following laryngectomy. *Ostomy/Wound Management, 39*,(8), 36–44.

Hazzard, W. R., Bierman, E. L., Blass, J. P., Ettinger, W. H., Jr., & Halter, J. B. (1994). *Principles of geriatric medicine and gerontology* (3rd ed.). New York: McGraw-Hill.

Karper, W. B., & Boschen, M. B. (1993, January-February). Effects of exercise on acute respiratory tract infections and related symptoms. *Geriatric Nursing, 14*(1), 15–18.

Konstantinides, N., & Lehmann, S. (1993). The impact of nutrition on wound healing. *Critical Care Nurse, October 93*, 25–33.

Kozier, B., Erb, G., Blais, K., & Wilkinson, J. M. (1995). *Fundamentals of nursing: Concepts, process, and practice* (5th ed.). Redwood City, CA: Addison-Wesley Nursing.

Lockhart, J., & Bryce, J. (1993). Restoring speech with tracheoesophageal puncture. *Nursing 93, 23*(1), 59–61.

Lockhart, J., Troff, J., & Artim, L. (1992). Total laryngectomy and radical neck dissection. *AORN Journal, 55*(2), 458–479.

Loftus, B., Blitzer, A., & Cozine, K. (1994). Epistaxis, medical history, and the nasopulmonary reflex: What is clinically relevant? *Otolaryngology: Head and Neck Surgery, 110*(4), 363–369.

Mabry, R. (1993). Therapeutic agents in the medical management of sinusitis. *Otolaryngologic Clinics of North America 26*(4), 561–571.

McCance, K. L., & Huether, S. E. (1994). *Pathophysiology: The biologic basis for disease in adults and children* (2nd ed.). St. Louis: Mosby-Year Book.

McGarvey, H. (1990, October 17). Making sense of endotracheal intubation. *Nursing Times, 86*(42), 35–37.

Meehan, M. (1992). Nursing Dx: Potential for aspiration. *RN, 55*(1), 30–34.

Miller, S. (1990). The role of the speech language pathologist in voice restoration after total laryngectomy. *CA-A Cancer Journal for Clinicians, 40*(3), 174–183.

Mohide, E., Archibald, S., Tew, M., Young, J., & Haines, T. (1992). Postlaryngectomy quality-of-life dimension identified by patients and health care professionals. *The American Journal of Surgery, 164*(16), 619–622.

Oleson, M., & King, T. (1990). Back to the beginning: Nursing care management of the older client with alaryngeal speech needs. *Journal of Gerontological Nursing, 16*(12), 27–29.

Porth, C. (1994). *Pathophysiology: Concepts of altered health states* (4th ed.). Philadelphia: Lippincott.

Price, S. A., & Wilson, L. M. (1992). *Pathophysiology: Clinical concepts of disease process* (4th ed.). St. Louis: Mosby-Year Book.

Rice, D. (1993). Chronic frontal sinus disease. *Otolaryngologic Clinics of North America, 26*(4), 619–622.

Rice, D. (1993). Endoscopic sinus surgery. *Otolaryngologic Clinics of North America, 26*(4), 613–618.

Rubenstein, E., & Federman, D. D. (Eds.). (1978–1994). *Scientific American medicine.* New York: Scientific American.

Ruth, T., Jr. (1995, January). Fielding the flu. *ADVANCE for Nurse Practitioners, 3*(1), 18–20, 34.

Sawyer, D., & Bruya, M. (1990). Care of the patient having radical neck surgery or permanent laryngostomy: A nursing diagnostic approach. *Focus on Critical Care, 17*(2), 166–173.

Schoemick, L., Katz, P., & Beam, T. (1991, September/October). The many guises of infection. *Geriatric Nursing, 12*, 223–224.

Shlafer, M. (1993). *The nurse, pharmacology, and drug therapy: A prototype approach* (2nd ed.). Redwood City, CA: Addison-Wesley Nursing.

Silver, C., & Moisa, I. (1990). The role of surgery in the treatment of laryngeal cancer. *CA-A Cancer Journal for Clinicians, 40*(3), 134–149.

Singer, M., & Blom, E. (1990). Medical techniques for voice restoration after total laryngectomy. *CA-A Cancer Journal for Clinicians, 40*(3), 166–173.

Smalley, P. J. (1990, September). Lasers in otolaryngology. *Nursing Clinics of North America, 25*, 645–656.

Spencer, R. T., Nichols, L. W., Lipkin, G. B., Henderson, H. S., & West, F. M. (1993). *Clinical pharmacology and nursing management* (4th ed.). Philadelphia: Lippincott.

Stankiewicz, J., Newell, D., & Park, A. (1993). Complications of inflammatory diseases of the sinuses. *Otolaryngologic Clinics of North America, 26*(4), 639–655.

Tange, R. (1991). Some historical aspects of the surgical treatment of the infected maxillary sinus. *Rhinology, 29*(2), 155–162.

Tierney, L. M., McPhee, S. J., & Papadakis, M. A. (Eds.). (1994). *Current medical diagnosis & treatment* (33rd ed.). Norwalk, CT: Appleton & Lange.

Tucker, S. M., Canobbio, M. M., Paquette, E. V., & Wells, M. F. (1992). *Patient care standards: Nursing process, diagnosis, and outcome* (5th ed.). St. Louis: Mosby-Year Book.

Wang, R., Bui, T., Sauris, E., Ditkoff, M., Anand, V., & Klatsky, I. (1991). Long-term problems in patients with tracheoesophageal puncture. *Archives of Otolaryngology: Head and Neck Surgery, 117*(11), 1273–1276.

Ward, C. (1992, November/December). Influenza: The unwanted visitor. *Geriatric Nursing, 13*, 329–331.

Way, L. W. (Ed.). (1994). *Current surgical diagnosis and treatment* (10th ed.). Norwalk, CT: Appleton & Lange.

Weilitz, P., & Dettenmeier, P. (1994). Back to basics: Test your knowledge of tracheostomy tubes. *AJN, 94*(2), 46–50.

Wilson, E., & Malley, N. (1990). Discharge planning for the patient with a new tracheostomy. *Critical Care Nurse, 10*(7), 73–79.

Wilson, J. D., Braunwald, E., Isselbacher, K. J., Petersdorf, R. G., Martin, J. B., Fauci, A. S., & Root, R. K. (Eds.). (1991). *Harrison's principles of internal medicine* (12th ed.). New York: McGraw-Hill.

Zinreich, J. (1993). Imaging of inflammatory sinus disease. *Otolaryngologic Clinics of North America, 26*(4), 535–547.

Nursing Care of Clients with Lower Respiratory Disorders

LEARNING OBJECTIVES

After completing this chapter, you will be able to

- Describe the pathophysiology of common disorders of the lower respiratory system.

- Relate manifestations of disorders of the lower respiratory system to their pathophysiologic processes.

- Identify laboratory and diagnostic tests used to diagnose disorders of the lower respiratory system.

- Discuss nursing implications for medications and treatments prescribed for clients with disorders of the lower respiratory system.

- Provide appropriate care for the client having thoracic surgery.

- Provide teaching to clients with disorders of the lower respiratory system and to their families.

- Use the nursing process to assess needs, plan and implement individualized care, and evaluate responses for a client with a disorder of the lower respiratory system.

Many clients in both acute and long-term care facilities experience acute or chronic disorders affecting the lower respiratory system. Respiratory disorders result in much lost work time and account for a significant portion of health care costs.

Normal function of the lower respiratory system depends on several organ systems: the central nervous system, which stimulates and controls breathing; chemoreceptors in the brain, aortic arch, and carotid bodies, which monitor the pH and oxygen content of blood; the heart and circulatory system, which provide for blood supply and gas exchange; the musculoskeletal system, which provides an intact thoracic cavity capable of expanding and contracting; and the lungs and bronchial tree, which allow air movement and gas exchange. Impaired function of any of these systems affects ventilatory and respiratory function, potentially resulting in tissue *hypoxia,* decreased available oxygen to support metabolic activity.

Conversely, disorders affecting the lower respiratory tract have both local and systemic effects. Local effects include cough, excess production of mucus, shortness of breath or dyspnea, *hemoptysis* (bloody sputum), and chest pain. Systemic effects may include fever, anorexia and malaise, cyanosis, edema, clubbing of fingers and toes, and other manifestations of impaired gas exchange. Disorders of the lower respiratory system discussed in this chapter include infectious or inflammatory conditions, obstructive and restrictive lung diseases, pulmonary vascular disorders, lung cancer, chest and respiratory trauma, and respiratory failure.

Infections and Inflammatory Disorders

A number of physiologic defense mechanisms protect the lower respiratory system from infection. The anatomic barriers of the epiglottis and the branching of the bronchial tree prevent the entry of microorganisms and other possible contaminants. The cilia and mucus that line the respiratory tract, along with the cough reflex, serve to trap and eliminate foreign matter. Organisms that make it past all these barriers usually are rapidly phagocytized in the alveolus by resident macrophages, then attacked by the inflammatory and immune defenses of the body (Wilson et al., 1991). When these defenses are impaired by structural or functional changes, the risk of infection of the lower respiratory tract increases. For example, drugs, alcohol, or neuromuscular disease may suppress the cough reflex; chronic lung disease impairs mucociliary responses; and the influenza virus can cause denuding of respiratory epithelium, increasing the likelihood of bacterial infection (Andreoli, Carpenter, Plum, & Smith, 1990). Even in healthy clients, microorganisms and other foreign material occasionally enter the bronchial tree and lung parenchyma, causing an infectious or inflammatory response.

A number of changes associated with aging and disease processes affect respiratory function and airway clearance, increasing the older adult's susceptibility to respiratory infections. The number of cilia decreases, and the cough weakens. Gag and cough reflexes diminish. The older adult is more susceptible to dehydration, resulting in thick, viscous mucus that is difficult to expectorate. Immune function declines with aging. These factors increase the risk of pulmonary infection and reduce the body's ability to respond appropriately to infectious processes or other lung insults.

Other factors may increase the risk and severity of lower respiratory infections in the older adult: immobility, smoking history, surgical procedures, the use of multiple medications, malnutrition, and such chronic diseases as chronic obstructive pulmonary disease (COPD) and heart disease (Foyt, 1992).

The Client with Acute Bronchitis

Bronchitis, inflammation of the bronchi, can occur as either an acute or chronic condition. Acute bronchitis is a relatively common disorder among adults. When the trachea is also involved, the disorder is called tracheobronchitis. Chronic bronchitis is a component of chronic ob-

structive pulmonary disease (COPD) and is discussed in that section of this chapter.

Pathophysiology

People with impaired physiologic defense mechanisms and cigarette smokers are more susceptible to bronchitis. In otherwise healthy adults, it typically follows an upper respiratory infection. Infectious bronchitis can be caused by either viruses or bacteria. Inhalation of toxic gases or chemicals can lead to inflammatory tracheobronchitis. In either case, the inflammatory response leads to vasodilation and edema of the mucosal lining of the bronchi. Mucosal irritation increases mucus production.

Acute bronchitis is typically heralded by a nonproductive cough that later becomes productive. The cough often occurs in paroxysms, and may be aggravated by cold, dry, or dusty air (McCance & Huether, 1994). Chest pain, often substernal, is common. Other manifestations include moderate fever and general malaise.

Collaborative Care

The diagnosis of acute bronchitis typically is based on the client's history and clinical presentation. A chest X-ray may be ordered to rule out pneumonia, because the presenting manifestations can be similar. Other laboratory and diagnostic testing is rarely indicated. Treatment is conservative and includes rest, increased fluid intake, and the use of aspirin or acetaminophen to relieve fever and malaise. Many physicians prescribe a broad-spectrum antibiotic such as erythromycin or penicillin, because approximately 50% of acute bronchitis is bacterial in origin. An expectorant cough medication is recommended for use during the day and a cough suppressant for night to facilitate rest.

Nursing Care

Clients with acute bronchitis are rarely hospitalized, so most nursing interventions are directed toward teaching. Educational needs for these clients relate to maintaining activities of daily living (ADLs), increasing fluid intake, the use and effects of prescribed medications, and, if the client is a smoker, the importance of smoking cessation. The following nursing diagnoses may be applicable for the client with acute bronchitis:

- *Knowledge Deficit* regarding the use of prescribed medications
- *Sleep Pattern Disturbance* related to coughing
- *Altered Health Maintenance* related to cigarette smoking

Table 34-1	Common Organisms Causing Pneumonia in Adults

Client Profile	Cause
Young, otherwise healthy adults	*Streptococcus pneumoniae, Mycoplasma pneumoniae,* viruses
Older adults	*Streptococcus pneumoniae,* influenza
Debilitated adults	*Streptococcus pneumoniae,* influenza, oral flora, gram-negative bacilli
Hospitalized adults	Oral flora, *Staphylococcus aureus,* gram-negative bacilli

Note: Adapted from *Cecil Essentials of Medicine* (2nd ed.) (p. 580) by T. E. Andreoli, C. C. J. Carpenter, F. Plum, and L. H. Smith, Jr., 1990, Philadelphia: W. B. Saunders.

The Client with Pneumonia

■ ■ ■

Inflammation of the lung parenchyma (the respiratory bronchioles and alveoli) is known as **pneumonia.** The source of inflammation can be either infectious or noninfectious. Bacteria, viruses, fungi, protozoa, and other microbes can lead to infectious pneumonia. Noninfectious causes include aspiration of gastric contents and inhalation of toxic or irritating gases.

In spite of significant advances in antibiotic therapy, the mortality rate from pneumonia remains significant. Along with influenza, pneumonia was the sixth leading cause of death in the United States in 1991, accounting for more than 77,500 deaths (Centers for Disease Control and Prevention [CDC], 1993b). It is a particularly significant disease in older adults and in people with debilitating diseases. Pneumonia currently accounts for about 10% of adult hospital admissions in the United States (Andreoli et al., 1990).

Pathophysiology

Microbes can enter the lung via a number of routes. They may be inhaled, enter through the bloodstream (the hematogenous route), or spread from an adjacent locus of infection. The most common means of entry, however, is aspiration of secretions containing microbes colonizing the naso-oropharynx (Andreoli et al., 1990; Wilson et al., 1991).

Different organisms are implicated in "community-acquired" and nosocomial (hospital-acquired) pneumonias. The most common causative organism for both community- and hospital-acquired pneumonia is *Streptococcus pneumoniae,* a gram-positive bacterium. This organism accounts for approximately 70% to 75% of all diagnosed

cases of pneumonia. *Mycoplasma pneumoniae, Haemophilus influenzae,* and the influenza virus are also among the leading causes of community-acquired pneumonia. *Staphylococcus aureus* and gram-negative bacteria such as *Klebsiella pneumoniae, Pseudomonas aeruginosa,* and enteric bacilli, including *Escherichia coli,* are often implicated as nosocomial causes of pneumonia. Other pneumonias such as Legionnaires' disease and *Pneumonocystis carinii* pneumonia are less common and often are limited to selected populations (McCance & Huether, 1994; Price & Wilson, 1992). Table 34-1 summarizes common pneumonia-causing organisms.

When the invading microorganisms colonize the alveoli, an inflammatory and immune response is initiated. Bronchial and alveolar mucous membranes are damaged by the antigen-antibody response and endotoxins released by some organisms, leading to inflammation and edema. Infectious debris and exudate can fill alveoli, interfering with ventilation and gas exchange (McCance & Huether, 1994).

The pathologic process, anatomic location, and manifestations of pneumonias vary according to the infective organism. The disease typically is classified as either acute bacterial, atypical, viral, or *Pneumocystis* pneumonia.

Acute Bacterial Pneumonia

The presentation of bacterial pneumonia is typically acute. In some instances, the client may experience a viral upper respiratory infection prior to the onset of pneumonia symptoms.

Of the bacterial pneumonias, the pathogenesis of pneumococcal (*Streptococcus pneumoniae*) pneumonia is best understood (Figure 34-1). The inflammatory response initiated by these organisms causes alveolar edema and the formation of exudate. As alveoli and respiratory bronchioles fill with serous exudate, blood cells, fibrin, and bacteria, consolidation (solidification) of lung tissue occurs. The lower lobes of the lungs are affected most often because of gravity. Consolidation of a large portion of an entire lung lobe is known as *lobar pneumonia.* This is the typical pattern for pneumococcal pneumonia. *Bronchopneumonia* is patchy consolidation involving several lobules. Other bacterial pneumonias often present with the patchy involvement of bronchopneumonia; pneumococcal pneumonia may also follow this pattern. The process resolves when macrophages predominate, digesting and removing inflammatory exudate from the infected lung.

The presentation of bacterial pneumonia is usually acute, with rapid onset of shaking chills, fever, and cough productive of rust-colored or purulent sputum. Chest aching or *pleuritic pain* (sharp localized chest pain that increases with breathing and coughing) are common. Limited breath sounds and fine crackles or rales are heard over the affected area of lung. A pleuritic friction rub also may be present. If the involved area is large, the client may be dyspneic and have a dusky skin color.

A more insidious onset with low-grade fever, cough, and scattered crackles can also occur in clients with bronchopneumonia. Dyspnea is less often present. In the older adult or debilitated client, manifestations of pneumonia may be atypical, with little cough, scant sputum, and minimal evidence of respiratory distress. Fever, tachypnea, and altered mentation or agitation may be the primary presenting symptoms.

Pneumococcal pneumonia typically resolves uneventfully; normal lung structure is restored on completion of the process. The infection can extend locally to involve the pleura; this is the most common complication. Bacteremia can result in the spread of the infection to other tissues, leading to meningitis, endocarditis, or peritonitis, and increasing the risk of mortality.

Pneumonias caused by *Staphylococcus aureus* and gram-negative bacteria often result in extensive parenchymal damage with necrosis, lung abscess, and empyema. **Empyema** is the accumulation of purulent exudate in the pleural cavity. Progressive destruction of lung tissue and functional impairment is a possible consequence of *Klebsiella* pneumonia (Price & Wilson, 1992).

Legionnaires' disease is a form of bronchopneumonia caused by *Legionella pneumophila,* a gram-negative bacterium widely found in water, particularly warm standing water. Legionnaires' disease occurs either sporadically or in outbreaks, such as that which occurred at an American Legion convention in 1976, when the disease was first recognized. Contaminated water-cooled air conditioning systems and other water sources have been implicated in its spread.

Smokers, older adults, and people with chronic diseases or impaired immune defenses are most susceptible to Legionnaires' disease. Symptoms develop gradually, beginning 2 to 10 days after exposure. Dry cough, dyspnea, general malaise, chills and fever, headache, confusion, anorexia and diarrhea, myalgias and arthralgias are common manifestations. Consolidation of lung tissue is patchy or lobar. The mortality rate in Legionnaires' disease is 15% to 30% in otherwise healthy people and up to 80% in immunocompromised populations (Andreoli et al., 1990; Porth, 1994; Price & Wilson, 1992).

Primary Atypical Pneumonia

Pneumonia caused by the bacterium *Mycoplasma pneumoniae* is generally classified as *primary atypical pneumonia* because its presentation and course are significantly different from those of other bacterial pneumonias. *Mycoplasma* infection often causes pharyngitis or bronchitis. When pneumonia develops, patchy inflammatory changes in the alveolar septum and interstitial tissue of the lung occur. Alveolar exudate and consolidation of lung tissue are not features of atypical pneumonia.

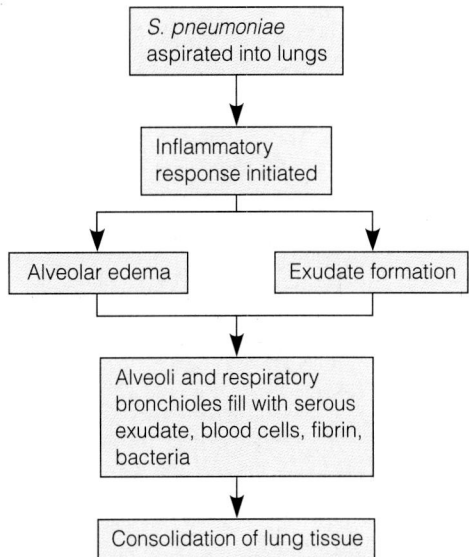

Figure 34-1 The pathogenesis of pneumococcal pneumonia.

Young adults, college students, and military recruits in particular, are the primary affected population. Primary atypical pneumonia is highly contagious. The manifestations resemble those of viral pneumonia; systemic manifestations of fever, headache, myalgias, and arthralgias often predominate. The cough associated with atypical pneumonia is dry, hacking, and nonproductive. Because of the typically mild nature and predominant systemic manifestations, mycoplasmal and viral pneumonia are often referred to as "walking pneumonias."

Viral Pneumonia

Approximately 10% of pneumonias in adults are viral in origin. Influenza and adenovirus are the most common organisms involved; however, cytomegalovirus (CMV) pneumonia is increasing in immunocompromised populations. Herpesviruses, such as those that cause chicken-pox and herpes simplex, and the measles virus also have been implicated in viral pneumonias. As in primary atypical pneumonia, lung involvement in viral pneumonia is limited to the alveolar septum and interstitial spaces.

Viral pneumonia is typically a mild disease that is more likely to affect older adults and people with chronic conditions. It usually occurs in community epidemics. Flu-like manifestations of headache, fever, fatigue, malaise, and muscle aching are common, along with a dry cough.

Pneumocystis carinii Pneumonia

As many as 75% to 80% of people with acquired immune deficiency syndrome (AIDS) develop an opportunistic pneumonia caused by *Pneumocystis carinii,* a common parasite found worldwide. Immunity to *P. carinii* is nearly universal, except in immunocompromised people.

Table 34–2 Clinical Manifestations of Infectious Pneumonias

Type	Onset	Respiratory Manifestations	Other Manifestations
Pneumococcal or lobar pneumonia	Abrupt	Cough productive of purulent or rust-colored sputum; pleuritic or aching chest pain; decreased breath sounds and crackles over affected area; possible dyspnea and cyanosis	Chills and fever
Bronchopneumonia	Gradual	Cough, scattered crackles; minimal dyspnea and respiratory distress	Low-grade fever
Legionnaires' disease	Gradual	Dry cough; dyspnea	Chills and fever; general malaise; headache; confusion; anorexia and diarrhea; myalgias and arthralgias
Primary atypical pneumonia	Gradual	Dry, hacking, nonproductive cough	Fever, headache, myalgias, and arthralgias predominate
Viral pneumonia	Sudden or gradual	Dry cough	Flulike symptoms
Pneumocystis carinii pneumonia	Abrupt	Dry cough; tachypnea and shortness of breath; significant respiratory distress	Fever

Opportunistic infection occurs in people treated with immunosuppressive or cytotoxic therapy for cancer or organ transplant. It also occurs in people with genetic or acquired immunodeficiency.

Infection with *P. carinii* produces patchy involvement throughout the lungs, causing affected alveoli to thicken, become edematous, and fill with foamy, protein-rich fluid. Gas exchange becomes severely impaired as the disease progresses (Porth, 1994).

P. carinii pneumonia (PCP) has an abrupt onset with fever, tachypnea and shortness of breath, and a dry, nonproductive cough. Respiratory distress can be significant, with intercostal retractions and cyanosis.

Manifestations of infectious pneumonias are compared in Table 34–2.

Aspiration Pneumonia

When gastric contents are aspirated into the lungs, the result is a chemical and bacterial pneumonia known as *aspiration pneumonia*. The risk for aspiration pneumonia is highest in clients undergoing emergency surgical or obstetric procedures and in those with depressed cough and gag reflexes or impaired swallowing. Older surgical clients are at particular risk for aspiration pneumonia. Clients receiving enteral nutrition by either nasogastric or gastric tube are also at increased risk for aspiration pneumonia. Vomiting is not always apparent; silent regurgitation of gastric contents may occur in the client with a depressed level of consciousness. Minimizing the use of preoperative medications, taking measures to enhance the elimination of anesthetics, and preventing nausea and gastric distention can reduce the risk of aspiration pneumonia.

The low pH of gastric contents results in a severe inflammatory response when they are aspirated into the respiratory tract. Pulmonary edema and respiratory failure may result. Common complications of aspiration pneumonia include abscesses, *bronchiectasis* (chronic dilation of the bronchi and bronchioles), and gangrene of pulmonary tissue (Price & Wilson, 1992).

Collaborative Care

Prevention is a key component in the management of pneumonia. Identifying vulnerable populations and instituting preventive strategies are important measures to reduce the mortality and morbidity associated with pneumonia.

With early identification of the infecting organism, appropriate intervention, and support of respiratory function, most clients recover uneventfully. However, pneumonia remains a serious disease with significant mortality, especially in aged and debilitated populations. See the accompanying box for collaborative care of the client with pneumonia.

Immunization

Vaccines offer some degree of protection against the most common bacterial and viral pneumonias.

Pneumococcal vaccine, made up of antigens from 23 types of pneumococcus, usually confers a lifetime immunity with a single dose. The vaccine is particularly recommended for people who have a high risk of adverse outcome from bacterial pneumonias: people over age 65; those with chronic cardiac or respiratory conditions, diabetes mellitus, alcoholism, or other chronic diseases; and immunocomprised people.

Collaborative Care: The Client with Pneumonia

Health Care Team	Client-Centered Care
Primary care physician	Assesses for signs and symptoms; orders diagnostic tests such as chest X-ray and arterial blood gases; oversees hydration and nutrition status, supplemental oxygen, respiratory treatments, analgesics, and antibiotics. Refers to pulmonologist if necessary. Manages health care following discharge.
Respiratory therapist	Manages mechanical ventilation if necessary, performs arterial blood gases, administers respiratory therapy including oxygen and aerosol nebulizers.
Dietitian	Develops a diet to ensure adequate hydration and nutrition. Teaches the client and family about an appropriate diet with consideration of risk factors.
Social worker	Coordinates discharge referrals for home care or community-based service with consideration of the client's fatigue, dyspnea, and social support. Makes arrangements for necessary equipment at home. Provides information about agencies such as the American Lung Association.
Registered nurse in charge of health care team communications	Reports evidence of increasing shortness of breath or dyspnea to physician. Discusses client's tolerance to activity with physician and respiratory therapist. Teaches client and family how to avoid upper respiratory tract infections and viruses. Collaborates with respiratory therapist regarding the timing of treatments and the need for postural drainage and/or percussion.

Influenza vaccine is also recommended for high-risk populations. Immunity from influenza vaccine is of shorter duration, because the predominant strain of the virus varies from year to year. A new vaccine formulation is developed yearly, incorporating antigens of the influenza strains predicted to be the most prevalent for the upcoming flu season (typically the winter months). Vulnerable populations for whom yearly vaccine is recommended include those listed above as well as health care workers and residents of long-term care facilities.

Laboratory and Diagnostic Tests

Laboratory and diagnostic testing for people with pneumonia is directed toward establishing a diagnosis, determining the extent of lung involvement, and identifying the causative organism.

The following laboratory studies may be ordered for the client with pneumonia:

- *Sputum gram stain* is ordered to obtain an initial determination of the causative organism and to direct therapy. Sputum culture and sensitivity testing for definitive diagnosis and treatment may not yield results for as long as 24 to 48 hours, and it is important to initiate therapy as soon as possible, especially in the immunocompromised or debilitated client. The gram stain, by contrast, can indicate whether the infecting organisms are gram-positive or gram-negative bacteria within minutes. Antibiotic therapy can then be directed at the predominant type of organism until culture and sensitivity results are obtained.

- *Sputum culture and sensitivity tests* are ordered to identify the infecting organism and determine the most effective antibiotic therapy. When obtaining sputum for culture, it is important to obtain secretions from the lower respiratory tract, not the mouth and nasal passages. See Procedure 34–1 on page 1384.

- *Complete blood count (CBC) with white blood cell (WBC) differential* is performed. In an acute bacterial pneumonia, the WBC is generally elevated to 15,000/mm^3 to 21,000/mm^3. The differential reveals a left shift with increased numbers of immature leukocytes in the circulation, indicating that less mature cells are being released from the bone marrow in response to the infectious process. White blood cell changes are minimal in viral and other pneumonias (Wilson et al., 1991).

- *Arterial blood gases (ABGs)* may be ordered to determine blood oxygen and carbon dioxide levels. Inflammation of the alveoli may interfere with gas exchange across the alveolar-capillary membrane, especially if exudate or consolidation is present. Respiratory secretions or pleuritic pain also can interfere with alveolar ventilation. An arterial oxygen tension (PO_2) of less than 75 to 80 mm Hg and PCO_2 of greater than 45 mm Hg may indicate poor alveolar gas exchange or impaired alveolar ventilation.

- *Pulse oximetry* is a noninvasive method of measuring arterial oxygen saturation. The SaO_2 is the percentage of arterial hemoglobin that is saturated or combined with oxygen; it normally is 95% or higher. An SaO_2 of less than 95% may indicate impaired alveolar gas exchange or ventilation.

Procedure 34–1 Obtaining a Sputum Specimen

SUPPLIES

- Sterile sputum container, specimen cup, or mucus trap
- Mouth care supplies
- Sterile suction kit, if necessary
- Gloves

PREPROCEDURE

If culture and sensitivity testing is to be performed for initial diagnosis, obtain the specimen before initiating oxygen and/or antibiotic therapy; results obtained after therapy has been initiated may not identify the infecting organism. Oxygen therapy also dries mucous membranes, making it more difficult for the client to produce a specimen. Unless otherwise specified, obtain the specimen early in the morning, just after the client awakens. Respiratory secretions tend to pool during sleep; it is easier to obtain a specimen before normal coughing and daily activity has cleared them.

Provide for privacy, and explain the procedure to the client. Emphasize the importance of coughing deeply to obtain sputum from the lower respiratory tract, avoiding expectoration of saliva. Increasing the client's fluid intake prior to obtaining the specimen can help liquefy secretions, making them easier to expectorate.

PROCEDURE

1. Follow universal precautions.
2. Provide or have the client perform mouth care prior to obtaining the specimen to reduce contamination by oral flora.
3. Instruct the client to cough deeply several times, expectorating mucus into container.
4. Close the container securely using aseptic technique.
5. Label the container with the client's name and other identifying data, the time and date, and any special conditions, such as antibiotic or oxygen therapy. Enclose the specimen container in a clean plastic bag, and take it to the laboratory or refrigerate as ordered to preserve the specimen.
6. To obtain a specimen by suctioning:

   - Provide mouth care as indicated above.
   - Obtain a sterile mucus trap. Using aseptic technique, attach the trap to the suction apparatus between the suction catheter and tubing.
   - Preoxygenate the client for suctioning as needed.
   - Perform tracheal suctioning using aseptic technique via either the nasotracheal route, endotracheal tube, or tracheostomy. Lubricate the catheter with sterile normal saline. Apply no suction as the catheter is being inserted into the trachea; apply suction for no longer than 15 seconds.
   - Detach the mucus trap from the suction apparatus; close and label. Clear the suction catheter and tubing with normal saline after removing the mucus trap. Dispose of equipment appropriately.

7. A sputum specimen may also be obtained during bronchoscopy procedure.

POSTPROCEDURE

Provide mouth care as needed for the client. Teach the client the importance of completing all ordered prescriptions for antibiotics to ensure complete eradication of microorganisms. Document the time and date the specimen was obtained, and note its color, consistency, and odor.

- *Blood cultures* may be performed to identify the presence of bacteremia and direct antibiotic therapy. Special precautions are taken in the procedure of drawing blood for culture to ensure no contamination by skin bacteria.

Diagnostic studies that may be ordered for the client with pneumonia include the following:

- *Chest X-ray* is performed to determine the extent and pattern of lung involvement. Fluid, infiltrates, consolidated lung tissue, and atelectasis (areas of alveolar collapse) appear as densities on the film. No special client preparation is required for this study, except removal of all jewelry and clothing from the chest and neck area.
- *Fiberoptic bronchoscopy* may be done to obtain a sputum specimen or remove secretions from the bronchial tree (Figure 34–2). In this procedure, a flexible fiberoptic bronchoscope is inserted through the mouth and larynx into the tracheobronchial tree, allowing direct visualization of tissues and collection of specimens for analysis. Nursing responsibilities related to caring for the client undergoing a bronchoscopy are summarized in the box on page 1386.

Table 34–3   Antibiotic Therapy for Selected Pneumonias

Causative Organism	Antibiotic of Choice	Alternative Antibiotic Therapy
Streptococcus pneumoniae	Penicillin G or V	Ampicillin/amoxicillin, erythromycin, clindamycin, tetracycline, chloramphenicol
Staphylococcus aureus	Penicillinase-resistant penicillin; vancomycin for methicillin-resistant organisms	Cephalosporins, vancomycin, clindamycin; ciprofloxacin, sulfa-trimethoprim
Mycoplasma pneumoniae	Tetracycline, erythromycin	
Klebsiella pneumoniae	Aminoglycoside + ceftazidime, penicillin + vancomycin	Aminoglycoside + 3rd generation cephalosporin, imipenem aztreonam or ciprofloxacin; ceftazidime + piperacillin
Legionella pneumophila	Erythromycin + rifampin	Sulfamethoxazole-trimethoprim + rifampin; doxycycline + rifampin; ciprofloxacin + rifampin
Pneumocystis carinii	Trimethoprim + sulfamethoxazole; trimethoprim + dapsone Prophylaxis: Trimethoprim + sulfamethoxazole	Pentamidine; aerosolized pentamidine

Note: Adapted from *Pocketbook of Infectious Disease Therapy* (pp. 186–187) by J. G. Bartlett, 1991, Baltimore, MD: Williams & Wilkins.

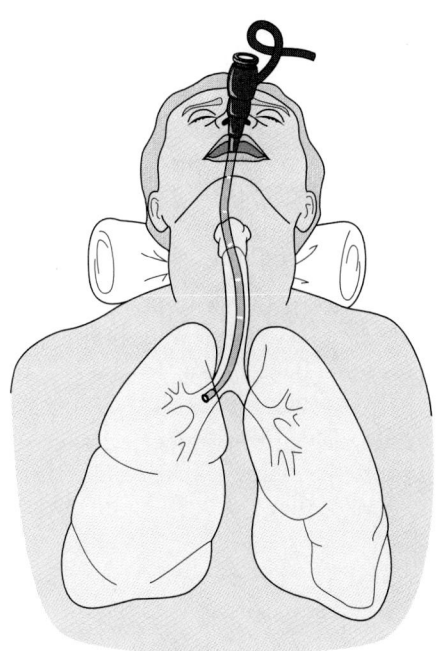

Figure 34–2 Fiberoptic bronchoscopy.

Pharmacology

Medications prescribed for the client with pneumonia may include antibiotics to eradicate the causative organisms and bronchodilators to reduce bronchospasm and facilitate ventilation.

Initial antibiotic therapy is based on the results of sputum gram stain and the pattern of lung involvement shown on the chest X-ray. Typically, a broad-spectrum antibiotic such as a penicillin, cephalosporin, erythromycin, or aminoglycoside is prescribed until the results of sputum culture and sensitivity tests are available (Wilson et al., 1991). Table 34–3 lists commonly prescribed antibiotics for selected pneumonias; nursing implications for these agents are summarized in the pharmacology box on page 257 of Chapter 8.

When a significant inflammatory response results in bronchospasm and constriction, bronchodilators may be ordered to improve ventilation and reduce hypoxia. Bronchodilators generally belong to one of two major groups: the sympathomimetic drugs, such as albuterol sulfate (Proventil) and metaproterenol (Alupent); or the methylxanthines, such as theophylline and aminophylline. The use of these drugs and related nursing implications are discussed in detail in the section on asthma.

An agent to "break up" mucus or reduce its viscosity may be prescribed for the client with pneumonia. Acetylcysteine (Mucomyst), potassium iodide, and guaifenesin (a common ingredient in expectorant cough syrups), all help to liquefy mucus, making it easier to expectorate. For many clients, however, increasing fluid intake is as effective a means of liquefying mucus.

Oxygen Therapy

Oxygen therapy may be indicated for the client with pneumonia if the client is tachypneic or if blood gas measurements reveal hypoxemia (Andreoli et al., 1990).

Inflammation of the alveolar-capillary membrane interferes with the diffusion of gases across the membrane. Diffusion is affected by several other factors, including the partial pressure of the gases. Increasing the percentage of inspired oxygen above that in room air (21%) increases the partial pressure of oxygen in the alveoli and enhances

Nursing Implications for Diagnostic Tests: Bronchoscopy

■ ■ ■

Nursing Responsibilities

- Ensure that the client has signed an informed consent. *Bronchoscopy is an invasive procedure requiring informed consent.*

- Provide and clarify information regarding the procedure, its purpose, and client expectations as needed. Notify the physician if the client needs further explanation. *The fully informed client will be less anxious and better able to cooperate during and after the procedure. If the client's questions and responses indicate a lack of understanding about the procedure and its risks, benefits, and alternatives, it is important to notify the physician because the client has not given true informed consent.*

- Maintain NPO status from midnight or for 6 to 8 hours before the procedure. *Keeping the gastrointestinal tract nearly empty and nondistended reduces the risk of aspiration.*

- Obtain a baseline physical assessment, including vital signs and heart and lung sounds. *Baseline assessment data are used for comparison during the postprocedure period.*

- Provide mouth care just prior to the bronchoscopy. *Mouth care reduces oral microorganisms and the risk of their introduction into the lungs.*

- Remove dentures and partial plates, glasses, and contact lenses, and store them in a safe place. *This helps prevent inadvertent damage to or loss of these items during the bronchoscopy.*

- Administer preprocedure medications as ordered. This may include sedation and local anesthetic preparations. *Medications are used to reduce the client's anxiety and pain perception.*

- Have resuscitation and suction equipment available at the bedside. *Laryngospasm and respiratory distress may occur following the procedure. The anesthetic suppresses the client's cough and gag reflexes, and secretions may be difficult for the client to handle.*

- On completion of the procedure, monitor the client's vital signs and respiratory status closely. *Possible complications of bronchoscopy include laryngospasm, bronchospasm, bronchial perforation with possible pneumothorax or subcutaneous emphysema,* hemorrhage, hypoxia, pneumonia or bacteremia, and cardiac stress *(Chernecky, Krech, & Berger, 1993).*

- Instruct the client not to eat or drink anything for approximately 2 hours, until the effects of the anesthesia have worn off and the cough and gag reflexes have returned. *The client is at high risk for aspiration if oral food or fluids are consumed when cough and gag reflexes are suppressed.*

- Provide an emesis basin and tissues for the client to expectorate sputum and saliva. *Until reflexes have returned, the client may be unable to swallow sputum and saliva safely.*

- Monitor the color and character of respiratory secretions. It is normal for secretions to be tinged with blood for several hours following a bronchoscopy, especially if biopsy has been performed. Notify the physician if sputum is grossly bloody. *Although blood-tinged sputum is an expected finding after bronchoscopy, grossly bloody sputum may indicate a complication.*

- Collect postbronchoscopy sputum specimens for cytologic examination as ordered. *A cytologic examination may be ordered if a tumor is suspected.*

Client and Family Teaching

- Fiberoptic bronchoscopy may be performed either at the bedside, in a special procedure room, or in the surgical suite. It requires approximately 30 to 45 minutes to complete.

- Usually, little pain or discomfort is associated with the procedure, because an anesthetic is given. You will be able to breathe during the bronchoscopy.

- Some hoarseness of the voice is common following the procedure. Throat lozenges or warm saline gargles may help relieve sore throat.

- Fever often develops within the first 24 hours as a result of an inflammatory response to the procedure.

- Persistent cough, bloody or purulent sputum, wheezing, shortness of breath, difficulty breathing, or chest pain may indicate a complication of the procedure. Report these manifestations to the physician.

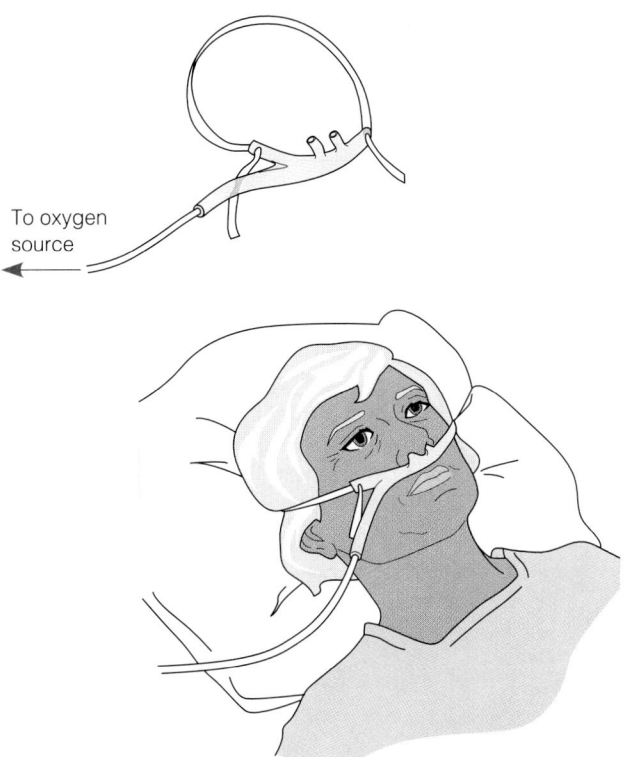

Figure 34–3   Nasal cannula.

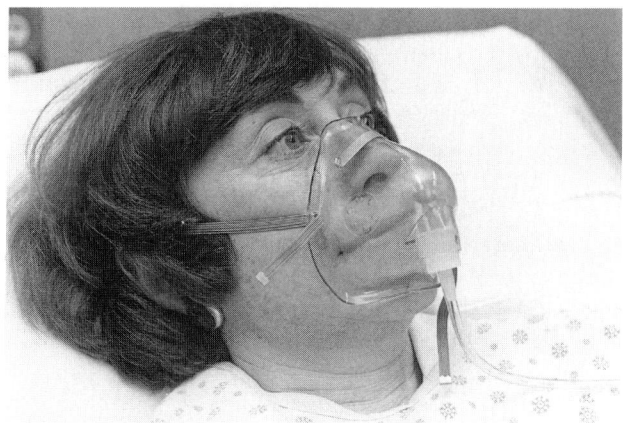

Figure 34–4   Simple face mask.

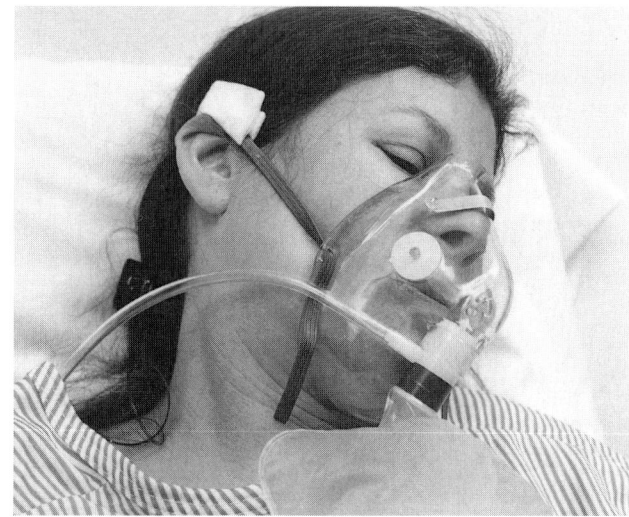

Figure 34–5   Nonrebreather mask.

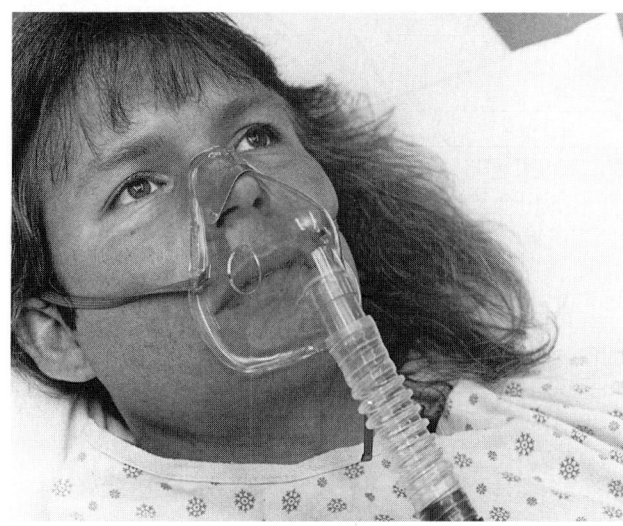

Figure 34–6   Venturi mask.

its diffusion into the capillaries. Thus, administering supplemental oxygen to hypoxemic clients with pneumonia will help improve oxygenation of the blood and tissues.

Depending on the degree of hypoxia, oxygen may be administered to the client by either a low-flow or high-flow system. Low-flow systems that may be used for the adult client with pneumonia include the nasal cannula, simple face mask, partial rebreathing mask, and nonrebreathing mask. The nasal cannula can deliver 24% to 45% oxygen concentration with flow rates of 2 to 6 liters per minute (Figure 34–3). The nasal cannula is comfortable and does not interfere with eating or talking. A simple face mask can deliver 40% to 60% oxygen concentration, with flow rates of 5 to 8 liters per minute (Figure 34–4). Up to 100 percent oxygen can be delivered by the nonrebreather mask, the highest concentration possible by any means other than mechanical ventilation (Figure 34–5). When the amount of oxygen delivered must be precisely regulated, a high-flow system is used. These systems regulate the ratio of oxygen to room air, allowing a measured percentage of oxygen. The Venturi mask is the most common high-flow system used for adult clients who do not need mechanical ventilation (Figure 34–6).

The percentage of oxygen delivered by Venturi mask can be precisely regulated, from 24% to 50%. The severely hypoxic client may require intubation and mechanical ventilation. Endotracheal intubation and methods of mechanical ventilation are discussed in the section on respiratory failure.

Other Therapies

When mucus secretions are thick and viscous or the client has a weak cough, assistive measures may be required. Increasing the client's fluid intake to 2500 to 3000 mL per day will help liquefy secretions, making them easier to cough up and expectorate. If the client is unable to maintain an adequate oral intake, intravenous fluids and nutrition may be required.

Chest physiotherapy, including percussion, vibration, and postural drainage, may be prescribed to reduce lung consolidation and prevent atelectasis. *Percussion* is performed by rhythmically striking or clapping the chest wall with cupped hands (Figure 34–7), using rapid wrist

flexion and extension. Cupping traps air between the palm and the client's skin, setting up vibrations through the chest wall that loosen respiratory secretions. The trapped air also provides a cushion, protecting the client from injury. When performed correctly, percussion produces a hollow, popping sound. Percussion may also be performed using a mechanical percussion cup. The breasts, sternum, spinal column, and kidney areas are avoided during percussion.

Vibration facilitates the movement of secretions into larger airways. It is generally combined with percussion, although it may be used when percussion is contraindicated or poorly tolerated by the client. Vibration is performed by repeatedly tensing the arm and hand muscles while maintaining firm but gentle pressure over the affected area with the flat of the hand (Figure 34–8).

Percussion and vibration are performed in conjunction with postural drainage. *Postural drainage* uses gravity to facilitate the removal of secretions from a particular lung segment. The client is positioned so that the segment to

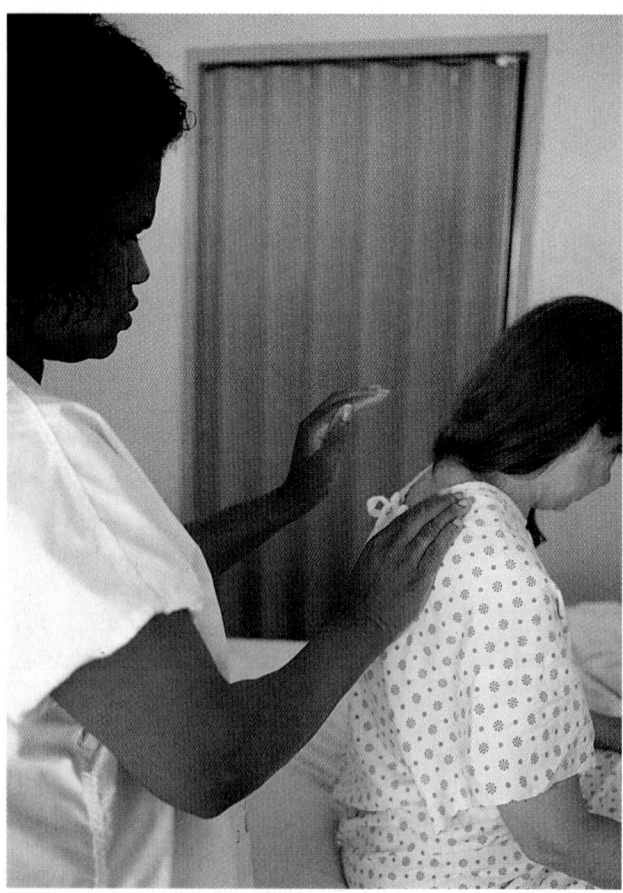

Figure 34–7   Percussing (clapping) the upper posterior chest. Notice the cupped position of the nurse's hands.

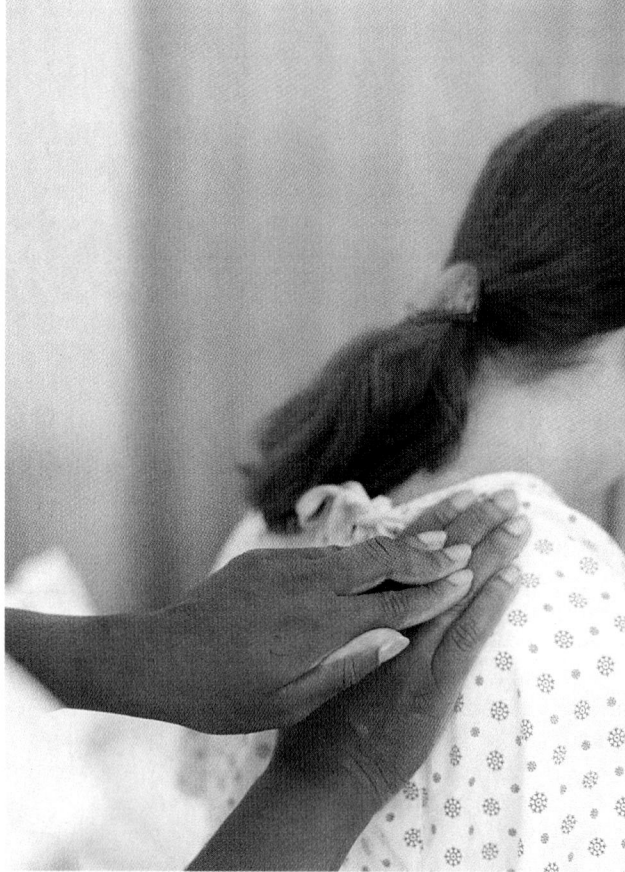

Figure 34–8   Vibrating the upper posterior chest.

be drained is superior to or above the trachea or mainstem bronchus. Drainage of all lung segments requires a variety of positions (Figure 34–9); however, few clients need to have all segments drained or to use all positions. Prior to performing postural drainage, the nurse administers bronchodilator medication or nebulizer treatments. It is best to perform postural drainage before meals to avoid nausea and vomiting.

Endotracheal suctioning may be required if the client is unable to cough effectively. This invasive technique is discussed in the section describing nursing care for the client with acute respiratory failure. On occasion, bron-

choscopy is used to perform pulmonary toilet and remove secretions (Andreoli et al., 1990).

Nursing Care

The client with pneumonia and other diseases or disorders affecting the lower respiratory system has multiple nursing care needs. Any disease affecting the lungs potentially can interfere with alveolar ventilation and the process of alveolar respiration. The end result of impaired ventilation and respiration is *hypoxemia*, low levels of oxygen in the blood, and tissue hypoxia. All body systems

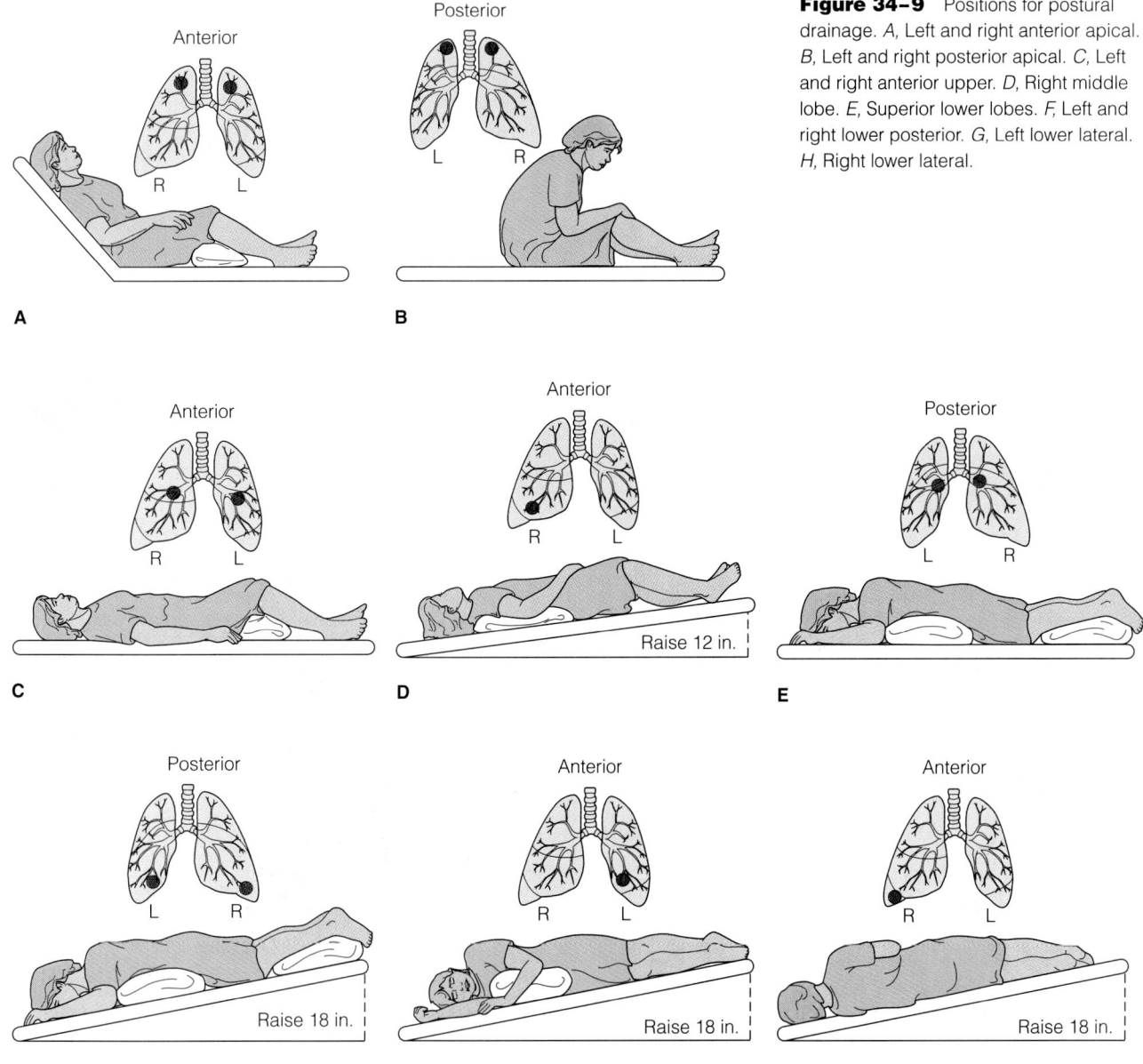

Figure 34–9 Positions for postural drainage. *A*, Left and right anterior apical. *B*, Left and right posterior apical. *C*, Left and right anterior upper. *D*, Right middle lobe. *E*, Superior lower lobes. *F*, Left and right lower posterior. *G*, Left lower lateral. *H*, Right lower lateral.

can be affected. Nursing care therefore is directed toward promoting optimal respiratory function and promoting rest to reduce the client's metabolic and oxygen needs.

In addition, nurses need to be aware of the increased risk for respiratory dysfunction and pneumonia in the older adult. Frequent pulmonary assessment and aggressive interventions will help prevent problems. Restoring and maintaining the older client's mobility will improve ventilation and help mobilize secretions. Promoting an adequate fluid intake liquefies secretions, making them easier to expectorate. A Critical Pathway for the hospitalized client with pneumonia begins on page 1391.

This section focuses on nursing needs related to maintaining clear airways and effective breathing patterns and reducing the body's metabolic demands.

Ineffective Airway Clearance

The body's inflammatory response to an infection leads to tissue edema and the formation of exudate. When this occurs in the lungs, narrowing and potential obstruction of the bronchial passages and alveoli is a possible result. Assessment findings that support this nursing diagnosis for the client with pneumonia include adventitious breath sounds, such as crackles (rales), rhonchi, and wheezes; dyspnea and tachypnea; coughing; and indicators of hypoxia, such as cyanosis, anxiety, and apprehension.

Nursing interventions with rationales follow:

- Assess the client's respiratory status, including vital signs, breath sounds, and skin color at least every 4 hours. *Early identification of beginning respiratory compromise allows intervention before tissue hypoxia is significant.*

- Assess cough and sputum (amount, color, consistency, and possible odor). *These assessments provide information about the effectiveness of respiratory secretion clearance, the infective organism, and the client's response to therapy.*

- Monitor arterial blood gas measurements and pulse oximetry readings; notify the physician of worsening hypoxemia or **hypercapnia,** increased blood levels of carbon dioxide. *Blood gas changes are an early indicator of impaired gas exchange, which may indicate airway narrowing or obstruction.*

- Position the client in Fowler's position. Encourage frequent turning, sitting at the bedside, and ambulation as allowed. *These measures promote lung expansion and facilitate the movement of secretions.*

- Assist the client to cough, deep breathe, and use assistive devices. Provide endotracheal suctioning using aseptic technique as ordered. *Coughing, deep breathing, and suctioning help clear airways.*

- Provide a fluid intake of at least 2500 to 3000 mL per day. *A liberal fluid intake helps liquefy secretions, facilitating their clearance.*

- Work with the physician and respiratory therapist to provide pulmonary hygiene measures, such as postural drainage, percussion, and vibration. *These techniques help mobilize and clear secretions.*

- Administer prescribed medications as ordered, and monitor their effects. *Antibiotic therapy must be tailored to the organism. If the infecting organism is resistant to the prescribed antibiotic, little improvement may be seen in the client's condition. Bronchodilators help maintain open airways but may cause adverse effects, such as anxiety and restlessness.*

- Administer oxygen therapy as ordered. *Oxygen therapy increases the alveolar oxygen concentration and facilitates its diffusion across the alveolar-capillary membrane.*

Ineffective Breathing Pattern

Pleural inflammation often accompanies pneumonia, causing sharp localized pain that increases with deep breathing, coughing, and movement. This can result in a rapid and shallow breathing pattern. Distal airways and alveoli may not expand optimally with each breath, increasing the possibility of atelectasis and decreasing gas exchange. Fatigue from the increased work of breathing is an additional problem for the client with pneumonia. This, too, can lead to decreased lung inflation and an ineffective breathing pattern.

Nursing interventions with rationales follow:

- Assess the client's respiratory rate, depth, and lung sounds every 4 hours or more frequently as indicated. *Tachypnea and diminished or adventitious breath sounds may be early indicators of respiratory compromise. Early intervention can prevent atelectasis and significant tissue hypoxia.*

- Place the client comfortably in an upright or semi-upright position. *This position promotes lung expansion and ventilation as well as comfort.*

- Provide for periods of rest. *Rest is important to reduce fatigue and the work of breathing.*

- Assess and document pleuritic discomfort. Provide analgesics as ordered. *Adequate pain relief minimizes splinting and promotes adequate ventilation.*

- Provide reassurance when the client is experiencing respiratory distress. *Hypoxia and respiratory distress produce high levels of anxiety in the client, which tends to further increase tachypnea and fatigue and decrease ventilation.*

- Administer oxygen as ordered. *Supplemental oxygen reduces hypoxia and associated anxiety.*

- Teach the client to use slow abdominal breathing. *This promotes lung expansion.*

- Teach the client how to use relaxation techniques, such as visualization and meditation. *These techniques help reduce anxiety and slow the client's breathing pattern.*

Text continues on page 1394

Critical Pathway for Client with Pneumonia		
	Date _____ **1st Day**	**Date _____** **2nd Day**	**Date _____** **3rd Day**
Expected length of stay: 5 days			
Daily outcomes	The client will ■ have stable vital signs. ■ verbalize understanding and demonstrate cooperation with turning and splinting. ■ cough and deep breathe purposefully q1–2h during day. ■ have a productive cough. ■ have an intake of 3000 mL/day (IV/PO). ■ verbalize ability to cope.	The client will ■ have stable vital signs and unlabored respirations at rest. ■ verbalize understanding and demonstrate cooperation with turning and splinting. ■ cough and deep breathe purposefully q1–2h during day. ■ have a productive cough. ■ have an intake of 3000 mL/day (IV/PO). ■ verbalize ability to cope.	The client will ■ be afebrile, have stable vital signs and unlabored respirations with activity. ■ verbalize understanding and demonstrate cooperation with turning and splinting. ■ cough and deep breathe purposefully q1–2h during day. ■ have a productive cough. ■ have an intake of 3000 mL/day (PO). ■ verbalize ability to cope. ■ verbalize beginning understanding of home care instructions.
Assessments, tests, and treatments	CBC with differential PA and lateral chest X-ray ABGs Blood culture × 2, if temperature is over 101 Sputum for gram stain and C & S Vital signs and O_2 saturation, q4h if stable Incentive spirometer q2h Nebulizer therapy q4h Chest physical therapy Intake and output every shift Assess respirations and respiratory movements q4h and prn. Encourage coughing and deep breathing q1–2h. Demonstrate effective coughing while splinting client's chest. Position client in semi-Fowler's or high Fowler's position. Assist with postural drainage 3 times daily. Assist with nebulizer treatments.	Vital signs and O_2 saturation, q4h if stable Incentive spirometer q2h Intake and output every shift Assess respirations and respiratory movements q4h and prn. Nebulizer therapy q4h Chest physical therapy Encourage coughing and deep breathing q1–2h. Demonstrate effective coughing while splinting client's chest. Position client in semi-Fowler's or high Fowler's position. Assist with postural drainage 3 times daily. Assist with nebulizer treatments. Maintain oxygen per nasal cannula at 5 liters. Assist with ADLs.	Vital signs and O_2 saturation, q4h if stable Incentive spirometer q2h Intake and output every shift Assess respirations and respiratory movements q4h and prn. Nebulizer therapy q4h Chest physical therapy Encourage coughing and deep breathing q1–2h. Position client in semi-Fowler's or high Fowler's position. Assist with postural drainage 3 times daily. Assist with nebulizer treatments. Maintain oxygen per nasal cannula at 2–5 liters to maintain pulse oximeter at 98%. Assist with ADLs. Check culture and sensitivities.

Critical Pathway for Client with Pneumonia (continued)

	Date _____ 1st Day	Date _____ 2nd Day	Date _____ 3rd Day
Assessments, tests, and treatments *continued*	Maintain oxygen per nasal cannula at 5 liters. Assist with ADLs. Monitor arterial blood gases/pulse oximeter.		
Knowledge deficit	Orient to room and routine. Review plan of care and importance of increased fluids, activity, turning, coughing, deep breathing, and incentive spirometer. Include family in teaching. Assess understanding of teaching.	Review plan of care and continued importance of increased fluids, activity, turning, coughing, deep breathing, and incentive spirometer. Include family in teaching. Assess understanding of teaching.	Reinforce earlier teaching regarding ongoing care. Begin discharge teaching regarding rest, activity, and diet. Include family in teaching. Assess understanding of teaching.
Psycho-social	Assess level of anxiety. Encourage verbalization of concerns. Provide information and ongoing support and encouragement to client and family.	Assess level of anxiety. Encourage verbalization of concerns. Provide information and ongoing support and encouragement to client and family.	Encourage verbalization of concerns. Provide ongoing support and encouragement to client and family.
Diet	Diet as tolerated providing small, frequent, nutritious feedings. Encourage fluid intake of 3000 mL/day.	Diet as tolerated providing small, frequent, nutritious feedings. Encourage fluid intake of 3000 mL/day.	Diet as tolerated providing small, frequent, nutritious feedings. Encourage fluid intake of 3000 mL/day.
Activity	Assess safety needs and provide appropriate precautions. Bathroom privileges with assistance. Provide rest periods.	Maintain safety precautions. Bathroom privileges with assistance Provide rest periods.	Maintain safety precautions. Ambulate 4 to 6 times with assistance. Provide rest periods.
Medications	IV fluids IV antibiotics Bronchodilators Tylenol 650 mg q4h PO for temperature over 101	IV fluids/intermittent IV device IV antibiotics Bronchodilators Tylenol 650 mg q4h PO for temperature over 101	Intermittent IV device — D/C if IV antibiotics D/C. IV/PO antibiotics Bronchodilators Tylenol 650 mg q4h PO for temperature over 101
Transfer/ discharge plans	Establish discharge goals with client and significant other. Consult with social service re: VNA Project home health care needs	Review progress toward discharge goals with client and significant other. Identify potential referrals.	Review progress toward discharge goals with client and significant other.

Critical Pathway for Client with Pneumonia (continued)

	Date _____ 4th Day	Date _____ 5th Day	
Daily outcomes	The client will ■ be afebrile, have stable vital signs and unlabored respirations with activity. ■ verbalize understanding and demonstrate cooperation with turning and splinting. ■ cough and deep breathe purposefully q1–2h during day. ■ have an intake of 3000 mL/day (PO). ■ verbalize ability to cope. ■ verbalize understanding of home care instructions.	The client will ■ be afebrile and have stable vital signs. ■ have unlabored respirations and lungs clear to auscultation. ■ be independent in self-care. ■ be fully ambulatory. ■ resume preadmission urine and bowel elimination pattern. ■ verbalize/demonstrate home care instructions. ■ tolerate usual diet and have an intake of 3000 mL/day. ■ verbalize ability to cope with ongoing stressors.	
Assessments, tests, and treatments	Vital signs and O_2 saturation, q4h if stable Incentive spirometer q2h Intake and output every shift Assess respirations and respiratory movements q4h and prn. Nebulizer therapy q4h Chest physical therapy Encourage coughing and deep breathing q1–2h. Position client in semi-Fowler's or high Fowler's position. Assist with postural drainage 3 times daily. Assist with nebulizer treatments. D/C oxygen if pulse oximeter 98% on room air	Vital signs and O_2 saturation, q4h if stable Incentive spirometer q2h Intake and output every shift Assess respirations and respiratory movements q4h and prn. Nebulizer therapy q4h Chest physical therapy Encourage coughing and deep breathing q1–2h. Position client in semi-Fowler's or high Fowler's position.	
Knowledge deficit	Reinforce earlier teaching regarding ongoing care. Review written discharge instructions with client and significant other. Include family in teaching. Assess understanding of teaching.	Reinforce earlier teaching regarding ongoing care. Complete discharge teaching to include diet, follow-up care, signs and symptoms to report, follow-up MD visit, activity, and medications: name, purpose, dose, frequency, route, dietary interactions, and side effects.	

➤

	Date _____ 4th Day	Date _____ 5th Day	
Knowledge deficit *continued*		Provide client with written discharge instructions. Include family in teaching. Assess understanding of teaching.	
Psycho-social	Encourage verbalization of concerns. Provide ongoing support and encouragement to client and family.	Encourage verbalization of concerns. Provide ongoing support and encouragement to client and family.	
Diet	Diet as tolerated, providing small, frequent, nutritious feedings. Encourage fluid intake of 3000 mL/day.	Diet as tolerated, providing small, frequent, nutritious feedings. Encourage fluid intake of 3000 mL/day.	
Activity	Ambulate independently at least 4 times. Maintain safety precautions.	Fully ambulatory	
Medications	PO antibiotics Bronchodilators Tylenol 650 mg q4h PO for temperature over 101	PO antibiotics Bronchodilators Tylenol 650 mg q4h PO for temperature over 101	
Transfer/discharge plan	Continue to review progress toward discharge goals. Finalize discharge plans.	Finalize plans for home care. Make appropriate referrals. Complete discharge teaching.	

Critical Pathway for Client with Pneumonia (continued)

Activity Intolerance

The client with pneumonia often has impaired gas exchange and other problems that interfere with the supply of oxygen to body cells. At the same time, the infectious process and the body's response to it increase the metabolic demands on the cells. The net result of this imbalance between oxygen delivery and oxygen demand is a lack of physiologic energy to maintain normal daily activities.

Nursing interventions with rationales follow:

- Assess the client's level of activity tolerance, noting any increase in pulse, respirations, dyspnea, diaphoresis, or cyanosis. *These assessment findings may indicate limited or impaired activity tolerance.*

- Assist the client with self-care activities, such as bathing. *Assistance with ADLs reduces the client's energy demands.*

- Schedule activities, planning for rest periods. *Rest periods minimize fatigue and improve activity tolerance.*

- Provide assistive devices, such as an overhead trapeze. *These assistive devices facilitate movement of the client and reduce energy demands.*

- Enlist the help of the family to minimize the client's level of stress and anxiety. *Stress and anxiety increase metabolic demands and can decrease activity tolerance.*

- Perform active or passive range-of-motion (ROM) exercises. *Exercises help maintain muscle tone, joint mobil-*

ity, and prevent contractures for the client on prolonged bed rest.

- Provide emotional support and reassurance that the client's strength and activity level will return to normal when the infectious process has resolved and the balance of oxygen supply and demand is restored. *The client may be concerned that activity intolerance will continue to be a problem after the acute infection is resolved.*

Other Nursing Diagnoses

Although nursing care needs vary from client to client, the following nursing diagnoses also may apply to the client with pneumonia:

- *Anxiety* related to impaired oxygenation
- *Ineffective Airway Clearance* related to mucus secretions
- *Altered Nutrition: Less Than Body Requirements* related to decreased oral intake and increased metabolic needs
- *Hyperthermia* related to infectious process
- *Risk for Noncompliance* with therapeutic regimen related to lack of information

Client and Family Teaching

Health teaching for pneumonia focuses not only on treatment but also on prevention. Make clients who are in high-risk groups aware of the benefits of immunizations against influenza and pneumococcal pneumonia: A single dose of pneumococcus vaccine is usually sufficient to produce immunity to most strains of pneumococcal pneumonia, although repeat doses may be needed for older adults and for people who are immunosuppressed. (Pneumococcus vaccine is contraindicated for people who are receiving immunosuppressive therapy, however.) Influenza vaccine, which needs to be administered yearly, is helpful in preventing pneumonia, because viral infection often precedes pneumonia.

Many clients with pneumonia are managed outside the acute care facility, unless their respiratory status is significantly compromised. Stress the importance of following the prescribed medication regimen and completing the entire prescription. Provide information about side effects and their management and possible hypersensitivity, toxic, and other effects. Teach the client to identify manifestations that necessitate stopping the drug and notifying the physician.

Instruct the client to limit activities and increase rest to conserve energy. Encourage the client to maintain an adequate fluid intake to keep mucus thin for easier expectoration, and explain that small, more frequent meals reduce the energy demand for eating and may be better tolerated. Recommend that the client and household members avoid smoking to prevent further irritation of the lungs and airway.

When pneumonia is managed at home, monitoring the effectiveness of therapy will fall to the client and family. Increasing shortness of breath, difficulty breathing, temperature, fatigue, headache, sleepiness, or confusion may indicate worsening condition and must be reported to the physician. Stress to the client the importance of keeping all follow-up appointments to ensure cure of the disease.

When the client is hospitalized, teaching for both the client and family focuses on medications, procedures, and equipment used in providing care. Teaching helps alleviate anxiety and thereby promotes rest. Teaching also promotes the client's cooperation and sense of control.

Applying the Nursing Process

Case Study of a Client with Pneumonia: Mary O'Neal

Mary O'Neal is a 35-year-old executive assistant who is attending college part-time in the evenings. She lives in a suburban area with her husband and two school-age children. On returning home from class one evening, she begins to feel a chill, as if she would never get warm. She alternates between chills and sweats all night. Staying home from work, she remains in bed most of the next day. Her fever continues, and she develops a cough and dull aching chest pain. When the cough becomes productive of rust-colored sputum the following day, she seeks medical treatment from her family doctor.

Assessment

Debby Kowalski, the family practice clinic nurse, admits Mrs. O'Neal to the clinic and performs an initial nursing assessment. Ms. Kowalski notes that Mrs. O'Neal describes herself as "Generally very healthy—sometimes I wish I could get sick for a day off!" She denies any previous history of respiratory diseases "other than the usual colds, flu, and such." She also denies any history of smoking or medication allergies. She says her symptoms had begun abruptly with the onset of the chills. She describes her chest pain as a dull ache that was initially located in the substernal area but that now seems to be localized in her lower lateral right chest. The pain increases with deep breathing, coughing, and moving. Her cough is increasing in frequency and severity, and her sputum appears rusty brown. Her vital signs are as follows: BP, 116/74; P, 104 and regular; R, 26; T 101.8 F (38.7 C). Her skin is warm and flushed, with no evidence of cyanosis.

On examination, Ms. Kowalski notes that Mrs. O'Neal's respirations are shallow and that her respiratory excursion is equal. She has faint but clear breath sounds throughout the anterior chest and upper posterior lung fields. Breath sounds in the lower posterior fields are diminished, and crackles are present in the right posterior and lateral base. A faint pleural rub is also present at the right midaxillary line. No other abnormal findings are noted in the examination. A STAT blood count shows a WBC count of 18,900/mm^3; differential shows a shift to the left. Ms. Kowalski has Mrs. O'Neal rinse her mouth with an antiseptic mouthwash and collect a sputum specimen for culture and gram stain prior to seeing the physician.

The physician orders a chest X-ray after examining Mrs. O'Neal. Based on her history, the examination, and the appearance of the chest X-ray, he makes the diagnosis of acute bacterial pneumonia, probably pneumococcal. Because Mrs. O'Neal shows no evidence of respiratory compromise at this time, he prescribes penicillin V, 500 mg to be administered orally every 6 hours for 10 days. He asks Mrs. O'Neal to return for a follow-up appointment in 10 days and sends her back to Ms. Kowalski for appropriate teaching.

Diagnosis

Ms. Kowalski develops the following nursing diagnoses for Mrs. O'Neal:

- *Ineffective Breathing Pattern* related to pleuritic chest pain
- *Hyperthermia* related to inflammatory process
- *Knowledge Deficit* about pneumonia and its treatment

Expected Outcomes

The expected outcomes established in the plan of care specify that Mrs. O'Neal will:

- Maintain normal pulmonary function.
- Be able to describe measures to minimize elevations in body temperature.
- Identify a schedule for taking her medication that will facilitate compliance with the regimen.
- Describe manifestations that should be reported to the physician.

Planning and Implementation

Ms. Kowalski plans and implements the following interventions for Mrs. O'Neal prior to her discharge from the family practice clinic:

- Assess the client's knowledge and understanding of pneumonia and its effects.
- Work with Mrs. O'Neal to develop a medication schedule that coincides with her normal daily routine.
- Teach about the following:
  a. Why it is important not to use a cough suppressant except at night to facilitate rest
  b. How increasing fluid intake will help reduce fever and keep the mucus liquid so that it can be expectorated easily

  c. The beneficial effects of rest, especially during the acute phase of her illness
  d. The safe use of aspirin and acetaminophen to reduce fever
  e. The importance of taking all prescribed medication doses on the prescribed schedule
  f. Common side effects of penicillin V and their management
  g. Early manifestations of penicillin allergy that necessitate stopping the medication and notifying the physician
  h. Signs of complications of pneumonia or worsening pneumonia to report

Evaluation

The sputum culture results confirm that *S. pneumoniae* is the cause of Mrs. O'Neal's pneumonia. When she returns for her follow-up visit at the clinic, she reports that she had begun to feel better after 2 days on the penicillin and returned to work the following Monday. Her examination reveals good breath sounds throughout with no adventitious sounds, and the follow-up sputum culture is free of pathogens. Mrs. O'Neal and Ms. Kowalski discuss the potential benefits of pneumococcal and influenza vaccine, but Mrs. O'Neal decides to wait until October to be immunized.

Critical Thinking in the Nursing Process

1. Are there any factors identified in the case study that increased Mrs. O'Neal's risk for acute bacterial pneumonia?

2. Mrs. O'Neal's WBC differential showed a shift to the left. Define what the term "left shift" means, and describe the process that causes it.

3. Even though Mrs. O'Neal had no history of medication allergies, anaphylactic shock is a potential risk for any client receiving penicillin. Describe the sequence of events leading to anaphylactic shock, its initial symptoms, and immediate nursing interventions.

4. Had Mrs. O'Neal required hospitalization to treat her acute pneumococcal pneumonia, interruption of her usual activities and responsibilities could lead to anxiety. Develop a care plan for this situation, using the nursing diagnosis *Altered Role Performance* related to hospitalization.

The Client with Lung Abscess

■ ■ ■

A **lung abscess** is a localized area of lung destruction or necrosis and pus formation. Although lung abscess can result from many causes, the most common cause is aspiration and resulting pneumonia (Way, 1994). Disorders that predispose the client to aspiration increase the risk of lung abscess. Altered levels of consciousness due to anesthesia, injury or disease of the central nervous system, seizure, excessive sedation, or alcohol abuse are major risk factors for lung abscess. Other risk factors include swallowing disorders, dental caries, and debilitation secondary to cancer or chronic disease. Lung abscess also may occur as a complication of some types of pneumonia, including those due to *Staphylococcus aureus, Klebsiella,* and *Legionella.*

A lung abscess forms after lung tissue becomes consolidated (that is, after alveoli become filled with fluid, pus, and microorganisms). Consolidated tissue becomes necrotic. This necrotic process can spread to involve the entire bronchopulmonary segment and progress proximally until it ruptures into a bronchus. With rupture, the contents of the abscess empty into the bronchus, leaving a cavity filled with air and fluid, a process known as *cavitation.* If the client is unable to expectorate the purulent material from the abscess, the infection may spread, leading to diffuse pneumonia or a syndrome similar to adult respiratory distress syndrome (ARDS, discussed later in this chapter).

Manifestations of lung abscess typically occur about 2 weeks after the precipitating event (aspiration, pneumonia, and so on). Their onset may be either acute or insidious. Early manifestations are those of pneumonia: productive cough, chills and fever, pleuritic chest pain, malaise, and anorexia. The temperature may be significantly elevated, 103 F (39.4 C) or higher. When the abscess ruptures, the client may expectorate large amounts of foul-smelling, purulent, and possibly blood-streaked sputum. Breath sounds are diminished, and crackles may be noted in the region of the abscess. A dull percussion tone is also present.

The diagnosis of lung abscess usually is based on the client's history and presentation. The CBC may indicate leukocytosis. Sputum culture may not show the organism involved unless rupture occurs. Chest X-ray may reveal a thick-walled, solitary cavity with surrounding consolidation; it can be difficult to differentiate lung abscess from consolidation until cavitation occurs, however.

Lung abscess is treated with antibiotic therapy, usually intravenous penicillin G or clindamycin (Cleocin), a broad-spectrum antibiotic with a wide range of activity against both aerobic and anaerobic bacteria. Postural drainage may be ordered to relieve obstruction and promote drainage. In some cases, bronchoscopy is used to drain the abscess. If the pleural space becomes involved, a chest tube (tube thoracostomy) may be used to drain the abscess. See the section on pneumothorax for further discussion of chest tubes.

Although most clients with lung abscess recover fully with appropriate antibiotic treatment, rupture and drainage of the abscess into a bronchus is a frightening experience. Nursing care needs of the client relate pri-marily to maintaining a patent airway and adequate gas exchange. The following nursing diagnoses may be appropriate for the client with lung abscess:

- *Risk for Ineffective Airway Clearance* related to large amounts of purulent drainage in bronchi
- *Impaired Gas Exchange* related to necrotic and consolidated lung tissue
- *Risk for Infection* related to the presence of pathogens in pulmonary system
- *Anxiety* related to copious amounts of purulent sputum

Teaching for the client with a lung abscess and his or her family focuses primarily on the importance of completing the prescribed antibiotic therapy. Most lung abscesses are successfully treated with antibiotics; however, treatment may last up to one month or more. The client must understand the need to complete the treatment prescribed in order to eliminate the infecting organisms. Teach the client about the medication, including its name, dose, desired, and adverse effects. Stress the need to contact the physician if symptoms do not improve or if they become worse: Infection from lung abscess can spread not only to lung and pleural tissue but also via the blood, causing systemic sepsis. If postural drainage is prescribed, teach the client and family members how to perform this procedure. When procedures such as bronchoscopy or thoracostomy are performed to drain the abscess, provide preoperative teaching as well as instruction on postoperative care.

The Client with Tuberculosis

■ ■ ■

Tuberculosis (TB) is a chronic, recurrent infectious disease that usually affects the lungs, although any organ can be affected. In 1989, the CDC announced a strategic plan to eliminate tuberculosis by the year 2010. Tuberculosis, caused by *Mycobacterium tuberculosis,* was at that time a disease that had almost been eradicated, its incidence having fallen to a low of 22,000 cases in the United States in 1985. Today, however, the picture is dramatically different: Approximately 27,000 new cases were reported in 1991; 1700 people died of tuberculosis in the United States that same year. It is estimated that by the year 2000, nearly 50,000 new cases will emerge in the United States each year. In New York City alone, the number of new cases is close to 4000 per year. Worldwide, tuberculosis kills between 2 and 3 million people yearly, and at least 10 million develop new active pulmonary disease (CDC, 1993a; DiFerdinando, 1993; Fein & Adler, 1993).

Tuberculosis today is primarily a disease of racial and ethnic minorities, the poor, and the homeless—the very

---

Applying Research to Nursing Practice: Screening for Tuberculosis in Older Adults

▪ ▪ ▪

Residents of long-term care facilities are at particular risk for tuberculosis. Primary disease that has long been quiescent can become active as the aging process and chronic diseases impair immune function and the body's ability to ward off infection. The older adult may not demonstrate the weight loss, productive cough, hemoptysis, anorexia, and evening temperatures that are typical of active tuberculosis: Changes in functional status and other nonspecific symptoms may be the only or predominant manifestations of disease.

A screening program to identify residents who are resistant to tuberculosis and those who are susceptible is vital in the prevention of outbreaks. In a study conducted in one long-term care facility, a protocol of screening all new residents and staff for tuberculosis both on entry into the facility and once a year thereafter was found to be effective in identifying new cases and preventing outbreaks (Wright & Staats, 1992).

All residents and staff were retested during the same week of the year. To track the findings, results were kept in a card file as well as in the medical record. Because the absence of immune system response to an antigen is not unusual in the older adult, even when antibodies have been previously formed, new residents with negative test results were retested within a 1- to-

2-week period. On retesting, 38% showed a positive result.

Implications for Nursing

When an older client is being tested, a negative result from a single PPD or Mantoux test may not be an accurate indicator of the client's immune response and tuberculosis status. This suggests that hospital and community screening programs should adopt a protocol of retesting older adults with negative test results.

Critical Thinking in Client Care

1. Why do older adults often demonstrate nonspecific manifestations, such as behavior changes, when tuberculosis infection is present?

2. Why is the older adult at risk for reactivation of tuberculosis? How does secondary tuberculosis differ from primary?

3. Why is the older adult more likely to demonstrate *anergy* (diminished reactivity to a specific antigen) than a younger adult?

4. Develop a teaching plan for a nursing assistant who requires prophylactic tuberculosis therapy for exposure and new conversion to a positive tuberculin test.

---

groups who are most likely to use the emergency department for primary care and who are most difficult to reach for preventive and continuing care. Although the incidence of tuberculosis continues to drop in non-Hispanic whites, Native Americans, and Alaska natives, it increased by 72% in Hispanic populations, 26% in non-Hispanic blacks, and 32% in Asian/Pacific islanders in 1991 (DiFerdinando, 1993). Poor urban areas are hit the hardest—areas that are also affected by the epidemics of injection drug use, homelessness, malnutrition, and poor living conditions. Overcrowded institutions also contribute to the spread of TB; transmission in hospitals, homeless shelters, drug treatment centers, prisons, and residential facilities has been documented. People with altered immune function, including older clients (see the accompanying research box and the gerontology box on page 1399) and people with AIDS are at particular risk for tuberculosis. In addition to increasing numbers of susceptible people, many strains of the infecting organism have developed resistance to available antimicrobials, contributing to the spread of the epidemic (Davidson, DiFerdinando, Reichman, & Snider, 1992; Fein & Adler, 1993).

M. tuberculosis is a relatively slow-growing, slender, rod-shaped, acid-fast organism with a waxy outer capsule which increases its resistance to destruction. Although the lungs are most often infected, tuberculosis can involve other organs as well (Porth, 1994). It is transmitted by *droplet nuclei*, airborne droplets produced when an infected person coughs, sneezes, speaks, or sings. Infection may occur when a susceptible host breathes in air containing droplet nuclei and the contaminated particle eludes the normal defenses of the upper respiratory tract to reach the alveoli.

A number of factors affect the risk for infection: characteristics of the infectious person; the amount of air contamination; the duration of exposure; and the susceptibility of the host. The number of microbes in the sputum, frequency and force of coughing, and client behaviors (such as covering the mouth when coughing) affect the production of droplet nuclei. In a small, closed, or poorly ventilated environment, droplet nuclei become more concentrated, increasing the risk of exposure. When contact is prolonged, as for people living in the same household, the risk increases. Less-than-optimal immune function, a problem for people in lower socioeconomic groups, injec-

Gerontologic Considerations: Care of the Older Adult Client with Tuberculosis

■ ■ ■

Up to 30% of all newly diagnosed tuberculosis cases occur among people over 65 years of age. Of these cases, approximately 90% occur due to reactivation of the dormant bacterium. Older adults are at increased risk for reactivation of tuberculosis due to age-related decreases in cell-mediated immunity. Chronic illnesses, poor nutrition, gastrectomy, alcoholism, or the long-term use of steroids and immunosuppressive agents may also reactivate dormant TB lesions.

Presenting symptoms of tuberculosis in the older adult are often vague. Older adults with tuberculosis may experience coughing, weight loss, anorexia, or periodic fevers. These signs and symptoms should not be dismissed as a normal part of aging.

Older adult residents in nursing homes are at increased risk for acquiring tuberculosis because of group living. Yearly tuberculin skin testing with purified protein derivative (PPD) is recommended and is often required by state health departments. If the older adult tests negative, a repeat PPD in 1 to 2 weeks is recommended. This improves sensitivity to the test so that silent cases of tuberculosis are not missed. A chest X-ray and sputum culture for acid-fast bacilli should be part of the diagnostic work-up for the older client with a positive PPD.

Successful treatment for tuberculosis includes taking at least two drugs to which the organisms are susceptible. The medications must be taken for at least 6 to 9 months to totally eradicate the organism. Older adults usually do not present with drug-resistant forms of tuberculosis, because they acquired the disease prior to the emergence of the drug resistant strains.

Older adults need to be educated about the anti-tuberculin drugs that are prescribed to them. Pyridoxine (Vitamin B6), may be given along with Isoniazid (INH), to minimize the side effect of peripheral neuropathy that may occur. Older adults taking INH are at greater risk for drug-induced hepatitis. They should be taught not to drink alcohol while taking INH. Rifampin, another drug that is used to treat tuberculosis, may also cause hepatitis. This drug may cause the saliva and urine to change to an orange-red color. Streptomycin may cause changes in hearing and balance that may be irreversible in the older adult. Streptomycin should be used with caution in older adults. If it is used, the client should be monitored closely for these side effects. Ethambutol, another drug used to treat tuberculosis, may cause loss of color discrimination (red-green) and decreased vision.

The older adult with active tuberculosis must be followed by a physician until the disease is resolved. Monthly sputum cultures are done until they are negative. While taking anti-tuberculin medications, clients will be monitored monthly for drug toxicity. Chest X-rays will be taken periodically during and following treatment.

Older adults with tuberculosis should be educated to follow instructions given by their health care provider, particularly those related to following their medical regime. Specific teaching for the older adult with tuberculosis includes:

- Keep all appointments with your physician.

- Do not stop taking the medication without first consulting your physician.

- Report medication side effects to your physician.

- To promote healing, eat a well-balanced diet with adequate fluids.

- Avoid exposure to people with infectious diseases.

- Get adequate rest and sleep.

---

tion drug users, the homeless, alcoholics, and people with HIV infection, increases the susceptibility of the host (DiFerdinando, 1993).

Pathophysiology

Pulmonary Tuberculosis

Minute droplet nuclei containing one to three bacilli that succeed in gaining entry to the lungs implant in an alveolus or respiratory bronchiole, usually in an upper lobe. As the bacteria multiply, they spread through the lymphatic system to regional lymph nodes, the bloodstream, and throughout the body, stimulating an immune response. Systemic and local inflammatory responses bring neutrophils and macrophages to the site of infection. These cells phagocytize and isolate the bacteria but cannot destroy them. A granulomatous lesion called a *tubercle* or *Ghon focus,* a sealed-off colony of bacilli, is formed. Within the tubercle, infected tissue dies, forming a cheese-like center, a process called caseation necrosis. Caseous granulomas may also form in lymph nodes of the affected lung. A combination of a primary lung lesion and lymph node granulomas is called *Ghon's complex.*

If the immune response is adequate, scar tissue develops around the tubercle, and the bacilli remain encapsu-

---

Clinical Manifestations of Pulmonary Tuberculosis

- Fatigue
- Weight loss
- Anorexia
- Low-grade afternoon fever and night sweats
- Cough: initially dry, later productive of purulent and/or blood-tinged sputum

---

lated. These lesions eventually calcify and are visible on X-ray. When the immune response is insufficient to contain the disease, primary tuberculosis can progress, causing extensive destruction of lung tissue. In *primary progressive tuberculosis,* granulomatous tissue may erode into a bronchus or into a blood vessel, allowing the disease to spread throughout the lung, to other organs, and to other people. A previously healed lesion also may be reactivated. This is known as *reactivation tuberculosis,* and it occurs when the immune system is suppressed as a result of age, disease, or the use of corticosteroids or other immunosuppressive agents. Fortunately, only about 5% of infected people develop active primary disease, and another 5% develop reactivation tuberculosis at a later time (DiFerdinando, 1993; McCance & Huether, 1994; Porth, 1994). The pathogenesis of tuberculosis is illustrated in Figure 34–10.

Clients infected with HIV are at high risk for developing clinically active tuberculosis, as a result of either primary infection or reactivation of latent disease. Fifty percent of HIV-infected people who contract TB will develop active disease within 60 days, in contrast to the usual rate of about 5% of people in 1 to 2 years (Berkow & Fletcher, 1992).

The inflammatory response evoked by the initial infection causes few symptoms and typically goes unnoticed until a positive response is noted on a tuberculin test or calcified lesions are visible on chest X-ray.

Clinical manifestations of primary progressive or reactivation tuberculosis often develop insidiously and are initially nonspecific (see the accompanying box). Fatigue, weight loss, anorexia, low-grade afternoon fever, and night sweats are common manifestations. A cough develops, which is dry initially and later becomes productive of purulent and/or blood-tinged sputum. It is often at this stage that the client seeks medical attention.

Tuberculosis empyema and bronchopleural fistula are the most serious complications of pulmonary tuberculosis. When a tuberculosis lesion containing bronchi ruptures, massive contamination of the pleural space and pneumothorax occurs as air enters the pleural space from the lung. This significant event requires prompt treatment to preserve respiratory function (Berkow & Fletcher, 1992).

Extrapulmonary Tuberculosis

Organs other than the lungs can become seeded by *M. tuberculosis* during a period of silent bacteremia that follows initial invasion of the lung. These distant metastases may produce an active lesion, or they may become dormant and reactivate at a later time. Extrapulmonary tuberculosis is especially prevalent in HIV-infected people. The skin, bones and joints, the gastrointestinal tract, or liver can be infected. Tuberculosis peritonitis or tuberculosis percarditis may develop.

Miliary Tuberculosis *Miliary tuberculosis* results when the primary tuberculosis lesion erodes into a blood vessel and the bacilli spread via the bloodstream throughout the body. The client generally presents with manifestations of chills and fever, weakness, malaise, and progressive dyspnea. Multiple lesions evenly distributed throughout the lungs are noted on X-ray; however, these characteristic findings may not be evident for several weeks. The sputum rarely contains organisms. The bone marrow is usually involved, leading to anemia, thrombocytopenia, and leukocytosis. Unless miliary tuberculosis is properly treated, the prognosis is poor.

Genitourinary Tuberculosis The kidney and genitourinary tract are common sites for extrapulmonary tuberculosis. The organism spreads to the kidney via the blood from the primary lesion in the lungs. An inflammatory process similar to that which occurs in the lungs serves to isolate the organism. Reactivation can occur at a later time, often years after the original infection. The small focus lesion may then enlarge and caseate, destroying a large portion of the renal parenchyma and eventually ulcerating into the renal calyces or pelvis. From the kidney, the infection can spread to involve other parts of the urinary tract, including the ureters and bladder. Scarring and strictures commonly result. In men, the prostate, seminal vesicles, and epididymis may be involved. In women, tuberculosis may affect the uterine tubes and ovaries.

Manifestations of genitourinary tuberculosis usually have an insidious onset. The client may have symptoms of a urinary tract infection, including malaise, dysuria, hematuria, and pyuria. Flank pain may be present. Men may have manifestations of epididymitis or prostatitis: perineal, sacral, or scrotal pain and tenderness; difficulty voiding; and fever. Women may have manifestations of pelvic inflammatory disease, impaired fertility, or ectopic pregnancy.

Tuberculosis Meningitis Tuberculosis meningitis results when tuberculosis spreads to the subarachnoid

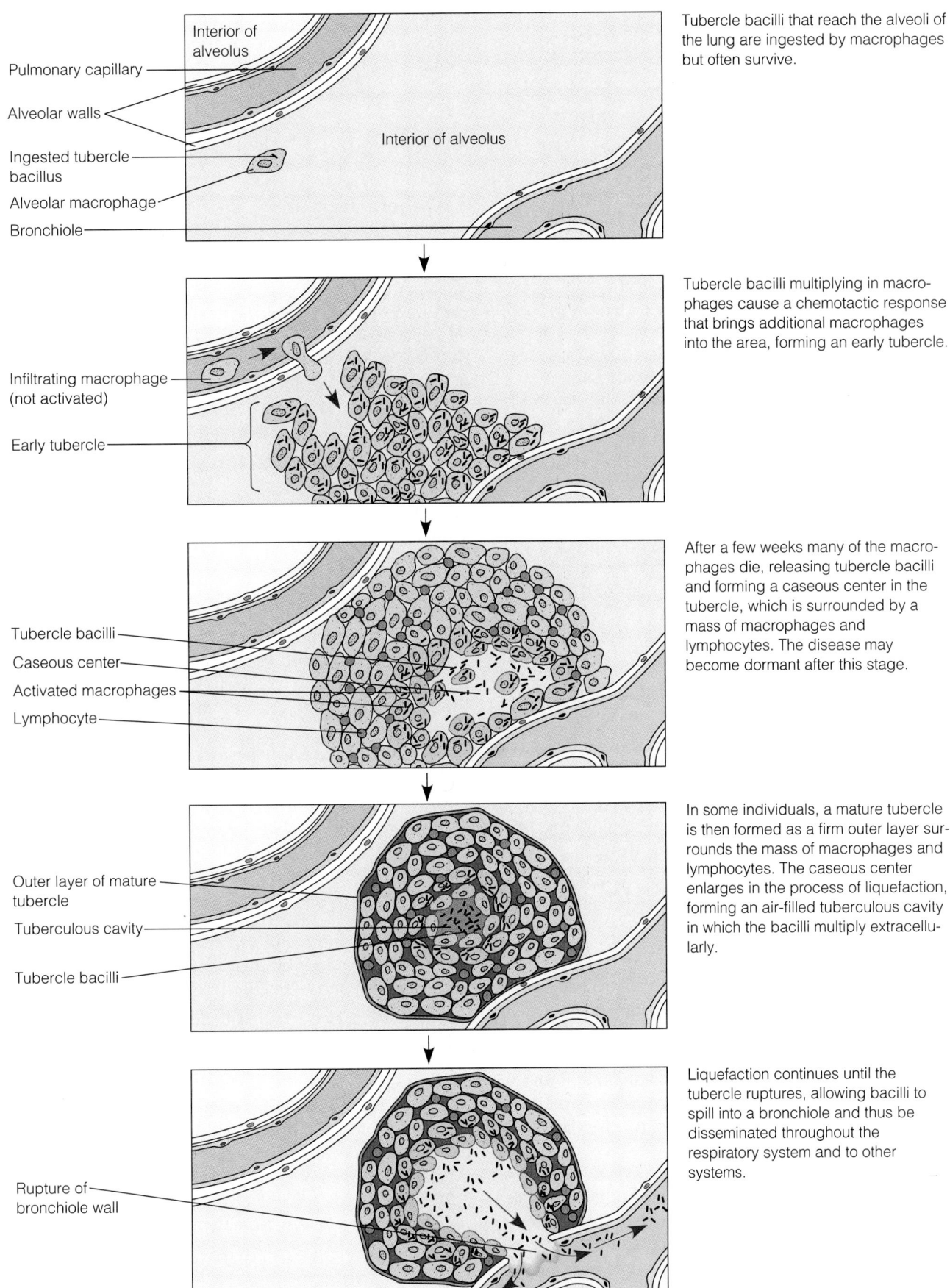

Tubercle bacilli that reach the alveoli of the lung are ingested by macrophages but often survive.

Interior of alveolus

Pulmonary capillary

Alveolar walls

Ingested tubercle bacillus

Alveolar macrophage

Bronchiole

Interior of alveolus

Tubercle bacilli multiplying in macrophages cause a chemotactic response that brings additional macrophages into the area, forming an early tubercle.

Infiltrating macrophage (not activated)

Early tubercle

After a few weeks many of the macrophages die, releasing tubercle bacilli and forming a caseous center in the tubercle, which is surrounded by a mass of macrophages and lymphocytes. The disease may become dormant after this stage.

Tubercle bacilli

Caseous center

Activated macrophages

Lymphocyte

In some individuals, a mature tubercle is then formed as a firm outer layer surrounds the mass of macrophages and lymphocytes. The caseous center enlarges in the process of liquefaction, forming an air-filled tuberculous cavity in which the bacilli multiply extracellularly.

Outer layer of mature tubercle

Tuberculous cavity

Tubercle bacilli

Liquefaction continues until the tubercle ruptures, allowing bacilli to spill into a bronchiole and thus be disseminated throughout the respiratory system and to other systems.

Rupture of bronchiole wall

Figure 34–10   The pathogenesis of tuberculosis.

Table 34–4	Interpreting Tuberculin Test Results
Area of Induration	**Significance**
Less than 5 mm	Negative response; however, does not rule out infection.
5 to 9 mm	Positive for people who: ■ Are in close contact with a client with infective TB. ■ Have an abnormal chest X-ray. ■ Have HIV infection. Negative for all others.
10 to 15 mm	Positive for people who have other risk factors: ■ Birth in a high-incidence country ■ Low socioeconomic status ■ African American, Hispanic, Asian American in poverty areas ■ Injection drug use ■ Residence in a long-term care facility ■ Identified local risk factors
Greater than 15 mm	Positive for all people

Note. Adapted from "Tuberculosis: An Epidemic Reemerges, 2. Current Diagnostic and Treatment Strategies" (pp. 159, 163–164, 167–168) by L. Raju, 1993, *Emergency Medicine, 25*(2).

space. In the United States, this complication occurs most often in older adults, usually from reactivation of a previously healed primary lesion. The onset of tuberculosis meningitis is usually gradual. Initial manifestations include listlessness, irritability, anorexia, and fever. Headache and behavior changes are common early manifestations in the older adult (Tierney et al., 1994). As the disease progresses, the client develops a severe, constant headache; vomiting; and a decreasing level of consciousness. Convulsions and coma may follow. Without appropriate treatment, neurologic effects may become permanent.

Skeletal Tuberculosis Tuberculosis of the bones and joints is most likely to occur when the primary disease is contracted during childhood, when bone epiphyses are open and their blood supply is rich (Berkow & Fletcher, 1992). The organisms spread via the blood to vertebrae, the ends of long bones, and joints. As with other forms of tuberculosis, the immune and inflammatory processes serve to isolate the bacilli, and the disease often becomes evident years or decades later.

Skeletal tuberculosis may present in several forms. Tuberculous spondylitis, or Pott's disease (tuberculosis of the spine), usually involves the thoracic vertebrae, causing erosion of the vertebral bodies and vertebral collapse. Significant kyphosis develops, and compression of the spinal cord may lead to paraplegia.

The large, weight-bearing joints, such as the hips and knees, are most often affected by tuberculous arthritis. Other joints, such as the wrist, hand, and elbow may be affected, particularly if they have been previously damaged by trauma. The joint is painful and warm and tender to the touch.

Collaborative Care

Tuberculosis was a major public health concern earlier in this century, before the development of effective pharmacologic treatment. It is reemerging as a potentially significant threat to public health. The development of drug-resistant strains, its prevalence in HIV-infected populations, and lack of adequate access to health care for high-risk populations all contribute to the reemergence of tuberculosis as a significant public health issue. Collaborative care, therefore, is directed toward the following:

- Early detection
- Accurate diagnosis
- Effective treatment of the disease
- Prevention of the spread of the disease to others

Clients with active tuberculosis rarely require hospitalization for treatment of the disease. With appropriate treatment, they become noninfective to others fairly rapidly. When a client with tuberculosis is hospitalized, respiratory isolation should be maintained to minimize the risk of infection to other clients and to the health care workers.

Noncompliance with the prescribed treatment regimen is a major problem in treating active tuberculosis: The client can continue to transmit the disease to others, and drug-resistant strains of bacteria often develop when treatment is incomplete. Continuing contact with clients who have active TB is vital to ensure effective cure. Tuberculosis is a disease that must be reported to local and state public health departments; the client's contacts are then identified and examined. People who share living or work environments with the client should receive testing and prophylactic treatment. The public health department may also assume responsibility for follow-up care of the infected client.

Screening Methods
The tuberculin test is used to screen for tuberculosis infection. People who are exposed to the tubercle bacillus develop a cellular, or delayed hypersensitivity, response to the bacillus within 3 to 10 weeks after the infection. Injection of a small amount of purified protein derivative (PPD) of tuberculin any time thereafter will activate this response, attracting macrophages to the area and resulting in a pronounced local inflammatory response. The amount of induration surrounding the injection site is

used to determine infection (see Table 34–4 and Figure 34–11). It is important to remember that a positive response indicates that the client has been infected and has developed antibodies to the tubercle bacillus; it does not mean that the client has active disease or is currently infectious.

Several methods are currently available for tuberculin testing:

- *Intradermal PPD (Mantoux) test:* 0.1 mL of PPD (5 tuberculin units, or TU) is injected intradermally into the dorsal aspect of the forearm. This test is read during peak reaction period, that is, within 48 to 72 hours, and recorded as the diameter of induration (raised area, not erythema) in millimeters.

- *Jet injection tuberculin test:* 5 TU of PPD is injected intradermally by high pressure or jet injection. The results are read and interpreted like the Mantoux test.

- *Multiple-puncture (tine) test:* A multiple-puncture device is used to introduce tuberculin into the skin. This test is less accurate than other testing methods. A vesicular reaction is considered positive; any other reaction must be confirmed using a Mantoux test (Porth, 1994; Price & Wilson, 1992).

Although it is impractical and unnecessary to screen the entire population, the CDC recommend screening for people in any of the following risk groups (Davidson et al., 1992):

- People with or at high risk for HIV infection

- Close contacts of people who have or are suspected of having infectious TB

- People with medical risk factors, such as silicosis, chronic malabsorption problems, end-stage renal failure, diabetes mellitus, immunosuppression, and hematologic and other malignancies

- People born in countries with a high prevalence of TB

- Low-income populations who are medically underserved, including racial and ethnic minorities

- Alcoholics and injection drug users

- Residents and staff of long-term residential facilities, such as long-term care facilities, correctional institutions, and mental health facilities

Laboratory and Diagnostic Tests

A positive tuberculin test alone does not indicate active disease. Sputum tests for the presence of the bacillus and chest X-rays are routinely used to diagnose and evaluate active disease.

Laboratory testing includes a series of three consecutive early morning sputum specimens sent for acid-fast bacilli smear and culture (see Procedure 34–1 on page 1384). *M. tuberculosis* resists decolorizing chemicals after staining. This property is called "acid-fast" (Chernecky et

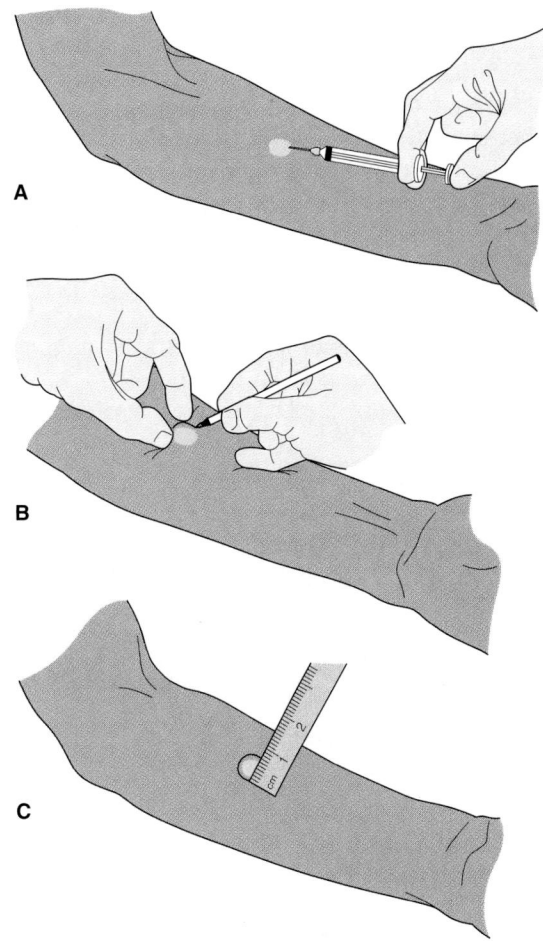

Figure 34–11   *A,* Intradermal injection for tuberculin testing. *B,* The injection causes a local inflammatory response (wheal). *C,* Measurement of induration following tuberculin testing.

al., 1993). The acid-fast smear provides a rapid indicator of the presence of the tubercle bacillus.

A culture positive for *M. tuberculosis* provides the definitive diagnosis of TB. However, the tubercle bacillus is slow-growing, and even newer culture methods require 10 or more days to obtain results. Once the organism has been cultured, drug sensitivity testing is performed to determine any resistance.

When obtaining sputum specimens from a client with suspected tuberculosis, it is important to use special procedures or personal protective devices. If possible, collect the specimens in a room equipped with air flow control devices such as fans or air filters, with ultraviolet light, or a combination of these. Alternatively, have the client step outside to collect the specimen (Raju, 1993). If this is not possible, wear a special mask capable of filtering droplet nuclei when collecting sputum specimens outside the above situations.

Aerosol therapy, chest clapping, and postural drainage may be helpful for the client who has difficulty producing a sputum specimen. For some clients, endotracheal suctioning may be necessary to obtain a culture.

Other laboratory studies that may be ordered include liver function testing if a hepatotoxic agent such as isoniazid (INH) is to be used to treat TB.

Diagnostic tests ordered for the client with suspected TB may include the following:

- *Chest X-ray* is a standard procedure used to diagnose and evaluate TB. Abnormalities typical of pulmonary TB include dense lesions in the apical and posterior segments of the upper lobe and possible cavity formation.

- *Fiberoptic bronchoscopy and bronchial washing* may be used to obtain culture specimens for the client who is unable to produce adequate sputum. In this procedure, the client's oropharynx is anesthetized, and a bronchoscope inserted through the larynx into the trachea and bronchial tree to visualize the tissues directly. When the scope has been inserted as far into the bronchiole as possible, sterile saline is instilled to "wash out" the alveoli, removed by suctioning, and sent for culture and cytologic examination. This procedure is helpful when the client is unable to obtain deep sputum specimens (Chernecky et al., 1993). Nursing care for the client undergoing bronchoscopy is outlined in the box on page 1386.

- *A thorough vision examination* will be ordered if the client is to be treated with ethambutol, a commonly used antituberculosis medication. Optic neuritis is an important potential adverse effect of this drug. A baseline vision evaluation is performed before therapy is initiated, and periodic examinations are conducted during the course of therapy.

- *Audiometric examination* is performed before streptomycin therapy is initiated. Ototoxicity is a significant adverse effect of streptomycin and other aminoglycoside antibiotics. The client's hearing is evaluated before the medication is started and periodically during the course of therapy. Tones are presented to the client's ear and vibrations through the bone to measure the frequencies the client is able to hear. With this method, the amount and type of any hearing loss can be determined (Chernecky et al., 1993).

Pharmacology

Chemotherapeutic medications are used both to prevent and treat tuberculosis infection. Goals for the pharmacologic treatment of TB are to

- Make the disease noncommunicable to other people.

- Reduce the symptoms of the disease.

- Effect a cure in the shortest possible time.

Prophylactic treatment is used to prevent the development of active tuberculosis. Clients demonstrating a recent skin test conversion from negative to positive are often started on prophylactic therapy, especially when other risk factors, such as HIV infection, age, chronic diseases, or close household contact with a person whose sputum is positive for bacilli, are present. Single-drug therapy is effective for prophylactic treatment, whereas treatment of active disease always involves two or more chemotherapeutic medications. For adults, isoniazid (INH), 300 mg per day for a period of 6 to 9 months, is commonly used to prevent active TB (Berkow & Fletcher, 1992).

When isoniazid prophylaxis cannot be used, bacilli Calmette-Guérin (BCG) vaccine may be prescribed. This vaccine, which is widely used in developing countries, is made from an attenuated strain of *M. bovis,* a closely related bacillus that causes tuberculosis in cattle. In the United States, BCG vaccine is used for people with a negative tuberculin test who are repeatedly exposed to untreated or ineffectively treated people with active disease (Berkow & Fletcher, 1992; Tierney et al., 1994).

The tuberculosis bacillus mutates readily to drug-resistant forms when only one anti-infective agent is used. Clients with active tuberculosis disease are *always* treated with concurrent use of at least two antibacterial medications to which the organism is sensitive. The primary antituberculosis drugs can prevent the development of resistance because all act by different mechanisms. However, the organism is protected within poorly vascularized lesions, and prolonged therapy of 6 to 9 months or more is necessary to eradicate it. For the client with HIV infection, therapy is continued for as long as the client can tolerate it (Berkow & Fletcher, 1992; Shlafer, 1993; Spencer et al., 1993).

In the United States, the newly diagnosed client with tuberculosis is started on three antitubercular drugs, isoniazid (INH), rifampin, and pyrazinamide, for the first 2 months of treatment. All these drugs are given orally on a daily basis. This initial regimen is followed by at least 4 additional months of therapy with isoniazid and rifampin, administered daily or twice weekly. Clients with HIV infection are continued on all three initial agents for 9 months or more (Davidson et al., 1992; Raju, 1993). The antituberculosis drugs most often used today are outlined in Table 34–5, and their nursing implications are discussed in the pharmacology box on page 1406.

If a drug-resistant strain is suspected, therapy is tailored to the resistance. In some cases, four or more anti-infective drugs may be used.

Antitubercular medications have many adverse and toxic effects; close monitoring of the client while therapy is continued is therefore necessary. Most of the medications have some degree of, or risk for, hepatotoxicity. For this reason, clients need to be cautioned not to use alcohol while taking these drugs and to avoid exposure to

Table 34–5	Antituberculosis Medications	
Drug and Dosage	**Adverse Effects**	**Nursing Implications**
Isoniazid (INH), oral: 300 mg daily or 900 mg twice weekly	Peripheral neuropathy Liver impairment	Administer pyridoxine (vitamin B_6) concurrently. Monitor liver function studies (AST and ALT); avoid other hepatotoxins.
Rifampin (RMP), oral: 600 mg daily or twice weekly	Hepatotoxicity Flulike syndrome; fever Colors body fluids—including sweat, urine, saliva, tears, and cerebrospinal fluid (CSF)— orange-red	As for INH. Do not miss or skip doses; flulike syndrome and fever occur when drug is resumed. Contact lenses may become discolored and should not be worn.
Pyrazinamide (PZA), oral: 15 to 30 mg/kg, up to 2 g daily; or 30 to 70 mg/kg twice weekly	Hyperuricemia Hepatotoxicity	Monitor uric acid levels. Monitor AST and ALT; avoid other hepatotoxins.
Ethambutol (EMB), oral: 15 to 25 mg/kg, up to 2.5 g daily; or 50 mg/kg twice weekly	Optic neuritis	Monitor red-green color discrimination and visual acuity.
Streptomycin (SM), intramuscular: 15 mg/kg, up to 1 g daily; or 25 to 30 mg/kg twice weekly	Ototoxicity Nephrotoxicity	Have periodic audiometric examinations conducted. Monitor renal function studies, including BUN and serum creatinine.

other potentially toxic chemicals. Baseline liver and renal function studies are done prior to initiating therapy. Audiometric testing may also be done before therapy is started or early in the course of therapy, because several commonly used medications can affect the ear. Although follow-up diagnostic and laboratory tests are not typically done on a routine basis, during visits to the health care facility the client is questioned carefully about manifestations of adverse effects. Further studies are then ordered if warranted. Although none of these drugs have been proved to be teratogenic, potential adverse effects on the fetus are weighed against the benefit to the mother before they are prescribed during pregnancy.

Compliance with the prescribed regimen also is evaluated during follow-up visits. The urine can be examined for color changes characteristic of rifampin and tested for metabolites of INH. When compliance is a problem, medications are administered under direct supervision. Twice-weekly therapy is more cost-effective in this instance, with a public health nurse watching the client take and swallow the prescribed medication.

Sputum specimens and chest X-rays are used to evaluate the effectiveness of therapy. In most clients, the sputum becomes negative for the tubercle bacillus within 3 months after the initiation of therapy. If this does not happen, reassessment of the sensitivity of the organism is necessary. Chest X-rays are performed monthly for the first 2 or 3 months and at the end of treatment. The final

X-ray serves as a baseline for comparison with future films (Raju, 1993).

Surgery
Surgical resection of infected lung tissue was a common treatment for tuberculosis earlier in the 20th century but is rarely employed today. Surgery may be indicated to remove a portion of lung when the disease is localized or cavitation has occurred and the infecting bacilli are resistant to several drugs (Berkow & Fletcher, 1992; Davidson et al., 1992). Care of the client having lung surgery is discussed in the section on lung cancer.

Nursing Care

Tuberculosis is a disease that today presents a greater threat to public health than it does to the individual. When the prescribed treatment regimen is adhered to, more than 90% of clients demonstrate negative sputum for the bacillus within 3 months (Raju, 1993). With current therapy, the relapse rate is less than 5%, and the principal cause of treatment failure is noncompliance (Tierney et al., 1994).

Nurses play a key role in maintaining public health. Documented outbreaks of drug-resistant tuberculosis in large cities and among people with HIV infection indicate that nursing care must focus primarily on infection control and compliance with prescribed treatment.

Nursing Implications for Pharmacology: The Client with Tuberculosis

ISONIAZID (INH, LANIAZID, NYDRAZID)

Isoniazid is the drug of choice for tuberculosis prophylaxis and a first-line drug in treatment of active disease. It is effective against both intracellular and extracellular organisms. Isoniazid is used alone as a prophylactic medication and in combination with rifampin, ethambutol, or both. A fixed-dose combination form with 150 mg of INH and 300 mg of rifampin (Rifamate) is available as well.

Nursing Responsibilities

- Administer isoniazid on an empty stomach 1 hour before or 2 hours after meals for maximal effect if tolerated by the client; INH may be given with meals to reduce gastrointestinal side effects.
- Monitor the client for adverse effects:
  a. Numbness and tingling of the extremities (most likely to occur in clients who are malnourished, alcoholic, or diabetic)
  b. Hepatotoxicity, as evidenced by abnormal liver function studies and scleral jaundice
  c. Hypersensitivity reactions, such as rash, drug fever, or evidence of anemia, bruising, bleeding, or infection related to agranulocytosis
- Isoniazid interferes with the metabolism of diazepam (Valium), phenytoin (Dilantin), and carbamazepine. Doses of these drugs may need to be reduced to prevent toxicity.

Client and Family Teaching

- Take the medication as prescribed for the entire duration of therapy to prevent incomplete eradication of the bacteria and development of resistant strains.
- Take the medication on an empty stomach. If this causes nausea and vomiting, take the medication with meals.
- If anorexia, nausea, vomiting, and jaundice (yellowing of the skin and the whites of the eyes) develop, notify the physician immediately.
- While taking INH, take pyridoxine as prescribed to prevent peripheral neuropathy.

- While taking INH, avoid alcohol and other agents that may be harmful to the liver.
- Notify the physician if signs of an allergic reaction, such as rash, fever, easy bruising, bleeding gums, or fatigue, develop.
- Use appropriate measures to prevent pregnancy while taking INH; this drug may be harmful to the developing fetus.

RIFAMPIN (RIFADIN, RIMACTANE)

Rifampin is another first-line antituberculosis agent that is commonly used in combination with INH and other antitubercular drugs. It is relatively low in toxicity, although it can cause hepatitis, a flulike immune response, and, rarely, renal failure. Rifampin stimulates the microsomal enzymes of the liver, increasing the rate of metabolism of many drugs and decreasing their effectiveness.

Nursing Responsibilities

- Administer rifampin on an empty stomach.
- Monitor CBC, liver function studies, and renal function studies for evidence of toxic effect.
- Rifampin reduces the effect of oral contraceptives, quinidine, corticosteroids, warfarin, methadone, digoxin, and hypoglycemics. Monitor the client for the effectiveness of these drugs.

Client and Family Teaching

- Rifampin causes body fluids, including sweat, urine, saliva, and tears, to turn red-orange. This is not harmful. Avoid wearing soft contact lenses while taking the drug because they may be permanently stained.
- Aspirin may interfere with the absorption of rifampin and should not be taken concurrently.
- Fever, flulike symptoms, excessive fatigue, sore throat, or unusual bleeding may indicate an adverse or allergic reaction to the drug and should be reported to the physician.

Knowledge Deficit

The client with tuberculosis needs adequate knowledge and information to manage the disease and prevent its transmission to others. It is vital that the client understand the reasons for prolonged drug therapy and the importance of complying with the regimen and follow-up. Antituberculosis drugs are relatively toxic, and the client needs to know what can be done to minimize this toxicity.

Nursing interventions with rationales follow:

Pharmacology: The Client with Tuberculosis (continued)

PYRAZINAMIDE (TEBRAZID)

Pyrazinamide typically is given with INH and rifampin for the first 2 months of tuberculosis treatment. Often, the concurrent use of pyrazinamide allows the course of therapy to be shortened to a total of 6 months rather than 12 to 18 months, as was once common. As with many of the antitubercular agents, pyrazinamide is toxic to the liver. Its other principal adverse effect is hyperuricemia. Gout, however, rarely results from the hyperuricemia.

Nursing Responsibilities

- Administer pyrazinamide with meals to reduce gastrointestinal side effects.
- Monitor liver function studies and serum uric acid levels. Notify the physician if changes are noted.

Client and Family Teaching

- Notify the physician if loss of appetite, nausea, vomiting, jaundice, or symptoms of gout (a painful, red, hot, swollen joint, often the great toe or elbow) develop.
- While taking this drug, avoid the use of alcohol or other substances that may be harmful to the liver.

ETHAMBUTOL (MYAMBUTOL)

Ethambutol is added to the initial treatment regimen or substituted for INH when an INH-resistant strain of TB is suspected. Ethambutol is a bacteriostatic drug that reduces the development of resistance to the bactericidal first-line agents. Its principal toxic effect is optic neuritis; fortunately, this is reversible. Early signs of optic neuritis include decreased visual acuity and loss of red-green discrimination. This drug may be safe for use in pregnancy.

Nursing Responsibilities

- Record a baseline visual examination prior to initiating therapy. Schedule periodic eye exams during the course of treatment.
- Administer ethambutol with meals to reduce gastrointestinal side effects.

- Monitor liver and renal function studies and neurologic status while the client is taking this drug. Notify the physician of abnormal findings or significant changes.

Client and Family Teaching

- Monitor vision daily by reading newspapers and looking at the same blue object (while using usual corrective lenses, if appropriate). Notify the physician if changes in vision or color perception occur.

STREPTOMYCIN

A member of the aminoglycoside class of antibiotics, streptomycin is highly effective in treating most mycobacterial infections, although resistance may develop if it is used alone. There are two primary drawbacks to streptomycin: (1) It must be administered parenterally because it is not absorbed in the gastrointestinal tract, and (2) it has toxic effects on the kidneys and ears.

Nursing Responsibilities

- Administer streptomycin by deep intramuscular injection into a large muscle mass, rotating sites to minimize tissue trauma.
- Monitor urine output, daily weight, and renal function studies (including BUN and serum creatinine) to detect early signs of nephrotoxicity. Report significant changes to the physician.
- Maintain the client's fluid intake at 2000 to 3000 mL per day to minimize the concentration of drug in the kidney tubules.
- Assess the client's hearing and balance frequently. Have audiometric testing performed as indicated.

Client and Family Teaching

- Maintain a daily fluid intake of at least 2½ to 3 quarts.
- Weigh yourself on the same scale at least twice a week, and report any significant weight gain to the physician.
- Notify the physician if hearing acuity decreases, ringing or buzzing sensations in the ear develop, or dizziness occurs.

- Assess the client's level of knowledge about the disease process; identify misperceptions and emotional reactions. *Basing teaching on previous learning enhances understanding and retention of information.*

- Assess the client's ability to learn and interest in learning, developmental levels, and obstacles to learning. *Assessment allows the nurse to present information in a manner that is tailored to the learning needs and style of the client. This will promote learning.*

- Identify the client's support systems, and include significant others in teaching. *Including significant others in the teaching will promote the client's understanding and retention of information, because the client has another person with whom to confirm his or her understanding. This person can also provide reinforcement and encouragement to the client.*

- Establish a relationship of mutual trust with the client and significant others. *An atmosphere of trust increases the client's receptiveness to teaching.*

- Develop mutually acceptable learning goals with the client and significant other. *Working with the client to identify learning needs and establish goals increases the client's "ownership" and interest in the process.*

- Select teaching strategies that are appropriate for the individual client. Use learning aids such as literature and visual materials that are appropriate for the client's age, level of education, and intellect. *Teaching that is tailored to the client is more effective and results in better learning.*

- Teach the client about tuberculosis and the prescribed treatment, including the following:
  a. Nature of the disease
  b. Purpose of treatment and follow-up procedures
  c. Respiratory isolation and its purpose
  d. Importance of maintaining good general health by eating a well-balanced, high-protein, high-carbohydrate diet, balancing exercise with rest, and avoiding crowds and people with upper respiratory infections
  e. Names, doses, purposes, and side effects of the prescribed medications
  f. Importance of avoiding alcohol and other substances that may damage the liver while taking chemotherapeutic drugs
  g. Fluid intake needs of 2½ to 3 quarts of fluid per day
  h. Prevention of the spread of disease to others
  i. Manifestations to report to the physician: chest pain, hemoptysis, or difficulty breathing; anorexia, nausea, or vomiting; yellow tint to skin or sclera; sudden weight gain, swollen feet, ankles, legs, or hands; hearing loss, tinnitus, or vertigo; change in vision or difficulty discriminating colors
  Tuberculosis is a chronic disease requiring lengthy treatment with antitubercular medications. The client with a good understanding of the disease, the prescribed treatment, and potential adverse effects of therapy is better prepared to manage his or her own care.

- Document teaching and the client's level of understanding. Provide reinforcement of information and learning as needed. *Until the client has demonstrated that he or she has learned the information, teaching is not complete.*

Ineffective Individual Therapeutic Regimen Management

The populations at highest risk for developing active tuberculosis—people with AIDS, the homeless, members of lower socioeconomic groups—are also at highest risk for being unable to manage the complex treatment regimen prescribed. The client is placed on three or more costly medications that may have unpleasant or even dangerous side effects. Frequent medical follow-up is required. The client feels the stigma of having an infectious disease and may wish to deny its seriousness. Clients who are alcoholics or injection drug users need to cope with withdrawal from their addiction to be successful in treating their disease. The client with HIV infection is facing a fatal disease and costly treatment that may well override concerns about tuberculosis management.

Nursing interventions with rationales follow:

- Assess the client's self-care abilities and support systems. *This assessment is necessary to develop an initial determination of the client's ability to follow the prescribed regimen.*

- Assess the client's level of knowledge and understanding of the disease, its complications, its treatment, and risks to others. Provide additional teaching and reinforcement as indicated. *A lack of understanding of tuberculosis and its risks presents a barrier to compliance with and management of the treatment regimen.*

- Work with the client to identify barriers or obstacles to managing the prescribed treatment. *In working together to identify potential problems, the nurse and the client gain insight into ways in which these barriers can be overcome.*

- Assist the client and significant others to develop a plan for managing the prescribed regimen. *Having the client develop a plan for implementation increases the sense of control and ownership and helps ensure that personal, cultural, and life-style factors are considered. This increases the likelihood of compliance.*

- In addition to verbal instructions, provide written instructions that are clearly written at the client's level of literacy, knowledge, and understanding. *Clearly written directions provide support and reinforcement for the client.*

- Make referrals as appropriate:
  a. Smoking cessation clinics or support groups
  b. Alcohol treatment facilities, Alcoholics Anonymous, other treatment programs or support groups
  c. Drug treatment facilities, Narcotics Anonymous, other outpatient or inpatient treatment programs or support groups
  d. Hospice or residential care facilities, support groups for people with AIDS (PWAs) or family members of PWAs

Counseling, support groups, and other community resources provide additional assistance and support for the client in managing the disease and its treatment.

■ Provide active intervention for homeless people, including shelter placement or other housing and ongoing follow-up by easily accessed health care providers (clinics and public health workers in the neighborhood that do not present transportation or access problems, either real or perceived). *Simple referral will not assure compliance, especially among disenfranchised populations. Active intervention is needed to make it possible for clients to comply with treatment.*

■ Refer clients who are unlikely to comply with the treatment regimen to the public health department for management and follow-up. *Because tuberculosis, especially multiple-drug-resistant TB, presents a significant public health risk, public health follow-up is essential. In some cases, it is necessary for nurses to administer the client's medication, watching them swallow all pills.*

Risk for Infection

The spread of tuberculosis is a risk in any facility housing many people. It is especially high in residential care facilities for older clients and for people with AIDS. With the disease's increasing incidence in homeless people and members of lower socioeconomic groups, the risk in hospitals, emergency departments, and public and urgent care clinics is growing. Because this disease is spread by microscopic airborne droplets, nurses need to use respiratory precautions to prevent its spread to other clients and to protect themselves.

Nursing interventions with rationales follow:

■ Place the client in a private room with air flow control that prevents air within the room from circulating into the hallway or other rooms. A negative flow room in which air is diluted by at least six fresh-air exchanges per hour is recommended. *A negative flow room and multiple fresh-air exchanges dilute the concentration of droplet nuclei within the room and prevent their spread to adjacent areas (Adler, 1993).*

■ Use universal precautions and tuberculosis isolation techniques as recommended by the CDC, including wearing masks and gowns when caring for clients who do not reliably cover the mouth when coughing. *These measures are important to prevent the spread of tuberculosis to others.*

■ Use personal protective devices to reduce the risk of transmission during client care. The Occupational Safety and Health Administration (OSHA), requires use of a HEPA-filtered respirator for protection against occupational exposure to tuberculosis. *Surgical masks are ineffective to filter droplet nuclei, necessitating the use of protective devices capable of filtering bacteria and particles smaller than 1 micron.*

■ Inform the client about the reasons for and importance of carrying out respiratory isolation procedures during initial hospitalization. For the client who was treated as an outpatient, provide instruction about avoiding crowds and close physical contact and maintaining ventilation in living facilities, particularly during the first 3 weeks of treatment. *These measures help protect others during initial treatment, when sputum is still likely to contain bacilli.*

■ Place a mask on the client when transporting the client to other parts of the facility for diagnostic or treatment procedures. *Covering the client's mouth during transport minimizes air contamination and the risk to visitors and personnel.*

■ Inform all personnel having contact with the client of the diagnosis. *This allows personnel to take appropriate precautions.*

■ Assist visitors to mask prior to entering the client's room. *Providing visitors with appropriate masks or respirators reduces their risk of infection.*

■ Teach the client about measures to limit the transmission of bacilli to others:
   a. Always cough and expectorate into tissues.
   b. Dispose of tissues properly, placing them in a closed bag. The client should dispose of tissues personally to avoid placing other people at risk.
   c. If the client is sneezing or otherwise unable to control respiratory secretions, he or she should wear a mask.
   d. Inanimate objects are not an important means of spread for tuberculosis, so no special precautions are required for eating utensils, clothing, books, or other objects that the client uses.
   Teaching appropriate precautions helps prevent the spread of tuberculosis to others while allowing the client as much freedom from restraints as possible.

■ Teach the client how to collect sputum specimens. If necessary, have the client step outside to collect a sputum specimen. *This minimizes the risk of exposure to health care personnel and provides for rapid dilution of any droplet nuclei produced and their exposure to ultraviolet light (which kills the bacteria).*

■ Teach the client about the importance of complying with prescribed treatment for the entire course of the regimen. *It is important that the client complete the entire course of therapy to reduce the risk of relapse and the creation of drug-resistant organisms.*

Other Nursing Diagnoses

Other nursing diagnoses which may be applicable for the client with active tuberculosis follow:

- *Activity Intolerance* related to tuberculosis pneumonitis
- *Ineffective Airway Clearance* related to mucopurulent secretions
- *Altered Nutrition: Less Than Body Requirements* related to anorexia and other effects of the disease
- *Risk for Noncompliance* related to lack of understanding

Client and Family Teaching

The increasing prevalence of multiple-drug-resistant strains of tuberculosis makes the disease a significant public health problem, especially for immunocompromised people, health care workers, prison guards, and other high-risk populations. This threat heightens the need for better public education and teaching of infected people.

Public health teaching includes increasing the public's awareness of tuberculosis as a reemerging threat among all populations, especially those who are at high risk. People need to know how to reduce the spread of TB by covering their mouths when coughing or sneezing and disposing of sputum appropriately. Because the client with tuberculosis is often infective for a prolonged period before the disease is diagnosed, these measures should be taught to all people. The benefit of screening programs to identify infected (though not necessarily *infective*) people also needs to be included in public health education.

Clients with TB and their families need teaching that will enhance their willingness and ability to comply with treatment. Teach them not only the means to prevent disease transmission to loved ones but also the importance of screening close contacts for infection and possibly prophylactic treatment. Explain the effect, dose, and timing for all medications, and potential side effects and their management. The client needs to understand the importance of long-term therapy in eradicating the disease.

Teach principles of good nutrition and provide dietary guidelines for a client with TB. In addition, introduce the client to other measures that help maintain good health, such as balancing rest with exercise.

Applying the Nursing Process

Case Study of a Client with Tuberculosis: Harry Facée

Harry Facée, a 53-year-old man, arrives at a public health clinic in a large metropolitan city. He complains of aching chest pain that has lasted for the past few days and says that now the sputum he is bringing up with coughing is bloody. He is afraid he might have lung cancer, so he feels he should see a doctor.

Assessment

Raj Kamil, the public health nurse at the clinic, obtains an admission history and conducts a physical examination of Mr. Facée. Mr. Kamil notes in his assessment that Mr. Facée is a homeless person who has lived on the streets and in various shelters for the past "10 years or so." He usually prefers to sleep outdoors, taking refuge in shelters only during very cold or very wet weather. He has a small disability income but usually scrounges for food or eats with other homeless people at soup kitchens.

On further questioning about his symptoms, Mr. Facée states that he has had a cough for a long time and has noticed that it has become worse recently and has become productive, especially in the mornings. He had thought little about it, attributing it to his homeless life-style. Mr. Facée also admits that he has recently been waking up drenched with sweat in the middle of the night and is more fatigued than usual. Mr. Facée's vital signs are as follows: BP, 152/86; P, 92; R, 20; and T, 100.2 F (37.8 C).

Although Mr. Facée's clothes are tattered, he appears fairly clean. He answers questions appropriately and intelligently. Mr. Kamil does not detect any odor of alcohol on Mr. Facée's breath. He appears very thin, almost emaciated. Other examination findings are essentially normal. Suspecting tuberculosis, Mr. Kamil has Mr. Facée obtain a sputum specimen for gram stain and culture, administers a tuberculin test, and sends him for a chest X-ray before Mr. Facée sees the clinic physician. Although the chest X-ray is inconclusive, the gram stain is positive for acid-fast bacillus, and the diagnosis of probable active pulmonary tuberculosis is made. The physician prescribes isoniazid, 300 mg orally; rifampin, 600 mg orally; and pyrazinamide, 1500 mg orally daily for 2 months, to be followed by twice weekly isoniazid 900 mg orally and rifampin 600 mg orally. The physician also orders weekly sputum cultures for the first month.

Diagnosis

Mr. Kamil develops the following nursing diagnoses for Harry Facée:

- *Altered Health Maintenance* related to homelessness
- *Risk for Noncompliance* with prescribed treatment related to lack of understanding and resources
- *Altered Nutrition: Less Than Body Requirements* related to increased metabolic needs associated with infection
- *Risk for Sensory-Perceptual Alteration: Kinesthetic* related to effects of isoniazid therapy

Expected Outcomes

The expected outcomes established in the plan of care specify that Mr. Facée will

- Keep all follow-up appointments as scheduled.

- Verbalize an understanding of his disease and its treatment.
- Follow the prescribed plan of care.
- Demonstrate measures to prevent bacterial spread to others.
- Gain 1 to 2 lbs of weight per week.
- Report promptly any symptoms of peripheral neuropathy, including numbness, tingling, or burning sensations

Planning and Implementation

Mr. Kamil plans the following interventions for Harry Facée to be initiated prior to his discharge from the clinic and continued during follow-up visits:

- Teach Mr. Facée about tuberculosis, and provide him with a client-education pamphlet about the disease.
- Instruct Mr. Facée in the prescribed medications, their possible adverse effects, and the importance of completing the entire prescribed regimen.
- Emphasize the importance of continued follow-up.
- Teach and demonstrate sputum and droplet control measures.
- Take Mr. Facée to the local incentive shelter program for directly observed medical therapy and meals.
- Identify verbally and in writing manifestations that Mr. Facée should report to the physician.

Evaluation

Mr. Kamil is successful in enrolling Harry Facée in the local incentive shelter program. In this program, a health care worker administers Mr. Facée's medications daily, watching him swallow them. He is assigned a small individual room and is able to eat all three daily meals at the shelter. He still prefers to sleep outside when the weather permits, but he complies with the requirement for supervised medication administration because he "likes the food there." Always a clean person, Mr. Facée is able to demonstrate appropriate sputum control measures and practices them faithfully. The sputum culture done after two months of treatment is negative for tubercle bacilli, and his chest X-ray indicates no disease progression.

Now, his 2 months of daily therapy having been completed, Mr. Facée moves out of the shelter, but he continues to come to the public health clinic to receive his medications twice weekly. He says this is easier than trying to get them at a drug store and keep them safe with his homeless life-style.

Critical Thinking in the Nursing Process

1. Many homeless people have schizophrenia or other mental diseases. How would you adapt the care plan for a homeless schizophrenic client with active tuberculosis? For an alcoholic client?
2. Mr. Kamil was fortunate in having access to an incentive shelter with health care workers to supervise medication compliance. Identify the resources that are available in your area for homeless clients infected with tuberculosis.
3. Develop a care plan for Mr. Facée for the nursing diagnosis *Ineffective Airway Clearance* related to mucopurulent sputum and weak cough.

The Client with a Fungal Infection

■　■　■

Fungal spores are endemic to the environment and present in the air everyone breathes. Normal respiratory defense mechanisms allow few of these spores ever to reach the lungs. When they do cause infection, it is typically mild and self-limiting. Most fungi are opportunistic, able to cause infection only in an immunocompromised host. For this reason, clients with AIDS, renal failure, leukemia, burns, or chronic diseases, as well as people receiving corticosteroids or immunosuppressants, are particularly susceptible to fungal diseases (Berkow & Fletcher, 1992; Porth, 1994).

In the United States, many fungal lung diseases demonstrate a geographic distribution. Histoplasmosis typically is seen in the East and Midwest, particularly in the valleys of the Ohio, Mississippi, and Missouri rivers. The San Joaquin Valley in central California is the primary site for coccidioidomycosis, also known as "valley fever" or "San Joaquin fever." Blastomycosis is found throughout North America, particularly in the southeast and south central regions (Berkow & Fletcher, 1992; Porth, 1994).

The course and manifestations of fungal lung diseases resemble those of tuberculosis. Lung lesions are slow to develop, and symptoms are mild. The fungus can disseminate from the lung to other organs.

Histoplasmosis

Histoplasmosis, an infectious disease caused by *Histoplasma capsulatum,* is the most common fungal infection in the United States. The organism is found in the soil and is linked to exposure to bird droppings and bats. Infection occurs when the spores are inhaled and reach the alveoli. Most infections develop into *latent asymptomatic disease,* much like tuberculosis, or *primary acute histoplasmosis,* a mild, self-limiting influenza-like illness. Initial chest X-rays are nonspecific; later ones show areas of calcification. *Chronic progressive disease,* usually seen in older adults, typically is limited to the lung but may involve any organ. Progressive lung changes and cavitation occur, with increasing dyspnea and eventual disabling pulmonary disease.

Regional lymph vessels spread the organism from the lungs to other parts of the body, much like the process that occurs in tuberculosis. In the healthy host, normal immune responses inactivate and remove the organism. In the immunocompromised host, by contrast, macrophages remove the fungi but are unable to destroy them; the result is *disseminated histoplasmosis*. This type of histoplasmosis is often fatal. Manifestations of fever, dyspnea, cough, weight loss, and muscle wasting are usual. Ulcerations of the mouth and oropharynx may be present, and the liver and spleen are enlarged (Berkow & Fletcher, 1992; Porth, 1994; Tierney et al., 1994).

The diagnosis of histoplasmosis is made by culturing the organism from sputum, lymph nodes, blood, bone marrow, or other tissue. Although skin sensitivity testing can be done, it typically yields negative results during the initial infection and is of little value for diagnosis and treatment.

Because the primary acute form of histoplasmosis is typically self-limiting, often no treatment is required. With disseminated forms, antifungal drugs are used. Itraconazole (Sporanox), a broad-spectrum antifungal agent, is very effective in treating both localized and disseminated histoplasmosis. It is administered orally for a period of 2 weeks to several months. For severely immunocompromised clients and those unable to tolerate oral medications, intravenous amphotericin B may be used (Tierney et al., 1994).

Clients with histoplasmosis have different nursing care needs, depending on the form of the disease and their immune status. For most clients, nursing care focuses on education. People living in high-prevalence areas or who are exposed to bird droppings (for example, by cleaning chicken coops, pigeon lofts, or barns where birds roost) need to have an awareness of the disease, its symptoms, and measures to reduce their risk. Clients with latent disease may need education about maintaining good general health to prevent reactivation. The client undergoing chemotherapy for the disease needs information about the drug and its side effects. When the severe disseminated form of the disease is present, direct supportive nursing care is also required.

The following nursing diagnoses may be appropriate for the client with histoplasmosis:

- *Knowledge Deficit* about the disease, risk factors, manifestations, and treatment
- *Altered Nutrition: Less Than Body Requirements* related to ulcerations of oral mucous membranes
- *Self-Care Deficit* related to severe manifestations of disseminated disease

Coccidioidomycosis

Coccidioidomycosis is an infectious disease caused by the fungus *Coccidioides immitis*. This mold grows in the soil of the arid Southwest, Mexico, and Central and South America. When inhaled, the fungus typically causes an acute, self-limiting pulmonary infection that often is asymptomatic and goes unrecognized. If manifestations do occur, they resemble those of influenza, with malaise, fever, body aches, and cough. The client may also develop pleuritic pain, skin rash, and arthritis of the knees and ankles. Disseminated disease, which may affect the lymph nodes, meninges, spleen, liver, kidney, skin, and adrenal glands, is rare in immunocompetent people. When it does occur, the mortality rate is high. Meningitis is the usual cause of death.

The diagnosis of coccidioidomycosis is made by identification of the parasite in sputum or biopsy specimens or by serologic testing for antibodies. Because the fungus is highly infectious when grown in culture, this procedure is considered too risky to use for diagnosis. Primary coccidioidomycosis does not require treatment, because clients typically recover uneventfully. Progressive disseminated disease is treated with the oral antifungal agents ketoconazole (Nizoral) or fluconazole (Diflucan), or with amphotericin B. Amphotericin B administered intrathecally for a prolonged period, possibly years, is used to treat meningitis (Berkow & Fletcher, 1992; Porth, 1994; Tierney et al., 1994). Nursing care measures are similar to those for histoplasmosis as well as those indicated for acute arthritis and/or meningitis.

Blastomycosis

The fungus *Blastomyces dermatitidis* causes the infectious disease blastomycosis. It occurs primarily in the south central and midwestern regions of the United States and in Canada. Men are affected more frequently than women. The lungs are the primary site for the disease, although it may spread to involve the skin, bones, genitourinary system, and, rarely, the central nervous system. Pulmonary symptoms include fever, dyspnea, pleuritic chest pain, and cough, which may become productive of bloody or purulent sputum. The diagnosis is established by direct visualization of the budding yeast fungus in sputum or other contaminated fluids or by culture. If untreated, the disseminated disease is slowly progressive and ultimately fatal. Itraconazole or ketoconazole, oral antifungal drugs, are the treatment of choice. Amphotericin B may also be used, especially if the central nervous system is involved (Berkow & Fletcher, 1992; Tierney et al., 1994). Nursing care is supportive and individualized to the client's manifestations of the disease.

Obstructive Disorders of the Airways

A number of varied disorders and diseases can affect the airways of the lungs, altering air flow. Although the pathophysiologic mechanism differs in these diseases, limited air flow is a characteristic of all. Air flow is limited when

- The elastic recoil of the lungs is reduced, decreasing the force to push air out.
- The lumen of the airway is obstructed by secretions, increasing resistance.
- Airway walls are thickened.
- Smooth muscle of the airways is activated, resulting in bronchoconstriction.
- Interstitial support that is necessary to maintain airway distention and patency is lost.

With aging, the number of alveoli decrease, and emphysematous changes (senile emphysema) reduce the gas exchange surface area. Alveoli become less elastic, and there is increased air trapping and dead space.

With air flow limitation, the work of breathing and the residual volume of the lungs increase as air becomes trapped behind narrowed or collapsed airways. Inspired air mixes with an abnormally large volume of residual air, effectively reducing the amount of oxygen available in the alveoli. Decreased alveolar ventilation further reduces oxygen available for exchange.

The Client with Asthma

Asthma is an inflammatory disease of the airways that is characterized by episodes of reversible airway obstruction and increased responsiveness of the airways to multiple stimuli. The widespread airway narrowing of asthma reverses either spontaneously or with treatment. Asthma is an episodic disease with acute exacerbations and symptom-free periods.

In the United States, approximately 10 million people have bronchial asthma. Although it is more common in children than adults, about 5% of the adult population is affected. The prevalence of asthma is increasing, as is its mortality rate (Berkow & Fletcher, 1992; Porth, 1994; Tierney et al., 1994).

Pathophysiology

During symptom-free periods, the airway inflammation of the client is subacute or quiet. An acute inflammatory response may be triggered by a variety of factors. When a trigger occurs, the hyperreactive airways that are charac-teristic of the disease constrict with an exaggerated response. The degree of hyperreactivity depends on the degree of inflammation. In addition to bronchoconstriction, the acute inflammatory response also stimulates mucus secretion, edema of the airway mucosa, and damage to the epithelium of the airways. The combination of bronchoconstriction, edema and inflammation, and mucus secretion causes narrowing of the airway. Airway resistance increases, air flow is limited, and the work of breathing increases. The sequence of events is outlined in Figure 34–12.

Asthma is often classified as either intrinsic or extrinsic. With *intrinsic asthma,* a trigger or stimulus such as cold air, emotional upset, or a bronchial irritant produces symptoms in people who are predisposed to bronchospasm. Asthma that occurs in response to such inflammatory triggers as allergens is known as *extrinsic asthma.* Many people with asthma demonstrate both intrinsic and extrinsic responses.

Stimuli that trigger an asthma attack may be either external or internal. Childhood asthma (which may continue into adulthood) is most often linked to the inhalation of specific allergens, such as pollen, animal dander, or household dust. Clients with allergic asthma often have a history of other allergies as well.

Environmental pollutants, such as tobacco smoke and irritant gases (e.g., sulfur dioxide, nitrogen dioxide, and

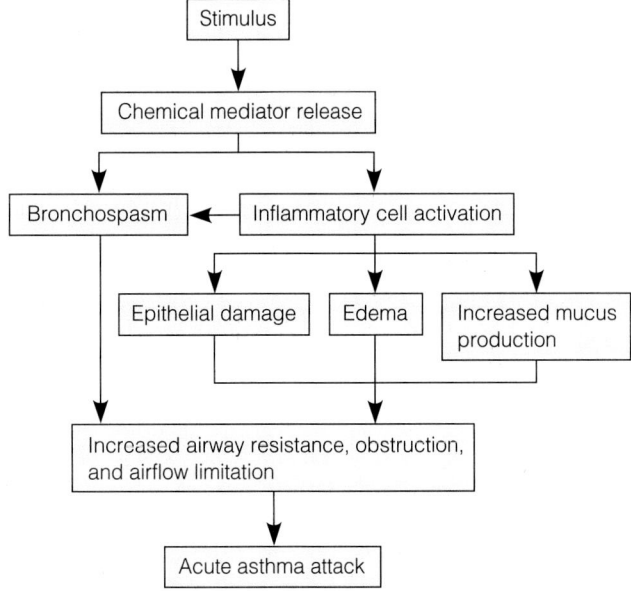

Figure 34–12   The pathogenesis of an acute episode of asthma.

Clinical Manifestations of Acute Asthma

■ ■ ■

- Chest tightness
- Dyspnea
- Wheezing
- Cough
- Tachypnea and tachycardia
- Anxiety and apprehension

---

ozone) can provoke asthma. Agents found in the workplace, such as noxious fumes and gases, chemicals, and organic and inorganic dusts, may cause occupational asthma.

Respiratory infections, viral in particular, are a common internal stimulus for an asthmatic attack. Exercise-induced asthma is also considered to be an internal stimulus, possibly related to heat or water loss from the bronchial surface. Exercise in cold, dry air increases the risk in clients with this type of asthma.

Emotional stress is a significant etiologic factor for attacks in as many as half of clients with asthma. Common pharmacologic triggers include aspirin and other nonsteroidal anti-inflammatory drugs (NSAIDs), sulfites (which are used as preservatives in wine, beer, fresh fruits, and salad), and beta-blockers (Tierney et al., 1994; Wilson et al., 1991).

An attack of asthma is characterized by a sensation of chest tightness, dyspnea, wheezing, and cough (see the accompanying clinical manifestations box). The frequency of attacks and severity of symptoms vary greatly from person to person. Although some clients experience infrequent, mild episodes, others have nearly continuous manifestations of cough and wheezing with periodic severe exacerbations. The onset of symptoms may be either abrupt or insidious, and an attack may subside rapidly or persist for hours or days (Berkow & Fletcher, 1992).

Physical examination findings vary with the severity of the episode. Tachycardia, tachypnea, and prolonged expiration are common. Diffuse wheezing is heard on auscultation. With more severe attacks, use of accessory muscles of respiration, intercostal retractions, loud wheezing, and distant breath sounds may be noted. Fatigue, anxiety, apprehension, and severe dyspnea, that allows the client to speak only one or two words before taking a breath, may occur if the condition progresses. The onset of respiratory failure is marked by inaudible breath sounds with reduced wheezing and an ineffective cough (Porth, 1994;

Wilson et al., 1991). Without careful assessment, this apparent reduction in symptoms can be misinterpreted as an improvement in the client's condition.

Status asthmaticus is severe, prolonged asthma that does not respond to routine treatment. Without aggressive therapy, status asthmaticus can lead to respiratory failure with hypoxemia, hypercapnia, and acidosis. The client may require intubation and mechanical ventilation along with aggressive pharmacologic treatment to sustain life (Andreoli et al., 1990; Porth, 1994; Tierney et al., 1994).

In addition to acute respiratory failure, other complications associated with acute asthma include dehydration, respiratory infection, atelectasis, pneumothorax, and cor pulmonale.

Collaborative Care

The diagnosis of asthma is based primarily on the client's history and manifestations. Laboratory studies and diagnostic tests are used to identify causative factors and the degree of airway involvement during and between acute episodes.

Treatment of the asthmatic client is twofold. Day-to-day management for the asthmatic focuses on controlling symptoms and preventing acute attacks. When an acute episode occurs, therapy is directed toward restoring airway patency and alveolar ventilation.

Laboratory and Diagnostic Tests

There is no single or conclusive test for asthma. The following laboratory tests may be ordered:

- *CBC with WBC differential* often shows a high eosinophil count. This finding is common even when allergies are not the trigger for attacks. The degree of eosinophilia may correlate with the severity of the asthma. The eosinophil count is also used as a measure of the adequacy of treatment with corticosteroids.

- *ABGs* are drawn during an acute attack to evaluate blood pH, oxygen tension, and carbon dioxide levels. ABGs initially show hypoxemia with a low P_{O_2}, and mild respiratory alkalosis with an elevated pH and low P_{CO_2} due to the client's tachypnea. When air flow and ventilation are severely compromised, significant hypoxemia and respiratory acidosis occur (pH less than 7.35 and P_{CO_2} greater than 42 mm Hg). Respiratory acidosis may indicate the need for mechanical ventilation.

- *Examination of the sputum* in a client with asthma shows the presence of many eosinophils and other white blood cells.

- *Skin testing* may be done to identify specific allergens if an allergic trigger is suspected for asthma attacks.

The following diagnostic studies may be performed:

- *Pulmonary function tests* are used to evaluate the degree of airway obstruction; to assess airway response to inhaled allergens, chemicals, and medications; and for long-term follow-up. Pulmonary function testing done before and after use of an aerosolized bronchodilator is valuable to determine the reversibility of airway obstruction. The residual volume (RV) of the lungs may be increased and vital capacity decreased or normal even during periods of remission. The forced expiratory volume (FEV_1) and peak expiratory flow rate (PEFR) are the most valuable pulmonary function studies to evaluate the severity of an asthma attack and the effectiveness of treatment measures.

- *Challenge or bronchial provocation testing* is used to confirm the diagnosis of asthma by detecting airway hyperresponsiveness. A substance such as methacholine or histamine or a nonpharmacologic stimulant such as cold air is inhaled, and pulmonary function testing is performed to evaluate airway responsiveness.

Preventive Measures

Nonpharmacologic treatment is used to prevent asthma attacks and in early management of an episode. Attacks of asthma often can be prevented by avoiding allergens and environmental triggers. Modifications in the household environment, such as controlling dust, removing carpets, covering mattresses and pillows to reduce dust mite populations, and installing air filtering systems may be useful. Clients with asthma may need to remove pets from the household. Eliminating all tobacco smoke in the house is also an important control measure. For the client with exercise-induced asthma, wearing a mask that retains humidity and warm air while exercising in cold weather may be a useful preventive measure. Early treatment of respiratory infections is vital to prevent asthmatic exacerbations.

Pharmacology

Medications are used to prevent airway obstruction and to treat it when an acute episode occurs. Both bronchodilators and anti-inflammatory drugs are used.

Bronchodilators Most asthmatics need bronchodilator therapy to control their symptoms. Inhalation of nebulized medication is the preferred means of administration, but it is not effective for all clients. The primary bronchodilators used include beta-adrenergic agonists or sympathomimetics, methylxanthines, and anticholinergic agents.

Beta-adrenergic agonists stimulate receptors on smooth muscle cells of the respiratory tract, causing smooth muscle relaxation and bronchodilation. Inhaled beta-agonists, administered by metered-dose inhalers, are the treatment of choice for bronchial asthma (see the accompanying client teaching box). Their onset is rapid,

---

Client Teaching: Using a Metered-Dose Inhaler

■ ■ ■

- Be sure a charged canister is firmly inserted into the outer shell or mouthpiece unit.

- Remove the mouthpiece cap, and shake the container for 3 to 5 seconds.

- Holding the canister upside down, place the mouthpiece in the mouth, closing lips around it.

- Exhale slowly and completely through the nose until no more air can be expelled from the lungs.

- Press the canister down on the mouthpiece while inhaling deeply and slowly through the nose (see figure).

- Alternatively, place the mouthpiece directly in front of the mouth; inhale, keeping the mouth open wide while pressing down on the canister to release the aerosol.

- Hold breath as long as possible, release pressure on the container, then exhale. Wait 30 seconds to 2 minutes before shaking the container a second time and repeating the above procedure for a second puff.

- Rinse the mouth after using the inhaler to minimize systemic absorption and drying the mucous membranes.

- Rinse the inhaler mouthpiece at least once per day.

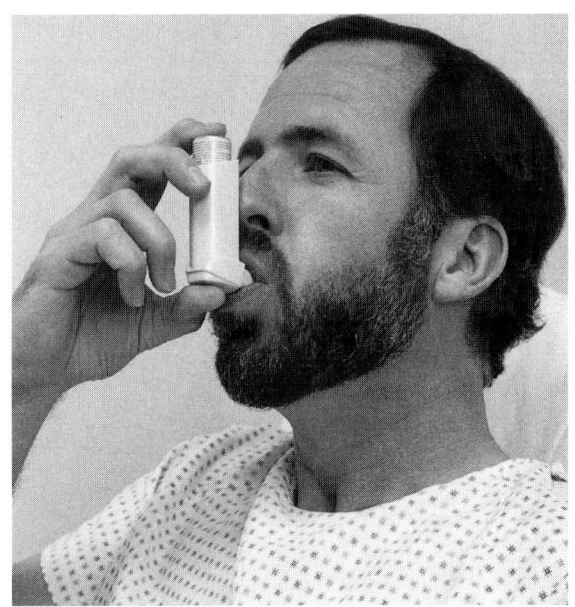

Use of a metered-dose inhaler.

taking effect within minutes, but their duration generally is short, lasting only 4 to 6 hours. The cardiac and neuromuscular side effects commonly seen when these drugs are administered orally or parenterally are minimal with inhalation therapy. Drugs in this group include epinephrine, isoproterenol, metaproterenol, terbutaline, isoetharine, albuterol, bitolterol, and pirbuterol. Salmeterol, a stronger beta-adrenergic agonist related to albuterol, has a longer duration of action, allowing twice-a-day dosing for maintenance therapy.

Theophylline is the primary methylxanthine used in asthma management. It relaxes bronchial smooth muscle and may also inhibit the release of chemical mediators of the inflammatory response. Once considered the treatment of choice for asthma, theophylline is now used as an adjunctive treatment. The sustained-release form may also be used for long-term asthma management. Monitoring of serum theophylline levels is necessary because of wide individual variations in metabolism and elimination of the drug.

Anticholinergic medications prevent broncho-constriction by blocking input from the parasympathetic nervous system via vagal pathways. Ipratropium bromide, an anticholinergic drug administered by metered-dose inhaler, is useful for clients whose asthma symptoms are poorly controlled by beta-adrenergic agonists alone.

Anti-Inflammatory Agents Both corticosteroids and NSAIDs are used to suppress airway inflammation and reduce asthma symptoms.

Corticosteroids block the late response to inhaled allergens and reduce bronchial hyperresponsiveness. Metered-dose inhaler is the route of choice for administration to minimize systemic absorption and reduce the adverse effects of prolonged steroid use (cushingoid effects). For a severe acute attack, oral or parenteral corticosteroids may be used to alleviate symptoms and induce remission.

Cromolyn sodium is an NSAID used to prevent acute episodes of asthma. It reduces airway hyperreactivity and inhibits the release of mediator substances. The primary drawbacks of cromolyn sodium are its cost and lack of effectiveness in treating an acute attack.

Nursing implications for medications used in the treatment of asthma are outlined in the accompanying pharmacology box.

Nursing Care

Nurses encounter clients with asthma both in the acute care setting during an acute exacerbation and as outpatients or in homes when the disease is quiescent. The priority nursing care needs differ with each setting. This section focuses on the client experiencing an acute attack of asthma. The section on client and family teaching addresses the needs of the client in remission.

An acute asthma attack is frightening for the client, because breathing becomes increasingly difficult and hypoxemia occurs. The anxiety in turn tends to increase the severity and manifestations of the attack. Priority nursing care needs are therefore related to reducing the client's fear or anxiety as well as improving airway clearance. Teaching the client about ways to prevent further attacks and home management must be postponed until adequate ventilation is restored.

Ineffective Airway Clearance

Bronchospasm and bronchoconstriction, increased mucus secretion, and airway edema all contribute to narrowing of air passages and impairment of air flow during an acute attack of asthma. Both inspiratory and expiratory volume are affected, resulting in decreased oxygen available at the alveolus for the process of respiration. Narrowed air passages increase the energy required for breathing, raising the metabolic rate and increasing tissue demand for oxygen. This then becomes a priority nursing problem.

Nursing interventions with rationales follow:

- Assess the adequacy of respirations frequently, every 1 to 2 hours. Assess respiratory rate and depth, chest movement or excursion, and breath sounds. *Respiratory status can change rapidly during an acute asthma attack, necessitating frequent assessment. Slowed, shallow respirations with significantly diminished breath sounds and decreased wheezing may indicate exhaustion and impending respiratory failure. Immediate intervention is necessary.*

- Assess the client's cough effort and sputum for color, consistency, and amount. *Ineffective cough with little sputum production may also be an indicator of impending respiratory failure.*

- With respiratory assessment, assess the client's skin color and temperature and level of consciousness every 1 to 2 hours or as indicated. *Cyanosis, cool clammy skin, and changes in level of consciousness (such as agitation, lethargy, or confusion) indicate worsening hypoxia.*

- Assess arterial blood gas results and pulse oximetry readings; notify the physician of abnormal values or changes in status. *These values provide information about gas exchange and the adequacy of alveolar ventilation.*

- Position the client in Fowler's, high-Fowler's, or orthopnea (with head and arms supported on the overbed table) position to facilitate breathing and lung expansion. *These positions reduce the work of breathing and increase lung expansion, especially of basilar areas.*

Nursing Implications for Pharmacology: The Client with Asthma

SYMPATHOMIMETICS OR BETA-ADRENERGIC AGONISTS

Epinephrine

Isoproterenol (Isuprel)

Metaproterenol (Alupent, Metaprel)

Terbutaline (Brethaire, Brethine)

Isoetharine (Bronkosol, Bronkometer)

Albuterol (Proventil, Ventolin)

Bitolterol (Tornalate)

Pirbuterol (Maxair)

Salmeterol (Serevent)

Sympathomimetics stimulate sympathetic nervous system receptors in the respiratory tract, resulting in relaxation of smooth muscle and bronchodilation. Administered by metered-dose inhalers (pressurized canisters that deliver a fixed dose of a drug), these drugs are the treatment of choice for bronchial asthma. Oral forms may be used for prophylaxis but are not effective in treating an acute attack because of their slow onset. When sympathomimetics are administered by either oral or parenteral routes, their systemic effect on the sympathetic nervous system can produce many undesirable and potentially harmful side effects, such as nervousness, irritability, tachycardia, and cardiac dysrhythmias.

Nursing Responsibilities

- Use these drugs with caution in clients who have hypertension, cardiovascular disease or dysrhythmias, hyperthyroidism, or diabetes.

- These drugs may not be effective when the client is hypoxemic and acidotic. Instead of producing bronchodilation, they can lead to potentially dangerous cardiac stimulation (Shlafer, 1993).

- Become familiar with the particular inhaler or nebulizer to ensure its proper use. When two puffs are ordered, wait 1 to 2 minutes between puffs to allow time for bronchodilation, permitting the second dose to reach distal airways.

- Observe the client for desired and adverse effects. Reduction in dyspnea and wheezing indicate beneficial effect. Central nervous system stimulation (anxiety, irritability, and insomnia) and tremor are common side effects.

Client and Family Teaching

- Use the prescribed inhaler or nebulizer according to the instructions provided.

- If you are taking a bronchodilator along with another medication by inhalation, use the bronchodilator first to open airways and enhance the effectiveness of the second medication.

- Rinse the mouth after using inhalers to reduce systemic absorption of the medication.

- When the drug is used over a long period of time, tolerance may develop. Keep a therapy log to track bronchodilator use. If you find that the drug has become less effective, or if you need a higher dosage or more frequent doses than prescribed, inform the physician.

- Report palpitations, irregular pulse, and other side effects to the physician.

METHYLXANTHINES

Theophylline (Bronkotabs, Quibron, Slo-Phyllin Theolair, Theo-Dur, others)

Aminophylline (Somophyllin)

Dyphylline (Dilor)

Oxtriphylline (Choledyl)

The methylxanthines are chemically related to caffeine. Once the drugs of choice for preventing and treating asthma attacks, they are now are used primarily to prevent nocturnal asthma in affected adult clients. Theophylline has a narrow margin of safety and high potential for toxicity. Because the metabolism and excretion of theophylline vary significantly from person to person—affected by such factors as age, smoking, genetic factors, alcoholism, and other chronic diseases—monitoring of serum levels is vital.

Nursing Responsibilities

- Sustained-release forms of these medications are not used until the client's response to regular preparations has been evaluated. Question orders that initiate therapy with sustained-release preparations.

- If the client has difficulty swallowing a sustained-release capsule, open the capsule and sprinkle the contents on a cold, semisolid food, such as custard, pudding, or applesauce. Do not crush or chew the

➤

Pharmacology: The Client with Asthma (continued)

medication; this can result in rapid absorption and toxicity (Shlafer, 1993).

- The therapeutic blood level for theophylline is 10 to 20 μg/mL.
- Monitor the client for manifestations of theophylline toxicity. Anorexia, nausea, vomiting, restlessness, insomnia, cardiac dysrhythmias, and seizures are early manifestations. Other manifestations include epigastric pain, hematemesis, diarrhea, headache, irritability, muscle twitching, palpitations, tachycardia, flushing, and circulatory failure (Spencer et al., 1993).
- Administer the medications with meals or a full glass of water or milk to minimize gastric irritation.
- Monitor the client closely for desired and/or toxic effects when administering theophylline concurrently with any of the following medications:
   a. Barbiturates, phenytoin, rifampin, and thyroid hormone stimulate metabolism of theophylline and may reduce its effectiveness.
   b. Beta-blockers, cimetidine, and some antibiotics inhibit theophylline's metabolism and increase the risk of toxicity.
   c. Sympathomimetic bronchodilators may increase the side effects of theophylline.
   d. Halothane (an inhaled general anesthetic) can cause fatal cardiac dysrhythmias when used concurrently with theophylline. Be sure the anesthesia staff is aware of the client's theophylline use prior to any surgical procedure (Shlafer, 1993).
- Intravenous aminophylline solutions are diluted in a solution of 5% dextrose in water or normal saline to a concentration of no more than 25 mg/mL.
- Aminophylline is incompatible with many other intravenous drugs. Use a separate line or flush the line with normal saline before and after administering any other preparation.

Client and Family Teaching

- Oral methylxanthines are not effective in treating an acute attack of asthma; do not delay other treatment by trying to alleviate acute symptoms with these drugs.
- Do not take any over-the-counter medications or other prescription drugs while on theophylline without checking with the physician first.
- Do not smoke while using this drug.
- Report adverse reactions, especially those associated with toxicity, to the physician.

ANTICHOLINERGICS

Atropine

Ipratropium bromide (Atrovent)

Anticholinergics are potent bronchodilators, acting to block input from the parasympathetic nervous system. Atropine is used infrequently because of its tendency to dry secretions of the mucous membranes and other side effects. It may be administered orally, by injection, or by inhalation. Ipratropium bromide is available only as an inhaler and has fewer side effects than atropine. Unlike atropine, it does not appear to affect mucus viscosity.

Nursing Responsibilities

- Assess the client for possible contraindications to the drug, including hypersensitivity, glaucoma, prostatic hypertrophy, or bladder neck obstruction.
- Assess the client for desired and/or adverse effects: improving or worsening symptoms of asthma; nausea, vomiting, abdominal cramping; anxiety, dizziness, headache.
- Provide the client with ice chips, fluids, or hard candy to relieve dry mouth.

- Administer oxygen as ordered. If a mask is used, monitor the client closely for feelings of claustrophobia or suffocation. *Supplemental oxygen reduces hypoxemia. Although the mask is a very effective delivery system for oxygen, it may increase the client's anxiety and actually worsen his or her condition.*
- Administer nebulizer treatments and provide humidification as ordered. *Nebulizer treatments are used to administer bronchodilators and other medications; humidity helps loosen secretions.*

- Initiate or assist with chest physiotherapy, including percussion and postural drainage. *Percussion and postural drainage facilitate the movement of secretions and airway clearance.*
- Increase the client's fluid intake. *Increasing fluids helps keep secretions thin.*
- Provide endotracheal suctioning as needed. *Endotracheal suctioning may be necessary to remove secretions and improve ventilation if the client is unable to clear secretions by coughing.*

Pharmacology: The Client with Asthma (continued)

Client and Family Teaching

- To avoid the risk of overdose, take no more than the prescribed number of doses per day.
- If the drug becomes less effective over time, notify the physician; an adjustment in dosage may be needed.

CORTICOSTEROIDS

Beclomethasone dipropionate (Vanceril, Beclovent)

Triamcinalone acetonide (Azmacort)

Flunisolide (AeroBid)

Dexamethasone sodium phosphate (Decadron Phosphate Respihaler)

The anti-inflammatory effect of corticosteroids is beneficial in both preventing and treating acute episodes. Corticosteroids are used to reduce the frequency and severity of asthma attacks and allow dosages of other drugs to be reduced (Shlafer, 1993). The cushingoid side effects of corticosteroids, always a major concern with their use, are minimized when they are administered by inhalation.

Nursing Responsibilities

- Administer ordered inhaler doses after bronchodilators to facilitate transit of the medication to distal airways.
- Assess the client for common side effects: sore throat, hoarseness, and oropharyngeal or laryngeal *Candida albicans* infection.
- Administer antifungal medications or gargles as ordered.

Client and Family Teaching

- Rinse the mouth after taking the medication and maintain good oral hygiene to reduce the risk of fungal infections.

- These medications are not effective in alleviating the symptoms of an acute attack and should not be used for that purpose.
- Several weeks of continued therapy may be required before a beneficial effect is experienced.
- Notify the physician if the following side effects occur: weight gain, fluid retention, muscle weakness, redistribution of fat, or mood changes.

NONSTEROIDAL ANTI-INFLAMMATORY DRUGS (NSAIDs)

Cromolyn sodium (Intal, Nasalcrom)

Cromolyn sodium prevents asthma attacks by preventing the release of histamine. Because cromolyn sodium is poorly absorbed when orally administered, it is inhaled by means of a nebulizer. There are few adverse effects of this medication, although it may cause wheezing, sneezing, or coughing, and, occasionally, bronchoconstriction.

Nursing Responsibilities

- Evaluate the client for potential adverse effects of wheezing and bronchoconstriction.

Client and Family Teaching

- Gargling or sipping water can decrease the throat irritation associated with nebulizer treatment.
- Use appropriate technique: Inhale deeply with head tipped back to open airways, hold breath, and then exhale. Repeat until all of the drug has been inhaled.
- This drug is used only to prevent asthma attacks; it is not effective in treating an acute attack.
- Several weeks may be required before a beneficial effect is noted.

Ineffective Breathing Pattern

The physiologic changes in lung ventilation that take place during an acute attack of asthma impair both lung expansion and emptying. Anxiety caused by hypoxia and difficulty breathing compounds the problem by causing a rapid respiratory rate. Combined with pharmacologic therapy, nursing interventions can help restore a more normal breathing pattern and adequate lung ventilation.

Nursing interventions with rationales follow:

- Assess respiratory rate, pattern, and breath sounds every 1 to 2 hours or as indicated. Look for manifestations of ineffective breathing, including rapid rate, shallow respirations, nasal flaring, use of accessory muscles, intercostal retractions, and diminished or absent breath sounds. *Early identification of ineffective respirations allows appropriate interventions to be initiated in a timely manner.*

- Monitor vital signs and laboratory results. *Increased respiratory and pulse rates, an elevated blood pressure, and increasing hypoxemia and hypercapnia are signs of compromised respiratory status.*

- Assist the client with ADLs as needed. *This allows the client to conserve energy.*

- Provide rest periods between scheduled activities and treatments. *Scheduled rest is important to prevent fatigue and reduce oxygen demands.*

- Assist the client to use techniques to control breathing pattern:
  a. Pursed-lip breathing
  b. Abdominal breathing
  c. Relaxation techniques including visualization, meditation, and others
  Pursed-lip breathing helps keep airways open by maintaining positive pressure, and abdominal breathing improves lung expansion. Relaxation techniques reduce anxiety and its effect on the respiratory rate.

- Administer medications, including bronchodilators and anti-inflammatory drugs, as ordered. Monitor for desired and possible adverse effects. *Medications are used to improve airway status and facilitate breathing.*

Anxiety

Clients experiencing acute episodes of asthma are often extremely anxious. The fear of not being able to breathe and the feeling of suffocation associated with acute asthma are significant. Financial or other concerns may cause the client to want to avoid hospitalization. The client who is experiencing increasingly frequent and severe episodes may fear the future. Hypoxia contributes to the feeling of anxiety as well, stimulating the sympathetic nervous system and the "fight or flight" response.

Nursing interventions with rationales follow:

- Assess the client's level of anxiety. *Interventions for the client with severe anxiety or panic differ from those for mild or moderate anxiety.*

- Assist the client to identify usual coping skills that have been successful in the past. *Successful coping helps the client regain control of the situation.*

- Provide physical and emotional support for the client. Remain with the client during acute episodes of severe anxiety; schedule time every 1 to 2 hours to be with the client who is mildly or moderately anxious, and reassure the client that the call light will be answered promptly. *The severely anxious client may fear being alone or believe that he or she will die if someone is not on hand. Knowing that nursing assistance is readily available and that the nurse will return whether help is needed or not reduces the client's anxiety.*

- Listen actively to the client's concerns; do not deny or negate the fear of dying or of being unable to breathe. *Active listening promotes trust and helps the client express concerns.*

- Provide clear, concise directions and explanations about procedures. Avoid presenting more information than the client is able to assimilate. *Anxiety interferes with the ability to learn. Explanations may need to be repeated frequently.*

- Include the client in care planning and decision making as appropriate, without making excessive demands on the client. *Including the client in decisions regarding care increases the client's sense of control. It is important, however, to avoid demanding that the client make decisions; this may increase the client's level of anxiety.*

- Reduce excessive environmental stimuli, and maintain a calm demeanor. *This promotes rest.*

- Allow supportive family members to remain with the client. *Significant others provide additional support for the client and can help reduce the client's anxiety.*

- Assist the client to use relaxation techniques, such as guided imagery, muscle relaxation, and meditation. *These techniques help restore psychologic balance and reduce the response of the autonomic nervous system (Sparks & Taylor, 1993).*

Ineffective Individual Therapeutic Regimen Management

Once an acute asthma attack is under control and effective respirations have been reestablished, it is important to help the client identify factors that may have contributed to the attack. In doing so, the nurse is helping the client to prevent future episodes.

Nursing interventions with rationales follow:

- Assess the client's level of understanding about asthma and the prescribed maintenance treatment regimen. Provide additional information and teaching as indicated. *Assessment will help identify and clarify misperceptions and factors in the disease management that pose difficulties for the client.*

- Discuss the client's perception of the illness and its effect on his or her life-style. *Open discussion can help identify conflicts between the client's life-style and the treatment regimen (Sparks & Taylor, 1993).*

- Work with the client to identify factors that contributed to development of the acute episode. *By identifying contributing factors, the client becomes more aware of his or her disease and how to prevent future exacerbations.*

- Assist the client and family or significant others to identify problems or difficulties in integrating the maintenance regimen into their life-style. *Modifications may need to be made in either the regimen or the client's life-style to accommodate the disease. Some modifications may impact family members significantly, for example, a need to eliminate cigarette smoking and pets in the house-hold, remove carpets, and/or perform daily damp-dusting to reduce dust mites.*

- Assess the client's knowledge and understanding of the use of prescribed medications as well as available over-the-counter preparations. *This is important to determine misperceptions or possible misuse of medications.*

- Provide written instructions in addition to verbal. *Written instructions provide further reinforcement and allow future reference.*

- Refer the client and significant others to counseling, support groups, or self-help organizations. *Counseling, support groups, and self-help organizations can help the client and family with required life-style changes and the demands of the treatment regimen.*

Other Nursing Diagnoses

Other nursing diagnoses that may apply to the client with an acute attack of asthma follow:

- *Activity Intolerance* related to asthmatic triggers
- *Ineffective Individual/Family Coping* related to chronic disease
- *Impaired Gas Exchange* related to airway narrowing and edema

Client and Family Teaching

Teaching is a vital component of nursing care for the client with asthma. This is a chronic disease that is best managed by the client with assistance from medical personnel.

In the acute care setting, the teaching needs of the client are related primarily to diagnostic and treatment procedures. Include teaching about the specific medications prescribed and their expected effects, both desired and potential adverse effects. Instruct the client about procedures such as pulmonary function testing, nebulizer treatments, and other respiratory therapy procedures, such as intermittent positive pressure breathing (IPPB) treatments, percussion, and postural drainage. When instruction is provided, the client will be better able to co-operate with the procedures, increasing their effectiveness. If the client or a family member is a smoker, this is an ideal time to initiate teaching about the effects of tobacco smoke on asthma.

To promote wellness and reduce the incidence of remissions, clients with asthma need additional teaching about home care. If specific triggers for asthma attacks have been identified, help the client find ways to avoid these triggers. Because exercise, particularly in cold weather, is often an initiating event, teach the client to warm up slowly before exercise. Wearing a special mask that retains air warmth and humidity while exercising in cold weather will also help avoid problems. If necessary, help the client identify indoor exercises that may be substituted. Respiratory infections also are associated with asthma attacks. Adequate rest, good nutrition, and stress management help maintain immune function, making the client better able to resist infection. Other recommendations include yearly influenza vaccines and immunization against pneumococcal pneumonia. Because physical and psychologic stress is also associated with the onset of asthma attacks, assist clients to identify stress management techniques they can incorporate into their lifestyles. Provide referral to a local or regional agency for further teaching and support as needed.

Teaching about prescribed medications is also important. Present information both verbally and in writing, to include the following:

- The name of the medication, its frequency, dose, and optimal use
- The desired effect of the medication and how the client can evaluate for this effect
- Potential adverse effects of the medication and their management, including effects that signal the need to notify the physician
- Potential interactions of this medication with other medications or with foods, including the necessity of avoiding over-the-counter medications
- If tolerance is known to occur with the medication: how the client can identify tolerance, and what to do about it

The Client with Chronic Obstructive Pulmonary Disease (COPD)

Clients with chronic air flow obstruction due to chronic bronchitis and/or emphysema are said to have **chronic obstructive pulmonary disease** or **COPD** (Wilson et al., 1991).

Approximately 10 million Americans are affected by COPD. In 1991, COPD became the fourth leading cause of death in the United States, preceded only by heart disease, cancer, and cerebrovascular disease (CDC, 1993a). In the past 30 years, the mortality rate of COPD has nearly tripled. In addition to the high mortality rate, morbidity is significant. In people under age 65, COPD is second only to heart disease as a cause of disability, resulting in an estimated 250 million lost work hours yearly (Bullock & Rosendahl, 1992; McCance & Huether, 1994; Tierney et al., 1994).

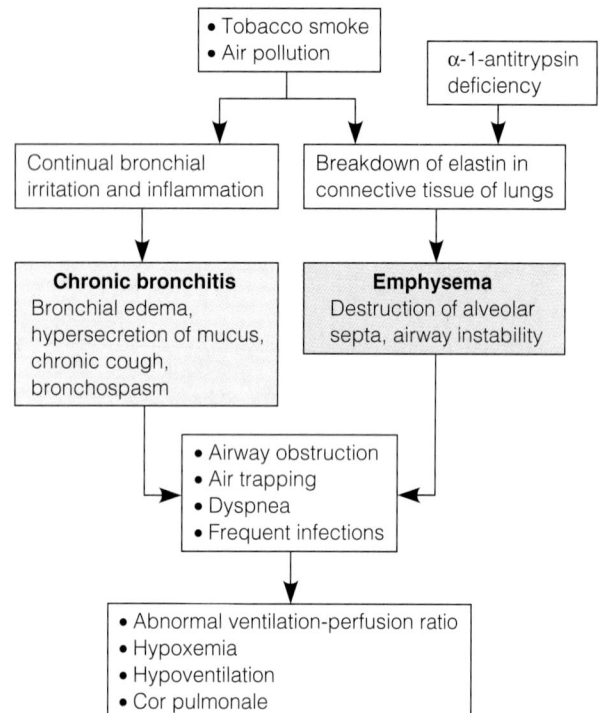

Figure 34–13 The pathogenesis of chronic obstructive pulmonary disease.

Pathophysiology

COPD is characterized by slowly progressive obstruction of the airways. The disease is one of periodic exacerbations, often related to a respiratory infection, with increased symptoms of dyspnea and sputum production. Unlike acute processes in which lung tissues recover, airways and lung parenchyma do not return to normal following an exacerbation; instead, they demonstrate progressive destructive changes (Andreoli et al., 1990; Bullock & Rosendahl, 1992).

Although one or the other may predominate, clients with COPD typically have components of both chronic bronchitis and emphysema, two distinctly different processes. Chronic asthma is also often present. Through different mechanisms, these processes cause airways to narrow, resistance to airflow to increase, and expiration to become slow or difficult (Figure 34–13). The result is a mismatch between alveolar ventilation and blood flow or perfusion, leading to impaired gas exchange (Wilson et al., 1991).

The clinical presentation of COPD varies from simple chronic bronchitis without disability to chronic respiratory failure and severe disability. Manifestations are typically absent or minor early in the disease. When the client does present, manifestations of productive cough, dyspnea, and exercise intolerance often have been present for as long as 10 years. The cough typically occurs in the mornings and often is attributed to "smoker's cough." Initially, dyspnea occurs only on extreme exertion; as the disease progresses, dyspnea becomes more severe and accompanies mild activity. Manifestations characteristic of chronic bronchitis and emphysema develop. The clinical features and manifestations of COPD are summarized in Table 34–6.

Chronic Bronchitis

Chronic bronchitis is a disorder of excessive secretion of bronchial mucus characterized by a productive cough lasting 3 or more months in 2 consecutive years (Tierney et al., 1994). Cigarette smoke is the major factor implicated in the development of chronic bronchitis.

Inhaled irritants lead to a chronic inflammatory process with vasodilation, congestion, and edema of the bronchial mucosa. Thick, tenacious mucus is produced in increased amounts. Narrowed airways and excess secretions obstruct air flow; expiration is affected first, then inspiration. Because ciliary function is impaired, normal defense mechanisms are unable to clear the mucus and any inhaled pathogens. Infection is common in clients with chronic bronchitis. An imbalance between ventilation and perfusion leads to hypoxemia, hypercapnia, and pulmonary hypertension. Many clients with chronic bronchitis develop right-sided heart failure as a result of the pulmonary hypertension.

Clinical manifestations of chronic bronchitis are a cough productive of copious amounts of thick, tenacious sputum, cyanosis, and evidence of right-sided heart failure, including distended neck veins, edema, liver engorgement, and an enlarged heart. Adventitious sounds, including loud rhonchi and possible wheezes, are prominent on auscultation.

Emphysema

Emphysema is characterized by destruction of the walls of the alveoli, with resulting enlargement of abnormal air spaces. As in chronic bronchitis, cigarette smoking is strongly implicated as a causative factor in most cases of

---

Obstructive lung disease typically affects middle and older adults. The incidence is higher in men, although it is increasing in women. Cigarette smoking is clearly implicated as the primary cause of COPD, even though it develops in only 10% to 15% of smokers (Tierney et al., 1994). Cigarette smoke and the irritants it contains impair ciliary movement, inhibit the function of alveolar macrophages, and cause mucus-secreting glands to hypertrophy. It also produces emphysema or airway destruction and constricts smooth muscle, increasing airway resistance. Other contributing factors include air pollution, occupational exposure to noxious dusts and gases, airway infection, and familial and genetic factors (Wilson et al., 1991).

Table 34–6 Clinical Features and Manifestations of COPD

	Feature	Chronic Bronchitis	Emphysema
History	Onset	After age 35; recurrent respiratory infections	After age 50; insidious progressive dyspnea
	Smoking	Usual	Usual
	Cough	Persistent, productive of copious mucopurulent sputum	Absent or mild with scant clear sputum, if any
Physical Examination	Appearance	Typically obese; edematous and cyanotic; distended neck veins and other symptoms of right-sided heart failure	Usually thin and cachectic; barrel chest; prominent accessory muscles of respiration
	Chest	Adventitious sounds with wheezing and rhonchi; normal percussion note	Distant or diminished breath sounds; hyperresonant percussion note
Other Features	Blood gases	Hypercapnia and hypoxemia; respiratory acidosis	Normal or mild hypoxemia; normal pH
	Pulmonary function studies	Normal or decreased total lung capacity; moderately increased residual volume	Increased total lung capacity; markedly increased residual volume
	Pulmonary hypertension	May be severe	Only when advanced

emphysema. Deficiency of alpha$_1$-antitrypsin, an enzyme that normally inhibits the activity of proteolytic enzymes and tissue destruction in the lungs, leads to an early onset of emphysema, often before age 40 (Bullock & Rosendahl, 1992; McCance & Huether, 1994).

With the destruction of alveolar walls, alveoli and air spaces enlarge, and portions of the pulmonary capillary bed are lost; the result is a reduction in the alveolar-capillary diffusing surface area. Elastic recoil is lost, reducing the volume of air that is passively expired. The loss of support tissue also affects airways, increasing the risk of expiratory collapse and further air trapping. Anatomically, either respiratory bronchioles or alveoli may be the primary tissue involved.

Emphysema is insidious in onset. Dyspnea is the initial presenting manifestation. Initially noted only on exertion, it may progress to become severe even when the client is at rest. Cough is minimal or absent. Air trapping and hyperinflation increase the anteroposterior chest diameter, causing barrel chest. The client is thin, tachypneic, uses accessory muscles of respiration and often assumes a position of sitting and leaning forward (Figure 34–14). The expiratory phase of the respiratory cycle is prolonged. On auscultation, breath sounds are diminished, and the percussion tone is hyperresonant (Bullock & Rosendahl, 1992; Wilson et al., 1991).

Collaborative Care

Although COPD can be prevented for the majority of clients, it is not a curable disease. Smoking cessation is

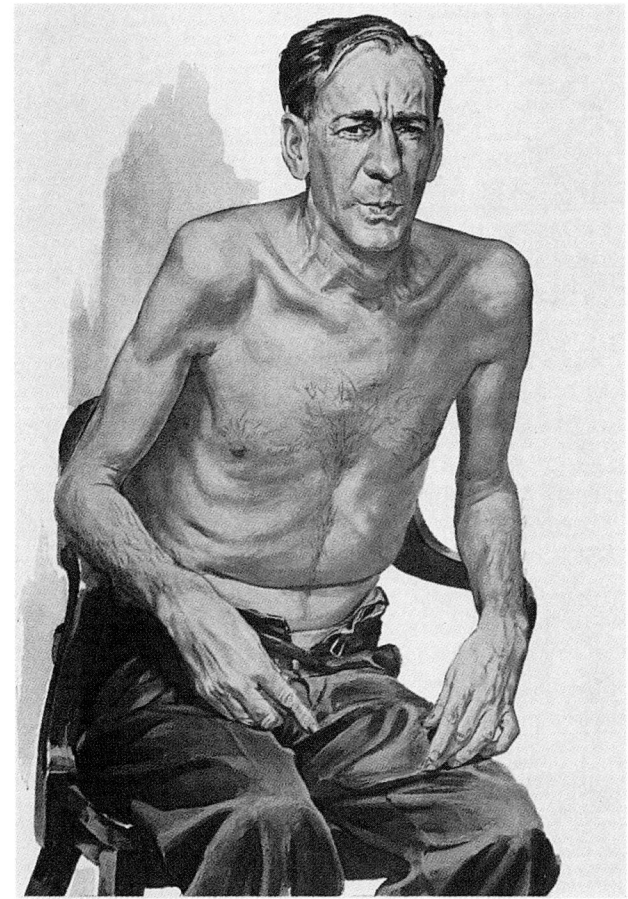

Figure 34–14 Typical appearance of a client with emphysema.

the only certain way to prevent COPD and to slow its progression. To a certain extent, airway obstruction can be reversed and disability minimized early in the disease. Treatment generally focuses on easing the symptoms and is based on the degree of obstruction and the extent of disability (Wilson et al., 1991).

Laboratory and Diagnostic Tests

Laboratory and diagnostic tests are used to help establish the diagnosis of chronic obstructive pulmonary disease and determine whether emphysema or chronic bronchitis is predominant. These procedures are used also to assess the client's status, direct treatment, and monitor the effectiveness of therapy.

Laboratory studies that may be ordered include the following:

- *CBC with WBC differential* may be performed. In COPD, the RBC and hematocrit often are increased (erythrocytosis) as the body attempts to compensate for hypoxia by increasing the blood's oxygen-carrying capacity. Polycythemia, with increased numbers of all blood cells, may be evident. If an acute infection is complicating the client's condition, increased numbers of WBCs with a shift to the left on the differential may be noted.

- *Serum alpha$_1$-antitrypsin levels* may be drawn. COPD clients with a family history of obstructive airway disease, those with an early onset, women, and nonsmokers should be screened for alpha$_1$-antitrypsin deficiency. With the availability of replacement therapy, some physicians may screen all clients with COPD for this deficiency. Normal adult serum alpha$_1$-antitrypsin levels range from 80 to 260 mg/dL (Chernecky et al., 1993). In most cases, it is not necessary for the client to fast prior to drawing the blood sample for this test.

- *ABGs* are drawn to evaluate the diffusing capacity of the client's lungs, particularly during acute exacerbations of the disease. Possible abnormal findings include hypoxemia, hypercapnia, and respiratory acidosis. Clients with predominant emphysema tend to have mild hypoxemia and normal or low carbon dioxide tension. They may actually demonstrate mild respiratory alkalosis due to the increased respiratory rate and maintain a normal skin color, because hemoglobin remains well saturated with oxygen. When chronic bronchitis and airway obstruction are predominant, marked hypoxemia and hypercapnia with respiratory acidosis are more likely. These clients are often cyanotic as a result of their marked hypoxemia. Chronically high blood levels of carbon dioxide diminish the stimulatory effect of CO_2 on breathing; these clients are at increased risk for sleep apnea and for respiratory arrest with oxygen administration because oxygen suppresses their hypoxic drive to breathe.

- *Pulse oximetry* is used to measure oxygen saturations of the blood. Clients with marked airway obstruction often have pulse oximetry readings of less than 95%. These measurements may be used continuously to assess the client's need for supplemental oxygen.

The following diagnostic tests may be ordered:

- *Pulmonary function testing* is a mainstay in establishing the diagnosis and evaluating the extent and progress of the disease. A number of different tests are used to evaluate lung ventilation and function, including measurements of volume and force of air flow and diffusing capacity. A signed consent is not required, nor is fasting; however, the client should not use any tobacco product or bronchodilator or eat a heavy meal for 4 to 6 hours prior to testing. Because results are based on calculated norms for each person by age, height, sex, and weight, these are recorded on the requisition form, as are any medications the client is currently taking; these may affect results. Specific pulmonary function tests with changes seen in COPD are outlined in the accompanying box.

- *Ventilation/perfusion scanning* or other studies of gas diffusion may be performed. A radioisotope is injected or inhaled, allowing areas of shunting and absent capillaries to be identified. In COPD, this test is useful to help determine the extent of ventilation/perfusion mismatch—that is, the extent to which lung tissue is ventilated but not perfused ("dead space"), or perfused but inadequately ventilated (physiologic shunting). As a result, inadequately oxygenated blood returns to the heart, resulting in hypoxemia (Figure 34–15).

- *Chest X-ray* may be performed. No specific changes are typically seen on the chest X-ray until late in the course of COPD. Flattening of the diaphragm due to hyperinflation may be present. Chest X-rays are also used to evaluate overlying pulmonary infections.

- *Thoracic computed tomography (CT) scan* may be ordered to localize emphysematous changes in the lungs but is of little practical value in guiding therapy.

- *Doppler echocardiography,* a noninvasive test that uses the echoes of an ultrasonic beam to provide a three-dimensional picture of the heart on an oscilloscope, provides a means of assessing cardiac hypertrophy and estimating pulmonary artery pressure when pulmonary hypertension is suspected (Tierney et al., 1994).

Pharmacology

Although medications cannot cure chronic obstructive pulmonary disease, they are used to help manage manifestations and slow the progression of the disease.

Clients with COPD are susceptible to respiratory infections, which in turn can lead to an exacerbation of the COPD. Immunization against pneumococcal pneumonia and yearly influenza vaccine are recommended. A broad-

Pulmonary Function Tests and COPD

■ ■ ■

Pulmonary function tests (PFTs) are performed in a pulmonary function laboratory. After preparing the client, a nose clip is applied and the unsedated client breathes into a spirometer or body plethysmograph, a device for measuring and recording on a graph lung volume in liters versus time in seconds. The client is given instructions in how to breathe for specific tests: for example, to inhale as deeply as possible and then exhale to the maximal extent possible. Using measured lung volumes, respiratory capacities are calculated to assess the client's pulmonary status. The specific values determined by PFT and illustrated in the figure include the following:

- The *total lung capacity (TLC)*, is the total volume of the lungs at their maximum inflation. Four values are used to calculate TLC:
  a. *Tidal volume (V_T)*, the volume inhaled and exhaled with normal quiet breathing.
  b. *Inspiratory reserve volume (IRV)*, the maximum amount that can be inhaled over and above a normal inspiration.
  c. *Expiratory reserve volume (ERV)*, the maximum amount that can be exhaled following a normal exhalation.
  d. *Residual volume (RV)*, the amount of air remaining in the lungs after maximal exhalation.

In COPD, TLC is increased as a result of overdistention of the lungs. Residual volume is increased, and tidal volume may also be increased. The inspiratory reserve volume however, is decreased.

- The *vital capacity (VC)* is the total amount of air that can be exhaled after a maximal inspiration. It is calculated by adding together the IRV, V_T, and the ERV.

- The *inspiratory capacity* is the total amount of air that can be inhaled following a normal quiet exhalation. It is calculated by adding the V_T and IRV.

- The *functional residual capacity (FRC)* is the volume of air left in the lungs after a normal exhalation. The ERV and RV are added together to determine the FRC. The overdistention of the lungs associated with COPD leads to an increased FRC.

- The *forced expiratory volume (FEV_1)* is the amount of air that can be exhaled in 1 second. Because of narrowed airways and resistance to airflow, FEV_1 is typically reduced in the client with COPD.

- The *forced vital capacity (FVC)* is the amount of air that can be exhaled forcefully and rapidly after maximum air intake. The FVC is decreased in obstructive lung disease because of increased resistance to expiratory airflow.

- The *minute volume (MV)* is the total amount or volume of air breathed in 1 minute.

In older clients, residual capacity is increased, and vital capacity is decreased. These age-related changes result from the following:

- Calcification of the costal cartilage and weakening of the intercostal muscles, which reduce movement of the chest wall.

- Vertebral osteoporosis, which decreases spinal flexibility and increases the degree of kyphosis, further increasing the anterior-posterior diameter of the chest.

- Diaphragmatic flattening and loss of elasticity.

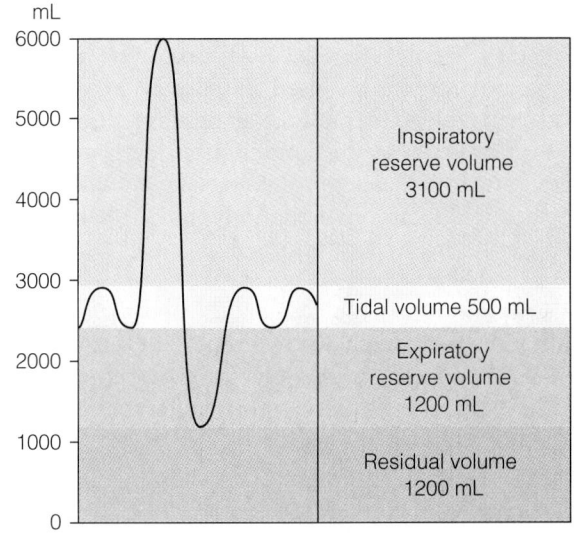
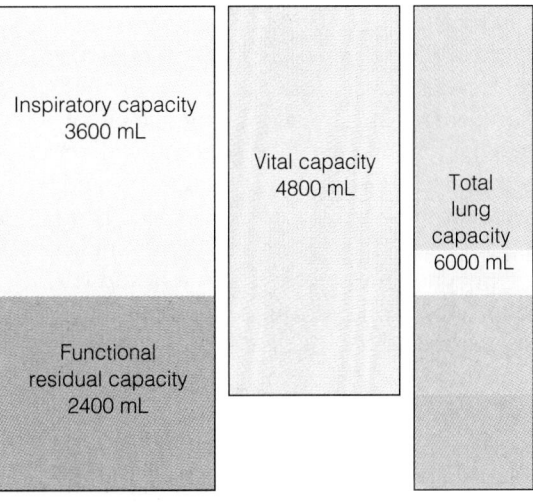

The relationship of lung volumes and capacities. Volumes (mL) shown are for an average adult male.

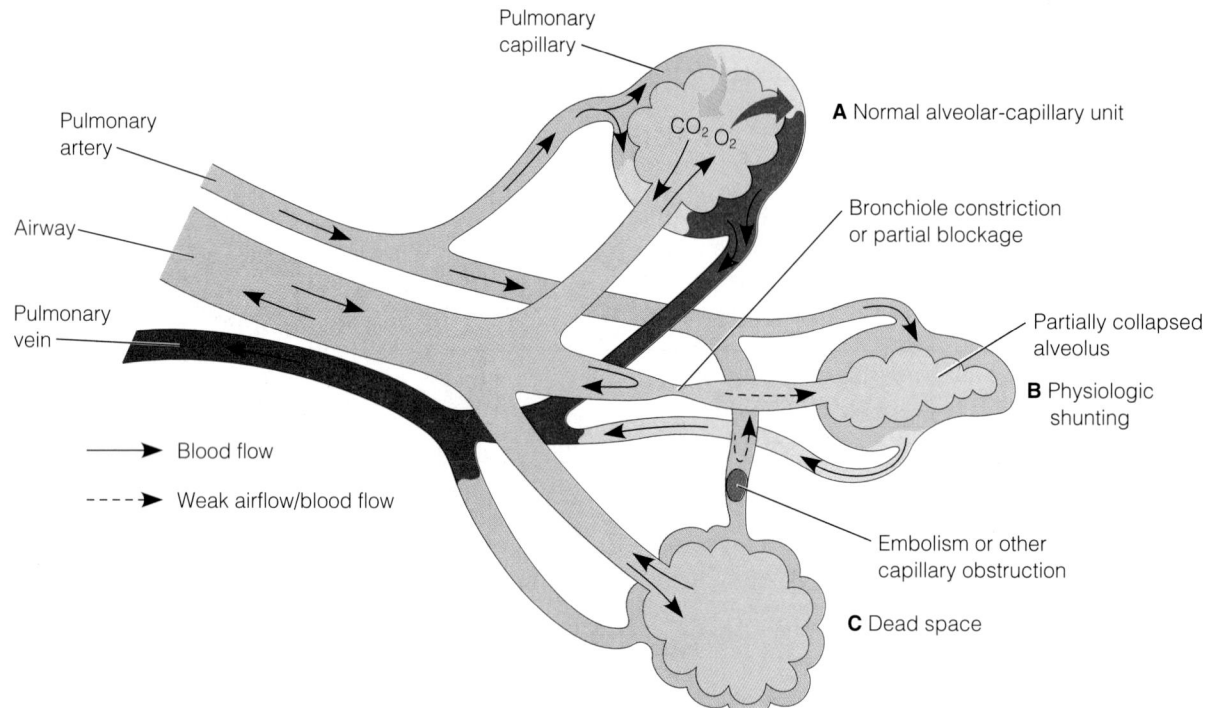

Figure 34–15 Ventilation-perfusion relationships. *A,* Normal alveolar-capillary unit with an ideal match of ventilation and blood flow. Maximum gas exchange occurs between alveolar wall and blood. *B,* Physiologic shunting: A unit with adequate perfusion but inadequate ventilation. *C,* Dead space: A unit with adequate ventilation but inadequate perfusion. In the latter two cases, gas exchange is impaired.

spectrum antibiotic such as amoxicillin, ampicillin, tetracycline, or trimethoprim-sulfamthoxazole is prescribed if infection is suspected. Recent studies indicate that clients with purulent sputum and increased dyspnea will likely benefit from antibiotic therapy, even if no other signs of infection are present. Prophylactic antibiotics are also of benefit for clients who experience four or more disease exacerbations per year (Murphy & Sethi, 1993; Tierney et al., 1994).

A therapeutic trial of bronchodilator therapy is initiated for all clients with symptomatic COPD. Because the reversibility of airway obstruction is variable in these clients, the effectiveness of treatment is monitored closely with spirometry. If little or no benefit is demonstrated, the drugs are discontinued. Ipratropium bromide, an anticholinergic agent administered by metered inhaler, is the bronchodilator of choice. It has a longer duration of action than the sympathomimetic bronchodilators and few side effects. Salmeterol, a longer-acting beta2-agonist, also may be used, particularly for clients with nocturnal symptoms. Oral theophylline, a methylxanthine, also may be prescribed for clients with sleep-related respiratory disturbances and those for whom neither ipratropium or sympathomimetics are effective or well tolerated. Theophylline has the additional advantage of strengthening the function of cardiac and respiratory

muscle, which may be beneficial for the COPD client (Andreoli et al., 1990; Wilson et al., 1991). Bronchodilators are discussed in further detail in the section on asthma, and their nursing implications are outlined in the box on page 1417.

Corticosteroid therapy is used primarily for clients who have asthmatic bronchitis as a component of their COPD and for those who have frequent exacerbations or disabling symptoms and who do not respond to bronchodilators (Tierney et al., 1994). Oral corticosteroids, such as prednisone, are used initially. If the client responds favorably to therapy, the amount is reduced to the lowest effective dose, preferably on an every-other-day schedule or by inhaler to minimize steroid side effects, such as altered carbohydrate and protein metabolism, fluid retention, hypertension, and fat redistribution (cushingoid effects).

Alpha1-antitrypsin replacement therapy is available for clients with emphysema due to a genetic deficiency of the enzyme. The efficacy of this therapy is as yet unknown, and it is expensive, requiring intravenous administration of the preparation at regular intervals.

Other Therapies

As noted previously, smoking cessation is vital to slow the progression of COPD. Clients may be referred to a smoking cessation clinic, self-help group, or counselor or therapist specializing in helping clients quit. Nicotine chewing gum or nicotine patches may be prescribed to help the client stop smoking. In addition to refraining from smoking, the client should avoid exposure to other airway irritants and allergens. During times of significant air pollution, the client may need to remain indoors to prevent exacerbations of the disease. Air filtering systems or air conditioning may be useful in urban areas.

Pulmonary hygiene measures, including hydration, effective cough, percussion, and postural drainage, are used to reduce the amount of secretions and enhance the client's ability to clear them. Maintaining adequate systemic hydration is essential to keep secretions thin. Forceful coughing is often less effective for clients than leaning forward and repeatedly "huffing," with relaxed breathing between huffs. Percussion and postural drainage generally are needed only when the client is unable to clear secretions by usual means. Cough suppressants and sedatives generally should not be used for clients with COPD; these agents may cause retention of secretions (Berkow & Fletcher, 1992; Tierney et al., 1994).

Unless the client has disabling cardiac disease, a regular exercise program is beneficial in

- Improving exercise tolerance.
- Enhancing the client's ability to carry out activities of daily living.
- Preventing deterioration of physical condition.

A program of aerobic physical exercise (e.g., walking for 20 minutes at least three times weekly) designed to gradually increase the client's exercise tolerance is recommended. In addition, activities that strengthen the muscles used for breathing and ADLs, such as swimming and golf, are beneficial.

In some clients, breathing exercises are useful in slowing the respiratory rate and relieving fatigue of accessory muscles. Pursed-lip breathing helps slow the respiratory rate and maintain open airways during exhalation by keeping positive pressure in the airways. Abdominal breathing helps relieve the work of the accessory muscles of respiration.

Clients with severe hypoxemia may require home oxygen therapy. Those who are most likely to benefit include clients with pulmonary hypertension, erythrocytosis, impaired cognitive function, exercise intolerance, nocturnal restlessness, or morning headache. Oxygen may be prescribed for use with exercise, at night, or continuously. Oxygen therapy has a positive impact on the long-term survival, need for hospitalization, and quality of life in clients with advanced COPD (Andreoli et al., 1990; Tierney et al., 1994; Wilson et al., 1991).

The client who is hospitalized with an acute exacerbation of COPD may require oxygenation and inspiratory positive-pressure assistance with a face mask or intubation and mechanical ventilation. Oxygen administered without intubation and mechanical ventilation requires caution in the COPD client. Chronic increased levels of carbon dioxide in the blood inhibit this normal stimulus to breathe, leaving only the stimulus of low blood oxygen tension. Oxygen administered at high flow rates or a high percentage can reduce this stimulus, leading to respiratory insufficiency or arrest.

For clients with end-stage obstructive disease for whom medical therapy is no longer effective, lung transplantation may be an option. Because organs for transplantation are scarce, candidates must be dependent on oxygen and likely to die within 12 to 18 months. Both single and bilateral transplants have been performed successfully, with a 2-year survival rate of 75% (Tierney et al., 1994; Way, 1994).

Nursing Care

Clients with chronic obstructive pulmonary disease, whether hospitalized with an acute exacerbation or maintaining day-to-day functioning at an optimal level at home, have multiple nursing care needs. Because of the obstructive nature of the disease, airway clearance is a high priority in either setting. Many clients, those with predominant emphysema in particular, experience a nutritional deficit that needs to be addressed. Because this chronic disease affects all areas of the client's life as it progresses, psychosocial issues are also of concern in planning nursing care. See the box on page 1428 for applying rehabilitation principles to chronic obstructive pulmonary disease.

Ineffective Airway Clearance

Both major components of COPD, chronic bronchitis and emphysema, can lead to problems in maintaining open airways. In chronic bronchitis, copious amounts of thick, tenacious mucus are produced. Ciliary action is impaired, making it difficult for the client to clear this mucus from the airways. The loss of supporting tissue that occurs with emphysema increases the likelihood that airways will collapse. In both cases, air is trapped distally, and less oxygen-rich air is available to the alveoli for diffusion. Normal respiratory defense mechanisms are impaired, and mucus-plugged airways provide an ideal environment for bacterial growth. Respiratory infection further impairs airway clearance and is often the cause of an acute exacerbation of the client's disease.

Nursing interventions with rationales follow:

- Perform respiratory assessment every 1 to 2 hours or as indicated. Assess rate and pattern; cough and secretions (color, amount, consistency, and odor); and breath sounds, both normal and adventitious. *Frequent and accurate respiratory assessment provides data about the client's condition and response to treatment. Adventitious sounds should decrease with effective intervention.*

Applying Rehabilitation Principles to Medical/Surgical Nursing: Chronic Obstructive Pulmonary Disease (COPD)

■ ■ ■

Applying rehabilitation principles such as maintaining function and facilitating the client's ability to perform activities of daily living can increase the quality of life for the client with COPD.

Mr. Andy Kerlick, a 50-year-old man, is admitted to your medical/surgical unit with shortness of breath. His vital signs are stable with the exception of his respiratory rate, which is 22 breaths per minute. He complains of feeling exhausted. He has a 5-year history of COPD.

Rehabilitation Principle

Conservation of existing function as well as prevention of further loss of function are central goals of rehabilitation nursing.

Rehabilitation Time Frame

Mr. Kerlick will stay in your unit for 5 days. Several energy conserving techniques as well as pursed lip breathing exercises can be taught to Mr. Kerlick in this time frame.

Nursing Diagnosis: Activity Intolerance

Clients with COPD find it difficult to perform many activities of daily living due to fatigue, which results from inadequate oxygenation. Rehabilitation techniques such as adapted devices, breathing exercises, and the proper pacing of activities can allow the client to regain independence in performing ADLs.

Rehabilitation Goals and Interventions

1. Teach the client how to pace activities by taking rests between activities as well as scheduling the activities. *Rest periods between activities allows the client to maintain adequate oxygenation.*

2. Provide the client with assistive devices such as a long shoe horn, elastic shoe laces, and a sock holder. *These devices allow the client to put his shoes and socks on without bending at the waist. This facilitates diaphragmatic breathing.*

3. Teach the client diaphragmatic breathing and pursed-lip breathing techniques. *Diaphragmatic breathing prohibits shallow breathing. Pursed-lip breathing slows the respiratory rate and enhances expiration.*

Diminished or absent breath sounds may indicate increasing airway obstruction and possible atelectasis.

- Assess skin color and mental status frequently, reporting any changes such as increasing cyanosis, confusion, or agitation. *Increasing cyanosis or an altered level of consciousness indicate significant hypoxemia, possibly related to airway obstruction.*

- Monitor arterial blood gas results. *Increasing hypercapnia, hypoxemia, and respiratory acidosis may be indicative of increasing airway obstruction.*

- Maintain pulse oximetry, and monitor values. *Decreasing levels of oxygen saturation may also be indicative of airway obstruction and impaired alveolar ventilation.*

- Assess hydration status by weighing the client daily, measuring intake and output, and monitoring status of mucous membranes and skin turgor. *Dehydration causes respiratory secretions to become thicker, more tenacious, and difficult to expectorate; fluid overload can further compromise respiratory status.*

- Encourage a fluid intake of at least 2000 to 2500 mL per day unless contraindicated. *Adequate fluid intake helps keep mucus secretions thin.*

- Position the client to facilitate maximal lung ventilation; encourage movement and activity to tolerance. *Placing the client in Fowler's to high-Fowler's position improves ventilation. Activity helps mobilize secretions and prevent them from pooling.*

- Assist the client to cough at least every 2 hours while awake. Position the client for optimal lung ventilation and energy conservation while coughing; usually, the client sits upright, leaning forward. *This position promotes chest expansion, increasing the effectiveness of coughing.*

- Provide tissues and a paper bag for disposal of expectorated sputum. *This is an important infection control measure to minimize the spread of respiratory organisms to other people.*

- Refer the client to a respiratory therapist, and assist with or perform percussion and postural drainage as needed. *Percussion helps loosen secretions in airways; postural drainage facilitates movement of these secretions out of the respiratory tract.*

- Provide endotracheal, oral, or nasopharyngeal suctioning as necessary. *Suctioning may be necessary to stimulate cough and help clear secretions.*

- Provide for rest periods between treatments and procedures. *The client with COPD becomes fatigued easily; adequate rest is important to conserve energy and reduce fatigue.*

- Administer expectorant and bronchodilator medications as ordered. Correlate timing with respiratory treatments. *Using expectorants and bronchodilators prior to coughing, percussion, and postural drainage increases their effectiveness in clearing airways.*

- Provide humidified oxygen therapy as ordered. *Oxygen therapy may be needed to maintain adequate blood and tissue oxygenation. Humidification of delivered oxygen decreases its drying effects on respiratory tissues.*

- Prepare for intubation and mechanical ventilation if the client's condition is deteriorating (as indicated by increasing hypoxemia and hypercapnia, decreased level of consciousness, cyanosis, or worsening airway obstruction). *Respiratory failure is a possible complication of an acute exacerbation of COPD and requires immediate intervention to preserve life.*

Altered Nutrition: Less Than Body Requirements

Clients with advanced COPD often become fatigued and dyspneic with minimal activity, including eating. They may not be able to consume a full meal without resting. At the same time, the increased work of breathing raises their metabolic demands, and more calories are required to meet their body's needs. The client may present with a cachectic (thin and wasted) appearance. Poor nutritional status further impairs the immune system and increases the risk of a complicating infection.

Nursing interventions with rationales follow:

- Assess the client's nutritional status, including diet history, weight and height comparison (check against reference tables of desired weights), and anthropometric (skinfold) measurements. *It is important to differentiate nutritional status from body type rather than assume a nutritional impairment.*

- Observe and document food intake, including types, amounts, and caloric intake. *This information can provide direction for supplementation, if needed.*

- Monitor laboratory measures of nutritional status, including serum albumin and electrolyte levels. *These values provide information about the adequacy of the client's nutritional intake, including protein.*

- Consult with a dietitian to plan meals and nutritional supplements that meet the client's caloric needs. *The client may need to consume more concentrated energy source foods to maintain caloric intake without excess fatigue.*

- Provide frequent, small feedings with between-meal supplements. *Frequent, small meals help maintain intake and reduce fatigue associated with eating.*

- Place the client in high-Fowler's position for meals. *High-Fowler's position promotes lung expansion and reduces dyspnea.*

- Assist the client to choose preferred foods from the menu; encourage family members to bring food from home if allowed. *Providing food to the client's preferences encourages eating.*

- Keep snacks at the client's bedside. *Snacks provide additional caloric intake for the client.*

- Provide mouth care prior to meals. *This helps enhance the client's appetite.*

- If the client is unable to maintain oral intake, consult with the physician about enteral or parenteral feedings. *Maintenance of caloric and nutrient intake is vital to prevent catabolism.*

Ineffective Family Coping

Chronic illness of one person affects the entire family structure. Roles and relationships change; the client's condition places additional demands on the family. Family members may be intolerant of the client's ailments and needs or have distorted perceptions about the client's health problem, even denying its existence. They may refuse to assist or participate in the client's care. The client may develop an attitude of helplessness or dependence or may demonstrate anger, hostility, or aggression (Sparks & Taylor, 1993).

Nursing interventions with rationales follow:

- Assess interactions between the client and family. *Assessment is important to identify potential destructive behaviors.*

- Assess the effect of the client's illness on the family. *This assessment is necessary to help plan appropriate interventions.*

- Help the client and family identify strengths for coping with the situation. *Identifying personal and family strengths helps the family regain a sense of control.*

- Provide information and teaching about COPD. *This can assist the family in gaining an understanding of the client's condition and needs.*

- Encourage the client and family to express their feelings. Avoid judging the feelings expressed or judging family members as "good" or "bad," "right" or "wrong." *It is important that the nurse remain objective to maintain the therapeutic relationship.*

- Help family members recognize behaviors and attitudes that may hinder effective treatment, such as continuing to smoke in the house when the client is present. *Family members may be unaware of the effect of their behavior on the client's ability to change habits and cope with a disabling disease.*

- Encourage family members to participate in the client's care. *This helps develop skills for use at home.*

- Initiate a care conference involving the client, family, and members of the health care team from a variety of disciplines. *This will aid in problem solving and facilitate communication (Lederer, Marculescu, Mocnik, & Seaby, 1993).*

- If dysfunctional family relationships interfere with measures to facilitate coping, assume the role of client advocate, reaffirming the client's right to make decisions. *Dysfunctional family relationships are not likely to change simply because the client is now ill. The nurse can better meet the client's needs by accepting his or her limitations in dealing with family members (Sparks & Taylor, 1993).*

- Provide a referral for the client and/or family to available support groups and pulmonary rehabilitation programs, if available. *Support groups and structured rehabilitation programs enhance coping abilities.*
- Arrange a social services consultation. *This can help the client and family identify care and support service needs.*
- Refer the client to community agencies or services such as home health, homemaker services, or Meals on Wheels as appropriate. *Agencies or community services may be necessary to provide additional support which is beyond the family's means or capability.*

Decisional Conflict: Smoking

Smoking is more than a habit; it is an addiction. The client who must quit is facing a significant loss, not only of nicotine but also of a life-style. Although the client may fully comprehend the consequences of continuing to smoke, the decision to give up a part of his or her life is not easy. This fear may be expressed in such concerns as "I'll gain weight," or "What will I do with my hands?" In addition to providing practical information, a plan, and assistance with nicotine withdrawal, the nurse must support the client's decision-making process to comply with an order to stop smoking.

Nursing interventions with rationales follow:

- Assess the client's knowledge and understanding of the choices involved and possible consequences for each. *The client must ultimately be the one to make the decision to quit smoking, so he or she needs a full understanding of the consequences of quitting or continuing to smoke.*
- Acknowledge the client's concerns, values, and beliefs; listen nonjudgmentally. *The nurse needs to avoid imposing his or her values and beliefs about smoking on the client.*
- Spend time with the client, allowing the client to express feelings. *This demonstrates acceptance of the client and his or her right to make the decision.*
- Help the client plan a course of action for quitting smoking and adapt it as necessary. *When the client develops the plan, he or she has more ownership in it and interest in making it work.*
- Demonstrate respect for the client's decisions and right to choose. *Respect supports the client's self-esteem and ability to cope.*
- Provide referral to a counselor or other professional as needed. *Counselors or other people trained to assist with smoking cessation can help the client make the decision.*

Other Nursing Diagnoses

As noted before, the client with COPD has numerous nursing care needs, both in and out of the acute care setting. Other nursing diagnoses that may be applicable follow:

- *Activity Intolerance* related to hypoxemia
- *Ineffective Breathing Pattern* related to use of accessory muscles
- *Impaired Home Maintenance Management* related to dyspnea
- *Caregiver Role Strain* related to lack of respite care availability
- *Hopelessness* related to chronic progressive disease
- *Risk for Infection* related to impaired respiratory defenses
- *Sleep Pattern Disturbance* related to nocturnal dyspnea
- *Inability to Sustain Spontaneous Ventilation* related to respiratory muscle fatigue
- *Sexual Dysfunction* related to fatigue and dyspnea

Client and Family Teaching

As with any chronic disease, teaching is vital to help the client with COPD attain and maintain optimal health. Although medical interventions are important to manage the symptoms, the client and family will have primary responsibility for disease management. Teaching focuses on effective coughing and breathing techniques, preventing exacerbations, and managing prescribed therapeutic interventions.

Pursed-lip and diaphragmatic breathing techniques may be useful for the client to minimize air trapping and fatigue. *Pursed-lip breathing* helps maintain open airways by maintaining positive pressures longer during exhalation. Teach the client to:

1. Inhale through the nose with the mouth closed.
2. Exhale slowly through pursed lips, as though whistling or blowing out a candle, making exhalation twice as long as inhalation (Tucker, Canobbio, Paquette, & Wells, 1992).

Diaphragmatic or *abdominal breathing* helps conserve energy by using the larger and more efficient muscles of respiration. Teach the client to

1. Place one hand on the abdomen, the other on the chest.
2. Inhale, concentrating on pushing the abdominal hand outward while the chest hand remains still.
3. Exhale slowly, while the abdominal hand moves inward and the chest hand remains still (Tucker et al., 1992).

Repeat these exercises as often as necessary until the techniques become incorporated into normal breathing.

Several different coughing techniques may be useful to teach the client. For *controlled cough technique,* teach the client to

1. Follow prescribed bronchodilator treatment, inhale deeply, and hold breath briefly.

2. Cough twice, the first time to loosen mucus, the second to expel secretions.

3. Inhale by sniffing to prevent mucus from moving back into deep airways.

4. Rest. Avoid prolonged coughing to prevent fatigue and hypoxemia (Tucker et al., 1992).

For *huff coughing,* teach the client to

1. While leaning forward, inhale deeply.

2. Exhale sharply with a "huff" sound. This helps keep airways open while mobilizing secretions.

Other home care techniques to teach the client and family include the following:

- Maintaining adequate fluid intake, at least 2 to 2½ quarts of fluid daily.

- Avoid respiratory irritants, including cigarette smoke, both primary and secondary, other smoke sources, dust, aerosol sprays, air pollution, and very cold dry air.

- Try to prevent exposure to infection, especially upper respiratory infections.

- Obtain a yearly influenza immunization.

- Follow the prescribed exercise program, and maintain activities as tolerated, balancing with rest periods.

- Maintain adequate food intake, eating small frequent meals and using nutritional supplements to provide adequate calories. If the client has pulmonary hypertension or cor pulmonale, a sodium restriction may be prescribed and should be included in the client's dietary teaching.

Teach the client and family to identify early signs of an infection or exacerbation of the disease so that early intervention can be implemented. Teach the client to report promptly any of the following signs or symptoms to the physician: fever, increase in sputum production, purulent (green or yellow) sputum, upper respiratory infection, increased shortness of breath or difficulty breathing, decreased activity tolerance or appetite, increased need for oxygen (Tucker et al., 1992).

Provide instruction about the prescribed medications, including their purpose, proper use, and expected effects. Instruct the client to avoid over-the-counter medications unless approved by the physician. Teach the client and family about other prescribed therapies, such as the use of home oxygen, percussion, postural drainage, and nebulizer treatments. If special equipment is required, be sure to include its use, cleaning, and maintenance in teaching.

Finally, advise clients who have COPD to wear an identification band and carry a list of their medications at all times to be readily available should an emergency occur.

Applying the Nursing Process

Case Study of a Client with COPD: Anna Mercurio

Anna Mercurio, known as "Happy" by all her friends, is an 83-year-old widow. She lives in her family home in the country with her two grown sons. Over the past 15 years, Mrs. Mercurio has noticed that she is becoming increasingly short of breath while gardening and walking, two favorite activities. She also has developed a chronic cough that is particularly bad in the mornings. Ten years ago, her family physician told her that she had emphysema. She has been admitted to the hospital with possible pneumonia and an acute exacerbation of her COPD.

Assessment

Jeff Harris, RN, admits Mrs. Mercurio to the nursing unit. In the nursing history, Mr. Harris notes that she denies any history of smoking but says that her husband and two sons have been smokers "for practically their whole lives." She says her health has always been good and that she had lived an active life before developing lung disease. She reports that her breathing and cough have progressed gradually to the point where she now must rest after just a few minutes of housework or other activity. Her cough is productive of moderate to large amounts of sputum, particularly in the mornings. She began having increasing shortness of breath and sputum 2 days ago; this morning, she was unable to complete her morning activities without resting, so she contacted her doctor.

On physical examination, Mr. Harris notes that Mrs. Mercurio's skin is very warm and dry, and her color is dusky. She pauses frequently while answering questions to catch her breath. Her respiratory rate is 36 and fairly shallow. She coughs frequently, producing large amounts of thick, tenacious green sputum. Other vital signs are as follows: P, 115 and irregular; BP, 186/60; T, 102.4 F (39 C). Mrs. Mercurio appears very thin, weighing 96 lb (43.6 kg) and standing 5 feet 3 inches (160 cm) tall. Her anteroposterior:lateral chest diameter is approximately 1:1, with moderate kyphosis. Her chest is hyperresonant on percussion. Auscultation reveals distant breath sounds with scattered wheezes and rhonchi throughout her lung fields. Her chest X-ray shows flattening of her diaphragm, slight cardiac enlargement, prominent vascular and bronchial markings, and patchy infiltrates. Her initial laboratory work reveals moderate erythrocytosis, low serum albumin, and the following arterial blood gas results: pH, 7.19; PO_2, 54 mm Hg; PCO_2, 59 mm Hg; and HCO_3^-, 30 mg/dL. Admitting orders include sputum specimen for culture; intravenous penicillin G, 2 million units every 4 hours; ipratropium bromide (Atrovent) inhaler, 2 puffs every 6 hours; beclomethasone diproprionate (Vanceril) inhaler, 2 puffs every 6 hours; bed rest with bathroom privileges; oxygen per nasal cannula at 2 L continuously; and regular diet.

Diagnosis

Mr. Harris develops the following nursing diagnoses for Mrs. Mercurio:

- *Ineffective Airway Clearance* related to pneumonia and COPD
- *Impaired Gas Exchange* related to lung disease, acute and chronic
- *Risk for Inability to Sustain Spontaneous Ventilation* related to loss of hypoxemic respiratory drive and respiratory muscle fatigue
- *Impaired Home Maintenance Management* related to activity intolerance

Expected Outcomes

The expected outcomes established in the plan of care specify that Mrs. Mercurio will

- Expectorate secretions effectively.
- Return to her level of pulmonary function prior to onset of pneumonia.
- Demonstrate an improvement in arterial blood gas values.
- Maintain spontaneous respirations without excess fatigue.
- Verbalize willingness to allow sons or a housekeeper to assist with daily household tasks.

Planning and Implementation

Mr. Harris plans and implements the following interventions for Mrs. Mercurio while she is hospitalized:

- Increase fluid intake to at least 2500 mL per day.
- Provide a bedside humidifier.
- Keep the head of bed elevated to at least 30 degrees at all times.
- Change position frequently, no less often than every 2 hours.
- Teach "huff" coughing technique.

- Administer medications as ordered; administer beclomethasone diproprionate inhaler after ipratropium bromide inhaler.
- Provide mouth care following inhaler treatments.
- Refer to respiratory therapy for possible percussion and postural drainage; schedule treatments after inhalers.
- Assess respiratory status and level of consciousness every 1 to 2 hours until Mrs. Mercurio's condition is stable, then at least every 4 hours.
- Monitor response to oxygen therapy carefully, including skin color, sputum consistency, and respiratory drive.
- Provide for uninterrupted rest periods following respiratory therapy treatments and other procedures.
- Assist with completion of all ADLs to minimize energy expenditure.
- Meet with Mrs. Mercurio and her sons to develop a postdischarge care plan.
- Refer Mrs. Mercurio to the home health department for nursing follow-up.
- Refer to social services for possible assistance with home maintenance tasks.

Evaluation

After the first day in the hospital, Mrs. Mercurio's condition begins to improve slowly. By the time she is discharged 6 days later, she is able to provide self-care with less fatigue and dyspnea. Her oxygen order has been changed to prn, and she is using it only at night, admitting that it is just for security. Although Mrs. Mercurio still has a few scattered wheezes and rhonchi throughout her lungs, her sputum is thinner, white, and easily expectorated. The physician has changed her medication order from intravenous penicillin G to oral penicillin V, which she will continue for an additional 10 days at home. She will also continue to use the Atrovent and Vanceril inhalers as prescribed at home. Although Mrs. Mercurio's sons have admitted they will probably never be able to quit smoking, they have agreed to smoke only in the garage or outside. Mr. Harris has arranged for the home health department to send a nurse to evaluate Mrs. Mercurio's progress three times weekly initially. Arrangements have also been made for a housekeeper to come twice a week in the mornings for cleaning and laundry. Mrs. Mercurio is glad to be returning home and grateful for the arrangements that have been made.

Critical Thinking in the Nursing Process

1. Mrs. Mercurio was not and had never been a smoker but had a long-term exposure to secondhand smoke.

How does secondhand smoke contribute to lung diseases in adults and children?

2. Mr. Harris's nursing care plan included the nursing diagnosis: *Risk for Inability to Sustain Spontaneous Ventilation* related to loss of hypoxemic respiratory drive and respiratory muscle fatigue. Identify the normal physiologic events that stimulate a client to breathe, and describe how these differ for the client with chronic hypoxemia and hypercapnia.

3. The client with an acute exacerbation of COPD is at risk for respiratory failure. What changes in Mrs. Mercurio's assessment findings could indicate this complication?

4. Develop a nursing care plan for Mrs. Mercurio for the nursing diagnosis *Diversional Activity Deficit* related to inability to continue preferred activities.

The Client with Cystic Fibrosis

■ ■ ■

Cystic fibrosis (CF) is an inherited disorder of the exocrine glands that results in the secretion of abnormal amounts of mucus. Although it can affect many organ systems, CF is particularly damaging to the lungs, resulting in chronic obstructive pulmonary disease in childhood and early adulthood. Respiratory manifestations of CF are the most common cause of morbidity and death from this disease. The gastrointestinal tract also is affected significantly, and exocrine pancreatic insufficiency is characteristic of CF. Abnormally high sweat electrolytes also occur in CF.

CF is the most common lethal genetic disease in Caucasian Americans, affecting about 1 in 2400 live births. It is less common in African Americans and rare in Asians. An autosomal-recessive pattern is seen in the inheritance of CF; the trait is carried by about 5% of the Caucasian population in the United States. Although the manifestations of CF develop in childhood, aggressive management strategies have prolonged the life span for people with CF, and adults now make up about 25% to 30% of the CF population in the United States (Berkow & Fletcher, 1992; Hardy, 1993; Tierney et al., 1994).

Pathophysiology

An abnormal gene on the long arm of chromosome 7 results in a lack of or abnormality in a protein involved in the transport of chloride across the surfaces of epithelial cells. As a result of defective chloride transport, water and sodium are reabsorbed to a greater extent than normal. Secretions in affected organs (those in which this protein is normally abundant) become thick and viscous, obstructing glands and ducts. This obstruction causes dilation of secretory glands and damage to exocrine tissue. The hallmark pathophysiologic manifestations of CF include the following (McCance & Huether, 1994):

■ Excess mucus production in the respiratory tract with impaired ability to clear secretions and progressive chronic obstructive pulmonary disease

■ Pancreatic enzyme deficiency and impaired digestion

■ Abnormal elevation of sodium and chloride concentrations in sweat

In the lungs, viscous mucus plugs small airways and impairs mucociliary clearance, resulting in atelectasis, infection, bronchiectasis, and dilation of distal airways. Acute and chronic involvement of the lung parenchyma causes loss of tissue and extensive scarring and fibrosis, involving the upper lobes to a greater extent than the lower lobes. Severe airway obstruction and chronic hypoxemia lead to pulmonary hypertension, right ventricular hypertrophy, and eventual cor pulmonale. Death usually results from a combination of these cardiovascular changes and respiratory failure (Berkow & Fletcher, 1992; Porth, 1994; Wilson et al., 1991).

Pancreatic insufficiency is a frequent component of CF. Its severity can range from slight dysfunction to complete absence of pancreatic activity resulting from obstruction of ducts with thick mucus and degenerative and fibrotic changes in the pancreas. Significant pancreatic insufficiency and impaired enzyme secretion leads to maldigestion of proteins, carbohydrates, and fats (McCance & Huether, 1994).

Clinical manifestations of cystic fibrosis include a history of chronic lung disease in a young adult. Growth and development are often retarded, resulting in small stature. Recurrent pneumonia, exercise intolerance, and chronic cough are typical of CF. Other pulmonary manifestations include clubbing of the fingers and toes, an increased anteroposterior chest diameter (barrel chest), a hyperresonant percussion tone, and basilar crackles on auscultation. Distended neck veins, ascites, and peripheral edema accompany right-sided heart failure. Abdominal pain and *steatorrhea* (excess fat in the stools, resulting in frequent, bulky, foul-smelling stool) are common manifestations of the pancreatic insufficiency associated with CF. Diabetes mellitus may be present.

Collaborative Care

Cystic fibrosis typically is diagnosed in infancy, but as many as 10% of clients with CF may not be diagnosed until adolescence or early adulthood. Once the diagnosis has been made, a multidisciplinary treatment plan can help lengthen survival and manage symptoms. Treatment goals include preventing or treating respiratory complications and maintaining adequate nutritional status. Psychosocial care must be included in the plan, along with genetic and occupational counseling (Berkow & Fletcher, 1992; Tierney et al., 1994).

Laboratory and Diagnostic Tests
Although evidence of lung disease, pancreatic insufficiency, and diabetes mellitus suggest CF, the diagnosis is usually based on an abnormal pilocarpine iontophoresis sweat chloride test. Pilocarpine (a parasympathomimetic agent) and a small electric current are used to increase sweat production on the forearm. Absorbent paper or gauze is used to collect the sweat, which is then analyzed. In CF, levels of sodium and chloride in sweat are significantly elevated (Porth, 1994; Tierney et al., 1994).

Arterial blood gas measurements show hypoxemia. Pulmonary function studies reveal reduced air flow, reduced forced vital capacity (see the box on page 1425), and reduced total lung capacity. The diffusion capacity of the lungs also is typically reduced.

Pharmacology
Immunization against respiratory infections is vital to maintain optimal health in the client with CF. Yearly influenza vaccine is recommended, along with measles and pertussis boosters as needed.

Bronchodilator inhalers may be used if the client has reversible airway obstruction. Antibiotic therapy is used to treat active pulmonary infections; the choice of antibiotic is determined by culture and sensitivity testing of the sputum. Antibiotics may also be prescribed for prophylactic use in clients with frequent respiratory exacerbations of the disease.

Other Therapies
Chest physiotherapy with percussion, vibration, postural drainage, and coughing has been an essential component of care to promote airway clearance. Newer airway clearance techniques include the use of the "huff" cough technique with specified breathing cycles or patterns. In one technique, the client uses a valved mask or mouthpiece to maintain a positive end expiratory pressure for approximately 20 breaths, followed by 3 to 5 "huff" coughs. This cycle is repeated for a total of 20 minutes. The *autogenic drainage technique,* a form of biofeedback, is also employed. In this technique, the client breathes at certain lung volumes with specific respiratory patterns to facilitate the movement of mucus into larger airways, where it can be cleared with the "huff" cough (Hardy, 1993).

Oxygen therapy may be required for hypoxemia. A liberal fluid intake helps reduce the viscosity of mucus secretions. A diet high in protein, fat, and calories is necessary to maintain the client's weight. Vitamins and minerals are supplemented to counteract excess losses in the sweat and stools. Enteral or parenteral nutrition may be required during acute exacerbations of the disease.

Genetic screening of family members of a CF client is recommended. This can detect 70% to 75% of carriers of the CF gene but is not recommended for use with the general population (Porth, 1994; Tierney et al., 1994). Gene therapy is being explored as a treatment for CF. Experiments involving inhalation of the normal human gene inserted into an attenuated adenovirus to replace the defective CF gene are under way. It is hoped that the gene will transfer into respiratory epithelial cells, normalizing mucus production (Hardy, 1993).

Lung transplantation currently offers the only definitive treatment for CF. With transplantation, clients are able to live longer and healthier lives. Single-lung, double-lung, and heart-lung transplants have been successful in CF clients. Because the donor lungs do not have the genetic abnormality that causes CF, they do not develop the pathophysiologic changes of CF (Hardy, 1993; Tierney et al., 1994). Although the other defects characteristic of CF remain, these can be managed with pharmacologic therapy.

Nursing Care

Although nursing care for the client with cystic fibrosis is much the same as that for any client with chronic obstructive pulmonary disease, the genetic component of the disease and the client's age are important considerations. Many clients who have chronic disability due to COPD are older adults of retirement age. By contrast, adults with CF are just entering their productive years and face a life span that is likely to be shortened significantly.

The following nursing diagnoses are all appropriate for the client with CF:

- *Ineffective Airway Clearance*
- *Ineffective Breathing Pattern*
- *Anxiety*
- *Ineffective Individual Therapeutic Regimen Management*
- *Altered Nutrition: Less Than Body Requirements*
- *Ineffective Family Coping*

Suggested interventions for each of these diagnoses are included in the nursing care sections for asthma and COPD.

Other diagnoses that should be considered for the client with CF follow:

- *Diversional Activity Deficit* related to exercise intolerance
- *Altered Family Processes* related to chronic genetic disease

- *Hopelessness* related to limited career options and opportunities
- *Altered Growth and Development* related to gastrointestinal and respiratory effects of CF

Client and Family Teaching

Adequate education of the client and family affected by cystic fibrosis is essential to maintaining optimal health. The adult whose disease was diagnosed in infancy or childhood has grown up with the disease as a fact of life and often has a much greater knowledge level than many caregivers. However, when the initial diagnosis is made as an adolescent or young adult, teaching needs are significant.

Respiratory care techniques, including percussion, postural drainage, and controlled cough techniques are a major component of the client's self-care activities. Teach specific procedures for breathing and coughing, as well as positions that facilitate drainage of various lung segments. Include in teaching the importance of avoiding respiratory irritants, such as cigarette smoke, air pollution, and occupational dusts and gases. Stress the need to take measures to prevent respiratory infection, such as maintaining immunization status and optimal general health and avoiding exposure to large crowds and infected people.

Refer the client to a dietitian for planning and instruction to maintain adequate nutrition and minimize gastrointestinal symptoms. Referral to community agencies and support groups is also helpful.

Teach the client and family members about the genetic transmission of cystic fibrosis. Provide counseling or referral for genetic testing. Help the client and family sort through the impact of the disease on future pregnancies and generations. Remember that the possibility of CF may present an ethical dilemma regarding future pregnancies for clients and their families. Provide support as needed.

The Client with Atelectasis

■ ■ ■

Atelectasis is not a pulmonary disease but a condition associated with many respiratory disorders. It is a state of partial or total lung collapse and airlessness that may be acute or chronic. The most common cause of atelectasis is obstruction of the bronchus ventilating the affected lung tissue. Obstruction may affect only a small segment of a lung or an entire lobe. Other causes include compression of the lung due to pneumothorax, pleural effusion, or tumor; or loss of pulmonary surfactant and inability to maintain open alveoli.

The manifestations of atelectasis depend on its size. Diminished breath sounds over the affected area may be the only sign of a small area of atelectasis. If a major portion of tissue is affected, the client may have a rapid pulse and respiratory rate, appear dyspneic and cyanotic, and demonstrate signs of hypoxemia. Chest expansion may be reduced and breath sounds absent on the affected side. Fever and other manifestations of infection may be present.

On chest X-ray, an area of airless lung is seen. CT scan may help determine the cause of atelectasis. Bronchoscopy may be ordered to remove an obstructive cause.

The primary therapy for atelectasis is prevention. Clients at high risk, such as those with COPD, smokers undergoing surgery, and people on prolonged bed rest or mechanical ventilation, should have vigorous chest physiotherapy to maintain open airways. Frequent assessment of respiratory status, including rate, breath sounds, spirometry, and chest X-ray findings allows for early detection and treatment.

When atelectasis does occur, treatment is directed at removing the underlying cause. Vigorous coughing and chest therapy may be effective in removing a mechanical obstruction. If not, bronchoscopy is used. Antibiotic therapy may be prescribed to treat any underlying infection.

Nursing care measures for both prevention and treatment of atelectasis are directed toward airway clearance. The client with atelectasis should be positioned on the unaffected side, with the involved side uppermost to promote drainage. Move the client frequently, and encourage coughing and deep breathing. Unless contraindicated, encourage fluids to help liquefy secretions.

Client and family teaching is important, especially for people in groups who have a high risk for developing atelectasis. Diligent attention to pulmonary care measures, fluid intake, and avoidance of infections prevent the conditions that predispose a client to atelectasis.

The Client with Bronchiectasis

■ ■ ■

Bronchiectasis is characterized by the permanent abnormal dilation of one or more large bronchi and destruction of bronchial walls, usually accompanied by infection. The destructive process of bronchiectasis is initiated by inflammation, usually as the result of recurrent infection of the airways. About half of all cases of bronchiectasis are related to cystic fibrosis. Other causes include infections, such as severe pneumonia, tuberculosis, or fungal infections; lung abscess; exposure to toxic gases; abnormal lung or immunologic defenses; and localized airway obstruction due to a foreign body or tumor. Inflammation and airway obstruction are common to all these processes. Bronchial walls become weakened and dilated as a result, leading to pooling of secretions and further infection and inflammation (Porth, 1994; Tierney et al., 1994; Wilson et al., 1991).

A chronic cough productive of large amounts of mucopurulent sputum is characteristic of bronchiectasis. Other manifestations include hemoptysis, recurrent pneumonia, wheezing and shortness of breath, malnutrition, right-sided heart failure, and cor pulmonale.

Collaborative care for the client with bronchiectasis focuses on maintaining optimal pulmonary function and preventing the disorder from progressing. The diagnosis is typically based on the client's history and presenting manifestations. Chest X-ray and CT scan may be ordered to help confirm the diagnosis and determine the extent of lung damage.

Antibiotics are prescribed at the first indication of an infection and may be used prophylactically, as well. Inhaled bronchodilators also may be ordered. Chest physio-therapy is another vital component of the continuing care of a client with bronchiectasis. Percussion and postural drainage help mobilize secretions. Oxygen may be prescribed if the client is hypoxemic. Bronchoscopy may be necessary to remove retained secretions or obstruction or to evaluate hemoptysis. If lung destruction is localized and unresponsive to conservative management, surgical lung resection may be performed.

Nursing care of the client with bronchiectasis is much the same as that for clients with other obstructive lung diseases. Airway clearance is a primary problem, as is ineffective breathing pattern. Other applicable nursing diagnoses may include *Impaired Gas Exchange, Altered Nutrition: Less Than Body Requirements* and *Self-Care Deficit* (Sparks & Taylor, 1993).

▪▪▪ Interstitial Pulmonary Disorders ▪▪▪

Many lung diseases result in damage to the interstitial or connective tissue of the lung. The occupational lung diseases and sarcoidosis fall into this group of disorders. Toxic drugs and radiation also cause interstitial damage. Table 34–7 identifies common causes of interstitial or fibrotic pulmonary disorders.

In these disorders, the alveolar epithelium undergoes damage that leads to an inflammatory process involving the alveoli and interstitial tissue of the lung. The inflammatory response produces further damage, and abnormal fibrotic (scar) tissue replaces or infiltrates normal lung tissue. As a result, the lungs become stiff and noncompliant. Lung dysfunction is characterized by diminished lung volumes, impaired diffusing capacity, and hypoxemia (Andreoli et al., 1990; Porth, 1994; Tierney et al., 1994).

These disorders may be acute or insidious in onset. They also vary from person to person in their rate of progression and the degree of disability they produce. The usual presenting symptoms are dry cough and exertional dyspnea. Respirations are often rapid and shallow. Fine inspiratory crackles at the lung bases may be noted on auscultation, as well as clubbing of the fingers and toes.

Pulmonary function testing shows a restrictive impairment in lung ventilation, with reduced vital capacity and reduced total lung capacity. The diffusing capacity of the lungs is also decreased. Blood gas analysis reveals hypoxemia, especially with exercise. The chest X-ray shows characteristic infiltrative patterns. A bronchoscopy may be performed to obtain tissue for biopsy, and specialized lung scans may be ordered to determine the extent of fibrosis (Porth, 1994; Tierney et al., 1994).

Care of the client with interstitial lung disease varies according to the underlying cause. Overall management goals are directed at

- Identifying and removing the causative agent.
- Reducing the inflammatory response.
- Preventing disease progression.
- Providing supportive care (Porth, 1994).

The Client with an Occupational Lung Disease

▪ ▪ ▪

The occupational lung diseases are a diverse group of disorders directly related to the inhalation of noxious substances in the work environment. There are two major classifications of occupational lung diseases:

- The *pneumoconioses,* chronic fibrotic lung diseases caused by the inhalation of inorganic dusts and particulate matter
- *Hypersensitivity pneumonitis,* allergic pulmonary diseases caused by exposure to inhaled organic dusts

Pathophysiology

When a noxious substance is inhaled, the body's response to that substance depends on several factors: the size of the particulate matter; its nature (organic or inorganic); where it deposits in the respiratory tract; and the susceptibility of the individual. Relatively large particles, those greater than 6 microns, are too big to reach the lower airways and often are deposited in the nose. Smaller particles can be carried with inspired air into the alveoli. Normal lung defenses, including alveolar macrophages, lymph channels, and the mucociliary escalator, attempt to remove particulate matter from the alveoli. These defenses may be impaired by cigarette smoking, alcohol ingestion, or hypersensitivity reactions (Porth, 1994; Tierney et al., 1994).

Asbestosis

The most frequent occupational lung diseases resulting from exposure to inorganic dust are related to asbestos. *Asbestosis* is a diffuse interstitial fibrotic disease involving the terminal airways, alveoli, and pleurae that results from the inhalation of asbestos fibers. Exposure occurs in the mining, milling, manufacturing, and application of asbestos products. Although symptoms may not become apparent until after 20 years of exposure, they tend to progress, even after exposure has ended. Asbestosis is also associated with an increased risk of bronchogenic carcinoma, especially in cigarette smokers, malignant *mesothelioma* (an uncommon tumor of serous membranes such as the pleura and peritoneum), and pleural plaques (Price & Wilson, 1992; Tierney et al., 1994; Wilson et al., 1991).

The clinical manifestations of asbestosis include exertional dyspnea, exercise intolerance, and inspiratory crackles. Diffuse, small, irregular or linear opacities appear on chest X-ray, primarily in the lower lobes. As the disease progresses, the client may ultimately develop respiratory failure and marked hypoxemia.

Silicosis

The inhalation of silica dust by hard-rock miners, foundry workers, sandblasters, pottery makers, and granite cutters can lead to a nodular pulmonary fibrosis known as *silicosis*. Silicosis affects between 1.2 and 3 million workers in the United States. It is generally associated with long-term exposure to silica, but it can develop in as little as 10 months of intense exposure (Wilson et al., 1991). In this disorder, the macrophages are destroyed as they engulf silica particles, releasing substances harmful to lung tissue and leading to fibrosis and scarring (Berkow & Fletcher, 1992; Porth, 1994). Silicosis increases the client's risk for developing tuberculosis (Tierney et al., 1994).

Clients with simple silicosis have no symptoms or demonstrable respiratory impairment. Complicated silicosis, by contrast, is characterized by large conglomerate densities in the upper lungs. These clients may be severely dyspneic and have a productive cough. Pulmonary function testing shows both restrictive or fibrotic and obstructive changes. Increasing size of the conglomerate masses can lead to severe disability, cor pulmonale, and death (Berkow & Fletcher, 1992; Tierney et al., 1994).

Coal Worker's Pneumoconiosis

The ingestion of coal dust by alveolar macrophages causes "coal macules" to form, resulting in *coal worker's pneumoconiosis,* or *"black lung disease."* This occupational lung dis-

Table 34–7	Causes of Interstitial Pulmonary Disorders
Cause	**Disorder**
Inorganic dusts	Pneumoconioses
■ Silica	■ Silicosis
■ Asbestos	■ Asbestosis
■ Coal	■ Black lung disease
■ Talc	■ Talcosis
■ Beryllium	■ Berylliosis
Organic dusts	Hypersensitivity pneumonitis
■ Cotton	■ Byssinosis
■ Sugar cane	■ Bagassosis
■ Moldy hay	■ Farmer's lung
Unknown Causes	■ Sarcoidosis
	■ Idiopathic pulmonary fibrosis
	■ Connective tissue disorders

Other Causes	**Examples**
Drugs	Antineoplastic agents, antibiotics, gold salts, phenytoin
Radiation	External radiation or inhaled radioactive materials
Infections	Widespread TB or fungal infections, viral or *Pneumocystis carinii* pneumonia
Poisons and noxious gases	Paraquat, nitrogen dioxide, chlorine, ammonia, sulfur dioxide
Systemic diseases	Uremia, pulmonary edema

ease affects 12% of all miners, with a higher incidence in the eastern United States than in the West (Wilson et al., 1991). Coal macules appear on chest X-ray as diffuse, small opacities that are especially prominent in the upper lungs (Berkow & Fletcher, 1992; Tierney et al., 1994).

Simple coal worker's pneumonconiosis (CWP) generally has no manifestations. A small percentage (1% to 2%) of clients with simple CWP develop *progressive massive fibrosis* with conglomeration and contraction in the upper lungs. Progressive, massive fibrosis destroys the pulmonary vascular bed and airways, resulting in symptoms similar to those of complicated silicosis (Berkow & Fletcher, 1992; Tierney et al., 1994).

Hypersensitivity Pneumonitis

Workers exposed to organic dusts and gases may develop *hypersensitivity pneumonitis,* an allergic pulmonary disease affecting the airways and alveoli. Byssinosis, which results from exposure to cotton dust, bagassosis, which results from exposure to moldy sugar cane fiber, farmer's lung, and bird-fancier's lung are examples of hypersensitivity pneumonitis.

Either acute or subacute illness can occur. Acute illness occurs 4 to 8 hours after exposure and is manifested by sudden onset of malaise, chills and fever, dyspnea, cough, and nausea. The subacute syndrome is characterized by an insidious onset of chronic cough, progressive dyspnea, anorexia, and weight loss. Diffuse fibrosis occurs after repeated exposure to the organic material, resulting in respiratory insufficiency (Tierney et al., 1994).

Collaborative Care

Prevention is a key treatment strategy in all the occupational lung diseases. Containing dust and wearing personal protective devices that limit the amount of inhaled particles are essential for people who work in industries with known risks.

In addition to a history of occupational exposure, chest X-ray, pulmonary function studies, bronchoscopy, and possibly lung biopsy are used to establish a diagnosis for the pneumoconioses. Characteristic patterns are seen for each disorder on X-ray. Pulmonary function studies help determine the extent of disability.

Eliminating further exposure to the offending agent is an important part of managing all occupational lung diseases. There is no specific therapy available. In some cases, anti-inflammatory drugs, such as corticosteroids, can reduce the inflammatory response and slow the progression of the disease. Generally, care is supportive, similar to that for clients with COPD.

Nursing Care

As with medical management, nursing care for clients with occupational lung diseases is much the same at that for a client with COPD.

Activity intolerance is a high-priority problem for many clients with pneumoconiosis. With severe dyspnea, the client's ability to carry out ADLs may be significantly impaired. Nursing measures to reduce energy expenditures and provide for rest are essential. Caregiver role strain, either actual or potential, must be considered when the client with severe disability is being cared for at home.

Ineffective individual and family coping may also place high on the list of priority nursing diagnoses. Many of these diseases develop after 20 to 30 years of exposure to the hazardous material. Clients who entered the industry following high school may develop evidence of disease in their 40s and face the possibility of changing their occupation or developing significant disability. The resulting role strain affects all other members of the family.

Other nursing diagnoses to consider for the client with an occupational lung disease follow:

- *Ineffective Breathing Pattern* related to restrictive lung disease
- *Anticipatory Grieving* related to potential loss of employment and income
- *Low Self-Esteem: Situational* related to change of occupation

Client and Family Teaching

Teaching about the dangers of occupational lung diseases and ways to reduce their risk needs to begin early, before evidence of the disease is present. Nurses in industrial and public health settings can begin by being alert to potential dangers in their areas and teaching workers about measures to reduce dust in their work area and the use of personal protective devices such as masks. Nurses working with affected families have an excellent opportunity to begin educating children about the risks associated with the occupation.

The affected client and family need instruction in how to avoid further damage to the lungs, for example, to avoid respiratory irritants such as cigarette smoke and heavy air pollution. Immunizations for influenza and pneumococcal pneumonia are recommended. Yearly tuberculin testing is recommended for clients with silicosis.

Teach the client and family about pulmonary hygiene measures, such as maintaining good fluid intake, coughing, and deep-breathing exercises. If the client requires oxygen therapy, teach about its use and care of the equipment. Always include teaching about the use and effects of any prescribed or recommended over-the-counter medications.

The Client with Sarcoidosis

■ ■ ■

Sarcoidosis is a systemic disease characterized by granulomas in the lungs, lymph nodes, liver, eyes, skin, and other organs. Its cause is unknown. Sarcoidosis primarily affects young adults between the ages of 20 and 40, and the incidence is highest in African Americans, followed by Caucasians. Women are affected at a slightly higher rate than men (Andreoli et al., 1990; Berkow & Fletcher, 1992; Porth, 1994).

Multiple granulomas with little or no necrosis form in sarcoidosis. These lesions may resolve spontaneously or proceed to fibrosis. The lungs are affected in about 90% of clients with sarcoidosis (Tierney et al., 1994). Sarcoidosis has a low mortality rate—less than 3%—but a relatively high rate (approximately 10%) of serious disability from ocular, respiratory, or other organ damage. Pulmonary hemorrhage and cardiac and respiratory failure from pulmonary fibrosis are the leading causes of death from sarcoidosis (Berkow & Fletcher, 1992).

The presentation of sarcoidosis varies, depending on the organ system affected. Many clients are asymptomatic, with the disease diagnosed by characteristic findings on a routine chest X-ray. Others present with a gradual onset of anorexia, fatigue, weight loss, fever, dyspnea, arthralgias, and myalgias. Skin lesions, uveitis, lymphadenopathy, hepatomegaly, or other manifestations may be noted.

Leukopenia, eosinophilia, and an elevated erythrocyte sedimentation rate (ESR) typically are noted in sarcoidosis. The chest X-ray helps determine the extent of pulmonary involvement; however, biopsy of a granulomatous lesion may be required to confirm the diagnosis of sarcoidosis. Pulmonary function tests reveal a restrictive pattern with decreased compliance and impaired diffusing capacity (Berkow & Fletcher, 1992; Tierney et al., 1994).

Treatment is reserved for clients with severe or disabling symptoms, because sarcoidosis often resolves spontaneously. Corticosteroid therapy is used for clients with severe manifestations, hepatic insufficiency, cardiac dysrhythmias, involvement of the central nervous system, ocular disease, or disfiguring skin lesions. Relapse frequently occurs when corticosteroids are discontinued (Berkow & Fletcher, 1992). Other anti-inflammatory or immune-modifier medications may also be used, including chloroquine, indomethacin, azathioprine, and methotrexate (Andreoli et al., 1990).

Nursing care for clients with sarcoidosis is directed by the organ systems involved and the related manifestations. Respiratory care is supportive and includes avoidance of respiratory irritants and maintenance of adequate ventilation. Refer the client for help to quit smoking as needed.

Clients with limited symptoms require little nursing intervention other than teaching about the disease and manifestations which should be reported to a health care provider. Teach the client to report shortness of breath, tearing and eye inflammation, chest pain or irregular pulse, skin lesions, and swollen and painful joints.

If corticosteroid therapy is prescribed, teach the client about the importance of taking the medication as prescribed and not stopping it abruptly. Include information about managing the side effects of corticosteroids by limiting sodium and increasing potassium in the diet, taking the medication with food or milk to minimize gastric irritation, and identifying early signs of infection.

◾◾◾ Pulmonary Vascular Disorders ◾◾◾

The cardiovascular and respiratory systems are closely interrelated. As blood flows through the capillary network of the pulmonary vascular system, oxygen diffuses into it, and carbon dioxide diffuses out. An effective match of ventilation and perfusion is essential to maintain this process and, ultimately, tissue oxygenation and adequate functioning of all organ systems. In the older adult, vascular and alveolar changes can alter gas exchange. Arteriosclerotic changes in the pulmonary vasculature reduce blood flow to the alveolus. Nearly all disorders of the lower respiratory system potentially can affect ventilation. Many also have a secondary effect on lung perfusion, because the breakdown or fibrosis of alveolar walls destroys the capillary network as well. This section discusses primary disorders affecting the pulmonary vascular system.

The Client with Pulmonary Embolism

◾ ◾ ◾

A **pulmonary embolism** is the sudden occlusion of a pulmonary artery resulting in disruption of blood supply to the lung parenchyma. *Thromboemboli*, or blood clots, arising in the venous system or right side of the heart are the most frequent causes of pulmonary embolism. Other potential sources of emboli include tumors that have entered the venous circulation, fat or bone marrow that enter the circulation following fracture or other trauma, amniotic fluid released into the circulation during childbirth, and intravenous injection of air or other foreign substances.

Pulmonary embolism is the most common acute pulmonary problem in hospitalized clients and a leading cause of morbidity and mortality. Deep vein thrombosis, the leading cause of pulmonary embolism, develops in approximately 5 million people per year in the United States. The incidence of pulmonary embolism probably exceeds 500,000 per year, resulting in 50,000 or more deaths (Bone, 1992; Wilson et al., 1991). Often pulmonary embolism is not accurately diagnosed and is found only on autopsy after an unexpected death. Ninety percent of fatalities from pulmonary embolism occur within the first 1 to 2 hours; thus it is a medical emergency. Because pulmonary embolism is difficult to diagnose and is a significant cause of death in hospitalized clients, prevention is the most effective treatment strategy.

Pathophysiology

More than 90% to 95% of pulmonary emboli originate as clots or thrombosis in the deep veins. The risk factors for pulmonary embolus therefore are those for deep vein

---

Clinical Manifestations of Pulmonary Embolism

■ ■ ■

Common

- Abrupt onset
- Dyspnea and shortness of breath
- Chest pain
- Anxiety and apprehension

- Cough
- Tachycardia and tachypnea
- Crackles (rales)
- Low-grade fever

Less Common

- Diaphoresis
- Hemoptysis
- Syncope

- Cyanosis
- S_3 and/or S_4 gallop

---

thrombosis: stasis of blood flow, damage to the vessel wall, and/or alterations in blood coagulation. Clinical risk factors include prolonged immobility or bed rest; trauma, including hip and femur fractures; surgery (orthopedic, pelvic, and gynecologic surgery in particular); myocardial infarction and congestive heart failure; obesity; and advanced age. Women who use oral contraceptives or estrogen therapy are at risk, as are women during pregnancy and childbirth.

Deep vein thrombosis is often not suspected until pulmonary embolism occurs. Obstruction of pulmonary blood flow results in both hemodynamic and pulmonary changes. Neurohumoral reflexes that follow obstruction cause vasoconstriction, increasing pulmonary vascular resistance. In severe cases, this can cause pulmonary hypertension and right ventricular heart failure. Bronchoconstriction occurs in the affected area of lung, along with wasted ventilation of alveoli that are not being perfused (dead space) and loss of alveolar surfactant. Pulmonary infarction and lung tissue necrosis is uncommon (Porth, 1994; Tierney et al., 1994; Wilson et al., 1991).

The manifestations of a pulmonary embolism depend on its size and location. Small emboli may be asymptomatic. There is no one sign or symptom or group of manifestations diagnostic of pulmonary embolism (see the accompanying box). Manifestations usually develop abruptly, over a period of minutes. The most common symptoms are dyspnea and pleuritic chest pain. Anxiety, a sense of impending doom, and cough are also common. The client may experience diaphoresis and hemoptysis. With a massive pulmonary embolus, syncope and cyanosis may occur. On examination, the client is tachycardic and tachypneic. Crackles may be heard on auscul-

tation of the chest, and a cardiac gallop (S_3 and possibly S_4) may be noted. The client may have a mild fever. It is difficult to differentiate pulmonary embolism from myocardial infarction or pneumonia by its manifestations.

Fat emboli are the most common nonthrombotic pulmonary emboli. A fat embolism usually occurs after fracture of long bone (typically the femur) releases bone marrow fat into the circulation. Adipose tissue or liver trauma may also lead to fat emboli. Characteristic manifestations of fat emboli include sudden onset of cardiopulmonary and neurologic symptoms: dyspnea, tachypnea, tachycardia, confusion, delirium, and decreased level of consciousness. Petechiae often develop on the chest and arms (Wilson et al., 1991).

Complications of pulmonary embolism include sudden death and *pulmonary infarction* with necrosis. Sudden death, the most significant potential complication, results from obstruction of a large pulmonary artery. Gas exchange is significantly reduced or prevented, and cardiac output falls dramatically as blood fails to move through the pulmonary vascular system and return to the left heart. Fewer than 10% of pulmonary emboli result in pulmonary infarction, which involves hemorrhagic consolidation of lung tissue and possible necrosis.

Collaborative Care

Most pulmonary emboli arise in the deep veins of the lower extremities, especially the large veins of the thigh (Bone, 1992). Accurate diagnosis of deep vein thrombosis (DVT) is difficult, although newer diagnostic studies are helpful. However, the risk factors for DVT are well known, making prevention the primary goal in treatment of pulmonary embolism.

Early ambulation of medical and surgical clients has been extremely effective in preventing venous stasis and reducing the incidence of pulmonary embolism. External pneumatic compression of the legs is a preventive measure used for clients undergoing neurosurgery, urologic surgery, or major surgery of the hip or knee. It is also helpful for clients for whom anticoagulant therapy is contraindicated. Other preventive measures include elevating the legs of immobilized clients and active and passive leg exercises.

When a pulmonary embolism occurs, treatment is supportive. Oxygen therapy is initiated, and analgesics may be ordered to relieve severe pleuritic pain and anxiety. Pulmonary artery and wedge pressures are monitored with a balloon (Swan-Ganz) catheter. Cardiac outputs also may be assessed. The client is placed on a cardiac monitor to detect dysrhythmias.

Laboratory and Diagnostic Tests

The studies performed to identify DVT differ from those used to diagnose a pulmonary embolism. Venography, impedance plethysmography, and duplex ultrasonography are useful to identify DVT. Venography, an X-ray study to identify and locate thrombi in the veins of the lower extremities, is the most accurate diagnostic tool for DVT, but it is invasive and can potentially cause clot formation. Duplex venography is a noninvasive test that is nearly as reliable as venography in diagnosing DVT (Bone, 1992). These studies are discussed in further detail in Chapter 30.

Routine laboratory tests provide little information in pulmonary embolism; however, the following tests may be ordered when one is suspected:

- *Arterial blood gas analysis* reveals hypoxemia (a PO_2 of less than 80 mm Hg) in the majority of clients with a pulmonary embolism. Although hypoxemia is characteristic, it does not necessarily confirm the diagnosis, particularly in the client with preexisting lung disease such as COPD. However, normal oxygen tension does not rule out a pulmonary embolus, particularly a small embolus. Respiratory alkalosis is also often noted and is due to tachypnea and hyperventilation.

- *Blood coagulation studies,* although not diagnostic for pulmonary embolism, are ordered to provide a baseline prior to instituting anticoagulation therapy and to monitor the client's response to therapy.
  a. *Activated partial thromboplastin time (APTT or PTT)* is used to assess the intrinsic clotting pathway. Because heparin works by interfering with this pathway, PTT values are useful to evaluate the response to heparin therapy. The normal APTT is 30 to 40 seconds; normal PTT 60 to 70 seconds. Desired levels with anticoagulant therapy are 1.5 to 2 times the control value. At levels less than 1.5 times the control, the risk of recurrent thromboembolism is high; with levels greater than 2 times the control, the risk for bleeding increases (Bone, 1992; Pagana & Pagana, 1992).
  b. *Prothrombin time (PT or Pro-time)* is used to assess the extrinsic clotting system. Oral anticoagulation with coumarin interferes with the production of vitamin K–dependent clotting factors, prolonging the PT. The normal prothrombin time is 10 to 12 seconds; the goal of anticoagulant therapy is to achieve a time that is 1.25 to 1.5 times the control time.

Diagnostic studies are more useful in confirming the size and presence of a pulmonary embolism. The following studies may be ordered:

- *Chest X-ray* often shows pulmonary infiltration and occasionally pleural effusion. Other changes may be evident, but none are specifically diagnostic for pulmonary embolus.

- *Electrocardiogram (ECG)* is ordered to rule out acute myocardial infarction as the cause of the client's symp-

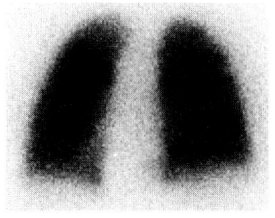 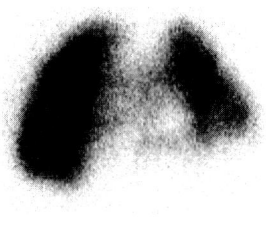

A   **B**

Figure 34–16   *A,* A normal perfusion lung scan showing smooth outlines and complete lung fields. *B,* Perfusion lung scan of a client with pulmonary embolus showing uneven densities in right lung, indicating impaired blood flow.

toms. ECG findings that are commonly associated with pulmonary embolism include tachycardia and nonspecific changes in the T wave.

- *Lung scans* provide more reliable evidence of pulmonary embolism. Perfusion and ventilation scans may be ordered, alone or in combination. In a perfusion lung scan, radiotagged albumin is injected intravenously and distributed in the lungs by the pulmonary blood flow. The lungs are then scanned for the distribution of this isotope. Homogeneous distribution of the particles that fills the pulmonary vasculature completely (a normal scan) rules out pulmonary embolism, making further diagnostic testing for the disorder unnecessary (Figure 34–16). For a ventilation scan, a radiotagged gas such as krypton or xenon-133 is inhaled; the client then holds his or her breath while the lungs are scanned for distribution of the gas. By combining perfusion and ventilation scans, it is possible to identify areas of the lungs that are ventilated but not perfused, a characteristic of pulmonary embolism (Pagana & Pagana, 1992; Porth, 1994).

- *Pulmonary angiography* is the definitive test for pulmonary embolism. It is possible to detect emboli as small as 3 mm in diameter with angiography. A contrast medium is injected into the pulmonary arteries, allowing visualization of the pulmonary vascular system. Although this procedure is expensive, invasive, and carries a higher risk for complications than others used to diagnose pulmonary embolism, it is used when establishing an absolute diagnosis is necessary. Pulmonary angiography may be ordered for clients who are at high risk from anticoagulation, such as older clients or clients with peptic ulcer disease. It is also required if any surgical procedure to prevent recurrent thromboemboli is planned (Pagana & Pagana, 1992; Tierney et al., 1994).

Pharmacology

Anticoagulant therapy is the standard treatment to prevent pulmonary emboli. It is often instituted in high-risk

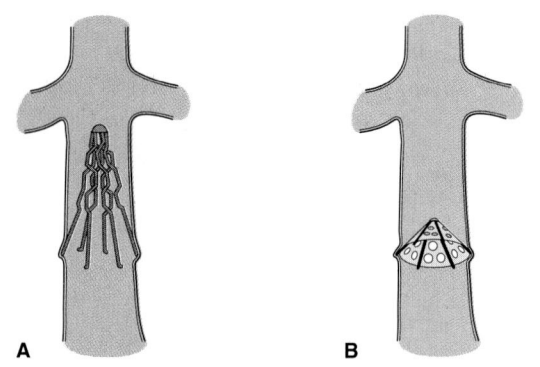

Figure 34–17 Examples of vena caval filters used to prevent emboli from reaching the pulmonary system. *A,* Greenfield filter. *B,* Umbrella filter.

clients who have no evidence of pulmonary embolism to prevent possible devastating effects. In the client with DVT or a pulmonary embolus, anticoagulants are administered to prevent further clotting and embolization.

Low-dose heparin, 5000 units every 12 hours, is administered subcutaneously after surgical procedures such as hip and other orthopedic surgery, gynecologic and urologic surgery, and extensive general surgery. Heparin can significantly reduce the incidence of DVT and pulmonary embolism in high-risk clients. Clients in intensive care units also benefit from the prophylactic administration of heparin. Low doses of heparin affect the PTT very little and carry only a small risk of bleeding (Bone, 1992).

For the client with a pulmonary embolus, heparin therapy is initiated with an intravenous bolus of 5000 to 10,000 units of heparin, followed by continuous infusion at the rate of 1000 to 1500 units per hour. The APTT or PTT is monitored frequently until it has stabilized, and the client is assessed for evidence of abnormal bleeding. Heparin therapy is typically continued for about 5 days or until oral anticoagulant therapy has become fully effective (Bone, 1992; Tierney et al., 1994).

Oral anticoagulant therapy with warfarin sodium (Coumadin) is initiated at the same time as heparin. Warfarin acts by altering the synthesis of vitamin K–dependent clotting factors and requires 5 to 7 days to be fully effective. Anticoagulant therapy is continued for 2 to 3 months for clients with few risk factors, such as surgery. Long-term anticoagulant therapy is used for clients with chronic disorders that increase their risk of thromboemboli.

Bleeding is a risk for any client on anticoagulant therapy. Although major hemorrhage is an uncommon side effect of therapy, it occurs in approximately 5% of clients receiving intravenous heparin. Cardiac, hepatic, and renal disease increase the risk of significant bleeding in clients receiving anticoagulant therapy. Clients over age 60 are also at increased risk. *Protamine,* a protein that combines with heparin to inactivate it, is used to stop the anticoagulant effect if major bleeding occurs. *Vitamin K* is administered to clients on warfarin who have bleeding complications.

Thrombolytic therapy may be instituted for clients with a massive pulmonary embolus and hypotension. Streptokinase, urokinase, or recombinant tissue plasminogen activator (t-PA) are used to lyse (disintegrate) the embolus, restoring pulmonary blood flow and reducing pulmonary artery and right heart pressures. Although thrombolytic therapy has not been proved to have a beneficial effect on mortality, it may reduce the incidence of pulmonary hypertension, which develops 3 to 5 years after an embolism. The risk of bleeding, particularly cerebral bleeding, is significantly increased when thrombolytic agents are used, however. Contraindications to thrombolytic therapy include intracranial disease, recent stroke, active bleeding or a bleeding disorder, pregnancy, severe hypertension, and recent surgery or trauma. Because of the increased risk of hemorrhage, invasive procedures are avoided after administration of thrombolytic agents (Andreoli et al., 1990; Bone, 1992; Tierney et al., 1994). See Chapter 28 for further discussion of thrombolytic therapy and its nursing implications.

Surgery

When anticoagulant therapy fails to prevent recurrent emboli or is contraindicated, surgical interruption of the inferior vena cava may be performed. The usual technique involves the insertion of an umbrella-like filter into the inferior vena cava via the percutaneous transjugular route. This device is designed to trap large emboli while allowing blood to flow through the inferior vena cava (Figure 34–17). Alternatively, a clip or suture ligation may be applied to the inferior vena cava distal to the renal veins to partially occlude the vessel and prevent the passage of large clots (Way, 1994).

Nursing Care

Nurses are involved in preventing pulmonary embolism. Encouraging clients with early ambulation after surgery or illness, applying compression stockings or pneumatic compression devices, having the client perform leg exercises, discouraging the use of pillows under the knees—all these measures help prevent DVT and subsequent pulmonary emboli.

When an embolus does occur, the client has different and urgent nursing care needs. The mismatch between pulmonary ventilation and circulation can be significant if the embolus is large, and it can result in a priority problem of impaired gas exchange. The client's cardiac output may be affected significantly by obstruction of pulmonary blood flow. With thrombolytic or anticoagulant therapy, there is a risk for injury due to bleeding. Anxiety accompanies pulmonary embolism almost universally.

Impaired Gas Exchange

With pulmonary embolism, an area or areas of the lung continue to be ventilated while they receive no capillary blood flow. If the embolus is large, resulting in a major segment of unperfused lung, gas exchange is significantly affected. Nursing interventions may not be able to restore adequate gas exchange but are directed toward compensating for this impairment.

Nursing interventions with rationales follow:

- Frequently conduct and record respiratory assessment, including rate, depth, effort, and lung sounds. *Any impairment of ventilation will further compromise gas exchange and worsen hypoxemia.*

- Monitor and record the client's level of consciousness, mental status, and skin color. *Hypoxemia often causes confusion and agitation; hypercapnia may reduce the client's level of consciousness. Cyanosis indicates significant hypoxemia.*

- Place the client in a Fowler's or high-Fowler's position, with the lower extremities dependent. *This position facilitates maximal lung expansion and reduces the venous return to the right side of the heart, lowering pressures there and in the pulmonary vascular system.*

- Start oxygen per nasal cannula or mask as ordered. *Supplemental oxygen is administered to increase alveolar and arterial oxygenation.*

- Monitor arterial blood gas results, reporting abnormal findings as indicated. Maintain pulse oximetry and arterial line, if in place. *ABGs and pulse oximetry are used to assess the adequacy of gas diffusion and tissue oxygenation. An arterial line may be inserted for monitoring arterial pressure and arterial blood sampling.*

- Administer vasopressors and other medications as ordered. *Drugs may be prescribed to maintain adequate arterial pressure and tissue perfusion.*

- Maintain bed rest. *Bed rest reduces metabolic demands.*

Decreased Cardiac Output

The impact of a large pulmonary embolus on the client's hemodynamic status can be significant. Pressures in the pulmonary vascular system and right heart increase; return to the left heart and cardiac output may significantly decrease. Nursing interventions are directed toward preserving an adequate blood pressure and organ function until the client's condition and cardiovascular status stabilize.

Nursing interventions with rationales follow:

- Assess and record vital signs frequently as indicated. Initially, assess the client every 15 to 30 minutes, then every 2 to 4 hours as the client's condition stabilizes. *It is important to institute early any necessary measures to maintain cardiovascular status to preserve organ functioning.*

- Auscultate heart sounds every 2 to 4 hours, reporting any abnormalities. *Sounds such as an S_3 or S_4 gallop may indicate cardiac compromise.*

- Monitor and record intake and output hourly. *Decreased urinary output may indicate impaired renal perfusion resulting from decreased cardiac output. Maintenance of renal perfusion is vital to maintain renal function and prevent acute renal failure.*

- Assess skin color and temperature. *These assessments are used to monitor tissue perfusion.*

- Place the client on a cardiac monitor. *Cardiac monitoring allows early detection and treatment of dysrhythmias.*

- Carefully monitor the rate and response to prescribed vasopressors. *These potent medications must be monitored carefully to evaluate the effect of therapy.*

- Monitor pulmonary artery and wedge pressures, neck vein distension, and peripheral edema. Report findings as indicated. *Right-sided heart failure is a potential complication of pulmonary embolism because of increased pulmonary artery pressures.*

- Maintain intravenous and arterial access sites as well as central lines. *The client with pulmonary embolism may be unstable and critically ill, requiring immediate interventions to maintain life.*

- Provide frequent skin care. *Skin care is important to maintain perfusion and prevent skin breakdown.*

- Instruct client to report any chest pain or other symptoms. *Decreased cardiac output and an increased workload due to pulmonary hypertension may result in anginal pain.*

Risk for Injury

The client who has received thrombolytic therapy or who is receiving anticoagulant therapy is at risk for hemorrhage due to alteration of normal clotting mechanisms. Although the risk may be low once therapy has stabilized, it is important to remain alert for evidence of bleeding during the initial period.

Nursing interventions with rationales follow:

- Monitor results of laboratory tests for coagulation. Report results outside the desired levels for anticoagulant therapy: PTT of 1.5 to 2 times the control time for heparin, and PT (Pro-time) of 1.25 to 1.5 times the control time for warfarin. *Levels below target times indicate insufficient anticoagulation and further risk of clot formation; levels above those targeted indicate risk for bleeding.*

- Assess frequently for overt and covert signs of bleeding:
  a. Bleeding gums
  b. Hematuria
  c. Obvious or occult blood in the stool or vomitus
  d. Incisional bleeding
  e. Bleeding from or bruising of injection sites

f. Bruising or hematoma formation

g. Joint pain or immobility

h. Abdominal or flank pain

The client receiving anticoagulant therapy requires close monitoring for signs of abnormal bleeding to prevent potential hemorrhage.

- Monitor neurologic status frequently. *Although cerebral bleeding is not evident externally, changes in the client's level of consciousness and other neurologic signs suggest it and should be reported immediately.*

- Have the following medications available: protamine sulfate for heparin therapy, and vitamin K for warfarin (Coumadin) therapy. *Bleeding or hemorrhage due to excess anticoagulant therapy may require administration of an antidote to rapidly reverse anticoagulant effects.*

- Assess the client's medication regimen for possible interactions with other drugs that could either potentiate or inhibit the anticoagulant effects. *Drug interactions can increase the client's risk for hemorrhage or further embolus formation.*

- Avoid invasive procedures, injections, and venous punctures as much as possible, particularly if the client has received thrombolytic therapy. *These procedures can increase the client's risk of bleeding.*

- Maintain firm pressure on injection and venipuncture sites. *This helps prevent bleeding into the tissues.*

- Monitor and maintain heparin infusion carefully, using an infusion device. *Use of an infusion pump or device with heparin infusion is vital to prevent administration of excess medication.*

- Maintain adequate fluid intake, and administer stool softeners as ordered. *These measures help prevent constipation and straining, which may precipitate bleeding of hemorrhoids.*

Anxiety

Pulmonary embolism is both a physiologic and psychologic threat to the client's safety and integrity. It is a major physiologic stressor, eliciting a strong neuroendocrine stress response. The feeling of suffocation and inability to catch one's breath that accompanies a pulmonary embolus is also a strong psychologic stressor. Fear, anxiety, and apprehension are common responses.

Nursing interventions with rationales follow:

- Assess the client's level of anxiety. *Appropriate interventions are determined by the client's level of anxiety.*

- Provide reassurance and emotional support, listening to the client's fears. Do not negate the client's fear of dying, but reassure the client that treatment is generally effective to restore respiratory function. *The client's fear of death is very real and must not be discounted; however, it is important to provide reassurance to alleviate excess anxiety.*

- Remain with the client as much as possible. *This helps reduce the client's fear.*

- Explain procedures and treatments, using short, simple sentences. *Providing clearly understood, simple instructions reduces the client's fear of the unknown.*

- Reduce environmental stimuli, and use a calm, reassuring manner. *These measures help reduce anxiety (for both the nurse and the client).*

- Allow family members to remain with the client as much as possible. *Calm, supportive family members provide further reassurance for the client.*

- Administer morphine sulfate as ordered. *Morphine is given to reduce pain and anxiety.*

Other Nursing Diagnoses

Other nursing diagnoses that may be appropriate for the client with pulmonary embolism include the following:

- *Activity Intolerance* related to altered pulmonary status

- *Ineffective Breathing Pattern* related to pain and anxiety

- *Altered Tissue Perfusion: Cardiopulmonary* related to embolus

Client and Family Teaching

Nurses can teach clients to reduce their risk for thrombus formation and pulmonary embolism. Teach clients to avoid the risks associated with such long periods of immobility as riding in an automobile or long airplane flights. On automobile trips, stopping every 1 to 2 hours for a brief stretch and walk helps restore venous circulation. While on a long flight, suggest to clients that they get up every hour or so and perform leg exercises and stretches in their seats. Sitting without crossing the legs helps prevent venous pooling. Regular exercise such as walking also reduces the risk of DVT. Instruct clients who must stand for long periods to use elastic hose or antiemboli stockings, being careful to avoid hose that bind around the knee or thigh.

Teach hospitalized clients the reasons for early ambulation and leg exercises while on bed rest. For clients on anticoagulant therapy, teach the client and family about the prescribed drug. Include teaching about manifestations of bleeding to report to the primary care provider. Instruct the client to use a soft toothbrush and to check urine, sputum, and stool for bleeding. Explain the need to avoid taking aspirin (unless prescribed) and other over-the-counter medications without first checking with the physician. Stress the importance of wearing a medical identification bracelet or tag to alert medical personnel about anticoagulant use.

Include teaching about symptoms that could indicate recurrent pulmonary embolism, such as sudden chest pain, shortness of breath, and possibly bloody sputum. Stress the need to avoid smoking to promote respiratory health.

The Client with Pulmonary Hypertension

■ ■ ■

The pulmonary vascular system is normally a high-flow, low-pressure, low-resistance system able to accommodate large increases in blood flow when necessary (e.g., during exercise). The normal mean arterial pressure in the pulmonary system is 12 to 15 mm Hg (25 to 28 systolic/8 diastolic). **Pulmonary hypertension** is a condition in which the pulmonary arterial pressure is elevated to an abnormal level (Porth, 1994; Tierney et al., 1994). This section discusses primary pulmonary hypertension, secondary pulmonary hypertension, and cor pulmonale, a condition associated with long-standing pulmonary hypertension.

Pathophysiology

Pulmonary hypertension can develop as a primary disorder, but it usually occurs secondary to another condition.

Primary Pulmonary Hypertension

Primary pulmonary hypertension is an uncommon disease that is characterized by increased pulmonary pressure and resistance with no apparent cause. Its etiologic origin is unknown. It affects primarily women in their 30s or 40s. Primary pulmonary hypertension is characterized by progressive dyspnea, fatigue, angina, and syncope with exertion. Clients typically demonstrate a steady decline to death within 3 to 4 years (Andreoli et al., 1990; Porth, 1994; Wilson et al., 1991).

Secondary Pulmonary Hypertension

Secondary pulmonary hypertension is more common than the primary type. The usual cause is a reduction in the size of the pulmonary vascular bed, which may be the result of vasoconstriction or widespread vessel destruction or obstruction. Hypoxemia is a potent pulmonary vasoconstrictor and a common initiating factor in pulmonary hypertension. Chronic lung diseases, sleep apnea, and hypoventilation due to obesity or neuromuscular disease can lead to hypoxemia. The alveolar wall destruction that occurs in emphysema leads to loss of pulmonary capillaries; large or multiple pulmonary emboli may cause significant obstruction. Other factors such as left ventricular failure or mitral stenosis also can lead to elevated pulmonary pressures. Once initiated, pulmonary hypertension becomes self-sustaining, because pulmonary vessels undergo changes that further narrow the pulmonary bed (Porth, 1994; Tierney et al., 1994).

Manifestations of secondary pulmonary hypertension typically are masked by those of the underlying disease. Dyspnea is usual; dull, retrosternal chest pain may also be present, along with fatigue and syncope on exertion (Tierney et al., 1994).

Cor Pulmonale

Cor pulmonale is a condition of right ventricular hypertrophy and failure that results from long-standing pulmonary hypertension. Chronic obstructive pulmonary disease is the most common cause of cor pulmonale.

The manifestations of cor pulmonale are those of the underlying pulmonary disorder and right-sided heart failure. Chronic productive cough, progressive dyspnea, and wheezing are common manifestations. With right-sided heart failure, peripheral edema and distended neck veins are seen. Skin is warm, moist and both ruddy and cyanotic because of increased numbers of red blood cells (RBCs) and hypoxemia.

Collaborative Care

Laboratory tests are not diagnostic for pulmonary hypertension. The CBC commonly shows *polycythemia,* increased numbers of red blood cells. Blood gas analysis reveals hypoxemia.

The chest X-ray shows enlargement of the right heart and dilation of the central pulmonary arteries. Typical ECG changes are those of right ventricular hypertrophy. An echocardiogram may be ordered to identify cardiac changes occurring either as a cause or result of pulmonary hypertension. Doppler ultrasonography provides a noninvasive means of estimating pulmonary artery pressure, but cardiac catheterization may be required for definitive diagnosis (Tierney et al., 1994; Wilson et al., 1991). Cardiac catheterization is discussed in detail in Chapter 28.

Treatment for primary pulmonary hypertension is not particularly effective in reversing or slowing the course of the disease. Current therapy involves using the calcium channel blockers nifedipine (Procardia) or diltiazem (Cardizem) to reduce pulmonary vascular resistance and improve cardiac output. Heart-lung transplant is the most effective long-term treatment for primary pulmonary hypertension (Tierney et al., 1994; Wilson et al., 1991).

Treatment of secondary pulmonary hypertension is directed toward the underlying disease process. The pulmonary hypertension often is advanced at the time of diagnosis and resistant to treatment. Supplemental oxygen may be ordered to reduce hypoxemia. Clients may be placed on long-term anticoagulation or calcium channel blockers. If polycythemia is present, phlebotomy is performed to reduce the viscosity of the blood.

When cor pulmonale is present, salt and water restrictions as well as diuretic therapy are added to the above regimen to manage the right-sided heart failure.

Nursing Care

Nursing care for the client with pulmonary hypertension or cor pulmonale is largely supportive and directed toward the underlying lung disease. Impaired gas exchange due to contraction of the pulmonary vascular system is a significant problem for the client and results in many secondary problems, such as activity intolerance, anxiety, fatigue, and others. Nursing interventions for impaired gas exchange are directed toward maintaining adequate alveolar ventilation, oxygenation, and perfusion and include the following measures:

- Monitoring breath sounds, respiratory rate, skin color, and use of accessory muscles
- Placing the client in Fowler's position for optimal lung expansion
- Coughing, deep breathing, and chest physiotherapy
- Administering prescribed vasodilators

It is important to assess the client's level of fatigue and dyspnea that occur with activities and to plan frequent rest periods. Assist the client with self-care activities as needed to preserve energy.

With primary pulmonary hypertension, anticipatory grieving and hopelessness are additional potential nursing diagnoses. When the client also has cor pulmonale, decreased cardiac output, fluid volume excess, and ineffective individual coping must be considered.

Client and Family Teaching

For the client and family who are facing these disorders, teaching is directed both at the underlying lung disease, if present, and the resultant hypertensive process. Teaching for the client with COPD, the most frequent cause of pulmonary hypertension and cor pulmonale, is outlined on pages 1430-1431.

Provide information about pulmonary hypertension and cor pulmonale (if appropriate) to the client and family. Include teaching about the disease process, its management, and the prognosis. Discuss the manifestations or changes in condition that should be reported to the physician, including change in activity tolerance, increased edema, and signs of respiratory infection or exacerbation. Talk about the importance of planned rest periods between activities and taking measures to conserve the client's energy, such as using a shower chair. Stress the importance of not smoking due to its irritant and vasoconstrictive effects. As always, include teaching about prescribed medications, both their use and their effects.

◾◾◾ Neoplastic Disorders ◾◾◾

The Client with Lung Cancer

◾ ◾ ◾

In 1991, an estimated 161,000 new cases of lung cancer were diagnosed in the United States; for 1994, the number of new cases may reach 170,000. Lung cancer accounted for 143,000 deaths in the United States in 1991, making it the leading cause of cancer deaths in both men and women. It is a major health problem with a grim prognosis: Most people with lung cancer die within one year of the initial diagnosis (Seale & Beaver, 1992; Tierney et al., 1994; Wilson et al., 1991).

The incidence of lung cancer varies from state to state and among nations. It increases with age, occurring most commonly in clients over age 50. Cigarette smoke, which contains 43 known chemical carcinogens and cancer promoters, is clearly the most important cause of lung cancer. An estimated 85% of lung cancer cases are related to smoking, and the disease is 10 to 30 times more common in smokers than nonsmokers. There is a dose-response relationship between smoking and lung cancer; the more the person smokes and the longer the person smokes, the greater the risk. Exposure to ionizing radiation and inhaled irritants, asbestos in particular, is also recognized as a risk factor for lung cancer (Andreoli et al., 1990; Porth, 1994; Seale & Beaver, 1992).

At the time of diagnosis, cancer of the lung typically is well advanced, with distant metastasis present in 55% of clients and regional lymph node involvement in another 25%. The prognosis is generally poor: the overall 5-year survival rate is only 10% to 15% (Tierney et al., 1994; Wilson et al., 1991).

Pathophysiology

The vast majority of primary lung lesions are bronchogenic carcinoma, tumors of the airway epithelium. These tumors are further differentiated by cell type: small-cell, or oat cell, carcinoma; and non-small-cell carcinomas, which include adenocarcinoma, squamous cell carcinoma, and large-cell carcinoma. Small-cell carcinomas, which account for approximately 25% of lung cancers, grow rapidly and spread early. These tumors have paraneoplastic properties; that is, they produce manifestations at sites that are not directly affected by the tumor. Small-cell lung carcinomas can synthesize bioactive products and hormones such as adrenocorticotropic hormones (ACTH), antidiuretic hormone (ADH), a parathor-

Table 34–8   Comparison of Lung Cancer Cell Types

	Cell Type and Prevalence	Presentation and Associated Manifestations	Spread
	Small-cell (oat cell) carcinoma: 20% to 25% of all lung cancers	Central lesion with hilar mass common, early mediastinal involvement, no cavitation; SIADH, Cushing's syndrome, thrombophlebitis	Aggressive tumor; more than 40% of clients have distant metastasis at time of presentation
	Non-small-cell cancers: 75% of all lung cancers	More than 25% of clients present with manifestations related to primary tumor, more than 30% with metastatic disease, and 33% with systemic manifestations	
	Adenocarcinoma 33% to 35% of all lung cancers	Peripheral mass involving bronchi; few local symptoms; hypertrophic pulmonary osteoarthropathy	Early metastasis to central nervous system, skeleton, and adrenal glands
	Squamous cell carcinoma 30% to 32% of all lung cancers	Central lesion located in large bronchi; client presents with cough, dyspnea, atelectasis, and wheezing; hypercalcemia common	Spreads by local invasion
	Large-cell carcinoma 15% to 20% of all lung cancers	Usually, peripheral lesion that is larger than that associated with adenocarcinoma and tends to cavitate; gynecomastia, thrombophlebitis	Early metastasis

mone-like hormone, and gastrin-releasing peptide. Non-small-cell carcinoma accounts for about 75% of lung cancers. Each cell type differs in its incidence, presentation, and manner of spread (Porth, 1994; Seale & Beaver, 1992). Table 34–8 outlines the incidence and unique characteristics of each cell type.

Bronchogenic cancer, regardless of cell type, tends to be aggressive, locally invasive, and have widespread metastatic lesions. Tumors begin as mucosal lesions that grow to form masses which obstruct the bronchi or invade adjacent lung tissue. All types frequently spread via the lymph system to nodes and other organs (Porth,

Table 34–9 Lung Cancer Staging

	Primary Tumor (T-Stage)	Regional Lymph Nodes (N)	Distant Metastasis (M)
Stage 0	T_0–No evidence of primary tumor T_X–Malignant cells in bronchopulmonary secretions, but no tumor visualized		MX–Presence of distant metastasis cannot be assessed
Stage I	T_1S–Carcinoma in situ T_1–Tumor that is 3 cm diameter or less, with no evidence of invasion	NO–No regional lymph node metastasis	MO–No distant metastasis
Stage II	T_2–Tumor that is greater than 3 cm diameter, or invades visceral pleura, or has associated atelectasis or pneumonitis	N_1–Metastasis or direct extension to peribronchial or ipsilateral hilar nodes	
Stage III	T_3–Tumor with direct extension into an adjacent structure, or any tumor with associated pleural effusion or atelectasis or pneumonitis of entire lung	N_2–Metastasis to ipsilateral mediastinal or subcarinal nodes	
Stage IV	T_4–Tumor that invades mediastinum or involves the heart, great vessels, trachea, esophagus, vertebral body, or carina; presence of malignant pleural effusion	N_3–Metastasis to contralateral mediastinal, scalene, or supraclavicular nodes	M_1–Distant metastasis present

1994). Lung cancer is staged by the tumor size, location, degree of invasion of the primary tumor, and the presence of metastatic disease. Lung cancer staging is summarized in Table 34–9.

The clinical manifestations of lung cancer are related to the location and spread of the tumor. Initial symptoms often are attributed to smoking or chronic bronchitis. Chronic cough is common, as is hemoptysis. Wheezing and shortness of breath occur as a result of airway obstruction. Dull, aching chest pain occurs as the tumor spreads to the mediastinum; pleuritic pain occurs when the pleura is invaded. Hoarseness and/or dysphagia indicates pressure of the tumor on the trachea or esophagus.

General manifestations and manifestations of paraneoplastic syndrome of lung cancer include weight loss, anorexia, fatigue, and weakness; bone pain, tenderness, and swelling; clubbing of the fingers and toes; and various endocrine, neuromuscular, cardiovascular, and hematologic manifestations. Local and general manifestations of lung cancer are summarized in the box on page 1449.

Lung cancer tends to metastasize to the lymph nodes, brain, bones, liver, and other organs. Confusion, disturbances of gait and balance, headache, and personality changes may be manifestations of brain metastasis. Tumor spread to the bone causes bone pain, pathologic fractures, and possible spinal cord compression, as well as thrombocytopenia and anemia if bone marrow is invaded. When the liver is affected, symptoms of liver dysfunction and biliary obstruction—including jaundice, anorexia, and upper right quadrant pain—are evident (Seale & Beaver, 1992; Wilson et al, 1991).

Superior vena cava syndrome, partial or complete obstruction of the superior vena cava, is a potential complication of lung cancer, particularly when the tumor involves the superior mediastinum or mediastinal lymph nodes. Either an acute or subacute onset of symptoms may be noted. The client develops edema of the neck and face, headache, dizziness, vision disturbances, and syncope. Veins of the upper chest and neck become dilated; flushing occurs, followed by cyanosis. Cerebral edema may alter the level of consciousness; laryngeal edema may impair respirations.

Collaborative Care

Because lung cancer typically has reached an advanced state at the time of diagnosis and the prognosis is generally poor, prevention of the disease must be a primary goal for all health care providers. With 85% of lung cancer related to cigarette smoking, reducing the use of tobacco products will make a significant impact on the death rate from lung cancer—a far greater impact than advances in treatment. The box on page 1450 discusses cigarette smoking and tobacco use.

Establishing an accurate diagnosis is the first step in treating lung cancer. Treatment decisions are based on the tumor location, type of cancer cell, staging of the tumor, and the client's ability to tolerate treatment. Surgical intervention provides the only significant chance for a cure in most forms of lung cancer.

Laboratory and Diagnostic Tests

The chest X-ray often provides the first evidence of lung cancer. Once a tumor mass has been identified, various studies are performed to determine the cell type, extent of local invasion, and spread to distant sites.

The following laboratory tests may be ordered for a client with lung cancer:

- *Cytologic examination of the sputum* provides a definitive diagnosis of lung cancer in 40% to 60% of clients. It is inexpensive and easily obtained, requiring only a simple sputum sample when the client arises in the morning. If malignant cells are identified in the sputum, the test is positive, and the client may be spared more expensive and invasive examinations. However, a negative result from sputum cytologic testing does not always mean that no tumor is present; it means only that the tumor is not shedding cells into mucus secretions.
- *CBC, liver function studies, and serum electrolytes* including calcium are conducted to evaluate the client for evidence of metastatic disease or paraneoplastic syndromes.

In addition to the above laboratory studies, the following diagnostic tests may be ordered:

- *Chest X-ray* is particularly valuable as a low-cost, noninvasive study that provides reliable evidence of lung cancer, especially when compared with a previous chest X-ray of the client. In high-risk populations, the chest X-ray may be used as a screening tool for lung cancer.
- *CT scan* is used to evaluate and localize tumors. It is especially valuable to assess tumors in the mediastinal structures, and it is also used prior to needle biopsy to localize the tumor. CT scanning is also used to detect distant tumor metastasis and evaluate tumor response to treatment with chemotherapy or radiation therapy.
- *Magnetic resonance imaging (MRI)* produces a high-resolution and high-quality image based on differences in the water content of tissues and proton activity. MRI

Clinical Manifestations of Lung Cancer

Local Manifestations

- Cough
- Hemoptysis
- Wheezing and dyspnea
- Chest pain, dull or pleuritic
- Hoarseness and dysphagia
- Pleural effusion
- Compression of the superior vena cava

General Manifestations

- Weight loss
- Anorexia
- Fever

Paraneoplastic Syndromes

Endocrine System

- Hypercalcemia
- Hyperphosphatemia
- Cushing's syndrome
- Syndrome of inappropriate antidiuretic hormone (SIADH) with water retention and hyponatremia

Connective Tissue

- Osteoarthropathy with clubbing and periosteal inflammation

Neuromuscular Effects

- Peripheral neuropathy
- Cerebellar degeneration
- Myasthenia-like muscle weakness

Cardiovascular System

- Thrombophlebitis
- Endocarditis

Hematologic Effects

- Anemia
- Disseminated intravascular coagulation (DIC)
- Eosinophilia

Cigarette Smoking and Tobacco Use

■ ■ ■

The use of tobacco reaches back to early civilizations, where it was used in religious ceremonies and as an offering of friendship. At one time, tobacco was thought to have medicinal qualities effective against all common diseases. Widespread use of tobacco among the male population of the industrialized world began during World War I.

Tobacco is now recognized as the leading cause of preventable illness in the world. In spite of this knowledge, aggressive marketing of the product continues, and its worldwide use is increasing, especially in underdeveloped countries.

The link between tobacco use and cancer was reported as early as 1912. In 1987, lung cancer became the leading cause of cancer-related death in the United States among both men and women. Between 1930 and 1985, lung cancer deaths among women increased by 500%!

Cigarette smoke contains approximately 4000 chemicals, including nicotine. Nicotine is a highly addictive psychoactive substance that is relatively cheap and readily available. It produces euphoria, which acts as a positive reinforcer for continued use. In North American society, tobacco is more acceptable than many other dependency-producing drugs.

Tar is the particulate matter in cigarette smoke that is responsible for the majority of its carcinogenic and pathologic effects on the lungs. Smoke also paralyzes the cilia, reducing their ability to remove tars from contact with the respiratory epithelium. The risk for cancer and other lung diseases is dose related, affected by the age at which the person started smoking, the number of cigarettes smoked per day, and the number of years the person smoked. Cessation of smoking reduces the risks associated with tobacco use. For some risks, such as the risk of coronary artery disease, quitting smoking yields rapid benefits. For others, the degree of risk reduction is affected by the number of years and amount the person smoked, the time since the person quit, and the person's health status at that time.

Nurses need to do more than simply tell clients they should quit smoking and inform them of the risks for continuing. Nurses can take an active role in smoking cessation. Beginning with the nursing history, identify the client's smoking habits, any smoking-related illnesses, and previous efforts to quit. Work with the client to identify barriers and obstacles to quitting. Teach the client that nicotine is an addictive substance, and explain that the manifestations of nicotine withdrawal may include anxiety, irritability, headache, and disturbed sleep. Develop a plan with the client that specifies a target date to quit and includes ways to deal with obstacles to quitting, withdrawal symptoms, and the temptation to resume smoking. Offer self-help material at a reading level that is appropriate to the client. Provide a referral to a counselor, physician, self-help group, or smoking-cessation clinic. If the client experiences a relapse, recognize that this is a normal occurrence in the process of rehabilitation from any addictive substance. Continue to provide support and encouragement, helping the client avoid further relapses.

Nurses can be especially effective in primary prevention of cigarette smoking and the diseases associated with it. Just as tobacco companies direct advertising at women and teens, nurses can target these populations, along with younger children, for programs to prevent smoking. In addition, nurses can and should become active in reducing minors' access to tobacco products, especially cigarettes and chewing tobacco (often the first product used by teenaged boys).

Nursing diagnoses that may be appropriate for the client related to smoking include the following:

- *Altered Health Maintenance* related to tobacco use

- *Decisional Conflict* related to tobacco use

- *Ineffective Denial* related to acknowledgment of substance abuse and dependence

Note. Data are from "Smoking" (pp. 631–642) by R. A. Franklin, 1992, *Nursing Clinics of North America, 27*(3).

uses a strong magnetic field and radiofrequency waves and has the advantage of not involving radiation. It is most useful to evaluate thoracic structures and separate normal tissue from possible malignant tissue in the hilum and mediastinum. The MRI is not as effective a tool for lung cancer diagnosis and evaluation as the CT scan; also, it is expensive and not available in all areas (Epps, 1992).

- *Bronchoscopy* is frequently performed to allow visualization of the tumor and tissue biopsy. For this procedure, a flexible fiberoptic bronchoscope is inserted through the mouth, larynx, and trachea into the bronchus. Once a tumor mass or suspicious tissue is identified visually, a cable-activated instrument can be used to obtain a biopsy specimen. If the tumor cannot be visualized, a saline solution can be used to flush the airways (bronchial washing), and cells obtained in this manner are sent for cytologic examination. Nursing care of the client undergoing a bronchoscopy is included in the box on page 1386.

■ *Other procedures* that may be used to obtain tissue or cells for biopsy and cytologic examination include aspiration of fluid from a pleural effusion, percutaneous needle biopsy, lymph node biopsy, and biopsy of metastatic sites. Depending on the location of the tissue to be obtained, these procedures may be done in an outpatient or in a surgical setting.

■ *Mediastinoscopy,* a procedure performed under general anesthesia with controlled ventilation, uses a scope passed through a suprasternal incision along the anterior aspect of the trachea to visualize the mediastinum and to biopsy lymph nodes or tumor. Although it is invasive, this procedure may allow the client to escape more extensive exploratory surgery to evaluate a tumor (Epps, 1992).

Pharmacology

Combination chemotherapy is the treatment of choice for small cell lung cancer because of its rapid growth, dissemination, and sensitivity to cytotoxic drugs. Used in combination, chemotherapeutic drugs allow tumor cells to be attacked at different parts of the cell cycle and in different ways, increasing the effectiveness of therapy. Fifty percent of clients with tumors at early stages achieve complete tumor remission with combination chemotherapy. When a complete tumor response is achieved in the first few cycles of chemotherapy, the chances for long-term survival are much greater (Pate, 1992).

Combination chemotherapy is used also as an adjunct to surgery or radiation therapy for lung cancer. It is often employed to lengthen survival time when metastases are known to be present. The size of advanced local cancers can be reduced prior to surgery to make them easier to remove (Pate, 1992; Wilson et al., 1991). See Chapter 9 for further discussion of chemotherapy.

Other medications that may be ordered for the client with lung cancer include bronchodilators to reduce airway obstruction and antibiotics to treat any infection. Analgesic therapy is necessary following surgery and for advanced cancers.

Surgery

Surgery offers the only real chance for a cure in non-small-cell lung cancer; however, at the time of diagnosis, the majority of clients have tumors that are either inoperable or only partially resectable. The goal of surgical in-

tervention is to remove all tumorous tissue, including involved lymph nodes. The 5-year survival rate for clients with resectable tumors is still only about 30% (Langston, 1992; Wilson et al., 1991).

The type of surgical procedure used depends on the location and size of the tumor, as well as the client's pulmonary and general health status. Although the goal of surgery is to remove all involved tissue, as much functional lung as possible is preserved. The surgical procedure of choice for tumors that are confined to a single lobe of the lung is a **lobectomy.** A significant amount of lung tissue is preserved when only a single lung lobe is removed. The space occupied by the resected lobe will be filled by the remaining lung. When a tumor is located in the lung periphery and there is no evidence of extension to the chest wall or metastasis, a *segmental resection,* the removal of an individual bronchovascular segment of a lobe, can be used. The most conservative surgical procedure used is a *wedge resection,* the removal of a small section of lung tissue that leaves intact the remaining part of the bronchovascular segment. This procedure may be used for clients with small, peripheral lesions and for those who are unable to tolerate more extensive lung surgery. A small lesion of a major bronchus may be removed in a *sleeve resection* or *bronchoplastic reconstruction* procedure. The section containing the lesion is resected and the remaining normal bronchus reattached, preserving lung function. Laser bronchoscopy is used to resect tumors localized in a main bronchus (Langston, 1992; Tierney et al., 1994).

Pneumonectomy, the removal of an entire lung, is the most extensive procedure used in the treatment of lung cancer. Pneumonectomy is done only when the tumor is widespread throughout the lung, involves the main bronchus, or is fixed to the hilum. This extensive surgery is considered only for clients with good pulmonary reserve and preoperative health. Following the surgery, the empty hemithorax gradually fills with fluid and eventually consolidates (Langston, 1992).

A **thoracotomy,** incision of the chest wall, is used to gain access to the lung for surgery. Surgical incisions used for lung resection include the posterolateral, anterolateral, median sterotomy, and axillary incision (Langston, 1992). Nursing care for the client having lung surgery is outlined in the box on page 1452.

Radiation Therapy

Radiation therapy involves the use of high-energy radioactive particles to destroy or weaken cancer cells. Radiation therapy is used either as curative or palliative treatment alone or in combination with surgery or chemotherapy. Prior to surgery, radiation therapy is used to "debulk" tumors. When cancer has spread by direct extension to other thoracic structures and surgery is not feasible or the client refuses surgery, radiation therapy may

Nursing Care of the Client Having Lung Surgery

PREOPERATIVE CARE

- Obtain a complete nursing history, paying particular attention to history of smoking, respiratory and cardiac diseases, and other chronic conditions. *These factors may affect the client's ability to tolerate the surgical procedure and postoperative course.*

- Assess the client's knowledge and understanding of the underlying disease process and the procedure to be performed. *The client who has a good understanding of why surgery is being performed and what is being done will be less anxious and better able to cooperate with preoperative and postoperative procedures.*

- Perform a baseline physical assessment. *The baseline assessment provides data for comparison in the postoperative period.*

- Provide emotional and psychologic support for the client and family. *In addition to facing surgery, the client may be adjusting to a new diagnosis of cancer and the possibility that surgical intervention will be only partially successful.*

- Provide instructions about postoperative procedures, including respiratory therapy, breathing exercises, and coughing techniques. Allow the client time to practice techniques. *Learning will be easier for the client in the preoperative period, when pain and anesthesia recovery are not affecting the client.*

- For the client who will return from the surgical procedure with an endotracheal tube and mechanical ventilation, establish a means of communication using hand or eye signals or a magic slate. *Establishing a means of communication is easier in the preoperative period and reduces the client's postoperative anxiety at being unable to speak.*

- If the client is to return to an intensive care unit, allow the client and family to see the unit and any machines, such as ventilators and monitors, that will be used. *The knowledge that the use of these machines is expected and does not indicate a complication of surgery reduces the client's and family's anxiety in the postoperative period.*

POSTOPERATIVE CARE

- Assess the client, and provide routine postoperative care as outlined in Chapter 7.

- Assess the client for adequate pain control, and provide analgesics as needed. *Incisional pain is a common cause of altered breathing patterns in the client who has undergone lung surgery.*

- Frequently assess the client's respiratory status, including color, respiratory rate and depth, chest expansion, lung sounds, percussion tone, oxygen saturation, and arterial blood gases. *In the client who has undergone lung surgery, it is especially important to maintain adequate ventilation and respiratory function to reduce the risk of mortality and morbity. Gas exchange may be impaired by many complications associated with lung resection, including pneumothorax, atelectasis, bronchospasm, pulmonary embolus, bronchopleural fistula, and adult respiratory distress syndrome (ARDS) (Langston, 1992).*

- Assist the client with effective coughing techniques, postural drainage, and incentive spirometry. Perform endotracheal suctioning as needed and/or prescribed while the client is intubated. *Surgical manipulation and anesthesia can increase the production of mucus, which can obstruct the client's airway. Aggressive pulmonary hygiene is important in preventing this complication.*

- Monitor and maintain effective mechanical ventilation. *This is vital to ensure adequate ventilation and gas exchange in the early postoperative period.*

- Maintain the patency of chest tubes and the integrity of closed drainage system. Monitor chest tube output every hour initially, then every 2 to 4 or 8 hours as indicated. Notify the physician if chest tube output exceeds 70 mL per hour and/or is bright red, warm, and free flowing. *Maintaining a patent, intact chest drainage system is vital to reestablishment of negative pressure within the chest cavity and reexpansion of the lungs. Increased amounts of warm, free-flowing blood indicate intrathoracic hemorrhage that may necessitate surgical intervention.*

- Assess the client for signs of infection involving the surgical wound or chest tube site(s). Use strict aseptic technique in caring for incisions and invasive monitoring devices. *The postoperative client is at risk for incisional infections, empyema in the chest cavity, and pneumonia.*

- Assist the client to turn in bed and ambulate as soon as possible. *Early mobility is an important measure in preventing possible complications, such as pulmonary embolus.*

- Maintain the client's nutritional status. If the client will require intubation and mechanical ventilation for an extended period, enteral or parenteral nutrition should be initiated early. Once the client is extubated, frequent small feedings may be necessary. *Maintaining nutritional status helps promote wound healing and prevent negative nitrogen balance. Frequent small feedings reduce the fatigue associated with eating.*

be the treatment of choice. It is also palliative for such manifestations as cough, hemoptysis, pain due to bone metastasis, and dyspnea from bronchial obstruction. Complications of lung cancer, such as superior vena cava syndrome, may be treated with radiation (Stewart, 1992; Tierney et al., 1994; Wilson et al., 1991).

Radiation therapy may be delivered by external beam to the primary tumor site or by intraluminal radiation, or brachytherapy. Other applications include hemibody radiation and whole-body irradiation with chemotherapy followed by bone marrow transplant. For the client with documented brain metastasis, high-dose radiotherapy to the whole brain may be used (Stewart, 1992; Tierney et al., 1994; Wilson et al., 1991). Radiation therapy is discussed further in Chapter 9. Nursing care of the client undergoing radiation therapy for lung cancer is described in the box on page 1454.

Other Therapies

Pleural effusion, a collection of fluid in the pleural space, is a frequent complication of lung cancer. As fluid collects, lung expansion and alveolar ventilation is impaired. A *thoracentesis* may be performed to remove this fluid from the pleural space. In this procedure, a needle is inserted into the pleural space to remove the excess fluid. See the section on pleural effusion for further discussion of this complication and its management.

Nursing Care

The client with lung cancer is facing invasive treatments with undesirable side effects, possibly surgery, and typically a poor prognosis for long-term survival. Nursing care needs of the lung cancer client are diverse, related to the client's respiratory status, to the cancer disease process and possible metastatic lesions, and to chosen therapeutic interventions. Priority nursing diagnoses related to respiratory function include ineffective breathing pattern and activity intolerance. Pain and anticipatory grieving also are likely to be high-priority problems.

Ineffective Breathing Pattern

The breathing pattern and effectiveness of ventilation in the client with lung cancer may be affected by the tumor itself or by therapy used to treat the tumor. The client who has had resectional surgery is at particularly high risk related to the thoracic incision and disruption of the muscles of respiration. Maintaining effective lung ventilation is particularly important for the postoperative client to reexpand remaining lung tissue and prevent complications associated with surgery.

Nursing interventions with rationales follow:

- Assess and document respiratory rate, depth, and lung sounds at least every 4 hours; more frequently in the immediate postoperative period or as indicated by the client's condition. *It is important to detect signs of respiratory compromise or adventitious lung sounds early for effective intervention.*

- Monitor pulse oximetry, oxygen saturation readings, and/or blood gas results, reporting changes from normal. *Changes in levels of blood oxygen may be an early indication of respiratory compromise.*

- Frequently assess and document the client's level of pain, providing analgesics as needed. *Pain and splinting can lead to rapid, shallow respirations and ineffective ventilation.*

- Elevate the head of the bed to 60 degrees. *Elevation of the head of the bed permits optimal lung expansion.*

- Assist the client to turn, cough, and deep breathe and/or use incentive spirometry. Help the client splint the chest with a pillow or blanket when coughing. *These measures promote airway clearance.*

- Administer oxygen as ordered. *Supplemental oxygen improves alveolar oxygenation and gas exchange.*

- Suction the client's airway as necessary. *Suctioning may be necessary to remove secretions that the client is unable to cough up and expectorate.*

- Maintain the integrity and patency of the chest tube by milking it as ordered and ensuring an uninterrupted gravity flow. *Chest tubes help reestablish negative pressure in the thoracic cavity, which allows the lung to fully reexpand.*

- If the client is on a mechanical ventilator, work with the respiratory therapist and use analgesia or sedation as needed to achieve synchronization of respirations with the ventilator. *Maximal effectiveness of mechanical ventilation requires that the client's respirations be coordinated with ventilator-delivered breaths.*

- Provide chest physiotherapy with percussion and postural drainage as needed or ordered. *Percussion and postural drainage help maintain airway patency and effective respirations.*

- Provide reassurance and emotional support. *These measures help relieve anxiety and promote an effective breathing pattern.*

Activity Intolerance

Both the client who has had resectional lung surgery and the client with inoperable lung cancer lose functional lung tissue and surface area for gas diffusion. This loss can cause an activity intolerance because the oxygen supply is insufficient to meet the body's oxygen demand.

Nursing interventions with rationales follow:

- Assess and document the client's physiologic responses to activity, including pulse, respiratory rate, dyspnea, and fatigue. *These assessments are good indicators of the client's level of activity tolerance.*

Nursing Implications for Management: The Client Receiving Radiation Therapy

■ ■ ■

Clients with lung cancer may be treated with radiation therapy, either alone or in combination with surgical resection or chemotherapy. Although radiation therapy is well controlled and specifically directed toward the tumor cells, some normal cells are also damaged in the process of treatment. Nursing care and client teaching help the client cope with uncomfortable side effects associated with radiation therapy.

Nursing Responsibilities

■ Assess the client for adverse effects of therapy, including skin breakdown.

■ Monitor the client for signs of radiation pneumonitis, such as dyspnea on exertion, dry cough, and fever.

■ Monitor the client for manifestations of pericarditis, including chest pain, pericardial friction rub, muffled heart sounds, paradoxical pulse, and ECG abnormalities. Notify the physician should symptoms occur.

■ Observe the client for evidence of esophagitis, including pain, sore throat, and difficulty swallowing.

■ Preserve indelible dye marks placed by the physician to identify the treatment field or port.

■ Use no soap, lotion, powders, or other preparation that may cause scattering of radiation on the area(s) to be irradiated. Clean the skin gently, using tepid water only.

■ If pain or drainage develops over the area being irradiated, notify the physician. Redness or darkening of the treatment field is normal.

■ Encourage adequate fluid intake to liquefy respiratory secretions.

■ Provide local analgesics and local anesthetics such as viscous lidocaine as ordered to relieve dysphagia and sore throat.

■ Offer small frequent meals of soft, cool foods and liquids to maintain nutritional status.

■ Provide antiemetics prior to meals if nausea is a problem.

Client and Family Teaching

■ Teach the client to wash the skin over treatment area gently, using no soaps, lotions, ointments, powders, bath oils, or perfumes unless prescribed by the physician.

■ Instruct the client in the importance of preserving the dye marks that define the treatment field.

■ For the client who develops dyspnea or pneumonitis, teach positioning, pursed-lip techniques, and relaxation exercises that can facilitate breathing.

■ Assure the client that pneumonitis is generally a self-limiting process and should resolve when the course of radiotherapy is completed.

■ Teach the client about the manifestations of pericarditis, which may develop during treatment or up to 1 year after its completion. Chest pain or pressure, rapid heartbeat, and fever may signal pericarditis; increasing fatigue, dyspnea, and lightheadedness can indicate a chronic process with pericardial effusion and possible cardiac tamponade.

■ Instruct the client in any prescribed medications or procedures such as pericardiotomy used to treat complications of radiation therapy.

■ Teach the client to eliminate hot, spicy, or acidic foods from the diet if esophagitis is a problem. Alcohol and tobacco should also be avoided.

■ Adequate rest and nutrition are important to alleviate the symptoms of radiation fatigue, which is common in clients receiving radiation therapy for lung cancer. The fatigue is generally temporary.

Note. Data are from "Trends in Radiation Therapy for the Treatment of Lung Cancer" (pp. 643–651) by G. S. Stewart, 1992, *Nursing Clinics of North America*, 27(3).

■ Plan rest periods interspersed with activities and procedures. *Rest periods reduce oxygen demands and fatigue.*

■ Assist the postoperative client to increase activities gradually. *Increasing activity levels gradually improves exercise tolerance.*

■ Teach the client measures to conserve energy while performing ADLs, such as sitting while showering and dressing and wearing slip-on shoes. *These energy-conserving measures reduce oxygen demand and allow the client to remain independent as long as possible.*

- Keep frequently used objects within easy reach for the client. *This helps conserve energy.*

- Administer oxygen therapy as prescribed and teach the client and family about the use of home oxygen if appropriate. *Supplemental oxygen can help improve the client's activity and exercise tolerance.*

- Encourage the client to maintain physical activity to tolerance. *Maintaining activity levels to the degree possible improves the client's physical and emotional well-being.*

- Allow family members to provide assistance as needed. *This helps the client conserve energy and allows the family to retain a sense of usefulness.*

Pain

Pain is a priority problem for any postoperative client as well as for clients in the terminal stages of cancer. Poorly managed pain prolongs recovery from surgery. In the terminal cancer client, chronic and acute pain must be managed effectively to allow a peaceful death.

Nursing interventions with rationales follow:

- Assess and document subjective and objective evidence of pain. *Remember that pain is a subjective experience in evaluating the client's reports of pain, its level, and intensity. Changes in vital signs as well as the client's ability to move in bed may indicate unreported pain.*

- Provide analgesics as needed to maintain comfort. *Postoperative recovery and restoration of function is facilitated by adequate pain management.*

- For the client experiencing cancer pain, maintain an around-the-clock medication schedule using narcotic, nonsteroidal anti-inflammatory drugs, and other medications as ordered. *Addiction is not a concern for the terminal cancer client; providing adequate pain relief that does not allow "breakthrough" pain is important.*

- Provide or assist the client with comfort measures, such as massage, positioning, distraction, and relaxation techniques. *These techniques promote relaxation and enhance pain relief.*

- Assist the client and family to plan and engage in activities that provide distraction from pain such as reading, television, and social interactions. *Distraction helps the client focus away from the pain.*

- Spend as much time with the client as possible; allow family members to remain with the client. *Physical presence of the nurse and family members provides emotional support for the client.*

Anticipatory Grieving

The client with lung cancer faces the very real prospect of death within 1 year of the diagnosis because of the advanced stage of most lung cancers at time of diagnosis. Grieving for the anticipated loss of life is a normal response as the client and family begin to adapt to the diag-

nosis. The goals of nursing interventions are to allow the client and family to express feelings and thoughts about the potential loss, to initiate grief work, to make decisions, and to use appropriate resources and coping mechanisms to deal with the loss.

Nursing interventions with rationales follow:

- Spend time with the client and family. *Time is necessary to develop a trusting, therapeutic relationship.*

- Answer questions honestly; do not deny the probable outcome of the disease. *Honesty reinforces reality and allows the client and family a sense of control over decisions to be made.*

- Encourage the client and family to express their feelings, fears, and concerns. *Open expression of feelings helps to promote understanding and acceptance.*

- Assist the client to understand the grieving process and to accept his or her feelings as normal. *Feelings of guilt, anger, or depression may cause the client to withdraw from others. Explanation of the grieving process enhances the client's understanding and ability to cope.*

- Help the client and family identify strengths and coping measures that have been used effectively in the past. Provide positive reinforcement for effective coping behavior. *Coping measures that have been effective for the client and family in the past can help them deal with the present situation and regain a sense of control.*

- Help the client and family make decisions regarding treatment and care. *This also is important to give them a sense of control.*

- Encourage the client and family to call upon other support systems, such as spiritual and social groups. Refer the client and family to support groups, social support services, and hospice care as indicated. Provide American Cancer Society literature and information as appropriate. *These support systems provide emotional support and help the client and family cope with the diagnosis.*

- Discuss advance directives (the living will) and power of attorney for health care with the client and family. *These documents give the client and family a sense of control over the extent of medical care provided in case the client is no longer able to express his or her own wishes.*

Other Nursing Diagnoses

Although the needs of clients differ, the following nursing diagnoses may be appropriate for the client with lung cancer:

- *Impaired Gas Exchange* related to loss of lung tissue

- *Ineffective Airway Clearance* related to the presence of obstructive tumor

- *Powerlessness* related to terminal disease

- *Impaired Physical Mobility* related to thoracic incision

Client and Family Teaching

A primary teaching need for the client and family affected by lung cancer is information about the disease itself, the expected prognosis, and planned treatment strategies. Provide honest information and answers; do not promote false hope.

Stress the importance of stopping smoking, especially if surgery has been performed. The client who already has lung cancer may have difficulty recognizing the need to stop smoking. Include information about the effects of nicotine and the tars in cigarette smoke on healing and already compromised lung tissue.

Provide information about planned treatments such as chemotherapy or radiation therapy, explaining the expected effects and usual side effects of each. Help the client develop strategies to cope with noxious effects. If the client has had surgery, provide information about activities and exercises to improve strength and regain function. Explain the need to continue coughing and deep-breathing exercises at home. Include information about manifestations that should be reported to the physician: fever, increasing or continued shortness of breath, cough, increased or purulent sputum, redness, pain, swelling, or incisional drainage.

Discuss the use of prescribed medications, including desired and potential side effects and interactions with other drugs or foods. Teach the client about the use of analgesics and other pain relief measures for postoperative or chronic pain.

Provide information about hospice services, home health, local cancer support groups for clients and caregivers, and American Cancer Society services.

Applying the Nursing Process

Case Study of a Client with Lung Cancer: James Mueller

After coughing up bloody sputum one morning, James Mueller, a 68-year-old retired millworker, makes an appointment to see his physician. The physician orders a chest X-ray which shows a suspicious density in the central portion of Mr. Mueller's right lung. Mr. Mueller agrees to be admitted to the hospital the following Monday for diagnostic tests.

Assessment

Anita Sarros, RN, admits Mr. Mueller to the oncology unit and obtains a nursing history. She notes that Mr. Mueller is married and has three grown children and ten grandchildren. He had worked in a local paper mill for 35 years before retiring at age 60. He describes himself as "pretty healthy," except for a chronic smoker's cough. When asked about his smoking history, he admits having started as a young man in the army. He has a 50 pack-year smoking history, having consumed one pack a day for 50 years, since age 18. Mr. Mueller says he had briefly quit smoking following a small heart attack 3 years ago but resumed smoking after 4 months. On further questioning, Mr. Mueller says his cough has been productive for the past few months, especially in the morning. He also admitted to getting shorter of breath than usual with physical activity.

Mr. Mueller examination shows the following: BP, 162/86; P, 78 and regular; R, 20; and T, 98.4 F (36.9 C). His color is good and his skin warm and dry. Ms. Sarros notes inspiratory and expiratory wheezes in Mr. Mueller's right chest but good breath sounds throughout. No other abnormal findings are noted on his examination. The physician orders early-morning sputum specimens to be attained over 3 days for cytologic examination and schedules a CT scan of the chest for the morning after admission. Mr. Mueller's CBC shows mild anemia, but the results of his chemistry panel are essentially normal. Sputum cytologic examination is positive for small-cell bronchogenic cancer. The CT scan shows a central mass approximately 4 cm in diameter with involved mediastinal and subclavicular lymph nodes. A small mass is also noted on Mr. Mueller's lumbar spine. After conferring with his physician and an oncologist, Mr. Mueller decides to undergo a trial course of chemotherapy. The oncologist recommends combination therapy with the CAV regimen: cyclophosphamide (Cytoxan), doxorubicin (Adriamycin), and vincristine (Oncovin).

Diagnosis

Ms. Sarros develops the following nursing diagnoses for Mr. Mueller:

- *Ineffective Airway Clearance* related to tumor mass
- *Risk for Altered Nutrition: Less Than Body Requirements* related to side effects of chemotherapy
- *Risk for Ineffective Family Coping: Compromised* related to new diagnosis of lung cancer
- *Knowledge Deficit* about lung cancer and aids to smoking cessation

Expected Outcomes

The expected outcomes established in Mr. Mueller's plan of care specify that he and/or his family will

- Maintain a patent airway.
- Maintain his current weight.
- Express feelings and concerns about the effect of cancer on the family unit.

- Participate in care.
- Contact appropriate support groups.
- Verbalize an understanding of his disease, its treatment, and prognosis.
- Develop a plan to stop smoking.

Planning and Implementation

Ms. Sarros plans and implements the following interventions for Mr. Mueller:

- Teach coughing, deep breathing, and hydration measures to facilitate airway clearance.
- Discuss symptoms that should be reported to the physician: increased dyspnea or hemoptysis, severe stridor or wheezing, chest pain.
- Discuss measures to relieve nausea associated with chemotherapy treatment, including premedication with a prescribed antiemetic.
- Have dietitian consult with Mr. and Mrs. Mueller to develop a diet plan for maintaining ideal weight.
- Discuss the possible effects of lung cancer with Mr. and Mrs. Mueller.
- Encourage Mr. and Mrs. Mueller to call a family conference to discuss the disease with their children and grandchildren.
- Evaluate family members' knowledge and understanding of lung cancer, correcting misinformation and teaching as needed.
- Ask an American Cancer Society volunteer to contact the family.
- Provide referral to local cancer care provider support group.
- Refer to home health department for follow-up and further teaching.

- Work with Mr. Mueller to develop a plan to stop smoking.
- Ask the physician to provide a prescription for nicotine patches or gum for Mr. Mueller.

Evaluation

Mr. Mueller had his first chemotherapy treatment in the hospital and was discharged 4 days after admission. After 3 months of chemotherapy, his tumor shows little regression, and a liver scan reveals the presence of further metastasis. He and his wife decide to stop chemotherapy treatments, a decision with which the children reluctantly agree. The physician has referred Mr. and Mrs. Mueller to hospice services. With the help of a hospice nurse and volunteer, Mr. Mueller is able to remain at home. His pain is managed initially with oral MS Contin, a sustained-release form of morphine sulfate, and later with an intravenous morphine infusion. Mr. Mueller dies at home with his family at his side 9 months after his diagnosis of lung cancer.

Critical Thinking in the Nursing Process

1. The oncologist prescribed a chemotherapy regimen of cyclophosphamide, doxorubicin, and vincristine. Describe how each of these drugs works against cancer cells, and discuss the rationale for using this combination.

2. Develop a care plan to deal with the specific side effects for the above treatment regimen.

3. Mr. Mueller had small-cell (oat cell) cancer. How would his presentation and treatment differ if the diagnosis had been non-small-cell adenocarcinoma, stage $T_2N_2M_0$?

▚ ▚ ▚   Disorders of the Pleura   ▚ ▚ ▚

The pleura is a thin membrane consisting of two layers: the visceral pleura, which overlies the lung surface, and the parietal pleura, which lines the inner chest wall. Between the layers of pleura is a potential space, the *pleural cavity,* which contains a thin layer of serous fluid. As the chest wall expands and the diaphragm flattens with breathing, the pressure in this space becomes negative in relation to atmospheric and alveolar pressure. The expansible lung is drawn out, and air rushes into the alveoli. When the pleura becomes inflamed or is affected by disease or injury, air or fluid can collect in the pleural cavity, restricting lung expansion and air movement.

The Client with Pleuritis

▪ ▪ ▪

When the pleura becomes inflamed, the sensory fibers of the parietal pleura become irritated, and the characteristic pain of **pleuritis** results. Pleural inflammation usually occurs secondarily to another process, such as a viral respiratory illness, pneumonia, or rib injury.

The onset of pleuritis is typically abrupt. The pain is unilateral and well localized and it is described as sharp or stabbing. The pain occasionally may refer to the neck or to the shoulder. Deep breathing, coughing, and move-

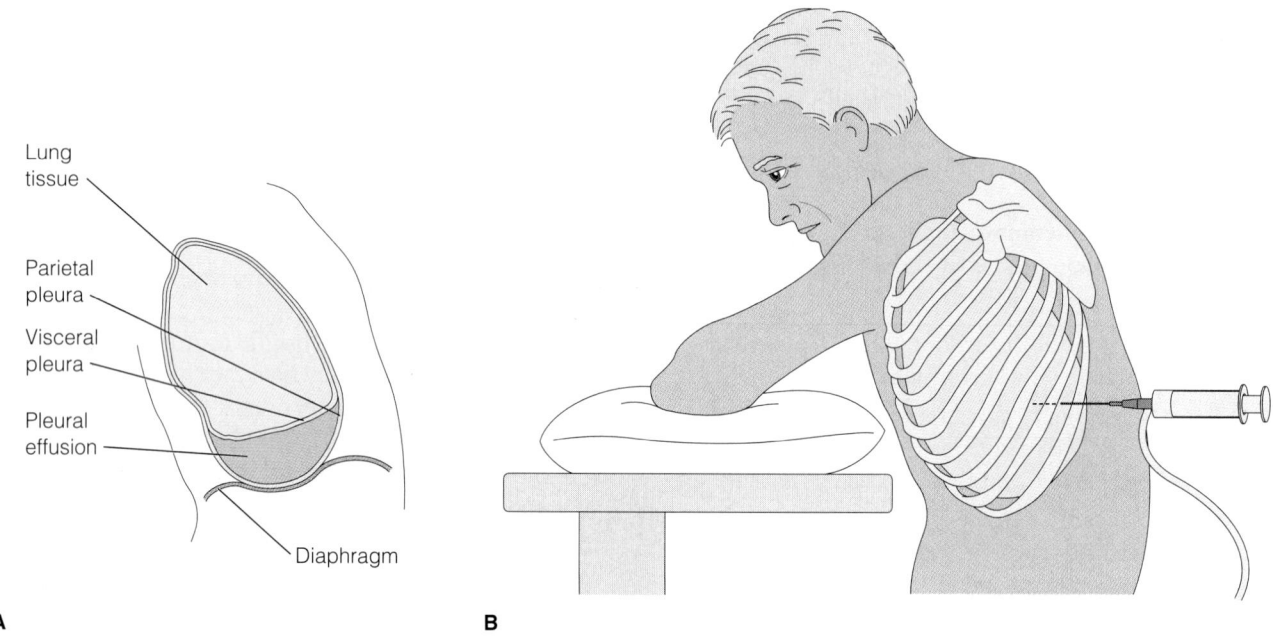

Figure 34–18   Thoracentesis. *A,* Region of pleural affusion formed between visceral and parietal pleura. *B,* With the client seated, a needle is inserted between the ribs into the pleural space to withdraw fluid.

ment aggravate the pain. The client's respirations are rapid and shallow, and the movement of the chest wall is limited on the affected side. The client's breath sounds are diminished, and a pleural friction rub may be heard over the site.

The diagnosis of pleuritis is based on presenting manifestations. Chest X-ray and ECG may be ordered to rule out other causes of chest pain. Treatment for pleuritis addresses the manifestations: Analgesics and NSAIDs, indomethacin (Indocin) in particular, are helpful in relieving the pain. Codeine may be ordered, both to relieve pain and to suppress the cough.

Nursing care for the client with pleuritis is directed toward providing comfort measures, including administration of NSAIDs and analgesics. Positioning and splinting the chest while coughing also can be helpful. Some clients obtain pain relief by wrapping the chest with 6-inch-wide elastic bandages; for some clients, however, this may restrict chest motion excessively.

Teach the client and family that pleuritis is generally a self-limited process of short duration. Discuss symptoms that should be reported to the physician: increased fever, productive cough, difficulty breathing, or shortness of breath. Provide information about prescription and nonprescription NSAIDs and analgesics, including the drug ordered, how to use it, and its desired and possible adverse effects.

The Client with a Pleural Effusion

The pleural space normally contains only about 10 to 20 mL of serous fluid. **Pleural effusion** is a collection of excess fluid in the pleural space. Excess fluid may be either *transudate,* formed when capillary pressure is high or plasma proteins are low, or *exudate,* the result of increased capillary permeability. Other pleural fluid collections include *empyema,* pus in the pleural cavity; *hemothorax,* the presence of blood in the cavity; and *hemorrhagic pleural effusion,* a mixture of blood and pleural fluid.

Pleural effusions result from either systemic or local disease. Systemic disorders associated with pleural effusion include congestive heart failure, liver or renal disease, and connective tissue disorders, such as rheumatoid arthritis and systemic lupus erythematosus. Pneumonia, atelectasis, tuberculosis, lung cancer, and trauma are local conditions that may cause pleural effusion.

A large pleural effusion compresses adjacent lung tissue. This results in the characteristic manifestation of dyspnea. Pain may also be present, although with inflammatory processes pleuritic pain is usually relieved by the formation of an effusion. Breath sounds are diminished or absent, and a dull tone is heard on percussion over the affected area. Movement of the chest wall may be limited.

Nursing Care of the Client Having a Thoracentesis

PREPROCEDURE CARE

- Ensure that the client has signed an informed consent form for the procedure. *This is an invasive procedure requiring informed consent.*

- Assess the client's knowledge and understanding of the procedure and its purpose; provide additional information as needed. *The client's cooperation is necessary because only local anesthesia is used during this procedure. An informed client will be less apprehensive and more able to cooperate during the thoracentesis.*

- Preprocedure fasting or sedation is not required. *Only local anesthesia is used in this procedure, and the gag and cough reflexes remain intact.*

- Administer a cough suppressant if indicated. *Movement and coughing during the procedure may result in inadvertent damage to the lung or pleura.*

- Obtain a thoracentesis tray, sterile gloves, injectable lidocaine, povidone-iodine, dressing supplies, and an extra overbed table or mayo stand. *These supplies are used by the physician performing the procedure.*

- Place the client in an upright position, leaning forward with arms and head supported on an anchored overbed table. *This position spreads the ribs, enlarging the intercostal space for needle insertion.*

- Inform the client that although local anesthesia will eliminate pain as the needle is inserted, the client may feel a sensation of pressure. *The pressure sensation occurs as the needle punctures the parietal pleura to enter the pleural space.*

POSTPROCEDURE CARE

- Monitor the client's pulse, color, and other signs during thoracentesis. *These are indicators of physiologic tolerance of the procedure.*

- Apply a dressing over the puncture site, and position the client on the unaffected side for 1 hour. *This allows the pleural puncture to heal.*

- Label the obtained specimen with the client's name, date, source, and diagnosis; send the specimen to the laboratory for analysis. *Fluid obtained during thoracentesis may be examined for abnormal cells, bacteria, and other substances to determine the cause of the pleural effusion.*

- During the first several hours after thoracentesis, frequently assess and document vital signs; respiratory status, including respiratory excursion, lung sounds, cough, or hemoptysis; and puncture site for bleeding or presence of crepitus. *Frequent assessment is important to detect possible complications of thoracentesis, such as pneumothorax.*

- Obtain a chest X-ray. *Chest X-ray is ordered to detect possible pneumothorax.*

- Normal activities generally can be resumed after 1 hour if no evidence of pneumothorax or other complication is present. *The puncture wound of thoracentesis heals rapidly.*

Chest X-ray often provides the first evidence of a pleural effusion. Because fluid typically seeks the dependent position, it is visible at the base of the affected lung on chest X-ray taken with the client in the upright position, and along the lateral wall when the client is positioned on the affected side. CT scans and ultrasonography also are used to localize and differentiate pleural effusions.

When a pleural effusion is detected and the cause is not apparent, a **thoracentesis** is performed. Thoracentesis is an invasive procedure in which fluid (or occasionally air) is removed from the pleural space with a needle. Aspirated fluid is analyzed for general appearance, cell counts, protein and glucose content, the presence of enzymes such as LDH and amylase, abnormal cells, and culture.

When pleural effusion is significant and interferes with respirations, thoracentesis to remove the fluid is usually the treatment of choice (Figure 34–18). Thoracentesis may be performed at the client's bedside, in a procedure room, or in the physician's office. Local anesthesia is used, and the procedure requires less than 30 minutes to complete. Percussion, auscultation, radiography, or ultrasonography is used to locate the effusion and needle insertion site. The amount of fluid removed is limited to 1200 to 1500 mL at one time to prevent the possibility of cardiovascular collapse from rapid removal of too much fluid. Pneumothorax is a possible complication of thoracentesis if the visceral pleura is punctured or a closed drainage system not maintained during the procedure. Nursing care for the client undergoing a thoracentesis is outlined in the accompanying box.

Because pleural effusion usually occurs secondarily to another disease or disorder, medical management also is directed toward treating the underlying condition to prevent further fluid accumulation. An empyema may require repeated drainage, as well as high doses of parenteral antibiotics. Occasionally, thoracotomy and surgical excision may be necessary. Recurrent pleural effusions, often due to cancer, may be prevented by instilling an irritant, such as tetracycline, into the pleural space to cause adhesion of the parietal and visceral pleura. Water-seal chest tube drainage is often employed for hemothorax (Berkow & Fletcher, 1992).

Nursing care for the client with a pleural effusion is directed toward supporting respiratory function and assisting with procedures to evacuate collected fluid. With a large pleural effusion resulting in partial lung collapse, impaired gas exchange and activity intolerance are high-priority nursing problems. A high risk for impaired gas exchange is also a priority problem during the initial period following thoracentesis.

Client and family teaching focuses on manifestations of recurrent effusion or complications following a thoracentesis that should be reported to the physician. Instruct the client to report increasing dyspnea or shortness of breath, cough, and hemoptysis. Pleuritic pain may be an early sign of effusion and also should be reported. Further teaching about any underlying condition also may be necessary; for example, the client with congestive heart failure may need to be taught to maintain a salt-restricted diet.

The Client with Pneumothorax

■ ■ ■

Accumulation of air in the pleural space is called **pneumothorax**. Pneumothorax can occur spontaneously, without apparent cause, as a complication of preexisting lung disease, as a result of blunt or penetrating trauma to the chest, or from an iatrogenic cause (e.g., following thoracentesis).

Pathophysiology

Pressure in the pleural space is normally negative in relation to atmospheric pressure. When either the visceral or parietal pleura is breached, air enters the pleural space, equalizing this pressure. The natural recoil tendency of the lung then causes it to collapse to a greater or lesser extent, depending on the size and rapidity of air accumulation (Figure 34–19).

Spontaneous Pneumothorax
Spontaneous pneumothorax involves the rupture of an air-filled bleb, or blister, on the lung surface, which allows air from the airways to enter the pleural space. Air accumulates in the pleural space until pressures are equalized or until collapse of the involved section causes the leak to seal (Porth, 1994). Spontaneous pneumothorax is further categorized as *primary (simple) spontaneous pneumothorax* or *secondary (complicated) spontaneous pneumothorax*.

Primary pneumothorax occurs in previously healthy individuals, affecting mainly tall, slender men between the ages 20 and 40. Although smoking and familial factors are thought to contribute, it is not known what causes the air-filled blebs to form and rupture. Usually the apices of the lungs are affected. This is considered to be a benign condition, although recurrences are not uncommon.

Secondary pneumothorax, generally caused by overdistention and rupture of an alveolus, is more serious and potentially life threatening (Wilson et al., 1991). It develops in clients with underlying lung disease, most often COPD. As such, it is predominantly a condition that affects middle and older adults. Besides COPD, secondary pneumothorax may be associated with asthma, cystic fibrosis, pulmonary fibrosis, tuberculosis, adult respiratory distress syndrome (ARDS), and other pulmonary diseases. A form of secondary pneumothorax called *catamenial pneumothorax* occurs in relation to the menstrual cycle; affected women develop manifestations within 24 to 48 hours of the onset of menstrual flow (Porth, 1994).

The manifestations of spontaneous pneumothorax vary according to the size of pneumothorax, extent of lung collapse, and any underlying lung disease. Typically, pleuritic chest pain and shortness of breath begin abruptly, often while the client is at rest. The respiratory rate increases, as does the heart rate. Chest wall movement may be asymmetrical, with the affected side showing less movement than the unaffected side. The percussion tone on the affected side is hyperresonant, and breath sounds may be diminished or absent. The client may be hypoxemic, although normal mechanisms that shunt blood flow to the unaffected lung often maintain normal oxygen saturation levels. Hypoxemia is more pronounced in the client with underlying lung disease.

Traumatic Pneumothorax
Traumatic injury to the chest wall and pleura can also lead to pneumothorax. Either blunt or penetrating trauma can cause pneumothorax. Blunt trauma may occur in a motor vehicle accident, fall, or during cardiopulmonary resuscitation (CPR). Fractured ribs penetrating the pleura are the leading cause of pneumothorax due to blunt trauma. Fracture of the trachea and a ruptured bronchus or esophagus are other possible results of blunt chest trauma leading to pneumothorax.

Open pneumothorax, or a *sucking chest wound,* results from penetrating chest trauma, as may occur with a stab wound, gunshot wound, or impalement injury. With an open pneumothorax, air moves freely between the pleural space and the atmosphere through the wound. Pressure on the affected side equalizes with the atmosphere, and

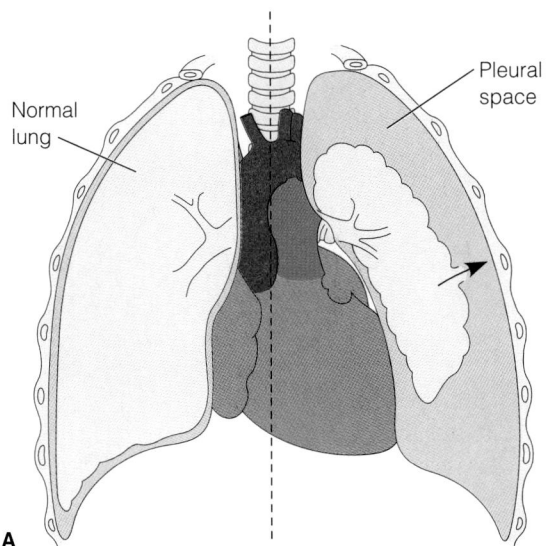

Normal lung

Pleural space

A

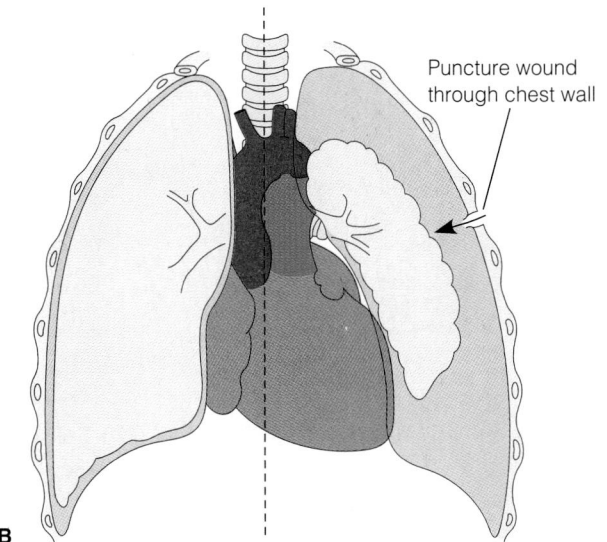

Puncture wound through chest wall

B

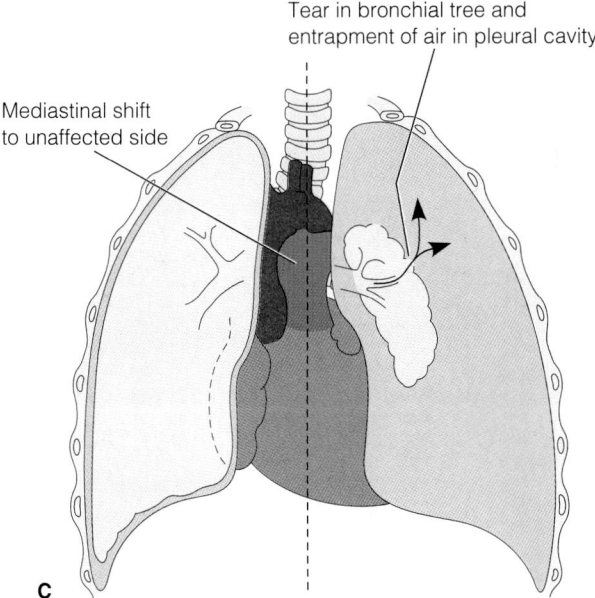

Tear in bronchial tree and entrapment of air in pleural cavity

Mediastinal shift to unaffected side

C

Figure 34–19   Pneumothorax. *A,* A spontaneous pneumothorax with an air leak from the lung into the pleural space. *B,* A traumatic or open pneumothorax (sucking chest wound) in which air enters the pleural space through a wound in the chest wall. *C,* A tension pneumothorax. Air enters the pleural space during inspiration but is unable to exit during expiration, resulting in rapid lung collapse and a shift of mediastinal structures toward the unaffected side.

the lung collapses rapidly. The result is significant hypoventilation that may be fatal (Way, 1994).

With traumatic pneumothorax, manifestations of pain and dyspnea may be masked or missed because of the client's other injuries. Tachypnea and tachycardia may also be attributed to the primary injury, making physical assessment for possible signs of a pneumothorax vital. Chest wall movement on the affected side is diminished, and breath sounds are absent. If a penetrating wound is present, air may be heard and felt moving through it with respiratory efforts. Hemothorax frequently accompanies traumatic pneumothorax.

Tension Pneumothorax

In a *tension pneumothorax,* injury to the chest wall or lungs allows air to enter the pleural space but prevents it from escaping. Pressure within the pleural space actually be-

comes positive in relation to atmospheric pressure as air accumulates rapidly with each breath. The lung on the affected side collapses, and pressure on the mediastinum causes thoracic organs to shift to the unaffected side of the chest, placing pressure on the opposite lung as well. Ventilation is severely compromised, and venous return to the heart is impaired. Tension pneumothorax is a medical emergency requiring immediate intervention to preserve respiration and cardiac output.

The client presents with hypotension and distended neck veins in addition to manifestations of a pneumothorax. The trachea is displaced toward the unaffected side as a result of the mediastinal shift. Signs of shock may be present.

Iatrogenic Pneumothorax

Iatrogenic pneumothorax is increasingly common. Iatrogenic pneumothorax may result from puncture or lacera-

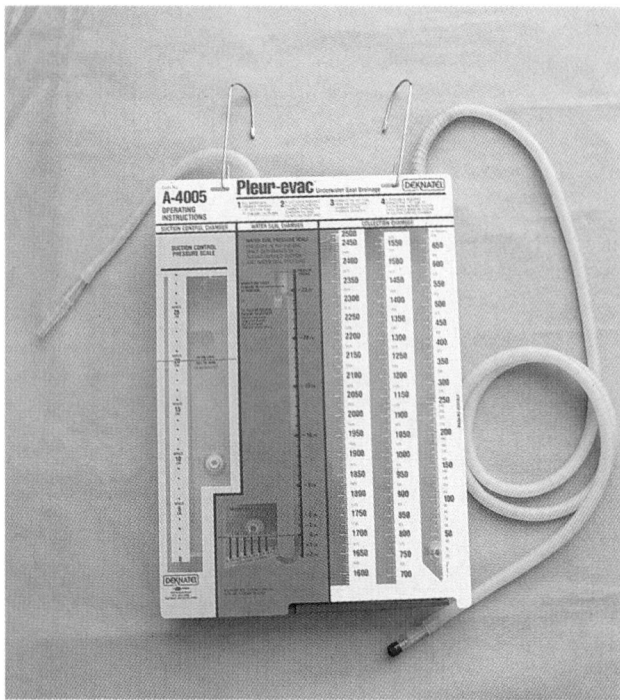

Figure 34-20 Disposable commercial chest drainage system.

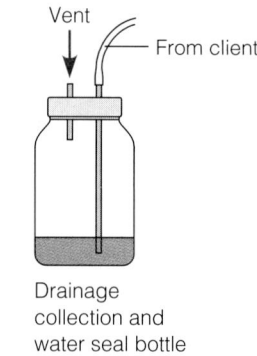

A Drainage collection and water seal bottle

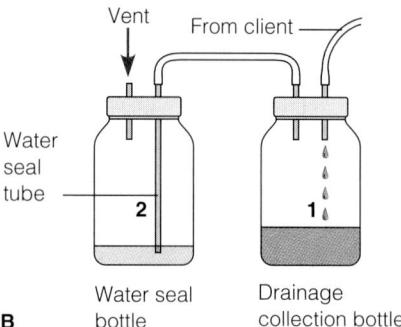

B Water seal bottle / Drainage collection bottle

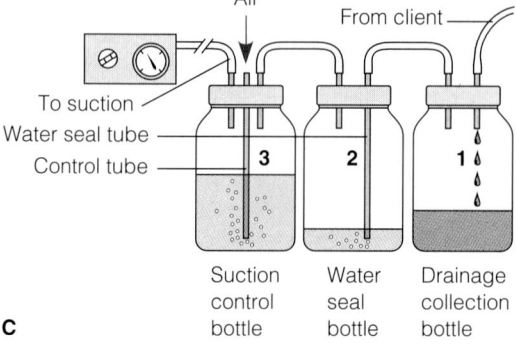

C Suction control bottle / Water seal bottle / Drainage collection bottle

Figure 34-21 Water-seal drainage system for chest tubes: *A,* one-bottle system; *B,* two-bottle system; *C,* three-bottle system.

tion of the visceral pleura during central line placement, thoracentesis, or lung biopsy. During bronchoscopy, the bronchi or lung tissue can be disrupted. Alveoli can become overdistended and rupture as a result of anesthesia, resuscitation procedures, or mechanical ventilation (Wilson et al., 1991). The manifestations of iatrogenic pneumothorax are those for a spontaneous pneumothorax.

Collaborative Care

Treatment of the client with pneumothorax depends on the severity of the problem. Clients with a small simple pneumothorax may be followed on an outpatient basis with serial X-rays. Air is absorbed from the pleural space, allowing most small pneumothoraces to resolve spontaneously without treatment. Clients with significant symptoms or a pneumothorax greater than 15%, by contrast, generally require *tube thoracostomy,* or the placement of chest tubes. Surgical intervention may be necessary for clients with recurrent spontaneous pneumothorax.

Laboratory and Diagnostic Tests

Most clients with pneumothorax require no laboratory testing for diagnosis or follow-up. Hypoxia may be evident on arterial blood gas analysis.

The chest X-ray is a simple and effective tool for diagnosing pneumothorax. In tension pneumothorax, air is visualized on the affected side, and mediastinal structures appear shifted to the opposite or unaffected side.

Chest Tubes

The treatment of choice for a pneumothorax is the placement of a chest tube with water-seal drainage and suction to allow the lung to reexpand. When a tube is placed in the pleural cavity to remove air or fluid, measures must be taken to prevent air from also entering the tube or, in essence, creating an open pneumothorax. Chest tubes are connected to a closed drainage system. The end of the drainage system has a "water-seal" that prevents air from entering the chest cavity during inspiration and allows air to escape during expiration. Applying a low level of suction to the system helps to reestablish negative pressure in the pleural space, allowing the lung to reexpand.

Nursing Care of the Client with Chest Tubes

PREPROCEDURE CARE

- Be sure that the client has signed an informed consent form for chest tube insertion. *This is an invasive procedure requiring informed consent.*

- Provide additional explanation to the client as indicated. Explain that local anesthesia will be used but that the client may feel pressure as the trochar is inserted. Reassure the client that breathing will be easier once the chest tube is in place and the lung begins to reexpand. *The client may be extremely dyspneic and anxious and needs reassurance that this invasive procedure will provide relief.*

- Gather all needed supplies, including a thoracostomy tray, injectable lidocaine, sterile gloves, chest tube drainage system (Pleurevac, Thoravac, others), sterile water, and a large sterile catheter-tipped syringe to use as a funnel for filling water-seal and suction chambers. *These supplies are used by the physician during the insertion procedure and by the nurse to establish the water-seal drainage system.*

- Position the client as indicated for the procedure. *The client may be placed in an upright position (as for a thoracentesis) or side-lying position, depending on the site of the pneumothorax.*

- Assist the physician with insertion of the chest tube as needed. The procedure may be performed in a procedure room, in the surgical suite, or at the client's bedside. *Although the insertion of the chest tube is a relatively simple procedure, nursing assistance is necessary to support the client and rapidly establish a closed drainage system.*

POSTPROCEDURE CARE

- Perform and document respiratory assessments at least every 4 hours. *Frequent assessment is necessary to monitor respiratory status and the beneficial effect of chest tube.*

- Maintain a closed system. Tape all connections, and secure the chest tube to the chest wall. *These measures are important to prevent inadvertent tube removal or disruption of the system's integrity.*

- Keep the collection apparatus below the level of the chest. *Pleural fluid drains into the collection apparatus by the flow of gravity.*

- If ordered, milk chest tubes every 1 to 2 hours. *Chest tubes may be milked to maintain patency and adequate drainage. This procedure does, however, increase the risk of tissue damage, so it should not be performed routinely without specific orders.*

- Check tubes frequently for kinks or loops. *These could interfere with drainage.*

- Check the water seal frequently. The water level should fluctuate with respiratory effort; if it does not, the system may not be patent or intact. Periodic air bubbles in the water seal chamber are normal and indicate that trapped air is being removed from the chest. *Frequent assessment of the system is important to ensure appropriate functioning.*

- Measure drainage every 8 hours, marking the drainage level on the drainage chamber. Report drainage that is cloudy, in excess of 70 mL per hour, or red, warm, and free flowing. *Red, free-flowing drainage indicates hemorrhage; cloudiness may indicate presence of an infection. Drainage must not be emptied because doing so would disrupt the integrity of the closed system.*

- Periodically assess the water level in the suction control chamber, adding water as necessary. *Adequate water in the suction control chamber prevents excess suction from being placed on delicate pleural tissue.*

- Help the client change positions frequently, and assist with sitting and ambulation as allowed. *The presence of chest tubes should not prevent the client from carrying out allowed activities. Care is needed to prevent inadvertent disconnection or removal of the tubes.*

- When the chest tube is removed, immediately apply a sterile occlusive petroleum jelly dressing. *An occlusive dressing prevents air from reentering the pleural space through the chest wound.*

A number of closed-drainage chest tube systems are available. Most are self-contained disposable systems (Figure 34–20) based on the old "three-bottle" water seal drainage system (Figure 34–21). Drainage from the chest tube is collected in the first bottle or collection chamber of a disposable system. This sealed bottle or chamber is connected to the water-seal chamber or bottle, which is in turn connected to the suction-control chamber or bottle. The accompanying box discusses nursing care of the client with chest tubes.

A large-bore needle or plastic intravenous catheter may be inserted through the chest wall as emergency treatment of a tension pneumothorax. This allows air to escape from the affected side, relieving pressure on mediastinal structures and the opposite lung (Way, 1994).

The client with severe respiratory compromise or underlying pulmonary disease may require intubation and mechanical ventilation until the size of the pneumothorax is reduced.

Surgery

The risk for recurrence of spontaneous pneumothorax increases with each attack (Way, 1994). Clients experiencing two spontaneous pneumothoraces on the same side may undergo surgical intervention to prevent future ruptures. A thoracotomy is performed to excise or oversew blebs (usually at the apices of the lungs). The overlying pleura is then roughened or irritated to induce scarring and adhesion to the surface of the lung.

Nursing Care

Maintaining or restoring adequate alveolar ventilation and gas exchange is of highest priority for the client with a pneumothorax. The presence of a chest tube may interfere with the client's physical mobility as well, contributing to a high risk for injury.

Impaired Gas Exchange

Loss of negative pressure in the pleural cavity and the resulting collapse of lung tissue can result in poor chest expansion and loss of alveolar ventilation. As the pneumothorax is removed or reabsorbed, ventilation and gas exchange improve.

Nursing interventions with rationales follow:

- Assess and document vital signs and respiratory status, including respiratory rate, depth, and lung sounds, at least every 4 hours. *Frequent assessment enables the nurse to monitor the adequacy of respirations and lung expansion.*

- Evaluate chest wall movement, position of the trachea, and neck veins frequently. *Early identification of signs of tension pneumothorax and appropriate intervention are vital to preserve cardiorespiratory function.*

- Place the client in Fowler's or high-Fowler's position. *This position facilitates lung expansion.*

- Administer oxygen as ordered. *Supplemental oxygen is administered to improve blood oxygen levels.*

- Provide emotional support, particularly in early stages and during chest tube insertion. *Dyspnea and hypoxemia can cause the client to be extremely anxious and apprehensive, impairing his or her ability to cooperate with procedures.*

- Monitor drainage and function of chest tube. *To function appropriately, chest tubes must remain patent and securely connected to the closed system.*

- Help the client change position frequently and ambulate as tolerated. *Movement facilitates ventilation of lungs.*

- Provide for rest periods. *Adequate rest is also important to conserve energy and reduce oxygen demand.*

Risk for Injury

Pain and the presence of chest tubes can reduce the client's perceived ability to ambulate and provide self-care. The client who does not have significant respiratory impairment can maintain a moderate level of physical activity while chest tubes are in place, as long as caution is exercised to maintain the integrity of the system. If the tube is inadvertently pulled out or the integrity of the system is disrupted, the client is at risk for increasing pneumothorax or infection.

Nursing interventions with rationales follow:

- Assess chest tube and drainage system frequently, at least every 2 hours. *The system must remain patent and intact to function effectively.*

- When turning the client or providing care, ensure that tension is not placed on chest tubes. *These measures help prevent the tubes from becoming dislodged.*

- Secure a loop of drainage tubing to the sheet or client's gown. *Looping the drainage tubing prevents direct pressure on the chest tube itself.*

- When turning the client to the affected side, be sure that neither the chest tube nor drainage tubing is kinked or occluded under the client. *This maintains the patency of the tubing.*

- Teach the client how to ambulate with the drainage system, keeping the system lower than the chest. In most cases, suction can be discontinued during ambulation. *Disposable chest tube drainage systems are portable to allow the client to ambulate while they are in place. Maintaining the drainage system lower than the chest facilitates continued drainage and prevents reflux.*

- Observe the insertion site for redness, swelling, pain, or drainage. Report any signs of infection, including fever, to the physician. *Interruption of skin integrity by insertion of a chest tube increases the client's risk for infection.*

- Should a connection come loose, reconnect it as soon as possible. *A closed system to water-seal drainage is vital to prevent air from entering the pleural space and an open pneumothorax.*

- For clients who have an open pneumothorax or have inadvertently removed a chest tube, seal the wound as soon as possible with a sterile occlusive dressing, such as gauze impregnated with petroleum jelly. If a sterile dressing is not available, other occlusive material such as foil or plastic wrap can be used. Tape the dressing on three sides only. *An occlusive dressing taped on three sides prevents the development of a tension pneumothorax by inhibiting air from entering the wound in inhalation but allowing it to escape during exhalation.*

Other Nursing Diagnoses

Other nursing diagnoses that may be appropriate for the client with a pneumothorax follow:

- *Ineffective Breathing Pattern* related to increased pressure in pleural cavity
- *Decreased Cardiac Output* related to mediastinal shift and impaired venous return
- *Risk for Infection* related to loss of chest wall integrity
- *Pain* related to chest wall trauma

Client and Family Teaching

Although all clients with pneumothorax need teaching about procedures and prescribed treatments during the acute period, clients who have experienced spontaneous pneumothorax also need education about their future risk. The risk of recurrence following spontaneous pneumothorax is 50%. Stress the importance of quitting smoking to reduce the risk. Other activities that can cause pneumothorax to recur include mountain climbing or other activities involving exposure to high altitudes, flying in unpressurized aircraft, and scuba diving (Tierney et al., 1994). The client also may be advised to avoid contact sports.

Following a pneumothorax, teach the client that exercise and activity can and should be increased gradually to previous levels. Stress the importance of follow-up care and monitoring. Discuss manifestations that should be reported to the physician: upper respiratory infections; fever, cough, or difficulty breathing; sudden, sharp chest pain; or redness, pain, swelling, tenderness, or drainage from the chest tube puncture wound.

The Client with Hemothorax

■ ■ ■

Hemothorax, or blood in the pleural space, usually occurs as a consequence of thoracic trauma or surgery. On rare occasion, it can occur spontaneously. When blood collects in the pleural space, pressure on the affected lung impairs ventilation and gas exchange. With significant hemorrhage, a risk of shock exists.

The client with hemothorax demonstrates symptoms similar to those of a pneumothorax. Lung sounds are diminished, and a dull percussion tone is noted over the collection of blood, typically at the base of the lung. Chest X-ray is used to confirm the diagnosis of hemothorax.

Thoracentesis or thoracostomy with chest tube drainage is used to remove blood from the pleural space. With significant hemorrhage, such as that which follows trauma or surgery, the blood may be collected in an autologous collection device for subsequent autotransfusion. Blood for autotransfusion should be collected and reinfused within 4 hours. Strict aseptic technique is used in collecting the blood. It is collected through a gross particulate filter into a container primed with anticoagulant and reinfused when the container is full or when the client's status indicates a need for transfusion. Air is removed from the blood container prior to reinfusion and a filter used to eliminate debris, such as degenerating blood cells, fat particles, and fibrin.

Nursing care for the client with hemothorax is related to assessment and maintenance of adequate respiratory status and cardiac output. The priority of care depends on the rate and extent of hemothorax. In a large, slow-developing hemothorax, ventilatory status may be affected significantly. For a client in this circumstance, the following nursing diagnoses should be considered:

- *Ineffective Breathing Pattern*
- *Impaired Gas Exchange*

When hemothorax develops rapidly and hemorrhage is significant, additional priority nursing diagnoses include the following:

- *Decreased Cardiac Output*
- *Risk for Fluid Volume Deficit*

The educational needs of the client with hemothorax typically are related to the acute period. Explain all procedures fully to the client to relieve anxiety and gain cooperation. If autotransfusion is used, discuss its benefits with the client. Teach the client about the reason for chest tubes and water-seal drainage. If hemothorax was spontaneous or related to trauma, discuss possible etiologic factors and prevention of future episodes.

▚ ▚ ▚ Trauma of the Chest or Lung ▚ ▚ ▚

Chest injury is second only to head injury as a cause of death from trauma, accounting for approximately 25% of all trauma deaths in the United States (Hammond, 1990; Hurst, 1992). It is commonly associated with motor vehicle accidents (MVA) and other trauma involving multiple injuries. Chest injuries can range from mild, such as a

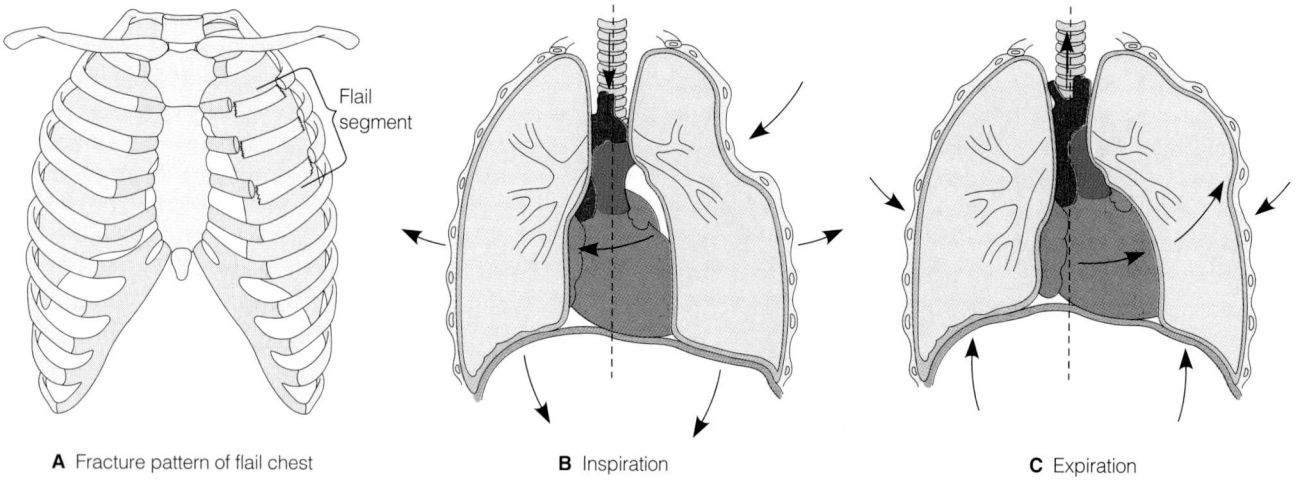

A Fracture pattern of flail chest   **B** Inspiration   **C** Expiration

Figure 34–22 Flail chest with paradoxic movement.

simple rib fracture, to severe and fatal. Traumatic injury to the chest may involve both the chest wall and underlying thoracic structures, including the lungs, heart, great vessels, and esophagus. Chest and lung injury can result from several different mechanisms: penetrating trauma, such as a stab or gunshot wound; blunt trauma, such as a fall, MVA, pedestrian accident, or crush injury; or inhalation injury, such as smoke inhalation or near drowning.

Assessment of the airway, breathing, and circulation (ABCs), is vital in the client with possible chest or lung injury. Chest trauma may disrupt normal mechanisms for maintaining any of these functions. Chest injuries considered to be life threatening include airway obstruction, tension pneumothorax, open pneumothorax, massive hemothorax, and flail chest with pulmonary contusion (Hurst, 1992).

The Client with a Chest Wall Injury

■ ■ ■

Injury to the chest wall may be minor, having little effect on respiratory status; one example is a simple fractured rib in a previously healthy client. A more significant risk exists when pain or instability of the chest wall results in a mechanical breathing impairment or when underlying lung tissue is damaged as a result of chest wall injury.

Pathophysiology

Simple rib fracture, usually involving a single rib, is the most common chest wall injury. A young, previously healthy client usually tolerates rib fracture well, healing

without complications. In the older client or person with preexisting lung disease, in contrast, a fractured rib may lead to significant complications, including pneumonia, atelectasis, and, potentially, respiratory failure. If fractured ribs are displaced, they may penetrate the pleura, leading to pneumothorax and possible hemothorax.

With a rib fracture, the client experiences pain on inspiration and coughing. This leads to voluntary splinting, with rapid, shallow respirations and inhibited cough. Bruising may be seen over the fracture site. On palpation, crepitus may be felt with respiratory movement. Breath sounds are diminished, especially in the bases, as a result of splinting. If pneumothorax is present, chest wall movement on the affected side may be reduced, and breath sounds absent or significantly diminished. A hyperresonant percussion tone usually is noted. Hemothorax also causes diminished or absent breath sounds on the affected side, with a dull percussion note.

Flail Chest

With multiple rib fractures, chest wall stability may be lost and normal chest wall function impaired. When two or more consecutive ribs are fractured in multiple places, a free-floating segment of the chest wall, or **flail chest**, results. The physiologic function of the chest wall is impaired as the flail segment is sucked inward during inhalation and moves outward with exhalation. This is known as *paradoxic movement* (Figure 34–22). Flail chest impairs lung expansion and increases the work of breathing. It is frequently associated with an underlying pulmonary contusion, which may be the primary cause of respiratory failure in clients with flail chest.

The client with flail chest is dyspneic and experiences pain, especially on inspiration. Paradoxic chest movement is evident with inspection. Chest expansion is unequal, and palpable crepitus is present. Breath sounds are diminished, and crackles may be heard on auscultation.

Pulmonary Contusion

Pulmonary contusion, or injury to lung tissue, is frequently associated with flail chest and other blunt chest trauma. It occurs in 75% of clients with flail chest and is the most common lethal chest injury in the United States (Hammond, 1990; Way, 1994).

Pulmonary contusion is thought to result from sudden compression of the chest and lung tissue followed by sudden decompression, as can occur with an MVA, significant fall, or crush injury. Alveoli and pulmonary arterioles rupture, leading to intra-alveolar hemorrhage and interstitial and bronchial edema. Increased capillary permeability in the damaged tissue contributes to edema. After several days, capillary permeability changes may also occur in the unaffected lung, probably because of the inflammatory response. The production of surfactant is reduced as well (Hurst, 1992). Airway obstruction, atelectasis, and impaired gas diffusion result. Associated chest wall injury impairs the client's ability to clear secretions effectively, and the work of breathing is significantly increased.

Manifestations of pulmonary contusion may not be evident until 12 to 24 hours after the injury (Way, 1994). Increasing shortness of breath, restlessness, apprehension, and chest pain are early signs. Copious sputum, which may be blood-tinged, is present. Later manifestations include tachycardia, tachypnea, dyspnea, and cyanosis. Even with appropriate therapy, approximately 15% of clients with pulmonary contusion die.

Collaborative Care

Chest X-ray is used to identify most chest wall injuries. Rib fractures are evident on X-ray. With pulmonary contusion, initial patchy opacifications may progress to diffuse opacification, or "white-out." Changes in arterial blood gas levels relate to the degree of ventilatory impairment and hypoxemia resulting from the injury.

Simple rib fractures typically heal uneventfully. Providing adequate analgesia to allow the client to breathe, cough, and move is the primary intervention. With multiple rib fractures, an intercostal nerve block may be used to ensure adequate ventilation. Rib belts, binders, and taping to stabilize the rib cage are *not* recommended, because they may interfere with ventilation and lead to atelectasis. Even with simple rib fracture, older clients and clients with preexisting lung disease require close monitoring to prevent and detect atelectasis, pneumonia, and other complications.

Intercostal nerve blocks or continuous epidural analgesia may be employed to manage the pain in a client with flail chest. For a small flail chest, analgesia combined

with supplemental oxygen therapy may be adequate. In some cases, internal or external fixation of the flail segment may be done.

The preferred treatment for flail chest is intubation and mechanical ventilation. This positive-pressure ventilation provides support and stabilization of the flail segment and improves ventilation and gas exchange. The work of breathing is decreased and healing improved.

Clients with pulmonary contusion typically are critically ill, requiring intensive care management. Treatment is supportive, directed at maintaining adequate ventilation and alveolar gas exchange. Endotracheal intubation and mechanical ventilation are necessary to manage most clients with pulmonary contusion. Repeated bronchoscopy may be performed to remove secretions and cellular debris, preventing atelectasis. Although adequate hydration is necessary to prevent shock, overhydration can increase pulmonary edema. Pulmonary arterial pressure monitoring with a Swan-Ganz catheter and frequent arterial blood gas measurement is required for optimal fluid replacement and management of ventilatory support.

The client with unilateral pulmonary contusion may present a unique management problem. Mechanical ventilation with positive end-expiratory pressure (PEEP) to maintain open alveoli and adequate gas exchange can actually increase damage to the affected lung and result in overdistention of the normal lung. Intubation with a double-lumen endotracheal tube, which permits independent ventilation of each lung, is one solution to this management problem.

Nursing Care

Chest wall trauma has the potential to interfere with adequate chest expansion and alveolar ventilation. When a pulmonary contusion is also present, gas exchange is affected as well. Priorities for nursing management include controlling pain, ensuring adequate ventilation, and taking measures to assess and prevent hypoxemia if possible.

With many chest wall injuries, pain interferes with adequate lung expansion and coughing, leading to such complications as pneumonia and atelectasis. Adequate pain management is a key component of the medical and nursing management for these clients. Analgesics are most effective when administered on a schedule to maintain pain control, rather than on an as-needed basis that allows pain to become severe between doses. Assess the client frequently for evidence of adequate pain control. An increased respiratory rate, shallow respirations, diminished breath sounds, and reluctance to move and cough are indicators of inadequate control in the client with a chest wall injury. It is also important to assess the client for possible respiratory depression resulting from narcotic analgesia. If pain relief is inadequate or if excess sedation and respiratory depression occur, the physician may use an intercostal nerve block. Nursing responsibilities related to this procedure are directed primarily toward support and positioning of the client. Following the procedure, assess for possible bleeding and check lung sounds.

Aggressive respiratory hygiene may be necessary to maintain open airways and adequate ventilation. Assess lung sounds and respiratory rate, depth, and effort frequently. Have the client cough, deep breathe, and change position every 1 to 2 hours, and encourage the client to use the incentive spirometer. Teach the client how to splint the affected area with a blanket or pillow when coughing. Suction the client's airway as indicated. Work with the respiratory therapist to maintain optimal mechanical ventilation. Secure the endotracheal tube to maintain appropriate position and ventilation of both lungs. This is especially important when a double-lumen endotracheal tube is in place, because malposition can occlude one main bronchus and prevent ventilation of the affected lung. Elevate the head of the bed to facilitate lung expansion. Promptly report to the physician signs of complications, such as diminished breath sounds, increasing crackles (rales) or rhonchi, dull or hyperresonant percussion tones, unequal chest movement, hemoptysis, chills or fever, or changes in vital signs.

Impaired gas exchange is of particular concern in the client with pulmonary contusion. Alveolar damage and pulmonary edema can significantly impair oxygenation of the blood and removal of carbon dioxide. Monitor the client's vital signs, skin color, oxygen saturation levels, and arterial blood gases for evidence of hypoxemia or hypercapnia. Assess for clinical manifestations, such as anxiety or apprehension, restlessness, confusion or lethargy, or complaints of headache. Maintain oxygen therapy and mechanical ventilation as ordered. Hyperoxygenate the client with 100% oxygen prior to suctioning to help maintain blood and tissue oxygenation. Assess the client's fluid status by keeping accurate measurements of intake and output, weighing the client daily, and using invasive monitoring, such as monitoring of central venous pressure and pulmonary artery pressure. Maintain any ordered fluid restriction. Help reduce the client's oxygen consumption by restricting activity and providing sedation as needed. Space procedures to allow for periods of uninterrupted rest.

Client and Family Teaching

The client with simple rib fracture or a minor chest wall injury often is managed as an outpatient. Teaching is a vital component of promoting optimal health for the client. The client needs to have a good understanding of pain management and its relationship to preventing respiratory complications. Instruct the client in the importance of coughing and deep breathing, and teach the client how

to splint the rib cage during coughing, being sure to explain the reasons for not taping or wrapping the chest continuously. Describe complications that should be reported to the physician: chills and fever, productive cough, purulent or bloody sputum, shortness of breath or difficulty breathing, and increasing chest pain. Emphasize the importance of avoiding respiratory irritants, such as cigarette smoke and occupational or environmental pollutants.

The client who requires hospitalization needs teaching about treatments and procedures used to manage chest and pulmonary trauma. Include information about pain management strategies such as patient-controlled analgesia (PCA), intercostal nerve block, or continuous epidural infusion. If intubation and mechanical ventilation are required, teach the client communication strategies. Explain the purpose of the ventilator, suctioning procedures, and bronchoscopy if ordered. Reassure the family that mechanical ventilation generally is required for no more than 2 to 3 weeks and that the client will be able to breathe without assistance once healing is under way.

With a significant pulmonary contusion, the client may have long-term respiratory insufficiency. This can require the client to modify his or her usual activity level and, possibly, to change occupations.

The Client with Inhalation Injury

∎ ∎ ∎

The internal environment of the lungs normally is protected from noxious substances by respiratory defense mechanisms. If these defenses are breached, inhaled agents, such as gases, fumes, toxins, and water, can result in internal trauma to the lungs.

Pathophysiology

Smoke Inhalation

Pulmonary injury due to the inhalation of hot air, toxic gases, or particulate matter is the leading cause of death in burn injury (Andreoli et al., 1990; Way, 1994). Smoke inhalation affects up to one-third of clients admitted to burn units (Tierney et al., 1994). Smoke inhalation can significantly affect normal respiratory function through three different mechanisms:

- Thermal damage to the airways, leading to impaired ventilation

- Carbon monoxide or cyanide poisoning, resulting in tissue hypoxia

- Chemical damage to the lung from noxious gases, which can impair gas exchange

Smoke inhalation is suspected whenever a burn occurs in a closed space; if there is evidence of burns on the face or upper torso or singed nasal hairs; if the client's sputum contains ashlike material; and when the client has such manifestations as dyspnea, wheezing, rales, or rhonchi.

The lower airways of the lungs typically are protected from thermal damage by cooling of the inhaled gases in the upper airway and laryngeal spasm. Upper airway obstruction due to tissue edema and laryngeal spasm can occur quickly, however, resulting in **asphyxiation,** or oxygen deprivation, without lung damage. Steam inhalation can result in thermal damage to tissues of the lower respiratory tract.

Inhalation of carbon monoxide or cyanide gas poses an immediate threat to life for the burn victim. Carbon monoxide is a colorless, odorless gas produced in a fire. It binds readily with hemoglobin; the affinity of carbon monoxide for hemoglobin is 200 to 250 times stronger than that of oxygen. Hemoglobin bound to carbon monoxide reduces the oxygen-carrying capacity of the blood and oxygen delivery to cells of the body. Carbon monoxide poisoning is suspected if the burn occurred in a closed space, if there is evidence of inhalation injury, or if the client is dyspneic.

The manifestations of carbon monoxide poisoning depend on the level of carboxyhemoglobin saturation. When the hemoglobin is 10% to 20% saturated with carbon monoxide, the client may experience headache, dizziness, dyspnea, and nausea. A characteristic "cherry-red" color of the skin and mucous membranes may be seen. With increasing levels, the client demonstrates confusion, visual disturbances, irritability, hallucinations, hypotension, seizures, and coma. Permanent neurologic deficit can occur in survivors of severe acute poisoning.

Many other toxic chemicals may be present in smoke, especially in a house fire or industrial plant fire. Hydrogen cyanide is a component of smoke that can be lethal when inhaled. The inhalation of toxic chemicals leads to bronchospasm and edema of the airways and alveoli. Adult respiratory distress syndrome may develop within 1 to 2 days. Sloughing of damaged mucosa leads to airway obstruction and atelectasis. Pneumonia is common following smoke inhalation.

Near-Drowning

Drowning is a leading preventable cause of accidental death in the United States. Approximately 5500 people die of drowning every year in the United States. Alcohol ingestion is a factor in one-fourth to one-third of adult drowning deaths (Tierney et al., 1994; Way, 1994). Asphyxia and aspiration are the primary problems associated with drowning and near-drowning. About 10% of victims do not aspirate water; in these victims, laryngeal spasm causes asphyxia. This is known as "dry drowning." In the majority of cases, however, asphyxia and hypox-

emia are the result of fluid aspiration. The effects of hypoxemia occur rapidly: Significant hypoxemia, with loss of consciousness, can occur within 3 to 5 minutes after total immersion; circulatory impairment, brain injury, and brain death can occur within 5 to 10 minutes. Immersion in very cold water and the *dive reflex,* a protective mechanism that slows the heartbeat, constricts peripheral vessels, and shunts blood to the brain and heart, may prolong survival.

Delayed death in the near-drowning victim can result from water aspiration. Respiratory and systemic effects differ, depending on whether fresh water or salt water has been aspirated. Fresh water is hypotonic; when aspirated, it is rapidly absorbed from the alveoli, resulting in significant hypervolemia and hemodilution. Hemolysis occurs as blood cells are subjected to a hypotonic environment, and serum electrolytes are diluted. Electrolyte imbalances can lead to cardiac irregularities and death; hemolysis can result in acute tubular necrosis and acute renal failure. Aspiration of fresh water impairs pulmonary surfactant and damages the alveolar-capillary membrane. Respiratory failure can result.

Nearly the opposite effects occur with salt water aspiration. As a hypertonic fluid, salt water causes fluid to be drawn into the alveoli, resulting in hypovolemia and hemoconcentration. Hemolysis is insignificant, and small elevations in serum sodium and chloride levels rarely cause life-threatening effects. With either type of near-drowning episode, inhaled microorganisms and debris can lead to the eventual development of pneumonia. The pathophysiologic changes associated with fresh water and salt water near-drowning are illustrated in Figure 34–23.

Clinical manifestations of near-drowning may include altered level of consciousness, restlessness, and apprehension. The client may complain of headache or chest pain. Other signs include vomiting, possible cyanosis, apnea, tachypnea, and wheezing. If pulmonary edema is present, pink froth may be visible in the mouth and nose. Other manifestations include tachycardia, dysrhythmias, hypotension, shock, and cardiac arrest. The client may be hypothermic.

The near-drowning victim who never loses consciousness or is conscious on admission to the emergency department has a good prognosis for recovery. The prognosis is less optimistic when neurologic damage has occurred.

Collaborative Care

With inhalation injuries, the most effective treatment is prevention. A working smoke detector (with functioning batteries) could prevent the majority of deaths from smoke inhalation occurring in the home. The line "A smoke detector was found, but the batteries had been

Figure 34-23 The pathogenesis of near-drowning, fresh water and salt water.

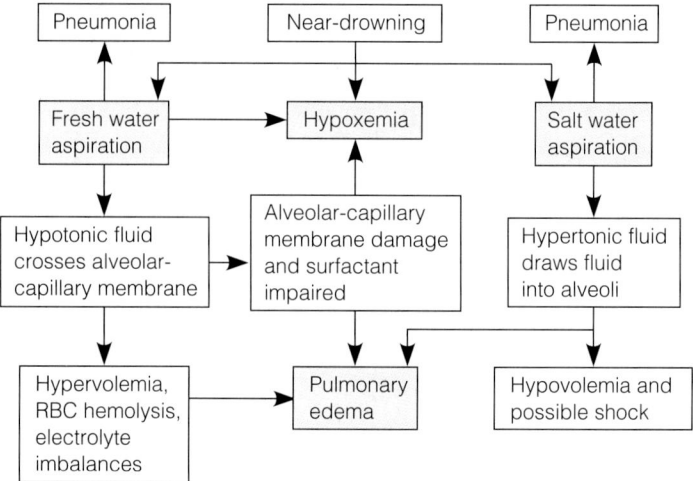

removed" is all too familiar in news reports of fire-related deaths.

To prevent drowning, life preservers and flotation vests or jackets should be worn on the body, not stored in the hold of the boat. These devices are designed to keep the head above water. Even accomplished swimmers should never enter the water alone in unguarded areas. Just as alcohol and driving do not mix, neither do alcohol and boating or other water sports.

The second most important line of defense against death or permanent injury from inhalation injuries is removing the victim from the area of the fire or water and administering effective cardiopulmonary resuscitation. In many cases, immediate restoration of effective breathing and circulation is key to preserving life. Hypoxemia progresses rapidly until breathing is restored; reversal of tissue hypoxia depends on adequate circulation. In both smoke inhalation and near drowning, intubation may be necessary to establish an airway. Oxygen is administered as soon as available. Attempts to drain water out of the lungs of the near-drowning victim waste time and are generally ineffective in restoring alveolar ventilation. External cardiac defibrillation may be necessary to reestablish an effective cardiac rhythm and circulation. When the victim is hypothermic, resuscitation measures are continued until the core body temperature reaches approximately 90 F (32 C). The basic "rule" in hypothermia is that the client is not considered to be dead until the body has been rewarmed and life signs remain absent.

Medical evaluation and possible hospital admission are necessary for clients with inhalation injuries. Laboratory and diagnostic tests which may be ordered include the following:

- *ABGs* are measured to determine the degree of hypoxemia. Respiratory and metabolic acidosis due to impaired gas exchange and hypoxemia may also be apparent. With effective ventilation and supplemental

oxygen, acidosis may reverse quickly, requiring no further treatment. With carbon monoxide poisoning, the arterial P_{O_2} may be normal, but measured oxyhemoglobin saturation less than normal.

- *Carboxyhemoglobin levels* are drawn in suspected carbon monoxide poisoning. Normal levels of carboxyhemoglobin are less than 5% in nonsmokers and less than 10% in smokers. Higher levels indicate carbon monoxide poisoning. Levels of less than 20% are considered mild poisoning; between 20% and 40% is moderate poisoning; and 40% to 60% is severe poisoning. Levels higher than 60% are generally fatal.

- *Serum electrolytes and osmolality* are measured, particularly in the client with near drowning. Expected levels vary according to the type of water aspirated. With fresh-water drowning, serum electrolyte levels may be significantly reduced, as is serum osmolality. With salt-water drowning, serum sodium and chloride may be somewhat elevated, and the osmolality is increased because of hypovolemia.

- *Chest X-ray* is performed, but it often does not demonstrate immediate changes. Frequently changes are not visible on the chest X-ray until 12 or more hours after the insult. Evidence of adult respiratory distress syndrome may be apparent 24 to 48 hours after inhalation injury.

- *Bronchoscopy* may be ordered to allow visualization of damaged lung tissue, particularly with smoke inhalation and possible thermal injury.

Medical management of the client with an inhalation injury is generally supportive. Endotracheal intubation and mechanical ventilation often are required to maintain the airway and provide adequate alveolar ventilation and oxygenation. All clients with inhalation injury require supplemental oxygen, even when intubation and ventilation are not necessary.

Other measures used for the client who has experienced inhalation injury may include bronchodilator therapy to manage bronchospasm. Bronchodilators can be delivered by either aerosol inhalation or intravenous administration. Coughing and suctioning is important to remove secretions and debris. Chest physiotherapy with percussion and postural drainage may be performed.

Intravenous fluids may be ordered; if significant hemolysis has occurred, packed red blood cells may be administered to improve the oxygen-carrying capacity of the blood. Fluid therapy is monitored carefully, using pulmonary artery or central venous pressures to reduce the risk of pulmonary edema.

With near-drowning victims, measures such as inducing hypothermia or barbiturate-induced coma and administering corticosteroids and osmotic diuretics may be employed to help prevent neurologic damage.

Throughout the course of treatment, the client is carefully monitored for signs of complications, such as pneumonia or adult respiratory distress syndrome. Frequent assessment of respiratory status, vital signs, and other factors is performed to allow early intervention should complications occur.

Nursing Care

Depending on the degree of pulmonary damage, the client with inhalation injury may be critically ill or simply require close observation for 2 to 3 days. In either case, priorities for nursing care are determined by the type of injury or damage. Airway clearance is a major concern in either smoke inhalation or near drowning, as is impaired gas exchange. Tissue hypoxia also can be a significant problem for the client with inhalation injury.

Nursing measures to maintain adequate airway clearance begin with careful and frequent assessment of respiratory status, including respiratory rate, depth, and effort as well as breath sounds. Note the amount, color, and consistency of sputum. Assist the client to cough frequently; suction the intubated client as needed to remove secretions. Generally, the client will be positioned with the head of the bed elevated to facilitate alveolar ventilation. Stabilize the endotracheal tube with tape and ties to prevent it from being displaced into a mainstem bronchus, which could result in ventilation of only one lung. Report changes in the character of secretions that may indicate complications: pink, frothy sputum, which may signal pulmonary edema, or purulent sputum, which may signal pneumonia. Administer bronchodilators as ordered. Perform percussion and postural drainage procedures.

Gas exchange is enhanced by the administration of supplemental oxygen, with or without mechanical ventilation. Assess the client's skin color and mental status frequently. Decreasing level of consciousness may be an early sign of hypoxemia. Monitor oxygen saturation levels, arterial blood gas results, and pulmonary artery pressures as ordered and indicated by the client's condition. Report changes to the physician. Maintain oxygen flow rates as ordered. Provide frequent mouth care to reduce the discomfort of dry mucous membranes and prevent tissue breakdown. Work with the respiratory therapist to maintain effective oxygen delivery with mechanical ventilation. Administer sedation as required. Maintain fluid restriction if ordered.

Impaired cerebral tissue perfusion is another priority problem especially with the near-drowning victim. Hypoxia and possible hypervolemia can lead to cerebral edema and increased intracranial pressure (IICP), further impairing blood flow. Monitor the client's vital signs and neurologic status frequently. A change in level of consciousness or behavior is typically the earliest sign of IICP. Changes noted on an intracranial pressure monitor also provide early evidence of IICP. Increasing systolic blood pressure and pulse pressure and slowed cardiac rate are late signs. Other manifestations may include pupillary changes and decreasing muscle strength. Report changes promptly to the physician. Position the client with the head of the bed elevated to facilitate drainage from the cerebral vault. Keep the head in a neutral position. Maintain effective ventilation and oxygenation; hypercapnia and hypoxemia increase cerebral edema. Administer barbiturate sedation, osmotic diuretics, or corticosteroids as ordered to reduce cerebral edema. Maintain fluid restriction. Space activities and promote rest to reduce metabolic demands.

Other nursing diagnoses may be applicable for the client with inhalation injury. The following are examples:

- *Anxiety* related to intubation and mechanical ventilation
- *Hypothermia* related to submersion in cold water
- *Fluid Volume Deficit* or *Fluid Volume Excess* related to aspiration of salt or fresh water
- *Risk for Infection* related to inhalation of bacteria and particulate matter
- *Inability to Sustain Spontaneous Ventilation* related to asphyxia
- *Altered Urinary Elimination* related to hemolysis of red blood cells and acute tubular necrosis

Client and Family Teaching

Education of clients and their families begins with prevention of inhalation injuries. Teach clients the value of a working smoke detector, especially in the sleeping areas of the house. Encourage families to develop an escape plan in case of fire and to use fire drills to rehearse getting out of the house. Smoldering cigarettes are a leading cause of house fires; help clients develop a plan to stop smoking. Teach clients to drop and roll should clothing catch fire. (Fire rises, increasing the risk of respiratory injury if the client remains upright.)

Learning to swim safely is important to prevent drowning. Teach clients never to swim alone, when fatigued, or immediately following a meal. Remind clients that knowing how to swim will not prevent drowning in very cold water or in large bodies of water, such as lakes, rivers, or the ocean. Encourage clients always to wear flotation devices while boating, water-skiing, surfing, or wind-surfing. Wet suits also help to prevent hypothermia during activities in very cold water. Advise clients to cover or fence household swimming pools, hot tubs, and ponds to prevent inadvertent entry and drowning.

A population well trained in effective, safe cardiopulmonary resuscitation (CPR) provides the best second line of defense against inhalation injury. Rapid restoration of breathing is essential to prevent hypoxia and brain damage. Encourage all clients and their families to become trained and maintain current CPR certification. Work with communities to increase the number of trained individuals. Refer clients to the local chapters of the American Red Cross or the American Heart Association for available classes.

The client with a minor inhalation injury who does not require hospitalization needs information about manifestations that may indicate a complication. Tell the client to notify the physician should he or she note increasing dyspnea, cough productive of purulent or pink frothy mucus, confusion, or other changes. Manifestations of respiratory damage may not be evident for 24 to 48 hours following the injury.

Clients requiring hospitalization and their families need support and education about their condition and prescribed treatments. Teach communication strategies to the client who is intubated. Explain the respirator, monitors, and alarms to reduce the client's anxiety. If sedative coma is being maintained or skeletal muscle paralysis is necessary for adequate ventilation, reassure the client and/or family that this is temporary and an effect of the prescribed medication. When the medication is discontinued, the effects will be reversed.

The client who has experienced significant hypoxia as a result of drowning or carbon monoxide poisoning may have permanent neurologic effects. Work with the family to develop communication techniques and identify remaining strengths. Help the family identify future care needs and means for meeting them, such as home health, personal care aids, or long-term care facilities. Provide social services and support group referrals.

Respiratory Failure

Many of the conditions discussed in this chapter, from pneumonia to adult respiratory distress syndrome (ARDS), can lead to **respiratory failure.** In respiratory failure, the lungs are unable to oxygenate the blood and remove carbon dioxide adequately to meet the body's needs, even at rest.

The Client with Acute Respiratory Failure

Respiratory failure is often defined by arterial blood gas values. An arterial oxygen level (PO_2) of less than 50 to 60 mm Hg and an arterial carbon dioxide level (PCO_2) of greater than 50 mm Hg are generally accepted as indicators of respiratory failure (Porth, 1994; Tierney et al., 1994). However, clients with chronic COPD may be alert and functional with blood gas values that would indicate respiratory failure in the client whose respiratory function was previously normal. In clients with COPD, respiratory failure is indicated by an acute drop in blood oxygen levels along with increased carbon dioxide levels (Bullock & Rosendahl, 1992; Wilson et al., 1991).

Pathophysiology

Respiratory failure is not a disease but a consequence of severe respiratory dysfunction. Respiratory failure can result from inadequate ventilation of the alveoli, impaired gas exchange, or a significant ventilation-perfusion mismatch. COPD is the most common cause of respiratory failure. Other lung diseases, chest injury, inhalation trauma, neuromuscular disorders, and cardiac conditions can also lead to respiratory failure. Selected causes of acute respiratory failure are identified in Table 34–10.

Respiratory failure may be either primarily hypoxemic in nature or involve a combination of hypoxemia and hypercapnia (Figure 34–24). In hypoxemic respiratory failure, PO_2 is significantly reduced, whereas PCO_2 remains normal or even lower than normal as a result of hyperventilation. The lower oxygen pressure experienced at high altitudes, hypoventilation, impaired diffusion across the alveolar-capillary membrane, and a ventilation-perfusion mismatch can result in a drop of arterial oxygen levels that is more rapid than the rise in carbon dioxide. Metabolic acidosis results from tissue hypoxia. With significant hypoventilation of the lungs, the carbon dioxide level of the blood rises rapidly, leading to respiratory acidosis. An accompanying fall in oxygen level occurs as

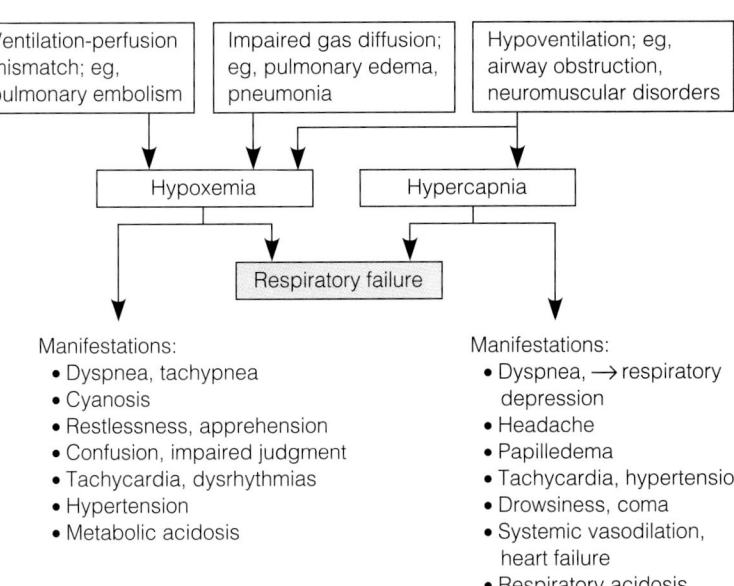

Figure 34–24   Respiratory failure, its causes and manifestations.

well. In summary, hypoxemia without a corresponding rise in carbon dioxide levels indicates a failure of oxygenation; hypoxemia with hypercapnia is the result of lung hypoventilation.

The manifestations of respiratory failure are those of hypoxia and hypercapnia along with those of the underlying disease process. The predominant manifestations of hypoxemia are dyspnea, along with neurologic manifestations of restlessness, apprehension, impaired judgment, and motor impairment. Tachycardia and hypertension develop as the heart increases the cardiac output in an effort to bring more oxygen to the tissues. Cyanosis is present. With progression of hypoxemia, cardiac rhythm disturbances, bradycardia, hypotension, and decreased cardiac output may be seen.

Increased carbon dioxide levels have a depressant effect on the central nervous system, as well as a vasodilator effect. Dyspnea is an early sign, as is headache. Other signs and symptoms include peripheral and conjunctival *hyperemia* (vasodilation), papilledema, neuromuscular irritability, and impaired consciousness. As hypercapnia worsens, the respiratory center may be depressed, reducing dyspnea and slowing respirations. When this occurs, the client has lost the usual carbon dioxide stimulus to breathe. A low level of oxygen in the blood remains the only active breathing stimulus. Administration of oxygen without ventilatory support may eliminate any drive to breathe, with dire consequences for the client.

The prognosis for acute respiratory failure varies, depending on the underlying disease process. The client with an uncomplicated drug overdose generally recovers readily from acute respiratory failure without long-term sequelae. The client with underlying respiratory disease may have a more prolonged course and less favorable outcome. Among adults requiring mechanical ventilation for

Table 34–10	Selected Conditions Leading to Respiratory Failure
Type of Dysfunction	**Examples**
Impaired ventilation:	
■ Airway obstruction	Laryngospasm, foreign body aspiration, airway edema
■ Respiratory disease	Asthma, COPD
■ Neurologic causes	Spinal cord injury, poliomyelitis, Guillain-Barré syndrome, drug overdose, stroke
■ Chest wall injury	Flail chest, pneumothorax
Impaired diffusion:	
■ Alveolar disorders	Pneumonia, pneumonitis, COPD
■ Pulmonary edema	Heart failure, adult respiratory distress syndrome (ARDS), near-drowning
Ventilation-perfusion mismatch	Pulmonary embolism

acute respiratory failure, it is estimated that 62% survive to be weaned from the ventilator, but only 43% survive to be discharged from the hospital, and 30% remain alive at one year after discharge (Tierney et al., 1994).

Collaborative Care

Treatment of the client with respiratory failure is directed toward correcting the underlying cause or disease process, supporting ventilation, and correcting hypoxemia and hypercapnia. Care related to disorders that can precipitate respiratory failure is discussed in the sections specific to each disorder.

Nursing Implications for Pharmacology: Neuromuscular Blockers

NONDEPOLARIZING NEUROMUSCULAR BLOCKERS

Tubocurarine (curare, Tubarine)

Pancuronium bromide (Pavulon)

Atracurium besylate (Tracrium)

Nondepolarizing neuromuscular blockers competitively block the action of acetylcholine (ACh) at the nicotinic receptors of skeletal muscle, preventing muscle depolarization and resultant contraction. Complete muscle paralysis is achieved within minutes of administration. Facial muscles, including those of the eye and mouth, are affected first, followed by muscles of the limbs, neck, and trunk. The muscles of respiration (the diaphragm and intercostal muscles) are least sensitive to the effects of neuromuscular blockers and are paralyzed last. After the medication is discontinued or an antagonist is administered, muscles recover their function in reverse order; respiratory function is recovered first (Shlafer, 1993).

Nursing Responsibilities

- Prior to administering the medication, assess the placement of the endotracheal tube, and ensure that the mechanical ventilator is functioning effectively. The risk of hypoxemia and organ damage is significant if respiratory muscles are paralyzed without adequate ventilatory support in place.
- Administer the prescribed drug by slow intravenous injection and/or intravenous infusion as prescribed.

- Keep an acetylcholinesterase (AChE) inhibitor such as neostigmine (Prostigmin) available at the client's bedside for rapid reversal of neuromuscular effects if needed.
- Administer the neuromuscular blocker with morphine sulfate, diazepam (Valium), or other antianxiety agent or sedative. Neuromuscular blockers provide no sedation or pain relief; muscle paralysis produces extreme anxiety in the client.
- Administer only fresh solution; do not store the solution in the syringe.
- Instill artificial tears every 2 to 4 hours for lubrication of eyes (the client is unable to blink).
- Suction oral cavity to remove saliva (the client is unable to swallow).
- *Never* turn off ventilator alarms on a client receiving neuromuscular blockers. Should the tubing become disconnected or plugged, the client will be unable to breathe independently and unable to call for help.

Client and Family Teaching

- Reassure the client that the ability to move and communicate will be restored when the medication is discontinued.
- Teach the client's family about the effects of the drug and the reason for its use. Tell them that although the client is unable to respond, he or she can hear and understand what is going on.

Laboratory and Diagnostic Tests

Because the manifestations of respiratory failure are not definitive and are often obscured by the underlying disease process, arterial blood gas values provide the best information for diagnosis and treatment. As noted previously, an arterial PO_2 of less than 50 to 60 mm Hg is indicative of respiratory failure in the client who does not have chronic obstructive pulmonary disease. In the COPD client, an acute drop of 10 to 15 mm Hg from previous levels indicates respiratory failure.

With hypoxemic respiratory failure, the PCO_2 may be normal, 38 to 42 mm Hg. If the client is tachypneic, a low PCO_2 may result from hyperventilation. A pH of less than 7.35 and low bicarbonate levels indicate metabolic acidosis, typical of hypoxemic respiratory failure.

In respiratory failure due to hypoventilation, the PCO_2 is elevated, usually greater than 50 mm Hg. With the ele-

vated carbon dioxide level, respiratory acidosis develops, demonstrated by a low pH. The client with hypoxemia and hypercapnia rapidly becomes acidotic because of the combined metabolic and respiratory effects. Correcting this acidosis by reversing hypoxemia and improving ventilation is a major goal of therapy for the client with respiratory failure.

Pharmacology

Pharmacologic management of acute respiratory failure consists primarily of bronchodilators to reverse airway spasm and constriction, and antibiotic therapy to treat infection.

Beta-adrenergic (sympathomimetic) or anticholinergic medications may be administered in aerosol form to promote bronchodilation. For the client who requires mechanical ventilation, the medications may be given by nebulizer attached to the ventilator. Methyxanthine bronchodilators (theophylline derivatives) may be administered intravenously. Bronchodilators are discussed in detail in the asthma section of this chapter, and their nursing implications are outlined in the box on page 1417. Corticosteriods may be prescribed to reduce airway edema. These also can be administered either in aerosol or intravenous forms.

On occasion, it is necessary to induce paralysis of the voluntary muscles to allow the ventilator to control respirations fully for maximal effectiveness. In some clients, spontaneous respiratory effort is insufficient to maintain effective ventilation and gas exchange, but it is strong enough to "fight" the ventilator, decreasing its effectiveness and increasing the work of breathing. Neuromuscular blocking agents such as tubocurarine (curare) or pancuronium bromide (Pavulon), commonly used in surgery, are administered to suppress the client's ability to breathe and allow the ventilator to control respirations. Nursing implications of neuromuscular blockers are described in the accompanying pharmacology box.

Oxygen Therapy

Oxygen therapy is vital to reverse the hypoxemia of acute respiratory failure. In general, the goal of oxygen therapy is to achieve an oxygen saturation of 85% to 90% (the percentage of hemoglobin saturated with oxygen) without oxygen toxicity. A P_{O_2} of 60 to 80 mm Hg usually allows adequate oxygen to meet the needs of body tissues. Higher levels do not significantly increase oxygen saturation and may lead to hypoventilation in clients with chronic hypercapnia (Berkow & Fletcher, 1992; Tierney et al., 1994). Clients with chronic COPD may require as little as 1 to 3 liters of oxygen per nasal cannula or 28% oxygen per Venturi mask to correct hypoxemia. Higher concentrations are necessary when gas diffusion is affected by disorders such as pneumonia or adult respiratory distress syndrome. In this case, concentrations of 40% to 60% may be required. Concentrations this high are used only for short periods to avoid oxygen toxicity. The development of oxygen toxicity depends on both the concentration of oxygen delivered and the duration of therapy. With continued high levels of oxygen delivery, surfactant synthesis is impaired, and the lungs become less compliant (more "stiff"). Adult respiratory distress syndrome can develop. Absorption atelectasis is another possible consequence (Holloway, 1993; Price & Wilson, 1992).

When hypoventilation is the cause of respiratory failure or an adequate level of oxygen cannot be maintained with oxygen delivery systems alone, it is necessary to intubate the client and initiate mechanical ventilation.

Airway Management

Clients who do not readily respond to supplemental oxygen therapy, who have an upper airway obstruction, or

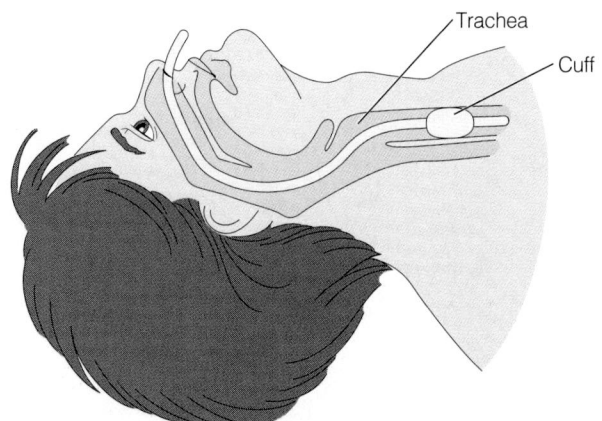

Figure 34–25 Nasal endotracheal (nasotracheal) intubation.

who need positive-pressure mechanical ventilation require intubation with an endotracheal tube extending from the mouth or nose into the trachea (Figure 34–25). Oral endotracheal intubation can be performed more rapidly and with less trauma than nasal intubation in an emergency situation, but it is less comfortable for the client. It is also more difficult to stabilize an orotracheal tube. Although nasotracheal tubes are more comfortable and better tolerated by the client, they are smaller and may be more difficult to clear with suctioning. Nasotracheal tubes can cause pressure necrosis of the nose or prompt purulent otitis media due to obstructed drainage of the auditory (eustachian) tube.

To maintain positive pressure ventilation, the tube is cuffed with an air-filled or foam sac just above the end of the tube. When the cuff is inflated, it obstructs the upper airway, preventing air from escaping back into the nose or mouth. Excess pressure of the cuff on tracheal walls can lead to ischemia and tissue necrosis. To minimize damage to the trachea, high-volume, low-pressure ("floppy") cuffs are used. Tubes with low-pressure cuffs may be left in place for 3 to 4 weeks, although there is a risk of laryngeal damage from tube motion.

A tracheostomy may be performed for the client who requires chronic ventilatory support. Although a tracheostomy is more comfortable for the client and easier to secure in place, complications such as cuff necrosis and increased risk of infection are associated with tracheostomy as well as endotracheal intubation.

When the client with acute respiratory failure no longer needs ventilatory support, the endotracheal tube is removed. Prior to its removal, the client must have been weaned from the ventilator; that is, he or she must be able to sustain effective spontaneous respirations. The client's gag, cough, and swallow reflexes must be intact to prevent aspiration. The client is oxygenated and suctioned, the cuff deflated, and the tube removed. Humidified oxygen is provided immediately following tube removal,

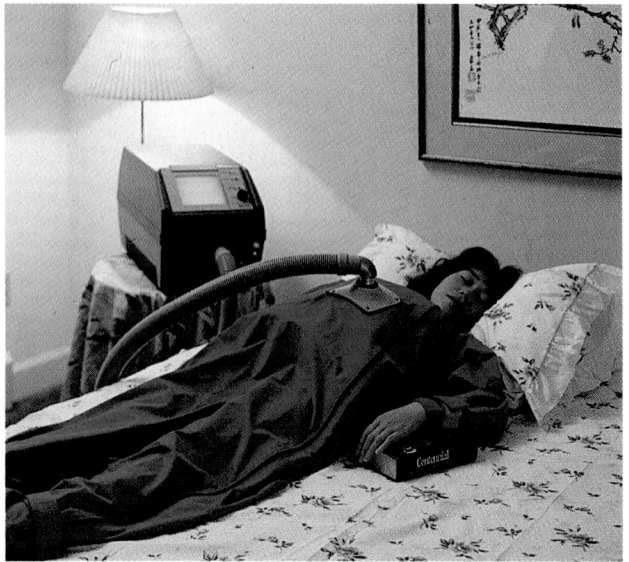

Figure 34-26 A negative-pressure ventilator.

and the client closely observed for signs of respiratory distress. Inspiratory stridor within the first 24 hours following removal is indicative of laryngeal edema. This may necessitate reintubation. Sore throat and a hoarse voice are common following extubation (Holloway, 1993). Oral intake is reinitiated slowly, with careful assessment of swallowing.

Mechanical Ventilation

Mechanical ventilation is indicated for acute respiratory failure when alveolar ventilation is inadequate to maintain blood oxygen and carbon dioxide levels. Specific indications for mechanical ventilation include apnea or acute ventilatory failure, hypoxemia unresponsive to oxygen therapy alone, and increased work of breathing leading to progressive client fatigue (Holloway, 1993; Tierney et al., 1994). Drug overdose, neural disorders, and chest wall injury such as flail chest can lead to acute ventilatory failure, as can airway problems such as severe asthma or COPD. In clients with disorders affecting alveolar-capillary diffusion, such as pulmonary contusion, pneumonia, and ARDS, mechanical ventilation may be required to achieve adequate oxygenation. Positive pressure ventilation increases lung volume, helps redistribute fluid from the alveolar to the interstitial space, and helps reduce the oxygen demand caused by increased work of breathing in many conditions leading to respiratory failure (Andreoli et al., 1990).

Types, Modes, and Settings Two broad general classifications of mechanical ventilators are available. *Negative-pressure ventilators* create subatmospheric pressure externally to draw the chest outward and air into the lungs,

mimicking spontaneous breathing. The iron lung, Curiass ventilator, and PulmoWrap are examples of negative-pressure ventilators (Figure 34–26).

Positive-pressure ventilators are much more commonly used today, especially in the treatment of acute respiratory failure. These ventilators push air into the lungs, rather than drawing it in like negative-pressure ventilators. An artificial airway is necessary for positive-pressure ventilation.

Two types of positive-pressure ventilators are available: pressure-cycled and volume-cycled. With a *pressure-cycled ventilator,* air is delivered until a preset airway pressure is reached. The volume of air delivered varies according to airway compliance and clearance. Pressure-cycled ventilators such as the Bird Mark 7 and Bennett PRII are rarely used today; however, pressure-support ventilation combines aspects of pressure-cycled ventilation with volume-cycled ventilation.

Volume-cycled ventilators deliver a preset volume of gas to the lungs over a preset range of pressures (Figure 34–27). Volume-cycled ventilators are more commonly used for adults than pressure-cycled ventilators. These ventilators are able to maintain tidal volume despite changes in airway compliance or resistance. The MA-1 and MA-2, Bennett 7200, Ohio 560, and Bear 5 are examples of volume-cycled ventilators. The Siemens Servo 900C can be used as either a volume-cycled or pressure-cycled ventilator.

A number of different modes or patterns of ventilation may be used with positive-pressure ventilators. Control, assist-control, intermittent mandatory ventilation (IMV), synchronized intermittent mandatory ventilation (SIMV), continuous positive airway pressure (CPAP), positive end-expiratory pressure (PEEP), pressure support ventilation (PSV), and inverse ratio ventilation are common modes of ventilation in use today.

With the *control mode,* all breaths are delivered by the ventilator at a preset frequency, volume or pressure, and inspiratory flow rate. The client has no control over breathing. This mode may be used for the client who has sustained a head injury and has no spontaneous respiratory effort. The control mode may also be used in conjunction with sedation and paralysis of voluntary muscles when the client's respiratory efforts interfere with the effectiveness of ventilation.

Assist-control is used more frequently than control mode. The client can trigger breaths to be delivered by initiating respiratory effort. If the client's respiratory rate falls below a present number (e.g., 14 breaths per minute), the ventilator will deliver mandatory breaths. All breaths, whether initiated by the client or the ventilator, are delivered at a specific tidal volume or pressure and inspiratory flowrate.

Using the *intermittent mandatory ventilation (IMV)* mode, mandatory or machine-controlled breaths are delivered at a set frequency and volume or pressure. Between mandatory breaths, the client can breathe spontaneously at any rate and depth desired, with no ventilator assistance. *Synchronized intermittent mandatory ventilation (SIMV)* allows client inspiratory effort to initiate mandatory breaths. With this mode, mandatory breaths are coordinated with the client's spontaneous breaths; with IMV, they are not. IMV and SIMV are widely used in the process of weaning the client from ventilator support.

With *continuous positive airway pressure (CPAP)*, positive pressure is applied to the airways of a spontaneously breathing client. CPAP may be used with either endotracheal intubation or a tight-fitting face mask. All breathing is spontaneous (client triggered) and pressure controlled. CPAP is used to help maintain open airways and alveoli, decreasing the work of breathing.

Positive end-expiratory pressure (PEEP) requires intubation and can be applied to any of the previously described ventilator modes. With PEEP, a positive pressure is maintained in the airways during exhalation and between breaths. By keeping alveoli open between breaths, there is less of a ventilation-perfusion mismatch, and diffusion across the alveolar-capillary membrane is improved. This allows better oxygenation of the blood using lower percentages of inspired oxygen. PEEP is particularly useful for clients with ARDS.

Two newer modes of ventilation are pressure support and inverse ratio ventilation. With *pressure support ventilation (PSV)*, the client's inspiratory effort is assisted by the ventilator to a certain level of pressure. The client initiates all breaths and controls the flow rate and tidal volume. This mode decreases the work of breathing for the client and increases comfort through increased control by the client. All breaths are mandatory (ventilator controlled) when *inverse ratio ventilation (IRV)* is used. Breaths are pressure limited and time cycled, and the inspiratory time is longer than the expiratory time (the opposite of the normal respiratory cycle, in which expiration is longer than inspiration).

High frequency jet ventilation (HFV) is another relatively new mode of ventilation in which small pulses or "jets" of air are delivered at a frequency of 60 to 100 times per minute. With HFV, alveoli remain open with low airway pressures. Modes of ventilator function are compared in Table 34–11.

In addition to the choice of the mode of ventilator operation, four main parameters are set to meet individual client needs when a volume-cycled ventilator is used:

- The rate or number of breaths per minute

- The tidal volume, or milliliters of air delivered with each breath

- Oxygen concentration of delivered air (FIO_2)

- Positive end-expiratory pressure (PEEP)

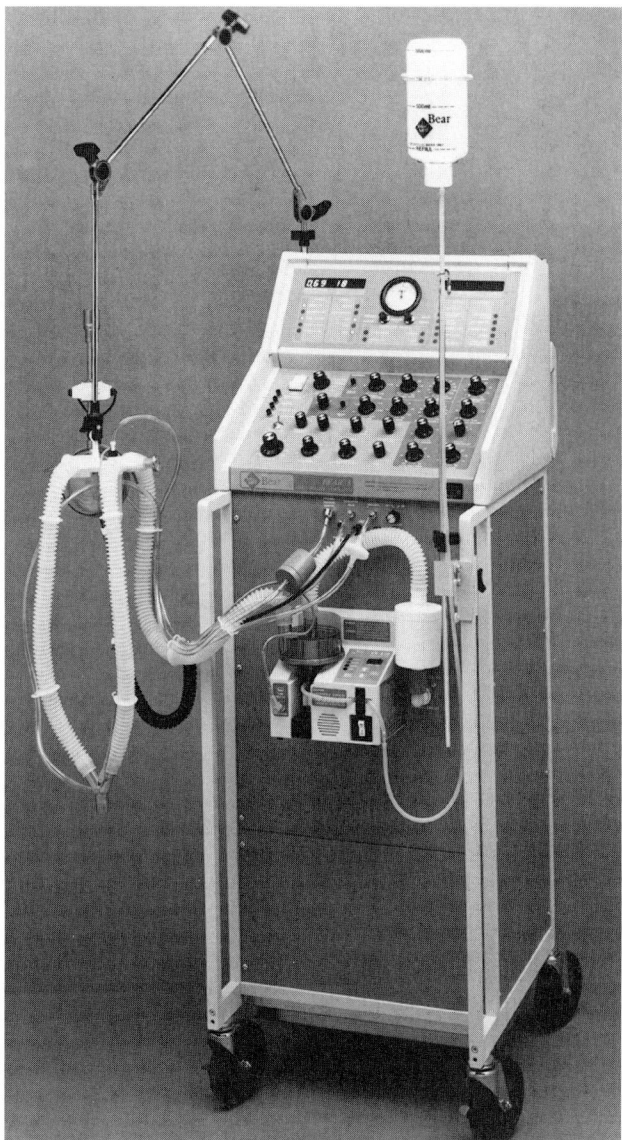

Figure 34–27   Volume-cycled ventilator.

For most adult clients, the rate is initially set at between 12 and 15 breaths per minute. In the control mode, the rate set on the ventilator will be the client's respiratory rate. With assist-control, IMV, or SIMV, the client's respiratory rate is generally going to be higher than that set on the ventilator as the client initiates spontaneous breaths. The rate may be adjusted, based on the client's PCO_2. If the PCO_2 falls below 40 mm Hg, indicating hyperventilation and respiratory alkalosis, the set rate is reduced. An increased PCO_2, above 40 mm Hg, indicates hypoventilation and a need to increase the respiratory rate.

The tidal volume setting controls the amount of gas to be delivered with each ventilator breath. For adults, the normal tidal volume at rest is 7 mL/kg of body weight, or

Table 34-11	Modes of Ventilator Operation	
Mode	**Description**	**Pattern**
Spontaneous breathing	Client has full control of rate, tidal volume, pressures.	
Control mode	Ventilator controls all breaths: rate, volume or pressure, and inspiratory flow rate are preset.	
Assist-control mode	Client can trigger ventilator to deliver breaths at preset volume or pressure and inspiratory flow rate; breaths will be delivered at preset rate if client does not initiate.	
Intermittent mandatory ventilation (IMV)	Ventilator delivers mandatory breaths at preset rate; client breathes spontaneously between mandatory ventilation.	

400 to 550 mL on average. With mechanical ventilation, the tidal volume is calculated using 10 to 15 mL/kg of body weight (650 to 1000 ml tidal volume) to compensate for tubing dead space and to minimize atelectasis (Way, 1994). Higher tidal volumes can result in trauma to the lung tissue.

The amount of oxygen delivered is adjusted by changing the oxygen percentage of the gas delivered with ventilator breaths. Because of the risk of oxygen toxicity and pulmonary fibrosis associated with prolonged administration of high oxygen concentrations, the FIO_2 is set at the lowest possible level for adequate tissue oxygenation. The PO_2 and arterial oxygen saturation levels are used to help determine oxygen concentration settings. For most clients, the goal is to maintain an oxygen saturation of

greater than 90%. Lower levels may be appropriate for clients with long-standing COPD.

When hypoxemia occurs despite oxygen concentrations of 50% or greater, PEEP is added to prevent alveolar collapse and increase alveolar-capillary diffusion. PEEP is maintained by placing a valve in the expiratory circuit of the ventilator that prevents airway pressure from falling below a preset level, even at the end of expiration (Way, 1994).

Complications   Although endotracheal intubation and mechanical ventilation can be life-saving measures for the client in respiratory failure, they are not without risk.

The intubated client is vulnerable to pressure necrosis of the nose, lip, or trachea due to the continued presence

Table 34–11	(continued)	
Mode	**Description**	**Pattern**
Synchronized intermittent mandatory ventilation (SIMV)	Mandatory breaths delivered by ventilator are synchronized with client's inspiratory effort.	
Continuous positive airway pressure (CPAP)	Positive pressure is maintained in airways; all breaths are spontaneous.	
Positive end-expiratory pressure (PEEP)	Used in conjunction with other ventilator modes; positive airway pressure is maintained throughout respiratory cycle.	
Pressure support ventilation (PSV)	Pressurized inspiratory flow supports the client's inspiratory effort, decreasing the work of breathing.	
Inverse ratio ventilation	Mandatory breaths are delivered in an inverse ratio, with inspiration longer than expiration.	
High frequency jet ventilation (HFV)	Small tidal volumes, pulses or "jets" of air, are delivered at a frequency of 60 to 100 times per minute, maintaining open alveoli with low airway pressures.	

of a moveable foreign object. A tracheal-esophageal fistula may form. Saliva production is reduced, and mouth care may be difficult, leading to ulcerations of oral mucosa. Improper placement or dislodging of the endotracheal tube can result in ventilation of one lung only, with resultant overdistention of the inflated lung and atelectasis and collapse of the uninflated lung.

Infection is a significant risk for the intubated client. The normal defense mechanisms of the upper respiratory tract (the nose, oropharynx, epiglottis, and larynx) have been bypassed. Humidification and trapping of bacteria and other foreign substances are lost. The gag reflex may be intact, but substances are allowed to enter the respiratory tree through the open epiglottis. Often, the cough reflex is inhibited or impaired by the underlying disease

process and the continued presence of a foreign object, the endotracheal tube. Unless suctioning and other respiratory procedures are carried out under strict aseptic conditions, bacteria can be introduced. Secretions often become thick and tenacious, increasing the risk of atelectasis. In addition, the warm, moist environment of the ventilator tubing provides a good place for bacteria to grow and multiply. Condensed moisture in the tubing should always be drained toward the ventilator (away from the client) and the tubing changed every 24 to 48 hours to reduce the risk of introducing infection from this source.

Complications directly associated with mechanical ventilation include respiratory alkalosis from hyperventilation, barotrauma, and decreased cardiac output.

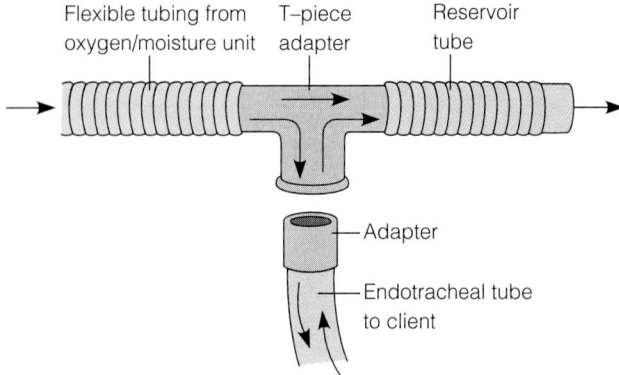

Flexible tubing from oxygen/moisture unit

T–piece adapter

Reservoir tube

Adapter

Endotracheal tube to client

Figure 34–28 The T-piece, or "blow-by" unit, for weaning from mechanical ventilation.

Barotrauma is lung injury due to pressure. The nature of positive-pressure ventilators places the client at risk for barotrauma. The use of large tidal volumes, high peak airway pressures, and PEEP are all associated with an increased risk of barotrauma in the mechanically ventilated client. Endotracheal tube displacement into the right mainstem bronchus with resulting overdistension of the right lung presents a significant risk for barotrauma. Subcutaneous emphysema, pneumothorax, and pneumomediastinum are possible manifestations of barotrauma. *Subcutaneous emphysema,* or air in the subcutaneous tissue, is not dangerous to the client with an artificial airway in place, but it is an indicator of damage resulting from barotrauma. Subcutaneous emphysema results in tissue swelling, which can be massive and involve the chest, neck, and face. A "crackling" or air-bubble-popping sensation is felt when areas of subcutaneous emphysema are palpated. With correction of the cause, the air is gradually reabsorbed.

Pneumothorax may result from alveolar rupture due to overdistension with mechanical ventilation. The client experiencing a pneumothorax shows signs of unequal chest expansion, a sudden loss or significant decrease in breath sounds on the affected side, and a hyperresonant percussion tone. Rapid chest tube insertion is necessary to prevent tension pneumothorax and impairment of cardiac function and the great vessels.

Pneumomediastinum is the presence of air in the mediastinum, the space between the lungs that contains the heart, great vessels, trachea, and esophagus. Air in the mediastinal space can interfere with the function of all these organs and lead to such complications as pneumopericardium (air in the pericardial sac). Few manifestations may be present initially with pneumomediastinum, but the presence of increased air in the space is evident on chest X-ray.

Pressure within the intrathoracic cavity increases when positive-pressure mechanical ventilation is used. This increased pressure can interfere with venous return to the heart and ventricular filling. As a result, clients on mechanical ventilation are at risk for decreased cardiac output, especially when high levels of PEEP are used.

Gastrointestinal complications also are associated with prolonged mechanical ventilation, most likely from the stress response. Gastrointestinal hemorrhage, typically painless, occurs in about 25% of clients on mechanical ventilation for a prolonged period (Holloway, 1993). Histamine H_2-receptor blockers, antacids, and sucralfate help prevent stress gastritis and resultant hemorrhage. Gastrointestinal secretions and feces are tested for occult blood for early detection of bleeding.

For all the above complications of mechanical ventilation, the best treatment is prevention. Reducing PEEP to the lowest possible levels to maintain oxygen saturation, keeping the tidal volume within appropriate parameters for the client's stature, and maintaining the proper placement of the endotracheal tube are vital components of mechanical ventilator management.

Weaning **Weaning** is the process of removing the client from ventilator support and reestablishing spontaneous, independent respirations. The process and length of weaning depend on a number of factors, including the client's preexisting lung condition, duration of mechanical ventilation, and the client's general condition, both physical and psychologic.

The client who has been on mechanical ventilation for only a short time may be removed from the ventilator and the airway attached to a T-piece connected to oxygen (Figure 34–28). The client is closely monitored for ability to tolerate the switch, using frequent assessment of vital signs and arterial blood gas results. An initial rise in respiratory rate, pulse, and blood pressure is expected. Oxygen saturation and P_{O_2} should remain within satisfactory limits. The endotracheal tube may be removed after the client has remained stable for several hours.

Clients who have been on ventilatory support for longer periods may require gradual withdrawal of the ventilator. In the *"wind sprint"* or *rest/exercise schedule* of weaning, the client is placed on the T-piece for short periods of time at first, 5 to 15 minutes, followed by a rest period of assist/control ventilation or IMV. The T-piece time is gradually increased, until full withdrawal of ventilator support is well tolerated and the client can be extubated.

Intermittent mandatory ventilation (IMV), synchronous IMV, and pressure-support ventilation (PSV) are very useful modes for weaning the client from mechanical ventilation. With IMV and SIMV, the set rate of mandatory breaths is gradually decreased, shifting the work of breathing back to the client. Higher rates may be used at night to provide respiratory muscle rest and facilitate

Table 34–12   Advantages and Disadvantages of Weaning Processes

Technique	Advantages	Disadvantages
T-piece trial	Does not require additional work of breathing to open ventilator demand valve.	There is no monitoring or ventilator alarms while client is on T-piece.
Continuous positive airway pressure (CPAP)	Client remains connected to ventilator circuits with alarms.	Additional work of breathing is required to open ventilator demand valve.
Intermittent mandatory ventilation (IMV)	Allows gradual transition from 100% mechanical to 100% spontaneous ventilation; may be better tolerated by less stable clients.	Additional work of breathing is required to open demand valve during spontaneous breaths; weaning rate may be slower.
Pressure support (PS)	Low levels of increased pressure decrease the work of spontaneous breathing; may be more comfortable for the client.	Tidal volumes may vary.

Note. Adapted from *Harrison's Principles of Internal Medicine* (12th ed.) by J. D. Wilson, E. Braunwald, K. J. Isselbacher, R. G. Petersdorf, J. B. Martin, A. S. Fauci, and R. K. Root, 1991, New York: McGraw-Hill.

sleep (Holloway, 1993). When the client is able to tolerate an IMV rate of 4 per minute, T-piece trial is initiated. If this is tolerated for 30 minutes, the client may be extubated. Continuous positive airway pressure (CPAP) is useful to help support the client during the initial period off ventilator and airway support.

Pressure support, which decreases the effort required by the client to initiate a spontaneous breath, is particularly useful for clients who have required long-term mechanical ventilation. Pressure support is used with IMV, gradually decreasing the rate of mandatory breaths.

Weaning methods are compared in Table 34–12. In all cases, the client's vital signs, respiratory rate, degree of dyspnea, blood gases, and clinical status are used to evaluate weaning and its progress.

For clients with a terminal illness or irreversible condition having a poor prognosis, terminal weaning may be requested by the client or family. *Terminal weaning* is the gradual withdrawal of mechanical ventilation from a client who is not expected to survive without assisted ventilation (Campbell, 1994). Unlike other instances of weaning, which are usually performed in the intensive care unit (ICU), the client is moved to a quiet medical-surgical room or even home prior to the initiation of terminal weaning. Family members are encouraged to stay with the client throughout the process. If possible, decisions about sedation and analgesia prior to and during the course of weaning are made with the client, as are decisions about hydration and nutritional support should the client survive after weaning. Ventilator support is gradually withdrawn using the same mechanisms described earlier (IMV, SIMV, PSV). Analgesia and sedation is administered to maintain comfort during weaning.

Other Therapies

In addition to respiratory support and efforts to prevent complications, attention must be paid to fluid and electrolyte status and adequate nutrition.

Mechanical ventilation increases the risk of sodium and water retention. As noted previously, positive-pressure ventilation decreases venous return to the heart, causing a reduced cardiac output. Renal perfusion is decreased, stimulating the renin-angiotensin-aldosterone system to retain sodium and water. A Swan-Ganz catheter is often placed to allow monitoring of pulmonary artery pressures and cardiac output. An arterial line permits repeated blood gas analysis and continuous arterial pressure monitoring. Serum electrolytes are drawn frequently, along with careful assessment of daily weight and intake and output.

While on mechanical ventilation, the client requires enteral or parenteral nutrition, because eating is not possible when an endotracheal tube is in place. An enteral feeding tube may be placed either through the nasal-esophageal route or percutaneously into the stomach or jejunum. For some clients, the jejunostomy is preferred to reduce the risk of regurgitation and aspiration.

Nursing Care

Clients in respiratory failure are generally clinically unstable and often critically ill. They need not only intensive medical care but also intensive nursing care. Obvious nursing care needs are those related to maintenance of ventilation and a patent airway. Perhaps less obvious, but no less critical, are nursing care needs related to preventing injury and managing anxiety.

Inability to Sustain Spontaneous Ventilation

The client with acute respiratory failure may become so fatigued from the work of breathing that it is not possible to maintain adequate ventilation. This is a concern not only prior to the initiation of mechanical ventilation, but also during attempts to wean the client off ventilatory support.

Nursing interventions with rationales follow:

- Assess and document respiratory rate and other vital signs every 15 to 30 minutes. *Frequent assessment is important to detect early signs of increasing respiratory distress and inability to sustain adequate breathing.*

- Assess the client for other signs of respiratory distress, including nasal flaring, use of accessory muscles, intercostal retractions, cyanosis, increasing restlessness, anxiety, or a decreased level of consciousness. *These signs may be apparent before vital sign changes are noted or become significant.*

- Monitor arterial blood gas results and pulse oximetry readings for evidence of improving or worsening respiratory status. Report changes promptly. *Close assessment of these values allows timely intervention as needed.*

- Administer oxygen as prescribed, monitoring the client's response. Observe closely for signs of respiratory depression, especially in the client with COPD. *Administration of oxygen may reduce the hypoxemic respiratory drive. In clients with chronic high P_{CO_2} levels, the respiratory center is depressed, and low oxygen levels may provide the only respiratory drive.*

- Place the client in Fowler's position. *Fowler's position improves lung ventilation and decreases the work of breathing.*

- Minimize activities and energy expenditures by assisting the client with care, spacing procedures and activities, and allowing uninterrupted rest periods. *Rest is vital to reduce oxygen and energy demands.*

- Avoid sedatives and respiratory depressant drugs. *These medications can further depress the respiratory drive, worsening respiratory failure.*

- Prepare for endotracheal intubation and mechanical ventilation:
  a. Obtain an intubation tray with a selection of sterile endotracheal tubes and laryngoscope with a variety of adult blades.
  b. Check laryngoscope lamp; replace battery pack or bulb as needed.
  c. Set up for endotracheal suction, keeping continuous suction head, container, tubing, sterile catheter and glove kits, and sterile normal saline at the bedside.
  d. Notify the respiratory therapy department to set up the ventilator in the client's room.

  e. Notify the radiology department that a portable chest X-ray will be needed on completion of the intubation procedure to verify correct placement of the endotracheal tube.

  The client with respiratory failure may be unable to sustain the work of breathing without mechanical assistance. Intubation and mechanical ventilation may need to be performed on an emergency basis.

- Explain the procedure and its purpose to the client, providing reassurance that this is a temporary measure to reduce the work of breathing and allow the client to rest. Tell the client that talking is not possible while the endotracheal tube is in place, and establish a means of communication. *Thorough explanation is important to relieve the client's anxiety.*

Ineffective Airway Clearance

With acute respiratory failure, ineffective airway clearance may be either a cause of the condition or a result of interventions. Impaired ventilation is one of the major factors leading to acute respiratory failure. The client with COPD who develops pneumonia or other respiratory infection or who is exposed to excess amounts of respiratory irritants is at particular risk. The thoracic trauma client is also at high risk for impaired airway patency as a result of pulmonary contusion and ineffective cough. Although an endotracheal tube or tracheostomy can be a life-saving intervention to open the airway, they also increase the risk of respiratory infection and ineffective secretion management.

Nursing interventions with rationales follow:

- Assess the client's respiratory status, including rate, ventilator settings, chest movement, and lung sounds frequently. *Placement of the client on a ventilator does not automatically ensure adequate oxygenation and ventilation.*

- Assess coordination of respiratory efforts with ventilator. Remember that with IMV, there will appear to be little coordination; be sure to count the client's respiratory rate, not that of the ventilator. *If the client is breathing too rapidly or "fighting" the respirator, sedation or voluntary muscle paralysis may be necessary to achieve an effective breathing pattern.*

- Monitor and assess oxygen saturations and ABGs. *These values provide indications of the effectiveness of mechanical ventilation.*

- Suction the client as needed to maintain a patent airway. Indicators for suctioning include crackles and rhonchi on auscultation, frequent coughing or setting off the high-pressure alarm, and increasing restlessness or anxiety. The procedure for endotracheal suctioning is outlined in Procedure 34–2. *Although clients with a tracheostomy are usually able to cough up secretions, the*

Procedure 34–2   Endotracheal Suctioning

SUPPLIES

- Functioning suction unit (wall unit or free-standing unit) with appropriate connecting tubing and connector at the client's bedside
- If the client does *not* have an in-line suction catheter:
  a. Sterile suction catheter and glove kit (separately if not available packaged together) with a 12 to 14 Fr thumb-control catheter
  b. Sterile normal saline to lubricate and clear catheter
- 3 to 5 mL of sterile normal saline suitable for instillation into the endotracheal tube to loosen secretions
- Personal protective devices as indicated: goggles, mask, gown

PREPROCEDURE

Explain the procedure and the reasons why it is being performed, being sure to tell the client that although suctioning is not painful, it is uncomfortable. While suction is being applied, the client will feel as though he or she is unable to breathe, but these periods will last only 10 seconds. Stress that suctioning allows the removal of secretions. Suctioning also stimulates coughing, which helps clear secretions from smaller airways that the catheter does not reach. Establish a means of communicating with the client; for example, tell the client to raise a finger or rapidly blink the eyes, if he or she is unable to tolerate suctioning.

PROCEDURE

1. Follow universal precautions.
2. Prepare the suction unit by turning it on and regulating it to no more than 120 to 140 mm Hg of suction.
3. Open sterile saline bottle, leaving the cap loosely in place.
4. Put on personal protective wear.
5. Disconnect the ventilator tubing from the endotracheal tube *briefly* while instilling 3 to 5 mL of sterile saline; if a port is available for instillation, use it instead.

With an In-Line Catheter

- Wearing exam gloves, attach the catheter to suction tubing.
- Adjust the oxygen percentage dial (FIO_2) to 100%; allow three breaths (See the research box on page 1484).
- Manipulating the catheter through the plastic shield (to maintain its sterility), insert the catheter without applying suction until resistance is met; apply suction while slowly withdrawing the catheter with a twirling motion.
- Suction for no longer than 10 seconds (count the seconds or watch the clock—the time passes more quickly than you think), then allow the client to rest for three to five breaths. Repeat the procedure as needed for a total of no more than three times.
- Remove the suction tubing from the catheter, clear the tubing, turn off the suction, and remove and discard gloves.

With a Separate Catheter-and-Glove Kit

- Open suction catheter/glove kit. Remove saline cup, and fill with sterile normal saline.
- Put on sterile gloves, and attach the catheter to suction tubing, keeping the dominant hand sterile; lubricate the catheter with sterile saline.

- Use the nondominant hand to adjust oxygen percentage dial (FIO_2) to 100%; allow three breaths.
- Using the nondominant hand, disconnect the ventilator tubing from the endotracheal tube; manipulating the suction catheter with the dominant (sterile) hand and the suction control valve with the nondominant (nonsterile) hand, insert the catheter, without applying suction, into the endotracheal tube until resistance is met. Then, apply suction while slowly withdrawing the catheter, using a twirling motion.
- Suction for no longer than 10 seconds. Reconnect the ventilator, and allow the client to rest for three to five breaths; clear the suction tubing with sterile saline.
- Repeat the above two steps as needed for a total of three times.
- Reconnect the ventilator tubing to the client's endotracheal tube.
- Clear the suction tubing, turn off suction, and remove the catheter, discarding it with the gloves.
6. Provide three additional breaths at 100% oxygen, then readjust it to the previous ordered level.
7. Note the color, quantity, consistency, and odor of sputum obtained.
8. Assess the client's lung sounds and tolerance of the procedure.
9. Wash hands.

POSTPROCEDURE

Document assessment findings before and after suctioning, along with the character of the sputum and the client's tolerance of the procedure. Report changes in sputum character, such as purulence or an odor that may indicate infection.

Applying Research to Nursing Practice: Endotracheal Suctioning

■ ■ ■

Although much research has been conducted on the effects of endotracheal suctioning on blood oxygen levels, no standard protocol for providing oxygen before endotracheal suctioning is used consistently from hospital to hospital. In one study, researchers investigated the effects of one oxygenation technique on a sample of critically ill adults requiring mechanical ventilation following traumatic or surgical injury (Lookinland & Appel, 1991). In this technique, clients received three breaths of 100% oxygen from the ventilator at a normal tidal volume. In these clients, arterial oxygen levels were maintained at presuctioning levels or higher throughout the procedure. By contrast, clients who did not receive preoxygenation experienced a drop in arterial oxygen levels that persisted for as long as 5 minutes.

Interestingly, pulse oximetry readings did not indicate the extent of the fall in arterial oxygen levels, whereas transcutaneous oxygen sensor readings correlated well with measured arterial blood gases (ABGs). Oxygen delivery at higher tidal volumes (hyperinflation) resulted in some complaints of dyspnea after suctioning and did not significantly change arterial oxygen levels.

Implications for Nursing
The technique used in this study involved delivering three breaths of 100% oxygen at the preset tidal volume on the ventilator prior to endotracheal suctioning. The time required is minimal, and no additional nurs-

ing assistance is needed, as with a bag technique. The benefits to the clients in preventing tissue hypoxia were significant.

The findings of the study suggest that in the absence of contraindicators, hyperoxygenation should be part of the standard endotracheal suctioning technique. Furthermore, transcutaneous oxygen measurement was shown to be an accurate indicator of blood oxygen levels and to be particularly advantageous because it provides a noninvasive means for monitoring blood gases. Eliminating unnecessary invasive procedures can significantly reduce the risk of infection in the critically ill client.

Critical Thinking in Client Care

1. The sample in this study consisted of critically ill adults who did not have preexisting lung disease. How might the results differ in the client with COPD?

2. How do pulse oximetry measurements differ from transcutaneous oxygen sensor measurements?

3. Why does the pulse oximetry reading for oxygen saturation not correlate well with arterial measurements of blood oxygen?

4. Develop a plan to teach your peers how to use the mechanical ventilator to hyperoxygenate the client prior to endotracheal suctioning.

---

length and diameter of endotracheal tubes makes this extremely difficult. Even with humidification, secretions often become thick and tenacious, which further inhibits their removal.

- Obtain a specimen for culture if the sputum appears purulent or develops an odor. *Culture is necessary to identify the presence of pathogens and guide antibiotic therapy.*

- Perform percussion, vibration, and postural drainage as ordered. *These techniques help loosen secretions and move them into larger airways, where they can be coughed up and suctioned out.*

- Use minimal occluding volume technique, minimal leak technique, or measured pressures of 20 to 25 mm Hg in the cuff of the endotracheal tube. To achieve the minimal occluding volume technique, inflate the cuff

just until no air leak is heard on auscultation during inspiration. For minimal leak technique, inflate the cuff as described for minimal occluding volume, then withdraw a small amount of air to allow a slight leak at maximal inspiration. *These techniques are used to minimize cuff pressure and reduce the risk of tracheal ischemia and damage.*

- Firmly secure endotracheal tube or tracheostomy tube. Provide adequate slack on ventilator tubing to prevent tension on endotracheal tube when turning, positioning, transferring, or getting the client out of bed. If necessary, loosely restrain the client's hands. *These measures are important to ensure proper placement of the endotracheal tube and prevent its inadvertent removal.*

- Assess the client's fluid balance, and maintain adequate hydration. *Adequate hydration helps liquefy secretions for easy removal.*

- Change the client's position frequently, using semi-Fowler's and Fowler's positions if tolerated. *Position changes facilitate ventilation of all lung areas and prevent atelectasis.*

Risk for Injury

Many factors increase the risk for injury in a client with acute respiratory failure. Hypoxemia and hypercapnia impair the client's level of consciousness and may lead to drowsiness and/or apprehension and agitation. Endotracheal intubation and mechanical ventilation carry risks of tracheal damage and trauma to the lungs. If neuromuscular blockade is being used, this is a significant risk for injury due to the client's inability to breathe spontaneously, communicate, and move.

Nursing interventions with rationales follow:

- Assess the client frequently, including a head-to-toe assessment in addition to a complete respiratory assessment. Pay particular attention to the following:
  a. Level of consciousness, orientation, and awareness
  b. Mucosa of the mouth and nose
  c. Respiratory status, including lung sounds, chest excursion, and ventilator pressures
  d. Cardiovascular status, including vital signs, skin color, capillary refill, and peripheral pulses
  e. Gastrointestinal status, including bowel sounds and the presence of occult blood in gastric secretions or feces
  f. Genitourinary status, including urine output
  g. Skin and extremities
  The client with acute respiratory failure is vulnerable to complications affecting many body systems. Frequent assessment is necessary for early identification and intervention.

- Do not bypass or turn off any ventilator alarms. *The intubated client is unable to communicate verbally and thus cannot call for help. If neuromuscular blockers have been administered, the client is also unable to breathe without ventilator support.*

- Report changes in the client's condition or response to mechanical ventilation, such as increasing air leak around the cuff and decreased breath sounds or chest movement. *These manifestations may indicate a complication of intubation and ventilation, such as tracheal necrosis, migration of the endotracheal tube into the right mainstem bronchus, pneumothorax, or atelectasis.*

- Turn and reposition the client frequently, taking care to stabilize the endotracheal tube during movement. *Frequent position changes help maintain tissue perfusion and prevent skin and tissue breakdown due to pressure.*

- Keep skin and linens clean, dry, and wrinkle-free. Lotion and massage pressure points frequently. *Because the client may not be able to perceive pain and pressure or move voluntarily, good skin care is mandatory.*

- Perform passive range-of-motion (ROM) exercises every 4 to 8 hours. *These exercises maintain joint flexibility and help prevent contractures associated with long-term immobility.*

- Keep side rails up and use soft restraints as needed. *These measures are important to prevent the client from falling out of bed, disconnecting the ventilator inadvertently, or pulling out the endotracheal tube.*

- Administer histamine H_2-blockers and antacids as ordered. *Stress gastritis and possible gastrointestinal hemorrhage are common, preventable complications of mechanical ventilation.*

Anxiety

Critical illness creates anxiety for any client. In the client with acute respiratory failure, this anxiety is compounded by the presence of an endotracheal tube or tracheostomy, mechanical ventilator, numerous monitors and equipment, and, potentially, neuromuscular blockade and paralysis of voluntary muscles. Additionally, the client may fear that he or she will always be dependent on the mechanical ventilator and unable to return to a normal life.

Nursing interventions with rationales follow:

- Monitor the client's level of anxiety frequently. *High levels of anxiety increase the use of oxygen and often interfere with the client's ability to work with the respirator. This can lead to increased hypoxemia and increased anxiety; intervention is necessary to break this cycle.*

- Stay with the client as much as possible. *The frequent presence of a caregiver provides reassurance that help is readily available.*

- Explain all monitors, procedures, unusual sounds, and machinery. *The client will be less anxious when he or she understands the purpose of items in the environment and the meaning of beeps, buzzers, and alarms.*

- Provide a simple means of communication for the client who is intubated, such as a slate, picture board, or alphabet board. For the client who is under the effects of neuromuscular blockade, use methods such as looking to the right for "yes" and left for "no." Reassure the client that the ability to speak will return once the endotracheal tube is removed. *The inability to speak and call out for help is frightening to the client. Providing an alternate means of communication helps reduce anxiety.*

- Encourage family visits as often as possible, especially if the time of visitations must be limited. Encourage the family to participate in care as much as possible. *Family visits help reduce the client's anxiety and feelings of abandonment. Allowing family members to participate in providing care helps reduce their anxiety as well as the client's.*

- Provide distraction with radio or television if allowed. *Distraction helps reduce the client's focus on machines and unusual sounds of monitors and alarms.*

- Attend to the client's physical needs promptly and completely. *This provides reassurance that needs will be met even though he or she is unable to ask for assistance.*

- Reassure the client that intubation and mechanical ventilation is a temporary measure to allow the lungs to rest and heal and that he or she will be able to breathe independently again. *The client may fear continued dependence on mechanical ventilation.*

- Provide sedation and antianxiety medications as needed, especially for the client with neuromuscular blockade. *Although neuromuscular blockade induces paralysis of the voluntary muscles, level of consciousness is unimpaired.*

Other Nursing Diagnoses

Although the needs of clients differ greatly, especially in critical illness, the following nursing diagnoses may be applicable for the client with acute respiratory failure:

- *Risk for Aspiration* related to presence of an endotracheal tube

- *Impaired Gas Exchange* related to underlying disease process

- *Powerlessness* related to inability to control environment

- *Impaired Verbal Communication* related to presence of endotracheal tube or tracheostomy

- *Risk for Suffocation* related to dependence on mechanical ventilation

- *Impaired Physical Mobility* related to the presence of multiple tubes, wires, and monitors

- *Self-Care Deficit: Total* related to critical illness

- *Risk for Impaired Skin Integrity* related to difficulty repositioning

Client and Family Teaching

For clients experiencing respiratory failure and their families, the teaching focuses primarily on the acute period. Provide explanations for all procedures, monitors, tubes, machines, and alarms. Explain all care with which they may not be familiar, such as suctioning and other respiratory hygiene measures. Teach the client alternative communication strategies. Explain to the family that although the client cannot speak and may not be able to respond, he or she can hear and understand. Emphasize the importance of talking to the client, not over or about the client. Encourage family members to talk about everyday things to help the client feel included and less isolated from his or her normal world. Explain that intubation and

Table 34–13	Conditions Associated with the Development of ARDS
Conditions	**Examples**
Shock	Hemorrhagic shock, septic shock
Inhalation injuries	Aspiration of gastric contents, smoke and toxic gases, near-drowning, oxygen toxicity
Infections	Gram-negative sepsis, viral pneumonias, *Pneumocystis cariniii* pneumonia, miliary tuberculosis
Drug overdose	Heroin, methadone, propoxyphene, aspirin
Trauma	Burns, head injury, lung contusion, fat emboli
Other	Disseminated intravascular coagulation (DIC), pancreatitis, uremia, amniotic fluid and air emboli, multiple transfusions, open heart surgery with cardiopulmonary bypass

mechanical ventilation is a temporary measure, and provide reassurance that the client will, in nearly all cases, be able to resume spontaneous breathing.

Prior to hospital discharge, teach the client about factors that precipitated respiratory failure and measures to prevent it in the future. The client with COPD needs to understand the impact of respiratory irritants on compromised lungs and be able to identify measures to prevent exposure to them. These measures may include remaining indoors with an air filter or air conditioning when pollution levels are high, obtaining influenza and pneumonia immunizations, and avoiding exposure to cigarette smoke. Teach effective coughing and pulmonary hygiene measures such as percussion, vibration, and postural drainage.

Clients who experience acute respiratory failure as a result of an acute insult such as pneumonia or near drowning often recover with few long-term sequelae. When COPD is the underlying disease precipitating respiratory failure, the prognosis is less optimistic. Clients with end-stage COPD may experience several episodes of acute respiratory failure, with a gradual loss of respiratory function and reserve. These clients may choose terminal weaning rather than face a future of further disability. Teach the client and family what to expect during the terminal weaning process. Discuss the use of sedation prior to and during the weaning process. Explain that medications will be used to reduce respiratory distress and dysp-

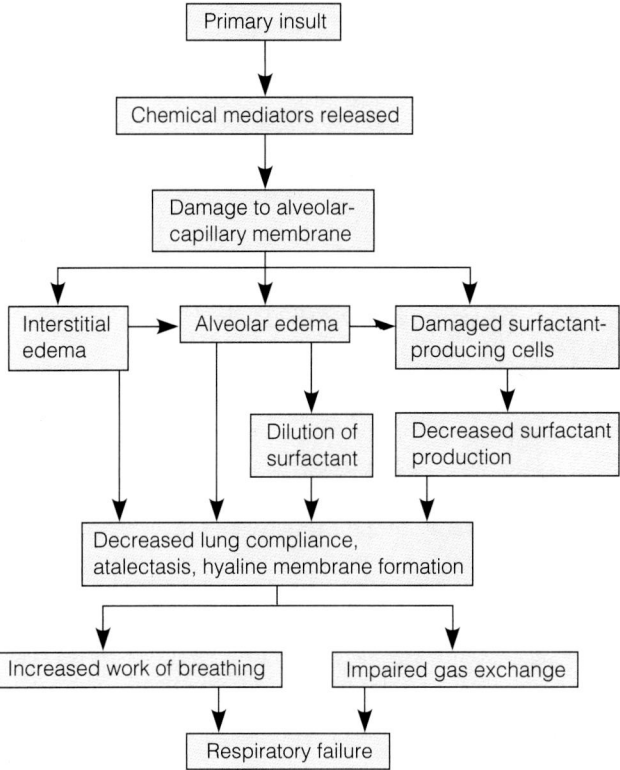

Figure 34–29   The pathogenesis of ARDS.

nea during weaning. Assure the client and family members that nursing support will be available continuously during the weaning process and that family and other support people such as clergy will be allowed to remain with the client.

The Client with Adult Respiratory Distress Syndrome (ARDS)

■ ■ ■

Adult respiratory distress syndrome, commonly known as **ARDS,** is characterized by noncardiac pulmonary edema and progressive refractory hypoxemia. First identified in 1967, ARDS has been known by various names, such as *shock lung, wet lung, Vietnam lung,* and *adult hyaline membrane disease.* It has become widely recognized as a severe form of acute respiratory failure that can follow a number of primary insults to the body. The mortality rate associated with Adult Respiratory Distress Syndrome remains greater than 50%, despite aggressive therapy (Steinberg, 1993).

Pathophysiology

Although the exact etiologic origin of ARDS is still unclear, it is clear that ARDS does not occur as a primary process but may follow a number of diverse conditions producing direct or indirect lung injury (see Table 34–13).

The underlying pathologic condition in ARDS is alveolar-capillary membrane damage (Figure 34–29). The figure on pages 1488 and 1489 illustrates the pathophysiology of ARDS. In many instances, it appears that chemical mediators released after acute injury, insult, or infection damage the microcapillaries of the pulmonary vascular system, initiating the process. The damaged capillary membranes allow plasma and blood cells to escape into the interstitial space. Increased interstitial pressure and damage to the alveolar membrane cause fluid to enter the alveoli. Within the alveolus, surfactant is diluted and inactivated by the fluid. In addition, surfactant-producing cells are damaged, leading to a deficit of surfactant, increased alveolar surface tension, and alveolar collapse with atelectasis. The lungs become less compliant, and gas exchange is impaired. As the syndrome progresses, hyaline membranes form, further reducing gas exchange and compliance. Finally, fibrotic changes occur in the lungs. Intra-alveolar septa thicken, and alveolar surface area for gas exchange is reduced. Hypoxemia becomes refractory or resistant to improvement with supplemental oxygen, and the P_{CO_2} rises as diffusion is further impaired.

The clinical manifestations of ARDS typically appear 24 to 48 hours after the initial insult. Dyspnea and tachypnea are the initial manifestations. The client demonstrates progressive respiratory distress with an increasing respiratory rate, intercostal retractions, and use of the accessory muscles of respiration. Cyanosis may be present and may not improve with oxygen administration (Berkow & Fletcher, 1992). Breath sounds are initially clear, but crackles (rales) and rhonchi develop later. As respiratory failure progresses, the client may become agitated and confused or lethargic.

For clients who survive ARDS, the long-term prognosis for recovery is good. However, as ARDS progresses, tissue hypoxia becomes significant, and metabolic acidosis develops. Carbon dioxide exchange is impaired as well as oxygen exchange, leading to a combined respiratory and metabolic acidosis. Sepsis and multiple organ system failure involving the kidneys, liver, gastrointestinal tract, central nervous system, and cardiovascular system are the leading causes of death in clients with ARDS.

Collaborative Care

The management of ARDS is directed toward identifying and treating the underlying cause of the syndrome. While the primary disorder is being treated, aggressive respiratory support must be provided to compensate for ARDS.

Adult Respiratory Distress Syndrome

Adult respiratory distress syndrome (ARDS) is a severe form of acute respiratory failure that occurs in response to pulmonary or systemic insults. ARDS is characterized by non-cardiogenic pulmonary edema caused by conditions that damage alveolar and capillary walls. Many disorders may result in ARDS.

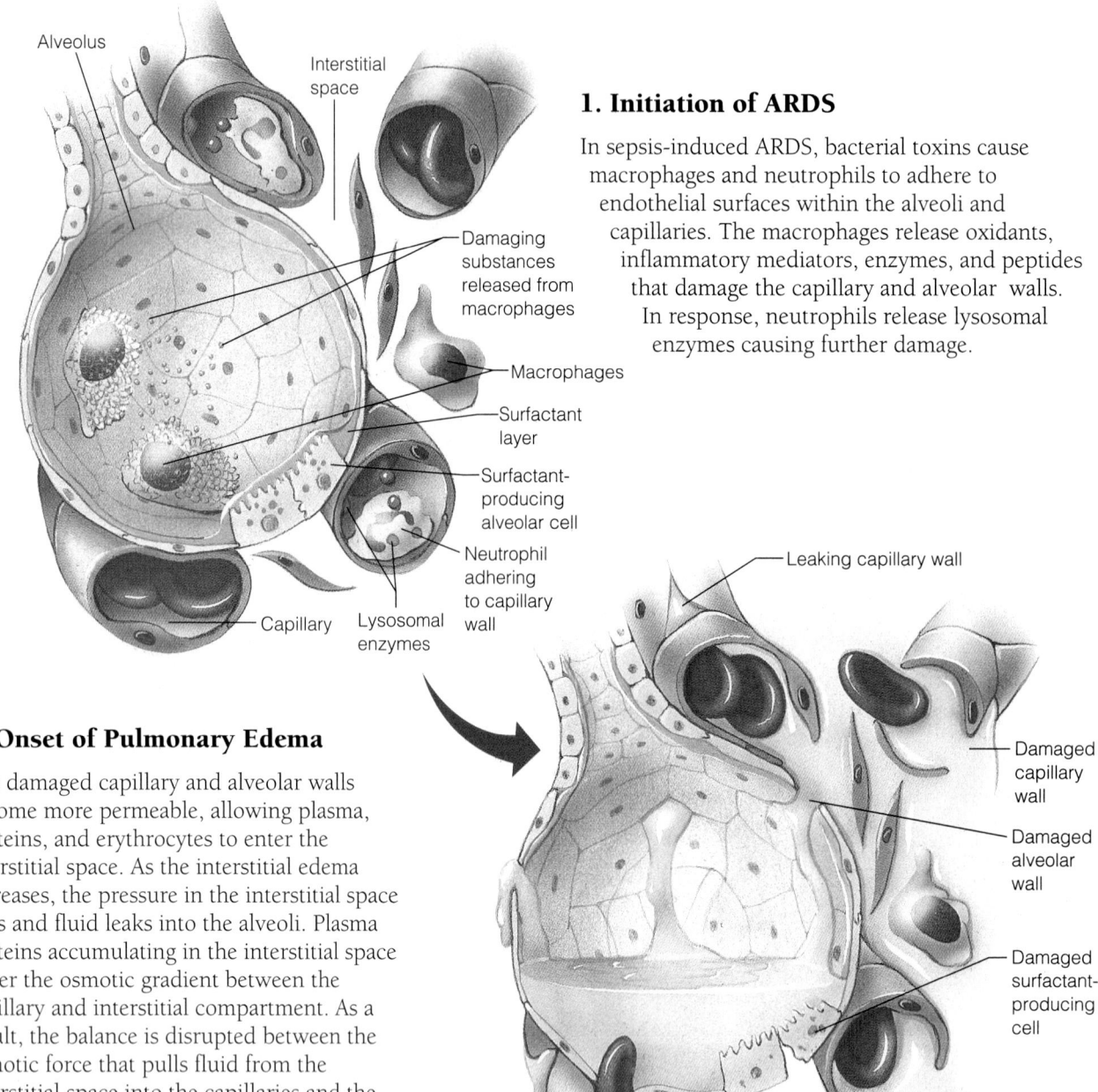

Alveolus

Interstitial space

Damaging substances released from macrophages

Macrophages

Surfactant layer

Surfactant-producing alveolar cell

Neutrophil adhering to capillary wall

Capillary

Lysosomal enzymes

Leaking capillary wall

Damaged capillary wall

Damaged alveolar wall

Damaged surfactant-producing cell

1. Initiation of ARDS

In sepsis-induced ARDS, bacterial toxins cause macrophages and neutrophils to adhere to endothelial surfaces within the alveoli and capillaries. The macrophages release oxidants, inflammatory mediators, enzymes, and peptides that damage the capillary and alveolar walls. In response, neutrophils release lysosomal enzymes causing further damage.

2. Onset of Pulmonary Edema

The damaged capillary and alveolar walls become more permeable, allowing plasma, proteins, and erythrocytes to enter the interstitial space. As the interstitial edema increases, the pressure in the interstitial space rises and fluid leaks into the alveoli. Plasma proteins accumulating in the interstitial space lower the osmotic gradient between the capillary and interstitial compartment. As a result, the balance is disrupted between the osmotic force that pulls fluid from the interstitial space into the capillaries and the normal hydrostatic pressure that pushes fluid out of the capillaries. This imbalance causes even more fluid to enter the alveoli.

4. End-Stage ARDS

Fibrin and cell debris from necrotic cells combine to form hyaline membranes, which line the interior of the alveoli and further reduce alveolar compliance and gas exchange. Because CO_2 cannot diffuse across hyaline membranes, PCO_2 levels now begin to rise while PO_2 levels continue to fall. Rising PCO_2 levels can lead to respiratory acidosis. Without respiratory support, the client will develop respiratory failure. Even with aggressive treatment, almost 50% of clients with ARDS die.

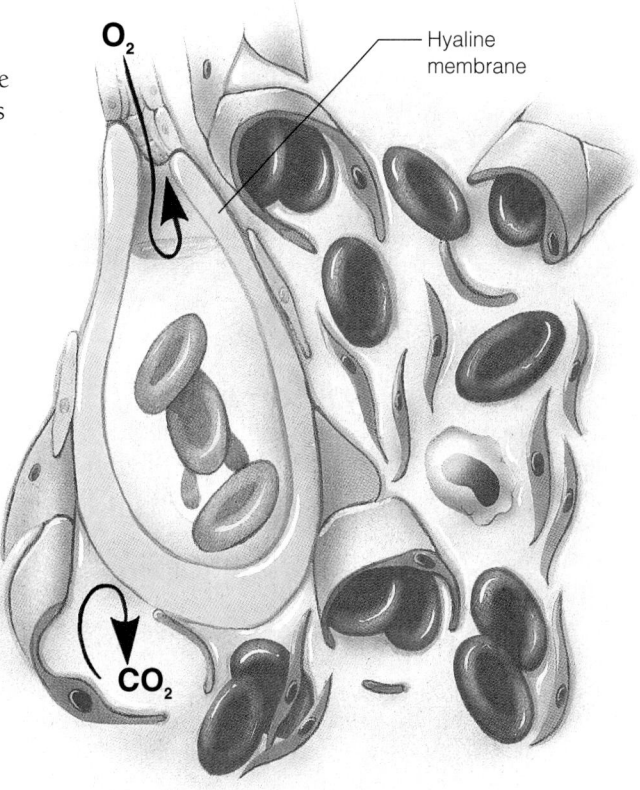

O_2

Hyaline membrane

CO_2

O_2

CO_2

3. Alveolar Collapse

Protein-rich fluid accumulates in the alveoli, inactivating surfactant and damaging type II alveolar cells that produce surfactant. (Surfactant is important in maintaining alveolar compliance—the ability of tissue to stretch or distend.) As active surfactant is lost, the alveoli stiffen and collapse, leading to atelectasis, which increases breathing effort.

Decreased alveolar compliance, atelectasis, and fluid-filled alveoli interfere with gas exchange across the alveolar-capillary membrane. Blood oxygen (PO_2) levels fall. Because carbon dioxide diffuses more readily than oxygen, however, blood carbon dioxide (PCO_2) levels also fall initially as the increased respiratory rate causes more CO_2 to be expired.

1489

Laboratory and Diagnostic Tests

The hallmark of ARDS is refractory hypoxemia, that is, hypoxemia that does not improve with the administration of oxygen therapy. Arterial blood gases initially reveal hypoxemia with a PO_2 of less than 50 mm Hg and respiratory alkalosis due to the rapid respiratory rate. Large amounts of albumin may be present in the sputum late in the course of the disease.

Changes in the chest X-ray often are not apparent for as much as 24 hours after the onset of symptoms of ARDS. Diffuse infiltrates are seen initially, progressing to a "white out" pattern. The heart size is normal, a finding that helps rule out cardiogenic pulmonary edema. Pulmonary function testing shows decreased lung compliance with reduced vital capacity, minute volume, and functional vital capacity (see the box on page 1424).

Pulmonary arterial pressure monitoring with a Swan-Ganz line shows normal pressures in ARDS, helping to distinguish ARDS from cardiogenic pulmonary edema.

Pharmacology

Surfactant therapy is the newest line of defense against ARDS. However, it is still in the research stage at this time and not in widespread use. Surfactant is a complex mixture of phospholipids, neutral lipids, and proteins. In normal lungs, it is produced constantly; an estimated 10% to 30% of the intra-alveolar surfactant pool is replaced every hour (Steinberg, 1993). This surfactant forms a thin layer atop a thin layer of water on the inner surface of the alveolus, reducing the surface tension within the alveoli. Surface tension tends to pull the walls of the alveoli together, increasing the likelihood of collapse during exhalation. Surfactant, by reducing the surface tension, helps maintain open alveoli, decreasing the work of breathing, improving compliance and gas exchange, and preventing atelectasis.

Natural surfactants from calf lungs (Survanta, beractant) and pig lungs (Curosurf) and artificial surfactants made of phospholipids (Exosurf) or phospholipids with recombinant protein are both being tested for use in clients with ARDS. Limited studies have demonstrated improved oxygenation with lower FIO_2 and an apparent improvement in mortality rate when aerosolized surfactant is administered to clients with ARDS (Steinberg, 1993). Still an experimental treatment for ARDS, surfactant therapy holds promise for the future.

Mechanical Ventilation

The mainstay of ARDS management is endotracheal intubation and mechanical ventilation. With ARDS, it is rarely, if ever, possible to maintain adequate tissue oxygenation with the administration of oxygen therapy alone.

With mechanical ventilation, the FIO_2 is set at the lowest possible level that will maintain a PO_2 of greater than 60 mm Hg and oxygen saturation of approximately 90%.

When the PO_2 cannot be maintained with inspired oxygen levels of 50% or less, there is a risk that oxygen toxicity will accentuate the ARDS process. Often it is necessary to add continuous positive airway pressure (CPAP) or positive end-expiratory pressure (PEEP) to mechanical ventilation settings to maintain adequate blood and tissue oxygenation. By maintaining open airways and alveoli, gas diffusion is enhanced and the ventilation-perfusion mismatch reduced. PEEP is associated with decreased cardiac output and an increased risk of pulmonary barotrauma, necessitating close monitoring of the client. Either the assist-control or IMV modes of ventilation may be used along with PEEP or CPAP in treating the client with ARDS.

It is important to remember that mechanical ventilation does not cure ARDS; it is simply a means of providing respiratory support while the underlying problem is being identified and treated.

Other Therapies

In addition to surfactant therapy and mechanical ventilation, care of the client with ARDS includes careful fluid replacement, attention to nutrition, treatment of any infection, and treatment of the underlying condition. A Swan-Ganz line is placed to monitor pulmonary artery pressures and cardiac output. Fluid replacement is carefully tailored to these measurements to avoid either hypovolemia or fluid overload, which may worsen hypoxia and ARDS. Enteral or parenteral feeding is necessary to maintain the client's nutritional status and prevent tissue catabolism. Intravenous antibiotic therapy is instituted, using preparations specific to the organism implicated in infection or sepsis. Heparin may be used to prevent thrombophlebitis and possible pulmonary embolus or to prevent or treat disseminated intravascular coagulation (DIC), a possible complication of ARDS.

Nursing Care

The client with ARDS has nursing care needs that are very similar to those of any client with acute respiratory failure. Maintaining adequate ventilation and respirations are of highest priority, along with preventing injury and managing anxiety. Refer to the section on acute respiratory failure for nursing care related to these diagnoses. Additional high-priority nursing care concerns for the client with ARDS are related to the effect of PEEP on cardiac output and potential problems of weaning the client off ventilatory support.

Decreased Cardiac Output

With positive pressure ventilation, cardiac output is decreased because of increased intrathoracic pressure. When PEEP is applied, the additional increase in intrathoracic pressure can significantly decrease venous return to the heart, ventricular filling, stroke volume, and cardiac output. Clinically, the client demonstrates a decrease in arterial pressure and a compensatory tachycardia as the heart attempts to compensate for the decreased stroke volume by increasing its rate. In the client who is already hypoxic because of ARDS, this drop in cardiac output can increase tissue damage. Urine output falls, and dysrhythmias may develop (Kidd & Wagner, 1992).

Nursing interventions with rationales follow:

- Monitor and record vital signs, including blood pressure and apical pulse, at least every 2 hours; assess the client more frequently immediately following initiation of mechanical ventilation or the addition of PEEP. Correlate measurements with baseline vital signs. *Frequent assessment is vital to detect early evidence of decreased cardiac output.*

- Measure and record urinary output hourly. *Because a significant portion of the cardiac output goes directly to the kidneys, a drop in urine output to less than 30 mL per hour is often the first sign of decreased cardiac output.*

- Assess the client's level of consciousness every 4 hours or more frequently. *Altered level of consciousness, confusion, and restlessness are early signs of cerebral hypoxia due to decreased cardiac output.*

- Monitor pulmonary artery pressures, central venous pressure, and cardiac output readings frequently, every 1 to 4 hours. *Changes in these measurements may indicate worsening cardiac status.*

- Assess heart and lung sounds frequently. *Increasing crackles or abnormal heart sounds may indicate heart failure.*

- Weigh the client daily at the same time. *Daily weight provides the best indicator of fluid status and is necessary to detect fluid retention.*

- Provide good skin care frequently, keeping the skin clean and dry and massaging pressure points. *Tissue hypoxia increases the risk of skin breakdown, which in turn increases the risk of infection and sepsis.*

- Maintain intravenous fluids as ordered. *Intravenous fluids are administered to maintain adequate vascular volume and prevent dehydration.*

- Administer analgesics, sedatives, and neuromuscular blockers as needed. *These medications may be prescribed to decrease the cardiac workload.*

Dysfunctional Ventilatory Weaning Response

The client with dysfunctional ventilatory weaning response has difficulty adjusting to lower levels of mechanical ventilator support, prolonging the weaning process. Airway congestion, inadequate rest or nutrition, pain, anxiety, and a nonsupportive environment are some of the factors that may contribute to difficulty weaning (Lederer et al., 1993). With ARDS, the pathologic processes of the disease and the severity of the impairment in gas ex-

change may be responsible for a prolonged or ineffective weaning process.

The following assessment findings indicate dysfunctional weaning (Lederer et al., 1993; Sparks & Taylor, 1993):

- Dyspnea
- Apprehension or agitation
- Changes in skin color, including cyanosis or pallor
- Diminished or adventitious breath sounds
- Increased blood pressure, pulse, and respiratory rate
- Use of accessory muscles
- Decreased level of consciousness
- Deteriorating arterial blood gas values
- Diaphoresis
- Shallow, gasping breaths or paradoxic abdominal breathing

Nursing interventions with rationales follow:

- Monitor and record vital signs every 15 to 60 minutes following changes in ventilator settings and during T-piece trials. *The vital signs may provide early signs of hypoxemia and poor tolerance of the weaning process.*

- Monitor arterial blood gas levels and pulse oximetry readings when the ventilator settings are changed. *These measurements are used to assess the adequacy of oxygenation.*

- Prior to changing ventilator settings, auscultate lung sounds, and hyperoxygenate and suction as needed. *Airway obstruction by mucus can significantly impair alveolar ventilation and impair weaning.*

- Place the client in Fowler's position. *Fowler's position facilitates lung expansion and reduces the work of breathing.*

- Fully explain all weaning procedures to the client, along with expected changes in the breathing sensation. *Adequate explanations help reduce anxiety and improve the client's ability to cooperate.*

- Remain with the client during initial periods following changes of ventilator settings or T-piece trials. *This provides reassurance and allows close monitoring of the client's response.*

- Limit procedures and activities during weaning periods. *The weaning process is facilitated by reducing energy expenditures for other activities.*

- Provide diversion, such as television or radio. *Diversional activities help distract the client's focus from breathing.*

- Start weaning procedures in the morning, when the client is well rested and alert; weaning may be discontinued overnight to provide for adequate rest. *The work of breathing is increased for the client during the weaning process; adequate rest is important.*

- When IMV is used for weaning, decrease the IMV rate by increments of 2 breaths per minute. *Slow reduction of ventilator support allows the client to gradually resume the work of breathing (Sparks & Taylor, 1993).*

- Avoid administering drugs that may depress respirations during the weaning process (except as ordered at night to facilitate rest while the client is on ventilator support). *Administration of sedatives or analgesics that depress respirations can put the client at risk for inadequate respirations during the weaning process.*

- Once the client has been weaned from the ventilator and the endotracheal tube removed, keep oxygen available at the bedside. *The client may continue to need supplemental oxygen to maintain adequate oxygen saturation and to meet tissue demands.*

- Provide pulmonary hygiene with percussion, vibration, and postural drainage. *Maintaining patent airways and adequate alveolar ventilation is vital for the client during the weaning process.*

- Continue to assess the client's respiratory status, including lung sounds, vital signs, level of consciousness, or complaints of dyspnea. *These assessments are important to detect deteriorating respiratory status.*

Other Nursing Diagnoses

The following nursing diagnoses may also be appropriate for the client with ARDS:

- *Ineffective Breathing Pattern* related to decreased lung compliance

- *Risk for Infection* related to invasive monitors and tubes

- *Ineffective Individual Coping* related to critical illness

- *Altered Tissue Perfusion: Cardiopulmonary* related to damaged alveolar-capillary membrane

- *Impaired Verbal Communication* related to endotracheal intubation

- *Sleep Pattern Disturbance* related to placement in critical care unit

Client and Family Teaching

As with acute respiratory failure, teaching for the client with ARDS focuses on the acute illness period. Explain all procedures, tubes, equipment, and therapeutic interventions to the client and the family as indicated. Reassure the client that endotracheal intubation and mechanical ventilation are temporary measures to support the client's lungs and respiratory function during the acute phase of the syndrome. Explain to the client and family that ARDS is not the result of something they did or did not do, but a consequence of serious illness. Provide factual information about ARDS and its prognosis, being careful to be realistic without being overly optimistic or pessimistic. Reassure the family that clients who survive the initial insult of ARDS generally recover without significant long-term adverse effects, although the recovery period to regain previous respiratory function may be prolonged. If the client has been a smoker, stress the importance of avoiding cigarette smoking in the future to preserve lung function.

Applying the Nursing Process

Case Study of a Client with ARDS: Peggy Adamson

Peggy Adamson is a 36-year-old single woman who works as a features editor for a sports magazine. Peggy is admitted to the hospital following a water-skiing accident and near-drowning in a local lake. On admission to the emergency department, Ms. Adamson is alert and oriented, having been rescued from the lake and resuscitated within 2 minutes of the accident. Rescuers report that she seems to have aspirated a significant amount of water. She is placed in the intensive care unit for observation. Oxygen is started per nasal cannula at 6 liters per minute, an intravenous infusion is initiated to correct electrolyte imbalances, and 40 mg of furosemide (Lasix) is administered intravenously for hypervolemia.

Assessment

Nadia Mucha is assigned to care for Ms. Adamson on the evening shift the day after her admission. Throughout her stay, Ms. Adamson has remained alert and oriented with stable vital signs. Her respiratory rate has been running at 20 to 24 per minute, with scattered crackles and oxygen saturation levels of around 94% and a PO_2 of 75 to 80 mm Hg on 6 L/min of oxygen. Her pulse has been 96 to 100 and regular. When Ms. Mucha does her initial assessment, she notes that Ms. Adamson seems apprehensive and anxious. Although her blood pressure is 116/74, unchanged from previous levels, her heart rate is up to 106 and respiratory rate up to 28 per minute. Her lungs have scattered crackles but good breath sounds throughout, unchanged from previous assessments. Ms. Adamson's oxygen saturation has fallen to 84%, so Ms. Mucha orders arterial blood gases to be drawn and increases the oxygen flow rate to 8 L/min. ABG results show a fall in PO_2 to 65 mm Hg, respiratory alkalosis with a pH of 7.48, and PCO_2 of 32 mm Hg.

Ms. Mucha orders a portable chest X-ray and notifies the physician of the arterial blood gas results and the change in Ms. Adamson's status. The physician orders a nonrebreather mask at flow of 8 L/min and ABG measurements to be repeated in 1 hour. The chest X-ray reveals scattered infiltrates and a normal heart size.

With Ms. Adamson on the rebreather mask, oxygen saturations continue to fall, and subsequent blood gases show a PO_2 of 55 mm Hg. The attending physician makes the diagnosis of probable ARDS and initiates procedures to insert a nasoendotracheal tube and place Ms. Adamson on mechanical ventilation.

Diagnosis

Ms. Mucha identifies the following nursing diagnoses for Ms. Adamson:

- *Ineffective Breathing Pattern* related to anxiety
- *Impaired Gas Exchange* related to effects of near-drowning
- *Anxiety* related to hypoxemia
- *Risk for Decreased Cardiac Output* related to mechanical ventilation
- *Risk for Injury* related to endotracheal intubation
- *Knowledge Deficit* about ARDS and respiratory care procedures

Expected Outcomes

As outcomes for the plan of care, Ms. Mucha indicates that Ms. Adamson will:

- Breathe effectively with the mechanical ventilator.
- Demonstrate improvement in arterial blood gases and oxygen saturations.
- Express her fears related to intubation and mechanical ventilation.
- Demonstrate reduced levels of anxiety (relaxed facial expression, ability to rest between procedures).
- Maintain adequate cardiac output and tissue perfusion.
- Tolerate endotracheal intubation and mechanical ventilation without evidence of infection or barotrauma.
- Demonstrate an understanding of ARDS and necessary procedures by cooperating with these procedures.

Planning and Implementation

Ms. Mucha plans and begins to implement the following nursing interventions:

- Prepare for endotracheal intubation and mechanical ventilation, notifying other departments as needed and obtaining all necessary supplies.
- Explain the purpose and procedure of intubation to Ms. Adamson, providing reassurance.
- Discuss means of communication while Ms. Adamson is intubated; obtain a magic slate.
- Administer analgesics and/or sedatives as ordered.
- Monitor oxygen saturation levels every 30 to 60 minutes initially after institution of mechanical ventilation; report changes to the physician.
- Obtain arterial blood gases as prescribed or indicated; monitor and report results.
- Suction via endotracheal tube as needed to maintain good breath sounds.

- Provide an opportunity for Ms. Adamson to express her fears related to intubation and mechanical ventilation prior to the procedure.
- Explain all activities and procedures fully.
- Schedule activities to allow periods of uninterrupted rest.
- Monitor vital signs every 1 to 2 hours.
- Perform quick physical assessment, noting skin color, capillary refill, and the presence of edema every 4 hours.
- Monitor urine output hourly; report output of less than 30 mL per hour.
- Change position at least every 1.5 to 2 hours; apply lotion to and massage bony prominences.
- Assess lung sounds and chest excursion every 1 to 2 hours.
- Ensure strict aseptic technique in suctioning and respiratory care.

Evaluation

Ms. Adamson is intubated and placed on a volume-cycled ventilator at 50% FIO_2 and a tidal volume of 1000 mL in the assist-control mode at 16 breaths per minute. She has difficulty working with the ventilator initially, so 50 units of tubocurarine chloride (Tubarine) is administered intravenously to induce voluntary muscle motor paralysis. Ms. Mucha administers 10 mg of intravenous morphine sulfate along with the tubocurarine to help reduce Ms. Adamson's anxiety. Ms. Adamson's oxygen saturations and arterial blood gas results do not begin to improve until 10 mm Hg of PEEP is added to the ventilator settings. After 3 days of mechanical ventilation with PEEP and aggressive fluid and diuretic therapy, Ms. Adamson begins to show improvement. She is placed on IMV, and over the course of another 3 days she is gradually weaned off the ventilator to a face mask with CPAP. She eventually recovers fully, with no apparent long-term effects of her near drowning and ARDS episode.

Critical Thinking in the Nursing Process

1. Endotracheal intubation and mechanical ventilation were effective in supporting Ms. Adamson's respiratory status as she recovered from ARDS. Discuss the possible sequence of events had her lungs continued to deteriorate and it had not been possible to wean her from the ventilator.

2. How might the presentation and management of an acute episode of respiratory failure due to ARDS differ from respiratory failure related to COPD?

3. What measures can nurses take to prevent the development of ARDS?

4. Develop a nursing care plan for Ms. Adamson for the nursing diagnosis *Powerlessness* related to endotracheal intubation and mechanical ventilation.

Bibliography

■ ■ ■

Adler, J. J. (1993). Tuberculosis: An epidemic reemerges, 3. Modern problems in TB management. *Emergency Medicine, 25*(2), 169–70, 174–75, 179.

Aldrich, J. (1994). Pulmonary edema: Preventing respiratory arrest. *Nursing94, 24*(10), 33.

American Association for Respiratory Care. (1992). Consensus statement of the essentials of mechanical ventilators—1992. *Respiratory Care, 37*(9), 1000–1008.

American Journal of Nursing. (1994). New drugs: For asthma, a twice-a-day inhaled bronchodilator. *94*(5), 63–64.

Andreoli, T. E., Carpenter, C. C. J., Plum, F., & Smith, L. H., Jr. (1990). *Cecil Essentials of medicine* (2nd ed.). Philadelphia: W. B. Saunders.

Andrews, L. (1994). Medical management of pulmonary emboli. *MEDSURG Nursing, 3*(1), 31–35.

Ashworth, L. J. (1990). Pressure support ventilation. *Critical Care Nurse, 10*(7), 20–22, 24–25.

Bartlett, J. G. (1991). *Pocketbook of infectious disease therapy.* Baltimore, MD: Williams & Wilkins.

Berkow, R., & Fletcher, A. J. (Eds.). (1992). *The Merck manual of diagnosis and therapy* (16th ed.). Rahway, NJ: Merck Sharp & Dohme Research Laboratories.

Bolton, P. (1994). Understanding modes of mechanical ventilation. *American Journal of Nursing, 94*(6), 36–42.

Bone, R. C. (1992). Pulmonary embolism: New approaches to a complex problem. *Emergency Medicine, 24*(14), 144–146, 149–152.

Branson, R. D., & Chatburn, R. L. (1992). Technical description and classification of modes of ventilator operation. *Respiratory Care, 37*(9), 1026–1044.

Bullock, B. L., & Rosendahl, P. P. (1992). *Pathophysiology: Adaptations and alterations in function* (3rd ed.). Philadelphia: Lippincott.

Campbell, M. L. (1994). Terminal weaning. *Nursing94, 24*(9), 34–38.

Carroll, P. (1994). Safe suctioning prn. *RN, 57*(5), 32–36.

Centers for Disease Control and Prevention (1993a). Advance report of final mortality statistics, 1991. *Monthly Vital Statistics Report, 42*(2, Supplement).

Centers for Disease Control and Prevention (1993b). Draft guidelines for preventing the transmission of tuberculosis in health-care facilities (2nd ed.). *Federal Register, 58*(195).

Centers for Disease Control and Prevention (1994, February 2). Draft guidelines for prevention of nosocomial pneumonia. *Federal Register, 59*(22).

Chernecky, C. C., Krech, R. L., & Berger, B. J. (1993). *Laboratory tests and diagnostic procedures.* Philadelphia: W. B. Saunders.

Dabbs, A. D. & Olslund, L. (1994). The new alternatives to intubation. *American Journal of Nursing, 94*(8), 42–45.

Davidson, P. T., DiFerdinando, G. T., Jr., Reichman, L. B., & Snider, D. E. (1992). TB: Coming soon to your town? *Patient Care, 26*(9), 40–44, 46, 51–52, 55–58, 61ff.

DiFerdinando, G. T., Jr. (1993). Tuberculosis: An epidemic reemerges, 1. The new face of an old disease. *Emergency Medicine, 25*(2), 141–144, 147–148, 157–158.

Epps, M. E. (1992). Diagnostic treating for patients with lung cancer. *Nursing Clinics of North America, 27*(3), 615–630.

Esler, R., Bentz, P., Sorensen, M., & Van Orsow, T. (1994). Patient-centered pneumonia care: A case management success story. *American Journal of Nursing, 94*(11), 34–38.

Fein, A. M., & Adler, J. (1993). Tuberculosis: An epidemic reemerges (Editorial). *Emergency Medicine, 25*(2), 6.

Foyt, M. M. (1992). Impaired gas exchange in the elderly. *Geriatric Nursing, 13*(5), 262–268.

Franklin, R. A. (September). Smoking. *Nursing Clinics of North America, 27*(3), 631–642.

Hammond, S. G. (1990). Chest injuries in the trauma patient. *Nursing Clinics of North America, 25*(1), 35–43.

Hardy, K. A. (1993). Advances in our understanding and care of patients with cystic fibrosis. *Respiratory Care, 38*(3), 282–289.

Hazzard, W. R., Bierman, E. L., Blass, J. P., Ettinger, W. H., Jr., & Halter, J. B., (Eds.). (1994). *Principles of geriatric medicine and gerontology* (3rd ed.). New York: McGraw-Hill.

Holloway, N. M. (1993). *Nursing the critically ill adult* (4th ed.) Redwood City, CA: Addison-Wesley Nursing.

Houston, S. J., & Kendall, J. A. (1992). Psychosocial implications of lung cancer. *Nursing Clinics of North America, 27*(3), 681–690.

Hurst, J. M. (1992). Thoracic trauma. *Respiratory Care, 37*(7), 708–717.

Johanssen, J. (1994). Chronic obstructive pulmonary disease: Current comprehensive care for emphysema and bronchitis. *Nurse Practitioner, 19*(1), 59–67.

Kidd, P. S., & Wagner, K. D. (1992). *High acuity nursing: Preparing for practice in today's health care settings.* Norwalk, CT: Appleton & Lange.

Langston, W. G. (1992). Surgical resection of lung cancer. *Nursing Clinics of North America, 27*(3), 665–679.

Lederer, J. R., Marculescu, G. L., Mocnik, B., & Seaby, N. (1993). *Care planning pocket guide: A nursing diagnosis approach* (5th ed.). Redwood City, CA: Addison-Wesley Nursing.

Lookinland, S., & Appel, P. L. (1991). Hemodynamic and oxygen transport changes following endotracheal suctioning in trauma patients. *Nursing Research, 40*(3), 133–138.

Marcinelli-Van Atta, J., & Beck, S. L. (1994). Endotracheal suctioning: Preventing hypoxemia and hemodynamic compromise. *Nursing94, 24*(10), 32.

McCance, K. L., & Huether, S. E. (1994). *Pathophysiology: The biologic basis for disease in adults and children* (2nd ed.). St. Louis: Mosby-Year Book.

McKinney, B. (1994). COPD and depression: Treat them both. *RN, 57*(4), 48–50.

Murphy, T. F., & Sethi, S. (1993). Preventing or treating COPD flare-ups. *Emergency Medicine, 25*(4), 65–66, 68.

Pagana, K. D., & Pagana, T. J. (1992). *Mosby's Diagnostic and laboratory test reference.* St. Louis: Mosby-Year Book.

Pasero, C., & Mccaffery, M. (1994). Avoiding opioid-induced respiratory depression. *American Journal of Nursing, 94*(4), 24–30.

Pate, R. W. (1992). The role of chemotherapy in the treatment of lung cancer. *Nursing Clinics of North America, 27*(3), 653–663.

Porth, C. M. (1994). *Pathophysiology: Concepts of altered health states* (4th ed.). Philadelphia: Lippincott.

Price, S. A., & Wilson, L. M. (1992). *Pathophysiology: Clinical concepts of disease processes* (4th ed.). St. Louis: Mosby-Year Book.

Raju, L. (1993). Tuberculosis: An epidemic reemerges, 2. Current diagnostic and treatment strategies. *Emergency Medicine, 25*(2), 159,163–164,167–168.

Repasky, T. M. (1994). Emergency! Tension pneumothorax. *American Journal of Nursing, 94*(9), 47.

Rule, C. (1994). Exposure control: Implementing OSHA regulations in home care. *Advance for Nurse Practitioners, 2*(8), 15–16, 30.

Seale, D. D., & Beaver, B. M. (1992). Pathophysiology of lung cancer. *Nursing Clinics of North America, 27*(3), 603–613.

Shlafer, M. (1993). *The nurse, pharmacology, and drug therapy: A prototype approach* (2nd ed.). Redwood City, CA: Addison-Wesley Nursing.

Sparks, S. M., & Taylor, C. M. (1993). *Nursing diagnosis reference manual* (2nd ed.). Springhouse, PA: Springhouse Corporation.

Spencer, R. T., Nichols, L. W., Lipkin, G. B., Henderson, H. S., & West, F. M. (1993). *Clinical pharmacology and nursing management* (4th ed.). Philadelphia: Lippincott.

Steinberg, K. P. (1993). Surfactant therapy in the adult respiratory distress syndrome. *Respiratory Care, 38*(4), 365–371.

Stewart, G. S. (1992). Trends in radiation therapy for the treatment of lung cancer. *Nursing Clinics of North America, 27*(3), 643–651.

Tierney, L. M., McPhee, S. J., & Papadakis, M. A., (Eds.). (1994). *Current medical diagnosis and treatment* (33rd ed.). Norwalk, CT: Appleton & Lange.

Tucker, S. M., Canobbio, M. M., Paquette, E. V., & Wells, M. F. (1992). *Patient care standards: Nursing process, diagnosis, and outcome* (5th ed.). St. Louis: Mosby-Year Book.

Turner, J. T. (1992). Nursing care of the terminal lung cancer patient. *Nursing Clinics of North America, 27*(3), 691–702.

Way, L. W. (Ed.). (1994). *Current surgical diagnosis and treatment* (10th ed.). Norwalk, CT: Appleton & Lange.

Wilson, J. D., Braunwald, E., Isselbacher, K. J., Petersdorf, R. G., Martin, J. B., Fauci, A. S., & Root, R. K. (1991). *Harrison's Principles of internal medicine* (12th ed.). New York: McGraw-Hill.

Wright, B. A., & Staats, D. O. (1992). Tuberculosis surveillance program: A nursing home experience. *Geriatric Nursing, 13*(5), 257–261.

Responses to Altered Musculoskeletal Function

Assessing Clients with Musculoskeletal Disorders

LEARNING OBJECTIVES

After completing this chapter, you will be able to

- Identify the major bones and muscles of the body.
- Describe the structure and function of bones, joints, muscles, ligaments, and tendons.
- Describe the normal movements allowed by synovial joints.
- Identify interview questions pertinent to the assessment of the musculoskeletal system.

- Identify physical assessment techniques for musculoskeletal function.
- Identify manifestations of impairment in the function of the musculoskeletal system.
- Describe variations in assessment findings for the older adult.

Review of Anatomy and Physiology

▪ ▪ ▪

The tissues and structures of the musculoskeletal system perform many different functions for the body, including support, protection, and movement. The musculoskeletal system is composed of two subsystems: the bones and joints of the skeleton, and the skeletal muscles. These subsystems work together to allow the body to perform both gross, simple movements, such as closing a door, and fine, complex movements, such as repairing a watch.

The Skeleton

The human skeleton is made up of 206 bones (Figure 35–1). The bones of the *axial skeleton* include the bones of the skull, the ribs and sternum, and the vertebral col-

umn. The *appendicular skeleton* consists of all of the bones of the limbs, the shoulder girdles, and the pelvic girdle.

Bones form the body's structure and provide support for soft tissues. They also protect vital organs from injury and serve to move body parts by providing points of attachment for muscles. Bones also serve as a storage site for fat and minerals and as a site for *hematopoiesis* (blood cell formation).

Bone Structure

Bone cells include *osteoblasts* (cells that form bone), *osteocytes* (cells that function to maintain bone matrix), and *osteoclasts* (cells that resorb bone). Bone *matrix* is the extracellular element of bone tissue; it is made up of collagen fibers, minerals (primarily calcium and phosphate), proteins, carbohydrates, and ground substance. *Ground substance* is a gelatinous material that facilitates diffusion of nutrients, wastes, and gases between the blood vessels and bone tissue. Bones are covered with *periosteum,* a double-layered connective tissue. The outer layer of the periosteum contains blood vessels and nerves, whereas the inner layer is anchored to the bone.

Bone Tissue

Bones are composed of a rigid connective tissue called *osseous tissue.* There are two types of osseous tissue: *Compact bone* is smooth and dense, whereas *spongy bone* contains spaces between meshworks of bone. Both types of bone contain the same elements and are found in almost all bones of the body.

The basic structural unit of compact bone is the *Haversian system* (also called an *osteon*). The Haversian system is made up of a central canal, called the *Haversian canal;* concentric layers of bone matrix, called *lamellae;* spaces between the lamellae, called *lacunae;* osteocytes within the lacunae; and small channels, called *canaliculi* (Figure 35–2).

Spongy bone does not have Haversian systems. Instead, the lamellae are arranged in concentric layers called *trabeculae* that branch and join to form meshworks. The spongy sections of long bones and flat bones contain tissue for hematopoiesis. In the adult, these sections, called *red marrow cavities,* are present in the spongy center of flat bones (especially the sternum) and in only two long bones: the humerus and the head of the femur. This red marrow is active in hematopoiesis in adults.

Bone Characteristics

Bones are classified by shape (Figure 35–3):

- *Long bones* are longer than they are wide. They have a midportion, or shaft, called a *diaphysis* and two broad ends, called *epiphyses.* The diaphysis is made of compact bone and contains the marrow cavity, which is lined with endosteum. Each epiphysis is made of spongy bone that is covered by a thin layer of compact bone. Long bones include the bones of the arms and legs, fingers, and toes.

- *Short bones,* also called *cuboid bones,* are made of spongy bone covered by compact bone. Short bones include the bones of the wrist and ankle.

- *Flat bones* are thin and flat, and most are curved. Their disc-like structure consists of a layer of spongy bone between two thin layers of compact bone. Flat bones include most bones of the skull, the sternum, and the ribs.

- *Irregular bones* are of various shapes and sizes and, like flat bones, are composed of plates of compact bone with spongy bone between. Irregular bones include the vertebrae, the scapulae, and the bones of the pelvic girdle.

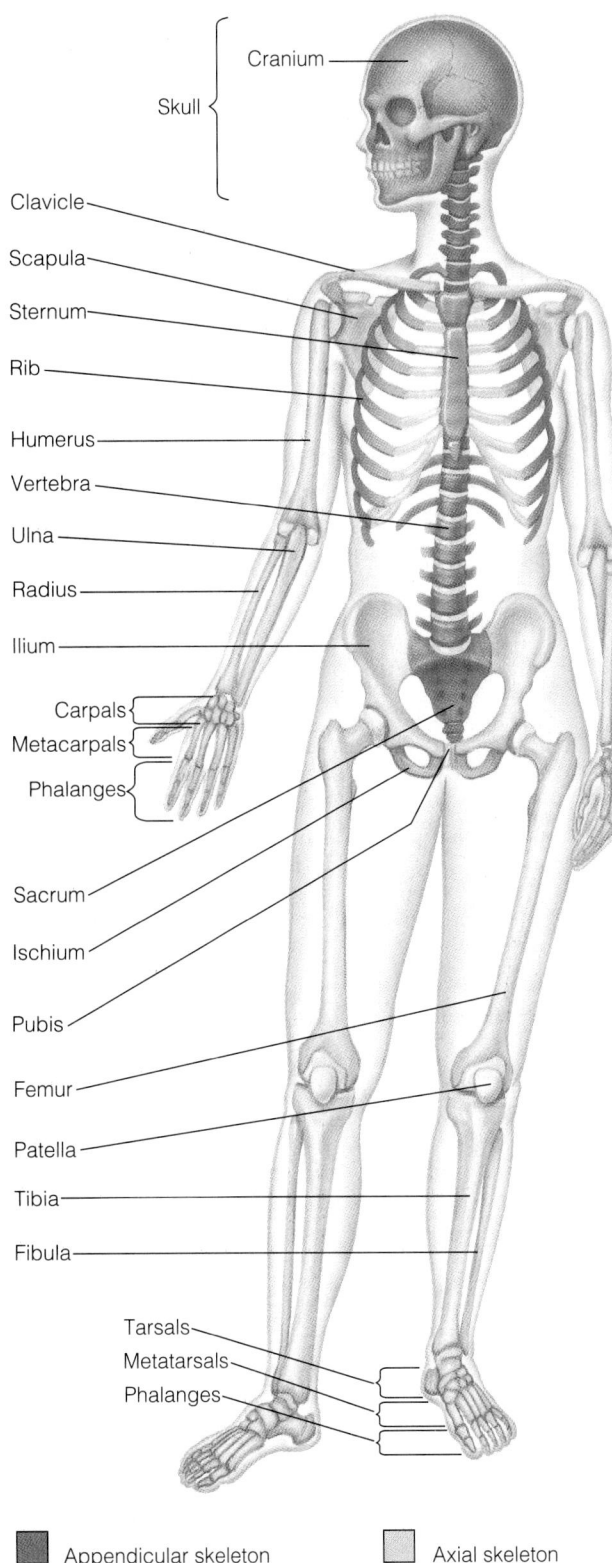

Figure 35–1   Bones of the human skeleton.

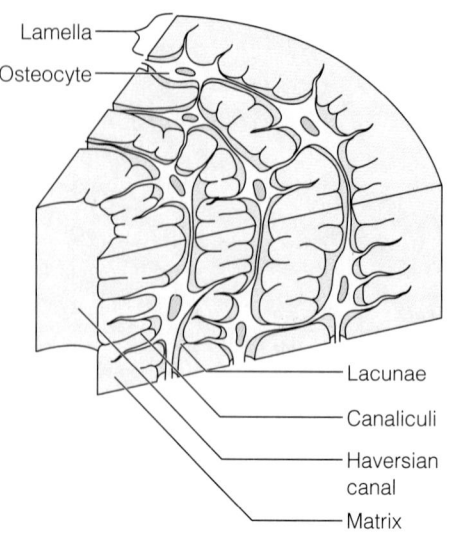

Lamella

Osteocyte

Lacunae

Canaliculi

Haversian
canal

Matrix

Figure 35-2   The microscopic structure of compact bone.

Bone Remodeling in Adults

Although the bones of adults do not normally increase in length and size, constant remodeling of bones, as well as repair of damaged bone tissue, does occur throughout life. *Bone remodeling* is a process whereby bone resorption and bone deposit occur at all periosteal and endosteal surfaces. This process, which involves a combined action of the osteocytes, osteoclasts, and osteoblasts, is regulated by hormones and by forces that put stress on the bones. Bones that are in use, and are therefore subjected to stress, increase their osteoblastic activity to increase ossification (the development of bone). Bones that are inactive undergo increased osteoclast activity and bone resorption.

The hormonal stimulus for bone remodeling is controlled by a negative feedback mechanism that regulates blood calcium levels. This stimulus involves the interaction of parathyroid hormone (PTH) from the parathyroid

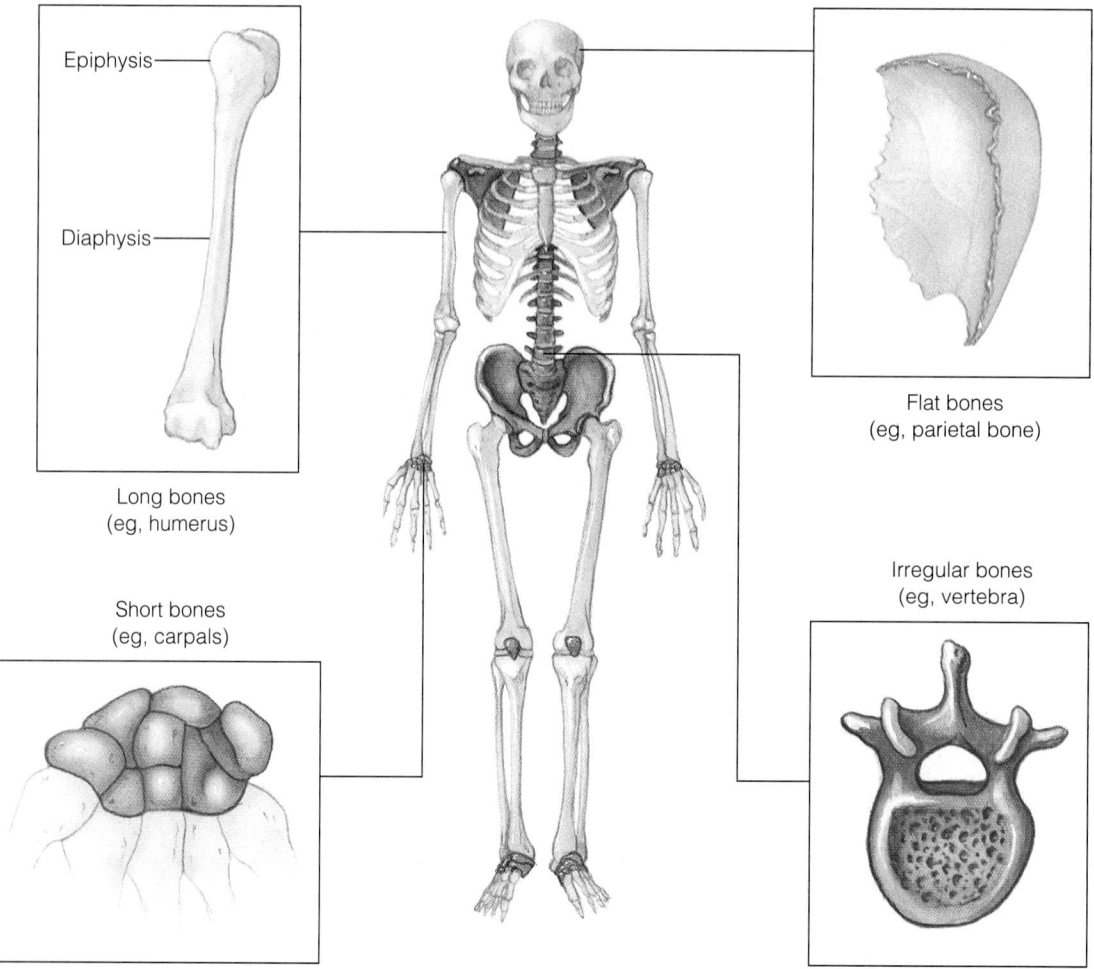

Epiphysis

Diaphysis

Long bones
(eg, humerus)

Short bones
(eg, carpals)

Flat bones
(eg, parietal bone)

Irregular bones
(eg, vertebra)

Figure 35-3   Classification of bones according to shape.

glands and calcitonin from the thyroid gland. When blood levels of calcium decrease, PTH is released; PTH then stimulates osteoclast activity and bone resorption so that calcium is released from the bone matrix. As a result, blood levels of calcium rise, and the stimulus for PTH release ends. As blood calcium levels rise, the secretion of calcitonin is stimulated, bone resorption is inhibited, and calcium salts are deposited in the bone matrix. Thus, bones serve as a regulator of blood calcium levels. Calcium ions are necessary for the transmission of nerve impulses, the release of neurotransmitters, muscle contraction, blood clotting, glandular secretion, and cell division. Of the body's 1200 to 1400 g of calcium, over 99% is present as bone minerals.

Bone remodeling is also regulated by the response of bones to gravitational pull and to mechanical stress from the pull of muscles. Although the exact mechanism is not fully understood, it is known that bones that undergo increased stress are heavier and larger. This finding supports Wolff's law, which states that bone develops and remodels itself to resist the stresses placed on it.

The process of bone repair following a fracture is discussed in Chapter 36.

Joints, Ligaments, and Tendons

Joints, also called *articulations,* are regions where two or more bones meet. Joints hold the bones of the skeleton together while allowing the body to move. Joints may be classified by function as synarthroses, amphiarthroses, or diarthroses. Table 35–1 describes each of these types.

Joints are also classified by structure as fibrous, cartilaginous, or synovial. *Fibrous joints* permit little or no movement, because the articulating bones are joined either by short connective tissue fibers that bind the bones together, as with the sutures of the skull, or by short cords of fibrous tissue called ligaments (discussed below), which permit slight "give" but no true movement.

Some *cartilaginous joints,* such as the sternocostal joints of the rib cage, are composed of hyaline cartilage growths that fuse together the articulating bone ends. These joints are immobile. In other cartilaginous joints, such as the intervertebral discs, the hyaline cartilage fuses to an intervening plate of flexible fibrocartilage. This structural feature accounts for the flexibility of the vertebral column.

Bones in *synovial joints* are enclosed by a cavity that is filled with synovial fluid, a filtrate of blood plasma. These joints are freely movable. Synovial joints are found at all articulations of the limbs. They have several characteristics:

- The articular surfaces are covered with articular cartilage.
- The joint cavity is enclosed by a tough, fibrous, double-layered articular capsule; internally, the cavity is lined with a synovial membrane that covers all surfaces not covered by the articular cartilage.

- Synovial fluid fills the free spaces of the joint capsule, enhancing the smooth movement of the articulating bones.

Synovial joints allow many different kinds of movements. Movements of synovial joints are listed and described in Table 35–2.

Table 35–1	Functional Classification of Joints	
Type	**Description**	**Examples**
Synarthrosis	Immovable joint	Skull sutures Epiphyseal plates Joint between first rib and manubrium of sternum
Amphiarthrosis	Slightly movable joint	Vertebral joints Joint of the pubic symphysis
Diarthrosis	Freely movable joint	Joints of the limbs Shoulder joints Hip joints

Table 35–2	Movements Allowed by Synovial Joints
Movement	**Description**
Abduction	Move limb away from body midline
Adduction	Move limb toward body midline
Extension	Straighten limbs at joint
Flexion	Bend limbs at joint
Dorsiflexion	Bend ankle to bring top of foot toward shin
Plantar flexion	Straighten ankle to point toes down
Pronation	Turn forearm to place palm down
Supination	Turn forearm to place palm up
Eversion	Turn out
Inversion	Turn in
Circumduction	Move in circle
Internal rotation	Move inward on a central axis
External rotation	Move outward on a central axis
Protraction	Move forward and parallel to ground
Retraction	Move backward and parallel to ground

Table 35–3 Types of Body Muscle

Type	Description	Examples
Skeletal	Striated, voluntary muscle (can consciously move)	Biceps, triceps, deltoid, gluteus maximus
Smooth	Nonstriated, involuntary muscle (cannot consciously move)	Muscles in the walls of the bladder, stomach, and bronchi
Cardiac	Striated, involuntary muscle	Heart muscle

The fibrous capsules that surround synovial joints are supported by *ligaments,* which are dense bands of connective tissue that connect bones to bones. Ligaments either limit or enhance movement, provide joint stability, and enhance joint strength. *Tendons* are fibrous connective tissue bands that connect muscles to the periosteum of bones and enable the bones to move when skeletal muscles contract. When muscles contract, increased pressure causes the tendon to pull, push, or rotate the bone to which it is connected.

Bursae are small sacs of synovial fluid that cushion and protect bony areas that are at high risk for friction, such as the knee and the shoulder. Tendon sheaths are a form of bursae, but they are wrapped around tendons in high-friction areas.

Muscles

There are three types of muscle tissue in the body: skeletal muscle, smooth muscle, and cardiac muscle (Table 35–3). This discussion focuses on skeletal muscle, the only muscle that allows musculoskeletal function.

Skeletal muscle cells have typical functional properties (Marieb, 1995):

- *Excitability:* the cell's ability to receive and respond to a stimulus. The stimulus is usually a neurotransmitter released by a neuron, and the response is the generation and transmission of an action potential along the plasma membrane of the muscle cell. (Chapter 39 discusses action potentials.)
- *Contractibility:* the cell's ability to respond to a stimulus by forcibly shortening.
- *Extensibility:* the cell's ability to respond to a stimulus by extending and relaxing; muscle fibers shorten when they contract and extend when they relax.
- *Elasticity:* the cell's ability to resume its resting length after it has shortened or lengthened.

Skeletal muscles are thick bundles of parallel multinucleated contractile cells called *fibers* (Figure 35–4). Each single muscle fiber is itself a bundle of smaller structures called *myofibrils.* The myofibrils have alternating light and dark bands that give skeletal muscle its *striated* (striped) appearance under an electron microscope. Myofibrils are strands of smaller repeating units called *sarcomeres,* which are composed of thick filaments of *myosin* and thin filaments of *actin,* proteins that contribute to muscle contraction.

Skeletal muscle movement is triggered when motor neurons release acetylcholine, a neurotransmitter that alters the permeability of the muscle fiber. Sodium ions enter the fiber, producing an action potential that causes muscle contraction. The more fibers that contract, the stronger the contraction of the entire muscle.

Prolonged strenuous activity causes continuous nerve impulses and eventually results in a buildup of lactic acid and reduced energy in the muscle, or *muscle fatigue.* However, continuous nerve impulses are also responsible for maintaining muscle tone. Lack of use results in muscle atrophy, whereas regular exercise increases the size and strength of muscles.

Skeletal muscles attach to and cover the bones of the skeleton. Skeletal muscles promote body movement, help maintain posture, and produce body heat. They may be moved by conscious, voluntary control or by reflex activity. There are approximately 600 skeletal muscles in the body (Figure 35–5).

Assessment of Musculoskeletal Function

■ ■ ■

The function of the musculoskeletal system is assessed by both a health assessment interview to collect subjective data and a physical assessment to collect objective data.

The Health Assessment Interview

This section provides guidelines for collecting subjective data through a health assessment interview specific to musculoskeletal function. Interview questions and leading statements for assessing musculoskeletal function also are provided.

Overview

A health assessment interview to determine problems with musculoskeletal function may be conducted as part of a health screening or as part of a total health assessment, or it may focus on a chief complaint (such as pain, swelling, or limited mobility). Health problems affecting the neurologic system may manifest as musculoskeletal function problems; an assessment of both systems may be necessary. (See Chapter 39 for assessment of the neurologic system.) If the client has a health problem involving the bones or muscles, analyze its onset, characteristics and course, severity, precipitating and relieving factors, and any associated manifestations, noting the timing and circumstances. For example, ask the client:

- Describe the pain you have had in your elbow. Does the pain increase with movement? Have you noticed any redness or swelling?

- Did you injure your ankle before you began to experience difficulty walking?

- Is your pain worse in the morning, or does it get worse through the day?

The primary manifestations of altered function of the musculoskeletal system are pain and limited mobility. Specific descriptors of the pain, its location, and its nature are important. Other significant information includes associated manifestations, such as fever, fatigue, changes in weight, rash, and/or swelling. Also collect information about the client's life-style: type of employment, ability to carry out activities of daily living (ADLs) and provide self-care, exercise or participation in sports, use of alcohol or drugs, and nutrition. Explore past injuries and measures to self-treat pain (such as over-the-counter medications, prescribed medications, application of heat or cold, splinting, wrapping, or rest).

Interview Questions

The following interview questions and leading statements are categorized by functional health patterns:

Health Perception–Health Management

- Have you ever had any muscle or bone injuries?

- Describe any surgery, physical therapy, or other treatments you have received for musculoskeletal problems.

- List any medications (e.g., muscle relaxants, anti-inflammatory agents) you use for musculoskeletal problems.

- What other medications are you taking?

Nutritional-Metabolic

- Describe your dietary intake for a 24-hour period. How much meat, dairy products, fruits, and vegetables do you consume? Do you take vitamins?

- Have you had any recent weight gain or loss? What do you see as your ideal body weight?

- Do you have any redness or swelling in your joints?

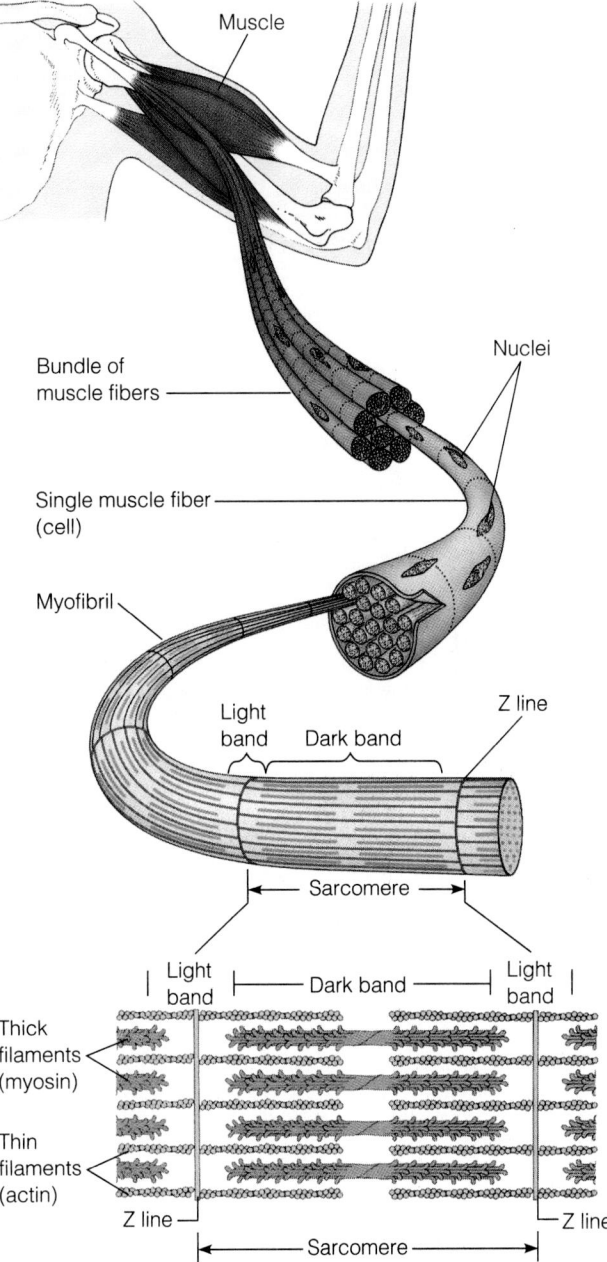

Figure 35–4 Anatomy of a skeletal muscle. A skeletal muscle is a bundle of muscle fibers, each of which is a bundle of myofibrils, made up of repeating units of sarcomeres that contain myosin and actin protein filaments active in muscle contraction.

Activity-Exercise

- Describe your normal activities for a 24-hour period.

- Describe any musculoskeletal problems (e.g., weakness, pain, stiffness) that limit your activities of daily living, such as driving, dressing, bathing, walking, climbing stairs, cooking, or cleaning.

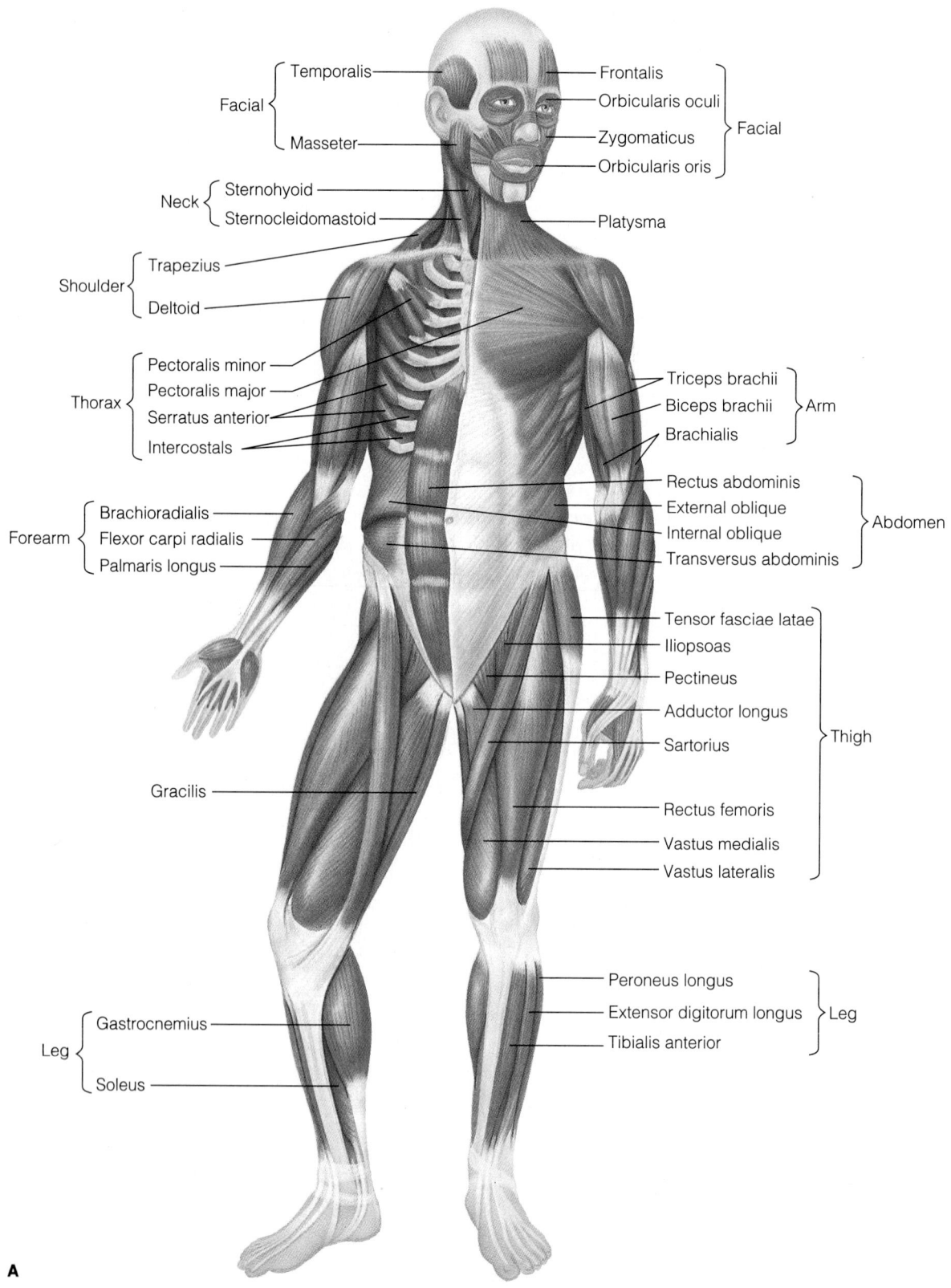

Facial
- Temporalis
- Masseter

Facial
- Frontalis
- Orbicularis oculi
- Zygomaticus
- Orbicularis oris

Neck
- Sternohyoid
- Sternocleidomastoid

Platysma

Shoulder
- Trapezius
- Deltoid

Thorax
- Pectoralis minor
- Pectoralis major
- Serratus anterior
- Intercostals

Arm
- Triceps brachii
- Biceps brachii
- Brachialis

Forearm
- Brachioradialis
- Flexor carpi radialis
- Palmaris longus

Abdomen
- Rectus abdominis
- External oblique
- Internal oblique
- Transversus abdominis

Thigh
- Tensor fasciae latae
- Iliopsoas
- Pectineus
- Adductor longus
- Sartorius
- Rectus femoris
- Vastus medialis
- Vastus lateralis

Gracilis

Leg
- Peroneus longus
- Extensor digitorum longus
- Tibialis anterior

Leg
- Gastrocnemius
- Soleus

A

Figure 35–5   *A*, Muscles of the anterior body. *B*, Muscles of the posterior body.

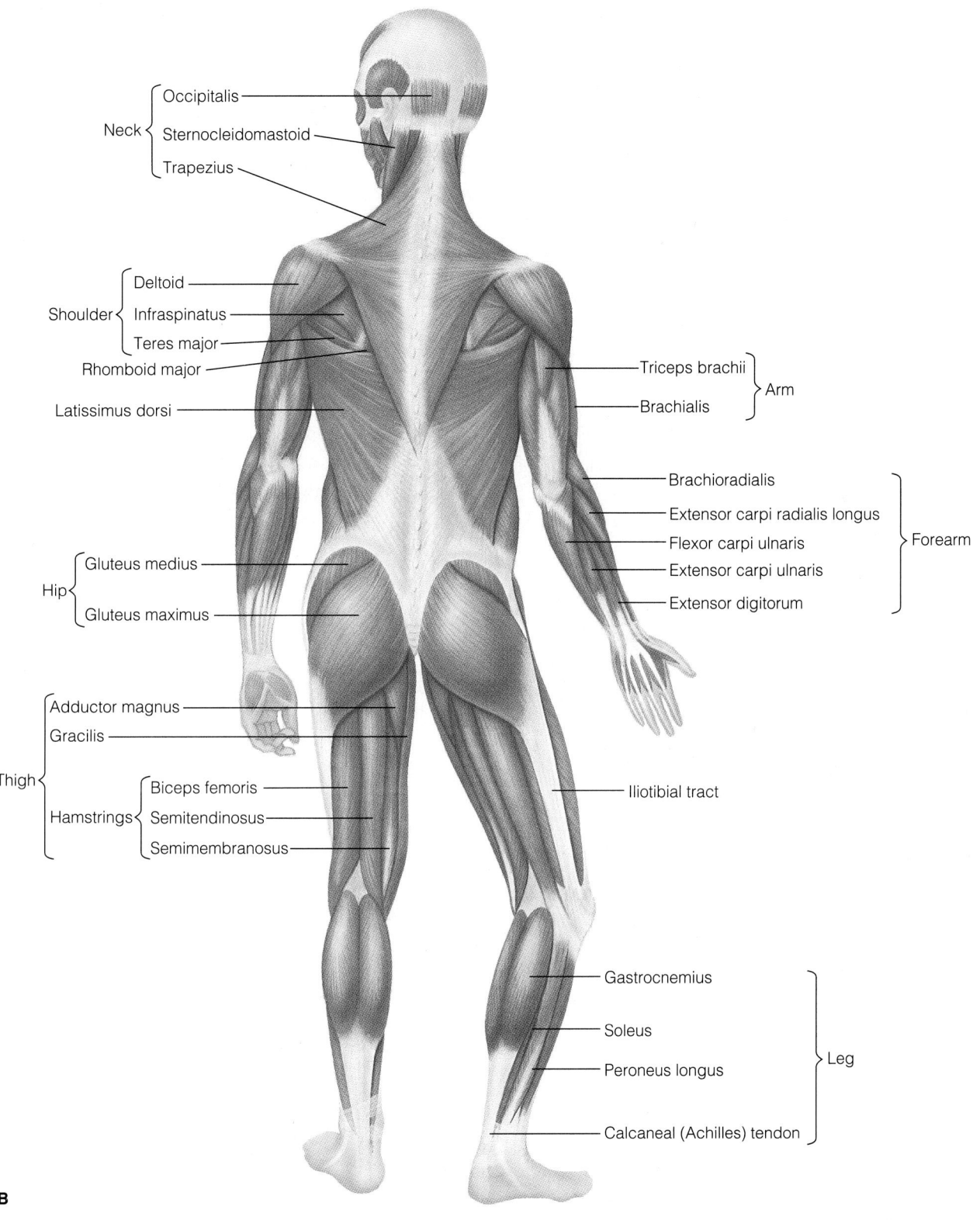

B

- Has there been a change in your level of mobility?
- Do you engage in any strenuous exercise or lifting? Explain.

Elimination

- Do you have difficulty getting to the bathroom in time to empty your bowel and bladder? Explain.

Sleep-Rest

- Have your normal patterns of sleep or rest been disturbed by any musculoskeletal pain, stiffness, or cramping?

Cognitive-Perceptual

- Describe any bone, joint, or muscle pain you are feeling. What relieves and/or aggravates the pain?
- Describe any changes in the temperature, color, or sensations of your extremities.
- Describe any muscular weakness you are experiencing.

Self-Perception–Self-Concept

- Describe how you feel about your musculoskeletal problem.
- Has your musculoskeletal problem affected how you feel about your appearance?
- Has your musculoskeletal problem affected how you feel about your life?

Role-Relationship

- Has anyone in your family had osteoporosis, arthritis, tuberculosis, or gout?

- Have you experienced any musculoskeletal injuries from family conflict?
- Have problems with your bones, joints, or muscles interfered with your work? Explain.

Sexuality-Reproductive

- Has your musculoskeletal problem altered your usual sexual activities? If so, explain.
- Describe how problems with your bones, joints, or muscles make you feel about yourself as a man or woman.

Coping-Stress

- How have you managed to cope with your musculoskeletal problem?
- What do you feel is the most stressful time you have had with your musculoskeletal problem?
- Has the condition created much stress for you? Explain. Describe what you do to cope with stress.
- Who or what will be able to help you cope with stress from this musculoskeletal problem?

Value-Belief

- Are there significant others, practices, or activities that help you cope with a musculoskeletal problem? Explain.
- Describe how you feel about the future with this musculoskeletal problem.

The Physical Assessment

Physical assessment of the musculoskeletal system is conducted through inspection, palpation, and measurement of muscle mass and range of motion. The client should be comfortably dressed in clothing that will allow the nurse to view the movement of all joints clearly. The client may be standing, sitting, or lying down; the sequence of the examination should be such that the client does not have frequent position changes. Musculoskeletal assessment of the older adult, the client in pain, or the client who is weak may take additional time.

The Musculoskeletal System: Preparation

The equipment necessary for conducting an assessment of the musculoskeletal system is a tape measure to determine muscle size and a goniometer to measure joint range of motion (ROM). Prior to the examination, collect all equipment and explain the techniques to decrease the client's anxiety.

The general sequence for a musculoskeletal examination follows:

The Physical Assessment (continued)

1. Begin the examination with an assessment of the client's gait and posture. Observe how the client walks, sits, and/or moves about in bed.

2. Inspect and palpate the client's bones for any obvious deformity or changes in size or shape. Palpation also will elicit tenderness or pain.

3. Measure the extremities for length and circumference. Before taking measurements, make sure the client is lying in a comfortable position. Remember to compare limbs bilaterally.

4. Assess muscle mass by first inspecting for obvious increase or decrease in size. Assess and document muscle strength on a scale of 0 to 5 (Table 35–4). The accompanying box provides client instructions for testing the strength of various muscles.

Table 35–4   Muscle Grading Scale

Grading Scale	Assessment Description
0	(No visible) contraction; paralysis
1	Can feel contraction of muscle but there is no movement of limb
2	Passive ROM
3	Full ROM against gravity
4	Full ROM against some resistance
5	Full ROM against full resistance

Guidelines for Determining Muscle Strength

■   ■   ■

In adults, muscles are usually strong and equally strong bilaterally. However, neuromuscular diseases, disuse, metabolic disorders, or infections can cause muscle weakness. Muscle strength is expected to be greater in the dominant arm and leg. In most instances (and especially when moving digits and extremities), the nurse provides resistance by pushing in the opposite direction.

The muscles listed below are routinely tested. Instructions for clients are also provided:

Muscle	Client Instructions	Muscle	Client Instructions
Ocular muscles and lids	Close eyes tightly.	Finger muscles	Shake hands. Make a fist. Spread fingers.
Facial muscles	Blow out cheeks. Stick out tongue.	Hip muscles	Raise straight leg while supine.
Neck muscles	Bend head forward and backward.	Gluteal and leg muscles	Alternately cross legs while sitting.
Deltoid muscles	Hold arms up.	Quadriceps muscle	Straighten leg.
Biceps muscle	Bend the arm.		
Triceps muscle	Straighten the arm.		
Wrist muscles	Bend hand forward and backward.	Ankle and foot muscles	Bend foot up and down.

5. Assess joints for swelling, pain, redness, warmth, crepitus, and ROM. The ROM of every joint is assessed only if the client has a specific musculoskeletal problem; however, the assessment of one or more joints is a common part of nursing care. A goniometer is used for precise measurements of joint ROM (Figure 35–6). This device has a pointer joined to a protractor at 0 degrees. These two arms are placed along articulating bones, and the angle of joint movement is recorded in degrees.

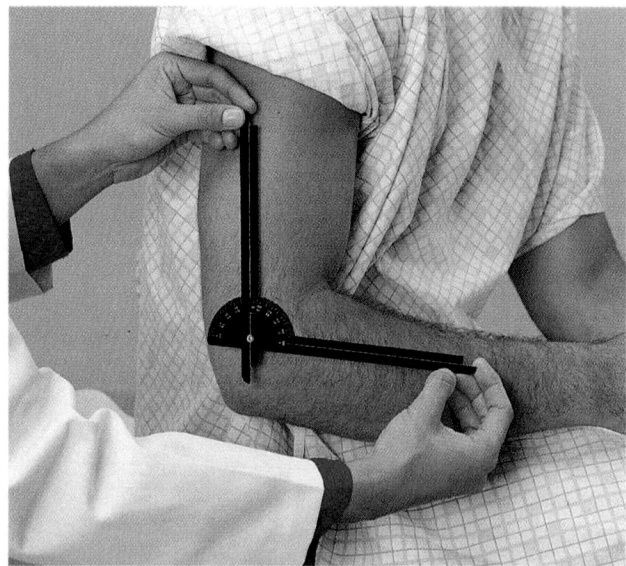

Figure 35–6 Using a goniometer to measure joint ROM.

ASSESSMENT TECHNIQUE	POSSIBLE ABNORMAL FINDINGS

Inspection
- **Inspect gait and body posture.**

Ask the client to walk around the room. Note the client's gait, posture, alignment, and any obvious deformities.

- **Inspect the spine for curvature.**

Ask the client to stand and bend back slowly as far as possible, bend slowly to the right and then the left as far as possible, turn slowly to the right and left in a circular motion, and bend forward slowly and try to touch fingers to toes.

Joint stiffness, pain, deformities, and muscle weakness can cause changes in gait and posture.

With herniated lumbar discs, the lumbar curve flattens and spinal mobility is decreased. An increased lumbar curve, called **lordosis,** may be seen in obesity or pregnancy. A lateral, S-shaped curvature of the spine is called **scoliosis.** *Functional scoliosis* usually is a compensatory response to painful paravertebral muscles, herniated discs, or discrepancy in leg length. It disappears with forward flexion. *Structural scoliosis* is often congenital and tends to appear during adolescence. It is accentuated with forward bending. **Kyphosis,** also called *hump-back,* is an exaggerated thoracic curvature of the spine common in older adults.

ASSESSMENT TECHNIQUE	POSSIBLE ABNORMAL FINDINGS

- **Inspect the joints for deformity, swelling, and redness.**

Diseases of the joints may be manifested by such deformities as tissue loss, tissue overgrowth, or *contractures,* irreversible shortenings of muscles and tendons. Edema in a joint may cause obvious bulging. Redness, swelling, and pain are evidence of an inflammation or infection in the joint. They are common in **arthritis,** a general term meaning inflammation of a joint.

Palpation
- **Palpate the joints for tenderness, warmth, crepitation, consistency, and muscle mass.**

Inflammation and injury cause joint pain. Arthritis, bursitis, tendinitis, and *osteomyelitis* (infection of a bone) result in painful, hot joints. *Crepitation* (a grating sound) is present in a joint when the articulating surfaces have lost their cartilage, such as in arthritis.

Assessment of Range of Motion (ROM)
Assess ROM by asking the client to follow the instructions listed for each expected ROM.

- **Temporomandibular joint.**

Open your mouth wide, and then close your mouth. (As the client opens and closes the mouth, palpate the temporomandibular joints with your index and middle fingers, as shown in Figure 35–7.)

Clicking or popping noises, decreased ROM, pain, and swelling may indicate temporomandibular joint syndrome or, in rare cases, osteoarthritis.

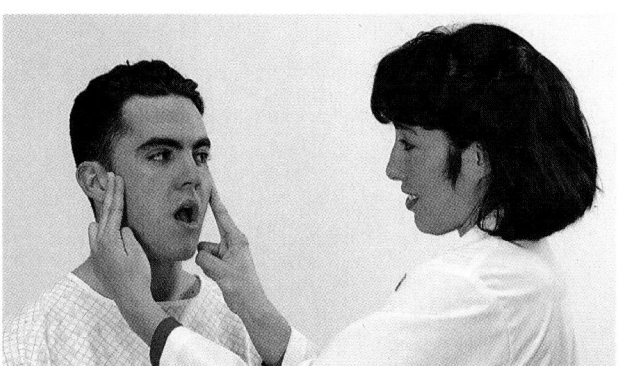

Figure 35-7   Palpating the temporomandibular joints.

- **Cervical spine.**
    45-degree flexion: Touch your chin to your chest.
    55-degree extension: Look at the ceiling.
    40-degree lateral bending: Try to touch your right ear to your right shoulder. Repeat with the left side.
    70-degree rotation: Try to touch your chin to each shoulder.

Neck pain and limited extension with lateral bending are seen with herniated cervical discs and in cervical spondylosis. An immobile neck with head and neck thrust forward is seen with **ankylosing spondylitis.**

- **Lumbar spine.**
    75- to 90-degree flexion: Touch your toes with your fingers (Figure 35–8, *A*).

Decreased movement or pain with movement may indicate an abnormal spinal curvature, arthritis, herniated

ASSESSMENT TECHNIQUE	POSSIBLE ABNORMAL FINDINGS

30-degree extension: Bend backward slowly.
35-degree lateral bending: Bend right and left (Figure 35–8, *B*).
30-degree rotation: Twist your shoulders right and left (Figure 35–8, *C*).

disc, or spasm of paravertebral muscles. A **strain** is a stretching or tearing of muscle fibers. Strains occur most commonly in the lumbar region of the spine.

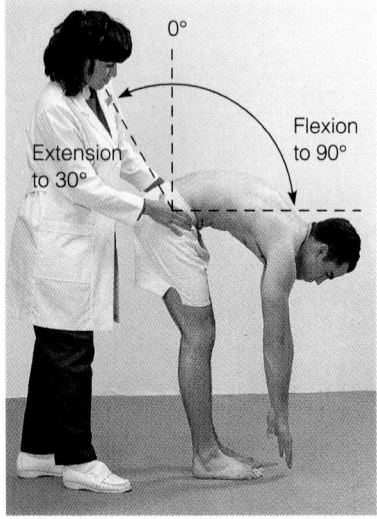

Figure 35–8 *A,* Forward flexion of spine. *B,* Lateral flexion of spine. *C,* Rotation of spine.

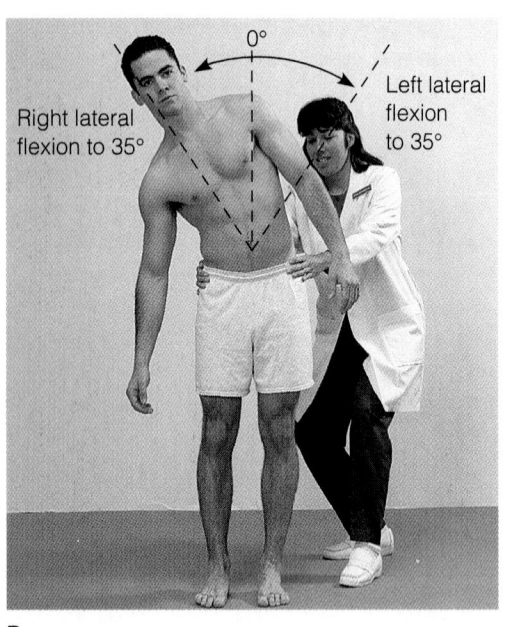

B

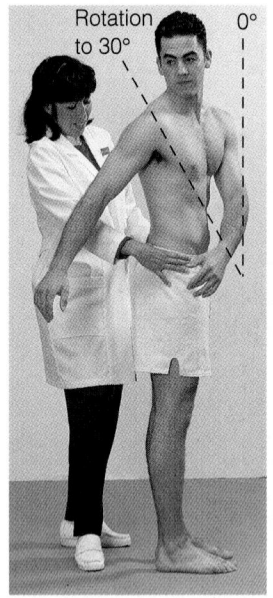

C

- **Fingers.**

  Flexion: Make a fist.
  Extension: Open your hand.
  Abduction: Spread your fingers.
  Adduction: Close your fingers.

Flexion and extension of fingers is decreased in arthritis. *Heberden's nodes* and *Bouchard's nodes* are hard, nontender nodules on the dorsolateral parts of the distal and proximal interphalangeal joints, respectively. They are common in osteoarthritis. Stiff, painful, swollen finger joints are seen in acute rheumatoid

ASSESSMENT TECHNIQUE	POSSIBLE ABNORMAL FINDINGS

arthritis. *Boutonnière* and *swan-neck deformities* are seen in chronic rheumatoid arthritis. Swollen finger joints with a white chalky discharge may be seen in chronic gout.

- **Wrists.**

  90-degree flexion: Bend wrist down.
  70-degree extension: Bend wrist up.
  55-degree ulnar deviation: Bend wrist toward little finger.
  20-degree radial deviation: Bend wrist toward thumb.

Bilateral chronic swelling in the wrist is seen in arthritis.

- **Elbows.**

  160-degree flexion: Touch your hands to your shoulders.
  180-degree extension: Straighten your elbows.
  90-degree supination: Bend your elbows 90 degrees, and turn hands palm up.
  90-degree pronation: Bend your elbows 90 degrees, and turn fists down.

Swollen, tender, inflamed elbows are apparent in gouty arthritis and rheumatoid arthritis. Pain and tenderness at the lateral epicondyle occurs in *tennis elbow.*

- **Shoulders.**

  180-degree flexion: Hold your arms straight up and out.
  50-degree hyperextension: Put your straight arm behind your back.
  90-degree internal rotation: Put your forearm behind your lower back.
  180-degree abduction: Raise your straight arm up and out to your side.
  50-degree adduction: Put your straight arm across your chest.

Pain and tenderness over the biceps tendon occurs with **tendinitis** (inflammation of a tendon). The client cannot abduct the arm fully when the supraspinatus tendon of the shoulder is ruptured. Pain and limited abduction is also seen with **bursitis** (inflammation of a bursa) and calcium deposits in this area.

- **Toes.**

  90-degree flexion: Walk on your toes.

The great toe is excessively abducted in *hallux valgus.* The joint above the great toe is swollen, inflamed, and painful in *gouty arthritis.* There is hyperextension of the metatarsophalangeal joint and flexion of the proximal interphalangeal joint with *hammer toes.*

- **Ankles.**

  20-degree dorsiflexion: Point your foot to the ceiling.
  45-degree plantar flexion: Point your foot to the floor.
  30-degree inversion: Walk on the outside of your feet.
  20-degree eversion: Walk on the inside of your feet.

Contractures of the Achilles tendon may occur in clients with rheumatoid arthritis following prolonged bed rest. Inflammation may indicate a **sprain,** a tearing or stretching of the ligaments. The ankle is the most commonly sprained joint in the body.

- **Knees.**

  130-degree flexion: Do a deep knee bend.
  180-degree extension: Sit down and hold your legs straight out in front of you.

Swelling over the suprapatellar pouch is seen with inflammation and fluid in the articular capsule of the knee. **Synovitis** is inflammation of the synovial membrane lining the articular capsule of a joint. It is common with knee trauma. Swelling over the patella is seen in bursitis.

ASSESSMENT TECHNIQUE	POSSIBLE ABNORMAL FINDINGS

■ **Hips.**
(The client is lying down.)
120-degree flexion: Bring bent knee up to your chest.
30-degree hyperextension: Lie on the abdomen, and lift up one leg at a time.
45-degree abduction: Hold your leg straight, and move it out to the side.
40-degree internal rotation: Bend your knee, and swing it toward your other leg.
45-degree external rotation: Bend your knee, and swing it out to the side.

Movement of the hip is limited and/or painful in arthritis. A **fracture** is a break in a bone usually due to trauma. Hip fracture (that is, fracture of the neck of the femur) occurs most commonly in older adults. It is often due to a fall, but it may occur spontaneously in clients with *osteoporosis,* a bone-wasting condition.

Special Assessments

■ **Perform Phalen's test.**

Ask the client to hold the wrist in acute flexion for 60 seconds (Figure 35–9).

Numbness and burning in the fingers during Phalen's test may indicate carpal tunnel syndrome.

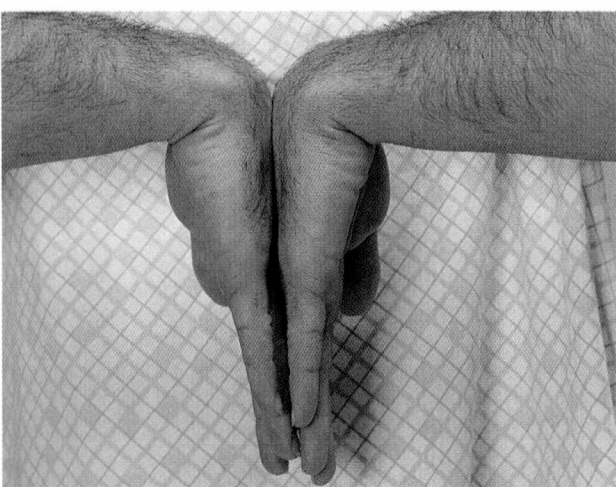

Figure 35–9 Phalen's test.

■ **Check for small amounts of fluid on the knee by assessing for a "bulge sign."**

Milk upward on the medial side of the knee, and then tap the lateral side of the patella (Figure 35–10).

A fluid bulge indicates increased fluid in the knee joint rather than soft tissue swelling.

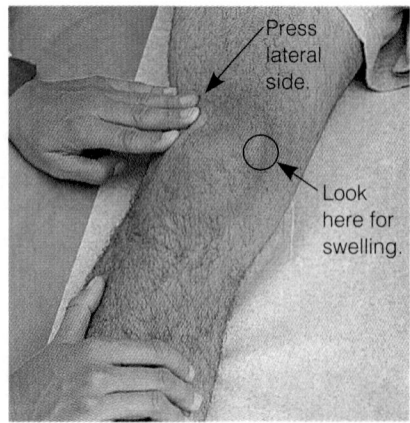

Milk upward on medial side.

Press lateral side.

Look here for swelling.

Figure 35–10 Checking for the bulge sign.

ASSESSMENT TECHNIQUE	POSSIBLE ABNORMAL FINDINGS

- **Check for larger amounts of fluid by assessing ballottement.**

Apply downward pressure on the knee with one hand while pushing the patella backward against the femur with the other hand (Figure 35–11).

Increased fluid will cause a tapping sound as the patella displaces the fluid and hits the femur.

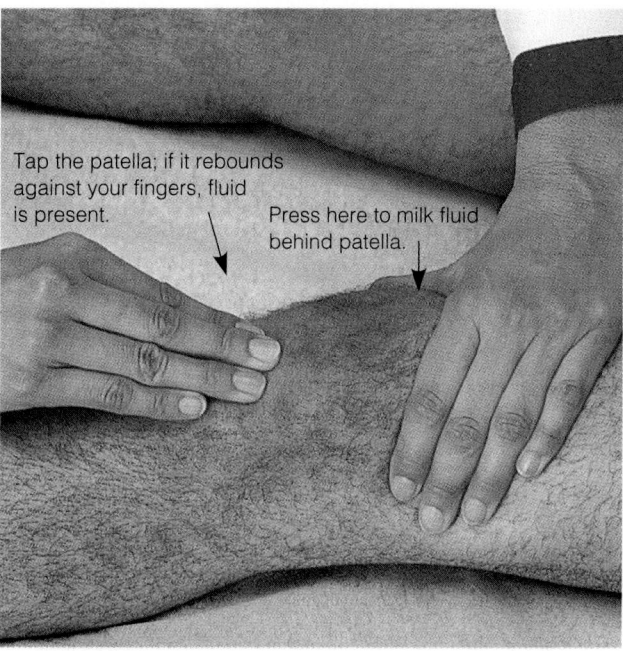

Tap the patella; if it rebounds against your fingers, fluid is present.

Press here to milk fluid behind patella.

Figure 35–11   Checking for ballottement.

- **Perform McMurray's test.**

With the client reclining, ask the client to turn the flexed knee toward the center of the body. Stabilize the knee with one hand, and apply pressure on the lower leg with the other hand (Figure 35–12).

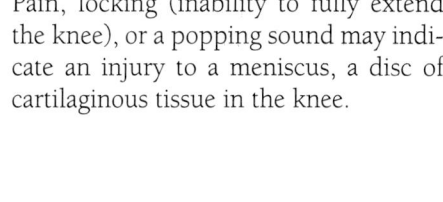

Pain, locking (inability to fully extend the knee), or a popping sound may indicate an injury to a meniscus, a disc of cartilaginous tissue in the knee.

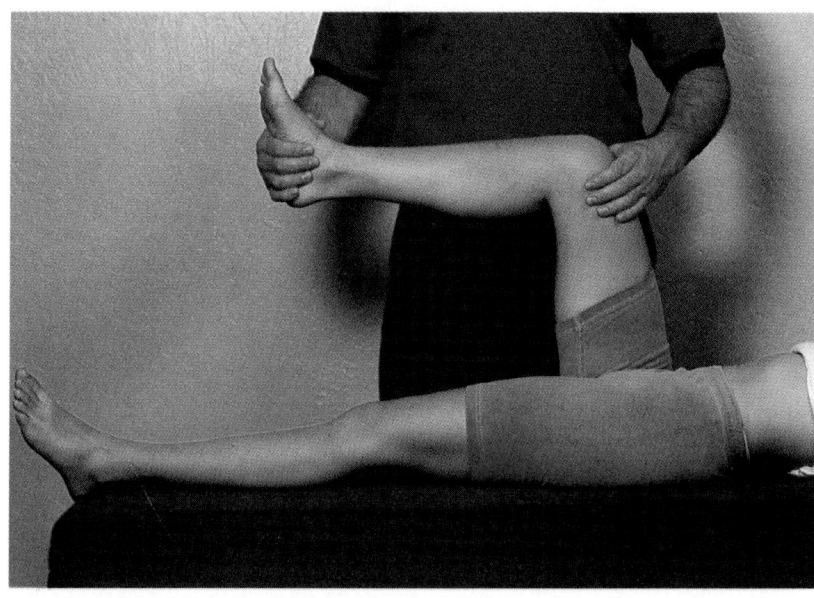

Figure 35–12   McMurray's test.

ASSESSMENT TECHNIQUE	POSSIBLE ABNORMAL FINDINGS

■ **Perform the Thomas test.**

Ask the client to lie down and extend one leg while bringing the knee of the opposite leg to the chest (Figure 35–13).

A hip flexion contracture will cause the extended leg to rise off the table.

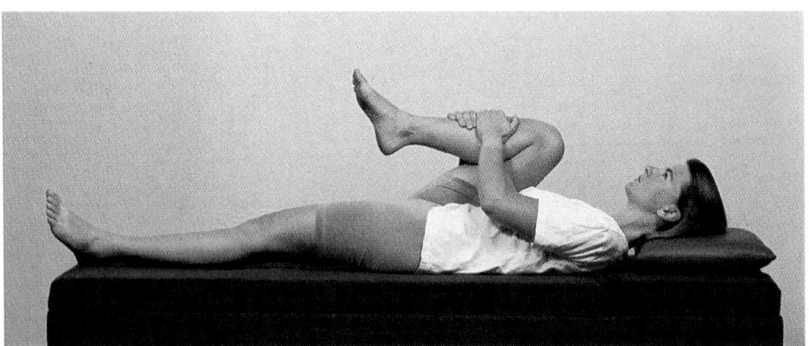

Figure 35–13 Thomas test for hip contracture.

Variations in Assessment Findings for the Older Adult

With aging, compact bone erodes and is replaced by spongy bone, resulting in an overall loss of bone density. Bone remodeling takes longer, and mineralization slows. There are fewer bone cells, because the bone marrow becomes fatty and unable to provide an adequate supply of precursor cells. Joint cartilage is less rigid and more fragile. Other changes include the following:

■ Muscle wasting and a slow decline in strength occur after the 50s, the results of a loss of muscle fibers. Muscle fiber loss is believed to be due to alterations in activity levels, decreased nutrition, atrophy of nerves, and/or cardiovascular disease.

■ Hormonal changes, especially in the postmenopausal woman, cause calcium to be drawn out of bones, resulting in thinning of bone. This condition, called *osteoporosis,* is more common in Caucasian women with small bones.

■ Height decreases as a result of thinning of the intervertebral discs and a loss of normal spinal curves.

■ Kyphosis commonly occurs as bone mass is lost from the vertebrae.

■ Joint stiffness, pain, and crepitation are common results of *osteoarthritis,* a degenerative form of arthritis.

Bibliography

■ ■ ■

Burke, M. (1993). Coping strategies and health states of elderly arthritic women. *Journal of Advanced Nursing, 18*(1), 7–13.

Carroll, P. (1993). Deep venous thrombosis: Implications for orthopedic nursing. *Orthopedic Nursing, 12*(3), 33–43.

Chang, B. L. (1990). Self-care deficit with etiologies: Reliability of measurement. *Nursing Diagnosis, 1*(1), 31–36.

Folcik, M. A. (1991). Meniscal injuries. *Nursing Clinics of North America, 26*(1), 181–198.

Jones-Watlow, P. (1990). Orthopedic nursing assessment. *Advancing Clinical Care, 5*(3), 22.

Keity, J. E. (1989). Emergent assessment of the multiple trauma patient. *Orthopedic Nursing, 8*(6), 29–32.

Leahey, J. L. (1988). "Signs" of altered gait. *CONA Journal, 10*(1), 7–9.

Marieb, E. N. (1995). *Human anatomy and physiology* (3rd ed). Redwood City, CA: The Benjamin/Cummings Publishing Company, Inc.

Martin, L., & Gupta, A. (1992). Hand assessment. *Plastic Surgical Nursing, 12*(3), 89–94, 106–107.

National Women's Health. (1992). Osteoporosis update: New research findings. *National Women's Health Report, 14*(6), 7.

National Women's Health. (1993). Women at risk: Osteoporosis. *National Women's Health Report, 15*(4): 1–5.

Olson, E., Johnson, B., & Thompson, L. (1990). The hazards of immobility. *American Journal of Nursing, 90*(3), 43–44, 46–48.

Osterman, H. M. (1990). The aging foot. *Orthopedic Nursing, 9*(6): 43–47, 76.

Portenoy, R. K. (1993). Back pain in the elderly patient. *Hospital Practice, 28*(4), 81–85, 88–90, 92.

Sedlak, C. A. (1991). Assessment of the surgical adult orthopedic client with Down syndrome. *Orthopedic Nursing, 10*(50), 27–36.

Sonzogni, J. (1990). Why is this shoulder painful? *Emergency Medicine, 22*(2), 56–60.

Sordana, R. (1992). Nutritional management of osteoporosis. *Geriatric Nursing, 13*(6), 315–319.

Spellbring, A. M. (1992). Assessing elderly patients at high risks for falls: A rehabilitative study. *Journal of Nursing Care Quality, 6*(3), 30–35.

Spratt, K., Lehmann, T., Weinstein, J., & Sayre, H. (1990). A new approach to the low-back physical examination: Behavioral assessment of mechanical signs. *Spine, 15*(2), 96–102.

Nursing Care of Clients with Musculoskeletal Disorders

LEARNING OBJECTIVES

After completing this chapter, you will be able to

- Describe the pathophysiology of common musculoskeletal disorders.
- Relate the manifestations of musculoskeletal disorders to the pathophysiologic processes.
- Discuss nursing implications for medications prescribed for the client with musculoskeletal disorders.

- Provide appropriate nursing care for the client in the preoperative and postoperative phases of musculoskeletal surgery.
- Use the nursing process as a framework for providing individualized care to clients with musculoskeletal disorders.

The musculoskeletal system may be subjected to various metabolic, structural, neoplastic, and infectious disorders. When these problems occur, clients may experience impaired physical mobility, altered body image, discomfort or pain, and the inability to perform self-care. Some musculoskeletal conditions are chronic. Nursing care for chronic conditions is directed toward meeting physiologic needs, providing education, and ensuring psychologic support for the client and family. A holistic approach is essential when planning and implementing nursing care.

The Client with Osteoporosis

■ ■ ■

Osteoporosis, literally defined as "porous bones," is a metabolic bone disorder in which the rate of bone resorption (**osteoclastic** activity) is greater than the rate of bone formation (**osteoblastic** activity). This imbalance causes a severe reduction of bone mass, which, in turn, causes skeletal weakness and places the person at risk for bone fractures and other degenerative changes.

Osteoporosis can be classified as primary or secondary. *Primary osteoporosis,* the most common form of the disease, occurs with aging and is not associated with a pathologic process. *Secondary osteoporosis* results from certain medical disorders or long-term use of certain drugs.

Osteoporosis affects an estimated 25 million Americans and occurs six to eight times more frequently in women than in men (Liscum, 1992). It is estimated that osteoporosis affects about 14 million women in the United States; 70% of these women are older than 60 (Cohen, 1990). Overall, 85% of the female population develop osteoporosis (American Academy of Orthopaedic Surgeons, 1988).

An estimated $7 to $10 billion is spent annually for the treatment of fractures, many of which are associated with osteoporosis (Peck et al., 1988). These national expenditures include inpatient and outpatient medical services as

---

Risk Factors for Osteoporosis

■ ■ ■

Unmodifiable Risk Factors

- Increasing age
- Female gender
- Postmenopausal status
- Caucasian race

- Pale complexion, light hair and eyes
- Long-term gluco- corticoid therapy

Modifiable Risk Factors

- Calcium deficiency
- Estrogen deficiency
- Smoking

- High caffeine intake
- High alcohol intake
- Sedentary life-style

---

well as nursing home care. Both the costs and incidence of fractures will increase as life expectancy increases. The significance of these numbers can be better appreciated by noting that the lifetime risk of a hip fracture (15% in white women and 5% in men) is equivalent to a woman's combined lifetime risk of developing breast, uterine, or ovarian cancer and about the same as a man's lifetime risk of developing prostate cancer (Berg & Cassells, 1992).

Although the cause of osteoporosis remains unclear, several risk factors have been identified. These risk factors can be described as unmodifiable (those that cannot be altered) or modifiable (ones that can be altered); see the accompanying box.

Unmodifiable Risk Factors

Both men and women are susceptible to osteoporosis as they age because the osteoblasts and osteoclasts (see Chapter 35) undergo alterations that diminish their activity. Osteoporosis occurs in about one-fourth of all older adults; the incidence of the disease is greater in women than men (at least 5:1). The reason for this greater incidence is that women's total bone mass is 10% to 25% less than that of men. Also, as women age, the level of estrogen decreases. Estrogen promotes osteoblastic activity, thereby increasing the growth of new bone. In addition, estrogen stimulates the thyroid gland to secrete calcitonin, which suppresses osteoclastic activity and increases osteoblastic activity. When estrogen levels decrease, therefore, bone loss occurs.

Caucasians are at a higher risk for osteoporosis than African Americans, who have greater bone density. There is some evidence that pale complexion, thin skin, and light-colored hair and eyes indicate an increased risk of developing osteoporosis. There is also a great deal of evi-

dence supporting the theory that a person can have a genetic predisposition to osteoporosis (Evans, Marel, Lancaster, Kos, Evans, & Wong, 1988).

Clients who are on long-term glucocorticoid therapy are also at risk for developing osteoporosis. Glucocorticoid therapy creates anti-inflammatory effects that are helpful for clients with hypersensitivity and inflammatory reactions, but it also inhibits the formation of new bone and has a negative indirect effect on bone through its actions on the kidney and the intestine. The long-term use of glucocorticoids causes the kidneys to excrete calcium and decreases the absorption of calcium in the intestine (Bockman & Weinerman, 1990).

Modifiable Risk Factors

Modifiable risk factors result from behaviors that directly conflict with current prevention and treatment efforts. Calcium deficiency is one of the most important modifiable risk factors causing osteoporosis. Calcium is an essential ingredient in the process of bone formation and other significant body functions. When there is an insufficient intake of calcium in the diet, the body compensates by removing calcium from the skeleton, resulting in a weakening of bone tissue. Also, an increase in protein intake leads to additional losses of calcium through the kidneys; this process promotes additional **demineralization** of the bone.

Smoking increases the incidence of osteoporosis; women who smoke frequently experience an earlier menopause than nonsmoking women. High caffeine intake can also increase the risk of osteoporosis because caffeine has a diuretic effect that causes calcium to be excreted more rapidly. High alcohol intake has also been identified as a risk factor for osteoporosis. Alcohol affects bone metabolism by altering intestinal absorption of calcium and assimilation of calcium into the bone **matrix.**

Estrogen deficiency is usually assumed to be the result of menopause; however, there are other modifiable factors that cause estrogen deficiency and amenorrhea. Amenorrhea caused by excessive exercise, anorexia, or bulimia places the individual at risk for osteoporosis. When menses resume, the risk of osteoporosis is reduced.

Sedentary life-style is another modifiable risk factor that can cause osteoporosis. Weight-bearing exercise, such as walking, influences bone metabolism in several ways. The stress of this type of exercise causes an increase in blood flow to bones, which brings growth-producing nutrients to the cells. Walking causes an increase in osteoblast growth and activity. An increase in estrogen and a lowering of adrenal hormones have also been proved to cause new bone to form.

Over the course of their lives, women may lose onethird of their original bone mass, which forms the shafts of limb bones and constitutes up to 80% of the skeleton

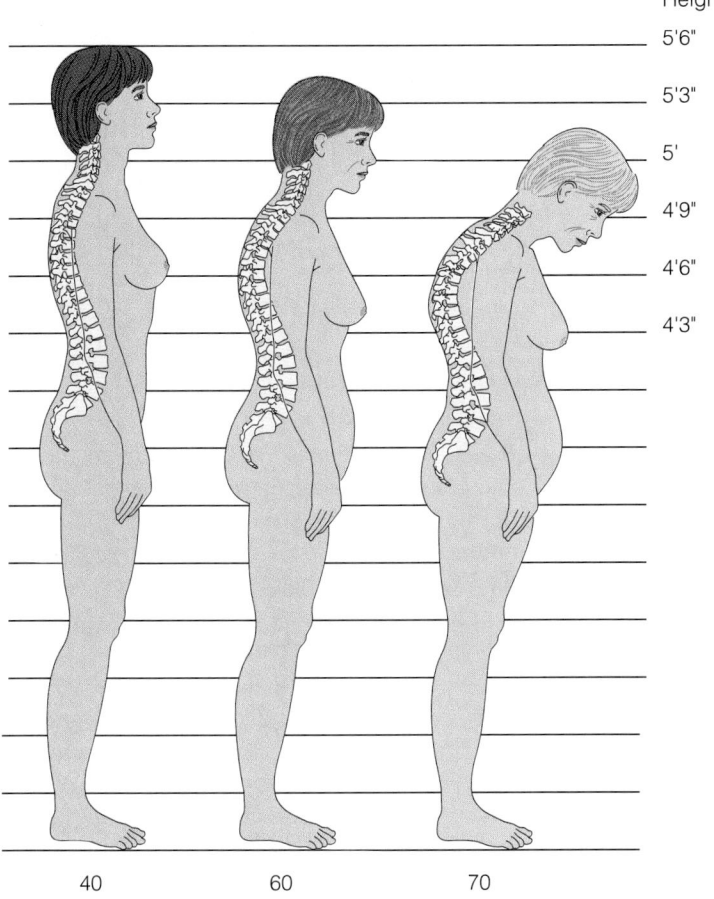

Height
5'6"
5'3"
5'
4'9"
4'6"
4'3"

Age   40   60   70

Figure 36-1   Spinal changes caused by osteoporosis. As the condition progresses, height can be reduced by as much as 7 inches. Increased flexion of the upper thoracic spine can result in "dowager's hump." The abdomen protrudes in an attempt to compensate by maintaining the center of gravity.

(Riggs & Melton, 1986). Because men's bone mass is 10% to 25% greater than that of women, age-related bone loss in men occurs 15 to 20 years later than in women and at a slower rate.

The loss of height due to compaction and degeneration of the vertebral discs in osteoporosis can be quite dramatic. The loss of 6 to 7 inches in height, as well as permanent flexion of the head and a protruding abdomen, can occur in clients with osteoporosis (Figure 36–1). There is also an increase of the flexion of the upper part of the thoracic spine, which is often referred to as a "dowager's hump." The abdomen usually protrudes as the body attempts to maintain its center of gravity.

The first indication of bone degeneration in the form of osteoporosis may be a report of low back pain or fractures of the forearm, hip, or spine. These three sites of fractures are most common because they contain more trabecular, or spongy, bone, which has more metabolic activity than cortical, or hard bone (Maher, Salmond, & Pellino, 1994).

There may be no obvious manifestations of osteoporosis until fractures occur. Some fractures are spontaneous, whereas others result from everyday activities. Most of the fractures related to osteoporosis, however, occur in con-

junction with falls (Berg & Cassels, 1992). Relatively few people are diagnosed in time for effective preventive therapy. See Chapter 37 for nursing care of the client with fractures.

Pathophysiology

The exact cause of osteoporosis is unknown. It is thought to result either from an increase in the activity of osteoclasts, whose function is to resorb bone, or from a loss of efficiency in osteoblasts, whose function is to form bones. As the person ages beyond 30, bone formation does not keep pace with resorption; the result is a reduction in bone mass and increased porosity of the skeleton (Cotran, Kumar, & Robbins, 1994). Whereas the normal bone formation cycle takes place over 4 months in a young adult, 2 years may be needed to complete the same cycle in the older adult (McCance & Huether, 1994). After age 25 or 30, loss of bone mass progressively increases to 0.5% each year; 1% or more is lost per year in menopausal women (Raisz, 1982).

Bone mineral density accounts for most of the strength of bone tissue; however, other skeletal factors are important. With increasing age, the body compensates for bone

---

Clinical Manifestations of Osteoporosis

■   ■   ■

- Loss of height
- Progressive curvature of the spine
- Low back pain
- Fractures of the forearm, hip, and spine

---

loss by increasing the diameter of the limb bones. This increase results in greater resistance to bending and twisting. However, this compensatory process is less marked at the ends of the limb bones and in the vertebrae; this is where the majority of fractures occur.

The most common clinical manifestations of osteoporosis are loss of height, progressive curvature of the spine, low back pain, and fractures of the forearm, hip, and spine (see the accompanying box). All of these conditions can also be attributed to the normal age-related changes of the musculoskeletal system, so further diagnostic studies are necessary to establish the diagnosis.

Fractures associated with osteoporosis may lead to disability and even death. The majority of people with hip fractures had been able to walk before the injury; however, only 50% of those individuals are able to walk again after the fracture (Miller, 1978). In addition, after age 75, the likelihood of death due to hip fracture increases, probably because many of these people have preexisting medical problems and experience other complications, such as pressure ulcers, pneumonia, or urinary tract infections. These problems complicate the rehabilitation posed by the fracture itself.

In contrast, reports of wrist fractures and spine fractures due to osteoporotic changes have not been shown to increase disability or mortality (Berg & Cassells, 1992). However, restricted activity, persistent pain, loss of function, neuropathies, posttraumatic arthritis, and posture changes due to these types of fractures may interfere with the person's activities of daily living (ADLs).

Collaborative Care

The care of the client with osteoporosis focuses on stopping or slowing the process, alleviating the symptoms, and preventing complications. The accompanying box describes the roles played by various members of the health care team in providing this care.

Laboratory and Diagnostic Tests

The manifestations of osteoporosis can mimic those of other bone disorders, so certain diagnostic tests are needed to differentiate osteoporosis from other problems. Formerly, it was impossible to diagnose osteoporosis early enough to prevent significant damage to the bone. Recent technologic advances, however, now permit early diagnosis of osteoporosis. Diagnostic tests include the following:

- *X-rays* provide a picture of skeletal structures; however, osteoporotic changes cannot be seen until over 30% of the bone mass has been lost (Maher et al., 1994).

- *Computed tomography (CT) scans* can be used to evaluate bone density.

- *Absorptiometry* is a newer radiographic technique to evaluate bone density.

- *Urinary hydroxyproline levels* provide an indication of bone resorption. A urine specimen is obtained after an overnight fast to determine the excretion of hydroxyproline. The total urinary hydroxyproline level is elevated in clients with osteoporosis; however, there are many other disease processes that also can cause elevated hydroxyproline excretion.

- *Serum bone Gla-protein,* also called *osteocalcin,* can be used as a marker of osteoclastic activity and therefore is an indicator of the rate of bone turnover. Serum bone Gla-protein tends to be elevated in clients who are actively losing bone mineral content.

- *Bone biopsy* may be performed when all of the above noninvasive measures have proven unreliable or when the client has not responded to treatment. A core of bone is removed from the anterosuperior iliac spine and is examined both biochemically and microscopically to determine the bone's structure and function. The sample provides important and useful information for proper management of osteoporosis as well as other bone disorders.

Pharmacology

Medications for osteoporosis include agents that block bone resorption, because there are no medications that can restore lost bone mass. Some commonly used medications are discussed in the accompanying box. Postmenopausal women and those who have had their ovaries removed have an estrogen deficiency, which results in bone loss and subsequent fractures. Therefore, hormonal replacement therapy is considered essential to preserve existing bone mass. Hormone replacement therapy is discussed in detail in Chapter 47.

Calcium supplements are frequently recommended because the average daily intake of calcium in the American woman is estimated to be about 500 mg, in contrast to the recommended levels of 800 to 1250 mg (Maher et al., 1994).

Calcium supplements are commercially available in many forms. A combination of vitamin D and a calcium

Collaborative Care: The Client with Osteoporosis

Health Care Team	Client-Centered Goals
Orthopedic physician	May be consulted if fractures occur and perform open or closed reduction as indicated.
Primary care physician	Manages health in both the inpatient and outpatient setting. Consults with orthopedist as needed. Evaluates osteoporosis with X-ray examinations, laboratory studies, and single-photon absorptiometry or CT scans. Orders calcium replacement, pain medications, and discusses the prevention of injury and further disability.
Social worker	Coordinates discharge referrals for home care and community-based services for nursing care, physical and occupational therapy. May need to coordinate continuing care in extended care facility.
Physical therapist	Assesses the client's rehabilitation potential. Develops and provides individualized physical therapy program. Teaches good body mechanics and strategies to prevent injury. Encourages walking program or daily regimen of weight-bearing exercises and muscle strengthening exercises. Makes recommendations about the use of assistive devices to prevent injuries.
Occupational therapist	Assesses client and plans interventions to assist the client to achieve maximum independence in self-care, work, and leisure activities. Assists client to modify activities to avoid strenuous lifting, sudden bending, or jarring motions.
Dietitian	Teaches the client about maintaining a well-balanced diet high in minerals and vitamins and avoiding caffeine and alcohol. Instructs client in strategies to increase dietary calcium.
RN and Health Care Team Communications	Discusses client's mobility and breathing problems with physician. Alerts physical and occupational therapist to mobility and self-care limitations. Discusses client's food likes and dislikes with dietitian and client's compliance with recommended calcium intake.

Nursing Implications for Pharmacology: The Client with Osteoporosis

ESTROGEN REPLACEMENT THERAPY

Esterified estrogen (Estratab, Menest)

Estradiol (Depogen, Estraderm)

Conjugated estrogens (Premarin)

Estrone (Aquest, Estrone-5, Femogen Forte)

Estrogens decrease osteoporosis, if they are taken with an adequate amount of calcium. Progestins are frequently given along with estrogens.

Nursing Responsibilities

- Review with client the anticipated benefits and possible side effects of estrogen replacement therapy.
- Caution patients taking estrogen to stop smoking; the risk of cardiovascular complications increases with amount of smoking (and age).

Client and Family Teaching

- Maintain the prescribed medication schedule. Withdrawal bleeding is normal and does not indicate return of fertility.

- If you miss a dose, take it as soon as you remember to do so, but do not double up to make up for missed doses.
- Perform breast self-examination every month, obtain a gynecologic examination every 6 months, and obtain a mammogram every year. If any abnormal vaginal bleeding occurs, notify the physician.
- If you are using a transdermal patch, apply it to clean, dry skin, preferably on the abdomen; press tightly about 10 seconds to get a good seal. Rotate sites so that at least 1 week elapses between applications to the same site.
- Estrogen decreases glucose tolerance; if you have diabetes, you may need a higher dose of hypoglycemic medication.

CALCIUM

Postmenopausal women, both those who do take replacement estrogens and those who do not, are encouraged to take calcium to prevent osteoporosis.

Pharmacology: The Client with Osteoporosis (continued)

Nursing Responsibilities

- Help clients maintain an adequate dietary intake of calcium. The best dietary source is milk and other dairy products, including yogurt.

- Postmenopausal women who take estrogens need the usual adult amount of calcium (1000 mg daily). Those who do not take estrogens need about 1500 mg daily to prevent or minimize osteoporosis.

- For clients who avoid or minimize the intake of dairy products because of the high caloric content, lactose intolerance, or vegetarian diet, identify alternate sources, such as skim milk and low-fat yogurt, oysters, canned sardines or salmon, beans, cauliflower, and dark-green leafy vegetables.

- Monitor for a history and ongoing presence of hypercalcemia or hypercalciuria.

Client and Family Teaching

- Take calcium carbonate in divided doses 30 to 60 minutes before meals to allow for absorption.

- Take calcium citrate with meals to minimize gastrointestinal distress.

CALCITONIN

Cibacalcin

Calcimar

Miacalin

In postmenopausal osteoporosis, calcitonin prevents further bone loss and increases bone mass if the client consumes adequate amounts of calcium and vitamin D.

Nursing Responsibilities

- Assess and record baseline data including renal function studies (BUN and serum creatinine) and serum electrolyte levels to detect adverse effects of calcitonin products.

- Review the client's medical history for existing or previous conditions that contraindicate use of calcitonin products: hypersensitivity to salmon calcitonin and lactation (calcitonin is secreted in breast milk and may inhibit lactation).

- Observe the client for side effects: nausea and vomiting, anorexia, mild transient flushing of the palms of the hands and the soles of the feet, and urinary frequency.

- Teach the client the proper technique for handling and injecting the drug at home.

Client and Family Teaching

- Take the medication in the evening to minimize side effects.

- Nausea and vomiting may occur during initial stages of therapy; they disappear as treatment continues.

- Continue taking the medication even when clinical symptoms have abated.

- While taking the medication, be sure to consume adequate amounts of calcium and vitamin D.

FLUORIDE

Fluoride is a mineral long recognized as essential for the normal formation of dentin and tooth enamel. Fluoride appears to decrease the solubility of bone mineral and therefore the rate of bone reabsorption. Its use in preventing and treating osteoporosis is relatively new but promising.

Nursing Responsibilities

- Assess and record baseline data to detect adverse effects of fluoride.

- Side effects include gastrointestinal upset and painful joints.

- Monitor serum fluoride levels every 3 months.

- Have bone mineral density studies conducted at 6-month intervals to document progress of bone growth.

- Do not administer oral doses of medication in the presence of dairy products; they impair absorption.

Client and Family Teaching

- Take sodium fluoride tablets after meals, and avoid milk or dairy products; these reduce gastrointestinal absorption of the medication.

- While taking fluoride, be sure to maintain an adequate calcium intake.

- Use fluoride mouth rinse immediately after brushing teeth and just before retiring at night. Do not swallow the rinse, and avoid eating or drinking for at least 30 minutes after use.

- Notify the physician if teeth become stained or mottled after repeated use of fluoride mouth rinse.

supplement is recommended, because vitamin D enhances the absorption of calcium (Einhorn, Levine, & Michel, 1990). This is very important for the older adult, whose skin is less able to synthesize vitamin D and whose intestine is less able to absorb vitamin D.

Calcitonin, which has been used for years to treat Paget's disease of bone, is now also used in treating osteoporosis. Calcitonin increases bone formation and decreases bone resorption. This medication may be used for women who are unable or unwilling to take estrogens; however, it is expensive and available only in parenteral form. Preliminary studies indicate that calcitonin in nasal spray form may be useful for treating osteoporosis.

Sodium fluoride in pill form has proved effective in the treatment of osteoporosis of the spine. Sodium fluoride enhances trabecular bone mass rather than cortical bone mass. However, the use of sodium fluoride remains controversial, and blood, urine, and bone density should be carefully monitored at regular intervals.

Nursing Care

Osteoporosis is both preventable and treatable; therefore, nursing care focuses primarily on planning and implementing interventions to prevent the disease itself, its manifestations, and the resulting injuries. An important aspect of preventing osteoporosis is educating clients under age 35. The accompanying box presents the findings of a research study that has implications for all nurses in promoting behaviors that prevent osteoporosis. Nursing management of clients who already have osteoporosis focuses on teaching about the disease process and helping maintain physical mobility, ingest nutritious meals, and solve problems associated with pain and injury.

Knowledge Deficit

Clients with osteoporosis must be taught about the common risk factors and how to modify them.

Nursing interventions with rationales follow:

- Teach school-age children the importance of calcium intake and weight-bearing exercises in building and maintaining strong bones. *Peak bone mass occurs around age 30. Children taught in early years can develop dietary and exercise habits that may prevent or delay the onset of osteoporosis.*

- Assess adolescents (especially females) for their exercise pattern, eating habits, and menstrual status. *Female gymnasts and dancers frequently consume a limited diet to remain in shape. They also have a vigorous exercise routine that may prevent the onset of menses. Female teenagers are also prone to develop bulimia. All of these factors lead to amenorrhea (resulting in lack of estrogen) and lack of calcium. Both of these factors make this age group susceptible to bone demineralization. Extensive*

Applying Research to Nursing Practice: Perceived Benefits of and Barriers to Osteoporosis Prevention

■ ■ ■

Researchers conducted a study to describe behaviors for preventing osteoporosis and to examine the perceived benefits of and barriers to performing them (Ali & Twibell, 1994). The study sample consisted of 100 Caucasian perimenopausal and elderly women. The behaviors reported were the use of dietary and supplemental calcium, exercise, and the use of estrogen replacement therapy. The investigators found that although the majority of the sample participated in regular exercise, most did not maintain an adequate daily intake of calcium and did not take estrogen replacement therapy. The researchers also concluded that perceived barriers influenced the subjects' failure to carry out these behaviors.

Implications for Nursing

The results of this study suggest that women are more likely to practice behaviors that help prevent osteoporosis if they are aware of the following:

- Age-related need for daily calcium intake and misconceptions about milk intake

- The risks, benefits, and duration of estrogen replacement therapy

- Benefits of exercise on bones and muscles

The investigators also recommended that nurses be aware that many older adults have limited incomes. It is therefore important that nurses provide information about less costly calcium-containing food products and estrogen products that delay or prevent osteoporosis.

Critical Thinking in Client Care

1. Identify 2 or 3 potential barriers in the female older adult for each of the following: exercise, calcium intake, and estrogen replacement therapy.

2. Discuss at least one nursing strategy for each barrier identified.

3. Develop an exercise program to reduce the risk of osteoporosis for a 72-year-old widow who lives alone in an unsafe neighborhood.

counseling may be necessary to help these clients balance their desire to remain thin and exercise with the body's physiologic need for adequate calcium to prevent bone loss.

■ Teach adults and older adults how to limit the severity of osteoporosis through diet, activity, and estrogen replacement therapy. *Food sources of calcium are believed to be more effectively absorbed and used by the body than most calcium supplements. Yogurt, low-fat cheeses, skim or low-fat milk, broccoli, collards, kale, and calcium-fortified orange juice are foods rich in calcium. The skeleton appears to benefit most from activities that resist the force of gravity. Walking, jogging, and using an exercise bike or mini trampoline can have a beneficial effect on bone density. Estrogen therapy is the only pharmacologic treatment approved by the Food and Drug Administration for the prevention of osteoporosis. Women who take estrogen have a lower risk of developing a postmenopausal bone fracture. Women should be encouraged to discuss the risks and benefits of estrogen with their physician. (Hormone replacement therapy is discussed in detail in Chapter 47.)*

■ Encourage clients not to smoke. *Smoking increases the incidence of osteoporosis. Women who smoke frequently experience an earlier menopause than women who do not smoke.*

■ Encourage clients to limit caffeine intake. *High caffeine intake increases the risk of osteoporosis because caffeine has a diuretic effect, causing calcium to be excreted more rapidly.*

■ Encourage clients to limit alcohol intake. *Alcohol affects bone metabolism by altering intestinal absorption of calcium and assimilation of calcium into the bone matrix.*

Impaired Physical Mobility

A major contributing factor in the development of osteoporosis is the lack of weight-bearing exercises. Age and the fear of falling also promote a sedentary life-style and, in turn, the risk of osteoporosis.

Nursing interventions with rationales follow:

■ Teach clients who are able to participate in weight-bearing exercises to perform exercises at least three times a week for a sustained period of 30 to 40 minutes. *The mechanical force of weight-bearing exercises promotes bone growth. Bones weaken and demineralize without exercise. Walking is an easy, low-impact form of exercise. Swimming (including walking on the bottom of the pool) does not provide the needed weight-bearing activity.*

■ Encourage older adults to use assistive devices to maintain independence in activities of daily living. *Walking sticks, canes, and other assistive devices encourage client independence and support activities that promote bone growth. A consultation with physical and occupational therapists is essential in helping the client maintain mobility and independence.*

■ Teach older clients about safety and fall precautions. *A simple assessment of the client's home for safety and fall risks may reduce the risk of fractures and, in turn, the cost of hospitalization and potential disability and/or death. The nurse is encouraged to read the many nursing research studies about preventing falls in both acute care and long-term care institutions.*

■ Evaluate and closely monitor the client's medications. *The reasons for, types of, and dosage of the client's medications should be evaluated, especially if the person has been falling frequently or has a change in mental status. Falls may be related to the number of both prescribed and over-the-counter medications the client is taking. Older adults may be taking as many as six to ten medications for their chronic diseases and other problems related to aging.*

Altered Nutrition: Less Than Body Requirements

Most Americans do not maintain the recommended daily intake of 1200 mg of calcium. Clients must therefore be made aware of the relationship between an adequate calcium intake and maintaining strong bones.

Nursing interventions with rationales follow:

■ Teach adolescents, pregnant or lactating women, and adults through the mid 30s to eat foods high in calcium, to maintain a daily calcium intake of 1200 mg. *The National Academy of Sciences (1989) recommends a daily calcium intake of 1200 mg, compared with the previous recommendation of 800 mg/day.*

■ Encourage postmenopausal women to maintain a calcium intake of 1500 mg daily, either through diet or a calcium supplement. *The National Academy of Sciences (1989) recommends a daily calcium intake of 1500 mg for postmenopausal women.*

■ Collaborate with the dietitian to help the client understand which foods and liquids prevent the absorption of calcium. *Diets high in caffeine, protein, fiber, sodium and carbohydrates diminish total body calcium stores and thus should be either avoided or ingested in low quantities.*

■ Provide current information regarding the absorption of supplemental calcium. *It is recommended that consumers test a calcium supplement by placing it in vinegar. If the supplement does not dissolve within 30 to 45 minutes, it is doubtful that the supplement will adequately dissolve in the client's stomach. Research indicates that brands of commercially available calcium supplements vary in their absorption rates (Carr & Shangraw, 1987).*

■ Teach clients taking calcium supplements the importance of taking the medication at the proper time and the side effects that may occur. *Free hydrochloric acid is needed for calcium absorption. Calcium carbonate supplement (e.g., Tums) should be taken 30 to 60 minutes before meals to allow adequate absorption. Calcium citrate sup-*

plements should be taken with meals to prevent gastrointestinal distress. All of the supplements should be taken in divided doses (two to three times daily) for improved distribution.

Pain

Advanced stages of osteoporosis can result in pain and immobilization. Acute pain usually results from a complicating fracture, especially a compression fracture of the vertebrae. Pain can be treated with many simple remedies so that the client can remain mobile.

Nursing interventions with rationales follow:

- Review activity tolerance and suggest modifications in exercise schedules as indicated. *Clients with osteoporosis should remain active and participate in weight-bearing exercises; however, the client's abilities and severity of the disease may warrant a modification in the exercise regimen.*

- Suggest anti-inflammatory pain medications for treatment of both acute and chronic phases of pain. *Continuous administration of ibuprofen or other nonsteroidal anti-inflammatory drugs (NSAIDs) can be useful to provide relief from pain. Clients should be instructed in the amount and frequency as noted on the manufacturer's labels.*

- Suggest the application of heat to relieve pain. *A heating pad may offer temporary pain relief. To avoid the "rebound effect," the heat should be removed every 20 to 30 minutes.*

Other Nursing Diagnoses

Examples of other nursing diagnoses that are appropriate for the client with osteoporosis follow:

- *Activity Intolerance* related to pain and impaired mobility
- *Anxiety* related to fear of fractures
- *Ineffective Individual Coping* related to alteration in body image and chronic disease progression
- *Sexual Dysfunction* related to back pain and deformity
- *Social Isolation* related to back pain, spinal deformity, and fear of falls
- *Constipation* related to inactivity and inadequate fluid intake
- *Ineffective Breathing Pattern* related to spinal deformities

Client and Family Teaching

As explained above, helping clients understand the risk factors for osteoporosis and ways to modify their behavior to lessen these risks or to decrease the progression of the disorder is a major part of nursing care.

Care of the Older Client

Of all the age-related changes that occur in the body, osteoporosis is one that is most likely to cause serious negative functional consequences. The older client may need a written handout that reinforces the importance of eating foods rich in calcium, taking adequate calcium supplements, and participating in weight-bearing exercises appropriate for their level of activity. Nurses may need to follow up on the suggested changes in the diet and exercise, because these changes may vary significantly from the client's lifelong habits. The older adult may also live alone, lack a family support system, and have reduced finances that influence compliance with the suggested changes.

Applying the Nursing Process

Case Study of a Client with Osteoporosis: Nancy Bauer

Nancy Bauer is a 53-year-old school teacher. She has been married for 36 years and has two children, ages 31 and 33. Mrs. Bauer says she is 65 inches tall. On inspection, it is noted she has a fair complexion and small bone structure. She has smoked 1 pack of cigarettes a day for 30 years and drinks 1 to 2 glasses of wine with dinner each evening. She does not routinely exercise. Mrs. Bauer has had symptoms of menopause for 8 years, including hot flashes in the early years and mood swings of late. She has never been on estrogen therapy.

Mrs. Bauer's mother died 1 year ago at age 78 after sustaining a hip fracture in a fall. Mrs. Bauer has a 60-year-old sister who was recently diagnosed with osteoporosis and who has had two vertebral compression fractures.

Mrs. Bauer is currently seeking medical advice for continuous low back pain. The pain is not relieved with an over-the-counter analgesic, and she frequently wakes up during the night because of the pain.

Assessment

The nurse practitioner notes that Mrs. Bauer's vital signs are all within normal limits. She has full range of motion of all extremities and is able to stand and bend over, but she reports discomfort when returning to the upright position. Mrs. Bauer has a slightly pronounced "hump" on her upper back and is 1 inch shorter than her stated height on admission. Her muscle strength is symmetric and strong.

Diagnosis

The nursing diagnoses for Mrs. Bauer include the following:

- *Pain* of the lower spine
- *Body Image Disturbance* related to curvature of the thoracic spine
- *Self-Care Deficit* related to knowledge deficit about osteoporosis and treatment to prevent further damage
- *Altered Nutrition: Less Than Body Requirements* related to inadequate intake of calcium
- *Risk for Injury* related to effects of change in bone structure secondary to osteoporosis

Expected Outcomes

The expected outcomes established in the plan of care specify that Mrs. Bauer will

- Experience a decrease in back pain.
- Have minimal anxiety about the effects of postural changes and be able to describe ways to treat her osteoporosis and prevent further complications.
- Verbalize an understanding of the current research and treatment regarding osteoporosis.
- Verbalize how cessation of smoking can help prevent further progression of osteoporosis.
- Seek consultation for self-administration of estrogen therapy as well as adequate intake of calcium and vitamin D.
- Maintain optimum physical activity to prevent complications of osteoporosis.
- Verbalize safety precautions to prevent fractures due to falls.

Planning and Implementation

The following interventions are planned and implemented in teaching Mrs. Bauer about the effects of osteoporosis:

- Teach the client about back-strengthening exercises.
- Enroll the client in an osteoporosis support group, if available, for psychosocial help in dealing with the effects of osteoporosis.
- Provide realistic, yet optimistic, feedback about loss of height and bone integrity and the potential outcomes of treatment.
- Assess the client's current knowledge base, and correct misconceptions regarding treatment of osteoporosis.
- Provide current educational literature regarding treatment of osteoporosis.
- Instruct the client in dietary and calcium supplements that help prevent effects of osteoporosis.
- Promote routine physical exercises that help prevent complications due to osteoporosis.
- Review safety and fall precautions, and provide literature regarding how to create a safe home environment.

Evaluation

On her return visit to the nurse practitioner 6 months later, Mrs. Bauer reports that she feels much better. She is no longer irritable and does not experience mood swings, because she is taking the prescribed estrogen replacements. She is also eating products rich in calcium and taking a daily supplement of calcium with vitamin D. Mrs. Bauer has reduced her wine intake to 1 glass in the evening and now drinks decaffeinated coffee and tea. She also states that since she stopped smoking, she has been walking 30 to 45 minutes every day and increasing her pace and distance.

Critical Thinking in the Nursing Process

1. What is the physiologic basis for Mrs. Bauer's decrease in height?
2. What is the rationale for stopping smoking and limiting caffeine and alcohol intake in the treatment of osteoporosis?
3. What foods would you encourage for clients at high risk for osteoporosis whose serum cholesterol and LDL/HDL ratios indicate a high risk for cardiovascular disease?
4. What physical activities would you consider beneficial in helping to prevent the effects of osteoporosis in the female client who is wheelchair-bound or has limited mobility?
5. Develop a care plan for Mrs. Bauer for the nursing diagnosis *Sleep Pattern Disturbance*.

The Client with Osteomalacia

■ ■ ■

Osteomalacia, often referred to as "softening of bones," is a metabolic bone disorder characterized by inadequate mineralization of bone matrix. Bone mineralization requires calcium and phosphorus. When there are inadequate amounts of calcium or phosphorus—or inadequate amounts of vitamin D to synthesize the calcium and phosphorus—the bone matrix is not mineralized and thus is unable to sustain weight-bearing. Marked deformities of weight-bearing bone and pathologic fractures therefore occur. Osteomalacia, which is frequently called the adult form of rickets, can be corrected with treatment.

Osteomalacia is a significant health problem in cultures whose diets tend to be deficient in calcium and vitamin D. Women in northern China, Japan, and northern India have a higher incidence of the disorder than men because of the combined effects of pregnancy, lactation, and more indoor confinement (Porth, 1994).

Osteomalacia has been almost nonexistent in the United States because many foods are fortified with vitamin D, but its incidence is increasing among older adults, very-low-birth-weight infants, and people who adhere to strict vegetarian diets (McCance & Huether, 1994).

The most common causes of osteomalacia in the United States are summarized in the accompanying box. The primary causes of osteomalacia are vitamin D deficiencies and poor phosphate metabolism. Other causes include long-term administration of medications that increase the degradation of vitamin D and diseases that impair intestinal absorption of calcium and phosphorus.

The major risk factors for vitamin D deficiency are a diet low in vitamin D, decreased endogenous production of vitamin D, intestinal malabsorption of vitamin D, renal tubular diseases, and long-term use of anticonvulsant drugs, such as phenytoin and phenobarbital (McCance & Huether, 1994). Other risk factors include gastrectomy (removal of the major portion of the stomach due to cancer or complications of ulcers), pancreatic insufficiency and hepatobiliary disorders (chronic biliary obstruction and cirrhosis), chronic renal disorders, and hyperparathyroidism.

In a majority of the gastrointestinal disorders, mucosal disruption caused by gastric or intestinal resection or intestinal disease hampers the transport of digested nutrients; vitamin D and calcium absorption are disrupted and lost through fecal elimination. Liver disease interferes with the metabolism of vitamin D, and diseases of the pancreas and biliary system cause a deficiency in bile salts, which are necessary for normal intestinal absorption of vitamin D (McCance & Huether, 1994).

Chronic renal failure frequently alters calcium and phosphate metabolism. As the serum phosphorous levels rise and calcium levels decrease, the release of parathyroid hormone is increased. This increase of hormone in turn stimulates the mobilization of calcium and phosphorus from the bones, thus demineralizing the bone matrix.

It is believed that long-term anticonvulsant therapy (e.g., phenobarbital and phenytoin) results in vitamin D deficiency. These drugs interfere with calcium absorption in the intestine and vitamin D metabolism in the liver. However, the exact mechanism of this interaction is not completely understood.

Pathophysiology

As stated above, the two main causes of osteomalacia are (1) insufficient calcium absorption in the intestine due to a lack of calcium or resistance to the action of vitamin D and (2) increased losses of phosphorus through the urine (Porth, 1994). In its natural form, vitamin D is obtained from certain foods and ultraviolet radiation of the sun. The function of vitamin D is to maintain adequate serum levels of calcium and phosphate for normal mineralization of the bone. A deficiency in vitamin D intake or resistance to its action disrupts the normal mineralization of the bone, which, in turn, causes softening of the bone.

Causes of Osteomalacia According to Pathophysiologic Mechanisms

■ ■ ■

Inadequate Synthesis and Dietary Lack of Vitamin D

- Dark-skinned individuals
- Inadequate exposure to sunlight
- Malnutrition
- Low-birth-weight infants
- Use of foods not fortified with vitamin D

Malabsorption of Fats

- Extrahepatic biliary tract obstruction
- Pancreatic insufficiency
- Celiac sprue
- Extensive small bowel disease (e.g., regional enteritis), gastrectomy

Inadequate Metabolism of Vitamin D

- Diffuse liver disease (e.g., cirrhosis)
- Chronic renal failure
- Long-term use of anticonvulsant drugs (phenytoin, phenobarbital) and rifampin
- Chronic use of antacids (e.g., Maalox, Mylanta) that bind to phosphate and interfere with vitamin D absorption

---

Vitamin D is inactive when it is absorbed from the intestine or synthesized from exposure to ultraviolet light. In order for vitamin D, a fat-soluble vitamin, to become active, a two-step process must occur. Vitamin D (and its metabolites) is transported in the blood to the liver, where it is converted to calcidiol. Calcidiol is then transported to the kidney and transformed to an active form, calcitriol.

The active form of vitamin D is needed for optimal absorption of calcium and phosphorus from the intestine. Calcium and phosphorus are transported in the blood to the bones for normal mineralization. If there is a lack of vitamin D, calcium and phosphorus are not absorbed from the intestine, and serum calcium and phosphorus levels therefore fall. A deficiency in these minerals in turn activates the parathyroid glands, thus causing mobilization of calcium and phosphorus from bone. The continued loss of concentration of calcium and phosphate in the bone disrupts bone mineralization and deprives the bone matrix of minerals.

Clinical Manifestations of Osteomalacia

■ ■ ■

- Bone pain: May be vague and generalized at first, becoming more intense with activity as the disease progresses; occurs most frequently in the pelvis, long bones of the extremities, spine, and ribs.
- Difficulty changing from lying to sitting position, sitting to standing position, and so on.
- Muscle weakness: Frequently an early sign in severe cases.
- Waddling gait: May be due to pain and muscle weakness.
- Dorsal kyphosis: May occur in severe cases.
- Pathologic fractures

Impairment of bone mineralization causes abnormalities in both spongy and compact bone. The **osteoid** (the soft, noncalcified part of the matrix) continues to be produced but is not mineralized. Ultimately, this abnormal buildup of demineralized bone leads to gross deformities of the long bones, spine, pelvis, and skull, because the bone is soft and unable to bear the weight and stress of body movement.

The clinical manifestations of osteomalacia include bone pain and tenderness (see the accompanying box). As the disease progresses, fractures occur (Porth, 1994). In contrast to osteoporosis, osteomalacia is not associated with a significant occurrence of hip fractures. Instead, pathologic fractures occur in the commonly weakened areas (e.g., distal radius and proximal femur).

Collaborative Care

Osteomalacia is a reversible condition. Once the specific cause is determined, appropriate therapy will correct the disorder. Osteomalacia may be difficult to differentiate from osteoporosis because the manifestations are very similar. Muscle weakness and bone pain, which are common manifestations of osteomalacia, may be also associated with arthritis or rheumatism. However, there are certain laboratory and diagnostic tests that can help pinpoint the diagnosis of osteomalacia.

Laboratory and Diagnostic Tests

In adults, laboratory evaluation and radiologic evidence of osteomalacia are often subtle; therefore, a clinical diagnosis is difficult. A history of inadequate dietary intake, renal failure, or some malabsorption states may suggest osteomalacia. Table 36–1 compares the laboratory and diagnostic findings of osteomalacia with those of osteoporosis and Paget's disease of bone. (Paget's disease is discussed later in this chapter). Laboratory and diagnostic tests for osteomalacia include the following:

- *X-ray examinations* demonstrate the effects of generalized bone demineralization, that is, trabecular bone loss, cyst formation, compression fractures, bowing and bending deformities of the long bones, and osteoid deposits, particularly in the vertebral bodies and pelvis. Looser's zones, known as pseudofractures or milkman's fractures, may be present. These are radiolucent narrow bands that lie either at right angles or obliquely to the cortical outlines of bones and often transect them (Cotran et al., 1994). These bands are frequently found on the femoral neck, pubic rami, ribs, clavicles, and lateral aspects of the scapulae (Pitt, 1991).
- *Serum calcium level* usually remains unchanged until osteomalacia becomes severe or late in its course. Hypocalcemia may indicate intestinal malabsorption of calcium or an impairment in the action of parathyroid hormone in maintaining bone calcium levels.
- *Serum phosphorus level* is usually evaluated when the serum calcium level is low (Corbett, 1992). Like calcium, phosphorus is controlled by the parathyroid hormone. A low or normal level of phosphorus may be present in the client with osteomalacia.
- *Serum parathyroid hormone* is frequently elevated as a compensatory response to hypocalcemia in clients with renal failure or vitamin D deficiency.
- *Serum alkaline phosphatase level* is decreased in malnourished adults, whereas a client who has liver or biliary tract dysfunction exhibits an increased level.

Pharmacology

Therapeutic management of osteomalacia depends on the cause of the vitamin D deficiency; however, vitamin D supplementation is very easy, and the client shows dramatic response in a few months (see the accompanying box). Calcium and phosphorus supplements may also be prescribed. Ultraviolet irradiation may be an adjunct therapy.

Nursing Care

Managing the client with osteomalacia includes assessing the client's current dietary intake of calcium and phosphorus and exposure to ultraviolet light and treating bone pain and tenderness, fractures, and muscle weakness. Nursing interventions for the client with osteomalacia focus on maintaining adequate nutrition, minimizing risk

Table 36–1 Differential Features of Osteoporosis, Osteomalacia, and Paget's Disease

Differentiating Features	Osteoporosis	Osteomalacia	Paget's Disease
Pathophysiology	Resorption greater than bone formation	Inadequate mineralization of bone matrix, due primarily to deficiency of vitamin D	Excessive osteoclastic activity and formation of poor-quality bone
Calcium level (serum)	Normal	Low or normal	Normal or elevated (especially in immobilized clients)
Phosphate level (serum)	Normal	Low or normal	Normal
Parathyroid hormone level (serum)	Normal	High or normal	Normal
Alkaline phosphatase level (serum)	Normal	Decreased in malnutrition, increased in liver disease	Increased; not a reliable test for clients who have liver disease or are pregnant
Hydroxyproline (urine)	Not applicable	Not applicable	Increased
Radiographic findings	Osteopenia, fractures	Pseudofractures, Looser's transformation zones, or milkman's fractures	"Punched-out" appearance of bone, increase in bone thickness, linear fractures, mosaic pattern of bone matrix

Nursing Implications for Pharmacology: The Client with Osteomalacia

VITAMIN D

The main action of vitamin D is to raise serum calcium levels by increasing intestinal absorption of dietary calcium and mobilizing calcium from the bone.

Nursing Responsibilities

- Assess and record baseline data, including serum electrolytes, and renal and liver function studies to detect adverse effects of vitamin D.

- Ensure that the client's diet is critically evaluated before vitamin D supplementation is initiated. Clients who eat fortified foods and receive normal exposure to sunlight may not need supplements.

- When supplements are given, observe the client for excessive accumulation of vitamin D, which produces manifestations of hypercalcemia.

Client and Family Teaching

- Keep the drug in a cool, dark place to ensure its stability.

- Discontinue the drug and notify physician if manifestations of hypervitaminosis D appear.

- Avoid excessive or indiscriminate use of vitamin D.

- Dosage levels will be adjusted as the deficiency abates.

- Improvement may develop slowly (over 7 to 10 days), and effects may persist for up to 30 days after therapy is terminated.

for injury and pain, promoting physical mobility, and providing information about the disorder.

Altered Nutrition: Less Than Body Requirements

Nursing actions focus on teaching the client about diet-related causes and treatment of osteomalacia.

Nursing interventions with rationales follow:

- Review with the client the dietary sources of calcium, phosphorus, and vitamin D. *Clients who have osteomalacia or may be prone to bone demineralization problems due to gastrointestinal or renal problems should be instructed to increase their intake of foods rich in vitamin D, calcium, and phosphorus. Coordination with a nutritionist may be necessary for in-depth dietary counseling.*

- Provide consultation with appropriate specialists, especially the dietitian and gastroenterologist. *Consultants are frequently necessary to inform the client about current, research-based treatment modalities that may not be familiar to nurses in general practice.*

- Teach clients about foods fortified with vitamin D. *An awareness of vitamin D-fortified foods and their costs encourages the client to include them in the diet.*

Risk for Injury and Pain

In the client with osteomalacia, the skeleton's inability to tolerate stress or weight-bearing increases the risk of traumatic injuries.

Nursing interventions with rationales follow:

- Evaluate the home setting of clients with a high risk of fractures. *The client's home should be evaluated for the presence of hazards. For example, the use of throw rugs should be discouraged, adequate lighting ensured, and extension cords properly placed or eliminated. The older person's vision should also be evaluated. Because Medicare does not provide coverage for an eye examination or a necessary new eyeglass prescription, older adults may be hesitant to give this recommendation a priority.*

- Document the client's use of analgesics. *The client's use of prescribed medications and over-the-counter self-administered medications should be evaluated by the primary caregiver. It is estimated that older adults in the community setting take an average of 8 to 11 prescribed medications daily. Therefore, the addition of over-the-counter analgesics should be closely monitored and evaluated prior to suggested treatment.*

- Teach the client safety measures and ways to acquire safety aids for home. *The use of grab bars and elevated toilet seats are just a few devices that should be encouraged.*

- Consult with physical therapist regarding use of ambulatory or gait devices. *Ambulatory aids (e.g., canes or walkers) should be evaluated for safe use. Canes should have rubber tips with sufficient tread. Instructions on the proper use of canes and walkers should be routinely reviewed and monitored. The nurse may consult a physical therapist to assist in this review.*

Impaired Physical Mobility

Muscle weakness may impair the physical mobility of the client with osteomalacia.

Nursing interventions with rationales follow:

- Instruct client to space activities to conserve energy. *Spacing activities allows clients to participate in many activities of daily living, which may increase self-esteem and participation in self-care and recreational activities.*

- Instruct client to use ambulatory or gait devices. *Ambulatory aids, such as walkers or canes, provide mobility in the client whose muscles are weak.*

Knowledge Deficit

The client with osteomalacia requires information about the various treatment methods that will be employed.

Nursing interventions with rationales follow:

- Encourage homebound and institutionalized clients to get brief exposure to the sun. *Extensive exposure to ultraviolet light can have deleterious effects. Instruct clients to use sunscreen, wear sunglasses to protect the eyes, and increase their exposure gradually. Older adults who are homebound or institutionalized can seek out a sunny area of the home or long-term care agency.*

- Instruct clients taking large doses of vitamin D about the potentially toxic effect of hypercalcemia. *Vitamin D supplementation can result in hypercalcemia. When vitamin D is prescribed and consistently taken, calcium and phosphorus are absorbed in the liver and kidneys and distributed throughout the body. Clients taking this fat-soluble vitamin should be advised to consult with their physician and continue follow-up appointments and necessary laboratory evaluation.*

- Instruct older adults to monitor their intake of fat while taking vitamin D. *In older adults, an increase of fat intake may reduce the distribution of vitamin D; as a result, osteomalacia may not be reversed in a timely fashion.*

Other Nursing Diagnoses

Examples of other nursing diagnoses that are appropriate for the client with osteomalacia follow:

- *Noncompliance* with exercise regimen and participation in treatment due to fatigability and depression

- *Impaired Physical Mobility* related to limited range of motion secondary to skeletal changes

- *Fear* related to unpredictable nature of chronic condition.

Client and Family Teaching

Client and family teaching for the client with osteomalacia focuses on meeting needs related to the cause and treatment of the disorder. These include diet and nutritional supplementation, safety concerns, mobility considerations, and support systems. Consultations with dietitians, gastroenterologists, and other members of the health care team are often required.

Care of the Older Client

The most common cause of osteomalacia in the older adult is vitamin D deficiency. Therefore, emphasize the importance of getting sun exposure for at least 5 minutes weekly, even in the summer and winter. Encourage the older adult to eat foods high in calcium and vitamin D, including milk and dairy products (e.g., ice cream or ice milk, yogurt, and cheese). Also encourage the older client to perform appropriate exercises on a regular basis (at least 3 times a week for 20 to 30 minutes).

The Client with Paget's Disease

■ ■ ■

Paget's disease of bone, also called osteitis deformans, is not a true metabolic disease, but rather a skeletal disorder that results from excessive osteoclastic activity. Paget's disease is characterized by bone deformity, especially of the long bones of the lower limbs, the pelvis, the lumbar vertebrae, and the skull. It is differentiated from osteoporosis (in which the rate of resorption is greater than that of bone formation) and osteomalacia (which is caused by inadequate mineralization of bone matrix, usually due to deficiency of vitamin D).

Paget's disease usually follows a two-stage process: an excessive amount of osteoclastic bone resorption, followed by excessive osteoblastic bone formation. The bone is at first hyperemic and soft, and bowing occurs. When this excessive bone cell activity decreases, the result is a gain in bone mass; however, the newly formed bone becomes hard and brittle. This brittleness may lead to fractures.

As with osteoporosis and osteomalacia, clients may not realize they have the disease until some sort of trauma occurs and X-ray studies taken to determine the effect of the injury demonstrate the characteristic changes of the disease.

Paget's disease is one of the most common chronic diseases of the skeleton (Eisenberg & Dennis, 1990). About 3% of the population over age 40 are affected, and the incidence increases to 10% in those over age 70 (Singer, 1987). Paget's disease occurs more frequently in whites in continental Europe, England, Australia, New Zealand, and North America. It has a familial tendency and is slightly more common in men than in women (ratio of 3:2) (Maher et al., 1994, p. 487).

The cause of Paget's disease is unknown; however, several theories have been proposed over the years, including a disorder of hormonal imbalance, vascular disorder, neoplasm, autoimmune disorder, and inborn error of connective tissue (Singer, 1994). A theory many hold is that the disease is caused by a viral infection. According to this thoery, osteoclastic capability contracted in young adulthood manifests itself 20 to 40 years later. Researchers have found respiratory and measles virus antigens in the osteoclasts of bone specimens removed from clients with the diagnosis of Paget's disease (Mills, Singer, Weiner, Suffin, Stabile, & Holst, 1984; Basle, Fournier, Rozenblatt, Rebel, & Bouteille, 1986).

Pathophysiology

In the initial phase of Paget's disease, there is an abnormal increase in osteoclasts. Resorption of spongy bone, or **cancellous bone,** occurs rapidly. As new bone tissue tries to replace the loss, fibrous tissue forms in the bone **marrow.** Heavy blue lines outline the disorganized fibrous tissue, creating a hallmark mosaic pattern in the mature (lamellar) bone that is visible both under a microscope and in radiographic studies. Histologically, these Paget's lesions also show increased vascularity and bone marrow fibrosis with intense cellular activity (Porth, 1994).

During the initial stage, the bones actually increase in size and thickness because of the acceleration in bone resorption and regeneration. The result is a thick layer of coarse bone with a rough and pitted outer surface that resembles pumice (Porth, 1994). Eventually, Paget's disease progresses to an inactive phase in which abnormal remodeling is minimal or absent. The disease varies in severity and may be present long before clinical evidence appears.

Most clients with Paget's disease are asymptomatic. Clinical manifestations are often vague and depend on the specific area involved (see the box on page 1528). The most common complaint is localized pain of the commonly affected bones, that is, long bones, spine, pelvis, and cranium (Cotran et al., 1994). The pain is described as a mild to moderate deep ache that is aggravated by pressure and weight-bearing. It is more noticeable at night or when the client is resting. The pain usually is due to metabolic bone activity, secondary degenerative osteoarthritis, fractures, or nerve impingement. Because of the increase in blood flow to pagetic bone, flushing and warmth of the overlying skin may be apparent.

Because of the overworked heart's attempts to pump more blood through the increased mass of blood vessels in active pagetic bone, the client with compromised cardiac conditions may develop complications, such as congestive heart failure. Other cardiovascular abnormalities that may be associated with Paget's disease include hypertension, arteriosclerosis, and systolic ejection murmurs (Maher et al., 1994).

Both benign and malignant bone tumors have been reported in a small percentage of clients with severe Paget's disease. These tumors arise in the same bones that are affected by Paget's disease, that is, the long bones, pelvis, skull, and spine. The most serious complication is the development of sarcoma. This life-threatening tumor occurs in approximately 5% to 10% of client's with severe Paget's disease. Bone tumors are discussed in detail later in this chapter.

Paget's disease is usually not a serious or life-threatening disease, provided that no malignant bone tumor is present. Most clients have mild symptoms that readily respond to medication.

Clinical Manifestations of Paget's Disease

Musculoskeletal Effects

- Pain (in the long bones of lower extremities or joints)
- Deformity (enlargement of skull, bowing of lower extremities, and deformity of elbows and knees)
- Chalkstick-type fractures of lower extremities
- Pathologic fractures (especially of the tibia)
- Compression fractures
- Collapse of the vertebrae, resulting in kyphosis and loss of height
- Muscle weakness

Neurologic Effects

- Hearing loss
- Spinal cord injuries
- Dementia
- Pain from spinal stenosis
- Bladder and/or bowel dysfunction

Cardiovascular Effects

- High cardiac output
- Congestive heart failure
- Increased skin temperature over affected extremities

Metabolic Effects

- Symptoms of hypercalcemia in immobilized clients
- Hypercalciuria and renal calculi

Collaborative Care

Care of the client with Paget's disease focuses on relieving pain, suppressing bone cell activity if necessary, and preventing or minimizing the effects of complications. Many clients with Paget's disease are asymptomatic and do not require treatment. For more severely affected clients, pharmacologic agents are usually effective. Occasionally, surgery may be required.

Laboratory and Diagnostic Tests

Many of the laboratory and diagnostic tests that are useful for the diagnosis of osteoporosis and osteomalacia are equally useful for clients with Paget's disease (see Table 36–1). These include the following:

- *X-rays.* In the early phase of the disease, detectable localized areas of demineralization create "punched out" areas that lend a coarse, irregular appearance to the bone. In the later phase, X-rays show enlargement of the bones, tiny cracks in the long bones, and/or bowing of the weight-bearing bones.

- *Bone scan.* A radioactive isotope with an affinity for bone is injected into the client's bloodstream. Areas of active Paget's disease tend to absorb most of the isotope. An inactive lesion in the later stages of Paget's disease will not show affinity for the isotope.

- *CT scans and magnetic resonance imaging (MRI).* These techniques can help identify possible causes of the client's pain, including degenerative problems, spinal stenosis, or nerve root impingement.

- *Serum alkaline phosphatase.* This is the most frequently used laboratory test for Paget's disease. Alkaline phosphatase is an enzyme located in the plasma membrane of osteoblasts. If a client with untreated Paget's disease has a series of serum alkaline phosphatase determinations, a steady rise of the phosphatase can be expected as the disease progresses; the serum alkaline phosphatase level (30 to 115 IU/L) may be elevated from a high normal to over 3000 IU/L (Wallach, 1982).

- *Urinary hydroxyproline.* Hydroxyproline is an amino acid present in clients with Paget's disease. It is released from the skeleton and excreted in the urine. A normal urinary hydroxyproline level is 26 to 65 mg/day; in Paget's disease, the level can range from high normal to over 700 mg/day (Wallach, 1982).

- *Urinary collagen pyridinoline.* A newly developed test, urinary collagen pyridinoline testing is a more reliable diagnostic measure than hydroxyproline because it is a more sensitive indicator of the rate of bone resorption (Ubelhart, Gineyts, Chapuy, & Delmas, 1990).

- *Bone biopsy.* A bone biopsy may be performed to differentiate Paget's disease from other problems, such as osteoporosis or osteomalacia.

Pharmacology

Clients who have mild symptoms often find relief using analgesics and nonsteroidal anti-inflammatory drugs (NSAIDs), such as ibuprofen (Motrin) and indomethacin (Indocin). Clients who are experiencing manifestations and whose diagnostic test results are elevated are usually treated with one of the following agents: salmon calcitonin, human calcitonin, or disodium etidronate (Singer, 1994). See the accompanying box.

Calcitonin is the preferred medication for Paget's disease because it inhibits osteoclastic resorption of bone. It also works as an analgesic for bone pain. There are two

Nursing Implications for Pharmacology: The Client with Paget's Disease

Medications used for calcium replacement in osteoporosis, calcitonin in particular, may also be prescribed for clients with Paget's disease. Other medications for Paget's disease (etidronate disodium and plicamycin) are discussed here.

ETIDRONATE DISODIUM (DIDRONEL)

Etidronate disodium is a calcium regulator that acts primarily on the bone to slow the accelerated bone turnover of Paget's disease. Bone pain is relieved, and the incidence of pathologic fractures may be reduced. Cardiac and vascular manifestations of the disease also improve.

Nursing Responsibilities

- Common side effects include nausea, altered taste, and loose stools. Significant adverse reactions include increased bone pain at previously asymptomatic sites, rash, pruritus, and electrolyte abnormalities.

- Monitor the client's renal status prior to and during treatment. Etidronate disodium is contraindicated if the serum creatinine drops below 5 mg/dL.

- Administer the drug with fruit juice or water 2 hours before meals. If gastrointestinal upset occurs, divide into two equal doses.

- Do not administer foods high in calcium, vitamins with mineral supplements, or antacids high in metals within 2 hours of doses.

- Provide easy access to bathroom facilities and small, frequent meals if gastrointestinal upset occurs.

- Expect the drug to be discontinued if a fracture occurs. It will be resumed only after the fracture heals completely.

Client and Family Teaching

- Food impairs the absorption of etidronate disodium. Take the medication on an empty stomach, 2 hours before meals, unless gastrointestinal distress is extreme.

- Expect the response to this medication to be gradual and to continue for months after the drug is stopped.

- Dosage is usually increased cautiously. If discontinued, treatment usually is not reinstituted until there is clear evidence of disease recurrence, and only after at least 3 drug-free months have elapsed.

- Maintain adequate intake of calcium and vitamin D through dietary sources, calcium supplementation, or both.

PLICAMYCIN (MITHRACIN)

Plicamycin is an antibiotic used to treat clients with Paget's disease whose condition is not responsive to conventional therapy. It is administered by intravenous infusion and has serious side effects.

Nursing Responsibilities

- This medication is to be administered only under the supervision of a physician familiar with its use.

- Assess platelet count, prothrombin time, and bleeding time prior to and frequently during administration of this drug. Plicamycin is contraindicated for use in clients with bleeding disorders as it may cause significant bleeding tendencies.

- Assess the client frequently for evidence of bleeding (epistaxis, bruising, bleeding gums, joint pain, petechiae); guaiac all stools. Stop the drug immediately and notify the physician if bleeding occurs.

- Assess the CBC, liver function studies (bilirubin, AST, ALT, LDH, serum albumin), and renal function studies (BUN and serum creatinine) prior to and frequently during administration of this medication.

- Administer the drug diluted in one liter of 5% dextrose in water or normal saline by slow intravenous infusion over 4 to 6 hours.

- Assess the injection site frequently during infusion for evidence of infiltration. Discontinue the infusion and restart at another site if infiltration occurs.

Client and Family Teaching

- Notify your physician immediately if you think you are pregnant. This drug may harm the fetus. Use effective methods of birth control while taking this medication.

- Notify your physician immediately should you develop a nosebleed or other evidence of bleeding.

derivatives of this medication: salmon (fish) and human. Salmon calcitonin (Calcimar) is generally preferred because it is inexpensive and widely available. Human calcitonin (Cibacalcin) is derived from human thyroid glands, which makes it more expensive and difficult to obtain.

Some clients are hypersensitive to salmon calcitonin; thus, skin testing is necessary prior to its use. In clients who are hypersensitive to the drug, a local inflammatory response occurs at the intradermal test site within 15 minutes. These clients should receive human calcitonin. Occasionally, some clients develop a resistance to calcitonin. In this event, a "drug holiday" is prescribed, usually for 6 months to a year, after which calcitonin therapy is resumed.

Diphosphonates are a second category of agents used in the treatment of Paget's disease. Disodium etidronate (EHDP, Didronel) blocks bone resorption and formation by coating the bone surfaces with a slippery, soaplike substance (Maher et al., 1994). These medications are available in an easy-to-administer oral form. Diphosphonates are useful in treating clients who have developed resistance to calcitonin. To reduce immediate side effects of etidronate disodium, such as nausea and vomiting, the client should take medication on an empty stomach and refrain from eating for 90 minutes.

Because it inhibits bone formation, etidronate disodium is usually not prescribed for immobilized clients or for clients with fractures. Clients should not take this drug for longer than 6 months. Prolonged use or large doses may cause osteomalacia and pathologic fractures.

A toxic cancer medication, plicamycin (Mithracin), is occasionally used for the treatment of Paget's disease. Like other cytotoxic (cell-destroying) medications, plicamycin has limited use because it is toxic to the liver, kidneys, and bone marrow. Therefore, the use of this medication is reserved for clients who fail to respond to other medications or the uncommon young Paget's client who may respond well to aggressive therapy when a long-term remission is desired.

Surgery

Total hip or knee replacement is usually required when the client with Paget's disease develops degenerative arthritis of the hip or knee. These surgical procedures are usually performed to address severe pain during weight bearing and impaired mobility (see Chapter 38). Neurologic manifestations related to spinal stenosis or nerve root compression may also require surgery. Spinal surgery is discussed later in this chapter.

Nursing Care

The nursing interventions for the client with symptomatic Paget's disease focus on pain control, prevention of injury or fractures, and education regarding the disease process and prescribed therapies.

Pain

The most common symptom of Paget's disease is bone pain. This usually is the manifestation that prompts the client to seek health care.

Nursing interventions with rationales follow:

- Assess the location and extent of client's pain to determine the bone areas involved. *Bone pain in Paget's disease is poorly localized and is frequently described as "aching and deep." Radiographic studies can help pinpoint the location of the client's pain.*

- Administer pain medications to keep the client comfortable prior to both activity and rest periods. *Pain is most noticeable at night or when the client is resting. The pain can become evident when it is aggravated by pressure and weight-bearing.*

- Ensure correct placement of prescribed brace or corset. *The client may be required to wear a light brace or corset to relive back pain and provide support when the client assumes an upright position. The client may need instruction in the correct application of the device and in the evaluation of pressure areas that may result from wearing the device.*

- Provide heat therapy and massage. *Heat therapy and massage can alleviate mild discomfort. Care should be taken when applying massage over areas prone to pathologic fractures.*

- Teach the client to take pain medications as prescribed. *Clients who are not receiving calcitonin and/or etidronate may need instruction regarding simple analgesics or anti-inflammatory medications. Clients should take over-the-counter medications only as recommended.*

Impaired Physical Mobility

Like clients with osteoporosis and osteomalacia, clients with Paget's disease need to maintain or improve mobility so that they can perform necessary self-care activities and prevent complications of immobility.

Nursing interventions with rationales follow:

- Provide an assistive device when the client ambulates. *During the active phase of Paget's disease, the client is prone to fractures. Bone deformities, activity intolerance, fear of falling, and pain are all factors that may make the client more prone to falls. An assistive device can provide both physical and psychologic support during ambulation, permit the client to ambulate further, and provide a device for resting during the ambulation session.*

- Teach the client good body mechanics. *The client with bone deformities should avoid activities that require lifting and twisting; these may result in fractures.*

- Plan and instruct the client in exercise protocols and activity regimens. *Exercise and activity protocols should be planned carefully to prevent injury and to minimize fatigue.*

Knowledge Deficit

Clients who have manifestations of Paget's disease require education during their treatment. The nurse is a primary resource for this information and can evaluate the clients' understanding as they progress during the treatment.

Nursing interventions with rationales follow:

- Maintain contact with the physician so that the client's progress can be evaluated. *Self-administration of medication for Paget's disease usually lasts approximately 1 year. During this time, clients need serial serum alkaline phosphatase measurements to monitor their progress.*

- Provide information regarding Paget's Disease Foundation. *Clients with Paget's disease can obtain knowledge about the current research and other information written for the layperson by requesting information from the Paget's Disease Foundation.*

- Provide information on medications for the treatment of Paget's disease (see the box on page 1529).

Other Nursing Diagnoses

Additional nursing diagnoses for clients with Paget's disease follow:

- *Body Image Disturbance* related to bone deformity
- *Anxiety* related to potentially fatal complications of the disease and selected treatment
- *Ineffective Individual and Family Coping* related to chronicity of the disease
- *Sensory/Perceptual Alterations (Auditory)* related to cranial nerve damage
- *Sleep Pattern Disturbance* related to headache and/or bone pain

Client and Family Teaching

Important nursing actions related to client and family teaching are included in the discussions of collaborative care and nursing care of the client with Paget's disease.

Care of the Older Client

As previously discussed, the incidence of Paget's disease increases with age. If the older client develops localized pain of the affected bones or other manifestations, help him or her adjust the dosage of analgesics to ensure comfort and, at the same time, prevent excessive sedation, which may make the person hesitate to ambulate or exercise and/or prone to falls.

Older adults must alert their primary physician regarding the over-the-counter medications they are taking (either alone or with other prescribed medications) for pain control or anti-inflammatory response.

The Client with Osteomyelitis

■ ■ ■

Osteomyelitis is an infection of the bone. Osteomyelitis is a severe problem and must be treated immediately to prevent extensive physical disability. With the advent of more sophisticated diagnostic measures and antibiotic therapies, the mortality from osteomyelitis has decreased but the complication rate remains about 5% (Maher et al., 1994).

A client with osteomyelitis requires immediate treatment for several reasons (McCance & Huether, 1994). First, when the microorganisms enter the microscopic channels in the bone, the body's natural defenses cannot follow immediately, and the bacteria multiply unimpeded. Second, the infection stimulates osteoclastic activity, and the resorption process weakens the structure of the bone. Finally, the microcirculation of bone is vulnerable to damage and destruction by bacterial toxins; vessel damage causes blockage of the small vessels, which in turn leads to necrosis (death) of bone.

The cause of osteomyelitis is usually bacterial; however, fungi, parasites, and viruses can also cause bone infection. *Staphylococcus aureus* is the most common infecting organism. Other organisms include *Escherichia coli, Pseudomonas, Klebsiella, Salmonella,* and *Proteus.*

Pathogenic organisms reach the bone by one of three routes. Organisms that enter bone from outside the body (e.g., through open fractures; penetrating wounds such as animal or human bites; or orthopedic surgical procedures) are known as *exogenous* infections. *Hematogenous* infections are caused by pathogens that are carried in the blood from sites of infection elsewhere in the body. Common examples of these infectious sites include abscessed teeth, burn infections, urinary tract infections, upper respiratory infections, and bacterial endocarditis. The third mode of entry for microorganisms that invade bone tissue is the *extension* from adjacent soft tissue infection. Clients with venous stasis or arterial ulcers of the lower extremities (see Chapter 30) or long-term complications of diabetes mellitus (see Chapter 21) are good candidates for this type of bacterial invasion.

Osteomyelitis can occur at any age, but children under age 12 and adults over age 50 are more commonly affected. Males have a higher incidence than females because they have a higher incidence of blunt trauma (Maher et al., 1994).

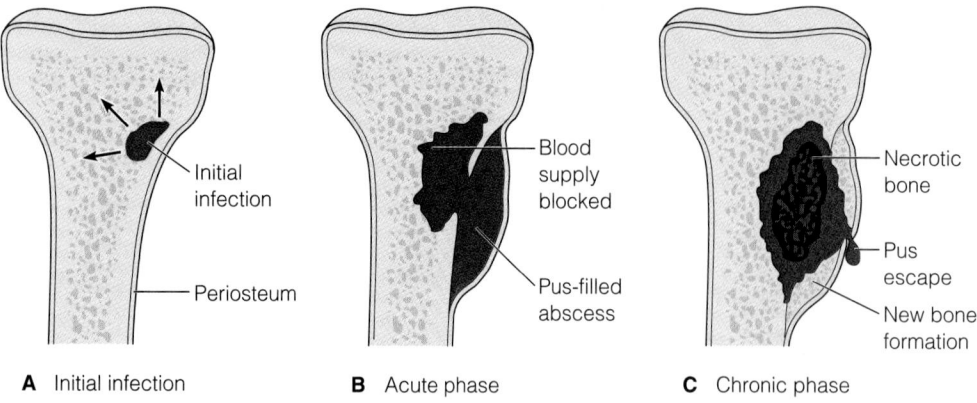

A Initial infection   **B** Acute phase   **C** Chronic phase

Figure 36–2   Osteomyelitis. *A,* site of initial infection. Bacteria enter and multiply in the bone, and the inflammatory response is initiated. *B,* Acute phase, in which infection spreads to other parts of the bone. Pus forms, edema occurs, and the vascular supply is compromised. If the infection reaches the outer margin of the bone, the periosteum is lifted, and ischemia and necrosis eventually occur. *C,* Chronic phase. Necrotic bone separates, a new layer of bone forms around the necrotic bone, and a sinus develops to allow the wound to drain.

Pathophysiology

In the acute phase of osteomyelitis, bacteria lodge and multiply in the bone, resulting in the inflammatory and immune system response. Pus forms, followed by edema and vascular congestion. The Haversian canals in the medullary (marrow) cavity of the bone allow the infection to travel to other segments of the bone. If the infection reaches the outer margin of the bone (Figure 36–2), it raises the periosteum of the bone, spreading along the surface a considerable distance (Eisenberg & Dennis, 1990). Lifting of the periosteum from the cortex disrupts the blood vessels that enter the bone. Pressure increases further compromising the vascular supply and leading to ischemia and, eventually, necrosis of the bone. Blood and antibiotics cannot reach the bone tissue once the pressure compromises the vascular and arteriolar systems. All of these factors support the need for immediate assessment and treatment when the client has a history or the manifestations of suspected osteomyelitis.

Chronic osteomyelitis results if initial treatment is omitted or inadequate. The necrotic bone separates from the living bone and becomes a medium for further growth of microorganisms. In addition, the osteoblasts, in an attempt to heal the infected bone, isolate the dead fragments and form a layer of new bone around the old dead bone. This layer of new bone also acts as a reservoir for chronic infection. Chronic infection reservoirs either remain localized or exit the body. If the infection travels to the periosteum, soft tissue abscesses and cutaneous sinus tracts develop, and the exudate drains from the body. Sinus tracts result in chronic wound drainage and create a port of entry for new microorganisms.

Osteomyelitis can also wall itself off and remain localized. When this occurs it is referred to as a Brodie's abscess. Pathologic fractures often occur at sites of severe bone destruction (McCance & Huether, 1994).

Age affects the progress of osteomyelitis. In children, the overlying periosteum is loosely attached, so the exudate can easily collect under the periosteum. In adults, by contrast, this process rarely occurs, because the periosteum is firmly attached and resists displacement.

Clinical manifestations of osteomyelitis vary according to the age of the client, the cause and site of involvement, and whether the infection is acute, subacute, or chronic (McCance & Huether, 1994). Clinical manifestations of osteomyelitis are summarized in the accompanying box.

Collaborative Care

The care of the client with osteomyelitis focuses on relieving pain, eliminating the infection, and preventing or minimizing complications. Early diagnosis is important to prevent progression of the infection. Diagnosis is facilitated by a thorough assessment of the client's injury and its manifestations and prompt preparation for radiographic studies.

Laboratory and Diagnostic Tests

The diagnosis of osteomyelitis is based on bone scans, magnetic resonance imaging, blood tests, and biopsy. Tests include the following:

- *Bone scan and gallium scan* are the most efficient imaging modalities for the early diagnosis of osteomyelitis (Eisenberg & Dennis, 1990). See the box on page 1534.

- *Magnetic resonance imaging (MRI)* is frequently used to assist in the diagnosis of osteomyelitis because it is able to distinguish soft tissue from bone marrow.

- *Plain radiographs* do not show changes in the bone due to osteomyelitis until about 10 days after the onset of symptoms. For this reason, plain radiographs are used initially to detect the presence of fractures. Later, they are used to evaluate the progress of treatment and to show definitive structural changes of the bone, that is, new bone formation or erosion.

- *Erythrocyte sedimentation rate (ESR)* is measured. The client with acute osteomyelitis will have an elevated ESR; the client with chronic osteomyelitis will have a normal ESR.

- *Differential white blood cell (WBC) count* is also measured. Clients with acute osteomyelitis will have an elevated WBC count; clients with chronic osteomyelitis will have a normal WBC count. When the client is diagnosed with acute osteomyelitis and bacteremia or septicemia are suspected, blood cultures are obtained. Venous blood specimens are collected and tested for both anaerobic and aerobic organisms.

Pharmacology

Pharmacologic therapy is mandatory to prevent acute osteomyelitis from progressing to the chronic phase. Parenteral antibiotic therapy begins as soon as cultures (blood and/or wound) are obtained. A penicillinase-resistant semisynthetic penicillin (e.g, methacillin, oxacillin) may be given until the culture and sensitivity results are known. These antibiotics are used initially because many cases of osteomyelitis are caused by *Staphylococcus aureus*. When the detailed sensitivity report is obtained from the cultures, more definitive antibiotics are prescribed.

The duration of parenteral antimicrobial therapy is a major variable influencing the resolution of osteomyelitis (Maher et al., 1994). For the client with acute or chronic osteomyelitis, intravenous antibiotics are administered for 4 to 8 weeks to ensure a sustained therapeutic level of the antibiotic within the bone tissue. After laboratory results reveal that parenteral therapy has substantially reduced the infectious process, a course of oral antibiotics is prescribed for another 4 to 8 weeks.

Surgery

Needle aspiration or *percutaneous needle biopsy* may be performed to obtain a specimen in acute osteomyelitis. Surgery may be performed to obtain a specimen of the infectious agent, to debride the area, or both.

Surgical debridement is the primary treatment for the client with chronic osteomyelitis. The periosteum is excised and the cortex is drilled to release the pressure from accumulated pus. During this procedure, cultures may be

---

Clinical Manifestations of Osteomyelitis

Cardiovascular Effects

- Tachycardia

Gastrointestinal Effects

- Nausea and vomiting
- Anorexia

Musculoskeletal Effects

- Limp in involved extremity
- Localized tenderness, especially in epiphyseal area

Integumentary Effects

- Drainage and ulceration at involved site
- Swelling, erythema, and warmth at involved site
- Lymph node involvement, especially in the involved extremity

Other Effects

- High temperature with chills
- Abrupt onset of pain
- Sleep disturbances
- Malaise

---

obtained and sent to the laboratory for analysis. The wound holes are irrigated, and the wound is then closed. In some cases, the cavity is kept clean by inserting drainage tubes that are connected to an irrigation and suction system.

Postoperatively, the nurse is responsible for instilling and removing dilute antibiotic solutions through the drainage tubes. See the nursing care box on page 1535 for additional information.

A musculocutaneous (myocutaneous) flap is another approach used for the treatment of the dead space caused by extensive debridement of the infected site. The flap obliterates the dead space left after debridement and provides a blood supply to the evacuated area. The procedure involves moving or rotating a muscle and the section of skin fed by the arteries from that muscle into the cavity created by the surgery. A skin graft is performed at a later time.

Nursing Implications for Diagnostic Tests: Bone Scan and Gallium Scan

■ ■ ■

Bone Scan

Client Preparation

■ Assess the client's understanding of the procedure, providing explanation, clarification, and emotional support as needed.

■ Radioactive material (technetium-99m phosphate) is injected intravenously for 2 to 3 hours so that it concentrates in the bone.

■ Observe the injection site for redness or swelling. If a hematoma forms, apply warm soaks to the area to relieve pain.

■ Have the client drink four to six glasses of water in the 2- to 3-hour waiting period before the procedure to facilitate renal clearance of the circulating radioactive material that is not picked up by the bone.

■ The client is not restricted to foods or fluids prior to the exam.

■ Have the client empty the bladder prior to testing; a full bladder will mask the pelvic bones.

■ If the client is in pain or debilitated, help the client void before the test so that he or she will remain still during the examination.

■ The scan takes about 30 to 60 minutes to complete. The client must remain still during the scanning.

■ The client may be as active as desired during the waiting period.

■ A sedative should be ordered and administered to any client who may have difficulty lying quietly during the scanning period.

Postprocedure Care

■ No special care needs to be provided after the bone scan is complete.

Client and Family Teaching

■ Remove jewelry or any metal objects that may obscure X-ray visualization of the bones.

■ The scanner machine moves back and forth over the body and detects radiation emitted by the skeleton. This information is then translated into X-ray film, thus showing a two-dimensional view of the skeleton. Many X-ray pictures are taken; the client may have to be repositioned several times during the test.

■ The scanning machine makes a clicking sound as it detects radioactivity.

■ Drinking liquids and frequent activity in the first 6 hours after the procedure help reduce excess radiation to the bladder and gonads.

■ The injected radionuclide will not affect the family, visitors, or other hospital staff members. The radioactive substance is usually excreted via the urine in 6 to 24 hours.

■ Family members will not be affected by the injected radionuclide, nor will the client's urine or feces need special handling before, during, or after the procedure.

Gallium Scan

Client Preparation

■ Prepare the client as for a bone scan.

■ Radioactive material, gallium-67, is injected intravenously 24 to 72 hours prior to the examination.

■ Gallium is used because of its high affinity for soft tissue abscesses.

Postprocedure Care

■ Additional imaging may be performed at 24-hour intervals to differentiate normal activity from pathologic concentrations.

■ No specific care is needed after the procedure.

Client and Family Teaching

■ Refer to bone scan discussion.

■ After a gallium scan, X-ray films may be obtained in 24-hour intervals for comparative results.

Nursing Care

Nursing diagnoses associated with acute osteomyelitis focus on preventing the transmission of infection and problems due to immobility. Providing comfort and client teaching are also very important.

The client with chronic osteomyelitis faces frequent and lengthy hospitalizations and/or treatment modalities. The prognosis is uncertain, and functional deficits and amputation are a constant concern. The ongoing expenses, loss of financial support, and role changes within the family are also nursing concerns.

Nursing Care of the Client Undergoing Surgical Debridement for Osteomyelitis

PREOPERATIVE CARE

- Discuss the impending surgery, the client's concerns regarding surgery and its risks, and what steps will be taken if surgery is ineffective. *Open discussion and active listening are important means of gaining the client's trust and encouraging the client to express concerns about the outcome of the surgery. Surgery is frequently performed when 36 to 48 hours of antimicrobial therapy yields no improvement and when prolonged bacteremia and evidence of an abscess formation are present. The periosteum is excised, allowing access to the purulent material in the infected area. If pus is not apparent, several holes may be drilled into the bone. In some cases, irrigation tubes are inserted and connected to an elaborate system for postoperative antimicrobial therapy.*

- Clients may need extensive antimicrobial treatment postoperatively if an irrigation system is surgically implanted. Before the procedure, explain to the client that bed rest and an extended period of treatment in the hospital are imperative. *Clients who understand the events that may occur postoperatively may be more accepting of the required restrictions.*

POSTOPERATIVE CARE

- Provide meticulous care of the dressing and/or irrigation set-up. *Frequently, the irrigation tubes are connected to a 3-way stopcock, which allows irrigation and drainage of the debrided area without separating the tube from the collection device. Nurses need to be extremely cautious and adhere to strict sterile technique.*

- Assess the client for manifestations of further infection. *Although the client will receive antimicrobial agents, it is important to assess the client continually for sudden spikes in temperature, pain at the involved site, and other indications of superinfection.*

CLIENT AND FAMILY TEACHING

- While receiving antimicrobial agents, be sure to drink adequate amounts of fluid and eat a high-calorie diet to minimize the risks for damage to the kidneys, yeast infection, and adverse gastrointestinal effects.

A Critical Pathway for the client with osteomyelitis is provided on page 1536.

Risk for Infection

Compromised immune status places the client with osteomyelitis at risk for superinfection. An inadequate kcal intake is an additional factor that contributes to the risk. Nursing interventions with rationales follow:

- Maintain strict hand-washing practices. *Meticulous hand washing helps prevent the spread of infection by minimizing the entry of organisms into susceptible clients.*

- Administer antimicrobial therapy at specified time intervals. *Optimal blood levels of antibiotic therapy are mandatory in clients with infectious processes.*

- Maintain the client's optimal dietary kcal and protein intake. *High kcal and protein intake provide the client with sufficient nutritional support for the body's needs during the stressful event of the inflammatory process.*

Hyperthermia

The inflammatory process can cause fever in the client with osteomyelitis. Nursing interventions with rationales follow:

- Monitor temperature every 4 hours and when client reports chills and/or fever. *Blood cultures are frequently ordered when an acute elevation of temperature occurs. A sudden rise in temperature in clients with either acute or chronic osteomyelitis may indicate inadequate antimicrobial management.*

- Maintain a cool environment and provide light clothing and bedding during temperature elevation. *Proper environmental conditions and clothing enhance the evaporative process during acute temperature elevation and promote comfort.*

- Ensure a daily fluid intake of 2000 to 3000 mL. *Dehydration may result from evaporative losses during acute temperature elevations. Furthermore, clients taking large doses of antibiotic therapy may experience fluid loss through excessive diarrhea, as a side effect of the therapy. Fluid replacement is necessary during this time to prevent further dehydration.*

Impaired Physical Mobility

Pain, infection, inflammation, and the use of immobilizers can all impair the mobility of the client with osteomyelitis. Nursing interventions with rationales follow:

Text continues on page 1539

	Date _____ Day 1	Date _____ Day 2	Date _____ Day 3
	Critical Pathway for the Client with Osteomyelitis		
Expected length of stay: 5 days			
Daily outcomes	The client ■ Has stable vital signs. ■ Verbalizes understanding of diagnosis and planned treatment. ■ Maintains a fluid intake of 3000 mL/day (IV/PO). ■ Demonstrates ability to cope.	The client ■ Has stable vital signs. ■ Maintains a fluid intake of 3000 mL/day (IV/PO). ■ Demonstrates ability to cope.	The client ■ Is afebrile and has stable vital signs. ■ Demonstrates ability to cope. ■ Verbalizes beginning understanding of home care instructions.
Tests, treatments, and assessments	CBC with differential Erythrocyte sedimentation rate Prepare for X-rays, bone scanning, CT, or MRI as ordered. Blood culture × 2, if temp over 101 F (38.3 C) Wound smear for gram stain and culture and sensitivity (C & S) Vital signs q4h if stable Assess respiratory status q4h and prn. Intake and output every shift Immobilize affected area. Assess distal pulses q2–4h and prn. Assess affected area for redness, swelling, drainage, and pain. Maintain sterile technique for any dressing changes. Assess pain level q2h and prn.	Vital signs q4h if stable Assess respiratory status q4h and prn. Immobilize affected area. Assess distal pulses q2–4h and prn. Assess affected area for redness, swelling, drainage, and pain. Maintain sterile technique for any dressing changes. Assess pain level q2h and prn.	Vital signs q4h if stable Assist with ADLs. Check C & S. Immobilize affected area. Assess distal pulses q2–4h and prn. Assess affected area for redness, swelling, drainage, and pain. Maintain sterile technique for any dressing changes. Assess pain level q2h and prn.
Knowledge deficit	Orient to room and hospital routine. Review plan of care and the importance of long-term antibiotic therapy. Include family in teaching. Assess understanding of teaching.	Review plan of care. Include family in teaching. Assess understanding of teaching.	Reinforce earlier teaching regarding ongoing care. Begin discharge teaching regarding the need for long-term antibiotic therapy at home, activity, and diet. Include family in teaching. Assess understanding of teaching.

	Date ——— **Day 1**	Date ——— **Day 2**	Date ——— **Day 3**
Psychosocial	Assess level of anxiety. Encourage verbalization of concerns. Provide information and ongoing support and encouragement to client and family.	Assess level of anxiety. Encourage verbalization of concerns. Provide information and ongoing support and encouragement to client and family.	Encourage verbalization of concerns. Provide ongoing support and encouragement to client and family.
Diet	Diet as tolerated, providing small, frequent, nutritious feedings. Encourage fluid intake of 2000 mL/day.	Diet as tolerated, providing small, frequent, nutritious feedings. Encourage fluid intake of 2000 mL/day.	Diet as tolerated, providing small, frequent, nutritious feedings. Encourage fluid intake of 2000 mL/day.
Activity	Assess safety needs, and provide appropriate precautions. Bathroom privileges with assistance Provide rest periods.	Maintain safety precautions. Bathroom privileges with assistance Provide rest periods.	Maintain safety precautions. Ambulate 4 to 6 times with assistance Provide rest periods.
Medications	IV fluids IV antibiotics Acetaminophen 650 mg q4h PO for temperature over 101 F (38.3 C)	IV fluids/intermittent IV device IV antibiotics Acetaminophen 650 mg q4h PO for temperature over 101 F (38.3 C)	Intermittent IV device IV antibiotics Acetaminophen 650 mg q4h PO for temperature over 101 F (38.3 C)
Transfer/ discharge plans	Establish discharge goals with client and significant other. Consult with social service regarding projected needs for home health care (if any).	Review progress toward discharge goals with client and significant other. Identify potential referrals.	Review progress toward discharge goals with client and significant other.

	Date ——— **Day 4**	Date ——— **Day 5**	
Daily outcomes	The client ■ Is afebrile and has stable vital signs. ■ Maintains a fluid intake of 3000 mL/day (PO). ■ Demonstrates ability to cope. ■ Verbalizes understanding of home care instructions.	The client ■ Is afebrile and has stable vital signs. ■ Is free of signs and symptoms of infection. ■ Has a WBC below 11,000/mm^3 and negative wound cultures. ■ Is independent in self-care. ■ Is fully ambulatory. ■ Has resumed preadmission urine and bowel elimination pattern.	

➤

	Critical Pathway for the Client with Osteomyelitis (continued)		
	Date _____ **Day 4**	**Date _____** **Day 5**	
Daily outcomes (continued)		■ Verbalizes/demonstrates home care instructions. ■ Demonstrates care of IV catheter and administers antibiotics correctly. ■ Tolerates usual diet and maintains a fluid intake of 3000 mL/day. ■ Demonstrates ability to cope with ongoing stressors.	
Tests, treatments, and assessments	Vital signs q4h if stable Assess respiratory status q4h and prn. Immobilize affected area. Assess distal pulses q2–4h and prn. Assess area for redness, swelling, drainage, and pain. Maintain sterile technique for any dressing changes. Assess pain level q2h and prn.	Vital signs q4h if stable Assess respiratory status q4h and prn. Immobilize affected area. Assess distal pulses q2–4h and prn. Assess area for redness, swelling, drainage, and pain. Maintain sterile technique for any dressing changes. Assess pain level q2h and prn.	
Knowledge deficit	Reinforce earlier teaching regarding ongoing care. Review instructions regarding care of the IV and antibiotic administration. Review written discharge instructions with client and significant other. Include family in teaching. Assess understanding of teaching.	Reinforce earlier teaching regarding ongoing care. Complete discharge teaching to include diet, follow-up care, signs and symptoms to report, follow-up MD visit, activity, and medications: name, purpose, dose, frequency, route, dietary interactions, and side effects. Provide client with written discharge instructions. Include family in teaching. Assess understanding of teaching.	
Psycho-social	Encourage verbalization of concerns. Provide support and encouragement to client and family.	Encourage verbalization of concerns. Provide support and encouragement to client and family.	
Diet	Diet as tolerated, providing small, frequent, nutritious feedings.	Diet as tolerated, providing small, frequent, nutritious feedings.	

	Date _____ Day 4	Date _____ Day 5	
Diet (continued)	Encourage fluid intake of 3000 mL/day.	Encourage fluid intake of 3000 mL/day.	
Activity	Ambulate independently at least 4 times. Maintain safety precautions.	Fully ambulatory	
Medications	IV antibiotics Acetaminophen 650 mg q4h PO for temperature over 101 F (38.3 C)	IV antibiotics Acetaminophen 650 mg q4h PO for temperature over 101 F (38.3 C)	
Transfer/ discharge plan	Continue to review progress toward discharge goals. Finalize discharge plans.	Finalize plans for home care if needed. Make appropriate referrals. Complete discharge teaching.	

- Maintain the affected limb in functional position when immobilized. *The client may hesitate to move the involved extremity because of continuous pain; therefore, the extremity must be maintained in functional position to avoid flexion contracture. Splints or immobilizers are useful for this purpose.*

- Maintain rest, and avoid subjecting the affected extremity to weight-bearing activities. *The involved extremity must be immobilized to avoid pathologic fractures caused by stress on the weakened bone.*

- Ensure active or passive range-of-motion (ROM) exercises every 4 hours. *Flexion contracture occurs when the client remains immobile or when there is only minimal joint movement. Consult a physical therapist for plan of exercises to avoid contracture.*

Pain

The client with osteomyelitis can experience pain due to swelling and tenderness.

Nursing interventions with rationales follow:

- Use a splint or immobilizer when the client experiences acute pain from swelling. *Splinting or immobilizing the involved extremity provides support and reduces pain caused by movement.*

- Offer analgesic medication 20 to 30 minutes prior to the expected time when movement is necessary. *The nurse frequently knows when the client is scheduled for a diagnostic procedure requiring transport. Medicate the client several minutes prior to transport to allow sufficient time for the medication to take effect. In addition, diagnos-*

tic procedures may require that the client's involved extremity remain immobile for the entire procedure. Ensure that the involved extremity is supported so that the client does not experience pain during the lengthy procedure.

- Ask the physician to order scheduled administration of narcotic and nonnarcotic analgesics on a 24-hour basis rather than as needed. *The use of 24-hour administration allows blood levels of pain-relieving medications to remain constant.*

- Use nonpharmacologic strategies (e.g., distraction, relaxation techniques) for pain management. *Pain of the muscles and joints may be controlled through nonpharmacologic interventions. Warm moist packs, warm baths, or heating pads to the involved extremity provide comfort due to vasodilation (Maher et al. 1994).*

- Have the client use assistive devices during ambulation. *Assistive devices can provide support to the involved extremity and remind the client to avoid weight-bearing when ambulating.*

- Avoid excessive manipulation of the involved area; handle the area gently. Carefully assess the client for guarding, limping, or unwillingness to move the affected part. Communicate to other health care professionals the client's preferences for assistive devices and means of manipulating the involved area. *Gentle handling and minimal manipulation help reduce pain.*

Anxiety and Powerlessness

The long-term nature of the disease can cause feelings of anxiety and powerlessness in the client with osteomyelitis. Nursing interventions with rationales follow:

- While the client is in the hospital, provide information regarding the disease process and diagnostic tests. *An understanding of the disease process and the diagnostic and treatment modalities minimizes anxiety. Nurses can frequently interpret information given to the client by repeating that information in language the client can understand.*

- Inform the client about ways to maximize the treatment phases for the disease process. *The nurse should enable the client to participate fully in the treatment plan so that maximum results can be obtained. Clients need to understand that their compliance with the prescribed antibiotic therapy is essential.*

Other Nursing Diagnoses

Other nursing diagnoses for the client with osteomyelitis may include the following:

- *Fear* related to outcome of disease process
- *Ineffective Individual Coping* related to nonacceptance of disease process
- *Ineffective Family Coping* related to long-term nature of disease process, potential threat to job security, and/or cost of hospitalization and treatment
- *Altered Nutrition: Less Than Body Requirements* related to side effects of medications used for treatment of disease process and/or inactivity secondary to prescribed bed rest

Client and Family Teaching

Instruct the client in the general principles of infection control in the hospital and/or home environment. The client needs to understand the importance of good hand washing to prevent further transmission of microorganisms, especially after toileting and after contact with wound drainage. It is important to provide information about the following as well:

- The importance of follow-up medical care
- Community agencies and social services that can provide financial assistance during the prolonged recuperative period
- The importance of shifting position to relieve pressure on skin areas while the client remains on bed rest
- Taking medication before the pain becomes too severe
- Maintaining the joint in a position of function as well as comfort
- Maintaining range of motion in unaffected and affected joint as directed by the physician

Care of the Older Client

The older adult who is incontinent, immobile, or cognitively impaired is prone to pressure ulcers and thus is a candidate for osteomyelitis. Pressure ulcers that cannot be staged and treated because of eschar formation pose a particular risk. It is therefore essential to perform a thorough assessment of the older adult's skin condition over bony prominences and note any changes. In addition, be aware that the first indication of an infection in these clients is often a change in cognitive status rather than the obvious manifestations of warm, flushed skin and rise in temperature.

Applying the Nursing Process

Case Study of a Client with Osteomyelitis: Quon Tanaka

Mr. Quon Tanaka, age 76, is a retired chef. He has been married for 52 years and has 4 children and 9 grandchildren. He has been a diabetic for 25 years and has been able to control the diabetes with dietary modifications. Five days ago, he cut his big toe while trimming his toenails. He treated the cut with warm epsom soaks several times a day, but the cut has not healed and is quite swollen and sore.

After visiting his physician, Mr. Tanaka is admitted to the hospital for an infected toe with possible osteomyelitis. Juanita Perez, RN, enters the room to complete the admission assessment and notes that Mr. Tanaka is very lethargic and that his skin is very warm to the touch.

Assessment

The admission history for Mr. Tanaka includes the following:

- Mr. Tanaka has not eaten for the last 12 hours because he has not felt well.
- Vital signs are as follows: T, 102.2 F (39 C); BP, 160/94; P, 110
- The right big toe is swollen, red, shiny, and hot to the touch.
- Mr. Tanaka describes the pain as constant, throbbing, and increasing with touch; range of motion is restricted by the pain.
- Pedal pulses are regular and bounding.
- Yellowish thick material is draining from a small opening near the nail.

Diagnostic tests yield the following abnormal findings:

Blood glucose: 368 mg/dL (normal range: 70 to 110 mg/dL)

Erythrocyte sedimentation rate (ESR): 40 mm/hr (normal range: < 20 mm/hr)

White blood cell (leukocyte) count: 15,000/mm^3 (normal range: 5,000 to 10,000/mm^3)

Blood culture: positive

Culture of wound drainage indicates presence of *Staphylococcus aureus*

Wound culture sensitive to cephalothin, clindamycin, oxacillin, and vancomycin

Bone scan showing acute inflammation and increased blood flow to right great toe area.

Bed rest and analgesics are ordered for Mr. Tanaka. The right leg is elevated, and continuous warm soaks are applied to the right foot. Vancomycin, 1 g, is administered "stat" and ordered for administration every 8 hours.

Diagnosis

The nursing diagnoses for Mr. Tanaka include the following:

- *Risk for Extended Infection* related to current infection in right toe and/or treatment
- *Pain* related to inflammatory process
- *Hyperthermia* related to osteomyelitis
- *Altered Nutrition: Less Than Body Requirements* related to inability to eat secondary to febrile condition
- *Risk for Injury* related to diabetic condition, decreased appetite, infection, and adverse effects of medications
- *Impaired Physical Mobility* related to inability to ambulate secondary to extremely painful right toe
- *Anxiety* related to lack of knowledge about disease process and long-term effects

Expected Outcomes

The expected outcomes established in the plan of care specify that Mr. Tanaka will

- Experience control of and improvement in infectious process.
- Control pain and other discomforts within an acceptable level.
- Experience a reduction in temperature, resulting in increased comfort.
- Maintain optimal range of motion of right foot and toes.
- Eat a diet that provides adequate nutrients for wound healing and adheres to the dietary restrictions imposed by diabetes.
- Have no further extension of infection.
- Have vital signs within an acceptable level.
- Understand the disease process and treatment.

Planning and Implementation

The following interventions are planned and implemented for Mr. Tanaka:

- Teach Mr. Tanaka to carry out good hand-washing technique, especially after toileting and after contact with wound drainage from toe.
- Explain the rationale behind any infection control precautions prompted by drainage from the infected toe wound.
- Monitor Mr. Tanaka for side effects of large doses of intravenous antibiotics.
- Upon discharge, inform Mr. Tanaka of the need to complete prescribed oral dosage of antibiotics.
- Place Mr. Tanaka's right foot in a position of comfort while maintaining optimal function.
- Use nonpharmacologic strategies for pain management.
- Collaborate with the physician regarding prescription of analgesics on a 24-hour basis rather than as needed so that constant blood levels are achieved.
- Monitor temperature elevation frequently, and administer medication for hyperthermia.
- Provide comfort measures during periods of hyperthermia.
- Monitor blood glucose results, and administer insulin according to a sliding scale.
- Monitor food intake to ensure adequate intake of food and fluids.
- Contact dietitian if Mr. Tanaka wants to change his diet plan to include his ethnic foods.
- Encourage Mr. Tanaka to eat foods high in protein and vitamin C.
- Monitor intravenous insertion site for signs of infiltration or phlebitis.
- Monitor white blood cell counts to determine effectiveness of antibiotics and wound care measures.
- Prior to discharge, reinforce teaching for Mr. Tanaka and/or family members regarding nail, foot, and wound care.
- Instruct Mr. Tanaka to report problems with sores in the oral cavity or excessive diarrhea that may result from large doses of antibiotics administered during hospitalization and upon discharge.
- Arrange home care nurse visits for wound care and for continuous assessment and monitoring of diabetes during rehabilitation phase.

Evaluation

Mr. Tanaka is discharged from the hospital after 6 days. A home health nurse monitors Mr. Tanaka's progress and administers doses of intravenous antibiotics at his home for another 6 weeks. Comprehensive teaching has prepared Mr. Tanaka to care for his wound and to assess the toe for the presence of healing and any indications of

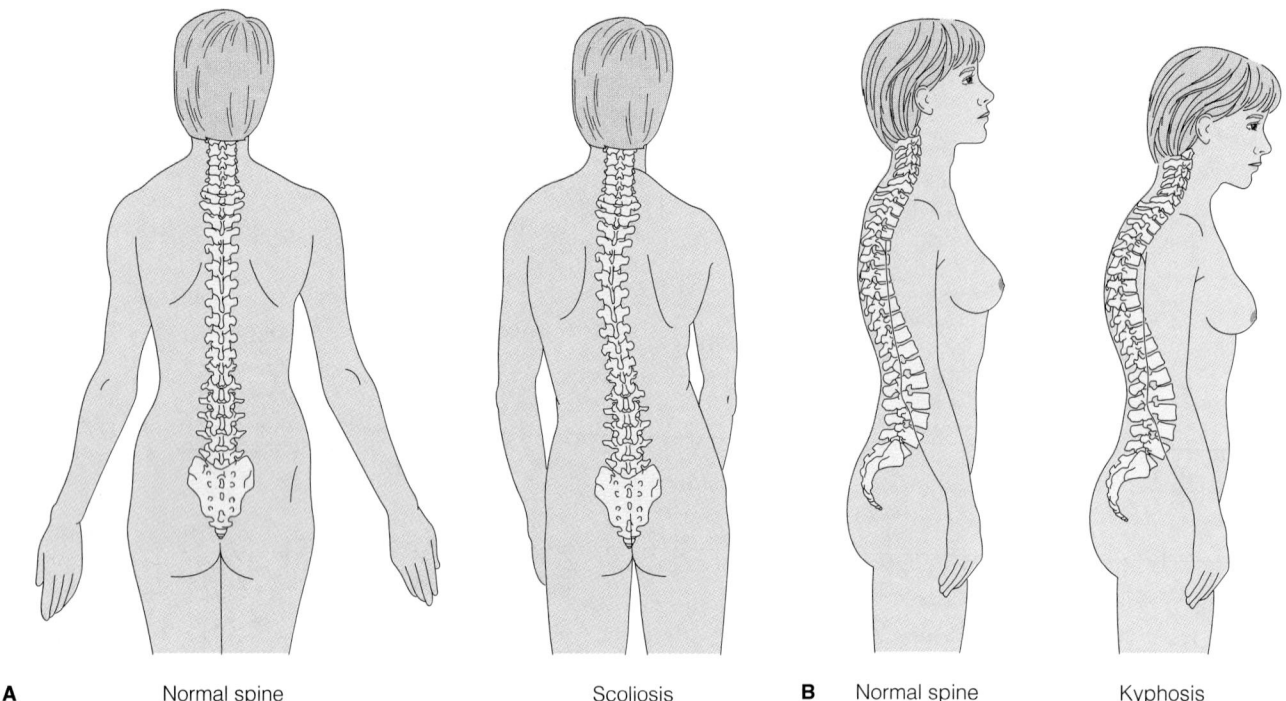

| A | Normal spine | Scoliosis | B | Normal spine | Kyphosis |

Figure 36–3   The two most common deformities of the spinal column: *A,* Scoliosis is a lateral curvature of the spine. *B,* Kyphosis is an exaggerated posterior curvature of the thoracic spine.

superinfection involving the administration of the antibiotics. He is able to inspect his feet and do routine nail care properly.

After the additional weeks of intravenous antibiotics, the erythrocyte sedimentation rate (ESR) and serial bone scans indicate that his infection is responding to treatment. Mr. Tanaka takes oral antibiotics for an additional 6 weeks, and his toe continues to heal.

Critical Thinking in the Nursing Process

1. What priority assessments would the nurse make to determine the cause of Mr. Tanaka's lethargy on admission?

2. What are the most important alterations in Mr. Tanaka's condition that the nurse must immediately report to the physician?

3. Describe the best method to ensure Mr. Tanaka's safety when assisting him to ambulate for the first time after his extended period of bed rest.

4. List the factors that are likely to provoke anxiety in Mr. Tanaka at the following periods of time: on admission to the hospital, during hospitalization, on discharge from the hospital, and on discharge from the care of the home health nurse. List nursing interventions that are appropriate for each of these situations.

5. Develop a care plan for Mr. Tanaka for the nursing diagnoses *Sleep Pattern Disturbance.*

The Client with Common Spinal Deformities

■ ■ ■

Scoliosis and kyphosis are the two most common deformities of the spinal column. *Scoliosis* is a lateral curvature of the spine. *Kyphosis* is excessive angulation of the normal posterior curve of the thoracic spine (Figure 36–3).

Scoliosis is classified as postural, structural, or idiopathic. *Postural scoliosis* is caused by muscoloskeletal factors apart from the spine itself, such as poor posture or unequal leg length. This form of scoliosis often can be corrected through bending or other exercises. *Structural scoliosis* is due to a defect in the spinal vertebrae. This form of scoliosis may result from a variety of congenital or neuromuscular disorders. *Idiopathic scoliosis,* in which the cause is not evident, accounts for the majority of cases. Both structural and idiopathic forms of scoliosis produce spinal deformities that cannot be corrected by bending or exercise.

Over 1 million Americans have scoliosis requiring treatment (Porth, 1994). Most cases are idiopathic scoliosis occurring among girls and young women.

Kyphosis is classified as postural if the client can voluntarily hyperextend and correct the excessive posterior curvature of the thoracic spine. Kyphosis arising from other disease processes is suspected if the client cannot hyperextend the back or if the curvature exceeds 45 degrees.

Like scoliosis, many cases of kyphosis are caused by a variety of congenital conditions or childhood disorders. Detailed discussions of the causes and treatment of scoliosis and kyphosis in younger clients can be found in pediatric nursing textbooks. This discussion focuses on the nursing care of adults with these disorders.

Pathophysiology

Scoliosis

The lateral curve that occurs in scoliosis is usually evident in the thoracic, lumbar, or thoracolumbar regions of the spine. The vertebral bodies in these spinal regions can be rotated as well as curved to one side or the other.

As scoliosis emerges, the soft tissue (muscles and ligaments) shorten on the concave side of the curvature. Over time, progressive deformities of the vertebral column and ribs develop, causing one-sided compression of the vertebral bodies. The degree of compression and twisting varies according to the location of each vertebra within the curved portion of the spine (McCance & Huether, 1994).

If the lateral curvature is less than 40 degrees when the client's spine reaches maturity, the risk of further progression during adult life is small. However, the spine becomes unstable if the lateral curvature is greater than 50 degrees, and curvature likely will worsen throughout the client's lifetime.

Scoliosis is usually first noted by the deformity it causes, such as one shoulder that is higher than the other, a prominent hip, or a projecting scapula. Pain is present in severe cases, usually in the lumbar region. Pain also may be caused by pressure on the ribs or the crest of the ilium. Shortness of breath may result from diminished chest expansion, and gastrointestinal disturbances because of crowding of the abdominal organs. See the accompanying clinical manifestations box.

Kyphosis

Like scoliosis, kyphosis may result from congenital malformations or pediatric disorders such as rickets or poliomyelitis. However, kyphosis also may emerge during adulthood from vertebral tuberculosis and Paget's disease or from metabolic disorders such as osteoporosis and osteomalacia. The condition can also result from the surgical removal or radiation of intervertebral discs for the treatment of spinal cord tumors or cysts.

The manifestations of kyphosis include moderate back pain and increased curvature of the thoracic spine as viewed from the side ("hunchback"). Impaired mobility

---

Clinical Manifestations of Spine Abnormalities: Scoliosis and Kyphosis

Scoliosis

- Asymmetry of shoulders, scapulae, waist creases
- Prominence of the thoracic ribs or paravertebral muscles on forward bend
- Lateral curvature and vertebral rotation on posteroanterior X-ray film

Severe scoliosis

- Back pain
- Shortness of breath
- Anorexia, nausea

Kyphosis

- Posterior rounding at the thoracic level
- Kyphotic curve of over 45 degrees on X-ray film

---

and respiratory problems may occur in cases of severe curvature. See the accompanying box.

Collaborative Care

Diagnosis of scoliosis and kyphosis is important to prevent severe spinal deformity in the adult. The client stands with the arms relaxed and hanging freely at the sides while the examiner evaluates the client from both the back and the front for symmetry of the shoulders, scapulae, waist creases, and the length of the arms. The client then bends forward, and the examiner observes for prominence of the thoracic ribs or vertebral muscles. The client is then viewed from the side while the screener looks for increased thoracic rounding or lumbar swayback.

A scoliometer is used to quantify the prominence of any curvatures noted during the examination. The scoliometer is placed at the apex of the curvature. A reading of greater than 5 degrees requires referral to a physician (Maher et al., 1994).

Diagnostic Tests

Upright posteroanterior and lateral radiographs are used to confirm the diagnosis of curvature of the spine. For the client with scoliosis, the degree of curve is measured by determining the amount of lateral deviation to the left or right. For the client with kyphosis, anteroposterior and lateral views typically reveal wedging of the vertebrae.

Conservative Treatment

Braces, electrical stimulation, and traction may be used to prevent progression of scoliosis and kyphosis in younger clients whose skeletons have not yet matured. Unfortunately, these approaches are ineffective in the adult client. Conservative treatment for adults with scoliosis and kyphosis may include weight reduction, active and passive exercises, and the use of braces for support.

Surgery

For adolescents and adults, the use of surgery to correct spinal deformities depends on factors such as the degree of curvature and the client's overall physical, emotional, and neurologic status. Even with surgery, it is not possible to correct the abnormal curvature completely. The surgical procedure involves attaching metal reinforcing rods to the vertebrae, and may be performed using a posterior or anterior approach.

The posterior surgical approach begins with the exposure of the malaligned spinous processes. One or more metal straightening devices are threaded through screw and staple units attached directly into the vertebral bodies. This provides a counteracting tension on the convex side of the curve, thus reducing the curvature and providing rotational stability. Bone grafts taken from the iliac crest are placed between the spinous process to provide further fusion.

The two types of straightening devices used most frequently are the Cotrel-Duboussedt (CD) system and the Harrington rod system. The CD system consists of two rods, multiple hooks, and a transverse coupling device. The CD system requires no postoperative mobilization, a distinct advantage for the client. The Harrington rod system consists of one rod, two hooks, and wiring along the spinous processes. The client needs to remain on bed rest and wear a brace postoperatively for an extended period when Harrington rods are used.

The anterior approach for correction of spinal curvature is used when additional stabilization is necessary. The spinous processes are fused or instrumentation is used to provide additional stabilization. Because this approach requires entry through the thorax or abdomen, the anterior approach poses a greater risk of complications to the client.

Nursing Care

The nurse provides secondary and tertiary preventive actions for clients who have been diagnosed with spinal deviation and who require correction of the spinal deviation. Nursing interventions focus on minimizing the risk for injury and neurologic impairment.

Risk for Injury

Clients with spinal deformities are at risk for injury from several sources, including structural aspects of bracing both prior to and after surgical intervention, dislocation of hooks and rods resulting from improper alignment or movement of the back, and changes in body position after prolonged immobilization.

Nursing interventions with rationales follow:

- Assess the environment for safety hazards. *Certain braces for spinal deviations do not allow the client to flex or hyperextend the spinal column. The client needs to learn to use the handrail on stairways and take precautions when walking on slippery surfaces, throw rugs, and so on.*

- Teach the clients ways to reduce irritation of skin surfaces beneath the brace: wearing a smooth cotton T-shirt or cotton tube under the brace at all times, changing undergarments at least once daily, and washing them with a mild soap. Undergarments should be changed more frequently in warmer weather. Avoid lotion and body powders; they may irritate the skin. *The client wearing a brace is especially prone to skin breakdown and must take precautions to prevent it.*

- Teach the client to loosen the brace during meals and for the first 30 minutes after each meal. *Clients have difficulty eating if the brace is tight. Loosening the brace after each meal will allow adequate nutritional intake and promote comfort.*

- Instruct the client in the importance of maintaining body alignment. *Fusion of the vertebral bodies requires extended time for healing. Clients requiring extended immobilization are frequently on bed rest for at least 3 to 4 weeks and must wear a brace for approximately 6 months to 1 year.*

- Turn clients by using the log-rolling technique. *Clients require a position change at least every 2 hours. The use of a turnsheet and sufficient assistance allow the nurse to maintain the client's proper body alignment during the turning procedure.*

- Use a fracture bedpan when the client needs to urinate or defecate. *The fracture bedpan provides minimal misalignment of spine and thus ensures comfort when it is necessary for the client to urinate or have a bowel movement.*

- Teach clients how to apply the brace, and explain ambulatory restrictions. *Clients requiring a brace need to learn how to apply the brace prior to ambulating. Ambulation is frequently restricted to walking rather than sitting for long periods.*

- Instruct the client who has been on extended bed rest to change slowly from a reclining position to a sitting position. *Postural hypotension occurs when the client who has been on extended bed rest changes from a reclining position to a sitting position. Slow movement can prevent or reduce this problem.*

- Instruct the client to sit on the edge of the bed for a few minutes prior to ambulating. *Postural hypotension can cause the client to faint and perhaps result in further injury.*

To prevent the client from falling and causing further injury, ensure that someone remains close when the client first ambulates.

Risk for Peripheral Neurovascular Dysfunction

Surgical procedures can lead to neurologic impairment in the client with a spinal deformity. Nursing interventions with rationales follow:

- Assess the movement and sensation of lower extremities every 2 hours for the first 8 hours then every shift and as needed. *Neurologic assessment related to sensation and movement of the lower extremities is necessary because the surgical procedure is in close proximity to spinal nerves. Swelling of the surgical site can impinge on the spinal nerves and cause a loss of sensation.*

The Client with Common Foot Disorders

■ ■ ■

Hallux valgus, hammertoe, and Morton's neuroma are common foot disorders that cause pain or difficulty in walking. All three disorders are usually caused by wearing poorly fitting or confining shoes. For this reason, these disorders are more prevalent among women.

Pathophysiology

Hallux Valgus

Hallux valgus, commonly called a *bunion,* is the enlargement and lateral displacement of the first metatarsal, that is, the great toe (Figure 36–4). Although bunions may be a congenital disorder, most are caused by wearing pointed, narrow-toed shoes or high heels. Bunions occur nine times more frequently among women than men (Maher et al., 1994).

Hallux valgus develops when chronic pressure against the great toe causes the connective tissue in the sole of the foot to lengthen so that the stabilizing action of the great toe is gradually lost. The toe bends laterally away from the midline of the body, and the metatarsophalangeal joint (MPJ) is exposed to friction during walking and becomes enlarged. As the deformity progresses, calluses form over the metatarsal head, and bursitis develops in the MPJ. In severe cases, the lateral displacement of the great toe may approach 70 to 90 degrees, and the second toe may be forced upward, causing hammertoe (Mann, 1989).

Hallux valgus is obvious on physical examination of the foot. The client may report an inability to fit into shoes. Often, the client may report joint pain or pain around calluses. In advanced or severe cases, the first metatarsal joint may have limited range of motion, particularly in dorsiflexion, and crepitus (crackling or popping) may occur during joint movement.

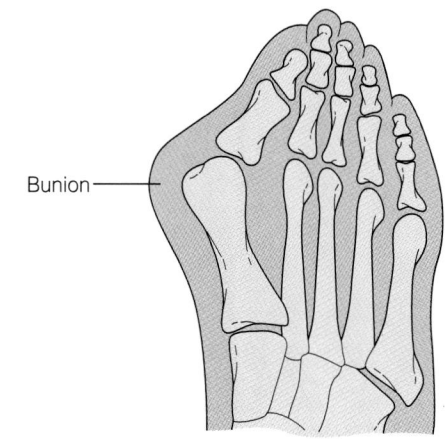

Figure 36–4   Hallux valgus (bunion).

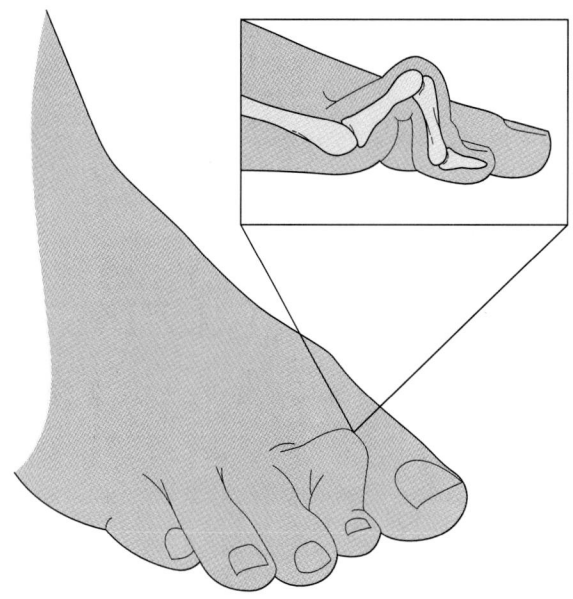

Figure 36–5   Hammertoe.

Hammertoe

Hammertoe (claw toe) is the dorsiflexion of the first phalanx with accompaning plantar flexion of the second and third phalanges (Figure 36–5). The condition may affect any toe, but the second toe is most commonly affected. As the deformity begins, clients experience mild inflammation of the synovial membranes of the involved joints. As the deformity progresses, the dorsiflexed joint rubs against the overlying shoe, causing painful corns to develop.

Morton's Neuroma

Morton's neuroma is a tumorlike mass formed within the neurovascular bundle of the intermetatarsal spaces (Figure 36–6). The neuromas usually occur in only one foot,

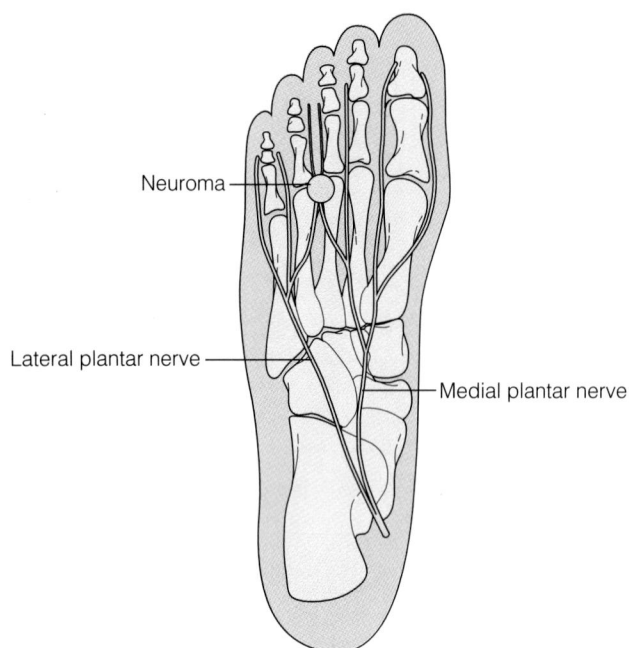

Neuroma

Lateral plantar nerve

Medial plantar nerve

Figure 36–6 Morton's neuroma.

most frequently in the third web space (Holman, Poehling, & Martin, 1994). Like other common foot disorders, Morton's neuroma usually is caused by wearing tight, confining shoes. The condition develops when repeated compression of the toes causes irritation and scarring of tissues surrounding the plantar digital nerve. The affected nerve becomes inflamed and swells. After repeated episodes of inflammation, the nerve fibers become fibrotic, and a neuroma forms.

Manifestations of Morton's neuroma include a burning pain at the web space of the affected foot that radiates into the tips of the involved toes. Weight-bearing usually worsens any symptoms; removing the shoe and massaging the foot often relieves the pain. The neuroma may present as a palpable mass between the affected toes. The area over the neuroma usually is tender.

Collaborative Care

Care of the client with common foot disorders such as hallux valgus, hammertoe, and Morton's neuroma focuses on relieving pain, correcting the structural deformity, and preventing reoccurrence. In most cases, all three conditions are diagnosed by inspection; X-ray films of the affected foot are taken if the need for surgery arises.

Conservative treatment for common foot disorders usually involves the use of corrective shoes. Orthotic devices that cushion and stretch the affected joints may be placed within shoes or between the client's toes. For Morton's neuroma, metatarsal pads are used to spread the client's toes and decompress the affected nerve. Anal-

gesics may be prescribed to relieve pain and inflammation. In severe cases, corticosteroid drugs may be injected into the affected joints or surrounding tissue to relieve acute inflammation.

Surgery is reserved for clients with intractable toe deformities or pain. Hallux valgus is treated with bunionectomy; ligaments are lengthened or shortened as needed, and pins are drilled into place so the toe remains in position. Similarly, the correction of hammertoe also involves straightening the affected toe and inserting pins to retain the correction. A cast may be applied over the foot following surgery to correct toe deformities. Surgery for Morton's neuroma causes loss of sensation to a portion of the foot because removing the neuroma involves cutting out a portion of the plantar nerve.

Nursing Care

Nursing care for clients with any of the three foot deformities discussed focuses on the same areas because the conservative treatment and preoperative and postoperative interventions are similar. Pain relief, prevention of infection, and client education are important components of the nursing care of these clients.

Pain

In the client with a foot deformity, constant pressure of footwear over the involved joint can cause pain. Nursing interventions with rationales follow:

- Instruct clients to wear corrective footwear to assist in the conservative treatment of foot problems. *Pain related to foot problems can result from improper footwear that does not provide proper toe room; in addition, heels higher than 1 inch can cause constant flexion and hyperextension problems. In some instances, the client must purchase special shoes to ensure correct fit and relief of symptoms. Shoes that fit well and provide enough foot space laterally and dorsally, such as running shoes, are recommended.*

- Provide clients with information about available resources that can help them obtain a proper shoe fit. *Shoe stores have devices for stretching the shoe at the pressure area, but the customer must purchase the shoe before the stretching is done. Shoe repair shops charge a reasonable fee for stretching a shoe. Fabric shoes are the most comfortable shoes for the aged client with bunions because fabric stretches more readily than leather or other synthetic materials (Ebersole & Hess, 1994).*

- Instruct clients to purchase appropriate pads to wear over painful bunions, calluses/corns, and the ball of the foot. *Protective pads are manufactured for specific foot problems; these include bunion pads, corn pads, and metatarsal pads.*

- Instruct clients to remove pads and inspect the skin every other day. *The client must inspect the area beneath the pad to ensure that the skin is intact. Clients who have difficulty reaching or observing the involved foot should ask another person to do the inspection for them. It is very important to emphasize the need for inspection to clients who have experienced loss of sensation of the feet due to such disorders as diabetes and chronic peripheral vascular disease.*

Risk for Infection

Like all surgeries, foot surgery carries a risk of infection. This risk may be increased because of impaired peripheral circulation and exposure of the feet to the environment. Nursing interventions with rationales follow:

- Teach clients proper care and cleaning of exposed pins implanted during the surgical procedure. *Pins inserted into soft tissue of the toes and bones are prone to becoming infected and can potentially result in osteomyelitis.*

- Teach clients how to keep pins and casts dry while bathing or ambulating in inclement weather. *Clients must wear a plastic bag over the cast or pins when bathing or walking in rain or snow. When casts or pins are exposed in water, infection may result.*

Care of the Older Client

The older adult that has bunions or hammertoe needs to be assessed for mobility problems and to guard against falls. The pain due to poorly fitting shoes may be corrected by cutting out sections of the client's shoe over the area of bony protrusion. The client or caregiver should assess the feet frequently to ensure that the "window" area in the shoe does not cause skin breakdown or other problems related to pressure.

The Client with Low Back Pain

■ ■ ■

Managing the care of the client with low back pain has changed significantly in the last 2 decades. In the past, the client was frequently hospitalized, and bed rest and pelvic traction were applied. Today, the client is usually treated conservatively on an outpatient basis. Hospital admission or surgical intervention is reserved for clients with neurologic complications.

Acute or chronic low back pain involves the lumbar, lumbosacral, or sacroiliac areas of the back. In most cases, low back pain is due to strains in the muscles and tendons of the back caused by abnormal stress or overuse. Low back pain caused by degenerative disc disease and herniated vertebral discs is covered in Chapter 41.

Low back pain has been reported to affect up to 80% of the population at some time during their life; however, 60% of the clients are back to work within 1 week, and

---

Risk Factors for Low Back Pain

■ ■ ■

Physiologic Risk Factors

- Age: late 20s to mid 50s
- Poor physical fitness
- Poor posture
- Morbid obesity
- Above-average height
- Severe scoliosis
- Spondylolisthesis
- Herniated nucleus pulposus
- Spondylolysis
- Spinal stenosis
- Osteoporosis
- Smoking

Environmental Risk Factors

- Prolonged sitting
- Bending and twisting
- Long exposure to vibrations
- Participation in sports (e.g., golf, tennis, gymnastics, football)

Psychosocial Risk Factors

- Work dissatisfaction
- Depression

Note. Data are from "Outpatient Management of Low Back Pain" (pp. 11–20, 43) by J. Chase, 1992, *Orthopaedic Nursing, 11(1);* and *Orthopaedic Nursing* by A. B. Maher, S. W. Salmond, and T. A. Pellino, 1994, Philadelphia: W. B. Saunders.

---

only about 10% have disabling back pain after 6 weeks (Olmarker & Rydevik, 1991). The age range in which low back pain is most prevalent is the late 20s to mid 50s. Both men and women are affected.

Several risk factors for low back pain, including physical, environmental, and psychosocial factors, have been identified. See the accompanying box. Certain client populations are more likely to develop low back pain than other populations. For example, clients engaged in occupations that require repeated lifting in the forward bent-and-twisted position, exposure to vibrations caused by vehicles or industrial machinery, and persons who smoke

---

Clinical Manifestations of Low Back Pain

■ ■ ■

Alterations in Gait and Flexion

- Walking in a stiff, flexed state
- Inability to bend at waist
- Limp, which may indicate impairment of the sciatic nerve

Neurologic Involvement

- When tested for light and deep touch with a pin and cotton ball, client may feel sensations in both limbs but experience a stronger sensation in the unaffected side
- Loss of both bowel and bladder control due to involvement of the sacral nerve

Pain

- Pain in the affected leg when the client walks on heel or toes
- Continuous, knife-like localized pain in muscles close to the affected disk
- Pain that radiates down posterior of leg
- Sharp, burning pain in the posterior thigh or calf
- Pain in middle of buttock
- Tenderness when muscle close to the affected disk is palpated
- Severe pain with straight leg-raising maneuver

---

have the highest incidence of low back pain (Frymoyer, 1988). Osteoporosis, degenerative disc disease, and genetic conditions (e.g., spondylolisthesis, spinal stenosis, and spondylolysis) also predispose the client to low back pain.

Pathophysiology

Any condition that puts pressure on the nerves branching out from the spinal cord or on the vertebral muscles may cause low back pain. Clients with low back pain report pain ranging from mild discomfort lasting a few hours to chronic debilitating pain. Clinical manifestations are presented in the accompanying box. Acute pain is usually caused when the client participates in an activity that is not usually pursued, such as unusual lifting or bending, playing an active sport, or shoveling snow.

Collaborative Care

Care of the client with low back pain focuses on relieving pain, correcting the condition if possible, preventing complications, and educating the client.

Diagnostic Tests

The choice of diagnostic tests for the client with low back pain depends on the suspected diagnoses, clinical findings, and history. Current guidelines of the Agency for Health Care Policy and Research (1994) recommend that radiography, CT scans, and MRI be used only when there are clinical signs of a potentially serious underlying condition. They also state that diagnostic testing may be considered if pain and other manifestations continue to limit the client after 4 weeks of conservative treatment.

Conservative Treatment

The majority of clients with acute low back pain need only a short-term treatment regimen (Chase, 1992). See the accompanying box. Only a few days of rest are recommended because of the deleterious effect of prolonged bed rest. There is no evidence that activity is harmful or aggravating to the source of pain. In fact, increased activity promotes bone and muscle strength and may increase endorphin levels. Therefore, active rehabilitation helps to restore function and reduce pain.

Ice therapy, such as ice packs or ice massage, can be applied or rubbed over the painful area for 15 minutes every hour or more. Moist, warm towels or a heating pad can be used as an alternative to ice therapy.

Exercise programs are helpful provided that the client begins gradually and increases activity gradually as the recovery process continues.

Physical therapy procedures include diathermy (deep heat therapy), ultrasonography, hydrotherapy, and transcutaneous electrical nerve stimulation (TENS) units. These therapies are used to reduce the muscle spasms and pain temporarily. They are frequently used in combination with exercise to provide early mobilization for the client.

Other treatments include chiropractic manipulation of the spine to reduce spasms and pain. Back school is a rehabilitation program that provides education for the client. The client is instructed on the anatomy of the spine and the appropriate techniques to decrease the probability of a recurrence of back injury. A well-organized program provides both instruction and supervision while the client performs the back exercises.

Pharmacology

The medications of choice for low back pain include NSAIDS and analgesics. NSAIDs block prostaglandin production and reduce inflammation, thus relieving the pain. Muscle relaxants, such as cyclobenzaprine (Flexeril), methocarbamol (Robaxin), or carisoprodol (Soma) may be used; however, there is little evidence to support their efficacy.

Epidural steroid injections may be used to help reduce intense, intractable pain. A steroid solution is injected into the epidural space, which helps decrease the swelling and inflammation of the spinal nerves.

Surgery

Surgery is recommended only for clients with low back pain due to degenerative disc disorders, and only when there is evidence of serious neurologic involvement. Surgery benefits only 1 in 100 clients with acute low back problems. Surgical procedures include percutaneous disc excision, removal of the lamina of the vertebrae (laminectomy), decompression of the disc, and fusion of the vertebrae (see Chapter 41).

Nursing Care

Nursing care of the client with low back pain focuses on relieving the pain. In addition, most clients have very little understanding of the anatomy of the spine, the reasons for the pain, the choices for treatment, and the importance of self management (Chase, 1992). Therefore, education is another essential aspect of treating low back pain.

Pain

Muscle spasms and inflammation are among the contributing factors of low back pain.

Nursing interventions with rationales follow:

- Provide comfort measures as appropriate. *Every client with low back pain has discomfort due to muscle spasms and/or inflammation due to nerve compression, surgery, or irritation from a brace.*

- Instruct the client to take NSAIDs or analgesics on a routine schedule rather than as needed. *Maintaining a constant blood level of the NSAIDs or analgesics reduces inflammation and provides continuous pain relief.*

Knowledge Deficit

The client with low back pain requires information regarding treatment modalities.

Nursing interventions with rationales follow:

- If the client is confined to bed rest, instruct the client to assume a side-lying position with the hips and knees flexed. Keep a pillow under or between the knees. Tell the client to use a footstool when seated to support the weight of the feet. *Flexion, maintaining a side-lying position with a pillow between the legs, and the use of a footstool reduce direct pressure on the protruding nucleus pulposus of the disc, thus relieving compression on the spinal nerves.*

Conservative Treatment of Low Back Pain

■ ■ ■

1. Short-term rest—no more than 2 days
2. Application of ice or heat
3. Medications
   - Nonsteroidal anti-inflammatory drugs (NSAIDs)
   - Muscle relaxants
   - Analgesics
4. Physical therapy
5. Exercise
6. Corset or brace
7. Manipulation
8. Back school
9. Transcutaneous electrical nerve stimulation (TENS) unit

Note. From "Outpatient Management of Low Back Pain" (pp. 11–20, 43) by J. Chase, 1992, *Orthopaedic Nursing, 11*(1).

- Encourage clients to remain on bed rest for a limited period. *There is little scientific evidence to show that bed rest is beneficial, and there is ample evidence about the adverse effects of bed rest (Chase, 1992). Prolonged rest can lead to depression, loss of work, and difficulty in initiating rehabilitation (Waddell, 1987).*

- Teach the client about the "rebound phenomenon" of prolonged heat or ice therapy. *Ice remaining on the skin longer than 15 minutes or heat longer than 30 minutes causes a reverse effect known as the rebound phenomenon. For example, heat produces maximum vasodilation in 20 to 30 minutes. Continuation of the application beyond 30 to 45 minutes causes tissue congestion, and the blood vessels constrict. Likewise, with cold application, maximum vasoconstriction occurs when the skin reaches a temperature of 60 F (15 C). Prolonged cold can create a drop in temperature, at which time vasodilation occurs.*

- Provide instructions about appropriate back exercises such as partial sit-ups with the knees bent and knee-chest exercises to stretch hamstrings and spinal muscles. Each exercise should be done five times and gradually increased to ten times. Advise the client to discontinue any exercise that is painful and to seek professional advice before continuing the exercise. *Repetition of prescribed back exercises, such as the pelvic tilt, partial sit-ups, and back rolls, will strengthen the muscles that protect the spine and thus prevent back strain.*

Impaired Adjustment

In the client with low back pain, the need for life-style changes may lead to impaired adjustment.

Nursing interventions with rationales follow:

- Teach the client to use appropriate body mechanics in lifting and reaching. *The client should be instructed to plan the lift, keep the object being lifted close to the body, and avoid twisting when lifting. Encourage the client to obtain help when lifting. An item is considered excessively heavy if it equals 35% of the lifter's body weight.*

- Instruct the client to modify the workplace or environment to minimize stress to the lower back. *Lumbar supports in chairs, adjustment of chair or table height, and rubber floor mats help prevent back strain or injury.*

- Encourage morbidly obese clients to lose weight. *The trunk of the body has to carry excess weight when the client is obese. Obese people are farther away from the objects they lift because of their greater abdominal girth. They may also have more difficulty squatting to lift. The greater the distance between an object and the client's center of gravity, the higher the risk for straining the lower back.*

- Encourage the client to stop smoking. *Research indicates that smoking decreases blood oxygenation to the disc and thereby interferes with repair of the disc and causes premature aging and degeneration. Smokers also cough frequently, which increases the number of pounds of pressure on the disc, increasing disc stress.*

- Instruct client to refrain from prolonged standing or sitting, lying prone, and wearing high heels. *These activities exacerbate back pain.*

Other Nursing Diagnoses

Other nursing diagnoses that may be appropriate for the client with low back pain include the following:

- *Risk for Altered Family Processes* related to impaired ability to meet role responsibilities (financial, home, social)

- *Risk for Ineffective Management of Therapeutic Regimen* related to insufficient knowledge of condition, exercise program, noninvasive pain relief methods, and proper posture and body mechanics

Client and Family Teaching

Important features that the nurse should include in client and family teaching regarding low back pain are included in the discussions of collaborative care and nursing care.

Care of the Older Client

Back pain is a common problem among the older adult. Spinal pain in the older adult is frequently due to osteoarthritis, disc degeneration, and back sprain. If the older adult continues to complain of acute back pain, encourage the person to seek medical advice.

The Client with Bone Tumors

■ ■ ■

Bone tumors may originate in the bone itself (*primary tumors*) or may invade the bone as a metastatic growth from a tumor elsewhere in the body (*metastatic* or *secondary tumors*). Like other tumors, bone tumors can be either benign or malignant.

Bone is the third most common site for malignant growths; the lung and liver are the first and second most common sites (Maher et al., 1994). Virtually every malignant tumor can metastasize to bone. However, the most common metastatic bone tumors originate from primary tumors of the prostate, breast, kidney, thyroid, and lung. The most frequent sites of metastatic bone tumors are the pelvis, spine, ribs, femur, and humerus.

Primary bone tumors arise from bone tissue itself, that is, cartilage (chondogenic), bone (osteogenic), collagen (collagenic), and bone marrow cells (myelogenic). The tissue type, neoplasm classification, sites, and incidence of the most common primary bone tumors are summarized in Table 36–2. Care of the client with primary bone tumors is the focus of the discussions in this section.

Pathophysiology

The etiologic origin of bone tumors is unknown; however, there is a connection between increased bone activity and the development of primary bone tumors. Bone tumors frequently occur when primary bone growth is at its peak (adolescence) or is overstimulated during disease (e.g., Paget's disease).

Primary tumors cause bone breakdown, called *osteolysis,* which weakens the bone, resulting in bone fractures. Normal bone adjacent to the tumor responds to tumor pressure by altering its normal pattern of remodeling. The bone's surface becomes altered, and the contours enlarge in the area of the tumor growth.

Malignant bone tumors invade and destroy adjacent bone tissue by producing substances that promote bone resorption or by interfering with a bone's blood supply. Benign bone tumors, unlike malignant ones, have a symmetric, controlled growth pattern. As they grow, they push against neighboring bone tissue. This weakens the bone's structure until it becomes unable to withstand the stress of ordinary use and frequently causes pathologic fracture.

The clinical manifestations of bone tumors are usually associated with a history of a fall or blow to the extremity that brings the mass to the client's attention. The injury, rather than the growth itself, usually causes the client to

| **Table 36–2** | Description of Common Primary Bone Tumors | | | |

Classification of Neoplasm

Tissue Type	Benign	Malignant	Site	Incidence
Chondrogenic (cartilage-forming tumors)	Osteochondroma— most common benign tumor		Pelvis, scapula, ribs	Higher in males
	Chondroma		Hands, feet, ribs, spine, sternum, or long bones	Age 30 to 50 Higher in males
		Chondrosarcoma	Femur, pelvis, ribs, head (epiphysis) of long bones	13% of malignant tumors Middle age and older Higher in males
Osteogenic (bone-forming tumors)	Osteoid Osteoma		Shaft (diaphysis) of long bones, i.e., femur, tibia	Age 20 to 30 Higher in males
		Osteosarcoma— most common malignant tumor	Long bones, knee	38% of malignant bone tumors Predominant in adolescents and people 50 to 60
Collagenic (collagen-forming tumors)		Fibrosarcoma	Femur, tibia	4% of malignant bone tumors Wide age distribution, but usually occurs in people 40 to 50 Higher in females
Myelogenic (tumors of bone marrow cells)	Giant cell tumor		Shaft (diaphysis) of long bones, i.e., femur, tibia, radius, humerus	4% to 5% of bone tumors Wide age distribution Higher in females

seek medical attention. Occasionally, the client seeks medical attention because of a pathologic fracture. Clinical manifestations of bone tumors are presented in the accompanying box.

Collaborative Care

Care of the client with bone tumors focuses on prompt diagnosis, removal of the tumor, prevention of complications, and client education.

Laboratory and Diagnostic Tests

The diagnosis of bone tumors is critical to the survival of the client and possible preservation of the affected limb. Because the client's symptoms are usually vague, diagnosis may be delayed. The following tests may be performed:

- *X-rays.* Conventional radiologic films show the location of the tumors and the extent of bone involvement. Benign tumors are characterized by sharp margins that are clearly separate from the surrounding normal

bone. Metastatic bone destruction has a characteristic "moth-eaten" pattern in which the growth has a less-defined margin that cannot be separated from the normal bone.

- *CT scan.* In areas where it is difficult to visualize an abnormal growth, such as the pelvis and vertebra, the CT scan is useful in evaluating the extent of tumor invasion into bone, soft tissues, and neurovascular structures.

- *MRI.* An MRI is used to determine the extent of tumor invasion of surrounding tissue, to determine the response of bone tumors to radiation or chemotherapy, and to detect recurrent disease.

- *Percutaneous needle biopsy or needle biopsy.* The exact type of bone tumor can be determined only by obtaining a biopsy at the time of surgery. Often, a bone tumor cannot be classified until it and the surrounding tissue are removed.

- *Serum alkaline phosphatase.* A client with a malignant bone tumor will have an elevated serum alkaline phosphatase.

Clinical Manifestations of Neoplasms of the Musculoskeletal System

Bony Sarcomas

Site

Upper or lower extremity or pelvis

Metaphysis of distal femur, proximal tibia, proximal humerus, and pelvis

Clinical Manifestations

- Worsening deep bony pain due to inflammation or weakness of bone
- Pain at night or during rest that may radiate and become severe
- Muscular weakness or atrophy due to pain
- Soft tissue mass extending from bone with erythematous or warm skin over tissue mass
- Alteration in ability to perform activities of daily living
- Fever

Soft Tissue Sarcomas

Site

Upper or lower extremity and pelvis

Thigh, shoulder, and pelvis

Pelvis

Clinical Manifestations

- Enlarging firm mass with irregular borders, which causes pain in surrounding soft tissue structures
- Erythema or warmth and venous dilation over skin
- Muscular weakness and atrophy with limited range of motion, alteration in ability to perform activities of daily living, and alteration in gait
- Paresthesia with neurologic involvement and distal swelling
- Palpable local lymph nodes resulting from inflammation of tumor
- Above clinical manifestations, plus altered bowel and bladder habits or pain with intercourse
- Weakening of muscles due to lumbosacral nerve involvement

- *Red blood cell (RBC) count.* A client with a malignant bone tumor will have an elevated RBC.
- *Serum calcium.* Serum calcium level will be elevated when there is massive bone destruction.

Chemotherapy

Chemotherapeutic agents are administered to shrink the tumor before surgery, to control recurrence of tumor growth after surgery, or to treat metastasis of the tumor. Chemotherapeutic agents used to treat bone tumors are listed in the accompanying box. See Chapter 9 for further discussion of chemotherapy and its nursing implications.

Radiation Therapy

Radiation therapy may be used in combination with chemotherapy. Radiation therapy is frequently applied to metastatic bone carcinomas as a method of pain control. It is also used to eliminate bony tumors or to eliminate any remaining tumor after a surgical procedure. Radiation therapy is discussed in Chapter 9.

Surgery

The goal of surgery for the treatment of primary bone tumors is to eliminate the tumor completely. Tumors are removed either by excising the tumor itself or by amputating the affected limb. The type of procedure varies from removing the tumor only, to removing the tumor along with a small margin of normal tissue surrounding the tumor, to removing the tumor and a wide zone of normal tissue, to removing the tumor and part or all of the bone in which it lies. When the tumor involves a joint, the limb must be amputated. Care of the client undergoing amputation is presented in Chapter 37.

Nursing Care

Nursing care for the client with bone tumors requires innovative actions from the time of diagnosis through the rehabilitation phase. In the acute phase, problems associated with pain, lack of knowledge, immobility, coping, and anxiety are foremost. If the client develops complications from treatment or if a malignancy metastasizes, problems related to home health maintenance management, self-concept, and prevention of further complications become more prominent in addition to those problems encountered in the acute phase.

Risk for Injury
In the client with a bone tumor, changes in bone tissue can cause pathologic fractures.

Nursing intervention with rationale follows:

■ Instruct clients in ways to avoid falls or injury to the tumor site. *Pathologic fractures may occur at the tumor site because bone destruction can weaken the area.*

Pain
In the client with a bone tumor, pain may be related to direct invasion of the tumor or to pathologic fractures.

Nursing interventions with rationales follow:

■ Develop strategies for controlling both acute pain (from surgery, fracture, or inflammation) and chronic pain (from progression of the disease). *Analgesics combined with nonpharmacologic methods of pain control provide optimum relief of pain. Chronic pain, when mild in nature, is best managed with NSAIDs or aspirin. Moderate pain is best managed with a combination of codeine and NSAIDs. Severe pain is best relieved with narcotic analgesics.*

■ Provide assistive devices (e.g., canes, walkers, crutches) when the client ambulates. *Assistive devices lessen the pain by supporting weight-bearing during ambulation.*

Activity Intolerance
Pain, recent surgical procedures, and effects of the disease process can cause activity intolerance in the client with a bone tumor. Nursing intervention with rationale follows:

■ Provide regular rest periods between therapeutic activities. *Therapy should be performed at a time of maximum comfort for the client to increase mobility.*

Knowledge Deficit
When surgical intervention is necessary, the client will need information about the postoperative routine. Nursing intervention with rationale follows:

■ Provide information about the postoperative routines related to wound care, drains, catheters, dressings, braces, casts, and timing of ambulation. *Cooperation from the postoperative client is essential to prevent complications.*

Impaired Physical Mobility
Pain, muscle wasting, or surgical procedures can impair the physical mobility of the client with a bone tumor. Nursing interventions with rationales follow:

> ### Chemotherapeutic Agents Used for Musculoskeletal Neoplasms
>
> **Alkylating Agents**
> Ifosfamide
> Cyclophosphamide
>
> **Antibiotics**
> Doxorubicin
> Bleomycin
>
> **Antimetabolites**
> Methotrexate
>
> **Plant Alkaloids**
> Vincristine
>
> **Synthetic Agents**
> Cisplatin

■ Begin muscle-strengthening and active and passive ROM exercises immediately after surgery. A continuous passive motion (CPM) machine may be used after surgical procedures to either upper or lower extremities. *Muscle strengthening exercises must be encouraged as soon as possible to prevent muscle wasting and shorten the rehabilitation period.*

■ For the client who has had an amputation, encourage active ROM exercises for all uninvolved joints. *Muscle-strengthening exercises must be encouraged because the client will need to ambulate using assistive devices until a prosthesis may be worn.*

■ Encourage exercises that help strengthen the triceps muscles. *The triceps are the major muscles in the arms and must be strengthened to assist in use of crutches or other devices.*

■ For the client who has undergone an amputation of a lower extremity, encourage quadriceps and gluteal setting exercises and leg raises. *These exercises will benefit the client when the rehabilitation period begins.*

■ Teach clients how to use the trapeze correctly. Clients can use the trapeze to reposition themselves while supine, get out of bed, and assist the nurse's efforts to reposition them in bed and perform other activities. *Use of the trapeze helps strengthen the biceps of the arm.*

Decisional Conflict
Knowledge deficit about diagnosis and treatment regimen can impair the client's ability to make informed decisions about the treatment plan. Nursing interventions with rationales follow:

■ Explain issues related to diagnosis, radiologic evaluation, biopsy, surgery, chemotherapy, radiation therapy, potential complications, alternative therapies, risks, benefits, nursing management, discharge plans, home care, and long-term treatment and follow-up. *The client requires this information in order to make informed decisions about treatment.*

Body Image Disturbance

The loss of limb and the effects of chemotherapy can alter the client's body image. Nursing interventions with rationales follow:

- Be supportive during the grieving period for the client who has lost a limb. *Changes in self-concept accompany physical changes due to surgery and the side effects of chemotherapy, especially the loss of hair.*

- Allow time for open discussions of the client's feelings about changes in body image and potential changes in social and personal life. *The client should be able to talk about the amputation and to view the stump prior to the rehabilitation process.*

Client and Family Teaching

Important aspects of teaching clients with bone tumors and their families are described in the collaborative care and nursing care sections.

Applying the Nursing Process

Case Study of a Client with Osteosarcoma: Harold Thompson

Harold Thompson, a 22-year-old African-American, is a quarterback for an Ivy League college. Mr. Thompson is 6 feet, 4 inches (193 cm) tall and weighs 230 lb (104.4 kg). He is majoring in pre-med and plans to become a veterinarian. He currently lives in a fraternity on campus.

After the fourth game of the football season, Mr. Thompson reports pain and swelling in his left knee and upper thigh that has subsided with the usual ice and hyperthermia treatments. He informs his coach that he has noticed that the swelling of the area has increased in size and tenderness since the beginning of the season. The coach is concerned and contacts the team's orthopedic physician for an evaluation.

Several diagnostic studies are ordered for Mr. Thompson after a thorough history and physical examination are conducted. After receiving results of the studies, the physician informs Mr. Thompson and his parents that the tentative diagnosis is osteogenic sarcoma.

This diagnosis is based on the results of the following studies:

- Serum alkaline phosphatase: 210 IU/L (normal range: 19 to 74 IU/L)

- Serum calcium: 18 mg/dL (normal range: 8.4 to 10.2 mg/dL).

- X-ray examination of left femur indicating a masslike structure at distal portion of left femur. Cortical breakthrough with the typical sunburst appearance of osteogenic sarcoma is also present. The mass shows poor margination, bone destruction, and the formation of irregular periosteal new bone at the edges of the growth.

- Total body bone scan: negative for metastasis.

Based on these data, Mr. Thompson and his parents decide that he should undergo the recommended radiation and chemotherapy treatments on an ambulatory basis at an outpatient department. Following recovery from the radiation and chemotherapy, he will be admitted for amputation of the involved extremity.

Assessment

The following week Mr. Thompson and his mother come to the outpatient department for his first chemotherapy treatment. Mike Tomei, RN, completes Mr. Thompson's admission assessment.

When performing the musculoskeletal assessment, Mr. Tomei notes the swelling at the distal femur area as well as limited range of motion of the left knee. Mr. Thompson confirms pain and tenderness when the nurse palpates the tumor area.

Mr. Tomei postpones the routine physical examination, knowing that Mr. Thompson and his parents had just learned about his diagnosis less than a week ago. Mr. Thompson tells the nurse that he did not think that the swelling in his knee was of any significance because he had been tackled several times in the last few games. Mr. Tomei listens very attentively and is able to obtain a thorough psychosocial history from Mr. Thompson.

After completing the necessary history and physical examination, Mr. Tomei reviews the procedure for administration of the prescribed chemotherapeutic agents with Mr. Thompson and his parents. Once the intravenous agent begins to infuse, he ensures that Mr. Thompson is comfortable and then visits with Mr. Thompson's parents to learn about their fears and anxieties about their son's condition and prognosis.

Diagnosis

The nursing diagnoses for Mr. Thompson include the following:

- *Pain* related to direct tumor invasion into soft tissue

- *Body Image Disturbance* related to effects of chemotherapy, radiation therapy, and surgery

- *Anticipatory Grieving* related to change in body image and possibility of impending death

- *Risk for Injury* related to bone demineralization secondary to bone tumor

- *Anxiety* related to lack of knowledge about disease process

- *Impaired Physical Mobility* related to size and extent of tumor and/or effects of terminal disease
- *Altered Role Performance* related to temporary or permanent inability to pursue professional career goals and/or maintain role in family or community

Expected Outcomes

The expected outcomes established in the plan of care specify that Mr. Thompson will

- Have a reduction in or alleviation of pain associated with the bone lesion.
- Work through the grieving process and accept the prognosis.
- Accept the physical changes that result from the effects of chemotherapy and radiation therapy.
- Prevent fracture of left leg by avoiding falls and minimizing trauma.
- Have a reduction in anxiety so that function is not impaired.
- Accept an altered role and the need to plan for different activities during his time in school.

Planning and Implementation

The following nursing interventions are planned and implemented for Mr. Thompson:

- Teach Mr. Thompson to take analgesics around the clock rather than on an as-needed basis to ensure that blood levels of medication remain constant.
- Teach Mr. Thompson about other forms of analgesic medications so that he can request these alternative forms if he is unable to take the medications orally.
- Be an active listener, and allow Mr. Thompson and the family to verbalize their feelings about the diagnosis and treatment.
- Refer Mr. Thompson and/or family members to counselors or members of the clergy to provide additional assistance to promote acceptance of the diagnosis, treatment, and, possibly, impending death.
- Help Mr. Thompson accept the body image alterations that result from the effects of chemotherapeutic agents and radiation therapy.
- Teach Mr. Thompson about precautions to take when walking to prevent fracture of the involved tumor site.
- Encourage Mr. Thompson to be an active participant in the decision-making aspects of care.
- Encourage Mr. Thompson to plan activities according to his present abilities rather than his former activities.

Evaluation

After completing the prescribed chemotherapy and radiation therapies, Mr. Thompson reports that his pain has been alleviated. He plans to continue attending the cancer support group, where he has met several other people his age with the same diagnosis. Members of the support group have helped him work through the body changes that occurred as a result of the therapies he received. He states that he is less anxious regarding his diagnosis, although he remains fearful about the upcoming surgical amputation of his leg.

Critical Thinking in the Nursing Process

1. List questions that the nurse can ask on first meeting Mr. Thompson to determine his state of anxiety and grieving related to the disease process.
2. Outline a teaching plan for Mr. Thompson that includes methods to alleviate the side effects following the administration of the chemotherapeutic agents used for osteosarcoma.
3. Compare and contrast the nursing interventions for a client receiving intravenous chemotherapeutic agents in the home with those for a client receiving chemotherapy on an outpatient basis.
4. List resources in your community that Mr. Thompson could use for support after he receives his chemotherapy, radiation, and amputation.

The Client with Muscular Dystrophy

■ ■ ■

Muscular dystrophy (MD) is a group of inherited muscular diseases that cause progressive muscle degeneration and wasting. The differences in the various types of MD relate to the age at onset, the gender affected by the disorder, the muscles involved, and the rate at which the disease progresses. These factors are summarized in Table 36–3.

In the majority of cases of MD, there is a positive family history. The most common form of MD, *Duchenne's muscular dystrophy,* is inherited as a recessive single gene defect on the X chromosome (a sex-linked recessive disorder), and is therefore transmitted from the mother to male children (Porth, 1994). This disorder affects males exclusively and occurs in 1 out of 3500 live male births. At this time, genetic counseling cannot be reliably used to prevent this disease because there is no way to determine if the woman carries the defective gene. The remainder of cases result from a new mutation of the gene; therefore, there is no evidence of family history that may alert parents to anticipate the disease.

Pathophysiology

The basic defect in MD is unknown; however three theories have been proposed. The vascular and neurogenic

Table 36–3   Types of Muscular Dystrophy

Type	Sex and Age at Onset	Clinical Manifestations	Progression
Duchenne	Males Age 3 to 5	Weakness of pelvic and shoulder girdles Waddling gait Toe walking Lordosis Cardiac abnormalities Low IQ in 50% of cases	Rapid; client usually confined to wheelchair by age 15; death occurs by age 20
Myotonic	Males & females Any age	Myotonia of hand muscles Muscular weakness of arms and legs Cardiac abnormalities Endocrine abnormalities Mental retardation (common)	Slow; death usually occurs in early 50s
Becker's	Males Age 5 to 20	Weakness of pelvic and shoulder girdles	Slow; client usually confined to wheelchair at 25 years after onset; normal life span
Facioscapulohumeral	Males and females Age 10 to 20	Weakness of face and shoulder girdles	Slow; normal life span
Limb-girdle	Males and females Age 20 to 40	Weakness of shoulder and pelvic girdles	Extremely variable; usually slow

theories suggest, respectively, that the cause is a lack of blood supply to the muscle or a disturbance in the interaction between the nerve and muscle. The most popular theory, the membrane theory, suggests that an alteration in the cell membranes of the muscle causes them to degenerate. Recent genetic studies have shown that there is a deficiency in the amount of a muscle membrane protein, called *dystrophin*, in clients with Duchenne MD. Dystrophin plays an important role in protecting the muscle against mechanical stresses.

All forms of MD exhibit clinical manifestations of muscle weakness (see Table 36–3). The specific muscles involved depend on the type of MD. As the disease progresses, the person develops difficulty with ambulation and eventually becomes wheelchair-bound and finally bed-bound. Depending on the type of MD, cardiac abnormalities, endocrine abnormalities, and mental retardation may also be involved.

Collaborative Care

Because there is no cure or specific treatment for MD, care focuses on preserving and promoting mobility as much as possible. A multidisciplinary approach, involving many members of the health care team, is necessary to meet the physical and psychologic needs of these clients and their families.

Diagnosis and classification of the muscular dystrophies are most often based on the clinical signs and the pattern of muscle involvement. Biochemical examination, muscle biopsy, and electromyography confirm the diagnosis. Tests include the following:

- *Creatine kinase (CK)*. CK is an enzyme found in high concentration in the heart, skeletal muscles, and brain. The laboratory study used to determine the possibility of muscular dystrophy is based on the isoenzyme found in skeletal muscle (CK-MM). When muscles are damaged, the enzyme is released from the cells. Thus, the client with suspected muscular dystrophy will have an elevated CK-MM.

- *Muscle biopsy*. A biopsy of the muscle of a client with muscular dystrophy will show fibrous connective tissue and fatty deposits that displace functional muscle fibers.

- *Electromyogram (EMG)*. EMG readings show a decrease in amplitude in clients with MD.

Nursing Care

Nursing care for a client with any form of muscular dystrophy focuses on promoting independence and mobility and providing psychologic support for both the client and family. A holistic approach is essential in planning and implementing care.

Self-Care Deficit

The progressive muscle weakness that is associated with MD impairs the client's ability to perform self-care. Nursing interventions with rationales follow:

- Provide clients and family with supportive care during the progress of the disease. *The goal of treatment is to prolong each functional stage and delay or prevent deformity. When transition from ambulation to a wheelchair occurs, depression and grief may occur. Constant medical, physical, and emotional involvement is required during these critical periods.*

- Promote independence as long as possible. Encourage tasks the client can accomplish rather than letting the client struggle with tasks that may prove frustrating. *All forms of muscular dystrophy result in progressive muscle weakness. Management of the disease is directed toward keeping the client as functional as possible while preventing any deformities.*

Other Nursing Diagnoses

Other nursing diagnoses that may apply follow:

- *Risk for Injury* related to unsteady gait and increasing weakness
- *Risk for Self-Esteem Disturbance* related to the effects of prolonged debilitating condition on life-style and development
- *Altered Family Processes* related to the nature of debilitating condition, role disturbances, and uncertain future
- *Risk for Diversional Activity Deficit* related to inability to perform job-related or diversional activities
- *Risk for Social Isolation* related to mobility difficulties and embarrassment associated with altered physical development
- *Anticipatory Grieving* related to the progressive, terminal nature of the disease

Client and Family Teaching

The important aspects of teaching clients and their family about muscular dystrophy have been described in collaborative care and nursing care sections.

Bibliography

■ ■ ■

Ali, N. S., & Twibell, K. R. (1994). Barriers to osteoporosis prevention in perimenopausal and elderly women. *Geriatric Nursing, 15*(4), 201–205.

American Academy of Orthopaedic Surgeons. (1988). *Osteoporosis.* Park Ridge, IL: Author.

Basle, M. F., Fournier, J. G., Rozenblatt, S., Rebel, A., Bouteille, M. (1986). Measles virus RNA detected in Paget's disease bone tissue by in situ hybridization. *Journal of General Virology, 67,* 907–913.

Berg, R. L. & Cassells, J. S. (Eds.). (1992). *The second fifty years: Promoting health and preventing disability.* Washington, D.C: National Academy Press.

Bockman, R. S. & Weinerman, S. A. (1990). Steroid-induced osteoporosis. *Orthopedic Clinics of North America, 21*(1), 97–107.

Carr, C. J. & Shangraw, R. F. (1987). Nutritional and pharmaceutical aspects of calcium supplementation. *American Pharmacy, 27*(2), 49–50, 54–57.

Chase, J. (1992). Outpatient management of low back pain. *Orthopaedic Nursing, 11*(1), 11–20, 43.

Cohen, L. D. (1990). Fractures of the osteoporotic spine. *Orthopedic Clinics of North America, 21*(1), 143–150.

Corbett, J. V. (1992). *Laboratory tests and diagnostic procedures with nursing diagnoses* (3rd ed.). Norwalk, CT: Appleton & Lange.

Cotran, R. S., Kumar, V., & Robbins, S. L. (1994). *Robbins pathologic basis of disease.* Philadelphia: Saunders.

Ebersole, P. & Hess, P. (1994). *Toward healthy aging: Human needs and nursing response* (4th ed.). St. Louis: Mosby.

Einhorn, T. A., Levine, B., & Michel, P. (1990). Nutrition and bone. *Orthopedic Clinics of North America, 21*(1), 43–50.

Eisenberg, R. L., & Dennis, C. A. (1990). *Comprehensive radiographic pathology.* St. Louis: Mosby.

Evans, R. A., Marel, G. M., Lancaster, E. K., Kos, S., Evans, M., & Wong, Y. P. (1988). Bone mass is low in relatives of osteoporotic patients. *Annals of Internal Medicine, 109,* 870–873.

Frymoyer, J. W., (1988). Back pain and sciatica. *New England Journal of Medicine, 318*(5), 291–300.

Frymoyer, J. W. & Cats-Baril, W. L. (1991). An overview of the incidence and costs of low back pain. *Orthopedic Clinics of North America, 22*(2), 263–271.

Holman, J. A., Poehling, G. G., & Martin, D. F. (1994). Common foot problems. In W. R. Hazzard, E. L. Bierman, J. P. Blass, W. H. Ettinger, Jr., & J. B. Halter (Eds.), *Principles of geriatric medicine and gerontology* (3rd ed.) (pp. 1297–1306). New York: McGraw-Hill.

Liscum, B. (1992). Osteoporosis: The silent disease. *Orthopaedic Nursing, 11*(4), 21–25.

Maher, A. B., Salmond, S. W., & Pellino, T. A. (1994). *Orthopaedic Nursing.* Philadelphia: W. B. Saunders.

Mann, R. A. (1989). The great toe. *Orthopedic Clinics of North America, 20*(4), 519–533.

McCance, K. L. & Huether, S. E. (1994). *Pathophysiology: The biologic basis for disease in adults and children* (2nd ed.). St. Louis: Mosby.

Miller, C. W. (1978). Survival and ambulation following hip fracture. *Journal of Bone and Joint Surgery, 60A,* 930–934.

Mills, B. G., Singer, F. R., Weiner, L. P., Suffin, S. C., Stabile, E., & Holst, P. (1984). Evidence for both respiratory syncytial virus and measles virus antigens in the osteoclasts of patients with Paget's disease of bone. *Clinical Orthopedics and Related Research, 183,* 303–311.

Olmarker, K., & Rydevik, B. (1991). Pathophysiology of sciatica. *Orthopedic Clinics of North America, 22*(2), 223–234.

Peck, W. A., Riggs, B. L., Bell, N. H., Wallace, R. B., Johnston, C. C., Gordon, S. L., & Shulman, L. E. (1988). Research directions in osteoporosis. *American Journal of Medicine, 84,* 275–282.

Pitt, M. (1991). Rickets and osteomalacia are still around. *Radiologic Clinics of North America, 29*(1), 97–118.

Porth, C. M. (1994). *Pathophysiology: Concepts of altered health states* (4th ed.). Philadelphia: Lippincott.

Raisz, L. G. (1982). Osteoporosis. *Journal of the American Geriatric Society, 30,* 127–138.

Riggs, B. L., & Melton, L. J. (1986). Medical progress: Involutional osteoporosis. *New England Journal of Medicine, 314*(26), 1676–1684.

Singer, F. R. (1987). Paget's disease of bone. In T. J. Martin & L. G. Raisz (Eds.). *Clinical endocrinology of calcium metabolism* (pp. 369–374). New York: Dekker.

Singer, F. R. (1994). Paget's disease of bone. In W. R. Hazzard, E. L. Bierman, J. P. Blass, W. H. Ettinger, Jr., J. B. Halteer, & R. Anders (Eds.), *Principles of geriatric medicine and gerontology* (pp. 929–934). New York: McGraw-Hill.

Uebelhart, D., Gineyts, E., Chapuy, M. C., & Delmas, P. D. (1990). Urinary excretion of pyridinium crosslinks: A new marker of bone resorption in metabolic bone disease. *Bone Mineral, 8*(1), 87–96.

Waddell, G. (1987). A new clinical model for the treatment of low-back pain. *Spine, 12*(7), 632–644.

Wallach, S. (1982). Treatment of Paget's disease. *Advances in Internal Medicine, 27,* 1–43.

Nursing Care of Clients with Musculoskeletal Trauma

LEARNING OBJECTIVES

After completing this chapter, you will be able to

- Discuss the factors that lead to musculoskeletal trauma.
- State how fractures are classified.
- Identify the laboratory and diagnostic tests used to assess the client who has experienced musculoskeletal trauma.
- Discuss collaborative interventions applied to clients who have experienced musculoskeletal trauma.
- Discuss common complications of fractures and nursing strategies to prevent their occurrence.

- Discuss the psychologic effects that are unique to amputation.
- Describe the difference between skin and skeletal traction.
- Develop a teaching plan for the client who has experienced musculoskeletal trauma.
- Use the nursing process as a framework for providing individualized care for clients who have experienced musculoskeletal trauma.

Trauma is an injury that results from excessive external force. The external source transmits more kinetic energy than the tissue can absorb, and injury results. The severity of the trauma depends not only on the amount of force but also on the location of the impact, because different parts of the body can withstand different amounts of force. For example, a small carpal bone in the hand cannot absorb as much energy as the femur. A wide variety of external sources can cause trauma, and the force involved can vary in severity; a step off the curb, a fall, being tackled in a football game, and a motor vehicle crash are a few examples.

Trauma is caused by either blunt or penetrating forces. A *blunt force* distributes energy over a large area and does not directly break the integrity of the skin. The chest hitting the steering wheel in a motor vehicle crash is one example of a blunt force. A *penetrating force*, by contrast, di-

rectly causes a break in the integrity of the skin. Common causes of penetrating trauma are guns and knives. It is important to remember that the size of the penetrating wound does not reflect the amount of energy exchanged; for example, an enormous amount of kinetic energy is dissipated when a bullet is fired. Trauma is the leading cause of death in people under age 44. Trauma is discussed in detail in Chapter 10.

Musculoskeletal injuries occur in 85% of people who sustain multiple trauma (Rosenthal, 1984). These injuries do not necessarily result in death; however, they often result in disability: Each year, approximately 80,000 Americans are permanently disabled as a result of traumatic injury (National Research Council, 1985).

Trauma prevention can save lives. Many communities are educating people of all ages, from grade-school children to older adults, in trauma prevention. Young adults face a high risk of sustaining trauma. They need to be taught the importance of safety equipment—such as automobile seat belts, bicycle helmets, football pads, proper footwear, protective eyewear, and hard hats—in preventing or decreasing the severity of injury from trauma. Young people also should be encouraged to avoid high-risk activities, such as diving into pools and drinking while operating heavy machinery.

Older clients are at higher risk for musculoskeletal trauma due to falls. For these clients, home assessments must be performed and potential hazards removed. Steps should be well lighted and have antislip treads and railings. Throw rugs and clutter should be removed from travel areas. Clients should always wear shoes with good treads to decrease the risk of slipping. The use of bath mats and other bathroom safety measures is also advisable.

Musculoskeletal trauma can result in mild injuries or very severe injuries. A patient may experience a soft tissue injury, a fracture, and/or a complete amputation. In addition, trauma to one part of the musculoskeletal system often produces dysfunction in adjacent structures. For example, a fracture of the femur prevents the adjacent muscles from abducting and adducting. Nursing care of clients with trauma is varied and complex. Nursing interventions focus on restoring homeostasis and may include administering pain medication and providing emotional support, education, and verbal assurance. Nursing care helps minimize the effects of trauma, prevents complications, and hastens restoration of function. The injury may require rehabilitation and changes in life-style, either temporary or permanent. This chapter focuses on nursing care of clients with fractures, amputations, soft tissue injuries, dislocations, and repetitive use injuries.

The Client with a Fracture

■ ■ ■

A **fracture** is any break in the continuity of a bone. Fractures vary in severity according to the location and the type of fracture. Fractures occur in all age groups and are more common in people who have sustained trauma and in older clients. Of the 32.8 million musculoskeletal injuries reported between 1985 and 1988, 18.8% were fractures (Praemer, Furner, & Rice, 1992). Risk factors and preventive measures are the same as those discussed above for musculoskeletal trauma in general.

Pathophysiology

A fracture occurs when the bone is subjected to more kinetic energy than it can absorb. Fractures may result from a direct blow, a crushing force (compression), a sudden twisting motion (torsion), a severe muscle contraction, or

disease that has weakened the bone (pathologic fracture). Two basic mechanisms produce fractures: direct force and indirect force. With direct force, the kinetic energy is applied at or near the site of the fracture. The bone cannot withstand the force. With indirect force, the kinetic energy is transmitted from the point of impact to a site where the bone is weaker. The fracture occurs at the weaker point.

Types of Fractures

Fractures are classified in a number of different ways (Table 37–1 on page 1562). One general classification is based on whether the skin is intact over the fractured bone(s). If the skin is intact, the fracture is considered a **closed fracture**, or *simple fracture*. If the skin integrity is interrupted, by contrast, the fracture is considered an **open fracture**, or *compound fracture*. An open fracture allows bacteria to enter the injured area and increases the risk of complications. Fractures are also classified as **complete fractures**, which involve the entire width of the bone, or **incomplete fractures**, which do not involve the entire width of the bone. Another classification of fractures is based on whether the anatomic alignment of the bone has been maintained. A **stable (nondisplaced) fracture** is a fracture in which the bones maintain their anatomic alignment. An **unstable (displaced) fracture** is a fracture in which the bones move out of correct anatomic alignment. If a fracture is displaced, immediate interventions are required. The bones must be placed back into proper alignment to prevent further damage to soft tissue, muscle, and bone and to promote healing. The direction of the fracture line is another important consideration used to classify fractures. The fracture line may be *oblique*, at a 45-degree angle to the bone, *spiral*, or along the lengthwise plane of the bone (*Greenstick* fracture).

Any of the 206 bones in the body can sustain a fracture. A fracture of the pelvis usually is considered the most serious; it often is accompanied by severe blood loss. One of the most common fractures is a hip fracture.

Fracture Healing

Regardless of the type, fracture healing progresses over three phases: the inflammatory phase, the reparative phase, and the remodeling phase (see the accompanying art). The inflammation that develops at the site of the fracture is accompanied by bleeding and initiates the **inflammatory phase**. A hematoma forms between the fractured bone ends and around the bone surfaces. The osteocytes at the bone ends die as the hematoma clots and deprives them of oxygen and nutrients. Necrosis of the cells heightens the inflammatory response, which in turn leads to vasodilation and edema. In addition, fibroblasts, lymphocytes, macrophages, and even osteoblasts from

Text continues on page 1562

Bone Healing

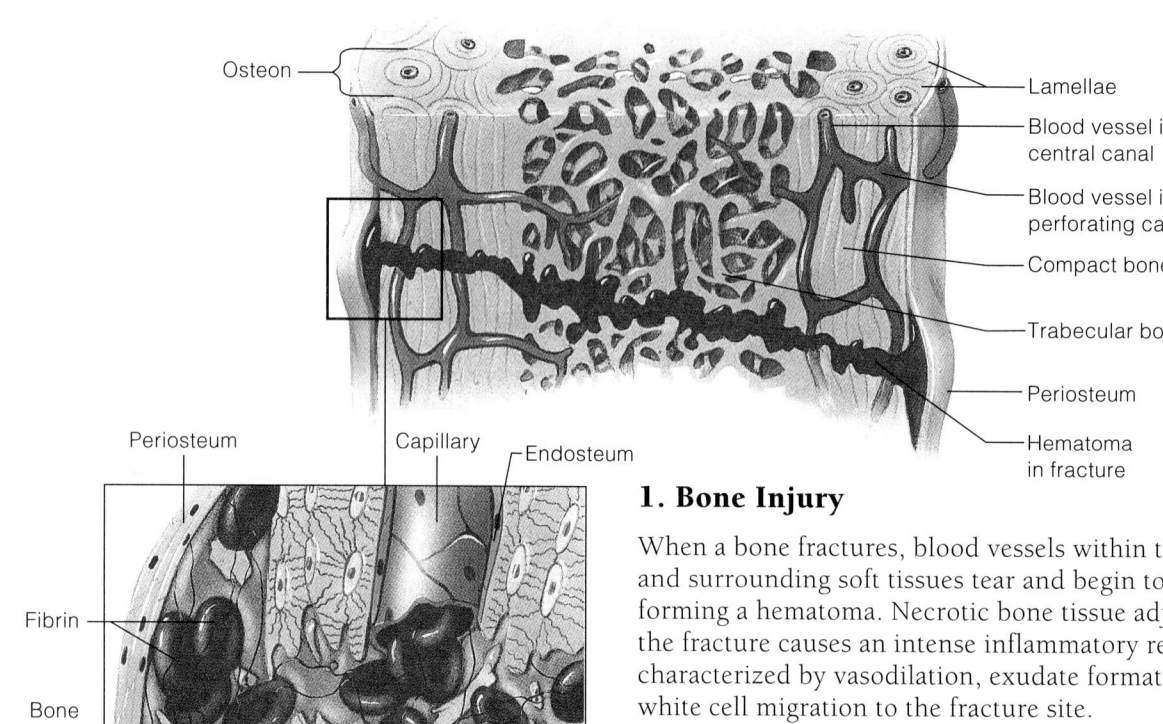

Osteon

Lamellae

Blood vessel in central canal

Blood vessel in perforating canal

Compact bone

Trabecular bone

Periosteum

Hematoma in fracture

Periosteum

Capillary

Endosteum

Fibrin

Bone fragment

Osteocyte

1. Bone Injury

When a bone fractures, blood vessels within the bone and surrounding soft tissues tear and begin to bleed, forming a hematoma. Necrotic bone tissue adjacent to the fracture causes an intense inflammatory response characterized by vasodilation, exudate formation, and white cell migration to the fracture site.

2. Fibrocartilaginous Callus Formation

Clotting factors within the hematoma form a fibrin meshwork. Within 48 hours, fibroblasts and new capillaries growing into the fracture form granulation tissue that gradually replaces the hematoma. Phagocytes begin to remove cell debris.

Osteoblasts, bone-forming cells, proliferate and migrate into the fracture site, forming a fibrocartilaginous callus. The osteoblasts build a web of collagen fibers from both sides of the fracture site that eventually unites to connect bone fragments, thus splinting the bone. Chondroblasts lay down patches of cartilage that provide a base for bone growth.

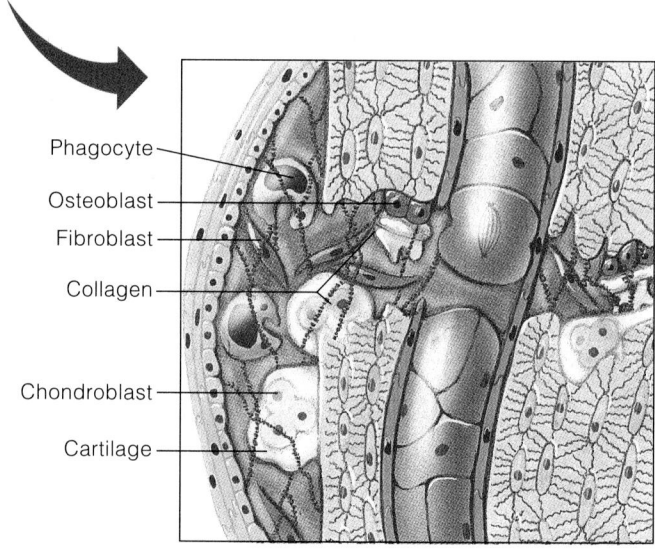

Phagocyte

Osteoblast

Fibroblast

Collagen

Chondroblast

Cartilage

4. Bone Remodeling

Osteoblasts continue to form new woven bone, which is in turn organized into the lamellar structures of compact bone. Osteoclasts resorb excess callus as it is replaced by mature bone.

As the bone heals and is subjected to the mechanical stress of everyday use, osteoblasts and osteoclasts respond by remodeling the repair site along the lines of force. This ensures that the repaired section of bone eventually resembles the structure of the uninjured part.

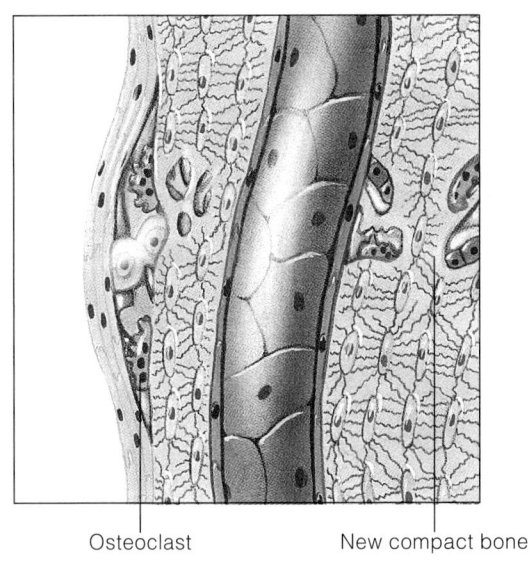

Osteoclast   New compact bone

3. Bony Callus Formation

Osteoblasts continue to proliferate and synthesize collagen fibers and bone matrix, which are gradually mineralized with calcium and mineral salts to form a spongey mass of woven bone. The trabeculae of woven bone bridge the fracture. Osteoclasts migrate to the repair site and begin removing excess bone in the callus. Bony callus formation usually continues for 2 to 3 months.

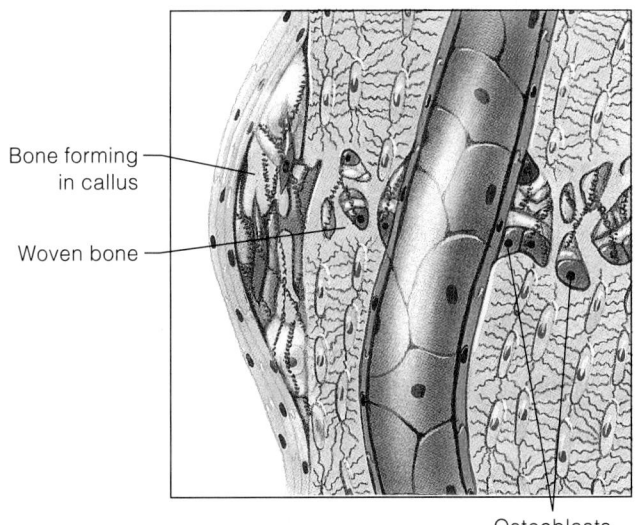

Bone forming in callus

Woven bone

Osteoblasts

Table 37–1   Common Fractures

Fracture Type	Description	Comments	Fracture Type	Description	Comments
Closed	Bone breaks cleanly but does not penetrate skin.	Also called a simple fracture.	Depressed	Broken bone is pressed inward.	Common in skull fractures.
Open	Broken ends of bone protrude through soft tissues and skin.	Serious; may result in osteomyelitis. Also called a compound fracture.	Spiral	Jagged break due to twisting force applied to bone.	Common fracture due to sports injuries.
Comminuted	Bone fragments into many pieces.	Common in the aged, whose bones are more brittle.	Greenstick	Bone breaks incompletely, much in the way a green twig breaks.	Common in children, whose bones have proportionally more organic matrix and are more flexible than those of adults.
Compression	Bone is crushed.	Common in clients with osteoporosis.			
Impacted	Broken ends of bone are forced into each other.	Commonly results from falls; also common in hip fracture.			

Note. Adapted from *Human Anatomy and Physiology* (3rd ed.) (p. 172) by E. N. Marieb, 1995, Redwood City, CA: Benjamin/Cummings.

the bone migrate to the fracture site. Fibroblasts form the fibrin meshwork. They promote the growth of granulation tissue and capillary buds. The lymphocytes and macrophages wall off the area, localizing and containing the inflammation. The capillary buds invade the fracture site and supply a source of nutrients to promote the formation of collagen. The collagen allows calcium to be deposited.

Once calcium is deposited, a callus begins to form. In this phase, referred to as the **reparative phase**, osteoblasts promote the formation of new bone, and osteoclasts destroy dead bone and assist in the synthesis of new bone. Collagen formation and calcium deposition continues. During the **remodeling phase**, excess callus is removed and new bone is laid down along the fracture line. Eventually, the fracture site is calcified, and the bone is reunited.

The age and physical condition of the client and the type of fracture sustained influence the healing of fractures. Other factors influence bone healing, either positively or negatively, and may be grouped according to

their local or systemic influence. See the accompanying box. Healing time varies with the individual. An uncomplicated fracture of the arm or foot can heal in 6 to 8 weeks. A fractured vertebra will take at least 12 weeks to heal. A fractured hip may take from 12 to 16 weeks.

Fractures are frequently accompanied by soft tissue injuries that involve muscles, arteries, veins, nerves, or skin. The degree of soft tissue involvement depends on the amount of energy or force transmitted to the area. Clinical manifestations and their causes are presented in the accompanying box. Fractures may be complicated by compartment syndrome, shock, fat embolism, deep vein thrombosis, infection, necrosis, delayed union, and reflex sympathetic dystrophy. The clinical implications of these complications are discussed in detail later in this chapter.

Collaborative Care

A fracture requires immediate treatment involving rapid transport to a healthcare provider, stabilization of the

---

Factors Influencing Bone Healing

■ ■ ■

Positive Factors

Local

- Immobilization
- Timely correction of displacement
- Application of ice
- Electrical stimulation

Systemic

- Adequate amounts of growth hormone, vitamin D, and calcium
- Adequate blood supply
- Absence of infection or diseases
- Younger age
- Moderate activity level prior to injury

Negative Factors

Local

- Delay in correction of displacement
- Open fracture (increases risk of infection)
- Presence of foreign body at fracture site

Systemic

- Immunocompromised status
- Decreased circulation (as in diabetes or peripheral vascular disease)
- Malnutrition
- Osteoporosis
- Advanced age

Clinical Manifestations of Fracture

■ ■ ■

Clinical Manifestation	Source
Deformity	Abnormal position of bones secondary to fracture and muscles pulling on fractured bone
Swelling	Edema from localization of serous fluid and bleeding
Pain/tenderness	Muscle spasm, direct tissue trauma, nerve pressure, movement of fractured bone
Numbness	Nerve damage or nerve entrapment
Guarding	Pain
Crepitus	Grating of bones or entrance of air in an open fracture. *Note:* Do not manipulate the extremity to elicit crepitus; doing so may cause additional damage.
Hypovolemic shock	Blood loss or associated injuries
Muscle spasms	Muscle contraction near the fracture
Ecchymosis	Extravasation of blood into the subcutaneous tissue

---

fractured bone(s), maintenance of bone immobilization, prevention of complications, and restoration of function. Frequent assessment and a variety of interventions are required of the health care team.

Prehospital/Emergency Care

Prehospital and emergency care of the client with a fracture includes immobilizing the fracture, maintaining tissue perfusion and sensation, preventing infection, and relieving pain. In the prehospital arena, the client must be safely removed from the scene of the trauma. Normal body alignment must be maintained and may involve cervical immobilization. Once the client is in a secure location, he or she is assessed for instability or deformity of the bone. If any deformity or instability is detected, the extremity is rapidly immobilized. Open wounds are covered with sterile dressings, and bleeding may be controlled with a pressure dressing. The extremities are assessed for the presence of pulses, movement, and sensation. The joint above and below the deformity is immobilized. Pulses, movement, and sensation are reevaluated after splinting.

The fracture is splinted to maintain normal anatomical alignment and prevent the fracture from dislocating. Splinting relieves pain and prevents further damage to the arteries, nerves, and bones. Splinting can be accomplished with military antishock trousers (MAST) and air splints. If equipment is not available, the limb may be secured to the body. For example, an arm may be secured with a sling, or one leg may be strapped to the other leg. In the emergency phase of care, the primary focus is to maintain the client's airway, breathing, and circulation. (See Chapter 10 for a full discussion of trauma.) After ensuring the adequacy of the client's breathing and circulation, the emergency department personnel perform a

Pain Management in the Client with a Fracture

∎ ∎ ∎

The client who has had musculoskeletal trauma from accident or surgery experiences pain from many different causes:

- The interruption in the continuity of the bone itself
- Damage to ligaments and tendons
- Swelling of tissues around the trauma site
- Muscle spasms
- Tissue anoxia from swelling inside a cast, splint, or the muscle fascia sheath
- Hematoma formation
- Pressure over bony prominences from casts or splints

The pain is often severe and may be described as sharp, aching, or burning. Carefully assess any complaint of pain; pain may be an indication of a serious complication, such as compartment syndrome, decreased tissue perfusion and neurovascular impairment, or pressure ulcers. Do not administer analgesics until the location, character, and duration of pain has been carefully assessed. After the cause of the pain has been identified, the following nursing interventions may be implemented.

1. Administer prescribed analgesics, which may include NSAIDs and narcotic analgesics. For serious fractures or following orthopedic surgery, PCA or epidural methods of providing pain relief may be used. If medications are used on an as-needed basis, tell the client to request the medication before the pain is severe; alternatively, offer the medications at regular intervals for the first 24 to 48 hours. Reassure the client that addiction does not result from taking medications to relieve fracture or surgical pain. Most clients require only oral analgesics by the third or fourth day after orthopedic surgery. Refer to Chapter 4 for information about narcotic and nonnarcotic pain medications.

2. Elevate the involved extremity, and apply cold (if prescribed) to help decrease swelling.

3. Monitor and drain the accumulated fluids in any drainage devices to ensure patency and to decrease the possibility of hematoma formation.

4. Encourage the client to wiggle fingers and toes on an extremity in a cast or traction to improve venous return and decrease edema.

5. Assist the client to change positions to relieve pressure and use pillows to provide support.

6. Teach the client alternative methods of pain management, such as relaxation and guided imagery.

7. Notify the physician of unrelieved pain, which may indicate a serious complication such as compartment syndrome or neurovascular impairment.

---

neurovascular assessment and then a general assessment (see Chapters 10 and 39). Once a thorough assessment is performed, the client undergoes diagnostic studies to confirm the presence of a fracture.

Laboratory and Diagnostic Tests

Diagnosis of a fracture begins with the history and initial assessment and usually is confirmed by radiographic tests. In the case of a severe open fracture, laboratory tests need to be completed so the client can proceed to the operating room. Less severe fractures may be immobilized with traction until the following day or until callus formation has begun. The following tests may be ordered:

- *X-rays.* X-rays are commonly used to assess bones for fractures. Anteroposterior and lateral views are often obtained. In children, the uninjured extremity is also X-rayed to allow comparison.
- *Bone scan.* A bone scan may be necessary to determine whether a fracture is present. A bone scan involves in-travenous administration of radioisotopes. An area of increased uptake, or a "hot" spot, may indicate a fracture.
- *Blood tests.* Blood chemistry studies, complete blood count (CBC), and coagulation studies are performed to assess blood loss, renal function, muscle breakdown, and the risk of excessive bleeding or clotting.
- *Urine myoglobin.* Urine myoglobin is measured to assess muscle breakdown.

Pharmacology

Most clients with a fracture require pharmacologic interventions. The first and foremost intervention focuses on alleviating discomfort. Initially, narcotics are administered intramuscularly. If surgery is required, the client may control postoperative pain with a patient-controlled analgesia (PCA) pump. This apparatus allows the client to receive medication intravenously at a continual rate (the basal rate) and to self-medicate with the press of a button up to

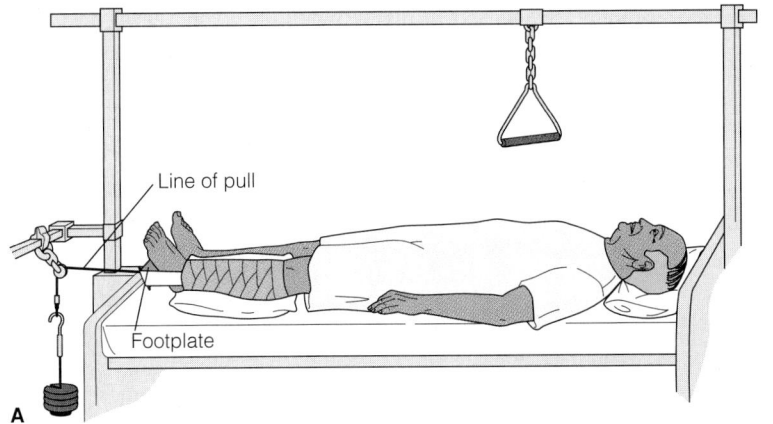

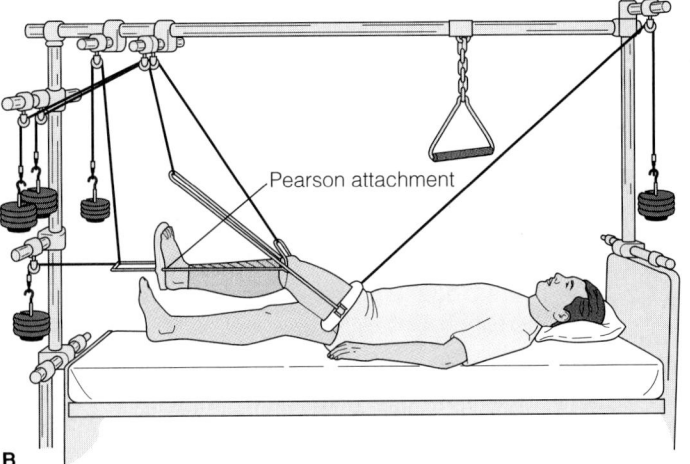

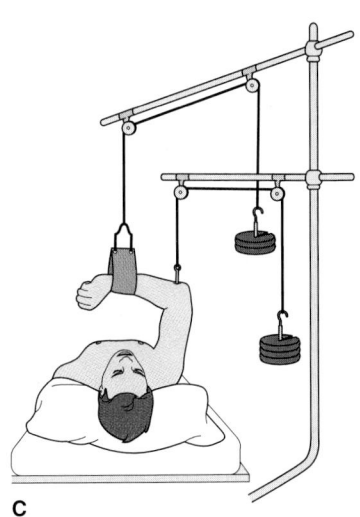

Figure 37–1 Traction is the application of a pulling force to maintain bone alignment during fracture healing. Different fractures require different types of traction. *A,* Skin traction (also called straight traction) such as Buck's traction shown here, is often used for hip fractures. *B,* Balanced suspension traction is commonly used for fractures of the femur. *C,* Skeletal traction, in which the pulling force is applied directly to the bone, may be used to treat fractures of the humerus.

a certain amount (the lock out rate). The PCA pump allows the client to have control over pain management and to prevent pain from peaking to unbearable levels. The client is weaned off the pump by first eliminating the continual dosage and then the self-administered dosage. The client then begins to take oral medication for pain. Pain management for the client with a fracture is described in the accompanying box.

Stool softeners may be administered or dietary fiber increased to decrease the risk of constipation secondary to narcotics and immobility. Clients who have sustained trauma are often placed on antiulcer medications such as histamine H_2 blockers or antacids. Nonsteroidal anti-inflammatory drugs (NSAIDs) may continue to be prescribed to decrease inflammation. Antibiotics may be administered prophylactically, particularly to clients with open or complex fractures. Pharmacologic interventions are individualized to the client's needs; for example, the client's hypersensitivities must be noted and the effectiveness of pain relief measures continually assessed.

Traction

Muscle spasms usually accompany fractures and may pull bones out of alignment. **Traction** is the application of a straightening or pulling force to return or maintain the fractured bones in normal anatomic position. Weights are applied to maintain the necessary force. There are several types of traction. In manual traction, the hand directly applies the pulling force. Physicians often utilize this type of traction when casting a fractured limb. Other common types of traction include straight traction, balanced suspension traction, skin traction, and skeletal traction (Figure 37–1).

Straight traction is a pulling force applied in a straight line to the injured body part resting on the bed. The most common type of straight traction is Buck's traction. In Buck's traction, the lower portion of the injured extremity is placed in a cradle-like sleeve. This sleeve is harnessed to itself, and a weight is hung from the bottom of a traction frame. The result is a force that pulls straight away from the body. This traction exerts its grabbing and pulling force through the client's skin. Therefore, this traction may be considered straight **skin traction.** The advantage of skin traction is the relative ease of use and ability to maintain comfort. The disadvantage is that the weight required to maintain normal body alignment or fracture alignment cannot exceed the tolerance of the skin, about 6 lb per extremity.

Nursing Implications for Clients Receiving Traction

■ ■ ■

- In skeletal traction, never remove the weights.

- In skin traction, remove weights only when intermittent skin traction has been ordered to alleviate muscle spasm.

- For traction to be successful, a countertraction is necessary. In most instances, the countertraction is the client's weight. Therefore, do not wedge the client's foot or place it flush with the footboard of the bed.

- Maintain the line of pull:
  a. Center the client on the bed.
  b. Ensure that weights hang freely and do not touch the floor.

- Ensure that nothing is lying on or obstructing the ropes. Do not allow the knots at the end of the rope to come into contact with the pulley.

- If a problem is detected, contact the physician to assist in repositioning. The area of the fracture must be stabilized when the client is repositioned.

- In skeletal traction:
  a. Frequent skin assessments should include pin care per hospital policy.
  b. Report signs of infection at the pin sites, such as redness, drainage, and increased tenderness, to the physician.
  c. The client may require more frequent analgesic administration.

- Perform neurovascular assessments frequently.

- Assess for common complications of immobility, including formation of pressure ulcers, formation of renal calculi, deep vein thrombosis, pneumonia, paralytic ileus, and loss of appetite.

- Instruct the client and family about the type and purpose of the traction.

Balanced suspension traction involves more than one force of pull. Several forces work in unison to raise and support the client's injured extremity off the bed and pull it in a straight fashion away from the body. The advantage of this type of traction is that it increases mobility without threatening joint continuity. It is easier to change linen and perform back care. The disadvantage is that the increased use of multiple weights makes the client more likely to slide in the bed.

Skeletal traction is the application of a pulling force through placement of pins into the bone. The client receives local anesthetic, and the pin is inserted in a twisting motion into the bone. This type of traction must be applied under sterile conditions because of the increased risk of infection. One or more pulling forces may be applied with skeletal traction. The advantage of this type of traction is that more weight can be used to maintain the proper anatomic alignment if necessary. The disadvantages include increased anxiety, increased risk of infection, and increased discomfort. Nursing implications for clients receiving traction are presented in the accompanying box.

Casts

Casts are applied on clients who have relatively stable fractures. A **cast** is a rigid device applied to immobilize the injured bones and promote healing. The cast is applied to immobilize the joint above and the joint below the fractured bone so that the bone will not move during healing. A fracture is first **reduced**, that is, placed in correct anatomic alignment, manually by the physician; a cast is then applied. The cast, which may be composed of plaster or fiberglass, is applied over a thin cushion of padding and molded to the normal contour of the body. The cast must be allowed to dry before any pressure is applied to it; simply palpating a wet cast with the fingertips will leave dents that may cause pressure sores. A plaster cast may require up to 48 hours to dry, whereas a fiberglass cast dries in less than 1 hour. The type of cast applied is determined by the location of the fracture (Figure 37–2). Nursing implications for clients with casts are presented in the accompanying box.

During follow-up appointments, the physician may X-ray the bone to assess alignment and healing, and possibly remove the cast for skin assessment.

Electrical Bone Stimulation

Electrical bone stimulation is the application of electrical current at the fracture site. It is used to treat fractures that are not healing appropriately. The electrical stress increases the migration of osteoblasts and osteoclasts to the fracture site. Mineral deposition increases, promoting bone healing. Electrical bone stimulation can be accomplished invasively or noninvasively (Figure 37–3). In invasive stimulation, the surgeon inserts a cathode and a lead wire at the fracture site. The lead wire is attached to an internal or external generator, which delivers electricity through the lead wire to the cathode 24 hours a day. In noninvasive inductive stimulation, a treatment coil encircles the cast or skin directly over the fracture site. The coil is attached to an external generator that runs on batteries.

Nursing Implications for Clients with Casts

Nursing Responsibilities

- Perform frequent neurovascular assessments.
- Palpate the cast for "hot spots" that may indicate the presence of underlying infection.
- Report any drainage to physician promptly.

Client and Family Teaching

- Do not place any objects in the cast.
- If the cast is made of plaster, keep it dry.
- If the cast is made of fiberglass, dry it with a blow dryer on the cool setting if it becomes wet.
- Assess the injured extremity for coolness, changes in color, increased pain, increased swelling, and/or loss of sensation.

- Use a blow dryer on the cool setting to relieve itching by blowing cool air into the cast.
- If a sling is used, it should distribute the weight of the cast evenly around the neck. Do not roll the sling; this can impair circulation to the neck.
- If crutches are used, arrange for physical therapist to teach correct crutch walking.
- When the cast is removed at follow-up appointments for skin assessments, an oscillating cast remover will be used. A guard prevents the cast remover from penetrating past the depth of the cast, so it will not cut the client. It is noisy, and the client will feel vibration. The client may wish to wash and thoroughly dry the extremity before reapplication of the cast.

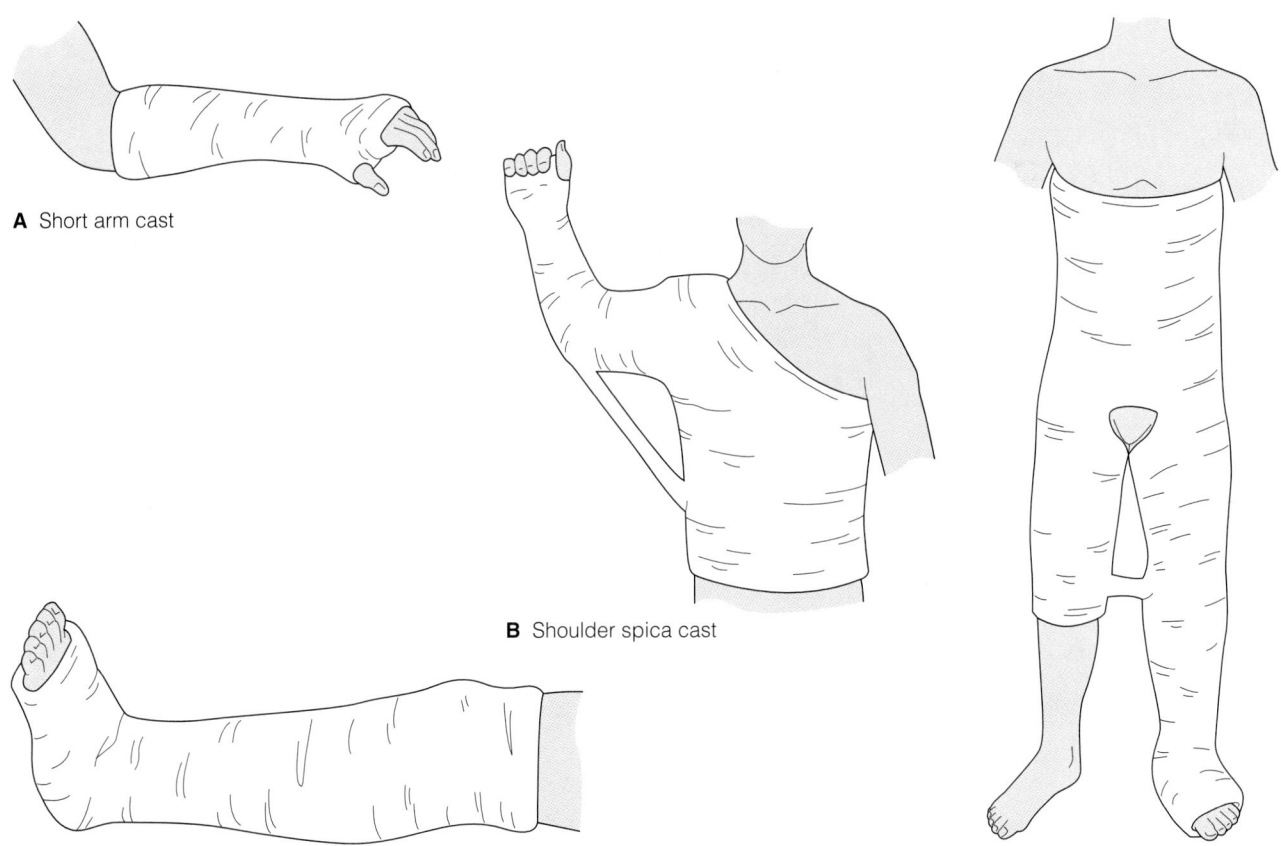

A Short arm cast

B Shoulder spica cast

C Long leg cast

D One-and-one half hip spica cast

Figure 37–2   Common types of casts used to immobilize fractures.

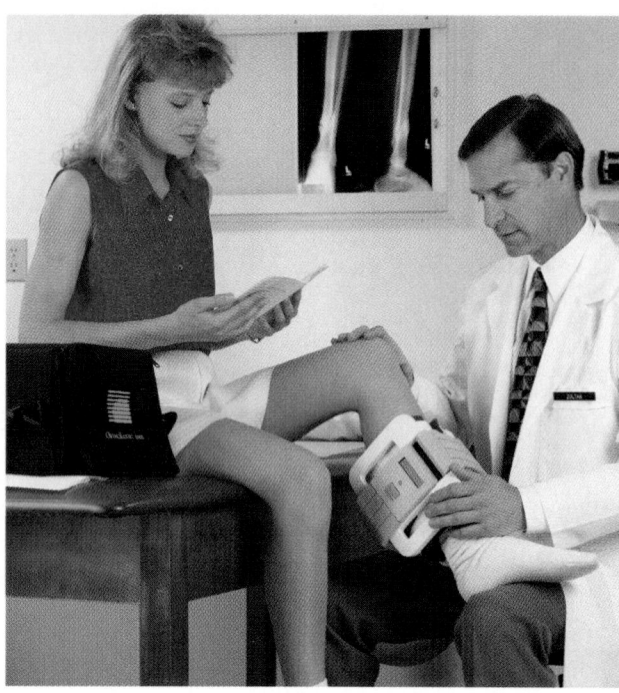

Figure 37–3 External electrical bone growth stimulator.

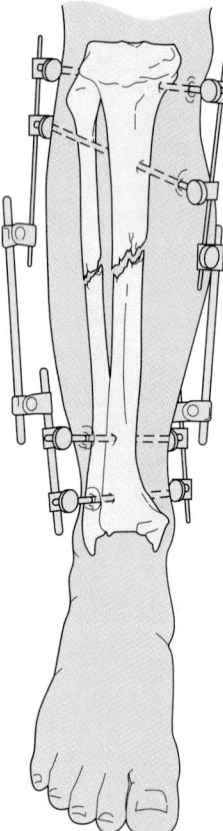

Figure 37–4 In external fixation, pins are placed through the bone above and below the fracture site to immobilize the bone. External fixation rods hold the pins in place.

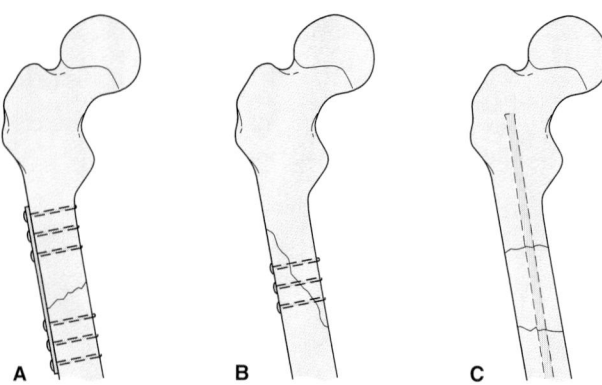

Figure 37–5 Internal fixation hardware is entirely within the body. *A,* Fixation of a short oblique fracture using a plate and screws above and below the fracture. *B,* Fixation of a long oblique fracture using screws through the fracture site. *C,* Fixation of a segmental fracture using a medullary nail.

The electricity goes through the skin to the fracture site. The physician specifies how long the fracture site is to be stimulated; the time period can vary from 3 to 10 hours per day. The client may be taught to self-administer the noninvasive electrical stimulation. Electrical bone stimulation is contraindicated in the presence of infection.

Surgery

Surgery is indicated in the client who has a fracture that requires direct visualization and repair, a fracture with common long-term complications, or a fracture that is severely comminuted and threatens vascular supply. The physician decides whether surgery is indicated and what type is needed. The accompanying collaborative care box describes the roles played by various members of the health care team in caring for the client requiring open reduction of a fractured leg.

The simplest form of surgery is the application of an external fixator device. An *external fixator* consists of a frame connected to pins that are inserted perpendicular to the long axis of the bone (Figure 37–4). The number of pins inserted varies with the type and site of the fracture, but in all cases the same number of pins is inserted above and below the fracture line. The pins require care similar to that of skeletal traction pins. The client is monitored for infection, and frequent neurovascular assessment is performed. The fixator increases independence while maintaining immobilization. It can lead to early discharge and decrease health care costs.

Internal fixation can be accomplished through a surgical procedure called an open reduction and internal fixation (ORIF). In this procedure, the physician directly reduces the fracture and uses a nail, screws, plates and screws, or pins to hold the bones in place (Figure 37–5). Open fractures of the arms and legs are most commonly

Collaborative Care: The Client Requiring Open Reduction of a Fractured Leg	
Health Care Team	**Client-Centered Goals**
Orthopedic surgeon	Provides emergency treatment of fractures. May use traction, casts, splints, rods, plates, and/or prostheses to immobilize the fracture. Performs open reduction. Monitors and manages for complications such as hemorrhage and infection. Prescribes pain medication.
Dietitian	Assesses and teaches age-appropriate diet to promote bone healing. Encourages intake of high-protein, high-kcal diet rich in vitamins and minerals.
Physical therapist	Teaches isometric, passive, and active exercise. Instructs client in the use of appropriate assistive devices and partial to full weight-bearing.
Home care coordinator	Arranges for continuation of physical therapy and support services as needed after discharge. Assesses home situation and arranges home health assistance for personal care.
RN and Health Care Team Communications Facilitator	Reports any change in neurovascular status, evidence of compartment syndrome, hemorrhage, or signs or symptoms of infection. Reports pain not controlled by ordered medications. Discusses food likes and dislikes with dietitian and develops strategies to enhance nutritional intake. Alerts social worker to home care needs during recuperation.

repaired in this way. Hip fractures in older clients are almost always repaired with ORIF to prevent complications and to allow early rehabilitation. Implications for postoperative nursing care are presented in the accompanying box. A Critical Pathway for the client following open reduction and internal fixation of a fracture of the lower leg is provided on page 1570.

Collaborative Care for Fracture Complications

Potential complications of fractures include compartment syndrome, shock, fat embolism, deep vein thrombosis, infection, necrosis, delayed union, and reflex sympathetic dystrophy.

Compartment Syndrome

A **compartment** is a space enclosed by a fibrous membrane. Compartments within the limbs may enclose and support bones, nerves, and blood vessels. **Compartment syndrome** occurs when external or internal pressure constricts the structures within a compartment, reducing tissue perfusion. An improperly fitted cast, bleeding, or edema within the structures enclosed by a cast are sources of pressure that can trigger compartment syndrome. The pressure results in entrapment of nerves, blood vessels, and muscles. Entrapment of the blood vessels limits tissue perfusion, beginning a cycle of events that may result in the loss of the limb. Inadequate oxygen supply causes cellular acidosis, which intensifies as cellular energy requirements are met through anaerobic metabolism. The capillaries inside the compartment dilate in an attempt to increase the supply of blood and oxygen. Additional blood and oxygen are not available, and plasma proteins leak out into the interstitial tissues. The interstitial tissue

---

Postoperative Nursing Implications for Clients with Internal Fixation

■ ■ ■

- Expect the client to have sutures and at least one Hemovac drain.
- Perform neurovascular assessments frequently.
- Also assess the following:
  a. Wounds for drainage
  b. Hemovac for drainage of serosanguineous fluid
  c. Bowel sounds
  d. Lung sounds
- Administer medications, such as analgesics and antibiotics, per physician's orders.
- In hip fractures, place an abductor pillow between client's legs to prevent dislocation of the hip joint.
- Arrange for physical and occupational therapy, as ordered.
- Assist with weight-bearing program, if ordered.
- Encourage early mobilization, coughing, and deep breathing, as appropriate, to help prevent complications.

then pulls fluid in to balance the protein load; as a result, edema within the compartment increases. The edema causes further compression of the vascular network, and the cycle continues. Uninterrupted, this cycle threatens

Text continues on page 1572

Critical Pathway for Client Following Open Reduction and Internal Fixation of a Lower Leg Fracture		
	Date _____ **Operative Day**	**Date** _____ **1st Postoperative Day**
	Expected length of stay: 3–4 days following surgery	
Daily outcomes	The client ■ Has stable vital signs. ■ Recovers from anesthesia: vital signs return to baseline; client is awake, alert, and oriented; lungs are clear. ■ Verbalizes understanding of and demonstrates cooperation with turning, coughing, deep breathing, and prescribed activity level. ■ Controls pain with ordered medication. ■ Tolerates ordered diet without nausea and vomiting. ■ Verbalizes ability to cope.	The client ■ Has stable vital signs, with clear lungs, and is alert, and oriented. ■ Verbalizes understanding of and demonstrates cooperation with turning, coughing, deep breathing, and prescribed activity level. ■ Controls pain with ordered medication. ■ Tolerates ordered diet without nausea and vomiting. ■ Verbalizes ability to cope.
Tests and treatments	Hct/Hgb Vital signs and O_2 saturation, neurovascular assessment, and cast assessment q15min $\times$ 4; q30min $\times$ 4 ; q1h $\times$ 4 and then q4h if stable. Head-to-toe assessment* q4–8 h Incentive spirometer q2h. Intake and output every shift	Vital signs and O_2 saturation, neurovascular assessment, and cast assessment q4h if stable Head-to-toe assessment every shift and prn Incentive spirometer q2h Intake and output every shift
Knowledge deficit	Orient to room and surroundings. Provide simple, brief instructions. Review plan of care and importance of specific postoperative care: turning, coughing, deep breathing, incentive spirometer, mobilization, possible tubes and intravenous, pain management (IV/PCA or IM prn medications). Include family in teaching. Assess understanding of teaching.	Review plan of care and importance of early mobilization. Begin discharge teaching regarding cast care and mobility. Include family in teaching. Assess understanding of teaching.
Psycho-social	Assess anxiety related to diagnosis and surgery. Assess fears of the unknown and surgery. Encourage verbalization of concerns. Provide information regarding surgical experience. Minimize external stimuli (e.g., noise, movement).	Assess level of anxiety. Encourage verbalization of concerns. Provide information. Provide ongoing support and encouragement.
Diet	Advance from clear liquids to full liquids to tolerance. Baseline nutritional assessment.	Advance from full liquids to regular diet as tolerated. Offer supplemental feedings high in protein and vitamins.

* Head-to-toe asessment: Assess major body systems affected by immobility, including the musculoskeletal, cardiovascular, respiratory, metabolic and nutritional, urinary, endocrine, gastrointestinal, integumentary, and neurosensory systems.

	Date _____ **Operative Day**	Date _____ **1st Postoperative Day**
Activity	Assess safety needs and provide appropriate precautions. Reposition q2h and prn. Assist client with full range of motion to all unaffected extremities 3 or 4 times daily. Teach the client isometric exercises for lower limb. Encourage client to participate in activities of daily living as much as possible. Provide overhead trapeze and encourage use q3h. Keep extremity elevated.	Maintain safety precautions. Reposition q2h and prn. Assist client with full range of motion to all unaffected extremities 3 or 4 times daily. Encourage the client to perform isometric exercises for lower limb. Encourage client to participate in activities of daily living as much as possible. Encourage use of overhead trapeze q3h. Keep extremity elevated.
Medications	IV/PCA or IM analgesic IV antibiotics IV fluids Antipyretics—prn	IV/PCA or IM analgesic IV antibiotics IV fluids or intermittent IV device Antipyretics—prn
Transfer/ discharge plans	Assess discharge needs and support system. Establish discharge goals with client and family.	Determine referral needs for time of discharge. Begin home care teaching.

	Date _____ **2nd Postoperative Day**	Date _____ **3rd to 4th Postoperative Day**
Daily outcomes	The client ▪ Has stable vital signs and clear lungs. ▪ Demonstrates cooperation with turning, coughing, deep breathing, and prescribed activity level. ▪ Controls pain with ordered medication. ▪ Tolerates ordered diet without nausea and vomiting. ▪ Ambulates with crutches 2 to 3 times per day. ▪ Verbalizes ability to cope. ▪ Verbalizes/demonstrates beginning understanding of home care instructions.	The client ▪ Is afebrile, has stable vital signs and clear lungs. ▪ Has intact neurovascular status to affected extremity. ▪ Manages pain with oral medications. ▪ Is independent in self-care. ▪ Is independent in transfers and ambulatory with crutches. ▪ Has resumed preadmission urine and bowel elimination pattern. ▪ Verbalizes/demonstrates home care instructions. ▪ Tolerates usual diet. ▪ Verbalizes ability to cope with ongoing stressors.
Tests and treatments	Vital signs q4h Neurovascular assessment q4h and prn Head-to-toe assessment every shift and prn Incentive spirometer q2h until client is fully ambulatory Intake and output every shift	Vital signs q4h Neurovascular assessment q4h and prn Head-to-toe assessment every shift Incentive spirometer q2h until fully ambulatory D/C intake and output if client is taking adequate fluids and input is balanced with output

➤

	Date _____ **2nd Postoperative Day**	**Date _____** **3rd to 4th Postoperative Day**
Knowledge deficit	Initiate discharge teaching regarding diet, signs and symptoms to report, and activity level. Consult with physical therapist for beginning instructions regarding crutch walking. Review written discharge instructions. Include family in teaching. Assess understanding of teaching.	Provide client with written discharge instructions that discuss (1) weight-bearing on affected extremity, (2) manifestations of infection related to internal fixation device, (3) regular follow-up care, (4) care of cast, (5) monitoring neurovascular status, and (6) use of assistive devices. Include family in teaching. Complete discharge teaching to include diet, follow-up care, manifestations to report, activity, and medications: name, purpose, dose, frequency, route, food interactions, and side effects. Assess understanding of teaching.
Psycho-social	Encourage verbalization of concerns. Provide ongoing support and encouragement.	Encourage verbalization of concerns. Provide ongoing support and encouragement.
Diet	Regular diet as tolerated. Encourage fluid intake of 2000 mL per day when IV fluids D/C. Offer supplemental feedings high in protein and vitamins.	Regular diet as tolerated Encourage fluids to 2000 mL/24 hours. Offer supplemental feedings high in protein and vitamins.
Activity	Maintain safety precautions. Assist client with full range of motion to all unaffected extremities 3 or 4 times daily. Encourage client to perform isometric exercises for lower limb. Encourage client to participate in activities of daily living as much as possible. Encourage client to use overhead trapeze q3h. Refer to physical therapist to begin non-weight-bearing crutch walking. Assist out of bed 2 to 3 times/day to tolerance. Keep extremity elevated.	Provide safety precautions. Assist client with full range of motion to all unaffected extremities 3 or 4 times daily. Encourage client to perform isometric exercises for lower limb. Encourage client to participate in activities of daily living as much as possible. Encourage client to use overhead trapeze q3h. Continue to work with physical therapy to promote non-weight-bearing crutch walking 4 times per day, and begin stair training.
Medications	IV/PCA, IM, or PO analgesics IV antibiotics Intermittent IV device	PO analgesic. D/C intermittent IV device.
Discharge plans	Complete discharge plans, including referrals. Continue home care instructions.	Complete discharge instructions and referrals.

the patient's limb and increases the risk of sepsis. Compartment syndrome usually develops within the first 48 hours of injury, when edema is at its peak. Clinical manifestations of compartment syndrome are shown in the accompanying box.

Compartment syndrome is best treated through prevention, by means of rest, ice, and elevation of the injured extremity. If compartment syndrome develops, the physician must be notified. Interventions to alleviate pressure will be implemented; often, these include removal of a tightly fitting cast. If the pressure is internal, a **fasciotomy**, a surgical intervention by which muscle fascia is cut to relieve muscle constriction or to reduce muscle contracture, may be necessary. After a fasciotomy, the incision is left open, and passive range-of-motion (ROM) exercises are performed on the extremity.

Volkmann's contracture, a common complication of elbow fractures, can result from unresolved compartment syndrome. Arterial blood flow decreases, leading to ischemia, degeneration, and contracture of the muscle. Arm mobility is impaired, and the client is unable to completely extend the arm.

Shock

Shock can result early from blood loss or from sepsis. In early stages, shock is usually secondary to severe blood loss. A pelvic fracture, for example, may result in a blood loss of up to 4½ liters. Table 37–2 lists the potential blood loss associated with fractures of various bones.

Associated injuries may also cause severe hypovolemia. The client initially presents with an increased cardiac rate and a decreased blood pressure. Administration of a fluid challenge with isotonic fluid, such as normal saline or lactated Ringer's solution, will improve the client's condition; however, only a blood transfusion and control of bleeding will correct it. If hypotension and hypovolemia continue untreated, the client may develop cardiac arrest with pulseless electrical activity (PEA). This dysrhythmia is corrected only by correcting the underlying mechanism, that is, replacing lost blood and controlling bleeding.

If infection develops in the fracture and remains untreated, bacteria can invade the bloodstream and cause sepsis. Bacteria may release endotoxins, vasodilators that cause blood pressure to fall and heart rate to increase. The client also develops a high fever, which further dilates blood vessels and increases heart rate. Sepsis requires adequate treatment with antibiotics. (Refer to Chapter 6 for a discussion of septic shock.)

Fat Embolism

A **fat embolism** is the occlusion of small blood vessels by fat globules. A major cause of death in clients with fractures, fat embolism can develop at any age but is more common in 20- to 40-year olds and in males. Up to 25% of people with long bone fractures will develop a fat embolism. Older people who experience hip fractures are also at risk for fat embolism.

When a bone is fractured, pressure within the bone marrow rises and exceeds capillary pressure; as a result, fat globules leave the bone marrow and enter the bloodstream. Another contributing factor may be the stress-induced release of catecholamine, which causes the rapid mobilization of fatty acids. Once the fat globules are released, they combine with platelets and travel to the

---

Clinical Manifestations of Compartment Syndrome

Early Manifestations

- Pain
- Decreased pulse

Later Manifestations

- Cyanosis
- Tingling
- Loss of sensation
- Severe pain, especially when the extremity is passively flexed
- Eventual renal failure (due to release of myoglobin into the blood stream; myoglobin molecule is too large for effective filtration and excretion by kidney and renal failure results)

Table 37–2	Fracture Site and Potential Blood Loss
Fracture Site	**Potential Blood Loss (Liters)**
Humerus	1.0 to 2.0
Elbow	0.5 to 1.5
Forearm	0.5 to 1.0
Pelvis	1.5 to 4.5
Hip	1.5 to 2.5
Femur	1.0 to 2.0
Knee	1.0 to 1.5
Tibia	0.5 to 1.5
Ankle	0.5 to 1.5
Spine/ribs	1.0 to 3.0

---

brain, lungs, kidneys, and other organs, occluding small blood vessels and causing tissue ischemia.

Manifestations usually develop within 24 to 48 hours of injury but can develop from a few hours to a week after injury. The manifestations result from the occlusion of the blood supply and the presence of fatty acids. If blood flow to the brain is occluded, confusion and alterations in mental status develop. If blood flow to the lungs is occluded, tachypnea, dyspnea, and hypoxia develop. If blood flow to the kidneys is occluded, renal failure may

Table 37–3	Precursors of Deep Vein Thrombosis
Precursor	**Implications for Fractures**
Decreased blood flow	Common in fracture clients, who are immobilized and less active. Bed rest alone can decrease venous flow by 50%.
Injury to blood vessel wall	May occur as a direct result of the force that caused the fracture or from surgical manipulation.
Altered blood coagulation	May result from active blood loss. The body's attempt to maintain homeostasis leads to increased production of platelets and clotting factor.

develop with resulting oliguria or anuria. A unique manifestation found with fat embolism is *petechiae*. Petechiae are pin-sized purple or red spots that appear on the skin, buccal membranes, conjunctival sacs, and fundus of the eye as the result of hemorrhages induced by fat emboli.

Treatment of fat emboli focuses first on prevention. Fractures need to be immobilized and stabilized quickly. Because hypovolemia may increase the risk, rapid fluid replacement and control of bleeding are essential. The nurse also needs to monitor clients with fractures closely for any change in mental status, which may indicate fat embolus. If fat embolus is suspected, respiratory support, including oxygen therapy and ventilator support, may be necessary.

Deep Vein Thrombosis

Fat emboli are sometimes confused with deep vein thrombosis. A **deep vein thrombosis (DVT)** is a blood clot that forms along the intimal lining of a vein. There are three definite precursors that have been linked to DVT formation: (1) venous stasis, or decreased blood flow, (2), injury to blood vessel walls, and (3) altered blood coagulation (Table 37–3). Any or all of these precursors can cause a DVT to form. A weakened area in the lining of the vein causes the platelets to aggregate or clump together, forming the thrombus. Fibrin, white blood cells (WBCs), and red blood cells (RBCs) begin to cling to the thrombus, and a tail forms. This tail or the entire thrombus may dislodge and move to the brain, lungs, or heart. Five percent of DVTs dislodge and enter the pulmonary circulation to form a pulmonary embolus. If the thrombus remains in the vein, it will decrease blood supply to that area. A decrease in the blood supply can inhibit healing.

The best treatment for DVT is prevention. Early immobilization of the fracture and early ambulation of the client are imperative. The extremity should be elevated above the level of the heart. Frequent assessments of the injured extremity may lead to early recognition of DVT and prevent the formation of pulmonary embolus. Prophylactic subcutaneous administration of heparin is also beneficial. Antiembolism stockings and compression boots also increase venous return and prevent stasis of blood. Constrictive clothing, however, should be avoided, as should the use of the knee gatch on the bed.

If a DVT is present, swelling, leg pain, tenderness, or cramping may be present. The client may complain of pain in the calf when the foot is dorsiflexed; this is referred to as a positive Homans' sign. Not all clients experience manifestations, however. For this reason, diagnostic tools, such as a venogram or Doppler ultrasound of lower extremities, may be required. A venogram requires intravenous administration of dye in the radiology department, whereas a Doppler ultrasound study is noninvasive and can be performed at the client's bedside. Doppler ultrasonography uses sound waves to form an image on a computer screen.

Regardless of the diagnostic tool used, the diagnosis of deep vein thrombosis requires rapid intervention. The client is placed on bed rest for 5 to 7 days to prevent dislodgment of the clot. Thrombolytic agents, which dissolve the clot, may be administered. Heparin may be administered intravenously to prevent more clots from forming. A vena cava filter may be placed to prevent the existing clot from entering the pulmonary circulation and forming a pulmonary embolus. In extreme cases in which anticoagulation therapy is contraindicated, a thrombectomy (surgical removal of the clot) may be necessary.

Infection

Infection is more likely to occur in an open fracture than a closed fracture, but any complication that decreases blood supply increases the risk of infection. Infection may result from contamination at the time of injury or during surgery. *Pseudomonas, Staphylococcus,* or *Clostridium* organisms may invade the wound or bone. *Clostridium* infection is particularly serious because it may lead to severe gas gangrene and cellulitis, but any infection may delay healing and result in *osteomyelitis,* infection within the bone that can lead to tissue death and necrosis. (See Chapter 36 for a complete discussion of osteomyelitis.)

Delayed Union

Infection, whether acute or chronic, can result in delayed union of fractures. **Delayed union** is defined as prolonged healing of bones beyond the usual time period. Many factors may inhibit bone healing; inadequate immobilization, prolonged reduction time, infection, necrosis, age, immunosuppression, and severe bone trauma resulting in multiple fragments are examples. Delayed union is diagnosed by means of serial X-ray studies. It is important to note that X-ray findings may lag 1 to 2 weeks behind the healing process; for example, a client may be completely healed by week 13, but this fact may not be apparent on the X-ray until week 14.

Delayed union may led to *nonunion,* which can cause persistent pain and movement at the fracture site. Nonunion may require surgical interventions, such as internal fixation and bone grafting. If infection is present, the bones are surgically debrided. Electrical stimulation of the fracture site may be as effective as bone grafting. Electrical current continually traversing the fracture site enhances mineral deposition and bone formation (see the previous discussion of electrical bone stimulation). It is important to note that electrical stimulation is not effective when infection is present.

Reflex Sympathetic Dystrophy

Reflex sympathetic dystrophy may occur after musculoskeletal trauma. This term refers to a group of poorly understood post-traumatic conditions involving persistent pain, hyperesthesias, swelling, changes in skin color and texture, changes in temperature, and decreased motion. The cause is unknown. Diagnosis is made by the client's history and physical examination. X-rays may demonstrate spotty osteoporosis, and bone scans may reveal increased uptake of radionucleide. Treatment with a sympathetic nervous system blocking agent often alleviates the symptoms.

Nursing Care

In planning and implementing nursing care for the client with fractures, the nurse should consider the client's response to the traumatic experience. Nursing care includes careful follow-up, client education, and early recognition of complications. Although each client has individual needs, nursing care commonly focuses on client problems with pain, impaired physical mobility, impaired tissue perfusion, and neurovascular compromise.

Frequent neurovascular assessment is an extremely important part of nursing care for these clients. Neurovascular assessement entails the five P's: pain, pulses, paresthesia, pallor, and paralysis. Assess pain in the injured extremity by asking the client to grade it on a scale of 0 to 10, with 10 as the most severe pain. Assess the medication's effectiveness in relieving the pain. Remember also that pain may be an early symptom of compartment syndrome. Assess distal pulses beginning with the unaffected extremity. Then compare the quality of pulses in the affected limb to those of the unaffected limb. Remember that some people are born without dorsalis pedis pulses. Assess sensation proximal and distal to the fracture. Ask the client if any change in sensation (paresthesia) has occurred. Check for pallor and skin color in the injured extremity. Coolness may indicate arterial compromise, whereas warmth and a bluish tinge may indicate

venous blood pooling. Assess motion distal to the fracture site. Documenting limited range of motion may help lead to early recognition of such problems as nerve damage and paralysis. It is also important to apply rehabilitation principles to care of the immobile client. See the box on page 1576.

Pain

Pain originates with the bone fracture and is compounded by muscle spasms and swelling.

Nursing interventions with rationales follow:

- Monitor baseline vital signs. *Some analgesics decrease respiratory effort and blood pressure. A client with a poor respiratory effort or very low blood pressure may not be able to receive some types of analgesics.*

- Ask the client to rate the pain on a scale of 0 to 10 (with 10 as the most severe pain) before and after any intervention. *This facilitates objective assessment of the effectiveness of the chosen pain relief strategy. Pain that increases in intensity or remains unrelieved with analgesics can indicate compartment syndrome.*

- Splint and support the injured area. *Splinting prevents additional injury by immobilizing the bone fragments.*

- Elevate the injured extremity 2 inches above the heart. *Elevating the extremity promotes venous return and decreases edema, which decreases pain.*

- Apply ice. *Ice causes vasoconstriction and decreases the pooling of blood in the injured area. Ice may also numb the tender area.*

- Move the client gently and slowly. *Gentle turning prevents the development of severe muscle spasms.*

- Encourage distraction. *Distraction prevents the client from focusing on the pain and lessens the intensity of pain.*

- Administer pain medications as prescribed. A PCA pump may be ordered by the physician. *Analgesics alleviate pain by stimulating opiate receptor sites. PCA pumps increase client control over and allow pain to be relieved before it intensifies.*

- Encourage deep breathing and relaxation exercises. *These techniques increase the effectiveness of analgesics and help diminish pain.*

Impaired Physical Mobility

The client who has experienced a fracture requires immobilization of the fractured bone(s). Immobilization alters normal gait and mobility. The client will need to use assistive devices such as crutches, canes, slings, or walkers.

Nursing interventions with rationales follow:

- Assist client with ROM exercises of the unaffected limbs. *ROM exercises help prevent muscle atrophy and maintain strength and joint function.*

Applying Rehabilitation Principles to Medical-Surgical Nursing: Immobility

■ ■ ■

Rehabilitation principles instituted early in your client's plan of care can decrease potential for health risks associated with immobility.

Case Example

Mrs. Janet Smith is 34 years old. She is admitted to your unit from the emergency room with a diagnosis of left tibia and fibula fracture. Mrs. Smith has been placed in skeletal traction. Her vital signs are stable, and she is alert and oriented. During your initial assessment, you notice bruises on both of her knees. She reports that she fell down her front steps and her left leg was caught in the railing.

Rehabilitation Principle

A primary goal of rehabilitation nursing is to maintain the maximum level of function. Immobility due to skeletal traction poses many potential risks to the client's health, such as contractures, pressure ulcers, constipation, and deconditioning.

Rehabilitation Time Frame

Mrs. Smith will remain in skeletal traction until bone healing occurs. This may take from 6 to 8 weeks. She will also need physical therapy after traction removal.

Nursing Diagnosis

■ *Risk for disuse syndrome.* Mrs. Smith will be partially immobile due to the skeletal traction. Her left let is completely immobilized, and she will remain in bed for the duration of the traction.

Rehabilitation Goals and Interventions

■ Maintain good skin care. *Pressure ulcers are a threat to immobile clients. Ulcers develop when any pressure on the skin is in excess of capillary pressure (32 mm Hg)* and exerted over time sufficient to cause cell death. Factors such as moisture, shearing, or poor nutrition put the client at risk for injury to the skin.

■ Assist the client to perform range of motion exercises on all joints not involved in the skeletal traction. *Range of motion exercises have been demonstrated to facilitate the maintenance of joint mobility, which will aid in the prevention of contractures.*

■ Place an overhead trapeze above the client's bed and instruct the client in its use. *Use of the trapeze will strengthen the client's upper body and will aid in toileting.*

■ Offer the client the bedpan on a regular basis (every 2 to 3 hours). *The client may be hesitant to call for the bedpan frequently and hold urine for a long period of time. An overlong period of time between voiding can cause overflow incontinence as well as urinary stasis, which could result in a urinary tract infection.*

■ Encourage the client to eat high fiber foods. Stool softeners may be necessary. *Immobility slows peristalsis which can result in constipation and/or impaction. High fiber foods help with peristalsis. Stool softeners will allow the client to empty the bowel more easily.*

■ Encourage the client to maintain a balanced diet. *Nutrition is a major factor in bone healing. Proteins, calcium, and vitamin C are necessary for bone healing.*

■ Encourage the client to perform independently as many activities of daily living as possible. *Client independence maintains self-esteem and is an asset to motivation. The client's performance of these activities also maintains muscle strength and tone. This can reduce the muscle deconditioning that often accompanies immobility.*

■ Teach isometric exercises, and encourage the client to perform them every 4 hours. *Isometric exercises help prevent muscle atrophy and force synovial fluid and nutrients into the cartilage.*

■ Encourage the client to ambulate when he or she is able to do so; provide assistance as necessary. *Ambulation maintains and improves circulation and helps prevent muscle atrophy.*

■ Teach and observe the client's use of assistive devices (canes, crutches, walkers, slings, and so forth) in conjunction with physical therapist, as appropriate. *Proper use of devices is necessary for safe ambulation and helps prevent the loss of joint function secondary to complications and falls.*

■ Encourage flexion and extension exercises of feet, ankles, elbows, shoulders, and knees. *Flexion and exten-*

sion exercises prevent the development of foot drop, wrist drop, or frozen joints.

- Turn the client on bed rest every 2 hours. If the client is in traction, teach the client to shift his or her weight every hour. *Turning and shifting weight increase circulation and help prevent skin breakdown.*

- Observe the client's ambulation. *As the client becomes comfortable with external immobilization devices, he or she may use them unsafely. Ensure that the client does not place weight on fixator or cast; this will disrupt healing of the fracture.*

Risk for Impaired Tissue Perfusion

In the client with a fracture, compartment syndrome or deep vein thrombosis can impair circulation and, in turn, tissue perfusion.

Nursing interventions with rationales follow:

- Assess pain, pulses, and pallor. *Unrelenting pain is an early sign of compartment syndrome. The presence of strong and equal pulses indicates that arterial circulation is not compromised. Pallor may indicate arterial obstruction.*

- Assess the cast for tightness. *Edema can cause the cast to become tight; a tightly fitting cast may lead to compartment syndrome.*

- If cast is tight, be prepared to assist the physician with **bivalving** (Figure 37–6). *Bivalving, the process of splitting the cast down both sides, alleviates pressure on the injured extremity.*

- If compartment syndrome is suspected, assist the physician in measuring compartment pressure. *Normal compartment pressure is 10 to 20 mm Hg. Elevation of the pressure indicates compartment syndrome.*

- Elevate the injured extremity 2 inches above the heart. *Elevating the extremity increases venous return and decreases edema.*

- Administer heparin per physician's order. *Prophylactic administration of heparin decreases the risk of clot formation.*

- Apply antiembolism stockings or pneumatic compression boots. *These devices increase venous return to the heart, decrease pooling of blood, and therefore decrease the risk of clotting.*

Risk for Sensory/Perceptual Alterations: Tactile

The client who has sustained a fracture is at risk for nerve injury from the initial trauma and such complications as compartment syndrome.

Nursing interventions with rationales follow:

- Assess the client for the presence of paresthesias and paralysis at least every 4 hours. *Paresthesias develop as a result of pressure on nerves and may indicate compartment syndrome. Paralysis is a late sign of nerve entrapment and requires that the physician be notified immediately.*

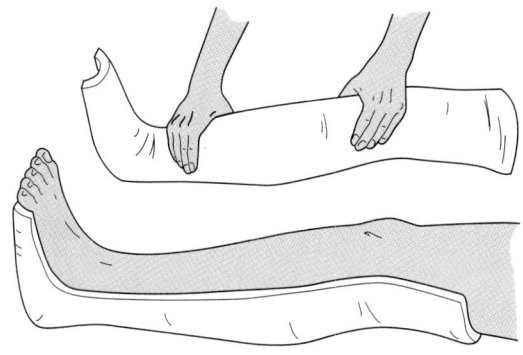

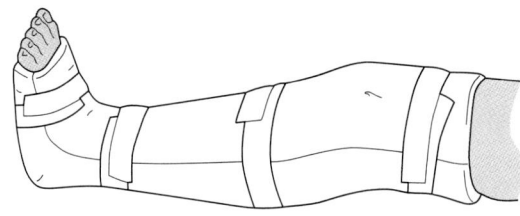

Figure 37–6   Bivalving is the process of splitting the cast down both sides to alleviate pressure on or allow visualization of the extremity.

- Elevate the injured extremity 2 inches above the heart. *Elevating the extremity decreases swelling and the risk of compartment syndrome and nerve entrapment.*

- Check the cast for fit. *A tightly fitting cast can cause compartment syndrome.*

- Support the injured extremity above and below the fracture site when moving the client. *Supporting the injured extremity above and below the fracture site helps prevent displacement of bony fragments and decreases the risk of further nerve damage.*

- Teach the patient to report any change in tactile sensation. *Decreased tactile sensation may indicate nerve impairment. Early intervention can lead to a more successful outcome.*

Other Nursing Diagnoses

Other nursing diagnoses that are appropriate for the client with fractures follow:

- *Activity Intolerance* related to pain and fatigue
- *Anxiety* related to traumatic nature of injury and feelings of loss of control
- *Body Image Disturbance* related to the presence of a cast, traction, splints, or external fixators
- *Risk for Constipation* related to decreased mobility and administration of narcotics

Gerontologic Considerations: Falling

■ ■ ■

Falling is the most common cause of musculoskeletal injury and fractures in older adults. Fall-related hip fractures are the leading cause of hospitalization for injuries in older adults. The clavicles and wrists are also common fracture sites. Fractures in older adults may lead to loss of functional ability or death. Fall-related deaths are seldom caused by the act of falling, but usually are related to complications from prolonged immobility during hospitalization.

Besides producing musculoskeletal trauma, falling can adversely affect the older adult's psychologic and social well-being. The shock of falling and the fear of falling again may result in anxiety and the restriction of activities, which in turn may lead to social isolation, dependence, and depression.

The nurse who works with older adults assesses for risk factors of falling in order to implement prevention strategies in the home and institutional setting. Assessment typically focuses on the following risk factors:

■ Neuromuscular status

■ Mental status

■ Urinary tract function

■ Use of medications

■ Living environment

■ Previous history of falling

Assessment of the neuromuscular system includes observing the client's gait, balance, and mobility, including muscle strength and range of motion. Based on assessment findings, exercise programs to improve the client's strength, flexibility, and endurance are prescribed. If the client has disorders that cause pain, joint deformity, or changes in gait and mobility (e.g., arthritis), these are addressed by the physician. Assess the feet for common deformities (e.g., hallux valgus) and, when necessary, refer the client to a podiatrist. Also, assess footwear for fit and comfort.

Urinary urgency and urinary incontinence can cause the client to rush to the bathroom, increasing the risk of falling. Consequently, it is important to assess the client's urinary status and bladder habits and to implement preventive interventions, such as toileting schedules, if warranted.

Conduct a thorough medication assessment to identify medications that might increase the client's risk for falling. Categories of medications that contribute to falling include those that affect blood pressure and mental alertness, as well as those that cause increased urinary frequency and dizziness. The greater the number of medications that the older adult takes, the greater the risk for drug interactions and side effects that may contribute to falling.

If the client is in a home setting, conduct a home safety assessment to identify conditions in the home that may increase the risk of falling. Specific areas to observe include stairs, hand rails, lighting, electrical cords, carpeting, and general clutter. Also, assess the bathroom to note whether grab bars and nonskid surfaces are present on the floor and in the tub or shower.

A history of previous falls is a reliable predictor of fall risk. Ask the client about a history of falls, including those that did not result in injury, and gather detailed information about the events leading up to the fall and the outcome of the fall.

Teach the client that falls are not a normal part of aging and that falls can be prevented. Include the following topics in client teaching to prevent falling:

■ Home safety measures

■ Exercise to improve strength, gait, and balance

■ Correct use of assistive devices

■ Use of properly fitting, comfortable footwear

■ Use of corrective glasses and hearing aids

■ Methods of changing position to prevent dizziness

■ Side effects of medications

Note: Data are from "Managing Falls: The Current Bases for Practice" (pp. 41–57) by C. Hogue, in *Key Aspects of Elder Care* by S. Funk, E. Tornquist, M. Champagne, and R. Wiese (Eds.), 1992, New York: Springer Publishing Company; and "Falling and the Elderly" (pp. 281–296) by J. Miller, in *Gerontological Nursing* by M. Stanley and M. Beare (Eds.), 1995, Philadelphia: F. A. Davis.

■ *Risk for Diversional Activity Deficit* related to bed rest and/or decreased mobility

■ *Altered Family Processes* related to inability to perform normal role secondary to impaired mobility

■ *Fatigue* related to stress and decreased mobility

■ *Risk for Impaired Gas Exchange* related to bed rest

■ *Impaired Home Maintenance Management* related to decreased physical mobility

- *Risk for Infection* related to surgery or open wounds
- *Knowledge Deficit* of traction care, crutch walking, use of cane or walker, and/or cast care
- *Post-Trauma Response* related to unexpected disruption in life caused by injury
- *Self-Care Deficit: Bathing, Feeding, Grooming, and/or Toileting*
- *Risk for Altered Sexuality Patterns* related to pain
- *Risk for Impaired Skin Integrity* related to decreased mobility, bed rest, and cast
- *Risk for Injury* related to disturbed gait

Client and Family Teaching

Client and family teaching focuses on individualized needs. The type of fracture and its location determine how much teaching the client and family will require. For example, a client who has a simple nondisplaced tibial fracture may need to be taught only cast care and crutch walking. An older client who has sustained a hip fracture and requires surgical intervention, by contrast, has a wider array of teaching needs, including the use of an abduction pillow, proper bending, and proper sitting. Referrals to visiting nurses and community services are more likely in older clients.

Regardless of the type of fracture, all clients must be instructed in the medications prescribed to them. Emphasize the importance of taking complete courses of antibiotics. The client also needs to know whether the fracture can withstand any weight. Initially, the client should avoid weight-bearing on any fracture to allow healing. Teach the client the importance of eating well-balanced meals. If assistive devices are necessary at home, show them to the client in the hospital, and teach their proper use.

Care of the Older Client

Older adults experience changes in the bone (e.g., osteoporosis), slowing of reflexes, and changes in sensation (e.g., altered vision). These factors predispose the older adult to falls, which are common causes of fractures and other musculoskeletal injuries in this age group; see the accompanying box.

When caring for older clients who have sustained fractures, remember that they do not metabolize and excrete drugs as rapidly as younger clients. Dosage should be adjusted according to renal and hepatic function. Also decreased circulation may prolong healing time in older clients, and underlying illnesses may increase the time required for rehabilitation.

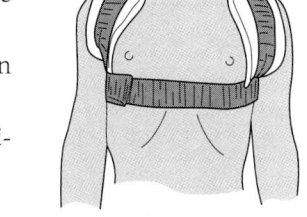
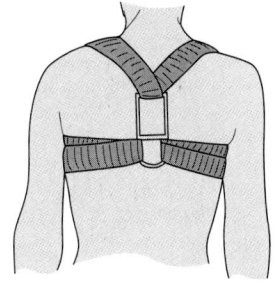

Figure 37-7   A clavicular strap is used to immobilize a clavicular fracture.

The Client with Fractures of Specific Sites

■ ■ ■

Clavicle

The clavicle, or collar bone, forms the anterior portion of each shoulder. A fracture of the clavicle commonly results from a direct blow or a fall. The most common clavicular fracture occurs at the middle of the clavicle. When a person sustains this type of fracture, he or she assumes a protective slumping position to immobilize the arm and prevent shoulder movement. A less common fracture occurs along the distal third of the clavicle. This type of fracture may be associated with ligament damage. If no ligament damage is present, a clavicular fracture usually requires only a sling. If there is ligament damage, an open reduction with internal fixation may be necessary. The surgeon manually aligns the fractured bone and repairs the ligament.

The diagnosis of a clavicular fracture is made by physical assessment and radiographic examination. Physical assessment reveals a lowering of the injured shoulder. A deformity may also be palpated along the clavicle. Treatment focuses on immobilizing the fractured bone in normal anatomic position by applying a figure-eight splint or clavicular strap (Figure 37-7). Nursing implications for clients with fractures of the clavicle are presented in the box on page 1580.

Injuries to the clavicle may be associated with skull or cervical fractures. The fractured bone, if displaced, may lacerate the subclavian vessels and result in hemorrhage. The fractured bone may also puncture the lung, resulting in a pneumothorax. Malunion may occur at the fracture site and result in asymmetry of the clavicles. Injury to the brachial plexus may result in numbness and decreased movement of the arm on the affected side.

Nursing Implications for Clients with Fractures of the Clavicle

■ ■ ■

- Perform neurovascular assessments of the affected arm frequently.

- Instruct the client not to elevate the arm above shoulder level.

- Encourage range-of-motion exercises for wrist and elbow.

- Instruct client in proper application of figure-eight splint or clavicular strap. Ensure that the splint or strap is not too tight under the axilla; excessive tightness can cause injury to the brachial plexus.

- Instruct the client in the proper use of prescribed medications.

- Instruct the client in the manifestations of complications.

Humerus

The humerus approximates with the shoulder proximally and the elbow distally. The exact location of the fracture, the presence of displacement, and the results of the neurovascular examination determine the severity of the fracture and the appropriate interventions. The diagnosis of a humeral fracture is made by physical assessment and radiographic examination. Treatment focuses on immobilizing the fractured bone in normal anatomic position. Common complications of humeral fracture include nerve and ligament damage, frozen or stiff joints, and malunion. Early interventions and follow-up may prevent permanent damage.

Fractures of the proximal humerus are common in older adults. A simple nondisplaced fracture of the proximal humerus (near the humeral head) with a normal neurovascular assessment can be safely treated with immobilization. A more complicated displaced fracture of the proximal humerus with bone fragmentation requires surgical interventions and preoperative nursing interventions. The more severe the fracture and damage to soft tissue, the more likely the range of motion of the shoulder will be impaired. Rehabilitative measures focus on increasing range of motion.

The humerus may also fracture along the shaft, usually as a direct result of trauma. If the humeral shaft fracture is simple and nondisplaced, a hanging arm cast is applied. This cast maintains alignment of the fracture by using the pulling force of gravity; therefore, the client must be in-structed not to rest the cast on anything to alleviate the weight. If the client is on bed rest, a hanging arm cast is not applied, because the arm would not be able to hang freely. Instead, the fracture is immobilized with external skeletal traction. This traction places the injured arm in an upright position over the face, and weights are hung off the distal portion of the humerus (see Figure 37-1c).

Nursing implications for clients with fractures of the humerus are presented in the accompanying box.

Elbow

The most common location of an elbow fracture is the distal humerus. Elbow fractures usually result from a fall or direct blow to the elbow. The client guards the injured extremity, holding the arm rigidly in a flexed position or an extended position. Diagnosis of the fracture is based upon physical assessment and radiographic examination. Because the radius, ulna, or humerus may be involved in the elbow fracture, all three bones must be visualized by X-ray.

Complications of an elbow fracture include nerve or artery damage and *hemarthrosis,* the collection of blood in the elbow joint. The most serious complication of an elbow fracture is *Volkmann's contracture,* which results from arterial occlusion and muscle ischemia. The client complains of forearm pain, impaired sensation, and loss of motor function. Rapid interventions are aimed at relieving pressure on the brachial artery and nerve and preventing muscle atrophy.

Nondisplaced elbow fractures are treated by immobilizing the fracture with a posterior splint or cast. The displaced fracture is first reduced and then immobilized.

Nursing interventions, as presented previously for other fractures, focus on alleviating pain, maintaining immobilization, and educating clients in neurovascular assessments.

Radius and Ulna

The radius and ulna form the forearm. Between 1985 and 1988, 88,000 people were hospitalized with a fractured radius and ulna, most of them between 18 and 44 years old (Praemer et al., 1992).

The diagnosis of a fractured radius and/or ulna is based on physical assessment and radiographic examination. If the client undergoes an open or closed reduction, a follow-up X-ray will be performed to evaluate the alignment of the bones.

The usual classification and treatment of radius fractures depend on the location. The proximal radial head may be fractured from a fall on an outstretched hand. Blood commonly collects in the elbow joint and must be aspirated. If the fracture is nondisplaced, a sling is applied. If the fracture is displaced, surgical intervention is required. After surgical repair of a displaced fracture, the arm is splinted with a posterior plaster splint. The client avoids movement for the first week and then initiates movement gradually. The client is instructed not to begin exercises until first checking with the physician.

Fractures of the shaft of the radius and/or ulna are more common in children. When both bones are broken, the fracture is usually displaced. The client complains of pain and inability to turn the palm of the hand up. A nondisplaced fracture is casted for about 6 weeks, and either a shorter cast or a brace is then applied for 6 more weeks. If the fracture is displaced, surgical intervention is performed. The physician reduces the fracture and may insert pins or screws to keep the bones in alignment. After the surgery, a cast is applied, and the client is encouraged to exercise the fingers.

Complications after a radius and/or ulna fracture include compartment syndrome, delayed healing, and decreased wrist and finger movement. After surgery, the client also has an increased risk of infection.

Nursing interventions, as discussed previously, focus on alleviating pain, maintaining immobilization, and educating clients in neurovascular assessments and the need to elevate the arm to decrease swelling. The client needs to be aware of the need to inform the physician of changes in sensation or an increase in pain.

Wrist and Hand

The wrist is formed by the approximation of the distal radius, distal ulna, and the carpal bones. Most commonly, the distal radius is involved in a wrist fracture. Wrist fractures often result from a fall onto an outstretched hand or onto the back of the hand. A common type of wrist fracture is Colles's fracture, in which the distal radius fractures after a fall onto an outstretched hand. The client with a wrist fracture presents with a bony deformity, pain, numbness, weakness, and decreased range of motion of the fingers. The capillary refill and sensation of the hand must be assessed.

The hand is composed of many bones. Most commonly, the metacarpals and phalanges are involved in a hand fracture. The injuring mechanism in a hand fracture varies greatly from striking an object with a closed fist to closing a hand in a door. The client presents with complaints of pain, edema, and decreased range of motion. The cause of the injury usually focuses the assessment on the hand. Circulation, sensation, and range of motion need to be assessed.

The diagnosis of a hand or wrist fracture is based on physical assessment, history of injury, and radiographic examination. Frequently, comparative X-rays are obtained to compare left and right wrists and hands. Complications of wrist and hand fractures are compartment syndrome, nerve damage, ligament damage, and delayed union.

Nursing Implications for Clients with Fractures of the Humerus

- Perform neurovascular assessments frequently.
- Administer prescribed medications to alleviate pain.
- Encourage exercises for clients with a hanging cast.
  a. Finger exercises: Move each finger of the affected arm through complete range of motion.
  b. Pendulum shoulder exercises: Dangle the affected arm at the side, and move it forward and backward about 30 degrees in each direction.
- If client is discharged, instruct the client and family in cast care and sling application, neurovascular assessments, exercises, prescribed pain medications, and manifestations of complications.
- If client is admitted to the hospital, provide preoperative teaching.

A wrist fracture is commonly treated with closed reduction, cast application, and elevation of the injured extremity. A hand fracture is splinted and elevated.

Nursing interventions focus on alleviating pain and educating the client in neurovascular assessments, the importance of elevation, and how to exercise the fingers to prevent stiffness. The client needs to be aware of the need to inform the physician of changes in sensation or an increase in pain. If the dominant hand is injured, the client will require assistance in performing activities of daily living (ADLs).

Rib

Rib fractures commonly result from blunt chest trauma. The location of the fracture and involvement of underlying organs determine the severity of the injury. Fractures of the first through third ribs may result in injury to the subclavian artery or vein. Fractures of the lower ribs may result in spleen and liver injuries.

The client presents with a history of recent chest trauma. Typically, the client complains of pain along the lateral portion of the rib. Palpation of the rib reveals a bony deformity and increases pain. Deep inspiration also increases pain. The skin over the fracture site may be ecchymotic. The diagnosis of rib fractures is based upon physical assessment and radiographic examination.

A complication of adjacent rib fractures is a flail chest, which results from the fracture of two or more adjacent ribs in two or more places and the formation of a free-floating segment that moves in the opposite direction of the rib cage. On inspiration, the rib cage expands, and the segment retracts. On expiration, the rib cage recoils, and the segment bulges. The segment impairs the client's ability to inhale and exhale. Treatment is aimed at stabilizing the flail segment and supporting respirations. Other complications of rib fractures include pneumothorax and/or hemothorax. The fractured rib may pierce the lung and injure it. The lower ribs may pierce the liver or spleen, resulting in intra-abdominal bleeding. Pneumonia may also develop from ineffective clearing of respiratory secretions.

A rib fracture alone is treated with pain medication and instructions for coughing, deep breathing, and splinting. The client is also instructed to return to the emergency room if shortness of breath develops.

Nursing interventions focus on alleviating pain and teaching the client about splinting. Because deep inspiration increases pain, clients frequently avoid it. The client may be instructed to splint the injured rib with the hand or a pillow and take deep breaths and cough to decrease the chance of developing atelectasis. Incentive spirometry is encouraged. With this device, the client takes a deep breath, and a ball rises. This allows clients to monitor their own progress and motivates them to increase the depth of inspiration.

Femur

The femur, the largest bone in the body, forms the upper portion of the leg. The most proximal portion of the femur approximates with the pelvis and forms the hip. Direct force may fracture the shaft of the femur. A large amount of force is required to fracture the femur; motor vehicle crashes, falls, or acts of violence are among the sources of such force.

The client with a fracture of the femoral shaft presents with an edematous, deformed, painful thigh. The client is unable to move the hip or knee. Initial assessment focuses on the circulation and sensation present in the affected extremity. Pedal pulses and capillary refill in the affected extremity are compared to that of the unaffected extremity. Secondary assessment focuses on associated injuries. Clients with femoral shaft fractures usually have associated multiple trauma.

Diagnosis is based on radiographic studies and physical assessment. Initially, skin traction is initiated to prevent further tissue trauma. Skeletal traction is applied. Treatment of the fracture focuses on separating the bony fragments and reducing and immobilizing the fracture.

After 1 to 2 weeks of traction, additional X-rays are obtained to evaluate healing. At this time, the surgeon decides whether to apply an external fixator or perform an open reduction and internal fixation. If the fracture is in the distal portion of the femoral shaft, a cast brace may be applied after 2 to 4 weeks. The cast brace allows the client to begin ambulating with limited weight-bearing.

Complications of a femoral shaft fracture include hypovolemia due to blood loss, fat embolism, dislocation of the hip or knee, muscle atrophy, and ligament damage.

The nurse assesses the client's vital signs for increased pulse rate and decreased blood pressure, which may indicate hypovolemia. The nurse also assesses circulation to the lower extremity and checks dorsalis pedis pulses and compares them bilaterally. Sensation is evaluated by asking whether the client can feel touch and discriminate sharp from dull objects. Nursing interventions include implementing pain-relief measures, providing reassurance and decreasing anxiety, and assisting with exercises of the lower legs, feet, and toes. After the orthopedic physician confirms that the knee joint is stable, the client begins ROM exercises of the knee to prevent joint stiffness.

Tibia and Fibula

Fractures of the lower extremities often result from a fall on a flexed foot, a direct blow, or a twisting motion. The client presents with edema, pain, bony deformity, and a hematoma at the level of injury. The client is assessed for the presence of circulation and sensation.

The diagnosis of the fracture is based upon physical examination and radiographic studies. Further assessment is needed to rule out common complications of the fracture, including damage to the peroneal nerve or tibial artery, compartment syndrome, hemarthroses, and ligament damage. Peroneal nerve damage may be indicated by the client's inability to point the toe on the affected side upward. Tibial artery damage may be the cause of an absent dorsalis pedis pulse on the affected side. Compartment syndrome may be present if the client develops pain on passive movement and paresthesias. An edematous knee may indicate collection of blood in the knee joint. Ligament damage may be present if the client cannot move the knee and/or ankle.

If the fracture is closed, a closed reduction and casting are performed. A long leg cast that allows for partial weight-bearing is used. Partial weight-bearing usually is prescribed by the orthopedic physician within 10 days of the fracture. A short leg cast will be applied in 3 to 4 weeks. If the fracture is open, either external fixation or open reduction and internal fixation will be performed. After surgery, a cast may be applied, and weight-bearing is begun according to the physician's orders, usually in about 6 weeks.

Nursing care is aimed at increasing comfort, assessing neurovascular status, and preventing complications. The nurse instructs the client in cast care, the use of assistive devices, how to perform neurovascular assessment, and when to follow-up with the orthopedic physician. The client also is instructed to rest, apply ice, and elevate the affected extremity.

Ankle and Foot

The client with an ankle or foot fracture presents with pain, hematoma, edema, and difficulty ambulating. The client with an ankle fracture is unable to perform ROM exercises with the affected ankle because of severe pain. The diagnosis of an ankle fracture is based on physical assessment and radiographic studies. Most ankle fractures are treated by closed reduction and casting. Open fractures are treated by surgical intervention and splinting. The physician evaluates the client for ligament injury.

The client with a foot fracture presents with similar symptoms; however, range of motion of the ankle is not usually affected. Most foot fractures are nondisplaced and treated with closed reduction and casting. More severe displaced foot fractures may require surgery and the placement of wires to maintain reduction of the fracture.

Nursing care focuses on increasing comfort, increasing mobility, and educating the client. Analgesia is given for pain. The extremity should be elevated, and ice can be applied. The client is taught cast care, neurovascular assessment, and crutch walking.

Skull

The skull can suffer a fracture as a result of a fall or as a result of a direct blow. A skull fracture is diagnosed on physical assessment and radiographic studies. The client must be assessed for neurologic damage, and any loss of consciousness must be documented. A complete neurologic assessment is conducted: Pupillary reaction to light, movement and strength of all extremities, complaints of nausea and vomiting, level of consciousness and orientation to person, place, and time are noted. A displaced skull fracture, which is referred to as *depressed,* may press on the brain and cause neurologic damage. Skull fractures are discussed further in Chapter 40.

Spine

The spine can be injured in many ways, including sports injuries, falls, and motor vehicle accidents. The spine can be fractured in the cervical, thoracic, lumbar, or sacral area. The client complains of pain and may lose the normal curvature of the spine.

The client who is suspected of having a spinal fracture is immobilized with a cervical collar or sandbags to pre-vent head movement and secured on a long flat board called a *spine board.* The client is assessed, and the diagnosis of spine fracture is based on radiographic studies. The nondisplaced spine fracture may be treated with a cervical collar fastened shut with plaster, a halo immobilizing brace, a thoracic brace, or a body cast. The displaced fracture is reduced by skeletal traction and, eventually, application of a brace and/or surgical stabilization of the bones with plates and screws. Immobilization after a spine fracture may last as long as 6 months.

The most severe complication of spine fracture is injury to the spinal cord. A fracture to the vertebrae may cause the bones to become displaced and apply pressure on the spinal cord. This pressure on the spinal cord may result in permanent paralysis.

The nurse needs to assess the client for numbness, sensation, and movement in each extremity. If the client cannot feel or move an area, the physician is notified. After airway, breathing, and circulation are assessed, the nurse focuses on relieving the client's anxiety, increasing comfort, and maintaining immobilization of the fractured bones. Spinal trauma is discussed further in Chapter 41.

Pelvis

The client with a pelvic fracture presents with pain in the back or hip area. Diagnosis is based on assessment and radiographic studies. A single fracture in the pelvis is treated conservatively with bed rest on a firm mattress. Log rolling increases client comfort. A pelvic fracture with two fracture sites is considered unstable and treated with surgery. An external fixator may be applied to stabilize the pelvis. In the client who is not stable for surgery, a pelvic sling may be used. The pelvic sling stabilizes the pelvis and allows the client to move in bed with less pain. Common complications include hypovolemia, spinal injury, bladder injury, kidney damage, and gastrointestinal trauma.

Nursing care focuses on alleviating discomfort, maintaining immobilization, and preparing the client for surgery if necessary. The nurse monitors the client for increased heart rate, decreased blood pressure, and decreasing hemoglobin levels. These findings may indicate impending hypovolemia due to bleeding into the pelvis. Any blood in the urine should be reported to the physician; this may indicate kidney or bladder damage.

Face

Fracture of the facial bones may result from a direct blow. The client presents with hematomas, complaints of pain, edema, and bony deformity. The diagnosis of facial fractures is based on assessment and radiographic studies. Nondisplaced fractures are usually monitored initially to ensure the airway is not compromised. The client is

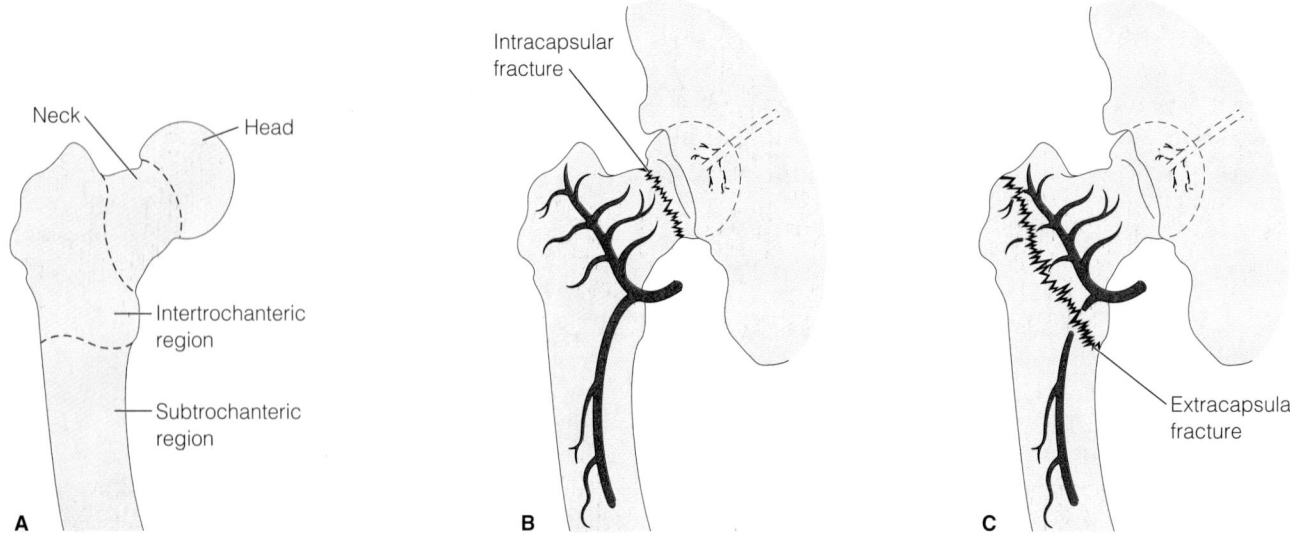

Figure 37–8   *A,* Regions where hip fractures may occur: the head of the femur, the neck of the femur, and the trochanteric regions of the femur. *B,* Intracapsular fractures occur across the head or neck of the femur. *C,* Extracapsular fractures occur across the trochanteric regions. Note how both intracapsular and extracapsular fractures disrupt the blood supply to the bone.

observed for any neurologic deficits, as described previously in the discussion of skull fractures. Severely displaced or multiple facial fractures are treated with open reduction and internal fixation with wires or plates.

Nursing care focuses on maintaining the airway by helping the client clear secretions from the oropharynx. The nurse monitors the client's breathing for increased effort or tachypnea and notifies the physician immediately if these findings are noted. Pain is treated with analgesics, and body image disturbances are addressed by allowing the client to discuss how he or she feels about the injury. If the client asks to see his or her face, the nurse should plan to stay with the client and answer questions while the client looks in a mirror. A plastic surgeon may also be present.

The Client with a Hip Fracture

■ ■ ■

The incidence of hip fractures is increasing. The National Institute of Aging predicts that by the year 2000, 300,000 people will sustain hip fractures every year. Other sources estimate the number at 500,000. The increase in the incidence of hip fractures can be attributed to an aging population: Increased life span, chronic illness, debilitation, and increased occupational and recreational risks for trauma are among the factors that predispose older adults to hip fracture. The nurse is challenged to deliver care to manage pain and ensure safety. In addition, the nurse should aggressively encourage rehabilitation to increase

the client's independence and promote the return to preinjury function.

Pathophysiology

A hip fracture refers to a fracture of the femur at the head, neck, or trochanteric regions (Figure 37–8). The head of the femur fits into the socket of the pelvis. The neck is the narrower area below the head. The trochanteric region is the area below the neck. Hip fractures are classified as intracapsular or extracapsular. *Intracapsular fractures* are fractures of the head or neck of the femur; *extracapsular fractures* are fractures of the trochanteric region. The majority of hip fractures involve the neck or trochanteric regions. The femoral head and neck lie within the joint capsule and are not covered in periosteum; thus, they do not have a large blood supply. Fractures here usually fragment and may further decrease blood supply, increasing the risk of nonunion and avascular necrosis. The trochanteric region is covered in periosteum and therefore has more blood supply than the head or neck.

Hip fractures are common in older adults as a result of decreases in bone mass and the increased tendency to fall. Whether the femur breaks spontaneously and causes the fall or whether the fall causes the fracture is not always clear; regardless of the cause of the fracture, however, rapid interventions are required to prevent bone necrosis.

Collaborative Care

The care of the client with a hip fracture does not differ from the care of a client with any other fracture. Prehospital interventions include splinting, assessing circulation and sensation, and observing for any other injury. Because a large amount of blood can be lost into the hip and pelvis, the client is observed for manifestations of hypovolemia, and intravenous access may be established.

On the client's arrival in the emergency department, the nurse and physician reevaluate circulation and sensation and observe for complications. The assessment also involves determining the cause of the fracture; myocardial infarction, transient ischemic attack, cerebrovascular accident, seizure, or hypoglycemic episode are among the possible causes of the fall. It is important to evaluate the client for associated injuries such as a concussion or head trauma. The client is asked whether he or she remembers falling and whether any other part of the body was hit. The secondary survey assesses the client for pain in any other area of the body.

Assessment findings commonly associated with a hip fracture are shortening of the affected lower extremity and external rotation. Rarely, the fracture dislocates posteriorly; if that occurs, the extremity may internally rotate.

Laboratory and Diagnostic Tests

The following laboratory and diagnostic tests may be ordered:

- *X-rays.* Radiographic films determine the presence of a fracture. If a fracture is present, preoperative studies, including a chest X-ray, are also ordered.

- *Laboratory analysis.* Baseline studies, such as a CBC, are performed to evaluate blood loss. If a fracture is present, preoperative laboratory studies, including blood chemistry, coagulation studies, and typing and cross-match, are conducted to prepare for a possible blood transfusion.

Pharmacology

Analgesics are key pharmacologic agents for the client with a hip fracture. The physician may order parenteral narcotics. Preoperatively, the client may also receive an intravenous antibiotic. Postoperatively, the client may receive oral medications to prevent constipation, ulcer formation, and muscle spasms.

Surgery

The orthopedic surgeon is called to evaluate the client and determine the appropriate treatment. Some surgeons initially order traction and then perform surgery, whereas others perform surgery immediately or within the first 24 hours. Traction prior to surgery decreases muscle spasm.

The goal of surgery is to reduce and stabilize the fracture, thereby increasing mobility, decreasing pain, and preventing complications. Surgery usually consists of open reduction and internal fixation of the fracture. Fixation is accomplished by securing the femur in place with

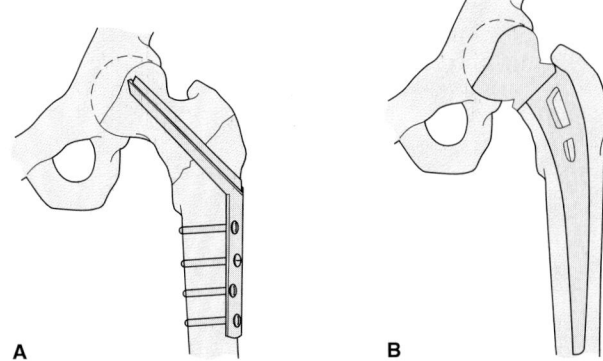

Figure 37–9 Surgical fixation of hip fractures. *A,* A surgical nail or screw used to stabilize an intertrochanteric fracture. *B,* Use of a hip prosthesis (artifical hip) to replace a damaged femoral head.

pins, screws, nails, or plates (Figure 37–9a). An open reduction and internal fixation works well for fractures in the trochanteric area. Fractures of the femoral neck frequently disrupt blood supply to the femoral head. If blood supply is disrupted, the surgeon will replace the femoral head with a prosthesis (Figure 37–9b). If the pelvic socket, called the acetabulum, has been damaged, the surgeon may insert a metal cup. Replacement of either the femoral head or the acetabulum with a prosthesis is called a **hemiarthroplasty.** Replacement of both the femoral head and the acetabulum is a **total hip arthroplasty (THA).** See Chapter 38.

If a client is at high risk for intraoperative complications, surgery may be delayed. Surgery may also be delayed for clients who suffered a fall due to another process, such as a myocardial infarction or cerebrovascular accident, and those who also suffered a head injury during the fall. Care is focused at treating the more severe injury; for example, only after the myocardial or cerebral processes are corrected will surgery be performed.

Nursing Care

The nursing care of a client with a hip fracture is challenging. Once a person passes age 50, the risk of hip fracture increases every year. Many clients with a hip fracture are older and have several underlying health problems. The nurse must deliver holistic care to the client, focusing on the hip fracture but also being aware of and addressing any other conditions that may be present. Nursing care focuses on alleviating pain, maintaining circulation to the injured extremity, and increasing mobility.

Pain

In a hip fracture, as with any fracture, swelling and muscle spasm cause pain. Clients with hip fractures do not

have the ability to splint the fracture site with the other extremity, so care must be taken when they are moved.
Nursing interventions with rationales follow:

- Monitor baseline vital signs. *Some analgesics decrease respiratory effort and blood pressure. A client with a poor respiratory effort or very low blood pressure may not be a candidate for these analgesics.*

- Ask the client to rate the pain on a scale of 0 to 10 (with 10 as the most severe pain) before and after any intervention. *This facilitates objective assessment of the effectiveness of the chosen pain relief strategy. Pain that increases in intensity or is unrelieved with analgesics can indicate the presence of compartment syndrome.*

- Place a pillow between the client's legs. *Placing a pillow between a client's legs helps minimize external rotation of the leg and decrease muscle spasms.*

- Apply Buck's traction per physician's orders. *Buck's traction immobilizes the fracture and decreases pain and additional trauma.*

- Move the client gently and slowly. *Gentle turning prevents the development of severe muscle spasms.*

- Encourage distraction. *Distraction prevents the client from focusing on the pain and lessens the intensity of pain.*

- Administer pain medications as prescribed. A PCA pump may be ordered by the physician. *Analgesics alleviate pain by stimulating opiate receptor sites. PCA pumps allow for increased client control and early relief of pain before it intensifies.*

- Encourage deep breathing and relaxation exercises. *These techniques increase the effectiveness of analgesics and modify the pain experience.*

- Assist the client with frequent position changes. *Change of position redistributes weight and alleviates discomfort.*

Impaired Physical Mobility

The client with a hip fracture has severe pain and therefore avoids moving. Once pain has subsided, however, it is important to address the client's mobility problems. Increasing mobility decreases the risk of pulmonary compromise, pressure sores, and deep vein thrombosis; it also increases self-esteem.
Nursing interventions with rationales follow:

- Assist the client with ROM exercises of the unaffected limbs. *ROM exercises help prevent muscle atrophy and maintain strength and joint function.*

- Teach isometric exercises, and encourage the client to perform them every 4 hours. *Isometric exercises help prevent muscle atrophy and force synovial fluid and nutrients into the cartilage.*

- Refer the client to a physical therapist for assistance in increasing activity per physician's instructions. *Postoperatively, the physician will order the amount of weight-bearing a client can place on the hip. The physical therapist will also provide any assistive devices necessary for the client, such as a walker.*

- Assist the client to get out of bed to a hip chair per physician's orders. *A hip chair (a chair with a high seat) helps prevent flexion of the hip. Sitting out of bed increases circulation and improves lung expansion.*

- Assist and encourage ambulation per physician's orders. *Ambulation helps prevent muscle atrophy.*

- Teach the client how to use assistive devices: canes, walkers, and so forth. Evaluate the client's ability to use these devices properly. *Proper use of devices is necessary for safe ambulation. It helps prevent the loss of joint functions secondary to complications and falls.*

- Encourage flexion and extension exercises of the feet, ankles, elbows, shoulders, and knees. *Flexion and extension exercises help prevent the development of foot drop, wrist drop, and frozen joints.*

- If the client is on bed rest, turn the client every 2 hours. If the client is in traction, teach the client to shift his or her weight every hour. *Turning and weight shifting increase circulation and help prevent skin breakdown.*

- Place a pillow between the client's legs when the client is at rest in bed or turning. *A pillow supports the legs and prevents adduction during turning. Adduction may dislocate the hip.*

Impaired Skin Integrity

The client who undergoes surgical repair will have a postoperative wound. Any break in skin integrity must be monitored for infection.
Nursing interventions with rationales follow:

- Monitor vital signs. *Increases in pulse rate, respiratory rate, and temperature may indicate infection.*

- Use sterile technique for dressing changes. *The initial postoperative dressing will be changed by the surgeon. The nurse must change all subsequent dressings without introducing organisms into the operative site.*

- Assess the wound for size, color, and the presence of any drainage. *Redness, swelling, and purulent drainage may indicate infection.*

- Administer antibiotics per physician's orders. *Prophylactic antibiotics inhibit bacterial reproduction and thereby help prevent skin flora from entering the wound.*

- If the client's vital signs are abnormal or if the wound has purulent drainage, notify the physician. *Prompt notification of the physician will lead to prompt treatment and may prevent the development of osteomyelitis.*

Risk for Altered Musculoskeletal Tissue Perfusion

The client with a hip fracture is at risk for compartment syndrome and vascular compromise. Nursing care is aimed at preventing this complication, but if it does occur, early recognition and rapid treatment may save the injured extremity.

Nursing interventions with rationales follow:

- Assess the affected extremity for color. *Pale skin may indicate decreased tissue perfusion. Cyanosis may indicate venous congestion.*

- Assess the temperature of the affected extremity. *Cool skin may indicate decreased tissue perfusion.*

- Assess toes for capillary refill. *Delayed capillary refill may indicate decreased tissue perfusion.*

- Assess the extremity for edema and swelling. *Excessive swelling and hematoma formation can compromise circulation.*

- Assess the client for deep, throbbing, unrelenting pain. *Pain that is not relieved by analgesics may indicate neurovascular compromise.*

- Assess pedal pulses in both feet. *Pedal pulses indicate arterial blood flow to the lower extremities.*

- Notify the physician of any abnormal findings. *Early treatment increases the chance of saving the limb.*

Other Nursing Diagnoses

For other possible nursing diagnoses for clients with fractures of the hip, refer to the section on nursing care of clients with fractures in general.

Client and Family Teaching

Explain to the client and family that surgery is being performed to increase mobility and decrease the complications that may result from immobility. The client will need preoperative teaching. Postoperatively, instruct the client and family in the amount of weight the client can place on the affected extremity. Explain that the client should sit only on high chairs to prevent excess flexion of the hip; a high toilet seat can be added to a regular toilet seat. Encourage the client and family to equip the shower with a rail to aid stability and prevent falls. If a walker is needed, teach the client its proper use. Explain that the client should not carry the walker, but rather lift it, advance it, and then take two steps. If a cane is needed, tell the client to use it on the affected side. Stress the importance of well-balanced meals, and explain all prescribed medications.

Care of the Older Client

The incidence of hip fractures is higher in older clients. Women are more predisposed to hip fractures because of age-related osteoporotic changes in the bones. Quadriceps muscles also weaken with age. Cerebral processes that occur in older clients, such as transient ischemic attacks, cerebrovascular accidents, carotid artery disease, dementia, and Parkinson's disease, increase the risk of falling and hip fractures. Medications may alter alertness and balance, and arthritis may cause an unsteady gait and alter balance. Rehabilitation needs to be initiated and mobility increased as soon as possible to prevent loss of independence. See the research box on page 1588.

Applying the Nursing Process

Case Study of a Client with a Fractured Hip: Stella Carbolito

Stella Carbolito is a 64-year-old Italian-American woman with a history of osteoporosis. She is a widow and lives alone in a two-story row home. She has a 40-year-old son and a 30-year-old daughter living in the same city. She has six grandchildren, whom she frequently watches for her children. Mrs. Carbolito is retired and depends on a pension check and Social Security for her income. She takes pride in making all her own food from scratch.

While walking to the market one day, Mrs. Carbolito falls and fractures her left hip. She is transported by paramedics to the nearest trauma center. On arrival in the emergency department, she is greeted by her nurse, Maria Davis, and a team of physicians.

Assessment

The paramedics report that they found Mrs. Carbolito lying near the curb. She states she had fallen only 5 minutes prior to their arrival. Ms. Davis immediately notices that Mrs. Carbolito's left leg is shorter than her right leg and is externally rotated. Distal pulses are present and bilaterally strong; both legs are warm. Mrs. Carbolito complains of severe pain but states that no numbness or burning is present. She is able to wiggle the toes on her left leg and has full movement of her right leg. Initial vital signs are as follows: T, 98.0 F (36.6 C); P, 100; R, 18; BP, 120/58. Diagnostic tests include CBC, blood chemistry, and X-ray studies of the left hip and pelvis. The CBC reveals a hemoglobin of 11.0 g/dL and a normal white blood cell count. Blood chemistry findings are within normal limits. The X-ray reveals a fracture of the left femoral neck. Mrs. Carbolito is admitted to the hospital with an order for 10 lb of straight leg traction. An ORIF is planned for the following day.

Diagnosis

Ms. Davis makes the following nursing diagnoses:

- *Pain* related to fractured left femoral neck, muscle spasms, and traction

Applying Research to Nursing Practice: Outcomes for Women with a Fractured Hip

■ ■ ■

Fracture of the hip, a common fracture among older women, often results in loss of independence and long-term disability. In one study, researchers evaluated the mood states and mobility outcomes in women with a fractured hip who were discharged either from the hospital to home or from the hospital to a long-term care facility. The latter were also evaluated according to their length of stay in the long-term care facility; one group stayed less than 1 month, and the other group stayed longer than 1 month (Williams, Oberst, & Bjorklund, 1994). Data on both variables (mood and mobility) were collected before discharge and at 2, 8, and 14 weeks after discharge. The women in the study who were in the long-term care facility for less than 1 month regained mobility as well as did those who went home, and both groups rated their overall recovery much the same. Mood distress was greater in women who stayed in the long-term care facility longer than 1 month. The researchers suggest that further study is needed to identify both client characteristics and institutional features that contribute to positive outcomes. The need is especially great because more women with hip fractures are being discharged to long-term care facilities for recovery.

Implications for Nursing

Although older women are more likely to live alone and have a greater incidence of hip fractures, little research has been conducted to determine the setting or length of stay that is most likely to promote rehabilitation and independent self-care. As more clients are discharged from the acute care setting early in the recovery period, health care providers must give more attention to promoting recovery in long-term care facilities as well as to meeting clients' needs in the home and community more effectively. Nurses in all settings must collaborate with other nurses and with other members of the health care team to facilitate continuity of care so that the client achieves maximum function and quality of life.

Critical Thinking in Client Care

1. Many people believe that once they are admitted to a nursing home, they will never again live at home. How can nurses change this perception?

2. If your client is an older woman who lives alone and has no available caregivers, what community resources can you recommend to provide care until she regains her independence?

3. This study suggests that nurses investigate features of long-term care facilities that promote positive outcomes in women with a fractured hip. What features do you believe should be examined?

4. You are assigned to care for an 84-year-old woman with a fractured hip who is being discharged to a nursing home. She begins to cry and says, "I know I will die there; please don't let them send me there." What would you say to her?

- *Impaired Physical Mobility* related to bed rest and fractured left femoral neck
- *Risk for Altered Tissue Perfusion* related to unstable bones and swelling secondary to left femoral neck fracture
- *Risk for Altered Sensory Perception: Tactile* related to the risk of nerve impairment

Expected Outcomes
The expected outcomes established in the plan of care specify that Mrs. Carbolito will

- Verbalize an increase in comfort and a decrease in pain.
- Maintain traction of her left leg.
- Verbalize the purpose of traction.
- Verbalize the purpose of any surgery.
- Demonstrate exercises.

- State the importance of reporting increased pain, pallor, paresthesia, or paralysis to the nurse.

Planning and Implementation
The following nursing interventions are planned and implemented for Mrs. Carbolito:

- Assess pain on a scale of 0 to 10 before and after implementing measures to reduce pain.
- Handle the injured leg gently.
- Administer narcotics per the physician's order.
- Assess for pain, pulses, paresthesia, paralysis, and pallor every 2 to 4 hours, and document findings.
- Apply straight leg traction per physician's order.
- Encourage deep breathing and relaxation techniques.
- Utilize distraction techniques.

- Apply pneumatic compression boots to lower extremities per physician's order.
- Administer subcutaneous heparin per physician's order.
- Teach Mrs. Carbolito the purpose of traction.
- Teach Mrs. Carbolito the purpose of any planned surgery.
- Teach Mrs. Carbolito the purpose of and the procedure for performing isometric and flexion/extension exercises.

Evaluation

Three days after surgery, Mrs. Carbolito is out of bed and in a hip chair. She verbalizes a decrease in pain and demonstrates isometric and flexion/extension exercises. She is able to state the purpose of traction in her initial care and the purpose of surgery. She verbalizes the need for heparin and compression boots to prevent deep vein thrombosis. Mrs. Carbolito was also able to state the reason for a hip chair: "This chair prevents me from knocking my hip back out. I have to be careful." Mrs. Carbolito will be discharged home tomorrow, and her family will care for her. A community nurse will visit, and the social worker at the hospital has ordered a trapeze for her bed, an elevated toilet set, an elevated cushion for her chair, and a walker.

Critical Thinking in the Nursing Process

1. What factors placed Mrs. Carbolito at risk for a fracture?
2. Develop a preoperative teaching plan for Mrs. Carbolito for an open reduction internal fixation on the hip.
3. Explain why Mrs. Carbolito was placed in traction when she was going to the operating room anyway.
4. List all the departments in the hospital that would have to collaborate in Mrs. Carbolito's care. Describe their roles.
5. Develop a care plan for Mrs. Carbolito for the nursing diagnosis *Sleep Pattern Disturbance*.

The Client with an Amputation

■ ■ ■

An **amputation** is the partial or total removal of a body part. Amputation may be the result of a chronic condition, such as peripheral vascular disease or diabetes mellitus, or it may be the result of an acute process, such as an accident. Regardless of the cause, the event is devastating to the client.

The loss of a limb is a serious condition that profoundly affects the client. The physical and psychosocial impact on the client and family can be devastating, and adaptation may take a long time and require much effort. The nursing challenges in helping a client with a new amputation are great; a multidisciplinary health care team is necessary to meet the client's physical, spiritual, cultural, and emotional needs.

Peripheral vascular disease (PVD) is the major cause of amputation of the lower extremities (see Chapter 30). Common risk factors for the development of PVD include hypertension, diabetes, smoking, and hyperlipidemia. The risk of PVD is four to five times higher in people with diabetes (Bild, Selby, Sinnock, Browner, Braveman, & Showstack, 1989). Peripheral neuropathy also places the person with diabetes at risk for amputation. In peripheral neuropathy, loss of sensation frequently leads to unrecognized injury and infection. Untreated infection may lead to gangrene and, hence, the need for amputation.

Trauma is the major cause of amputation of the upper extremities. An upper extremity amputation represents a more serious threat to independence, because they perform more specialized functions. The incidence of traumatic amputations is highest among young men. Most amputations in this group result from motor vehicle crashes or accidents involving machinery at work. Traumatic amputations differ from chronic amputations in that the surgeon does not have as much say in the level of amputation. The client presents to the trauma center with an injury that may be life-threatening; significant loss of blood and tissue may have already occurred, and shock may develop. (See Chapter 10 for a discussion of trauma.) The area is debrided, and the level of amputation determined by the amount of healthy tissue that remains.

Pathophysiology

Amputations result from or are necessitated by interruption in blood flow, either acute or chronic. In acute trauma situations, the limb is partially or completely severed, and tissue death ensues. There have been recent advances in the replantation of fingers and small body parts, but not in limb attachment. The body may recognize a partially amputated nonfunctional body part as a threat, and sepsis may develop. In such cases, the body part is removed to prevent death of the client. Clients facing this situation require counseling; they may not be willing to sacrifice a limb, even a nonfunctional one, to ensure life.

In the chronic disease processes, circulation is impaired, venous pooling begins, proteins leak into the interstitium, and edema develops. Edema increases the risk of injury and further decreases circulation. Stasis ulcers develop and readily become infected because impaired healing and altered immune processes allow bacteria to proliferate. The presence of progressive infection further compromises circulation and ultimately leads to gangrene (tissue death), which requires amputation.

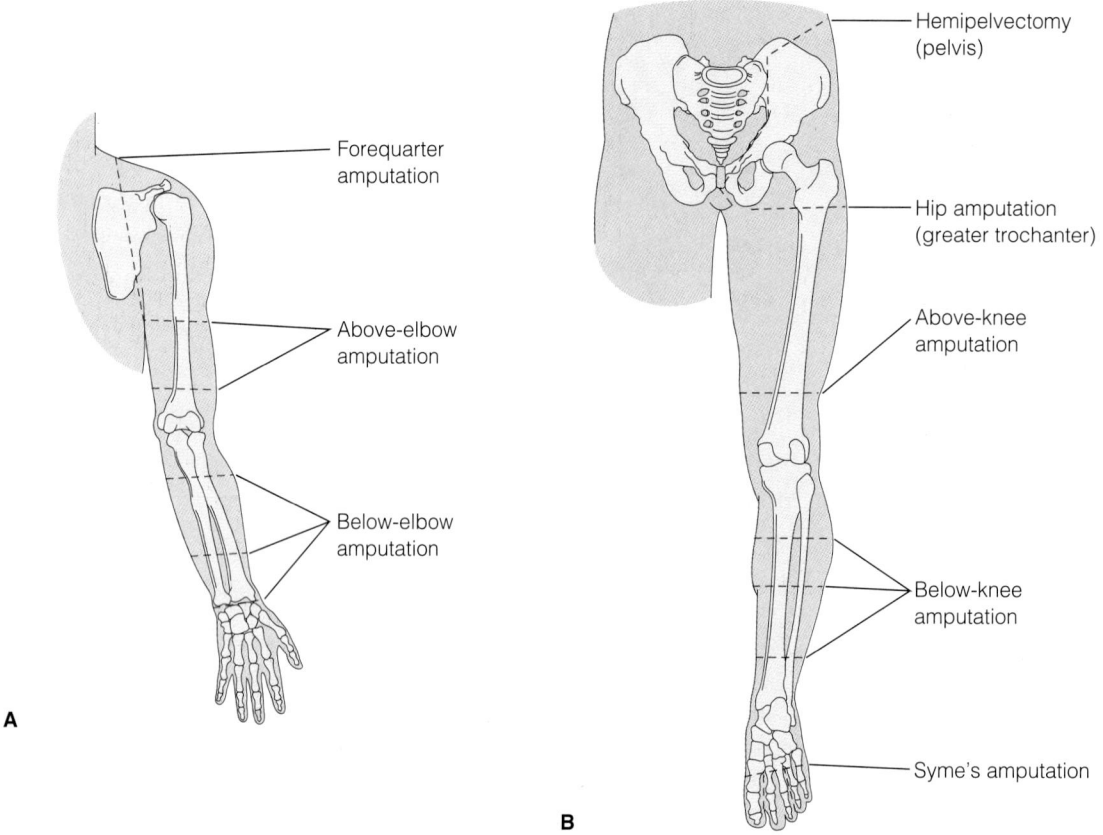

Figure 37–10   Common sites of amputation. *A,* The upper extremities. *B,* The lower extremities. The surgeon determines the level of amputation based on blood supply and tissue condition.

Levels of Amputation

The level of amputation is determined by the surgeon. The goal is to alleviate symptoms, to maintain healthy tissue, and to increase functional outcome. When possible, the joints are preserved because they allow for greater function of the extremity. The surgeon must also consider the prosthesis fit. Figure 37–10 illustrates common sites of amputation.

Types of Amputation

Amputations may be open (*guillotine*) or closed (*flap*). Open amputations are performed when infection is present. The wound is not closed but remains open to drain. When infection is no longer present, surgery is performed to close the wound. In closed amputations, the wound is closed with a flap of skin that is sutured in place over the stump. Terms used to refer to amputations are presented in Table 37–4.

Healing of the Amputation Site

For the prosthesis to fit well, the amputation site must heal properly. To promote healing, a rigid or compression dressing is applied to prevent infection and minimize edema. A rigid dressing is made by placing a cast on the stump and molding the stump to fit a prosthesis. A soft compression dressing is applied when frequent wound checks are necessary. When this type of dressing is used, a splint is sometimes applied to help mold the extremity to fit the prosthesis. After the wound is dressed, the client is encouraged to toughen the stump skin by pushing it into first soft and then harder surfaces. The stump is wrapped in an Ace bandage to allow a conical shape to form and prevent edema. The bandage is applied from the distal to the proximal (Figure 37–11).

Complications

Complications that may ensue after an amputation include infection, delayed healing, and contracture.

Infection   Generally, the client who suffers a traumatic amputation has a greater risk of infection than the person who has a planned amputation. However, even planned amputations carry a risk of infection; the client who is older, has diabetes, or suffers peripheral neurovascular compromise is at a particularly high risk for infection. Infection may present itself either locally or systemically. Local manifestations of infection include drainage, odor,

Table 37–4	Amputation Terms
Term	**Meaning**
Arm	Amputation of a portion of the arm, either above or below the elbow
Disarticulation	Amputation through a joint
Forequarter	Removal of the entire arm and disarticulation of the shoulder
Closed (flap)	Amputation in which a flap of skin is formed to cover the end of the wound
Open (guillotine)	Perpendicular cutting of the extremity in which the wound is left open; used when infection is present
Leg	Amputation below the knee
Thigh	Amputation above the knee
Finger or Toe	Amputation of one or all of the fingers or toes
Syme	Modified disarticulation of the ankle
Foot	Amputation of part of the foot and toes

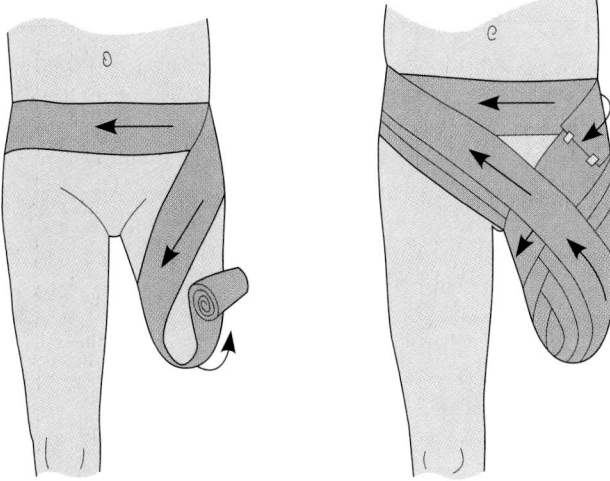

Figure 37–11   Stump dressings increase venous return, decrease edema, and help shape the stump for a prosthesis. With an above-knee amputation, a figure-eight bandage is started by bringing the bandage down over the stump and back up around the hips.

redness, positive wound cultures, and increased discomfort at suture line. Systemic manifestations include fever, an increased heart rate, a decrease in blood pressure, chills, and perhaps even positive blood cultures. If any of these manifestations develop, the physician should be immediately notified. In the client with diabetes, a sudden elevation in blood glucose levels sometimes precedes the onset of these manifestations. Pneumonia also may develop; the client complains of a productive cough, pain on deep inspiration, and possibly malaise. Nursing measures to prevent infection include maintaining asepsis during wound care, providing routine skin care, administering antibiotics per physician's orders, monitoring respiratory status, and encouraging coughing and deep breathing.

Delayed Healing   If infection is present or if the circulation remains compromised, delayed healing will result. **Delayed healing** is healing that occurs at a slower rate than expected. In older clients, other preexisting conditions can increase the risk of delayed healing. In clients of any age, electrolyte imbalances can contribute to delayed healing, as can a diet that lacks the proper nutrients to meet the body's increased metabolic demands. Smoking may also compromise healing by causing vasoconstriction and decreasing blood flow to the stump. Deep vein thrombosis and compromised venous return, which may result from prolonged immobilization, are other potential factors. Decreased cardiac output decreases blood flow and thus also delays healing.

The nurse must carefully assess the wound for healing. If the wound does not appear well approximated or if the stump is cool, the physician should be notified. Early mobilization of the client is encouraged, and preventing infection is imperative.

Contractures   A **contracture** is an abnormal flexion and fixation of a joint caused by muscle atrophy and shortening. Contracture of the joint above the amputation is a common complication. The client needs to be taught to extend the joint. The client with an above-the-knee amputation should lie prone for periods throughout the day. The client with a below-the-knee amputation should elevate the stump, keeping the knee extended. The same principles apply to the upper extremity. All joints should receive either active or passive ROM exercises every 2 to 4 hours. A trapeze frame should be added to the bed to encourage the client to change position every 2 hours. The client who has an upper extremity amputation should exercise both shoulders. Postural exercises can help prevent the client from hunching over secondary to the loss of weight on the affected side. The client with a thigh amputation should be discouraged from sitting for prolonged periods of time; prolonged sitting can lead to hip contracture.

Collaborative Care

Multidisciplinary care is necessary for the client who has sustained an amputation. Physical therapy and occupational retraining are necessary, and the client may also benefit from the presence of clergy. The entire health care team needs to view the positive as well as the negative effects of amputation, that is, to look on amputation as a means to increase the client's independence and relieve symptoms. The client should be given opportunities to become familiar with the members of the health care team and their roles; this allows the client greater control over his or her care and rehabilitation and promotes independence.

Laboratory and diagnostic tests are necessary to prepare the client for surgery. Pharmacologic agents are necessary during the entire operative phase.

Laboratory and Diagnostic Tests

Preoperatively, the client may need the following routine tests:

- *CBC* is performed to measure the WBC count and hemoglobin and hematocrit levels.
- *Serum electrolytes* are performed to assess the client's fluid balance.
- *Prothrombin time (PT)* and *partial thromboplastin time (PTT)* are ordered to assess the blood's ability to clot.
- *Urinalysis* is performed to detect the presence of WBCs, RBCs, or protein, which may indicate infection.
- *Electrocardiogram (ECG)* is ordered to assess the heart for signs of injury or ischemia.
- *Chest X-rays* help identify the presence of infection in the lungs, such as pneumonia.

These tests provide a baseline for future tests and determine whether the client is in the best possible health to undergo surgery.

The client may also undergo amputation-specific studies, such as:

- *Doppler flowmetry* evaluates blood flow in the extremity.
- *Segmental blood pressure determinations* evaluate the blood flow and vessel pressures in the extremity.
- *Transcutaneous partial pressure oxygen readings* measure the oxygen delivery by blood vessels in the affected extremity.

These tests are performed to assess the circulation present in the limb at different levels. They assist the physician in determining the level of viable tissue. If revascularization with a bypass is planned in conjunction with the amputation, angiography is also performed.

Postoperative diagnostic tests include the following:

- *CBC* is performed to determine the client's hemoglobin and hematocrit levels. A sudden drop in these values may indicate hemorrhage. The WBC count is also monitored with a CBC; a sudden increase in the WBC may indicate the presence of infection.

- *Blood Chemistry:* Measures electrolytes and reflects fluid balance. During surgery, clients often receive intravenous fluids and develop postoperative diuresis.
- *Vascular Doppler ultrasonography* may be performed if a client is suspected of having a DVT.

Pharmacology

The client receives pharmacologic agents preoperatively, intraoperatively, and postoperatively. Preoperatively, the physician may prescribe intravenous antibiotics. Intraoperatively, anesthetic agents are administered. It also may be necessary to administer agents to control blood pressure during the surgery. Postoperatively, the client resumes any routinely prescribed medications and in addition may receive antibiotics and analgesics, such as narcotics. Steroids may be administered to decrease swelling. A histamine H_2 antagonist may also be ordered to decrease the risk of peptic ulcer formation. Stool softeners may be administered to prevent constipation.

Nursing Care

The goals of nursing care for a person with an amputation are to relieve pain, promote healing, prevent complications such as infection, and support the client and family during the process of grieving and adaptation to alterations in body image, and restore mobility. Care is individualized, and the circumstances that led to the amputation (e.g., traumatic injury or disease) also must be addressed. Applying rehabilitation principles to nursing care is also an important consideration; see the accompanying box.

Pain

The client who has sustained an amputation experiences pain. Pain originates with the suture site and can be compounded by muscle spasms, swelling, and phantom pain. **Phantom pain** is a real pain that the client develops in the area of the amputation as a result of trauma to the nerves. In phantom pain, the brain receives messages that cause the client to feel that the missing extremity feels numb, crushed, trapped, twisted, or burning.

Nursing interventions with rationales follow:

- Monitor baseline vital signs. *Some analgesics decrease respiratory effort and blood pressure. A client with a poor respiratory effort or very low blood pressure may not be able to receive these analgesics.*
- Ask the client to rate the pain on a scale of 0 to 10 (with 10 being the most severe pain) before and after any intervention. *This facilitates objective assessment of the effectiveness of the chosen pain relief strategy. Pain that increases in intensity or remains unrelieved with analgesics can indicate compartment syndrome.*

Applying Rehabilitation Principles to Medical/Surgical Nursing: Lower Limb Amputation

■ ■ ■

Rehabilitation principles for the amputee can ease the transition from the hospital setting to home. Exercises and positioning techniques help prepare the stump for a prosthesis.

Case Example

Mr. Jake Binden, 56 years old, has diabetes and a history of peripheral vascular disease. He is admitted to the unit postoperatively after undergoing a below-the-knee amputation of his right leg. An IV is infusing in his left hand. Mr. Binden's vital signs are stable, and he is alert and talking.

Rehabilitation Principle

Preparing the client for a prosthesis as well as for the change in body image that occurs following amputation is an important component of rehabilitation. Maintaining the client's self-esteem and motivation is critical.

Rehabilitation Time Frame

Mr. Binden will stay in the unit for 3 to 5 days before being transferred to a rehabilitation unit. It is during these days that the acute-care nurse can play an invaluable role in facilitating the successful rehabilitation of the client.

Nursing Diagnoses

- *Impaired Physical Mobility* secondary to amputation
- *Powerlessness* related to grieving and inability to maintain self-care

Because of his amputation, Mr. Binden has difficulty ambulating. He also faces a grieving process in adjusting to the loss of a body part. This grieving, in combination with his difficulty in caring for himself, may lead to a sense of helplessness. The nurse can implement a plan of care that encourages the client to regain control.

Rehabilitation Goals and Interventions

- Allow Mr. Binden time to verbalize his feelings concerning his surgery. *Verbalization of fears has been demonstrated to decrease the anxiety that accompanies fears. A decrease in anxiety facilitates the teaching/learning process, which is a necessary component of rehabilitation.*

- Encourage the client to participate in the care of his stump. *Active participation not only builds the client's self-esteem but also reinforces the importance of good stump care. Visualization of the amputation also desensitizes the client to the amputation.*

- Teach the client the proper wrapping technique for stump care. *Proper wrapping of the stump helps to shape the stump in preparation for prosthetic fitting.*

- Caution the client not to prop the stump and/or allow the stump to dangle while sitting. *Propping the stump can cause a contracture, thereby preventing proper fitting of a prosthetic device. Dangling the stump while sitting can also cause a knee contracture, which will interfere with the client's ability to ambulate.*

- Teach the client how to perform stump exercises: range of motion exercises of the knee; and pushing down on the bed to a count of 5 and releasing. *These exercises maintain joint mobility and muscle tone and thereby prepare the stump to accept a prosthetic device.*

- Encourage the client to ambulate as soon as possible. Consult a physical therapist to obtain a walker or possibly a pylon as soon as possible. *Early ambulation provides increased client motivation and self-esteem.*

- Splint and support the injured area. *Splinting prevents additional injury by immobilizing the stump and decreasing edema while molding the stump for a good prosthetic fit.*

- Elevate the stump on a pillow for 24 hours. *Elevating the stump promotes venous return and decreases edema, which will decrease pain.*

- Move the client gently and slowly. *Gentle turning prevents the development of severe muscle spasms.*

- Encourage distraction. *Distraction prevents the patient from focusing on the pain, lessens the intensity of pain, and helps diminish phantom pain.*

- Administer pain medications as prescribed. A PCA pump may be ordered by the physician. *Analgesics alleviate pain by stimulating opiate receptor sites. PCA pumps increase client control over and allow early relief of pain before it intensifies.*

- Encourage deep breathing and relaxation exercises. *These techniques increase the effectiveness of analgesics and modify the pain experience.*
- Reposition client every 2 hours; turn the client from side to side and onto abdomen. *Repositioning alleviates pressure from one area and distributes it throughout the body and helps prevent cramping of muscles. Lying prone prevents further pain from hip contracture.*

Risk for Infection

The client who has an amputation is at risk for wound infection. Early recognition of infection can lead to early treatment and prevention of wound dehiscence.

Nursing interventions with rationales follow:

- Assess the wound for redness, drainage, temperature, edema, and suture line approximation. *Redness is normal in the immediate postoperative period; if it persists, however, it can indicate infection. A hot area over the incision or drainage may also indicate infection. Poor suture approximation can complicate all of these manifestations.*
- Take the client's temperature at least once every 4 hours. *Abnormal body temperatures may develop as the body attempts to eradicate infection.*
- Monitor white blood cell count for elevation. *The white blood cell count rises as the body tries to rid itself of infection.*
- Elevate the stump for the first 24 hours after surgery. *Elevating the stump increases venous return and prevents the pooling of blood.*
- Change the wound dressing as ordered, using aseptic technique. *Aseptic technique prevents the contamination of the wound with bacteria.*
- Administer antibiotics as ordered. *Antibiotics inhibit bacterial cell replication and help prevent or eradicate infection.*
- Teach the client stump-wrapping techniques. *Correctly wrapping the stump from the distal to the proximal increases venous return and prevents pooling of fluid, thereby reducing the chance of infection.*

Risk for Dysfunctional Grieving

The patient who has lost a limb is at risk for dysfunctional grieving. Denial of the need for surgery and the inability to discuss feeings compound this risk.

Nursing interventions with rationales follow:

- Encourage verbalization of feelings. Ask the client open-ended questions. *Asking open-ended questions allows the client to discuss his or her feelings and communicates the listener's willingness to listen.*
- Actively listen. *Active listening communicates respect for what the client is expressing.*

- Maintain eye contact. *Eye contact communicates respect for the client.*
- Reflect on the client's feelings. *Reflection statements, such as "You seem angry," allow the client to recognize feelings and perhaps develop a plan for resolution.*
- Allow the client to have unlimited visiting hours, if possible. *Unlimited visiting hours allow for increased social supports.*

Body Image Disturbance

Although amputation is a reconstructive surgery, the client's body image will be disturbed. Risk for body image disturbance is higher in young trauma clients, in whom body image is a particularly important component of self-image.

Nursing interventions with rationales follow:

- Encourage verbalization of feelings. *This allows the client to communicate his or her fears and lets the client know the nurse is willing to listen.*
- Allow the client to wear clothing from home. *Familiar clothing provides emotional comfort and helps the client retain a sense of his or her own identity.*
- Encourage the client to look at the stump. *Looking at and touching the stump helps the client face his fear of the unknown and move from denial to acceptance.*
- Encourage the client to bathe and participate in care of the stump. *Active participation in care increases self-esteem and independence.*
- Offer to have a fellow amputee visit the client. *A support person who has experienced the same change gives the client the hope that he or she can regain independence.*
- Encourage active participation in rehabilitation. *Active participation in rehabilitation increases independence and mobility.*

Impaired Physical Mobility

If time allows, the client should begin strengthening of muscles preoperatively. If the amputation is the result of an emergency, exercises begin within 24 to 48 hours of surgery. The return of independent mobility boosts self-esteem and promotes adaptation to amputation.

Nursing interventions with rationales follow:

- Elevate the stump for the first 24 hours postoperatively. *Elevating the stump promotes venous return and decreases edema, which will increase mobility.*
- Perform ROM exercises on all joints. *ROM exercises help prevent the development of joint contractures that limit mobility.*
- Maintain postoperative dressing (rigid or compression). *Postoperative dressings mold the stump and decrease edema by increasing venous return.*

- Turn and reposition the client every 2 hours. The client with a lower extremity amputation should lie prone every four hours. *Repositioning increases blood flow to muscles, forces synovial fluid into joints, and helps prevent contractures.*

- Teach crutch walking or the use of assistive devices. *These devices increase mobility by balancing the client and allowing ambulation.*

- Encourage active participation in physical therapy. *Physical therapy will fatigue the client in the early stage of healing. Encouragement may increase the client's participation in the physical therapy regimen and thereby increase activity tolerance.*

Other Nursing Diagnoses

Other nursing diagnoses that are appropriate for the client with an amputation follow:

- *Activity Intolerance* related to pain and fatigue

- *Anxiety* related to traumatic nature of injury and feelings of loss of control

- *Body Image Disturbance* related to cast, traction, splints, or external fixators

- *Ineffective Individual Coping* related to loss of control and weak coping strategies

- *Risk for Constipation* related to decreased mobility and narcotic administration

- *Risk for Diversional Activity Deficit* related to bed rest and/or decreased mobility

- *Altered Family Processes* related to inability to perform normal role secondary to impaired mobility

- *Fatigue* related to stress and decreased mobility

- *Risk for Impaired Gas Exchange* related to bed rest

- *Impaired Home Maintenance Management* related to decreased physical mobility

- *Knowledge Deficit* regarding stump care, crutch walking, and use of prosthesis

- *Post-Trauma Response* related to traumatic interruption in life resulting from injury

- *Self-Care Deficit: Bathing, Feeding, Grooming, and/or Toileting*

- *Risk for Altered Sexuality Patterns* related to pain and altered body image

- *Risk for Impaired Skin Integrity* related to decreased mobility and prosthesis

- *Risk for Injury* related to disturbed gait

- *Risk for Ineffective Individual Coping* related to perceived effect of amputation on role performance

- *Hopelessness* related to chronic disease process and view of amputation as a failure

Client and Family Teaching

Client and family teaching focuses on stump care, prosthesis fitting and care, medications, assistive devices, exercises, rehabilitation, counseling, support services, and follow-up appointments. The depth of teaching depends on the cause and site of the amputation and the needs of the client.

Care of the Older Client

Holistic nursing care is especially important for the older client with an amputation. The normal aging process decreases renal and liver function; hence, medications have longer half-lives. Altered circulation prolongs wound healing, and slowing of reflexes and alterations in gait may disrupt balance. The nurse must consider these factors when providing care: Medications should be administered at low doses and gradually increased, and assistive devices must be introduced in stages. A walker may be more appropriate than crutches, because older clients have less strength in the upper extremities. Safety issues, such as decreasing the risk for recurrent falls, must be addressed. The nurse should also assess the client's need for in-home assistance and make appropriate referrals to visiting nurses and home health aides.

Applying the Nursing Process

Case Study of a Client with a Left Below-the-Knee Amputation: John Rocke

John Rocke is a 45-year-old divorced man with no children. He has a history of diabetes mellitus and poor control of blood glucose levels. Mr. Rocke is unemployed and currently receives unemployment compensation. He lives alone in a second-floor apartment. Mr. Rocke had developed gangrene in the toe and failed to seek prompt medical attention; as a result, a left below-the-knee amputation was necessary.

Mr. Rocke is in his second postoperative day and his vital signs are stable. The stump is splinted and has a soft dressing. The wound is approximating well without signs of infection. He has not performed ROM exercises or turning since his surgery, complaining of severe pain. When the nurse goes into the room, he yells, "Get out! I don't want anyone to see me like this." No one has visited him since his hospitalization. He is tolerating an 1800-kcal American Diabetes Association diet and is using a urinal independently. He has an order for meperidine (Demerol), 100 mg IM every 4 hours prn for pain, and cefazolin (Ancef), 1 g IV every 8 hours. He is on blood glucose coverage with regular insulin subcutaneously.

Assessment

Jane Simmons, the nurse who has just come on duty, notes that the client is upset and angry. He will not let anyone enter the room to give him medication or assess his vital signs.

Diagnosis

Ms. Simmons makes the following nursing diagnoses for Mr. Rocke:

- *Ineffective Individual Coping* related to altered body image
- *Body Image Disturbance* related to amputation of a limb
- *Dysfunctional Grieving* related to anger and loss of limb
- *Self-Esteem Disturbance* related to appearance
- *Risk for Injury* due to infection and contractures related to refusal of care
- *Pain* related to surgery

Expected Outcomes

The expected outcomes established in the plan of care specify that Mr. Rocke will

- Verbalize his feelings about the amputation.
- Allow the staff to monitor his vital signs and administer medications.
- Be allowed to control his pain with a PCA pump.
- Verbalize a decrease in pain.
- Verbalize the importance of turning.
- Turn every 2 hours.

Planning and Implementation

The following interventions are planned and carried out with Mr. Rocke:

- Encourage verbalization of feelings.
- Have a psychiatrist see the client if ordered.
- Actively listen to the client.
- Offer to arrange a visit with a fellow amputee.
- Ask the physician if the client can be placed on a PCA pump.
- Teach the client the importance of turning every 2 hours to prevent contractures.
- Encourage turning and lying prone.
- Teach the client the importance of antibiotics in preventing and treating infection.

Evaluation

One week after his surgery, Mr. Rocke is actively participating in his care. He has apologized for his behavior and has explained to Ms. Simmons that he was angry about the loss of his limb. He states, "I thought I knew what to expect, but I didn't."

Critical Thinking in the Nursing Process

1. What is the effect of pain on normal coping mechanisms?
2. Develop a care plan for an angry client who is refusing medications.
3. Once Mr. Rocke is ready to assist with his stump care, how would you proceed? Would you give him full responsibility for care and dressings, or would you gradually increase his participation? Why?
4. Do you expect Mr. Rocke to follow up on care after his discharge? Why or why not?
5. Mr. Rocke states, "Why should I exercise this leg—it was already cut off!" How would you respond? What is the purpose of exercising the stump?

The Client with Soft Tissue Trauma

▪ ▪ ▪

Contusions, sprains, and strains are common soft tissue injuries. Soft tissue trauma accounts for about 50% of all reported occupational injuries. The most common occupational strain or sprain is injury to the lower back. Only about 19% of reported sprains and strains involve the knee or ankle (Praemer et al., 1992). It is important to remember, however, that these statistics reflect only reported occupational injuries. Many soft tissue injuries are not work related, and many soft tissue injuries, both those that are work related and those that are not, are not reported.

Pathophysiology

A **contusion,** the simplest form of musculoskeletal injury, is bleeding into soft tissue that results from a blunt force, such as a kick or blow with an object. The force causes small blood vessels to rupture and bleed into soft tissues. A contusion with a large amount of bleeding is referred to as a hematoma. The clinical manifestations of a contusion include a history of a blow or blunt force and swelling and discoloration of the skin. The blood in the soft tissue initially results in a purple and blue color commonly referred to as a "black-and-blue" mark or bruise. As the blood begins to reabsorb, the mark becomes brown and then yellow, until it disappears.

A **sprain** is an injury to a ligament that results from a twisting motion. Forces going in opposite directions cause the ligament to overstretch and/or tear. There is bleeding into the soft tissues, and tenderness and edema develop. The most familiar type of sprain is an ankle sprain. Ankle sprains usually result from ankle inversion or external rotation (Clark & Bonfiglio, 1994). The sprain is a result of the ankle's moving in one direction while the rest of the body twists in the opposite direction. Clinical manifestations include joint instability, pain, edema, and swelling. Motion increases the joint pain.

A **strain** is a microscopic tear in the muscle that results in bleeding into the tissues. A strain usually results from overexertion and is commonly referred to as a "pulled muscle." A muscle that is forced to extend past its elasticity will become strained. Strains can be caused by lifting heavy objects without bending the knees, or a sudden acceleration-deceleration, as in a motor vehicle crash. The clinical manifestations of a strain include a sharp or dull pain that increases with isometric contraction of the muscle, swelling, and local tenderness. A comparison of sprains and strains is presented in the accompanying box.

Collaborative Care

The client with soft tissue trauma complains of severe pain and impaired range of motion. It is necessary to rule out a fracture before any further treatment is rendered. The degree of force can cause serious debilitating injuries to muscles, ligaments, and tendons.

Soft tissue trauma is treated with measures that decrease swelling, alleviate pain, and encourage rest. The client is instructed to avoid using the injured area. A splint may be applied to rest the injured area. Ice is applied for the first 48 hours, after which heat can be applied. A compression dressing, such as an Ace bandage, may be applied. The injured extremity should be elevated to the level of the heart to increase venous return and decrease swelling. If the lower extremity is injured, crutches are provided. A knee injury also requires a knee immobilizer. If the upper extremity is injured, a sling is provided. The client needs instruction in the purpose and use of any assistive devices.

Diagnostic Tests
The following diagnostic tests may be ordered when soft tissue trauma is suspected:

- *X-rays.* The diagnosis of a contusion, strain, or sprain requires a thorough physical examination, followed by X-ray studies. The physician first rules out a fracture before making a diagnosis of soft tissue injury.

- *Magnetic resonance imaging (MRI).* If traditional treatment does not alleviate the manifestations of a soft tissue injury, the client may require MRI studies for further assessment.

Pharmacology
Pharmacologic agents used to treat soft tissue trauma include nonsteroidal anti-inflammatory drugs (NSAIDs) and analgesics, including narcotics. See the previous box on pain management, page 1564.

Comparison of Sprains and Strains
■ ■ ■

Sprain

- Defined as an injury to a ligament that results from a twisting motion.
- Can cause joint instability.
- Pain, edema, and swelling are present.
- Motion increases the joint pain.

Strain

- Defined as a microscopic tear in the muscle.
- Sharp or dull pain is present.
- Pain increases with isometric contraction of the muscle.
- Swelling and local tenderness are present.

Nursing Care

The nursing care of each client is individualized and holistic. A strain or sprain may not be as devastating to a businessman as it is to a professional athlete; therefore, the nurse should determine what the injury means to the particular client. Nursing diagnoses focus on alleviating pain and returning physical mobility to preinjury levels.

Pain
The pain that results from soft tissue trauma is due primarily to the injury to the muscle or ligament and secondarily to bleeding and edema at the injury site.

Nursing interventions with rationales follow:

- Assess vital signs. *Some analgesics decrease respiratory effort and blood pressure. The client's ability to tolerate the medication must be established.*

- Ask the client to rate the pain on a scale of 0 to 10 (with 10 being the most severe pain) before and after any intervention. *This facilitates objective assessment of the effectiveness of the chosen pain relief strategy.*

- Instruct the client to rest the injured extremity. *Rest allows the injured muscle or ligament to heal.*

- Apply ice to the injured extremity. *Ice causes vasoconstriction and decreases the pooling of blood in the injured area. Ice may also numb the tender area.*

- Maintain a compression dressing, such as an Ace bandage. *A compression dressing can decrease the formation of edema and thereby decrease pain.*

Clinical Manifestations of Hip and Shoulder Dislocations

■ ■ ■

Anterior Hip Dislocation

- Shortening of thigh
- External rotation
- Pain

Posterior Hip Dislocation

- Shortening of thigh
- Internal rotation
- Pain

Anterior Shoulder Dislocation

- Bone deformity
- Inability to shrug
- Lengthening of arm
- Pain

Posterior Shoulder Dislocation

- Inability to rotate shoulder externally
- Inability to elevate arm
- Pain

- Elevate the extremity 2 inches above the heart. *Elevating the extremity promotes venous return and decreases edema which will decrease pain.*

- Teach the client the acronym RICE to remember how to care for the injury (rest, ice, compression, elevation). *Acronyms help people remember things. Knowing the treatment plan will decrease anxiety and lessen pain.*

- If pain is still present after several days, instruct the client to apply heat. *Heat is used after several days to increase blood flow and venous return and thereby decrease edema and pain.*

Impaired Physical Mobility

Pain causes the client to avoid using or bearing weight with the injured extremity.

Nursing interventions with rationales follow:

- Teach the client correct use of crutches, canes, or slings if prescribed. *An awareness of the correct technique increases safety and encourages the client to use these devices.*

- Remind the client to rest the injured extremity. *Using the extremity before it heals can lead to long-term complications.*

- Encourage the client to follow up with the primary physician. *Severe sprains may require further testing to determine whether surgical intervention is indicated.*

Other Nursing Diagnoses

Other diagnoses that might apply to a client with soft tissue trauma follow:

- *Anxiety* related to fear of not knowing what is wrong with the injured extremity

- *Knowledge Deficit* regarding appropriate activity, medication, and assistive device use

- *Activity Intolerance* related to pain and fatigue

Client and Family Teaching

Teach the client and family the purpose of any medications, splints, dressings, and assistive devices, and specify when to schedule a follow-up appointment with the physician. Explain that activity limitations will be re-addressed at the follow-up appointment. Emphasize the importance of rest to allow complete healing, and instruct the client to report any further complications, such as numbness, coolness of the limb, or severe pain, to the physician immediately. Warn the client that severe edema may also result in compartment syndrome (see previous discussion of compartment syndrome).

Care of the Older Client

Any client with a soft tissue injury that may also involve a fracture should be evaluated with radiographic studies. Because the risk of fractures is higher in older adults, these clients require particularly careful evaluation to rule out fractures; clients should not assume they have a soft tissue injury until a fracture has been ruled out. The nurse also needs to educate older clients about the importance of early accurate diagnosis and treatment to prevent long-term complications.

Always observe the client's use of assistive devices; if the device is inappropriate, the client can face a greater risk of falling. For example, as a person ages, muscle mass in the upper extremities declines. As a result, the older client with a sprained ankle may not be able to use crutches, because crutches require that the person distribute body weight along the upper extremities. Older clients may therefore find a walker more useful.

The Client with a Joint Dislocation or Subluxation

■ ■ ■

Pathophysiology

Joint dislocations and subluxations occur most frequently in people 18 to 41 years old. A **dislocation** is a separation of contact between two bones of a joint. A **subluxation** is a partial separation (or dislocation) of the bones of a joint.

Dislocations may be congenital, spontaneous, or traumatic: Congenital dislocations are present at birth; spontaneous dislocations result from disease of the joint; traumatic dislocations result from sudden force. A dislocation can occur in any joint. The most common dislocations are hip dislocations and shoulder dislocations.

The clinical manifestations of a dislocation include pain, change in shape of the joint, change in length of the extremity, immobility, and change in the axis of the bone. See the box on page 1598.

Collaborative Care

Care of the client with a dislocation focuses on relieving pain, correcting the dislocation, and preventing complications. The diagnosis of dislocation is made by physical examination and X-ray examination. The client is assessed for the manifestations discussed above and for any neurovascular compromise. Once the diagnosis is made, the joint is reduced by means of manual traction. The client receives muscle relaxants and sedatives to ease the reduction. Conscious sedation, the administration of medications to achieve an altered state of consciousness, may be used; see the accompanying box. Narcotics may be administered for pain.

When the shoulder is dislocated, it is placed back in the joint by manual traction and immobilized in a sling for 3 weeks, at which time rehabilitation can begin.

A hip dislocation is the most common type of dislocation. It is also the most severe type. A dislocated hip requires immediate reduction in the emergency room. After reduction, the physician immobilizes the hip with bed rest and, depending on the age of the client, perhaps a cast. In some cases, traction is needed for several weeks. Immobilization allows time for the tendons and ligaments to heal. After a follow-up examination, the physician assesses the stability of the hip and may allow exercises under the supervision of a physical therapist. The therapist will perform ROM exercises of the joint to prevent stiffness. The nurse assesses the extremity after therapy to ensure the hip did not dislocate. If deformity is found, the physician is called.

If a displaced hip is not reduced within 6 hours of injury, necrosis of the femoral head may result. The dislocated hip also threatens the sciatic nerve posteriorly and the femoral nerve anteriorly. Movement, sensation, pallor, and pulses must be assessed frequently. If a hip dislocation is accompanied by a fracture, the client will undergo surgery to increase mobility, decrease complications, and rapidly stabilize the joint.

Nursing Care

Nursing care of the client with a dislocation or subluxation is holistic and individualized to the client. The nurse

---

Nursing Implications for Clients Receiving Conscious Sedation

■ ■ ■

Conscious sedation is the administration of medications to achieve an altered level of consciousness. Drugs commonly administered for this purpose include midazolam (Versed), propofol (Diprivan), diazepam (Valium), and lorazepam (Ativan).

Nursing Responsibilities

- Closely monitor the client.

- Have an emergency airway cart available whenever a client receives conscious sedation.

- Ensure that the client is on continuous oximetry.

- Monitor the client's vital signs every 5 minutes during the reduction.

- Monitor ECG readings.

- The client will be discharged when fully awake and alert.

- Ensure that a family member or friend will drive the client home.

- Observe the client's gait for impairment.

---

considers the cause of injury, the type of dislocation, and the age of the client. Nursing diagnoses focus on relieving pain and preventing complications.

Pain
The client with a dislocation or subluxation experiences pain related to swelling and pressure on the nerves.

Nursing interventions with rationales follow:

- Closely monitor the client's vital signs. *Some analgesics decrease respiratory effort and blood pressure. The client's ability to tolerate the medication must be established.*

- Ask the client to rate the pain on a scale of 0 to 10 (with 10 being the most severe pain) before and after any intervention. *This facilitates objective assessment of the effectiveness of the chosen pain relief strategy.*

- If the client is receiving conscious sedation for the reduction, follow the guidelines in the box above.

- Administer narcotics per physician's orders. *Narcotics decrease pain by depressing the central nervous system at various receptor sites.*

- Maintain traction per physician's orders. *Traction maintains joint alignment and prevents pain due to movement of inflamed tissues.*

Risk for Injury

The client with a dislocation requires frequent assessments to ensure that neurovascular compromise does not develop.

Nursing interventions with rationales follow:

- Assess pain, pulses, pallor, paralysis, and paresthesia. *Any abnormality should be reported to the physician.*

- Maintain immobilization after reduction. *Immobilization prevents the joint from dislocating again.*

Client and Family Teaching

Teach the client and family the purpose of medications and immobilization. Explain that maintaining joint alignment and resting the extremity promote joint healing.

Care of the Older Client

Many older clients have preexisting mobility problems that compound the problems associated with a joint dislocation. Arthritis, for example, is a common cause of mobility problems in older adults. The client may assume a posture that alleviates pain by decreasing the weight borne by an arthritic joint. The altered posture or gait, when further compromised by a joint dislocation, may threaten the client's safety. Nurses should therefore observe the client's ambulation for steadiness.

The effects of narcotics last longer in an older person because of decreased liver and renal function. Dosages must therefore be increased only gradually. If the client is receiving other medications, the nurse must check each medicine for drug interactions.

The Client with a Repetitive Use Injury

∎ ∎ ∎

Clients with repetitive use injuries pose a challenge to the health care team. Often these clients appear puzzled as they relate a history of manifestations that have worsened over time. They emphatically deny abrupt trauma and often worry about the ability to return to work. Repeatedly twisting and turning the wrist, pronating and supinating the forearm, kneeling, or raising arms over the head can result in repetitive use injuries. Common repetitive use injuries include carpal tunnel syndrome, bursitis, and epicondylitis.

Repetitive use injuries are extremely common, and the number of worker's compensation claims for repetitive use injuries is steadily growing. In Ohio, for example, the number of claims for carpal tunnel syndrome, bursitis, and epicondylitis increased from 1712 to 3543 in only 4

> ### Carpal Tunnel Syndrome
> ∎ ∎ ∎
>
> - Repetitive use causes irritation of the tendon sheath, resulting in irritation of the median nerve.
> - More common in women.
> - Characterized by numbness or tingling of the thumb, index finger, and lateral ventral surface of the middle finger.
> - Treatment includes rest, immobilization, splinting, and, in extreme cases, surgery.

years (Praemer et al., 1992). The increase is believed to be a result of technology advances in the workplace.

Pathophysiology

Carpal Tunnel Syndrome

The carpal tunnel is a canal through which flexor tendons and the median nerve pass from the wrist to the hand. The syndrome develops from narrowing of the tunnel and irritation of the median nerve. **Carpal tunnel syndrome** involves compression of the median nerve as a result of inflammation and swelling of the synovial lining of the tendon sheaths. The client complains of numbness and tingling of the thumb, index finger, and lateral ventral surface of the middle finger. See the accompanying box. The client may also complain of pain in this area that wakes the person at night and is alleviated by shaking or massaging the hand and fingers. As symptoms persist, the affected hand may be weak and the client may be unable to hold utensils or perform activities that require precision.

Carpal tunnel syndrome is one of the three most common work-related injuries. The incidence is believed to be related directly to the number of people using computers. The incidence of carpal tunnel syndrome is higher in women, especially postmenopausal women.

Bursitis

Bursitis is an inflammation of a bursa. A bursa is an enclosed sac found between muscles, tendons, and bony prominences. The bursae that commonly become inflamed are in the shoulder, hip, leg, and elbow. Constant friction between the bursa and the musculoskeletal tissue around it causes irritation, edema, and inflammation. Clinical manifestations develop as the sac becomes engorged. The area around the sac is tender, and extension and flexion of the joint near the bursa produce pain. The inflamed bursa is hot, red, and edematous. The client guards the joint to decrease pain and may point to the area of the bursa when identifying joint tenderness.

Epicondylitis

Epicondylitis is the inflammation of the tendon at its point of origin into the bone. Epicondylitis is also referred to as *tennis elbow* or *golfer's elbow.* The exact pathophysiology of epicondylitis is unknown. Current theories attribute inflammation of the tendon to microvascular trauma. Tears, bleeding, and edema are thought to cause avascularization and calcification of the tendon. Clinical manifestations of epicondylitis include point tenderness, pain radiating down the dorsal surface of the forearm, and a history of repetitive use.

Collaborative Care

The health care team works to alleviate pain and increase client mobility. Once the diagnosis is made, treatment can range from conservative measures, such as rest and pharmacologic agents, to aggressive measures, such as surgery.

Diagnostic Tests

Carpal tunnel syndrome is diagnosed by the client's history and physical examination. History may reveal an occupation that involves computer work, jackhammer operation, mechanical work, gymnastics, or percussive devices. History of a radial bone fracture or rheumatoid arthritis also increases the risk of carpal tunnel syndrome. Tests specific for carpal tunnel include the Phalen test (see Figure 35–9 on page 1510).

Bursitis and epicondylitis are diagnosed by history and physical examination.

Conservative Management

The first steps in the care of all repetitive use injuries are to immobilize and rest the joint involved. The client must be made aware of the potential for serious scarring and complications if rest does not occur. The joint may also be splinted, and ice may be applied in the first 24 to 48 hours to decrease pain and inflammation. Ice application may be followed by heat application every 4 hours.

Pharmacology

The client with a repetitive use injury usually receives NSAIDs. Narcotics also may be administered for acute flare-ups and severe pain. For the client who has epicondylitis or carpal tunnel syndrome, the physician may decide to inject corticosteroids into the joint.

Surgery

Surgery is usually reserved for the client who does not obtain relief with conservative treatment. Surgery for carpal tunnel syndrome includes resection of the carpal ligament

to enlarge the tunnel. In epicondylitis and bursitis, calcified deposits may be removed from the area surrounding the tendon or bursa.

Nursing Care

The nursing care of a client with a repetitive use injury focuses on alleviating pain, teaching about the disease process and treatment, and improving physical mobility.

Pain

Swelling and nerve inflammation lead to pain in the client with a repetitive use injury. Nursing interventions with rationales follow:

- Ask the client to rate the pain on a scale of 0 to 10 (with 10 being the most severe pain) before and after any intervention. *This facilitates objective assessment of the effectiveness of the chosen pain relief strategy.*
- Encourage the use of immobilizers. *Splinting maintains joint alignment and prevents pain due to movement of inflamed tissues.*
- Apply ice. *Ice causes vasoconstriction and decreases the pooling of blood in the inflamed area. Ice may also numb the tender area.*
- Apply heat. *Heat decreases swelling by increasing venous return.*
- Administer NSAIDs per physician's orders. *NSAIDs decrease swelling by inhibiting prostaglandins.*
- Inform the client not to discontinue treatment abruptly. *Abrupt discontinuation of treatment may cause reinflammation of the injured area.*

Impaired Physical Mobility

In the client with a repetitive use injury, joint pain and swelling can impair mobility. Nursing interventions with rationales follow:

- Provide care to alleviate pain. *If the joint is pain free, the client will be more likely to take an active role in therapy.*
- Consult the physical therapist for exercises per physician's orders. *The physical therapist can assist the client with exercise to prevent joint stiffness.*
- Suggest occupational rehabilitation to the client and physician. *Occupational therapy can help the client learn new ways to perform old tasks to prevent the symptoms from recurring.*

Client and Family Teaching

Teach the client about the repetitive use injury and its causes and treatments. Rehabilitation may be necessary to allow the client to return to a state of independence. Help the client find ways to avoid unnecessary exposure to the things that increase risk of redeveloping the injury. An understanding of the condition can promote the client's compliance with treatment.

Bibliography

■ ■ ■

Amell, A. (1992). *Orthopedic nursing: An illustrated perspective.* Harrisburg: Community General Osteopathic Hospital.

Barden, R., & Sinkora, G. (1991). Bone stimulators for fusions and fractures. *Nursing Clinics of North America, 26*(1), 89–103.

Belsole, R. J. & Hess, A. V. (1993). Concomitant skeletal and soft tissue injuries. *Orthopedic Clinics of North America, 24*(2), 327–331.

Bild, D., Selby, J., Sinnock, P., Browner, W., Braveman, P., & Showstack, J. (1989). Lower-extremity amputations in people with diabetes: Epidemiology and prevention. *Diabetes Care, 12*(1), 24–31.

Campbell, C. (1984). *Nursing diagnosis and interventions in nursing practice* (2nd ed.). New York: John Wiley & Sons.

Carter, P. R., Hamlin, C., & Uehara, D. T. (1990). Early care for hand injuries. *Patient Care, 24*(12), 166–172, 180, 182.

Clark, C., & Bonfiglio, M. (1994). *Orthopedics.* New York: Churchill Livingstone.

Collins, D. C. (1993). Management and rehabilitation of distal radius fractures. *Orthopedic Clinics of North America, 24*(2), 365–378.

Dykes, P. (1993). Minding the five P's of neurovascular assessment. *American Journal of Nursing, 93*(6), 38–39.

Fleischer, E., & LeBel, L. A. (1993). Fat embolism syndrome. *Nurse Anesthesia, 4*(1), 18-27.

Gallapsy, J. G. (1994). Management of traumatic injuries in the workplace. *AAOHN Journal, 42*(1), 33–41.

Gerding, D. N., Piziak, V. K., & Rowbotham, J. L. (1991). Saving the diabetic foot. *Patient Care, 24*(4), 84–88, 90, 97–98.

Greenspan, S. L., Myers, E. R., Maitland, L. A., Resnick, N. M., & Hayes, W. C. (1994). Fall severity and bone mineral density as risk factors for hip fractures in ambulatory elderly. *Journal of the American Medical Association, 271*(2), 128–133.

Harrahill, M. (1994). Open pelvic fracture: The lethal injury. *Journal of Emergency Nursing, 20*(3), 243–245.

Heafey, M. L., Golden-Baker, S. B., & Mahoney, D. W. (1994). Using nursing diagnoses and interventions in an inpatient amputee program. *Rehabilitation Nursing, 19*(3), 163–168.

Herron, D. G., & Nance, J. (1990). Emergency department nursing management of patients with orthopedic fractures resulting from motor vehicle accidents. *Nursing Clinics of North America, 25*(1), 71–83.

Kelsy, J. L. (1989). Risk factors for osteoporosis and associated fractures. *Public Health Reports,* September-October Supplement, 14–20.

Liddel, D. (1985). An in-depth look at osteoporosis. *Orthopedic Nursing, 4*(3), 23–33.

MacLean, N., & Fick, G. H. (1994). The effect of semi-rigid dressings on below-knee amputations. *Physical Therapy, 74*(7), 668–673.

Monk, H. L. (1993). Fractures are never simple. *RN, 56*(4), 30–36.

Mourad, L. (1991). *Orthopedic Disorders.* Philadelphia: Mosby.

National Research Council (1985). *Injury in America: A continuing public health problem.* Washington, DC: National Academy Press.

Neff, J. & Kidd, P. (1993). *Trauma nursing: The art and science.* Philadelphia: Mosby.

Pederson, P., & Damholt, V. (1994). Rehabilitation after amputation following lower limb fracture. *Journal of Trauma, 36*(2), 195–197.

Pellino, T. A. (1994). How to manage hip fractures. *American Journal of Nursing, 94*(4), 46–50.

Praemer, A., Furner, S., & Rice, D. (1992). *Musculoskeletal conditions in the United States.* Illinois: American Academy of Orthopedic Surgeons.

Resnick, B. (1994). Die from a broken hip? *RN, 57*(7), 22–27.

Rosenthal, R. E. (1984). Emergency department evaluation of musculoskeletal injuries. *Emergency Medicine Clinics of North America, 2,* 219–244.

Sheehy, S., Marvin, J., & Jimmerson, C. (1989). *Manual of clinical trauma care.* St. Louis: Mosby.

Slye, D. A. (1991). Orthopedic complications: Compartment syndrome, fat embolism syndrome, and venous thromboembolism. *Nursing Clinics of North America, 26*(1), 113–132.

Titinalli, J., Krome, R., & Ruiz, E. (1992). *Emergency medicine: A comprehensive study guide.* New York: McGraw-Hill.

Whatley-Brown, L. K. (1990). Traumatic amputation: Mechanisms of injury, treatment, and rehabilitation. *AAOHN Journal, 38*(10), 483–486.

Williams, M., Oberst, M., & Bjorklund, B. (1994). Early outcomes after hip fracture among women discharged home and to nursing homes. *Research in Nursing and Health, 17*(3), 175–183.

Wyshak, G. (1993). Dietary animal fat intake, calcium intake, and bone fractures in women 50 years and older. *Journal of Women's Health, 2*(4), 329–334.

CHAPTER 38

Nursing Care of Clients with Arthritic and Connective Tissue Disorders

LEARNING OBJECTIVES

After completing this chapter, you will be able to

- Compare the pathophysiology of common arthritic and connective-tissue disorders.

- Relate manifestations of arthritic and connective-tissue disorders to the pathophysiologic process.

- Discuss laboratory and diagnostic tests used to diagnose arthritic and connective-tissue disorders.

- Relate nursing implications for medications and treatments prescribed for clients with arthritic and connective-tissue disorders.

- Provide appropriate care for clients experiencing joint replacement and other surgical interventions for arthritic and connective-tissue disorders.

- Provide teaching to clients with arthritic and connective-tissue disorders and their families.

- Use the nursing process to assess needs, plan and implement individualized care, and evaluate responses for a client with an arthritic or connective-tissue disorder.

The term **arthritis,** which literally means inflammation of a joint, is often used generically to refer to any disorder causing pain and stiffness of the musculoskeletal system. Many laypeople use the terms arthritis and rheumatism synonymously. *Rheumatism* is actually a broader term than arthritis, used to identify a variety of diseases and disorders involving inflammation, degeneration, or derangement of connective-tissue structures, including joints and related tissues. More than 100 rheumatic disorders have been identified. They range in severity from mild, localized, and self-limiting disorders to severe, potentially fatal systemic processes (Porth, 1994).

Arthritis and related rheumatic disorders are widespread, affecting more than 37 million people in the United States (National Institutes of Health, 1993). Arthritic disorders are a leading cause of disability. However, their very prevalence may lead the public and health care professionals to treat them as normal aging processes or discount the validity of the pain and disability experienced by the person with arthritis.

The etiology of most rheumatic disorders is not clear; in many cases, the pathophysiologic processes involved are often complex and poorly understood. Many are primary disorders; others occur as secondary processes associated with another disease. The wear-and-tear of aging, autoimmune processes, metabolic disorders, genetic factors, and infection are all implicated as causative factors in some forms of rheumatic disease. A classification system of rheumatic disorders developed by the American

Rheumatism Association groups rheumatic disorders into broad general categories (Table 38–1). This chapter is organized according to these categories.

Regardless of the etiology or pathophysiologic process involved, arthritic disorders can cause problems with mobility, deformity, and disability.

▪ ▪ ▪ Degenerative Joint Disease ▪ ▪ ▪

Degenerative changes in the joints occur with such frequency in older adults that they have often been considered part of the "normal" aging process. It is now better understood that aging of itself does not cause degenerative joint disease, rather, it is a separate entity. Both primary and secondary forms are seen. Primary or idiopathic osteoarthritis occurs without a clear precipitating factor. It is the most common type. Secondary osteoarthritis is associated with an identifiable cause. For instance, it may be related to trauma to a joint, inflammation, skeletal disorders such as congenital hip dysplasia, or metabolic disorders. Degenerative joint disease may be iatrogenic in origin, resulting from multiple intra-articular corticosteroid injections, a common management strategy.

The Client with Osteoarthritis

▪ ▪ ▪

Osteoarthritis is degenerative joint disease characterized by degeneration and loss of articular cartilage in synovial joints. The terms *osteoarthritis (OA)* and *degenerative joint disease (DJD)* are often used synonymously. OA also may be called noninflammatory arthritis because it is not accompanied or caused by a systemic inflammatory process.

Osteoarthritis is the most common arthritic or rheumatic disorder affecting humans and the leading cause of disability in the aged. It affects between 20 and 40 million adults in the United States (Hazzard et al., 1994; Tierney et al., 1994). The incidence of OA increases with age. By age 40, nearly 90% of adults show changes characteristic of OA in the weight-bearing joints. Virtually everyone over the age of 70 years has manifestations of OA (Berkow & Fletcher, 1992).

The etiology of the primary form of this disease is unknown, although genetic and immunologic factors appear to play a role in its development. The prevalence of osteoarthritis in older adults leads to the belief that it is part of the aging process; however, there are significant differences in the tissues of normal aged joints and those affected by osteoarthritis. A number of other risk factors have also been identified. Obesity is a risk factor, particularly for OA of the knee. Repetitive mechanical joint overuse (as evidenced by shoulder and elbow changes in, for instance, baseball pitchers and tennis players) has long been recognized as a risk factor for OA.

Pathophysiology

The cartilage that lines joints serves two important functions: (1) it provides a smooth surface, so that the bones of the joint glide over one another without friction, and (2) it distributes the load from one bone to the next, dissipating the mechanical stress that occurs with joint loading. This cartilage normally contains more than 70% water. More than 90% of its dry weight is *collagen,* which provides strength, and *proteoglycans,* which provide elasticity and stiffness to compression. Cartilage cells, the chondrocytes, nest in this meshwork of collagen and proteoglycans. Normal articular cartilage exudes some of its water with compression, providing lubrication for joint surfaces. This water is reabsorbed during relaxation of the joint.

In osteoarthritis, proteoglycans and collagen are lost from the cartilage as a result of enzymatic degradation. The water content of the cartilage increases as the collagen matrix is destroyed. With the loss of proteoglycans and collagen fibers, the cartilage becomes yellow or brownish gray and loses its tensile strength. Surface ulcerations occur, and fissures develop in deeper layers of the cartilage. Eventually, large areas of articular cartilage are lost, and underlying bone is exposed. The bone thickens in exposed areas, reducing its ability to absorb energy in joint loading. Cysts can also develop in the bone. Cartilage-coated *osteophytes* (bony outgrowths) change the anatomy of the joint. As these spurs or projections enlarge, small pieces may break off, leading to mild **synovitis,** inflammation of the synovial membrane.

The onset of osteoarthritis is usually gradual and insidious, and the course slowly progressive. Individuals rarely have symptoms before the age of 40 years, even though joint changes may be evident in X-ray studies. Pain is the most common and usually the initial manifestation of OA. The pain is localized to the affected joints and may be described as a deep ache. It typically is aggravated by use or motion of the joint and relieved by rest, although it may become persistent as the disease progresses. Following periods of immobility (e.g., on awakening in the morning or after an automobile ride), involved joints may stiffen. Usually only a few minutes of activity are necessary to relieve the stiffness. Range of motion of the joint decreases as the disease progresses, and grating or *crepitus* may be noted during movement. Bony overgrowth may cause joint enlargement, and flexion contractures may oc-

Table 38–1	Classification of the Rheumatic Diseases
Classification	**Examples**
I. Diffuse connective-tissue diseases	▪ Rheumatoid arthritis ▪ Systemic lupus erythematosus ▪ Systemic sclerosis ▪ Polymyositis/dermatomyositis ▪ Vasculitis ▪ Sjögren's syndrome
II. Arthritis associated with spondylitis	▪ Ankylosing spondylitis ▪ Reiter's syndrome ▪ Psoriatic arthritis ▪ Arthritis associated with inflammatory bowel disease
III. Degenerative joint disease	▪ Osteoarthritis
IV. Arthritis associated with infectious agents	▪ Bacterial, viral, fungal, or parasitic arthritis ▪ Rheumatic fever ▪ Hepatitis B
V. Metabolic and endocrine diseases with associated arthritis	▪ Crystal-induced conditions (gout, pseudogout) ▪ Amyloidosis ▪ Scurvy ▪ AIDS
VI. Neoplasms	▪ Primary neoplasms of the joint ▪ Multiple myeloma
VII. Neuropathic disorders	▪ Charcot's joints ▪ Carpal tunnel syndrome
VIII. Bone and cartilage disorders with associated arthritis	▪ Osteoporosis ▪ Osteomalacia ▪ Hypertrophic osteoarthropathy
IX. Nonarticular rheumatism	▪ Fibromyalgia ▪ Low back pain ▪ Tendinitis and bursitis
X. Miscellaneous disorders	▪ Trauma ▪ Pancreatic disease ▪ Sarcoidosis ▪ Chronic active hepatitis

Note. Modified from *Primer on the rheumatic diseases* (9th ed.). Atlanta: Arthritis Foundation.

Table 38–2	Manifestations of Osteoarthritis
Affected Site	**Manifestations**
Interphalangeal joints	▪ *Heberden's nodes*—bony enlargements of the DIP joints; may cause pain, redness, swelling (See the accompanying figure.) ▪ *Bouchard's nodes*—bony enlargement of PIP joints
First carpometacarpal	▪ Swelling, tenderness at base of thumb ▪ Crepitus with movement ▪ "Squared" appearance of joint
Spine	▪ Localized pain and stiffness ▪ Muscle spasm ▪ Limited range of motion ▪ Nerve root compression with radicular pain and motor weakness
Hips	▪ Pain referred to inguinal area, buttock, thigh, or knee ▪ Loss of internal rotation ▪ Limited extension, adduction, and flexion
Knees	▪ Pain and bony enlargement ▪ Effusions ▪ Crepitus ▪ Instability and deformity with advanced disease

Typical interphalangeal joint changes associated with osteoarthritis. Note the presence of Heberden's nodes on the DIP joints and Bouchard's nodes on the PIP joints.

cur because of joint instability. In OA, enlarged joints are characteristically bony-hard and cool on palpation.

The hips, knees, lumbar and cervical vertebrae, proximal and distal interphalangeal (PIP and DIP) joints of the fingers, first carpometacarpal joint of the wrist, and first metatarsophalangeal (big toe) joint of the foot are affected most frequently by osteoarthritis. Manifestations specific to affected joints are outlined in Table 38–2.

Osteoarthritis of the spine may involve either the vertebral bodies and intervertebral disks, the diarthrodial joints, or both. *Spondylosis* is degenerative disk disease. As the intervertebral disks degenerate, disk space between the vertebrae is lost. Degenerative disk disease may be complicated by *herniated disk,* the protrusion of the nucleus pulposus of the disk. Herniation usually occurs in a lateral direction, potentially compressing nerve roots and causing *radicular* (distributed along the nerve) pain and muscle weakness. See Chapter 41 for further discussion of disk disorders.

Disk degeneration and joint space narrowing alter the mechanics of the spinal column, promoting osteoarthritic changes in the articular processes (the facet joints) of the vertebrae. The cartilage covering the inferior and superior articular processes degenerates, causing localized pain, stiffness, muscle spasm, and limited range of motion. Osteophytes may form on articular processes, further contributing to pain and muscle spasm.

The presentation of osteoarthritis in older clients is similar to that in younger adults. However, in this population, the risk of debilitation because of OA is greater, and the disease may progress faster. In addition, pain, stiffness, and limited range of motion increase the risk of falls in the older adult, with a subseqent risk of fracture (Hazzard et al., 1994).

Collaborative Care

Osteoarthritis is a slowly progressive process. At this time, no treatment is available to arrest this process of joint degeneration. Appropriate management is, however, important to relieve pain and maintain the client's function and mobility.

Laboratory and Diagnostic Tests

The diagnosis of osteoarthritis is generally based on the client's history and physical and radiologic examination of affected joints.

In primary OA, laboratory studies are normal because the disease is not systemic. The erythrocyte sedimentation rate (ESR) is a general indicator of systemic inflammatory processes. In OA, the ESR remains within the normal range of less than 20 mm per hour.

Characteristic changes of OA are visible in X-ray studies of affected joints. Initially, irregular joint space narrowing is seen. Progressive changes include increased density of *subchondral* (under cartilage) bone, osteophyte formation at the joint periphery, and the formation of cysts in the bone.

Pharmacology

The pain of osteoarthritis often can be managed through the use of simple analgesics such as aspirin or acetaminophen. Acetaminophen is generally preferred for use in older clients because it has fewer toxic side effects. Nonsteroidal anti-inflammatory drugs (NSAIDs) may also be prescribed. These medications are discussed in more detail in the section of this chapter on rheumatoid arthritis. Stronger analgesics such as narcotic preparations are rarely necessary for a client with OA.

Potent anti-inflammatory medications, such as systemic corticosteroids, are seldom used for clients with osteoarthritis, although intra-articular corticosteroid injections may be used. With intra-articular injections, a long-acting corticosteroid medication, often mixed with a local anesthetic such as lidocaine, is injected directly into the joint space of the affected joints. Although this procedure may provide marked pain relief, it can hasten the rate of cartilage breakdown if performed more frequently than every 4 to 6 months.

Surgery

Surgical procedures can provide dramatic results for clients with significant chronic pain and loss of joint function. Although elective surgical procedures are frequently avoided in the older adult, even aged clients can benefit significantly if they do not have a chronic medical condition that contraindicates surgery.

Arthroscopy may be employed for clients with osteoarthritis of the knee. In this procedure, an arthroscope is introduced into the knee joint through a small stab incision. The scope allows visual inspection of joint structures, debridement of damaged cartilage, and removal of loose bodies and osteophytes. Arthroscopy often relieves pain and improves function. Joint *lavage,* or irrigation, may also be performed to flush debris out of the joint space.

Osteotomy, an incision into or transection of the bone, may be performed to realign an affected joint, particularly when significant bony overgrowth or osteophyte formation has occurred. This procedure may also be employed to shift the joint load toward areas of less severely damaged cartilage. Although osteotomy does not halt the process of osteoarthritis, it may have a beneficial effect on joint function and pain, delaying the need for a joint replacement by several years (Way, 1994).

Joint **arthroplasty**, reconstruction or replacement of a joint, has tremendously improved the management of clients with severe and disabling osteoarthritis. Arthroplasty is usually indicated when the client has severely restricted joint mobility and pain at rest. Pain is virtually eliminated, and the function of the joint is generally improved. Arthroplasty may involve partial joint replacement or reshaping of the bones of a joint. For most clients with osteoarthritis, both surfaces of the affected joint are replaced with prosthetic parts in a procedure known as a *total joint replacement.* The hip joint prosthesis, the first to be developed, remains the most successful joint replacement procedure. Arthroplasty is also commonly performed on the knee joint. Other joints that may be replaced include the shoulder, elbow, ankle, wrist, and joints of the fingers and toes.

In a total joint replacement, some or all of the synovium, cartilage, and bone on both sides of the joint are removed. A metallic prosthesis is inserted to replace one joint surface (generally the load-end or distal portion of a weight-bearing joint). The other joint surface is replaced by a silicone-lined ceramic or plastic prosthesis.

The average life span of a prosthetic joint is approximately 10 years, although it is improving continually. Currently, most prosthetic joints are *uncemented,* that is, made of porous ceramic and metal components inserted so that they fit tightly into existing bone. The implant is secured by new bone growth into the prosthesis, a process that requires approximately 6 weeks. Although a longer non-weight-bearing period is necessary initially until the prosthesis is fixed in place by the bony growth, the implant appears to have a longer useful life span than cemented prostheses. In a *cemented* joint replacement, methyl methacrylate (a pliable polymer that hardens to hold the prosthesis in place) is used to secure the prosthesis to existing bone. Although the client is able to resume normal activities more rapidly following a cemented joint replacement, methyl methacrylate initiates an inflammatory response, and the joint eventually loosens.

In a *total hip replacement,* the articular surfaces of the acetabulum and femoral head are replaced. The entire head of the femur and part of the femoral neck are removed and replaced with a prosthesis made of cobalt-chrome alloy, stainless steel, or titanium (Figure 38–1). The acetabulum is remodeled, and a prosthesis of high-molecular-weight polyethylene is inserted. The success rate for total hip replacement is reported to be greater than 90%, but its long-term reliability has not been established. For this reason, it is usually not performed on people under the age of 50 years (Way, 1994).

Potential problems associated with a total hip replacement include dislocation within the prosthesis, loosening of joint components from surrounding bone, and infection. If recurrent or ineffectively treated, these complications may necessitate removal of the prosthesis, resulting in severe shortening of the extremity and an unstable hip joint. If the prosthesis is removed, the client must use a crutch for ambulation indefinitely (Way, 1994).

A *total knee replacement* is performed if the client has intractable pain and X-ray films show evidence of arthritis of the knee. Several prosthetic devices involving removal of varying amounts of bone are available for knee joint replacement (Figure 38–2). The femoral side of the joint is replaced with a metallic surface, and the tibial side

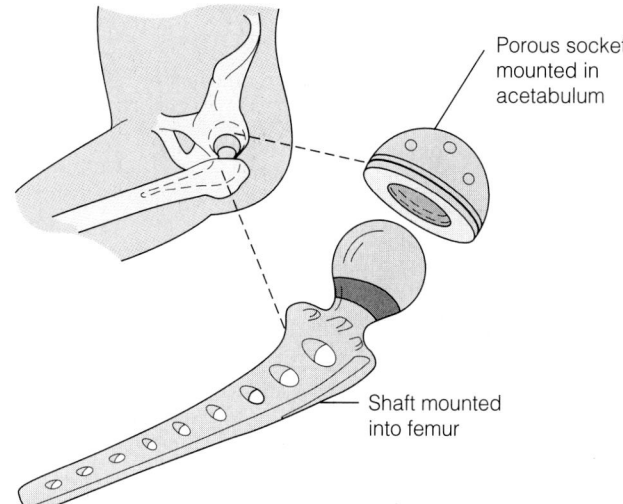

Figure 38–1   Total hip prosthesis.

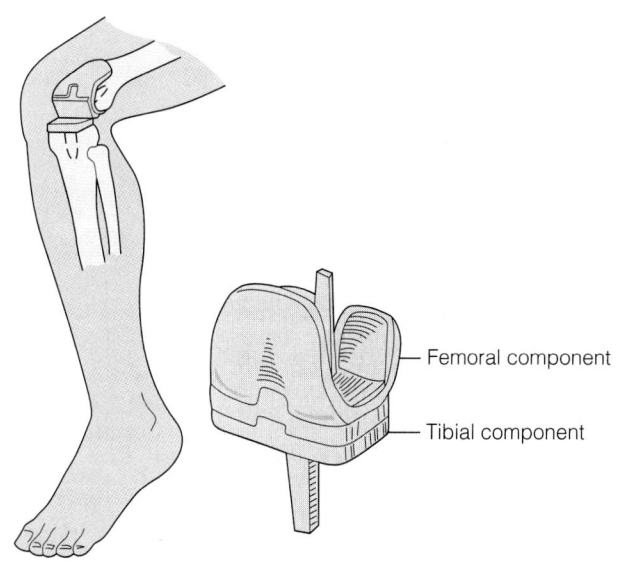

Figure 38–2   Total knee replacement.

with polyethylene. More than 80% of clients obtain significant or total relief of pain with a total knee replacement. They must, however, be prepared to engage in a vigorous program of rehabilitation to achieve the best results. The box on page 1608 gives the goals of collaborative care for the client undergoing total knee replacement.

Joint failure is more common with knee replacement than with a total hip replacement. Loosening of joint components, often on the tibial side, is the most common cause of failure. Infection, impaired healing, and nerve

Collaborative Care: The Client with a Total Knee Replacement	
Health Care Team	**Client-Centered Goals**
Orthopedic surgeon	Conducts preoperative assessment including X-ray films and physical examinations to evaluate pain, disability, and range of motion. Explains surgical options and performs surgery. Orders active flexion of knee following surgery. Orders progressive ambulation and weight-bearing limits. Following discharge, monitors for complications including infection and loosening of components.
Physical therapist	Assesses client's rehabilitation potential. Provides isometric and passive and active exercises. Provides CPM and monitors active flexion. Instructs regarding proper use of recommended assistive devices. Develops and provides individualized physical therapy program.
Respiratory therapist	Assesses client's respiratory status and provides respiratory care including incentive spirometry until client is fully ambulatory.
Social worker	Coordinates discharge referrals for home care and community-based services such as home health aide and physical therapist. Arranges for CPM at home. May need to arrange skilled care until client is independent in ambulation and self-care.
RN and Health Care Team Communications	Reports uncontrolled pain, changes in neurovascular status, evidence of compartment syndrome, and excessive wound drainage or bleeding. Reports signs and symptoms of fat embolism, deep venous thrombosis, and infection. Collaborates with physical therapy to promote mobility and maintain safety. Consults with social worker to determine needs at time of discharge. Discusses possibility of skilled care versus home care with social worker and physical therapist.

palsy are other complications associated with a total knee replacement.

Unremitting pain and marked limitation of range of motion because of arthritic involvement of both the humeral and glenoid joint surfaces of the shoulder are indications for a *total shoulder replacement.* Shoulder prostheses may be either *nonconstrained,* with separate glenoid and humeral components, or *constrained,* with a fixed fulcrum in a ball-and-socket design. The nonconstrained joint allows freer movement and a full range of motion; in a constrained joint, movement is somewhat limited, but the risk of dislocation is less. The joint is immobilized in a sling or abduction splint for 2 to 3 weeks following arthroplasty. Dislocation, loosening of the prosthesis, and infection are potential problems associated with total shoulder replacement.

Total elbow replacement involves replacement of the humeral and ulnar surfaces of the elbow joint with a metal and polyethylene prosthesis. Pain and disabling stiffness of the joint are indications for an elbow arthroplasty. Complications, including dislocation, fracture, triceps weakness, loosening, and infection, occur frequently (Way, 1994).

Infection is the major complication associated with total joint replacement. Not only does infection interfere with healing and prolong recovery, but also it may necessitate removal of the prosthesis and may lead to loss of joint function. Other potential complications include circulatory impairment to the affected limb, thromboembolism, nerve damage, and dislocation of the joint.

The accompanying box outlines nursing care for the client undergoing total joint replacement. Refer to Chapter 7 for further discussion of care for the client undergoing surgery and see the accompanying Critical Pathway.

Nursing Care

Osteoarthritis is a chronic process for which there is no cure. Although severely affected joints may be surgically repaired or replaced, many clients continue to experience pain and stiffness in other joints as the process progresses. The focus of nursing care for the client with osteoarthritis is providing comfort, helping maintain mobility and ADLs, and assisting with adaptations to maintain life roles.

Chronic Pain

Pain is a primary manifestation of osteoarthritis. As joint tissues degenerate and changes in joint structure occur, the amount of discomfort generally increases. The pain associated with OA increases with activity and tends to be relieved with rest. Because of the noninflammatory and chronic nature of this disease, nonpharmacologic comfort measures are appropriate, with mild analgesics used to supplement these as needed.

Nursing interventions with rationales follow:

- Assess the client's level of pain, including intensity, location, quality, and aggravating and relieving factors. *Accurate assessment of pain provides a basis for evaluation of the effect of interventions.*

Text continues on page 1614

Nursing Care of the Client Undergoing Total Joint Replacement

PREOPERATIVE CARE

- Assess the client's knowledge and understanding of the planned operative procedure. Provide further explanations and clarification as needed. *It is important that the client have a clear and realistic understanding of the surgical procedure and expected results. Knowledge decreases anxiety and increases the client's ability to assist with postoperative care procedures.*

- Obtain a nursing history and physical assessment, including range of motion of the affected joints. *This information not only allows nurses to tailor care to the needs of the individual but also serves as a baseline for comparison of postoperative assessment data.*

- Explain necessary postoperative activity restrictions. Teach the client how to use the overhead trapeze for changing positions. *The client who learns and practices moving techniques before surgery can use them more effectively in the postoperative period.*

- Provide or reinforce teaching of postoperative exercises specific to the joint on which surgery is to be performed. *Exercises are prescribed postoperatively to (a) strengthen muscles providing joint stability and support, (b) prevent muscle atrophy and joint contractures; and (c) prevent venous stasis and possible thromboembolism.*

- Teach respiratory hygiene procedures such as the use of incentive spirometry, coughing, and deep breathing. *Adequate respiratory hygiene is imperative for all clients undergoing joint replacement to prevent respiratory complications associated with immobility and the effects of anesthesia. In addition, many clients undergoing total joint replacement are elderly and may have reduced mucociliary clearance.*

- Discuss postoperative pain control measures, including use of patient-controlled analgesia (PCA) or epidural infusion as appropriate. *It is important for the client to understand the purpose and use of postoperative pain control measures to allow early mobility and reduce complications associated with immobility.*

- Teach or provide prescribed preoperative skin preparation such as shower, shampoo, and skin scrub with antibacterial solution. *These measures help reduce transient bacteria that may be introduced into the surgical site.*

- Administer intravenous antibiotic as ordered. *Antibiotic therapy is initiated before or during surgery and continued postoperatively to further reduce the risk of infection.*

POSTOPERATIVE CARE

- Check vital signs, including temperature and level of consciousness, every 4 hours or more frequently as indicated. Report significant changes to the physician. *These routine assessments provide information about the client's cardiovascular status and can give early indications of complications such as excessive bleeding, fluid volume deficit, and infection.*

- Perform neurovascular checks (color, temperature, pulses and capillary refill, movement, and sensation) on the affected limb hourly for the first 12 to 24 hours, then every 2 to 4 hours. Report abnormal findings to the physician immediately. *Surgery can disrupt the blood supply to or innervation of the affected extremity. If so, rapid intervention is important to preserve the function of the extremity.*

- Monitor incisional bleeding by emptying and recording suction drainage every 4 hours and assessing the dressing frequently. *Significant blood loss can occur with a total joint replacement, particularly a total hip replacement.*

- Reinforce the dressing as needed. *The dressing is usually changed 24 to 48 hours after surgery but may need reinforcement if excess bleeding occurs.*

- Maintain intravenous infusion and accurate intake and output records during the initial postoperative period. *The client is at risk for fluid volume deficit in the initial postoperative period because of blood and fluid loss during surgery, as well as the effects of the anesthetic.*

- Maintain bed rest and prescribed position of the affected extremity using a sling, abduction splint, brace, immobilizer, or other prescribed device. *Proper positioning of the affected extremity is vital in the initial postoperative period so that the joint prosthesis does not become dislocated or displaced.*

- Help the client shift position at least every 2 hours while on bed rest. *Shifting of position helps prevent pressure sores and other complications of immobility.*

- Remind the client to use the incentive spirometer, to cough, and to breathe deeply at least every 2 hours. *These measures are important to prevent respiratory complications such as pneumonia.*

- Assess the client's level of comfort frequently. Maintain PCA, epidural infusion, or other prescribed analgesia to promote comfort. *Adequate pain management promotes healing and mobility.*

➤

Nursing Care of the Client Undergoing Total Joint Replacement (continued)

- Help the client get out of bed as soon as allowed (usually 24 to 48 hours postoperatively). Teach and reinforce the use of techniques to prevent weight-bearing on the affected extremity, such as the overhead trapeze, pivot turning, and toe-touch. *Early mobility prevents complications such as pneumonia and thromboembolism, but appropriate techniques must be used to prevent injury to the operative site.*

- Initiate physical therapy and exercises as prescribed for the specific joint replaced, such as quadriceps setting, leg raising, and passive and active range-of-motion exercises. *These exercises help prevent muscle atrophy and thromboembolism and strengthen the muscles of the affected extremity so that it can support the prosthetic joint.*

- Use sequential compression devices or antiembolism stockings as prescribed. *These help prevent thromboembolism and pulmonary embolus for the client who must remain immobile following surgery.*

- For the client with a total hip replacement, prevent hip flexion of greater than 90 degrees or adduction of the affected leg. Provide a seat riser for the toilet or commode. *These measures prevent dislocation of the joint.*

- Assess the client with a total hip replacement for signs of prosthesis dislocation, including pain in the affected hip or shortening and internal rotation of the affected leg.

- For the client with a total knee replacement, use a continuous passive range-of-motion (CPM) device or range-of-motion exercises as prescribed. *Dislocation is not a problem with a knee replacement, and more emphasis is placed on range-of-motion exercises in the early postoperative period.*

- Maintain fluid intake and encourage a high-fiber diet. Administer stool softeners or rectal suppositories as needed. *Immobility contributes to the potential problem of constipation; these measures help maintain regular fecal elimination.*

- Encourage consumption of a well-balanced diet with adequate protein. *Adequate nutrition promotes tissue healing.*

- Teach or reinforce postdischarge exercises and activity restrictions. Emphasize the importance of scheduled follow-up physician visits. *Clients are discharged from the acute care facility before healing is complete. Exercises are prescribed and activities are resumed gradually to protect the integrity of the joint replacement and prevent contractures.*

- For those clients needing additional direct care after discharge, arrange placement in a long-term care or rehabilitation facility. *Activity restrictions may preclude discharge to home for some clients.*

- Make referrals as needed to home health agencies and physical therapy. *Clients often require home health care for both nursing care needs and continued physical therapy following discharge from acute or long-term care.*

Critical Pathway for Client Following Total Hip Replacement

	Date _____ 1st 24 Hours postoperative	Date _____ 2nd Postoperative day	Date _____ 3rd Postoperative day
Expected length of stay: 6–7 days			
Daily outcomes	Client will ■ Have stable vital signs. ■ Have a clean wound with edges well-approximated,	Client will ■ Have stable vital signs. ■ Have a clean wound with edges well-approximated,	Client will ■ Be afebrile. ■ Have a clean wound with edges well-approximated, healing by first intention.

	Date _____ **1st 24 Hours postoperative**	Date _____ **2nd Postoperative day**	Date _____ **3rd Postoperative day**
Daily outcomes *(continued)*	■ Recover from anesthesia as evidenced by return of vital signs to baseline; remain awake, alert, and oriented. ■ Verbalize understanding and demonstrate cooperation with turning, coughing, deep breathing, and splinting. ■ Tolerate ordered diet without nausea and vomiting. ■ Verbalize understanding and demonstrate cooperation with hip precautions. ■ Demonstrate ability to use PCA. ■ Verbalize control of incisional pain. ■ Pivot to chair with two assists morning after surgery. ■ Demonstrate ability to cope.	■ Be awake, alert, and oriented. ■ Demonstrate cooperation with turning, coughing, deep breathing, and splinting. ■ Tolerate ordered diet without nausea and vomiting. ■ Demonstrate cooperation with hip precautions. ■ Demonstrate ability to use PCA. ■ Verbalize control of incisional pain. ■ Pivot to chair with two assists three times with steps as tolerated. ■ Demonstrate ability to cope.	■ Have stable vital signs. ■ Demonstrate cooperation with turning, coughing, deep breathing, and splinting. ■ Tolerate ordered diet without nausea and vomiting. ■ Demonstrate cooperation with hip precautions. ■ Demonstrate ability to use PCA. ■ Verbalize control of incisional pain. ■ Ambulate 10 feet with walker three or four times. ■ Demonstrate ability to cope.
Tests and treatments	Vital signs and O_2 saturation, neurovascular assessment, dressing and Hemovac assessment q15min × 4; q30min × 4; q1h × 4; q4h × 24 hours and prn Incentive spirometer q2h O_2 as indicated Assess calves for redness, tenderness, swelling, heat, edema q4h TED stockings: remove and replace every shift. Intake and output every shift Empty Hemovac q8h and prn. Assess Foley catheter or voiding; use suggestive voiding techniques and/or catheterize q8h or prn if unable to void. Reinfuse drainage via blood retrieval system as ordered. Transfuse as ordered. Hemoglobin and hematocrit Prothrombin time A & P X-ray of hip in PACU Maintain dry, sterile dressing.	Vital signs and O_2 saturation, neurovascular assessment, dressing and Hemovac assessment q4h and pm Intake and output every shift Empty Hemovac q8h & prn. Assess Foley catheter or voiding; catheterize q8h or prn if unable to void. Hemoglobin and hematocrit Prothrombin time Incentive spirometer q2h O_2 as indicated Assess calves for redness, tenderness, swelling, heat, edema every shift. TED stockings: remove and replace every shift. Maintain dry, sterile dressing. Assess wound and change dressing per MD order.	Vital signs and O_2 saturation, neurovascular assessment, dressing assessment q4h Intake and output every shift Hemovac removed if drainage less than 30 mL shift Change dressing and assess would healing. Prothrombin time Incentive spirometer q2h O_2 as indicated Assess calves for redness, tenderness, swelling, heat, edema every shift. TED stockings: remove and replace every shift.

➤

Critical Pathway for Client Following Total Hip Replacement (continued)

	Date _____ 1st 24 Hours postoperative	Date _____ 2nd Postoperative day	Date _____ 3rd Postoperative day
Knowledge deficit	Orient to room and postoperative routine including hip precautions. Include family in teaching. Review care and plan early mobilization. Review importance of coughing, deep breathing, splinting incision, incentive spirometer, mobilization, and any drainage tubes, intravenous, and pain management. Assess understanding of teaching.	Review importance of early progressive exercise. Review plan of care with client and family. Reinforce hip precautions and safety measures for transfers and ambulation. Assess understanding of teaching.	Review plan of care. Include family in teaching. Initiate discharge teaching regarding wound care, activity, and diet. Assess understanding of teaching.
Diet	NPO to clear liquids to tolerance	If clear liquids are tolerated, advance to full liquids or regular diet as tolerated; 2000 mL fluid/day.	Regular diet as tolerated; 2000 mL fluid/day Encourage diet high in fiber, vitamin C, iron, and protein. Consider dietary consult.
Activity	Use abductor pillow when supine and with turning; check MD order regarding turning. The morning after surgery pivot to chair with two assists on affected side. Turn, cough, and deep breathe q2h. Encourage muscle strengthening exercises: quadriceps, gluteal sets, plantar flexion, and leg lifts q2h. Assess safety needs and maintain appropriate precautions.	Continue day 1 activities. From affected side, pivot to chair with two assists one to three times; steps as tolerated (weight-bearing per physical therapy). Maintain safety precautions.	Continue day 1 activities. Ambulate 10 feet with walker three to four times (weight-bearing per physical therapy). Maintain safety precautions.
Medications	Analgesics (PCA/IV) or epidural IV antibiotics Stool softener Antipyretics prn Evening of surgery: initiate aspirin or warfarin therapy IV fluids	Analgesics (PCA or IV) or epidural IV antibiotics Stool softener Antipyretics prn Laxative if no BM in 3 days Warfarin or aspirin therapy IV fluids as ordered	D/C antibiotics D/C PCA or epidural and/or wean to oral analgesics Stool softener Warfarin or aspirin therapy Intermittent IV device, if needed
Transfer/ discharge plan	Conduct home assessment if not previously completed.	Review with client and family discharge objectives regarding activity and home care.	Review with client and significant others progress toward discharge objectives.

	Date _____ **1st 24 Hours postoperative**	Date _____ **2nd Postoperative day**	Date _____ **3rd Postoperative day**
Transfer/ discharge plan (*continued*)	Consult with social service re- garding projected needs for home health care, including home health aides, visiting nurse, physical and occupa- tional therapy. Establish discharge objectives with client and family.	Consult and collaborate with physical therapy.	Collaborate with physical therapy.

	Date _____ **4th Postoperative day**	Date _____ **5th Postoperative day**	Date _____ **6th–7th Postoperative day**
Daily outcomes	Client will ■ Be afebrile. ■ Have a clean wound with edges well-approximated, healing by first intention. ■ Have stable vital signs. ■ Demonstrate cooperation with turning, coughing, deep breathing, and splinting. ■ Tolerate ordered diet with- out nausea and vomiting. ■ Demonstrate cooperation with hip precautions ■ Verbalize control of inci- sional pain. ■ Ambulate 20 to 30 feet with walker four times. ■ Demonstrate ability to cope.	Client will ■ Be afebrile. ■ Have a clean wound with edges well-approximated, healing by first intention. ■ Have stable vital signs. ■ Demonstrate cooperation with turning, coughing, deep breathing, and splinting. ■ Tolerate ordered diet with- out nausea and vomiting. ■ Demonstrate cooperation with hip precautions. ■ Verbalize control of inci- sional pain. ■ Ambulate 30 to 50 feet with walker four times. ■ Demonstrate ability to cope.	Client will ■ Be afebrile. ■ Have a dry, clean wound with edges well-approximated, healing by first intention. ■ Have stable vital signs. ■ Manage pain with nonphar- macologic measures. ■ Be independent in self-care. ■ Be independent in transfers and ambulates 50 to 70 feet qid with ordered assistive devices. ■ Resume preadmission urine and bowel elimination pat- tern. ■ Demonstrate home care in- structions. ■ Tolerate usual diet. ■ Demonstrate ability to cope with ongoing stressors.
Tests and treatments	Vital signs bid Change dressing every day and prn. Assess wound healing. Prothrombin time TED stockings: remove and replace every shift. Assess calves for redness, ten- derness, swelling, heat, ede- ma every shift. Intake and output every shift; assess urine output.	Vital signs bid Change dressing every day and prn. Assess wound healing. Hemoglobin and hematocrit Transfuse if ordered. Prothrombin time	Vital signs Remove dressing Assess wound Prothrombin time
Knowledge deficit	Review plan of care. Include family in teaching.	Review plan of care with cli- ent and family.	Client and family verbalize un- derstanding of discharge

➤

Critical Pathway for Client Following Total Hip Replacement (continued)

	Date _____ 4th Postoperative day	Date _____ 5th Postoperative day	Date _____ 6th–7th Postoperative day
Knowledge deficit *(continued)*	Continue discharge teaching regarding wound care, activity, and diet. Assess understanding of teaching.	Continue discharge teaching regarding wound care, activity, and diet. Review safety measures for transfers and ambulation or home care. Assess understanding of teaching.	teaching including wound care, activity, safety measures, diet, signs and symptoms to report, follow-up care and MD appointment, medications (name, purpose, dose, frequency, route, dietary interactions, and side effects), and home care arrangements. Assess understanding of teaching.
Diet	Regular diet as tolerated; 2000 mL fluids/day. Encourage high-fiber diet, rich in vitamin C and high in protein.	Regular diet as tolerated; 2000 mL fluids/day. Encourage high-fiber diet, rich in vitamin C and high in protein.	Regular diet as tolerated; 2000 mL fluids/day. Encourage high-fiber diet, rich in vitamin C and high in protein.
Activity	Continue day 1 activities. Ambulate 20 to 30 feet qid (weight-bearing and assistive devices per physical therapy).	Continue day 1 activities. Ambulate 30 to 50 feet qid (weightbearing and assistive devices per physical therapy).	Continue day 1 activities. Ambulate 50 to 70 feet qid (weight-bearing and assistive devices per physical therapy).
Medications	Analgesics PO Stool softener Aspirin or warfarin therapy D/C intermittent IV device	Analgesics (PO) Stool softener Laxative if no BM in 3 days Warfarin or aspirin therapy	Analgesics (PO) Stool softener Warfarin or aspirin therapy
Transfer/ discharge plan	Review with client and family discharge objectives regarding activity and home care. Collaborate with physical therapy.	Review with client and family discharge objectives regarding activity and home care. Collaborate with physical therapy. Complete referrals for home health care.	Discharge with referrals for home health care including nursing, physical, and occupational therapy.

- Administer prescribed analgesic or anti-inflammatory medication as needed. *Analgesics reduce the perception of pain and may decrease muscle spasm as well. Anti-inflammatory medication may be ordered to decrease local inflammatory response in affected joints.*
- Encourage rest of painful joints. *The pain of OA is often relieved by joint rest.*
- Apply heat to painful joints using the shower, a tub or sitz bath, warm packs, hot wax baths, heated gloves, or *diathermy,* which uses high-frequency electrical currents to generate heat. *Heat application reduces accompanying muscle spasm, relieving pain. Moist heat penetrates deeper than dry heat; diathermy delivers heat directly to lesions in deeper body tissues.*
- Emphasize the importance of proper posture and good body mechanics for walking, sitting, lifting, and moving. *Good body mechanics and posture reduce stress on affected joints.*

- Encourage the overweight client to reduce. *Excess weight places abnormal stress on joints, particularly the knees.*

- Teach the client to use splints or other devices on affected joints as needed. *These assistive devices help maintain the correct anatomic position of the joint and relieve stress.*

- Encourage the client to use nonpharmacologic pain-relief measures such as progressive relaxation, meditation, visualization, and distraction. *These adjunctive pain-relief measures can reduce the client's reliance on analgesics and increase comfort.*

Impaired Physical Mobility

As intra-articular cartilage degenerates and joint structures are altered, the client with OA experiences pain, stiffness, and decreased range of motion in affected joints. When the spine, large weight-bearing joints of the hips and knees, or the ankles and feet are affected, physical mobility can be significantly reduced.

Nursing interventions with rationales follow:

- Assess the range of motion of affected joints. *Assessment of joint mobility is important as a basis for planning appropriate interventions.*

- Perform a functional mobility assessment, evaluating the client's gait, ability to sit and rise from sitting, ability to step into and out of the tub or shower, and negotiation of stairs. *The functional assessment provides vital data about the client's ability to maintain ADLs.*

- Teach the client active and passive range-of-motion exercises as well as isometric, progressive resistance, and low-impact aerobic exercises. *Active range-of-motion exercises help maintain muscle tone and mobility of affected joints and prevent contractures. Isometric and progressive resistance exercises improve muscle tone and strength; aerobic exercise improves endurance and cardiovascular fitness.*

- Provide analgesics or other pain-relief measures prior to exercise or ambulation. *With decreased pain, the client is able to perform exercises better and ambulate greater distances.*

- Teach the client the importance of proper posture and good body mechanics when moving. Encourage the client to avoid heavy lifting. *Good posture and body mechanics reduce the stress on joints and decrease pain and fatigue with activity.*

- Encourage the client to plan periods of rest during the day. *Rest helps reduce fatigue, pain, and joint stress.*

- Teach the client how to use ambulatory aids such as a cane or walker as ordered. *These devices help relieve some weight-bearing and stress on affected joints.*

- Assess the client's home for hazards to safe mobility, such as scatter rugs. Encourage installation of safety devices such as hand rails and grab bars. *Simple assistive devices can prolong independence in performing ADLs.*

Self-Care Deficit

Just as OA of the lower extremities can reduce the client's mobility, OA of the upper extremities (the wrist, hand, and finger joints in particular) can significantly interfere with performance of ADLs such as cooking and brushing the hair. When the lower extremities are affected, bathing and toileting can be difficult.

Nursing interventions with rationales follow:

- Perform a functional assessment of the upper and lower extremities. For upper extremities, assess the ability to touch the back of the head, and to hold and use small items such as eating utensils. *The functional assessment provides important data about the client's ability to provide self-care.*

- Assess the client's home setting to determine the need for assistive devices such as hand rails, grab bars, walk-in shower stall, or shower chair and hand-held shower head. *Many assistive devices are relatively easy and inexpensive to obtain and can significantly improve the client's independence in performing ADLs.*

- Assist the client to obtain other assistive devices such as long-handled shoehorns, zipper grabbers, long-handled tongs or grippers for retrieving items from the floor, jar openers, and special eating utensils. *These devices can prolong independence in performing ADLs.*

Other Nursing Diagnoses

The following nursing diagnoses may also be appropriate for the client with osteoarthritis:

- *Risk for Disuse Syndrome* related to pain with movement

- *Impaired Home Maintenance Management* related to mobility restrictions

- *Risk for Injury* related to restricted joint range of motion

When the client has undergone surgical repair or replacement of an arthritic joint, the following nursing diagnoses should be considered:

- *Risk for Infection* related to disruption of skin integrity and joint structures

- *Risk for Injury* related to limited weight-bearing ability of affected extremity

- *Risk for Noncompliance* with activity restrictions and positioning recommendations related to lack of understanding

Client and Family Teaching

Because of the chronicity of osteoarthritis, clients and their families need appropriate teaching to manage the disease and its consequences effectively. Much of the teaching focus is on preservation of joint function and mobility.

Teach the client about the disease process and its chronic degenerative nature. Stress that OA is not a systemic disease but a localized one affecting selected joints. Educate the client in ways to slow joint destruction and preserve function:

- Exercise, including range of motion, isometric, postural, stretching, and strengthening, maintains healthy cartilage, preserves range of motion, and develops supportive muscles and tendons. A walking program is beneficial for clients with OA of the knee.

- Do not overuse or stress affected joints with heavy lifting, excessive stair climbing or bending, or other repetitive actions.

- Balance exercise with rest of affected joints through the use of whole body rest (relaxing in a chair or in bed every 4 to 6 hours during the day), splints, or assistive devices.

- If obese, reduce weight to decrease stress on weight-bearing joints, the knees in particular.

- Sit in a straight chair without slumping; avoid soft chairs or recliners.

- Sleep on a firm mattress or use a bed board.

Teach the client about prescribed or over-the-counter analgesic medications. Include instructions about their safe use, side effects, and any particular precautions specific to the medication. Discuss nonpharmacologic pain-relief measures such as heat, rest, massage, relaxation, and meditation.

Teaching needs for the client who has undergone a total joint replacement vary according to the joint replaced. Reinforce instructions regarding the use and weight-bearing of the affected limb. Teach the client about the proper use of splints, braces, slings, or other devices to maintain the desired limb position during healing. Discuss appropriate environmental modifications, such as an overhead trapeze for getting out of bed, elevated toilet seats, and types of chairs to use and avoid when sitting. Assist the client to learn and perform prescribed exercises. Observe and provide instructions as needed about the use of assistive devices for ambulation, such as crutches or a walker.

In addition, teach the client about the use of any prescribed medications, their purpose, and their potential side effects. Discuss possible complications, including signs of infection or dislocation, and instruct the client to notify the physician promptly if these occur.

Provide referrals to home care, physical or occupational therapy, or other community agencies as indicated for the client with osteoarthritis.

Applying the Nursing Process

Case Study of a Client with Osteoarthritis: Robert Cerulli

Robert Cerulli is a 72-year-old retired commercial fisherman who has experienced arthritic pain in his hips for the past 10 to 15 years. Over the past year, the pain in his right hip has become severe, limiting his ability to engage in activities such as gardening and sports fishing, and prompting him to seek medical attention. Significant degenerative changes in both hip joints are noted on X-ray films. The physician recommends a total replacement of the right hip, and total replacement of the left hip to follow in 6 to 12 months. Mr. Cerulli is admitted the day before surgery for final preoperative teaching and preparation.

Assessment

Christie Phlaugh, RN, completes a nursing history and examination of Mr. Cerulli on his admission to the orthopedic unit. Reviewing his medical record, she notes that Mr. Cerulli has mild Parkinson's disease and is taking carbidopa/levodopa (Sinemet 25-100) four times a day to control his symptoms. No other chronic medical conditions have been reported. Mr. Cerulli says he has been essentially healthy his entire life. He has no known allergies to medications, has never smoked, and consumes only small amounts of alcohol, averaging no more than two to three drinks per month.

On examination of Mr. Cerulli, Ms. Phlaugh notes that he is alert and oriented. His speech is soft but clear. His vital signs are BP, 116/64; P, 68 regular; R, 18; T, 97.4 F (36.3 C) PO. His color is good, and his skin is warm and moist. Peripheral pulses are strong and equal in the upper extremities, and slightly weaker but equal in the lower extremities. His feet are cool to touch but have good capillary refill. Ms. Phlaugh notes some resistance to passive range-of-motion and cogwheel movement in Mr. Cerulli's extremities. He has full ROM of his shoulders, elbows, and wrists, with only minor restriction of flexion and extension noted in his fingers. She notes that Mr. Cerulli's distal interphalangeal (DIP) and proximal interphalangeal (PIP) joints appear swollen, although they are cool, hard, and nontender to palpation with no apparent inflammation present. Several Heberden's nodes are present over DIP joints of both hands. Ms. Phlaugh notes a slight pill-rolling tremor of his hands at rest. The ROM of both hips is significantly restricted, with flexion, abduction, and rotation particularly affected. Hip flexion beyond 90 degrees prompts pain on both sides. Both flexion and extension of the knees are limited slightly. Mr. Cerulli walks with a limp, favoring his right hip, and has a shuffling gait, lifting his feet only slightly off the floor. No other abnormal assessment findings are noted on the remainder of his exam.

Preoperative laboratory studies including CBC, coagulation studies, chemistry panel, and urinalysis show a serum creatinine of 1.7 mg/dL and BUN of 30 mg/dL, with no other abnormal values noted. His ECG and chest X-ray show no apparent pathologies. The physician ordered 4 units of packed blood cells typed and cross-matched. Cefazolin (Ancef) 500 mg is to be administered intravenously at 0600 prior to surgery, and Mr. Cerulli is to shower and shampoo with antibacterial soap at bedtime. The physical therapist meets with Mr. Cerulli to evaluate his mobility and begin teaching him about postoperative weight-bearing restrictions. Mr. Cerulli is also evaluated by a respiratory therapist who initiates instruction in the use of an incentive spirometer.

Diagnosis

Ms. Phlaugh develops the following nursing diagnoses for Mr. Cerulli:

- *Pain* related to surgical incision
- *Impaired Physical Mobility* related to activity and weight-bearing restrictions
- *Risk for Infection* related to disruption in skin integrity
- *Risk for Altered Peripheral Tissue Perfusion,* right leg, related to vascular disruption and edema
- *Risk for Injury* related to manifestations of Parkinson's disease

Expected Outcomes

The expected outcomes for Mr. Cerulli's plan of care are that he will

- Maintain an adequate level of comfort postoperatively as demonstrated by
  - The ability to move easily within restrictions
  - Compliance with instructions to cough and breathe deeply
  - Verbal expressions of comfort
  - A relaxed facial expression
- Remain free of adverse consequences of immobility such as pneumonia, pressure areas, thromboembolism, or contracture.
- Remain free of infection.
- Maintain adequate perfusion of affected leg.
- Remain free of injury postoperatively.

Planning and Implementation

Ms. Phlaugh plans and implements the following nursing interventions for Mr. Cerulli:

- Assess Mr. Cerulli's pain at least hourly during first 24 to 48 hours postoperatively, and as needed thereafter.
- Instruct Mr. Cerulli in the use of patient-controlled analgesia (PCA) and monitor its effectiveness.
- Help Mr. Cerulli to change position at least every 2 hours; encourage the use of the overhead trapeze to shift positions frequently.
- Maintain sequential compression device and antiembolic stocking as ordered; remove for 1 hour daily.
- Encourage the use of the incentive spirometer hourly for first 24 hours, then at least every 2 hours while awake.
- Assist Mr. Cerulli out of bed three times a day after the first 24 hours. Use the two-person assist technique to get him out of bed; use the post technique with no weight-bearing on the affected leg.
- Maintain abduction of the right hip with pillows.
- Perform passive ROM exercises of unaffected extremities every shift.
- Encourage frequent quadriceps-setting exercises and plantar and dorsiflexion of feet.
- Assess the surgical site frequently; report signs of excess bleeding or inflammation.
- Monitor temperature every 4 hours.
- Assess pulses, color, movement, and sensation of right foot hourly for the first 24 hours, then every 2 hours for 24 hours, then every 4 hours.
- Assess level of consciousness (LOC) and orientation every shift.

Evaluation

Mr. Cerulli returns to the orthopedic unit from the postanesthesia care unit. He becomes confused and disoriented during the first 36 hours after surgery, but his orientation and thought processes gradually clear. His family has stayed with him, and he has not experienced injury or other adverse consequences from his confusion. Otherwise, Mr. Cerulli has had an uneventful postoperative recovery. Six days after surgery, he is transferred to an extended care rehabilitation facility for further therapy until he is able to ambulate with partial weight-bearing on his affected leg. He returns home 5 weeks after surgery, able to use a walker for ambulation. Arrangements are made for an overbed trapeze, elevated toilet seat, and shower chair in his home. A home health nurse and physical therapist visit Mr. and Mrs. Cerulli weekly for a month following his discharge. During this time he gradually resumes full weight-bearing. Mr. Cerulli expresses pleasure with the relief of his hip pain and says he has no fear of having his left hip replaced in the future.

Critical Thinking in the Nursing Process

1. What are the mechanisms restricting the range of motion of Mr. Cerulli's arthritic joints?

2. Mr. Cerulli's preoperative laboratory work showed a modest elevation in his serum creatinine and BUN. What are these studies indicative of? How might these changes affect nursing responsibilities related to medication administration for Mr. Cerulli?

3. Mr. Cerulli became confused postoperatively. What factors in his history might have alerted the nurses to this possibility? How might anesthesia and postoperative analgesics have contributed to his confusion?

4. Develop a care plan for Mr. Cerulli using the nursing diagnosis *Acute Confusion.*

▪ ▪ ▪ Crystal-Induced Arthritis ▪ ▪ ▪

Certain crystals can precipitate out of body fluids in the synovium, within the synovial cavity, or in tissues surrounding the joint, leading to an acute inflammatory response. Deposition of monosodium urate crystals leads to gout, the most common form of crystal-induced arthritis. Pseudogout is the result of the precipitation of other crystals, such as calcium pyrophosphate dihydrate.

The Client with Gout

▪ ▪ ▪

Gout is a metabolic disorder characterized by an elevated serum uric acid concentration and deposition of urate crystals in synovial fluid and surrounding joint tissues. Approximately 0.15% to 0.40% of people in the United States are affected by gout. It is more prevalent in men than in women, and its incidence increases with age. It rarely occurs before age 30, peaking in incidence in the 5th decade of life (Rubenstein & Federman, 1992; Wilson et al., 1991).

Gout may occur as either a primary or secondary disorder. *Primary gout* is characterized by elevated serum uric acid levels resulting from either an inborn error of purine metabolism or a decrease in renal uric acid excretion due to an unknown cause. Purines are part of the structure of the nuclear compounds DNA and RNA; they also may be synthesized by the body. Impaired uric acid excretion leads to elevated serum levels (*hyperuricemia*) in the majority of people with primary gout. Heredity appears to play a role in its development, with approximately 18% or more of people with gout reporting a positive family history of the disease.

In *secondary gout,* hyperuricemia occurs as a result of another disorder or treatment with certain medications. Disorders associated with rapid cell turnover, such as some malignancies (leukemia in particular), hemolytic anemia, and polycythemia, can increase purine metabolism. Chronic renal disease, hypertension, starvation, and diabetic ketoacidosis can interfere with uric acid excre-tion, as can certain drugs, including some diuretics (such as furosemide, ethacrynic acid, and chlorothiazide), pyrazinamide, cyclosporin, ethambutol, and low-dose salicylates. Ethanol ingestion appears to interfere with uric acid excretion and to accelerate its synthesis.

Pathophysiology

Uric acid is the breakdown product of purine metabolism. Normally, a balance exists between its production and excretion, with approximately two-thirds of the amount produced each day excreted via the kidneys and the rest in the feces. The serum uric acid level is normally maintained between 3.4 and 7.0 mg/dL in men and 2.4 and 6.0 mg/dL in women. At levels greater than 7.0 mg/dL, the serum is saturated, and monosodium urate crystals may form. Crystals tend to form in peripheral tissues of the body, where lower temperatures reduce the solubility of the uric acid. Other factors that can precipitate crystal formation and tissue deposition include a decrease in extracellular fluid pH and reduced plasma protein binding of urate crystals. Tissue trauma and a rapid change in uric acid levels may also lead to crystal deposition. A rapid increase in uric acid may occur with tissue trauma and release of cellular components; administration of a drug that rapidly lowers serum uric acid can rapidly decrease uric acid levels.

Unless treated, gout progresses in four stages. The first stage is *asymptomatic hyperuricemia,* with serum levels averaging 9 to 10 mg/dL. Most people with hyperuricemia do not progress to further stages of the disease; only about 5% to 20% go on to develop an acute attack of gout. The risk of progression increases with increasing serum levels and duration (Price & Wilson, 1992; Wilson et al., 1991).

Acute gouty arthritis is the second stage of the disease. The acute attack, usually affecting a single joint, occurs unexpectedly, often beginning at night. It may be triggered by trauma, alcohol ingestion, dietary excess, or a stressor such as surgery. It is often precipitated by an abrupt or sustained increase in uric acid levels. Urate crystals precipitate within a joint (and often, surrounding

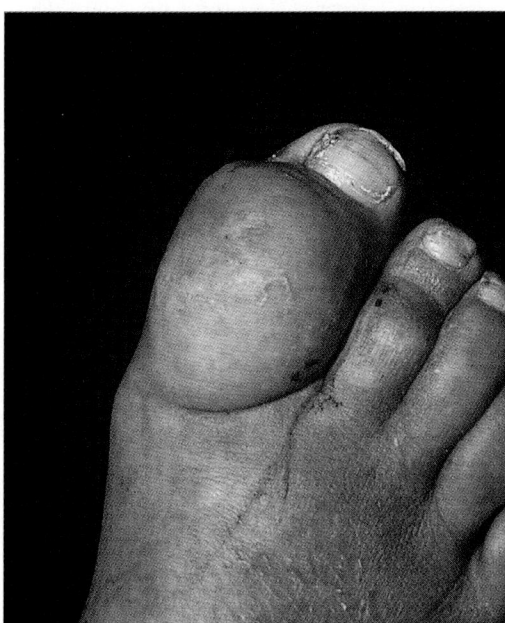

Figure 38–3   Acute gouty arthritis of the great toe.

Clinical Manifestations of Gout

Acute Gouty Arthritis

- Abrupt onset
- May be precipitated by trauma, overindulgence in food or alcohol, stress
- Usually monoarticular, affecting metatarsophalangeal joint of great toe, instep, ankle, knee, wrist, or elbow
- Acute pain
- Red, hot, swollen, and tender joint
- Fever, chills, malaise
- Elevated WBC and sedimentation rate

Chronic Tophaceous Gout

- Tophi evident on joints, bursae, tendon sheaths, pressure points, helix of ear
- Joint stiffness, limited ROM, and deformity
- Ulceration of tophi with chalky discharge

tissues), initiating an acute inflammatory response. Polymorphonuclear leukocytes (PMNs) infiltrate the joint and phagocytize the urate crystals, resulting in the death of the PMNs and the release of lysosomal enzymes and other inflammatory mediators into the tissues. The affected joint becomes red, hot, swollen, and exquisitely painful and tender.

Approximately 50% of initial attacks of acute gouty arthritis occur in the metatarsophalangeal joint of the great toe (Figure 38–3). Other sites for acute attacks include the instep of the foot, ankles, heels, knees, wrists, fingers, and elbows. The pain peaks within several hours and may be accompanied by systemic signs such as fever and an elevated WBC and sedimentation rate (see the accompanying clinical manifestations box).

Acute attacks of gouty arthritis last from days up to several weeks and typically subside spontaneously. There are no long-lasting sequelae, and the client enters an asymptomatic period called the *intercritical period*. The intercritical period may last up to 10 years; however, approximately 60% of people experience a recurrent attack within 1 year. Successive attacks tend to last longer, occur with increasing frequency, and resolve less completely than the initial attack.

Tophaceous or *chronic gout* occurs when hyperuricemia continues untreated. The urate pool expands, and monosodium urate crystal deposits known as *tophi* develop in cartilage, synovial membranes, tendons, and soft tissues. Tophi appear as firm, movable, cream-colored or reddened nodules. They are often evident in the helix of the ear; in tissues surrounding joints and bursae, especially around the elbows and knees; along tendons of the finger, toes, ankles, and wrists; on ulnar surfaces of the forearms; along the shins of the legs; and on other pressure points. The skin over tophi may ulcerate, exuding chalky material containing inflammatory cells and urate crystals. Tophi can also develop in the tissues of the heart and spinal epidura. Although tophi themselves are not painful, they may restrict joint movement and cause deformities of the hands and feet.

Kidney disease, *nephropathy,* may occur in clients with untreated gout, particularly when hypertension is also present. Urate crystals are deposited in renal interstitial tissue. Uric acid crystals also form in the collecting tubules, renal pelvis, and ureter, forming stones. Uric acid stones can potentially obstruct urine flow and lead to acute renal failure.

Collaborative Care

The classic presentation of acute gouty arthritis is so distinctive that the diagnosis can often be based on the client's history and physical examination. Treatment is directed toward termination of an acute attack, prevention of recurrent attacks, and reversal or prevention of complications resulting from crystal deposition in tissues and formation of uric acid kidney stones.

Laboratory and Diagnostic Tests

Laboratory and diagnostic testing is performed to establish an accurate diagnosis and direct long-term therapy.

The following laboratory tests may be ordered:

- *Serum uric acid* is nearly always elevated, usually above 7.5 mg/dL. This is indicative of hyperuricemia, due to excess uric acid production or impaired excretion.

- The *white blood cell (WBC) count* shows significant elevation, reaching levels as high as 20,000/mm^3 during an acute attack. During asymptomatic periods, the WBC count remains within normal limits of 5,000 to 10,000/mm^3.

- *Eosinophil sedimentation rate (ESR or sed rate)* is also elevated during an acute attack. The elevated rate is indicative of the acute inflammatory process that accompanies urate crystal deposition in a joint.

- A *24-hour urine specimen* is collected and examined to determine uric acid production and excretion. Normally, a person excretes 250 to 750 or 800 mg/24 hours of uric acid in the urine. When uric acid production is increased, these levels are higher. A value of less than 800 mg/24 hours indicates impaired uric acid excretion in the client with an elevated serum uric acid level. Instruct the client to save all urine and avoid contaminating urine with feces or toilet tissue during the collection period. Usually a normal diet is recommended during the collection period, although occasionally a purine-free diet may be ordered.

- *Analysis of fluid* aspirated from the acutely inflamed joint or material aspirated from a tophus shows typical needle-shaped urate crystals, providing the definitive diagnosis of gout.

The following diagnostic test may be ordered:

- *Radiologic examination* of affected joints typically shows no changes early in the disease. As the disease progresses, punched-out areas may be seen in the bone underlying the joint synovium.

Pharmacology

As noted at the beginning of this section, the primary goals of treatment are to terminate an acute attack, prevent further attacks, and reduce serum uric acid levels to prevent long-term sequelae of the disease. It is important to treat the acute attack of gouty arthritis before initiating treatment to reduce serum uric acid levels, because an abrupt decrease in serum uric acid may lead to further acute manifestations. Pharmacologic therapy is a mainstay of treatment in achieving these goals.

Acute Attack   Nonsteroidal anti-inflammatory drugs (NSAIDs) are the treatment of choice for an acute attack of gout. Indomethacin (Indocin) is the most frequently used NSAID for gout, although others are equally effective. During an acute attack, indomethacin is usually prescribed at 50 mg every 8 hours until the client's manifestations have resolved. Other NSAIDs which may be prescribed include ibuprofen (Motrin, others), naproxen (Naprosyn, Anaprox), tolmetin sodium (Tolectin), piroxicam (Feldene), and sulindac (Clinoril). While extremely effective, NSAIDs are contraindicated for use in clients with active peptic ulcer disease, impaired renal function, or a history of hypersensitivity reactions to the drugs. These drugs are discussed further in the section dealing with rheumatoid arthritis, later in this chapter.

Colchicine can dramatically affect the course of an acute attack. Joint pain begins to diminish within 12 hours of the initiation of treatment and disappears within 2 days. Colchicine apparently acts by interrupting the cycle of urate crystal deposition and inflammation in an acute attack of gout. It has no anti-inflammatory effect in other forms of arthritis, and its use is limited to gout. The use of colchicine is limited by significant side effects. When administered orally, the majority of clients develop significant abdominal cramping, diarrhea, nausea, or vomiting. Intravenous administration is limited by potential toxic effects including local pain, tissue damage if extravasation occurs during injection, bone marrow suppression, and disseminated intravascular coagulation (DIC). It is contraindicated for clients who have significant gastrointestinal, renal, hepatic, or cardiac disease.

Corticosteroids may also be prescribed for the client with acute gouty arthritis. If possible, the intra-articular route is preferred for monoarticular arthritis to avoid the multiple systemic effects of steroid therapy. When gout is polyarticular, corticosteroids may be administered either orally or intravenously.

Analgesics may also be prescribed during an acute episode of gouty arthritis. Either codeine, 30 to 60 mg, or meperidine (Demerol), 50 to 100 mg, may be administered orally every 4 hours to manage the client's pain. Aspirin is avoided because it may interfere with uric acid excretion.

Intercritical Period   In clients at high risk for future attacks of acute gout, prophylactic therapy with daily colchicine may be initiated. Prophylaxis is particularly useful during the first 1 to 2 years of treatment with antihyperuricemic agents. Although colchicine does not affect the serum uric acid directly, it reduces the frequency of attacks by preventing crystal deposition within the joint. The doses required to achieve this effect are small, and few side effects are associated with therapy.

Treatment to reduce serum uric acid levels is typically initiated for clients with recurring gout, tophi, or renal

Nursing Implications for Pharmacology: The Client with Gout

COLCHICINE

Colchicine may be used to terminate an acute attack of gouty arthritis and to prevent recurrent episodes of the disease. Although its mechanism of action is unclear, colchicine appears to interrupt the cycle of urate crystal deposition and inflammatory response. Colchicine does not alter serum uric acid levels. This drug may be administered either by mouth or intravenously. Colchicine is also available as a fixed-dose combination with a uricosuric agent, probenecid. Only plain colchicine is used to treat an acute attack of gout; combination therapy is employed to prevent further attacks.

Nursing Responsibilities

- Assess the client for possible contraindications to colchicine therapy, including serious gastrointestinal, renal, hepatic, or cardiac disease.
- Note CBC values prior to the initiation of the drug for subsequent comparison during therapy.
- Administer the following as ordered:
  a. Intravenous doses into an intact, properly positioned intravenous line with no leakage into surrounding tissue. Colchicine may be given undiluted or diluted in up to 20 mL sterile normal saline for injection. Administer over a period of 2 to 5 minutes.
  b. Oral doses on an empty stomach to facilitate absorption.
  c. No more than 4 mg for termination of an acute attack; do not administer further colchicine for 7 days after a full 4 mg course of intravenous colchicine has been given.
- If extravasation occurs, application of heat or cold to the affected area may help reduce pain, although no specific treatment is available to prevent tissue damage.

- Evaluate for desired or adverse effects, including abdominal cramping, nausea, vomiting, and diarrhea.
- Report nausea, vomiting, or diarrhea to the physician promptly, because these side effects may necessitate discontinuation of the drug.

Client and Family Teaching

- Drink 3 to 4 quarts of liquid per day.
- Report adverse responses, including gastrointestinal disruptions, fatigue, bleeding, easy bruising, or recurrent infections, to the physician.
- While taking colchicine, avoid the use of alcohol or other central nervous system depressants unless they are prescribed by the physician.

URICOSURIC DRUGS

Probenecid (Benemid)

Sulfinpyrazone (Anturane)

Probenecid is a uricosuric drug that inhibits the tubular reabsorption of urate, promoting the excretion of uric acid and decreasing serum uric acid levels.

Sulfinpyrazone is a uricosuric drug that potentiates the renal excretion of uric acid, reducing serum uric acid levels. It is used to prevent recurrent attacks of acute gouty arthritis and treat chronic gout.

The nursing responsibilities and client and family teaching are different for these two drugs.

Nursing Responsibilities for Probenecid

- Assess the client for prior hypersensitivity responses to this drug.
- Do not initiate probenecid therapy during an acute attack of gouty arthritis.
- Administer after meals or with milk to minimize gastric distress.

---

damage. Asymptomatic hyperuricemic clients require no treatment. Uricosuric agents are used for clients who do not eliminate uric acid adequately; allopurinol is prescribed for clients who produce excessive amounts of uric acid.

Uricosuric drugs block the tubular reabsorption of uric acid, promoting its excretion and reducing serum levels. These drugs reduce the frequency of acute attacks, particularly when administered with colchicine. Probenecid

(Benemid) and sulfinpyrazone (Aprazone, Anturane, Zynol) are the primary uricosuric drugs employed.

Allopurinol is a xanthine oxidase inhibitor that lowers plasma uric acid levels and facilitates the mobilization of tophi. Because of its effectiveness in lowering serum uric acid levels, it may trigger an attack of acute gout. The nursing implications for medications used commonly in the treatment of gout are included in the accompanying box.

Pharmacology: The Client with Gout (continued)

- Monitor intake and output. Increase fluid intake to at least 3 liters per day to prevent the formation of uric acid kidney calculi.

- Administer sodium bicarbonate or potassium citrate as ordered to maintain an alkaline urine.

- Do not administer aspirin to clients receiving probenecid because salicylates interfere with the action of the drug.

- Monitor clients receiving the following drugs concurrently with probenecid for increased or toxic effects: penicillin and related antibiotics, indomethacin, acetaminophen, naproxen, ketoprofen, meclofenamate, lorazepam, and rifampin.

- Assess for the desired effect of decreased serum uric acid levels.

- Evaluate for possible adverse effects including headache, dizziness, hepatic necrosis, nausea and vomiting, renal colic, bone marrow depression, anaphylaxis, fever, hives, and pruritus.

Client and Family Teaching for Probenecid

- Do not take aspirin or products containing aspirin while taking probenecid. Use acetaminophen for relief of mild pain.

- Drink at least 3 quarts of fluids per day to minimize the risk of kidney stone formation.

Nursing Responsibilities for Sulfinpyrazone

- Assess for contraindications to therapy with sulfinpyrazone, including active peptic ulcer disease, a history of hypersensitivity to phenylbutazone or other pyrazoles, or blood dyscrasias.

- Administer with meals or antacid to minimize gastric distress.

- Monitor clients receiving other sulfa drugs for increased or toxic effects.

- Monitor for hypoglycemia in clients receiving insulin or oral hypoglycemics concurrently.

- Monitor for bleeding or increased anticoagulant effect in clients receiving warfarin concurrently.

- Encourage a fluid intake of at least 3 liters per day and administer urinary alkalinizing agents as ordered to prevent formation of renal uric acid calculi.

- Do not administer aspirin or salicylate-containing products concurrently.

- Report signs of peptic ulcer disease to the physician promptly.

Client and Family Teaching for Sulfinpyrazone

- Drink at least 3 quarts of fluid per day while taking sulfinpyrazone.

- Take the drug with meals to minimize gastric distress.

- Do not take aspirin or other preparations containing aspirin; use acetaminophen for relief of mild pain.

- Report epigastric pain, nausea, or black stools to the physician promptly. Discontinue the drug immediately.

ALLOPURINOL (ZYLOPRIM)

Allopurinol acts on purine metabolism, reducing the production of uric acid and decreasing serum and urinary concentrations of uric acid. It is used for clients with manifestations of primary or secondary gout,

---

Diuretics that inhibit renal excretion of uric acid, including thiazide diuretics and furosemide, are avoided in clients with gout. Nicotinic acid and low doses of aspirin also promote hyperuricemia and should be avoided.

Other Therapies

During an acute attack of gouty arthritis, bed rest is prescribed. It is continued for approximately 24 hours after the attack has subsided, because early ambulation may bring about recurrence of acute manifestations (Tierney et al., 1994). The affected joint may be elevated, and hot or cold compresses may be applied for comfort.

A liberal fluid intake (3 or more liters per day) is prescribed to reduce the risk of urinary stone formation. Urinary alkalinizing agents, such as sodium bicarbonate or potassium citrate, may be prescribed as well to minimize the risk of uric acid stones. It is important to monitor clients receiving these preparations carefully for signs of fluid and electrolyte or acid-base imbalances.

Dietary purines contribute only slightly to uric acid levels in the body, and no specific diet may be recommended. The obese client is advised to lose weight, but fasting is contraindicated for clients with gout. Alcohol intake and specific foods that tend to precipitate attacks are avoided.

Pharmacology: The Client with Gout (continued)

including acute attacks, tophi, joint destruction, urinary stones, and nephropathy. It is *not* indicated for use in the treatment of asymptomatic hyperuricemia.

Nursing Responsibilities

- Monitor intake and output on clients receiving allopurinol. Increase fluid intake to approximately 3 liters per day.

- Continue prescribed antigout medications such as colchicine or NSAIDs because attacks may occur more frequently during the initial stages of allopurinol therapy.

- Monitor for desired effect of decreased serum uric acid levels, and for adverse effects such as nausea, diarrhea, and rash.

- Assess BUN and creatinine levels prior to the initiation of and during treatment with allopurinol. Report signs of impaired renal function such as an elevated BUN and creatinine, decreased urine output, and dilute or frothy urine to the physician.

- Administer with meals to minimize gastric distress.

- Administer with caution to clients with pre-existing liver disease. Monitor liver function tests during therapy.

- Monitor the client's CBC periodically because allopurinol therapy may cause bone marrow depression.

- In clients receiving warfarin concurrently, monitor prothrombin times and be alert to evidence of bleeding, because allopurinol prolongs the half-life of warfarin.

- Monitor clients receiving chlorpropamide, cyclophosphamide, hydantoin, theophylline, vidarabine, or ACE inhibitors concurrently for increased drug effects.

- Discontinue the drug and notify the physician immediately if the client develops a rash. Rash and hypersensitivity responses occur more frequently in clients receiving ampicillin, amoxicillin, or thiazide diuretics.

Client and Family Teaching

- Discontinue the drug and report any skin rash, painful urination, blood in the urine, eye irritation, or swelling of the lips or mouth to the physician immediately.

- Take the medication after meals to minimize gastric distress.

- Drink 3 to 4 liters of fluid daily to maintain a urinary output greater than 2 liters per day.

- Report signs of abnormal bleeding, frequent bruising, fatigue, pallor, or sore throat or frequent infections to the physician promptly.

- Acute gouty attacks may occur during the initial stages of allopurinol therapy; continue therapy prescribed for attacks (such as colchicine) as ordered to minimize acute episodes.

- Do not take a double dose of medication if you miss a dose.

- Use caution when driving, operating machinery, or performing other activities that require alertness, because allopurinol may cause drowsiness.

Nursing Care

Pain is a primary focus for nursing interventions in the client experiencing an acute attack of gouty arthritis. The client's mobility is also impaired during an acute attack, both because of discomfort and prescribed activity limitations.

Acute Pain

The pain associated with an attack of acute gouty arthritis is intense and accompanied by exquisite tenderness of the affected joint. Measures to alleviate the pain are vital in the initial period until anti-inflammatory medications be-

come effective and the acute inflammatory response is relieved.

Nursing interventions with rationales follow:

- Have the client rate the pain on a scale of 0 to 10. Note the location and quality of the pain, as well as factors that aggravate or alleviate it. *An accurate assessment of the client's pain is necessary for appropriate and effective intervention.*

- Position the client and affected joint for comfort. Elevate the joint or extremity (usually the great toe) on a pillow, maintaining alignment. *Elevation and normal body alignment facilitate blood return from the affected joint, alleviating some of the edema.*

- Protect the affected joint from pressure, placing a foot cradle on the bed to keep bed covers off the foot. *Affected joints are so tender that even the weight of a sheet can be unbearable for the client.*

- Administer prescribed anti-inflammatory and antigout medications as ordered. In the initial period, colchicine may be given hourly. *These medications reduce the acute inflammatory response, gradually relieving discomfort.*

- Administer analgesics as prescribed. *Supplemental analgesia may be necessary in the acute period until the inflammatory response is mediated.*

- Monitor the client for desired and adverse effects of medications. Report adverse effects to the physician. *Anti-inflammatory and antigout medications can have significant side effects that may necessitate a change of therapy.*

- Maintain bed rest. *It is important to immobilize the affected joint and promote rest to prevent exacerbation of joint inflammation.*

Impaired Physical Mobility

Bed rest is ordered during the period of acute joint inflammation and for a period of approximately 24 hours after it has begun to subside. Rest is important to prevent further urate mobilization and joint inflammation as well as to protect the affected joint.

Nursing interventions with rationales follow:

- Assist the client to maintain ADLs while on bed rest. *The client's ability to bathe, toilet, and perform other ADLs may be impaired by prescribed bed rest and pain.*

- Encourage the client to perform active and passive range-of-motion exercises of joints and muscle-tensing exercises on unaffected limbs. *These exercises help maintain joint mobility, muscle tone, and the client's sense of well-being.*

- When ambulation is allowed, help the client use a walker or cane as needed. *Weight-bearing on the affected limb may be restricted until the inflammation is totally relieved.*

- Encourage the client to resume normal activities as allowed by the physician. *Initial acute attacks of gouty arthritis do not cause permanent damage to the affected joint, and the client can resume usual activities once the attack has subsided.*

Other Nursing Diagnoses

The following nursing diagnoses may also be appropriate for the client with gout:

- *Activity Intolerance* related to pain and acute inflammation

- *Body Image Disturbance* related to presence of tophi

- *Altered Nutrition: More Than Body Requirements* related to lack of knowledge about dietary needs

- *Noncompliance* with cessation of alcohol use related to lack of understanding about the effects of alcohol on gout

Client and Family Teaching

Clients with gout are rarely managed in the acute care setting except for treatment of an acute episode. Once the acute inflammatory response has been relieved, the client often has no further manifestations of the disease. Without appropriate treatment, however, recurrences are likely. For these reasons, teaching is a vital component of nursing care for the client with gout.

Teach the client about the disease and its manifestations. Tell the client that initial attacks cause no permanent damage but that recurrent attacks can lead to permanent damage and joint destruction. Discuss other potential effects of continued hyperuricemia, including tophaceous deposits in subcutaneous and other connective tissues. Teach the client about the potential for kidney damage and kidney stones.

Instruct the client about the rationale for and use of prescribed medication. Stress the need to continue the medication until the physician discontinues it, even though the client is free of manifestations of gout. Teach the client about potential side effects of the medications and their management. Instruct the client to drink approximately 3 quarts of fluid per day and to avoid the use of alcohol. Tell the client to avoid over-the-counter medications without first consulting the physician. Encourage the client to keep scheduled follow-up appointments.

The Client with Pseudogout

■ ■ ■

Pseudogout, or calcium psyrophosphate dihydrate (CPPD) crystal deposition disease, is a joint disease characterized by intermittent attacks of acute arthritis mimicking the acute attacks of gout. In pseudogout, calcium-containing salt crystals are present in articular cartilage and synovial fluid. Its etiology is unknown, but calcium crystal deposits may be related to degenerative or metabolic changes in joint cartilage (Berkow & Fletcher, 1992). This condition is commonly associated with a number of metabolic disorders including hyperparathyroidism, diabetes mellitus hypothyroidism, and true gout. Pseudogout usually affects people over the age of 60 years. It typically affects larger peripheral joints, primarily the knees and wrists. Attacks may be intermittent with no intervening manifestations, or the client may have continued low-grade inflammation.

Aspiration of the affected joint shows the presence of CPPD crystals in synovial fluid. The serum uric acid is generally within normal limits. Colchicine and NSAIDs are also used in the management of pseudogout. No effective treatment is currently available to prevent crystal deposition, and joint destruction can result.

Nursing care and teaching needs for the client with pseudogout are closely related to those for the client with gout.

Diffuse Connective-Tissue Disorders

Connective tissue is the most abundant and widely distributed body tissue. It not only connects body parts but also provides support; forms bones, cartilage, and the walls of blood vessels; and attaches muscles to bones. Connective tissue is composed of three elements, *long fibers* embedded in a noncellular *ground substance,* and *cells* specific to the class of connective tissue. Fibers made up primarily of collagen, a protein, are the most abundant in connective tissue.

Connective-tissue disorders, also known as *collagen diseases,* are a group of immune-mediated disorders. Although they appear to have a genetic component, their cause is unknown. Because connective tissue and collagen are widely distributed in many varied tissues, these are systemic diseases with diverse manifestations. Rheumatoid arthritis and systemic lupus erythematosus are the most prevalent of the connective-tissue disorders; others include scleroderma, polymyositis, vasculitis, Sjögren's syndrome, and mixed connective tissue disorders.

The Client with Rheumatoid Arthritis

Rheumatoid arthritis is a chronic, systemic inflammatory disorder characterized by persistent synovitis of multiple joints. Rheumatoid arthritis (RA) is found worldwide, affecting approximately 1% of the total population and all races. It affects three times as many women as men. The onset of RA occurs most frequently between the ages of 30 and 50 years. Its course and severity are variable, and the range of manifestations is broad. Manifestations of RA may be minimal, with mild inflammation of only a few joints and little structural damage, or relentlessly progressive, with multiple inflamed joints and marked deformity. Most clients exhibit a pattern of symmetric involvement of multiple peripheral joints and periods of remission and exacerbation.

The cause of rheumatoid arthritis is unknown. A genetic link has been demonstrated; however, environmental factors are also thought to play a role in its development. It is speculated that Epstein-Barr virus (EBV) may play a role in initiating the autoimmune processes present in RA.

Pathophysiology

Although the etiology of rheumatoid arthritis is unknown, it is characterized by persistent immunologic activity. T lymphocytes or T cells infiltrate the synovial membrane, proliferating in the synovium and initiating an immune response. (See Chapter 8 for further discussion of T cells and immune processes.) Many of the inflammatory features of RA appear to result from the release of cytokines, which further stimulate macrophage activity. Through the complex interaction of immune system components, B cells are stimulated to produce autoantibodies to IgG, a class of immunoglobulin. The antibodies produced, known as *rheumatoid factors,* are the hallmark of the disease, demonstrable in nearly all clients with RA. Antigen-antibody interaction leads to the formation of immune complexes with activation of complement and attraction of polymorphonuclear leukocytes (PMNs), monocytes, and lymphocytes to the area. These cells phagocytose immune complexes. In the process, lysosomal enzymes that can destroy joint tissue are released.

The immune response characteristic of rheumatoid arthritis leads to an increase in the number and size (hyperplasia and hypertrophy) of cells lining the synovium, microvascular injury with thrombosis and neovascularization, and infiltration of the synovium by phagocytic cells. Vasodilation due to the inflammatory response causes tissues to become warm and red. Increased capillary permeability leads to swelling of the affected area.

Rheumatoid arthritis destroys joints by means of an extensive network of new blood vessels (vascular granulation tissue known as *pannus*) in the synovial membrane. The pannus erodes the cartilage and bone of affected joints and invades surrounding tissues, including ligaments and tendons (Figure 38–4).

Joint Manifestations

The onset of rheumatoid arthritis is typically insidious, although it may be abrupt. Joint manifestations are often

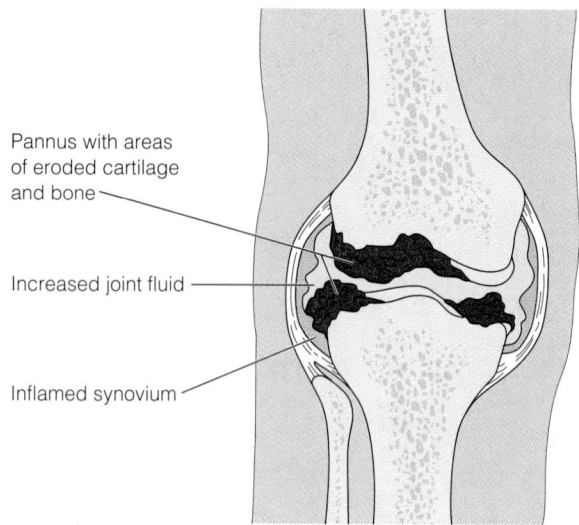

Figure 38–4   Joint inflammation and destruction in rheumatoid arthritis. Note synovial inflammation with pannus formation and the erosion of cartilage and underlying bone.

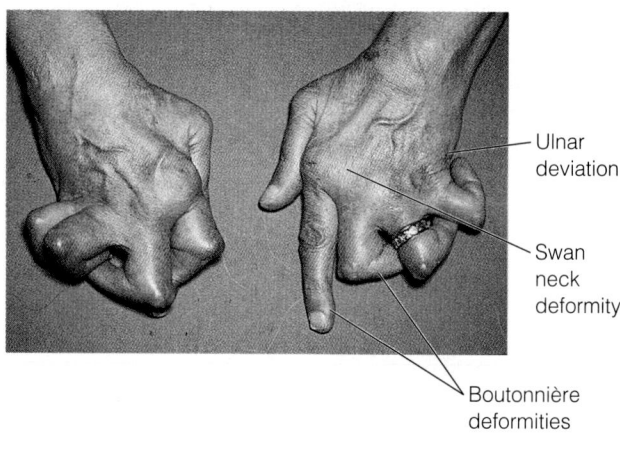

Figure 38–5   Typical hand deformities associated with rheumatoid arthritis.

preceded by systemic manifestations of inflammation, including fatigue, anorexia, weight loss, and nonspecific aching and stiffness. Clients report joint swelling with associated stiffness, warmth, tenderness, and pain. The pattern of joint involvement is typically *polyarticular* (involving multiple joints) and symmetric. The proximal interphalangeal (PIP) and metacarpophalangeal (MCP) joints of the fingers, the wrists, the knees, the ankles, and the toes are most frequently involved, although RA can affect any joint. Stiffness is most pronounced in the morning, lasting more than 1 hour. It may also occur with prolonged rest during the day and may be more severe following strenuous activity. Swollen, inflamed joints feel "boggy" or spongelike on palpation because of synovial edema. Range of motion is limited in affected joints, and weakness may be evident.

The persistent inflammation of RA causes deformities of the joint itself and supporting structures such as ligaments, tendons, and muscles. As the joint is destroyed, ligaments, tendons, and the joint capsule are weakened or destroyed. Joint cartilage and bone are also destroyed. Weakening or destruction of these supporting structures results in lack of opposition to muscle pull, causing deformity (Wilson et al., 1991).

Characteristic changes in the hands and fingers include ulnar deviation of the fingers and subluxation at the MCP joints. *Swan-neck deformity* is characterized by hyperextension of the PIP joint with compensatory flexion of the distal interphalangeal (DIP) joints. A flexion deformity of the PIP joints with extension of the DIP joint is called a *boutonnière deformity* (Figure 38–5). The ability to effect a pinch is limited by hyperextension of the inter-

phalangeal joint and flexion of the MCP joint of the thumb.

Wrist involvement is nearly universal, leading to limited movement, deformity, and carpal tunnel syndrome. Inflammation of the elbows often causes flexion contracture.

The knees are frequently affected in rheumatoid arthritis, with visible swelling often obliterating normal contours. Instability of the knee joint along with quadriceps atrophy, contractures, and valgus (knock-knee) deformities can lead to significant disability. Ambulation may be limited by pain and deformities when the ankles and feet are involved. Typical deformities of the feet and toes include subluxation, *hallux valgus* (deviation of the great toe toward the other digits of the foot), lateral deviation of the toes, and cock-up toes (turned-up toes).

Spinal involvement is usually limited to the cervical vertebrae. Neck pain is common, and neurologic complications can occur.

Extra-Articular Manifestations

As noted previously, rheumatoid arthritis is a systemic disease with a variety of extra-articular manifestations. These are seen particularly in clients with high levels of circulating rheumatoid factor (autoantibodies). Fatigue, weakness, anorexia, weight loss, and low-grade fever are common when the disease is active. Anemia resistant to iron therapy frequently affects clients with RA. Skeletal muscle atrophy is common, usually most apparent in the musculature around affected joints.

Rheumatoid nodules may develop, usually in subcutaneous tissue in areas subject to pressure, e.g., on the fore-

---

**Diagnostic Criteria for
Rheumatoid Arthritis**

▪ ▪ ▪

- Morning stiffness lasting for at least 1 hour and persisting over at least 6 weeks
- Arthritis with swelling or effusion of three or more joints persisting for at least 6 weeks
- Arthritis of wrist, MCP, or PIP joints persisting for at least 6 weeks
- Symmetric arthritis with simultaneous involvement of corresponding joints on both sides of the body
- Rheumatoid nodules
- Positive serum rheumatoid factor
- Characteristic radiologic changes of rheumatoid arthritis noted in hands and wrists

---

arm, olecranon bursa, over the MCP joints, and on the toes. Rheumatoid nodules are granulomatous lesions that are firm and either moveable or fixed. They may also be found in viscera, including the heart, lungs, intestinal tract, and dura.

Other possible extra-articular manifestations of rheumatoid arthritis include vasculitis, pleural disease, pericarditis, episcleritis or scleritis of the eye, Sjögren's syndrome (covered later in this chapter), and *Felty's syndrome*. Felty's syndrome is splenomegaly, neutropenia, and occasional anemia and thrombocytopenia (from increased splenic activity) associated with RA (Wilson et al., 1991). The multisystem effects of RA are illustrated in Figure 38–6 on page 1628.

The course of rheumatoid arthritis is variable and fluctuating. Remissions are most likely to occur in the first year of the disease. The rate at which joint deformities develop is not constant. Disease progression is fastest during the first 6 years, slowing thereafter. RA contributes to a shortened life expectancy, with death often attributed to infection and gastrointestinal bleeding (typically resulting from the long-term use of anti-inflammatory drugs and thrombocytopenia).

Collaborative Care

The diagnosis of rheumatoid arthritis is based on the client's history, physical assessment, and laboratory studies. Diagnostic criteria developed by the American Rheumatism Association are used as well (see the accompanying box). At least four of seven criteria must be present to establish the diagnosis.

Once the diagnosis of rheumatoid arthritis has been established, the goals of therapy are to

- Relieve pain
- Reduce inflammation
- Preserve joint function
- Resolve pathologic processes
- Facilitate healing (Wilson et al., 1991)

No cure currently exists for rheumatoid arthritis; the goal of treatment is to relieve its manifestations. A multidisciplinary approach is used, with a balance of rest, exercise, physical therapy, and suppression of the inflammatory processes.

Because a cure is not available and traditional therapies are not always fully effective, the client with rheumatoid arthritis is vulnerable to quackery. Many nontraditional treatments, including diets, topical preparations, vaccines, hormones, plant extracts, and copper bracelets, have been put forth. These treatments are often costly, and none has been shown to be effective.

Laboratory and Diagnostic Tests

Laboratory and diagnostic testing is used to help establish the diagnosis of rheumatoid arthritis, although no test specific to the disease is available. Testing is also used to rule out other forms of arthritis and connective tissue disorders.

The following laboratory tests may be ordered for the client with suspected rheumatoid arthritis:

- *Rheumatoid factors (RF),* autoantibodies to IgG, are present in approximately 70% of people with RA. They are not specific, however, and may also be found in healthy individuals and people with chronic liver disease, subacute bacterial endocarditis, and other disorders. High levels of RF are often associated with progressive disease and a poorer prognosis.
- *CBC* often shows anemia in clients with RA.
- *Erythrocyte sedimentation rate (ESR)* is typically elevated, often markedly, in clients with RA. The ESR is often used as an indicator of disease and inflammatory activity in evaluating the effectiveness of treatment.
- *Synovial fluid* is aspirated from inflamed joints and sent for laboratory analysis. Inflammatory changes are seen in the synovial fluid, including increased turbidity (cloudiness), decreased viscosity, increased protein levels, and 3000 to 50,000 WBCs per microliter with PMNs predominating.

The following diagnostic study may be performed:

- *Radiologic (X-ray) examination* of affected joints. Early in the disease, few changes may be evident other than soft-tissue swelling and joint effusions. As the disease progresses, joint changes, including osteoporosis

Figure 38–6 Multisystem effects of rheumatoid arthritis.

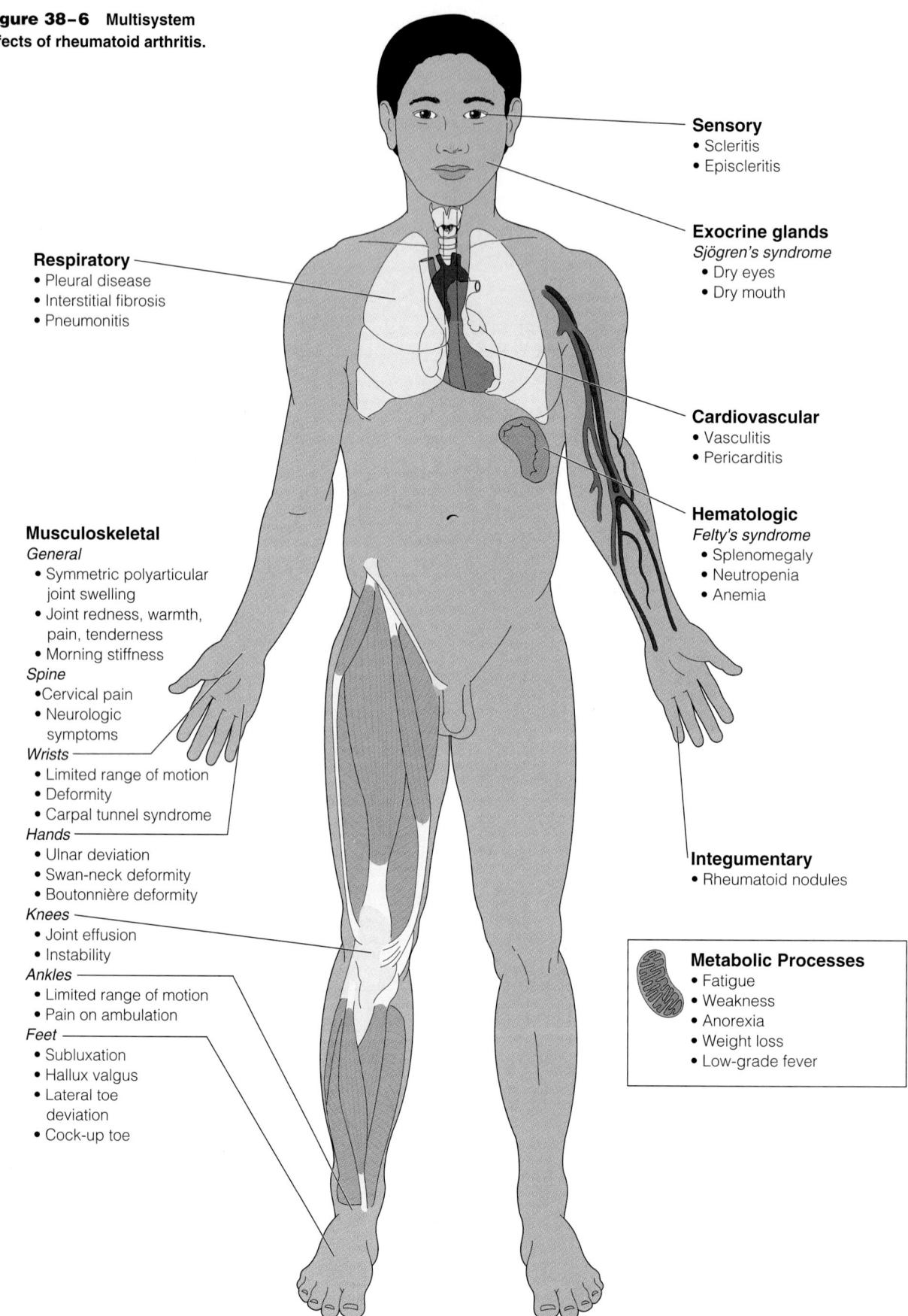

Sensory
- Scleritis
- Episcleritis

Exocrine glands
Sjögren's syndrome
- Dry eyes
- Dry mouth

Cardiovascular
- Vasculitis
- Pericarditis

Hematologic
Felty's syndrome
- Splenomegaly
- Neutropenia
- Anemia

Integumentary
- Rheumatoid nodules

Respiratory
- Pleural disease
- Interstitial fibrosis
- Pneumonitis

Musculoskeletal
General
- Symmetric polyarticular joint swelling
- Joint redness, warmth, pain, tenderness
- Morning stiffness

Spine
- Cervical pain
- Neurologic symptoms

Wrists
- Limited range of motion
- Deformity
- Carpal tunnel syndrome

Hands
- Ulnar deviation
- Swan-neck deformity
- Boutonnière deformity

Knees
- Joint effusion
- Instability

Ankles
- Limited range of motion
- Pain on ambulation

Feet
- Subluxation
- Hallux valgus
- Lateral toe deviation
- Cock-up toe

Metabolic Processes
- Fatigue
- Weakness
- Anorexia
- Weight loss
- Low-grade fever

around the joint, joint space narrowing, and erosions, are seen. These characteristic changes, as well as the symmetric pattern of joint involvement, support the diagnosis of RA.

Rest and Exercise

A balanced program of rest and exercise is an important component in the management of clients with rheumatoid arthritis.

During an acute exacerbation of the disease, the client may be hospitalized, or a short period of complete bed rest may be prescribed. For most clients, regular rest periods during the day are beneficial to reduce manifestations of the disease. Additionally, splinting of inflamed joints reduces unwanted motion and provides local joint rest. A variety of orthotic devices are available to reduce joint strain and help maintain function.

Rest must be balanced with a program of physical therapy and exercise to maintain muscle strength and joint mobility. Range-of-motion exercises are prescribed to maintain joint function and prevent contractures. Isometric exercises are used to improve muscle strength without increasing joint stress. Isotonic exercises also help improve muscle strength and preserve function. Low-impact aerobic exercises, such as swimming and walking, have been shown to benefit clients with RA without adversely affecting joint inflammation or prompting acute episodes (Porth, 1994; Rubenstein & Federman, 1992; Wilson et al., 1991).

Pharmacology

Three general approaches are used in the pharmacologic management of clients with rheumatoid arthritis. Aspirin and other nonsteroidal anti-inflammatory drugs, and mild analgesics are used to reduce the inflammatory process and manage the signs and symptoms of the disease. If necessary, low-dose corticosteroids are added to the regimen. Although these drugs may relieve manifestations of RA, they appear to have little effect on disease progression (Wilson et al., 1991). The second approach is the employment of a diverse group of drugs classified as disease-modifying drugs. These drugs, which include gold compounds, D-penicillamine, antimalarial agents, and sulfasalazine, appear to alter the course of the disease, reducing its destruction of joints. Immunosuppressive and cytotoxic drugs are the third approach to RA management. These agents are similar in effect to disease-modifying agents (Wilson et al., 1991).

Aspirin   Aspirin is usually the first drug prescribed in the treatment of rheumatoid arthritis unless its use is contraindicated for the client. Aspirin is an inexpensive and effective anti-inflammatory and analgesic agent. The dose of aspirin required to achieve a therapeutic blood level of 15 to 30 mg/dL and its full anti-inflammatory effect is ap-

proximately 4 g per day in divided doses (three or four 5 gr [325 mg] tablets qid). This effective dose is just under the toxic dose, which produces tinnitus and hearing loss. The client may be instructed to increase the dose of aspirin gradually until either maximal improvement or toxicity occurs. If tinnitus develops, the client reduces the dose by two to three tablets per day until the tinnitus stops.

Gastrointestinal side effects and interference with platelet function are the greatest hazards of aspirin therapy. Clients are instructed to take aspirin with meals, milk, or antacids to minimize gastrointestinal distress and reduce the risk of GI bleeding. Enteric-coated forms of aspirin and nonacetylated salicylate compounds produce less gastric distress than plain or buffered aspirin and reduce the risk of gastric ulceration, but they are more expensive. Salsalate (Disalcid, Mono-Gesic, Salflex) and choline magnesium trisalicylate (Trilisate, Tricosal) are examples of nonacetylated salicylate products. All salicylate products are contraindicated for clients with a history of aspirin allergy.

Other Nonsteroidal Anti-Inflammatory Drugs   A number of other nonsteroidal anti-inflammatory drugs (NSAIDs) are available for use in the management of rheumatoid arthritis if aspirin is not tolerated or effective. All NSAIDs act by inhibiting prostaglandin synthesis. Although the efficacy of all NSAIDs, including aspirin, is equivalent, client responses are individual. Several trials of different NSAIDs may be necessary to find the most effective drug.

Some NSAIDs are considerably more expensive than aspirin but may cause less gastrointestinal distress and require fewer doses per day. Gastric irritation, ulceration, and bleeding remain the most common toxic effects of NSAIDs. They can also affect the lower intestinal tract, leading to perforation or aggravation of inflammatory bowel disorders. All NSAIDs can also be toxic to the kidneys (Tierney et al., 1994).

NSAIDs commonly prescribed for clients with rheumatoid arthritis are listed in Table 38–3. Nursing implications of their administration are summarized in the box on page 1631.

Corticosteroids   Systemic corticosteroids can dramatically relieve the symptoms of rheumatoid arthritis. Like NSAIDs, they do not, however, alter the course of the disease or halt joint destruction. The long-term use of corticosteroids is associated with multiple side effects, such as poor wound healing, increased risk of infection, osteoporosis, and gastrointestinal bleeding. Severe rebound manifestations can occur when these medications are discontinued. For these reasons, the use of systemic corticosteroids is limited to low dosages, 5.0 to 7.5 mg of prednisone daily, when other measures are contraindi-

Table 38–3   Selected Nonsteroidal Anti-inflammatory Drugs Used to Treat Rheumatoid Arthritis

Drug	Average Dose	Comments and Precautions
Aspirin	600–900 mg 4 to 6 times daily	Least expensive NSAID; associated with risk of GI ulceration, bleeding, and possible hemorrhage; may cause hepatotoxicity
Diclofenac (Voltaren)	50 mg tid or qid; or 75 mg bid	Expensive; risk of hepatotoxicity
Fenoprofen (Nalfon)	300–600 mg tid or qid	Should not be administered to clients with impaired renal function; risk of GU effects such as dysuria, cystitis, hematuria, acute interstitial nephritis, and nephrotic syndrome
Flurbiprofen (Ansaid)	50–100 mg tid or qid, not to exceed 300 mg/day	Expensive
Ibuprofen (Motrin, Advil, others)	300 mg qid; 400–800 mg tid or qid	Available in prescription and over-the-counter forms; less gastric distress reported than with aspirin or indomethacin; discontinue if visual disturbances develop
Indomethacin (Indocin)	25–50 mg bid or tid	A potent NSAID used for moderate to severe RA and acute episodes of chronic disease; higher incidence of adverse GI effects and CNS effects such as headache, dizziness, and depression
Ketoprofen (Orudis)	50–75 mg tid or qid	Expensive; older adults and clients with renal insufficiency require lower doses
Meclofenamate sodium (Meclomen)	100 mg bid to qid	Increased risk of adverse effects in older adults; GI effects include diarrhea and abdominal pain; anemia may develop during therapy
Nabumetone (Relafen)	1000–2000 mg per day	Most common adverse effects include diarrhea, dyspepsia, and abdominal pain
Naproxen (Aleve, Anaprox, Naprosyn)	250–500 mg bid	Available in prescription and over-the-counter preparations
Oxaprozin (Daypro)	1200 mg daily	Expensive; risk of severe hepatotoxicity; rash may occur
Piroxicam (Feldene)	20 mg daily in a single or divided dose	Expensive; GI side effects including stomatitis, anorexia, and gastric distress may occur more frequently than with other NSAIDs
Sulindac (Clinoril)	150–200 mg bid	May be safer for use than other NSAIDs in clients with chronic renal disease; rare fatal hypersensitivity reaction with fever, liver function abnormalities, and severe skin reaction
Tolmetin (Tolectin)	200–600 mg tid	Expensive; may have higher rate of side effects including GI distress, headache, dizziness, elevated blood pressure, edema, and weight gain

cated or ineffective. The nursing implications for corticosteroid therapy are outlined in the pharmacology box on page 1633.

Disease-Modifying Drugs   When 3 to 4 months of treatment with rest, physical therapy, and NSAIDs fail to produce a reduction in morning stiffness, fatigue, and joint swelling in the client with rheumatoid arthritis, additional medications may be employed. These medications fall into one of two groups: disease-modifying drugs (sometimes called slow-acting drugs) and immunosuppressive drugs.

Disease-modifying drugs are a diverse group of med-

ications including gold salts, antimalarial agents, sulfasalazine, and D-penicillamine (Table 38–4 on page 1634). They do, however, share characteristics that make them useful in the treatment of rheumatoid arthritis. Although beneficial effects are not apparent for several weeks or months following the initiation of therapy, they can produce not only clinical improvement but also evidence of decreased disease activity. Because their anti-inflammatory effect is minimal, NSAIDs are continued during therapy.

Gold salts may be administered by mouth, but the intramuscular route is preferred because it is more effective

Nursing Implications for Pharmacology: Nonsteroidal Anti-Inflammatory Drugs

ASPIRIN

Acetylsalicitic Acid, aspirin, Ecotrin, Empirin, others

Aspirin is a nonsteroidal anti-inflammatory drug (NSAID) with analgesic, antipyretic, and antiplatelet effects. Aspirin inhibits prostaglandin synthesis and activity, reducing inflammation. This also provides an analgesic and antipyretic effect by reducing prostaglandin stimulation of peripheral sensory nerves and the hypothalamus. In very low doses (as little as 80 mg per day), aspirin inhibits platelet aggregation and normal blood clotting. Doses of up to 3.6 to 4.8 g per day are required to achieve maximal anti-inflammatory effect.

Nursing Responsibilities

- Before administering aspirin, assess the client for a history of aspirin allergy, bleeding disorders, peptic ulcer disease, gastritis, liver disease, or allergic asthma.
- Assess the client's prescribed regimen for other drugs that may interact with aspirin. Concurrent administration of any other anticoagulant such as warfarin or heparin, or a thrombolytic such as streptokinase greatly increases the risk of bleeding. Concurrent administration of aspirin with other NSAIDs diminishes the antiarthritic effect of both drugs (Shlafer, 1993).
- Administer aspirin crushed or whole with food or milk to prevent gastric irritation.
- Do not crush enteric-coated or sustained-release forms.
- Evaluate for the desired response, e.g., reduction of pain, fever, and inflammation.
- Discontinue the drug and notify the physician if the following occur:
  a. Signs of a hypersensitivity response, including rash, urticaria, or anaphylaxis.
  b. Evidence of gastrointestinal bleeding including coffee-ground emesis, black or overtly bloody stools, or anemia.
- Continue the drug and notify the physician if ototoxicity with tinnitus (ringing in the ears) develops. A reduction in dose may relieve this toxic effect.

Client and Family Teaching

- Take the medication as prescribed. Even though it is available over the counter, aspirin is an effective medication with potentially serious side effects.

- Always take aspirin with food or milk to avoid gastric irritation.
- Do not substitute acetaminophen (Tylenol) for aspirin; acetaminophen does not have the anti-inflammatory effects that aspirin does.
- If gastric irritation and nausea is a problem, try using enteric-coated aspirin.
- Report any dark stools, hematemesis, abnormal bleeding, blurred vision, ringing in the ears, rashes, or difficulty breathing to the physician.
- Check the labels of other over-the-counter drugs carefully; many contain aspirin.
- Do not use alcohol while taking aspirin because the combination of these two greatly increases the risk of gastrointestinal bleeding.
- If you are also taking oral hypoglycemics, monitor your blood glucose levels frequently, because the risk of hypoglycemia is increased.

OTHER NONSTEROIDAL ANTI-INFLAMMATORY DRUGS (NSAIDS)

Diclofenac (Voltaren)

Fenoprofen (Nalfon)

Flurbiprofen (Ansaid)

Ibuprofen (Motrin, others)

Indomethacin (Indocin)

Ketoprofen (Orudis)

Meclofenamate sodium (Meclomen)

Nabumetone (Relafen)

Naproxen (Anaprox, Naprosyn)

Oxaprozin (Daypro)

Piroxicam (Feldene)

Sulindac (Clinoril)

Tolmetin (Tolectin)

Although the drugs in the NSAID class are not salicylates, they have many of the same effects and side effects as aspirin. NSAIDs are widely used to manage arthritis and other causes of inflammation. Although their chemical composition differs, all inhibit prostaglandin synthesis, thus effecting an anti-inflammatory response. All are more costly than aspirin. Their advantage may be in longer duration of action and reduced daily doses to achieve the desired effect. Indomethacin (Indocin) is one of the most effective inhibitors of prostaglandin synthesis and therefore an extremely

➤

Pharmacology: Nonsteroidal Anti-inflammatory Drugs (continued)

effective NSAID. However, the short- and long-term side effects of indomethacin limit its use to short-term therapy for an acute inflammatory response.

Nursing Responsibilities

- Assess the client for possible contraindications to NSAID therapy, including aspirin allergy (cross-sensitivity between these drugs and aspirin is common), asthma of allergic origin, peptic ulcer disease or gastritis, pre-existing renal impairment, anticoagulant therapy, or antihypertensive therapy with beta-blockers or ACE inhibitors.

- Obtain baseline weight and vital signs prior to initiating therapy, because all these drugs potentially can cause sodium and water retention.

- Determine if the client is taking other drugs that may interact with the prescribed NSAID. Although the specific effects of NSAIDs differ, monitor the following clients receiving NSAID therapy closely:
  a. Elderly clients who are most likely to have chronic diseases, organ dysfunction, or multiple prescriptions.
  b. Clients on digoxin or an aminoglycoside antibiotic and with diminished renal function. The kidneys may not clear these drugs effectively, increasing the risk of toxicity.
  c. Clients on lithium or methotrexate, because these drugs may not be cleared effectively.
  d. Clients receiving diuretic therapy. NSAIDs may reduce its effectiveness, increasing the risk of edema and possible heart failure. In clients taking potassium-sparing diuretics, the risk of hyperkalemia is increased (Spencer et al., 1993).

- Administer these medications with food or milk to minimize their gastric effects.

- Evaluate the client for the desired anti-inflammatory effect, including decreased pain, swelling, redness, and increased mobility.

- Assess for possible adverse effects of therapy, including evidence of GI bleeding; impaired renal function; and CNS effects such as drowsiness, dizziness, headache, nervousness, or sedation. Indomethacin may cause severe headache, confusion, or psychosis. It is also associated with possible bone marrow depression and leukopenia, anemia, and thrombocytopenia.

Client and Family Teaching

- Take these medications as prescribed, because you need to maintain a therapeutic blood level for the most beneficial effect. Do not use them as pain-relief agents.

- It may take several weeks of continuing therapy for you to feel the full anti-inflammatory effect.

- Do not take these drugs on an empty stomach; take with food or milk.

- Weigh yourself at least weekly while taking these medications. Report any sudden weight gain of more than 3 to 5 pounds to the physician.

- Do not drive or operate machinery if you notice drowsiness while taking NSAIDs.

- Report these to the physician promptly: changes in vision, hearing, or mood; a change in urination or bloody urine, coffee-ground emesis; or blood in the stool.

- Avoid the use of alcohol while taking NSAIDs because of the increased risk of CNS depression and gastric bleeding.

- Use acetaminophen as needed for pain relief; avoid aspirin.

(Tierney et al., 1994). The mode of action of gold is unknown, but it may produce clinical remission in some clients and decrease new bony erosions. Weekly therapy is continued until significant improvement is noted unless toxic reactions occur. Clients experiencing benefit from gold therapy may be continued on monthly injections for several years. About 30% of clients on gold therapy experience toxic reactions, including dermatitis, stomatitis, bone marrow depression, and proteinuria. Mild skin reactions do not always necessitate discontinuation of therapy.

CBC and urinalysis are monitored throughout treatment with gold to assess for more severe toxic responses.

Hydroxychloroquine (Plaquenil) is an antimalarial agent sometimes employed in the treatment of rheumatoid arthritis. Three to six months of therapy is required to achieve the desired response, and many clients do not experience significant benefit. Although hydroxychloroquine has a relatively low toxicity, it can cause pigmentary retinitis and vision loss. Clients receiving this drug require a thorough vision examination every 6 months.

Nursing Implications for Pharmacology: Corticosteroids

Methylprednisolone (Medrol, Solu-Medrol)

Prednisolone (Delta-Cortef)

Prednisone

Glucocorticoids are hormones normally produced by the cortex of the adrenal glands. These hormones affect the metabolism of carbohydrates, proteins, and fat in the body, and are necessary for the stress response. Cortisol, the main glucocorticoid, has significant anti-inflammatory effects. As pharmacologic agents, the corticosteroids are used to treat many acute inflammatory and allergic conditions. Because of their multiple and significant side effects, their use as anti-inflammatory agents is limited to clients having acute episodes and clients for whom other anti-inflammatory medications are ineffective.

Nursing Responsibilities

- Assess the client for conditions that may be adversely affected by corticosteroid administration: peptic ulcer disease, glaucoma or cataracts, diabetes, or psychiatric disorders.

- Obtain baseline vital signs and weight; monitor both routinely while the client is on corticosteroid therapy. Hypertension and weight gain may result from salt and water retention.

- Monitor intake and output; assess for edema.

- Administer as ordered. If taken daily, corticosteroids should be administered in the morning, when physiologic glucocorticoid levels are highest, to reduce adrenal cortisone suppression.

- Administer oral preparations with food to decrease gastrointestinal side effects. Antacids or histamine-receptor blocking agents such as cimetidine (Tagamet) may be prescribed while the client is on corticosteroid therapy.

- Monitor for desired effects of reduced inflammation and pain with increased mobility.

- Monitor for adverse effects, including the following:
  a. Increased susceptibility to infection and masking of early signs of infection.
  b. Hyperglycemia.
  c. Hypokalemia. Muscle weakness, nausea, vomiting, and cardiac rhythm disturbances are potential signs of hypokalemia.
  d. Edema, hypertension, and signs of cardiac failure due to fluid overload.
  e. Peptic ulcer formation and possible gastrointestinal hemorrhage. Monitor for abdominal pain, black or tarry stools, and signs of bleeding.
  f. Changes in mental status including depression, euphoria, aggression, and behavioral changes.
  g. With long-term use, cushingoid effects such as abnormal fat deposits in the face (moon facies) and trunk (buffalo hump), muscle wasting and thin extremities, thinning of the skin, and osteoporosis.

Client and Family Teaching

- Take the drug as prescribed; do not change the dose or time of day. Do not stop the medication abruptly. The dose will be tapered down gradually when the drug is discontinued.

- Notify the physician if you experience adverse or cushingoid effects.

- Take the medication with food or at mealtimes to decrease the gastrointestinal effects.

- Monitor your body weight. If you gain more than 5 pounds, notify the physician.

- Moderate your salt intake and avoid foods high in sodium, such as processed meats and snacks like potato chips. Increase high-potassium foods, such as fruits, vegetables, and lean meats, in your diet.

- Carry a card, or wear a bracelet or tag at all times, stating that you are taking corticosteroids.

Sulfasalazine, a drug regularly prescribed for chronic inflammatory bowel disease, may also be prescribed for rheumatoid arthritis. See Chapter 23 for further discussion of this drug and its nursing implications. For clients not responding to the above preparations, penicillamine may be prescribed. Although this agent may be effective in the management of RA, toxic reactions are common

and can be severe, including bone marrow suppression, proteinuria, and nephrosis.

Immunosuppressive Therapy Immunosuppressive or cytotoxic drugs are increasingly employed in the management of rheumatoid arthritis. Indeed, many now consider methotrexate the treatment of choice for clients with

Table 38–4 Disease-Modifying Drugs Used to Treat Rheumatoid Arthritis

Class/Medications	Usual Dose	Adverse Effects	Comments/Nursing Responsibilities
Gold salts: Gold sodium thiomalate (Myochrysine) Aurothioglucose (Solganal) Auranofin (Ridaura Capsules)	Parenteral: 1st dose 10 mg; 2nd dose 25 mg, then 50 mg weekly IM Oral: 6 mg daily	■ Pruritus, dermatitis ■ Stomatitis, metallic taste ■ Renal toxicity ■ Blood dyscrasias ■ Gastrointestinal distress	■ Frequent UA and CBC ■ Monitor client after injection for flushing, fainting, dizziness, sweating, possible anaphylactic reaction
Antimalarial: Hydroxychloroquine (Plaquenil)	200–600 mg daily with meals	■ CNS reactions including irritability, nightmares, psychoses ■ Retinopathy ■ Alopecia, pruritus ■ Blood dyscrasias ■ GI disturbances	■ Should not be used during pregnancy ■ Regular ophthalmologic examination required
Sulfasalazine (Azulfidine)	2 g/day in divided doses with meals	■ Anorexia, nausea, vomiting, gastric distress ■ Decreased sperm count ■ Headache ■ Rash ■ Blood dyscrasias ■ Hypersensitivity responses including Stevens-Johnson syndrome ■ CNS, liver, and renal toxicity	■ Administer in evenly divided doses ■ Maintain high fluid intake ■ May cause yellow-orange skin or urine discoloration ■ Regular CBCs necessary
Penicillamine (Cuprimine, Depen Titratable)	125–250 mg/day initially, slowly increased to a total of 1000–1500 mg/day	■ Skin rashes ■ Fever ■ Gastrointestinal distress ■ Oral ulcers, loss of taste ■ Fever ■ Bone marrow depression with thrombocytopenia, leukopenia, anemia ■ Renal toxicity ■ May induce immune complex disorders such as Goodpasture's syndrome and myasthenia gravis	■ Regular CBC and UA necessary ■ Administer on an empty stomach ■ Discontinue during pregnancy ■ May require 2 to 3 months of therapy before benefit is seen

severe RA who do not respond to NSAIDs (Tierney et al., 1994). A weekly dose can produce a beneficial effect in as few as 2 to 4 weeks. Gastric irritation and stomatitis are the most frequent side effects associated with methotrexate. Alcoholism, diabetes, obesity, advanced age, and renal disease increase the risk of toxic effects (hepatotoxicity, bone marrow suppression, interstitial pneumonitis) (Rubenstein & Federman, 1992).

Other immunosuppressive agents such as cyclosporine, azathioprine, and monoclonal antibodies have also been employed in the treatment of clients with severe, progressive, crippling disease who have failed to re-

spond to other measures. See the box on page 1644 for further discussion of immunosuppressive agents and their nursing implications.

Surgery

Surgical intervention may be employed for the client with rheumatoid arthritis at a variety of disease stages. Early in the course of the disease, *synovectomy,* excision of synovial membrane, can provide temporary relief of inflammation, relieve pain, and slow the destructive process, helping to preserve joint function. Arthroscopic surgery may be performed on arthritic knees to remove frayed menisci and loosen fragments of cartilage from the joint. *Arthrodesis*, joint fusion, may be used to stabilize joints such as cervical vertebrae, wrists, and ankles. Arthroplasty, or total joint replacement, may be necessary in cases of gross deformity and joint destruction. Total joint replacement and nursing care needs of clients undergoing this surgery are discussed in this chapter in the preceding section on osteoarthritis.

Other Therapies

Several newer treatments that are not yet in widespread use may be employed in clients with progressive rheumatoid arthritis. These experimental therapies are directed toward ameliorating the underlying immunologic process. Plasmapheresis has been used to remove circulating antibodies, moderating the autoimmune response. Total lymphoid irradiation decreases total lymphocyte levels, although serious adverse effects are associated with this treatment, and its continued efficacy has not been established.

For most clients with rheumatoid arthritis, an ordinary, well-balanced diet is recommended. Some clients may benefit from substitution of usual dietary fat with omega-3 fatty acids found in certain fish oils.

Nursing Care

Clients with chronic, progressive, systemic disorders such as rheumatoid arthritis have multiple nursing care needs involving all functional health patterns. Physical manifestations of the disease often result in acute and chronic pain, fatigue, impaired mobility, and difficulty performing routine tasks. The disease also has many psychosocial effects. The client has an incurable chronic disease that may lead to severe crippling. Pain and fatigue can interfere with the client's ability to perform expected roles, such as home maintenance or job responsibilities. Even though the client's hands may appear swollen, other people may not understand the systemic nature of the disease or realize the difference between rheumatoid arthritis and osteoarthritis.

Many nursing diagnoses may be appropriate for the client with rheumatoid arthritis. This section focuses on those related to its predominant manifestations and their effect on the client's life.

Pain

Pain is a constant feature of rheumatoid arthritis when the disease is active. Pain accompanies both acute inflammation as well as lower levels of chronic inflammation. Some clients say the pain in joints and surrounding tissue is like a deep, constant toothache. Pain can significantly affect the client's ability to provide self-care and maintain daily activities. It also contributes to the client's fatigue.

Nursing interventions with rationales follow:

- Assess the level of pain and duration of morning stiffness. *Pain and morning stiffness are indicators of disease activity. Increased pain may necessitate changes in the therapeutic treatment plan.*

- Encourage the client to relate pain to activity level and adjust activities accordingly. Teach the client the importance of joint and whole-body rest in relieving pain. *Pain is an indicator of excess stress on inflamed joints. Increasing pain indicates a need to decrease activity levels.*

- Teach the use of heat and cold applications to provide pain relief. The client may apply heat by showering or taking tub baths, or using warm compresses or other local applications such as paraffin dips. For clients who find that heat increases pain and swelling during periods of acute inflammation, cold packs may be more effective. *Both heat and cold have analgesic effects and can help relieve associated muscle spasms.*

- Teach the client about the use of prescribed anti-inflammatory medications and the relationship of pain and inflammation. *Anti-inflammatory agents reduce chemical mediators of inflammation and swelling, relieving pain.*

- Encourage the client to use other nonpharmacologic pain-relief measures such as visualization, distraction, meditation, and progressive relaxation techniques. *These techniques can reduce muscle tension and help the client focus away from the pain, decreasing the intensity of the pain experience. See Chapter 4 for further discussion of adjunctive pain-relief measures.*

Fatigue

The pain and chronic inflammatory processes associated with rheumatoid arthritis lead to fatigue. Other factors contribute as well. Discomfort often disrupts the client's sleep patterns. Anemia, muscle atrophy, and poor nutrition also play a role in the development of fatigue. The client with RA may experience depression or hopelessness, with associated manifestations of fatigue (see the research box on page 1636).

Nursing interventions with rationales follow:

- Encourage the client to balance periods of activity with periods of rest. *Both joint and whole-body rest are important to reduce the inflammatory response.*

- Stress the importance of planned rest periods during the day. *Rest is vital during acute exacerbations of the disease but also important to maintain the client in remission.*

- Help the client prioritize activities, performing the most important ones early in the day. *Assigning priorities helps the client avoid performing relatively unimportant activities at the expense of more meaningful and important ones.*

Applying Research to Nursing Practice: The Client with Rheumatoid Arthritis

■ ■ ■

A group of researchers (Belza et al., 1993) have examined the presence of fatigue in clients with rheumatoid arthritis and explored the relationship of fatigue to disease activity, pain, quality of sleep, gender, activity level, duration of disease, and the presence of other medical conditions.

Study results show that adults in this sample with a relatively long duration of rheumatoid arthritis report significant and relatively constant daily fatigue affecting activities of daily living. Respondents reporting high fatigue levels have greater disease activity, as demonstrated by more physician visits. In this study, female gender, greater overall pain, poor sleep quality, the presence of other medical conditions, and more functional limitations correlated positively with increased fatigue. Participants who engaged in less physical activity were more likely to experience fatigue as well.

Implications for Nursing

Fatigue is known to be a systemic manifestation of rheumatoid arthritis. This study appears to bear out the correlation between increased levels of fatigue and increased disease activity as well as with other factors. Nurses who work with clients with rheumatoid arthritis would do well to monitor the client's fatigue levels as one indicator of disease activity. Measures to promote comfort and restful sleep can reduce fatigue as well. Encourage the client to maintain a regular schedule of approved exercise such as walking, swimming, or other activities that place relatively little stress on joints. These can reduce fatigue and improve functional capacity.

Critical Thinking in Client Care

1. How can regular physical exercise reduce fatigue in the client with RA?

2. Develop an exercise/activity plan for a client with RA that takes the disease manifestations into consideration and minimizes stress on affected joints.

3. What measures can the nurse recommend to promote comfort and uninterrupted, restful sleep for the client with RA?

- Encourage the client to engage in regular physical activity in addition to prescribed ROM exercises. *Aerobic exercise promotes a sense of well-being and restful sleep patterns.*

- Refer the client to counseling or support groups. *Counseling and support groups can help the client develop effective coping strategies and deal with depression and hopelessness.*

Altered Role Performance

Fatigue, pain, and the crippling effects of rheumatoid arthritis can interfere with the client's ability to pursue a career and fill other life roles, such as parent, spouse, or homemaker. As the client's role changes, so must the roles of other family members. This can contribute to changes in family processes, increased stress in the family, and further difficulty coping with the effects of the disease.

Nursing interventions with rationales follow:

- Discuss the effects of the disease on the client's career and other life roles. Encourage the client to identify changes brought on by the disease. *Discussion helps the client to accept the changes and begin to identify strategies for coping with them.*

- Encourage the client and family to discuss their feelings about role changes and grieve lost roles or abilities. *Verbalization allows family members to validate and accept feelings about losses and changes, thus helping them to move into new roles.*

- Listen actively to concerns expressed by the client and family members; acknowledge the validity of concerns about the disease, prescribed treatment, and the prognosis. *Demonstrating acceptance of these feelings and concerns promotes trust and validates their reality.*

- Help the client and family identify strengths they can use to cope with role changes. *Identifying strengths helps the client and family to consider role changes that maintain self-esteem and dignity.*

- Encourage the client to make decisions and assume personal responsibility for disease management. *Clients who assume a personal and active role in managing their disease maintain a greater sense of self-control and self-esteem.*

- Encourage the client to maintain life roles as far as the disease allows. *Maintaining roles helps the client continue to feel useful and stay in contact with other people (Sparks & Taylor, 1993).*

Body Image Disturbance

The acute and long-term effects of rheumatoid arthritis can affect the client's body image, leading to feelings of hopelessness and powerlessness, social withdrawal, and difficulty adapting to changes. When inflammation and joint deformity occur despite compliance, the client may have difficulty accepting the need to continue therapeutic measures, particularly those that have side effects or are costly or time-consuming. In addition, unproven alternative treatment strategies and quackery may become increasingly attractive to the client.

Nursing interventions with rationales follow:

- Demonstrate a caring, accepting attitude toward the client. *This attitude helps the client accept the physical changes brought on by the disease.*

- Encourage the client to talk about the effects of the disease, both physical effects and effects on life roles. *Verbalization helps the client identify feelings and gives the nurse opportunity to validate these feelings.*

- Involve the client in decision making and provide choices whenever possible. *Autonomy enhances the client's sense of control.*

- Encourage the client to maintain self-care and usual roles to the extent possible. Discuss the use of clothing and adaptive devices that promote independence. *Independence enhances the client's self-esteem.*

- Provide positive feedback for self-care activities and adaptive strategies. *Positive reinforcement encourages the client to continue adaptive measures and maintain independence.*

- Refer the client to self-help groups, support groups, and the Arthritis Foundation and other agencies that provide assistive devices and literature. *These groups and agencies can help the client develop adaptive strategies to cope with the effects of rheumatoid arthritis, enhancing the client's self-concept, body image, and independence.*

Other Nursing Diagnoses

The following nursing diagnoses may also be appropriate for the client with rheumatoid arthritis:

- *Activity Intolerance* related to systemic inflammatory process

- *Ineffective Individual/Family Coping* related to chronic disease process

- *Altered Family Processes* related to changes in family roles caused by disabling disease

- *Impaired Home Maintenance Management* related to fatigue and chronic pain

- *Altered Nutrition: Less Than Body Requirements* related to anorexia and chronic inflammation

- *Self-Care Deficit* related to joint deformities

- *Altered Sexuality Patterns* related to pain and fatigue

- *Ineffective Management of Therapeutic Regimen: Individual* related to lack of knowledge and understanding

Client and Family Teaching

Rheumatoid arthritis is typically a chronic, progressive disease. As with most diseases of this nature, involvement of the client and family in its management is vital. Education is an important nursing role in caring for clients with RA and their families.

Teach the client and family members about the disease. Stress that although the effects of rheumatoid arthritis are usually most evident in the joints, the disease is systemic, having multiple effects such as stiffness, fatigue, anorexia, and weight loss. Discuss the importance of compliance with all aspects of the treatment plan in managing the disease. Encourage the client and family to become actively involved in planning care with the treatment team. Assist the client to identify strategies for balancing rest and exercise. Discuss the need to reduce exercise and increase rest if pain and stiffness increase. Teach the client about the use of heat and cold to promote comfort and activity.

Instruct the client about prescribed medications. If the physician prescribes aspirin, the client may feel that the physician has not taken the complaints of pain and stiffness seriously. Stress that although aspirin is an over-the-counter medication, its anti-inflammatory effects make it an ideal drug for rheumatoid arthritis. Emphasize the need to take the medication as prescribed, and not on an as-needed basis for pain. Encourage the client to take aspirin and other NSAIDs with food or milk to minimize gastric distress and to report significant GI symptoms or black stools to the physician promptly. Teach the client taking an NSAID to monitor weight routinely, because these medications may cause fluid retention. If a salt-restricted diet has been recommended, instruct the client in foods to avoid and low-salt cooking techniques. Refer the client and family to a dietitian as needed. Emphasize the importance of keeping regular follow-up appointments with the physician to monitor the disease and effectiveness of treatment.

Educate family members about the disease and effects of treatment to help them understand why the client may not be able to engage in all usual activities despite appearing well. Help them identify ways in which they can assist the client to comply with recommended therapy.

Discuss the use of assistive devices to maintain independence. Include ambulatory aids, such as canes and walkers, and self-care aids, such as hand-held showers, long-handled brushes and shoe horns, and eating utensils with over-sized or special handles. Discuss clothing options to help the client remain independent, such as elastic waist pants without zippers, Velcro closures, zippers with large pull-tabs, and slip-on shoes. Provide referrals to local and community agencies as indicated.

It is important to remember the vulnerability of the client with rheumatoid arthritis to quackery and

Table 38–5 Manifestations of Rheumatoid Arthritis and Osteoarthritis

Feature	Rheumatoid Arthritis	Osteoarthritis
Onset	Usually insidious, may be abrupt	Insidious
Course	Generally progressive, characterized by remissions and exacerbations	Slowly progressive
Pain and stiffness	Predominant on arising, lasting >1 hour; also occurs after prolongued inactivity	Pain with activity; stiffness following periods of immobility generally relieved within minutes
Affected joints	• Appear red, hot, swollen; "boggy" and tender to palpation; decreased ROM, weakness • Multiple joints affected in symmetric pattern; PIP, MCP, wrists, knees, ankles, and toes often involved	• Affected joints may appear swollen; cool and bony hard on palpation; decreased ROM • One or several joints affected including hips, knees, lumbar and cervical spine, PIP and DIP, wrist, and 1st MTP joint
Systemic manifestations	Fatigue, weakness, anorexia, weight loss, fever; rheumatoid nodules; anemia	Fatigue

unproven alternative treatment strategies. Maintain open lines of communication to encourage the client to discuss these options and possible experimental therapies with the treatment team.

Care of the Older Client

The incidence of rheumatoid arthritis increases with age up to about 70 years (Hazzard et al., 1994). Although the onset and manifestations of RA are much the same in older and younger clients, differentiating between RA and osteoarthritis in the older adult may be difficult at times. It is important to establish an accurate diagnosis, however, because the management of these disorders differs significantly. Clinical features distinguishing RA from osteoarthritis are listed in Table 38–5.

For older clients, rheumatoid arthritis is managed much as it is for younger people. However, prolonged bed rest or inactivity is not prescribed for acute episodes, because it may result in irreversible immobility in the older adult. Also, pharmacologic therapy is used with greater caution because of the increased risk of toxicity. In many cases, less emphasis is placed on preventing joint deformity and more emphasis on maintaining function for the older client with rheumatoid arthritis.

The nursing care and teaching needs of the older adult with rheumatoid arthritis are essentially the same as those of younger people. Several additional nursing diagnoses may be considered for the older adult, including these:

■ *Risk for Disuse Syndrome* related to pain, stiffness, and joint deformity

■ *Caregiver Role Strain* related to debility of client

■ *Risk for Injury* related to adverse effects of prescribed medications

Adapt teaching strategies to the needs of the older adult, limiting the duration of teaching sessions, providing good lighting, minimizing distractions, and reinforcing teaching with written instructions and repeated sessions.

Applying the Nursing Process

Case Study of a Client with Rheumatoid Arthritis: Janice James

Janice James is a 42-year-old high school science teacher referred to a local rheumatology clinic for evaluation of arthritic symptoms. Three months ago, Mrs. James began noticing vague arthralgias, fatigue, poor appetite, and general malaise, which she initially attributed to a case of the flu. However, her symptoms have continued, and she reports feeling very stiff in the mornings, often taking until 10:00 or 11:00 a.m. to begin to feel "normal." She has begun to call this her "morning sickness." She then began to notice aching in her hands and wrists, which she attributed to the quilting she loves to do in the evenings. She makes an appointment with her family physician when she notices that her knuckles and finger joints are not just achy but also swollen and hot. Noting that Mrs. James has lost 10 pounds since her last visit and has mild anemia and a significantly elevated sedimentation rate (ESR), the physician refers her to the rheumatology clinic for further evaluation. Following examination, laboratory, and radiologic testing, the rheumatologist establishes a diagnosis of rheumatoid arthritis and initiates a multidisciplinary team conference to plan the management of Mrs. James's rheumatoid arthritis.

Assessment

Cathy Greenstein, RN, completes a nursing assessment of Mrs. James. She notes that Mrs. James is well groomed and answers questions readily but appears fatigued and ill. Mrs. James relates the history of her present illness, adding that her job has been extremely stressful because teacher lay-offs have resulted in larger class sizes and fewer teaching assistants. She also has been assigned to teach an advanced ecology science section, a new area for her. Despite her symptoms, she has continued to teach full-time but say she feels unable to keep up with her responsibilities either at school or home due to her fatigue.

Mrs. James states that she is allergic to penicillin. Her past medical history reveals only the usual childhood diseases and three uncomplicated pregnancies, resulting in the births of her children, ages 14, 11, and 9 years.

Ms. Greenstein obtains the following vital signs: BP, 124/78; P, 82 regular; R, 18; T, 100.2 F (37.8 C) PO. She notes no unusual findings in completing respiratory, cardiac, abdominal, and neurologic assessments of Mrs. James. Ms. Greenstein finds swelling of the PIP and MCP joints of both hands. In addition, she notes that the 2nd and 3rd PIP and 2nd MCP joints of her right hand appear red and shiny, and are hot, spongy, and tender to palpation. Ms. Greenstein notes the ring size of the thumb and all PIP joints on both hands for future comparisons. Mrs. James is able to extend her fingers to 180 degrees but cannot make a complete fist with either hand, with flexion limited to less than 90 degrees. Her grip strength is weak bilaterally. Wrist ROM is limited in all directions. Mrs. James's knees also appear swollen, and flexion is slightly limited. Ms. Greenstein elicits a positive *bulge sign* in the right knee by milking the medial aspect of the joint to displace fluid, then tapping laterally and observing the fluid "bulge" medially. Although Ms. Greenstein notes some tenderness of other joints, she finds no other obvious swelling or inflammation during the remainder of Mrs. James's musculoskeletal assessment.

Blood work completed prior to Mrs. James's appointment shows an ESR of 52 mm/hr and a hematocrit of 30%. She is positive for rheumatoid factor. Few changes other than soft tissue swelling are evident on hand and wrist X-rays.

Diagnosis

Ms. Greenstein develops the following nursing diagnoses for Mrs. James based on her nursing history:

- *Pain* related to joint inflammation
- *Altered Home Maintenance Management* related to fatigue
- *Activity Intolerance* related to the effects of inflammation
- *Risk for Noncompliance* with therapeutic regimen related to lack of information and understanding

Expected Outcomes

The expected outcomes are that Mrs. Greenstein will

- Verbalize effective pain-management strategies.
- Contact the Arthritis Foundation regarding assistive devices to minimize joint stress with activities of daily living.
- Verbalize a plan to reduce her responsibilities for home maintenance.
- Express a willingness to plan rest breaks during the day.
- Demonstrate understanding of the prescribed therapeutic regimen and the importance of compliance for both short and long-term benefit.

Planning and Implementation

Ms. Greenstein plans the following nursing interventions and implements them over the first 6 weeks of Mrs. James's care by the treatment team:

- Teach techniques for relieving pain and morning stiffness, including
  a. Scheduling NSAIDs at equal intervals throughout the day
  b. Taking morning NSAID dose with milk and crackers approximately 30 minutes before arising
  c. Performing ROM exercises in shower or bathtub
  d. Applying local heat with paraffin dip or compress; using cold packs as needed
  e. Using supplemental acetaminophen as needed for pain relief
- Teach techniques to minimize joint stress while performing ADLs.
- Provide Arthritis Foundation literature and information.
- Discuss ways to delegate household tasks to other family members.
- Explore ways to incorporate 30-minute rest breaks into Mrs. James's work schedule.
- Provide and reinforce teaching as needed about
  a. The disease process and its manifestations
  b. Prescribed NSAIDs, including information about dose, scheduling, desired effects, possible adverse effects, and management of adverse effects
  c. The importance of balancing rest and exercise

Evaluation

The initial treatment regimen of aspirin, rest, exercise, and physical therapy has succeeded in partially relieving the acute manifestations of rheumatoid arthritis in Mrs. James. Her "morning sickness" now lasts only about 45 minutes. However, complete remission has not been achieved. She has had difficulty scheduling rest periods at work and has had to struggle to delegate household tasks.

"I don't look sick to the kids, and they seem to think housecleaning is a terrible imposition on their time. It's often easier to just do it myself than to fight about it. Besides, that way it gets done right." Mrs. James has faithfully followed the prescribed medication regimen and exercise routines, and she has kept her scheduled appointments and maintained contact with the treatment team.

Critical Thinking in the Nursing Process

1. When a complete remission had not been achieved after 9 months of treatment with NSAIDs, the rheumatologist puts Mrs. James on methotrexate 7.5 mg PO once a week. Develop a plan to teach Mrs. James about this drug, including its mechanism of action, potential adverse effects and their management, as well as potential toxic effects and their manifestations.

2. Explain the normal inflammatory process and relate this to the inflammatory joint changes Mrs. James experienced. Discuss the systemic effects of inflammation on Mrs. James as well.

3. Develop a nursing care plan for Mrs. James using the nursing diagnosis *Altered Family Processes* related to changing roles and responsibilities.

The Client with Systemic Lupus Erythematosus

■ ■ ■

Systemic lupus erythematosus (SLE) is a chronic inflammatory connective-tissue disease of probable autoimmune origin. The manifestations of SLE are widely variable, thought to result from cell and tissue damage caused by deposition of antigen-antibody complexes in connective tissues. SLE affects multiple body systems, and it can range from a mild, episodic disorder to a rapidly fatal disease process.

Approximately 1 person in 2000 is affected by SLE, with females predominating by a ratio of 8:1 to 9:1 over men (Porth, 1994; Price & Wilson, 1992; Tierney et al., 1994). The disease usually affects women of childbearing age, but it can occur at any age. It is more common and more severe in people of African ancestry; it is also more prevalent in Asians and Hispanics than in the rest of the population (Wilson et al., 1991).

Although the exact etiology of SLE is unknown, genetic, environmental, and hormonal factors play a role in its development. Twin studies and a familial pattern of the disease point to a genetic component, as does an increased incidence of other connective-tissue diseases in relatives of people with SLE. Certain human leukocyte antigen (HLA) genes are seen more frequently in people

with SLE. Environmental factors such as viruses, bacterial antigens, chemicals, drugs, or ultraviolet light may play a role in activation of the pathologic mechanisms of the disease. In addition, it is felt that sex hormones may influence the development of SLE. Women with SLE have reduced levels of several active androgens that are known to inhibit antibody responses. Estrogens have been shown to enhance antibody responses and have an adverse effect in clients with SLE.

Pathophysiology

The pathophysiology of SLE involves the production of a large variety of autoantibodies against normal body components such as nucleic acids, erythrocytes, coagulation proteins, lymphocytes, and platelets. Autoantibody production results from hyperreactivity of B cells (humoral response) because of disordered T-cell function (cellular immune response). The most characteristic autoantibodies in SLE are produced in response to nucleic acids, including DNA, histones, ribonucleoproteins, and other components of the cell nucleus (McCance & Huether, 1994; Wilson et al., 1991).

SLE autoantibodies react with their corresponding antigen to form immune complexes, which are then deposited in the connective tissue of blood vessels, lymphatic vessels, and other tissues. Their deposition prompts an inflammatory response leading to local tissue damage (Porth, 1994). The kidneys are a frequent site of complex deposition and damage; other tissues affected include the musculoskeletal system, brain, heart, spleen, lung, GI tract, skin, and peritoneum (McCance & Huether, 1994). The autoantibodies produced and their target tissue determine the clinical manifestations of SLE.

Typical early manifestations of SLE mimic those of rheumatoid arthritis, including systemic manifestations of fever, anorexia, malaise, and weight loss, and musculoskeletal manifestations of multiple arthralgias and symmetric polyarthritis. Joint symptoms affect more than 90% of clients with SLE. Although synovitis may be present, the arthritis associated with SLE is rarely deforming.

Most people affected by SLE have skin manifestations at some point during their disease. In fact, SLE was originally described as a skin disorder and named for the characteristic red *butterfly rash* across the cheeks and bridge of the nose (Figure 38–7). This rash was thought to resemble the bite of a wolf, hence *lupus* (wolf) *erythematosus* (red). Many clients with SLE are photosensitive; a diffuse maculopapular rash on skin exposed to the sun is also common. Other cutaneous manifestations include *discoid lesions* (raised, scaly, circular lesions with an erythematous rim), hives, erythematous fingertip lesions, and splinter hemorrhages. Alopecia is common in clients with SLE, although the hair usually grows back. Painless mucous membrane ulcerations may occur on the lips or in the mouth or nose.

Approximately 50% of people with SLE experience renal manifestations of the disease, including proteinuria, cellular casts, and nephrotic syndrome. Up to 10% develop renal failure as a result of their disease.

Hematologic abnormalities such as anemia, leukopenia, and thrombocytopenia are common with SLE. Cardiovascular disorders such as pericarditis, vasculitis, and Raynaud's phenomenon often occur. Less frequently, myocarditis, endocarditis, and venous or arterial thrombosis may develop. Pleurisy, pleural effusions, and lupus pneumonitis are common pulmonary manifestations of SLE.

Many clients with SLE develop transient nervous system involvement, often within the first year of the disease. Organic brain syndrome manifestations include decline in intellect, memory loss, and disorientation. Other possible neurologic manifestations include psychosis, seizures, depression, and stroke. Ocular manifestations of SLE include conjunctivitis, photophobia, and transient blindness due to retinal vasculitis.

Gastrointestinal symptoms of SLE, such as anorexia, nausea, abdominal pain, and diarrhea, may affect up to 45% of clients with the disease. The liver may be enlarged, and liver function tests may yield abnormal results.

Clients with SLE who become pregnant may experience abrupt onset of hypertension, edema, and proteinuria (a syndrome similar to pregnancy-induced hypertension). Midtrimester fetal death may result (Rubenstein & Federman, 1993).

The multisystem effects of SLE are illustrated in Figure 38–8.

The course of SLE is mild and chronic in most clients, with periods of remission and exacerbation. The number and severity of exacerbations tend to decrease with time. In some clients, however, SLE is a virulent disease with significant organ system involvement. Clients with active disease have an increased risk for infections, often opportunistic and severe. Infections such as pneumonia and septicemia are the leading cause of death in clients with SLE, followed by the effects of renal or central nervous system involvement (Tierney et al., 1994).

Drug-Induced Lupus

A number of drugs can cause a syndrome that mimics lupus in clients with no other risk factors for the disease. Procainamide (Procan SR, Pronestyl, others) and hydralazine (Apresoline, Hydralyn) are the most common drugs implicated, along with isoniazid (INH). Renal and CNS manifestations of SLE rarely occur with drug-induced lupus, but arthritic and other systemic symptoms are common. Manifestations of drug-induced lupus usually resolve when the medication is discontinued.

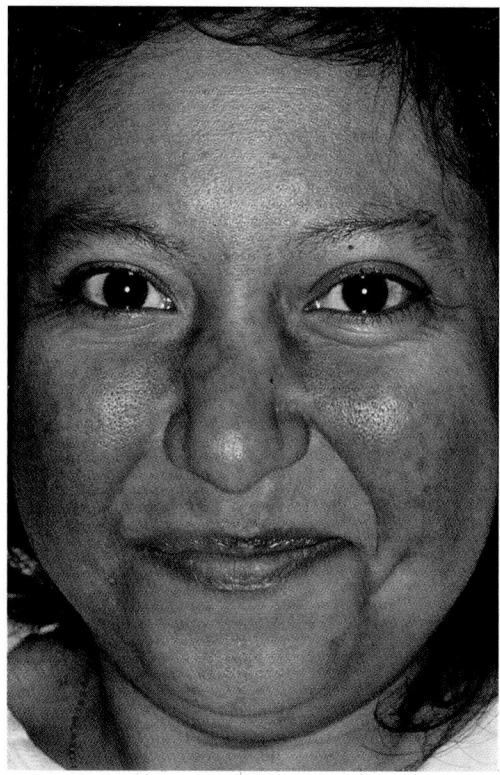

Figure 38–7   The butterfly rash of systemic lupus erythematosus.

Collaborative Care

Because of the diversity of organ system involvement and manifestations of SLE, its identification can be difficult. No one specific test is available that confirms the presence of this disease in all people suspected of having it. Instead, the diagnosis is based on the client's history and physical assessment, as well as laboratory studies.

As with rheumatoid arthritis, effective management of SLE requires teamwork, with active participation by both the client and the physician. Communication, trust, and emotional support are especially important. Although there is no cure for SLE, the 10-year survival rate is greater than 85% among clients with this disease, which was once considered fatal in most cases.

Laboratory and Diagnostic Tests

The multiple autoantibodies produced in SLE cause a number of abnormalities in laboratory studies.

- *Antinuclear antibody (ANA)* tests are the most frequently ordered laboratory study. A negative result, with no antinuclear antibodies found at a 1:20 dilution of serum, is normal. Although virtually all clients with SLE have positive ANA tests, so do many clients with conditions such as rheumatoid arthritis, pulmonary fi-

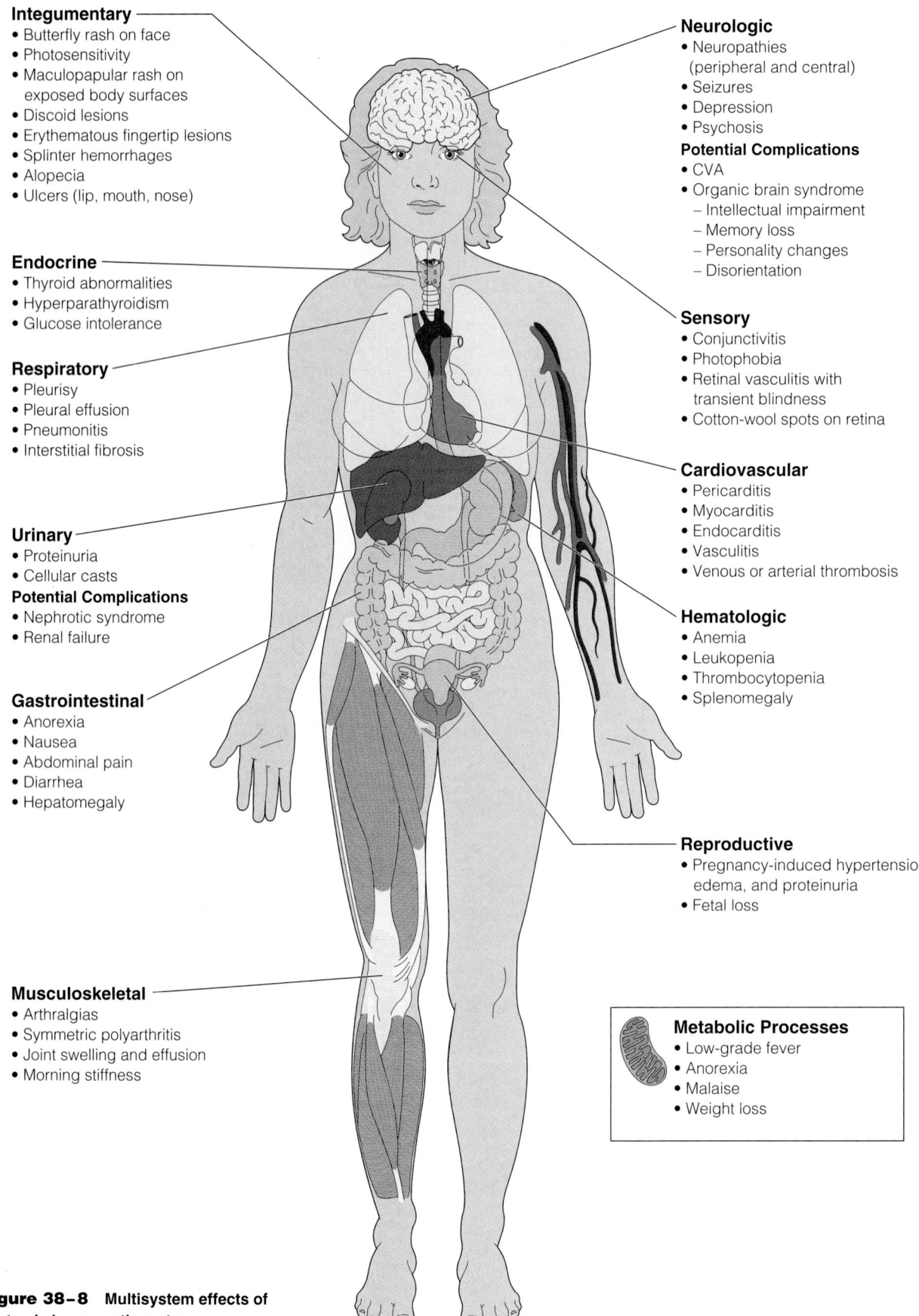

Integumentary
- Butterfly rash on face
- Photosensitivity
- Maculopapular rash on exposed body surfaces
- Discoid lesions
- Erythematous fingertip lesions
- Splinter hemorrhages
- Alopecia
- Ulcers (lip, mouth, nose)

Endocrine
- Thyroid abnormalities
- Hyperparathyroidism
- Glucose intolerance

Respiratory
- Pleurisy
- Pleural effusion
- Pneumonitis
- Interstitial fibrosis

Urinary
- Proteinuria
- Cellular casts

Potential Complications
- Nephrotic syndrome
- Renal failure

Gastrointestinal
- Anorexia
- Nausea
- Abdominal pain
- Diarrhea
- Hepatomegaly

Musculoskeletal
- Arthralgias
- Symmetric polyarthritis
- Joint swelling and effusion
- Morning stiffness

Neurologic
- Neuropathies (peripheral and central)
- Seizures
- Depression
- Psychosis

Potential Complications
- CVA
- Organic brain syndrome
  - Intellectual impairment
  - Memory loss
  - Personality changes
  - Disorientation

Sensory
- Conjunctivitis
- Photophobia
- Retinal vasculitis with transient blindness
- Cotton-wool spots on retina

Cardiovascular
- Pericarditis
- Myocarditis
- Endocarditis
- Vasculitis
- Venous or arterial thrombosis

Hematologic
- Anemia
- Leukopenia
- Thrombocytopenia
- Splenomegaly

Reproductive
- Pregnancy-induced hypertension, edema, and proteinuria
- Fetal loss

Metabolic Processes
- Low-grade fever
- Anorexia
- Malaise
- Weight loss

Figure 38–8   Multisystem effects of systemic lupus erythematosus.

brosis, chronic active hepatitis, and other diseases. *Anti-DNA antibody testing* is a more specific indicator of SLE, bcause these antibodies are rarely found in any other disorder.

- *Eosinophil sedimentation rate (ESR or sed rate)* is typically elevated, occasionally to >100 mm/hr, in the presence of active SLE.

- *Serum complement levels* are usually decreased in SLE as complement is consumed or "used up" by the development of antigen-antibody complexes.

- *CBC* abnormalities include moderate to severe anemia, leukopenia and lymphocytopenia, and possible thrombocytopenia.

- *Urinalysis* shows mild proteinuria, hematuria, and blood cell casts during exacerbations of the disease when the kidneys are involved. Renal function tests including a serum creatinine and blood urea nitrogen (BUN) may also be ordered to evaluate the extent of renal disease.

In addition to laboratory testing, the following diagnostic test may be ordered for the client with SLE:

- A *kidney biopsy* to assess the severity of renal lesions and guide therapy. Many clients with SLE develop mild glomerulonephritis without deterioration of renal function; however, clients with more severe active or chronic lesions may develop renal failure (Wilson et al., 1991).

Pharmacology

The client with mild or remittent lupus erythematosus may need little or no therapy other than supportive care. Arthralgias, arthritis, fever, and fatigue can often be managed with aspirin or other nonsteroidal anti-inflammatory drugs. Aspirin is particularly beneficial for clients with SLE because its antiplatelet effects help prevent thrombosis. It may, however, cause liver toxicity and hepatitis. The pharmacology box on page 1631 outlines nursing responsibilities for clients taking aspirin or NSAIDs.

Skin and arthritic manifestations of SLE may be treated with antimalarial drugs such as hydroxychloroquine (Plaquenil). Hydroxychloroquine has also been shown to be effective in reducing the frequency of acute episodes of SLE in people with mild or inactive disease. Retinal toxicity and possibly irreversible blindness are the primary concerns with this drug. For this reason, the client taking hydroxychloroquine undergoes ophthalmologic exam every 6 months.

Clients with severe and life-threatening manifestations of SLE (such as nephritis, hemolytic anemia, myocarditis, pericarditis, or CNS lupus) require corticosteroid therapy in high doses. Such clients may require 40 to 60 mg of prednisone per day initially. The dosage is tapered down as rapidly as the client's disease allows, although lowering the dosage may precipitate an acute episode. Some clients with SLE require long-term corticosteroid therapy to manage symptoms and prevent major organ damage. These clients are at increased risk for corticosteroid side effects, such as cushingoid effects, weight gain, hypertension, infection, accelerated osteoporosis, and hypokalemia. The nursing implications of corticosteroid therapy are outlined in the pharmacology box on page 1633.

Immunosuppressive agents such as cyclophosphamide or azathioprine may be employed to treat clients with active SLE or lupus nephritis. They may be used alone or in combination with corticosteroids. When these agents are used in combination, lower, less toxic doses of each drug can be used. The client receiving immunosuppressive agents is at increased risk for infection, malignancy, bone marrow depression, and toxic effects specific to the drug prescribed. The nursing implications for these drugs are outlined in the pharmacology box on page 1644.

Other Therapies

Because of the photosensitivity associated with SLE, the client should be cautioned to avoid sun exposure. Clients should use sunscreens with a sun protection factor (SPF) rating of 15 or higher when out of doors. Topical corticosteroids may be used to treat skin lesions. Some physicians recommend avoiding the use of oral contraceptives, because estrogen can trigger an acute episode.

Clients with lupus nephritis who progress to develop end-stage renal disease are treated with dialysis (hemodialysis or peritoneal dialysis) and kidney transplantation. These treatment strategies are discussed in depth in Chapter 26.

Nursing Care

The nursing care needs for the client with mild SLE may be limited to teaching. The client with severe disease, however, has many diverse nursing needs, which vary according to the organ systems involved. Because of the close link between rheumatoid arthritis and SLE, many of the nursing problems and interventions identified for the client with arthritis may be appropriate for the client with lupus. The client with lupus nephritis or end-stage renal disease has the nursing care needs outlined in the sections of Chapter 26 related to glomerulonephritis and chronic renal failure. This section focuses on the unique needs of the client related to the dermatologic manifestations of lupus, the client's increased risk for infection, and health maintenance problems.

Impaired Skin Integrity

Skin lesions are a common manifestation of lupus erythematosus. A rash or discoid lesion interrupts the integrity

---

Nursing Implications for Pharmacology: Immunosuppressive Agents

CYTOTOXIC AGENTS

Azathioprine (Imuran)

Cyclophosphamide (Cytoxan)

Cyclosporine (Sandimmune)

Certain cytotoxic or antineoplastic drugs are effective as immunosuppressive agents. They act by decreasing the proliferation of cells within the immune system and are widely used to prevent rejection following a tissue or organ transplant. They are usually administered concurrently with corticosteroid therapy, allowing lower doses of both preparations, and resulting in fewer side effects.

Nursing Responsibilities

- Monitor the client's blood count, with particular attention to the white blood cell (WBC) and platelet counts. Notify the physician if WBCs fall below 4000 or platelets below 75,000.

- Monitor renal and liver function studies including creatinine, BUN, creatinine clearance, and liver enzyme levels. Report any abnormal levels to the physician.

- Administer the drug as ordered. Oral preparations should be administered with food to minimize gastrointestinal effects. Antacids may be ordered.

- Increase fluids to maintain good hydration and urinary output.

- Monitor intake and output.

- Monitor for signs of abnormal bleeding: bleeding gums, bruising, petechiae, joint pain, hematuria, and black or tarry stools.

- Use meticulous hand washing and other appropriate measures to protect the client from infection. Assess for signs of infection.

- Pulmonary fibrosis is a potential adverse effect of cyclophosphamide. Therefore, monitor the results of pulmonary function studies and be alert to clinical signs of dyspnea or cough.

Client and Family Teaching

- Avoid large crowds and situations where you might be exposed to infections.

- Report signs of infection such as chills, fever, sore throat, fatigue, or malaise to the physician.

- Use contraceptive measures to prevent pregnancy while you are taking these drugs because they cause birth defects.

- Avoid the use of aspirin or ibuprofen while taking these drugs. Report any signs of bleeding to the physician.

- You may stop menstruating while you are taking cyclophosphamide. The menses will resume after the drug is discontinued.

- If you are taking cyclophosphamide, be sure to report difficulty breathing or cough to the physician.

---

of the skin and the first line of protection against infection, increasing the client's already high risk of infection. These lesions, which usually appear on exposed parts of the skin, can also be disfiguring and cause the client emotional distress.

Nursing interventions with rationales follow:

- Assess the client's knowledge of systemic lupus erythematosus and its possible effects on the skin. *Assessment allows the nurse to base teaching and information on the client's existing knowledge, improving learning and retention.*

- Discuss the relationship between sun exposure and disease activity, both dermatologic and systemic. *It is important for the client to understand that sun exposure*

may not only cause dermatologic manifestations but also trigger an acute episode.

- Help the client identify strategies to limit sun exposure:
  a. Avoid being out of doors during hours of greatest sun intensity (10:00 a.m. to 3:00 p.m.).
  b. Use sunscreen with an SPF of 15 or higher when sun exposure cannot be avoided.
  c. Reapply sunscreen after swimming, exercising, or bathing.
  d. Wear loose clothing with long sleeves and wide-brimmed hats when out of doors (Carpenito, 1991).

These strategies can help the client maintain a normal lifestyle while helping to prevent acute episodes.

- Keep skin clean and dry; apply therapeutic creams or ointments to lesions as prescribed. *These measures promote healing and reduce the risk of infection.*

Altered Protection

Altered protection can be a problem for the client with lupus erythematosus. The client with lupus is at increased risk for infection and multiple organ system problems because of the disease; in addition, treatment with corticosteroids or immunosuppressive agents further impairs immune responses and the ability to fight infection.

Nursing interventions with rationales follow:

- Wash hands on entering the client's room and before providing direct care. *Hand washing removes transient organisms from the skin, reducing the risk of transmission to the client.*

- Use strict aseptic technique in caring for intravenous lines and indwelling urinary catheters or performing any wound care. *Aseptic technique offers protection against external and resident host microorganisms.*

- Assess the client frequently for signs and symptoms of infection. Monitor temperature and vital signs every 4 hours. Assess for signs of cellulitis, including tenderness, redness, swelling, and warmth. Report signs of infection to the physician promptly. *The client with lupus is susceptible to infection, and the usual signs and symptoms may not be evident. Therapy can suppress usual responses, such as elevated temperature and inflammation. The fever of infection may be mistaken for the fever commonly associated with lupus. The client receiving immunosuppressive therapy for the disease has an even higher risk for infection.*

- Monitor laboratory values, including CBC and tests of organ function; report changes to the physician. *An elevation in the WBC count with a shift to the left (increased numbers of immature leukocytes in the blood) may be an early indication of infection. Changes in liver function studies, renal function studies, myocardial enzymes, or other laboratory values may indicate organ system involvement.*

- Initiate reverse or protective isolation procedures as indicated by the client's immune status. *These procedures provide further protection from infection for the severely immunocompromised client.*

- Instruct family members and visitors to avoid contact with the client when they are ill. *A "minor" upper respiratory infection can be a significant illness for the client with SLE.*

- Help ensure an adequate nutrient intake, offering supplementary feedings as indicated or maintaining parenteral nutrition if necessary. *Adequate nutrition is important for healing and immune system function.*

- Teach the client the importance of good hand washing after using the bathroom and before eating. *Hand washing reduces the risk of infection with endogenous organisms.*

- Provide good mouth care. *Good oral hygiene reduces the population of microorganisms in the mouth and helps to keep oral mucous membranes intact.*

- Monitor for potential adverse effects of medications including
  a. Thrombocytopenia and possible bleeding
  b. Fluid retention with edema and possible hypertension
  c. Loss of bone density, osteoporosis, and possible pathologic fractures
  d. Renal or hepatic toxicity
  e. Cardiac effects, particularly in the client with fluid retention and hypervolemia

  Medications used to treat SLE have many potential adverse effects that can impair normal protective and homeostatic mechanisms.

Altered Health Maintenance

As with other chronic diseases, much of the responsibility for maintaining optimal health rests with the client. Disease manifestations such as fatigue, arthralgias, arthritis, and increased risk for infection can interfere with the client's ability to maintain health. Psychosocial issues can also be a significant factor in health maintenance for the client with lupus. These issues may include denial of the significance of the disease, poor coping, lack of financial and other resources, and an inadequate support system.

Nursing interventions with rationales follow:

- Assess the client's ability to maintain optimal health, identifying physical and psychosocial factors that may affect health maintenance. *Before intervening to improve the client's health maintenance, the nurse must identify and understand factors affecting it.*

- Provide care and teaching in a nonjudgemental manner. *To intervene effectively, the nurse must accept the client and family as they are.*

- Encourage the client and family members to discuss the impact of the disease on their lives. *Open discussion helps the client and the nurse to identify barriers to health maintenance and to begin exploring alternative strategies.*

- Initiate a multidisciplinary care conference with the client and family (Lederer et al., 1993). *In this care conference, a number of perspectives can be expressed, improving the planning of strategies for health maintenance activities.*

- Refer the client and family to counseling as needed. *Counseling may help the client and family develop the necessary coping skills to accept and deal with the disease.*

- Refer the client and family to community and social service agencies, and local support groups. *These groups and agencies are valuable resources for the client.*

Other Nursing Diagnoses

Because of the systemic and chronic nature of lupus, multiple nursing diagnoses may be appropriate for the client, including these:

- *Altered Tissue Perfusion* related to the vascular effects of the disease
- *Body Image Disturbance* related to skin rash or lesions
- *Ineffective Individual Coping* related to chronic, incurable disease
- *Noncompliance* with medical regimen related to side effects of medications
- *Social Isolation* related to concerns about appearance

Client and Family Teaching

Unlike rheumatoid arthritis, the arthritis associated with systemic lupus erythematosus is rarely crippling, but the chronic nature and multiple systemic effects of the disease make teaching a vital component of care.

Teach the client about the disease and its potential effects. Promote an optimistic outlook, stressing that the majority of clients do not require long-term corticosteroid therapy and that the disease may improve over time.

Discuss the importance of skin care with the client. Teach the client to avoid irritating soaps, shampoos, or chemicals (e.g., hair dyes and permanent wave solution) to prevent excessive drying of the skin. Encourage the client to use hypoallergenic products. Discuss the need to limit sun exposure, particularly between 10:00 a.m. and 3:00 p.m. Encourage the client to use sunscreen with an SPF of at least 15 and to wear long sleeves and wide-brimmed hats. For clients with hair loss, discuss the use of wigs, turbans, or other head coverings. Provide encouragement by reminding the client that the hair will regrow during periods of remission.

Stress the importance of avoiding exposure to infection. Encourage the client to avoid crowds and infectious individuals. Teach the client that getting adequate rest and nutrition and avoiding stress increase resistance to infection.

Stress the need to follow the prescribed treatment plan, including rest and exercise, medications, and follow-up appointments. Discuss manifestations of an acute episode, including fever, chills, rash, increased fatigue and malaise, arthralgias, arthritis, urinary manifestations such as oliguria or dysuria, chest pain, cough, or neurologic symptoms. Stress the importance of contacting the physician promptly if any of these symptoms occur.

Encourage the client to wear a medical alert bracelet or tag identifying their condition and therapy such as corticosteroids or immunosuppressives.

Discuss family planning with the client and spouse. The use of oral contraceptives may be contraindicated for the client; if appropriate, provide information about alternative means of birth control. Pregnancy is not contraindicated for most women with lupus. However, the pregnant client requires close monitoring because acute episodes sometimes accompany pregnancy.

Refer the client and family to national and community agencies for additional support and education.

Care of the Older Client

While the onset of SLE is typically during young adulthood, "late onset" SLE does occur. Because older adult clients often present with nonspecific symptoms such as fever, multiple arthralgias, fatigue, and weight loss, the diagnosis may be delayed. Manifestations of lupus in the older adult may vary from those seen in younger people, with an increased incidence of pulmonary disease seen in older clients. Management of the disease is similar, although immunosuppressive drugs are used less frequently (Hazzard et al., 1994).

Applying the Nursing Process

Case Study of a Client with Systemic Lupus Erythematosus: Susan Do

Susan Do is a 28-year-old administrative assistant for a large metropolitan corporation. Approximately 3 months ago she developed chronic fatigue and vague muscle and joint achiness. She has become increasingly concerned because the joints of her fingers have begun to swell and she has developed a red rash across her cheeks and the bridge of her nose. She is referred to a rheumatologist/immunologist by her primary care nurse practitioner, and a tentative diagnosis of systemic lupus erythematosus is made. Because she has acute manifestations of the disease, her physician admits her to the hospital and places her on bed rest with bathroom privileges.

Assessment

Donna Thorne-Taleporos, RN, admits Ms. Do to the medical care unit and completes her nursing history. Ms. Do states that she has been healthy all her life, having experienced only chickenpox and occasional earaches as childhood diseases. Her family history is unremarkable except for a maternal aunt with rheumatoid arthritis. She also remarks that ending up in the hospital seems "to fit," because over the past year she has lost her mother to cancer, has had a sister enter treatment for alcohol abuse, and has been in the process of trying to end an abusive relationship with her ex-boyfriend. She states she has lost 15 pounds over the past few months but attributed the weight loss to poor eating habits due to stress.

During the physical assessment, Mrs. Thorne-Taleporos notes that Ms. Do has a red maculopapular rash on her face and a few scattered lesions on her lower arms. Several DIP joints on both hands are red, swollen, warm, and slightly tender to touch. Ms. Do complains of pain in her knees and feet, although no swelling is noted. Her vital signs are within normal limits, and no other significant changes are apparent in the remainder of her examination.

Laboratory studies show a strongly positive ANA titer, negative rheumatoid factor, mild anemia (hemoglobin 11 g/dL and hematocrit 33%), and leukopenia (white cell count 3800). Urinalysis and chemistry panels are all within normal limits. Ms. Do is started on buffered aspirin, 15 gr q4h with food, and 1% cortisone cream applied tid to her rash.

Diagnosis

Mrs. Thorne-Taleporos develops the following nursing diagnoses for Ms. Do:

- *Fatigue* related to disease process
- *Impaired Skin Integrity* related to rash of SLE
- *Ineffective Individual Coping* related to multiple life stressors
- *Knowledge Deficit* related to lack of information about SLE and its management

Expected Outcomes

The expected outcomes of the plan of care are that Ms. Do will

- Acknowledge the relationship between fatigue and SLE.
- Identify measures to reduce her fatigue.
- Demonstrate healing and intact skin.
- Develop a plan for dealing with identified stressors, including illness.
- Demonstrate knowledge of her disease and its management.
- Express an understanding of the importance of achieving and maintaining disease remission.

Planning and Implementation

Mrs. Thorne-Taleporos plans and implements the following interventions for Ms. Do:

- Teach about SLE and its varied manifestations. Explain the relationship between stress and acute episodes of the disease.

- Help Ms. Do to identify strengths that she can use to cope with stressors.
- Help identify personal support systems.
- Refer Ms. Do to a local lupus support group.
- Teach her the proper use of topical cortisone cream and sunscreens.
- Educate her about the use of aspirin and its importance in reducing inflammation. Stress the need for regular follow-up with her physician.

Evaluation

After 5 days of hospitalization, Ms. Do is discharged with instructions to stay home from work for 2 more weeks. She expresses interest in learning more about her disease and says that she is eager to talk to others who have lupus to get ideas about how to cope with it. She says she needs to let her sister deal with her alcoholism because she cannot take responsibility for her sister's disease. Ms. Do also says that the hardest part of the next few months will be not to let her ex-boyfriend persuade her to resume their relationship, because she still really cares for him. She states, "He's really a nice guy when he doesn't drink, and I know he loves me a lot. He's always so sorry after he hits me."

Critical Thinking in the Nursing Process

1. Discuss possible assessment findings that would have indicated lupus nephritis. What signs and symptoms of this potential problem should Ms. Do report to her physician if they occur? (Refer to Chapter 26 as needed.) How might her plan of care (medical and nursing) differ if lupus nephritis develops?

2. SLE can affect other organ systems, such as the heart and nervous system. How would the involvement of these systems be identified?

3. Suppose Ms. Do tells Mrs. Thorne-Taleporos that she really wants to have a baby within the next 2 to 3 years, "before my biological alarm clock rings." How should Mrs. Thorne-Taleporos respond? What does Ms. Do need to know about her disease and its treatment before becoming pregnant?

4. Develop a nursing care plan for Ms. Do using the nursing diagnosis *Risk for Violence* related to a history of abusive relationship.

The Client with Systemic Sclerosis (Scleroderma)

■ ■ ■

Systemic sclerosis, also known as **scleroderma,** is a chronic disease characterized by the formation of excess fibrous connective tissue and diffuse fibrosis of the skin

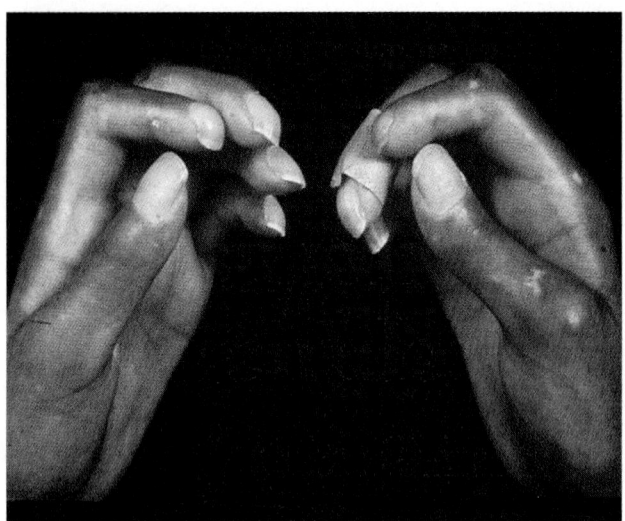

Figure 38–9 Characteristic skin changes of scleroderma.

and internal organs. The cause of scleroderma is unknown, although genetic, immune, and environmental factors are thought to play a role. Although this uncommon disease is distributed worldwide, a higher incidence is noted in coal and gold miners and in people exposed to certain chemicals such as polyvinyl chloride, epoxy resins, and aromatic hydrocarbons. It affects women more often than men by a ratio of approximately 3:1. The onset of scleroderma typically occurs between the ages of 20 and 40 years.

Pathophysiology

Abnormalities in cellular immune function are believed to contribute to the development of scleroderma. Abnormal proliferation of fibrous connective tissue occurs in affected tissues, including the skin, blood vessels, lungs, kidneys, and other organs.

Scleroderma may be either *localized,* affecting the skin only, or *generalized (systemic sclerosis),* with both skin and visceral organ involvement. Eighty percent of people with generalized disease have limited involvement, frequently manifested by *CREST syndrome,* a combination of calcinosis (abnormal calcium salt deposition in the tissues), Raynaud's phenomenon, esophageal dysfunction, sclerodactyly (localized scleroderma of the fingers), and telangiectasia. The remainder of clients with generalized systemic sclerosis have a diffuse form of the disease and a higher risk of visceral organ involvement.

The initial manifestations of systemic sclerosis are usually noted in the skin, which thickens markedly. Diffuse, nonpitting swelling also is noted. As the disease progresses, the skin begins to atrophy, becoming taut, shiny, and hyperpigmented (Figure 38–9). Facial skin tightening leads to loss of skin lines and a pursed-lip appearance.

Skin tightness may limit mobility, particularly of the face and hands. Other skin manifestations include telangiectasias (flat, red areas caused by dilation of small blood vessels, usually noted on the face, hands, and in the mouth) and calcium deposits, usually noted around joints.

Arthralgias and Raynaud's phenomenon also are common early manifestations of systemic sclerosis. Raynaud's phenomenon, intermittent attacks of small artery vasospasm, is characterized by pallor of the fingers followed by cyanosis, and then reactive hyperemia with redness. Attacks are usually triggered by cold temperatures (Rubenstein & Federman, 1994).

The client with visceral organ involvement may have varied symptoms. Dysphagia is common, because the motility of the esophagus is affected. Pulmonary involvement can lead to exertional dyspnea due to impaired gas exchange and right-sided heart failure due to pulmonary hypertension. Involvement of the heart may cause manifestations of pericarditis and dysrhythmias. Diarrhea or constipation, abdominal cramping, and malabsorption can occur when the GI tract is affected. Renal effects can lead to proteinuria, hematuria, hypertension, and renal failure (Price & Wilson, 1992).

The prognosis for localized and limited scleroderma is good; many clients have a normal life span. The course of diffuse systemic sclerosis is highly variable. This disease is usually progressive; complete remission is rare. Clients with diffuse disease have a 5-year survival rate of approximately 50% (Rubenstein & Federman, 1994).

Collaborative Care

The clinical manifestations of systemic sclerosis often allow diagnosis with little or no testing. No cure is currently available; treatment is symptomatic and supportive.

No single test is specific for systemic sclerosis. The ESR is typically elevated because of the chronic inflammatory process. The client may be anemic because of the chronic disease process and its effects on various organs. Approximately half of all clients with systemic sclerosis have high levels of gammaglobulin. Many also have antinuclear antibodies, and some demonstrate rheumatoid factor in low levels. Other autoantibodies may also be found in clients with systemic sclerosis, but these are not specific to the disease. Skin biopsy may be performed to confirm the diagnosis.

Medications to treat systemic sclerosis are chosen based on the client's symptoms. Unlike rheumatoid arthritis and SLE, systemic sclerosis is not responsive to corticosteroids and immunosuppressive agents. Penicillamine may be used to treat scleroderma and pulmonary fibrosis. Calcium channel blockers such as nifedipine (Procardia) or alpha-adrenergic blockers such as prazosin (Minipress) may be prescribed for clients with Raynaud's phenomenon. When manifestations of esophagitis accompany systemic sclerosis, H_2-receptor blockers such as cimetidine (Tagamet) or ranitidine (Zantac), antacids, or omeprazole (Prilosec), which blocks all gastric secretion, may be ordered. Tetracycline or another broad-spectrum antibiotic may be prescribed to suppress intestinal flora and relieve symptoms of malabsorption. Clients with kidney disease are usually treated with angiotensin-converting enzyme (ACE) inhibitors such as captopril (Capoten) to control hypertension and preserve renal function. End-stage kidney disease is managed with dialysis and transplantation.

Physical therapy is an important part of the management of systemic sclerosis to maintain mobility of affected tissues, the hands and face in particular. Because the mouth opening becomes increasingly smaller as the disease progresses, stretching and strengthing of facial muscles can be vital to maintaining oral food intake.

Nursing Care

Nursing care needs of clients with systemic sclerosis may be quite varied, depending on the effects and manifestations of the disease.

Skin manifestations are present to some degree in nearly all clients with scleroderma. Nursing care related to the skin focuses on maintaining skin integrity and flexibility. Measures to maintain supple skin are important, because elasticity cannot be regained once it is lost. Apply moisturizers to prevent dryness and cracking. Protect the skin where it is stretched taut over joints or bony prominences. Perform range-of-motion exercises to help prevent joint contractures due to increasingly tight skin.

Difficulty swallowing and recurrent esophagitis may interfere with the client's nutritional status. Provide small, frequent meals. Consult with the dietitian and the client to determine which foods are easy to swallow. Keep the client in a sitting or Fowler's position after meals to minimize esophageal reflux. Elevate the head of the bed at night as well.

The dermatologic and systemic effects of the disease may have significant psychologic effects on the client, leading to feelings of helplessness and hopelessness, and self-esteem disturbance. Establish an atmosphere of trust with the client. Listen actively and acknowledge concerns about the disease and its effects on the client's life and appearance. Encourage the client to share these concerns with family members and significant others. Provide referral to social services or counseling as appropriate.

The client with predominant pulmonary disease has nursing care needs similar to those of other clients with restrictive respiratory disorders (see Chapter 34). If the client with systemic sclerosis has impaired renal function, nursing care is similar to that for clients with chronic renal failure (see Chapter 26).

Client and Family Teaching

Teach the client with systemic sclerosis about the disease and introduce measures to help manage its effects. Stress the importance of good skin care and physical therapy exercises to maintain mobility, particularly of the hands and face. Discuss the need to avoid chilling (local and whole-body) to prevent episodes of Raynaud's phenomenon. Teach the role of proper dress: loose, warm clothing, gloves, and warm stockings in the winter. Stress the need to stop smoking because of the vasoconstrictive effect of nicotine and the respiratory effects of the disease. Provide the client with information about manifestations of disease progression and organ involvement. Teach the client to report new or worsening symptoms to the physician.

The Client with Polymyositis

Polymyositis is a systemic connective-tissue disorder characterized by inflammation of connective tissue and muscle fibers leading to muscle weakness and atrophy. When muscle fiber inflammation is accompanied by skin lesions, the disease is known as *dermatomyositis*. Polymyositis is an autoimmune disorder of unknown cause that affects more women than men by a ratio of 2:1. The onset of the disease typically occurs between the ages of 40 and 60 years, although a childhood-onset form is also seen.

The immune mechanism causing the inflammatory response in polymyositis is not clear, but autoantibodies can be identified in the majority of people with the disease. The activation of complement is thought to contribute to the inflammatory process. Inflammation leads to muscle fiber necrosis and degeneration.

Initial manifestations of polymyositis include muscle pain, tenderness, and weakness; rash; arthralgias; fatigue; fever; and weight loss. Skeletal muscle weakness is the predominant manifestation. Its onset may be either insidious or abrupt. Muscle weakness tends to progress over weeks to months. Muscles of the shoulder and pelvic girdles are particularly affected, making it difficult for the client to get out of chairs, climb stairs, and reach overhead (Rubenstein & Federman, 1989). Weakness of neck flexor muscles may make it difficult to raise the head from a pillow. Affected muscles may also be tender and painful. A characteristic dusky red rash may be present on the face and upper trunk. Other manifestations include Raynaud's phenomenon, dysphagia, dyspnea, and cough (due to interstitial pneumonitis). The risk of malignancy is increased, particularly in clients with dermatomyositis.

There is no specific test to diagnose polymyositis. Autoantibodies may be identified in blood serum. Serum levels of muscle enzymes are elevated, particularly creatine kinase (CK) and aldolase levels. Biopsy of involved muscle shows patchy muscle fiber necrosis and the presence of inflammatory cells.

A combination of rest and corticosteroid therapy is prescribed for the client with polymyositis. Long-term corticosteroid therapy may be necessary to manage the disease. Immunosuppressive agents such as methotrexate, cyclophosphamide, and azathioprine may be used for clients who do not respond well to treatment with corticosteroids.

The nursing role in caring for the client with polymyositis is supportive. Measures to promote the client's comfort are important. Muscle weakness may interfere with the client's ability to provide self-care and manage health and home. The client may have difficulty with speech because of pharyngeal muscle weakness. Provide alternate means of communication as needed, and use patience in listening. Observe closely while the client eats, because aspiration is a potential problem. Modify the client's diet as needed to maintain nutrition and safety.

Education of the client and family is an important component of care. Emphasize the need to balance periods of rest and activity. Discuss skin care to prevent dryness and infection. Teach the client about prescribed medications and their short- and long-term side effects. Provide information about safety measures while eating. Encourage family members to become trained in performance of the Heimlich maneuver and CPR. Discuss signs of respiratory infection and other possible complications of polymyositis, including renal failure and malignancy.

The Client with Sjögren's Syndrome

■ ■ ■

Sjögren's syndrome is an autoimmune disorder that causes inflammation and dysfunction of the exocrine glands. It is thought to be the second most common autoimmune rheumatic disease, preceded only by rheumatoid arthritis. Sjögren's syndrome affects more women than men by a 9:1 ratio; an estimated 15% to 25% of normal older adults experience some manifestations of the disorder (Hazzard et al., 1994). The majority of people affected by Sjögren's syndrome have another rheumatic disease such as rheumatoid arthritis, systemic lupus erythematosus, or systemic sclerosis, although it can occur as a primary disorder.

In Sjögren's syndrome, exocrine glands in many areas of the body are destroyed by the infiltration of lymphocytes and deposition of immune complexes. The salivary and lacrimal glands are particularly affected, leading to the characteristic manifestations of *xerophthalmia* (dry eyes) and *xerostomia* (dry mouth). Clients often experience dry, gritty-feeling eyes and may develop corneal ulcerations. Mucosal dryness affects taste, smell, chewing, and swallowing and leads to increased dental caries. Parotid gland enlargement is common. Excess dryness can also affect the nose, throat, larynx, bronchi, vagina, and skin. Systemic effects of Sjögren's syndrome include arthritis, dysphagia, pancreatitis, pleuritis, neurologic manifestations including migraine, and vasculitis. Nephritis may occur, but renal failure rarely results. Clients with Sjögren's syndrome have a greatly increased risk of developing malignant lymphoma.

The diagnosis of Sjögren's syndrome is often based on the client's history and clinical presentation. *Schirmer's test,* which measures the quantity of tears secreted in a 5-minute period in response to irritation, ocular staining, and slit-lamp examination of the eye may be performed. A definitive diagnosis can be made by biopsy of either the lacrimal or salivary glands.

Treatment is supportive. Artificial tears are used to decrease eye irritation and dryness. The client can keep the mouth moist by drinking fluids, using a saliva substitute, and chewing sugarless gum. Medications that increase mouth dryness, such as atropine and decongestants, should be avoided.

Nurses caring for clients with Sjögren's syndrome need to promote and teach measures to protect the client's eyes and oral mucosa. Instill artificial tears as needed. Encourage the client to sip fluids throughout the day. Provide frequent oral hygiene, particularly before and after meals. Ensure that the client has sufficient fluids to drink during meals, because fluids help with chewing and swallowing.

The Client with Fibromyalgia

■ ■ ■

Fibromyalgia, also known as *fibrositis*, is a common rheumatic syndrome characterized by musculoskeletal pain, stiffness, and tenderness. It usually affects women between the ages of 20 and 50, and it may be precipitated or aggravated by stress, sleep disorders, trauma, or depression. It closely resembles chronic fatigue syndrome, except that musculoskeletal pain is predominant in fibromyalgia, whereas fatigue is a more significant feature of chronic fatigue syndrome.

The cause of fibromyalgia is unknown, and its pathophysiology is unclear. No objective evidence of inflammation is seen in fibromyalgia, although muscle biopsy has shown subtle histochemical abnormalities (Tierney et al., 1994).

A gradual onset of chronic, achy muscle pain is typical of fibromyalgia, although the onset may be sudden, occasionally following a viral illness. The pain may be localized or involve the entire body. The neck, shoulders, lower back, and hips are often affected; tenderness is present, usually in small, localized trigger points. Local tightness or muscle spasm may also occur. Systemic manifestations of fibromyalgia include fatigue, sleep disruptions, headaches, and an irritable bowel. Pain and fatigue are aggravated by exertion.

The diagnosis of fibromyalgia is based on the history and physical assessment. There are no laboratory or diagnostic tests for the disorder, although tests may be performed to rule out other rheumatic disorders, such as rheumatoid arthritis or systemic lupus erythematosus. Fibromyalgia also may occur as a complication of hypothyroidism, so thyroid function studies are performed.

This disorder may resolve spontaneously or become chronic and recurrent. The client with fibromyalgia needs reassurance of the benign nature of the disorder along with validation of its reality. Other therapeutic measures include local heat applications, massage, stretching exercises, and sleep improvement. Amitriptyline, a tricyclic antidepressant, has been shown to promote better sleep and relieve manifestations of fibromyalgia. NSAIDs have not been effective in its treatment.

Nursing care for clients with fibromyalgia is supportive and educational, provided in community settings such as clinics and other primary care settings. It is important to validate clients' concerns and reassure them that their symptoms are not "all in the head." This syndrome is recognizable and manageable; its course is not progressive. Teach clients about the disorder, and reassure them that it resolves uneventfully in most instances. Provide verbal and written instructions about the use of heat, exercise, stress-reduction techniques, and prescribed medications to relieve its manifestations. Instruct the client to take prescribed medications at bedtime, because they may make the client drowsy. Caution the client about driving while taking the medication. The following nursing diagnoses may be appropriate for the client with fibromyalgia:

- *Pain* related to muscle tension and stress
- *Fatigue* related to fibromyalgia syndrome and sleep disruptions

Arthritis Associated with Spondylitis

The arthritic disorders in this grouping, including ankylosing spondylitis, reactive arthritis, psoriatic arthritis, and arthritis associated with inflammatory bowel disease, have several common features. These arthritic disorders, often called *spondyloarthropathies*, tend to affect the spine (hence the prefix *spondyl,* referring to the vertebrae or spinal column), sacroiliac joints, and large peripheral joints. They are also known as *seronegative* because autoantibodies are not present in the serum. A strong genetic component is evident; many clients affected by these disorders have a common antigen called HLA-B27 (human leukocyte antigen-B27).

The Client with Ankylosing Spondylitis

■ ■ ■

Ankylosing spondylitis is a chronic inflammatory arthritis that primarily affects the axial skeleton, leading to pain and progressive stiffening of the spine. Although its exact prevalence is unknown, ankylosing spondylitis is thought to affect nearly as many people as rheumatoid arthritis does. Unlike rheumatoid arthritis, however, it affects more men than women by a 3:1 ratio. Men also tend to have more significant disease manifestations. It is common in people of European ancestry and certain Native American tribes; it's rare in African Americans and people of Japanese descent.

The cause of ankylosing spondylitis is unknown. As with the other spondylarthropathies, there is a strong genetic component. Approximately 90% of people with ankylosing spondylitis have the HLA-B27 antigen; about 8% of the general population have this antigen (Porth, 1994).

Pathophysiology

In ankylosing spondylitis, early inflammatory changes often are first noted in the sacroiliac joints. As the cartilage erodes, joint margins ossify and are replaced by scar tissue. The joints of the spine are also affected, with inflammation of the cartilaginous joints, and gradual calcification and ossification that leads to *ankylosis,* or joint consolidation and immobility. Other organ systems may be affected as well, including the eyes, lungs, heart, and kidneys.

The onset of ankylosing spondylitis is usually gradual and insidious. Clients may complain of persistent or intermittent bouts of low back pain. The pain is worse at night, followed by morning stiffness that is relieved by activity. Pain may radiate to the buttocks, hips, or down the legs. As the disease progresses, back motion becomes limited, the lumbar curve is lost, and the thoracic curvature is accentuated (Figure 38–10). In severe cases, the entire spine becomes fused, preventing any motion. Clients with ankylosing spondylitis may also experience some peripheral arthritis, primarily affecting the hip, shoulders,

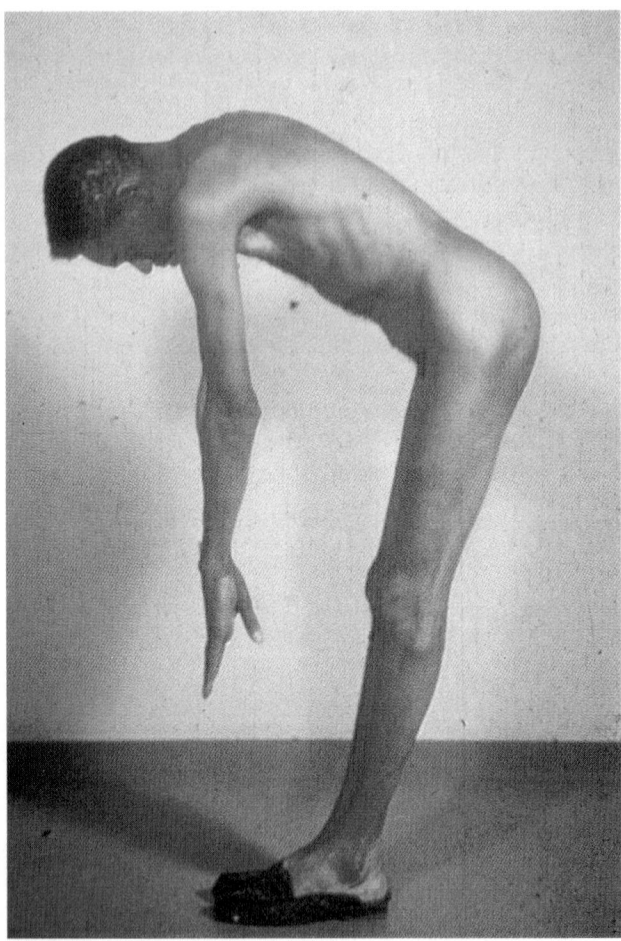

Figure 38–10 A client with ankylosing spondylitis. Note the flattened lumbar curve, exaggerated thoracic curvature, and flexion deformity of the neck.

and knee joints. Systemic manifestations include anorexia, weight loss, fever, and fatigue. Many clients develop *uveitis*, inflammation of the iris and the middle, vascular layer of the eye.

For most clients with ankylosing spondylitis, the disease is intermittent with mild to moderate acute episodes. These clients have a good prognosis with little risk of severe disability.

Collaborative Care

Laboratory testing shows an elevated ESR during periods of active disease and typically a positive HLA-B27 antigen. Neither of these tests is specific, however. The diagnosis of ankylosing spondylitis is usually confirmed with X-ray examination of the sacroiliac joints and spine. The sacroiliac joint becomes blurred and gradually obliterated. As the disease progresses, vertebrae become squared, and disc spaces narrow.

As with other forms of arthritis, the management of ankylosing spondylitis is multidirectional. Physical ther-

apy and daily exercises are important to maintain posture and joint range of motion. Nonsteroidal anti-inflammatory drugs relieve pain and stiffness and allow the client to perform necessary exercises. Indomethacin (Indocin) is the NSAID most commonly used to treat ankylosing spondylitis. It may, however, have many adverse effects, including headache, nausea and vomiting, depression, and psychosis. See the pharmacology box on page 1631 for nursing implications of NSAIDs. Other drugs that may be employed include sulfasalazine (Azulfidine) and topical or intra-articular corticosteroids. Severe hip joint arthritis may necessitate total hip arthroplasty.

Nursing Care

As with other chronic arthritic disorders, the primary nursing role in ankylosing spondylitis is one of providing supportive care and education. To promote mobility, administer NSAIDs at regular intervals throughout the day with food, milk, or antacid. Encourage the client to maintain a fluid intake of 2500 mL or more per day. Allow the client to perform exercises in the shower because warm, moist heat prompts mobility.

The client with uveitis may experience photophobia and blurred vision in the affected eye. Provide indirect lighting and a darkened room for the client with photophobia. If vision is significantly impaired, employ measures appropriate for the client with reduced vision, as follows:

- Orient the client to the surroundings; do not move furniture or place objects in usual pathways.
- Introduce yourself verbally when you enter the client's room. Tell the client what you are doing during procedures.
- Assist the client while ambulating by allowing the client to hold your elbow.

See Chapter 44 for further discussion of care for the client with uveitis.

Client and Family Teaching

The client with ankylosing spondylitis needs education about the disease and the importance of appropriate management. With attention to therapeutic strategies, most clients remain mobile, suffering little or no long-term disability.

Teach the client about the prescribed medication and its use. Discuss possible adverse effects and their management. Instruct the client to maintain close contact with the physician for continuing care. Discuss manifestations of adverse drug effects and acute episodes, both of which should be reported to the physician. Stress the importance of following the prescribed physical therapy and exercise program to maintain mobility.

The Client with Reactive Arthritis

■ ■ ■

An acute, nonpurulent inflammatory arthritis that complicates a nonarticular infection is known as **reactive arthritis.** The best known form of reactive arthritis is *Reiter's syndrome,* a group of clinical manifestations that includes arthritis, urethritis, conjunctivitis, and mucocutaneous lesions.

Although the cause is unknown, Reiter's syndrome nearly always occurs in people who have the HLA-B27 antigen and is precipitated by a sexually transmitted or dysenteric infection. *Chlamydia, Shigella, Campylobacter, Salmonella,* and *Yersinia* bacterial infections and HIV infection are associated with its development. Reactive arthritis is typically self-limited, although it can be recurrent or progressive.

Nonbacterial urethritis is often the initial manifestation of Reiter's syndrome. In women, urethritis and cervicitis may be asymptomatic. Conjunctivitis and inflammatory arthritis follow. The arthritis is usually asymmetric, affecting large weight-bearing joints like the knees and ankles, the sacroiliac joints, or the spine. Mouth ulcers, inflammation of the glans penis, and skin lesions may occur. The heart and aorta may also be affected.

The diagnosis of reactive arthritis is generally based on the client's history and presenting symptoms. No test is specific for the disorder. Urethral or cervical cultures are obtained to rule out gonococcal infection. When *Chlamydia* is suspected, the client and sexual partner are treated with tetracycline or erythromycin. Reactive arthritis is treated symptomatically, usually with NSAIDs.

Clients with reactive arthritis usually are seen in primary care settings such as a clinic or physician's office, making the nursing role primarily one of education. Teach the client about the association of the arthritis with the precipitating infection (if identified). Stress the importance of treating the infection effectively if it is still present. Use this opportunity to provide information about sexually transmitted diseases and protective measures to prevent their transmission. Discuss the usual self-limited nature of reactive arthritis, the appropriate use of prescribed NSAID preparations, and symptomatic relief measures such as application of heat and rest.

The Client with Psoriatic Arthritis

■ ■ ■

Up to 20% of people with psoriasis, usually those with severe skin disease (see Chapter 17), develop arthritis similar to rheumatoid arthritis. Skin manifestations of psoriasis typically precede the development of arthritis. Although psoriatic arthritis usually affects only a few joints, it can be destructive. The distal interphalangeal (DIP) joints of the fingers and toes are particularly affected; however, large and small joints, including the spine and sacroiliac joints, also can be affected.

Management of psoriatic arthritis is directed toward both the skin manifestations of psoriasis and the arthritic symptoms. NSAIDs are employed, as may be gold therapy (see the preceding section on rheumatoid arthritis), sulfasalazine, or methotrexate. Antimalarial agents are not used because they tend to exacerbate skin lesions.

Nursing care is supportive and educative, stressing the importance of complying with prescribed therapy. It is important for the client to understand that the skin and joint manifestations are part of the same disease because the severity of the arthritis tends to mirror the severity of skin lesions.

The Client with Enteropathic Arthritis

■ ■ ■

Approximately 20% of people with inflammatory bowel disease (ulcerative colitis or Crohn's disease) develop arthritis as well. The arthritis associated with inflammatory bowel disease may take one of two forms: acute migratory polyarthritis, usually affecting the larger weight-bearing joints, or sacroiliitis and ankylosing spondylitis. The course of migratory arthritis tends to mirror that of the bowel disease, with increased symptoms during periods of active bowel disease. Management of this form involves the use of NSAIDS and control of the bowel disease (see Chapter 23). Sacroiliitis and spondylitis, by contrast, tend to follow a course independent from that of the bowel disease, and are managed like primary ankylosing spondylitis.

▪▪▪ Arthritis Associated with Infectious Agents ▪▪▪

A number of infectious agents are associated with the development of arthritis. The joint itself may be infected by the organism, or arthritis may be a manifestation of a systemic disease, such as HIV infection or disseminated gonococcal infection. Many viral infections may have acute arthritic manifestations, including mumps, rubella, and hepatitis B. *Mycobacterium tuberculosis* infection can cause a chronic arthritis (see Chapter 34). This section focuses on septic arthritis with infection of a joint, and Lyme disease, a bacterial infection transmitted by ticks.

The Client with Septic Arthritis

■ ■ ■

Septic arthritis can develop if a joint space is invaded by a pathogen. The primary risk factors for septic arthritis are persistent *bacteremia* (bacteria in the blood, e.g., due to use of injectable drugs, endocarditis) and previous joint damage (e.g., due to trauma or rheumatoid arthritis). Bacteria usually spread to the joint by the hematogenous route. Arthroscopic surgery and total joint replacements which allow potential direct contamination of the joint are additional risk factors (Tierney et al, 1994).

Pathophysiology

The most common bacteria implicated in septic arthritis include gonococci, *Staphylococcus aureus,* and streptococci. Infections by gram-negative bacteria such as *Escherichia coli* and *Pseudomonas* are seen with increasing frequency, particularly in people who inject recreational drugs and in immunocompromised people (Tierney et al., 1994).

Infection of the joint leads to inflammation with resulting synovitis and joint effusion. Abscesses may form in synovial tissues or bone underlying joint cartilage. If not treated promptly and effectively, septic arthritis can lead to destruction of the affected joint. A single joint, often the knee, is usually affected. Septic arthritis may also affect other joints such as the shoulder, wrist, hip, fingers, or elbow.

The onset of septic arthritis is typically abrupt, marked by pain and stiffness of the infected joint. The joint appears red and swollen, and is hot and tender to the touch. Effusion (increased fluid within the joint space) is usually present. Systemic manifestations of infection, such as chills and fever, often accompany local manifestations, although these may be muted if the client is taking anti-inflammatory medications.

Collaborative Care

Septic arthritis is a medical emergency requiring prompt treatment to preserve joint function. When it is suspected, the affected joint is aspirated and fluid sent for gram stain and culture. Cultures also are obtained from all likely sources of the infection, including blood, sputum, or wounds. The synovial fluid culture is always positive in nongonococcal septic arthritis but often is negative for bacteria in early gonococcal arthritis. Infected synovial fluid usually is cloudy, with a high white blood cell count and a low glucose level. Joint X-ray films are often normal in the initial stages but soon show demineralization, bony erosions, and joint space narrowing.

The infected joint is treated with rest, immobilization, and elevation along with systemic antibiotic therapy. Therapy with a broad-spectrum parenteral antibiotic is initiated before the results of culture are obtained. The medication may be changed or adjusted once the organism has been identified. Antibiotic therapy is continued for at least 2 weeks after inflammatory signs and symptoms have abated. Frequent joint aspirations may be performed to remove excess fluid and pus, and to evaluate for the continued presence of bacteria. Surgical drainage may be performed if the hip joint is involved (because of the difficulty of aspirating this joint) or when medical therapy does not rapidly eliminate bacteria from the synovial fluid. Physical therapy is implemented during the recovery period to ensure maintenance of optimal joint function.

Nursing Care

Septic arthritis can be frightening to the client who experiences a sudden onset of joint pain and swelling and is faced with the possibility of rapid functional loss of movement. Nursing care is both supportive and educative. Clients may be hospitalized for initial treatment with intravenous antibiotics. It is important to monitor the client's response to therapy, including systemic manifestations such as fever. Position the affected joint appropriately, using pillows to elevate it as needed. Splints or traction may be used to immobilize the joint. Warm compresses may be ordered for comfort. Active range-of-motion exercises preserve joint mobility and should be initiated as soon as the physician allows.

Client and Family Teaching

The client with septic arthritis needs information about the disorder, its etiology, and its treatment. Teach the client how organisms may gain entry into the joint space. Discuss the role that the use of injected drugs and sexually transmitted diseases play in septic arthritis, and means to prevent infection as appropriate (e.g., using clean "works," practicing safer sex). Refer the client to a drug treatment program if necessary. Emphasize the importance of complying with all aspects of the treatment plan to prevent joint destruction and disability.

Teach the client with rheumatoid arthritis how to differentiate between an acute episode of the disease (multiple joint involvement, increasing morning stiffness, increased fatigue and malaise) and the early manifestations of septic arthritis (single joint involvement, usually the knee, chills and fever).

The Client with Lyme Disease

■ ■ ■

Lyme disease is an inflammatory disorder caused by a spirochete, *Borrelia burgdorferi,* which is transmitted primarily by ticks. This disease was first recognized in 1975, and is named for Lyme, Connecticut, where a cluster of cases was recognized. It is now the most commonly reported tick-borne illness in the United States (Berkow & Fletcher, 1992). Although Lyme disease is most often seen in children, adults also can be affected. Geographically, Lyme disease is more prevalent in the Northeast, Upper Midwest, and along the Pacific Coast, although it has been identified in most areas of the country (Tierney et al., 1994). It has also been reported throughout Europe, Asia, and Australia. Ticks that act as vectors for Lyme disease, primarily *Ixodes dammini, Ixodes pacificus,* and *Ixodes scapularis* in the United States, are usually carried by mice or deer, although other animals may be infected. The most frequent time of onset is the summer months.

Pathophysiology

Borrelia burgdorferi enters the skin at the site of the tick bite. After an incubation period of up to 30 days, it migrates outward in the skin, forming a characteristic lesion called *erythema migrans.* It may also spread via lymph or blood to other skin sites, nodes, or organs. Its manifestations often are seen in the skin, musculoskeletal system, and central nervous system. The inflammatory joint changes associated with Lyme disease closely resemble those of rheumatoid arthritis (vascular congestion, tissue infiltration by inflammatory cells, possible pannus formation, and erosion of cartilage and bone).

Erythema migrans is the initial manifestation of Lyme disease. This flat or slightly raised red lesion at the site of the tick bite expands over several days (up to a diameter of 50 cm), with the central area clearing as it expands. Systemic symptoms such as fatigue, malaise, fever, chills, and myalgias often accompany the initial lesion. As the disease spreads, secondary skin lesions develop, as do migratory musculoskeletal symptoms, including arthralgias, myalgias, and tendinitis. Persistent fatigue is common during this stage of the disease. Headache and stiff neck are characteristic neurologic manifestations.

With untreated infection, late manifestations can develop months to years after the initial infection. Chronic recurrent arthritis, primarily affecting large joints (especially the knee), is common. Permanent disability may result. Other effects that may be seen weeks to months after the initial infection include meningitis, encephalitis, and neuropathies, as well as cardiac manifestations including myocarditis and heart block.

Collaborative Care

Both clinical manifestations and laboratory studies are used to establish the diagnosis of Lyme disease. Culture of the organism from tissues and body fluids is difficult and slow. Antibodies to *B. burgdorferi* can be detected by either ELISA (enzyme-linked immunosorbent assay) or Western blot methods within 2 to 4 weeks of the initial skin lesion.

A number of antibiotics may be employed to treat Lyme disease, including doxycycline (Doxy-Caps, Vibramycin, others), tetracycline, amoxicillin (Amoxil, others), cefuroxime axetil (Ceftin), or erythromycin. Therapy may be continued for up to 1 month to ensure eradication of the organism from affected tissues. The nursing implications for various classes of antibiotics are summarized in the pharmacology box on page 257 of Chapter 8.

In addition to antibiotic treatment, aspirin or another NSAID may be prescribed for relief of arthritic symptoms. The affected joint may be splinted to rest the joint. When the knee is involved, weight-bearing may be restricted and the use of crutches indicated.

Nursing Care

The nursing role in treatment of the client with Lyme disease is primarily educative. Teach the client about the disease and its transmission. Emphasize the importance of complying with prescribed antibiotic therapy for the full course of treatment. Discuss possible adverse effects of treatment and their appropriate management. Teach the client with arthritic manifestations about the use of NSAIDs, including the importance of maintaining a consistent schedule of doses rather than taking the medication only as needed for pain.

Client and Family Teaching

Nurses can take a major role in educating the public about Lyme disease and its prevention. Teach clients how to avoid contact with the tick that spreads the disease and what to do if a tick bite occurs. See the box on page 1656 for specific information to include.

Bibliography

■ ■ ■

Abrahamson, I. A., & Abrahamson, R. I. (1993). Eye signs of systemic disease. *Emergency Medicine, 25*(2), 95–96, 101–103, 107–108.

Abrams, W. B., & Fletcher, A. J. (Eds.). (1990). *The Merck manual of geriatrics.* Rahway, NJ: Merck Research Laboratories.

Arnett, F. C. (1990). Revised criteria for the classification of rheumatoid arthritis. *Orthopaedic Nursing, 9*(2), 58–64.

Ball, K. (1990). *Lasers: The perioperative challenge.* St. Louis: Mosby.

Bates, B., Bickley, L. S., & Hoekelman, R. A. (1995). *A guide to physical examination and history taking* (6th ed.). Philadelphia: Lippincott.

Belza, B. L., Henke, C. J., Yelin, E. H., Epstein, W. V., & Gilliss, C. L. (1993, March/April). Correlates of fatigue in older adults with rheumatoid arthritis. *Nursing Research, 42*(2), 93–99.

Berkow, R., & Fletcher, A. J. (Eds.). (1992). *The Merck manual of diagnosis and therapy* (16th ed.). Rahway, NJ: Merck Research Laboratories.

Bertino, L. S., & Lu, L. (1993). The bite of a wolf: Systemic lupus erythematosus. *Rehabilitation Nursing, 18*(3), 173–178.

Birchenall, J. M., & Streight, M. E. (1993). *Care of the older adult* (3rd ed.). Philadelphia: Lippincott.

Prevention of Lyme Disease

■ ■ ■

- Avoid tick-infested areas, particularly tall grasses and dense brush.

- When walking or working in potentially infested areas, wear clothing that covers the extremities completely, e.g., long pants tucked into boot tops or long socks, and long-sleeved shirts tucked into pants.

- Use an insect repellent such as diethyltoluamide (DEET) or permethrin on skin and clothing.

- Inspect skin and clothing for ticks after you have been outside.

- Protect pets with tick collars and inspect them frequently for ticks.

- Remove any ticks found on the body or on pets immediately. Grasp the mouth portion of the tick with fine tweezers where it enters the skin, and pull steadily and firmly until the tick releases. Do not twist or jerk.

- Put the tick in alcohol and save it for future examination in case you develop symptoms. Do not crush the tick.

- Wash the affected area thoroughly with soap and water; apply an antiseptic.

- If you develop flulike symptoms or a "bull's eye" rash around the tick bite, notify a physician immediately.

Carpenito, L. J. (1991). *Nursing care plans and documentation: Nursing diagnoses and collaborative problems.* Philadelphia: Lippincott.

Chase, J. A. (1991, March). Spinal stenosis: When arthritis is more than arthritis! *Nursing Clinics of North America, 26*(1), 53–64.

Dale, K. G., Orr, P. M., & Harrell, P. B. (1992). Total elbow replacement. *Orthopaedic Nursing, 11*(5), 23–29.

Dolan, M. B. (1990). *Community and home health care plans.* Springhouse, PA: Springhouse.

Dykes, P. C. (1993). Minding the five Ps of neurovascular assessment. *American Journal of Nursing, 93*(6), 63–65.

Eden-Kilgour, S., & Miller, B. (1993). Understanding neurovascular assessment. *Nursing, 23*(8), 56–58.

Halverson, P. B., & Holmes, S. B. (1992). Systemic lupus erythematosus: Medical and nursing treatments. *Orthopaedic Nursing, 11*(6), 17–25.

Hayden, R. J. (1993, April). Chronic wrist pain: A primary care challenge. *Clinician Reviews, 3*(4), 51–54, 59–65.

Hazzard, W. R., Bierman, E. L., Blass, J. P., Ettinger, W. H., Jr., & Halter, J. B. (Eds.). (1994) *Principles of geriatric medicine and gerontology* (3rd ed.). New York: McGraw-Hill.

Johnson, R. L. (1993). Total shoulder arthroplasty. *Orthopaedic Nursing, 12*(1), 14–20.

Keel, T. A. (1994, September) Bone and joint infections: Guidelines to diagnosis, antibiotic therapy, and surgical indications. *Clinician Reviews, 4*(8), 49–52, 54–56, 60–62.

Kuper, B. C., & Failla, S. (1994, November). Shedding new light on lupus. *American Journal of Nursing, 94*(11), 26–32.

Lash, A. A. (1993). Systemic lupus erythematosus, part 2: Diagnosis, treatment modalities, and nursing management. *MEDSURG Nursing, 2*(5), 375–385.

Lederer, J. R., Marculescu, G. L., Mocnik, B., & Seaby, N. (1993). *Care planning pocket guide: A nursing diagnosis approach* (5th ed.). Redwood City, CA: Addison-Wesley Nursing.

Marieb, E. N. (1992). *Human anatomy and physiology* (2nd ed.). Redwood City, CA: Benjamin/Cummings.

Marlow, S. M. (1994, January). It's time to stop treating arthritis generically. *ADVANCE for Nurse Practitioners, 2*(1), 11–12, 26.

Mayers, M., & Pancratz, C. (1995). *McGraw-Hill Clinical care plans: Medical-surgical nursing.* New York: McGraw-Hill.

McCance, K. L., & Huether, S. E. (1994). *Pathophysiology: The biologic basis for disease in adults and children* (2nd ed.). St. Louis: Mosby-Year Book.

Mooney, N. E. (1991, March). Pain management in the orthopedic patient. *Nursing Clinics of North America, 26*(1), 73–87.

National Institutes of Health. (1993). *Arthritis, rheumatic diseases, and related disorders* (Publication No. 93-3413). Washington, DC: Department of Health and Human Services, National Institute of Arthritis and Musculoskeletal and Skin Diseases.

Needham, J. F. (1995). *Gerontological nursing.* Albany, NY: Delmar Publishers.

Neuberger, G. B., Kasal, S., Smith, K. V., Hassanein, R., & DeViney, S. (1994). Determinants of exercise and aerobic fitness in outpatients with arthritis. *Nursing Research, 43*(1), 11–17.

Oldaker, S. M. (1992). Live and learn: Patient education for the elderly orthopaedic client. *Orthopaedic Nursing, 11*(3), 51–56.

O'Toole, M. (Ed.). (1992). *Miller-Keane Encyclopedia & dictionary of medicine, nursing, & allied health* (5th ed.). Philadelphia: Saunders.

Panush, R. S., Greer, J. M., & Morshedian, K. K. (1993). What is lupus? What is not lupus? *Rheumatic Disease Clinics of North America, 19*(1), 223–234.

Paparone, P. (1990, June) The summer scourge of Lyme disease. *American Journal of Nursing, 90*(6), 44–47.

Physicians' desk reference (48th ed.). (1994). Montvale, NJ: Medical Economics Data Production Company.

Porth, C.M. (1994). *Pathophysiology: Concepts of altered health states* (4th ed.). Philadelphia: Lippincott.

Price, S. A., & Wilson, L. M. (1992). *Pathophysiology: Clinical concepts of disease processes* (4th ed.). St. Louis: Mosby-Year Book.

Riggins, R. S. (1993). Getting comfortable with joint aspiration and injection. *Emergency Medicine, 25*(4),75–76,85–88, 93.

Roitt, I. (1994). *Essential immunology* (8th ed.). Oxford: Blackwell Scientific Publications.

Rubenstein, E., & Federman, D. D. (Eds.). (1986–1994). *Scientific American Medicine.* New York: Scientific American.

Shlafer, M. (1993). *The nurse, pharmacology, and drug therapy: A prototype approach* (2nd ed.). Redwood City: Addison-Wesley Nursing.

Slye, D. A. (1991). Orthopedic complications: Compartment syndrome, fat embolism syndrome, and venous thromboembolism. *Nursing Clinics of North America, 26*(1), 113–132.

Smith, J. E. (1990). Applying the continuous passive motion device. *Orthopaedic Nursing, 9*(3), 54–56.

Sparks, S. M., & Taylor, C. M. (1993). *Nursing diagnosis reference manual* (2nd ed.). Springhouse, PA: Springhouse.

Spencer, R. T., Nichols, L. W., Lipkin, G. B., Henderson, H. S., & West, F. M. (1993). *Clinical pharmacology and nursing management* (4th ed.). Philadelphia: Lippincott.

Thompson, J. M., McFarland, G. K., Hirch, J. E., & Tucker, S. M. (1993). *Mosby's Clinical nursing* (3rd ed.). St. Louis: Mosby-Year Book.

Tierney, L. M., Jr., McPhee, S. J., & Papadakis, M. A. (Eds.). (1994). *Current medical diagnosis and treatment* (33rd ed.). Norwalk, CT: Appleton & Lange.

Tucker, S. M., Canobbio, M. M., Paquette, E. V., & Wells, M. F. (1992) *Patient care standards: Nursing process, diagnosis, and outcome* (5th ed.). St. Louis: Mosby-Year Book.

Way, L. W. (Ed.). (1994). *Current surgical diagnosis and treatment* (10th ed.). Norwalk, CT: Appleton & Lange.

Wilson, J. D., Braunwald, E., Isselbacher, K. J., Petersdorf, R. G., Martin, J. B., Fauci, A. S., & Root, R. K. (Eds.). (1991). *Harrison's principles of internal medicine* (12th ed.). New York: McGraw-Hill.

Yeomans, A. C. (1991). Assessment and management of gouty arthritis. *Nurse Practitioner, 16*(4), 20–21, 25–26.

Cognitive and Perceptual Patterns

Responses to Altered Neurologic Function

Assessing Clients with Neurologic Disorders

LEARNING OBJECTIVES

After completing this chapter, you will be able to

- Describe the structure of neurons and discuss transmission and regulation of nerve impulses.

- Identify the major structures and functions of the central and peripheral nervous systems.

- Identify interview questions pertinent to the assessment of neurologic function.

- Describe physical assessment techniques for neurologic function, including examinations of mental status, cranial nerves, sensory nerves, motor nerves, cerebellar function, and reflexes.

- Describe special neurologic examinations for clients with suspected meningeal irritation and for comatose clients.

- Identify manifestations of impairment in neurologic function.

- Describe variations in assessment findings for the older adult.

The nervous system is a highly complex series of organs, tissues, and cells that regulate and integrate all body functions, mental abilities, and emotions. It collects information from the internal and external environment as sensory input, processes and interprets the input, and causes responses that are manifested as motor or sensory output.

▗▗▗ Review of Anatomy and Physiology ▗▗▗

The nervous system is divided into two regions: the central nervous system (CNS), which consists of the brain and spinal cord, and the peripheral nervous system (PNS), which consists of the cranial nerves, the spinal nerves, and the autonomic nervous system. These two regions are highly integrated, and both are made up of just two types of cells: *neurons,* which receive impulses and send them on to other cells, and *neuroglia,* which protect and nourish the neurons.

Structure and Function of Neurons

Neural Cells

Each neuron is made up of three parts: a dendrite, a cell body, and an axon. The *dendrite* is a short projection from the cell body that conducts impulses toward the cell body in what is called an *afferent* process. *Cell bodies,* most of which are located within the central nervous system, are clustered together in *ganglia* or *nuclei.* The *axon,* a long projection, conducts impulses away from the cell body in what is called an *efferent* process. Many axons are covered with a *myelin sheath,* a white lipid substance. The myelin sheath is interrupted at intervals in unmyelinated areas called *nodes of Ranvier,* which allow movement of ions between the axon and the extracellular fluid.

Neurons are supported by four types of neuroglia: *oligodendroglia,* which produce the myelin sheath for the CNS axons; *astroglia* or *astrocytes,* which maintain the electrical potential of the neuron and play a role in the blood–brain barrier; *ependyma,* which assist in the production of cerebrospinal fluid (CSF); and *microglia,* which remove traumatic and metabolic wastes.

Transmission and Regulation of Nerve Impulses

Neurons are excitatory; that is, they are highly responsive to stimuli. When a neuron reaches a certain level of stimulation, an electrical impulse is generated and conducted along the length of its axon. The movement of impulses to and from the CNS is made possible by afferent and efferent neurons. *Afferent,* or *sensory, neurons* have receptors in skin, muscles, and other organs and relay impulses to the CNS. *Efferent,* or *motor, neurons* transmit impulses from the CNS to cause some type of action.

Nerve impulses occur when a stimulus reaches a point great enough to generate a change in electrical charge across the cell membrane of a neuron. A neuron that is not involved in impulse conduction is in a resting, or *polarized,* state, in which the number of positive ions in the fluid outside of the cell membrane is greater than in the fluid within the cell. The chief regulators of membrane potential are sodium and potassium: Sodium is the major positive ion in the extracellular fluid, and potassium is the major positive ion inside the cell. Normally, sodium cannot diffuse across the cell membrane, but in response to an electrical stimulus, the cell membrane becomes permeable for an instant, and sodium flows into the cell. This changes the polarity of the cell membrane, and the neuron is said to *depolarize.* This event stimulates the neuron to send an *action potential,* or a nerve impulse, over the axon. When the charges and ions return to their original resting state, the neuron is *repolarized.*

The action potential is generated only at the point of the stimulus, but once generated, it is propagated along the entire length of the axon whether the stimulus continues or not. Conduction of the impulse is rapid in myelinated fibers, with the action potential "jumping" from one node of Ranvier to the next. The conduction of the impulse is slower in unmyelinated fibers.

When the action potential reaches the presynaptic terminal (at the end of the axon of a presynaptic neuron), a *neurotransmitter* is released and travels across the synaptic cleft to bind with receptors in the postsynaptic neuron dendrite or cell body. The neurotransmitter may either be inhibitory or excitatory. The excitatory neurotransmitter

is almost always *acetylcholine (ACh),* which is rapidly degraded by the enzyme acetylcholinesterase. *Norepinephrine (NE)* is another major neurotransmitter. It may be either excitatory or inhibitory.

Nerves that transmit impulses through the release of ACh are called *cholinergic.* Receptors that bind ACh are found in the viscera, skeletal muscle cells, and the adrenal medulla (where they stimulate the release of epinephrine). The effect of ACh binding may be either to stimulate or to inhibit a response.

Nerves that transmit impulses through the release of NE are called *adrenergic.* Receptors that bind NE are found in the heart, lungs, kidneys, blood vessels, and all target organs stimulated by the sympathetic division except the heart. Adrenergic receptors are further divided into alpha and beta types. Alpha-adrenergic receptors help control such varied functions as arterial vasoconstriction and pupil dilation. Beta-adrenergic fibers may be either beta-1 or beta-2 receptors. Beta-1 receptors are found only in the heart, where they regulate the rate and force of contraction. Beta-2 receptors are found in receptor cells of the lungs, arteries, liver, and uterus; they help regulate bronchial diameter, arterial diameter, and glycogenesis. Generally, binding of NE to alpha receptors stimulates a response, whereas binding to beta receptors inhibits a response.

Other neurotransmitters include *gamma aminobutyric acid (GABA),* which inhibits CNS function; *dopamine,* which may be inhibitory or excitatory and helps control fine movement and emotions; and *serotonin,* which is usually inhibitory and controls sleep, hunger, and behavior and also affects consciousness.

The Central Nervous System

The *central nervous system (CNS)* consists of the brain and spinal cord, highly evolved clusters of neurons which act to accept, interconnect, interpret, and generate a response to nerve impulses originating throughout the body.

The Brain

The *brain* is the control center of the nervous system. It also generates thoughts, emotions, and speech. A large, complex mass of tissue that averages 3 to 4 lb in weight, the brain is surrounded by the skull, a bony structure that provides support and protection.

Anatomical Structures of the Brain The brain consists of four major regions: the cerebrum, the diencephalon, the brain stem, and the cerebellum (Figure 39–1). The general functions of these regions are summarized in Table 39–1.

Cerebrum Two *cerebral hemispheres* make up the *cerebrum,* the most superior part of the brain. The cerebrum accounts for almost 60% of brain weight. The surface of

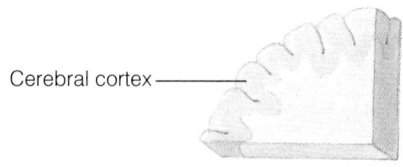

Cerebral cortex

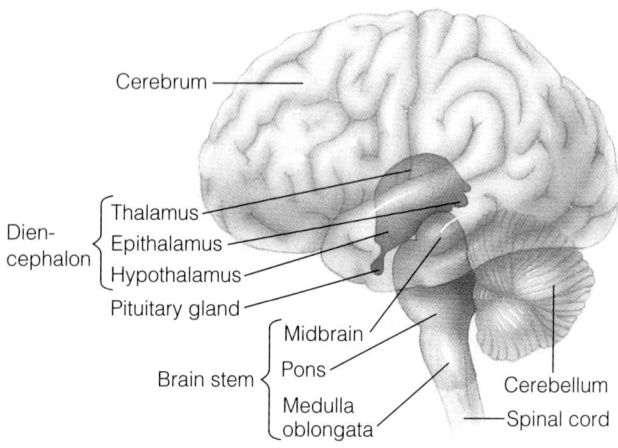

Cerebrum

Dien-cephalon
Thalamus
Epithalamus
Hypothalamus
Pituitary gland

Brain stem
Midbrain
Pons
Medulla oblongata

Cerebellum
Spinal cord

Figure 39–1   The four major regions of the brain.

Table 39–1	General Functions of the Four Regions of the Brain
Region	**Functions**
Cerebrum	Interprets sensory input. Controls skeletal muscle activity. Processes intellect and emotions. Contains skills memory.
Diencephalon	Conducts sensory and motor impulses. Regulates autonomic nervous system. Regulates and produces hormones. Mediates emotional responses.
Brain stem	Serves as conduction pathway. Serves as site of decussation of tracts. Contains respiratory nuclei. Helps regulate skeletal muscles.
Cerebellum	Processes information. Provides information necessary for balance, posture, and coordinated muscle movement.

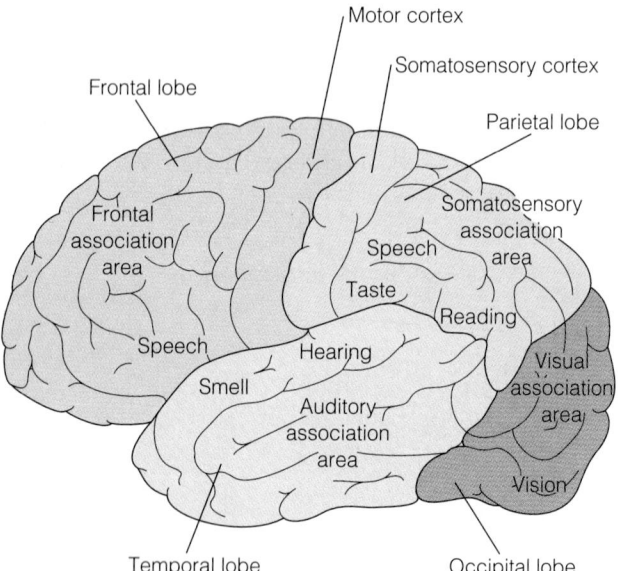

Motor cortex
Somatosensory cortex
Parietal lobe
Frontal lobe
Frontal association area
Somatosensory association area
Speech
Taste
Reading
Speech
Hearing
Visual association area
Smell
Auditory association area
Vision
Temporal lobe
Occipital lobe

Figure 39–2   Lobes of the cerebrum and functional areas of the cerebral cortex.

the cerebrum is folded into elevated ridges of tissue called *gyri,* which are separated by shallow grooves called *sulci.* The surface of the cerebrum is further divided by deep grooves called *fissures.* The *longitudinal fissure* separates the *hemispheres,* and the *transverse fissure* separates the cerebrum from the cerebellum. In addition, each cerebral

hemisphere is divided into *frontal, parietal, temporal,* and *occipital lobes* (Figure 39–2).

The two cerebral hemispheres are connected by a thick band of nerve fibers called the *corpus callosum,* which allows the two hemispheres to communicate with each other. Each cerebral hemisphere receives sensory and motor impulses from the opposite side of the body. One of the cerebral hemispheres tends to develop more than the other. Most people have a more highly developed left hemisphere, which is responsible for the control of language. The right hemisphere has greater control over nonverbal perceptual functions.

The *cerebral cortex* is the outer surface of the cerebrum. It is made up of neuron cell bodies, unmyelinated fibers, neuroglia, and blood vessels. The cerebral cortex is responsible for such functions as memory, speech, perception, voluntary movement, consciousness, logistics, and emotions. The functions of the different lobes of the cerebrum and the specific areas of the cerebral cortex are shown in Figure 39–2 and listed in Table 39–2.

Diencephalon   The *diencephalon,* or *interbrain,* is embedded in the cerebrum superior to the brain stem. It consists of the thalamus, hypothalamus, and epithalamus. The *thalamus* begins to process sensory impulses before they ascend to the cerebral cortex. It serves as a sorting, processing, and relay station for inputs into the cortical region. The *hypothalamus* is located inferior to the thalamus. It regulates temperature, water metabolism, appetite, emotional expressions, part of the sleep-wake cycle, and thirst. The *epithalamus* forms the dorsal part of the diencephalon and includes the pineal body, which is part of the endocrine system that affects growth and development.

Brain Stem   The *brain stem* consists of the midbrain, pons, and medulla oblongata. The *midbrain*, located between the diencephalon and the pons, is a center for auditory and visual reflexes. In addition, it functions as a nerve pathway between the cerebral hemispheres and lower brain. The *pons* is located just below the midbrain. It consists mostly of fiber tracts, but it also contains nuclei that control respiration. The *medulla oblongata*, located at the base of the brain stem, is continuous with the superior portion of the spinal cord. It also contains fiber tracts. Nuclei of the medulla oblongata play an important role in controlling cardiac rate, blood pressure, respirations, and swallowing.

Cerebellum   The *cerebellum* is connected to the midbrain, pons, and medulla. Like the cerebrum, it has two hemispheres. Its functions include coordination of skeletal muscle activity, maintenance of balance, and control of fine movements.

Ventricles   Within the brain are four *ventricles*, chambers filled with cerebrospinal fluid (CSF). They are linked by ducts that allow the CSF to circulate. One *lateral ventricle* is located within each hemisphere. These communicate with the *third ventricle* through the foramen of Monro. The third ventricle communicates with the *fourth ventricle* through the cerebral aqueduct that runs through the midbrain. The *cerebral aqueduct* is continuous with the central canal of the spinal cord.

Cerebrospinal Coverings   The central nervous system is covered and protected by three connective tissue membranes called *meninges*. The meninges form divisions within the skull, enclose venous sinuses, and contain CSF.

The meninges consist of three layers (Figure 39–3). The outermost layer is the *dura mater*. The dura mater has a double layer; the outermost layer is attached to the inner surface of the skull, and the innermost layer is the most external brain covering. The *arachnoid mater* is the middle layer of meninges. It forms a space that contains CSF and is the site of all major cerebral blood vessels. The innermost *pia mater* clings to the brain itself, and is filled with small blood vessels.

Cerebrospinal Fluid   *Cerebrospinal fluid (CSF)*, a clear and colorless liquid, is formed by the *choroid plexus*, groups of capillaries located in the brain ventricles. CSF circulates from the lateral ventricles of the cerebral hemispheres into the third ventricle of the diencephalon through the midbrain into the fourth ventricle. Some of this CSF flows down the center of the spinal cord as the rest of it circulates into the subarachnoid space and returns to the blood through the arachnoid villi.

Table 39–2	Functions of Lobes of the Cerebrum and Areas of the Cerebral Cortex
Area	**Functions**
Parietal lobe (somatic sensory area of cerebral cortex)	Promotes recognition of pain, coldness, and light touch. The left side receives input from the right side of the body, and vice versa.
Occipital lobe	Receives and interprets visual stimuli.
Temporal lobe	Receives and interprets olfactory and auditory stimuli.
Frontal lobe	Controls movements of voluntary muscles.
Primary motor area	Facilitates voluntary movement of skeletal muscles.
Speech area	Promotes understanding of spoken and written words.
Motor speech area (Broca's area)	Promotes vocalization of words.

CSF forms a cushion for the brain tissue, protects the brain and spinal cord from trauma, helps provide nourishment for the brain, and removes waste products of cerebrospinal cellular metabolism. The usual amount of CSF ranges from 80 mL to 200 mL, averaging about 130 mL, and is replaced several times each day. It is absorbed by arachnoid villi. CSF is normally produced and absorbed in equal amounts.

Blood Supply to the Brain   The cerebral hemispheres of the brain receive their blood supply from the anterior and middle internal cerebral arteries. These two arteries are branches of the common carotid arteries. The brain stem and cerebellum receive their blood supply from the *basilar artery*. The posterior cerebrum receives blood from the *posterior cerebral arteries*. These major arteries are connected by small anterior and posterior communicating arteries, which form a circle of connected blood vessels called the *circle of Willis*. This circle serves as a protective device, providing alternative routes for brain tissues to receive their blood supply.

The brain receives about 750 mL of blood each minute and uses 20% of the body's total oxygen uptake. The large oxygen demand is necessary for metabolism of glucose, which is the brain's sole source of energy.

The Blood–Brain Barrier   The capillaries in the brain have low permeability because the cells that compose their walls join at very tight junctions. As a result, the brain is protected from many harmful substances in the blood. This *blood–brain barrier* allows only glucose, some amino acids, respiratory gases, and water to pass through

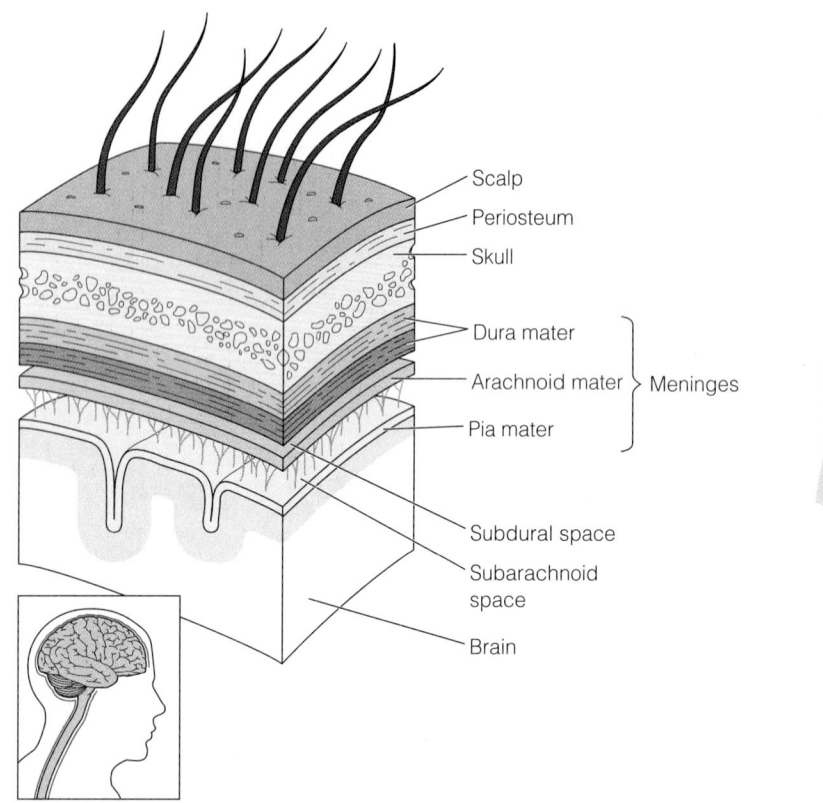

Figure 39–3 Anatomy of the meninges.

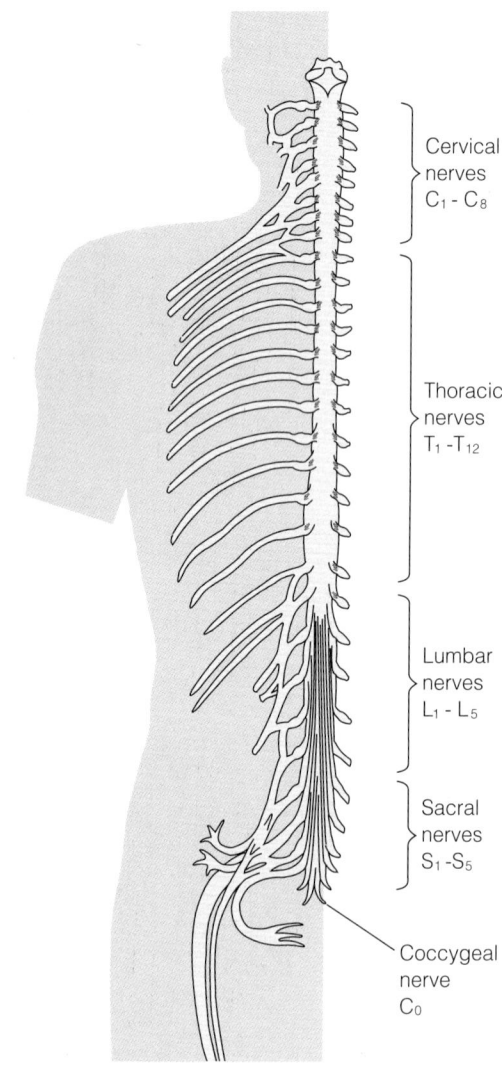

Figure 39–4 Distribution of spinal nerves.

it, thus maintaining a controlled environment. Substances such as urea, creatinine, proteins, some toxins, and most antibiotics cannot pass this barrier and enter brain tissue. However, injury to the brain may cause a localized breakdown of the barrier.

The Limbic System and the Reticular Formation

The limbic system and the reticular formation are functional brain systems. These systems, made of networks of neurons, communicate across areas of the brain.

The *limbic system* consists of structures that form a ring of tissue in the medial side of each hemisphere, surrounding the upper portion of the brain stem and corpus callosum. The limbic system integrates and modulates input to make up the affective part of the brain, providing emotional and behavioral responses to environmental stimuli.

The *reticular formation* is located through the central core of the medulla oblongata, pons, and midbrain. This system has widespread connections throughout the brain and relays sensory input from all body systems to all levels of the brain. A part of the reticular formation is the *reticular activating system (RAS)*. The RAS is a stimulating system for the cerebral cortex, keeping it alert and responsive to incoming sensory stimuli while filtering out repetitive or unwanted stimuli. Activity of the RAS is inhibited by the sleep center and may be depressed by

drugs and alcohol. Other parts of the reticular formation include motor nuclei that help maintain muscle tone and coordinated movements through interconnections with spinal nerves, and the vasomotor and cardiovascular regulatory centers, a part of autonomic regulation of the cardiovascular system.

The Spinal Cord

Accessory Structures The spinal cord is surrounded and protected by 33 vertebrae, including 7 cervical, 12 thoracic, 5 lumbar, 5 sacral, and 4 fused vertebrae, which form the *coccyx*. Each vertebra consists of a *body* and a *vertebral arch* formed by projections from the body. This arch encloses a space called the *vertebral foramen*. The vertebral foramina of all the vertebrae form the *vertebral canal* through which the spinal cord passes. *Intervertebral foramina* are spaces between the vertebrae through which spinal nerve roots pass as they exit the vertebral column.

Ascending (sensory) tracts

Descending (motor) tracts

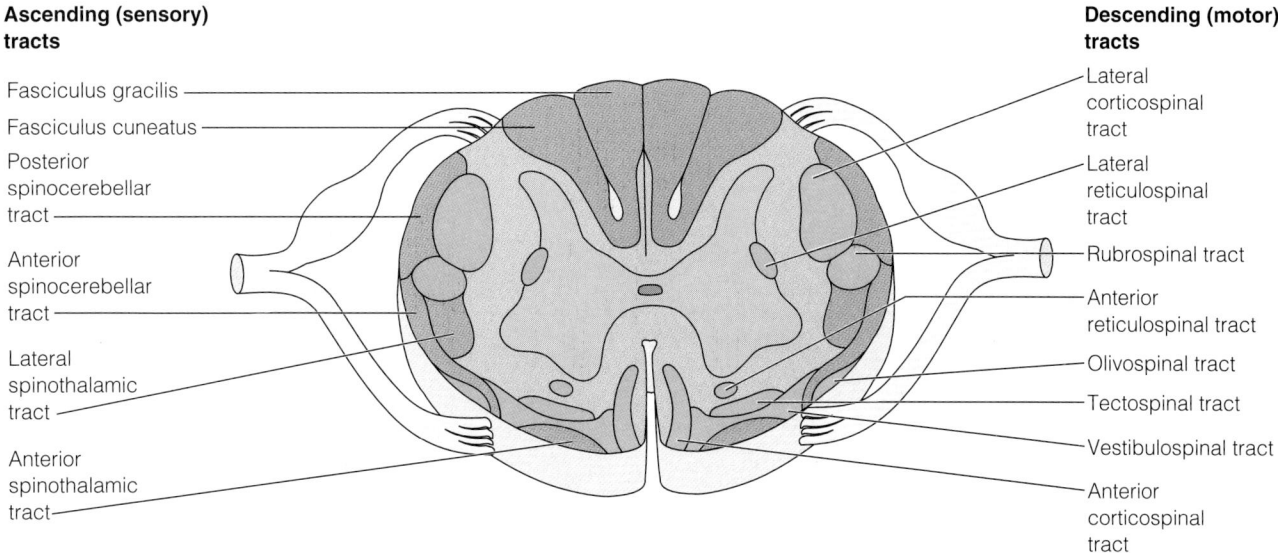

Figure 39–5 Ascending and descending tracts of the spinal cord.

Intervertebral discs are located between each of the moveable vertebrae. Each disc is made of a thick capsule surrounding a gelatinous core called the *nucleus pulposus.* The vertebral column is surrounded by ligaments that provide mobility and protection. The vertebral column is discussed in greater detail in Chapter 41.

Anatomy of the Spinal Cord The *spinal cord* extends from the medulla to the level of the first lumbar vertebra (Figure 39–4). It serves as a center for conducting messages to and from the brain and as a reflex center. The spinal cord is about 17 inches (42 cm) long and 3/4 inch (1.8 cm) thick. The cord is protected by the vertebrae, the meninges, and cerebrospinal fluid. The gray matter of the cord is on the inside, and the white matter is on the outside (the reverse of the arrangement in the brain).

Spinal Roots The roots of 31 pairs of spinal nerves, divided into the cervical, thoracic, and lumbar nerves, arise from the cord (see Figure 39–4). Each separates into posterior (sensory) and anterior (motor) roots. Damage to the posterior roots results in loss of sensation, whereas damage to the anterior root results in flaccid paralysis.

Functions of the Spinal Cord and Spinal Roots Messages to and from the brain are conducted via ascending (sensory) pathways and descending (motor) pathways. The major ascending tracts are the lateral and anterior *spinothalamic tracts,* which carry sensations for pain, temperature, and crude touch; and the posterior tracts, called the *fasciculus gracilis* and *fasciculus cuneatus,* which carry sensations for fine touch, position, and vibration (Figure 39–5).

The lateral and anterior *corticospinal (pyramidal) tracts* are descending tracts consisting of fibers that originate in the motor cortex of the brain and travel to the brain stem and then down the spinal cord. They mediate voluntary purposeful movements and stimulate certain muscular actions while inhibiting others. They also carry fibers that inhibit muscle tone. The rubrospinal, anterior and lateral reticulospinal, and *tectospinal (extrapyramidal) tracts* include the pathways between the cerebral cortex, basal ganglia, brain stem, and spinal cord outside the pyramidal tract. They maintain muscle tone and gross body movements.

Upper and Lower Motor Neurons
Upper motor neurons, such as those of the corticospinal and extrapyramidal tract, carry impulses from the cerebral cortex to the anterior gray column of the spinal cord. Damage to upper motor neurons results in increased muscle tone, decreased muscle strength, decreased coordination, and hyperactive reflexes. *Lower motor neurons,* such as the peripheral and cranial nerves, begin in the anterior gray column of the spinal cord and end in the muscle. These are the "final common pathways." Damage to lower motor neurons results in decreased muscle tone and loss of reflexes.

The Peripheral Nervous System

The *peripheral nervous system (PNS)* links the central nervous system with the rest of the body. It is responsible for receiving and transmitting information from and about the external environment. The PNS is made up of nerves, ganglia (groups of nerve cells), and sensory receptors located outside—or peripheral to—the brain and spinal cord. The PNS is divided into a *sensory,* or *afferent, division* and a *motor,* or *efferent, division.* Most nerves of the PNS contain fibers for both divisions and all are classified regionally as either spinal nerves or cranial nerves.

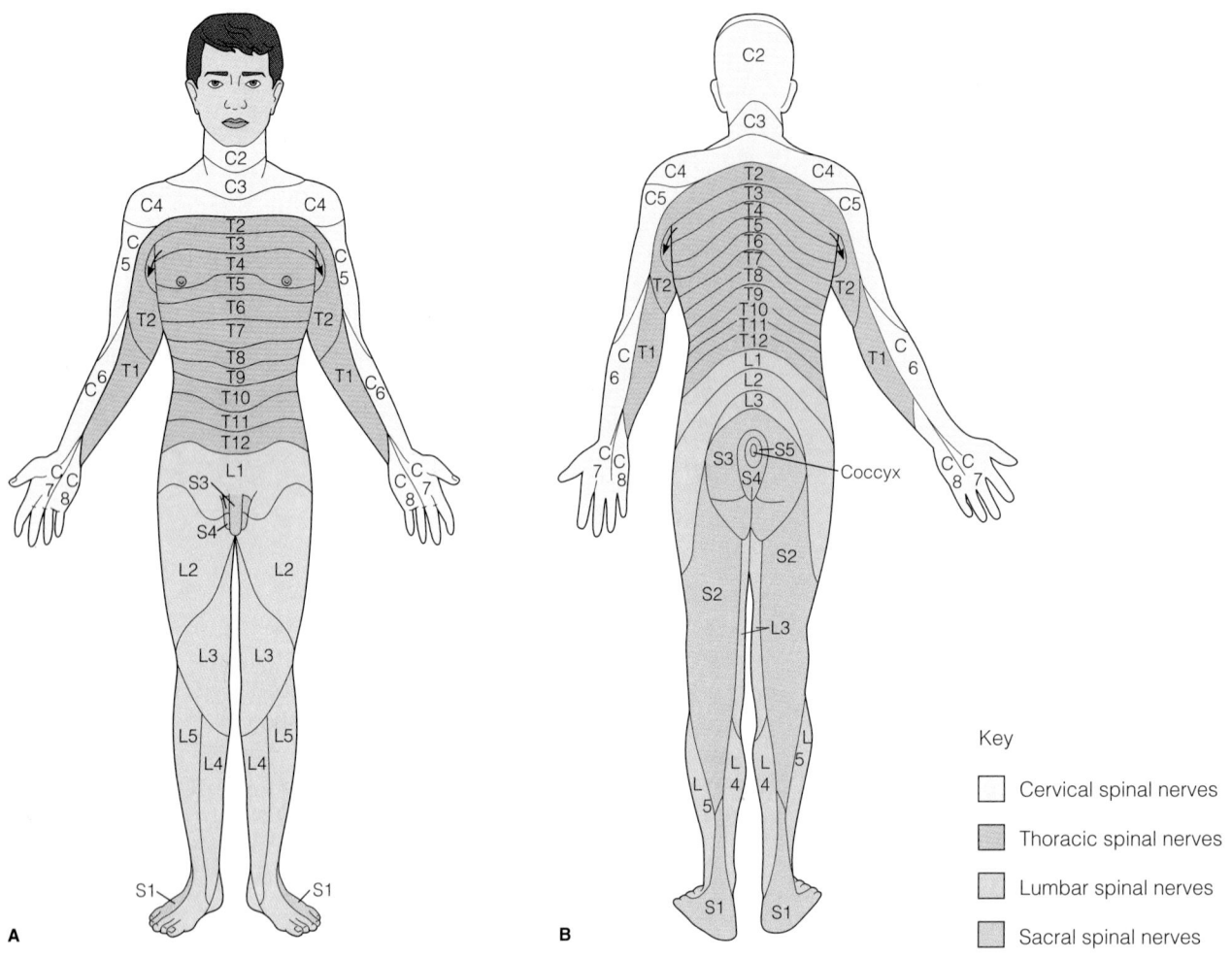

Figure 39–6   *A,* Anterior and *B,* posterior dermatomes of the body.

Spinal Nerves

As mentioned earlier, there are 31 pairs of spinal nerves (see Figure 39–4). These nerves are named by their location:

- Cervical: 8 pairs (C_1 to C_8)
- Thoracic: 12 pairs (T_1 to T_{12})
- Lumbar: 5 pairs (L_1 to L_5)
- Sacral: 5 pairs (S_1 to S_5)

Spinal nerves exit the vertebral column through intervertebral foramina to travel to the body regions they serve. The spinal cord does not reach the end of the vertebral column; as a result, the lumbar and sacral nerve roots travel inferiorly through the vertebral canal for some distance before exiting the vertebral column through their associated intervertebral foramina. This collection of descending nerve roots is called the *cauda equina.*

Each spinal nerve contains both sensory and motor fibers. The sensory fibers are located in the dorsal root, and their cell bodies are located within the *dorsal root gan-*

glion. The motor fibers are located in the ventral root, and their cell bodies are located within the spinal cord. The dorsal and ventral roots merge outside the vertebral canal just past the dorsal root ganglion, forming a spinal nerve. Each spinal nerve further divides into branches called *rami.*

The ventral rami of the cervical, brachial, lumbar, and sacral regions form complex clusters of nerves called *plexuses.* The main spinal nerve plexuses innervate the skin and the underlying muscles of the arms and legs. For example, the cervical plexus innervates the diaphragm through the phrenic nerve; the brachial plexus innervates the upper extremities through the median, ulnar, and radial nerves; and the lumbar plexus innervates the anterior thigh through the femoral nerve.

An area of skin innervated by cutaneous branches of a single spinal nerve is called a **dermatome.** The dorsal roots of the spinal nerves carry sensations from these specific dermatomes. Dermatomes provide anatomical landmarks that are useful for locating neurologic lesions. Figure 39–6 illustrates the dermatomes.

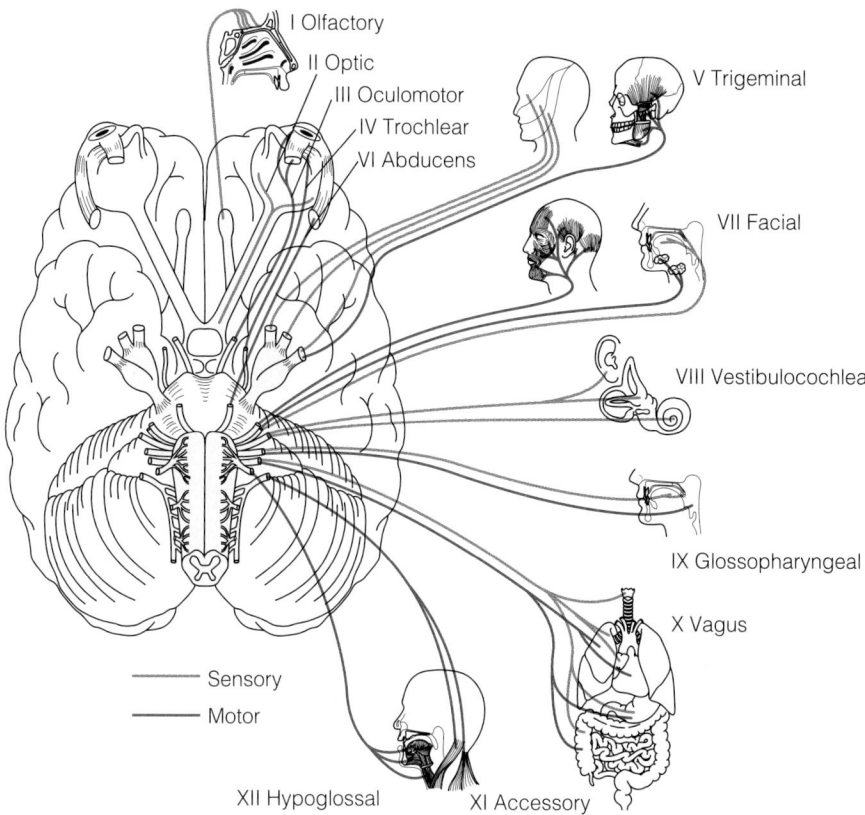

I Olfactory
II Optic
III Oculomotor
IV Trochlear
VI Abducens

V Trigeminal

VII Facial

VIII Vestibulocochlear

IX Glossopharyngeal

X Vagus

——— Sensory
——— Motor

XII Hypoglossal   XI Accessory

Figure 39–7   Cranial nerves.

Cranial Nerves

Twelve pairs of cranial nerves originate in the forebrain and brain stem (Figure 39–7). The vagus nerve extends into the ventral body cavity, but the eleven other pairs innervate only head and neck regions. Although most are mixed nerves, three pairs (olfactory, optic, and vestibulocochlear) are solely sensory. The cranial nerves and their related functions are listed in Table 39–3.

Reflexes

A *reflex* is a rapid, involuntary, predictable motor response to a stimulus (Marieb, 1995). Reflexes are categorized as either somatic or autonomic. Somatic reflexes result in skeletal muscle contraction; autonomic reflexes activate cardiac muscle, smooth muscle, and glands. A reflex occurs over a pathway called a *reflex arc.*

The essential components of a reflex arc are a receptor, a sensory neuron to carry afferent impulses to the CNS, an integration center in the spinal cord or brain, a motor neuron to carry efferent impulses, and an effector (the tissue that responds by contracting or secreting) (Figure 39–8).

Somatic reflexes mediated by the spinal cord are called *spinal reflexes.* Many spinal reflexes occur without impulses traveling to and from the brain, with the cord serving as the integration center; others require brain activity and modulation. Commonly assessed reflexes include stretch, deep-tendon, flexor, and superficial reflexes.

Stretch reflexes, caused by muscle contraction in response to increased muscle length, are elicited by striking a skeletal muscle or tendon; they include the patellar, or knee-jerk, reflex. *Deep-tendon reflexes (DTRs)* occur in response to muscle contraction and cause muscle relaxation and lengthening. DTRs depend on intact sensory and motor nerve roots, functional synapses in the spinal cord, a functional neuromuscular junction, and a competent muscle. Thus, an abnormal deep-tendon reflex could indicate a variety of problems, including a lesion of a spinal nerve.

Flexor, or *withdrawal, reflexes* are caused by actual or perceived painful stimuli and result in withdrawal of the part of the body that is threatened. *Superficial responses* result from gentle cutaneous stimulation. These responses depend on functional upper motor pathways and on an intact reflex arc. Examples of superficial responses are the plantar reflex, elicited by stroking the sole of the foot (the normal response is to curl the toes downward), and the abdominal reflex, elicited by stroking the skin of the abdomen (which normally causes the skin of the abdomen to contract).

The Autonomic Nervous System

The *autonomic nervous system (ANS)* is a division of the PNS that regulates the internal environment of the body. It is also called the *general visceral motor system,* because it is made up of motor neurons that innervate the body's vis-

Table 39–3	Cranial Nerves
Name	**Function**
I Olfactory	Sense of smell
II Optic	Vision
III Oculomotor	Eyeball movement Raising of upper eyelid Constriction of pupil Proprioception
IV Trochlear	Eyeball movement
V Trigeminal	Sensation of the upper scalp, upper eyelid, nose, nasal cavity, cornea, and lacrimal gland Sensation of the palate, upper teeth, cheek, top lip, lower eyelid, and scalp Sensation of the tongue, lower teeth, chin, and temporal scalp Chewing
VI Abducens	Lateral movement of the eyeball
VII Facial	Movement of facial muscles Secretions of lacrimal, nasal, submandibular, and sublingual glands Sensation of taste
VIII Vestibulocochlear	Sense of equilibrium Sense of hearing
IX Glossopharyngeal	Swallowing Gag reflex Secretions of parotid salivary gland Sense of taste Touch, pressure, and pain from pharynx and posterior tongue Pressure from carotid arteries Receptors to regulate blood pressure
X Vagus	Swallowing Regulation of cardiac rate Regulation of respirations Digestion Sensation from thoracic and abdominal organs Proprioception Sense of taste
XI Accessory	Movement of head and neck Proprioception
XII Hypoglossal	Movement of tongue for speech and swallowing

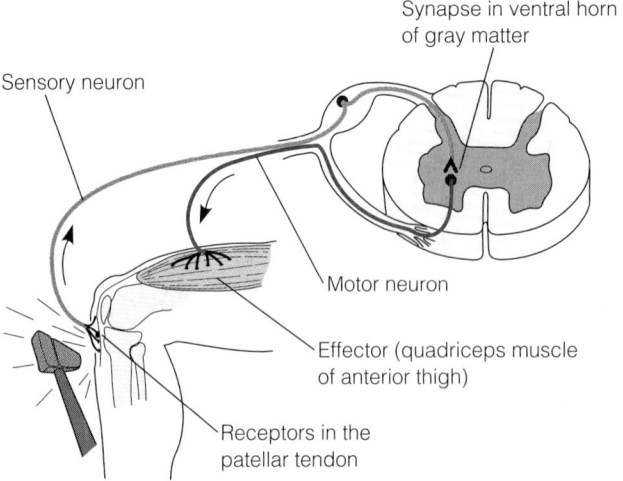

Figure 39–8   A typical reflex arc of a spinal nerve. In the two-neuron reflex arc, the stimulus is transferred from the sensory neuron directly to the motor neuron at the point of synapse in the spinal cord.

cera. Whereas skeletal muscle activity is regulated by a division of the PNS called the somatic nervous system, the ANS regulates the activity of cardiac muscle, smooth muscle, and glands.

The reticular formation in the brain stem is the primary controller of the ANS. Stimulation of centers in the medulla initiates reflexes that regulate cardiac rate, blood vessel diameter, and gastrointestinal function.

The ANS has sympathetic and parasympathetic divisions. Although fibers from both divisions affect the same structures, the actions of the two divisions are opposite in effect, and they serve to counterbalance each other.

The major neurotransmitters for impulse transmission in the ANS are acetylcholine (ACh) and norepinephrine (NE). ACh is the primary neurotransmitter of the parasympathetic division. NE is the primary neurotransmitter of the sympathetic division.

Sympathetic Division   The *sympathetic division* of the ANS prepares the body to handle situations that are perceived as harmful or stressful and to participate in strenuous activity. Cell bodies for this division arise in the lateral horns of the spinal cord in the area from T_1 through L_2. The fibers separate after leaving the cord, and form a chain of ganglia that extend from the neck to the pelvis. Long fibers then extend to the organs that are supplied by the sympathetic division.

Stimulation of the sympathetic division can exert the following effects on target organs or tissues:

- Dilated pupils
- Inhibited secretions
- Copious production of sweat
- Increased rate and force of heartbeat

- Vasodilation of the coronary arteries
- Dilation of the bronchioles
- Decreased digestion
- Increased release of glucose by the liver
- Decreased urine output
- Vasoconstriction of arteries to increase blood pressure
- Vasoconstriction of abdominal and skin blood vessels to increase systemic circulation
- Increased blood clotting
- Increased metabolic rate
- Increased mental alertness

Parasympathetic Division The *parasympathetic division* of the ANS operates during nonstressful situations. It conserves the body's energy as it regulates digestion, elimination, and other activities. Cell bodies for this division are located in the brain stem (for the cranial nerves) and in the lateral gray matter of S_2 through S_4. Other than the fibers supplying the cranial nerves III, VII, IX, and X, the fibers are carried by the vagus nerve to body tissues, thoracic organs, and visceral organs.

Stimulation of the parasympathetic division of the ANS produces the following effects:

- Constriction of pupils
- Stimulation of glandular secretions
- Decreased heart rate
- Vasoconstriction of coronary arteries
- Constriction of the bronchioles
- Increased peristalsis and secretion of gastrointestinal fluid

Assessment of Neurologic Function

■ ■ ■

Function of the neurologic system is assessed both by a health assessment interview to collect subjective data and a physical assessment to collect objective data.

The Health Assessment Interview

This section provides guidelines for collecting subjective data through a health assessment interview specific to the functions of the neurologic system. Interview questions and leading statements for assessing neurologic function are also provided. If the client's level of consciousness is altered, the nurse may need to rely on family members for information. The client's level of consciousness may be assessed by using the Glasgow Coma Scale, found in Table 39–4.

Table 39–4	Glasgow Coma Scale	
Assessment	**Response**	**Score**
Eyes open (Record C if eyes are closed by swelling.)	Spontaneously	4
	To speech	3
	To pain	2
	No response	1
Best motor response (Record best upper arm response.)	Obeys commands	6
	Localizes pain	5
	Flexion-withdrawal	4
	Abnormal flexion	3
	Abnormal extension	2
	No response	1
Best verbal response (Record T if an endotracheal or tracheostomy tube is in place.)	Oriented	5
	Confused	4
	Inappropriate words	3
	Incomprehensible sounds	2
	No response	1
Total Score:		_____

Overview

An interview to assess neurologic function may focus on a chief complaint or may be done as part of a total health assessment. If the client has a health problem involving any component of neurologic function, analyze its onset, characteristics and course, severity, precipitating and relieving factors, and any associated symptoms, noting the timing and circumstances. For example, ask the client:

- Describe the location and intensity of the pain you have experienced in your left leg. Is it made worse by coughing, sneezing, or walking?
- When did you first notice that you were having numbness in your fingers?
- Describe the difficulty you have when you try to walk.

Questions about present health status include information about numbness, tingling sensations, tremors, problems with coordination or balance, or loss of movement in any part of the body. Ask the client about difficulty with speaking, seeing, hearing, tasting, or detecting odors. In addition, elicit information about memory, feeling state (such as anxiety or depression), recent changes in sleep patterns, ability to perform self-care and activities of daily living, sexual activity, and weight. If the client is taking prescribed or over-the-counter medications, ask about the type and purpose, as well as the frequency and duration of use.

Ask about any past history or seizures, fainting, dizziness, headaches and any trauma, tumors, or surgery of the brain, spinal cord, or nerves. Discuss other illnesses that may cause neurologic manifestations, including cardiac disease, strokes, pernicious anemia, sinus infections, liver disease, and/or renal failure. Also ask the client whether there is a family history of neurologic health problems, diabetes mellitus, hypertension, seizures, or psychiatric problems.

Question the client about occupational hazards, such as exposure to toxic chemicals or materials, use of protective headgear, and the amount of time spent performing repetitive motions (e.g., data entry and assembly). Ask questions about self-care to assess the client's diet and use of tobacco, drugs, or alcohol, and ask whether the client wears a helmet when riding a bike or motorcycle or participating in contact sports.

Interview Questions

The following interview questions and leading statements are categorized by functional health patterns:

Health Perception–Health Management

- Have you ever had a neurologic illness, injury, or surgery, including seizures, stroke, brain or spinal cord injury, infection, tumor, meningitis, or encephalitis?
- Have you ever had problems with your ability to move body parts? Explain.
- Would you say you think clearly? Explain.
- Are you having any problems in your ability to see, hear, taste, or smell? Explain.
- If you have answered yes to any of these questions, describe how you were treated for these problems.
- Have you ever had diagnostic tests for a neurologic problem (EEG, EMG, nuclear scan, MRI, spinal tap)? When and for what?
- Do you take medications for seizures, headaches, or any other neurological problem? If so, what type and how often?
- Do you smoke tobacco or drink alcohol? If so, what type, how much, and for how long?

Nutritional-Metabolic

- Describe your usual dietary intake for a 24-hour period. Do you eat foods from all the food groups?
- Do you have difficulty chewing or swallowing your food?

Elimination

- Has there been a change in your usual pattern of urination or bowel elimination? If so, explain.
- Do you use laxatives, suppositories, or enemas to assist with bowel elimination? If so, what type and how often?

- Are you able to go to the bathroom independently? If not, describe your usual routine.

Activity-Exercise

- Describe your typical activities in a 24-hour period.
- Do you have difficulty with balance, coordination, or walking? Do you use an assistive device when you walk (such as a cane, crutches, or a walker)?
- Do you have any weakness in your arms or legs?
- Are you able to move all parts of your body? Explain.
- Do you trip or fall easily?
- If you have seizures, can you identify precipitating factors? Describe where the seizures begin in your body. What are you told happens during a seizure? How do you feel after the seizure?
- Have you experienced any shakiness or tremors? Where?

Sleep-Rest

- Does this health problem interfere with your ability to sleep and rest? If so, how?
- Do you ever have pain that awakens you at night? Explain.
- Describe your energy level. Does rest or sleep restore your energy and strength?

Cognitive-Perceptual

- Describe any headaches you experience, including frequency, type, location, and precipitating or relieving factors.
- Do you ever feel dizzy or faint? Do you ever feel that the room is spinning? Explain.
- Do you ever experience any numbness, burning, or tingling sensations? If so, where and when?
- Do you ever have visual problems, such as double vision, blurring, or blind spots?
- Do you ever have problems with hearing? Explain.
- Has there been a change in your ability to taste or smell? Explain.
- Do you have difficulty remembering things? Describe.

Self-Perception–Self-Concept

- How has this neurologic problem affected the way you feel about yourself?
- How has this neurologic problem affected the way you feel about your normal life?
- How do you feel about any impairment you might have from a neurologic problem?

Role-Relationship

- Is there a history of neurologic problems in your family (such as brain tumors, Alzheimer's disease, epilepsy)?
- Do you have difficulty expressing yourself and making others understand you? Explain.
- Has having neurologic problems affected your role in your family? If so, how?
- Has having neurologic problems affected interactions with others in your family? With friends? At work? In social activities?
- Has having neurologic problems affected your ability to work? Explain.

Sexuality-Reproductive

- Have your usual sexual activities been altered by a neurologic problem?
- Have you ever received information on alternative methods of sexual expression if a neurologic problem impairs your usual sexual activity?
- Describe how having neurologic problems makes you feel about yourself as a man or a woman.

Coping-Stress

- Describe what you do to cope with stress.
- How has this neurologic problem affected the way you normally cope with stress?
- Does increased stress make the neurologic problem more severe?
- What do you believe is the most stressful time you have had with this neurologic problem?
- Who or what will be able to help you cope with stress from this problem?

Value-Belief

- Are there significant others, practices, or activities that help you cope with this problem? Explain.
- What do you see as your greatest source of inner strength at this time?
- How do you perceive the future with this health problem?

The Physical Assessment

Physical assessment of the client begins when the nurse first meets the client and makes an overall evaluation of the client's mental and physical status. The mental status examination is conducted with both the nurse and the client seated. The rest of the neurologic examinations may be performed with the client either sitting or standing.

The neurologic system is assessed through inspection, palpation, and percussion (with a reflex hammer). When conducting the mental status and cognitive portions of the examination, be aware that fatigue or illness may alter findings. When interpreting findings, consider the client's age, educational background, and cultural orientation.

The Neurologic Examination: Preparation

The assessment should take place in a private, comfortable setting. Ask the client to remove outer clothing, shoes, and stockings. Provide a gown for the client to wear.

Prior to the examination, collect all the equipment necessary for this assessment: a cottonball and safety pin, tongue blade, tuning fork, ophthalmoscope, reflex hammer, pencil and paper, printed materials, and substances to test the senses of smell and taste.

It is important to explain to the client that the neurologic examination is lengthy and may consist of questions and requests that seem strange to the client. Explain to the client the rationale for each of the examinations.

This is a detailed and comprehensive examination that requires a considerable amount of time to perform. A shorter version of this physical assessment, often referred to as a *neuro check,* may be performed in a shorter time period when a client requires frequent ongoing assessments of his or her neurologic status. The box on page 1672 outlines an abbreviated neurologic assessment.

The Physical Assessment (continued)

Abbreviated Neurologic Assessment ("Neuro Check")

■ ■ ■

1. Assess level of consciousness (client's response to auditory and/or tactile stimulus).
2. Obtain vital signs (BP, P, R).
3. Check pupillary response to light.
4. Assess strength of hand grip and movement of extremities.
5. Determine ability to sense touch/pain in extremities.

Mental Status Examination

The mental status examination consists of observing the client's verbal and nonverbal responses to questions and specific requests. First, observe the client's appearance and behavior. Then, question the client to determine his or her cognitive functioning, thought processes, and perceptions.

ASSESSMENT TECHNIQUE	POSSIBLE ABNORMAL FINDINGS
■ **Assess the client's appearance.** Observe dress, hygiene, and grooming.	**Unilateral neglect** (inattention to one side of body) may occur with some cerebral vascular accidents (CVAs) of the middle cerebral artery. Poor hygiene and grooming may be seen in clients with organic brain syndrome.
Observe gait and posture.	Abnormal gait and posture may be seen in transient ischemic attacks (TIAs) and clients with CVAs.
■ **Assess the client's behavior.** Observe client's actions and affect.	Emotional swings or changes in personality may be observed with CVAs of the anterior cerebral artery. The face appears masklike (very little expressive movement of facial muscles) in clients with Parkinson's disease. Apathy is seen in organic brain disease.
Note the content and quality of speech.	**Aphasia** (defective or absent language function) may occur in TIAs. *Receptive aphasia* (inability to understand verbal or written language) is often noted in CVAs of the posterior or anterior cerebral artery. Aphasias are seen with damage to the left cerebral cortex. Aphasias are more often seen with CVAs of the right hemisphere than the left hemisphere. **Dysphonia** (change in the tone of the voice) is common in CVAs of the poste-

ASSESSMENT TECHNIQUE	POSSIBLE ABNORMAL FINDINGS
	rior inferior cerebral artery. Dysphonia is seen with paralysis of the vocal cords (cranial nerve X).
	Dysarthria (difficulty speaking) is seen with lesions of upper and lower motor neurons, the cerebellum, and the extrapyramidal tract. It is also seen in CVAs of the anterior inferior and superior cerebral arteries.
Note level of consciousness. Use the Glasgow Coma Scale (see Table 39–4) to document findings. Scores may range from 3 (deeply comatose) to 15 (alert and oriented).	Damage to the brain stem and/or cerebral cortex may alter one's level of consciousness. Drowsiness and decreased level of consciousness may be associated with TIAs and CVAs. Level of consciousness is usually altered and may progress to coma with CVA of the middle cerebral artery. Confusion and coma may be seen in clients with CVAs affecting the vertebralbasilar arteries.
■ **Assess cognitive functioning.** Note the client's orientation to time, place, and person.	Disorientation to time and place may occur in clients with CVAs of the right cerebral hemisphere.
Note the client's attention span and recent and remote memory. Ask the client to 1. Repeat 5 to 7 numbers. 2. Recall 3 items after 5 minutes. 3. Recall his or her address, breakfast, or birthday.	Memory deficits are often seen with CVAs of the anterior cerebral artery and vertebralbasilar artery.
Assess the client's thought processes (both content and perceptions) by noting responses to questions.	Perceptual deficits may be seen in CVAs of the middle cerebral artery.
Note the client's ability to understand what is said and to express thoughts.	Communication ability may be impaired with CVAs of the middle cerebral artery. Receptive aphasia may be associated with CVAs of the posterior cerebral arteries.
Note the client's ability to make logical and safe judgments.	Impaired cognition is often noted with CVAs of the middle cerebral artery.

Cranial Nerve Examination

The cranial nerve (CN) examination is the second part of the neurologic assessment.

ASSESSMENT TECHNIQUE	POSSIBLE ABNORMAL FINDINGS
■ **Test CN I (olfactory).** Assess client's ability to smell scents (e.g., soap, coffee) with each nostril. This test is usually done only if the client has reported a problem with the ability to smell.	**Anosmia** (an inability to smell) may be seen with lesions of the frontal lobe. Also occurs with impaired blood flow to the middle cerebral artery.

ASSESSMENT TECHNIQUE	POSSIBLE ABNORMAL FINDINGS

■ **Test CN II (optic).**

Assess vision with Snellen chart. (See Chapter 43 for guidelines.)

Blindness in one eye may be seen with CVAs of the internal carotid artery or with TIAs. Impaired vision or blindness in one side of both eyes *(homonymous hemianopia)* is associated with blockage of the posterior cerebral artery. Impaired vision may also be seen with CVA of the anterior cerebral artery.

Blindness or double vision may be noted with involvement of the vertebral-basilar arteries. Double or blurred vision may also occur with TIAs. Papilledema occurs with increased intracranial pressure.

■ **Test CN III, IV, and VI (oculomotor, trochlear, and abducens).**

Assess extraocular movements by having client follow your finger as you write an "H" in the air (see Chapter 43).

Nystagmus (involuntary eye movement) may be seen with CVA of the anterior, inferior, and superior cerebellar arteries.

Assess *perrla* (pupils equally round and reactive to light and accommodation) by covering one eye at a time and shining a bright light directly into the uncovered eye (use a penlight or the ophthalmoscope).

Constricted pupils are associated with impaired blood flow to the vertebral-basilar arteries.

Assess for **ptosis** (droopy eyelids).

Ptosis (also called *Horner's syndrome*), occurs with CVA of the posterior inferior cerebellar artery, myasthenia gravis, and palsy of CN III.

■ **Test CN V (trigeminal).**

Assess the client's ability to feel light, dull, and sharp facial sensations. With the client's eyes closed, check whether sensation is the same on both sides of the face. Stroke the cheek with a wisp of cotton for light touch, with a closed safety pin for dull touch, and with a tongue blade for sharp touch. If the sharp point of a safety pin is used to assess sharp touch, be sure to avoid scratching the surface of the skin, and discard the pin after it is used.

Changes in facial sensations are noted with impaired blood flow to the carotid artery. Decreased sensations to the face and cornea on the same side of the body occur with CVA of the posterior inferior cerebral artery. Lip and mouth numbness occur with CVAs of the vertebral-basilar artery. Loss of facial sensation or contraction of the masseter and temporal muscles is seen with lesions of CN V. Severe facial pain is seen with trigeminal neuralgia (tic douloureux).

Assess the corneal reflex by touching the corneal surface with a wisp of cotton. This reflex is tested on *unconscious* clients. Normally, the client blinks.

The corneal reflex may be impaired with lesions of CN V or VII.

■ **Test CN VII (facial).**

Assess the client's ability to taste sweet, sour, and salt on the anterior two-thirds of the tongue: Ask the client to project the tongue. Apply a salty, sweet, or sour substance.

Loss of ability to taste may occur with brain tumors or deficits or with nerve impairment.

Assess the client's ability to frown, show teeth, blow out cheeks, raise eyebrows, smile, and close eyes tightly.

Asymmetry or decreased movement of facial muscles is noted with lesions of the upper and lower motor neurons. Paralysis of the lower motor neurons results in the inability to close eyes, a flat nasolabial fold, paralysis of lower face,

ASSESSMENT TECHNIQUE	POSSIBLE ABNORMAL FINDINGS
	and inability to wrinkle forehead. Paralysis of the upper motor neurons results in weakness of eyelids and paralysis of lower face.
	Pain, paralysis, and sagging of facial muscles is seen on the affected side in Bell's palsy.
■ **Test CN VIII (acoustic).** Assess the client's ability to hear the ticking of a watch and whispered and spoken words (see Chapter 43).	Decreased hearing or deafness may occur with CVAs of the vertebralbasilar arteries and/or tumors of CN VIII.
■ **Test CN IX and X (glossopharyngeal and vagus).** Observe as the client swallows a small amount of water. Observe for a symmetrical rise of the soft palate and uvula as the client says "ah." Assess gag reflex by touching back of client's throat with tongue blade. Assess the client's ability to taste salty, sweet, and sour substances on the posterior third of the tongue (see previous description).	**Dysphagia** (difficulty swallowing) is common with impaired blood flow to the vertebralbasilar arteries and to the posterior inferior, anterior inferior, or superior cerebellar arteries. Unilateral loss of the gag reflex occurs with lesions of CN IX and X.
■ **Test CN XI (spinal accessory).** Assess the client's ability to shrug the shoulders and turn head against resistance: Ask the client to turn the head to one side against the resistance of your hand; ask the client to shrug the shoulders while you exert downward pressure. Observe symmetry, strength, and size of muscles.	Muscle weakness is noted with lower motor neuron disease. Contralateral hemiparesis is seen with CVAs affecting the middle or internal carotid artery.
■ **Test CN XII (hypoglossal).** Assess the client's ability to project the tongue and move the tongue from side to side against resistance of tongue blade.	Atrophy and fasciculations of the tongue are seen in lower motor neuron disease. The tongue may deviate towards involved side of the body.

Sensory Examination

Testing for sensation is the third part of the neurologic examination. Have the client close the eyes, and scatter stimuli (sharp, dull, hot, cold, light touch, and vibration) over all dermatomes.

ASSESSMENT TECHNIQUE	POSSIBLE ABNORMAL FINDINGS
■ **Assess the client's ability to perceive various sensations.** Touch both sides of various parts of the body (the chest, abdomen, arms, and legs) with one or more of the following: 1. Cotton wisp 2. Sharp object 3. Dull object 4. Test tubes of hot and cold water 5. Vibrating tuning fork placed on bony prominences	Decreased sensation of pain occurs with injury to the spinothalamic tract. Decreased vibratory sensations are seen with injuries to the posterior column tract. Transient numbness of face, arm, or hand is seen with TIAs. Sensory loss on one side of the body is seen with lesions of higher pathways to

ASSESSMENT TECHNIQUE	POSSIBLE ABNORMAL FINDINGS

the spinal cord. Bilateral sensory loss is seen in polyneuropathy. Sensations are impaired with CVAs.

Lesions of the posterior column of the spinal cord may affect sense of position.

- **Assess the client's sense of position (kinesthesia).**

Move the client's finger or big toe up or down while the client keeps the eyes closed. Ask the client to describe the movement.

- **Assess the client's ability to discriminate fine touch.**

Ask the client to identify the following:

1. Object in hand, such as a coin or key (tests *stereognosis*).

2. Number written on hand (tests *graphesthesia*) (Figure 39–9).

Inability to discriminate fine touch (stereognosis, graphesthesia, two points, point localization and extinction) may occur with injury to the posterior columns or sensory cortex.

Figure 39–9
Testing graphesthesia.

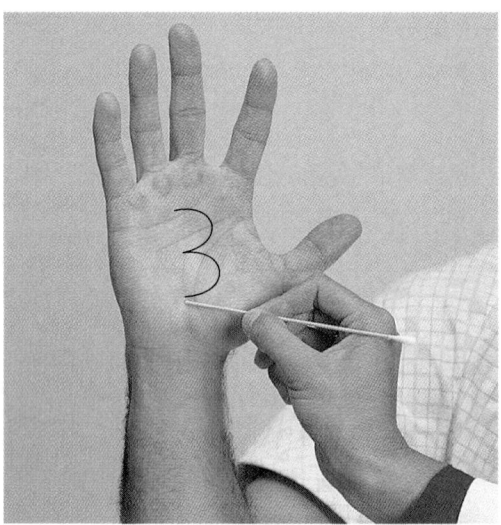

3. Two points of simultaneous pinpricks on the hand (tests *two-point discrimination*) (Figure 39–10).

Figure 39–10
Testing two-point discrimination.

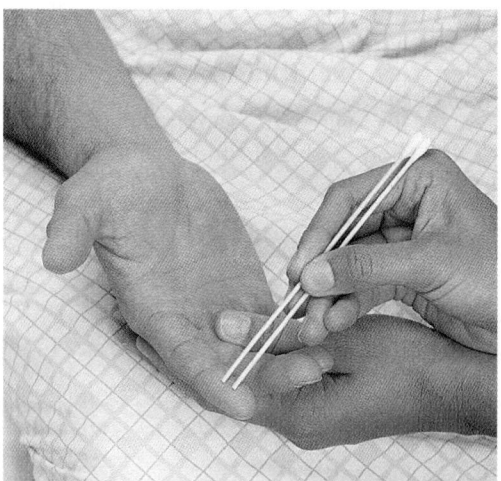

4. Where he/she is being touched (tests *localization*).

5. How many sensations are felt when touched simultaneously on both sides of the body (tests *extinction*).

The Physical Assessment (continued)

Motor Examination

Examination of the motor system requires inspection of the size, tone, movement, and strength of all body muscles and includes bilateral comparisons. Muscle tone and strength is assessed by having the client move each of the major muscle groups against resistance. The following criteria for recording the grading of muscle strength are often used:

0 = no contraction

1 = trace of contraction

2 = active movement with gravity

3 = active movement against gravity

4 = active movement against gravity and resistance

5 = normal power

ASSESSMENT TECHNIQUE	POSSIBLE ABNORMAL FINDINGS
■ **Assess bilateral symmetry and size of muscles.**	Atrophy of muscles is seen with disease of the lower motor neurons.
■ **Assess for tremors and fasciculations.** Observe movements as client is at rest (not making a purposeful movement) and with activity (making a purposeful movement, such as reaching for a glass of water).	**Tremors** (rhythmic movements) that occur with activity are seen in multiple sclerosis and disease of the cerebellar system. Tremors that occur at rest and disappear with movement are common in Parkinson's disease. **Fasciculations** (twitching) occur in disease of the lower motor neurons.
■ **Assess for muscle tone.**	Muscle tone is decreased (*flaccidity*) in disease of the lower motor neurons and early CVAs. Muscle tone is increased (*spasticity*) in disease of the corticospinal motor tract. Muscles are rigid in disease of the extrapyramidal motor tract. Muscles move in small, regular jerky movements (*cogwheel rigidity*) in Parkinson's disease.
■ **Assess bilateral muscle strength and movement.** Ask the client to: 1. Squeeze your hands. 2. Push his/her feet against the resistance of your hands. 3. Raise both legs off the bed.	Weakness of the arms, legs, or hands is often seen with TIAs. Hemiplegia is noted with CVAs of the internal carotid artery and posterior cerebral artery. Weakness of extremities is often noted with CVAs of the vertebralbasilar arteries. Flaccid paralysis is noted with CVA of the anterior spinal artery. Paralysis or decreased movement is seen in multiple sclerosis and myasthenia gravis. There is total loss of motor function below the level of injury in complete spinal cord transection and in injuries to the anterior portion of the spinal cord.

Assessment Technique	Possible Abnormal Findings
	A variety of motor losses is seen with injury to the cauda equina. Spasticity of muscles may occur as a result of incomplete spinal cord injuries, which may result in contraction of muscles.

Cerebellar Examination

To assess the client's cerebellar function, test the client's ability to keep his or her balance and to perform coordinated movements.

Assessment Technique	Possible Abnormal Findings
■ **Assess the client's gait.** Ask the client to walk normally, then in a heel-to-toe fashion, then on toes, and finally on heels.	The following abnormalities of gait may be observed: ■ **Ataxia** is a lack of coordination and a clumsiness of movements. Gait is staggering, wide-based, and imbalanced. Ataxia is often seen with anterior CVAs and cerebellar tumors. Swaying and falling is seen in cerebellar ataxia. Inability to walk on toes, then heels may indicate disease of the upper motor neurons. ■ *Spastic hemiparesis* is often associated with CVA or upper motor neuron disease. The client walks with one leg stiffly dragging while the other leg circles out and forward. One arm is held flexed and close to the side. ■ *Steppage gait* is noted with disease of the lower motor neurons. The client drags or lifts the foot high, then slaps the foot onto the floor. The client cannot walk on the heels. *Sensory ataxia* may be associated with polyneuropathy or damage to the posterior columns. The client walks on the heels before bringing down the toes. The feet are held wide apart. The client staggers and watches the floor while walking. Gait worsens with the eyes closed. *Parkinsonian gait* is often seen in Parkinson's disease. The client stoops over while walking and shuffles the feet. The arms are held close to the side.
Perform Romberg's test: Ask the client to stand with the feet together and eyes closed. Stand close to client to prevent falling. There should be minimal swaying for up to 20 seconds.	A positive Romberg's test may be seen in cerebellar ataxia.

ASSESSMENT TECHNIQUE	POSSIBLE ABNORMAL FINDINGS

■ **Assess the client's coordination.**

Observe the client's ability to pat knees, alternating front and back of hands and increasing speed.

Observe the client's ability to touch each finger of one hand to the thumb.

Observe the client's ability to touch the nose, then one of your fingers, then the nose again.

Observe the client's ability to run each heel down each shin, while in a supine position (Figure 39–11).

Ataxic movements are apparent in cerebellar disease.

Figure 39–11
Heel-to-shin test.

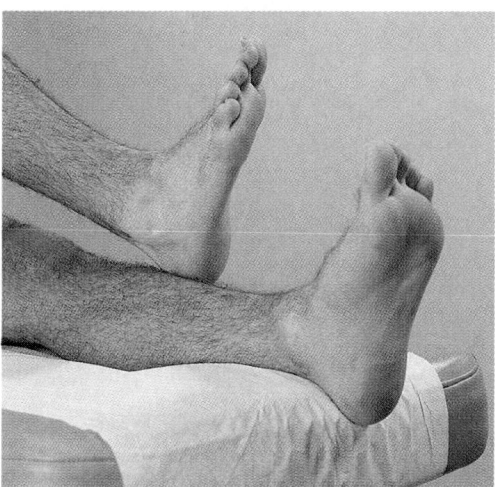

Reflex Examination

The last part of the neurologic examination is the testing of reflexes. A reflex hammer is used to strike the tendon of various reflex sites. To test deep-tendon reflexes, ask the client to lock the fingers of both hands together and then pull; this encourages relaxation and promotes reflexes of lower extremities. Superficial reflexes are elicited by lightly stroking the area to be assessed with the end of a tongue blade. The following criteria for recording reflexes are often used. A score of 2 is considered normal.

0 = absent or no response

1 = hypoactive; weaker than normal (+)

2 = normal (++)

3 = stronger than normal (+++)

4 = hyperactive (++++)

ASSESSMENT TECHNIQUE	POSSIBLE ABNORMAL FINDINGS

■ **Assess the following deep-tendon reflexes** (Figure 39–12):

1. Patellar
2. Biceps
3. Brachioradialis
4. Triceps
5. Achilles

Hyperactive reflexes are present with lesions of upper motor neurons as in CVAs. Decreased reflexes are present with lower motor neuron involvement, as in spinal cord injuries.

ASSESSMENT TECHNIQUE

POSSIBLE ABNORMAL FINDINGS

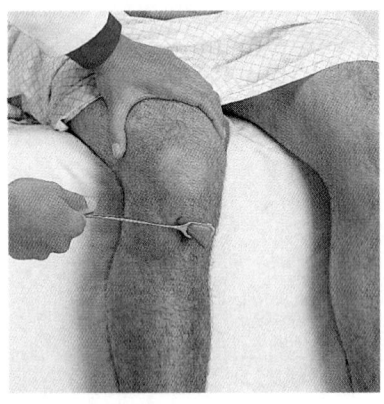

A

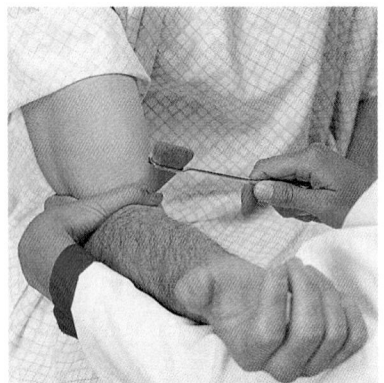

B

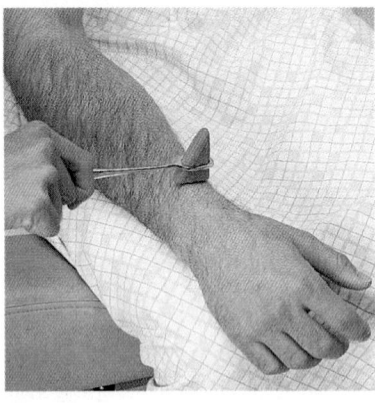

C

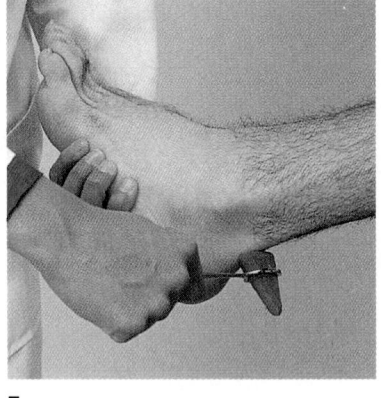

D

Figure 39–12   Deep-tendon reflexes.
A, Using reinforcement technique to test
the patellar reflex. *B,* Biceps reflex.
C, Brachioradialis reflex. *D,* Triceps reflex.
E, Achilles reflex.

E

- **Assess for clonus.**

Dorsiflex the client's foot.

A hyperactive, rhythmic dorsiflexion and plantar flexion of the foot are noted with upper motor neuron disease.

- **Assess the superficial abdominal and cremasteric reflexes.**

1. Abdominal reflex: Lightly stroke the abdomen with a tongue blade from the side to the midline. Normally, the side of the abdomen being stroked will contract (Figure 39–13).

Superficial reflexes may be absent with disease of the lower and upper motor neurons.

Figure 39–13 Location of superficial abdominal reflexes.

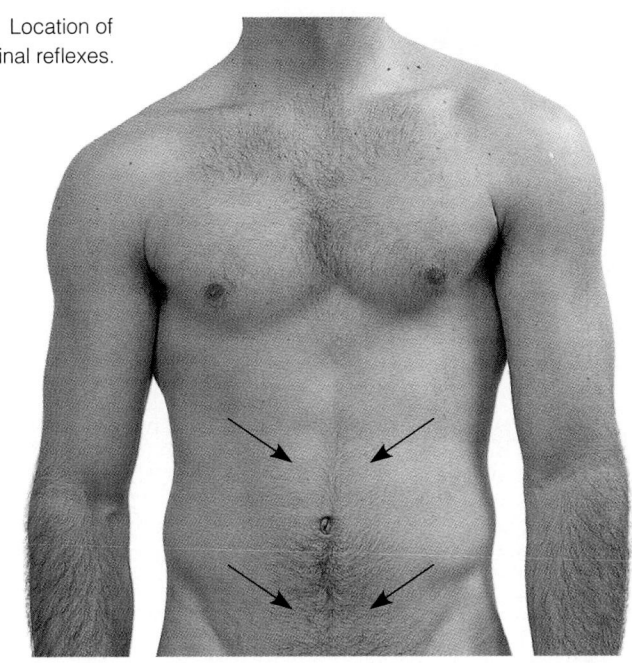

2. Cremasteric reflex: Lightly stroke the inner thigh of the male client with a tongue blade. Normally, the testicle on the side being stroked will rise.

■ **Assess the Babinski reflex** (Figure 39–14).

Dorsiflexion of the big toe and fanning of the other toes is seen with upper motor neuron disease of the pyramidal tract.

Figure 39–14 Testing for the Babinski reflex.

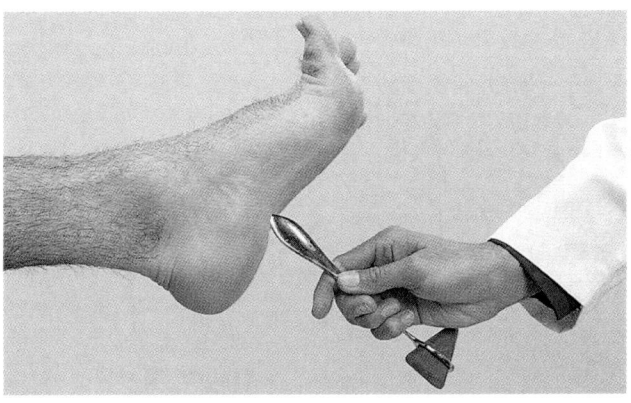

Special Neurologic Examinations

Brudzinski's and Kernig's signs are assessed in the presence of suspected meningeal irritation (as when the client has meningitis). Abnormal postures are assessed in comatose clients.

■ **Assess for Brudzinski's sign.**

With the client supine, flex the head to the chest (Figure 39–15).

Pain, resistance, and flexion of hips and knees occur with meningeal irritation.

ASSESSMENT TECHNIQUE	POSSIBLE ABNORMAL FINDINGS

Figure 39–15
Testing for
Brudzinski's sign.

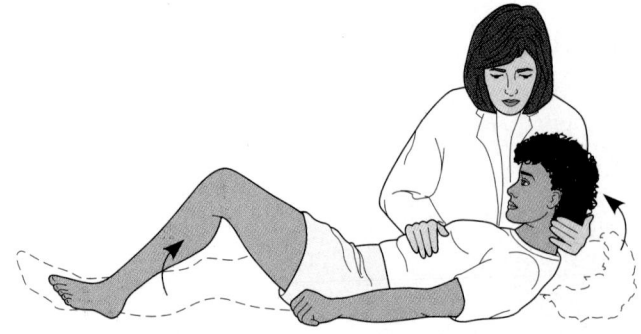

■ **Assess for Kernig's sign.**

With the client supine, flex the knees and hips, then straighten the knee (Figure 39–16).

Excessive pain and/or resistance occurs with meningeal irritation.

Figure 39–16   Testing for
Kernig's sign.

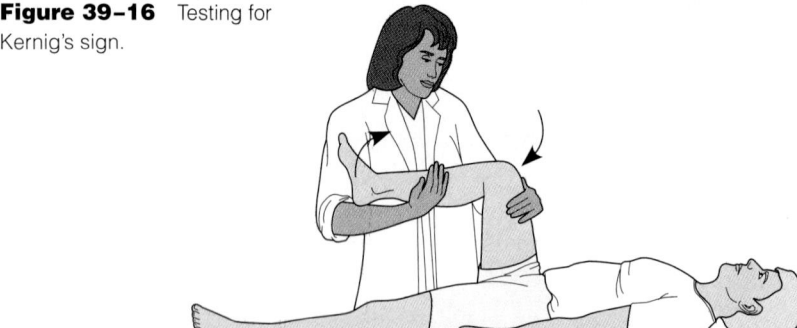

■ **Assess for abnormal postures.**

Observe for *decorticate posturing,* in which the upper arms are close to the sides; the elbows, wrists, and fingers are flexed; the legs are extended with internal rotation; and the feet are plantar flexed (Figure 39–17).

Decorticate posturing occurs with lesions of the corticospinal tracts.

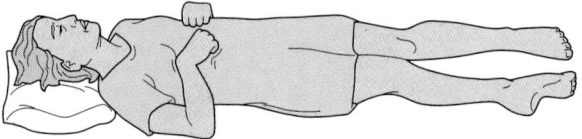

Figure 39–17   Decorticate rigidity.

Observe for *decerebrate posturing,* in which the neck is extended, with the jaw clenched; the arms are pronated, extended, and close to the sides; the legs are extended straight out; and the feet are plantar flexed (Figure 39–18).

Decerebrate posturing occurs with lesions of the midbrain, pons, or diencephalon.

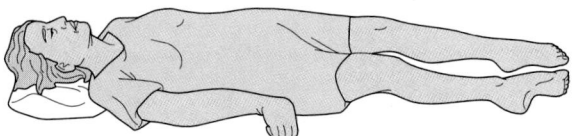

Figure 39–18   Decerebrate rigidity.

Variations in Assessment Findings for the Older Adult

As one ages, neurons continue to die without being replaced, and the weight and mass of the brain decline. However, intellectual function continues at a nearly optimal level, unless disease impairs the function of the brain; for example, arteriosclerosis and hypertension may lead to a CVA that causes brain damage. Older people respond to questions more slowly, and sensations, reflexes, and motor coordination decline. Thus, when interviewing the older client, it is important to ask questions slowly and clearly and to allow adequate time for the client to respond. When testing the client's ability to perceive various tactile stimuli, be prepared to use more pressure before the client perceives the sensation. Although sensation may be decreased, it should be symmetrical. Other age-related changes include the following:

- All reflexes may be decreased, and the abdominal and plantar reflexes may be absent. Often, the ankle reflex is the first tendon reflex lost with aging.

- It may be difficult for the older client to perform alternating movements.

- Senile tremors at rest may be observed in the hands; the head may nod, and the tongue may protrude. However, this type of senile tremor is benign and does not have any associated rigidity, as occurs in Parkinson's disease.

- The older client usually walks with a gait that is slower and more deliberate than that of the younger client, and the posture may be stooped.

- Motor strength may decrease slightly.

- Vibratory sensation, especially in the feet and ankles, decreases.

- There is a progressive decrease in the ability to taste and smell.

- Visual acuity and color vision decrease.

- The pupil may respond more slowly to light.

Bibliography

■ ■ ■

Barber, E., & Moore, K. (1992). Perfecting the art: Neurological assessment, *RN, 55*(4), 28–34.

Barker, E, & Moore, K. (1992). Cranial nerve assessment. *RN, 55*(4), 62–69.

Boss, B. J. (1991). Attention and memory systems: Nursing assessment. *AXON, 12*(4), 89–94.

Braverman, B. G. (1990). Eliciting assessment data from the patient who is difficult to interview. *Nursing Clinics of North America, 25*(4), 743–750.

Crosby, L. et al. (1989). Clinical neurological assessment tool: Development & testing of an instrument to index neurological status. *Heart & Lung, 18*(2), 121–129.

Dykes, P. C. (1993). Minding the five Ps of neurovascular assessment. *American Journal of Nursing,93*(6), 38–39.

Ellis, A., & Cavanagh, S. (1992). Aspects of neurosurgical assessment using the Glasgow Coma Scale. *Intensive & Critical Care Nursing, 8*(2), 94–99.

Hogstel, M. O. (1991). Assessing mental status. *Journal of Gerontological Nursing, 17*(5), 42–43.

Lower, J. (1992). Rapid neuro assessment. *American Journal of Nursing, 92*(6), 38–45, 47–48.

McHugh, J., & McHugh, W. (1990). How to assess deep tendon reflexes. *Nursing 90, 20*(8), 62–64.

Marieb, E. N. (1995). *Human anatomy and physiology* (3rd ed.). Redwood City, CA: Benjamin/Cummings.

Neatherlin, J. S. (1991). Neurologic assessment: You can make a difference in cost. *Journal of Neuroscience Nursing, 23*(2), 107–110.

Phipps, M. A. (1991). Assessment of neurological deficits in stroke: Acute care and rehabilitation implications. *Nursing Clinics of North America, 26*(4), 957–970.

Purath, J. (1991). Assessing headache pain. *RN, 54*(10), 26–31.

Rubin-Terrado, M. (1991). Don't choke on this: A swallowing assessment. *Geriatric Nursing: American Journal of Care for the Aging, 12*(6), 288–291.

Sullivan, J. (1990). Neurological assessment. *Nursing Clinics of North America, 25*(4), 795–809.

Nursing Care of Clients with Intracranial Disorders

LEARNING OBJECTIVES

LEARNING OBJECTIVES

After completing this chapter, you will be able to

- Describe the pathophysiology of altered level of consciousness, increased intracranial pressure, seizures, and headaches.
- Describe the pathophysiology of craniocerebral trauma, cranial infections, and tumors.
- Identify laboratory and diagnostic tests used to diagnose intracranial disorders.

- Discuss nursing implications for specific medications prescribed for the client with intracranial disorders.
- Discuss collaborative care measures for clients with intracranial disorders.
- Describe nursing interventions in the preoperative and postoperative care of the client having intracranial surgery.
- Use the nursing process as a framework for providing individualized care to clients with intracranial disorders.

The client with an intracranial disorder presents a unique challenge to the nurse. Problems that the client experiences in the acute stage of the disorder are often a prelude to long-term problems requiring ongoing management. These long-term problems range from alterations in the body's basic functioning to dysfunctions in the complex processes of the human mind. Systemic neurologic problems may accompany or develop secondary to an intracranial disorder. Intracranial disorders may affect not only the client's quality of life but also that of the client's family. The complex nature of intracranial disorders requires an astute and accurate nursing assessment that may mean the difference between life and death for the client.

This chapter begins with a discussion of manifestations of altered intracranial function. Further discussion focuses on craniocerebral trauma, cranial infections, inflammations, and neoplasms. General principles related to the care of the client having neurosurgery also are described.

Altered Intracranial Function

Manifestations of altered intracranial function may include an altered level of consciousness, increased intracranial pressure, headache, and seizure activity. These manifestations may occur alone or as part of a systemic disease process.

The Client with an Altered Level of Consciousness

Many disorders discussed in this chapter and the chapters that follow may affect the client's level of consciousness

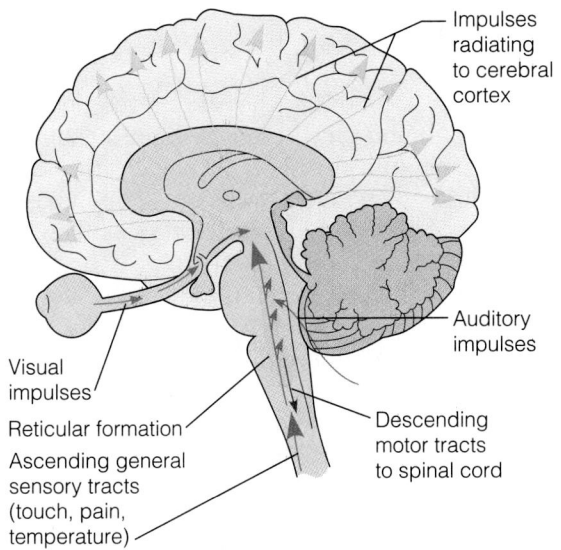

Figure 40–1 The reticular formation extends the length of the brain stem. The reticular activating system, a system of cells within the reticular formation, maintains arousal.

(LOC). Consciousness is a condition in which the person is aware of self and the environment and is able to respond appropriately to stimuli. Full consciousness requires both normal arousal and full cognition:

- Arousal, or alertness, depends on the reticular activating system (RAS), a diffuse system of neurons in the thalamus and upper brain stem.

- Cognition is a more complex process involving all mental activities controlled by the cerebral hemispheres, including thought processes, memory, perception, problem solving, and emotion.

These two components of consciousness depend on the normal physiologic function of and connection between the arousal mechanisms of the reticular formation and the cognitive functions of the cerebral hemispheres.

Because arousal and cognition are independent components of consciousness, each can act separately on stimuli. For example, the RAS reacts to the discomfort caused by a full bladder by waking the person in the middle of the night. Once awake, however, the frontal cortex is what alerts the person that the bladder is full and prompts the person to go to the bathroom and empty it.

The physiologic seat of consciousness, the *reticular formation,* is a diffuse structure extending the length of the brain stem (Figure 40–1). The axons of reticular neurons are exceptionally long and branch outward to cells in the hypothalamus, thalamus, cerebellum, and spinal cord. A system of reticular neurons within the reticular formation, the **reticular activating system (RAS),** passes steady streams of impulses through thalamic relays in order to stimulate the cerebral cortex into wakefulness. Furthermore, the body's sensory tracts interact with RAS neu-

Table 40–1	Terms Used to Describe Level of Consciousness
Term	**Characteristics of Client**
Full consciousness	Alert; oriented to time, place, and person; comprehends spoken and written words
Confusion	Unable to think rapidly and clearly; easily bewildered, with poor memory and short attention span; misinterprets stimuli; judgment is impaired
Disorientation	Not aware of or not oriented to time, place, or person
Obtundation	Lethargic, somnolent; responsive to verbal or tactile stimuli but quickly drifts back to sleep
Stupor	Generally unresponsive; may be briefly aroused by vigorous, repeated, or painful stimuli; may shrink away from or grab at the source of stimuli
Semicomatose	Does not move spontaneously; unresponsive to stimuli, although vigorous or painful stimuli may result in stirring, moaning, or withdrawal from the stimuli, without actual arousal
Coma	Unarousable; will not stir or moan in response to any stimulus; may exhibit nonpurposeful response (slight movement) of area stimulated but makes no attempt to withdraw
Deep coma	Completely unarousable and unresponsive to any kind of stimulus, including pain; absence of brain stem reflexes, corneal, pupillary, and pharyngeal reflexes and tendon and plantar reflexes

rons; this interrelationship helps control the strength of the RAS's rousing effect on the cerebrum (Marieb, 1995).

Conditions that affect either the reticular activating system or the function of the cerebral hemispheres can interfere with the normal level of consciousness. Although terms such as *stupor, obtundation,* or *coma* are commonly used to refer to altered LOC (see Table 40–1), lack of standardization of these terms makes them less useful in the clinical setting. Nurses should remember that consciousness is a dynamic state: A client may pass from full consciousness to coma within hours or experience a slow diminishment of consciousness that does not become evident for weeks or months. The nurse can help provide effective care for a client with an altered level of consciousness by looking beyond the diagnostic labels of consciousness and accurately assessing the client's behavior and response to stimuli.

Pathophysiology

Level of consciousness may be altered by processes that affect the arousal functions of the brain stem, the cognitive functions of the cerebral hemispheres, or both. Coma usually is due to one of two causes (Wilson, Braunwald, Isselbacher, Petersdorf, Martin, Fauci, & Root, 1991):

- Damage to or suppression of the RAS by direct damage to the brain stem, by ischemia, or by a metabolic disorder; or
- Bilateral damage to the cerebral hemispheres or suppression of their function by drugs or toxins

When the RAS is damaged, the person's ability to maintain wakefulness and arousal is impaired. Cerebrovascular disease is the most common cause of RAS destruction. Other causes include demyelinating diseases such as multiple sclerosis, tumors, abscesses, and head injury. Function of the RAS may be suppressed by compression of the brain stem, which produces edema and ischemia. Pressure and compression of the brain stem may be due to tumors, increased intracranial pressure, hematomas or hemorrhage, or aneurysm (McCance & Huether, 1994). Although it is possible to assess level of consciousness or arousal in the client with RAS damage, the impairment in arousal may make it impossible to assess cognitive function.

The function of the brain, especially the cerebral hemispheres, depends on continuous blood flow with unimpeded supplies of oxygen and glucose. Processes that disrupt this flow of blood and nutrients may cause widespread damage to the cerebral hemispheres, impairing arousal and cognition. Bilateral hemispheric lesions, such as global ischemia, or metabolic disorders, such as hypoglycemia, are the most common causes of altered LOC related to cerebral dysfunction of the hemispheres. Localized masses, such as a hematoma or cerebral edema, that displace normal structures and cause direct or indirect pressure on the opposite hemisphere or brain stem can also affect LOC (Wilson et al., 1991). The client who has widespread damage to the cerebral hemispheres but an intact RAS has sleep-wake cycles and may rouse in response to stimuli; the client cannot be said to be alert, however, because cognition is impaired.

Both localized neurologic processes and systemic disorders can alter LOC. Processes occurring within the brain, which may directly destroy or compress neurologic structures, including the following:

- Head trauma
- Increased intracranial pressure
- Cerebrovascular accident (CVA), or stroke
- Hematoma
- Intracranial hemorrhage
- Tumors
- Infections
- Demyelinating disorders

Any systemic condition that affects the delivery of blood, oxygen, and glucose to the brain or alters cell membranes may also alter LOC. As noted earlier, normal brain metabolism and function require continuous supplies of oxygen and glucose. If cerebral blood flow is impaired or the client becomes hypoxic or hypoglycemic, cerebral metabolism deteriorates, and level of consciousness declines rapidly. Clients at particular risk include those with poorly controlled diabetes and those with cardiac or respiratory failure.

Other metabolic alterations that can affect LOC include fluid and electrolyte imbalances, such as hyponatremia or hyperosmolality, and acid-base alterations, such as hypercapnia (an elevated PCO_2). Accumulated waste products and toxins from liver or renal failure can affect neuronal and neurotransmitter function, altering LOC. Drugs that depress the central nervous system (e.g., alcohol, analgesics, anesthetics) suppress metabolic and membrane activities in the RAS and cerebral hemispheres, thereby affecting LOC.

Seizure activity, abnormal electrical discharges from a local area of the brain or from the entire brain, commonly affects LOC. It appears that the spontaneous, disordered discharge of activity that occurs during a seizure exhausts energy metabolites or produces locally toxic molecules altering LOC for a period of time following the seizure. Consciousness returns when the metabolic balance of the neurons is restored (Wilson et al., 1991).

Manifestations

Except in the case of direct damage to the brain stem and RAS, brain function deterioration and changes in LOC usually follow a predictable rostral to caudal progression, that is, a pattern in which higher levels of function are impaired initially, progressing to impairment of more primitive functions. Altered LOC and behavior changes are early manifestations of the deterioration of the function of the cerebral hemispheres. Structures in the midbrain and brain stem are affected sequentially, with characteristic changes in motor function, pupillary response, and breathing patterns (Porth, 1994). Manifestations of progressive deterioration of brain function are outlined in Table 40–2.

Arousal As the impairment of brain function progresses, more stimuli are required to elicit a response from the client. Initially, the client may rouse to verbal stimuli and respond appropriately to questions, remaining oriented to time, place, and person. With deterioration of neurologic function, the client becomes more difficult to rouse and may become agitated and confused when awakened. Orientation to time is lost initially, followed by orientation to place and then to person. Contin-

Table 40–2 Progression of Deteriorating Brain Function

Level of Consciousness	Pupillary Response	Oculomotor Responses	Motor Responses	Breathing
Alert; oriented to time, place, and person	Brisk and equal; pupils regular	Eyes move as head turns Caloric testing (ear irrigation) produces nystagmus	Purposeful movement; responds to commands	Regular pattern with normal rate and depth
Responds to verbal stimuli; decreased concentration; agitation, confusion, lethargy; disoriented	Small and reactive	Roving eye movements; doll's eyes positive, with gaze fixed straight ahead; eye deviation away from cold caloric stimulus and toward warm stimulus	Purposeful movement in response to pain stimulus	Yawning, sighing respirations
Requires continuous stimulation to rouse			Decorticate positioning with upper extremity flexion	Cheyne-Stokes respirations with crescendo-decrescendo pattern in rate and depth followed by period of apnea
Reflexive positioning to pain stimulus	Pupils fixed (nonreactive) in midposition	Caloric testing produces nystagmus	Decerebrate positioning with adduction and rigid extension of upper and lower extremities	Central neurogenic hyperventilation with rapid, regular, and deep respirations; apneustic breathing with prolonged inspiration and pauses at full inspiration and following expiration
No response to stimuli	Pupils fixed in midposition	No spontaneous eye movement or nystagmus	Extension of upper extremities with flexion of lower extremities; flaccidity	Cluster or ataxic breathing with irregular pattern and depth of respirations; gasping respirations or apnea

uous stimulation or vigorous shaking is required to maintain wakefulness as LOC decreases. Eventually, no response is obtained, even with deep painful stimuli.

Pupillary and Oculomotor Responses A predictable progression of pupillary and oculomotor responses also occurs as level of consciousness deteriorates toward coma. If the lesion or process affecting neurologic function is localized, effects may initially be seen in the ipsilateral pupil (the pupil on the same side as the lesion). With generalized or systemic processes, pupils are affected equally. If the pupils are small and equally reactive, metabolic processes affecting LOC may be present. With compression of cranial nerve III at the midbrain, the pupils may become oval or eccentric (off center) (Wilson et al., 1991). As the level of functional impairment progresses, the pupils become fixed (unresponsive to light) and, eventually, dilated.

In deteriorating LOC and coma, spontaneous eye movement is lost and reflexive ocular movements are altered. Normally, both eyes move simultaneously in the same direction; injury to the cranial nerve nuclei in the midbrain and pons can impair normal movement. *Doll's eye movements* are reflexive movements of the eyes in the opposite direction of head rotation; they are an indicator of brain stem function (Figure 40–2). As a result of the oculocephalic reflex, the eyes move upward with passive flexion of the neck; with passive extension, they move downward. *Doll's eyes present* is the normal response to passive head movement. As brain stem function deteriorates, this reflex is lost. The eyes fail to turn together and, eventually, remain fixed in the midposition as the head is turned. This response is called *doll's eyes absent* (Hickey, 1992; McCance & Huether, 1994).

The oculovestibular response is tested by instilling cold water into the ear canal (cold caloric testing).

Head in neutral position

Head rotated to client's left

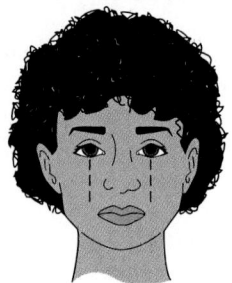

Eyes midline

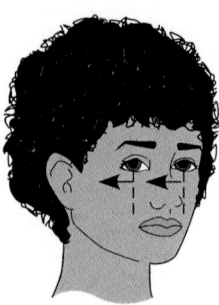

Doll's eyes present:
Eyes move right in
relation to head.

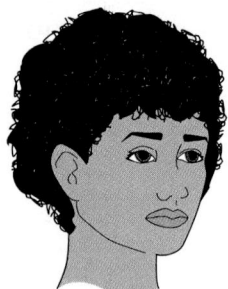

Doll's eyes absent:
Eyes do not move
in relation to head.
Direction of vision follows
head to left.

Figure 40–2 Doll's eye movements characteristic of altered level of consciousness.

Normally, this stimulus causes nystagmus (lateral tonic deviation of the eyes) toward the stimulus. This reflex is also lost as brain function deteriorates.

Motor Responses In altered LOC, motor responses to stimuli range from an appropriate response to a command (e.g., "squeeze my hand"; "push my hands away with your feet") to flaccidity. Initially, the client may be able to move purposefully away from a noxious stimulus, for example, to brush the examiner's hand away from the face. As function declines, movements become more generalized (withdrawal, grimacing) and less purposeful. Reflexive motor responses may occur, including decorticate movement with flexion of the upper extremities accompanied by extension of the lower extremities. With further decline, decerebrate posturing is seen, with adduction and rigid extension of the upper and lower extremities. Without intervention, the client eventually becomes flaccid, with little or no motor response to stimuli.

Breathing Progressive impairment of neural function also causes predictable changes in breathing patterns as respiratory centers become affected. These patterns are described and illustrated in Table 40–3.

The prognosis for clients with altered levels of consciousness and coma varies according to the underlying cause and pathologic process. Age and general medical condition also play a role in determining outcome. Young adults may fully recover following deep coma from head injury, drug overdose, or other cause. In general, the prognosis is poor for clients who lack pupillary reaction or reflex eye movements 6 hours after the onset of coma (Wilson et al., 1991). The Glasgow Coma Scale (see Chapter 39) is helpful in predicting the outcome of altered LOC but does not provide absolute evidence about the chances for recovery.

Possible outcomes of altered LOC and coma include full recovery with no long-term residual effects, recovery

with residual damage (such as learning deficits, emotional difficulties, or impaired judgment), or more severe consequences such as persistent vegetative state (cerebral death) or brain death.

Persistent Vegetative State
Persistent vegetative state, or *cerebral death,* is loss of function of the cerebral hemispheres while the brain stem and cerebellum remain intact and functional. While the homeostatic regulatory functions of the brain continue, the ability to respond meaningfully to the environment is lost (McCance & Huether, 1994).

The client in persistent vegetative state has sleep-wake cycles and retains the ability to chew, swallow, and cough but cannot interact with the environment. When awake, the client's eyes may wander back and forth across the room, but they cannot track an object or person.

Persistent vegetative state is usually the result of severe head injury or global anoxia. With appropriate supportive care, the client may remain in this state for many years. If the condition lasts for more than a few months, improvement or recovery is unlikely (Berkow & Fletcher, 1992).

Brain Death
Brain death is the cessation of cerebral blood flow with global brain infarction and permanent loss of all brain function (McCance & Huether, 1994). Although the exact criteria for establishing brain death may vary somewhat from state to state, it is generally agreed that brain death has occurred when there is no evidence of cerebral or brain stem function for an extended period (usually 6 to 24 hours) in a client who has a normal body temperature and is not affected by a depressant drug or alcohol poisoning. Generally recognized criteria follow:

- Unresponsiveness with absent motor and reflex movements (deep tendon reflexes may remain intact if the reflex loop to the spinal cord is unaffected)

Table 40–3	Breathing Patterns Characteristic of Altered Level of Consciousness

Pattern		Description
Cheyne-Stokes respirations	~wwwWWwww—wwWWWw~	A regular crescendo-decrescendo pattern with increasing then decreasing rate and depth of respirations followed by a period of apnea
Central neurogenic hyperventilation	ΛΛWWWWWWWWWWWW	A sustained pattern of rapid, regular, deep respirations (hyperpnea)
Apneustic breathing	⎍_⎍_⎍_	Prolonged inspiration with a pause at full inspiration followed by expiration and a possible pause following expiration
Cluster breathing	⅃ₗ_ₗₗₗₗ_ₗₗₗₗ_ₗₗ_ₗₗₗ	Clusters of several breaths with irregular periods of apnea between clusters
Ataxic respirations	⌃⌃⌃⌃⌃⌃	Respirations that are completely irregular in pattern and depth with irregular periods of apnea

- Pupils fixed (unresponsive to light) and dilated
- Absent corneal reflexes and ocular responses to head turning and caloric stimulation
- Apnea
- Lack of cerebral circulation

Apnea in the comatose client is established by removing the ventilator while maintaining oxygenation by tracheal cannula and allowing the P_{CO_2} to increase to 60 mm Hg or higher. This level of carbon dioxide is high enough to stimulate respiration if the brain stem is functional. The electroencephalogram (EEG) may be used to establish the absence of brain activity when brain death is suspected. A flat or isoelectric EEG over a period of 6 to 24 hours in a client who is not hypothermic or under the influence of drugs that depress the central nervous system is generally accepted as an indicator of brain death (McCance & Huether, 1994). Evidence of absent cerebral circulation may be established by brain scan, cerebral angiography, or transcranial Doppler measurements.

Locked-In Syndrome

Locked-in syndrome is distinctly different from persistent vegetative state. In locked-in syndrome, the client is alert and fully aware of the environment and has intact cognitive abilities but is unable to communicate through speech or movement because of blocked efferent pathways from the brain (McCance & Huether, 1994). Motor paralysis affects all voluntary muscles, although the upper cranial nerves (I through IV) may remain intact, allowing the client to communicate through eye movements and blinking (McCance & Huether, 1994). In essence, the client is "locked" inside a paralyzed body in which he or she remains fully conscious of self and environment. In-

farction or hemorrhage of the pons that disrupts outgoing nerve tracts but spares the RAS is the usual cause of locked-in syndrome. Locked-in syndrome may also result when the corticospinal tracts between the midbrain and pons are interrupted. Disorders of the lower motor neurons or muscles, such as acute polyneuritis, myasthenia gravis, or amyotrophic lateral sclerosis (ALS), may also paralyze motor responses, leading to locked-in syndrome.

Psychogenic Coma

Although uncommon, psychogenic disorders such as hysteria, catatonia, and severe depression can cause apparent alterations in a client's level of consciousness. Despite outward appearances, however, the person is physiologically awake (Berkow & Fletcher, 1992). Other manifestations of psychogenic coma vary markedly from the physiologic alterations that are present in LOC. For example, a client with catatonia may exhibit abnormal motor responses, often maintaining distorted postures for long periods of time. For a complete description of psychogenic disorders that produce apparent alterations in level of consciousness, consult a textbook in psychiatric nursing.

Collaborative Care

The neurologic assessment required for a client with an altered level of consciousness is the key to developing the plan of care. Five categories of neurologic function are examined: (1) level of consciousness; (2) vital signs, particularly the airway and breathing pattern; (3) pupillary reactions; (4) ocular movements; and (5) skeletal motor responses. See Chapter 39 for a complete presentation of neurologic assessment procedures.

Clients whose level of consciousness is altered because of acute processes require frequent and repeated assessments. The Glasgow Coma Scale (see Table 39–4 on page 1669) is an objective measurement tool used to evaluate changes in LOC. Although the Glasgow Coma Scale is valuable to track LOC, complete neurologic assessment requires assessment of the client's pupillary and oculomotor responses and breathing pattern.

Management of the client with an altered LOC or coma must begin immediately, even before assessment is complete. The focus of management is to identify the underlying cause, preserve function, and prevent deterioration if possible. Airway and breathing must be maintained during the initial acute stage until the diagnosis and prognosis can be established. Intravenous fluids are used to support circulation and to correct fluid, electrolyte, and acid-base imbalances. Treatment protocols to reduce increased intracranial pressure or control seizure activity (discussed later in this chapter) may be initiated. Changes in LOC associated with craniocerebral trauma, such as hematomas, often require immediate surgical intervention.

Laboratory and Diagnostic Tests

Although the client's history and physical examination findings often indicate the cause of coma and other alterations in LOC, several laboratory and diagnostic tests may be useful to establish the diagnosis. The following laboratory tests may be ordered to evaluate for possible metabolic, toxic, or drug-induced disorders:

- *Blood glucose* is measured immediately when coma is of unknown origin and hypoglycemia is suspected or possible. The brain contains minimal stores of glucose and is dependent on a continuous supply for metabolism. When the blood glucose falls to less than 40 to 50 mg/dL, cerebral function declines rapidly. The client with insulin-dependent diabetes is at particular risk for hypoglycemia-induced coma. Elevated blood glucose levels in the client with diabetes may also alter level of consciousness because of the effect of hyperglycemia on serum osmolality. In either diabetic ketoacidosis or hyperglycemic, hyperosmotic, nonketotic coma (HHNC), blood glucose levels may be greater than 400 mg/dL.

- *Serum electrolytes*—sodium, potassium, bicarbonate, chloride, and calcium in particular—are measured to assess for metabolic disturbances and guide intravenous therapy as needed. Hyponatremia, in which serum sodium levels are below 115 mEq/L (normal level: 135 to 145 mEq/L) is associated with coma and convulsions, especially if it develops rapidly (Wilson et al., 1991). Hyponatremia may be indicative of syndrome of inappropriate antidiuretic hormone (SIADH), in which the normal feedback mechanism

fails; that is, ADH secretion continues despite a decrease in serum osmolarity (see Chapter 20).

- *Serum osmolality* is evaluated. Both hyperosmolar and hypo-osmolar states may be associated with coma. Hyperosmolality (above 320 mOsm/kg H_2O), as occurs with diabetic ketoacidosis or HHNC, causes cellular dehydration of brain tissue as fluid is drawn into the vascular system by osmosis. Hypo-osmolality (less than 250 mOsm/kg H_2O), by contrast, leads to cerebral edema and swelling, impairing consciousness.

- *Arterial blood gases (ABGs)* are drawn to evaluate arterial oxygen and carbon dioxide levels as well as acid-base balance. Hypoxemia is a frequent cause of altered LOC; increased levels of carbon dioxide are also toxic to the brain and can induce coma, particularly when the onset of hypercapnia is acute.

- *Serum creatinine* and *blood urea nitrogen (BUN)* are measured to evaluate renal function. Although the exact cause of encephalopathy (altered brain function) in renal failure is not clearly understood, retained toxins have a detrimental effect on brain metabolism and function.

- *Liver function tests,* including bilirubin, AST, ALT, LDH, serum albumin, and serum ammonia levels are determined to evaluate hepatic function. High ammonia levels seen in hepatic failure interfere with cerebral metabolism and neurotransmitters, affecting level of consciousness (Wilson et al., 1991).

- *Toxicology screening* of blood and urine is done to determine whether altered LOC is the result of acute drug or alcohol toxicity. Serum alcohol levels are measured and the blood is assessed for the presence of substances such as barbiturates, carbon monoxide, or lead. Urine toxicology tests may include tests for illicit drugs.

- *Complete blood count (CBC) with differential* is drawn to assess for possible anemia or infectious causes of coma.

Diagnostic studies for the client with an altered level of consciousness include the following:

- *Computed tomography (CT) and magnetic resonance imaging (MRI) scanning* are done to detect neurologic damage due to hemorrhage, tumor, cyst, edema, myocardial infarction, or brain atrophy. These tests may also identify displacement of brain structures by large or expanding lesions. It is important to remember, however, that not all lesions or causes of altered LOC can be determined by CT scan or MRI.

- *Electroencephalogram (EEG)* is used to evaluate the electrical activity of the brain. The EEG is particularly valuable in identifying unrecognized seizure activity as a cause of altered LOC and is also useful in identifying certain infectious and metabolic causes of altered LOC.

A normal EEG in an unresponsive client may identify locked-in syndrome. In addition to the baseline EEG, evoked responses may also be determined. The EEG is monitored as an auditory tone or other sensory stimulus is provided to assess the brain's responsiveness (Wilson et al., 1991).

- *Radioisotope brain scan* is performed to identify abnormal lesions in the brain and evaluate cerebral blood flow.

- *Cerebral angiography* allows radiographic visualization of the cerebral vascular system. A radiopaque dye is injected into the carotid or vertebral arteries, followed by fluoroscopic and serial X-ray evaluation of the cerebral circulation. Lesions such as aneurysms, occluded vessels, or tumors can be identified. This exam may also be used to determine cessation of cerebral blood flow and brain death.

- *Transcranial Doppler studies* use an ultrasound velocity detector that records sound waves reflected from RBCs in blood vessels to assess cerebral blood flow.

- *Lumbar puncture with CSF analysis* is a vital diagnostic test when infection and possible meningitis are suspected as a cause of altered LOC.

Pharmacology

Pharmacologic treatment is used to support homeostasis and normal function for the client with altered LOC, as well as to treat specific underlying disorders. An intravenous catheter is inserted, and fluid balance is maintained using isotonic or slightly hypertonic solutions, such as normal saline or lactated Ringer's solution. The client's response to fluid administration is monitored carefully for evidence of increased cerebral edema.

If hypoglycemia is suspected, glucose is administered intravenously to restore cerebral metabolism rapidly. Conversely, insulin is administered to the client with hyperglycemia to reduce the blood glucose level and thus the serum osmolality. With suspected narcotic overdose or coma of unknown cause, naloxone is administered. Naloxone is a narcotic antagonist that competes for narcotic receptor sites, effectively blocking the depressant effect of the narcotic. Thiamine is usually administered with glucose, particularly if the client is malnourished or known to be an alcoholic, to prevent exacerbation of Wernicke's encephalopathy, a hemorrhagic encephalopathy due to thiamine deficiency and associated with chronic alcoholism (Wilson et al., 1991).

Any underlying fluid and electrolyte imbalance is corrected by administering medications or appropriate electrolytes. For the client who is hyponatremic and has a low serum osmolality, furosemide (Lasix) or an osmotic diuretic such as mannitol may be administered to promote water excretion. In acute processes causing coma, intravenous corticosteroids may be administered to reduce inflammation and swelling. Appropriate antibiotics are administered intravenously to the client with suspected or confirmed meningitis.

Surgery

Although surgery is not indicated for the majority of clients with altered LOC and coma, it may be necessary if the cause of coma is a tumor, hemorrhage, or hematoma. Surgical intervention is discussed later in this chapter, in the section on brain tumors. When there is a risk of increased intracranial pressure, the client is monitored continuously. These measures are discussed in the section on increased intracranial pressure.

Other Therapeutic Measures

Support of the airway and respirations is vital in the client with an altered LOC. The client who is drowsy but rousable may require little more than an oral pharyngeal airway. With more severe alterations in consciousness, the client may require endotracheal intubation to maintain airway patency, particularly if the cough and gag reflexes are absent. Mechanical ventilation is indicated when hypoventilation or apnea is present. Unless a do-not-resuscitate (DNR) order is in effect, mechanical ventilation should be initiated even if it has not been established that the disorder is reversible; without ventilatory support, cerebral anoxia develops rapidly, and brain death may ensue. ABGs are monitored frequently to determine the adequacy of ventilation. Hyperventilation may be used to reduce PCO_2 and promote cerebral vasoconstriction to reduce cerebral edema.

In clients with long-term alterations in consciousness, such as persistent vegetative state or locked-in syndrome, measures to maintain nutritional status are initiated. Enteral feedings with a gastrostomy tube are preferred if the client is unable to take food by mouth in adequate amounts without aspirating. In some cases, parenteral nutrition may be used.

Nursing Care

Nursing care of the client with an altered level of consciousness must anticipate a wide variety of client responses. Nursing diagnoses discussed in this section are directed toward the unconscious client and focus on problems with airway maintenance, skin integrity, contractures, and nutrition.

Ineffective Airway Clearance

Ineffective airway clearance related to loss of the cough reflex and the inability to expectorate is a major problem for the unconscious client. The cough reflex may be absent or impaired when conditions that produce coma depress the function of the medullary centers.

Nursing interventions with rationales follow:

- Assess the client's ability to clear secretions. Monitor breath sounds, rate and depth of respirations, dyspnea, and the presence of cyanosis. *The client's ability to clear secretions serves as the initial assessment base for developing further interventions.*

- In clients who are unconscious or who do not have an intact cough reflex, maintain an open airway by periodic suctioning, limiting the time of suctioning to 15 seconds or less. If the client has a basilar skull fracture or cerebral spinal fluid draining from the ears or nose, never suction nasally. *Periodic suctioning may be necessary to clear the airway of mucus, blood, or other drainage. Suctioning for more than 15 seconds in the client with increased intracranial pressure may cause hypercapnia, which in turn vasodilates cerebral vessels and further increases intracranial pressure (Hickey, 1992).*

- Turn the client from side to side every 2 hours, and maintain a side-lying position with the head of the bed elevated. Do not position the unconscious client on the back. *Turning the client from side to side facilitates respirations, prevents the tongue from obstructing the airway, and helps prevent pooling of secretions in one area of the lungs (thus decreasing the risk of pneumonia).*

- If the client has a tracheostomy, provide tracheostomy care every 4 hours and suction when secretions are present. (See Chapter 33.) *The client may be unable to maintain an open airway without a tracheostomy.*

Risk for Aspiration

The unconscious client with a depressed or absent gag and swallowing reflex is at high risk for aspiration. Drainage, mucus, or blood may obstruct the airway and interfere with oxygenation. Pooling of aspiration secretions in the lungs also increases the risk of pneumonia.

Nursing interventions with rationales follow:

- Assess swallowing and gag reflexes every shift as appropriate to the client's level of consciousness. *Deepening levels of unconsciousness may cause a loss in swallow and gag reflexes.*

- Monitor for and report manifestations of aspiration: crackles and wheezes, dullness to percussion over an area of the lungs, dyspnea, tachypnea, cyanosis. *Early recognition of these manifestations facilitates prompt intervention.*

- Provide interventions to prevent aspiration in the unconscious client:
  a. Maintain NPO status.
  b. Place the client in the side-lying position.
  c. Provide oral hygiene and suctioning as needed.
  Unconscious clients are never given oral food and fluids because of the risk of aspiration. The side-lying position allows secretions to drain from the mouth rather than into the pharynx. Oral hygiene and suctioning remove secretions that might otherwise be aspirated.

- Monitor the results of arterial blood gas analysis and pulse oximetry. Maintain records of trends. *The analysis of arterial blood gases and of pulse oximetry provides a direct measure of the oxygen content of blood and is a good indicator of the lungs' ability to oxygenate the blood.*

Risk for Impaired Skin Integrity

The unconscious client is at risk for impaired skin integrity as a result of immobility and the inability to provide self-care. On average, healthy people change positions during sleep every 11 minutes; the unconscious client often is unable to maintain the movement needed to prevent pressure on the skin, especially over bony prominences. As a result, the skin and subcutaneous tissues may become ischemic and prone to develop pressure ulcers. Perspiration and incontinence of urine and stool may exacerbate the problem. Nursing interventions are directed to maintaining the integrity not only of the skin, but also of the lips and mucous membranes.

Nursing interventions with rationales follow:

- Assess skin every shift, especially over bony prominences and around genitals and buttocks. *The large surface area of the skin bears weight and is in constant contact with the surface of the bed. The skin, subcutaneous tissue, and muscles, especially those tissues over bony prominences, undergo constant pressure. This impairs normal capillary blood flow, which interferes with the exchange of nutrients and waste products. Tissue ischemia and necrosis may result and lead to the development of pressure ulcers. Other contributing factors are moisture from bed linens and the forces of friction and shear. Continuous assessment provides the data necessary to develop an alternative plan of care. (For more information, see Chapter 17.)*

- Provide proper positioning. Reposition bed-ridden clients at least every 2 hours if this is consistent with the overall treatment goals. Keep the head of the bed elevated no higher than 30 degrees. Provide special pads and mattresses that distribute weight more evenly (e.g., silicone-filled pads, egg-crate cushions, turning frames, flotation pads). Lift the client instead of dragging the client across the sheet. *When the head of the bed is elevated above 30 degrees, the client's torso tends to slide down toward the foot of the bed. Friction and perspiration cause the skin and superficial fascia to remain fixed against the bed linens while the deep fascia and skeleton slide downward. When a person is pulled rather than lifted, the skin remains fixed to the sheet while the fascia and muscles are pulled upward.*

- Provide interventions to prevent breakdown of the skin and mucous membranes:
  a. Keep bed linens clean, dry, and wrinkle free.
  b. Provide daily bath with mild soap.
  c. Cleanse the skin following urine and fecal soiling with a mild cleansing agent.

d. Provide oral care and lubricate the lips every 2 to 4 hours.

e. Maintain accurate intake and output records.

f. Maintain accurate intravenous fluid administration.

g. Keep the cornea moist by instilling methyl cellulose solution (0.5% to 1%) and apply protective eye shields or close the eyelids with adhesive strips if the corneal reflex is absent.

Keeping linens clean, dry, and wrinkle free decreases the risk of injury from the shearing force of bed rest and protects against environmental factors that cause drying. Adequate hydration of the stratum corneum appears to protect the skin against mechanical insult. The prevention of dehydration improves the circulation. It also decreases the concentration of urine, thereby minimizing skin irritation in people who are incontinent. Proper eye care prevents corneal abrasion and irritation.

Impaired Physical Mobility

Clients who are unconscious are unable to maintain normal musculoskeletal movement and are at high risk for contractures related to decreased movement. Because the flexor and adductor muscles are stronger than the extensors and abductors, flexor and adductor contractures develop quickly if preventive measures are not instituted. Passive range-of-motion (ROM) exercises must be performed routinely to maintain muscle tone and function, to prevent additional disability, and to aid in restoration of impaired motor function.

Nursing interventions with rationales follow:

■ Maintain extremities in functional positions by providing proper support devices. Remove support devices every 4 hours for skin care and passive ROM exercises. Provide pillows for the axillary region; rolled washcloths may be placed in elevated hands; ask family to supply hightop shoes. *Pillows in the axillary region help prevent adduction of the shoulder. Rolled washcloths help decrease edema and flexion contracture of the fingers. Hightop shoes are useful in preventing plantar flexion. These support devices need to be removed every 4 hours to increase circulation to the area.*

■ Perform passive ROM exercises (unless contraindicated, as for the client with increased intracranial pressure) at least 4 times a day, keeping the following principles in mind:

a. Place one hand above the joint being exercised. The other hand gently moves the joint through its normal range of motion.

b. Move the body part to the point of resistance, and stop.

Placing one hand above the joint provides support against gravity and prevents unwanted movement. ROM exercises help prevent contractures by stretching muscles and tendons and maintaining joint mobility.

Risk for Altered Nutrition: Less Than Body Requirements

The unconscious client is at risk for an alteration in nutrition related to a reduced or complete lack of ability to eat. This is especially true for the client who is unconscious as the result of an infection or trauma, both of which increase metabolic requirements.

Nursing interventions with rationales follow:

■ Monitor nutritional status through daily weights (on bed scales) and laboratory data. *For accuracy, weigh the client at the same time each day, using the same scales. Ensure that the client wears the same clothing. Changes in laboratory data with decreased nutrition include a decrease in the levels of serum albumin and serum transferrin.*

■ Assess the need for alternative methods of nutritional support (tube feeding or total parenteral nutrition) through collaboration with dietitian. *Clients who are unable to take oral food will need parenteral nutrition or liquid feedings through a nasogastric, gastrostomy, or jejunostomy tube. Needs for protein, calories, zinc, and vitamin C increase during wound healing (refer to Chapter 7 for further details).*

Other Nursing Diagnoses

Other nursing diagnoses that may be appropriate for the client with an altered level of consciousness follow:

■ *Risk for Infection* related to retention of secretions in lungs

■ *Constipation* related to the inability to perceive the need to defecate

■ *Diarrhea* related to the inability to tolerate tube feedings

■ *Functional Urinary Incontinence* related to the inability to perceive the need to void

■ *Altered Protection* related to neurosensory alteration

■ *Self-Care Deficit: Bathing/Hygiene* related to unconscious state

Client and Family Teaching

Family members of a client with an altered level of consciousness are often very anxious. It is difficult for the family to deal with the uncertainty involved in the client's prognosis. They may experience various conflicting emotions, such as guilt and anger. Reinforce information provided by the physician, and encourage the family to talk to the client as though he or she were able to understand. Explain that this communication may initially seem awkward, but in time it will feel appropriate. Evaluate the family's readiness to receive explanations regarding the client's treatment and care. The presence of many tubes (e.g., intravenous line, catheter, ventilator) may be overwhelming to the family. Misperceptions of the seriousness of the situation can occur if a thorough explanation is not given. Include the family in the client's care as much as they wish to be involved.

Allow significant others to stay with the client whenever possible. Reinforce the need for family members to care for themselves by encouraging adequate meals and rest. Offer to contact support services, such as friends, neighbors, and social services that the hospital may provide. Ask family members to leave a telephone number where they can be reached, and assure them that they will be called if any significant changes occur. Encourage family members to call if they have questions or concerns.

Applying the Nursing Process

Case Study of a Client with an Altered Level of Consciousness: Martin Straight

Martin Straight is a physically active 52-year-old stockbroker. While jogging in the park during his lunch hour, Mr. Straight suddenly falls to his knees and then collapses on the pavement. A fellow runner sees that Mr. Straight is not breathing and is "turning blue." He initiates CPR, which is continued successfully by paramedics called to the scene.

Assessment
When Mr. Straight arrives at the coronary care unit 2 hours later, the nurse, Antonio Petrucci, performs the initial assessment. Mr. Petrucci finds that Mr. Straight's cardiopulmonary status is stable, with normal sinus rhythm and occasional unifocal premature ventricular contractions. Oxygen is administered through a face mask. His blood pressure is 90/60, and vasopressors are not required. His temperature is normal.

Mr. Straight does not open his eyes to command, noise, or pain. There is no purposeful movement, that is, no withdrawal from or localization of painful stimulation. His pupils are equal, round, 2 millimeters in diameter, and nonreactive to light. His deep tendon reflexes are symmetrically hyperactive, and he has bilateral positive Babinski responses. The neurologist diagnoses a coma due to acute anoxia following cardiopulmonary arrest, and feels it is too soon to predict Mr. Straight's chances for recovery.

Diagnosis
Mr. Petrucci makes the following diagnoses for Mr. Straight:

- *Ineffective Airway Clearance* related to altered level of consciousness
- *Risk for Aspiration* related to inability to cough

- *Risk for Impaired Skin Integrity* related to immobility
- *Risk for Altered Nutrition: Less Than Body Requirements* related to altered level of consciousness and inability to eat

Expected Outcomes
The expected outcomes for the plan of care specify that Mr. Straight will

- Maintain a clear airway.
- Demonstrate clear lung sounds.
- Maintain skin integrity.
- Maintain adequate nutritional status.

Planning and Implementation
The following interventions are planned and implemented for Mr. Straight:

- Assess Mr. Straight's ability to clear secretions.
- Turn Mr. Straight side to side every 2 hours, and maintain side-lying position with the head of the bed elevated 30 degrees.
- Listen for shrill or harsh respirations, and observe for obvious increase in efforts to breathe.
- Assess gag reflex every shift.
- Keep suction equipment available, and suction Mr. Straight's posterior pharynx and upper trachea as needed. In addition, monitor closely for dysrhythmias.
- Assess breath sounds every hour. Document results.
- Monitor and document the results of Mr. Straight's arterial blood gas analysis and pulse oximetry.
- Place Mr. Straight in a side-lying position while performing mouth care. Inspect his mouth every shift. Keep his lips moist with a water-soluble lubricant. Use toothettes to clean his tongue, gums, and roof of the mouth. Do not use agents containing lemon or alcohol.
- Maintain NPO status.
- Assess skin every shift, especially over bony prominences and around genitals and buttocks.
- Lift Mr. Straight when moving instead of dragging him across the sheet.
- Provide all physical care: Keep bed linens clean, dry, and wrinkle free; cleanse skin after episodes of urinary and fecal soiling with a mild cleansing agent; provide hair care. Provide adequate hydration as indicated. Keep the cornea moist by instilling methyl cellulose solution (0.5% to 1%) and apply protective eye shields or close the eyelids with adhesive strips.
- Assess fluid status and document intake and output.
- Monitor Mr. Straight for signs of nutritional deficit.

Evaluation

Ten hours after Mr. Straight is admitted to the CCU, Mr. Petrucci notices that Mr. Straight's neurologic status begins to change. Mr. Straight continues to be unresponsive to verbal stimuli but begins responding to painful stimulation. When pressure is applied to the nail bed, purposeful movement of each arm is noted. The pupils are 4 mm and minimally reactive to light. Corneal responses are present but depressed. The arterial blood gas analysis is within normal limits.

Critical Thinking in the Nursing Process

1. Mr. Straight was found unconscious. What assessments would you make at the scene, and what would you do to help maintain an open airway at the scene?

2. Mr. Straight's wife is understandably very upset. She says, "I know he's going to die." A nurse says "Oh, no, we have the best doctors in town here—they won't let him die." Was this an accurate response? Why or why not?

3. For clients who are unconscious, an indwelling urinary catheter usually is inserted. Clients who are unconscious are at risk for renal calculi. Explain how these two statements are related.

4. Design a care plan for Mr. Straight for the nursing diagnosis *Fluid Volume Deficit*.

The Client with Increased Intracranial Pressure

■ ■ ■

Intracranial pressure (ICP) is the pressure within the cranial cavity, usually measured as the pressure within the lateral ventricles (Porth, 1994). ICP normally is less than 15 mm Hg or 180 mm H_2O. Transient increases occur with normal activities such as coughing, sneezing, straining, or bending forward. These transient increases are not harmful; however, sustained increases in intracranial pressure can result in significant tissue ischemia and damage to delicate neural tissue. Cerebral edema is the most frequent cause of sustained increases in ICP. Other causes include head trauma, tumors, abscesses, stroke, inflammation, hemorrhage, and a number of other pathologic conditions.

In the adult, the rigid cranial cavity created by the skull is normally filled to capacity with three essentially noncompressible elements: the brain (80%), cerebrospinal fluid (10%), and blood (10%). A state of dynamic equilibrium exists; if the volume of any of the three components increases, the volume of the others must decrease to maintain normal pressures within the cranial cavity. This

is known as the *Monro-Kellie hypothesis*. Displacement of some cerebrospinal fluid (CSF) to the spinal subarachnoid space and increased CSF absorption are early compensatory mechanisms. The low-pressure venous system is also compressed, and cerebral arteries constrict to reduce blood flow. The ability of brain tissue to accommodate to change is relatively restricted (Porth, 1994). The relationship between the volume of the intracranial components and intracranial pressure is known as *compliance*. When the capacity to compensate for increased intracranial pressure is exceeded, intracranial hypertension develops. *Intracranial hypertension* is a sustained state of increased ICP and is potentially life-threatening. Aggressive treatment of increased ICP is thought to improve survival and function in clients who have sustained a head injury or other condition associated with intracranial hypertension (Wilson et al., 1991).

Pathophysiology

Cerebral blood flow and perfusion are important concepts for understanding the development and effects of intracranial hypertension. Whereas blood and CSF contribute an equal percentage to normal intracranial volume, vascular factors account for twice the amount of increase in ICP that CSF does (Hickey, 1992). The brain requires a constant supply of oxygen and glucose to meet its metabolic demands; 15% to 20% of the resting cardiac output goes to the brain to meet its metabolic needs (Dasch, 1994). Interruption of the cerebral blood flow leads to ischemia and disruption of the cerebral metabolism. Cerebral blood flow is controlled by both systemic and local factors.

The *cerebral perfusion pressure (CPP)* is the difference between the mean arterial blood pressure (MAP) and ICP:

$$CPP = MAP - ICP$$

In adults, the normal CPP range is 70 to 100 mm Hg. CPP may be reduced by either a drop in MAP or an increase in ICP. Brain tissue ischemia develops when the CPP falls below 60 to 70 mm Hg and the risk of neuronal hypoxia and necrosis increases; when ICP is equal to MAP, the cerebral perfusion pressure is 0 and cerebral blood flow ceases (Hickey, 1992).

Autoregulation is a compensatory mechanism in which cerebral arterioles change diameter to maintain cerebral blood flow when ICP increases. There are two forms of autoregulation: pressure autoregulation and chemical, or metabolic, autoregulation.

In pressure autoregulation, stretch receptors within small blood vessels of the brain cause smooth muscle of the arterioles to contract. Increased arterial pressure stimulates these receptors, leading to vasoconstriction; when arterial pressure is low, stimulation of these receptors decreases, causing relaxation and vasodilation.

Chemical, or metabolic, autoregulation works in much the same way as pressure autoregulation. In this case, the stimulus is a buildup of metabolic by-products of cell metabolism, including lactic acid, pyruvic acid, carbonic acid, and carbon dioxide. Carbon dioxide and increased hydrogen ion concentration are potent cerebral vasodilators that may act locally or systemically to increase cerebral blood flow. Conversely, a fall in PCO_2 causes cerebral vasoconstriction. Arterial oxygen tension (PO_2) also affects cerebral blood flow, although it is a less powerful mechanism than that exerted by carbon dioxide and hydrogen ions.

The ability of autoregulatory mechanisms to maintain cerebral blood flow is limited. When autoregulation fails, cerebrovascular tone is reduced and cerebral blood flow becomes dependent on changes in blood pressure. Autoregulation may be lost either locally or globally because of several factors (Hickey, 1992):

- ICP of greater than 40 to 50 mm Hg
- Local or diffuse cerebral tissue injury, ischemia, or inflammation
- MAP of greater than 60 to 130 mm Hg
- Hypercapnia or hypoxia
- Prolonged hypotension
- Drugs causing cerebral vasodilation such as halothane, nitrous oxide, histamines, ketamines, and nitroprusside

With the loss of autoregulation, intracranial pressure continues to rise and cerebral perfusion falls. Cerebral tissue becomes ischemic, and manifestations of cellular hypoxia appear. Because the neurons of the cerebral cortex are most sensitive to oxygen deficit, changes in cortical function are the earliest manifestations of increasing ICP (Porth, 1994). Behavior and personality changes occur; the client may become irritable and agitated. Memory and judgment are impaired, and speech pattern changes may be noted. The client's level of consciousness declines. As cerebral hypertension and hypoxia progress, the level of consciousness continues to decline in a predictable pattern to coma and unresponsiveness.

Pressure on the pyramidal tract often causes weakness or hemiparesis on the contralateral side early in increased ICP. As ICP continues to increase, hemiplegia and abnormal motor responses, such as decorticate or decerebrate positioning, develop (Hickey, 1992).

Altered vision is an early manifestation of increased ICP because of pressure on the visual pathways and cranial nerves. Blurred vision, decreased visual acuity, and diplopia are common. Pupillary and oculomotor responses are affected as well. Because the cause of increased ICP is often localized initially, pupillary changes, including gradual dilation and sluggish response to light, may initially be limited to the ipsilateral side (Hickey, 1992).

Additional manifestations of increased ICP include headache, particularly on rising, that worsens with position changes. Headache is more common in clients with slowly developing increased ICP and occurs because of pressure on pain-sensitive structures, such as the middle meningeal arteries, the venous sinuses, and the dura at the base of the skull (Hickey, 1992). Papilledema, or edema and swelling of the optic disk, may be noted on fundoscopic examination. Vomiting, often projectile and occuring without warning, may develop (Price & Wilson, 1992).

Ischemia of the vasomotor center in the brain stem triggers the CNS ischemic response, a late sign of increased ICP. Neuronal ischemia in the vasomotor center causes a marked increase in the MAP, with a significant increase in systolic blood pressure and increased pulse pressure. The increased MAP causes reflexive slowing of the cardiac rate. This trio of manifestations (increased MAP, increased pulse pressure, and bradycardia) is known as *Cushing's response* or *triad,* and represents the brain stem's final effort to maintain cerebral perfusion (Porth, 1994). The respiratory pattern also changes, often in the predictable progression outlined in Table 40–3 on page 1689. Although the temperature is usually normal in early stages, as ICP continues to increase, hypothalamic function is impaired and the temperature may rise dramatically (Hickey, 1992).

The manifestations of increased ICP are listed in the accompanying box.

Cerebral Edema

Cerebral edema is an increase in the volume of brain tissue due to abnormal accumulation of fluid. Cerebral edema is often associated with increased intracranial pressure; it may occur as a local process in the area of a tumor or injury, or it may affect the entire brain. Three types of cerebral edema have been identified. More than one type may be present in the client with intracranial hypertension.

- *Vasogenic edema* is due to an unusual increase in the capillary permeability of cerebral vessels. The process allows a plasmalike filtrate to leak into the interstitial spaces of the brain's white matter. Vasogenic edema is the most common form of cerebral edema causing intracranial hypertension (Hickey, 1992). A variety of insults, such as abscesses, brain tumors, and toxins, may cause the increase in capillary permeability. The rate and extent of spreading of edema are influenced by the site of the brain injury, the level of increase in capillary permeability, and the client's systemic blood pressure.
- *Cytotoxic edema* involves changes in the functional or structural integrity of cell membranes due to intracra-

nial hypoxia and ischemia. As oxygen and nutrients are depleted, intracranial cells switch to anaerobic metabolism, and the sodium-potassium pump in the cell walls is impaired. Sodium diffuses into the cells, pulling fluid after it. The cells swell, and intracranial pressure rises. Accumulated metabolic waste products, such as lactic acid, contribute to a rapid deterioration of cell function (Hickey, 1992). Cytotoxic cerebral edema occurs most often in gray matter. Causes of cytotoxic cerebral edema include trauma, destructive lesions in brain tissue resulting in cerebral hypoxia, conditions causing sodium depletion, and syndrome of inappropriate antidiuretic hormone (see Chapter 20).

- *Interstitial cerebral edema* is an increase in interstitial fluids. The brain does not have a lymphatic system linked to the rest of the body. Therefore, the interstitial fluid within the brain drains by bulk flow into CSF circulation, where it eventually is reabsorbed into the blood through the arachnoid villi. In a client with interstitial cerebral edema, the drainage of fluid is compromised.

Cerebral edema tends to be proportional to the extent of the insult precipitating it. Cerebral edema reaches maximal levels in approximately 48 to 72 hours, then begins to subside gradually (Hickey, 1992). Brain function is not disrupted by cerebral edema unless it causes an increase in ICP. When cerebral edema does increase ICP, a vicious cycle can ensue. Cerebral edema increases ICP, which in turn decreases cerebral blood flow. Brain tissue becomes hypoxic and ischemic, increasing toxic metabolic byproducts, hydrogen ion concentration, and carbon dioxide levels in the tissue. Autoregulatory mechanisms cause vasodilation and increase cerebral blood flow, further increasing cerebral edema and intracranial pressure. Without effective intervention, the client's condition can deteriorate rapidly; intracranial pressure increases to the point where brain structures herniate.

Hydrocephalus

Hydrocephalus is an increase in volume of CSF within and dilation of the ventricular system. Hydrocephalus may increase ICP when it develops acutely in the adult client (Porth, 1994). Hydrocephalus occurs when the production of CSF exceeds its absorption. It is generally classified as either noncommunicating or communicating hydrocephalus. *Noncommunicating hydrocephalus* occurs when CSF drainage from the ventricular system is impaired. It may develop when a mass or tumor, inflammatory response, or congenital malformation obstructs the ventricular system. *Communicating hydrocephalus* is a condition in which CSF is not effectively reabsorbed through the arachnoid villi. It may occur secondarily to subarachnoid hemorrhage or infection (Hickey, 1992; Porth,

---

Clinical Manifestations of Increased Intracranial Pressure

- Decreased level of consciousness. *Early:* Confusion, restlessness, lethargy; disorientation, first to time, then to place and person. *Late:* Comatose with no response to painful stimuli.
- Pupillary dysfunction. Sluggish response to light progressing to fixed pupils; with a localized process, pupillary dysfunction is first noted on the ipsilateral side.
- Oculomotor dysfunction. Inability to move eye(s) upward; ptosis (drooping) of the eyelid.
- Visual abnormalities. Decreased visual acuity, blurred vision, diplopia.
- Papilledema. May be late sign.
- Motor impairment. *Early:* Hemiparesis or hemiplegia of the contralateral side. *Late:* Abnormal responses such as decorticate or decerebrate positioning; flaccidity.
- Headache. Uncommon but may occur with processes that slowly increase ICP; worse on rising in the morning and with position changes.
- Projectile vomiting without nausea
- Cushing's response. Increased systolic blood pressure, widening pulse pressure, bradycardia. Respirations. Altered respiratory pattern related to level of brain dysfunction (see Table 40–3 on page 1689).
- Temperature. May be significantly elevated as compensatory mechanisms fail.

1994). In adults, manifestations of hydrocephalus depend on the rate of its development. They may be mild and insidious in onset, presenting as progressive dementia or gait disruptions. If the process causing hydrocephalus is an acute one, the manifestations are those of increased ICP.

Brain Herniation

If increased ICP is not treated, cerebral tissue is displaced toward a more compliant area. This can result in *brain herniation,* the displacement of brain tissue from its normal compartment under dural folds of the falx cerebri or through the tentorial notch or incisura of the tentorium cerebelli (Porth, 1994). Herniation of the cerebellum through the tentorium exerts pressure on the brain stem,

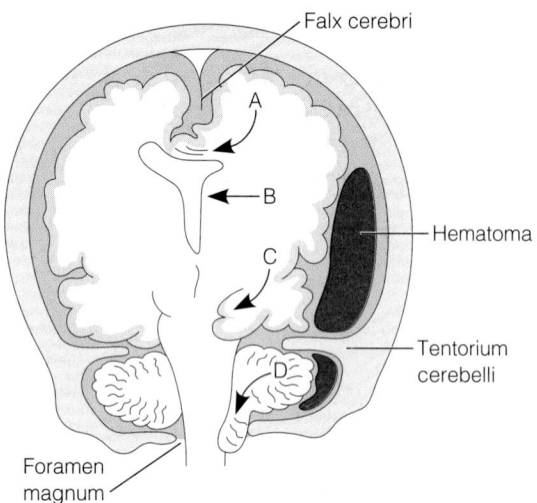

Figure 40–3 Forms of brain herniation due to intracranial hypertension. *A,* Cingulate herniation occurs when the cingulate gyrus is compressed under the falx cerebri. *B,* Central herniation occurs when a centrally located lesion compresses central and midbrain structures. *C,* Lateral herniation occurs when a lesion at the side of the brain compresses the uncus or hippocampal gyrus. *D,* Intratentorial herniation occurs when the cerebellar tonsils are forced downward, compressing the medulla and top of the spinal cord.

with subsequent herniation through the foramen magnum. This is a lethal complication of increased ICP because of pressure on the vital centers of the medulla (Hickey, 1992).

Brain herniation syndromes are generally categorized as supratentorial or infratentorial, depending on their location above or below the tentorium cerebelli (Figure 40–3). *Supratentorial herniation syndromes* include cingulate herniation, central or transtentorial herniation, and uncal or lateral transtentorial herniation.

- *Cingulate herniation* (Figure 40–3, *A*) occurs when the cingulate gyrus is displaced under the falx cerebri. Local blood supply and cerebral tissue are compressed, resulting in ischemia and further increases in intracranial pressure. This type of herniation is common but difficult to identify by specific manifestations (Hickey, 1992; Porth, 1994).

- *Central* or *transtentorial herniation* is the downward displacement of brain structures, including the cerebral hemispheres, basal ganglia, diencephalon, and midbrain through the tentorial incisura (Figure 40–3, *B*). With central herniation, the client's neurologic signs may deteriorate rapidly, with decreased LOC progressing to coma, Cheyne-Stokes respirations progressing to central neurogenic hyperventilation, and pupils progressing from small and reactive to midsize and fixed. The client may demonstrate abnormal motor responses with unilateral decorticate positioning.

- *Uncal* or *lateral transtentorial herniation* is the most common herniation syndrome (Hickey, 1992). It typically occurs when a lateral mass displaces cerebral tissue centrally, forcing the medial aspect of the temporal lobe under the edge of the tentorial incisura (Figure 40–3, *C*). The oculomotor nerve (cranial nerve III) often becomes trapped between the uncus and the tentorium, causing ipsilateral pupillary dilation. Other manifestations include alterations in LOC, motor deficits (which may occur on the same side as the herniation because of compression of the cerebral peduncle on the opposite side), decreased sensation, respiratory changes, abnormal positioning, and eventual respiratory arrest.

- *Infratentorial herniation* results from increased pressure within the infratentorial compartment. Herniation may occur either upward, in which structures are displaced through the tentorial incisura, or downward, with displacement through the foramen magnum (Figure 40–3, *D*). Downward displacement causes compression of the medulla, including its centers for controlling vital functions. Manifestations associated with medullary compression include coma, altered respiratory patterns, fixed pupils, and decorticate or decerebrate positioning. Respiratory or cardiac arrest may occur.

Collaborative Care

Care of the client with increased ICP is directed to identifying and treating the underlying cause of the disorder, and controlling ICP. Unless increased ICP is treated aggressively, herniation syndrome may result. Increased ICP is a medical emergency, and there is little time to complete lengthy diagnostic tests. The diagnosis must be made on the basis of observation and neurologic assessment; even subtle changes may be clinically significant.

Increased ICP affects all body systems. Management of the client with increased ICP thus involves supporting other body systems and preventing complications.

Laboratory and Diagnostic Tests

Laboratory and diagnostic studies focus on identifying the presence of increased ICP and its underlying cause. The diagnostic tests discussed previously for the client with an altered level of consciousness also are used for the client with increased ICP. CT scanning or MRI is generally the initial test. These diagnostic tests can be used to identify the possible causes of increased ICP (such as space-occupying lesions, hydrocephalus, and so on) and to evaluate therapeutic options. In general, a lumbar puncture is not performed when increased ICP is suspected because of the possibility of cerebral herniation due to the sudden release of the pressure in the skull.

Laboratory tests are performed to augment and monitor individual treatment approaches. In addition to the tests discussed for the client with an altered level of consciousness, the following specific tests are ordered and their results closely monitored:

- *Serum osmolality* is an indicator of hydration status in the client with increased ICP. The test measures the number of dissolved particles (electrolytes, urea, glucose) in the serum. The normal range for the adult is 280 to 300 mOsm/kg H_2O. In addition to the restriction of fluids in the client with increased ICP, serum osmolality is maintained at a slightly elevated level (325 mOsm/kg H_2O) to draw excess intracellular fluid into the vascular system.

- *Arterial blood gases* are monitored frequently to assess pH and levels of oxygen and carbon dioxide. As noted previously, hydrogen ions and carbon dioxide are both potent vasodilators; hypoxemia also causes vasodilation, although to a lesser degree. The client with increased ICP may be hyperventilated and kept in a state of slight respiratory alkalosis to minimize cerebral vasodilation.

Pharmacology

Pharmacologic therapy plays an important role in the management of the client with increased ICP. Diuretics, particularly osmotic diuretics, and corticosteroids are commonly used to reduce ICP and are the mainstays of pharmacologic treatment.

Osmotic diuretics work by increasing the osmolarity of the blood, thereby drawing water out of edematous brain tissue and into the vascular system for elimination via the kidneys. The effects of these drugs vary with the type of injury. Regardless of the agent used, the optimal dose is the lowest that reduces ICP (Wilson, Shannon, & Stang, 1995). Mannitol is the most commonly employed osmotic diuretic. Glucose, urea, and glycerol are other osmotic diuretics that may be employed.

Loop diuretics, such as furosemide (Lasix) and ethacrynic acid (Edecrin), may be prescribed for some clients with increased ICP. These diuretics act on the renal tubule and are extremely effective in promoting diuresis. Additionally, loop diuretics may be used to manage the rebound effect that may occur with mannitol administration (Hickey, 1992).

Corticosteroids, dexamethasone (Decadron) in particular, are often used to treat increased ICP. Although the exact mechanism of action of corticosteroids in reducing ICP is unclear, they are particularly effective in treating vasogenic edema associated with brain tumors (Hickey, 1992). The use of corticosteroids to treat cerebral edema following trauma is more controversial (Holloway, 1993). Corticosteroid therapy is associated with multiple side effects, including gastrointestinal ulceration and hemorrhage and elevation of blood glucose.

Calcium channel blockers are relative newcomers in the management of increased ICP. These drugs block the influx of calcium into the cell during depolarization. This prevents excess levels of calcium from reaching injured areas of the brain and causing cell death by entering hyperexcitable neurons. Calcium channel blockers also prevent cerebral vasospasm, reducing ischemia.

To treat clients with severe, persistent intracranial hypertension that is refractory to other therapy, barbiturates may be used to induce coma. The mechanism of action of this controversial therapy is unclear, but it is thought to reduce metabolic demands in the injured brain. Because neurologic signs are masked, close monitoring of the client in induced coma is vital (Holloway, 1993).

Nursing implications for these medications are described in the pharmacology box on page 1700.

Anticonvulsants are often required to manage seizure activity associated with brain injury and increased ICP. Other drugs that may be administered include histamine-H_2 blockers, such as cimetidine or ranitidine, or antacids to prevent gastrointestinal irritation and hemorrhage.

Intravenous fluids are usually necessary to maintain the client's fluid and electrolyte balance as well as vascular volume. If the client's blood pressure is unstable, vasoactive medications may be administered to maintain the MAP in a range that supports cerebral perfusion while minimizing increases in ICP. When enteral feeding is not possible, total parenteral nutrition may be administered.

Surgery

Clients with increased ICP may undergo various intracranial surgical techniques to treat the underlying cause (see the discussion in the section on brain tumor). In addition, infarcted or necrotic tissue may be resected to reduce brain mass. A drainage catheter or shunt may be inserted laterally via a burr hole into a ventricle to drain excess cerebrospinal fluid and reduce hydrocephalus. The removal of even a small amount of CSF may dramatically reduce ICP and restore cerebral perfusion pressure.

ICP Monitoring

For clients with increased ICP, the use of intracranial pressure monitors facilitates continual assessment of ICP and is more precise than relying on often vague clinical manifestations. With these devices, the effects of medical therapy and nursing interventions on ICP can also be monitored. In addition, cerebral perfusion pressure (the difference between MAP and ICP) can be readily calculated, allowing more precise manipulation of therapeutic measures to maintain cerebral perfusion and thereby prevent ischemia.

Basic monitoring systems include an intraventricular catheter, subarachnoid screw, and epidural probe (Figure 40–4 on page 1702). A newer device is an intraparenchymal fiberoptic transducer-tipped catheter, which can be placed in various locations. The choice of monitor depends on both the suspected disorder and the physician's

Nursing Implications for Pharmacology: The Client with Increased Intracranial Pressure

OSMOTIC DIURETICS

Mannitol (Osmitrol)

Glycerol

Urea

Osmotic diuretics (hyperosmotic agents) draw fluid out of brain cells by increasing the osmolality of the blood. The effects of these drugs vary with the type of injury. Mannitol therapy is often initiated if the client's ICP has exceeded 15 to 20 mm Hg for at least 10 minutes. Both intravenous bolus and continuous infusion techniques are used. Repeated use of mannitol can lead to continual elevations in serum osmolality, with attendant risk of seizures and serious fluid and electrolyte imbalance. Urea is seldom administered intravenously because a severe local reaction may result if leakage occurs at the injection site. Mannitol and urea are used cautiously if renal disease is present.

Note: Because the client with increased intracranial pressure often has an altered level of consciousness, client and family teaching is not discussed in this box.

Nursing Responsibilities

- Monitor vital signs, urinary output, central venous pressure (CVP), and pulmonary artery pressures (PAP) before and every hour throughout administration.
- Assess client for manifestations of dehydration.
- Assess client for muscle weakness, numbness, tingling, paresthesia, confusion, and excessive thirst.
- Assess client for pulmonary edema while administering the medication.
- Monitor neurologic status and intracranial pressure readings.
- Monitor renal function and serum electrolytes throughout therapy.

- Do not administer the medication if crystals are present in solution. Administer with an in-line filter. Observe infusion site frequently for infiltration.
- Do not administer mannitol solution with blood.
- Do not discontinue medication abruptly. Rebound migraine headaches may occur.

LOOP DIURETICS

Furosemide (Lasix)

Ethacrynic acid (Edecrin)

Loop diuretics such as furosemide and ethacrynic acid inhibit sodium and chloride reabsorption at the ascending loop of Henle. They cause a reduction in the rate of CSF production, thus reducing the ICP.

Nursing Responsibilities

- Monitor vital signs and electrolyte values closely.
- Assess fluid status throughout therapy.
- Monitor blood pressure and pulse before and during administration.
- Monitor renal laboratory studies closely.
- Use infusion pump to ensure accurate dosage.

STEROIDS

Dexamethasone (Decadron)

Dexamethasone is effective in reducing vasogenic edema and ICP and improving neurologic status. Steroid therapy has been shown to be most effective in clients with focal chronic lesions. The exact mode of action by which steroids work is unknown, but it is thought that they act by stabilizing the cell membrane, which prevents the pulling of fluids into the cell.

preference. Once the intracranial sensor is implanted, it is connected to a transducer that converts the impulses to a signal that the recording device can translate into an oscilloscope tracing, digital value, or graphic recording (Hickey, 1992). Factors that put the client at higher risk for infection during ICP monitoring are listed in the box on page 1703.

Nursing Care

The nursing care of clients with increased intracranial pressure involves identifying the client at risk and managing factors that are known to increase intracranial pressure. A major focus is to protect the client from sudden increases in ICP or a decrease in cerebral blood flow. Nursing management includes performing neurologic as-

| **Pharmacology: The Client with Increased Intracranial Pressure (continued)** |

Nursing Responsibilities

- Monitor intake and output closely.
- Assess level of consciousness throughout therapy.
- Monitor respiratory status and lung sounds.
- Monitor serum electrolytes and glucose level.

CALCIUM CHANNEL BLOCKER

Nimodipine (Nimotop)

Nimodipine inhibits the movement of calcium ions across cell membranes in the smooth muscle of the blood vessels; its effect is greatest on cerebral arteries. Nimodipine improves neurologic deficits due to spasm of cerebral vessels.

Nursing Responsibilities

- Assess level of consciousness and neurologic status prior to and throughout therapy.
- Monitor for bradycardia.
- Assess skin for dermatitis or flushing.

ANTICONVULSANTS

Phenytoin (Dilantin)

Pentobarbital

Diazepam (Valium, Valrelease, Apo-Diazepam)

Seizures increase metabolic requirements, cerebral blood flow, cerebral blood volume, and ICP. Phenytoin, pentobarbital, and diazepam may be useful to control or treat seizures. Diazepam may be used to stop muscle activity, whereas phenytoin and pentobarbital depress motor nerve function.

Nursing Responsibilities

- Monitor neurologic status frequently.

- Monitor blood pressure, pulse, and respiratory rate frequently throughout therapy.
- Administer phenytoin through a large vein, at a rate not to exceed 50 mg/min. Do not piggy-back phenytoin through dextrose solutions, because precipitation will occur. Assess the infusion site frequently.
- Ensure that resuscitation equipment is available when administering these drugs intravenously.
- Do not dilute or mix with any other drugs.
- Administer intravenous dosages very slowly.

INTRAVENOUS FLUIDS

Keeping the client moderately dehydrated to maintain serum osmolality can be effective in reducing cerebral edema. When giving intravenous fluids, closely monitor the osmolality of the solutions; if clients with increased ICP are given hypoosmolar solutions, increased cerebral edema can occur. Preferred solutions include 0.45% to 0.9% sodium chloride solutions.

Nursing Responsibilities

- Monitor fluid status closely.
- Monitor neurologic status closely.
- Avoid administering hypoosmolar solutions, such as 5% dextrose in water.
- Half-strength normal saline (0.45% sodium chloride) is considered a suitable fluid for a client who has increased intracranial pressure.
- Take care not to restrict fluids excessively in clients receiving dehydrating agents (such as osmotic or loop diuretics).
- Report significant findings to the physician immediately.

sessments, maintaining the patency of the airway, ensuring adequate ventilation, positioning and moving, instituting seizure precautions, and monitoring fluids and electrolytes. Additionally, both client and family need emotional support during this period. The client with increased intracranial pressure exhibits a variety of responses to actual or potential changes in physiologic

processes. Nursing diagnoses discussed in this section focus on altered cerebral tissue perfusion and risk for infection.

Altered Cerebral Tissue Perfusion

A number of disorders may lead to increased intracranial pressure, including cerebral edema, hydrocephalus,

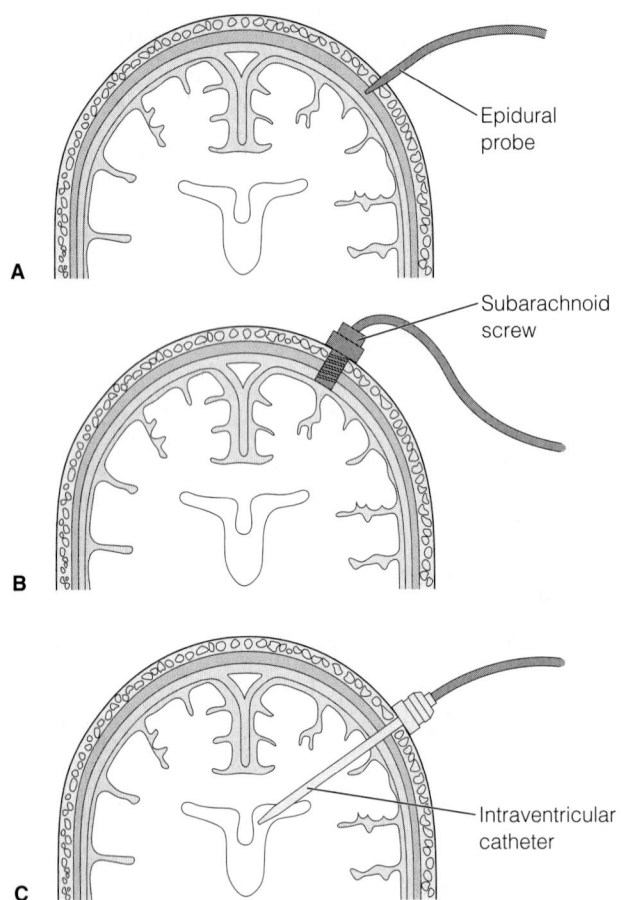

Figure 40–4   Types of intracranial pressure monitoring. *A,* Epidural probe. *B,* Subarachnoid screw. *C,* Intraventricular catheter.

Epidural probe

Subarachnoid screw

Intraventricular catheter

space-occupying lesions and hemorrhage, herniation syndromes, and changes in carbon dioxide concentrations. Increasing intracranial pressure alters cerebral perfusion and oxygenation of brain cells. The client with increased intracranial pressure requires intensive care, and often requires ventilator assistance.

Nursing interventions with rationales follow:

- Assess for and report any of the indicators of increasing ICP every 1 to 2 hours and as necessary. Assessment areas include level of consciousness, behavior, motor/sensory functions, pupillary size and reaction to light, and vital signs, including temperature. *Assessment of neurologic status establishes the client's clinical condition and provides a baseline to measure changes. Sudden changes in neurologic signs often indicate deterioration. Often, the earliest manifestations of a change in intracranial pressure are alterations in the level of consciousness and respirations. Look for trends, because vital signs alone do not correlate well with early deterioration. An elevated*

temperature with increased oxygen consumption further increases intracranial pressure. Pupillary responses mirror the status of the midbrain and pons. Pressure on the brain stem may compromise the function of cranial nerves IX and X and protective mechanisms, such as the gag and cough reflexes.

- For the client on a ventilator: Maintain patency of the airway; preoxygenate and hyperventilate client with 100% oxygen before suctioning; limit suctioning to 10 seconds; suction gently. *Oxygenation prevents carbon dioxide from accumulating and further increasing intracranial pressure. Suctioning stimulates the cough reflex and Valsalva maneuver. Correct suctioning minimizes the risk of hypoxemia.*

- Monitor arterial blood gases (ABGs). *ABGs provide a reliable indicator of oxygen and carbon dioxide levels. If oxygen concentration is low, oxygen may be given or increased. $Paco_2$ may be maintained at 25 to 30 mm Hg by deliberately hyperventilating the client on a ventilator (by increasing the rate and tidal volume). The resulting mild vasoconstriction reduces cerebral blood volume and ICP.*

- Elevate head of the bed to 30 to 45 degrees; maintain the alignment of the head and neck to avoid hyperextension or exaggerated neck flexion; avoid prone position. *Keeping the head of the bed elevated facilitates venous drainage from cerebrum. Obstruction of jugular veins can impede venous drainage from the brain.*

- Maintain head and neck in neutral plane (avoid flexion, extension, or lateral rotation). *Turning the head to the lateral position (especially left lateral) decreases jugular venous drainage. The left jugular vein connects to the subclavian vein at a right angle and may be more easily stenosed or kinked. In addition, the left jugular vein is narrower than the right jugular vein (Drummond, 1990; Germon, 1988).*

- Assess for bladder distention and bowel constipation. Administer stool softeners and use the Credé technique to empty the bladder. If the Credé technique is not effective, evaluate the pros and cons of urinary catheterization if the bladder remains distended. *Constipation and bladder distention increase intrathoracic or intra-abdominal pressure and place the client at risk for impaired venous drainage from the brain.*

- Assist the client to move up in bed. Do not ask the client to push with heels or arms or push against a footboard. Avoid the use of a footboard or restraints. *Moving up in bed requires pushing. Assisting the client with moving prevents initiation of the Valsalva maneuver, which increases intracranial pressure.*

- Plan nursing care so that activities are not clustered together; avoid turning the client, getting the client on the bedpan, or suctioning within the same time period. Individualize nursing care to provide rest periods be-

---

Risk Factors for Infection Associated with Intracranial Pressure Monitoring
■ ■ ■

Factor	Rationale
Intraventricular catheter	Is more invasive than other monitoring devices
Open head trauma or neurogsurgery	Disrupts protective skin and skeletal barriers
Intracranial hemorrhage	Necessitates frequent flushing of catheter to maintain patency
Older adult	Tends to have impaired immune defenses
Monitoring for more than 3 to 5 days; or open system or frequent irrigation	Offers increased opportunity for pathogens to enter and grow

---

tween procedures. *Multiple procedures, including certain nursing care activities, can increase ICP. Constant stimulation tends to increase ICP. Individualized nursing care ensures optimal spacing of activities and rest.*

- Provide a quiet environment, limiting noxious stimuli. Avoid jarring the bed. Try to limit situations that cause the client to become emotionally upset; maintain a calm, reassuring manner; caution family members to refrain from unpleasant conversations or conversations that may be emotionally stimulating to the client (Baker, 1990). *Noxious stimuli and emotional upsets cause an elevation in ICP (Acom & Roberts, 1992).*

- Maintain fluid limitations, if prescribed. *Restricting fluids helps decrease cerebral edema by reducing total body water.*

Risk for Infection
Although any client with an open head wound is at risk for infection, the interventions discussed here are for the client with an intracranial monitoring device. There is a risk for infection related to the intracranial monitor devices. Most clinical units have written protocols for managing these systems. The following nursing actions serve only as a general guide.

- Keep dressings over the catheter dry, and change dressings on a prescribed basis (usually every 24 to 48 hours). *Wet dressings are conducive to bacterial growth. Once inside the body, the organism begins to reproduce. As the pathogens reproduce, immune cells are destroyed, even if no clinical manifestations of disease appear.*

- Monitor the insertion site for leaking CSF, drainage, or infection. Monitor for physical manifestations of infection, including changes in vital signs, chills, increased white blood cell (WBC) counts, and positive cultures of drainage. *Close monitoring facilitates detection of the earliest signs of infection and helps prevent major compli-*

cations. *Fever is usually considered the key assessment. However, fever in a client with a neurologic disorder may be due to damage to the hypothalamus. Headache, generalized muscle aches, shivering, and chills may also be seen in the client with infection. Assessment of vital signs usually reveals increased pulse, blood pressure, and respiratory rate.*

- Use strict aseptic technique when in contact with the device. Check drainage system for loose connections. *The use of aseptic technique and monitoring drainage systems for loose connections helps prevent nosocomial infections. Most nosocomial infections are transmitted by health care workers who fail to wash their hands properly, to change gloves between clients, or to follow aseptic technique protocols. Invasive procedures provide an excellent opportunity for microbes to enter the body. Loose connections cause leaking and contamination of the system and CSF.*

Other Nursing Diagnoses
Other nursing diagnoses that may be appropriate for the client with or at risk for increased intracranial pressure follow:

- *Ineffective Breathing Pattern* related to compression of brain by increased intracranial pressure secondary to expanding intracranial lesion

- *Ineffective Airway Clearance* related to loss of cough reflex from increased intracranial pressure

- *Sensory/Perceptual Alterations* related to neurologic deficits secondary to increased intracranial pressure

- *Altered Family Processes* related to actual or perceived loss of client's well-being

- *Hyperthermia* related to effects of increased intracranial pressure

- *Risk for Injury* related to seizure activity and environmental hazards

■ *Risk for Fluid Volume Deficit* related to osmotic diuretic therapy or fluid restriction

Client and Family Teaching

Teach the client who is at risk for increased intracranial pressure (and who is able to follow instructions) to avoid coughing, blowing the nose, straining to have a bowel movement, pushing against the bed rails, or performing isometric (muscle contracting) exercises. Advise the client to maintain head and neck alignment when turning in bed and to take rest periods.

Encourage the family to talk to the client, but maintain a quiet environment with a minimum of stimuli. Inform family members that upsetting the client may increase intracranial pressure and that therefore they should avoid discussions that may distress the client. For clients who are unable to make decisions about treatment and to sign informed consent, the family must carry out these functions.

Applying the Nursing Process

Case Study of a Client with Increased Intracranial Pressure: Hubert McAllen

Hubert McAllen is a 65-year-old manager of a communications department in a Fortune 500 company. Mr. McAllen underwent a left lung lobectomy 5 months ago for large-cell anaplastic carcinoma; up until approximately 1 month ago, he had been feeling fine. At that time, Mr. McAllen began having right-sided headaches and increasing irritability, and during the past week, he has had difficulty concentrating and staying alert. Today, during a video shoot of the president of the company, Mr. McAllen becomes so confused and drowsy that the shoot is cancelled. The president of the company, concerned about Mr. McAllen's condition, directs the video assistants to contact the nurse practitioner at the company clinic. After a brief assessment, the nurse practitioner calls for an ambulance to transfer Mr. McAllen to a nearby medical center. Mr. McAllen's wife and son join him there.

Assessment

The admission assessment at the medical center reveals that Mr. McAllen is emaciated and lethargic, opens his eyes spontaneously, moves all extremities on command (the right side is stronger than the left), and is oriented to person only. Both pupils are 3 mm in diameter and demonstrate both direct and consensual reflex reactions to light. Testing of cranial nerves III, IV, and V reveals normal findings, except for a decreased corneal reflex in the left eye; testing of cranial nerves IX and X reveals a depressed gag reflex. Motor reflexes are normal on the right

side; the left reflexes are hyperactive and show a positive Babinski reflex. Visualization of the optic discs reveals papilledema of both discs. CT scan of the skull demonstrates a large bifrontal mass with surrounding edema. Mr. McAllen is started on dexamethasone and prepared for surgery immediately.

Diagnosis

The nurses caring for Mr. McAllen include the following nursing diagnosis and collaborative problem in the plan of care:

■ *Altered Cerebral Tissue Perfusion* related to cerebral edema and increased intracranial pressure
■ Risk for herniation of brain tissue related to cerebral edema and increased intracranial pressure

Expected Outcomes

The expected outcomes established in the plan of care specify that Mr. McAllen will

■ Maintain adequate cerebral tissue pressure.
■ Show reduced cerebral edema.
■ Maintain a patent airway.
■ Maintain an effective breathing pattern.

Planning and Implementation

The following nursing interventions are planned and implemented for Mr. McAllen:

■ Use conservative measures to reduce cerebral circulatory volume:
   a. Elevate head of bed to 30 to 45 degrees to promote venous return.
   b. Position the client to avoid flexion of the hips, waist, and neck.
   c. Prevent rotation of the neck (especially to the right).
   d. Provide a calm, nonstimulating environment as much as possible.
   e. Group care from all disciplines to allow adequate rest.
■ Prepare for surgery (see the discussion on craniotomy, in the section on brain tumors).
■ Prepare for postoperative intracranial pressure monitoring.
■ Inform family members about the need to keep the conversation very general and not discuss topics that may upset Mr. McAllen.

Evaluation

A right frontal craniotomy was performed that evening, with partial tumor removal. Twelve hours after surgery, Mr. McAllen's vital signs are stable. Neurologic assessment at this time shows spontaneous eye opening; he is restless and moves all extremities, and the right limbs continue to be stronger than the left limbs. He speaks incomprehensible sounds. There are no other focal neurologic signs. Approximately 20 hours after surgery, Mr. McAllen's left pupil (4 mm) reacts to light slightly, and his right pupil (6 mm) does not react to light at all. He demonstrates bilateral extension of his extremities to painful stimulation. His respiratory rate is 12 and irregular. He is intubated and hyperventilated; drugs administered at this time include furosemide, mannitol, and dexamethasone. A CT scan reveals herniation secondary to edema formation. Pharmacologic and nursing management to treat the cerebral edema improve Mr. McAllen's preoperative status only slightly, and he remains in critical condition.

Critical Thinking in the Nursing Process

1. If you were the nurse at the company clinic, what assessments would you have made? Describe abnormal findings that indicate increased intracranial pressure.

2. Mr. McAllen's wife begins to cry and says, "I feel so guilty . . . I should have insisted he go to the doctor." What would be your response, and why?

3. What is the significance of Mr. McAllen's motor strength being stronger on the right than on the left?

4. What assessments would indicate that the medications are effective in treating the increased intracranial pressure?

5. Develop a plan of care for Mr. McAllen's family related to the nursing diagnosis *Anticipatory Grieving.*

The Client with a Seizure Disorder

■ ■ ■

A **seizure** is an episode of excessive and abnormal discharge of electrical activity within the central nervous system. This abnormal electrical activity, which may involve all or part of the brain, causes a disturbance in skeletal motor function, sensation, autonomic function of the viscera, behavior, or consciousness (Hickey, 1992).

Isolated seizure episodes may occur in otherwise healthy people for a variety of reasons, including an acute febrile state, head injury, infection, metabolic or endocrine disorder (such as hypoglycemia), or exposure to toxins. If the seizure activity is chronic, by contrast, the client is diagnosed as having **epilepsy,** a syndrome of recurrent, paroxysmal episodes of seizure activity. Epilepsy is categorized as a paroxysmal disorder because its manifestations are discontinuous; that is, minutes, days, weeks, or even years may elapse between seizures. Epilepsy may be idiopathic (that is, it may have no identifiable cause), or it may occur secondarily to birth injury,

infection, vascular abnormalities, trauma, or tumors (Hickey, 1992).

It is estimated that 2 to 4 million people in the United States have epilepsy, many of them children (Hickey, 1992). The incidence of epilepsy is increasing. Researchers have suggested that the increase may be due to technologic advances in obstetric and pediatric care that allow extremely high risk neonates to survive and to other technologic advances that have improved survival rates associated with craniocerebral trauma (Hartshorn & Byers, 1992). The onset of epilepsy occurs before age 20 in most clients.

Pathophysiology

Normally, when the mind is actively working, electrical activity in the brain is unsynchronized; when the mind is at rest, electrical activity is mildly synchronized. It is believed that most seizures arise from a few unstable neurons within the brain that are hypersensitive and hyperreactive. During a seizure, these neurons produce a rhythmic and repetitive hypersynchronous discharge. Although the exact initiating factor for seizure activity has not been identified, several theories have been proposed (Porth, 1994):

- Alterations in the permeability of or ion distribution across cell membranes

- Alterations in the excitability of neurons resulting from glial scarring or decreased inhibition of activity in the cerebral cortex or thalamic region

- Imbalances of excitatory and inhibitory neurotransmitters such as acetylcholine (ACh) or gamma-aminobutyric acid (GABA)

All people have a seizure threshold; when this threshold is exceeded, a seizure may result. In some people, the seizure threshold may be abnormally low, increasing their risk for seizure activity; in other people pathologic processes may alter the seizure threshold (Porth, 1994). The neurons that initiate seizure activity are called the *epileptogenic focus.* Abnormal neuronal activity may remain localized, causing a partial or focal seizure, or it may spread to involve the entire brain, causing generalized seizure activity (Wilson et al., 1991).

Metabolic needs of the brain increase dramatically during seizure activity. The demand for adenosine triphosphate (ATP), the energy source of the brain, increases by approximately 250%. Consequently, the demand for glucose and oxygen (which are needed to produce ATP) increases, and oxygen consumption increases by about 60%. To supply this increased oxygen need and remove carbon dioxide and other metabolic by-products, cerebral blood flow increases to about $2\frac{1}{2}$ times that of the normal rate. As long as oxygenation, blood glucose levels, and

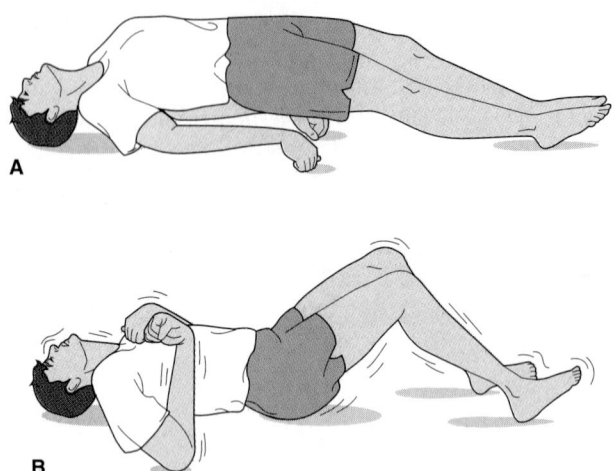

Figure 40–5 Tonic-clonic contractions in grand mal seizures. *A,* Tonic phase. *B,* Clonic phase.

cardiac function remain normal, cerebral blood flow can respond to this increased metabolic demand of the brain. If cerebral blood flow cannot meet these needs, however, cellular exhaustion and cellular destruction may result (Hickey, 1992).

As noted earlier, seizure activity may involve only a portion of the brain, or it may involve all neurons. Seizures are thus typically classified as either partial (or focal) or generalized.

Partial Seizures

Partial or *focal seizures* begin in one area of the cerebral cortex. The manifestations of partial seizures vary, depending on the area of cortex involved. A partial seizure accompanied by no alteration in consciousness is called a simple partial seizure; one in which consciousness is impaired is called a complex partial seizure.

Simple partial seizures are usually limited to one cerebral hemisphere. Manifestations may include alterations in motor function, sensory signs, or autonomic or psychic symptoms. Typically, the motor portion of the cortex is affected, causing recurrent muscle contractions of a contralateral part of the body, such as a finger or hand, or the face. This motor activity may remain confined to one area or spread sequentially to adjacent parts, a phenomenon known as a *Jacksonian march* or *Jacksonian seizure*. Manifestations of a simple partial seizure involving the sensory portion of the brain may include abnormal sensations or hallucinations. Disruptions in the function of the autonomic nervous system, with resulting tachycardia, flushing, hypotension, hypertension, and so on, or psychic manifestations, such as a sense of déjà vu or inappropriate fear or anger, may also be experienced during a simple partial seizure (Porth, 1994; Wilson et al., 1991).

During a *complex partial seizure,* consciousness is impaired and the client may engage in repetitive, nonpur-

poseful activity, such as lip smacking, aimless walking, or picking at clothing. These behaviors are known as *automatisms*. During the seizure, the client loses conscious contact with the environment; amnesia is common after the seizure, and several hours may elapse before the client regains full consciousness. Complex partial seizures (formerly known as temporal lobe or psychomotor seizures) usually originate in the temporal lobe and may be preceded by an *aura,* such as an unusual smell, a sense of déjà vu, or a sudden intense emotion.

The seizure activity of partial seizures may spread to involve both hemispheres and the deeper structures of the brain. When this occurs, it is known as a *secondarily generalized partial seizure.*

Generalized Seizures

Generalized seizures involve both hemispheres of the brain as well as deeper brain structures, such as the thalamus, basal ganglia, and upper brain stem. Consciousness is always impaired with generalized seizures. Absence and tonic-clonic seizures are the common forms of generalized seizure activity; they occur more frequently (especially in children) than partial seizures.

Absence Seizures *Absence seizures,* also known as *petit mal seizures,* are characterized by a sudden brief cessation of all motor activity accompanied by a blank stare and unresponsiveness. Absence seizures are much more common in children than in adults. The seizure typically lasts only 5 to 10 seconds, although some may last for 30 seconds or more. Movements such as eyelid fluttering or automatisms such as lip smacking may occur during an absence seizure. Seizure activity may vary from occasional episodes to several hundred per day.

Tonic-Clonic Seizures *Tonic-clonic seizures,* or *grand mal seizures,* are the most common type of seizure activity in both adults and children. This type of seizure activity follows a typical pattern. An aura may precede generalized seizure activity. The aura may be a vague sense of uneasiness or an abnormal sensation (such as a smell of burning rubber or seeing bright light). Often, however, the seizure occurs without warning.

The onset of the seizure begins with a sudden loss of consciousness and sharp *tonic* muscle contractions. With this muscle contraction, air is forced out of the lungs, and the client may emit a cry. Postural control is lost, and the client falls to the floor in the *opisthotonic* posture (Figure 40–5, *A*). Muscles are rigid, with the arms and legs extended; the jaw is clenched. Urinary incontinence is common; bowel incontinence may also occur. Breathing ceases and cyanosis develops during the tonic phase of a seizure. The pupils are fixed and dilated. The tonic phase lasts an average of 15 seconds, although it may persist for up to a minute (Hickey, 1992).

The *clonic* phase, which follows the tonic phase, is characterized by alternating contraction and relaxation of the muscles in all the extremities along with hyperventilation (Figure 40–5, *B*). The eyes roll back, and the client froths at the mouth. The clonic phase varies in duration and subsides gradually. The entire tonic-clonic portion of the seizure generally lasts no more than 60 to 90 seconds.

Following the clonic phase of seizure activity, the client remains unconscious and unresponsive to stimuli. The client is relaxed and breathes quietly. This period is known as the *postictal period* or phase. The client regains consciousness gradually and may be confused and disoriented on waking. Clients often experience headache, muscle aches, and fatigue following the seizure, and many sleep for several hours. Amnesia of the seizure is usual; the client also may not recall events just prior to the seizure activity.

Because of the lack of warning with tonic-clonic seizures, the client may experience injury. Head injury, fractures, burns, or motor vehicle accidents may occur secondarily to seizure activity.

Status Epilepticus

A condition known as **status epilepticus** can develop during seizure activity. Status epilepticus is considered a life-threatening medical emergency that requires immediate treatment. In this case, the seizure activity becomes continuous, with only very short periods of calm occurring between intense and persistent seizures. The repetitive seizures may be of any type, although they are usually generalized tonic-clonic (Porth, 1994). Repeated seizures have a cumulative effect. This cumulative effect produces muscular contractions that can interfere with respirations. The client is in great danger of developing hypoxia, acidosis, hypoglycemia, hyperthermia, and exhaustion if the convulsive activity is not halted.

Collaborative Care

Initial treatment focuses on controlling the seizure; the long-term goal is to determine the cause and prevent future seizures. Collaborative care includes diagnostic testing, pharmacologic treatment, and, in some cases, surgery.

Laboratory and Diagnostic Tests

Diagnostic testing is performed to confirm the seizure diagnosis and to determine any treatable causes and precipitating factors.

The following diagnostic tests may be ordered:

- *Complete neurologic exam* to determine the focal neurologic deficit or the focus or origin of seizure activity

---

Nursing Implications for Diagnostic Tests: Electroencephalogram (EEG)

■ ■ ■

An EEG is used to detect abnormal brain function. It provides a graphic record of the brain's electrical activity (brain waves) and is useful in evaluating seizure activity.

Client Preparation

- Explain the procedure to the client, emphasizing the importance of cooperation.

- Withhold fluids, foods, and medications (as prescribed) that may stimulate or depress brain waves. These include anticonvulsants, tranquilizers, depressants, and caffeine-containing foods (e.g., coffee, tea, colas, and chocolate). Medications are usually withheld for 24 to 48 hours before the test.

- Help the client wash the hair before the test.

Client and Family Teaching

- The test takes about an hour.

- The test is painless and will be performed while you sit in a comfortable chair or lie on a stretcher.

- The electrodes are applied to the scalp with a thick paste.

- During the test, you will first be asked to breathe in and out deeply for a few minutes. Then, you will close your eyes while a light is flashed on them and, finally, you will lie quietly with your eyes closed.

- After the test, the nurse will help you wash the paste out of your hair.

- *Electroencephalogram (EEG)* to help confirm the seizure diagnosis and localize any lesion(s). See the accompanying box for the nursing implications of EEG.

- *Skull X-ray studies* to identify possible fractures, deformities in bony structures, or calcification

- *CT scan* to determine the presence of a tumor, congenital lesions, edema, infarct, hemorrhage, arteriovenous malformation, or a structural deviation, such as ventricular enlargement

- *Lumbar puncture* to determine the presence of infection (meningitis), elevated protein levels in the CSF, or the presence of increased intracranial pressure

Nursing Implications for Pharmacology: Drugs Used to Treat Seizures

ANTICONVULSANTS

Phenytoin (Dilantin)	Valproic acid (Depakene)
Phenobarbital	Ethosuximide (Zarontin)
Primidone (Mysoline)	Clonazepam (Klonopin)
Carbamazepine (Tegretol)	

Anticonvulsant agents are used to control chronic seizures and involuntary muscle spasms or movements characteristic of certain neurologic diseases. These drugs act in the motor cortex of the brain to reduce the spread of electrical discharges from the rapidly firing epileptic foci in this area. These agents cannot cure convulsive disorders, but they do control seizures without impairing the normal functions of the CNS. Drugs effective against one type of seizure may not be effective against another; anticonvulsant therapy must be individualized.

Nursing Responsibilities

- Monitor blood pressure, pulse, and respirations. Observe for manifestations of impending seizures.
- Note evidence of CNS side effects, such as complaints of blurred vision, dimmed vision, slurred speech, nystagmus, or confusion. Gingival hyperplasia may be noted in clients taking phenytoin.
- Recognize that if clients are to be on prolonged therapy, they may need a diet rich in vitamin D.

- Check the serum calcium level as ordered; phenytoin can contribute to demineralization of bone.
- When administering anticonvulsants intravenously, monitor the client closely for respiratory depression and cardiovascular collapse.

Client and Family Teaching

- Take the exact dosage prescribed. Do not increase, decrease, or discontinue the dosage without obtaining the primary care provider's approval; doing so may lead to convulsions.
- Avoid hazardous tasks until the drug has been regulated. Anticonvulsant drugs may at first decrease mental alertness and cause drowsiness, headache, dizziness, and incoordination of muscles. These effects are usually dose related and may disappear with a change of dosage or continued therapy.
- If you are taking phenytoin (Dilantin), maintain good oral hygiene: Use a soft toothbrush, massage the gums, and floss daily.
- It is very important to obtain liver function studies regularly as ordered by the primary care provider. This will help detect early signs of hepatitis and other liver problems. Report for all scheduled laboratory studies, including complete blood count, kidney and liver function studies, and drug levels.
- Carry identification indicating the type of seizures for which you are being treated.

- *Blood studies* to monitor electrolytes, blood urea, and blood glucose
- *Electrocardiogram (ECG)* to rule out underlying cardiac dysrhythmias

Pharmacology

Most seizure activity can be reduced or controlled through the use of anticonvulsant medications. These medications do not cure the disorder; they only manage its manifestations. Anticonvulsant medications generally act in one of two ways: by raising the seizure threshold or by limiting the spread of abnormal activity within the brain.

The goals of pharmacologic treatment for epilepsy are to protect the client from harm and to reduce or prevent seizure activity without impairing cognitive function or producing undesirable side effects (Wilson et al., 1991).

Ideally, the lowest possible dose of a single medication that will control the client's seizures is prescribed; often, however, several medications must be tried before the most effective is identified, and a combination of drugs may be needed to manage the client's seizures. Therapy is individualized, based on the type of seizure activity and the client's response to the medication. Nursing implications for these drugs are described in the accompanying pharmacology box; important drug interactions are presented in the box at the top of the following page.

Status epilepticus is a medical emergency that requires immediate intervention to preserve life. Establishing and maintaining the airway is a priority. A solution of 50% dextrose is administered intravenously to prevent hypoglycemia. Diazepam (Valium) is the drug of choice to stop seizure activity. It is administered intravenously, and the dose repeated in 10 minutes if necessary. Phenytoin is

Important Drug Interactions with Anticonvulsants

■ ■ ■

- *Valproic acid (Depakene) and phenobarbital.* Blood levels of phenobarbital may rise significantly when valproic acid is added to the client's medication regimen.
- *Phenobarbital and digoxin.* This combination may increase the metabolism of digoxin, resulting in decreased digoxin levels.
- *Phenobarbital and sodium warfarin (Coumadin).* Phenobarbital may decrease the absorption of sodium warfarin from the gastrointestinal tract and decrease the drug's anticoagulant response.

- *Disulfiram (Antabuse) and phenobarbital.* This combination may inhibit the metabolism of the anticonvulsant drug and increase the incidence of side effects associated with the anticonvulsant drug.
- *Other drugs.* Other drugs reported to interact with anticonvulsant drugs include aspirin, certain antibiotics, isoniazid, acetazolamide (Diamox), antacids, folic acid, and narcotics.

Nursing Care of the Client with Seizures Having Surgery

PREOPERATIVE CARE

- For most clients, anticonvulsant medications are withheld the morning or evening of the day before surgery. *Anticonvulsant medications may interfere with intraoperative EEG monitoring.*
- For clients with frequent and/or severe seizures, however, a partial dose of medication may be administered. *This prevents seizures or status epilepticus during surgery.*
- A low dose of analgesics is administered before surgery. *The client must remain awake throughout the lengthy procedure to respond to commands during EEG recording.*

POSTOPERATIVE CARE

- Anticonvulsant medications are administered parenterally until the client can tolerate oral fluids; medications are then continued orally. *It is common for the client to have seizures in the early postoperative period.*
- Steroids are administered for the first 3 days after surgery and are tapered and then discontinued during the following week. *Steroids are given to decrease cerebral edema.*

also administered intravenously for longer-term control of seizures. Phenobarbital may also be administered to clients in status epilepticus.

Surgery

When all attempts to control the client's seizures fail, excision of the tissue involved in the seizure activity may be an effective and safe treatment alternative. It is estimated that approximately 5% of clients with epilepsy may be candidates for surgery. The goal of surgery is to reduce the client's uncontrollable seizures.

To be selected as a candidate for surgery, the client must be highly motivated and psychologically prepared. A psychologic screening is required because the preoperative preparation is extensive and time-consuming and

because the surgery is long and requires that the client remain awake during surgery so that he or she can cooperate and respond to commands. The EEG is monitored during surgery to identify the epileptogenic focus and evaluate the effect of surgical intervention.

General postoperative care for the client with intracranial surgery follows the nursing management guidelines outlined later in the chapter. Specific preoperative and postoperative care for a client with a seizure disorder is described in the accompanying box.

The use of vagal nerve stimulation as an alternative mode of treatment for intractable partial seizures is currently being evaluated in selected centers nationwide. The vagus nerve (cranial nerve X) has both efferent (motor) and a large number of afferent (sensory) components. It is

Table 40–4	Nursing Observations Before, During, and After a Seizure

Observation	Rationale
What was the client's level of consciousness? If consciousness was lost, at what point?	Indicates area of brain involved and type of seizure.
What was the client doing just before the attack?	May suggest precipitating factors.
In what part of the body did the seizure start?	May indicate the site of seizure activity in the brain tissue; for example, if jerking movements were first observed in right hand, the seizure focus may be in left motor cortex in the area of the hand.
Was there an epileptic cry?	Usually indicates the tonic stage of a generalized tonic-clonic seizure.
Were any automatisms, such as eyelid fluttering, chewing, lip smacking, or swallowing, observed?	Often seen in complex, partial, and absence seizures.
How long did movements last? Did the location or character change (tonic to clonic)? Did movements involve both sides of the body or just one?	Indicates areas in which focal activity originated.
Did the head and/or eyes turn to one side and, if so, which side?	Helps localize the focus of the seizure. During the seizure, the head and eyes typically will turn away from the side of the epileptogenic focus.
Were there changes in pupillary reactions?	Indicates involvement of the autonomic nervous system.
If the client fell, was the head hit?	Skull X-ray studies may be needed to rule out subdural hematoma or fracture.
Was there foaming or frothing from the mouth?	Usually indicates a tonic-clonic seizure.

believed that vagal nerve stimulation desynchronizes the electrical activity of the brain, yielding an antiepileptic effect (Michael, 1992).

Nursing Care

Nursing management of clients with a seizure disorder focuses on providing care during and immediately after the seizure and on client teaching. The most important data used in determining an accurate diagnosis are descriptions of manifestations obtained from nursing assessments before, during, and after a seizure. Table 40–4 lists the most important nursing assessments. The client with seizures has a wide variety of responses to actual or potential changes in health status; interventions discussed in this section focus on facilitating physical and psychologic comfort and safety.

Risk for Ineffective Airway Clearance

During a seizure, the tongue may fall back and obstruct the airway, the gag reflex may be depressed, and secretions may pool at the back of the throat. All of these effects of altered neurologic function place the client at risk for an obstructed airway. Most seizures occur in the home or community; the interventions described are also taught to the family of the client.

Nursing interventions with rationales follow:

- Provide interventions during a seizure to maintain a patent airway:
  a. Loosen clothing around the neck.
  b. Turn the client on the side.
  c. Do not force anything into the client's mouth.
  d. If prescribed and available, administer oxygen by mask to clients who are very ill or debilitated.
  Although it was at one time believed that it was necessary to place a padded tongue blade in the client's mouth during a seizure, this is no longer recommended; an improperly placed tongue blade can obstruct the airway. Turning the client on the side allows secretions to drain from the mouth.

- Teach family members or significant others how to care for the client during a seizure to prevent airway obstruction. *Family members are often the only people present to provide this emergency intervention.*

Risk for Injury

The client with a seizure disorder is at risk for injury. Protecting the client from trauma involves identifying the client at risk for seizures, using seizure precautions, and implementing nursing interventions both during and after a seizure to prevent injury.

Nursing interventions with rationales follow:

- Obtain information about past seizures: age when the client's first seizure occurred, most recent seizure, factors precipitating a seizure, any warning signs (aura), prophylactic anticonvulsant therapy, and specific concerns the client may have about the seizures. Include family members in the discussion. *Information will help with diagnosis and planning of care and teaching to decrease the risk of injury.*

- Provide interventions during a seizure to reduce the risk of injury:

a. Maintain the bed in low position and keep side rails up.
b. If the client is sitting or standing at the onset of the seizure, assist the client to ease to the floor.
c. Place a folded towel or pillow under the client's head.
A low bed position helps the client avoid falls and injuries. Side rails help the client remember not to get up alone and help prevent the client from falling out of bed should a seizure occur. The loss of consciousness at the onset of the seizure could precipitate falling.

- Teach client and family members measures to prevent injury at home:
a. Avoid smoking when alone or in bed.
b. Avoid alcohol.
c. Avoid becoming excessively tired.
d. Install grab bars in the shower and tub area.
e. Do not lock doors of the bedroom or bathroom.
f. Avoid an excessive intake of caffeine.
Cigarette smoking creates a fire hazard. Alcohol may produce a reaction when taken with anticonvulsant medications and precipitate seizure activity. Excessive fatigue and caffeine can precipitate a seizure. Grab bars provide an area of support. Doors should remain unlocked so that family members may enter if a seizure occurs.

Anxiety

The client with a seizure disorder is understandably anxious about the future, with questions about ability to go to school, work, have a family, and drive a car. Feelings of embarrassment about having a seizure in public and rejection by others are common and also increase the client's anxiety.

Nursing interventions with rationales follow:

- Provide support by explaining that the client's concerns are normal. *It is important to be sensitive to the effect of seizures on the client's self-concept and body image; alterations in these areas of one's being not only increase anxiety but also cause withdrawal from socialization with others. Demonstrating acceptance of the client's concerns allows further discussion.*

- Stress the importance of following the treatment plan. *Carefully following the prescribed treatment plan can lessen or prevent seizure activity.*

- Help the client identify leisure activities that are nonhazardous. *Worrying about being hurt if a seizure occurs may cause the client to withdraw from social activities that are pleasurable.*

- Discuss sharing the diagnosis with family members, friends, and co-workers. *Openly sharing the possibility of a seizure decreases anxiety about how others will react and also provides others with the knowledge they will need in order to help if a seizure occurs.*

- Provide information about information sources and support groups. *Sharing information with other people with similar health problems allows for a more realistic viewpoint; accurate information can clear misconceptions that cause anxiety.*

- Provide accurate information about hiring practices and legal limitations on driving or operating heavy or dangerous machinery. *Accurate information decreases anxiety about the unknown. The American Disabilities Act prohibits discrimination; however, there are legal limitations on driving until the person is proved free of seizures.*

Other Nursing Diagnoses

Other nursing diagnoses that may be appropriate for the client with or at risk for seizure activity follow:

- *Risk for Aspiration* related to glottal obstruction and depressed level of consciousness
- *Knowledge Deficit* about seizures, treatment, precipitating factors, preventive measures, and community resources
- *Ineffective Individual Coping* related to chronic nature of disease, feelings of helplessness regarding seizures, and social stigma associated with seizure disorders
- *Ineffective Breathing Pattern* related to neuromuscular impairment secondary to tonic phase of seizure
- *Social Isolation* related to embarrassment about having seizures
- *Powerlessness* related to inability to control seizure activity
- *Ineffective Management of Therapeutic Regimen* related to lack of knowledge of effects of anticonvulsant medications, environmental hazards, and community resources

Client and Family Teaching

Teaching follows a systematic assessment of the needs of both the client and family. Include family members so that they can learn seizure management, including the care and observations necessary before and during a seizure. Stress the importance of safety and keeping the airway patent. Explain specific anticonvulsant medication protocols and side effects.

Help both the client and family to adjust to a diagnosis of epilepsy (see the research box on page 1712). The following recommendations assist the client and family with adjustment:

- Correct misconceptions, common fears, and myths about epilepsy.
- Encourage both the client and family to express their feelings. Feelings of shame, fear, and anxiety are common.

Applying Research to Nursing Practice: Learning Needs of Clients with Epilepsy

∎ ∎ ∎

In one study, researchers investigated the learning needs of clients with epilepsy (Dilorio, Faherty, & Manteuffel, 1993). In the study, clients, nurses, and physicians were asked to rank 41 items grouped into 5 categories: anatomy and physiology, psychologic factors, medication information, seizure information, and general life-style information. Each category consisted of 6 to 10 items to be rated. Study participants included 59 clients, 85 nurses, and 38 physicians.

Medication information was identified as the most important category of learning needs. All three groups ranked seizure information as the second most important learning need; psychologic factors were ranked third. Specific items within the medication category included "what to do if there is a problem" and "side effects of medications." Clients also expressed interest in obtaining information about reducing the risk of seizures.

Implications for Nursing

Teaching is an important component of the care of clients with seizures. Teaching sessions should include both general information about medication therapy and actions to take when problems arise (e.g., running out of medication while on vacation). Stress-reduction strategies, such as relaxation training and biofeedback, may be appropriate in some teaching plans. Teaching plans should be individualized and should follow an assessment of specific learning needs.

Critical Thinking in Client Care

1. Why do people have different types of seizures?
2. How do seizures affect the brain?
3. Identify strategies to help clients with seizures remember to take their anticonvulsant medication.
4. Why should the client learn about maintaining blood levels of anticonvulsant medications?

∎ Provide the name and location of community and national resources, such as the Epilepsy Foundation of America. Information about the latest treatment modalities, research, and audiovisual materials can provide support and reassurance and facilitate social-

ization with others who are facing the same type of crisis.

∎ Stress the importance of follow-up care and keeping medical appointments.
∎ Review any state and local laws that apply to people with seizure disorders. Driving a motor vehicle is usually prohibited for 6 months to 2 years after a seizure episode. Usually, a driver's license can be reinstated or obtained after a seizure-free period and a letter from the nurse practitioner or physician.
∎ Refer the client to employment or vocational counseling as needed.
∎ Stress the importance of wearing a MedicAlert band or carrying a medical alert card at all times.
∎ Emphasize the importance of aura identification and the course of action to take.
∎ Stress the importance of continuing to take anticonvulsant medications as prescribed even when no seizures are experienced.
∎ Stress the importance of avoiding physical and emotional stress.
∎ Help the client focus on the positive aspects of life.
∎ In general, alcoholic beverages should be avoided completely and coffee intake should be limited. Showers, rather than tub baths, should be taken because the client may drown during a generalized seizure.
∎ Discuss factors that may trigger a seizure (abrupt withdrawal from medication, constipation, fatigue, excessive stress, fever, menstruation, sights and sounds such as television, flashing video, and computer screens) in the overall teaching plan.

Applying the Nursing Process

Case Study of a Client with a Seizure Disorder: Janet Carlson

Janet Carlson is a 19-year-old college student who lives with her parents and one younger sister. Although Ms. Carlson had seizures while she was in grade school, they have been controlled with medication. However, she had a tonic-clonic seizure yesterday and immediately made an appointment with her family physician. She is currently taking phenytoin (Dilantin) 300 mg/day as a maintenance medication to prevent seizures. At her office visit, measurement of serum phenytoin level is included in the laboratory orders.

Assessment

Evita Farias, RN, completes a health history for Ms. Carlson. During the history, Ms. Carlson tells Ms. Farias that she has been under stress because of difficulties in completing her course requirements this semester. She has not been sleeping as many hours per night, and sometimes she forgets to take her medication. Ms. Carlson's serum phenytoin level is 8 μg/mL. Therapeutic level is 10-20 mg/ml.

Diagnosis

Ms. Farias makes the following nursing diagnoses for Ms. Carlson:

- *Risk for Injury* related to recurrence of generalized tonic-clonic seizure activity and low serum phenytoin levels
- *Knowledge Deficit* of activities that may trigger seizure occurrence, the effect of stress on seizures, and medication information

Expected Outcomes

The expected outcomes for the plan of care specify that

- Ms. Carlson's seizures will be controlled or minimized.
- Ms. Carlson and her family will verbalize precipitating and triggering factors related to the onset of seizures.
- Ms. Carlson and her family will verbalize the relationship between emotional and physical stress and seizures.
- Ms. Carlson and her family will verbalize the importance of taking anticonvulsant medications.

Planning and Implementation

Ms. Farias plans and implements the following nursing interventions for Ms. Carlson:

- Teach Ms. Carlson and her family the following:
  a. Current information about seizures
  b. Care during and after a seizure
  c. Medication protocols
  d. Factors and activities that can trigger seizures
  e. The importance of follow-up care
- Refer Ms. Carlson and her family to a local epilepsy support group.
- Recommend that she purchase and wear a MedicAlert bracelet.

Evaluation

Ms. Carlson is instructed to continue taking Dilantin 300 mg/day. Ms. Carlson verbalizes the importance of nutrition, rest, and measures to reduce stress. She also verbalizes the importance of maintaining the proper blood levels of her medication, stating that too little or too much of the medication could cause problems. Ms. Carlson recognizes that the seizure problems had recurred during a busy time in school during which she had forgotten to take her medication. Ms. Carlson's parents verbalize the steps to take if Ms. Carlson has another seizure. Ms. Carlson is now wearing a MedicAlert bracelet. Ms. Farias pro-

vides the Carlsons with the telephone number of the local chapter of the Epilepsy Foundation of America.

Critical Thinking in the Nursing Process

1. If you were Ms. Carlson's nurse, would your teaching differ if Ms. Carlson were living alone? If so, how?

2. Ms. Carlson tells you that although she knows she should not drive a car, she often drives her friend to work. How would you approach this problem?

3. What would your response be if Ms. Carlson called two weeks later and stated that she was having problems with her vision and some slurring of her words?

4. Ms. Carlson states that "it's embarrassing to wear a MedicAlert bracelet." How would you respond, and what recommendation(s) would you make?

5. Develop a care plan for Ms. Carlson for the nursing diagnosis *Risk for Social Isolation*.

The Client with Headaches

∎ ∎ ∎

Headache is pain within the cranial vault (Hickey, 1992). Headache is one of the most common symptoms people experience across the life span, although its cause is frequently unknown. Headaches may occur as a result of benign or pathologic conditions, intracranial or extracranial conditions, diseases of other body systems, stress, musculoskeletal tension, or a combination of these factors.

The majority of headaches are mild in severity, transient, and relieved by a mild analgesic. However, some headaches are chronic, intense, and recurrent. Clinical manifestations of headache vary according to the cause, type, and precipitating symptoms.

Pathophysiology

Most selected structures within the cranial vault are sensitive to pain. Pain-sensitive structures include supporting structures, such as the skin, muscles, and periosteum; the nasal cavities and sinuses; portions of the meninges, cranial nerves II, III, IV, V, VI, IX, and X; and cerebral vessels, including extracranial arteries and the venous sinuses. Most facial and scalp structures are sensitive to pain. Stretching (traction), inflammation, pressure compression, and dilation of the pain-sensitive structures of the cranial vault, scalp, and face can produce a headache. The most common types of headaches are migraine, cluster, and tension headaches. Migraine and cluster headaches are associated with disturbances of cranial circulation, whereas tension headaches result from muscle contraction (Table 40–5).

Table 40–5 Comparison of Migraine, Cluster, and Tension Headaches

Type	Risk Factors	Frequency and Duration	Description	Prodromal and Associated Manifestations
Migraine	Female sex. Family history of migraine headache. Age not a risk factor.	Episodic: ■ Tends to occur with stress and crisis. ■ Often correlates with menstrual cycle. ■ Can last hours to days.	Slow onset; pain becomes more severe, involving one side of head more than other.	Prodromal manifestations: visual defects, confusion, parenthesias. Associated manifestations: nausea, vomiting, chills, fatigue, irritability, sweating.
Cluster	Male sex. Use of alcohol or nitrates. May begin in early childhood.	Episodes are clustered together in rapid succession for a few days or weeks with remissions that last for months. Can last a few minutes to a few hours.	May begin in infraorbital region and spread to head and neck; throbbing, deep pain, often unilateral.	Prodromal manifestations: uncommon. Associated manifestations: flushing, tearing of eyes, nasal congestion, sweating and swelling of temporal vessels.
Tension	Related to tension and anxiety. No family history. Often begins in adolescence.	Episodic: ■ Varies with amount of stress. ■ Duration also varies; can be constant.	Tight, pressing, viselike; may involve neck and shoulders.	Prodromal manifestations: uncommon. Associated manifestations: sustained contraction of neck muscles.

Migraine Headaches

Migraine headache is the most common type of vascular headache. The classification of migraine headache includes headaches that differ in intensity, duration, and frequency. Migraine headaches are often familial, affecting females more often than males. It is thought that the underlying physiology of migraine changes involves dysfunction of the endothelial cells of the blood vessels (Porth, 1994).

Classic Migraine Headache The classic migraine headache has three stages: the *aura stage* (also called the prodromal stage), the *headache stage* (or period of throbbing), and the *postheadache stage*. The aura or prodromal stage is characterized by sensory manifestations, usually visual disturbances such as bright spots or flashing lights zig-zagging across the visual fields. This stage lasts approximately 15 to 30 minutes. Less common sensory symptoms include numbness or tingling of the face or hand, paresis of an arm or leg, mild aphasia, confusion, drowsiness, and lack of coordination. Additionally, some clients experience a premonition the day prior to an attack. Nervousness or other mood changes may occur. The aura period corresponds with the initial physiologic change of vasoconstriction. Serotonin levels also increase during this stage (Hickey, 1992).

Vasodilation, a decline in serotonin levels, and the onset of throbbing headache signal the headache phase. It appears that the pain is related to increased vessel permeability and polypeptide exudation by perivascular nerve endings rather than the vasodilation itself (Porth, 1994). Cerebral arteries are dilated and distended, with walls that are edematous and rigid. Beginning unilaterally, the headache eventually may involve both sides as it increases in intensity during the next several hours. Nausea and vomiting often occur; the headache is therefore often referred to as a "sick headache." The client may be acutely ill and is often extremely irritable. The sensory organs often become hypersensitive, and the client withdraws from sound and light. The scalp is tender. The headache may last from several hours to a day or two.

During the postheadache phase, the headache area is sensitive to touch, and a deep aching is present. The client experiences exhaustion. Vessel size and serotonin levels return to normal.

A variety of factors are believed to trigger the vasoconstriction. Rapid changes in blood glucose levels, stress, emotional excitement, fatigue, hormonal balance changes due to menstruation, stimuli such as bright lights, and food high in tyramine or other vasoactive substances (e.g., aged cheese, nuts, chocolate, and alcoholic beverages) have been associated with migraine attacks. Hypertension and febrile states may make the disorder worse.

Common Migraine Headache Another type of migraine headache is called a *common migraine*. This type is associated with hereditary factors. The prodromal stage is often absent; some clients are aware only that a headache is coming on. The headache develops gradually, lasting hours to days, and may occur during periods of premenstrual tension and fluid retention. Chills, nausea and vomiting, fatigue, and nasal congestion are often present.

Cluster Headache

The **cluster headache** (or atypical migraine headache) is a form of vascular headache predominantly experienced by older men. The headache typically begins 2 to 3 hours after the person falls asleep. Prodromal signs are absent. Intense unilateral pain around or behind one eye wakes the client. The pain is accompanied by rhinorrhea, lacrimation, flushing, sweating, facial edema, and possible miosis or ptosis on the affected side. Headaches last 30 minutes to a few hours and abate abruptly.

The attacks tend to occur frequently, in clusters, for weeks or a few months. The headaches often occur in the spring and fall and then disappear for an extended period. The same side of the head is involved in each cluster of attacks. The physiologic mechanism underlying cluster headaches is not well understood but is attributed to a vascular origin.

Tension Headache

Tension headache, or muscle contraction headache, is a poorly localized headache characterized by ill-defined bilateral head aching, tightness, pressure, or a viselike feeling. Sharply localized painful spots (trigger points) may be present. The onset is gradual, and the intensity, frequency, and duration of the attack vary greatly. This type of headache is caused by sustained contraction of the muscles of the head and neck. It is often precipitated by stressful situations and anxiety. Secondary causes include disorders of the eyes, ears, sinuses, or cervical vertebrae. Abnormal posture associated with occupations that require bending over a desk (e.g., office workers, students) often precipitates tension headache. Additionally, slouching while reading or watching television can lead to muscle contraction. The majority of headaches are tension-type headaches.

Collaborative Care

Identifying the underlying cause(s) of the headache is the initial focus of collaborative care. If the underlying cause is treatable, manifestations of the headache will often decrease or disappear. An accurate diagnosis of the type of headache is key to the treatment.

Therapeutic management for migraine headache includes a combination of client teaching, drug therapy, and measures to control contributing factors. Dietary changes such as eliminating caffeine, cured meats, monosodium glutamate (MSG), and foods containing tyramine (red wine, aged cheese, and others) may be necessary. Stress management or biofeedback are also part of the overall strategy. Treatment protocols for cluster headache include the elimination of aggravating factors (e.g., consumption of alcohol). The management of muscle contraction (tension) headaches is directed toward reducing the client's level of stress. Behavioral techniques such as meditation, biofeedback, psychotherapy, and other methods to reduce anxiety may help the client. Improving poor posture and initiating comfort measures such as gentle massage or heat may also help.

Laboratory and Diagnostic Tests

Diagnosis and treatment are based on history, the identification of triggering or precipitating events, and the type of headache. A thorough history and physical examination are integral parts of the assessment. Neurodiagnostic testing may be done to rule out a structural disease process. Testing may include a brain scan, MRI, X-ray studies of the skull and cervical spine, EEG, or lumbar puncture for CSF if inflammation is suspected. Serum metabolic screens and hypersensitivity testing also may be performed if systemic problems are suspected.

Pharmacology

Pharmacologic management of headache depends on the specific type of headache experienced by the client. The goals of treatment are to reduce the frequency and severity of headaches and to limit or abolish a headache that is beginning or in progress.

The management of migraine includes administering medications to prevent headaches (prophylactic therapy) as well as drugs to stop (or abort) a headache in progress. The client with frequent migraine headaches is a candidate for prophylactic therapy. Drugs used to reduce the frequency and severity of migraine follow:

- Methysergide maleate (Sansert) is a serotonin antagonist that competitively blocks serotonin receptors in the central nervous system and is also a potent vasoconstrictor.

- Propranolol hydrochloride (Inderal) is a beta-blocker that prevents dilation of vessels in the pia mater and inhibits serotonin uptake.

- Verapamil (Isoptin) and nifedipine (Procardia) are calcium channel blockers that are thought to prevent migraine by controlling cerebral vasospasms.

- Amitriptyline hydrochloride (Elavil) is a tricyclic antidepressant that blocks the uptake of serotonin and catecholamines; it is often used for combination migraine and tension headaches (Hickey, 1992).

When the manifestations of migraine are recognized early, several medications may be used to abort or limit the severity and duration of the headache. Ergotamine tartrate (Cafergot) is a complex drug that reduces extracranial blood flow, decreases the amplitude of cranial artery pulsation, and decreases basilar artery hyperperfusion. Administered at the onset of an attack, ergotamine is effective in controlling up to 70% of acute attacks. Sumatriptan (Imitrex) is a new medication available for subcutaneous autoinjection. It binds with serotonin receptors and is rapidly effective in aborting the headache.

Once an attack of migraine is in progress, a narcotic analgesic such as codeine or meperidine (Demerol) may be required. Antiemetics such as promethazine hydrochloride (Phenergan) may be prescribed to control nausea and vomiting.

Many of the same medications used for migraine are used to prevent or treat cluster headache. Because the onset of cluster headaches is abrupt, abortive therapy is not possible. Medications such as ergotamine tartrate may be given in suppository form at bedtime to prevent headache during attacks. Clients may find inhalation of 100% oxygen for 15 minutes at the onset of an attack effective in relieving headache (Tierney et al., 1994).

Simple analgesics such as aspirin or acetaminophen may be effective in relieving tension headaches. Additionally, tranquilizers such as diazepam may be employed to reduce muscle tension.

Nursing implications for drugs commonly prescribed for headache are described in the accompanying box.

Nursing Care

Nursing care of the client with headache includes obtaining a detailed history and description of the headaches' characteristics to help identify triggering or precipitating factors. Assessment also includes investigating the effects of recurring headaches on the client's life-style, activities of daily living (ADLs), and role performance. Nursing interventions are developed to help the client identify strategies for controlling the pain and discomfort of the headache. The primary response of the client requiring nursing interventions is pain.

Pain

Headaches originate from both intracranial and extracranial sources and range in severity from benign, transient discomfort to severe, incapacitating pain. Interventions focus on teaching the client self-care measures to control or relieve the pain, and reducing any associated problems, such as nausea and vomiting or anxiety.

Nursing interventions with rationales follow:

- Teach the client to maintain a diary of headaches, including duration, onset, location, relation to menstruation or food intake, and related manifestations such as factors that relieve or intensify the pain. *A thorough assessment of the headache is essential for both the client and*

the health care provider to identify the circumstances and patterns of headache occurrence.

- Ask the client to rate the pain or discomfort on a scale of 0 to 10 (with 10 being the worst pain). *Using a scale to rate the pain provides an objective measure of the client's subjective experience of the pain or discomfort. The scale can also be used to evaluate the effectiveness of pain relief measures.*

- Teach the client to minimize light, noise, and activity and rest in a quiet, nonstimulating environment when experiencing a headache. *Manipulating the environment helps reduce noxious stimuli that may increase pain.*

- Teach the client to use noninvasive and nonpharmacologic pain relief measures such as deep breathing or relaxation to facilitate self-management of pain (see Chapter 4). *Alternative strategies to control pain can help reduce tension and may help to increase the client's sense of control over the pain.*

- If appropriate, teach the client to apply cold compresses or dry heat to the head and neck. *The application of cold can cause vasoconstriction, which helps reduce pain in vascular headaches. Application of heat can reduce muscle tension and improve circulation.*

- Teach the client to follow good nutrition guidelines, get regular exercise and sleep, and practice a life-style that minimizes stress. *Headaches are more likely to occur when ill, tired, or under stress (Hickey, 1992).*

Other Nursing Diagnoses

Additional nursing diagnoses appropriate for the client with or at risk for headache follow:

- *Ineffective Individual Coping* related to severe pain and stress and changes in life-style
- *Sensory/Perceptual Alterations* related to visual, tactile alterations
- *Knowledge Deficit* related to a lack of understanding about headaches and treatment protocols, strategies
- *Fear* related to pain and inability to control the pain
- *Sleep Pattern Disturbance* related to pain, nausea, vomiting, and medication
- *Altered Role Performance* related to pain and medication side effects

Client and Family Teaching

In addition to relieving pain and implementing comfort measures, client education has a high priority. Develop a teaching plan to help the client learn how to limit attacks (for example, by avoiding precipitating factors) and reduce the effects of the headache. Specific information about prescribed medications should be provided. Referrals for methods of stress reduction may be necessary for clients with long-term or migraine headaches.

Nursing Implications for Pharmacology: The Client Having Headaches

BETA-BLOCKERS

Propanolol hydrochloride (Inderal)

Nadolol (Corgard)

Atenolol (Tenormin)

Timolol maleate (Blocadren)

Beta-blockers are effective in the prophylactic treatment of headache. Although the mechanisms involved are not clear, they act by combining with beta-adrenergic receptors to block the response to sympathetic nerve impulses, circulating catecholamines, or adrenergic drugs.

Nursing Responsibilities

- Note indications for therapy and carefully assess client's mental status.
- Before beginning therapy, determine pulse and blood pressure in both arms with client lying, sitting, and standing.
- Assess baseline and monitor serum glucose level, CBC, electrolytes, and liver and renal function studies.
- Note any history of diabetes or impaired renal function.
- Note the rate and quality of respirations; drugs in this category may cause dyspnea and bronchospasm.
- Administer the drug with meals to prevent gastrointestinal disturbances.
- Be alert that beta-blockers cause bradycardia and the heart rate may not rise in response to stress, such as exercise or fever. Notify the primary health care provider if pulse falls below 50 or if blood pressure changes significantly.
- Teach the client or family member how to take a pulse and blood pressure reading.

Client and Family Teaching

- Take the medication with meals to provide a coating for the gastrointestinal tract and prevent gastrointestinal disturbances.
- Return for blood work as prescribed.
- Take the last dose of the day at bedtime.
- Rise from a sitting or lying position to a standing position slowly to avoid dizziness and falls.

- Take pulse and blood pressure each day and maintain a record of readings.
- Avoid excessive intake of alcohol, coffee, tea, or cola. Consult with the health care provider before taking any over-the-counter medications.
- Report any cough, nasal stuffiness, or feelings of depression to the health care provider.

TRICYCLIC ANTIDEPRESSANTS

Imipramine hydrochloride (Tofranil)

Amitriptyline hydrochloride (Elavil)

Nortriptyline hydrochloride (Pamelor)

The tricyclic antidepressants were used first to treat depression. More recently, they have been successful in the prophylaxis of cluster and migraine headaches. Although the exact mechanism is not known, they do prevent the reuptake of norepinephrine or serotonin, or both. They are chemically related to the phenothiazines, and as such they exhibit many of the same pharmacologic effects (e.g., anticholinergic, antiserotonin, sedative, antihistaminic, and hypotensive effects).

Nursing Responsibilities

- Assess baseline CBC and liver function studies, heart sounds, and neurologic status before initiating prescribed therapy.

Client and Family Teaching

- Make position changes slowly.
- Chew sugarless gum to relieve dry mouth.
- Do not abruptly quit taking the medication.

ERGOT ALKALOID DERIVATIVES

Methysergide maleate (Sansert)

Methysergide is an ergot alkaloid derivative structurally related to LSD. It acts by stimulating smooth muscle, leading to vasoconstriction. It is thought that methysergide prevents headaches by blocking the effects of serotonin, a powerful vasodilator believed to play a role in vascular headaches. It also inhibits the release of histamine from mast cells and prevents the release of serotonin from platelets.

➤

Pharmacology: The Client Having Headaches (continued)

Nursing Responsibilities

- Note any history of renal or hepatic disease. Obtain baseline liver and renal function studies.
- Before initiating therapy, assess the client's behavior.
- Obtain baseline eosinophil and neutrophil counts before beginning therapy.
- Administer the drug with meals or milk to minimize gastrointestinal irritation due to increased hydrochloric acid production.
- Assess for renal, central nervous system, and cardiovascular complications.
- Drug dosage should be gradually reduced over 2 to 3 weeks to prevent rebound headaches. A drug-free interval of 3 to 4 weeks is required with each 6-month course of therapy to prevent complications.
- Monitor for signs of ergotism, such as coldness or numbness of the fingers and toes, nausea, vomiting, headache, muscle pain, and weakness. Vasoconstriction may further impair peripheral circulation and increase blood pressure.

Client and Family Teaching

- Take the medication with meals or milk to minimize gastrointestinal upset.
- Report to the primary care provider nervousness, weakness, rashes, hair loss, or swelling of the extremities.
- Weigh daily and report any unusual weight gain to the primary care provider.
- Return to the primary care provider for a checkup at least every 6 months or as instructed. Do not take the drug on a regular basis for longer than 6 months, but do not abruptly stop taking it.
- Return for follow-up blood work as ordered.

SEROTONIN SELECTIVE AGONIST

Sumatriptan succinate injection (Imitrex)

Sumatriptan is rapidly absorbed when administered subcutaneously. It binds to vascular receptors to vasoconstrict cranial blood vessels and relieve migraine headache.

Nursing Responsibilities

- Assess the client for history of peripheral vascular disease, renal or hepatic problems, and pregnancy.

- Evaluate relief of migraine headache, and assess for side effects of photophobia, sound sensitivity, and nausea and vomiting.

Client and Family Teaching

- Do not use more than 2 injections in a 24-hour period, and allow at least 1 hour between injections.
- Use the autoinjector to administer the medication, and follow instructions for proper method of giving the injection and disposing of the syringe.
- Report wheezing, heart palpitations, skin rash, swelling of the eyelids or face, or chest pain to the health care provider immediately.

CALCIUM CHANNEL BLOCKERS

Verapamil (Isoptin)

Nifedipine (Procardia)

Although the exact mechanism is not known, it is thought that the calcium channel blockers may have value in controlling cerebral vasospasms by two mechanisms: inhibiting the influx of calcium into the cerebral artery and interfering with the destruction of erythrocytes and aggregation of platelets.

Nursing Responsibilities

- These drugs cause peripheral vasodilation. Therefore, monitor blood pressure and pulse during the initial administration of the drug. Any excessive hypotensive response and tachycardia may precipitate angina. Request written parameters for safe drug administration.
- Monitor intake and output and daily weights. Assess for manifestations of congestive heart failure: weight gain, peripheral edema, dyspnea, rales, and jugular vein distention.
- Teach client and family members how to take pulse and blood pressure readings.

Client and Family Teaching

- Take the medication with meals to reduce gastrointestinal irritation.
- Take pulse and blood pressure before taking medications each day at the same time, and follow instructions regarding when to withhold medication and when to contact the provider. Keep a record of pulse and blood pressure readings.

Pharmacology: The Client Having Headaches (continued)

- Report any side effects, such as dizziness, vertigo, unusual flushing, facial warmth, or headaches, to the primary care provider.

- Report immediately any swelling of the hands or feet, pronounced dizziness, or chest pain accompanied by sweating, shortness of breath, or severe headaches.

NONSTEROIDAL ANTI-INFLAMMATORY DRUG (NSAID): SALICYLATE

Acetylsalicylic acid (Ecotrin, Bufferin)

Acetylsalicylic acid, or aspirin, is a nonnarcotic analgesic, antipyretic, anti-inflammatory agent used to relieve headache pain. The mechanism of action is not known fully, but the analgesic effects are partly attributable to improvement of the inflammatory condition.

Nursing Responsibilities

- Determine the type and pattern of pain. Determine whether the pain is unusual or recurs. Use a rating scale of 0 to 10 to assess the level of pain (with 10 being the worst pain). If aspirin was used in the past for pain control, note its effectiveness.

- Note any history of peptic ulcers or other conditions that may suggest potential problems with the use of salicylates.

- Assess clients receiving anticoagulant therapy for bruises, bleeding of the mucous membranes, or blood in the urine or stool.

Client and Family Teaching

- Take aspirin after meals or before meals with an antacid and a full glass of water to minimize gastric irritation.

- Report ringing in the ears, unusual bleeding of gums, bruising, or black tarry stools to the primary health care provider.

- Monitor blood glucose levels carefully (if you have diabetes), and report hypoglycemia if it occurs.

ERGOTAMINE

Caffeine-ergotamine tartrate combination (Cafergot)

Ergotamine tartrate (Gynergen)

Ergot alkaloids vasoconstrict the cerebral blood vessels, decreasing the amplitude of the pulsations of the cranial arteries. The major use of ergot alkaloids is the treatment of migraine headaches. Cafergot has the same actions as Gynergen; in addition, the caffeine it contains provides a vasoconstrictive action, enhancing the effects of ergotamine.

Nursing Responsibilities

- Because the drug accumulates in the body and is eliminated slowly, ergotamine poisoning may occur. Sepsis, renal and vascular disease, heavy smoking, malnutrition, pregnancy, contraceptive hormones, and fever can increase the risk of ergotamine poisoning.

- These drugs are contraindicated in clients with diabetes mellitus, sepsis, hepatic or renal disease, peripheral and coronary artery disease, hypertension, and pregnancy.

Client and Family Teaching

- Take the drug immediately at onset of headache.

- Report the following to your health care provider: pain in the leg muscles, weakness, and coldness or numbness of fingers or toes.

- A dose of Cafergot taken late in the day may prevent sleep because of the effects of caffeine.

Applying the Nursing Process

Case Study of a Client with a Migraine Headache: Betty Friedman

Betty Friedman is a 25-year-old grade-school teacher. Her friends and the other teachers regard Ms. Friedman as an enthusiastic person who sets high standards for herself and strives for perfection. During the spring semester, Ms. Friedman begins to miss work more often than usual and sometimes appears very nervous. One day, another teacher notices Ms. Friedman running down the hall and into the restroom; the teacher finds Ms. Friedman vomiting. As she washes up, Ms. Friedman tells the other teacher that she has been having headaches off and on since she began menstruating but that they have never been as intense and frequent as during this past year. They even wake her from her sleep at night. Ms. Friedman agrees to see the nurse practitioner, Jane Schickadanz, at the school clinic for evaluation.

Assessment
During the interview, Ms. Friedman reveals that each month before her menstrual cycle, she becomes nervous and sees flashing lights. She also has difficulty expressing herself and thinking clearly. The next day she develops a "sick headache." She states that the headache can last 1 to 2 days and that afterwards she cannot brush her hair because her scalp hurts. Ms. Friedman attributes these symptoms to PMS and adds that she thinks she is allergic to cheese and nuts because she gets very sick after eating them. After a complete assessment, and in consultation with the physician, Ms. Schickadanz diagnoses Ms. Friedman's problem as a classic migraine headache. Sumatriptan succinate (Imitrex) injections are prescribed.

Diagnosis
Ms. Schickadanz makes the following nursing diagnoses for Ms. Friedman:

- *Pain* related to vasodilatation of cerebral vessels and a decreased serotonin level
- *Knowledge Deficit* of ways to manage pain
- *Altered Role Performance* related to pain

Expected Outcomes
The expected outcomes for the plan of care specify that Ms. Friedman will

- Experience reduced frequency and duration of pain.
- Verbalize understanding of the therapy regimen.
- Identify the available resources for helping with self-management of pain.

Planning and Implementation
The following nursing interventions are planned and implemented for Ms. Friedman:

- Ask Ms. Friedman to keep a diary of her headaches for the next month, noting times of their occurrence, location and duration of pain, and factors that trigger the onset, such as her menstrual period or certain foods.
- Teach Ms. Friedman techniques for administering the subcutaneous injection and for disposing of the syringe and guidelines for administration (e.g., take no more than 2 injections within 24 hours, and space injections by at least 1 hour). Teach her to take the medication at the first awareness of an impending attack.
- Suggest that Ms. Friedman make an appointment with a counselor to learn methods of relaxation and stress relief.
- Discuss with Ms. Friedman the importance of good nutrition and regular exercise.
- Request dietary referral for elimination of foods that might precipitate headaches.

Evaluation
Four weeks after beginning medication therapy with Imitrex and relaxation techniques, Ms. Friedman has noted a decrease in the intensity of the headaches. She reports that the medication has stopped the headaches, which, she has noted, tend to occur more frequently immediately before her menstrual period. She is walking for 30 minutes each day and has made changes in her usual diet. Ms. Friedman states that she feels "good about going to work with her kids at school and knowing she can control her pain."

Critical Thinking in the Nursing Process

1. List the questions you would include in a health history that would identify physical and psychologic stressors consistent with migraine headaches.

2. Develop a teaching plan for Ms. Friedman that includes methods of reducing fluid retention before her menstrual period, as well as a suggested diet based on the Food Guide Pyramid.

3. Design a plan of care for Ms. Friedman for the nursing diagnosis *Sleep Pattern Disturbance.*

Craniocerebral Trauma

Craniocerebral trauma, traumatic injury to the brain or cranial vault, is a leading cause of death and disability in the United States. Craniocerebral traumas, or head injuries, are among the most frequent and serious neurologic disorders. It is estimated that 10 million people in the United States experience head injuries every year; about 20% of these result in brain damage (Wilson et al., 1991). Trauma is the leading cause of death between age 1 and 44; head injury contributes to mortality in more than half these trauma victims (Hickey, 1992). Motor vehicle accidents (MVAs) are a major cause; elevated blood alcohol levels contribute significantly to the risk of MVA and subsequent injury. Other causes of head injury include falls, sports injuries, occupational injuries, assaults, and gunshot wounds (Hickey, 1992). Many clients who survive craniocerebral trauma are left with a deficit that precludes a resumption of their previous life-styles. It is estimated that two-thirds of these clients are below age 30, with males outnumbering females.

Specific damage following craniocerebral injuries is related to the mechanism of the injury (how it occurs), the nature of the injury (type), and the location of the injury (where it occurs).

Injuries to the head can occur through several mechanisms:

- An acceleration injury is sustained when the head is struck by a moving object, such as a swinging bat.

- A deceleration injury occurs when the head hits a stationary object, such as a concrete wall.

- An acceleration-deceleration injury (also called a coup-contrecoup phenomenon) occurs when the head hits an object and the brain "rebounds" within the skull (Figure 40–6). Injury to the brain occurs at the point of impact and on the opposite side of the impact. Two or more areas of the brain can be injured as a result of this phenomenon.

- Deformation injuries are those in which the force results in deformation and disruption of the integrity of the impacted body part. An example is skull fracture. Head injuries can also be classified as blunt or penetrating.

There are several types of craniocerebral trauma: injuries to the skull, including fractures; injuries to the brain, including concussion and contusion; and intracranial hemorrhage, including hematomas. Brain damage can result either from the direct effects of the trauma on brain tissue or from secondary responses to trauma, such as cerebral edema, hematoma, swelling, or increased intracranial pressure.

The Client with a Skull Fracture

■ ■ ■

A *skull fracture* is a break in the continuity of the skull. It occurs in approximately 7% of the clients who have craniocerebral trauma. It may occur with or without damage to the brain; however, intracranial lesions occur with approximately ⅔'s of skull fractures (Wilson et al., 1991). The considerable force which occurs on impact significantly increases the risk of underlying hematoma formation. Disruption of the skull can also cause cranial nerve

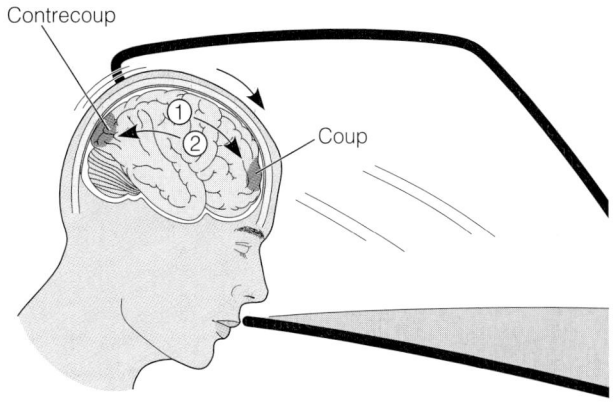

Figure 40–6   Coup-contrecoup head injury. Following the initial injury (coup), the brain rebounds within the skull and sustains additional injury (contrecoup) in the opposite part of the brain.

injury, allow bacteria to enter the cranial vault, or allow CSF to leak out.

Pathophysiology

Skull fractures are classified as open or closed. In an open fracture, the dura is torn, and in a closed fracture, the dura is not torn. Skull fractures are further classified into one of four categories: linear, comminuted, depressed, or basilar (Table 40–6).

Linear fractures are the most common type of skull fracture, accounting for 80% of all skull fractures. They typically extend from the point of impact toward the base of the skull (Wilson et al., 1991). Although the risk of infection or CSF leakage is minimal with this type of fracture because the dura usually remains intact, subdural or epidural hematomas frequently underlie the fracture. A hematoma (discussed later in this chapter) places pressure on underlying brain tissue, increasing both intracranial pressure and the risk of brain damage.

Comminuted and *depressed skull fractures* increase the risk of direct damage to brain tissue from contusion and bone fragments. In contrast, however, the risk of secondary brain injury may be reduced in these fractures because in breaking the bone, the traumatic impact energy is distributed and dissipated (Wilson et al., 1991). If the skin overlying the fracture is lacerated or the dura is torn, the risk of infection is greater.

Basilar skull fractures involve the base of the skull and usually are extensions of adjacent fractures, although they may occur independently. Although most basilar skull fractures are uncomplicated, they may involve the sinuses of the frontal bone or the petrous portion of the temporal bone (middle ear). If the dura is disrupted, CSF may leak through the tear. Manifestations of CSF leakage may in-

Table 40–6	Types of Skull Fractures
Type	**Description**
Linear (simple)	Simple, clean break in skull. Occurs with low-velocity injuries.
Comminuted	Bone is crushed into small, fragmented pieces. Usually seen with high-impact injuries.
Depressed	Inward depression of bone fragments. Usually due to a powerful blow to the skull. The dura may or may not be intact. Bone fragments may penetrate into the brain tissue.
Basilar	Occurs at the base of the skull. May be linear, comminuted, or depressed.

clude *rhinorrhea* (CSF leakage through the nose) or *otorrhea* (CSF leakage from the ear). Basilar skull fractures can be difficult to identify on X-ray film, but certain clinical manifestations may be associated with the fracture. For example, blood may be visible behind the tympanic membrane (hemotympanum), or ecchymosis may be noted over the mastoid process (known as Battle's sign). Bilateral periorbital ecchymosis (raccoon eyes) is another possible manifestation of basilar skull fracture. If CSF leakage is present, the risk of infection is high. Other complications of basilar skull fractures include injury to the internal carotid artery and compression of cranial nerve II, VI, or VII.

Collaborative Care

Treatment of a client with a skull fracture depends on the type and location of the fracture. Skull fracture may be only one of several head injuries.

A simple linear fracture generally requires bed rest and observation for underlying injury to brain tissue or hematoma formation. No specific treatment is required. Depressed skull fractures require surgical intervention, usually within 24 hours of the injury, to debride the wound completely and remove bone fragments, which may become embedded in brain tissue or cerebral blood vessels. If the bone is depressed deeply, the depressed bone may be elevated. If cerebral edema is not present, a cranioplasty with insertion of acrylic bone may be performed. If there is concern about infection, this procedure may be postponed for 3 to 6 months. Basilar skull fractures do not require surgery unless CSF leakage persists. Regular neurologic assessments and observation for manifestations of meningitis are required for the hospitalized client. Dexamethasone (Decadron) may be administered to reduce cerebral edema. Antibiotics may be administered prophylactically even if surgery is postponed.

Nursing Care

The client with a craniocerebral trauma, depending on its location and extent, may have many different responses and health care needs. Many of those problems with related nursing interventions are discussed in other sections of this chapter, including seizures, increased intracranial pressure, and bleeding within the brain. This section discusses the risk for infection, a problem common to the client with an open head wound from a skull fracture.

Risk for Infection

The client who sustains a fracture of the skull is at high risk for infection related to possible access to the cranial contents through a tear in the dura. In an open, depressed fracture, the wound may be contaminated by dirt, hair, or other debris. The nurse assesses for CSF leakage (which indicates a dural tear), monitors for manifestations of infection, and provides care to prevent infection.

Nursing interventions with rationales follow:

- Observe the client for otorrhea or rhinorrhea. *Open fractures of the skull increase the possibility of leakage of CSF from the ears or nose.*

- Test drainage of clear fluid from ear and nose for glucose by using a glucose reagent strip, such as Dextrostix. If drainage contains blood, it will test positive for glucose. *Clear drainage that tests positive for glucose indicates leakage of CSF.*

- Observe blood-tinged fluid for "halo" sign. *CSF contains glucose and dries in concentric rings on gauze or tissues.*

- Keep the nasopharynx and the external ear clean. Place a piece of sterile cotton in the ear, or tape a sterile cotton pad loosely under the nose; change dressings when they become wet. *Wet dressings facilitate movement of organisms.*

- Instruct client not to blow nose, cough, or inhibit sneeze; sneeze through open mouth. *Blowing the nose and coughing increase ICP. Withholding a sneeze forces bacteria backward.*

- Use aseptic technique at all times when caring for the client, such as when changing head dressings or ICP monitor dressings and insertion sites. *Using aseptic technique reduces the possibility of introducing infection.*

Other Nursing Diagnoses

Other nursing diagnoses that may be appropriate for the client with craniocerebral trauma follow:

- *Pain* related to traumatic skull injury

- *Risk for Ineffective Breathing Pattern* related to altered level of consciousness and inadequate respiratory function
- *Risk for Altered Cerebral Tissue Perfusion* related to increased intracranial pressure secondary to craniocerebral trauma
- *Risk for Ineffective Thermoregulation* related to damage or pressure on the hypothalamus
- *Altered Thought Processes* related to memory deficit or altered LOC secondary to cerebral trauma

Client and Family Teaching

The client and family need to be informed about the amount of damage that has occurred with the skull fracture. The client with a linear fracture, who may not be hospitalized, will need discharge planning that focuses on the need to monitor progress closely. To prevent complications after discharge, advise the client and family to go to the emergency room if the client experiences any of the following:

- Growing drowsiness or confusion
- Difficulty waking (instruct a family member to wake the client every 2 hours during the first night home)
- Vomiting
- Blurred vision
- Slurred speech
- Prolonged headache
- Blood or clear fluid leaking from the ears or nose
- Weakness in an arm or leg
- Stiff neck
- Convulsions

The Client with a Brain Injury

■   ■   ■

Even when the skull and other structures overlying the brain remain intact, a blow to the head can cause significant brain damage. Closed head injuries may result in either diffuse or focal damage to the brain. They range in severity from mild to severe. Concussion and diffuse axonal injury are classified as diffuse injuries; focal injuries include contusion, intracerebral hemorrhage, and brain stem injuries (Hickey, 1992).

Pathophysiology

Brain damage can result from a primary injury or from a secondary injury to the head. The primary injury is brain damage due to the impact; secondary injury to the brain may be due to swelling, bleeding (hematomas), infection, cerebral hypoxia, or ischemia that follows the primary injury. Secondary damage may develop rapidly, within hours of the primary injury (Porth, 1994).

The neurons require a constant supply of nutrients in the form of glucose and oxygen and are very susceptible to metabolic injury when supplies are cut off. As a result, the cerebral circulation may lose its ability to regulate the available circulating blood volume, causing ischemia of certain areas within the brain.

Concussion

A **concussion** is defined as a momentary interruption of brain function, with or without loss of consciousness, due to a blow to the head (blunt trauma) or acceleration-deceleration injury (Hickey, 1992). A concussion usually involves no structural brain damage and is considered the most benign form of brain injury (also called minor or mild). The exact pathophysiology of concussion is not clearly understood. It is believed that loss of consciousness results when shearing stress on the reticular activating system of the midbrain causes transient electrophysiologic dysfunction as the cerebral hemispheres rotate on the relatively fixed brain stem (Hickey, 1992; Wilson et al., 1991). Although no gross or microscopic changes in brain structure are apparent following injury, biochemical changes, including depletion of ATP and local disruption of the blood–brain barrier, can be detected (Wilson et al., 1991).

A concussion may be associated with an immediate, brief loss of consciousness on impact. Altered consciousness may last only seconds or persist for several hours. In a severe concussion, a brief seizure and respiratory arrest may occur; transient pallor, bradycardia, and hypotension may accompany loss of consciousness. Amnesia for events immediately preceding and following the injury (retrograde and antegrade amnesia) is common. Other manifestations of concussion include headache, drowsiness, confusion, dizziness, and visual disturbances such as diplopia or blurred vision (Hickey, 1992). See the clinical manifestations box on page 1724.

Following concussion, clients may develop *postconcussion syndrome* with persistent headache, dizziness, irritability, insomnia, impaired memory and concentration, and learning problems. Postconcussion syndrome may last for several weeks or, rarely, up to a year.

Contusion

A **contusion** is defined as a bruise of the brain. A contusion typically is accompanied by small, diffuse venous hemorrhages. Both white and gray matter may have a bruised, discolored appearance. A decrease in pH, with accumulation of lactic acid and decreased oxygen consumption, may hinder cell function. Contusions occur when the brain strikes the inner skull, often with a coup

---

Clinical Manifestations of Concussion

- Immediate loss of consciousness (lasting usually no longer than 5 minutes)
- Amnesia for events surrounding injury
- Headache
- Drowsiness, confusion, dizziness
- Visual disturbances
- Possible brief seizure activity with transient apnea, bradycardia, pallor, and hypotension

Postconcussion Syndrome

- Persistent headache
- Dizziness
- Irritability and insomnia
- Impaired memory and concentration, learning problems

(point of impact) lesion and a contrecoup lesion on the opposite side of the brain. Contusions occur most frequently near bony prominences of the skull. The tissue has a soft, pulpy quality. Cerebral edema can follow contusion, resulting in increased ICP. Contusions; small, diffuse venous hemorrhages; and brain swelling are at their peak 12 to 24 hours after injury.

Manifestations of contusion depend on the size and location of the brain injury. An initial loss of consciousness occurs; level of consciousness may remain altered, and behavior changes such as combativeness persist for an extended period. Full consciousness may be regained extremely slowly, and residual deficits may persist; in some clients, full level of consciousness never really returns. Focal effects of the contusion may cause hemiparesis or abnormal posturing. Manifestations of increased ICP (discussed earlier in this chapter) may be apparent if cerebral edema develops.

Diffuse Axonal Injury

Diffuse axonal injury (DAI) is a brain injury in which a high-speed acceleration-deceleration injury, typically associated with motor vehicle accidents, causes widespread disruption of axons in the white matter. Focal lesions may be found in the corpus callosum, midbrain, and brain stem. There is an immediate loss of consciousness with DAI. The prognosis is poor; most clients with DAI either die or remain in persistent vegetative state (Hickey, 1992).

Brain Stem Injury

Brain stem injury may accompany DAI. Although hemorrhage is not always detectable, rotational forces and shearing of vessels in the upper midbrain can cause acute midbrain hemorrhage. The client with brain stem injury presents with deep coma from the moment of impact, abnormal posturing (decerebration) or flaccidity, nonreactive pupils, impaired oculomotor responses, and abnormal respiratory patterns (Hickey, 1992; Wilson et al., 1991).

Collaborative Care

Concussion, diffuse axonal injury, and contusion are usually diagnosed by the history and mechanism of injury and the physical examination. Care is supportive, directed toward reducing the risk of secondary injury or identifying it as early as possible.

There are no specific laboratory or diagnostic tests to establish these diagnoses. Laboratory testing may be done to monitor the client's hemodynamic status and detect conditions that may contribute to cerebral edema. Arterial blood gases are analyzed, with particular attention to oxygen and carbon dioxide levels. Adequate oxygenation is vital to maintain cerebral metabolism; carbon dioxide is a potent vasodilator, and increased levels may contribute to cerebral edema and increased ICP. The blood count, serum glucose and electrolyte levels, and serum osmolarity are also assessed to monitor for infection or conditions that can affect cerebral blood flow or metabolism. A CT scan is ordered to detect contusions and focal lesions associated with diffuse axonal injury. CT scan shows normal findings in concussion but characteristic lesions with contusion and DAI. Other diagnostic tests may include an MRI, EEG, and possibly a lumbar puncture to assess for bleeding.

Following a concussion, the client may be observed for an hour or two in the emergency department, then discharged home with instructions for further observation to detect manifestations of secondary injury. If the loss of consciousness extended more than 2 minutes, the client may be admitted to the hospital for observation.

Clients who have experienced either DAI or contusion usually require hospital admission and close observation for secondary effects. An intracranial pressure monitor probe may be inserted to assess ICP and monitor therapy to reduce cerebral edema and maintain cerebral perfusion. A corticosteroid such as hydrocortisone or dexamethasone may be administered to reduce inflammation. Osmotic diuretics such as mannitol may also be employed to reduce cerebral edema.

Clients with severe head injuries may require additional care measures to maintain normal body functions and prevent long-term disability. These measures include intravenous fluids, enteral or parenteral feedings, and positioning and range-of-motion exercises to prevent contractures and maintain mobility.

Nursing Care

The client who has sustained a concussion or contusion requires close observation for the development of manifestations of increased cerebral edema leading to increased intracranial pressure. Many of the nursing diagnoses that apply to the client with an altered level of consciousness or increased ICP (see previous discussions) also apply to the client with a concussion or contusion. The following nursing diagnoses also commonly apply to the client with a concussion or contusion.

- *Risk for Ineffective Breathing Pattern* related to increased intracranial pressure
- *Pain* related to traumatic skull injury
- *Impaired Thought Processes* related to impaired memory and altered LOC secondary to cerebral trauma
- *Altered Tissue Perfusion* related to cerebral injury
- *Impaired Verbal Communication* related to cerebral injury
- *Bowel Incontinence* or *Urinary Incontinence* related to perceptual impairment secondary to cerebral trauma
- *Sleep Pattern Disturbance* related to frequent assessments and loss of REM sleep

Client and Family Teaching

The client and family should be informed that a postconcussion syndrome sometimes occurs. If the client experiences persistent headaches and dizziness, is uncharacteristically emotional, seems overly tired, or has difficulty paying attention or remembering, the health care provider should be notified. Explain that these manifestations may persist for some time. Rehabilitation may help the client compensate for memory impairment and attention deficits.

The Client with an Intracranial Hemorrhage

■ ■ ■

An intracranial hemorrhage is defined as an escape of blood within the cranium. It is the most common serious complication of blunt craniocerebral trauma. The hemorrhage may cause rapid deterioration in the injured client's condition.

Pathophysiology

Intracranial hemorrhage can result directly from the trauma (e.g., beneath a fracture) or from shearing forces

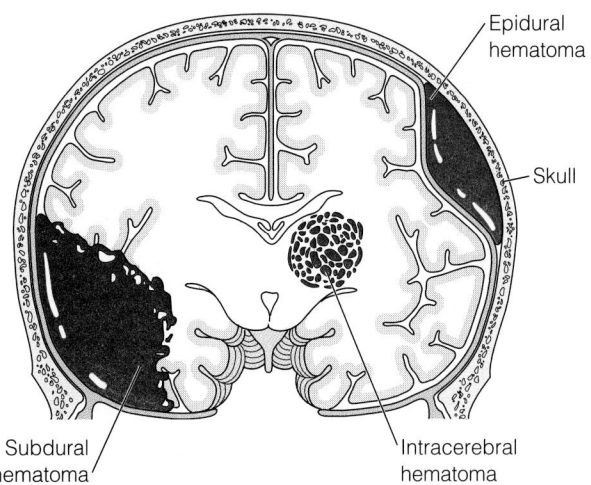

Figure 40–7   Three types of hematomas: epidural hematoma, subdural hematoma, and intracerebral hematoma.

on cerebral arteries and veins that occur with acceleration-deceleration. Depending on the site and rate of bleeding, manifestations may appear immediately or may not become evident for hours or even months (Hickey, 1992). Intracranial hemorrhages and the hematomas they cause place pressure on surrounding structures, causing manifestations of an expanding focal lesion. They also cause increased intracranial pressure, leading to such manifestations as altered levels of consciousness and potential complications such as herniation syndromes. Intracranial hemorrhages are classified by their location as epidural, subdural, or intracerebral. Table 40–7 compares the frequency, locations, common sites, precipitating factors, and clinical manifestations of intracranial hematomas; Figure 40–7 illustrates their locations.

Epidural Hematoma

An *epidural hematoma,* also called an extradural hematoma, develops in the potential space between the dura and the skull, which normally adhere to one another. As the blood collects, the expanding hematoma strips the dura away from the skull. Epidural hematomas affect young adults more frequently than older adults, because the dura becomes more tightly attached to the skull with aging.

Epidural hematomas usually result from a torn artery, often the middle meningeal artery. Because they are arterial in origin, they tend to develop rapidly. The client may lose consciousness with the initial injury, then have a brief lucid period before the level of consciousness rapidly declines from drowsiness to coma as the hematoma expands, stripping the dura away from the skull and placing pressure on brain tissue. Other manifestations of epidural hematomas include headache; a fixed, dilated pupil on

Table 40–7   Comparison of Intracranial Hematomas

	Location/Common Site	Precipitating Factors	Clinical Manifestations
Epidural Hematoma 2% to 3% of head injuries	Located in the space between the skull and the dura mater\n\nCommon site: the temporal bone (over the middle meningeal artery)	Skull fractures\nContusion	Momentary loss of consciousness followed by a lucid period lasting from a few hours to 1 to 2 days\nRapid deterioration in level of consciousness (drowsiness to confusion to coma)\nSeizures\nHeadache\nHemiparesis (may be ipsilateral or contralateral)\nFixed dilated ipsilateral pupil\nRise in blood pressure with decreases in pulse and respirations indicates a rapidly increasing hematoma
Subdural Hematoma 10% to 15% of head injuries	Located in the space below the dural surface (between the dura and arachnoid and pia mater layers of meninges)\n\nCommon site: may occur any place in cranium	Closed head injury\nAcceleration-deceleration injury\nCerebral atrophy (seen in older adults)\nChronic alcoholism\nUse of anticoagulants\nContusion	Acute:\n■ Headache\n■ Drowsiness\n■ Agitation\n■ Slowed thinking\n■ Confusion\nSubacute:\n■ Same as those of acute subdural hematoma but develop more slowly\nChronic:\n■ Manifestations may not appear until weeks to months after injury\n■ Confusion, slowed thinking, drowsiness
Intracerebral Hematoma 2% to 3% of all types of head injuries	Located directly in the brain tissue\n\nCommon sites: frontal or temporal region	Gunshot wounds\nDepressed bone fractures\nStab injury\nLong history of systemic hypertension\nContusions	Headache\nDeteriorating consciousness to deep coma\nHemiplegia on contralateral side\nDilated pupil on the side of the clot

the same side as the hematoma (ipsilateral); hemiparesis or hemiplegia; and possible seizures.

Because epidural hematomas usually develop rapidly, timely intervention is vital to prevent significant increases in ICP and herniation.

Subdural Hematoma

Subdural hematomas, which form between the dura mater and the arachnoid-pia mater layers of the meninges, are more common than epidural hematomas. These hematomas are often venous in origin, although they may involve bleeding from small arteries as well. Subdural hematomas may form without direct trauma or contusion; acceleration-deceleration forces may tear the bridging veins that connect veins on the surface of the cerebral cortex to the dural sinuses. As blood collects, it places direct pressure on underlying brain tissue. Subdural hema-

tomas are classified as acute, subacute, and chronic, depending on their rate of development.

Acute subdural hematomas develop rapidly following head injury. Although a lucid period may occur, the client commonly develops drowsiness, confusion, and enlargement of the ipsilateral pupil within minutes or hours of the injury. If responsive, the client may complain of a unilateral headache. Hemiparesis may be noted.

Subacute subdural hematomas are often associated with less severe head injury. The older adult is particularly vulnerable to subacute subdural hematoma. These hematomas are often diagnosed when the client fails to regain consciousness following a closed head injury.

Chronic subdural hematomas are often associated with relatively minor trauma such as a fall. Weeks to months may elapse before manifestations of the hematoma occur; the initial trauma may have been forgotten. Chronic subdural hematomas may also occur spontaneously in the older adult or in clients with bleeding disorders. Manifestations of the hematoma develop slowly and may be mistaken for the onset of dementia in the older adult. Slowed thinking, confusion, drowsiness, or lethargy are common early manifestations. Other manifestations include headache, dilation and sluggishness of the ipsilateral pupil, and possible seizures (Hickey, 1992).

Intracerebral Hematoma

Intracerebral hematomas, bleeding into the brain tissue itself, may occur in any location but usually are found in the frontal or temporal lobes. They may result from closed head trauma, particularly contusion or shearing of small blood vessels deep within the hemispheres. Intracerebral hematomas can also accompany other types of head trauma such as lacerations. Older adults and alcoholics are particularly vulnerable to intracerebral hemorrhage because cerebral blood vessels are more friable (fragile and easily torn).

The manifestations of intracerebral hematoma vary according to the location of the hematoma. Headache may develop, along with decreasing level of consciousness, hemiplegia, and dilation of the ipsilateral pupil. The expanding clot increases intracranial pressure, and herniation may occur.

Collaborative Care

Management of the client with a suspected intracranial hemorrhage focuses on establishing an accurate diagnosis rapidly and initiating appropriate interventions to prevent further deterioration in the client's condition.

Laboratory testing is of little value in establishing the diagnosis of intracranial hemorrhage. CT scans and MRI are used extensively to locate and identify hematomas as well as assess their size and rate of expansion.

Small subdural hematomas can frequently be reabsorbed and may be treated conservatively, with close observation and supportive care (Hickey, 1992). However, the treatment of choice for epidural hematomas and large acute or subacute subdural hematomas is surgical evacuation of the clot. This can often be performed through burr holes made into the skull (Figure 40–8). In an epidural hematoma, the bleeding vessel can also be ligated during this procedure, preventing further bleeding. Rebleeding may occur following evacuation of an acute subdural hematoma in older adults and clients with chronic alcoholism. A craniotomy is necessary to evacuate chronic subdural hematomas because the hematoma tends to solidify, making it difficult or impossible to remove through burr holes (Hickey, 1992). Surgery is less successful in treating intracerebral hematomas because of widespread tissue damage. Supportive care to manage in-

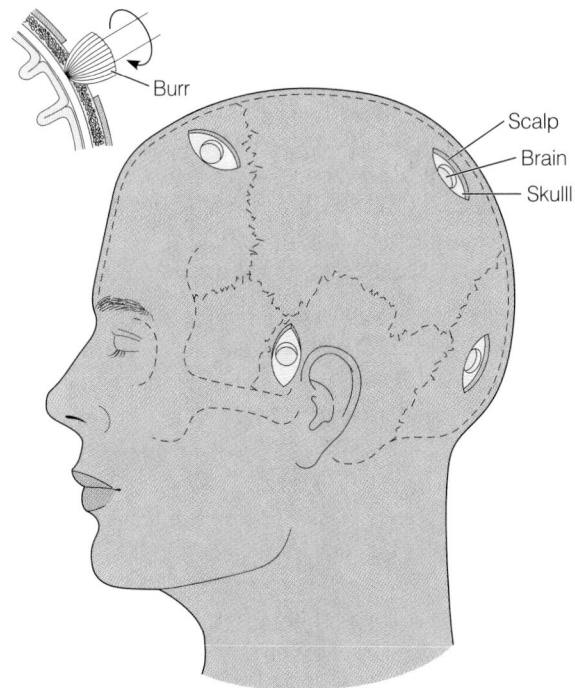

Figure 40–8   Possible locations of burr holes.

tracranial pressure and prevent complications is provided.

Nursing Care

A history of the injury is helpful in understanding the nature of the craniocerebral trauma. Knowing if a loss of consciousness occurred assists the nurse in planning care. Nursing care of the client in the acute care phase initially focuses on maintaining an effective airway and breathing pattern. Nursing care is also directed toward continuous assessment and monitoring of neurologic function as well as other body systems. This close monitoring provides early recognition and treatment of problems and complications, and initiation of aggressive forms of therapy that may be needed.

Many nursing diagnoses associated with intracranial hematomas correspond with those outlined previously in the section on the client with increased intracranial pressure. Specific nursing diagnoses discussed in this section focus on problems with airway clearance and breathing patterns.

Ineffective Airway Clearance

The primary objective in the care of any trauma client is maintaining a patent airway to prevent hypoxia. However, in the initial acute care phase, the risk of cervical vertebral fractures and spinal cord injury may complicate the process of establishing a patent airway. In addition, other multisystem injuries may complicate the interpretation of vital signs. In general, all unconscious people with a head injury should be intubated with an endotracheal tube to prevent aspiration (Hickey, 1992). Clients with head trauma may also require a tracheostomy to provide an airway and be placed on a ventilator.

Nursing interventions with rationales follow:

- Assess neurologic signs on a regular schedule. *Changes in neurologic signs may indicate increased intracranial pressure, with the risk of further depression of the respiratory system and respiratory arrest.*

- Maintain client's head and neck in immobilized position. *Immobilization is necessary to prevent spinal cord injury in suspected or actual fractures of the cervical spine; spinal cord injury at this level would further impair respiratory function.*

- Clear the client's nose and mouth of mucus and blood. *This ensures patency of the airway.*

- Suction the airway as needed, limiting suctioning time to no more than 15 seconds at one time. Do not suction the nasal passages until a dural tear has been ruled out. *Suctioning is usually necessary to maintain a patent airway.*

Ineffective Breathing Pattern

The client with an intracranial hematoma is at high risk for ineffective breathing pattern related to increased ICP. If ICP increases dramatically, tentorial herniation may occur, leading to sudden respiratory arrest.

Nursing interventions with rationales follow:

- Monitor the respiratory pattern for rate, depth, and rhythm every 2 hours if the client is not on a ventilator. Assess breath sounds, presence of cyanosis, restlessness, and use of accessory respiratory muscles. Monitor blood gas levels. *Head injuries may cause alterations in respirations. An increased respiratory rate may indicate hypoxia. A decrease in respiratory rate may be the result of depression of the medullary respiratory center. In general, an initial increase in intracranial pressure causes respirations to slow; as the pressure continues to increase, respirations become rapid.*

- Monitor ICP readings. *Continuous measurement of ICP is used to diagnose and monitor increased intracranial pressure. As ICP increases, herniation may occur, leading to respiratory arrest and death.*

- If the client is not intubated, prepare for oxygen administration and/or tracheal intubation if respiratory distress occurs. *Supplying oxygen prevents hypoxia until the hematoma can be evacuated, relieving pressure on the respiratory center.*

- Prepare for cranial surgery if deteriorating respiratory pattern and neurologic changes are noted. *Surgical intervention usually consists of placing several burr holes in the skull or performing a craniotomy to remove the hematoma. (Intracranial surgery is discussed later in the chapter.) However, the cerebral edema and increased intracranial pressure may cause death even if surgery is performed.*

Other Nursing Diagnoses

Other nursing diagnoses that may be appropriate for the client with an intracranial hematoma follow:

- *Altered Cerebral Tissue Perfusion* related to increased intracranial pressure secondary to hemorrhage and edema (see previous discussion of increased ICP)

- *Sleep Pattern Disturbance* related to frequent assessments and loss of sleep

- *Risk for Injury* related to seizures secondary to increased intracranial pressure

- *Self-Care Deficit: Bathing/Hygiene* related to decreased level of consciousness

- *Inability to Sustain Spontaneous Ventilation* related to increased intracranial pressure secondary to expanding hematoma

Client and Family Teaching

The client with an intracranial hematoma (if conscious) and the family need to be informed of the possible need for surgery to evacuate the hematoma. In many cases, the client is unconscious and the client's family must sign the consent for surgery.

Applying the Nursing Process

Case Study of a Client with a Subdural Hematoma: Wong Lee

Wong Lee is a 50-year-old tug boat mechanic who is married and has three sons. Although Mr. Lee has been through rehabilitation twice for alcoholism, he has not been able to quit drinking. His physician has explained the physical consequences as well as the possible interaction between alcohol and the anticoagulant Mr. Lee is taking for chronic atrial fibrillation. While attending a family reunion, during which he eats a large meal and drinks several beers, Mr. Lee joins a game of softball. Mrs. Lee is concerned that Mr. Lee has consumed too much alcohol to play ball in the heat. She asks her sons to try to talk their father out of playing, but Mr. Lee is adamant and states that he wants to pitch. During the end of the second inning, the batter hits a ball that strikes Mr. Lee in the head. Mr. Lee stumbles and drops to the ground, holding his head. He does not lose consciousness and gets up on his own. His sons and wife try to persuade him to go to the hospital, but Mr. Lee insists he feels fine, that the injury was only a tap on the head.

Two months later, after an evening of consuming several mixed drinks, Mr. Lee develops a headache. He attributes the headache to a hangover, but instead of improving the next day, the headache becomes steadily worse. He becomes confused and disoriented. His wife, concerned that his drinking is increasing again, calls the physician, who admits Mr. Lee to the detoxification center at the local hospital. A CT scan and MRI are performed after the nurse conducts her initial assessment. The diagnosis of a subdural hematoma is made, and Mr. Lee is transferred to the neurology unit.

Assessment
When Saundra Knight, the nurse on the neurology unit, enters the room, she notices that Mr. Lee is sitting in bed, laughing and giddy. As she begins to talk to Mr. Lee, he states, "Don't ask me anything—I can't think. My headache is getting worse." Over the next few hours, the giddiness subsides, and Mr. Lee becomes drowsy. Ms. Knight reports a Glasgow Coma Scale score of 11. An ICP monitor is inserted and reveals increased intracranial pressure. Mr. Lee is scheduled to have burr holes and hematoma evacuation the following morning.

Diagnosis
Ms. Knight identifies the following nursing diagnoses for Mr. Lee:

- *Risk for Ineffective Breathing Pattern* related to pressure on respiratory center by intracranial hematoma
- *Altered Cerebral Tissue Perfusion* related to increased intracranial pressure secondary to cerebral edema

Expected Outcomes
The expected outcomes established in the plan of care specify that Mr. Lee will

- Maintain a respiratory rate and rhythm within normal limits.

- Maintain adequate cerebral perfusion, as evidenced by stable vital signs, stable neurologic status, and no decrease in level of consciousness.

Planning and Implementation
Ms. Knight plans and implements the following nursing interventions for Mr. Lee:

- Perform neurologic assessment every 2 hours or as needed.
- Monitor vital signs every 2 hours or as needed.
- Explain to the family the procedure for intracranial surgery.
- Prepare for intracranial surgery and evacuation of the clot.

Evaluation
The first day postoperatively, Mr. Lee begins breathing on his own without ventilatory support. His respiratory rate and rhythm are within normal limits, with no signs of abnormal breath sounds. The ICP monitor readings are appropriate, and Mr. Lee shows significant improvement in level of consciousness, with a Glasgow Coma Scale score of 15. Mr. Lee continues to improve and is discharged to home 6 days after surgery.

Critical Thinking in the Nursing Process

1. Describe the similarities and differences between Mr. Lee's disorder and the manifestations of other types of intracranial hematomas.
2. How would knowing whether Mr. Lee lost consciousness assist Ms. Knight in planning his care?
3. Why was Mr. Lee at risk for developing an ineffective breathing pattern?
4. Mr. Lee kept trying to pull out his ICP line. You know he should not be restrained, because pulling against restraints increases restlessness and increases intracranial pressure. What would you do?
5. Write a care plan for Mr. Lee for the nursing diagnosis *Acute Confusion*.

Cranial Infections, Inflammation, and Neoplasms

The Client with Meningitis

Meningitis is an inflammation of the meninges of the brain and spinal cord. Infection of the pia mater, arachnoid, and CSF is the usual cause of meningitis, although chemical meningitis may also occur (Porth, 1994).

Meningitis may be acute or chronic, and it may be bacterial, viral, fungal, or parasitic in origin.

The incidence of meningitis in the United States is highest in children under 5 years old, although it can affect people of all ages. Children and young adults have the highest incidence of meningococcal meningitis, a disease that may occur in epidemics among people who are

---

Clinical Manifestations of Bacterial Meningitis

- Restlessness, agitation, and irritability
- Severe headache
- Signs of meningeal irritation:
  a. Nuchal rigidity (stiff neck)
  b. Positive Brudzinski's sign
  c. Positive Kernig's sign
- Chills and high fever
- Confusion, altered LOC
- Photophobia (aversion to light), diplopia
- Seizures
- Signs of increased ICP (widened pulse pressure and bradycardia, respiratory irregularity, decreased LOC, headache, and vomiting)
- Petechial rash (in meningococcal meningitis)

---

in close contact with one another, such as military recruits. Pneumococcal meningitis, in contrast, primarily affects the very young and very old. A number of risk factors for meningitis can be identified: basilar skull fracture, otitis media, sinusitis or mastoiditis, neurosurgery or other invasive procedures, systemic sepsis, and impaired immune function (Porth, 1994).

Pathophysiology

In meningitis, the infecting organisms usually reach the CNS in one of two ways: by direct extension, such as can occur after cranial trauma or invasive procedures (e.g., ICP monitoring devices or neurosurgery); or through the bloodstream secondary to another infection in the body.

The organism responsible for meningitis must overcome nonspecific and specific host defense mechanisms to invade and replicate in the CSF. These defenses include the skin barrier, the blood–brain barrier, the nonspecific inflammatory response, and the immune response. Host response to the particular pathogen is responsible for the manifestations of clinical meningitis. The organisms that initiate the host response in meningitis demonstrate an affinity for the nervous system. They colonize and invade the nasopharyngeal mucosa, survive intravascularly, and penetrate the CNS if the blood–brain barrier is damaged, as can happen during surgery, the inflammatory response, or cerebral edema.

Infection of the CSF and meninges causes an inflammatory response in the pia, arachnoid, and CSF. Because

the meninges and subarachnoid space are continuous around the brain, spinal cord, and optic nerves, the infection and inflammatory response is always cerebrospinal, involving both the brain and the spinal cord (Wilson et al., 1991).

Bacterial Meningitis

The common pathogens that cause bacterial meningitis usually reside in the upper respiratory tract without causing disease. The bacteria most frequently implicated include *Neisseria meningitidis* (meningococcal meningitis), *Streptococcus pneumoniae,* and *Haemophilus influenzae.* A predisposing factor such as an upper respiratory infection, dental procedure, or basilar skull fracture with CSF leakage typically precedes invasion of the blood and CSF by the bacteria. Once the pathogen enters the central nervous system, it or its toxins initiate an inflammatory response in the meninges, CSF, and ventricles. Meningeal vessels become engorged, and their permeability increases. Phagocytic white blood cells migrate into the subarachnoid space, forming a purulent exudate that thickens and clouds the CSF and interferes with its flow. Rapid exudate formation causes further inflammation and edema of meningeal cells. Blood vessel engorgement, exudate formation, impaired CSF flow, and cellular edema cause the intracranial pressure to increase. Secondary infection of the brain may also occur (McCance & Huether, 1994).

The client with bacterial meningitis typically presents with fever and chills, headache, back and abdominal pain, and nausea and vomiting. Meningeal irritation causes nuchal rigidity, with a very stiff neck and positive Brudzinski's sign (flexion of the neck that causes the hip and knee to flex) and positive Kernig's sign (inability to extend the knee while the hip is flexed at a 90-degree angle). Photophobia is present; the client may also experience diplopia. With meningococcal meningitis, a rapidly spreading petechial rash involving the skin and mucous membranes may be noted. The client may also demonstrate signs of increased ICP, including decreased LOC, seizures, changes in vital signs and respiratory pattern, and papilledema. The clinical manifestations of bacterial meningitis are listed in the accompanying box.

Complications of bacterial meningitis include arthritis, cranial nerve damage, and hydrocephalus. Cranial nerve VIII, the auditory nerve, is frequently affected, with resulting nerve deafness. Thrombophlebitis may develop in cerebral vessels, with infarction of surrounding tissues (Porth, 1994).

Viral Meningitis

Acute *viral meningitis,* also referred to as aseptic meningitis, is a less severe disease than bacterial meningitis. It can be caused by a variety of viruses, such as herpes simplex, herpes zoster, Epstein-Barr virus, or cytomegalovirus

(CMV). Viral meningitis most often appears after a case of mumps. Although viral infection also triggers the inflammatory response, the course of the disease is benign and of short duration. Recovery is uneventful.

The clinical manifestations of viral meningitis are similar to those of bacterial meningitis, although usually milder. The client may have a mild flulike illness prior to the onset of meningitis. Headache is intense and is accompanied by malaise, nausea, vomiting, and lethargy. Photophobia may be present. The client generally remains oriented, although he or she may be drowsy. Temperature is mildly elevated. Neck stiffness, positive Brudzinski's sign, and positive Kernig's sign are usually present.

Collaborative Care

Bacterial meningitis is a medical emergency that, if not treated immediately, can be fatal within days. Successful management depends on rapidly establishing an accurate diagnosis and providing aggressive treatment to eradicate the infecting organism and support vital functions. The client may be placed in strict or respiratory isolation until the organism has been identified, depending on hosptial policy. Universal precautions apply to CSF as well as blood.

Treatment for viral meningitis focuses on managing client symptoms and is supportive. The manifestations of viral meningitis are generally milder than those of bacterial meningitis and more flulike. Antipyretics and analgesics may provide relief. Antibiotic therapy is not indicated, and specific isolation precautions are not required.

Laboratory and Diagnostic Tests
The diagnosis of bacterial or viral meningitis is based principally on the clinical presentation of the client. Diagnostic tests are evaluated in combination with the clinical manifestations.

The following diagnostic tests may be ordered:

- *Lumbar puncture* is the definitive diagnostic measure for bacterial meningitis. Data that indicate bacterial meningitis include turbid, cloudy fluid; a markedly increased white blood cell count and protein content; and a decreased glucose content. Also, the opening pressure on the lumbar puncture is greater than 180 mm water. (*Note:* A lumbar puncture should *not* be performed in the presence of increased ICP. This procedure may cause downward herniation of the brain tissue onto the medulla, leading to cardiopulmonary arrest.)
- *Gram's stain and culture reports on CSF* are performed. Gram's stain is used to discern rapidly whether a bacterial infection is present. Culture has been used to determine the specific agent; no bacteria are cultured

from the CSF in viral meningitis. Unfortunately, culture results take several days, and the Gram's stain is often negative in bacterial meningitis. Counterimmunoelectrophoresis (CIE) is a laboratory test that may be ordered to determine the presence of viruses or protozoa.

- *Cultures from the blood, urine, throat, and nose* are performed to identify a possibly bacterial source of infection. It is recognized that organisms colonize and invade the nasopharyngeal mucosa, survive intravascularly, and penetrate the CNS if the blood–brain barrier is damaged.

Pharmacology
Immediate administration of a broad-spectrum antibiotic that crosses the blood–brain barrier into the subarachnoid space is instituted in cases of bacterial meningitis. Once culture reports identify the causative organism, drug therapy is continued for at least 10 days, using the most effective drug or drugs specific to that bacterium. High doses of penicillins and third-generation cephalosporins are preferred agents. Antibiotics are given intravenously; their dosage is not reduced as the client improves because the blood–brain barrier recovers as inflammation resolves and high doses are required in order to reach the CSF. Anticonvulsant medications such as phenytoin (Dilantin) are often prescribed to prevent or control seizure activity. Antipyretic and analgesic medications may provide symptomatic relief; however, analgesics that have a depressant effect on the CNS (such as opiates) are avoided to prevent masking of early manifestations of deteriorating LOC. The client initially may require antiemetics to control nausea and vomiting. Fluid and electrolyte status is maintained through intravenous fluid replacement until the client is able to resume oral intake.

Surgery
An intraventricular method of medication administration uses an Ommaya reservoir that has been surgically implanted into a lateral ventricle of the brain (Figure 40–9). This device is used to enhance CSF absorption of antibiotics and to maintain treatment over an extended period of time. The device is also used with clients receiving chemotherapy for CNS tumors.

Nursing Care

In planning and implementing nursing care for the client with bacterial or viral meningitis, the client's prognosis may depend on the supportive care given. The client with bacterial meningitis is very ill, and the combination of fever, dehydration, and cerebral edema may predispose the client to seizures. Airway obstruction, respiratory

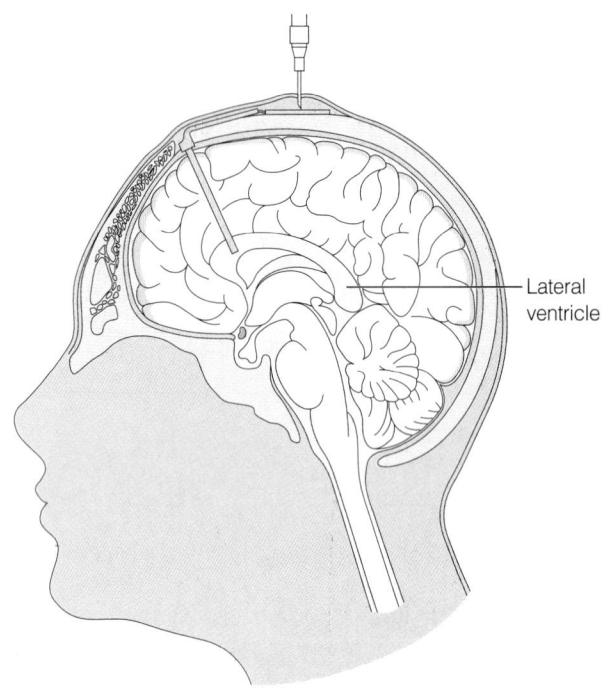

Lateral ventricle

Figure 40–9 Ommaya reservoir for medication administration.

arrest, or cardiac dysrhythmias may ensue. Nursing interventions in this section focus on altered protection and fluid volume deficit.

Altered Protection

Clients with meningitis are less able to protect themselves against insults from both internal and external sources. The effects of the inflammation and resulting pathophysiologic processes may include pain, fever, altered levels of consciousness, seizures, increased intracranial pressure, and cranial nerve dysfunction. In addition, pathophysiologic effects on the brain from toxins or thrombosis of a cerebral vessel may lead to permanent neurologic deficits, such as loss of motor function and dementia.

The nurse monitors the client for manifestations of altered protection and reports abnormal findings so that treatment can be instituted to prevent further complications.

Nursing interventions with rationales follow:

■ Assess neurologic status on a regular basis. *Many of the complications of meningitis are evidenced by changes in neurologic signs.*

■ Assess vital signs, including temperature, on a regular basis. *The client with bacterial meningitis often has a high temperature throughout the illness, ranging from 101 F (38 C) to 105 F (40.5 C). Hyperthermia may result from*

increased intracranial pressure, while an increased temperature can also increase ICP.

■ Assess for and report decreasing levels of consciousness. Assess levels of orientation, memory, attention span, and response to stimuli. *Early in the infection, the client often has problems with memory and orientation. There may be problems with following commands, restlessness, irritability, and combativeness. As the illness progresses, the level of consciousness decreases to lethargy and finally into deep coma (Hickey, 1992).*

■ Assess for and report manifestations of seizure activity, and institute seizure precautions:
    a. Monitor the client for twitching of hands or face and tonic-clonic movements.
    b. Have an oral airway and suction equipment readily available.
    c. Pad side rails.
    d. Maintain bed in low position and keep side rails up. *Irritation of the cerebral cortex secondary to meningeal inflammation initiates the development of seizures. Careful monitoring and seizure precautions are necessary to prevent injury.*

■ Assess for and report manifestations of cranial nerve damage; monitor extraocular movements, facial movement, dizziness, ability to hear, double vision, drooping upper eyelids (ptosis), and pupillary changes. *Cranial nerve dysfunction may result from inflammation or vascular changes in the brain.*

■ Assess for and report manifestations of increased intracranial pressure: decreased pulse, increased blood pressure, widening pulse pressure, respiratory changes, and vomiting. *Meningitis causes increased intracranial pressure from infectious or inflammatory exudate, cerebral edema, and hydrocephalus.*

■ Administer prescribed medications, and maintain prescribed fluid restrictions. *Diuretics are often prescribed to prevent increases in ICP, anticonvulsants are prescribed to prevent or control seizures, and antibiotics are prescribed to eradicate the bacteria. Fluids are often restricted to help prevent increased ICP.*

Risk for Fluid Volume Deficit

The client with meningitis is at risk for fluid volume deficit related to increased metabolic rate, diaphoresis, and fluid restrictions.

Nursing interventions with rationales follow:

■ Assess for presence, or worsening, of fluid volume deficit.
    a. Measure and compare intake and output every 2 to 4 hours.
    b. Monitor daily body weights.
    c. Monitor skin turgor and tongue turgor.

d. Monitor condition of mucous membranes.
e. Monitor concentration of urine.
f. Monitor BUN:creatinine ratio.
g. Monitor body temperature at least every 4 hours.

An acute weight loss of 1 lb represents a fluid loss of approximately 500 mL. The elastic property of the skin depends partially on interstitial fluid volume. If there is a fluid volume deficit, skin flattens more slowly after a pinch is released. Also, there will be additional longitudinal furrows on the tongue, and the tongue will be smaller. In fluid volume deficit, urine specific gravity is greater than 1.020, and BUN will rise out of proportion to serum creatinine. Temperature will drop below normal when isotonic fluid volume deficit is moderate or severe, unless infection is present.

■ When administering fluids, either orally or parenterally, consider other illnesses that are occurring concurrently. *For example, clients with increased intracranial pressure or renal failure require complex management. See Chapter 5 for a further discussion of fluid volume deficit.*

Other Nursing Diagnoses

Other nursing diagnoses that might be appropriate for the client with meningitis follow:

■ *Hyperthermia* related to infection and abnormal temperature regulation by the hypothalamus

■ *Pain* related to headache, muscle, neck pain, joint aches, and malaise secondary to meningeal irritation

■ *Altered Cerebral Tissue Perfusion* related to increased ICP or cerebral edema

■ *Risk for Injury* related to seizures and changes in mentation and level of consciousness

■ *Decreased Adaptive Capacity: Cranial* related to intracranial hypertension

Client and Family Teaching

On discharge, teach the client and family the names and purposes of all medications that may be prescribed. The importance of taking all medication until completely gone is a major focus of client teaching because some clients may think it is acceptable to stop the medication as soon as they feel better.

The importance of preventive measures, such as recognizing predisposing conditions, is another major focus for client education. People who have had close contact with the client with meningitis should be assessed for fever, headache, or neck stiffness. Some physicians believe that those closest to the client are candidates for antimicrobial prophylaxis. The client and family are taught to report any signs or symptoms of ear infection, sore throat, or upper respiratory infection.

Case Study of a Client with Bacterial Meningitis: Monty Cook

Monty Cook is a 22-year-old musician who plays in a local rock band. He is unmarried and lives with his parents. He is known by everyone in the community as a quiet, low-key, easygoing person and an excellent guitar player. During a performance 2 days ago, he had difficulty playing his guitar, complaining of bright stage lights blazing in his eyes. When he tried to keep his head down to prevent the lights from hurting his eyes, he noticed his neck was very stiff. After the performance, one of the newest members of the band remarked that it certainly was not their best performance. Mr. Cook responded angrily that maybe the new members of the group needed more practice. Then he stomped out and went home to bed.

He wakes at 4:00 a.m. with a severe headache, sweating, and chills; his temperature is 102 F, and he cannot bend his neck without severe pain. His mother recognizes that he is agitated and irritable and that this is not his normal behavior. Frightened, she rushes him to the hospital emergency room. A lumbar puncture performed in the emergency room reveals turbid, cloudy fluid, a markedly increased white blood cell count, and protein with a decreased glucose content. Bacterial meningitis is the medical diagnosis. Mr. Cook is admitted to the hospital for treatment and care.

Assessment

When the nurse, Mr. Aldi, enters Mr. Cook's room, he sees Mr. Cook thrashing about in the bed, talking incoherently, and becoming more agitated. On assessment, Mr. Aldi notes dry mucous membranes, cracked lips, and small petechiae over the upper torso and abdomen. Mr. Cook's temperature was 104 F. Kernig's sign is positive. Intravenous broad-spectrum antibiotics are prescribed and initiated. After the first 2 hours on duty, Mr. Aldi notes a decrease in Mr. Cook's level of consciousness.

Diagnosis

The following nursing diagnoses are made by Mr. Aldi for Mr. Cook:

■ *Hyperthermia* related to infection and abnormal temperature regulation by hypothalamus

■ *Altered Thought Processes* related to intracranial infection

■ *Altered Protection* related to progression of illness

Expected Outcomes

The expected outcomes of the plan of care are that Mr. Cook will

- Have a decrease in body temperature.
- Become less restless and agitated.
- Remain free of injury.

Planning and Implementation

The following nursing interventions are planned and implemented by Mr. Aldi for Mr. Cook:

- Monitor vital signs every 2 hours.
- Provide sponge baths if temperature continues to rise.
- Provide a quiet, nonstimulating environment with the shades drawn.
- Provide oral care every 4 hours.
- Measure and compare intake and output every 2 hours.
- Perform neurologic checks every 2 to 4 hours.
- Monitor for and report seizure activity and decreasing level of consciousness.
- Pad side rails, and keep bed in low position with side rails elevated.
- Administer prescribed intravenous antibiotics.

Evaluation

After 4 days of antibiotic therapy, Mr. Cook's temperature has returned to near normal. Mr. Aldi notes that Mr. Cook has begun opening his eyes and visually tracking Mr. Aldi as he moves about the room. Mr. Cook responds to a request to squeeze Mr. Aldi's fingers and after several hours asks Mr. Aldi what had happened. On day 5, Mr. Cook states that he feels better and his headache is gone. He asks for sips of juice and begins urinating on a regular basis. Seven days after admission, Mr. Cook is discharged and is able to go home with his mother. He has some weakness in his legs, but otherwise has no evidence of neurologic deficits.

Critical Thinking in the Nursing Process

1. Discuss the pathogenic process of the organisms that entered Mr. Cook's nervous system and related structures.
2. What strategies should the nurse use to decrease the environmental stimuli for Mr. Cook, and what is the rationale behind reducing the environmental stimuli?
3. If you were caring for Mr. Cook in the initial phase of the illness and he became combative, what would you do?
4. Develop a plan of care for Mr. Cook for the nursing diagnosis *Pain*. Consider the effect of narcotics on respiratory function in designing the plan.

The Client with Encephalitis

■ ■ ■

Encephalitis is an acute inflammation of the parenchyma of the brain or spinal cord. It is almost always caused by a virus, but it may also be caused by bacteria, fungi, and other organisms. More than 25 different viruses have been implicated in encephalitis, some of which are endemic to particular geographic regions or have a seasonal occurrence (Hickey, 1992; Porth, 1994). See Table 40–8 for a list of the most common causes of encephalitis.

Pathophysiology

Viruses depend on living tissue for reproduction and become very destructive when they invade brain tissue. The inflammatory response extends over the cerebral cortex, the white matter, and the meninges, with degeneration of the neurons. The pathologic picture of encephalitis includes local necrotizing hemorrhage, which ultimately becomes generalized, with prominent edema. There is progressive degeneration of nerve cell bodies. The inflammatory response in encephalitis does not cause exudate formation as it does in meningitis. Certain viruses show a propensity for certain areas of the brain (e.g., herpes simplex virus involves frontal and temporal lobes). The virus gains access to the CNS via the bloodstream or along peripheral or cranial nerves, or it may already be present in the meninges in the client with meningitis (Porth, 1994).

The clinical manifestations of viral encephalitis vary, depending on the organism and area of the brain affected. Usual manifestations are similar to those of meningitis, including fever, headache, seizures, stiff neck, and altered LOC. The client may be disoriented, agitated and restless, or lethargic and drowsy. As the disease progresses, the LOC deteriorates, and the client may become comatose. Focal manifestations may also develop with viral encephalitis, including aphasia, hemiparesis, or facial weakness (Hickey, 1992).

Collaborative Care

Because many of the clinical manifestations are similar to those of other neurologic diseases, including meningitis and brain abscess, the diagnosis of encephalitis is complicated. Thus, a complete history and physical assessment are essential components of the collaborative care of the client. In acute uncomplicated viral encephalitis, supportive and preventive care during the early phase of the illness is the major focus of therapy. There is no specific medical treatment for encephalitis. The treatment for this disorder is similar to that for meningitis, with the exception of drug therapy. Pharmacologic therapy is focused to the specific organism. Isolation is not necessary, because encephalitis is not transmitted from person to person.

Table 40–8	Causes of Encephalitis
Cause	**Comments**
Arboviruses	Transmitted by bites from ticks and mosquitoes.
	Bites from ticks occur more frequently in spring.
	Bites from mosquitoes occur in middle to late summer.
	Most common types are St. Louis and eastern and western equine encephalitis.
	May destroy major parts of the lobe or hemisphere.
	Two-thirds of clients who develop eastern equine encephalitis either die or develop severe residual disabilities (e.g., seizures, blindness, deafness, speech disorders, or mental retardation).
	The incubation is 5 to 15 days.
	Mortality rates associated with arboviruses higher than those associated with enteroviruses.
Enteroviruses, such as echovirus, coxsackievirus, poliovirus, paramyxovirus (the virus that causes mumps) and varicella-zoster (the virus that causes chickenpox)	Infection occurs more frequently in summer (except infection by the mumps virus, which occurs more frequently in early winter).
	Some degree of protection can be afforded by immunization against measles, mumps, and poliomyelitis.
	Mortality rates are lower than those associated with herpes simplex type 1 virus.
Herpes simplex type 1 virus	Most common nonepidemic encephalitis in North America.
	Can occur any time of year and throughout the world.
	Has an affinity for the inferomedial portions of the frontal and temporal lobes.
	Prognosis is grave but not hopeless: Mortality rate can be as high as 40%, and client may die within 2 weeks.
Amebic meningoencephalitis due to infection by *Naegleria* and *Acanthamoeba* protozoa	Both protozoa are found in warm fresh water.
	Enter the nasal mucosa of people swimming in ponds or lakes.
	May also be found in soil and decaying vegetation.
	Incidence of infection is increasing in North America.
Exogenous poisoning	May occur after ingestion of lead or arsenic or inhalation of carbon monoxide.

Laboratory and Diagnostic Tests

The same diagnostic tests done for meningitis are also instituted with encephalitis, including lumbar puncture, Gram's stain, and culture reports on CSF (see the discussion on meningitis).

Pharmacology

Treatment for encephalitis consists of administering antiviral drugs and preventing complications. Vidarabine (Vira-A) and acyclovir (Zoviran) are most effective if used before the client becomes stuporous or comatose, which usually occurs within 4 to 6 days after the appearance of initial neurologic symptoms. Osmotic diuretics and corticosteroids may also be used to control cerebral edema.

Nursing Care

Nursing interventions for the client with encephalitis are similar to those for meningitis (see the previous discussion). Nursing care is primarily supportive. A careful history to elicit symptoms and a physical assessment to determine the extent of deficits are essential. Additionally,

the nurse monitors vital signs and intracranial pressure (as discussed previously). Nursing diagnoses appropriate for the client with encephalitis include the following:

- *Pain* related to inflammation of the brain and irritation of pain receptors
- *Altered Cerebral Tissue Perfusion* related to cerebral edema
- *Sleep Pattern Disturbance* related to agitation and restlessness
- *Risk for Altered Skin Integrity* related to prolonged bed rest
- *Risk for Injury* related to potential for seizures and decreased level of consciousness

Client and Family Teaching

The client with permanent neurologic deficits that result from encephalitis is usually discharged to a rehabilitation setting or a long-term care facility. For arboviral infections, the client and family need to be aware that prevention includes destruction of the insect larvae and elimination of breeding places, such as pools of stagnant water. Control includes avoiding bites of the mosquito or tick through use of protective clothing and insect repellents.

The Client with a Brain Abscess

■ ■ ■

A **brain abscess** is an infection with a collection of purulent material within the brain tissue. Approximately 75% of brain abscesses are found in the cerebrum; 25% are found in the cerebellum. Approximately 40% of all brain abscesses extend into the brain by traveling from middle ear and mastoid infections along the wall of the cerebral veins. Sinus infections, direct trauma to the brain, and neurosurgery allow immediate access and are responsible for approximately 10%. The remaining 50% are the result of infections in other sites within the body that cause septic emboli to travel via the bloodstream to the brain. Common sources of septic emboli include the lungs (lung abscess), the heart (bacterial endocarditis), the pelvis (pelvic abscesses), skin infections, and complications associated with some forms of meningitis.

Pathophysiology

A brain abscess results from the presence of microorganisms in the brain tissue. Occasionally, the abscess does not become encapsulated; instead, it spreads through the brain tissue to the subarachnoid space and ventricular system. If the abscess is encapsulated, it has the ability to enlarge and, therefore, behave as a space-occupying lesion within the cranium. This predisposes the client not only to the systemic effects of the inflammatory process but also to the serious consequences of increased intracranial pressure.

Initially, the client exhibits the general symptoms associated with an acute infectious process, such as chills, fever, malaise, and anorexia. Because brain abscess generally forms after infection, the client may consider these signs to be an exacerbation of that illness. As the abscess enlarges, neurologic signs may increase.

Collaborative Care

Treatment of the client with a brain abscess focuses on the prompt initiation of the antibiotic therapy. Other manifestations are treated symptomatically, as with the client diagnosed with meningitis or encephalitis. If pharmacologic management is not effective, the abscess may be drained or, if it is encapsulated, removed.

Laboratory and Diagnostic Tests

Diagnosis of a brain abscess can present some difficulties because of the lack of definitive symptoms and a somewhat confusing clinical picture. The following diagnostic tests may be helpful in identifying a primary cause:

- *X-ray films* of the chest, skull, and sinuses may help identify a primary source of infection.
- *Lumbar puncture* reveals a markedly elevated pressure (200 to 300 mm water), with elevated protein content and elevated white blood cell count. Glucose content is normal, and culture and sensitivity are negative because the bacteria are encapsulated.

Pharmacology

Antimicrobial therapy is the primary treatment for brain abscess. Anticonvulsant medications may be given as prophylaxis against seizures.

Surgery

Surgical drainage of an encapsulated abscess is considered somewhat controversial. The decision to perform surgery is based on the client's general condition, the stage of abscess development, and the site of the abscess.

Nursing Care

A careful history and nursing assessment is important to assist in identifying brain abscess. Nursing diagnoses and interventions are generally the same as those previously discussed for clients with meningitis and increased intracranial pressure.

The Client with a Brain Tumor

■ ■ ■

Brain tumors are growths within the cranium, including tumors in brain tissue, meninges, pituitary gland, or blood vessels. Because clients with brain tumors present with diverse and confusing symptoms, diagnosis can be difficult.

The cause of brain tumors is unknown. Although a number of chemical and viral agents can cause brain tumors in laboratory animals, there is no evidence that these agents cause tumors in humans. There may be a hereditary factor; 16% of clients with primary brain tumors have a family history. Cranial irradiation and exposure to some chemicals may lead to an increased incidence of both astrocytomas and meningiomas (Porth, 1994).

It has been estimated that 36,000 new cases of brain tumors are diagnosed in the United States each year. The incidence of brain tumors in the general population has been estimated to be approximately 4.5 per 100,000 (Mc-Dermott & Wilson, 1992). Although brain tumors can occur in any age group, the highest incidence is among young children and among adults ages 50 to 70 (Willis, 1991). In the adult population, the most common tumor is glioblastoma multiforme, followed by meningioma and cytoma. Glioblastomas represent more than one-half of all primary intracranial lesions.

Brain tumors may be classified as benign or malignant, based on the tissue type and characteristics of the cells. The use of the term *benign* may be misleading. A tumor that is benign by histologic examination but is surgically inaccessible may continue to expand, increasing intracranial pressure and causing neurologic deficits, herniation, and finally death. In discussions of brain tumors, the term *malignant* is used to describe the lack of cell differentiation, the invasive nature of the tumor, and its ability to metastasize.

Brain tumors also may be classified as primary or secondary (metastatic), depending on their origin (Table 40–9). Primary tumors arise from the cells and structures that are found within the brain. They can be intracerebral or extracerebral. Gliomas are intracerebral tumors. The primary extracerebral tumors arise from the supporting structures; these include meningiomas, acoustic neuromas, and pituitary tumors. Primary brain tumors rarely metastasize outside the central nervous system.

Secondary brain tumors originate from structures outside the brain, such as the breasts and lungs. They then metastasize to the brain. Secondary brain tumors that originate from primary lesions of the lung, breast, and prostate contribute most significantly to metastatic lesions in the brain.

Brain tumors may be classified according to their anatomic location. They also may be classified according to the regional location of the lesion (e.g., frontal lobe, temporal lobe, cerebellum, and so on).

Pathophysiology

Focal disturbances take place when there is compression of brain tissue and infiltration or direct invasion of brain parenchyma with destruction of neural tissue. As the tumor grows, edema develops in adjacent tissues. The mechanism is not completely understood, but it is thought that an osmotic gradient causes absorption of fluid by the tumor. Some tumors may cause hemorrhage. Venous obstruction and edema due to breakdown of the blood–brain barrier increase intracranial volume and intracranial pressure. Obstruction of the circulation of CSF from the lateral ventricles to the subarachnoid space causes hydrocephalus (Price & Wilson, 1992).

Multiple clinical manifestations can develop as a result of the growth of the tumor, while others are related to the location of the lesion; see the accompanying box. Some of the more common manifestations include changes in cognition or consciousness, headache that is usually worse in the morning, seizures, and vomiting. Compression of brain tissue and the invasion of the brain tumor into the cerebral tissue may lead to changes typically seen with cerebral edema and increased ICP. Cerebral blood supply may diminish as the tumor compresses blood vessels. Shifts in brain tissue can occur, leading to brain herniation syndromes and, if untreated, death.

Collaborative Care

Treatment for a brain tumor may involve chemotherapy, radiation therapy, surgery, or any combination of these.

Clinical Manifestations of Brain Tumors

Frontal Lobe Tumors

- Inappropriate behavior
- Personality changes
- Inability to concentrate
- Impaired judgment
- Recent memory loss
- Headache
- Expressive aphasia
- Motor dysfunctions

Parietal Lobe Tumors

- Sensory deficits: paresthesia, loss of two-point discrimination, visual field deficits

Temporal Lobe Tumors

- Psychomotor seizures

Occipital Lobe Tumors

- Visual disturbances

Cerebellum Tumors

- Disturbances in coordination and equilibrium

Pituitary Tumors

- Endocrine dysfunction
- Visual deficits
- Headache

Table 40–9   Classification of Brain Tumors

Tumor Type	Tumor	Characteristics
Primary Tumors Intracerebral tumors Account for 40% to 50% of all brain tumors	*Glioma*	
	■ Astrocytoma	Most common glioma Graded I to IV according to degree of cell differentiation
Originates from neuroglia and invades brain tissue Most common type of brain tumor	■ Glioblastoma multiforme	Most malignant form Fast growing
	■ Ependymoma	Tumor that develops from lining of ventricles Graded I to IV according to degree of cell differentiation Slow growing
	■ Oligodendroglioma	Rare, slow-growing May be encapsulated
	■ Astroblastoma	Benign
Extracerebral tumors Tumors arising from the supporting structures of the nervous system Account for 10% to 15% of all brain tumors	Medulloblastoma	Fast growing and malignant Occurs primarily in children; can occur in adults Found in cerebellum
	Meningioma	Slow growing Develops in meninges (especially dura) Firm and encapsulated
	Acoustic neuroma	Slow growing Benign Originates from Schwann cells of the cranial nerve XIII May also affect cranial nerves V, VII, IX, and X Also called neurofibromatosis Genetic origin due to autosomal dominant mendelian trait Firm, encapsulated lesions attached to nerve
Congenital (developmental) tumors Account for 4% to 8% of all brain tumors	Hemangioblastoma	Vascular tumor Slow growing
	Craniopharyngioma	Originates from Rathke's pouch Solid or cystic tumor Compresses pituitary gland Presses on the third ventricle and may cause blockage of cerebrospinal fluid (CSF)
Pituitary adenomas Slow growing Account for 8% to 12% of all brain tumors	Chromophobic	Account for 90% of pituitary tumors Nonsecreting tumor
	Eosinophilic	Secreting tumors that produce growth hormone
	Basophilic	Secreting tumors that produce adrenocorticotropic hormone Fast growing
Secondary Tumors Metastatic brain tumors Slow-growing tumors that arise from other parts of the body Account for 10% of all brain tumors		
Tumors of the lung, breast, lower gastrointestinal tract, pancreas, kidney, skin		Usually well differentiated from the brain

Several variables are considered when selecting the appropriate treatment modality: the size and location of the tumor, the type of tumor, related symptoms (such as neurologic deficits), and the overall condition of the client.

Laboratory and Diagnostic Tests

A variety of tools are used to aid in the diagnosis of a brain tumor:

- *CT scan* or *MRI* is often ordered. Following a thorough neurologic examination, these diagnostic tests can locate and define the size of the tumor.

- *EEG* is ordered if seizures are present.

- *Pneumoencephalogram and ventriculogram* may be used to rule out the presence of a lesion of the ventricles and cisternal system, although the availability of CT scans has made them less common. The pneumoencephalogram involves a lumbar puncture or cisternal tap with injection of a contract medium (air or oxygen). It is never done in the presence of increased ICP because of the danger of herniation. In a ventriculogram, burr holes are made into the lateral ventricles and air is introduced directly via the ventricles.

- *Endocrine studies* are conducted if a pituitary tumor is suspected.

Pharmacology

The use of chemotherapy to treat brain tumors is still emerging. An intraventricular method of medication administration uses an Ommaya reservoir that has been surgically implanted into a lateral ventricle of the brain (see Figure 40–9 on page 1732).

Various chemotherapeutic agents are used in the treatment of brain tumors. The choice of drug is based on the type of tumor, its location, and the client's response to therapy.

Radiation Therapy

Radiation therapy may be administered alone or as adjunctive therapy with surgery. Radiation is often the treatment of choice for tumors that are surgically inaccessible; it may also be used to decrease the size of a tumor prior to surgery. Tumors that were not completely excised by surgery may also be treated with radiation.

Intracranial Surgery

Neurosurgery is used to remove tumors, to reduce the size of the tumor, or for symptom relief (palliation). The type of procedure, the surgical approach, and the timing of surgery (emergency procedure versus planned) influence the overall nursing management of the client having intracranial surgery.

Some of the more common intracranial neurosurgical procedures follow:

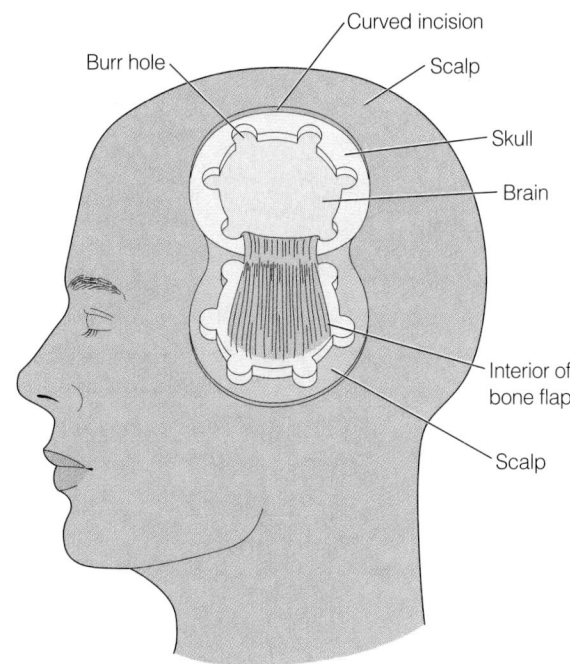

Figure 40–10   In a craniotomy, a portion of the skull and overlying scalp is removed to allow access to the brain.

- *Burr hole.* A hole made in the skull with a special drill. The hole may facilitate the evacuation of an extracerebral clot, or a series of holes may be made in preparation of craniotomy (see Figure 40–8).

- *Craniotomy.* A surgical opening into the cranial cavity (Figure 40–10). For a craniotomy, a series of burr holes are made. The bone between the holes is then cut with a special saw called a craniotome. The tumor is excised, and the bone flap is turned down. A craniotomy may also be performed to repair defects associated with traumatic head injuries or to repair a cerebral aneurysm.
  a. A *supratentorial craniotomy* refers to surgery above the tentorium. It provides access to the frontal, temporal, parietal, and occipital lobes. The incision for this procedure is usually within the hairline over the area involved.
  b. An *infratentorial craniotomy* refers to surgery below the tentorium. Access is provided to lesions in the cerebellum and the brain stem. The incision is made at the nape of the neck, around the occipital lobe.
  The Collaborative Care box on page 1740 describes the role of each health care team member caring for a client requiring a craniotomy for a brain tumor. A Critical Pathway for a client following a craniotomy for a brain tumor begins on page 1741.

- *Craniectomy.* An excision of a portion of the skull and complete removal of the bone flap. This procedure may be done to provide decompression after cerebral edema.

Collaborative Care: The Client Requiring a Craniotomy for a Brain Tumor

Health Care Team	Client Centered Care
Neurosurgeon	Assesses client's neurological status. Orders diagnostic tests such as CT scan and MRI. Removes tumor, orders anticonvulsants, diuretics, and steroids, monitors neurologic progress.
Oncologist	Collaborates with neurosurgeon and makes recommendations regarding chemotherapy and/or radiation therapy.
Primary care physician	Orders initial diagnostic tests for presenting neurologic signs and symptoms. Refers to neurosurgeon and/or manages medical care after discharge.
Physical therapist	Plans early mobilization activities. With team input, determines self-care deficits and assistive devices that are required.
Respiratory therapist	Assesses for respiratory complications, helps to maintain patent airway, administers oxygen for adequate air exchange to maintain pulse oximeter at 90% or greater.
Dietitian	Determines calorie requirements, recommends tube feeding type, strength and rate if necessary. Eventually plans and teaches adequate oral intake.
Speech therapist	Evaluates speech, swallowing ability, and plans interventions depending on needs.
Social worker	Coordinates discharge referrals for home care or community-based services. Arranges home health care and follow-up services including physical therapy. Consults with the family regarding discharge plans if extended care of hospice is required.
RN and Health Care Team Communications	Reports increased ICP, fluid and electrolyte imbalances, changes in neurologic status, hyperthermia or hypothermia, or seizures. Notifies family or significant other(s) about client's condition. Alerts social worker of discharge needs and assists in making arrangements for chemotherapy or radiation therapy if necessary. Collaborates with physical therapist to initiate rehabilitation planning.

Pressure on the brain structures is lessened by providing space for expansion.

- *Cranioplasty.* Plastic repair to the skull in which synthetic material is inserted to replace the cranial bone that was removed. This procedure may be performed after a large craniectomy. The plastic repair restores the contour and integrity of the cranium.

Specialty Procedures

Technologic advances—including the development of special instruments, the use of stereotaxic techniques for localizing a specific target, and the use of the laser beam—have greatly advanced neurosurgical practice. Microsurgery involves an operating microscope with microinstruments and supportive illumination equipment. With stereotaxic techniques, the client is positioned to allow location of discrete areas of the brain that control specific functions and exact locations of deep brain lesions. The use of a laser beam for excision of a tumor results in less damage to surrounding tissue and less postoperative swelling. A new tool to assist with therapy is the gamma knife, which can apply radiation to a precise area of the brain, destroying tumor tissue while limiting damage to

the surrounding normal brain tissue (Willis, 1991). The gamma knife, which is not actually a knife but a gamma unit, consists of a heavily shielded helmet containing 201 sources of cobalt-60, which is capable of destroying deep and inaccessible lesions in a single treatment session.

Nursing Care

The nursing care of the client with a brain tumor includes support during the diagnostic period and specific management as directed by the selected treatment modality. The foundation for care is data from the health history, which includes identifying neurologic deficits. This information provides direction for planning and implementing care. Many of the alterations in health commonly experienced by the client with a brain tumor have been discussed throughout this chapter, including altered level of consciousness, increased intracranial pressure, and seizures. The client will require intensive care in the immediate postoperative period. This section of the chapter focuses on nursing interventions for the client who has intracranial surgery. The nursing diagnoses discussed are *Anxiety, Risk for Infection, Altered Protection, Pain,* and *Self-Esteem Disturbance.*

Critical Pathway for Client Following Craniotomy for Brain Tumor

	Date _____ **1st 24 hours postoperative**	Date _____ **48 hours postoperative**	Date _____ **3 to 4 days postoperative**
	Expected length of stay: 3 to 4 days		
Daily outcomes	Client will ■ Maintain adequate cerebral blood flow as evidenced by stable vital signs, being alert and oriented, and maintaining usual sensory and motor function. ■ Maintain cranial nerve function. ■ Have stable vital signs and B/P within specified range. ■ Have lungs clear to auscultation. ■ Have unlabored respirations and maintain oxygen saturation above 92%. ■ Have clean, dry dressing. ■ Recover from anesthesia. ■ Verbalize understanding and demonstrate cooperation with turning and deep breathing. ■ Tolerate ordered diet without nausea and vomiting. ■ Verbalize control of incisional pain with ordered medications. ■ Demonstrate ability to cope.	Client will ■ Maintain adequate cerebral blood flow as evidenced by stable vital signs, being alert and oriented, and maintaining usual sensory and motor function. ■ Maintain cranial nerve function. ■ Have stable vital signs and B/P within specified range. ■ Have lungs clear to auscultation. ■ Have unlabored respirations and maintain oxygen saturation above 92%. ■ Have clean, dry wound with edges well-approximated, healing by first intention. ■ Demonstrate cooperation with turning and deep breathing. ■ Tolerate ordered diet without nausea and vomiting. ■ Ambulate 4 times per day. ■ Verbalize control of incisional pain. ■ Demonstrate ability to cope. ■ Verbalize/demonstrate beginning understanding of home care instructions.	Client will ■ Be afebrile. ■ Maintain adequate cerebral blood flow as evidenced by stable vital signs and being alert and oriented. ■ Maintain usual sensory and motor function. ■ Maintain cranial nerve function. ■ Have stable vital signs and B/P within specified range. ■ Have lungs clear to auscultation and unlabored respiration with an oxygen saturation above 92%. ■ Have clean, dry wound with edges well-approximated, healing by first intention. ■ Manage pain with oral medications and/or non-pharmacologic measures. ■ Be independent in self-care. ■ Be fully ambulatory. ■ Resume preadmission urine and bowel elimination pattern. ■ Verbalize ability to cope with changes to body image and utilize strategies to cope with shaved scalp, scars, indentations, and any neurologic deficits. ■ Verbalize/demonstrate home care instructions. ■ Tolerate ordered diet without nausea or vomiting. ■ Demonstrate ability to cope with ongoing stressors including current illness and any neurologic deficits.
Assessments, tests, and treatments	Vital signs O₂ saturation Neurovascular and mental status assessment	Vital signs Neurovascular and cranial nerve assessment O₂ saturation	Vital signs Neurovascular and cranial nerve assessment O₂ saturation

	Critical Pathway for Client Following Craniotomy for Brain Tumor (continued)		
	Date _____ **1st 24 hours postoperative**	**Date _____** **48 hours postoperative**	**Date _____** **3 to 4 days postoperative**
Assessments, tests, and treatments *continued*	Dressing and wound drainage assessment q15min × 4; q30min × 4; q1h × 24 and prn Ventilator care and weaning per protocol ABGs as indicated EKG monitoring Head of the bed up 30 to 45 degrees Avoid flexion, extension, and rotation of head and neck. Monitor for seizures and protect from injury. ICP monitoring per clinical protocol Maintain patency of any drains. Assess cranial nerve function q2–4 h and prn. Monitor for bleeding, cerebral edema, and/or cerebral ischemia. Incentive spirometer q2h Intake and output every shift Foley catheter Assess coping status of client and family. Provide ongoing emotional support to client and family. Allow for client's input regarding sequence of care. When extubated: Oxygen as ordered to maintain O_2 saturation >92%	Dressing and wound drainage assessment q2–4h and prn Head of the bed up 30 to 45 degrees Avoid flexion, extension, and rotation of head and neck. Monitor for seizures and protect from injury. Monitor for bleeding, cerebral edema, and/or cerebral ischemia. Assess respiratory status q4h and prn. Incentive spirometer q2h until fully ambulatory Intake and output every shift Remove catheter and assess voiding—if unable to void, try suggestive voiding techniques or catheterize q8h or prn. Dressing change and wound assessment BID and prn Assess coping status of client and family. Encourage client and family to verbalize feelings regarding any changes in appearance and functional abilities. Provide ongoing emotional support to client and family.	Dressing and wound drainage assessment q4–8h and prn Assess respiratory status q4–8h. Assess wound and apply dry sterile dressing q day and prn. Encourage client to verbalize feelings regarding any changes in appearance and functional ability. Assist the client and family to identify any resources or strategies to cope with changes in appearance and functional ability. Assess coping status and provide appropriate emotional support.
Knowledge deficit	Orient to room and surroundings. Provide simple, brief instructions. Include family in teaching. Review specific postoperative care: turning, deep breathing, incentive spirometer, mobilization, intravenous, pain management (prn medications).	Review plan of care and importance of early mobilization. Begin discharge teaching regarding wound care/dressing change, diet, and activity. Review written discharge instructions with client and significant other.	Complete discharge teaching to include wound care, diet, follow-up care and appointment, signs and symptoms to report, activity, and medication: name, purpose, dose, frequency, route, food interactions, and side effects. Provide client with written discharge instructions regarding home care.

	Date _____ **1st 24 hours postoperative**	Date _____ **48 hours postoperative**	Date _____ **3 to 4 days postoperative**
Knowledge deficit *continued*	Instruct client regarding the importance of supporting head and neck during position changes. Assess understanding of teaching.		
Diet	Prior to offering fluids, assess return of gag and ability to chew and swallow. HOB up for all meals Maintain fluid restriction. When fully awake, clear liquids as tolerated.	Full liquids to diet as tolerated	Diet as tolerated
Activity	Assess safety needs and provide adequate precautions. HOB up 30 degrees, support head and neck when changing positions Dangle/chair evening of surgery if stable.	Maintain safety precautions. Fully ambulatory in room with required assistance Walk in hall 4 to 6 times with required assistance.	Maintain safety precautions. Fully ambulatory
Medications	IV fluids Antiepilepsy medications as ordered Glucocorticosteroids as ordered Diuretics as ordered Analgesics as ordered H_2-receptor antagonists as ordered Stool softeners, antitussives, and antiemetics as ordered Antihypertensives as ordered.	Intermittent IV device Antiepilepsy medications as ordered. Glucocorticosteroids as ordered Diuretics as ordered Analgesics as ordered H_2-receptor antagonists as ordered. Stool softeners, antitussives, and antiemetics as ordered	PO analgesics. D/C IV device. Other medications as ordered.
Transfer/ discharge plans	Establish discharge objectives with client and family. Determine discharge needs and support system with client and significant others. Begin home care instructions.	Review progress toward discharge goals. Make appropriate referrals. Finalize discharge plans.	Finalize any home care arrangements. Complete discharge instructions.

Anxiety

The diagnosis of a brain tumor often brings anxiety and feelings of uncertainty about the future. Both the client and family members are likely to be apprehensive and require education and emotional support.

Nursing interventions with rationales follow:

- Assist client through routine medical procedures, including blood work and radiologic studies. *Baseline laboratory and radiologic studies are needed to ensure that the client has no other preexisting medical condition. Explaining the procedures and assisting the client through this process helps decrease anxiety.*

- Reinforce, clarify, and repeat information that has been provided. *Both client and family may have limited understanding of the scheduled diagnostic tests, procedures, and treatment modalities. The client may be confused or have altered thought processes as a result of the tumor. Information may need to be repeated or reexplained.*

- Encourage client and family to verbalize feelings, questions, and fears; provide realistic information appropriate to their level of understanding. *Verbalization helps reduce anxiety and fear.*

- Review the client's and family's strengths and effective coping skills. *Personal strengths, support systems, and coping skills can aid in the development of appropriate strategies to reduce anxiety.*

- Arrange for a member of the clergy to visit if the client so desires. *Faith in a higher being is often a strong source of strength and support.*

- Assess the family's knowledge and response to hospitalization and impending surgery. *The need for surgery frequently produces anxiety in the family.*

- Provide preoperative teaching, including the following information:
  a. Type of anesthesia and surgery.
  b. Time surgery will begin.
  c. Where the client will be taken after surgery (CCU, ICU). If possible, show the client and family the CCU or ICU and introduce them to the nurse who will be in charge of the client's care after the surgery.
  d. Expected length of time for the surgery.
  e. Where family can wait during and following surgery.
  f. Appearance of the client after surgery, which may include swollen, bruised eyelids and other facial features; a large dressing covering the head; and a tracheostomy or endotracheal tube.
  g. Behavior of the client after surgery, which will differ depending on the site of surgery; however, cognitive and behavioral changes are common following intracranial surgery.

Information about what to expect reduces anxiety.

- Allow time for client and family to be together. *Clients and families need quiet time together to support each other and prepare emotionally for surgery.*

Risk for Infection

The client who has had intracranial surgery is at risk for infection from multiple invasive lines, the scalp wound, and an introduction of bacteria into the operative area. The nurse provides interventions to monitor for manifestations of infection and also to prevent infection.

Nursing interventions with rationales follow:

- Assess and report leakage of CSF:
  a. Presence of glucose in clear drainage from ears, nose, or wound
  b. Complaints of "something dripping down the back of the throat"
  c. Constant swallowing
  These manifestations indicate an opening in the dura, which provides an avenue for an ascending infection.

- Provide interventions to prevent contamination of area leaking CSF:
  a. If leaking from the nose: Keep head of bed elevated 20 degrees unless contraindicated; do not suction nasally; do not clean nose; tell client not to put finger in nose; do not insert packing.
  b. If leaking from the ear: Position client on side of leakage unless contraindicated; do not clean ear; tell client not to put finger in ear; do not insert packing.
  c. Place a sterile dressing over the area of drainage and change as soon as it becomes damp.
  Leakage of CSF indicates a break in the dura and increases the risk of an ascending infection. Surgery may be necessary to repair the break; however, the leak usually heals spontaneously in about a week.

- Assess and report manifestations of infection:
  a. Take and record temperature on a regular basis.
  b. Assess insertion sites for redness, swelling, drainage, and pain.
  c. Assess scalp wound for redness, swelling, bulging, drainage, and pain.
  d. Assess for manifestations of meningitis:
     - Fever and chills
     - Increasing headache
     - Neck stiffness
     - Positive Kernig's or Brudzinski's sign
     - Photophobia
  e. Monitor laboratory reports for increased white blood count
  Intact skin is the first line of defense against infection. Any break in the skin increases the risk of infection. Intracranial surgery increases the risk of meningitis, with infectious agents ascending into the brain.

- Implement interventions to prevent infection:
  a. Use strict aseptic technique when changing dressings and when caring for wound drains and ICP monitor lines.
  b. Keep the client's hands away from drains and dressings; use mitten restraints if necessary.
  c. Administer prescribed antibiotics.
  The use of sterile technique decreases the risk of introducing infection into a wound. Antibiotics are usually prescribed prophylactically to prevent infection.

Altered Protection

The client who has intracranial surgery is not able to provide normal human defenses against changes in intracranial pressure and is also at risk from cerebral edema and a shift of intracerebral contents. In addition, the surgery may cause cerebral bleeding or hematoma formation.

Nursing interventions with rationales follow:

- Monitor for manifestations of increased intracranial pressure:
  a. Restlessness, agitation, and decreasing level of consciousness
  b. Headache
  c. Vomiting
  d. Seizures
  e. Decreasing sensory and motor function
  f. Changes in pupil size and reaction
  g. Changes in vital signs: altered respiratory rate or depth, increasing pulse pressure, decreasing pulse rate, increasing blood pressure
  h. Abnormal posturing
  Increasing intracranial pressure is manifested by alterations in the functions and centers controlled by the brain.

- Implement interventions to decrease the risk of increased intracranial pressure:
  a. Elevate the head of the bed 15 to 30 degrees (unless contraindicated).
  b. Avoid neck flexion or rotation; keep head in midline position unless a large bone flap or mass was removed; then position the client on unoperated side to decrease venous congestion in the operative area.
  c. Do not take rectal temperatures.
  d. Avoid clustering activities that increase intracranial pressure: suctioning, turning, bathing.
  e. Administer medications to prevent vomiting.
  f. Do not suction for more than 10 to 15 seconds at one time.
  g. Teach the client (if possible) to avoid coughing, sneezing, and straining to have a bowel movement.
  h. Maintain fluid restrictions as prescribed.
  i. Administer diuretics as prescribed.
  j. Maintain patency of any drains or shunts.

- For internal shunts: avoid pressure on the shunt, reservoir, or tubing. Pump the shunt as prescribed.

- For external shunts: avoid kinks in tubing, and maintain the drainage collecting device and client's head at the prescribed levels.
  Keeping the head of the bed slightly elevated facilitates venous drainage from the brain. Neck flexion or rotation disrupts circulation to and from the brain. Rectal stimulation, suctioning, turning, bathing, coughing, sneezing, and straining to have a bowel movement all initiate Valsalva's maneuver, which constricts the jugular veins and impairs venous return from the brain. Fluid restriction may be prescribed to dehydrate the client slightly and lessen ICP; diuretics are prescribed to decrease cerebral edema.

- Maintain (as much as possible) a quiet, calm, softly lighted environment. Avoid excessive sensory stimulation. *These interventions promote rest and decrease stimulation, thereby reducing ICP.*

- Implement interventions to prevent seizures or, if they occur, to prevent injury to the client:
  a. Pad side rails of the bed.
  b. Place bed in lowest position, and keep side rails up.
  c. Carry out interventions to prevent and treat increased intracranial pressure.
  d. Have an oral airway and suction equipment immediately available.
  e. Administer prescribed anticonvulsants.
  f. If a seizure occurs: Maintain a patent airway; do not restrain client; do not force anything into the client's mouth; provide physical and emotional support.
  These interventions promote safety and help prevent injury. Anticonvulsants are often prescribed prophylactically to prevent seizures following intracranial surgery.

- Carefully monitor hydration status. Compare trends in intake and output, laboratory results of serum osmolality, and urine specific gravity and osmolality. *Changes in fluid balance and osmolality may result from excess intravenous fluids, osmotic diuretics, surgically induced diabetes insipidus or syndrome of inappropriate antidiuretic hormone secretion (see Chapter 20), fever, diarrhea, tube feedings, or hyperglycemia.*

Pain

The client who has intracranial surgery has pain, manifested as a headache, as a result of either compression or displacement of brain tissue or from increased intracranial pressure. A headache may also be a manifestation of meningitis.

Nursing interventions with rationales follow:

- Assess the location, duration, and intensity of the pain, using a scale of from 0 (no pain) to 10 (worst pain) in the client who can verbally communicate. *The client is the best source of information about pain.*

- Implement interventions to reduce the pain:
  a. Raise the head of the bed slightly.

b. Reduce noise and bright lights in the room.

c. If allowed, loosen head dressing.

d. Administer narcotic analgesics with caution.

Nonpharmacologic measures may be used to reduce increased intracranial pressure and headache. Narcotic analgesics mask changes in eye signs and depress respirations.

Self-Esteem Disturbance

The client who has intracranial surgery has many alterations that affect self-esteem and body image. Physical changes include a loss of hair on the scalp, swelling and bruising in the eyelids and face, and perhaps an indentation in the skull. The client is no longer independent in self-care but must depend on others to meet basic needs. There are often long-term neurologic deficits, affecting areas such as speech, vision, and motor abilities, which require changes in roles and relationships.

Nursing interventions with rationales follow:

- Assess for verbal and nonverbal manifestations of negative self-esteem:
  a. Denial of changes
  b. Preoccupation with changes
  c. Refusal to look in the mirror
  d. Withdrawal from family and friends
  e. Expressions of grief and loss (see Chapter 11)
  Low self-esteem can be initiated by stressful situations and changes in body image.

- Provide interventions to improve self-concept:
  a. Limit negative self-assessment.
  b. Help client focus on positive areas of life.
  c. Help client identify sources of support and strength.
  d. Help client identify and use helpful coping methods.
  e. Encourage significant others to visit.
  f. Encourage independence in self-care.
  Self-esteem is derived from one's own perceptions of competence and from the responses of others. When one's self-concept and self-ideal are congruent, self-esteem is enhanced.

Other Nursing Diagnoses

Other nursing diagnoses that might be appropriate for the client who has had intracranial surgery follow:

- *Hyperthermia* related to increased intracranial pressure
- *Ineffective Breathing Patterns* related to increased intracranial pressure
- *Risk for Impaired Skin Integrity* related to loss of motor function
- *Altered Role Performance* related to neurologic deficits following craniotomy
- *Altered Sexuality Patterns* related to feelings of inadequacy following intracranial surgery with residual neurologic deficits
- *Spiritual Distress* related to inability to accept diagnosis

- *Ineffective Denial* related to unwillingness to accept neurologic deficits
- *Body Image Disturbance* related to indentatation in skull
- *Powerlessness* related to inability to provide self-care

Client and Family Teaching

Both the client and family members have teaching needs that should be addressed in an individualized plan of care as discussed above. Generally, information should be provided about the overall treatment plan, management of deficits and/or disabilities, and future needs.

Some specific teaching topics follow:

- Safety measures for motor deficits, sensory deficits, lack of coordination, seizures, and cognitive deficits
- Comfort measures for nausea, vomiting, and pain
- Measures for communication if aphasia is present
- Measures to improve vision if visual deficits are present
- How to buy wigs and hairpieces
- Referrals to support groups and community resources

The effect of the possible outcomes following the surgery often produces fear in both client and family, interfering with their ability to retain information. Also, the client may have cognitive or neurologic deficits that interfere with learning. Family members must be assessed as well for their ability to cope with the stress of the surgery. Information may have to be repeated several times.

Clients and their families who have experienced intracranial surgery require emotional support. The process of recovery is often extended and may involve adaptation to change in body image and management of any motor or sensory deficits. The family should be involved in the care of the client. If family members are willing, they may begin to assist with activities of daily living while the client is in the hospital, such as assisting the client with personal hygiene and meals. Clients should also be encouraged to take an active role in their own care. Discharge planning includes a discussion of the following topics: medication information; wound care; the use of wigs, turbans, or colorful scarves; and the importance of follow-up visits. In addition, emphasize the importance of reporting manifestations such as stiff neck, increasing headache, elevated temperature, new motor or sensory deficits, vision changes, or seizures.

Applying the Nursing Process

Case Study of a Client with a Brain Tumor: Claire Lange

Claire Lange is a 44-year-old television announcer. During one night's broadcast, she confuses several major news items so badly that her co-anchor tries to correct her. Ms. Lange responds angrily that she does not need any help and then rises and storms off the set. As she leaves the camera area, she limps noticeably and appears to drag her left leg. The show's producer asks her what is wrong; she screams that nothing is wrong—she simply has another headache. He follows her to her dressing room and inquires about her headaches. She tells him that they come and go but have been getting worse lately. He then asks her if she has injured her left leg; she responds that the leg was weak because she was tired. As the producer leaves the dressing room, Ms. Lange begins to shake and collapses on the floor. The producer recognizes that she is having a seizure and calls for an ambulance.

Ms. Lange is admitted to the neurology floor of the local hospital for evaluation. A CT scan, MRI study, and EEG are completed and identify an intracranial mass. A biopsy of the mass is positive for malignant cells. A glioma in the frontal lobe is identified, and surgery is scheduled for later in the week.

Assessment

When Clara Rosetti, RN, enters Ms. Lange's room, she sees Ms. Lange looking at her shoulder-length hair in the mirror. Ms. Lange tells Ms. Rosetti that she has never in her life worn her hair any shorter, and "Now you're going to cut it all off!" She paces the room and makes the statement, "I guess the hair isn't really important if I survive this situation." She also says that she has a headache.

Diagnosis

Ms. Rosetti identifies the following nursing diagnoses for Ms. Lange:

- *Pain* (headache) related to tumor and increase in intracranial pressure
- *Body Image Disturbance* related to upcoming hair loss and cranial incision
- *Anxiety* related to unknown future following surgery

Expected Outcomes

The expected outcomes for the plan of care are that Ms. Lange will

- Verbalize a reduction in headache.
- Verbalize the causes of pain.
- Verbalize an understanding of the changes in body appearance that are associated with the scheduled intracranial surgery (e.g., shaving of the head prior to surgery, cranial incision, facial swelling postoperatively).
- Identify measures that will help minimize the impact of the hair loss.
- Verbalize a reduction in anxiety.

Planning and Implementation

Ms. Rosetti plans and implements the following nursing interventions for Ms. Lange:

- Assess level of discomfort using a rating scale of 0 to 10.
- Provide a quiet, nonstimulating environment.
- Position the client for comfort, keeping the head of the bed elevated to promote venous drainage.
- Explain reasons for headache pattern.
- Assess level of consciousness for potential increases in ICP.
- Assess Ms. Lange's awareness of and reactions to body changes.
- Encourage Ms. Lange to verbalize feelings about the surgery.
- Suggest measures that may help minimize the hair loss, such as the use of turbans, scarves, hats, and wigs.
- Suggest relaxation techniques to decrease anxiety.

Evaluation

By the time of surgery, Ms. Lange has recognized the relationship between the brain tumor and the headache. She states that lying in a flat position and coughing increase the headache. The head of the bed is kept at a 30- to 45-degree angle. Daily activities are spaced to provide periods of rest. Ms. Lange demonstrates no significant changes in level of consciousness (Glasgow Coma Scale score = 15). She has talked about the effect of the hair loss and her television responsibilities. Ms. Lange has learned that the hair preparation would be done in surgery and that the hair would be saved for her. She states she has already consulted her hair stylist and that "scarves and turbans are on the way." The possibility of making a wig from her own hair is also discussed.

Critical Thinking in the Nursing Process

1. Outline interventions to decrease intracranial pressure both before and after surgery.

2. When making your initial assessments on the morning of surgery, you find that Ms. Lange has a decreased pulse and increased blood pressure. She tells you her headache is worse and suddenly vomits. What do you do now?

3. Ms. Lange asks you to be sure that she has absolutely no visitors after surgery, because she knows how ugly she will look. How would you respond?

4. Outline a preoperative teaching plan for Ms. Lange, including both general preoperative care and care specific to a craniotomy.

5. Design a plan of care for Ms. Lange for the nursing diagnosis *Powerlessness*.

Bibliography

■ ■ ■

Acom, S., & Roberts, E. (1992). Head injury: Impact on the wives. *Journal of Neuroscience Nursing, 24*(6), 324–328.

Adams, B., Clancey, J., & Eddy, M. (1991). Malignant glioma: Current treatment perspectives. *Journal of Neuroscience Nursing, 23*(1), 15–19.

Alfaro-Lefevre, R. (1994). *Applying the nursing process: A step by step guide* (3rd ed.). Philadelphia: Lippincott.

American Academy of Neurology. (1989). Position of the American Academy of Neurology on certain aspects of the care and management of the persistent vegetative state patient. *Neurology, 39,* 125–126.

Ammons, A. M. (1990). Cerebral injuries and intracranial hemorrhages as a result of trauma. *Nursing Clinics of North America, 25*(91), 23–33.

Arbour, R. (1993). Stereotactic localization and resection of intracranial tumors. *Journal of Neuroscience Nursing, 25*(1), 14–21.

Aumick, J. (1991a). Head trauma. *RN, 54*(4), 27–32.

Aumick, J. (1991b). Head trauma: Guidelines for care. *RN, 54*(5), 27–31.

Bachman, D. (1992). The diagnosis and management of common neurologic sequelae of closed head injury. *Journal of Head Trauma Rehabilitation, 7*(2), 50–59.

Baggerly, J. (1991). Sensory perceptual deficits following stroke. *Nursing Clinics of North America, 26,* 997–1005.

Baker, J. (1990). Family adaptation when one member has a head injury. *Journal of Neuroscience Nursing, 22*(4), 232–237.

Barclay, L. (1993). *Clinical geriatric neurology.* Philadelphia: Lea & Febiger.

Barker, E., & Moore, K. (1992a). Perfecting the art of neurological assessment. *RN, 55*(4), 28–35.

Barker, E., & Moore, K. (1992b). Perfecting the art of cranial nerve assessment. *RN, 55,* 62–68.

Bauman, C., & Zumwalk, C. (1989). Intracranial neoplasms: An overview. *AORN Journal, 50,* 240–256.

Berkow, R., & Fletcher, A. (1992). *The Merck manual of diagnosis and therapy.* New Jersey: Merck Research Laboratories.

Caine, R., & Bufalino, P. (1991). *Applying nursing diagnosis: Nursing care planning guides for adults* (2nd ed.). Baltimore: Williams & Wilkins.

Campbell, C. H. (1988). Needs of relatives and helpfulness of support groups in severe head injury. *Rehabilitation Nursing, 13*(6), 320–325.

Carpenito, L.J. (1995a). *Nursing care plans and documentation: Nursing diagnosis and collaborative problems.* Philadelphia: Lippincott.

Carpenito, L.J. (1995b). *Nursing diagnosis: Application to clinical practice* (6th ed.). Philadelphia: Lippincott.

Chenitz, W., Stone, J., & Salisburn, S. (1991). *Clinical gerontological nursing.* Philadelphia: W. B. Saunders.

Cheung, R. (1992). Responsiveness. In P. S. Kidd & K. D. Wagner (Eds.), *High acuity nursing* (pp. 277–297). Norwark, CT: Appleton & Lange.

Chipps, E., Clanin, N., & Campbell, V. G. (1992). *Neurologic disorders.* St. Louis: Mosby.

Crobett, J. V. (1992). *Laboratory tests and diagnostic procedures with nursing diagnosis* (3rd ed.). Norwalk, CT: Appleton & Lange.

Cox, H., Hinz, M., Lukino, M., Newfield, S., Ridernaur, N., Slater, M., & Sridaramont, K. (1993). *Clinical applications of nursing diagnosis* (2nd ed.). Philadelphia: F. A. Davis.

Crosby, J., & Parsons, L. (1992). Cerebrovascular response of closed head injured patients to a standardized endotracheal tube suctioning and manual hyperventilation procedure. *Journal of Neuroscience Nursing, 24*(1), 40–49.

Davis, M., & Lucatorto, M. (1992). The false localizing signs of increased intracranial pressure. *Journal of Neuroscience Nursing, 24,* 245–250.

Dilorio, C., Faherty, B., & Manteuffel, B. (1993). Learning needs of persons with epilepsy: A comparison of perceptions of persons with epilepsy, nurses and physicians. *Journal of Neuroscience Nursing, 25*(1), 22–29.

Drummond, B. (1990). Preventing increased intracranial pressure: Nursing care can make the difference. *Focus on Critical Care, 17*(2), 116–122.

Engli, M., & Kirsivalia-Farmer, K. (1993). Needs of family members of critically ill patients with and without acute brain injury. *Journal of Neuroscience Nursing, 25*(2), 78–85.

Fischback, F. (1992). *A manual of laboratory & diagnostic tests* (4th ed.). Philadelphia: Lippincott.

Gerdner, L., & Buckwater, K. (1994). Assessment and management of agitation. *Journal of Gerontological Nursing, 20*(4), 11–20.

Gilman, S. (1992a). Advances in neurology. Part 1. *New England Journal of Medicine, 326,* 1610–1616.

Gilman, S. (1992b). Advances in neurology. Part 2. *New England Journal of Medicine, 326,* 1617–1666.

Gilman, S., & Winan-Newman, S. (1992). *Manter and Gatz's Essentials of clinical neuroanatomy and neurophysiology* (8th ed.). Philadelphia: F. A. Davis.

Godbole, K., Berbiglia, V., & Goddard, L. (1991). A head-injured patient: Caloric needs, clinical progress and nursing care priorities. *Journal of Neuroscience Nursing, 23*(5), 290–294.

Guyton, A. C. (1991). *Textbook of medical physiology* (8th ed.). Philadelphia: W. B. Saunders.

Hachinski, V. (1992). *Challenges in neurology.* Philadelphia: F. A. Davis.

Hanak, M. (1992). *Rehabilitation nursing for the neurologic patient.* New York: Springer.

Hartshorn, J., & Byers, V. (1992). Impact of epilepsy on quality of life. *Journal of Neuroscience Nursing, (24),* 24–29.

Hickey, J. V. (1992). *The clinical practice of neurological and neurosurgical nursing.* Philadelphia: Lippincott.

Jackson, S. (1992). Assessing a head injury. *Nursing92, 22*(6), 49.

Kerr, M. E., Rudy, E. B., Brucia, J., & Stone, K. (1993). Head injured adults: Recommendations for endotracheal suctioning. *Journal of Neuroscience Nursing, 25*(2), 86–91.

Lower, J. (1992). Rapid neurological assessment. *American Journal of Nursing, 92*(6), 38–45.

Marieb, E. N. (1995). *Human anatomy and physiology* (3rd ed.). Redwood City, CA: Benjamin/Cummings.

Mass-Clum, N., Cole, M, McCort, T., & Eifler, D. (1991). Locked-in syndrome: A team approach. *Journal of Neuroscience Nursing, 23*(5), 273–286.

McCance, K., & Huether, S. E. (1994). *Pathophysiology: The biologic basis for disease in adults and children* (2nd ed.). St. Louis: Mosby

Michael, J. E. (1992). Vagal nerve stimulation in treatment of intractable partial seizures: Nursing implications. *Journal of Neuroscience Nursing, 24*(1), 19–23.

Moak, E. (1992). Preoperative care of the craniotomy patient: A review. *Today's O.R. Nurse, 14*(1), 9–14.

Parker, C. (1995). Emergency! Fast action for subarachnoid hemorrhage. *American Journal of Nursing, 95*(1), 47.

Porth, C. (1994). *Pathophysiology: Concepts of altered health status* (4th ed.). Philadelphia: Lippincott.

Price, S., & Wilson, L. (1992). *Pathophysiology: Clinical concepts of disease processes.* St. Louis: Mosby.

Purath, J. (1992). Assessing headache pain. *RN, 54*(10), 26–30.

Ridgeway, G., & Like, M. (1991). Demystifying tonic-clonic seizures. *Nursing91, 21*(11), 63–64.

Ross, A. M., Pitts, L. H., & Kobayashi, S. (1992). Prognosticators of outcome after major head injury in the elderly. *Journal of Neuroscience Nursing, 24*(2), 88–93.

Skidmore-Roth, L. (1993). *Mosby's nursing drug reference.* St. Louis: Mosby.

Spratto, G., & Woods, A. (1995). *RN Magazine's NDR-95.* New York: Delmar.

Twomey, C. (1992). Brain abscess: An update. *Journal of Neuroscience Nursing, 24*(91), 34–39.

Voss, H. (1993). Making headway with intracranial hypertension. *American Journal of Nursing, 93*(2), 28–35.

Willis, D. (1991). Intracranial astrocytoma: Pathology, diagnosis and clinical presentation. *Journal of Neuroscience Nursing, 23*(1), 7–14.

Wilson, J. D., Braunwald, E., Isselbacher, K. J., Petersdorf, R. G., Martin, J. B., Fauci, A. S., & Root, R. K. (Eds.). (1991). *Harrison's Principles of internal medicine* (12th ed.). New York: McGraw-Hill.

Wilson, B., Shannon, M., & Stang, C. (1995). *Nurses drug guide.* Norwalk, CT: Appleton & Lange.

Nursing Care of Clients with Cerebral Blood Flow Disorders and Spinal Cord Disorders

LEARNING OBJECTIVES

After completing this chapter, you will be able to

- Identify factors responsible for disorders in cerebral blood flow.
- Discuss the pathophysiologic effects of alterations in cerebral blood flow due to thrombi, emboli, and hemorrhage.
- Describe the manifestations of a cerebral vascular accident.
- Describe the pathophysiologic effects of a ruptured intracranial aneurysm.
- Provide nursing care for clients with a ruptured intracranial aneurysm.

- Describe an arteriovenous malformation.
- Identify factors responsible for spinal cord injuries.
- Discuss the pathophysiologic effects of injuries of the spinal cord by level of injury.
- Describe the causes and manifestations of a cervical and lumbar herniated intervertebral disk.
- Provide nursing care for the client having a laminectomy.
- Discuss the types and manifestations of a spinal cord tumor and describe appropriate client care.
- Use the nursing process as a framework for providing individualized care to clients with cerebral blood flow and spinal cord disorders.

The health problems discussed in this chapter result from alterations in cerebral blood flow and from disorders of the spinal cord. Clients with disorders of cerebral blood flow and the spinal cord experience a wide variety of neurologic deficits that affect cognitive and perceptual health patterns.

The nursing care that is planned and implemented for clients with these disorders is tailored to meet the needs of the client and individualized according to the client's responses to alterations in cranial and spinal cord structure and function. Discussion of nursing care includes consideration of acute and long-term health care needs.

Disorders of Cerebral Blood Flow

The brain, which makes up only 2% of the total body weight, receives approximately 20% of the cardiac output each minute (about 750 mL) and accounts for 20% of the body's oxygen consumption. Brain function depends on a consistent blood and oxygen supply. When cerebral blood flow is decreased or interrupted, the resulting ischemia may lead to death of brain cells and pathophysiologic alterations (Porth, 1994).

Overview of Cerebral Blood Flow

The brain is supplied with blood from the internal carotid arteries (anteriorly) and the vertebral arteries (posteriorly). The branches of these arteries and the areas to which they supply blood are outlined in Table 41–1. These systems connect at the base of the brain at the circle of Willis; this joining of arteries may allow uninterrupted blood flow if one of the major blood vessels is occluded.

Two sets of veins drain cerebral blood into venous plexuses and dural sinuses and then into the internal jugular veins at the base of the skull. The veins in the cerebral system do not have valves; therefore, the direction of flow depends on gravity or pressure differences between the venous sinuses and the extracranial veins. Activities that increase intrathoracic pressure (such as sneezing, coughing, straining to have a bowel movement, or vomiting) also briefly increase intracranial pressure. This increased intracranial pressure occurs because the increased intrathoracic pressure is transmitted through the internal jugular veins and the dural sinuses.

Cerebral blood flow, especially in the deep cerebral vessels, is largely self-regulated by the brain to meet metabolic needs. This self-regulation (also called autoregulation) allows the brain to maintain a constant blood flow despite changes in systemic blood pressure. However, autoregulation is not effective when systemic blood pressure falls below 60 mmHg or rises above 140 mmHg. In the latter case, the increased systemic pressure (as in hypertension) causes an increase in cerebral blood flow with resultant overdistention of cerebral vessels.

The superficial and major cerebral vessels are innervated by the sympathetic nervous system. This innervation pattern is especially significant in the presence of increased arterial pressure when sympathetic response constricts, and possibly thus protects, the smaller vessels (Porth, 1994). Cerebral blood flow is affected by concentrations of carbon dioxide, oxygen, and hydrogen ions. Cerebral blood flow increases in response to increased carbon dioxide concentrations, increased hydrogen ion concentrations, and decreased oxygen concentrations.

This section of the chapter addresses cerebral vascular accidents, cerebral aneurysms, and arteriovenous malformations.

Table 41–1	Areas Supplied by Cerebral Arteries and Branches	
Artery and Branches		**Area Supplied**
External Carotid Arteries	Superior thyroid artery	Thyroid gland Larynx
	Lingual artery	Tongue
	Facial artery	Skin and muscles of anterior face
	Occipital artery	Posterior scalp
	Maxillary and superficial temporal arteries	Lower jaw Chewing muscles Mucosa of the nose and pharynx Lateral face Scalp Dura mater
Internal Carotid Arteries	Ophthalmic arteries	Eye socket structures Anterior scalp Nasal cavity
	Anterior cerebral arteries	Medial surface of the cerebral hemisphere
	Middle cerebral arteries	Lateral temporal and parietal lobes
Vertebral Arteries	Basilar artery	Cerebellum Pons Inner ear structures
	Right and left posterior cerebral arteries	Occipital lobes Inferior temporal lobes of the cerebral hemispheres
	Posterior communicating arteries	Unites the anterior and posterior blood supply

The Client with a Cerebral Vascular Accident (CVA)

■ ■ ■

A *cerebral vascular accident (CVA),* often referred to as a *stroke,* is a condition in which neurologic deficits occur as a result of decreased blood flow to a focal (localized) area of brain tissue. The neurologic deficits caused by ischemia and the resultant necrosis of cells in the brain vary according to the area of the brain involved, the extent of the involvement, and the length of time blood flow is decreased or stopped. A major loss of blood supply to the brain can cause severe disability or death. When the duration of decreased blood flow is short and the anatomical area involved is small, the person may not even be aware that damage has been done.

CVAs are the third leading cause of death in North America. The highest incidence occurs in persons over 65 years of age. However, 1 of every 7 cerebral vascular accidents occurs in people under the age of 65, and CVAs occur in every age group. Familial predisposition is a risk factor, and they occur more frequently in men than women. They are also more common in the African-American population, probably because of an increased incidence of hypertension in individuals of African descent (McCance & Huether, 1994). Approximately 500,000 people suffer a CVA each year in North America. Of those, 150,000 die, and more than 2 million North Americans are currently disabled because of this disorder (Hickey, 1992; Purtilo & Purtilo, 1989).

Certain pathophysiologies and life-style habits increase the risk of a CVA, including the following:

- *Hypertension.* Increased systolic and diastolic blood pressure is associated with damage to all blood vessels, including the cerebral vessels.

- *Diabetes mellitus.* Diabetes leads to vascular changes in both the systemic and cerebral circulation and increases the risk of hypertension.

- *Sickle cell disease.* Changes in the shape of the red blood cells increase blood viscosity and produce erythrocyte clumps that may occlude small cerebral vessels.

- *Substance abuse.* The injection of unpurified substances increases the risk for a CVA, and abuse of certain drugs can decrease cerebral blood flow and increase the risk for intracranial hemorrhage. Substances associated with CVA incidence include alcohol, nicotine, heroin, amphetamines, and cocaine (Bronstein, Popovich, & Stewart-Amidei, 1991).

- *Atherosclerosis.* Occlusion of cerebral vessels by atherosclerotic plaque impairs or obstructs blood flow to specific areas of the brain.

Other risk factors include a previous history of CVA, a familial history of CVA, obesity, a sedentary life-style, hyperlipidemia, cardiac disease, and oral contraceptive use.

Pathophysiology

A CVA is characterized by a gradual or rapid onset of neurologic deficits due to a decrease in blood flow and resultant ischemia of a focal area of the brain. This broad diagnostic label encompasses compromised cerebral blood flow due to a variety of factors, including transient ischemic attack (TIA), cerebral thrombosis, cerebral embolism, and cerebral hemorrhage. CVAs are either ischemic (due to cerebral thrombosis or embolism) or hemorrhagic.

When blood flow to and oxygenation of cerebral neurons are decreased or interrupted, pathophysiologic changes at the cellular level take place in 4 to 5 minutes. Cellular metabolism ceases as glucose, glycogen, and adenosine triphosphate (ATP) are depleted and the sodium-potassium pump fails. Cells swell as sodium draws water into the cell. Cerebral blood vessel walls also swell, further decreasing blood flow. Even if circulation is restored, vasospasm and increased blood viscosity can continue to impede blood flow. Severe or prolonged ischemia leads to cellular death and loss of consciousness. Other neurologic deficits vary greatly according to the severity, location, and duration of ischemia.

The neurologic deficits that occur as a result of a CVA can often be used to identify its location. Because the sensory-motor pathways cross at the junction of the medulla and spinal cord (decussation), CVAs lead to loss or impairment of sensory-motor functions on the side of the body opposite the side of the brain that is damaged. This effect, known as a *contralateral deficit,* causes a CVA in the right hemisphere of the brain to be manifested by deficits in the left side of the body (and vice versa).

Transient Ischemic Attack

A *transient ischemic attack (TIA)* is a brief period of localized cerebral ischemia that causes neurologic deficits lasting for less than 24 hours (Porth, 1994). The deficits may be present for only minutes or may last for hours. TIAs are often warning signals of an ischemic thrombotic CVA: about 30% of clients with a thrombotic CVA have a history of one or more TIAs (Tierney, McPhee, & Papadakis, 1994). A CVA may be preceded by one or many TIAs, with the time between the TIA and a CVA ranging from hours to months.

The causes of TIA include inflammatory artery disorders, sickle cell anemia, atherosclerotic changes in cerebral vessels, thrombosis, and emboli. Transient cerebral ischemia may also occur as a result of *subclavian steal syndrome,* a relatively rare pathophysiologic process in which blood, which normally flows from the vertebral arteries into the circulation of the brain, changes direction and flows from the vertebral arteries into the arteries of the arm. This reverse flow occurs when the arm is exercised and the subclavian artery is occluded.

Neurologic manifestations of a TIA vary according to the location and size of the cerebral vessel that is involved. The manifestations are of sudden onset and often disappear within minutes. Commonly occurring neurologic deficits include contralateral numbness or weakness of the hand, forearm, and corner of the mouth (due to middle cerebral artery involvement); aphasia (due to ischemia of the left hemisphere); and visual disturbances such as blurring (due to involvement of the posterior cerebral artery) (Porth, 1994).

Thrombotic CVA
A *thrombotic CVA* is caused by occlusion of a vessel by a thrombus (a blood clot) on the interior wall of an artery. About 50% of all CVAs are thrombotic (American Heart Association, 1993). Thrombotic CVAs most often occur in people over the age of 50 who are resting or sleeping. During sleep, the blood pressure is lower, there is less

pressure to push the blood through a narrowed arterial lumen, and ischemia results.

Thrombi tend to form in large arteries that bifurcate and have narrowed lumens as a result of deposits of atherosclerotic plaque. The plaque involves the intima of the arteries, causing the internal elastic lamina to become thin and frayed with exposure of underlying connective tissue. This structural change causes platelets to adhere to the rough surface and release the enzyme adenosine diphosphate. This enzyme initiates the clotting sequence, and the thrombus forms. A thrombus may remain in place and continue to enlarge, completely occluding the lumen of the vessel, or a part of it may break off and become an embolus.

The most common locations of thrombi are the internal carotid artery, the vertebral arteries, and the junction of the vertebral and basilar arteries (McCance & Huether, 1994). Thrombotic CVAs affecting the smaller cerebral vessels are called *lacunar strokes* because the infarcted areas slough off, leaving a small cavity or "lake" in the brain tissue. A thrombotic CVA usually affects only one region of the brain that is supplied by a single cerebral artery.

A thrombotic CVA occurs rapidly but progresses slowly. It often begins with a TIA, then continues to worsen during a 1-to-2 day period during which the condition is called a *stroke-in-evolution*. When maximum neurologic deficit has been reached, usually in 3 days, the condition is called a *completed stroke*. At that time, the damaged area is edematous and necrotic.

Embolic CVA

An *embolic CVA* occurs when a blood clot or clump of matter traveling through the cerebral blood vessels becomes lodged in a vessel too narrow to permit further movement. About 30% of all CVAs are embolic in origin (American Heart Association, 1993). This type of CVA is seen in clients who are younger than those experiencing thrombotic CVAs and occurs when the client is awake and active.

Because of blockage by the embolus, the area of the brain supplied by the vessel becomes ischemic. The most frequent sites of cerebral emboli are at bifurcations of vessels, particularly those of the carotid and middle cerebral arteries.

Many embolic CVAs originate from a thrombus in the left chambers of the heart, formed during atrial fibrillation. Emboli result when parts of the thrombus break off and are carried through the arterial system to the brain. Cerebral emboli may also be due to carotid artery atherosclerotic plaque, bacterial endocarditis, recent myocardial infarction, rheumatic heart disease, and fat emboli from the fracture of long bones.

An embolic CVA is of sudden onset and causes immediate deficits. If the embolus breaks up into smaller fragments and is absorbed by the body, symptoms will disap-

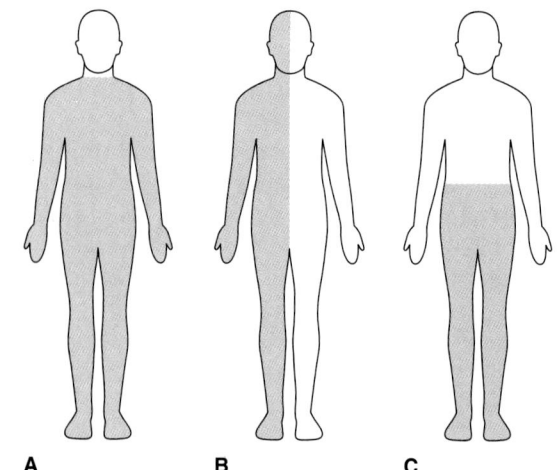

Figure 41–1 Types of paralysis. *A,* Quadriplegia is complete or partial paralysis of the upper extremities and complete paralysis of the lower part of the body. *B,* Hemiplegia is paralysis of one-half of the body when it is divided along the median sagittal plane. *C,* Paraplegia is paralysis of the lower part of the body.

pear in a few hours to a few days. If the embolus is not absorbed, symptoms will persist. Even if the embolus is absorbed, the vessel wall where the embolus lodges may be weakened, increasing the potential for cerebral hemorrhage.

Hemorrhagic CVA

A *hemorrhagic CVA,* or intracranial hemorrhage, occurs when a cerebral blood vessel ruptures. Hemorrhagic CVAs account for about 10% of all strokes (American Heart Association, 1993). It occurs most often in older adults who have long-term, poorly controlled hypertension (Hickey, 1992). Intracranial hemorrhage usually occurs suddenly, often when the affected person is engaged in some activity. Although hypertension is the most common cause, a variety of factors may contribute to a hemorrhagic CVA, including ruptured intracranial aneurysms, embolic CVA, tumors, arteriovenous malformations, anticoagulant therapy, liver disease, brain tumors, and blood disorders. (Ruptured intracranial aneurysms and subarachnoid hemorrhage are discussed in the next section of the chapter.) Of all forms of CVA, this form is most often fatal.

As a result of the blood vessel rupture, blood enters the brain tissue, the cerebral ventricles, or the subarachnoid space, compressing adjacent tissues and causing blood vessel spasm and cerebral edema. Blood in the ventricles or subarachnoid space irritates the meninges and brain tissue, causing an inflammatory reaction and impairing absorption and circulation of cerebral spinal fluid.

The onset of manifestations from a hemorrhagic CVA is rapid. Loss of consciousness occurs in about half of all clients (Tierney et al., 1994). The person may vomit and sometimes has a headache. Flaccid hemiplegia is common. If the hemorrhage continues, the pressure on the brain tissue from increased intracranial pressure may cause coma and death.

Manifestations and Complications

The manifestations and complications of a CVA vary according to the cerebral artery involved and the area of the brain affected. The various deficits associated with involvement of a specific cerebral artery are collectively referred to as stroke syndromes, although the deficits often overlap, as shown in the accompanying box. Typical manifestations include motor deficits, elimination disorders, sensory-perceptual deficits, language disorders, and behavioral changes. These manifestations may be transient or permanent, depending on the degree of ischemia and necrosis. As a result of the neurologic deficits, the client with a CVA has manifestations that involve many different body systems. (See the accompanying manifestations box.)

Motor Deficits

Body movement is the result of a complex interaction between the brain, the spinal cord, and the peripheral nerves. The motor areas of the cerebral cortex, the basal ganglia, and the cerebellum initiate voluntary movement by sending messages to the spinal cord, which then transmits the messages to the peripheral nerves. A CVA may interrupt the central nervous system component of this relay system and produce effects ranging from mild weakness to severe limitation of any kind of movement.

Depending on the area of the brain involved, CVAs may cause weakness, paralysis, and/or spasticity. The deficits include

- *Hemiplegia:* paralysis of the left or right half of the body (see Figure 41–1).
- *Hemiparesis:* weakness of the left or right half of the body.
- *Flaccidity:* absence of muscle tone (hypotonia).
- *Spasticity:* increased resistance to the stretching of the extremities, with resistance increasing as the extremity is stretched.
- *Rigidity:* increased resistance to stretching of the extremity that is uniform throughout the stretching.

As previously described, a CVA causes contralateral deficits. The affected arm and leg is initially flaccid and then becomes spastic within 6 to 8 weeks. Spasticity often causes characteristic body positioning: adduction of the shoulder, pronation of the forearm, flexion of the fingers, and extension of the hip and knee.

The motor deficits may result in altered mobility, further impairing body function. The complications of im-

---

Clinical Manifestations of a CVA by Involved Cerebral Vessel

Internal Carotid Artery

- Contralateral paralysis of the arm, leg, and face
- Contralateral sensory deficits of the arm, leg, and face
- If the dominant hemisphere is involved: aphasia
- If the nondominant hemisphere is involved: apraxia, agnosia, unilateral neglect
- Homonymous hemianopia

Middle Cerebral Artery

- Drowsiness, stupor, coma
- Contralateral hemiplegia of the arm and face
- Contralateral sensory deficits of the arm and face
- Global aphasia (if dominant hemisphere involved)
- Homonymous hemianopia

Anterior Cerebral Artery

- Contralateral weakness or paralysis of the foot and leg
- Contralateral sensory loss of the toes, foot, and leg
- Loss of ability to make decisions or act voluntarily
- Urinary incontinence

Vertebral Artery

- Pain in face, nose, or eye
- Numbness and weakness of the face on involved side
- Problems with gait
- Dysphagia
- Dysarthria

---

mobility involve multiple body systems and include orthostatic hypotension, increased thrombus formation, decreased cardiac output, impaired respiratory function, osteoporosis, formation of renal calculi, contractures, and decubitus ulcer formation (Olson, 1967/1990; Rubin, 1988).

Clinical Manifestations and Complications of CVA by Body System

Integument

- Decubitus (pressure) ulcers

Neurologic

- Hyperthermia
- Neglect syndrome
- Seizures
- Agnosias
- Communication deficits
  a. Expressive aphasia
  b. Receptive aphasia
  c. Global aphasia
  d. Agraphia
- Visual deficits
  a. Homonymous hemianopia
  b. Diplopia
  c. Decreased acuity
- Cognitive changes
  a. Memory loss
  b. Short attention span
  c. Distractibility
  d. Poor judgment
  e. Poor problem-solving ability
  f. Disorientation
- Behavioral changes
  a. Emotional lability
  b. Loss of social inhibitions
  c. Fear
  d. Hostility
  e. Anger
  f. Depression

- Increased intracranial pressure
- Alterations in consciousness
- Sensory loss (touch, pain, heat, cold, pressure)

Respiratory

- Respiratory center damage
- Airway obstruction
- Decreased ability to cough

Gastrointestinal

- Dysphagia
- Constipation
- Stool impaction

Genitourinary

- Incontinence
- Frequency
- Urgency
- Urinary retention
- Renal calculi

Musculoskeletal

- Hemiplegia
- Contractures
- Bony ankylosis
- Disuse atrophy
- Dysarthria

Elimination Disorders

Disorders of bladder and bowel elimination are common in the client who has had a CVA. A CVA may cause partial loss of the sensations that trigger bladder elimination, resulting in urinary frequency, urgency, or incontinence. Control of urination may be altered as a result of cognitive deficits. Changes in bowel elimination are common and are the result of changes in level of consciousness, immobility, and dehydration (Hickey, 1992).

Sensory-Perceptual Deficits

A CVA may cause alterations in the ability to integrate, interpret, and attend to sensory data as a result of pathologic changes in neurologic pathways. Following a CVA, the client may experience deficits in vision, hearing, equilibrium, taste, and sense of smell. The ability to perceive vibration, pain, warmth, cold, and pressure may be impaired, as may proprioception (the body's sense of its position) (Bronstein et al., 1991). The loss of these sensory abilities increases the risk for injury.

Sensory/perceptual deficits that may occur because of a CVA include:

- *Hemianopia*: the loss of half of the visual field of one or both eyes; when the same half is missing in each eye, the condition is called *homonymous hemianopia* (Figure 41–2).

- *Agnosia*: the inability to recognize one or more subjects that were previously familiar; agnosia may be visual, tactile, or auditory.

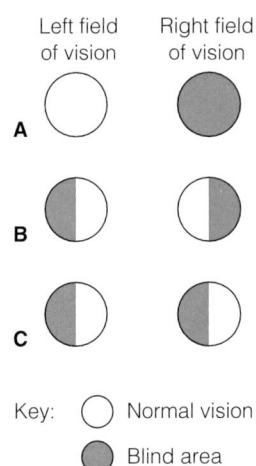

Left field of vision   Right field of vision

Key: ○ Normal vision
        ● Blind area

Figure 41-2   Abnormal visual fields. *A,* Normal left field of vision with loss of vision in right field. *B,* Loss of vision in temporal half of both fields (bitemporal hemianopia). *C,* Loss of vision in nasal field of right eye and temporal field of left eye (homonymous hemianopia).

- *Apraxia:* the inability to carry out some motor pattern (e.g., drawing a figure, getting dressed) even when strength and coordination are adequate.

Another form of sensory-perceptual deficit is the *neglect syndrome* (or unilateral neglect), in which the client has a disorder of attention. In this syndrome, the person cannot integrate and use perceptions from the affected side of the body or from the environment on the affected side, and that part is ignored. In severe cases, the client may even deny the paralysis. This deficit is more common following a CVA of the right hemisphere where damage to the parietal lobe (a center for mediation of directed attention) results in perceptual deficits.

Language Disorders
Communication is a complex process, involving motor functions, speech, language, memory, reasoning, and emotions. Communication problems are usually the result of a CVA affecting the dominant hemisphere. The left hemisphere is dominant in about 95% of right-handed people and 70% of left-handed people (Porth, 1994).

Many different impairments of communication may occur following a CVA. Disorders of communication affect both speech (the mechanical act of articulating language through the spoken word) and language (the vocal or written formulation of ideas to communicate thoughts and feelings). Language involves oral and written expression and auditory and reading comprehension. Among these disorders are:

- *Aphasia:* the inability to use or understand language; aphasia may be expressive, receptive, or mixed (global).

- *Expressive aphasia:* a motor speech problem in which one can understand what is being said but can respond verbally only in short phrases; also called *Broca's aphasia.*

- *Receptive aphasia:* a sensory speech problem in which one cannot understand the spoken (and often written) word. Speech may be fluent but with inappropriate content; also called *Wernicke's aphasia.*

- *Mixed or global aphasia:* language dysfunction in both understanding and expression.

- *Dysarthria:* any disturbance in muscular control of speech.

Cognitive and Behavioral Changes
A change in consciousness, ranging from mild confusion to coma, is a common manifestation of a CVA. It may result from tissue damage following ischemia or hemorrhage involving either the carotid or vertebral arteries. Altered consciousness may also be the result of swelling of brain tissue following the CVA, causing increased intracranial pressure.

Behavioral changes due to a CVA include emotional lability (in which the client may laugh or cry inappropriately), loss of self-control (manifested by behavior such as swearing or refusing to wear clothing), and decreased tolerance for stress (resulting in anger or depression).

The client who had a CVA may also have intellectual changes. These changes include memory loss, decreased attention span, poor judgment, and an inability to think abstractly.

Collaborative Care

The client with a CVA may receive pharmacologic and/or surgical treatment. The focus in the acute care phase is on diagnosing the type and cause of the CVA and on supporting cerebral circulation and controlling or preventing further deficits.

Laboratory and Diagnostic Tests
There are no laboratory tests specifically for detecting a cerebral vascular accident. However, the following diagnostic tests may be ordered to detect increased risk for a CVA or to identify pathophysiologic changes after a CVA has occurred:

- *Computed tomography (CT)* may be performed to demonstrate the presence of hemorrhage, tumors, aneurysm, ischemia, edema, and tissue necrosis. A CT scan can also demonstrate a shift in intracranial contents and is useful in distinguishing the type of CVA (for example, a hemorrhagic CVA results in an increase in density). Nursing interventions for the client having a CT scan of the head are described in the box on page 1756.

Nursing Implications for Diagnostic Tests: Computed Tomography (CT) of the Head

■ ■ ■

Preparation of Client

- Ensure that client or family signs a consent form (this consent may be obtained as part of the general consent given on admission to the hospital).

- Check hospital policy on withholding food and fluids. Clients are usually on NPO status (except for the medications ordered as part of the test) for 8 hours before the test if it is done in the morning. If the test is done in the afternoon, the client may have a liquid breakfast.

- Give medications up to 2 hours before test.

- Assess for possible reaction to iodine dye (by asking about allergy to seafood). Document any allergy and inform the physician and radiology department.

- Remove hairpins, clips, and earrings.

Client and Family Teaching

- (*If applicable*) Do not drink or eat anything before the test except for the ordered medications.

- You may be given an intravenous infusion. When the contrast dye is injected, you may feel warm and have a metallic taste in the mouth.

- The exam lasts from 30 to 90 minutes.

- Your head will be positioned in a cradle, and a wide rubber strap will be applied snugly across the forehead during the test (to keep your head immobilized).

- The CT scanner is circular with a round opening. You are strapped to a special table, and the scanner revolves around the body part to be examined. The scanner makes a clicking noise.

- The test is painless.

- Someone is always immediately available during the test.

- *Arteriography* of cerebral vessels is performed to demonstrate abnormal vessel structures, vasospasm, loss of vessel wall integrity, and stenosis of the carotid arteries.

- *Ultrasound Doppler* studies are used to evaluate the blood flow through the carotid arteries and provide information about partial or complete occlusion. These noninvasive studies include Doppler ultrasonography and carotid ultrasonography.

- A *magnetic resonance imaging test (MRI)* may be conducted to detect shifting of brain tissues as a result of hemorrhage or edema.

- *Magnetic resonance angiography* may be performed to detect occlusive disease of the large cerebral vessels.

- *Positron emission tomography (PET)* and *single-photon emission computed tomography (SPECT)* are used to examine cerebral blood flow distribution and metabolic activity of the brain. Both of these tests use very short-lived radionuclides that emit radioactive energy as they move through the circulation. PET allows the identification of the location and size of the CVA; SPECT provides information about the metabolism of and blood flow through the brain tissue affected by the CVA.

- A *lumbar puncture* may be performed to obtain cerebrospinal fluid for examination if there is no danger of increased intracranial pressure. (Removal of cerebrospinal fluid when intracranial pressure is increased can result in herniation of the brainstem.) A thrombotic CVA may elevate cerebrospinal fluid pressure; after a hemorrhagic CVA frank blood may be seen in the cerebrospinal fluid. Nursing interventions for the client having a lumbar puncture are described in the accompanying box.

Pharmacology

Pharmacologic management is instituted to prevent a CVA in clients with TIAs or a previous CVA, and to treat the client during the acute phase of a CVA.

Prevention Antiplatelet agents are often used to treat clients with TIAs or who have had a previous CVA. Platelets are concentrated in high blood flow arteries, they adhere to endothelial tissue damaged by atherosclerosis, and occlude the vessel. The drugs that are used to prevent clot formation and blood vessel occlusion are aspirin, prostacyclin, dipyridamole, and ticlopidine hydrochloride.

The daily use of low-dose aspirin does reduce TIA occurrence and stroke risk by interfering with platelet aggregation (Biller, 1992). Prostacyclin, currently under study, is both an antiaggregant and vasodilator. Dipyridamole (Persantine) prevents platelet aggregation but is more expensive and has little known benefit over aspirin. Ticlopidine hydrochloride (Ticlid) is a newer platelet-aggregation inhibitor that has shown reduction in stroke risk during two major clinical trials (Whitney, 1994).

Treatment During Acute CVA Pharmacologic agents are used to treat the client during the acute phase of a CVA to prevent further thrombosis formation, increase cerebral blood flow, and protect cerebral neurons. The type of medication used varies according to the type of CVA.

Nursing Implications for Diagnostic Tests

■　■　■

Lumbar Puncture

Preparation of the Client

- Ensure that a consent form has been signed (this consent may be obtained as part of the general consent given on admission to the hospital or agency).
- Ask the client to empty the bladder before the procedure begins.
- Help the client to assume a lateral recumbent position near the side of the bed. The client should assume the fetal position (knees flexed toward the head, head bent toward the chest), with the hands clasped around the knees.

Client and Family Teaching

- A local anesthetic is injected into the skin over the area of the needle insertion. This medication may cause a burning sensation.
- A long, thin needle is inserted into the lower back below the level of the spinal cord. Cerebrospinal fluid is withdrawn.
- The cerebrospinal fluid pressure is measured with a calibrated tube called a manometer.
- There may be slight pain down one leg during the procedure.
- It is important to remain still during the procedure.
- A small dressing is used to cover the place where the needle was inserted.

- After the procedure, remain flat in bed for the number of hours prescribed by the physician (this ranges from 4 to 24 hours). The nurses will take your vital signs and look under the small dressing at regular intervals.
- Drink fluids so that your body can replace the fluid that was withdrawn.
- If you have a headache or backache, ask for medications for pain.
- Notify your health care provider if you notice increased pain or drainage from the area where the procedure was done.

Post-Procedure Nursing Care

- Take and record vital signs as indicated by agency standards.
- Monitor neurologic status at least every 4 hours for 24 hours following the procedure.
- Monitor the puncture site for leakage of cerebrospinal fluid or hematoma formation.
- Ensure that the client voids within 8 hours of the procedure.
- Encourage increased intake of fluids (up to 3000 mL in 24 hours).
- Administer analgesics as prescribed for pain.

Anticoagulant drug therapy (discussed in Chapter 28) is often ordered for thrombotic CVA during the stroke-in-evolution phase but is contraindicated in completed stroke because it may increase the risk of cerebral hemorrhage (Swonger & Matejski, 1988). Anticoagulants are never administered to a client with a hemorrhagic CVA. Anticoagulants do not dissolve an existing clot but prevent further extension of an existing clot and formation of new clots. Sodium heparin may be given subcutaneously or by continuous IV drip, or warfarin sodium (Coumadin) may be given orally. Newer drugs include urokinase, streptokinase, tissue plasminogen activator (tPA), ancrod, and pentoxifylline, all which promote fibrinolysis to dissolve formed clots.

Antithrombotic drugs, which inhibit the platelet phase of clot formation, have been used as a preventive measure for clients at risk for embolic and thrombotic CVA. Both aspirin and dipyridamole have been used for this purpose. These drugs are sometimes also used in combination with other drugs during acute treatment. Antiplatelet agents are contraindicated in the client with a hemorrhagic CVA.

Calcium channel blockers, such as nimodipine (Nimotop), are under investigation and have been used in clinical trials to reduce cerebral vasospasm. They act by relaxing the smooth muscle of vessel walls, thereby decreasing damage to cerebral neurons. Nimodipine has been approved by the FDA for treatment of subarachnoid hemorrhage but is not yet recommended for routine use in the management of CVAs.

If the client with a CVA has increased intracranial pressure, hyperosmolar solutions (such as mannitol) or diuretics (such as furosemide) may be administered. Anticonvulsants, such as phenytoin (Dilantin), and barbiturates may be prescribed if increased intracranial pressure causes seizures.

Surgery

Surgery may be performed to prevent the occurrence of a CVA or to restore blood flow when a CVA has already occurred. In people who have had TIAs or are in danger of having another CVA, a carotid endarterectomy at the carotid artery bifurcation may be performed to remove atherosclerotic plaque (Meeker & Rothrock, 1991) (Figure 41–3). Nursing care for the client in the initial postoperative period following a carotid endarterectomy is described in the box on page 1759. The client having this surgery is often cared for in the intensive care unit for the first 24 hours after surgery. See the accompanying box outlining collaborative care on page 1759 for the client following a carotid endarterectomy as well as the accompanying Critical Pathway on page 1760 for this client.

When an occluded or stenotic vessel is not directly accessible, an extracranial-intracranial bypass may be performed. Bypass of the internal carotid, middle cerebral, or vertebral arteries may be required. The indications for the bypass are symptoms of ischemia caused by TIAs or a mild completed CVA. The procedure reestablishes blood flow to the affected area of the brain.

Surgery may also be performed to prevent a CVA in clients with a cerebral aneurysm or arteriovenous malformation. These disorders and surgeries are discussed later in the chapter.

Nursing Care

Even though many people who have a CVA have full recovery, a substantial number are left with disabilities that affect their physical, emotional, interpersonal, and family status. The nursing care that is required is often complex and multidimensional, requiring consideration of continuity of care for clients in acute care settings, long-term care settings, rehabilitation centers, and the home.

Nurses caring for clients who have had a CVA require knowledge and skill to meet client needs during both the acute and the rehabilitative phases of care. The client with a CVA often has multiple losses: loss of mobility, ability to provide self-care, communications, concept of self, and interpersonal or intimate relationships with others. Nursing care that is holistic and individualized is essential in all settings and focuses on promoting the achievement of maximum potential and quality of life. Teaching the family as well as the client how to participate in the recovery process facilitates meeting goals and outcomes outlined in the plan of care.

Because a CVA has the potential to affect so many dimensions of an individual, a wide variety of nursing diagnoses may be appropriate. It is important to remember that each person will be affected differently, depending on the degree of ischemia and the area of the brain involved. Nursing diagnoses discussed in this section focus on problems with cerebral tissue perfusion (specific to nursing care during the acute phase) and physical mobility,

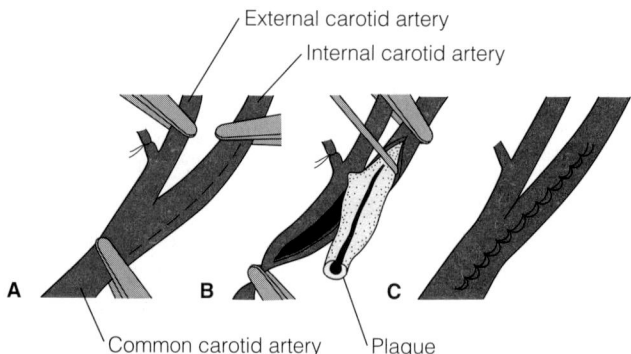

Figure 41–3 Carotid endarterectomy. *A*, The occluded area is clamped off and an incision is made in the artery. *B*, Plaque is removed from the inner layer of the artery. *C*, To restore blood flow through the artery, the artery is sutured, or a graft is completed.

self-care, communication, sensory-perceptual deficits, bowel and urine elimination, and swallowing (specific to prevention of complications and rehabilitation).

Altered Cerebral Tissue Perfusion

The acute phase of a CVA is most often the time from admission to the hospital until the client is stabilized; usually 24 to 72 hours after admission (Hickey, 1992). Depending on the severity of the CVA, the client may be admitted to the intensive care unit. Regardless of the hospital setting, the nurse provides interventions to maintain body functions and prevent complications. Assessments should be conducted on a frequent, regular, and ongoing basis.

Nursing interventions with rationales follow:

- Monitor respiratory status and airway patency.
  a. Suction as necessary, using care to suction no longer than 10 to 15 seconds at any one time, and using sterile technique.
  b. Place client in a side-lying position.
  c. Monitor respiratory status. Auscultate pulmonary sounds and monitor respiratory rate and results of studies of arterial blood gases.
  d. Administer oxygen as prescribed.
  The client with a CVA is often unconscious, and breathing may be impaired because of damage to cerebral tissue. Suctioning removes secretions that not only obstruct air flow but also pose the risk for aspiration and pneumonia. Suctioning for longer than 15 seconds at a time may increase intracranial pressure (Hickey, 1992). Positioning the client on the side allows secretions to drain out of the mouth, helping to prevent aspiration. Respiratory complications develop rapidly, as manifested by crackles and wheezes, rapid respirations, and respiratory acidosis. The administration of oxygen decreases the risk for hypoxia and hypercapnia, which can increase cerebral ischemia and intracranial pressure.

Postoperative Nursing Care of the Client Having a Carotid Endarterectomy

■ ■ ■

- Position the client on the unoperated side and either maintain a flat position or elevate the head of the bed 30 degrees as prescribed. Maintain head and neck alignment and avoid rotating, flexing, or hyperextending head. *Pressure on the wound is undesirable. Elevating the head decreases edema in the operative site. Maintaining head and neck alignment prevents additional tension or pressure on the operative side.*

- Support the head when changing the client's position. Teach the client to support the head with the hands when able to move about. *Supporting the head helps prevent stress on the operative site (which may cause bleeding and hematoma formation); it also helps reduce stress on the suture line.*

- Perform focused assessments to monitor for complications:
  a. *Hemorrhage.* Assess the dressing and the area under the client's neck and shoulders for drainage. Monitor the operative site for swelling and the dressing for tightness. Take and record vital signs at least every hour; assess for increased pulse and decreased blood pressure. *The most common cause of respiratory problems is pressure on the trachea from a hematoma formation.*

  b. *Respiratory distress.* Assess respiratory rate, rhythm, depth, and effort. Observe for restlessness. Keep a tracheostomy tray at the bedside. *Respiratory distress may result from edema and hematoma formation, which may compress the trachea.*

  c. *Cranial nerve impairment.* Observe and record any facial drooping, tongue deviation, hoarseness, dysphagia, or loss of facial sensation. *Cranial nerves may be stretched during surgery, leading to temporary deficits in cranial nerve function.*

  d. *Hypertension or hypotension.* Take and record blood pressure at least hourly. Report any changes immediately and implement orders for medications to treat hypertension or hypotension. *About one-half of all clients having a carotid endarterectomy develop unstable blood pressure related to surgical denervation of the carotid sinus. Uncontrolled hypertension may precipitate a CVA. The most common problem is hypotension, possibly related to stimulation of the carotid body baroreceptors, which are exposed during surgery. Hypotension may result in myocardial ischemia.*

Collaborative Care for the Client Following a Carotid Endarterectomy

Health Care Team	Client-Centered Care
Vascular surgeon	Orders and evaluates diagnostic tests. Removes atherosclerotic plaque from the inner lining of the carotid artery after a CVA or TIA or as preventive surgery.
Primary care physician	Assesses the progression of atherosclerosis by monitoring diagnostic studies and risk factors, initiates conservative measures, refers to surgeon, and manages medical care following discharge.
Dietitian	Assesses client's weight and caloric, fat, and fluid intake. Teaches about low-fat, low-salt diet and appropriate caloric intake.
Physical therapist	Develops a plan of care to maintain physical mobility and safety. Assesses any self-care deficits related to mobility and develops individualized rehabilitation plan.
Social worker	Assesses adequacy of social support and home environment and availability of assistance during recovery period. Consults with home health agencies for discharge home or long-term facilities for transitional care.
RN and health care team communications	Reports to physician any changes in strength, mentation, speech, and level of consciousness. Notifies physician of bleeding in the incisional area and swelling of the neck or complaints of dysphagia. Collaborates with physical therapy to promote independence and implement activity/exercise program. Alerts dietitian of food likes and dislikes and compliance to recommended diet.

Critical Pathway for Client Following Carotid Endarterectomy

	Preoperative	Date _____ 1st 24 hours postoperative
Expected length of stay 3–4 days		
Daily outcomes	Client verbalizes understanding of preoperative teaching including TCDB, IV therapy, JP drain, mobilization, telemetry, O₂, PCA for pain management. Client demonstrates ability to cope. Client verbalizes understanding of procedure. Obtain informed consent.	Client will ■ Maintain adequate cerebral blood flow as evidenced by stable vital signs, being alert and oriented, maintaining usual sensory and motor function. ■ Maintain cranial nerve function. ■ Have stable vital signs and B/P within specified range. ■ Have lungs clear to auscultation. ■ Have unlabored respirations and maintain oxygen saturation above 92%. ■ Have clean, dry dressings ■ Recover from anesthesia. ■ Verbalize understanding of and demonstrate cooperation with turning, deep breathing, coughing, and splinting. ■ Tolerate ordered diet without nausea and vomiting. ■ Verbalize control of incisional pain with ordered medications. ■ Demonstrate ability to cope.
Assessments, tests, and treatments	CBC, urinalysis CXR, EKG Arteriogram Carotid ultrasound Baseline physical assessment with focus on respiratory, cardiovascular, and neurologic function	Vital signs and O₂ saturation, neurovascular assessment, dressing and wound drainage assessment q15min × 4; q30min × 4; q1h × 24 and prn Maintain patency of drain. Assess cranial nerve function q2–4h and prn Monitor for bleeding and cerebral ischemia. Assess respiratory status q4h and prn. Oxygen as ordered to maintain oxygen saturation > 92%. Incentive spirometer q2h Intake and output every shift Assess voiding; if client cannot void, try techniques to stimulate voiding or catheterize q8h or prn. Assess coping status of client and family. Provide ongoing emotional support to client and family. Allow for client's input regarding sequence of care.

	Preoperative	**Date** _____ **1st 24 hours postoperative**
Knowledge deficit	Orient to surroundings and room. Provide simple, brief instructions. Preoperative teaching as ordered	Orient to room and surroundings. Provide simple, brief instructions. Include family in teaching. Review specific postoperative care: turning, coughing, deep breathing, incentive spirometer, mobilization, intravenous lines, pain management (prn medications or PCA). Instruct client regarding the importance of supporting head and neck during position changes. Assess understanding of teaching.
Psycho-social	Assess anxiety regarding impending surgery. Assess fears of unknown and surgery. Offer emotional support. Encourage verbalization of concerns. Provide information regarding surgical experience. Minimize external stimuli (noise, movement).	Assess level of anxiety. Encourage verbalization of concerns. Provide information and ongoing support and encouragement to client and family.
Diet	NPO Baseline nutritional and hydration assessment	Prior to offering food or fluids, assess return of gag reflex and ability to chew and swallow. Elevate head of bed for all meals unless contraindicated. Clear liquids as tolerated.
Activity	Assess potential safety needs and provide appropriate safety measures.	Assess safety needs and provide adequate precautions. Elevate head of bed 30 degrees, support head and neck when changing positions. Dangle legs or sit in chair evening of surgery if client is stable. Encourage finger, wrist, and elbow movement and use of affected arm for ADLs and personal hygiene.
Medications	Preoperative medications per anesthesiologist	IM or IV analgesics IV fluids Antihypertensives as ordered
Transfer/ discharge plans	Assess potential discharge needs and support system. Establish discharge goals with client and family.	Establish discharge objectives with client and family. Determine discharge needs and support system with client and significant others. Begin home care instructions.

➤

Critical Pathway for Client Following Carotid Endarterectomy (continued)

	Date _____ 48 hours postoperative	Date _____ 3rd–4th day postoperative
Daily outcomes	Client will ■ Maintain adequate cerebral blood flow as evidenced by stable vital signs, being alert and oriented, maintaining usual sensory and motor function. ■ Maintain cranial nerve function. ■ Have stable vital signs and B/P within specified range. ■ Have lungs clear to auscultation. ■ Have unlabored respirations and maintain oxygen saturation above 92%. ■ Have clean, dry wound with edges well-approximated, healing by first intention. ■ Demonstrate cooperation with turning, deep breathing, coughing, and splinting. ■ Tolerate ordered diet without nausea and vomiting. ■ Ambulate four times per day in hallway. ■ Verbalize control of incisional pain. ■ Demonstrate ability to cope. ■ Verbalize/demonstrate beginning understanding of home care instructions.	Client is afebrile. Client maintains adequate cerebral blood flow as evidenced by stable vital signs, being alert and oriented, maintaining usual sensory and motor function. Client maintains cranial nerve function. Client has stable vital signs and B/P within specified range. Client has lungs clear to auscultation and unlabored respiration with an oxygen saturation above 92%. Client has clean, dry wound with edges well-approximated, healing by first intention. Client manages pain with oral medications and/or nonpharmacologic measures. Client is independent in self-care. Client is fully ambulatory. Client has resumed preadmission urine and bowel elimination pattern. Client verbalizes/demonstrates home care instructions. Client tolerates low-salt, low saturated fat, and low-cholesterol diet or ordered diet. Client demonstrates ability to cope with ongoing stressors.
Assessments, tests, and treatments	Vital signs, neurovascular and cranial nerve assessment, O_2 saturation, and dressing and wound drainage assessment q2–4h and prn Monitor for bleeding and cerebral ischemia. Assess respiratory status q4h and prn. Incentive spirometer q2h until fully ambulatory Intake and output every shift Assess voiding pattern each shift. Dressing change and wound assessment BID and prn Assess coping status of client and family. Provide ongoing emotional support to client and family.	Vital signs, neurovascular and cranial nerve assessment, O_2 saturation, and dressing and wound drainage assessment q4–8h and prn Assess respiratory status q4–8h. Assess wound. Assess coping status and provide appropriate emotional support.

	Date _____ **48 hours postoperative**	**Date** _____ **3rd–4th day postoperative**
Knowledge deficit	Review plan of care and importance of early mobilization. Begin discharge teaching regarding wound care, dressing change, diet, and activity. Review written discharge instructions with client and significant other.	Complete discharge teaching to include wound care, diet, follow-up care and appointment, signs and symptoms to report, strategies to slow the progression of arteriosclerosis, activity, and medication (name, purpose, dose, frequency, route, food, interactions, and side effects) Provide client with written discharge instructions.
Psycho-social	Assess level of anxiety. Encourage verbalization of concerns. Provide information and ongoing support and encouragement to client and family.	Assess level of anxiety. Encourage verbalizations of concerns. Provide information and ongoing support and encouragement to client and family.
Diet	Ordered diet or low-salt, low saturated fat, and low-cholesterol diet to tolerance Dietary consult for diet teaching	Ordered diet, or low-salt, low saturated fat, and low-cholesterol diet to tolerance Provide written copy of diet.
Activity	Maintain safety precautions. Fully ambulatory in room with required assistance Walk in hall 4 to 6 times with required assistance.	Maintain safety precautions. Fully ambulatory
Medications	PO analgesics Intermittent IV device Aspirin or anticoagulant therapy if ordered	PO analgesics D/C IV device Aspirin or anticoagulant therapy if ordered
Transfer/ discharge plans	Review progress toward discharge goals. Make appropriate referrals. Finalize discharge plans.	Finalize any home care arrangements. Complete discharge instructions.

■ Monitor neurologic status.
  a. Assess mental status and level of consciousness: restlessness, drowsiness, lethargy, inability to follow commands, unresponsiveness.
  b. Monitor strength and reflexes, and assess for pain, headache, decreased muscle strength, sluggish pupillary reflexes, absent gag or swallowing reflexes, hemiplegia, Babinski's sign, and decerebrate or decorticate posturing.
Frequent monitoring of neurologic status is necessary to detect changes. Alterations in mental status, level of consciousness, movement, strength, and reflexes are indications of increased intracranial pressure, the major cause of death in the acute phase of a CVA.

■ Continuously monitor cardiac status, observing for dysrhythmias. *A CVA may cause cardiac dysrhythmias, including bradycardia, PVCs, tachycardia, and AV block*

(Whitney, 1994). Characteristic ECG changes include a shortened PR interval, peaked T waves, and a depressed ST segment.

■ Monitor body temperature. *Hyperthermia may develop if a CVA affects the hypothalamus.*

■ Maintain accurate intake and output records; measure urinary output via a Foley catheter. *A CVA may damage the pituitary gland, resulting in diabetes insipidus and the possibility of dehydration from greatly increased urinary output.*

■ Monitor the client for seizures. Pad the side rails, and administer prescribed anticonvulsants. *Seizures may be the result of cerebral tissue damage or increased intracranial pressure. Side rails are padded to prevent injury if a seizure occurs. Anticonvulsants are administered to prevent or treat seizures.*

Impaired Physical Mobility

The broad goals of care for clients with impaired mobility from a CVA are to maintain and improve functional abilities (by maintaining normal function and alignment, preventing edema of extremities, and reducing spasticity) and to prevent complications.

Nursing interventions with rationales follow:

- Encourage active range-of-motion exercises for unaffected extremities and perform passive range-of-motion exercises for affected extremities every 4 hours during day and evening shifts and once during the night shift. Support the joint during passive range-of-motion exercises. *Active range-of-motion exercises maintain or improve muscle strength and endurance, and help to maintain cardiopulmonary function. Passive range-of-motion exercises do not strengthen muscles but do help maintain joint flexibility. Both active and passive exercises increase venous return.*

- Turn the client every 2 hours around the clock, following a posted schedule for side-to-side and supine-to-prone position changes (verify prone positioning with the physician). Maintain body alignment and support extremities in proper position with pillows. *Turning on a regular basis, accompanied by proper positioning, maintains joint function, alleviates pressure on bony prominences that can lead to skin breakdown, decreases dependent edema in hands and feet, and lessens the risk of complications resulting from immobility (Figure 41–4).*

- Monitor the lower extremities each shift for symptoms of thrombophlebitis. Assess for Homans's sign; assess for increased warmth and redness in calves; measure the circumference of the calves and thighs. *Clients on bed rest (especially those with loss of muscle strength and tone) are particularly prone to the development of deep vein thrombosis. Symptoms of thrombophlebitis should be promptly reported.*

- Do not use a footboard; use hand splints only as directed by the physician and physical therapist to prevent flexion contractures of the fingers and wrists. *The use of footboards is no longer recommended and may actually cause increased dorsiflexion as the client slides down in bed; hand splints may in some instances increase spasticity (Bronstein et al., 1991).*

- Collaborate with the physical therapist as the client gains mobility, using consistent techniques to move the client from the bed to the wheelchair and to help the client ambulate. *The use of consistent techniques facilitates rehabilitation.*

Self-Care Deficit

The client who has had a CVA may have a self-care deficit as a result of impaired mobility or mental confusion. It is important for clients to perform as much of their own

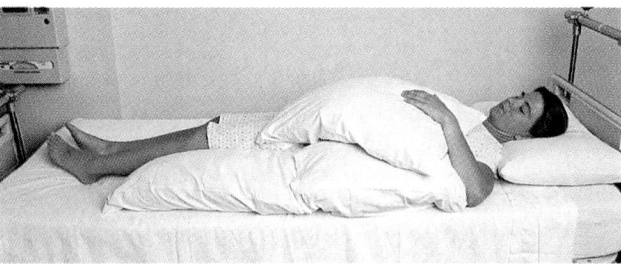

A

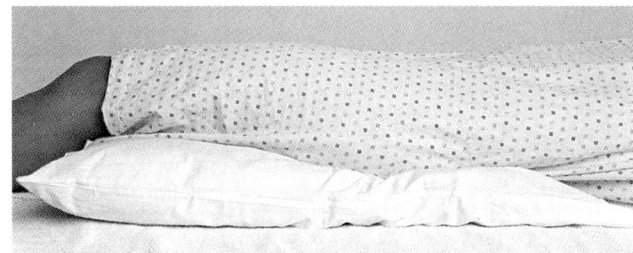

B

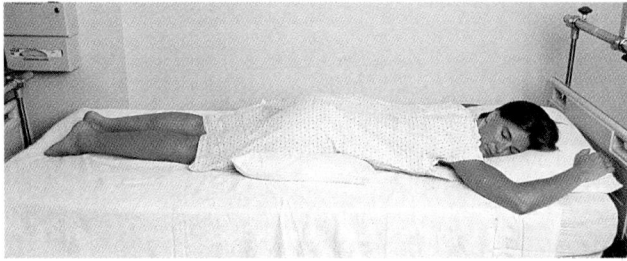

C

Figure 41–4   Positioning the client with hemiplegia is important in preventing deformity of the affected extremities. *A,* With the client in a supine position, place a pillow in the axilla (to prevent adduction) and under the hand and arm, with the hand higher than the elbow (to prevent flexion and edema). *B,* When the client is lying supine, use a pillow from the iliac crest to the middle of the thigh to prevent external rotation of the hip. *C,* When the client is in the prone position, place a pillow under the pelvis to promote hip hyperextension.

physical care and grooming as possible to promote functional ability, increase independence, decrease feelings of powerlessness, and improve self-esteem.

Before establishing a plan to increase self-care, the nurse should determine which hand was dominant before the CVA. If the client's dominant side is affected by the CVA, self-care will be more difficult.

Nursing interventions with rationales follow:

- Encourage the client to use the unaffected arm to bathe, brush teeth, comb hair, dress, and eat. *Use of the unaffected arm promotes functional ability and independence.*

- Teach the client and family to put on clothing by first dressing the affected extremities and then dressing the unaffected extremities. *This technique facilitates self-dressing with minimal assistance.*

- Collaborate with the occupational therapist in scheduling times for training for upper extremity functioning necessary for activities of daily living. Encourage the use of assistive devices (if required) for eating, physical hygiene, and dressing. *Following a regular schedule in daily routines promotes learning. The use of assistive devices promotes independence and decreases feelings of powerlessness. Optimal grooming facilitates positive self-concept.*

Impaired Verbal Communication

The client who loses communication abilities because of a CVA requires intensive speech therapy and emotional support. It is important to determine the specific nature of the impairment so that the nurse can plan individualized interventions and help family members to understand the specific problem. Although the speech therapist is usually most involved with the client's speech rehabilitation, nurses must plan interventions to meet communication needs during all phases of care.

Nursing interventions with rationales follow:

- Use the following guidelines when communicating with the client:
  a. Approach and treat the client as an adult.
  b. Do not assume that the client who does not respond verbally cannot hear. Do not raise the voice when addressing the client.
  c. Allow adequate time for the client to respond.
  d. Face the client and speak slowly.
  e. When you do not understand the client's speech, be honest and say so.
  f. Use short, simple statements and questions.
  Accepting the client and providing dignity and respect enhances the nurse-client relationship. Allowing adequate response time and using short verbal statements or questions while facing the client motivates the client to communicate and decreases frustration.

- Accept client's frustration and anger as a normal reaction to the loss of function. *Anger represents the client's frustration at the inability to control the loss of function.*

- Try alternate methods of communication, including writing tablets, flash cards, computerized talking boards. *Clients who are unable to communicate verbally may use other methods effectively.*

Sensory/Perceptual Alterations

Nursing interventions with rationales follow:

- Keep the environment free of clutter and well lighted. Keep the bed at a low position with the side rails ele-

vated. *Keeping the client's environment clutter-free and well lighted decreases risk for injury. Having the bed in the low position and keeping side rails elevated lessens the potential for falls.*

- Teach self-care by breaking down each activity into small steps and using verbal cues and pictures. *Clients may be able to carry out complex tasks by breaking them down into simple steps. Clients with apraxia may understand pictures and not verbal instructions.*

- Encourage self-care by placing items on the unaffected side. *Clients with a visual field deficit may ignore items on the affected side of the body.*

- Teach the client to turn the head and move the eyes toward the direction of the affected field of vision or side of body. *Turning the head and moving the eyes in one direction (called scanning) enhances self-care abilities, facilitates mobility, and helps decrease the risk of injury.*

- Alternate sides when positioning the client in a side-lying position. *Alternating positions stimulates muscle tone and may facilitate bilateral weight bearing as mobility increases (Passarella & Gee, 1987).*

Altered Urinary Elimination and Constipation

The client who has a CVA is at increased risk for alterations in urinary and bowel elimination. Elimination may be altered because of neurologic deficits due to the CVA or because of impaired mobility, cognitive impairment, communication deficits, or pre-existing problems (especially if the client is an older adult, as is usual). Other causes include changes in food and fluid intake and side effects of medications.

Urinary incontinence or retention and constipation and fecal impaction are the usual manifestations. Most clients, however, can reestablish normal bowel and urinary elimination patterns.

Nursing interventions with rationales follow:

- Assess for urinary frequency, urgency, incontinence, nocturia, and voiding in small amounts. In addition, assess client's ability to respond to the need to void, the ability to use the call light, and the ability to use toileting equipment. *The nurse must identify the underlying problem before beginning a teaching program.*

- Establish bladder retraining through one or more of the following:
  a. Have the client void every 2 hours.
  b. Encourage bladder training by having client void on schedule rather than in response to the urge to void.
  c. Teach the client to perform Kegel exercises (10 repetitions three times a day). To perform Kegel exercises, the client contracts the perineal muscles as though stopping urination, holds the contraction for 5 seconds, and then releases.

d. Use positive reinforcement (verbal praise) for successful management of urinary elimination.
Voiding every 2 hours or on schedule promotes bladder tone and urine storage. Kegel exercises increase pubococcygeal muscle tone and bladder control, decreasing incontinence. Positive reinforcement can be a useful part of the teaching program.

- Discuss pre-CVA bowel habits, as well as the pattern of bowel elimination since CVA, with the client and family. Establish a bowel routine.
  a. If client is able to swallow without difficulty, encourage the client to drink fluids (up to 2000 mL per day) and eat a high-fiber diet.
  b. Increase physical activity as tolerated.
  c. Help the client to use toilet facilities at the same time each day (based on usual patterns of bowel elimination), ensuring privacy and having client sit in upright position if at all possible.
  d. Administer prescribed stool softeners if the client is following a bowel elimination routine or is not drinking sufficient fluids.
  Increased fluids, fiber, and activity stimulate intestinal motility. Establishing a regular daily time for bowel movements in the upright position and in privacy promotes normal bowel elimination. Stool softeners help prevent the formation of hard stool that is more difficult to expel.

Impaired Swallowing

A CVA may impair the client's ability to swallow. Weakness or lack of coordination of the tongue, attention deficits, and deficits involving the swallowing reflex all play a role. Dysphagia (difficulty swallowing) may result in choking, drooling, aspiration, or regurgitation (Bronstein et al., 1991). Nursing care focuses on maintaining safety by preventing aspiration and on ensuring adequate nutrition.

Nursing interventions with rationales follow:

- Ensure safety when the client eats.
  a. Make sure the client is sitting upright.
  b. Be sure client's neck is slightly flexed.
  c. Order puréed or soft food.
  d. Feed the client or teach client to eat by putting food behind the front teeth on the unaffected side of mouth and tilting the head slightly backward. Teach client to swallow one bite at a time.
  e. When the client has finished eating, check the mouth for "pocketing" of food, especially in the affected cheek.
  f. Have suction equipment available at the bedside in case of choking or aspiration.
  Sitting upright with the head and neck first slightly flexed and then tilted back helps the client swallow. The client can usually swallow puréed or soft foods more easily than liquid or solid foods. Using the unaffected side of the mouth helps

prevent food from collecting in the mouth and makes swallowing safer; in addition, food is less likely to fall out of the mouth.

- Minimize distractions and, if necessary, give step-by-step instructions for eating. *Distractions increase the risk of aspiration. Complex activities are easier to perform when broken down into small steps.*

Other Nursing Diagnoses

The following nursing diagnoses may also be appropriate for the client who has had a CVA:

- *Ineffective Airway Clearance* related to decreased mobility and inability to cough effectively
- *Impaired Skin Integrity* related to urinary incontinence and prolonged pressure from bed rest
- *Altered Thought Processes:* impaired memory and impulsive responses related to damage from cerebral ischemia
- *Risk for Injury* related to potential for falls from visual deficit and weakness
- *Self-Esteem Disturbance* related to hemiplegia, facial droop, and urinary incontinence
- *Ineffective Individual Coping* related to anxiety, frustration, and feelings of powerlessness
- *Social Isolation* related to impaired ability to communicate verbally
- *Powerlessness* related to a change in role status and to loss of income

Client and Family Teaching

The family of a person who has had a CVA is often faced with many changes (see the research box for a discussion of caregiver burden). The young to middle-aged adult with a family member who has had a CVA may be faced with economic difficulties and social isolation. The middle-aged adult family member may become the caretaker for an older parent, in essence switching roles with the parent. An older adult may not be able to care for a spouse who has had a CVA and may have to accept placement of the spouse in a nursing home. In addition, the older adult who has no family may have to struggle alone to regain the ability to function independently. Although not all of these problems are amenable to nursing solutions, the nurse is most often the health care provider who assesses and identifies the needs of each individual and provides information and referrals to clients and families to help meet those needs.

Discharge planning assessments should include the areas of education, equipment, and psychosocial needs. The following questions should be addressed in discharge planning:

- What does the client and family know about prevention of CVA, neurologic deficits, physical care, and medications?

- Have the client and family participated in prescribed health care activities while in the hospital?

- What learning style is best for the client and family?

- Is the home environment furnished in such a way that the client and family will be able to use any necessary equipment (for example, a wheelchair or walker)?

- Can the necessary items for physical care be secured; if so, does the client/family know how to use them?

- How have the client and family members responded to home care and the need for support?

Critical areas of client and family education include

- Education about CVA and CVA prevention
  a. What is a CVA; causes of CVA
  b. Symptoms of TIA and CVA
  c. Prevention of CVA

- Psychologic support
  a. Involvement in self-care
  b. Coping skills
  c. Realistic expectations
  d. Time off for the caregiver

- Home and equipment modifications (for example, a raised toilet seat, grab bars in the bathroom, a bath chair, a vise lid opener, a long-handled shoehorn).

- Physical care (activities of daily living, exercises, transfer techniques, skin care).

- Community resources
  a. Referral to a home health care agency for the client who is returning home
  b. Specific communications with a long-term care facility about the established plan of care if the client is going to such a setting for rehabilitation or care
  c. Meals on Wheels, nutrition centers
  d. Eldercare (day-care for older adults)
  e. Outpatient clinics
  f. Community health services
  g. Special services for the visually and hearing impaired (for example, telephone services)
  h. Literature from the American Heart Association, Easter Seals Society, National Stroke Association, and U.S. Department of Health and Human Services on a variety of topics specific to CVA
  i. Support groups, stroke clubs
  j. Respite care
  k. Emergency alerting systems through a local hospital or agency

Throughout the rehabilitation process, it is important to encourage self-care by the client as much as possible but also to involve family members in the plan of care.

Applying Research to Nursing Practice: The Effects of Home Care on Caregivers

■ ■ ■

One researcher has examined the effects of long-term home care on female caregivers whose husbands have debilitating neurologic disorders, including Parkinson's disease, multiple sclerosis, and cerebrovascular disorders (Gaynor, 1990). Feelings of perceived burden were higher among women who had given care at home for an extended period of time, especially after 4 years. In addition, long-term caregivers had a greater incidence of illnesses, most commonly arthritis and hypertension. The investigator concluded from this sudy that as years of caregiving continue, home care becomes more stressful, especially when the caregiver is frail or disabled.

Implications for Nursing

In today's health care system, clients are sent home for rehabilitation and recovery or, if recovery is not possible, for life-long care by the family. As the majority of CVAs occur in older men, the family member most likely to provide care is an older female spouse. Nurses must include that spouse in all aspects of care, including teaching, and should involve the spouse during the acute stage of illness. It is critical that the discharge plan include referrals to community agencies for nursing care, appropriate support services, and respite care.

Critical Thinking in Client Care

1. Consider how the following factors would increase caregiver burden in long-term care:
   a. Loss of home health services
   b. Loss of support systems
   c. Decrease in income
   d. Illness of the caregiver

2. Is care of elderly parents a responsibility of adult children?

3. How does caregiver burden compare to burnout?

4. Describe the advantages and disadvantages of a federally mandated caregiver tax credit.

Stress that activities of daily living may take twice as long as they did before the CVA. Emphasize that physical function may continue to improve for up to 3 months, and speech may continue to improve for even longer (Moore, 1994).

Applying the Nursing Process

Case Study of a Client with a CVA: Orville Boren

Orville Boren is a 68-year-old male of African ancestry who had a CVA due to right cerebral thrombosis 1 week ago. He is a history instructor in the local community college. His hobby is wood carving, and he spends hours each week working in his garden. Mr. Boren is also an active member of his church. For the past 2 years, Mr. Boren has been taking medication for hypertension, but his wife Emily reports that he often forgets to take it and that his blood pressure was high at his last physical examination. Mrs. Boren tells the staff that she has never had to worry about her husband's health before and that she wants to learn everything she can to care for him at home. However, she says that her husband was always the one to make the decisions and pay the bills. Mrs. Boren adds that all the children, grandchildren, neighbors, and family pastor want to see Mr. Boren back at home as soon as possible.

Assessment

Carol Merck, RN, the primary care nurse assigned to Mr. Boren, completes a health history and physical assessment, with Mrs. Boren providing information for the history. Mrs. Boren reports that her husband did have several spells of dizziness and blurred vision the week before his CVA, but they lasted only a few minutes and he believed them to be due to "old age and working out in the sun." On the morning of admission, Mr. Boren woke up and could not move his left arm or leg; he also could not speak sensibly. Mrs. Boren called 911, and an ambulance took her husband to the hospital.

Physical assessment findings include the following: Mr. Boren is drowsy but responds to verbal stimuli. Although he does not respond verbally, he can nod his head to indicate "yes" when asked questions. Flaccid paralysis is present in his left arm and left leg, with no response noted to touch in those extremities (he is left-handed). Visual fields are decreased in a pattern consistent with homonymous hemianopia. A CT scan, negative on admission, is repeated on the third day after admission and confirms the medical diagnosis of a right-brain CVA due to a thrombus of the middle cerebral artery. Mr. Boren's medical treatment includes heparin sodium administered by continuous intravenous drip, with a partial thrombo-

plastin time (PTT) test to be performed every 4 hours and the dose adjusted accordingly.

Diagnosis

Ms. Merck identifies the following nursing diagnoses for Mr. Boren:

- *Feeding Self-Care Deficit* related to loss of the ability to use the left hand and arm
- *Impaired Physical Mobility* related to neurologic deficits causing left hemiplegia
- *Risk for Impaired Skin Integrity* related to inability to change position
- *Sensory/Perceptual Alterations: Visual* related to changes in visual fields
- *Impaired Verbal Communication* related to cerebral injury

Expected Outcomes

The expected outcomes for the plan of care are that Mr. Boren will

- Learn to use his right hand to feed himself.
- Participate in exercises necessary to maintaining muscle strength and tone.
- Maintain skin integrity.
- Indicate understanding that visual fields may improve in a few weeks.
- Practice and implement speech-therapy activities while at the same time using alternative methods of communication.

Planning and Implementation

The following interventions are planned and implemented for Mr. Boren:

- Arrange mealtimes so that Mr. Boren is sitting up by the window in a clean and private environment.
- Provide adaptive devices (silverware with thick handles and nonslip plates) for Mr. Boren to use.
- Encourage Mrs. Boren to visit at mealtimes, to assist Mr. Boren with meals, and periodically to bring a favorite food from home.
- Provide passive range-of-motion exercises for his left arm and leg; schedule active range-of-motion exercises for his right extremities as well as quadriceps and gluteal sets every 4 hours during waking hours.
- Keep his skin clean and dry at all times.
- Establish and maintain a regular schedule for turning Mr. Boren when he is in bed.
- Place objects (e.g., call bell, tissues) on Mr. Boren's unaffected side and approach him from that side.

- Support Mr. Boren's attempts to communicate verbally; when he is not understood, he prefers to use a large marker and tablet.

Evaluation

Mr. Boren is discharged to his home after being in the hospital for 10 days. During the first 2 months after discharge, Martha Grimes, the home health nurse, visits Mr. and Mrs. Boren at home. At the end of 2 months, Mr. Boren is using his right hand to feed himself. He has regained partial use of his left arm and leg and is using a walker to move around the house and yard; he is even able to work in his flower garden. His skin has remained intact, and his vision is back to normal. He is slowly relearning speech; this has been the most difficult change for him to accept; once he writes on his tablet "I think God has forgotten me."

Critical Thinking in the Nursing Process

1. Hypertension is sometimes referred to as "the silent killer." Provide justifications for this statement.
2. The functional changes Mr. Boren has experienced may make a return to teaching difficult. What other uses of his knowledge and abilities might you suggest?
3. What would be your reply if, after you had completed passive ROM on Mr. Boren's left arm, he wrote: "I just ignore that part of my body—it doesn't work anyway."
4. Develop a teaching plan to improve Mr. Boren's compliance with his regimen of antihypertensive medication.
5. Design a nursing care plan for Mr. Boren for the diagnosis *Spiritual Distress.*

The Client with an Intracranial Aneurysm

■ ■ ■

An *intracranial aneurysm* is a saccular outpouching of a cerebral artery that occurs at the site of a weakness in the vessel wall. The weakness may be the result of atherosclerosis, a congenital defect, trauma to the head, aging, or hypertension. A ruptured cerebral aneurysm is the most common cause of a hemorrhagic CVA.

Approximately 5 million North Americans have intracranial aneurysms; most of these people go through life without any manifestations of bleeding. However, it is estimated that 28,000 people will have a rupture of an intracranial aneurysm each year, that more than 50% will die within 3 months of the hemorrhage, and that half of the survivors will have serious disabilities (Hickey, 1992; Porth, 1994).

Intracranial aneurysms are most common in adults of ages 35 to 60, with about 20% of affected people having multiple aneurysms (Tierney et al., 1994). The exact etiology is unknown, but theories of cause include (1) a developmental defect in the vessel wall and (2) degeneration or fragility of the vessel wall due to conditions such as hypertension, atherosclerosis, connective-tissue disease, or abnormal blood flow (Porth, 1994). Hypertension and cigarette smoking may be predisposing factors (Way, 1994).

Intracranial aneurysms tend to occur at the bifurcations and branches of the carotid arteries and the vertebrobasilar arteries at the circle of Willis, with most aneurysms (85%) located anteriorly. They range in size from smaller than 15 mm to larger than 50 mm. Intracranial aneurysms tend to enlarge with time, making the vessel wall thin and increasing the probability of rupture.

There are several different types of intracranial aneurysms (Figure 41–5):

- A *berry aneurysm* is probably the result of a congenital abnormality of the tunica media of the artery. These berry-shaped aneurysms are the most common type, occurring primarily at the junctures of vessels in the circle of Willis. The sac that is formed at the site of weakness grows over time, with the saccular dilation forming above a stem. The aneurysm usually ruptures without warning.
- A *saccular aneurysm* is defined as any aneurysm with a saccular outpouching, which distends only a small portion of the vessel wall. This type of aneurysm is often caused by trauma.
- In a *fusiform aneurysm,* the entire circumference of a blood vessel swells to form an elongated tube. Most aneurysms of this type occur as a result of the changes of arteriosclerosis. Fusiform aneurysms act as space-occupying lesions.
- In a *dissecting aneurysm,* the tunica intima pulls away from the tunica media of the artery, and blood is forced between the two layers. They may result from atherosclerosis, inflammation, or trauma.

Pathophysiology

Intracranial aneurysms typically rupture from the dome rather than the base, forcing blood into the subarachnoid space at the base of the brain. However, the aneurysm may also rupture and force blood into brain tissue, the ventricles, or the subdural space. This discussion focuses on intracranial hemorrhages due to rupture of a cerebral aneurysm. See Chapter 40 for further discussion of types of intracranial hemorrhage.

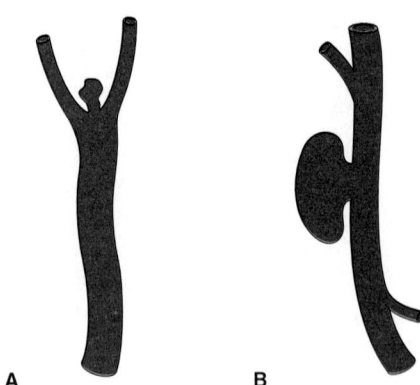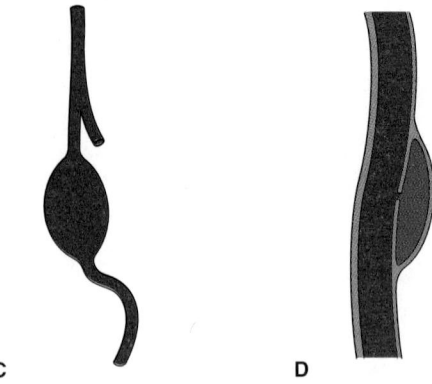

Figure 41–5 Types of aneurysms. *A*, A berry aneurysm is a small sac on a stem (or stalk). *B*, A saccular aneurysm is formed from a distended small portion of the vessel wall. *C*, A fusiform aneurysm is an enlarged area of the entire blood vessel. *D*, A dissecting aneurysm is formed when blood fills the area between the tunica media and the tunica intima.

Fibrin and platelets seal off the bleeding point, but the escaped blood forms a clot that irritates the brain tissue. The resulting inflammatory response causes cerebral edema, and both the edema and the hemorrhage increase intracranial pressure (Hickey, 1992). Bleeding into the subarachnoid space also causes meningeal irritation.

An intracranial aneurysm is usually asymptomatic until it ruptures, although very large aneurysms may cause headache and/or neurologic deficits due to pressure on adjacent intracranial structures. Small leakages of blood may occur periodically, causing headache, nausea, vomiting, and pain in the neck and back. The client may also have prodromal manifestations before the rupture occurs, such as headache, eye pain, visual deficits, and a dilated pupil.

The manifestations of a ruptured intracranial aneurysm (and subsequent subarachnoid hemorrhage) include a sudden, explosive headache; loss of consciousness; nausea and vomiting; a stiff neck and photophobia (due to meningeal irritation); cranial nerve deficits; stroke syndrome manifestations; and pituitary malfunctions (that result primarily from changes in ADH secretion).

The severity of the rupture is often inferred from the manifestations of the subarachnoid hemorrhage. In the system developed by Hunt and Hess (1968), severity ranges from grade I, in which the client has no symptoms or a slight headache with some stiffness of the neck, to grade V, in which the client is in a deep coma with decerebrate posturing.

The major complications of a ruptured intracranial aneurysm are rebleeding, vasospasm, and hydrocephalus. Hypothalamic dysfunction and seizures are also potential complications. The deficits caused by these complications make a ruptured intracranial aneurysm a serious health problem.

The greatest risk for rebleeding is within the first 48 hours after the initial rupture, and again in 7 to 10 days (when the initial clot breaks down). Rebleeding is manifested by a sudden severe headache, nausea and vomiting, decreasing levels of consciousness, and new neurologic deficits (Hickey, 1992). The mortality from rebleeding is as high as from the initial rupture.

Cerebral vasospasm is a common but dangerous complication that occurs between 4 and 12 days after a subarachnoid hemorrhage. It is associated with a large number of deaths and disability. A cerebral vasospasm is a narrowing of the lumen of one or more cerebral vessels, causing ischemia and infarction of tissue supplied by the affected vessels (Armstrong, 1994). The actual cause is unknown, but it occurs in blood vessels surrounded by thick blood clots, suggesting that some substance in the clot initiates the spasm. The manifestations of vasospasm vary according to the degree of spasm and the area of brain affected; regional alterations may cause focal deficits (such as hemiplegia), whereas global alterations cause loss of consciousness.

Hydrocephalus, which is an abnormal accumulation of cerebrospinal fluid (CSF) within the cranial vault and dilation of the ventricles, is a potential complication of a ruptured intracranial aneurysm. Hydrocephalus is thought to be the result of obstruction of reabsorption of CSF through the arachnoid villi. The obstruction is caused by an increased protein content of the CSF because of lysis of blood in the subarachnoid space (Porth, 1994). The accumulation of cerebrospinal fluid increases intracranial pressure. Initial manifestations of hydrocephalus are typically nonspecific but commonly include decreasing levels of consciousness.

Collaborative Care

The care of the client with a ruptured intracranial aneurysm includes determining the location of the aneurysm, treating the manifestations of the hemorrhage, and preventing rebleeding and vasospasm. Surgery is the treatment of choice to repair the bleeding artery.

Laboratory and Diagnostic Tests

The following diagnostic tests may be conducted to identify the site and extent of a ruptured intracranial aneurysm, as well as rebleeding:

- A *CT scan* of the brain demonstrates blood in the subarachnoid space in most clients within the first 24 to 48 hours after rupture.

- A *lumbar puncture* may be performed to withdraw cerebrospinal fluid for analysis. The presence of blood in the cerebrospinal fluid confirms a subarachnoid hemorrhage. However, this procedure poses a risk of rebleeding and brain herniation (Porth, 1994).

- Bilateral *carotid* and *vertebral cerebral angiography* may be conducted to determine the site and size of an aneurysm. A contrast medium is injected into an artery, and X-ray films are taken to visualize the cerebral vessels. This diagnostic test is not conducted unless the client's condition is stable enough for surgery (Tierney et al., 1994).

Diagnostic tests used to determine a vasospasm include CT cerebral angiography. A CT scan is used to rule out other causes of neurologic deficit (such as rebleeding or hydrocephalus) and determine the presence of thick blood clots, which may precipitate vasospasm. Angiograms are used to diagnose this complication definitively. The vasospasm is visualized as a narrowing of the column of dye in the affected artery (Armstrong, 1994).

Pharmacology

If surgery is not possible because of the client's condition, medications may be used to reduce the risk of rebleeding and vasospasm until surgery is feasible.

Aminocaproic acid (Amicar, Epsikapron) is a fibrinolysis inhibitor used to treat excessive bleeding in acute, life-threatening situations. It prevents the lysis of any blood clot that has formed near the site of a rupture. This drug is used in the first 2 weeks after aneurysm rupture (or until the client has surgery) to reduce the risk of rebleeding. The drug is administered intravenously the first week and orally thereafter. Potential complications include pulmonary embolism, venous thrombosis, and focal ischemic neurologic deficits.

Calcium channel blockers, such as nimodipine (Nimotop), are used to improve neurologic deficits due to vasospasm following subarachnoid hemorrhage from ruptured intracranial aneurysms. The drug is administered orally for 3 weeks after the hemorrhage. It has been found to reduce the incidence of ischemic deficits without side effects (Tierney et al., 1994).

Other medications that may be prescribed include

- Anticonvulsants, such as phenytoin (Dilantin), to prevent seizures if the client has increased intracranial pressure

- Steroids, such as dexamethasone (Decadron) or methylprednisolone (Solu-Medrol), to treat cerebral edema and meningeal irritation

- Analgesics (e.g., acetaminophen or codeine) for headache

Surgery

Surgery is performed for the treatment of intracranial aneurysm either to prevent rupture or to isolate the vessel to prevent further bleeding. Clients with good neurologic status may have surgery soon after the rupture. In clients with significant neurologic deficits, surgery may be delayed until they are more stable and less at risk for vasospasm.

There are several different types of surgery to repair a ruptured intracranial aneurysm or to prevent the rupture of an existing large aneurysm. The skull is opened (*craniotomy*), and the aneurysm is located. The neck of the aneurysm may be clipped with a metal clip (preventing the entry of blood into the aneurysm), or the involved artery may be clipped both proximally and distally to the aneurysm to isolate the affected area. Other forms of surgical treatment include wrapping the body of the aneurysm with a reinforcing material or performing endovascular surgery (Way, 1994).

Nursing Care

Nursing care is planned and implemented for the client with a ruptured intracranial aneurysm to prevent rebleeding as well as to meet needs resulting from neurologic deficits. Client responses to an intracranial hemorrhage with related nursing interventions are described earlier in the chapter in the discussion of nursing care for the client with a CVA.

Altered Cerebral Tissue Perfusion

This discussion focuses on the care of the client immediately after the intracranial aneurysm ruptures. The expected outcome of care is preventing rebleeding and improving cerebral tissue perfusion.

Nursing interventions with rationales follow:

- Institute aneurysm precautions to prevent rebleeding, as follows:
  a. Keep the client in a private, quiet, darkened room. Disconnect or remove the telephone. Avoid using bright overhead lights. *A quiet environment helps prevent an increase in blood pressure, which could precipitate rebleeding. The client may experience photophobia (abnormal sensitivity to light) if hemorrhage has damaged the oculomotor nerve.*

b. Elevate the head of the bed 30 to 45 degrees; follow prescribed activity orders (usually complete bed rest, but in some cases bathroom privileges may be approved). *Elevating the head of the bed promotes venous return from the brain and thus decreases intracranial pressure. Decreasing activity reduces the likelihood of increases in blood pressure.*

c. Limit visitors to two family members at any one time, and limit the duration of visits. Monitor client response to visitors and decrease interactions if the client becomes agitated or upset. *Psychologic stress may increase blood pressure and the risk of rebleeding; however, social isolation may increase anxiety and stress. Each client (and family) must be individually evaluated.*

d. Allow reading, watching television (if available), or listening to the radio (if available) to promote relaxation. *Although these passive activities were previously contraindicated for the client on aneurysm precautions, current therapy is based on the belief that these activities promote relaxation and help control blood pressure.*

e. Prevent constipation and straining to have a bowel movement. Administer stool softeners as prescribed. Collaborate with the client and physician about use of a bedside commode or the bathroom. Do not administer enemas. *The client is at risk for constipation as a result of decreased mobility and the administration of narcotics (such as codeine) for headache. When straining to have a bowel movement, the client uses the Valsalva maneuver, which increases intracranial pressure and may precipitate rebleeding.*

f. If the client is alert, and depending on physician preferences, allow the client to feed self and provide own personal care. *In many instances, self-care causes less anxiety and stress than care provided by the nurse. The extent of care provided varies according to client condition and physician preferences.*

- Monitor vital signs and neurologic status as indicated by client condition (frequency of assessments may range from every 15 minutes to every 4 hours). Neurologic assessment includes
  a. Level of consciousness
  b. Pupillary response
  c. Strength, movement, and sensation
  d. Communication ability
  e. Pain (headache, face, neck)

Vital signs and neurologic assessments provide ongoing data for evaluation of changes indicative of increasing intracranial pressure and decreasing neurologic function. Any change should be reported immediately to the physician.

- Maintain seizure precautions: have suction equipment and an oropharyngeal tube at the bedside, maintain the bed in the low position, and keep the side rails padded and raised. *Applying suction and inserting an oropharyngeal airway may be necessary to maintain an open airway in case of seizure. The bed is lowered and the side rails are padded and kept raised to prevent injury if a seizure occurs.*

- Avoid positioning and activities that increase intracranial pressure such as coughing, sneezing, vomiting, sharply flexing the neck, blowing the nose, enemas, moving self up in bed, or cigarette smoking. *These measures help to prevent increasing intracranial pressure and rebleeding.*

Other Nursing Diagnoses

Other nursing diagnoses that may be appropriate for the client with a ruptured intracranial aneurysm include:

- *Anxiety* related to sudden hospitalization and unknown future
- *Body Image Disturbance* related to inability to move one side of the body
- *Impaired Verbal Communication* related to the presence of expressive aphasia secondary to cerebral tissue damage
- *Pain* related to severe headache
- *Risk for Impaired Skin Integrity* related to inability to change position secondary to hemiplegia
- *Altered Thought Processes* related to decreased cerebral perfusion

Client and Family Teaching

Although teaching for the client and family with a CVA has previously been discussed, the following points, described by Hickey (1992), are essential to developing a teaching plan to provide a calm environment for the client who is on aneurysm precautions:

- Orient the client to time, place, and person frequently. If possible, have a calendar and a clock in the room.
- Describe the environment to the client and the family.
- Assess the client and family for signs of anxiety or concern. Take time to address concerns when they arise.
- Provide information to clarify misconceptions; use short, simple sentences when speaking to the client and allow time for the client to respond.
- Allow the client to make simple decisions about care.
- Report any problems the client or family is having with the restrictions imposed by aneurysm precautions to the physician, and discuss modifications.
- Remain supportive and helpful to the family throughout the period of hospitalization.

The Client with an Arteriovenous Malformation

∎ ∎ ∎

An *arteriovenous (AV) malformation* is a congenital intracranial lesion, formed by a tangled collection of dilated arteries and veins, that allows blood to flow directly from the arterial into the venous system, bypassing the normal capillary network. Most AV malformations (90%) are located in the cerebral hemispheres; the remainder are found in the cerebellum and brain stem.

AV malformations account for 8.6% of subarachnoid hemorrhages with resultant CVAs. Clients with this condition develop manifestations between the ages of 20 and 40 years of age (Hickey, 1992). The manifestations are the result of spontaneous bleeding from the lesion into the subarachnoid space or brain tissue. Mortality from bleeding is about 10% to 15% (Way, 1994).

Pathophysiology

AV malformations displace rather than encompass normal brain tissue (Hickey, 1992). The pathophysiologic effects of an AV malformation are the result of the shunting of blood from the arterial to the venous system and of altered perfusion of cerebral tissue near the malformation. The shunting of arterial blood directly into the venous system within the malformation transfers the higher arterial pressure directly into the lower-pressure venous system. This increased pressure is likely to cause spontaneous bleeding or progressive expansion and rupture of a blood vessel. Altered cerebral perfusion results when blood flow through a large, high-flow malformation is diverted from the normal cerebral circulation, causing tissue ischemia of the area surrounding the malformation. This is sometimes called a *vascular "steal" phenomenon.*

AV malformations range in size from very small to very large. Large malformations are usually initially manifested by seizure activity. In contrast, the manifestations of a small malformation are more often due to a hemorrhage that causes neurologic deficits. In both instances, the client may have recurrent headaches that do not respond to treatment.

Collaborative Care

AV malformations are diagnosed with the same diagnostic tests (CT scan, MRI, angiography) used to diagnose an intracranial aneurysm.

If the malformation is accessible, the ideal treatment is excision of the malformation and removal of any hematoma. Large malformations may be treated by embolization; in this procedure, substances such as Gelfoam or metallic pellets are introduced into the involved area of the cerebral circulation, where they form emboli and gradually obstruct blood flow in the malformation. Inaccessible malformations are also treated with radiation therapy or laser therapy, to coagulate blood in and thicken vascular elements of the malformation, eventually obstructing it. When the malformation is excised or obstructed, blood flow is no longer shunted, and cerebral perfusion improves.

Nursing Care

Nursing care for the client with an AV malformation depends on the condition of the malformation. If hemorrhage has not occurred, the client is taught to avoid activities that raise blood pressure or could cause injury. The client is usually given medications to control blood pressure and prevent seizures (Hickey, 1992).

If the malformation ruptures and causes an intracranial hemorrhage, nursing care is the same as for any client who has had a hemorrhagic CVA (discussed earlier in this chapter).

▚▚▚ Spinal Cord Disorders ▚▚▚

The spinal cord, the vertebrae, the intravertebral disks, the spinal nerves, the ligaments, and the surrounding soft-tissue structures are in such close anatomic proximity that any condition or injury affecting one structure may well affect any one or all of the other structures. The conditions with the most critical effects are disorders affecting the spinal cord. Disorders and injuries of the spinal cord have the potential to affect movement, perception, sensation, sexual function, and elimination.

Nursing care of clients with disorders of the spinal cord takes place from the acute management phase through ongoing rehabilitation in a variety of settings. Although priorities of care may change depending on the client and setting, care focuses on maximizing function to preserve quality of life. The nurse provides independent care and also cooperates with other health care professionals to meet this goal.

This section of the chapter discusses spinal cord injury, herniated intravertebral disk, and spinal cord tumors.

The Client with a Spinal Cord Injury

∎ ∎ ∎

A *spinal cord injury* is usually due to trauma. Although spinal cord injuries occur in people of all ages, they are most often seen in adolescent and young adult males between the ages of 16 and 30; 60% of all people with cord injuries are males in this age group. The majority of the injuries are due to motor vehicle accidents (45.5%), other causes include falls, violent acts, and sports injuries. Each year, 15,000 spinal cord injuries occur in the United States, with the average cost of care for one client from the initial injury to death exceeding $500,000 (Way, 1994).

Overview

This overview presents the basic structure and function of the spinal cord, the mechanism of injury to the spinal cord, and classifications of spinal cord injury.

Structure and Function of the Spinal Cord

The spinal cord runs through the vertebral canal of the vertebral column from the foramen magnum to the L-1 or L-2 level. The cord provides a two-way pathway for the conduction of impulses and information to and from the brain and the body, serves as a major reflex center, and (through its attached spinal nerves) is involved in the sensory and motor innervation of the entire body below the head.

The cord is made of an outer region of white matter and an inner region of gray matter. The gray matter makes up the central canal of the cord, the posterior horns, the anterior horns, and the lateral horns. It is divided into a sensory half (dorsally) and a motor half (ventrally) and innervates somatic and visceral regions of the body. The white matter is made up of tracts or pathways that convey information. The ascending (sensory) pathways carry information about proprioception, fine touch, discrimination, pain, temperature, deep pressure, and touch. The descending (motor) pathways carry information about movement. The pyramidal tracts control skilled voluntary movements (such as writing). The extrapyramidal tracts (all tracts other than the pyramidal tracts) bring about all other body movements.

Mechanisms of Injury

Spinal cord injuries are the result of the application of excessive force to the spinal column. The most common cause of abnormal spinal column movements are acceleration and deceleration (forces that are applied to the body, for example, in automobile accidents and falls). Acceleration occurs when external force is applied in a rear-end collision; the upper torso and head are forced backward and then forward. Deceleration occurs in a head-on collision; the external force is applied from the front. The head and body move forward until they meet a stationary object and then are forced backward. The following forces and movements (Figure 41–6) may cause a variety of spinal cord injuries, with the extent of injury depending on the amount and direction of motion, and the rate of application of force (Porth, 1994):

- Hyperflexion, or forcible forward bending, may compress vertebral bodies and disrupt ligaments and intervertebral disks.

- Hyperextension, or forcible backward bending, often disrupts ligaments and causes vertebral fractures. A *whiplash* injury is a less severe form of hyperextension, with injury to soft tissues but no vertebral or spinal cord damage.

- Axial loading, a form of compression, is the application of vertical force to the spinal column (for instance, by falling and landing on the feet or buttocks or by diving into shallow water).

- Excessive rotation, in which the head is excessively turned, may tear ligaments, fracture articular surfaces, and cause compression fractures.

The alteration of the spinal cord and soft tissues caused by these abnormal movements is called deformation. In addition, the spinal cord may be penetrated by bullets and other foreign objects (e.g., sharp objects used as weapons, shrapnel from explosions). Penetrating injuries may cause vertebral fractures, tear ligaments and muscles, or cut through a part or all of the spinal cord. Complete severing of the cord is rare.

These injuries occur most often in the lumbar and cervical regions. The most frequent sites of injury of the cord are at the first, second, and fourth to sixth cervical vertebrae (C-1, C-2, C-4 to C-6); and the eleventh thoracic to second lumbar vertebrae (T-11 to L-2) (Porth, 1994). Because the cervical spine has a wider range of movement than the rest of the spine, the cervical portion is more likely to be affected by externally applied forces. In addition, the cord fills most of the vertebral canal in the cervical and lumbar regions and thus is more easily injured. Damage to the vertebrae and ligaments causes the spinal column to become unstable, increasing the possibility of compression or stretching of the spinal cord with any further movement.

Classifications of Injury

Spinal cord injuries are classified according to systems, for instance (1) as complete or incomplete cord injury, (2) by cause of injury, and (3) by level of injury. In clinical practice, these classifications often overlap.

In a complete spinal cord injury, the motor and sensory neural pathways are completely interrupted (*transected*), resulting in total loss of motor and sensory function below the level of the injury. In an incomplete spinal cord injury, the motor and sensory pathways are only partially interrupted, with variable loss of function below the level of injury. Incomplete spinal cord injuries are further classified into syndromes as outlined in Table 41–2 on page 1776.

The major causes of spinal cord injury are concussion, contusion, laceration, transection, hemorrhage, and damage to blood vessels that supply the spinal cord (Hickey,

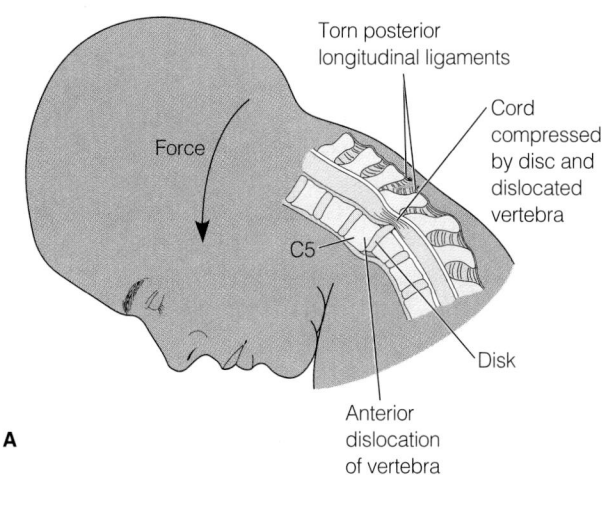

Torn posterior longitudinal ligaments

Force

Cord compressed by disc and dislocated vertebra

C5

Disk

Anterior dislocation of vertebra

A

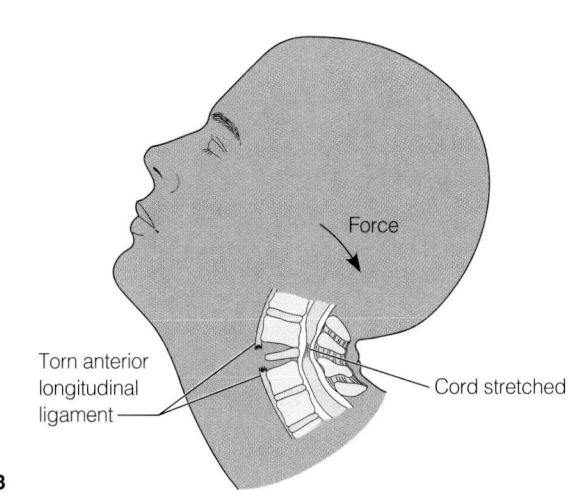

Force

Torn anterior longitudinal ligament

Cord stretched

B

Figure 41-6   Spinal cord injury mechanisms. *A*, Hyperflexion. *B*, Hyperextension. *C*, Axial loading, a form of compression.

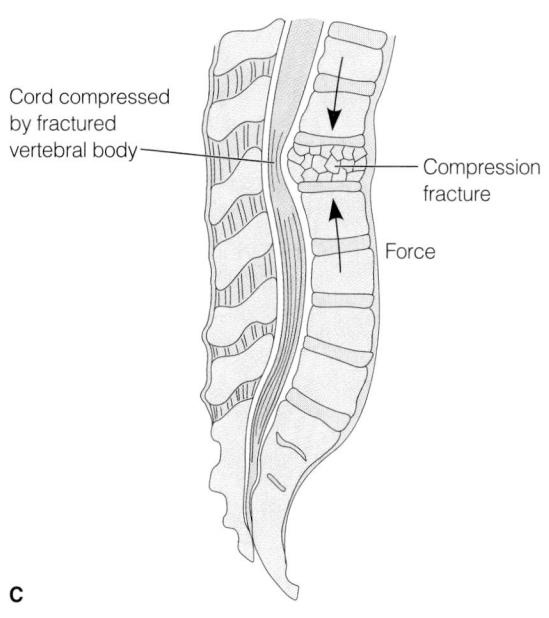

Cord compressed by fractured vertebral body

Compression fracture

Force

C

1992). If vertebrae are fractured and ligaments are torn, bony fragments can damage the cord and make the spinal column unstable. Injury to blood vessels supplying the cord can cause permanent damage.

The injury is identified by vertebral level. For example, a C-6 spinal cord injury is present at the sixth cervical vertebra.

Risk Factors

Three major risk factors for spinal cord injuries are age, gender, and alcohol or drug abuse. Young men are more prone to take risks than women are, and to do so under the influence of mind-altering chemicals. Older adults are more likely to have spinal cord injuries from even minor trauma as a result of age-related vertebral degeneration.

Pathophysiology

The initial injury causes microscopic hemorrhages in the gray matter of the cord and edema of the white matter of the cord. These initial pathologic changes are followed by other mechanisms that increase the area of injury. The hemorrhages extend, eventually involving the entire gray matter. Microcirculation to the cord is impaired by edema and hemorrhage. The injured tissue releases norepinephrine, serotonin, dopamine, and histamine; these vasoactive substances cause vasospasm and further decrease microcirculation. As a result, vascular perfusion and oxygen tension of the affected area is decreased, which leads to ischemia.

When ischemia is prolonged, necrosis of both gray and white matter begins within a few hours, and within 24 hours the function of nerves passing through the injured area is lost. Although circulation returns to the white matter of the cord in about 24 hours, decreased circulation in the gray matter continues (McCance & Huether, 1994). Because edema extends the level of injury for two cord segments above and below the affected level, the extent of injury cannot be determined for up to 1 week.

Tissue repair occurs over a period of 3 to 4 weeks. Phagocytes enter the area in 36 to 48 hours after the initial injury. Neurons degenerate and are removed by mi-

Table 41–2 Incomplete Spinal Cord Injury Syndromes

Type	Cause	Location	Deficits
Central syndrome	Cord transection Hyperextension	Cervical	Spastic paralysis of the upper extremities Variable paralysis of the lower extremities Variable effects on the bowel, the bladder, and sexual function
Anterior syndrome	Damage to the anterior spinal artery Infarction of the anterior spinal artery Hyperflexion	Anterior two-thirds of the cord	Paralysis below the level of injury Loss of temperature and pain sensation below the level of injury
Posterior syndrome	Vertebral dislocation Herniated disk Compression	Nerve roots	Weakness in isolated muscle groups Tingling, pain Decreased or absent reflexes in the involved area Bowel or bladder dysfunction
Brown-Séquard syndrome	Penetrating trauma	Hemisection of the anterior and posterior cord	Paralysis below the level of injury on the ipsilateral (same) side of the body Contralateral loss of temperature and pain sensation below the level of injury Ipsilateral loss of proprioception below the level of injury
Horner's syndrome	Incomplete cord transection	Cervical sympathetic nerves	Ipsilateral ptosis of the eyelid, constricted pupil, and facial anhidrosis (inability to perspire)

Table 41–3 Losses in Functional Abilities by Level of Injury to the Spinal Cord

Level	Function	ADL	Elimination	Mobility
C-1	No control of head, neck, and diaphragm.	D*	D*	Limited
C-4	Sensation in head and neck; some control of neck and diaphragm.	D	D	Limited
	Movement of head, neck, and diaphragm	D	D	Wheelchair/WA (electric)
C-5	Controls head, neck, and shoulders; flexes elbows.	I/WA	WA	Wheelchair/WA
C-6	Uses shoulder, extends wrist.	I or WA	I or WA	Wheelchair; self-transfer
C-7 to C-8	Extends elbow, flexes wrist, has some use of fingers.	I	I	I/wheelchair (manual)
T-1 to T-5	Has full hand and finger control, full use of thoracic muscles.	I	I	I/wheelchair (manual)
T-6 to T-10	Controls abdominal muscles, has good balance.	I	I	I/wheelchair (manual)
T-11 to L-5	Flexes and abducts the hips; flexes and extends the knees.	I	I	WA/ambulation
S-1 to S-5	Has full control of legs; has full innervation of muscles needed for bowel and bladder control and sexual function.	I	I	I/ambulation

*D=Dependent, I=Independent, WA=With Assistance

crophages in the first 10 days after the injury. Red blood cells disintegrate, and the hemorrhages are reabsorbed. Eventually the area of injury is replaced by acellular collagenous tissue, and the meninges thicken (McCance & Huether, 1994).

The alterations in function that occur as the result of a spinal cord injury vary greatly depending on the amount of tissue damage and the level of the injury. Table 41–3 describes alterations in functional abilities by injury level. The client may have deficits in motor abilities, sensory abilities, and reflex activity; these are discussed in the accompanying clinical manifestations box.

Spinal Shock

Spinal shock is the temporary loss of reflex function (called *areflexia*) below the level of injury. It is an immediate response to spinal cord injury. This response begins immediately after complete transection of the spinal cord, when connections between the brain and the spinal cord are interrupted and the cord does not function at all. The response also occurs (although in varying degrees) after partial transection as well as after spinal cord contusions, compression, and ischemia.

The exact cause of spinal shock is unknown. However, it is known that it involves the motor pathways, with loss of motor function, tendon reflexes, and autonomic function (Porth, 1994). Of particular concern is the effect on pulse and blood pressure; the parasympathetic system dominates in spinal shock, causing bradycardia and hypotension.

Spinal shock may begin within 1 hour of the injury. The condition may last from a few minutes to several months (although it usually lasts from 1 to 6 weeks), and then reflex activity returns. Spinal shock ends slowly, with the gradual reappearance of reflexes, hyperreflexia (increased reflex responses), muscle spasticity, and reflex bladder emptying.

The manifestations of acute spinal shock (which vary in degree) include the following:

- Bradycardia
- Hypotension
- Flaccid paralysis of skeletal muscles
- Loss of sensations of pain, touch, temperature, and pressure
- Absence of visceral and somatic sensations
- Bowel and bladder dysfunction
- Loss of the ability to perspire

The individual with a cervical cord injury may also have neurogenic shock, resulting in cardiovascular changes. These changes are due to the inability of higher centers in the brain stem to modulate reflexes. As a result, vascular beds dilate, and the cardiac accelerator reflex is

---

Clinical Manifestations and Complications of Spinal Cord Injury by Body System

Integument

- Decubitus (pressure) ulcers

Neurologic

- Pain
- Areflexia
- Hypotonia
- Autonomic dysreflexia

Cardiovascular

- Spinal shock
- Paroxysmal hypertension
- Orthostatic hypotension
- Cardiac dysrhythmias
- Decreased venous return
- Hypercalcemia

Respiratory

- Limited chest expansion
- Decreased cough reflex
- Decreased vital capacity

Gastrointestinal

- Stress ulcers
- Paralytic ileus
- Stool impaction
- Stool incontinence

Genitourinary

- Urinary retention
- Urinary incontinence
- Neurogenic bladder
- Impotence
- Testicular atrophy
- Inability to ejaculate
- Decreased vaginal lubrication

Musculoskeletal

- Joint contractures
- Bone demineralization
- Osteoporosis
- Muscle spasms
- Muscle atrophy
- Pathologic fractures
- Paraplegia
- Quadriplegia

---

suppressed. The client experiences orthostatic hypotension and bradycardia. Other symptoms may include respiratory insufficiency due to loss of innervation of the diaphragm in C-1 to C-4 injuries, hypothermia, paralytic ileus, urinary retention, and oliguria.

Both bradycardia and hypotension may persist even after the spinal shock resolves. In addition to losing sympathetic control of the heart rate, the client with a high-level spinal cord injury experiences decreased peripheral resistance and loss of muscle activity. These changes result in sluggish blood flow and decreased venous return, increasing the risk for thrombophlebitis.

Upper and Lower Motor Neuron Deficits

Injuries to the spinal cord are often classified as either upper motor neuron lesions or lower motor neuron lesions. Motor neurons are functional units that carry motor impulses. The upper motor neurons (located in the cerebral cortex, thalamus, brain stem, and corticospinal and corticobulbar tracts) are responsible for voluntary movement. When these motor pathways are interrupted, the client experiences spastic paralysis and hyperreflexia and may be unable to carry out skilled movement.

Lower motor neurons (located in the anterior horn of the spinal cord, the motor nuclei of the brain stem, and the axons that reach the motor end plate of skeletal muscles) are responsible for innervation and contraction of skeletal muscles. Interruption of lower motor neurons results in muscle flaccidity and extensive muscle atrophy, with loss of both voluntary and involuntary movement. If only some of the motor neurons supplying a muscle are affected, the client experiences partial paralysis (*paresis*); if all motor neurons to a muscle are affected, the client experiences complete paralysis. Hyporeflexia is also present.

Paraplegia and Quadriplegia

Two of the common neurologic deficits resulting from spinal cord injury are paraplegia and quadriplegia (see Figure 41–1). *Paraplegia* is paralysis of the lower portion of the body, sometimes involving the lower trunk. Paraplegia occurs when the thoracic, lumbar, and sacral portions of the spinal cord are injured, causing loss or impairment of sensory and/or motor function. *Quadriplegia,* which is also called *tetraplegia,* occurs when cervical segments of the cord are injured, impairing function of the arms, trunk, legs, and pelvic organs (American Spinal Injury Association, 1992).

Autonomic Dysreflexia

Autonomic dysreflexia (also called *autonomic hyperreflexia*) is an exaggerated sympathetic response that occurs in approximately 85% of all clients with spinal cord injuries at or above the T-6 level. This response, which is seen after recovery from spinal shock, occurs as a result of a lack of control of the autonomic nervous system by higher centers. When stimuli (such as a full bladder) are unable to ascend the cord, mass reflex stimulation of the sympathetic nerves below the level of the injured cord area occurs, triggering massive vasoconstriction. In response, the vagus nerve causes bradycardia and vasodilation above the level of injury. If untreated, autonomic dysreflexia can cause seizures, a CVA, or a myocardial infarction (Hickey, 1992). The complications of untreated dysreflexia are potentially fatal.

Autonomic dysreflexia is triggered by stimuli that would normally cause abdominal discomfort (a full bladder is the most common cause), by stimulation of pain receptors, and by visceral contractions (Porth, 1994). Causes include fecal impaction, bladder infections or stones, acute abdominal disorders, intrauterine contractions, ejaculation, and stimulation from pressure ulcers or ingrown toenails.

The manifestations of this condition include pounding headache; bradycardia; hypertension (with readings as high as 300/160); flushed, warm skin with profuse sweating above the lesion and pale, cold, and dry skin below it; and anxiety (Ceron & Rakowski-Reinhardt, 1991; Porth, 1994). Dysreflexia is a neurologic emergency and requires immediate treatment.

Collaborative Care

The client with an acute spinal cord injury requires emergency assessment and care and medications; sometimes the client also requires immobilization and surgery. The client is first assessed and stabilized at the scene of the accident, initially treated in the emergency room, and then admitted to the hospital intensive care unit.

Emergency Care at the Scene

The danger of death from spinal cord injury is greatest when there is damage to or transection of the upper cervical region. When the injury is at the C-1 to C-4 level, respiratory paralysis is common, and the client who survives requires ventilator assistance to breathe. Injuries below C-4 may increase the risk of respiratory failure if edema ascends the cord. It is of critical importance not to complicate the initial injury by allowing the fractured vertebrae to damage the cord further during transport to the hospital. Although at one time injuries to the high cervical cord were almost always fatal, advances in trauma care have greatly improved the survival rate.

All people who have sustained trauma to the head or spine, or who are unconscious, should be treated as though they have a spinal cord injury. It is estimated that as many as 25% of cervical spine injuries result in permanent neurologic deficits because the person was improperly handled during removal from a vehicle, during transport, or in the emergency department (Metcalf, 1986). Here are some guidelines for emergency care (Dossey, Guzzetta, & Kenner, 1990):

- Avoid flexing, extending, or rotating the neck.
- Immobilize the neck, using rolled towels or blankets, or apply a cervical collar before moving the person onto the stretcher.
- Secure the head by placing a belt or tape across the forehead and securing it to the stretcher.
- Maintain the client in the supine position.
- Transfer the person directly from the stretcher to the type of bed that will be used in the hospital.

Emergency Department Management

Assessment findings at the scene of the accident or in the emergency room vary according to the level of injury. These findings indicate cervical injury:

- Paralysis or weakness of extremities
- Respiratory distress manifested by changes in arterial blood gas studies, cyanosis, flaring of the nostrils, use of accessory muscles of respiration, and restlessness
- Pulse rate below 60 and systolic BP below 80
- Decreased peristalsis

This finding indicates thoracic and lumbar injury:

- Paralysis or weakness of extremities

These findings indicate acute spinal shock:

- Loss of skin sensation
- Flaccid paralysis, areflexia
- Absent bowel sounds
- Bladder distention
- Decreasing blood pressure
- Absence of the cremasteric reflex in males (retraction of the left or right testicle in response to stimulation of the skin of, respectively, the inner left or right thigh)

The client in the emergency department with a suspected or identified spinal cord injury is also treated for respiratory problems, paralytic ileus, atonic bladder, and cardiovascular alterations. Respiratory distress in the client with a cervical level injury is treated by placing the client on a ventilator. Oxygen is administered to the client with a thoracic level injury. Paralytic ileus (obstruction of the intestines due to lack of peristalsis) is common in clients with a spinal cord injury and is treated by the insertion of a nasogastric tube with connection to suction. To prevent overdistention of an atonic bladder, an indwelling catheter is inserted and connected to dependent drainage. Cardiovascular status is assessed on a continuous basis by inserting invasive monitoring devices, such as a Swan-Ganz catheter, and attaching the client to a cardiac monitor.

The client also may be given methylprednisolone (Medrol) on admission to the emergency department. Clinical research indicates that the use of this adrenocorticosteroid is effective in preventing secondary spinal cord damage from edema and ischemia. The medication must be administered intravenously within 8 hours of the injury to be effective in preventing secondary damage. A loading dose is administered initially and a maintenance dose is continued for 23 hours. The drug is contraindicated in clients who are pregnant, have uncontrolled diabetes mellitus, are allergic to the medication, have other serious injuries, or were injured more than 8 hours before medical care (Nolan, 1994).

The use of other steroids and naloxone (an opioid antagonist) has not proven to be as effective, but research is ongoing. Other agents to treat acute spinal cord injury and prevent secondary injury are being used in clinical trials. These drugs (WIN 44, 441-3; nalmefene; U-50488h; and norbinaltophimine) are specific opioid antagonists, believed to promote blood flow in the spinal cord. Other drugs that show promise for clients with acute spinal cord injury include the glutamate antagonists (especially MK-801), which decrease the influx of calcium into the neuron, thereby helping prevent cellular ischemic damage and enhancing neuronal growth and possible regeneration (Nolan, 1994).

Laboratory and Diagnostic Tests

No specific laboratory tests are used in the diagnosis of spinal cord injury. Arterial blood gases are measured to establish a baseline or to identify problems due to respiratory insufficiency.

The following diagnostic studies are used to diagnose injuries of the spinal cord:

- *X-ray films* of the spine are taken to visualize any fracture, deformity, displacement of vertebrae, or hematomas. However, significant cord damage can be present even if X-ray films show none.
- A *CT scan* or *MRI study* illustrates changes in the vertebrae, spinal cord, and tissues around the cord.
- Following the acute phase, *electromyography (EMG)* or *evoked potential* studies may be done to locate the level of spinal cord injury. In these tests, peripheral nerves are stimulated and response times are measured.

Pharmacology

The pharmacologic treatment of the client with a spinal cord injury is symptomatic. It is directed primarily toward decreasing edema from the injury, treating hypotension and bradycardia, and treating spasticity.

- Specific corticosteroids, discussed earlier in this section, may be used to decrease or control edema of the cord.
- Vasopressors are used in the immediate critical care phase to treat bradycardia or hypotension due to spinal shock (see Chapter 6).
- Muscle relaxants are used to treat spasticity in clients with spinal cord injury. Both baclofen (Lioresal) and dantrolene sodium (Dantrium) may be used. A discussion of nursing implications of treatment with these medications is found in the accompanying pharmacology box.
- Analgesics (such as nonsteroidal anti-inflammatory agents) and tricylic antidepressants (such as amitriptyline [Elavil] and imipramine [Tofranil]) are administered to reduce pain.

Nursing Implications for Pharmacology: Muscle Relaxants in Spinal Cord Injury

Baclofen (Lioresal)

Chlorzoxazone (Paraflex)

Cyclobenzaprine hydorchloride (Flexeril)

Dantrolene sodium (Dantrium)

Orphenadrine citrate (Norflex)

These drugs depress the central nervous system and inhibit the transmission of impulses from the spinal cord to skeletal muscle. They are used to control muscle spasm and pain associated with acute or chronic musculoskeletal conditions. They are not always effective in controlling spasticity resulting from cerebral or spinal cord conditions.

Nursing Responsibilities

- Assess the client's spasticity and involuntary movements to obtain baseline data for comparison of results of therapy.

- Do not expect therapy to have effects for 1 week.
- Administer oral medications with food to decrease gastrointestinal symptoms.

Client and Family Teaching

- These drugs may cause drowsiness, diplopia, and impotence.
- Take your medications with meals to decrease gastric irritation.
- Physical improvement may take several weeks.
- Report slurred speech, drooling, or inability to carry out normal functions to the physician.

- Histamine H_2 antagonists (e.g., ranitidine [Zantac]) are often administered to prevent stress-related gastric ulcers, a common complication in spinal cord injury.
- Anticoagulants (heparin or warfarin) may be given to prevent thrombophlebitis.
- Stool softeners may be administered as part of a bowel-training program.

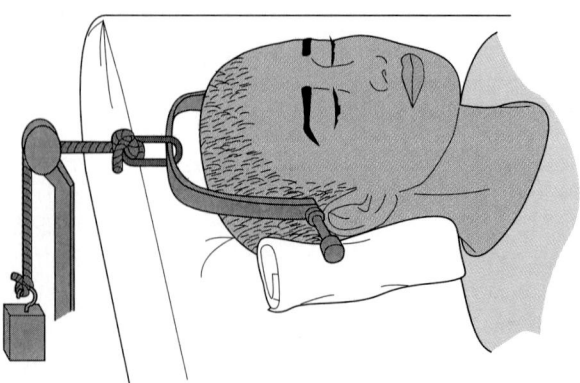

Figure 41–7 Cervical traction may be applied by several methods, including Gardner-Wells tongs.

Stabilization and Immobilization

The client who has a spinal cord injury as a result of one or more dislocations or fractures of the cervical vertebrae is usually immobilized by being placed in some type of traction or external fixation device to stabilize the vertebral column and prevent any further damage. Traction may also be used to stabilize the spinal column for clients who are not yet in a condition to have surgery or who have severe bleeding and edema of the injured cord. The physician applies the traction or fixation device; the nurse is responsible for assessments and interventions following the application.

There are various devices to provide cervical traction. Gardner-Wells tongs are often used (Figure 41–7). When this type of traction is used, the physician applies the pins to the skull, approximately 1 cm above each ear, and weights are attached to the device. The amount of weight is usually 5 pounds per level of cervical injury; for example, a client with a fracture of C-6 to C-7 would begin with 30 pounds of weight (Nolan, 1994).

The client may be placed on a special bed, such as a kinetic bed, CircOlectric bed, or Stryker frame to allow movement or turning while keeping the spinal column in alignment.

The halo external fixation device may be used to provide stabilization if there is no significant involvement of the ligaments (Figure 41–8). It is most often used to provide stability for fractures of the cervical vertebrae without cord damage. This device allows greater mobility, self-care, and participation in rehabilitation programs. This device is secured through four pins inserted into the skull, two in the frontal bone and two in the occipital bone. The halo ring is then attached to a rigid plastic vest lined with sheepskin (Ohman & Spaniol, 1990). Nursing interventions for the client using a halo fixation device are described in the accompanying box.

Surgery

Surgical treatment may be necessary if there is evidence of compression of the spinal cord by bone fragments or a hematoma. Surgery may also be done to stabilize and support the spine. However, many clients are treated with stabilization devices and do not require surgery. Surgeries that may be performed include a decompression laminectomy, a spinal fusion, and insertion of metal rods. Surgeries of the spine are discussed later in the chapter.

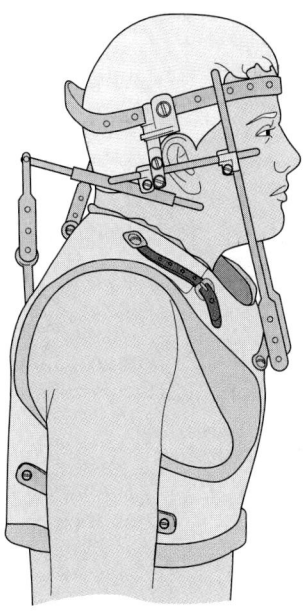

Figure 41–8   The halo external fixation device.

Nursing Care of the Client in Halo Fixation

NURSING RESPONSIBILITIES

- Maintain the integrity of the halo external fixation device.
  a. Inspect pins and traction bars for tightness, report loosened pins to physician.
  b. Tape the appropriate wrench to the head of the bed for emergency intervention.
  c. Never use the halo ring to lift or reposition the client.
  Loosening of the apparatus poses the risk of further damage to the cord. It is the responsibility of the nurse to maintain the integrity of the apparatus and the safety of the client.

- Assess muscle function and skin sensation every 2 hours in the acute phase and every 4 hours thereafter.
  a. Assess motor function on a scale of 0 to 5, with 0 being no evidence of muscle contraction and 5 being normal muscle strength with full range of motion.
  b. Assess sensation by comparing touch and pain, moving from impaired to normal areas, and testing both the right and left sides of the body.

Monitoring muscle function and skin sensation allows early identification of potential neurologic deficits.

- Monitor the pin sites each shift and follow hospital policy for pin care. Here are some general guidelines:
  a. Assess the pin sites for redness, edema, and drainage.
  b. Depending on policy, clean pin site with a sterile applicator dipped in hydrogen peroxide, apply a topical antibiotic, and cover with sterile 2-inch split gauze squares.
  Organisms can enter the body through the pin-insertion site; assessments and care are provided to detect signs of and prevent infection.

- Maintain skin integrity.
  a. Turn the immobile client every 2 hours.
  b. Inspect the skin around edges of the vest every 4 hours.
  c. Change the sheepskin liner when it is soiled and at least once each week.

These interventions prevent skin injury and irritation.

Nursing Care

The client with a spinal cord injury has, both during the acute phase and the rehabilitative phase, complex needs that involve all members of the health care team. Because these injuries are more common in younger clients, consideration of life-long effects on both the client and the family is essential. The nurse coordinates client care and develops and implements a care plan that is individualized to each client and family. The focus of the plan is to prevent the secondary complications of immobility and altered body functions, to promote self-care, and to educate the client and family (Drayton-Hargrove & Reddy, 1986).

Because a spinal cord injury has many possible effects, many nursing diagnoses may be appropriate. Nursing diagnoses discussed in this section focus on problems with physical mobility, gas exchange, dysreflexia, bowel and bladder elimination, sexual dysfunction, and self-esteem.

Impaired Physical Mobility

The client with a spinal cord injury initially experiences a period of spinal shock. After this phase, the client regains spinal reflex activity and muscle tone that is not under the control of higher centers. Clients with injuries above the level of T-12 experience involuntary spastic movements of skeletal muscles. These movements reach a peak about 2 years after the injury and then gradually subside (Porth, 1994). Spasms impair the ability to carry out the activities of daily life and work. In addition, the paraplegia or quadriplegia increases the potential for impaired skin integrity, thrombophlebitis, and contractures.

The goals of care for clients with impaired mobility due to a spinal cord injury are to reduce the effects of spasticity and to prevent complications involving the skin, the cardiovascular system, and joint function.

Nursing interventions with rationales follow:

- Perform passive range-of-motion exercises for all extremities at least twice a day. Identify stimuli that cause spastic movements and either avoid the stimuli (such as certain exercises) or teach the client to expect the movements. *Range-of-motion exercises help prevent contractures and stretch spastic muscles, promoting rehabilitation.*

- Maintain skin integrity by turning the client every 2 hours, assessing pressure points at least once each shift, and using a special bed if necessary. *Immobility compresses soft tissues and promotes the development of decubitus ulcers. The lack of sensory warning mechanisms and of voluntary motor control of skin dermatomes further increases the risk for altered skin integrity.*

- Assess the lower extremities each shift for symptoms of thrombophlebitis. Observe for redness and for increased heat every shift; measure thigh and calf circumference daily. If antiembolic stockings (TEDs) are ordered, remove for 30 to 60 minutes each shift. Assess for skin impairment and provide skin care while TEDs are removed. *Clients with neurologic deficits are at high risk for deep vein thrombosis as a result of immobility, vasomotor dysfunction, and decreased venous return with venous stasis. Antiembolic stockings help to prevent the pooling of blood in the lower extremities and increase venous return, lessening the risk for venous stasis and thrombus formation. Removing them from time to time not only promotes healthy skin but also lets the nurse assess skin integrity.*

Impaired Gas Exchange

Injuries at the level of C-8 to C-5 leave the phrenic nerve intact, but the innervation of intercostal muscles is affected, compromising respiratory function. In addition, because the abdominal muscles are paralyzed, the client cannot expel secretions by coughing. (Clients with cord injuries at C-3 or above have paralysis of the respiratory muscles and cannot breathe without a ventilator.)

- Monitor vital capacity and respiratory effectiveness, assessing for tachycardia, restlessness, PaO_2 less than 60 mm Hg, $PaCO_2$ greater than 50 mm Hg, and vital capacity less than 1 liter. *Clients with cervical cord injuries frequently require ventilatory support because of reduced vital capacity and inability to expel secretions by coughing. Changes in arterial blood gases and vital capacity signal respiratory insufficiency.*

- Monitor for signs of ascending edema of the spinal cord, including difficulty in swallowing or coughing, respiratory stridor, use of accessory muscles of respiration, bradycardia, and increased motor and sensory loss. *Hemorrhage and edema can further impair respiratory function.*

- Help the client to cough, as follows: Place the hand between the umbilicus and xiphoid process and push in and up as the client exhales and coughs (Metcalf, 1986). *The client who is unable to cough effectively and has decreased ventilatory capacity may develop atelectasis, pneumonia, and respiratory failure.*

Ineffective Breathing Patterns

Respiratory function is impaired in the client with a spinal cord injury in the cervical and thoracic levels if the diaphragm (innervated by C-1 to C-4), the intercostal muscles (innervated by C-5 to C-8), and the abdominal muscles are affected (Hickey, 1992: Porth, 1994). In clients with injury at higher levels, assisted ventilation and a tracheostomy are necessary; when the injury is at lower levels, the client's ability to take a deep breath and cough is diminished. The goal of nursing interventions is to maintain normal respiratory rate (16 to 20 breaths per minute) and to prevent pulmonary complications such as atelectasis and pneumonia.

Nursing interventions with rationales follow:

- Assess respiratory rate, rhythm, and depth every 4 hours (or more frequently if needed). Auscultate breath sounds as a part of respiratory assessment. *Injury to the cord in the cervical or thoracic regions can decrease respiratory function and increase the risk for respiratory problems.*

- Monitor results of oxygen saturation and arterial blood gas studies. *Arterial blood gas studies provide information about gas exchange; decreasing Ph, oxygen, and oxygen saturation levels, and increasing carbon dioxide levels signal respiratory acidosis.*

- Help the client turn, cough, and deep breathe at least every 2 hours. Use assisted coughing as necessary by placing the hand between the umbilicus and the xiphoid process and applying firm pressure with the heel of the hand during the cough (Metcalf, 1986). *Paralysis of intercostal or abdominal muscles decreases the ability to expel secretions by coughing; retained secretions increase the risk for pneumonia and atelectasis.*

- Increase fluids given by mouth to 3000 mL per day (if oral intake is approved), according to client preference for type of liquids and predicated on the client's ability to swallow. *Increased fluid intake thins secretions, which can more easily be expelled and expectorated.*

Dysreflexia

Autonomic dysreflexia is an emergency that requires immediate assessment and intervention to prevent complications of extremely high blood pressure.

Nursing interventions with rationales follow:

- Elevate the head of the client's bed and remove TEDs. *These measures increase pooling of blood in the lower extremities and decrease venous return, thus decreasing blood pressure.*

- Assess blood pressure every 2 to 3 minutes while at the same time assessing for stimuli that initiated the response (such as a full bladder, impacted stool, or skin pressure). *The most serious danger in dysreflexia is elevated blood pressure, which could precipitate a CVA, myocardial infarction, dysrhythmias, or seizures. If the client has a Foley catheter, ensure that there are no kinks in the tubing. If the client does not have a Foley catheter, drain the bladder with a straight catheter. If symptoms persist, assess for a fecal impaction. If an impaction is present, insert Nupercaine cream into the anus, wait 10 minutes, and manually remove the impaction (Buchanan & Nawoczenski, 1987).*

- If blood pressure remains dangerously elevated, the physician may prescribe intravenous administration of diazoxide (Hyperstat). Other medications that may be used include nifedipine (Procardia) and hydralazine (Apresoline). *Diazoxide is an antihypertensive drug used in emergency situations to lower blood pressure in adults with dangerously high readings. Nifedipine and hydralazine are peripheral vasodilators that are administered to decrease the elevated blood pressure.*

Altered Urinary Elimination and Constipation

Depending on the level of the injury, the client with a spinal cord injury may have alterations in bowel and bladder function. Clients with injuries to the spinal cord at or above the S-2 to S-4 levels will have a neurogenic bladder, with deficits in control of micturition. Voluntary and involuntary bowel control is affected in the client with a lower motor neuron injury. Both bowel and bladder retraining are possible; if not, some form of assisted elimination is necessary. Although an indwelling catheter may be used in the acute phase of care, the goal is to reestablish a catheter-free state.

Nursing interventions with rationales follow:

- Monitor for manifestations of a full bladder. *Overdistention stretches the bladder and can lead to backflow of urine into the ureters and kidney; stasis of urine in an incompletely emptied bladder increases the risk for infection.*

- Teach client to use trigger voiding techniques prior to straight catheterization. These techniques include stroking the inner thigh, pulling the pubic hair, tapping on the abdomen over the bladder, and (in females) pouring warm water over the vulva. *These trigger voiding techniques stimulate parasympathetic nerve fibers to cause reflex activity and may facilitate voiding.*

- Teach self-catheterization to clients who will be able to carry out the procedure alone or with minimal assistance (Procedure 41–1 on page 1784). *Straight catheterization at regular intervals is part of bladder training because periodic distention and relaxation of the muscles of the bladder promote reflex bladder activity. In addition, self-care fosters independence.*

- Monitor residual urine throughout the bladder retraining program. *A residual urine amount of less than 80 mL after a triggered voiding is considered satisfactory (Drayton-Hargrove & Reddy, 1986).*

- Institute a bowel retraining program as follows:
  a. Assess usual patterns of bowel elimination to establish best times for individualized program.
  b. Maintain a high-fluid, high-fiber diet.
  c. Use stool softeners as prescribed; rectal suppositories and enemas may be used 30 minutes after meals to stimulate stronger peristalsis and facilitate evacuation.
  d. Maintain upright position if at all possible and ensure privacy.
  e. If client is unable to evacuate, digital stimulation or manual removal on a regular basis may be the most effective long-term management.

Procedure 41–1 Client Self-Catheterization

Self-catheterization on an intermittent basis (usually a part of client self-care at home) is a clean rather than a sterile procedure. The hands should be washed before and after the procedure, and the urinary meatus should be cleaned by washing with soap and water.

FEMALE SELF-CATHETERIZATION

- Attempt to void. If urine is not of sufficient quantity (at least 100 mL) or if you cannot void at all, do self-catheterization. *A large amount of residual urine means that more frequent catheterizations (every 4 to 6 hours) are necessary.*

- While sitting on the wheelchair or the commode, locate the urethra. Visualize the urethra by looking in a mirror, or palpate the urethra with a fingertip. *Visualization or palpation of the meatus is necessary for proper catheter insertion.*

- Lubricate the meatus with a water-soluble lubricant. *Lubrication facilitates the insertion of the catheter and reduces trauma to tissues.*

- Take a deep breath and insert the catheter tip 2 to 3 inches or until urine flows. *The catheter enters the bladder more easily when the sphincter is relaxed. The deep breath relaxes the sphincter. The female urethra is 1½ to 2½ inches long.*

- Hold the catheter securely and allow urine to drain until the flow stops. *Withdrawing and reinserting the catheter increase the risk of infection.*

- Withdraw the catheter and wash it with soap and water. Store the catheter in a clean container. *The catheter can be reused until it is too soft or too hard to be directed into and through the urinary meatus. Clean rather than sterile technique is usually used for self-catheterization at home.*

MALE SELF-CATHETERIZATION

- Attempt to void. If urine is not of sufficient quantity (for example, less than 100 mL) or if you cannot void at all, do self-catheterization. *A large amount of residual urine means that more frequent catheterizations (every 4 to 6 hours) are necessary.*

- Sit either on the commode or in the wheelchair. Hold the penis with slight upward tension and extend it to its full length. *Extending the penis straightens the urethra.*

- Lubricate the catheter from the tip to about 6 inches downward. *Lubrication is especially important for male catheterization because of the length of the urethra.*

- Take a deep breath and insert the catheter 6 to 7 inches or until urine flows. *The catheter enters the bladder more easily when the sphincter is relaxed. The deep breath relaxes the sphincter. The male urethra is about 6 inches long.*

- Hold the catheter securely and allow urine to drain until flow has stopped. *Withdrawing and reinserting the catheter increase the risk of infection.*

- Withdraw the catheter and wash it with soap and water. Store the catheter in a clean container. *The catheter can be reused until it is too soft or too hard to be directed into and through the urethra. Clean rather than sterile technique is usually used for self-catheterization at home.*

A bowel retraining program to regulate the bowel through reflex activity may be instituted in clients with upper motor neuron injuries. The client with a lower motor neuron injury loses the defecation reflex, and bowel retraining is more difficult.

Sexual Dysfunction

Sexual intercourse is often still possible for the client with a spinal cord injury. In men, the general rule is that the higher the level of injury the greater the potential to have reflexogenic erections, although ejaculation or orgasm may not occur, and fertility is usually lower. However, ejaculation may be stimulated and the sperm used to inseminate the client's partner, so that fatherhood is a possi-

bility. Men who have sacral level injuries do not have reflexogenic erections but may have psychogenic erections (Poorman, 1988). They are also more likely to remain fertile.

Women with spinal cord injury generally do not have sensation during sexual intercourse, but pregnancy is possible. However, pregnant women with a spinal cord injury are at increased risk for autonomic dysreflexia during labor and delivery. Birth control options should be discussed prior to discharge from the acute care setting.

A client with a spinal cord injury may be deeply concerned about alterations in sexual function. These concerns may lead to lowered self-esteem, altered self-image, or changes in feelings about self as an attractive and desirable person. The nurse should assess concerns and provide a climate that is receptive to discussion about sexuality and sexual function. Examples of objectives for sexual counseling for the client with a spinal cord injury are that the client will

- Understand how the injury has altered sexual functioning.
- Be aware of alternative ways of achieving sexual pleasure.
- Have a positive self-concept and body image (Spica, 1989).

Nursing interventions with rationales follow:

- Include data about sexuality when obtaining the nursing history and data base. *Sexuality is a private matter for most people, and the client may not discuss it unless the nurse introduces the topic.*
- Provide accurate information about the effect of the spinal cord injury on sexual function. *Accurate information gives the client a realistic picture of how the injury will affect sexuality.*
- Initiate a discussion with the client and partner of alternative means of gaining sexual satisfaction; these include the use of vibrators, and oral-genital and manual stimulation. *Alternatives to intercourse can meet sexual needs and help maintain the relationship with a significant other.*
- Refer the client for sexual counseling if appropriate, or to local support groups where questions can be answered by others with similar concerns. *Knowing that others have had similar experiences can decrease social isolation and provide a means of learning alternative methods of sexual functioning (Carpenito, 1994).*

Self-Esteem Disturbance

A spinal cord injury is often the result of sudden trauma. Within moments, a formerly independent, fully functioning individual is suddenly unable to move and faces enormous adjustments in social, economic, and personal roles and relationships. Body image, self-esteem, and role performance are all affected by the damage. As a result, the client often demonstrates behaviors that may be difficult for the nurse to handle: depression, denial, and anger are often seen in the period immediately after the injury. In addition to these responses, the young adult client may act out by making sexually overt statements.

Nursing interventions with rationales follow:

- Encourage the client to verbalize feelings about all aspects of physical function and care. *Talking provides a safe outlet for fears and frustrations and also increases self-awareness. Acceptance of self facilitates rehabilitation.*
- Encourage self-care and independent decision making. *Participation in self-care can promote positive coping; making decisions decreases feelings of powerlessness.*

- Help the client identify strategies to increase independence in desired roles; include both short- and long-term goals. Discuss assistive devices (such as hand-operated automobiles). *Identifying strategies to increase independence in the future fosters a positive self-concept and motivates the client to achieve rehabilitation goals.*
- Include family members and important others in discussions. *The realization that others do care and will continue to provide support is important in fostering positive self-regard.*
- Refer the client and family to support groups or for psychologic counseling. *Adjustment to change is more likely when the client and family seek peer and professional assistance.*

Other Nursing Diagnoses

The following nursing diagnoses may also be appropriate for the client with a spinal cord injury:

- *Self-Care Deficit* related to complete paralysis of lower extremities and weakness of upper extremities
- *Anxiety* related to unknown future following cervical cord injury
- *Risk for Disuse Syndrome* related to spasticity
- *Risk for Injury* related to impaired peripheral vision secondary to presence of halo traction
- *Impaired Skin Integrity* related to presence of pins in skull for traction placement
- *Risk for Impaired Skin Integrity* related to paralysis of all extremities and inability to change position
- *Altered Peripheral Tissue Perfusion* related to thrombophlebitis in leg secondary to immobility and loss of vasomotor tone
- *Powerlessness* related to hospitalization, inability to carry out self-care activities, and loss of normal role
- *Impaired Home Maintenance Management* related to paraplegia, use of wheelchair, and lack of finances to make modifications in home
- *Risk for Self-Directed Violence* related to inability to accept paralysis of lower extremities

Client and Family Teaching

Rehabilitation of the client with a spinal cord injury is an ongoing process that moves from intensive care through intermediate care to rehabilitation and then home care. Nursing interventions are necessary at all points in the process to prevent the complications of altered physical mobility and body functions, and to teach the client and family measures that promote independence in self-care. The research box on page 1786 discusses life satisfaction of individuals with spinal cord injury with implications for nursing care.

Discharge planning should be addressed even in the initial plan of care while the client is in the critical care

**Applying Research to Nursing Practice:
Life Satisfaction and Spinal Cord Injury**

■ ■ ■

This study of 31 individuals with spinal cord injuries was conducted to examine the widely held assumption that individuals with spinal cord injuries have less life satisfaction than the general population and would be better off not living (Dunnum, 1990). Data were collected through telephone interviews and were used to determine if correlations exist between life satisfaction and physical functioning. Results supported that life goals and financial situations were the major areas of concern of respondents but that satisfaction with one's life was not correlated with the neurologic deficits resulting from the spinal cord injury.

Implications for Nursing

Based on these findings, it is suggested that nurses in the acute care setting make referrals to social services and rehabilitation counselors as soon as possible after admission to help the client reassess life goals and to identify financial resources. Collaboration with these services may enhance the discharge planning process. In addition, nurses themselves should initiate discussion about life goals held prior to the injury and help the client set realistic goals for the future. Last, nurses should listen actively to the client's expressions of frustration, and should refer the client to support groups.

Critical Thinking in Client Care

1. What are the difficulties of planning interventions to help the client meet realistic goals? Consider the usual age and developmental level of these clients.

2. What resources are available in your area, and how can they be contacted?

3. Do you agree with the general assumption that individuals with spinal cord injury have less life satisfaction than the general population does? Why or why not?

- Self-care activities (activities of daily living, exercises, bowel and bladder programs, skin care)
- Mobility (use of assistive devices: wheelchair, crutches, special automobiles)
- Preparation of the home
  a. If the client is in a wheelchair, will steps, stairs, doors, or carpeted floors present physical barriers?
  b. If a special bed is necessary, have arrangements been made, and is it in the home?
- Psychologic support
  a. Independent activities
  b. Information about support groups
  c. Coping skills for client and caregiver
- Community resources
  a. Referral to a home-health agency for the client who is returning home
  b. Communication of the plan of care to the rehabilitation center if the client is entering this setting after leaving the acute care setting
  c. Physical rehabilitation
  d. Job retraining programs
  e. Rehabilitation resources and programs. For example, The National Spinal Cord Injury Foundation provides peer support and educational resources. The Regional Model Spinal Cord Injury Systems provides medical services, education, vocational training and job placement assistance, counseling, and follow-up services. The National Paraplegic Foundation provides counseling and information on resources. State vocational rehabilitation programs provide vocational retraining and job placement services. The National Wheelchair Association provides scheduled athletic activities.

Applying the Nursing Process

Case Study of a Client with a Spinal Cord Injury: Jim Valdez

Jim Valdez, a 19-year-old college sophomore, is admitted to the hospital by ambulance following an automobile accident. His family (father, mother, and sister) live 100 miles away and cannot visit often, although they are very concerned. His fraternity brothers have been to visit, but most of them seem uncomfortable and don't know what to say when they visit. On admission to the hospital, a CT scan of the spine shows a fracture and partial laceration of the cord at the C-7 level. Mr. Valdez stays in the intensive care unit for a week and is then transferred to the neurologic unit of the hospital. He is in halo traction. One night, he tells the nurse: "I wish I had just died when I got hurt. I don't think I can stand to live like this."

setting. Advance planning ensures continuity of care when the client leaves the hospital setting and either returns home or enters a rehabilitation center.

The following should be included in teaching the client and family about care at home:

Assessment

When Mr. Valdez is admitted to the intensive care unit, he has flaccid paralysis involving all extremities. He has no sensation below the clavicle or in portions of his arms and legs. His bladder is distended and bowel sounds are absent. Other assessment findings include BP, 90/56; P, 50; T, 97 F (36.1 C); arterial blood gases Ph 7.4, PaO_2 96, $PaCO_2$ 37, SaO_2 96%. Oxygen per nasal cannula is given at 2 liters per minute, and halo traction is applied. A Foley catheter is inserted into his bladder, and a nasogastric tube is inserted into his stomach and attached to low-pressure continuous suction.

After 7 days, Mr. Valdez is moved from the intensive care unit to the neurosurgical unit for continuing care and planning for transfer to a rehabilitation hospital in his home town. His vital signs have stabilized and are normal for his age; respirations and oxygenation are normal. Other neurologic assessments remain the same. He refuses to eat at mealtime, saying repeatedly, "I hate this food."

Diagnosis

The following nursing diagnoses are made by the nurses caring for Mr. Valdez:

- *Impaired Physical Mobility* related to paralysis of lower and upper extremities secondary to C-7 injury
- *Bowel Incontinence* related to lack of voluntary sphincter control secondary to C-7 injury
- *Grieving* related to loss of the use of his arms and legs and the effect of that loss on finishing school and getting a job
- *Risk for Altered Nutrition: Less Than Body Requirements* related to increased metabolic needs for body repair, depression, and refusal to eat hospital food

Expected Outcomes

The expected outcomes for the plan of care are that Mr. Valdez will

- Be actively involved in exercise programs.
- Have a soft, formed stool every second or third day.
- Verbally express his grief to parents and staff.
- Increase oral intake of foods sufficient to maintain body weight and nitrogen balance.

Planning and Implementation

The following interventions are planned and implemented for Mr. Valdez:

- Conduct passive exercises on all extremities four times a day.
- Provide progressive mobilization by initially raising the head of the bed 90 degrees (repeat two to three times during the first day of movement); if blood pressure remains normal, dangle Mr. Valdez for 5 minutes before transferring him to a chair.
- His usual time for a bowel movement is after breakfast; schedule retraining program for that time.
- Encourage a diet high in fiber and fluids. Mr. Valdez likes whole-wheat bread, orange juice, and cola. He does not like water.
- Promote grief work by providing time for Mr. Valdez and his family to express feelings. Explain to the family that his denial and anger are a part of a process that must be worked through before grief can be resolved.
- Determine food likes and dislikes and order preferred foods from the menu. Encourage his friends to bring in his favorite foods periodically.
- Take and record Mr. Valdez's weight every third day, using the bed scales.
- Monitor results of calorie counts and nitrogen levels conducted by the dietitian.

Evaluation

By the time Mr. Valdez is transferred to the rehabilitation hospital he is looking forward to learning how to use special equipment and getting his own motorized wheelchair. He is able to sit up in a chair without dizziness or hypotension. The use of ordered stool softeners combined with a high-fiber diet and fluid intake of 2000 to 3000 mL per day has maintained bowel elimination. Mr. Valdez and his parents have spent 3 hours talking about their feelings about the accident and Jim's future. Although the discussion is emotionally difficult, all three say they now feel much better. Mr. Valdez still has episodes of angry outbursts and tears, but he is more optimistic about what can be done and believes he can finish college. He selects foods from the menu each day and eats most of his meals, but he especially enjoys the times his friends bring in pizza or hamburgers. His weight has remained within normal limits for his height.

Critical Thinking in the Nursing Process

1. Considering Mr. Valdez's age and developmental level, do you think his emotional responses to his injury were appropriate? Why or why not?

2. Issues of sexuality are obviously important for the client with a spinal cord injury. How would you approach Jim Valdez about this topic?

3. What would be your response as a male or female nurse if Mr. Valdez would allow only male nurses to provide care.

4. Develop a care plan for Mr. Valdez for the nursing diagnosis *Post-Trauma Response*.

5. Outline a teaching program to help Mr. Valdez meet long-term urinary elimination needs.

The Client with a Herniated Intervertebral Disk

■ ■ ■

The intervertebral disks, located between the vertebral bodies, are made of an inner nucleus pulposus and an outer collar (the annulus fibrosus). The disks allow the spine to absorb compression by acting as shock absorbers.

A **herniated intervertebral disk**, also called a *ruptured disk, herniated nucleus pulposus,* or a *slipped disk,* is a rupture of the cartilage surrounding the intervertebral disk with protrusion of the nucleus pulposus (Figure 41–9). Perhaps few neuro-orthopedic disorders are as challenging as those involving the intervertebral disks. Clients with herniation (rupture) of a disk have not only excruciating pain but also limited mobility. These problems may in turn cause alterations in role function, coping, and the ability to perform activities of daily living.

A herniated intervertebral disk may occur at any adult age. However, it is more common as people enter middle age and age-related changes occur. The nucleus pulposus loses fluid content, and the disks are less able to absorb shocks. The disks become smaller and slip out of place more easily. Aging causes degeneration in the annulus fibrosus and the posterior longitudinal ligaments, and the vertebrae and disks are less able to respond to movement and are more easily injured.

Herniated intervertebral disks are more common in men than women. Most clients are between the ages of 30 and 50. The majority of herniated disks occur in the lumbar region (L-4 or L-5 to S-1); when disks herniate in the cervical region, they most commonly do so at C-6 to C-7. Multiple herniations are not common, occurring in only about 10% of all clients (Hickey, 1992).

Pathophysiology

A herniated intervertebral disk occurs when the nucleus pulposus protrudes through a weakened or torn annulus fibrosus of an intervertebral disk. This protrusion may occur anywhere along the vertebral column, but herniation of thoracic disks is uncommon. The protrusion may occur spontaneously or as a result of trauma, with trauma (such as lifting heavy objects or falling) causing about half of all cases. Rupture of the disk allows herniation of the nucleus pulposus in a posterolateral direction, with compression of the associated nerve root. The resulting pressure on adjacent spinal nerves causes characteristic manifestations, which vary with the location and the amount of protruding disk material (see the accompanying clinical manifestations box). Occasionally the herniation is central rather than posterolateral, with pressure on the spinal cord.

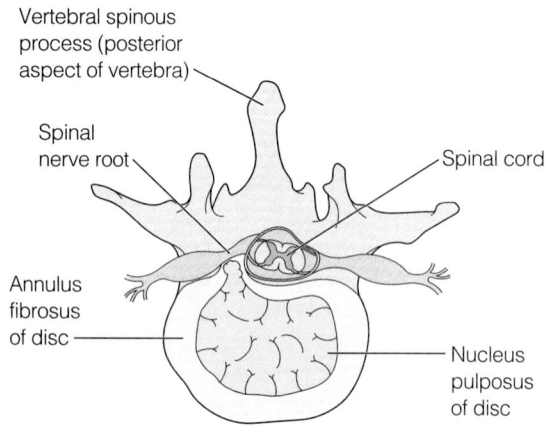

Figure 41–9 A herniated intervertebral disk. The herniated nucleus pulposus is applying pressure against the nerve root.

The herniation may be abrupt or gradual. Lifting incorrectly or suddenly twisting the spine can cause rupture with immediate intense pain and muscle spasms. Gradual herniation is the result of degenerative changes, osteoarthritis, or ankylosis spondylitis. Clients with a gradual herniation have a slow onset of pain and neurologic deficits.

Lumbar Disk Manifestations

The classic manifestation of a ruptured lumbar disk is recurrent episodes of pain in the lower back. The pain typically radiates across the buttock and down the posterior leg, although it may be experienced only in the leg. *Sciatica* is a term used to describe lumbar back pain that radiates down the posterior leg to the ankle and is increased by sneezing or coughing (the result of pressure on nerve roots L-4, L-5, S-1, S-2, or S-3, which give rise to the sciatic nerve). Sciatica may be elicited by straight-leg raising: the client feels pain when lifting one leg while dorsiflexing the foot of that leg. Sciatica pain varies in intensity, ranging from mildly uncomfortable to excruciating. It is aggravated by a variety of positions and activities, including sitting, straining, coughing, sneezing, climbing stairs, and walking or riding in a car.

Other manifestations include postural deformity, motor deficits, sensory deficits, and changes in reflexes. In about 60% of clients with ruptured lumbar disks, the normal lumbar lordosis is absent. When standing, the client typically has a slight forward tilt to the trunk, scoliosis of the lumbar spine, slight flexion of the hip and knee on the affected side, and paravertebral muscle spasms (Hickey, 1992). Motor deficits include weakness and in some clients problems with sexual function and urinary elimination. Sensory deficits include paresthesias and numbness. Knee and ankle reflexes are decreased or absent.

Cervical Disk Manifestations

Cervical disks that herniate laterally cause pain in the shoulder, neck, and arm. Other manifestations of lateral cervical herniation include paresthesias, muscle spasms and stiff neck, and decreased or absent arm reflexes. Central cervical herniations result in mild, intermittent pain; however, the client may also experience lower extremity weakness, unsteady gait, muscle spasms, urinary elimination problems, altered sexual function, and hyperactive lower extremity reflexes.

Collaborative Care

Considerations for the client with a ruptured intervertebral disk include identifying the location of herniation and determining whether conservative treatment or surgery is indicated. Nursing care is directed toward preparing clients for diagnostic tests and providing teaching and care for the client who has either medical or surgical interventions.

Laboratory and Diagnostic Tests

No laboratory tests provide the specific diagnosis of a ruptured intervertebral disk. Diagnostic tests are used to differentiate the cause of back pain; for example, back and leg pain is also caused by spinal tumors, degenerative processes, or abdominal disease. Assessing pain is an important part of diagnosis.

The following diagnostic tests may be ordered:

- Flat-plate *X-ray films* may be taken of the lumbosacral or cervical area to identify skeletal deformities and narrowing of the disk spaces.

- *CT scans* are used to identify disk rupture or protrusion and may provide definitive diagnosis. However, if the client has had previous back surgery or if more than one disk is involved, a CT scan may not clearly identify the ruptured disk (Way, 1994).

- An *MRI study* is used to image the vertebral elements, thecal sac, disks, cerebrospinal fluid, nerve roots, and spinal cord. This noninvasive examination is increasingly being used to provide initial diagnosis.

- *Myelography* with contrast medium illustrates areas of herniation but does not provide the detail found with CT or MRI. However, myelography is diagnostic in 80% to 90% of all cases and is used both to rule out tumors and locate the herniation (Way, 1994).

This examination is a fluoroscopic and radiologic examination of the subarachnoid space of the spinal canal, using air or a radiopaque contrast agent. The radiopaque agent may be either water-soluble (e.g., metrizamide) or oil-based (e.g., iophendylate) and contains iodine dye. If the client is allergic to iodine, air is used for the procedure. The client is taken to the radiology department and

---

Clinical Manifestations of a Ruptured Intervertebral Disk

L-4 to L-5 Level (Affects 5th Lumbar Nerve Root)

- Pain in hip, lower back, posterolateral thigh, anterior leg, dorsal surface of foot, great toe
- Muscle spasms
- Paresthesia over lateral leg and web of great toe
- Footdrop (rare)
- Decreased or absent ankle reflex
- Cauda equina syndrome (with complete nerve root compression): bowel and bladder incontinence, paralysis of lower extremities

L-5 to S-1 Level (Affects 1st Sacral Nerve Root)

- Pain in mid-gluteal region, posterior thigh, calf to heel, plantar surface of the foot to the 4th and 5th toes
- Paresthesias in posterior calf and lateral heel, foot, and toes
- Difficulty walking on toes

C-5 to C-6 Level (Affects 6th Cervical Nerve Root)

- Pain in neck, shoulder, anterior upper arm, radial area of forearm, thumb
- Paresthesia of forearm, thumb, forefinger and lateral arm
- Decreased biceps and supinator reflex
- Triceps reflex normal to hyperactive

---

placed on a fluoroscopy table. A spinal needle is inserted in the lower lumbar area, a small amount of cerebrospinal fluid is removed (to provide space for the contrast agent), and the dye or air is injected. The table is then tilted (head downward), and films are taken.

If an oil-based contrast agent is used, it must be removed at the end of the test. The client is positioned to allow the agent to move downward by gravity (because it is heavier than spinal fluid, it does not mix), and the agent is withdrawn. Water-based agents do not have to be removed, but the client must remain in a high-Fowler's position (the head of the bed is elevated 60 degrees) for at least 8 hours. Nursing implications for the care of a client having a myelogram are outlined in the accompanying box.

- *Electromyography (EMG)*, which measures electrical activity of skeletal muscles at rest and during voluntary contraction, may be conducted to identify specific muscles that are affected by the pressure of the herniation on the nerve roots.

Pharmacology

The client with a ruptured intervertebral disk is treated with medications to relieve pain and reduce swelling and muscle spasms. Pain is usually managed with non-

steroidal anti-inflammatory drugs (see Chapter 4). Muscle spasms are treated with muscle relaxants (see the box on page 1780).

Conservative Management

A ruptured intervertebral disk is usually managed conservatively with bed rest and medication unless the client is experiencing severe neurologic deficits. The goals of treatment are pain relief and healing of the involved disk by fibrosis. Conservative treatment is usually prescribed for a period of from 2 to 6 weeks. After that time, surgery may be considered.

Nursing Implications for Diagnostic Studies: Myelography

■ ■ ■

Preparation of the Client

- Ensure that client or family signs the informed consent form.

- Clients are usually NPO for 4 to 8 hours prior to the examination. The client may eat a light breakfast if the myelogram is scheduled for the afternoon.

- Assess for possibility of reaction to iodine dye (ask about allergy to seafood); document and communicate any allergy to the physician and radiology department.

- Administer enemas or laxatives as ordered to ensure visualization of lumbar spine.

- Administer prescribed pre-test medications, such as a sedative or diazepam (Valium).

Client and Family Teaching

- You won't be able to drink or eat anything for several hours before the test.

- The examination lasts about 1 hour.

- The position used to perform the examination will depend on the physician. You may have to lie on your stomach, sit and lean forward, or sit with the knees to the chest.

- A strap may be used to prevent falls, and the table will be tilted during the examination.

- A lumbar puncture ("spinal tap") is performed to inject the dye. A local anesthetic is used where the needle will be inserted. There may be a feeling of pressure during needle insertion. The needle is inserted below the level of the spinal cord.

- You may feel warmth or a burning sensation briefly as the dye is injected.

- Tell the physician if you experience pain.

- If an oil-based dye is used, it is important to remain flat in bed for at least 8 hours (the length of time will depend on physician preference and hospital policy).

- If a water-based dye is used, it is important to stay in bed with the head of the bed elevated for at least 6 hours (the length of time will depend on physician preference and hospital policy).

- The nurse will check your blood pressure, pulse, and respirations. The nurse will also check your ability to feel and move at least every 4 hours (or more often) after the examination.

Post-Examination Nursing Care

- Take and record vital signs and assess neurologic status as prescribed (and at least every 4 hours) for 24 hours post-examination. Record and report any changes.

- Assess the site of the lumbar puncture for leakage of cerebrospinal fluid or bleeding every 4 hours. Notify the physician of leakage or bleeding.

- Encourage increased intake of oral fluids to replace that withdrawn during the examination. (This may also help decrease a postmyelogram headache).

- Make sure that the client voids within 8 hours after the examination. If policy permits, allow male clients to stand at the bedside, or clients of either gender to use the bathroom. Notify the physician if the client has not voided within 8 hours.

- Administer analgesics as prescribed for postexamination pain, headache, or muscle spasms.

The treatment regimen depends on the severity of the manifestations but usually includes one or more of the following (Hickey, 1992):

- Remaining on bed rest
- Avoiding flexion of the spine (e.g., do not lift, bend, or twist)
- Wearing a support garment, such as a corset or cervical collar
- Following a prescribed exercise program
- Using a firm mattress
- Taking prescribed medications for pain, inflammation, and muscle spasms

Some clients achieve pain relief with *transcutaneous electrical stimulation (TENS)* or *transcutaneous neural stimulation (TNS)*. Electrodes are placed on the skin to stimulate the skin over the painful area.

Another pain-relief intervention is bed rest. It is important that the client use a firm mattress. The client should lie so that the pull on the affected nerve is reduced. Clients with lumbar involvement should usually flex the knees and elevate the head of the bed to about 30 degrees.

Although traction is of limited therapeutic value for clients with herniated lumbar disks, it may be ordered to encourage bed rest and limit activity (Mankin, 1991). Some clients report decreased muscle spasms while on traction.

After this period of bed rest, the client follows an exercise program designed by the physical therapist. This program includes the teaching of proper body mechanics and positioning, exercises to strengthen the back and decrease muscle spasms, massage, and the application of heat. Most clients report a good recovery after conservative management.

Surgery

Surgery is indicated for clients who do not respond to conservative management or have serious neurologic deficits. Several surgical interventions are used to treat a ruptured intervertebral disk. The type of surgery chosen depends on the location of the disk and the stability of the spinal column.

- *Laminectomy* is the removal of a part of the vertebral lamina. The surgery is done to relieve pressure on the nerves. It is often combined with removal of the protruding nucleus pulposus (*nuclectomy*). This is the type of surgery most often performed. Nursing care for the client having a laminectomy is discussed in the box on page 1792.
- *Diskectomy* is the removal of the nucleus pulposus of an intervertebral disk. Diskectomy may be performed alone or along with a laminectomy.

- *Spinal fusion* is the insertion of a wedge-shaped piece of bone or bone chips between the vertebrae to stabilize them. The bone is usually taken from a client donor site, such as the iliac crest.
- *Foraminotomy* is an enlargement of the opening between the disk and the facet joint to remove bony overgrowth compressing the nerve.
- *Chemonucleolysis* is the injection of the enzyme chymopapain (extracted from the papaya plant) into the nucleus pulposus. The enzyme hydrolyzes the nucleus pulposus, decreasing the size of the protruding herniation. This procedure has had several periods of popularity over the years but has never proven to be as successful as the more invasive types of surgery.

The location and size of the incision vary according to the surgeon's preference and the location and size of the ruptured disk. The posterior approach is taken for lumbar surgery. Either the posterior or the anterior approach may be taken for cervical disks.

A *microdiskectomy,* in which microsurgical techniques are used, is performed through a very small incision. This type of surgery decreases the possibility of trauma to surrounding structures during surgery and allows earlier postoperative mobility as well as a shorter hospital stay. See the Critical Pathway on page 1794 for a client following a microdiskectomy.

Nursing Care

Nursing care for clients with a herniated intervertebral disk focuses largely on pain management, both during conservative management and after surgery. Another problem clients often experience is constipation.

Pain

Clients with a ruptured intervertebral disk experience both acute and chronic back pain. Acute pain may be related to preoperative muscle spasms or nerve root compression. After surgery, the client may have pain at the site of the incision and in the surgical area.

Nursing interventions with rationales follow:

- Encourage discussion of pain. Assess the degree of pain and identify contributing and relieving factors. *Pain is a subjective experience. The nurse needs to assess it thoroughly before initiating interventions.*
- Maintain bed rest as prescribed. Teach the client how to logroll (to turn the body without bending the spine) when changing positions. *Restricting activity and proper positioning may prevent muscle spasms.*
- Use a firm mattress or place a board under the mattress. *A firm bed supports the spinal column and muscles.*
- Teach the client to avoid turning or twisting the spinal column and to assume positions that decrease stress on the vertebral column (for example, when in the supine

Nursing Care of the Client Having a Posterior Laminectomy

PREOPERATIVE TEACHING

- Demonstrate and ask the client to practice logrolling; explain that it will be done by the nurses for the first day or two, and then the client can do it alone. *To ensure healing, the spinal column must remain in alignment when turning and moving.*

- Explain the importance of taking pain medications regularly and of asking for them before the pain is severe. Include information about the possibility of the pain being much the same after surgery. *Pain is easier to control if medications are taken before the pain is severe. Pain may be the same following surgery for a herniated intervertebral disk because edema due to surgery irritates and compresses the nerve roots.*

- Demonstrate the use of a fracture bedpan and ask the client to practice its use. *The client usually must remain flat in bed for a period of time following surgery. A fracture bedpan is more comfortable for clients who must lie flat.*

- Explain that the client may need to eat while lying flat. *This position prevents flexion of the spine.*

- Demonstrate and ask the client to practice deep breathing, the use of the incentive spirometer, and leg exercises. Ask the client to practice these skills. *These measures prevent respiratory and circulatory complications.*

POSTOPERATIVE CARE

- Maintain the client in a position that minimizes stress on the surgical wound. For clients with cervical laminectomy:
  a. Elevate the head of the bed slightly.
  b. Position a small pillow under the neck.
  c. Maintain the position of the cervical collar.

  For clients with lumbar laminectomy:
  a. Keep the bed flat or elevate the head of the bed slightly.
  b. Place a small pillow under the head.
  c. Place a small pillow under the knees, or use a pillow to support the upper leg when the client lies on one side.
  These positions minimize stress on the surgical wound and suture line. A cervical collar provides stability and prevents flexing or twisting the neck.

- Turn the client every 2 hours, using the logrolling technique. Teach the client not to use the side rails to change position. Maintain proper body alignment in all positions. *The client's body is turned as a single unit (usually with a turning sheet) to avoid movement of the operative area. Pulling on the side rails puts stress on the operative area and may also cause misalignment of the vertebral column.*

- Monitor the client for signs of nerve root compression.
  a. Cervical laminectomy: Assess hand grips and arm strength, ability to move the fingers, and ability to detect touch.
  b. Lumbar laminectomy: Assess leg strength, ability to wiggle the toes, and ability to detect touch.

  Compare bilateral findings. Report muscle weakness or sensory impairment to the physician immediately. *Loss of motor and sensory function may indicate nerve root compression.*

- Assess for hematoma formation as manifested by severe incisional pain that is not relieved by analgesics and decreased motor function. Report these findings to the surgeon immediately. *A hematoma may form at the surgical site. If untreated, it may cause irreversible neurologic deficits, including paraplegia and bowel/bladder dysfunctions (Hickey, 1992).*

- Assess for leakage of cerebrospinal fluid. Assess the dressing for increased moisture. Check the sheets for wetness when the client is lying supine; check for clear liquid running down the back when the client is sitting or standing. Gently palpate the sides of the wound to detect a bulge. Use a Dextrostrix strip to assess any leakage for the presence of glucose, a positive indicator of cerebrospinal fluid. *Although uncommon, leakage of cerebrospinal fluid greatly increases the risk for infection of the wound and of the meninges.*

- Assess for nerve root injury. Assess the client's ability to dorsiflex the foot (lumbar laminectomy) and the client's grip strength (cervical laminectomy). Assess the client who has had a cervical laminectomy for hoarseness. Report hoarseness to the physician and further assess the client's ability to swallow. *Nerve root compression may cause permanent damage, resulting in footdrop (in lumbar laminectomy clients) and hand weakness (in cervical laminectomy clients). Damage to the laryngeal nerve may cause permanent hoarseness. Impaired ability to swallow puts the client at risk for aspiration.*

Nursing Care of the Client Having a Posterior Laminectomy (continued)

- Assess for urinary retention. The client should void within 8 hours after surgery. If the physician allows, let males stand to void. Compare intake and output for each 8-hour period. *All clients who have received a general anesthetic are at risk for urinary retention. The client who has had a lumbar laminectomy may have even more difficulty voiding as a result of stimulation of sympathetic nerves during surgery.*

- Assess for pain using a scale from 0 (no pain) to 10 (severe pain). Administer prescribed analgesics on a regular basis, or teach client to use PCA analgesia, if prescribed. Discuss client concerns about pain that is unrelieved by surgery. *Compression of the nerve root over time results in edema and inflammation. Because of surgery-induced edema, the client is likely to experience either the same pain or perhaps more severe pain in the period immediately after surgery. This pain usually persists for several weeks after surgery. In addition, many clients who have had a lumbar laminectomy have muscle spasms in the lower back, abdomen, and thighs for the first few days after surgery.*

- Assess for infection by taking and recording vital signs at least every 4 hours; report increased body temperature. Assess the wound and dressing for signs of infection: increased redness, drainage, pain, and pus. Use sterile technique to change dressings. *The surgical client is always at risk for infection; the*

client with a laminectomy is also at risk for arachnoiditis. This inflammation of the arachnoid layer of the spinal meninges results from wound infection or contamination during surgery and may cause the formation of painful adhesions.

- Encourage deep breathing and the use of the incentive spirometer every 2 hours; coughing may be discouraged. *Anesthesia and immobility depress respiratory function. Coughing may be discouraged because it can disrupt healing tissues, especially in clients having a cervical laminectomy.*

- Increase mobility as prescribed. (The time frame for ambulation is prescribed by the physician; the routine here is representative.) Clients often sit on the side of the bed and dangle their legs the evening after surgery or the first day thereafter. Many clients ambulate the first or second postoperative day. To help the client out of bed, first elevate the head of the bed. Then bring the client's legs over the side of the bed at the same time that the upper body moves into the upright position. Clients should not ambulate without assistance until they are no longer dizzy or weak. *Early ambulation increases respiratory and circulatory function and decreases the risk of thrombophlebitis of the lower extremities. The vertebral column should remain in alignment while the client sits and stands. Safety must be considered throughout care.*

position, flex the hips slightly). A small pillow may be placed under the knees (for clients with a herniated lumbar disk) or under the neck (for clients with a herniated cervical disk). *Correct body positions can decrease intradisk pressure.*

- Provide analgesic medications on a regular basis around the clock. *Intense pain can increase muscle spasms; maintaining serum levels of analgesics often prevents severe pain.*

Chronic Pain

The client with a ruptured intervertebral disk often has pain for an extended period of time. Despite conservative treatment or previous surgery, pain may be ongoing or intermittent. If previous surgery has not relieved the pain, the client may be depressed or angry. Caring for a client with chronic pain is frustrating, and the client is often regarded as difficult. The following interventions are useful for the client with chronic pain (McCaffery & Beebe, 1989, pp. 241–251):

- Treat the client's reports of pain with respect. *The client is the person experiencing the pain and is thus the expert about it.*

- Do not refer to the client as being addicted to pain medication. *All types of pain medications may be used legitimately to manage pain. Although the client may develop tolerance to a narcotic analgesic, tolerance does not imply addiction.*

- Monitor the client carefully for any changes in condition. *Significant changes in the client's condition may go unrecognized when pain is present for a prolonged period of time.*

- Ensure that the client understands the reason for the pain experienced. *It is important for the client to know what is causing the pain and what is being done to try to manage it.*

- Do not withdraw pain medications abruptly; suggest a gradual withdrawal for clients who have been taking narcotic or sedative medications for longer than 3

Critical Pathway for Client Following Microdiskectomy

	Preoperative	Date _____ 1st 24 hours postoperative
Expected length of stay: less than 24 hours		
Daily outcomes	Client verbalizes understanding of preoperative teaching including turning, deep breathing, incentive spirometer, mobilization, and pain management. Client demonstrates ability to cope. Obtain informed consent.	Client has stable vital signs and is alert and oriented. Client has a dry, clean wound with edges well-approximated, healing by first intention. Client has intact neurovascular assessments. Client manages pain with non-pharmacologic measures and/or oral medications. Client is independent in self-care with minimal assistance. Client is fully ambulatory. Client has resumed preadmission urine and bowel elimination pattern. Client verbalizes/demonstrates home care instructions. Client verbalizes strategies to prevent re-herniation. Client tolerates usual diet. Client demonstrates ability to cope with ongoing stressors.
Assessments, tests, and treatments	CBC, urinalysis Baseline physical assessment with a focus on respiratory status and gastrointestinal and urinary function Measure for anti-emboli stockings and apply. Anesthesia consult	Vital signs, O_2 saturation, mental status exam, dressing and wound drainage assessment q15min × 4; q30min × 4; q1h × 4 and then q4h and prn Neurovascular assessments to include distal pulse checks, capillary refill, skin color and temperature, muscle strength, movement, and sensation. Monitor for any numbness, tingling, or neurologic impairment. If there is serous drainage on the dressing, assess for presence of absence of glucose. Maintain dry, sterile dressing and reinforce prn.

	Preoperative	**Date _____** **1st 24 hours postoperative**	
Assessments, tests, and treatments (*continued*)		Monitor very carefully for changes in bladder/bowel function and check for distention. Assess lung sounds q4–8h. Assess gastrointestinal and urinary function q2–4h and prn. Intake and output every shift. Assess voiding—if unable to void, try suggestive voiding techniques or catheterize q8h or prn if unable to void. Remove and replace anti-emboli stockings for 30 minutes q8h	
Knowledge deficit	Orient to room and surroundings. Include family in teaching. Provide simple, brief instructions. Review preoperative preparation including hospital and surgical routines. Reinforce preoperative teaching regarding specific postoperative care: turning, deep breathing, incentive spirometer, mobilization, and pain management. Assess understanding of teaching.	Reorient to room and postoperative routine. Include family in teaching. Review plan of care and importance of early mobilization, as well as any activity restrictions. Complete discharge teaching regarding wound care/dressing change, follow-up care and appointment, signs and symptoms to report, medications: name, purpose, dose, route, frequency, food interactions, side effects, and diet. Instruct regarding the importance of a progressive exercise program with frequent rest periods and avoiding heaving lifting or driving until okayed by health care provider. Assess understanding of teaching.	
Psycho-social	Assess anxiety related to pending surgery. Assess fears of the unknown and surgery. Encourage verbalization of concerns. Provide emotional support to client and family.	Assess level of anxiety. Encourage verbalization of concerns. Provide emotional support to client and family. Provide information and on-going support and encouragement.	

➤

		Critical Pathway for Client Following Microdiskectomy (continued)

	Preoperative	Date _____ 1st 24 hours postoperative
Psycho-social *(continued)*	Provide information regarding surgical experience. Minimize external stimuli (noise, movement).	
Diet	NPO Baseline nutritional assessment	Advance to clear liquids; if tolerated, advance to full liquids/regular diet morning following surgery.
Activity	QOB ad lib until premedicated for surgery. Assess safety needs and implement appropriate precautions.	Maintain safety precautions. Instruct regarding log-rolling, and the importance of avoiding flexion, extension, stretching, flexing, twisting, and jarring movements. Bathroom privileges with assistance evening after surgery and begin progressive ambulation to tolerance morning following surgery, until fully ambulatory.
Medications	NPO except preoperative medications	IM, IV, or PCA analgesics Muscle relaxants Non-steroidal anti-inflammatory drugs Antibiotics if ordered IV fluids until adequate PO intake then intermittent IV device. Discontinue prior to discharge.
Transfer/discharge plans	Assess potential discharge needs and availability of support system. Establish discharge goals with client and family.	Probable discharge within 24 hours of surgery. Complete discharge instructions when fully awake and oriented and before discharge. Provide a written copy of discharge instructions. Make referral to physical therapy for progressive exercise program on an outpatient basis.

weeks. *Although the client may want to stop medications abruptly, abrupt cessation most often leads to further frustration when the pain again becomes severe.*

- Follow recommended guidelines for administering pain medications (see Chapter 4).

- Maintain written plans of care for pain management that are individualized and ensure continuity of care. *When the client makes several visits (for instance, to an emergency department or a pain clinic), written records help caregivers determine what is effective in managing pain and what is not.*

- Teach the client alternative methods of pain management. Consider the client's coping style when recommending methods. *Clients who have a passive coping style are often better able to manage pain by depending on others, taking medications, and resting. Clients with an active coping style are probably better able to manage pain by learning self-management methods, taking part in activities, and staying busy.*

- Develop effective methods of improving rest and sleep. *Problems with rest and sleep make pain management more difficult. Sleeping poorly at night contributes to decreased motivation, confused thinking, depression, and muscle aches.*

- Encourage the client to take part in regular physical and mental activities. *Physical and mental activities distract attention from pain and increase feelings of self-worth.*

- Include family members in the plan of care. *Family members often feel helpless to decrease the pain experienced by their loved one. Help the family to understand that the pain should not dictate what the family does and that the client is in control of pain management. The most important actions the family can take are to believe what the client says, not to argue with the client, and to validate that it is indeed difficult to cope with ongoing pain.*

- Identify client support systems and encourage their use. *Support systems include family members, friends, health care providers, church groups, support groups, and coworkers.*

- Refer the client to a physical therapist for an exercise program, if appropriate. *The client needs to know exactly what exercises to do, how many repetitions are recommended, for how long, and how often. The client should not exercise to the point of causing increased pain.*

- Assess the need for referrals (and make them if necessary) for the client who is depressed or anxious. *Anxiety and depression often are a part of long-term chronic pain, making pain management more difficult. Suggest that referrals for help with the frustration (rather than "depression") may make a significant difference in the client's ability to manage pain.*

Constipation

The client with a ruptured intervertebral disk often has problems with constipation because of reduced mobility and bed rest. Nursing interventions to alleviate and prevent constipation are important because straining to have a bowel movement can increase intradisk pressure, thus increasing pain.

Nursing interventions with rationales follow:

- Assess the client's usual bowel routine, including diet, fluid intake, and the use of laxatives or enemas. *Effective interventions are based on individualized needs.*

- Encourage a fluid intake of 2500 to 3000 mL per day unless contraindicated by the presence of renal or cardiac disease. *Adequate fluid intake facilitates the passage of feces.*

- Increase fiber and bulk in the diet. If the client is unable to tolerate increased fiber, consult with the physician about the use of stool softeners or bulk-forming agents. *Bulk and fiber promote regularity by retaining water in the large intestine.*

- Place the client on the bedpan or (if allowed) help the client to the bathroom or bedside commode at the usual time of bowel movements. Provide privacy. *Following normal bowel elimination routines and providing privacy contribute to regularity.*

Other Nursing Diagnoses

The following nursing diagnoses may also be appropriate for the client with a ruptured intervertebral disk:

- *Bathing/Hygiene Self-Care Deficit* related to pain
- *Risk for Disuse Syndrome* related to immobility
- *Situational Low Self-Esteem* related to dependence on others for care
- *Anxiety* related to the need for surgery and an unknown future
- *Altered Role Performance* related to the inability to work secondary to severe back pain

Client and Family Teaching

Clients with a ruptured intervertebral disk often have chronic pain. It is the nurse's responsibility to teach the client and family about chronic pain control, including specific interventions to alleviate pain. The nurse's role may be that of advocate and creative problem solver. Often the goal is to control pain so that the client can perform normal activities of daily living, rather than to reach a pain-free state.

It is important for nurses not to judge the client, and to experiment with a variety of pain-control measures until pain is relieved. Nonpharmacologic methods of pain management include relaxation techniques, guided

---

Client Teaching: Ruptured Intervertebral Disk

■ ■ ■

- Sleep on a firm mattress; use a bedboard if necessary.

- When lying in the supine position, flex the knees to approximately a 45-degree angle with a small pillow and use a small pillow under the head.

- Avoid any activities that flex the spine, such as bending or lifting, and do not twist the back.

- Follow your diet to maintain body weight or to lose weight if needed.

- Follow the prescribed exercise program.
  a. Lie flat on your back on the floor. Tighten your abdominal and buttock muscles and tilt your pelvis forward so that your lower back is flat on the floor (this is called a *pelvic tilt*). Hold the position for 3 seconds and repeat for prescribed number of times.
  b. Lying on the back on a firm surface, press the feet to the floor, tighten the abdominal muscles, and lift the upper half of the body off the floor. Hold the position for 3 seconds, and repeat as prescribed.
  c. Lying on your back on a firm surface, bring your knees up to the chest. Put your hands around your knees and raise the buttocks off the floor. Repeat as prescribed.
  d. Sit upright on the floor or a firm surface. Keep one leg straight and bend the other knee. Reach for the toes of the straightened leg. Switch legs. Repeat as prescribed.
  e. Stand upright. Squat down, flexing the hips and knees. Straighten your back. Stand upright by straightening the knees. Repeat as prescribed.

- Wear flat-heeled shoes that provide good support.

- Use proper lifting techniques. For instance, squat and use your thigh muscles to lift an object from the floor, and spread your feet to get a wide base of support when you lift while you are standing.

---

imagery, distraction, hypnosis, and music. Joining a support group may be an effective intervention in coping with and managing pain (Lewis, Frain, & Donnelly, 1993). Decreasing anxiety also may help decrease pain.

Another aspect of teaching involves the scheduling of analgesics. Although many people continue to believe that the use of analgesic medications causes addiction, it is now widely accepted that providing medications on a routine schedule is the preferred administration method. Clients are monitored for effectiveness of prescribed analgesics, and dosages are adjusted as necessary. Sometimes, rather than increasing the dose of an analgesic, adding another medication (such as an NAISD or anti-anxiety agent) may provide relief. Listening to the client is of utmost importance in determining methods of pain management.

A component of pain management is body positioning and body mechanics. Clients may be referred to a physical therapist for education about body mechanics and back-strengthening exercises. The accompanying box outlines information about back-strengthening exercises for use in teaching clients. Nurses should have the client demonstrate the exercises as a way of reinforcing teaching. Family members should be encouraged to participate in the exercises and learn healthy back habits.

Applying the Nursing Process

Case Study of a Client with a Ruptured Intervertebral Disk: Maree Ivans

Maree Ivans is a 50-year-old lawyer who lives in Montana. She sustains ruptured intervertebral disks at C-5 and C-6 when she is thrown over the handlebars of her bicycle while mountain biking. Mrs. Ivans is the mother of two young adults; her husband operates a small business.

Assessment

Immediately after the accident, Mrs. Ivans is taken to the nearest hospital by ambulance and evaluated by a neurosurgeon. Diagnostic tests include a CT scan, an MRI study, and X-ray films of the cervical vertebrae. The results demonstrate damaged ligaments and herniation of the C-7 disk. Mrs. Ivans is sent home wearing a cervical collar to stabilize the area and is instructed to limit activity. Twisting or turning the neck is prohibited. After 2 weeks at home, Mrs. Ivans complains of having no appetite, being unable to sleep at night, and having acute pain in the neck and shoulders. She also has numbness and tingling in several fingers of her left (dominant) hand. A major concern is whether she will be able to return to work and resume her usual activities. A cervical laminectomy with spinal fusion is being discussed.

Diagnosis

The nursing diagnoses for Mrs. Ivans are:

- *Pain* related to edema and muscle spasms

- *Impaired Mobility* related to altered comfort
- *Sleep Pattern Disturbance* related to pain with movement
- Risk for *Ineffective Family Coping: Compromised* related to altered life-style and lack of knowledge about the injury

Expected Outcomes

The expected outcomes for the plan of care are that Mrs. Ivans will

- State that her pain is decreased to the point of tolerance.
- Experience restful sleep as evidenced by statements of increased energy.
- Collaborate with her husband in discussing the injury and planning how best to meet household needs.

Planning and Implementation

The following interventions are planned and implemented for Mrs. Ivans through teaching:

- Take prescribed analgesics around the clock (when awake) to manage pain. Take prescribed muscle relaxants to control muscle spasms.
- Keep the cervical collar on at all times. Do not lift objects or bend or twist the neck.
- Follow a regular bedtime routine, sleeping on a firm mattress with a small pillow under the neck if desired.
- Drink 6 to 8 full glasses of water each day.
- Increase fiber and bulk in the diet.
- Eat several small meals each day rather than three large meals.

Evaluation

Following the acute care period, Mrs. Ivans's physical symptoms have decreased. She is able to manage her pain with oral analgesics and is sleeping better at night. She has begun a program of physical therapy and has continued to wear the cervical collar. After 2 months, Mrs. Ivans is so much improved that she begins to work half days. Her family has taken over cooking and cleaning responsibilities, and they remain supportive and understanding.

Critical Thinking in the Nursing Process

1. Discuss the rationale for taking Mrs. Ivans to the hospital by ambulance after the bicycle accident.
2. Mrs. Ivans has grown children and a husband who provided help and support. How might the teaching you provide differ if the client who sustained this injury were a young single mother of two small children?
3. Outline specific assessments that would be part of a nursing care plan for the diagnosis *Sensory/Perceptual Alterations: Tactile.*
4. Design a teaching plan for Mrs. Ivans for the diagnosis *Dressing/Grooming Self-Care Deficit.*

The Client with a Spinal Cord Tumor

■ ■ ■

Spinal cord tumors may be benign or malignant, primary or metastatic. They may arise at any level of the spinal column. Fifty percent of all spinal cord tumors are thoracic, 30% are cervical, and 20% are lumbosacral. They constitute about 0.5% to 1% of all tumors, and 15% are malignant (Hickey, 1992). Tumors of the spinal cord are seen equally in men and in women, and they most often occur between the ages of 20 and 60. They are rarely seen in the older adult.

Spinal cord tumors are classified by anatomic location as either *intramedullary* tumors or *extramedullary* tumors. Intramedullary tumors, which make up about 10% of spinal tumors, arise from within the neural tissues of the spinal cord; those that occur include astrocytomas, ependymomas, glioblastomas, and medulloblastomas (Tierney et al., 1994). Extramedullary tumors arise from tissues outside the spinal cord, with commonly occurring tumors including neurofibromas, meningiomas, sarcomas, chordomas, and vascular tumors.

Extramedullary tumors are further categorized as *intradural* (arising from the nerve roots or meninges within the subarachnoid space) or *extradural* (arising from epidural tissue or the vertebrae outside the dura). Extradural tumors are more common, occurring in 55% of all spinal tumors; 40% are intradural, and only 5% are intramedullary (McCance & Huether, 1994).

Tumors of the spinal cord are also classified as either primary or secondary (metastatic). Primary tumors, arising from the epidural vessels, spinal meninges, or glial cells, have an unknown cause. Secondary tumors are metastatic in origin, most commonly the result of malignancies of the lung, breast, prostate, gastrointestinal tract, or uterus.

Pathophysiology

Depending on their anatomic location, spinal cord tumors result in pathologic changes as a result of compression, invasion, or ischemia secondary to arterial or venous obstruction. Extramedullary tumors (whether benign or malignant) alter normal function through compression of the spinal cord, with destruction of white matter and eventual filling of the space around the spinal cord. Cord compression interferes with normal blood flow and membrane potentials, altering afferent and efferent motor, sensory, and reflex impulses. Compression of the spinal cord also causes edema, which can ascend the cord and cause further neurologic deficits. Intramedullary tumors both compress and invade. As the tumor grows within the cord, the cord also enlarges and white matter is distorted.

Neurologic deficits are related to how rapidly or slowly the tumor grows and to whether it is a soft or hard tumor.

Clinical Manifestations of Spinal Cord Tumors

Cervical Cord Tumors

- Ipsilateral arm motor involvement, followed by ipsilateral and contralateral leg involvement, followed by contralateral arm involvement
- Paresis of the arms and legs
- Stiffness of the neck
- Paraplegia
- Pain in the shoulders and arms
- Hyperactive reflexes

Thoracic Cord Tumors

- Paresis and spasticity of one leg, followed by paresis and spasticity of the other leg
- Pain in the back and chest
- Positive Babinski reflex
- Bowel and bladder dysfunction
- Sexual dysfunction

Lumbosacral Cord Tumors

- Paresis and spasticity of one leg, followed by paresis and spasticity of the other leg
- Pain in the lower back, radiating to the legs and perineal area
- Loss of sensation in the legs
- Bowel and bladder dysfunction
- Sexual dysfunction
- Decreased or absent ankle and knee reflexes

If the tumor grows very slowly, the cord may adapt to the neoplasm, with only minimal deficits. If the tumor is metastatic or rapidly growing, it often causes edema and rapidly occurring deficits. Soft tumors are of the same consistency as the spinal cord. If they grow slowly, they tend to elongate. Thus, the vascular supply remains constant, and the tumor is not affected by movement of the spinal column or normal changes in blood flow. Hard tumors do not conform to the available space and respond to vascular changes and spinal column movement by causing ischemia and irreversible cord damage (Hickey, 1992).

The manifestations of a spinal cord tumor depend on the anatomic location, level of occurrence, type of tumor, and spinal nerves involved. However, the general manifestations of a spinal cord tumor include pain, motor and sensory deficits, and changes in bowel and/or bladder elimination and sexual function. Pain is discussed here; specific manifestations by anatomic level are outlined in the accompanying box.

Pain is often the first manifestation of a spinal cord tumor. It is caused by compression of the spinal cord, tension on the spinal nerves, or tumor attachment to the proximal dura. The pain may be either localized or radicular. Localized pain is felt when pressure is applied over the spinous process of the involved area; this type of pain often accompanies metastatic tumors involving the vertebrae. Radicular pain is felt along the course of a nerve as a result of compression, irritation, or tension of a nerve root. The pain is often made worse by any activity that causes intraspinal pressure, such as sneezing or coughing.

Motor manifestations resulting from a spinal cord tumor include paresis and paralysis below the level of the tumor, spasticity, and hyperactive reflexes. The Babinski reflex may be positive. These deficits are the result of involvement of the corticospinal tracts.

Many different sensory manifestations may occur, depending on the location and level of the tumor. Lateral tumor growth and compression affect the lateral spinothalamic tracts, causing pain, numbness, tingling, and coldness. If the tumor involves the posterior columns, the senses of vibration and proprioception of body parts are affected.

Bladder and bowel elimination and sexual function are often affected. Bowel elimination deficits include constipation that may progress to paralytic ileus. Initial bladder elimination deficits include frequency, urgency, and difficulty in voiding and progress to urinary retention and a neurogenic bladder. In addition, the male client may be impotent.

Syringomyelia is a complication of some spinal cord tumors. In this condition, a fluid-filled cystic cavity forms in the central intramedullary gray matter. This syndrome causes pain, motor weakness, and spasticity (Hickey, 1992).

Collaborative Care

The medical management of the client with a spinal cord tumor focuses first on diagnosis. The type of treatment depends on the type of tumor, its location, and the client's condition.

Laboratory and Diagnostic Tests

The client with a spinal cord tumor undergoes many of the same diagnostic tests as does the client with a ruptured intervertebral disk. The following tests are often used to identify the tumor:

- A flat-plate *X-ray film* of the spine illustrates bony changes, such as erosion of the vertebral pedicles. Destruction of bone is usually the result of metastatic tumors.
- A *CT scan* or *MRI study* is used to visualize the tumor and may also demonstrate the site of cord compression.
- A *myelogram* may demonstrate complete blockage of cerebrospinal fluid circulation at the level of the tumor.
- *Electromyography (EMG)* may be performed to determine motor deficits.
- A *lumbar puncture* may be performed to obtain cerebrospinal fluid for analysis. The cerebrospinal fluid in the client with a spinal cord tumor is commonly *xanthochromic* (having a yellow color), has increased protein, has few to no cells, and clots immediately (this cluster of findings is called *Froin's syndrome*).

Pharmacology

The client with a spinal cord tumor is given medications to relieve pain and control edema. If the pain is severe and the result of a metastatic tumor, an epidural catheter may be inserted for narcotic analgesic administration. Pain management for clients with a spinal cord tumor is provided by narcotic analgesics (see Chapter 4).

Steroids, such as dexamethasone (Decadron), are administered to control edema of the cord. The steroids are given in high doses for 3 days and then are rapidly tapered off (Tierney et al., 1994).

Surgery

Intramedullary and intradural tumors are surgically excised whenever possible. Advances in microsurgical techniques and laser surgery have increased the possibility of tumor excision. Metastatic tumors may be partially excised to reduce cord compression; rapidly growing metastatic lesions may require surgical decompression to preserve motor, bowel, or bladder function.

The surgical excision is made through a laminectomy. The client with a tumor involving more than two vertebrae often has a spinal fusion and may also have rods inserted to stabilize the spinal column.

Radiation Therapy

Radiation therapy is used to treat metastatic spinal cord tumors for several different reasons. It may be used on an emergency basis to treat the client with rapidly progressing neurologic deficits. It may be used to reduce pain. Radiation may also be used following surgical excision of as much tumor mass as possible.

However, radiation of the spinal cord may cause the development of radiation-induced myelopathy. This complication of radiation exposure occurs over time, with manifestations of a Brown-Séquard syndrome developing about 12 to 15 months after therapy. The manifestations may progress to paraplegia, sensory loss, and loss of bowel and bladder control (Hickey, 1992).

Nursing Care

Nursing care for the client with a spinal cord tumor is individualized in accordance with the type of tumor and the type of treatment. The client with a benign tumor that is removed by surgery has different health care needs than does the client with a metastatic tumor, even though they may have similar neurologic deficits. However, the client with a spinal cord tumor (regardless of type) requires nursing care to monitor for neurologic changes, to provide pain management, and to manage motor and sensory deficits in order to preserve quality of life.

The assessments and nursing interventions for the client with a spinal cord tumor are similar to those described for the client who has a spinal cord injury or who is undergoing surgery for a ruptured intervertebral disk. The following nursing diagnoses may be appropriate for the client with a spinal cord tumor:

- *Anxiety* related to a diagnosis of malignant spinal cord tumor
- *Constipation* related to the effects of spinal cord compression.
- *Impaired Physical Mobility* related to weakness of lower extremities
- *Pain* related to compression of spinal nerve roots
- *Sexual Dysfunction* related to effects of spinal cord compression
- *Sensory/Perceptual Alterations: Kinesthetic and Tactile* related to edema and compression of the spinal cord
- *Sleep Pattern Disturbance* related to chronic pain
- *Urinary Retention* related to the effects of spinal cord compression

Following surgical treatment, the client may be transferred to a rehabilitation center or may go home for the recovery period. Referrals for home care, occupational therapy, and physical therapy often help the client regain functional abilities. Family members should be taught how to move the client in the bed and from the bed to a chair. They should also be taught how to provide physical care, care for any appliances (such as an indwelling catheter), and prevent or treat constipation.

Bibliography

■ ■ ■

Alfaro-LeFevre, R., Blicharz, M. E., Flynn, N. M., & Boyer, M. J. (1992). *Drug handbook: A nursing process approach.* Redwood City, CA: Addison-Wesley Nursing.

American Heart Association. (1993). *1993 heart and stroke facts.* Dallas: American Heart Association.

American Spinal Injury Association. (1992). *Standards of neurological and functional classification of spinal cord injury.* Chicago: American Spinal Injury Association.

Armstrong, S. (1994). Cerebral vasospasm: Early detection and intervention. *Critical Care Nurse, 14*(4), 33–37.

Barker, E. (1990). Action stat! Spinal cord injury. *Nursing, 20*(11), 33.

Biller, J. (1992). Medical management of acute cerebral ischemia. *Neurologic Clinics, 10*(1), 63–85.

Bronstein, K. S., Popovich, J. M., & Stewart-Amidei, C. (1991). *Promoting stroke recovery: A research-based approach for nurses.* St. Louis: Mosby.

Browner, C. M., Hadley, M. N., Sonntag, V., & Mattingly, L. (1987). Halo immobilization brace care: An innovative approach. *Journal of Neuroscience Nursing, 19*(1), 24–29.

Bryant, G. (1992). When your patient needs back surgery. *RN, 55*(7), 46–52.

Buchanan, L. E., & Nawoczenski, D. A. (1987). *Spinal cord injury: Concepts and management approaches.* Baltimore: Williams & Wilkins.

Cailliet, R. (1988). *Low back pain syndrome.* Philadelphia: F. A. Davis.

Carpenito, L. J. (1995). *Nursing care plans and documentation: Nursing diagnosis and collaborative problems.* Philadelphia: Lippincott.

Carpenito, L. J. (1992). *Nursing diagnosis: Application to clinical practice* (4th ed.). Philadelphia: Lippincott.

Ceron, G. E., & Rakowski-Reinhardt, A. C. (1991) Action stat! Autonomic dysreflexia. *Nursing, 21*(2), 33.

Crowell, R. W. (1986). Surgical management of cerebrovascular disease. *Nursing Clinics of North America, 21*(2), 297.

DiIorio, C., & Price, M. C. (1990). Swallowing: An assessment guide. *American Journal of Nursing, 90*(7), 38–41.

Dossey, B. M., Guzzeta, C. E., & Kenner, C. V. (1990). *Essentials of critical care nursing: Body-mind spirit.* Philadelphia: Lippincott.

Drayton-Hargrove, S., & Reddy, M. A. (1986). Rehabilitation and long-term management of the spinal cord injured adult. *Nursing Clinics of North America, 21*(4), 599–610.

Dunnum, L. (1990). Life satisfaction and spinal cord injury: The patient perspective. *Journal of Neuroscience Nursing, 22*(1), 43–47.

Esberger, K. K., & Hughes, Jr., S. T. (Eds.). (1989). *Nursing care of the aged.* Norwalk, CT: Appleton & Lange.

Fode, N. C. (1988). Subarachnoid hemorrhage from ruptured intracranial aneurysm. *American Journal of Nursing, 88*(5), 673–680.

Gaynor, S. E. (1990). The long haul: The effects of home care on caregivers. *IMAGE: Journal of Nursing Scholarship, 22*(4), 208–212.

Guthkelch, A. V., & Fleischer, A. S. (1987). Patterns of cervical spine injury and their associated lesions. *American Journal of Medicine, 147*, 428–431.

Halm, M. A. (1990). Elimination concerns with acute spinal cord trauma: Assessment and nursing interventions. *Critical Care Nursing Clinics of North America, 2*(3), 385–398.

Hickey, J. V. (1992). *The clinical practice of neurological and neurosurgical nursing* (3rd ed.). Philadelphia: Lippincott.

Hunt, W., & Hess, R. (1968). Surgical repair as related to time of intervention in the repair of intracranial aneurysms. *Journal of Neurosurgery, 28*, 14–20.

Kee, J. L. (1991). *Laboratory and diagnostic tests with nursing implications.* Norwalk, CT: Appleton & Lange.

Kidd, P. S. (1990). Emergency management of spinal cord injuries. *Critical Care Nursing Clinics of North America, 2*(3), 349–356.

Laskowski-Jones, L. (1993). Acute SCI: How to minimize the damage. *American Journal of Nursing, 93*(12), 22–32.

Lewis, D., Frain, K., & Donnelly, M. (1993). Chronic pain management support group: A program designed to facilitate coping. *Rehabilitation Nursing, 18*(5), 318–320.

Loebl, S., Spratto, G. R., Matejski, M. P., & Woods, A. L. (1991). *The nurse's drug handbook* (6th ed.). Albany, NY: Delmar.

Mankin, H. (1991). Back and neck pain. In J. D. Wilson, E. Braunwald, J. Isselbacher, R. Petersdorf, J. Martin, A. Fauci, & R. Root (Eds.), *Harrison's principles of internal medicine* (12th ed.) (pp. 116–124). New York: McGraw-Hill.

McCaffery, M., & Beebe, A. (1989). *Pain: Clinical manual for nursing practice.* St. Louis: Mosby.

McCance, K. L., & Huether, S. E. (1994). *Pathophysiology: The biologic basis for disease in adults and children* (2nd ed.). St. Louis: Mosby.

Meeker, M. H., & Rothrock, J. C. (1991). *Alexander's care of the patient in surgery* (9th ed.). St. Louis: Mosby.

Metcalf, J. A. (1986). Acute phase management of persons with spinal cord injury: A nursing diagnosis perspective. *Nursing Clinics of North America, 21*(4), 589–598.

Moore, K. (1994). Stroke: The long road back. *RN, 57*(3), 50–55.

Moore, K., & Trifiletti, E. (1994). Stroke: The first critical days. *RN, 57*(2), 22–28.

National Spinal Cord Injury Statistical Center. (1990). *Spinal cord injury fact sheet.* Birmingham, AL: University of Alabama at Birmingham.

Nolan, S. (1994). Current trends in the management of acute spinal cord injury. *Critical Care Nursing Quarterly, 17*(1), 64–78.

Ohman, K., & Spaniol, D. (1990). Halo immobilization: Discharge planning and patient education. *Journal of Neuroscience Nursing, 22*(6), 351–357.

Olson, E. V. (1967/1990). The hazards of immobility. *American Journal of Nursing, 90*(3), 43–48.

Passarella, P., & Gee, Z. (1987). Starting right after stroke. *American Journal of Nursing, 87*(6), 803–808.

Poorman, S. G. (1988). *Human sexuality and the nursing process.* Norwalk, CT: Appleton & Lange.

Porth, C. M. (1994). *Pathophysiology: Concepts of altered health status* (4th ed.). Philadelphia: Lippincott.

Purtilo, D. T., & Purtilo, R. B. (1989). *A survey of human diseases* (2nd ed.). Boston: Little, Brown.

Richmond, T. S. (1990). Spinal cord injury. *Nursing Clinics of North America, 25*(1), 57–69.

Rubin, M. (1988). The physiology of bedrest. *American Journal of Nursing, 88*(1), 50–58.

Schwenker, D. (1990). Spinal cord injury: Cardiovascular considerations in the critical care phase. *Critical Care Nursing Clinics of North America, 2*(3), 363–367.

Spica, M. M. (1989). Sexual counseling standards for the spinal cord injured. *Journal of Neuroscience Nursing, 21*(1), 56–60.

Swarczinski, C., & Graham, P. (1990). From ICU to rehabilitation: A checklist to ease the transition for the spinal cord injured. *Journal of Neuroscience Nursing, 22*(2), 89–91.

Swearingen, P. L. (1990). *Manual of nursing therapeutics: Applying nursing diagnoses to medical disorders* (2nd ed.). St. Louis: Mosby.

Swearingen, P. L., & Keen, J. H. (1991). *Manual of critical care: Applying nursing diagnoses to adult critical illness.* St. Louis: Mosby.

Swonger, A. K., & Matejski, M. P. (1988). *Nursing pharmacology: An integrated approach to drug therapy and nursing practice.* Glenview, IL: Scott, Foresman.

Tierney, Jr., L., McPhee, S., & Papadakis, M. (Eds.). (1994). *Current medical diagnosis & treatment.* Norwalk, CT: Appleton & Lange.

Walleck, C. A. (1990). Spinal cord injury: Neurologic considerations in the critical care phase. *Critical Care Nursing Clinics of North America, 2*(3), 357–361.

Way, L. (Ed.). (1994). *Current surgical diagnosis & treatment.* Norwalk, CT: Appleton & Lange.

Whitney, F. (1994). Drug therapy for acute stroke. *Journal of Neuroscience Nursing, 26*(2), 111–117.

Zejdlik, C. P. (1992). *Management of spinal cord injury* (2nd ed.). Boston: Jones and Barlett.

Nursing Care of Clients with Degenerative Neurologic, Neuromuscular, and Cranial Nerve Disorders

LEARNING OBJECTIVES

After completing this chapter, you will be able to

- Describe the pathophysiology of common degenerative neurologic, neuromuscular, and cranial nerve disorders.
- Identify laboratory and diagnostic tests used to diagnose these disorders.
- Discuss the nursing implications of the major categories of drugs used to treat clients experiencing neurologic disorders.

- Provide appropriate preoperative and postoperative care to clients undergoing neurologic surgery.
- Provide appropriate teaching to clients with a degenerative neurologic disorder and to their families.
- Use the nursing process as a framework for providing individualized care to clients with degenerative neurologic, neuromuscular, and cranial nerve disorders.

Degenerative neurologic disorders can affect the central nervous system and the peripheral nerves. By progressively disrupting cognitive processes or motor functions, disorders such as Alzheimer's disease and Parkinson's disease strike at the core of the client's sense of personal autonomy and well-being and can be psychologically and emotionally devastating to the client's family and caregivers. The long-term medical and custodial care that these clients require often cause financial ruin.

Ongoing medical research into degenerative neurologic disorders offers an increasing measure of hope to clients and their families. The discovery of genetic or biochemical markers associated with some of these disorders is leading to the development of effective screening and diagnostic tools. Also, the availability of new drugs may make it possible to halt the progression of the disorders in some clients, transforming the disorders into manageable conditions.

The nurse caring for a client with a degenerative neurologic disorder must plan and implement short-term and long-term holistic interventions for the client and the client's family. Acute exacerbations of degenerative neurologic disorders often require intensive, supportive nursing interventions directed at the client's immediate physical and psychosocial responses to illness. Equally important, the nurse can facilitate the long-term support of these clients by providing the client and family teaching and referrals to follow-up care in the community.

This chapter discusses major degenerative disorders of the central nervous system, the peripheral nervous system, and the cranial nerves. It also discusses toxic and infectious neuropathies, such as rabies and postpolio syndrome. Although rare, these neurologic disorders require intensive nursing care and support when they do occur.

▚ ▚ ▚   Disorders of the Central Nervous System   ▚ ▚ ▚

Alzheimer's disease, multiple sclerosis, Parkinson's disease, Huntington's disease, and amyotropic lateral sclerosis are considered the most physically and psychologically devastating of the degenerative neurologic disorders. Most of these disorders are believed to have a genetic or autoimmune cause. Despite ongoing research, the exact causes and pathophysiologic processes of these disorders are not fully understood.

The Client with Alzheimer's Disease

■ ■ ■

Alzheimer's disease (AD) is a form of **dementia** characterized by progressive, irreversible deterioration of the general intellectual functioning. Affecting an estimated 4 million adults in the United States, Alzheimer's disease is the most common degenerative neurologic illness and the most common cause of cognitive impairment (Porth, 1994).

There are two forms of Alzheimer's disease, distinguished by the age of onset. When the disease occurs in people over age 65, it is called *senile dementia of the Alzheimer's type (SDAT)*. When it occurs in people under age 65, it is called *presenile dementia*. Alzheimer's disease usually affects older adults, and more than 50% of cases are of the senile type. Presenile dementia occurs less frequently.

Although the incidence of AD increases with age, aging in and of itself is not the cause. The specific etiologic origin of AD is unknown. Genetic factors have been implicated, specifically, a defect on chromosome 21; this type of AD is considered a familial form of the disorder (Pallett & O'Brien, 1985). The role of neurotransmitters, such as somastostatin, norepinephrine, and dopamine, is also under investigation.

Memory loss is usually the first sign of Alzheimer's disease. Memory deficits are initially subtle, and family members and friends may not suspect a problem until the disease progresses and symptoms become more noticeable. Family members may also deny the symptoms and cover up the client's deficits until the client exhibits unsafe or extremely unusual behavior. Progression of the disease varies, but the course is one of deteriorating cognition and judgment with eventual physical decline and total inability to perform activities of daily living (ADLs).

Generally, presenile dementia progresses faster than SDAT. With the loss of the ability to perform even the most basic ADLs, the burden of meeting the client's needs shifts to the caregiver.

Pathophysiology

Several structural and chemical changes in the brain occur with AD, especially in areas of high cholinergic activity found in the hippocampus and the frontal and temporal lobes of the cerebral cortex. Characteristic findings in the brains of AD clients are loss of nerve cells and the presence of *neurofibrillary tangles* and *neuritic plaques* (Figure 42–1). These changes are manifested as progressive degeneration of the dendrites of the cortical cells and clustering and clumping of the axons. The neuritic plaques are microscopically visible atrophied cells. The

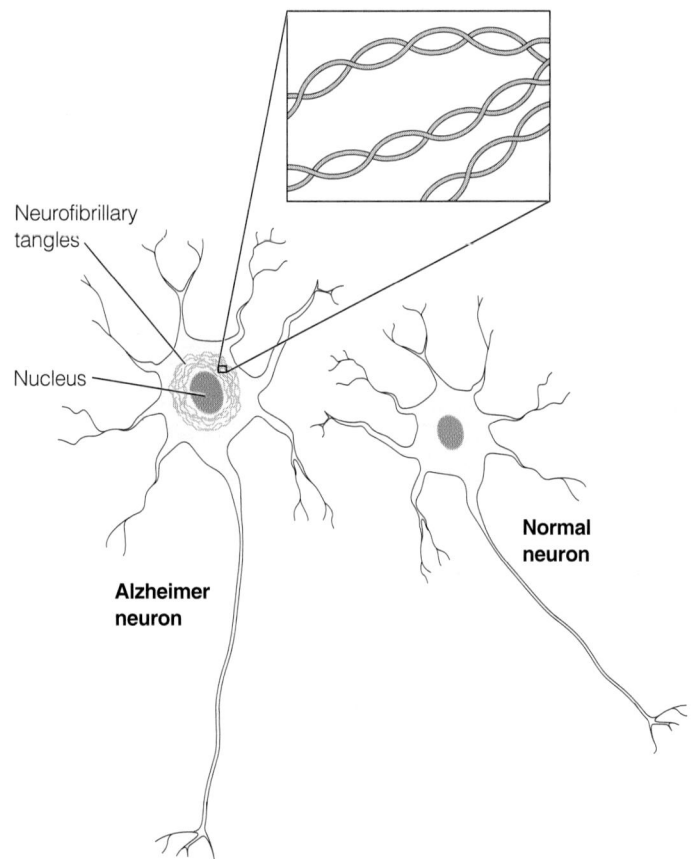

Figure 42–1   Neuron with neurofibrillary tangles seen in Alzheimer's disease.

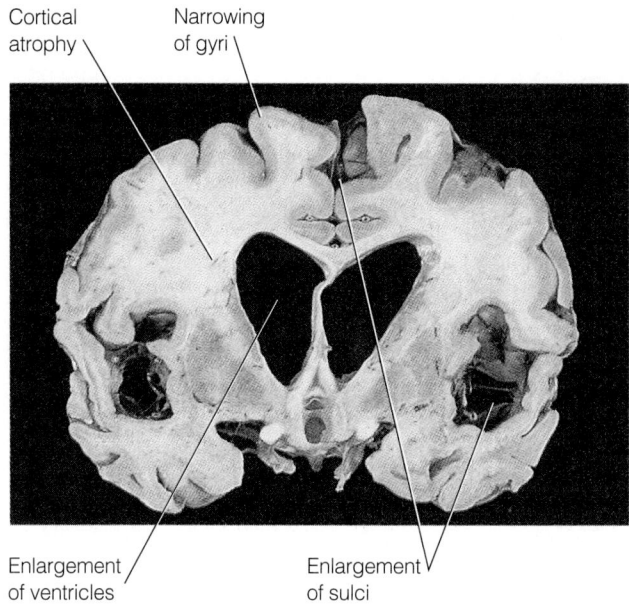

Cortical atrophy

Narrowing of gyri

Enlargement of ventricles

Enlargement of sulci

Figure 42–2   Changes in neuroanatomy associated with Alzheimer's disease. Note areas of cortical atrophy, narrowing of the gyri, enlargement of sulci, and ventricular dilation.

brain atrophies, and corresponding enlargement of ventricles and sulci is evident (Figure 42–2). Blood flow to the affected areas of the brain is decreased.

Chemical changes that occur with AD are related to decreases of neurotransmitters, such as **acetylcholine**, norepinephrine, serotonin, and somatostatin. These substances function in the transmission of nerve impulses. Loss of acetylcholine usually is evident first in the hippocampus, the area associated with recent memory and acquisition of new information. **Amyloid,** a starchlike protein, accumulates in brain tissue in clients with AD. Another metabolic change is decreased glucose use in affected areas of the brain.

As AD progresses, more areas of the brain are affected, with symptoms correlating to the affected areas of the brain. For example, neuronal and neurotransmitter losses in the parietal lobe result in problems with perception and interpretation of environmental stimuli; deficits in the frontal lobe cause changes in personality and emotional lability.

Alzheimer's disease is classified into three stages based on the client's manifestations and abilities, as outlined in the box on page 1806. It is important to note that the progression of AD varies for each individual and may not precisely follow the model. In the early stage of AD, a client typically appears physically healthy and alert; the client's cognitive deficits can go undetected unless thorough and periodic evaluations are performed. Usually, family members are the first to notice lapses in memory, subtle changes in personality, or problems in doing simple calculations. AD clients and families may consciously

or unconsciously compensate for cognitive deficits by adjusting schedules and routines. Clients may seem restless, forgetful, or uncoordinated.

In the middle stage of AD, memory deficits are more apparent, and the client is less able to behave spontaneously. Clients may wander and get lost, even in their own homes. Although progression of manifestations continues and orientation to place and time deteriorates, AD clients may still have periods of mental lucidity and engage in time-oriented conversations. Generally, however, clients exhibit increasing confusion and loss of their sense of time, which lead to changes in sleeping patterns, agitation, and stress. AD clients exhibit a decrease in the ability to make even simple decisions, and they are less able to adapt to environmental changes. Some AD clients develop severe attacks related to seemingly minor events; this reaction may result from a progressively lowered stress threshold (Hall & Buckwalter, 1987).

Sundowning is another observed behavioral change among AD clients. This behavior is characterized by increased agitation, time disorientation, and wandering behaviors during afternoon and evening hours; it is accelerated on overcast days.

Language deficits are common in the middle stage. They include *paraphasia,* use of the wrong word; *echolalia,* repetition of words or phrases; and scanning speech, in which the client appears to search for words. Eventually, total *aphasia,* absence of speech, may occur. Frustration and depression are common among AD clients as the full extent and implications of the deficits become obvious.

The AD client slowly loses the ability to perform simple tasks required for hygiene or eating because sequencing of tasks is lost. For example, the client may open a can of soup but not remember to pour it into a pan to heat it. Instead, the client might place the can directly on the burner and leave the heat on high even after a smoke alarm sounds. The AD client may falsely interpret the smoke alarm as a telephone ringing, a tornado warning siren, or an ambulance siren. Thus, safety is a high priority for the client in stage 2.

Sensorimotor deficits in the second stage of AD include *apraxia,* the inability to perform purposeful movements and use objects correctly; *astereognosis,* the inability to identify objects by touch; and *agraphia,* the inability to write.

Problems related to malnutrition and decreased fluid intake, such as anemia and constipation, may be evident. Sleep pattern disturbances are also common and are related to the loss of time orientation, sundowning phenomenon, and depression.

Stage 3 AD brings increasing dependence, with inability to communicate, loss of continence, and progressive loss of cognitive abilities. Common complications include pneumonia, dehydration, malnutrition, falls, depression, delusions, and paranoid reactions (Butler, 1990). The

---

Clinical Manifestations of Alzheimer's Disease

Stage 1: Lasting Approximately 1 to 3 Years

- Short-term memory loss: Client forgets location and names of objects and has difficulty learning new information; long-term memory is unaffected.

- Decreased attention span.

- Subtle personality changes: Client lacks spontaneity; denial, irritability, and depression are possible.

- Mild cognitive deficits: Client attempts to adjust to and cover up memory loss.

- Visuospatial deficits: Client has some problems with depth perception.

Stage 2: Lasting Approximately 2 to 10 Years

- Impaired cognition: Obvious memory deficits and confusion; loss of abstract thinking; astereognosis and agraphia; inability to do math calculations; loss of ability to tell time and time disorientation, manifested as "sundowning"; wandering behavior.

- Personality changes: Client becomes easily agitated and irritable; may have delusions or hallucinations.

- Visuospatial deficits: Client is unable to dress self; has poor spatial orientation.

- Impaired motor skills: Client paces and is restless at times; motor apraxia is evident when the client uses familiar objects.

- Impaired judgment: Diminished social skills; inability to drive a car; inability to make decisions (e.g., choose clothing).

Stage 3: Lasting Approximately 8 to 10 Years

- Cognitive abilities grossly decreased or absent: Client is usually disoriented to time, place, and person.

- Communication skills usually absent: Client is frequently mute.

- Motor skills grossly impaired or absent: Limb rigidity and posture flexion; bowel and bladder incontinence.

---

prognosis of a client with AD is poor, with an average life expectancy of 7 years from time of diagnosis. Death frequently occurs from pneumonia secondary to aspiration.

Collaborative Care

Following a thorough evaluation, AD clients and their families require extensive follow-up and support. Nurses in the community are frequently asked about changes family members notice in their older relatives. Teaching involves exposing the myth that older people inevitably have memory problems and show signs of confusion—normal aging does not entail progressive decline in cognitive functioning. Referral to the primary care provider for evaluation is indicated as soon as manifestations suggesting AD are discovered.

There is no existing cure for AD, and the main objective of care is to provide an environment that matches the client's functional abilities. Nurses, physicians, physical therapists, and social workers collaborate with the client's family to provide the AD client with the least restrictive environment in which the client can safely function.

Laboratory and Diagnostic Tests

Alzheimer's disease is diagnosed by ruling out causes for the client's symptoms. The only definitive method of diagnosis is postmortem examination of brain tissue.

An extensive workup is especially important, because the dementia may be due to a condition that is reversible or treatable. For example, misuse of medications by the older client can lead to overdosing and resulting confusion. Other categories of conditions that are excluded in the evaluation for AD which need to be considered and ruled out include the following:

- Psychologic causes: depression, delirium

- Infections: urinary tract infection (UTI), pneumonia

- Endocrine disorders: hypothyroidism

- Nutritional problems and fluid or electrolyte imbalances: hypokalemia, hyperglycemia, acidosis, dehydration, anemia

- Conditions causing hypoxia: congestive heart failure (CHF), chronic obstructive pulmonary disease (COPD), dysrhythmias

- Miscellaneous causes: pain, general anesthesia, trauma

The following laboratory and diagnostic tests are performed:

- *Complete blood count (CBC)* may reflect anemia from malnutrition, which develops when AD clients are not able to cook for themselves or feed themselves.

- *Electroencephalogram (EEG)* may reveal a slowed pattern in the later stages of the disorder.

- *Magnetic resonance imaging (MRI) and computed tomography (CT) scan* of the brain demonstrates enlarged ventricles and subarachnoid space.

- *Positron emission tomography (PET) scan* can show diminished glucose metabolism in the affected areas of the brain, notably the parietal and temporal lobes (Beal, Richardson, & Martin, 1991).

- *Psychometric evaluation* using the Folstein Mini-Mental Status Examination form (Figure 42–3) or a similar instrument reflects the loss of memory and other cognitive skills over time.

A new test for AD currently under investigation offers possible detection of AD before clinical manifestations become evident. The test involves measuring the speed of pupillary dilation in response to tropicamide, an eye medication commonly used to produce mydriasis and cycloplegia (Sciento et al., 1994).

Other tests may be performed, depending on the client's manifestations. For example, if the client has hypertension and memory changes, cerebral vascular studies are indicated to exclude multi-infarct dementia or other problems. Ruling out reversible dementia disorders requires evaluation of specific laboratory studies, such as thyroid function studies and measurement of electrolyte and vitamin levels.

Mini Mental Status Examination Form

Maximum Score	Score	
		Orientation
5	( )	• What is the (year) (season) (date) (day) (month)?
5	( )	• Where are we: (state) (county) (town) (hospital) (floor)?
		Registration
3	( )	• Name 3 objects: 1 second to say each. Then ask the patient all 3 after you have said them. Give 1 point for each correct answer. Then repeat them until the patient learns all 3. Count trials and record.
		Trials _____
		Attention and calculation
5	( )	• Serial 7s. 1 point for each correct answer. Stop after 5 answers. Alternatively, spell "world" backwards.
		Recall
3	( )	• Ask for 3 objects repeated above. Give 1 point for each correct answer.
		Language
9	( )	• Name a pencil and watch. (2 points)
		• Repeat the following "No ifs, and, or buts." (1 point)
		• Follow a 3-stage command: "Take a paper in your right hand, fold it in half, and put it on the floor." (3 points)
		• Read and obey the following: "Close your eyes." (1 point)
		• Write a sentence. (1 point)
		• Copy design. (1 point)

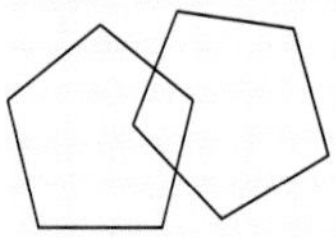

Points achieved/
out of 30 possible

Assess level of consciousness
along a continuum.

Alert   Drowsy   Stupor   Coma

Figure 42–3   The Mini-Mental Status Examination Form is an assessment instrument used for evaluating clients with cognitive impairment. The highest possible score is 30 points: Clients with scores less than 24 need further evaluation for dementia, depression, delirium, or schizophrenia. A score of less than 20 usually indicates presence of one of the disorders noted.

Pharmacology

Tacrine hydrochloride (Cognex) is the first medication specifically approved for the treatment of mild to moderate Alzheimer's disease. It has undergone clinical study since the mid 1980s; refer to the accompanying box for nursing implications of this medication. Tacrine is not a cure for Alzheimer's disease, but it does seem to improve memory in about 40% of patients. Ergoloid mesylate (Hydergine) has been prescribed for clients in stage 1 AD with limited success.

Frequently, depression accompanies AD and is treated with the appropriate medication. Antihistamines and tricyclic antidepressants that have high anticholinergic activity are usually avoided because they can actually increase AD symptoms. Optimally, the lowest effective dose is prescribed and administered.

Occasionally clients with AD require tranquilizers to manage severe agitation. For these clients, thioridazine (Mellaril) or haloperidol (Haldol) may be prescribed. It is important that these medications be used cautiously because of their potentially serious side effects.

Nursing Care

During the early stage of AD, nursing care focuses on assisting the client in making minor adaptations to his or her environment. As the client becomes progressively unable to manage self-care tasks, more adaptations are required. Equally important, the caregiver needs much support—both physical and psychosocial—as the client becomes increasingly dependent.

Nursing diagnoses discussed in this section include *Altered Thought Processes, Anxiety, Hopelessness,* and *Caregiver Role Strain.* However, safety measures and preventing nutritional problems associated with increasing incapacitation are also major areas of concern. For example, potential nutritional deficiencies and dehydration require that food and fluid intake be monitored.

Altered Thought Processes

Clients with AD often have memory deficits that make it difficult for them to function in a nonstructured environment. Many of the nursing interventions for this diagnosis need to be modified over time as the client continues to lose cognitive function.

Nursing interventions with rationales follow:

- Label rooms, drawers, and other items as needed. *Visual cues promote the highest degree of independence for the client possible.*

- Keep environmental stimuli to a minimum: Decrease noise levels; speak in a calm, low voice; and take an unhurried approach. *Minimizing sensory input and maintaining a calm manner may decrease anxiety.*

- Limit questions to those which require a simple yes or no response. *Questions need to be appropriate to the client's ability as decision-making and verbal skills decline.*

- Orient the client to the environment, person, and time as able; place large, easy-to-read calendars and clocks in the client's line of vision. Make references to the season or day of the week when conversing with the client. *Orient the client according to his or her level of ability; attempting to orient to precise time may not be possible in the later stages of AD.*

- Provide continuity in nursing staff. *This not only promotes consistency of care for the client but also allows the nurse to determine more accurately changes in the client's condition.*

- Repeat explanations simply and as needed to decrease anxiety. *Loss of short-term memory leads to loss of a point of reference; eventually, AD clients think they are experiencing everything for the first time.*

Anxiety

Managing the AD client's behaviors associated with anxiety, restlessness, and confusion is a major challenge confronting nurses and caregivers. Frequently, clients are relatively calm in the morning hours, only to experience increasing periods of agitation in the afternoon and evening hours. The AD client may even waken from the night's sleep with confusion, fearfulness, or panic attacks.

Nursing interventions with rationales follow:

- Assess for and note on care plan early behaviors of fatigue and agitation. *Early assessment of problems results in prompt intervention to promote rest or to remove the client from the situation causing anxiety.*

- Remove client from situations that are causing increased anxiety, such as noisy activities involving large groups. *High-stimulus situations may increase anxious feelings and agitation.*

- Keep daily routine as consistent as possible. *Providing a structured day enhances feelings of familiarity and decreases stress.*

- Schedule rest periods or quiet times throughout the day. *Fatigue contributes to anxiety and lowers the stress threshold.*

Hopelessness

As the client and family recognize the impact of AD on their lives, they may feel a sense of hopelessness and powerlessness. They may not have the coping skills to enable them to deal effectively with the diagnosis and anticipated problems. The increasingly degenerative, irreversible nature of the disorder tends to diminish hope; only the ability to adapt to the many problems can restore it.

Nursing Implications for Pharmacology: The Client with Alzheimer's Disease

TACRINE HYDROCHLORIDE (COGNEX)

Tacrine affects AD by blocking the breakdown of acetylcholine, thus causing an increase in the concentration of acetylcholine. Reasoning and memory improve in approximately 40% of clients receiving the medication. Tacrine may cause liver toxicity, jaundice, and increased gastric acid secretion because of its cholinergic properties.

Nursing Responsibilities

- Administer tacrine on an empty stomach; however, if nausea occurs, the client can ingest the drug at mealtime.

- Monitor for jaundice, increased bilirubin levels, and other signs of liver involvement, such as rising serum aminotransferase levels (AST, ALT). Therapy is usually decreased when the enzyme level exceeds 4 times normal limits and discontinued when the level reaches 5 times normal.

- Observe for gastrointestinal bleeding and gastric ulcer pain.

- Report other cholinergic-related problems: bladder outlet obstruction, seizures, and slowed cardiac rate.

- The dose of tacrine is titrated according to the client's tolerance. Initial dose is 10 mg four times daily for 6 weeks. Then, at 6-week intervals, an additional 10 mg four times daily is given until the maximum dose of 160 mg/day is reached. For the first 18 weeks, liver enzymes are monitored and the dose adjusted according to the client's tolerance to the medication. If the client tolerates the medication, ALT and AST levels need be monitored only every 3 months.

- Assess for improvement in AD symptoms, especially an improvement in reasoning, memory, and functioning in daily activities.

Client and Family Teaching

- Avoid suddenly stopping the medication; this can cause behavioral problems.

- Notify the physician promptly if jaundice, seizures, slowed heart rate, or difficulty urinating occurs.

- Smoking decreases the serum levels of tacrine; if the client smokes, the dose may need to be increased.

Nursing interventions with rationales follow:

- Assess the client's and family's response to the diagnosis and understanding of AD; encourage expression of feelings. *Understanding the client/family's perspective enables the nurse to dispel myths about AD.*

- Provide realistic information about the disorder; provide information at the client/family's level of understanding. Client and family may need to have separate sessions. *Factual information provides a foundation for decision making.*

- Avoid criticizing or judging expressed feelings. *An environment accepting of the expression of real feelings promotes both further expression of feelings and willingness to discuss other issues.*

- Support positive family bonds and enhance communication among family members; promote mutual positive regard. *Strong family relationships can provide direc-*

tion for living and convey a willingness to share the burden (Miller, 1990).

- Encourage the client to make as many decisions as he or she can. *Self-determination enhances a feeling of control over a situation and may give a sense of hope.*

- Encourage the client and family to seek spiritual guidance that previously inspired hope. *The client's church is a legitimate support system. Belief in God can inspire hope beyond present circumstances* (Carpenito, 1995).

Caregiver Role Strain

Most caregivers of clients with AD are spouses or other family members. Because AD is a chronic and eventually debilitating disorder, caregivers may feel overwhelmed by their responsibilities. The caregiving spouse faces not only the responsibility for the client's multiple physical demands but also economic and psychosocial stressors. Fear of the future, loss of income, loss of companionship

Caring for the Client with Alzheimer's Disease: Safety Considerations

■ ■ ■

Decreasing the Risk of Falls

- Assess the client's usual environment for hazards, such as throw rugs, electrical cords, and slick floors.
- Observe areas of special concern, such as the bathroom, kitchen, and stairs, and modify as needed; for example, provide skidproof surfaces, and mark stairs to show depth.
- Evaluate the client's muscle strength and gait; consult a physical therapist to plan exercises to increase strength and balance.
- Check the client's shoes for fit and support.
- Inquire about alcohol use and medications that affect balance or cause mobility problems; for example, antihypertensive agents can cause dizziness with position changes.
- Use night-lights and increase daytime lighting in dark areas, such as hallways.
- Keep traffic areas free from clutter.

Decreasing the Injuries Related to Cognitive Impairments

- Secure items that may be mistakenly ingested, such as cleaning preparations and house plants.
- Modify potentially unsafe areas, such as unenclosed porches.
- Provide double lock systems to outside doors and doors to rooms that are off-limits.
- Protect the client from fire hazards; for example, make matches and cigarettes inaccessible.
- Fence the yard with a locked gate to prevent the client from wandering.
- Modify the controls on the oven and stove.
- Adjust the water heater to a safe temperature.

General Safety Considerations

- Plan a calling system for emergencies; have children call at about the same time every day as a check.
- Ensure that the cognitively impaired family member has no access to objects in the home such as knives and guns.

and a mate—combined with fatigue—make the caregiver vulnerable.

Caregivers may become physically and mentally exhausted and socially isolated because of the overwhelming responsibilities of providing total care to the incapacitated family member. Nurses need to be especially vigilant when evaluating family situations. Many of the nursing interventions for this diagnosis relate to assisting caregivers with physical care of the client, providing referrals, and making realistic plans.

Nursing interventions with rationales follow:

- Teach the caregivers self-care techniques, such as taking rest periods and avoiding fatigue. *Fatigue adds to stress and potentially leads to poor decision making.*
- Have the caregivers list and partake regularly in activities they enjoy, such as walking. *Regular physical exercise decreases stress.*
- Refer the caregivers to local AD support groups and to the national AD association. Suggest books pertinent to the subject. *Explicit suggestions in locating support systems and providing specific information promotes coping.*
- Refer the caregivers to Meals-on-Wheels, home health, and other community services. *Community agencies can relieve some of the daily care burdens, thus providing time for other activities.*

Other Nursing Diagnoses

Many other nursing diagnoses may apply to clients and families dealing with Alzheimer's disease, among them:

- *Sleep Pattern Disturbance* related to frequent awakenings
- *Impaired Verbal Communication* related to cognitive impairment secondary to Alzheimer's disease
- *Risk for Injury* related to loss of ability to attend to details and tendency to wander
- *Self-Care Deficit* related to cognitive changes
- *Altered Role Performance* related to cognitive changes
- *Altered Nutrition: Less Than Body Requirements* related to inability to buy and prepare food
- *Altered Sexuality Patterns* related to cognitive impairment

Client and Family Teaching

Teaching for clients and families centers initially on explaining the disorder and exploring available support systems. Anticipate the need to reexplain the disorder and its consequences, partially because clients and families may be in shock or denial during the initial period of the disease.

If the client will be cared for at home, address safety considerations (see the accompanying box) as well as the caregivers' ability to meet the client's basic needs, such as maintaining hygiene and other ADLs. Adapt nursing interventions and teaching to the stage of Alzheimer's disease the client is experiencing.

In addition to explaining the anticipated changes with AD, suggest practical solutions to identified problems. It is important to evaluate both the client and caregivers; interventions need to be appropriate for the family's situation and resources. Maintaining the least restrictive environment that promotes safety for the client is a major goal of teaching. Using memory cues, such as labeling drawers to indicate the specific types of clothing and labeling rooms, can help orient the client and foster independence. Consistency in the environment and daily routine is an essential part of care.

Emphasizing realistic expectations means adjusting care and communication techniques to the client's level of ability; see the accompanying box.

Suggest obtaining a MedicAlert bracelet or pendant for the client in case the client wanders and is unable to identify himself or herself.

Evaluate caregivers for their ability to provide consistent care over a long period of time. Community services, including home health nursing, Meals-on-Wheels, and adult day care help caregivers manage the overwhelming responsibilities that caring for a client with AD presents. Periodic respite care during the initial stages, with plans for increasing assistance to meet the client's daily needs as the disease progresses, may be sufficient. Referrals to the appropriate agency for long-term care, including skilled nursing facilities, may be indicated. Family members may need assistance with adjusting to the idea of extended care but may be relieved to relinquish the physical care needs.

Communication Techniques for the Client with Alzheimer's Disease

■ ■ ■

- Face the client and talk directly to him or her; call the client by name.

- When first approaching the client, identify yourself.

- Use simple sentences and words with few syllables.

- Match speaking style to client's needs; that is, speak more slowly, clearly enunciating words.

- Ask one question at a time. Use questions that require only a yes or no response.

- Keep nonverbal communication relaxed and parallel to the verbal communication.

- Avoid giving the impression of being in a hurry; try to have a relaxed approach.

- Observe for anxiety—wringing hands, pacing, darting eye movements—and alter your approach to decrease anxiety.

- Avoid arguing with clients; do not insist on orienting client to reality; the client's point of reference may not be based in reality.

- Give plenty of time for the client with AD to process what you are trying to say; do not expect clients to perform skills beyond their abilities.

Note. Modified from "When your patient has Alzheimer's disease" (pp. 34–40) by J. M. Stolley, 1994, *American Journal of Nursing,* 94(8).

Applying the Nursing Process

Case Study of a Client with AD Who Lives at Home: Arthur Joste

Arthur and Ruth Joste have been married for 47 years; he is a retired history teacher, and she has been a homemaker. Both are 73 years of age. They have four children; two live in the same town, and two live out of state. For approximately 9 months, Arthur has noticed that he is having problems remembering friends' names and phone numbers; his wife has been asking him if he is driving in the correct direction when they go shopping.

Mrs. Joste has severe osteoarthritis and is unable to lift heavy objects or perform all but light housekeeping tasks. For about 18 months, Mrs. Joste has been aware of her husband's progressive cognitive decline, including forgetting current news from last night's newspaper; miscalcu-

lating checkbook balances; neglecting his hygiene needs; and confusing their children's and grandchildren's names. The Jostes are referred to a neurologist for evaluation.

Assessment

Ms. Martha Spital, RN, initially assesses Mr. Joste at the neurologist's office. She notes that he is unable to recall his home address without prompting, to name correct date (although he does know the day of the week), to subtract serial 7s more than twice, and to recall two of three objects. He is alert to his surroundings. Mr. Joste scores 21 of a possible 30 points on the Mini-Mental Status Examination. Mrs. Joste states that the problems seem to be getting worse with time and that she has had to "cover up" mistakes for her husband; as a result, they have limited their socializing over the past few months. Mr. Joste seems easily agitated, and his wife reports that his sleep habits are "jumbled"; he has long periods of wakefulness in the nighttime hours.

Following a thorough evaluation and diagnostic testing that ruled out other possible disorders, Dr. George informs the couple that Mr. Joste has senile dementia of the Alzheimer's type. Both have feared this diagnosis; they want to know how they can be sure that Mr. Joste has this disease and what they can do to prevent further decline. Both are obviously much saddened, and they verbalize their feelings of being overwhelmed. They do not want to tell their children, who nonetheless have made comments about "Dad" and his changed behaviors. The Jostes intend to remain in their home "for as long as we can."

Diagnosis

Nursing diagnoses for Mr. Joste and his family include the following:

- *Altered Thought Processes* related to deterioration of brain function and dementia
- *Self-Care Deficit* related to forgetfulness and declining physical abilities
- *Risk for Injury* related to decreased orientation
- *Caregiver Role Strain* related to multiple losses
- *Anticipatory Grieving* related to altered role performance secondary to loss of memory
- *Sleep Pattern Disturbance* related to time disorientation and daytime sleeping

Expected Outcomes

The Jostes are referred to Mr. Dixon Montane, a home health nurse. The expected outcomes of care specify that Mr. Joste will

- Remain free of injury.
- Navigate his home environment with modifications as needed.
- Attend with family members the available community support group for clients and families with AD.
- Participate at his maximum level in grooming and hygiene activities with prompting and supervision.
- Obtain a minimum of 7 uninterrupted hours of sleep a night.
- Mrs. Joste will participate in a minimum of two out-of-home activities a week.

Planning and Implementation

Mr. Montane makes a home visit to evaluate the environment, assess available support, and determine needs. He meets two of the Jostes' children, Dawn and Jay, who re-side in the same community; they are willing to participate as much as possible in providing care and modifying the home. Throughout the evaluation and planning process, Mr. Montane takes a realistic approach and encourages the family to plan for both short-term and anticipated long-term needs.

Mr. Montane discusses the importance of establishing and maintaining a consistent daily routine. He encourages Mr. Joste to take part in activities, such as walking and simple cooking, to decrease daylight sleep time and stimulate memory. Mr. Montane emphasizes the importance of matching activities to Mr. Joste's mental abilities in order to avoid frustration and increased agitation. Mr. Montane recommends labeling drawers with their contents, such as Mr. Joste's sock drawer. Labeling rooms may eventually be necessary.

Because his inability to comprehend and process information distresses and agitates Mr. Joste, Mr. Montane teaches the family to modify their communications to fit Mr. Joste's cognitive ability, such as using simple, direct statements and directions. Eventually, Mr. Joste will need much guidance with even the simplest activities; fewer and fewer options will be available to him. Mr. Montane recommends that family members keep background noise to a minimum because this may be a source of confusion. For example, turning the television off unless the family is watching a specific show.

After touring the home, Mr. Montane makes the following recommendations about safety:

- Remove throw rugs from hallways, and tack down any remaining carpets.
- Secure the kitchen, bathroom, and workshop cabinets as well as the controls on the oven and stove.
- Modify the doors so that negotiating locks requires a two-step system of unlocking, such as with a deadbolt and a key.
- Provide extra lighting in dark areas, especially a night-light in the bathroom.

Mr. Montane explains that Mrs. Joste will need assistance with housekeeping as Mr. Joste continues to decline. Mr. Montane provides referrals to community services, including Meals-on-Wheels, which can supply a daily meal. He also suggests that the Jostes obtain the services of a home health aide to provide daily hygiene care. Most of the remaining home maintenance needs can be met with the children's assistance.

Mr. and Mrs. Joste and the two children attend the weekly local support group meetings for Alzheimer's disease and related disorders for approximately 3 months; thereafter, Mrs. Joste attends with her daughter.

Mr. Montane makes monthly home visits to reevaluate Mr. Joste's disease progression and the family's abilities to meet his needs as well as their own. Mr. Montane stresses the importance of ongoing medical evaluation.

Evaluation

Six months after the initial home visit and family planning session, Mr. Montane's follow-up evaluation reveals that Mr. Joste

- Has not had a fall, burn, or other injury.

- Has periods of confusion when outside his home, but 90% of the time is oriented to place when inside his home.

- Attended several support group meetings until 3 months ago. Currently, his wife attends weekly, and she is occasionally accompanied by a daughter. She has continued to participate in their church and maintains contact with a few close friends. She is having increasing difficulty leaving her husband unattended for even a few minutes.

- Is able to clean and dress himself with prompting; he is not able to choose his own clothing articles. If the hygiene articles are "set-up" (e.g., if the toothpaste is placed on the toothbrush), he remembers to perform the hygiene activity. The children have been replacing buttons and zippers with Velcro closures on his clothing.

- Sleeps an average of 6½ hours a night with a half-hour nap in the afternoon; this pattern is consistent with his previous sleep pattern.

- Has for the past month seemed to be more easily agitated. He wanders from room to room, apparently looking for something. These behaviors are worse in the evening and on cloudy days. Mrs. Joste acknowledges her progressive inability to care for her husband.

Another family conference is held to discuss options. Mrs. Joste and the children want to carry out Mr. Joste's wish to remain at home; however, this is becoming more and more difficult. Mr. Montane offers options regarding placing Mr. Joste in a local adult day care setting, increasing the use of home health assistance, and placing Mr. Joste in a long-term care facility. The nurse adjusts the client's goals to reflect Mr. Joste's changing care needs, with special focus on preventing complications related to immobility and malnutrition.

Critical Thinking in the Nursing Process

1. Develop a tool to teach safety needs for the client and family with Alzheimer's disease.

2. List five interventions to decrease agitation in cognitively impaired older adults; give three additional examples of activities suited to an older adult with AD who has osteoarthritis.

3. You are caring for a client in stage 2 Alzheimer's disease. She is 5 feet, 5 inches (165 cm) tall and weighs 132 lb (59.9 kg); she has lost 3 pounds within the past month. The client has difficulty focusing on eating and is easily agitated. Describe your plan for ensuring that she takes in enough nutrition to meet her needs.

4. Contact the local department of human services and at least one home nursing agency; determine their criteria for qualifying for home care assistance for a person with AD from a home health aide. What is the cost of these services? Compare these costs to the cost of nursing home placement and day care services.

The Client with Multiple Sclerosis

■ ■ ■

Multiple sclerosis (MS) is a degenerative disease of the central nervous system (CNS) primarily affecting the white matter. MS damages the myelin sheath that surrounds nerves and eventually scars neuronal axons. The disease has acute and chronic forms. The symptoms of MS vary according to the area of the nervous system affected; the initial onset may be followed by a total remission, making diagnosis difficult. MS is characterized by periods of exacerbation, when symptoms are highly pronounced, followed by periods of remission. The end result, however, is progression of the disease with increasing loss of function.

Approximately 500,000 people in the United States have MS. Females are more frequently affected than males, and the incidence is highest in young adults (age 20 to 40). The disease occurs more commonly in temperate climates, including the northern United States. This association is established by approximately age 15, and moving to or from a temperate climate after that age does not change it. The annual incidence of MS is about 10 new cases per 100,000 people between 20 and 50 years. The risk is increased approximately 15-fold for close relatives of people with MS.

Because the disease affects young adults in the prime of life, the psychosocial and economic impact can be devastating. People with MS have to make adjustments to the body image changes while simultaneously adapting to the altered relationships and decreased earnings usually encountered with the disease. A once-healthy spouse becomes wheelchair-bound; a person once independent may eventually become dependent for even the most basic ADLs. The unpredictable course of MS is a challenge for long-term planning. There are four possible courses that MS may take, as described in the box on page 1814.

Although the precise etiologic mechanism is unknown, slow-acting viral agents combined with altered immune responses are being investigated. There is evidence of lymphocytes in the area of degeneration

Possible Clinical Courses of Multiple Sclerosis

■ ■ ■

- *Benign (20%):* Minimum deficits from few mild exacerbations; total or nearly total return to previous functioning.

- *Exacerbating-remitting (25%):* Attacks are more frequent and begin earlier; remissions are marked by less clearing of manifestations compared to the benign course; remissions last longer with stable manifestations.

- *Chronic-relapsing (40%):* Remissions fewer and symptoms more disabling and cumulative between exacerbations compared to the exacerbating remitting form. More symptoms are evident with each exacerbation.

- *Chronic-progressive (15%):* Onset insidious; no remissions; disabilities steadily more severe; similar to chronic-relapsing course, but slower in its progression.

Note. Adapted from *Merritt's Textbook of Neurology* (8th ed.) by L. Rowland (Ed.), 1989, Philadelphia: Lea & Febiger.

(demyelination), implicating an inflammatory response. Various stressors have been suggested as triggers for MS, including febrile states, pregnancy, extreme physical exertion, and fatigue. These precipitating factors can also cause a relapse of the symptoms during the course of the disease (Chipps et al., 1992).

Pathophysiology

The **myelin** sheaths are fatty, segmented wrappings that normally protect and insulate nerve fibers and increase the speed of transmission of nerve impulses. In multiple sclerosis, these myelin sheaths are destroyed in patches, called *plaques,* along the axon. See the Pathophysiology Illustrated art for Multiple Sclerosis on pages 1816-1817.

This **demyelination** of nerve fibers slows conduction of nerve impulses and sometimes results in the total absence of nerve transmission. Significantly more energy is required to conduct an impulse over a demyelinated nerve fiber than over a healthy nerve. Some research findings reveal that as much as 200 times the normal amount of energy is required to conduct an impulse past injured areas (Pallet & O'Brien, 1985). The neurons usually affected by MS are located in the spinal cord, brain stem, cerebral and cerebellar areas, and the optic nerve.

Clinical manifestations of MS vary according to the areas destroyed by demyelination and the affected body system (Figure 42–4). Fatigue is a common symptom of MS. Fatigue is often part of a group of manifestations related to spinal cord involvement. Other manifestations related to the spinal cord syndrome include weakness of the legs (frequently described as heaviness), weakness of the arms; paresthesia; and bowel and bladder problems. Foot drop, or *talipes equinus,* becomes evident with plantar flexion and increased muscle weakness of the lower extremities. Additional manifestations include *Uhthoff's sign,* a sudden worsening of motor symptoms following a hot shower or tub bath, and *Lhermitte's sign,* a bilateral "shocklike" sensation that is felt down the back, arms, and lower trunk when the client's neck is flexed. The client may have any of these manifestations.

Optic manifestations are frequently the first complaint and are part of the *cerebral syndrome.* Clients with optic nerve involvement report visual changes, such as partial blindness, blurred vision, and diplopia (double vision). Visual disturbances, notably clouded vision and blindness in part of the visual field, result from optic neuritis. The cerebral syndrome also includes memory deficits, personality changes, seizures, and hemiparesis.

Brain stem syndrome is another presentation of MS and involves changes in cranial nerves III through XII. Dysarthria presents with slurred speech. Explosive speech and scanning speech, in which the client seems to search for words, are later manifestations. Eye pain, nystagmus, and decreased visual acuity are common. The *cerebellar syndrome* is characterized by **ataxia**, uncoordinated, irregular gait and muscle movement; weakness; and **intention tremor**, tremor that occurs or is intensified when the client attempts voluntary movements.

About 20% of patients have a benign form of MS with only a few mild attacks that do not result in progressive deficits. Some people have MS and are not diagnosed until autopsy, when sclerotic lesions are noted. The course of MS is highly individualized and difficult to generalize because of its unpredictable nature. Most clients are able to live a relatively normal life span.

Cause of death related to MS is usually an infectious process, such as pneumonia or urinary tract infection. In rare instances, a rapid, acute onset of the disease occurs, usually in middle age, with sudden progression of neurologic symptoms, such as headaches, convulsions, coma, and death within 1 to 2 years.

Collaborative Care

Care of the client with MS varies according to the severity of symptoms present. The focus is on retaining the optimal level of functioning possible, given the degree of disability. Rehabilitation—physical, occupational/vocational, and psychosocial—is a cornerstone of a team

Text continues on page 1818

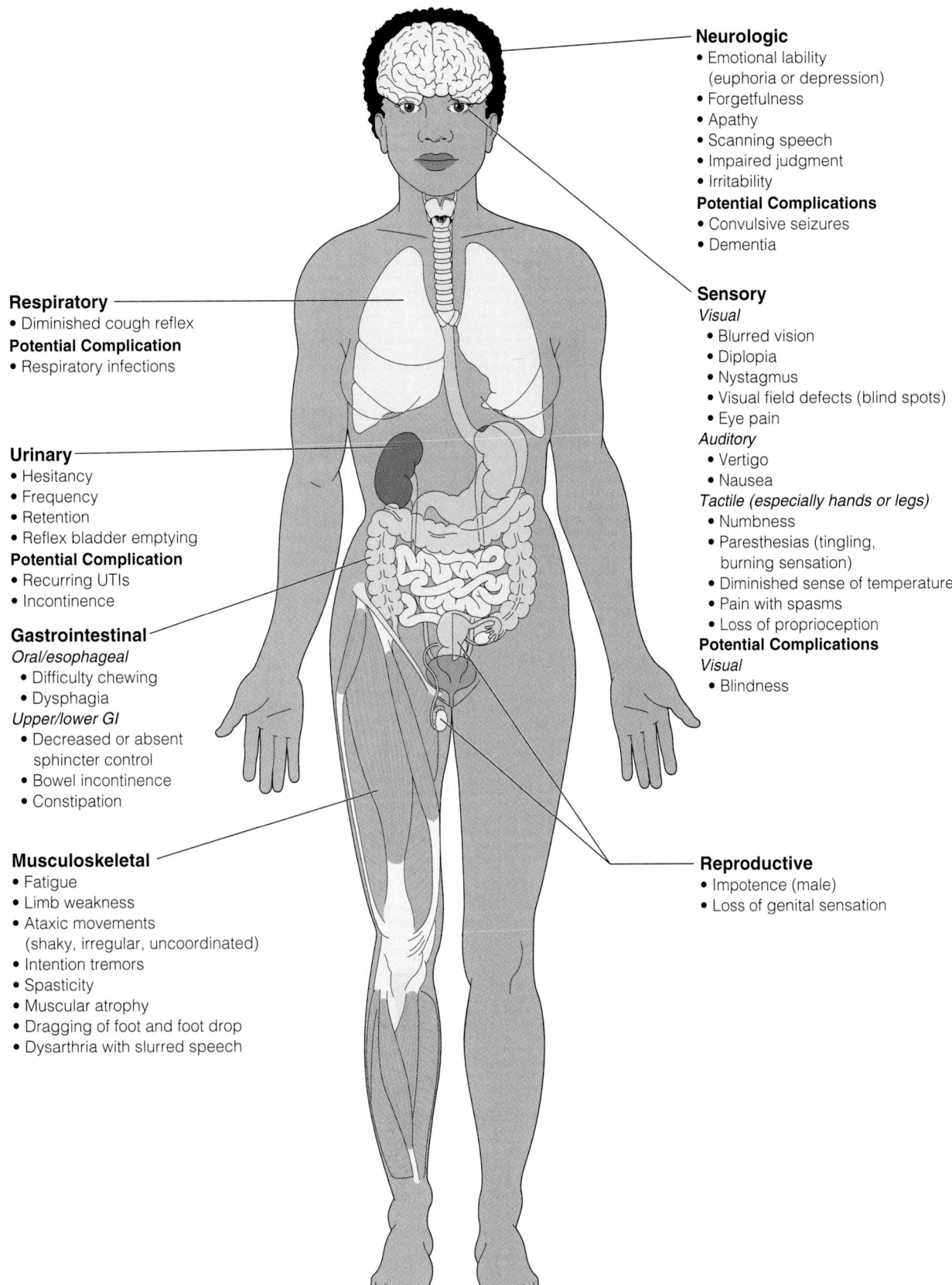

Neurologic
- Emotional lability
  (euphoria or depression)
- Forgetfulness
- Apathy
- Scanning speech
- Impaired judgment
- Irritability
Potential Complications
- Convulsive seizures
- Dementia

Sensory
Visual
- Blurred vision
- Diplopia
- Nystagmus
- Visual field defects (blind spots)
- Eye pain
Auditory
- Vertigo
- Nausea
Tactile (especially hands or legs)
- Numbness
- Paresthesias (tingling,
  burning sensation)
- Diminished sense of temperature
- Pain with spasms
- Loss of proprioception
Potential Complications
Visual
- Blindness

Respiratory
- Diminished cough reflex
Potential Complication
- Respiratory infections

Urinary
- Hesitancy
- Frequency
- Retention
- Reflex bladder emptying
Potential Complication
- Recurring UTIs
- Incontinence

Gastrointestinal
Oral/esophageal
- Difficulty chewing
- Dysphagia
Upper/lower GI
- Decreased or absent
  sphincter control
- Bowel incontinence
- Constipation

Musculoskeletal
- Fatigue
- Limb weakness
- Ataxic movements
  (shaky, irregular, uncoordinated)
- Intention tremors
- Spasticity
- Muscular atrophy
- Dragging of foot and foot drop
- Dysarthria with slurred speech

Reproductive
- Impotence (male)
- Loss of genital sensation

Figure 42–4   Multisystem effects of multiple sclerosis.

Multiple Sclerosis

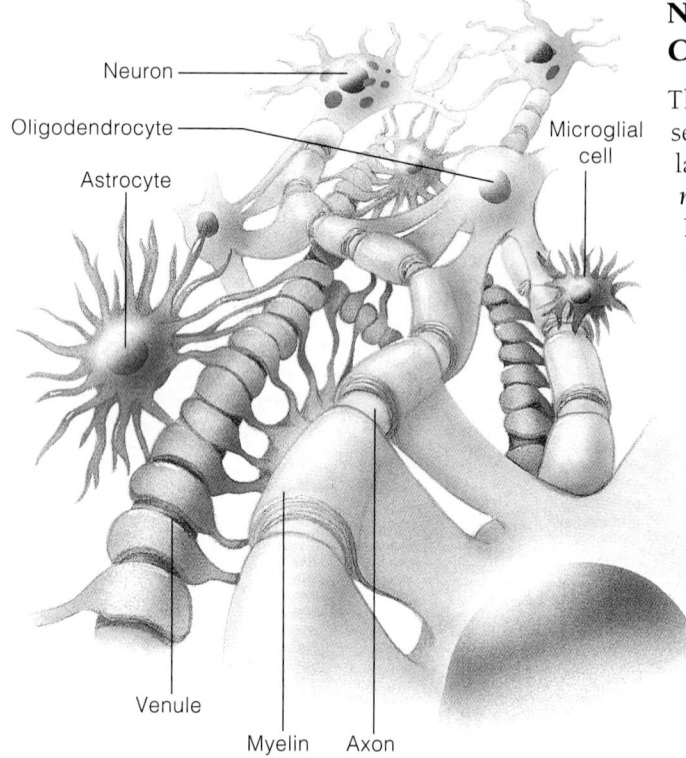

Neuron

Oligodendrocyte

Astrocyte

Microglial cell

Venule

Myelin sheath

Axon (Node of Ranvier)

Normal Anatomy of the Central Nervous System

The central nervous system (CNS) is composed of several cell types arranged in a dense, interconnected lattice. The basic functional cell of the CNS is the *neuron*, which transmits electrochemical impulses. Dendrites, thin projections extending from the neuron body, receive impulses that are passed down the neuronal axon for transmission to other cells. Myelin, a lipid-protein substance, surrounds the axons, insulating them and speeding nerve impulse transmission.

Neurons are surrounded by a network of neuroglial cells:

- *Astrocytes* support neurons and connnect them to surrounding capillaries and venules.
- *Microglia* are motile phagocytic cells.
- *Oligodendrocytes* wrap concentric layers of myelin around nearby axons.

Acute Attack

Multiple sclerosis (MS) is a demyelinating disease in which axonal myelin in the central nervous system is eroded, destroyed, and replaced by scar tissue.

An autoimmune process apparently triggered by genetic and environmental factors is believed to cause inflammation of venules in the CNS. This disrupts the blood-brain barrier, allowing lymphocytes to enter CNS tissue. These lymphocytes proliferate and produce IgG, an antibody that attacks and damages myelin and causes the release of inflammatory chemicals and edema. As the inflammation subsides, the myelin regenerates and manifestations of the disease subside.

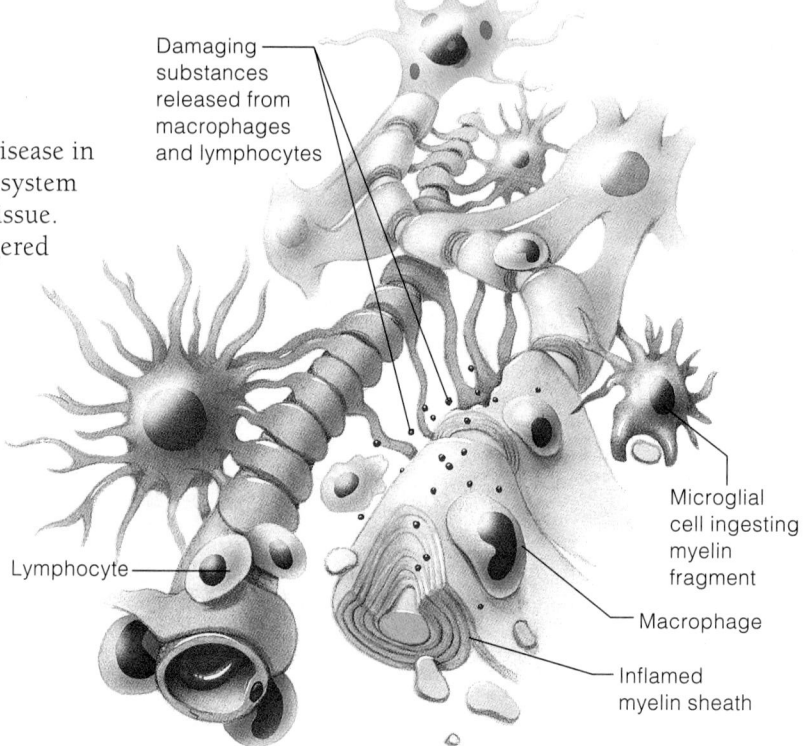

Damaging substances released from macrophages and lymphocytes

Lymphocyte

Microglial cell ingesting myelin fragment

Macrophage

Inflamed myelin sheath

Chronic Lesion

After repeated inflammatory attacks, myelin is irreparably damaged. Segments of axons become totally demyelinated and may degenerate. Astrocytes proliferate in damaged regions of the CNS (a process call *gliosis*), forming plaques. The plaques are scattered throughout the CNS, appearing as gray or pinkish lesions. The relapsing-remitting character of MS and the scattered areas of damage within the CNS account for the variable nature of MS manifestations.

Proliferating astrocytes

Damaged oligodendrocyte

Demyelinated axon

Abnormal Nerve Impulse Transmission

In an undamaged neuron, nerve impulses travel down the axon by "leaping" from one node of Ranvier to the next, thus greatly increasing the speed of impulse transmission. When nerve impulses travel down an axon damaged by MS, they are significantly slowed and weakened as they pass across the surface of demyelinated areas. Impulses may be blocked entirely when axons degenerate. The weakening or interruption of the transmission of nerve impulses and plaque formation within the CNS cause the manifestations of MS, including extremity weakness, paresthesias, visual disturbances, bladder dysfunction, and vertigo.

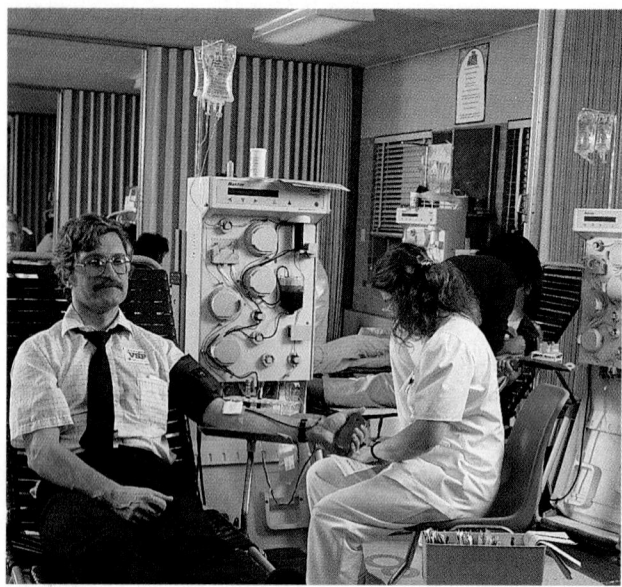

Figure 42-5 Plasmapheresis is a procedure used to separate the blood's cellular components from plasma. About 50 mL per minute is withdrawn to the centrifuge in the plasmapheresis machine. The plasma is replaced with donor plasma or colloids and returned to the client.

approach to treatment. During exacerbations, interventions shift to symptom control with a quick return to remission.

Laboratory and Diagnostic Tests

Diagnosis of MS is challenging because of the lack of uniform presentation of the disease. Initially, a thorough history and physical examination are completed, and their importance in establishing a diagnosis cannot be overemphasized. Diagnostic tests vary with the presenting complaints. MRI is the most definitive test available; however, several other laboratory and diagnostic tests are performed when establishing the diagnosis.

The following laboratory and diagnostic tests may be ordered:

- *Cerebral spinal fluid (CSF) analysis* reveals an increased number of T lymphocytes that are reactive with antigens, indicating the presence of an immune response in the client. Eighty percent of MS patients have elevated levels of immunoglobulin G (IgG) in the CSF. IgG may not be increased during the initial period of the disease.

- *MRI* studies are performed. Cerebral MRI detects multifocal lesions in the white matter. Serial MRIs may be performed to chart the course of the disease. MRI of the spinal cord or optic nerves can detect lesions in these areas.

- *CT* scan of the brain shows atrophy and white matter

lesions. In about 25% of clients with MS, enlarged ventricles are visible on CT.

- *Positron emission tomography (PET) scan* measures brain activity. In MS clients, the scan reveals areas with changes in glucose metabolism.

- *Evoked response testing* of visual, auditory, or somatosensory impulses shows sensitivity to delayed conduction.

- *EEG* is performed to determine brain activity. During the acute stage of MS, 35% of clients have slowed conduction time.

Pharmacology

A new medication, Interferon beta-1B, is being used for ambulatory patients with relapsing-remitting MS. It is administered every other day and appears to decrease the number of exacerbations. See the accompanying pharmacology box.

Pharmacotherapeutics during an exacerbation are aimed at decreasing inflammation to inhibit manifestations and induce remission. Frequently, the combination of adrenocorticotrophic hormone (ACTH) and glucocorticoids is used to decrease inflammation and suppress the immune system. Immunosuppressive agents, including azathioprine (Imuran) and cyclophosphamide (Cytoxan), are also used. Some centers are administering cyclophosphamide on a monthly basis to prevent exacerbations (Hickey, 1992).

Other medications are prescribed for treating the manifestations of MS, such as medications to relieve muscle spasms. More information on specific medications is presented in the accompanying box. Anticholinergics are sometimes administered for bladder spasticity; cholinergics are given if the client has a problem with urinary retention related to flaccid bladder.

Plasmapheresis

Some clinicians have successfully induced remission by using plasmapheresis in combination with ACTH therapy or other pharmacologic therapies. **Plasmapheresis,** also called *plasma exchange,* is a procedure that removes the plasma component from whole blood. The goal of this therapy is to remove inflammatory agents, such as T lymphocytes, through exchanging plasma while suppressing the immune response and inflammation.

An artery and a vein are accessed through two injection sites or by using a shunt, similar to hemodialysis. A blood cell separator removes antibodies from plasma via the arterial port. During the procedure, the nurse must be alert to signs of hypersensitivity reactions and fluid volume decrease. The blood then passes through a blood separator, where the plasma is removed (Figure 42-5). The cellular blood components are then retransfused using fresh-frozen plasma or albumin in place of the re-

Nursing Implications for Pharmacology: The Client with Multiple Sclerosis

IMMUNE SYSTEM-REGULATING MEDICATION

Interferon beta-1B (Betaseron)

Interferon beta-1B seems to reduce both the number and degree of relapses experienced by ambulatory clients with relapsing-remitting MS. Interferon beta-1B produces a decrease in the MS lesions in some clients. Some clients, however, develop a decrease in the absolute neutrophil count and increases in the levels of liver enzymes. Anxiety, confusion, and depression with suicidal tendencies also have been reported.

Other adverse reactions include pain, inflammation, hypersensitivity at the injection site, and generalized flulike manifestations. Some women experience menstrual disorders. However, these reactions decrease over time. Pregnant women should not take this medication.

Nursing Responsibilities

- Assess baseline parameters to evaluate drug side effects: psychologic profile, liver function tests, and CBC with differential.
- Evaluate client's baseline neurologic, sensory, and motor function. Monitor changes in condition and function.
- Monitor CBC and liver function tests every 3 months or as physician orders.
- Report if client is pregnant or breast-feeding.

Client and Family Teaching

- This drug may cause depression and thoughts of suicide; report these feelings immediately to the physician.
- The medication is reconstituted and should be discarded if it becomes discolored or precipitates out. Administer the medication within 3 hours of reconstitution. Rotate injection sites, and avoid any areas that are red or show other skin reactions.
- Seek follow-up care to monitor neurologic changes, CBC, and liver function.

ADRENOCORTICOSTEROID THERAPY

Adrenocorticotropic hormone (ACTH) (Acthar)

Prednisone (Deltasone, Meticorten, Orasone)

Methylprednisolone (Medrol, Solu-Medrol)

Adrenocorticosteroids are used both to sustain a remission and to treat exacerbations of MS. ACTH is usually given to induce a remission; it is administered intravenously for 1 week and may be followed by oral prednisone therapy. Another protocol involves administering ACTH intravenously for 3 days followed by intramuscular injections every 12 hours for 1 week (Hickey, 1992). The drugs are given to suppress the immune system, which has been implicated in the etiologic origin of MS. If the drug is used long term, the usual steroid precautions are indicated, such as monitoring for glucose intolerance, osteoporosis, and cataract formation. The drugs are used with caution in pregnant and lactating women (see Chapter 20).

Nursing Responsibilities

- Assess and record baseline data: vital signs, weight, motor and sensory function, mental status.
- Report cushingoid effects, weight gain, hypertension, or edema.
- Give oral corticosteroids with meals to prevent ulcer formation.

Client and Family Teaching

- Take medications as directed. Do not stop them abruptly.
- Consult the physician before receiving immunizations; live vaccines should not be used.
- Avoid people who have infections, and report early signs of an infection.
- Report tarry or dark stools to physician; avoid using medications, such as aspirin or other nonsteroidal anti-inflammatory drugs (NSAIDs) when taking corticosteroids.

MUSCLE RELAXANTS

Baclofen (Lioresal)

Dantrolene (Dantrium)

Diazepam (Valium)

Muscle relaxants are given to clients with MS to relieve muscle spasms. Baclofen and diazepam act by suppressing CNS reflexes that regulate muscle activity; neither drug affects muscle strength. Baclofen therapy should be discontinued over 1 to 2 weeks; sudden withdrawal may cause seizures and paranoid ideation. In contrast to diazepam and baclofen, dantrolene acts

➤

Pharmacology: The Client with Multiple Sclerosis (continued)

directly on skeletal muscles, and it may affect muscle strength. Dantrolene may cause hepatotoxicity and should not be administered when hepatitis or cirrhosis is present.

Nursing Responsibilities

- Evaluate baseline muscle strength and spasticity, range of motion (ROM), and dexterity.
- Maintain safety or fall precautions; dizziness and drowsiness are common side effects.
- For the client taking dantrolene, monitor liver function tests (enzymes and bilirubin) for signs of hepatotoxicity.
- Do not abruptly stop the administration of diazepam or baclofen.

Client and Family Teaching

- These drugs may cause sedative effects. Take appropriate safety measures; for example, avoid driving.
- Avoid CNS depressants (antihistamines, alcohol); they can increase the sedative effects of the medication.
- Continue follow-up care; if you are taking dantrolene, for example, liver function will need to be monitored.
- If you are taking baclofen, do not suddenly stop the medication.
- Increase fiber and fluids in the diet to prevent constipation.
- Change positions slowly to minimize dizziness and other effects of orthostatic hypotension.

IMMUNOSUPPRESSANTS

Azathioprine (Imuran)

Cyclophosphamide (Cytoxan)

Immunosuppressants are given to clients with MS because of the autoimmune component of the disease. Both medications can cause bone marrow suppression and increase the risk of cancer. Azathioprine may produce hepatitis. Toxic effects of cyclophosphamide include hemorrhagic cystitis, sterility, and stomatitis.

Nursing Responsibilities

- Monitor baseline parameters: CBC with platelet count and differential, urinalysis, liver function tests, hepatitis profile.
- Assess the client for signs of anemia: fatigue, lethargy, pallor.
- Watch for signs of bleeding.
- Protect against and observe for subtle signs of infection.

Client and Family Teaching

- Report signs of infection, bleeding, and anemia immediately.
- Drink at least 2 liters (about 2 quarts) of fluid a day, and observe urine for blood.
- Report jaundice immediately.
- Check oral cavity daily for changes or ulcers.
- Avoid becoming pregnant while taking these drugs.
- Obtain follow-up care, including frequent blood tests.

moved plasma. Nursing implications for clients undergoing plasmapheresis are presented in the accompanying box.

Surgery

Surgery may be indicated for clients who experience severe spasticity and deformity. However, physical therapy can prevent most severe problems. Foot drop from severe plantar flexion can be relieved with an Achilles tenotomy, a surgical procedure in which the Achilles tendon is transected.

Diet Therapy

Diet therapy is not used to treat MS, although several diets involving manipulation of fats are currently under investigation (Asbeck & Burns, 1992). Clients with MS may be overweight because of their inability to ambulate; depression may contribute to the problem because depressed people tend to eat more and burn fewer calories. Ideally, the client should maintain a weight as close to that recommended for the client's height and body type.

As MS progresses, the client's ability to prepare and ingest food is compromised. Changes in muscle tone, tremor, weakness, and ataxia all contribute to nutritional problems. Dysphagia also is a common problem. In particular, the diet must be adapted to accommodate changes in the client's ability to chew and swallow.

Rehabilitation

Physical and rehabilitative therapies are individualized to the client's level of functioning. The long-term goal is to enable the client to retain independence to the extent possible. One major intervention is to maintain and increase existing muscle strength.

Spasticity is managed with stretching exercises, gait training, and the use of braces, splints, or other assistive devices. To maintain balance, the client is encouraged to widen the base of support by standing with the feet slightly further apart. Walkers and canes may be weighted to provide support and balance for the ataxic client (Hickey, 1992).

A team approach to rehabilitation will provide for supportive services: speech therapy for problems with phonation, occupational therapy to maintain strength in the upper extremities and carry out ADLs, and occupational counseling. Consultations with a urologist are indicated for problems with urinary incontinence, urinary tract infections, retention, and impotence. Consultation with a respiratory therapist may be needed if the client develops chronic respiratory infections from inability to cough, move secretions, or breathe deeply, especially with increased debilitation.

Nursing Care

Care is individualized to client and family needs. Interventions vary with the acuity of exacerbations and the presenting problems. Many of the physiologic nursing diagnoses for a client with MS relate to the inability to

---

Nursing Care of the Client Undergoing Plasmapheresis

PREPROCEDURE CARE

- Teach the client about the procedure and what to expect, including what the machine looks like, the need for arterial and venous insertion sites, and the length of time of the procedure (2 to 5 hours). *Preparing the client by giving information, answering the client's questions, and addressing concerns decreases anxiety.*

- Check with physician about holding medications until after the procedure. *Medications may be removed from the body as an incidental part of the plasmapheresis process.*

- Assess the client's vital signs and weight. *Baseline parameters are necessary to evaluate for fluid imbalances and response to therapy.*

- Assess CBC, platelet count, and clotting studies. *Clients undergoing plasmapheresis are at high risk for anemia and coagulation problems secondary to hemolysis of cells.*

- Check blood type and crossmatch for replacement blood products. *Hypersensitivity reactions can occur, and close monitoring is important.*

CARE DURING THE PROCEDURE AND POSTPROCEDURE

- Observe the client for dizziness or hypotension. *Hypovolemia is a complication of plasma exchange,* especially during the procedure when up to 15% of the client's blood volume is in the cell separator.

- Apply pressure dressing to access site(s). *Direct pressure helps decrease or prevent bleeding.*

- Monitor for infection and bruises at the intravenous port site. *The site of vascular access is at risk for complications and must be routinely and carefully assessed for signs of infection and for bleeding or hematoma formation.*

- Monitor electrolytes and signs of electrolyte loss. Report imbalances, and replace electrolytes as ordered. Observe for circumoral tingling, Chvostek's and Trousseau's signs if calcium levels are low, and cardiac dysrhythmias and leg cramps if potassium levels are low. *Hypocalcemia and hypokalemia may occur. Hypocalcemia occurs because the anticoagulant citrate dextrose binds with calcium.*

- Reevaluate preprocedure laboratory data, especially CBC, platelet count, and clotting times. *The cell-separating process can damage cells; anticoagulation is part of the procedure.*

perform ADLs: for example, *Self-Care Deficit, Impaired Home Maintenance Management,* and *Powerlessness.* Others reflect problems with musculoskeletal changes or altered nerve conduction, for example, *Impaired Physical Mobility, Ineffective Breathing Pattern, Social Isolation, Bowel Incontinence,* and *Urinary Incontinence.* The nursing diagnoses discussed in this section are *Fatigue* and *Self-Care Deficit.*

Fatigue

Fatigue affects every aspect of the MS client's life—the ability to remain independent and perform self-care, sexual function, mobility, airway clearance and, ultimately, self-concept and coping. A great deal of teaching is needed to assist the client and family in understanding fatigue and how to adapt. Clients and families need assistance in confronting fatigue in a society in which energy and vigor are highly valued.

Nursing interventions with rationales follow:

- Encourage the client to discuss fatigue; assess degree of fatigue and identify contributing factors. *Fatigue is a subjective experience that needs to be evaluated thoroughly BEFORE planning can begin (Carpenito, 1995). Contributing factors can be modified to help clients enhance their ability to perform self-care.*

- Arrange daily activities to include rest periods. *Rest is essential to manage feelings of fatigue; periods of relaxation can replenish energy reserves.*

- Help the client set priorities. Ask the client to consider which activities are really necessary. *Prioritizing activities promotes independence and self-control (Hubsky & Sears, 1992).*

- Encourage the client to perform tasks in the morning hours. *Biorhythm studies indicate that people usually have greater energy reserves in the morning hours and diminished reserves in the afternoon (Freal, Kraft, & Coryell, 1984).*

- Advise the client to avoid temperature extremes, such as hot showers or exposure to cold. *Maintaining a relatively constant body temperature may avoid exacerbation of the disorder. Heat can delay impulse transmission across demyelinated nerves, which contributes to fatigue (Roohi & Cook, 1987).*

- Refer the client and family to the appropriate professionals to manage fatigue: stress management groups, support groups, occupational or physical therapist, as indicated. *The more nurses can anticipate problems, the sooner the problem can be addressed and managed, thus decreasing anxiety and improving coping.*

Self-Care Deficits

Clients with MS may need assistance with bathing, toileting, dressing, grooming, and feeding. The assistance needed can range from minimal guidance to total dependence. The client's ability to perform self-care activities is the gauge by which family members and caregivers need to adjust assistance. Self-care encompasses both the decisions about care and the provision of care; most clients are capable of making decisions even after physical limitations prevent physical self-care. The need to maintain self-determination cannot be overemphasized and must be incorporated into each intervention. See the accompanying nursing research box about the importance of maintaining a client's locus of control.

Nursing interventions with rationales follow:

- Fully assess the extent of the client's self-care deficit; refer to other health team members for assessment as appropriate. For example, refer to a speech pathologist to assess swallowing and gag reflex, if indicated. *An accurate assessment is crucial to individualizing interventions.*

- Help the client to maintain as much independence in activities as possible; modify self-care tasks with client input. *Powerlessness can be decreased through allowing the client control over and input about decisions that directly affect the client's daily routine.*

- Assist with daily hygiene needs; modify toothbrush, comb, and so on, as indicated. Provide adaptive devices, such as arm or wrist braces, as needed. Maintain privacy. *Meeting hygiene needs is essential for positive self-concept, self-esteem, and socialization (Carpenito, 1995).*

- Assist the client with feeding needs: Teach the client to use assistive devices, such as plate guards; to modify consistency of foods; and to eat when energy level is high. If the client is unable to buy and prepare meals, provide referral to Meals-on-Wheels. *Proper nutrition is basic to health; adapting utensils and foods can ensure that nutritional needs are met.*

- Assist with bathing needs and individualize care as indicated. Avoid extremes of temperature. *Hot or extremely cold water may cause manifestations to worsen.*

- Teach routine inspection of skin. *Altered sensation, spasticity, and decreased mobility put the client with MS at high risk for skin breakdown.*

- Teach interventions related to altered bowel and bladder function: fluid intake of at least 2000 mL daily, bowel routine as indicated to prevent constipation, self-catheterization skills as necessary. *Maintaining optimal bowel and bladder function decreases the chance of urinary tract infection and bowel impaction.*

Other Nursing Diagnoses

A myriad of nursing diagnoses may apply to clients with MS. Examples of selected diagnoses follow:

- *Ineffective Airway Clearance* related to effects of limited lung expansion and decreased cough mechanism

Applying Research to Nursing Practice: The Client with Multiple Sclerosis

■ ■ ■

In one study, 100 respondents with MS were randomly selected to be interviewed and respond to a brief, 11-item questionnaire for determining locus of control. This questionnaire is called the Health Locus of Control Scale.

Findings indicated that respondents with an internal locus of control had more knowledge of their disease and practiced more self-care than respondents with an external locus of control. These respondents also had a more benign course of the disease (Wassem, 1991).

Implications for Nursing
Nursing interventions may be adjusted according to whether the client has an internal or external locus of control. For example, clients with an external locus of control seem to prefer receiving advice from an authority figure; clients with an internal locus of control, in contrast, would rather take a more active role in learning. The Health Locus of Control Scale can be administered as part of an initial assessment in a rehabilitation setting.

Critical Thinking in Client Care

1. How can nurses determine a client's locus of control?

2. How could you modify your teaching approach according to a client's locus of control?

3. What, if any, benefits do you perceive in assessing a client's locus of control?

- *Altered Nutrition: Less Than Body Requirements* related to inability to control spasticity and coordination while eating
- *Risk for Altered Sexuality Patterns* related to sensory and motor changes, anxiety, and altered body image
- *Impaired Verbal Communication* related to fatigue
- *Ineffective Individual Coping* or *Ineffective Family Coping* related to inability to effectively manage symptoms of MS

Client and Family Teaching

To promote the client's highest level of wellness, the nurse adapts teaching approaches based on the MS client's needs. The inconsistent and erratic nature of the disease can make teaching difficult and challenging. Initial teaching focuses on a realistic explanation of MS. Referral to a support group early in the course of the disease also is indicated. Social support can make a positive difference in a client's ability to cope with MS (Hastings, 1992).

Following an overview of the disorder, the client needs to understand how to prevent fatigue and exacerbations. Teach the client to avoid stress, extremes of cold and heat, high humidity, physical overexertion, and infections. Because pregnancy can also exacerbate symptoms, counseling about this risk also is indicated. Preventive measures to avoid risk of respiratory and urinary tract infections are other areas that must be addressed.

Various treatment options and their side effects should be reviewed and reinforced in collaboration with the physician. Provide clients and families with information about medications, particularly steroid use, and about possible interactions with prescription or over-the-counter medications.

Safety is an important consideration in medication administration, ambulation, and hygiene. For example, ascertain that the client and family take steps to make the home safe, such as removing throw rugs and using hand rails in the shower.

Follow-up care is indicated and is essential to promoting optimal adaptation as the disease progresses. Ongoing care from nurses, counselors, and physical, occupational, and speech therapists, as well as the physician and community health nurse is indicated. As the disease progresses, remember to allow time to clarify information and allow both the client and family to verbalize feelings.

Applying the Nursing Process

Case Study of a Client with Multiple Sclerosis: George McMurphy

George McMurphy, a 45-year-old Irish Catholic from northern Minnesota, was diagnosed with MS approximately 5 years ago. He states that he probably had mild symptoms as long ago as 10 years. He works as a manager with a large grocery store chain near his home. He lives at home with his wife and two children, ages 12 and 15. Recently, Mr. McMurphy has had increasing problems with chest congestion, urinary incontinence, lack of energy, weakness, extreme fatigue, and altered mobility from spasticity in his leg muscles. He is admitted to the hospital for evaluation and treatment of pneumonia and exacerbation of his MS.

Assessment

Denise Miller, primary care nurse, is assigned to care for Mr. McMurphy. His major complaint is the inability to "bring up all this sputum; I feel rotten from being so congested. I hate not being able to get to work and for my wife having to tend to my personal needs." Vital signs are as follows: BP, 134/84; P, 94; R, 30; T, 102 F (38.8 C). Mr. McMurphy is admitted for an acute exacerbation of the disorder, probably triggered by pneumonia. He will be treated with ACTH and intravenous antibiotics during this admission.

Diagnosis

Ms. Miller makes the following nursing diagnoses for Mr. McMurphy:

- *Ineffective Airway Clearance* related to decreased ability to cough
- *Activity Intolerance* related to fatigue and spasticity
- *Self-Care Deficit: Toileting, Feeding, and Grooming* related to muscle weakness
- *Powerlessness* related to inability to perform role function

Expected Outcomes

The expected outcomes established in Mr. McMurphy's plan of care specify that he will

- Be able to clear airway.
- Have breath sounds clear to auscultation and pulse oximetry readings above 95%.
- Be able to ambulate using assistive devices, if needed.
- Perform self-care activities without becoming overly fatigued and tired.
- Verbalize methods to adapt daily routine to his level of tolerance.
- Identify resources and methods to assist him in controlling situations.

Planning and Implementation

Ms. Miller plans and implements the following interventions, which included Mr. McMurphy's wife and children in care and teaching as appropriate:

- Initiate pulmonary hygiene measures (e.g., incentive spirometry, turning, deep breathing and coughing, breathing exercises, and postural drainage) at least every 2 hours. Assess lung sounds, oxygen saturation, and ability to clear airway.
- Teach the importance of maintaining an oral fluid intake of at least 2000 mL per day to prevent tenacious sputum and to prevent urinary tract infections. Teach signs and symptoms of urinary and respiratory infections.
- Allow Mr. McMurphy to participate in decision making about his care.
- Assist client with ADLs only as needed, based on his level of fatigue and muscle weakness.

- Plan self-care activities so that they are performed during periods of Mr. McMurphy's peak level of energy; intersperse rest periods throughout the day.
- Refer Mr. McMurphy and his family to an MS support group, if they are not already attending one.
- Refer to physical and occupational therapists for counseling regarding control of spasticity and possible splinting of spastic muscles.
- Consult a urologist for assessment of bladder incontinence; teach intermittent catheterization. Alternatively, the use of an external condom catheter may be indicated.

Evaluation

Mr. McMurphy is discharged 7 days following admission. He states that he feels stronger; on discharge, he has no problem clearing his airway. Although he continues to pace his activities to avoid fatigue, his muscle strength and "tiredness" have improved. He is able to complete ADLs unassisted.

Pulmonary function has returned to normal, prehospitalization levels: ABGs and pulse oximetry are within normal limits. Both Mr. McMurphy and his wife have listed several methods of modifying their daily routine to allow more rest and decreased stress. Follow-up visits to his primary care physician have been arranged, and they have been provided with information about the local MS support group.

Critical Thinking in the Nursing Process

1. Describe approaches the nurse could take to ensure that Mr. McMurphy does not exceed his activity tolerance.
2. How could the nurse explain Mr. McMurphy's symptoms and illness to his children?
3. What are the nursing implications of the various drugs used to treat exacerbations of MS?
4. Develop a teaching plan for Mr. McMurphy to help prevent future respiratory infections.
5. Develop a care plan for Mr. McMurphy for the nursing diagnosis *Risk for Injury* related to fatigue, muscle weakness, and spasticity caused by MS.

The Client with Parkinson's Disease

■ ■ ■

Parkinson's disease is a progressive, degenerative neurologic disease characterized by nonintention tremor, bradykinesia, and muscle rigidity. It is one of the most common neurologic disorders affecting older adults; approximately 1 to 1½ million people are affected. The symptoms of Parkinson's disease are sometimes initially mistaken as signs of the normal aging process. Most people with this disorder are diagnosed between ages 50 and 60; it is somewhat more common among males (Hickey, 1992).

The chronic and eventually debilitating nature of Parkinson's disease poses many challenges to clients, families, and health care professionals. Dependence due to declining physical and mental abilities is of major concern. In the early stages, most clients are able to remain at home, with the family assisting with or providing many of the client's ADL needs. As the disease progresses and the burden of care increases, the client and family may prefer placement in a long-term care facility.

Parkinson's-like manifestations, called *secondary parkinsonism* or *parkinsonian syndrome,* may be present in clients taking tranquilizers, such as the phenothiazines. Secondary parkinsonism can also be caused by carbon monoxide or cyanide poisoning. This discussion focuses on primary parkinsonism, that is, Parkinson's disease, whose cause is unknown.

Pathophysiology

Coordinated, voluntary, body movement is achieved through the actions of neurotransmitters in the basal ganglia of the brain. Some neurotransmitters facilitate the transmission of excitatory nerve impulses, while other neurotransmitters inhibit their transmission. Together, this system allows control of movement. When the normal balance between excitatory and inhibitory neurotransmitters is disturbed, disorders of voluntary motor function occur.

In Parkinson's disease, there is atrophy of the neurons of the substantia nigra that produce **dopamine,** a neurotransmitter that helps regulate nerve impulses involved in motor function. As a result of this atrophy, levels of dopamine in the basal ganglia decrease. The usual balance of neurotransmitter activity in the brain is disrupted when dopamine production decreases; acetylcholine is no longer inhibited by dopamine. The failure to inhibit acetylcholine is the underlying basis for the clinical manifestations of the disorder (Marieb, 1995).

Parkinson's disease begins with subtle symptoms. Clients complain of feeling tired and seem to move more slowly; a slight tremor may accompany the fatigue. In a small percentage of clients, dementia is the initial presenting symptom. Parkinson's disease has several stages; see the accompanying box.

Clinical manifestations related to motor and postural effects include uncoordinated movements, bradykinesia, tremors, and rigidity. Posture reflexes are lost, and the client exhibits an unsteady gait with a forward bend of the upper body. Gait disturbances range from inability to be-

---

Stages of Parkinson's Disease

■ ■ ■

I Unilateral involvement only, usually with minimal or no functional impairment.

II Bilateral or midline involvement, without impairment of balance.

III First sign of impaired righting reflexes, evidenced as unsteadiness as the client turns or demonstrated when the client is pushed from standing equilibrium with the feet together and eyes closed. Functionally, the client is somewhat restricted in activities but may have some employment potential, depending on the type of employment. Clients are physically capable of leading independent lives, and their disability is mild to moderate.

IV Fully developed, severely disabling disease; the client is still able to walk and stand unassisted but is markedly incapacitated.

V Client is confined to bed or wheelchair unless aided.

Note. From "Parkinsonism: Onset, Progression, and Mortality" (pp. 151–166) by M. Hoehn and M. Yahr, 1967, *Neurology, 17.*

---

gin movement to *festination,* an involuntary, short, rapid shuffling. *Retropulsion,* or walking backwards, also occurs.

The cardinal signs of Parkinson's disease are bradykinesia, nonintention tremor, and muscle rigidity. **Bradykinesia,** slowed movements due to muscle rigidity, may be pronounced. Clients describe being "frozen" in place as voluntary movement is lost (*akinesia*). Slowed or delayed movements affect the eyes, mouth, and voice, causing a masklike face and softened or muffled voice. A staring gaze with minimal change in expression is evident (Figure 42–6).

Nonintention tremors affect hand movement. These tremors show a "pill rolling" characteristic of the thumb and fingers and occur when the client is at rest. The nonintention tremor may be controlled with purposeful, voluntary movement. Clients have progressive impairment in performing skills that require dexterity and fine muscle control, such as writing and eating.

Many manifestations result from the loss of functions controlled by the autonomic nervous system. Elimination problems include constipation and urinary hesitation or frequency. Drooling occurs as a result of impaired swallowing secondary to hypopharyngeal neuromuscular dysfunction; the dysphagia eventually interferes with

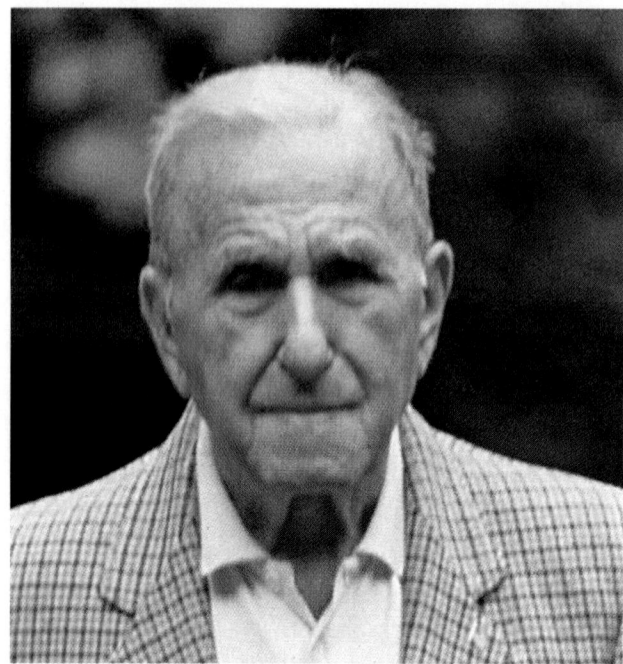

Figure 42-6 In Parkinson's disease, the client's face lacks expression or animation.

nutrition. Clients may experience problems related to orthostatic hypotension, including dizziness with position change. Eczematous skin changes are related to the increase in sweat gland activity secondary to increased sebotropic hormone production (Hickey, 1992). The clinical manifestations of Parkinson's disease are presented in the accompanying box.

Clients with Parkinson's disease also have sleep disturbances. The ability to initiate and maintain sleep is affected because of the effect of acetylcholine, an excitatory neurotransmitter. Muscle rigidity may compromise sleep because the client has lost the ability to change position. This lack of muscle movement causes the client to awaken and consciously shift position.

There are multiple contributing factors to some of the manifestations that clients with Parkinson's disease experience. For example, clients with Parkinson's disease have constipation because of decreased peristalsis. However, decreased peristalsis is not the only cause: The client's immobility, tremors (unable to drink from a glass easily), and dietary changes from dysphagia all contribute to the problem of constipation. Signs of dementia may be related to the primary disorder or to dopamine therapy. Alterations in sleep are associated with increased levels of acetylcholine, tremors that disrupt sleep, side effects of L-dopa (levodopa), and depression.

Several possible complications are associated with Parkinson's disease:

- Oculogyric crisis, in which the eyes become fixed with a lateral and upward gaze
- Paranoia and hallucinations, which may accompany the dementia
- Impaired communication due to changes in speech, handwriting, and expressiveness
- Falls from balance, posture, motor changes
- Infections, such as pneumonia, related to immobility
- Malnutrition related to dysphagia and inability to prepare meals
- Altered sleep patterns due to loss of dopamine, L-dopa side effects (nightmares, dreams), or side effects of anticholinergics (hyperreflexia, muscle twitching), depression (Miller, 1995)
- Skin breakdown and pressure ulcers associated with urinary incontinence and malnutrition; sweat reflex changes
- Depression and social isolation

Prognosis is poor owing to the progressive degeneration that ultimately affects multiple physiologic systems and their function. Approximately 25% of clients eventually experience dementia. Psychosocial effects are equally devastating, and the need for family support increases as the client's debilitation increases.

Collaborative Care

Diagnosis is based primarily on a thorough history and physical examination. Interventions vary with the clinical stage of the disorder and include medication, surgery, and rehabilitation (physical, occupational, speech, and psychosocial) to retain the optimal level of functioning possible. A team approach is essential for these clients. Clients who have Parkinson's disease require substantial supportive care.

Laboratory and Diagnostic Tests
Laboratory and diagnostic studies may support a potential diagnosis of Parkinson's disease; however, there is no test that clearly differentiates Parkinson's disease from other neurologic disorders. Thus, tests are commonly performed to rule out disorders that produce secondary parkinsonism.

The following laboratory tests may be ordered:

- *CBC* is frequently ordered and may show low hemoglobin and hematocrit levels due to anemia.
- *Chemistry profile* may reflect low protein and albumin levels related to the client's inability to buy and prepare meals.
- *Drug screens* may be performed to determine the presence of medications or toxins that cause secondary

parkinsonism, such as methyldopa, reserpine, or carbon monoxide.

The following diagnostic tests may be ordered:

- *Electroencephalogram (EEG)* may indicate slowed pattern and disorganization.
- *Upper GI X-ray series with small bowel follow-through* shows delayed emptying, distention, and possibly megacolon with severe constipation.
- *Video fluoroscopy* of the client swallowing barium is monitored on a fluoroscopic screen (Corbett, 1992). A slowed response of the cricopharyngeal muscles when swallowing is typical in Parkinson's disease.

Pharmacology

The goal of drug therapy is to control symptoms to the extent possible. Generally, medications vary with the stage of the disease; however, individual response is variable and guides the selection of medications. Types of drugs used include monoamine oxidase (MAO) inhibitors, dopaminergics, dopamine agonists, and anticholinergics. Specific information and nursing implications for these drugs are presented in the box on page 1828.

Initially clients are treated with selegiline, amantadine, or anticholinergics. As the disease progresses, levodopa in combination with carbidopa is used. Because levodopa eventually loses its effectiveness, dopamine agonists are added to increase the effectiveness of levodopa. Throughout the disease process, various drug combinations may be tried in order to achieve and maintain optimal symptom control with the fewest adverse reactions. Eventually, pharmacotherapeutic agents lose their efficacy, and the disease continues to progress despite treatment. Response to the drugs fluctuate; this phenomenon is called the "on-off" response (Beal et al., 1991). Other problems may include dyskinesia (impairment in voluntary movement), akinesia, and the need to increase doses of medication to achieve a therapeutic response.

Other medications may be used to treat problems related to Parkinson's disease. Antidepressants, notably amitriptyline (Elavil), may be prescribed. Propranolol (Inderal) may be used to treat tremors; it should be used cautiously when clients have orthostatic hypotension.

Surgery

Pallidotomy is the most recent surgical technique for Parkinson's disease, and its results have been dramatic for many clients. In this procedure, the neurosurgeon locates the affected areas of the globus pallidus and destroys the involved tissue. As a result, clients who could not previously ambulate are able to walk, and tremors cease. The long-term effects are still being evaluated.

Clinical Manifestations of Parkinson's Disease

Manifestations Related to Motor Dysfunction

- Nonintention tremor
- Bradykinesia or akinesia
  a. Slowed movements; inability to initiate voluntary movements
  b. Slowed speech, low amplitude
  c. Poor articulation
  d. Decreased eye movements (i.e., blinking)
  e. Masklike, expressionless face
- Rigidity
- Posture and gait disturbances
  a. Trunk tilted forward
  b. Shuffling gait, propulsive at times
  c. Retropulsion
- Complications: falls, fractures, impaired communication, social isolation

Manifestations Related to Autonomic System Dysfunction

- Skin problems
  a. Seborrhea
  b. Excess sweating on face and neck, absence of sweating of trunk and extremities
  c. Mottled skin
- Heat intolerance
- Postural hypotension
- Constipation
- Complications: skin breakdown, dizziness, falls, constipation

Manifestations Related to Cognitive and Psychologic Dysfunction

- Dementia
  a. Memory loss
  b. Lack of insight and problem-solving ability
  c. Declining intellectual abilities
- Anxiety
- Depression
- Complications: loss of ability to function, social isolation

Nursing Implications for Pharmacology: The Client with Parkinson's Disease

MONOAMINE OXIDASE (MAO) INHIBITORS

Selegiline (Eldepryl, Deprenyl)

Selegiline works by selectively inhibiting the enzyme that inactivates dopamine in the brain. It is used in stage I and II Parkinson's disease because it has been shown to slow the disease progression. Insomnia may occur when the drug is used alone. The second use is as an adjunct therapy with levodopa: Selegiline inhibits the enzyme system that would otherwise break down and destroy dopamine. This synergistic effect lasts approximately 1 to 2 years. The combination of selegiline and levodopa increases the adverse reactions of dopamine; nurses must be alert for orthostatic hypotension, changes in movement, hallucinations, and confusion. These responses can be modified by lowering the dose of levodopa. Because it is highly selective for the MAO-A enzyme, selegiline does not have antidepressant effects like the MAO-B inhibitors. The risk of severe hypertension is low.

Nursing Responsibilities

- Establish baseline functional abilities: motor control and movements, position changes, mental status.
- Monitor sleeping patterns.
- Assess for orthostatic hypotension; look for unsteadiness with position change and complaints of dizziness.
- Assess for hypertension, which can occur with higher than usual doses.

Client and Family Teaching

- It is very important to take the medication as directed, especially dose and time of administration.
- Notify the practitioner if insomnia occurs.
- Report signs of orthostatic hypotension, changes in ability to move, or psychologic changes.
- Change positions slowly, especially when moving from a sitting to standing position.
- Keep follow-up appointments for evaluation of the medication's effectiveness.

DOPAMINERGICS

Levodopa (Larodopa, Dopar)

Carbidopa-Levodopa (Sinemet)

Amantadine (Symmetrel)

Whereas dopamine cannot cross the blood–brain barrier, levodopa can; therefore, levodopa is used to treat Parkinson's disease. Once transported to the brain, levodopa is converted to dopamine in the presence of the catalytic enzyme decarboxylase. Most of the body's concentrations of this enzyme are active in peripheral tissues, so most of the levodopa administered is broken down before it reaches the brain. Large doses are required to provide symptom relief, and as a consequence, adverse reactions frequently occur. Vitamin B_6 (pyridoxine) is also given, because decarboxylase is more effective in its presence. Levodopa is reserved for stages III and IV or after other medications have been tried because it can have severe side effects and usually is effective in controlling symptoms over the long term.

Carbidopa prevents decarboxylase from converting levodopa to dopamine in the peripheral tissues; therefore, carbidopa is frequently given in combination with levodopa. The dose of levodopa can be decreased by up to 75% when administered with carbidopa (Moore et al., 1994). Various fixed combinations of the two drugs are available in the medication Sinemet.

Levodopa is avoided in clients with narrow-angle glaucoma, severe angina pectoris, transient ischemic attacks, or melanoma. The "on-off" phenomenon occurs after the client takes levodopa for several years; this phenomenon is characterized by unexpected dyskinesias and lack of symptom control.

Common side effects are nausea and vomiting; darkening of urine and sweat; dyskinesias, especially in the first few months of therapy; dysrhythmias; orthostatic hypotension; and psychologic reactions, such as hallucinations and vivid dreams. Older adults are particularly susceptible to psychologic disturbances.

Amantadine is an antiviral agent that was only incidentally found to control symptoms of Parkinson's disease. It works by releasing dopamine from dopaminergic terminals in the brain. Although it acts more quickly than levodopa, its period of effectiveness is limited, usually lasting only a few months if the drug is given continuously. For this reason, levodopa is administered for only 2 to 3 weeks initially and during periods of increased symptoms. Adverse effects include urinary retention, blurred vision, dry mouth, constipation, anxiety, and confusion. Use with anticholinergics increases these effects.

Pharmacology: The Client with Parkinson's Disease (continued)

Nursing Responsibilities

- Establish the client's baseline functional abilities in performing ADLs and administering the medication; assess motor control and coordination.

- To avoid adverse reactions, assess the client's overall health status before initiating therapy.

- Monitor medications known to cause adverse drug interactions: anticholinergics, pyridoxine, and antipsychotic agents alter the effectiveness of levodopa; MAO-B inhibitors can cause severe hypertension because of their vasoconstrictive effects.

- Withhold levodopa for 8 hours prior to administering Sinemet to avoid potentiating the effects of the circulating levodopa.

Client and Family Teaching

- Levodopa may not take effect for several weeks to months.

- Do not alter dosages of medications; taking more of a medication may not result in better symptom control and can cause severe side effects.

- Always tell health care providers about other medications currently being taken.

- Levodopa may cause a change in color of urine; this is harmless, however.

- To prevent side effects:
  a. Prevent nausea by taking medication with food.
  b. Change position slowly to avoid orthostatic hypotension.
  c. Prevent constipation by increasing fluid intake and exercising regularly.

- Notify practitioner if difficulty making voluntary movements or cardiac or psychologic symptoms develop.

- Watch for the "on-off" phenomenon, in which periods of symptom control alternate with periods when the drug fails to control symptoms.

DOPAMINE AGONISTS

Bromocriptine (Parlodel)

Pergolide (Permax)

Dopamine agonists act by directly activating dopamine receptors in the brain. They are frequently used in combination with levodopa therapy: When dopamine agonists are given with levodopa, they in-

crease the therapeutic effects of levodopa and reduce fluctuations in motor symptoms. Adverse reactions are similar to those of levodopa: nausea, orthostatic hypotension, and psychologic disturbances are common. Nursing responsibilities and client and family teaching information are similar to those that apply to the dopaminergics.

ANTICHOLINERGICS

Trihexyphenidyl (Artane)

Benztropine (Cogentin)

Biperiden (Akineton)

Procyclidine (Kemadrin)

Anticholinergics are effective in Parkinson's disease because they block the excitatory action of the neurotransmitter acetylcholine. They are frequently used during the early stages of the disease or when the client can no longer take levodopa. They may be given in combination with carbidopa-levodopa therapy. These medications ease drooling, tremors, and rigidity; however, side effects are common and may include blurred vision, dry mouth, constipation, delayed gastric emptying, urinary retention, photophobia, and tachycardia. Older adults are especially susceptible to heat stroke and psychologic side effects, including confusion, depression, delusions, and hallucinations. Anticholinergics should be tapered slowly when discontinued to avoid enhancing parkinsonian symptoms. The use of anticholinergics with Parkinson's disease is decreasing because of the appearance of newer medications that are more effective and have fewer side effects.

Nursing Responsibilities

- Perform baseline assessment for presence of glaucoma, cardiac dysfunction, and prostatic hypertrophy.

- Document effects of anticholinergics on Parkinson's symptoms.

- Note the client's use of other medications, including over-the-counter medications, that have anticholinergic effects, such as antihistamines and tricyclic antidepressants.

- Monitor for side effects, especially changes in vision, elimination, gastric emptying, and mentation.

➤

Pharmacology: The Client with Parkinson's Disease (continued)

Client and Family Teaching

- Inform practitioner if you begin taking any new medications or notice any new symptoms.

- Avoid overexposure to heat, and take precautions to avoid heat stroke: Drink fluids, keep cool, and avoid strenuous activity on hot days.

- Drink adequate amounts of fluid to minimize the effects of dehydration that are associated with anticholinergics, especially constipation.

- Practice home safety to prevent falls associated with blurred vision.

- Avoid taking over-the-counter antihistamines or sleeping aids; these have anticholinergic activity.

- Have the eyes examined annually to check for glaucoma; wear dark glasses if photophobia develops.

- Do not suddenly stop taking anticholinergics.

Stereotaxic thalamotomy (an X-ray is taken during neurosurgery to guide the insertion of a needle into a specific area of the brain) has been used only for clients who do not respond to medications—generally, younger people with extreme unilateral tremor. The surgeon destroys a small amount of tissue by creating a lesion in the ventrolateral nucleus of the thalamus. The result of this surgery is a decrease in tremors and rigidity in the contralateral extremity.

Autologous adrenal medullary transplant is another procedure performed on clients who do not achieve sufficient control of symptoms through medications. The client must be a good surgical risk and free of dementia and end-stage cardiac, pulmonary, or renal disease. First an adrenalectomy and then a craniotomy are performed. Care of the client undergoing craniotomy has been presented in Chapter 40. Small portions of the adrenal medulla are grafted to the basal ganglia; a subdural catheter is positioned for intracranial pressure monitoring.

Fetal tissue transplantation is a controversial surgical procedure limited to select medical centers. In this procedure, tissue of the substantia nigra is transplanted into the client's caudate nucleus.

Rehabilitation

Depending on their individual needs, clients frequently benefit from rehabiliation therapy with a physical therapist, social worker, psychologist and/or speech therapist.

Physical therapists (PT) can implement an individual exercise program to improve coordination, balance, gait, and transfers. Preventing contractures is an important goal of exercise therapy. It is crucial that family and health care personnel permit the client adequate time to perform not only exercise regimens but also ADLs. Activities should not be rushed.

Occupational therapists (OT) assist the client to adapt to changing abilities pertinent to work, self-care, and recreational activities. Some rehabilitation centers assign OT personnel the responsibility of addressing the client's upper extremity functions while assigning PT personnel to manage lower extremity problems. For example, skills related to cooking and grooming would be supervised by the OT, whereas mobility and posture skills would be supervised by PT.

Speech therapists frequently address not only the client's speech but also chewing and swallowing. These therapists evaluate clients and plan treatment regimens. The challenge with clients who have Parkinson's disease is that they not only have vocalization problems, but also dexterity deficits; speech therapists therefore must evaluate the potential benefits of assistive devices, such as a magic slate, voice synthesizer, or computer, on an individual basis.

Community health nurses may be contacted to visit the client's home and evaluate it for potential safety hazards. Poor lighting and throw rugs are examples of hazards that contribute to falls.

Nursing Care

Clients with Parkinson's disease have complex and, ultimately, multisystem needs. Deficits in mobility and self-care are common. As the disorder progresses, nutritional and airway-related problems are common.

Major considerations in caring for clients taking medications for Parkinson's disease are conducting baseline assessments, controlling side effects, monitoring for adverse reactions, and teaching.

Psychosocial needs may include problems related to ineffective coping, powerlessness, and body image disturbance. In addition, nursing diagnoses relevant to clients with other neurologic disorders may be pertinent to clients with Parkinson's disease. Refer to the nursing care sections throughout this chapter for discussions of *Fatigue, Self-Care Deficit, Ineffective Airway Clearance,* and other pertinent diagnoses. This section focuses on the nursing diagnoses *Impaired Physical Mobility, Impaired Ver-*

bal Communication, Altered Nutrition: Less Than Body Requirements, and *Sleep Pattern Disturbance.*

Impaired Physical Mobility

Clients with Parkinson's disease have impaired mobility for several reasons, including tremors, gait pattern disturbances, and alterations in body positioning, such as forward bending of the trunk. Poor self-esteem may contribute to the client's lack of motivation and willingness to be mobile. Safety considerations related to immobility are addressed in this section.

Nursing interventions with rationales follow:

- Perform ROM exercises at least twice a day, emphasizing the trunk, neck, arms, hips, and legs. *Maintaining joint mobility promotes better function and strength, improving gait pattern. Contractures can be prevented with consistent ROM exercises.*

- Consult with a physical therapist to develop an individualized exercise program. *A program specific to the client supplies motivation as well as helping the client maintain muscle tone, flexibility, and mobility.*

- Ambulate at least four times a day. *Exercise fosters independence and self-esteem (Carpenito, 1995).*

- Incorporate assistive devices, such as canes, splints, or braces, as indicated. *Adaptive equipment improves balance, protects joints, and promotes proper anatomic positioning.*

- The following interventions are recommended when safety is a concern:
  a. Slightly elevate the back legs of chairs and raise the toilet seat to help the client rise to a standing from a sitting position.
  b. Wear shoes with Velcro closures.
  c. Remove potential hazards, such as unanchored throw rugs, from the home environment.
  d. Install hand rails and nonskid surfaces to bathing area.
  e. Ensure adequate lighting throughout the home and in outside areas, especially in areas where transfers are common. Check garage, carports, and sidewalks.
  Safety measures prevent potential complications that may result from falls or other accidents and promote self-esteem through self-care. Parkinson's disease is a disorder common in older adults, who are at greater risk for falls resulting from orthostatic hypotension, osteoporosis, poor vision, and other problems causing disorientation and confusion, such as Alzheimer's disease.

Impaired Verbal Communication

Diminished vocal amplitude and loss of muscular control can impair the client's ability to speak. Both health care givers and family members need to remember that clients require sufficient time for self-expression; an unhurried approach is recommended. Seek input from family members when determining alternative methods of communicating with the client.

Nursing interventions with rationales follow:

- Assess the client's current communication abilities—speech, hearing, writing. *Assessment forms the basis for planning appropriate care. Communication involves both sending and receiving messages.*

- Develop methods of communication appropriate to client's coordination abilities, such as a write-on, wipe-off slate; flash cards with common phrases; pointing to objects. *Individualizing a method of communication decreases anxiety and isolation.*

- Consult with a speech pathologist to develop oral exercises and interventions that will facilitate speaking. *The muscles of speech and swallowing are affected by the Parkinson's disease process.*

- Remind the client to speak more loudly, if possible. *A low, monotonous voice is characteristic of the client with Parkinson's disease; verbal cues remind clients to alter behavior.*

Altered Nutrition: Less Than Body Requirements

Tremors, altered gait, and impaired chewing and swallowing can cause nutritional problems in the client with Parkinson's disease. As the disorder progresses, interventions for ensuring optimal nutrition need to be adapted to the client's functional abilities. Assess the client's swallow reflex prior to initiating any feeding program. During the initial stages of the disorder, some clients may have a nursing diagnosis of *Altered Nutrition: More Than Body Requirements* if kcal intake exceeds energy expenditure.

Nursing interventions with rationales follow:

- Assess the client's nutritional status and self-feeding abilities; consult with occupational therapist or speech therapist, if needed. *An initial assessment of abilities ensures that interventions are individualized to the client's current functional abilities.*

- Provide foods of proper consistency as determined by the client's swallowing function. *Food that is too liquid can be aspirated by the client.*

- Weigh the client weekly. *Early recognition of weight loss allows for intervention.*

- Teach eating methods to decrease tremors, such as holding a piece of bread in the hand that is not holding an eating utensil. *Nonintention tremor may be reduced through purposeful activity.*

- Monitor diet for foods high in bulk and fluids. *Several anti-Parkinson's medications can cause constipation.*

Sleep Pattern Disturbance

Rigidity and weakness can cause clients with Parkinson's disease to lose the ability to move and change positions during sleep. The resulting discomfort causes periods of wakefulness. Medications to treat Parkinson's disease contribute to sleep pattern disturbance; for example, levodopa can cause vivid dreams. Nurses can assist in accurately assessing the sleep pattern disturbance and in planning interventions to improve or increase sleep time. Other interventions address the anxiety associated with this diagnosis. Family members may also experience sleep pattern disturbance and seek the nurse's input. Whenever possible, the family should be included in the plan of care.

Nursing interventions with rationales follow:

- Thoroughly assess the client's sleep pattern and existing conditions that may affect sleep, such as depression. *Clients experiencing anxiety, depression, and dementia have a difficult time falling asleep and may have more awakenings during sleeptime (Miller, 1995). Lack of adequate pain control may interfere with sleep.*

- Explain the disease process and the effects of decreased dopamine on the sleep-wake cycle. *Depending on the dosage, levodopa causes less REM sleep and deep sleep.*

- Review the client's medication. *Bromocriptine and levodopa, especially if used with an anticholinergic, can cause vivid dreams. Other medications (diuretics, theophylline, hypnotics) also may interfere with sleep (Miller, 1995).*

- Modify life-style activities that affect sleep:
  a. Institute a routine of activities with limited rest periods during the day; avoid napping close to bedtime. Avoid strenuous exercise in the evening. *Daytime sleeping may contribute to decreased nighttime sleeping. Vigorous exercise just before bedtime may act as a stimulant.*
  b. Incorporate diet modifications, such as limiting caffeine and alcohol intake. *Caffeine is a stimulant, and alcohol may cause early-morning awakenings, increased daytime sleepiness, and nightmares (Miller, 1995).*
  c. Avoid nicotine products in the evening. *Nicotine is a stimulant that may delay falling asleep and cause nighttime awakenings.*
  d. Drink a glass of milk before bedtime. *Milk contains L- tryptophan, which produces sedative effects by shortening the time taken to fall asleep (sleep latency).*
  e. Assess and modify the environment to aid in sleep; for example, darken the room, and decrease noises. *Reducing environmental stimuli decreases external sleep disturbances.*

Other Nursing Diagnoses

Additional nursing diagnoses that may apply to the client with Parkinson's disease follow:

- *Risk for Aspiration* related to effects of changes in neuromuscular functioning

- *Self-Care Deficit: Grooming, Bathing, Toileting* related to joint immobility and inability to manage tremors
- *Risk for Sexual Dysfunction* related to altered self-concept
- *Ineffective Individual Coping* or *Ineffective Family Coping* related to loss of hope and lack of support systems
- *Risk for Impaired Skin Integrity* related to effects of immobility and increased sebaceous secretions

Client and Family Teaching

Teaching preventive measures is extremely important when working with clients who have Parkinson's disease. Preventing malnutrition, falls and other environmental accidents, constipation, skin breakdown from incontinence or immobility, and joint contracture requires much teaching and reinforcement.

In addition to incorporating information about safety needs (discussed previously under the nursing diagnosis *Impaired Physical Mobility*), teach ways to prevent orthostatic hypotension when the client changes positions; some clients may also benefit from wearing elastic hose (Hickey, 1992). In addition, address safety considerations regarding proper administration of medications. Refer to the box on page 1828 for teaching related to specific medications.

Teach gait training and exercises for improving ambulation, speech, swallowing, and performance of self-care. In addition to coordinating referrals from speech therapy, physical therapy, and occupational therapy, reinforce information and incorporate specific interventions that the various therapists initiate. For example, incorporate specific oral exercises to improve eating and speaking.

The Client with Huntington's Disease

■ ■ ■

Huntington's disease, also called *Huntington's chorea,* is a progressive, degenerative, inherited neurologic disease characterized by increasing dementia and **chorea** (jerky, rapid, involuntary movements). It is a single-gene autosomal-dominant inherited disease that affects the neurons of the basal ganglia (Porth, 1994). Each child born to a parent who has the disease has a 50% chance of inheriting Huntington's disease. It affects approximately one in every 18,000 to 25,000 people; males and females are equally affected (Bullock & Rosendahl, 1992). Although carriers can be identified, there is no cure for the disease. Huntington's disease, like Parkinson's disease, involves an imbalance between the excitatory and inhibitory neurotransmitters in the brain that causes progressive chorea, speech problems, and dementia.

Because the client is usually asymptomatic until age 30 to 40, he or she may already have passed the gene to the next generation. The psychologic impact is devastating to clients and their families. The family not only experiences guilt from passing the disease from one generation to the next but also is faced with the overwhelming long-term care needs of those affected. It is common for several family members to be afflicted with the disease.

Nurses are faced with a multitude of challenges when caring for families who have Huntington's disease, including physiologic, psychosocial, and ethical problems. Physiologic problems are related to the progressive and eventually debilitating nature of the disease. Psychosocial concerns occur as a result of the client's personality and mental changes, the family's responsibility for providing care, and the guilt implicit in a genetically transmitted disease. Ethical difficulties relate to the genetic nature of the disease: DNA testing for the marker on chromosome 4 can determine whether the person is a carrier of the disease before he or she begins to exhibit manifestations (Martin, 1987). Children of people with Huntington's disease are thus faced with the choice of finding out whether they will eventually be affected. If they choose not to be tested, they may pass the disease on to yet another generation. And if a fetus is affected, they may face the decision of whether to undergo an abortion.

Pathophysiology

Huntington's disease causes destruction of cells in the caudate nucleus and putamen areas of the basal ganglia (Pallett & O'Brien, 1985). Other areas of the brain, such as the frontal lobes, may selectively atrophy. Several neurotransmitters and their receptors are decreased including gamma-aminobutyric acid (GABA) and acetylcholine. The neurotransmitter dopamine is not affected in Huntington's disease, but the decrease in acetylcholine results in a relative excess of dopamine in the basal ganglia. The resulting imbalance among the neurotransmitters is a suspected underlying cause of the manifestations (Porth, 1994). Whereas in Parkinson's disease a deficit of dopamine causes slow movement or lack of movement, in Huntington's disease the opposite occurs: There is a relative excess of dopamine, causing excessive, uncontrolled movement.

Clinical manifestations primarily affect movement and posture, swallowing and speech, cognition, and personality; see the accompanying box. The progression and sequence of manifestations varies somewhat; however, initially the psychologic manifestations are more debilitating than the choreiform movements (Beal, Richardson, & Martin, 1991).

Early signs of personality change include severe depression, memory loss with decreased ability to concentrate, emotional lability, and impulsiveness. The client

---

Clinical Manifestations of Huntington's Disease

Motor Effects

Early

- Restlessness
- "Fidgety" feeling
- Minor gait changes—unsteady on feet
- Posture and positioning disturbances, frequent falls
- Inability to keep the tongue from protruding
- Slurred speech with poor articulation
- Complications: increasing problem with self-care activities, such as bathing, grooming, eating

Late

- Chorea—severely altered gait with irregular, uncontrollable movement; the distal extremity is most affected; shoulders shrug arrhythmically
- Facial grimacing—raising of eyebrows, uncontrollable protrusion of the tongue
- Dysphagia
- Unintelligible speech
- Impaired diaphragmatic movement
- Complications: immobility, aspiration, choking, and, eventually, total dependence, poor oxygenation, emaciation, and cachexia

Psychosocial Effects

Early

- Irritability
- Outbursts of rage alternating with euphoria
- Depression
- Complication: suicide

Late

- Decreasing memory
- Loss of cognitive skills
- Eventual dementia
- Complication: total dependence

experiences frequent mood swings ranging from uncontrollable periods of anger to apathy. Eventually, signs of dementia, including disorientation, confusion, and lack of sense of time, become evident and interfere with self-care.

Motor symptoms usually parallel personality and mood changes. The motor symptoms worsen with environmental stimuli and emotional stress but are absent when the client is sleeping (Pallatt & O'Brien, 1985). Initially movement problems are described as "fidgeting," or restlessness followed by progressive worsening of abnormal movements. The dyskinesias are manifested by facial grimaces, tongue protrusion, jerky movement of the distal arms or legs, and a rhythmic, lurching gait that almost resembles a dance. (The term *chorea* comes from *choreia*, the Greek word for "dance.") Gait changes cause incoordination and contribute to frequent falls.

The muscles of swallowing, chewing, and speaking are affected, leading to dysphagia and dysarthria and associated problems with communication and nutrition. The client's constant movement and difficulty in swallowing contribute to weight loss and eventual cachexia. Breathing is impaired because the diaphragm is unable to move effectively.

The manifestations slowly progress over approximately 15 to 20 years after initial symptoms. Prognosis is poor, with inevitable debilitation and total dependence. Death usually results from aspiration pneumonia or another infectious process.

Collaborative Care

There is no cure for Huntington's disease, and treatment addresses the disease's manifestations. Nurses provide care to clients with Huntington's disease in a variety of community settings. Initially, clients and families can manage care needs at home, but as the disease progresses, the client requires constant supervision, such as that provided in day care facilities. Eventually, skilled long-term care is needed. Clients who develop acute problems may be hospitalized until the crisis is managed. Because of the inevitable total multisystem debilitation of clients with Huntington's disease, nurses and other care givers face many challenges.

Laboratory and Diagnostic Tests

Genetic testing is the only test available to diagnose clients suspected of having Huntington's disease. Both blood and amniotic fluid may be tested for the presence of chromosome 4 using DNA analysis. The test can predict with 95% accuracy which offspring have the disease.

Pharmacology

The following medications are given for palliation of the symptoms of Huntington's disease.

- Antipsychotics, specifically, phenothiazines and butyrophenones, are effective in Huntington's disease because they block dopamine receptors in the brain. The therapeutic goal is to restore the balance among the neurotransmitters.
- Antidepressants are prescribed in the early stage of the disease; however, medications are no substitute for intense follow-up counseling for clients and families.

Nursing Care

Initially, much of the nursing care focuses on teaching about the disease, psychologic support, and genetic counseling. As manifestations become more severe, nursing considerations center on problems related not only to immobility and altered nutrition but also to the increasing self-care deficits. Families and clients experiencing Huntington's disease face many psychosocial issues. Nurses must be prepared to listen actively as well as to provide comfort and encouragement throughout the lengthy illness. There are many possible nursing diagnoses for the client with Huntington's disease; this section focuses on nursing diagnoses related to aspiration, altered nutrition, impaired skin integrity, and impaired communication.

Risk for Aspiration

Uncoordinated movements and swallowing and chewing problems put the client at high risk for aspiration.

Nursing interventions with rationales follow:

- Maintain the client in an upright position while the client eats; support the head. *Proper positioning may preventing aspiration during mealtime.*
- Review the Heimlich maneuver frequently with caregivers and family members. *Aspiration is a real possibility; caregivers must be prepared to reestablish the client's airway.*
- Provide food that is small and thick enough to manage, such as thick soups, mashed potatoes, stews, or casseroles. *These foods are more readily tolerated and manipulated by the tongue than liquids.*
- Make sure client has swallowed prior to giving another spoonful of food. *The automatic phase of swallowing may be disrupted in the client with Huntington's disease; providing adequate time and smaller bites may improve the ability to manipulate foods.*
- Provide a calm, relaxing eating environment. *Stress worsens choreiform movements and inappropriate behaviors.*

Altered Nutrition: Less Than Body Requirements

Clients with Huntington's disease have unpredictable choreiform movements of the extremities and decreased ability to control muscles involved with chewing and swallowing. Families and caregivers are challenged to provide sufficient calories to maintain the client in positive nitrogen balance. The nursing diagnosis *Impaired Swallowing* also is commonly applicable.

Nursing interventions with rationales follow:

- Evaluate the client's current weight and nutritional status, including serum albumin and transferrin levels. *Establishing a baseline is crucial for meeting individual caloric, protein, vitamin, and mineral needs.*

- Assess client's ability to swallow and manipulate eating utensils. *Aspiration is an ever-present danger that must be avoided; utensils may need to be adapted to client's abilities, if client is able to assist at all.*

- Continue feeding even if the client physically turns away from the meal. *Involuntary choreiform movements should not be interpreted as a refusal to eat.*

- Provide high-kcal, nutritious foods and sufficient snacks; seek input from a dietitian. *The constant movement of Huntington's disease increases caloric requirements.*

- Avoid milk; provide frequent oral hygiene. *Milk tends to thicken secretions. Decreasing thick secretions may improve ability to swallow and enable the client to ingest more calories.*

Impaired Skin Integrity

Skin integrity is only one component of the client's general need for protection and avoidance of injury. Several factors increase the client's risk for impaired skin integrity, including poor nutritional status, eventual total immobility, and incontinence. Although the client's mobility may not be drastically impaired early in the disease, total decline eventually results.

Nursing interventions with rationales follow:

- Evaluate the client's skin for actual and potential areas of breakdown. *Establishing a baseline is necessary in order to modify care and provide prophylactic protection of high-risk pressure areas.*

- Determine the client's nutritional status, especially serum albumin level and vitamin, mineral, and kcal intake. *Optimal nutritional status and positive nitrogen balance help prevent skin breakdown and formation of pressure ulcers.*

- Turn the client and inspect the skin at least every 2 hours, giving special consideration to areas that are most prone to breakdown, such as heels. *Pressure points are particularly susceptible to skin breakdown; prompt reporting of reddened areas helps ensure early treatment.*

- Provide ROM exercises when turning, if client is not independently moving all extremities. *Movement stimulates circulation, which provides oxygenation and allows nutrients to reach muscles and skin.*

- Keep the skin clean and dry; pay particular attention to the perineal area if the client is incontinent. If the client is incontinent, determine hydration status. *Skin in close proximity to perineal area, such as the sacral area, is highly susceptible to breakdown due to exposure to wet, acidic urine and fecal material.*

- Place client on an alternating-pressure mattress with foot board. *Decreasing pressure on bony prominences and preventing shearing forces serve to prevent skin breakdown.*

- Pad side rails and headrests of special chairs; have the client wear a football-type helmet. *The client's violent movements can cause trauma to the head and extremities.*

Impaired Verbal Communication

The client's inability to control muscles related to speech, swallowing, and facial movement contributes to problems of verbal communication. Because Huntington's disease affects fine motor movement, especially the distal portion of the extremities, the hands are not effective in communication. As the disease progresses, the client's mental abilities are also compromised, making both receptive and expressive communication impossible.

Nursing interventions with rationales follow:

- Choose alternative methods of communication while the client is able to participate. *Anticipatory planning may facilitate communication and decrease anxiety.*

- Continue to incorporate therapeutic communication techniques, even though client is not responsive:
  a. Maintain eye contact.
  b. Use touch.
  c. Talk directly to the client rather than to others in the room.
  These techniques enhance the individual's dignity and worth.

- Seek input from family regarding client's usual preferences and how they are communicated; be alert for subtle cues. *Nonverbal communication techniques may be individualized and more readily recognized by the family member or caregiver who usually provides care.*

- Continue talking to the client, even though there is no apparent response. *Hearing may not be impaired, even though the client cannot speak.*

Other Nursing Diagnoses

Additional nursing diagnoses for the early stage of Huntington's disease might include:

- *Impaired Physical Mobility* related to loss of motor control and chorea

- *Altered Role Performance* related to inability to carry out motor skills and communicate effectively

- *Altered Family Processes* related to need for constant care and supervision

- *Self-Esteem Disturbance* related to loss of control of facial movements and ability to verbally communicate
- *Ineffective Individual Coping* related to response to diagnosis
- *Fear* related to inevitable total loss of function

Additional nursing diagnoses that might apply to the client and family with later-stage Huntington's disease include:

- *Bathing/Hygiene Self-Care Deficit* related to total debilitation
- *Ineffective Management of Therapeutic Regimen* related to acceleration of disease manifestations
- *Urinary Incontinence* or *Bowel Incontinence* related to physical effects of the disease
- *Ineffective Airway Clearance* related to decreased function of the diaphragm
- *Powerlessness* related to inability to stop progression of the disease
- *Hopelessness* related to deteriorating condition

Client and Family Teaching

Clients and families who experience Huntington's disease know how devastating the illness is; they probably have cared for a parent or other close family member who has suffered through the illness. Many families are overwhelmed with just the thought of the physical and psychosocial debilitation that the disease brings. Fear, anxiety, and hopelessness leading to depression are common reactions. Teaching methods to cope effectively with the psychosocial and physical changes is an integral part of the nurse's responsibilities. Referrals to appropriate agencies, such as the national Huntington's Disease Foundation and local support groups or psychologist, should be part of the nursing plan. Because suicide is many times higher in this population, nurses need to intervene early with suicide prevention measures.

Another aspect of client teaching concerns the genetic transmission of Huntington's disease; clients and family members are referred to a geneticist. Nurses are frequently involved with clarifying information, especially concerning the transmission, course of illness, and prognosis. A caring, sensitive approach is crucial. Information about transmission of an autosomal-dominant trait is presented in the accompanying box.

Presymptomatic individuals have fear of the unknown and must decide whether to undergo genetic testing to determine presence of the marker on chromosome 4. Some might argue that knowledge of the trait's existence allows for time to prepare for the inevitable; others might argue that such knowledge would negatively impact the person's ability to enjoy life in the present. Parental guilt

---

Inheritance of an Autosomal Dominant Trait

- - -

- The abnormal trait is dominant over the normal characteristics—in the case of Huntington's disease, neurologic functioning.
- People affected usually have at least one parent who also is affected.
- Each offspring has a 50% risk of being affected. In other words, transmission of the dominant trait is independent of number of children who may or may not already have the disease.
- Both sexes are equally affected because the inheritance is autosomal dominant, not X-linked.
- Children who are not affected will not genetically transmit the disease to their children.

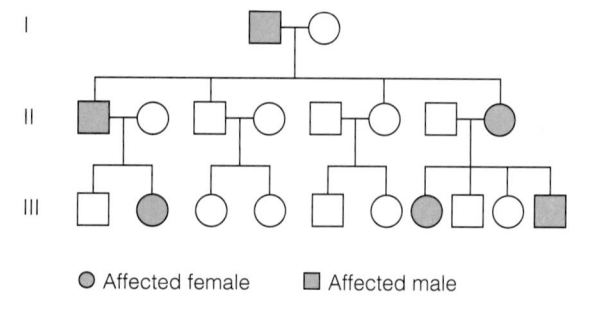

○ Affected female   ■ Affected male

---

compounds the devastation of diagnosis. Ethical questions surrounding genetic counseling include the client's feelings about abortion of an affected fetus.

Nurses in the community are often the professionals with whom families have the most contact. Teaching family members ways to prevent injury from falls (see the interventions discussed in the previous section on Parkinson's disease) and methods to avoid malnutrition are part of holistic care. Measures to assist with incontinence are instituted when indicated (see Chapters 23 and 25). If dementia is present, teach safety considerations (see the discussion of Alzheimer's disease).

The Client with Amyotrophic Lateral Sclerosis

■ ■ ■

Amyotrophic lateral sclerosis (ALS) is a progressive, degenerative neurologic disease characterized by weakness and wasting of the involved muscles, without any accompanying sensory or cognitive changes. The cause is unknown, but ALS involves loss of motor neurons in the spinal cord and brain stem. The name is derived from the pathophysiologic processes of muscle atrophy (*amyotrophy*) and the hardness of the affected tissues (*sclerosis*). Most people are between 40 and 70 years of age at diagnosis, with men having a slightly higher incidence. Many people know this disorder as *Lou Gehrig's disease,* named after the famous baseball player who contracted ALS. ALS is the most common motor neuron disease. In the United States, approximately 30,000 people have ALS; the incidence is approximately 4 per 100,000. Most of the physiologic problems a client with ALS encounters are related to swallowing and managing secretions, communication, and dysfunction of the muscles used in respiration.

Pathophysiology

ALS results from the degeneration and demyelination of motor neurons in the anterior horn of the spinal cord, brain stem, and cerebral cortex. It involves both upper and lower motor neurons. The upper motor neurons are located in the cerebral cortex and conduct impulses within the central nervous system. When upper motor neuron function is interrupted, the affected muscles become spastic, weak, and have increased deep-tendon reflexes. Lower motor neurons originate in the gray matter of the spinal cord or the brain stem cranial nerves and innervate skeletal muscles. A disruption in lower motor neuron transmission results in muscle flaccidity, weakness, paralysis, and atrophy.

Weakness and paresis are common early complaints. The weakness may initially affect only one muscle group (Chipps et al., 1992). Clinical manifestations vary according to the particular muscle group involved; **fasciculations,** or focal twitching, of involved muscles are common in the early stage of the disorder. With the loss of muscle innervation, the muscles atrophy, and paralysis results (Beal et al., 1991). Clinically, the muscle mass decreases, and clients complain of progressive fatigue. Typically, the disease first affects the hands, then the shoulders, upper arms, and finally the legs.

With increasing brain stem involvement, there is progressive atrophy of the tongue and facial muscles with eventual dysphagia and dysarthria. Emotional lability and loss of control occur, but dementia is not part of the pathologic progression of ALS. The senses of vision, hearing, and sensation as well as cognitive ability usually remain intact (Hickey, 1992). A summary of clinical manifestations is presented in the accompanying box.

About 50% of clients die within 3 to 5 years of diagnosis, but the course of the disease varies (Stone, 1987). Eventually, the client faces total debilitation and dependence. Death frequently results from aspiration pneumonia, another infectious process, or respiratory failure.

Clinical Manifestations of Amyotrophic Lateral Sclerosis

Musculoskeletal System

- Weakness and fatigue
- "Heaviness" of legs
- Fasciculations
- Uncoordinated movements, loss of fine motor control in hands
- Spasticity
- Paresis
- Hyperreflexia
- Atrophy
- Problems with articulation
- Complications: paralysis, loss of ability to perform ADLs, total immobility, aspiration, loss of verbal communication

Respiratory System

- Dyspnea
- Difficulty clearing airway
- Complications: pneumonia, eventual respiratory failure

Nutritional Effects

- Difficulty chewing
- Dysphagia
- Complication: malnutrition

Emotional Effects

- Loss of control, lability
- Complication: depression

Collaborative Care

Because there are many treatable disorders that may cause manifestations similar to those that appear in the initial stage of ALS, a thorough evaluation is required. Once ALS is diagnosed, the primary goal is to support the client and family in meeting physical and psychosocial needs, particularly as the disease progresses.

Medical and nursing care for clients with ALS is primarily supportive. Referral to community health nurses for home health management is indicated. Occupational, physical, speech, and respiratory therapy are major supportive and rehabilitative treatments. As the disorder progresses and swallowing becomes ineffective, a gastrostomy tube may be indicated to provide adequate nutritional intake (Rabin, 1986). Ventilatory assistance should be discussed with clients before the need occurs.

Laboratory and Diagnostic Tests

A number of disorders may mimic early ALS, including hyperthyroidism, hypoglycemia, compression of the spinal cord, toxic agents, infections, and neoplasms. In addition to diagnostic studies that are performed to rule out other suspected conditions, the following tests may be ordered:

- *EMG* is done to differentiate a neuropathy from a myopathy. Fibrillations of the muscle at rest supports the diagnosis of ALS.
- *Muscle biopsy* reflects tissue changes consistent with atrophy and loss of muscle fiber.
- *Serum creatine kinase (CK) enzyme levels* are usually elevated; however, this finding is not specific to ALS.
- *Pulmonary function studies* may be ordered if there is respiratory involvement.

Nursing Care

Nursing care focuses on the client's current problems and on anticipating the client's future difficulties. As with other disorders causing incapacitation and dependence, individualized nursing goals and interventions relate to decreasing complications, especially those associated with loss of muscular function and immobility; promoting independence to the extent possible; initiating referrals, particularly to a support group for both client and family; and providing physical and psychosocial support as indicated (see the previous discussions of nursing care in this chapter).

Of special consideration is planning for the client's eventual inability to communicate. Because the client's eye muscles and movements remain intact, signals can be prearranged prior to the loss of speech. Two nursing diagnoses that frequently apply to clients with ALS are: *Disuse Syndrome* and *Ineffective Breathing Pattern.*

Disuse Syndrome

Clients with ALS are at risk for developing problems associated with bed rest not only because they cannot move and reposition themselves but also because they frequently have altered nutritional and hydration status. Nursing interventions focus on preventing skin breakdown and infections, such as urinary tract infections.

Nursing interventions with rationales follow:

- Assess current condition for baseline parameters, particularly skin over bony prominences, lung sounds,

and vital signs. *Knowledge of the client's current condition allows for accurate future assessment and realistic planning.*
- Lubricate and inspect skin; obtain an alternating-pressure mattress. *Pressure points are at risk for breakdown; early detection is crucial to instituting appropriate care.*
- Institute active ROM exercises, as the client is able. Perform passive ROM exercises every 2 hours, when the client is turned. *Contractures can develop within a week because extensor muscles are weaker than flexor muscles (Carpenito, 1995).*
- Maintain positive nitrogen balance and hydration status: monitor albumin levels, hemoglobin and hematocrit levels, and urine specific gravity. *Adequate protein is required to maintain osmotic pressure and prevent edema; positive nitrogen balance promotes optimal body functioning.*
- Monitor client for manifestations of infection; for example, assess urinalysis, especially if a urinary catheter is present. *Urinary catheters place clients at high risk for developing sepsis; bed rest places the client at greater risk for urinary stasis.*

Ineffective Breathing Pattern

As the muscle weakness of ALS continues, clients become less able to breathe. The respiratory muscles are affected, and clients eventually may require ventilatory assistance. The nurse must initiate measures to support the existing respiratory effort.

Nursing interventions with rationales follow:

- Obtain a baseline assessment of breathing pattern, air movement, and oxygen saturation. *Assessments indicating the client's current condition provide data to plan individualized interventions.*
- Turn the client at least every 2 hours. *Mobility enhances the client's ability to move pulmonary secretions and prevents stasis.*
- Elevate the head of the bed at least 30 degrees, suction as indicated, and provide oxygen. *This supports ventilation and enhances lung expansion as the client's condition changes.*
- Assess the client's temperature and lung sounds routinely; obtain sputum culture as indicated. *Early detection of a possible infectious process leads to prompt treatment.*

Other Nursing Diagnoses

Additional possible nursing diagnoses follow:

- *Fatigue* related to muscle weakness
- *Risk for Aspiration* related to inability to manage secretions and effects of changes in neuromusculature

- *Self-Care Deficit: Bathing/Hygiene, Feeding, Dressing/ Grooming, Toileting* related to inability to control motor functions
- *Impaired Verbal Communication* related to weakness of muscles used in articulation
- *Ineffective Family Coping* related to altered abilities and role functions
- *Risk for Altered Sexuality Patterns* related to impaired communication and motor deficits

Also refer to Chapter 41 (on spinal cord injuries) for interventions appropriate for clients who face incapacitation and total care needs.

Client and Family Teaching

Initial teaching centers on explaining the disease process, expected course, and prognosis. Clients and families require assistance with realistic planning. Referral to a social worker to determine home care needs and financial assistance also is helpful. Counseling and referrals to a community health nurse, dietitian, and physical, speech,

and occupational therapists can help the family meet the client's changing needs and abilities. The necessity for realistic anticipation of needs cannot be overemphasized.

As the client becomes more debilitated, family members or other care providers focus on preventing complications. For example, family members need to know how to suction the client and perform the Heimlich maneuver to prevent aspiration. Teaching the family how to prevent problems related to immobility is a primary consideration for the nurse.

Another focus of teaching is basic care needs, such as care required to meet elimination needs. Families are taught methods to establish a bowel routine, considerations related to a urinary catheter, and symptoms of constipation or infection to report promptly.

Throughout the early stage and continued care of the client and family with ALS, much consideration is given to psychosocial concerns. Depression, anger, and denial may be initial reactions; refer the client and family to an ALS support group, social worker, psychologist, or psychiatrist as indicated. Nurses are in a unique position to coordinate care and evaluate the effectiveness of home care.

Disorders of the Peripheral Nervous System

There are many etiologic agents responsible for peripheral nervous system disorders. Autoimmune disorders, viruses, environmental toxins such as heavy metals, and nutritional deficiencies can all affect the peripheral nervous system. Although there are various other peripheral nervous system disorders, this section discusses myasthenia gravis and Guillain-Barré syndrome. Nursing care for clients experiencing these disorders focuses on problems of immobility, ineffective breathing, and self-care deficits.

The Client with Myasthenia Gravis

■ ■ ■

Myasthenia gravis is a chronic, progressive neuromuscular disorder characterized by fatigue and severe weakness of skeletal muscles. Clients experience periods of remission and exacerbation, and mild forms of the disorder exist. Weakness may remain limited to a few muscle groups, especially the ocular muscles, or may become generalized with all muscles eventually becoming weakened.

Myasthenia gravis is believed to be an autoimmune disease. It occurs in approximately 1 in 10,000 people, and women are more frequently affected than men. The age of onset for most women is between ages 20 and 40,

whereas the age of onset for most men is between ages 50 and 60 (Drachman, 1991). Treatment with anticholinesterase medications has greatly improved the prognosis and symptom management.

Pathophysiology

The axons of motor neurons divide as they enter skeletal muscles, and each axonal ending forms a neuromuscular junction. Although the axonal ending and the muscle fiber are extremely close, they are separated by a space, the synaptic cleft. The transmission of nerve impulses from the nerve to the muscles occurs at the neuromuscular junctions. The neurotransmitter acetylcholine is released from the axonal ending, crosses the synaptic cleft, attaches to acetylcholine receptors on the muscle fiber, and stimulates the muscle.

In myasthenia gravis, antibodies destroy or block neuromuscular junction receptor sites, resulting in a decrease in the number of acetylcholine receptors. There are also structural changes that result in diminished acetylcholine uptake (Pallett & O'Brien, 1985). The net result is a decrease in the muscle's ability to contract despite a sufficient amount of acetylcholine. A comparison of a normal neuromuscular junction and one affected by myasthenia gravis is shown in Figure 42–7.

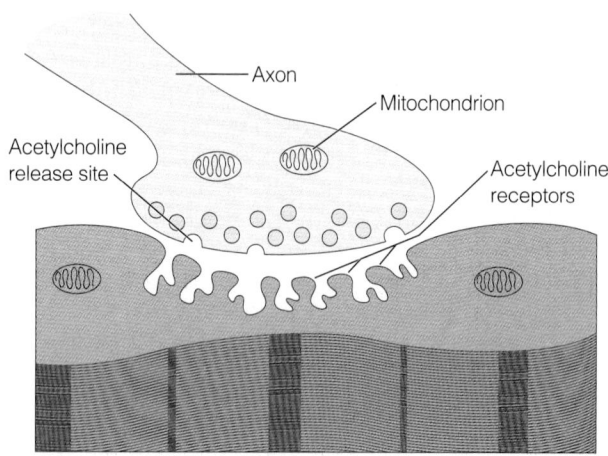

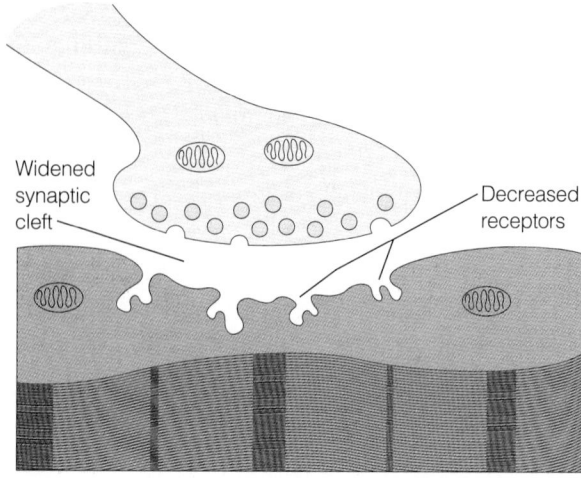

A Normal neuromuscular junction

B Myasthenia gravis

Figure 42–7   *A,* A normal neuromuscular junction and *B,* one showing the changes seen in myasthenia gravis. These changes interfere with the transmission of nerve impulses to the muscle.

In about 75% of clients with myasthenia gravis, the thymus gland, which is usually inactive after puberty, continues to produce antibodies because of hyperplasia of the gland or because of tumors. It is believed that the thymus is a source of autoantigen that triggers an autoimmune response in myasthenia gravis (Drachman, 1991). The exact mechanism and reason for the thymus gland's antibody production is unknown.

The clinical manifestations of myasthenia gravis correspond to the muscles involved. Initially, the eye muscles are affected and the client experiences either **diplopia** (unilateral or bilateral double vision) or **ptosis** (drooping

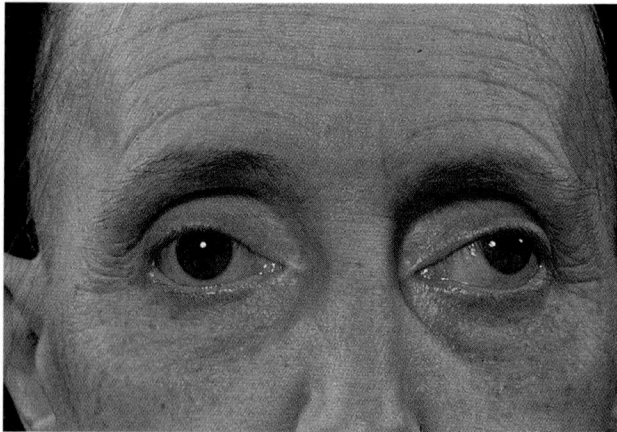

Figure 42–8   In myasthenia gravis, the client experiences unilateral weakness of the facial muscles. Note the drooping of one eyelid.

of the eyelid) (Figure 42–8). Next, the facial, speech, and mastication muscles become weak, and clients may have periods of dysarthria and dysphagia. Fatigue is evident even when the client tries to eat a meal; the muscles of chewing tire, and the client is forced to stop eating momentarily. A smile becomes a snarl or grimace, and the voice is weak with a muffled nasal quality.

As the disease progresses, the muscles of the neck and extremities become affected; in some clients, problems in performing fine motor movements of the hands, such as writing, appear early in the disease. As the muscles of the neck become affected, the head juts forward (Hickey, 1992). For many clients, weakness in their legs when climbing stairs is the first manifestation. Deep-tendon reflexes are usually normal, however, even in weak muscles. Fatigue and weakness are exacerbated with stress, fever, overexertion, and exposure to heat and are relieved by rest. Symptoms vary on a daily basis, and the disease is characterized by remissions and exacerbations. Clinical manifestations of myathenis gravis are listed in the accompanying box.

Complications are directly related to the degree of muscle weakness and the specific muscles involved. For example, when the pharyngeal and palatal muscles are affected, the client is not able to manage swallowing and may aspirate food or fluids. The client is at increased risk for pneumonia because weakness of the diaphragm and muscles of respiration compromises gas exchange.

Clients with myasthenia gravis can develop life-threatening emergencies. A *myasthenic crisis* is a sudden exacerbation of motor weakness exposing the client to the risk of respiratory failure and aspiration. Myasthenic crisis most often is due to undermedication, missed doses of medication, or a developing infection (Chipps, 1991). Manifestations of myasthenic crisis include tachycardia, tachypnea, severe respiratory distress, dysphagia, restlessness, impaired speech, and anxiety. *Cholinergic crisis* is the result of overdosage with anticholinesterase (cholinergic) medications used to treat myasthenia gravis (Price & Wilson, 1992). Gastrointestinal symptoms, severe muscle weakness, vertigo, and respiratory distress are signs of cholinergic crisis. Both types of crises are emergency, life-threatening situations; clients frequently require ventilatory assistance. Differentiation is based on the client's response to Tensilon. In myasthenic crisis the test is positive, and in cholinergic crisis the test is negative (see discussion below).

Collaborative Care

Care of the client with myasthenia gravis focuses on providing appropriate treatment, preventing complications, and supporting the client and family in meeting physical and psychosocial needs, especially as the disease progresses.

Laboratory and Diagnostic Tests

Laboratory and diagnostic tests are performed following a thorough history and physical examination, with special attention to the facial, oculomotor, laryngeal, and respiratory muscles. Diagnostic tests include the following:

- *Tensilon test.* The client is injected with edrophonium chloride (Tensilon), a short-acting anticholinesterase. In clients with myasthenia gravis, there is a significant improvement in muscle strength that lasts approximately 5 minutes. This test is also used to differentiate myasthenic crisis (caused by insufficient medication, so the client shows improvement with the drug) from cholinergic crisis (caused by overmedication, so the client does not show improvement).
- *EMG studies* demonstrate a reduced amplitude of the action potential in response to electrical stimulation when myasthenia gravis is present.
- *Antiacetylcholine receptor antibody serum levels* are increased in about 80% of clients with myasthenia gravis; this test is also useful in follow-up of effectiveness of therapy (Drachman, 1991).
- *CT scan* of the chest may demonstrate abnormalities in the thymus.
- *Pulmonary function tests* assess the degree of respiratory involvement and establish a baseline. Maximum inspiratory pressure (MIP) is highly selective to respiratory muscle weakness (Hoffman, 1987).
- *Other tests* may be performed to rule out specific disorders causing similar presenting symptoms, for example, CT or MRI scans of the head may document the presence of a tumor causing the ocular complaints.

Clinical Manifestations of Myasthenia Gravis

Ocular and Facial

- Ptosis
- Diplopia
- Facial weakness
- Dysphagia
- Dysarthria
- Complications: difficulty closing eyes, aspiration, impaired communication and nutrition

Musculoskeletal

- Weakness and fatigue
- Decreased function of hands, arms, legs, and neck muscles
- Complications: inability to perform ADLs and self-care activities, complications related to immobility, myasthenic and cholinergic crises

Respiratory

- Weakening of intercostal muscles
- Decrease in diaphragm movement
- Breathlessness and dyspnea
- Poor gas exchange
- Complications: decreasing ability to walk, eat, and perform other ADLs, pneumonia

Nutritional

- Inability to chew and swallow
- Decreasing ability to move tongue
- Impairment of fine motor movements: inability to feed self
- Complications: weight loss, dehydration, malnutrition, aspiration

---

Pharmacology

The primary group of medications used to treat myasthenia gravis is the *anticholinesterases.* These drugs act at the neuromuscular junction and allow acetylcholine to concentrate at the receptor sites, thus promoting muscle contraction. Pyridostigmine (Mestinon) is the most commonly used *acetylcholinesterase* inhibitor for myasthenia gravis. The client's decrease in symptoms guides dosage.

Nursing Implications for Pharmacology: The Client with Myasthenia Gravis

ANTICHOLINESTERASES/CHOLINESTERASE INHIBITORS

Neostigmine (Prostigmin)

Ambenonium (Mytelase Caplets)

Pyridostigmine (Mestinon, Regonol)

For diagnosis: edrophonium chloride (Tensilon)

Cholinesterase inhibitors are used in myasthenia to enhance the effects of acetylcholine at the remaining skeletal muscle receptors. Cholinesterase inhibitors do not cure or change the underlying pathophysiologic processes, but they can provide effective, lifelong improvement of symptoms. Because the cholinesterase inhibitors are nonselective, the neuromuscular, muscarinic, and ganglionic junctions are each affected.

Adjusting the dose to obtain maximum benefit with minimal side effects is a major consideration when administering cholinesterase inhibitors. Initially, small doses are given followed by incremental increases until optimal muscle strength is obtained. The dose may need to be adjusted when activities result in symptoms of undermedication, such as increased ptosis. Severe undermedication results in myasthenic crisis. Although a sustained release form of pyridostigmine is available for bedtime use, it should not be used during the day because of its inconsistent absorption.

When the client takes an overdose of anticholinesterase inhibitors, a cholinergic crisis occurs. Clients and family members must be taught the symptoms and actions to take in each crisis. The oral dose of neostigmine is approximately 30 times greater than parenteral doses.

Cholinesterase inhibitors should not be administered to clients experiencing obstruction of the intestinal or urinary tract. Caution is advised when administering these drugs to clients with asthma, hyperthyroidism, bradycardia, or peptic ulcer disease. Cholinesterase inhibitors can cross the placenta; reproductive counseling is indicated (Flagg, 1991).

Nursing Responsibilities

- Obtain a baseline assessment of muscle strength and abilities, concentrating on swallowing and ptosis.
- Administer the medication parenterally if the client has dysphagia.

- Check the dose of the medication carefully when changing from oral to parenteral routes.
- Evaluate the effectiveness of the medication and document the response, for example, time when fatigue occurs in relation to activities.
- Promptly recognize and respond to manifestations of excessive stimulation of muscarinic receptors: excess salivation, urinary urgency, bradycardia, gastrointestinal hypermotility, diaphoresis. Atropine can be administered to combat these manifestations. Respiratory depression and failure can occur and requires mechanical ventilation.
- Have a muscarinic antagonist (e.g., physostigmine) readily available to treat poisoning.

Client and Family Teaching

- Balancing symptom control with dosage is crucial; record time of dose and response in a journal. Note the time of day when fatigued and any adverse effects, such as excess salivation, sweating, slow heartbeat, and diarrhea.
- Take the medication about 30 minutes prior to meals to enhance swallowing and chewing.
- Report manifestations of myasthenic crisis immediately: severe muscle weakness, fast heartbeat, restlessness, difficulty breathing, increasing difficulty swallowing or speaking.
- Report manifestations of cholinergic crisis immediately: slow heartbeat, increased salivation or sweating, decreased blood pressure.
- Review possible causes of myasthenic crisis: physical or emotional stress, infection, or reduction in the medication dosage.
- Wear or carry MedicAlert identification.

IMMUNOSUPPRESSANTS

Corticosteroids: prednisone (Deltasone, Meticorten), methylprednisolone (Solu-Medrol)

Azathioprine (Imuran)

Cyclosporine (Cytoxan)

Immunosuppressants are administered to inhibit the body's autoimmune response. Because symptoms may not improve for several weeks, clients need to be encouraged to continue therapy despite little change in

Pharmacology: The Client with Myasthenia Gravis (continued)

muscle weakness. Precautions related to steroid therapy include infection, adrenal insufficiency, osteoporosis, glucose intolerance, and cataract formation. Clients are warned about the probable body changes secondary to iatrogenic Cushing's syndrome. See the discussion of steroid therapy in multiple sclerosis for more information related to immunosuppressive therapy.

Immunosuppression with glucocorticoids, typically prednisone, is another pharmacologic therapy aimed at improving muscle strength. Clients need to be aware of the need to stay on the drug at the prescribed dose to determine the least amount required for efficacy. If clients do not respond to prednisone alone, it may be combined with other immunosuppressive agents, such as cyclosporine or azathioprine (Imuran). Nursing implications for medications used to treat myasthenia gravis are presented in the accompanying box.

Surgery

Approximately 75% of clients with myasthenia gravis have dysplasia of the thymus gland (Drachman, 1991); therefore, **thymectomy** is often recommended within the first 2 years of diagnosis. The two surgical approaches used are the transcervical approach, which is considered less invasive, and the transternal approach. The latter approach allows a more extensive removal of the gland. However, it also poses more potential complications because it involves splitting the sternum (Pallett & O'Brien, 1985).

Preoperatively, clients may be tapered from steroid therapy. Usually, pyridostigmine is administered to prevent muscular manifestations during the perioperative period. Postoperative nursing care focuses on preventing complications and controlling pain. Nursing implications for the client undergoing thymectomy are presented in the accompanying box. Remission is obtained in about 40% of clients but may take several years to achieve. Refer to Chapter 34 for care of the client having a thoracotomy and chest tubes.

A tracheostomy may be required when the diaphragm or intercostal muscles are involved.

Nursing Care of the Client Undergoing a Thymectomy

PREOPERATIVE CARE

- Reinforce the physician's explanation of the procedure, and prepare the client for chest tubes and tracheostomy. *Realistic preparation of what to expect postoperatively encourages compliance and allays anxiety.*

- Anticipate the need for alternative communication. *The client may have a tracheostomy; preoperative planning facilitates communication after surgery.*

- Allow sufficient time for questions. *Thymectomy is a major surgery requiring either a thoracotomy and sternal split or transcervical approach. The client is usually anxious, and adequate time must be allocated to preoperative instruction.*

POSTOPERATIVE CARE

- Provide meticulous pulmonary hygiene: turning, deep breathing, and coughing at least every 2 hours; use an incentive spirometer. *Regardless of surgical approach, measures are aimed at preventing pulmonary complications of atelectasis and pneumonia.*

- Clients with a thoracotomy and sternal split procedure will require care of the anterior chest tube. Observe for complications, such as pneumothorax. *Air may enter the thoracic cavity—be alert for sudden chest pain and dyspnea, decreased breath sounds, and early signs of shock, such as restlessness.*

- Manage pain with scheduled analgesic therapy. *Maintaining a therapeutic blood level of analgesic provides better pain control than waiting until the client requests medication, as on a prn basis.*

Plasmapheresis

Plasma exchange in myasthenia gravis may be used in conjunction with other therapies; for example, it may be performed prior to surgical intervention. The goal of therapy is to remove the antiacetylcholine receptor antibodies, thus improving severe muscle weakness, fatigue, and other symptoms. The procedure is frequently performed when respiratory muscle involvement is evident. Approximately four daily exchanges every other day are performed (Hickey, 1992). Refer to the discussion on plasmapheresis, earlier in this chapter.

Nursing Care

Nursing care of clients with myasthenia gravis focuses not only on present problems but also on anticipated needs. Preventing myasthenic and cholinergic crises and providing psychologic support to clients and families are two important aspects of care. Individualized care depends on the specific therapy instituted. This section discusses the nursing diagnoses *Ineffective Airway Clearance* and *Impaired Swallowing;* other nursing diagnoses that commonly apply, such as *Fatigue,* are addressed in other sections of this chapter.

Ineffective Airway Clearance

The underlying causes for ineffective airway clearance for the person with myasthenia gravis include poor cough mechanism, decreased rib cage expansion, diminished diaphragm movement, and decreased expiratory effort (Hoffman, 1987). The interventions listed below require particular attention if the client undergoes a thymectomy.

Nursing interventions with rationales follow:

- Assist the client with turning, deep breathing, and coughing at least every 2 hours. Teach proper coughing techniques; use an incentive spirometer every 2 hours while the client is awake. *Position changes promote lung expansion; coughing aids in clearing secretions from the tracheobronchial tree.*

- Use the semi-Fowler's position. *This position expands the lungs and alleviates pressure from the diaphragm, especially important considerations if the client is obese.*

- Maintain the client's hydration status and monitor for dehydration; use a humidifier as needed. If needed, teach family how to perform percussion, postural drainage and suction. *Interventions to liquefy secretions, such as ensuring a daily fluid intake of up to 2500 mL (perhaps via feeding tube or parenteral route) helps the client mobilize and expectorate sputum.*

- Assess lung sounds, the rate and character of respirations, and pulse oximetry readings at least every 4 hours or as indicated by client's condition. *Monitoring*

for hypoxia and worsening of client's ability to move air alerts the nurse to early signs of arteriovenous shunting.

Impaired Swallowing

Clients with myasthenia gravis have weakness of the laryngeal and pharyngeal muscles involved with swallowing. Alterations in swallowing place the client at risk for poor nutrition as well as for possible aspiration. Family members need to be included in teaching, particularly the person who prepares and assists with meals.

Nursing interventions with rationales follow:

- Assess the client's ability to manage safely various consistencies of foods; consult with a speech pathologist for evaluation. *Dysphagic clients are at risk for aspiration; matching food consistency to the client's ability to swallow enhances safety.*

- Plan meals to promote medication effectiveness. *Pyridostigmine should be given 30 minutes before the meal to provide optimal muscle strength for swallowing and chewing (Hickey, 1992).*

- Have the client eat slowly, using small bites of food. Schedule meals during periods when the client is adequately rested; develop a daily schedule incorporating rest periods. *Fatigue may add to dysphagia, putting the client at greater risk for aspiration.*

- If necessary, give cues while eating to remind client of task: "Chew your food thoroughly; swallow." *Keeping client focused may enhance swallowing (Carpenito, 1995).*

- Teach caregivers the Heimlich maneuver and how to suction. *Knowing specific measures to take in the event of aspiration decreases both the client's and family's anxiety and promotes confidence in managing potential problems.*

If the above interventions do not ensure adequate swallowing and maintain body weight, a consultation with the physician may be necessary for further evaluation. Alternative feeding methods, such as a gastrostomy tube, may be indicated.

Other Nursing Diagnoses

Clients who have myasthenia gravis need to be assessed for problems in meeting self-care needs. Families are at risk for problems related to inability to cope with the multiple difficulties the person with myasthenia gravis presents.

Possible nursing diagnoses follow:

- *Activity Intolerance* related to fatigue
- *Altered Role Performance* related to immobility
- *Impaired Social Interaction* related to changed body image
- *Self-Care Deficit: Bathing/Hygiene, Feeding, Dressing/ Grooming* related to muscle weakness
- *Risk for Injury* related to altered swallowing and loss of motor control

Client and Family Teaching

Teaching the client and family with myasthenia gravis focuses on prevention and recognition of crisis situations, understanding the disorder, and methods for coping with both physical and psychosocial problems. Setting realistic goals with the client and family provides opportunities for self-assessment and promotes active participation in rehabilitation (Diehl, 1989).

Preventing myasthenic and cholinergic crises includes stressing the importance of maintaining consistency in medication dosage and management. Teach about side effects and scheduling, and instruct the client to avoid nonprescription medications without first consulting the physician. Manifestations of both types of crisis are part of teaching.

Clients and family members need to know what myasthenia gravis is and what they must realistically expect. Incorporate methods to avoid fatigue and undue stress in the teaching plan; specific measures for avoiding upper respiratory infections and exposure to extreme heat or cold also are important. Birth control measures or referral for counseling may be indicated because pregnancy can cause exacerbation of symptoms; also, medications used to control myasthenia gravis, such as neostigmine bromide (Prostigmin), cross the placenta (Flagg, 1991).

Referral to support groups is one intervention for enhancing coping. Assess both formal and informal support systems prior to referral.

Keeping goals realistic to the client's current capabilities promotes self-esteem. Because avoiding fatigue is a major part of teaching, it is important to incorporate interventions to enhance rest and conserve energy; see the accompanying box. Suggest that client sit while preparing meals and while performing hygiene and grooming, for example (Rhynsburger, 1989). Anticipating problems, such as impaired communication, and developing alternative solutions can be helpful in promoting independence.

Applying the Nursing Process

Case Study of a Client with Myasthenia Gravis: Kirsten Avis

Kirsten Avis, a 44-year-old homemaker and mother of two teenage sons, was diagnosed with myasthenia gravis 2 years ago. She takes an anticholinesterase medication, pyridostigmine (Mestinon), four times a day. Over the past month she has been experimenting with decreasing the dose of her pyridostigmine because she has "felt so good." She was prescribed 60 mg of pyridostigmine three times a day before meals and one-half of a long-acting 180-mg pyridostigmine tablet at night.

Client and Family Teaching to Avoid Weakness in Myasthenia Gravis

- Promote periods of rest and avoid stress; conserve energy when possible.
- Avoid cigarette smoke, alcohol, and beverages with quinine (e.g., tonic water).
- Take medications as prescribed. If manifestations change, consult the physician; the dose may need to be adjusted.
- Avoid extremes of temperature; an environment that is too hot or too cold may cause an exacerbation of myasthenia gravis.
- Avoid people with upper respiratory infections; infections can result in an exacerbation and extreme weakness.

Three days ago, she began having chills and fever and her myasthenic symptoms became markedly worse. Mrs. Avis is easily fatigued and has been experiencing increasing weakness, bilateral ptosis, and mild dysphagia in the late afternoon and evenings.

Assessment

Lela Silva, RN, is caring for Mrs. Avis. Physical examination of Mrs. Avis reveals severe muscle weakness bilaterally in her hands, arms, and thorax. Her voice is nasal, and she speaks slowly; the longer she speaks, the more difficult it becomes to understand her. She is anxious and dyspneic. Her complaints of weakness, dysphagia, dysarthria, problems with mobility, and ptosis are more pronounced later in the day. Vital signs are as follows: BP, 138/88; P, 88; R, 28; T, 102.4 F (39 C).

Some clinical improvement in muscle weakness is noted following a restful night's sleep; however, the respiratory distress is more evident, and Mrs. Avis is increasingly restless. She is moved to the intensive care unit for advanced monitoring and possible ventilatory assistance. The physician's diagnosis is myasthenic crisis secondary to pulmonary infection.

Diagnosis

Ms. Silva identifies the following nursing diagnoses:

- *Impaired Gas Exchange* related to ineffective breathing pattern and muscle weakness
- *Risk for Aspiration* related to difficulty swallowing
- *Fatigue* related to increased energy needs from muscular involvement

- *Ineffective Management of Therapeutic Regimen* related to insufficient knowledge

Expected Outcomes

The expected outcomes established in the plan of care specify that

- Pulse oximetry readings will be maintained at 92% or above.

- No aspiration will occur.

- Mrs. Avis will verbalize decreasing fatigue when performing ADLs.

- Mrs. Avis will state the correct method of medication dosing and demonstrate how she will maintain schedule.

- Mrs. Avis will state potential reasons for myasthenic crisis and list ways to avoid crisis.

Planning and Implementation

Mrs. Avis's clinical manifestations improve following administration of edrophonium (Tensilon) to verify myasthenic crisis. She is placed on oxygen mask and suctioned as needed; equipment for possible intubation and ventilation is made readily available.

Mrs. Avis receives careful monitoring while her blood level of pyridostigmine returns to a therapeutic range. She is placed in a semi-Fowler's position, and vital signs are assessed every 5 minutes during the acute exacerbation. Marilyn Holland, RN, and other nurses in the intensive care unit remain in constant attendance throughout the crisis period and provide explanations to Mrs. Avis in an effort to decrease her stress and to avoid further severity of manifestations.

Three days after the crisis period, Mrs. Avis is moved to a progressive nursing care unit. Nurses follow up on teaching her the manifestations of both myasthenic and cholinergic crisis. They discuss the need to wear Medic-Alert identification and reviewed medication administration techniques with Mrs. Avis. The nurses emphasize in particular that Mrs. Avis must not split time-released medications.

Within 5 days, Mrs. Avis's condition stabilizes, and her weakness decreases sufficiently to allow discharge home. Although her temperature has returned to normal and her respiratory status has improved, she still has a productive cough. Oral antibiotics are prescribed for a 2-week period, after which she will have a follow-up visit with her primary care provider. Nurse Holland carefully instructs Mrs. Avis to seek treatment promptly if respiratory symptoms or temperature indicate recurrence of infection.

Evaluation

Mrs. Avis is discharged without developing aspiration pneumonia or any symptoms of aspiration. Her airway was maintained throughout the myasthenic crisis, and her pulse oximetry readings remained above 92% once oxygen therapy was initiated. On discharge, pulse oximetry is above 95% without oxygen therapy. Mrs. Avis states that her fatigue and weakness have significantly improved.

Both Mrs. Avis and her husband are able to explain the difference between myasthenic and cholinergic crises and to identify methods to avoid both problems. Mrs. Avis correctly relates her proper medication regimen and makes an appointment for a follow-up visit with her physician.

Critical Thinking in the Nursing Process

1. Mrs. Avis has a 12-year-old niece, who asks you what is happening to her aunt; explain myasthenia gravis and myasthenic crisis to a preteen of average intelligence.

2. Provide Mrs. Avis and her husband with several realistic methods to relieve stress, taking into account their busy schedules and family responsibilities.

3. What is the rationale for administering Tensilon to evaluate a myasthenic crisis?

4. Develop a plan to teach Mrs. Avis how to avoid fatigue when preparing and eating meals.

5. Develop a nursing care plan for Mrs. Avis for the nursing diagnosis *Altered Role Performance*.

The Client with Guillain-Barré Syndrome

■ ■ ■

Guillain-Barré syndrome (GBS) is an acute demyelinating disorder of the peripheral nervous system characterized by progressive, usually rapid muscle weakness and paralysis. Other names for Guillain-Barré syndrome are *postinfection polyneuritis, acute demyelinating polyneuropathy,* and *acute idiopathic polyneuritis.*

Guillain-Barré syndrome is one of the most common peripheral nervous system disorders; its incidence is approximately 1.3 per 100,000 (Rowland, 1989). It usually follows a viral respiratory or gastrointestinal infection. Cytomegalovirus, herpes zoster, and even general anesthesia have been associated with development of the disease (Rowland, 1989). An outbreak of Guillain-Barré syndrome occurred in the United States following the 1976 to 1977 immunization program for swine flu. The cause of the increase in the number of cases has not been discovered (Asbury, 1991).

Clients with Guillain-Barré syndrome have muscle pain, sensory changes, and symmetric paralysis (Pallett & O'Brien, 1985); the client may become quadriplegic.

Interventions during the acute phase (1 to 3 weeks) focus primarily on ensuring oxygenation via ventilatory assistance and preventing complications from immobility. Rehabilitation time to regain muscle strength and function varies; most people return to full presyndrome muscle function within 6 months to 2 years.

The cause of Guillain-Barré syndrome is not known, but an autoimmunologic response is thought to be responsible for the demyelination.

Pathophysiology

Four different clinical presentations of Guillain-Barré syndrome are possible, as outlined in the accompanying box. The primary pathophysiologic process in Guillain-Barré syndrome is the destruction of myelin sheaths covering the axons of peripheral nerves. The demyelination is thought to be an autoimmune response. The loss of myelin results in poor conduction of nerve impulses, causing sudden muscle weakness and loss of reflex response. Other clinical manifestations occur when nerve conduction to various muscles is interrupted. The stages of Guillain-Barré syndrome and their usual clinical manifestations are presented in the box on page 1848.

Muscles, sensory nerves, and cranial nerves are commonly affected in clients with Guillain-Barré syndrome. Most people experience symmetric muscle weakness, initially in the lower extremities; the weakness and sensory loss then ascends to the upper extremities, torso, and cranial nerves (Chipps et al., 1992). Sensory involvement includes severe pain, paresthesia, and numbness. Cognition and level of consciousness are not affected. Facial nerve involvement results in the inability to change facial expressions and close the eyes. Muscles involved with chewing, swallowing, and speaking may be affected.

Altered respiratory function due to paralysis of intercostal and diaphragmatic muscles occurs in almost one-fourth of clients with Guillain-Barré syndrome (Pallett & O'Brien, 1985). These clients require ventilatory assistance and supportive care. Involvement of the autonomic nervous system is characterized by fluctuating blood pressure, cardiac dysrhythmias and tachycardia, paralytic ileus, syndrome of inappropriate antidiuretic hormone secretion (SIADH), and urinary retention (Hickey, 1992).

Although the mortality rate is approximately 4%, the overall prognosis is good; almost 85% of clients recover completely or nearly completely (Asbury, 1991); rehabilitation may require 2 years, however. Women who have had Guillain-Barré syndrome are at increased risk for relapse in the first trimester of pregnancy (Rowland, 1989).

Collaborative Care

Care of the client with Guillain-Barré syndrome requires a team approach. From the initial acute phase through re-

---

Clinical Presentations of Guillain-Barré Syndrome

■ ■ ■

Ascending

- Most common presentation.
- Weakness and numbness begin in the legs, then progress upward to the trunk, arms, and cranial nerves.
- Motor deficits: paresis to quadriplegia; deficits are symmetric.
- Sensory deficits: mild numbness, which is worse in toes.
- Reflexes: diminished or absent.
- Respiratory insufficiency occurs in about 50% of clients.

Descending

- Motor deficits: initial weakness in the cranial nerves (facial, glossopharyngeal, vagus, and hypoglossal nerves); weakness then progresses downward.
- Sensory deficits: numbness occurs distally, more often in the hands than in the feet.
- Reflexes: diminished or absent.
- Rapid respiratory involvement.

Miller-Fisher Variant

- Rare presentation.
- Seen as a triad of ophthalmoplegia, areflexia, and pronounced ataxia.
- Usually no sensory loss.
- Rarely, respiratory involvement occurs.

Pure Motor

- Identical to ascending form; sensory manifestations are absent, however.
- May be a mild form of ascending Guillain-Barré syndrome.
- Muscle pain is generally not present.

---

habilitation, many members of the health care team are involved. An accurate and rapid diagnosis is needed to ensure prompt supportive treatment, particularly if there

---

Stages of Guillain-Barré Syndrome

■ ■ ■

I. Acute Stage

- Characterized by severe and rapid weakness, especially in the lower extremities; loss of muscle strength progressing to quadriplegia and respiratory failure; decreasing deep-tendon reflexes; decreasing vital capacity; paresthesias, numbness; pain, especially nocturnal; facial muscle involvement (inability to wrinkle forehead or change expressions).

- Involvement of the autonomic nervous system manifested by bradycardia, sweating, fluctuating blood pressure, notably hypotension, which may last for 2 weeks.

II. Stabilizing/Plateau Stage

- Occurs 2 to 3 weeks after initial onset.
- Marks the end of changes in condition; characterized by a "leveling off" of symptoms.
- Generally, the labile autonomic functions stabilize.

III. Recovery Stage

- May take from several months to 2 years.
- Marked by improvement in symptoms.
- Generally, muscle strength and function return in descending order.

---

is respiratory involvement combined with widespread paralysis.

Laboratory and Diagnostic Tests

Diagnosis of Guillain-Barré syndrome is made after a thorough history and clinical examination. It must be differentiated from several disorders, among them influenza, heavy metal poisoning, Lyme disease, and cranial hemorrhage (Penrose, 1993). Although there is no specific test to diagnose this syndrome, several findings support and confirm the diagnosis.

The following tests may be ordered:

- *CSF analysis* shows decreased protein concentration in the initial phase, followed by a rapid, severe rise in protein. This elevation is caused by active demyelination (Corbett, 1992).

- *EMG studies* reflect decreased nerve conduction with fibrillations during the severe stage of the syndrome.

- *Pulmonary function tests and arterial blood gases* are performed when respiratory function is compromised. Results reflect the decreased ventilatory function.

Pharmacology

There are no pharmacologic agents available for the specific treatment of Guillain-Barré syndrome. Some controversy exists over the use of corticosteroid therapy. High-dose steroids may be administered intravenously during the acute phase; as the client's condition improves and the ability to swallow returns, smaller doses are given orally. Immunosuppressive agents, such as azathioprine (Imuran) and cyclophosphamide (Cytoxan), may also be used (Chipps, 1992).

Other medications may be prescribed to provide support or prophylaxis, or to combat concurrent problems; for example, antibiotics may be prescribed for urinary tract or respiratory infections. Morphine is commonly administered to control muscle pain and for clients on ventilators. Anticoagulation therapy is usually instituted to prevent thromboembolic complications, such as deep vein thrombosis and pulmonary embolism, which are associated with prolonged bed rest. If hypotension is a problem, vasopressors are prescribed.

Surgery

Tracheostomy is performed if respiratory failure is present. Clients who require ventilatory support are usually able to be weaned after 2 to 3 weeks, but the time frame varies greatly. When the client's vital capacity reaches 8 to 10 mL/kg, he or she may be weaned from the ventilator (Hickey, 1992). Nursing care for the client with a tracheostomy is described in Chapter 33. Insertion of a temporary pacemaker may be indicated for bradycardia. See Chapter 28 for care of a client undergoing pacemaker insertion.

Plasmapheresis

Plasma exchange has been beneficial, particularly when performed within the first 2 weeks of the syndrome's development (Asbury, 1991). Along with the removal of the antibodies, immunosuppressive agents are administered concurrently. Clients typically have five exchanges during an 8- to 10-day period. For more information about plasmapheresis, see the section on multiple sclerosis.

Diet Therapy

Nutritional support for the client who is immobilized for prolonged periods of time is crucial. Maintaining positive nitrogen balance, ensuring sufficient fluid intake and electrolyte balance, and ensuring recommended caloric intake are goals of therapy. When swallowing problems occur, total parenteral nutrition may be indicated if feeding via a nasogastric or gastrostomy tube is ineffective.

Rehabilitation Therapy

Long-term physical and occupational therapy is crucial to recovery. Clients with Gullain-Barré syndrome usually require prolonged rehabilitation care. Rehabilitation begins during the acute phase and focuses on preventing complications and limiting the effects of immobility. The severe muscle atrophy and loss of muscle tone require that clients relearn many functions and skills, such as walking. Compromise in respiratory function may delay physical rehabilitation; clients need positive reinforcement when they make even small gains in their progress. Continued attention to pain control is essential because paresthesia and pain can interfere with physical therapy.

Nursing Care

Many of the nursing interventions for clients with this syndrome involve assessing neurologic function, preventing problems of immobility, ensuring adequate hydration and nutrition, promoting respiratory function, and providing psychosocial support. Anticipating needs of both the client and family is an important aspect of care. For example, developing an alternative method of communication before one is necessary may decrease anxiety. Refer to the discussion of Huntington's disease for interventions related to the nursing diagnosis *Impaired Verbal Communication*.

Anxiety and powerlessness are major nursing considerations. Clients and family members are frequently stunned by the rapid deterioration of function and fear that the paralysis will be permanent. Teaching must be regularly reinforced because the client's high anxiety level may interfere with listening and understanding. Whenever possible, include the client and family in decision making. For example, seek their input when planning a daily schedule of care that incorporates various therapies.

Referrals to appropriate therapists is a component of anticipating needs; speech, nutritional, occupational, and physical therapists are an integral part of rehabilitation. Another focus of care is teaching both the client and family; incorporate explanations for interventions aimed at promoting self-care.

Teaching the rationales for preventive measures reinforces the client's and family's understanding and may promote compliance during the lengthy rehabilitation. For example, because of autonomic nerve involvement, clients need to be monitored for cardiac dysrhythmias and taught to avoid changing position suddenly to prevent orthostatic hypotension. Refer to previous nursing care sections in this chapter for interventions related to *Altered Nutrition, Impaired Swallowing, Impaired Verbal Communication* and *Ineffective Airway Clearance*. This sec-

tion focuses on managing the nursing diagnoses *Pain* and *Risk for Impaired Skin Integrity*.

Pain

Pain experienced with Guillain-Barré syndrome varies. Frequently, there is a "stocking-glove" pattern, with pain in the hands, feet, and legs. Pain and tenderness in muscles can be severe; interventions must be individualized to client needs. The intense pain combined with altered sensations leads to anxiety; nursing interventions can make a difference in breaking the cycle of increasing pain that leads to increased anxiety and in turn causes more pain.

Nursing interventions with rationales follow:

- Listen to the client's description of pain; determine presence of triggers or a pattern. *Acknowledging the client's perception of pain is a basis for treatment; listening establishes trust.*

- Use a pain scale for determining extent of pain. *Consistent measurement is essential to evaluate degree of pain and effectiveness of intervention.*

- Provide alternatives for managing pain:
  a. Application of heat/cold
  b. Guided imagery
  c. Relaxation techniques
  d. Massage
  e. Medications
  Presenting options for managing pain gives the client control over the situation and helps reduce anxiety. Noninvasive interventions may augment the therapeutic benefit of medications (Carpenito, 1995).

- Provide analgesics as indicated; administer on a regular schedule rather than waiting until pain becomes severe. *Anticipating and managing pain before it becomes severe decreases anxiety and averts the cycle of increased anxiety leading to increased pain.*

- Monitor for side effects of analgesics, particularly depression of respirations; assess respirations and lung sounds. Perform routine pulmonary hygiene measures and watch for signs of aspiration. *Clients with Guillain-Barré syndrome have a weakened thoracic musculature; frequent respiratory monitoring is indicated.*

Risk for Impaired Skin Integrity

During the acute and plateau stages of Guillain-Barré syndrome, clients are at risk for problems related to immobility and malnutrition. Impaired skin integrity is one such problem. Preventing areas of skin breakdown is important. Prophylactic interventions will help ensure that ingested protein and calories are used to maintain ideal body weight and other body functions rather than to heal an avoidable problem. Implicit in the following interventions is maintenance of adequate nutrition.

Nursing interventions with rationales follow:

- Inspect bony prominences and provide skin care at least every 2 hours. Reposition the client and clean, dry, and lubricate the skin as needed. *These activities stimulate circulation and ensure even distribution of body weight; proper assessment is indicated to obtain baseline observations and to discover early signs of altered integrity.*

- Pad bony prominences, such as sacral area, heels, and elbows. *This decreases shearing tears on these pressure points.*

- Use an alternating-pressure mattress or water bed. *Relieving pressure stimulates circulation and promotes oxygenation of tissues.*

- Monitor for incontinence and provide thorough skin care following each episode of incontinence. *Urine is caustic to the skin, and the moisture promotes skin breakdown.*

Other Nursing Diagnoses

Additional nursing diagnoses that may be appropriate for the client with Guillain-Barré syndrome follow:

- *Anxiety* related to loss of mobility and sensory changes, loss of ability to communicate, and ventilatory support

- *Self-Care Deficit* related to effects of altered neuromuscular function

- *Body Image Disturbance* related to inability to control body functions

- *Altered Protection* related to sensory impairments and immobility

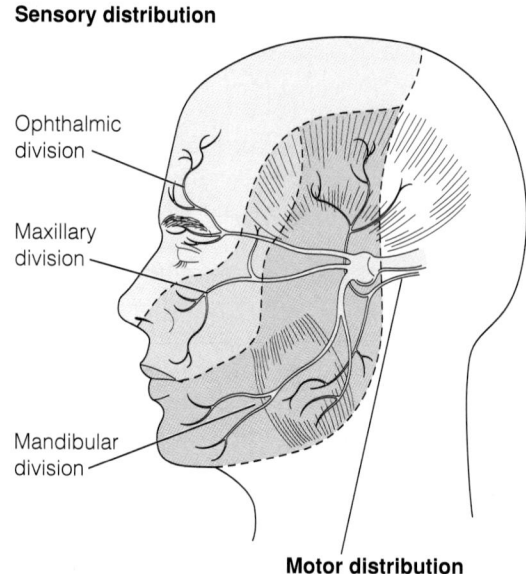

Sensory distribution

Ophthalmic division

Maxillary division

Mandibular division

Motor distribution

Figure 42–9 Sensory and motor distribution of the trigeminal nerve. There are three sensory divisions: ophthalmic, maxillary, and mandibular.

- *Impaired Verbal Communication* related to altered cranial nerve function

- *Ineffective Airway Clearance and Risk for Aspiration* related to changes in neuromuscular functioning

▰▰▰ Disorders of the Cranial Nerves ▰▰▰

Disorders of the cranial nerves may be caused by intracranial trauma or by pathologic processes. The pairs of cranial nerves, described in Chapter 39, are numbered in the order in which they arise in the brain and are named according to their anatomic characteristic or primary function. The most common cranial nerve disorders are those affecting the trigeminal (cranial nerve V) and the facial (cranial nerve VII) nerves. These disorders, discussed in the following sections, result primarily in pain or loss of sensory or motor function.

The Client with Trigeminal Neuralgia

▰ ▰ ▰

Trigeminal neuralgia, also called *tic douloureux,* is a chronic disease of the trigeminal cranial nerve (cranial nerve V) that causes severe facial pain. The trigeminal

nerve has three divisions: the ophthalmic, the maxillary, and mandibular (Figure 42–9). The ophthalmic division supplies the forehead, eyes, nose, temples, meninges, paranasal sinus, and part of the nasal mucosa. The maxillary division supplies the upper jaw, teeth, lip, cheeks, hard palate, maxillary sinus, and part of the nasal mucosa. The mandibular division supplies the lower jaw, teeth, lip, buccal mucosa, tongue, part of the external ear, and the meninges. Sensory fibers of the nerve conduct impulses for touch, pain, and temperature; motor fibers innervate the temporal and masseter muscles used for chewing and lateral movement of the jaw. The maxillary and mandibular divisions are the divisions of the trigeminal nerve affected in almost all cases of this disorder.

Trigeminal neuralgia occurs more commonly in middle and older adults and affects women more often than men. The actual cause is unknown; however, contributing factors include irritation from flulike illnesses, trauma or infection of the teeth or jaw, and pressure on the nerve by an aneurysm, a tumor, or arteriosclerotic changes of an artery close to the nerve (Hickey, 1992).

Pathophysiology

Trigeminal neuralgia is characterized by brief (lasting a few seconds to a few minutes), repetitive episodes of sudden severe facial pain. The pain may occur as often as hundreds of times a day to as infrequently as a few times a year. The pain is unilateral and is experienced over the surface of the skin. It most often begins near one side of the mouth and rises toward the ear, eye, or nostril on the same side of the face. Motor or sensory deficits rarely occur. Clients describe the pain as stabbing or lightning-like and often respond to the pain by wincing or grimacing.

Specific areas of the face, called *trigger zones,* may initiate the onset of pain when they are stimulated. These trigger zones usually parallel the distribution of the nerve and typically follow a track leading from just over the eyebrow to the ridge of the cheekbone, along the nasolabial fold, around the corner of the mouth, and down the side of the chin. The episodes of pain are set off by many factors, including light touch, eating, swallowing, talking, sneezing, shaving, chewing gum, brushing the teeth, or washing the face. Other factors that may trigger a pain episode include changes in temperature and exposure to wind. In an attempt to control the pain, clients may refuse to wash, shave, eat, or talk.

The episodes of pain may recur for several weeks or months. The disease then spontaneously goes into remission, and the client is free of pain for periods lasting from days to years. As the client grows older, the remissions tend to become shorter, and a dull ache may be present between episodes of acute pain.

Collaborative Care

There are no specific laboratory or diagnostic tests for trigeminal neuralgia. The disorder is diagnosed by the characteristic location and type of pain. The disorder is treated by pharmacologic or surgical interventions.

Pharmacology

The drug most useful in controlling the pain is the tricyclic anticonvulsant carbamazepine (Tegretol). If carbamazepine is ineffective, the anticonvulsant phenytoin (Dilantin) may be used. These drugs are administered to decrease paroxysmal afferent impulses and thus stop the pain. Drugs in this category may cause side effects of dizziness, nausea, and drowsiness. In addition, liver function, bone marrow function, and blood levels of the medications should be monitored on a regular basis. Another pharmacologic agent that may be administered alone or in conjuction with either of the other two drugs is baclofen (Lioresal), a skeletal muscle relaxant (Tierney, McPhee, & Papadakis, 1994).

Surgery

If pharmacologic treatment is not successful in controlling the pain, surgical procedures may be performed, including various types of **rhizotomy,** the surgical severing of a nerve root. Closed surgical interventions by *percutaneous rhizotomy* involve inserting a needle through the cheek into the foramen ovale at the base of the brain and partially destroying the trigeminal nerve with glycerol (an alcohol), by radiofrequency-induced heat, or by balloon compression of the trigeminal ganglion (Way, 1994). These procedures carry less risk and result in shorter hospital stays than do open procedures, but there is a possibility of recurrence of pain. Following surgery, the client may have some facial numbness, but there usually is no residual paralysis (Victor & Martin, 1991). The involved side of the face is insensitive to pain. The client will have some loss of facial sensation (for example, to temperature and/or touch) and is at risk for loss of the corneal reflex. Closed procedures provide long-term pain relief and are well tolerated by the older adult. Nursing care of the client undergoing a percutaneous rhizotomy is presented in the accompanying box.

Total severing of the sensory root of the trigeminal nerve through a *retrogasserian rhizotomy* (surgical resection of the dorsal root of a nerve to relieve pain) may be performed but is done less often than in the past. This procedure is conducted by opening the skull in a craniotomy. This surgery results in permanent anesthesia of the involved facial areas but may cause sensory changes, such as burning or itching. In addition, the procedure places the client at risk for facial paralysis and loss of the corneal reflex. Nursing care of the client undergoing a craniotomy is discussed in Chapter 40.

More recently, it has been found that some structural abnormalities (such as an artery or vein compressing the nerve) may cause the neuralgia, and if so, decompression and separation of the blood vessel from the nerve root produces lasting relief of the pain (Tierney et al., 1994). The *Jannetta procedure* involves locating and lifting the involved vessel and placing a small piece of silicone sponge between the vessel and the nerve. Possible complications of the procedure include headache and facial pain.

Nursing Care

Nursing care for the client with trigeminal neuralgia involves teaching self-management at home after medical or surgical intervention. Primary client concerns are managing pain, maintaining nutrition, and preventing injury.

Interventions for managing pain and improving nutritional intake are addressed here; teaching to prevent injury following surgery is discussed under client and family teaching.

Pain

The client with trigeminal neuralgia has excruciating pain and often avoids ADLs and socializing with others in an attempt to prevent the onset of pain. Pain management is fully discussed in Chapter 4. Nursing interventions for

Postoperative Nursing Care of the Client Undergoing Percutaneous Rhizotomy for Trigeminal Neuralgia

- Follow routine postoperative interventions for clients having surgery (see Chapter 7).
- Monitor cranial nerve function every 2 to 4 hours:
  a. Assess the corneal reflex by lightly touching the cornea with a wisp of cotton. If the reflex is intact, the client will blink. *Severing the ophthalmic division of the trigeminal nerve destroys the corneal reflex and leaves the cornea at risk for dryness and injury.*
  b. Assess the facial nerve by asking the client to blow out the cheeks, wrinkle the forehead, frown, wink, and close both eyes tightly. Test taste by placing bitter, salty, and sweet substances on the anterior portion of the tongue. *Facial weakness is evidenced by changes in movement in the involved side of the face. The facial nerve also innervates the anterior two-thirds of the tongue.*
  c. Assess the function of the oculomotor muscles by asking the client to follow your finger through the cardinal positions of vision (see Chapter 39). *The eyes should move together; alterations in movement indicate an abnormal response.*
  d. Assess the motor portion of the trigeminal nerve by asking the client to clench the teeth while you palpate the tightness of the contracted masseter and temporal muscles. *Loss of motor function is indicated by loss of bulk and tightness of these muscles.*
  e. Apply, as prescribed, an ice pack to the jaw on the operative site. *Cold decreases bleeding and swelling.*
  f. Teach the client to avoid rubbing the eye on the involved side. *Loss of the corneal reflex removes protection because the client no longer has the sensation of pain in the involved eye. Rubbing the eye could cause corneal abrasions.*

---

pain in clients with this disorder focus on strategies for self-management.

Nursing interventions with rationales follow:

- Identify factors that trigger an attack, and discuss with the client strategies to avoid these precipitating factors. *Most clients can clearly identify trigger zones and triggering factors. Identification is the first step in controlling the pain.*
- Determine the client's usual response to pain. *Sensitivity and reaction to pain are influenced by previous experiences with pain, age, gender, emotional factors, and cultural background.*
- Assess factors that affect the client's ability to influence pain tolerance, including the knowledge and cause of the pain, the meaning of the pain, the ability to control the pain, the client's cultural background, and the client's support systems. *Pain tolerance, which is the duration and intensity of pain a person is willing to endure, differs greatly among individuals and may also vary within an individual client in different situations (Acute Pain Management Guideline Panel, 1992).*
- Monitor the effects of the medication prescribed for the neuralgia. *If the prescribed medication does not provide relief, other medications or methods of treatment may be used to control the pain.*

Risk for Altered Nutrition: Less Than Body Requirements

Clients often refuse to eat during periods of pain attacks, fearing that the movements of chewing may precipitate the pain. In addition, the chronic nature of the illness often causes depression, which may depress the appetite.

Nursing interventions with rationales follow:

- Monitor dietary intake and weight loss at each visit, and ask the client to keep a record of weekly weight measurements. *Ongoing assessments are necessary for early detection of nutritional deficiencies.*
- Discuss with the client the temperature and consistency of foods eaten, and suggest referral to a dietitian if necessary. *Hot or cold foods may trigger an attack; soft, warm, or cool foods are less likely to act as triggers.*
- Suggest that the client chew on the unaffected side of the mouth. *Chewing on the unaffected side is less likely to trigger an attack of pain and so facilitate food intake.*
- If the client is unable to tolerate oral food, tube feedings may be necessary. *Provision of adequate kcal and nutrients for metabolic processes is essential.*

Other Nursing Diagnoses

Other nursing diagnoses that may be appropriate for the client with trigeminal neuralgia follow:

- *Impaired Verbal Communication* related to onset of pain when speaking
- *Fatigue* related to interruption of sleep by attacks of facial pain
- *Hopelessness* related to chronic and ongoing nature of disease process and chronic pain
- *Self-Care Deficit: Bathing/Hygiene* related to fear of initiating an attack of pain

Client and Family Teaching

The client with trigeminal neuralgia who is receiving medical treatment and providing self-care at home requires teaching about the disease process, the medication(s) being taken, and methods of reducing the incidence of attacks or pain. Diet teaching and assistance with self-management of pain are also important. For example, if the home setting is drafty and attacks of pain are triggered by wind blowing across the face, it may be necessary to encourage the client to put weather stripping around windows and doors. Family members are also included in teaching.

Clients treated with surgery are at risk for injury as a result of deficits in the corneal reflex and the loss of sensation in the involved side of the face. Teaching focuses on the following topics:

Eye Care

- Do not rub the eyes; use artificial tears 4 times a day if the eyes are dry or irritated.
- Wear an eyepatch at night.
- Wear protective sunglasses or goggles when outside, when working in dusty areas, when mowing the lawn, and when using any type of spray material (e.g., hair spray, cleaning materials, paint, insecticides).
- Remember to blink frequently.
- Check your eyes for redness or swelling each day.
- Schedule regular eye examinations.

Face and Mouth Care

- Chew on the unaffected side of the mouth.
- Avoid eating hot foods or drinking hot liquids.
- After every meal, brush your teeth and inspect the inside of your mouth for food that may collect between the gums and cheek.
- Have regular dental examinations; you will not be able to feel pain associated with gum infection or tooth decay.
- Use an electric razor to shave.
- Protect your face from very cold or windy conditions.

> ### Clinical Manifestations of Bell's Palsy
>
> - Paralysis of the facial muscles on one side of the face
> - Paralysis of the upper eyelid with loss of the corneal reflex on the affected side
> - Loss or impairment of taste over the anterior portion of the tongue on the affected side
> - Increased tearing from the lacrimal gland on the affected side

The Client with Bell's Palsy

Bell's palsy, also called *facial paralysis,* is a disorder of the facial nerve (seventh cranial nerve), characterized by unilateral paralysis of the facial muscles. The facial nerve is primarily a motor nerve that supplies all the muscles associated with expression on one side of the face. The sensory component innervates the anterior two-thirds of one side of the tongue.

This disorder can occur at any age but is seen most often in adults between 20 and 60. The incidence is equal in men and women (Hickey, 1992). The exact cause of the disorder is unknown, although inflammation of the nerve and a relationship to the herpes simplex virus have been suggested (Tierney et al., 1994).

Pathophysiology

The onset of Bell's palsy is usually sudden and almost always involves one side of the face. Pain behind the ear or along the jaw may precede the paralysis. Clinical manifestations of Bell's palsy are listed in the accompanying box.

The client initially notices numbness or stiffness of one side of the face that distorts the appearance. As the disease progresses, the distortion becomes more obvious, and the face appears asymmetric. The facial paralysis causes the entire side of the face to droop, and the client can not wrinkle the forehead, close the eye, or pucker the lips on the affected side. When the client attempts to smile, the lower facial muscles are pulled to the opposite side of the face. Some clients have only mild manifestations, whereas others have complete facial paralysis (Figure 42–10).

Eighty percent of clients recover completely within a few weeks to a few months (and three-fourths recover without any treatment). Of those remaining, 15% recover some function but have some permanent facial paralysis; these clients are usually older, have diabetes mellitus, or

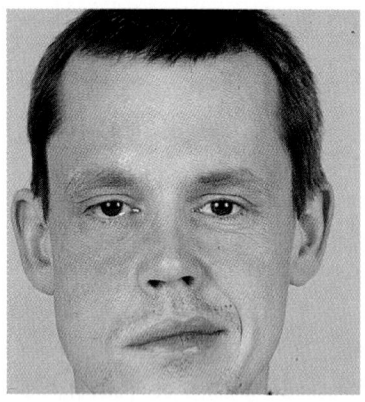

Figure 42–10   The client with Bell's palsy shows the typical drooping of one side of the face.

have more severe manifestations, such as vertigo, a sensitivity to noise, and deep head pain.

Collaborative Care

There are no definitive laboratory or diagnostic tests, nor are there any specific treatments. The only medical treatment that influences outcome is the use of corticosteroids, but their use has also been questioned. There is no evidence that surgical decompression of the facial nerve is of value (Tierney et al., 1994). Care of the client with Bell's palsy is supportive, as described below.

Nursing Care

Although most clients provide self-care at home, the nurse plays a key role in teaching the client and family about the disease and how to prevent injury and maintain nutrition. The client is often anxious about his or her appearance and may require counseling if any deficits in facial expression become permanent.

The loss of the corneal reflex and the inability to close the eyelid increase the risk of corneal dryness and abrasion, with possible loss of vision. The client is taught to use artificial tears 4 times a day to lubricate the eye and to wear an eye patch or tape the eye shut at night. Other strategies to prevent eye injury include wearing sunglasses or goggles when outside, when working in dusty conditions, and when using any type of spray. The client should be taught how to instill the eyedrops and to inspect the eye each day for redness or swelling.

If the client experiences pain, analgesics can be prescribed. Massage combined with warm, moist heat often is effective in relieving the pain.

The facial paralysis makes it difficult for the client to chew and swallow food or drink liquids. Drooling from the affected side is common. Most clients are better able to tolerate a soft diet that does not require chewing and often prefer to eat 6 small meals a day rather than 3 large meals. Chewing slowly on the unaffected side and avoiding hot foods help prevent injury to the lining of the mouth. To prevent infection and tooth decay, the client must clean the mouth and carefully inspect the area between the gums and cheek for food after each meal.

To maintain muscle tone, the client is taught to massage the affected side of the face and manually close the eyelid several times a day. As function returns, the client should practice wrinkling the forehead, closing the eyes, blowing air out of the puckered mouth, and whistling for 5 minutes three or four times a day. A facial sling may be worn during meals and to prevent muscle stretching. Electrical nerve stimulation may be used to stimulate the affected muscles and prevent sagging of the affected side of the face.

Examples of nursing diagnoses that may be appropriate for the client with Bell's palsy follow:

- *Risk for Altered Nutrition: Less Than Body Requirements* related to inability to chew food
- *Risk for Injury* related to loss of corneal reflex
- *Body Image Disturbance* related to distorted facial appearance

Client and Family Teaching

Client and family teaching is discussed above.

▚▚▚   Toxic and Infectious Neurologic Disorders   ▚▚▚

The Client with Rabies

· ■ ·

A variety of disorders of the nervous system may have toxic or infectious causes. Although these disorders are not common, those included here require significant nursing care when they do occur. The disorders discussed in this section include rabies, tetanus, botulism, postpolio syndrome, and Creutzfeldt-Jakob disease.

Rabies is a viral (rhabdovirus) infection of the central nervous system transmitted by infected saliva that enters the human body through a bite or an open wound. This is a critical illness that almost always causes death. The rabies virus is carried by both wild and domestic animals, including bats, skunks, foxes, raccoons, cats, and dogs. After an incubation period that may last from 10 days to many years (but that usually lasts 3 to 7 weeks), the virus travels to the brain of the infected animal via the nerves. It multiplies and migrates to the salivary glands.

Pathophysiology

The client with rabies usually has a history of an animal bite but may also become infected through an abrasion or open wound that is exposed to the infected saliva. The virus spreads from the wound to local muscle cells and then invades the peripheral nerves. It eventually travels to the central nervous system. The incubation period in humans varies according to the severity and location of the bite. For example, bites on the face may result in manifestations in 10 days to a few weeks, whereas bites on the lower extremities may incubate for as long as 1 year.

The manifestations occur in stages. During the initial, or prodromal, stage, the site of the wound is painful and then exhibits various paresthesias. The infected person experiences a feeling of anxiety and is irritable and depressed. General manifestations of infection (such as headache, loss of appetite, and sore throat) may appear. The person may also have increased sensitivity to light and sounds, and the skin is especially sensitive to changes in temperature.

The prodromal stage is followed by an excitement stage. The infected person has periods of excitement that alternate with periods of quiet. Attempts to drink cause such painful larynogospasms that the person refuses to drink (a phenomenon called *hydrophobia*). Large amounts of thick, tenacious mucus are present. The client experiences convulsions, muscle spasms, and periods of apnea. Death occurs approximately 7 days from the onset of manifestations and is usually due to respiratory failure.

Collaborative Care

Animals who bite are kept under observation, if possible, for 7 to 10 days to detect rabies manifestations. Sick animals should be euthanized and their brains examined for presence of the rabies virus, which is detected by fluorescent antibody testing. The blood of an infected person can also be tested with the same diagnostic study to demonstrate the presence of rabies antibodies.

Because the disease is almost always fatal, the best intervention is prevention. Preventive activities follow:

- Immunization
  a. Immunize household dogs and cats.
  b. Immunize people who are exposed to animals.
- Local treatment of animal bites and scratches
  a. Carefully and thoroughly clean and flush wounds with soap and water to remove the saliva and dilute the viral exposure.
  b. Immediately take the person with the bite for emergency treatment.
- Postexposure care
  a. Rabies immune globulin (RIG) is administered for passive immunization. Up to 50% of the globulin is infiltrated around the wound, and the rest is administered intramuscularly. At the same time, an inactivated human diploid cell rabies vaccine (HDCV) is administered intramuscularly, with 1 mL given on the day of exposure and on days 3, 7, 14, and 28 after exposure (Tierney et al., 1994). Rabies immune globulin and rabies vaccine (HDCV) should never be given in the same syringe or at the same site. Local and mild systemic reactions include itching, tenderness, headaches, muscle aches, and nausea.
  b. If rabies immune globulin is not available, equine rabies antiserum may be administered after testing the client for horse serum sensitivity.

Nursing Care

Nursing care for clients with rabies is provided in an intensive care unit, with the client in a quiet, darkened room to decrease stimulation as much as possible. The client requires interventions to maintain the airway, maintain oxygenation, and control seizures. Universal blood and body fluid precautions are essential, because the rabies virus is present in the saliva of the client. If an open wound of a health care provider is contaminated with infected saliva, the provider must receive postexposure immunizations.

Client and Family Teaching

Client and family teaching focuses on the importance of immunizing pets, providing proper care of wounds, seeking immediate medical attention for animal bites, and obtaining treatment after any suspicious bite.

The Client with Tetanus

■ ■ ■

Tetanus, more commonly called *lockjaw,* is a disorder of the nervous system caused by a neurotoxin elaborated by *Clostridium tetani*. This anaerobic bacillus lives in the soil. Spores of the bacillus enter the body through open wounds contaminated with dirt, street dust, or feces (animal or human). The wounds may result from scratches or abrasions, bee stings, abortions, surgery, trauma, burns, or intravenous drug use. Incidence is highest among people who have never been immunized, older adults whose immunity has been lost, and women. The majority of cases occur in people over age 50 (Wesche & Overfield, 1992). Tetanus has a high mortality rate, with death occurring in over 40% of all cases. Lesions of the head and face that are contaminated are more dangerous than those in other parts of the body.

Pathophysiology

When the spores of *Clostridium tetani* enter the open wound, they germinate and produce a toxin called *tetanospasmin*. The incubation period averages 8 to 12 days but can range from 5 days to 15 weeks (Tierney et al., 1994). The toxins are absorbed by the peripheral nerves and carried to the spinal cord, where they block the action of inhibitory enzymes at spinal synapses and interfere with transmission of neuromuscular impulses. As a result, even minor stimuli cause uncontrolled muscle spasms.

The clinical manifestations often begin with pain at the site of the infection. The infected person presents with stiffness of the jaw and neck and dysphagia. There is often profuse perspiration and drooling from increased salivation. As the infection progresses, the person experiences hyperreflexia, spasms of the jaw muscles (*trismus*) or facial muscles, and rigidity and spasms of the abdominal, neck, and back muscles. Generalized tonic seizures are caused by even minor stimuli, and the person assumes a typical opisthotonic position during the seizures: The head is retracted, the back is arched, and the feet are extended. The muscle spasms are painful. The person may be unable to breathe from spasms of the glottis and respiratory muscles. Despite these physical effects, the client has no change in mental status.

The complications of tetanus include urinary retention and airway obstruction from the spasms. Cardiac and respiratory failure are late, life-threatening complications.

Collaborative Care

There are no specific laboratory or diagnostic tests for tetanus. The diagnosis is based on the clinical manifestations. Tetanus is completely preventable by active immunization. Immunization for children includes tetanus toxoid, administered as part of the diphtheria-tetanus-pertussis (DPT) immunization series. In adults, immunization is obtained by administering tetanus toxoid as two doses 4 to 6 weeks apart, with a third dose in 6 to 12 months. All individuals should have a booster dose every 10 years throughout life or at the time of a major injury if the last booster dose was given more than 5 years prior to the injury.

If a wound is contaminated or if the person's immunization status is uncertain, passive immunization with tetanus immune globulin is administered. Active immunization with tetanus toxoid is begun at the same time.

The wound is carefully and thoroughly debrided and antibiotics administered.

The client with tetanus requires intensive care in an area of minimal stimulation. Penicillin and metronidazole hydrochloride (Flagyl) are administered to all clients to help destroy the toxin-producing organism. Muscle spasms and seizures are controlled by chlorpromazine (Thorazine) or diazepam (Valium), often combined with a sedative. Anticoagulants may be prescribed to prevent venous thrombosis. In severe cases, seizures and spasms are controlled with paralysis by a curare-like medication, and airway obstruction is managed by mechanical ventilation.

Nursing Care

Nursing care for the client with tetanus is intensive and focuses on assessments and interventions to promote safety, prevent injury, maintain nutrition, and maintain pulmonary and cardiovascular function. The client ususally requires in-hospital care for 2 to 5 weeks. The nursing care plan commonly includes the following:

- Place the client in a quiet, darkened room to decrease stimuli that cause muscle spasms and seizures. Care of the client with seizures is discussed in Chapter 40.
- Provide only necessary physical care, and do so during periods of maximal sedation to decrease tactile stimulation that causes muscle spasms.
- Maintain oxygenation through mechanical ventilator and frequent suctioning of secretions. Chapters 33 and 34 discuss intensive respiratory care measures.
- Maintain intravenous access for the administration of fluids and medications.
- Administer prescribed antibiotics, anticonvulsants, and sedatives. In the case of cardiovascular complications, administer prescribed beta-adrenergic blocking agents such as propranolol (Inderal).
- Provide adequate nutrition through prescribed nutritional support, such as total parenteral nutrition.
- Monitor respiratory and cardiovascular status and provide immediate interventions for respiratory or cardiovascular failure.
- Monitor fluid and electrolyte status. Ensure adequate fluid intake to maintain hydration and urinary output.
- Monitor urinary output, which should be maintained at 1.5 to 2 liters per day.
- Monitor for the hazards of immobility, including constipation, pneumonia, deep vein thrombosis, and pressure ulcers.

Client and Family Teaching

Tetanus is a preventable disorder, and nurses have a major role in promoting immunizations for all children and for educating adults about the need for booster doses.

The older population is especially as risk for never having been immunized or for letting immunizations lapse. Information for this age group can be provided through activities such as community health fairs and programs at senior citizen groups.

It is also necessary to teach the proper care of wounds. All wounds, no matter how small, should be thoroughly washed with soap and water. All foreign material should be carefully flushed out or removed from a wound, and medical care should be sought for wounds that are more extensive or contaminated.

The Client with Botulism

Botulism is food poisoning caused by ingestion of food contaminated with a toxin produced by the bacillus *Clostridium botulinum*. This anaerobic spore-forming bacillus is found in the soil. Most cases of botulism occur from eating improperly canned or cooked foods, especially home-canned vegetables and fruits, smoked meats, and vacuum-packed fish. The mortality rate is high if the disease is untreated.

Pathophysiology

The toxins liberated by *Clostridium botulinum* are absorbed by the gastrointestinal tract and bound to nerve tissues. They block the release of acetylcholine from nerve endings and thus cause respiratory paralysis from paralysis of skeletal muscles. Manifestations usually appear 12 to 36 hours after ingestion of the contaminated food.

The manifestations of botulism usually begin with visual disturbances such as diplopia, loss of accommodation, and fixed, dilated pupils. Ptosis is often present. Gastrointestinal manifestations include nausea and vomiting, diarrhea, dysphagia, and dry mouth. Involvement of the larynx is manifested by dystonia (impaired muscle tone). Paralysis of all muscle groups progresses throughout the body, with respiratory paralysis causing death if the client is not placed on a mechanical ventilator. There is no effect on mental status.

Collaborative Care

Infection with the *Clostridium* toxin is verified by laboratory analysis of the serum and stool and of suspected food, if possible. If botulism is suspected, the state health department and the Centers for Disease Control and Prevention should be notified for assistance with laboratory assays and procuring botulism antitoxin. All people who may have eaten the contaminated food must be located and observed.

Any toxins in the gastrointestinal system are removed by cathartics, enemas, and gastric lavage. The client with respiratory paralysis is placed on a mechanical ventilator and may require a tracheostomy. Botulism antitoxin is administered to eradicate toxins in the circulation. Nutritional support is often provided with total parenteral nutrition. Intravenous fluids are administered to prevent dehydration and renal failure. If ventilation can be maintained, the client often recovers without further neurologic deficits.

Nursing Care

The client with botulism is hospitalized, and interventions focus on monitoring for respiratory failure and providing ventilatory assistance if necessary. Chapters 33 and 34 discuss intensive respiratory care measures. Ongoing assessments are also made for manifestations of paralytic ileus and urinary retention. The client will be NPO until able to swallow and breathe; therefore, hydration and nutritional status are monitored.

Client and Family Teaching

Teach the client and family that fatigue and weakness may persist for up to a year. During this time, the client may need to modify ADLs and take rest periods throughout the day.

Education of the public to prevent botulism is important. The following topics should be addressed at health fairs and community programs and explained to rural residents who do home-canning:

- Home-canned foods must be processed in a pressure cooker rather than in boiling water because the organism is difficult to kill.
- Do not eat home-processed foods that have a change in color, are soft, contain gas bubbles, or have a bad odor.
- Always heat both home-processed and commercial foods at temperatures over 248° F (120° C) or boil for 10 minutes before tasting or eating them.
- Discard home-processed or commercially canned or bottled foods with defective seals.
- Discard commercially prepared canned foods that are damaged or have bulging sides or leaking contents.

The Client with Postpolio Syndrome

Postpolio syndrome is a complication of a previous infection by the poliomyelitis virus. This disease was epidemic in the 1940s and 1950s but has largely been eradicated through immunization with oral live trivalent virus vaccine. However, it is estimated that nearly one-half of the estimated 1.63 million people in the United States who had the disease are reexperiencing manifestations of the acute illness (Kuehn & Winters, 1994).

The poliomyelitis virus destroys some of the motor cells of the anterior horn cells of the spinal cord, causing neuromuscular effects that range from mild to severe flaccid paralysis and atrophy. The primary cause of death is respiratory arrest (Tierney et al., 1994).

Manifestations of motor neuron degeneration and weakness may emerge years after the initial infection. This complex of manifestations is not infectious, however. Most clients with postpolio syndrome are between the ages of 45 and 65, initially had a more severe case of polio and required hospitalization, contracted the disease after the age of 10, required ventilator assistance for respiration, and had paralysis in all four extremities (Stice & Cunningham, 1995). The incidence is slightly higher in women. As the population ages, it is projected that the number of older adults with postpolio syndrome will increase. The actual cause of postpolio syndrome is unknown.

Pathophysiology

The pathophysiologic process in postpolio syndrome is not known. The manifestations of postpolio syndrome include fatigue, muscle and joint weakness, loss of muscle mass, respiratory difficulties, and pain. These manifestations typically begin 25 to 35 years after the initial illness. The manifestations are most often seen in muscles affected by the initial infection, but new muscle groups may also be affected. In addition to neuromuscular manifestations, the client may experience cold intolerance, dizziness, headaches, urinary incontinence, and sleep disorders.

Collaborative Care

Postpolio syndrome is diagnosed by a previous history of polio and the current manifestations. Current physical status is determined through diagnostic studies of nerve conduction, muscle strength, and pulmonary function. Treatment addresses the manifestations, and often involves physical therapy and pulmonary rehabilitation programs.

Nursing Care

The client with postpolio syndrome faces the challenge of unexpected physical changes. Clients are often anxious about how others will react or what the future holds. Respiratory dysfunction may result in the need for oxygen. Muscular weakness and decreased pulmonary function may make walking difficult, if not impossible. Activities of daily living, independent self-care, and careers are threatened.

Many clients have not fully recovered psychologically from having polio and may respond to a recurrence of symptoms with denial and disbelief. Older clients may not know they had polio as small children. Nurses are responsible for assessing and identifying the manifestations of postpolio syndrome. It is essential to question middle to older adults about a past history of polio when conducting the health history and to ask specific questions about manifestations that the client may be experiencing.

Nursing care is provided in a variety of settings, including clinics, rehabilitation centers, and the client's home. The plan of care is developed collaboratively with other health care providers, and is individualized to the client's physical, emotional, and social needs. The number of support groups for people with postpolio syndrome is increasing; information about available groups should be provided to the client and family.

Nursing diagnoses that may be appropriate for the client with postpolio syndrome follow:

- *Knowledge Deficit* related to onset of postpolio syndrome
- *Ineffective Breathing Pattern* related to decreased function of respiratory muscles
- *Impaired Gas Exchange* related to decreased vital capacity
- *Risk for Disuse Syndrome* related to muscle weakness
- *Altered Family Processes* related to onset of disability from postpolio syndrome
- *Altered Sexuality Patterns* related to altered body function
- *Defensive Coping* related to denial of onset of manifestations
- *Impaired Physical Mobility* related to loss of lower extremity function and decreased respiratory function
- *Self-Esteem Disturbance* related to changes in physical abilities and need to use wheelchair
- *Hopelessness* related to recurrence of manifestations of polio and uncertain future

Client and Family Teaching

To promote the client's highest level of wellness, the nurse individualizes teaching to meet the physical and psychosocial needs of the client and family. Provide candid explanations, and teach the client how to prevent fatigue, promote optimal respiratory function, meet self-care needs, modify ADLs, and maintain safety. Follow-up care with nurses, physicians, physical therapists, respiratory therapists, and couselors is indicated. Referral to a support group can make a positive difference in the client's and family's ability to cope with the disorder.

The Client with Creutzfeldt-Jakob Disease

■ ■ ■

Creutzfeldt-Jakob disease is a rare, progressive neurologic disease that causes brain degeneration without inflammation. The disease is transmissible and progressively fatal. It was first reported in 1969, and as yet the exact causative agent has not been identified (Belcaster, 1994). It may possibly be a slow virus (one that causes transmissible disease but has a long, asymptomatic incubation period). Transmission has been traced to corneal transplantation from infected people, to infected dura mater grafts from cadavers, and to growth hormone generated from human pituitary glands.

In the United States, the annual incidence of Creutzfeldt-Jakob disease is estimated to be between 0.9 and 31.3 cases per million people. It primarily affects adults over the age of 50; men and women are affected equally. The peak age for onset is between the ages of 55 and 74 (Wallace, 1993).

The disease occurs worldwide, but clusters occur in several areas, more often in England, Chile, and Italy. It is also prevalent in Jewish immigrants to Israel and Libya and in Tunisian and Algerian immigrants to France (Wood & Anderson, 1988).

Pathophysiology

Creutzfeldt-Jakob disease is characterized by degeneration of the gray matter of the brain. The spongiform degeneration (involving the formation of tiny holes and resembling a sponge) produces severe dementia, myoclonus (muscle contractions), and characteristic changes in brain waves. On autopsy or biopsy of brain tissue, the brain shows loss of neurons and a proliferation of astrocytes (indicating destruction of nearby neurons).

The mode of transmission is unknown, but areas of greatest infection have been found in the brain, CSF, and spinal cord tissue. Indications of the infectious process have also been found in the liver, lung, lymph nodes, kidneys, blood, and urine. Whatever the causative agent, it is not easily destroyed. The current theory is that the only method of transmission among humans is by percutaneous contact.

The disease, which is often fatal within 3 to 12 months of diagnosis, has characteristic stages and manifestations. The onset is characterized by memory changes, an exaggerated startle reflex, sleep disturbances, and nervousness. The person then experiences rapid deterioration in motor, sensory, and language function. Tremors, hyperreflexia, rigidity, and a positive Babinski reflex are often present, and confusion progresses to dementia in almost all cases. Clients in the terminal state are comatose and exhibit decorticate and decerebrate posturing.

Collaborative Care

The disease is diagnosed by a thorough neurologic examination, specific electroencephalographic changes, and a CT scan. However, the final diagnosis of Creutzfeldt-Jakob disease can be made only by postmortem examination. It is often difficult to differentiate this disease from Alzheimer's disease, especially in the early stages.

There is no specific treatment available to stop or slow the progression of Creutzfeldt-Jakob disease. Collaborative interventions focus on the disease's manifestations.

Nursing Care

The nurse may identify the manifestations of Creutzfeldt-Jakob disease when conducting a health history and total physical assessment. Questions about familial history, cultural and geographic risk, and high-risk occupations or procedures should be included in the history. Assessment of mental function, reflexes, and cranial nerve function may provide information to assist in diagnosis.

Nursing care focuses on maximizing comfort, preventing injury, preventing transmission, and providing support. The following guidelines are useful in designing the plan of care:

- Although comfort is difficult to assess in clients with impaired cognitive function, interventions that provide a quiet environment and analgesia are important.

- Communication is essential, even if the client is unable to respond.

- Institute seizure precautions, and pad side rails.

- Provide skin care, changes in position, and pressure-relief mattresses to decrease the risk of pressure ulcers, venous stasis, and pneumonia.

- Use universal precautions for blood and body fluids when providing care. Disinfect surfaces with a solution of 5% bleach. Sterilize contaminated equipment by autoclave, or soak in 5% bleach solution for 1 hour. Label all specimens as biohazardous. Label lines as biohazardous. Teach staff members and family members guidelines for care, including careful handwashing. It is not necessary to place the client in isolation, however.

- Provide time for family members to verbalize grief and loss, which may be manifested as anger and frustration with the health care system.

- Provide information to family members about all procedures and the plan of care.

- Refer family members to sources of support, such as social services and the appropriate clergy.

Bibliography

■ ■ ■

Acute Pain Management Guideline Panel. (1992). *Acute pain management in adults: Operative procedures. Quick reference guide for clinicians* (AHCPR Pub. No. 92-0019). Rockville, MD: Agency for Health Care Policy and Research, Public Health Service, US Department of Health and Human Services.

Asbeck, C., & Burns, B. (1992). Nutritional care in diseases of the nervous system. In L. K. Mahan & M. T. Arlin (Eds.), *Krause's food, nutrition & diet therapy* (8th ed.) (pp. 671–690). Philadelphia: Saunders.

Asbury, A. K. (1991). Diseases of the peripheral nervous system. In J.D. Wilson, E. Braunwald, J. K. Isselbacher, R. G. Petersdorf, J. B. Martin, A. S. Fauci, & R. K. Root (Eds.). (1991). *Harrison's principles of internal medicine* (12th ed.) (pp. 2096–2108). New York: McGraw-Hill.

Beal, M. F., Richardson, E. P., & Martin, J. B. (1991). Degenerative diseases of the nervous system. In J. D. Wilson, E. Braunwald, J. K. Isselbacher, R. G. Petersdorf, J. B. Martin, A. S. Fauci, & R. K. Root (Eds.), *Harrison's principles of internal medicine* (12th ed.) (pp. 2060–2076). New York: McGraw-Hill.

Beck, C., & Heacock, P. (1988). Nursing interventions for patients with Alzheimer's disease. *Nursing Clinics of North America, 23*(1), 95–124.

Belcaster, A. (1994). Creutzfeldt-Jakob disease: A family-centered approach. *Critical Care Nurse, 14*(4), 38–43.

Breton, D. (1994). These patients go through life without smiling. *RN, 57*(11), 69.

Bullock, B. & Rosendahl, P. (1992). *Pathopathology: Adaptations and alterations in function.* (3rd ed.). Philadelphia: Lippincott.

Burns, E. M., & Buckwalter, K. C. (1988). Pathophysiology and etiology of Alzheimer's disease. *Nursing Clinics of North America, 23*(1), 11–30.

Carpenito, L. J. (1995). *Nursing diagnosis: Application to clinical practice* (6th ed.). Philadelphia: Lippincott.

Chipps, E. (1991). Myasthenia gravis: The patient in crisis. *Critical Care Nurse, 11*(7), 18–26.

Chipps, E., Clanin, N., & Campbell, V. (1992). *Yearbook of Neurologic Disorders.* St. Louis: Mosby-Year Book.

Corbett, J. V. (1992). *Laboratory tests and diagnostic procedures with nursing diagnoses* (3rd ed.). Norwalk, CT: Appleton & Lange.

Cummings, J. L., & Benson, D. F. (1992). *Dementia: A clinical approach.* Boston: Butterworth-Heinemann.

Diehl, L. N. (1989). Client and family learning in the rehabilitation setting. *Nursing Clinics of North America, 24*(1), 257–264.

Drachman, D. B. (1991). Myasthenia gravis. In J. D. Wilson, E. Braunwald, J. K. Isselbacher, R. G. Petersdorf, J. B. Martin, A. S. Fauci, & R. K. Root (Eds.), *Harrison's principles of internal medicine* (12th ed.) (pp. 2118–2120). New York: McGraw-Hill.

Folstein, M. E., & Folstein, S. E. (1975). Mini-mental state: A practical method for grading the cognitive state of patients for the clinician. *Journal of Psychiatric Research, 12,* 189–198.

Freal, J. D., Kraft, G. H., & Coryell, J. K. (1984). Symptomatic fatigue in multiple sclerosis. *Archives of Physical Medicine and Rehabilitaiton, 65,* 135–138.

Gulick, E. E. (1992). Model for predicting work performance among persons with multiple sclerosis. *Nursing Research, 41*(5), 266–272.

Hagan, N. A. (1991). Action stat! Myasthenic crisis. *Nursing91, 21*(6), 33.

Hall, G. R. (1988). Care of the patient with Alzheimer's disease living at home. *Nursing Clinics of North America, 23*(1), 31–46.

Hall, G., & Buckwalter, K. (1987). Progressively lowered stress threshold: A conceptual model for care of adults with Alzheimer's disease. *Archives of Psychiatric Nursing, 1,* 399–406.

Hastings, D. (1992). Adjustment, coping resources, and care of the patient with multiple sclerosis. In J. F. Miller (ed.), *Coping with chronic illness: Overcoming powerlessness* (2nd ed.) (pp. 222–254). Philadelphia: F. A. Davis.

Hickey, J. (1992). *The clinical practice of neurological and neurosurgical nursing* (3rd ed.). Philadelphia: Lippincott.

Hoffman, L. A. (1987). Ineffective airway clearance related to neuromuscular dysfunction. *Nursing Clinics of North America, 22*(1), 151–166.

Hubsky, E. P., & Sears, J. H. (1992). Fatigue in multiple sclerosis: Guidelines for nursing care. *Rehabilitation Nursing, 17*(4), 176–180.

Kuehn, A., & Winters, R. (1994). A study of symptom distress, health locus of control, and coping resources of aging post-polio survivors. *IMAGE: Journal of Nursing Scholarship, 26*(4), 325–331.

Mace, N. L., & Rabins, P. V. (1981). *The 36-hour day: A family guide to caring for persons with Alzheimer's disease.* Baltimore: Johns Hopkins University Press.

Marieb, E. N. (1995). *Human anatomy and physiology* (3rd ed.). Redwood City, CA: Benjamin/Cummings.

Martin, J. B. (1987). Huntington's disease: Pathogenesis and management. *New England Journal of Medicine, 315,* 1267–1276.

Matteson, M. A., & McConnell, E. S. (1988). *Gerontological nursing: Concepts and practice.* Philadelphia: W. B. Saunders.

Miller, C. A. (1995). *Nursing care of older adults: Theory and practice.* (2nd ed.). Philadelphia: Lippincott.

Pallett, P. J., & O'Brien, M. T. (1985). *Textbook of neurological nursing.* Boston: Little, Brown.

Penrose, N. J. (1993). Guillain-Barré syndrome: A case study. *Rehabilitation Nursing, 18*(2), 88–90.

Porth, C. M. (1994). *Pathophysiology: Concepts of altered health states.* Philadelphia: Lippincott.

Price, S. A., & Wilson, L. M. (1992). *Pathophysiology: Clinical concepts of disease processes* (4th ed.). St. Louis: Mosby-Year Book.

Rabin, D. (1986). Practical tips for patients with A.L.S. *Nursing, 16*(2), 47–49.

Reisberg, B. (1986). Dementia: A systematic approach to identifying reversible causes. *Geriatrics, 41*(4), 30–46.

Rhysnburger, J. (1989). How to fight MG fatigue. *American Journal of Nursing, 89,* 337–340.

Roohi, F., & Cook, A. W. (1987). The effect of raising body temperature on peripheral nerve conduction and neuromuscular transmission in patients with multiple sclerosis. *Electromyography and Clinical Neurophysiology, 27,* 437–441.

Rowland, L. (Ed.). (1989). *Merritt's textbook of neurology,* (8th ed.). Philadelphia: Lea & Febiger.

Sciento, L.; Daffner, K., Dressler, D., Ransil, B., Rentz, D., Weintraub, S., Mesulan, M., & Potter, H. (1994). A potential noninvasive neurobiologic test for AD. *Science, 266* (Nov. 11), 1051–1054.

Snyder, M. (Ed.). (1983). *A guide to neurological and neurosurgical nursing.* New York: John Wiley & Sons.

Stewart, K. (1994). Tetanus: Protecting the airway and preventing toxin spread. *Nursing94, 24*(5), 51.

Stice, K., & Cunningham, C. (1995). Pulmonary rehabilitation with respiratory complications of postpolio syndrome. *Rehabilitation Nursing, 20*(1), 37–42.

Stone, N. (1987). Amyotrophic lateral sclerosis: A challenge for constant adaptation. *The Journal of Neuroscience Nursing, 19*(3) 166–185.

Tierney, L., McPhee, S., & Papadakis, M. (1994). *Current medical diagnosis & treatment.* Norwalk, CT: Appleton & Lange.

Victor, M., & Martin, J. B. (1991). Disorders of the cranial nerves. In J. D. Wilson, E. Braunwald, J. K. Isselbacher, R. G. Petersdorf, J. B. Martin, A. S. Fauci, & R. K. Root (Eds.), *Harrison's principles of internal medicine* (12th ed.) (pp. 2076–2081). New York: McGraw-Hill.

Wallace, M. (1993). Creutzfeldt-Jakob disease: Assessment and management. *Journal of Gerontological Nursing, 19*(11), 15–22.

Wassem, R. (1991). A test of the relationship between health locus of control and the course of multiple sclerosis. *Rehabilitation Nursing, 16*(4), 189–193.

Way, L. (1994). *Current surgical diagnosis & treatment.* Norwalk, CT: Appleton & Lange.

Weeks, D. (1991). Washing the blood. *RN, 54*(5), 60–63.

Wesche, H., & Overfield, T. (1992). Tetanus immunity in older persons. *Public Health Nursing, 9*(2), 125–127.

Wineman, N. M. (1990). Adaptation of multiple sclerosis: The role of social support, functional disability, and perceived uncertainty. *Nursing Research, 39*(5), 294–299.

Wood, M., & Anderson, M. (Eds.). (1988). *Neurological infections* (pp. 574–577). Philadelphia: W. B. Saunders.

Responses to Altered Visual and Auditory Function

CHAPTER 43
Assessing Clients with Eye or Ear Disorders

CHAPTER 44
Nursing Care of Clients with Eye and Ear Disorders

Assessing Clients with Eye or Ear Disorders

● ●

LEARNING OBJECTIVES

After completing this chapter, you will be able to

- Identify the major structures of the eye and the ear.
- Describe the physiologic processes involved in vision, hearing, and equilibrium.
- Identify interview questions pertinent to the assessment of the eye and the ear.

- Describe physical assessment techniques for eye and ear function.
- Identify manifestations of impairment in the function of the eye and the ear.
- Describe variations in assessment findings for the older adult.

Vision and hearing are special senses that allow us to experience the world in which we live. The eyes allow us to see by providing a pathway for visual stimuli to reach the brain. The ears allow us to hear by providing a pathway for auditory stimuli to reach the brain. In addition, specialized structures within the ear help maintain position sense and equilibrium. Deficits in any of these functions may limit self-care, mobility, independence, communication, and relationships with others. Assessment of the structure and function of the eye and the ear is necessary for both health promotion and health restoration.

Review of Anatomy and Physiology

■ ■ ■

The Eye and Vision

The eyes are complex structures, containing 70% of the sensory receptors of the body. Each eye is a sphere measuring about 1 in (2.5 cm) in diameter, surrounded and

protected by a bony orbit and cushions of fat. The primary functions of the eye are to encode the patterns of light from the environment through photoreceptors and to carry the coded information from the eyes to the brain. The brain gives meaning to the coded information, allowing us to make sense of what we see. Both extraocular and intraocular structures are considered a part of the eye.

Extraocular Structures

Extraocular or accessory structures of the eye are those portions of the eye outside the eyeball yet vital to its protection. These structures are the eyebrows, the eyelids, the eyelashes, the conjunctiva, the lacrimal apparatus, and the extrinsic eye muscles (Figure 43–1).

The *eyebrows* are short, coarse hairs located above the eyes over the superior orbital ridges of the skull. The eyebrows shade the eyes and keep perspiration away from them.

The *eyelids* are thin, loose folds of skin covering the anterior eye. They protect the eye from foreign bodies, regulate the entry of light into the eye, and distribute tears by blinking.

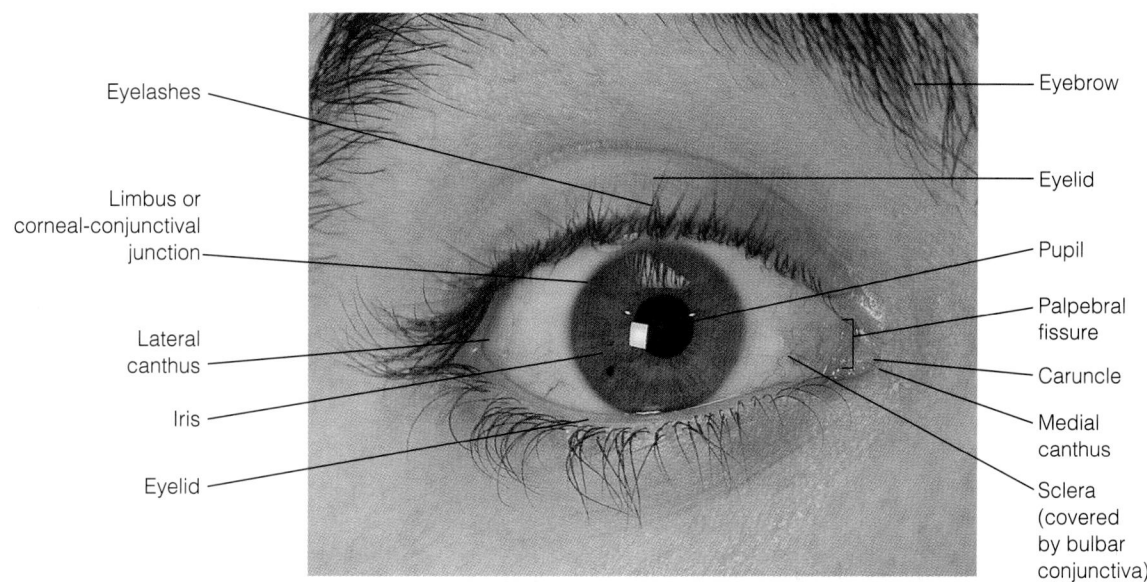

Figure 43–1 Accessory and external structures of the eye.

The *eyelashes* are short hairs that project from the top and bottom borders of the eyelids. When anything touches the eyelashes, the blinking reflex is initiated to protect the eyes from foreign objects.

The *conjunctiva* is a thin, transparent membrane that lines the inner surfaces of the eyelids and also folds over the anterior surface of the eyeball. The *palpebral conjunctiva* lines the upper and lower eyelids, whereas the *bulbar conjunctiva* loosely covers the anterior sclera (the white part of the eye). The conjunctiva is a mucous membrane that lubricates the eyes.

The *lacrimal apparatus* is composed of the *lacrimal gland,* the *puncta,* the *lacrimal sac,* and the *nasolacrimal duct.* Together, these structures secrete, distribute, and drain tears to cleanse and moisten the eye's surface.

The six extrinsic eye muscles control the movement of the eye, allowing it to follow a moving object. The muscles also help maintain the shape of the eyeball. The cranial nerves control the extrinsic muscles (Figure 43–2 on page 1864), which allow precise movement of the eyeball.

Intraocular Structures

The intraocular structures transmit visual images and maintain homeostasis of the inner eye. Those lying in the anterior portion of each eyeball are the sclera and the cornea (forming the outermost coat of the eye, called the *fibrous tunic*), the iris, the pupil, and the anterior cavity (Figure 43–3 on page 1865).

The white *sclera* lines the outside of the eyeball. The functions of the sclera are to protect and give shape to the eyeball.

The sclera gives way to the *cornea* over the iris and pupil. The cornea is transparent, avascular, and very sensitive to touch. The cornea forms a window that allows light to enter the eye and is a part of its light-bending apparatus. When the cornea is touched, the eyelids blink (the corneal reflex) and tears are secreted.

The *iris* is a disc of muscle tissue surrounding the pupil and lying between the cornea and the lens. The iris gives the eye its color and regulates light entry by controlling the size of the pupil.

The *pupil* is the dark center of the eye through which light enters. The pupil constricts when bright light enters the eye and when it is used for near vision; it dilates when light conditions are dim and when the eye is used for far vision. In response to intense light, the pupil constricts rapidly in the pupillary light reflex.

The *anterior cavity* is made up of the *anterior chamber* (the space between the cornea and the iris) and the *posterior chamber* (the space between the iris and the lens). The anterior cavity is filled with a clear fluid called the *aqueous humor.* Aqueous humor is constantly formed and drained to maintain a relatively constant pressure of from 15 to 20 mm Hg in the eye. The *canal of Schlemm,* a network of channels that circle the eye in the angle at the junction of the sclera and the cornea, is the drainage system for fluid moving between the anterior and posterior chambers. Aqueous humor provides nutrients and oxygen to the cornea and the lens.

The intraocular structures that lie in the internal chamber of the eye are the posterior cavity and vitreous humor, the lens, the ciliary body, the uvea, and the retina.

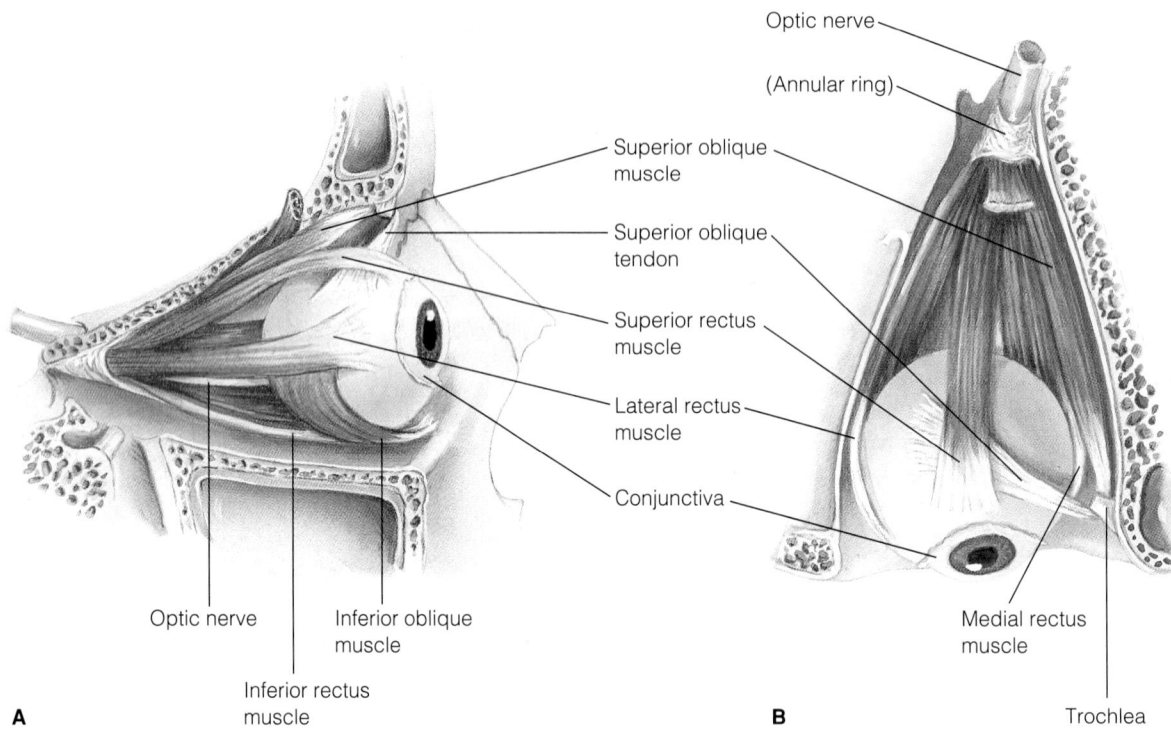

Name	Controlling cranial nerve	Action
Lateral rectus	VI (abducens)	Moves eye laterally
Medial rectus	III (oculomotor)	Moves eye medially
Superior rectus	III (oculomotor)	Elevates eye or rolls it superiorly
Inferior rectus	III (oculomotor)	Depresses eye or rolls it inferiorly
Inferior oblique	III (oculomotor)	Elevates eye and turns it laterally
Superior oblique	IV (trochlear)	Depresses eye and turns it laterally

C

Figure 43-2 Extraocular muscles. *A*, Lateral view of the right eye. *B*, Superior view of the right eye. *C*, Innervation of the extraocular muscles by the cranial nerves.

The *posterior cavity* lies behind the lens. It is filled with a clear gelatinous substance called the vitreous humor. *Vitreous humor* supports the posterior surface of the lens, maintains the position of the retina, and transmits light.

The *lens* is a biconvex, avascular, transparent structure located directly behind the pupil. It can change shape to focus and refract light onto the retina.

The *uvea*, also called the *vascular tunic,* is the middle coat of the eyeball. This pigmented layer has three components: the iris, ciliary body, and choroid. The *ciliary body* encircles the lens, and along with the iris, regulates the amount of light reaching the retina by controlling the

shape of the lens. Most of the uvea is made up of the *choroid,* which is pigmented and vascular. Blood vessels of the choroid nourish the other layers of the eyeball. Its pigmented areas absorb light, preventing it from scattering within the eyeball.

The *retina* is the innermost lining of the eyeball. It has an outer pigmented layer and an inner neural layer. The outer layer, next to the choroid, serves as the link between visual stimuli and the brain. The transparent inner layer is made up of millions of light receptors in structures called rods and cones. *Rods* allow for vision in dim light as well as for peripheral vision. *Cones* allow for vision in bright

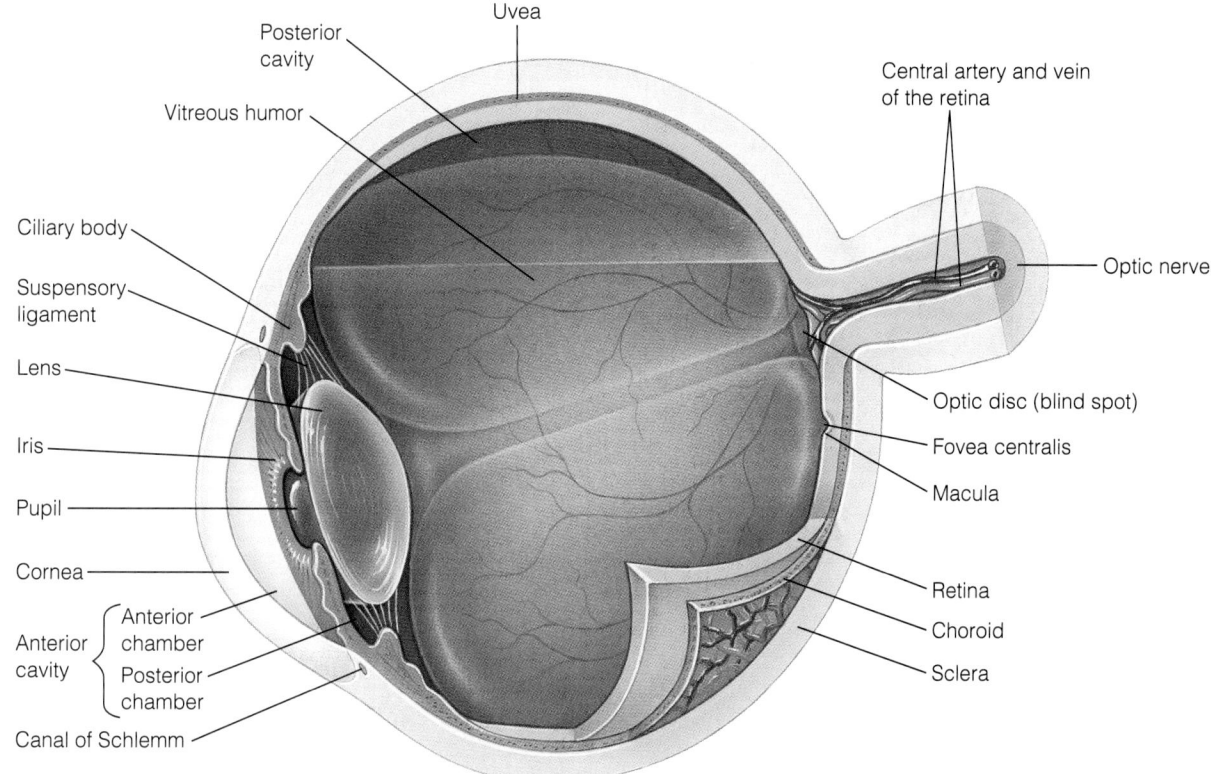

Figure 43–3 Internal structures of the eye.

light and for the perception of color. The *optic disc,* a cream-colored round or oval area within the retina, is the point at which the optic nerve enters the eye. The slight depression in the center of the optic disc is often called the *physiologic cup.* Located laterally to the optic disc is the *macula,* which is a darker area with no visible blood vessels. The macula contains primarily cones. The *fovea centralis* is a slight depression in the center of the macula that contains only cones and is a main receptor of detailed color vision.

The Visual Pathway

The *optic nerves* are cranial nerves formed of the axons of ganglion cells. The two optic nerves meet at the *optic chiasma,* which is just anterior to the pituitary gland in the brain. At the optic chiasma, axons from the medial half of each retina cross to the opposite side to form pairs of axons from each eye. These pairs continue as the left and right *optic tracts* (Figure 43–4 on page 1866). The crossing of the axons results in each optic tract carrying information from both eyes. The left optic tract carries visual information from the lateral half of the retina of the left eye and the medial half of the retina of the right eye, whereas the right optic tract carries visual information from the lateral half of the retina of the right eye and the medial half of the retina of the left eye.

The ganglion cell axons in the optic tracts travel to the thalamus and create synapses with neurons, forming pathways called *optic radiations.* The optic radiations terminate in the *visual cortex* of the occipital lobe. Here the nerve impulses that originated in the retina are interpreted.

The visual fields of each eye overlap considerably, and each eye sees a slightly different view. Because of this overlap and the crossing of the axons, information from both eyes reaches each side of the visual cortex, which then fuses the information into one image. This fusion of images accounts for the ability to perceive depth; however, depth perception depends on visual input from two eyes that both focus well.

Refraction

Refraction is the bending of light rays as they pass from one medium to another medium of different optical density. As light rays pass through the eye, they are refracted at several points: as they enter the cornea, as they leave the cornea and enter the aqueous humor, as they enter the lens, and as they leave the lens and enter the vitreous humor. At the lens, the light is bent so that it converges at a single point on the retina. This focusing of the image is called *accommodation.* Because the lens is convex, the image projected onto the retina (the *real image*) is upside down and reversed from left to right. This real image is

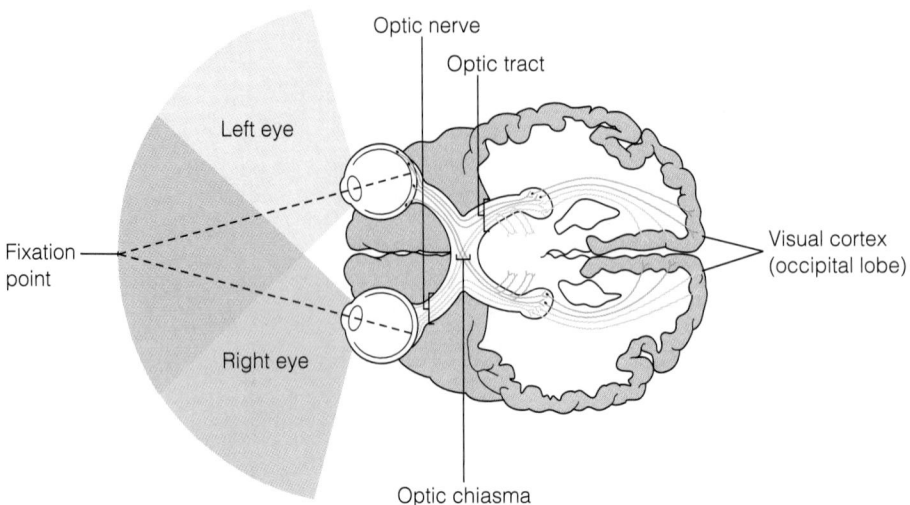

Figure 43–4   The visual fields of the eye, and the visual pathways to the brain.

coded as electric signals that are sent to the brain. The brain decodes the image so that the person perceives it as it occurs in space.

The eyes are best adapted to see distant objects. Both eyes fix on the same distant image and do not require any change in accommodation. For people with *emmetropic* (normal) *vision,* the distance from the viewed object at which the eyes require no accommodation is 20 ft (6 m). This point is called the *far point of vision.* To focus for near vision, the eyes must instantly accommodate the lens, constrict the pupils, and converge the eyeballs. Accommodation is accomplished by contraction of the ciliary muscles. This contraction reduces the tension on the lens capsule so that it bulges outward to increase the curvature. This change in shape also achieves a shorter focal length, another requirement for the focusing of close images on the retina. The closest point on which a person can focus is called the *near point of vision;* in young adults with normal vision this is usually 8 to 10 in. (20 to 25 cm). Pupillary constriction helps eliminate most of the divergent light rays and sharpens focus. *Convergence* (the medial rotation of the eyeballs so that each is directed toward the viewed object) allows the focusing of the image on the retinal fovea of each eye.

The Ear and Hearing

As a sensory organ, the ear has two primary functions— hearing and maintaining equilibrium. Anatomically, the ear is divided into three areas, the external ear, the middle ear, and the inner ear (Figure 43–5). Each area has a unique function. All three are involved in hearing but only the inner ear is involved in equilibrium.

The External Ear

The *external ear* consists of the auricle (or pinna), the external auditory canal, and the tympanic membrane.

The *auricles* are made up of elastic cartilage covered with thin skin. They contain sebaceous and sweat glands and sometimes hair. Each auricle has a rim (the *helix*) and a lobe. The auricle serves to direct sound waves into the ear.

The *external auditory canal,* which is about 1 in. (2.5 cm) long, extends from the auricle to the tympanic membrane. The canal is lined with skin that contains hair, sebaceous glands, and ceruminal glands. The external auditory canal serves as a resonator for the range of sound waves typical of human speech and actually increases the pressure on the tympanic membrane of sound waves in this frequency. The canal's ceruminal glands (which are modified apocrine glands) secrete a yellow to brown waxy substance called **cerumen** (earwax). Cerumen traps foreign bodies; it also has bacteriostatic properties, protecting the tympanic membrane and the middle ear from infections.

The *tympanic membrane* (eardrum) lies between the external ear and the middle ear. It is a thin, semitransparent, fibrous structure covered with skin on the external side and mucosa on the inner side. The membrane vibrates as sound waves strike it; these vibrations are transferred as sound waves to the middle ear.

The Middle Ear

The *middle ear* is an air-filled cavity in the temporal bone. The middle ear contains three auditory ossicles: the *malleus,* the *incus,* and the *stapes.* These bones extend

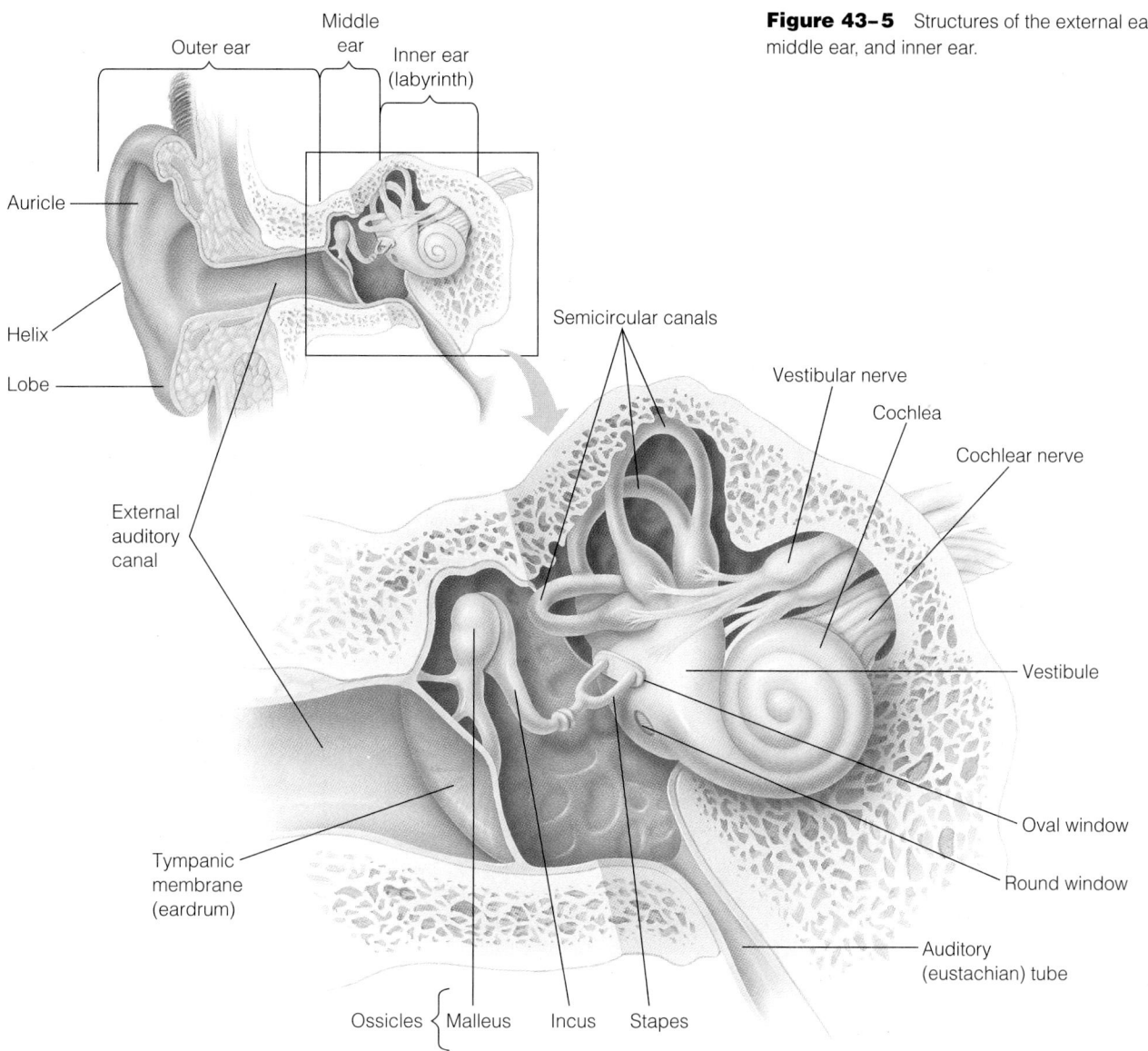

Figure 43–5 Structures of the external ear, middle ear, and inner ear.

across the middle ear. The medial side of the middle ear is a bony wall containing two membrane-covered openings: the oval window and the round window. The posterior wall of the middle ear contains the *mastoid antrum*. This cavity communicates with the *mastoid sinuses* (or *air cells*), which help the middle ear adjust to changes in pressure. It also opens into the *auditory tube* (or *eustachian tube*), which connects with the nasopharynx. The auditory tube helps to equalize the air pressure in the middle ear by opening briefly in response to differences between middle ear pressure and atmospheric pressure. This action also ensures that vibrations of the tympanic membrane remain adequate. The mucous membrane lining the middle ear is continuous with the mucous membranes lining the throat.

The malleus attaches to the tympanic membrane and articulates with the incus, which in turn articulates with the stapes. The stapes fits into the oval window. When the tympanic membrane vibrates, the vibrations are conducted across the middle ear to the oval window by the ossicles. The vibrations then set in motion the fluids of the inner ear, which in turn stimulate the hearing receptors. Two small muscles attached to the ossicles contract reflexively in response to sudden loud noises, thus decreasing the vibrations and protecting the inner ear.

The Inner Ear

The *inner ear,* also called the *labyrinth,* is a maze of bony chambers located deep within the temporal bone, just behind the eye socket. The labyrinth is further divided into two parts: the *bony labyrinth,* a system of open channels that houses the second part, the *membranous labyrinth.* The bony labyrinth is filled with a fluid similar to cerebrospinal fluid called *perilymph,* which bathes the membranous labyrinth. Within the chambers of the membranous labyrinth is a fluid called *endolymph.*

The bony labyrinth has three regions: the vestibule, the semicircular canals, and the cochlea. The *vestibule* is the central portion of the inner ear, one side of which is a bony wall containing the oval window. Two sacs within the vestibule (the *saccule* and the *utricle*) join the vestibule with the cochlea and the semicircular canals. The saccule and the utricle contain receptors for equilibrium that respond to changes in gravity and changes in position of the head. The three *semicircular canals* each project into a different plane (anterior, posterior, and lateral). Each canal contains a *semicircular duct* that communicates with the utricle of the vestibule. Each duct has an enlarged area at one end containing an equilibrium receptor that responds to angular movements of the head.

The *cochlea* is a tiny bony chamber that houses the *organ of Corti,* the receptor organ for hearing. The organ of Corti is a series of sensory hair cells, arranged in a single row of inner hair cells and three rows of outer hair cells. The hair cells are innervated by sensory fibers from cranial nerve VIII. The organ of Corti is supported in the cochlea by the flexible basilar membrane, which has fibers of varying lengths that respond to different sound wave frequencies.

Sound Conduction

Hearing is the perception and interpretation of sound. Sound is produced when the molecules of a medium are compressed, resulting in a pressure disturbance evidenced as a sound wave. The intensity or loudness of sound is determined by the amplitude (height) of the sound wave, with greater amplitudes causing louder sounds. The frequency of the sound wave in vibrations per second determines the pitch or tone of the sound, with higher frequencies resulting in higher sounds. The human ear is most sensitive to sound waves with frequencies between 1000 and 4000 cycles per second but can detect sound waves with frequencies between 20 and 20,000 cycles per second (Spence, 1990).

Sound waves enter the external auditory canal and cause the tympanic membrane to vibrate at the same frequency. The ossicles not only transmit the motion of the tympanic membrane to the oval window but also amplify the energy of the sound wave. As the stapes moves against the oval window, the perilymph in the vestibule is set in motion. The increased pressure of the perilymph is transmitted to fibers of the basilar membrane and then to the organ of Corti (directly above the basilar membrane). The up-and-down movements of the fibers of the basilar membrane pull the hair cells in the organ of Corti, which in turn generates action potentials that are transmitted to cranial nerve VIII and then to the brain for interpretation.

There are several brain stem auditory nuclei that transmit impulses to the cerebral cortex. Several fibers from each ear cross, with each auditory cortex receiving impulses from both ears. Auditory processing is so finely tuned that a wide variety of sounds of different pitch and loudness can be heard at any one time. In addition, the source of the sound can be localized.

Maintenance of Equilibrium

The inner ear also provides information about the position of the head. This information is used to coordinate body movements so that equilibrium and balance are maintained. The types of equilibrium are *static balance* (affected by changes in the position of the head) and *dynamic balance* (affected by the movement of the head).

Changes in the position of the head are detected by receptors called *maculae* in the utricle and the saccule of the vestibule. Maculae are made up of groups of hair cells; these cells have protrusions covered with a gelatinous substance. Embedded in this gelatinous substance are tiny particles of calcium carbonate called *otoliths* (ear stones), which make the gelatin heavier than the endolymph that fills the membranous labyrinth. As a result, when the head is in the upright position, gravity causes the gelatinous substance to bear down on the hair cells. When the position of the head changes, the force on the hair cells also changes, bending them and altering the pattern of stimulation of the neurons. Thus, a different pattern of nerve impulses is transmitted to the brain, where stimulation of the motor centers initiates actions that coordinate various body movements according to the position of the head.

The receptor for dynamic equilibrium is in the *crista,* a crest in the membrane lining the ampulla of each semicircular canal. The cristae are stimulated by rotatory head movement (acceleration and deceleration) as a result of changes in the flow of endolymph and of movement of hair cells in the maculae. The direction of endolymph and hair cell movement is always opposite to the motion of the body.

Assessment of Eye and Ear Function

■ ■ ■

Data about the function of the eyes and the ears, including vision and hearing, are gathered both during the health assessment interview (subjective data) and the physical assessment (objective data).

The Health Assessment Interview

This section provides guidelines for collecting subjective data about the functions of the eye and ear through a health assessment interview. Interview questions and leading statements for assessing eye and ear function also are provided.

The Eye and Vision

A health assessment interview to determine problems with the eyes and vision may be part of a health screening, may focus on a chief complaint (such as blurred vision or an eye infection), or may be part of a total health assessment. If the client has a health problem involving one or both eyes, the nurse analyzes its onset, characteristics and course, severity, precipitating and relieving factors, and any associated symptoms, noting the timing and circumstances. For example, the nurse may ask the client the following questions:

- Describe the type of pain you experience in your eyes. When did it begin? How long does it last?
- Have you noticed rings of color around street lights at night?
- When did you first notice having difficulty reading the paper?

Throughout the interview, be alert to nonverbal behaviors (such as squinting or abnormal eye movements) that suggest problems with eye function. Explore problems such as watery, irritated eyes or changes in vision. Assess the client's use of corrective eyewear and care of eyeglasses or contact lenses. If the client uses eye medications, ask about the type and purpose as well as the frequency and duration of use. When obtaining the history, elicit information about eye trauma, surgery, or infections, as well as the date and results of the last eye examination. In addition, ask the client about a medical history of diabetes, hypertension, thyroid disorders, glaucoma, cataracts, and eye infections. Include questions about a family history of nearsightedness or farsightedness, cancer of the retina, color blindness, and any other eye or vision disorders.

Finally, collect information about environmental or work exposure to irritating chemicals, participation in sports or hobbies that pose the risk of eye injury, and the use of protective eyewear during dangerous activities.

The Ear and Hearing

The health history assessment to collect subjective data about the ears and hearing may also be part of a health screening, may focus on a chief complaint (such as hearing problems or pain in the ear), or may be part of a total health assessment. If the client has a problem involving one or both ears, the nurse analyzes its onset, characteristics and course, severity, precipitating and relieving factors, and any associated symptoms, noting the timing and circumstances. For example, the nurse may ask these questions:

- Have you noticed any difficulty hearing high-pitched sounds, low-pitched sounds, or both?
- When did you first notice the ringing in your ears?
- Is your place of work very noisy? If so, do you wear protective ear equipment at work?

Throughout the examination, be alert to nonverbal behaviors (such as inappropriate answers or requests to repeat statements) that suggest problems with ear function. Explore changes in hearing, ringing in the ears (*tinnitus*), ear pain, drainage from the ears, or the use of hearing aids. When obtaining the history, elicit information about trauma, surgery, or infections of the ear as well as the date of the last ear examination. In addition, ask the client about a medical history of infectious diseases, such as meningitis or mumps, as well as the use of medications that may affect hearing. Because ear problems tend to run in families, ask about a family history of hearing loss, ear problems, or diseases that could result in such problems. If the client has a hearing aid, ascertain the type and assess measures for its care.

Interview Questions

The following interview questions and leading statements are categorized by functional health patterns.

Health Perception–Health Management

- Describe your vision. Rate it on a scale of 1 to 10, with 10 being excellent vision. Is it the same in both eyes? If not, which eye is better?
- Describe your hearing. Rate it on a scale of 1 to 10, with 10 being excellent hearing. Is it the same in both ears? If not, which ear is better?
- Describe your current vision (hearing) problems. How have these been treated?
- What eye (ear) medications do you use? How often?
- Have you ever had eye (ear) surgery? Explain.
- Describe the type of corrective lenses (hearing aid) that you use. Are you satisfied with these appliances? How do you care for them?
- Describe how you care for your eyes (ears).
- When was your last eye (ear) examination? Have you been tested for glaucoma?

Nutritional-Metabolic

- Do you have any redness, swelling, watering, or dryness of your eyes?

- Do you have any swelling or tenderness of the ears, or drainage from your ears?

Activity-Exercise

- Does your vision (hearing) impairment interfere with your usual activities of daily living (such as walking, cooking, grooming, driving, shopping, socializing)? Explain.
- Do you wear protective goggles or earplugs when you engage in activities that increase the risk of injury to the eyes or ears?

Sleep-Rest

- Does your eye (ear) problem interfere with your ability to sleep or rest (for example, because of pain or ringing in the ears)?

Cognitive-Perceptual

- Do you have any difficulty focusing on objects?
- Is your vision blurred? Do you see halos around lights? Do you see "floaters" or flashes of light? Do you see double?
- Do you have pain in or around your eyes (ears)? If so, describe its location, intensity, aggravating factors, and duration. How do you treat it?
- Do you have trouble hearing conversations either in person or on the telephone? Do you have trouble hearing the television? Do you have trouble hearing conversations when you are in crowds?
- Do you have buzzing, ringing, or crackling in your ears?
- Do you feel dizzy?

Self-Perception–Self-Concept

- How has this problem with your eyes (ears) affected how you feel about yourself?

- How has this problem with your eyes (ears) affected how you feel about your normal life?
- How do you feel about wearing corrective lenses or a hearing aid?

Role-Relationship

- Has your eye (ear) problem affected your role in your family? If so, how?
- Has your vision (hearing) loss affected your interactions with others in your family? With friends? At work? In social activities?
- Has your eye (ear) problem interfered with your work? Explain.

Sexuality-Reproductive

- Have your usual sexual activities been altered by problems with your eyes (ears)?
- Describe how these problems with your eyes (ears) have affected how you feel about yourself as a man (woman).

Coping-Stress

- How have you managed with your eye (ear) problem?
- What do you feel is the most stressful time you have had with your eye (ear) problem?
- Describe what you do to cope with stress.
- Who or what will be able to help you cope with the stress caused by your eye (ear) problem ?

Value-Belief

- Are there significant others, practices, or activities that help you cope with a vision (hearing) impairment? Explain.
- How do you think this health problem will affect your future?

The Physical Assessment

The Eye and Vision: Preparation

Physical assessment of the eyes and of visual acuity may be performed as part of a total assessment or separately for clients with known or suspected problems of the eyes. The eyes and vision are primarily assessed through inspection of external structures and assessment of visual fields and visual acuity, extraocular muscle function, and internal structures. Palpation (e.g., of a blocked lacrimal duct) may be used if a problem is identified. Prior to the examination, collect all necessary equipment—visual acuity charts, an opaque eye cover, a pen, a penlight, a cotton-tipped applicator, and an ophthalmoscope—and explain the techniques to the client to decrease anxiety. The client may sit or stand during the assessment.

The Physical Assessment

Visual acuity is assessed by using the Snellen chart or the E chart for testing distance vision and the Rosenbaum chart for testing near vision.

- The *Snellen chart* contains rows of letters in various sizes, with standardized numbers at the end of each row. The number at the end of the row indicates the visual acuity of a client who can read the row at a distance of 20 feet. (If the client is unable to read or does not read English, you can use the E chart to test visual acuity.) The top number at the end of the row is always 20, representing the distance between the client and the chart. The bottom number is the distance (in feet) at which a person with normal vision can read the line. A person with normal vision can read the row marked 20/20.

  To conduct the assessment, ask the person to stand 20 feet from the chart in a well-lit area. Ask the client to cover one eye with an opaque cover (Figure 43–6). Then ask the client to read each row of letters, moving from largest letters to the smallest ones that the client can see. Measure visual acuity in the other eye in the same way, and then assess visual acuity while the client has both eyes uncovered. You may test the client who wears corrective lenses with and without the lenses.

- The *Rosenbaum chart* is held at a distance of from 12 to 14 inches from the eyes, with visual acuity measured in the same manner as with the Snellen chart (Figure 43–7). A gross estimate of near vision may also be assessed by asking the person to read from a magazine or newspaper.

Visual fields are tested to assess the functioning of the macula and peripheral vision. The visual fields of the examiner (which must be normal to perform this assessment) are used as the standard. To measure visual fields, sit directly opposite the client at a distance of 18 to 24 inches. Ask the client to cover one eye with the opaque cover while you cover your own eye opposite to the client (for example, if the client covers the right eye, you cover your left eye). Ask the client to look directly at you. Move the penlight from the periphery toward the center from right to left, above and below, and from the middle of each of these directions. Both you and the client should see the penlight enter the field of vision at the same time.

Assess extraocular muscle function by examining the six cardinal fields of vision and using the cover-uncover test.

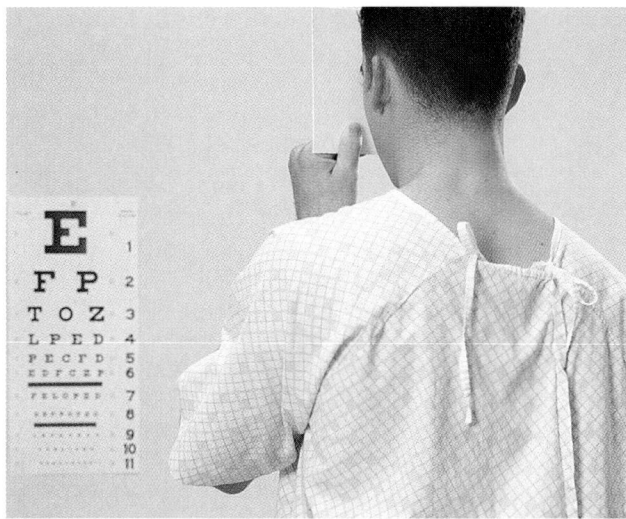

Figure 43–6 Testing distant vision using the Snellen eye chart.

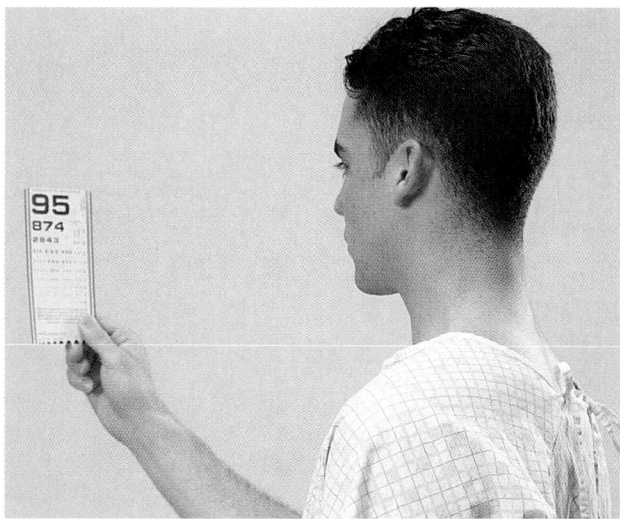

Figure 43–7 Testing near vision using Rosenbaum eye chart.

The Physical Assessment (continued)

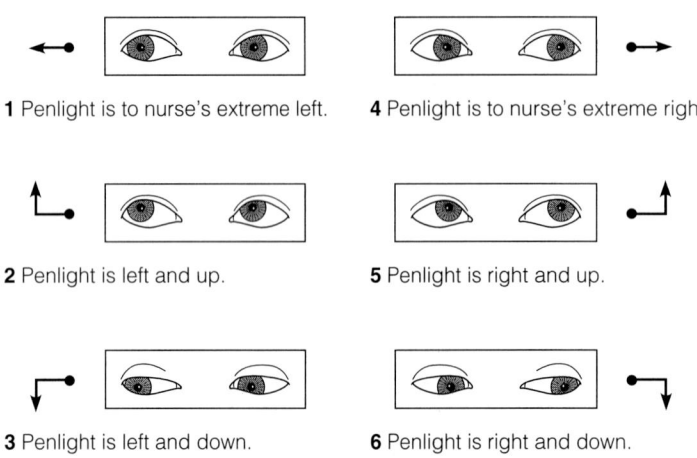

1 Penlight is to nurse's extreme left.

4 Penlight is to nurse's extreme right.

2 Penlight is left and up.

5 Penlight is right and up.

3 Penlight is left and down.

6 Penlight is right and down.

Figure 43–8 The six cardinal fields of vision.

- Assess the *cardinal fields of vision* to gain information about extraocular eye movements. Ask the client to follow a pen or your finger while keeping the head stationary. Move the pen or your finger through the six fields one at a time, returning to the central starting point before proceeding to the next field (Figure 43–8). The eyes should move through each field without involuntary movements.

- The *cover-uncover test* is a test for *strabismus*, a weakening of a muscle that causes one eye to deviate from the other when the person is focusing on an object. To conduct the test, hold a pen or your finger about 1 foot from the eyes and ask the person to focus on that object. Cover one of the client's eyes and note any movement in the uncovered eye; as you remove the cover, assess for movement in the eye that was just uncovered. Repeat the procedure with the other eye.

Assess internal structures of the eye by using the ophthalmoscope, an instrument that allows visualization of the lens, the vitreous humor, and the retina.

ASSESSMENT TECHNIQUE	POSSIBLE ABNORMAL FINDINGS
Vision - **Assess distant vision.** Using a Snellen chart or E chart, test each eye separately and both eyes together.	Changes in distant vision are most commonly the result of **myopia** (nearsightedness). For example, a reading of 20/100 indicates impaired distance vision. A person has to stand 20 feet from the chart to read a line that a person with normal vision could read 100 feet from the chart.
- **Assess near vision.** Hold either a Rosenbaum chart or a card with newsprint 12 to 14 inches from the client's eyes. Ask the client to read the chart or card.	Changes in near vision, especially in clients over 45, can indicate **presbyopia,** impaired near vision resulting from a loss of elasticity of the lens related to aging. In younger clients, this condition is referred to as **hyperopia** (farsightedness).

ASSESSMENT TECHNIQUE	POSSIBLE ABNORMAL FINDINGS
Eye Movement and Alignment ■ **Assess convergence.** Ask the client to follow an object as you move it toward the client's eyes; normally both eyes converge toward the center.	Failure of the eyes to converge equally on an approaching object may indicate a neuromuscular disorder or improper eye alignment.
■ **Assess extraocular movements.** Ask the client to hold the head steady and to follow an object as you move it through the six cardinal fields of vision.	Failure of one or both eyes to follow the object in any given direction may indicate extraocular muscle weakness or cranial nerve dysfunction. An involuntary rhythmic movement of the eyes, *nystagmus,* is associated with neurologic disorders and the use of some medications.
■ **Perform the cover-uncover test.** Ask the client to look straight ahead. Cover one eye with an opaque card. Watch for movement of the uncovered eye. Then test the other eye.	Movement of the uncovered eye when covering one eye indicates strabismus.
■ **Assess the corneal light reflex.** Direct a light source onto the bridge of the nose from 12 to 15 inches. Observe for equal reflection of the light from each eye.	Reflections of the light from different sites on the eyes reveal improper alignment.
Pupil Size, Response, and Accommodation ■ **Observe pupil size and equality.**	Pupils that are unequal in size may indicate a severe neurologic problem, such as increased intracranial pressure. However, a small number of healthy people have a slight inequality in pupil size called *benign anisocoria,* a congenital anomaly.
■ **Assess direct and consensual pupil response.** Ask the client to look straight ahead. Shine a light obliquely into one eye at a time. Observe for constriction of the pupil in the illuminated eye. Test both eyes.	Failure of the pupils to respond to light may indicate degeneration of the retina or destruction of the optic nerve. Paralysis of the oculomotor nerve may be present in a client who has one dilated and unresponsive pupil. Note that pupillary reactions are normal in benign anisocoria.
To test consensual pupil response, again shine a light obliquely into one eye at a time as the client looks straight ahead. Observe constriction of the pupil in the opposite eye.	Some eye medications may cause unequal dilation, constriction, or inequality of pupil size. Morphine and similar drugs may cause small, unresponsive pupils, and anticholinergic drugs such as atropine may cause dilated, unresponsive pupils.
■ **Test for accommodation.** Hold an object at a distance of a few feet from the client. The pupils should dilate. Ask the client to follow the object as you bring it to within a few inches of the client's nose. The pupils should constrict and converge as they change focus to follow the object.	Failure of accommodation along with lack of pupil response to light may signal a neurologic problem. Lack of response to light with appropriate response to accommodation is often seen in clients with diabetes or syphilis.

ASSESSMENT TECHNIQUE	POSSIBLE ABNORMAL FINDINGS

Visible Structures

■ **Inspect the eyelids.**

Unusual redness or discharge may indicate an inflammatory state due to trauma, allergies, or infection. Drooping of one eyelid, called *ptosis,* may be the result of a CVA, indicate a neuromuscular disorder, or be congenital (Figure 43–9).

Figure 43–9
Ptosis.

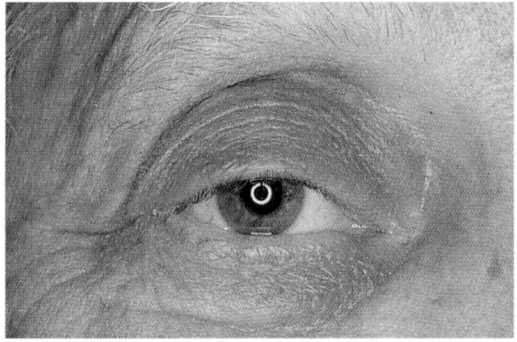

Unusual widening of the lids may be due to *exophthalmos,* protrusion of the eyeball due to an increase in intraocular volume. Exophthalmos is often associated with hyperthyroid conditions (see Chapter 20).

Yellow plaques noted most often on the lid margins are referred to as *xanthelasma* and may indicate high lipid levels.

Figure 43–10
Hordeolum.

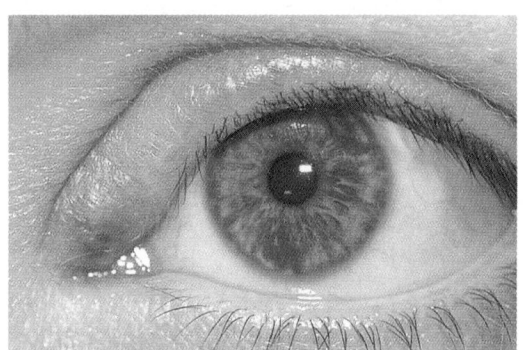

An acute localized inflammation of a hair follicle is known as a *hordeolum* (sty) and is generally caused by staphylococcal organisms (Figure 43–10).

A *chalazion* is an infection or retention cyst of the meibomian glands (Figure 43–11). The swelling is firm and not painful.

Figure 43–11
Chalazion.

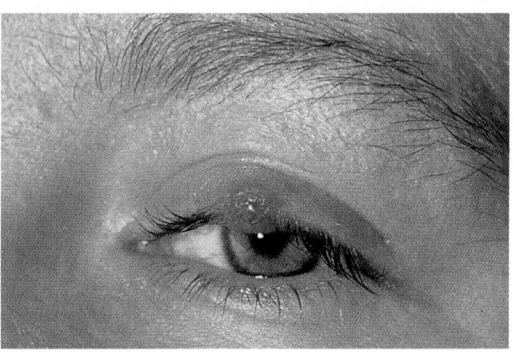

■ **Inspect the puncta.**

Unusual redness or discharge from the puncta may indicate an inflammatory state due to trauma, infection, or allergies.

■ **Inspect the bulbar and palpebral conjunctiva.**

Increased erythema or the presence of exudate may indicate acute conjunctivitis. A cobblestone appearance is often associated with allergies.

ASSESSMENT TECHNIQUE	POSSIBLE ABNORMAL FINDINGS
	A fold in the conjunctiva, called a *pterygium,* may be seen as a clouded area that extends over the cornea. This is an abnormal growth of the bulbar conjunctiva, usually seen on the nasal side of the cornea. It may interfere with vision if it covers the pupil.
▪ **Inspect the sclera.**	Unusual redness may indicate an inflammatory state as a result of trauma, allergies, or infection. Yellow discoloration of the sclera may be seen in conditions involving the liver, such as hepatitis. Bright red areas in the sclera are often subconjunctival hemorrhages and may indicate trauma or bleeding disorders. They may also occur spontaneously.
▪ **Inspect the cornea.**	Dullness, opacities, or irregularities of the cornea may be abnormal. Corneal arcus is a thin grayish white arc seen toward the edge of the cornea. It is normal in older clients.
▪ **Assess corneal sensitivity.** Lightly touch a wisp of cotton to the client's cornea. This action should cause a blink reflex.	Failure of the blink reflex may indicate a neurologic disorder.
▪ **Inspect the iris.**	Lack of clarity of the iris may indicate a cloudiness of the cornea. An iridectomy is a surgical incision in the iris used to treat glaucoma. It is seen more commonly in older clients. Constriction of the pupil accompanied by pain and circumcorneal redness is indicative of acute iritis.
Internal Structures (See the box on page 1876 for guidelines on using the ophthalmoscope.) ▪ **Inspect for the red reflex.**	Absence of a red reflex often indicates improper position of the ophthalmoscope but also may indicate total opacity of the pupil by a cataract or a hemorrhage into the vitreous humor.
▪ **Inspect the lens and vitreous body.**	A *cataract* is an opacity of the lens, often seen as a dark shadow on ophthalmoscopic examination. It may be due to aging, trauma, diabetes, or a congenital defect.
▪ **Inspect the retina.**	Areas of hemorrhage, exudate, and white patches may be a result of diabetes or long-standing hypertension.

ASSESSMENT TECHNIQUE	POSSIBLE ABNORMAL FINDINGS
■ **Inspect the optic disc.**	Loss of definition of the optic disc, as well as an increase in the size of the physiologic cup, results from papilledema and is a sign of increased intracranial pressure.
■ **Inspect the blood vessels of the retina.**	Glaucoma often results in displacement of blood vessels from the center of the optic disc due to increased intraocular pressure. Hypertension may cause an apparent narrowing of the vein where an arteriole crosses over. Engorged veins may occur with diabetes, atherosclerosis, and blood disorders.
■ **Inspect the retinal background.**	Variations in color or a pale color overall may indicate disease.
■ **Inspect the macula.**	Absence of the fovea centralis is common in older clients. It may indicate macular degeneration, a common cause of loss of central vision.
■ **Palpate over the lacrimal glands, puncta, and nasolacrimal duct.**	Tenderness over any of these areas or drainage from the puncta may indicate an infectious process. (Wear gloves if you see any drainage.) Excessive tearing may indicate a blockage of the nasolacrimal duct.

Guidelines for Using the Ophthalmoscope

■   ■   ■

The ophthalmoscope has a head and a handle. (See the accompanying figure.) The head contains a focus wheel (also called a lens selector dial) located on the side, lenses of varying magnification, and an opening through which the eye structures are visualized. The focus wheel adjusts the lens refraction, which is measured in diopters. The diopter measurements range from 0 to +40 when the lens is rotated clockwise, and from 0 to −25 when the lens is rotated counterclockwise. By moving the focus wheel, the examiner can converge or diverge light rays to visualize the retina.

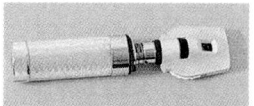

An ophthalmoscope.

The handle usually contains batteries that can be plugged into a wall socket for recharging.

Before the examination, explain the procedure to the client. Assemble the ophthalmoscope. Wash your hands and wear disposable gloves if the client has any drainage from the eyes. Darken the room (to allow the pupils of the client to dilate), and ask the client to look straight ahead, focusing on a fixed point such as an object on the wall. Hold the ophthalmoscope in one hand, resting the index finger on the focus wheel. (See the figure on page 1877.)

1. Turn on the ophthalmoscope light, and set focus wheel to 0 diopters. Hold the ophthalmoscope in your right hand with your index finger on the focus wheel. Standing in front of the client, position

Guidelines for Using the Ophthalmoscope (continued)

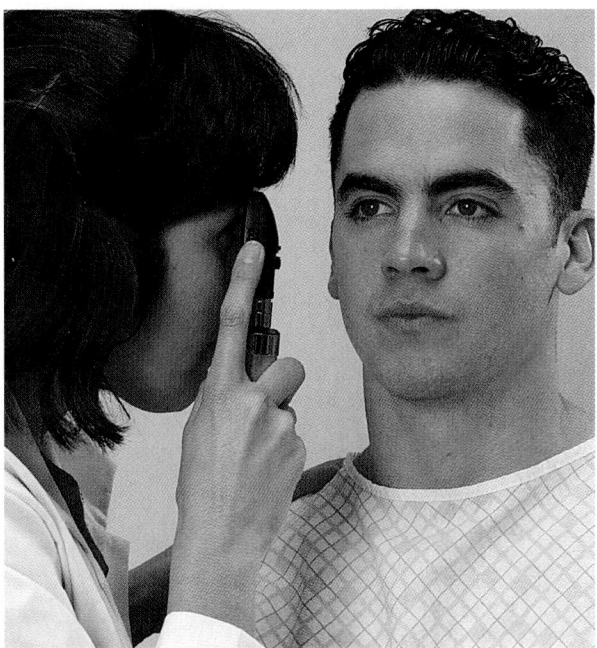

Technique for holding an ophthalmoscope.

yourself at a 15-degree angle to the client's line of vision.

2. Hold the opening of the ophthalmoscope up to your right eye and direct the light toward the client's right eye from a distance of about 12 inches.

3. As the beam of light falls on the client's pupil, observe for the red reflex, which appears as a sharply outlined orange glow from within the pupil. This glow is the reflection of the light from the retina.

4. Move closer to the client, turning the focus wheel clockwise toward the positive numbers as needed to maintain clear focus.

5. Examine the lens and the vitreous body, both of which should be clear.

6. Gradually rotate the focus wheel counterclockwise toward the negative numbers as needed, focusing on a structure of the retina (such as the disc or a blood vessel). Turn the focus wheel until the image is clear. Examine the structures of the retina as follows:

   a. The optic disc (see the accompanying figure). Assess for size, shape, color, distinct margins, and the physiologic cup. The disc is round to slightly oval and about 1.5 mm in diameter. It has a yellow to pink color that is lighter than the retina itself. The margins should be sharp and clear. The physiologic cup is a small depression that occupies about one-third of the optic disc, lying temporal to the center of the disc.

   b. The vessels of the retina. Assess for color, arteriolar light reflex, ratio of arterioles to veins, and arteriovenous crossings. The arterioles are red, brighter than the veins, and about one-fourth smaller. The arterioles normally have a narrow light reflex from the center of each vessel; veins do not have this light reflex. The ratio of arterioles to veins is usually 2:3 or 4:5. The vessels normally cross and become smaller toward the periphery.

   c. The retinal background. Assess color and changes in color. The retina is normally reddish orange and regular in color.

   d. The macula. Assess size and color. To assess the macula, ask the client to look directly into the ophthalmoscope light. The macula is temporal to the optic disc, appears slightly darker than the retina, and has no visible vessels. The fovea centralis may be seen as a bright spot of light. Because looking directly into the light causes some discomfort, conduct this portion of the examination last. The macula is often difficult to visualize.

7. Using the same technique, examine the left eye.

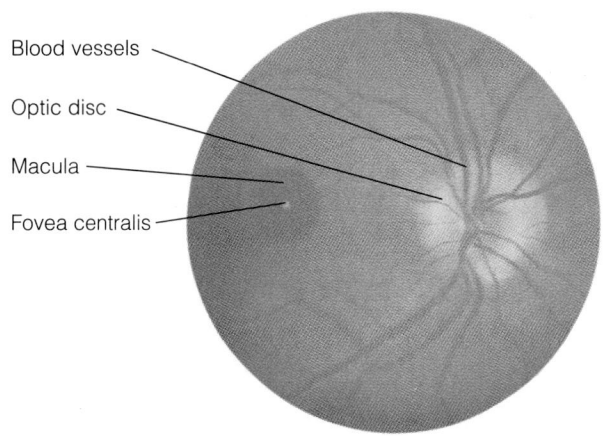

Blood vessels
Optic disc
Macula
Fovea centralis

The optic disc.

The Physical Assessment

Physical assessment of the ear and hearing may be performed as part of a total health assessment or separately for clients with known or suspected problems with the ears. The ears and hearing are assessed primarily through inspection of external structures, the external auditory canal, and the tympanic membrane. Hearing acuity is assessed by voice tests and tuning fork tests. The external structures may be palpated.

Equipment includes an otoscope and a tuning fork. The client should be sitting, and the examiner's head should be level with the head of the client. Prior to the assessment, collect all necessary equipment and explain the techniques to the client to decrease anxiety.

The auditory canal and tympanic membrane are inspected with the otoscope. Guidelines for use of the otoscope are listed in the accompanying box.

Tuning forks are used to determine whether a hearing loss is conductive or perceptive (sensorineural) (Figure 43–12). The tuning fork is held at the base and made to ring softly by stroking the prongs or by lightly tapping them on the heel of the opposite hand. The vibrating tuning fork emits sound waves of a particular frequency, measured in Hertz (Hz). Tuning forks with a frequency of 512 to 1024 Hz are preferred for auditory evaluation because that range corresponds to the range of normal speech.

Figure 43–12   A tuning fork.

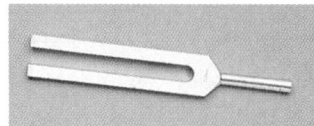

ASSESSMENT TECHNIQUE	POSSIBLE ABNORMAL FINDINGS

Hearing
- **Perform the Weber test.**

Place the base of a vibrating tuning fork on the midline vertex of the client's head (Figure 43–13). Ask whether the client hears the sound equally in both ears or better in one than the other. Sound is normally heard equally in both ears.

Figure 43–13
Performing the
Weber test.

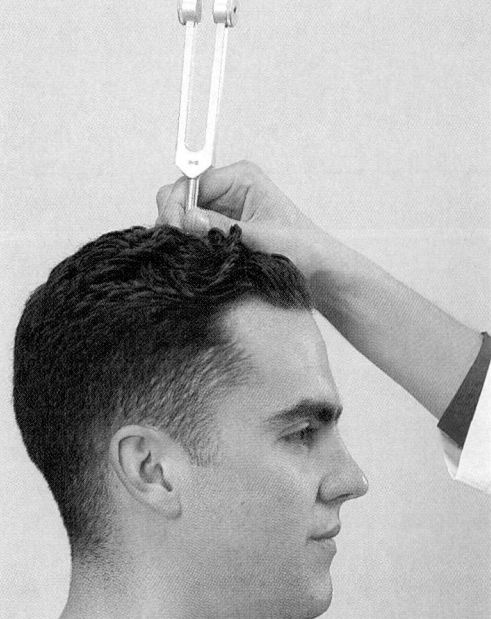

Sound heard in, or lateralized to, one ear indicates either a conductive loss in that ear or a sensorineural loss in the other ear. Conductive losses may be due to a buildup of cerumen, an infection such as otitis media, or perforation of the eardrum.

ASSESSMENT TECHNIQUE	POSSIBLE ABNORMAL FINDINGS

■ Perform the Rinne test.

Place the base of a vibrating tuning fork on the client's mastoid bone. Ask the client to indicate when the sound is no longer heard. When the client does so, quickly reposition the tuning fork in front of the client's ear close to the ear canal. Ask whether the client can hear the sound. If the client says yes, ask the client to indicate when the sound is no longer heard. The client with no conductive hearing loss will hear the sound twice as long by air conduction as by bone conduction. (Figure 43–14).

Bone conduction is greater than air conduction in the ear with a conductive loss. The normal pattern is AC>BC (air conduction greater than bone conduction).

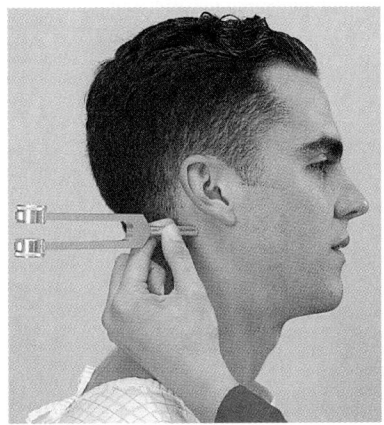 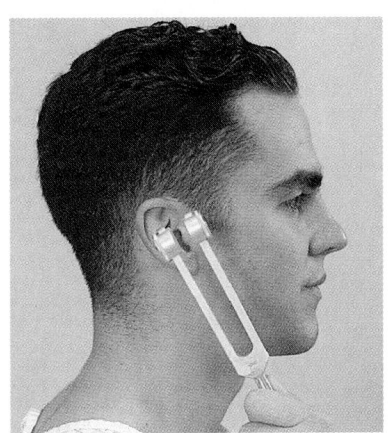

Figure 43–14 Performing the Rinne test.

■ Perform the whisper test.

Ask the client to occlude one ear with a finger. Stand 1 to 2 feet away from the client, on the side of the unoccluded ear. Softly whisper numbers and ask the client to repeat them. Repeat the procedure, having the client occlude the other ear. Note whether you need to raise your voice or to stand closer to make the client hear you.

This is a rough estimate of hearing loss.

The Ears
■ Inspect the auricle.

Unusual redness or drainage may indicate an inflammatory response to infection or trauma. Scales or skin lesions around the rim of the auricle may indicate skin cancer. Small, raised lesions on the rim of the ear are known as *tophi* and indicate gout (Figure 43–15).

ASSESSMENT TECHNIQUE	POSSIBLE ABNORMAL FINDINGS

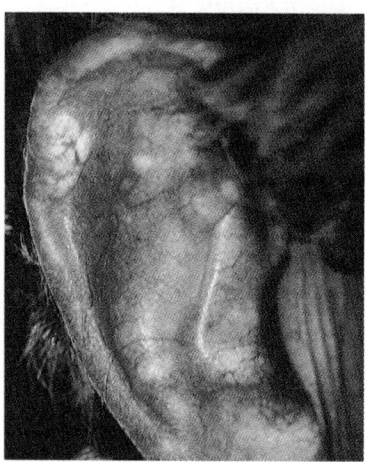

Figure 43–15 Tophi.

■ **Inspect the external auditory canal.**
(See the box on page 1881 for guidelines on the use of an otoscope.)

Unusual redness, lesions, or purulent drainage may indicate an infectious process.
Cerumen varies in color and texture, but hardened, dry, or foul-smelling cerumen may indicate an infection or an impaction of cerumen that requires removal. People with darker skin colors tend to have darker cerumen.

■ **Inspect the tympanic membrane.**

White, opaque areas on the tympanic membrane are often scars from previous perforations (Figure 43–16).
Inconsistent texture and color may also be due to scarring from previous perforation caused by infection, allergies, or trauma.
Bulging membranes can be detected by noting a loss of bony landmarks and a distorted light reflex. Such bulges may

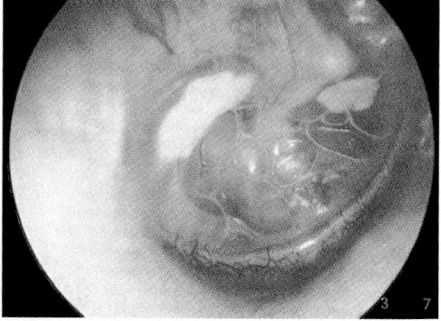

Figure 43–16 Scarring of the tympanic membrane.

ASSESSMENT TECHNIQUE	POSSIBLE ABNORMAL FINDINGS
	be the result of otitis media or malfunctioning auditory tubes.
	Retracted tympanic membranes can be detected by noting accentuated bony landmarks and a distorted light reflex. Such retraction is often due to an obstructed auditory tube.
■ **Palpate the auricles and over the mastoid process.**	Tenderness, swelling, or nodules may indicate inflammation of the external auditory canal or mastoiditis.

Guidelines for Using the Otoscope

■ ■ ■

The otoscope has a handle that contains batteries for the light and various specula that fit onto the handle. (See the accompanying figure.) This instrument is used to inspect the auditory canal and the tympanic membrane. A pneumatic otoscope is used to determine the mobility of the tympanic membrane. A pneumatic otoscope has an attached rubber bulb that can be squeezed to inject air into the auditory canal, causing a normal tympanic membrane to move in and out.

Before the examination, explain the procedure to the client. Assemble the otoscope, using the largest speculum that will fit into the client's auditory canal without discomfort. Wash your hands; wear disposable gloves if the client has any drainage from the ears. Turn on the otoscope light. Ask the client to tip the head slightly toward the shoulder opposite the ear being examined. When the client is in this position, the auditory canal is aligned with the speculum.

1. Hold the handle of the otoscope in your dominant hand. If the client is restless, hold the otoscope handle upward, resting the hand against the client's head. If the client is cooperative, hold the handle downward.

2. For adult clients, grasp the superior portion of the auricle and pull up, out, and back to straighten the auditory canal. (See the accompanying figure.)

3. Insert the speculum into the ear and advance it gently. Assess the walls of the auditory canal while advancing the speculum, inspecting for color, obstructions, hair growth, and cerumen. Old cerumen is very dark and may obstruct visualization of part or all of the tympanic membrane.

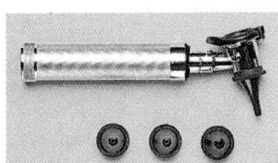
An otoscope.

4. Move the otoscope so that you can see the tympanic membrane. You may need to realign the auditory canal by gently continuing to pull up and back on the auricle. A normal membrane is semi-transparent, allowing visualization of a portion of the auditory ossicles. The concave nature of the tympanic membrane and its oblique position in the auditory canal account for the triangular light

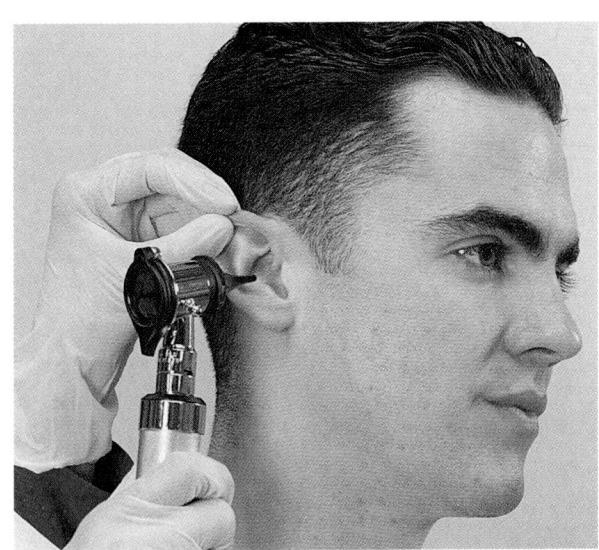
Technique for using an otoscope.

Guidelines for Using the Otoscope (continued)

reflex (cone of light) seen on otoscopic examination.

5. Note the color and surface of the membrane. The normal tympanic membrane is pearly gray, shiny, and semitransparent. The surface should be continuous, intact, and either flat or concave.

6. Identify the landmarks of the tympanic membrane (see the accompanying figure):
   a. The cone of light, located over the anteroinferior quadrant.
   b. The malleus, pars tensa, annulus, pars flaccida, and malleolar folds.

7. Assess movement of the tympanic membrane. If the auditory tube is patent, the membrane moves in and out when air is injected (or when the client performs the Valsalva maneuver).

8. Gently withdraw the speculum. If the speculum is soiled with drainage or cerumen, use a clean speculum for the other ear.

9. Using the same technique, examine the other ear.

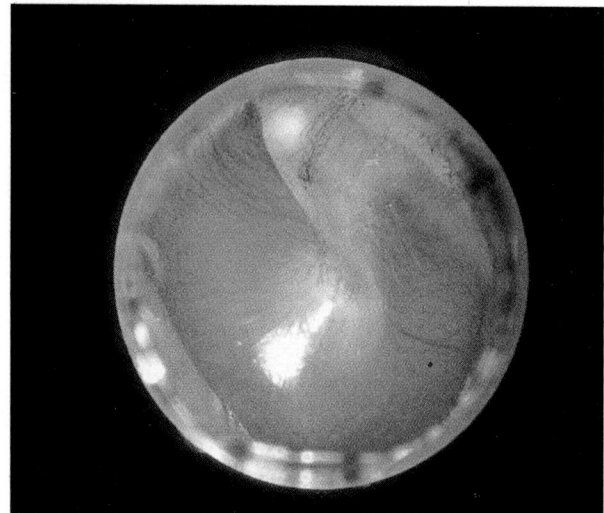

Structures of the tympanic membrane visible through the otoscope.

Variations in Assessment Findings for the Older Adult

The Eyes of the Older Adult

Age-related changes in the eyes affect not only the structures of the eye but also vision. As a result, many older adults must wear corrective lenses. The following changes are often seen in the older client:

- Loss of fat from the orbit causes the eyes to appear sunken.

- The muscles that allow the lids to close tightly lose strength, resulting in a turning out of the lower lid, called *ectropion* (Figure 43–17). *Entropion,* the turning inward of the lower lid, is the result of muscle spasm (Figure 43–18). Entropion may cause constant irritation of the eye by the eyelashes. Ptosis is common as the muscles that hold the upper lid open become weaker.

- Dry eye syndrome often develops as the cells that lubricate the conjunctiva decrease in number. The older

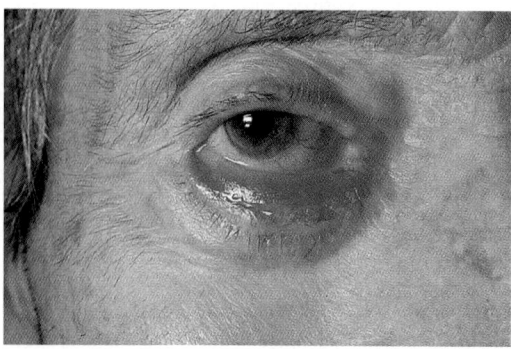

Figure 43–17 Ectropion.

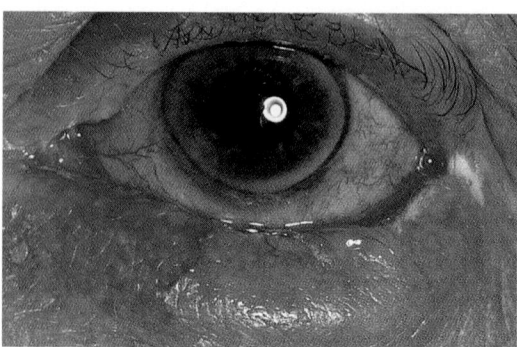

Figure 43–18 Entropion.

adult with this chronic condition experiences red, irritated eyes that feel scratchy.

- *Arcus senilis* is an accumulation of calcium and cholesterol salts around the limbus, creating a gray halo around the outer edge of the cornea. This condition does not affect vision.

- The cornea becomes thicker and less curved, increasing astigmatism.

- The pupil constricts more slowly in bright light and dilates more slowly in dim light, reducing adaptation of vision to a dark room.

- The lens loses elasticity and becomes firmer and more opaque. As a result, there is a decrease in refraction, decreased color vision, and a decrease in accommodation for near vision. This loss of accommodation, called presbyopia, usually increases after age 40.

- The anterior chamber decreases in size and volume as the lens thickens, increasing the risk for glaucoma.

- The retina loses rods at the periphery. Thus, the older adult needs more light to see and may lose some peripheral vision.

The Ears of the Older Adult

Age-related changes affect the outer ear, the middle ear, and the inner ear. Alterations in hearing also occur with age, and the older client may need a hearing aid. The following changes are often seen:

- The skin on the outer ear becomes dry and less resilient, and some connective tissue is lost.

- Coarse, wiry hair often grows along the periphery of the helix and tragus of the pinna.

- The pinna becomes longer and wider, and the earlobes are elongated.

- Less cerumen is produced, drying the auditory canal and increasing the risk for impaction of cerumen.

- Degenerative changes occur in the joints of the ossicles. These changes do not appear to affect hearing.

- **Presbycusis,** an age-related loss of the ability to hear high-frequency sounds, may occur because of cochlear hair cell degeneration or loss of auditory neurons in the organ of Corti. This condition decreases the client's ability to hear normal speech.

- The ability to discriminate the localization of sound decreases, most often for high-frequency sounds.

Bibliography

■ ■ ■

Andresen, G. (1989). A fresh look at assessing the elderly. *RN, 33*(6), 28–40.

Barker, E., & Moore, K. (1992). Perfecting the art: Cranial nerve assessment. *RN, 55*(5), 62–69.

Boyd-Monk, H. (1990). Assessing acquired ocular disease. *Nursing Clinics of North America, 25*(4), 811–822.

Braverman, B. (1990). Eliciting assessment data from a patient who is difficult to interview. *Nursing Clinics of North America, 25*(4), 743–750.

Kain, C. (1990). The older adult: A comparative assessment. *Nursing Clinics of North America, 25*(4), 833–848.

Marieb, E. N. (1994). *Human anatomy and physiology* (2nd ed.). Redwood City, CA: Benjamin/Cummings.

McCance, K. L., & Huether, S. E. (1994). *Pathophysiology: The biologic basis for disease in adults and children* (2nd ed.). St. Louis: Mosby.

McConnell, E. (1988). Seeing your patient as a mosaic. *Nursing '88, 18*(12), 50–51.

Sapira, J. D., & Schneiderman, H. (1990). The fundascopic examination: How to make the most of it. *Consultant, 30*(6), 22–27.

Spence, A. P. (1990). *Basic human anatomy* (3rd ed.). Redwood City, CA: Benjamin/Cummings.

Swartz, M. (1989). *Textbook of physical diagnosis: History and examination.* Saunders: Philadelphia.

Nursing Care of Clients with Eye and Ear Disorders

LEARNING OBJECTIVES

After completing this chapter, you will be able to

- Describe the pathophysiology of commonly occurring disorders of the eyes and ears, relating their manifestations to the pathophysiologic process.
- Identify diagnostic tests used to diagnose eye and ear disorders.
- Discuss the nursing implications for medications prescribed for clients with eye and ear disorders.
- Provide appropriate care for the client having eye or ear surgery.
- Use the nursing process to assess needs, plan and implement individualized care, and evaluate responses for the client with impaired vision or hearing.

The special senses provide the primary means of input for much of what we know about the world. The ability to receive and organize information orients us to our surroundings (Maas et al., 1991). Our interactions with others are facilitated by these senses. They allow us to communicate easily, give us access to information, and let us derive pleasure from the arts and from the sights, smells, and sounds of the world around us. The special senses also warn us of danger and protect us from injury.

Diseases and disorders that affect the eyes and ears threaten this access and early warning system. Loss of vision or hearing is a potential result of eye and ear disorders. Nurses care for clients with visual or hearing deficits as well as those with eye or ear disorders. This chapter discusses conditions affecting the eyes and ears. Nursing care planning focuses on clients with vision and hearing deficits that can result from the disorders presented.

◼◼◼ Eye Disorders ◼◼◼

Any portion of the eye and its protective structures may be affected by an acute or chronic condition. Although many eye disorders do not pose a threat to vision, the client may perceive a threat, causing anxiety. Disorders and diseases of the outer, visible portion of the eye often cause discomfort and may have cosmetic effects. The effect on vision can often be prevented or reversed with proper treatment of the disorder. The client who has had eye surgery or minor trauma may have either temporary or permanent visual impairment. Disorders affecting the internal structures or the function of the eye are more likely to have adverse effects on vision. Although these disorders often cannot be prevented or cured, some can be controlled and vision corrected to normal or near-normal. Not all conditions affecting the eye are pathologic; some are associated with normal aging.

Table 44–1	Age-Related Changes in the Eye and Vision	
Physiologic Change	**Conditions**	**Effect on Vision**
Changes that lead to altered protection of the eye	■ Senile entropion: Inversion of the lid margins ■ Senile ectropion: Eversion of the eyelid margin ■ Decreased corneal sensitivity ■ Decreased tear secretion	■ Lashes may cause corneal irritation and damage ■ Conjunctival exposure and possible inflammation ■ Increased potential for damage due to foreign body or trauma ■ Increased potential for infection or damage due to environmental pollution
Changes that affect vision	■ Flattening of the cornea ■ Pupillary constriction ■ Decreased lens elasticity and increased lens density ■ Loss of sensory cells at the periphery of the retina	■ Reduced refractory power and decreased visual acuity ■ Reduction in the amount of light reaching the retina to approximately one-third of previous amount (in younger years) ■ Decreased visual acuity, affecting close vision especially ■ Increased problems with glare (scattering of light rays) ■ Decreased color perception, especially in blue, green, and violet spectra ■ Decreased visual fields (peripheral vision)
Mechanical changes that may affect vision	■ Senile enophthalmos: Sinking in of the eyes giving a "hollow-eyed" appearance ■ Decreased eye motility	■ May limit peripheral vision in all directions: to the sides, upward, and downward ■ Increased difficulty with looking upward and convergence
Cosmetic changes	■ Yellowing of the sclera due to fatty deposits ■ Arcus senilis: Formation of a grayish yellow ring at the corneal margin	■ None ■ None

The Client with Age-Related Changes in Vision

■ ■ ■

A number of changes in the eye and vision are attributed to the aging process. The pupil decreases in size and does not dilate readily, reducing the amount of light that reaches the retina. Night vision is affected, and increased light intensity is necessary for reading and handwork. The lens becomes less elastic, making it increasingly difficult to focus for near vision. Clients notice that their arms have become too short to read the newspaper comfortably. With aging, the lens discolors and opacifies, causing it to absorb more of the short wavelengths of light, resulting in a decrease in color perception. This change affects the green, blue, and violet hues in particular. Clients may tend to choose brighter colors of clothing and decor as color perception changes.

Other effects of aging on the eye include changes in the vitreous humor, atrophy of the choroid, thinning of the retina, and degenerative changes in the optic nerve (Hazzard et al., 1994). Depth perception and the ability to see lines of demarcation (e.g., the edges of steps or a change in direction of walls) diminish with age.

As the aging client loses subcutaneous tissue, the eyes may recess into the eye sockets, creating tissue folds on the upper lids. These structural changes, along with a decrease in eye mobility, can limit the older adult's vision upward and to the sides. Nurses can help the client by placing signs at eye level, not above. Checking for low-hanging objects that the client may not see can prevent head injuries.

Changes of the eye and vision commonly associated with the aging process are summarized in Table 44–1.

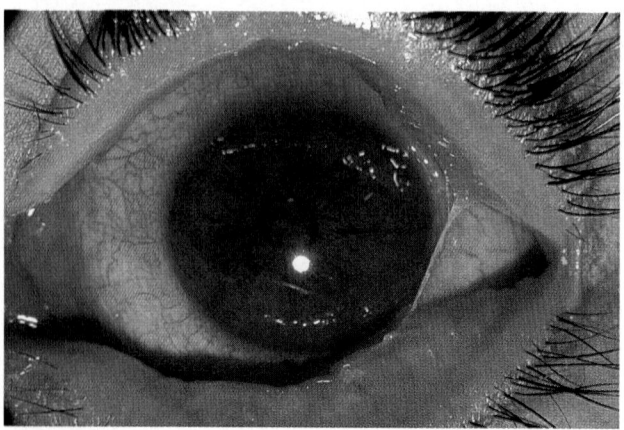

Figure 44–1   The appearance of an eye with conjunctivitis.

The Client with an Infectious or Inflammatory Eye Disorder

■ ■ ■

The extraocular structures—the eyelids, eyelashes, and conjunctiva in particular—are vulnerable to inflammation and infection because of their constant exposure to the environment. When inflamed, these normally protective structures may perform their functions less effectively and may cause discomfort and changes in the client's appearance. The corneal reflex and tears (which contain antibodies and *lysozyme,* an antibacterial enzyme) protect the eye against most hazards. As tear production decreases with aging, the risk increases.

Conjunctivitis, inflammation of the conjunctiva, is the most common eye disease (Tierney et al., 1994). Bacterial or viral infections are the most common causes of conjunctivitis. These are usually transmitted to the eye by direct contact (e.g., hands, tissues, towels). Allergens, chemical irritants, and exposure to radiant energy such as ultraviolet light from the sun or tanning devices can also lead to this common condition.

Pathophysiology

Eyelid Infections and Inflammations
The most common disorder affecting the eyelids is **marginal blepharitis,** an inflammation of the glands and lash follicles on the margins of the eyelids. This inflammatory disorder can be caused by a staphylococcal infection or it may be seborrheic in origin; commonly, both types are present. Seborrheic blepharitis is nearly always associated with seborrhea (dandruff) of the scalp or eyebrows. Irritation, burning, and itching of eyelid margins are common manifestations of blepharitis. The eye appears red-rimmed with mucus discharge, and there is crusting or scaling of lid margins. Lid margins may ulcerate, resulting in a loss of eyelashes.

Infection of one or more of the sebaceous glands of the eyelid may cause a **hordeolum (sty).** Hordeolum is a staphylococcal abscess that may occur on either the external or internal margin of the lid (see Figure 43–10 on page 1874). An external hordeolum is characterized by initial pain, redness, and acute tenderness of the lid margin. A small tender raised area is visible. The client may also experience photophobia, tearing, and the sensation of a foreign body in the affected eye. Internal hordeola are seen on the conjunctival side of the lid and may have more severe manifestations.

Chronic inflammation of a meibomian gland may lead to formation of a **chalazion,** a granulomatous cyst or nodule of the lid (see Figure 43–11 on page 1874). It presents as a hard swelling on the lid, and surrounding conjunctival tissue is reddened. Chalazion may also follow a hordeolum that was inadequately treated. Unlike a hordeolum, a chalazion is painless. It may slowly increase in size and eventually require removal, but most resolve within several months.

Conjunctivitis
The conjunctiva lines the inner lid and covers the outer portion of the eye to the margin of the cornea. Introduction of an infectious agent, allergen, toxin, or other irritant into the eye can initiate an inflammatory process in this fragile membrane. Its severity can range from mild irritation with redness and tearing to conjunctival edema, hemorrhage, or a severe necrotizing process with tissue destruction.

Acute Conjunctivitis   Infectious conjunctivitis may be bacterial, viral, or fungal in origin. Adenovirus infection is the leading cause of conjunctivitis in adults. Systemic infections that may affect the eyes include herpes simplex and other viral infections. Contact with genital secretions infected with gonococcus can cause gonococcal conjunctivitis, a medical emergency that can lead to corneal perforation.

Redness and itching of the affected eye are common manifestations of acute conjunctivitis (Figure 44–1). The client may also complain of a scratchy, burning, or gritty sensation. Pain is not common; however, photophobia may occur. Tearing and discharge accompany the inflammatory process. The discharge may be watery, purulent, or mucoid, depending on the cause of conjunctivitis. The client may have associated manifestations such as pharyngitis, fever, malaise, and swollen preauricular lymph nodes (Tierney et al., 1994).

Trachoma   Trachoma, a chronic conjunctivitis caused by *Chlamydia trachomatis,* is a significant preventable cause of blindness worldwide that remains endemic in north and sub-Saharan Africa, the Middle East, and parts of Asia. Trachoma is contagious, transmitted primarily by close personal contact (eye-to-eye, hand-to-eye) or by fomites such as towels, handkerchiefs, and flies. Certain forms of trachoma are transmitted from the genital tract to the eye (Berkow & Fletcher, 1992; Wilson et al., 1991).

Bilateral conjunctivitis with congestion of the conjunctiva, eyelid edema, tearing, and photophobia is an early manifestation of trachoma. Small conjunctival follicles develop, usually on the upper lids. The inflammation also affects the upper portion of the cornea, causing superficial corneal vascularization and infiltration with granulation tissue. Scarring of the conjunctival lining of the lid causes *entropion,* inversion or inward turning of the lid. The lashes then abrade the cornea, eventually causing ulceration and scarring. The scarred cornea is opaque, resulting in loss of vision (Grimes et al., 1992; Wilson et al., 1991).

Corneal Infections and Inflammations

The clear cornea allows light rays to enter the eye and transmits images onto the retina. It helps to focus light on the retina and protects the internal eye structures. The cornea has three major layers: The outermost epithelium consists of five or six layers of cells that are constantly being renewed; the stroma, which makes up 90% of corneal tissue; and the single-cell thickness endothelium adjacent to the aqueous humor of the anterior chamber. The cornea is avascular tissue; the central cornea is dependent on atmospheric oxygen to meet its metabolic needs. Because there is no blood supply, immune defenses have difficulty fending off infections of the cornea. Corneal scarring or ulceration are two major causes of blindness worldwide.

Keratitis   **Keratitis** is an inflammation of the cornea. Keratitis may be caused by many of the microorganisms that cause conjunctivitis. Other causes include hypersensitivity reactions, ischemia, tearing defects, trauma, and interrupted sensory innervation of the cornea (Porth, 1994). When the inflammatory process involves both the conjunctiva and the cornea, the term *keratoconjunctivitis* may be used. Inflammation that involves only the epithelial layer of the cornea is nonulcerative and does not destroy the cornea or its clarity.

Corneal Ulcer   A **corneal ulcer,** local necrosis of the cornea, may be caused by infection, exposure trauma, or the misuse of contact lenses (Porth, 1994). A frequent cause is bacterial infection following trauma or contact lens overuse. Herpes viruses, including herpes simplex and herpes zoster, are a leading cause of ulcerative corneal disease. Corneal ulcers may also complicate bacterial conjunctivitis, trachoma, gonorrhea, and other acute infections. Clients who are immunosuppressed because of disease or drug therapy are at particular risk for developing corneal ulcers due to infection.

In corneal ulceration, a portion of the epithelium and/or stroma is destroyed. Ulcers may be superficial or deep, penetrating underlying layers and posing a risk of perforation. Fibrous tissue may form during healing, resulting in scarring and opacity of the cornea. Perforation can lead to infection of deeper eye structures or extrusion of eye contents. Partial or total vision loss may result.

The cornea is extremely sensitive tissue, serving as a mechanism to protect the eye and vision. When it becomes inflamed, the client commonly experiences photophobia and discomfort, ranging from a gritty sensation in the eye to severe pain. Tearing (lacrimation) is extensive, and a discharge may be present, especially if the conjunctiva is also inflamed. Visual acuity may be decreased, and *blepharaospasm* (spasm of the eyelid and inability to open the eye) may be present. Corneal ulceration may be visible on direct examination.

Uveitis and Iritis

The middle vascular layer of the eye, including the choroid, the ciliary body, and the iris, is known as the uvea and uveal tract. **Uveitis** is inflammation of all or part of this vascular layer. **Iritis,** inflammation of the iris only, occurs more commonly than uveitis.

Uveitis is usually a disease limited to the eye; it may be idiopathic (of unknown origin), or caused by an autoimmune process, infection, parasitic disease, or trauma. Approximately 40% of cases can be linked to a systemic disease, often an arthritic or autoimmune disorder such as ankylosing spondylitis, Reiter's syndrome, rheumatoid arthritis, or sarcoidosis (see Chapter 38 for further discussion of these disorders). Uveitis has also been linked with systemic infections such as tuberculosis and syphilis.

Manifestations of uveitis include pupillary constriction and erythema around the limbus. The client may complain of severe eye pain and photophobia, as well as blurred vision.

Collaborative Care

Management of the client with an infectious or inflammatory eye disorder is directed toward establishing an accurate diagnosis and prompt treatment to reduce the risk of permanent vision deficit.

The history and physical assessment are key in diagnosing these disorders. The diagnosis can often be made based on clinical manifestations, and no laboratory or diagnostic procedures are required. Accurate diagnosis of conjunctivitis is especially important because other potentially vision-threatening conditions, such as acute uveitis or acute angle-closure glaucoma, can cause a red eye. Although many eye disorders can be treated in the community, the client with a severe corneal infection or ulcer may require hospitalization. Corneal ulcers are medical emergencies, requiring prompt referral to an

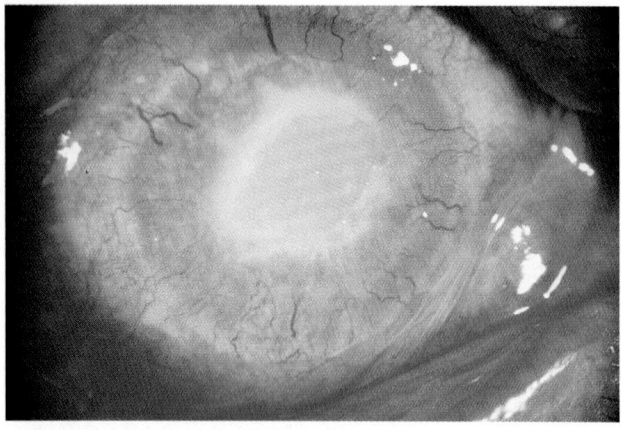

A

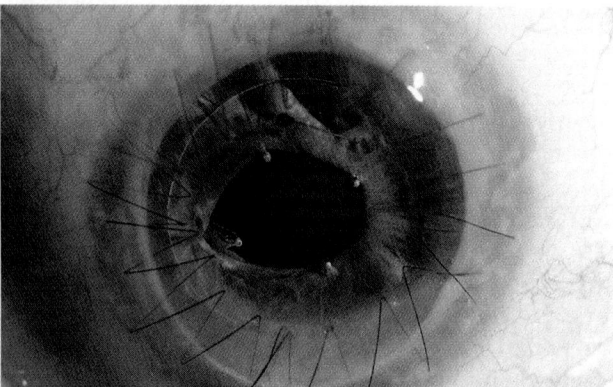

B

Figure 44–2 Corneal transplant. *A,* The diseased, opaque cornea. *B,* The diseased cornea is removed and a corneal graft is sutured in place using material finer than a human hair.

ophthalmologist for treatment. Pressure dressings may be applied to both eyes for comfort and to reduce the risk of perforation and loss of eye contents.

Laboratory and Diagnostic Tests

The following tests may be ordered to identify the cause and extent of eye infections or inflammations:

- *Fluorescein stain with slit lamp examination* allows visualization of any corneal ulcerations or abrasions, which appear green with staining.

- *Conjunctival or ulcer scrapings* are examined microscopically or cultured to identify the organisms.

Additional laboratory testing such as blood counts or antibody titers may be used to identify any underlying infectious or autoimmune processes.

Pharmacology

Infectious processes involving the lids, conjunctiva, or cornea are treated with antibiotic or antiviral therapy as appropriate. Topical anti-infectives applied as either eye

drops or ointment may include erythromycin, gentamicin, penicillin, bacitracin, sulfacetamide sodium, amphotericin B, or idoxuridine. For very severe infections, central ulcers, or cellulitis, anti-infectives may be administered by subconjunctival injection and/or systemic intravenous infusion.

Antihistamines are used to minimize symptoms of conjunctivitis when an allergic response underlies the inflammatory process. Corticosteroids may be prescribed for keratitis related to systemic inflammatory disorders or trauma; however, it is important to avoid their use with local infections to avoid suppressing the immune and inflammatory responses. Immunosuppressive therapy with azathioprine (Imuran) or cyclosporine (Sandimmune) may be employed to suppress the inflammatory response in clients with severe uveitis. Atropine may also be prescribed for the client with associated inflammation of the iris. The client may require analgesics such as acetaminophen and/or codeine for pain management.

Corneal Transplant

Once the cornea has become scarred and opaque, no treatment can restore its clarity. The first successful *corneal transplant* (or *keratoplasty*), replacement of diseased cornea by healthy corneal tissue from a donor, was performed in 1906. Current corneal transplant procedures have a success rate of approximately 90%.

Corneas are harvested from the cadavers of uninfected adults who were under the age of 65 and who died as a result of acute trauma or illness. After harvesting, the cornea can be stored in a tissue-culture medium for up to 4 weeks before being used as a graft. Corneal transplantation is usually an elective surgery, although emergency transplantation may be required for perforation of the cornea.

Corneal transplant may be either lamellar or penetrating. In a *lamellar keratoplasty,* the superficial layer of cornea is removed and replaced with a graft. The anterior chamber remains intact. In a *penetrating keratoplasty,* a button or full thickness of cornea is removed and replaced by donor tissue (Figure 44–2). The graft is then sutured in place using suture finer than human hair and a continuous or interrupted stitch. Because the cornea is avascular, these sutures remain in place for up to a year to ensure healing.

Most corneal transplants are performed on an outpatient basis, and clients do not generally require hospitalization. The eye is patched for 24 hours following surgery. Narcotic analgesia may be required initially, because the cornea is extremely sensitive. Antiemetic medications and stool softeners are prescribed to prevent vomiting or straining at stool, activities that increase intraocular pressure. The client is also cautioned to avoid other activities that may increase intraocular pressure, such as bending over and lifting or pushing heavy objects. Corticosteroid eye drops are ordered to reduce the inflammatory response to surgery, preventing edema of the graft. Antibiotic drops may also be prescribed to prevent infection.

The risk of transplant rejection is low in this procedure. Because the cornea is avascular, there is little exposure of the transplanted corneal tissue to the host's immune defenses (Porth, 1994). When rejection does occur, it occurs within 3 weeks of the transplant, beginning with inflammation at the edge of the grafted tissue and spreading to involve the entire graft.

See the box on page 1896 for nursing care of the client undergoing eye surgery.

Other Therapeutic Measures

Careful cleansing of the lid margins using a "no-tears" baby shampoo is often recommended for marginal blepharitis. Soaking the lids with warm saline compresses prior to cleansing facilitates the removal of crusts and exudate in blepharitis or conjunctivitis. Frequent eye irrigations may be ordered to remove the copious purulent discharge associated with conjunctivitis. Local heat applications may be used to treat hordeolum or chalazion; excision and drainage may be required if this is not effective.

Nursing Care

The nursing role in management of clients with infections and inflammatory eye disorders may involve direct care, but more often focuses on prevention and providing education. Nurses working in clinics and outpatient surgical settings care for clients undergoing corneal transplant. The priority nursing diagnoses for clients with infectious and inflammatory eye disorders include risk for altered vision, pain, and risk for injury.

Risk for Sensory/Perceptual Alteration: Visual

Disorders affecting the conjunctiva or cornea have the potential to disrupt the integrity or clarity of these structures. Because the cornea plays a vital role in focusing light on the retina, corneal damage can affect vision, impairing visual acuity and even causing legal blindness.

Nursing interventions with rationales follow:

- Assess the client's vision with and without corrective lenses. *Assessment provides a baseline to evaluate possible changes in vision resulting from the inflammatory disorder or therapy.*

- Instruct the client to wash the hands thoroughly before inserting or removing contact lenses or instilling any eye medications. Teach the client to avoid touching or rubbing the eyes. *Hand washing is the single most important measure to prevent transmission of infection to the eye. Touching or rubbing the eyes increases the risk of infection and corneal trauma.*

- Emphasize the importance of proper care of contact lenses. Reinforce the need to follow directions for periodic lens removal and appropriate cleaning, specific to the type of lens used. *Extended wearing times and improper cleaning of contact lenses are major risk factors for corneal damage. Clients who wear hard contact lenses must remove them daily because the central cornea needs exposure to atmospheric oxygen. Although soft and extended-wear lenses allow the cornea to "breathe," improper cleaning carries a major risk for infection.*

- Teach clients about the importance of using eye protection when engaging in potentially dangerous activities. *Trauma increases the risk of infection and scarring of the cornea.*

- Suspect corneal perforation if the client complains of sudden, severe eye pain and photophobia. Place the client in the supine position, close the eye, and cover it with a dry, sterile dressing. Notify the physician immediately. *Corneal perforation may occur without warning in clients with corneal ulcers and places the client at risk for loss of eye contents. Emergency measures are taken to reduce intraocular pressure and maintain eye integrity to preserve vision.*

Pain

The cornea of the eye is extremely sensitive. Corneal disorders frequently cause significant pain. Pain, in turn, increases the client's stress response and interferes with rest, potentially impairing healing.

Nursing interventions with rationales follow:

- Assess the client's pain, using verbal and nonverbal cues. *Pain is a subjective experience and can be evaluated only by the client's response and in terms of its effect on the client.*

- Administer prescribed analgesia routinely in the first 12 to 24 hours after corneal surgery. *Routine administration of analgesics prevents pain from reaching a level of severity at which it becomes difficult to relieve.*

- Patch both eyes if necessary. *Patching both eyes reduces eye movement and irritation of the affected eye.*

- Teach the client to apply warm compresses to reduce inflammation and pain. *Warm compresses for 15 minutes, three to four times a day, promote comfort for clients with keratitis or corneal injury.*

- Instruct the client to use dark sunglasses with appropriate UV protection when out of doors, even on cloudy days. *True photophobia, often associated with corneal disorders, causes eye pain with increased light intensity.*

- Teach the client to instill prescribed eyedrops as ordered. *Prescribed medications may reduce inflammation and eliminate infection, reducing discomfort.*

Risk for Injury

The client who has undergone corneal transplantation has an increased risk for injury for several reasons. The eye on which surgery was performed is patched for 24 hours after surgery, changing the client's depth perception and increasing the risk for falls. Increased intraocular pressure or trauma to the eye may damage the graft, resulting in graft rejection.

Nursing interventions with rationales follow:

- Instruct the client to call for help before getting up or ambulating after surgery. Ensure access to the call light. *It may take time for the client to adjust to changes in depth perception caused by the eye patch. Assistance helps prevent falls that may not only injure the client but also traumatize the operative site.*

- Administer prescribed analgesics and antiemetics postoperatively. *These medications promote comfort and reduce the risk of vomiting, which can significantly increase intraocular pressure, damaging suture lines.*

- Help the client to deep breathe and use the incentive spirometer to promote lung expansion. *These are important postoperative measures to prevent pulmonary complications. Coughing is avoided because it increases intraocular pressure.*

- Teach the client how to apply an eye shield at night after the eye patch is removed. *The physician may recommend an eye shield at night to prevent inadvertent rubbing or trauma to the eye during sleep.*

- Instruct the client not to rub or scratch the eye. *Rubbing or scratching may disrupt suture lines or damage the grafted tissue.*

- Reinforce the importance of using eye protection during hazardous activities. *Following a corneal transplant, the client has the same risk of eye injury that other people performing hazardous activities do.*

Other Nursing Diagnoses

The following nursing diagnoses may also be appropriate for the client with an infectious or inflammatory eye disorder:

- *Risk for Infection* related to disrupted corneal epithelium

- *Anxiety* related to possible visual impairment

- *Altered Role Performance* related to pain and visual deficit

Client and Family Teaching

Education is a vital strategy for preventing infectious and inflammatory eye disorders. All clients should be taught about proper eye care, including the importance of avoiding rubbing or scratching the eyes, to prevent trauma and infection. Teach contact lens users appropriate care and cleaning techniques. Stress the importance of periodic removal of lenses, even extended-wear lenses. In general, lenses should be removed at night, even though manufacturers may claim it is safe to wear them while sleeping. Emphasize the need to follow cleaning instructions precisely to avoid bacterial contamination of lenses and possible corneal infection. If the client experiences a corneal abrasion or keratitis, instruct the client to avoid wearing contact lenses until the cornea has healed completely.

If cleansing of lid margins is recommended, emphasize the importance of safety and medical asepsis. Instruct the client to wash the hands thoroughly before providing eye care and to use a new, clean cotton-tipped swab or cotton ball for each eye. Teach clients how to instill prescribed eye drops and ointments. If an eye patch is ordered, be sure the client or a family member knows how to apply it and where to obtain necessary supplies.

Encourage clients with photophobia to wear sunglasses when outdoors, even on cloudy days. Eye rest also promotes comfort; encourage the client to avoid excessive reading or other close tasks while inflammation is acute.

Following corneal transplant surgery, stress the importance of maintaining regular contact with the physician or clinic for follow-up. Teach the client about signs of graft rejection, including inflammation, cloudiness of the graft, and increased pain. Instruct the client and family to report these signs to the physician promptly so that treatment to save the graft can be instituted. Teach the client that it is important to avoid straining, coughing, sneezing, bending over, lifting heavy objects, and other activities that increase intraocular pressure until the physician says it is safe to do so.

The Client with Eye Trauma

■ ■ ■

Over two million eye injuries occur each year (Kitt & Kaiser, 1990). Many eye injuries are minor, but without timely and appropriate intervention, even a minor injury can threaten vision. For this reason, all eye injuries should be considered medical emergencies requiring immediate evaluation and intervention.

Pathophysiology

Any part of the eye, especially the exposed parts, may be affected by trauma. Foreign bodies, abrasions, and lacerations are the most common types of eye injury. Traumatic injury may also be due to a burn, penetrating objects, or blunt force.

Corneal Abrasion

Disruption of the superficial epithelium of the cornea is termed a *corneal abrasion*. Objects commonly causing corneal abrasion include contact lenses, eyelashes, small foreign bodies such as dust and dirt, and fingernails. Drying of the eye surface and chemical irritants may also result in a corneal abrasion (Thompson et al., 1993).

Superficial abrasions of the cornea are extremely painful but generally heal rapidly without complication or scarring. Photophobia and tearing are also commonly present. When the stroma is damaged by a deep abrasion or laceration, there is an increased risk of infection, slowed healing, and scar formation.

Burns

The outer surface of the eye may be subjected to burns caused by heat, radiation, or explosion, but chemical burns are the most common. Either acid or alkaline substances may burn the eye. Ammonia, products that contain lye (such as oven and drain cleaners), and acids from car batteries or other sources are often implicated in eye injuries (Kitt & Kaiser, 1990). Burns caused by alkaline substances are particularly serious because tiny particles of the chemical may remain in the conjunctival sac causing progressive damage. Acid causes rapid damage to the eye but generally causes less serious burns than alkalis do (Way, 1994).

Explosions and flash burn injuries pose the greatest risk for thermal burns of the eye. Ultraviolet rays can also cause corneal damage ranging in severity from mild to extensive. Depending on the source of the ultraviolet light, these burns may be known by various names such as snow-blindness, welder's-arc burn, or flash burn (Way, 1994).

In addition to giving a history of face and eye contact with a caustic substance or other burning agent, the client complains of eye pain and decreased vision. Eyelids are often swollen. Burns may be present on the face or lids. The appearance of the eye may vary, depending on the type of burn. The conjunctiva is reddened and edematous; sloughing may be seen, particularly with chemical burns. The cornea often appears cloudy or hazy, and ulcerations may be evident.

Penetrating Trauma

Perforation of the eye occurs from a variety of causes. Metal flakes or other particles produced by high-speed drilling or grinding, glass shards, or other substances may penetrate the eye. Gunshots (including BBs), arrows, and knives can penetrate the eye. In a *penetrating injury,* the layers of the eye spontaneously reapproximate after entry of a sharp-pointed object or small missile into the globe. These injuries may not be readily apparent with inspection of the eye. In a *perforating injury,* the layers of the eye do not spontaneously reapproximate, resulting in rupture of the globe and potential loss of ocular contents (Way, 1994).

Penetrating injuries may be hidden because of tissue swelling or missed when the client has other significant injuries that command attention. When there is a laceration or puncture wound to the eyelid, it is vital to inspect the underlying eye tissue for possible damage. Eye perforations cause pain, partial or complete loss of vision, and possibly bleeding or extrusion of eye contents.

Blunt Trauma

Sports injuries are a common cause of blunt trauma to the eye: It may be struck with a ball (baseball, tennis, racketball, and handball are frequently implicated) or injured in contact sports such as basketball, football, boxing, or wrestling. Motor vehicle accidents, falls, and physical assault are examples of other causes of blunt eye trauma.

Blunt trauma may lead to a minor eye injury such as lid ecchymosis (black eye) or subconjunctival hemorrhage, caused by rupture of a blood vessel in the conjunctiva. A well-defined bright area of erythema appears under the conjunctiva. No pain or discomfort is associated with the hemorrhage and no treatment is necessary. The blood typically reabsorbs within 2 to 3 weeks.

Hyphema, bleeding into the anterior chamber of the eye, is another potential result of blunt eye trauma. When the highly vascular uveal tract of the eye is disrupted by blunt force, hemorrhage may result, filling the anterior chamber. The client complains of eye pain, decreased visual acuity, and seeing a reddish tint. Blood is visible in the anterior chamber.

An orbital blow-out fracture is another potential result of blunt eye trauma. Although any part of the eye orbit may be fractured, the ethmoid bone on the orbital floor is the most likely site. Orbital contents, including fat, muscles, and the eye itself may herniate through the fracture into the underlying maxillary sinus. The client complains of diplopia (double vision), pain with upward movement of the affected eye, and decreased sensation on the affected cheek. The eye appears sunken (**enophthalmos**) and has limited movement on examination (Kitt & Kaiser, 1990).

Collaborative Care

When trauma to the eye is known or suspected, a thorough examination is necessary to determine the type and extent of the injury. Unless immediate treatment is indicated, as with a chemical burn, vision is evaluated initially. If the client normally wears corrective lenses, vision assessment is performed while the client wears glasses. The initial examination also includes evaluation of eye movement (unless a penetrating object is present) and inspection for lid and conjunctival lacerations. The examiner inspects the eye using strong light and magnification using a headband loupe or slit lamp. Topical anesthesia may be necessary prior to inspection if eye pain and photophobia make it difficult for the client to keep the eye open. Fluorescein staining can help identify the presence of foreign bodies and abrasions. Any conjunctival or anterior chamber hemorrhage is noted, as is the presence or absence of the red reflex. Ophthalmoscopic examination is used to detect hemorrhage or trauma to the interior chamber.

Facial X-rays and CT scans are used to identify orbital fractures or the presence of foreign bodies within the globe. Ultrasonography may be employed to determine the presence of a detached retina or vitreous hemorrhage.

Foreign bodies are removed using irrigation, a sterile cotton-tipped applicator, or a sterile needle or other instrument. Antibiotic ointment—erythromycin or sulfacetamide sodium—is applied after their removal. In clients with corneal abrasions and large foreign bodies in the eye, an eye patch is applied firmly after the antibiotic application to keep the eye closed for approximately 24 hours.

The immediate priority of care for clients with chemical burns is flushing the affected eye with copious amounts of fluid. Normal saline is preferred; however, water may be used if saline is not available. A special contact lens irrigating unit or a bottle of irrigant with intravenous tubing held to flush all eye surfaces may be useful. The eyelid is everted to identify and remove material from the conjunctival fornix (sac). A topical anesthetic, such as tetracaine drops, helps relieve pain, making inspection and irrigation easier. During irrigation, fluid is directed from the inner canthus of the eye to the outer. Tipping the client's head slightly to the affected side prevents contamination of the unaffected eye. Irrigation is continued until the pH of the eye is normal, in the range of 7.2 to 7.4 (Kitt & Kaiser, 1990). Following irrigation, a topical antibiotic ointment such as gentamicin ophthalmic is applied.

Penetrating wounds of the eye generally require surgical intervention by an ophthalmic surgeon. Immediate care focuses on relieving pain and protecting the eye from further injury. To prevent loss of intraocular contents, it is vital not to place pressure on the eye itself. It may be gently covered with a sterile gauze or an eye pad. If a foreign body is embedded in or sticking out of the eye, no attempt is made to remove it. The object should be immobilized and the eye protected with a metal eye shield until an ophthalmologist can see the client. A paper cup or other protective device may be used if the object is too large to use an eye shield. Patching the unaffected eye as well decreases ocular movement (Kitt & Kaiser, 1990). Pain is managed using narcotic analgesics such as morphine or meperidine (Demerol). The client may also require sedation (e.g., diazepam) and antiemetic medications to prevent vomiting. Vomiting increases intraocular pressure and may damage the eye further. Antibiotics such as intravenous cefazolin (Ancef) or gentamicin (Garamycin) are prescribed to prevent infection.

Interventions for the client with blunt trauma to the eye include placing the client on bed rest in semi-Fowler's position and protecting the eye from further injury with an eye shield. The unaffected eye is also patched to minimize eye movement. A carbonic anhydrase inhibitor such as acetazolamide (Diamox) or dichlorphenamide (Daranide) may be prescribed to reduce intraocular pressure.

Nursing Care

The nursing role involves educating people about the prevention of eye injuries and providing direct care to clients with eye injuries.

Impaired Tissue Integrity: Ocular

All types of eye trauma pose the risk of violating the integrity of the eye, threatening vision. The goals of nursing care measures, therefore, are preserving the integrity of the eye, preserving vision, and preventing further damage.

Nursing interventions with rationales follow:

- Evaluate the client's vision on entry into the emergency department or physician's office. Assess and record the client's vision in each eye and both eyes, with and without corrective lenses. *This initial assessment provides valuable information about the effect of the injury on the client's vision and a baseline for future comparisons.*

- Assess the client's eye(s) carefully for evidence of foreign bodies, burns, penetrating injury, or blunt trauma. Pay particular attention if lacerations, burns, or other trauma are evident in tissues surrounding the eye. *Eye trauma may be hidden by other injuries and, as a result, remain untreated.*

- In cases of burns or foreign bodies in the eye, the nurse may instill anesthetic drops and perform eye irrigation before or after the physician evaluates the client. *Blepharism (spasm of the eyelid) and eye pain may impair assessment of the injured eye. If there is a possibility of a chemical burn of the eye, irrigation to remove the chemical is of higher priority than assessment of the eye.*

- Loose foreign bodies may be removed using a moist, sterile, cotton-tipped applicator. *Prompt removal of foreign bodies may prevent corneal abrasion.*

- In cases of severe or penetrating injury, have the client rest and stabilize the injured eye by applying an eye pad or gauze dressing loosely over both the affected and unaffected eye. Stabilize any penetrating object if possible. *These measures reduce eye movement and can help preserve the client's vision.*

- Following treatment, apply eye drops or ointment as prescribed and apply an eye pad or shield if ordered. *An eye pad is often applied to the affected eye to reduce pain and photophobia and to promote healing.*

Other Nursing Diagnoses

The following nursing diagnoses may also be appropriate for the client with eye trauma:

- *Pain* related to disruption of sensitive eye structures
- *Risk for Injury* related to impaired vision
- *Sensory-Perceptual Alteration: Visual* related to eye trauma
- *Risk for Infection* related to impaired eye tissue integrity

Client and Family Teaching

Teaching related to eye injuries focuses on strategies for prevention, first-aid measures, and home care following an injury.

Through community-based care, the nurse teaches individuals and groups how to prevent eye injuries. Education is particularly important for people involved in hazardous occupations and activities. Teach employees and participants in high risk sports or activities how and when to use eye-protection devices. Stress the importance of using seat belts and air bags (if available) to prevent eye injury in automobile accidents. Teach clients what immediate care to give to prevent permanent loss of sight. Teach clients to immediately flush the eye with copious amounts of water if a chemical splash occurs. Loose, visible foreign bodies can be removed using a clean, moistened cotton-tipped swab. If an abrasion, penetrating, or blunt injury is suspected, the eye should be covered loosely with sterile gauze and medical attention sought immediately. Instruct clients not to remove objects that penetrate the eye.

Following an injury, the client and family need information about follow-up treatment. Instruct the client about prescribed medications, including techniques for instilling eye drops and ointments. Discuss possible adverse effects of prescribed medication and their management. Stress the need to avoid further trauma to the eye, protecting it with an eye pad or shield if ordered and avoiding rubbing or scratching the eye. Teach the client or family how to apply the eye pad or shield. The client who has experienced penetrating or blunt eye trauma may need to avoid activities that increase intraocular pressure, such as lifting, straining, or bending over. Stress the importance of complying with prescribed activity restrictions to prevent further eye damage.

The Client with Cataracts

■ ■ ■

A **cataract** is an opacification (clouding) of the lens of the eye. This opacification can significantly interfere with light transmission to the retina and the ability to perceive images clearly (Porth, 1994; Wilson et al., 1991).

Pathophysiology

Cataracts are a common and significant cause of visual deficits in the elderly. It is estimated that 95% of people over the age of 65 have some degree of cataract formation; however, only a small percentage of those have impaired vision as a result of the cataract (Burke & Walsh, 1992). This population accounts for more than 1.25 million cataract surgeries in the United States yearly (Ruehl & Schremp, 1992).

The majority of cataracts are *senile cataracts,* formed as a result of the normal aging process. As the lens ages, its fibers and proteins change and degenerate, losing clarity (Bullock & Rosendahl, 1992; Porth, 1994). This process generally begins at the periphery of the lens, gradually spreading to involve the central portion. As the cataract continues to develop, the entire lens may become opaque. When only a portion of the lens is affected, the cataract is called *immature.* A *mature cataract* is opacity of the entire lens.

Although senile cataracts are by far the most common, cataracts also may be congenital or acquired in origin. Eye trauma, including injury to the lens capsule by a foreign body, blunt trauma, or exposure to heat or radiation, can precipitate cataract formation. Other factors implicated include inflammation of the eye and some systemic diseases. Diabetes mellitus, a metabolic disorder involving carbohydrate metabolism, is associated with earlier development of cataracts, especially when the blood glucose level is not carefully controlled at normal or near normal levels. Certain drugs, taken systemically, may also prompt the formation of cataracts. These medications include corticosteroids, chlorpromazine (Thorazine), and busulfan (Myleran) (Bullock & Rosendahl, 1992; Porth, 1994; Wilson et al., 1991).

Cataracts tend to occur bilaterally unless related to eye trauma. Fortunately, their development is usually not symmetric, and one cataract generally matures more rapidly than the other. As a cataract matures and interferes with light transmission through the lens, the client begins to experience symptoms. Visual acuity gradually declines, affecting both close and distance vision. Details become obscured. Light rays are scattered as they pass through the lens, causing the client to experience increased difficulty with glare. Because of the increased glare, the client also has more difficulty adjusting between light and dark environments. In the client with a mature cataract, the pupil may appear cloudy gray or white rather than black.

Collaborative Care

The diagnosis of a cataract is made based on the history and eye examination, including ophthalmoscopy. As the cataract matures, the red reflex is lost. It is possible to

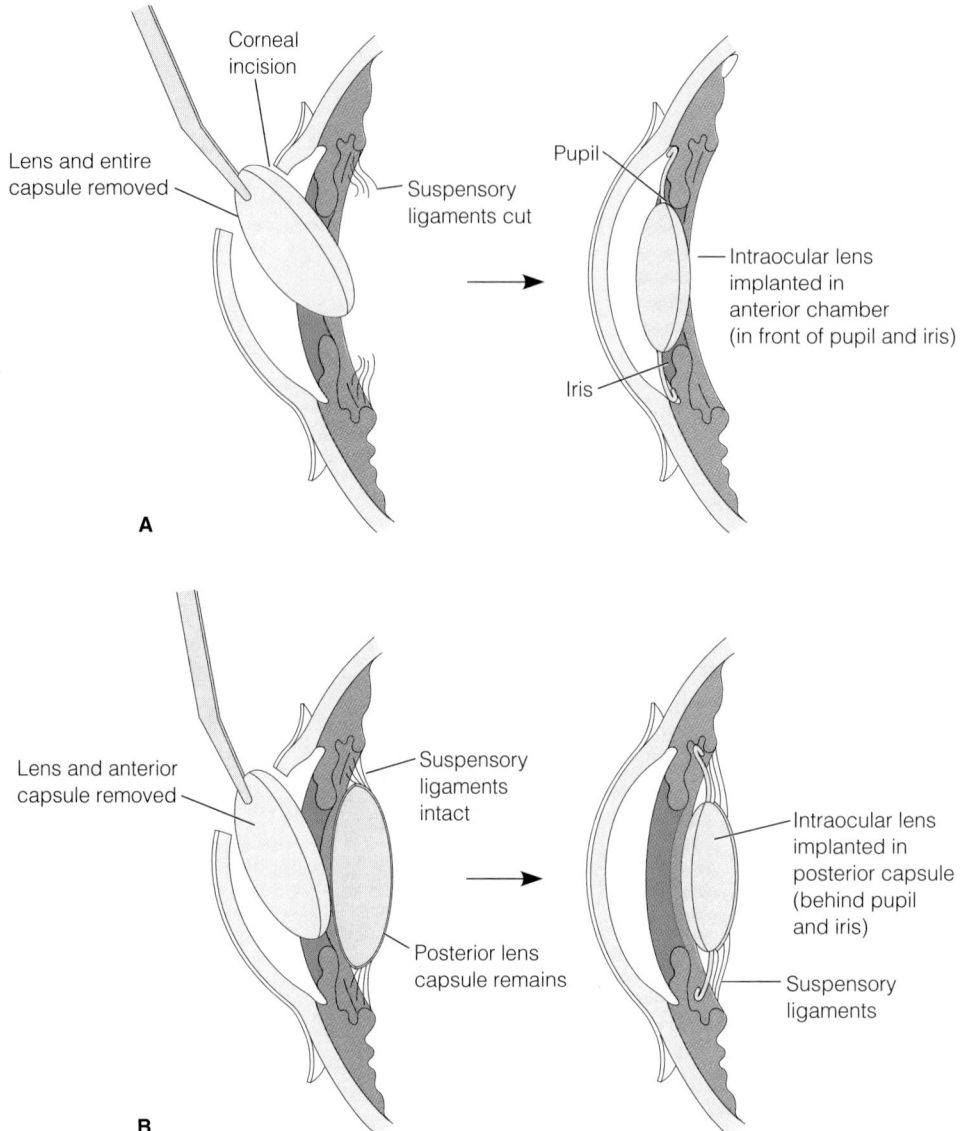

Figure 44-3 Cataract removal with intraocular lens implant. *A*, Intracapsular cataract extraction with removal of the entire lens and capsule. The intraocular lens is implanted in the eye's anterior chamber. *B*, Extracapsular cataract extraction with removal of the lens and anterior capsule, leaving the posterior capsule intact. The intraocular lens is implanted within posterior capsule.

identify the location and extent of cataract formation with ophthalmoscopic examination. No special diagnostic or laboratory procedures are required for diagnosis.

Surgical removal is the only treatment used at this time for cataracts; no medical treatment is available to prevent or treat them. If an intraocular lens (an artificial lens to replace the diseased lens of the eye) is to be implanted during surgery, the corneal curvature and anteroposterior diameter of the eye are measured prior to surgery to determine the lens power needed for the intraocular lens implant (Ruehl & Schremp, 1992).

Surgical removal of the cataract and lens is indicated when the cataract has developed to the point that vision and activities of daily living are affected. A mature cataract may also be removed when it causes a secondary condition such as glaucoma or uveitis (Porth, 1994).

Cataract surgery is usually done on an outpatient basis, using local anesthesia. If general anesthesia is required, the client may be hospitalized overnight. Using an operating microscope, the surgeon makes a small incision at the edge of the cornea and extracts the lens using either forceps or a supercooled probe (*cryoextraction*), or emulsification and aspiration. In the latter technique, ultrasound vibrations are used to break the lens material into fragments (phacoemulsification), which are then suctioned out of the eye.

The entire lens and its surrounding capsule may be removed in a procedure called *intracapsular extraction* (Figure 44–3, *A*). *Extracapsular extraction* is the most common procedure presently used to treat cataracts. It involves removal of the nucleus and cortex of the lens, leaving the posterior capsule intact (Figure 44–3, *B*). The remaining capsule supports the lens implant and protects the retina (Ruehl & Schremp, 1992). An additional advantage to extracapsular lens removal is the smaller incision required.

After removal of the lens, the eye can no longer focus light on the retina, and vision is seriously affected. Usually a polymethylmethacrylate (PMMA or Plexiglas) intraocular lens is implanted at the time of surgery to provide for light refraction and restore visual acuity. This implant rapidly restores binocular vision and depth perception. An anterior chamber lens implant is used following intracapsular lens removal. In an anterior chamber implant, the lens is lodged in the anterior chamber of the eye, resting over the pupil. In a posterior implant, the lens is positioned in the posterior capsule to restore vision following an extracapsular lens extraction (Way, 1994). The posterior chamber lens is positioned behind the iris and stabilized by the remaining posterior capsule.

For some clients, thick convex corrective lenses or contact lenses may be used instead of intraocular lens implants to correct vision after cataract removal. Although contact lenses can provide excellent vision correction following cataract surgery, they may be difficult for some clients to adapt to or manipulate. The client with a preexisting refractive error may continue to require corrective lenses and often needs a prescriptive change after surgery.

Cataract surgery is typically uncomplicated, with a reported 2% to 5% rate of surgical complications. Vitreous humor may be lost through the incision during surgery. Corneal edema, increased intraocular pressure, hemorrhage, inflammation or infection, retinal detachment, and displacement of the implanted lens are other potential complications. Up to 35% of clients who undergo extracapsular extraction may develop opacification of the remaining posterior capsule. Vision can be restored using *laser capsulotomy* (creating an opening for light to pass through the opacified capsule) or surgical incision into the posterior capsule to allow light to reach the retina (Ruehl & Schremp, 1992; Way, 1994).

Nursing Care

The client with cataracts has few physical care nursing needs. Patient advocacy, psychologic and emotional support, and teaching/learning needs are typically of higher priority for these clients.

With the initial diagnosis of a cataract, the nurse often becomes an important resource for the client. The nurse can explain the nonemergent nature of the condition and help the client to determine the extent to which the cataract is affecting daily life. In so doing, the nurse helps the client decide when to proceed with surgery. The nurse can also provide information about cataracts and their surgical removal to assist the client with decision making. A preoperative nursing evaluation of the client's ability to perform necessary postoperative care is helpful. If the client has a chronic condition, such as arthritis, that may make administration of eye drops difficult, a family member may need teaching to perform this intervention. If visual limitations in the initial postoperative period are likely to interfere with the client's other care needs, such as insulin injections, arrangements may need to be made for home health coverage or other assistance (Ruehl & Schremp, 1992).

Fear of blindness is second only to fear of cancer for many clients (Ruehl & Schremp, 1992). Careful listening, teaching, and a caring, understanding attitude by the nurse can help the client deal with this fear prior to surgery.

As cataract surgery is often performed on an outpatient or same-day basis, postoperative nursing care focuses on maintaining client safety and patient teaching. If local anesthesia was used, the client is often discharged within 1 hour after surgery. The box on page 1896 outlines nursing care of the client having eye surgery.

The following nursing diagnoses may be appropriate for the client with cataracts:

- *Sensory/Perceptual Alteration: Visual* related to effect of lens opacification
- *Risk for Injury* related to altered vision and depth perception
- *Knowledge Deficit* related to lack of information about cataracts, treatment options, and postoperative care
- *Risk for Ineffective Management of Therapeutic Regimen: Individual* related to difficulty in administering eye medications or inserting contact lenses

Client and Family Teaching

With the initial diagnosis of cataract, teaching focuses on the nature of the condition, indications for intervention, and options for replacement lenses following cataract removal. Teaching adaptive strategies to deal with the alteration in vision and depth perception is also useful.

When the client makes the decision to proceed with cataract surgery, the nurse begins teaching about surgery and postoperative care. The client and, if possible, a

---

Nursing Care of the Client Having Eye Surgery

PREOPERATIVE CARE

- Assess the client's knowledge and understanding of the procedure to be performed, providing clarification as needed. Notify the physician if further explanation is necessary for complete understanding by the client. *The client's understanding of the procedure, operative and postoperative course, and his or her role in the recovery process reduces anxiety and promotes cooperation.*

- Assess the visual acuity of the client's unaffected eye prior to surgery. *The client with limited visual acuity in the unaffected (nonoperative) eye may need additional assistance and attention in the postoperative period to ensure safety and maintain activities of daily living (ADLs).*

- Assess the client's support systems and the possible effect of impaired vision on life-style and ability to perform ADLs in the postoperative period. *Vision in the operative eye may be impaired during the postoperative period, limiting the client's depth perception and mobility. Safety measures such as installing handrails and removing throw rugs in the client's home are often useful, especially if the client has limited vision in the unaffected eye.*

- Orient the client to the room environment, including the floor plan, bathroom, call bell, and personal effects. *A thorough preoperative orientation to the environment helps ensure safety in the postoperative period.*

- Teach the client measures to prevent eye injury postoperatively. The client should avoid vomiting, straining at stool, coughing, sneezing, lifting more than 5 pounds, and bending over at the waist. *These activities increase intraocular pressure temporarily and may be associated with postoperative complications.*

- Remove all eye makeup and contact lenses or glasses prior to surgery. Store them in a safe place. Have glasses readily available for the client on return from surgery. *Maintaining visual acuity in the unaffected eye helps reduce the client's fear and maintain safety.*

- Administer preoperative medications and eye drops or ointments as prescribed. *Mydriatic (pupil-dilating) or cycloplegic (ciliary-paralytic) drops and drops to lower intraocular pressure may be prescribed preoperatively. Preanesthetic medications may also be ordered.*

POSTOPERATIVE CARE

- Perform and document a physical assessment, including vital signs, level of consciousness, and status of the eye dressing on return from surgery. *The client who has had local anesthesia should have few constitutional changes from the preoperative period. Assess dressings for the presence of bleeding or drainage from the eye, as either could indicate a surgical complication.*

- Maintain the eye patch or eye shield in place. *The eye patch or shield helps prevent inadvertent injury to the operative site.*

- Place the client in a semi-Fowler's or Fowler's position, having the client lie on the unaffected side. *These positions reduce intraocular pressure in the affected eye.*

- After surgery for a detached retina, the client is positioned so that the detachment is dependent or inferior. For example, if the outer portion of the left retina is detached, the client is positioned on the left side. *Positioning so that the detachment is inferior maintains pressure on that area of the retina, improving its contact with the choroid.*

---

family member or friend are taught how to instill eye drops. The time of surgery, instructions for fasting, and other preoperative care are included in teaching.

During the immediate postoperative period, teaching may be limited to instructions for care during the operative day and night. Include a significant other in the teaching, and reinforce information with written instructions. Instruct the client to avoid reading, lifting, or strenuous activity, leave the eye dressing in place, and take prescribed medications during the initial 24-hour period. The client should avoid sleeping on the operative side to reduce edema and intraocular pressure. A mild analgesic

such as acetaminophen may be used for discomfort. During the return visit the following day for evaluation and dressing removal, teaching focuses on activity limitations to prevent increased intraocular pressure, protection of the operative eye, and manifestations of postoperative complications. The client learns to report symptoms such as eye pain, decreased visual acuity or other change in vision, headache, nausea, or itching and redness of the affected eye to the physician (Ruehl & Schremp, 1992). After eye surgery, the client needs to know what medications have been prescribed and why, how, and when to instill eye drops, and how to use the eye patch or shield.

Nursing Care of the Client Having Eye Surgery (continued)

- Assess the client, and medicate or assist to avoid vomiting, coughing, sneezing, or straining as needed. *These activities increase intraocular pressure.*

- Assess comfort and medicate as necessary for complaints of an aching or scratchy sensation in affected eye. Immediately report any complaint of sudden, sharp eye pain to the physician. *An abrupt increase in or onset of eye pain may indicate hemorrhage or other ocular emergency requiring immediate intervention to preserve sight.*

- Assess for potential surgical complications.
  a. Pain in or drainage from the affected eye.
  b. Hemorrhage with blood is evident in the anterior chamber of the eye.
  c. Retinal detachment causes the client to experience flashes of light, floaters, or the sensation of a curtain being drawn over the eye.
  d. Corneal edema is evidenced by a cloudy appearance to the cornea.
  Evidence of any of the above manifestations or unusual complaints by the client should be reported to the physician at once. *Early intervention is often necessary to preserve sight.*

- Approach the client on the unaffected side. *This approach facilitates eye contact and communication.*

- Place all personal articles and the call bell within easy reach. *These measures prevent stretching and straining by the client.*

- Assist with ambulation and personal care activities as needed. *Assistance may be necessary to maintain safety.*

- Administer antibiotic, anti-inflammatory, and other systemic and eye medications as prescribed. *Medications are prescribed postoperatively to prevent infec-*

tion or inflammation of the operative site, maintain pupil constriction, and control intraocular pressure.

- Administer antiemetic medication as needed. *It is important to prevent vomiting to maintain normal intraocular pressures.*

- Teach the client and family about home care.
  a. The proper way to instill eye drops
  b. The name, dosage, schedule, duration, purpose, and side effects of postoperative medications
  c. The proper use of the eye patch and eye shield.
  d. The need to avoid scratching, rubbing, touching, or squeezing the affected eye
  e. Measures to avoid constipation and straining, and activity limitations
  f. Symptoms that should be reported to the physician, including eye pain or pressure, redness or cloudiness, drainage, decreased vision, floaters or flashes of light, or halos around bright objects
  g. The need to wear sunglasses with side shields when outdoors. *Photophobia is common after eye surgery.*

- Remind the client that vision may not stabilize for several weeks following eye surgery. New corrective lenses, if necessary, are not prescribed until vision has stabilized. The client should make and keep recommended follow-up appointments with the physician. *Clients may be alarmed that vision seems worse after surgery than before and need reassurance that visual acuity usually improves with time and healing of the affected eye.*

- Provide referral to a community home health agency for assistance with home care after discharge as needed.

If contact lenses have been prescribed to restore the client's vision, instruction should be provided on their care, insertion, and removal. Have the client redemonstrate lens care, and emphasize the importance of maintaining a regular schedule of cleaning using good technique to prevent eye infections or corneal abrasion.

The client receiving eyeglasses for vision restoration needs additional instruction in the visual changes associated with these thick-lensed glasses. The client's visual field is narrowed because of the shape of the lenses, requiring the client to turn the head from side to side, rather than simply looking to the side. Depth perception

also changes, affecting the client's ability to drive safely and negotiate stairs.

The Client with Glaucoma

Glaucoma is a condition characterized by increased intraocular pressure of the eye and a gradual loss of vision (Bullock & Rosendahl, 1992). Glaucoma is a "silent" thief of vision. The client typically does not experience any manifestations other than narrowing of the visual field,

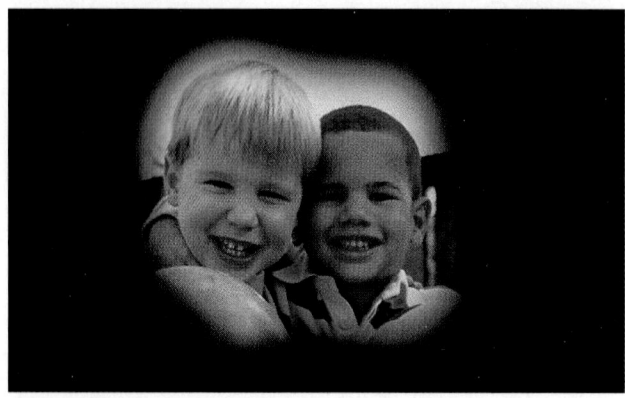

Figure 44–4   Narrowing of visual fields typical of untreated glaucoma.

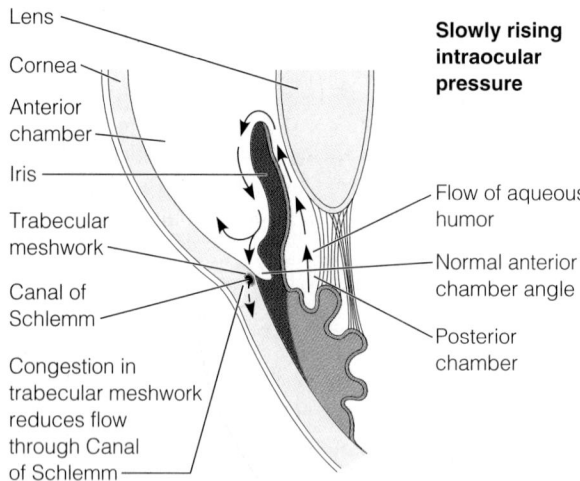

Lens
Cornea
Anterior chamber
Iris
Trabecular meshwork
Canal of Schlemm
Congestion in trabecular meshwork reduces flow through Canal of Schlemm

Slowly rising intraocular pressure

Flow of aqueous humor
Normal anterior chamber angle
Posterior chamber

A

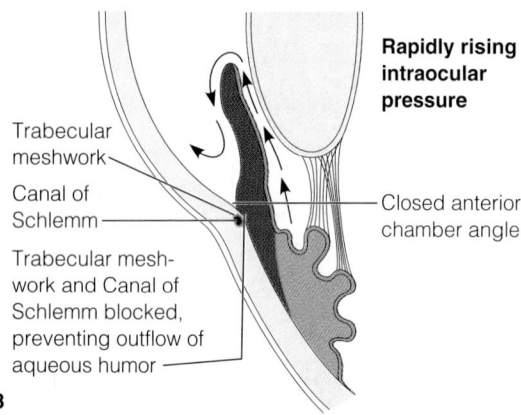

Trabecular meshwork
Canal of Schlemm
Trabecular meshwork and Canal of Schlemm blocked, preventing outflow of aqueous humor

Rapidly rising intraocular pressure

Closed anterior chamber angle

B

Figure 44–5   Forms of primary adult glaucoma. *A,* In chronic open-angle glaucoma, the anterior chamber angle remains open, but drainage of aqueous humor through the canal of Schlemm is impaired. *B,* In acute angle-closure glaucoma, the angle of the iris and anterior chamber narrows, obstructing the outflow of aqueous humor.

which occurs so gradually that it often is not noticed until late in the disease process.

Glaucoma affects about 2% of the population over the age of 40 in the United States; it remains undetected in approximately 25% of these cases. It accounts for 13% of all blindness worldwide (Porth, 1994; Tierney et al., 1994; Wilson et al., 1991).

Glaucoma usually exists as a primary condition without identified precipitating cause. Primary glaucoma is most common in adults over the age of 60, but may be a congenital condition in infants and children. Secondary glaucoma can develop as a result of infection or inflammation of the eye, cataract, tumor, hemorrhage, or eye trauma (Bullock & Rosendahl, 1992; Porth, 1994).

Pathophysiology

Aqueous humor, a thick fluid, occupies both the anterior and posterior chambers of the eye. The normal intraocular pressure of 12 to 20 mmHg is maintained by a balance between the production of aqueous humor in the ciliary body, its flow through the pupil from the posterior to the anterior chamber of the eye, and its outflow or absorption through the trabecular meshwork and canal of Schlemm (see Figure 43–3, page 1865). When this balance is disrupted, usually because of a decrease in the outflow or absorption of aqueous humor, the intraocular pressure increases. Increased intraocular pressure causes ischemia of the neurons of the eye and degeneration of the optic nerve. The ischemic neurons die beginning at the periphery of the retina, causing a painless, progressive narrowing of the visual field (Figure 44–4) and eventual blindness (Bullock & Rosendahl, 1992; Wilson et al., 1991). Vision loss is often significant before the client seeks treatment and the diagnosis of glaucoma is made.

Primary glaucoma in adults has two major forms: *open-angle glaucoma* and *angle-closure glaucoma*. Both terms refer to the angle formed at the point where the iris meets the cornea in the eye's anterior chamber (Figure 44–5). Forms of primary glaucoma are compared in Table 44–2.

Open-Angle Glaucoma

Open-angle glaucoma, often called chronic simple glaucoma, is the most common form in adults, accounting for approximately 90% of all glaucoma. Its cause is unknown; it is thought to have a hereditary component, but no clear inheritance pattern can be identified. Open-angle glaucoma occurs more frequently and at an earlier age in African-Americans (Tierney et al., 1994).

In open-angle glaucoma, the anterior chamber angle between the iris and cornea is normal (Figure 44–5, *A*), hence the term "open-angle." However, the flow of aqueous humor through the trabecular meshwork and into the canal of Schlemm is relatively obstructed; the cause of

Table 44–2 A Comparison of Open-Angle and Angle-Closure Glaucoma

	Open-Angle Glaucoma	Angle-Closure Glaucoma
Incidence	■ Common ■ Accounts for 90% of all cases of glaucoma	■ Uncommon
Risk Factors	■ Over age 35 ■ Genetic link ■ African-American ancestry	■ Narrow anterior chamber angle ■ Aging ■ Asian ancestry
Pathophysiology	■ Impaired aqueous outflow through the canal of Schlemm ■ Cause unknown ■ Gradual, consistent increase in intraocular pressure ■ Usually bilateral	■ Pupil dilation or lens accommodation causes already narrowed angle to close, blocking aqueous outflow ■ Rapid rise in intraocular pressure ■ Usually unilateral
Manifestations	■ No initial manifestations ■ Frequent lens changes in glasses ■ Impaired dark adaptation ■ Halos around lights ■ Gradual reduction of visual fields with preservation of central vision until late in the disease ■ Mild to severe increased intraocular pressure	■ Abrupt onset of eye pain, headache ■ Decreased visual acuity ■ Nausea and vomiting ■ Reddened conjunctiva ■ Cloudy cornea ■ Fixed pupil ■ Rapid, significant increase in intraocular pressure
Management	■ Topical medications such as miotics, beta-blockers ■ Carbonic anhydrase inhibitors ■ Laser trabeculoplasty	■ Topical miotics or beta-blockers ■ Systemic osmotic agents, carbonic anhydrase inhibitors ■ Laser iridotomy or peripheral iridectomy

this obstruction is unknown. Restricted outflow leads to an increased amount of fluid in the eye and increased intraocular pressure. Open-angle glaucoma tends to be a chronic, gradually progressive disease. The trabecular meshwork increasingly inhibits the outflow of aqueous humor, and the intraocular pressure gradually increases. The result is neuronal ischemia and optic nerve degeneration, leading to gradual loss of vision.

Open-angle glaucoma typically affects both eyes, although the pressures and progression may not be symmetric.

The manifestations of open-angle glaucoma are vague, and often the client is unaware of them. Along with loss of peripheral vision, the client may complain of mild headaches, have difficulty adapting to the dark, see halos around lights, and have some difficulty focusing on near objects. As intraocular pressure continues to increase, visual acuity is reduced.

Angle-Closure Glaucoma
Acute angle-closure (also called narrow-angle or closed-angle) glaucoma is the other, less common, form of primary glaucoma in adults. It accounts for approximately 5% to 10% of all cases of glaucoma (Porth, 1994).

Approximately 1% of people over the age of 35 have narrowed anterior chamber angles; the incidence is higher in older adults and in people of Asian ancestry. Narrowing of the anterior chamber angle occurs because of corneal flattening or bulging of the iris into the anterior chamber. When the lens thickens during accommodation or the iris thickens during pupil dilation, this angle can close completely. Closure of the angle blocks the outflow of aqueous humor through the trabecular meshwork and canal of Schlemm, and the intraocular pressure rises abruptly (Figure 44–5, B). This abrupt increase in intraocular pressure damages the neurons of the retina and the optic nerve, leading to a rapid and permanent loss of vision if not treated promptly.

Episodes of angle-closure glaucoma are typically unilateral. However, in clients who have experienced angle-closure glaucoma of one eye, the other eye is at increased risk for angle-closure glaucoma in the future.

Because of the effect of pupil dilation on aqueous outflow in angle-closure glaucoma, episodes often occur in association with darkness, emotional upset, or other factors that cause the pupil to dilate (Porth, 1994). Clients may experience intermittent episodes of several hours duration prior to experiencing a more typical prolonged attack of angle-closure glaucoma. For clients with a history of angle-closure glaucoma, it is *vital* to avoid medications such as atropine and other anticholinergics, which have a mydriatic or pupil-dilating effect.

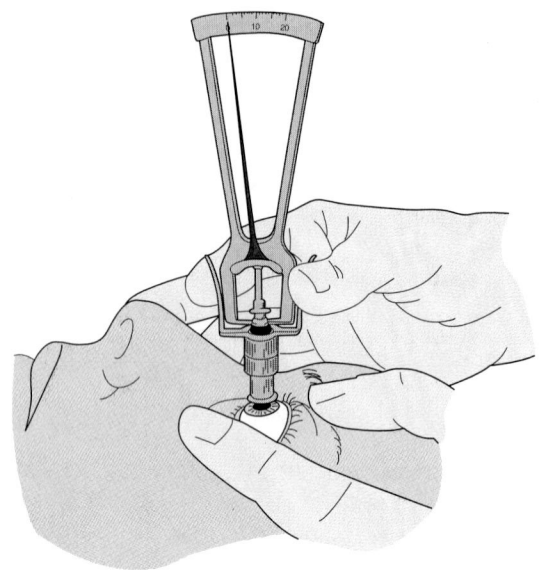

Figure 44–6 The Schiøtz tonometer for measuring intraocular pressure.

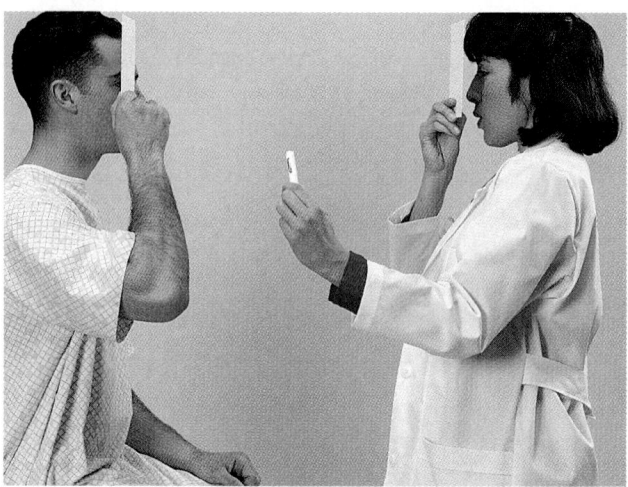

Figure 44–7 Visual field testing. Peripheral vision or visual fields are assessed by testing the client's ability to detect an object brought into the line of vision from the periphery. The client's peripheral vision is compared to the nurse examiner's. Each eye is tested separately.

Symptoms such as severe eye and face pain, general malaise, nausea and vomiting, seeing colored halos around lights, and an abrupt decrease in visual acuity are associated with acute episodes of angle-closure glaucoma. The conjunctiva of the affected eye may be reddened and the cornea clouded with corneal edema. The pupil may be fixed (nonreactive to light) at midpoint (Wilson et al., 1991).

Collaborative Care

Although glaucoma cannot at this time be predicted, prevented, or cured, in most cases it can be controlled and vision preserved if diagnosed early. Because the most prevalent type of glaucoma, open-angle, has few symptoms, routine eye examinations are recommended for early detection. Measurement of intraocular pressure, fundoscopy to assess the optic disk, and visual field testing are used for diagnosis and monitoring of treatment effectiveness.

Laboratory and Diagnostic Tests

The following diagnostic studies are used to detect and evaluate for the presence, severity, type, and effects of glaucoma:

- *Tonometry* is an indirect measurement of the intraocular pressure. Either contact or noncontact tonometry may be used. In *contact tonometry*, the eye is anesthetized, and the force needed to produce an indentation in the cornea is measured using a Schiøtz tonometer (Figure 44–6) or a Goldmann applanation tonometer. *Noncontact tonometry* measures the time required to flatten the cornea with a blast of air to determine the intraocular pressure (Porth, 1994). No anesthesia is required for noncontact tonometry. Routine tonometry screening is recommended for all people over the age of 40. A single elevated pressure reading does not warrant a diagnosis of glaucoma; variations in intraocular pressure occur throughout the day, much as variations in blood pressure do.

- The angle of the anterior chamber of the eye is assessed with *gonioscopy*. The gonioscope is a special instrument used to measure the depth of the anterior chamber. This test is performed to differentiate open-angle from angle-closure glaucoma.

- *Visual field testing,* illustrated in Figure 44–7, is used to identify the degree of visual field narrowing and peripheral vision loss resulting from uncontrolled or poorly controlled glaucoma. The visual field is the entire area seen by the eye when focused on a central point. Testing of visual fields is typically done by confrontation. Facing one another approximately 2 feet apart, the examiner and examinee each cover an eye directly opposite the other (i.e., if the examiner covers the left eye, the examinee covers the right eye). The examiner brings an object from the periphery into the field of vision on a plane midway between them, with the client indicating when the object is seen. This provides an estimate of the client's visual fields in most directions. The temporal and inferotemporal fields of both examiner and examinee likely extend beyond the reach of testing (Bates, 1995).

Pharmacology

Although medications cannot cure glaucoma, many clients with open-angle glaucoma are able to control intraocular pressure and preserve vision indefinitely with drug therapy. Medications are used alone or in combination with the timing and dosage individually determined by pressure measurements. The primary classes or groups of pharmacologic agents used to treat glaucoma are the miotics, beta-adrenergic blocking agents, and carbonic anhydrase inhibitors.

Miotics (pilocarpine, carbachol) are typically cholinergic agents that cause contraction of the sphincter of the iris, constricting the pupil. In addition, these agents cause contraction of the ciliary muscle that promotes accommodation for near vision. The net effect is to facilitate aqueous humor outflow by increasing drainage through the trabecular meshwork in open-angle glaucoma. In angle-closure glaucoma, pupillary constriction flattens the iris, opening the angle and the canal of Schlemm. Miotics are administered topically as drops, with the dose and frequency dependent on the preparation prescribed and the client response.

The adrenergic agonist epinephrine may be prescribed along with miotics to counteract the effect of the miotic on accommodation. In addition, epinephrine decreases the production of aqueous humor by the ciliary body, further reducing the intraocular pressure.

Timolol (Timoptic) is a beta-adrenergic blocking agent that also acts to decrease the production of aqueous humor in the ciliary body. Timolol and other beta-adrenergic blockers have the advantage of a longer duration of activity than the miotics, allowing fewer doses per day. Also, the beta-blockers have less effect on visual acuity than the miotics do. When administering beta-blockers or teaching a client about their use, it is important to remember that ophthalmic preparations can produce the systemic effects of other beta-blockers, including bronchospasm, bradycardia, and hypotension. Compressing the lacrimal sac by pinching the bridge of the nose for 1 minute after the instillation of the drops minimizes the systemic absorption and effects of the drug.

Acetazolamide (Diamox) is a systemic agent that is also used to decrease the production of aqueous humor and reduce intraocular pressure. This drug is a diuretic in the carbonic anhydrase inhibitor group. Acetazolamide is administered by mouth or parenterally in doses of 250 mg to 1 g per day.

Nursing implications for the medications used to control chronic glaucoma are outlined in the pharmacology box on page 1902.

In acute angle-closure glaucoma, diuretics may be administered intravenously to achieve a rapid decrease in intraocular pressure prior to surgical intervention. Both the carbonic anhydrase inhibitor acetazolamide and osmotic diuretics, such as mannitol, are used. Fast-acting miotic drops, such as acetylcholine, are also administered to constrict the pupil and draw the iris away from the angle and from the canal of Schlemm.

Surgery

Surgical intervention is indicated for clients with acute angle-closure glaucoma and for clients with chronic open-angle glaucoma that is not effectively controlled by medication.

Surgical management of chronic open-angle glaucoma involves improving the drainage of aqueous humor from the anterior chamber of the eye. *Trabeculoplasty* and trabeculectomy filtration surgery are the most commonly used procedures.

In a *laser trabeculoplasty,* an argon laser is aimed through a gonioscope to create multiple laser burns spaced evenly around the trabecular meshwork. As the burns heal, the scars they create cause tension, stretching and opening the meshwork. This noninvasive technique is the treatment of choice because it requires no incision and can be performed as an outpatient procedure.

Trabeculectomy is a type of filtration surgery in which a permanent fistula is created to drain aqueous humor from the anterior chamber of the eye. A portion of trabecular meshwork is removed, and a flap of sclera is left unsutured to create a channel or fistula between the anterior chamber and the subconjunctival space. Aqueous humor is able to drain into the space under the conjunctiva, where it can be absorbed into the systemic circulation. A trabeculectomy is usually performed under general anesthesia and requires hospitalization of the client.

If these procedures are not fully effective, surgical intervention to reduce the production of aqueous humor by the ciliary body may be indicated. Either *photocoagulation* using an argon laser (heat) or *cyclocryotherapy* using a probe to freeze tissue may be employed to destroy portions of the ciliary body. This tissue destruction reduces the production of aqueous humor, subsequently reducing intraocular pressure.

Surgical procedures used in the treatment of acute angle-closure glaucoma include gonioplasty, laser iridotomy, and peripheral iridectomy.

In *gonioplasty,* the healing and scarring of microscopic lesions created at the periphery of the iris draws the iris away from the cornea, widening the anterior chamber. This widening of the chamber increases the angle and opens drainage channels for aqueous humor.

Laser iridotomy is a noninvasive procedure using a laser to create multiple small perforations in the iris of the eye. These perforations allow aqueous humor to drain from the posterior chamber to the anterior chamber and out through the trabecular meshwork and the canal of Schlemm.

During an *iridectomy,* a small segment of the iris is removed to facilitate the flow of aqueous humor between

Text continues on page 1904

Nursing Implications for Pharmacology: The Client with Glaucoma

MIOTICS

Acetylcholine (Miochol)

Carbachol (Isopto Carbachol)

Pilocarpine (Isopto Carpine, Ocusert-Pilo)

The miotics in general use are all cholinergic drugs. The ocular effect of these drugs is to constrict the pupil and block the sympathetic nervous system input, which causes the pupil to dilate in low light. In addition, they contract the ciliary muscle, allowing the lens to accommodate for near vision. The effect of miosis and ciliary muscle contraction is to stretch or open the trabecular meshwork, facilitating the absorption of aqueous humor into the canal of Schlemm and reducing intraocular pressure. Pilocarpine is the most widely used of these drugs (Shlafer, 1993).

Nursing Responsibilities

- Assess the client for contraindications to therapy with miotic or parasympathomimetic agents, including bronchial asthma, peptic ulcer disease, intestinal obstruction, urinary retention, hypotension or bradycardia, corneal abrasion, or acute iritis.

- The primary drug interactions to consider when miotics are administered are with anticholinergic drugs such as atropine and drugs with anticholinergic side effects. These drugs can block the desired effect.

- After administering drops, have the client gently squeeze the lacrimal sac for 1 to 2 minutes to increase the local effect and decrease systemic absorption.

- Follow this procedure for the administration of pilocarpine with the Ocusert system.
  a. Pilocarpine may blur vision. Apply at bed time, as the greatest effect is within the first few hours after administration.
  b. Place Ocusert-Pilo in the conjunctival sac, preferably under the upper lid.
  c. Notify the physician if the client develops signs of conjunctival irritation with redness and increased mucous secretion that do not clear within several days of the initial use of Ocusert.
  d. Remove and replace the system weekly or if the client develops signs of an unexpected increase in drug action.

- Assess the client for possible side effects including increased lacrimation, brow pain, and headache.

Client and Family Teaching

- Follow these steps when administering eye drops:
  a. Wash your hands prior to administration.
  b. Do not touch the dropper to the eye or lid, or with the hands.
  c. Squeeze the bridge of the nose gently after administration to prevent systemic absorption.
  d. Keep the eye closed for 1 to 2 minutes after administration to enhance the effect of the medication.

- If you are using the Ocusert system, follow a special procedure. (See the procedure in the preceding section, "Nursing Responsibilities.")

- Avoid medications that may block the effect of the miotics, including many over-the-counter cold and sleep preparations.

- Visual acuity may be decreased during the initiation of therapy. Avoid tasks requiring sharp vision.

- Night vision will be affected. Providing night lights in halls and baths is helpful. Avoid night driving.

- Report adverse effects such as abdominal pain, wheezing, difficulty breathing, sweating, or flushing to the physician.

MYDRIATIC

Epinephrine (Epitrate, Mytrate/Epifrin)

Epinephrine is a sympathomimetic drug acting to dilate the pupil, reduce the production of aqueous humor, and increase its absorption, effectively reducing intraocular pressure in open-angle glaucoma.

Nursing Responsibilities

- Assess the client for contraindications and adverse reactions to epinephrine, including acute angle-closure glaucoma, hypertension, cardiac dysrhythmias, and coronary artery disease.

- Monitor blood pressure, pulse, and respirations.

- Assess for central nervous system side effects of anxiety, nervousness, and muscle tremors. If these side effects are severe, the drug may need to be discontinued.

- Assess for signs of a hypersensitivity reaction, including itching, lid edema, and discharge from the eyes. Notify the physician if you notice these signs.

- Instruct the client about the drug, its dose and administration, desired and side effects.

Pharmacology: The Client with Glaucoma (continued)

Client and Family Teaching

- Report any change in visual acuity or eye pain. (Eye pain may indicate an attack of angle-closure glaucoma and should be reported to the physician immediately.)
- Avoid over-the-counter sinus and cold medications. (Drugs that have a sympathomimetic activity, such as pseudoephedrine and phenylephrine, may accentuate the side effects associated with epinephrine.)

BETA-ADRENERGIC RECEPTOR BLOCKERS

Betaxolol (Betoptic)   Metipranolol (Opti-Pranolol)
Levobunol (Betagan)   Timolol (Timoptic)

Selected beta-adrenergic receptor blocking agents are used to reduce intraocular pressure by reducing the production of aqueous humor in the ciliary body. Because beta-blockers do not affect pupil size and lens accommodation, they do not have the adverse effects on visual acuity that miotics and mydriatics do. An additional advantage is a longer duration of action, allowing twice-a-day dosing.

Nursing Responsibilities

- Assess the client for allergies or contraindications to beta-blocker therapy, including asthma, chronic obstructive pulmonary disease (COPD), heart block, and heart failure.
- Maintain pressure over the lacrimal sac after administration to prevent systemic absorption.
- Assess for therapeutic effect and side effects such as bradycardia, hypotension, wheezing, and difficulty breathing.
- Teach the client the dose, administration, therapeutic and side effects of the medication.

Client and Family Teaching

- Put pressure on the lacrimal sac, at the corner of the eye near the bridge of the nose, to keep the drug from entering your system.
- Your vision may be blurred during the initial period of therapy, but it will improve as you continue to use the drug.
- Report adverse effects, including worsening vision, difficulty breathing, reduced exercise tolerance, and sweating or flushing, to the physician.

CARBONIC ANHYDRASE INHIBITORS

Acetazolamide (Diamox)   Methazolamide
Dichlorphenamide (Daranide)   (Neptazane)

The carbonic anhydrate inhibitors are systemic medications that reduce the production of aqueous humor and lower intraocular pressure. They are typically administered orally and used primarily as adjunctive therapy. Administered intravenously, acetazolamide reduces intraocular pressure preoperatively for the client with angle-closure glaucoma.

Nursing Responsibilities

- Assess for allergies or other contraindications to the use of carbonic anhydrase inhibitors, including known allergy to sulfa, severe renal or hepatic disease, and electrolyte or acid-base imbalances.
- Monitor for drug interactions. Carbonic anhydrase inhibitors increase the activity of amphetamines, procainamide, quinidine, tricyclic antidepressants, and the sympathomimetics ephedrine and pseudoephedrine. Electrolyte and fluid depletion may occur when taken with other diuretics.
- Assess daily weight, intake and output, and vital signs for potential volume depletion.
- Assess skin for adverse reactions including rash and pruritus, purpura, pallor, and bleeding.
- Monitor serum electrolytes, blood gases, and renal and liver function tests for possible adverse effects, including hyponatremia, hypokalemia, metabolic acidosis, and renal or liver insufficiency or failure.
- Administer in the morning to prevent sleep disruption because of the diuretic effect. The drug may be administered with food if nausea occurs.
- Teach the client the name of the drug, its dosage and administration, and the desired and potential adverse effects.

Client and Family Teaching

- Maintain a fluid intake of 2 to 3 liters per day.
- Rise slowly from lying or sitting positions because you may feel dizzy when you first stand (orthostatic hypotension).
- Notify the physician if you have fever, a sore throat, easy bleeding or bruising, numbness and tingling, tremors, flank pain, or a skin rash (Skidmore-Roth, 1993).

the posterior and anterior chambers and to open the anterior chamber angle. Iridectomy, iridotomy, and gonioplasty are all effective in reducing intraocular pressure for the client with angle-closure glaucoma. Because of the high risk for a future attack of angle-closure glaucoma in the unaffected eye, these procedures are often performed prophylactically.

Nursing Care

When planning and implementing nursing care for the client with glaucoma, the nurse needs to consider both the specific pathophysiology and related needs affecting the client, and the actual or potential effects on the client's vision, life-style, safety, and psychosocial well-being. In the hospitalized client, glaucoma is typically a complicating factor rather than the primary reason for seeking care, unless the diagnosis is acute angle-closure glaucoma. Nursing care planning focuses on problems associated with the temporary or permanent visual impairment, the resultant increased risk for injury, and the psychosocial problems of anxiety and coping.

Risk for Sensory/Perceptual Alteration: Visual

Whether glaucoma and resulting impaired vision is the client's primary problem or a pre-existing condition in a client with another disorder, it must be a primary consideration in nursing care planning.

Nursing interventions with rationales follow:

- Address the client by name and identify yourself with each interaction. Orient the client to time, place, person, and situation as indicated. Tell the client the purpose of your visit. *The client with impaired vision must rely on input from the other senses. A lack of visual cues increases the importance of verbal ones, e.g., the visually impaired client cannot see the nurse checking an intravenous infusion and needs a verbal explanation of who is in the room and why. When the client's normal daily routine is disrupted by illness or hospitalization, additional sensory input such as a radio, television, and explanations of the routine and activities may be necessary to help maintain the client's orientation.*

- Provide any visual aids that the client routinely uses. Keep them in close proximity, making sure that the client knows where they are and can reach them easily. *Easy access encourages the client to use these items and enhances the ability to provide self-care.*

- Orient the client to the environment. Explain the location of the call bell, personal items, and the furniture in the room. If the client is able, provide a walking tour of the client's room and immediate facilities, including the bathroom and sink. Do not rearrange the physical environment without reorienting the client to the

changes. Keep traffic areas free of clutter. *Visually impaired clients are usually very capable of providing self-care in a known environment. However, placing a stool or overbed table in an unexpected location can be a hazard and lead to injury.*

- Provide other tools or items that can help compensate for diminished vision:
  a. Bright, nonglare lighting
  b. Books, magazines, and instructions in large print
  c. Books on tape
  d. Telephones with oversize pushbuttons
  e. A clock with numbers and hands that can be felt

- Assist the client with meals by:
  a. Reading menu selections to the client and marking choices.
  b. Describing the position of foods on a meal tray according to the clock system, for example, "On the plate, the peas are at 9 o'clock, the mashed potatoes at 1 o'clock, and the chicken breast at 6 o'clock. The milk glass is at 2 o'clock on the tray above the plate, and coffee is at 11 o'clock."
  c. Placing the utensils in a readily accessible position.
  d. Assisting the client further by removing lids from containers, buttering the bread, and cutting meat, as needed.
  e. If the visual impairment is new or temporary, the client may need feeding or continued assistance during the meal.
  Careful assessment and provision of needed assistance in eating is important to maintain the client's nutritional status. The client may be ashamed of needing help or embarrassed to request it and may respond by not eating or by claiming not to be hungry.

- Assist the client with mobility and ambulation as needed:
  a. Have the client hold your arm or elbow, and walk slightly ahead, to guide the client. Do not hold the client's arm or elbow.
  b. Describe the surroundings and progress as you proceed. Warn the client in advance of potential hazards, turns, and steps.
  c. Have the client feel the chair, bed, or commode with the hands and the back of the legs before sitting.
  These measures help ensure the client's safety while providing for mobility and helping prevent complications associated with immobility.

- If the vision loss is unilateral and recent, provide instructions related to unilateral vision loss and change in depth perception:
  a. Caution about the loss of depth perception and teach safety precautions, such as reaching slowly for objects and using visual cues as to distance, especially when driving.

b. Teach the client to scan, turning the head fully toward the affected side to identify potential hazards and looking up and down to compensate for the loss of depth perception.
The client with a unilateral vision loss is often unaware of its effect on peripheral vision and depth perception. The client needs to learn techniques to accommodate to these changes.

- Provide referral to community, state, and national agencies and resources specializing in information and assistive devices for the visually impaired. *These local and national agencies can provide additional teaching, adaptive resources, and support for the client with a visual deficit.*

Risk for Injury

The client who experiences a sudden loss of vision due to acute angle-closure glaucoma is at high risk for traumatic injury while adapting to the loss of visual input. The client with significant visual impairment as a result of untreated chronic glaucoma who is placed in an unfamiliar environment is also at an increased risk for injury. An additional risk exists for clients who have experienced surgical interventions for glaucoma.

Nursing interventions with rationales follow:

- Assess the client's ability to provide for self-care in activities of daily living. *Clients may be reluctant to request assistance, believing that they should be able to perform these familiar tasks. Careful assessment and provision of needed assistance help prevent injury and maintain the client's self-esteem.*

- Provide for a safe environment by removing furniture and other objects from traffic pattern areas. Orient the client to the environment. Be sure that frequently used items are readily accessible. *Maintaining a safe environment helps ensure client safety and promotes independence.*

- Notify housekeeping and place a sign on the client's door to alert all personnel not to change the arrangement of the client's room. *The visually impaired client is at high risk for falling when in an unfamiliar environment. It is important to maintain a safe, familiar room when the client is hospitalized.*

- Raise the side rails on the client's bed. *The raised rails help remind clients to ask for assistance in ambulating until they are familiar with the environment.*

- Work with the client and family to identify changes in the home environment to help the client remain as independent as possible and prevent falls or other injuries. *Often minor changes in the home environment, such as removing scatter rugs and small items of furniture, allow the client to navigate safely in this already familiar environment.*

- Refer to a local home health agency, senior services, or community resources for the blind to assist in identifying assistive devices and modifications of the home environment.

Anxiety

The actual or potential loss of sight threatens the client's self-concept, role functioning, patterns of interaction, and, potentially, environment. The visually impaired client who functions well in a familiar environment will experience anxiety when placed in the unfamiliar setting of a hospital or care facility.

Nursing interventions with rationales follow:

- Assess the client for verbal and nonverbal indications of level of anxiety and for normal coping mechanisms. Repeated expressions of concern or denial that the vision change will affect the client's life are indicators of anxiety. Nonverbal indicators include tension, difficulty concentrating or thinking, restlessness, poor eye contact, and changes in vocalization (rapid speech, voice quivering). Physical indicators include tachycardia, dilated pupils, cool and clammy skin, and tremors. *Anxiety is defined as a vague, uneasy feeling without a specific or known source (Lederer, 1993). The client may not recognize this feeling as anxiety. Identifying and acknowledging the anxiety state can help the client recognize and deal with it.*

- Encourage the client to verbalize fears, anger, and feelings of anxiety. *Verbalizing helps externalize the anxiety and allows fears to be addressed.*

- Discuss the client's perception of the eye condition and its effects on life-style and roles. *Discussion provides an opportunity to correct misperceptions and introduce alternative activities and assistive devices for the visually impaired.*

- Introduce yourself whenever entering the room, explain all procedures fully before and as they are being performed, and use touch to convey proximity and caring. *The visually impaired client must rely on the other senses to make up for the loss of sight. Because the client cannot see what you are doing, complete explanations of even simple tasks such as refilling a water glass help to relieve anxiety.*

- Help the client to identify coping strategies that have been useful in the past and to adapt these strategies to the present situation. *Previously successful coping strategies may be employed to increase the client's sense of control.*

Other Nursing Diagnoses

The following nursing diagnoses may also be appropriate for the client with glaucoma:

- *Impaired Adjustment* related to sudden loss of vision

- *Altered Health Maintenance* related to visual impairment
- *Knowledge Deficit* related to a lack of information about glaucoma, its management, and available resources
- *Altered Role Performance* related to loss of vision
- *Impaired Social Interaction* related to vision deficit

Client and Family Teaching

Clients with glaucoma require teaching about the medications prescribed, including the name of the medication, dose, expected and potential adverse effects, and proper way to instill drops. They need to know that certain prescription and over-the-counter medications can cause increased intraocular pressure and should not be taken without consulting a physician. These clients need to understand the importance of lifetime therapy and periodic eye examinations with intraocular pressure measurement in controlling the disease and preventing blindness.

The client who has experienced an episode of acute angle-closure glaucoma is taught about the risks, warning signs, and management of future attacks. If surgery is planned to prevent further episodes, information about possible options for treatment, the procedure, and pre- and postoperative care is included. If a permanent visual impairment has resulted, the client needs information on achieving the maximum possible independence while maintaining safety. Referral to local, state, and national agencies is useful for both the client and family.

Applying the Nursing Process

Case Study of a Client with Glaucoma and Cataracts: Lila Rainey

Lila Rainey is an 80-year-old widow who lives alone in the house she and her late husband built 50 years ago. She has worn glasses for nearsightedness since she was a young girl and was diagnosed 4 years ago with chronic open-angle glaucoma, for which she takes timolol maleate (Timoptic) 0.5%. Recently she has noticed difficulty reading and watching television despite a new lens prescription. She has stopped driving at night because the glare of oncoming headlights makes it very difficult for her to see. Mrs. Rainey's ophthalmologist has told her that she has cataracts but that they don't need to come out until they bother her. Although her glaucoma is still controlled with timolol maleate 0.5%, one drop in each eye twice a day, her intraocular pressure measurements have been gradually increasing. Mrs. Rainey has taken 5 gr of aspirin daily since a TIA 8 years ago. She is being admitted to the outpatient surgery unit for a cataract removal and intraocular lens implant in her right eye.

Assessment

Lila Rainey is admitted to the eye surgery unit by Susan Schafer, RN. In her assessment, Ms. Schafer finds Mrs. Rainey to be alert and oriented, though apprehensive about her upcoming surgery. Assessment findings include BP, 134/72; P, 86; R, 18. Mrs. Rainey's neurologic, respiratory, cardiovascular, and abdominal assessments are essentially normal. Mrs. Rainey's pupils are round and equal, and react briskly to light and accommodation. Her conjunctivae are pink; sclera and corneas, clear. Using the opthalmoscope, Ms. Schafer notes that the red reflex in Mrs. Rainey's right eye is diminished. Ophthalmic examination shows visual acuity of 20/150 OD (right eye) and 20/50 OS (left eye) with corrective lenses. Her intraocular pressures are 21 mmHg OD and 17 mmHg OS. On fundoscopic exam, no disease of the blood vessels, retina, macula, or disc is found. Ms. Schafer reviews the operative procedure with Mrs. Rainey, answering her questions and telling her what to expect after surgery. Following preoperative protocols, Mrs. Rainey is prepared and transported to surgery.

Diagnosis

Ms. Schafer develops the following nursing diagnoses for Mrs. Rainey:

- *Sensory/Perceptual Alteration: Visual* related to myopia and lens extraction
- *Anxiety* related to anticipated surgery
- *Knowledge Deficit* related to a lack of information regarding postoperative care
- *Impaired Home Maintenance Management* related to activity restrictions and impaired vision

Expected Outcomes

The expected outcomes for the plan of care are that Mrs. Rainey will

- Adapt to an increased vision deficit in the immediate postoperative period.
- Regain sufficient visual acuity to maintain activities of daily living, including reading and watching television for enjoyment.
- Demonstrate a reduced level of anxiety.
- Demonstrate the procedure for instilling eye drops postoperatively.
- Demonstrate knowledge of the home care she will require after surgery, signs of complications, and actions to take if complications occur.
- Use appropriate resources to assist with home maintenance until vision stabilizes and activity restrictions are lifted.

Planning and Implementation

Ms. Schafer plans and implements the following interventions for Mrs. Rainey:

- Provide a safe environment, placing the call light and personal care items within easy reach.
- Encourage Mrs. Rainey to express her fears about surgery and its potential effect on vision.
- Explain all procedures related to surgery and recovery.
- Instruct her to avoid shutting the eyelids tightly, sneezing, coughing, laughing, bending over, lifting, or straining to have a bowel movement.
- Teach her to wear glasses during the day and an eye shield at night to prevent injury to the surgical site.
- Inform her that it may take several days or weeks for her vision to stabilize before she can be fitted with new prescription lenses.
- Explain and demonstrate the procedure for administering eye drops.
- Provide verbal and written instructions about postoperative care, including a schedule of follow-up examinations, potential complications, and actions to take in response.
- Help her to identify hazards that may interfere with her ability to maintain her home.
- Refer Mrs. Rainey to a discharge planner or social worker to help establish a plan for home maintenance.

Evaluation

Mrs. Rainey is discharged the morning after her surgery. She is visibly relieved when the eye patch is removed because her vision in the operated eye is better than before surgery, even without her glasses. She is able to relate the recommended activity restrictions and measures to take to avoid lifting, bending, and straining. Mrs. Rainey administers her own eye drops before discharge and relates an understanding of the prescribed postoperative care and safety precautions. Mrs. Rainey's daughter plans to visit her mother two to three times a week to help with laundry and vacuuming until Mrs. Rainey is able to resume all her household activities. Mrs. Rainey expresses relief that this surgery is over with and says that she won't "be so scared when I need my other eye done." She understands the chronic nature of her glaucoma and says that her vision is too important for her to neglect her timolol drops and routine eye exams.

Critical Thinking in the Nursing Process

1. Why did it become more difficult to control Mrs. Rainey's intraocular pressure as her cataract matured?
2. Identify medications that are commonly prescribed following cataract surgery. What are the risks of interactions between these medications and Mrs. Rainey's timolol drops?
3. How does Mrs. Rainey's daily aspirin affect her operative and postoperative risk of complications?
4. Develop a care plan for the nursing diagnosis *Self-Care Deficit: Dressing/Grooming* related to visual impairment and restricted bending.

The Client with a Retinal Detachment

■ ■ ■

The retina contains the photoreceptors of the eye, which allow the perception of light and initial processing of images and stimuli for transmission to the optic center of the brain. Disruption of this neural layer of the eye by trauma or disease interferes with light perception and image transmission, potentially resulting in blindness.

Both primary eye conditions and systemic diseases can affect the retina and interfere with vision. Retinal tears or detachments can occur either spontaneously or as a result of trauma.

Pathophysiology

Separation of the retina or sensory portion of the eye from the choroid, the pigmented vascular layer, is known as a **retinal detachment**. Although retinal detachment may be precipitated by trauma, it usually occurs spontaneously. The vitreous humor normally adheres to the retina at the optic disk, the macula, and the periphery of the eye. With aging, the vitreous humor shrinks and may pull the retina away from the choroid. Aging therefore is a common risk factor, as are myopia and *aphakia*, absence of the lens (e.g., following lens removal for cataracts) (Bullock & Rosendahl, 1992; Porth, 1994).

The retina may actually tear and fold back on itself, or the retina may remain intact but no longer adhere to the choroid (Figure 44–8). A break or tear in the retina allows fluid from the vitreous cavity to enter the defect. This, along with fluid that escapes from choroid vessels, the pull of gravity, and traction exerted by the vitreous humor, separates the retina from the choroid. The detached area may rapidly increase in size, increasing loss of vision. Unless contact between the retina and choroid is reestablished, the neurons of the retina become ishemic and die, causing permanent vision loss. For this reason, retinal detachment is a true medical emergency, requiring prompt ophthalmologic referral and treatment.

When the retina detaches, the client experiences floaters, or "spots," and lines or flashes of light in the visual field. Often the client describes the sensation of having a curtain drawn across the vision, much like a curtain being drawn over a window (Figure 44–9). The area of

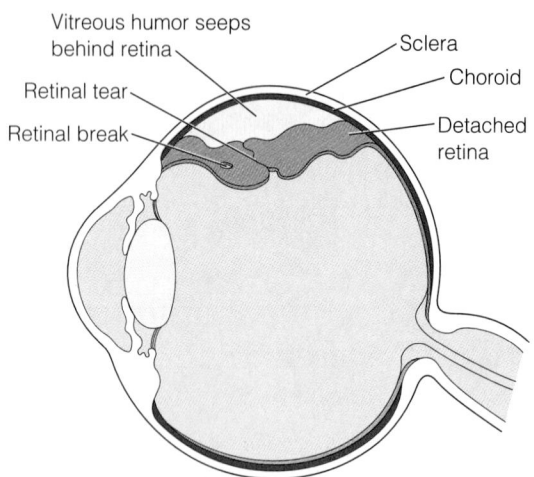

Figure 44–8 Retinal detachment.

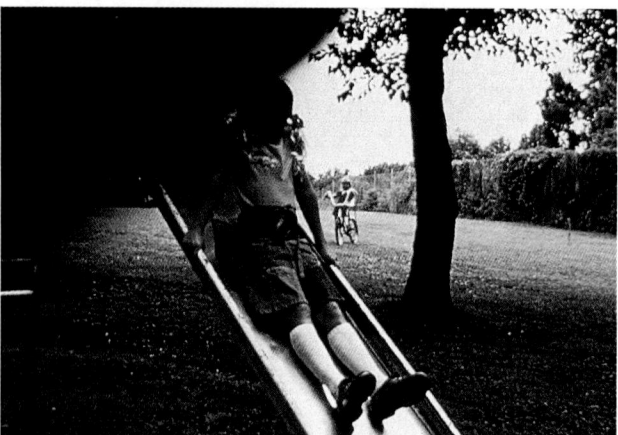

Figure 44–9 Vision deficit associated with detached retina.

Clinical Manifestations of Retinal Detachment

■ ■ ■

- Floaters: irregular, dark lines or spots in the field of vision
- Flashes of light
- Blurred vision
- Progressive deterioration of vision
- Sensation of a curtain or veil being drawn across the field of vision
- If the macula is involved, loss of central vision

---

the visual field affected is directly related to the area of detachment. For example, because light rays cross as they pass through the lens, a retinal tear in the superior portion of the eye results in a deficit in the lower part of the visual field. No pain is experienced, and the eye appears normal to visual inspection. The accompanying box lists common manifestations of retinal detachment.

Collaborative Care

The clinical manifestations and examination of the ocular fundus by ophthalmoscopy establish the diagnosis of retinal detachment. Early diagnosis and intervention are vital. If the condition is left untreated, the detached portion will become necrotic because of separation from the vascular supply of the choroid. The result is permanent blindness in that portion of the eye. If an ophthalmologist is not readily available, the client's head is positioned so that gravity pulls the detached portion of the retina into closer contact with the choroid.

Interventions are directed toward bringing the retina and choroid back into contact and reestablishing the blood and nutrient supply to the retina. Either *cryotherapy*, using a supercooled probe, or *laser photocoagulation* may be employed to create an area of inflammation and adhesion to "weld" the layers together.

A surgical procedure called *scleral buckling* also may be employed. In this procedure, an indentation or fold is created in the sclera, bringing the choroid into contact with the retina. Contact is maintained by use of a local implant on the sclera or an encircling strap or "buckle." Air may also be injected into the vitreous cavity, a procedure called *pneumatic retinopexy*. The client is positioned so that the air bubble pushes the detached portion of the retina into contact with the choroid.

With a retinal tear, it may be necessary to use surgical instruments to manipulate the detached section of retina into place. Air or a liquid is then injected into the vitreous to maintain retinal contact with the choroid, or laser therapy used to create a bond.

Nursing Care

The nursing focus for the client with a detached retina is on early identification and treatment. Because early intervention is vital to preserve the client's sight, nurses need to be able to recognize early manifestations of retinal detachment and intervene appropriately to obtain definitive treatment for the client. Priority interventions are directed toward maintaining optimal contact of the retina with the choroid and preventing further detachment if possible. Retinal detachment is often successfully treated on an outpatient basis, often in an ophthalmologist's office. For these clients, the nursing focus is on education.

Altered Tissue Perfusion: Retinal

Restoring contact between the retina and choroid is a priority of nursing and medical care for the client with retinal detachment. Vitreous humor may leak through a retinal tear, and fluid exudate may collect behind the tear, causing further retinal detachment. If the macula is detached, central vision is lost, and the client's prognosis for full vision restoration is poorer.

Nursing interventions with rationales follow:

- Carefully assess the client who complains of a sudden change in vision. *Most disorders affecting vision cause a gradual loss of vision; those that cause a rapid loss are often medical emergencies requiring immediate intervention to preserve vision.*

- Assess the client for other manifestations of eye disease. *Retinal detachment is a painless process and has no outward manifestations. The client with a red eye or cloudy cornea may be experiencing acute angle-closure glaucoma rather than retinal detachment.*

- Notify the client's physician and the ophthalmologist immediately if the client has an acute painless vision loss in one eye, often described as a curtain coming down (or up) over the field of vision. *This is the typical presentation of retinal detachment.*

- Position the client so the area of detachment is inferior. For instance, for a superior temporal retinal detachment of the right eye (with corresponding vision loss in the inferior medial visual field of that eye), place the client supine with the head turned to the right. *Correct positioning allows the contents of the posterior portion of the eye to place pressure on the detached area, bringing the retina in closer contact with the choroid.*

Anxiety

The client with retinal detachment experiences a rapid decline in vision in the affected eye, often occurring spontaneously and without pain. Unless the client has had previous episodes, he or she usually does not know what is causing the problem. Anxiety and fear of complete vision loss are common, expected reactions.

Nursing interventions with rationales follow:

- Maintain a calm, confident attitude while carrying out priority interventions. *Administering care in a calm although urgent manner helps reassure the client that the problem, while serious, is treatable and that appropriate measures are being taken to institute treatment.*

- Reassure the client that most retinal detachments are successfully treated, usually on an outpatient basis. *This reassurance can help allay the client's fear of permanent vision loss.*

- For spontaneous detachments, assure clients that they did nothing to cause the detachment to occur. *The client may believe that the detachment is related to a specific activity and feel guilty for "causing" this loss of vision.*

- Explain all procedures fully, including the reason for positioning. *Explanations facilitate the client's understanding and help relieve anxiety in unfamiliar settings.*

- Allow supportive family members or friends to remain with the client as much as possible. *Additional support helps lower the client's anxiety level.*

Other Nursing Diagnoses

The following nursing diagnoses may also be appropriate for the client with retinal detachment:

- *Sensory/Perceptual Alteration: Visual* related to loss of contact between the retina and choroid

- *Risk for Injury* related to altered vision in the affected eye

Client and Family Teaching

Teaching for the client undergoing surgical repair of retinal detachment is similar to that provided for clients experiencing other types of eye surgery. See the box on page 1896. Emphasize the importance of positioning as prescribed by the ophthalmologist; following treatment for retinal detachment, the client may be positioned with the affected area of the eye inferior to maintain contact between the retina and choroid.

The client who has experienced a spontaneous retinal detachment has a 20% to 25% risk of future retinal detachment in the other eye (Way, 1994). Teach the client about early manifestations and emphasize the importance of seeking immediate treatment should they occur. Emphasize the need to maintain follow-up treatment with the ophthalmologist; approximately 15% of clients with retinal detachment require repeated therapy (Tierney et al., 1994). The client whose retina remains detached needs instructions about the change in peripheral vision or other visual fields and changes in depth perception caused by the loss of vision.

The Client with Macular Degeneration

■ ■ ■

The leading cause of blindness in people over the age of 75 is **macular degeneration** (Porth, 1994). The macula is the area of the retina that receives light from the center of the visual field and that has the greatest visual acuity. Destructive changes in the macula may be the result of injury, infection, inflammation, or a hereditary condition; however, they occur most often as a response to the aging

Figure 44-10 *A,* The visual distortion of straight lines typical of early macular degeneration. *B,* Loss of central vision with advanced macular degeneration.

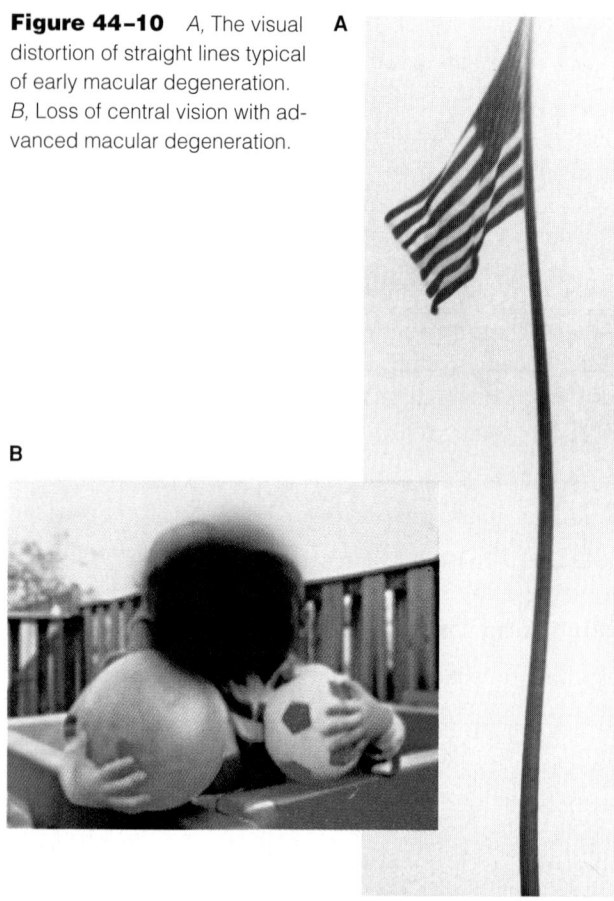

generation, serous fluid or blood leaks into the retina, separating the pigmented retina from the choroid or separating the neurosensory retina (innermost layer) from the pigmented retina. This form of macular degeneration is often associated with neovascularization, growth of fibrovascular tissue from the choroid between it and the retina (Hazzard et al., 1994; Tierney et al., 1994).

When the macula is damaged, central vision becomes blurred and distorted, but peripheral vision remains intact. Distortion of vision in one eye is a common initial manifestation; straight lines appear wavy or distorted (Figure 44–10, *A*) (Hogstel, 1992). With the loss of central vision, activities that require close central vision, such as reading and sewing, are particularly affected (Figure 44–10, *B*).

There is currently no effective treatment for atrophic macular degeneration. Laser photocoagulation may slow the exudative form if performed early in the course of the disease to seal leaking capillaries and stop exudation. Large-print books and magazines, the use of a magnifying glass, and high-intensity lighting can help the client to cope with the reduced vision of macular degeneration.

Nurses should be alert for clients demonstrating new and rapid onset manifestations of macular degeneration and promptly refer these clients for ophthalmologic evaluation. Early intervention may preserve a greater degree of vision and slow the progress of the disease. For clients with slowly progressive manifestations, the nursing focus is on helping the client and family members adapt to the gradual decline in vision by recommending visual aids and other coping strategies.

The Client with Retinitis Pigmentosa

· · ·

Retinitis pigmentosa is a hereditary degenerative disease characterized by retinal atrophy and loss of retinal function progressing from the periphery to the central region of the retina. It is inherited as an autosomal dominant, autosomal recessive, or X-linked trait and may be associated with other genetic defects (Berkow & Fletcher, 1992; Bullock & Rosendahl, 1992; Porth, 1994).

In retinitis pigmentosa, the genetic defect appears to cause production of an unstable form of *rhodopsin,* the receptor protein of rod cells in the retina. Rod cells degenerate, initially at the periphery of the retina. The areas of degeneration and cell death slowly expand, causing vision to narrow. Central vision is finally lost as well (Montgomery, 1995).

The initial manifestation of retinitis pigmentosa, difficulty with night vision, is often noted during childhood. As the disease progresses, there is slow loss of visual

process. The onset of macular degeneration typically occurs at around age 65; it affects males and females equally and is seen more frequently in people of European ancestry.

Gradual failure of the outer pigmented layer of the retina (the retinal layer adjacent to the choroid), which removes cellular waste products and keeps the retina attached to the choroid, is believed to be the cause of age-related macular degeneration. This failure causes photoreceptor (sensory) cells to be lost at an increasing rate. In addition, waste and toxins from cell breakdown further damage the cells of the outer pigmented retinal layer. Serous fluid may enter the subretinal space, leading to retinal detachments and deprivation of oxygen and nutrients from sensory cells, increasing cell death. The process is typically bilateral and slowly progressive (Porth, 1994; Thompson et al., 1993; Woods, 1992).

Two forms of macular degeneration have been identified. *Atrophic degeneration* causes gradual and progressive vision loss because of atrophy and degeneration of the outer pigmented retinal layer (Tierney et al., 1994). Vision loss is more rapid and severe in *exudative degeneration;* this form accounts for 90% of people who are legally blind because of macular degeneration. In exudative de-fields, photophobia, and disrupted color vision. The progression to tunnel vision and blindness is gradual; the client may be totally blind by age 40 (Bullock & Rosendahl, 1992; Montgomery, 1995; Porth, 1994).

Currently, there is no effective treatment for retinitis pigmentosa. Research into the role that defective rhodopsin plays in the disease holds future promise for the development of therapy that may at least slow its progress.

Clients with retinitis pigmentosa may benefit from low-vision aids, much like those for the client with macular degeneration. Additionally, information about the disease and its progress is vital so the client can plan for the eventual total loss of sight. Clients with retinitis pigmentosa should be referred for genetic counseling prior to starting a family to determine the risk of transmitting the disease to their children.

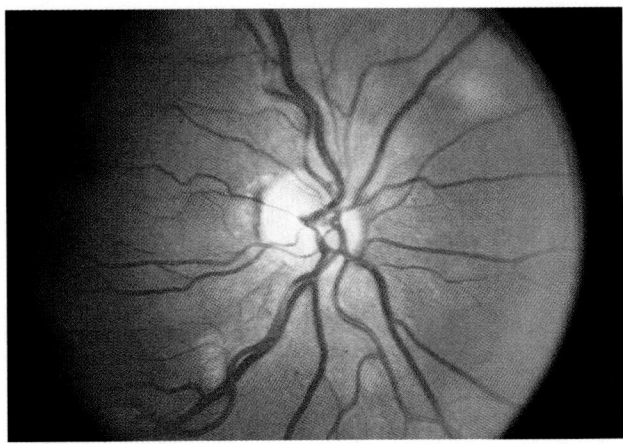

Figure 44–11   Appearance of the ocular fundus in diabetic retinopathy.

The Client with Diabetic Retinopathy

■ ■ ■

In the United States, **diabetic retinopathy** is the leading cause of blindness in people between the ages of 20 years and 74 years and the third leading cause of new blindness in all age groups. In the diabetic, the extent of retinopathy is reflective of the length of time the client has had the disease and the degree of control that has been maintained (Porth, 1994; Smith, 1992). Nursing care of the client with diabetes is discussed in Chapter 21.

Diabetic retinopathy is a vascular disorder affecting the capillaries of the retina. The capillaries become sclerotic and lose their ability to transport sufficient oxygen and nutrients to the retina (Smith, 1992). Retinopathy is seen in both insulin-dependent diabetes and noninsulin-dependent diabetes. The degree of retinopathy present appears to be related more to the duration of the disease than to its stability or control (Berkow & Fletcher, 1992).

Diabetic retinopathy has two major forms: *nonproliferative* or *background retinopathy* and *proliferative retinopathy*. Nonproliferative retinopathy is typically the initial form seen. The venous capillaries of the eye dilate and develop microaneurysms that may then leak, causing retinal edema, or rupture, causing small hemorrhages into the retina. On ophthalmoscopic examination, yellow exudates, cotton-wool patches indicative of retinal ischemia, and red-dot hemorrhages are observed (Figure 44–11). When the peripheral retina is involved, the client may experience few symptoms other than light glare. Edema of the macula or a large hemorrhage may cause vision loss.

Diabetic retinopathy may progress to the proliferative form. This disease is marked by large areas of retinal ischemia and the formation of new blood vessels (neovascularization) spreading over the inner surface of the retina and into the vitreous body. These vessels are fine and fragile, making them permeable and easily ruptured. Blood and blood protein leakage contribute to retinal edema, and hemorrhage into the vitreous body may occur. The vessels gradually become fibrous and firmly attached to the vitreous body, increasing the risk of retinal detachments.

Clients with diabetes should be examined regularly by an ophthalmologist. Yearly retinal examination is recommended for all adults with diabetes; the development of any new visual manifestations is an additional indication for prompt ophthalmologic examination.

Laser photocoagulation is used to treat both the nonproliferative and proliferative forms of diabetic retinopathy. Leaking microaneurysms are sealed and proliferating vessels destroyed, reducing the risk of hemorrhage, retinal edema, and retinal detachment. This treatment also slows the progress of aneurysm and new vessel formation; however, it does not cure the disorder. Clients with severe proliferative retinopathy may undergo vitrectomy to remove vitreous hemorrhage or treat associated retinal detachments (Tierney et al., 1994).

As with many other eye disorders, the nursing care focus for diabetic retinopathy is primarily educational. The newly diagnosed diabetic client needs to understand the importance of regular eye examinations beginning approximately 5 years after the onset of insulin-dependent diabetes and at the time of onset of noninsulin-dependent diabetes. Changes of diabetic retinopathy may already be present when noninsulin-dependent diabetes is diagnosed.

Teach the client to report promptly any new visual manifestation, including blurred vision; black spots (floaters), cobwebs, or flashing lights in the visual field; or a sudden loss of vision in one or both eyes (Berkow & Fletcher, 1992).

Emphasize to the client that careful blood glucose control may help prevent diabetic retinopathy from developing; it may also slow its progress. The client's blood pressure should also be maintained within normal limits to prevent further damage to retinal vessels. Although diabetic retinopathy cannot be halted or cured, its progress can be slowed with aggressive management. Much of the burden for this management falls on the client, increasing the importance of good teaching.

The Client with HIV Infection

■ ■ ■

Seventy-five percent of people infected with the human immunodeficiency virus (HIV) develop an infectious or noninfectious ocular condition related to the HIV infection (Plona & Schremp, 1992).

HIV retinopathy manifested as cotton-wool spots around the optic nerve is the most common noninfectious ophthalmic lesion in AIDS. Cotton-wool spots indicate areas of retinal ischemia. Microaneurysms and dot-, blot-, or flame-shaped hemorrhages may also be seen in HIV retinopathy.

Neoplasms common in the client with AIDS can also affect the eye. Kaposi's sarcoma may affect the external surface or anterior segment of the eye or the eyelids. Kaposi's lesions vary in color (red, brown, or purple) and in size, shape, and location. Conjunctival lesions resemble a benign subconjunctival hemorrhage. Kaposi's lesions of the lid may cause **ptosis** (drooping of the lid) and abnormal lid function. Non-Hodgkin's lymphoma can affect the eye orbit or the central nervous system. Vision or eye position and movement may be affected by the tumor or by the effect of increased intracranial pressure on the cranial nerves (Plona & Schremp, 1992; Wilson et al., 1991).

The most serious and frequent opportunistic eye infection associated with HIV infection is cytomegalovirus (CMV) retinitis. CMV retinitis develops in 10% to 15% of people with AIDS. Initially unilateral, CMV retinitis commonly progresses to become bilateral because of the systemic nature of the infection. CMV invades the retina of the eye directly, producing exudate and cotton-wool spots, hemorrhage, cell death, and necrosis. Visual field deficits develop and can progress to eventual blindness (Plona & Schremp, 1992).

Corneal ulcers from opportunistic bacterial, fungal, protozoal, or viral infections are also associated with HIV infection. Toxoplasmic and fungal retinal infections may occur (Plona & Schremp, 1992; Wilson et al., 1991).

The client with an HIV-associated ocular condition may complain of a change in visual acuity, blurring, floaters, or gaps in the field of vision. Extensive retinal damage may cause retinal detachment and symptoms of flashing lights, multiple floaters, and a loss of vision.

Because the observed changes in the retina are nonspecific, it is important for the examining physician to have knowledge of the client's HIV-positive status in order to make an accurate diagnosis.

In addition to the general treatment of HIV infection with zidovudine (AZT), didanosine (ddI), or zalcitabine (ddC), specific therapies may be directed toward the ocular manifestations of the disease. CMV retinitis is commonly treated with the antivirals ganciclovir (Cytovene) and foscarnet sodium (Foscavir) (Plona & Schremp, 1992).

Although treatment of ocular Kaposi's sarcoma is usually not indicated, conjunctival lesions may be excised for comfort or cosmetic reasons. Lid lesions may be treated with radiation or intralesional chemotherapy.

The Client with an Enucleation

■ ■ ■

Occasionally surgical removal of an eye is necessary because of trauma, infection, glaucoma, intractable pain, or malignancy. This procedure is known as **enucleation.**

Enucleation is performed under local or general anesthesia. After the globe is removed, the conjunctiva and eye muscles are sutured to a round implant inserted into the orbit to maintain its shape. A pressure dressing is left in place for 24 to 48 hours. The client is permitted out of bed on the day of surgery. Hemorrhage and infection are the most commonly seen complications.

Postoperative nursing care includes teaching, psychologic support, and observation for potential complications. The client may be instructed to apply warm compresses and instill antibiotic ointment or drops postoperatively.

Within 1 week, a temporary prosthesis called a conformer is fitted into the empty socket. The permanent prosthesis is individually designed to closely resemble the client's other eye. The prosthesis can be fitted 1 to 2 months after surgery. Often it is difficult to discern which eye is functional and which is the prosthesis. Don't make the mistake of charting "Pupils equal and readily react to light and accommodation (PERRLA)" on a client with an eye prosthesis. Procedure 44–1 outlines the proper way to remove and reinsert an eye prosthesis when the client is unable to do so.

The Client Who Is Blind

■ ■ ■

Visual impairment exists on a continuum from blindness to decreased visual acuity that can be corrected with refractive lenses to normal or near normal. The legal definition of blindness is visual acuity no better than 20/200 in

Procedure 44–1 Removing and Reinserting a Prosthetic Eye

SUPPLIES

- Gloves
- Clean basin or plastic denture cup
- Sterile normal saline or soap and water for cleaning the prosthesis
- Gauze squares or cotton cloth for cleaning the socket
- A bulb syringe for irrigation if necessary

BEFORE THE PROCEDURE

Most clients who have an artificial eye provide self-care and require little assistance. However, it may be necessary for the nurse to remove an eye prosthesis from the unconscious or debilitated client. Explain the procedure to the client and provide for privacy.

PROCEDURE

- Follow universal precautions.
- Wash the hands and put on clean exam gloves.
- To remove the prosthesis, either
  - Pull down the lower lid and gently exert outward and upward pressure on the lower edge of the prosthesis. This pressure usually causes the prosthesis to slip out.
  - Pull down the lower lid and apply a moistened suction cup to the prosthesis by squeezing the device. Twist gently to remove the prosthesis from the socket.
- Wash the prosthesis using mild soap and water or normal saline. Rinse thoroughly. Do not use abrasives or chemicals for cleaning.
- If the prosthesis is not immediately replaced in the eye socket, store it in a clearly labeled plastic container lined with a soft cloth or gauze squares. Avoid scratching or damaging the prosthesis. Store it in a safe place to prevent loss.
- If irrigation of the eye socket is ordered, have the client lean over a sink or basin if possible, or position on the affected side with a clean emesis basin to hold the irrigant as it flows out of the socket. Gently hold the lids open and irrigate the socket using a bulb syringe and clean warm water.

- Reinsert the prosthesis.
  a. Moisten the prosthesis with warm normal saline or water.
  b. Gently hold the lids open, inserting the upper edge of the prosthesis under the upper lid first, then the lower edge under the lower lid using slight pressure.
  c. If a suction device is used, attach it to the cleaned prosthesis over the pupil. Holding the lids open, insert the prosthesis using the above procedure, then remove the suction cup by squeezing it gently and exerting slight pressure on the edge of the cup with the lower lid.

AFTER THE PROCEDURE

- Ensure that the client is comfortable. Chart the procedure and any abnormal findings, such as drainage or inflammation.

---

the better eye with optimal correction, or a visual field of less than 20 degrees (compared to the normal of 180 degrees). Total blindness usually indicates that the client has no light perception at all. In practical terms, a person with a visual deficit sufficient to need assistive devices or aid from other people for normal activities of daily living is considered blind (Grimes et al., 1992; Thompson et al., 1993).

Ten to twelve million people in the United States have a visual impairment that cannot be corrected. More than 500,000 Americans are legally blind. Worldwide, between 40 and 50 million people have visual impairment significant enough to be considered blind (Grimes et al., 1992; Vader, 1992).

The major worldwide causes of blindness are:

1. Cataracts
2. Trachoma
3. Glaucoma
4. Onchocerciasis (river blindness), a parasitic infection transmitted by flies that causes opacification of the cornea, inflammation of the iris and choroid (uveitis), and eventual destruction of vision
5. Nutritional deficiencies including xerophthalmia and keratomalacia due to vitamin A deficiency
6. Trauma

Pathophysiology

Although approximately two-thirds of all cases of blindness worldwide are either preventable or curable, it continues to be prevalent because of lack of access to care, fear of surgery or other treatment, poor sanitation and nutrition, and ignorance of need. In the United States, sanitation measures, better access to health care, and a higher level of nutrition have reduced the threat of infectious disorders to vision. However, glaucoma and cataract remain significant causes of blindness. Other major causes of blindness in the United States include retinal diseases such as diabetic retinopathy, macular degeneration, and congenital disorders (Grimes et al., 1992; Thompson et al., 1993; Vader, 1992).

Nursing Care

Blind people need to cope not only with the loss of a significant sense but often also with societal attitudes that make them feel inferior, helpless, and inadequate. The idea of losing the sense of vision is uniformly feared, leaving sighted people unable to understand the magnitude and impact of the loss in those who have experienced it. Because of this fear and confusion, sighted people are unsure of what is expected by the blind (Vader, 1992).

The adjustment of the person who is born blind and raised to become an independent member of society differs from that of the person who has been sighted and becomes blind. The person who has been blind from birth has developed numerous adaptive strategies that the newly blind person has yet to learn.

Although adaptation may be easier for the client who has experienced a gradual loss of vision than for someone with an abrupt loss, grieving the lost sense is necessary for both. The blind client needs to grieve the lost body part as well as the loss of mobility, self-sufficiency, perhaps economic security, and, to a certain extent, contact with reality as it has been perceived (Vader, 1992). The client's self-concept and self-esteem are threatened. Anger, denial, remorse, and self-pity are not uncommon in the initial period following loss of sight. Interpersonal relationships and roles are affected. Communication patterns change with the loss of the ability to perceive many nonverbal cues. Expressions of sexuality may be impaired.

Acceptance of the change from sighted to blind is characterized by releasing the hope that vision will be regained. Self-esteem increases as the client attempts and masters activities of self-sufficiency such as completing ADLs, cooking, and becoming mobile outside the known home environment (Vader, 1992).

Health professionals often confuse the role of the blind person with the role of the patient, seeing them as helpless, dependent, and lacking in personal identity and control. Although nurses need to take blindness into account in planning care and maintaining client safety, it is vital to give the blind client the same respect and decision-making power that all clients deserve. Nurses who have dealt with their own emotions and responses to vision loss are better prepared to help the client adapt.

Nurses can foster independence in the hospitalized client with a significant vision deficit by doing the following:

- Orient the client to the environment verbally and physically. Describe the client's room using a central point such as the bed. Lead the client around the room, identifying chairs, sink, bathroom, and other landmarks. Be sure that objects such as chairs, personal items, and clothing are not moved within the client's room unless the client moves them. Leave doors either fully open or closed as the client wishes, but, to preserve the client's safety, do not leave doors partially open. Keep the room and hallways where the client will be ambulating free of clutter.

- Use verbal communication freely. Describe activities going on around the client. Introduce yourself as you enter the room and let the client know when you are leaving.

- Provide other sensory stimuli such as radio and television as desired by the client.

- Orient the client to food trays, describing the position of food items on the plate and tray using the face of a clock as a reference (unless the client has always been blind and cannot visualize a clock face).

- When assisting with ambulation, allow the client to hold your arm as you walk slightly ahead. Do not hold the client's arm. Verbally describe the environment, such as, "There will be two steps up 5 feet ahead."

- Do not be afraid to ask the client what assistance he or she desires.

For the client with a new loss of sight, referral to available services is appropriate. Counseling can help the client cope with and eventually adapt to the loss of sight. Persons who are blind are eligible for mobility training, assistance with relearning self-care activities, education in the use of braille to communicate, and vocational and other forms of rehabilitation. State, local, and national agencies help coordinate services for the blind. Many assistive devices are available, including guide or pilot dogs, computer services, talking books and tape players, and low-vision aids.

Although each client with a significant vision deficit has individualized needs, the following nursing diagnoses may be appropriate for the blind client:

- *Sensory/Perceptual Alteration: Visual* related to trauma or disease process

- *Self-Care Deficit: Bathing/Hygiene, Dressing/Grooming, Feeding* related to impaired vision

- *Knowledge Deficit* related to lack of information about available resources

- *Hopelessness* related to loss of vision

- *Grieving* related to loss of a body part

- *Self-Esteem Disturbance* related to significant change in body image

Ear Disorders

For a person to hear, sound waves must enter the external auditory meatus and travel through the ear canal to vibrate the tympanic membrane and bony structures of the middle ear, which in turn activate the receptors of the cochlea. Trauma or disease involving any portion of this pathway can affect hearing. **Tinnitus,** the perception of sound such as ringing, buzzing, or roaring in the ears, is another potential result of problems affecting the auditory system (Andreoli et al., 1990).

Disorders of the external ear, including the auricle, auditory meatus, and ear canal, can affect the conduction of sound waves and hearing. Obstruction of the external auditory canal or damage to the tympanic membrane, which separates the outer from the middle ear, may lead to conductive hearing loss (Bullock & Rosendahl, 1992). Infection or inflammation, trauma, and obstruction of the ear canal with cerumen (wax) or a foreign body are the most common conditions affecting the external ear.

Disorders of the middle ear, the area between the internal tympanic membrane and the cochlea, may be either acute or chronic. Unless these disorders are treated promptly and effectively, damage and scarring of middle ear structures can result in a permanent conductive hearing loss. Infectious or inflammatory disorders such as otitis media and mastoiditis are the most common conditions affecting the middle ear. Otosclerosis, a genetic condition, may also affect the structures of the middle ear.

The Client with External Otis

■ ■ ■

External otitis is a common inflammation of the ear canal. Commonly known as *swimmer's ear,* it is most prevalent in people who spend significant time in the water. Competitive athletes, including swimmers, divers, and surfers, are particularly prone to external otitis. Wearing a hearing aid or ear plugs, which hold moisture in the ear canal, is an additional risk factor. Although *Pseudomonas aeruginosa* or other bacterial infection is the most common cause, external otitis may also be due to fungal infection or a local hypersensitivity reaction (Andreoli et al., 1990; Porth, 1994; Schelkun, 1991).

Pathophysiology

Disruption of the normal environment within the external auditory canal typically precedes the inflammatory process. Retained moisture, cleaning, or drying of the ear canal remove the protective layer of cerumen, an acidic, water-repellent substance with antimicrobial properties. Its removal leaves the skin of the ear canal vulnerable to invasion and infection. For surfers, the presence of *exos-*

toses, bony growths in the ear canals resulting from prolonged exposure to cold, predisposes to impaction and retained moisture within the canal (Schelkun, 1991).

The client with external otitis often complains of a feeling of fullness in the ear. Ear pain typically is present and may be severe. The pain of otitis externa can be differentiated from that associated with otitis media by manipulation of the auricle or tragus. In external otitis this maneuver increases the pain, whereas the client with otitis media experiences no change in pain perception. Odorless watery or purulent drainage may be present. The ear canal appears inflamed and edematous on examination.

Collaborative Care

Management of the client with an external ear disorder focuses on restoring the normal balance of the external ear and canal and teaching the client how to prevent future problems.

For otitis externa, the following steps are recommended in treatment (Schelkun, 1991):

- Thorough cleansing of the ear canal, particularly if drainage or debris is present
- Treatment of the infection with local or, if necessary, systemic antibiotic agents
- Medication to relieve the pain and itching
- Teaching on the prevention of future episodes of swimmer's ear

The recurrent nature of otitis externa in swimmers, divers, and surfers makes the last step of the treatment plan a vital one. The box on page 1916 outlines the teaching for clients who are at risk for external otitis.

A topical antibiotic is often prescribed for the treatment of otitis externa. A topical corticosteroid may be ordered in combination with the antibiotic to provide immediate relief of the pain, swelling, and itching. Polymyxin B-neomycin-hydrocortisone (Cortisporin Otic) is a typical combination preparation used to treat external otitis; these antibiotics are effective against *Pseudomonas,* the most common infective organism. It is important to identify known sensitivity to any of the drugs in this preparation prior to initiating therapy. Clients who are sensitive to neomycin may develop dermatitis, which necessitates stopping the drug. Other preparations such as 1% tolnaftate solution (Tinactin) may be prescribed for a fungal infection of the ear canal (Schelkun, 1991).

Nursing Care

External otitis can cause the client to experience severe pain and discomfort. Although the disorder is rarely serious enough to require hospitalization, the nurse teaches

Teaching to Prevent External Otitis

■ ■ ■

- Stay out of the water until the acute inflammatory process is completely resolved. Ideally, allow 7 to 10 days before resuming water activities.

- Take precautions to keep the ear canal dry while in the water.
  a. Use silicone earplugs, which can keep water out of the ear without reducing hearing significantly.
  b. Wear a tight-fitting swim cap or wet suit hood, especially in cold ocean water. Although these do not prevent water from entering the ear, they protect the ear from the cold and possibly slow the formation of bony growths in the ears. They also protect the ear from sand and other water debris.

- Immediately after swimming, dry the ear canal. Allow water to drain by tilting the head and jumping to shake water out of the ear. Dry the outer ear with a towel, then use a hair dryer on the lowest setting several inches from the ear to dry the canal.

- Do not insert cotton swabs or other objects into the ear canal to dry it. This removes the protective layer of cerumen and may damage the skin of the canal, increasing the risk of bacterial infection. In addition, if debris such as sand is present, the swab may actually push debris further into the canal, forming an impacted mass.

- Use a drying agent in the ear canal after swimming. A 2% acetic acid solution or 2% boric acid in ethyl alcohol is effective in drying the canal and restoring its normal acidic environment.

- If it is necessary to remove impacted debris from the ear canal, irrigate the ear with warm tap water. A bulb syringe available over the counter or a 20 mL syringe attached to a short Teflon intravenous catheter (with the needle removed) is effective. With the head tilted toward the affected side, direct a stream of warm water toward the upper wall of the ear canal, allowing the water to run out into a bowl or sink. Repeated instillations may be necessary to break up and flush out impacted wax and debris.

Adapted from: Swimmer's Ear: Getting Patients Back in the Water by P. H. Schelkun in *The Physician and Sports Medicine*, 19(7), 85–88, 90.

the client about the disorder, comfort measures, and prevention of future episodes.

Impaired Tissue Integrity

External otitis may result from attempts to clean the ear canal with a toothpick, cotton-tipped applicator, or other implement that damages the skin, allowing an infectious organism to invade the tissue. Even if the canal is not damaged by attempts to clean it, the cleaning process often interrupts normal mechanisms, causing cerumen and debris to collect in the canal. This collected debris, in turn, tends to trap water within the canal, causing maceration of the skin.

Nursing interventions with rationales follow:

- Inform clients that ear canals rarely need cleansing beyond washing of the external meatus with soap and water. Teach clients of all ages not to clean ear canals with any implement. *"Cleaning" increases the risk of tissue damage and impairs the normal mechanism that clears the canal of accumulated cerumen and debris.*

- Teach the client (and, if necessary, a family member or friend) how to instill prescribed ear drops:
  a. Wash the hands.
  b. Warm the medication briefly by holding the container in the hand or placing it in a pocket for approximately 5 minutes before instilling the drops. *Warming the medication promotes comfort.*
  c. Lie on the unaffected side; if sitting, tilt the head toward the unaffected side. *This position allows gravity to assist in moving the medication to the inner portion of the ear canal.*
  d. Partially fill the ear dropper with medication.
  e. Using the nondominant hand, straighten the ear canal by pulling the pinna of the ear up and back. *Straightening helps the medication travel along the length of the canal.*
  f. Administer the prescribed number of drops into the ear canal. *It is important that the full amount of prescribed medication be administered to penetrate the length of the canal and achieve full effectiveness.*
  g. Remain in the side-lying position for approximately 5 minutes after the instillation of drops. *This position allows the medication to penetrate into deeper portions of the canal and prevents it from running out when the head is moved upright.*
  h. Loosely place a small piece of cotton in the auditory meatus for 15 to 20 minutes. *The cotton helps retain the medication within the canal.*

- Teach the client to avoid getting water in the affected ear until it is fully healed. Cotton balls may be used while showering to prevent water from entering the ear canal. The client should refrain from water sports and activities until approved by the primary care provider. *Retained moisture in the ear canal can further impair skin integrity, increasing inflammation.*

Applying Research to Nursing Practice: Ear-Cleaning Practices and Hearing Loss

■ ■ ■

A descriptive study of the incidence of cerumen impaction, ear-cleaning practices, and hearing loss in three groups of adults over the age of 60 included people living independently and participating in senior citizen center activities, and clients in personal care homes and nursing homes (Ney, 1993). The researchers found that individuals living independently had significantly fewer cerumen impactions than those in the other groups. This finding may reflect the higher level of activity of the independent adults, facilitating the natural drainage of cerumen from the ear canal, or better hygiene practices of that group. Approximately one-third of the subjects inserted an object (usually a cotton-tipped applicator) into the ear canal for the purpose of cleaning on a regular or periodic basis.

Some degree of hearing deficit was demonstrated in two-thirds of the subjects, with 18% of the population unable to hear any tone presented. Loss at the highest frequency was the most common deficit noted.

Implications for Nursing

This study demonstrates the potential role nurses can play in identifying hearing deficits, preventing further conductive deficit from impacted cerumen, and teaching clients about appropriate ear-hygiene measures.

The higher incidence of impacted cerumen in residents of personal care homes and nursing homes demonstrates the need for routine assessment of the ear canal and cleaning as necessary. Clients who routinely clean the ear canals using an object such as a cotton-tipped swab, hairpin, paper clip, or nail need to be taught alternative methods. Several subjects in this study used alcohol or hydrogen peroxide to soften cerumen; only one used a commercial product specifically for that purpose. Nurses can have a positive impact by increasing awareness of acceptable alternatives.

Critical Thinking in Client Care

1. Why is the resident of a personal care home or nursing home at higher risk for developing a cerumen impaction?

2. How can nurses in these settings prevent cerumen from accumulating to this degree?

3. How can the nurse in a long-term care setting screen the hearing of the residents to identify possible deficits?

Other Nursing Diagnoses

The following nursing diagnoses may also be appropriate for the client with external otitis:

- *Pain* related to acute inflammatory process
- *Sleep Pattern Disturbance* related to ear discomfort
- *Risk for Noncompliance* with water activity restrictions related to desire to continue training

Client and Family Teaching

The client is ultimately responsible for carrying out the prescribed treatment regimen in external otitis and for implementing measures to prevent future episodes. Teaching is vital. Provide verbal and written instructions on use of the prescribed medications. Teach the client care measures to prevent recurrent episodes (see the box on page 1916).

Cellulitis of the surrounding tissue is a possible complication of external otitis. Instruct the client to report to the primary care provider any increase in pain, swelling, or redness of surrounding tissues; fever; or other manifestations of infection such as malaise or increased fatigue.

The Client with Impacted Cerumen and Foreign Bodies

■ ■ ■

The external auditory canal can be obstructed by cerumen or foreign bodies. The curved shape and narrow lumen of the canal make it particularly vulnerable to obstruction.

As cerumen dries, it moves down and out of the ear canal. In some individuals it tends to accumulate, narrowing the canal. Aging is a risk factor for cerumen impaction, because less is produced and it is harder and drier. The accumulation of cerumen is often aggravated by attempting to remove it using cotton-tipped swabs or hairpins, which pack it more deeply into the ear canal. The accompanying box summarizes a study of cerumen impaction, common ear-cleaning practices, and hearing acuity in a population of older adults.

A variety of objects become foreign bodies in the ear canal. In adults, implements used to clean the ear canal may break and become lodged. Insects also may enter the ear canal and be unable to exit.

When the ear canal becomes occluded with either cerumen or a foreign body, the client experiences a conductive hearing loss in the affected ear. The client reports a sensation of fullness, along with tinnitus and coughing due to stimulation of the vagal nerve. The foreign body or impacted cerumen may be visualized on otoscopy. Impacted cerumen appears as a yellow, brown, or black mass in the canal (Porth, 1994).

Treatment focuses on clearing the canal. If there is no evidence of tympanic membrane perforation, irrigation of the canal is often the initial therapy.

Impacted wax, objects, or insects may require physical removal using an ear curet, forceps, or right-angle hook inserted via an otoscope and ear speculum. Mineral oil or topical lidocaine drops are used to immobilize or kill insects prior to their removal from the ear. When an organic foreign body such as a bean or an insect is suspected, water should not be instilled into the ear canal, because it may cause the object to swell, making its removal more difficult. Smooth, round objects present the biggest challenge to remove from the ear canal. Suction applied using a piece of soft intravenous tubing may be effective.

Nurses are often involved in identifying and relieving obstructions of the ear canal, especially in outpatient and community settings. Any client with evidence of a new conductive hearing loss or complaints of discomfort and fullness in one ear should be evaluated for possible obstruction. Inability to visualize the tympanic membrane or observation of a dark, shiny mass obstructing the canal may indicate a need for an irrigation or other procedure to clear the canal. It is important to determine that the tympanic membrane is intact prior to irrigation procedures; assessment by a physician or advanced practitioner may be necessary if a ruptured membrane is suspected.

Because obstruction of the ear canal with cerumen or a foreign body is generally preventable, teaching is a key component of nursing care. Clients need to know appropriate care measures for the external ear. Although the ear canal rarely needs cleaning, the client prone to cerumen impaction needs teaching about the use of mineral oil or commercial products to soften wax and of irrigation to remove it. All clients should understand the importance of not inserting anything smaller than a finger wrapped with a washcloth into the ear canal to avoid trauma to the canal or eardrum. Stress the risk of impacting cerumen against the tympanic membrane when using cotton-tipped swabs to clean the ear canal. Additionally, the swab may break and lodge in the canal. If ear drops have been prescribed, teach the client and a family member how to instill them.

The Client with Otitis Media

■ ■ ■

Otitis media, inflammation or infection of the middle ear, primarily affects infants and young children but may also occur in adults. The tympanic membrane, which separates the middle ear from the external auditory canal, protects the middle ear from the external environment. The auditory (eustachian) tube connects the middle ear with the nasopharynx to help equalize the pressure in the middle ear with the atmospheric pressure. Unfortunately, this connecting tube also provides a route by which infectious organisms enter the middle ear from the nose and throat, causing otitis media, the most common disease of the middle ear.

Pathophysiology

There are two primary forms of otitis media: (1) serous and (2) acute or suppurative. Both forms are associated with upper respiratory infection and auditory tube dysfunction. The auditory tube is narrow and flat, normally opening only during yawning and swallowing. Allergies or upper respiratory tract infections can cause edema of the tube lining, impairing its function. Air within the middle ear is trapped and gradually absorbed, creating negative pressure in this space.

Serous Otitis Media

Serous otitis media occurs when the auditory tube is obstructed for a prolonged time, impairing equalization of air pressure in the middle ear. Air within the middle ear space is gradually absorbed; the tube obstruction prevents more air from entering the middle ear. The resulting negative pressure in the middle ear causes sterile serous fluid to move from the capillaries into the space, forming a sterile effusion of the middle ear.

Upper respiratory infection or allergies such as hay fever predispose the client to serous otitis media. Clients with narrowed or edematous auditory tubes may also be subject to *barotrauma* or *barotitis media*. In these clients, the middle ear cannot adapt to rapid changes in barometric pressure as occur during air travel or underwater diving. Barotrauma tends to occur during descent in an airplane, because negative pressure within the middle ear causes the auditory tube to collapse and lock. However, underwater diving places even greater stress on the auditory tube and middle ear (Tierney et al., 1994).

Typical manifestations of serous otitis media include decreased hearing in the affected ear and complaints of "snapping" or "popping" in the ear. On examination, the tympanic membrane demonstrates decreased mobility and may appear retracted or bulging. Fluid or air bubbles are often visible behind the drum. Severe pressure differences as occur with barotrauma may cause acute pain, hemorrhage into the middle ear, rupture of the tympanic membrane, or even rupture of the round window with sensory hearing loss and severe vertigo (Berkow & Fletcher, 1992; Tierney et al., 1994). Hemotympanum, bleeding into or behind the tympanic membrane, may be observed on otoscopic examination.

Acute Otitis Media

The auditory tube also provides a route for the entry of pathogens into the normally sterile middle ear, resulting in *acute* or *suppurative otitis media*. Acute otitis media typically follows an upper respiratory infection. Edema of the auditory tube impairs drainage of the middle ear, causing mucus and serous fluid to accumulate. This fluid is an excellent environment for the growth of bacteria, which may enter from the oronasopharynx via the auditory tube. Although a viral upper respiratory infection may predispose the client to a middle ear infection, the bacteria *Streptococcus pneumoniae, Haemophilus influenzae,* and *Streptococcus pyogenes* account for most cases of otitis media in adults. Invasion and colonization of the middle ear by bacteria and the resultant migration of white blood cells cause pus formation. Accumulated pus can increase middle ear pressure sufficiently to rupture the tympanic membrane. The bacterial infection may also migrate internally, causing mastoiditis, brain abscess, or bacterial meningitis. A more common complication of otitis media is a persistent conductive hearing loss, which typically resolves when the middle ear effusion clears (Porth, 1994; Wilson et al., 1991).

The client with acute otitis media experiences pain, which may be severe, in the affected ear. The client's temperature is often elevated. Diminished hearing, dizziness, **vertigo** (a sensation of whirling or rotation), and tinnitus are common associated complaints. Pus within the mastoid air cells often causes mastoid tenderness in acute otitis media. On otoscopic examination, the tympanic membrane appears red and inflamed or dull and bulging (Figure 44–12). Decreased movement of the membrane is demonstrated by tympanometry or air insufflation. Spontaneous rupture of the tympanic membrane releases a purulent discharge. **Myringotomy** (an incision of the tympanic membrane) may be performed to relieve the pressure.

Collaborative Care

The diagnosis of otitis media is usually based on the client's history and the physical examination. The tympanic membrane may be visualized with a pneumatic otoscope that allows a puff of air to be instilled into the ear canal so that the examiner can evaluate the mobility of the tympanic membrane. Generally, the tympanic membrane moves slightly when air is instilled or the client performs the Valsalva maneuver. Less movement is seen in clients with auditory tube dysfunction and acute otitis media with effusion.

Laboratory and Diagnostic Tests

Impedance audiometry, also known as tympanometry, is an accurate diagnostic test for otitis media with effusion. In this test, an audiometer with a sealed probe tip is used to

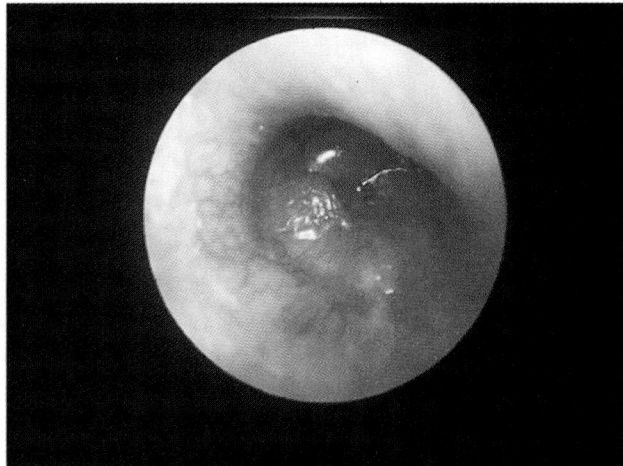

Figure 44–12   A red, bulging tympanic membrane of otitis media.

deliver a continuous tone to the tympanic membrane. The instrument also records the energy reflected from the surface of the tympanic membrane, allowing measurement of the compliance of the tympanic membrane and middle ear system. With middle ear effusion, compliance is reduced (Way, 1994).

A CBC may be performed to assess for an elevated WBC indicative of acute bacterial infection. If the tympanic membrane has ruptured or a tympanocentesis or myringotomy is performed, drainage is cultured to determine the infecting organism.

Pharmacology

Auditory tube dysfunction and serous otitis media are treated with decongestants and autoinflation of the middle ear. Decongestants are used to reduce the mucosal edema of the auditory tube and improve its patency. They may be administered either systemically or by intranasal spray. Antihistamines may be used to relieve obstruction in clients with allergies. Refer to Chapter 33 for further discussion and the nursing implications of these medications.

The client with auditory tube dysfunction may be taught to autoinflate the middle ear by performing the Valsalva maneuver or by forcefully exhaling against closed nostrils. Additionally, the client is advised to avoid air travel and underwater diving.

Acute otitis media is treated with antibiotic therapy, often in combination with decongestants. Penicillin, erythromycin, amoxicillin, trimethoprim-sulfamethoxazole, or cefaclor are commonly prescribed and effective against most organisms infecting the middle ear. Therapy may be continued for 12 to 14 days to ensure eradication of the infective organism. Nursing care of the client receiving antibiotic therapy is included in the pharmacology box on page 257 of Chapter 8. Symptomatic relief may be provided by analgesics, antipyretics, and local application of heat.

Surgery

A myringotomy or tympanocentesis may be performed to relieve excess pressure in the middle ear and prevent spontaneous rupture of the eardrum. To perform a *tympanocentesis,* the physician inserts a 20-gauge spinal needle through the inferior portion of the tympanic membrane, allowing aspiration of fluid and pus from the middle ear to relieve pressure and, if necessary, obtain a specimen for culture. Myringotomy, or surgical drainage of the middle ear, may be performed to relieve severe pain or when complications of acute otitis media, such as mastoiditis, are present. As soon as the pressure is released, pain subsides and hearing improves (Porth, 1994; Wilson et al., 1991).

Clients who do not respond to antibiotic therapy may require myringotomy with insertion of ventilation (tympanostomy) tubes. Indications for ventilation tube insertion include

- Failure of the infection to respond to 3 months of antibiotic therapy with amoxicillin-clavulanate potassium (Augmentin) or sulfamethoxazole

- Persistent and severe negative middle ear pressures

- Impending cholesteatoma (See the next section of this chapter.)

These small tubes are inserted into the inferior portion of the tympanic membrane, providing for ventilation and drainage of the middle ear during healing. The tube is eventually extruded from the ear, and the tympanic membrane heals. While the tube is in place, it is important to avoid getting any water in the ear canal and potentially into the middle ear space.

Nursing Care

Clients with otitis media are commonly seen and treated in outpatient and community settings. The nursing role is primarily one of support and education. Pain can be a significant problem for clients with otitis media, as well as the risk of damage to delicate tissues of the middle ear by the infectious and inflammatory processes.

Pain

Tissue edema, effusion of the middle ear, and the inflammatory response can affect the pain-sensitive tissues of the middle ear in otitis media, causing acute discomfort. This discomfort is increased by pressure changes, such as those that occur during air travel or underwater diving.

Nursing interventions with rationales follow:

- Assess the client's pain for severity, quality, and location. *A thorough assessment is important to determine the source of the pain. The pain of otitis media, unlike that of external otitis, is not aggravated by movement of the external ear.*

- Instruct the client to use mild analgesics such as aspirin or acetaminophen every 4 hours as needed to relieve pain and fever. *These nonprescription medications are effective in reducing the perception of pain. Aspirin also has anti-inflammatory properties that may help relieve the inflammation of the ear.*

- Advise the client to apply heat to the affected side unless contraindicated. *Heat dilates blood vessels, promoting the reabsorption of fluid and reducing swelling.*

- Instruct the client to avoid air travel, rapid changes in elevation, or diving. *A rapid change in barometric pressure can increase the client's pain significantly.*

- Instruct the client to report promptly an abrupt relief of pain to the primary care provider. *Pain that subsides abruptly may indicate spontaneous perforation of the tympanic membrane with relief of pressure within the middle ear.*

Impaired Tissue Integrity

Altered pressures within the middle ear and the inflammatory process affect delicate tissues of the middle ear. In acute otitis media, pus forms within the middle ear space and mastoid air cells. Unless the condition is treated, the tympanic membrane may rupture or chronic otitis media may develop. In chronic otitis media, mucosal changes occur, granulation (scar) tissue may develop, and changes in the ossicular chain may result.

Nursing interventions with rationales follow:

- Stress the importance of completing the full prescribed dose of antibiotic therapy. *Completion of the full course of antibiotic is important to ensure eradication of the infecting organisms and prevent development of antibiotic-resistant forms of the microbe.*

- Discuss the desired and potential adverse effects of the prescribed antibiotic. Tell the client to report any adverse effects to the physician. Stress the importance of not discontinuing the medication unless the primary care provider so advises. *If the client develops manifestations of an allergy or adverse response to the medication, or if the desired effect is not achieved, a different antibiotic may be prescribed.*

- Inform the client that antibiotic therapy may cause diarrhea, vaginitis, or thrush because these drugs destroy normal body flora. Unless contraindicated, instruct the client to consume 8 oz of yogurt containing live bacterial cultures daily while antibiotic therapy continues. *Live yogurt cultures help restore normal gastrointestinal and body flora, preventing superinfection.*

- Stress the importance of complying with recommended follow-up examinations. *Follow-up is impor-*

tant to confirm cure of the infection and prevent chronic otitis media.

- Instruct the client who has tubes inserted to avoid swimming, diving, or submerging the head while bathing as long as the tubes are in place. *Water can enter the ear canal and the middle ear through the ventilation tubes.*
- Instruct the client to avoid air travel, rapid changes in elevation, or diving. *A rapid change in barometric pressure can cause bruising, hematoma, or hemorrhage of the middle ear.*
- Encourage the client to rest, drink ample amounts of fluid, and consume a nutritious diet. *These general health measures enhance the function of the client's immune system and hasten resolution of the infection.*

Other Nursing Diagnoses

The following nursing diagnoses may also be appropriate for the client with otitis media:

- *Sensory/Perceptual Alteration: Auditory* related to conductive hearing loss associated with middle ear effusion
- *Risk for Noncompliance* with prescribed therapeutic regimen related to lack of understanding
- *Risk for Injury* related to potential perforation of tympanic membrane

Client and Family Teaching

The client who has otitis media needs teaching about the disorder, its causes and prevention, and any specific treatment recommended or prescribed.

When antibiotic therapy is prescribed, teach the client about the drug, its effects, recommended administration (with or without food, doses evenly spaced throughout the day), and possible side effects. The client also needs to know about symptoms of allergic or adverse reactions that should be reported to the physician. Stress the importance of completing all ordered doses of the medication to ensure eradication of the infection.

If surgical intervention is necessary, teach the client and family members about the surgery and postoperative care. Provide instruction about any special postoperative precautions, such as avoiding water in the ear canals or avoiding sudden changes in air pressure.

The Client with Acute Mastoiditis

■ ■ ■

The mastoid process is a portion of the temporal bone of the skull lying adjacent to the middle ear. It is full of air cavities called *mastoid air cells* or *mastoid sinuses*. The infection of acute otitis media always extends into the mastoid air cells; effective treatment of acute otitis media eliminates the infection from the mastoid cells as well. When treatment of acute otitis media is ineffective, pus remains in the mastoid air cells, and acute **mastoiditis,** bacterial infection of the mastoid process, may develop.

Pathophysiology

In acute mastoiditis, the bony septa between mastoid air cells are destroyed and cells coalesce to form large spaces. Portions of the mastoid process are eroded. With chronic infection, an abscess may form, or bony sclerosis of the mastoid may result. Acute mastoiditis increases the risk of meningitis because only a very thin bony plate separates mastoid air cells from the brain (Marieb, 1992). Fortunately, this complication is rare since the advent of effective antibiotic therapy for treating otitis media.

Manifestations of acute mastoiditis usually develop approximately 2 to 3 weeks after an episode of acute otitis media and include recurrent earache and hearing loss on the affected side. The pain is persistent and throbbing; tenderness is present over the mastoid process (behind the ear). It may also be red and inflamed. Swelling of the process can cause the auricle of the ear to protrude more than normal. Fever may be present. Tinnitus and headache may also be present. Profuse drainage from the affected ear may be noted.

Collaborative Care

In addition to the clinical manifestations of acute mastoiditis, loss of septa between mastoid air cells may be noted on radiologic examination. Acute mastoiditis is treated aggressively with antibiotic therapy. Intravenous penicillin, ceftriaxone (Rocephin), or metronidazole (Flagyl) may be used initially, with therapy tailored to the specific organism once culture results are obtained. Antibiotics are continued for at least 14 days. Infections that do not respond to medical therapy or that pose a high risk of spreading to the brain may necessitate *mastoidectomy,* surgical removal of the infected mastoid air cells, bone, and pus, and inspection of the underlying dura for possible abscess. The extent of tissue destruction determines the extent of surgery required. In a modified mastoidectomy, as much tissue is preserved as possible to avoid disruption of hearing. A radical mastoidectomy involves removal of middle ear structures including the incus and malleus as well as the diseased portions of the mastoid process. Unless reconstruction is performed at the time of surgery, this surgery results in conductive hearing loss. **Tympanoplasty,** surgical reconstruction of the middle ear, can restore or preserve hearing.

Nursing Care

The primary focus of collaborative and nursing care related to mastoiditis is on its prevention. Adequate, effective antibiotic treatment of acute otitis media prevents mastoiditis in nearly all instances. It is vital, therefore, that clients understand the importance of complying fully with prescribed antibiotic therapy and recommendations for follow-up.

Following surgical intervention, the wound and drainage are assessed carefully for evidence of infection or other complications. The client's hearing may be temporarily or permanently affected, depending on the extent of the surgery. If the client has impaired hearing in the unaffected ear as well, develop a means of communication with the client prior to surgery if possible. If the hearing is preserved in the unaffected ear, position the client with that ear toward the door. Speak slowly and clearly; do not shout or increase the volume of the voice. Be sure that family and staff know about the client's hearing loss and use appropriate communication techniques. Assist the client with ambulation initially, because dizziness and vertigo are not unusual following surgery. Nursing care of the client having ear surgery is included in the accompanying box.

Client and Family Teaching

When teaching about acute mastoiditis, stress the importance of complying with the prescribed antibiotic therapy. Instruct the client and family to report any adverse reactions to the primary care provider so that therapy can be adjusted if necessary. Teach the client and family how to change the surgical dressing if necessary using aseptic technique. Provide referrals to appropriate community agencies for the client with a new hearing loss resulting from mastoiditis or its treatment.

The Client with Chronic Otitis Media

■ ■ ■

Chronic otitis media involves permanent perforation of the tympanic membrane, with or without recurrent pus formation and often accompanied by changes in the mucosa and bony structures (ossicles) of the middle ear. Chronic otitis media is usually a consequence of recurrent acute otitis media and auditory tube dysfunction but may also result from trauma or other diseases.

Marginal perforations, which usually occur in the posterior-superior portion of the tympanic membrane, are associated with more complications than central perforations. With marginal perforations, squamous epithelium may migrate from the ear canal into the middle ear, where

it begins to desquamate and accumulate, forming a *cholesteatoma* (a cyst or mass filled with epithelial cell debris). Its incidence is highest in young adults. The desquamating epithelium continues to accumulate and remains infected, producing collagenases (enzymes) that destroy adjacent bone. The inflammatory process compromises blood supply to the stapes, causing its destruction and conductive hearing loss. Cholesteatomas are benign and slow-growing tumors, which can enlarge to fill the entire middle ear. Untreated, the cholesteatoma can progressively destroy the ossicles and erode into the inner ear, causing profound hearing loss (Way, 1994).

Systemic antibiotics are prescribed for exacerbations of purulent otitis media. The tympanic membrane perforation is repaired with a tympanoplasty to restore sound conduction and the integrity of the middle ear. Cholesteatoma requires more extensive surgery. A radical mastoidectomy may be performed with removal of the tympanic membrane, ossicles, and tumor. The mastoid air cells and middle ear are converted into an open cavity, which can be inspected and cleaned as necessary.

As with other complications of acute otitis media, a priority of nursing care is prevention of chronic otitis media and cholesteatoma. For clients with chronic otitis media, education is vital. The client needs to understand various treatment options and their risks and benefits, as well as the long-term risk of not treating a perforated tympanic membrane.

Do not irrigate the ear when the tympanic membrane is known or suspected to be perforated. Instill ear drops as prescribed, and clean the external auditory meatus as needed.

If surgical treatment of chronic otitis media will affect the client's hearing, include this information in preoperative teaching. Teach the client and family how to use alternative means of communication if this will be necessary postoperatively. When an assistive device is prescribed, teach both the client and a family member about its use and care.

The Client with Otosclerosis

■ ■ ■

Otosclerosis is a common cause of conductive hearing loss. Abnormal bone formation in the osseous labyrinth of the temporal bone causes the footplate of the stapes to become fixed or immobile in the oval window. The result is a conductive hearing loss.

Otosclerosis is a hereditary disorder with an autosomal dominant pattern of inheritance. It occurs most commonly in Caucasians and in females. The progressive hearing loss typically begins in adolescence or early adulthood and seems to be accelerated by pregnancy. Although both ears are affected, the rate of hearing loss is asymmetric. Because bone conduction of sound is retained, the

Nursing Care of the Client Having Ear Surgery

PREOPERATIVE CARE

- Ensure that the client has signed a consent form specific to the surgical procedure to be performed. *The presence of a signed consent on the chart verifies that the surgery to be performed as well as its risks, benefits, and alternative therapies have been explained to the client.*

- Assess the client's and family's knowledge and understanding of the procedure to be performed. Provide clarification as needed. *Adequate teaching in the preoperative period decreases anxiety and shortens the recovery period.*

- Assess the client's hearing or verify documentation of preoperative hearing assessment. *These data are important in evaluating the results of the surgical procedure.*

- Agree on a means of communication to be used after surgery. *Hearing may be impaired after surgery.*

- Explain postoperative expectations and precautions. Blowing of the nose, coughing, and sneezing are restricted to prevent pressure changes in the middle ear and potential disruption of the surgical site. Provide instructions on activities to be avoided and suggestions for minimizing them. If the client needs to cough or sneeze, leaving the mouth open minimizes pressure changes in the middle ear. *Providing teaching and the opportunity to practice before surgery promotes the client's cooperation in the postoperative period.*

- Perform preoperative procedures and administer medications as prescribed.

POSTOPERATIVE CARE

- Assess the client for bleeding or drainage from the affected ear. Note color, character, and amount of any drainage. *Infection and hemorrhage are possible complications.*

- Assess for nausea and vomiting; medicate with antiemetics as ordered. *Both the surgery and the effects of anesthesia/analgesia may cause nausea. Vomiting may increase the pressure in the middle ear, disrupting the surgical site.*

- Elevate the head of bed and have the client lie on the unaffected side. *This position minimizes the pressure in the middle ear.*

- Assess for vertigo or dizziness, especially with ambulation or movement in bed. Avoid unnecessary movements such as turning. Take measures to ensure safety when the client gets up and ambulates. *Surgery on the ear may disrupt the client's equilibrium, increasing the risk of falling.*

- Assess the client's hearing postoperatively. Stand on the client's unaffected side to communicate and use other measures such as written messages as needed for effective communication with the hearing-impaired client. Reassure the client that decreased hearing acuity immediately after surgery is expected. *Hearing improvement, if an expected result of the ear surgery, typically does not occur until ear plugs are removed, and edema and drainage at the operative site have resolved. If no reconstruction of the middle ear is done or the cochlea is involved, permanent hearing loss in the affected ear may be an expected result.*

- Remind client to avoid coughing, sneezing, or blowing the nose. *These increase pressure in the middle ear.*

- Provide instructions for home care.
  a. To prevent contamination of the ear canal, avoid showers, shampooing, and immersing the head until the physician says you can do so.
  b. Keep the outer ear plug clean and dry, changing it as needed. Do not remove inner ear dressing until the physician so orders.
  c. Avoid blowing the nose; if you need to cough or sneeze, keep the mouth open.
  d. Do not swim or dive without physician approval. Check with the physician regarding air travel.
  e. Meclizine hydrochloride (Antivert) or other antiemetic/antihistamine medication may be necessary for up to 1 month following surgery.
  f. Fever, bleeding, increased drainage, increased dizziness, or decreased hearing after discharge may indicate a complication. Notify the physician if any of these occur.

client may be able to use the telephone but have difficulty conversing in person. Tinnitus may also be associated with otosclerosis.

On examination, a reddish or pinkish-orange tympanic membrane may be noted because of increased vascularity of the middle ear. The Rinne test (see Chapter 43) shows bone sound conduction to be equal to or greater than air conduction, an abnormal finding.

Clients with otosclerosis may choose conservative treatment, relying on a hearing aid to improve their ability to hear and interact with others. Sodium fluoride may be prescribed to slow bone resorption and overgrowth. Surgical treatment for otosclerosis involves a stapedectomy and middle ear reconstruction or a stapedotomy. A *stapedectomy* is a microsurgical technique for removing the diseased stapes. A metallic prosthesis is then inserted, with one end connected to the incus and the other inserted into the oval window. *Stapedotomy* involves creation of a small hole in the footplate of the stapes and insertion of a wire or platinum ribbon prosthesis. An argon, KTP, or CO_2 laser may be employed for surgery (Bullock & Rosendahl, 1992; Porth, 1994; Way, 1994). Surgery usually restores hearing for the client with otosclerosis.

Education and referral of the client to appropriate community agencies are important nursing care priorities for the client with otosclerosis. For the client who chooses to undergo surgical treatment, nursing care is similar to that for other clients undergoing ear surgery (see the box on page 1923). The following nursing diagnoses may be appropriate:

- *Risk for Injury* related to hearing loss or postoperative vertigo
- *Sensory/Perceptual Alteration: Auditory* related to bony sclerosis of the stapes
- *Impaired Verbal Communication* related to hearing loss
- *Anxiety* related to concern about transmission of genetic disorder to children

The Client with an Inner Ear Disorder

■ ■ ■

Disorders affecting the inner ear are much less common than disorders of the outer or middle ear. Inner ear disorders affect equilibrium and may also affect sensorineural hearing, the perception of sound. Labyrinthitis and Meniere's disease are the most common diseases of the inner ear. Vertigo may be a disorder of the inner ear itself or a manifestation of other disorders.

Pathophysiology

The inner ear (also called the labyrinth) contains the cochlea and the semicircular canals. The hair cells and neurons that allow sound perception and transmission to the auditory center of the brain are in the cochlea. The semicircular canals filled with endolymph are the primary organs involved in maintaining equilibrium. Disruption of this portion of the ear by an inflammatory process or excess endolymph not only affects balance but may also result in permanent hearing loss.

Labyrinthitis

Labyrinthitis, also called *otitis interna,* is an inflammation of the inner ear. It is an uncommon disorder, because the bony protection of the membranous labyrinth makes it difficult for organisms to enter the inner ear. However, bacteria, viruses, and other organisms may enter and infect the inner ear through the oval window during acute otitis media, through the cochlear aqueduct during meningitis, or through the blood. Viral labyrinthitis is suspected when the client has a sudden onset of symptoms after an upper respiratory infection or when there is no evidence of concurrent otitis media.

Inflammation of the labyrinth typically causes vertigo, sensorineural hearing deficit, and **nystagmus** (rapid involuntary eye movements).

Vertigo, a sensation of motion when there is none, or an exaggerated sense of motion in response to movement, is the hallmark manifestation of inner ear disorders (Tierney et al., 1994). The vertigo of labyrinthitis is severe and often accompanied by nausea and vomiting. Any movement can aggravate the vertigo, and falling is a significant risk if the client attempts to stand. Vertigo lasts days to weeks in labyrinthitis, making client education a vital component of care.

Hearing loss in the ear affected by labyrinthitis may be temporary or permanent. If the inflammatory process results in tissue destruction of the membranous labyrinth, the hearing loss may be complete and permanent.

The involuntary rhythmic eye movements of nystagmus may not be present in all clients with labyrinthitis. When present, the eye movement is typically horizontal. Applying positive or negative pressure to the tympanic membrane of the affected ear may stimulate nystagmus, as will caloric testing (irrigating the ear canal with warm or cool water). Although nystagmus may also be a symptom of brain stem or cerebellar dysfunction, no vertigo or hearing loss is typically associated with those disorders.

Meniere's Disease

Meniere's disease, also known as *endolymphatic hydrops,* is a chronic disorder of unknown cause characterized by attacks of vertigo with tinnitus and a progressive unilateral hearing loss. This disorder affects an estimated 2.4 million Americans (Cleveland & Morris, 1990). It affects men and women equally, with adults between the ages of 35 and 60 in the highest risk group.

The cause of Meniere's disease is unclear. It is brought about by an overaccumulation of endolymph, the fluid in the membranous labyrinth of the inner ear. The lymphatic channels dilate in response, resulting in labyrinthine dysfunction (Porth, 1994; Tierney et al., 1994; Way, 1994). It is unclear whether this excess fluid results from an overproduction or decreased absorption of endolymph. Autonomic nervous system control of labyrinthine circulation may be impaired, or damage to the inner ear from severe otitis media or a head injury can precipitate Meniere's disease. A family history of the disease increases risk, suggesting a possible genetic link in some clients. In many clients, however, it is idiopathic.

The onset of Meniere's disease may be gradual or sudden. It is characterized by recurrent attacks of vertigo and gradual loss of hearing. The sensorineural hearing loss and associated tinnitus is usually unilateral. However, clients with Meniere's disease of one ear are at increased risk of developing it in the other. Attacks of severe rotary vertigo occur abruptly and often unpredictably, lasting from minutes to hours. In some cases, an attack may be linked to increased sodium intake, stress, allergies, vasoconstriction, or premenstrual fluid retention. Often no precipitating factor can be identified. The frequency and severity of attacks vary. As the disease continues and hearing loss progresses, episodes of vertigo often become less frequent and severe.

Although episodic, the vertigo of Meniere's disease can be severe enough to cause immobility, nausea, and vomiting. The client may relate a feeling of fullness in the ears, and a roaring or ringing sensation. Attacks are often accompanied by hypotension, sweating, and nystagmus.

Vertigo

Balance and posture are normally maintained by the integration of input from the labyrinths, eyes, muscles, joints, and neural centers. This input and integration can be affected by disorders of the labyrinth, vestibular nerve or nuclei, eyes, cerebellum, brain stem, or cerebral cortex, causing vertigo. Vertigo is a disorder of equilibrium. The sensation of whirling, rotation, or movement is described as either subjective or objective.

Clients with *subjective vertigo* report the sensation of being in motion in a stable environment. This is not always a sense of spinning; the client may have a sense of tumbling or falling forward or backward (Tierney et al., 1994). The sensation is reversed in *objective vertigo;* clients report a sensation of stability in a moving environment. This motion may be perceived as the room spinning around the client or the ground rocking beneath the client's feet. *Dizziness,* which may be mistaken for vertigo, is a sensation of unsteadiness, lack of balance, lightheadedness, or movement within the head. The person who is dizzy does not have the rotational sensation felt with vertigo.

Vertigo may be disabling, resulting in falls, injury, and difficulty walking. Attacks of vertigo are often accompanied by nausea and vomiting, nystagmus, and autonomic symptoms such as pallor, sweating, hypotension, and salivation (Bullock & Rosendahl, 1992; Porth, 1994).

Collaborative Care

The manifestations associated with inner ear disorders are very similar, making testing necessary to establish a diagnosis. Once the diagnosis is determined, collaborative care is directed toward managing symptoms and preventing permanent hearing loss.

The following diagnostic studies may be ordered for the client with symptoms of an inner ear disorder:

- *Electronystagmography* is a series of tests used to evaluate the vestibulo-ocular reflex by identifying eye movements (nystagmus) in response to specific stimuli. Caloric testing, the best known portion of this test battery, involves the direct instillation of water into the ear canal so that it contacts the tympanic membrane while eye motion is recorded. In clients with impaired vestibular function, the normal nystagmus response is blunted or absent. This portion of the test is contraindicated in clients who have a perforation of the tympanic membrane.

- The *Rinne and Weber tests* of hearing (see Chapter 43) show decreased air and bone conduction on the affected side if a sensorineural hearing loss is present. In Meniere's disease, audiology shows sensorineural hearing loss involving the low tones.

- *X-rays* and *CT scans* of the petrous bones are used to evaluate the internal auditory canal. In clients with Meniere's disease, the vestibular aqueducts may be shorter and straighter than normal.

- A hyperosmolar substance such as glycerin and urea or a fast-acting diuretic such as intravenous furosemide or acetazolamide may be administered to the client to decrease fluid pressure in the inner ear. An acute temporary hearing improvement is considered diagnostic for Meniere's disease.

Once the diagnosis is established for the client, specific treatments can be ordered. Clients with labyrinthitis or an acute attack of Meniere's disease may require hospitalization to manage the vertigo and its effects. Atropine is used to decrease the parasympathetic nervous system response. A central nervous system depressant such as diazepam (Valium) or lorazepam (Ativan) may be an alternative to atropine. Parenteral droperidol (Inapsine) provides both a sedative and antiemetic effect, making it a useful drug for acute attacks. Antivertigo/antiemetic medications such as meclizine (Antivert), prochlorperazine (Compazine), or hydroxyzine hydrochloride (Vistaril) are prescribed to reduce the whirling sensation and nausea. If the nausea and vomiting are severe, intravenous fluids may be necessary to maintain fluid and electrolyte balance. Bed rest in a quiet, darkened room with minimal sensory stimuli and minimal movement provides the most comfort for the client.

Large doses of antibiotics, often administered intravenously, are prescribed for labyrinthitis when the cause is thought to be bacterial. No specific therapy is indicated for viral labyrinthitis.

Management of the client between acute attacks of Meniere's disease is directed at preventing future attacks and preserving hearing. A low-sodium diet and an oral diuretic such as furosemide (Lasix) or hydrochlorothiazide/triamterene (Dyazide) help maintain a lower labyrinthine pressure. The Furstenberg diet, a salt-free neutral ash diet, may be prescribed if moderate sodium restriction is ineffective in controlling attacks. Tobacco, which causes vasoconstriction and can precipitate an attack, should be avoided, along with alcohol and caffeine.

When medical interventions are ineffective in controlling episodes of vertigo in Meniere's disease, surgical intervention may be necessary. Several procedures are available, which offer varying degrees of relief and hearing preservation.

Surgical *endolymphatic decompression* relieves the excess pressure in the labyrinth; a shunt is then inserted between the membranous labyrinth and the subarachnoid space to drain excess fluid away from the labyrinths and maintain lower pressure. This procedure preserves hearing for the majority of the clients. Vertigo is relieved in approximately 70% of clients, but the sensations of fullness and tinnitus remain for about 50% of people after the surgery.

Destruction of a portion of the acoustic nerve is an alternative to shunting procedures. In a *vestibular neurectomy,* the portion of the cranial nerve VIII controlling balance and sensations of vertigo is severed. This procedure relieves vertigo for up to 90% of clients. Although there is a risk of damage to the cochlear portion of the nerve and resultant hearing loss, for most clients hearing loss stabilizes after neurectomy, even improving for some.

The surgery of last resort for Meniere's disease is a **labyrinthectomy.** The labyrinth is completely removed, destroying cochlear function. This procedure is used only when hearing loss is nearly complete and vertigo is persistent. Although labyrinthectomy relieves vertigo in nearly all cases, the client may remain unsteady and have continued problems with balance (Cleveland & Morris, 1990; Porth, 1994).

Following surgery on the inner ear, the client is positioned to minimize ear pressure and vertigo. Movement of the client is restricted, and assistance is provided when the client gets up. Antiemetics and antivertigo medications are used to manage the symptoms resulting from disruption of the inner ear. Complications include infection and leakage of cerebral spinal fluid.

Nursing Care

The client with an inner ear disorder has multiple nursing care needs related to the manifestations of the disorder. The risk for trauma in clients with inner ear disorders is great. Attacks of vertigo may occur without warning and can be so severe that the client is unable to remain upright. Nausea and vomiting often accompany attacks of vertigo; the client's nutrition may be compromised if attacks are frequent. Constant or intermittent tinnitus can interfere with sleep and rest. Finally, because nearly all inner ear disorders are associated with some degree of hearing loss, which may be progressive, the client has significant psychosocial needs.

Risk for Trauma

Because of the unpredictable nature of attacks, the client with vertigo due to Meniere's disease, labyrinthitis, or another cause needs to learn strategies for dealing with an acute episode. Attacks may be debilitating, leaving the client unable to remain upright, and may be accompanied by nausea and vomiting. Poorly controlled vertigo may interfere with the client's ability to work and lead to social isolation. Because vertigo tends to be chronic except in acute viral labyrinthitis, the emphasis is on helping the client develop strategies to reduce the frequency of attacks and the risk of injury.

Nursing interventions with rationales follow:

- Assess the client for manifestations of vertigo, nystagmus, nausea and vomiting, and hearing loss. *Assessment is important to determine the severity of impairment, the duration of attacks, and the client's ability to predict an impending attack. The client who is able to predict an impending attack is more able to prevent trauma associated with an attack of acute vertigo.*

- Place the client experiencing an acute attack of vertigo on bed rest with the side rails elevated and the call light readily accessible. Instruct the client not to get up without assistance. *Movement should be restricted during an acute attack of vertigo to reduce the risk of falling and to minimize the associated nausea and vomiting.*

- Teach the client to avoid sudden head movements or position changes. *Sudden movement may precipitate an attack of vertigo.*

- Administer prescribed medications as ordered, including antiemetics, diuretics, and sedatives. *These medications may reduce the frequency, severity, and duration of vertigo attacks.*

- Instruct the client who senses an impending attack to respond by taking the prescribed medication and lying down in a quiet, darkened room. *These measures help protect the client from injury and may shorten the duration and reduce the severity of the attack.*

- Advise the client to pull to the side of the road and wait for the symptoms to subside if an attack occurs while the client is driving. *Perception and judgment necessary for safe driving may be impaired during an acute attack; pulling off the road is vital to protect the safety of the client and others.*

- Discuss the importance of wearing a medical alert bracelet or necklace. *A medical alert bracelet or tag may be essential to ensure appropriate medical intervention for the client who is debilitated by an acute attack of vertigo or who has experienced severe hearing loss as a result of an inner ear disorder.*

- Discuss the effect of unilateral hearing loss on the client's ability to identify the direction from which sounds come. To ensure safety, encourage the client to use other senses (e.g., when crossing the street). *Just as depth perception changes when vision is lost in one eye, sound perception and differentiation of direction change when hearing is lost unilaterally.*

Sleep Pattern Disturbance

The tinnitus often associated with inner ear disorders may be loud and continuous, interfering with the client's ability to concentrate, relax, and sleep. The sound perceived in tinnitus varies by individual and the mechanism causing it. It may be perceived as a continuous high-pitched whine, buzzing, ringing, or humming sound. In some clients, it may have a pulsatile quality.

Nursing interventions with rationales follow:

- Assess the client's tinnitus, including reported pitch, tone, quality, and duration. Refer the client for a complete hearing and ear examination if one has not been performed. *Although most tinnitus is associated with hearing loss, often due to noise exposure, it may also be associated with treatable conditions such as impacted cerumen, hypertension, cerebrovascular disorders, and other conditions.*

- Discuss options for masking tinnitus to promote concentration and sleep.
  a. Ambient noise from a radio or sound system
  b. A masking device or white-noise machine
  c. A hearing aid that produces a tone to mask the tinnitus
  d. A hearing aid that amplifies ambient sound
  These techniques or devices help mask the subjective perception of tinnitus, allowing the client to focus on something other than the sound.

- Discuss the possible risks and benefits of medications to treat tinnitus. *Many medications have been used to treat tinnitus; at this time, oral antidepressants such as nortriptyline (Aventyl, Pamelor) taken at bedtime have been shown to be most effective.*

Other Nursing Diagnoses

Although clients with inner ear disorders have individualized needs, the following additional nursing diagnoses may be appropriate:

- *Impaired Home Maintenance Management* related to unexpected attacks of vertigo
- *Sensory/Perceptual Alteration: Auditory* related to inflammation of the inner ear structures

- *Ineffective Individual Coping* related to disabling vertigo and hearing loss
- *Anticipatory Grieving* related to progressive unilateral hearing loss
- *Impaired Physical Mobility* related to vertigo

Client and Family Teaching

Because disorders of the inner ear disrupt balance, safety is a primary focus of teaching. Teach the client to change positions slowly, especially when ambulating. Turning the whole body rather than just the head helps to prevent the onset of vertigo; however, attacks can be unpredictable. The client should not ambulate alone unless in a safe environment. Teach the client to sit down immediately with the onset of vertigo and lie down if possible. Instruct the client about using prescribed antiemetic and antivertigo medications effectively to prevent episodes.

The client who is to have surgical intervention on the inner ear needs information about the surgical procedure, the immediate postoperative period, and the long-term effects of the surgery. If vertigo is expected in the initial postoperative period, inform the client. Teach techniques to minimize vertigo and associated nausea. Surgical intervention may result in permanent hearing loss in the affected ear. Teach alternative communication strategies for the client to use postoperatively.

The Client with an Acoustic Neuroma

■ ■ ■

An **acoustic neuroma** is a benign tumor of cranial nerve VIII. It typically occurs in adults between the ages of 40 and 50. Acoustic neuromas are among the most common intracranial tumors, accounting for 7% to 8% of intracranial tumors (Tierney et al., 1994; Way, 1994).

These tumors usually occur in the internal auditory meatus, compressing the auditory nerve where it exits the skull to the inner ear. Both the vestibular and cochlear branches are affected; however, the tumor arises from the vestibular division of the auditory nerve twice as often. If allowed to grow, the tumor eventually destroys the labyrinth, including the cochlea and vestibular apparatus. As the tumor expands, it erodes the wall of the internal auditory meatus. The tumor may eventually impinge on the inferior cerebellar artery, which provides blood to the lateral pons and medulla, the brain stem, and the cerebellum. An obstructive hydrocephalus can also occur. Cranial nerves VII (facial) and V (trigeminal) are often affected by the expanding tumor; the tumor frequently wraps around the facial nerve.

Early manifestations of an acoustic neuroma are those associated with disorders of the inner ear: tinnitus, unilateral hearing loss, and nystagmus. Dizziness or vertigo may occur. As the tumor expands and occupies increasing amounts of space in the closed cranium, the client experiences neurologic signs related to the area of the brain affected.

The presence of the tumor can generally be identified on CT or MRI scans. X-ray films of the petrous pyramid of the temporal bone may show erosion caused by the tumor.

The treatment of choice for an acoustic neuroma is surgical excision. In surgery, every effort is made to preserve this nerve and its function as well as other cranial nerves that may be affected. Small tumors of the vestibular division of the acoustic nerve may be excised using microsurgical techniques; hearing can often be preserved. A translabyrinthine approach provides good access to the tumor and allows the facial nerve to be preserved. However, this approach destroys hearing in the affected ear, and it is usually used only when the tumor is large or little effective hearing remains in the affected ear. Larger tumors require craniotomy for removal; facial nerve paralysis is a common result of surgery.

Postoperative nursing care focuses on preserving cerebral function. The client is positioned to minimize cerebral edema and monitored frequently for signs of increased intracranial pressure. Because the gag reflex may be affected, the client must be assessed carefully before food and fluids are allowed by mouth. Speech therapy is often prescribed for the client after surgery. Because deficits may not resolve for a long time after surgery, education and support are vital components of nursing care for the client. Further discussion of care for the client undergoing craniotomy is included in Chapter 40.

The Client with a Hearing Loss

■ ■ ■

It is estimated that approximately ten million adults in the United States are hearing impaired. The problem of hearing loss is particularly significant in older adults, affecting an estimated 13% to 27% of people over the age of 65 years and 38% to more than 50% of people over the age of 75 years (Burke & Walsh, 1992; O'Rourke et al., 1993). As many as 90% of nursing home residents have impaired hearing (Taylor, 1993).

Lesions in the outer ear, middle ear, inner ear, or central auditory pathways can result in hearing loss. The process of aging also can affect the structures of the ear and hearing. Hearing loss is classified as conductive, sensorineural, or mixed, depending on what portion of the auditory system is affected. Profound deafness is often a congenital condition.

Clients with a hearing loss, whether conductive or sensorineural, may display signs that caregivers can recognize. The voice volume of the hearing-impaired client frequently increases, and the client positions the head with the better ear toward the speaker. The client frequently may ask people to repeat what they have said or respond inappropriately to questions or statements. A question may elicit a blank look if the client has not heard or understood its content.

Pathophysiology

Hearing loss impairs the ability to communicate in a world filled with sound and hearing individuals. A hearing deficit can be partial or total, congenital or acquired. It may affect one or both ears. In some types of hearing loss, the ability to perceive sound at specific frequencies is lost. In others, hearing is diminished across all frequencies.

Conductive Hearing Loss

Anything that disrupts the transmission of sound from the external auditory meatus to the inner ear results in a conductive hearing loss. The most common cause of conductive hearing loss is obstruction of the external ear canal. Impacted cerumen, edema of the canal lining, stenosis, and neoplasms all may lead to canal obstruction. Other etiologic factors for conductive loss include a perforated tympanic membrane, disruption or fixation of the ossicles of the middle ear, fluid, scarring, or tumors of the middle ear (Andreoli et al., 1990; Porth, 1994; Wilson et al., 1991).

With conductive hearing loss, there is an equal loss of hearing at all sound frequencies. If the level of sound is greater than the threshold for hearing, speech discrimination is good (Andreoli et al., 1990). Because of this, the client with a conductive hearing loss is able to benefit from amplication by a hearing aid.

Sensorineural Hearing Loss

Disorders that affect the inner ear, the auditory nerve, or the auditory pathways of the brain may lead to a sensorineural hearing loss. In this type of hearing loss, sound waves are effectively transmitted to the inner ear. In the inner ear, however, lost or damaged receptor cells, changes in the cochlear apparatus, or auditory nerve abnormalities decrease or distort the ability to receive and interpret stimuli. Causes of acquired sensorineural hearing loss include trauma, vascular lesions or insufficiency, infections, and ototoxic medications (Porth, 1994).

Damage to the hair cells of the organ of Corti is a significant cause of sensorineural hearing deficit. In the United States, noise exposure is the major cause. Exposure to a high level of noise (for example, standing close to the stage or speakers at a rock concert) on an intermittent or continuing basis damages the hair and supporting cells of the organ of Corti. Ototoxic drugs also damage the hair cells; when combined with high noise levels, the damage is greater and resultant hearing loss more profound. Ototoxic drugs include the salicylates, furosemide (Lasix), the aminoglycoside antibiotics, antimalarial drugs, and some chemotherapeutic medications such as cisplatin (Platinol) and vancomycin (Vancocin) (Andreoli et al., 1990; Porth, 1994). When ototoxic drugs are administered concurrently (e.g., when the client is receiving both furosemide and an aminoglycoside antibiotic), the risk of sensory hearing loss is increased. Other potential causes of sensory hearing loss include viral infections, meningitis, trauma, Meniere's disease, and aging.

Tumors such as acoustic neuromas, vascular disorders, demyelinating or degenerative diseases, infections (bacterial meningitis in particular), or trauma may affect the central auditory pathways and produce a neural hearing loss (Wilson et al., 1991).

Sensorineural hearing losses typically affect the perception of high-frequency tones more than of low-frequency tones. This loss makes speech discrimination difficult, especially in a noisy environment. Hearing aids are often not very useful, because they amplify both speech and background noise. The increased sound intensity may actually cause discomfort for the client (Andreoli et al., 1990).

Presbycusis

With aging, the hair cells of the cochlea degenerate, producing a gradually progressive hearing loss. In presbycusis, hearing acuity begins to decrease in early adulthood and progresses as long as the individual lives. This is a type of sensorineural loss. As with noise-induced hearing loss, higher tones are lost initially (Andreoli et al., 1990; Porth, 1994).

Because the hearing loss of presbycusis is gradual, the client and family may not realize the extent of the deficit. The hearing-impaired individual may be described as unsociable or paranoid. The family may worry that the person is becoming increasingly forgetful, absent minded, or perhaps "senile." Depression, confusion, inattentiveness, tension, and negativism have all been noted in hearing-impaired older adults. Functional problems such as poor general health, reduced mobility, and impaired interpersonal communication are also associated with hearing loss (Taylor, 1993). Caregivers need to be alert for signs of impaired hearing such as cupping an ear, difficulty understanding verbal communication when the person cannot see the speaker's face, difficulty following conversation in a large group, and withdrawal from social activities. The research box on page 1930 describes a protocol for hearing screening for older adults.

Hearing aids and other amplification devices are useful for most clients with presbycusis.

Tinnitus

Tinnitus is the perception of sound or noise in the ears without stimulus from the environment. The sound may be steady, intermittent, or pulsatile and is often described as a buzzing, roaring, or ringing.

Tinnitus is usually associated with hearing loss (conductive or sensorineural); however, the mechanism producing the sound is poorly understood. It is often an early symptom of noise-induced hearing damage and drug-related ototoxicity. Tinnitus is especially associated with salicylate, quinine, or quinidine toxicity. Other etiologic conditions include obstruction of the auditory meatus, presbycusis, inflammations and infections of the middle or inner ear, otosclerosis, and Meniere's disease. Most tinnitus, however, is chronic and has no pathologic importance (Andreoli et al., 1990; Wilson et al., 1991).

Tinnitus that is intermittent or slight enough to be masked by environmental sounds is often well tolerated. When it is loud, continuous, and not responsive to treatment, tinnitus can be a significant stressor. It can interfere with activities of daily living, sleep, and rest.

Collaborative Care

The best treatment for hearing loss is prevention. Clients need to know the potential for hearing damage and how to prevent it. Awareness of the effects of noise exposure, especially when combined with the ototoxic effects of aspirin or other drugs, is important to prevent sensorineural hearing loss. Health care personnel can be instrumental in promoting the use of ear protectors and in the early detection and treatment of disorders affecting hearing.

Assessment of the client with a hearing loss begins with evaluation of the external ear canal, tympanic membrane, and upper respiratory tract. It is important to rule out obstructive, infectious, or inflammatory causes of hearing loss. Treatment may restore or preserve hearing. Associated symptoms such as vertigo, tinnitus, unsteadiness, or imbalance should be evaluated. Cranial nerve function is also assessed.

Laboratory and Diagnostic Tests

Hearing evaluation includes gross tests of hearing (such as the whisper test), the Rinne and Weber tests, and audiometry.

- The *Rinne and Weber tests* compare air and bone sound conduction. When bone conduction of sound is better than air conduction, the hearing deficit is a conductive loss. The Rinne test is able to identify even mild conductive hearing losses. If both air and bone conduction are impaired, a sensorineural loss is indicated. (See Chapter 43.)

Applying Research to Nursing Practice:
Meeting the Needs of Older Adults with Hearing Loss

■ ■ ■

The population is aging. Because hearing deficits become more severe and prevalent with aging, hearing loss can potentially become a more significant problem than it is currently. Nurses are often the primary care providers for the older people in their homes or extended care facilities. Screening for hearing deficits is an important nursing responsibility.

One study (O'Rourke, Britten, Gatschet, & Krien, 1993) has demonstrated that a hearing-screening protocol is an effective means of identifying hearing deficits in the elderly. The researchers used an abbreviated case history with questions related to recent episodes of ear discharge, dizziness, ear pain, and a change in hearing along with otoscopic visual inspection of the ears and a pure-tone screening test. The researchers were able to identify all but 3 individuals out of a group of 60 who had a hearing deficit or were at risk.

Implications for Nursing

Nurses can identify clients who are at risk for a hearing deficit by incorporating questions about the ears and recent changes in hearing in the nursing history, routinely inspecting the ears as part of the physical assessment, and either performing or referring the client for audiometric testing. This screening allows for earlier intervention and referral of the client. In addition, when the client is identified as having or being at risk for a hearing loss, nurses can use communication techniques that enhance the client's understanding. Recommendations for safety and alternatives for socialization can be provided as well.

Critical Thinking in Client Care

In this study, subjects were also interviewed using the Hearing Handicap Inventory for the Elderly—Screening Version. This inventory asks questions related to the client's perception of a hearing problem interfering with meeting new people, causing frustration in talking to family members, causing arguments, hampering the client's personal or social life, and so on. This tool did not identify 15 subjects to be at risk who were identified on other parts of the protocol, and identified as at risk only 3 not otherwise identified. What may have contributed to the apparent lack of effectiveness of this tool?

- *Audiometry* is used to quantify hearing deficits further. Specific sound frequencies are presented to each ear by either air or bone conduction. In this manner, it is possible to identify the type and pattern of hearing loss.
- *Speech audiometry* is used to identify the intensity at which speech can be recognized and interpreted.
- *Tympanometry* is an indirect measurement of the compliance and impedance of the middle ear to sound transmission. The external auditory meatus is subjected to neutral, positive, and negative air pressure while the resultant sound energy flow is monitored.

Amplification

A hearing aid or other amplification device can help many clients with hearing deficits. These assistive devices do nothing to prevent, minimize, or treat the hearing loss itself, but they amplify the sound presented to the hearing apparatus of the ear. Amplification may bring the level of sound above the hearing threshold for the client, allowing more accurate perception and interpretation of its meaning. For the client with distorted sound perception, the hearing aid may be less helpful, because it simply amplifies the sound.

Unfortunately, only 18% of older clients with a hearing deficit have a hearing aid. Denial of the deficit, other health problems, poor visual acuity, decreased manual dexterity, and cost all contribute to this low usage (Taylor, 1993). With the exception of the assistive listening device (described shortly), hearing aids must be individually prescribed by an audiologist. Proper design, proper fit, and regular maintenance are necessary for their effectiveness.

Hearing aids are available in a variety of styles, each with advantages and disadvantages. The newest and least noticeable style fits entirely in the ear canal. This small and unobtrusive device allows use of the telephone and can be worn during exercise. Because of its small size, the client must have good manual dexterity to insert it, clean it, and change the batteries. For this reason, older clients or clients with impaired dexterity may be unable to use it.

The in-ear style of aid fits into the external ear and is more visible than the in-canal aid (Figure 44–13). Its larger size makes manipulation somewhat easier, although it still may be difficult for less dextrous individuals. A greater degree of amplification is possible with the in-ear aid. Many have a toggle switch for telephone usage.

With both the in-canal and in-ear style, cleaning is important. Small portals may become plugged with cerumen, interfering with sound transmission.

The behind-ear hearing aid allows finer adjustment of the level of amplification and is easier for the client to manipulate (Figure 44–14). For the client who wears glasses, this style can be modified, with all components fitting into the temple of the eyeglasses.

Clients with profound hearing loss may require a body hearing aid. The microphone and amplifier of this aid are contained in a pocket-sized case that the client clips onto clothing, slips into a pocket, or carries in a harness. The receiver is attached by a cord to the case and clips onto the ear mold, which delivers the sound to the ear canal.

For the client who does not have a hearing aid, an *assistive listening device,* or "pocket talker," with a microphone and "Walkman" type earpieces, is useful. Pocket talkers are available over the counter or through an audiologist and are relatively inexpensive. The earpiece requires no special fitting, and the external microphone allows the client to focus on the desired sound rather than simply amplifying all sounds. Assistive listening devices may also be used in conjunction with a hearing aid.

Clients with tinnitus may find a "white-noise" masking device helpful to promote concentration and rest. These devices conduct a pleasant sound to the affected ear, allowing the client to block out the abnormal sound.

Surgery

Reconstructive surgeries of the middle ear, such as a stapedectomy or tympanoplasty, may be useful for the client with a conductive hearing loss. Stapedectomy is the removal and replacement of the stapes. This procedure is used for clients with a conductive hearing loss related to otosclerosis.

In a tympanoplasty, the structures of the middle ear are reconstructed to improve conductive hearing deficits. Chronic otitis media with necrosis and scarring of the middle ear is a common precipitating factor.

For the client with a sensorineural hearing loss, a cochlear implant may be the only hope for restoring sound perception. Two types of cochlear implant are available. The first uses an electrode implanted in the cochlea to stimulate remaining, intact, excitable auditory neurons (Figure 44–15). A small processor carried outside the body receives sound through a microphone and sends a signal to a transmitter mounted behind the ear. The transmitter then sends the signal to a receiver implanted under the skin, which in turn transmits it to the electrode implanted in the cochlea.

The second type of cochlear implant is used when no excitable auditory nerve fibers are available. The external microphone-transmitter sends the signal to an implanted receiver, which transmits the stimulus via an electrode

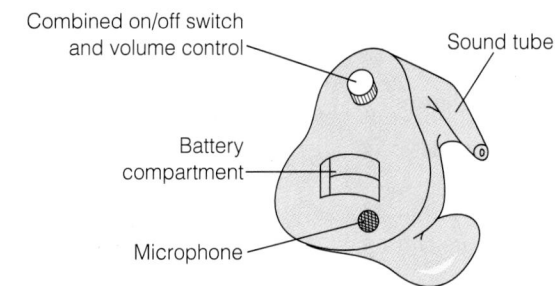

Figure 44–13   An in-ear hearing aid.

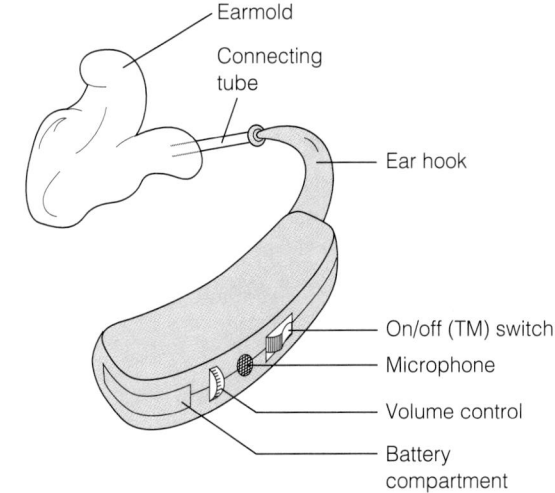

Figure 44–14   A behind-ear hearing aid.

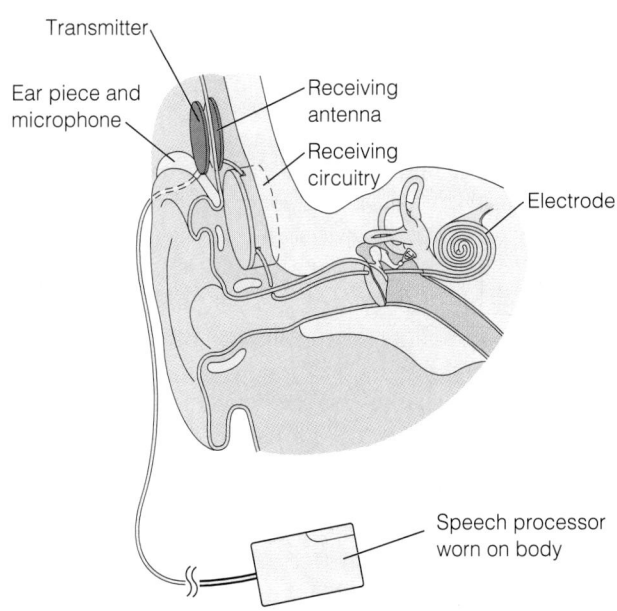

Figure 44–15   A cochlear implant for sensorineural hearing loss.

implanted in the brain stem over the cochlear nucleus (Thompson et al., 1993).

Cochlear prostheses provide the client with the perception of sound but not normal hearing. The client is able to recognize warning sounds such as automobiles, sirens, telephones, and doors opening or closing. They also receive stimuli to alert them to incoming communication so they can focus on the person speaking (Porth, 1994). Many clients can learn to interpret the perceived sounds as words, especially with newer implant devices.

Nursing Care

In planning and implementing nursing care for the client with a hearing deficit, the nurse needs to consider the following factors:

- The type and extent of hearing loss
- Its duration and the adaptation of the client to the loss
- The availability of assistive hearing devices and the client's ability and willingness to use them

This section focuses on the problems of the hearing deficit, impaired communication, and social isolation for the hearing-impaired client.

Sensory/Perceptual Alteration: Auditory

Whether the client's hearing deficit is partial or total, impaired sound perception is the primary problem. The client needs to understand what causes the deficit and what to expect for the future. Nursing interventions focus on maximizing available hearing and preventing further deterioration to the extent possible.

Nursing interventions with rationales follow:

- Assess the client's degree of hearing loss. *This information helps the nurse tailor interventions to the specific needs of the client.*
- Encourage the client to talk about the loss of hearing and its effect on activities of daily living. *Hearing loss affects each individual in a different way. The client may be denying the extent of the deficit or grieving the loss. Listening to the client and providing support encourage the client to develop coping strategies.*
- Provide information about the type of hearing loss to the client and family. Refer to an audiologist for evaluation of the hearing loss and possible exploration of amplification devices. *With improved understanding of the deficit, the client can plan ways to compensate.*
- Replace batteries in hearing aids on a regular and as-needed basis. *Hearing aid batteries last approximately 1 week. If a battery is old or has been improperly stored, the life may be reduced further.*
- If the hearing aid has a toggle switch for microphone/telephone, be sure it is in the appropriate position.

Check hearing aids for patency, cleaning out cerumen as necessary. *A hearing aid plugged with cerumen does not transmit sound well.*

Impaired Verbal Communication

A hearing deficit impairs the client's ability to receive and interpret verbal communication. A hearing loss affects the client's ability to follow conversations, use the telephone, and enjoy television or other forms of entertainment.

Nursing interventions with rationales follow:

- Get the client's attention before beginning to speak. A wave of the hand or tap on the shoulder may be used. *Prepare the client to receive incoming communication.*
- When speaking, face the client and keep the hands away from the face. Avoid making the client look into glare or standing so that your face is in shadow. Mustaches should be trimmed so the lips are visible. *Hearing-impaired individuals often supplement their sound perception by conscious or unconscious lip-reading, making good visibility of the speaker's face necessary.*
- When speaking to the client, use a low voice pitch with normal loudness. *The voice, particularly of women, tends to increase in pitch with increasing loudness. Because the perception of higher tones is typically lost with presbycusis and other types of hearing loss, lowering the pitch of the voice brings it into the hearing range of the client.*
- Speak at a normal rate, and do not overarticulate. Use shorter sentences and pause at the end of each sentence. *Changing the pace of speech and consciously overarticulating make it more difficult for the client to follow the flow and to lip-read. Using short sentences and pausing gives the client time to interpret the message.*
- If the client has a hearing aid, be sure that it is properly in place, turned on, and has fresh batteries. *The client may not be aware that the hearing aid is not functioning well.*
- Reduce the noise in the environment before speaking with the client. *Excessive environmental noise interferes with the client's ability to perceive the message.*
- Use nonverbal and written communication to enhance the client's understanding of the message. Provide a magic slate for written communication. *Providing nonverbal cues and written messages makes it easier for the client to understand. The client has a greater sense of control when unimpaired senses are used to enhance hearing.*
- Leave the postoperative client's dominant hand free of intravenous catheters. *The client may need to use that hand to write.*
- Rephrase sentences when the client has difficulty understanding. *Because hearing losses often are not uniform across all sound tones, some words are more difficult to comprehend than others. Using alternative words and*

phrases may make it possible for the client to perceive the message.

- When you provide client teaching, ask the client to repeat important information. *The nurse thus makes sure that the client understood the information.*

- Communicate with other staff about the client's hearing deficit and effective strategies for communication. *Consistent use of effective strategies for communication decreases the client's frustration.*

Social Isolation

The client with impaired hearing often becomes socially isolated. This isolation may be self-imposed because of the client's difficulty in communicating, especially in a group. Often, however, the isolation comes about gradually and without intention. The client finds social settings such as family dinners or community gatherings increasingly difficult. Friends and family become frustrated trying to communicate with the hearing-impaired person, and invitations to participate in social activities dwindle.

Nursing interventions with rationales follow:

- Work with the client to determine the extent and cause of the social isolation. Help the client differentiate the reality of the isolation and its cause from the client's perception of isolation. *Hearing-impaired clients may be unaware that they are isolated. Identifying factors that contribute to the isolation helps clients to confront the cause. Clients with a hearing deficit may also experience paranoid thinking as a result of the impaired communication. The client may believe that friends and family have purposely begun to avoid interactions. Identifying the hearing deficit as a contributing factor may provide the impetus the client needs to remedy the hearing loss.*

- Encourage the client to interact with friends and family on a one-to-one basis in quiet settings. *Clients with impaired hearing are more successful in understanding conversations that take place in small groups and quiet settings.*

- Treat the client with dignity and remind friends and family that a hearing deficit does not mean loss of mental faculties. *Inappropriate responses due to a hearing deficit can cause others to perceive the client as "stupid" or demented.*

- Involve the client in activities that do not require acute hearing, such as checkers and chess. *The client has an opportunity to interact socially without the stress of straining to hear.*

- Obtain a pocket talker or encourage the client and family to do so.

- Refer the client to an audiologist for evaluation and possible hearing-aid fitting.

- Refer to resources such as support groups and senior citizen centers. *These groups provide new social outlets.*

Other Nursing Diagnoses

The following nursing diagnoses may also be appropriate for the client with a hearing deficit:

- *Ineffective Individual Coping* evidenced by denial of hearing deficit
- *Diversional Activity Deficit* related to hearing deficit
- *Knowledge Deficit* regarding available assistive devices related to lack of information
- *Altered Role Performance* related to inability to hear
- *Self-Esteem Disturbance* related to difficulty interacting with others

Client and Family Teaching

Teaching is a primary intervention in preventing hearing loss. Teaching for primary prevention focuses on

- Care of the ears and ear canals, including cleaning and treatment of infection
- The use of plugs to protect the ears during swimming or diving
- Protection from injury in sports
- Protecting the hearing from damage by intermittent or frequent exposure to loud noise

For the client with a permanent hearing loss, teaching relates to managing the deficit and developing coping strategies. The nurse can refer the client to an audiologist to evaluate the usefulness of a hearing aid. The client with a hearing aid may need instruction on proper use, care, and maintenance. Strategies for coping with the hearing deficit include acknowledging the deficit and asking people to speak clearly and repeat statements as needed. Voicing a preference for individual visits and small group interactions rather than large social functions can help the client to remain connected to friends and family.

Providing referral to appropriate agencies is an important part of teaching for the hearing-impaired client and the family. National, state, and local agencies can provide education and assistance. Local and regional agencies are often listed in the telephone book. An audiology center may also have a list of local resources.

| Applying the Nursing Process |

Case Study of a Client with Presbycusis: Carl Aaron

Carl Aaron is a 74-year-old retired logger. For the past 5 years, Mr. Aaron has been caring for his wife, who has been disabled by a stroke. She recently has had another stroke, making her unable to help with her ADLs. Mr. Aaron has degenerative arthritis, which makes it difficult for him to lift and care for Mrs. Aaron. Mr. Aaron and the family decide that the best solution is to move to a care center where his wife can receive the care she needs and where he can reside in the assistive living wing.

Assessment

Mr. Aaron is admitted to the assistive living center by the gerontology nurse specialist, Etta Marks. In her assessment, Ms. Marks notes that Mr. Aaron frequently asks her to repeat questions during their interview. Occasionally, his answers are not appropriate to the question asked, but his mental status examination is normal. Observing Mr. Aaron at lunch, she notices that he seems to ignore the conversation at his table. During her physical assessment, Ms. Marks performs the Rinne and Weber tests. The Weber test shows no lateralization of sound, but the Rinne test shows decreased air and bone sound conduction. She makes an appointment for Mr. Aaron with the audiologist. Audiometric testing confirms that Mr. Aaron has a significant hearing loss consistent with presbycusis. In-ear hearing aids are prescribed and ordered.

Diagnosis

Ms. Marks develops the following nursing diagnoses for Mr. Aaron:

- *Sensory/Perceptual Alteration: Auditory* related to presbycusis

- *Diversional Activity Deficit* related to a change of residence and difficulty with social interactions

- *Knowledge Deficit* related to lack of information about the use and care of hearing aids

- *Risk for Impaired Adjustment* to hearing aids related to poor manual dexterity due to degenerative arthritis

Expected Outcomes

The expected outcomes of the plan of care for Mr. Aaron are that he will

- Understand instructions and other verbal communications from staff.

- Interact with other residents on a one-on-one basis.

- Participate in scheduled activities in small groups.

- Use headphones to hear the television and radio.

- Obtain and use hearing aids.

- Demonstrate the ability to insert, turn on, and clean the hearing aid and to change its battery.

Planning and Implementation

Ms. Marks plans the following interventions to be implemented with Mr. Aaron:

- Use effective communication techniques for hearing-impaired individuals.
  a. Face Mr. Aaron when speaking with him.
  b. Speak distinctly in a low voice.
  c. Supplement verbal communcation with nonverbal communication.
  d. Provide a magic slate.

- Use a pocket talker as needed until hearing aids are obtained.

- Facilitate one-on-one interactions between Mr. Aaron and other residents.

- Provide Mr. Aaron with a schedule of activities, highlighting those that are limited to small groups or that provide for individual interactions.

- Have Mr. Aaron's family obtain headphones for radio and television use.

- Ensure that the audiologist considers Mr. Aaron's limited manual dexterity when ordering hearing aids.

- Teach Mr. Aaron how to use and care for hearing aids.

Evaluation

After using the pocket talker, Mr. Aaron is surprised and pleased at the difference he notes in his ability to hear and understand conversations. He decides that a hearing aid is a good investment, in spite of the cost. The audiologist orders a hearing aid with easily manipulated switches and battery cover, allowing Mr. Aaron to care for it himself. As Mr. Aaron becomes more comfortable with the hearing aid, he begins to interact with other residents more and seems to adjust well to the assistive living center.

Critical Thinking in the Nursing Process

1. What factors contributed to Mr. Aaron's lack of recognition of a hearing deficit?

2. Discuss additional interventions for the identified diversional activity deficit.

3. Identify techniques for teaching Mr. Aaron to use and care for his hearing aid despite his limited manual dexterity.

4. Develop a care plan for the nursing diagnosis *Ineffective Individual Coping* related to change of role and residence.

Bibliography

■ ■ ■

Abrams, W. B., & Berkow, R. (Eds.). (1990). *The Merck manual of geriatrics*. Rahway, NJ: Merck Sharp & Dohme Research Laboratories.

Andreoli, T. E., Carpenter, C. C. J., Plum, F., & Smith, L. H., Jr. (1990). *Cecil essentials of medicine* (2nd ed.). Philadelphia: Saunders.

Andrews, J. F., & Wilson, H. F. (1991, December). The deaf adult in the nursing home. *Geriatric Nursing, 12,* 279–283.

Armitage, J., & Easty, D. (1993, June 23). Bankable assets. *Nursing Times, 89*(25), 36–37.

Bates, B. (1995). *A guide to physical examination and history taking* (6th ed.). Philadelphia: Lippincott.

Berkow, R., & Fletcher, A. J. (Eds.). (1992). *The Merck manual of diagnosis and therapy* (16th ed.). Rahway, NJ: Merck Research Laboratories.

Brookbank, J. W. (1990). *The biology of aging.* New York: Harper & Row.

Bullock, B. L., & Rosendahl, P. P. (1992). *Pathophysiology: Adaptations and alterations in function* (3rd ed.). Philadelphia: Lippincott.

Burke, M. M., & Walsh, M. B. (1992). *Gerontologic nursing: Care of the frail elderly.* St. Louis: Mosby-Year Book.

Carpenito, L. J. (1991). *Nursing care plans and documentation: Nursing diagnoses and collaborative problems.* Philadelphia: Lippincott.

Chernecky, C. C., Krech, R. L., & Berger, B. J. (1993). *Laboratory tests and diagnostic procedures.* Philadelphia: Saunders.

Clark, J. B. F., Queener, S. F., & Karb, V. B. (1993). *Pharmacologic basis of nursing practice* (4th ed.). St. Louis: Mosby-Year Book.

Cleveland, P. J., & Morris, J. (1990, August). Meniere's disease: The inner ear out of balance. *RN, 53*(8), 28–32.

Cox, H. C., Hinz, M. D., Lubno, M. A., Newfield, S. A., Ridenour, N. A., Slater, M. M., & Sridaromont, K. (1993). *Clinical applications of nursing diagnosis: Adult, child, women's, psychiatric, gerontic and home health considerations* (2nd ed.). Philadelphia: F.A. Davis.

Easterbrook, M. (1992, July). Getting patients to protect their eyes during sports. *The Physician and Sportsmedicine, 20*(7), 165–166, 169–170.

Erie, J. C. (1991, November). Eye injuries: Prevention, evaluation, and treatment. *The Physician and Sportsmedicine, 19*(11), 108–112, 115–116, 119–120+.

Grimes, M. R., Scardino, M. A., & Martone, J. F. (1992, September). Worldwide blindness. *Nursing Clinics of North America, 27,* 807–816.

Hayes, P. L. (1981, September). Treatment and nursing care of corneal disease. *Nursing Clinics of North America, 16*(3), 383–392.

Hazzard, W. R., Bierman, E. L., Blass, J. P., Ettinger, W. H., Jr., & Halter, J. B. (1994). *Principles of geriatric medicine and gerontology* (3rd ed.). New York: McGraw-Hill.

Hogstel, M. O. (Ed.). (1992). *Clinical manual of gerontological nursing.* St. Louis: Mosby-Year Book.

Kitt, S., & Kaiser, J. (1990). *Emergency nursing: A physiologic and clinical perspective.* Philadelphia: Saunders.

Kozier, B., Erb, G., & Bufalino, P. M. (1989). *Introduction to nursing.* Redwood City, CA: Addison-Wesley Nursing.

Lederer, J. R., Marculescu, G. L., Mocnik, B., & Seaby, N. (1993). *Care planning pocket guide: A nursing diagnosis approach* (5th ed.). Redwood City, CA: Addison-Wesley Nursing.

Lee, D. J., Carlson, D. L., Lee, H. M., Ray, L. A., & Markides, K. S. (1991, November). Hearing loss and hearing aid use in Hispanic adults: Results from the Hispanic health and nutrition examination survey. *American Journal of Public Health, 81,* 1471–1474.

Maas, M., Buckwalter, K. C., & Hardy, M. (1991). *Nursing diagnoses and interventions for the elderly.* Redwood City, CA: Addison-Wesley Nursing.

Macleod, J. (1994, June 29). Pre-admission clinics for corneal graft patients. *Nursing Times, 90*(26), 35–36.

Marieb, E. N. (1992). *Human anatomy and physiology,* 2nd ed. Redwood City, CA: The Benjamin Cummings Publishing Company, Inc.

Montgomery, G. (1995) Breaking the code of color. *Seeing, hearing, and smelling the world: New findings help scientists make sense of our senses.* Chevy Chase, MD: Howard Hughes Medical Institute.

Ney, D. F. (1993, March/April). Cerumen impaction, ear hygiene practices, and hearing acuity. *Geriatric Nursing, 14,* 70–73.

O'Rourke, C. M., Britten, C. F., Gatschet, C. A., & Krien, T. L. (1993, March/April). Effectiveness of a hearing screening protocol for the elderly. *Geriatric Nursing, 14,* 66–69.

O'Toole, M. (Ed.). (1992). *Miller-Keane encyclopedia and dictionary of medicine, nursing, and allied health* (5th ed.). Philadelphia: Saunders.

Physician's desk reference (48th ed.). (1994). Montvale, NJ: Medical Economics Data Production Company.

Plona, R. P., & Schremp, P. S. (1992, September). Nursing care of patients with ocular manifestations of human immunodeficiency virus infection. *Nursing Clinics of North America 27,* 793–805.

Porth, C. M. (1994). *Pathophysiology: Concepts of altered health states* (4th ed.). Philadelphia: Lippincott.

Potter, P. A., & Perry, A. G. (1993). *Fundamentals of nursing: Concepts, process and practice* (3rd ed.). St. Louis: Mosby-Year Book.

Ruehl, C. A., & Schremp, P. S. (1992, September). Nursing care of the cataract patient: Today's outpatient approach. *Nursing Clinics of North America 27,* 727–743.

Schelkun, P. H. (1991, July). Swimmer's ear: Getting patients back in the water. *The Physician and Sportsmedicine, 19* (7), 85–88, 90.

Shlafer, M. (1993). *The nurse, pharmacology, and drug therapy: A prototype approach* (2nd ed.). Redwood City, CA: Addison-Wesley Nursing.

Skidmore-Roth, L. (1995). *Mosby's 1995 Nursing drug reference.* St. Louis: Mosby-Year Book.

Smith, S. C. (1992, September). Diabetic retinopathy. *Nursing Clinics of North America 27,* 745–759.

Stevens, J. (1994, June 29). Treating keratoconus. *Nursing Times, 90*(26), 36–39.

Taylor, K. S. (1993, March/April). Geriatric hearing loss: Management strategies for nurses. *Geriatric Nursing, 14,* 74–76.

Thompson, J. M., McFarland, G. K., Hirsch, J. E., & Tucker, S. M. (1993). *Mosby's clinical nursing* (3rd ed.). St. Louis: Mosby-Year Book.

Tierney, L. M., Jr., McPhee, S. J., & Papadakis, M. A. (Eds.). (1994). *Current medical diagnosis and treatment* (33rd ed.). Norwalk, CT: Appleton & Lange.

Tucker, S. M., Canobbio, M. M., Paquette, E. V., & Wells, M. F. (1992). *Patient care standards: Nursing process, diagnosis, and outcome* (5th ed.). St. Louis: Mosby-Year Book.

Vader, L. A. (1992, September). Vision and vision loss. *Nursing Clinics of North America, 27,* 705–714.

Way, L. W. (Ed.). (1994). *Current surgical diagnosis and treatment* (10th ed.). Norwalk, CT: Appleton & Lange.

Wesorick, B. (1990). *Standards of nursing care: A model for clinical practice.* Philadelphia: Lippincott.

Wilson, J. D., Braunwald, E., Isselbacher, K. J., Petersdorf, R. G., Martin, J. B., Fauci, A. S., & Root, R. K. (Eds.). (1991). *Harrison's principles of internal medicine* (12th ed.). New York: McGraw-Hill.

Woods, S. (1992, September). Macular degeneration. *Nursing Clinics of North America 27,* 761–775.

Sexuality and Reproductive Patterns

Responses to Altered Sexual and Reproductive Function

Assessing Clients with Reproductive Disorders

LEARNING OBJECTIVES

After completing this chapter, you will be able to

LEARNING OBJECTIVES

After completing this chapter, you will be able to

- Identify the major structures of the reproductive systems of men and women.

- Identify the functions of the reproductive organs in men and women.

- Describe the functions of the sex hormones of men and women.

- Identify interview questions pertinent to the assessment of reproductive function in men and women.

- Describe physical assessment techniques for reproductive function in men and women.

- Identify manifestations of impairment in reproductive function in men and women.

- Describe normal variations in assessment findings for older men and women.

Although the reproductive organs in men and women are very different, they do share common functions: providing for sexual pleasure and producing children. The reproductive organs, in conjunction with the neuroendocrine system, also produce hormones that are important in biologic development and sexual behavior. Parts of the reproductive organs also enclose and are integral to the function of the urinary system. The assessment of the reproductive and urinary systems is often difficult for both the beginning nurse and the client and requires skill on the part of the nurse when asking questions about sensitive topics that the client may be hesitant to talk about. Skill in conducting physical examinations of an area of the body usually considered to be private is also required. This chapter discusses the assessment of the reproductive system for both men and women.

Review of Anatomy and Physiology

■ ■ ■

The Reproductive System in Men

The reproductive system in men consists of the paired testes, the scrotum, ducts, glands, and penis (Figure 45–1). The location and function of the male reproductive organs are summarized in Table 45–1.

The Testes

The *testes* develop in the abdominal cavity of the fetus and then descend through the inguinal canal into the scrotum. They are homologous to the female's ovaries. These paired organs are each about 1.5 inches (4 cm) long and 1 inch (2.5 cm) in diameter. They are suspended in the scrotum by the spermatic cord. Each is surrounded by two coverings: an outer *tunica vaginalis* and an inner *tunica albuginea*. Each testis is divided into 250 to 300 lobules, with each lobule containing one to four *seminiferous*

Table 45–1   Location and Function of the Male Reproductive Organs

Male Reproductive Organ	Location	Function
Scrotum	Hangs from body at root of penis.	Contains testes, epididymis, and portions of the vas (ductus) deferens.
Testes	In the scrotal sac.	Produce sperm and testosterone.
Epididymis	Posterolateral to upper aspect of each testis.	Stores sperm. Promotes sperm maturation. Transports sperm to vas deferens.
Vas deferens (ductus deferens)	Between the epididymis and the seminal vesicle forming the ejaculatory duct.	Stores sperm. Transports sperm.
Penis	Attached to front and sides of the pubic arch. Proximal, ventral surface is directly continuous with the scrotum.	Excretes semen and urine. Deposits sperm in female reproductive tract.
Urethra	Begins at bladder and passes through prostate and penis.	Serves as passageway for urine or semen.
Prostate gland	Encircles the urethra at the neck of the bladder.	Contributes to ejaculatory volume. Enhances sperm motility and fertility.
Seminal vesicles	Lie on posterior bladder wall.	Contribute to ejaculatory volume. Contain nutrients to sustain sperm and prostaglandins to facilitate sperm motility.
Bulbourethral (Cowper's) glands	Inferior to the prostate.	Secrete mucus into urethra. Neutralize traces of acidic urine in the urethra.

tubules. The testes function to produce sperm and testosterone.

The seminiferous tubules are responsible for sperm production. *Leydig's cells* (or *interstitial cells*) lie in the connective tissue surrounding the seminiferous tubules. They produce testosterone.

The Ducts and Semen

The seminiferous tubules lead into the efferent ducts and become the *rete testis.* From the rete testis, 10,000 to 20,000 efferent ducts join the *epididymis,* a long coiled tube that lies over the outer surface of each testis. The epididymis is the final area for the storage and maturation of sperm. When a man is sexually excited, the epididymis contracts to propel the sperm through the *vas deferens* to the *ampulla,* where they are stored until ejaculation.

The *seminal vesicles* at the base of the bladder produce about 60% of the volume of *seminal fluid.* Seminal fluid is also made of secretions from the accessory sex organs, the epididymis, the prostate gland, and Cowper's glands. Seminal fluid nourishes the sperm, provides bulk, and increases its alkalinity. (An alkaline pH is essential to mobilize the sperm and ensure fertilization of the ova.) Sperm mixed with this fluid is called *semen.* Each seminal vesicle joins its corresponding vas deferens to form an *ejaculatory*

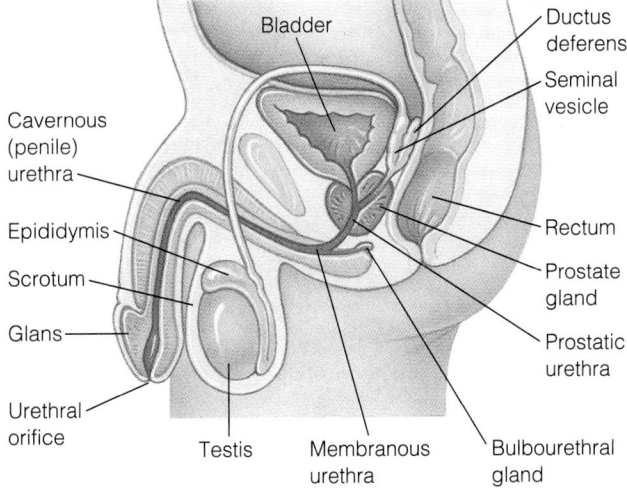

Figure 45–1   The male reproductive system.

duct, which enters the prostatic urethra. During ejaculation, seminal fluid mixes with sperm at the ejaculatory duct and enters the urethra for expulsion.

The total amount of semen ejaculated is 2 to 4 mL, although the amount varies. The sperm count of the total ejaculate of a healthy male is from 100 to 400 million.

The Scrotum

The *scrotum* is a sac or pouch made of two layers. The outer layer is continuous with the skin of the perineum and thighs. The inner layer is made of muscle and fascia. The scrotum hangs at the base of the penis, anterior to the anus. The scrotum regulates the temperature of the testes. The optimum temperature for the production of sperm is about 2 to 3 degrees below body temperature; when the testicular temperature is too low, the scrotum contracts to bring the testes up against the body. When the testicular temperature is too high, the scrotum relaxes to allow the testes to lie further away from the body.

The Prostate Gland

The *prostate gland* is about the size of a walnut. It encircles the urethra just below the urinary bladder (see Figure 45–1). It is made of 20 to 30 tuboloalveolar glands surrounded by smooth muscle. Secretions of the prostate gland make up about one-third of the volume of the semen. These secretions enter the urethra through several ducts during ejaculation.

The Penis

The *penis* is the genital organ that encloses the urethra (see Figure 45–1). It is homologous to the clitoris of the female. The penis is composed of a *shaft* and a tip called the *glans*, which is covered in the uncircumcised man by the *foreskin* (or *prepuce*). The shaft contains three columns of erectile tissue: the two lateral columns are called the *corpora cavernosa*, and the central mass is called the *corpus spongiosum*.

Erection occurs when the penile masses become filled with blood in response to a reflex that triggers the parasympathetic nervous system to stimulate arteriolar vasodilation. The erection reflex may be initiated by touch, pressure, sights, sounds, smells, and/or thoughts of a sexual encounter. After ejaculation, the arterioles vasoconstrict, and the penis becomes flaccid.

Spermatogenesis

Spermatogenesis is the series of physiologic events that generate sperm in the seminiferous tubules. This process begins with puberty and continues throughout a man's life, with several hundred million sperm being produced each day (Marieb, 1995).

The inner layer of the seminiferous tubules is composed of *sustentacular cells* (or *Sertoli's cells*), which contain the spermatocytes and sperm in different stages of development. Sertoli's cells secrete a nourishing fluid for the developing sperm, as well as enzymes that help convert spermatocytes to sperm. The events in spermatogenesis, which takes 64 to 72 days, are as follows:

1. The spermatogonia (sperm stem cells) undergo rapid mitotic division. As these cells multiply, the more mature spermatogonia divide into two daughter cells. These daughter cells grow and become the primary spermatocytes (and eventually become sperm).

2. Primary spermatocytes divide by meiosis to form two smaller secondary spermatocytes, which in turn divide to form two spermatids. This process occurs over several weeks.

3. The spermatids elongate into a mature sperm cell with a head and a tail. The head contains enzymes essential to the penetration and fertilization of the ova. The flagellar motion of the tail allows the sperm to move. The sperm cells then move to the epididymis to mature further and develop motility.

Male Sex Hormones

The male sex hormones are called *androgens*. Most androgens are produced in the testes, although the adrenal cortex also produces a small amount of androgens. *Testosterone*, the primary androgen produced by the testes, is essential for the development and maintenance of sexual organs and secondary sex characteristics. It also promotes metabolism, growth of muscles and bone, and libido (sexual desire).

The Reproductive System in Women

The reproductive system in women consists of the paired ovaries and fallopian tubes, uterus, vagina, mons pubis, labia majora, labia minora, and clitoris. The breasts are also a part of women's reproductive organs. In women, the urethra and urinary meatus are separated from the reproductive organs; however, they are in such close proximity that a health problem with one often affects the other. The location and function of the female reproductive organs are summarized in Table 45–2.

The Internal Genitalia

The ovaries, fallopian tubes, uterus, and vagina make up the internal organs of the female reproductive system (Figure 45–2). The ovaries are the primary reproductive organs in women and also produce female sex hormones. The fallopian tubes, uterus, and vagina serve as accessory ducts for the ovaries and a developing fetus.

The Vagina   The *vagina* is a fibromuscular tube about 3 to 4 inches (8 to 10 cm) in length located posterior to the bladder and urethra and anterior to the rectum. The upper end contains the uterine cervix in an area called the *fornix*. The walls of the vagina are made of membranes that form folds, called *rugae*. These membranes are composed of mucus-secreting stratified squamous epithelial cells. The vagina serves as a route for the excretion of secretions, including menstrual fluid, and also is an organ of sexual response.

Table 45–2   Location and Function of the Female Reproductive Organs

Female Reproductive Organ	Location	Function
Mons pubis (mons veneris)	Anterior and superior to the pubis.	Enhances sexual sensations. Protects and cushions pubic symphysis during intercourse.
Labia majora	Extend from mons pubis to perineum.	Protect labia minora, urethral and vaginal openings. Enhance sexual arousal.
Labia minora	Enclosed by the labia majora.	Protect clitoris. Inferiorly, merge to form posterior ring of vaginal introitus (fourchette). Lubricate vulva. Enhance sexual arousal.
Vestibule	Area enclosed by labia minora.	Contains openings for urethra, vagina, Bartholin's glands, and Skene's glands.
Bartholin's (greater vestibular) glands	Posterior on each side of the vaginal orifice. Open onto the sides of the vestibule in the groove between the labia minora and hymen.	Secrete clear, viscid mucus during intercourse.
Skene's (lesser vestibular, paraurethral) glands	Open onto the vestibule on each side of the urethra.	Drain urethral glands. Produce lubricating mucus.
Clitoris	Small bud of erectile tissue just below the superior joining of the labia minora.	Stimulates and elevates levels of sexual arousal.
Perineum	Skin-covered muscular area between vaginal opening and anus.	Provides support for pelvic organs.
Mammary glands	Contained within breasts. Anterior to pectoral muscles of thorax.	Produce human milk. Play a role in sexual arousal.
Ovaries	Lie on each side of the uterus below and behind the uterine tubes.	Produce and secrete ova. Produce the hormones estrogen and progesterone.
Fallopian tubes (uterine tubes, oviducts)	One tube extends medially from the area of each ovary and empties into the upper portion (fundus) of the uterus.	Transport ova.
Uterus (adnexa of the uterus are composed of the uterine tubes and ovaries)	Anterior to the rectum and posterior/superior to the bladder.	Receives, retains, and nourishes the fertilized ovum. Contracts rhythmically to expel infant. Cyclically sheds lining when ovum is not fertilized.
Cervix	Lower portion of uterus extending into the vagina.	Connects uterine cavity with vagina. Opens to allow passage of menstrual flow and infant.
Vagina	Extends from the external orifice in the vestibule to the cervix.	Receives penis and semen during intercourse. Passageway for menstrual flow and expulsion of infant at birth.

The walls of the vagina are usually moist and maintain a pH ranging from 3.8 to 4.2. This pH is bacteriostatic and is maintained by the action of estrogen and normal vaginal flora. Estrogen stimulates the growth of vaginal mucosal cells so that they thicken and have increased glycogen content. The glycogen is fermented to lactic acid by the action of Döderlein's bacilli (lactobacilli that normally inhabit the vagina), slightly acidifying the vaginal fluid.

The Uterus   The *uterus* is a pear-shaped muscular organ with thick walls located between the bladder and the

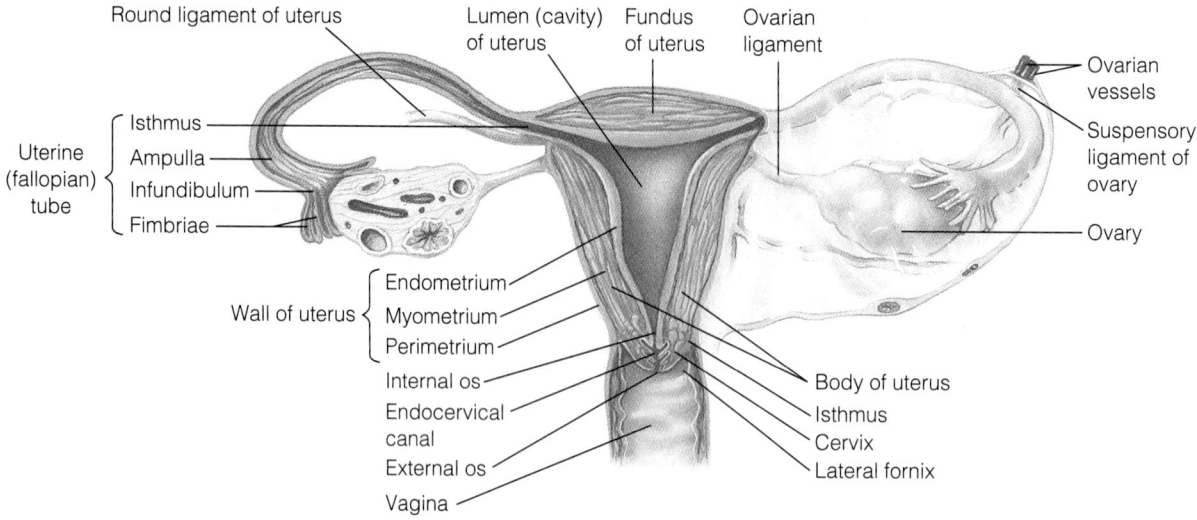

Figure 45–2   The internal organs of the female reproductive system.

rectum. The uterus is made up of three parts: the fundus, the body, and the cervix. It is supported in the abdominal cavity by the broad ligaments, the round ligaments, the uterosacral ligaments, and the transverse cervical ligaments. The uterus functions to receive the fertilized ovum and provides a site for growth and development of the fetus.

The uterine wall has three layers. The *perimetrium* is the outer serous layer that merges with the peritoneum. The *myometrium* is the middle layer and makes up most of the uterine wall. This layer has muscle fibers that run in various directions, allowing contractions during **menstruation** (the periodic shedding of the uterine lining in a woman of childbearing age who is not pregnant) or childbirth and expansion as the fetus grows. The *endometrium* lines the uterus. Its outermost layer is shed during menstruation.

The *cervix* projects into the vagina and forms a pathway between the uterus and the vagina. The uterine opening of the cervix is called the *internal os;* the vaginal opening is called the *external os.* The space between these openings, the *endocervical canal,* serves as a route for the discharge of menstrual fluid and the entrance for sperm. The cervix is a firm structure that softens in response to hormones during pregnancy. It is protected by mucus from glandular tissue; this mucus changes consistency and quantity during the menstrual cycle and during pregnancy.

The Fallopian Tubes   The *fallopian tubes* (or *uterine tubes*) are thin cylindrical structures about 4 inches (10 cm) long and 1 cm in diameter. They are attached to the uterus on one end and are supported by the broad ligaments. The lateral ends of the uterine tubes are open and

made of projections called *fimbriae* that drape over the ovary. The fimbriae pick up the ovum after it is discharged from the ovary.

The uterine tubes are made of smooth muscle and are lined with ciliated, mucus-producing epithelial cells. The movement of the cilia and contractions of the smooth muscle move the ovum through the tubes toward the uterus. Fertilization of the ovum by the sperm usually occurs in the outer portion of one of the fallopian tubes.

The Ovaries   The *ovaries* in the adult woman are flat, almond-shaped structures located on either side of the uterus below the ends of the fallopian tubes. They are homologous to the male's testes. They are attached to the uterus by a ligament and are also attached to the broad ligament. The ovaries store the female germ cells and produce the female hormones estrogen and progesterone. A woman's total number of ova is present at her birth.

Each ovary is divided into a medulla and a cortex. It contains many small structures called *ovarian follicles.* Each follicle contains an immature ovum, called an *oocyte.* Each month, several follicles are stimulated by *follicle-stimulating hormone* (*FSH*) and *luteinizing hormone* (*LH*) to mature. The developing follicles are surrounded by layers of follicle cells, with the mature follicles called *graafian follicles.* The graafian follicles produce estrogen, which stimulates the development of endometrium. Each month in the menstruating woman, one or two of the mature follicles ejects an oocyte in a process called **ovulation.** The ruptured follicle is then changed into a structure called the *corpus luteum.* The corpus luteum produces both estrogen and progesterone to support the endometrium until conception occurs or the cycle begins again (Porth, 1994). The corpus luteum slowly degenerates, leaving a scar on the surface of the ovary.

The External Genitalia

The external genitalia collectively also are called the *vulva.* They include the mons pubis, the labia, the clitoris, the vaginal and urethral openings, and glands (Figure 45–3).

The *mons pubis* is a pad of adipose (fat) tissue covered with skin. It lies anterior to the symphysis pubis. After puberty, the mons is covered with hair with a diamond-shaped distribution.

The labia are divided into two structures. The *labia majora* are outermost, located from the base of the mons pubis to the anus. They are folds of skin and adipose tissue covered with hair. The *labia minora* are enclosed by the labia majora, and are located between the clitoris and the base of the vagina. They are made of skin, adipose tissue, and some erectile tissues. They are usually light pink and hairless.

The area between the labia is called the *vestibule,* and contains the openings for the vagina and the urethra as well as the *Bartholin's glands.* These glands secrete lubricating fluid during the sexual response cycle. *Skene's glands* open onto the vestibule on each side of the urethra.

The *clitoris* is an erectile organ that is analogous to the penis in the male. It is formed by the joining of the labia minora. Like the penis, it is highly sensitive and distends during sexual arousal.

The vaginal opening, called the *introitus,* is the opening between the internal and the external genitals. The introitus is surrounded by a connective tissue membrane called the *hymen,* which determines the size and shape of the opening.

The Breasts

The *breasts* (or *mammary glands*) are located between the 3rd and 7th ribs on the anterior chest wall. They are supported by the pectoral muscles and are richly supplied with nerves, blood, and lymph (Figure 45–4). A pigmented area called the *areola* is located slightly below the center of each breast and contains sebaceous glands and a nipple. The *nipple* is usually protrusive and becomes erect in response to cold and stimulation. The primary purpose of the breasts is to supply nourishment for the infant.

The breasts are made of adipose tissue, fibrous connective tissue, and glandular tissue. *Cooper's ligaments* support the breast and extend from the outer breast tissue to the nipple, dividing the breast into 15–25 lobes. Each lobe is made of alveolar glands connected by ducts which open to the nipple.

Female Sex Hormones

The ovaries produce estrogens, progesterone, and androgens in a cyclic pattern.

Estrogens are steroid hormones that occur naturally in three forms: estrone (E_1), estradiol (E_2), and estriol (E_3). *Estradiol* is the most potent and the form secreted in greatest amount by the ovaries. Although estrogens are

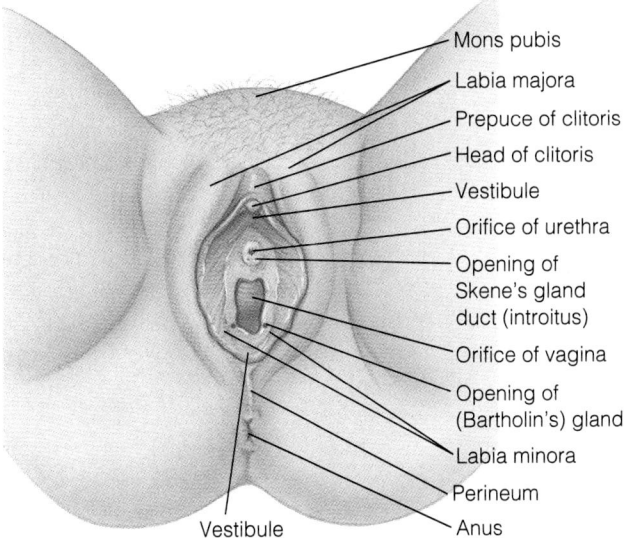

Figure 45–3   The external organs of the female reproductive system.

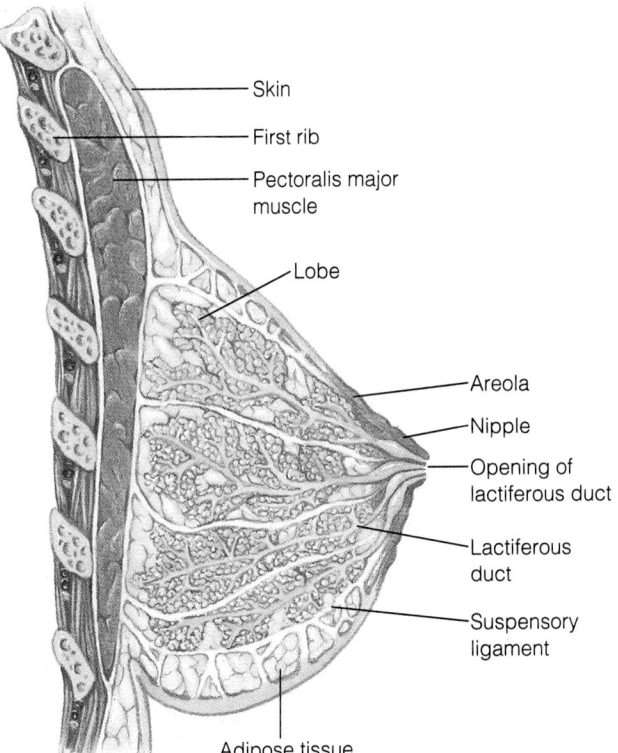

Figure 45–4   Structure of the female breast.

secreted throughout the menstrual cycle, they are at a higher level during certain phases of the cycle, discussed shortly.

Estrogens are essential for the development and maintenance of secondary sex characteristics, and in conjunction with other hormones, stimulate the female reproductive organs to prepare for growth of a fetus. Estrogens are responsible for the normal structure of skin and blood vessels. They also decrease the rate of bone resorption, promote increased high-density lipoproteins, reduce cholesterol levels, and enhance the clotting of blood. Estrogens also promote the retention of sodium and water.

Progesterone primarily affects the development of breast glandular tissue and the endometrium. During pregnancy, progesterone relaxes smooth muscle to decrease uterine contractions. It also increases body temperature. *Androgens* are responsible for normal hair growth patterns at puberty and may also have metabolic effects.

Oogenesis and the Ovarian Cycle

As mentioned earlier, all of a woman's ova are present as primary oocytes in primordial ovarian follicles at her birth. Each month from puberty until menopause, the remaining events of **oogenesis,** the production of ova, occur. Collectively, these events are known as the *ovarian cycle.*

The ovarian cycle has three consecutive phases that occur cyclically each 28 days (although the cycle normally may be longer or shorter). The *follicular phase* lasts from the 1st to the 10th day of the cycle; the *ovulatory phase* lasts from the 11th to the 14th day of the cycle and ends with *ovulation;* and the *luteal phase* lasts from the 14th to the 28th days.

The follicular phase encompasses the development of the follicle and the maturation of the oocyte. These processes are controlled by the interaction of FSH and LH. On day 1 of the cycle, gonadotropin-releasing hormone (Gn-RH) from the hypothalamus increases and stimulates increased production of FSH and LH by the anterior pituitary. FSH and LH stimulate follicular growth, and the oocyte increases in size. The structure, now called the *primary follicle,* becomes a multicellular mass surrounded by a fibrous capsule called the *theca folliculi.* As the follicle continues to increase in size, estrogen is produced and a fluid-filled space (the *antrum*) forms within the follicle. The oocyte is enclosed by a membrane, the *zona pellucida.* By about the 10th day, the follicle is a mature graafian follicle and bulges out from the surface of the ovary. There are always follicles at different stages of development in each ovary, but usually only one follicle becomes dominant and matures to ovulation, while the others degenerate.

The ovulatory phase begins when estrogen levels reach a level high enough to stimulate the anterior pituitary, and a surge of LH is produced. The LH stimulates meiosis in the developing oocyte, and its first meiotic division occurs. The LH also stimulates enzymes that act on the bulging ovarian wall, causing it to rupture and discharge the antrum fluid and the oocyte. The oocyte is expelled from the mature ovarian follicle in the process called ovulation.

During the luteal phase, the surge in LH also stimulates the ruptured follicle to change into a corpus luteum and then stimulates the corpus luteum to begin immediately to produce progesterone and estrogen. The increase of progesterone and estrogen in the blood has a negative-feedback effect on the production of LH, inhibiting the further growth and development of other follicles.

If pregnancy does not occur, the corpus luteum begins to degenerate, and its hormone production ceases. The declining production of progesterone and estrogen at the end of the cycle allows the secretion of LH and FSH to increase, and a new cycle begins. The ovarian cycle is compared to the menstrual cycle in Figure 45–5.

The Menstrual Cycle

The endometrium of the uterus responds to changes in estrogen and progesterone during the ovarian cycle to prepare for implantation of the fertilized embryo. The endometrium is receptive to implantation of the embryo for only a brief period each month, coinciding with the time when the embryo would normally reach the uterus from the uterine tube (usually 7 days).

The cycle begins with the *menstrual phase,* lasting from days 1 to 5. The inner endometrial (functionalis) layer detaches and is expelled as menstrual fluid (fluid and blood) for 3 to 5 days. As the maturing follicle begins to produce estrogen (days 6 to 14), the *proliferative phase* begins. In response, the functionalis layer is repaired and thickens, while spiral arteries increase in number and tubular glands form. Cervical mucus changes to a thin, crystalline substance, forming channels to help the sperm move up into the uterus.

The final phase, lasting from days 14 to 28, is the *secretory phase.* As the corpus luteum produces progesterone, the rising levels act on the endometrium, causing increased vascularity, changing the inner layer to secretory mucosa, stimulating the secretion of glycogen into the uterine cavity, and causing the cervical mucus again to become thick and block the internal os. If fertilization does not occur, hormone levels fall. Spasm of the spiral arteries causes hypoxia of the endometrial cells, which begin to degenerate and slough off. As with the ovarian cycle, the process begins again with the sloughing of the functionalis layer.

Assessment of Reproductive Function

■ ■ ■

The function of the reproductive systems in men and women is assessed both by a health assessment interview to collect subjective data and a physical assessment to collect objective data. The following section provides guidelines for collecting data through the health assessment interview. Interview questions and leading statements for assessing reproductive system function are also provided.

When assessing the male or female reproductive systems, the nurse considers the psychologic, social, and cultural factors that affect sexual activity and sexuality. Thus, the nurse uses words that the client understands, and is not embarrassed by the client's terminology. The client may perceive the interview as less threatening if the discussion begins with more general questions and then progresses to questions specific to the reproductive system. For example, the nurse may first ask a female client about menstrual and childbirth histories before asking questions about sexually transmitted diseases. Interview questions are also less threatening if they are asked in a way that gives the client permission to report behaviors and manifestations. For example, rather than asking a man if he has difficulty achieving or maintaining an erection, the nurse asks him to describe any changes he has noticed in having an erection.

Health Assessment Interview for Men

Overview

The health assessment for the male reproductive system is often a part of the assessment of the urinary system (see Chapter 24). Before asking questions about sexual history, explain that this information is a part of a general health assessment. If a health problem is identified, collect information specific to its onset, characteristics, duration, frequency, precipitating or relieving factors, treatment and/or self-care, and outcome. For example, ask the client:

- When did you first notice that you were having difficulty urinating?

- Did you use a different brand of condoms before you noticed the rash on your penis?

- Describe the changes that occurred in your ability to have an erection after you started taking medicine for high blood pressure.

In questioning the client about past medical history, ask about chronic illnesses such as diabetes, chronic renal failure, cardiovascular disease, multiple sclerosis, spinal cord tumors or trauma, or thyroid disease. The effects of these illnesses as well as the treatment of the illnesses may cause **impotence** (inability to achieve or maintain an erection). For example, the following drugs may cause sexual function problems: antihypertensives, antidepressants, antispasmodics, tranquilizers, sedatives, and hista-

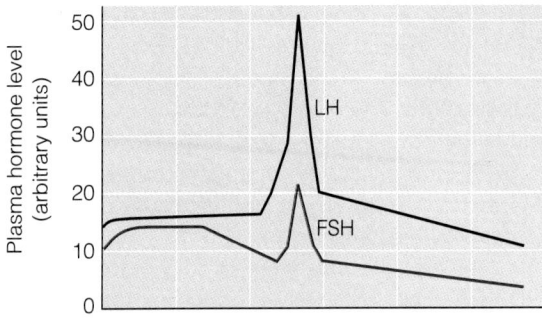

A Fluctuation of gonadotropin levels

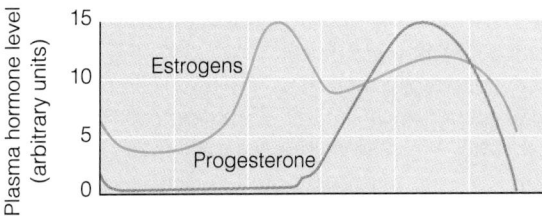

B Fluctuation of ovarian hormone levels

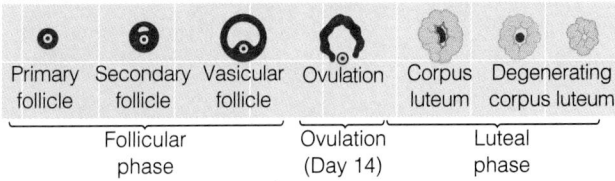

C Ovarian cycle

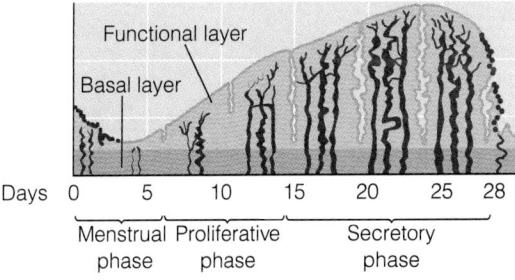

D Uterine cycle

Figure 45–5 Comparison of the ovarian and uterine cycles. *A,* Fluctuating levels of follicle stimulating hormone (FSH) and luteinizing hormone (LH), the pituitary gonadotropins regulating the ovarian cycle. *B,* Fluctuating levels of ovarian hormones that cause endometrial changes during the uterine cycle. *C,* Changes in the ovarian follicles during the 28-day ovarian cycle. *D,* Corresponding changes in the endometrium during the uterine cycle.

mine$_2$-receptor antagonists. Psychosocial stressors also may contribute to impotence.

If the man was born to a woman treated during pregnancy with diethylstilbestrol (DES), a drug used in the

1940s and 1950s to prevent miscarriage, congenital deformities of the urinary tract as well as decreased semen levels may be present. If the man had mumps as a child, sterility is possible. The risk for testicular cancer is greatest in men who have a history of an undescended testicle, an inguinal hernia, testicular swelling with mumps, a history of maternal use of DES or oral contraceptives, and a family history of testicular cancer.

Explore the life-style and social history of the man; the use of alcohol, cigarettes, or street drugs may affect sexual function. Frequent sexual intercourse, especially if unprotected, increases the potential for sexually transmitted diseases including HIV infection. Sexual intercourse with same-sex partners further increases the risk for acquired immune deficiency syndrome (AIDS). Other questions about sexuality may include number of sexual partners; history of premature ejaculation, impotence, or other sexual problems; any history of sexual trauma; use of condoms or other contraceptives; and current level of sexual satisfaction.

Interview Questions

The following interview questions and leading statements are categorized by functional health patterns.

Health Perception–Health Management

- Have you ever had any problems with your reproductive organs (penis, testicles, prostate gland)? Explain.

- How was the problem treated? Medications? Surgery?

- Have you ever had surgery on your reproductive organs or your urinary organs? Explain. What was the outcome?

- Have you ever noticed any swelling or pain in your breasts? Explain.

- Have you ever had a sexually transmitted disease? What was it, and how was it treated?

- Do you practice safer sex? Explain.

- Do you practice testicular self-examination? How often?

- Do you smoke? If so, how much and for how long?

Nutritional-Metabolic

- Describe your usual dietary intake for a 24-hour period.

Elimination

- Do you now have or have you ever had a discharge from your penis? Describe the color, consistency, odor, amount, and frequency.

- Have you had any bleeding from your penis? Explain.

- Have you noticed any changes in urination (burning, frequency, urgency, difficulty starting the stream, size of the stream, dribbling, getting up at night)? Explain.

Activity-Exercise

- Describe your usual activities of daily living for a 24-hour period.

- Do you participate in sports or heavy lifting? If so, do you wear a protective cup, truss, or athletic support?

Sleep-Rest

- Describe the quality of your rest and sleep.

Cognitive-Perceptual

- Describe any pain you have had in the groin area, testicles, penis, or scrotum. Where is it? Do you experience it in other parts of your body? How long does it last? What precipitates and relieves it?

- Has there been a change in the condition or color of the skin on your penis or scrotum? Explain.

Self-Perception–Self-Concept

- Do you feel that your needs for intimacy and affection are being met?

- How has this health problem made you feel about yourself as a man?

Role-Relationship

- Has there been any history of infertility or other reproductive problems in your family?

- Are you satisfied with your relationship with your sexual partner?

- How has this health problem affected your relationship with your sexual partner or others close to you?

- Has there been any change in your sexual relationship(s)? Explain.

Sexuality-Reproductive

- Are you currently sexually active?

- Have you fathered any children?

- Are you satisfied with your current level of sexual functioning?

- Has there been a change in your sexual functioning?

- Have you ever had difficulty in achieving or maintaining an erection or ejaculation during sexual activity? Explain.

Coping-Stress

- On a scale of 1 to 10 (with 10 being the greatest amount), describe the amount of stress you are experiencing from this health problem.
- How have you coped with this health problem?

Value-Belief

- What is most important in your life?
- Who or what has been most helpful and supportive to you in dealing with this problem?
- Does your religious or cultural background influence your sexual activities? Explain.

Health Assessment Interview for Women

Overview

The focused interview for the female reproductive system is usually extensive. However, the questions may in many instances be tailored to the specific health problem of the client. As with the assessment of other body systems, analyze and document the onset of the problem, its duration, frequency, precipitating and relieving factors, any associated symptoms, treatment, self-care, and outcome. For example, ask the client:

- Did you notice that you had increased vaginal bleeding after intercourse?
- Does the over-the-counter medication relieve the vaginal itching and discharge?
- How many pads do you use during each period?
- Have you had any fever or abdominal pain with this vaginal infection?

Ask about menstrual history, obstetric history, use of contraceptives, sexual history, use of medications, and reproductive system examinations. Also assess the use of condoms during intercourse; unprotected sexual intercourse increases the risk of sexually transmitted diseases, including HIV infection. Also ask about smoking; a history of smoking increases the risk of circulatory problems in the woman who is taking oral contraceptives. Smoking also increases the risk for cancer of the cervix.

Chronic illnesses may affect the function of the female reproductive system. Diabetes increases the risk of vaginal infections and vaginal dryness, both of which interfere with sexual pleasure. Chronic heavy menstrual flow may result in anemia. Thyroid and adrenal disorders may affect secondary sex characteristics, the menstrual cycle, and the ability to become pregnant.

Obtaining any family history of cancer is important. The risk for endometrial cancer is higher in women with a family history of endometrial, breast, or colon cancer; the risk for ovarian cancer is higher in women with a family history of ovarian or breast cancer; and the risk for breast cancer is higher in women with a family history of breast cancer. Exposure to diethylstilbestrol (DES) in utero increases the risk of cancer of the cervix and vagina. Exposure to asbestos poses a risk of cancer of the ovary. The risk for breast cancer is also greater if the client has a history of fibrocystic disease.

Carefully explore any history of vaginal bleeding and vaginal discharge. Ask about the onset of vaginal bleeding, any related factors, the color (pink, red, dark red, brown), the character (thin, watery, presence of mucus, size and number of clots), the amount (spotting, how many pads or tampons in a specific amount of time) and relationship to menstrual cycle. Regarding vaginal discharge, ask about the onset, color (white, green, gray), character (thin, curdlike, infected), odor, itching, and rash.

Questions about sexuality may include number of sexual partners; history of **anorgasmia** (absence of orgasm), **dyspareunia** (painful intercourse), or other problems; any history of sexual trauma; use of condoms or other contraceptives, and current level of sexual satisfaction.

Interview Questions

The following interview questions and leading statements are categorized by functional health patterns. The age and reproductive status of the woman being interviewed determine which of the questions will be asked.

Health Perception–Health Management

- Have you ever had any problems with your reproductive organs (menstruation, ovaries, tubes, uterus, vagina)? Explain.
- How was the problem treated? Medications? Surgery?
- Have you noticed any lumps in your breasts or discharge from you nipples? Explain.
- Do you take oral contraceptives? What type and for how long?
- Describe any other medications you take.
- When was your last gynecologic examination? Pap smear? How often do you have these done?
- Have you ever had a breast examination and/or mammogram? When? How often do you have these done?
- Do you practice breast self-examination? When and how often do you do this?
- What do you do to provide self-care if you have mood swings or menstrual cramps?
- Have you ever had a sexually transmitted disease or an infection of the reproductive organs? Explain.

- If you are sexually active, do you use protection against sexually transmitted diseases?
- Do you use douches or vaginal sprays? If so, what type and how often?
- What type of underwear do you wear?
- Do you smoke? If so, how much and for how long?

Nutritional-Metabolic

- Do you ever have an increase or a decrease in your appetite during or before your menstrual period?
- Have you noticed a change in your appetite or weight since menopause?
- Describe your usual dietary intake for a 24-hour period.

Elimination

- When was your last menstrual period?
- At what age did you start/stop having menstrual periods?
- Describe the length, amount of flow, and clotting with your menstrual periods. Do you ever bleed between periods? If so, describe the type and amount.
- Describe any unusual vaginal discharge you have had (color, amount, consistency, odor, associated itching and/or rash).
- Have you noticed any changes in urination (frequency, urgency, burning)?

Activity-Exercise

- Describe your usual activities of daily living.
- Do your activities of daily living change before or during your menstrual periods? If so, how?
- Have your activities of daily living changed since menopause? If so, how?

Sleep-Rest

- Describe the quality of your rest and sleep.
- Do menstrual cramps waken you at night?
- Do you have night sweats? How often?

Cognitive-Perceptual

- Do you have pain or other symptoms (headache, mood swings, irritability, bloating, constipation or diarrhea, breast tenderness) before your menstrual periods? Describe these.
- Do you have cramping before or during your menstrual period? Describe the type of cramping, how long it lasts, and what relief measures you use.
- Do you have any pain in the genital area?

- Do you ever have vaginal itching, pain, or dryness during or after intercourse?
- Do you have any concerns or questions about sexual activity or reproduction?

Self-Perception–Self-Concept

- Describe how the problem with your reproductive system makes you feel as a woman.
- Do you believe your needs for intimacy and affection are being met?
- How has menopause made you feel about yourself?

Role-Relationship

- Are you satisfied with your current sexual relationship?
- Are you satisfied with your communication with your partner?
- How has having a problem with reproductive health affected your relationship with your spouse or sexual partner?

Sexuality-Reproductive

- Is there a history of reproductive problems in your family? Explain.
- Are you currently participating in a sexual relationship? If so, have there been any changes in your interest in or ability to enjoy sexual activities?
- Are you able to have an orgasm?
- Have you ever been pregnant? How many times? Did you have any complications?
- Have you ever had a miscarriage or abortion?
- Have you ever had problems getting pregnant? If so, did you have fertility studies?
- Are you planning or avoiding pregnancy at this time? Explain.

Coping-Stress

- How have you coped with this health problem?
- On a scale of 1 to 10 (with 10 being the greatest), rate how stressful this current reproductive problem has been for you.

Value-Belief

- What is most important in your life?
- What or who has been most helpful and supportive to you in dealing with this health problem?
- Does your religious or cultural background influence your sexual activities or your feelings about yourself as a woman? Explain.

Physical Assessment

Physical assessment of the reproductive system usually is conducted as part of a scheduled screening (e.g., for an annual Papanicolaou smear) or for a specific reproductive health problem. If conducted as part of a total physical assessment, this is usually the final system to be assessed. The nurse must feel comfortable with the examination of clients of the opposite gender; if either the nurse or the client is not comfortable, a nurse of the same gender should be asked to conduct this part of the assessment.

The reproductive system is assessed by inspection and palpation. Ask the client to void before having the examination. Prior to the examination, collect all necessary equipment and explain the techniques to the client to decrease anxiety. Put on rubber gloves before beginning the examination and wear them throughout the examination.

The Male Reproductive System: Preparation

The equipment necessary for assessing the male reproductive system includes disposable latex gloves, a flashlight, sterile cotton swabs, and culture media. Explain the procedures for the examination thoroughly; if the man is unfamiliar with his internal genitalia, charts may be used to demonstrate the parts that will be examined.

Ask the client to remove his clothing from the waist down. The assessment may be done with the client sitting or standing. Ensure that the examining room is warm and private.

ASSESSMENT TECHNIQUE	POSSIBLE ABNORMAL FINDINGS

The Breasts
(Note: Assessment of male breasts is less complicated than assessment of female breasts but should not be overlooked.)
■ **Inspect and palpate both breasts, including areola and nipple.**

A smooth, firm, mobile, tender disc of breast tissue behind the areola indicates **gynecomastia,** abnormal enlargement of the breast(s) in men. Gynecomastia requires additional investigation to determine cause. A hard, irregular nodule in the nipple area suggests carcinoma.

■ **Palpate the axillary lymph nodes.**

Enlarged axillary nodes are common with infections of the hand or arm but can be caused by cancer. Enlarged supraclavicular nodes may indicate metastases.

External Male Reproductive Organs
■ **Inspect and palpate the inguinal and femoral area for bulges.**
Ask the client to bear down or cough as you palpate (Figure 45–6).

A bulge that increases with straining suggests a hernia.

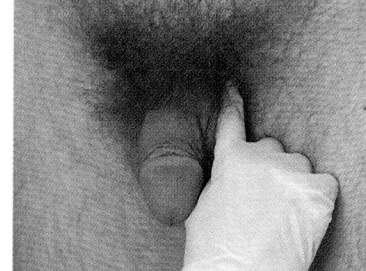

Figure 45–6 Palpating the male inguinal area for bulges.

■ **Inspect the penis.**
If the client is uncircumcised, retract the foreskin or ask the client to do so.

Phimosis (tightness of prepuce that prevents retraction of foreskin) may be congenital or due to recurrent *balanoposthitis* (generalized infection of glans penis and prepuce). Narrow or inflamed foreskin can cause *paraphimosis,* retraction

ASSESSMENT TECHNIQUE	POSSIBLE ABNORMAL FINDINGS

of the foreskin that causes painful swelling of the glans. *Balanitis* (inflammation of the glands) is associated with bacterial or fungal infections. Ulcers, vesicles, or warts suggest sexually transmitted diseases. Nodules or sores seen in uncircumcised men may be cancer.

- **Inspect the external urinary meatus.**

Press the glans between the thumb and forefinger (Figure 45–7). Replace the foreskin if appropriate.

Erythema or discharge indicates inflammatory disease. Further assessment is required.

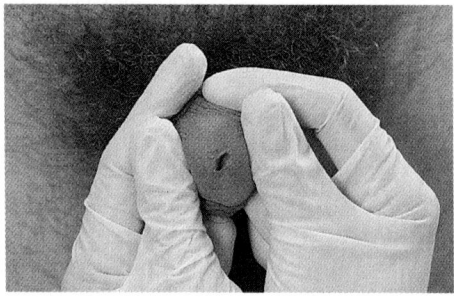

Figure 45–7 Inspecting the external urinary meatus of the male.

- **Inspect the skin around the base of the penis.**

Excoriation or inflammation suggests lice or scabies.

- **Palpate the shaft of the penis.**

Induration with tenderness along with ventral surface suggests urethral stricture with inflammation.

- **Inspect the scrotum.**

Any swelling in the scrotum should be further assessed using transillumination: Darken the room and place a lighted flashlight against the skin of the scrotum. The normal scrotum and epididymis appear as dark masses with regular borders.

A unilateral or bilateral poorly developed scrotum suggests *cryptorchidism* (failure of one or both testes to descend into the scrotum). Swelling of the scrotum may indicate indirect inguinal hernia, *hydrocele* (accumulation of fluid in the scrotum), or scrotal edema. Swellings containing serous fluid will transilluminate. Swellings containing blood or tissue will not transilluminate.

- **Palpate each testis and epididymis.**

Tender, painful scrotal swelling occurs in acute epididymitis, acute orchitis, torsion of the spermatic cord, and strangulated hernia. A painless nodule in the testis is associated with testicular cancer.

Internal Male Reproductive Organs
(*Note: The prostate gland is assessed by digital rectal examination. See Chapter 22 for technique for palpation of the rectal wall.*)

- **Palpate the posterior surface of the prostate gland.**

With a gloved index finger, palpate the anterior rectal wall for the rounded, two-lobed structure of the posterior prostate.

Enlargement (1-cm protrusion into the rectum) with obliteration of the median sulcus suggests benign prostatic hypertrophy. Enlargement with asymmetry and tenderness suggests prostatitis. A hard irregular nodule is seen in carcinoma.

Physical Assessment

The Female Reproductive System: Preparation

The equipment necessary for assessing the female reproductive system includes disposable latex gloves, a good light source, sterile cotton swabs, a spatula, water-soluble lubricant, slides, cytologic fixative, and specula of various sizes. If cultures are to be taken, culture media is necessary. Carefully explain the procedure for the examination, and show the speculum to the woman. If the woman is unfamiliar with her genitalia, charts may be used to demonstrate the parts that will be examined.

Ask the client to remove her clothing and put on a gown. Ensure that the examining room is private and warm.

The examination usually begins with examination of the breasts with the client in the sitting and supine positions. The nurse then assists the client to move to the lithotomy position on the examining table, with the feet in the stirrups and the buttocks even with the foot of the table. Older or frail clients may not be able to tolerate this position. In this case, the client is examined in the supine position. Draping should be used throughout the examination so that only the part of the body being examined is exposed. Although the entire examination is described here, the internal examination is conducted only by a nurse with advanced practice in the procedure. Guidelines for use of the vaginal speculum and for conducting the bimanual pelvic examination are outlined in the boxes on pages 1958 and 1959.

ASSESSMENT TECHNIQUE	POSSIBLE ABNORMAL FINDINGS

The Breasts

- **Inspect both breasts simultaneously with the client seated in the following positions:**

    1. Arms at sides
    2. Arms overhead
    3. Hands pressed on hips
    4. Leaning forward.

Inspect breast size, symmetry, contour, skin color, texture, venous patterns, and lesions. Lift the breasts, and inspect the lower and lateral aspects.

- **Inspect the areolae and nipples.**

- **Palpate both breasts, axillae, and supraclavicular areas.**

Figure 45–8 illustrates a possible pattern for breast palpation. Various palpation patterns may be used provided that every part of each breast is palpated, including the axillary tail (also called *tail of Spence*), which is the breast tissue that extends from the upper outer quadrant toward and into the axillae. Ask the client to assume a supine position with a small pillow under the shoulder and the arm over the head, and repeat the systematic palpation sequence. Findings of nonpathologic breast enlargement, nodularity, and tenderness are more common the week preceding and during menstrual flow. Describe identified masses by location, size, shape, consistency, tenderness, mobility, and delineation of borders.

Retractions, dimpling, and abnormal contours suggest underlying malignancy. These findings may also be due to benign lesions. Thickened, dimpled skin with enlarged pores (called *peau d'orange,* orange peel, or pig skin) and unilateral venous patterns are also associated with malignancy. Redness may be seen with infection or carcinoma.

Peau d'orange may be noted first in the areola. Recent unilateral inversion of the nipple or asymmetry in the directions in which the nipples point suggests cancer.

Tenderness may be related to premenstrual fullness, fibrocystic disease, or inflammation. Tenderness may also indicate cancer. Nodules in the tail of the breast may be enlarged lymph nodes. Hard, irregular, fixed unilateral masses that are poorly delineated suggest carcinoma. Bilateral, single or multiple, round, mobile, well-delineated masses are consistent with fibrocystic breast disease or fibroadenoma. Swelling, tenderness, erythema, and heat may be seen with mastitis.

| ASSESSMENT TECHNIQUE | POSSIBLE ABNORMAL FINDINGS |

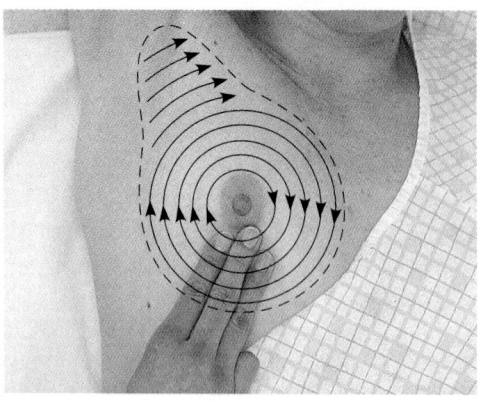

Figure 45–8 Possible pattern for palpation of the breast.

- **Palpate the nipple.**

Palpate the nipple, then compress it between the thumb and index finger. Note the color of any discharge.

Loss of nipple elasticity is seen in cancer. Bloody or serous discharge is associated with intraductal papilloma. Milky discharge not due to prior pregnancy and found on both sides suggests **galactorrhea** (lactation not associated with pregnancy or nursing), which is sometimes associated with a pituitary tumor. Unilateral discharge from one or two ducts can be seen in fibrocystic breast disease, intraductal papilloma, or carcinoma.

- **Inspect the skin of the axillae.**

Rash may be due to allergy or other causes. Signs of inflammation and infection may be due to infection of the sweat glands.

- **Palpate all sections of both axillae for palpable nodes.**

Palpate the axillary lymph nodes (Figure 45–9).

Enlarged axillary nodes are most often due to infection of the hand or arm but can be caused by malignancy. Enlarged supraclavicular nodes are associated with lymphatic metastases from abdominal or thoracic carcinoma.

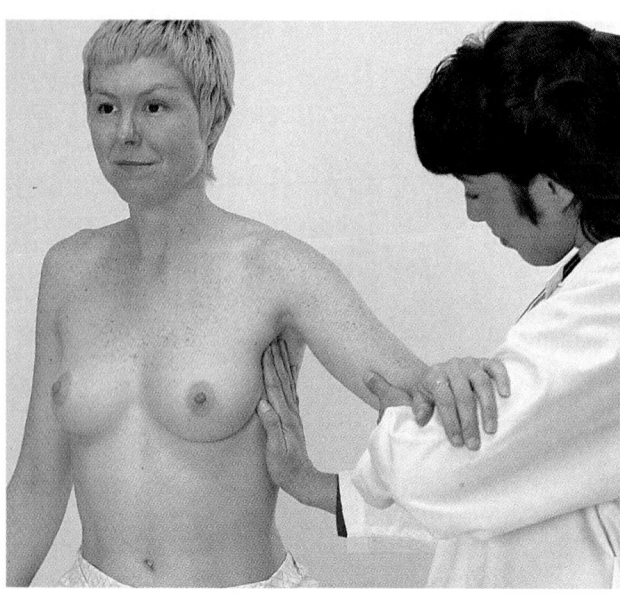

Figure 45–9 Palpating the axillary lymph nodes.

ASSESSMENT TECHNIQUE	POSSIBLE ABNORMAL FINDINGS

The External Female Reproductive Organs
Help the client to the lithotomy position with the knees flexed and separated.

- **Inspect and palpate the labia majora.**

Excoriation, rashes, or lesions suggest inflammatory or infective processes. Bulging of the labia that increases with straining suggests a hernia. Varicosities may be present on the labia.

- **Inspect the labia minora.**

Use a gloved hand to separate the labia majora for better visualization.

Inflammation, irritation, excoriation, or caking of discharge in tissue folds suggests vaginal infection or poor hygiene. Ulcers or vesicles may be symptoms of sexually transmitted diseases.

- **Palpate the inside of the labia minora between gloved thumb and forefinger.**

Small, firm, round cystic nodules in labia suggest sebaceous cysts. Wartlike lesions suggest condylomata acuminata (genital warts). Firm, painless ulcers suggest chancre of primary syphilis. Shallow, painful ulcers suggest herpes. Ulcerated or red raised vulvar lesions in older women suggest vulvar carcinoma.

- **Inspect the clitoris for size and length.**

Enlargement may be a symptom of a masculinizing condition.

- **Inspect the vaginal opening.**

Swelling or discoloration may be caused by trauma. Discharge or lesions may be symptoms of infection. Fissures or fistulas may be related to injury, infection, spreading of a malignancy, or trauma.

- **Palpate Skene's glands.**

Using a gloved index finger, "milk" Skene's glands on both sides and over the urethra and inspect for possible discharge (Figure 45–10).

Discharge from Skene's glands and/or tenderness suggests infection.

Figure 45–10   Palpating Skene's glands.

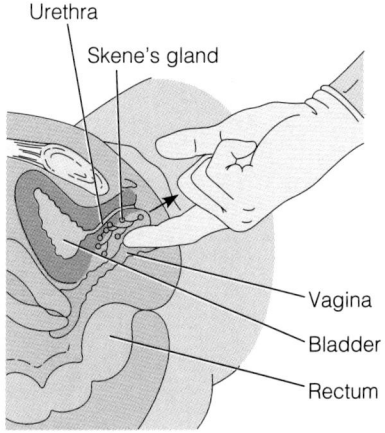

Urethra

Skene's gland

Vagina

Bladder

Rectum

ASSESSMENT TECHNIQUE	POSSIBLE ABNORMAL FINDINGS

■ Palpate Bartholin's glands.

Palpate Bartholin's glands at the posterior labia majora (Figure 45–11).

A nontender mass in the posterolateral portion of the labia majora is indicative of a Bartholin's cyst. Swelling, redness, or tenderness, especially if unilateral, may indicate abscess of Bartholin's glands.

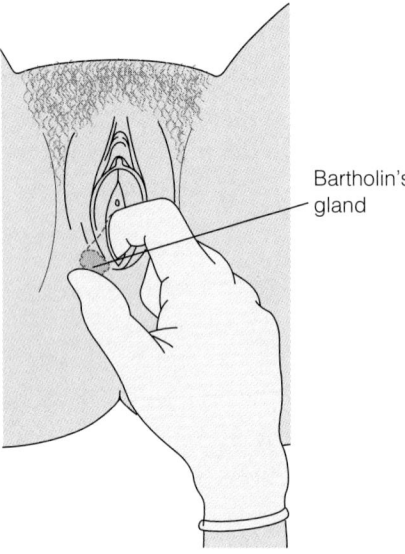

Bartholin's gland

Figure 45–11 Palpating Bartholin's glands.

■ Inspect the vaginal orifice for bulging and urinary incontinence.

Ask the client to strain or "bear down."

Bulging of the anterior vaginal wall and urinary incontinence suggest a cystocele. Bulging of the posterior wall suggests a rectocele. Protrusion of the cervix or uterus into the vagina indicates uterine prolapse.

■ Inspect and palpate the perineum.

Episiotomy scarring may be apparent. Inflammation, lesions, and growths may be seen in infections or cancer. Fistulas may be the result of injury, trauma, infection, or spreading of a malignancy.

Internal Female Reproductive Organs
■ Use a vaginal speculum to inspect the vaginal walls and cervix.

See the guidelines in the box on page 1958.

Bluish color of the cervix and vaginal mucosa may be a sign of pregnancy. A pale cervix is associated with anemia. A cervix located to the right or left of the midline may indicate a pelvic mass, uterine adhesions, or pregnancy. Projection of the cervix more than 3 cm into the vaginal canal may indicate a pelvic or uterine mass.

Transverse or star-shaped cervical lacerations reflect trauma causing tearing of the cervix. An enlarged cervix is associated with infection. An *ectropion* (eversion of columnar epithelium lining the cervical canal) appears plush red around the central cervical os and may bleed easily. *Nabothian cysts* (small, white, or yellow raised, round areas on the cervix) are considered normal but may become infected. Cervical polyps may be cervical or endometrial in origin.

ASSESSMENT TECHNIQUE	POSSIBLE ABNORMAL FINDINGS
Bimanual Pelvic Examination ■ **Palpate the cervix, uterus and ovaries.** See the guidelines in the box on page 1959.	The uterus may be retroverted (tilted backward) or retroflexed (angled backward). Pain on movement of the cervix during manual examination suggests pelvic inflammatory disease (PID). Softening of the uterine isthmus (Hegar's sign), softening of the cervix (Goodell's sign), and uterine enlargement may be objective signs of pregnancy. Firm, irregular nodules that vary greatly with size and are continuous with the uterine surface are likely to be myomas (fibroids). Unilateral or bilateral smooth, compressible adnexal masses are found in ovarian tumors. Profuse menstrual bleeding is seen with endometrial polyps, dysfunctional uterine bleeding (DUB), and use of an intrauterine device. Irregular bleeding may be associated with endometrial polyps, DUB, uterine or cervical carcinoma, or oral contraceptives. Postmenopausal bleeding is seen with endometrial hyperplasia, estrogen therapy, and endometrial cancer.

Variations in Assessment Findings in the Older Adult

Aging affects the reproductive system in both men and women, although the physiologic changes are more pronounced in women. With age, women lose their reproductive capacity but retain sexual capacity; men retain both reproductive and sexual capacity. It is important to remember that both men and women remain sexual beings all of their lives.

The Older Male

The primary age-related change in the reproductive system of men is a decrease in its efficiency. Although production of male sex hormones gradually declines with age, the decline starts later than it does in women, and hormone production does not totally cease. Other age-related changes include the following:

■ The testes become smaller and less firm.

■ The prostate gland enlarges.

■ The penis decreases in size.

■ Responses to sexual stimulation undergo changes: It takes longer to attain erection and ejaculation; the amount and force of ejaculate decrease; and the time between orgasm and another erection increases.

The Older Female

The gradual cessation of ovarian function and a decline in estrogen results in the final reproductive marker for women that is known as *menopause*. Although some estrogens are produced by the adrenal glands, their levels are not sufficient to maintain secondary sex characteristics at a level experienced during the menstruating years. This aging process brings about the following changes:

■ Absence of menstruation, called *amenorrhea* (usually around age 50).

■ Vasomotor instability, resulting in hot flashes and night sweats.

■ Atrophy of the vaginal mucosa, causing vaginal dryness and dyspareunia.

■ Atrophy of the urethra, causing stress incontinence.

■ Scanty body hair, but increased facial hair.

■ Loss of elasticity and subcutaneous fat in the skin and breasts.

■ Loss of bone from osteoporosis.

■ Altered responses to sexual stimulation: decreased breast engorgement and nipple erection, decreased engorgement of the clitoris and vulva, decreased vaginal secretions, and less intense contractions during orgasm.

Guidelines for Intravaginal Assessment and Use of the Vaginal Speculum
■ ■ ■

The size of the speculum that is used for an internal examination of the female reproductive system depends on the age of the woman and size of the vagina. Two types of specula are available. The Graves speculum, used most often for examinations of adult women, is available in lengths of 3½ to 5 inches and widths of ¾ to 1½ inches. The Pederson speculum, which is narrower, may be used to examine adolescents or adult women who are virgins, who have never had a baby, or who are postmenopausal with vaginal atrophy. The speculum should be warm: A heating pad is used in many institutions. If cultures or smears are to be obtained, neither water nor gel should be used either to warm or to lubricate the speculum.

If cells are to be taken for cytologic studies, the client should not douche, use vaginal medications, or take a tub bath for 24 hours before the examination. Finally, the examination is usually deferred if the client is menstruating or has a vaginal infection.

The general procedure is as follows:

1. Place the index and middle finger of one hand into the vagina, just inside the introitus, and press the fingers toward the rectum. Hold the speculum in the other hand.

2. Ask the client to bear down, and insert the closed blades of the speculum into the vagina at an oblique angle until the ends of the blades reach the fingertips (see the accompanying figure). Withdraw the fingers and rotate the speculum to a transverse position.

3. Continue to insert the speculum until it reaches the end of the vagina. Depress the lever of the speculum to open the blades. If the cervix is not in full view, try closing the blades, withdrawing the speculum about halfway, and inserting it again at a more downward angle. When the cervix is in full view, fix the depressed lever to an open position.

4. Inspect the cervix. The normal cervix is pink and midline. Assess color, position, size, projection into the vagina, surface and shape, and any discharge.

If a Papanicolaou (Pap) smear to collect cervical cells for cytologic studies is done, the following procedure may be used:

1. To collect cells from the vaginal pool, roll a sterile cotton-tipped applicator on the vaginal wall below the cervix. Paint the smear on the slide, and spray the slide with fixative.

2. To collect endocervical cells, place the groove of the spatula snugly against the cervical os, and rotate it 360 degrees. In a single stroke, spread the material from both sides of the spatula on a slide, and immediately spray with fixative.

If cultures are to be done, take a specimen from the vagina and/or cervix with a sterile, cotton-tipped applicator, and then either spread the specimen on a culture plate or place it in a culture container. Follow institutional protocols for preparing specimens for vaginal infections from suspected organisms.

At the end of the examination, loosen the lever control and slowly withdraw the speculum, closing the blades slowly and rotating the speculum while observing all areas of the vaginal wall. Assess the color of the mucosa and the color and appearance of any discharge.

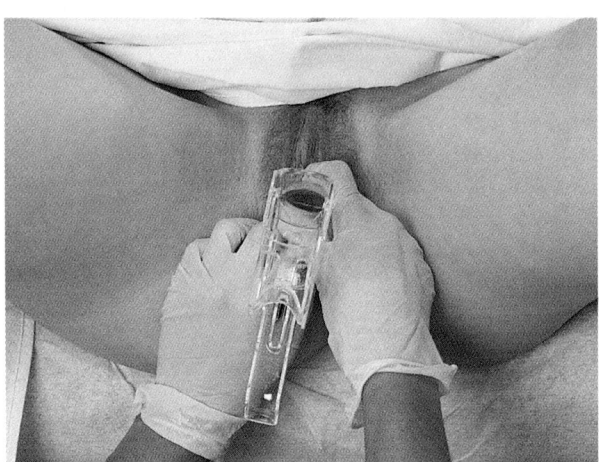

Inserting the vaginal speculum.

Guidelines for Bimanual Pelvic Examination

■ ■ ■

The bimanual pelvic examination is done to palpate the cervix, uterus, and ovaries. The examiner's hand that will be used intravaginally is held with the index and middle fingers extended, the thumb abducted, and the fourth and fifth fingers folded on the palm of the hand. The extended fingers are lubricated.

The general procedure is as follows:

1. Spread the labia with the thumb and finger of the opposite hand and insert the lubricated fingers into the vagina with the palm upward.

2. Place the opposite hand on the abdomen; it is used to press on the abdomen and gently move the internal genitals toward the intravaginal fingers (see the accompanying figure).

3. Ask the client to take deep breaths to relax the abdominal wall.

4. Palpate the cervix, assessing size, contour, position, surface, consistency, tenderness, and mobility. The cervix should be freely movable and non-tender.

5. Palpate the uterus by pressing downward on the abdomen while placing the intravaginal fingers in the anterior fornix and gently lifting against the abdominal hand. Assess the size, shape, surface, consistency, position, mobility, and tenderness of the uterus. The normal uterus is freely movable and nontender.

6. Palpate the adnexal areas, which surround the uterus and contain the fallopian tubes and ovaries.

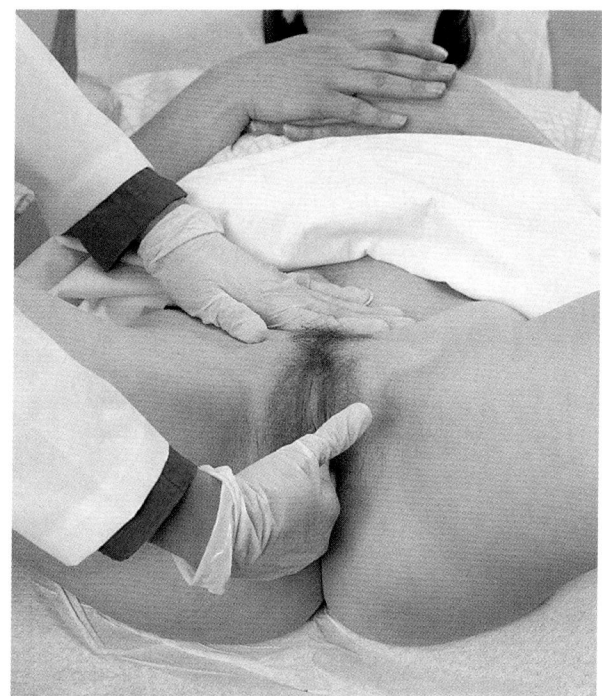

Bimanual pelvic examination.

Because these structures are small, palpation may not be possible. If the ovaries are palpable, they should be smooth and firm. The normal ovary is sensitive to touch, firm, and highly movable.

7. Withdraw the fingers. Provide tissues for the client's use in wiping the genital area.

Bibliography

■ ■ ■

Blair, K. (1990). Aging: Physiological aspects and clinical implications. *The Nurse Practitioner: The American Journal of Primary Health Care, 15*(2), 14–28.

Clark-Coller, T. (1991). Dysfunctional uterine bleeding and amenorrhea: Differential diagnosis and management. *Journal of Nurse Midwifery, 36,* 49–62.

Dubin, S. (1992). The physiologic changes of aging. *Orthopaedic Nursing, 11*(3), 45–50.

Fishbein, E. (1992). Women at midlife: The transition to menopause. *Nursing Clinics of North America, 27,* 951–957.

Hortobagyi, G., McLelland, R. & Reed, F. (1990). Your key role in breast cancer screening. *Patient Care, 24*(13), 82–87, 90, 93.

Marieb, E. (1995). *Human anatomy and physiology* (3rd ed.). Redwood City, CA: Benjamin/Cummings.

Norwood, S. (1990). Fibrocystic breast disease. *Journal of Obstetric, Gynecologic, and Neonatal Nursing, 19,* 116–121.

Porth, C. M. (1994). *Pathophysiology: Concepts of altered health states* (4th ed.) Philadelphia: J. B. Lippincott Company.

Willson, P. (1991). Testicular, prostate, and penile cancers in primary care settings. *The Nurse Practitioner: The American Journal of Primary Health Care, 16*(11), 18–26.

Nursing Care of Male Clients with Reproductive System Disorders

LEARNING OBJECTIVES

After completing this chapter, you will be able to

- Describe the pathophysiology of commonly occurring disorders of the male reproductive system.
- Identify laboratory and diagnostic tests used to diagnose disorders of the prostate gland, penis, testes, and scrotum.
- List the clinical manifestations of commonly occurring disorders of the prostate gland, penis, testes, and scrotum.
- Discuss nursing implications for medications prescribed for clients with disorders of the male reproductive system.
- Provide appropriate nursing care for the client in the preoperative and postoperative phases of surgery of the male reproductive system.
- Use the nursing process as a framework for providing individualized care to clients with disorders of the male reproductive system.

Men are subject to disorders of the prostate gland, scrotal contents, and the penis. As men age, problems with the prostate gland become common. Many of the disorders pose significant risk to the client's fertility and sexual and urinary function, and some are life threatening.

The nurse must provide sensitive care in a variety of roles, including advocate, educator, caregiver, and coordinator of care. These roles are fulfilled in health care settings such as clinics, acute care hospitals, skilled care facilities, home care, public health facilities, and hospices.

◆◆◆ Disorders of the Prostate Gland ◆◆◆

The Client with Prostatic Cancer

■ ■ ■

Cancer of the prostate is the most common type of cancer in North American men and the second leading cause of cancer death, following lung cancer. It is primarily a dis-ease of older men, increasing in incidence with age, and rarely occurring before age 50 (Sagalowsky & Wilson, 1994). In 1995, approximately 244,000 men will be diagnosed with prostate cancer, and 40,400 will die of it (Wingo, Tong, & Bolden, 1995). The threat to men's health increases as the average male's life span continues to increase. There has been a 65% increase in the incidence of prostate cancer between 1973 and 1991 (Demers, Swanson, Weiss, & Kau, 1994). Approximately 1 of 11 men will experience prostate cancer.

The cause of prostate cancer is unknown; however, in its early stages, the tumor is androgen dependent. **Testosterone,** the major androgen, is converted in the prostate to androgen 5-alpha dihydrotestosterone (DHT). Androgen receptors in the cell nuclei bind to DHT and over time lead to **hyperplasia,** an increase in the number of cells in a tissue. Although long associated with benign prostatic hyperplasia (BPH, discussed later in this chapter), DHT may also be a factor in prostatic carcinogenesis (Greco & Kulawiak, 1994). One fact supporting this hypothesis is that men who undergo *orchiectomy* (surgical removal of the testicles) before puberty never develop adenocarcinoma of the prostate.

The progression of prostate cancer is slow, and there may be two forms of the disease: a clinically unimportant, latent stage and a clinically important, aggressive form of the disease. It is estimated that 23% of men who have latent prostate cancer at age 50 will develop the disease with significant symptoms, and 7% will die of the disease (Hanks et al., 1993).

Pathophysiology

The prostate gland is a doughnut-shaped structure that surrounds the urethra at the base of the bladder (see Chapter 45). Most of the prostate gland is composed of glandular epithelial cells; therefore, virtually all cancers arising from the prostate are **adenocarcinomas.**

Prostate cancer usually begins in the peripheral tissue, in the posterior or posterolateral portions of the gland. In the early stages, there are usually no symptoms. As the tumor grows larger, it may compress the urethra, obstructing urinary flow. The tumor may metastasize and involve the seminal vesicles or bladder by direct extension. Despite its proximity to the rectum, metastasis to the bowel is uncommon because a tough sheet of tissue, Denonvilliers' fascia, acts as an effective physical barrier (Davis, 1994).

Metastasis via lymph and venous channels is common. Although the pelvic lymph nodes are the most frequently involved, other lymph nodes in the region may harbor metastatic lesions even when pelvic nodes are negative (Hanks et al., 1993). The major site of distant metastasis is bony tissue, in particular the pelvic bones and spinal column, although the clavicles, ribs, humerus, and skull may be involved as well. Prostate cancer may also spread to the liver and lungs. Clinical manifestations are summarized in the accompanying box. Death usually occurs secondary to debility caused by multiple sites of skeletal metastasis, especially to the vertebrae. Compression fractures of the spine are common, resulting in the possible loss of mobility and bowel and bladder function. Tumors

---

Clinical Manifestations of Prostate Cancer

Genitourinary

- Dysuria
- Frequency of urination
- Reduction in urinary stream
- Nocturia
- Nocturia
- Hematuria
- Abnormal prostate on digital rectal examination

Musculoskeletal

- Bone or joint pain
- Migratory bone pain
- Back pain

Neurologic

- Nerve pain
- Bilateral lower extremity weakness
- Bowel or bladder dysfunction
- Muscle spasms

Systemic

- Weight loss
- Fatigue

---

may eventually involve bone marrow, resulting in severe anemias and impaired immune function.

Collaborative Care

Care of the client with prostate cancer involves many members of the health care team and focuses on diagnosis, elimination or containment of the cancer, and prevention or treatment of complications. There are currently no proven clinical strategies to prevent the development of prostate cancer. Therefore, strategies for early detection remain the major emphasis for control of this disease (see the nursing research box on page 1962). The controversies over prostate cancer screening center on cost-versus-benefit issues. Currently, the screening method recommended by the American Cancer Society is the annual digital rectal examination (DRE) after age 40, and an annual prostate-specific antigen (PSA) check after age 50 (Mettlin, Jones, Averette, Gusberg, & Murphy, 1993). The National Cancer Institute recommends only the annual DRE. Many experts recommend adding annual PSA testing after age 50, and follow-up with transrectal ultrasonography if either PSA or DRE are positive.

The treatment of prostate cancer is complex and depends on the grade and stage of the cancer as well as the age, general health, and preference of the client. In some

Applying Research to Nursing Practice:
Methods to Increase Participation in Prostate Cancer Screening

■ ■ ■

In the absence of knowledge about prevention, early detection of prostate cancer is believed to be the most effective method to reduce mortality from this disease. Certainly, men diagnosed with early prostate cancer have a much higher survival rate. One researcher examined factors that might increase the likelihood that men will participate in prostate cancer screening (McKee, 1994). The classic Health Belief Model, introduced by Becker, served as the theoretical framework for this descriptive study. A major component of this model is that appropriate health behavior can be triggered by a "cue" to action. A random sample of 200 subjects selected from men in a high-risk category were surveyed by questionnaire (Prostate Screening Follow-Up Questionnaire, or PSFQ) after undergoing cancer screening. Subjects were asked to rate, on a 5-point Likert scale, the importance that 13 items had on their decision to seek prostate cancer screening. The men ranked appointment scheduling and reminder cards as the two most important factors in increasing adherence to prostate cancer screening. Having a friend or family member with cancer, newspaper promotions, and flyers at seniors programs were also identified as important.

Implications for Nursing

As nursing adapts to changing trends in national health care and becomes increasingly involved in community health, providing clients with information to avoid or minimize illness will receive increased attention. The National Cancer Institute has established a goal of reducing prostate cancer mortality by 50% by the year 2000. Education by nurses about the early detection of prostate cancer can play a significant part in meeting this goal.

Critical Thinking in Client Care

1. This study examined one part of the Health Belief Model (cues to action) in influencing participation in prostate cancer screening. How might other parts of the model, such as demographic variables (e.g., age, race, education) and perceived susceptibility to prostate cancer influence a client to seek screening?

2. Can the results of this study be generalized? If women were studied using the same research technique and questionnaire for breast cancer screening, would the results be the same?

3. If you were asked to develop a flyer for a seniors program advertising a community screening effort for prostate cancer, how would you go about it? What information about screening and prostate cancer would you include? How would you alter the design and information to accommodate your audience's age-related changes in vision?

---

cases, no treatment may be recommended but rather to monitor the cancer carefully. Possible treatments for prostate cancer include surgery, radiation therapy, hormone therapy, and chemotherapy.

Laboratory and Diagnostic Tests

Although an increasing number of clients are now diagnosed with asymptomatic prostate cancer, over 50% of clients with prostate cancer have either locally advanced cancer or distant metastasis at the time of diagnosis. The definitive diagnosis can be made only by biopsy; however, other tests may suggest the presence of prostate cancer.

The following laboratory and diagnostic tests may be used:

■ *Prostate-specific antigen (PSA)* levels may be an effective method of detecting asymptomatic prostate cancer, al-

though false positive results (e.g., because of BPH) can be a problem. Sexual activity or rectal manipulation of the prostate does not increase PSA levels (Greco & Blank, 1993).

■ *Transrectal Ultrasonography (TRUS)* is used when the DRE is abnormal or if the PSA is elevated. Cancerous tissue does not produce as strong an echo as normal tissue. This difference can be detected by placing an ultrasonic probe in the client's rectum. TRUS is not recommended as a first-line screening procedure.

■ A *tissue biopsy* must be performed and interpreted before the diagnosis of prostate cancer can be established. If the lesion is visible only on ultrasonography, or if the physician is uncertain about the location of the abnormality, a transrectal ultrasound-guided biopsy is performed. Implications for the nursing care of these clients are presented in the accompanying box.

Nursing Implications for Diagnostic Tests:
Transrectal, Ultrasound-Guided Biopsy of the Prostate

■   ■   ■

Preparation of the Client

- Assess the client's understanding of the procedure. The procedure is becoming common, and many men will have heard about it from friends or family and may have significant anxiety. Especially if the client has experienced uncomfortable or perhaps painful rectal examinations in the past, the prospect of a needle advanced through the rectum into the gland can be frightening. Be sure to describe the procedure fully, and explain what the client will feel. Inform the client that he will be awake and lying on his side. (The examination can also be performed in the sitting, supine, or lithotomy position.) A local anesthetic (2% lidocaine jelly) will be applied to the rectum to minimize pain caused by stretching of the rectal wall. Because the pain receptors in the rectum respond only to stretch, the client will feel no pain as the needle penetrates the rectal wall. The ultrasound probe is inserted in the rectum approximately 10 cm, and then a balloon covering the probe is inflated with water to visualize the prostate. The client will feel a sensation of rectal fullness and possibly pain. Many clients describe it as very uncomfortable. The biopsy instrument is inserted next to the probe. Clients may feel a sharp pain (a "pinch") as the biopsy is obtained. Reassure

the client that the nurse will be with him throughout the procedure to provide support.

- A signed consent should be in the client's chart, as this procedure is invasive.

- Some urologists require a preoperative bleeding profile and complete blood count. The client is often advised to avoid aspirin products and nonsteroidal anti-inflammatory agents for a week before the biopsy.

- An enema is usually administered prior to the examination to ensure a clean rectum.

Client and Family Teaching

- You will be monitored for approximately 1 hour after the examination to ensure that your vital signs are stable and that you can urinate without difficulty.

- Avoid any strenuous activity for the rest of the day.

- Hematuria (blood in the urine) and some bloody streaks in the stool are expected for 24 to 48 hours after the procedure. You can also expect hematospermia (blood in the ejaculate) for a few days to 2 weeks afterward, depending on how often you ejaculate.

- Report any signs of unusual bleeding, such as blood clots in your urine or bloody stools, or infection, such as rectal pain, dysuria, and urgency.

- The *grade* and *stage* help to determine prognosis and guide treatment decisions. The grade (cancer cell differentiation) is determined by the pathologist. Prostate cancer is staged with a variety of tests. Table 46–1 shows treatment options according to the stage of the cancer.

Pharmacology

Hormone Therapy   Hormone therapy is used to treat metastatic prostate cancer. Many cells in the growing tumor are androgen dependent and either cease to grow or die if deprived of androgens. Unfortunately, other cancer cells thrive without androgen and are unaffected by therapy to reduce circulating androgens. Therefore, the effects of hormone manipulations vary from complete but temporary regression of the tumor to no response at all. Studies indicate that deprivation of androgens (including testosterone) does not cure prostate cancer and may not

prolong life if the disease is far advanced and there is extensive bone metastasis. When this therapy is offered to men with minimal bone involvement and no symptoms, a survival advantage of up to 2 years is possible. Regardless of when offered, the therapy may improve the quality of life (Hanks et al., 1993). Strategies to induce androgen deprivation vary from orchiectomy to oral administration of hormonal agents. Table 46–2 lists hormone therapies and the advantages and disadvantages of each.

Surgery

Surgery for clients with prostate cancer includes several types of prostatectomies and transurethral resection of the prostate (Figure 46–1 on page 1965). For clients with stage I or II prostate cancer, prostatectomy can be used for control and sometimes cures the cancer.

A *retropubic* approach is most often performed because it allows adequate control of bleeding, visualization of the prostate bed and bladder neck, and access to pelvic lymph nodes. A *suprapubic prostatectomy* is used only rarely, usually when problems with the bladder are expected. Control of bleeding is more difficult because the surgical approach is through the bladder. The *perineal prostatectomy* is often preferred for older men or men who are poor surgical risks. This approach requires less time,

and there is less bleeding (Nagle, 1991; Sagalowsky & Wilson, 1994).

For very early disease in older men, cure may be achieved with a *simple prostatectomy,* which is removal of only the prostate tissue. A *radical prostatectomy* involves removal of the prostate, prostatic capsule, seminal vesicles, and a portion of the bladder neck. Many clients experience varying degrees of urinary incontinence and erectile dysfunction. Nursing care for these problems are discussed in the section on the client with prostate problems and the section on erectile dysfunction. Surgical intervention is now available for men with urinary sphincter insufficiency, which is the major cause of incontinence after prostatectomy. An artificial urinary sphincter is surgically implanted (Figure 46–2). To be eligible, the client must be able to manipulate the pump placed in the scrotum and have adequate cognitive function to know when a problem with the appliance occurs. Men with total incontinence report a high rate of satisfaction; most gain full control, and the rest note substantial improvement (Gundian, Barrett, & Parulkar, 1993). The box on page 1966 outlines the nursing care for clients undergoing prostatectomy.

For clients with stage III, locally advanced (beyond the prostatic capsule) cancer, surgery is controversial because of the likelihood of hidden lymph node metastasis and relapse. *Transurethral prostatic resection* is not performed as curative therapy but may be used to relieve urinary obstruction for men with advanced disease (stage III or IV). This procedure is discussed in detail in the later section on benign prostatic hyperplasia.

Table 46–1	Treatment Options for Prostate Cancer According to Stage

Stage	Treatment Options

I	If over 70 or in poor health:
	    Close follow-up
	    Simple prostatectomy
	 If under 70:
	    Radical prostatectomy
	    External radiation therapy

II	Radical prostatectomy External radiation therapy
III	External radiation therapy Prostatectomy plus postoperative external radiation External radiation and brachytherapy
IV	Hormone therapy Radiation therapy Chemotherapy Investigational agents

Table 46–2	Surgical and Hormone Therapy in the Management of Advanced Prostate Cancer

Treatment	Advantages	Disadvantages
Orchiectomy	Inexpensive Immediate effect; i.e., clients report diminished pain from metastasis in the recovery room	Body image problems due to loss of testicles
Estrogen compounds (diethylstilbestrol)	Inexpensive Effects reversible	Increased risk of cardiovascular problems More likely to cause gynecomastia, hypertrophy of breast tissue
Luteinizing hormone-releasing hormone agonist (LHRH) (leuprolide)	Effects reversible No cardiovascular risk Monthly administration	Very expensive Subcutaneous injection route Slow onset: up to 4 weeks
Steroidal antiandrogens (megestrol [Megace])	Effects reversible No cardiovascular risk Inexpensive	May not drop testosterone levels sufficiently Weight gain
Nonsteroidal antiandrogens (flutamide; often used in conjunction with LHRH)	Does not alter circulating androgens Blocks some side effects of LHRH May be effective if other methods fail	Very expensive

All hormonal manipulations have the potential disadvantage of loss of libido, erectile dysfunction, hot flashes, and gynecomastia.

Radiation Therapy

Radiation therapy has many uses for clients with prostate cancer. External beam radiation is one of the options for cure of stage I or II disease. Five-year survival rates are comparable to those of men treated with radical prostatectomy. External beam radiation therapy may be the only effective treatment for clients with stage III or IV disease. This therapy is also an option for men in poor health who cannot tolerate surgery (Davis, 1994). Table 46–3 compares the possible complications of radiation therapy with those of surgery.

Radiation therapy has a palliative role for clients with metastatic prostate cancer, reducing the size of bone metastasis, controlling pain and restoring function, such as continence or the ability to ambulate for clients with spinal cord compression.

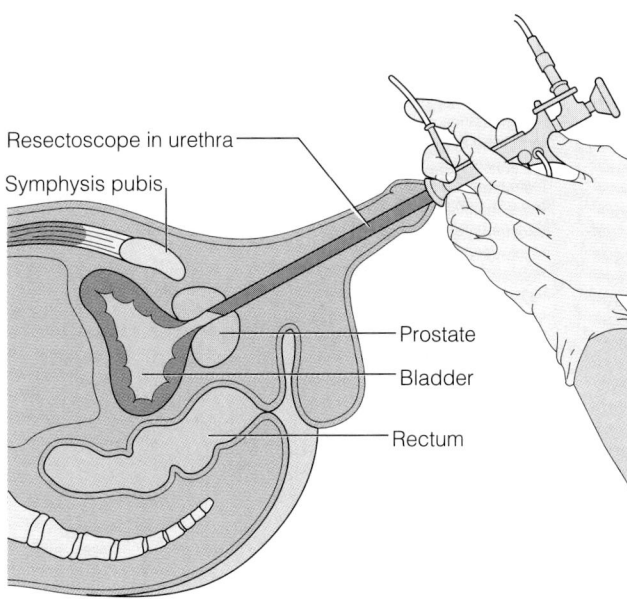

A   Transurethral resection of the prostate

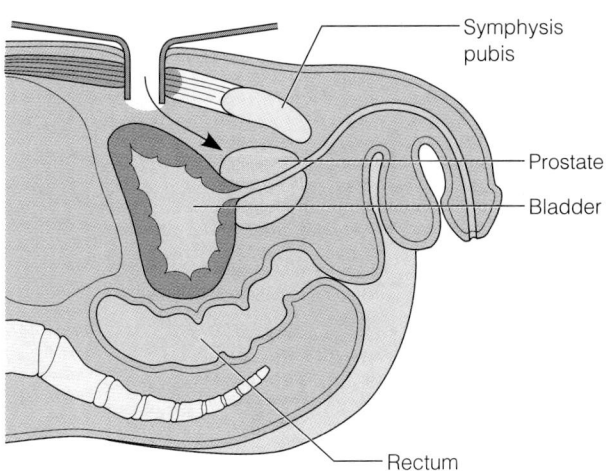

B   Retropubic prostatectomy

Figure 46–1   *A,* In a transurethral resection of the prostate (TURP), a resectoscope inserted through the urethra is used to remove excess prostate tissue. *B,* In a retropubic prostatectomy, prostate tissue is removed through an abdominal incision.

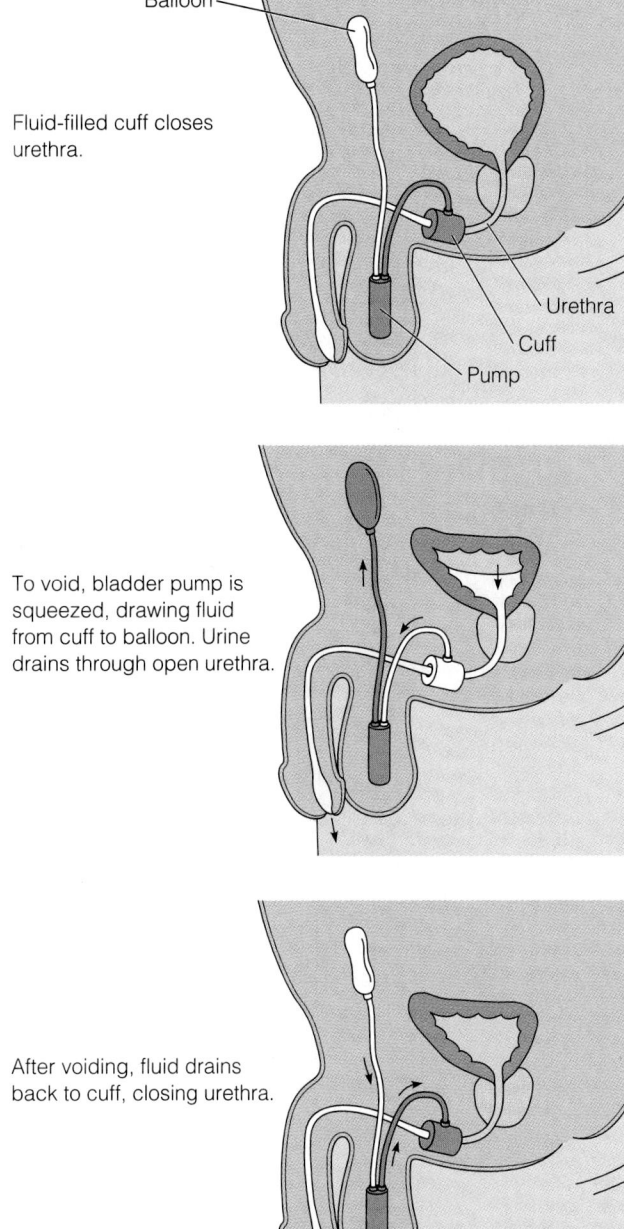

Figure 46–2   Method of operation of an artificial urinary sphincter.

Nursing Care of the Client Undergoing Prostatectomy for Prostate Cancer

PREOPERATIVE NURSING CARE

- Assess the client's and family's knowledge about the surgery. *Some clients are confused about the surgical approach, because there are several, quite different, methods.*

- Inform the client that he will have a Foley catheter when he returns from surgery, and he may have a drain(s) in his incision. The client should also be prepared for the likelihood that he will be wearing sequential pneumatic compression stockings. *This knowledge can reduce the client's anxiety postoperatively and increase his cooperation with postoperative care.*

- Ensure that a signed consent form is in the chart and that all other preoperative tasks outlined in Chapter 7 are done.

- Ask about the client's decisions in regard to blood transfusions. *Many clients donate their own blood before the surgery.*

- Bowel preparation with a 2% neomycin enema may be ordered. *This cleanses the bowel if a perineal approach will be used.*

- Communicate willingness to address any client concerns or anxiety. *Many clients are not sure of the extent of their cancer at the time of surgery.*

POSTOPERATIVE CARE

- Provide routine postoperative nursing care as described in Chapter 7. Assess vital signs, airway patency, bleeding, and wound complications. Inspect the abdomen for distention, and listen for bowel sounds. Measure intake and output, including wound drainage. Provide respiratory support and pain control. *Surgery performed in the lower pelvis causes problems similar to those experienced by clients with abdominal surgery. However, because these surgeries involve the urinary tract and disturb structures in close proximity to the rectum, clients present with special needs.*

- Assess the patency of the Foley catheter. *The catheter may become occluded by blood clots or kinks. Continuous bladder irrigation (CBI) through a three-lumen Foley catheter minimizes problems with patency. Continuous bladder irrigation is usually maintained for 24 to 48 hours after surgery.*

- Assess bleeding by inspecting the dressing and the color of the urine (see Table 46–4). *If bleeding into the urinary tract is heavy, the physician may wish to apply traction to the catheter. The passage of hard stool and straining to defecate may increase bleeding. As soon as the client can tolerate liquids, he is started on stool softeners or a mild laxative.*

- Assist the client to manage pain through assessment and intervention. *The client may have at least three types of pain: incisional pain, bladder spasms, and abdominal cramps due to intestinal gas. Pain from bladder spasms can be excruciating and difficult to control with the usual doses of narcotic analgesics. Spasms may also be accompanied by strong urges to void and the spurting of urine from around the catheter. Bladder spasms are frequently treated with belladonna and opium suppositories. Ketorolac, a nonsteroidal anti-inflammatory drug, diminishes the need to use narcotics for incisional pain.*

- Assist the client with dorsiflexion exercises, ambulation by the first postoperative day, and either graduated compression stockings or sequential pneumatic compression stockings. *These measures are important to prevent the development of thromboembolic complications.*

- Provide careful wound and catheter care. Teach the client to perform perineal irrigations with sterile normal saline daily and after each bowel movement as needed. *In the client having a perineal prostatectomy, the incision is very close to the rectum, and special wound care is needed to prevent infection.*

- Encourage the client to maintain a fluid intake of at least 2 to 3 liters a day. *A liberal fluid intake reduces the risk of urinary tract infection.*

- If the client is to be discharged with an indwelling catheter, provide home care instructions:
  a. Change from the daytime leg drainage bag to a larger night drainage bag. Teach the client not to strap the leg bag on too tightly. *A tight leg bag can decrease venous return and increase risk for thromboembolic complications.*
  b. Place a soft cloth between the leg bag and thigh. *The cloth decreases friction and absorbs dampness under the bag.*
  c. Empty the leg bag every 3 to 4 hours. *This prevents possible reflux of urine into the bladder.*

Table 46–3   Potential Complications Related to Radical Prostatectomy and Radiation Therapy

Radical Prostatectomy	Radiation Therapy
Erectile dysfunction	Erectile dysfunction*
Urethral stricture	Urethral stricture
Fistula/rectal injury	Rectal/anal stricture*
Urinary incontinence	Cystitis
Surgical/anesthetic risk	Diarrhea
	Proctitis
	Rectal ulcer
	Bowel obstruction*
	Urinary incontinence

*Delayed complications; may appear months or years after completion of therapy.

Table 46–4   Significance of Character of Urine After Prostatectomy and Related Nursing Care

Urine Color	Nursing Implications
Light red to red	Normal day of surgery and first postoperative day
Very dark red	May indicate increased venous bleeding or inadequate dilution. Catheter at risk for occlusion. Increase flow rate of irrigant. If urine does not clear, notify physician.
Bright red	May indicate arterial bleeding. Increase flow rate of irrigant, monitor vital signs, and notify physician.
Contains blood clots	Occasional blood clot normal. If clots are frequent, catheter may become obstructed. Increase flow rate of irrigant.
Clear to light pink	Normal throughout hospitalization.

Nursing Care

The nursing care of clients with prostate cancer must be holistic, sensitive, and individualized to meet client needs. Although many nursing diagnoses may be appropriate, this section focuses on problems related to the course of the disease and nonsurgical treatment. The box on page 1966 outlines nursing care of the client undergoing prostatectomy. See also Chapter 9 for a general discussion of the client with cancer.

Altered Urinary Elimination (Stress Incontinence, Urge Incontinence)

Urinary incontinence is a disturbing complication following treatment for prostate cancer. Both radical prostatectomy and external beam radiation therapy can cause incontinence ranging from a drop or two when the client lifts a heavy object, to no control at all.

The majority of incontinence is **stress incontinence,** which is loss of usually less than 50 mL of urine occurring with increased abdominal pressure (Cox et al., 1993).

Many clients will have had voiding problems prior to treatment, especially because most clients with prostate problems are older. Stress incontinence is rare in older men who have not had pelvic surgery. Older men may also experience **urge incontinence,** the involuntary passage of urine soon after a strong sense of urgency to void (Resnick & Yalla, 1992). Loss of urinary control while in bed is classified as *total incontinence.* The man's reaction to incontinence may be severe even if the incontinence is not great. Many men have significant anxiety at the prospect of an incontinent episode in public, because they feel shame and often guilt about the loss of control.

Nursing interventions with rationales follow:

- Assess the client for the degree of incontinence and its impact on life-style. *The nurse needs to determine the client's previous urinary patterns and the type of incontinence currently being experienced to plan appropriate interventions.*

- Teach the client exercises designed to help restore continence. *Pelvic muscle exercises, sometimes called Kegel exercises, can often either eliminate or improve stress incontinence.*

- Teach the client methods to control dampness and odor from stress incontinence.
  a. Teach the client not to attempt to prevent accidental voiding by restricting fluids. *Not only will the client continue to have incontinent episodes, but his urine will become concentrated, exacerbating the problem with odor.*
  b. Teach the client to control occasional episodes (one to three small volume accidents per day) with absorbent pads worn inside the underwear and changed as needed. Most pads are made with a polymer gel that controls odor. *Appropriate measures help promote good hygiene, decrease anxiety, and increase comfort.*

- Explore options with the client who has total incontinence.

- Help the client verbalize his feelings about the impact of incontinence on his quality of life. *The degree of incontinence does not necessarily correlate to the client's perceived level of suffering. Listening to these concerns with sensitivity can help the client work through these feelings and may allow him to move toward a healthy adaptation to his disability.*

Sexual Dysfunction

Surgical treatment for prostate cancer may cause erectile dysfunction and changes in ejaculatory function. These disorders are discussed in detail later in this chapter. Hormone therapy for advanced prostate cancer lowers libido and may also cause erectile dysfunction. The diagnosis of cancer and body image changes caused by hormone therapy may lower self-esteem, which in turn can diminish sexual desire and willingness to interact sexually with a partner. Because most men with prostate problems are older, some have sexual disabilities unrelated to the prostate. Most older men, however, are active sexually and fully capable of sustaining an erection. They are likely to fear the effect of treatment on their sexual health. They may allow this concern to guide their decision about the treatment course, or they may refuse all therapy because of this fear. Assessment may identify men who are having difficulty coping with anxiety, as well as men who may have lost erectile function in the past and thus are not concerned about this possible complication.

Hormone therapy almost always results in erectile dysfunction. Surprisingly, a few men can maintain satisfying erections despite extremely low testosterone levels. Orchiectomy causes permanent erectile dysfunction. The effects of medications can be reversed, although they usually last for several weeks or months. Because hormone therapy prolongs life a few months and does not cure the cancer, the client and his partner must carefully weigh the benefits versus the negative effect on quality of life. Client reactions vary greatly, and the nurse must maintain a non-judgmental approach to education and support.

Nursing interventions with rationales follow:

- Assess the client's pretreatment sexual function. *Knowledge of previous sexual function is necessary to plan appropriate interventions.*
- Teach the client about the impact of therapy on sexual function. *The incidence of erectile dysfunction varies with different therapies for prostate cancer.*

Pain

The causes of pain in clients with advanced prostate cancer are many. It is not unusual for a client to have three or four distinct pains simultaneously, all from different sources. The most common cause of pain is metastasis to the spinal column, usually the thoracic spine (Held & Peahota, 1993). Other sources of pain include fractures, lymphedema of the lower extremities, gynecomastia, and muscle spasms. Because most clients are over the age of 65, many also have pain associated with pre-existing conditions, such as osteoarthritis, unrelated to the cancer.

Nursing interventions with rationales follow:

- Assess the intensity, location, and quality of the client's pain. *Careful assessment of the client's pain often reveals its source. A cardinal rule of successful pain management is the importance of reducing or eliminating the cause of the pain. Appropriate interventions are based on a careful assessment of the client's pain.*
- Teach the client and family methods of pain control. *Various modalities can be successful in alleviating pain or reducing its perception, thus enhancing the comfort of the client. Nonpharmacologic and pharmacologic pain-control methods are discussed in Chapters 4 and 9.*

Other Nursing Diagnoses

The following nursing diagnoses may also be appropriate for the client with prostate cancer:

- *Risk for Injury* related to weakness and disability
- *Urinary Retention* related to extension of cancer to the bladder
- *Altered Role Performance* related to weakness and disability
- *Powerlessness* related to a diagnosis of cancer
- *Self-Esteem Disturbance* related to the effects of therapy
- *Body Image Disturbance* related to change in appearance and sexual function

Client and Family Teaching

Shortly after diagnosis, the client, with the help of his family, must make a decision about treatment. The client and his family, still trying to cope with the news of the diagnosis, must deal with often conflicting advice from a number of sources. Advice may come from the urologist, medical and radiation oncologists, friends, the media, and advocate groups (Montie, 1994). To make the decision that is right for himself, the client usually needs assistance from the nurse. Accurate information about the efficacy of treatments and their impact on his life helps the client make a decision. The nurse must be prepared to provide information about the types of treatment and their side effects, and to listen to client concerns.

The client's current life-style is often the deciding factor in his decision. Clients must consider long-term implications of the decision. Unbiased information is essential to this decision-making process. Another source of information and support is prostate cancer support groups, hosted by many larger hospitals. Men struggling with treatment choices may attend and learn about the options from men who have experience. The location of support groups can be obtained through the American Cancer Society (ACS).

Once the client has received primary therapy for prostate cancer, he requires careful follow-up for recurrence of the disease. The nurse emphasizes the impor-

---

Discharge Instructions for Clients after Prostate Surgery

■ ■ ■

Activity

The healing period lasts from 4 to 8 weeks. Avoid strenuous activity and heavy lifting. Do not drive for 2 weeks, except for short rides. Do take long walks, but take stairs slowly and carefully. Continue dorsiflexion exercises that you did in the hospital to prevent blood clots in the legs. You can take showers, but avoid tub baths while the catheter is in place.

Bleeding

Bleeding can occur any time after surgery. It is fairly common after a bowel movement, coughing, or increased exercise. If you notice blood in the urine, increase fluids and rest until the urine is clear. If heavy bleeding plugs the channel, call the care provider immediately. Avoid aspirin and nonsteroidal anti-inflammatory medications for at least 2 weeks.

Bowel Movements

Keep bowel movements regular and soft to avoid pressure on the prostate area. Drink fruit juices and take mild laxatives or stool softeners as ordered.

Diet

Resume your normal diet. Increase fluids to ten, 8-ounce glasses daily. Avoid alcohol unless otherwise advised by your physician.

Sexual Intercourse

Do not have sex for 6 weeks after surgery to avoid bleeding. You may still have erections even with the catheter in place. When you resume sex, ejaculate flows back into the bladder, so you will express little or no semen.

Urination

After your catheter is removed, you may experience some burning, stinging, or leakage for several weeks, and you may pass small blood clots occasionally. These symptoms will disappear as the area heals. It is best to use pads to control leakage.

Work

If work is not strenuous, you may return in 4 weeks; otherwise, wait 6 to 8 weeks.

Please Call Immediately If:

- You are unable to urinate.
- Bleeding is not controlled by fluids and rest, or is excessive.
- You have chills and fever or severe abdominal pain.
- Your scrotum becomes swollen and tender.
- You have pain in one calf, chest pain, or difficulty breathing.

---

tance of keeping appointments with care providers. Usually the client undergoes yearly PSA and rectal examinations only. However, if the chance of recurrence is high, or if the client has symptoms associated with bone involvement, then bone scans are also performed. Recurrence is associated with a poor prognosis. Most clients know this and may be reluctant to keep follow-up appointments. The nurse needs to point out the benefits of early detection of metastasis or local recurrence: longer life of better quality.

Because of the high incidence of prostate cancer metastasis to the spinal cord, clients need to be taught early warning symptoms of spinal cord compression. For most clients, the first manifestation is back pain, which may be intermittent and aggravated by activity. Many clients report that they ignored this early symptom, associating the pain with "muscle strains," or "ligament problems." The next manifestation is often weakness of the lower extrem-

ities, which usually alerts clients to the need to seek medical attention. Early detection of spinal cord compression is important because early, symptomatic treatment may prevent irreversible damage to spinal nerves, thus avoiding permanent loss of function. (Peterson, 1993).

Following surgery, clients are provided with specific instructions related to diet, resumption of activities, and possible complications. These discharge instructions are outlined in the accompanying box. The family should be included whenever possible in client teaching. There is much to learn, and the family may remember important details that the client forgets. The family is also better able to support the client in adjusting to his illness when they understand the rationale for continued follow-up appointments and the importance of detecting spinal cord compression early.

Nurses are also in a unique position to increase public awareness about strategies for detecting prostate cancer early. Every encounter with male clients and their families—in clinics, hospital units, or in the home—is an opportunity to assess knowledge about early detection and identify needs. The American Cancer Society has designated September as Prostate Cancer Awareness Month, and it presents special programs to the public at that time. The ACS also has free pamphlets about early detection of prostate cancer.

Applying the Nursing Process

Case Study of a Client with Prostate Cancer: William Turner

William Turner is a 71-year-old African-American man who lives with his wife in a small retirement community. He has been in good health for most of his life, reporting only a touch of "arthritis" in his hips and hands that causes moderate difficulty in manipulating objects, and a gradual onset of urinary urgency over the past 2 years. He says, "When I've got to go, I've got to go!" He reports no actual incontinence. His other major concern is his wife, who had a stroke and needs his help in taking care of the house. During a routine physical assessment, his nurse practitioner performs a digital rectal examination and palpates a hard nodule on the surface of the prostate. After the PSA is found to be elevated, he is referred to a urologist, who diagnoses the cancer. After being informed of his options, Mr. Turner chooses surgery. Other staging tests, such as bone scans, are negative. A radical retropubic prostatectomy and pelvic lymphadenectomy are performed. The lymph nodes are negative for cancer, and the tumor is confined to the prostatic capsule. Mr. Turner's immediate hospital recovery goes well; however, his surgical nurse becomes concerned because Mr. Turner's arthritis makes it difficult for him to care for his indwelling catheter. The nurse is aware that Mr. Turner's wife is disabled and cannot help. Since Mr. Turner is being discharged with the catheter in place, the surgical nurse initiates a home health consultation to ensure that Mr. Turner can manage his care at home.

Assessment

Two days after his discharge, Mr. Turner greets the home health nurse, Ms. Wendy Lyle, with a friendly smile and an apology that his wife is ill and cannot come out to meet her. Ms. Lyle notes that the home is clean and neat. Mr. Turner is fully dressed and still wearing his large night urinary drainage bag, although it is one o'clock in the afternoon. Mr. Turner says his main problem is getting out of the house to get groceries, because he is embarrassed to be seen with the large drainage bag. Some church mem-

bers have helped with groceries. He says he has been unable to remove the drainage bag and attach the leg bag because of his arthritis. A physical assessment reveals vital signs within normal range. The pelvic incision is healing with no evidence of infection. His calves are not tender, and he denies chest pain or shortness of breath. Lung sounds are clear. His urine is pale yellow, with no special odor, and he reports no problems with voiding around the catheter. Ms. Lyle learns that he is uncertain about the need for perineal muscle and dorsiflexion exercises as he is no longer in the hospital. Mr. Turner also expresses the belief that he is cured of his cancer and questions the need for follow-up appointments.

Diagnosis

Ms. Lyle establishes the following nursing diagnoses for Mr. Turner:

- *Risk for Stress Incontinence* related to surgery
- *Altered Health Maintenance* related to inability to care for the urinary drainage system, knowledge deficit of postoperative exercises and follow-up care related to lack of information

Expected Outcomes

The expected outcomes for the plan of care are that Mr. Turner will:

- Regain urinary continence after the catheter has been removed.
- Change the urinary drainage bag with appropriate assistance.
- Verbalize the rationale for performing postoperative exercises at home.
- Verbalize the need for continued follow-up care.

Planning and Implementation

Ms. Lyle plans and implements the following nursing interventions for Mr. Turner:

- Prepare Mr. Turner for the possibility of stress incontinence after the catheter is removed.
- Reinforce the need for perineal muscle exercises while the catheter is still in place.
- Explore Mr. Turner's support system to identify people who could assist him with catheter care, and arrange a teaching session with them and Mr. Turner as appropriate.
- Teach Mr. Turner about postoperative complications that can occur after discharge, relating it to the need for dorsiflexion exercises.
- Teach Mr. Turner, in words that he can understand,

about the importance of follow-up care, relating the need for care to the natural history of the disease.

Evaluation

When the catheter is removed, Mr. Turner is alert to the possibility of stress incontinence. He understands the need for perineal muscle exercises, and correctly describes how to perform them. Mr. Turner expresses interest in learning more about how to control the problem. Ms. Lyle asks about close friends or relatives who could assist him with his catheter care. Mr. Turner mentions that one of his nephews is interested in nursing and might be willing to help. A teaching session is scheduled with Mr. Turner and his nephew for the following day. Mr. Turner's nephew quickly learns the essentials of changing the drainage bag, although the client seems upset about the "personal" care and the fact that he can't do it himself. Still, he says it's "worth the trouble to get out of the house again." He has less difficulty accepting the need for continued dorsiflexion exercises, and is doing them when the nurse leaves. Efforts to help him understand the need for continued long-term follow-up care are not so successful. Mr. Turner states that he believes he is cured and needs no further care beyond that needed to recover from surgery. The nurse does not pursue the issue at this time but plans to approach him again on another home visit and to inform other members of the health care team about this concern.

Critical Thinking in the Nursing Process

1. Mr. Turner initially reported a problem with urge incontinence and no other urinary symptoms. What was the likely cause of this problem? Was this problem related to his prostate cancer?

2. How would the nurse teach Mr. Turner about perineal muscle exercises? What other information might he require about stress incontinence?

3. Explain Mr. Turner's reluctance to allow his nephew to assist in his catheter care. What might be the outcome if he does not receive adequate catheter care?

4. What coping mechanism was Mr. Turner using when he stated his belief that the cancer was cured? What rationale did the nurse use when she chose to avoid direct confrontation with the client?

The Client with Benign Prostatic Hyperplasia

■ ■ ■

Enlargement of the prostate gland, **benign prostatic hyperplasia (BPH)**, is the most common disorder in the aging male client. The prostate, very small at birth, grows at

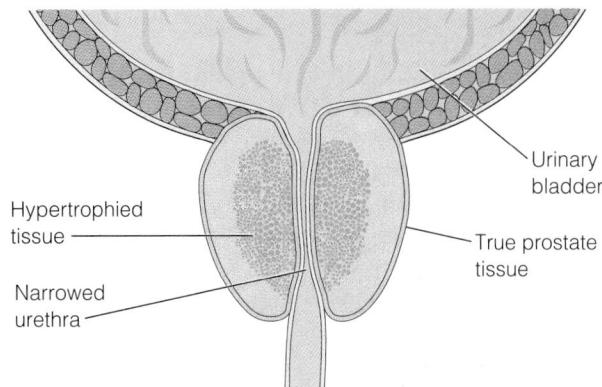

Figure 46–3   Benign prostatic hyperplasia.

puberty, reaches adult size around age 20, and grows again in most men in the fifth decade. The incidence of BPH increases with age. Approximately 75% of men over the age of 50 have some symptoms of BPH (Carney et al., 1995). There is a 78% probability that a man who survives to the age of 80 will have physical signs of BPH, and there is a 30% chance that he will require surgery (Walsh, 1992).

The cause of BPH is not well understood. Various relationships between diet, obesity, sexual activity, and ethnic origin have been explored; however, none of these provide insight into its etiology. Family history of BPH may be a risk factor for the development of BPH in younger (age 55 to 65) men (Sanda et al., 1994).

There are two necessary preconditions for BPH: age of 50 or greater and the presence of testes. Men who are castrated before puberty do not develop BPH. The androgen that mediates prostatic growth at all ages is dihydrotestosterone (DHT), which is formed in the prostate from testosterone. Although androgen levels decrease in aging men, the aging prostate appears to become more sensitive to available DHT. Clients with BPH often have higher estrogen levels, and estrogen may act with DHT to produce BPH. Although the exact mechanisms are obscure, there is clear evidence that BPH is under endocrine control (Walsh, 1992).

Pathophysiology

BPH begins as small nodules in the transition zone of the prostate, which is next to the urethra. The nodules, which are glandular, form the main mass of hyperplastic tissue. The expanding tissue compresses surrounding tissue, narrowing the urethra (Figure 46–3). Whether or not BPH compresses the urethra and causes symptoms depends in part on the strength of the prostatic capsule. If the capsule is strong, the gland expands less, and the urethra is more likely to become obstructed (Carney et al.,

---

Clinical Manifestations of Benign Prostatic Hyperplasia

- Diminished force of urinary stream
- Hesitancy in initiating voiding
- Postvoid dribbling
- Sensation of incomplete emptying
- Urinary retention

- Nocturia
- Frequency
- Urgency
- Urge incontinence
- Dysuria
- Hematuria

1995). Narrowing of the prostatic urethra causes the symptoms of BPH, as summarized in the accompanying box. The detrusor muscles hypertrophy to compensate for increased resistance to urinary flow; however, eventually decreased bladder compliance and bladder instability result in symptoms. **Nocturia**, excessive urination at night, is frequently associated with early BPH. If not treated, increased pressure in the bladder leads to reflux of urine into the ureters, called **vesicoureteral reflux.** This problem can eventually lead to hydroureter and hydronephrosis, which can compromise renal function. Fortunately, these complications are rare, because the symptoms associated with BPH force most men to seek help before they develop.

Collaborative Care

Care of clients with BPH focuses on diagnosing the disorder, correcting or minimizing the urinary obstruction, and preventing or treating complications. The medical and surgical management of BPH is currently undergoing rapid change, with many new treatment modalities under investigation. Men present for medical care with a wide range of manifestations varying in severity. Some men are diagnosed with BPH during a routine physical examination before symptoms develop. Others, because of fear or embarrassment, wait until the discomfort from dysuria, urgency, and urinary retention become almost unbearable before seeking care.

Laboratory and Diagnostic Tests
The following laboratory and diagnostic tests may be performed for the client with BPH:

- A routine *urinalysis* is indicated, and if the client has symptoms such as dysuria, a *urine culture* is obtained as well.

- *Serum creatinine* and *blood urea nitrogen* levels are determined to estimate renal function.
- *Acid phosphatase* and *prostate-specific antigen (PSA)* levels are obtained to establish a baseline value and to help rule out prostate cancer.
- Urodynamic tests are used to evaluate the degree of urinary obstruction. *Uroflowmetry* measures the urine flow rate. If the urine flow rate is severely obstructed, no further urodynamic tests are necessary (Walsh, 1992). Other urodynamic tests that may be ordered include *cystometry* and *pressure flow* studies.
- *Ultrasonography* is used to provide images of the urinary tract. If hematuria is present, or if the prostatic obstruction is of long duration and serum studies indicate the possibility of upper urinary tract problems such as hydronephrosis, then *intravenous urography* may be necessary.
- *Cystoscopy* is direct visualization of the urinary tract with a flexible scope. This study is performed when the diagnosis is uncertain. Nursing implications for cystoscopy are presented in the box on page 887 in Chapter 25.

Pharmacology
Pharmacologic management of BPH is based on two considerations: the hyperplastic tissue is androgen dependent, and smooth muscle contraction within the prostate can exacerbate urinary obstruction. The first consideration is usually addressed by treatment with finasteride (Proscar), which inhibits the conversion of testosterone to DHT in androgen-sensitive tissue. Unfortunately, finasteride is only minimally effective in relieving symptoms in many men. Gonadotropin-releasing hormone analogues and antiandrogens are also used to reduce androgen levels and are far more effective; however, because they cause loss of libido and erectile dysfunction in almost all men, this option is rarely used (Oesterling, 1995).

Excessive smooth muscle contraction in BPH may be blocked with the adrenergic-antagonist, terazosin. Its long-term effectiveness is still under study (Lepor, 1995). Rapid progress can be expected in the medical management of BPH, but for the present, surgical management remains the primary therapy.

Surgery
Surgery for BPH includes transurethral resection of the prostate, simple prostatectomy, and transurethral incision of the prostate. Transurethral resection of the prostate (TURP) (see Figure 46–1) is the second most common surgery of any type performed in the United States (Carney et al., 1995). One of the problems associated with TURP is that much of the prostatic tissue remains and may regrow after a few years, causing another obstruction, particularly if the gland is quite large.

The primary reasons for performing prostatectomy are manifestations of prostatism, significant residual urine, and acute urinary retention (Mebust, 1992). Types of prostatectomies, complications, and implications for nursing care are discussed in the previous section on prostate cancer.

There are a number of less invasive surgical treatments under investigation. One is the transurethral incision of the prostate (TUIP). In this surgery, small incisions are made in the prostate to enlarge the prostatic urethra and relieve obstruction. The procedure can often be performed on an outpatient basis. TUIP is less likely than TURP to result in postoperative bladder neck contractures in men with small prostates. In addition, normal ejaculatory function is preserved in most clients. All of the newer approaches to treatment are being studied for long-term effectiveness in managing symptoms of BPH, and most can be performed on an outpatient basis.

Nursing Care

There are many similarities in the nursing care of men with BPH to that of men with prostate cancer (see the previous section). Nursing approaches to problems of urinary incontinence, sexual dysfunction, and body image disturbance, as well as nursing care for clients undergoing prostatectomies, are discussed there. However, there are important differences, and these are discussed below under the nursing diagnoses *Ineffective Management of Therapeutic Regimen* and *Fluid Volume Excess.*

Ineffective Management of Therapeutic Regimen

Most men are aware that noncancerous problems with the prostate gland are very common. Nevertheless, most men are unsure of the function of the prostate gland and even the prostate's exact location, though its relationship to sexual and urinary function is at least generally known. This lack of knowledge, coupled with the growing number of treatment options, is confusing to many men. The treatment options depend on the severity of symptoms and the age and condition of the client.

Nursing interventions with rationales follow:

- Assess the client's severity of symptoms. *This information is necessary in order to determine the most appropriate treatment.*

- Provide information about treatment options. *To make decisions, clients need to know the intended effects of treatments as well as their effectiveness and possible negative effects.*

- Teach the client methods to minimize symptoms and prevent infection. *Many clients with mild to moderate symptoms of BPH choose to wait, often for many years, before seeking definitive therapy.*

- Advise the client to drink 2 to 3 liters of fluids daily, unless contraindicated by preexisting cardiac problems. *Fluids help prevent urinary tract infections and lessen dysuria.*

- Advise the client to restrict alcohol intake, especially late at night, to minimize problems with nocturia. *Nocturia can pose a safety risk for older men who may have age-related changes in vision, muscular strength, and coordination. It is not unusual for men to suffer falls and fractured hips while ambulating to the bathroom in the middle of the night.*

Fluid Volume Excess

Fluid volume excess with resulting hyponatremia, also known as *transurethral syndrome,* is a complication that can occur during or after TURP. The incidence is approximately 2%. Transurethral syndrome is of special concern in the older client, who may have diminished pulmonary and cardiac reserve. These clients may decompensate rapidly if they develop acute volume overload or pulmonary edema. During the surgery, the surgeon must continually irrigate the bladder with a nonhemolytic irrigating solution to maintain visualization of the bladder and to wash out resected prostatic tissue. Because venous sinuses in the prostate are opened during surgery, some of the irrigating solution is absorbed. The amount absorbed depends on the length of the surgery, the volume of prostatic tissue resected, and the height of the irrigating solution above the client (increased height means increased pressure) (Koch & Hall, 1994). It is possible that the average client absorbs approximately 1000 mL of fluid during TURP (Mebust, 1992).

Nursing interventions with rationales follow:

- Assess the client for manifestations of fluid volume excess and dilutional hyponatremia. *Careful assessment is necessary for early detection of the problem (see Chapter 5).*

- Monitor fluid balance. The client's intake and output, including irrigating fluid used during and after surgery, should be carefully monitored. Weigh daily. *Frequent assessments aid in the early detection of fluid volume excess. The irrigating solution, normal saline, used postoperatively in intermittent or continuous bladder irrigation, is not absorbed by the client as it enters and leaves the bladder via an indwelling catheter. Careful measurement of this fluid is important to arrive at an accurate measurement of urine output. Weight is an effective indicator of fluid volume status.*

- Restrict fluids and administer diuretics as ordered. *Fluid restriction conserves sodium, and diuretics decrease total fluid load.*

- Administer replacement therapy as ordered. *Sodium replacement therapy may be used to correct hyponatremia.*

Clinical Manifestations of Prostatitis and Prostatodynia

■ ■ ■

Acute Bacterial Prostatitis

- Onset (may be abrupt): obstruction, irritation, or pain upon voiding; frequency; and urgency
- Positive cultures of infectious organism
- Nonurinary symptoms: chills, fever, low back and pelvic floor pain

Chronic Bacterial Prostatitis

- Urinary symptoms sometimes similar to those of the acute form, except less sudden, less dramatic, or even absent
- Positive cultures of causative organism not always obtainable

Nonbacterial Prostatitis

- Perineal, suprapubic, low back, or genital pain
- Irritation upon voiding
- Postejaculatory pain
- Negative cultures of organisms

Prostatodynia

- Pelvic, low back, or perineal pain
- Irritation or obstruction upon voiding
- No evidence of inflammation in the prostate
- No urinary tract infections
- Normal prostatic secretions

Other Nursing Diagnoses

The following nursing diagnoses may also be appropriate for the client with BPH:

- *Risk for Injury* related to neurologic changes secondary to hyponatremia
- *Sexual Dysfunction* related to retrograde ejaculation secondary to transurethral surgery
- *Stress Incontinence* related to sphincter damage during surgery

Client and Family Teaching

Clients with BPH require information about the disease process and treatment options. Preoperative and postoperative teaching for clients undergoing TURP is usually performed in the urologist's office. In the absence of complications, the client may be discharged within 2 days after surgery. Outpatient TURP is now a reality. Clients have surgery in the morning in an outpatient ambulatory surgery center and are discharged home in the afternoon with their indwelling catheter in place after the irrigation has been discontinued. Admission to the hospital may be necessary, usually because of persistent hematuria (Klimberg et al., 1994). Discharge instructions after prostate surgery are given in the box on page 1966.

The Client with Prostatitis or Prostatodynia

■ ■ ■

Prostatitis, inflammation of the prostate gland, is one of the more common genitourinary problems, accounting for about 25% of office visits (Moul, 1993). The types of prostatitis are acute bacterial, chronic bacterial, and nonbacterial. Nonbacterial prostatitis is the most common of these disorders (Meares, 1992).

Prostatodynia is a condition in which the client experiences the symptoms of prostatitis but shows no evidence of inflammation or infection.

Acute bacterial prostatitis is often associated with lower urinary tract infections. The infecting organism is most commonly *Escherichia coli*, but species of *Proteus*, *Klebsiella*, *Pseudomonas*, *Enterobacter*, and *Serratia* may also invade the prostate. Infected urine may reflux into the prostatic ducts, or perhaps organisms may ascend the urinary tract. There is evidence that meatal contamination during vaginal or anal sexual intercourse may play a role in ascending infections (Meares, 1992).

The etiology of chronic bacterial prostatitis is often difficult to determine. Chronic urinary tract infections, infected prostatic calculi, and inadequately treated acute bacterial prostatitis may be part of the cause.

The causes of nonbacterial prostatitis and prostatodynia are unknown. Various organisms, such as fungi, parasites, and viruses have been studied as infectious agents in nonbacterial prostatitis, with no definitive results. Possible causes of prostatodynia include increased tension of the urinary sphincter and pelvic floor muscles. Many clinicians have suggested a psychologic etiology, but recent studies have failed to confirm that hypothesis (De la Rosette et al., 1993). Clinical manifestations of prostatitis and prostatodynia are summarized in the accompanying box.

Collaborative Care

Care of clients with prostatitis focuses on diagnosis, elimination of any bacterial infections, and measures to relieve pain and promote comfort.

Laboratory and Diagnostic Tests

It is often difficult to diagnose prostatitis. The following laboratory and diagnostic tests may be performed:

- *Urine* and *prostatic secretion cultures* to determine the presence and type of bacteria

- *X-ray studies* and *ultrasound* to visualize organs

Pharmacology

Both types of bacterial prostatitis are treated with appropriate antibiotics. Clients with the chronic form must take antibiotics for a much longer period, often up to 4 months, and may still relapse as soon as the antibiotic is discontinued. Nonbacterial prostatitis does not usually respond satisfactorily to drug therapy, although relief from symptoms is possible. Nonsteroidal anti-inflammatory drugs are useful for pain, and anticholinergics may reduce voiding symptoms. Prostatodynia is also treated symptomatically to relieve muscle tension, usually with alpha-adrenergic blocking agents or muscle relaxants (Meares, 1992).

Surgery

In some cases of bacterial prostatitis, TURP (see the previous section on BPH) may be necessary to remove infected prostatic calculi to achieve a cure (Moul, 1993).

Nursing Care

Holistic nursing care of clients with prostatitis includes extensive, sensitive client and family teaching. Clients with acute and chronic bacterial prostatitis should be taught to increase fluid intake to around 3 liters daily and to void often. These measures help decrease irritation upon urination. Promotion of regular bowel habits helps ease pain associated with defecation. Local heat, such as sitz baths, may be helpful to relieve pain and irritation (Giroux, 1995). It is very important to teach the client to finish the course of antibiotic therapy. Otherwise, acute prostatitis may develop into chronic prostatitis, or chronic prostatitis may recur.

Symptoms associated with nonbacterial prostatitis and prostatodynia vary in severity over time. During severe episodes, sitz baths, increased fluids, and avoidance of alcohol and spicy foods may help. In clients with nonbacterial prostatitis, frequent ejaculation may help to decrease the congestion in the gland (Giroux, 1995). In this situation, prostatic massage may be helpful. Frank discussion with clients is important. It sometimes helps clients to conceptualize the disorder much as they would other chronic inflammatory conditions, such as arthritis. Misconceptions about the disease should be addressed with both the client and his partner. Sexual intercourse is actually helpful, and men cannot "infect" their partners. There is no relationship between these conditions and cancer of the prostate.

◣ ◣ ◣ Disorders of the Testes and Scrotum ◣ ◣ ◣

The Client with Testicular Cancer

◼ ◼ ◼

Testicular cancer accounts for only 1% of all cancers in men; however, it is the most common cancer in men between the ages of 15 and 35, and it the third leading cause of cancer death in young men. In 1995, approximately 7100 men will be diagnosed with this cancer, and 310 men will die from it (Wingo et al., 1995). The lifetime chance of developing testicular cancer is 0.2% for Caucasian men and less for African-American men. In the last 20 years, there has been a dramatic change in the cure rate for this cancer, from only 10% in the 1970s to over 80% for men with all stages of the disease and nearly 100% for men with early-stage disease. This change is due to improved diagnostic techniques and treatment (Einhorn, Richie, & Shipley, 1993).

The etiology of testicular cancer is unknown; however, there are suggested risk factors. There is a relationship between **cryptorchidism,** undescended testicles at birth,

and testicular cancer. Men who have had this problem have 48 times the risk of developing testicular cancer than men who have not (Richie, 1992). Men exposed to exogenous estrogens—diethylstilbestrol (DES) and oral contraceptives—taken by the mother during the first two months of fetal life are also at increased risk. Other factors marginally associated with increased risk include a history of excessive maternal nausea during the first 2 months of fetal life, low birth weight, prematurity, and family history (Klimaszewski & Karlowicz, 1995). Unfortunately, even when all these risk factors are considered, the majority of men who develop testicular cancer have no risk factors. Therefore, beginning at the age of 15, all men should perform monthly testicular self-examination, as described in the box on page 1976.

Pathophysiology

Testicular cancer grows within the testicle, eventually replacing most of the normal parenchymal tissue. Local spread to the epididymis or spermatic cord is inhibited by

Procedure for Testicular Self-Examination

■ ■ ■

- Examine your testicles when you are taking a warm shower or bath, or just after if you prefer to use a mirror to compare size.

- The scrotum, testicles, and hands should be soapy to allow easy manipulation of the tissue.

- Gently roll each testicle between the thumb and fingers of each hand. If one testicle is substantially larger than the other, or if you feel any hard lumps, consult your physician immediately.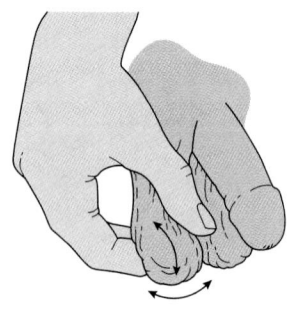

- Normal scrotal contents may be confusing. Just above and behind the testicle is the epididymis. It feels soft and tender overall, although parts of it may be rather firm. This is normal. The spermatic cord, a small, round, moveable tube, extends up from the epididymis. It feels firm and smooth. Of greatest concern is any hard lump felt directly on the testicle, even if it is painless.

- Choose a day out of each month on which to examine yourself. Most men choose an easy day to remember, such as the first or last day of the month. Star this day on your calendar to help you remember.

the outer covering of the testicles, the tunica albuginea. Therefore, spread by lymphatic and vascular channels to other organs often causes distant disease before large masses develop in the scrotum. Lymphatic dissemination usually leads to disease in retroperitoneal lymph nodes, whereas vascular dissemination can lead to metastasis in the lungs, bone, or liver. Bilateral presentation of testicular cancer is unusual. The classic presenting symptom of testicular cancer is a painless hard nodule. Other clinical manifestations are summarized in the accompanying box.

Collaborative Care

Care focuses on diagnosis, elimination of the cancer, and prevention or treatment of metastasis. Once testicular cancer is suspected, the client undergoes a number of screening tests to help determine the likelihood of the

disease and its stage. If the disease is confined to the testicle, it is classified as stage I. Stage II disease is limited to the testicle and regional lymph nodes. Stage III disease involves metastasis above the diaphragm or extensive visceral involvement. Often, the client does not undergo biopsy before the beginning of treatment but instead receives a definitive diagnosis after surgery (orchiectomy). Preoperative tests can provide sufficient information to allow considerable certainty about the diagnosis.

Laboratory and Diagnostic Tests

The following laboratory tests may be ordered for the client with testicular cancer:

- *Serum studies* for tumor markers. Germ cell tumors, which account for 95% of testicular cancers, produce primitive proteins that can be measured using radioimmunoassay techniques. Elevated levels provide strong evidence of testicular cancer. These markers are also measured after surgery to help determine the presence of residual disease, perhaps in lymph nodes, that remains undetected by other means. Persistent elevation may indicate the need for further therapy (Einhorn et al., 1993).

- *Serum lactic acid dehydrogenase (LDH)* levels help determine the presence of bulky disease outside of the testicle. Because this enzyme is also produced by the lungs, liver, kidneys, and brain, this marker is less useful than tumor markers.

- *Liver function tests* may be performed to evaluate the possibility of metastasis to the liver.

- *Computed tomography* of the chest and abdomen is performed to evaluate the possibility of metastasis to the lungs or abdominal organs.

Pharmacology

Progress in chemotherapy to treat testicular cancer is one of the chief reasons that most men survive the disease. The client with advanced disease receives platinum-based combination chemotherapy. Two frequently used combinations are (1) cisplatin, vinblastine, and bleomycin and (2) cisplatin, VP-16, and bleomycin (Einhorn et al., 1993).

Surgery

Radical orchiectomy (removal of the testicle) is the treatment used in all forms and stages of testicular cancer. Retroperitoneal lymph node dissection also may be performed. Complications of surgery are discussed under nursing care.

Radiation Therapy

Radiation therapy is used for stage I seminoma to treat cancer in the retroperitoneal lymph nodes, the most frequent site for distant metastasis. The best way to treat stage I seminoma—with radiation therapy or with careful observation—is currently under study. The client may experience temporary diarrhea, nausea, or a decline in bone marrow function, such as thrombocytopenia or leukopenia. These problems are usually mild and respond well to symptomatic treatment or time. Damage to the contralateral testicle is minimized by careful shielding. Pretreatment and posttreatment analysis of sperm number and function is necessary. The most common long-term complication is dyspepsia or ulcer disease (Einhorn et al., 1993).

Nursing Care

Nursing care of the client with testicular cancer is complex. The nurse takes into account the client's and his family's reactions to the diagnosis, the change in body image accompanying treatment, and sexual and reproductive issues. Although chances of a cure are excellent, the long-term effect on quality of life may be extensive, requiring a change in life goals.

Knowledge Deficit

The nurse often initiates client teaching about what to expect after radical orchiectomy. The client's knowledge about surgery is assessed, and postoperative routines such as early ambulation are explained (see Chapter 7).

Nursing interventions with rationales follow:

- Teach the client methods to control pain. In addition to the usual analgesics used to control postoperative incisional pain, ice bags may be applied to the scrotum. A scrotal support provides relief, especially when the client ambulates. *Surgery results in incisional pain, and the scrotum is tender and slightly swollen.*

- Teach the client the signs and symptoms of complications. The incision is closed with Steri-Strips or staples, and, although rare, wound dehiscence is possible. If the incision gaps open, or if there is bleeding beyond slight oozing after 24 hours, the client should call the surgeon. Another rare complication is a hematoma in the scrotum caused by bleeding from the spermatic cord stump. Rapid onset of scrotal edema is a sign of this problem (Klimaszewski & Karlowicz, 1995). *Because the client is usually discharged early, complications may not become apparent until the client is at home.*

- Reinforce knowledge concerning the effect of surgery on sexuality. *If the treatment involves only an orchiectomy, there should be no lasting effects on the client's sexual or reproductive function.*

Altered Sexuality Patterns

The effect of testicular cancer and its treatment on sexual and reproductive function is complex, and there is great

---

Clinical Manifestations of Testicular Cancer

Common

- Painless swelling of one testicle
- Painless nodule on one testicle

Occasional

- Dull ache in pelvis or scrotum

Uncommon (10%)

- Acute pain in scrotum

Metastatic symptoms

- Neck mass
- Respiratory symptoms
- Gastrointestinal disturbance
- Lumbar back pain

Rare (5%)

- Infertility
- Gynecomastia

---

variation in responses among men. Erectile and climactic function is rarely affected.

Nursing interventions with rationales follow:

- Assess the client's prediagnosis sexual function. To assess this area, the nurse must establish an atmosphere of openness and permission to discuss sexual concerns. After the initial shock of the diagnosis, clients report intense concern about sexual and reproductive issues, which can be relieved only by information. *Knowledge of the client's usual sexual function can guide teaching.*

- Discuss the possibility of preserving sperm in a bank. *The possibility is avilable to the client who wishes to father children.*

- Help the client cope with his feelings about altered sexual function and appearance. *Many clients, whether they are in a significant relationship or not, deeply grieve the loss of the ability to father children.*

Other Nursing Diagnoses

The following nursing diagnoses may also be appropriate for the client with testicular cancer:

- *Altered Role Performance* related to loss of reproductive ability

- *Body Image Disturbance* related to loss of testicle
- *Ineffective Family Coping: Compromised* related to threat to reproductive function

Client and Family Teaching

Families need to be included in teaching for a variety of reasons. If the client is of reproductive age, his partner will have significant anxiety and will require information. If the client is a teenager, his parents need information about the effect on sexual function and are often very involved in postoperative care. The client needs the support of the people he loves, and knowledgeable loved ones can give more effective support.

The client and family need careful teaching and reinforcement of the need for follow-up, especially if the retroperitoneal lymph nodes were not surgically explored. For clients with a risk for recurrence, surveillance with periodic physical examinations, chest X-ray films, tumor markers, and CT scans of the retroperitoneal nodes could continue for a minimum of 5 years and possibly 10 years after orchiectomy.

The Client with Testicular Torsion

■ ■ ■

Testicular torsion, or twisting of the testes and spermatic cord, is a potential medical emergency. The three types of torsion and their clinical manifestations are listed in the accompanying box. The cause of the condition, occurring almost always between birth and age 20, is not well understood. Elevated hormone levels and abnormal attachment of the testicles to the scrotum have been suggested. Trauma to the scrotum may precipitate the condition, but only in clients who are already predisposed.

Testicular torsion is usually diagnosed by history and physical examination. Testicular scanning may be used to determine if blood flow to the testicle is reduced, a usual result of this condition. Treatment, which involves detorsion of the testicle and fixation to the scrotum, must begin as quickly as possible. Compromised blood flow to the testicle may eventually lead to testicular ischemia and necrosis. If the testicle is necrotic or has sustained significant damage, it will be removed.

An episode of torsion is a frightening experience for the adolescent male. He is usually very embarrassed by the problem and may imagine that early sexual activity or even fantasies that result in erections are responsible. Because he is not likely to volunteer his concerns, the nurse should give information to relieve some of these anxieties. Postoperative nursing care is similar to that for clients

---

Clinical Manifestations of Testicular Torsion

■ ■ ■

Intravaginal Torsion*

- Sudden onset of scrotal pain, which may or may not be related to trauma
- Nausea and vomiting
- Past history of scrotal pain
- Cremasteric reflex depressed or absent

Extravaginal Torsion†

- Symptoms similar to those of intravaginal torsion

Torsion of the Appendix Teste‡

- Symptoms are not as severe
- Cremasteric reflex present

---

*Twisting of the testicle within its outer coat
†Strangulation of the spermatic cord at the external inguinal ring
‡Twisting of one of the four testicular appendages

---

with scrotal surgeries, discussed previously in the section on testicular cancer.

The Client with Cryptorchidism

■ ■ ■

Cryptorchidism is the failure of one or both testes to descend through the inguinal ring during months 7 or 8 of gestation. Most undescended testes lodge along the inguinal canal and descend without intervention in the first year of life. Occasionally, the testicle may be in the abdomen or femoral area. It is primarily a problem with children, although on rare occasions it is missed and discovered later in adolescent or adult life. The usual treatment is surgery, orchiopexy, which is performed between the ages of 1 and 10.

Although this condition is described as a childhood problem, the adult male must be cognizant of the fact that he had cryptorchidism and be aware of the implications. The relationship between undescended testes and testicular cancer has been noted previously. In addition, because spermatogenesis is decreased in the testicle, even after corrective therapy, the client may have fertility problems. Men who have this problem in their medical history should be especially vigilant about testicular self-exami-

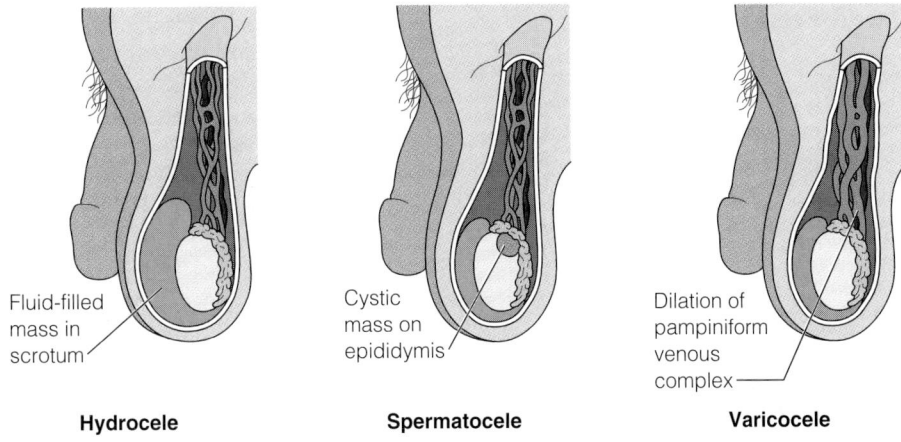

Fluid-filled mass in scrotum

Hydrocele

Cystic mass on epididymis

Spermatocele

Dilation of pampiniform venous complex

Varicocele

Figure 46–4   Common disorders of the scrotum. Hydroceles and spermatoceles do not usually require treatment unless they become large and cause pain. Varicoceles are usually treated to prevent infertility.

nation, and practitioners should be thorough when examining the testicles.

The Client with Scrotal Masses or Trauma

■ ■ ■

Most scrotal masses are benign and can be managed in a manner that is satisfactory to the client. The most common are hydroceles, spermatoceles, and varicoceles (Figure 46–4). These disorders, as well as scrotal trauma and vasectomy-related problems, are reviewed here.

Hydrocele

A **hydrocele** is a fluid-filled mass within the scrotum. The cause is not always clear, but an imbalance between production and reabsorption of fluid within the layers of the scrotum is thought to be responsible. Hydroceles can be differentiated from solid masses by transillumination of the scrotum. Ultrasound studies are occasionally performed if doubt remains about the type of mass. Treatment is usually not necessary. If the hydrocele becomes large enough to cause the client embarrassment or significant pain, a hydrocelectomy may be performed.

Spermatocele

A **spermatocele** is a mobile, usually painless mass containing dead spermatozoa that forms in the epididymis. The cause is thought to be leakage of sperm due to

trauma or infection. Treatment is usually not necessary. If the spermatocele becomes large enough to cause the client embarrassment or significant pain, a spermatocelectomy may be performed.

Varicocele

A **varicocele** is a dilation of the pampiniform venous complex of the spermatic cord. The dilated veins form a soft mass that can cause pain. A major concern with this condition is that it can decrease the sperm count and cause atrophy of the testicle, resulting in infertility. The cause is thought to be incompetent venous valves or obstruction of the gonadal vein. Varicoceles can be felt by scrotal palpation. Sonography is also frequently used for diagnosis. Varicoceles are usually treated, especially in younger clients, to prevent infertility. Surgery is performed to ligate the spermatic vein.

Scrotal Trauma

Scrotal trauma is usually minor, resulting in temporary hematomas caused by minor crushing or straddle type injuries. More severe crush injuries can rupture the testicles. Occasionally, the client's clothing and scrotal skin can be trapped in moving machinery, resulting in avulsion injuries. Such an accident can tear the skin away from the penis and scrotum, sometimes extruding scrotal contents. The client can also suffer penetrating injuries to the scrotum due to knife or gunshot wounds. Treatment of scrotal trauma varies greatly according to the extent of damage and the type of scrotal contents involved (Reilly, 1995).

Vasectomy-Related Problems

The most common surgery of the scrotum is **vasectomy**, a sterilization procedure in which a portion of the spermatic cord is removed. This surgery rarely results in long-term complications; however, some clients develop granulomas that cause chronic pain. Other complications include chronic testicular pain and epididymal obstruction (Goldstein, 1992).

Nursing Care

Clients with scrotal disorders require health education. For clients who have scrotal surgery, the nurse is concerned about the reduction of preoperative anxiety, pain management, and control of possible bleeding (see the section on testicular cancer). Clients should be assessed for anxiety. Almost all men are aware of the possible pain associated with scrotal manipulation. They need information and reassurance about pain management during and after surgery. External bleeding is minimal after surgery; however, some men do develop scrotal hematomas. The nurse observes for scrotal edema and a purple discoloration, which can indicate a problem. Rarely, severe internal bleeding may require reoperation. Clients who have had a varicocelectomy need to be taught that their fertility status may be compromised.

The Client with Epididymitis

■ ■ ■

Epididymitis is an infection or inflammation of the epididymis. It is the most common intrascrotal infection. The problem is usually caused by spread of a bladder or urethral infection down the vas deferens, but it may also be caused by trauma. Early manifestations include pain and local edema; symptoms can progress to erythema and edema of the entire scrotum, especially on the side of the involved epididymis. Late complications of the disorder include occlusion of the epididymis and sterility. Severe epididymitis is treated with intravenous antibiotics and hospitalization. Less acute forms of the disease can be treated with outpatient antibiotic therapy. Nursing care involves symptomatic relief. Ice packs may be applied to the scrotum to relieve pain. A scrotal support is usually applied. The client should be told about the possibility of infertility, as he may wish to seek evaluation for this problem at a later date.

The Client with Orchitis

■ ■ ■

Orchitis is an infection or inflammation of the testicle. It most commonly occurs in concert with epididymitis and is the most common complication of epididymitis. Infection may reach the testicle through the vas deferens and the lymphatic and vascular channels. Trauma, including vasectomy and other scrotal surgeries, may cause inflammation of the testes. Many different organisms may cause infection, including viruses, bacteria, parasites, and fungi. Orchitis can also be related to other diseases, such as malaria, influenza, and infectious mononucleosis; however, the incidence is rare. Clinical manifestations include pain and edema. Inflammation and infection of the testes can lead to testicular abscesses, atrophy, fibrosis, and infertility (Giroux, 1995). Treatment may be symptomatic; antibiotic therapy is used if urine cultures are positive. Rarely, severe damage to the testicle may require surgical drainage or orchiectomy. Nursing care is very similar to that of the client with epididymitis and other scrotal disorders.

▚ ▚ ▚ Disorders of the Penis ▚ ▚ ▚

The Client with Cancer of the Penis

■ ■ ■

Cancer of the penis is a very rare cancer in North America, accounting for less than 1% of all male cancers. However, penile cancer is a significant problem in areas of the world where circumcision is not usually practiced and hygiene is poor (Fair, Fuks, & Scher, 1993). The mean age for the development of penile cancer is approximately 60.

Cancer of the penis is associated with the presence of foreskin, the irritative effects of **smegma** (a natural product of sebaceous glands), and poor hygiene or any condition that causes problems with adequate hygiene. Other risk factors include infection or exposure to human papillomavirus, current cigarette smoking, genital warts, a history of multiple sexual partners (30 or more), and a history of a penile rash (Holly & Palefsky, 1993). The relationship of these risk factors to actual malignant change is not well understood.

Pathophysiology

Cancer of the penis originates at the distal end of the penis, spreads through lymph channels to the inguinal nodes, and very late in the disease may spread to the bone, liver, or lungs. If the lesion is treated before inguinal node involvement, chances for a cure are good. Clients usually die within 6 months after discovery of distant metastasis (Klimaszewski & Karlowicz, 1995). Clinical signs of this cancer include a mass or persistent sore or ulcer at the distal end of the penis, involving the glans or foreskin. Most of these lesions are painless; however, there may be significant ulceration and bleeding. Purulent, foul-smelling discharge may be evident under the foreskin. Occasionally, clients may present with enlarged inguinal lymph nodes (Fair et al., 1993).

Collaborative Care

Cancer of the penis is diagnosed by a biopsy of the lesion, including any suspicious inguinal lymph nodes. The cancer is staged according to the size of the tumor, extent of invasion, status of inguinal lymph nodes, and presence or absence of distant metastasis. Treatment for small lesions includes wide excision and sometimes inguinal node dissection. Larger lesions require a partial or total penectomy. One alternative for small lesions for selected clients is external beam radiation therapy, which preserves the penis. This treatment is controversial, as controlled studies are nonexistent in this rare cancer. Chemotherapy is offered to clients with metastatic disease, but often has poor results (Fair et al., 1993).

Nursing Care

Nurses help clients deal with the problems of a shortened or absent penis, including the potentially devastating effect on body image and self-concept. If a total penectomy is performed, the surgeon creates a perineal urethrostomy, preserving urinary continence. However, the client must void in the sitting position, reinforcing the feeling of loss. Dribbling of urine after voiding may be a problem for a few weeks. The client should be taught to perform careful perineal hygiene upon discharge, using mild soap and water. Sitz baths may be helpful to relieve pain and to promote healing. If an inguinal lymph node dissection was performed, the client may experience persistent lymphedema of the lower extremities.

Client and Family Teaching

Client and family teaching can help prevent this disease or provide early detection. Nurses need to teach parents who decide against circumcision how to minimize the risks. Parents need to teach their children proper hygiene as soon as they are capable of understanding. School health programs can reinforce this practice. Some authors (Klimaszewski & Karlowicz, 1993) advocate monthly self-examination of the penis for uncircumcised clients.

Factors Implicated in the Etiology of Veno-Occlusive Priapism

■ ■ ■

Illnesses/Conditions

- Sickle cell disease
- Leukemia
- Metastatic cancer
- Spinal cord trauma

Drugs

- Papaverine
- Psychotropic drugs
- Alcohol
- Marijuana

The Client with Priapism

■ ■ ■

Priapism is a sustained, painful erection that lasts at least 4 hours and is not associated with sexual arousal. The exact incidence is uncertain; however, the condition is unusual. There are two types of this disorder, arterial high-flow priapism and veno-occlusive priapism. *High-flow priapism* occasionally follows trauma to the perineal area which has torn the cavernous artery. Blood flows unregulated into the lacunar spaces, causing the erection. The cause of *veno-occlusive priapism* is unclear but seems to be related to certain conditions or drugs (see the accompanying box). Somehow, the contributing factor causes obstruction or venospasm of the small veins draining the corpus cavernosum. Blood trapped in the corpora causes the sustained erection. The erection is abnormal in that it is usually harder than normal and very painful because of ischemia. As the condition continues, there is danger of penile necrosis and urinary tract obstruction.

Collaborative Care

Ice to the perineum and vasoconstrictive drugs can provide temporary relief. Embolization of the cavernous artery may be needed to provide permanent relief. Data are sketchy; however, some authors report that most clients regain erectile function (Bastuba et al., 1994). Veno-occlusive priapism must be treated quickly and aggressively. Noninvasive measures, such as ice packs to the penis, warm or ice water enemas, or vigorous prostatic massage may be tried. Local anesthetic infiltration of the penis may provide relief. If none of these measures is successful, alternately aspirating blood from the penis and irrigating with fluid may achieve detumescence. If this measure is not effective, surgery is required. Under local anesthesia, a large needle is passed through the glans penis down to the distal shaft, and a core of tissue is removed. This procedure is repeated to create several fistulas from which blood can drain. The skin is closed with sutures after the procedure. Operative complications are not common but can include hematoma, stricture, gangrene, and sepsis (Bates, 1995).

Nursing Care

Nursing care focuses on assessing the penis, assessing urinary output, helping the client with anxiety and pain control, and teaching the client about effects on sexual function. Assessment of the penis includes inspection for degree of erection and changes in color due to ischemia, and palpation of the penis for firmness and degree of rigidity. Monitor urine output, assessing for oliguria or signs of acute urinary retention. Pain is treated with analgesics. Hypotension as a side effect of narcotics may be helpful in this situation. The client usually has moderate to severe anxiety related to pain, the treatment, and the threat to his sexual function. To the client, the treatment may sound bizarre and painful, especially since the area is already extremely sensitive. He needs to know not only the rationale for the treatment but also how it will feel. The client may be acutely embarrassed by the erection and needs reassurance that the nurse understands that the erection is not within his control.

The Client with Phimosis

Phimosis is constriction of the foreskin so that it cannot be retracted over the glans penis. It is an uncommon problem. Phimosis may be congenital, or it may be related to chronic infections under the foreskin, which lead to adhesions. The major problems with this condition are that it prevents adequate hygiene, which may lead to malignant changes of the penis, and it interferes with erections. The condition is treated with antibiotics and warm soaks. Eventually, circumcision may be necessary (Bates, 1995). Following a circumcision, the nurse assists the client with care of the incision. He should be aware that even though he is now circumcised, late circumcision places him at risk for penile cancer, and he should perform self-examination of the penis.

Disorders of Sexual Function

The Client with Erectile Dysfunction

Erectile dysfunction is defined as the inability of the male to attain and maintain an erection sufficient to permit *satisfactory* sexual intercourse. Satisfaction is, of course, a subjective concept. Many men do not require an erect penis to experience a satisfactory sexual relationship.

The incidence of erectile dysfunction is quite high. When men with partial erectile dysfunction are included in the statistics, about 30 million in the United States have this condition. Most are older than 65. A prevalence of 5% is noted at age 40, increasing to approximately 25% at age 65 or older. Thirty-three percent of clients receiving ambulatory care at a veteran's facility reported erectile problems (NIH Consensus Report, 1993).

Nurses in almost any health care setting may encounter clients with erectile dysfunction, either through routine examinations, or through careful assessment of clients' conditions and treatments that may incidentally cause erectile dysfunction. Nurses employed in clinics, operating rooms, and surgical units with urological services commonly encounter men under treatment for erectile dysfunction. Nurses in a variety of settings, including long-term care, encounter men who have had surgical interventions, such as penile implants.

There are many possible causes of erectile dysfunction (Table 46–5). At least 90% of men with erectile dysfunction over the age of 60 have a strong physiologic basis for their problem (Kaiser, 1994). Because this is a problem primarily of aging men, the discussion of pathophysiology focuses on this age group.

Pathophysiology

Age-related changes in sexual function involve cellular and tissue changes in the penis, decreased sensory activity, hypogonadism, and the effects of chronic illness. In the penis, a change from elastic collagen to a more rigid collagen results in decreased distensibility (a less rigid erection). This, in turn, interferes with the veno-occlusive mechanism. The veno-occlusive mechanism prevents blood from "leaking" out of the penis into the general vasculature prematurely. Problems with this mechanism result in incomplete erections. Vibrotactile sensation over the skin of the penis declines with age. This decline may explain why some older men have difficulty achieving erections, that is, why they require longer stimulation to achieve an erection. Hypogonadism, common in aging men, results in decreased testosterone levels. There may

Table 46–5   Causes of Erectile Dysfunction

Major Pathologic Causes		Major Iatrogenic Causes	
		Medications	**Procedures and Infections**

Neurogenic
    Spinal cord injury
    Cerebrovascular accident
    Parkinson's disease
    Multiple sclerosis
Endocrinologic
    Diabetes mellitus
    Hypogonadism
    Hypothyroidism
Inflammatory
    Prostatitis
    Cystitis
Activity Intolerance
    Pulmonary problems
    Anemias
    Myocardial infarction
    Congestive heart failure
    Hepatic diseases
    Renal failure
Substance Dependency
    Alcohol
    Marijuana
    Narcotics
    Sedatives
    Tobacco
Compulsive Food Disorders
    Compulsive overeating
    Anorexia nervosa
    Bulimia
	Arterial
	    Atherosclerosis
	    Hypertension
	    Aortic aneurysm
	    Sickle cell anemia
	Mechanical
	    Decreased penile
	    distensibility
	    Congenital disorders
	    Morbid obesity
	    Hydrocele
	    Hip or pelvic fractures
	Psychogenic
	    Depression
	    Stress
	    Fatigue
	    Fear of failure
		Antihypertensives
		    Hydrochlorothiazide
		    Spironolactone
		    Methyldopa
		    Clonidine
		    Prazosin
		    Propranolol
		    Reserpine
		Psychotropic Agents
		    Phenothiazines
		    Butyrophenones
		    Tricyclic antidepressants
		    MAO inhibitors
		    Diazepam
		    Chlorodiazepoxide
		Endocrinologic Agents
		    LHRH agonists
		    Estrogen compounds
		    Progesterone
		Other
		    Antiparkinsonian agents
		    Anticholinergic agents
		    Immunosuppressive agents
		    Antihistamines
			Surgery
			    Coronary artery bypass
			    Pelvic lymphadenectomy
			    Radical prostatectomy
			    Radical cystectomy
			    Abdominal perineal resection
			    Sympathectomy
			    Aortic aneurysm repair
			    Transplant surgeries
			Other
			    Severe nosocomial infection
			    Radiation therapy to pelvis

be a relationship between lower androgen levels and erectile function, and this relationship is under study. It may be that the primary relationship is between decreased testosterone and a generally lower libido rather than between decreased testosterone and erectile dysfunction (Donatucci & Lue, 1994). Many illnesses affect erectile function. Diabetes mellitus is the leading cause of organic erectile dysfunction, affecting approximately 2 million men (Lue, 1992). Given the aging changes on erectile function, the increased incidence of chronic illness, and the multiple treatments required to manage those illnesses, it is not surprising that older men have significant difficulty in this area of function.

Collaborative Care

The medical management of clients with erectile dysfunction is growing in importance and scale, because the inci-

dence increases as the population ages. Another factor is the gradual change in the willingness of men and their partners to be forthcoming about sexual concerns. Although sexuality is still a very sensitive and private area for most people, the knowledge that help is available is causing men to seek answers. Many older men are coming to believe that loss of erectile function is not an inevitable part of aging.

Laboratory and Diagnostic Tests

The following laboratory tests may be ordered for the client with erectile dysfunction:

- *Blood profiles,* including chemistry and testosterone, prolactin, thyroxin, and PSA levels, are performed to identify metabolic and endocrine problems that may be causing the dysfunction.

Nursing Care of the Client Using a Vacuum Constrictive Device (VCD)

Use of the VCD requires careful teaching for the client and partner. The physician, usually the urologist, determines the correct size of the device. There are several types. Some create vacuums with a hand-held pump, and others use an electric motor.

Nursing interventions with rationales follow:

- Assess the client's comfort level with the device. Practice is helpful. If the client wishes, the partner can help apply the lubricant and prepare the cylinder. *Most clients have not heard of the VCD and display some anxiety over its effectiveness.*

- Teach the client the technique for practice. The client will not experience an immediate erection, and daily practice sessions are necessary. The client should pump the device slowly until he feels a slight tightness, then release the vacuum. Gradually, he is able to build up to a complete, comfortable erection. *Conditioning of the corpora is necessary.*

- Help the client identify and solve potential problems. Examples of problems include no erection, rapid loss of erection, discomfort during intercourse, and the sensation of cold in the penis. The sensation of cold is caused by constriction of blood in the penis. The simple remedy is to warm the lubricant before use. *Although there may be many problems, almost all are simple and can be easily remedied.*

- Arrange follow-up appointments. If the client uses the device regularly, he may take as long as 3 months to reach maximum comfort with the device. He should call the nurse or physician if any problems develop. *Reassessment is necessary to determine the client's progress in using the device.*

- *Nocturnal penile tumescence and rigidity (NPTR)* monitoring helps differentiate between psychogenic and organic causes. These tests can be performed in a sleep laboratory; home testing with portable devices is an alternative. The number and quality of erections occurring during REM sleep can be determined. The client must spend 2 to 3 nights in the sleep lab. Although home testing is less expensive, many urologists believe that it is not reliable (Karacan, Moore & Gokcebay, 1994).

- *Cavernosometry* and *cavernosography* of the corpora are used to measure intracavernous pressure and venous outflow. These tests can reveal the precise nature of venous leaks.

- *Doppler studies with ultrasonography* are performed to help rule out calcifications or plaques.

- Vibrotactile sensation over the penis can be measured in the physician's office with a *biothesiometer.*

Pharmacology

Erectile dysfunction can be treated with oral medications, self-administered intracavernous injections, or by topical agents. Injections and topical agents have shown the most promise. Papaverine is the drug most commonly used. When injected directly into the penis, papaverine relaxes the arterioles and smooth muscles of the cavernosum, thus inducing tumescence. An erection usually develops that lasts from 30 minutes to 4 hours. The most common side effect (5%) is intracavernous fibrosis (Andersson, 1994). Prostaglandin E functions much as papaverine does but has fewer side effects. One problem with this treatment is its mode of delivery. There is a high attrition rate, and clients report dissatisfaction with lack of spontaneity, loss of interest in sex, physical limitations, cost, and occasionally, pain (Irwin & Kata, 1994).

Topical agents are under investigation. Transdermal nitroglycerin paste, the same paste that is used to treat coronary artery disease, has restored erectile function to a few men when applied directly to the penis. The mechanism of action is probably arteriolar dilation. Another arteriolar dilator undergoing investigation is minoxidil, applied topically to the penis. Oral drugs under investigation include naloxone, an opioid antagonist and dopamine (Andersson, 1994).

Mechanical Devices

The most frequently prescribed treatment for erectile dysfunction is the vacuum constriction device (Nadig, 1994). The vacuum constriction device (VCD) draws blood into the penis with a vacuum, trapping it there with a constricting band at the base of the penis. After the device is removed for intercourse, a single small band, often called an "O-ring," is left at the base of the penis to maintain the erection. If the man can attain an erection but cannot maintain it, then an O-ring alone can be used. Implications for nursing care of a client using a VCD are presented in the accompanying box.

Surgery

Surgical treatment for erectile dysfunction involves either revascularization procedures or implantation of prosthetic devices. Venous or arterial procedures are generally

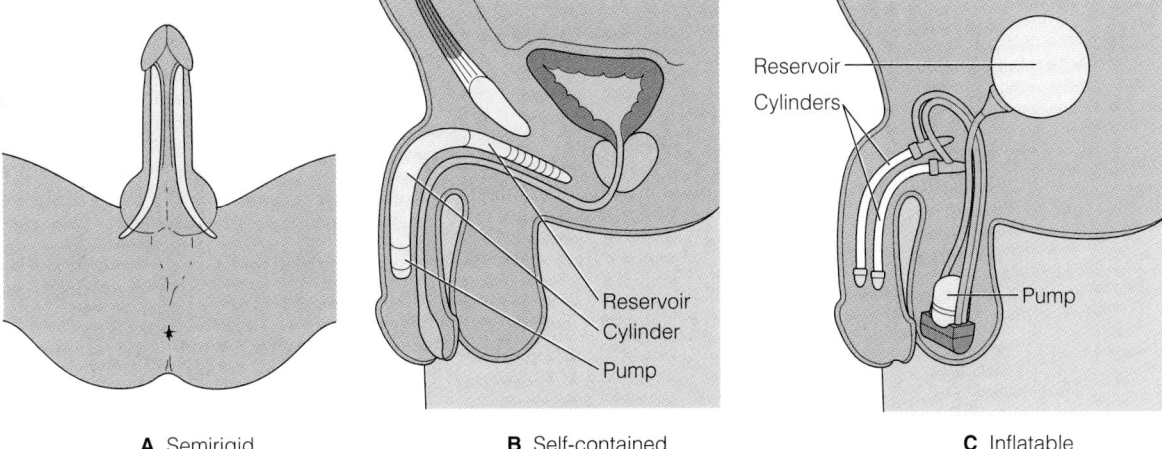

A Semirigid   **B** Self-contained   **C** Inflatable

Figure 46–5   Types of penile implants. *A,* With semirigid rods implanted in the corpora cavernosa, the penis is always in a state of semi-erection, which may not be acceptable to the client. *B,* With a self-contained penile implant, the penis remains flaccid until the client compresses a pump at the head of the penis, which transfers fluid from a reservoir to a cylinder within the penis to achieve an erection. The client presses a release valve to return the fluid to the reservoir. *C,* With an inflatable penile implant, the penis remains flaccid until the client compresses a pump in the scrotum, which transfers fluid from an abdominal reservoir to cylinders in the corpora cavernosa to achieve an erection. Pressing a release valve returns the fluid to the reservoir.

not successful. The result is often temporary, because the underlying cause of the vascular insufficiency is usually not corrected (Stief et al., 1994). Implantation of penile prostheses is now quite common (Figure 46–5). Clients are generally satisfied with their prostheses, and they rank the inflatable type highest. Partners are also more likely to report satisfaction with the penile implant, although not to the same degree as clients. Some partners report that the implanted penis is harder than a normal erect penis and therefore causes pain. Also, the man can have intercourse for a prolonged period of time, and some partners do not find prolonged penetration enjoyable. Client and partner teaching is mandatory. Counseling by a sex therapist may be needed to facilitate adaptation to the implant.

Nursing Care

Because nurses are usually accessible, they are most likely to discover problems of erectile dysfunction. Once a problem is known, nurses are involved in giving information, providing emotional support, and referring clients to physicians or counselors. Although there are many possible nursing diagnoses, this section focuses on nursing care related to sexual dysfunction.

Sexual Dysfunction

Many clients who lose erectile function are not aware of the cause. Often the client blames the loss on unrelated factors, such as age, a medication for an illness, a dangerous illness, or his sexual partner. Not knowing causes anxiety, which may disrupt the relationship with his part-

ner or lead the man to discontinue an important medication.

Nursing interventions with rationales follow:

- Assess the client for risk factors for erectile dysfunction. Be especially alert to clients who have recently begun medications or had recent surgeries that could cause erectile dysfunction. It may not be possible to assess all clients for risk factors for erectile dysfunction. *Awareness of risk factors helps the nurse to prioritize care, although nurses must remember that almost all aging clients have at least one risk factor.*

- Assess the client for sexual dysfunction. Men have shown increasing willingness to discuss sexual concerns and expect nurses to be aware of the physiologic effects of their disease and side effects of treatment on all aspects of their health. Still, most clients will not volunteer information unless asked. *If a problem exists, information obtained in a sexual assessment guides the nurse in deciding if the next step should be client teaching, referral, or both.*

- Perform a detailed assessment of client's current sexual practices. *It is essential for health care providers to understand the client and partner's sexual pattern in order to provide appropriate, individualized care.*

- Discuss client's previous methods of coping with erectile dysfunction. *Awareness of coping strategies can provide insight for the nurse and guide teaching.*

- Give client information about treatment options. *Clients need to know the details of the intervention, the chances for success, and the possible complications.*

Other Nursing Diagnoses

The following nursing diagnoses may also apply to clients with erectile dysfunction:

- *Self-Esteem Disturbance* related to loss of erectile function
- *Altered Role Performance* related to perceived loss of masculinity
- *Ineffective Family Coping: Compromised* related to loss of usual sexual pattern

Client and Family Teaching

Many nurses find that men with erectile dysfunction and their partners have lived in isolation with the problem for many years. The partner may even be unaware of the problem. The partner may believe that the client is seeing someone else or that the client has lost his attraction to the partner. The client may have kept his problem a secret because of an intense feeling of shame. He is unable to admit that he cannot perform sexually. Many clients greet the information about the high incidence of erectile dysfunction with a sense of relief. They are not alone in having this problem. All clients and their partners also need to be aware of support services available to them.

Applying the Nursing Process

Case Study of a Client with Erectile Dysfunction: Donald Lawton

Donald Lawton is a 68-year-old carpenter living in a rural area about 50 miles from a major metropolitan area. He has been married for 40 years, and his three children have graduated and moved out of the area. At the age of 52, he was diagnosed with insulin-dependent diabetes mellitus. He has frequently ignored his diet, resulting in blood sugar levels over 200. Two years ago, he began to notice a problem of incomplete penile erections. At first, the erections were simply not as rigid as normal, but gradually the problem has worsened until, about 1 year ago, he could no longer attain an erection adequate for sexual penetration. He has not experienced any kind of erection in the last 4 months, although his libido remains unaffected. He experiences shame and embarrassment because of this problem, and is not able to discuss it with anyone, including his wife.

Assessment

Mr. Lawton brings the problem to the attention of his family physician after his wife threatens to leave him, claiming neglect. He is referred to a urologist who specializes in the treatment of sexual dysfunction. In the physician's office, the nurse, Stephen Thomas, RN, performs the initial assessment of the client's sexual function. Mr. Thomas learns that Mr. Lawton places high value on his relationship with his wife, and that sexual intimacy has been an important part of their relationship. He says that their sexual activity has always been limited to foreplay and sexual intercourse, expressing mild distaste about other forms of sexual intimacy. As the problem became worse, he was unable to discuss the difficulty with his wife because of fear and shame. He reports that it felt as if he were no longer a man and that he was ashamed that he could no longer satisfy her. "I would not be surprised if she has found someone else, because I sure can't help her," he states. Gradually, even nonsexual shared activities have become emotionally painful and he has withdrawn, communicating only about essential aspects of maintaining their home.

Mr. Lawton's serum testosterone levels are normal. Nocturnal penile tumescence and rigidity monitoring in the sleep laboratory reveals an absence of erections during REM sleep. Because the primary problem is viewed as neurologic rather than vascular, cavernosometry is not performed. The urologist determines that Mr. Lawton might benefit from a vacuum constrictive device and couples counseling. Teaching sessions are scheduled with Mr. Thomas and the client. It is hoped that Mrs. Lawton can join the teaching sessions as soon as possible.

Diagnosis

Mr. Thomas makes the following nursing diagnoses for Mr. Lawton:

- *Sexual Dysfunction* related to disease process (diabetes)
- *Altered Sexuality Patterns* related to lack of knowledge and poor communication patterns with wife
- *Situational Low Self-Esteem* related to loss of male sexual role
- *Body Image Disturbance* related to change in erectile function

Expected Outcomes

The expected outcomes for the plan of care are that Mr. Lawton will

- State satisfaction with and acceptance of alternative sexual practices for himself and his wife.
- Demonstrate the ability to discuss sexual concerns with his wife.
- State acceptance of the change in his erectile function.
- Demonstrate the use of a vacuum constriction device.

Planning and Implementation

The following interventions are planned and implemented during care of Mr. Lawton:

- Listen to Mr. Lawton's concerns as he begins to learn about the vacuum constrictive device.

- Encourage discussion about alternative sexual practices.

- With Mr. Lawton's permission, include his wife in discussions and teaching sessions.

- Encourage Mr. and Mrs. Lawton to enter couples counseling.

- Listen to Mr. and Mrs. Lawton's concerns about the severity of the sexual problem, and encourage communication.

- Reinforce positive statements from Mr. Lawton concerning his change in erectile function.

- Teach the use of the vacuum constriction device.

- Provide information about other forms of sexual intimacy, remaining sensitive to client's cultural, religious, and developmental level.

Evaluation

Mr. Lawton experiences an atmosphere of acceptance about his sexual issues. He begins to express himself more freely about his sexual and relationship problems, and he begins to attend counseling with Mrs. Lawton. When Mrs. Lawton attends the teaching sessions with her husband, Mr. Thomas learns about the impact of her husband's sexual difficulties on her feelings. Mrs. Lawton states that she was afraid that her husband no longer found her attractive and that he had found another woman. She greets the knowledge of the true nature of the problem with relief and concern. Mrs. Lawton's ability to communicate her feelings with Mr. Lawton's support is viewed as an indication that the couple is progressing. Privately, Mr. Lawton tells Mr. Thomas that he feels his marriage is improving and that even though "things" will never be the same, he is beginning to look forward to some mutual exploration. Mr. Lawton masters the vacuum constriction device with little difficulty, and 4 months later reports that he and his wife are "90% satisfied with the result."

Critical Thinking in the Nursing Process

1. Mr. Lawton's erectile dysfunction was directly related to his diabetes. Describe the patholophysiology of diabetes-induced erectile dysfunction (see Chapter 21).

2. How does the nocturnal penile tumescence and rigidity test differentiate between organic and psychologic causes of erectile dysfunction?

3. When introduced to the vacuum constrictive device for the first time, Mr. Lawton states that he hopes it will work well enough for tonight. What does this statement imply about Mr. Lawton's teaching needs related to the early use of this device?

4. Discuss the importance of Mr. and Mrs. Lawton's lack of communication on the development of their sexual problems. Include possible reasons for their difficulty in discussing sexual concerns.

The Client with Ejaculatory Dysfunction

■ ■ ■

There are many types of ejaculatory dysfunction. *Premature ejaculation* is usually psychogenic in origin, although diabetes can cause the problem as well. *Delayed ejaculation* can be related to aging changes, such as decreased vibrotactile sensation over the penis or decreased libido secondary to hypogonadism. Delayed ejaculation and inability to ejaculate at all may be caused by certain medications, such as antihypertensives, antidepressants, anxiolytics, and narcotics (Bates, 1995). *Retrograde ejaculation* may develop in aging men (Kaiser, 1994) but is usually related to treatment of prostatic conditions or testicular cancer. Assessment of the problem may reveal the cause and direct treatment.

Among these problems, premature ejaculation has proved most responsive to medical management. The client can experiment with ways (such as wearing condoms) to decrease sensitivity. The man can remove the condom when he and his partner wish to experience ejaculation. Use of relaxation and guided imagery can delay sexual excitement. Mechanical devices, such as constrictive rings around the base of the penis can can help the man delay ejaculation and sustain an erection.

Nursing care focuses on assessment of the problem and client teaching. The client's partner can be included and taught how to avoid excessive stimulation until ejaculation. If the problem persists, the client can be referred to a specialist.

Bibliography

■ ■ ■

Aikey, C. (1992). Erectile dysfunction. *Urologic Nursing, 12,* 96–103.

Andersson, K. (1994). Pharmacology of erection: Agents which initiate and terminate erection. *Sexuality and Disability, 12,* 53–79.

Andriole, G. L., Smith, D. S., Rao, G., Goodnough, L., & Catalona, W. J. (1994). Early complications of contemporary anatomical radical retropubic prostatectomy. *Journal of Urology, 152,* 1858–1860.

Asplund, R., & Aberg, R. (1991). Diurnal variation in the levels of antidiuretic hormone in the elderly. *Journal of Internal Medicine, 229,* 131–134.

Basile, G., & Goldstein, I. (1994). Medical treatment of neurogenic impotence. *Sexuality and Disability, 12,* 81–94.

Bastuba, M. D., TeJada, I. S., Dinlenc, C. Z., Sarazen, A., Krane, R. J., & Goldstein, I. (1994). Arterial priapism: Diagnosis, treatment, and long-term followup. *Journal of Urology, 151,* 1231–1237.

Bates, P. (1995). External genital disorders. In K. A. Karlowicz (Ed.), *Urologic nursing: Principles and practice* (pp. 311–331). Phildadelphia: Saunders.

Brawn, P., Johnson, E., Kuhl, D., Riggs, M., Speights, V., Johnson, C., Pandya, P., Lind, M., & Bell, N. (1993). Stage at presentation and survival of white and black patients with prostate carcinoma. *Cancer, 71,* 2569–2573.

Brendler, C. B., & Walsh, P. C. (1992). The role of radical prostatectomy in the treatment of prostate cancer. *CA: A Cancer Journal for Clinicians, 42,* 212–222.

Cabot, A. T. (1986). The question of castration for enlarged prostate. *Annals of Surgery, 24,* 265.

Carney, S., Karlowicz, K. A., Meredith, C., Pear, S. M., Reilly, N. J., Swibold, L., Toner, M. L., & Wagner, J. D. (1995). Urinary tract obstructions. In K. A. Karlowicz (Ed.), *Urologic nursing: Principles and practice* (pp. 107–140). Philadelphia: Saunders.

Carter, H. B., & Coffey, D. S. (1990). The prostate: An increasing medical problem. *Prostate, 16,* 39–48.

Chang, S. W., Fine, R., Siegel, D., Chesney, M., Black, D., & Hulley, S.B. (1991). The impact of diuretic therapy on reported sexual function. *Archives of Internal Medicine, 151,* 2402–2408.

Chisholm, G. D., Rana, A., & Howard, G. C. W. (1993). Management options for painful carcinoma of the prostate. *Seminars in Oncology, 20*(3 Suppl. 2), 34–37.

Cisek, L. J., & Walsh, P. C. (1993). Thromboembolic complications following radical retropubic prostatectomy. *Urology, 42,* 406–408.

Cox, H. C., Hinz, M. D., Lubno, M. A., Newfield, S. A., Ridenour, N. A., Slater, M. M., & Sridaromont, K. (1993). *Clinical applications of nursing diagnosis.* Philadelphia: F. A. Davis.

Curn, C. A. (1992). Erectile dysfunction. *Urologic Nursing, 12,* 96–103.

Davis, M. (1994). Genitourinary cancers. In S. Otto (Ed.), *Oncology nursing* (pp. 168–220). St. Louis: Mosby.

De la Rosette, J. J. M. C., Ruijgrok, M. C. M., Jeuken, J. M. G., Karthaus, H. F. M., & Debruyne, F. M. J. (1993). Personality variables involved in chronic prostatitis. *Urology, 42,* 654–662.

Demers, R., Swanson, M., Weiss, L., & Kau, T. (1994). Increasing incidence of cancer of the prostate: The experience of black and white men in the Detroit metropolitan area. *Archives of Internal Medicine, 154,* 1211–1216.

Donatucci, C. F., & Lue, T. F. (1994). Management of impotence. In P. O'Donnell (Ed.), *Geriatric urology* (pp. 345–355). Boston: Little, Brown.

Einhorn, L. H., Richie, J. P., & Shipley, W. U. (1993). Cancer of the testes. In V. T. DeVita, S. Hellman, & S. A. Rosenthal (Eds.), *Cancer: Principles and practice of oncology* (pp. 1126–1150). Philadelphia: Lippincott.

Epstein, B. E., & Hanks, G. E. (1992). Prostate cancer: Evaluation and radiotherapeutic management. *CA: A Cancer Journal for Clinicians, 42,* 223–240.

Fair, W. R., Fuks, Z. Y., & Scher, H. I. (1993). Cancer of the urethra and penis. In V. T. DeVita, S. Hellman, & S. A. Rosenthal (Eds.), *Cancer: Principles and practice of oncology* (pp. 1114–1125). Philadelphia: Lippincott.

Garnick, M. (1993). Prostate cancer: Screening, diagnosis, and management. *Annals of Internal Medicine, 118,* 804–818.

Giovannucci, E., Tosteson, T., Speizer, F., Ascherio, A., Vessey, M., & Colditz, G. (1993). A retrospective cohort study of vasectomy and prostate cancer in U.S. men. *Journal of the American Medical Association, 269,* 878–882.

Giroux, J. A. (1995). Urinary tract infections in adults. In K. A. Karlowicz (Ed.), *Urologic nursing: Principles and practice* (pp. 141–176). Philadelphia: Saunders.

Goldstein, M. (1992). Surgery of male infertility and other scrotal disorders. In P. C. Walsh, A. B. Retik, T. A. Stamey, & E. D. Vaughan (Eds.), *Campbell's urology* (pp. 3114–3143). Philadelphia: Saunders.

Greco, K. E., & Blank, B. (1993). Prostate-specific antigen: The new early detection test for prostate cancer. *Nurse Practitioner, 18*(5), 30–38.

Greco, K. E. & Kulawiak, L. (1994). Prostate cancer prevention: Risk reduction through life-style, diet, and chemoprevention. *Oncology Nursing Forum, 21,* 1504–1511.

Gundian, J. C., Barrett, D. M., & Parulkar, B. G. (1993). Mayo clinic experience with the AS800 artificial urinary sphincter for urinary incontinence after transurethral resection of the prostate or open prostatectomy. *Urology, 41,* 318–321.

Hanks, G., Myers, C., & Scardino, P. (1993). Cancer of the prostate. In V. DeVita, S. Hellman, & S. A. Rosenthal (Eds.), *Cancer: Principles and practice of oncology* (pp. 1073–1113). Philadelphia: Lippincott.

Hayes, R. B., de Jong, F. H., Raatgever, J., Bogdanovicz, J., Schroeder, F. H., Van der Maas, P., Oishi, K., & Yoshida, O. (1992). Physical characteristics and factors related to sexual development and behavior and the risk for prostatic cancer. *European Journal of Cancer Prevention, 1,* 239–245.

Held, J. L., Osborne, D. M., Volpe, H., & Waldman, A. R. (1994). Cancer of the prostate: Treatment and nursing implications. *Oncology Nursing Forum, 21,* 1517–1529.

Held, J. L., & Peahota, A. (1993). Nursing care of the patient with spinal cord compression. *Oncology Nursing Forum, 20,* 1507–1516.

Holly, E. A., & Palefsky, J. M. (1993). Factors related to risk of penile cancer: New evidence from a study in the Pacific northwest. *Journal of the National Cancer Institute, 85,* 2–3.

Irwin, M. B., & Kata, E. J. (1994). High attrition rate with intracavernous injection of prostaglandin e1 for impotency. *Urology, 43,* 84–87.

Kaiser, F. E. (1994). Sexuality. In P. D. O'Donnell (Ed.), *Geriatric urology* (493–516). Boston: Little, Brown.

Karacan, I., Moore, C. A., & Gokcebay, N. (1994). Nocturnal penile tumescence (NPT) and rigidity monitoring in neurogenic impotence: Interpretations and limitations. *Sexuality and Disability, 12,* 39–51.

Klimaszewski, A. D., & Karlowicz, K. A. (1995). Cancer of the male genitalia. In K. A. Karlowicz (Ed.), *Urologic nursing: Principles and practice* (pp. 271–308). Philadelphia: Saunders.

Klimberg, I. W., Locke, D. R., Leonard, E., Madore, R., & Klimberg, S. R. (1994). Outpatient transurethral resection of the prostate at a urological ambulatory surgery center. *Journal of Urology, 151,* 1547–1549.

Koch, M. O., & Hall, M. C. (1994). Perioperative fluid and electrolyte management. In P. D. O'Donnell (Ed.), *Geriatric urology* (pp. 69–81). Boston: Little, Brown.

La Follette, S., Wettlaufer, J., & Karlowicz, K. A. (1995). Perioperative care of the urologic patient. In K. A. Karlowicz (Ed.), *Urologic nursing: Principles and practice* (pp. 86–103). Philadelphia: Saunders.

Lepor, H. (1995). Long-term efficacy and safety of terazosin in patients with benign prostatic hyperplasia. *Urology, 45,* 406–413.

Lewis, J. H. (1993). Nursing management for patients using external vacuum devices: A unique opportunity. *Urologic Nursing, 13,* 80–85.

Littrup, P. J., Lee, F., & Mettlin, C. (1992). Prostate cancer screening: Current trends and future implications. *CA: A Cancer Journal for Clinicians, 42,* 198–211.

Loescher, L. J. (1994). Prostate cancer: Controversies surrounding risk, screening, and management—Introduction. *Oncology Nursing Forum, 21,* 1503–1504.

Lue, T. F. (1992). Physiology of erection and pathophysiology of impotence. In P. C. Walsh, A. B. Retik, T. A. Stamey, & E. D. Vaughan, (Eds.), *Campbell's urology* (pp. 709–726). Philadelphia: Saunders.

Matzkin, H., & Soloway, M. (1993). Cigarette smoking: A review of possible associations with benign prostatic hyperplasia and prostate cancer. *Prostate, 22,* 277–290.

Maxwell, M. B. (1993). Cancer of the prostate. *Seminars in Oncology Nursing, 9,* 237–251.

McKee, J. M. (1994). Cues to action in prostate cancer screening. *Oncology Nursing Forum, 21,* 1171–1176.

Meares, E. M. (1992). Prostatitis and related disorders. In P. C. Walsh, A. B. Retik, T. A. Stamey, & E. D. Vaughan (Eds.), *Campbell's urolology* (pp. 807–822). Philadelphia: Saunders.

Mebust, W. K. (1992). Transurethral surgery. In P. C. Walsh, A. B. Retik, T. A. Stamey, & E. D. Vaughan (Eds.), *Campbell's urology* (pp. 2900–2922). Philadelphia: Saunders.

Meredith, C. E. (1995). Erectile dysfunction. In K. A. Karlowicz (Ed.), *Urologic nursing: Principles and practice* (pp. 332–359). Philadelphia: Saunders.

Mettlin, C., Jones, G., Averette, H., Gusberg, S.B., & Murphy, G. P. (1993). Defining and updating the American Cancer Society guidelines for the cancer-related checkup: Prostate and endometrial cancers. *CA: A Cancer Journal for Clinicians, 43,* 42–46.

Mettlin, C., & Murphy, G. (1994). The national cancer data base report on prostate cancer. *Cancer, 74,* 1640–1648.

Montie, J. E. (1994). Counseling the patient with localized prostate cancer. *Urology, 43*(2 Suppl.), 36–40.

Moul, J. W. (1993). Prostatitis: Sorting out the different causes. *Postgraduate Medicine, 94,* 191–194.

Nadig, P. W. (1994). Vacuum constriction devices in patients with neurogenic impotence. *Sexuality and Disability, 12,* 99–105.

Nagle, G. M. (1991). Genitourinary surgery. In M. H. Meeker & J. C. Rothrock (Eds.), *Alexander's care of the patient in surgery* (pp. 331–412). St. Louis: Mosby-Year Book.

NIH Consensus Conference: Impotence. (1993). *Journal of the American Medical Association, 270,* 83–90.

Oesterling, J. E. (1995). Benign prostatic hyperplasia: Medical and minimally invasive treatment options. *New England Journal of Medicine, 332,* 99–107.

Peterson, R. (1993). A nursing intervention for early detection of spinal cord compressions in patients with cancer. *Cancer Nursing, 2,* 113–116.

Reilly, N. J. (1995). Genitourinary trauma. In K. A. Karlowicz (Ed.), *Urologic nursing: Principles and practice* (pp. 411–435). Philadelphia: Saunders.

Resnick, N. M., & Yalla, S. V. (1992). Evaluation and medical management of urinary incontinence. In P. C. Walsh, A. B. Retik, T. A. Stamey, & E. D. Vaughan (Eds). *Campbell's urology* (pp. 643–658). Philadelphia: Saunders.

Richie, J. P., (1992). Neoplasms of the testis. In P. C. Walsh, A. B. Retik, T. A. Stamey, & E. D. Vaughan (Eds.), *Campbell's urology* (pp. 1222–1261). Philadelphia: Saunders.

Ronk, L. L., & Kavitz, J. M. (1994). Perioperative nursing implications of radical perineal prostatectomy. *AORN Journal, 60,* 438–445.

Sagalowsky, A., & Wilson, J. (1994). Hyperplasia and carcinoma of the prostate. In K. Isselbacher, E. Braunwald, J. Wilson, J. Martin, A. Fauci, & D. Kasper, (Eds), *Harrison's principles of internal medicine* (pp. 1862–1866). New York: McGraw-Hill.

Sanda, M. G., Beaty, T. H., Stutzman, R. E., Childs, B., & Walsh, P. C. (1994). Genetic susceptibility of benign prostatic hyperplasia. *Journal of Urology, 152,* 115–119.

Scher, H. I., & Chung, L. W. K. (1994). Bone metastases: Improving the therapeutic index. *Seminars in Oncology, 21,* 630–656.

Spear, K. A., Bollard, G. A., & Summers, J. L. (1994). Early discharge of transurethral prostatectomy patients with an indwelling Foley catheter. *Urology, 43,* 333–336.

Stief, C. G., Djamilian, M., Truss, M. C., Tan, H., Thon, W. F., & Jonas, U. (1994). Prognostic factors for the postoperative outcome of penile venous surgery for venogenic erectile dysfunction. *Journal of Urology, 151,* 880–883.

Tiemann, D., Shea, L., Klutke, C. G., Gaehle, K., & Moore, S. (1993). Artificial urinary sphincters: Treatment for post-prostatectomy incontinence. *AORN Journal, 57,* 1366–1379.

Walsh, P. C. (1992). Benign prostatic hyperplasia. In P. C. Walsh, A. B. Retik, T. A. Stamey, & E. D. Vaughan, E.D. (Eds.), *Campbell's urology* (pp. 1009–1027). Philadelphia: Saunders.

Walsh, P. C., Partin, A. W., & Epstein, J. I. (1994). Cancer control and quality of life following anatomical radical retropubic prostatectomy: Results at 10 years. *Journal of Urology, 152,* 1831–1836.

Wilson, M. (1994). Testicular prosthesis: Effect of the silicone controversy. *Urologic Nursing, 14,* 170–172.

Wingo, P. A., Tong, T., & Bolden, S. (1995). Cancer statistics, 1995. *CA: A Cancer Journal for Clinicians, 45,* 8–30.

Nursing Care of Female Clients with Reproductive System Disorders

LEARNING OBJECTIVES

After completing this chapter, you will be able to

- Describe the pathophysiology of common disorders of the female reproductive system.

- Identify laboratory and diagnostic tests used to diagnose disorders of the female reproductive system.

- Discuss nursing implications for medications pre-scribed for the client with disorders of the female reproductive system.

- Provide appropriate preoperative and postoperative nursing care for the client having gynecologic surgery.

- Use the nursing process as a framework for providing individualized care to clients with disorders of the female reproductive system.

Disorders of the female reproductive system range from the minor discomfort of menstrual cramps to life-threatening diseases, such as ovarian cancer. Many of these disorders can occur at any point in a woman's adult life. They may affect her ability to bear children, her sexuality, and her sense of well-being as a woman.

Women who experience problems with the reproductive system require a holistic approach to meet their physiologic, psychologic, and educational needs. Because the ability to reproduce affects self-esteem, feelings of femininity, and general health, sensitivity and understanding of caregivers are essential. Providing personal medical and family history and undergoing diagnostic tests often require clients to disclose personal, intimate information, which they may find embarrassing and uncomfortable. Effective care of the client may entail education and perhaps treatment of her sexual partner. When planning and implementing care, nurses must consider the client within the context of her culture, socioeconomic and educational level, and life-style. It is also important that the nurse not make assumptions or judgments about the client's sexual orientation.

This chapter discusses disorders of menstruation and menopause, structural disorders of the female reproductive system, disorders of female reproductive tissue, infections of the female reproductive system, and disorders of sexual expression. Disorders of the breast are presented in Chapter 48, and sexually transmitted diseases common to both males and females are discussed in Chapter 49. Detailed presentations of contraception, sterilization, abortion, infertility, pregnancy, and lactation are beyond the intended scope of this book; extensive coverage of these topics can be found in maternal-newborn or maternal-child health texts.

◾ ◾ ◾   **Disorders of Menstruation and Menopause**   ◾ ◾ ◾

Monthly menstruation normally involves some minor discomfort, including breast tenderness, a feeling of heaviness and congestion in the pelvic area, uterine cramping, and lower backache. Many women, however, experience more serious effects, both physiologic and psychologic. This section discusses premenstrual syndrome, dysmenorrhea, abnormal uterine bleeding, and menopausal symptoms.

The Client with Premenstrual Syndrome

◾ ◾ ◾

Premenstrual syndrome (PMS) is a complex of symptoms characterized by irritability, depression, edema, and breast tenderness preceding the monthly menses. It is estimated that PMS affects more than half of all women during their reproductive years: that is, approximately 9 to 12 million women in the United States. Major life stressors, age greater than 30, and depression are risk factors associated with PMS. Premenstrual syndrome can be a factor in absenteeism at school or work, decreased productivity, interpersonal relationship difficulties, and lifestyle disruption. The actual cause of PMS is unknown, but it is thought that imbalances of estrogen and progesterone are involved.

Pathophysiology

Although the pathophysiology of PMS is not clearly understood, it is believed that falling estrogen and progesterone levels and rising aldosterone levels during the luteal phase of the menstrual cycle may contribute to the problem. Increased production of aldosterone results in sodium retention and edema. Decreased levels of monamine oxidase in the brain are associated with depression, and reduced levels of serotonin can lead to mood swings.

Manifestations of PMS occur only during the luteal phase of the menstrual cycle (7 to 10 days prior to the onset of the menstrual flow), abating when the menstrual flow begins. The multisystem effects of PMS are shown in Figure 47–1. Although PMS may produce a host of physiologic and psychologic manifestations, the exact nature of these manifestations and their intensity vary remarkably for each client with this disorder.

Collaborative Care

Care of the client with PMS must first rule out any organic cause for the manifestations. If no cause can be identified, the goals of care are to relieve manifestations and to help the client develop self-care patterns that will help her anticipate and cope more effectively with future episodes of PMS.

There are no definitive diagnostic tests for PMS. When underlying organic causes for the symptoms have been ruled out, the regular recurrence of symptoms preceding the onset of menses leads to a diagnosis of PMS.

If the manifestations of PMS are severe or incapacitating, ovulation may be suppressed by the use of gonadotropin-releasing hormone (GRH) agonists, oral contraceptives, or danazol. Progesterone and antiprostaglandin agents such as NSAIDs may help relieve cramping. Diuretics, antidepressants, and tranquilizers may be prescribed to relieve bloating and depression.

Nonpharmacologic measures for the client with PMS focus on diet, exercise, relaxation, and stress management. A diet high in complex carbohydrates with limited simple sugars and alcohol is recommended to minimize reactive hypoglycemia, which can contribute to the manifestations of PMS. Reduced sodium intake helps to minimize fluid retention. Caffeine is also restricted to reduce irritability. Increased intake of calcium, magnesium, and vitamin B$_6$ may be helpful. Exercise is beneficial, but adequate rest also is necessary; the client needs to balance periods of activity and rest. Techniques for relaxation and stress management include deep abdominal breathing, meditation, muscle relaxation, and guided imagery.

Nursing Care

Nursing care for the client with PMS focuses on relieving the manifestations. Each plan of nursing care must be individualized; however, most women experiencing PMS will require interventions to manage pain and enhance coping.

Pain

The client with PMS has pain related to headache (including possible migraine), cramps, excessive fluid retention, breast swelling, or backache.

Nursing interventions with rationales follow:

- Teach effective pharmacologic and nonpharmacologic self-care measures to relieve pain: application of heat, relaxation techniques (such as breathing exercises, imagery techniques, or meditation), and exercise. *Heat relieves muscle spasms and causes blood vessels to dilate, increasing blood supply to the pelvis and uterine muscles. Relaxation and exercise aid the release of naturally produced pain relievers called endorphins.*

- Review daily activities with the client and suggest ways to balance rest periods and activity. *During rest periods,*

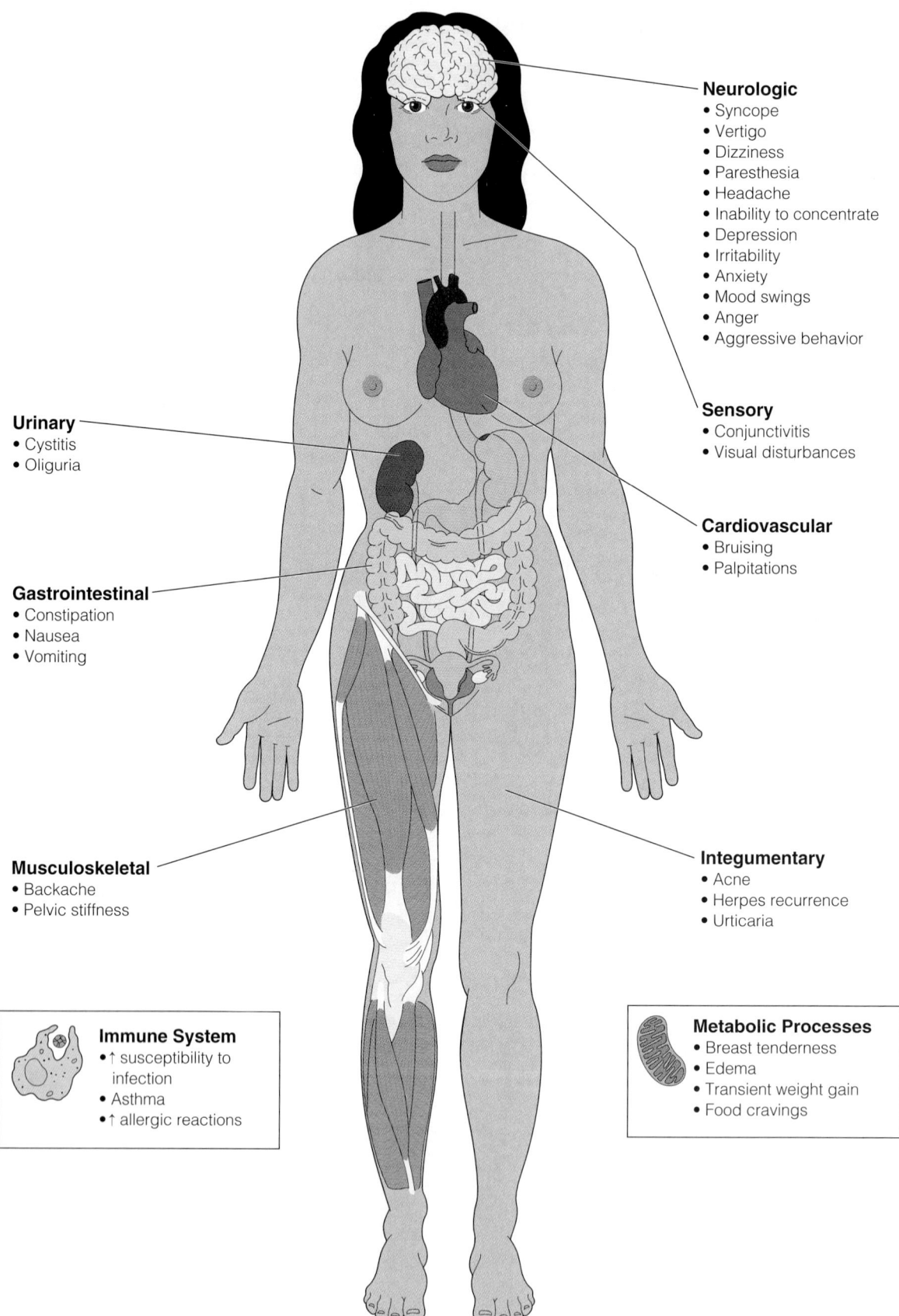

Neurologic
- Syncope
- Vertigo
- Dizziness
- Paresthesia
- Headache
- Inability to concentrate
- Depression
- Irritability
- Anxiety
- Mood swings
- Anger
- Aggressive behavior

Sensory
- Conjunctivitis
- Visual disturbances

Cardiovascular
- Bruising
- Palpitations

Urinary
- Cystitis
- Oliguria

Gastrointestinal
- Constipation
- Nausea
- Vomiting

Musculoskeletal
- Backache
- Pelvic stiffness

Integumentary
- Acne
- Herpes recurrence
- Urticaria

Immune System
- ↑ susceptibility to infection
- Asthma
- ↑ allergic reactions

Metabolic Processes
- Breast tenderness
- Edema
- Transient weight gain
- Food cravings

Figure 47–1   Multisystem effects of premenstrual syndrome.

energy and oxygen requirements decrease, increasing the amount of energy and oxygen available to muscles.

- Review manifestations with the client and, if possible, correlate these with dietary patterns and activity levels. Encourage the client to keep a diary of PMS manifestations. *Maintaining a diary of PMS manifestations, activity, and foods eaten can provide data to identify modifiable causes of discomfort (see the accompanying nursing research box).*

Ineffective Individual Coping

Many women experience wide mood swings during episodes of PMS, sometimes exhibiting self-destructive or aggressive behaviors toward others. These mood swings can interfere with a woman's ability to manage her responsibilities at home or at work.

Nursing interventions with rationales follow:

- Encourage the client to keep a journal of her menstrual cycle and to document her mood changes in the 7 to 10 days prior to menstruation. *Recognizing the signs and timing of PMS is the first step in developing methods to cope with the problem.*

- Explore possible ways in which the client can rearrange or reschedule activities when she is experiencing PMS. For example, family members may perform duties usually done by the client, and the client may schedule work meetings for non-PMS days, when possible. *Planning ahead enables the client to assume more control and promotes coping methods.*

- Explore with the client what, if any, self-care measures have helped her cope with mood alterations in the past. Encourage healthful coping mechanisms, such as relaxation techniques and exercise. *Some women may rely on alcohol or other drugs during PMS, which only exacerbate the manifestations.*

Other Nursing Diagnoses

Additional nursing diagnoses for the client with PMS follow:

- *Alterated Nutrition: More (or Less) Than Body Requirements* related to changes in appetite resulting from PMS

- *Sleep Pattern Disturbance* related to manifestations of PMS

- *Altered Thought Processes* related to changes in neurotransmitter levels associated with PMS

Client and Family Teaching

To promote the client's highest level of wellness, inform the client and family that PMS is not caused by a pathologic process but is a physiologic response to hormonal

---

Applying Research to Nursing Practice
Effect of Premenstrual Education on Premenstrual Symptoms

In one study, an investigator examined how a PMS education program can affect the manifestations of women experiencing the disorder (Seideman, 1990). A menstrual symptomatology questionnaire was administered to 47 women reporting premenstrual manifestations ranging from moderate to severe in intensity. Participants kept a menstrual symptom diary, and demographic and life-style data were also gathered. The subjects recorded symptoms for 1 month and then were randomly divided into control and experimental groups. The experimental group attended two 45-minute classes on PMS, which included suggestions for dietary and exercise interventions, stress management techniques, and hormone therapy. Both groups continued to keep a symptom diary for 2 more months. The investigator found that the experimental group experienced less severe manifestations than the control group: less edema, less anxiety, and less change in appetite. Manifestations also persisted longer in the control group.

Implications for Nursing

Teaching clients self-care measures may be a key component in reducing and relieving symptoms of PMS. This study suggests that women who understand how their bodies work may have a greater sense of well-being and control. Further investigation is needed comparing the effectiveness of various educational methods (written versus lecture or multimedia presentation) in populations of various ages, cultures, and socioeconomic levels.

Critical Thinking in Client Care

1. Do you think keeping a diary may heighten the client's focus on the manifestations of PMS, thus exaggerating their actual severity? Why or why not?

2. What effects might PMS have on a client's family members?

3. Does health locus of control affect PMS symptomatology?

Clinical Manifestations of Primary Dysmenorrhea

■ ■ ■

- Abdominal pain beginning with onset of menses and lasting 12 to 48 hours
- Pain radiating to lower back and thighs
- Headache
- Nausea
- Vomiting
- Diarrhea
- Fatigue
- Breast tenderness

---

changes of the menstrual cycle. With an understanding of the condition, the client is better able to manage anxiety and to become actively involved in techniques to reduce the manifestations. Client and family teaching should also include dietary measures, relaxation techniques and exercise, stress reduction techniques, and support systems.

The Client with Dysmenorrhea

■ ■ ■

Dysmenorrhea, pain associated with menstruation, is experienced by up to 75% of menstruating women. Approximately 15% of menstruating women miss work or school because of menstrual pain. There are two types of dysmenorrhea: **Primary dysmenorrhea** occurs without specific pelvic pathology, whereas **secondary dysmenorrhea** is related to identified pelvic disease, such as endometriosis or pelvic inflammatory disease.

Pathophysiology

In primary dysmenorrhea, excessive production of prostaglandins stimulates uterine muscle fibers to contract. These contractions can range from mild cramping to severe muscle spasms. As the muscles contract, uterine circulation is compromised, resulting in uterine ischemia and pain. Psychologic factors, such as anxiety and tension, may contribute to dysmenorrhea. Childbirth tends to decrease the incidence and severity of manifestations, possibly because of dilation of the internal cervical os.

Clinical manifestations of primary dysmenorrhea are presented in the accompanying box. They may be severe enough to disrupt activities of daily living, sexual function, and even fertility.

Secondary dysmenorrhea is related to underlying organic conditions that involve scarring or injury to the reproductive tract. Endometriosis, fibroid tumors, pelvic inflammatory disease, or ovarian cancer may result in painful menses. These conditions are discussed later in this chapter.

Collaborative Care

Care of the client with menstrual pain focuses on identifying the underlying cause, reestablishing functional capacity, and managing pain.

A careful history and physical are performed to rule out any underlying organic cause of dysmenorrhea. If no organic cause can be found, the diagnosis is primary dysmenorrhea. In addition, attitudes and expectations about menstruation and life-style disruption are identified and explored.

Laboratory and Diagnostic Tests

Various laboratory and diagnostic tests are performed to identify structural abnormalities, hormonal imbalances, and pathologic conditions that could cause menstrual pain:

- *Pelvic examination,* including a Papanicolaou (PAP) smear and cervical and vaginal cultures, is performed to detect structural abnormalities, malignancy, or infections.
- *Follicle-stimulating hormone (FSH) and luteinizing hormone (LH) levels* are measured to assess the function of the pituitary gland. The results are correlated with the time of the menstrual cycle.
- *Progesterone and estradiol levels* are measured to assess ovarian function.
- *Thyroid function tests (T_3 and T_4)* are performed to assess thyroid function.
- *Vaginal or pelvic ultrasonography* is used to detect the presence of space-occupying lesions, including fibroid tumors, cysts, abscesses, and neoplasms; see the accompanying box.
- *Computed tomography (CT) scan or magnetic resonance imaging (MRI)* can be used to detect pelvic tumors.
- *Laparoscopy* is used to diagnose structural defects and blockages caused by scarring, endometriosis, tumors, and cysts (Figure 47–2); see the accompanying box.
- *Dilation and curettage (D&C)* of the uterus is performed to obtain tissue for evaluation or to relieve dysmenorrhea and heavy bleeding. (This procedure is presented later in this chapter in the discussion on surgery.)

If it is determined that a client has secondary dysmenorrhea (that is, dysmenorrhea due to an underlying organic cause), therapeutic measures are directed at the specific condition.

Nursing Implications for Diagnostic Tests: Ultrasound Examination

■ ■ ■

- If indicated, ensure that the client's bladder is full by forcing fluids and instructing the client not to void. If the client is NPO, a Foley catheter may be inserted into the bladder and sterile water instilled. The catheter is then clamped to prevent the water from leaving the bladder. The full bladder lifts the pelvic organs higher into the abdomen and improves visualization.

- Explain to the client that she will be allowed to empty her bladder as soon as possible.

- Coat the abdomen with ultrasonic transducing gel. The gel provides a better image when the scanner is applied to the abdomen. For vaginal ultrasound, a transducer is covered with a condom or vinyl glove, coated with transducing gel, and introduced into the vagina.

- Explain the procedure to the client, indicating that she can watch the procedure and ask questions about the images on the screen. If appropriate, point out landmarks on the screen to the client.

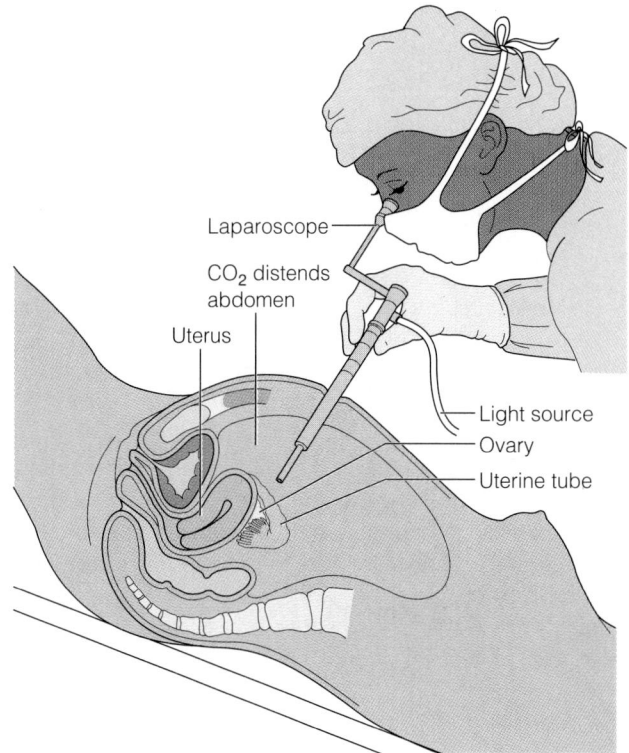

Figure 47–2   Laparoscopy. In this surgical procedure, a flexible, lighted instrument (laparoscope) is inserted through a periumbilical incision. Laparoscopy allows visualization of the pelvic cavity.

Nursing Care of the Client Undergoing Laparoscopy

PREOPERATIVE CARE

- Instruct the client to douche with povidone-iodine (Betadine) solution and to scrub the periumbilical area with Phisohex soap or povidone-iodine on the night before or morning of the procedure.

- Instruct the client to empty the bladder prior to the surgical procedure.

- Explain to the client that referred shoulder pain or expulsion of gas through the vagina may occur postoperatively. *During the procedure, the client's abdomen is insufflated with carbon dioxide gas to distend the abdomen and facilitate visualization of the pelvic organs. The surgical table is then tilted so that the intestines will fall away from the pelvic organs. Some carbon dioxide gas may remain in the abdomen after the procedure.*

- Explain that pain should be minimal. Instruct the client to report excessive pain to the nurse or physi-

cian at once. *Excessive pain signals infection or other postoperative complication.*

POSTOPERATIVE CARE

- Monitor vital signs. Report to the physician any elevation of temperature greater than 101 F (38.3 C) in the postoperative period.

- Apply a perineal pad. Teach the client proper perineal hygiene, emphasizing the need to change pads at least every 4 hours. Keep a pad count. *Proper perineal hygiene reduces the risk of postoperative infection. Pad count is an indication of blood loss.*

- Explain that the client may experience hiccups in the postoperative period. If it becomes a problem, prochlorperazine maleate (Compazine) can be ordered.

Nursing Implications for Pharmacology: The Client with Dysmenorrhea

ORAL CONTRACEPTIVES:

Norethindrone and ethinyl estradiol (Brevicon, Norinyl)

Norgestrel and ethinyl estradiol (Ovral)

Oral contraceptives inhibit ovulation and help reduce cramping and bleeding. Side effects of oral contraceptives include breast tenderness, weight gain, nausea, midcycle bleeding, mood swings, depression, chloasma (skin discoloration) on the face and chest, hypertension, vascular complications, vaginal candidiasis, migraines, and glucose intolerance. Oral contraceptives are contraindicated in women with personal or family history of breast cancer in first-degree relatives, hypertension, history of stroke or transient ischemic attack (TIA), smoking, history of estrogen-dependent cancer, pregnancy, liver disease, or thrombophlebitis.

Nursing Responsibilities:

- Assess the client for potential contraindications to drug therapy.

Client and Family Teaching

- Take the drug as prescribed until the physician indicates otherwise or until side effects prevent you from continuing to take them.

- If you are taking oral contraceptives, be sure to take them at the same time every day.

- Report to the physician suspected pregnancy and any side effects such as nausea, rash, drowsiness, stomach pain, ringing in the ears, tenderness in the calf of the leg, and shortness of breath.

- Do not smoke while taking oral contraceptives.

Pharmacology

Dysmenorrhea may be treated with analgesics, prostaglandin inhibitors such as NSAIDs, or oral contraceptives; see the accompanying box.

Additional Therapeutic Measures

Nonpharmacologic measures for the client with primary dysmenorrhea are related to diet, exercise, relaxation, and stress management. As noted in the PMS section, dietary measures, including reducing intake of sodium, sugar, caffeine, and alcohol; decreasing fluid consumption; and increasing intake of protein, calcium, magnesium, and vitamin B_6 may be helpful to relieve the manifestations of dysmenorrhea. Exercise is beneficial, but adequate rest also is necessary; the client needs to balance periods of activity and rest. Techniques for relaxation and stress management include deep abdominal breathing, meditation, muscle relaxation, and guided imagery. Use of a heating pad also helps reduce pain.

Nursing Care

Nursing care for the client with primary dysmenorrhea focuses on relieving pain and other manifestations and providing education about the normal physiology of the menstrual cycle and self-care measures. Care of the client with secondary dysmenorrhea varies according to the underlying cause and is discussed within sections on specific disorders. Although the plan of care must be individualized for each client, nursing interventions for the

client with primary dysmenorrhea commonly address problems with pain.

Pain

The ischemia produced by excessive uterine cramping can cause mild to severe pain that can incapacitate the client.

Nursing interventions with rationales follow:

- Teach effective pharmacologic and nonpharmacologic self-care measures to relieve pain. These include heat, relaxation, and exercise as well as medications (see the previous discussion of PMS).

- Teach the client to evaluate the character and severity of pain and to select relief measures accordingly. *If nonpharmacologic measures, such as relaxation techniques, can relieve minor pain, medications may be unnecessary.*

Other Nursing Diagnoses

Additional nursing diagnoses for the client with primary dysmenorrhea may include the following:

- *Altered Nutrition: More* (or *Less*) *Than Body Requirements* related to appetite-altering effect of primary dysmenorrhea

- *Altered Role Performance* related to manifestations of primary dysmenorrhea

- *Sleep Pattern Disturbance* related to severe uterine cramping

Client and Family Teaching

To promote the client's highest level of wellness, provide information about the benign nature of the disorder and its management, including pharmacologic and nonpharmacologic measures for pain relief. Teach methods of increasing rest and exercise, improving diet, and managing stress, as discussed above. Discuss the appropriate use of heat to relieve discomfort. Provide information about engaging in sexual intercourse, explaining that orgasm may help relieve the client's symptoms.

The Client with Abnormal Uterine Bleeding

■ ■ ■

Dysfunctional uterine bleeding (DUB), frequently referred to as *abnormal uterine bleeding,* refers to vaginal bleeding that is usually painless but abnormal in amount, duration, or time of occurrence. Disorders of DUB include primary and secondary amenorrhea, oligomenorrhea, menorrhagia, metrorrhagia, and postmenopausal bleeding.

Amenorrhea is the absence of menstruation. *Primary amenorrhea,* absence of menarche by age 17, may be caused by structural abnormalities, hormonal imbalances, polycystic ovary disease, or an imperforate hymen. Because a certain percentage of body fat is required in order for menstruation to occur, anorexia nervosa or excessive athletic activity or training can also cause primary amenorrhea.

Secondary amenorrhea, absence of menses in a previously menstruating female, may also be caused by anorexia nervosa, excessive athletic activity or training, or a large weight loss. Other causes include hormonal imbalances and ovarian tumors. Normal, or physiologic, secondary amenorrhea occurs during pregnancy, breastfeeding, and menopause.

Oligomenorrhea, scant menses, usually is related to hormonal imbalances. **Menorrhagia,** excessive or prolonged menstruation, may result from thyroid disorders, endometriosis, pelvic inflammatory disease, functional ovarian cysts, or uterine fibroids or polyps. Clotting disorders and anticoagulant medications also can cause menorrhagia. A single heavy or long cycle is not in itself a cause for concern; however, repetitive long or heavy cycles can lead to excessive blood loss, fatigue, anemia, hemorrhage, and sexual dysfunction.

Metrorrhagia, bleeding between menstrual periods, may be caused by hormonal imbalances, pelvic inflammatory disease, cervical or uterine polyps, uterine fibroids, or cervical or uterine cancer. Because cancer is a possible cause of metrorrhagia, early evaluation and treatment are extremely important. *Mittleschmerz* (midcycle spotting associated with ovulation) occurs in many women and is not considered metrorrhagia.

Postmenopausal bleeding may be caused by endometrial polyps, endometrial hyperplasia, or uterine cancer. The possibility of cancer makes early evaluation and treatment essential.

Dysfunctional uterine bleeding is the most frequently reported health care problem in women and the leading cause of hysterectomy. The problem increases with age: approximately 20% of cases of DUB occur in adolescents; 30% in women ages 20 to 40, and more than 50% in women over age 40.

A number of risk factors have been identified that may predispose a woman to DUB. These factors include stress, extreme weight changes, use of oral contraceptive agents or intrauterine devices (IUDs), and postmenopausal status. Dysfunctional uterine bleeding is usually related to hormonal imbalances or pelvic neoplasms, either benign or malignant.

Pathophysiology

Hormonal imbalances, especially progesterone deficiency with relative estrogen excess, results in endometrial hyperplasia. Estrogen stimulates endometrial proliferation. However, without the support provided by progesterone, sloughing occurs, resulting in vaginal bleeding that may be irregular, prolonged, or profuse. Defects in the follicular phase shorten the proliferative phase of the menstrual cycle, resulting in spotting and breakthrough bleeding. Defects during the luteal phase result in excessive amount or duration of flow due to persistence of the corpus luteum. This leads to a deficiency of progesterone, resulting in vaginal bleeding. *Anovulation,* absence of ovulation, is associated with both estrogen and progesterone deficiencies. Emotional upsets or stress also can cause hormonal imbalances and thus affect menstruation.

Pelvic neoplasms can also cause abnormal bleeding; they are discussed in later sections of this chapter.

Collaborative Care

The care of the client with DUB focuses on identifying and treating the underlying disease. A careful history and physical examination are performed. Abdominal and pelvic examinations are performed to rule out abdominal masses.

Laboratory and Diagnostic Tests
Laboratory and diagnostic tests that may be ordered for the client with DUB include the following:

- *Complete blood count (CBC)* is performed to rule out systemic disease as a contributing factor to DUB and to evaluate its effects.

Nursing Care of the Client Undergoing Dilation and Curettage (D&C)

PREOPERATIVE CARE

- If ordered, ask the client to come in 24 hours before surgery for insertion of a laminaria tent. *This device absorbs cervical secretions and slowly dilates the cervix.*

- Ensure that the client remains NPO after midnight on the day of surgery.

POSTOPERATIVE CARE

- Monitor circulation and sensation in the legs, and avoid compression of the popliteal area. *The lithotomy position requires the client's legs to be elevated in stirrups, which can impair circulation.*

- Instruct the client to use perineal pads and avoid tampons for 2 weeks. *This reduces the risk of infection and allows tissues to heal.*

- Explain that the onset of the next menstrual period may be delayed.

- Explain that intercourse should be avoided until after the postoperative checkup and after vaginal discharge has ceased. *This precaution reduces the risk of infection.*

- Instruct the client to rest for several days after surgery, avoid heavy lifting, and report any bleeding that is bright red or exceeds that of a normal menstrual period. *Vigorous activity, lifting, or straining interferes with healing and may cause hemorrhage.*

- *Thyroid function studies,* including measurement of triiodothyronine (T_3), thyroxine (T_4), and thyroid-stimulating hormone (TSH) levels are performed to rule out hyper- or hypothyroidism as a cause of DUB.

- *Endocrine workup* is done to evaluate pituitary and adrenal function. Hormones of the pituitary gland control the secretion of many other hormones. Pituitary dysfunction may first be manifested by menstrual irregularities.

- *Serum progesterone levels*

- *Pap smear* to rule out cervical carcinoma

- *Serum human chorionic gonadotropin (hCG) levels*

- *Pelvic ultrasound* to identify luteal cysts

- *Hysteroscopy* to detect abnormalities of the uterine cavity

- *Endometrial biopsy* to obtain endometrial tissue for histologic examination

The client may need to keep a menstrual history and basal body temperature chart for several months to determine whether ovulation is occurring.

Pharmacology

For many clients, menstrual irregularities can be corrected with hormonal agents. For anovulatory DUB, oral contraceptives may be prescribed for 3 to 6 months. Progesterone or medroxyprogesterone also may be prescribed to regulate uterine bleeding.

Ovulatory DUB may be treated with the administration of progestins during the luteal phase. Oral iron supplements may be prescribed to replace iron lost through menstrual bleeding.

Surgery

Surgical intervention emphasizes the least invasive method that proves effective, beginning with a therapeutic dilation and curettage (D&C), then endometrial ablation, and, finally, hysterectomy.

Therapeutic D&C In a *therapeutic D&C,* the cervical canal is dilated and the uterine wall is scraped. D&C, the most frequently performed minor gynecologic surgical procedure, is used to diagnose and treat DUB and other disorders of the female reproductive system. It may be performed to correct excessive or prolonged bleeding. D&C is contraindicated in any client who has been taking anticoagulant drugs or whose condition precludes the use of regional or general anesthesia. Nursing care of the client undergoing D&C is described in the accompanying box.

Endometrial Ablation In an *endometrial ablation,* the endometrial layer of the uterus is permanently destroyed using laser surgery or electrosurgical resection. It is performed in women who do not respond to pharmacologic management or D&C. The client needs to understand that this procedure ends menstruation and reproduction.

Hysterectomy *Hysterectomy,* or removal of the uterus, may be performed when medical management of bleeding disorders is unsuccessful or malignancy is present, particularly if the woman no longer wishes to bear children. In premenopausal women, the ovaries are usually left in place; in postmenopausal women, a total hysterectomy, or panhysterectomy, may be performed; this procedure involves removal of the uterus, uterine (fallopian) tubes, and ovaries.

Nursing Care of the Client Undergoing a Hysterectomy

PREOPERATIVE CARE

- Assess the client's understanding of the procedure. Provide explanation, clarification, and emotional support as needed. Reassure the client that the anesthesia will eliminate any pain during surgery and that medication will be administered postoperatively to minimize discomfort. *The client who understands about the procedure to be performed and what to expect after surgery will be less anxious.*

- Cleanse the abdominal and perineal area, and, if ordered, shave the perineal area.

- If ordered, administer a small cleansing enema and ask the client to empty her bladder. *This precaution helps prevent contamination from the bowel or bladder during surgery.*

- Administer preoperative medications as ordered.

- Check the chart to ensure that the consent form has been signed.

POSTOPERATIVE CARE

- Assess the client for signs of hemorrhage. *Hemorrhage is more common after vaginal hysterectomy than after abdominal hysterectomy.*

- Monitor vital signs every 4 hours, auscultate lungs every shift and measure intake and output. *These data are important indicators of the client's hemodynamic status and complications.*

- Connect the urinary catheter to gravity drainage. Clean the catheter with soap and water during the bath.

- Once the catheter has been removed, measure the amount of urine the client voids.

- Assess for complications, including infection, ileus, shock or hemorrhage, thrombophlebitis, and pulmonary embolus.

- Assess vaginal discharge; instruct the client in perineal care.

- Assess incision and bowel sounds every shift.

- Encourage turning, coughing, deep breathing, and early ambulation.

- Encourage fluid intake.

- Keep the incision clean and dry.

- Teach client to splint the abdomen and cough deeply. Teach the use of the incentive spirometer.

- Instruct the client to restrict physical activity for 10 to 14 days. Heavy lifting, stair climbing, douching, tampons, and sexual intercourse should be avoided. The client should shower, avoiding tub baths, until bleeding has ceased. *Infection and hemorrhage are the greatest postoperative risks; restricting activities and preventing the introduction of any foreign material into the vagina helps reduce these risks.*

- Explain to the client that she may feel tired for several days after surgery and needs to rest periodically.

- Explain that appetite may be depressed and bowel elimination may be sluggish. *These are aftereffects of general anesthesia, handling of the bowel during surgery, and loss of muscle tone in the bowel while empty.*

- Teach the client to recognize signs of complications that should be reported to the physician or nurse:
  a. Temperature greater than 100 F (37.7 C)
  b. Vaginal bleeding that is greater than a typical menstrual period or is bright red
  c. Urinary incontinence, urgency, burning, or frequency
  d. Severe pain

- Encourage the client to express feelings that may signal a negative self-concept. Correct any misconceptions. *Some women believe that hysterectomy means weight gain, the end of sexual activity, and the growth of facial hair.*

- Provide information on risks and benefits of hormone replacement therapy, if indicated. *If the ovaries have also been removed, the woman is immediately thrust into menopause and may want or need hormone replacement therapy.*

- Reinforce the need to obtain gynecologic examinations regularly even after hysterectomy.

Hysterectomy may involve either an abdominal or a vaginal approach. The choice depends on the underlying disorder, the need to explore the abdominal cavity, and the preference of the surgeon and client. Nursing care of the client undergoing a hysterectomy is described in the accompanying box.

Abdominal hysterectomy is performed when a preexisting abdominal scar is present, when adhesions are thought to be present, or when a large operating field is necessary. For example, the woman with endometriosis is more likely to have an abdominal hysterectomy because endometrial tissue implants that may be present on other abdominal organs need to be removed. The surgical incision may be either longitudinal, made in the midline from umbilicus to pubis, or a *pfannenstiehl incision,* also known as the *bikini cut.* A Critical Pathway for the client following abdominal hysterectomy is provided on page 2001.

Vaginal hysterectomy, removal of the uterus through the vagina, is desirable when the uterus has descended into the vagina or if the urinary bladder or rectum have prolapsed into the vagina. Vaginal hysterectomy leaves no visible abdominal scar. However, the vaginal approach increases the risk of postoperative infection. To reduce this risk, the vagina is usually cleansed with povidone-iodine (Betadine) douches for several nights prior to surgery, and sexual activity is avoided during this time.

Nursing Care

Dysfunctional uterine bleeding usually causes the client great anxiety. Her self-image, sexuality, or reproductive capacity may be threatened, and she may fear the possibility of cancer. She may be embarrassed to discuss her menstrual history and hygiene practices.

Nursing care for the client undergoing a hysterectomy has been discussed above. Although each nursing care plan must be individualized, interventions for the client with DUB commonly address problems with coping and sexual function.

Ineffective Individual Coping

The anxiety associated with abnormal uterine bleeding can be intense. Until the cause of the bleeding is identified and has been addressed, the client may fear cancer or other life-threatening conditions.

Nursing interventions with rationales follow:

- Discuss the results of tests and examinations with the client face-to-face. *This allows for open exchange of information.*
- Provide information about the causes, treatment modalities, risks, long-term effects of treatments, and prognosis. *This allows the client to assume responsibility for her own health and become involved in her own treatment plan.*
- Evaluate coping strategies and psychosocial support systems. Teach coping strategies if indicated. *The possibility of surgery or cancer represents a crisis for the client and her support system. Support groups can provide assistance for the client through crisis intervention.*

Sexual Dysfunction

The client with DUB may feel inhibited to express herself sexually, particularly if bleeding is frequent or heavy. Additionally, fatigue may prevent her from participating in sexual activity.

Nursing interventions with rationales follow:

- Offer information about engaging in sexual intercourse during menstruation. Explain that conception is possible during this time and that orgasm may help relieve symptoms. *Some women mistakenly believe that birth control measures are unnecessary during menstruation. Orgasm causes a release of tension and vascular congestion and frequently provides at least temporary relief of symptoms.*
- Provide an opportunity for the client to express concerns related to alterations in life-style and sexual functioning. *Some women have had a prolonged period of sexual abstinence related to DUB. Allowing women to verbalize concerns can assist them in working collaboratively with the health care provider to minimize the impact of illness and optimize function.*
- Encourage frequent rest periods. *This conserves energy and may allow sexual function to resume.*
- Provide information about alternative methods of sexual expression. *Methods of sexual expression other than vaginal intercourse may satisfy the needs of both partners.*

Other Nursing Diagnoses
Other possible nursing diagnoses for the client with DUB follow:

- *Activity Intolerance* related to fatigue and blood loss
- *Decreased Cardiac Output* related to decreased circulating blood volume
- *Altered Family Processes* related to client's illness
- *Fluid Volume Deficit* related to blood loss
- *Self-Esteem Disturbance* related to alterations in role performance and body image

Client and Family Teaching

To promote the client's highest level of wellness, provide support, appropriate reassurance, and information to help the client and her family better understand her disorder and the therapeutic interventions indicated. Teaching also includes self-care measures that help minimize the effects of DUB on the daily functioning of the client.

Discuss self-medication with oral contraceptives, iron supplements, or other agents, including dosage and side effects. Nutritional counseling should center on the need to maintain a balanced diet, increasing iron-rich foods, such as eggs, beans, liver, beef, and shrimp. Inform the client that while orange juice may improve the absorption of iron, foods high in calcium and oxalic acid, such as spinach, may reduce its absorption. Encourage the client to maintain a fluid intake of 2000 to 3000 mL a day. Emphasize the need to report recurring episodes of DUB, particularly in postmenopausal women, to the health care provider immediately.

Critical Pathway for the Client Following Abdominal Hysterectomy		
	Date _____ **Preoperative**	**Date _____** **1st Day Postoperative**
	Expected length of stay: 3 days	
Daily outcomes	The client ■ Verbalizes understanding of preoperative teaching, including turning, coughing, deep breathing, incentive spirometer, mobilization, possible tubes, pain management (PCA or prn medications). ■ Verbalizes ability to cope. ■ Signs informed consent form.	The client ■ Is afebrile. ■ Has clean, dry wound with well-approximated edges healing by first intention. ■ Recovers from anesthesia: Vital signs return to baseline; client is awake, alert, and oriented. ■ Verbalizes understanding and demonstrates cooperation with turning, coughing, deep breathing, and splinting. ■ Tolerates ordered diet without nausea and vomiting. ■ Verbalizes control of incisional pain. ■ Verbalizes ability to cope.
Tests and treatments	CBC Urinalysis Baseline physical assessment with a focus on respiratory status and gastrointestinal function Betadine douche if ordered Fleet enema a.m. of admission	CBC Assess vital signs and O_2 saturation, neurovascular status, dressing, wound, and vaginal drainage q15min × 4; q30min × 4; qh × 4 and then q4h if stable. Assess respiratory status and urinary and gastrointestinal function q4h and prn. Incentive spirometer q2h Intake and output every shift Assess voiding; if client is unable to void, try suggestive voiding techniques or catheterize q8h or prn.
Knowledge deficit	Orient to room and surroundings. Provide simple, brief instructions. Include family in teaching. Review preoperative preparation, including hospital and surgical routines. Discuss surgery and specific postoperative care: turning, coughing, deep breathing, incentive spirometer, mobilization, possible drainage tubes and intravenous lines, pain management (PCA or prn medications). Assess understanding of teaching.	Reorient to room and postoperative routine. Include family in teaching. Review plan of care and importance of early mobilization. Begin discharge teaching regarding wound care/dressing change. Assess understanding of teaching.
Psychosocial	Assess anxiety related to diagnosis and surgery. Assess fears of the unknown and surgery. Provide support to client and family. Encourage verbalization of concerns regarding loss of reproductive capability. Provide information regarding surgical experience. Minimize stimuli (e.g., noise, movement).	Assess level of anxiety. Encourage verbalization of concerns. Provide information. Provide ongoing support and encouragement to client and family.

➤

Critical Pathway for the Client Following Abdominal Hysterectomy (continued)

	Date _____ Preoperative	Date _____ 1st Day Postoperative
Diet	NPO after midnight. Baseline nutritional assessment	Advance to clear liquids.
Activity	Assess safety needs. Implement appropriate precautions. Bed rest or bathroom privileges with assistance	Maintain safety precautions. Bathroom privileges with assistance Dangle legs evening of surgery and ambulate 4 times with assistance.
Medications	Preoperative medications as ordered	IM or IV/PCA analgesics IV fluid
Transfer/ discharge plans	Assess discharge plans and support system at home. Identify potential referral needs.	Determine needs at time of discharge. Make appropriate referrals. Begin home care teaching.

	Date _____ 2nd Day Postoperative	Date _____ 3rd Day Postoperative
Daily outcomes	The client ■ Is afebrile. ■ Has clean, dry wound with well-approximated edges healing by first intention. ■ Demonstrates cooperation with turning, coughing, deep breathing, and splinting. ■ Tolerates ordered diet without nausea and vomiting. ■ Ambulates 4 times per day. ■ Verbalizes control of incisional pain. ■ Verbalizes ability to cope. ■ Verbalizes beginning understanding of home care instructions.	The client ■ Is afebrile. ■ Has a dry, clean wound with well-approximated edges healing by first intention. ■ Manages pain with nonpharmacologic measures. ■ Is independent in self-care. ■ Is fully ambulatory. ■ Has resumed preadmission urine and bowel elimination pattern. ■ Verbalizes home care instructions. ■ Tolerates usual diet. ■ Verbalizes ability to cope with ongoing stressors.
Tests and treatments	Assess vital signs, dressing, wound, and vaginal drainage q4h. Assess respiratory status and urinary and gastrointestinal function q4h. Incentive spirometer q2h until fully ambulatory Intake and output every shift Assess voiding pattern every shift	Assess vital signs, dressing, wound, and vaginal drainage q4h. Assess respiratory status and urinary and gastrointestinal function.
Knowledge deficit	Initiate discharge teaching regarding wound care, diet, and activity. Include family in teaching. Review written discharge instructions. Assess understanding of teaching.	Complete discharge teaching to include wound care, diet, follow-up care, manifestations to report, activity allowed, and medications: name, purpose, dose, frequency, route, dietary interactions, and side effects. Include family in discharge teaching. Provide written discharge instructions. Assess understanding of teaching.

	Date _____ **2nd Day Postoperative**	Date _____ **3rd Day Postoperative**
Psycho-social	Encourage verbalization of concerns. Provide ongoing support and encouragement to client and family. Continue to explore issues related to perceived body image changes.	Encourage verbalization of concerns. Provide ongoing support and encouragement.
Diet	If tolerating clear liquids, advance diet to full liquids to regular diet to tolerance.	Regular diet as tolerated
Activity	Maintain safety precautions. Ambulate independently at least 4 times. Shower/shampoo	Fully ambulatory
Medications	PO analgesics Stool softener, laxative, or suppository as ordered	PO analgesics Stool softener
Transfer/discharge plans	Complete discharge plans. Continue home care instructions.	Complete discharge instructions.

The Client with Menopausal Manifestations

■ ■ ■

Menopause denotes the permanent cessation of menses. The **climacteric,** or menopausal period, denotes the period of time during which reproductive function gradually ceases. For most women, the menopausal period lasts several years. It begins with a decline in the production of the hormone estrogen, includes the permanent cessation of menstruation due to loss of ovarian function, and extends for 1 year after the final menstrual period, at which time a woman is said to be *postmenopausal.* The average woman will live one-third of her life after menopause.

Menopause is neither a disease nor a disorder but a normal physiologic process. However, the hormonal changes that occur can be accompanied by unpleasant side effects. There is wide variation in how individual women experience these side effects. For some women, the menopausal period is an extremely disruptive and difficult time; for others, it is just one more midlife event.

In the United States, menopause occurs at approximately age 50. Certain health risks increase after menopause, including heart disease, osteoporosis, and breast cancer. During the 1990s, approximately 50 mil-

lion women will be older than 50 and therefore experiencing or at risk for the disorders associated with the postmenopausal period (United States Bureau of the Census, 1992).

Pathophysiology

The menopausal period marks the natural biologic end of reproductive ability. Surgical menopause occurs when the ovaries are removed in premenopausal women, dramatically reducing the production of estrogen and progestins. Chemical menopause often occurs during cancer chemotherapy, when cytotoxic drugs arrest ovarian function.

As ovarian function decreases, the production of **estradiol** (E2), the most biologically active estrogen, decreases and is ultimately replaced by **estrone** as the major ovarian estrogen. Estrone is produced in small amounts and has only about one-tenth the biologic activity of estradiol (Wentz, 1988). With decreased ovarian function, the second ovarian hormone, progesterone, which is produced during the luteal phase of the menstrual cycle, also is markedly reduced.

Clinical manifestations of the menopausal period are listed in the box on page 2004. These manifestations vary widely, however: Some women experience severe

---

Clinical Manifestations of the Menopausal Period

■ ■ ■

- Menstrual cycles become erratic. Menstrual flow varies widely in amount and duration and eventually ceases.

- Vaginal, vulval, and urethral tissues begin to atrophy.

- Vaginal pH rises, predisposing the client to bacterial infections.

- Vaginal lubrication decreases, and vaginal rugae decrease in number. This may result in dyspareunia (pain during sexual intercourse), injury, and fungal infections.

- Vasomotor instability due to a decrease in estrogen may result in hot flashes and night sweats. A hot flash starts in the chest and moves upward toward the face and may last from seconds to several minutes.

- Psychologic symptoms may include moodiness, nervousness, insomnia, headaches, irritability, anxiety, inability to concentrate, and depression.

---

symptoms, others experience moderate symptoms, and some women experience few or no symptoms at all.

High levels of estrogen have protective effects against cardiovascular disease and osteoporosis. Thus, postmenopausal status places a woman at higher risk for these disorders (see Chapters 28 and 36).

Collaborative Care

Care of the client experiencing menopausal symptoms focuses on relieving the symptoms, educating the client about the physiology of the menopausal period and the postmenopausal phase of life, and minimizing postmenopausal health risks.

Laboratory and Diagnostic Tests
As estrogen secretion diminishes, levels of FSH (follicle-stimulating hormone) and LH (luteinizing hormone) rise and remain elevated.

Pharmacology
Pharmacologic intervention is directed at alleviating symptoms caused by decreased estrogen and progesterone levels. Hormone replacement therapy (HRT) can alleviate many menopausal symptoms but is not without risk (see the accompanying box). The predominant bene-

fit of HRT seems to be the prevention of cardiovascular disease and osteoporosis.

Cardiovascular Benefits of HRT Although heart attack is rare in premenopausal women, more than 50% of deaths in postmenopausal women are related to cardiovascular disease (Philosophe & Seibel, 1991).

Research indicates that HRT appears to lower the risk of coronary artery disease in postmenopausal women by as much as 50% (Barrett-Connor & Bush, 1991; Stampfer & Colditz, 1991; Stampfer, Colditz, Willet et al., 1991), particularly when the client maintains life-style habits that are consistent with cardiovascular health and curtails high-risk behavior, such as smoking.

Skeletal Benefits of HRT High levels of circulating estradiol reduce the risk of bone loss and osteoporosis, whereas estrogen deficiency and early menopause accelerate bone loss (Christiansen, 1991). The decline in estrogen levels thus places some postmenopausal women at risk for fractures. It is estimated that initiating estrogen replacement early in the menopausal period and sustaining therapy for 5 years may reduce hip and wrist fractures by 50% and vertebral fractures by 80% (Lindsay, 1991).

Risks and Side Effects of HRT Common side effects of HRT include changes in vaginal bleeding pattern, breast tenderness and engorgement, increased risk of gallbladder disease, gastrointestinal distress, headache, depression, and chest pain. The presence of estrogen unopposed by progesterone also increases the risk of endometrial cancer by four to ten times, depending on the duration and dosage (Bush, 1992; Thomas, 1990); it also increases the risk of fatal ovarian cancer (Rodriguez et al., 1995). Thus, HRT for women who have not had a hysterectomy or an oophorectomy must include progesterone. In addition, long-term use of replacement estrogen therapy is associated with an increase in the risk of breast cancer (Brinton & Schairer, 1993). Absolute contraindications for HRT include the following:

- Liver or gallbladder disorders
- Acute or active vascular thrombotic disorders
- Neuro-ophthalmologic vascular disease
- Undiagnosed vaginal bleeding
- Known or suspected estrogen-dependent cancer of the breast, ovary, uterus, cervix, or vagina
- Thromboembolic disorders associated with previous estrogen use

Other Therapeutic Measures
Nonpharmacologic measures (such as calcium-rich diet, weight-bearing exercise, and not smoking) are also known to be effective in relieving menopausal symptoms (Heany, 1991; Lindsay, 1991).

Nursing Implications for Pharmacology: Hormone Replacement Therapy

SYSTEMIC AGENTS

Oral conjugated estrogen (Premarin)

Oral estradiol (Estrace)

Transdermal estradiol (Estraderm)

Oral medroxyprogesterone acetate (Provera)

Oral conjugated estrogen (Premarin) is the most commonly prescribed drug in the United States, and has ranked among the 50 most prescribed drugs since 1966. It helps relieve hot flashes and vaginal dryness; it is also believed that estrogen reduces the risk of osteoporosis.

Nursing Responsibilities

- Assess the client for potential contraindications to therapy, including liver or gallbladder disease, thromboembolic disorders, estrogen-dependent cancers, or undiagnosed vaginal bleeding.

Client and Family Teaching

- Have a mammogram *before* you begin HRT.
- Have an annual mammogram and an annual clinical breast examination by your primary care provider; perform breast self-examination (BSE) every month.
- Monitor your blood pressure closely if you have a history of high blood pressure.
- Effects of long-term HRT (that is, HRT that lasts more than 2 years) remain controversial. The most common side effects include vaginal bleeding, nausea and vomiting, migraine headache, dizziness, edema, breast tenderness, depression, and chest pain. More serious side effects include increased risk of gallbladder disease, stroke (particularly if you smoke), and breast cancer.
- Take the medication as prescribed, and report any adverse effects to the physician.

Nursing Care

Nursing care during and after the menopausal period focuses on minimizing the symptoms associated with hormonal changes, reducing the risk of cardiovascular disease and osteoporosis, and educating the client about life-style changes important to health and well-being. Although each nursing care plan must be individualized, interventions often focus on problems with lack of information, sexuality, and self-esteem.

Knowledge Deficit

Because menopausal manifestations vary widely, it is difficult to predict their effect on individual women. However, the well-informed client is better prepared to deal with whatever symptoms she experiences.

Nursing interventions with rationales follow:

- Discuss physiologic manifestations, such as hot flashes, that the client is experiencing, and suggest therapeutic measures (see the box on page 2006). *Many physiologic effects of menopause are amenable to nonpharmacologic methods of relief, such as life-style changes.*
- Provide information about dietary recommendations. *The client who is not on HRT needs 1500 mg of calcium each day; with HRT, the requirement is 1000 mg. Some women will need to use over-the-counter calcium supplements or calcium-containing antacid tablets.*

- Emphasize the importance of weight-bearing exercise. *Weight-bearing exercise reduces the rate of bone loss, helps maintain optimum weight, and reduces cardiovascular risk.*
- Provide information about the benefits and risks of hormone replacement therapy. *Not every woman will need or want HRT. Every woman needs to understand both the risks and the benefits before deciding whether to undergo hormone replacement therapy.*

Altered Sexuality Patterns

Vaginal dryness and atrophy, together with the emotional impact of menopause, can interfere with sexual expression and satisfaction. Suggesting measures to help the client and her partner cope with these changes can enable them to continue or resume a mutually satisfying sexual relationship.

Nursing interventions with rationales follow:

- Encourage the woman to express her feelings and concerns about how menopause is changing her sex life. *Midlife and older women may not be comfortable in discussing their intimate sexual behavior.*
- Suggest ways to increase vaginal lubrication, such as spending more time in foreplay and/or using water-soluble gels (e.g., Replens) for vaginal lubrication. *A more leisurely approach to sexual activity can be mutually*

Self-Help for Hot Flashes

■ ■ ■

- *Keep track.* Chart your hot flashes in relation to your menstrual periods and other events. Understanding your pattern will help you manage better.

- *Keep talking.* Stay comfortable by letting people know when you're having a hot flash and reaffirm that it's nothing to be ashamed of.

- *Keep learning.* Join or start a group. Women learning from and supporting each other counteract fears and uncertainties and ease the "change of life."

- *Keep calm.* Be aware of the connection between stress and the onset of a hot flash. Look into relaxation techniques such as meditation, guided imagery, prayer, massage.

- *Keep involved.* Get together with others to work on social and economic problems. A feeling of empowerment both relieves stress and enhances self-confidence.

- *Keep moving.* Activity relieves hot flashes, stress, and depression and helps you sleep better. Exercise tones the body, improves cardiovascular health, and keeps bones and muscles strong.

- *Keep away from hot-flash triggers.* Alcohol, caffeine, sugar, spicy foods, hot soups and drinks, and very large meals may trigger hot flashes.

- *Keep cool.* Dress in layers. When you feel a hot flash starting, take off a layer. Natural fibers may be more comfortable. Go to a cooler spot, stand by an open window, take a few deep breaths. Fan yourself. Drink something cool. Place something cool on your wrists, temples and forehead. Lower the thermostat, especially when you sleep.

Note. Reprinted from "Managing Menopause: New Thinking on an Old Subject," by Paula B. Doress-Worters and Diana Laskin Siegal, in *Modern Maturity,* May-June, 1995, pp. 40–42. Reprinted by permission.

---

gratifying for both the client and her partner. Use of water-soluble gels can prevent vaginal pain and irritation and improve the quality of the sexual experience.

Self-Esteem Disturbance

Each woman responds to the aging process in her own way, and most women have coping skills that adequately equip them to deal with the gradual changes associated with aging. Among the factors that may provoke a self-esteem disturbance are the loss of youth, a sense of emptiness as children leave home, and the need to redefine one's self-concept and roles as parenting becomes less important. Women who place a high value on their physical attractiveness may experience a painful psychologic response to the physical changes of menopause.

Nursing interventions with rationales follow:

- Encourage the client to express fears and concerns related to changes in interpersonal and family functions. *Many women associate aging with "uselessness" and unattractiveness.*

- Encourage volunteer activities or employment for the woman who has extra time. *This enables the woman to feel that she is still a contributing member of society. Volunteering for activities involving young people can help reduce anxiety about the loss of reproductive ability or any late regrets about not having had children.*

- Discuss the importance of a healthy life-style in maintaining physical attractiveness. Identify risk factors and high-risk behaviors. *Life-style habits and behaviors affect many body systems and physical appearance. For example, cigarette smoking and overexposure to the sun make the skin age faster, contributing to wrinkles. Active women who exercise and eat a well-balanced diet look better and feel better.*

Other Nursing Diagnoses

Additional nursing diagnoses for the client experiencing menopausal symptoms may include the following:

- *Anxiety* related to variability and unpredictability of menopausal symptoms

- *Sleep Pattern Disturbance* related to night sweats

- *Body Image Disturbance* related to the effects of menopause

- *Altered Role Performance* related to the perceived effects of menopause

- *Dysfunctional Grieving* related to loss of reproductive ability

Client and Family Teaching

To promote the client's highest level of wellness, emphasize that menopause is a normal physiologic process, not a disease or an illness, and that symptoms are temporary and manageable. Discuss ways to minimize undesirable side effects, and explain to the client and family that making healthy life-style changes and reducing risk behaviors may reduce the need for hormone replacement therapy. Health maintenance and self-care are increasingly important: Encourage the client to obtain yearly mammograms, clinical breast examinations, and Pap tests, and to perform monthly breast self-examination and self-monitoring for vaginitis.

Applying the Nursing Process

Case Study of a Client with Menopausal Symptoms: Maria Villagrana

Maria Villagrana, a 49-year-old married history teacher, has reported reluctantly for her annual checkup. She feels that it is no longer necessary to have yearly examinations, but she is concerned because she has been experiencing palpitations, hot flashes, night sweats, and periods of nervousness and insomnia. Over the past year, her menstrual periods have become short and erratic, and she has not menstruated for the past three months. Her most recent period lasted only one day.

Assessment

Norma Murphy, RN, conducts an assessment interview with Mrs. Villagrana. Mrs. Villagrana tells Ms. Murphy that she often feels as though her "heart is running away with her." Mrs. Villagrana states that she hates the thought of growing older and that she feels her husband is losing interest in sex. Early in their marriage, she and her husband decided not to have children, and now she wonders whether they made the right decision.

Mrs. Villagrana adds, "Sometimes at work, I just break down in tears for no reason. Last week I saw some children playing in the park, and the tears just flooded. I don't understand it." She also reports absentmindedness and difficulty concentrating. Ms. Murphy encourages Mrs. Villagrana to talk of her feelings about the loss of reproductive ability and sexual activity.

Ms. Murphy notes that Mrs. Villagrana's vital signs are as follows: BP, 140/70; P, 74; R, 18; T, 98.2 F (36.7C). Mrs. Villagrana smokes one pack of cigarettes daily and weighs 152 lb (69 kg), approximately 25% over her ideal body weight.

There is no history of uterine or breast cancer in Mrs. Villagrana's family. A 24-hour review of her nutritional intake reveals a diet heavy in fat and carbohydrates and low in protein and fiber. Calcium intake is less than 30% of the recommended level.

Ms. Murphy also obtains a complete menstrual history on Mrs. Villagrana, including age at menarche, regularity of past menstrual periods, and sexual history. She administers a mental/psychologic status examination and reviews the findings of the following tests: CBC, urinalysis, ECG, serum FSH level, and thyroid hormone levels. Thyroid hormone levels are normal, ruling out dysfunction of the thyroid gland as the source of Mrs. Villagrana's palpitations. The FSH level is elevated, confirming Mrs. Villagrana's suspicion that the menopausal period is occurring. All other laboratory findings are within normal ranges.

Diagnosis

Ms. Murphy makes the following nursing diagnoses for Mrs. Villagrana:

- *Risk for Injury* related to overweight, smoking, potential coronary artery disease, and osteoporosis
- *Knowledge Deficit* of menopausal physiology and risks and benefits of hormone replacement therapy
- *Anticipatory Grieving* related to perceived loss of physical attractiveness, reproductive ability, and sexual function

Expected Outcomes

Expected outcomes of plan of care specify that Mrs. Villagrana will

- Verbalize understanding of the risk for cardiovascular disease due to overweight, smoking, and high-fat diet.
- Verbalize understanding of need to maintain a low-fat, calcium-rich diet.
- Discuss the risks and benefits of hormone replacement therapy.
- Cope effectively with the physical and psychologic changes associated with menopause.
- Show acceptance of physical and structural changes associated with aging and loss of reproductive function as normal biologic events.
- Develop effective coping skills for dealing with situational changes related to physical stamina and ability.

Planning and Implementation

In collaboration with Mrs. Villagrana, Ms. Murphy plans and implements the following interventions:

- Teach the client about factors that increase the risk of coronary artery disease and injury.
- Refer the client to a smoking cessation program in the community.
- Arrange for consultation with a registered dietitian concerning the need for increasing calcium and decreasing fat in the diet.
- Explain the risks and benefits of hormone replacement therapy.
- Arrange for consultation with a physical therapist to evaluate Mrs. Villagrana's fitness level, and teach her the benefits of moderate weight-bearing exercise.

- Refer Mrs. Villagrana to a midlife women's support group at the local community center.
- Arrange for sexual counseling with Mr. and Mrs. Villagrana regarding techniques, positions, and modifications to accommodate midlife changes.

Evaluation

Three months later, Mrs. Villagrana reports that she is feeling better, even though she is still adjusting to the low-fat diet. "I miss those morning doughnuts," she says, "but bagels are tasting better all the time." Mrs. Villagrana has begun walking to and from school, almost 2 miles each day. By increasing her exercise level and limiting fat intake, she has lost 10 lb (4.5 kg). These measures have also helped reduce her stress level and lowered her low-density lipoprotein (LDL) levels to an acceptable range. She is using over-the-counter antacid tablets for calcium supplementation, and her food diary shows an overall increase in calcium intake. She has also given up smoking. She has begun hormone replacement therapy. She will continue to be monitored periodically for cardiovascular status and osteoporosis risk and will return annually for a mammogram, clinical breast examination, and a Pap smear.

Mrs. Villagrana indicates that sexual activity has become more pleasurable and less painful since she and her husband began using K-Y Jelly as a lubricant. She and her husband are able to discuss their relationship and have agreed to try new positions and approaches to improve the quality of their sexual life.

The women's midlife support group has proved very helpful and reassuring to Mrs. Villagrana. She finds that her concerns and symptoms are very similar to those of the other women in the group. Being able to express herself with women her own age has boosted her self-esteem and reduced her sense of loss. Her body image perception has improved markedly.

Critical Thinking in the Nursing Process

1. Mrs. Villagrana had a common misconception about the relationship of menopause to sexual functioning. What is the basis for this misunderstanding? How can nurses help correct these common misconceptions?

2. Discuss the relationship of hormone levels to the symptoms a woman experiences during the menopausal period.

3. What assessments help determine a woman's risk for osteoporosis?

4. What factors should continue to be assessed while Mrs. Villagrana is taking hormone replacement therapy?

5. Develop a teaching plan for Mrs. Villagrana that will allow her to maintain an optimal level of functioning during her menopausal period.

Structural Disorders of the Female Reproductive System

Structural disorders of the female reproductive system include displacement disorders and fistulas. The most common displacement disorders are

- Uterine displacement, either within the pelvic cavity or into the vagina. The latter is known as **uterine prolapse.**
- **Cystocele,** herniation of the bladder into the vagina.
- **Rectocele,** herniation of the rectum into the vagina.

Fistulas are abnormal openings between two internal body cavities or between a body cavity and the outside of the body.

The Client with a Displacement Disorder

Uterine displacement can occur in either of two forms. The first involves displacement of the uterus within the pelvic cavity. The second type involves descent of the uterus into the vaginal canal.

Displacement of the uterus within the pelvic cavity is classified according to the direction of the displacement (Figure 47–3). *Retroversion* of the uterus is a backward *tilting* of the uterus toward the rectum. *Retroflexion* involves a *flexing* or bending of the uterine corpus in a backward manner toward the rectum. *Anteversion* is an exaggerated forward tilting of the uterus, while *anteflexion* is a flexing or folding of the uterine corpus upon itself.

Prolapse of the uterus into the vaginal canal can vary from mild to complete prolapse outside of the body. *First-degree,* or mild, *prolapse* involves a descent of less than half the uterine corpus into the vagina. *Second-degree,* or marked, *prolapse* involves the descent of the entire uterus into the vaginal canal, so that the cervix is at the introitus to the vagina. *Third-degree prolapse,* or **procidentia,** is complete prolapse of the uterus outside the body, with inversion of the vaginal canal (Figure 47–4). Prolapse of the uterus is also often accompanied by cystocele or rectocele.

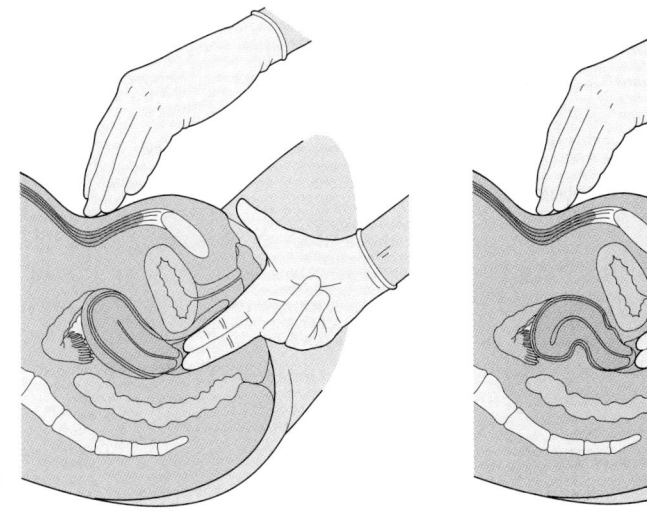

A Retroversion

B Retroflexion

C Anteversion

D Anteflexion

Figure 47–3 Displacements of the uterus within the uterine cavity. *A,* Retroversion is a backward tilting. *B,* Retroflexion is a backward bending. *C,* Anteversion is a forward tilting. *D,* Anteflexion is a forward bending.

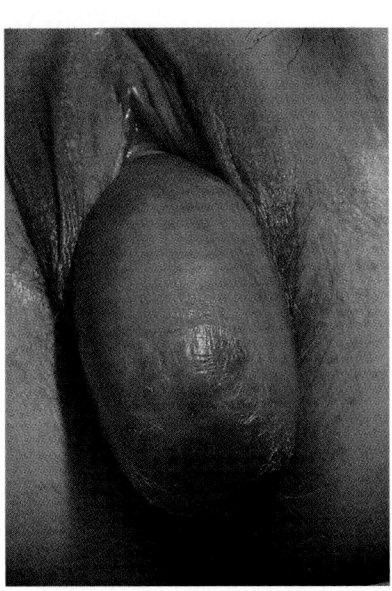

Figure 47–4 Prolapse of the uterus can vary from mild to complete. In third-degree uterine prolapse, or procidentia, the uterus prolapses completely outside the body, with inversion of the vagina.

Pathophysiology

Displacement or prolapse of the uterus, bladder, or rectum can be a congenital or acquired condition. Congenital tilting or flexion of the uterus is rare. More commonly, tilting or flexion disorders in which the uterus remains within the pelvic cavity are related to scarring and inflammation of pelvic inflammatory disease, endometriosis, pregnancy, trauma (rarely), and tumors.

Downward displacement of the pelvic organs into the vagina results from weakened pelvic musculature, usually attributable to stretching of the supporting ligaments and muscles during pregnancy and childbirth. Unrepaired lacerations from childbirth, rapid deliveries, multiple pregnancies, or congenital weakness may contribute to these disorders. Loss of elasticity and muscle tone related to the aging process also contributes to the development

of all these disorders. The clinical manifestations of displacement disorders are listed in the box on page 2010.

Collaborative Care

Care of the client focuses on identifying the cause of the structural disorder, correcting or minimizing the condition, relieving pain, preventing or treating infection, and supporting and educating the client.

A careful history and physical examination are performed. Diagnosis of uterine displacement is made after physical examination. If prolapse of the rectum or bladder is suspected, the client is asked to bear down or cough during examination so that the prolapse can be palpated and any leakage of urine or feces visualized. A history of infections, multiple pregnancies in rapid succession, and rapid labors support this diagnosis.

Clinical Manifestations of Pelvic Displacement Disorders

■ ■ ■

Uterine Displacement within the Pelvic Cavity

- Dysmenorrhea
- Dyspareunia
- Backache
- Infertility

Uterine Prolapse

- Backache
- Bearing-down sensation
- Constipation
- Urinary incontinence
- Hemorrhoids
- Dyspareunia

Cystocele/Rectocele

- Bearing-down sensation
- Constipation
- Hemorrhoids
- Urinary incontinence
- Fecal incontinence

Treatment may include Kegel exercises to strengthen weakened pelvic muscles. Kegel exercises can be useful in the early stages of downward displacement. These exercises are presented in the box on page 932 of Chapter 25.

Several surgical procedures are commonly used to repair structural disorders. For clients presenting with a cystocele, anterior *colporrhaphy* (repair of the cystocele) is the most common procedure. The anterior repair shortens the pelvic muscles, providing tighter support for the bladder. The Marshall-Marchetti-Krantz procedure involves resuspension of the urinary bladder in correct anatomic position; other procedures that may be used to correct cystocele include the Stamey, Raz, and Burch procedures.

A rectocele is repaired with a posterior colporrhaphy, which shortens the pelvic muscles, providing a tighter support for the rectum.

A prolapsed uterus may be surgically repositioned and the supporting muscles shortened to provide greater support. In postmenopausal clients or clients with procidentia, hysterectomy is the preferred treatment. For a retroflexed uterus, surgical suspension to realign the uterus may be attempted.

Surgical intervention is usually effective in repairing these structural disorders. However, anterior and posterior colporrhaphy shorten the overall length of the vagina and may result in dyspareunia in some cases.

When surgery is contraindicated or refused by the client, a *pessary* may be inserted into the vagina to provide temporary support for the uterus or bladder. At regular intervals, the pessary is removed, cleaned, and reinserted. The client is also examined for manifestations of irritation or infection.

Nursing Care

Nursing care focuses on client education about the disorder and proposed treatments and self-care measures for relief of symptoms. Although each nursing care plan must be individualized, possible nursing interventions for the client with a displacement disorder address problems with urinary incontinence and anxiety.

Stress Incontinence

Relaxation of the pelvic floor can lead to stress incontinence, a common problem in postmenopausal women. This can prove both troublesome and embarrassing and can increase the incidence of urinary tract infection.

Nursing interventions with rationales follow:

- Teach the client how to perform Kegel exercises (see Chapter 25). *These exercises strengthen perineal muscle tone, minimize urinary leakage, and minimize descent of the bladder and rectum into the vagina. In postmenopausal women, estrogen supplements also can improve muscle tone in the perineal area.*

- Discuss the possible benefits and risks of HRT with the client.

- Suggest the use of perineal pads to absorb urine leakage. *Depending on the seriousness of the problem, the thickness of these pads may range from thin pantiliners to full-thickness incontinence pads.*

- Instruct the client on perineal care and proper use of perineal pads. *Cleansing the perineum from front to back, and applying and removing perineal pads the same way minimizes cross infection from the anus to the vaginal and urethral openings. Incontinence pads need to be changed frequently to minimize surface bacterial counts.*

- Suggest reducing or eliminating caffeine intake. *Reducing caffeine intake can reduce urinary frequency and urgency.*

Anxiety

Anxiety is common among clients with a displacement disorder. Moreover, many women have only a cursory understanding of their reproductive anatomy. This lack of knowledge often compounds the anxiety the client may already be experiencing. The nurse can use drawings and models to explain the nature of structural disorders and treatment options available.

Nursing interventions with rationales follow:

- Encourage questions from the woman and her partner. *This helps assess the client's level of understanding so that teaching can be more effective.*

- Explain that the relief from discomfort and fatigue may positively influence sexual expression, and reassure the client that the capacity for orgasm will not be affected. *Many women and their partners have major concerns about the effects of the disorder and its treatment on their sex life and capacity for sexual pleasure.*

- Explore coping mechanisms that have been previously successful. *This can help relieve anxiety and boost self-esteem.*

Other Nursing Diagnoses

Additional nursing diagnoses that may be appropriate for the client follow:

- *Body Image Disturbance* related to manifestations of organ displacement

- *Pain* related to backache caused by organ displacement

- *Self-Esteem Disturbance* related to stress incontinence secondary to cystocele

Client and Family Teaching

If surgery is the treatment of choice, client and family teaching centers on how to manage the manifestations and what to expect in the preoperative and postoperative periods. If medical treatment is attempted initially, teaching focuses on measures to relieve the manifestations, such as Kegel exercises, use of incontinence pads, or the use, care, and insertion of a pessary.

Because obesity is a risk factor associated with relaxation of the pelvic and abdominal muscles, dietary counseling may be indicated. Preoperatively, a diet high in fiber may alleviate constipation, a particular concern during the postoperative period.

The Client with a Vaginal Fistula

■ ■ ■

A **fistula** is an abnormal opening or passage between two organs or spaces that are normally separated or an abnormal passage to the outside of the body. There are two types of vaginal fistulas:

- *Vesicovaginal fistula,* an abnormal opening between the urinary bladder and the vagina, leading to incontinent leakage of urine through the vagina.

- *Rectovaginal fistulas* (less common), an abnormal opening between the rectum and vagina, causing incontinent leakage of stool or flatus through the vagina.

Fistulas between the bladder and the vagina or between the rectum and the vagina may develop as a complication of childbirth, gynecologic or urologic surgery, or radiation therapy for gynecologic cancer. Cancer of the bladder is also sometimes involved. Urine or stool and flatus enter the vagina through this abnormal opening. The client with a vaginal fistula often presents with a complaint of involuntary leakage of urine or gas and symptoms of infection.

Fistulas are diagnosed by pelvic examination. Diagnosis of vesicovaginal fistula can be made by instilling dye into the urinary bladder by means of a catheter and observing the vagina for leakage. If no leakage is detected, a tampon or vaginal pack is inserted into the vagina, and the client is asked to ambulate. If an abnormal opening is present, the tampon will absorb the dye. Dye may also be injected intravenously because it is excreted by the kidneys. Urine and vaginal cultures may be performed to rule out infections. Antibiotics are administered if infection is present.

Often, a small vaginal fistula will resolve spontaneously. Otherwise, surgery is performed after inflammation has subsided, often a period of several months. Rarely, in the presence of a large, highly inflamed rectovaginal fistula, a temporary colostomy is performed, allowing inflammation and irritation to subside (see Chapter 23).

Nursing care for the client with repair of a vaginal fistula is similar to the nursing care for the client with a displacement disorder. Possible nursing diagnoses specifically related to the client with a fistula include *Risk for Impaired Tissue Integerty* and *Body Image Disturbance.*

Client and family teaching is an important component of nursing care for the client with a vaginal fistula. Stress the importance of careful perineal cleansing to reduce irritation and prevent further tissue breakdown. Suggest perineal irrigation or sitz baths for cleansing. Perineal pads may be used to absorb urine or fecal drainage. For the client with a rectovaginal fistula, provide information about avoiding gas-forming foods to minimize embarrassment from odor.

▪▪▪ Disorders of Female Reproductive Tissue ▪▪▪

Both benign and malignant tissue disorders affect the female reproductive system. Benign tumors and cysts include Bartholin's gland cysts, cervical polyps, endometrial cysts and polyps, ovarian cysts, and uterine leiomyomas (fibroids). Endometriosis is a usually benign condition in which endometrial tissue implants in various locations in

Table 47–1 Benign Cysts and Polyps of the Female Reproductive System

Site	Type	Etiologic Origin	Clinical Manifestations
Ovary	Functional cysts	Ovulation—include follicular cysts and corpus luteum cysts	Asymptomatic; may resolve spontaneously; can cause pain, menstrual irregularity, or amenorrhea
	Inflammatory cysts	Infection of ovary or uterine tube	Elevated WBC count; low-grade fever, pain, excessive menstrual flow
Vulva	Bartholin cysts	Obstruction or infection of Bartholin's gland	Pain, redness, perineal mass, dyspareunia
Endometrium	Chocolate cysts	Endometrial overgrowth; filled with old blood	
	Endometrial polyps	Unknown	Bleeding between periods
Cervix	Cervical polyps	Unknown	Bleeding after intercourse or between periods

the pelvic cavity outside the uterus. Malignant tumors of reproductive tissue include cervical cancer, endometrial cancer, ovarian cancer, and vulvar cancer.

The Client with Cysts or Polyps

■ ■ ■

A *cyst* is a fluid-filled sac. A *polyp* is a highly vascular solid tumor attached by a pedicle, or stem. Cysts or polyps of the female reproductive system can occur in the vulva, cervix, endometrium, or ovaries.

Pathophysiology

Bartholin's gland cysts are the most common cystic disorder of the vulva. These cysts are caused by the infection or obstruction of Bartholin's gland.

Cervical polyps are the most common benign cervical lesion in women of reproductive age. These polyps tend to occur in women over age 40 who have borne several children and have a history of using oral contraceptives. It is possible that cervical polyps develop from endocervical hyperplasia. The polyp develops at the vaginal end of the cervix, has a stem, and is very vascular.

Endometrial cysts and *polyps* are caused by endometrial overgrowth and are often filled with old blood. Endometrial cysts are the result of endometrial implants on the ovary and are associated with endometriosis. They are also known as chocolate cysts. Endometrial polyps, in contrast, are intrauterine overgrowths, similar to cervical polyps, and usually have a stalk.

Ovarian cysts are classified as inflammatory or functional. *Inflammatory cysts* develop as a result of infection of the ovary or uterine tube. *Functional cysts* are associated with ovulation; the two most frequently occurring types

are follicular cysts and corpus luteum cysts. *Follicular cysts* develop as a result of failure of the mature follicle to rupture or failure of an immature follicle to reabsorb fluid after ovulation. *Corpus luteum cysts* develop as a result of increased hormone secretion by the corpus luteum after ovulation. Most functional cysts regress spontaneously within two or three menstrual cycles. The causes and clinical manifestations of benign cysts and polyps of the female reproductive system are presented in Table 47–1. Complications associated with these disorders include infection, rupture, infertility, hemorrhage, and recurrence.

Collaborative Care

Care focuses on identifying and correcting the disorder and preventing its recurrence. A careful history and physical examination are performed, including inspection and visualization. Examination of the reproductive tract reveals the presence of most cysts and polyps. The menstrual history may reveal menstrual irregularities.

Laboratory and Diagnostic Tests

The following laboratory and diagnostic tests may be used to diagnose cysts and polyps of the female reproductive system:

■ *White blood cell (WBC) count* and *luteinizing hormone (LH) level* are measured. Elevations are associated with infections and functional cysts on the corpus luteum.

■ *Pregnancy test* is performed to rule out early pregnancy when luteal cysts are suspected.

■ *Laparoscopy* is performed to visualize ovarian cysts.

■ *Culture and sensitivity tests* are carried out if an abscess of Bartholin's gland is present.

■ *Ultrasonography* or *X-ray examination* is performed to differentiate cysts from solid tumors.

Pharmacology

Pharmacologic intervention includes antibiotic treatment of any infection and, for functional ovarian cysts, regulation of ovarian hormones through adminstration of oral contraceptives to achieve regression of the cyst. Mild analgesics are given for pain. Prophylactic antibiotics may be given before removal of cysts or polyps. If infection or abscess is present, antibiotics are administered and in many cases are continued after the client is discharged.

Surgery

Cervical polyps are readily visible through a vaginal speculum and usually are removed with a clamp, using a twisting motion. To remove endometrial cysts or polyps, in contrast, a transcervical approach is used. The specimen is sent to the laboratory for evaluation, and chemical or electrical cauterization is applied after cyst removal. For Bartholin's gland cysts and any abscesses, the lesion is incised and drained, and a drainage device is left in place.

Cystectomy may be performed on functional ovarian cysts that do not regress. Rarely, oophorectomy is performed if the cysts are very large.

Nursing Care

Nursing care focuses on relieving pain, implementing measures to correct the disorder, and preventing recurrence and complications. For the client with Bartholin's gland cysts, bed rest in semi-Fowler's position and moist heat promote drainage. Follow-up examinations for ovarian cysts to document regression are necessary. Although each nursing care plan must be individualized to the client, possible nursing interventions for the client with cysts or polyps are presented below.

Pain

Cysts vary in size from quite small to the size of an orange. As the cyst enlarges, pressure on regional nerves causes pain. Surgery subjects tissues and organs to manipulation, stress, and trauma, exacerbating pain.

Nursing interventions with rationales follow:

- Administer pharmacologic pain control measures, including acetaminophen or nonsteroidal anti-inflammatory drugs (NSAIDs). *Over-the-counter NSAIDs act on the pain center in the brain to reduce the perception of pain or act directly by reducing inflammation.*
- Apply warmth to the abdominal area. *Warmth relieves muscle spasm and increases circulation.*
- Apply moist heat via sitz baths. *The sitz bath cleanses, increases circulation, and promotes healing.*

Other Nursing Diagnoses

Other possible nursing diagnoses for the client experiencing problems with polyps or cysts in the reproductive tract follow:

- *Anxiety* related to concern over the development of carcinoma
- *Sexual Dysfunction* related to discomfort
- *Alterated Patterns of Urinary Elimination* related to mechanical obstruction
- *Constipation* related to mechnical obstruction
- *Ineffective Individual Coping* related to ineffective role performance

Client and Family Teaching

To promote the client's highest level of wellness, explain to the client and family the condition, its treatment, and measures to relieve pain. Emphasize the importance of keeping follow-up appointments. In preoperative teaching, include measures to prevent the development of thrombophlebitis during the postoperative period, including early ambulation and leg exercises. In postoperative follow-up, ensure that the client can recognize manifestations of infection and is aware of the need to notify the physician should they occur. If cervical polypectomy is performed, instruct the client to use external pads for a period of 1 week. The client must be able to state the signs of excessive bleeding and recognize that saturating more than one pad in an hour indicates the need for immediate followup.

The Client with a Uterine Fibroid Tumor (Leiomyoma)

■ ■ ■

Fibroid tumors, or **uterine leiomyomata,** are solid, pedunculated benign tumors. Leiomyomata are more common in African-American women: 40% to 50% of African-American women between ages 30 and 60 develop fibroid tumors, whereas only 20% of white women in this age group develop them. Increasing age is also a risk factor, although fibroid tumors normally shrink after menopause unless the woman is taking hormone replacement therapy.

Fibroid tumors are classified as intramural, subserous, or submucous (Figure 47–5). Intramural fibroid tumors lie within the uterine wall. Subserous fibroid tumors lie beneath the serous lining of the uterus and project into the peritoneal cavity. Submucous fibroid tumors lie beneath the endometrial lining of the uterus.

The actual cause of fibroid tumors is not clearly understood, but the association with estrogen stimulation is strong. Small tumors may be asymptomatic. Large uterine fibroid tumors can crowd other organs, leading to pelvic pressure, pain, dysmenorrhea, menorrhagia, and fatigue. Depending on the location of the tumor, constipation and urinary urgency and frequency are common.

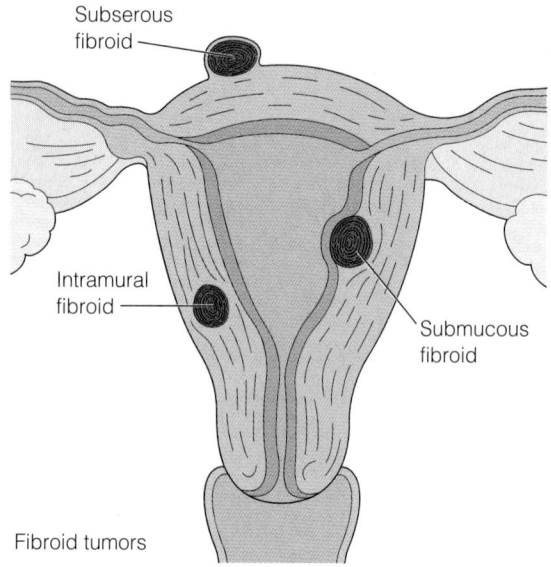

Figure 47–5 Types of uterine fibroid tumors (leiomyomata). Intramural fibroid tumors lie within the uterine wall. Subserous fibroid tumors lie beneath the serous lining of the uterus and project into the peritoneum. Submucous fibroid tumors lie beneath the endometrial lining of the uterus.

Fibroid tumors can cause enlargement of the uterus and pain during examination. Excessive bleeding often results in anemia, and compression of circulation may result in tissue necrosis.

Care of the client with uterine fibroids depends on the size and location of the tumors, the severity of the manifestations, and the age and childbearing status of the client. Tests used to diagnose uterine fibroids may include an ultrasound to differentiate leiomyomas from endometriosis and a laparoscopy to visualize subserosal leiomyomas.

In asymptomatic women who wish to bear children, the fibroid tumors are monitored. Follow-up two to three times per year to monitor growth and client response is recommended.

Leuprolide acetate (Lupron) is used to decrease the size of the tumor if surgery is contraindicated or not desired. Gonadotropin-releasing hormone (GRH) agonists are also administered.

Myomectomy, removal of the tumor without removing the entire uterus, is the surgical procedure of choice for young women who wish to retain reproductive capability. Laparoscopic laser technique is used for many women. Abdominal and vaginal approaches are less frequently used. Surgery is usually scheduled during the proliferative phase of the menstrual cycle. Hysterectomy is performed if tumors are large, and in perimenopausal and postmenopausal women.

Possible nursing diagnoses for the client with fibroids follow:

- *Pain* related to pressure from tumors
- *Stress Incontinence* related to pressure from tumors
- *Fatigue* related to uncompensated iron loss through bleeding
- *Fear* and *Anxiety* related to uncertain diagnosis and potential hysterectomy
- *Anticipatory Grieving* related to loss of the uterus and childbearing ability
- *Constipation* related to mechanical obstruction of the gastrointestinal tract by fibroids or anesthesia during surgery
- *Altered Family Processes* related to unexpected hospitalization
- *Body Image Disturbance* related to diagnosis of uterine disease

If surgery is deferred, client and family teaching emphasizes the importance of regular follow-up assessments to monitor tumor growth. If surgery is chosen, teaching emphasizes pain control techniques and appropriate preoperative and postoperative teaching (see the previous discussion of the client undergoing a hysterectomy). Dietary modifications to increase iron intake, prevent constipation, and promote healing are important.

The Client with Endometriosis

∎ ∎ ∎

Endometriosis is a condition in which multiple, small, usually benign implantations of endometrial tissue develop throughout the pelvic cavity. Endometriosis affects from 5% to 15% of women of childbearing age and is responsible for 30% to 45% of all cases of female infertility. Risk factors for endometriosis include nulliparity (never having had a child) and a history of the condition in the client's mother, sisters, or first-degree female relatives. Endometriosis occurs most frequently in Caucasian women.

Pathophysiology

The cause of endometriosis is unclear, but several theories have been proposed. The *metaplasia* theory asserts that endometrial tissue develops from embryonic epithelial cells as a result of hormonal or inflammatory changes. The theory of *retrograde menstruation* suggests that menstrual tissue backs up through the uterine tubes during menses, implants on various pelvic structures, and survives. The *transplantation* theory asserts that endometrial implants spread via lymphatic or vascular routes.

In endometriosis, the abnormally located endometrial tissue responds to cyclic ovarian hormone stimulation, and bleeding occurs at the sites of implantation. Scarring, inflammation, and adhesions may develop. Endometriosis is a slowly progressive disease, responsive to ovarian hormone stimulation. Thus, the implants regress during pregnancy and atrophy at menopause unless the woman is receiving hormone replacement therapy. Because progressive scarring may interfere with the client's ability to conceive, women with significant endometriosis are encouraged to have their children early in life and avoid delaying childbearing unnecessarily.

Clinical manifestations of endometriosis, which usually present during the luteal phase of the menstrual cycle, are summarized in the accompanying clinical manifestations box.

Clinical Manifestations of Endometriosis

- Heavy, throbbing pain of the lower abdomen and pelvis, radiating down the thighs and around the back. (The degree of pain, however, is not indicative of the severity of the disease.)
- Feeling of rectal pressure and discomfort when having a bowel movement
- Dyspareunia
- Dysfunctional uterine bleeding
- Infertility

Collaborative Care

Care of the client with endometriosis begins with careful history and physical examination, which reveals the presence of firm, tender nodules in the pelvic cavity. Retroflexion of the uterus is common. Interventions depend on the severity of symptoms, the extent of the disease, and the client's age and desire for childbearing. Treatment may include pharmacologic interventions to suppress ovarian function and/or surgical interventions to remove implants. The multidisciplinary health team may include a gynecologist, an endocrinologist, a nurse, and a psychiatrist or psychologist.

Laboratory and Diagnostic Tests

Diagnostic and laboratory tests may include:

- *Pelvic ultrasonography* to rule out other causes for pain and discomfort, including space-occupying masses
- *CBC with differential* to rule out pelvic abscesses and infectious processes as a potential cause. A low hemoglobin and hematocrit may be noted if menorrhagia accompanies endometriosis or tissue implants bleed significantly during the menses.
- *Laparoscopy* to visualize implants

Pharmacology

Pharmacologic management includes analgesics to control pain and prostaglandin synthesis inhibitors such as NSAIDs. Hormone therapy may include oral contraceptives or progesterone to induce pseudopregnancy, or danazol to induce pseudomenopause. Prolonged use of danazol, however, may result in irreversible masculinizing effects. Gonadotrophin-releasing hormone (GRH) is used to elevate levels of estrogen and progesterone and minimize bleeding.

Surgery

Surgical interventions include electrocautery of adhesions and endometrial implants or ablation of implants using a laser. Refractory endometriosis may be treated with total hysterectomy, including the ovaries and uterine tubes.

Nursing Care

Nursing care includes providing pain relief, providing education about the condition and the treatment options, and helping the client cope with treatment outcomes. The severity of the disease and its manifestations are not necessarily related: Advanced disease may exhibit few manifestations, whereas early disease may be quite painful. Although each nursing care plan must be individualized, nursing diagnoses that often apply to the client experiencing endometriosis are described below.

Pain

Endometrial tissue implants bleed with the menstrual cycle. The presence of blood in the peritoneal cavity is irritating, resulting in inflammation and scarring. Clients with endometriosis have varied manifestations of the disorder; the intensity and location of pain also vary.

Nursing interventions with rationales follow:

- Evaluate the severity of the pain, and provide information about a range of pain control measures. *Depending on the severity of the pain, the client may achieve relief through nonpharmacologic measures, such as heat to the abdomen or back, relaxation techniques (e.g., yoga and meditation), exercise, and biofeedback.*
- Suggest that the client and her partner explore alternative positions for sexual intercourse. *Different positions may reduce dyspareunia associated with endometriosis.*

Anxiety

Anxiety about the unsure prognosis related to infertility is a particular problem for young women who plan to have a family in the near or distant future.

Nursing interventions with rationales follow:

- Encourage the client to express her fears and anxiety about infertility, and answer her questions honestly. *Knowledge helps relieve anxiety and fear.*

- If surgery can be deferred, discuss the advantages of having children soon and in rapid succession, using oral contraceptives between pregnancies to minimize bleeding. *Knowledge about the disease and its prognosis diminishes anxiety and gives the woman a greater sense of control.*

- Provide information on fertility awareness methods, including measurement of basal body temperature and other techniques for recognition of ovulation. *Understanding these techniques helps the client and her partner optimize the conditions for conception to occur.*

Other Nursing Diagnoses

Other potential nursing diagnoses related to the client with endometriosis follow:

- *Ineffective Individual Coping* related to discomfort and the chronic nature of the disease

- *Activity Intolerance* related to pain and discomfort

- *Altered Role Performance* related to sexuality problems and possible infertility

Client and Family Teaching

To promote the client's highest level of wellness, explain to the client and family the cause of the disorder and the various treatment options, including their side effects. Discuss fertility awareness methods and the risks and benefits of long-term use of oral contraceptives. Stress the importance of exercise, smoking cessation, and weight control. If surgical treatment is chosen, provide preoperative and postoperative teaching.

Applying the Nursing Process

Case Study of a Client with Endometriosis: Angela Hall

Angela Hall is a 31-year-old married accountant, who relates a history of severe dysmenorrhea and menorrhagia, a feeling of pelvic heaviness and pain which radiates down her thighs. Because of her discomfort, her husband has complained about the quality of their sex life and has expressed concerns about their plans for having children. Sexual intercourse has become increasingly painful. Mrs.

Hall reports being so tired she doesn't care whether she has sex or not, and, in fact, would really prefer not to: "Sex hurts so much, I just can't stand it." Endometriosis is suspected, and a diagnostic laparoscopy has been scheduled.

Assessment

Christine Brigham, RN, interviews Mrs. Hall and makes the following assessments: BP, 110/70; P, 68; R, 18; T, 98.2 F (36.7C). Mrs. Hall's weight is 130 lb (59kg) and within normal limits for her height. Review of laboratory findings indicate a hemoglobin level of 9.8 g/dL (normal range: 12 to 16 g/dL) and a hematocrit of 33.1% (normal range: 35% to 45%). Physical examination reveals pelvic tenderness on manipulation of the cervix, and small masses that are palpable on abdominal/pelvic examination.

Diagnosis

Ms. Brigham makes the following nursing diagnoses for Mrs. Hall:

- *Pain* related to endometrial pelvic implants

- *Anxiety* related to effect of endometriosis on fertility

- *Knowledge Deficit* related to diagnosis and treatment options

- *Altered Sexuality Patterns* related to the manifestations of endometriosis and their effects on role functioning

Expected Outcomes

The expected outcomes for the plan of care specify that Mrs. Hall will

- Develop effective self-care measures to deal with her pain and discomfort.

- Experience decreased anxiety.

- Demonstrate understanding of the disease and treatment options.

- Verbalize an improvement in sexual functioning and a decrease in interpersonal stress between herself and her husband.

Planning and Implementation

The following interventions are planned and implemented during care of Mrs. Hall:

- Identify the location, type, duration, and history of the pain.

- Recommend analgesics and heat therapy.

- Provide information on biofeedback, relaxation, and imagery to lessen pain.

- Discuss with Mr. and Mrs. Hall the causes of endometriosis and its manifestations.

- Explain the use of medications, and review their side effects.

- Encourage the Halls to discuss their feelings about the impact of the disease on their sex life, life-style, and fertility.

- Refer the couple to the local mental health center for in-depth communication therapy.

Evaluation

Two years after the initiation of treatment, Mr. and Mrs. Hall have become parents of a baby girl. Mrs. Hall states that the discomfort and other manifestations of endometriosis have eased. Relaxation and imagery have effectively minimized her pain and brought about improvement in her function as wife, mother, and sexual partner. Counseling has improved the interpersonal and sexual relations between the Halls. Dietary management has improved her anemia, although the menorrhagia persists. The Halls are trying to have a second child, understanding the need for rapid succession of pregnancies. They will be followed in the nursing clinic and referred to an infertility clinic if conception does not occur within 1 year.

Critical Thinking in the Nursing Process

1. Explain the pathophysiologic basis for Mrs. Hall's anemia.

2. Describe how various hormone therapies may be effective in the treatment of endometriosis.

3. How would you handle the situation if Mr. and Mrs. Hall were extremely uncomfortable and embarrassed about discussing their sexual problems?

4. Develop a plan to teach Mrs. Hall about nonpharmacologic measures for pain relief.

5. Develop a plan of care for Mrs. Hall for the nursing diagnosis *Self-Esteem Disturbance* related to the manifestations of endometriosis.

The Client with Cervical Cancer

■ ■ ■

Cervical cancer is the third most common gynecologic cancer, following endometrial and ovarian cancer (American Cancer Society, 1993). Effective screening with the Papanicolaou smear (Pap test) has reduced the death rate by 70% over the last 40 years. Although the incidence of cervical carcinoma in situ (preinvasive carcinoma) has not diminished, early detection and intervention have

Table 47–2	FIGO Staging Classification for Cervical Cancer
Stage	**Description**
0	Carcinoma in situ, intraepithelial carcinoma
I	Carcinoma that is strictly confined to the cervix
II	Involvement of the vagina, limited to the upper two-thirds of the vagina, or infiltration of the parametria (connective tissue surrounding the uterus) but not the side wall of the pelvis
III	Involvement of the lower third of the vagina or extension to the pelvic side wall
IV	Extension outside the reproductive tract

substantially reduced the incidence of invasive cervical cancer.

The cause of cervical cancer is unknown; however, risk factors have been identified. These include early sexual experience, multiple sex partners, multiple pregnancies, human papilloma virus (HPV) infections, genital herpes infections, and cigarette smoking.

Pathophysiology

Most cervical cancers (90%) are squamous cell carcinomas that begin as neoplasia in the cervical epithelium. These cancers are called *cervical intraepithelial neoplasia (CIN)*. These preinvasive lesions are most common in women in their 20s. Squamous cell cancers spread by direct invasion of accessory structures, including the vaginal wall, pelvic wall, bladder, and rectum. Although metastasis is most frequently confined to the pelvic area, distant metastasis may occur through the lymphatic system. Clinical staging is based upon the FIGO (International Federation of Gynecology and Obstetrics) system; see Table 47–2.

Preinvasive cancer is limited to the cervix and rarely causes symptoms. Invasive cancer, which has spread to other pelvic organs, produces bleeding and leukorrhea (whitish discharge from the vagina), which increase as the cancer progresses. Other manifestations include referred pain in the back or thighs, hematuria, bloody stools, anemia, and weight loss.

Collaborative Care

Care is multidisciplinary, involving the gynecologist, radiologist, nurse, and oncologist. The goals of treatment are to eradicate the cancer and minimize complications and metastasis. Initial physical examination may yield normal

Nursing Implications for Diagnostic Tests: Papanicolaou (PAP) Test

■ ■ ■

The Papanicolaou smear (Pap test) is used to screen for cervical intraepithelial neoplasia (CIN) and cervical cancer. It can also be used to assess the client's hormonal status and identify the presence of sexually transmitted diseases, such as human papilloma virus (HPV) infection. For clients who have two consecutive negative Pap smears taken a year apart, the American Cancer Society recommends Pap tests be performed every 3 years thereafter. Pap tests may be performed more often if the client's risk factors so dictate; for example, DES daughters (daughters of women who took the drug diethylstilbestrol during pregnancy) may be screened every 6 months.

With the client in the lithotomy position, a speculum is inserted to visualize the cervix. A plastic or wooden spatula is used to scrape the cervical os and any suspicious-looking areas, and the material is transferred to a slide for histologic analysis. A cotton-tipped applicator or cytobrush is used to obtain a specimen from the endocervix; this specimen is then transferred to a second slide.

Client Preparation

- Instruct the client to empty her bladder.
- Explain that the test should be painless and quick, although slight cramping may be experienced when the endocervical specimen is obtained.

Client and Family Teaching

- Teach the client about recommended frequency of screening, every 3 years until age 65 after two successive negative results a year apart or more frequently if the client has specific risk factors for cervical cancer.
- Teach the client to schedule the Pap test for a time when she is not menstruating. Blood interferes with interpretation of the smear.
- Teach the client to avoid intercourse, douching, or placing of any medication in the vagina for 36 hours prior to the test.

findings unless substantial spread of the tumor has occurred.

Laboratory and Diagnostic Tests

Tests used in the diagnosis of cervical cancer include the following:

- *Pap test* is the primary screening tool for cervical carcinoma (see the accompanying box). If the results show atypical cells, the test is repeated. Pap test results may be reported in descriptive terms with abnormal cells described as benign, which may include infectious, inflammatory, atrophic, or other cell changes, or as epithelial cell abnormalities, including atypical squamous cells to squamous cell carcinoma, and atypical glandular cells to adenocarcinoma. Older reporting systems still in place may report Pap test results in terms of cervical intraepithelial neoplasia (CIN):

  CIN 1 – mild and mild-to-moderate dysplasia

  CIN 2 – moderate and moderate-to-severe dysplasia

  CIN 3 – severe dysplasia and carcinoma in situ
  (Pagana & Pagana, 1995)

- *Colposcopy and biopsy* of the suspicious area may be performed if the second Pap test yields abnormal findings (see the accompanying box).

- *MRI or CT of the pelvis, abdomen, or bones* may be performed to detect the spread of the tumor.

Pharmacology

Chemotherapy is used for tumors not responsive to other therapy, tumors that cannot be removed, or as adjunct therapy if metastasis has occurred (see Chapter 9).

Radiation Therapy

Radiation therapy is used to treat invasive cervical cancer. External radiation beam therapy is often performed initially to decrease the size of the tumor. Radioactive implants of needles, tubes, or seeds into the uterine cavity (brachytherapy) are used to treat tumors that have extended beyond the pelvic wall.

Surgery

When combined with colposcopy, laser surgery is a viable treatment method provided that the cancer is limited to the cervical epithelium. Cryosurgery, which involves the use of a probe to freeze tissue, causing necrosis and sloughing, is also utilized for noninvasive lesions. Conization (Figure 47–6) is performed to treat microinvasive carcinoma when colposcopy cannot define the limits of the invasion. For invasive lesions, hysterectomy or radical hysterectomy (removal of the uterus, uterine tubes, lymph nodes, and ovaries) is performed.

A *pelvic exenteration,* the removal of all pelvic contents, including the bowel, vagina, and bladder, is performed if

---

Nursing Implications for Diagnostic Tests: Cervical Biopsy

■   ■   ■

Cervical biopsy is performed for women whose Pap smear findings indicate possible cervical cancer or cervical intraepithelial neoplasia (CIN). The biopsy is also used to screen women at high risk for vaginal and cervical cancers due to intrauterine DES exposure. With the client in the lithotomy position, the cervix is cleaned with 3% acetic acid, and tissue samples are taken for biopsy. Afterward, the area is cleaned and a perineal pad applied.

Client Preparation

- Explain the procedure, indicating that the test usually involves minimal discomfort although a cramping sensation may be experienced as the cervix is dilated to obtain the specimen.

- Have the client empty her bladder prior to the procedure.

Client and Family Teaching

- Explain to the client that minor bleeding and vaginal discharge are expected following this procedure. Perineal pads should be used and tampons avoided for at least one week.

- Caution the client to avoid sexual intercourse until discharge has stopped.

- Instruct the client to notify the physician if heavy bleeding or manifestations of infection (pain, foul smelling discharge, fever, malaise) occur.

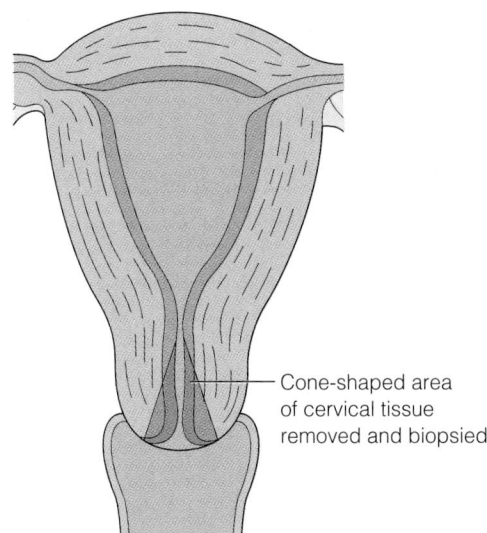

Cone-shaped area of cervical tissue removed and biopsied

Figure 47–6   Conization, the surgical removal of a cone-shaped section of the cervix, is used to treat microinvasive carcinoma of the cervix.

the cancer recurs without involvement of the lymphatic system. An *anterior exenteration* is the removal of the uterus, ovaries, uterine tubes, vagina, bladder, urethra, and lymphatic vessels and nodes. An ileal conduit is created for excretion of urine (see Chapter 25). A *posterior exenteration* is the removal of the uterus, ovaries, uterine tubes, bowel, and rectum. A colostomy is created for excretion of feces (see Chapter 23).

Nursing Care

Nursing care involves helping the client deal with the physical and psychologic effects of a potentially life-threatening illness, providing information needed to make informed decisions, and minimizing the adverse effects of therapy. Pain relief measures are important (see Chapter 4), as is grief work on the part of the client and family. The client should be encouraged to perform self-care activities and resume normal everyday activities and sexual functioning to the extent possible. Although each nursing care plan must be individualized, nursing diagnoses that often apply to the client with cervical cancer are presented below.

Risk for Impaired Tissue Integrity

Surgery interrupts the integrity of the skin surface, providing a potential portal of invasion for bacteria. Radiation therapy causes an inflammatory response in the skin and mucous membranes within the field of radiation, creating further risk of tissue reaction and breakdown.

Nursing interventions with rationales follow:

- Teach wound and skin care, particularly if pelvic exenteration is performed. *Irrigations with saline or solutions of saline and hydrogen peroxide are performed at intervals, with dry heat applied thereafter to dry the area. Open and damaged tissue increases the risk for infection. Meticulous skin and wound care is necessary to prevent infection and further tissue destruction.*

- If appropriate, teach stoma care, and care for the skin surrounding the stoma. (These procedures are discussed in Chapters 23 and 25.) *Urine and stool are irritating to the skin. Without proper care, the skin surrounding the stoma can become excoriated.*

- Apply non-oil-based lotions to skin surface. *This may minimize itching and help maintain integrity. Oil-based lotions are not recommended for tissue undergoing radiation.*

- Instruct the client not to remove the markings used to localize the radiation beam to the target area. *Markings are used in future radiation treatments.*

- Observe the client for evidence of fistula formation, and teach the client to do the same. *Fistula formation is a potential complication of radiation to the pelvic or abdominal cavities. Vaginal fistulas may form between the vagina and the bladder or rectum. Fistulas may also develop between the bladder and rectum, resulting in the expulsion of stool in the urine or loss of urine through the anus.*

Fear

Many clients believe that cancer equals death. Although this may be true for clients with late-stage diagnosis, cancer is now considered a chronic disease. For cervical cancer that is diagnosed at an early stage, the 5-year survival rate is 90%. If the disease is in situ, the rate is nearly 100%.

Nursing interventions with rationales follow:

- Explain that 66% of all women with cervical cancer survive for 5 years or more and that the earlier the cancer is detected, the better the prognosis. *This gives the client hope, an essential ingredient in recovery.*

- Allow adequate time for the client and her partner to express their feelings and fears and to ask questions. *Unexpressed feelings and fears and lack of understanding may cause the client to view the situation as worse than it is.*

- Refer to counselor or support groups for additional information. *Cancer survivors who visit clients in the hospital provide living proof that people can survive the diagnosis and treatment of cancer and lead normal, productive lives.*

Other Nursing Diagnoses

Other possible nursing diagnoses that may apply to the client with cervical carcinoma follow:

- *Alterated Patterns of Urinary Elimination* related to radiation therapy or diversional conduit

- *Fluid Volume Deficit* related to diarrhea

- *Altered Nutrition: Less Than Body Requirements* related to increased metabolic demands

- *Ineffective Individual Coping* related to changes in health status

Client and Family Teaching

Client and family teaching varies according to the stage of the cancer and the treatment selected. Provide information concerning radiation, chemotherapy, or surgery, as indicated. Preoperative teaching focuses on postoperative expectations, including management of urinary or fecal diversion, if indicated (see Chapters 23 and 25). Help the client and family recognize signs of infection and understand the importance of follow-up care.

Care of the Older Client

Many postmenopausal women do not receive regular gynecologic screening for cervical carcinoma. It is critical that nurses educate their clients and the public about the importance of screening for these cancers throughout life, not just during the reproductive years.

Applying the Nursing Process

Case Study of a Client with Cervical Cancer: Anna Eliza Gillam

Anna Eliza Gillam is a 45-year-old divorced woman with four children ranging in age from 16 to 23. She was married at age 18 and had several sexual partners prior to her marriage. She has had three sexual partners since her marriage ended. Last year she was treated with cryosurgery for venereal warts. The Pap smear taken 2 weeks ago showed atypical cells, and she has come in for a repeat test.

Assessment

Judy Davis, the admitting nurse, interviews Mrs. Gillam. Ms. Davis notes the following assessment findings: BP, 130/80; P, 72; R, 18; T, 99.2 F (37.3 C). Ms. Gillam weighs 142 lb (64.5 kg), approximately 15% over her ideal body weight. She has reduced her smoking to less than 1/2 pack per day, and she does not drink alcohol.

Ms. Gillam is extremely fearful and anxious and has told no one about her abnormal Pap smear. She reveals that she has had back pain radiating down her thighs for several months and a foul vaginal discharge that increases after intercourse. Until 2 weeks ago, she had not had a Pap smear for 5 years. Ms. Davis performs the repeat Pap smear and reviews the findings of CBC, chest X-ray, and vaginal cultures. Examination of the cervix reveals a large necrotic lesion at the 7 o'clock position.

The repeat Pap smear result is positive for squamous cell carcinoma of the cervix. A CT scan and lymphangiography are scheduled. Laparoscopy shows the disease to be widespread in the pelvic cavity.

Diagnosis

The nursing diagnoses for Ms. Gillam include the following:

- *Decisional Conflict* related to treatment options

- *Pain* related to metastasis and surgery
- *Risk for Impaired Skin Integrity* and *Risk for Impaired Tissue Integrity* related to radiation
- *Fear* and *Anxiety* related to diagnosis of cervical cancer
- *Ineffective Individual Coping* and *Anticipatory Grieving* related to potential loss of life

Expected Outcomes

The expected outcomes for the plan of care specify that Ms. Gillam will

- Gain knowledge to make informed decisions about treatment options.
- Develop strategies for pain control.
- Maintain skin and tissue integrity during radiation treatment.
- Express her feelings about the fear of cancer and death.
- Develop effective coping strategies for dealing with life-threatening illness and pain.

Planning and Implementation

The following interventions are planned and implemented during the care of Ms. Gillam:

- Explore treatment alternatives with Ms. Gillam, including the prognosis with each option.
- Administer pain medications as ordered.
- Inspect skin surfaces daily before and after radiation therapy.
- Perform routine preoperative and postoperative care.
- Provide information on biofeedback training and relaxation techniques for control of moderate pain.
- Review the side effects of prescribed medications.
- Refer Ms. Gillam to a local cancer support group so that she can interact with cancer survivors.
- Refer Ms. Gillam and her children to a mental health worker in preparation for Ms. Gillam's altered level of functioning.
- Assess at each visit Ms. Gillam's response to treatment and understanding of her disease.
- Arrange for dietary consultation regarding a low-residue diet.
- Weigh the client every 2 weeks.
- Recommend a high-protein, high-carbohydrate diet.

Evaluation

Ms. Gillam has begun radiation therapy following pelvic extenteration. She controls her pain with relaxation and imagery techniques, requiring only occasional analgesics.

She uses a water-based lotion to soothe the skin surface and is careful not to remove the skin markings. Ms. Gillam seems optimistic and has quit smoking. She and her family have continued to attend the cancer support group meetings. She is planning for the future and has talked with her family about what it means to live with cancer.

Critical Thinking in the Nursing Process

1. Develop guidelines for reducing modifiable risks for cervical cancer.
2. What health maintenance interventions are necessary for the client who is at risk for cervical cancer?
3. Explain the terms "noninvasive" and "invasive" in relation to cervical cancer and its methods of treatment.
4. Develop a teaching plan to help Ms. Gillam cope with the effects of radiation.

The Client with Endometrial Cancer

■ ■ ■

Endometrial carcinoma is the most frequently diagnosed gynecologic cancer in the United States. Each year, 33,000 women are diagnosed with endometrial cancer, and 5700 die from this disease. Endometrial carcinoma occurs most frequently between ages 50 and 70 (American Cancer Society, 1993).

Risk factors for endometrial carcinoma include early menarche, late menopause, history of infertility, failure to ovulate, extended use of tamoxifen or unopposed estrogen therapy (without progestins), obesity, and diabetes. Most of these risk factors suggest that endometrial carcinoma is related to increased exposure to estrogen.

All perimenopausal and postmenopausal women need annual pelvic examinations. Those in high-risk groups are advised to have endometrial biopsies every 2 years. Any vaginal bleeding in postmenopausal women should be reported at once to the physician. With early diagnosis and treatment, the 5-year survival rate for endometrial cancer exceeds 80%.

Pathophysiology

Most endometrial malignancies are adenocarcinomas that are slow to grow and metastasize. Endometrial hyperplasia is a precursor of endometrial cancer. Tumor growth usually begins in the fundal area of the uterus, invades the vascular myometrium, and spreads throughout the female reproductive tract. Metastasis occurs by means of the lymphatic system, through the uterine tubes to the peritoneal cavity, and to the rest of the body via the blood-

Table 47–3 FIGO Staging Classification for Endometrial Cancer

Stage	Description
I	Tumor limited to endometrium or myometrium
II	Endocervical glandular involvement or invasion of cervical stroma
III	Metastasis or invasion of serosa, adnexae, vagina, and pelvic or para-aortic lymph nodes
IV	Tumor invasion of bladder or bowel mucosa; distant metastases

stream. Target areas for metastasis include the lungs, liver, and bone. The FIGO classification of endometrial cancer is presented in Table 47–3.

The client usually presents with abnormal uterine bleeding after menopause. This bleeding is usually painless but may be moderate to large in amount. In advanced disease, lymph node enlargement, pleural effusion, abdominal masses, and ascites may be present.

Collaborative Care

As with most cancers, care of the client with endometrial cancer is multidisciplinary, involving the gynecologist, oncologist, radiologist, and nurse. The goals of care are to eradicate the cancer and minimize complications and metastasis.

A complete history is taken, including a menstrual and reproductive history. Physical examination includes a pelvic examination, which reveals an enlarged boggy uterus or the presence of a discrete mass.

Laboratory and Diagnostic Tests
Tests used in the diagnosis of cancer of the endometrium include the follow:

- *Vaginal ultrasonography* is sometimes used to determine endometrial thickening, which may indicate hypertrophy or malignant changes.
- *CBC* is used to determine the extent of blood loss.
- *Endometrial biopsy* (see the accompanying box) or *D&C* provides definitive diagnosis.
- *Other tests* to determine the extent of the disease include chest X-ray, intravenous urography, cystoscopy, sigmoidoscopy, and MRI.
- *Staging of the cancer* is based on surgical and histologic evaluation.

Pharmacology
Although the treatment of choice for primary endometrial carcinoma is surgery, progesterone therapy is used for recurrent disease. About one-third of clients respond favorably, primarily those with well-differentiated tumors. Chemotherapy is less effective than other forms of therapy, although cisplatin or combination chemotherapy may be used for clients with disseminated disease.

Surgery
Once diagnosis has been established, a total abdominal hysterectomy and bilateral salpingo-oophorectomy (panhysterectomy) is performed. A radical hysterectomy with node dissection is performed if the disease is stage II or beyond.

Radiation Therapy
Treatment with external and internal radiation may be performed as a preoperative measure or as adjuvant treatment in advanced cases.

Nursing Care

Nursing care involves helping the client deal with the physical and psychologic effects of a potentially life-threatening illness, make informed decisions, and minimize the adverse effects of therapy. Pain relief is a key component of care, as is grief work on the part of the client and family. The client should be encouraged to perform self-care and resume normal activities of daily living. Although each nursing care plan must be individualized, nursing diagnoses that often apply to the client with endometrial cancer are described below.

Pain
Total abdominal hysterectomy can involve severe and prolonged pain, not only from the surgical incision but also from the manipulation of internal organs during surgery. Abdominal viscera are highly vascular and easily bruised by handling.

Nursing interventions with rationales follow:

- Administer analgesics as ordered. *This affords pain relief and promotes early ambulation.*
- Insert a rectal tube, if ordered. *This relieves flatus, which can cause distention as well as discomfort.*
- Apply heat to the abdomen, and recommend that the client use a heating pad at home. *Heat causes dilation of blood vessels, increasing blood supply to the pelvis.*

Body Image Disturbance
For many women, the harsh side effects of cancer treatment can be almost as difficult and painful as the disease itself. Although side effects of the different therapies vary among individuals, the client's body image and quality of

life are always affected. Such side effects as alopecia (hair loss), nausea, vomiting, fatigue, diarrhea, stomatitis, and surgical scarring understandably disturb body image.

Nursing interventions with rationales follow:

- Review the side effects of the treatment regimen proposed, and assist the client to develop a plan to deal with these effects. *This promotes a sense of control.*
- Remind the client and family that side effects are usually manageable and temporary. *Over-the-counter agents can be used to alleviate stomatitis. Frequent rest periods can relieve fatigue. Medications can be prescribed for nausea, vomiting, and diarrhea.*

Altered Sexuality Patterns

Altered sexuality may result from a feeling of unattractiveness, fatigue, or pain and discomfort. The client's partner may fear that sexual activity will harm the client.

Nursing interventions with rationales follow:

- Encourage the client and partner to express feelings about the impact of cancer on their lives and sexual relationship. *Communication of the feelings relieves stress and maximizes relaxation.*
- Suggest that the couple explore alternative sexual positions and coordinate sexual activity with rest periods and periods that are relatively free from pain. *This creates a more favorable environment for satisfying sexual activity.*

Other Nursing Diagnoses

Other possible nursing diagnoses related to the diagnosis of endometrial carcinoma follow:

- *Impaired Skin Integrity* and *Imparied Tissue Integrity* related to surgery or radiation
- *Constipation* related to space-occupying lesion
- *Diarrhea* related to radiation
- *Alterated Nutrition: Less Than Body Requirements* related to side effects of radiation and cancer
- *Ineffective Individual Coping* and *Ineffective Family Coping* related to situational crisis of life-threatening illness

Client and Family Teaching

To promote the client's highest level of wellness, provide information about the specific treatment and prognosis for the client's cancer. To clients receiving radiation therapy, emphasize the importance of keeping appointments, and, if necessary, help them arrange for transportation to and from the facility. Explain the expected side effects of radiation implant therapy (see Chapter 9). Pain control measures are also an essential part of the teaching plan (see Chapter 4).

Nursing Implications for Diagnostic Tests: Endometrial Biopsy

■ ■ ■

Endometrial biopsy is performed to detect endometrial cancer or hyperplasia. With the client in the lithotomy position, the cervix is cleaned with iodine solution and the biopsy specimen is taken from the endometrial lining, using a transcervical approach and either curettage or vacuum aspiration.

Client Preparation

- Explain to the client that this procedure is uncomfortable but that postprocedure pain medication can offer relief.
- Explain that the procedure causes vaginal bleeding, and instruct the client to use perineal pads rather than tampons.
- When the physician has informed the client about the results of the biopsy, encourage the client to ask questions and express her feelings and concerns.

Client and Family Teaching

- Instruct the client to avoid intercourse until advised by the physician.
- Provide information about treatment options or health maintenance activities related to regular examinations and health screening.

The Client with Ovarian Cancer

■ ■ ■

Ovarian cancer is the most lethal of the gynecologic cancers, killing an estimated 14,000 women in the United States each year. Approximately 23,000 women in the United States are diagnosed with ovarian cancer each year, the majority of whom are over age 50 (American Cancer Society, 1993). Ovarian cancer is more common in white women than in African-American women; however, the mortality rate is higher in African-American women.

Ovarian cancer is often asymptomatic; 70% of those diagnosed have disease that has metastasized beyond the ovaries and the pelvis at the time of diagnosis (Gant & Cunningham, 1993). For these women, the prognosis is poor. The 5-year survival rate for those with regional metastases is 37%; for those with distant metastases, the 5-year survival rate is 18%.

Ovarian cancer is most common in industrialized countries of Western Europe and North America and least common in developing countries and in Japan. This fact suggests that environmental factors or diet may be related to the cause of ovarian cancer; however, the relationship remains unclear. Risk factors related to increased incidence include a family history of first-degree relatives with ovarian, colon, or breast cancer, advancing age, late first pregnancy, nulliparity, previous diagnosis of breast cancer, long-term use of estrogen replacement therapy (ERT); and regular use of products containing talc (feminine hygiene powder, body powder, baby powder, and condoms). Talc is closely related to asbestos, and studies have shown a strong link between frequent use of talc in the female genital area and ovarian cancer (Kasper & Chandler, 1995; Harlow, Cramer, Bill, & Welch, 1992; Cramer, Welch, Scully, & Wojciechowski, 1982; Rosenblatt, Szklo, & Rosenstein, 1992).

A recent study found that women who underwent ERT for 6 years or more increased their risk of fatal ovarian cancer by 40%; those who underwent ERT for at least 11 years increased their risk by 70%, compared with those who never underwent ERT (Rodriguez, 1995). There is evidence to suggest that use of oral contraceptives may offer some protective effect against ovarian cancer.

Pathophysiology

About 85% of ovarian cancers are epithelial tumors, 8% to 10% are germ cell tumors, and 4% are stromal tumors. The ovaries can also be sites for metastasis from other cancers, including those of the breast, endometrium, colon, and stomach.

There are five types of epithelial ovarian cancers: serous, mucinous, endometroid, undifferentiated, and clear cell. Approximately 50% are serous adenocarcinomas; these tumors are generally bilateral and grow aggressively.

Ovarian cancer can spread by way of the peritoneal fluid throughout the pelvis to adjacent organs, including the intestine, bladder, and mesentery, and through the lymphatic system and circulatory system to the liver and lungs.

In early stages, ovarian cancer generally causes no warning signs or manifestations. When manifestations do develop, they are often vague and mild, such as indigestion, urinary frequency, abdominal bloating, and constipation. Menstrual irregularities are rare; abnormal vaginal bleeding occurs in only about 15% of cases. Pelvic pain sometimes occurs. An enlarged abdomen with ascites signals later-stage disease.

Table 47–4	FIGO Staging Classification for Ovarian Cancer

Stage	Description
I	Growth limited to the ovaries
II	Growth involving one or both ovaries with pelvic extension
III	Tumor involving one or both ovaries, with peritoneal implants outside the pelvis or positive retroperitoneal or inguinal nodes
IV	Growth involving one or both ovaries with distant metastasis

Collaborative Care

Collaborative care involves the surgeon, gynecologist, and oncologist in addition to the nursing team. The history may elicit vague gastrointestinal symptoms and a positive family history. Physical examination may or may not be revealing, but a palpable ovary in a postmenopausal woman is a highly suspicius finding, particularly if the client has a positive family history. Staging for ovarian cancer is based on surgical and histologic evaluation (Table 47–4). Postsurgical treatment is aggressive and includes chemotherapy, radiation therapy, and, often, second-look surgery to assess the tumor and inspect for metastasis.

Laboratory and Diagnostic Tests

Tests used in the diagnosis of ovarian cancer may include the following:

- *Laparoscopy* is performed to determine definitive diagnosis and organ involvement.

- *Pap smears* are abnormal in up to 30% of women with ovarian cancer.

- *CA125 antigen level* can sometimes be useful in detecting ovarian cancer. CA125 is a tumor marker that is highly specific to epithelial ovarian cancer. Increased levels (above 35U/mL) may indicate peritoneal diseases such as endometriosis; significant elevations are usually found in ovarian cancer.

- *Barium enema, proctosigmoidoscopy, and intravenous pyelogram* are used to detect space-occupying lesions.

- *Ultrasonography* is used to indicate the location and size of the mass.

- *CT scans and X-ray films* can reveal areas of metastasis.

Pharmacology

While surgery is the treatment of choice for ovarian cancer, chemotherapy may be used to achieve remission of the disease. Chemotherapy is not curative for ovarian cancer. Combination chemotherapy regimens using cyclophosphamide and cisplatin or other agents may be employed. Recent evidence indicates that paclitaxel (Taxol), a relatively new chemotherapeutic agent, may be effective in achieving and maintaining remission. Close monitoring of bone marrow and renal function is vital while the client is on chemotherapy because these drugs have significant toxic effects.

Surgery

In young women with stage I disease who wish to bear children, treatment may be limited to removal of one ovary. Usually, however, total hysterectomy with bilateral salpingo-oophorectomy (removal of the ovaries and uterine tubes), and removal of the omentum are performed. Second-look surgery may be done at 6-month or yearly intervals to monitor for possible tumor recurrence.

Radiation Therapy

Radiation therapy using external beam or intracavitary implants is performed for palliative purposes only and is directed at shrinking the tumor at selected sites (see Chapter 9).

Nursing Care

Nursing care for the client with ovarian cancer is similar to the nursing care for clients with other gynecologic cancers. The side effects of treatment and generally poor prognosis diminish the client's quality of life and involve major psychosocial implications (see Chapter 9).

Client and Family Teaching

Client and family teaching includes preparation for and recovery from hysterectomy, as described earlier. In addition, the woman receiving chemotherapy or radiation needs information to help her cope more effectively with side effects.

Care of the Older Client

No postmenopausal woman should ignore feelings of abdominal bloating and constipation. The reproductive organs in the older woman are quite small, and the ovaries should not be palpable. If an abdominal mass is palpable, the woman should be evaluated for the possibility of ovarian cancer. Caution is warranted in treating the older woman with cytotoxic drugs and pain medications because the liver does not detoxify them as quickly and medications may rapidly build up to toxic levels.

The Client with Cancer of the Vulva

∎ ∎ ∎

Cancer of the vulva is the fourth most common gynecologic cancer, occurring most often in women between the ages of 60 and 70. The cause of vulvar cancer is unknown, but there is evidence to associate it with sexually transmitted diseases, particularly human papilloma virus. Nearly 85% of malignant and premalignant cervical and vulvar lesions have been found to contain HPV DNA, HPV structural antigens, or both (Scott et al., 1994). Herpes simplex type 2 (HSV2) infection has also been associated with vulvar cancer. Other risk factors include advanced age, diabetes, and a history of leukoplakia.

The prognosis of vulvar carcinoma depends on the degree of invasion, general health status of the client, presence of chronic diseases, and ability to withstand treatment. The 5-year survival rate for early vulvar carcinoma without lymphatic involvement is 85% to 90%.

Pathophysiology

Most vulvar cancers are epidermoid or squamous cell carcinomas. The primary site is usually the labia majora, but vulvar cancer is also found on the labia minora, clitoris, vestibule, and occasionally in multicentric locations. Metastasis occurs by direct extension into the vagina, perineal skin, anus, and urethra. The cancer also spreads through the lymphatic system via the superficial and deep inguinal and femoral nodes, and then to the pelvic lymph nodes.

The staging of vulvar cancer is based on surgical and histologic examination of the primary tumor and metastasis to adjacent organs and inguinal lymph nodes. More than 50% of cases are stages I and II, that is, limited to the vulva or perineum, at diagnosis. As with most cancers, the earlier the stage, the more favorable the prognosis.

The client with vulvar cancer is usually asymptomatic, and lesions are discovered on routine examination or self-examination. Discoloration can vary from white macular patches to red painless sores. Lesions may be exophytic (proliferating outwardly), endophytic (proliferating inwardly), ulcerative, or verrucous (resembling a wart).

Pruritus is the most common symptom; often the client has had a history of prolonged vulvar irritation. Perineal pain and bleeding indicate large tumors and advanced disease. In very advanced disease, dysuria related to urethral involvement may be the presenting symptom.

Collaborative Care

The client's report of itching, burning, or a sore or lesion on the vulva merits careful investigation and biopsy of

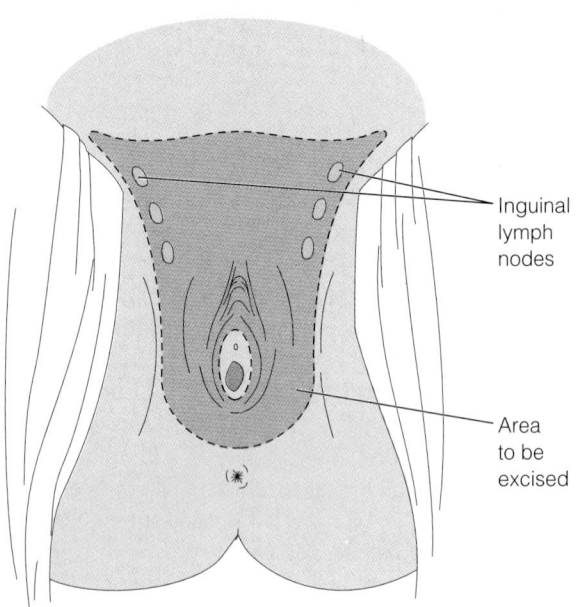

Figure 47–7 Vulvectomy for vulvar carcinoma. A radical vulvectomy involves removal of the vulva, labia majora, labia minora, clitoris, prepuce, subcutaneous tissue, and regional lymph nodes.

any lesions found. Inguinal lymph nodes may be enlarged. The goal of care is to eradicate the lesion and reduce the risk of recurrence. Surgical resection is the preferred treatment. If lymph nodes are involved, radiation therapy is used postoperatively. Chemotherapy is reserved for clients with distant metastases.

Diagnosis is based on the results of an excisional biopsy of the lesion. Metastasis, if suspected, can be evaluated by chest X-ray examination, barium enema, intravenous pyelogram, cystoscopy, CT and MRI scans, and proctoscopy. Lymphangiography can also be an important tool.

Surgery is the most common treatment for vulvar cancer. The specific procedure depends on the stage of the cancer. Early, noninvasive lesions may be treated with laser surgery, cryosurgery, or electrocautery. For more advanced disease, *vulvectomy* may be performed (Figure 47–7). A *skinning vulvectomy* is the removal of only the vulvar skin, which is then replaced with skin grafts, minimizing the effect on sexual appearance and function. A *simple vulvectomy* involves the removal of the vulva, labia majora and minora, clitoris, and prepuce. This surgery is indicated for carcinoma in situ if a skinning vulvectomy is not indicated. A *radical vulvectomy* is performed if invasion is suspected. This procedure involves removal of all the tissue in a simple vulvectomy, as well as the subcutaneous tissue and regional lymph nodes.

Nursing Care

Nursing care is similar to that for the client with endometrial cancer (see previous discussion). The client fears death as the ultimate outcome as well as the possible pain and suffering that surgery and other treatments may cause. Many older women (the age group most affected by vulvar cancer) are still sexually active, and radical surgery represents a great loss to them. Disruption of perineal tissues is a priority nursing problem for these clients.

Impaired Tissue Integrity

The client who has undergone a vulvectomy is at high risk for infection and inpaired healing because of proximity of the surgical site to urinary and anal orifices. In addition, clients are often older and may have age-related changes in healing and immune function.

Nursing interventions with rationales follow:

- Teach the client to wear support hose and elevate the legs at frequent intervals. *This improves circulation and reduces the risk of postoperative emboli.*

- Teach the client and/or her partner or other family member the procedure for irrigation of the vulvectomy. If neither is able to perform this procedure, arrange for home health nursing. *Irrigation helps prevent skin breakdown and infection.*

- After irrigation, apply dry heat using a heat lamp positioned about 18 inches from the area; emphasize safety precautions, including use of a low-wattage bulb (40 to 60 watts). *Dry heat helps promote healing and comfort.*

- Provide information on maintaining a diet high in protein, iron, and vitamin C. *These nutrients promote collagen formation and wound healing.*

Client and Family Teaching

Teaching for the client undergoing a vulvectomy should emphasize the potential for skin breakdown, particularly with radiation therapy. Explain that removal of lymph nodes leads to lymphedema and that recurrent cellulitis and sexual dysfunction are common complications of vulvar cancer.

Review prescribed medications with the client and family members. If an analgesic is prescribed, teach safety precautions related to balance, mental alertness, and the risk for falls.

Care of the Older Client

Vulvar cancers, like many other cancers, are managed with a treatment regimen that includes both pain medications and chemotherapy agents. In older clients, however, caution is warranted because the liver does not detoxify agents as quickly and these agents may build up rapidly to toxic levels.

■ ■ ■   Infections of the Female Reproductive System   ■ ■ ■

Infections affecting the female reproductive tract may be local or systemic. Many are sexually transmitted infections, which are discussed in Chapter 49. The most common local gynecologic infections are vaginal infections, including simple vaginitis, candidiasis, and trichomoniasis. Systemic infections involving the female reproductive system include pelvic inflammatory disease, toxic shock syndrome, and HIV/AIDS (see Chapter 8).

The Client with a Vaginal Infection

■ ■ ■

Vaginal infections are a common disorder of the female reproductive system. They are classified according to causative agent and may be either fungal, as in candidiasis, protozoan, as in trichomoniasis, or bacterial, as in simple (*Gardnerella*) vaginosis infections.

Risk factors include the use of oral contraceptives or broad-spectrum antibiotics, obesity, diabetes, pregnancy, unprotected sexual activity, multiple sexual partners, and poor personal hygiene. Menstruation provides a growth medium for pathogenic organisms, contributing to the development of toxic shock syndrome. Sexual activity and swimming in contaminated water are implicated in the transmission of trichomoniasis.

Preventive measures include educating women about personal hygiene practices and safer sex. Women need to avoid frequent douching and wearing nylon underwear and/or tight pants. Unprotected sexual activity, particularly with multiple partners, greatly increases the risk of vaginal infections and chronic or fatal sexually transmitted diseases.

Pathophysiology

The low pH of vaginal secretions, normal vaginal flora, and estrogen provide protection against vaginal infections. Thus, alterations in pH, changes in the normal flora, and low estrogen levels are conducive to the development of vaginal infections. When conditions are favorable, microorganisms invade the vulva and vagina. *Simple vaginitis*, also known as bacterial vaginosis, is the most common cause of manifestations of vaginal infection in women of reproductive age. *Gardnerella vaginalis* is the causative organism in many cases. Microscopic examination of vaginal discharge reveals the presence of characteristic "clue cells."

Candidiasis (**moniliasis** or yeast infection) is caused by the organism *Candida albicans*, which has several strains of different virulence. *Candida* organisms are part of the normal vaginal environment, causing problems only when they multiply rapidly. When increased estrogen levels, antibiotics, fecal contamination, or other factors alter the normal vaginal flora, the organism proliferates, resulting in a yeast infection.

Trichomoniasis, a protozoan infection, is caused by *Trichomonas vaginalis* and is frequently carried asymptomatically by the male partner.

Most vaginal infections are manifested by vaginal discharge, itching or burning, and dysuria (Table 47–5). Secondary infections also can occur. Some vaginal infections can injure the fetus or newborn of an infected woman.

Collaborative Care

Care of the client focuses on identifying and eliminating the infection and preventing recurrence. The client who presents with an unidentified vaginal discharge needs careful evaluation. The history may reveal frequent, troublesome infections and any self-care measures taken. Repeated vaginal yeast infections may be a manifestation of diabetes or HIV infection and must be evaluated in depth. (Women constitute the most rapidly growing segment of the population with AIDS.)

Laboratory and Diagnostic Tests

Laboratory and diagnostic tests vary with the suspected organism. The following laboratory tests may be ordered:

- *Culture of vaginal secretions* is performed and discharge is examined microscopically for the presence of "clue cells" if bacterial vaginitis is suspected.
- *"Wet mount" or "wet prep" with potassium hydroxide (KOH)* is prepared. If bacterial vaginitis is present, a fishy odor can be detected. If candidiasis is suspected,

Table 47–5 Vaginal Infections

Infection	Type of Discharge	Typical Manifestations	Treatment	Nursing Care
Candidiasis (*Monilia,* yeast)	Thick white patches adhering to cervix and vaginal wall, resembling cottage cheese; little odor	Itching of vulva and vaginal area, redness, painful intercourse	Miconazole, clotrimazole, or terconazole creams or suppositories; povidone-iodine (Betadine) or vinegar douches	Teach perineal hygiene and proper use of vaginal applicators. Instruct the client to complete the entire treatment.
Simple vaginalis (baterial vaginosis, *Gardnerella* vaginosis)	Thin, white, "milk-like," or gray with fishy odor, especially when mixed with potassium hydroxide	None to mild itching or burning in vulvar area; clue cells on microscopic examination	Oral metronidazole for client; topical metronidazole or clindamycin for client's sexual partner	Teach proper perineal hygiene. Instruct client to complete treatment. Teach client relationship of infection to PID.
Trichomoniasis	Frothy, yellow or white, foul odor	Burning and itching of vulva	Oral metronidazole for client and sexual partner	Teach perineal hygiene
Atrophic vaginitis (Senile vaginitis)	Thin, opaque discharge, occasionally blood-tinged, odorless; pale, smooth, thin, dry vaginal walls	Painful intercourse, itching, vaginal dryness	Use of topical estrogen cream; use of water-soluble lubricant for intercourse. Evaluate need for HRT and antibiotic therapy	Counsel client on symptoms of menopause and sexual techniques to minimize trauma

a KOH wet prep is examined microscopically to detect hyphae (filaments or threads) and *Candida* spores.

- *Normal saline wet prep* is used to detect the presence of protozoa if trichomoniasis is suspected
- *Glucose tolerance tests or HIV screening* are performed at the time of the initial assessment, if indicated.
- *Pregnancy tests* are performed if pregnancy is suspected, because certain treatments are contraindicated during pregnancy.

Pharmacology

The pharmacologic treatment varies with the organism, as shown in Table 47–6. The sexual partner must also be treated to prevent reinfection. Some antifungal agents are available without prescription, which can lead to self-medication with the incorrect agent or allow repeated infections to go unreported.

Mild vinegar douches or povidone-iodine douches may be prescribed but should not be used routinely. Frequent douching washes away normal flora, depleting the natural defense mechanism of the body against bacterial invasion.

Nursing Care

Nursing care focuses on teaching the client and, if necessary, her sexual partner to comply with the treatment regimen, use safer sex practices, and prevent future transmission of the infection. Careful history taking may also reveal high-risk sexual practices that require intervention, particularly if the client has had repeated yeast infections. The initial presenting symptom for many HIV-positive women is vaginal candidiasis, which may be refractory to over-the-counter treatments (Kelly & Holman, 1993). Treatment with some antibiotics destroys normal vaginal flora, resulting in superinfection with yeast. Although each nursing care plan must be individualized, nursing diagnoses that often apply to clients with vaginal infections are presented below.

Knowledge Deficit

Many women are unaware of the causes of vaginal infections and the self-care measures to prevent and treat these infections.

Nursing interventions with rationales follow:

- Explain to the client and her partner how the infection is transmitted. Many infections are transmitted most easily during certain times of the menstrual cycle; some can also be transmitted by towels or other inanimate objects, or by certain types of sexual activity. *A frank discussion of disease transmission and prevention with the woman and her partner can reduce the risk of reinfection.*

- Teach the client and her partner about the need for both of them to complete the course of treatment. *Many infections are asymptomatic in one partner. Incomplete treatment allows for recurrence of the infection and reinfection of the partner.*

Pain

The symptoms of vaginitis can lead to dysuria or painful excoriation or ulceration of tissue. Often these symptoms can be relieved by relatively simple self-care measures.

Nursing interventions with rationales follow:

- Suggest the use of cool compresses and vinegar or povidone-iodine douches. *Cool compresses relieve itching. Vinegar and iodine are fungicidal and bactericidal in effect.*
- Recommend sitz baths to alleviate discomfort. *Sitz baths cleanse the perineal area and wash away infectious discharge.*

Client and Family Teaching

To promote the highest level of wellness, client and family teaching focuses on eradicating the infection, preventing further disease transmission, and relieving discomfort associated with the condition. Educating the client and her partner(s) about safer sex and improved genital hygiene practices can reduce the incidence of recurrence. Unless contraindicated, encourage the client with repeated mild candidiasis infections to consume 8 oz of yogurt containing live active cultures daily to help restore normal vaginal flora.

Care of the Older Client

Many postmenopausal women experience atrophic vaginitis due to thinning and drying of the vaginal mucosa that result from lack of estrogen. These clients should be taught about the use of topical estrogen creams to restore vaginal tissue, the use of water-soluble lubricants for intercourse, and other methods of minimizing the undesirable effects of menopause.

Applying the Nursing Process

Case Study of a Client with Candidiasis: Vanessa Cook

Vanessa Cook, 17 years old, has come to the clinic complaining of severe itching and burning in the genital area. She has a history of diabetes mellitus that is frequently out of control. She also was recently treated with ampicillin for an ear infection.

Assessment

Ms. Cook's vital signs are as follows: BP, 100/70; P, 84; R, 20; T, 100.2 F (37.8 C). Her weight is 102 lb (46.3 kg), which is approximately 20% below her ideal weight. Jan Burroughs, RN, notes that Ms. Cook has a moderately severe case of acne. Ms. Cook tells Ms. Burroughs that she never "had anything like this before, and I haven't been having sex lately." Ms. Cook has been taking oral contraceptives for 2 years, has only one sexual partner, and douches several times a week. She is very athletic and wears tight-fitting spandex exercise clothes and nylon underclothing.

Physical examination reveals a thick, cheesy white discharge that adheres to the vaginal walls with erythema on the vulvar surface. A vaginal culture, HIV screen, and fasting blood sugar are performed. The culture is positive for yeast; the HIV screen is negative; and the fasting blood sugar is 144 mg/dL (normal range 70–105 mg/dL).

Diagnosis

Ms. Burroughs makes the following nursing diagnoses for Ms. Cook:

- *Altered Health Maintenance* related to lack of knowledge about the prevention of yeast infections
- *Altered Skin Integrity* related to irritation from vaginal discharge
- *Altered Nutrition: Less Than Body Requirements* related to lack of understanding about relationship of diabetes, diet, and exercise.

Expected Outcomes

The expected outcomes for the plan of care specify that Ms. Cook will

- Verbalize an understanding of the relationship between the use of antibiotics and the development of yeast infections.
- Modify her perineal hygiene to avoid developing vaginal yeast infections.
- Verbalize an understanding of the need to treat yeast infections completely.
- Use self-care measures that will minimize yeast overgrowth.
- Demonstrate an understanding of the importance of adequate diabetes control in preventing yeast infections and other sequelae.

Planning and Implementation

The following interventions are planned and implemented during the care of Ms. Cook:

- Teach Ms. Cook about the relationship between douching and use of antibiotics on normal vaginal flora and yeast superinfection.
- Teach Ms. Cook about showering after athletic activities and wearing cotton underclothing, without pantyhose, to allow for air circulation and evaporation of moisture.
- Refer Ms. Cook to the diabetes educator for teaching related to blood glucose control.
- Teach Ms. Cook about over-the-counter medications for yeast infections, proper usage and storage of the medications, and the necessity for professional follow-up should infections recur.

Evaluation

Two weeks after her first visit to the clinic, Ms. Cook is free of infection. She reports having used clotrimazole for 1 week. She says she uses proper perineal hygiene and has stopped regular douching. Ms. Cook has kept her follow-up appointments with the diabetes educator, and Ms. Burroughs notes that Ms. Cook has gained 3 lb (1.3 kg), and has a random blood sugar level of 118 mg/dL. Her acne shows noticeable improvement, and she reports that she has switched to cotton underclothing and wears spandex tights only during actual exercise periods.

Critical Thinking in the Nursing Process

1. What modifiable and nonmodifiable risk factors for vaginal infection are in Ms. Cook's history?
2. What is the rationale for testing Ms. Cook for HIV?
3. Develop a plan to teach women how to prevent yeast infections.
4. Develop a plan of care for the nursing diagnosis *Self-Care Deficit.*

The Client with Pelvic Inflammatory Disease

■ ■ ■

Pelvic inflammatory disease (PID) is an umbrella term used to describe infection of the pelvic organs, including the uterine tubes (salpingitis), ovaries (oophoritis), cervix (cervicitis), endometrium (endometritis), pelvic peritoneum, and the pelvic vascular system. PID can be caused by one or more infectious agents, including *Neisseria gonorrhoeae, Chlamydia trachomatis, Escherichia coli, Mycoplasma hominis,* and a variety of other organisms. The infection results in scarring and obstruction of the uterine tubes, making PID a major cause of female infertility.

Pelvic inflammatory disease results in nearly 180,000 hospitalizations annually in the United States. More than 1 million episodes are reported annually, 15,000 of which require surgery, such as removal of one or both uterine tubes. Among women of childbearing age in the United States, 1 in 7 reports being treated for PID (Aral, Mosher, & Cates, 1991).

Risk factors for PID include use of IUDs, history of sexually transmitted disease, multiple sexual partners, and previous PID. PID is most common in sexually active women age 15 to 24. The prognosis depends on the number of episodes, promptness of treatment, and modification of risk-taking behaviors. Prevention includes educating women, especially young women, regarding the causes and transmission of infection and methods of self-protection, such as appropriate personal hygiene and avoiding unprotected sexual activity.

Pathophysiology

Pelvic inflammatory disease is usually polymicrobial (caused by more than one microbe) in origin. Pathogenic microorganisms enter the vagina and travel to the uterus during intercourse or other sexual activity. They can also gain direct access to the uterus during childbirth, abortion, or surgery of the reproductive tract. The infection then spreads through the uterine tubes, obstructing them with scar tissue, and fulminates on the ovary, causing tubo-ovarian abscess. It can also enter the lymphatic system or bloodstream, leading to systemic infection.

Clinical manifestations of PID include high fever, vaginal discharge, severe lower abdominal pain, nausea, malaise, and dysuria. Scarring of the uterine tubes can result in infertility and increased risk of ectopic pregnancy, pelvic abscess, dyspareunia, and dysmenorrhea. If symptoms are not acute, PID may not be identified until an infertility workup is performed.

Collaborative Care

The goals of care are to eliminate the infection and prevent complications and recurrence. The history may reveal recent infection or insertion of an IUD. The physical examination may reveal abdominal pain and tenderness.

Laboratory and Diagnostic Tests

Tests used in the diagnosis of PID may include the following:

- *CBC with differential* reveals a markedly elevated WBC in PID.
- *Culdocentesis* (aspiration of fluid from the rectouterine space) can reveal the presence of pus and microorganisms. Gram's stain and culture and sensitivity of culdocentesis fluid identifies the causative organism.

■ *Ultrasonography* is performed to rule out ectopic pregnancy.

■ *Laparoscopy* or *laparotomy* may reveal inflammation, edema, or hyperemia of the uterine tubes, or tubal discharge and, possibly, generalized pelvic involvement, abscesses, and scarring.

Pharmacology

Combination antibiotic therapy with broad-spectrum antibiotics is the typical treatment for PID. If PID is not acute, outpatient antibiotic therapy is prescribed. In acute cases, however, the client is hospitalized. Analgesics are given, and antibiotics and fluids are administered intravenously. Commonly prescribed antibiotics include the following:

■ Doxycycline (Vibramycin), a tetracycline compound with a broad spectrum of activity

■ Cefoxitin (Mefoxin), a cephalosporin active against gram-positive and some gram-negative organisms

■ Clindamycin (Cleocin), an agent used for major infections with gram-positive and mixed anaerobic organisms

■ Gentamicin (Garamycin), an aminoglycoside antibiotic used for serious gram-negative infections

■ Ofloxacin (Floxin), a broad-spectrum fluoroquinolone

■ Metronidazole (Flagyl), an antiprotozoal agent that is also effective against most anaerobic bacteria

■ Ceftriaxone (Rocephin), a cephalosporin antibiotic

Nursing implications for these drugs are discussed in the pharmacology box on page 257 of Chapter 8.

Surgery

The surgeon may insert a drain into an abscess, if present, and remove any adhesions. If the client does not respond to conservative therapy, surgical removal of the uterus, uterine tubes, and ovaries may be necessary.

Nursing Care

The goals of nursing care are to treat the infection and to prevent complications, such as scarring and infertility. The client who is hospitalized maintains bed rest in semi-Fowler's position to promote drainage and localize the infectious process in the pelvic cavity. Although each nursing care plan must be individualized, nursing diagnoses that often apply to the client with PID are described below.

Risk for Injury

PID can have severe, even life-threatening, complications. Scarring of uterine tubes can lead to ectopic pregnancy or pelvic abscess. Infertility is a common complication, as are recurrent or chronic PID, chronic abdominal pain, pelvic adhesions, premature hysterectomy, and depression.

Nursing interventions with rationales follow:

■ Administer antibiotic therapy as ordered, and monitor closely for adverse effects (see the box on page 257, Chapter 8). *Antibiotics used in acute PID are potent agents; some can have life-threatening side effects.*

■ Teach the client to recognize and report side effects of medications, as well as manifestations of ectopic pregnancy. *The client may notice drug reactions before they become apparent to the nurse. Ectopic pregnancy can be life-threatening if not treated promptly.*

■ Practice thorough hand washing and strict adherence to universal precautions when handling perineal pads and linens. Appropriate disinfection of bedpans, toilet seats, linens, and utensils is also important. Teach client about these practices. *These practices help avoid disseminating the infection to others.*

Knowledge Deficit

PID is most common in young women, many of whom have limited understanding of their own anatomy and physiology, and of sexually transmitted disease. Diagnosis and treatment of PID offer an opportunity to increase that understanding, thereby preventing complications and recurrent infection.

Nursing interventions with rationales follow:

■ Explain how infection is spread and what measures to take to prevent future infection. *Understanding can improve compliance with treatment regimens and perhaps change high-risk behavior.*

■ Explain the need to complete the treatment regimen and the importance of follow-up visits. *If the client or partner fails to take all of the medication as prescribed, the infection may not be completely cured. Noncompliance and recurrence are common, particularly if follow-up appointments are not kept.*

■ Teach proper perineal care, especially wiping from front to back. *This reduces transmission of fecal organisms to reproductive tissues and reduces the incidence of urinary tract infections.*

■ Caution the client about using tampons, particularly if they previously have caused problems. Instruct the client to change tampons or pads at least every 4 hours. *Menstrual flow and other discharges provide a favorable environment for microorganisms to multiply.*

■ Provide information about safer sex practices and family planning. *Instruct the client to remove diaphragms within 6 hours after use. IUDs are contraindicated. Latex condoms offer the most effective protection against infection. These measures help prevent recurrence of infection.*

- Teach the client to report any unusual vaginal discharge or odor to the health care provider. *Treatment is most effective early in the disease process.*

Other Nursing Diagnoses

Additional nursing diagnoses that may apply to the client with PID follow:

- *Diarrhea* or *Constipation* related to space-occupying abscess or side effects of antibiotic therapy
- *Ineffective Individual Coping* related to pain and depression
- *Altered Health Maintenance* related to infection and systemic effects
- *Sexual Dysfunction* related to pain and treatment regimen
- *Anticipatory Grieving* related to possible effects of infection or its treatment on fertility

Client and Family Teaching

To promote the client's highest level of wellness, teach the client and family measures to eradicate the infection and prevent recurrence, and help the client deal with the physical and psychosocial implications of treatment, including possible infertility. Provide general information related to sexually transmitted diseases (see Chapter 49). Inform the client that the patency of the uterine tubes can be evaluated after several menstrual cycles, to allow for complete resolution of the inflammatory process.

The Client with Toxic Shock Syndrome

∎ ∎ ∎

Toxic shock syndrome (TSS) is a rare but acute illness caused by *Staphylococcus aureus* infection. It affects 1 to 3 per 100,000 menstruating women (Hatcher et al., 1994). Generally associated with tampon use during menstruation, TSS can also result from staphylococcal infection of the breast and endometrium following childbirth and from abdominal surgical wounds. TSS also has been associated with the use of vaginal barrier contraceptives such as the sponge, the diaphragm, and the cervical cap. The incidence related to barrier contraceptives is low, however, estimated at 2.25 cases per 100,000 in which these methods were used. Although TSS has been reported in children and in men (usually, those who have undergone surgery), 90% of cases are in women of childbearing age.

The incidence of TSS began to increase in 1977, when super-absorbent tampons were introduced. Since that time, certain products have been withdrawn from the market, and all tampon products carry a warning label

> ### Clinical Manifestations of Toxic Shock Syndrome
> ∎ ∎ ∎
>
> - High fever
> - Fatigue
> - Foul-smelling vaginal discharge
> - Gastrointestinal complaints
> - Sore throat
>
> If untreated, TSS progresses to:
>
> - Shock
> - Coma
> - Death

about TSS and a description of the manifestations. Unless TSS is diagnosed and treated promptly, the mortality rate is approximately 15%. Because TSS is better understood and more readily recognized and treated at this time, mortality has been reduced to 2% to 3%.

Pathophysiology

TSS is caused by virulent strains of *Staphylococcus aureus* that gain access to the vascular system through open blood vessels during the menses, a placental site after childbirth, or other open wound. Once inside the body, the organism produces toxins that result in vasodilation, hemodynamic instability, and shock. The clinical manifestations of TSS are presented in the accompanying box.

Collaborative Care

Care of the woman with toxic shock syndrome requires a multidisciplinary approach, often involving infectious disease specialists, the primary physician, respiratory and hemodynamic support, and nursing care. Goals of care include restoring hydration, administering antistaphylococcal medications, managing renal or cardiac insufficiency, and removing sources of infection (e.g., removing tampons or barrier contraceptives, draining an abscess). Prognosis depends on the severity and duration of infection, the degree of renal compromise, and the client's compliance with treatment and health teaching.

Laboratory and Diagnostic Tests
Tests used in the diagnosis of TSS may include the following:

- *WBC count* is markedly elevated in TSS.
- *Blood urea nitrogen (BUN) and serum creatinine* are elevated, particularly if renal involvement is severe.
- *SGOT and SGPT levels* are elevated.
- *Platelet count* is low.

- *Vaginal cultures* are positive for *Staphylococcus aureus.*
- *Blood cultures* are negative because the manifestations are caused by the toxin, not the invasive character of the organism (Tierney, McPhee, & Papadakis, 1994).

Pharmacology

Beta-lactamase-resistant antibiotics, such as nafcillin, cefoxitin, cefazolin, or cephalothin, are administered intravenously. If skin rash and urticaria appear, corticosteroids are used. Electrolyte imbalances are corrected as indicated. Blood products are administered as indicated to replace platelets.

Nursing Care

Nursing care focuses on administering the treatment regimen, preventing life-threatening complications, and teaching the client to prevent recurrence. In obtaining a history from the client with suspected TSS, the nurse elicits information about manifestations and the use of tampons, diaphragm, or vaginal barrier contraceptive devices. The compromised status of the client may mask reactions to medications and blood products; careful monitoring by the nurse is essential to detect any untoward effects. Although each nursing care plan must be individualized, nursing diagnoses that may apply to the client experiencing TSS are described below.

Altered Tissue Perfusion

Replacement of blood platelets and fluids is essential in preventing shock, coma, and death.

Nursing interventions with rationales follow:

- Administer plasma volume expanders as ordered. *Dilation of the vascular bed causes blood to pool rather than to flow to and perfuse the organ systems and tissues. Increasing the intravascular volume improves venous return, cardiac output, and tissue perfusion.*
- Administer oxygen as indicated. *Increasing the oxygen content of blood will increase the level of oxygen reaching the peripheral tissues.*

Decreased Cardiac Output

In the client with TSS, low circulating blood volume may lead to a decrease in cardiac output. Careful monitoring and appropriate measures are necessary to prevent life-threatening complications.

Nursing interventions with rationales follow:

- Administer inotropic agents if indicated. *Inotropic agents increase the force of myocardial contraction, thus increasing the ejection fraction and minute stroke volume.*
- Monitor vital signs hourly or more often, as indicated. *As shock ensues, blood pressure rises briefly and then decreases as the blood vessels become unable to respond to neural stimuli. As a compensatory measure, cardiac and respiratory rates increase.*
- Monitor urinary output hourly; notify the physician if urinary output falls below 30 mL per hour. *Urinary output falls as a reflection of renal perfusion, and renal perfusion is a mirror of total perfusion. Extremities become cool and clammy as blood is diverted to the vital organs. Temperature rises, increasing the metabolic rate and requirement for oxygen.*
- Monitor pulmonary function. *If the amount of fluid administered exceeds the heart's ability to pump, pulmonary edema may result. Adult respiratory distress syndrome (ARDS or noncardiac pulmonary edema) is a possible complication of TSS.*

Knowledge Deficit

Despite warnings in the media and on packages of tampons, many women remain unaware or unconcerned about the potential development of TSS. More responsible health behaviors can greatly reduce the incidence of this disorder.

Nursing interventions with rationales follow:

- Educate the client and the public about the causes and manifestations of TSS; see the box on page 2034. *Clients, as well as health professionals, need to be aware of the manifestations of TSS so that it can be identified and treated quickly.*
- Teach the client self-care measures to prevent recurrence of TSS. *More than 30% of women with TSS have recurrent episodes.*

Client and Family Teaching

Education of the client focuses on the causes of TSS and self-care measures to prevent future infection, as discussed above. The client needs to understand the importance of completing the prescribed course of antibiotics and keeping follow-up appointments, even after manifestations have subsided. Advise women who have had TSS to avoid using tampons and vaginal barrier contraceptives.

▪▪▪ Disorders of Sexual Expression ▪▪▪

The normal female sexual drive can persist well into the eighth and ninth decade. The body maintains the capacity for sexual activity and orgasm long after the climac-teric; see the gerontologic considerations box on page 2035 for a discussion of age-related changes in the female sexual response.

Client Teaching: Minimizing the Risks of Toxic Shock Syndrome

■ ■ ■

- Using sanitary pads instead of tampons almost entirely eliminates your risk for TSS, but even if you do use tampons, the risk is low.

- If you use tampons, choose the lowest absorbency that meets your menstrual flow needs, and be sure to change tampons at least every 4 hours. If possible, allow a tampon-free interval every day. For example, use sanitary pads at night.

- Wash your hands with soap before inserting anything into your vagina (for example, a tampon, your diaphragm, a contraceptive sponge, or vaginal medication).

- Follow instructions for vaginal contraceptive products carefully. Do not leave a sponge or your diaphragm or cervical cap in place in your vagina longer than the recommended time, and do not use these products during a menstrual period.

- During the first 12 weeks after childbirth, do not use tampons or contraceptive sponges or a cervical cap. It may be best to avoid using a diaphragm, as well.

- Watch for the danger signs of TSS, especially during menstrual periods. If you think you may have mild TSS, remove your tampon and see your clinician. Early manifestations of TSS can resemble those of influenza.

- If you have had TSS, it is safest to stop using tampons entirely and to avoid contraceptive sponges, diaphragms, and cervical caps.

- Be aware of the danger signs if TSS:
  a. Fever (temperature of 101 F [38.3 C] or more)
  b. Vomiting
  c. Diarrhea
  d. Dizziness
  e. Feeling faint or weak
  f. Muscle aches
  g. Rash-like sunburn

- In severe cases, TSS can cause shock, and even death.

Note. Modified from *Contraceptive Technology* (16th ed.) by R. A. Hatcher et al., 1994, New York: Irvington Publishers.

In a typical sexual event, two physiologic sexual responses occur: vasocongestion and myotonia. Sexual stimulation results in vasocongestion of the blood vessels surrounding the vagina, causing engorgement, increased lubrication, and genital swelling and enlargement. Arousal, or myotonia, increases muscular tension, resulting in voluntary and involuntary muscle contraction.

The sexual response cycle has four phases: excitement, plateau, orgasm, and resolution. These phases always occur in the same sequence; however, the duration of each phase may vary. Sexual arousal typically ends in orgasm, or climax, but sometimes fails to do so. The refractory period, or period in which the sexual organs are incapable of responding to stimulus, does not occur in the female. Multiple orgasms are physically possible in all women.

The Client with Inhibited Sexual Desire

■ ■ ■

Inhibited sexual desire may be a result of pathophysiologic processes or may be psychogenic in origin. A general sexual dysfunction is said to exist when a woman derives no sexual pleasure from sexual stimulation. Under normal circumstances, sexual desire can persist throughout life, although sexual expression may have to be modified to allow for changes associated with aging.

Sexual desire has many stimuli, including visual, auditory, tactile, olfactory, and gustatory. The inability to use any of the five senses or to freely process sexual thoughts can interfere with sexual desire. Often, inhibited sexual desire is rooted deeply in childhood teaching or experiences that may be to painful to recall. Cultural and religious values can also affect the processing of sexual stimuli. Fear of pregnancy or sexually transmitted diseases, and depression also contribute to decreased libido.

The successful treatment of inhibited sexual response frequently requires a multidisciplinary approach. Once physiologic inhibitors are ruled out, a psychologic counselor and spiritual counselor often may become involved in the therapy. It is important that the partner be included at appropriate intervals.

Nursing care for the client experiencing inhibited sexual desire focuses on identifying the cause(s) and educating the client about human sexuality. The initial assessment and interview are done sensitively and in privacy. A nonjudgmental attitude is essential; the client must feel free to express her feelings to the health care provider. Additionally, nurses must feel comfortable with their own sexuality in order to deal effectively with clients. The client may have many residual taboos from childhood that may be difficult to reveal and to unseat. If she does

Gerontologic Considerations: Female Sexual Function

■   ■   ■

Myths, taboos, and stereotypes held by society may foster the belief that older women are no longer interested in expressing their sexuality. Two commonly held myths are that menopause is the death of a woman's sexuality and that hysterectomy results in the inability to function sexually. Loss of sexual function is not an inevitable result of aging, although physical changes related to aging do affect the female sexual response. These physical changes, along with chronic conditions common in aging women, may alter a woman's sexual function. In addition, some medications used to treat the chronic conditions associated with aging can also alter the sexual response. It is the role of the nurse to educate women about the myths and misinformation about changes in sexual functioning and to provide information about ways to achieve optimal sexual health.

Physiologic Changes

Changes in aging women's sexual function begin in the perimenopausal period as estrogen levels decrease. Estrogen-sensitive cells are found throughout the central nervous system and the cardiovascular system. These cells are involved in the female sexual response. With menopause comes a decrease in the levels of estradiol, which affects nerve transmission and the response in the peripheral vascular system. As a result, the timing and degree of vasocongestion during the sexual response are affected.

Specific changes in the female sexual response occur in all phases. During the plateau phase, the capacity for vasocongestion decreases, as does muscle tension. In the orgasmic phase, the contractions are fewer and less intense. During the resolution phase, vasocongestion subsides more quickly.

Nursing Care

The nurse's role in assisting aging women to reach optimal sexual functioning centers on teaching them about the physiologic and psychologic changes associated with menopause. In addition, the nurse should instruct the client in how the effects of chronic illness and the medications used to treat these illnesses affect sexual functioning. The client should be taught the importance of maintaining a healthy life-style, which includes a balanced diet, weight-bearing and aerobic exercises, stress management, and routine health examinations.

For problems related to vaginal dryness and dyspareunia, the nurse can recommend that the client use water-soluble vaginal lubricants or vaginal gels before intercourse. Intercourse on a regular basis and estrogen replacement therapy can also be recommended for these problems. Women who experience joint pain or other musculoskeletal pain due to conditions such as arthritis can benefit from instruction in how to adapt positions for intercourse.

Note. Adapted from "Sexuality and Aging" (pp. 426–438) by B. K. Johnson in *Gerontological Nursing* by M. Stanley and P. Beare, 1995, Philadelphia: F. A. Davis.

---

not feel attractive to her partner, is fatigued or feels overworked, or considers her partner sexually unattractive, open communication must be established before these issues can be effectively addressed. Although each nursing care plan must be individualized, the following nursing diagnoses may apply to the client with inhibition of sexual desire:

- *Altered Sexuality Patterns* related to infrequency of and failure to achieve sexual satisfaction through intercourse
- *Sexual Dysfunction* related to inability to progress through phases of sexual response cycle
- *Knowledge Deficit* of normal sexual response and technique

- *Ineffective Family Coping* related to unrelieved sexual tension
- *Anxiety* related to lack of understanding about sexual functioning and expression of sexual desire

To promote the highest level of wellness, teach the client and significant other about varied normal and acceptable sexual responses. The goal is to increase self-awareness and understanding of communication and their relationship to sexual desire. Explain the differences in the behaviors men and women consider sexually stimulating. Training in autostimulation techniques (masturbation) is often undertaken after inhibitions against this practice are discussed. Group therapy may be encouraged to help the woman discuss her problem and to decrease the sense of isolation it gives her.

The Client with Orgasmic Dysfunction

■ ■ ■

Inhibited female orgasm (*anorgasmia*) is the most prevalent sexual problem among women. However, fewer than 20% of cases are physiologic in origin. It is estimated that from 8% to 15% of women have never experienced an orgasm in the waking state. Psychogenically induced anorgasmia may result from unresolved conflicts about sexual activity. Organic causes of anorgasmia include the presence of disease that results in general debilitation or that affects the sexual response cycle, and the use of drugs that depress the central nervous system.

Anorgasmia may be primary or secondary. *Primary anorgasmia* exists when a woman has never experienced an orgasm during the waking state, either through self-stimulation or intercourse. *Secondary anorgasmia* exists when a woman who previously experienced orgasms is no longer able to do so.

A number of situational and environmental factors can inhibit orgasmic response. The use of alcohol, barbiturates, narcotics, or any depressant can interfere with sexual functioning. Inflammatory, infectious, or painful gynecologic disorders, anxiety about "being heard by the children," stress, fatigue, and ignorance of sexual techniques on the part of either partner contribute to this disorder. With treatment, 80% to 90% of women become able to achieve orgasm, at least through self-stimulation.

Nursing care focuses on identifying the type of orgasmic dysfunction through a thorough history, including the onset, duration, frequency, and context or situation in which the problem occurs. The goal of nursing care is to increase self-awareness and teach effective self-stimulation techniques. When teaching masturbation techniques, suggest the use of a mirror at home. The woman's partner should be included in discussions whenever possible. Discontinuation of CNS-depressing drugs or oral contraceptive agents may be indicated.

Allowing free expression of feelings in a supportive environment is key to achieving success. Referral to a sex therapist may be necessary. Possible nursing diagnoses for these clients are similar to those that apply to the client with inhibited sexual desire.

The Client with Dyspareunia

■ ■ ■

The client with **dyspareunia** (pain during intercourse) may find it difficult to express her feelings to her partner. This condition is more likely to manifest itself as decreased desire or inhibited orgasm. The causes of dyspareunia range from organic to psychogenic.

Physical conditions, such as imperforate hymen, vaginal scarring, or *vaginismus,* may cause dyspareunia. Vaginismus is a rare condition in which the vaginal muscles at the introitus contract so tightly that an erect penis cannot be inserted. An early traumatic event, such as sexual abuse, fear of men, rape, or ignorance of sexual functioning contribute to this disorder. However, it is estimated that 90% of dyspareunia is psychogenic in origin. The woman develops an anxiety-fear-guilt cycle in which negative thoughts become associated with the act of vaginal penetration, initiating a conditioned involuntary reflex. Sexual activity, other than vaginal penetration, may be quite pleasurable.

If the cause of sexual dysfunction is psychogenic, a multifaceted approach including a psychologist, psychiatrist, or sex therapist may be indicated. A careful history and physical examination are performed to identify any physiologic causes for the dyspareunia (see Chapter 45, Assessing Clients with Reproductive Disorders).

Nursing care begins with a complete history. The client's complaints of pain on intercourse or the inability to insert a tampon must be fully explored. Fear related to penetration and pregnancy should be discussed openly, allowing the client adequate time to express her feelings in a nonthreatening atmosphere. Opportunity must also be provided for the partner to express possible feelings of frustration and rejection.

The client's response to physical examination and bimanual examination may yield important information. Frequently, pelvic examination results in involuntary muscle contraction that prevents bimanual examination or limits it to the insertion of only one finger. Should this occur, the clinician can make the client aware of this response. Graduated dilators and the use of fingers or tampons by the client herself and then her partner may be used to overcome the spasms and fear of pain upon penetration. Psychoanalysis, behavior modification, and sex therapy may be useful tools to decrease the phobic reaction to penetration.

One nursing goal is to assist the woman in modifying her conditioned response to vaginal penetration. This may be accomplished through guided imagery, biofeedback, and hypnosis/autosuggestion techniques. Open communication between the woman and her sexual partner is also necessary to overcome this disorder. The nurse may also demonstrate manual penetration of the vagina and the proper use of dilators.

Although each nursing care plan must be individualized, possible nursing diagnoses that may apply to the client with dyspareunia follow:

- *Fear* related to vaginal penetration
- *Sexual Dysfunction* related to vaginismus
- *Pain* related to vaginal penetration

Most women can be helped by desensitization therapy and gradual, progressive dilation. Psychotherapy to resolve underlying conflicts and sex therapy are useful adjuncts to nursing intervention. Education about normal sexual functioning should be included to minimize recurrence at a later time.

Bibliography

■ ■ ■

American Cancer Society. (1993). *Cancer Facts & Figures 1993.* Atlanta: Author.

American College of Obstetricians and Gynecologists. (1992). *Hormone Replacement Therapy.* (Technical Bulletin No. 166). Washington, D.C.: Author.

Aral, S. O., Mosher, W. D., Cates, W., Jr. (1991). Self-reported pelvic inflammatory disease in the United States, 1988. *Journal of the American Medical Association, 266:* 2570–2573.

Barrett-Connor, E., & Bush, T. L. (1991). Estrogen and coronary heart disease in women. *Journal of the American Medical Association, 265,* 1861–1867.

Bilezikian, J. P., & Silverberg, S. J. (1992). Osteoporosis: A practical approach to the postmenopausal woman. *Journal of Women's Health, 1,* 21–27.

Bourguet, C., Hamrick, G., & Gilchrist, V. (1991). The prevalence of osteoporosis risk factors and physician intervention. *Journal of Family Practice, 323,* 265.

Brinton, L. A., & Schairer, C. (1993) Estrogen replacement therapy and breast cancer risk. *Epidemiologic Reviews, 15*(1), 66–79.

Bush, T. L. (1992). Feminine forever revisited: Menopausal hormone therapy in the 1990's. *Journal of Women's Health, 1,* 1–4.

Centers for Disease Control. (1992, July). *HIV/AIDS Surveillance Report.* Atlanta: U.S. Department of Health and Human Services.

Christiansen, C. (1991). Introduction—Consensus Development Conference on Osteoporosis. *American Journal of Medicine, 91,* Supplement 1S.

Corson, S. L. (1991). Physiology of menopause and update on hormone replacement therapy. In A. McCormick (Ed.), *Clinical issues in perinatal and women's health nursing* (pp. 483–496). Philadelphia: Lippincott.

Cramer, D., Welch, W. R., Scully R. E., & Wojciechowski, C. A. (1982). Ovarian cancer and talc: A case-control study. *Cancer, 50,* 372–376.

Devor, M., Barrett-Connor, E., Renvall, M., Feigal, D., & Ramsdell, J. (1991). Estrogen replacement therapy and the risk of venous thrombosis. *American Journal of Medicine, 92,* 275–282.

Doress, P. B., & Siegal, D. L. (1995). *Ourselves, growing older.* New York: Touchstone/Simon & Schuster.

Dougherty, J., & Knutesen, P. (1995). The female reproductive system and its problem in the elderly. In M. Stanley & P. Beare (Eds.), *Gerontological Nursing* (pp. 225–264). Philadelphia: F. A. Davis.

Ebersole, P., & Hess, P. (1994). *Toward healthy aging: Human needs and nursing response* (4th ed.). St. Louis: Mosby-Year Book.

Fackelmann, K. S. (1992, September 19). Excess iron linked to heart disease. *Science News.*

Gambrell, R. D. (1990). *Estrogen replacement therapy* (2nd ed.). Dallas, TX: Essential Medical Systems, Inc.

Gant, N. F., & Cunningham, F. G. (1993). *Basic gynecology and obstetrics.* Norwalk, CT: Appleton & Lange.

Harlow, B. L., Cramer, D. W., Bell, D. A., & Welch, W. R. Perineal exposure to talc and ovarian cancer risk. (1992). *Obstetrics and Gynecology, 80,* 19–26.

Hatcher, R. A., et al. (1994). *Contraceptive technology* (16th ed.). New York: Irvington Publishers.

Heany, R. P. (1991). Effects of calcium on skeletal development, bone loss and risk of fractures. *American Journal of Medicine, 91* (Suppl.), 23S–28S.

Hunter, M., Battersby, R., & Whitehead, M. (1986). Relationships between psychological symptoms, somatic complaints and menopausal status. *Maturitas, 8,* 217–228.

Johnson, B. K. (1995). Sexuality and aging. In M. Stanley and P. G. Beare, *Gerontological Nursing.* Philadelphia: F. A. Davis.

Kasper, C. S., & Chandler, P. J., Jr. (1995). Not-so-safe "safe sex." *Journal of the American Medical Association, 273*(11), 846–847.

Kelly, P. J., & Holman, S. (1993). The new face of AIDS. *American Journal of Nursing, 93,* 26–32.

Lindsay, R. (1991). Estrogens, bone mass, and osteoporotic fracture. *American Journal of Medicine, 91* (Suppl.), 10S–13S.

Lufkin, E. G., Carpenter, P. C., Ory, S. J., Malkasian, G. D., & Edmonton, J. H. (1988). Estrogen replacement therapy: Current recommendations. *Mayo Clinic Proceedings, 63,* 453–460.

McCrea, F. (1983). The politics of menopause: The "discovery" of the deficiency disease. *Social Problems, 31,* 111–123.

McKeon, V. A. (1994). Hormone replacement therapy: Evaluating the risks and benefits. *Journal of Obstetric, Gynelogic, and Neonatal Nursing, 23*(8), 647–657.

McKinlay, S., & Jefferys, M. (1974). The menopausal syndrome. *British Journal Preventive Social Medicine, 28,* 108–115.

Meldrum, D. R. (1987). Treatment of hot flashes. In D. Mishell (Ed.), *Menopause: Physiology and pharmacology.* (pp. 141–150). Chicago: Yearbook Medical Publishers.

Miller, V. T., Muesing, R. A., LaRosa, J. C., Stoy, D. B., Phillips, E. A., & Stillman, R. J. (1991). Effects of conjugated equine estrogen with and without three different progestogens on lipoproteins, high-density lipoprotein subfractions, and apolipoprotein A-I. *Obstetrics and Gynecology, 77,* 235–240.

Miller, V. T., Ravnikar, V. A., & Timmons, M. C. (1990). ERT: Weighing the risks and benefits. *Patient Care, 24,* 30–48.

Morbidity and Mortality Weekly Report. (1992, January 17). The second 100,000 cases of acquired immunodeficiency syndrome—United States, June 1981–December 1991. *MMWR, 41,* 28–29.

Pagana K. D., & Pagana, T. J. (1995) *Mosby's diagnostic and laboratory test reference* (2nd ed.) St. Louis: Mosby-Year Book.

Philosophe, R., & Seibel, M. (1991). Menopause and cardiovascular disease. In A. McCormick (Ed.), *Clinical issues in perinatal and women's health nursing.* (pp. 441–451). Philadelphia: Lippincott.

Rinzler, C. A. (1993). *Estrogen and breast cancer: A warning to women.* New York: Macmillan.

Rodriguez, C., et al. (1995). Estrogen replacement therapy and fatal ovarian cancer. *American Journal of Epidemiology, 141*(8), 829–835.

Rosenblatt, K. A., Szklo, M., & Rosenshein, N. B. (1992). Mineral fiber exposure and the development of ovarian cancer. *Gynecologic Oncology, 45,* 20–25.

Samsoie, G. (1992). Introduction to steroids in the menopause. *American Journal of Obstetrics and Gynecology, 166,* 1980–1985.

Scott, J. R., et al. (1994). *Danforth's obstetrics and gynecology* (7th ed.). Philadelphia: Lippincott.

Seideman, R. Y. (1990). Effects of a premenstrual education program on premenstrual symptomatology. *Health Care for Women International, 11*(4), 491.

Stampfer, M. J., & Colditz, G. A. (1991). Estrogen replacement therapy and coronary heart disease: A quantitative assessment of the epidemiologic evidence. *Preventive Medicine, 20,* 47–63.

Stampfer, M. J., Colditz, G. A., Willett, W. C., Manson, J. E., Rosner, B., Speizer, F. E., & Hennekens, C. (1991). A meta-analysis of the effect of estrogen replacement therapy on the risk of breast cancer. *Journal of the American Medical Association, 265,* 1985–1990.

Thomas, D. B. (1990). Estrogen replacement therapy and cancer: Endometrial, breast and ovarian. In S. Korenman (Ed.), *The Menopause.* Norwell, MA: Serono Sumposia.

Tierney, L. T., McPhee, S. J., & Papadakis, M. A. (1994). *Current medical diagnosis & treatment, 1994.* Norwalk, CT: Appleton & Lange.

United States Bureau of the Census. (1992). *Population trends in the 1980's.* (Special Studies Series, p–23, No. 175). Washington, D.C.: U. S. Government Printing Office.

Wentz, A. C. (1988). Management of the menopause. In H. W. Jones, A. C. Wentz, & L. S. Burnett (Eds.), *Novak's textbook of gynecology* (11th ed.), (pp. 397–342). Baltimore: Williams & Wilkins.

Whitehead, M. I., Hillard, T. C., & Crook, D. (1990). The role and use of progestogens. *Obstetrics and Gynecology, 75* (Suppl.), 59S–76S.

Nursing Care of Clients with Breast Disorders

LEARNING OBJECTIVES

After completing this chapter you will be able to:

- Describe the pathophysiology of commonly occurring disorders of the breast.
- Identify laboratory and diagnostic tests used to diagnose disorders of the breast and the associated nursing implications.
- Compare and contrast the manifestations of benign and malignant disorders of the breast.

- Discuss nursing implications for medications prescribed for the client with disorders of the breast.
- Provide appropriate nursing care for the client receiving chemotherapy or radiation therapy.
- Provide appropriate nursing care for the client in the preoperative and postoperative phases of a mastectomy.
- Use the nursing process as a framework for providing individualized care to clients with disorders of the breast.

Breast disorders are common conditions that primarily affect women. When a woman discovers a breast lump, her first response is often fear: of breast cancer, of losing her breast, and perhaps of losing her life. Breast disorders, particularly breast cancer, are poorly understood by many people; their knowledge may be imprecise and anecdotal. Because American society views the breast as a significant component of feminine beauty, any problem that threatens the breast often strikes at the core of a woman's self-image.

Nurses play a critical role in the care of clients experiencing breast disorders by providing education, support, and advocacy. Part of the nurse's role is educating clients about normal breast tissue, common benign breast disorders, available screening techniques and risk factors for breast cancers, and breast self-examination. Nurses can make a difference in clients' lives by referring them to health care providers and participating in the care of the client with breast cancer and benign breast disorders.

Malignant Disorders of the Breast

The Client with Breast Cancer

Breast cancer strikes 1 woman every 3 minutes and kills 1 woman every 12 minutes. It is estimated that in 1995, 182,000 women were diagnosed with breast cancer and

46,000 died of it. Breast cancer also strikes men, although rarely. In 1995, about 1000 men were diagnosed with breast cancer and 300 died of it (Boring et al., 1994). Among cancer-related deaths in Caucasian women, breast cancer is second only to lung cancer as the cause, and it is the leading cause of cancer deaths in African-American women. Despite a steady increase in the incidence of breast cancer since World War II, the breast cancer mortality rate remained relatively stable for more than 50 years. Between 1989 and 1992, breast cancer mortality in white women dropped nearly 5% but rose 2.6% among African-American women (Broder, 1995).

Breast cancer is not one disease entity, but many, depending on the affected breast tissue, the tissue's estrogen dependency, and the age of the person at onset. Only 7% of all breast cancers occur in clients under the age of 40 (Ciatto et al., 1987; Taylor, 1994).

The psychosocial impact of breast cancer extends beyond the fear and threat of death. The diagnosis may transform the client's sense of self and lead to reintegration or negotiation of family relationships.

Risk Factors

The two most significant risk factors for breast cancer are female gender and age, with over 78% of breast cancer occurring in women over the age of 50 (Hankey et al., 1994). A history of the disease in a first-degree relative, such as a mother or sister, increases the risk, especially if the cancer occurred before menopause. Hereditary cancer is consistent with the presence of an autosomal dominant factor and actually accounts for less than 10% of familial clustering of breast cancer.

In September 1994, a researcher identified **BRCA1**, the so-called breast cancer gene, on chromosome 17. Women who carry this gene are believed to have a 50% chance of developing breast cancer before menopause and an 85% chance of developing it before age 70. This gene also greatly increases the risk of ovarian cancer (Futreal et al., 1994). The type of hereditary breast cancer caused by BRCA1 and other breast cancer genes account for only about 5% of all breast cancers. The cause of the remaining 95% of breast cancers is unclear.

A personal history of breast cancer in one breast increases the likelihood of cancer in the other breast. Women (particularly premenopausal women) with a history of a benign breast disorder called atypical hyperplasia are at higher risk (London et al., 1992). Women who have never had a child and women who bear a first child after the age of 30 are also at increased risk.

Early menarche and late menopause are believed to increase the risk of breast cancer, primarily because of the woman's increased exposure to unopposed estrogen, a hormone that promotes tumor growth. Although the relationship between estrogen and breast cancer is not fully understood, recent studies show that early (before age 15) or prolonged use (4 years or more) of either oral contraceptives or estrogen-replacement therapy increases the risk of breast cancer (Brinton, 1994; Thomas, 1991).

Exposure to environmental carcinogens such as ionizing radiation (as in X-rays and fluoroscopy) and pesti-

Table 48–1	Factors Associated with Increased Risk for Breast Cancer
Gender	Female
Race	White
Family History	Breast cancer in mother or sister (especially bilateral or premenopausal)
Medical History	Endometrial cancer Atypical hyperplasia Cancer in other breast
Menstrual History	Early menarche (under age 12) Late menopause (after age 50)
Reproductive History	First birth after age 25 Early or prolonged use of oral contraceptives Prolonged use of estrogen-replacement therapy
Radiation Exposure	Chest X-rays, fluoroscopic examination, particularly before age 30
Life-Style	High-fat diet Alcohol intake greater than two drinks daily Obesity High socioeconomic status Smoking Breast trauma

cides and other chemicals is also associated with increased risk of breast cancer and other cancers. Cancer caused by radiation exposure may take from 10 to 40 years to develop; thus, women who were treated for scoliosis as adolescents and monitored with X-ray studies and fluoroscopy have a much higher rate of breast cancer in their 30s and 40s than women who were not treated.

A growing body of evidence suggests that exposure to a class of chemicals known as organochlorines (including many pesticides, herbicides, and household cleaning products) is associated with an increased risk of breast cancer and other cancers. Controversy exists on this issue, however, because research has focused primarily on detecting and treating breast cancer rather than identifying its causes and ways to prevent it.

Other factors associated with increased risk of breast cancer are dietary fat, alcohol consumption, breast trauma, higher socioeconomic status, obesity, and smoking (ACOG, 1991; Smith, 1993).

Table 48–1 summarizes risk factors for breast cancer.

Pathophysiology

Breast cancer is the unregulated growth of abnormal cells in breast tissue. The majority of carcinomas of the breast occur in the ductal areas of the breast. Carcinomas of the

---

Clinical Manifestations of Breast Cancer

- Breast mass or thickening
- Unusual lump in the underarm or above the collarbone
- Persistent skin rash near the nipple area
- Flaking or eruption near the nipple
- Dimpling, pulling, or retraction in an area of the breast
- Nipple discharge
- Change in nipple position
- Burning, stinging, or pricking sensation

---

breast are classified as **noninvasive** (in situ) or **invasive.** Invasiveness refers to penetration of the tumor into surrounding tissue. Two atypical types of breast cancer are inflammatory carcinoma and Paget's disease.

The clinical manifestations of breast cancer may include a nontender lump in the breast (most often in the upper outer quadrant), abnormal nipple discharge, a rash around the nipple area, nipple retraction, dimpling of the skin, or a change in the position of the nipple (see the accompanying box). Breast cancer is usually painless, but some women report a burning or stinging sensation. Many women with breast cancer have no symptoms, and their tumors are detected by mammography. However, 90% of breast cancers are found by the women themselves (during breast self-examination or a shower) or by their partners while making love.

Noninvasive (In Situ) Carcinoma

Noninvasive, or in situ, carcinoma of the breast may be either ductal or lobular. Noninvasive carcinoma of the breast represents the proliferation of malignant cells within the ducts or lobules without the invasion of surrounding tissue.

Noninvasive ductal carcinoma is typically diagnosed on the basis of clinically occult mammographic calcifications instead of a breast mass or nipple discharge. The nipple and the subareolar region are commonly involved. *Noninvasive lobular carcinoma* is characterized by a solid proliferation of small cells with distinct borders within the lobules in multiple areas of the breast (Harris et al., 1992). These noninvasive cancers appear to increase the risk for invasive carcinoma of the breast (Way, 1994).

Invasive Carcinoma

Most breast cancers are adenocarcinomas and appear to arise in the terminal section of the breast ductal tissue.

There are five common invasive types of breast cancer, three of which (tubular, medullary, and mucinous) are variations of infiltrating ductal carcinoma. There is only a slight difference in prognosis among these various histologic types; the stage of the cancer is a more accurate predictor of prognosis.

Infiltrating ductal carcinoma is characterized by a stony hardness when palpated and commonly metastasizes to the axillary lymph nodes. This is the most common type of breast cancer, accounting for approximately 75% of cases. The prognosis is poorer than for most other histologic types (Harris et al., 1992).

Tubular carcinoma, also called "well differentiated" or "orderly cancer," occurs in less than 2% of clients with breast cancer. This cancer may occur with other cancers.

Medullary carcinoma is a well-circumscribed lesion that accounts for approximately 5% to 7% of all breast carcinomas. The tumor is often bulky and large; if small, the tumor may be mistaken for a fibroadenoma or a cyst.

Mucinous carcinoma occurs in approximately 3% of clients with breast cancer. This cancer is slow growing and can become bulky. This tumor may have sharp edges and may also be confused with a fibroadenoma (Harris et al., 1992; Navin, 1990).

Infiltrating lobular carcinoma is relatively uncommon, occurring in only 5% to 10% of clients with breast cancer. The most common clinical finding associated with this carcinoma is a thickened, ill-defined area of the breast. As in infiltrating ductal carcinoma, there is likelihood of metastasis to the axillary lymph nodes (Harris et al., 1992).

Inflammatory Carcinoma

Inflammatory carcinoma of the breast, a systemic disease, is the most malignant form of breast cancer. The client presents with a diffuse skin erythema and redness, warmth, and induration of the breast. Edema of the skin (peau d'orange) is usually present (Figure 48–1). At least half of these clients report tenderness and pain. Frequently, there is no discrete mass. Diagnosis of this cancer is based on clinical signs and symptoms and not by the pathologic tissue examination alone. Often the inflammatory changes are mistaken for an infectious process. Prognosis for these clients is poor, regardless of treatment.

Paget's Disease

Paget's disease (Paget's carcinoma) is a rare type of breast cancer involving infiltration of the nipple epithelium (Figure 48–2). Initial symptoms are itching or burning of the nipple with superficial erosion, crusting, or ulceration. Diagnosis is based on biopsy of the affected area. Like inflammatory breast cancer, Paget's disease is often misdiagnosed as an infection. If cancerous changes are confined to the nipple, however, Paget's disease has an excellent prognosis.

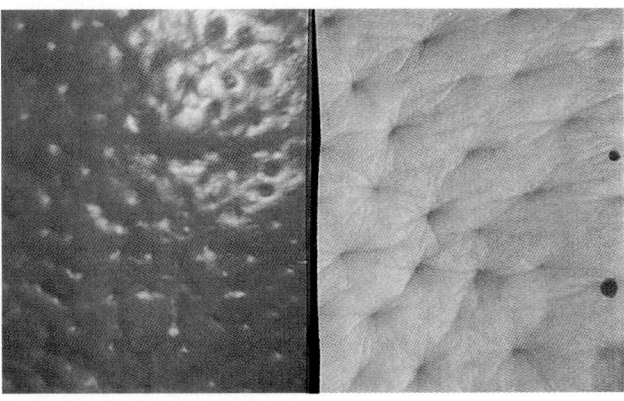

Figure 48–1 *Left,* Orange peel; *Right,* Peau d'orange sign.

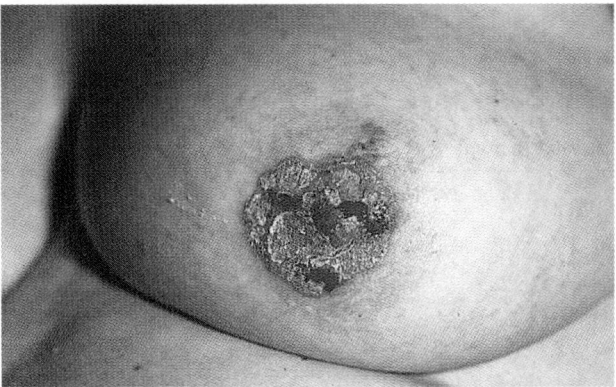

Figure 48–2 Paget's disease of the nipple.

Table 48–2 Staging of Breast Cancer

Stage	Tumor	Node	Metastasis
0	Tis–Carcinoma in situ or Paget's disease of the nipple	N0–No regional lymph node metastasis	M0–No evidence of distant metastasis
I	T1–Tumor no larger than 2 cm	N0	M0
IIA	T0–No evidence of primary tumor T1	N1–Metastasis to movable ipsilateral axillary nodes	M0
	T2–Tumor no larger than 5 cm	N0	M0
IIB	T2	N1	M0
	T3–Tumor larger than 5 cm	N0	M0
IIIA	T0 T1 T2	N2–Metastasis to ipsilateral fixed axillary nodes	M0
	T3	N1 N2	M0 M0
IIIB	T4–Tumor of any size with direct extension to chest wall or skin	Any N	M0
	Any T	N3–Metastasis to ipsilateral internal mammary lymph nodes	M0
IV	Any T	N0 and N1	M1–Distant metastasis

Metastasis of Breast Cancer

Breast cancer can metastasize to other sites through the bloodstream or lymphatic system. At least half the women diagnosed with breast cancer develop metastatic disease and die within 10 years. Metastatic breast cancer may be a chronic disease or a rapidly progressive terminal disease (Knobf, 1990). The common sites of metastasis of breast cancer are bone, brain, lung, liver, skin, and lymph nodes.

Staging of Breast Cancer

Staging is a system of classifying cancer according to the size of the tumor, involvement of lymph nodes, and metastasis to distant sites. Each stage is determined by the detection/size of the tumor, the presence/absence of nodal involvement, and the presence/absence of distant metastasis (Table 48–2). A classification of Stage 0 indicates that carcinoma in situ exists and that there is no nodal involvement or distant metastasis. Stage I indicates that the

Table 48–3   Staging of Breast Carcinoma and Survival

Histologic Staging	Crude Survival (%) 5 Years	10 Years
All patients	63	46
Negative axillary lymph nodes	78	65
Positive axillary lymph nodes	46	25
1 to 3 positive axillary lymph nodes	62	38
>4 positive axillary lymph nodes	32	13
Distant Metastasis	5	2

Note. From *Current Surgical Diagnosis and Treatment* (9th ed.) by L. W. Way, 1991, Norwalk, CT: Appleton & Lange.

tumor is 2 cm or less in greatest dimension and that no nodal involvement or distant metastasis is present.

In Stages II and III, tumor size is taken into consideration as well as the amount of nodal involvement. In Stage IV, tumor size is noted, nodal involvement is present, and distant metastasis has occurred. The staging of the breast cancer provides important information for making decisions about treatment options.

Staging of breast cancer is also used as a basis for prognosis. Seventy percent of clients with Stage I tumors survive for 10 years with accepted forms of therapy (Way, 1991). Table 48–3 gives survival percentages for other stages.

Collaborative Care

Diagnosis of breast cancer begins with detection, either detection of asymptomatic lesions discovered through screening or symptomatic lesions discovered by the client. Any palpable mass requires evaluation. Once the diagnosis is made, a number of treatment options are available. The choice of treatment depends on several factors, such as the stage of the cancer, the age of the woman, and the woman's preferences.

The standard treatment for breast cancer focuses on containment and removal of the cancer and prevention of recurrence. Care of the woman with breast cancer involves a team of health care professionals that can include a primary physician, mammography technician, radiologist, surgeon, medical oncologist, respiratory therapist, radiation oncologist, plastic surgeon, psychologist, social worker, dietitian, and several nurse specialists.

The client has three major therapeutic options from which to choose: surgery, radiation therapy, and chemotherapy and/or hormone therapy. These treatments have only recently begun to include biologic therapies, that is,

treatments that interrupt the cancer process and draw on the client's immune system to arrest the disease. For the most part, however, most biologic therapies are still undergoing clinical trials.

For many years, radical mastectomy was the only treatment available for breast cancer. Now, however, studies have shown that lumpectomy followed by radiation therapy, referred to as **breast-conservation treatment,** offers outcomes similar to that of mastectomy. Though it is impossible to remove all of the breast tissue surgically, radiation can treat a far greater area; thus, in a sense, lumpectomy plus radiation is a more thorough treatment. For various reasons, many women still choose mastectomy, however. In some cases—for instance, when there is a large tumor in a small breast or there are microcalcifications throughout the breast—breast-conserving surgery is not an option. Some women choose mastectomy to avoid radiation therapy, either because of its inconvenience (daily treatment for 6 weeks or more) or concern about its long-term effects. It is important for women to know that although radiation therapy does reduce the risk of local recurrence, it has not been shown to increase survival (Lichter & Findlay, 1988).

Breast cancer was once thought to be a localized disease, and radical surgery was believed to be the most effective treatment. Today, however, breast cancer is recognized as a systemic disease; once it has metastasized beyond the breast, systemic treatment is required.

The choice of systemic treatment depends on the woman's age, stage of cancer, and other individual factors. Breast cancer tends to be more aggressive in premenopausal women, probably because of hormonal factors. Thus treatment regimens for premenopausal women are also more aggressive and may even include autologous bone marrow transplant (ABMT) with high-dose chemotherapy.

The earlier breast cancer is detected, the more likely that treatment will be effective in extending survival. Unfortunately, most tumors detected by mammography have been in the body for 8 to 10 years before they are discovered.

Breast Cancer Screening

Optimal screening for breast cancers includes a triad of screening techniques: clinical examination, mammography, and breast self-examination (White & Spitz, 1993). Usually, these techniques are used in combination (Table 48–4). Controversy surrounds mammography. Screening women under age 50 has not been shown to be beneficial; women ages 50 to 74, however, had a 26% reduction in breast cancer deaths compared with those who were not screened (Kerlikowske et al., 1995).

Factors such as discomfort, perceived effectiveness, lack of knowledge, perceived importance, and the desire for control over health have been documented as vari-

Table 48–4	Recommendations for Breast Cancer Screening
Breast self-examination	Performed monthly for all women, beginning at age 20
Clinical breast examination	Performed annually by a physician or nurse practitioner for all women, beginning at age 20
Mammography	Baseline mammogram between ages 40 to 49; annual mammogram after age 50

ables affecting compliance with screening (Kurtz et al., 1993). Some women do not perform breast self-examination because they fear what they will find; indeed, finding a lump that turns out to be malignant seems like negative reinforcement.

Educational messages about breast cancer screening need to be culturally sensitive to the intended audience. Media campaigns promoting mammography often show young white women, an approach that has proved ineffective among women of color. (See the accompanying research box.) By working with women leaders in different racial and cultural groups, nurses can help make breast cancer education more meaningful to women in these groups.

The challenge for nurses is teaching women to learn the landscape of their breasts so that they can recognize any changes. Nurses can help women understand the importance of finding breast cancer at the earliest possible stage. In spite of educational programs, however, not all clients comply with recommended screening guidelines (Sharp, 1993).

Breast Clinical Examination   Clinical breast examination (CBE) is the inspection and palpation of the breasts and axillae performed by a trained health professional. The physical examination includes inspection, palpation, and a check for nipple discharge. This examination is described in detail in Chapter 45.

Screening Mammography   Mammography is a low-dose X-ray study of the breast used to detect breast lesions before they can be felt. Although mammography can detect breast tumors 2 years before they reach palpable size, most of these tumors have been present for 8 to 10 years.

Mammography is not diagnostic; only biopsy can determine whether a lesion is malignant or benign.

Although controversy exists about the ability of screening mammography to improve mortality rates for women under 50, there is a clear benefit for women over 50. Despite this fact, as of 1990, 40% of women over the age of

Applying Research to Nursing Practice: Breast Cancer Screening in African-American Women

■ ■ ■

Because breast cancer is the leading cause of cancer mortality in African-American women, researchers have studied development of culturally sensitive approaches to enhance compliance with recommendations for breast self-examination and mammography screening (Brown & Williams, 1994). Suggestions to increase compliance with screening techniques include reducing cost, increasing accessibility and availability, increasing knowledge, recommending that screening be done, and involving the community.

For older African-American women, other health concerns were of more concern than breast cancer. Black women did not recognize age as a risk factor. The fear of actually finding the cancer and the cancer's social consequences were perceived as barriers to screening.

Implications for Nursing

Nurses need to be aware of cultural beliefs about cancer in general and breast cancer in particular. Working with health professionals from different racial and cultural groups and with women in the affected community can help nurses become more culturally competent in their caregiving.

Critical Thinking in Client Care

1. What is the most effective way to encourage breast cancer awareness among older African-American women?

2. How can an African-American woman cope with the breast cancer experience if her culture treats cancer as a taboo subject?

3. What measures might be necessary to start a breast health program for African-American women based in the community and involving community members in the direction of the program?

50 had never had a screening mammogram (U.S. Department of Health and Human Services, 1992).

Mammography involves compression of breast tissue. Some people may experience pain as a result of this compression, depending on the size of the breast tissue, the

Teaching Breast Self-Examination (BSE)

Step 1   Teach the client to observe her breasts in front of a mirror and in good lighting. Tell her to observe her breasts in four positions:

With her arms relaxed and at her sides

With her arms lifted over her head

With her hands pressed against her hips

With her hands pressed together at her waist, leaning forward

Instruct her to look at each breast individually, and then to compare them. She should observe for any visible abnormalities, such as lumps, dimpling, deviation, recent nipple retraction, irregular shape, edema, discharge, or asymmetry.

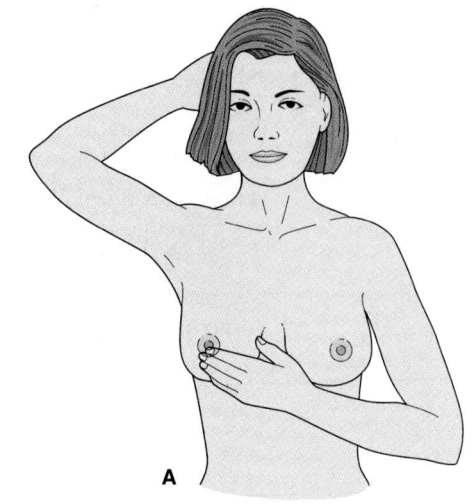

A

Step 2   Teach the client to palpate both breasts while standing or sitting, with one hand behind her head (Figure A). Tell her that many women palpate their breasts in the shower because water and soap make the skin slippery and easier to palpate. Show the woman how to use the pads of her fingers to palpate all areas of her breast, using the concentric circles technique (Figure B). Tell her to press the breast tissue gently against the chest wall, and to be sure to palpate the axillary tail.

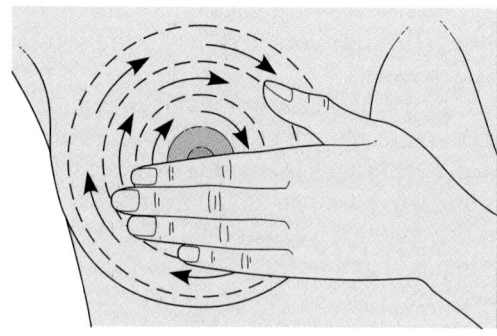

B

Step 3   Instruct the client to palpate her breasts again while lying down, as described in Step 2. Suggest that she place a folded towel under the shoulder and back on the side to be palpated. The arm on the examining side should be over the head, with the hand under the head (Figure C).

Step 4   Teach the client to palpate the areola and nipples next. Show her how to compress the nipple to check for discharge (Figure D).

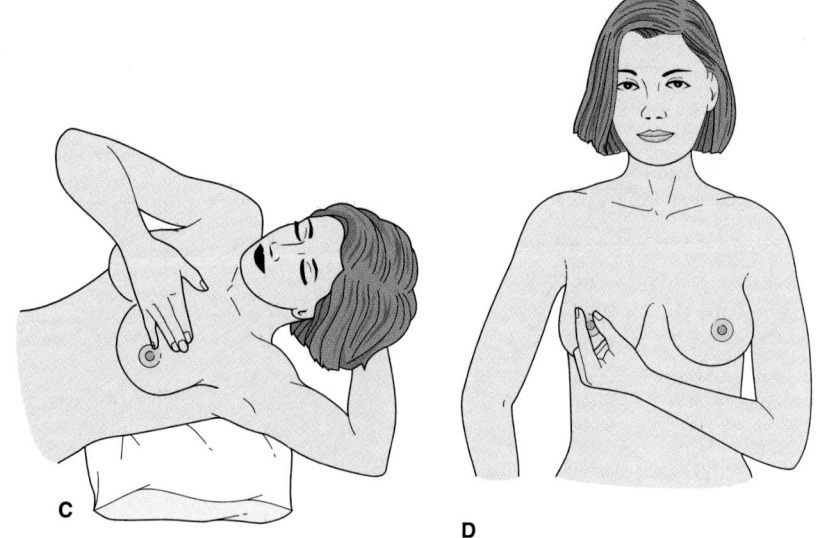

Step 5   Remind the client to use a calendar to keep a record of when she performs BSE. Teach her to perform BSE at the same time each month, usually 5 days after the onset of menses, when there is less hormonal influence on tissues.

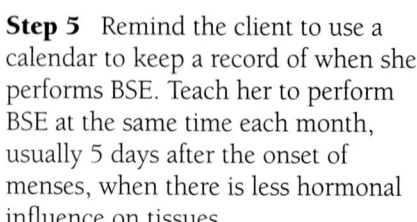

C

D

Figure 48–3

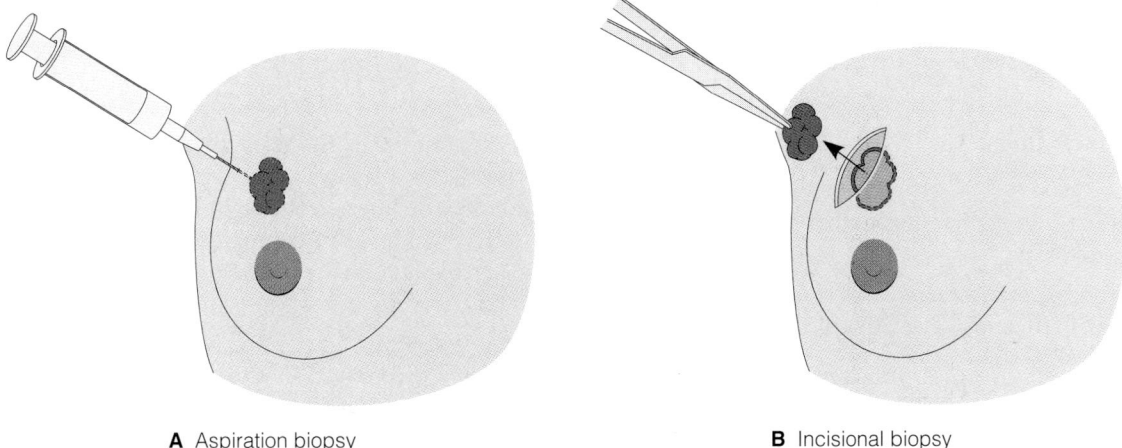

A Aspiration biopsy   **B** Incisional biopsy

Figure 48–4   Types of breast biopsy. *A*, In an aspiration biopsy, a needle is used to aspirate fluid or tissue from the breast. *B*, In an incisional biopsy, tissue from the breast lesion is removed surgically.

degree of breast tenderness, and the person's pain tolerance. Client teaching and preparation for mammography are generally the responsibility of the radiologic technician rather than the nurse.

A mammogram is usually interpreted in one of three ways:

- *Normal,* that is, no suspicious areas seen
- *Indeterminate,* which may indicate that an asymmetric area is suspicious and that a repeat examination is recommended within 3 to 6 months
- *Suspected breast cancer,* which shows findings (such as a mass, an area of microcalcification, or thickening) that suggest malignancy

Breast Self-Examination   Breast self-examination (BSE) is recommended as a means of detecting breast cancer. Almost all breast cancers are detected by the women themselves, often through BSE (Porth, 1994). All women should be taught to perform BSE monthly (Figure 48–3). Premenopausal women should perform BSE after their menstrual period because hormonal changes increase breast tenderness and lumpiness prior to menses. Following inspection of the breasts and nipples for symmetry, breast tissue is palpated in a systematic manner.

Diagnostic Tests

A combination of diagnostic techniques is used to assess breast lesions for possible malignancy. The definitive diagnosis of breast cancer is made by histologic examination of tissue removed from the breast lesion. The following diagnostic studies may be used.

- *Diagnostic mammography* provides a radiographic image of a palpable breast lesion. Depending on the age of the client and the density of her breast tissue, mammography may fail to show the lesion, even though it is palpable.

- *Ultrasonography* uses high-frequency sound waves to obtain a cross-sectional view of the breast. This technique is most useful for distinguishing between solid and cystic masses. It can also aid in interpretation of mammograms by helping to locate lesions within dense breast tissue (Love, 1995).

- *Magnetic resonance imaging (MRI)* uses radiopaque dye, administered intravenously, which is absorbed more thoroughly and quickly in cancers than in benign lesions. Like mammography, MRI is not foolproof, and it is difficult and expensive.

- *Positive emission tomography (PET)* is now being studied for its possible role in detecting breast cancer, particularly its metastasis to distant sites. Before a PET scan, the client is injected with radioactively labeled glucose molecules. These molecules are absorbed much more thoroughly and quickly by cancers than by benign tissues. Like MRI, PET scanning is expensive, and its usefulness in diagnosing breast cancer is still being explored (Love, 1995).

- In a *biopsy,* tissue is removed from the breast lesion for histologic examination to determine if it is cancerous. There are four types of biopsy. Two require only needles, and two require surgical incisions.
  a. In *aspiration biopsy* or *fine-needle aspiration biopsy,* a fine needle is used to remove cells or fluid from the breast lesion (Figure 48–4A). In many facilities, fine-needle aspiration biopsies are performed using a stereotactic biopsy device; mammography and a computer are used to guide the needle.
  b. In *incisional biopsy,* a larger piece of tissue from the breast lesion is removed surgically (Figure 48–4B).
  c. In *excisional biopsy,* the entire breast lesion, plus a margin of tissue surrounding the lesion, is removed surgically.

Nursing Implications for Diagnostic Studies: The Client Undergoing Breast Biopsy

■ ■ ■

Preparation of the Client
All Biopsies

■ Ensure that the client or family member signs an informed consent form.

■ Acknowledge that preoperative anxiety is normal. It is important to remember that 80% of all breast lesions are benign.

■ Ensure continuity of care by taking the client to the operating room and introducing her to the surgical nurse who will be with her during the procedure.

Client and Family Teaching
Aspiration Biopsy (Fine-Needle Aspiration Biopsy)

■ A needle will be used to remove tissue and/or fluid from the breast lesion. This procedure may be done in the surgeon's office and takes only a few minutes.

■ Aspirated tissue is sent for histologic examination to determine whether it is cancerous. Results are sent to the surgeon within a few days.

■ Mild analgesics are usually sufficient to relieve post-biopsy pain.

Stereotactic Core Biopsy (Tru-Cut Biopsy)

■ The client lies face down on a special stereotactic biopsy table with a hole through which her breast protrudes. The breast is anesthetized, the lesion located by mammography, and a computer-guided hollow-core needle enters the breast at high speed and withdraws a core of tissue.

■ The tissue is sent for histologic examination to determine whether it is cancerous. Results are available within 36 hours.

■ Mild analgesics are usually sufficient to relieve post-biopsy pain.

Incisional or Excisional Biopsy

■ The needle-wire localization procedure provides a guide for the surgeon to follow. This procedure involves a mammogram followed by insertion of a hollow needle and one or more wires into the lesion. Dye may be injected through the hollow needle; the dye may cause a stinging sensation. The woman is then taken to the operating room with the wires in place for the biopsy.

■ The biopsy is generally performed in an ambulatory surgery center using local anesthesia. If the client has large breasts or is at high risk for complications, the surgeon may prefer to use the standard operating room.

■ In an incisional biopsy, a section of tissue is removed from the breast lesion and sent for histologic examination.

■ In an excisional biopsy, the entire lesion is removed along with a surrounding margin of normal-looking tissue. The specimen is then sent for mammographic and histologic analysis, to be sure that the entire lesion has been removed and to determine whether it is cancerous.

■ A screen shields the operative area from the client's view. A nurse stands within view of the client to explain what's happening, answer questions, and offer emotional support.

■ If there is any painful sensation, the client needs to ask for additional anesthesia.

■ The surgeon closes the internal incision with absorbable sutures and secures the skin with sutures or tape. A gauze dressing is applied to protect the area.

■ Postoperative pain, bruising, or scarring varies according to the surgeon's technique and the client's tissue. It is helpful to wear a bra and to apply ice packs periodically. Mild analgesics are generally sufficient to control pain.

■ Results of the biopsy are usually available within a few days.

---

d. *Tru-cut* or *core biopsy* is a comparatively new technique. A stereotactic biopsy device is fitted with a large, hollow-core needle to remove one or more cores of tissue from the breast lesion. This technique is rapidly gaining acceptance among surgeons and clients because it is faster, less painful, and more cost effective than conventional incisional or excisional biopsy. Results of the biopsy are available within 36 hours (Love, 1995).

See the accompanying box for the nursing implications of caring for clients undergoing a breast biopsy.

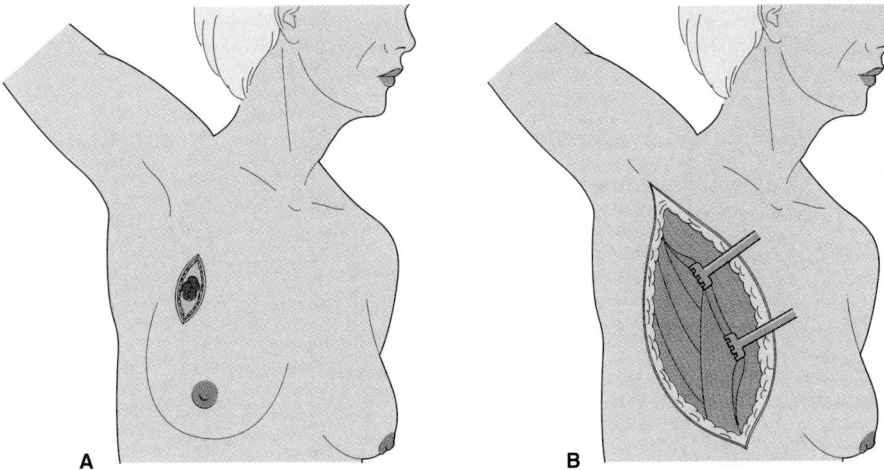

Figure 48–5   Types of mastectomy. *A,* In a lumpectomy, only the tumor and a small margin of surrounding tissue are removed. *B,* In a modified radical mastectomy, all breast tissue and the underarm lymph nodes are removed, but the underlying muscles remain.

■ *Risk Profile Analysis.* New tests are being used at major cancer centers to determine which women might benefit from aggressive therapy. Not all physicians order this series of tests, known collectively as a breast cancer risk profile.

   a. In *the hormone receptor assay,* a tumor is tested to find out whether the cells respond to either estrogen or progesterone. A positive response indicates that the cancer is less aggressive; a negative response indicates a more aggressive cancer. Breast cancer in younger women is more often estrogen-receptor negative; in postmenopausal women, breast cancer is more often estrogen-receptor positive.

   b. *Histologic type* is determined by the microscopic appearance of cancer cells. If cells are more irregular in size and shape, the cancer is more aggressive.

   c. *Nuclear grade* is based on the microscopic appearance of the nucleus of the cancer cell. The more abnormal it appears, the more aggressive the cancer.

   d. In *DNA flow cytometry,* DNA is studied to see whether cells have extra pieces of chromosomes and whether they are synthesizing new DNA quickly. If a high percentage of cells are in the DNA S-phase, early relapse is predicted.

   e. *HER-2 neu* is a protein that is overexpressed by cancers with a high rate of recurrence, particularly in younger women. A monoclonal antibody currently in clinical trials appears to block malignant cell growth.

   f. *Cathepsin D* is a protein secreted by cancer cells to help them metastasize. Oversecretion of this protein is a marker of aggressive cancer.

Radiation Therapy

Radiation therapy is typically used following breast cancer surgery to destroy any remaining cancer cells that could cause recurrence or metastasis. If a tumor is unusually large, radiation may be used to shrink the tumor prior to surgery. Radiation therapy is most commonly used in combination with lumpectomy for early stage (I or II) breast cancer (Osteen & Smith, 1990; Pierce & Harris, 1991; Weissberg, 1990). Palliative radiation therapy is also used to treat chest wall recurrences and some bone metastases to help control pain and prevent fractures. Radiation therapy is administered by means of an external beam or tissue implants.

Surgery

Until recently, the treatment of choice for breast cancer was a radical mastectomy. The recent trend is toward more conservative surgery, although mastectomy is still the treatment of choice in many parts of the country. Surgery is now combined with chemotherapy, hormone therapy, or radiation, depending on the stage of the tumor and the age of the client.

Mastectomy   There are various types of mastectomy for breast cancer. **Radical mastectomy** is the removal of the entire affected breast, the underlying chest muscles, and the lymph nodes under the arms. **Modified radical mastectomy** is the removal of the breast tissue and lymph nodes under the arm (axillary node dissection), leaving the chest wall muscles intact (Figure 48–5B). **Simple mastectomy** is the removal of the complete breast only. **Segmental mastectomy** or **lumpectomy** (Figure 48–5A) is the removal of the tumor and the surrounding margin of breast tissues (ACOG, 1991). See the accompanying

Nursing Care of the Client Having a Mastectomy

NURSING RESPONSIBILITIES

- Ensure that the client or family member signs informed consent form.
- Check hospital policy on withholding food and fluids.
- Administer preoperative medications (analgesics, tranquilizers).
- Provide teaching about turning, coughing, and deep breathing exercises.
- Assess client's pain tolerance using the pinch test and ask her to rate the severity of the pain on a 0 to 10 scale with 10 being the most severe.
- Determine whether client would like to have religious or spiritual support and refer to counselor as appropriate.
- Offer emotional support and continuity of care by accompanying the client to the operating room and introducing her to the surgical nurse.

CLIENT AND FAMILY TEACHING

- Deep-breathing exercises are important because after general anesthesia, it is difficult for air to reach the lungs, particularly with the restrictive surgical dressing that decreases chest expansion.
- A suction apparatus will be placed in the wound to allow drainage of excess body fluids that accumulate when the lymph nodes are removed. This device is usually removed 3 to 5 days after surgery.

- An IV line may be in place for fluid replacement and antibiotics to reduce the risk of postoperative infection.
- Pain can be controlled by analgesics and with proper positioning.
- Note any signs of bleeding on the dressing or on the bedding.
- Numbness or feelings of "pins and needles" in the axillary area are common.
- Lying on one's back or on the side not operated on helps fluid drain from the site.
- Moving the arm on the operated side helps regain mobility; specific exercises will be prescribed for increasing mobility after the incisions have healed.
- If fluid builds up after the drains have been removed, it can be aspirated by the surgeon.
- Use caution about lifting heavy objects with the arm on the operated side.
- Be careful about injury and infection on the affected side; wear rubber gloves when washing dishes, garden gloves when working outside.
- Feelings of anxiety, sadness, and fear of looking at the incision are normal; mastectomy means abrupt change in body image. It is normal to mourn the loss of a breast and to fear the loss of one's life after a cancer diagnosis.
- Sexual intimacy can be affected by mastectomy; it often helps to be able to discuss potential sexual problems with one's partner, with a counselor, or with a breast cancer support group.

box for the nursing implications of caring for the client undergoing mastectomy.

Axillary node dissection is generally performed with all invasive breast carcinoma to stage the tumor. Because this surgery can cause lymphedema, nerve damage, and adhesions, and because of the role of the lymph nodes in immune system function, nonsurgical methods of detecting lymph node involvement are being investigated.

Breast-conservation treatment may be defined as excision of the primary tumor and adjacent breast tissue followed by radiation therapy (NIH Consensus Committee, 1991). Many women are candidates for this procedure; however, women who have multicentric breast neoplasms and those who have large tumors in relation to their breast size are examples of unsuitable candidates.

Selection of clients for this procedure is guided by the need for local control of the lesion, good cosmetic results, and client preference (NIH Consensus Conference, 1991).

Breast Reconstruction Surgery   After a mastectomy, some women may choose to have their breast reconstructed. Some clients report that surgical reconstruction of the breast simplifies their lives and restores their sense of body integrity. Other women choose to use a removable breast prosthesis, and some women are comfortable without reconstruction or a prosthesis.

Breast reconstruction may be performed at the time of the mastectomy or at any time thereafter, depending on the woman's preference. A number of procedures may be used for the breast reconstruction (Figure 48–6). These

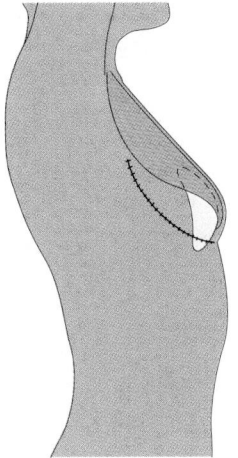
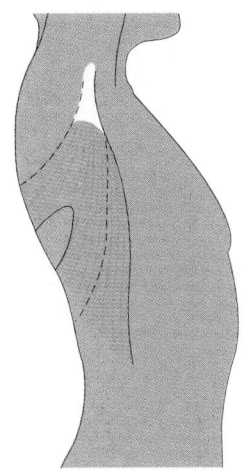
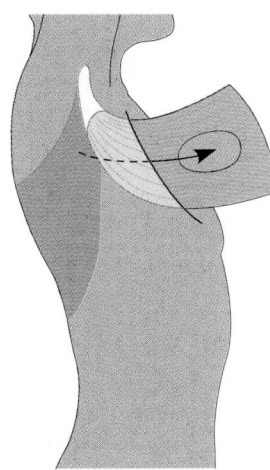

A Implant

B Latissimus dorsi musculocutaneous flap

Figure 48–6   Types of breast reconstruction surgeries. *A*, A breast implant is inserted under the pectoris muscle. *B*, Autogenous procedures transfer a flap of skin, muscle, and fat from the donor site on the client's body to the mastectomy site. The most frequently used donor muscle sites are the latissimus dorsi and the rectus abdominis (the TRAM-flap or trans-rectus abdominis muscle flap).

include placement of a submuscular implant, the use of a tissue expander followed by an implant, the transposition of muscle and blood supply from the abdomen or back, or the creation of a free tissue flap using the gluteus maximus muscle (Henderson, 1991). Nursing implications for the care of clients undergoing breast reconstruction surgery are summarized in the box on page 2050.

Pharmacology

Systemic therapy (chemotherapy, hormone therapy, or biologic therapy) has been used to delay the recurrence of breast cancer in all client groups. Systemic approaches to treatment require individual evaluation of the woman's age, menopausal status, hormone receptor status, and other tumor characteristics.

Chemotherapy   Chemotherapy is the use of cytotoxic drugs to destroy cancer cells. However, these drugs can also interfere with normal cell functions and have many serious side effects. **Adjuvant chemotherapy** has become the standard of care for the majority of breast cancer cases with axillary node involvement. In late metastatic disease, chemotherapy becomes the primary treatment to prolong the client's life. Nursing implications of the use of chemotherapy are presented in Chapter 9.

Hormone Therapy   The purpose of hormone therapy is to shrink the tumor and to delay postsurgical recurrence among women who have cancer that is sensitive to

estrogen or progesterone. Hormone therapy may also be used for clients with metastatic disease; quality of life is often better than with cytotoxic chemotherapy. Nursing implications of the use of hormone therapy are presented in the box on page 2050.

Biologic Therapy   The goal of biologic therapies is to interrupt or reverse the cancer process and boost the body's immune system. For example, to grow beyond 1 cm, a tumor must develop its own blood supply, a process called angiogenesis. If angiogenesis can be interrupted, the tumor cannot grow or spread. Thus anti-angiogenesis drugs are one avenue of hope for the treatment of breast cancer.

Metastasis of Breast Cancer

Once breast cancer has metastasized to other body sites, the primary focus of treatment is palliation of the disease, extending life, and ensuring the comfort of the client. It is important that each woman be given complete, current information about treatment options so that she can make an informed choice that is right for her. In some instances, quality of life takes precedence over quantity of life.

Treatment of metastatic disease involves a number of therapies such as radiation therapy, hormone therapy, chemotherapy, or surgery. These therapies may be used in combination for palliative treatment, depending on the sites of metastases (Hindle, 1990). Clients with bone

Nursing Care of the Client Having Breast Reconstruction Surgery

NURSING RESPONSIBILITIES

- Ensure that the client or family member signs the informed consent form.
- Check hospital policy on withholding food and fluids.
- Administer preoperative medications (analgesics, tranquilizers).
- Provide teaching about turning, coughing, and deep breathing exercises.

CLIENT AND FAMILY TEACHING

- Controversy exists about the health effects of silicone, and research studies are underway to better determine what those health effects are. Since even saline-filled implants are in a silicone shell, some risk may still exist. Symptoms of adverse effects include arthritis, joint pain, or other rheumatic disorders, memory loss, and inability to concentrate.
- Reconstruction can be done immediately after a mastectomy, or at any time later on. Some surgeons believe that delayed reconstruction offers better cosmetic results.
- Reconstructive surgery can create a natural looking breast that makes clothes fit better. Since it has no nerve endings, however, the reconstructed breast has no feeling or sensations.

- If a simple mastectomy is done, an implant approximately the same size as the other breast is placed under the pectoral muscle on the operative side. This creates a breast mound that closely resembles the natural breast in shape and softness. If the implant is placed over the pectoral muscle, a high degree of firmness may occur.
- With a simple mastectomy or modified radical mastectomy, a tissue expander may be used to replace the breast. The tissue expander is placed under the pectoral muscle and gradually expanded with saline injections every two to three weeks to stretch the overlying skin and create a pocket. After a period of time, usually one to two months, the tissue expander is exchanged for a saline implant (Cohen & Turner, 1987).
- With more extensive surgery such as radical mastectomy, a flap of skin, fat, or muscle is transferred from a donor site to the operative area. A new nipple may be created by using tissue from the opposite nipple or from the inner thigh.
- Reconstructive surgery may require multiple surgeries, including all the risks associated with anesthesia. As the complexity of the procedures increases, so does the risk of complications such as infection.
- To decrease the risk of a fibrous capsule forming around the implant, it is important to perform breast massage as instructed.

Nursing Implications for Pharmacology: Clients Receiving Hormone Therapy for Breast Cancer

SYSTEMIC AGENTS

Tamoxifen (Nolvadex)

Tamoxifen is the most widely prescribed breast cancer drug, commonly given to prevent recurrence of estrogen-positive breast cancer in postmenopausal women. It inhibits tumor growth by blocking the estrogen receptor sites of cancer cells.

NURSING RESPONSIBILITIES

- Assess the client for potential contraindications to therapy.

CLIENT AND FAMILY TEACHING

- If you can have children, use a nonhormonal, barrier form of contraception; tamoxifen has shown DES-like effects on the developing fetus.
- Take the drug as prescribed until the physician indicates otherwise or until side effects preclude the continuation of therapy.
- Report any adverse effects to the physician: vaginal bleeding or spotting if you are postmenopausal, vision changes, leg pain (indicating possible thromboembolic disease). Annual endometrial biopsies are recommended for women taking tamoxifen along with regular liver function tests.

Applying Research to Nursing Practice: How Breast Cancer in Young Women Affects Interpersonal and Family Relations

■ ■ ■

Breast cancer is a stressful experience for all women, but according to the findings of this study, young women may be particularly at risk (Northouse, 1994). Diagnosed with a life-threatening illness, they may also need to cope with children, a spouse, and often employment outside the home. A diagnosis of breast cancer and the subsequent treatment affect the young woman in all of her roles as wife, mother, homemaker, and employee. Studies show that young husbands reported more difficulty and stress in adjusting to changed roles than older husbands. Children's ability to adjust after their mother's breast cancer diagnosis depends on the developmental level of the child. Adolescent daughters appeared to be at special risk for relationship problems, perhaps because of the daughter's fear of inheriting the disease.

Implications for Nursing

Unless a woman lives alone, breast cancer is always a family issue. The younger the woman's age at diagnosis, the more difficult it is for her to confront the possibility of losing her breast and, most importantly, her life. Nurses need to remember to include the spouse whenever possible in all aspects of care (including teaching) and all phases of the disease, provided both partners are willing. It is also important to involve other family members, particularly any children old enough to assist with caregiving or filling in for the mother while she is recovering. Nurses can provide a vital link between the woman, her family, and community resources.

Critical Thinking in Client Care

1. Consider how the diagnosis of breast cancer affects a 35-year-old single parent with two small children for whom she is the sole financial support.

2. How does breast cancer affect the marital relationship from the woman's perspective? From the man's perspective?

3. How can breast cancer treatment affect sex and intimacy?

4. What emotions might an adolescent daughter feel when she learns that her mother has breast cancer? How would you help her cope with those feelings?

---

metastasis may experience pathologic fractures, chronic pain, and hypercalcemia. Clients with pulmonary metastasis may experience alterations in lung ventilation. Brain metastasis may cause alterations in sensory perception (Nielson & East, 1990).

Nursing Care

In planning and implementing holistic nursing care for the client with breast cancer, the nurse must consider the client's individual needs. This section addresses possible nursing diagnoses for the woman, both preoperatively and postoperatively.

Although each client has individual needs, nursing diagnoses prior to surgery are concerned with anxiety, decisional conflict, knowledge deficit, and sometimes anticipatory grief over the loss of a breast. Because the typical hospital stay is short, usually 2 to 3 days, preoperative teaching is done on an outpatient basis.

Anxiety

The client with breast cancer is at risk for anxiety because of the fear of surgery, the outcome of surgery if nodal involvement is found, the cancer itself, and the possible changes in sexual and family relationships. Studies show that young women with breast cancer, a growing population, are particularly vulnerable for anxiety and other psychosocial effects, as are their spouses and their children. See the accompanying box.

Nursing interventions with rationales follow:

- Provide opportunities for the client to express her thoughts and feelings. *In this process, the woman can name her fears. Once the fears are named, the nurse may simply listen, educate, or dispel fears that stem from lack of understanding.*

- Discuss with the client her knowledge of breast cancer. *Assessing the client's knowledge of breast cancer helps the nurse plan more effective client teaching.*

- Have the client discuss her immediate concerns about resuming her life at home and the changes she must make. *Anticipatory guidance can help the client plan for and cope with changes in her life and relationships.*

- Explain the surgical procedure. Tell the client what to expect regarding preoperative medications, anesthesia, and recovery. *Knowing what to expect helps to decrease anxiety.*

- Discuss that it is normal to have decreased sensation in the surgical area. *Severed or damaged nerves reduce sensation.*

Decisional Conflict

The woman with breast cancer must make life-changing decisions about treatment within a relatively brief and highly stressful time. Her age, menopausal status, and stage of cancer are only some of the factors that affect her decisions. Culture, values, life-style, socioeconomic status, and self-esteem also are considered.

Nursing interventions with rationales follow:

- Provide an opportunity for the client to ask questions; answer questions as simply and directly as possible. Make eye contact with the client and pay attention to body language. *During this time, the client can process information and make informed decisions.*

- Focus on immediate concerns, and provide up-to-date written material for the client to review. *Written material provides easy reference to information not processed immediately because of anxiety and stress.*

- Listen to the client in a nonjudgmental manner during her decision-making process. *Nonjudgmental, empathic listening helps the client process information and make informed decisions. Only she knows the context of her life.*

- If the client wishes, provide opportunities for her to meet with other women who have had breast cancer surgery. *Not all clients are ready to meet others in their situation, but opening the door to this resource is appropriate. The client may choose to talk with these women after the surgery.*

- Facilitate a team approach with the surgeon, anesthesiologist, oncologist, plastic surgeon, and other health professionals. *Being the client's advocate during this time of anxiety and decision making reduces the stress of coordinating multiple health care provider schedules.*

Anticipatory Grieving

Breast surgery, even lumpectomy, alters the appearance of the breast. This loss is expressed through grief.

Nursing interventions with rationales follow:

- Listen attentively to client's expression of grief and watch for nonverbal cues (failure to make eye contact, crying, silence). *Not all women will express grief clearly; sometimes unspoken grief is the most painful. Grief is relieved only when expressed in a nonthreatening environment.*

- Allow time to interact with client; do not rush interactions. *Taking time to be with the client communicates caring.*

- Explain that it is normal to have periods of depression, anger, and denial after breast surgery. *All these feelings are appropriate expressions of grief.*

- If the client wishes, involve the partner in helping the woman cope with her grief. Remember that the partner may also be grieving. *Not all clients want to share their grief, and not all partners are interested and supportive.*

Recovery from breast cancer surgery, regardless of the surgical procedure performed, requires time and energy. Nursing care focuses on maximizing rest and supporting the client. After discharge, the client is encouraged to engage in self-care.

Risk for Infection

Like any surgical client, the woman who has breast surgery is at risk for infection. Removal of lymph nodes and the presence of a draining wound increase the risk.

Nursing interventions with rationales follow:

- Assess the surgical dressings for bleeding, drainage, color, and odor every 4 hours for 24 hours and document your findings. Circle any visible bleeding and drainage on the dressing as a baseline for subsequent assessment. *Excessive bleeding or drainage signals postoperative complications that may require emergency attention.*

- Observe the incision and IV sites for pain, redness, swelling, and drainage. Assess the drainage system for patency and adequate suction; note the color and amount of drainage. *Careful observation for any signs of infection is essential because the client's immune system is compromised. IV catheters should be placed on the uninvolved side only to minimize risk of infection.*

- Change dressings and IV tubing using aseptic technique and document. *Moist dressings and intravenous tubing provide sites for bacterial growth. Routine dressing and IV tubing changes using aseptic technique reduce the risk for infection.*

- Encourage the client to eat a protein-rich diet. Discuss the client's nutritional status with the dietitian and request a consultation for the client. *Adequate nutrition promotes healing and boosts the immune system.*

- Teach the client how to care for the drainage system, (clean the site, empty the device, and record the amount, color, and type of drainage). *The client is often discharged prior to removal of the drainage system and dressings and needs teaching to provide self-care.*

- At discharge, teach the client to watch for signs and symptoms of infection: fever, redness or hardness at the surgical site, or purulent drainage. Any of these manifestations should be reported to the physician/surgeon. *Knowing the signs and symptoms of infection prepares the client to seek prompt treatment if infection occurs.*

- Explain that the client may experience scaling, flaking, dryness, itching, rash, or dry desquamation of the skin, particularly after radiation therapy. *Impaired skin integrity increases the risk of infection.*
- Tell the client to avoid deodorants and talcum powder on the affected side until the incision is completely healed. *These substances may irritate the skin and impede healing.*

Risk for Injury

Removal of the lymph nodes puts the client at risk for injury and long-term complications such as lymphedema and infection.

Nursing interventions with rationales follow:

- When obtaining blood pressure readings, use the non-surgical side. *Compression of the arm on the surgical side may cause lymphedema.*
- Elevate the affected arm on a pillow. *Elevating the arm permits drainage, prevents swelling, and promotes circulation.*
- Measure the circumference of the affected arm and document any numbness or tingling. *Measurements provide a baseline for subsequent assessment; numbness or tingling indicates nerve damage, some of which may resolve in time.*
- Elevate the affected arm higher than shoulder, but do not abduct it; the hand should be higher than the elbow. *This position helps ensure adequate lymph drainage.*
- Encourage range-of-motion exercises in the affected arm. *Exercise helps develop collateral drainage.*
- Teach the client to protect the affected arm and hand: avoid constricting sleeves, avoid lifting heavy objects, use a heavy oven mitt or potholder when cooking, and promptly apply antibiotic ointment to any cut or burn. Wear gloves when working in the yard or garden to prevent skin injury. *These measures help prevent infection and lymphedema.*

Risk for Body Image Disturbance

Breast surgery can change the client's sense of body image. The surgical changes may be compounded by weight gain and other side effects of chemotherapy or hormone therapy. Self-esteem also affects adjustment to a changed body image.

Nursing interventions with rationales follow:

- Encourage the client to verbalize her thoughts and feelings. *Talking about her thoughts and feelings helps the client work through the changes that have happened and will continue to happen.*
- Assess how the woman views her body. *Discuss with the client what image of herself she had prior to surgery. Self-image is related to self-esteem. Discuss whether her self-image has changed.*

- Explain that redness and swelling will fade with time. *The knowledge that the scar will fade may give the client a more realistic view of the changes.*
- Include the partner and family if possible when discussing the plan of care and ADLs. Request consultation with a psychologist or other professional if client is interested. *Discussion with the partner and family can facilitate the client's emotional healing process.*
- Offer pamphlets and suggest books and videos that might increase the client's understanding of what lies ahead; document her response. *Knowing what to expect can help the client cope.*
- Offer referral to support groups with women experiencing similar problems. Some women may prefer one-on-one counseling. *Support is sometimes best provided by people who share a similar experience.*
- Encourage the client to look at her incision when she feels ready; often the reality is not as frightening as the client had imagined. Explain that it is normal to be afraid to look. *Reassurance that her behavior is normal decreases the client's anxiety.*
- Make it clear that it is up to the client to decide whether and how she will involve others in her care. *Only she knows when she is ready to share this experience with others.*
- Let the client know that there is no rush in deciding about a prosthesis or reconstruction; she may choose neither. *She needs time to heal, physically and emotionally, before making these decisions.*
- If the client is interested in breast reconstruction, provide written material and encourage her to talk with a plastic surgeon and with women who have had reconstruction. *She should be fully informed about available options.*

Other Nursing Diagnoses

The following nursing diagnoses may also be appropriate for clients with breast cancer:

- *Pain* related to surgery
- *Self-Esteem Disturbance* related to loss of a breast
- *Sleep Pattern Disturbance* related to pain

Client and Family Teaching

Postoperative Exercises

Early and limited postoperative exercises are important and should be started within 24 hours after surgery. The client should begin with hand and wrist extension and flexion. She should also extend the elbow hourly.

Encourage the client to perform ADLs, such as eating, combing her hair, and washing her face. If wound drains are present, tell the client not to abduct the arm or raise

Figure 48–7 Postmastectomy exercises. *A,* Wall climbing: Stand facing wall with toes 6 to 12 inches from wall. Bend elbows and place palms against wall at shoulder level. Gradually move both hands up the wall parallel to each other until incisional pulling or pain occurs. (Mark that spot on wall to measure progress.) Work hands down to shoulder level. Move closer to wall as height of reach improves. *B,* Overhead pulley: Using operated arm, toss 6-foot rope over shower curtain rod (or over top of a door that has a nail in the top to hold the rope in place for the exercise). Grasp one end of rope in each hand. Slowly raise operated arm as far as comfortable by pulling down on the rope on opposite side. Keep raised arm close to your head. Reverse to raise unoperated arm by lowering the operated arm. Repeat. *C,* Rope turning: Tie rope to door handle. Hold rope in hand of operated side. Back away from door until arm is extended away from body, parallel to floor. Swing rope in as wide a circle as possible. Increase size of circle as mobility returns. *D,* Arm swings: Stand with feet 8 inches apart. Bend forward from waist, allowing arms to hang toward floor. Swing both arms up to sides to reach shoulder level. Swing back to center, then cross arms at center. Do not bend elbows. If possible, do this and other exercises in front of mirror to ensure even posture and correct motion.

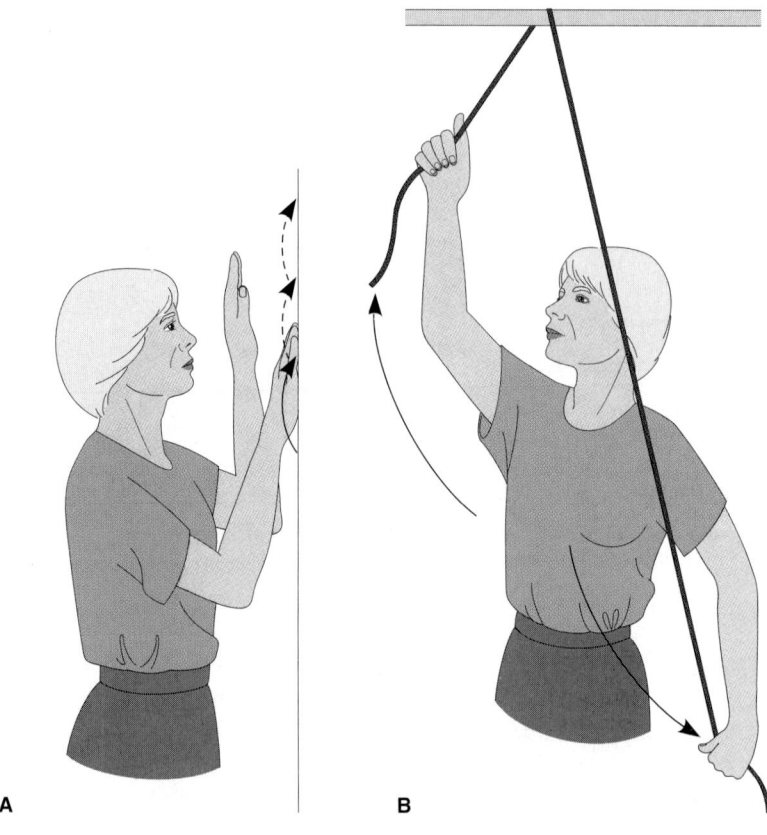

A

B

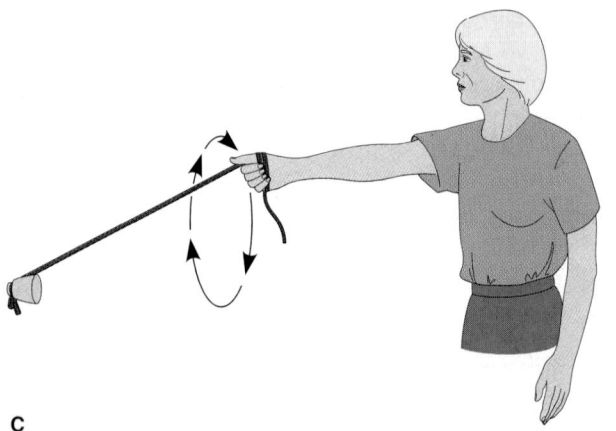

C

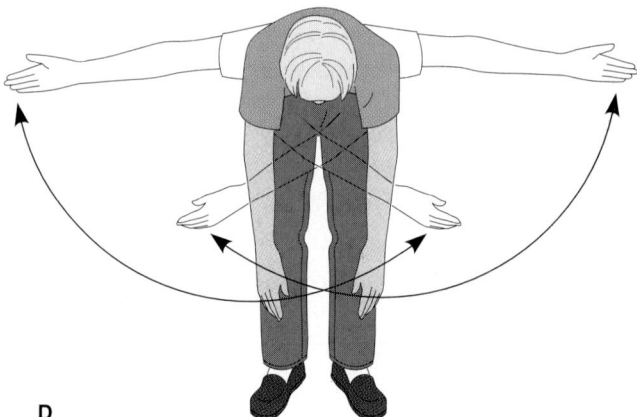

D

the elbow above the shoulder height until the drains are removed.

When the wound healing is complete and axillary drains have been removed, abduction and external rotation of the upper arm may begin. Activities that encompass complete range of motion include vacuuming and dusting. Postmastectomy exercises—wall climbing, overhead pulley, rope turning, and arm swings—have similar benefits (Figure 48–7). Forward and lateral elevation of

the arms may also increase function. Exercises should be discussed with physicians and physical therapists.

Self-Care

Adequate rest and emotional support remain important to promote healing and recovery. Both radiation and chemotherapy can cause fatigue and other symptoms. Learning what relieves those symptoms is part of self-care.

Participation in a breast cancer support group offers the opportunity to share thoughts, feelings, experiences, and information about treatments, side effects, insurance problems, and other practical aspects of living with breast cancer. Women with access to computers find on-line information services and bulletin boards to be helpful sources of education and support.

Inherent in a diagnosis of breast cancer is the possibility of recurrence, either as a second primary tumor or as metastasis of cancer cells from the original site. Recognizing the signs of possible recurrence allows the client to seek prompt treatment and prevent disease progression.

Breast cancer most often metastasizes to the lungs, liver, and bones. A dry, persistent cough or shortness of breath could signal lung metastasis. Metastasis to the liver tends to be asymptomatic until the cancer is advanced; occasionally, jaundice or pain in the upper right quadrant of the abdomen may occur. Pain in the hips, thighs, back, or ribs may indicate bone metastasis. In addition, any lumps in the area of the incision, around the collarbone, or under the arm should be promptly investigated.

Nutrition

A wholesome, balanced diet helps the client to recover strength and energy and also to deal with the effects of treatment, particularly chemotherapy. Maintaining body weight while on chemotherapy can be difficult because of the resultant nausea and vomiting, but women have learned some practical solutions. For example, many women on chemotherapy find that cold foods are more appetizing and more easily digested than hot foods.

Vitamin supplements can also help promote healing and recovery. Vitamins A, C, and E, the anti-oxidant vitamins, have been shown to have significant protective effects against cancer in research studies and should be considered in cancer treatment as well. Vitamin C has also been shown to be beneficial for people undergoing radiation and chemotherapy (Hanck, 1988; Okunieff, 1990).

Prosthesis Management

Some women may elect not to have breast reconstructive surgery and choose to use a prosthesis instead. Women should be advised that a temporary lightweight prosthesis may be worn immediately after the drains and sutures have been removed from the surgical site.

Because prostheses are expensive, a permanent prosthesis should not be purchased until the wound has completely healed. Prostheses are available at medical stores and many larger department stores. Most private and government insurance policies pay for the first prosthesis.

Gerontologic Considerations

Although the incidence of breast cancer is increasing among premenopausal women, it is still primarily a disease of older women. The risk increases with age; more than 60% of all breast cancers are diagnosed in women age 50 and older. However, the needs of older women with breast cancer have been inadequately addressed in the professional literature and in the popular media (Ludwick et al., 1994).

Women between the ages of 50 and 65 are the group most likely to benefit from annual screening mammography, yet many women in this age group have never had a mammogram. Failure of physicians to refer older women for mammography is the reason most frequently cited for this statistic; female physicians are more likely to refer women for mammography (Lurie et al., 1993). Promotional campaigns for mammography send a confusing message by showing images of women in their 20s and 30s for whom mammography is largely ineffective, rather than women in older age groups who are more likely to benefit from mammography.

For too long, mastectomy was perceived as the only treatment option open to most older women with breast cancer, even those with early-stage disease. Slowly that perception is changing as breast-conservation treatment gains greater acceptance. One study found that breast-conserving surgery was performed on 36% of clients under age 30 but only on 30% of clients over age 50. Modified radical mastectomy was performed on 51% of women under age 30 but on 65% of women over 50 (Osteen et al., 1994). The choice of surgical treatment, particularly for older women, is highly individual. Many older women wish to preserve their breasts.

Although older women with breast cancer may experience co-existing chronic illnesses and impaired physical function, the limited research available suggests that they show lower levels of emotional distress than younger women (Mor, Malin, & Allen, 1994). Obviously the need for services such as personal care, shopping, housekeeping, and transportation increases as the ages of the client and the caregiver increase.

Applying the Nursing Process

Case Study of a Client with Breast Cancer: Rachel Clemments

Rachel Clemments is a 42-year-old mother of two, Sarah, age 12, and Jennifer, age 18. Because of a family history of breast cancer, she has been closely monitored (annual mammograms and clinical breast examination, monthly BSE, a needle aspiration biopsy with negative findings) for 4 years prior to her diagnosis. In spite of careful monitoring, however, an incisional biopsy reveals invasive lobular carcinoma in the left breast. Modified radical mastectomy is performed; histologic examination shows a 3-cm tumor; axillary node dissection shows that 4 of 16 lymph nodes are positive.

Assessment

During the history, Laura Nelson, RN, the nurse admitting Rachel Clemments, learns that Ms. Clemments's mother, two of her aunts, and one sister had been diagnosed with breast cancer. Her mother and one of the aunts died before age 45. Painfully aware of her elevated risk, Ms. Clemments has consulted a leading breast surgeon for early, regular monitoring of her breast health. Physical assessment findings include T, 98.5 (37.0 C); BP, 110/62; P, 65; R, 14. Her weight is 120 lb (54 kg); she is 5'6" (168 cm) tall. A doctoral student in sociology and a competitive runner, she had just finished running a marathon the week before she discovered a thickened area in her left breast while performing BSE. Even though annual mammograms have shown no evidence of disease and needle aspiration biopsy shows no cancerous cells, an incisional biopsy reveals the malignancy. One week later, a modified radical mastectomy and axillary node sampling are performed. Ms. Clemments is debating whether to have reconstructive breast surgery. Also, her oncologist has recommended a 6-month course of adjuvant chemotherapy, and she is concerned about side effects. One of her greatest concerns is how her illness will affect her ability to support and care for her daughters. She is afraid that recovering from the mastectomy and completing the chemotherapy regimen will limit her ability to keep her part-time job, complete her academic work, and continue to meet the needs of her daughters. Also, this breast cancer diagnosis seems part of the family legacy. She wonders, "When will it happen to Jennifer? To Sarah?"

Diagnosis

Ms. Nelson identifies the following nursing diagnoses for Rachel Clemments:

- *Risk for Infection* related to surgical incision
- *Altered Tissue Perfusion* related to edema
- *Pain* related to surgery
- *Body Image Disturbance* related to loss of breast
- *Decisional Conflict* about treatment related to concerns about risks and benefits
- *Altered Family Processes* related to effect of surgery and therapy on family roles and relationships
- *Fear* related to disease process/prognosis

Expected Outcomes

The expected outcomes for the plan of care are that Ms. Clemments will

- Remain free of infection.
- Maintain adequate tissue perfusion.
- Experience minimal pain or discomfort during her recovery.

- Maintain a positive body image, regardless of her decision about reconstruction.
- Evaluate the treatment options in relation to personal values and decide on a course of action.
- Together with her daughters, acknowledge the need for a change in family roles during her illness and identify new coping patterns.
- Identify the sources of her fear and demonstrate behaviors that may reduce fears.

Planning and Implementation

The following nursing interventions are planned and implemented for Ms. Clemments:

- Teach her about postoperative turning, coughing, and deep breathing.
- Discuss the postoperative drainage device and its management after she goes home.
- Assess her pain tolerance and administer preoperative and postoperative medications as ordered.
- Teach her to use caution when moving the arm on the operated side, to avoid lifting heavy objects, and to wear gloves when gardening.
- Encourage her to discuss her thoughts and feelings about her body changes.
- Suggest that she talk with a Reach to Recovery volunteer about her thoughts and feelings.
- Assess her interest in spiritual/religious support and refer if appropriate.
- Discuss medication and dietary changes that will minimize the effects of chemotherapy; request a consultation with the dietitian.
- Provide a list of educational resources about chemotherapy and breast reconstruction.
- Discuss the use of a temporary prosthesis and later the fitting of a permanent prosthesis (6 to 8 weeks after surgery), the need to be fitted by an experienced person, and insurance reimbursement for the prosthesis.
- Encourage Ms. Clemments to discuss reconstructive surgery with a plastic surgeon, emphasizing that it can be done at any time after the mastectomy.
- Discuss the possibility of attending a breast cancer support group where she can draw on the experiences of other women who have undergone mastectomy, chemotherapy, or radiation.
- Refer her and her daughters to social services for a consultation about the changed family roles during her recovery and treatment.
- Encourage her to verbalize her fears about her own prognosis and about her daughters' future risk of

breast cancer; assess the need/interest for referral to psychologic counseling.

■ Teach her about dietary and life-style changes that can help reduce the risk of breast cancer for her daughters (low-fat, high-fiber diet; regular exercise; avoidance of obesity, alcohol, and oral contraceptives).

Evaluation

At discharge, Ms. Clemments has no signs of physical complications and is looking forward to being at home with her daughters as temporary caregivers. Together they decide to try a vegetarian diet and buy a new vegetarian cookbook. Ms. Clemments has met with a Reach to Recovery volunteer, who brought her a temporary prosthesis and booklets about postmastectomy exercises, chemotherapy, and breast reconstruction. The volunteer also referred her to a local breast cancer support group. Ms. Clemments has talked about her concerns related to breast reconstruction, which center on the possible health risks of silicone. "I want to wait and talk with women who

have had TRAM-flap reconstruction before I decide," she said. "I want to avoid anything that would increase the risk of complications. The possibility of recurrence and my fear for my daughters' future health are more than enough to worry about."

Critical Thinking in the Nursing Process

1. How can a vegetarian diet help reduce the risk of breast cancer?

2. What role could genetic counseling play in helping Ms. Clemments and her daughters better understand the daughters' risk of breast cancer?

3. Describe the types of mastectomies and their implications for nursing care.

4. What medications might help minimize the side effects of chemotherapy?

5. Develop a plan of care for Ms. Clemments for the nursing diagnosis *Sleep Pattern Disturbance*.

▪ ▪ ▪ Benign Disorders of the Breast ▪ ▪ ▪

Benign breast disorders occur frequently in women and are a source of anxiety. Changes in a woman's breast tissue often correspond to hormonal changes of the menstrual cycle. Most women notice increased tenderness and lumpiness prior to menses. (For this reason, it is best to perform BSE after the menstrual period.) Breast tissue is always changing in response to hormonal, nutritional, physical, and/or environmental stimuli (Porth, 1994). More than half of all women who menstruate regularly will find a lump in the breast; 80% of these lumps are not cancerous. Benign breast disorders include fibrocystic breast changes, fibroadenomas, intraductal papillomas, duct ectasia, fat necrosis, and mastitis (Table 48–5).

The Client with Fibrocystic Breast Changes

▪ ▪ ▪

Pathophysiology

Fibrocystic changes, which include swelling, pain, tenderness, and lumpiness, are collectively called "fibrocystic disease." These benign changes in the female breast are not a disease but a natural result of aging and hormonal changes in breast tissue. Fibrocystic changes are common in women 30 to 50 years of age (Way, 1994) and rare in postmenopausal women.

Women experience bilateral or unilateral pain or tenderness in the upper, outer quadrants of their breasts. Clients report that their breasts feel particularly thick and lumpy the week prior to menses. Nipple discharge may be present. Pain is due to edema of the connective tissue of the breast, dilation of the ducts, and some inflammatory response; some women report an increase in breast size (ACOG, 1991b). Multiple, mobile cysts may form, usually in both breasts (Figure 48–8). Fluid aspirated

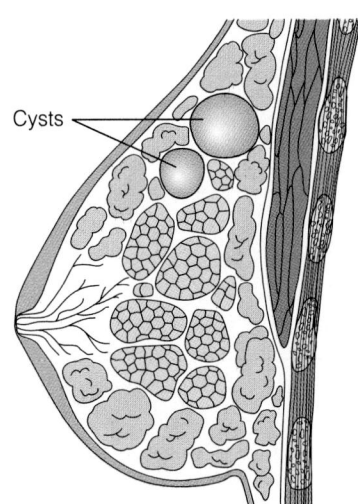

Cysts

Figure 48–8 Fibrocystic breast changes.

Table 48-5 Summary of Common Breast Disorders

Condition	Age	Pain	Nipple Discharge	Location	Consistency and Mobility	Diagnosis and Treatment
Duct ectasia	35 to 55 years; median age 40	Burning around nipple	Sticky, multi-colored; usually bilateral	No specific location	Retroareolar mass with advanced disease	Open biopsy; local excision of diseased portion of breast
Fibroadenoma	15 to 39 years; median age 20	No	No	No specific location	Mobile, firm, smooth, well delineated mass	Mammography, surgical or needle biopsy; excision of the tumor
Fibrocystic breast disease	20 to 49 years; median age 30 (may subside with menopause)	Yes	No	Upper outer quadrant	Bilateral multiple lumps influenced by the menstrual cycle	Needle aspiration; observation; biopsy if there is an unresolved mass or mammographic changes
Intraductal papilloma	35 to 55 years; median age 40	Yes	Serous or sanguineous; usually unilateral from one duct	No specific location	Usually soft, poorly delineated mass	Pap smear of nipple discharge; biopsy; wedge resection
Mastitis, acute	Childbearing years	Tenderness, pain	No	No specific location	Generalized redness of overlying skin	Antibiotic therapy; incision and drainage if mastitis progresses to an abscess
Mastitis, chronic	Any age	Tenderness, pain; headache; high fever	No	No specific location	Generalized redness and swelling	Antibiotics, usually penicillin
Fat necrosis	Any age	Tenderness	No	No specific location	Firm, irregular, palpable	Surgical biopsy to rule out cancer

from these cysts ranges in color from milky white to yellow, brown, or green. Unless the fluid is tinged with blood, there is no reason to suspect malignancy.

Fibrocystic changes may be classified as nonproliferative changes, proliferative changes without atypical cells, and proliferative changes with atypical cells.

Nonproliferative changes may be cystic or fibrous. Cystic change refers to the dilation of ducts in the subareolar, lobular, or lobe areas. Cysts often go unnoticed unless there is pain and tenderness associated with the menses. Fibrous changes are very infrequent but can occur during the menstrual years. A firm, palpable mass, 2 to 3 cm in size, is typically located in the upper outer

breast quadrant following an inflammatory response to ductal irritation (ACOG, 1991b).

Proliferative changes without atypical cells do not increase a woman's risk of developing breast cancer. Proliferative changes with atypical hyperplasia can occur; these changes are associated with an increased risk of developing breast cancer.

Collaborative Care

Diagnosis of fibrocystic breast changes is based on complete history, physical examination, and imaging studies. A biopsy may be required for diagnosis.

Several types of treatment have been tried to palliate the symptoms of fibrocystic changes. Oral contraceptives, progesterone, synthetic androgen, tamoxifen, vitamin E, and special diets have been tried, but none has emerged as a definitive treatment (Reifsnider, 1990; Love, 1995). Some women report that eliminating caffeine and chocolate from the diet ameliorates symptoms; both contain methylxanthines, believed to contribute to fibrocystic changes. Women who smoke report a reduction in breast lumps when they quit smoking. Aspirin, mild analgesics, and local heat or cold also are recommended (Hockenberger, 1993; Porth, 1994). Some clients report that the extra support of a well-fitted bra affords relief.

Nursing Care

When a woman presents with a breast mass, nursing responsibilities include taking a careful history and facilitating follow-up care. If a palpable mass is present, it is important to ask how long the lesion has been present and whether the client has noticed any pain associated with the mass, any change in its size, and any changes in association with the menstrual cycle.

In many cases, definitive diagnosis of the breast disorder requires surgical biopsy to rule out cancer. During the diagnostic process, the nurse can provide emotional support and education about diagnostic and therapeutic procedures, self-care and comfort measures, and resources to help the woman cope with the experience.

Applying the Nursing Process

Case Study of a Client with Fibrocystic Breast Changes: Sharon Turner

Sharon Turner is a 36-year-old single woman who is vice-president of a biotechnology company. She reports frequent breast tenderness and swelling prior to menses and has discovered a lump in the upper outer quadrant of her right breast. No fluid is apparent on aspiration biopsy of the lesion, and a mammogram shows no abnormalities. The surgeon has scheduled an excisional biopsy to rule out malignancy.

Assessment

Jane Martin, RN, the nurse admitting Sharon Turner, takes the history, which shows no known cancer in Ms. Turner's family. Menarche occurred at age 12, followed by an uncomplicated menstrual history. Ms. Turner has never been pregnant; she took oral contraceptives during college but has not taken them since age 22. She works out at a gym twice a week and eats a well-balanced diet, but she calls herself a "chocoholic" and drinks several cups of coffee during the day. She has had a history of breast tenderness and lumpiness. "My doctor calls it fibrocystic disease." Cysts were aspirated on three separate occasions to rule out cancer. "This new lump feels different, harder than the others. Maybe I'm scared because a close friend my age was just diagnosed with breast cancer," she states.

Diagnosis

The following nursing diagnoses are established by the nurses caring for Ms. Turner:

- *Risk for Infection* related to interrupted skin integrity
- *Pain* related to cystic breast changes
- *Anxiety* related to possible cancer diagnosis
- *Knowledge Deficit* regarding factors contributing to cystic breast changes

Expected Outcomes

The expected outcomes for the plan of care are that Ms. Turner will

- Remain free of infection.
- Experience minimal postoperative discomfort.
- Verbalize a decrease in anxiety if the breast lesion proves to be benign.
- Demonstrate understanding of dietary changes, nutritional therapies, and comfort measures that could help relieve the symptoms of fibrocystic breast changes.

Planning and Implementation

The nursing care measures described for the client having a biopsy, outlined in the box on page 2046, apply to Ms. Turner. In addition, these interventions are planned and implemented for Ms. Turner:

- Tell Ms. Turner that anxiety before a biopsy is normal and that 80% of breast lumps are benign. Explain that, unless the biopsy shows atypical cells, fibrocystic changes have not been shown to increase the risk of breast cancer.
- Explain that fibrocystic changes are not a "disease" but normal changes, probably influenced by hormonal cycles and aging, that are common in premenopausal women.
- Teach her that eliminating caffeine and chocolate from her diet, especially right before her menstrual period, and taking a vitamin E supplement (400 IU) may offer relief of the swelling and tenderness.
- Suggest that if dietary measures do not help, there are medications (danazol or tamoxifen) that might prove effective. Both these drugs can have serious side effects: danazol has virilizing effects, and tamoxifen can induce premature menopause. Long-term effects of tamoxifen in premenopausal women have not yet been determined.

Evaluation

At discharge, Ms. Turner is still anxious because the surgeon has not received the pathology report. When the report arrives the following day, however, it brings good news: Benign. Much relieved, Ms. Turner expresses her willingness to try decreasing or eliminating caffeine and chocolate from her diet and adding a vitamin E supplement. "I'm willing to make sacrifices if it will make a difference," she says. "Biopsies are too expensive and too nerve-wracking to repeat."

Critical Thinking in the Nursing Process

1. Describe the types of nonproliferative and proliferative fibrocystic breast changes.

2. Why are fibrocystic breast changes rare in postmenopausal women?

3. Why might oral contraceptives offer some relief for fibrocystic disease?

4. What pharmacologic action do danazol and tamoxifen have in common that relieves fibrocystic symptoms?

5. Develop a care plan for Ms. Turner for the nursing diagnosis *Body Image Disturbance* related to fibrocystic breast changes.

The Client with a Fibroadenoma

■ ■ ■

Fibroadenomas are overgrowths of periductal stromal connective tissue compressing ducts into well-defined lumps with circumscribed edges and smooth boundaries. Fibroadenomas are mobile, firm, and nontender lumps. They occur most often in women under the age of 25, and they tend to occur earlier in African-American women.

Treatment for fibroadenoma is surgical excision under local anesthesia, done as an outpatient procedure. The specimen is sent for histologic examination to rule out cancer.

The nurse can offer emotional support to the client as well as suggestions for dealing with postoperative discomfort. See the box on page 2046.

The Client with an Intraductal Papilloma

■ ■ ■

An **intraductal papilloma** is a tiny wartlike growth on the inside of the peripheral mammary duct that causes discharge from the nipple. The discharge may be clear and sticky or bloody. When more than one of these growths is present, the condition is called intraductal papillomatosis. This condition is most common in women in their 30s and 40s. The lesion is not palpable but must be investigated to rule out malignancy.

When intraductal papilloma is suspected, the nipple discharge is sent for laboratory analysis. A mammogram may also be ordered if the client is 30 or older. Some physicians order a ductogram; the radiologist inserts a fine plastic catheter into the duct, injects radiopaque dye, and then takes an X-ray. The ductogram provides a guide for the surgeon who performs the biopsy under local anesthesia on an outpatient basis. The blood-filled duct is removed and a specimen is sent for analysis.

Nursing care is the same as previously discussed for any breast biopsy.

The Client with Mammary Duct Ectasia

■ ■ ■

Mammary duct ectasia, also called plasma cell mastitis, is a palpable lumpiness found beneath the areola. Duct ectasia involves periductal inflammation, dilation of the ductal system, and accumulation of fluid and dead cells that block the involved ducts. The condition usually occurs in perimenopausal or late premenopausal women and is difficult to differentiate from cancer (Bland & Love, 1992).

Symptoms of mammary duct ectasia include sticky, thick nipple discharge with burning and itching around the nipple, and inflammation. The discharge may be green, greenish brown, or bloody. Nipple retraction often is associated with duct ectasia in postmenopausal women.

Mammary duct ectasia is diagnosed by open biopsy and treated with local excision of the involved ducts.

Nursing care is the same as for any open biopsy, with emphasis on cleanliness of the nipple area to reduce the risk of infection. It is also important to reassure the woman that duct ectasia is not related to breast cancer.

The Client with Mastitis

■ ■ ■

Mastitis is inflammation of the breast. Women with mastitis typically present with tenderness, induration, and redness of the breast. Mastitis may be either acute or chronic. Acute mastitis occurs most often in lactating women and is generally caused by staphylococcal and streptococcal organisms from the infant's nose and throat. Chronic mastitis in women who are not lactating is associated with galactorrhea, an increase in prolactin.

Mastitis requires prompt antibiotic therapy; the route is determined by the severity of the infection. Increasing fluid intake, wearing a supportive bra, and taking mild analgesics, such as aspirin or ibuprofen, help relieve symptoms. If lactating, the woman should continue to breast-feed from the unaffected breast and express milk from the affected breast (ACOG, 1991b).

Nursing care of the woman with mastitis includes education about the importance of hand washing, breast and nipple care, and, in lactating women, regular, thorough emptying of the breasts to prevent engorgement.

▪▪▪ Breast Disorders in Males ▪▪▪

The Client with Gynecomastia

▪ ▪ ▪

Gynecomastia is the abnormal enlargement of the male breast, thought to result from a high ratio of estradiol to testosterone. It is common during puberty, affecting as many as 50% of adolescent males, but usually resolves within 1 to 2 years. Any condition that increases estrogen activity or decreases testosterone production can contribute to gynecomastia. Conditions that increase estrogen activity include obesity, testicular tumors, liver disease, and adrenal carcinoma; conditions that decrease testosterone production include chronic illness such as tuberculosis or Hodgkin's disease, injury, and orchitis. Drugs such as digitalis, opiates, and chemotherapeutic agents are also associated with gynecomastia (Sharlip, 1992).

No treatment is necessary for the transient gynecomastia of puberty. If the condition becomes chronic, however, creating psychologic discomfort, surgery may be necessary to remove the subcutaneous breast tissue. When related to an underlying disorder such as tuberculosis, treatment of that disorder is required. In severe cases, tamoxifen is given to decrease estrogen activity.

Gynecomastia is usually bilateral. If it is unilateral, biopsy may be necessary to rule out breast cancer.

Nursing care for the client with gynecomastia includes education about the cause and treatment of the condition, and emotional support for the psychosocial implications of this feminizing condition.

The Male Client with Breast Cancer

▪ ▪ ▪

Although male breast cancer is rare, accounting for about 1% of all breast cancer cases, it is as serious to the men who have it as it is to women. About 1000 men in the United States were diagnosed with breast cancer in 1994, and about 300 men died from breast cancer.

The etiology of male breast cancer is unclear; hormonal, genetic, and perhaps environmental factors appear to be important.

Male breast cancer is clinically and histologically similar to female breast cancer, although lobular cancer is rare in males. Most tumors are estrogen-receptor positive (Hecht & Winchester, 1994). Because many men believe that breast cancer is only a woman's disease, they often delay seeking medical attention for symptoms and thus may present with advanced disease.

Treatment of male breast cancer is much like the treatment of female breast cancer, beginning with modified radical mastectomy, node dissection, and staging to determine the therapeutic options. Radiation, chemotherapy, or hormonal therapy (usually tamoxifen), are the conventional adjuncts to surgery. Approximately 21% of men with breast cancer stop taking prescribed tamoxifen because of its undesirable side effects; in comparison, only 4% of women with breast cancer discontinue tamoxifen for this reason (Anelli et al., 1994).

Nursing care for the man with breast cancer derives from the basic principles outlined earlier; however, the nurse has an opportunity to help the man and his family cope with the psychosocial effects of having breast cancer. He may feel embarrassment or shame about his condition as well as fear about the life-threatening nature of the disease. His family may share those feelings. By listening with understanding and empathy, the nurse can help the client and family resolve their feelings and move toward healing.

Bibliography

▪ ▪ ▪

ACOG Technical Bulletin. (1991a). *Carcinoma of the breast* (Number 158). An educational aid to obstetrician-gynecologists. Washington, D. C.: American College of Obstetricians and Gynecologists.

ACOG Technical Bulletin. (1991b). *Nonmalignant conditions of the breast* (Number 156). An educational aid to obstetrician-gynecologists. Washington, D. C.: American College of Obstetricians and Gynecologists.

American Joint Committee on Cancer. (1992). *Manual for staging of cancer* (3rd ed.). Philadelphia: Lippincott.

Anelli, T. F., Anelli, A., Tan, K. N., Lebwohl, D. E., & Borgen, P. I. (1994). Tamoxifen administration is associated with a high rate of treatment-limiting symptoms in male breast cancer patients. *Cancer, 74*(1), 74–77.

Baines, C., Miller, A., & Bassett, A. (1989). Physical examination: Its role as a single screening modality in the Canadian national breast screening study. *Cancer, 63,* 1816–1822.

Beisecker, A., Helmig, L., Graham, D., & Moore, W. (1994). Attitudes of oncologists, oncology nurses, and patients from a women's clinic regarding medical decision making for older and younger breast cancer patients. *Gerontologist, 34*(4), 505–512.

Bland, K., & Love, N. (1992). Evaluation of common breast masses. *Postgraduate Medicine, 92*(5), 95–112.

Boring, C., Squires, T., Tong, T., & Montgomery, S. (1994). Cancer statistics, 1994. *CA: A Cancer Journal for Clinicians, 44*(1), 7–8.

Breo, D. J. (1993). Altered fates: Counseling families with inherited breast cancer. *Journal of the American Medical Association, 269,* 2017–2022.

Brinton LA. (1994). Ways that women may possibly reduce their risk of breast cancer. *Journal of the National Cancer Institute, 86*(18), 1371–1372.

Broder, S. (1995). Address to the National Cancer Advisory Board, January 10, 1995. Washington, D. C.

Brown-Daniels, C. J., & Blasdell, A. (1990). Early stage breast cancer: Adjuvant drug therapy. *American Journal of Nursing, 90*(11), 32–33.

Brown, L., & Williams, R. (1994). Culturally sensitive breast cancer screening programs for older black women. *Nurse Practitioner, 19*(3), 21–32.

Cawley, M., Kostic, J., & Cappello, C. (1990). Informational and psychosocial needs of women choosing conservative surgery/primary radiation for early stage breast cancer. *Cancer Nursing, 13*(2), 90–94.

Ciatto, S., Smith, A., Di Maggio, C., Pescarini, L., Lattanzio, E., Ancona, A., Punzo, C., De Leo, G., Burke, P., Bonomini, M., & Melaranci, P. (1987). Breast cancer diagnosis under the age of forty years. *Tumori, 73,* 457–461.

Davis, D., & Love, S. (1994). Mammographic screening. *Journal of the American Medical Association, 271*(2), 152–153.

Donegan, W. (1991). Cancer of the breast in men. *Cancer, 41*(6), 339–354.

Ellerhorst-Ryan, J., & Goeldner, J. (1992). Breast cancer. *Nursing Clinics of North America, 27*(4), 821–833.

Entrekin, N., & McMillan, S. (1993). Nurses' knowledge, beliefs, and practices related to cancer prevention and detection. *Cancer Nursing, 16*(6), 431–439.

Evens, R. (1992). Factors affecting mammographic visualization of the breast after augmentation mammoplasty. *Journal of the American Medical Association, 268*(14), 1913–1917.

Feig, S. (1992). Breast masses: Mammographic and sonographic evaluation. *Radiology Clinics of North America, 30*(1), 67–92.

Futreal, P. A., et al. (1994). BRCA1 mutations in primary breast and ovarian carcinomas. *Science, 266*(5182), 120–122.

Glickstein, J. (1992). Understanding cancer of the breast. *Focus on Geriatric Care and Rehabilitation, 6*(2), 1–8.

Gofman, J. (1995). *Preventing breast cancer.* San Francisco: Committee for Nuclear Responsibility.

Gossage, J. (1990). Early stage breast cancer: How nurses help. *American Journal of Nursing, 90*(11), 31.

Guiliano, A. E. (1993). The breast. In L. T. Tierney, et al., *Current medical diagnosis and treatment 1993* (p. 546). Norwalk, CT: Appleton & Lange.

Haffty, B. G., et al. (1993). Breast conservation therapy without axillary dissection. *Archives of Surgery, 128,* 1315–1319.

Hanck, R. (1988). Vitamin C and cancer. In G. Tryflates & K. N. Prasad (Eds.), *Nutrition, growth and cancer.* New York: Alan R. Liss.

Hankey, B. F., et al. (1994). Trends in breast cancer in younger women in contrast to older women. *Journal of the National Cancer Institute Monographs, 16,* 7–14.

Harris, J., Lippman, M., Veronesi, U., & Willett, W. (1992). Medical progress. *New England Journal of Medicine, 327*(6), 390–398.

Hecht, J. R., & Winchester, D. J. (1994). Male breast cancer. *American Journal of Clinical Pathology, 102*(4 Suppl. 1) S25–30.

Henderson, I. C. (1991). Breast cancer therapy: The price of success. *New England Journal of Medicine, 325,* 1774–1775.

Hindle, W., (Ed.) (1990). *Breast disease for gynecologists* (pp. 179–195). Norwalk, CT: Appleton & Lange.

Hockenberger, S. (1993). Fibrocystic breast disease: Every woman is at risk. *Plastic Surgical Nursing, 13*(1), 37–40.

Homer, J. (1987). Imaging features and management of characteristically benign and probably benign breast lesions. *Radiology Clinics of North America, 25*(5), 939–951.

Ivey, C., & Gordon, S. I. (1994, July). Breast reconstruction: New image, new hope. *RN, 48,* 54.

Jacob, T., Penn, N., Kulik, J., & Spieth, L. (1992). Effects of cognitive style and maintenance strategies on breast self-examination (BSE) practice by African-American women. *Journal of Behavioral Medicine, 15*(6), 589–609.

Janes, R. H., & Bouton, M. S. (1994). Initial 300 consecutive stereotactic core-needle breast biopsies by a surgical group. *American Journal of Surgery 168*(6), 533–537.

Johnson, J. (1994, May). Caring for the woman who's had a mastectomy. *American Journal of Nursing 94*(5), 25–32.

Kaplan, H. S. (1992). Adjuvant treatment in breast cancer. *Lancet, 339,* 424.

Kerlikowske, K., Grady D., Rubin, S. M., Sandrock, C., & Ernster, V. (1995). Efficacy of screening mammography: A meta-analysis. *Journal of the American Medical Association, 273*(2), 149–154.

Knobf, M. T. (1991). Breast cancer. In S. B. Baird et al. (Eds.), *Cancer nursing: A comprehensive textbook* (pp. 425–451). Philadelphia: Saunders.

Knobf, M. T. (1990). Early-stage breast cancer: The options. *American Journal of Nursing, 90,*(11), 28–30.

Koroltchouck, V., & Stjernsward, S. (1990). The control of breast cancer: A World Health Organization perspective. *Cancer, 65,* 2803–2810.

Kurtz, M., Given, B., Given, C., & Kurtz, J. (1993). Relationships of barriers and facilitators to breast self examination, mammography and clinical breast examination in a worksite population. *Cancer Nursing, 16*(4), 251–259.

Lerner, M. (1994). *Choices in healing: Integrating the best of conventional and complementary approaches to cancer.* Cambridge, MA: MIT Press.

Lichter, A. S., & Findlay, P. A. (1988). Radiation therapy as an adjuvant to surgery in the treatment of operable breast cancer. In M. E. Lippman, A. S. Lichter, & D. N. Danforth (Eds.), *Diagnosis and management of breast cancer* (p. 348). Philadelphia: Saunders.

Lierman, L., Young, H., Powell-Cope, G., Georgiadou, F., & Benoliel, J. (1994). Effects of education and support on breast self-examination in older women. *Nursing Research, 43*(3), 158–163.

London, S., Connolly, J., Schnitt, S., & Colditz, G. (1992). A prospective study of benign breast disease and the risk of breast cancer. *Journal of the American Medical Association, 267*(7), 941–944.

Longman, A., Saint-Germain, M., & Modiano, M. (1992). Use of breast cancer screening by older Hispanic women. *Public Health Nursing, 9*(2), 118–124.

Loomis, D. P. (1992). Cancer of breast among men in electrical occupations. *Lancet 339,* 1482–1483.

Love, S. (1995). *Dr. Susan Love's breast book* (2nd ed.). Reading, MA: Addison-Wesley.

Ludwick, R., Rushing, B., & Biordi, D. L. (1994). Breast cancer and the older woman: Information and images. *Health Care Women International 15*(3), 235–242.

Lurie, N., et al. (1993). Preventive care for women: Does the sex of the physician matter? *New England Journal of Medicine, 329*(7), 478–482.

Mandelblatt, J., Wheat, M., Monane, M., Moshief, R., Hollenberg, J., & Tang, J. (1992). Breast cancer screening for elderly women with and without comorbid conditions. *American College of Physicians, 116*(9), 722–730.

Marwick, C. (1994). NCI changes its stance on mammography. *Journal of the American Medical Association, 271*(2), 96.

McCool, W. (1994). Barriers to breast cancer screening in older women. *Journal of Nurse Midwifery, 39*(5), 283–299.

McKenzie, I. (1965). Breast cancer following multiple fluoroscopies. *British Journal of Cancer, 19*(3), 1–8.

Miller, A., Baines, C., & Turnball, C. (1991). The role of the nurse examiner in the National Breast screening study. *Canadian Journal of Public Health, 82,* 162–167.

Miller, A., Baines, C., To, T., & Wall, C. (1992). Canadian National Breast screening study: Breast cancer detection and death rates among women aged 40-49 years. *Journal of the Canadian Medical Association, 147*(10), 1459–1476.

Mittra, I. (1994). Breast screening: The case for physical examination without mammography. *Lancet, 343,* 342–344.

Mor, V., Malin, M., & Allen, S. (1994). Age differences in the psychosocial problems encountered by breast cancer patients. *Journal of the National Cancer Institute Monographs, 16:* 191–197.

Nachtigall, M., Smilen, S., Nachtigall, R., Nachtigall, R., & Nachtigall, L. (1992). Incidence of breast cancer in a 22-year study of women receiving estrogen-progestin replacement therapy. *HRT and Breast Cancer, 80*(5), 827–830.

National Cancer Institute. (1992). *Office of cancer communications: Lifetime probability of breast cancer in American women.* (Cancer Information Service Cancer Facts Series). Bethesda, MD: National Cancer Institute.

National Cancer Institute. (1991). *Radiation therapy: A treatment for early stage breast cancer* (NIH Publication No. 91-659). Washington, D. C.: National Cancer Institute.

National Cancer Institute. (1990). *Radiation therapy and you* (NIH Publication No. 91-2227). Washington, D. C.: National Cancer Institute.

Newcomb, P., Storer, B., Longnecker, M., Mittendorf, R., Greenberg, R., Clapp, R., Burke, K., Willett, W., & MacMahon, B. (1994). Lactation and a reduced risk of premenopausal breast cancer. *New England Journal of Medicine, 330*(2), 81–87.

Nielsen, B., & East, D. (1990). Advances in breast cancer: Implications for nursing care. *Nursing Clinics of North America, 25*(2), 365–375.

NIH Consensus Conference. (1991). Treatment of early-stage breast cancer. *Journal of the American Medical Association, 265*(3), 391–395.

Northouse, L. L. (1994). Breast cancer in younger women: Effects on interpersonal and family relationships [Monograph]. *Journal of the National Cancer Institute, 16,* 183–190.

Okunieff, P. (1990). Interactions between ascorbic acid, radiation therapy, and misoidazole. Meeting abstract, Ascorbic acid: Biological functions and relation to cancer. Bethesda, MD: National Institutes of Health.

Olds, S., London, M., & Ladewig, P. (1992). *Maternal-newborn nursing* (4th ed.). Redwood City, CA: Addison-Wesley Nursing.

Olsen, S., & Frank-Stromborg, M. (1993). Cancer prevention and early detection in ethnically diverse populations. *Seminars in Oncology Nursing, 9*(3), 196–209.

O'Malley, M., & Fletcher, S. (1987). Screening for breast cancer with breast self examination: A critical review. *Journal of the American Medical Association, 257*(16), 2197–2203.

Osteen, R. T., Cady, B., Friedman, M., et al. (1994). Patterns of care for younger women with breast cancer. *Journal of the National Cancer Institute Monographs, 16,* 43–46.

Osteen, R. T., & Smith, B. L. (1990). Results of conservative surgery and radiation therapy for breast cancer. *Surgical Clinics of North America, 70*(5), 1005–1021.

Page, J. K., Mansel, R. E., & Hughes, S. E. (1985). Clinical experience of drug treatment for mastalgia. *Lancet, 2,* 373.

Parker, S. H. (1994). Percutaneous large core breast biopsy. *Cancer, 74*(Suppl. 1), 256–262.

Pierce, S. M., & Harris, J. R. (1991). Role of radiation therapy in the management of primary breast cancer. *CA: A Cancer Journal for Clinicians, 41*(2), 85–96.

Porth, C. M. (1994). *Pathophysiology: Concepts of altered health states,* 4th ed. Philadelphia: J. B. Lippincott Company.

Reifsnider, E. (1990). Educating women about benign breast disease. *AAOHN Journal, 38*(3), 121–126.

Roberts, M., Alexander, F., Anderson, T., Chetty, V., Donnan, P., & Forrest, P. (1990). Edinburgh trial of screening for breast cancer mortality at seven years. *Lancet, 335,* 241–246.

Salazar, M., & Carter, W. (1993). Evaluation of breast self examination beliefs using a decision model. *Western Journal of Nursing Research, 15*(4), 403–421.

Seoub, M., Johnson, J., & Weed, J. (1993). Gynecologic tumors in tamoxifen-treated women with breast cancer. *Obstetrics and Gynecology, 82*(2), 165–169.

Sharlip, I. (1992). Male reproductive disorders. In P. Fitzgerald, *Handbook of clinical endocrinology* (2nd ed.) (pp. 388–391). Norwalk, CT: Appleton & Lange.

Sharp, P. (1993). Breast cancer education for patients' relatives. *Health Values, 17*(4), 28–34.

Sickles, E., Filly, R., & Callen, P. (1984). Benign breast lesions: Ultrasound detection and diagnosis. *Radiology, 151*(2), 467–470.

Smith, P. (1993). Breast cancer prevention and detection update. *Seminars in Oncology Nursing, 9*(3), 150–154.

Steele, G., Osteen, R., Winchester, D., Murphy, G., & Menck, G. (1994). Clinical highlights from the National Cancer Data Base: 1994. *CA: A Cancer Journal for Clinicians, 44*(2), 71–80.

Stefanek, M. (1992). Psychosocial aspects of breast cancer. *Current Opinion in Oncology, 4,* 1055–1060.

Taylor, M. (1994). *Topics in breast disease: Problem management, breast cancer risk factors and mammography.* Keystone, CO: Presentation.

Tessaro, I., Eng, E., & Smith, J. (1994). Breast cancer screening in older African-American women: Qualitative research findings. *American Journal of Health Promotion, 8*(4), 286–293.

Thomas, D. B. (1991). Oral contraceptives and breast cancer: Review of the epidemiologic literature. *Contraception, 43,* 597–642.

U.S. Department of Health and Human Services, Public Health Service. (1992). *Treatment of early-stage breast cancer* (NIH Publication 90-3187). Bethesda, MD: National Cancer Institute, J National Cancer Institute Monograph 11.

U.S. Department of Health and Human Services, Public Health Service. (1990). Mammography and clinical breast examinations among women aged 50 years and older: Behavioral risk factor surveillance system. *Morbity and Mortality Weekly Reports, 42,* 737–741.

Way, L. W. (1994). *Current surgical diagnosis and treatment* (10th ed.). Norwalk CT: Appleton & Lange.

White, L., & Spitz, M. (1993). Cancer risk and early detection assessment. *Seminars in Oncology Nursing, 9*(3), 188–197.

Wilson, J., Braunwald, E., Isselbacher, K. J., Petersdorf, R. G., Martin, J. B., Fauci, A. S., & Root, R. K. (Eds.), (1991). *Harrison's principles of internal medicine* (12th ed.). New York: McGraw-Hill.

Winchester, D. (1990). Evaluation and management of breast abnormalities. *Cancer, 66*(September 15 Suppl.), 1345–1347.

Nursing Care of Clients with Sexually Transmitted Diseases

LEARNING OBJECTIVES

After completing this chapter, you will be able to

- Describe the pathophysiology of the most common sexually transmitted diseases (STDs).

- Identify laboratory and diagnostic tests used for STDs.

- Identify general measures to prevent and treat common STDs.

- List the signs and symptoms of the most common STDs.

- Discuss nursing implications for medications prescribed for clients with STDs.

- Use the nursing process as a framework for providing individualized care to clients with STDs.

Any infection transmitted by sexual contact, including vaginal, oral, and anal intercourse, is referred to as a **sexually transmitted disease (STD).** Each year, 1 of 20 people in the United States is infected with a non-AIDS sexually transmitted disease. One of six people in the United States already has such a disease, an estimated total of 30 to 40 million people. Every sexually active person is at risk for STDs, and some of these diseases can be life-threatening, particularly for women and infants.

Sexually transmitted diseases include the five *classic venereal diseases* (syphilis, gonorrhea, chancroid, granuloma inguinale, and lymphogranuloma venereum) plus such disorders as chlamydial infections, genital herpes, genital warts, and HIV/AIDS (Table 49–1 on pages 2066 to 2067). These disorders can be transmitted from a pregnant woman to her fetus during pregnancy or delivery. Sexually transmitted pathogens also have been implicated in enteritis, proctitis, ocular infections, and pharyngitis.

STDs have reached epidemic proportions in the United States (Figure 49–1) and continue to increase worldwide. They are the most frequent infections encountered by professionals in the field of reproductive health. The esti-

mated number of people newly infected each year with symptomatic non-AIDS STDs is approximately 13 million (Quinn & Cates, 1992). Syphilis, one of the most dangerous STDs, is at the highest level in 40 years: more than 50,000 new cases are reported annually.

Many people believe that STDs affect only certain groups (such as prostitutes) and do not consider themselves at risk for infection. For example, one 1994 survey found that 84% of U.S. women think they are safe from STDs, but 66% admit they know almost nothing about such diseases (EDK Associates, 1994). Such ignorance and lack of awareness have caused STD rates to soar. STDs inflict pain and suffering on people of all ages and socioeconomic levels and cost U.S. society more than $315 billion annually (Centers for Disease Control CDC, 1991).

Several factors help explain the escalating incidence of STDs. Penicillin and other antibiotics were widely and effectively used during the 1940s and 1950s against syphilis and gonorrhea, both of which declined dramatically. Although penicillin still seems to be effective against syphilis, several strains of penicillin-resistant gonorrhea have developed, making it more difficult to treat. The so-called sexual revolution of the 1960s and 1970s, fueled by "the pill" and the freedom from unplanned pregnancy, led to a more permissive attitude about sexuality and increases in sexual activity and the number of sexual partners. In addition, since oral contraceptives were introduced to American women in 1961, they have replaced the condom as a birth-control method for many couples. However, oral contraceptives do not protect against STDs, a fact of increasing importance in the age of HIV/AIDS. Indeed, by making the vaginal environment less acidic, oral contraceptives predispose women to infection.

Finally, the emergence of HIV/AIDS has created a kind of "epidemiologic synergy" among all STDs (Wasserheit, 1992). Other STDs, such as syphilis, HSV, and chancroid, facilitate the transmission of HIV/AIDS, and the immune suppression caused by HIV potentiates the infectious process of other STDs.

The incidence of STDs is concentrated in sociogeographic clusters, called "core populations" (Potterat, 1992), affected by poverty and ignorance. The incidence is highest among people of color in urban populations of lower socioeconomic status and lower educational attainment (CDC, 1993). People in these groups generally have little information about prevention of STDs and limited access to medical care, two factors that often delay diagnosis and treatment and sometimes limit compliance. Drug abuse, unprotected sexual activity, and sexual activity with multiple partners also are associated with increased incidence of STDs.

Two-thirds of all STDs occur in people under age 25; however, people of all ages are at risk. Anyone who is sexually active can be infected with STDs, and infants can be infected by their mothers in utero or during delivery. Children can be infected through incest or sexual abuse. Victims of sexual assault are also at risk.

All states require that cases of AIDS, the five classic STDs, and viral hepatitis be reported to state and federal agencies. Some states also require reporting of chlamydial infections, genital herpes, and genital warts. This uneven

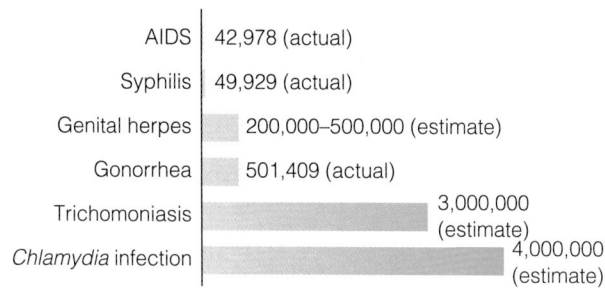

Figure 49–1   Incidence of STDs in the United States, 1993.

reporting of cases, however, means that the exact incidence of STDs is unknown.

Although sexually transmitted diseases are caused by many different organisms, they have several characteristics in common:

- Most can be prevented by the use of latex condoms.
- They can be transmitted during both heterosexual and homosexual activities.
- For treatment to be effective, sexual partners of the infected person must also be treated.
- Two or more STDs frequently coexist in the same client.

Some STDs can be cured through appropriate early treatment with antibiotics. Others, such as genital herpes and genital warts, are chronic conditions that can be managed but not cured. The most serious STD is AIDS, which is incurable and ultimately fatal. HIV/AIDS is discussed in Chapter 8. Treatment guidelines for STDs are updated regularly and are available from the Division of STD, Centers for Disease Control, Atlanta, Georgia. Nurses have a critical role in the prevention of STDs by teaching clients about these diseases, their prevention, treatment, and potential complications. See the box on page 2068.

▚▚▚ STDs Producing Ulcers or Chancres ▚▚▚

Two of the most common STDs produce one or more ulcers or chancres: syphilis, a classic systemic STD, and genital herpes, a chronic STD.

The Client with Syphilis

■ ■ ■

Syphilis is a complex systemic STD caused by a spirochete, *Treponema pallidum,* which may infect almost any body tissue or organ. It is transmitted from open lesions during any sexual contact (genital, oral-genital, or anal-genital). The organism is highly susceptible to heat and drying but can survive for days in fluids; thus it may also be transmitted by infected blood or other body fluid such as saliva. The average incubation period is 20 to 30 days, but ranges from 10 to 90 days. If not treated appropriately, syphilis can lead to blindness, paralysis, mental illness, cardiovascular damage, and death. Syphilis often occurs with one or more other STDs, such as HIV/AIDS or chlamydial infection. Pregnant women with syphilis can also infect the fetus, causing eye damage, dental and bone deformities, blindness, brain damage, and death.

Table 49–1 Selected Sexually Transmitted Diseases*

Condition / Organism	Signs & Symptoms	Medical Treatment†	Complications
Syphilis‡ *Treponema pallidum*	**Primary:** Painless chancre at site of exposure; regional lymphadenopathy	Benzathine penicillin G IM in a single injection *or* doxycycline PO for 14 days	Disease progression and transmission
	Secondary: Skin rash; oral mucous patches; generalized lymphadenopathy; condyloma lata; fever; malaise; patchy alopecia	Syphilis of indeterminate length or more than 1 year's duration: benzathine penicillin G IM weekly for 3 weeks *or* doxycycline PO for 28 days	Disease progression and transmission
	Tertiary (late): Infiltrating tumors of skin, bone, liver; *cardiovascular changes:* aortitis, aneurysms; *central nervous system degeneration:* paresthesias, shooting pains, abnormal reflexes, dementia, psychoses		Disease progression and transmission Heart failure, blindness, paralysis, skin ulcers, liver failure, mental illness
Gonorrhea‡ *Neisseria gonorrhoeae*	**In females:** Often asymptomatic, but can include abnormal vaginal discharge, abnormal menses, dysuria **In males:** Dysuria, increased urinary frequency, purulent urethral discharge	Ceftriaxone IM in a single injection *plus* doxycycline PO for 7 days to treat possible coexisting chlamydia	**In females:** Pelvic inflammatory disease (PID), sterility, ectopic pregnancy, abdominal adhesions **In males:** Prostatitis, urethritis, nephritis, epididymitis, sterility
Chancroid‡ (rare in U.S.) *Haemophilus ducreyi*	**In females:** Frequently asymptomatic **In males:** Painful penile ulcers and lymphadenopathy	Azithromycin PO once *or* ceftriaxone IM once *or* erythromycin PO for 7 days	Secondary infection of lesions, fistulas, chronic ulcers
Granuloma inguinale‡ (donovanosis) (rare in U.S.) *Calymmatobacterium granulomatis*	Single or multiple subcutaneous nodules that erode to form painless, bleeding, enlarging ulcers	Tetracycline for 21 days or until lesion heals	Secondary infection of lesions, keloid formations on genitals, tissue necrosis, fever, malaise, secondary anemia, cachexia, and death
Lymphogranuloma venereum‡ (LGV) (rare in U.S.) *Chlamydia trachomatis* (immunotypes L1, L2, or L3)	Painless vesicle or nonindurated ulcer, followed by regional lymphadenopathy, inguinal abscess	Doxycycline for 21 days *or* tetracycline for 21 days	Ruptured inguinal or perianal abscesses producing draining sinuses or fistulas, nephropathy, hepatomegaly, or phlebitis
Chlamydial infections *Chlamydia trachomatis*	**In females:** Asymptomatic but can include dysuria, mucopurulent vaginal or cervical discharge, vaginal bleeding or pelvic pain **In males:** Sometimes asymptomatic but can include dysuria, white or clear urethral discharge, testicular pain (epididymitis)	Doxycycline PO for 7 days or azithromycin PO once	**In females:** Pelvic inflammatory disease (PID), infertility, pelvic absces-ses, spontaneous abortion, still-birth, postpartum endometritis **In neonates:** Ophthalmia neonatorum or pneumonia **In males:** Nongonococcal urethritis, epididymitis, prostatitis, disease transmission

*This table does not include the following STDs discussed in other chapters: AIDS/HIV, viral hepatitis, sexually transmitted enteritis and proctitis, and ectoparasitic infections.

†Treatment recommendations are based on 1993 STD treatment guidelines by the Centers for Disease Control and Prevention.

‡Reporting to state and federal agencies required by law.

Table 49–1 (continued)

Condition / Organism	Signs & Symptoms	Medical Treatment†	Complications
Genital herpes Herpes simplex virus, usually type 2 but rarely type 1	Single or multiple vesicles, on the genitals with associated pruritus, followed by painful ulcers	No cure; acyclovir PO for 7–10 days or until symptoms resolve	**In females:** Potentially fatal infection of fetus or neonate; possible cervical cancer **In neonates:** Neonatal herpes affecting eye, skin, mucous membranes, and possibly central nervous system **In males:** Neuralgia, meningitis, ascending myelitis, urethral strictures, lymphatic suppuration **In both males and females:** Herpes keratitis, a severe eye infection, caused by autoinoculation
Genital warts (Condyloma acuminatum) Human papillomavirus (HPV)	Single or multiple painless warts on genitals or perianal area	No cure, recurrence in 80% of cases; cryotherapy with liquid nitrogen or cryoprobe, *or* podophyllin 10%–25% in tincture of benzoin compound applied to wart, *or* carbon dioxide laser surgery	**In females:** Enlargement during pregnancy and obstruction of the birth canal; transmission to fetus or neonate; increased risk of cancer of the cervix, vagina, vulva, and anus **In neonates:** Respiratory papillomatosis, a chronic condition requiring multiple surgeries **In males and females:** Urinary obstruction and bleeding
Bacterial vaginosis *Gardnerella vaginalis, Mycoplasma hominis*	Excessive or foul-smelling vaginal discharge; erythema, edema, and pruritus of the external genitals	Metronidazole PO *or* clindamycin cream 2% intravaginally for 7 days	Recurrent infections; increased risk of PID
Mucopurulent cervicitis *Chlamydia trachomatis, Neisseria gonorrhoeae*	Mucopurulent cervical discharge	Depends on causative organism; *Chlamydia* involved in 50% of cases	**In females:** Pelvic inflammatory disease (PID), infertility, pelvic abscesses, spontaneous abortion, stillbirth, postpartum endometritis **In neonates:** Opthalmia neonatorum or pneumonia
Nongonococcal urethritis (NGU) *Chlamydia trachomatis, Urea plasma urealyticum, Trichomonas vaginalis,* herpes simplex	Dysuria, urinary frequency, mucoid to purulent urethral discharge; some men asymptomatic	Depends on causative organism	Urethral strictures or epididymitis; if transmitted to female partners, may result in mucopurulent cervicitis and PID; if female is pregnant, can cause neonatal ophthalmia or pneumonia
Pelvic inflammatory disease (PID) *Chlamydia trachomatis, Neisseria gonorrhoeae, Mycoplasma hominis,* and others	Asymptomatic or can include pain and tenderness in lower abdomen, uterus and adnexa, possibly with fever, chills, and elevated white blood count and erythrocyte sedimentation rate	Combined drug therapy based on broadest possible spectrum of pathogens; may require hospitalization	Ectopic pregnancy, pelvic abscess; infertility, recurrent or chronic PID, chronic abdominal pain, pelvic adhesions, depression
Trichomoniasis *Trichomonas vaginalis*	**In females:** Asymptomatic or can include frothy, excessive vaginal discharge, erythema, edema and pruritus **In males:** Usually asymptomatic but can include urethritis, penile lesions, or inflammation	Metronidazole PO for 7 days	**In females:** Recurrent infections, salpingitis, low birth weight infants, prematurity

---

Preventing STDs: A Checklist for Clients

■ ■ ■

- You can eliminate your risk entirely by not having sex with anyone (abstinence) or by having sex only with a noninfected partner who has sex only with you (mutual monogamy).

- The more sexual partners you have, the greater your risk of contracting an STD.

- Many STDs have no symptoms, so people often don't know they're infected. If you are not sure that your partner is free of infection, use protection during sex. Latex condoms (rubbers), used properly from start to finish each time you have sexual intercourse, are the best protection. Spermicidal foams and jellies offer additional protection. They are best used along with condoms, not in place of them.

- Diaphragms used with spermicide and contraceptive sponges offer some protection. They are less reliable than condoms and best used *along with* condoms.

- If you suspect you've been exposed to an STD, see a doctor or clinic right away. Encourage your partner to seek treatment, too.

- Follow the doctor's instructions carefully and take *all* the medicine prescribed for you. Continue the medication even when the symptoms go away. (The infection sometimes remains active after symptoms go away.)

- Go back to your doctor for a follow-up exam according to his or her instructions.

- Don't have sex until you *and* your partner are completely cured.

From *Condoms, Contraceptives, and Sexually Transmitted Disease,* American Social Health Association, 1989. Reprinted by permission.

With the advent of penicillin in the 1940s and 1950s, the incidence of syphilis plummeted. Like most STDs, however, syphilis has increased in incidence since the 1970s and is now the third most commonly reported communicable disease in the United States. Between 1985 and 1990, the number of reported cases of syphilis rose to more than 50,000 cases annually. The greatest increase has been among adolescents and young adults. As the incidence of syphilis has increased among women of childbearing age, the incidence of congenital syphilis has increased correspondingly, occurring in 1 in 10,000 pregnancies (CDC, 1988).

Pathophysiology

Any break in the skin or mucous membrane is vulnerable to invasion by the spirochete. Once it has entered the system, the spirochete is spread through the blood and lymphatic system. Congenital syphilis is transferred to the fetus through the placental circulation. Syphilis is generally characterized by three clinical stages: primary, secondary, and tertiary. Each stage has characteristic clinical manifestations (see the accompanying box). The client with syphilis also may experience a latency period when no signs of the disease are evident.

Primary Syphilis

The primary stage of syphilis is characterized by the appearance of a chancre (Figure 49–2) and by regional lymphadenopathy; little or no pain accompanies these warning signs. The chancre appears at the site of inoculation (genitals, anus, mouth, breast, finger) 3 to 4 weeks after the infectious contact. In women, a genital chancre may go unnoticed, disappearing within 4 to 6 weeks. In both primary and secondary stages, syphilis remains highly infectious, even if no symptoms are evident.

Secondary Syphilis

Manifestations of secondary syphilis may appear any time from 2 weeks to 6 months after the initial chancre disappears. These symptoms can include a *skin rash,* especially on the palms of the hands (Figure 49–3) or soles of the feet, *mucous patches* in the oral cavity; *sore throat; generalized lymphadenopathy; condyloma lata* (flat, broad-based papules, unlike the pedunculated structure of genital warts) on the labia, anus or corner of the mouth; *flulike symptoms;* and *alopecia.* These manifestations generally disappear within 2 to 6 weeks, and an asymptomatic latency period begins.

Latent Stage Syphilis

The latent stage of syphilis begins 2 or more years after the initial infection and can last up to 50 years. During this stage, no symptoms of syphilis are apparent, and the disease is not transmissible by sexual contact. It can be transmitted by infected blood, however; thus all prospective blood donors must be screened for syphilis. In two-thirds of all cases, the latent stage persists without further complications. Unless treated, the remaining one-third of infected people progress to late stage or tertiary syphilis. In the presence of HIV infection, disease progression seems to be hastened.

Tertiary Syphilis

Two types of late stage syphilis occur. *Benign late syphilis,* of rapid onset, is characterized by localized development

Clinical Manifestations of Syphilis

Reproductive

Primary

- Genital chancre (may be internal in female)

Secondary

- Condyloma lata

Integumentary System

Secondary

- Rash on palms and soles

Tertiary

- Granulomatous lesions involving mucous membranes and skin

Gastrointestinal System

Secondary

- Anorexia
- Oral mucous patches

Neurologic System

Secondary

- Asymptomatic
- Headache
- Meningitis
- Cranial neuropathies

Tertiary

- Asymptomatic
- Neurosyphilis
- Tabes dorsalis
- Seizures, hemiparesis, hemiplegia

- Personality changes, hyperactive reflexes, Argyll Robertson pupil, decreased memory, slurred speech, optic atrophy

Musculoskeletal System

Secondary

- Arthralgia
- Myalgia
- Bone and joint arthritis
- Periostitis

Tertiary

- Gummas

Cardiovascular System

Tertiary

- Aortic insufficiency
- Aortic aneurysm
- Stenosis of openings to coronary arteries

Renal System

Secondary

- Glomerulonephritis
- Nephrotic syndrome

Other

Primary

- Regional lymphadenopathy

Secondary

- Generalized lymphadenopathy
- Fever
- Hepatitis
- Malaise
- Alopecia

---

of infiltrating tumors (*gummas*) in skin, bones, and liver, generally responding promptly to treatment. Of more insidious onset is a *diffuse inflammatory response* that involves the central nervous system and the cardiovascular system. Though the disease can still be treated at this stage, much of the cardiovascular and central nervous system damage is irreversible.

Collaborative Care

The goals of treatment are to inactivate the spirochete and educate the client about how to prevent reinfection or further transmission. Treatment includes antibiotic therapy and identification and referral of partners for testing and treatment if necessary, follow-up testing, and educa-

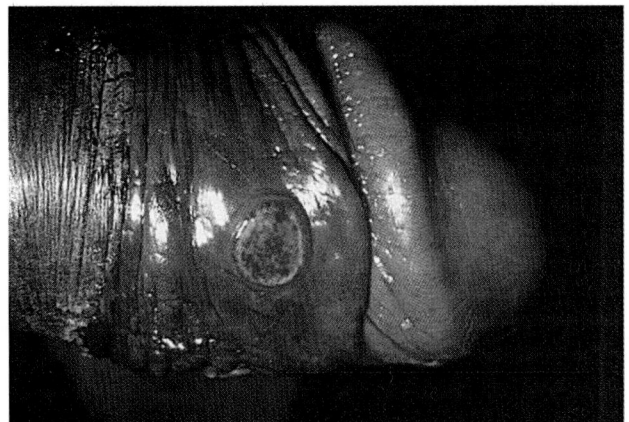

Figure 49–2   Chancre of primary syphilis on the penis.

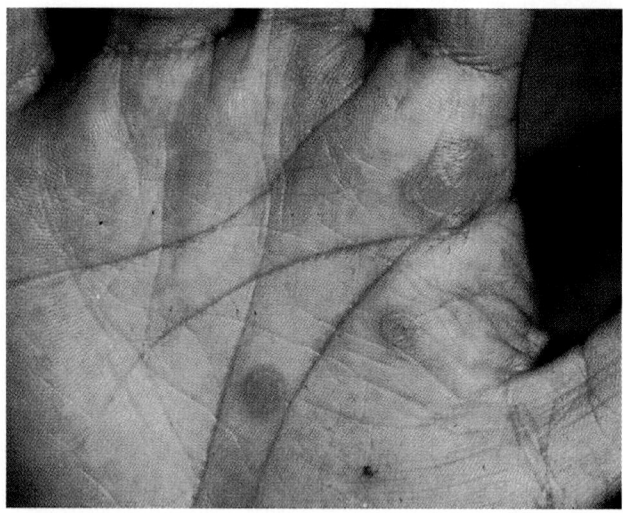

Figure 49–3   Palmar rash of secondary syphilis.

tion about condom use to prevent reinfection of self and transmission of disease to partners. In addition, clients should be screened for chlamydial infection and advised to have an HIV test.

Laboratory and Diagnostic Tests

Diagnosis of syphilis is complex because it mimics many other diseases. A careful history and physical examination are obtained, as well as laboratory evaluations of lesions and blood. The following tests are widely used:

- The *VDRL (Venereal Disease Research Laboratory)* and *RPR (rapid plasma reagin)* blood tests measure antibody production. People with syphilis become positive about 4 to 6 weeks after infection. However, these tests are not specific for syphilis, and other diseases may also cause positive results. Additional tests are required for definitive diagnosis.

- The *FTA-ABS (fluorescent treponemal antibody absorption)* test is specific for *T. pallidum* and can be used to confirm VDRL and RPR findings. It may be used for clients whose clinical picture indicates syphilis but who have negative VDRL results.

- *Immunofluorescent staining.* In this test, a specimen obtained from early lesions or aspiration of lymph nodes is specially treated and examined microscopically for the presence of *T. pallidum.*

- *Darkfield microscopy.* In this test, a specimen from the chancre is examined for the presence of *T. pallidum* using a darkfield microscope.

Pharmacology

The treatment of choice for primary and secondary syphilis is benzathine penicillin G, given intramuscularly

(IM) in a single dose. For syphilis of indeterminate length or more than 1 year's duration, the total dosage is increased and given in 3 weekly injections. Clients allergic to penicillin are given oral doxycycline. The length of therapy depends on the estimated duration of infection. If the client cannot tolerate doxycycline, oral erythromycin is substituted. The nursing implications of antibiotic therapy are presented in the box on page 257 of Chapter 8.

Treatment of syphilis in pregnant women may result in a severe reaction called the Jarisch-Herxheimer reaction, involving fever, musculoskeletal pain, tachycardia, and sometimes hypotension. This is not a reaction to the penicillin itself but to the sudden and massive destruction of spirochetes by the penicillin and the resulting release of toxins into the bloodstream. The Jarisch-Herxheimer reaction generally begins within 24 hours of treatment and subsides in another 24 hours. Treatment should not be discontinued unless symptoms become life-threatening.

Nursing Care

In planning and implementing holistic nursing care for the client with syphilis, the nurse needs to consider the client's age, life-style, access to health care, and educational level. Although each client has individualized needs, nursing diagnoses for the client with syphilis would be the same as for any client with an STD (see the accompanying box). Nursing diagnoses discussed in this section focus on high risk for injury, anxiety, and self-esteem.

Risk for Injury

If syphilis is not diagnosed and treated promptly and effectively, it can have devastating effects on all body systems, particularly the neurologic and cardiovascular systems, eventually leading to a painful death.

Nursing interventions with rationales follow:

- Teach the importance of taking any prescribed oral medication. *Completion of the prescribed course of antibiotic is important to ensure eradication of the infecting organism.*

- Encourage the client to refer any sexual partners for evaluation and any necessary treatment. *Without treatment of both partners, reinfection can occur or the disease may be transmitted to other people through sexual activity.*

- Teach the client to abstain from sexual contact until client and partners are cured and to use condoms to prevent future infections. *Abstinence until the organism is eradicated prevents reinfection. Condoms provide barrier protection, reducing the risk of infection during sexual activity.*

- Emphasize the importance of returning for follow-up testing at 3- and 6-month intervals for early syphilis, and 6- and 12-month intervals for late latent syphilis.

Follow-up testing is performed to assure eradication of the disease.

- Provide information about signs and symptoms of re-infection. *Successful treatment of the disease does not prevent possible subsequent infections.*

Anxiety

The diagnosis of syphilis understandably causes the client anxiety, not only about personal well-being but about the well-being of partners and, in the expectant woman, her fetus.

Nursing interventions with rationales follow:

- Emphasize that syphilis can be effectively treated, preventing the serious complications of late-stage disease. *This information gives the client a sense of control and helps decrease anxiety.*

- Teach the pregnant client that taking medications as directed and returning each month for follow-up testing will help ensure the well-being of her baby. *Knowing that treatment can reduce the risk to her baby relieves anxiety and possibly increases compliance.*

Self-Esteem Disturbance

Living with any chronic disease can be damaging to a person's self-esteem. However, the client with syphilis or any STD needs additional support to cope with the stigma of this kind of infection. Unfortunately, the populations most affected by STDs often lack family and other social support networks.

Nursing interventions with rationales follow:

- Create an environment where the client feels respected and safe to discuss questions and concerns about the disease and its effect on the client's life. *Being treated with respect helps enhance self-esteem.*

- Provide privacy and confidentiality. *Clients are often embarrassed to discuss the intimate details of their sex lives.*

- Let the client know that the nurse and other health care providers care about the client and the successful treatment of the disease. *Feeling valued enhances self-esteem.*

Client and Family Teaching

Education is an essential part of nursing care for the client with any STD, and syphilis is no exception. The nurse emphasizes that syphilis is a chronic disease that can be spread to others even though no symptoms are evident. Clients need to understand the importance of (1) taking any and all prescribed medication, (2) referring sexual partners for evaluation and treatment, (3) abstaining from all sexual contact for a minimum of 1 month after treatment, and (4) using a condom to avoid transmitting or

---

Selected Nursing Diagnoses for Clients with Sexually Transmitted Disease

■ ■ ■

- *Risk for Injury* related to manifestations of the disease process

- *Noncompliance* related to lack of understanding of treatment and/or importance of partner follow-up

- *Impaired Skin Integrity* related to the presence of lesions

- *Impaired Tissue Integrity* related to the the presence of disease lesions

- *Altered Health Maintenance* related to lack of knowledge about transmission, disease process, or treatment regimen

- *Pain* related to the infectious process

- *Ineffective Individual Coping* related to shame, guilt, or anger

- *Sexual Dysfunction* related to fear of transmission

- *Impaired Social Interaction* related to social stigma

- *Anxiety* related to possible infertility resulting from the STD

- *Self-Esteem Disturbance* related to the effects of having an STD

- *Fear* related to possible surgical intervention

---

contracting infections in the future (see the box on page 2068). They should also understand the need for follow-up testing (at 3 and 6 months for clients with primary or secondary syphilis, and at 6 and 12 months for those with late stage disease). If clients are HIV-positive, follow-up visits are recommended at 1, 2, 3, 6, 9, and 12 months after treatment.

Applying the Nursing Process

Case Study of a Client with Syphilis: Eddie Kratz

Eddie Kratz, a 22-year-old man, lives in a major metropolitan area on the East Coast. Mr. Kratz works as a bellman at a large hotel. For the past year, he has shared a small apartment with Marla Jones, a young woman who is 7 months pregnant with his child. Although he intends to marry Ms. Jones before the baby is born, he has continued a previous relationship with a woman named Justine

Simpson. His sexual activities with Ms. Simpson have increased in frequency as Ms. Jones's pregnancy has advanced. Recently Mr. Kratz has noticed a swelling in his groin and a sore on his penis.

Assessment

When Mr. Kratz comes to the community clinic, he is interviewed by the nurse practitioner, Sally Morovitz. Ms. Morovitz takes a thorough medical and sexual history, including questions about drug use, allergies, difficulty with urination, urinary frequency, itching or discharge from the penis, recent sexual activities, precautions taken against infection, history of STDs, and sexual function. She determines that Mr. Kratz has been having unprotected sex with Ms. Jones and Ms. Simpson. He believes that Ms. Jones is not having sex with anyone except him, but he is not sure.

Physical assessment reveals a classic syphilitic chancre on the shaft of the penis and regional lymphadenopathy. A specimen of exudate from the chancre is sent for dark-field examination. Ms. Morovitz discusses with Mr. Kratz the likelihood that he has syphilis and the need to tell both Ms. Jones and Ms. Simpson so that they can be tested and, if necessary, treated. Mr. Kratz has no prior history of STD or of intravenous drug use. Ms. Morovitz also suggests that Mr. Kratz be tested for HIV since he has been having unprotected sex with two women, at least one of whom may be sexually active with other partners. He agrees, and blood is drawn for an ELISA test.

Darkfield analysis of the chancre exudate confirms the diagnosis of syphilis, but the ELISA results are negative for HIV.

Diagnosis

Ms. Morovitz makes the following nursing diagnoses for Mr. Kratz:

- *Risk for Injury* to the client, his partners, and the infant related to the disease process
- *Altered Health Maintenance* related to a lack of knowledge about the disease process, its transmission, and the need for treatment
- *Altered Family Processes* related to the effects of the diagnosis of syphilis on the couple's relationship
- *Anxiety* related to the effects of the infection on the unborn child

Expected Outcomes

The expected outcomes for the plan of care are that

- Prompt treatment will cure the syphilis in Mr. Kratz, his partners, and the infant.
- Mr. Kratz and his partners will understand the need to abstain from sexual contact during treatment, com-

plete all medications, return for follow-up visits, and use condoms to prevent reinfection.

- Supportive counseling will help Mr. Kratz and Ms. Jones cope with the impact of diagnosis and treatment on their relationship.
- Education and reassurance that treatment for syphilis reduces the risk of harm to the infant will help relieve the couple's anxiety.

Planning and Implementation

The following interventions are planned and implemented during care of Mr. Kratz:

- Administer IM injection of benzathine penicillin G as ordered, and document.
- Discuss the importance of abstaining from sexual activity until he and his partners are cured, and of using condoms to prevent reinfection.
- Explain the need for Mr. Kratz to return for follow-up testing in 3 months and again at 6 months. Provide a copy of the STD prevention checklist, and document that reminders need to be sent at 3- and 6-month intervals.
- Notify Ms. Jones and Ms. Simpson that they need to come to the clinic for testing.
- Refer Mr. Kratz and Ms. Jones to a social worker for counseling about the impact of the disease on their relationship.
- Teach the couple about the importance of treatment to the health of their infant.

Evaluation

At the 3-month follow-up visit, the chancre on Mr. Kratz's penis has healed, and he reports that he is using a condom any time he has sex. Ms. Jones has also tested positive for syphilis and negative for HIV, so she, too, is given benzathine penicillin G, and verbal and written follow-up instructions, including monthly follow-up until the infant is born. The couple is meeting every other week with the social worker and say that their relationship is improving. Ms. Simpson has received similar test results and is given a prescription for doxycycline because she is allergic to penicillin.

Critical Thinking in the Nursing Process

1. What signs and symptoms might a client with early syphilis experience?

2. List some appropriate questions for taking a sexual history when you suspect the presence of one or more STDs.

3. How might you counsel Mr. Kratz to help him break the news of the diagnosis and his infidelity to Ms. Jones?

4. Develop a nursing care plan for Mr. Kratz for the nursing diagnosis *Impaired Social Interaction* related to social stigma.

The Client with Genital Herpes

■ ■ ■

Genital herpes (herpes genitalis) is caused by the herpes simplex virus, usually type 2 (HSV-2), and is spread by vaginal, anal, or oral-genital contact. The incubation period for genital herpes is 3 to 7 days.

Although not a new disease, genital herpes cases skyrocketed during the 1970s. Genital herpes is chronic and, in many people, largely asymptomatic. Currently, it is incurable.

Estimates suggest that 10 to 30 million people in the United States have genital herpes (about 1 in 6), and between 200,000 and 500,000 more people are infected each year (Johnson et al., 1989). The incidence of genital herpes, like that of other STDs, is highest among adolescents and young adults.

Up to 80% of infected people experience frequent, painful recurrences (Price & Wilson, 1992). Other than recurrences, however, men are not likely to experience serious physical complications of genital herpes. Women, however, face concerns about childbearing (and infection of the newborn during delivery, resulting in death for 6 of 10 infants) and possible cervical cancer, although the risk of malignancy is not clearly established (Trimble, 1986).

Pathophysiology

Within a week after exposure to genital herpes, painful red papules appear in the genital area. In men, the lesions generally occur on the glans or shaft of the penis. In women, the lesions commonly occur on the labia, vagina, and cervix. Anal intercourse may result in lesions in and around the anus.

Soon after the papules appear, they form small painful blisters filled with clear fluid containing virus particles (Figure 49–4). The blisters break, shedding the highly infectious virus and creating patches of painful ulcers that last 6 weeks (or longer if they become infected). Touching these blisters and then rubbing or scratching in another place can spread the infection to other areas of the body (*autoinoculation*).

The first outbreak of herpes lesions is called *first episode infection,* with a mean duration of 12 days. Subsequent occurrences, usually less severe, are termed *recurrent infections* (mean duration of 4 to 5 days). The period between episodes is called *latency,* during which time the person remains infectious even though no symptoms are present. During latency, the virus withdraws into the

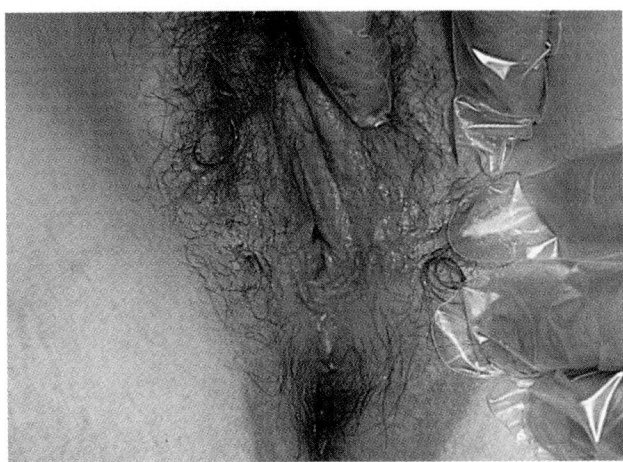

Figure 49–4   Genital herpes blisters as they appear on the labia.

Clinical Manifestations of Genital Herpes

■ ■ ■

- Herpetic lesions
- Regional lymphadenopathy
- Headache
- Fever
- General malaise
- Dysuria
- Urinary retention
- Vaginal discharge
- Urethral discharge (men)

---

nerve fibers that lead from the infected site to the lower spine, remaining dormant until recurrence, at which time it retraces its path to the genital area.

The clinical manifestations of genital herpes are presented in the accompanying box. *Prodromal symptoms* (warning signals or clues) of recurrent outbreaks of genital herpes can include burning, itching, tingling, or throbbing at the sites where lesions commonly appear. These sensations may be accompanied by pain in the legs, groin, or buttocks. Some authorities believe that prodromal symptoms signal increased levels of infectiousness, during which sexual contact should be avoided.

In rare cases, the herpes virus spreads to the brain, causing *herpes encephalitis,* a life-threatening disorder. Prompt treatment with acyclovir can cure the encephalitis, but more than 60% of survivors have permanent neurologic damage.

Applying Research to Nursing Practice: Physical and Psychosocial Effects of Genital Herpes

■ ■ ■

Researchers studied 70 young adults to determine the physical and psychosocial effects of living with genital herpes (Swanson, Dibble, & Chenitz, 1995). Stress was found to be the major cause of recurrence, headaches the major stress symptom, and acyclovir the major treatment. Findings indicated that young adults with genital herpes had lower self-concept, more psychopathology, greater frequency of daily hassles, and less intense emotional uplifts than nonpatient control subjects. The researchers found no differences between the two groups in scores on depression.

Implications for Nursing

Clients with genital herpes need psychosocial support and counseling as well as education in self-care measures to deal with physical effects of the disease. Teaching stress-management techniques and suggesting alternatives to sexual intercourse, such as masturbation, may be useful. Allowing clients to express feelings and perceptions about how genital herpes has affected their lives can be an important part of counseling. Teaching safer sex practices and communication skills to use with a partner needs to be part of the care of all clients with STDs.

Critical Thinking in Client Care

1. Do you believe that the threat of contracting genital herpes or another chronic STD will change established sexual behavior patterns among high school and college students? Why or why not?

2. Do people with genital herpes who take appropriate precautions have the right to enter into sexual relationships without revealing that they are infected? Why or why not?

3. Why would the presence of genital herpes increase the likelihood of contracting other STDs?

Collaborative Care

Because there is no cure for genital herpes, treatment focuses on relieving symptoms and preventing spread of the infection. Client education is essential to prevent further transmission of the disease and to help clients integrate management of a chronic disease into their life-styles.

Presumptive diagnosis of genital herpes is based on history and physical examination of the client, including lesions and patterns of recurrence. Definitive diagnosis requires isolation of the virus in tissue culture. Ideally, tissue specimens should be obtained within 48 hours of the appearance of the blisters.

Acyclovir helps reduce the length and severity of the first episode and is the treatment of choice for genital herpes. The oral form is considered most effective for first episode as well as recurrences and is given for 7 to 10 days or until lesions heal. It may also be administered intravenously. Evidence shows that some strains of HSV are becoming resistant to acyclovir, particularly in HIV-positive people. In those cases, foscarnet is used.

Nursing Care

In planning and implementing holistic nursing care for the client with genital herpes, the nurse needs to consider both short-term and long-term implications. Although the immediate priority is symptom relief and prevention of further transmission, the client needs assistance to deal with the life-changing diagnosis of a chronic disease (see the accompanying box). Nursing diagnoses discussed in this section focus on pain, sexual dysfunction, and anxiety regarding childbearing and possible malignancy.

Pain

Herpetic lesions are very painful and can become infected. Because the virus resides in the nerve ganglia, pain may also occur in the legs, thighs, groin, or buttocks. Although acyclovir diminishes the pain of herpes and accelerates the healing process, additional measures can relieve the discomfort further.

Nursing interventions with rationales follow:

- Teach the client to keep herpes blisters clean and dry. A solution of warm water, soap, and hydrogen peroxide can be used to cleanse the lesions two or three times daily. Burrow's solution can also be used. Lesions should be dried using a hair dryer turned to a cool setting. It is important to wear loose cotton clothing that will not trap moisture; panty hose and tight jeans are to be avoided. *Keeping the lesions clean and dry reduces the possibility of secondary infection and speeds the healing process.*

- For clients experiencing dysuria, suggest pouring water over the genitals while urinating. Drinking additional fluids also helps dilute the acidity of the urine; however, fluids that increase acidity, such as cranberry juice, should be avoided. *These measures dilute the acid content of urine and thereby reduce the burning sensation.*

Sexual Dysfunction

Clients who learn that they are infected with an incurable STD may believe they can no longer have a normal sex life. Fortunately, many people have learned to live with and manage genital herpes without infecting their partners or their children.

Nursing interventions with rationales follow:

- Provide a supportive, nonjudgmental environment for the client to discuss feelings and ask questions about what this diagnosis means to future sexual relationships. *Feelings of guilt, shame, and anger are natural responses to such a diagnosis and can lead to a total avoidance of sexual intimacy.*

- Offer information about support groups and other resources for people with herpes such as the National Herpes Information Hotline. *Information about how others cope with this disease can offset feelings of shame and hopelessness.*

Anxiety

The woman with genital herpes faces two serious potential complications: elevated risk of cervical cancer and infection of her neonate during delivery. Some evidence suggests that the risk of cervical cancer is higher among women with genital herpes (Trimble et al., 1986), although a direct causal link has not been identified. There is no question about the risk of neonatal infection from a mother with herpes, however, and such infection can range from asymptomatic to widely disseminated fatal disease. Transmission occurs during passage through the birth canal. The risk is highest during the first episode of infection.

Nursing interventions with rationales follow:

- Advise the client about need for regular Papanicolaou (Pap) smears; some authorities suggest Pap smears every 6 months for women with genital herpes. *Careful monitoring will detect cervical dysplasia at a time when treatment is most likely to be effective.*

- Discuss with women of childbearing age that cesarean delivery can prevent transmission of infection to the neonate. In women without signs or symptoms of recurrence, vaginal delivery is possible (Prober et al., 1988). *Understanding that infection of the neonate can be prevented helps relieve anxiety.*

Client and Family Teaching

Health teaching for clients with genital herpes involves helping them manage this chronic disease with the least possible disruption in life-style and relationships. Understanding the disease process and factors that affect it helps the client regain a sense of control and see the potential for future sexual intimacy without transmission of infection. The nurse discusses how to recognize prodromal symptoms of recurrence and factors that seem to trigger recurrences (such as emotional stress, acidic food, sun exposure) and explains the need for abstinence from sexual contact from the time prodromal symptoms appear until 10 days after all lesions have healed. If lesions become infected, topical acyclovir may prove useful. Painful lesions can be protected with sterile vaseline or aloe vera gel. It is important to emphasize the use of latex condoms and careful hygiene practices (such as not sharing towels or other personal items) even during latency periods.

◾◾◾   STDs Primarily Infecting Epithelial Surfaces   ◾◾◾

Sexually transmitted diseases that infect epithelial surfaces include gonorrhea (a classic, reportable STD), chlamydial infections, and genital warts (also known as condyloma acuminatum). Gonorrhea and chlamydial infections are caused by bacteria, and genital warts by a virus. These diseases cause many similar manifestations, and clients may be infected with more than one of them. For example, 45% of people with gonorrhea also are infected with *Chlamydia*.

The Client with Gonorrhea

◾ ◾ ◾

Gonorrhea, also known as *GC* or *clap,* is caused by *Neisseria gonorrhoeae,* a gram-negative diplococcus, strains of which have become increasingly resistant to antibiotics,

particularly penicillin. The incubation period is 2 to 8 days after exposure. Gonorrhea is transmitted by direct sexual contact and during delivery as the neonate passes through the birth canal. Gonorrhea is the most commonly reported communicable disease in the United States. More than 700,000 cases of gonorrhea were reported in 1992, and the CDC estimates that an equal or larger number of cases go unreported, making the actual total between 2 and 3 million cases annually. Like most STDs, gonorrhea is most commonly found in people 15 to 34 years old in urban ethnic minority populations (Schwebke, 1991).

Pathophysiology

The organism initially targets the cervix and the male urethra. Without treatment, the disease ultimately disseminates to other organs. In men, gonorrhea can cause acute, painful inflammation of the prostate, epididymis, and periurethral glands and can lead to sterility. In women, it can cause pelvic inflammatory disease (PID), endometritis, salpingitis, and pelvic peritonitis. In the neonate, gonorrhea can cause ophthalmia neonatorum, rhinitis, or anorectal infection.

Manifestations of gonorrhea in men include dysuria and serous, milky, or purulent discharge. Some men also experience regional lymphadenopathy. About 20% of men and 80% of women remain asymptomatic until the disease is advanced. Those women with symptoms experience dysuria, urinary frequency, or abnormal vaginal discharge.

Collaborative Care

The goals of treatment for the client with gonorrhea include eradication of the organism and any coexisting disease, and prevention of reinfection or transmission. It is important to emphasize the importance of taking all medications as prescribed and abstaining from sexual contact until the infection is cured in both client and partners. Condom use to prevent future infections is essential, particularly for pregnant women whose partners may be infected.

Laboratory and Diagnostic Tests

Diagnosis of gonorrhea is based on history and physical assessment, plus laboratory tests. A gonorrhea diagnosis can usually be confirmed in men by obtaining a smear of urethral discharge. Cultures are not necessary unless Gram stains of smears are negative despite typical clinical symptoms of gonorrhea.

Diagnosis of gonorrhea in women is more complex because organisms resembling *N. gonorrhoeae* are normally found in the female genital tract. Thus, Gram stains of cervical discharge smears are not conclusive, and cultures are necessary. Because culture studies involve 24- to 48-hour delays, treatment is usually begun on presumptive diagnosis.

The likely coexistence of multiple STDs in one client makes it important also to test for syphilis and to suggest that the client be tested for HIV. Any sexual partners should be examined and screened as well.

Pharmacology

Because there are now many penicillin-resistant strains of *N. gonorrhoeae,* an alternative antibiotic, ceftriaxone, is recommended for treatment of gonorrhea. Ceftriaxone is given in a single intramuscular injection. In addition, doxycycline is usually given orally for 7 days to treat any existing chlamydial infection. Infected sexual partners also need to be treated.

Nursing Care

In planning and implementing care for the client with gonorrhea, the nurse considers the possible coexistence of other STDs such as syphilis and HIV, the impact of the disease and its treatment on the client's life-style, and the likelihood of noncompliance. Nursing diagnoses discussed in this section focus on noncompliance and impaired social interaction.

Noncompliance

Although one-time treatment with ceftriaxone is highly effective in curing gonorrhea, noncompliance with the doxycycline regimen may leave any coexisting chlamydial infection unresolved. Noncompliance with recommendations for abstinence, follow-up, or condom use fosters a high rate of reinfection. Failure to refer partners for examination and treatment also leads to reinfection.

Nursing interventions with rationales follow:

- Help the client understand the need for taking all medications as directed and keeping follow-up appointments to be sure no reinfection has occurred. Discuss the prevalence of gonorrhea and the potential complications if it is not cured. *The client who understands the complications of incomplete or failed treatment is more likely to comply with the medication regimen.*

- Discuss with the client the importance of sexual abstinence until the infection is cured, referral of partners, and condom use to prevent reinfection. *Understanding that cure is possible and reinfection is avoidable helps the client cope with the disease and its treatment and is likely to increase compliance.*

Impaired Social Interaction

Diagnosis of any STD can make clients feel "dirty," ashamed, and guilty about their sexual behaviors, and unworthy to be with others.

Nursing interventions with rationales follow:

- Provide privacy, confidentiality, and a safe, nonjudgmental environment for client to express concerns. Help the client understand that gonorrhea is a consequence of sexual behavior, not a "punishment," and that it can be avoided in the future. *Being treated with respect and privacy helps the client realize that the disease does not change an individual's worth as a person. This knowledge enhances the client's ability to relate to others.*

Client and Family Teaching

Health teaching focuses on helping clients understand the importance of (1) taking any and all prescribed medication, (2) referring sexual partners for evaluation and treatment, (3) abstaining from all sexual contact until the client and partners are cured, and (4) using a condom to avoid transmitting or contracting infections in the future. Clients also need to understand the need for a follow-up visit 4 to 7 days after treatment is completed.

Applying the Nursing Process

Case Study of a Client with Gonorrhea: Janet Cirit

Janet Cirit, a 33-year-old legal secretary, lives in a suburban midwestern community. She is unmarried but dating a man named Jim Adkins, who lives in an adjacent suburb. Ms. Cirit visits her gynecologist because her periods have become irregular and she is experiencing pelvic pain and an abnormal amount of vaginal discharge. Recently she has developed a sore throat. The pelvic pain has begun to disrupt her sleeping pattern, and she is concerned that she might have cancer because her mother recently died of ovarian cancer.

Assessment
When Ms. Cirit arrives for her appointment at the gynecologist's office, she is interviewed by Marsha Davidson, the nurse practitioner. Ms. Davidson completes a thorough medical and sexual history, including questions about her menstrual periods, pain associated with urination or sexual intercourse, urinary frequency, most recent Pap smear, birth control method, history of STD and drug use, and types of sexual activity. Ms. Cirit reports her symptoms and her concern about ovarian cancer. She also indicates that she is taking oral contraceptives and therefore sees no need for Mr. Adkins to use a condom because she believes their relationship is monogamous.

Physical examination reveals both pharyngeal and cervical inflammation, and lower abdominal tenderness. Ms. Cirit's temperature is 98.5 F (37.0 C). There are no signs or symptoms of pregnancy.

The gynecologist orders a Pap smear and cultures of the cervix, urethra, and pharynx to evaluate for gonorrhea and chlamydial infection. Blood is drawn for WBC. Test results are positive for gonorrhea and negative for *Chlamydia*. The WBC is slightly elevated, indicating possible salpingitis. Because Mr. Adkins has been Ms. Cirit's only sexual partner, it is clear that he is the source of infection and needs to be treated as well.

Diagnosis
Ms. Davidson makes the following nursing diagnoses for Ms. Cirit:

- *Pain* related to the infectious process
- *Anxiety* related to fear about possible cancer

- *Self-Esteem Disturbance* related to shame and guilt because of having an STD
- *Altered Sexuality Patterns* related to the impaired relationship and fear of reinfection

Expected Outcomes
The expected outcomes are that Ms. Cirit will

- Experience relief of pain, indicating that the infection had been eradicated.
- Express relief that the Pap smear showed no abnormal cells.
- Verbalize that she has nothing to be ashamed of and that she has been wise to seek treatment as soon as symptoms occurred.
- Verbalize that she will insist her partner use condoms during future sexual activity.

Planning and Implementation
The following interventions are planned and implemented during care of Ms. Cirit:

- Administer ceftriaxone IM as ordered and document.
- Emphasize the need for regular Pap smears and pelvic examinations because of the family history of ovarian cancer.
- Discuss with Ms. Cirit her feelings and concerns about the diagnosis of gonorrhea. Remind her that such a diagnosis does not reflect on her self-worth as a person.
- Teach Ms. Cirit how she might talk with a future sexual partner about condom use.

Evaluation
A week later during her follow-up visit, Ms. Cirit states that she is feeling much better and sleeping well at night since the pain has ended. She has terminated her relationship with Mr. Adkins and is considering joining a health club in the hope of increasing her level of fitness and perhaps meeting someone new.

Critical Thinking in the Nursing Process

1. What signs might have caused Ms. Cirit to suspect that Mr. Adkins had gonorrhea?

2. How are Ms. Cirit's signs and symptoms related to the infectious process of gonorrhea?

3. How might Ms. Cirit convince a future sexual partner to use condoms during sexual activity without spoiling the romantic aspect?

4. Should the nurse have suggested that Ms. Cirit also be tested for HIV? Why or why not?

5. Develop a care plan for Ms. Cirit for the nursing diagnosis *Impaired Social Interaction*.

Risk Factors for Chlamydial Infection

■ ■ ■

- Personal or partner history of STD
- Pregnancy
- Adolescent sexual activity
- Oral contraceptive use
- Unprotected sexual activity
- Multiple sexual partners

The Client with a Chlamydial Infection

■ ■ ■

Chlamydial infections are caused by *Chlamydia trachomatis,* a bacterium that behaves like a virus, reproducing only within the host cell. It is spread by any sexual contact and to the neonate by passage through the birth canal of an infected mother. The incubation period is from 1 to 3 weeks; however, chlamydial infection may be present for months or years without producing noticeable symptoms in women.

In addition to causing a diverse group of genital infections, *C. trachomatis* causes *trachoma,* a chronic, contagious type of conjunctivitis and the leading cause of preventable blindness. Trachoma is prevalent in Asia and Africa.

Chlamydial infections are thought to be the most common STDs in the United States and the leading cause of pelvic inflammatory disease (PID) (see Chapter 47). Not all states require reporting of chlamydial infections; thus, accurate statistics are not available. However, the CDC estimates that 3 to 5 million men, women, and infants develop a chlamydial infection each year. Incidence is highest among sexually active teenagers. Young women using oral contraceptives appear to be at especially high risk for contracting chlamydial infection if exposed (Áral & Holmes, 1991). Risk factors for chlamydial infection are listed in the accompanying box.

Because chlamydial infections are asymptomatic in most women until they have invaded the uterus and uterine tubes, treatment is delayed, resulting in devastating long-term complications. Nearly a third of men with urethral chlamydial infection are also asymptomatic. Chlamydial infection is a leading cause of preventable blindness, particularly in the newborn.

Pathophysiology

Chlamydial infections typically invade the same target organs as gonorrhea (cervix and male urethra) and result in similar manifestations (dysuria, urinary frequency, and discharge). Clients may be asymptomatic; however, they are still potentially infectious.

If chlamydial infections in women are not treated, they ascend into the upper reproductive tract, causing such complications as PID, which includes endometritis, salpingitis, and chronic pelvic pain. These infections are a major cause of infertility and ectopic pregnancy, a potentially life-threatening disorder in women. Complications of chlamydial infections in men include epididymitis, prostatitis, sterility, and Reiter's syndrome.

Collaborative Care

Although *C. trachomatis* is similar to a virus in its intracellular growth, it is like a bacterium in its susceptibility to treatment with inexpensive antibiotics. Its prevalence, particularly in younger populations, makes widespread screening necessary if the disease is to be controlled.

Because chlamydial infections are often asymptomatic, treatment is often begun on a presumptive basis. The CDC recommends screening asymptomatic women who are at high risk for chlamydial infection.

Laboratory and Diagnostic Tests

Definitive diagnosis of chlamydial infection requires cultures of tissue from the female endocervix and urethra, or from the male urethra. This is an expensive test involving special media; thus, diagnosis may be based on ruling out gonorrhea on a urethral Gram's stain and culture, and on a complete history and physical assessment.

Three recently developed rapid tests are available for diagnosis of chlamydial infection, using specimens of urogenital secretions: (1) Enzyme immunoassay (EIA) chlamydiazyme or test patch (Abbott), (2) direct immunofluorescence (MicroTrak), and (3) polymerase chain reaction (PCR) assay (Bowie et al., 1994). Urine tests for chlamydia using PCR and LCR (ligase chain reaction) are more sensitive than cultures and expected to be widely available in early 1996 (Hook et al., 1995).

Pharmacology

The drug of choice for chlamydial infections in men and nonpregnant women is oral doxycycline given twice daily for 7 days. For pregnant women, erythromycin is the alternative therapy. Other alternatives include azithromycin given in a single dose or ofloxacin given twice daily for 7 days. Nursing implications for these antibiotics are presented in the box on page 257 of Chapter 8.

Nursing Care

Nursing care of the client with a chlamydial infection focuses on eradication of the infection, prevention of future infections, and management of any chronic complica-

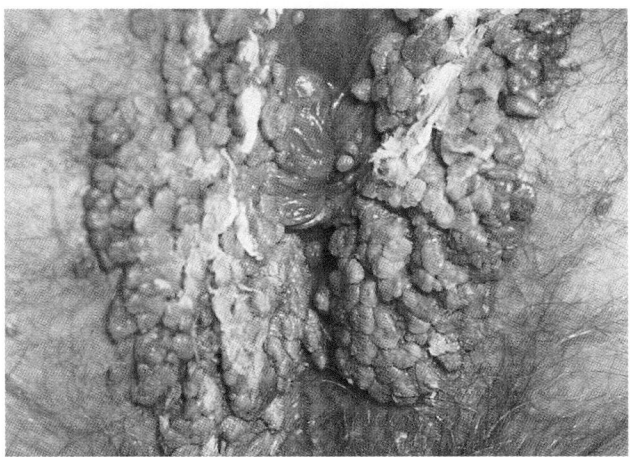
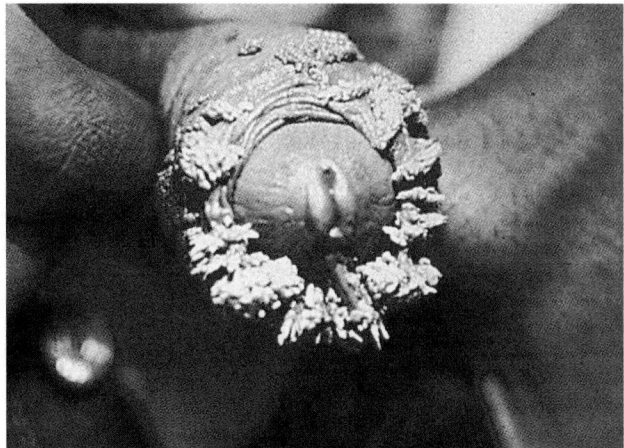

Figure 49–5   Genital warts (condyloma acuminatum) on the vulva and penis.

tions. Nursing diagnoses for the client with a chlamydial infection are the same as for clients with any STD (see the box on page 2071). Interventions are similar to those previously discussed for gonorrhea and genital herpes.

Client and Family Teaching

Health teaching for the client with a chlamydial infection centers on the need to comply with the treatment regimen, refer partners for examination and necessary treatment, and the use of condoms to avoid reinfection. If the infection has progressed to PID, the client needs additional information on self care and health promotion (see Chapter 47).

The Client with Genital Warts

■ ■ ■

Genital and anal warts, also known as *condyloma acuminatum* or venereal warts, are caused by human papillomavirus (HPV) and are transmitted by all types of sexual contact. The incubation period for genital warts ranges from 3 weeks to 18 months, with an average of 3 months. There are more than 70 types of HPV, several of which cause chronic genital infections (Wikström et al., 1992).

Genital warts are the most common symptomatic viral non-AIDS STD in the United States (Zazove et al., 1991). They account for more than one million physician office visits annually. Research suggests a strong association between HPV and cancers of the cervix, vagina, vulva, penis, and anus (Bauer et al., 1991; Cusick et al., 1992, Zazove et al., 1991).

Like most STDs, genital warts are most commonly found in young, sexually active adults and are associated with early onset of sexual activity and multiple sexual partners. An estimated 3 million cases are diagnosed each year. Studies indicate that 20 million or more women in the United States are infected with HPV and that three of four sexual partners of infected women are also infected (Zazove et al., 1991).

Pathophysiology

Although some people may carry HPV virus without symptoms, most exhibit characteristic manifestations: single or multiple painless, cauliflower-like growths on the vulvovaginal area, perineum, penis, urethra, or anus (Figure 49–5). In women, the growths may appear in the vagina or on the cervix and be apparent only during a pelvic examination.

Potential complications of genital warts include obstruction of the urethra, causing bleeding, and transmission of the virus to the fetus during pregnancy or delivery (Fletcher, 1991). Infants infected with HPV virus can develop *respiratory papillomatosis*, a respiratory condition causing chronic distress and requiring multiple surgeries.

Collaborative Care

Treatment is directed at removal of the warts, relief of symptoms, and health teaching to reduce the risk of recurrence and future transmission. The HPV is considered chronic, however, with recurrence experienced in 80% of those infected.

Laboratory and Diagnostic Tests

Genital and anal warts are diagnosed primarily by clinical appearance or by examination of Pap smear specimens. However, therapy is not determined until a VDRL test for syphilis and a gonorrheal culture have been done. Because HPV infection has been associated with various genital and anal cancers, biopsy is performed if lesions bleed.

Nursing Implications for Pharmacology: The Client with Genital Warts

TOPICAL APPLICATIONS

Podophyllin resin (Pod-Ben-25, podofilox 0.5% solution)

Trichloroacetic acid

Although cryotherapy using liquid nitrogen or a cryoprobe is more commonly used to treat genital warts, podophyllum preparations or trichloroacetic acid are sometimes used. Podophyllin resin, 25% in compound tincture of benzoin, is applied topically to the warts by the physician once weekly for 3 to 5 weeks.

Podophyllin resin is contraindicated during pregnancy; the alternative is cryotherapy or topical treatment with trichloroacetic acid. Podophyllin resin is also contraindicated in cervical, urethral, oral, or anorectal warts. It is important to avoid contact of podophyllin resin with the eyes.

Adverse effects of podophyllin resin include local irritation, severe ulceration of surrounding tissue, nausea, diarrhea, lethargy, paralysis, and coma.

Nursing Responsibilities

- Establish baseline data, including mental status, vital signs, and weight.

- Document and report any existing lesions (genital, anal, or oral).
- Cover the tissue surrounding the warts with petrolatum or a paste of baking soda and water to protect the tissue from the caustic treatment solution.

Client and Family Teaching

- Wash off the treated area thoroughly within 1 to 4 hours after the first application; gradually increase this period to 6 to 8 hours after the second and subsequent applications.
- Return for regular treatment until warts are gone.
- Refer partners for examination and any necessary treatment.
- Report any adverse effects (nausea, diarrhea, local irritation, lethargy, numbness)
- Avoid sexual activity until you and your partners have been free of disease for 1 month.
- Use condoms to prevent future infections.
- Return for an annual Pap smear.

Pharmacology

Topical agents used to treat genital warts include podofilox, 0.5% solution for self-treatment, or podophyllin, 10%–25% in compound tincture of benzoin. Podophyllin is contraindicated during pregnancy and can have serious side effects in any client, ranging from nausea, diarrhea, and lethargy to paralysis and coma (see the accompanying box).

Other Techniques

Genital warts may also be removed by cryotherapy, electrocautery, or surgical excision. Carbon dioxide laser surgery is becoming increasingly common for removal of extensive warts.

Nursing Care

Nursing care for the client with genital or anal warts includes pretreatment teaching, treatment of the lesions, health teaching for self-care, and health promotion. Nursing diagnoses discussed in this section focus on impaired tissue integrity and fear.

Impaired Tissue Integrity

Genital warts can enlarge and destroy normal tissue. They can also enlarge and block the urethra. The highly vascular lesions enlarge during pregnancy and may obstruct the birth canal, necessitating cesarean delivery. The increased risk of cervical cancer makes an annual Pap smear essential for women with genital warts.

Nursing interventions with rationales follow:

- Discuss the need for prompt treatment and the necessity for sexual abstinence until lesions have healed. *This reduces the risk of reinfection and further transmission of the disease.*
- Discuss the increased risk of cervical cancer and the importance of an annual Pap smear. *Understanding the risk, the client will be more motivated to seek annual screening.*

Fear

Surgery engenders some degree of fear in most clients: fear of the procedure itself, of pain and possible complications. Surgery or cryotherapy in the genital area involves all these fears plus fear of possible impaired sexual function.

Nursing interventions with rationales follow:

- Allow the client to express specific fears and feelings about the procedure. Explain the procedure, approximate recovery time, possible complications and ways to avoid them, and ways to cope with complications that do occur. *Knowing what to expect reduces the client's fear and helps the client feel a greater sense of control.*

- Explain that the procedure is performed with only local anesthesia. *Being awake during surgery gives the client a greater sense of participation in the treatment process.*

Client and Family Teaching

Health teaching emphasizes the need for the client and infected partners to return for regular treatment until lesions have resolved, and to use condoms to prevent reinfection. Because of the increased risk of cervical cancer, annual Pap smears are essential for female clients.

Bibliography

■ ■ ■

Althaus, F. A. (1991). An ounce of prevention: STDs and women's health. *Family Planning Perspectives, 23*(4),173–177.

Aral S. O., & Holmes K. K. (1991). Sexually transmitted diseases in the AIDS era. *Scientific American, 264*(2), 62–69.

Bauer, H. et al. (1991). Genital human papillomavirus infection in female university students as determined by a PCR-based method. *Journal of the American Medical Association, 265,* 472–477.

Bowie, W. R., Hammerschlag, M. R., & Martin, D. H. (1994). STDs in '94: The new CDC guidelines. *Patient Care, 28*(7), 29–53.

Cates, W., Jr. (1990). Sexually transmitted diseases: The scale of the problem in the developed and developing world. In N. Job-Spira, B. Spencer, J. P. Moatti, & E. Bouvet (Eds.). *Public health and sexual transmission of diseases: Directions for future research and health policy* (pp. 26–32). Paris: John Libbey.

Centers for Disease Control. (1988). Policy guidelines for the prevention and control of congenital syphilis. *Morbidity and Mortality Weekly Report, 37* (Suppl. S-1), 1–13.

Centers for Disease Control. (1990). Risk for cervical disease in HIV-infected women: New York City. *Morbidity and Mortality Weekly Report, 39,* 846–849.

Centers for Disease Control. (1991). Notifiable diseases. *Morbidity and Mortality Weekly Report, 40,*(51,52), 899–901.

Centers for Disease Control. (1992) Summary of notifiable diseases, United States, 1991. *Morbidity and Mortality Weekly Report, 41*(53), 1–41.

Centers for Disease Control. (1993). Sexually transmitted diseases treatment guidelines. *Morbidity and Mortality Weekly Report, 42*(RR 14), 1–102.

Cusick, J. et al. (1992). Human papillomavirus type 16 DNA in cervical smears as predictor of high-grade cervical cancer. *Lancet, 339,* 959–960.

Detmer, W. M., McPhee, S. J., Nicoll, D., & Chou, T. (1992). *Pocket guide to diagnostic tests.* Norwalk, CT: Appleton & Lange.

EDK Associates. (1994). *Women and sexually transmitted diseases: The dangers of denial.* New York: Campaign for Women's Health.

Fletcher, J. (1991). Perinatal transmission of human papillomavirus. *American Family Physician, 43,* 143–148.

Grimes, D. A. (1986). Deaths due to sexually transmitted diseases: The forgotten component of reproductive mortality. *Journal of the American Medical Association, 255*(13), 1727–1729.

Hatcher, R. A. et al. (1994). *Contraceptive technology* (16th ed.). New York: Irvington Publishers.

Hook, E. W., III, Sondheimer, S., & Zenilman, J. (1995). Today's treatment for STDs. *Patient Care,* February 28, 40–56.

Johnson, R. E. et al. (1989). A seroepidemiological survey of the prevalence of herpes simplex virus type 2 in the United States. *New England Journal of Medicine, 321*(1), 7–12.

Judson, F. N. (1990). Gonorrhea. *Medical Clinics of North America, 74*(6), 1353–1366.

Katzung, B. G. (1991). *Drug therapy: A Lange clinical manual.* Norwalk, CT: Appleton & Lange.

Killion, C. (1994). Pregnancy: A critical time to target STDs. *Maternal-Child Nursing, 19*(3), 156–161.

Libbus, M. K. (1992). Condoms as primary prevention in sexually active women. *Maternal-Child Nursing, 17*(5), 256–260.

Netting, S. L., & Kauffman, F. H. (1990). Diagnosis and management of sexually transmitted genital lesions. *Nurse Practitioner, 15*(1), 20.

Potterat, J. J. (1992). "Socio-geographic space" and sexually transmissible disease in the 1990s. *Today's Life Science,* December, 16–31.

Price, S. A. & Wilson, L. M. (1992). *Pathophysiology: Clinical concepts of disease processes,* 4th ed. St. Louis: Mosby Year Book.

Prober, C. G. et al. (1988). Use of routine viral cultures at delivery to identify neonates exposed to herpes simplex virus. *New England Journal of Medicine, 318*(14), 887–891.

Quinn, T. C., & Cates, W., Jr. (1992). Epidemiology of sexually transmitted disease in the 1990s. In T. C. Quinn, J. I. Gallin, & A. S. Fauci (Eds.). *Advances in host defense mechanisms: Sexually transmitted diseases* (Vol. 8.) (pp. 1–37). New York: Raven Press.

Rolfs, R. T., & Nakashima, A. K. (1990). Epidemiology of primary and secondary syphilis in the United States, 1981 through 1989. *Journal of the American Medical Association, 264*(11), 1432–1437.

Schwarcz, S. et al. (1992). Crack cocaine and the exchange of sex for money or drugs. *Sexually Transmitted Diseases, 19,* 7–13.

Schwebke, J. (1991). Gonorrhea in the '90s. *Medical Aspects of Human Sexuality.* March, 43–46.

Straus, M., & Baron, L. (1983, November). *Sexual stratification, pornography, and rape in American states.* Paper presented at the annual meeting of the American Society of Criminology, Denver, CO.

Swanson, J. M., Dibble, S. L., & Chenitz, W. C. (1995). Clinical features and psychosocial factors in young adults with genital herpes. *Image: Journal of Nursing Scholarship, 27*(1), 16–22.

Talashek, M., Tichy, A., & Epping, H. (1990). Sexually transmitted diseases in the elderly: Issues and recommendations. *Journal of Gerontological Nursing, 16*(4), 33–40.

Tierney, L. M., McPhee, S. J., & Papadakis, M. A. *Current medical diagnosis and treatment 1994.* Norwalk CT: Appleton & Lange.

Tinkle, M. B. (1990). Genital human papillomavirus infection: A growing health risk. *Journal of Obstetric, Gynecologic & Neonatal Nursing, 19*(6), 501.

Tortora. G. J., Funke, B. R., & Case, C. L. (1995). *Microbiology: An introduction* (5th ed.). Menlo Park, CA: Benjamin/Cummings.

Trimble J., Gay H., & Docherty J. (1986). Characterization of the tumor-associated 38-kd protein of herpes simplex virus type II. *Journal of Reproductive Medicine, 31* (Suppl.), 399–409.

Washington, A. E., & Katz P. (1991). Cost of and payment source for pelvic inflammatory disease: Trends and projections, 1985 through 2000. *Journal of the American Medical Association, 266*(18), 2565–2569.

Wasserheit, J. N. (1992). Epidemiological synergy. Interrelationships between human immunodeficiency virus infection and other sexually transmitted diseases. *Sexually Transmitted Diseases, 19*(2), 61–77.

Wasserheit, J. N., & Holmes, K. K. (1992). Reproductive tract infection: Challenges for international health policy, programs, and research. In A. Germain, K. K. Holmes, P. Piot, & J. N. Wasserheit (Eds.). *Reproductive tract infections: Global impact and priorities for women's reproductive health* (pp 7–33). New York: Plenum Press.

Wikström, A. et al. (1992). The acetic test in evaluation of subclinical genital papillomavirus infection: A comparative study on peroscopy, histopathology, virology and scanning electron microscopy findings. *Genitourinary Medicine, 68,* 90–99.

Zazove, P., Caruthers, B., & Reed, D. (1991). Genital human papillomavirus infection. *American Family Physician, 43,* 1279–1291.

Zenilman, J. M. (1993). Gonorrhea: Clinical and public health issues. *Hospital Practice,* February, 31–50.

APPENDIX A

UNIVERSAL PRECAUTIONS

Universal precautions apply to blood and body fluids containing visible blood. They also apply to body tissues and to the following specific body fluids: Vaginal secretions, seminal secretions, cerebrospinal fluid, synovial fluid, pleural fluid, peritoneal fluid, amniotic fluid, saliva in dental procedures, and body fluids in situations where it is difficult to differentiate among body fluids. Universal precautions do not apply to feces, urine, nasal secretions, sputum, saliva, sweat, tears, or vomitus unless they contain visible blood.

Health care workers are at risk of exposure to blood-borne pathogens, i.e., hepatitis B virus, (HBV), hepatitis C virus (HCV), and human immunodeficiency virus (HIV). Health care workers should consider all clients as potentially infected with bloodborne pathogens and must follow the infection control precautions for all clients.

The Centers for Disease Control recommend the following specific precautions to reduce the risk of exposure to potentially infective materials:

Handwashing

- Wash your hands thoroughly with warm water and soap (a) immediately, if contaminated with blood or other body fluids to which universal precautions apply, or potentially contaminated articles; (b) between clients; and (c) immediately after gloves are removed, even if the gloves appear to be intact. When hand washing facilities are not available, use a waterless antiseptic hand cleaner in accordance with the manufacturer's directions.
- If you have an exudative lesion or weeping dermatitis, refrain from all direct client care and from handling client care equipment until the condition resolves.

Gloves

- Wear gloves when touching blood and body fluids containing blood, as well as when handling items or surfaces soiled with blood or body fluids as mentioned above.
- Wear gloves for all invasive procedures (i.e., any surgical entry into tissues, cavities, or organs or repair of major traumatic injuries).
- Change gloves after client contact.

- Wear gloves (a) if you have cuts, scratches, or other breaks in the skin; (b) in situations where hand contamination with blood may occur, e.g., with an uncooperative client; and (c) when you are performing venipuncture and other vascular procedures.

Other Protective Barriers

- Wear masks and protective eyewear (glasses, goggles) or face shields to protect the mucous membranes of your mouth, nose, and eyes during all invasive procedures and/or any procedure that is likely to generate droplets of blood or other body fluids to which universal precautions apply.
- Wear a disposable plastic apron or gown during procedures that are likely to generate splatters of blood or other body fluids (e.g., peritoneal fluid) and soil your clothing.

Sharps Disposal

To prevent injuries, place used disposable needle-syringe units, scalpel blades, and other sharp items in puncture-resistant containers for disposal. Discard used needle-syringe units *uncapped* and *unbroken*. Place puncture-resistant containers as close as practicable to use areas.

Laundry

Handle soiled linen as little as possible and with minimum agitation to prevent gross microbial contamination of the air and of persons handling the linen. Place linen soiled with blood or body fluids in leakage-resistant bags at the location where it is used.

Specimens

Put all specimens of blood and listed body fluids in well-constructed containers with secure lids to prevent leakage during transport. When collecting specimens, take care to avoid contaminating the outside of the container.

Blood Spills

Use a chemical germicide that is approved for use as a hospital disinfectant to decontaminate work surfaces after there is a spill of blood or other applicable body fluids. In the absence of a commercial germicide, a solution of sodium hypochlorite (household bleach) in a 1:100 dilution is effective.

Infective Wastes

- Follow agency policies for disposal of infective waste, both when disposing of, and when decontaminating, contaminated materials.
- Carefully pour bulk blood, suctioned fluids, and excretions containing blood and secretions, down drains that are connected to a sanitary sewer.

Sources U.S. Department of Health and Human Services, Public Health Service, Update: Universal precautions for prevention of transmission of human immunodeficiency virus, hepatitis B virus, and other bloodborne pathogens in health care settings, *Morbidity and Mortality Weekly Report,* June 24, 1988; 37: 377-382, 387-388; *Morbidity and Mortality Weekly Report,* June 23, 1989, 38/No. S-6: 9-18.

APPENDIX B

NURSING DIAGNOSES

North American Nursing Diagnosis Association, 1995

Activity Intolerance
Activity Intolerance, Risk for
Adaptive Capacity: Intracranial, Decreased
Adjustment, Impaired
Airway Clearance, Ineffective
Anxiety
Aspiration, Risk for
Body Image Disturbance
Body Temperature, Risk for Altered
Breastfeeding, Effective
Breastfeeding, Ineffective
Breastfeeding, Interrupted
Breathing Pattern, Ineffective
Caregiver Role Strain
Caregiver Role Strain, Risk for
Communication, Impaired Verbal
Community Coping, Potential for Enhanced
Confusion, Acute
Confusion, Chronic
Constipation
Constipation, Colonic
Constipation, Perceived
Decisional Conflict (Specify)
Decreased Cardiac Output
Defensive Coping
Denial, Ineffective
Diarrhea
Disorganized Infant Behavior
Disorganized Infant Behavior, Risk for
Disuse Syndrome, Risk for
Diversional Activity Deficit
Dysfunctional Grieving
Dysfunctional Ventilatory Weaning Response
Dysreflexia
Energy Field Disturbance
Environmental Interpretation Syndrome, Impaired
Family Coping: Compromised, Ineffective
Family Coping: Disabling, Ineffective
Family Coping: Potential for Growth
Family Process: Alcoholism, Altered
Family Processes, Altered
Fatigue
Fear
Fluid Volume Deficit

Fluid Volume Deficit, Risk for
Fluid Volume Excess
Gas Exchange, Impaired
Grieving, Anticipatory
Grieving, Dysfunctional
Growth and Development, Altered
Health Maintenance, Altered
Health-Seeking Behaviors (Specify)
Home Maintenance Management, Impaired
Hopelessness
Hyperthermia
Hypothermia
Incontinence, Bowel
Incontinence, Functional
Incontinence, Reflex
Incontinence, Stress
Incontinence, Total
Incontinence, Urge
Infant Feeding Pattern, Ineffective
Infection, Risk for
Injury, Risk for
Knowledge Deficit (Specify)
Loneliness, Risk for
Management of Therapeutic Regimen: Community, Ineffective
Management of Therapeutic Regimen: Families, Ineffective
Management of Therapeutic Regimen: Individual, Effective
Management of Therapeutic Regimen: (Individuals), Ineffective
Memory, Impaired
Noncompliance (Specify)
Nutrition: Less than Body Requirements, Altered
Nutrition: More than Body Requirements, Altered
Nutrition: Potential for More than Body Requirements, Altered
Oral Mucous Membrane, Altered
Organized Infant Behavior, Potential for Enhanced
Pain
Pain, Chronic
Parent/Infant/Child Attachment, Risk for Altered
Parental Role Conflict
Parenting, Altered
Parenting, Risk for Altered
Perioperative Positioning Injury, Risk for
Peripheral Neurovascular Dysfunction, Risk for

Personal Identity Disturbance
Physical Mobility, Impaired
Poisoning, Risk for
Post-Trauma Response
Powerlessness
Protection, Altered
Rape-Trauma Syndrome
Rape-Trauma Syndrome: Compound Reaction
Rape-Trauma Syndrome: Silent Reaction
Relocation Stress Syndrome
Role Performance, Altered
Self-Care Deficit
    Bathing/Hygiene
    Feeding
    Dressing/Grooming
    Toileting
Self Esteem, Chronic Low
Self Esteem, Situational Low
Self Esteem Disturbance
Self-Mutilation, Risk for
Sensory/Perceptual Alterations (Specify) (visual, auditory, kinesthetic, gustatory, tactile, olfactory)
Sexual Dysfunction
Sexuality Patterns, Altered
Skin Integrity, Impaired
Skin Integrity, Risk for Impaired
Sleep Pattern Disturbance
Social Interaction, Impaired
Social Isolation
Spiritual Distress
Spiritual Well-Being, Potential for Enhanced
Suffocation, Risk for
Sustain Spontaneous Ventilation, Inability to
Swallowing, Impaired
Thermoregulation, Ineffective
Thought Processes, Altered
Tissue Integrity, Impaired
Tissue Perfusion, Altered (Specify Type) (renal, cerebral, cardio-pulmonary, gastrointestinal, peripheral)
Trauma, High Risk for
Unilateral Neglect
Urinary Elimination, Altered
Urinary Retention
Violence, High Risk for: Self-Directed or Directed at Others

Index

continued

continued

continued

continued

continued

continued

continued

continued

Photographic Credits

Chapter 1: 1–1, 1–6: © Richard Tauber/Benjamin/Cummings. 1–2, 1–7: © Alain McLaughlin/Benjamin/Cummings.

Chapter 2: 2–3: © Richard Tauber/Benjamin/Cummings. 2–7: © Alain McLaughlin/Benjamin/Cummings.

Chapter 3: 3–1: © Keystone View Co./FPG. 3–2: © Richard Tauber/Benjamin/Cummings. 3–3: © Alain McLaughlin/Benjamin/Cummings.

Chapter 4: 4–7: Courtesy of Baxter Healthcare Corporation. 4–9: © William Thompson/Benjamin/Cummings.

Chapter 7: Box on page 191: © Elena Dorfman/Benjamin/Cummings. 7–4: © Alain McLaughlin/Benjamin/Cummings. 7–6: © Richard Tauber/Benjamin/Cummings.

Chapter 8: 8–18: © SUI/Photo Researchers, Inc. 8–21: © Alain McLaughlin/Benjamin/Cummings/Reaction Images. 8–22: Zeva Delbaum/Peter Arnold.

Chapter 9: 9–7: Simon Fraser/SPL/Photo Researchers, Inc. 9–9a, b: Courtesy of Bard Access Systems, Salt Lake City, UT. 9–9c: Courtesy SIMS Deltec, Inc., St. Paul, MN. 9–9d: Courtesy of Norfolk Medical, Skokie, IL.

Chapter 10: 10–6: Courtesy of University Air Care/University of Cincinnati Hospital. 10–7: © Spencer Grant/Photo Researchers, Inc. 10–9: Courtesy of Kinetic Concepts Inc.

Chapter 11: 11–1, 11–2: © Richard Tauber/Benjamin/Cummings.

Chapter 12: 12–6, 12–7: © Elena Dorfman/Benjamin/Cummings. 12–8, 12–12, 12–14a, b, 12–15: © Richard Tauber/Benjamin/Cummings.

Chapter 13: 13–1: Courtesy of Biodynamic, Seattle. 13–4: Photo Researchers/© Biophoto Associates.

Chapter 14: 14–7: SPL/Photo Researchers, Inc.

Chapter 16: Table 16–4, top to bottom: © Science Photo Library/Photo Researchers, Inc., © NMSB/Custom Medical Stock Photography., Biophoto Associates., S. Lissau/Medichrome., Michael English, MD/Medical Images, Inc., Copyright © 1994, Carroll H. Weiss. All rights reserved., DeGrazia/Custom Medical Stock Photography., © Science Photo Library/Custom Medical Stock Photography., 16–4: © Alain McLaughlin/Benjamin/Cummings. 16–7: Copyright © 1994, Carroll H. Weiss. All rights reserved. 16–9, 16–11: © Custom Medical Stock Photography. 16–10: © Photo Researchers, Inc.

Chapter 17: Box on page 609: Courtesy of Karen Lou Kennedy, RN, FPN. 17–1, 17–4, 17–5, 17–7, 17–8, 17–10, 17–11, 17–12, 17–13, 17–17, 17–18, 17–19, 17–21, 17–22, 17–23, 17–24, 17–25: © Carroll Weiss/Camera M.D. Studios. 17–2, 17–6, 17–9, 17–14, 17–28: © Custom Medical Stock Photography. 17–3, 17–20, 17–26, 17–27: American Academy of Dermatology. 17–15: © Biophoto Associates/Photo Researchers, Inc. 17–16: © NMSB/Custom Medical Stock Photography. 17–31: © Elena Dorfman/Benjamin/Cummings. 17–32: Leonard Morse/Medical Images, Inc.

Chapter 18: 18–4, 18–5, 18–8, 18–9, 18–10, 18–11, 18–12: Dr. William Dominic, Valley Medical Center.

Chapter 19: 19–4: © Richard Tauber/Benjamin/Cummings.

Chapter 20: 20–2: University of Illinois/Custom Medical Stock Photography. 20–3: © Custom Medical Stock Photography. 20–5: Courtesy Dr. Charles Wilson, University of California, San Francisco. 20–6: Clinical Pathological Conference, American Journal of Medicine.

Chapter 21: 21–4: © Harry Przekop/Medichrome. 21–5: © Photo Researchers, Inc.

Chapter 23: 23–5: © Photo Researchers, Inc. 23–7: Courtesy of Carol Williams, R.N., B.S./UC Davis Medical Center. 23–9a, b: © William Thompson/Benjamin/Cummings.

Chapter 24: 24–7: © Richard Tauber/Benjamin/Cummings.

Chapter 25: 25–3a: Courtesy of Dornier Medical Systems.

Chapter 26: 26–1: A. Glauberman/Photo Researchers, Inc. 26–3: Dr. P. Marazzi/Science Photo Library/Photo Researchers, Inc.

Chapter 28: Box on page 1051: © Richard Tauber/Benjamin/Cummings. 28–10, 28–30c: Courtesy of Medtronics, Inc. 28–30a, d: Courtesy of Baxter. 28–30b: Courtesy of St. Jude Medical.

Chapter 29: 29–7, 29–8a, 29–9: © Richard Tauber/Benjamin/Cummings.

Chapter 30: 30–5: Photo Researchers, Inc./Dr. P. Marazzi/Science Photo Library. 30–7: MNSB/Custom Medical Stock Photography.

Chapter 31: 31–8: © Lennart Nilsson/Boehringer Ingelheim International GmbH.

Chapter 32: 32–9, 32–10, 32–11, 32–12: © Richard Tauber/Benjamin/Cummings.

Chapter 33: 33–1a, 33–02a: © Richard Tauber/Benjamin/Cummings. 33–4: Courtesy of Respironics, Inc. 33–8a, 33–9a: Courtesy of Luminaud, Inc.

Chapter 34: 34–4, 34–6: © William Thompson/Benjamin/Cummings. 34–5, 34–7, 34–8: © Richard Tauber/Benjamin/Cummings. 34–11a–c: CDC. 34–14: Ciba–Geigy Corporation. 34–16a, b: Courtesy of University of California, Davis, Medical Center. 34–20: © Elena Dorfman/Benjamin/Cummings. 34–26: Courtesy of Life Care Corporation. 34–27: Courtesy Bear Medical Systems, Inc.

Chapter 35: 35–6, 35–7, 35–8a–c, 35–9, 35–10a, b, 35–11: © Richard Tauber/Benjamin/Cummings. 35–12, 35–13: Todd Hammond.

Chapter 37: 37–3: Courtesy of Orthologic, Inc.

Chapter 38: 38–1, 38–8, 38–10, 38–11: American College of Rheumatology. 38–4: Copyright © 1994, Carroll H. Weiss. All rights reserved. 38–6: Biophoto Associates/Photo Researchers, Inc.

Chapter 39: 39–9, 39–10, 39–11, 39–12a–e, 39–13, 39–14: © Richard Tauber/Benjamin/Cummings.

Chapter 41: 41–4a–c: Todd Hammond

Chapter 42: 42–2: Courtesy of Churchill Livingstone. 42–5: Courtesy of Baxter. 42–6: © Yoav Levy/Phototake NYC. 42–8: © Custom Medical Stock Photography. 42–10: NIH/Phototake, NYC.

Chapter 43: Box on page 1876: Don Wong/Science Source/Photo Researchers, Inc./Nea Hanscomb. 43–6, 43–7, 43–10, 43–16, 43–19, 43–20: © Richard Tauber/Benjamin/Cummings. 43–9, 43–15, 43–18: © Elena Dorfman/Benjamin/Cummings. 43–12: Leonard Lessen/Peter Arnold, Inc. 43–13, 43–24: Science Photo Library/Photo Researchers, Inc. 43–14: Custom Medical Stock Photography. 43–17: Dr. R. Buckingham. 43–21: Brenda Spriggs, MD. 43–22: Professor Tony Wright, Institute of Laryncology and Otology/SPL/Photo Researchers, Inc. 43–23: Dr. P. Marazzi/Science Photo Library/Photo Researchers, Inc.

Chapter 44: 44–1: Buddy Crofton/Medical Images, Inc. 44–2a: Custom Medical Stock Photography. 44–2b: © Herbert Gould/Medichrome. 44–4, 44–9, 44–11: National Eye Institute. 44–7: © Richard Tauber/Benjamin/Cummings. 44–10a, b: Courtesy of Prevent Blindness America. 44–12: Janet Hayes/Medical Images, Inc.

Chapter 45: Box on page 1958, Box on page 1959, 45–6, 45–7, 45–8, 45–9: © Richard Tauber/Benjamin/Cummings.

Chapter 47: 47–4: © 1991, Mike English, MD/Custom Medical Stock Photography.

Chapter 48: 48–1: CNRI/Phototake. 48–2: Copyright © 1994, Carroll H. Weiss. All rights reserved.

Chapter 49: 49–2, 49–4: Biophoto Associates/Photo Researchers, Inc. 49–3: © Camera M. D. Studios. 49–5a: Kenneth Greer/Visuals Unlimited. 49–5b: National A V Center.

Art Credits

Chapter 1: 1–3: Betty Gee. 1–4, 1–5: The Left Coast Group.

Chapter 2: 2–1, 2–2, 2–4: The Left Coast Group. 2–5: Nea Hanscomb/Valerie Felts. 2–6: Robert Voigts/Valerie Felts.

Chapter 4: Box on page 85, Figures 4–1a–c, 4–3, 4–8: Christopher Burke. 4–2, 4–5: Nea Hanscomb. 4–4: Precision Graphics, 4–10, 4–12: GTS Graphics. 4–11: Michele Mangelli.

Chapter 5: Box on page 106: Christopher Burke. 5–1, 5–2, 5–3, 5–4, 5–5, 5–6, 5–8a–c, 5–9, 5–12, 5–13, 5–14, 5–15a, b, 5–16a, b: Nea Hanscomb. 5–7, 5–11: Biomed Arts Associates/Wendy Hiller Gee/Kristin N. Mount. 5–10a–c: The Left Coast Group.

Chapter 6: 6–1: Biomed Arts Associates/Wendy Hiller Gee/Kristin N. Mount. 6–2: The Left Coast Group. 6–3, 6–4: Precision Graphics.

Chapter 7: Box on page 192, Table 7–5: Precision Graphics. Box on page 206: Linda Harris/Valerie Felts/Nea Hanscomb. 7–1, 7–2, 7–3, 7–5, 7–8, 7–11: The Left Coast Group. 7–7a–h: Precision Graphics. 7–9, 7–10a, b: Christopher Burke.

Chapter 8: Box on page 255, Box on page 284, Figures 8–7, 8–8, 8–9, 8–13, 8–20: Precision Graphics. 8–1, 8–2, 8–3, 8–4, 8–5a–d, 8–6, 8–10a, b, 8–14, 8–15, 8–16, 8–17, 8–19: Christopher Burke. 8–11: Precision Graphics/Kristin N. Mount/Romaine LoPrete 8–12: Nea Hanscomb.

Chapter 9: 9–1, 9–2, 9–3, 9–4, 9–8: Precision Graphics. 9–5, 9–6: Christopher Burke. 9–10: Kristin N. Mount.

Chapter 10: Box on page 381: Nea Hanscomb. 10–1, 10–2a, b, 10–3a, b, 10–8: Kristin N. Mount. 10–4: Precision Graphics. 10–5a–d: Christopher Burke.

Chapter 11: 11–3: The Left Coast Group.

Chapter 12: 12–1, 12–2: Todd A. Buck/Valerie Felts. 12–3: Christopher Burke. 12–4a–d: Precision Graphics. 12–5: Romaine LoPrete. 12–13a, b: Kristin N. Mount.

Chapter 13: 13–2: Biomed Arts Associates/Wendy Hiller Gee/Kristin N. Mount 13–3, 13–5, 13–6, 13–7a, b, 13–8, 13–9: Kristin N. Mount.

Chapter 14: Box on page 498, Table 14–2, 14–1, 14–4, 14–10: Kristin N. Mount. 14–2, 14–5, 14–9: Christopher Burke. 14–3, 14–6, 14–8: Precision Graphics.

Chapter 15: 15–1, 15–2, 15–4a–d, 15–5, 15–6a, b, 15–7, 15–8a–d, 15–9, 15–10a, b: Kristin N. Mount. 15–3 Biomed Arts Associates/Wendy Hiller Gee/Kristin N. Mount.

Chapter 16: Table 16–2, Table 16–3, 16–2, 16–6, 16–8: Kristin N. Mount. 16–1: Biomed Arts Associates/Wendy Hiller Gee. 16–3: Barbara Cousins. 16–5: Romaine LoPrete.

Chapter 17: 17–29, 17–30: Christopher Burke.

Chapter 18: 18–1, 18–2: Nea Hanscomb. 18–3: Christopher Burke. 18–6, 18–7: Precision Graphics.

Chapter 19: 19–1, 19–2, 19–3: Kristin N. Mount.

Chapter 20: 20–1, 20–4: Biomed Arts Associates/Wendy Hiller Gee/Kristin N. Mount.

Chapter 21: Box on page 729, Table 21–5, Figure 21–2: Nea Hanscomb. 21–1a, b: Kristin N. Mount. 21–3: Biomed Arts Associates/Wendy Hiller Gee/Kristin N. Mount. 21–6: Precision Graphics.

Chapter 22: 22–1, 21–2: Christopher Burke. 22–3: Kristin N. Mount.

Chapter 23: 23–1, 23–2, 23–6, 23–8, 23–17: Christopher Burke. 23–3, 23–4, 23–10: Nea Hanscomb. 23–11, 23–12, 23–14, 23–15, 23–16: Kristin N. Mount. 23–13: Linda Harris.

Chapter 24: 24–1a, b, 24–2 Biomed Arts Associates/Wendy Hiller Gee/Nea Hanscomb. 24–3: Christopher Burke. 24–4: Kristin N. Mount. 24–5, 24–6: Nea Hanscomb.

Chapter 25: Box on page 893, Figures 25–1, 25–4, 25–5, 25–6: Kristin N. Mount. 25–2, 25–3b: Christopher Burke. 25–7: The Left Coast Group.

Chapter 26: 26–2, 26–5, 26–7, 26–8: Nea Hanscomb. 26–4a–c, 26–6, 26–10, 26–11: Precision Graphics. 26–9: Biomed Arts Associates/Wendy Hiller Gee/Kristin N. Mount. 26–12, 26–13: Kristin N. Mount.

Chapter 27: 27–1a, b, 27–4: Romaine LoPrete. 27–1c, 27–2: Biomed Arts Associates/Wendy Hiller Gee/Nea Hanscomb. 27–3, 27–7: Todd A. Buck/Valerie Felts. 27–5a, b, 27–6: Kristin N. Mount. 27–9: Romaine LoPrete/Kristin N. Mount.

Chapter 28: Box on page 1051: Precision Graphics. Table 28–1, 28–11a–c: GTS Graphics/Kristin N. Mount. Table 28–2: GTS Graphics/Kristin N. Mount/Nea Hanscomb. Table 28–10: Romaine LoPrete. Table 28–12, Figures 28–5, 28–12, 28–13a–d, 28–14a–c, 28–16, 28–17a, b, 28–18a, b, 28–19, 28–20, 28–23a–c, 28–24, 28–25, 28–26, 28–27, 28–28, 28–29: Kristin N. Mount. 28–1: Nea Hanscomb. 28–2a, b, 28–3 a–c, 28–7, 28–8, 28–9, 28–15, 28–21, 28–22, 28–31: Precision Graphics. 28–4, 28–6 © Addison-Wesley Nursing. 28–15: Precision Graphics/Kristin Mount. Pathophysiology Illustration: Wendy Hiller Gee/Biomed Arts Associates.

Chapter 29: Box on page 1776, Figures 29–5, 29–8b: Romaine LoPrete. Box 29–3: Linda Harris. 29–1, 29–2, 29–3: © Addison-Wesley Nursing. 29–4: Kristin N. Mount.

Chapter 30: 30–1: Nea Hanscomb. 30–2a, b: Christopher Burke. 30–3a–c, 30–6a, b: Precision Graphics. 30–4a–c: Kristin N. Mount.

Chapter 31: 31–1, 31–4: Christopher Burke. 31–2, 31–6, 31–9, 31–10, 31–11: Nea Hanscomb. 31–3, 31–7: Kristin N. Mount. 31–5: Biomed Arts Associates/Wendy Hiller Gee/Kristin N. Mount. 31.12: Precision Graphics. Pathophysiology Illustration: Wendy Hiller Gee/Biomed Arts Associates.

Chapter 32: 32–1: Todd A. Buck. 32–2: Christopher Burke. 32–4: Barbara Cousins. 32–5a, 32–6, 32–7: Kristin N. Mount. 32–5b: Romaine LoPrete. 32–8: Nea Hanscomb.

Chapter 33: 33–1b, 33–2b: Precision Graphics. 33–3a, b, 33–5, 33–10: Christopher Burke. 33–6, 33–7a, b: Kristin Mount. 33–8b, 33–9b: Precision Graphics. 33–11a–e: Linda Harris.

Chapter 34: Box on page 1425, Table 34–11, Figures 34–1, 34–12, 34–13, 34–21, 34–23, 34–24, 34–28, 34–29: Nea Hanscomb. Table 34–8, Figures 34–2, 34–3, 34–9a–h: Precision Graphics. 34–10, © Addison-Wesley Nursing. 34–15, 34–17a, b, 34–18a, b, 34–19a–c, 34–22a–c, 34–25: Kristin N. Mount. Pathophysiology Illustration: Wendy Hiller Gee/Biomed Arts Associates.

Chapter 35: 35–1, 35–4, 35–5a, b: Todd A. Buck/Nea Hanscomb. 35–2: Christopher Burke. 35–3: Biomed Arts Associates/Wendy Hiller Gee/Nea Hanscomb.

Chapter 36: 36–1, 36–3: Kristin N. Mount. 36–2a–c: Christopher Burke. 36–4, 36–5, 36–6: Precision Graphics.

Chapter 37: Table 37–1, Figures 37–1a–c, 37–2, 37–4, 37–5a–c, 37–6a, b, 37–7, 37–9a, b, 37–11a, b: Precision Graphics. 37–8a–c, 37–10a, b: Kristin N. Mount. Pathophysiology Illustration: Wendy Hiller Gee/Biomed Arts Associates.

Chapter 38: 38–2, 38–3: Precision Graphics. 38–5: Christopher Burke. 38–7, 38–9: Biomed Arts Associates/Wendy Hiller Gee/Kristin N. Mount.

Chapter 39: 39–1: Biomed Arts Associates/Wendy Hiller Gee/Nea Hanscomb. 39–2, 39–8: Romaine LoPrete. 39–3, 39–5: Christopher Burke. 39–4, 39–7: Kristin N. Mount. 39–6, 39–15, 39–16, 39–17, 39–18: Precision Graphics.

Chapter 40: Table 40–3: Nea Hanscomb. 40–1, 40–2, 40–5a, b: Precision Graphics 40–3, 40–4, 40–8, 40–9, 40–10: Kristin N. Mount. 40–6, 40–7: Christopher Burke.

Chapter 41: 41–1, 41–7, 41–8: Precision Graphics. 41–2, 41–3, 41–5a–d: Nea Hanscomb. 41–6a–c, 41–9: Kristin N. Mount.

Chapter 42: Box on page 1836: Nea Hanscomb. 42–1, 42–4, 42–7a, b, 42–9: Kristin N. Mount. 42–3: The Left Coast Group. Pathophysiology Illustration: Wendy Hiller Gee/Biomed Arts Associates.

Chapter 43: 43–1, 43–5: Todd A. Buck/Nea Hanscomb. 43–2a, b: Biomed Arts Associates/Wendy Hiller Gee/Nea Hanscomb. 43–3: Barbara Cousins/Nea Hanscomb. 43–4, 43–8: Romaine LoPrete.

Chapter 44: 44–3a, b, 44–5a, b, 44–8, 44–15: Kristin N. Mount. 44–6: Precision Graphics. 44–13, 44–14: Nea Hanscomb.

Chapter 45: 45–1, 45–3: Barbara Cousins/Nea Hanscomb. 45–2, 45–4: Biomed Arts Associates/Wendy Hiller Gee/Nea Hanscomb. 45–5, 45–10, 45–11: Kristin N. Mount.

Chapter 46: Box on page 1976, 46–1a, b, 46–2, 46–3, 46–4, 46–5a–c: Christopher Burke.

Chapter 47: 47–1: Biomed Arts Associates/Wendy Hiller Gee/Kristin N. Mount. 47–2: Christopher Burke. 47–3, 47–5, 47–6, 47–7: Kristin N. Mount.

Chapter 48: 48–3a–d: Precision Graphics. 48–4a, b, 48–5a, b, 48–6a, b, 48–7a–d: Kristin N. Mount. 48–8: Romaine LoPrete.

Chapter 49: 49–1: Kristin N. Mount.

Community Resource Directory

Al-Anon Family Group Headquarters
P.O. Box 862, Midtown Station
New York, NY 10018
(212) 302-7240

Alcoholic's Anonymous
475 Riverside Drive
New York, NY 10163
(212) 870-3400
  or
234 Eglinton Avenue E, Suite 502
Toronto, Ontario M4P 1K5
CANADA
(416) 487-5591

Alexander Graham Bell Association for the
  Deaf, Inc.
3417 Volta Place NW
Washington, DC 20007
(202) 337-5220

Alzheimer's Association
919 N. Michigan Avenue, Suite 1000
Chicago, IL 60611
(312) 335-8700/(800) 272-3900
In Illinois: (800) 572-6037

Alzheimer's Society of Canada
1320 Yonge Street, Suite 302
Toronto, Ontario M4T 1X2
CANADA
(416) 925-3552

American Amputee Foundation
P.O. Box 250218, Hillcrest Station
Little Rock, AR 72225
(501) 666-2523

American Anorexia/Bulimia Association,
  Inc. (AABA)
418 E. 76th Street
New York, NY 10021
(212) 734-1114

American Association of Retired
  Persons (AARP)
601 E Street, N.W.
Washington, DC 20049
(202) 434-2227

American Board of Nutrition
9650 Rockville Pike
Bethesda, MD 20814
(301) 530-7050

American Burn Association
c/o William Curreri, MD
New York Hospital
Cornell Medical Center
New York, NY 10021

American Cancer Society
1599 Clifton Road NE
Atlanta, GA 30329
(404) 320-3333

American Council of the Blind
1155 15th Street NW, Suite 720
Washington, DC 20005
(202) 467-5081

American Diabetes Association
1660 Duke Street
Alexandria, VA 22314
(703) 549-1500

American Dietetic Association
216 West Jackson Boulevard, Suite 800
Chicago, IL 60606
(312) 899-0040

American Foundation for AIDS Research
5900 Wilshire Boulevard, 2nd Floor
Los Angeles, CA 90036
(213) 857-5900

American Foundation for the Blind
15 W. 16th Street
New York, NY 10011
(212) 620-2000/(800) 232-5463

American Gastroenterological Association
7910 Woodmont Avenue, Suite 914
Bethesda, MD 20814
(301) 654-2055

American Heart Association
7272 Greenville Avenue
Dallas, TX 75231
(214) 373-6300

American Holistic Medical Association
4101 Lake Boone Triangle, Suite 201
Raleigh, NC 27607
(919) 787-5146

American Lateral Sclerosis Association
15300 Ventura Boulevard, Suite 315
Sherman Oaks, CA 91403

American Liver Foundation
1425 Pompton Avenue
Cedar Grove, NJ 07009
(201) 256-2550/(800) 223-0179

American Lung Association
1740 Broadway
New York, NY 10019
(215) 315-8700

American Optometric Association
4330 East West Highway, Suite 1117
Bethesda, MD 20814
(301) 718-6574

Medic-Alert Organ Donor Program
2323 Colorado
Turlock, CA 95381-1009
(209) 668-3333
(800) ID-ALERT

American Narcolepsy Association
425 California Street, Suite 201
San Francisco, CA 94104
(415) 788-4793

American Osteopathic Association
142 East Ontario Street
Chicago, IL 60611
(312) 280-5800

American Pain Society
5700 Old Orchard Road, 1st Floor
Skokie, IL 60077-1024
(708) 966-5595

American Parkinson Disease Association
60 Bay Street, Suite 401
Staten Island, NY 10301
(718) 981-8001/(800) 223-APDA

American Psychiatric Association
1400 K Street, N.W.
Washington, DC 20005
(202) 682-6000

American Public Health Association
1015 15th Street, NW
Washington, DC 20005
(202) 789-5600

American Red Cross
431 18th Street, N.W.
Washington, DC 20006
(202) 737-8300

American Sleep Disorders Association
1610 14th Street, N.W., Suite 300
Rochester, MN 55901
(507) 287-6006

American Society for Gastrointestinal
  Endoscopy
P.O. Box 1565
13 Elm Street
Manchester, MA 01944
(508) 526-8330

American Society of Geriatric Dentistry
211 E. Chicago Avenue
Chicago, IL 60611
(313) 440-2661

American Speech-Language-Hearing
  Association
10801 Rockville Pike
Rockville, MD 20852
(301) 987-5700

American Thoracic Society
1740 Broadway
New York, NY 10019
(212) 315-8700

American Tinnitus Association
P.O. Box 5
Portland, OR 97207
(503) 248-9985

American Venereal Disease Association
Box 1753
Baltimore, MD 21203-1753

Amyotrophic Lateral Sclerosis Association
21021 Ventura Boulevard, Suite 321
Woodland Hills, CA 91364
(818) 340-7500

Arthritis Foundation
1314 Spring Street, N.W.
Atlanta, GA 30309
(800) 283-7800

Arthritis Society
250 Bloor Street E, Suite 401
Toronto, Ontario M4W 3P2
CANADA
(416) 967-1414

Asthma and Allergy Foundation of America
1125 15th Street NW, Suite 502
Washington, DC 20005
(202) 466-7643/(800) 7-ASTHMA

Braille Institute
741 North Vermont Avenue
Los Angeles, CA 90029

Canadian AIDS Society
170 Laurier Avenue W, Suite 1101
Ottawa, ON K1P 5V5
CANADA
(613) 230-3580

Canadian Coalition on Organ Donor
 Awareness
c/o Pharmaceutical Manufacturer's
 Association of Canada
1111 Prince of Wales Drive, Suite 302
Ottawa, Ontario K2C 3P2
CANADA
(613) 727-1380

Canadian Council of the Blind
P.O. Box 2310, Station "D"
Ottawa, Ontario K1P 5W5
CANADA
(613) 567-0311

Canadian Diabetes Association
78 Bond Street
Toronto, Ontario M5B 2J8
CANADA
(416) 382-4440

Canadian Dietetic Association
480 University of Avenue, Suite 601
Toronto, Ontario M3G 1V2
CANADA

Canadian Foundation for Ileitis and Colitis
21 St. Clair Avenue E, Suite 301
Toronto, Onataria M4T 1L9
CANADA
(416) 920-5035

Canadian Liver Foundation
1320 Yonge Street, Suite 301
Toronto, Ontario M4T 1X2
CANADA
(416) 964-1953

Canadian Pain Society
c/o Dr. H. Merskey
London Psychiatric Hosptial
850 Highbury Avenue
P.O. Box 2532, Station A
London, Ontario N6A 4H1
CANADA
(519) 455-5110

Cancer Information Service
National Cancer Institute
9000 Rockville Pike
Building, 31, Room 10A16
Bethesda, MD 20892-0001
(301) 496-4000/(800) 4-CANCER

Centers for Disease Control
1600 Clifton Road, N.E.
Atlanta, GA 30333
(404) 639-3534

Council on Stroke
American Heart Association
7320 Greenville Avenue
Dallas, TX 75231
(214) 373-6300

Cystic Fibrosis Foundation
6931 Arlington Road, #200
Bethesda, MD 20814
(301) 951-4422

DES Action, USA
1615 Broadway, Suite 510
Oakland, CA 94617
(510) 465-4011

Dying With Dignity
175 St. Clair Avenue, West
Toronto, Ontario M4V 1P7
CANADA

Endometriosis Association
8585 N. 76th Place
Milwaukee, WI 53223
(414) 355-2200

Epilepsy Foundation of America
4351 Garden City Drive
Landover, MD 20785-2267
(301) 459-3700/(800) 332-1000

Eye Bank Association of America
1001 Connecticut Avenue NW, Suite 601
Washington, DC 20036
(202) 775-4999

Fibromyalgia Network
5700 Stockdale Highway, Suite 100
Bakersfield, CA 93309
(805) 631-1950

Food and Drug Administration (FDA)
Office of Consumer Affairs
Public Inquiries
5600 Fishers Lane (HFE-88)
Rockville, MD 20857
(301) 443-3170

Guide Dogs for the Blind
P.O. Box 1200
San Rafael, CA 94915
(510) 479-4000

Guillain-Barre-Syndrome Foundation
 International
P.O. Box 262
Wynnewood, PA 19096
(215) 667-0131

Heart and Stroke Foundation of Canada
160 George Street, Suite 200
Ottawa, Ontario K1N 9M2
CANADA
(613) 237-4381

Heart Information Center
National Heart Institute
U.S. Public Health Service
9000 Rockville Pike
Bldg. 31, Room 4A21
Bethesda, MD 20892

The Hemlock Society
P.O. Box 11830
Eugene, OR 97440-4030

Hemophilia Foundation
110 Greene Street, Suite 303
New York, NY 10012
(212) 219-8180

Hereditary Disease Foundation
1427 7th Street, Suite 2
Santa Monica, CA 90401
(310) 458-4183

Herpes Resource Center
13827 Research Triangle Park
Raleigh, NC 27709
(919) 361-8400

Huntington's Disease Foundation of America
140 West 22nd Street, 6th Floor
New York, NY 10011
(212) 242-1968/(800) 345-4372

Impotence Anonymous
119 S. Ruth Street
Maryville, TN 37802
(615) 926-7025

Independent Living for the Handicapped
1301 Belmont Street, NW
Washington, DC 20009
(202) 797-9803

International Association for Enterostomal
 Therapy
2755 Bristol Street, Suite 110
Costa Mesa, CA 92626
(714) 476-0268/(800) 228-4238

Juvenile Diabetes Foundation
432 Park Avenue South
New York, NY 10016
(212) 889-7575/(800) 223-1138

Kidney Foundation of Canada
4060 St. Catherine Street W, Suite 555
Montreal, PQ H3Z 2Z3
CANADA
(514) 934-4806

Leukemia Society of America, Inc.
600 Third Avenue
New York, NY 10016
(212) 573-8484

Living Bank
P.O. Box 6725
Houston, TX 77265
(713) 961-9431 in Texas
(800) 528-2971

Look Good, Feel Better
c/o American Cancer Society
1599 Clifton Road NE
Atlanta, GA 30329
(404) 320-3333

Lupus Foundation of America
4 Research Plaza, Suite 180
Rockville, MD 20850-2226
(301) 670-9292/(800) 558-0121

Lyme Disease Foundation
1 Financial Plaza, 18th Floor
Hartford, CT 06103
(203) 871-2900

Make-A-Wish Foundation
2600 North Central Avenue, Suite 936
Phoenix, AZ 85004
(602) 240-6600

Malignant Hyperthermia Association of the
 United States (MHAUS)
P.O. Box 191
Westport, CT 06881-0191

March of Dimes Birth Defects Foundation
Public Health Education Foundation
1275 Mamaroneck Avenue
White Plains, NY 10605
(914) 428-7100

Medic-Alert Foundation
2323 Colorado Street
Turlock, CA 95380
(209) 668-3333/(800) 344-3226